e-Learning Resources

COMPANION CD

Body Spectrum Electronic Anatomy Coloring Book

Fluids and Electrolytes Tutorial

English/Spanish Audio Glossary

Animations

Abdominal Examination
Abruptio Placentae
Adrenal Function
Alzheimer's Disease
Anatomy of Eye
Ankle Fracture
Antibiotics
Antibodies
Appendicitis, Symptoms
Asthma
Brain Anatomy
Brain Lobes
Cardiopulmonary Resuscitation (CPR)
Chemotherapy
Congestive Heart Failure
Cranial Nerves
Fertilization to Implantation
Fetal Circulation
Fetal Development in the First Trimester
Fetal Development in the Second Trimester
Function of the Heart
Hemolytic Disease
Hemothorax
Hip Fracture, Femur Fracture, Femoral Fracture
Inflammatory Response
Lymphocyte Function
Meningitis
Nasogastric Tube Placement
Organ Systems
Osteomyelitis
Parkinson's Disease
Passage of Food through Digestive Tract
Pelvic Inflammatory Disease
Pneumonia
Pressure Ulcers
Pulse
Radiation Therapy
Renal Anatomy and Function
Respiration
Retinal Detachment
Sickle Cell Anemia
Simple Pneumothorax and Tension Pneumothorax
Structure of the Heart
Thrombocytopenia
Types of Joint Movements
Visual Pathway

Video Clips

Auscultation: Abdomen, Bowel Sounds
Auscultation: Cardiac, with Diaphragm and Bell
Auscultation: Carotid Artery
Dressing Changes: Wet to Dry
Inspection: External Genitalia
Inspection: Fine Motor Coordination, Lower Extremities
Inspection: Fine Motor Coordination, Upper Extremities
Inspection: Speculum Examination
Inspection and Palpation: Breathing and Respiratory Excursion, Anterior Chest
Inspection and Palpation: Cardiac, Anterior Chest
Inspection and Palpation: Cardiac Auscultatory Landmarks
Inspection and Palpation: Muscular Development
Inspection and Palpation: Pulses, Lower Extremities
Intramuscular Injections
Midstream Urine Collection
Palpation: Abdomen Superficial and Deep
Percussion: Abdomen
Percussion: Liver
Percussion: Spleen
Pulse: Measuring an Apical Pulse
Sputum Specimen
Subcutaneous Injections

Audio Clips

Aortic Ejection Sound Related to S_1
Breath Sounds: Bronchial
Breath Sounds: Bronchovesicular
Breath Sounds: Vesicular
Crackles, High-Pitched
Crackles, Low-Pitched
Diastolic Murmur
Midsystolic Click Sound Related to S_1
Murmurs: Blowing, Harsh or Rough, and Rumble
Murmurs: High, Medium, Low
Paradoxical Split Sound Related to S_2
Pericardial Friction Rub
Pericardial Friction Sounds
Pleural Friction Rub
Pulmonic Ejection Sound Related to S_1
S_1 at Various Locations
S_2 at Various Locations
Stridor
Systolic Murmur
The Fourth Heart Sound (S_4)
The Fourth Heart Sound (S_4) with Bell Held Lightly then Applied Firmly
The Third Heart Sound (S_3)
Wheeze, High-Pitched
Wheeze, Low-Pitched
Wide Split Sound Related to S_2

EVOLVE

In addition to the resources available on the Companion CD, the following resources are also available on the evolve website at **http://evolve.elsevier.com/Christensen/foundationsadult.**

Review Questions for the NCLEX® Examination (for each chapter)

Concept Map Creator

Calculators

Body Mass Index (BMI)
Body Surface Area Calculator
Fluid Deficit
Glasgow Coma Scale
IV Dosage Calculator: Infusion of a Dose
Units Conversion

Additional Animations

Bacteria
Brain Abscess
Breast Cancer Spread; Metastasis
Cardiac Arrest, Ventricular Fibrillation, External Heart Monitor
Chest Pain Radiating to Arm
Chickenpox
Eye: Aqueous Humor, Vitreous Humor
Fungi
Generalized Seizure
Intussusception
Normal Cardiopulmonary Physiology
Normal Cardiopulmonary System
Protozoa
Simple Pneumothorax and Tension Pneumothorax
Spine Structures
Subarachnoid Hemorrhage
TIA, Transient Ischemic Attack; CVA, Cerebrovascular Accident; Stroke; Brain Blood Clot
Vascular Tree: Heart, Aorta, Major Branches
Viruses

Additional Video Clips

Evaluation: Pupil Responses, Direct and Accommodation, Cranial Nerves III, IV, VI—Oculomotor, Trochlear, and Abducens Nerves
Evaluation: Pupil Responses, Direct and Consensual
Inspection: Ear Canal
Inspection: Gait
Inspection: General Muscular Strength
Inspection: Nose
Inspection and Palpation: Cardiac, Anterior Chest
Inspection and Palpation: Cardiac Auscultatory Landmarks
Inspection and Palpation: External Ear
Inspection and Palpation: External Eye
Inspection and Palpation: Muscular Development
Inspection and Palpation: Standing Position
Intradermal Medications
Palpation: Tactile Fremitus, Posterior Chest
Percussion: Anterior Thorax
Respirations: How to Measure Respirations

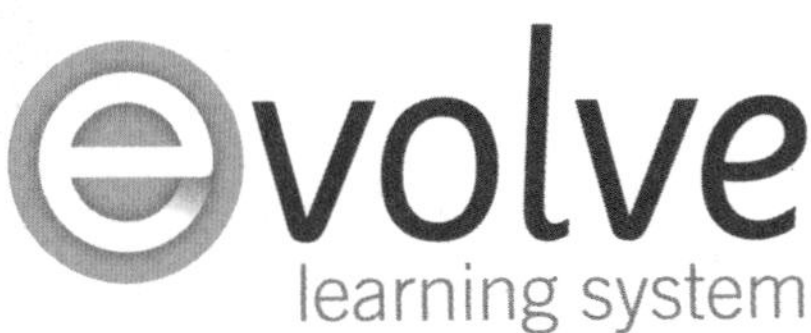

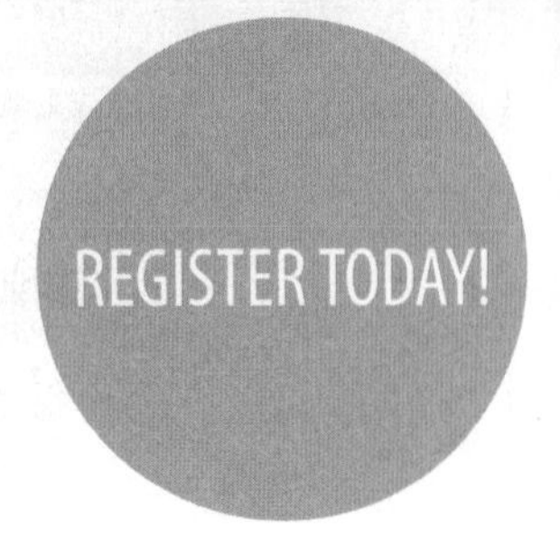

To access your Student Resources, visit:

http://evolve.elsevier.com/Christensen/foundationsadult

The following resources are available to help you:

- **Prepare for Class, Clinical, or Lab**

  Animations, Video Clips, Audio Clips, English/Spanish Audio Glossary, Concept Map Creator, Body Spectrum Electronic Anatomy Coloring Book, Fluids and Electrolytes Tutorial, Calculators (Body Mass Index, Body Surface Area Calculator, Fluid Deficit, Glasgow Coma Scale, IV Dosage, Units Conversion), and more!

- **Prepare for Exams**

  Review Questions for the NCLEX® Examination—More than 550 questions with rationales for correct and incorrect answers help you review and apply content and prepare for class tests and the NCLEX® Examination.

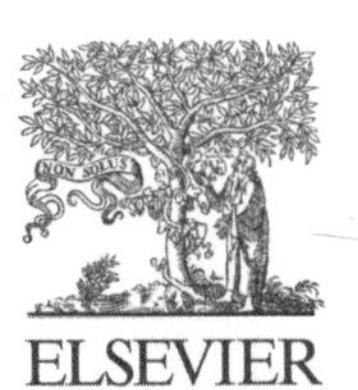

Foundations and Adult Health Nursing

Barbara Lauritsen Christensen, RN, MS
Formerly, Nurse Educator
Mid-Plains Community College
North Platte, Nebraska

Elaine Oden Kockrow, RN, MS
Formerly, Nurse Educator
Mid-Plains Community College
North Platte, Nebraska

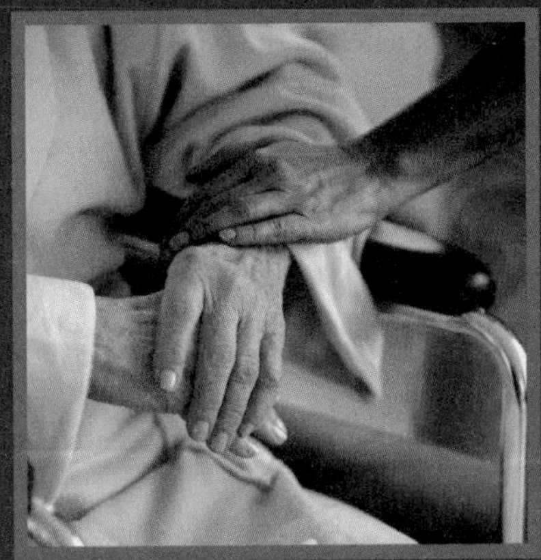

6th Edition

MOSBY

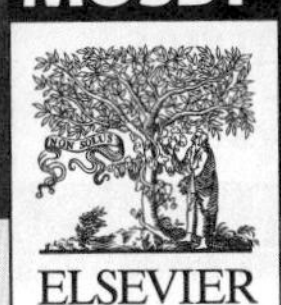

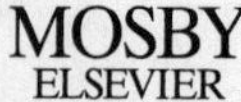

3251 Riverport Lane
St. Louis, Missouri 63043

FOUNDATIONS AND ADULT HEALTH NURSING ISBN: 978-0-323-05728-8

Notices

Knowledge and best practice in this field are constantly changing. As new research and experience broaden our understanding, changes in research methods, professional practices, or medical treatment may become necessary.

Practitioners and researchers must always rely on their own experience and knowledge in evaluating and using any information, methods, compounds, or experiments described herein. In using such information or methods they should be mindful of their own safety and the safety of others, including parties for whom they have a professional responsibility.

With respect to any drug or pharmaceutical products identified, readers are advised to check the most current information provided (i) on procedures featured or (ii) by the manufacturer of each product to be administered, to verify the recommended dose or formula, the method and duration of administration, and contraindications. It is the responsibility of practitioners, relying on their own experience and knowledge of their patients, to make diagnoses, to determine dosages and the best treatment for each individual patient, and to take all appropriate safety precautions.

To the fullest extent of the law, neither the Publisher nor the authors, contributors, or editors, assume any liability for any injury and/or damage to persons or property as a matter of products liability, negligence or otherwise, or from any use or operation of any methods, products, instructions, or ideas contained in the material herein.

The Publisher

Previous editions copyrighted 2006, 2003, 1999, 1995, 1991

Library of Congress Cataloging-in-Publication Control Number 2010921516

Vice President and Publisher: Tom Wilhelm
Managing Editor: Jill Ferguson
Developmental Editor: Tiffany Trautwein
Associate Developmental Editor: Jennifer Hermes
Publishing Services Manager: Jeffrey Patterson
Senior Project Manager: Mary G. Stueck
Book Designer: Margaret Reid

Printed in Canada

Last digit is the print number: 9 8 7 6 5 4 3 2

To my children and grandchildren: Jason Heath, Jennifer Holly, David Joseph,
Alexander Edison, Emma Elizabeth, Ava Louise, Jessica Heather, Eigo, Gus, and Mirabella.
Your love and support make my life a most pleasurable journey.

To my siblings: Shirlee, Ann, Lowell Chris, and Garnet.
A great joy in my life is the unconditional friendship of each of my siblings.

Barbara Lauritsen Christensen, RN, MS

To the brilliant health care providers who were responsible for the miraculous recovery
from my illness in 2008 and my continued good health:

North Platte, Nebraska
Janet Bernard, MD

Fort Walton Beach, Florida
Gregory Candell, MD
Patrick Anastasio, MD
Samuel Capra, MD
Christopher Dali, MD
Justin Philpott, MD
Larry Schatz, MD

Elaine Oden Kockrow, RN, MS

Acknowledgments

This edition has been completed through diligent research and response to reviewers, nurse educators, and student nurses. We are indebted to the nurse educators and student nurses who have used our text to assist in the achievement of excellence in the practice of nursing. We are grateful for the success of the past five editions and look forward to continuing to contribute to the education of student nurses.

For the completion of a textbook, one must have the cooperation of gifted and creative individuals. We wish to recognize those persons who have assisted with this text.

This text would not be possible without the superior effort of the talented editorial and production staff at Elsevier: Robin Richman, Managing Editor, Philadelphia, for her cheerfulness and keen observations; Jacqueline Twomey, Developmental Editor, Philadelphia, for her attention to detail; Jill Ferguson, Managing Editor, St. Louis, for her gracious assistance in coordination and development; Jennifer Hermes, Associate Developmental Editor, St. Louis, for her thoroughness and punctuality; Tiffany Trautwein, Developmental Editor, St. Louis, for her patience and accuracy; and Mary Stueck, Senior Project Manager, St. Louis, for her kind forbearance, organizational skills, and conscientious effort.

We are particularly grateful for the positive feedback and constructive reviews provided by our contributors and reviewers throughout the completion of this edition.

We wish to acknowledge Debbie Beebout, our typist, for her diligence and heedfulness to detail.

We would like to thank the administrators at Great Plains Regional Medical Center for their generous use of various GPRMC forms.

We wish to thank our siblings, children, and grandchildren for their love, kindness, and encouragement that provided us with vigor and inspiration to complete this labor of love.

Last, we wish to express to each other our gratitude for the gift of 35 years of friendship that is unique and has provided us with fortitude, stability, ardor, and purpose. We both share a love of family, community, teaching and the wonderful world of nursing.

Barbara Lauritsen Christensen
Elaine Oden Kockrow

Contributors and Reviewers

CONTRIBUTORS

Sharon K. Duffy, MS, RN, CRRN
Coordinator of Integrative Health and Medicine
Madonna Rehabilitation Hospital
Lincoln, Nebraska

Diane D. Kathol, MEd, MSN
Dean of Allied Health
BryanLGH College of Health Sciences
Lincoln, Nebraska

Kristen Kartchner Maughan, MS, RD, LD
Lecturer
Iowa State University
Ames, Iowa
Health/Fitness Specialist
Mary Greeley Medical Center Rehabilitation and Wellness
Story City, Iowa

Craig E. Nielsen, MS, NP, BC, ACRN
Assistant Professor of Medicine
Division of Infectious Disease
University of Colorado Denver
Aurora, Colorado

Linda North, PhD, RN
Dean of Health Sciences
Southern Union State Community College
Opelika, Alabama

Elaine U. Polan, PhD, RNC
Supervisor
Vocational Education and Extension Board Practical Nursing Program
Uniondale, New York

Anne W. Ryan, MSN, MPH, RNC
Associate Professor, MGW Nursing Program
Chesapeake College/MGW Nursing Program
Wye Mills, Maryland

Alita K. Sellers, MSN, PhD, RN
Chairperson, Health Sciences Division
West Virginia University at Parkersburg
Parkersburg, West Virginia

Martha E. Spray, MS, BSN, RN
Formerly, Practical Nursing Instructor
Mid-East Ohio Vocational School District
Zanesville, Ohio

Toni C. Wortham, MSN, RN
Professor
Madisonville Community College
Madisonville, Kentucky

REVIEWERS

Tonia Dandry Aiken, RN, BSN, JD
Nurse Attorney Institute
NurseLaw.com
New Orleans, Louisiana

Mary Ann Cosgarea RN, BSN, BA
Practical Nursing /Health Coordinator
Portage Lakes Career Center
W. Howard Nicol School of Practical Nursing
Green, Ohio

Brenda G. Holmes MSN/ED, RN
Assistant Professor
South Arkansas Community College
El Dorado, Arkansas

Laura Bevlock Kanavy, RN, BSN, MSN
Career Technology Center of Lackawanna County Practical Nursing Program
Scranton, Pennsylvania

Tammy Camille Killough, RN, BSN
Pearl River Community College-Forrest Co. Campus
Hattiesburg, Mississippi

Gloria Liefer, RN, MA
Associate Professor
Nursing Riverside Community College
Riverside, California

Sue Parker, MSN, APN, FNP-BC, CNOR
Assistant Professor
University of Arkansas—Fort Smith
Fort Smith, Arkansas

Trena L. Rich, MSN, ARNP, BC, CIC
Riverside County Regional Medical Center
Moreno Valley, California

Mary Russo, MSN, RN
Lincoln Land Community College
Springfield, Illinois

Barbara M. Schlager, RN, BSN, JD
Lincoln Technical Institute
Mount Laurel, New Jersey

Ann Leiphart Unholz, RN, MS
Adjunct Instructor
J. Sargeant Reynolds Community College
Richmond, Virginia

Rebecca S. Utz, RN, BSN
University of Arkansas Community College at Batesville
Batesville, Arkansas

Diane Trace Warlick, RN, BSN, JD
Continuing Education Faculty
Louisiana State University Health Sciences Center, School of Nursing
New Orleans, Louisiana

LPN Advisory Board and Consultant

LPN ADVISORY BOARD

Shirley Anderson, MSN
Kirkwood Community College
Cedar Rapids, Iowa

M. Gie Archer, MS, RN, C, WHCNP
Dean of Health Sciences
LVN Program Coordinator
North Central Texas College
Gainesville, Texas

Mary Brothers, MEd, RN
Coordinator, Garnet Career Center School of Practical Nursing
Charleston, West Virginia

Patricia A. Castaldi, RN, BSN, MSN
Union County College
Plainfield, New Jersey

Mary Ann Cosgarea, RN, BSN
PN Coordinator/Health Coordinator
Portage Lakes Career Center
Green, Ohio

Dolores Ann Cotton, RN, BSN, MS
Meridian Technology Center
Stillwater, Oklahoma

Lora Lee Crawford, RN, BSN
Emanuel Turlock Vocational Nursing Program
Turlock, California

Ruth Ann Eckenstein, RN, BS, MEd
Oklahoma Department of Career and Technology Education
Stillwater, Oklahoma

Gail Ann Hamilton Finney, RN, MSN
Nursing Education Specialist
Concorde Career Colleges, INC
Mission, Kansas

Pam Hinckley, RN, MSN
Redlands Adult School
Redlands, California

Deborah W. Keller, RN, BSN, MSN
Erie Huron Ottawa Vocational Education
School of Practical Nursing
Milan, Ohio

Patty Knecht, MSN, RN
Nursing Program Director
Center for Arts & Technology
Brandywine Campus
Coatesville, Pennsylvania

Lieutenant Colonel (RET) Teresa Y. McPherson, RN, BSN, MSN
LVN Program Director
Nursing Education
St. Philip's College
San Antonio, Texas

Frances Neu, MS, BSN, RN
Supervisor, Adult Ed Health
Butler Technology and Career Development Schools
Fairfield Township, Ohio

Dianna Danced Scherlin, MS, RN
National Director of Nursing
Lincoln Educational Services
West Orange, New Jersey

Beverley Turner, MA, RN
Director, Vocational Nursing Department
Maric College, San Diego Campus
San Diego, California

C. Sue Weidman, RN BSN
Brown Mackie College Nurse Specialist
Forest, Ohio

Sister Ann Wiesen, RN, MRA
Erwin Technical Center
Tampa, Florida

CONSULTANTS

Emily Cannon, RN, MSN
Associate Professor of Nursing
Ivy Tech Community College
Terre Haute, Indiana

Kim D. Cooper, MSN
Nursing Department Program Chair
Ivy Tech Community College
Terre Haute, Indiana

Kelly Gosnell, RN, MSN
Associate Professor of Nursing
Ivy Tech Community College
Terre Haute, Indiana

To the Instructor

The sixth edition of *Foundations and Adult Health Nursing* was developed to educate the practical/vocational nursing student and provide the knowledge required to care competently and safely for a wide variety of patients in various settings. As the level of knowledge and responsibility increases for LPN/LVNs in all health care settings from acute to community-based care, it is essential that a text such as *Foundations and Adult Health Nursing* be available to educate the student for the growing demands of this profession.

This full-color text provides all of the fundamentals and skills, maternal and neonatal, pediatric, geriatric, mental health, community, and anatomy and physiology content needed in the LPN/LVN curriculum. Accessible, clearly written, and user-friendly, this new edition was revised to incorporate the most current and clinically-relevant information available on the following topics:

- Historical, legal, and ethical aspects of nursing
- Communication
- Physical assessment
- Nursing process and critical thinking
- Cultural and ethical considerations in nursing interventions
- Growth and development across the life span
- Death and dying
- Safety, including terrorism and bioterrorism interventions
- Pain management, comfort, rest, and sleep
- Complementary and alternative therapies
- Basic nutrition and nutritional therapy
- Fluids and electrolytes
- Mathematics review and medication administration
- Emergency nursing interventions
- Maternal, neonatal, and pediatric care
- Gerontologic nursing and care of the older adult
- Mental health and community health
- Role of the LPN/LVN and leadership

Finally, it is our belief that nursing will always be both an art and a science. This philosophy is reflected throughout the text.

ORGANIZATION AND STANDARD FEATURES

The organization of the sixth edition continues to follow the strengths of the previous edition, based on positive comments from educators and students. The basic nursing skills are provided throughout the text and with special emphasis in Chapter 20. Medical-surgical nursing—with an overview of anatomy and physiology and a separate chapter on care of the surgical patient—is discussed in Unit Nine: Adult Health Nursing.

TABLE OF CONTENTS

The text is divided into 10 units with 58 chapters. Units are organized for easy, logical association of content. New and additional content has been added to ensure that students have access to the most current information. The following are just a few of the many recent advancements in treatment and nursing care described in this new edition: recognizing blood loss in vital sign changes, new technologies including capsule endoscopy for diagnosis of gastrointestinal disorders and for clot-retrieval in patients with acute stroke, C-reactive protein testing for coronary artery disease and biventricular pacing to improve outcomes for heart failure, new insulin and insulin-enhancing drugs, current procedures for cardiopulmonary resuscitation (CPR) and hands-only CPR, revised mammogram and breast self-examination guidelines, computer-controlled dispensing systems for medications, and current immunization schedules and new vaccines to help prevent cervical cancer.

CHAPTER ORGANIZATION

Disorders chapters typically are organized in the following format for more effective learning:

- Etiology/Pathophysiology
- Clinical Manifestations
- Assessment (with subjective and objective data)
- Diagnostic Tests
- Medical Management
- Nursing Diagnoses and Interventions (including relevant medications)
- Patient Teaching
- Prognosis

NURSING PROCESS

The nursing process as applied to specific disorders is integrated throughout. A special nursing process summary section appears at the end of appropriate chapters, enabling the reader to see more clearly its application to the chapter content as a whole. We have emphasized the role of the LPN/LVN in the nursing process as follows:

- The LPN/LVN will participate in planning care for the patient based on the patient's needs
- The LPN/LVN will review the patient's plan of care and recommend revisions as needed

- The LPN/LVN will follow defined prioritization for patient care
- The LPN/LVN will use clinical pathways, care maps, or care plans to guide and review patient care

REFERENCES AND SUGGESTED READINGS

These are grouped by chapter and listed at the end of the book for easy access. **Additional Resources** such as websites and agencies are included where applicable.

In appendixes, **The Joint Commission's Lists of Dangerous Abbreviations, Acronyms, and Symbols** promotes safety in clinical practice in such areas as avoiding dosage errors, and **Common Abbreviations** and **Laboratory Reference Values** provide quick access to important information. **Answers to the Review Questions for the NCLEX® Examination** are provided in Appendix D.

LPN THREADS

The sixth edition of *Foundations and Adult Health Nursing* shares some features and design elements with other Elsevier LPN/LVN textbooks. The purpose of these *LPN Threads* is to make it easier for students and instructors to use the variety of books required by the relatively brief and demanding LPN/LVN curriculum. *LPN Threads* include the following:

- A **reading level evaluation** is performed on every manuscript chapter during the book's development to increase the consistency among chapters and ensure the text is easy to understand.
- **Full-color design, cover, photos,** and **illustrations** are visually appealing and pedagogically useful.
- **Objectives** (numbered) begin each chapter. Chapter objectives provide a framework for content and are especially important in providing the structure for the TEACH Lesson Plans for the textbook.
- **Key Terms** with phonetic pronunciations and page number references are listed at the beginning of each chapter. Key terms appear in color in the chapter and are defined briefly, with full definitions in the **Glossary.** Simple phonetic pronunciations accompany difficult medical, nursing, or scientific terms or other words that may be difficult for students to pronounce. The goal is to help the student reader with limited proficiency in English to develop a greater command of the pronunciation of scientific and nonscientific English terminology. It is hoped that a more general competency in the understanding and use of medical and scientific language will result.
- A wide variety of **special features** related to critical thinking, clinical practice, care of the older adult, health promotion, safety, patient teaching, complementary and alternative therapies, communication, home health care, delegation and assignment, and more. Refer to the To the Student section of this introduction on pages xiii to xv for descriptions and examples of features from the pages of this textbook.
- **Critical Thinking Questions** with each Nursing Care Plan give students opportunities to practice critical thinking and clinical decision-making skills with realistic patient scenarios. Answers are provided in the Instructor Resources section on the Evolve website.
- **Key Points,** located at the end of chapters, follow the chapter objectives and serve as a useful chapter review.
- A full suite of **Instructor Resources** including TEACH Lesson Plans and Lecture Outlines, PowerPoint Lecture Slides, Test Bank, Image Collection, and Open Book Quizzes. Each of these teaching resources is described in detail below.
- In addition to consistent content, design, and support resources, these textbooks benefit from the advice and input of the **Elsevier LPN/LVN Advisory Board.**

TEACHING AND LEARNING PACKAGE

FOR STUDENTS

- A media-rich **Companion CD** is included with every book. Helpful features include animations and audio clips depicting physiologic processes, physical assessment video clips, an English/Spanish glossary with definitions and audio pronunciations, an anatomy coloring book, and a fluids and electrolytes tutorial.
- An **Evolve website** provides free student resources, including additional review questions for the NCLEX Examination for every chapter, calculators (Body Mass Index, IV Dosage, Unit Conversion, to name a few), and animations and video clips in addition to those provided on the book's Companion CD. All assets from the Companion CD are also available on the Evolve website.
- The ***Study Guide for Foundations and Adult Health Nursing*** is designed to promote learning, understanding, and application of the content in the textbook. Each chapter ties specific activities to specific objectives rather than simply listing objectives and activities separately. Illustrations from the textbook are incorporated into some of the exercises. Activities include hundreds of labeling, matching, and fill-in-the-blank questions, each with textbook page references; critical thinking questions with clinical scenarios; multiple-choice and alternate-format questions for NCLEX review; and performance checklists for every skill in the textbook. The complete answer key is provided to instructors in the Instructor Resources section of the Evolve website. *Sold separately.*

- *Virtual Clinical Excursions* is an interactive workbook/CD-ROM package that guides the student through a multifloor virtual hospital in a hands-on clinical learning experience. Students can assess and analyze information, diagnose, set priorities, and implement and evaluate care. NCLEX®-style review questions provide immediate testing of clinical knowledge. *Sold separately.*

FOR INSTRUCTORS

The comprehensive **Evolve Resources with TEACH Instructor Resource** provides a rich array of teaching tools that includes the following:

- **TEACH Lesson Plans with Lecture Outlines**, based on the textbook learning objectives, provide ready-to-use lesson plans that tie together all of the text and ancillary components provided for *Foundations and Adult Health Nursing*.
- A collection of more than 1200 text and graphic **PowerPoint Lecture Slides** are specific to the text.
- A **Test Bank**, delivered in ExamView and Partest, provides approximately 2000 multiple-choice and alternate-format NCLEX-style questions. Each question includes the correct answer, rationale, topic, objective, cognitive level, step of the nursing process, and NCLEX category of client needs, as well as corresponding textbook page references.
- An **Image Collection** contains nearly 800 images from the textbook. Images are suitable for incorporation into classroom lectures, PowerPoint presentations, or distance-learning applications.
- An **Open-Book Quiz** for every chapter includes textbook page references for each question.
- **Answer Keys** are provided for the Critical Thinking Questions in Nursing Care Plans and for the activities in the Study Guide.

To the Student

Designed with you in mind, *Foundations and Adult Health Nursing* presents fundamentals, skills, and medical-surgical nursing concepts in a visually-appealing and easy-to-use format. Here are some of the numerous special features that will help you understand and apply the material.

READING AND REVIEW TOOLS

Objectives introduce the chapter topics.

Key Terms are listed with page number references, and difficult medical, nursing, or scientific terms are accompanied by simple phonetic pronunciations. Key terms are in color the first time they appear in the narrative and are briefly defined in the text, with complete definitions in the Glossary.

Each chapter ends with a ***Get Ready for the NCLEX® Examination!* section.**

1 **Key Points** follow the chapter objectives and serve as a useful chapter review.

2 An extensive set of **Review Questions for the NCLEX® Examination** provide immediate opportunity for testing your understanding of the chapter content. **Answers** are located in the Appendix D in the back of the book.

ADDITIONAL LEARNING RESOURCES

3 The **Companion CD** included with your textbook contains Animations, Video Clips, Audio Clips, an English/Spanish Audio Glossary, a Body Spectrum Anatomy Coloring Book, and a Fluids and Electrolytes Tutorial. Your free online **Evolve Resources** at **http://evolve.elsevier.com/Christensen/foundationsadult** gives you access to all this *and* even more Review Questions for the NCLEX Examination, a Concept Map Creator, and much more.

CHAPTER FEATURES

4 **Skills** are presented in a logical step-by-step format with accompanying full-color illustrations. Clearly defined **nursing actions** followed by **rationales** in italicized type show you how and why skills are performed. These Skills also emphasize the importance of accurate, effective documentation of data.

5 **Nursing Care Plans,** developed around specific case studies, include nursing diagnoses with an emphasis on patient goals and outcomes and questions to promote **critical thinking.** These sample care plans are valuable tools that can be used as a guideline in the clinical setting. The critical thinking aspect empowers you to develop sound clinical decision-making skills.

6 **Nursing diagnoses and interventions** are screened and set apart in the text in a clear, easy-to-understand format to help you learn to participate in the development of a nursing care plan. The most current NANDA International–approved nursing diagnoses are used.

7 **Evidence-Based Practice boxes,** ***new to this edition,*** summarize the latest research findings and highlight how they apply to LPN/LVN practice.

8 **Safety Alert! boxes** emphasize the importance of maintaining safety in patient and resident care to protect patients, family, health care providers, and the public from accidents and the spread of disease.

9 **Health Promotion boxes** emphasize a healthy lifestyle, preventive behaviors, and screening tests to assist in the prevention of accidents and disease.

10 **Coordinated Care** boxes throughout the text promote comprehensive patient care with other members of the health care team, focusing on prioritization, assignment, supervision, collaboration, and leadership topics.

11 **Medication tables** developed for specific disorders provide quick access to action, dosage, side effects, and nursing considerations for commonly used medications.

Complementary and Alternative Therapies boxes give a breakdown of specific nontraditional therapies, along with precautions and possible side effects. A complete discussion of complementary and alternative therapies is given in Chapter 17.

Cultural Considerations boxes explore select specific cultural preferences and how to address the needs of a culturally diverse patient and resident population when planning nursing care.

12 **Communication boxes** focus on communication strategies with real-life examples of nurse-patient dialogue.

13 **Patient Teaching boxes** appear frequently in the text to help develop awareness of the vital role of patient/family teaching in health care today.

14 **Life Span Considerations for the Older Adult boxes** bring a gerontologic perspective to nursing care, focusing on the nursing interventions unique to the older adult patient or resident.

15 **Home Care Considerations** discuss the issues facing patients and caregivers in the home setting.

Get Ready for the NCLEX® Examination!

1

Key Points

- Discuss safety measures for coping with violence in the workplace.
- Preventing falls, electrical injuries, fires, burns, and accidental poisoning is key to maintaining a safe environment.
- Left-handed patients need special considerations to cope in a right-handed hospital environment.
- Infants, young children, older adults, and the ill or injured patient are at risk for falling.
- Proper patient orientation includes information about the use of the call light and bed controls. Place frequently used items within reach of patients.
- Question all patients regarding allergies. It is imperative to ask specifically about food and latex allergies.
- Keep adjustable beds in the low position except when care is given.
- Gait belts are an added safety feature to use when assisting patients to ambulate.
- Consider designing a restraint-free environment before applying an SRD.
- Make sure your priority is patient safety or the safety of others when applying an SRD.
- SRD use has the potential to result in increased restlessness, disorientation, agitation, anxiety, and feelings of powerlessness.
- Once SRDs are applied to a patient, it is mandatory to document the position of the device, circulation, physical and mental status, and ongoing need for the device.
- When extremity SRDs are applied, place gauze or padding around the extremity and secure the ends of the ties to the bed frame, not to the side rails.
- Remove SRDs at least every 2 hours and assess the skin. Do not leave the patient unattended during this time.
- Know agency policy and procedures regarding SRD use and documentation.
- Electrical accidents are often prevented by reporting frayed or broken electrical cords or any shocks felt when using equipment.
- It is possible to reduce fire-related injuries by knowing the location of exits, fire alarm boxes, and fire extinguishers.
- By remembering the formula RACE (**R**escue patients, sound the **A**larm, **C**onfine the fire, and **E**xtinguish or **E**vacuate), you will be prepared when safety is threatened by a fire.
- Participation in fire and disaster drills helps staff become familiar with established protocols.
- Poison control centers are valuable sources of information when poisoning is suspected or has occurred.
- A terrorist attack is a potential environmental health threat.
- Bioterrorism, or the use of biological agents to create fear and threat, is the most likely form a terrorist attack will take.
- Several national organizations, including OSHA, NIOSH, and the CDC, provide guidelines that help reduce safety hazards in the workplace.

Additional Learning Resources

3

Go to your Companion CD for an audio glossary, animations, video clips, and more.

evolve Be sure to visit the Evolve site at http://evolve.elsevier.com/Christensen/foundations/ for additional online resources.

Review Questions for the NCLEX® Examination

2

1. On the transfer sheet of a patient admitted to a health care facility is the order "restrain prn." SRDs are used in the hospital setting to prevent patient injury. Which statement is correct?
   1. SRDs often decrease anxiety because the patient feels safer.
   2. All older adult patients need some type of SRD at night.
   3. Allow as much freedom of movement as possible when applying SRDs.
   4. When using soft SRDs to prevent injury from falling out of bed, tie them to the side rail.
2. In the situation of question 1, what is an appropriate goal (expected outcome) for the patient requiring a physical restraint?
   1. Patient will remain free of injury.
   2. Patient will allow SRDs to be used.
   3. Nurse will check SRD every 30 minutes.
   4. Use least restrictive form of SRD possible.
3. Documentation related to use of an SRD is required to include:
   1. the nurse's feelings about having used the SRD.
   2. the specific type of SRD used.
   3. confirmation of a prn order for use of the SRD.
   4. evidence that the patient was assessed every 8 hours.
4. When caring for the patient who requires the use of an SRD, the nurse remembers that an appropriate nursing intervention when caring for a patient who needs an SRD is to:
   1. monitor the skin for signs of impairment.
   2. remove the SRD once every 24 hours.
   3. secure the ends of the ties to the side rails.
   4. ensure that the SRD is in place at all times.
5. The nurse discovers smoke in a soiled utility room and remembers that the initial step taken to protect the patient in the event of a fire is to:
   1. notify the fire department.
   2. disconnect the oxygen supply.
   3. use any extinguisher on the fire.
   4. remove the patient from the area.

Performing hand hygiene (Skill 12-1) will provide the necessary protection before you care for a patient. To effectively clean hands soiled with dirt or organic matter, or if you have handled a contaminated article, soap or detergents that contain antiseptic and water are required. The standard is to wash for 15 to 30 seconds using hospital approved soap, running hands under warm water (both cold and very hot water increase the risk of drying and chapping the skin). Box 12-7 contains an overview of the CDC hand hygiene guidelines, and Box 12-8 addresses the use of alcohol-based waterless antiseptics for hand hygiene. All forms of health care–associated infections can result from improper hand hygiene and use of contaminated equipment.

The CDC has pointed out the need for the health care worker in contact with patients to remove all artificial fingernails to maintain infection control principles (see Evidence-Based Practice box).

4

Skill 12-1 Performing Hand Hygiene Using Soap and Water

Nursing Action *(Rationale)*

1. Inspect hands, observing for visible soiling, breaks, or cuts in the skin and cuticles. *(Poor personal hygiene and an open area of the skin provide areas in which microorganisms are able to grow.)*
2. Determine amount of contaminant of hands. *(Determines the type of hand hygiene needed.)*
3. Assess areas around the skin that are contaminated. *(Prevents contamination of hands during and after hand hygiene procedure.)*
4. Remove jewelry (except plain wedding band), and push watch and long sleeves above wrist. *(Microorganisms collect in jewelry and watch bands; removing jewelry makes it easier to wash all areas of hands and wrists.)*
5. Adjust the water to appropriate temperature and force. *(Water that is too hot or too cold can chap skin, and too much force will cause splashing and spread microorganisms to other areas, especially your clothing.)*
6. Wet hands and wrists under the running water, always keeping hands lower than elbows. *(Hands are the most contaminated part of the upper extremities; water should flow from the wrists [least contaminated area] over the hands, and then down the drain.)*
7. Lather hands with liquid soap (about 1 teaspoon). *(Soap lather emulsifies fat and aids in cleansing.)*
8. Wash hands thoroughly using a firm, circular motion and friction on back of hands, palms, and wrists. Wash each finger individually, paying special attention to areas between fingers and knuckles by interlacing fingers and thumbs and moving hands back and forth, causing friction (see illustration). *(Helps to loosen soil and microorganisms, both resident [normally present] and transient [acquired from contamination].)*
9. Wash for 15 to 30 seconds, rinse thoroughly, relather, and wash another minute, using continuous friction. *(Rinsing removes the loosened microorganisms, and relathering ensures more thorough cleaning. The greater the contamination, the more need for longer washing.)*

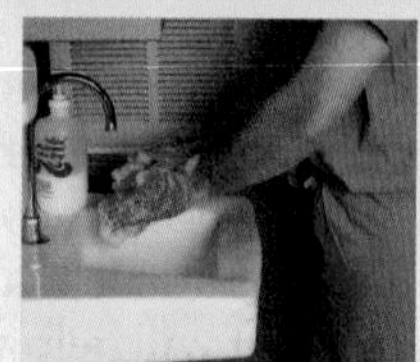

Step 8

10. Rinse wrists and hands completely, again keeping hands lower than elbows (see illustration). *(Water should run from cleaner area [the wrists] over the hands, and then down the drain, rinsing the dirt and microorganisms away.)*
11. Clean fingernails carefully under running water, using fingernails of other hand or blunt end of an orange stick. *(Reduces chance of microorganisms remaining under nails.)*

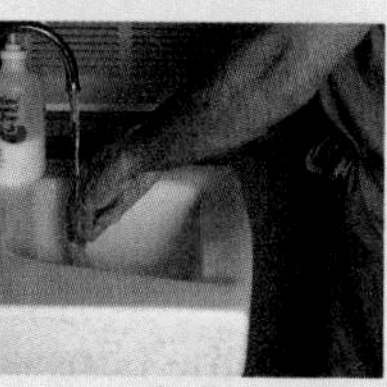

Step 10

5

Patient Teaching

Urostomy Care

- Teach patient and caregivers to avoid touching the stoma with adhesive solvents to prevent irritating the stoma.
- Teach patient and caregivers to wick the urine with an absorbent, lint-free material to prevent a constant flow of urine while changing the appliance.
- Teach patient and caregivers to remove hair from the stomal area with scissors or an electric razor to prevent hair follicles from becoming irritated when the pouch is removed. Suggest that the procedure be performed in the morning before fluids are consumed and when urine flows more easily.
- Teach patient and caregivers that the properly applied appliance is able to remain in place 3 to 5 days.
- Teach patient and caregivers to empty appliance through the drain valve when it is one third to one half full to prevent the weight of the urine from loosening the seal around the stoma.
- Teach patient and caregivers to connect the appliance to a urine-collection container at night to prevent urine from stagnating in the appliance.
- Teach sanitary and dietary measures that will protect the peristomal skin and control odor.
- Offer positive reinforcement and written instructions, perhaps even videos.

See Patient Teaching box on ostomy care for further instructions.

Coordinated Care

6

Collaboration

OSTOMY CARE

- The skill of pouching a stoma requires the critical thinking and knowledge application unique to a nurse. Some agencies permit delegation of the pouching of an established ostomy. In this case, instruct the care provider in the expected amount, color, and consistency of drainage from the ostomy. In addition, teach the care provider to report changes in the stoma and surrounding skin integrity.
- The skill of pouching an incontinent urinary diversion (see Chapter 10 in *Adult Health Nursing*) requires the critical thinking and knowledge application unique to a nurse. In some agencies, a stoma nurse specialist is available to provide this care. Assistive personnel who provide personal care receive instructions to report any leakage of urine and/or breakdown of skin integrity to the nurse.
- The skill of irrigating a newly established colostomy requires the critical thinking and knowledge application unique to a nurse. However, in some settings assistive personnel are trained to perform irrigations on established ostomies. Review agency policy.

7

Home Care Considerations

Ostomy Care

- Provide a referral to a home health agency or a visiting nurse before patient's hospital discharge.
- Pouches that wear well in the hospital will not necessarily wear well when the patient resumes a normal routine.
- A visiting nurse is often able to help achieve compliance with irrigation routine and assist in problem solving when necessary (colostomies are no longer routinely irrigated). A typical suggestion from the visiting nurse perspective is to hang the irrigation solution container from a hook on the wall or from a shower curtain rod instead of an intravenous pole.
- Urostomy, colostomy, and ileostomy products are usually available for purchase at local pharmacies.
- Encourage the patient to become involved with local ostomy organizations.
- Teach the patient and caregivers to routinely inspect the appearance of the stoma and the surrounding skin. The proper appearance of the stoma is moist, shiny, and dark pink to red, with minimal if any bleeding around it. Teach to report excessive bleeding, abnormal color, or swelling to you or the physician.
- Teach the patient and caregivers to avoid using alcohol around the stoma because alcohol dilates capillaries, causing bleeding.
- Teach the patient and caregivers not to use cold creams around the stoma because they tend to prevent pouches from adhering.
- Teach the patient and caregivers not to use peroxide on or around the stoma because it irritates tissue.
- Instruct the patient and caregivers to wash skin with mild soap and water. (Be certain to rinse thoroughly because soap is often irritating to the peristomal skin.) Pat or blot dry the skin thoroughly.
- Evaluate the patient's home toileting facilities. Evaluation includes the following:
  - —The presence of adequate functioning and accessible toileting facilities
  - —Number and location of toileting facilities
  - —Number of other people living with the patient who have to share the toileting facilities
  - —Identification of the pattern of use of the toileting facilities by the other people living with the patient (time of day and amount of time spent in bathroom)
- Evaluate the patient ostomy routine in relationship to usual lifestyle after discharge.
- Caution the patient that it is not possible to flush most ostomy pouches and barriers down the toilet; they clog the system. Dispose of used ostomy pouches according to local sanitation regulations.
- Make sure patient understands that it is not necessary to use sterile gauze to cleanse the stoma. Using a washcloth made of any soft material is fine.
- Review the patient's dietary pattern. Help patient and family members learn the types of foods to avoid so as to prevent problems with effluent (discharge or drainage of liquid, solid, or gas from the stoma) or odor.
- Teach patients that if water is not drinkable, they should not use it for irrigations (e.g., patients traveling to another country).

8

Communication

Developmental Considerations: Communicating Effectively with Young Children

INFANTS

- Consider your body language, such as gestures and posture, as well as pitch, intonation, and intensity of your voice.
- Nonverbal approaches work especially well for infants, with cuddling, patting, or some other form of gentle physical contact often quieting them.
- Maintain a calm voice and avoid sudden, loud noises. The actual words spoken are not as important as the way they are spoken.
- Because infants often begin fearing strangers at ages as young as 6 months, holding out the hands and asking the older infant to "come over" is seldom successful. If handling is necessary, the best approach is to pick up the infant firmly without using gestures.
- Infants are usually more at ease when upright and in visual contact with and proximity to their parents.

PRESCHOOL AND YOUNG SCHOOL-AGE CHILDREN

- Avoid quick approaches with preschool and young school-age children. Let them make the first move whenever possible.
- Broad smiles and other facial contortions sometimes have a threatening appearance.
- Avoid extended eye contact until after the child is comfortable.
- Position yourself at the child's eye level. You will appear less threatening to the child, and you will play down the child's smallness.
- Children are often more responsive when remaining close to the parent, such as sitting on the parent's lap.
- New or intimidating situations, such as hospitalization, are potentially stressful and make it even more difficult for children to grasp the new words they will encounter in this environment, as well as even simple words that express unfamiliar ideas. Avoid using expressions with dual meanings, such as "put to sleep."
- Substitute words that have potentially threatening interpretations with words that are less emotionally charged, such as replacing "stick" with "gently slide," or "hurt" with "feel uncomfortable."

OLDER SCHOOL-AGE CHILDREN

- Give children an opportunity to express their thoughts, concerns, and feelings. Listen and respond to underlying messages rather than just verbal content. Be attentive, try not to interrupt, and avoid making comments that convey disapproval or surprise.
- Avoid prying, asking embarrassing questions, and lecturing when giving advice.

ADOLESCENTS

- Be prepared to deal with a wide range of emotions and behaviors with adolescents. Give concrete explanations that focus on the teenager's concerns, even though the adolescent's capacity to think in abstract terms increases with age.
- It is not necessary to be fluent in teen jargon, but ask for clarification when necessary.
- To enhance communication, exchange information without using questions that back the teenager into a corner. Initially confine discussions to less threatening topics to allow time for trust to develop.
- Ask broad, open-ended questions before specific questions, such as "How's school?" before asking, "What is the best (or worst) thing about school?"

Modified from Clutter, L., et al. (1987). Communicating effectively with young children. *Child Nurse*, 5(4), 1.

Adequate preparation makes the transition from the security of a home to the unfamiliar atmosphere of a hospital less difficult. When it is best to begin preparation and how much information is right to give will vary. The age of the child will have a significant influence. A physician provides a family with details about a treatment plan, the length of stay, and expected results or outcomes. Parents are then able to reinforce the information by providing explanations to the child, using simple, age-appropriate terms. Usually there is time and opportunity before the actual admission for the child to talk about what is going to occur.

PREADMISSION PROGRAMS

Many hospitals have orientation programs for children who are to be admitted. In some hospitals, nurses conduct preadmission programs; other hospitals use **child life specialists** (health care professionals with extensive knowledge of child growth and development and the special emotional needs of children who are hospitalized).

The programs are based on the child's level of understanding and stage of development, with the purpose of familiarizing the child with hospital surroundings. These programs help to dismiss the child's fantasies and correct misconceptions. The programs include tours and audiovisual aids, such as movies, videos, and puppet shows. The child is given simple explanations of equipment used during surgery and hospitalization.

It is helpful for children to handle some of the items they will see while hospitalized, such as masks and gowns, stethoscopes, anesthesia masks, and syringes (without the needles attached). Make sure there is time for questions. Encourage children to talk about what they have seen or heard. By doing so, you will be able to identify problem areas or areas of concern. Some hospitals distribute coloring books or storybooks that focus on the information covered in the orientation program. This material reinforces information and also helps parents answer their children's questions. Many programs send the parents away with a brochure that describes hospital routines and lists items the hospital permits children to bring with them to the hospital. Keep written information simple, clear, and at an understandable level.

Timing of the orientation is important. There has to be enough advance time for the child to be able to assimilate the information after the program, but not so

1

Nursing Care Plan 47-1 The Patient with Leukemia

Ms. May is a 26-year-old patient diagnosed with acute lymphocytic leukemia. She is married and the mother of a 3-year-old daughter. Ms. May has been receiving chemotherapy and is immunocompromised, with a differential white blood cell (WBC) count revealing a neutrophil count of 22%. Her hemoglobin is 8.8 g/dL, and her platelets are 55,000/mm^3. Her mouth appears edematous, and she complains of oral tenderness.

NURSING DIAGNOSIS *Risk for infection, related to leukopenia*

Patient Goals and Expected Outcomes	Nursing Intervention	Evaluation/Rationale
Patient or caregiver will identify measures to prevent or control infection	Inspect all body sites for infection at least daily; note and report fever, sore throat, purulent exudate, chills, cough, burning with urination, erythema, edema, tenderness, and pain.	Patient will remain free of infection.
Patient or caregiver will verbalize and report signs and symptoms of infection	Monitor vital signs. Obtain cultures as ordered. Monitor WBC counts and culture reports. Administer antibiotics on time as ordered. Promote and maintain hygiene integrity of skin and mucous membranes. Use aseptic technique in treatments. Teach the patient and family: • Necessity of avoiding crowds or people with infections while WBC count is <1000/mm^3 • Personal hygiene measures • Signs and symptoms of infection	Patient demonstrates no signs or symptoms of infection; temperature and WBC count are within normal range.

NURSING DIAGNOSIS *Ineffective coping, related to diagnosis and disease process*

Patient Goals and Expected Outcomes	Nursing Intervention	Evaluation
Patient and family will demonstrate measures to effectively cope by verbalizing role of family, significant others, and support groups in therapeutic coping	Assess coping capabilities of patient and significant others. Discuss disease process and expectations. Alleviate knowledge deficit. Encourage questions and self-expression: listen actively, demonstrate compassion, reassure with touch and personal contact. Assess fear of threat of death: allow time for personal expression and provide one-on-one discussion opportunity.	Patient and family express factors that are causing anxiety and powerlessness.

Critical Thinking Questions

1. What should the nurse do if a visitor with an obvious upper respiratory tract infection is seen approaching Ms. May's room?
2. What nursing interventions would be most appropriate in providing therapeutic oral hygiene for Ms. May?
3. What kind of a bath and activities of daily living would be most beneficial for Ms. May?

Clinical Manifestations

Skin and mucous membrane manifestations include petechiae and ecchymoses. Epistaxis and gingival bleeding are common. Circulatory hypovolemia is noted through hypotension; pallor; cool, clammy skin; and tachycardia. GI tract bleeding is common, with abdominal flank pain caused by internal bleeding. CNS involvement ranges from altered response and malaise to loss of consciousness or affected speech.

Assessment

Subjective data include a history of bleeding after surgical or dental procedures. Exposure to toxic or hazardous agents or to radiation may be revealed. Complaint of headache, extremity pain, and numbness is noted. Medications taken (e.g., aspirin) may lead to suspicion of toxicity.

Collection of **objective data** involves observation of pain on pressure to the abdomen, revealing liver and spleen tenderness and perhaps enlargement. Skin and mucous membranes may have petechiae, ecchymoses, and occasionally hematoma. Emesis and stool may show signs of bleeding. Joint examination reveals motion pain.

Diagnostic Tests

The platelet count is low. The RBC count is low with a decreased hemoglobin level. Coagulation time is altered. Bone marrow studies show abnormal cells.

orrhoids or marked protrusion. Surgical removal may be done by cautery, clamp, or excision. After removal of the hemorrhoid, wounds can be left open or closed, although closed wounds are reported to heal faster. Hemorrhoidectomy is not considered a major procedure, but pain may be acute, requiring opioids and analgesic ointments. Complications include hemorrhage, local infection, pain, urinary retention, and abscess.

Nursing Interventions and Patient Teaching

Rectal conditions can be embarrassing to the patient, and the nurse's direct but concerned attitude can decrease this embarrassment. Assess the knowledge level by asking patients about their condition, what they have been told about treatment, and what treatments have been done before surgery and why.

Observe the patient with a prolapsed hemorrhoid for edema, thrombosis, and ischemia. Ischemic tissue will be dark red to necrotic (black). Explain that a low-bulk diet can produce chronic constipation (see Evidence-Based Practice box).

For the surgical patient, take vital signs frequently for the first 24 hours to rule out internal bleeding. Sitz baths are given several times daily. Early ambulation and a soft diet facilitate bowel elimination. The patient may have a great deal of anxiety concerning the first defecation; open a discussion on this and provide an analgesic before the bowel movement to reduce discomfort. A stool softener such as docusate (Colace) is usually ordered for the first few postoperative days.

Nursing diagnoses and interventions for the patient with hemorrhoids include but are not limited to the following:

2

Nursing Diagnoses	Nursing Interventions
Pain, related to edema, prolapse, and surgical interventions	Instruct patient to wash anal area after defecation and pat dry. Sitz baths or local heat applied to site may be soothing. Use of local anesthetics (dibucaine ointment or Tucks pads) may give relief. Reinforce need for high-residue diet. Instruct patient on manual reduction of external hemorrhoids. Apply ice packs to hemorrhoids if thrombosed to prevent edema and pain. Use cushion for sitting postoperatively.
Anxiety, related to: • previous experiences • fear of first bowel movement postoperatively • lack of knowledge regarding diet	Establish a supportive relationship with patient. Explain need for high-residue diet. Administer laxatives and oil-retention enema as ordered. Give analgesics before first bowel movement and a sitz bath for pain relief.

3

Evidence-Based Practice Treatment of Chronic Constipation in Older Adults

Evidence Summary

The combined effect of decreased activity, change in diet, multiple diseases, and multiple drugs all put older adults at increased risk for constipation. Constipation is diagnosed when a person has two of the following criteria for 12 weeks during the past year: straining, pelletlike stools, sensation of incomplete evacuation, sensation of anal blockage, or using manual maneuvers, all for more than 25% of bowel movements; or having fewer than three bowel movements per week. Data are too limited in the older adult population to recommend one treatment over another. Because constipation in older adults is more likely to be a result of multiple physical and pathologic conditions, there is no consensus that fits all older adults. From a pharmacologic perspective, the ideal drug is selected in terms of effectiveness, tolerance, adverse effects, drug interactions, and cost-effectiveness.

Application to Nursing Practice

- When possible, replace a medication causing constipation with a substitute.
- Encourage older adults to increase physical activity when feasible.
- Give attention to the potential risk of fluid overload in older adult clients with congestive heart failure or renal failure.
- Encourage fiber intake of 20 g/day of wheat bran to start. Observe for bloating and flatulence in older adults.
- Stool softeners are no longer recommended for constipation.
- Fiber and bulk-forming laxatives are the first step in treating constipation in older adults.
- Osmotic laxatives are effective in the treatment of constipation in older adults because they are well tolerated and have no known interactions with other drugs.
- Stimulant laxatives are more effective than placebo, but concern remains regarding their adverse effects on older adults.
- Older adults who have mobility problems often need enemas to avoid an impaction. The tap water enema is the safest for regular use. Glycerol suppositories trigger the defecatory reflex and are sometimes useful in treating older adults.

From Potter, P.A., & Perry, A.G. (2009). *Fundamentals of nursing: concepts, process, and practice.* (7th ed.) St. Louis: Mosby. Adapted from Bosshard, W., Dreher, R., Schnegg, J.F., (2004). The treatment of chronic constipation in elderly people: an update, *Drugs Aging, 21*(14), 911-930.

4

Table 55-2 Medications for Immune Disorders

Generic (Trade)	Action	Side Effects	Nursing Implications
Diphenhydramine (Benadryl)	Antihistamine	Drowsiness, confusion, nasal stuffiness, dry mouth, photosensitivity, urine retention	Use cautiously with central nervous system depressants, including alcohol; give with food; it is a safe hypnotic for older adults; tell patient to avoid driving or hazardous activity due to drowsiness.
Loratadine (Claritin)	Nonsedating antihistamine	Slight sedation (more common with increased doses)	Store in tight container at room temperature. Teach patient and family to avoid driving or other hazardous activities if drowsiness occurs.
Fexofenadine (Allegra)	Nonsedating antihistamine	Headache, drowsiness, blurred vision, hypotension, bradycardia, tachycardia, dysrhythmias (rare), urinary retention, pancytopenia	
Dexamethasone (Decadron)	Corticosteroid		Do not use for extended period; use cautiously with patients with diabetes or peptic ulcers.
Flunisolide (AeroBid)	Corticosteroid (inhaled)	Headache, transient nasal burning, epistaxis, nausea, vomiting	Not effective for acute episodes; use regularly; teach care and cleaning of inhaler; if symptoms do not improve in 3 weeks, consult physician.
Epinephrine (Adrenalin Chloride, Sus-Phrine, EpiPen)	Bronchodilator	Nervousness, tremor, headache, hypertension, tachycardia, ventricular fibrillation, stroke	Do not use with monoamine oxidase inhibitor; use cautiously in patients with hyperthyroidism, hypertension, diabetes, and heart disease.

as leukotriene-receptor blockers, and zileuton (Zyflo) inhibits the production of leukotrienes.

Nursing Diagnoses

Nursing diagnoses for patients with hypersensitivity include (1) *risk for injury,* related to exposure to allergen; (2) *activity intolerance,* related to malaise; and (3) *risk for infection,* related to inflammation of protective mucous membranes.

Patient Teaching

Patient teaching should revolve around the specific diagnosis. Advise the patient with seasonal allergies to avoid offending allergens, and ensure he or she understands the therapeutic medication plan. Focus on health promotion and health teaching for self-care management (see Safety Alert box).

5

Safety Alert!

Treating the Patient with a Hypersensitivity Reaction

- List all of a patient's allergies on the chart, the nursing care plan, and the medication record.
- After an allergic disorder is diagnosed, therapeutic treatment is aimed at reducing exposure to the offending allergen; treating the symptoms; and, if necessary, desensitizing the person through immunotherapy.
- All health care workers must be prepared for the rare but life-threatening anaphylactic reaction, which requires immediate medical and nursing interventions.
- Instruct the patient to wear a medical-alert bracelet listing the particular drug allergy.
- For a patient allergic to insect stings, commercial bee sting kits contain epinephrine and a tourniquet. Teach the patient to apply the tourniquet and self-inject the subcutaneous epinephrine. The patient should wear a medical-alert bracelet and carry a bee sting kit whenever going outdoors.

toms. The major difficulty in symptomatic patients is gastroesophageal reflux, manifested as pyrosis (heartburn) after overeating. Complications of strangulation, infarction, or ulceration of the herniated stomach are serious and require surgical intervention. Factors contributing to the development of these hernias include obesity, trauma, and a general weakening of the supporting structures as a result of aging (see Life Span Considerations box).

Medical Management

The physician may perform (1) a posterior gastropexy, in which the stomach is returned to the abdomen and sutured in place; or (2) a laparoscopically performed Nissen fundoplication, in which the fundus is wrapped around the lower part of the esophagus and sutured in place (Figure 45-16). The use of laparoscopic techniques has reduced the overall morbidity, complications, and the cost of hospitalization associated with a thoracic or open abdominal approach. However, a thoracic or open abdominal approach may be used in selected cases.

Nursing Interventions

Nursing care of the patient after surgery is similar to that after gastric surgery or thoracic surgery, depending on the procedure performed.

6

Life Span Considerations

Older Adults

Gastrointestinal Disorders

- Loss of teeth and resultant use of dentures can interfere with chewing and lead to digestive complaints.
- Dysphagia is commonly seen in the older adult population and may be caused by changes in the esophageal musculature or by neurologic conditions.
- Hiatal hernias and esophageal diverticuli are significantly increased with aging because of changes in musculature of the diaphragm and esophagus.
- Older adults have decreased secretion of hydrochloric acid (hypochlorhydria and achlorhydria) from the parietal cells of the stomach. This results in an increased incidence of pernicious anemia and gastritis in the older adult population.
- Peptic ulcers are common, but often the symptoms are vague and go unrecognized until there is a bleeding episode. Medications such as aspirin, nonsteroidal antiinflammatory drugs, and steroids that are taken for the chronic degenerative joint conditions common with aging should be used with caution because they can contribute to ulcer formation.
- Frequency of diverticulosis and diverticulitis increases dramatically with aging and can contribute to malabsorption of nutrients.
- Constipation is a problem for many older adults. Inactivity, changes in diet and fluid intake, and medications can contribute to this problem. Monitor bowel elimination and establish a bowel regimen to prevent impaction.

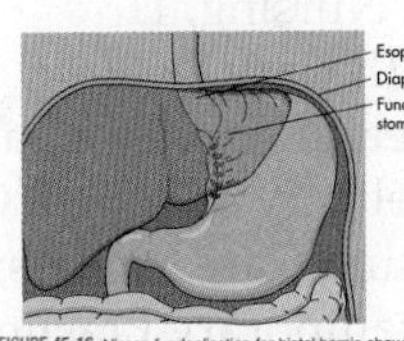

FIGURE 45-16 Nissen fundoplication for hiatal hernia showing fundus of stomach wrapped around distal esophagus and sutured to itself.

Prognosis

The prognosis for hernias is good because surgical intervention is usually successful. The result can be altered if the patient is a poor surgical risk or has other complications.

INTESTINAL OBSTRUCTION

Etiology and Pathophysiology

Intestinal obstruction occurs when intestinal contents cannot pass through the GI tract; it requires prompt treatment. The obstruction may be partial or complete. The causes of intestinal obstruction are classified as mechanical or nonmechanical.

Mechanical Obstruction

Mechanical obstruction may be caused by an occlusion of the lumen of the intestinal tract. Most obstructions occur in the ileum, which is the narrowest segment of the small intestine. Mechanical obstructions account for 90% of all intestinal obstructions. Mechanical obstructions include adhesions (Figure 45-17, *A*) or incarcerated hernias. Adhesions can develop after abdominal surgery. Other causes include impacted feces, diverticular disease, tumor of the bowel, intussusceptions, volvulus (Figure 45-17, *B*) (a twisting of bowel onto itself), or the strictures of inflammatory bowel disease. Residues from foods high in fiber, such as raw coconut or fruit pulp, can also obstruct the small bowel.

Nonmechanical Obstruction

Nonmechanical obstruction may result from a neuromuscular or vascular disorder. The cause is something that decreases the muscle action of the bowel and affects the ability of fecal matter and fluid to move through the intestines (Kent, 2007). Paralytic (adynamic) ileus (lack of intestinal peristalsis and bowel sounds) is the most common form of nonmechanical obstruction. It occurs to some degree after any abdominal surgery. Other causes include inflammatory responses (e.g., acute pancreatitis, acute appendicitis), electrolyte abnormalities (especially hypokalemia), and thoracic or lumbar spinal

Contents

44 Care of the Patient with a Musculoskeletal Disorder, 1345

Martha E. Spray

45 Care of the Patient with a Gastrointestinal Disorder, 1411

Barbara Lauritsen Christensen

53 Care of the Patient with a Visual or Auditory Disorder, 1837

Barbara Lauritsen Christensen

chapter 1

The Evolution of Nursing

evolve

Elaine Oden Kockrow

http://evolve.elsevier.com/Christensen/foundationsadult

Objectives

1. Describe the evolution of nursing and nursing education from early civilization to the twentieth century.
2. Discuss the significant changes in nursing in the twenty-first century.
3. Discuss societal influences on nursing.
4. Identify the major leaders of nursing history in America.
5. Identify the major organizations in nursing.
6. Define the four purposes of National Association for Practical Nurse Education and Service (NAPNES) and National Federation of Licensed Practical Nurses (NFLPN).
7. List the major developments of practical and vocational nursing.
8. Identify the components of the health care system.
9. Identify the participants in the health care system.
10. Describe the complex factors involved in the delivery of patient care.
11. Define practical and vocational nursing.
12. Describe the purpose, role, and responsibilities of the practical or vocational nurse.

Key Terms

accreditation (ă-CRĔD-ĭ-TĀ-shŭn, p. 9)
approved program (p. 9)
certification (sŭr-tĭ-fĭ-KĀ-shŭn, p. 6)
health (p. 2)
health care system (p. 11)
holistic (hō-LĬS-tĭk, p. 2)
holistic health care (p. 11)
illness (p. 1)
licensure (LĪ-sĕn-shŭr), p. 5)
medicine (p. 2)
patient (p. 2)
wellness (p. 11)

Nursing is one of today's most exciting and challenging careers. Each nurse receives a formal education in an institution with a set curriculum that has been approved by the state board of nursing. On completion of the program, the graduate takes an examination to become licensed as a nurse. The profession hasn't always been seen to have such an organized body of knowledge, however. To understand the position of nursing and nursing education today, first look back at the history of nursing and nursing education.

THE HISTORY OF NURSING AND NURSING EDUCATION

Nursing has evolved over many hundreds of years. Many influences have led to changes in nursing and nursing education: how we as a society care for the sick, the way people live, the relationship of people with their environment, the search for knowledge and truth through education, and technologic advances. Nursing evolves as society and health care needs and policies change. The field responds and adapts to these changes, meeting new challenges as they arise.

CARE OF THE SICK DURING EARLY CIVILIZATION

Early records from around 5000 BC make little reference to nursing as we understand it. **Illness** (an abnormal process in which aspects of the social, emotional, or intellectual condition and function of a person are diminished or impaired) was considered to be an indicator of how one stood with God; it was understood as a direct outcome of divine disfavor. Primitive people believed that a person became sick when an evil spirit entered the body and that the presence of a good spirit kept disease away.

Medicine men performed witchcraft and rituals to induce the bad spirits to leave the body of the ailing person. Some of their methods involved the use of frightening masks, noises, incantations, vile odors, charms, spells, and even sacrifices. Acting directly on the body or the affected part, they used purgatives and emetics, application of hot and cold substances, cautery, cupping, blistering, and massage. Although others assisted the medicine men in treating illnesses, few were women. Women mostly assisted other women in childbirth.

Babylonians

The Babylonians were intellectually, socially, and scientifically well developed, but ordinary people suffered from the misery, illness, and injury caused by frequent warfare. There is evidence that some form of medical service existed and that laypersons provided this service. It is believed that these caregivers were usually men. If they were women, they were probably of low status because Babylonian women were dominated by men.

Ancient Hebrews

The ancient Hebrews, according to the Talmud and the Old Testament, attributed their misfortunes and illnesses to God's wrath. They depended on God to restore them to **health** (a condition of physical, mental, and social well-being and the absence of disease or other abnormal conditions) when they were sick. Their religious beliefs dictated certain health and dietary practices, and these they combined with the hygienic practices that they acquired during their captivity in Babylon. In the Jewish religion, kosher dietary law requires strict separation of dairy- and meat-containing foods, careful slaughtering and inspection of all meats, and the meticulous selection and preparation of all foods. The Jews prevented the spread of communicable disease by burning infected garments, isolating ill persons, and scrubbing the homes of those infected with disease. In what appears to be the first incidence of public health or home care, nurses are mentioned occasionally in the Talmud as persons caring for the sick in their homes.

Ancient Egyptians

Ancient records of early Egyptian civilization describe nursing procedures such as feeding a **patient** (a recipient of a health care service) who had tetanus and dressing wounds.

The custom of embalming enabled the Egyptians to become well acquainted with organs of the body. From clinical observation, they learned to recognize some 250 different diseases. To treat them, they developed a number of drugs and procedures such as surgery. Evidence from the period includes detailed instructions for daily nursing care, which included recording the pulse, using splints and bandages, and using hollow reeds as catheters. Egyptian physicians were considered skillful at treating fractures.

Ancient Indians

Records of pre-Christian India report the establishment of hospitals that cared for the sick. The reports describe a corps of attendants, who were probably male, as clever, skillful, and endowed with kindness, and distinguished by their good behavior and their purity and cleanliness of habit. They bathed patients, made beds, and kept themselves at the disposal of the sick.

Ancient Greeks

By 500 BC, the Hellenic civilization showed keen intellect, independent thinking, democratic action, and a thirst for knowledge and truth. The basis of **medicine** (the art and science of the diagnosis, treatment, and prevention of disease and the maintenance of good health) progressed from the belief that demons and spirits caused human ills to the establishment of temples suitable for rest and the restoration of health. These temples, often referred to as hospitals, resembled our health centers of today: They had spas, mineral springs, baths, gymnasiums, as well as treatment and consultation rooms. The religious influence was still present in the form of prayer, thanks offerings, and rituals. Priestesses served as attendants and cared for the sick. Pregnant women and persons with incurable diseases were not admitted.

Hippocrates, born in 460 BC on the island of Cos in the Mediterranean, was a brilliant, progressive physician and teacher. He rejected the belief in the supernatural origin of disease. Integral to the system of patient care he developed and we still use are physical assessment, observation, and record keeping. As his patient-centered care approach and medical ethics were adopted, Hippocrates came to be called the "Father of Medicine" and is credited with the first ethical guide for medical conduct, the Hippocratic Oath that is still taken by physicians today. The work of Hippocrates is the basis for the **holistic** (of or pertaining to the whole; taking into consideration all factors, as **holistic medicine**) approach to patient care.

Early Christians

The Greek influence changed the approach to the care of the sick from one of mysticism to one based on issues of public health and safety. Still predominantly religious in the early years of Christianity, medicine placed an emphasis on the care of the poor, the sick, the widowed, and children. Roman bishops designated deacons and deaconesses to assist the church by providing services such as visiting sick women in their homes, visiting and tending to the needs of prisoners, and watching over the sick in the hospitals. One of the first deaconesses, Phoebe, took on the duties of what we today call a visiting nurse, attending the sick and poor in their homes in about AD 60. Another Roman woman, Fabiola, spent her wealth and time nursing the sick and poor. She is credited with providing the first free hospital in Rome in AD 390.

Monastic and Military Influences

Monastic and military orders were charged with caring for the sick over the next 1000 years. Knowledge was limited, however, and the rise and fall of feudalism in central Europe blocked widespread application of the progress made in Greece and Rome. Famine, disease, war, and the emphasis on survival resulted in an increased need to care for the sick and poor, but the ongoing battles between church and state hindered the development of any one approach to patient care. Care of the sick was performed by both men and women. Female religious orders concerned themselves with the care of the sick and needy, but religious problems took priority. Male military personnel served the medical needs of soldiers on the battlefield.

NURSING EDUCATION IN THE NINETEENTH CENTURY

In the early nineteenth century, hospitals were dirty and overcrowded, crammed with patients with open wounds. Workers used poor hygienic practices, and infection ran unchecked. The hospital was a place to contract diseases rather than be cured of them. There was a lack of trained and qualified people who were interested in caring for the sick and the infirm. Because women of "proper upbringing" did not work outside the home in this period, the ranks of nurses were filled with lower-class women who drank heavily and engaged in prostitution. The best source of nurses was the religious nursing orders, but these orders could not begin to meet the ever-increasing need for nursing services.

Under the guidance of Theodor Fliedner, a German pastor in Kaiserswerth, Germany, the Lutheran Order of Deaconesses established the first school of nursing. The reputation of the school soon spread throughout Europe. It reached a young woman in England whose interest in nursing spurred her to overcome the opposition of her family, her friends, and the social class to which she belonged.

Florence Nightingale (1820–1910)

Florence Nightingale (Figure 1-1), a strong-minded, intelligent, and determined young woman, joined the Kaiserswerth program in 1851 at age 31. Armed with the education and training she received at Kaiserswerth and with her administrative and organizational skills, in 1853 Nightingale became the superintendent of a charity hospital for ill governesses. The quality of patient care improved, but the governing board of the hospital was not always pleased with the changes and innovations she made and the guidance she gave her uneducated nurses.

In the following year, she was preparing to become superintendent of King's College Hospital in London. Shocking news reached England of the number of casualties and deaths among soldiers in the Crimean War, as well as the atrocious conditions suffered by the wounded. Nightingale sent the secretary of war, a long-standing friend, a letter offering her services; ironically, it crossed with his request for her to lead a group of nurses to Scutari, Turkey, to care for the wounded. Within a week of receiving the secretary's letter, she and 38 other nurses were on their way.

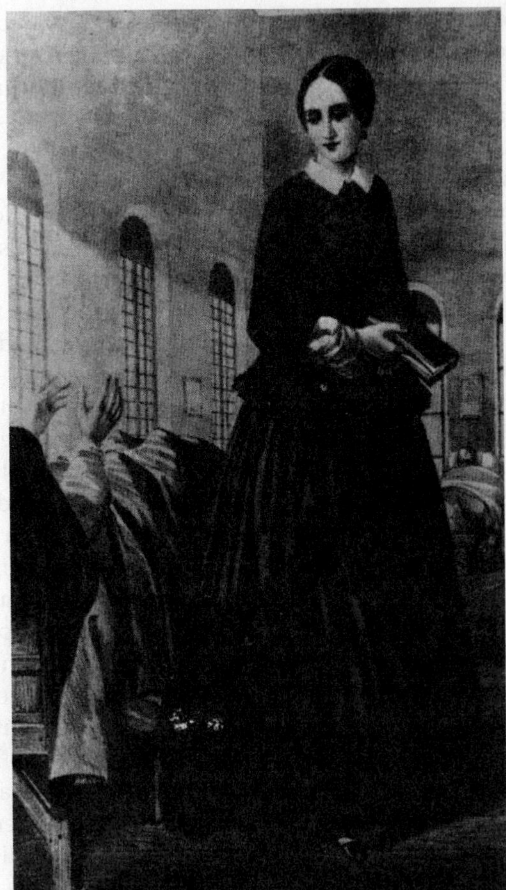

FIGURE 1-1 Florence Nightingale, the first nursing theorist.

Once again Florence Nightingale applied the principles of nursing she had learned at Kaiserswerth. These concepts, coupled with her dedication and leadership, turned the tide at the Barrack Hospital. The hospital units were cleaned. Clothes were washed regularly. Sanitary conditions, nonexistent before her arrival, were established. The mortality rate among the casualties dropped significantly. The changes did not end with the physical environment of the hospital, however. Through Nightingale's patience, dedication, and empathic treatment of the soldiers, a psychological change took place as well. The soldiers grew to respect her and looked forward to her presence on the wards. They looked for her smile and took strength from her personality. When she made her rounds late at night through the rows of the injured and sick, she carried a lamp to light her way. Soon she was known as the "Lady with the Lamp." The small lamp became her trademark and continues to be the symbol of the nursing profession around the world.

The standards of nursing care Florence Nightingale established gained the respect of the medical community and led to improved care for the sick and a much improved image of nursing in general. She is credited as the first nursing theorist. The need for educated and trained nurses had become painfully evident, and the time was right for a shift in the approach to nursing education.

Nursing from Occupation to Profession

In 1860, Florence Nightingale began the reformation of nursing from occupation to profession by establishing the nursing school at Saint Thomas Hospital in London. With a reputation as a progressive medical facility, it was the ideal place to promote the new standards of nursing in which she so strongly believed.

The nursing program operated separately from the hospital. It was financially independent to ensure that the major emphasis of its activity was squarely placed on educating nursing students (Figure 1-2). Students had to pass strict procedures for admission, and a residence was provided for them. The nurses' training lasted 1 year and included both formal instruction and practical experience. Complete records were kept on each student's progress. This practice became known as the "Nightingale Plan," which was to become the model for nursing education in the twentieth century. After the students graduated, records were also kept on where they were employed. The "register" that resulted was the beginning of a movement to exercise control over the nursing graduate and to establish a standard for the practicing nurse.

Students admitted into the nursing program at Saint Thomas had to provide excellent character references, show a strong commitment to a career in nursing, and demonstrate that they were intellectually capable of passing the course of study before them. The new "Nightingale nurses" improved patient care by such measures as good hygiene and sanitation, patient observation, accurate record keeping, nutritional improvements, and the introduction and use of new medical equipment. The demand for their services was overwhelming.

Development of Nursing Education in the United States

At the same time Florence Nightingale was active in Europe, circumstances in America were creating the same kinds of patient care problems. Both the American Revolution and the Civil War were characterized by severe casualties, disease, infected wounds, and archaic medical care. As in the Crimean War, nurses were scarce, and those who were available were poorly trained to handle the horrors of war.

In 1849, the same Pastor Theodore Fliedner of Germany who had established Nightingale's alma mater traveled to the United States with four of his highly trained nurse-deaconesses. Here he was instrumental in the establishment of the first Protestant hospital on these shores. Located in Pittsburgh, Pennsylvania, it was called the Pittsburgh Infirmary. Under the name Passavant Hospital, it is still in existence today. While Fliedner was busy with the hospital, his deaconesses began the first formal education of nurses in the United States.

As hospitals in the large cities grew to meet the demands for health care, a shortage of nurses developed. Most early nursing programs were supported by these large hospitals. In 1869, the American Medical Association recommended that every large hospital should establish and support its own school of nursing to meet the need for patient care. Schools of nursing would be established by the turn of the century, all modeled after the Nightingale Plan.

In May 1873, the Bellevue Hospital School of Nursing in New York established itself as the foremost proponent of the Nightingale Plan in America. In October of that same year, the Connecticut Training School opened in New Haven. In November, the Boston Training School began operating at the Massachusetts General Hospital.

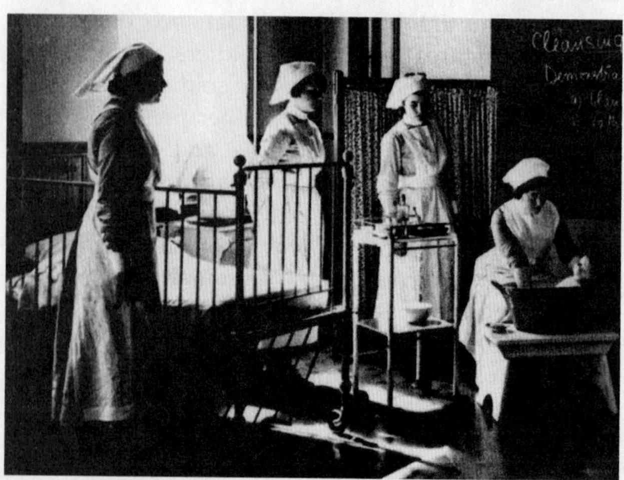

FIGURE 1-2 Nurses in a preliminary training school.

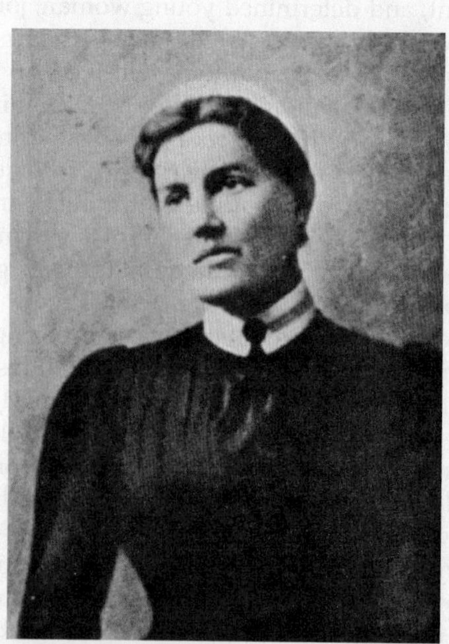

FIGURE 1-3 Isabel Hampton Robb.

Table 1-1 **Leaders in the Development of Nursing in America**

NURSE	CONTRIBUTION TO NURSING
Dorothea Dix (1802–1887)	Pioneer crusader for elevation of standards of care for the mentally ill Superintendent of Female Nurses of the Union Army
Clara Barton (1821–1912)	Developed the American Red Cross in 1881
Mary Ann Ball (1817–1901)	One of the greatest nurse heroines of the Civil War Championed the rights and comforts of the soldiers; organized diet kitchens, laundries, ambulance service; and supervised the nursing staff
Linda Richards (1841–1930)	First trained nurse in America Responsible for the development of the first nursing and hospital records Credited with the development of our present-day documentation system
Isabel Hampton Robb (1860–1910)	Organized the first graded system of theory and practice in the schools of nursing One of the founders of the *American Journal of Nursing*
Lavinia Dock (1858–1956)	Responsible, with Robb, for the organization of the American Society of Superintendents of Training Schools, which evolved into the National League for Nursing Education
Mary Eliza Mahoney (1845–1926)	Graduated from the New England Hospital for Women and Children in 1879, becoming the first African-American professional nurse Worked for acceptance of African-Americans in the nursing profession
Lillian D. Wald (1867–1940)	Responsible for the development of public health nursing in the United States through the founding of the Henry Street Settlement in New York City
Mary Adelaide Nutting (1858–1947)	A leader in nursing education Developed curriculum concepts and guidelines for student nurses Assisted in the development of the International Council of Nurses
Mary Breckenridge (1881–1965)	Pioneer in nurse-midwifery Established the Frontier Nursing Service to deliver obstetric care to mothers in the hills of Kentucky; these nurses traveled on horseback to reach the mothers

Isabel Hampton Robb (Figure 1-3) and Lavinia Dock organized the American Society of Superintendents of Training Schools of Nursing in 1894. The major goal of these dedicated women was to set educational standards for nurses. The structure of the organization was modeled after that of the American Medical Association. The society adopted a code of ethics for nurses, still subscribed to by the nursing profession and known today as the Nightingale Pledge (see Box 2-7). See Table 1-1 for a list of American nursing leaders.

CHANGES IN NURSING DURING THE TWENTIETH CENTURY

Like the superintendents, who operated at the national level, the graduates of the training schools also attempted to establish standards, in their case establishing the Alumnae Association for the actual practice of nursing at the local level.

Licensing

In 1903 the first laws governing nursing **licensure** (the granting of permission by a competent authority [usually a government agency] to an organization or individual to engage in a practice or activity that would otherwise be illegal) were passed in North Carolina, New Jersey, New York, and Virginia to protect the public. The nursing organizations recognized the need to amend their purpose and redirect their focus. As part of the reorganization that followed, in 1903 the American Society of Superintendents of Training Schools became the Education Committee of the National League for Nursing Education. In 1911 the Alumnae Association became the American Nurses Association.

At the same time, Isabel Hampton Robb and Mary Adelaide Nutting were developing a program at Columbia University to train and develop teachers of nursing. They were convinced that nurses needed not only a college education and experience in clinical practice, but also specific training in theoretic knowledge. The idea that nurses needed such a balance of liberal arts education and nursing practice skills brought a new, balanced perspective to the profession of nursing.

World War I

World War I brought an increased demand for nurses. The newly formed Army and Navy Nurse Corps sought nurses who certifiably demonstrated "good moral character and professional qualifications." The available supply of nurses could not meet the demand, so once again untrained women volunteered their services to their country. Nursing leaders, concerned that these untrained personnel would be caring without adequate training for wounded and ailing soldiers, moved quickly to establish the Army School of Nursing.

After the war, most of the women who had served as military nurses returned to their homes and their previous jobs and careers. The image attached to professional nurses still posed a problem for most women, and few had the desire to remain in nursing as civilians. Furthermore, they were disenchanted because nurses' training still focused heavily on "service to the patient" rather than on a comprehensive professional education. This was far removed from what the Nightingale Plan had proposed for aspiring nurses.

World War II

Twenty-five years later, World War II once again escalated, almost overnight, the demand for trained nurses. Although medicine had advanced, so had the art of war, and the casualties were numerous. Early in the war, the Cadet Nurse Corps was established to provide an abbreviated training program designed to meet the needs of the war effort. In addition, federally subsidized programs in nursing were developed and implemented to offer women and—for the first time—men an education and a career in nursing while serving their country in the war.

After the war, many of the nurses trained by these programs remained in military service. Prestige, pay, and the opportunity for advancement were much greater in military service than for civilian nurses. In the major hospitals, particularly in urban areas, civilian nurses received low pay and worked long shifts under atrocious conditions. These conditions were hardly likely to attract those who became nurses as a result of the war and who, ironically, enjoyed a certain lifestyle that war invariably provides. As a result, the shortage of nurses in the United States and other countries that had accumulated through the effects World War I, the Great Depression, and World War II grew steadily worse.

Further, state boards of nursing, which had licensure responsibility, came under increasing pressure to mandate requirements for nurses. State-administered licensing examinations no longer seemed adequate for the country's needs. The parochial state examinations were in no way standardized and allowed persons with a wide spectrum of competence to enter nursing. National norms of competence were sorely needed.

Contemporary Nursing

The characteristics of health care changed rapidly as health care became an industry. Growth and diversity became the major emphasis as the industry became increasingly lucrative. The need for nurses, particularly well-educated nurses, increased at a rate much greater than could be met. This was the beginning of contemporary nursing, with specialized nursing care adapted to areas such as private duty, school nursing, industrial nursing, nurse anesthesia, and nurse-midwifery.

The nursing organizations continued to deliberate on the future of nursing as a profession. In 1965 the American Nurses Association (ANA) took a position recommending that nursing education take place in institutions of learning within the general system of education, much as Robb and Nutting had proposed in 1903. Their position paper set the baccalaureate degree in nursing as the minimum acceptable preparation for the beginning professional nurse and the associate degree in nursing as the minimum for technical nursing practice. Assistants to nurses, they said, should have preservice programs in vocational education rather than just on-the-job training. This position has had a profound effect. Since 1965, many hospitals have disbanded their nursing programs, and an increasing number of colleges and universities have established baccalaureate and associate degree nursing programs. The intent is obviously to change the trend from "training" nurses to "educating" nurses (see Figure 1-2).

Certification

Since 1976, the ANA has offered certification testing for registered nurses (RNs). **Certification** is a process by which the nurse is granted recognition for competency in a specific area of nursing. To be eligible for certification testing, the RN is required to have a current license, have a minimum of 2 years' experience as an RN in the designated area, and be currently practicing in the designated area. Some types of certification for the RN include gerontologic nurse, medical-surgical nurse, psychiatric and mental health nurse, and adult nurse practitioner. The ANA continues to monitor the education and the role of the nurse in today's health care system. The organization also publishes numerous position papers to keep the nursing profession current and well informed of changes and events that affect the quality of nursing care.

Nursing Caps, Uniforms, and Pins

Originally, nurses wore the practical white, pleated cap and the apron of the maidservant, signifying respectability, cleanliness, and servitude. As the nursing profession gained recognition, nurses' caps became less utilitarian and more symbolic, a badge of office and achievement.

Since the Second World War, the nurse's cap has lost much of its significance. The "capping ceremony," a ritual in which a junior nurse receives her first cap, has virtually disappeared. Today there is controversy within the medical profession about nursing uniforms altogether. Many nurses do not approve of mandatory dress codes. They argue that other health care professionals do not depend on uniforms for their authority.

But looking professional is nonetheless important. Patients feel more comfortable and confident when they are easily able to find and distinguish nurses from other staff members. Most facilities require staff members to wear nametags and sometimes a badge with an identifying picture of the staff member. Some facilities are now requiring fingerprint scans to gain access into the record-keeping system.

Most schools of nursing continue to award a nursing pin to the graduate nurse. Many of these pins bear the Nightingale lamp as a common component, along with an emblem of the school of nursing.

SIGNIFICANT CHANGES IN NURSING FOR THE TWENTY-FIRST CENTURY

Nursing practice is affected by various societal factors, along with developments that are more internal to the field. Demographics of the population, women's health care issues, men in nursing, rising numbers of persons with fewer socioeconomic advantages seeking health care, and bioterrorism threats are a few of the societal factors that are influencing nursing today.

Demographic Changes

Because the demographics of the population are changing, nursing is also facing the need to change. Life expectancy of the population as a whole is rising, which is resulting in increased numbers of older adults seeking health care. There is a higher prevalence of chronic illnesses, and rising numbers of health care centers are located in inner-city rather than rural areas. This means that the profession is called on to alter practice standards and implement more appropriate approaches for providing care to individuals, as well as educating its members to adapt.

Women's Health Care Issues

Today's society is more sensitive to the unique health care needs of women. Research studies specific to these needs have increased, in part as a result of federal mandates requiring inclusion of women in studies. In addition, new health care specialties continue to emerge that deal with women's health care issues, including management of menopause, immunizations (such as the human papilloma virus [HPV] vaccine), preventive health care for women, and oncologic subspecialties (Potter & Perry, 2009).

Nursing is responding in two ways to women's health care issues and the women's movement. Nurses, most of whom are women, are increasingly asserting their equal rights as human beings, employees, and health care professionals. Encouraged by the women's movement, they have sought greater autonomy and responsibility in providing care. In addition, the women's movement has helped women to become more aware of their own unique needs. Nurses have learned to encourage female patients to seek more responsibility for and control over their bodies, health, and lives in general.

Men in Nursing

Men have had a role in nursing throughout its history. But as nursing evolved, it became essentially a profession of women. From the Civil War to the Korean War of the 1950s, men were not allowed to serve as nurses in the military. As of today, however, men have regained their historical position in the nursing profession. As nursing progresses, men and women will continue to practice side by side (see Chapter 58).

Human Rights

Nursing advocates for the rights of all individuals. But going even beyond this basic requirement, the profession has promoted the rights of specific segments of the population through the creation of bills of rights. Such bills address the rights of hospitalized patients, those who are dying, older adults, and pregnant women. These bills of rights speak to the need to respect all patients as unique individuals and ensure quality care for all.

Medically Underserved

Soaring rates of unemployment, homelessness, and the working poor, combined with the enormous rise in health care costs, have led to an increased number of individuals in the United States who are unable to afford health care. Some of these individuals receive federal aid such as Medicaid; others, however, are not aware of Medicaid assistance or earn just over the allowed maximum income to receive assistance. Lack of access to health care is another problem, especially relevant to many individuals with mental health disorders and individuals living in rural areas. Staffing rural-based and community-based clinics provides one of the solutions, allowing nurses to focus on health promotion and management of disease processes (Potter & Perry, 2009).

Frequently, nurses working in these settings have a higher degree of training and function as advanced practice nurses, giving them the capability to provide direct health care. This area of nursing is rapidly expanding as more nurses are seeking to work with this underserved population.

Threat of Bioterrorism

Recent acts of terrorism have prompted all communities and health care agencies to improve their bioterrorism response plans. Nurses are very involved in the disaster preparedness plans in the event of nuclear, chemical, or biological attack. Nursing is directly involved in the response to bioterrorism through various means, such as triage of casualties, crisis response teams, and vaccination research (Potter & Perry, 2009) (see Chapter 24).

DEVELOPMENT OF PRACTICAL AND VOCATIONAL NURSING

ATTENDANT NURSES

The first school for training practical nurses started in Brooklyn, New York, in 1892 under the auspices of the Young Women's Christian Association (YWCA). The Ballard School, as it was known, gave a course that lasted approximately 3 months and trained its students to care for the chronically ill, invalids, children, and the elderly. The main emphasis was on home care and included cooking, nutrition, basic science, and basic nursing procedures. Graduates of this program were referred to as **attendant nurses.**

Two other programs were patterned after the Ballard School. In 1907, the Thompson Practical Nursing School opened in Brattleboro, Vermont (still in operation and accredited by the National League for Nursing [NLN]), and in 1918 the Household Nursing Association School of Attendant Nursing (later changed to the Shepard-Gill School of Practical Nursing) opened in Boston. The focus of these programs continued to be on home nursing care and light housekeeping duties. Hospital experience was not a part of the training in the early programs.

PRACTICAL NURSING PROGRAMS

Practical nursing programs developed slowly during the first half of the twentieth century (Table 1-2). A total of 36 schools opened during that period. Practical nursing schools before 1940 had few controls, little educational planning, and minimal supervision. The increased demand for nursing services in World War II and the postwar years, combined with the excellent bedside nursing care demonstrated by the practical nurse, resulted in the opening of 260 practical and vocational nursing programs between 1948 and 1954. These programs varied in administrative design. Some were affiliated with hospitals or chronic care institutions, whereas others aligned themselves with private agencies or private schools. Students in these pro-

Table 1-2 Milestones of Practical and Vocational Nursing

YEAR	MILESTONE
1892	The Ballard School at the YWCA in Brooklyn, New York, established the first school to train practical nurses.
1907	The Thompson Practical Nursing School in Brattleboro, Vermont, was the second practical nursing school to be established.
1914	The Mississippi State Legislature was the first political body to pass licensing laws controlling practical nurses.
1917	The Smith-Hughes Act was passed. It provided federal funding for vocationally oriented practical nursing programs.
	Nursing requirements for practical nursing were standardized by the National League for Nursing Education, now the National League for Nursing (NLN).
1918	The Household Nursing Association School of Attendant Nursing in Boston, Massachusetts, later called the Shepard-Gill School of Practical Nursing, was the third practical nursing school established.
1920	Acute shortage of practical nurses; many military nurses did not return to nursing after World War I.
1938	New York was the only state to have mandatory licensure.
1920 to 1940	Most practical nursing was limited to public health agencies and visiting nurse associations.
1940	The number of practical nurses peaked at 150,009.
1941	The Association of Practical Nurse Schools was founded. It set standards for practical nursing education.
1942	The Association of Practical Nurse Schools became the National Association of Practical Nurse Education (NAPNE).
1944	The U.S. Department of Vocational Education commissioned an intensive study to differentiate tasks of the practical nurse.
1949	The National Federation of Licensed Practical Nurses (NFLPN) was founded by Lillian Kuster. The association is the official membership organization for licensed practical and vocational nurses, and membership is limited to LVNs and LPNs.
1951	*Journal of Practical Nursing* published by NAPNES (now *Practical Nursing Today*).
1952	Approximately 60% of the nurse workforce was made up of practical nurses.
1957	NLN established a council of practical nursing programs. Through this council, schools of practical nursing could be accredited.
1959	The National Association of Practical Nurse Education (NAPNE) changed its name to the National Association for Practical Nurse Education and Service (NAPNES).
1965	The American Nurses Association (ANA) first moves toward two specific levels of nursing—professional and technical.
1979	NLN publishes the first list of competencies for practical and vocational nursing programs.
1980s	Nursing shortage continues. Creation of American Licensed Practical Nurse Association (ALPNA).
1990s	Unlicensed personnel are used for patient care. The number of hospital jobs decreases. Primary employment sites move into the community (e.g., physicians' offices and long-term care facilities).
1994	NCLEX-PN® is available to practical and vocational nursing graduates.
1995	Full-time nursing positions in hospitals decrease; the patient/nurse ratio increases. Primary employment in the community continues.
1996	Long-term care certification examination is available to LPN/LVNs.
2000	Demand increases for LPN/LVNs in long-term care and extended care facilities but decreases in hospitals.

grams provided nursing services while they were obtaining their education and training. This apprentice training emphasized vocational and technical education. Federal funds allocated for training practical and vocational nurses helped recruit men and women.

ORGANIZATIONAL INFLUENCE

By mid-century, practical nursing programs were increasing rapidly. The need to establish standards again became a major issue. The Association of Practical Nurse Schools was founded in 1941 and was dedicated exclusively to practical nursing. Its membership was multidisciplinary and included licensed practical nurses, registered nurses, physicians, hospital and nursing home administrators, students, and public figures. Together they planned the first standard curriculum for practical nursing. By 1942, they saw the need to change the name to the National Association of Practical Nurse Education (NAPNE). They broadened their focus to include education and practice and established an accrediting service for schools of practical and vocational nursing in 1945. The association changed its name once more in 1959 to the National Association for Practical Nurse Education and Service (NAPNES).

In 1949, the National Federation of Licensed Practical Nurses (NFLPN) was founded by Lillian Kuster. This association is the official membership organization for licensed practical nurses and licensed vocational nurses (LPN/LVNs), and membership is limited to LVNs and LPNs.

These two organizations, NAPNES and NFLPN, set standards for practical and vocational nursing practice, promote and protect the interests of LPN/LVNs, and educate and inform the general public about practical and vocational nursing.

In 1961, the NLN broadened its scope of service because of the growth of practical and vocational nursing programs. The NLN established the Department of Practical Nursing Programs and developed an accreditation service for these programs, which is now called the Council of Practical Nursing Programs.

For 20 years, both the NLN and NAPNES provided accreditation services. Nursing programs had the option of seeking accreditation from either organization. In recent years, however, NAPNES has discontinued this service.

ADDITIONAL CREDENTIALING

NAPNES currently offers additional credentialing to LPN/LVNs, the Certification Examination for Practical and Vocational Nurses in Long-Term Care (CEPN-LTC). To be eligible to sit for the test, the LPN/LVN must have completed 2000 hours or 3 years in long-term care employment. This test is composed of 150 questions that evaluate the knowledge, the skills, and the abilities of the nurse experienced in the delivery of long-term care. Nurses who pass the CEPN-LTC become certified by NAPNES and may use the initials "CLTC" following LPN, their legal title, to signify their status.

Accreditation of a program differs from program approval. Approval is required for a program to operate. An **approved program** is one that satisfies minimum standards set by the state agency responsible for overseeing educational programs—for example, it meets the needs of the student, has adequate course content and qualified faculty, is of sufficient length, has adequate facilities, and provides clinical experience. To protect the welfare of the public, the state requires programs to demonstrate all these elements for graduates to be eligible for licensure. **Accreditation** is a higher standard: It signifies that the accrediting organization has judged that a program has met its preestablished criteria. The administrators of the program seeking accreditation submit voluntarily to the accreditation process; they do so because of the recognition of quality it confers. Often the standards established by professional organizations that give accreditation are far higher than those established by the state. Although graduates of nonaccredited programs can take the licensure examination required in most states, accreditation is extremely important when programs seek federal funding.

CONTEMPORARY PRACTICAL AND VOCATIONAL NURSING EDUCATION

Practical and vocational nursing programs have continued to proliferate, and by the 2003–2004 school year, 1100 practical and vocational nursing programs in the United States were producing thousands of graduates. Various organizations still offer nursing programs, such as high schools, trade or technical schools, hospitals, junior and community colleges, colleges and universities, and private education agencies. Health care corporations such as the Galen Health Institutes (formerly Humana Health Institute) also offer practical and vocational programs. However, they are all required to meet minimum state standards. The length of the programs is usually 12 to 18 months; there is a focus on nursing skills and theory that is correlated with clinical practice. On completing the program, the graduate is eligible to take the National Council Licensing Examination for Practical Nursing (NCLEX-PN®).

Educational programs in nursing today offer various creative approaches to educating student LPN/LVNs. The combination of practical and vocational nurse education with associate degree programs in 2-year colleges is available. At the successful completion of the first academic year, the student can either exit and take the licensure examination for practical or vocational nursing or continue for another year and earn an associate degree in nursing, becoming eligible to take the licensure examination for registered nursing. Many other programs offer other combinations of education and degrees throughout the United States. Most states have some type of articulation plan.

Articulation allows nursing programs to plan their curricula collaboratively; the purpose is to lessen duplication of learning experiences and support a process of progressive buildup. This means that one program becomes the foundation for another program. The LPN/LVN may receive as much as 50% credit toward the associate degree; the associate degree–prepared RN may receive as much as 50% credit toward the bachelor of science in nursing (BSN) degree. This process is sometimes referred to as a 1-plus-1 program or a 2-plus-2 program, respectively. Articulation acknowledges the student's existing knowledge base and permits the student to continue her or his advancement in education without repeating previous course work.

CAREER ADVANCEMENT

The career ladder is a model that some institutions follow for nurses' advancement. A career ladder serves to recognize the clinical expertise of the nurse and provide a mechanism for financial compensation and opportunities for advancement. Each institution clearly lists and defines its criteria for advancement on the ladder. Items generally included are adherence to attendance policies, completion of mandatory inservice programs, and demonstration of excellent clinical skills.

FACTORS THAT CHANGED PRACTICAL AND VOCATIONAL NURSING

Before 1860, nursing care in the United States was provided generally by people who were self-taught and who gained what knowledge they could through experience. Registration, licensing, and title differentiation were not clear or were nonexistent. Duties and responsibilities were not clearly defined. The term *nurse* was used only in the broadest sense as "a person who takes care of the sick."

The Need for Trained Caregivers

Practical nursing in the United States evolved from the need for caregivers who could be trained and ready for service in a short time. The cost of the services provided by these caregivers was expected to be reasonable and easily affordable by the patient. There was also the need to provide a vocation for the many unskilled women who were migrating to the larger cities to seek better lives. At the time, women generally were not skilled or trained for jobs other than manual labor. The YWCA in New York City started the first practical nursing program in the late 1800s to address these needs.

World War I

World War I caused the need for trained nurses abroad to grow, and in the United States the Spanish influenza epidemic strained the resources of the nursing community. The Smith-Hughes Act was passed in 1917 to provide vocational and public education. Federal funding then provided the means for vocational-based practical and vocational nursing programs throughout the country. Even with these resources, the demand for nurses caused by the war and the epidemic could not be met.

The Self-Taught Practical Nurse

By 1940, thousands of self-taught "practical nurses" were working to meet the needs of the country. However, they lacked the education and experience that is obtainable only under supervision in an established program. It was not really possible to call them practical or vocational nurses or grant them state licensure. In fact, few states even had minimum standards for the practice of practical and vocational nursing. Only 19 states and one territory had considered or passed legislation dealing with practical or vocational nurses, and at the end of 1945, licensing was mandatory in only one state. There was no agreement on the duties, the role, or the responsibilities of practical or vocational nurses, and they were known by many job descriptions and titles. This confusion and the absence of standards and licensing practices created difficulties.

The Great Depression

Even before the United States entered World War II, the Great Depression caused a huge demand for nurses. The Cadet Navy Corps and the American Red Cross were an expedient means of providing training in nursing. Practical nursing programs flourished throughout the country. Although there was a huge need for skilled medical care personnel, the need to prepare people for nursing in the shortest time took precedence. A 1-year program provided the minimal amount of training for practical and vocational nursing. As the shortage of nurses in the hospitals and other health care facilities became critical, practical and vocational nurses who were practicing in the home environment were hired to work in those institutions.

Duties of Licensed Practical Nurses and Licensed Vocational Nurses

In 1944, the U.S. Department of Vocational Education commissioned an intensive study of practical and vocational nursing tasks. The outcome of this study differentiated the tasks performed by the LPN/LVN in relation to those tasks performed by the RN. As a result of this study, individual state boards of nursing began to specify the duties and responsibilities that could be accomplished by each group of nurses.

Position Paper of the American Nurses Association

The 1965 position paper of the ANA was another influence bringing about a change in attitude toward practical and vocational nursing. This position paper clearly defined two levels of nursing practice: that of the registered nurse and that of the technical nurse. The term **practical nurse** was not included in this position paper. Practical and vocational nurses have nonetheless certainly proved their worth. Under the supervision of a registered nurse or physician, they provide excellent bedside nursing skills in many areas of service.

LICENSURE FOR PRACTICAL AND VOCATIONAL NURSING

Licensing laws have been passed to protect the public from unqualified practitioners in most fields and professions. These laws are put into effect through state agencies, usually the boards of nursing and the nurse practice acts, in their respective jurisdictions (areas such as states, which have the legal power to regulate nursing licensure and practice).

Laws that Monitor the Licensed Practical Nurse and the Licensed Vocational Nurse

Licensing for practical nurses in the United States began in 1914 when the state legislature in Mississippi passed the first laws pertaining to that group. This followed the passage of laws on licensing RNs by 11 years. The passage of such laws governing practical and vocational nursing in other states was slow in coming. Only six states passed such laws between 1920 and 1940. This may have been because not many practical nurses' training programs were initiated during that period. After the outbreak of World War II and the opening of a large number of practical and vocational nurses' training programs, all the states were forced to pass legislation concerning their licensure. By 1955 all states had passed laws in this area in consonance (agreement) with the standards set by NAPNE. The State Board Test Pool of the NLN Education Committee established a testing mechanism for all states and administered the examination several times a year throughout the country. Graduates of a state-approved practical or vocational nursing education program were eligible to sit for the examination; if they passed, they became LPNs, or LVNs, as they are called in Texas and California. Each state set its own required passing score on the examination.

Currently, graduates of an approved LPN/LVN education program are eligible to take the licensure examination. On completing the computerized examination with a "pass" score (numerical scores are no longer given), the graduate is issued a license to practice as an LPN or an LVN.

All states now have licensing laws for nursing. It is your responsibility to keep informed regarding licensure in the jurisdiction in which you reside or intend to practice. There is interstate endorsement (reciprocity between states), and you can obtain licensing for practice in other jurisdictions without repeating the licensure examination if you meet resident state requirements.

HEALTH CARE DELIVERY SYSTEMS

LPN/LVNs practice within the health care delivery system as a whole. To practice to your fullest capacity, be aware of the complexity of this system and your vital role in its functioning.

HEALTH CARE SYSTEM DEFINED

The **health care system** is the complete network of agencies, facilities, and providers involved with health care in a specified geographic area. Many types of health care professionals operate within this system, including the LPN/LVN, and interact with their external environment. This environment includes the patient, the patient's family, the community in which the system is operating, the current technology, governmental agencies, the medical profession in the community, third-party participants (e.g., insurance companies), and many other forces that affect the patient's care. The major goal of the system is to achieve optimal levels of health care for a defined population; the means of achieving this goal is provision of adequate and appropriate health care services. The LPN/LVN is an integral member of the team of health care professionals who will provide these services within the scope of practice as defined by the state's nurse practice act.

Wellness-Illness Continuum

The wellness-illness continuum of the consumer, as well as the environment where the consumer obtains health care, determines what services the LPN/LVN actually provides.

The **wellness-illness continuum** is defined as the range of a person's total health. An individual's position on this continuum is ever-changing and is influenced by the individual's physical condition, mental condition, and social well-being. At one end of the spectrum is **wellness** (a dynamic state of health in which an individual progresses toward a higher level of functioning, achieving an optimal balance between internal and external environment). Wellness represents the highest level of optimal health. Illness, at the opposite end of the spectrum, represents a diminished or impaired state of health (Figure 1-4).

A balance of all aspects of life is the key to maintaining one's health. Consider a number of interrelated factors when providing health care to the consumer, so you can help each individual achieve this equilibrium. Such factors include age, sex, family relationships, cultural influences, and economic status. This comprehensive approach to health care is known as **holistic health care** (a system of comprehensive or total patient

Wellness - Illness

Highest level of optimal health — Diminished or impaired state of health

FIGURE 1-4 Wellness-illness continuum.

care that considers the physical, emotional, social, economic, and spiritual needs of a person).

Maslow's Model of Health and Illness

Several models of the wellness-illness continuum have been developed, and they can help you to understand where your patient stands on it. The most common model was developed in the 1940s by Abraham Maslow. He believed that an individual's behavior is formed by the individual's attempts to meet essential human needs, which he identified as physiologic, safety and security, love and belongingness, and esteem and self-actualization. Maslow placed these needs into a conceptual hierarchy, or pyramid, that ranks them according to how basic each one is. A person has to meet needs at the base of the pyramid before advancing to the more noble or lofty needs higher on the pyramid. Remember that each patient may view or prioritize individual needs according to his or her own value system (Figure 1-5).

Health Promotion and Illness Prevention

From the earliest recorded civilizations to the twentieth century, the primary focus of health care was on the care of the sick. This has changed as the focus has broadened. Today, health care providers also seek to determine the cause of illness and prevent its spread.

In contrast to their origins as dirty, unsanitary, and ill-kept institutions where unsuspecting patients acquired diseases, hospitals have slowly become clean, sterile, well-kept places where patients are fairly well assured that their disease or illness will be attended to and, it is hoped, cured, without exposing them to the risk of additional medical problems. Think back to the dramatic decrease that took place in the phenomenal death rates in hospitals during the Crimean War when Florence Nightingale had the hospital units cleaned and imposed strict sanitary requirements.

More and better standards have been established and adhered to, and health statistics gathered by the U.S. Department of Public Health now help identify what types of diseases are most prevalent, which age-groups seem to be affected by certain illnesses, and which illnesses predominate in various parts of the country. These statistics identify problem areas for researchers and health care providers, who then direct their efforts at developing treatment for the illness, isolating its cause, and establishing methods to decrease its spread. Among the many lessons learned through study of these statistics are the following: childbirth without prenatal care increases the mortality rates of infant and mother; lack of milk in an infant's diet affects bone development and contributes to crippling deformities; and coal miners' constant exposure to coal dust and contaminated air in the mines causes their lungs to deteriorate.

Once cause-and-effect relationships like these become clear, prevention for these problems and others is, of course, the next step. In other words, the thrust of health care efforts has shifted form cure to prevention. By decreasing the risk factors for a given illness or disease and thereby preventing it, medicine has, in general, enhanced the quality of life and life expectancy in the United States. General medical research and specific research for the cause and cure of cancer, lung disease, acquired immunodeficiency syndrome (AIDS), heart disease, and many other life-threatening conditions continue to be integral parts of the health care system in this country.

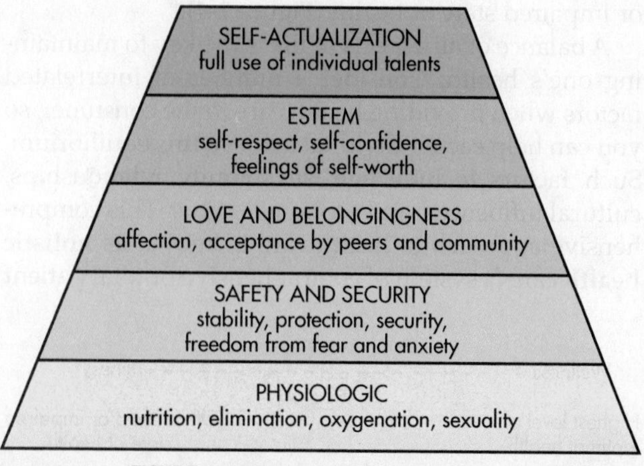

FIGURE 1-5 Maslow's hierarchy of needs.

Continuity of Care

The patient is the focus of the health care system. However, many factors in our holistic health care system determine what actually happens in the care of each patient. The number of health care providers and health care agencies involved in the care and treatment of a single patient is extensive. Increased specialization by health care providers and health care institutions, reimbursement procedures by third-party payors (e.g., insurance companies), cumbersome federal regulatory organizations, and state health care regulatory agencies all affect the consumer (the patient) and the type and quality of care provided.

One of the greatest challenges for the consumer of medical care in this health care delivery maze is to maintain autonomy and obtain continuity of care. Patients who are already bewildered and frightened by medical conditions that threaten their well-being are further discouraged to learn of yet another, often impossible task they face: that of understanding what procedures are done, why, and by whom. The right to choose which method of care will be provided or who will provide that care becomes a terrifying dilemma, and often the patient is unable to resolve it alone.

DELIVERY OF PATIENT CARE

Caring for patients comes down to the delivery of services by human beings to human beings. This humanistic enterprise involves not only the treatment of disease and injury but many other tasks as well: preventing disease, restoring optimal wellness through rehabilitation, maintaining a desirable level of wellness through such procedures as kidney dialysis, caring for the chronically ill, assisting the patient in the arduous process of self-care, and educating patients and families.

To identify individual needs of the patient and to plan a systematic approach to meet those needs, you will participate in developing an individualized care plan by using the nursing process (discussed in Chapter 6). The purpose of the care plan is to meet the expressed needs of the patient. Its development involves the patient and all health care providers who, through a coordinated and cooperative effort, work toward meeting the patient's total needs in a holistic, caring manner.

Participants in the Health Care System

Professional Health Care Specialists

The patient, the recipient of health care services, is the central focus of those activities performed by more than 200 types of health care providers identified in the health care system in the United States. Physicians, dentists, osteopathic physicians, surgeons, psychiatrists, and other professional health care specialists must pass examinations in their specialty to become **board certified** and obtain legal permission to practice in their area of specialization. In many cases, physicians employ people who have specialized training to function in cooperation with the physician: physician's assistants and nurse practitioners.

Registered Nurses

The RN, a direct health care provider, has completed one of three types of nursing education programs: a 4-year baccalaureate degree program, a 2-year associate degree program, or a 3-year diploma program. On satisfactory completion of one of these programs, the graduate nurse is eligible to take the National Council Licensing Examination for Registered Nurses (NCLEX-RN®). RNs practice in a variety of settings. The RN's duties and tasks vary according to educational background and the state's nurse practice act.

Licensed Practical Nurses and Licensed Vocational Nurses

The LPN/LVN practices under the supervision of the RN, the medical physician, the osteopathic physician, or the dentist. Working together, they are the direct patient caregivers in most institutions. Nursing recognizes the benefit of having this bedside caregiver on the health care team. What the LPN/LVN does on the job is based on the scope of practice outlined in a given state's nurse practice act.

Other Caregivers

There are other caregivers who are also required to be registered and to have the specialized education and training dictated by their professional organizations. A patient will often receive a referral to such other professionals or agencies for specific care and treatment. For example, a social worker is trained to counsel patients who have social, emotional, or environmental problems. A physical therapist, on the other hand, uses precise methods of massage, exercise, and hydrotherapy to help restore physical function of the body. A dietitian is trained to determine the foods that will meet the nutritional requirements of the patient. A respiratory therapist assists the patient by administering oxygen, monitoring and maintaining ventilators, drawing blood for blood gas analysis, and performing other pulmonary function tests.

Technologists, Medical Technicians, and Paraprofessionals

Technologists and medical technicians are among the group of laboratory, radiology, and other diagnostic personnel who are prepared to assist the medical professional staff in their attempt to diagnose and treat disease and injury. The term ***technologist*** refers to those who have a baccalaureate degree, whereas the term ***technician*** refers to those who have an associate degree or less. Paraprofessionals are those people educated to assist the professional in providing care for patients. A nursing assistant is educated in basic nursing techniques and performs under the supervision of the RN. A ward clerk is mainly a unit secretary, preparing and maintaining patients' records, ordering supplies, scheduling diagnostic tests, performing receptionist duties, and directing the flow of traffic in the patient care unit. These are only a sampling of the health care participants in the health care system. Each participant has a valuable contribution to make toward ensuring the safety and well-being of the patient.

Economic Factors Affecting Health and Illness

Rising Health Care Costs

Health care costs have reached a critical limit; national health care expenditures are projected to total $2.6 trillion by 2010. Some of the factors driving the rise in costs are an aging population, an increase in the use of technology, the rising cost of private health care insurance, and the rising cost of medical malpractice insurance.

Our aging population. The demands for health care usually increase as normal wear and tear on the body progresses. Many diseases are associated with aging—heart disease, diabetes, and osteoporosis, to name a few. In addition, some of our older adults need nursing home care, which is also costly and is usually not covered by private health insurance.

Advances in technology. Advances in technology have led to better diagnosis and treatment of illness, but such progress carries a large price tag. Research and the development of technology costs millions of dollars, a price that is passed on to the patient in the cost of the individual tests or treatments.

Health care insurance. Private health care insurance was initially developed to defray some or all of the cost of health care. It made health care more affordable, but also raised the demand for it. As more individuals sought care, the price of health care services and insurance costs spiraled. This trend continues at an alarming and seemingly uncontrollable speed. In particular, runaway costs are creating hardship for those who are underinsured or not insured at all. Often the deciding factor in determining who receives care and who does not, affordability and coverage is becoming an ethical issue at all levels of the health care delivery system.

Malpractice insurance. Nurses and doctors carry medical malpractice insurance to protect themselves in the event a malpractice claim is filed against them. As malpractice claims have increased in frequency and amount, the premiums for this insurance have also risen, particularly for physicians. Physicians, in turn, sometimes resort to practicing "defensive medicine." That is, they become overly cautious out of fear of a claim, ordering more and more costly tests and procedures not because they are medically necessary, but to protect themselves. These behaviors have resulted in higher medical costs for the patient.

Miscellaneous factors. To further compound the economic problems, more than 35 million people in the United States are without health care coverage. These people avoid preventive and routine care and are seen only in crisis situations.

These issues are alarming for health care providers. As a nurse, you can help keep the costs to the patient to a minimum by using materials and time economically and providing knowledgeable, efficient care.

Changes in Delivery System

Hospitals throughout the United States are changing delivery systems to make care more cost effective. Case management and cross-training are two of the more common ways they are reconfiguring care delivery.

Case management. Case management nursing revolves around the use of **clinical pathways**, which map out expectations of the hospitalization according to a designated time frame. The RN functions as a case manager, coordinating and planning the care of a group of patients, or caseload. An LPN/LVN works with the RN to assist the patient in attaining desired outcomes of care. Case management–style nursing has proven to reduce the length of stay for the patient, which in turn reduces the overall cost of the patient's health care.

Cross-training. Cross-training is a method of using staff resources to their fullest. Individuals receive training to perform duties that vary according to the needs at a given time. It can be as narrowly defined as medical training to care for surgical patients or as broadly defined as housekeeping personnel training to give basic morning care to patients. The scope of cross-training is usually defined by the individual institution. This practice often makes a reduction possible in the number of employees without compromising the quality of patient care.

Other trends. Other trends affecting the economics of health care include the development of multisystem health care chains that may include several hospitals, clinics, nursing homes, and pharmacies. These systems share expenses and generally achieve an overall reduction in operating expenses. Health maintenance organizations (HMOs) or group health care practices provide health care to members for a fixed prepaid rate. This service includes medical care, nursing care, diagnostic tests, hospitalization, and various inpatient and outpatient treatments. This service has demonstrated a high quality of low-cost health care.

Environmental Factors Affecting Health and Illness

Social and physical environmental factors do not necessarily cause illness, but they do influence the development or progression of an illness. Personal financial hardship, lifestyle, social pressures, and major societal issues (e.g., AIDS, abortion, and drug abuse) are some of the more obvious social factors. Stress, conflict, smoking, excessive weight, and alcoholism are among the physical factors.

Reactions to these factors vary from patient to patient. When people fear illness and dehumanization, loss of identity, and loss of control, their mental state often suffers. An imbalance in body functions can affect one's physical condition. Although we tend to separate social factors from physical factors, remember that the two areas affect each other reciprocally.

Early recognition of the effect of environmental factors on a patient and prompt intervention by family, health care providers, or the patients themselves can decrease or keep any negative impact to a minimum.

Expectations of the Patient and Health Care Team

Each patient is special, possessing a unique personality, background, lifestyle, and level of education. The patient's needs, expectations, and response to health care are influenced by all these factors.

Health Promotion

Most people in the United States believe that everyone has a right to health care, regardless of race, color, creed, or economic status. This health care includes the treatment of disease, as well as health promotion and preventive medicine. In many cases, treatment of illness is less of a concern than its prevention. The acute awareness of preventive medicine has resulted in today's emphasis on education about issues such as smoking, heart disease, drug and alcohol abuse, weight control, stress syndrome, and social diseases.

At the other end of the wellness-illness continuum, many people believe that they are no longer in control of their health when they do become ill and seek medical attention. Ironically, the presumption is that the care they receive will be highly satisfactory and lead to a cure. They expect health care providers to provide service in a knowledgeable, safe, and expeditious manner and to work in a cooperative manner for their benefit. They also expect the cost of care to be reasonable and, most importantly, paid by somebody else (an insurance company or the government).

Patients' Rights

There is one more vital expectation that you, together with all health care workers, must recognize and fulfill. Patients expect to be treated with dignity and compassion and to have their rights respected. In 1972, the American Hospital Association (AHA) issued the Patient's Bill of Rights in an effort to make sure these expectations are fulfilled. The Patient's Bill of Rights was replaced in 2003 when the AHA adopted the Patient Care Partnership (Box 1-1). Under the terms of this document, patients are assured that they can

Box 1-1 The Patient Care Partnership: Understanding Expectations, Rights, and Responsibilities

When you need hospital care, your doctor and the nurses and other professionals at our hospital are committed to working with you and your family to meet your health care needs. Our dedicated doctors and staff serve the community in all its ethnic, religious, and economic diversity. Our goal is for you and your family to have the same care and attention we would want for our families and ourselves.

The sections below explain some of the basics of how you can expect to be treated during your hospital stay. They also cover what we will need from you to care for you better. If you have questions at any time, please ask them. Unasked or unanswered questions can add to the stress of being in the hospital. Your comfort and confidence in your care are very important to us.

WHAT TO EXPECT DURING YOUR HOSPITAL STAY

- **High quality hospital care.** Our first priority is to provide you the care you need, when you need it, with skill, compassion, and respect. Tell your caregivers if you have concerns about your care or if you have pain. You have the right to know the identity of doctors, nurses, and others involved in your care, as well as when they are students, residents, or other trainees.
- **A clean and safe environment.** Our hospital works hard to keep you safe. We use special policies and procedures to avoid mistakes in your care and keep you free from abuse or neglect. If anything unexpected and significant occurs during your hospital stay, you will be told what happened, and any resulting changes in your care will be discussed with you.
- **Involvement in your care.** You and your doctor often make decisions about your care before you go to the hospital. Other times, especially in emergencies, those decisions are made during your hospital stay. When decision making takes place, it should include the following:
  1. *Discussing your medical condition and information about medically appropriate treatment choices.* To make informed decisions with your doctor, you need to understand the following:
     - The benefits and risks of each treatment
     - Whether your treatment is experimental or part of a research study
     - What you can reasonably expect from your treatment and any long-term effects it might have on your quality of life
     - What you and your family will need to do after you leave the hospital
     - The financial consequences of using uncovered services or out-of-network providers

     Please tell your caregivers if you need more information about treatment choices.
  2. *Discussing your treatment plan.* When you enter the hospital, you sign a general consent to treatment. In some cases, such as surgery or experimental treatment, you may be asked to confirm in writing that you understand what is planned and agree to it. This process protects your right to consent to or refuse a treatment. Your doctor will explain the medical consequences of refusing recommended treatment. It also protects your right to decide if you want to participate in a research study.
  3. *Getting information from you.* Your caregivers need complete and correct information about your health and coverage so that they can make good decisions about your care. That includes the following:
     - Past illnesses, surgeries, or hospital stays
     - Past allergic reactions
     - Any medications or dietary supplements (such as vitamins and herbs) that you are taking
     - Any network or admission requirements under your health plan
  4. *Understanding your health care goals and values.* You may have health care goals and values or spiritual beliefs that are important to your well-being. They will be taken into account as much as possible throughout your hospital stay. Make sure your doctor, your family, and your care team know your wishes.
  5. *Understanding who should make decisions when you cannot.* If you have signed a health care power of attorney stating who should speak for you if you become unable to make health care decisions for yourself, or a "living will" or "advance directive" that states your wishes about end-of-life care, give copies to your doctor, your family, and your care team. If you or your family need help making difficult decisions, counselors, chaplains, and others are available to help.

Adapted from American Hospital Association. (2003). *The patient care partnership: Understanding expectations, rights, and responsibilities.* Chicago: AHA. Reprinted with permission from the American Hospital Association.

Continued

Box 1-1 The Patient Care Partnership: Understanding Expectations, Rights, and Responsibilities—cont'd

WHAT TO EXPECT DURING YOUR HOSPITAL STAY—cont'd

6. *Protection of your privacy.* We respect the confidentiality of your relationship with your doctor and other caregivers, and the sensitive information about your health and health care that are part of that relationship. State and federal laws and hospital operating policies protect the privacy of your medical information. You will receive a Notice of Privacy Practices that describes the ways that we use, disclose, and safeguard patient information and that explains how you can obtain a copy of information from our records about your care.
7. *Preparing you and your family for when you leave the hospital.* Your doctor works with hospital staff and professionals in your community. You and your family also play an important role in your care. The success of your treatment often depends on your efforts to follow medication, diet, and therapy plans. Your family may need to help care for you at home. You can expect us to help you identify sources of follow-up care and to let you know if our hospital has a financial interest in any referrals. As long as you agree that we share information about your care with them, we will coordinate our activities with your caregivers outside the hospital. You can also expect to receive information and, where possible, training about the self-care you will need when you go home.
8. *Help with your bill and filing insurance claims.* Our staff will file claims for you with health care insurers or other programs such as Medicare and Medicaid. They will also help your doctor with needed documentation. Hospital bills and insurance coverage are often confusing. If you have questions about your bill, contact our business office. If you need help understanding your insurance coverage or health plan, start with your insurance company or health benefits manager. If you do not have health coverage, we will try to help you and your family find financial help or make other arrangements. We need your help with collecting needed information and other requirements to obtain coverage or assistance.

While you are here, you will receive more detailed notices about some of the rights you have as a hospital patient and how to exercise them. We are always interested in improving. If you have questions, comments, or concerns, please contact: ___________.

expect high-quality hospital care, a clean and safe environment, and involvement in their care and the decision-making process.

Health Care Providers' Rights

The delivery of health care has to be a process of mutual exchange between patients and health care providers. Patients expect their rights as just outlined to be respected, but health care workers have expectations as well. Health care professionals expect that patients will do the following to actively participate in their care as much as possible: take an active role in the planning process, have an understanding of the care and the treatment given, ask questions, follow the treatment plan prescribed, act responsibly with respect to their own conditions, and give health care workers the same respect to which patients are entitled.

Interdisciplinary Approach to Health Care

The primary goal of the health care team is the optimal physical, mental, and social well-being of the patient. This goal is achieved by promoting and restoring health within the wellness-illness continuum. It is imperative that health care personnel, when working to meet the needs of the patient, work together as a health care team. Following this interdisciplinary approach to treatment prevents the fragmentation of patient care. Just as the plan of care for patients is developed in a holistic manner, so is the actual delivery of health care. It is imperative for all health care providers to remember that the central focus of all their activity is the patient.

Each member of the team is responsible for coordinating her or his activity with every other member of the team by developing a comprehensive care plan, effectively communicating, and keeping accurate records (Figure 1-6).

Care Plan

A care plan is a document that outlines the individual needs of the patient and the approach of the health care team to meet these needs. It is developed in cooperation with the patient and, in some cases, the patient's family. It further identifies who will assist in treating the patient. The document guides and directs the activities surrounding the patient's care; it ensures continuity and consistency of care and eliminates duplication

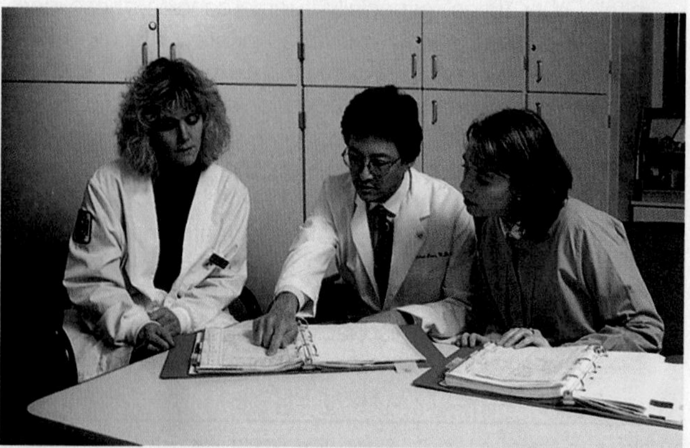

FIGURE 1-6 A nurse collaborating with other members of the interdisciplinary health care team.

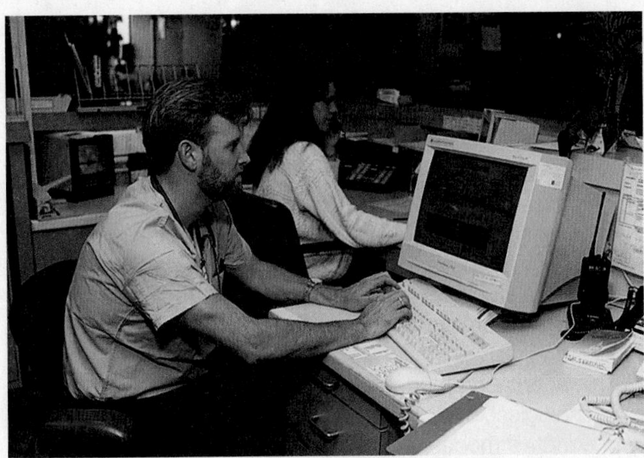

FIGURE 1-7 A nurse documenting patient care at a computer terminal.

of services. (See Chapter 6 for further discussion of using the nursing care plan in the nursing process.)

Communication

Good communication is essential for the exchange of information among the members of the health care team. Communication is the prerequisite for meeting the needs of the patient or, if necessary, making appropriate changes to do so. (See Chapter 3 for further discussion of communication.)

Documentation

Documentation in any form is the permanent record of the patient's progress and treatment. It constitutes the formal and legal record of care received by the patient and the patient's response to that care (Figure 1-7). The information recorded during the entire course of treatment serves many purposes. It provides a progress record of treatment so that all the involved health care members are aware of what treatment the patient is receiving. It also provides a history of events, which is frequently valuable in the future treatment of the same condition. (See Chapter 7 for further discussion of documentation.)

NURSING CARE MODELS

Since the time of Florence Nightingale, nursing and health care technology have continued to change to meet the needs of the patient. Initially, nursing education was like an apprenticeship. Experienced nurses demonstrated skills, and the student nurse practiced these skills until a smooth technical performance was achieved. Little emphasis was placed on development of a knowledge base to enable the nurse to solve problems down the road, or to adapt the skills learned to various complex situations that would be encountered later. Through research, nursing theorists have developed several models to assist you today with problem solving and organization of care. Many schools of nursing loosely base their curriculum or philosophy on a specific nursing model to help their students learn about and understand the nursing process (see Chapter 6).

As early as the 1970s, nursing leaders identified four major concepts that were the basis for all nursing models of care:

- **Nursing**—encompasses the roles and actions of the nurse
- **Patient**—the individual receiving the care
- **Health**—the area along the wellness-illness continuum that the patient occupies
- **Environment**—the setting for the nurse-patient interaction

Several leading nurse theorists have developed nursing models of care, and their work is ongoing. Table 1-3 shows six examples of nursing theories that incorporate those basic concepts.

CONTEMPORARY PRACTICAL AND VOCATIONAL NURSING CARE

As shown, the existence of the LPN/LVN in the health care delivery system is not new. What is new is the expansion of the LPN/LVN's role and responsibilities from bathing patients and doing light housekeeping to performing skilled tasks needed to provide health care to people along the wellness-illness continuum.

The ongoing evolution of your role is influenced by the various states' nurse practice acts, individual changes within the health care agencies, the availability of health care workers, and the needs of patients. LPN/LVNs are finding careers in hospitals, clinics, outpatient agencies, home health agencies, long-term care facilities, insurance companies, physicians' offices, and the military services.

Your career rests on a foundation comprised of nursing history and today's health care delivery system.

PRACTICAL AND VOCATIONAL NURSING DEFINED

Practical and vocational nursing is defined as the activity of providing specific services to patients under the direct supervision of a licensed physician or dentist, an RN, a podiatrist, or some combination. The services are provided in a structured setting surrounding the caring for the sick, the rehabilitation of the sick and injured, and the prevention of sickness and injury. This definition is adapted from NAPNES and several states' nurse practice acts.

The nurse has a unique function: to assist individuals, sick or well, in the performance of those activities contributing to health, to their recovery, or to a peaceful death—activities that patients would perform unaided if they had the necessary strength, will, or knowledge—and, if feasible, to do this in such a way as to help patients gain independence as rapidly as possible. The practical or vocational nurse is educated to be a responsible member of a health care team, performing basic

Table 1-3 Examples of Nursing Theories

THEORIST	NURSING OBJECTIVE	SETTING
Nightingale (1860)	To facilitate "the body's reparative processes" by arranging the patient's environment	Patient's environment is arranged; includes appropriate noise control, nutrition, hygiene, lighting, comfort, socialization, and hope.
Orem (1971)	To care for and help patient attain total self-care	This is self-care deficit theory. Nursing care becomes necessary when patient is unable to fulfill biologic, psychological, developmental, or social needs.
Leininger (1978)	To provide care consistent with nursing's emerging science and knowledge, with caring as central focus	In this transcultural care theory, caring is the central and unifying domain for nursing knowledge and practice.
Roy (1979)	To identify types of demands placed on patient, assess adaptation to demands, and help patient adapt	This adaptation model is based on the physiologic, psychological, sociologic, and dependence-independence adaptive modes.
Parse (1981)	To focus on man as living unity and man's qualitative participation with health experience (nursing as science and art)	Man continually interacts with environment and participates in maintenance of health. Health is a continual, open process rather than a state of well-being or absence of disease.
Benner and Wrubel (1989)	To focus on patient's needs for caring as a means of coping with stressors of illness	Caring is central to the essence of nursing. Caring creates the possibilities for coping and enables possibilities for connecting with and concern for others.

therapeutic, rehabilitative, and preventive care for anyone who needs it. Currently, more than 692,000 LPN/LVNs are employed in the health care field.

The practice of discharging patients from acute care facilities for continued recuperation in extended care units and nursing homes—places of employment for LPN/LVNs—is evident in the increasing number of patients requiring more complex care. Every 3 years, the National Council of State Boards of Nursing performs a job analysis. This analysis helps to determine the content areas for the NCLEX-PN®. The findings of the latest job analysis indicate that newly licensed LPN/LVNs are continuing to provide care in all types of settings, with the majority continuing to be employed in long-term care settings. No statistically significant changes have occurred in work settings since the last job analysis.

OBJECTIVES AND CHARACTERISTICS OF PRACTICAL AND VOCATIONAL NURSING EDUCATION

The objectives for practical and vocational nursing education are the following:

- To acquire the specialized knowledge and skills needed to meet the health care needs of patients in a variety of settings
- To be a graduate of a state-approved practical or vocational nursing program
- To take and pass the NCLEX-PN® Examination
- To acquire a state license to practice

To accomplish these objectives, students must assume responsibility for their own education, intensive study, and dedication to duty. Organizing time effectively helps accomplish these objectives and ultimately assures the patient of safe and competent care.

Distinguishing characteristics, roles, and responsibilities for the LPN/LVN are shown in Box 1-2.

Box 1-2 Characteristics, Roles, and Responsibilities of the Practical or Vocational Nurse

- Is a responsible and accountable member of the health care team
- Maintains a current license
- Practices within the scope of the nurse practice act
- Practices under the supervision of a medical physician, RN, osteopathic physician, dentist, or podiatrist
- Participates in continuing education activities
- Is an effective member of the health care team
- Uses the nursing process to meet patients' needs
- Promotes and maintains health, prevents disease, and encourages and assists in rehabilitation
- Maintains a professional appearance
- Subscribes to recognized ethical practices
- Performs within legal parameters
- Participates in activities of professional organizations
- Assists in developing the role of the LPN/LVN of tomorrow

ROLES AND RESPONSIBILITIES

In 1981, NAPNES issued the following statement of responsibilities required for practice as an LPN/LVN:

- Recognizes the LPN/LVN's role in the health care delivery system and articulates that role with those of other health care team members
- Maintains accountability for one's own nursing practice within the ethical and legal framework
- Serves as a patient advocate
- Accepts the LPN/LVN's role in maintaining developing standards of practice in providing health care
- Seeks further growth through educational opportunities

LPN/LVNs are required to be aware of the content of the nurse practice act of the state in which they are employed. The LPN/LVN's role is found in this law, and the law differs from state to state. Regardless of the site of employment, LPN/LVNs provide care in basic and complex situations under the general supervision of an RN, a physician, a podiatrist, or a dentist.

A major criterion in differentiating between the roles of the RN and the LPN/LVN is that the LPN/LVN never functions independently. LPN/LVNs are responsible for functioning safely and are accountable for their actions. You should assume responsibility only for nursing actions that are within your legal role and that you feel safe in carrying out.

LPN/LVNs function interdependently when they offer input to the RN about the effectiveness of care or offer suggestions to improve the patient's care. Because LPN/LVNs provide actual care at the bedside in acute care situations, the data you collect while engaged in giving care is valuable in determining whether progress is being made to meet patient goals.

Practical and vocational nursing is an exciting, challenging career that provides an opportunity to care for others while receiving personal satisfaction. The focus is on bedside and personal care of patients in a variety of settings. To perform in a responsible, accountable manner calls for knowledge, skill, and expertise.

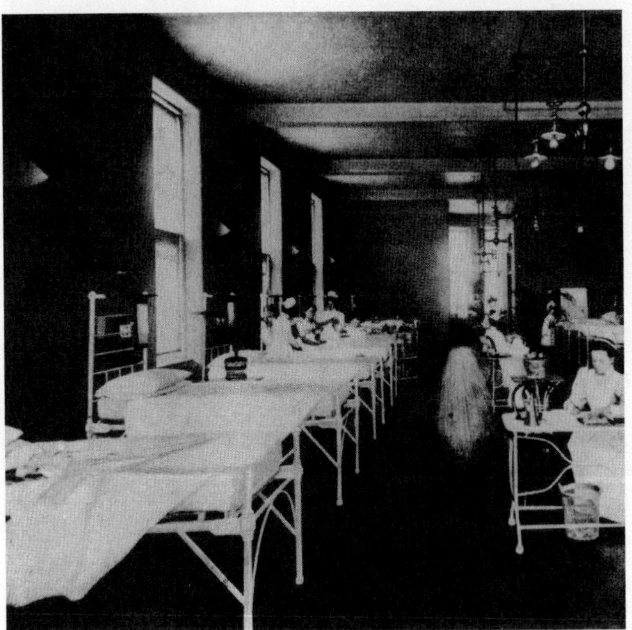

FIGURE 1-8 An early women's surgical ward.

The following job description was given to floor nurses by a hospital in 1887*:

> In addition to caring for your 50 patients, each nurse will follow these regulations:
>
> - Daily sweep and mop the floors of your ward, dust the patient's furniture and windowsills. Maintain an even temperature in your ward by bringing in a scuttle of coal for the day's business.
> - Light is important to observe the patient's condition. Therefore, each day fill kerosene lamps, clean chimneys, and trim wicks. Wash the windows once a week.
> - The nurse's notes are important in aiding the physician's work. Make your pens carefully; you may whittle nibs to your individual taste.
> - Each nurse on day duty will report every day at 7 AM and leave at 8 PM, except on the Sabbath, on which day you will be off from 12 noon to 2 PM.
> - Graduate nurses in good standing with the director of nurses will be given an evening off each week for courting purposes or two evenings a week if you go regularly to church.
> - Each nurse should lay aside from each payday a goodly sum of her earnings for her benefits during her declining years so that she will not become a burden. For example, if you earn $30 a month, you should set aside $15.
> - Any nurse who smokes, uses liquor in any form, gets her hair done at a beauty shop, or frequents dance halls will give the director of nurses good reason to suspect her worth, intentions, and integrity.
> - The nurse who performs her labors and serves her patients and doctors without fault for 5 years will be given an increase of 5 cents a day, providing there are no hospital debts outstanding.

It is interesting to compare current practical and vocational nursing tasks with those that were expected in 1887. Practical and vocational nursing has indeed come a long way (Figure 1-8).

---

*From Hill, S.S., & Howlett, H.A. (2005). *Success in practical/vocational nursing: from student to leader* (5th ed.). Philadelphia: Saunders.

Get Ready for the NCLEX® Examination!

Key Points

- The evolution of nursing was greatly influenced by the way care was given to the sick and injured.
- The influence of Florence Nightingale on nursing practice and nursing education was highly significant in the nineteenth century.
- Nursing practice and education in the United States were significantly influenced by the activities of Florence Nightingale.
- The Association of Practical Nurse Schools was organized in Chicago in 1941 to address the needs of practical nursing education. Its name was changed in 1942 to the National Association of Practical Nurse Education (NAPNE).
- NAPNE changed its name again, in 1959, to the National Association for Practical Nurse Education and Service (NAPNES).
- In 1949, the National Federation of Licensed Practical Nurses (NFLPN) was founded by Lillian Kuster.
- Mandatory licensure laws were established for practical and vocational nursing education and practice.
- The wellness-illness continuum is a range and comprises the entirety of a person's health.
- Prevention of illness and injury and continuity of patient care are integral components of holistic health care.
- The practical or vocational nurse is one of many of the large groups of health care workers who provide health care services.
- The practical and vocational nursing community functions in accordance with the several states' nurse practice acts.
- Roles and responsibilities of the nurse are varied and complex and evolve with new technologies and research advances.
- Ongoing education is valued, expected, and required for continued licensure.

Additional Learning Resources

Go to your Companion CD for an audio glossary, animations, video clips, and more.

evolve Be sure to visit the Evolve site at http://evolve.elsevier.com/Christensen/foundations/ for additional online resources.

Get Ready for the NCLEX® Examination

1. The student interested in attending an accredited school for practical nursing knows that an accredited program:
   1. voluntarily seeks a review by a given organization to determine whether the program meets that organization's preestablished criteria.
   2. is one that meets the minimal standards set by the respective state agencies responsible for overseeing educational programs.
   3. is necessary before the graduate is eligible to take the National Council Licensing Examination for Practical Nursing (NCLEX-PN®).
   4. is a federally funded health care program that educates practical nurse students.
2. The acute awareness by the health care consumer of preventive medicine has resulted in an increase in:
   1. anxiety over diagnostic workups such as colonoscopies or gynecologic examinations.
   2. the number of admissions for inpatient services.
   3. the length of a hospitalization stay.
   4. knowledge and services to promote health and prevent illness (wellness-illness continuum).
3. The factor that best advanced the practice of nursing in the first century was the:
   1. growth of cities.
   2. better education of nurses.
   3. teachings of Christianity.
   4. improved conditions for women.
4. Nursing education programs may seek voluntary accreditation by the appropriate council of the:
   1. American Nurses Association.
   2. International Council of Nurses.
   3. Congress for Nursing Practice.
   4. National League for Nursing.
5. When developing a definition of "health," a person should consider that health is:
   1. a condition of physical, mental, and social well-being and absence of disease.
   2. the ability to pursue activities of daily living.
   3. a function of the physiologic state.
   4. a static condition; the absence of pathology.
6. Comprehensive or total patient care that considers the physical, emotional, social, economic, and spiritual needs of the person, as well as the person's response to the illness and the impact of the illness on the person's ability to meet self-care needs is a philosophy referred to as:
   1. the wellness-illness continuum.
   2. the Patient Care Partnership.
   3. holistic nursing.
   4. the health care delivery system.
7. The student nurse reviewing the history of nursing knows that the "Lady with the Lamp" is:
   1. Clara Barton.
   2. Florence Nightingale.
   3. Phoebe.
   4. Lavinia Dock.

8. The American Society of Superintendents of Training Schools of Nursing was established in 1894. The major goal of this organization was:
   1. to promote development of new schools of nursing.
   2. to train nursing leaders.
   3. to set educational standards for nurses.
   4. to develop standards for licensure.

9. The ancient Hebrews, according to the Talmud and the Old Testament, documented several health and disease practices. They are also attributed with:
   1. the first practice of public health and home health.
   2. the first school of nursing in Europe.
   3. the first understanding of the wellness-illness continuum.
   4. the first nursing organization.

10. The student nurse who is studying the history of health care recognizes that Hippocrates is credited with the development of:
    1. the first text on health care.
    2. the first ethical guide for medical conduct.
    3. the first medical society.
    4. the first nursing care guide.

11. Care delivered by RNs and LPNs is legally defined as their scope of practice, which is determined by:
    1. the nursing process.
    2. the nurse in charge.
    3. the Hippocratic Oath.
    4. the nurse practice act.

12. The nursing student knows that the first nursing theorist was:
    1. Phoebe.
    2. Clara Barton.
    3. Florence Nightingale.
    4. Sister Calista Roy.

13. The most commonly used model that assists in the understanding of the patient's place on the wellness-illness continuum is:
    1. Abraham Maslow.
    2. Dorothea Dix.
    3. Clara Barton.
    4. Theodore Fliedner.

14. The first nurse to train in America was:
    1. Lavinia Dock.
    2. Linda Richards.
    3. Clara Barton.
    4. Mary Breckenridge.

15. The first school dedicated to the training of the practical nurse in the United States was:
    1. the Ballard School.
    2. the YWCA.
    3. the Thompson Practical Nursing School.
    4. the Shepard-Gill School.

16. Health is:
    1. the absence of illness.
    2. a state of complete physical, mental, and social well-being.
    3. a condition between disease and good health.
    4. the opposite of disease.

17. Men in nursing:
    1. are not permitted to serve in the military.
    2. became prominent during the Civil War.
    3. are becoming fewer and fewer.
    4. are regaining their historical position in the profession as nurses.

chapter

2 Legal and Ethical Aspects of Nursing

evolve

http://evolve.elsevier.com/Christensen/foundationsadult

Barbara Lauritsen Christensen and Katherine Parker-Feliciano

Objectives

1. Summarize the structure and function of the legal system.
2. Discuss the legal relationship existing between the nurse and the patient.
3. Explain the importance of maintaining standards of care.
4. Give examples of ways the nursing profession is regulated.
5. Explain nursing malpractice.
6. Give examples of ways the licensed practical/vocational nurse can avoid being involved in a lawsuit.
7. Give examples of legal issues in health care.
8. Explain the meaning of a code of ethics.
9. Summarize how culture affects an individual's beliefs, morals, and values.
10. Differentiate between a legal duty and an ethical duty.
11. Identify how values affect decision making.
12. Distinguish between ethical and unethical behavior.
13. Explain the nurse's role in reporting unethical behavior.
14. Give examples of ethical issues common in health care.
15. Discuss federal regulations of HIPAA privacy rule and its impact on the health care system.

Key Terms

accountability (ăk-kŏŭnt-ă-BĬL-ĭ-tē, p. 24)
advocate (p. 24)
deposition (p. 23)
doctrine of informed consent (p. 27)
ethical dilemmas (p. 31)
ethics (p. 31)
euthanasia (ū-thă-NĀ-zhă, p. 29)
laws (p. 23)
liability (lī-ă-BĬL-ĭ-tē, p. 24)
liable (LĪ-ă-bl, p. 23)
malpractice (p. 26)
nonmaleficence (p. 33)
standards of care (p. 24)
value clarification (p. 31)
values (p. 31)
verdict (p. 23)

Today's health care system is a dynamic, complex system that has gone through significant changes over the past years. It is an aspect of society and as such is bound by established laws, rules, regulations, and ethical principles. Societal concerns about the rising cost of health care, the quality of care, and growing consumer awareness have an impact on health care and the practice of nursing. Rapid advances in the technology and communication fields present new challenges on an ongoing basis. There is an increased focus on managed care, community health, and home health care, which is providing new practice opportunities for the licensed practical nurse and the licensed vocational nurse (LPN/LVN).

Guiding the LPN/LVN's practice of nursing is a combination of legal principles, established laws, moral standards, and ethical principles. It is important for you to understand how legal standards and ethical principles affect nursing practice. The law sets an obligatory minimum standard in any given situation. Ethical principles, which evolve out of society and culture, frequently impose an even higher duty. These legal standards and ethical principles serve as a support for all members of the health care system, and help protect the rights of all members of society.

LEGAL ASPECTS OF NURSING

The legal relationship that exists between the nurse and the patient is influenced by the existing laws, rules, and regulations that govern nursing practice. Acting outside the established scope of practice or failing to meet the established standard of care has the potential to result in injury to the patient and give rise to legal liability. It is crucial that you inform yourself of the scope of nursing practice and the standards of care that constitute your professional duties; acquisition of this knowledge, along with compliance with licensing requirements, is your responsibility.

There are many legal issues related to health care, and health care–related litigation involving nurses is common. Patients are more educated, are more aware of their rights, and have higher expectations regarding the care they receive. An understanding of the legal process and some of the ways you as a nurse will perhaps come into contact with the legal system, as well as familiarity with common legal issues in nursing, will serve you in good stead during your career.

OVERVIEW OF THE LEGAL SYSTEM

The legal system is a complex set of rules and regulations that has developed in response to the needs of society. **Laws** prescribe proper behavior in society; they sanction acceptable behavior and prohibit unacceptable behavior. It is important for you to have a basic understanding of the legal system, which serves both to mandate and to protect: The law assigns fundamental legal duties, and also provides protection for all members of the health care system.

There are two basic categories of law: **criminal** and **civil** (Box 2-1). Laws of both types are established in one of two ways: (1) federal, state, and local governments **develop statutory law;** and (2) **common law,** or case law, evolves in response to specific legal questions that come before the court and usually follows **precedent** (previous rulings on an issue).

OVERVIEW OF THE LEGAL PROCESS

Civil litigation (a lawsuit in a civil court) begins when the **plaintiff** (the complaining party) contacts an attorney. Depending on the specific state law, there is sometimes a prelitigation panel or tribunal that precedes the actual filing in court. Such panels have the purpose of weeding out the frivolous cases and decreasing the burden on the court systems. If this process results in a finding that litigation in this case has a legal basis, the plaintiff writes a statement called a **complaint** and files it in the appropriate court. The complaint names the **defendant** (the person alleged to be **liable** [legally responsible]), states the facts involved in the case, defines the legal issues the case raises, and outlines the **damages** (compensation that the plaintiff is seeking). The defendant is served a **summons** (a court order that notifies the defendant of the legal action), which constitutes the necessary legal notice, and the defendant usually hires an attorney to represent him or her in the lawsuit. The attorney will prepare and file an **answer** (a detailed response to the charges outlined in the complaint) in which the defendant either admits to or denies any or all of the allegations made in the complaint.

The next step in the litigation is a phase called **discovery** (a pretrial process allowing both sides to interview witnesses and look at documents). You will sometimes be involved in the discovery stage of a lawsuit. If you are a defendant or fact witness, the plaintiff will often take your **deposition.** A deposition is a question-and-answer session under oath during which attorneys ask the witness questions relating to the issues of the lawsuit. A court reporter records every word the witness says. A transcript of the testimony becomes part of the evidence.

Other tools also serve the process of discovery. The **interrogatory** is a written question that one party sends to the other party, to which an answer is obligatory. A **Request for Production of Documents and Things** is an instrument for discovering and obtaining such documents as policies and procedures, standards of care, medical records, assignment sheets, personnel files, equipment maintenance records, birth certificates, marriage certificates, medical bills, and other documents pertinent to the issues at hand. A fourth discovery technique is the admission of facts. This tool requests the party to admit or deny certain statements in order to streamline the factual presentation of the case; for example, the following questions:

- Do you admit or deny that Andrea Ali was admitted to Shirley Anthony Hospital on November 18, 2009?
- Do you admit or deny that signs and symptoms of sepsis can include elevated white blood cells (WBCs), deteriorating vital signs, elevated temperatures, and change in mental status?

Once the evidence has been presented, the court will render a **verdict** (a decision) based on the facts of the case, the evidence and testimony presented, the credibility of the witnesses, and the laws that pertain to the issue(s). Either party has the right, in case of disagreement with the outcome of the lawsuit, to file an **appeal** (request a review of the decision) asking that a higher court review the decision. The outcome of litigation is never certain.

In a criminal trial, the question is whether the defendant (the person accused of the crime) is answerable for a crime against the People (since criminal law concerns crimes against society rather than individuals). At trial, the People's attorney and the defendant's attorney present their cases. The judge or the jury (if a jury trial) then **deliberate** (consider and decide) the guilt or innocence of the defendant. If the judge or jury reaches a verdict of *not guilty*, the defendant is free to go. If the verdict is *guilty*, the judge passes a **sentence** (penalty) based on the severity of the crime, the defen-

Box 2-1 Characteristics of Criminal and Civil Law

CRIMINAL

- Conduct at issue is offensive to society *in general.*
- Conduct at issue is detrimental to society as a *whole.*
- The law involves *public* offenses (such as robbery, murder, assault).
- The law's purpose is to *punish* for the crime and deter and *prevent* further crimes.

CIVIL

- Conduct at issue violates a *person's* rights.
- Conduct at issue is detrimental to that *individual.*
- The law involves an offense that is against an *individual.*
- The law's purpose is to *make the aggrieved person whole again,* to restore the person to where he or she was.

dant's past criminal record, and applicable laws. The defendant who receives a guilty verdict may appeal if there has been an error either (1) in the process in which the conviction was obtained or (2) by the court during the proceedings *(Verdict Lawyers, Verdict Attorneys: The Verdict).*

See Box 2-2 for common legal terminology.

LEGAL RELATIONSHIPS

In the past, nurses did not hold legal liability for alleged harm suffered by a patient while receiving medical care, but rather the physician or the hospital did, and sometimes both. As nurses gained recognition for their expertise and gained more autonomy, dissatisfied patients (and their attorneys) began to look at nurses as potential defendants and to seek to hold nurses accountable under the law. **Accountability** (being responsible for one's own actions) is a concept that gives rise to a legal duty, and thus **liability** (legal responsibility), in nursing. Indeed, the nurse today is not immune from liability in the practice of nursing. It is possible for you to be charged with civil or criminal wrongdoing and, depending on the particular circumstances surrounding the case, held liable.

Box 2-2 Common Legal Terminology

abandonment of care	Wrongful termination of providing patient care
assault	An intentional threat to cause bodily harm to another; does not have to include actual bodily contact
battery	Unlawful touching of another person without informed consent
competency	A legal presumption that a person who has reached the age of majority can make decisions for herself or himself unless proved otherwise (if she or he has been legally declared incompetent)
defamation	Spoken or written statements made maliciously and intentionally that may injure the subject's reputation
harm	Injury to a person or the person's property that gives rise to a basis for a legal action against the person who caused the damage
libel	A malicious or untrue writing about another person that is brought to the attention of others
malpractice	Failure to meet a legal duty, thus causing harm to another
negligence	The commission (doing) of an act or the omission (not doing) of an act that a reasonably prudent person would have performed in a similar situation, thus causing harm to another person
slander	Malicious or untrue spoken words about another person that are brought to the attention of others
tort	A type of civil law that involves wrongs against a person or property; torts include negligence, assault, battery, defamation, fraud, false imprisonment, and invasion of privacy

When you assume the responsibility for a patient's care, a relationship comes about—the nurse-patient relationship. This relationship, beyond its more personal human component, has a legal basis: your duty to provide professional care. A failure to provide care to the expected level of expertise gives rise to legal liability (see the discussion in the next section of standards of care). Furthermore, in the nurse-patient relationship, the nurse accepts the role of advocate for the patient. An **advocate** is one who defends or pleads a cause or issue on behalf of another. A nurse advocate has a legal and ethical obligation to safeguard the patient's interests.

A landmark case that addressed nursing liability was *Darling v. Charleston Community Memorial Hospital.* In this case, an 18-year-old man fractured his leg and had a cast applied in the hospital. He was admitted to a room, and the nurses caring for the patient noticed that the toes on his casted leg were edematous and discolored. The patient complained to the nursing staff about decreased feeling in his toes. Over the next few days, gangrene developed, and the man's leg had to be amputated. The Illinois Supreme Court heard the case and held that the nurses were liable, along with the physician, because the nursing staff had *failed to adhere to the standards of care.* This case established a precedent that almost every state has adopted.

REGULATION OF PRACTICE

Standards of care define acts whose performance is required, permitted, or prohibited. These standards of care derive from federal and state laws, rules, and regulations, and codes governing other professional agencies and organizations such as the American Nurses Association (ANA) and the Canadian Nurses Association (CNA). These organizations regularly evaluate existing standards and revise them as needed. Standards of care coupled with the **scope of nursing practice** give direction to you as a practicing nurse, spelling out what you have the obligation to do, what you have permission to do, and what you are prohibited from doing for patients. You are duty-bound to know and follow these standards; failure to adhere to them gives rise to legal liability. Ignorance of the requirements and limitations does not absolve you from liability.

Nursing liability falls into several areas: practice, monitoring, and communication. Box 2-3 shows common breaches of the standards of care. The legal test is the comparison with the hypothetical actions under similar circumstances of a reasonably **prudent** (careful, wise) nurse of similar education and experience. You are held to the standards of care in the state or

Box 2-3 Common Breaches of the Standard of Care

PRACTICE
Failure to use proper judgment
Failure to properly assess
Failure to properly administer medication
Failure to protect patients from burns
Failure to properly maintain the airway
Failure to restock crash cart
Failure to honor advance directives
Failure to take an accurate and thorough history
Failure to provide a safe environment
Failure to properly administer injections
Failure to go through hierarchy to get the care needed
Failure to detect that the patient has an allergy
Failure to protect the patient from abuse
Failure to prevent abuse, neglect, or injury by other patients
Failure to obtain physician orders—practicing outside the scope of nursing practice by writing orders
Failure to practice safely (by using drugs or alcohol while working)
Failure to protect and prevent falls

MONITORING
Failure to properly monitor
Failure to recognize and report signs and symptoms of patient's deteriorating condition
Failure to properly use monitoring equipment
Failure to protect against injuries from monitoring equipment
Failure to detect and/or prevent decubitus ulcers
Failure to monitor and detect polypharmacy effects on patient
Failure to detect signs and symptoms of a medical condition in a timely and proper fashion
Failure to detect signs and symptoms of drug toxicity
Failure to properly use restraints

COMMUNICATION
Failure to document in a timely and proper fashion
Failure to notify physician of lab values in a timely and proper fashion
Failure to report child or elder abuse
Failure to notify physician of a change in status
Failure to communicate with other health care personnel about advance directives
Failure to properly give discharge instructions
Failure to document patient's status or condition in a timely and proper fashion
Failure to document communications between health care providers in a timely and proper fashion
Failure to document the need for restraints in a timely and proper fashion
Failure to properly document (precharting)

province in which you practice. However, real-life application of the standards is not always easy. Nursing shortages in some states have led to a need for individual nurses to work harder. Personnel cutbacks often leave units short-staffed, and nurses feel pressure to take on expanded duties; this raises their risk for liability considerably. In addition, special challenges face entry-level licensed nurses when they enter the workforce. Orientation programs often fail to adequately cover all the skills needed to be a competent practitioner. It is your responsibility to seek additional instruction and supervision when faced with an unfamiliar practice or procedure. Remember that it is not possible for you to meet every single patient's needs.

The laws formally defining and limiting the scope of nursing practice are called **nurse practice acts.** All state, provincial, and territorial legislatures in the United States and Canada have adopted nurse practice acts, although the specifics they contain often vary. It is your responsibility to know the nurse practice act that is in effect for your geographic region. Write to the board of nursing in a given state, or access its website, to obtain a free copy of the state's nurse practice act.

Basic legal mandates to practice as an LPN/LVN are the following: apply for licensure in the state or province in which they wish to practice, meet all licensing requirements, pass the computerized licensing examination, and maintain a current license. Once licensed, you are allowed to apply to another state for a license by endorsement, which follows upon confirmation that you have fulfilled the new state's licensing criteria. To streamline this process, a growing number of states have entered into a legal agreement, called an **interstate compact,** which allows multistate practice of nursing. If the nurse (registered nurse or LPN/LVN) is licensed in her or his home state, then privileges are granted to practice in other states that have signed the interstate compact. It remains the nurse's obligation to know and follow all the applicable rules, regulations, and standards for the state in which he or she practices.

Besides limitations made by the applicable nurse practice act, your employing institution will often place limitations on your practice. The institution has the right to specify what you are and are not allowed to do, as long as this does not conflict with established laws, rules, and regulations. When a question comes before the court regarding whether the standard of care was met in a particular situation, the court will use a variety of resources to answer the question (Box 2-4).

LEGAL ISSUES

Many legal issues affect the LPN/LVN and influence the level of care delivered to the patient. Statutory and common law both play important roles in defining the rights and responsibilities of the patient and the nursing professionals. The patient has a right to expect the nurse to act in the patient's best interest by providing care that meets and is consistent with the established legal standards and principles.

Box 2-4 Evidence of Nursing Standards

Practice protocols, contracts, practice agreements, employment agreements, personnel or employee manuals
Agency policy and procedure manuals
State nurse practice acts and regulations
American Nurses Association Code for Nurses (2001)
American Nurses Association Standards of Practice (1995)
Accreditation criteria of the Joint Commission (formerly the Joint Commission on Accreditation of Healthcare Organizations [JCAHO])
Other accreditation standards depending on the practice setting (e.g., National League for Nursing, National Association of Home Care)
State and federal licensing laws and regulations governing health care agencies; state, professional, and occupational legislation and regulations
Nursing specialty standards of care and certification
Nursing literature, textbooks, and journals
Education, continuing education, staff development, and orientation
Experience
Expert nurse witness, other experts, and peers
Customs and usual community practices

Malpractice

You are liable for acts of **commission** (doing an act) and **omission** (not doing an act) performed in the course of your professional duty, and a charge of **malpractice** (professional **negligence**) is one possible legal action against you. The following elements must be present for you to be held liable, that is, for a court to uphold the charge of malpractice:

1. **Duty** exists—the nurse-patient relationship establishes a duty, defined by the standards of care
2. **Breach** of the duty—failure to perform the duty in a reasonable, prudent manner
3. **Harm** has occurred—this does not have to be physical injury
4. The breach of duty was the **proximate cause** of the harm—the occurrence of harm depended directly on the occurrence of the breach

If the court finds that malpractice has occurred, you are subject to legal punishment and/or restitution as the court determines. The best way to avoid being charged with malpractice is to practice within the rules and regulations, the standards of care, and the employing agency's policies and procedures. The nurse-patient relationship is also very important; strive to maintain a positive relationship. A poor nurse-patient relationship has been identified as a leading factor determining whether a patient will seek legal action.

Patients' Rights

Patients have expectations regarding the health care services they receive. In 1972, the American Hospital Association (AHA) developed the Patient's Bill of Rights. Since its inception, the Patient's Bill of Rights has undergone revisions; the modified version of 2003 is called The Patient Care Partnership: Understanding Expectations, Rights, and Responsibilities (see Box 1-1). The AHA encourages health care institutions to adapt the template bill of rights to their particular environments. This involves considering the cultural, religious, linguistic, and educational backgrounds of the population the institution serves. In 1980, the Mental Health Patient's Bill of Rights and the Pregnant Patient's Bill of Rights were adopted into law. The goal of the AHA is to promote the public's understanding of their rights and responsibilities as consumers of health care. In addition, the Joint Commission (TJC) has developed a statement on the rights and responsibilities of patients. TJC is the organization that accredits health care facilities and monitors them to ensure that they are in compliance with all applicable laws, rules, and regulations. The Patient Self-Determination Act (included in the Omnibus Budget Reconciliation Act of 1990, U.S. Code vol. 42, sec. 1395cc[a][1]) regulates any institution receiving federal funding. The Patient Self-Determination Act requires that institutions maintain written policies and procedures regarding advance directives (including the use of life support if incapacitated), the right to accept or refuse treatment, and the right to participate fully in health care–related decisions.

On April 14, 2003, the Health Insurance Portability and Accountability Act of 1996 (HIPAA) took effect, and these federal regulations have had an impact on the field of health care. One important area of HIPAA relates to health care providers' duty to protect the confidentiality of all health information. Some of the rights that health care institutions are obligated to provide are the following: the right to have access to health care without any prejudice; the right to be treated with respect and dignity at all times; the right to privacy and confidentiality; the right to personal safety; and the right to complete information about one's own condition and treatment.

Health care providers who maintain and transmit health care information are required to maintain reasonable and appropriate administrative, technical, and physical safeguards on a patient's health information. The law sets rules and limits on who has permission to look at and receive health information, and assigns specific penalties for wrongful disclosure of individually identifiable health information. It is imperative that all health care providers be knowledgeable about the HIPAA standards and protect the privacy rights of patients and residents (www.hhs.gov/ocr/hipaa).

Patients also have responsibilities to the health care institution; for instance, to provide accurate information about themselves, to give information regarding their known condition(s), and to participate in decision making regarding treatment and care.

Informed Consent

The Patient Care Partnership establishes the patient's right to make decisions regarding his or her health care. The **doctrine of informed consent** refers to full disclosure of the facts the patient needs to make an intelligent (informed) decision before any invasive treatment or procedure is performed (Figure 2-1). The patient has the right to accept or reject the proposed care, but only after understanding fully what is being proposed, that is, the benefits of the treatment, the risks involved, any alternative treatments, and the consequences of refusing the treatment or procedure. The explanation of the procedure has to be in nontechnical terms and in a language the patient can understand. Failure to secure informed consent may result in civil liability for battery. **Civil battery** (also called technical battery) is the unlawful touching of a person; an intent to harm is not necessary.

It is the duty of the physician or nurse practitioner who is performing the procedure or treatment to obtain informed consent. As a nurse, if you see the patient sign the consent after receiving informed consent, you are only witnessing the signature. You are not providing informed consent. Do not discuss with the patient the elements of disclosure that the physician or the nurse practitioner are required to make, or you become potentially liable for failing to or negligently getting informed consent. Answers to any unanswered questions that the patient has about the procedure are the responsibility of the health care provider who will perform the procedure.

Confidentiality

You have a duty to protect information about a patient no matter how you come to have that information. Guard the information you receive about a patient, and restrict access to it to only those health care personnel who have a legitimate need to know it. Failure to maintain patient confidentiality gives rise to legal liability, and legal remedies exist to address breaches of confidentiality. Whether on duty or off duty, you are prohibited from breaching a patient's confidence. The duty does not end when the patient is discharged. If you have questions regarding the disclosure of patient information, follow the policies of the institution that employs you.

Medical Records

Laws govern the collection, maintenance, and disclosure of information in medical records. Each health care institution also has policies and procedures regarding patients' medical records. Medical records are not public documents, and the information they contain is to be kept secure. Breaches in the confidentiality of information kept in the patient's medical record give rise to legal liability.

In a lawsuit, both parties are permitted to use the patient's medical record to argue facts of the case. Entries made in the chart often show whether the standards of care were met in a given situation. It is essential that you follow the policies and procedures of the employing institution regarding the patient's medical record. All entries in the medical record must be permanent, accurate, complete, and legible. Two current trends are potentially going to affect patient confidentiality. Many smaller health care organizations are merging to form large corporations in an effort to save resources while continuing to provide services. In addition, computer-based health care records are becoming common. Together, these two trends have the potential to vastly expand the numbers of people with access to confidential patient information. Those implementing these trends have the mandate to take federal HIPAA privacy standards into consideration and prevent unauthorized disclosure of medical records and patient information.

Invasion of Privacy

The legal concept of invasion of privacy involves a person's right to be left alone and remain anonymous if he or she chooses. The patient does not waive the right to privacy by giving you consent to care for him or her. Do not expose the patient's body parts unnecessarily, discuss the patient inappropriately, or disclose information about the patient; you risk legal liability by doing so. Using any patient information (name, photograph, specific facts regarding an illness, and so on) without authorization is a violation of the patient's legal rights. Safeguard the patient's right to privacy at all times.

Reporting Abuse

There are exceptions to the right to privacy. The law stipulates that the health care professional is required to report certain information to the appropriate authorities. The report should be given to a supervisor or directly to the police, according to agency policy. When acting in good faith to report mandated information (e.g., certain communicable diseases or gunshot wounds), the health care professional is protected from liability.

Indeed, in response to the enormous problem of child abuse, the federal Child Abuse Prevention Treatment Act of 1973 made the reporting of child abuse **mandatory.** Be alert for signs of abuse. Because health care professionals are mandated reporters, you face possible fines, imprisonment, or both if you fail to report suspected cases of child abuse to the appropriate authorities. Withholding medical treatment to an infant born with serious, life-threatening handicaps is a form of child abuse. Congress enacted the Child Abuse Amendments in 1984 to protect the rights of these handicapped newborns to proper treatment and care. These regulations make any institution receiving federal funds legally responsible to investigate the with-

AUTHORIZATION FOR AND CONSENT TO OPERATION. ADMINISTRATION OF ANESTHETICS, SPECIAL DIAGNOSTIC OR THERAPEUTIC PROCEDURES AND THE RENDERING OF OTHER MEDICAL SERVICES

Patient Barbara McVey Date January 9, 2010 Time 0800

1. **Operation or Procedure and Alternatives**
   a. I hereby authorize Dr. Jennifer H. Christensen and whomever she may designate as her assistants to perform the following procedure and/or alternative procedure necessary to treat my condition: (state nature of procedure(s) to be performed).
   Right total hip replacement
   OK for blood transfusion
   (LIST PROCEDURE(S))
   b. I understand the reason for the procedure is: to replace my right hip joint and the head of my right hip bone. OK to receive blood transfusion
   c. For the purpose of advancing medical education and care, I consent to the admittance of observers to the operating room.
   d. It has been explained to me that conditions may arise during this procedure whereby a different procedure or an additional procedure may need to be performed and I authorize my physician and her assistants to do what they feel is needed and necessary.
   e. I understand that no guarantee or assurance has been made as to the results of the procedure and that it may not cure the condition.
   f. I consent to the examination and disposal by hospital authorities of any tissues or body parts that may be removed.
2. **Risks:** This authorization is given with the understanding that any operation or procedure involves some risks and hazards. The more common risks include: infection, bleeding nerve injury, blood clots, heart attack, allergic reactions, and pneumonia. These risks can be serious and possibly fatal. Specific risks for this procedure and alternative methods of care have been explained to me by my physician.
3. **Anesthesia:** The administration of anesthesia also involves risks, most importantly a rare risk of reaction to medications causing severe injury or death. I consent to the use of such anesthetics as may be considered necessary by the person responsible for these services.
4. **Photography:** I consent to the photographing of operations to be performed, including appropriate portions of my body for medical, scientific, or educational purposes, providing my identity is not revealed by the pictures or by the descriptive texts accompanying them.
5. **Patient's Consent:** I have read and fully understand this consent form, and I understand I should not sign this form if all items, including all my questions, have not been explained or answered to my satisfaction or if I do not understand any of the terms or words contained in this consent form.

IF YOU HAVE ANY QUESTIONS AS TO THE RISKS OR HAZARDS OF THE PROPOSED SURGERY OR TREATMENT, OR ANY QUESTIONS CONCERNING THE PROPOSED SURGERY OR TREATMENT ASK YOUR SURGEON NOW! **BEFORE SIGNING THIS CONSENT FORM.**

DO NOT SIGN UNLESS YOU HAVE READ AND THOROUGHLY UNDERSTAND THIS FORM!

6. I certify that I have read and fully understand the above consent after adequate explanations were made to me, and after all blanks were filled in or crossed out before I signed.

Dr. J.H. Christensen
(Witness to Signature only)

Signed Barbara McVey
(Patient, Parent, or Legal Guardian's Signature)

Betty Berg RN
(Second Witness Signature if needed)
(i.e., Telephone Consent)

(Doctor Signature)

AUTHORIZATION AND CONSENT

Great Plains Regional Medical Center
601 West Leota - P.O. Box 1167
North Platte, Nebraska 69103-1167
308-534-9310

NS-81 (Rev. 2/01)

LABEL

4532

FIGURE 2-1 Sample consent form for a special procedure.

holding of medical treatment to an infant. Note that in general, withholding lifesaving treatment and care is a form of passive **euthanasia** (letting a person die) and medical neglect, and carries the risk of professional neglect (medical malpractice) charges.

Like child abuse, spousal and elder abuse is often hidden behind closed doors. There are more reports of women as victims of spousal abuse than men, and older adults are a population at high risk (see Life Span Considerations box for Older Adults). Most states have responded to the issue of spousal and elder abuse by enacting laws to protect victims, but individual laws vary. Fines, restraining orders that prohibit contact by the abusing person, and even imprisonment are some of the ways often attempted to protect the victims of abuse. Unfortunately, only a portion of abuse cases are ever reported. You have a duty to know the signs of abuse and the procedures for reporting suspected cases. Especially if you work in a community health center or for a home health agency, you will sometimes see firsthand evidence of abuse; be prepared to act on the victim's behalf.

Workplace violence is another form of abuse that occurs at times in the health care setting. This form of violence includes verbal abuse, emotional abuse, sexual harassment, physical assault, and threatening behavior. Health care institutions are implementing policies and procedures to promote a safe work environment, and education is an important component of the awareness and prevention measures. Strategies to provide adequate supervision, employ security personnel, monitor work areas, and facilitate reporting of incidents represent efforts to decrease the incidence of workplace violence.

HOW TO AVOID A LAWSUIT

Your best defense against a lawsuit is to provide compassionate, competent nursing care. This means that the nurse-patient relationship is one that is based on

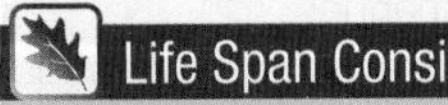

Life Span Considerations

Older Adults

Elder Abuse

Factors that put older adults at risk for physical, emotional, or financial abuse include the following:

- Declining physical health
- Declining mental ability
- Decreased strength and mobility
- Loss of independence
- Isolation
- Loss of loved ones, friends, and relatives

These factors often make the older adult feel helpless and frightened. Impaired communication, decreased hearing acuity, and anxiety will make assessment of an older adult more difficult, but make sure nonetheless to watch for the signs of abuse.

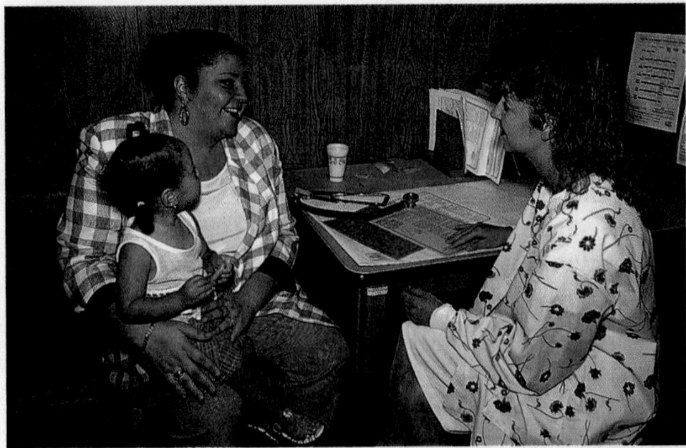

FIGURE 2-2 A patient-nurse relationship built on trust and open communication is the best way to prevent a lawsuit.

trust and respect. Open and honest communication is the key to building a therapeutic relationship and often helps resolve patient dissatisfaction before the patient resorts to legal action (Figure 2-2). A patient who feels that you really care about him or her as an individual is less likely to sue you for an error. If you follow the standards of care and adhere to the scope of practice for an LPN/LVN, you are also less likely to be sued.

Some laws, such as Good Samaritan laws, provide immunity from liability in certain circumstances. The goal of this protection (except in cases of gross negligence) is to encourage assistance in emergencies occurring outside of a medical facility. State and provincial laws vary, so it is important for you to know the Good Samaritan laws that apply where you practice.

Proper documentation in the medical record is another important factor in reducing your liability. The medical record will be thoroughly examined in the event of a lawsuit, and its use is permitted to prove in court that the standard of care was met (or not met). An important legal presumption to remember is, "Care was not given if it was not charted." No one will be convinced that something was or was not done merely because you say so. The court will look to the legal record of the patient's care for documentation of the care the patient received.

INSURANCE

Obtaining insurance is an important part of being a professional and protecting your personal assets or garnishment of wages.

Professional Liability Insurance

Even though your employer will carry insurance for the institution as a whole, many nurses choose to purchase individual coverage. You are well advised to have professional liability insurance to cover you while performing your nursing duties, job, or obligations. It is important to carefully review any policy before purchasing it to ensure that the terms of the policy meet your needs. There are two types of policies:

- **Claims Made Policy:** This type of policy protects you when the claim(s) for nursing or negligence is made while the policy is in force (during the policy period or during extended coverage).
- **Occurrence Basis Policy:** This type of policy protects you against claims made about event(s) that occurred during the policy period or extended coverage period.

A **"tail" agreement** offers extended coverage for periods when a nurse is exposed to professional liabilities but no longer has a claims made policy.

Disciplinary Defense Insurance

Disciplinary defense insurance or license protection insurance provides the following in the event that you are brought before the LPN/LVN Board of Nursing for disciplinary actions and problems with your license:

- Qualified nurse attorney or attorney to represent you
- Wage loss reimbursement
- Travel, food, lodging reimbursement
- Legal fees paid or reimbursement for payment

THE DISCIPLINARY PROCESS

If you receive a letter from your Board of Nursing alleging breaches of the standards of care or infractions of patient safety practices, it is best to seek legal representation. Every state has a variation of the disciplinary process. The process plays on various levels, such as investigation of the allegations, meeting with investigators, hearings with the board, and appeals through the court system. Licensure issues fall under administrative law (Box 2-5).

What Can Happen To Your License

Any of the following may result from investigation of a claim by the State Board of Nursing regarding licensure issues or disciplinary actions:

- Dismissed charge
- Investigations agreement
- Letter of reprimand—formal or informal
- Probation with stipulations (e.g., education, fines, monitoring fees, evaluation by psychiatrist, psychologist, and drug addiction specialists)
- Mandated diversion program for drug- or alcohol-related charges or based on mental condition

Box 2-5 Common Grounds for Licensure Proceedings

- Committing Medicare/Medicaid fraud
- Patient abuse
- Diverting or stealing narcotics
- Failure to use good nursing judgment
- Documentation errors
- Aiding and abetting a criminal
- Falsifying information on your renewal or application
- Failure to report previous criminal actions
- Practicing outside the scope of the nurse practice act
- Practicing without a valid license
- Attempting to sell or selling, or falsely obtaining or providing a nursing diploma of license to practice as a registered nurse
- Being convicted of a crime or offense that shows the inability of a nurse to practice without due regard for the safety and health of patients or clients
- Entering a plea of guilty or nolo contendere to a criminal charge regardless of the disposition of the proceeding, e.g., expungement
- Failure to practice nursing according to the legal standards of nursing practice
- Failure to maintain confidentiality of patient information
- Failure to exercise technical competence
- Having a mental or physical impairment that interferes with nursing skills, abilities, judgment, or a combination of these
- Falsifying records
- Misappropriating patient, facility, or individual items
- Performing duties when competency has not been attained, maintained, or achieved
- Failure to properly delegate or assign nursing care, treatment, or duties
- Failure to properly notify appropriate person when leaving or refusing an assignment
- Failure to report to the State Board of Nursing that you are a carrier of HIV or Hepatitis B when participating in or performing exposure-prone procedures
- Being guilty of moral turpitude
- Having a license in nursing or in another health care profession that has been revoked, suspended, probated, denied, or restricted
- Failure to report health care providers who are practicing in an illegal, unethical, or incompetent manner
- Failure to properly cooperate with the State Board of Nursing
- Using, when on duty, alcohol, illegal drugs, or drugs that impair nursing judgment
- Sexual misconduct
- Aiding and abetting someone in violating the Nurse Practice Act
- Being found to be legally insane or mentally incompetent by the courts
- Violating state or federal law relating to nursing practice
- Violating state or federal narcotics or controlled substance laws
- Violating rule(s) or orders(s), adopted by the State Board of Nursing

- Suspension with stipulations
- Revocation of license

ETHICAL ASPECTS OF NURSING

The science of ethics studies the relationships between moral actions and values and how these affect society. The word **ethics** refers to values that influence a person's behavior and the individual's feelings and beliefs about what is right or wrong. Nursing ethics involve moral values and principles that affect personal and professional conduct. As previously mentioned, you have a responsibility as an LPN/LVN to practice within the legal and ethical boundaries of nursing practice. Nursing ethics propose the duties and obligations of nurses to their patients, other health care professionals, the profession itself, and society.

DEVELOPMENT OF ETHICAL PRINCIPLES

Values are personal beliefs about the worth of an object, an idea, a custom, or an attitude. Values vary among people and cultures; they develop over time and undergo change in response to changing circumstances and necessity. Each of us adopts a value system that will govern what we feel is right or wrong (or good and bad) and will influence our behavior in a given situation.

Values influence our everyday decisions. Each of us has many values, and at times we have to choose between competing or conflicting values. Some values will be more important than others, and the choices we make will be based on the priority we place on each particular value. A person's values are learned through experience, observation, and reasoning. Some values we consciously choose; others we adopt unconsciously. When we are children, society has a strong influence on how we behave and what values we learn. Acceptable behavior is rewarded and unacceptable behavior is punished. We accept or reject values as we mature, eventually developing an individual value system that largely reflects our culture (see Cultural Considerations box).

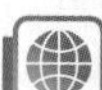 Cultural Considerations

Culture and Ethics

People of different cultural backgrounds often define health and illness in different ways. Culture is learned as the individual grows up and is influenced (usually subconsciously) by the environment surrounding him or her. Be aware of cultural differences and avoid (1) transferring your own expectations to the patient, (2) making generalizations based on your own views, (3) assuming a patient can understand what is being said just because he or she speaks English, and (4) treating each patient the same. To meet the individual's needs, you need to have respect for a patient's cultural heritage.

It is important to reflect on and assess the values you hold. **Value clarification** is the process of self-evaluation that helps you gain insight into your personal values. When you assess the values you hold, you are better able to make choices when faced with a decision. To clarify values, do the following: (1) select the belief or behavior and consciously examine it, (2) decide its value, and (3) incorporate the value into your set of everyday responses and behaviors. In doing this, you exercise your freedom of choice and determine which values are most important to you. You have the ability to assist the patient in value clarification, as well, by encouraging the patient to express feelings and thoughts related to a situation, without contributing your own opinion. The patient needs to act on his or her own values, not yours. Sometimes the patient may be referred to a clergy member or other professional who can help deal with ethical issues. Most health care institutions have an ethics committee to help resolve ethical questions that arise, and it is a good resource for you, as well, from which to seek advice on ethical issues.

Ethical dilemmas are situations that do not have a clear right or wrong answer (Box 2-6). They are complex, confusing, and often frustrating situations that call for careful, rational analysis. First you will have to identify the problem as an ethical one. This means that it will not be possible to answer the question presented by applying external laws, rules, policies, and procedures. Many situations present a combination of legal and ethical questions. It is important to sort out the questions and seek guidance as needed. The next step is to assess the situation completely, gathering as much information as possible to aid in the decision-making process. Before finalizing a decision, consider any ethical principles that might apply to the situation. Ethical

Box 2-6 Ethical Dilemmas: What Would You Do?

The following are scenarios with an ethical dilemma. What would you do or say in each one?

1. You see a nursing assistant stealing the patient's ring. She says she needs money to pay her house note or the bank will foreclose. What should you do?
2. The patient has a Do Not Resuscitate Order and a living will. He has not designated a health care proxy or representative. The patient goes into arrest, and the daughter who hasn't seen Dad in 10 years yells, "Do something, or I will sue you if he dies!" Whose wishes should you follow?
3. You know your friend at work is diverting drugs. You have confronted her but she says it is not for her but for a friend. What should you do?
4. You suspect elder abuse by a family member of one of your relatives. What should you do?
5. You made a mistake, and your charge nurse tells you to just rewrite the nurse's notes to protect the unit and the hospital. What should you do?

principles are general in nature, but they provide a framework for decision making.

ETHICAL PRINCIPLES IN NURSING PRACTICE

In health care, several common ethical principles are important for you to consider when confronted with an ethical question. The first, most fundamental principle is **respect for people.** This principle leads us to view all human life as sacred, with each individual having inherent worth as a person. To the nurse, this principle means that no one person is more important than another; each patient has the same worth and is always entitled to respect. **Autonomy** is another ethical principle; it refers to freedom of personal choice, a right to be independent and make decisions freely. It is correct and appropriate for you to assist the patient in the decision-making process, but you do not have the authority to make a decision for the patient. **Beneficence** means doing good or acting for someone's good; this principle is one of primary importance to nurses. The nurse has an ethical duty to protect life and promote the well-being of all patients. Another ethical principle is **nonmaleficence,** which means to do no harm. You have, as a nurse acting in the patient's best interest, an ethical as well as a legal duty to do nothing that has a harmful effect on the patient. Finally, there is the principle of **justice,** or the concept of what is fair. In the context of nursing, justice means that all patients have the same right to nursing interventions. You have an obligation to allocate your time among all the assigned patients to meet their needs.

Your challenge is to balance these ethical principles when they seem in conflict. You will rarely find the options you are weighing to be black and white. Your decision will often come down to choosing what seems more right and less wrong, more good and less bad.

CODES OF ETHICS

As a member of society and the health care community, you will use both personal and professional ethical principles to inform your professional practice. Professional organizations have developed codes of ethics for the nursing profession, which serve as a way to regulate the nurses' actions and give guidelines for ethical behavior. By helping health care practitioners become more competent, trustworthy, and accountable, such codes of ethics help safeguard society. The National Federation of Licensed Practical/Vocational Nurses (NFLPN) has developed a code for LPN/LVNs. This code specifies what will be expected of you: (1) to know and function within the scope of practice for a licensed LPN/LVN, (2) to maintain patient confidences, (3) to provide health care without discrimination, (4) to maintain a high degree of professional and personal behavior, and (5) to take an active role in the development of the LPN/LVN profession. The ANA and the CNA have also developed codes of ethics that specify the ethical duties required of the nursing professional. Both the Nightingale Pledge by Gretter (Box 2-7) and the Practical Nurse's Pledge (Box 2-8) challenge the nurse to practice nursing with the highest ethical standards.

Box 2-7 The Nightingale Pledge*

I solemnly pledge myself before God and in the presence of this assembly:

To pass my life in purity and to practice my profession faithfully;

I will abstain from whatever is deleterious and mischievous and will not take or knowingly administer any harmful drug;

I will do all in my power to maintain and elevate the standard of my profession, and will hold in confidence all personal matters committed to my keeping and all family affairs coming to my knowledge in the practice of my calling;

With loyalty will I endeavor to aid the physician in his work, and devote myself to the welfare of those committed to my care.

*Composed by Lysta E. Gretter and committee at the Farrand Training School for Nurses, Detroit, Michigan in 1893.

REPORTING UNETHICAL BEHAVIOR

Like each member of the nursing profession, you have a duty to report behavior you witness that does not meet the established standards. Unethical behavior involves failing to perform the duties of a competent, caring nurse. When reporting unethical behavior, always follow the proper chain of command and explain the facts as clearly as possible. Make sure any documentation of the incident is objective and accurately states what occurred, when and where it occurred, and any other pertinent facts. Reporting a co-worker is never an easy task. Always remember, however, that a nurse's first duty is to the patient's health, safety, and well-being.

Box 2-8 The Practical Nurse's Pledge

Before God and those assembled here, I solemnly pledge:

To adhere to the code of ethics of the nursing profession;

To cooperate faithfully with the other members of the nursing team and to carry out faithfully and to the best of my ability the instructions of the physician or the nurse who may be assigned to supervise my work;

I will not do anything evil or malicious and I will not knowingly give any harmful drug or assist in malpractice;

I will not reveal any confidential information that may come to my knowledge in the course of my work;

And I pledge myself to do all in my power to raise the standards and the prestige of practical nursing.

May my life be devoted to service, and to the highest ideals of the nursing profession.

ETHICAL ISSUES

Ethical issues are difficult for the nurse, as for everyone, because there is no absolutely right or absolutely wrong answer to the question the issue presents. Like many other issues in health care, ethical issues change as society changes. Some of the current ethical issues in nursing include practitioner-assisted suicide (PAS), the right to refuse treatment, the nurse's right to refuse to provide care, and genetic research.

Practitioner-Assisted Suicide

Health care professionals and patient advocacy groups on both sides of the issue are debating the ethics of PAS. Also called physician-assisted suicide, this is a form of active euthanasia in which a health care provider takes an active role in ending a patient's life. Two cases, *Vacco v. Quill* and *Washington v. Glucksberg*, were brought before the U.S. Supreme Court regarding the legality of state bans on assisted suicide. The Supreme Court ruled in 1997 that there is no constitutional right to assisted suicide. This ruling allows each state to decide whether to legalize or ban assisted suicides. The ANA has taken a firm stand on the issue of PAS, holding that PAS is not consistent with the philosophy of nursing. ANA's specific objections to PAS are based on the principle of **nonmaleficence** (to do no harm) and beneficence, the duty to protect life.

In 1944, the ANA adopted a position statement concerning PAS. The ANA wrote that such an act is in violation of the *Code of Ethics for Nurses* and the ethical tradition of the profession. Nurses have an obligation to provide compassionate end-of-life care that includes providing comfort and pain relief. Proponents of PAS, however, cite the ethical principles of the right to autonomy and the right to self-determination in support of their position.

Right to Refuse Treatment

In the context of health care, competent adults have the right to refuse treatment. This right derives from their right to determine what is done, or not done, to them. Medicine's technical capacity to sustain life and postpone death further complicates this complex issue. It is the right of the patient to accept or refuse a treatment, even if the refusal has the potential or is certain to result in death. To exercise the right to refuse treatment, many patients prepare advance directives. Living wills, one kind of advance directive, become effective when the patient is incapacitated and is not able to make his or her own wishes known; these documents specify which lifesaving treatments are acceptable and which are not. Some patients choose to designate a **health care proxy** (assign durable power of attorney) to make decisions regarding medical treatment in the event that the patient becomes unable to make them. The proxy is another person who will speak for the patient and make decisions regarding the patient's care. The proxy is obligated to act on the patient's behalf according to the patient's expressed wishes. State laws vary on the legalities of the various forms of advance directives, and you need to know the applicable laws in your state.

Do Not Resuscitate Orders

The patient is not usually involved directly at the time a **do not resuscitate (DNR) order** is written. Although many people make their wishes regarding DNR status known in an advance directive, at this stage the patient is usually incapacitated with little hope for recovery. The physician, after consultation with the patient's family, will write the DNR order in the medical record. The physician is responsible for following the applicable policies and procedures for writing DNR orders. When a DNR order is written in the chart, you have the duty to follow the order.

Refusal to Treat

Refusal to treat is an issue that arises when you encounter a patient whose care requires you to do something that conflicts with your own moral beliefs. A typical example of this dilemma involves assisting in or caring for a woman having an abortion. There is a legal right to abortion, but this does not establish whether abortion is morally right or wrong. If you have a strong moral or religious belief regarding abortion, it is imperative that you communicate with the appropriate supervisor and explain your moral dilemma. Do not abandon the patient; instead, ask for another assignment. It is important to remember that your right to disqualify yourself from assisting with an abortion does not extend to excusing yourself from providing care to the patient after the abortion. You do not have the right to refuse to care for a patient because you disagree with decisions the patient makes.

Likewise, you do not have a legal right to refuse to care for a person with an infectious disease, including those infected with the human immunodeficiency virus (HIV). The rationale is that the need for standard precautions (infection control measures) applies to every patient, and therefore you are at no greater risk for infection from one patient than from another. The ethical principle of respect for all people without discrimination underlies this issue. The patient has the right to receive care, and the nurse has the responsibility to provide nursing interventions.

CONCLUSION

There are no easy, quick answers to legal or ethical issues. You and other health team members have the charge of working together when faced with these difficult situations. Today's health care system is facing many challenges, as is the profession of nursing. The health care system will continue to undergo changes in response to the enormous problem of containing health care costs while improving quality of care. The nursing profession will be called on to adjust and adapt to these changes. The legal system is also undergoing changes. Members of the legal community and the health care system have to work together to ensure that the legal and ethical rights of all individuals are considered and protected.

Get Ready for the NCLEX® Examination!

Key Points

- Laws regulate the practice of the LPN/LVN.
- The Patient Care Partnership and other legislative directives outline what the patient can expect from the health care system.
- As an LPN/LVN, you are legally and ethically obligated to know the scope of practice and the standards of care that apply in the state or province where you are licensed.
- Every patient has the right to receive care that meets the established standards of care.
- Malpractice (professional negligence) is when the health care professional fails to meet the standard of care.
- Prevention is the best defense to a lawsuit. A competent, caring nurse who follows the standards of care is less likely to be sued.
- Values systems have developed over the history of civilization.
- Ethical decisions regarding health care are influenced by a person's culture, beliefs, attitudes, and values.
- A code of ethics and ethical principles helps guide you in the practice of nursing.
- On April 14, 2003, the Health Insurance Portability and Accountability Act of 1996 (HIPAA) for regulating patient privacy standards took effect, and these federal regulations have had an impact on the field of health care.

Additional Learning Resources

Go to your Companion CD for an audio glossary, animations, video clips, and more.

evolve Be sure to visit the Evolve site at http://evolve.elsevier.com/Christensen/foundations/ for additional online resources.

Review Questions for the NCLEX® Examination

1. The newly licensed practical nurse (LPN) carefully reads the nurse practice act (NPA) of the state in which she will practice. The primary purpose of the NPA is to:
   1. determine the quality of nursing care.
   2. enforce the standards of nursing practice.
   3. define the scope of nursing practice.
   4. set the nurse's educational requirements.

2. The nurse working in a nursing home knows that one of his duties is to be an advocate for his patients. A primary duty of an advocate is to:
   1. complete all nursing responsibilities on time.
   2. maintain the patient's right to privacy.
   3. safeguard the well-being of every patient.
   4. act as the patient's legal representative.

3. The health care provider's order read "assist the patient with walking." The nurse caring for the older adult patient let her walk by herself and the patient fell, fracturing her humerus. The nurse could:
   1. be found guilty of malpractice.
   2. only be guilty of misconduct.
   3. be charged with technical battery.
   4. not be found liable for any harm.

4. The patient refused to take the medication his doctor ordered for relief of pain. The LPN knows this is a patient right established by:
   1. the principle of beneficence.
   2. the doctrine of negligence.
   3. specific nurse practice acts.
   4. the Patient Self-Determination Act.

5. The LPN/LVN knows that one of the best defenses against a lawsuit is for a nurse to:
   1. work only in a large hospital or nursing home.
   2. provide for every patient's needs as quickly as possible.
   3. promote a positive nurse-patient relationship.
   4. carry individual professional liability insurance.

6. The nurse believes that all patients should be treated as individuals. The ethical principle that this belief reflects is:
   1. autonomy.
   2. beneficence.
   3. nonmaleficence.
   4. respect for people.

7. LPN/LVNs have a code of professional and personal ethics to follow. The purpose of a code of ethics is to:
   1. establish penalties for any unethical behavior.
   2. promote trustworthy, accountable LPN/LVNs.
   3. make certain that all nurses are competent and always honest.
   4. give the nurse guidelines for ethical decision making.

8. The patient admitted for surgery has a lump in her breast. The patient's daughter asks the LVN if her mother should have the surgery. Which issue must the LVN consider before answering?
   1. Confidentiality and invasion of privacy
   2. Informed consent, beneficence, and respect
   3. Respect for people and personal autonomy
   4. Nonmaleficence, justice, and liability

9. The nurse's first job as an LPN is on a unit that cares for terminally ill children. Before helping families deal with their children's illnesses, the nurse will need to:
   1. study the nurse practice act to find rules relating to the medical care of terminally ill children.
   2. spend time performing value clarification to aid in identifying her feelings about this new role.
   3. evaluate her own personal mores and customs that may affect the practice of nursing in general.
   4. review the state and federal laws that prescribe how a child may be treated when near death.

10. The LPN knows that the purpose of an advance directive is to:
   1. help every person exercise the right to die with dignity.
   2. encourage a person to determine how he or she will die.
   3. allow a patient to exercise the right of autonomy.
   4. provide a means to prevent medical maltreatment.

11. The nurse knows that all patients have the right to nursing interventions regardless of their race, religion, or sex. The ethical principle that best describes this concept is:
   1. nonmaleficence.
   2. justice.
   3. autonomy.
   4. beneficence.

12. An alert adult patient has refused an intramuscular injection. The nurse waits until the patient is asleep and gives the injection anyway. The nurse could be charged with:
   1. civil battery.
   2. malicious homicide.
   3. criminal negligence.
   4. invasion of privacy.

13. The nurse is licensed to practice nursing in New York. She just received a license by endorsement from Ohio. The nurse knows that when she works in Ohio, she must follow the:
   1. Nurse Practice Act of the United States.
   2. Nurse Practice Act of New York.
   3. Universal Nurse Practice Act.
   4. Nurse Practice Act of Ohio.

14. The nurse loves photography and brings his camera to work at the nursing home. He takes a picture of one of his co-workers walking a patient. The nurse has just:
   1. violated the patient's right to privacy.
   2. failed to get proper medical clearance.
   3. performed an act of nursing malpractice.
   4. legally obtained a realistic picture.

15. The nurse gets a report, puts his patient assignment notebook in his pocket, and goes on break. His notebook has very specific information about his patients and is missing from his pocket when he returns to the unit. The book is found later on the floor in the cafeteria by a visitor and is returned to the information desk. The nurse:
   1. may have breached the Patient Self-Determination Act.
   2. is guilty of criminal misconduct.
   3. could be fired for malpractice.
   4. has violated the Health Insurance Portability and Accountability Act of 1996 (HIPAA), which took effect April 14, 2003.

16. The newly licensed nurse starting her first job is assigned to catheterize a male patient but has never done this procedure before. Her best first action is to:
   1. quickly call her supervisor and disqualify herself from performing the procedure.
   2. find and read the procedure for male catheterization in the procedure book on her unit and ask another experienced nurse to supervise her during the procedure.
   3. immediately advise the charge nurse that someone else will need to take over this patient.
   4. promptly notify the staff development office that an instructor needs to do this procedure.

chapter

3 Communication

evolve

http://evolve.elsevier.com/Christensen/foundationsadult

Diane D. Kathol

Objectives

1. Recognize that communication is inherent in every nurse-patient interaction.
2. Discuss the concepts of verbal and nonverbal communication.
3. Discuss the impact of nonverbal communication.
4. Recognize assertive communication as the most appropriate communication style.
5. Use various therapeutic communication techniques.
6. Recognize trust as the foundation for all effective interaction.
7. Identify various factors that have the potential to affect communication.
8. Discuss potential barriers to communication.
9. Apply the nursing process to patients with impaired verbal communication.
10. Apply therapeutic communication techniques to patients with special communication needs.

Key Terms

active listening (p. 41)
aggressive communication (p. 39)
altered cognition (p. 49)
assertive communication (p. 39)
assertiveness (p. 39)
clarifying (p. 45)
closed posture (p. 38)
closed question (p. 42)
communication (kŏ-MYŪ-nĭ-KĀ-shŭn, p. 36)
connotative meaning (kŏn-nō-TĀ-tĭv, p. 37)
denotative meaning (dĭ-nō-TĀ-tĭv, p. 37)
expressive aphasia (ă-FĀ-zhă, p. 52)
focusing (p. 45)
gestures (p. 38)
jargon (JĂR-gŏn, p. 37)
minimal encouragement (p. 42)
nontherapeutic communication (nŏn-thĕr-ă-PYŪ-tĭk, p. 40)
nonverbal communication (p. 37)
one-way communication (p. 37)
open-ended question (p. 44)
open posture (p. 38)
paraphrasing (p. 45)
passive listening (p. 41)
posture (p. 38)
receive, receiver (p. 36)
receptive aphasia (p. 52)
reflecting (p. 45)
restating (p. 45)
send, sender (p. 36)
therapeutic communication (p. 40)
two-way communication (p. 37)
unassertive communication (p. 39)
verbal communication (p. 37)

Communication is essential to the delivery of nursing care. Some form of communication occurs each time an interaction takes place. These interactions are sometimes between two parties, such as you and the patient or you and a family member, a physician, or a co-worker, or any number of other combinations; and sometimes communication takes place among many parties all at once or over time. However, the message that is intended is not always the message that is received. Remember to strive at all times to communicate effectively and minimize miscommunication.

Communication is the reciprocal process in which messages are sent and received between people (Riley, 2008). Communication takes both verbal and nonverbal forms and conveys varied types of messages (e.g., information, emotions, humor, acceptance, or rejection). Many variables have an impact on how effective communication is.

OVERVIEW OF COMMUNICATION

For communication to occur, a sender and a receiver of a message are both necessary. The **sender** is the person conveying the message, whereas the **receiver** is the individual or individuals to whom the message is conveyed. The individual receiving the message is sometimes the intended receiver, and sometimes an unintended receiver. Consider the following scenario:

The night nurse, reporting to the day nurse outside Ms. B.'s room: "Ms. B. was on her call light all night. She's a real complainer!"

Ms. B. overhears the exchange.

The day nurse is the intended receiver, or the one with whom the night nurse means to communicate regarding Ms. B.'s behavior. However, since Ms. B. also hears the statement, she becomes an unintended receiver. Consider the possible effect of this message on the relationship between Ms. B. and the night nurse. Negative consequences for the relationship between Ms. B. and the day nurse are another possible outcome, if Ms. B. believes that the day nurse shares the night nurse's view of her.

Both one-way or two-way communication are possible, and which actually occurs partly depends on the roles of the people in the interaction. One-way communication is highly structured; the sender is in control and expects and gets very little response from the receiver. A lecture to a large audience is an example of one-way communication. **One-way communication** has very little place in the nurse-patient relationship. **Two-way communication** requires that both the sender and the receiver participate in the interaction. It allows for exchange between you and the patient, and its purpose is to meet the needs of both of you and to establish a trusting relationship. In other words, rather than talking at the patient, seek and accept the patient's input and feedback.

VERBAL COMMUNICATION

Verbal communication involves the use of spoken or written words or symbols. You might think that there is little room for misunderstanding or misinterpretation of the intended message as long as the receiver understands the language and symbols being used. Frequently, however, this is not the case. Sometimes words have very different meanings, or connotations, for different people. The **connotative meaning** of a word is subjective and reflects the individual's perception or interpretation. Be aware of the potential for miscommunication that lies in such subjective variation. Take, for example, the word *stable:* perhaps, if you tell family members that their loved one's condition is stable, they will understand that for the moment, the patient's condition is not deteriorating. On the other hand, it is also very possible they will hear a different message, and not the one you meant to give, namely that the patient is doing well and is out of danger.

Denotative meaning refers to the commonly accepted definition of a particular word. For example, the word *telephone* will mean essentially the same thing to anyone who is familiar with the English language. The key word here is *familiar.* There is no guarantee that both parties know the word, let alone assign the same definition to it. Consider the situation in which you ask the patient when he last voided or had a stool. It is possible that the patient will have no idea that you want to know when he last urinated or had a bowel movement, even though any nurse will know exactly what your question means. This is an example of hospital jargon. **Jargon** is commonplace "language" or terminology unique to people in a particular work setting, such as a hospital, or to a specific type of work, such as nursing. It is as though you and the patient have different dictionaries for what you think is the language you share. However, jargon is not part of the general, shared language, and it won't appear in the patient's dictionary. Be aware of the terminology you choose in communicating with patients. To promote understanding and prevent misinterpretation, avoid the use of hospital jargon.

NONVERBAL COMMUNICATION

Messages transmitted without the use of words (either oral or written) constitute **nonverbal communication.** Nonverbal cues include tone and rate of voice, volume of speech, eye contact, physical appearance, and use of touch (Table 3-1). Some degree of nonverbal communication almost always, if not always, accompanies verbal communication.

Voice

Aspects of the voice affect nonverbal messages, among them tone and volume and the rate of speech. Characteristics of people's voices vary depending on such things as their emotions, their familiarity with a situation, confidence, and geographic and cultural influences. It is not possible to interpret meaning accurately on the basis of tone, rate, and volume alone. For example, a high-pitched, loud voice and rapid speech often indicate that an individual is afraid, but people also speak that way out of excitement or enthusiasm; in fact, some people always tend to this speech pattern and thus no conclusions are appropriate at all. Be careful to consider the voice characteristics in the context of the situation as a whole so your interpretation of the message is accurate.

Eye Contact

Eye contact is responsible for much communication and much miscommunication. Generally, making eye contact communicates an intention to interact. However, the nature of the interaction and the results of eye contact are not necessarily always positive. Extended eye contact sometimes implies aggression and arouses anxiety; on the other hand, the person who maintains eye contact for 2 to 6 seconds during interaction helps involve the other person in what is said without being threatening or intimidating. An absence of eye contact communicates many things: shyness, lack of confidence, disinterest, embarrassment, or hurt, or, in contrast, deference and respect. Sensitivity to one's own eye contact and that of others will help you perceive what is actually occurring in an interaction. Culture significantly affects how people interpret eye contact.

Table 3-1 Nonverbal Cues

ATTRIBUTE OR BEHAVIOR EXHIBITED BY SENDER (CUE)	COMPONENTS	POSSIBLE INTERPRETATION OR PERCEPTION BY RECEIVER
Voice	Tone, volume, pitch, rate of speech	Fear, excitement, enthusiasm, stress, anger, comfort, concern, confidence, calmness
Eye contact	Extended (longer than 6 sec) Brief but direct (2-6 sec) Absent or fleeting	Aggression, intimidation, disrespect Interest, respect, caring Shyness, lack of confidence, low self-esteem, disinterest, anxiety, fear, uneasiness, hurriedness, or deference or respect (culture-specific)
Physical appearance	Size, color of skin, dress, grooming, body carriage, age, sex	Professional or nonprofessional, trust or distrust, respect or disrespect, comfort or intimidation, interest or disinterest, competence or incompetence
Gestures	Distinct movements of hands, head, body	Emphasis, clarification, pleasure, helpfulness, anger, threat, disrespect
Posture	Open—relaxed stance, facing receiver, uncrossed arms and legs, slight shift toward receiver, direct eye contact, smile	Warmth, acceptance, caring
	Closed—formal, distant stance; arms and possibly legs tightly crossed	Disinterest, coldness, nonacceptance, authority, control, intimidation, condescension

Physical Appearance

The physical appearance of the participants in an interaction has the potential to greatly influence the perceptions they form of each other. Physical appearance includes attributes of size, color of skin, dress, grooming, posture, and facial expression. Although often these attributes have absolutely nothing to do with any messages the sender intends to convey, it is very possible for them to have a major impact on the receiver's interpretation. Take for example, the patient with a personal bias against individuals with a particular attribute, such as being overweight. The patient is likely to negatively distort messages from an overweight nurse, who will then have more difficulty than a nurse of average weight in establishing a trusting and therapeutic relationship with this patient. Similarly, at times an older adult will not consider a young-looking nurse to be experienced enough to be a competent professional, and will thus discount what the nurse says or does.

A professional appearance conveys pride and competence. How you choose to dress while on duty sends a strong message to the patient. If you choose to wear ill-fitting clothing or sloppy shoes, you risk sending the message that the patient is not worth the time it would take for you to look professional, and leading the patient to view you as uncaring and incompetent.

Gestures

Gestures are movements people use to emphasize the idea they are attempting to communicate. Gestures also play a useful role in clarifying. A patient is often better able to express where pain is on the body by pointing to a particular area than trying to describe it in words. However, many gestures affect communication negatively. For example, frequently looking at your watch while interviewing a patient conveys to the patient that you are in a hurry and have no real desire to spend the time to listen to him or her. Also, gestures often have very different meanings from individual to individual and from culture to culture. It is essential to be constantly aware of gestures the participants use during interaction and consider the implication of your gestures to the patient.

Posture

The way that an individual sits, stands, and moves is called *posture*. **Posture** has the potential to convey warmth and acceptance or distance and disinterest. You have an **open posture** when you take a relaxed stance with uncrossed arms and legs while facing the other individual. A slight shift in your body position toward an individual, a smile, and direct eye contact are all consistent with open posturing and convey warmth and caring (Riley, 2008). **Closed posture** is a more formal, distant stance, generally with the arms, and possibly the legs, tightly crossed. A person will often interpret closed posture as disinterest, coldness, and even nonacceptance. Standing at the bedside looking down at the patient in the bed places the nurse in a position of authority and control. The patient is likely to experience this as intimidating and condescending. Whenever possible, place yourself level with the patient; this is especially important with pediatric patients. Sitting at the bedside in a relaxed and open posture is one example (Figure 3-1).

Consistency of Verbal and Nonverbal Communication

Nonverbal communication is very powerful. If nonverbal cues are inconsistent or incongruent with the verbal message, the nonverbal message will most

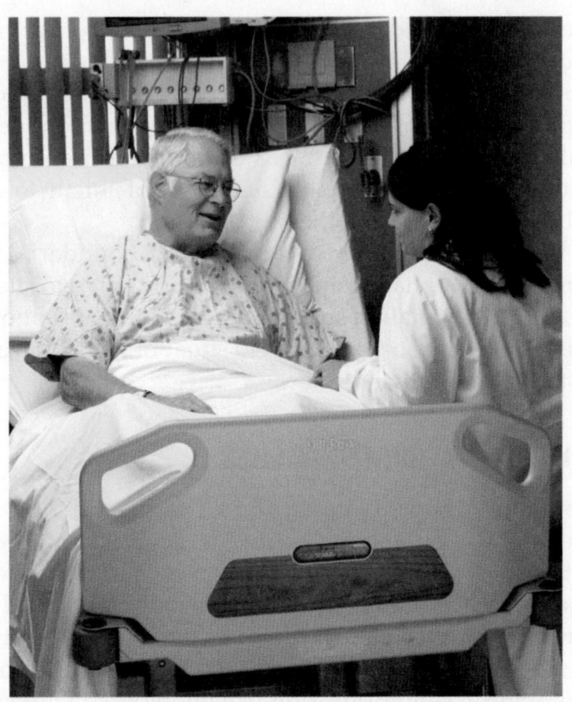

FIGURE 3-1 Whenever possible, place yourself level with the patient.

likely be the one received. At the very least, this incongruence is frequently the cause of misinterpretation and misunderstanding. In the following example, you will see incongruence between what the nurse is stating and what she is demonstrating.

> Nurse M. has been having a very busy morning. While trying to get Ms. D. ready to go to surgery, Nurse M. has been interrupted several times by staff members asking for help or advice. Now Mr. R., a patient also assigned to Nurse M., has put on his call light. As she enters Mr. R.'s room in an obvious hurry, Mr. R. states, "I'm very sorry to bother you, but could you refill my water pitcher?" Nurse M. grabs the pitcher from the bedside stand and takes it to the sink, while muttering through tight lips, "It's no bother, Mr. R. I'm happy to do it!"

The words Nurse M. used are quite appropriate. However, Nurse M.'s nonverbal cues are "speaking" much louder than her words, and Mr. R. is sure to pick up on her anger and frustration from her posture, tone of voice, and facial expression. How is it possible for him to really believe that he has not been a bother and that Nurse M. is "happy" to help him?

STYLES OF COMMUNICATION

The manner, or style, in which a message is communicated will greatly affect the mood and the overall outcome of an interaction. Every time you interact with a patient, you exert an influence on the patient. What influence will that be? You will determine that by the words you choose (verbal communication), as well as by the quality of your voice and your personal appearance, stance, eye contact, and gestures (nonverbal communication). Your style of communication is often what makes the difference between a positive or negative interaction.

ASSERTIVE COMMUNICATION

Assertiveness is your ability to confidently and comfortably express thoughts and feelings while still respecting the legitimate rights of the patient. An **assertive communication** style is interaction that takes into account the feelings and needs of the patient, yet honors your rights as an individual (Box 3-1). It makes interactions more even-sided and has positive benefits for all involved (Riley, 2008).

AGGRESSIVE COMMUNICATION

Aggressive communication is when you interact with another in an overpowering and forceful manner to meet your own personal needs at the expense of the other. Aggressive communication is destructive, often highly so. In the situation just described, Nurse M. responds to Mr. R. in an aggressive manner. Neither party benefits from such an interaction. After the fact, Nurse M. most likely feels guilty and disrespectful for having responded to Mr. R. in this harsh manner, and Mr. R. undoubtedly feels humiliated and unworthy.

UNASSERTIVE COMMUNICATION

Another choice for Nurse M., albeit not a favorable one, was to respond unambiguously to Mr. R. but in an **unassertive communication** style. In this style, the nurse agrees to do what the patient requests, even though doing so will create additional problems for

Box 3-1 Assertive Communication for Nurses

Communicating assertively means:

- Being skilled in a variety of communication strategies and able to express your thoughts and feelings in a way that simultaneously protects your rights and those of others
- Having a positive attitude about communicating directly and honestly
- Feeling comfortable and in control of anxiety, tenseness, shyness, or fear
- Feeling confident that you can conduct yourself in a self-respecting way while still respecting others
- Honoring the fact that you and the other person both have rights

An assertive nurse:

- Appears self-confident and composed
- Maintains eye contact
- Uses clear, concise speech
- Speaks firmly and positively
- Speaks genuinely, without sarcasm
- Is unapologetic
- Takes initiative to guide situations
- Gives the same message verbally and nonverbally

From Riley, J.B. (2008). *Communication in nursing* (6th ed.). St. Louis: Mosby.

the nurse. Use of this style sacrifices your legitimate personal rights to the needs of the patient, and there is a price to pay: resentment.

Imagine that Nurse M. had responded like this to Mr. R.'s request to have his water pitcher refilled:

> "Well, I'm really busy right now, but . . . well, I guess I can do it if I hurry. I just don't know how I'm ever going to get my other patient ready for surgery in time. Here, give me your pitcher."

This interaction is much like the previous one, although more out in the open. Who is benefiting? Obviously, no one! Mr. R. now has fresh water, but probably feels like he has imposed on the nurse unduly. Perhaps he even feels angry thinking that his needs are not as important as those of another patient. Nurse M. will now be even further behind than before and is likely to feel resentment toward Mr. R., as well as feeling as guilty or ashamed as before for giving Mr. R. the impression he is a "bother."

The most effective way for Nurse M. to address the situation is with an assertive communication style. Perhaps the interaction will sound like this:

> "Mr. R., if you can wait about 10 minutes, I will be glad to fill your water pitcher. If you need it filled before that, I can ask one of the nursing assistants to fill it for you now."

By using assertive communication, the needs of both Nurse M. and Mr. R. can be met, with neither of them feeling unworthy, belittled, resentful, or guilty.

ESTABLISHING A THERAPEUTIC RELATIONSHIP

A therapeutic nurse-patient interaction is one in which the nurse demonstrates caring, sincerity, empathy, and trustworthiness. If the patient senses that you are not being genuine in conveying these feelings, a therapeutic, trusting relationship will not develop. If you appear hurried or detached from the interaction, you will send a message that the patient is not as important as the other things on your mind, and will very likely leave the patient feeling frustrated and diminished in self-worth.

Make the *patient* the focus of each interaction, not the equipment or the task. Upon entering a patient's room, look at and address the patient before assessing or adjusting any equipment. Also be diligent in following through with commitments. For example, if you have promised to give the patient a bath in 15 minutes, make sure it happens. If that is not going to be possible, explain this to the patient and establish another mutually agreeable plan for completing the bath. Failure to follow through on commitments will undermine the relationship and erode trust.

Trust is essential to effective nurse-patient interaction. Much of the information that the patient shares with you is personal and is often highly sensitive. It is essential that the patient be able to trust you to treat the information confidentially and share it only with those individuals who need it to provide safe and competent care for the patient. Always give high priority to maintaining confidentiality! However, confidentiality has certain limits. For example, you are obligated to report a patient's statement of intent to do self-harm or to harm others.

Be careful to maintain professional boundaries in nurse-patient relationships. It is not advisable to share personal information such as your address and phone number. Doing so often leads to situations that you are not prepared to handle.

COMMUNICATION TECHNIQUES

Communication in nursing has the potential to be therapeutic or nontherapeutic. **Therapeutic communication** is the ideal. It consists of an exchange of information that facilitates the formation of a positive nurse-patient relationship and actively involves the patient in all areas of her or his care. In contrast, **nontherapeutic communication** usually blocks the development of a trusting and therapeutic relationship.

There are specific communication techniques to use to facilitate the development of therapeutic interaction. Some techniques are verbal, and others nonverbal. Individual nurses will be more or less comfortable with the various techniques, and you should choose a communication technique that fits both your style and the patient's, as well as a given situation. The use of therapeutic communication techniques does not guarantee that therapeutic communication will occur. Therapeutic communication requires you to have an awareness of the patient's feelings and the ability to respond to the patient's needs through the use of verbal and nonverbal communication skills (see Coordinated Care box).

NONVERBAL THERAPEUTIC COMMUNICATION TECHNIQUES

Listening

Listening is an acquired skill. One of the most effective methods of therapeutic communication, it is also one

 **Coordinated Care**

Supervision

COMMUNICATION SKILLS

- Nurses who have many years of education and experience are still working on developing effective communication skills, particularly cross-cultural communication.
- New and inexperienced assistive personnel (AP) often need guidance to make their communication skills more effective.
- It is a responsibility of the supervising nurse to monitor how effective the nursing assistants are when communicating with patients.
- Two methods to help nursing assistants become better communicators are role modeling effective communication techniques and inservice education programs.

of the most difficult to master (Table 3-2). It often feels awkward and uncomfortable at first. This nonverbal communication technique is a behavior that conveys interest and caring toward the patient. It is not always the result that counts the most: It is possible to *hear* without *listening*.

Listening is sometimes active and sometimes passive. **Active listening** requires full attention to what the patient is saying. You hear the message, interpret its meaning, and give the patient feedback indicating your understanding of the message. The patient has an opportunity to validate that you received or didn't receive the message as intended.

In **passive listening**, you indicate that you are listening to what the patient is saying either nonverbally, through eye contact and nodding, or verbally, through encouraging phrases such as "Uh-huh" and "I see" (Riley, 2008). However, it is not possible for the patient to be sure that you have accurately received or understood the message. Therefore, it is better to avoid passive listening.

Your level of confidence will affect your ability to listen attentively. As a novice nurse, for example, perhaps you will be "thinking ahead" to the most appropriate response to the patient and, by so doing, miss what the patient is really trying to communicate. As you gain experience and confidence, you will be able to give full attention to the patient's message, thus allowing for more appropriate intervention.

Silence

Maintaining silence is an extremely effective therapeutic communication technique, and yet tends to be quite underused. Because silence often feels awkward in American society, people tend to feel the need to "fill" it. This impulse does not always allow the people involved in an interaction time to organize their thoughts sufficiently to communicate what they would like. It is common for a person to need several seconds after hearing a verbal message to interpret what has been stated and to formulate the most appropriate response. Unfortunately, the receiver often does not get this amount of time before a response is necessary. In many cases, the sender becomes uncomfortable with the silence and begins speaking again before the receiver has had an opportunity to formulate a response and is really ready to deliver it.

The ability to use silence effectively requires skill and timing. It is easy for prolonged periods of misunderstood silence to cause uneasiness and tension. However, in many cases, purposeful use of silence conveys respect, understanding, caring, and support, and it is often used in conjunction with therapeutic touch. Silence is a particularly useful tool to use when a patient is faced with a difficult decision or a highly emotional issue. Consider the patient who has just been diagnosed with a terminal illness. The nurse who sits silently and attentively while the patient tries to sort through this devastating news conveys an understanding of the complexity of the patient's situation and feelings, and a compassionate willingness to wait for the patient to think. This silence also allows the time for private thought and does not place demands on the patient for a particular response. After a quiet pause, the patient is likely to be readier to talk and more able to express feelings clearly (Potter & Perry, 2009). Maintaining silence also allows you to observe the patient's nonverbal messages, which often more accurately convey the patient's thoughts and feelings than words.

In some cases, it is helpful for you to give verbal permission to the patient to not talk, and convey that you are willing to just sit and wait until the patient feels ready to respond. However, it is important that your nonverbal cues are congruent with this willingness to wait. Fidgeting, writing, or busying yourself with tasks at hand will communicate the opposite message. Therapeutic silence requires that you practice the skill to acquire it and make a conscious effort to use it.

Table 3-2 Therapeutic Communication Techniques: Nonverbal

NONVERBAL TECHNIQUES	BENEFITS
Active listening	Conveys interest and caring; gives patient full attention; allows feedback to verify understanding of the message
Maintaining silence (often used in conjunction with touch)	Allows time to organize thoughts and formulate an appropriate response; often conveys respect, understanding, caring, and support; allows observation of patient's nonverbal responses
Minimal encouragement by nodding occasionally and maintaining eye contact (usually also involves brief verbal comments, e.g., "Yes, go on" or "Then what happened?")	Communicates to the patient that the nurse is interested and wants to hear more
Touch	Often conveys warmth, caring, comfort, support, and understanding
Conveying acceptance (usually also involves a verbal component)	Demonstrates acceptance of patient's rights to current beliefs and practices without condoning them; nonjudgmental, therefore encourages honesty and openness on the part of the patient; provides an opportunity to bring about change in health behaviors while still maintaining the patient's personal integrity

Touch

Touch is another form of nonverbal communication that is inherent in the practice of nursing. Nearly every nursing intervention for the purpose of providing physical care calls for touch. This touch is frequently of a highly personal or intimate nature (e.g., giving a bed bath, assisting a patient on or off a bedpan, inserting a urinary catheter). Because of the intimate nature of touch in the nursing context, it is necessary to use it with great discretion to fit into sociocultural norms and guidelines. Some nurses are uncomfortable with touch because of a fear of its seeming inappropriate or being misinterpreted. When you are comfortable with physical contact with a patient, touch has great potential for conveying warmth, caring, support, and understanding (Figure 3-2). For you to convey warmth, it is absolutely necessary for the nature of your touch to be sincere and genuine. However, if you are not comfortable with touch, or you touch the patient in a manner that communicates hesitancy or reluctance, a very strong negative message, such as rejection, will be sent.

Interpretation of touch is dependent on several factors such as the duration and intensity of the contact; the body part touched; the culture, sex, and age of both the patient and the nurse; the environment; and the stage of development of the relationship. Holding the hand of a patient who does not speak English during a difficult procedure will be much more effective and comforting than efforts to communicate verbally. A small child who is frightened by the hospital environment will respond better to being cuddled than to a verbal explanation of what is taking place. Older adult patients frequently reach out to touch the person caring for them. Many patients who are sad find a warm embrace to be very comforting. A back rub for the patient who is in pain often promotes relaxation and eases the pain. However, because of sociocultural differences, it is crucial that you are always alert to and aware of the possible variations in interpretation of touch. When used appropriately, touch has powerful potential as a communication technique.

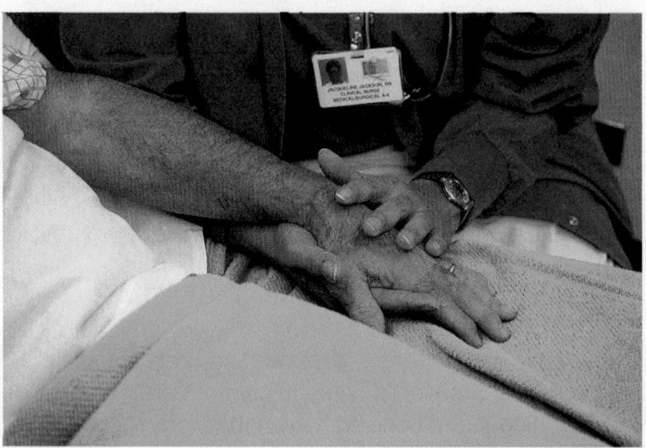

FIGURE 3-2 Touch has great potential to communicate caring and comfort.

VERBAL THERAPEUTIC COMMUNICATION TECHNIQUES

Conveying Acceptance

Many issues in the nurse-patient relationship are of a highly personal nature. Some patients are hesitant to give you complete information, particularly as it relates to values, beliefs, lifestyles, and practices. Often this reluctance has to do with a fear that you will disapprove of the patient's values, beliefs, or practices, or even reject the individual as a person.

Your acceptance is your willingness to listen and respond to what a patient is saying without passing judgment on the patient. It is likely that, given variances in sociocultural influences (e.g., economic status, religion, upbringing, cultural background, and age, to mention only a few) a patient's values, beliefs, and practices will differ from yours. Be careful not to allow these differences to become disapproval, or to communicate disapproval nonverbally through gestures or facial expressions.

Minimal encouragement is a subtle therapeutic technique that communicates to the patient that you are interested and want to hear more. It indicates your acceptance of the patient as a person. It usually involves nonverbal cues, such as maintaining appropriate eye contact and nodding occasionally, and verbal comments, such as "Yes, go on," to encourage the patient to continue.

You will often be confronted with a patient whose practices are detrimental to a healthy lifestyle, and you will sometimes feel, perhaps strongly, that accepting these practices is also detrimental. Acceptance and agreement are not synonymous, however. Your challenge is to facilitate changes in the patient's health behaviors while helping the patient to maintain his or her personal integrity. One approach to accomplishing this is to remember that all of us, including both the patient and yourself, have the right to our own beliefs. You can demonstrate acceptance of the patient's right to his or her present beliefs and practices without condoning them. The next step is to communicate a healthier alternative to the present behavior and assist the patient in initiating the new behavior.

Questioning: Closed

Much of the information that you gather about a patient comes from questioning the patient directly. The type of information that you are seeking will determine what type of questioning is most appropriate (Table 3-3). A **closed question** is focused and seeks a particular answer. For example, when interviewing a newly admitted patient with diabetes, you ask, "What time do you usually take your insulin?" A specific question with a specific answer, it is typical of closed questions, which generally require only one or two words in response. This direct type of questioning is useful if this is the type of information desired. How-

Table 3-3 Therapeutic Communication Techniques: Verbal

VERBAL TECHNIQUES	BENEFITS	EXAMPLES
CLOSED QUESTIONING Focused and seeks a particular answer; usually requires and elicits only a "yes" or "no" or one- to two-word answer	Provides a very specific answer to a very specific question	"How old are you?" "How many children do you have?" "Have you had a tetanus shot in the past 5 years?"
OPEN-ENDED QUESTIONING Does not require a specific answer and cannot be answered by "yes," "no," or a one-word response; usually begins with words like "how," "what," "can you tell me about," "in what way"	Allows the patient to elaborate freely; useful in assessing feelings; elicits the patient's thoughts without influencing the response	"How do you feel about having surgery tomorrow?" "What concerns do you have about going home?" "How are these symptoms different from the last time you were ill?"
RESTATING Repeating to the patient what the nurse believes to be the main point that the patient is trying to communicate; tone of voice rises slightly at the end of the phrase as if asking a question	Lets the patient know if the nurse heard what was said; encourages the patient to offer additional information	Patient: "I'm not sure how I will manage the housework when I get home. My husband will expect me to do the cooking and cleaning just like always, and I don't think I'll be able to do it so soon after my surgery." Nurse: "Your husband will expect you to do the cooking and cleaning when you get home?" Patient: "Yes. I don't think he understands how difficult this surgery has been for me, and how weak and tired I feel."
PARAPHRASING Restatement of the patient's message in the nurse's own words	Verifies that the nurse's interpretation of the message is correct	Patient: "I wish I was having a general anesthetic instead of a spinal. My neighbor had a relative who had a spinal anesthetic and never walked again." Nurse: "You are concerned that you might have complications from the spinal anesthetic?" Patient: "I sure am." Nurse: "I can have the anesthesiologist come talk to you some more about the risks and benefits of a spinal anesthetic. Would that be helpful?" Patient: "Oh, yes. Would you do that, please?"
CLARIFYING Seeks to understand the patient's message by asking for more information or for elaboration on a point; expressed as a question or statement followed by a restatement or paraphrasing of part of the patient's message	Allows the patient to verify that the message received is accurate; particularly useful when the message is ambiguous or not easily understood	Nurse: "How are you getting along with the new blood pressure medication?" Patient: "Well, the doctor told me to take one every day, but they are so darned expensive, I've only been taking them every other day. It seems to be working out okay." Nurse: "Let me make sure I understand this correctly. The cost of the medication is keeping you from being able to take it each day?" Patient: "Yes, I just can't afford it on my fixed income."
FOCUSING The nurse encourages the patient to select one topic over another as the primary focus of discussion	Allows the nurse to gather more specific information when the patient's message is too vague; focuses on specific data	Patient: "Don't let them give me any morphine. The last time they gave me that I almost died!" Nurse: "Will you please tell me as accurately as you can, what you experienced the last time you were given morphine?"

Continued

Table 3-3 Therapeutic Communication Techniques: Verbal—cont'd

VERBAL TECHNIQUES	BENEFITS	EXAMPLES
REFLECTING		
Assists the patient to reflect on inner feelings and thoughts rather than seeking answers and advice from another	Promotes independent decision making; allows the patient to see that her or his ideas and thoughts are important	Patient: "Sometimes I think my family is falling apart. All we ever do is fight and argue. My kids don't take responsibility for themselves, much less help out around the house. This makes my husband furious, and we all end up in a shouting match with everyone feeling miserable. What should I do? Sometimes I just feel like walking out." Nurse: "What do you think you should do?" Patient: "I don't know. I would like for us to go to counseling, but I'm afraid my husband won't hear of it." Nurse: "Have you discussed this with him?" Patient: "No. I suppose that is where I need to start."
STATING OBSERVATIONS		
The nurse makes observations of the patient during an interaction and communicates these observations back to the patient	Allows for clarification of the intended message when verbal cues do not match nonverbal cues; allows for more accurate interpretation of patient concerns	(Ms. C. denies having any concerns about her upcoming hysterectomy. However, the nurse notes that Ms. C.'s posture and facial expression are tense, her eye contact is brief and darting, and she is fidgeting about in bed. The nurse shares these observations with Ms. C.) Nurse: "Ms. C., you seem to understand the information about your surgery that we have discussed, but you still seem to be quite tense and anxious. Can you tell me what is bothering you?" Ms. C.: "Well, it's just that my husband and I always wanted to have one more child and now that will never happen. It all seems so final."
OFFERING INFORMATION		
Nurse provides the patient with relevant data and asks for feedback to determine the patient's level of understanding	Useful for patient teaching; promotes informed decision making	Preoperative teaching Diabetes education Discharge instruction
SUMMARIZING		
Concise review of main ideas from a discussion	Focuses on key issues and allows for additional information that was perhaps omitted; particularly useful when interaction has been lengthy or has covered several topics	"We've covered a lot of information in the past few minutes. The main things to keep in mind are ________________________."

ever, if you want the patient to give more details on a subject, this technique will be essentially useless. An **open-ended question** would be a more effective communication technique.

Questioning: Open-Ended

Open-ended questions do not require a specific response and allow the patient to elaborate freely on a subject. This type of question is useful in assessing feelings. Consider the different responses required to the following statements.

Closed: "Mr. A., are you worried about your scheduled surgery?"

Open-ended: "How you are feeling about having surgery tomorrow, Mr. A.?"

The closed question requires only a yes or no answer and will probably elicit little more. The open-ended question invites Mr. A. to elaborate in whatever direction he chooses with regard to his feelings about having surgery. Given the opportunity to explore his feelings, it is very possible that Mr. A. will reveal information about other aspects of his life, which will in turn allow you to provide better care. Open-ended questions also convey the message that you are interested in the patient as an individual, not just in obtaining a set of data.

Restating

When you use the technique of **restating**, you repeat to the patient what you believe to be the main point that the patient is trying to convey. It is another way of letting the patient know that you are listening. Simply by repeating the central theme of the patient's comments, you encourage the patient to open up further and provide more information. If you also allow the tone of your voice to rise slightly at the end of your restatement, the patient will probably take this as a signal that you hope to hear more details.

Restating often feels awkward to the nurse who is not experienced in using this technique. Perhaps you will feel that it sounds odd for the nurse to be "parroting" what the patient is saying. Indeed, if restating is overused, the patient is likely to share this perception. However, used selectively, restating is a valuable technique to encourage the patient to offer helpful information.

Paraphrasing

Although **paraphrasing** bears some similarity to restating, it differs in intent. Paraphrasing is the restatement of the patient's message in your own words to verify that your interpretation of the message is correct.

Clarifying

Clarifying takes restating and paraphrasing a step further, and is useful when the patient's message is incomplete, confusing, or does not go deeply enough into the area you are exploring. When clarifying, you suggest some of your own ideas about what the patient is trying to communicate back to the patient, in a manner that asks the patient to verify that your enhanced version of the message is accurate. This technique is helpful when you need to assess whether a patient is following a prescribed health regimen appropriately. If not, clarifying often helps you to identify the reason the patient is not following the regimen as prescribed and to intervene to correct the situation.

Focusing

The technique of **focusing** is also used when more specific information is needed to accurately understand the patient's message. It is quite possible that the patient is giving you some extremely important information. However, if the message is too vague it will not be useful, and you will have to seek further information and focus on specific data to provide safe nursing interventions to the patient.

Reflecting

Reflecting is like restating, but it involves inner feelings and thoughts more than facts. You use this therapeutic technique to assist patients to explore their own feelings, often about a choice that lies before them, rather than seeking answers or advice from someone else, such as the nurse. You allow for the expression of the patient's feelings but, rather than offering advice, reflect the thoughts back to the patient. This empowers the patient to verbalize a possible solution and at the same time places the patient in a position of control and promotes self-esteem.

Reflecting allows patients to see that their ideas and thoughts are important and have worth. The patient gains confidence in his or her own decision making instead of feeling the need to relegate it to others.

Stating Observations

You will observe the patient during every interaction. Communicating your observations to the patient is called **stating observations** and is often useful in validating the accuracy of your observations. This technique can be especially helpful when the patient's verbal message does not seem to match the nonverbal behaviors you witness. By describing the patient's observed behavior, you provide feedback and invite the patient to verify that the message you received was the one the patient intended to send. Having clarified the confusion between verbal and nonverbal cues, you are in a position to address the patient's concerns more effectively.

Offering Information

Much of the communicating that the nurse does takes the form of **offering information.** Preparing a patient for what to expect before, during, and after an invasive diagnostic procedure is one example of how you will use this communication technique. Discharge teaching to prepare the patient for self-care at home is another example. Be careful, when communicating this way, to make the interaction go in both directions. Use the patient's feedback to determine whether the information you give has been understood. Also consider what you learn from the feedback about the patient's likelihood of accepting and ability to follow the instructions you have given. Do not confuse offering information with giving advice. Giving advice takes decision making away from the patient and puts the nurse-patient relationship at risk.

Summarizing

Summarizing means providing a review of the main points covered in an interaction. You will use this technique most often after a lengthy interaction or one that has covered several issues, for example, at the end of a patient teaching session. It helps the patient to separate the essential information from the "nice to know" information and gives a sense of closure to the session.

Use of Humor

One of the most powerful tools at your disposal in promoting the well-being of an individual is humor. Apply that old phrase, "laughter is the best medicine," to help patients deal with stress and illness. Laughter provides a psychological and physical release (Figure 3-3). With humor, you have the ability to enhance feelings of well-being, reduce anxiety, and encourage a sense of hope.

Some ways to appropriately use humor are to share funny experiences or tell jokes in good taste. This helps the patient to see you as a human being, which in turn helps promote a trusting relationship. Humor helps put both you and the patient at ease, easing communication as well, not to mention enhancing its effectiveness.

A note of caution is warranted, however. Although humor is frequently effective and helpful, make sure to use it with caution and discretion. It is never appropriate to laugh *at*—only *with*—a person. Humor that makes fun of a person or his or her ways is neither funny nor appropriate. In general, you'll find that you need to know the patient fairly well before using humor. If you are perceptive and smart, you will take cues from the patient or the patient's significant others to predict how the patient might respond to humor. In some situations, remember to be especially cautious with the use of humor: when the patient is from a different culture or background, for example, or is confused or cognitively impaired. Another pitfall to watch out for is using humor to sidestep issues. Rather than allowing yourself or the patient to resort to humor to mask fears and other difficult emotions, try to find a more appropriate technique that helps the patient communicate effectively. Humor is certainly effective and therapeutic in some situations, but it becomes a hindrance, and potentially destructive, if it is the only tool in your communication toolbox.

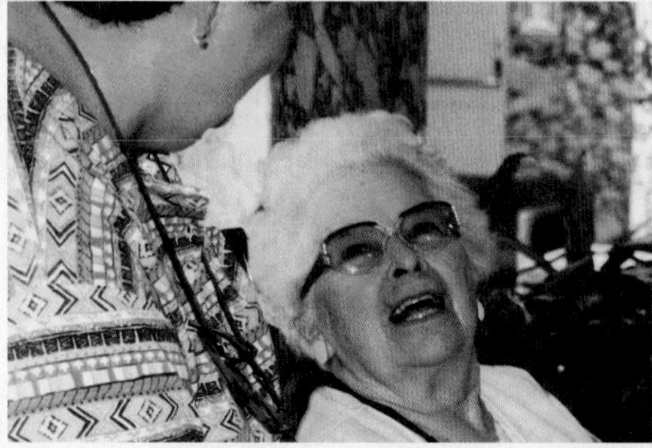

FIGURE 3-3 Help reduce stress and support a therapeutic relationship by sharing a joke or laughing with patients.

FACTORS AFFECTING COMMUNICATION

POSTURING AND POSITIONING

Where and how you sit or stand conveys a message to the patient. Standing at the bedside while the patient lies in the bed sends the message that you have power and the patient does not. Crossing your arms over your chest or crossing your legs while sitting conveys a lack of openness to the patient. Assuming a position of total relaxation, such as leaning back into the chair, possibly even slouching, sends a message of disinterest.

Your most therapeutic posture and positioning is the same position and level as the patient, or as close to it as feasible. For example, if the patient is lying in bed, sit on a chair at the bedside facing the patient. Keep the head of the bed elevated, unless contraindicated, so the patient feels at your level. If you sit in a comfortable position, with neither arms nor legs crossed, and lean slightly forward toward the patient, you convey a message of interest and openness.

SPACE AND TERRITORIALITY

An invisible line marks an area surrounding each of us and sets the boundaries of our "territory," the intangible personal space that is often called the **comfort zone.** Maintaining the distance between ourselves and others necessary to keep this comfort zone inviolate protects us against feelings of personal threat or intimidation. This distance is dynamic and varies with the individual, the situation, and cultural factors.

As a rule, in Western cultures we recognize four zones of personal space. From touching us to 18 inches away is the **intimate zone.** By necessity, a majority of nursing interventions provided to a patient occur in the intimate zone. Bathing, inserting urethral catheters, and changing dressings are just a few examples. Entrance into the intimate zone carries a high potential for causing uneasiness in both you and the patient. Approach these interventions, therefore, in a professional manner with gentleness and tact (Figure 3-4). The **personal zone** comprises the area from 18 inches to 4 feet away from a person. Sitting and talking with a patient is an example of an interaction in the personal zone. Both you and the patient are more at ease when this zone forms the setting of an interaction because your presence is less intimidating. The **social zone** (4 to 12 feet) is appropriate when speaking to a small group of people, and the **public zone** (12 feet or more) is primarily used for public speaking (Potter & Perry, 2008).

ENVIRONMENT

The general environment surrounding an interaction often has a significant impact on the interaction's effectiveness. It is extremely difficult to have a therapeutic interaction in the midst of chaos. Make every attempt to provide a calm, relaxed atmosphere for the

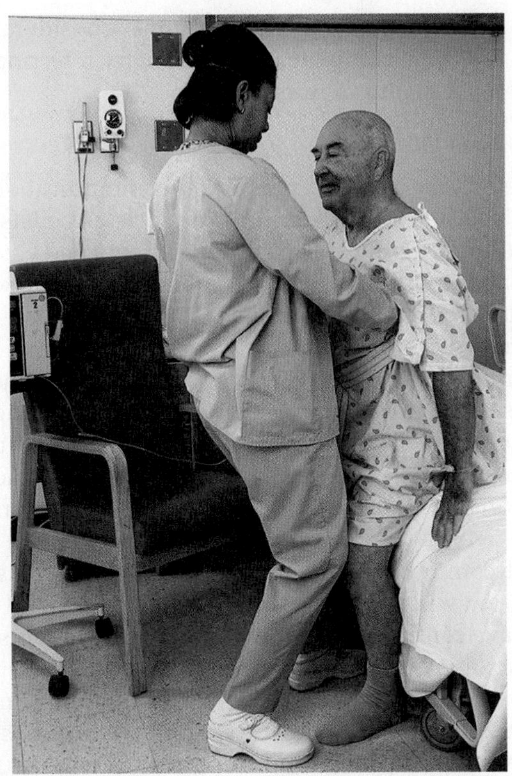

FIGURE 3-4 Much of the nursing care provided to a patient occurs in the intimate zone.

interaction. Another key aspect of the environment is privacy, or its lack; a private room with the door closed is ideal. However, this degree of privacy is often not possible. If the patient has a roommate, taking the patient to a private conference room is sometimes a good option, depending on the status of the patient and the nature of the interaction. At the very least, pull the privacy curtain between the two patients.

LEVEL OF TRUST

A trusting relationship is essential to effective nurse-patient interaction. Without trust, interaction will not progress past superficial social interaction. First, gain the patient's trust before expecting to have a meaningful or therapeutic interaction. One way to foster trust is by demonstrating confidence and competence. It is often difficult to establish a trusting relationship with a patient who has had negative encounters with other health care providers. Be sensitive to the patient's previous experiences, and demonstrate a genuine effort to make the current situation a positive experience for the patient.

LANGUAGE BARRIERS

Obviously, if the patient's primary language is different from yours, there is great potential for ineffective communication. Think how frightening the health care system probably is to a person who depends on but is unable to understand or speak to you. Make every attempt to find an interpreter. If no interpreter is available and the patient seems to have some understanding of the language, it is often helpful to use gestures and pictures and act out the message you want to convey. Keep messages simple and do not use extraneous words. It is especially important to avoid medical jargon and abbreviations.

It is hoped that your health care institution keeps resources such as translation dictionaries in the languages most common to its geographic location (Boxes 3-2 and 3-3). Use this resource with caution, however: There is a high risk of mispronouncing words or using the wrong ones, and doing so will convey unintended or inaccurate meanings and result in misunderstanding or even distress. Handbooks with summaries of cultural practices and beliefs of a variety of cultures are often very useful.

Use family members as interpreters only with great caution. Depending on cultural norms, it often creates discomfort for both family member and patient to discuss certain information together. Sometimes the family member will edit the message instead of relaying it as you intended. Never use children as interpreters.

CULTURE

Nursing is concerned with holistic care of the patient. Culture is a significant component of a patient's psychosocial well-being. Definitely make an effort to seek specific information regarding cultural practices and beliefs, especially when the patient is from a different culture than you. The effect of culture on communication is immense, and a complete discussion is beyond the scope of this chapter. Riley (2008) offers useful guidelines when relating to patients of different cul-

Box 3-2 Guidelines for Communicating with Patients Who Are Partially Fluent in English

- Assess the patient's nonverbal as well as verbal communication.
- Keep your eyes at approximately the same level as the patient's. This will probably mean you will sit. Assess whether the patient is comfortable with eye contact.
- Speak slowly, and never loudly (unless the patient has a hearing impairment).
- Use pictures when possible. (Remember: A picture is worth a thousand words.)
- Avoid using technical terms.
- Ask for feedback. Provide the patient with paper and pencil.
- Remember that patients understand more than they can express—and they need time to think in their own language.
- Remember that stress interferes with the patient's ability to think and speak in English.

Adapted from Riley, J.B. (2008). *Communication in nursing* (6th ed.). St. Louis: Mosby.

Box 3-3 Guidelines for Communicating with Non–English-Speaking Patients

If an interpreter is available:
- Use dialect-specific interpreters, not translators.
- Give the patient and interpreter time alone together.
- Build in time for translation and interpretation.
- Avoid using children and relatives as interpreters.
- Select same-age and same-sex interpreters.
- Address your questions to the patient, not the interpreter.

If an interpreter is **not** available:
- Use a translator.
- Determine if there is a third language that both you and the patient speak. In many cultures, it is common for patients to speak several languages.
- Remember that nonverbal communication is more important than verbal communication.
- Be attentive to both your own and the patient's nonverbal messages.
- Pantomime simple words and actions.
- Remember: A picture is worth a thousand words. Use paper and pencil.
- Talk with your institution's administration about the importance of using trained medical interpreters when caring for the non–English-speaking patient.
- Until medical interpreters are available, use both formal and informal networking to locate a suitable interpreter. If all else fails, owners of ethnic restaurants and grocery stores are possible resources to use to locate interpreters or translators.

Adapted from Riley, J.B. (2008). *Communication in nursing* (6th ed.). St. Louis: Mosby.

tures than your own (see Cultural Considerations box). For more complete information, try referring to a text on transcultural nursing.

AGE AND GENDER

The effects of **age** and **gender** on communication are largely influenced by cultural or societal beliefs and attitudes. A significant age difference between you and the patient will, in some cases, raise a barrier to communication. If you have had little experience with children, it is possible that you will have difficulty communicating effectively with a child in the health care setting. Teenagers present a unique challenge to many. Their vocabulary and expressions are often unique to their age-group—jargon, in a manner of speaking. If you are not clued in to the meaning of these words and expressions, you run a real risk of miscommunication. At the other end of the spectrum you will sometimes find an older adult who does not have confidence in a very young nurse or has some physiologic or cognitive impairment that hampers effective communication. Strive to understand as much about patients across the life span as possible to select the most appropriate communication techniques for a variety of circumstances (see Life Span Considerations for Older Adults box).

Male and female patterns of communication are often closely related to cultural, familial, and lifestyle patterns developed over a lifetime. The beliefs, values, and attitudes that an individual or a society in general, holds regarding male or female status and expecta-

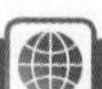 **Cultural Considerations**

Communicating with Patients of Different Cultures from Your Own

DOMINANT LANGUAGE AND DIALECTS
- Identify the dominant language of the group.
- Identify dialects that have the potential to interfere with communication.
- Explore contextual speech patterns of the group. What is the usual volume and tone of speech?

CULTURAL COMMUNICATION PATTERNS
- Explore the willingness of individuals to share thoughts, feelings, and ideas.
- Explore the practice and meaning of touch in the given society; within the family, among friends, with strangers, with members of the same sex, with members of the opposite sex, and with health care providers.
- Identify typical personal spatial and distancing characteristics during one-to-one communication. Explore how distancing changes with friends compared to strangers.
- Explore the use of eye contact within the group. Does avoidance of eye contact have special meanings? How does eye contact vary among family, friends, and strangers? Do eye contact practices change when communication occurs between members of different socioeconomic groups?
- Explore the meaning of various facial expressions. Do specific facial expressions have special meanings? Do people tend to smile a lot? How are emotions displayed or not displayed in facial expressions?
- Are there acceptable ways of standing and greeting outsiders?

ATTITUDES TOWARD TIME AND TEMPORAL ISSUES
- Explore attitudes in the group toward time. Are individuals primarily oriented to the past, present, or future? How do individuals see the context of past, present, and future?
- Identify differences in the interpretation of social time versus clock time.
- Explore how time factors are interpreted by the group. Are individuals expected to be punctual in arrival to jobs, appointments, and social engagements?

FORMAT FOR NAMES
- Explore the format for personal names.
- How does the individual expect to be greeted by strangers and health care practitioners?

From Riley, J.B. (2008). *Communication in nursing* (6th ed.). St. Louis: Mosby.

Life Span Considerations

Older Adults

Tips for Improved Communication with Older Adults Who Have Communication Needs or Barriers

- Get the patient's attention before speaking.
- Check for hearing aids and glasses.
- Introduce yourself.
- Be sure your face is visible to the patient, and use facial expressions and gestures.
- Choose a quiet, well-lit environment with minimal distractions.
- Do not shout; it distorts sounds. Speak clearly at a moderate speed.
- Allow time for the patient to respond. Do not assume the patient is being uncooperative if he or she does not reply or takes a long time to reply.
- Give the patient a chance to ask questions.
- Do not talk to the patient like a child. Use words appropriate to the patient's developmental level.

From Potter, P.A., & Perry, A.G. (2009). *Fundamentals of nursing* (7th ed.). St. Louis: Mosby.

tions are likely to affect how messages are sent and received (Riley, 2008).

Nursing remains a female-dominated profession, whereas medicine is predominantly male. Since in traditional gender roles the female is subordinate to the male, the (female) nurse has historically been viewed as a subordinate by the (male) physician rather than as an equal colleague on the health care team. Understandably, this has placed a strain on the nurse-physician relationship. Effective communication is difficult across stereotypes, particularly when either or both parties view one as more powerful than the other. Your attitudes regarding gender and those of your patients will also be a factor in the effectiveness of your interactions.

PHYSIOLOGIC FACTORS

There are many physiologic factors in the patient's experience that interfere with effective communication. **Pain** is a common example. While a patient is experiencing pain, all available energy is focused on coping with the pain; it is difficult, if not impossible, to communicate about anything except the pain. This is a poor time to try to accomplish discharge teaching with the patient, for example. Address the patient's pain before proceeding with any other interaction with the patient.

Altered cognition is another physiologic factor that frequently hinders effective communication. If the patient lacks the cognitive ability to receive, process, and send information, communication is derailed. Several factors have the potential to affect a patient's cognitive ability. Stroke (brain attack), sedative effects of medication, dementia, and developmental delays are examples of such factors.

Careful assessment of a patient's level of cognitive function is important when beginning any interaction. Keep the patient's sensory abilities operating at their maximum potential. For example, if the patient wears glasses or a hearing aid, make sure these assistive devices are in place to help the patient to process information accurately. If there is decreased ability to comprehend, keep the environment quiet when communicating. Be sure to get the patient's attention before trying to communicate (Ackley & Ladwig, 2008). Box 3-4 lists additional strategies for communicating with patients who are cognitively impaired.

Impaired hearing is common in the older adult. Obviously, do not expect a patient who is unable to hear what is being said to understand a spoken message. See Box 3-5 for strategies for communicating with the hearing-impaired patient.

PSYCHOSOCIAL FACTORS

A multitude of factors place patients under **stress.** The patient might be frightened, in pain, deprived of sleep, nauseated, or experiencing a host of other unpleasant things. These feelings make the patient feel vulnerable. The normal human response to feelings of vulnerability is one of self-defense. Unfortunately, the patient's usual means of responding to a threat is frequently not an option in the present situation. Thus the patient resorts to alternative coping mechanisms that are or are possibly not productive or healthy. Some patients become angry or verbally abusive, whereas others become depressed and withdrawn.

Box 3-4 Communicating with Patients Who Are Cognitively Impaired

- Reduce environmental distractions while conversing.
- Get patient's attention before speaking.
- Use simple sentences and avoid long explanations.
- Ask one question at a time.
- Allow time for patient to respond.
- Be an attentive listener.
- Include family and friends in conversations, especially in subjects known to patient.

Modified from Potter, P.A., & Perry, A.G. (2009). *Fundamentals of nursing* (7th ed.). St. Louis: Mosby.

Box 3-5 Communicating with Patients Who Have Hearing Impairment

- Check for hearing aids and glasses.
- Reduce environmental noise.
- Get patient's attention before speaking.
- Face patient with your mouth visible.
- Do not chew gum.
- Speak at normal volume—do not shout.
- Rephrase rather than repeat if misunderstood.
- Provide a sign language interpreter if indicated.

Modified from Potter, P.A., & Perry, A.G. (2009). *Fundamentals of nursing* (7th ed.). St. Louis: Mosby.

When the patient is experiencing stress, especially extreme stress, you will need to modify communication methods. You will find it helpful to keep information simple, basic, and concrete; offer only essential information; let the patient direct the conversation; and be supportive of the patient through words and presence.

An illness is often accompanied by some degree of **grieving** as a result of actual or perceived loss. There are many possible forms for this loss to take, including role or lifestyle change, physical change, altered function, terminal prognosis, and anticipated or actual loss of a loved one.

Nurses often feel uncomfortable interacting with a grieving patient for fear of not knowing what to say or saying the wrong thing. Because of this uneasiness, you probably find yourself sometimes saying nothing or avoiding the subject entirely. Your challenge in dealing with patients and their loved ones who are grieving is to attempt communication with them despite any feelings of personal inadequacy you have. A silent presence is often all that is necessary. You facilitate the grieving process by using therapeutic touch, warm and caring behaviors, and open-ended statements to listen and assist those who are grieving to understand their own feelings and behaviors.

BLOCKS TO COMMUNICATION

Just as therapeutic techniques enhance the quality of an interaction, barriers to communication block its effectiveness. The list of possible responses that block communication is long. The most common are presented in Table 3-4.

❖ NURSING PROCESS

The nursing diagnosis of **impaired verbal communication** is used to describe "decreased, delayed, or absent ability to receive, process, transmit, and use a system of symbols" (Ackley & Ladwig, 2008).

■ Assessment

Any of the factors affecting communication discussed earlier in this chapter is potentially related to impaired verbal communication. Defining characteristics indicating impaired verbal communication include absence of eye contact; inability to speak; willful refusal to speak; difficulty in comprehending and/or maintaining usual communication pattern; difficulty expressing thoughts verbally; difficulty forming words or sentences; difficulty in selective attending; difficulty or inability in use of body or facial expressions; disorientation to person, space, or time; inability to speak language of caregiver; difficult or inappropriate verbalization; and slurring or stuttering (Ackley & Ladwig, 2008).

■ Nursing Diagnosis

If one or more of the defining characteristics are present, you will perhaps make the nursing diagnosis of impaired verbal communication. For example, Mr. W. has an endotracheal tube in place to relieve respiratory distress that occurred following thoracic surgery. He is currently unable to speak because of the presence of the endotracheal tube. Because of his inability to speak, the nursing diagnosis of impaired verbal communication is appropriate.

■ Expected Outcomes and Planning

The goal for any patient experiencing impaired verbal communication is that the patient will be able to communicate effectively with others in the environment by sending and receiving clear, concise, and understandable messages. The desired outcomes you establish with the patient have to be specific and realistic for the patient and address the patient's needs and concerns. In general, the desired outcomes will state that the patient will:

- Report improved satisfaction with ability to communicate
- Demonstrate increased ability to understand
- Demonstrate improved ability to express self
- Use alternative methods of communication, as indicated (Carpenito-Moyet, 2008)

■ Implementation

Nursing interventions appropriate to the patient with impaired verbal communication will depend on the type of communication problem that exists, as well as the factors contributing to the problem. Thus it is possible for nursing interventions to vary greatly from one patient to the next. See Box 3-6 for examples of helpful nursing interventions related to specific types of impaired communication.

■ Evaluation

You will evaluate the effectiveness of communication based on the patient's ability to meet the established goals and outcomes. A good way to accomplish this is by observing the patient's response to an interaction and considering what kind of message you are receiving from the patient's verbal and nonverbal communication. Does the patient appear to have received your message, and is the patient satisfied with it, or not? If the expected outcomes have been achieved but the impairment is ongoing, continue with the current plan of care. If the impairment no longer exists, on the other hand, consider the nursing diagnosis resolved. If the outcomes have not been met, reexamine the phases of the nursing process to determine what revisions are necessary.

COMMUNICATION IN SPECIAL SITUATIONS

The communication techniques discussed thus far are generally applicable to any type of nurse-patient interaction. Some patients have unique communication needs. Three examples of such situations follow.

Table 3-4 Responses that Block Communication

CATEGORY OF RESPONSE	EXPLANATION OF CATEGORIES	EXAMPLES	OUTCOME
False reassurance	Using falsely comforting phrases in an attempt to offer reassurance	"It will be okay." "Don't worry. Everything will be just fine." "You'll be fine."	You promise something that will not occur or is unrealistic
Giving advice or personal opinions	Making a decision for a client; offering personal opinions; telling a patient what to do with phrases such as "should do," "ought to"	"If I were you I would …" "I think you should …" "Why don't you …"	Takes decision making away from the patient; inhibits spontaneity; impairs decision making; creates doubt
False assumptions	Making an assumption without validation; jumping to conclusions	"You're just afraid to give your own injection." "Your husband isn't very supportive." "You aren't really trying."	Easily leads to a wrong conclusion; often viewed as accusatory or argumentative
Approval or disapproval	Trying to impose the nurse's own attitudes, values, beliefs, and moral standards on a patient about what is right and wrong	"Abortion is wrong!" "Having cosmetic surgery is frivolous." "You shouldn't even think that." "He really is a good doctor."	Easily leads the patient to doubt personal values; creates feelings of guilt and resentment; causes friction between you and the patient
Automatic responses	Stereotyped or superficial comments that do not focus on what the client is feeling or trying to say	"You can't win them all." "Isn't that nice?" "I don't make the rules; I just follow them." "The doctor knows best."	Tends to belittle the individual's feelings and minimize the importance of the message; communicates the message that you are not taking the patient's concerns seriously
Defensiveness	Responding negatively to criticism; often in response to feelings of anger or hurt on your part; usually involves making excuses	"I'm doing the best I can." "Oh, I'm sure the night nurse wouldn't have done that." "You must not have heard me right."	Implies that the patient has no right to an opinion; often you end up ignoring or minimizing the patient's concerns because you are focusing on defense of yourself or others
Arguing	Challenging or arguing against the patient's statements or perceptions	"How can you say you didn't sleep a wink, when I heard you snoring all night long?" "How could your pain level be so high? You were just talking and laughing with your visitor."	Denies that the patient's perceptions are real and valid; implies that the patient is lying, misinformed, or uneducated
Asking for explanations	Asks the patient to explain her or his actions, beliefs, or feelings with "why" questions	"Why aren't you taking your medicine the way the doctor prescribed it?" "Why do you feel that way?" "Why didn't you go to the doctor sooner?"	Frequently viewed by the patient as accusatory; patient often thinks you know the answer and are testing her or him; risks causing resentment, insecurity, and mistrust
Changing the subject	Inappropriately focusing the discussion on something other than the patient's concern	"We'll worry about that later. It's time for your bath now." "Let's talk about something else. Talking about having cancer is making you too sad."	Rude and shows lack of empathy; blocks further communication, and sometimes makes patient feel uncomfortable about expressing feelings; interrupts thoughts, and often inhibits the sharing of important information

Adapted from Potter, P.A., & Perry, A.G. (2009). *Fundamentals of nursing* (7th ed.). St. Louis: Mosby; and Arnold, E., & Boggs, K.U. (2003). *Interpersonal relationships: Professional communication skills for nurses* (4th ed.). Philadelphia: Saunders.

Box 3-6 Nursing Interventions for Patients with Impaired Verbal Communication

1. Determine language spoken; obtain language dictionary or interpreter if possible and accepted by the patient.
2. Listen carefully. Validate verbal and nonverbal expression, particularly when dealing with pain.
3. Anticipate patient's needs until effective communication is possible.
4. Use simple communication, speak in a well-modulated voice, and smile and show concern for the patient.
5. Maintain eye contact at patient's level and read patient's eyes as able, if culturally appropriate.
6. Use touch as appropriate, if culturally appropriate. Holding a patient's hand or stroking the arm is a simple, unintrusive way of showing empathy and concern.
7. Spend time with the patient, allow time for responses, and make the call light readily available.
8. Explain all health care procedures.
9. Determine the patient's literacy status.
10. Obtain communication equipment such as electronic devices, letter boards, picture boards, and magic slates as indicated.
11. Using an individualized approach, establish an alternative method of communication such as writing or pointing to letters, words, phrases, picture cards, or simple drawings of basic needs.
12. If there is a comprehension deficit, keep environment quiet when communicating and get the patient's attention before attempting to communicate (e.g., touch patient's shoulder, call patient's name).
13. Give praise for progress noted. Ignore mistakes and watch for frustration or fatigue.
14. Never raise your voice or shout at a patient.
15. Be persistent in deciphering what the patient is saying, and do not pretend to understand when the message is unclear.

Modified from Ackley, B.J., & Ladwig, G.B. (2008). *Nursing diagnosis handbook: An evidence-based guide to planning care* (8th ed.). St. Louis: Mosby.

VENTILATOR-DEPENDENT PATIENTS

Patients who receive mechanical ventilation via endotracheal tube or tracheostomy will experience an inability to speak because the trachea is obstructed by the tube. Patients will often find this inability to speak devastating, and it will deal a real blow to their sense of well-being and control. When the patient is unable to produce sound, is essential to identify and implement **alternative methods of communication.**

To determine which communication method is most appropriate, carefully assess the patient's ability to use a particular alternative (e.g., cognitive level, literacy, visual acuity, consciousness level, primary language, gross motor skills, and fine motor skills). One valuable tool is a **communication board.** Depending on the patient's literacy, a communication board includes the alphabet, commonly used phrases, pictures, or a combination of all three. If able to point, the patient points to pictures or phrases on the board to communicate a need or thought. If the desired picture or phrase is not on the board, the patient points to the letters that spell out the message. This is not feasible, however, for the patient who does not read or cannot see well enough to select from the board.

If the patient is unable to move well enough to point, alternative selection methods will be necessary. Possibilities include setting up a "signal" system, such as one eye blink for "yes" and two blinks for "no." The receiver (e.g., you or a family member) systematically points to items or letters on the board, and the patient "signals" when the correct item is selected. This is a slow and rather cumbersome process for communicating and requires patience on the part of both the patient and the receiver of the message. In many cases, it is also very tiring for the patient. However, it has the potential to be a helpful tool when no other means of communicating is available or feasible. Box 3-7 lists additional alternative methods of communication to use with the patient who is unable to speak.

APHASIC PATIENTS

Aphasia is a deficient or absent language function resulting from ischemic insult to the brain, such as stroke (brain attack), brain trauma, or anoxia. Some patients experience **expressive aphasia,** in which they are unable to **send** the desired verbal message; and some suffer **receptive aphasia,** or an inability to recognize or

Box 3-7 Alternative Methods of Communicating with Patients Who Are Unable to Speak

- Lip reading: Patient mouths words to be interpreted by the receiver
- Sign language: Hand and finger signals used to indicate letters; used throughout the world for hearing-impaired patients
- Paper and pencil or magic slate: Patient writes messages to communicate needs
- Picture board: Patient points to pictures on a board or poster of typical patient needs
- Word or picture cards: 3 × 5 cards with words or pictures on them; patient picks appropriate card or sorts cards into short phrases or sentences
- Magnetic boards with plastic letters: Patient moves letters around on board to spell words or phrases
- Eye blinks: Predetermined system in which the number of times a patient blinks in response to a question indicates yes or no answer
- Computer-assisted communication: Patient uses keyboard to type messages
- Clock face communicator: Messages placed at intervals around the clock face; clock hand scans the messages, and the patient presses a button to stop the hand on the desired message

interpret the verbal message being **received.** Communication methods recommended for the patient with aphasia are summarized in Box 3-8.

UNRESPONSIVE PATIENTS

It is not certain if, or how much, the unresponsive patient is able to hear or interpret verbal stimuli. Some patients, after regaining consciousness, have reported hearing actual statements that were made in the room while the patient was still in an unconscious state. Because of this, it is important for anyone interacting with the unresponsive patient to assume that all sound and verbal stimuli have the potential of being heard by the patient. Caution people nearby about making negative or anxiety-producing statements. Encourage health care providers, as well as family and friends, to speak to the unresponsive individual as if he or she is awake. This sometimes feels awkward, and family members and friends in particular often need support and encouragement to talk with the patient as they would have before the illness or accident. Talking about daily activities and reading books, cards, and newspapers is beneficial. Also, always explain to the patient any procedure or activity that involves the patient. Remember not to converse with other health care providers about topics that do not place the patient at the center of the discussion or that might cause stress or anxiety if the patient were to hear it.

Box 3-8 Communicating with Patients with Aphasia

- Listen to the patient, and wait for the patient to communicate.
- Do not shout or speak loudly (hearing loss is not the problem).
- If the patient has problems with comprehension, use simple, short questions and facial gestures to give additional clues.
- Speak of things familiar and of interest to the patient.
- If the patient has problems speaking, ask questions that require simple yes or no answers or blinking of the eyes. Offer pictures or a communication board the patient can point to.
- Give the patient time to understand; be calm and patient; do not pressure or tire the patient.
- Avoid patronizing and childish phrases.
- Collaborate with a speech pathologist.
- Encourage the patient to speak as much as possible, not to provide just yes or no answers.
- Use communication aids (see Box 3-7).

Modified from Potter, P.A., & Perry, A.G. (2009). *Fundamentals of nursing* (7th ed.). St. Louis: Mosby.

CONCLUSION

No interaction takes place that does not result in communication. Every time you interact with a patient, there is opportunity for a positive or negative outcome. By becoming familiar with therapeutic communication techniques and practicing them to become proficient in their use, you have the ability to promote a helping relationship with the patient. By also being aware of factors that affect communication and of blocks to communication, you will succeed in preventing interactions that might negatively affect the patient's self-esteem and sense of worth.

Get Ready for the NCLEX® Examination!

Key Points

- All interactions result in the occurrence of some form of communication.
- Communication is both verbal and nonverbal.
- Nonverbal communication is very powerful.
- The manner, or style, in which a message is communicated will greatly influence the mood and the overall outcome of an interaction.
- Communication in nursing should be therapeutic.
- Trust is essential to effective nurse-patient interaction.
- Active listening is one of the most effective methods of therapeutic communication.
- Touch is a form of nonverbal communication that is inherent to the practice of nursing.
- Humor is potentially a powerful tool in promoting the well-being of an individual.
- Numerous factors affect communication.

Additional Learning Resources

Go to your Companion CD for an audio glossary, animations, video clips, and more.

evolve Be sure to visit the Evolve site at http://evolve.elsevier.com/Christensen/foundations/ for additional online resources.

Review Questions for the NCLEX® Examination

1. The patient is fearful concerning upcoming surgery. Which statement by the nurse would be most therapeutic?
   1. "Sometimes anxiety is not easy to deal with. Can you tell me what is bothering you the most?"
   2. "Don't worry. Everyone has some anxiety about having surgery."
   3. "Just try to think about the positive results from the surgery. You'll recover quickly."
   4. "I had surgery once and it still scares me to think about it, so I know how you feel."

2. During an admission interview, the patient refers several times to "all the problems I had last time." The most appropriate communication technique for the nurse to use in this situation is:
   1. reflection.
   2. paraphrasing.
   3. minimal encouragement.
   4. focusing.

3. The patient states, "I'm so nervous about being hospitalized." Which statement would be the nurse's best response to get the patient to elaborate?
   1. "It's normal to be nervous, but we'll take good care of you."
   2. "You're feeling especially nervous?"
   3. "How many times have you been hospitalized?"
   4. "There will be nurses here all the time to check on you."

4. The nurse is talking with the patient about her husband's death 2 years ago. Tears form in the patient's eyes, and she stops talking. A therapeutic response by the nurse would be to:
   1. change the subject to something less difficult for the patient.
   2. remain silent and hold the patient's hand.
   3. leave the room to provide privacy.
   4. pretend not to notice the tears and continue the conversation.

5. Which of the following is an example of clarification?
   1. "You will take your medicine now, won't you?"
   2. "Does this headache have anything in common with your previous headaches?"
   3. "In other words, you feel that your stomachaches are associated with stress at work?"
   4. "What do you mean by that?"

6. The newly admitted Vietnamese patient speaks almost no English. The nurse needs to obtain a urine specimen for culture and sensitivity from him. An interpreter is not readily available. The best approach to obtaining the specimen would be to:
   1. speak very slowly and distinctly.
   2. show the patient the equipment and illustrations of the process.
   3. obtain a physician's order to catheterize the patient to collect the specimen.
   4. delay the collection of the specimen until an interpreter can be found.

7. Abdominal surgery has revealed that the patient, a young mother, has advanced metastatic colon cancer. While the nurse is changing her dressing, the patient begins to cry and states, "If I had just gone to the doctor sooner, my kids wouldn't have to grow up without a mother." Which response by the nurse would be most therapeutic?
   1. "It's natural to blame yourself in situations like this."
   2. "Is their father available to care for the children?"
   3. "Don't give up. The chemotherapy and radiation might be very effective."
   4. "You feel that if you had been diagnosed earlier, the situation might be different?"

8. During his admission interview, an older patient states, "I can't hear you very well." After determining that the patient does not have a hearing aid, the nurse should:
   1. speak in a higher-pitched voice.
   2. speak loudly into his "good" ear.
   3. exaggerate lip movement while speaking.
   4. face the patient and speak slowly and distinctly.

9. Which statement by the student nurse is an example of assertive communication?
   1. "It's time for your bath now. Would you prefer to use the shower chair or do you think you are strong enough to stand during your shower today?"
   2. "I'd like you to take your shower now, but if you'd rather do it later, I guess that would be okay."
   3. "It would be best if you took your bath now, but since you want to wait until tonight, I'll ask my instructor if that would be okay."
   4. "I'm sure you'll feel better after you have your bath. Will you please take it now?"

10. The patient has a long history of smoking and has just been diagnosed with lung cancer. He states to the nurse, "There's no point in trying to stop smoking now. I might as well enjoy the time I have left." The best response by the nurse would be:
    1. "You're probably right. It won't do much good to stop smoking now."
    2. "You feel that there is no reason to stop smoking now?"
    3. "It's never too late to stop smoking."
    4. "I know it's hard, but if you stop smoking now, your condition might improve."

11. The patient tells the nurse that he is frightened about having cancer. Which response by the nurse would be most effective in getting the patient to ventilate his concerns?
    1. "Fear is a common reaction to having cancer."
    2. "Tell me more about being frightened by having cancer."
    3. "Have you told your wife you are afraid?"
    4. "Would you like me to call the chaplain to visit with you?"

12. The nurse is admitting a patient with long-standing type 1 diabetes. Which communication technique would be most efficient in ascertaining the number of units of insulin the patient usually takes?
    1. Closed question
    2. Reflection
    3. Minimal encouragement
    4. Paraphrasing

13. The patient is being seen in the clinic for a follow-up visit after fracturing her ankle. The nurse notes that she is not using her crutches correctly. Which statement by the nurse would be most appropriate?

1. "You are not using your crutches correctly."
2. "Let me show you some ways to make crutch walking easier for you."
3. "Who taught you to use your crutches like that?"
4. "Do your crutches seem to fit you properly?"

14. Which method would be most appropriate for communicating with an alert patient on a ventilator with an endotracheal tube in place?

1. Open-ended questions
2. Communication board
3. Reflection
4. Restatement

15. The patient is in a coma following a motor vehicle accident. Which statement regarding communication with the patient is most appropriate?

1. Speak to the patient as if he can hear what is being said.
2. Avoid verbal stimulation because of its potential to trigger excitability.
3. Encourage family members to limit visitation to no more than 5 minutes per hour.
4. Turn on the television to stimulate the patient.

16. Which statement is true?

1. Use of therapeutic communication techniques will guarantee that a therapeutic interaction takes place.
2. Some form of communication takes place each time there is an interaction between individuals.
3. The intended receiver is always the person receiving the communication.
4. Verbal communication is more effective than nonverbal communication.

17. Which communication technique is always considered appropriate?

1. Active listening
2. Silence
3. Touch
4. Eye contact

18. The nurse is providing discharge instructions to a patient. Which action would provide the most accurate assessment of understanding by the patient?

1. Asking the patient if he understands the instructions
2. Repeating the instructions a second time
3. Providing the patient with written instructions
4. Asking the patient to repeat the instructions

19. Which nurse-patient interaction usually occurs in the "personal zone" of space surrounding the patient?

1. Urethral catheterization
2. Complete bed bath
3. Discharge instructions
4. Enema administration

20. Which approach would be most appropriate for effective communication with a patient with cognitive impairment?

1. Repeating a phrase until the patient indicates understanding
2. Asking friends and family to step out of the room to decrease distraction
3. Using simple sentences and avoiding detailed explanations
4. Directing communication to significant others rather than the patient

chapter

4 Vital Signs

evolve

http://evolve.elsevier.com/Christensen/foundationsadult

Elaine Oden Kockrow

Objectives

1. Discuss the importance of accurately assessing vital signs.
2. Identify the guidelines for vital signs measurement.
3. Accurately assess oral, rectal, axillary, and tympanic temperatures.
4. List the various sites for pulse measurement.
5. Accurately assess an apical pulse, a radial pulse, and a pulse deficit.
6. Describe the procedure for determining the respiratory rate.
7. Accurately assess the blood pressure.
8. State the normal limits of each vital sign.
9. List the factors that affect vital signs readings.
10. Accurately assess the height and weight measurements.
11. Discuss optimal frequency of vital signs measurement.
12. Discuss methods by which the nurse can ensure accurate measurement of vital signs.
13. Identify the rationale for each step of the vital signs procedures.
14. Describe the benefits of and the precautions to follow for self-measurement of blood pressure.
15. Accurately record and report vital signs measurements.

Key Terms

apical pulse (ĀP-ĭ-căl PŬLS, p. 73)
auscultate (ĂW-skŭl-tāt, p. 70)
blood pressure (p. 77)
bradycardia (brād-ĭ-KĂR-dē-ă, p. 70)
bradypnea (brād-ĭp-NĒ-ă, p. 77)
Cheyne-Stokes respirations (CHĀN STŌKS, p. 77)
diastolic (dī-ă-STŎL-ĭk, p. 78)
dyspnea (DĬSP-nē-ă, p. 77)
dysrhythmia (dĭs-RĬTH-mē-ă, p. 71)
febrile (FĔB-rīl, p. 61)
hypertension (hī-pŭr-TĔN-shŭn, p. 79)
hyperthermia (hī-pŭr-THŬR-mē-ă, p. 61)
hypotension (hī-pō-TĔN-shŭn, p. 79)
hypothermia (hī-pō-THŬR-mē-ă, p. 62)
Korotkoff sounds (kŏ-RŎT-kŏf, p. 80)
orthostatic hypotension (ŏr-thō-STĂT-ĭk hī-pō-TĔN-shŭn, p. 79)
pulse (p. 70)
pulse deficit (p. 73)
pulse pressure (p. 78)
respiration (p. 75)
sphygmomanometer (sfĭg-mō-mă-NŎM-ĕ-tŭr, p. 80)
stethoscope (STĔTH-ō-skōp, p. 69)
systolic (sĭs-TŎL-ĭk, p. 78)
tachycardia (tăk-ĭ-KĂR-dē-ă, p. 70)
tachypnea (tăk-ĭp-NĒ-ă, p. 76)
temperature (p. 61)
tympanic (tĭm-PĂN-ĭk, p. 68)
vital signs (p. 56)

Vital signs include temperature, pulse, respirations, and blood pressure. The ability to obtain accurate measurements of vital signs is critical. Because vital signs are an indication of basic body functioning, it is appropriate to begin the physical assessment by obtaining these data. They are called **vital signs** because of their importance.

The skills required to measure vital signs are simple, but never allow them to become routine. Vital signs and other physiologic measurements often provide the basis for problem solving. Careful technique ensures accurate findings.

Many facilities have begun using a fifth vital sign—pain level or comfort level (see Chapter 16). See Figure 4-1 for an example of how to document levels of pain. You will use a more descriptive format for documentation in your notes.

Your assessment of vital signs enables you to identify nursing diagnoses, to implement planned interventions, and to evaluate success when vital signs have returned to acceptable values (see Health Promotion box).

Consider including a cultural assessment in the overall assessment for all patients. This will provide you with a better understanding of each patient as an individual and thus assist with administering appropriate nursing care to all patients. See Chapters 5 and 8 for a more thorough discussion (see Cultural Considerations box).

GRAPHIC RECORD

DATE	9-8-04						9-9-04						9-10-04						9-11-04						9-12-04					
HOUR	24	04	08	12	16	20	24	04	08	12	16	20	24	04	08	12	16	20	24	04	08	12	16	20	24	04	08	12	16	20
Relief acceptable (Y/N)			N		Y	Y	N	Y	Y	Y	Y		N	Y	Y	Y														
BLOOD PRESSURE			160/92	152/88	150/86	148/84	150/88	148/84	136/82	140/80	138/78	142/84	144/86	140/82	130/70	120/70														

CONNECT ALL DOTS

TEMPERATURE: 105, 104, 103, 102, 101, 100, 99, 98.6, 98, 97 (R) (AX)

PULSE: 140, 130, 120, 110, 100, 90, 80, 70, 60 (AP)

RESPIRATIONS: 40, 30, 20

Pain Intensity: 10, 5, 0

	9-8-04			9-9-04			9-10-04			9-11-04	9-12-04
PHYSICIAN VISITS 1)	Dr. D. Bradley			Dr. D. Bradley			Dr. D. Bradley				
2)	Dr. J. Heath			Dr. J. Heath			Dr. J. Heath				
WEIGHT/HEIGHT	136 lb/64"										
BOWEL MOVEMENT		†				†					
INTAKE ORAL		NPO	NPO	200	800	500	300	1000			
INTAKE IV		1000	960	1000	980	970	1000	Dc'd			
INTAKE TOTAL (shift)		1000	960	1200	1780	1470	1300	1000			
INTAKE TOTAL 24 hrs.											
OUTPUT CATHETER		750	700	900	1000	1200	980	Dc'd			
CBI		—	—	—	—	—	—	—			
VOIDED		—	—	—	—	—	—	800			
INCONTINENT		—	—	—	—	—	—	—			
		—	—	—	—	—	—	—			
Emesis		170	—	—	—	—	—	—			
Davol		60	50	20	03	Dc'd	—	—			
OUTPUT TOTAL (shift)		980	750	920	1003	1200	980	800			
OUTPUT TOTAL 24 hrs.											
NURS. INITIALS		B.C.	E.K.	G.J.	S.D.	P.S.	J.C.	B.M.			

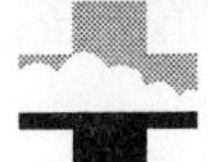

Great Plains Regional Medical Center

NORTH PLATTE, NEBRASKA

N-73 (Rev. 9/00)

LABEL

FIGURE 4-1 Vital signs documented on flow sheet.

Health Promotion

Vital Signs

- Demonstrate measurement of vital signs on self or family member. (Using patient for demonstration prevents patient from being able to observe entire procedure.)
- Explain rationale for each step during demonstration.
- Instruct patient and family in proper cleaning and storage of the thermometer in the home.
- Instruct patient not to take temperature after smoking or eating hot or cold foods for 30 minutes.
- Use caution in recommending aspirin use by patients whose conditions contraindicate it (e.g., gastric ulcer, bleeding tendencies, risk of Reye's syndrome, aspirin allergy).
- Instruct patient or primary caregiver to use fingertips, never thumbs, for counting the pulse. (The thumb has its own pulse.)
- Instruct in use of gentle pressure; reinforce not to press hard over the pulses, which will obliterate the pulse.
- Instruct in use of watch with a second hand to assess pulses.
- Patients who demonstrate decreased ventilation often benefit from being taught deep-breathing and coughing exercises.
- Advise family member to count patient's respiratory rate when patient is unaware of being observed. (If patient is aware of the assessment, respiratory rate is sometimes altered.)
- Instruct family member to notify physician if unusual fluctuations in respiratory rate occur.
- Educate patient about risks for hypertension. People with family history of hypertension are at significant risk. Obesity, cigarette smoking, heavy alcohol consumption, high blood cholesterol levels, and continued exposure to stress are factors linked to hypertension.
- Patients with hypertension should learn about blood pressure values, long-term follow-up care and therapy, the usual lack of symptoms that is responsible for hypertension's being called *the silent killer* (it cannot be felt), therapy's ability to control but not cure it, and the benefits of a consistently followed treatment plan.
- Instruct primary caregiver to take blood pressure at same time each day and after patient has had a brief rest. Take blood pressure sitting or lying down; use same position and arm each time pressure is taken. (Advise patient not to cross legs.)
- Place arm on a table or desk that is raised to the level of the heart.
- Instruct caregiver that if it is difficult to hear the pressure, it is possible that the cuff is too loose, not big enough, or too narrow; the stethoscope is over arterial pulse; cuff was deflated too quickly or too slowly; or cuff was not pumped high enough for systolic readings. Wait 5 minutes and try again.
- Patients often learn to take their own blood pressure.
- Positioning and selection of arm site are potential causes of inaccurate readings.
- Teach patient risk factors for hypothermia and frostbite: fatigue; malnutrition; hypoxemia; cold, wet clothing; and alcohol intoxication.
- Teach patient risk factors for heat stroke: strenuous exercise in hot, humid weather; tight-fitting clothing in hot environments; exercising in poorly ventilated areas; sudden exposure to hot climates; and poor fluid intake before, during, and after exercise.
- Patients undergoing cardiac rehabilitation should learn to assess their own pulse rates to determine their response to exercise. Pulses should be taken before, during, and after exercise.
- Instruct patients on the importance of appropriate-size and placement of blood pressure cuff for home use.
- Teach patient signs and symptoms of hypoxemia: headache; somnolence; confusion; dusky color; shortness of breath; dyspnea.
- Teach patient effect of high-risk behaviors such as cigarette smoking on oxygen saturation.

Cultural Considerations

Vital Signs

- It is a belief in many cultures that certain substances protect one's health.
- Some Italians, Greeks, and Native Americans believe that garlic or onions eaten raw or worn on the body will prevent an illness such as high blood pressure.
- Provide privacy when taking the apical pulse, especially for female patients of Asian, Middle Eastern, Hispanic, and African cultures and their elders.
  —Use same-sex providers or family members to take rectal temperatures and touch the patient's chest.
  —Procedures that are normally noninvasive can produce anxiety because of cultural variables regarding touch, privacy, and gender.
- Consult the physician and the family decision maker regarding giving information to the patient about abnormal vital signs.
  —Collectivistic cultures (e.g., Hispanics, Africans, and Asians) demonstrate their caring for ill members by protecting them from bad news about their health and well-being.
  —Document in the patient's chart what information is given.
  —Communicate the family decision to the physician.
- Determine the patient's understanding of new procedures being performed.
- Use an interpreter if needed, and demonstrate the procedure to promote patient's understanding.

Data from Perry, A., & Potter, P. (2006). *Clinical nursing skills and techniques* (6th ed.). St. Louis: Elsevier.

GUIDELINES FOR OBTAINING VITAL SIGNS

Vital signs are a part of the database that you obtain during assessment. The procedure for assessing vital signs is not routine; part of your task is to individualize the procedure to each patient's needs and condition. Make sure your skills include all of the following:

- Measure vital signs correctly
- Understand and interpret the values
- Communicate findings appropriately
- Begin interventions as needed

Whether and how frequently vital signs are measured (Box 4-1) depends on your judgment of the need, the patient's condition, and physician orders.

If there is a possibility of contact with body secretions, wear gloves while obtaining vital signs.

WHEN TO ASSESS VITAL SIGNS

Although this chapter presents temperature, pulse, respiration, and blood pressure as separate procedures, you will usually assess all of them at the same time and at set intervals. A set of vital signs is taken when a patient is admitted to a facility, and then as prescribed by the physician or as policy dictates, for example, every 4 hours, once a shift, or even weekly in some extended-care facilities (Box 4-2).

The more ill the patient, the more frequently you will take vital signs. Use your judgment in cases in which the

Box 4-1 Guidelines for Measurement of Vital Signs

- The nurse who cares for the patient is ideally the one to assess vital signs, interpret their significance, and participate in decisions about care.
- Make sure equipment used to measure vital signs (e.g., thermometer, stethoscope, sphygmomanometer) is in proper working condition to ensure accuracy of findings.
- Use standard precautions and make sure equipment is clean. Be aware of the normal range for all vital signs. This knowledge will help you detect abnormalities.
- Be aware of the patient's normal range of vital signs. The normal range of some patients differs from the standard range. These values serve as a baseline for comparison with findings obtained later.
- It is wise to know the patient's medical history, therapies, and medications prescribed. Some illnesses or treatments cause predictable changes in vital signs.
- Keep environmental factors that have potential to affect vital signs to a minimum. If you are not able to control these factors, values that are not true indicators of the patient's condition are likely to result; for example, if you assess the patient's pulse after ambulation or an emotional trauma or obtain a temperature reading in a warm, humid room.
- Approach the patient in a calm, caring manner while demonstrating proficiency in handling supplies needed for vital sign measurements.
- Use an organized, systematic approach when obtaining vital signs.
- The nurse and the physician decide the frequency of vital signs measurement on the basis of the patient's condition. Most acute care facilities have a policy of assessing patient's vital signs at least once every shift. However, certain conditions dictate more frequent measurement of vital signs. For instance, after a patient has had surgery or a major diagnostic procedure, take frequent measurements until vital signs stabilize to the patient's baseline before the procedure. If a patient's physical condition begins to worsen, take vital signs more frequently, perhaps every 5 to 10 minutes.
- Evaluate the results of vital sign measurement. Vital signs are only one measurement of the patient's condition. It is also necessary to assess other signs and symptoms and be aware of the patient's ongoing health status. Vital signs are only a part of the assessment of the patient's physical and psychological condition.
- Verify and communicate significant changes in vital signs. The baseline measurement allows you to identify changes in vital signs. Report significant changes in vital signs to the physician. Also record and report any changes to the nurses working the oncoming shift.
- Before examination of a patient by the primary provider in an outpatient setting, you or appropriate health care personnel measure the vital signs.
- Report abnormalities in vital signs to the physician.

Box 4-2 When to Assess Vital Signs

- During admission and discharge to a health care facility
- On a routine schedule as determined by physician's order or agency policy
- Before and after surgical procedures
- Before and after invasive diagnostic procedures
- Before and after administering certain medications, especially those that affect cardiovascular, respiratory, and temperature control function
- When the patient's general condition changes (loss of consciousness, hemorrhage, cardiac dysrhythmias, or the onset of intense pain)
- Before and after certain nursing interventions (when a patient ambulates for the first time or after tracheal suctioning)
- When the patient reports nonspecific symptoms of physical distress (complaints of "feeling funny" or "different")
- Routinely as part of a procedure (e.g., blood transfusion, liver biopsy, paracentesis, thoracentesis)
- When assessing patient during home health visit
- Pain is considered the fifth vital sign. Pain must be evaluated and documented each time other vital signs are taken. Refer to Chapter 16 for a more in-depth discussion of pain and the interventions available for pain control.

Table 4-1 Age-Related Variations in Vital Signs

AGE-GROUP	HEART RATE (PER MINUTE)	RESPIRATORY RATE (PER MINUTE)	BLOOD PRESSURE (mm Hg)*
Neonate	120-160	36-60	Systolic 20-60
Infant	125-135	40-46	Systolic 70-80
Toddler	90-120	20-30	Systolic 80-100
School-age (6-10 years)	65-105	22-24	Systolic 90-100 Diastolic 60-64
Adolescent (10-18 years)	65-100	16-22	Systolic 100-120 Diastolic 70-80
Adult	60-100	12-20	Systolic 100-120 Diastolic 70-80
Older adult	60-100	12-18	Systolic 130-140 Diastolic 90-95

*NOTE: A blood pressure reading of 120/80 mm Hg is now considered prehypertension.

Life Span Considerations

Older Adults

Taking Vital Signs

- An active older adult generally maintains a core body temperature within the accepted norms for younger adults. After age 75, core temperature averages 97.2° F (36° C).
- Environmental temperature plays a more significant role in older than in younger adults and is more likely to contribute to hypothermia and hyperthermia.
- Older adults often have occlusive amounts of cerumen (earwax) in one or both ear canals. Consider this when assessing an older adult's tympanic temperature reading.
- Pulse irregularities are more commonly seen in older adults. Apical pulses should be auscultated as part of a thorough assessment.
- Pulses can be easily occluded in older adults; therefore, apply only gentle pressure.
- With aging, depth of respirations typically decreases. Respiratory rate often increases to compensate.
- Often a standard adult cuff is too large for an older individual who has lost upper arm mass. Incorrect cuff sizing potentially results in significant errors.
- The skin of an older adult is more fragile and susceptible to cuff pressure when blood pressure measurements are frequent, as during the use of repeated electronic measurement. Perform more frequent assessment of the skin area under the cuff or rotation of blood pressure sites.
- Accurate measurement of blood pressure is essential for older adults receiving antihypertensive medication.
- Orthostatic hypotension (a sudden drop in blood pressure with positional change) is commonly observed in inactive older adults, particularly when rising after a period of bed rest.
- Closely monitor older adults receiving antihypertensives and vasodilators for orthostatic hypotension.
- Older adults often have a baseline temperature that is not typical of the adult patient, so it is important to know each patient's baseline.
- The older adult with an infection is often afebrile. In fact, do not assume that an infection in an older adult will cause an elevated temperature. Be aware of other signs and symptoms of infection in the older adult.
- Manifestations of delayed or diminished febrile response to infection are subtle and variable and very difficult to assess. Be especially attentive to subtle temperature changes and other manifestations of fever in this population, such as tachypnea, anorexia, falls, delirium, and overall functional decline.
- The older adult has a decreased heart rate at rest.
- Once elevated, the pulse rate of an older adult takes longer to return to normal resting rate.
- When assessing older adult women with sagging breasts, the breast tissue is gently lifted and the stethoscope placed at the fifth intercostal space (ICS) or the lower edge of the breast.
- Heart sounds are often muffled or difficult to hear in older adults because of an increase in air space in the lungs.
- An older adult's blood pressure often elevates with age. However, do not consider such elevations a normal aspect of aging, and monitor minor elevations.
- Older adults have an increase in systolic pressure related to decreased vessel elasticity. The diastolic pressure remains the same, resulting in a wider pulse pressure.
- Older adults are instructed to change position slowly and wait after each change to avoid postural hypotension and prevent injuries.
- Decreased efficiency of respiratory muscles results in breathlessness at low exercise levels.
- Responses to hypoxia are reduced 50% in older adults as compared with the young, limiting the ability of older adults to respond to hypoxia with respiratory changes.
- It is often difficult to identify an acceptable pulse oximeter probe site on older adults owing to the possible presence of peripheral vascular disease, decreased cardiac output, cold-induced vasoconstriction, and anemia.

patient's condition worsens, at which times it is always necessary to obtain vital signs more frequently. Vital signs readings are interrelated. A rise in temperature of 1° F has potential to cause an increase in pulse rate of four beats per minute. Respiratory rate and blood pressure readings likewise increase with a rise in temperature; however, when blood pressure falls because of hemorrhage, the pulse and respirations increase and the temperature usually decreases. It is also important to recognize the age-related differences in vital signs (Table 4-1) (see Home Care Considerations and Life Span Considerations for Older Adults boxes).

RECORDING VITAL SIGNS

Most facilities have graphic flow sheets for charting vital signs; Figure 4-1 shows an example. As you read about the different procedures for vital signs measurement and assessment in the following sections, consider how you will document your findings. In some facilities, a rectal temperature will be indicated with a small circled *R,* and axillary temperature with a small circled *Ax* (see Figure 4-1) next to the reading. Always write blood pressures with the systolic first and the diastolic beneath: 120/80 mm Hg. A final /0 may be added (120/80/0) if the beat is clearly heard until the end. When charting the pulse on a graphic flow sheet, note that the pulse was an apical measurement by writing *ap* next to the number (e.g., 78 ap). Immediately report any abnormal findings to the nurse-manager or physician. In addition to actual vital signs values, record in your nurses' notes any accompanying or precipitating signs and symptoms such as chest pain, vertigo, shortness of breath, flushing, and diaphoresis. Document any interventions initiated as a result of vital signs measurement, such as tepid sponging (for temperature elevation).

Home Care Considerations

Vital Signs

- Assess temperature and ventilation of environment to determine existence of any conditions that have the potential to influence patient's temperature.
- Assess home noise level to determine the room that will provide the quietest environment for assessing pulse and blood pressure (BP).
- Assess family's financial ability to afford a sphygmomanometer for performing BP evaluation on a regular basis.
- Consider an electronic BP cuff with large digital display for home if patient or caregiver has hearing or vision difficulties.
- It is wise for patients taking certain prescribed cardiotonic or antidysrhythmic medications to learn to assess their own pulse rates to detect side effects of medications.
- Assess for environmental factors in the home that have the potential to influence patient's respiratory rate, such as secondhand smoke, inadequate ventilation, or gas fumes.
- Instruct patients who are using mercury-in-glass thermometers at home on their proper use, safety factors, and hazards (see Box 4-8).
- Monitor the effectiveness of home oxygen therapy by the noninvasive method of pulse oximetry.

TEMPERATURE

THE BODY'S REGULATION OF TEMPERATURE

The body strives to maintain a **temperature** (a relative measure of sensible heat or cold) of 98.6° F (37° C) (Box 4-3) that is considered normal. However, we usually consider variations from 97° F to 99.6° F (36.1° C to 37.5° C) to be within normal range. Many factors have the potential to cause body temperature variances, including the environment, the time of day, the patient's state of health and activity levels, and the stage of the patient's monthly menstrual cycle (Box 4-4).

Regulation of body temperature is the job of the hypothalamus, which is located in the brain, forming the floor and part of the lateral wall of the third ventricle. The hypothalamus helps maintain a balance between heat lost and heat produced by the body. A rise in metabolism, as occurs with exercise and digestion, is the primary mechanism the body uses to generate heat. Constriction of peripheral vessels prevents loss of heat through the skin surface and thus helps conserve heat.

Body temperature falls into two categories: **core temperature,** which is the temperature of the deep tissues of the body, and **surface temperature,** which is the temperature of the skin. Apart from pathologic disturbances, core temperature remains relatively constant unless a person is exposed to severe extremes in environmental temperature. Surface temperature, on the other hand, often varies a great deal in response to the environment.

Temperature elevations are frequently the first sign of illness (Box 4-5). The terms *pyrexia, febrile,* and ***hyperthermia*** describe the condition of above-normal body temperature. Fever is actually a body defense. Elevated body temperature will destroy invading bac-

Box 4-3 Normal Body Temperatures According to Measurement Sites

	Oral	*Rectal*	*Axillary*	*Tympanic*
Fahrenheit (F)	98.6°	99.5°	97.6°	98.6°
Centigrade (C)	37.0°	37.5°	36.4°	37.0°

When it is necessary to convert temperature readings, there are formulas to use. To convert Fahrenheit to centigrade, subtract 32° from the Fahrenheit reading and multiply the results by 5/9:

$$C = (F - 32° \times 5/9)$$

To convert centigrade to Fahrenheit, multiply the centigrade reading by 9/5 and add 32° to the reading:

$$F = (9/5 \times C) + 32°$$

Box 4-4 Factors Affecting Body Temperature

AGE
The neonate's temperature normally ranges from 96° to 99.5° F (35.5° to 37.5° C). Temperature regulation is labile (unstable) during infancy because of immature physiologic mechanisms. This often continues to be the case until puberty. In older adults, the normal range commonly lowers, and a body temperature of 95° F (35° C) is not unusual for some older patients in cold weather. With aging, sensitivity to temperature extremes develops because of deteriorating control mechanisms.

EXERCISE
Any form of exercise can increase body temperature. Prolonged strenuous exercise has the potential to temporarily raise body temperatures to as high as the 103.2° to 105.8° F (40° to 41° C) range.

HORMONAL INFLUENCES
Women generally have greater variations in body temperature than men. Hormonal changes during ovulation and menopause cause body temperature fluctuations.

DIURNAL (DAILY) VARIATIONS
Body temperatures normally change throughout the day, with the lowest reading occurring between 1 AM and 4 AM (97.7° F [36.5° C] on average). The temperature usually peaks around 4 PM to 6 PM. Interestingly, the temperature patterns in people who work at night and sleep during the day do not automatically reverse themselves. It generally takes 1 to 3 weeks for the cycle to reverse.

STRESS
Physical or emotional stress, such as anxiety, often raises body temperature.

ENVIRONMENT
Environmental temperature extremes have potential to raise or lower the body temperature. The changes depend on the extent of exposure, air humidity, and the presence of convection currents.

INGESTION OF HOT AND COLD LIQUIDS
Drinking hot or cold liquids can cause variations in oral temperature readings, for instance, by 20.2° to 21.6° F after drinking iced water.

SMOKING
Smoking cigarettes or cigars sometimes alters body temperature measurement (±0.2° F).

Box 4-5 Signs and Symptoms of Elevated Body Temperature

Thirst
Anorexia
Flushed, warm skin
Irritability
Glassy eyes or photophobia (sensitivity to light), or both
Headache
Elevated pulse and respiratory rates
Restlessness or excessive sleepiness
Increased perspiration
Disorientation, progressing to convulsions in infants and children

teria. Unfortunately, temperatures exceeding 105° F (40.5° C) also have the potential to damage normal body cells, and therefore intervention is often necessary (Box 4-6).

Fevers are classified as constant, intermittent, or remittent. Constant fevers remain elevated consistently and fluctuate very little. Intermittent fevers rise and fall; for example, temperature is normal or subnormal in the morning and "spikes" (is elevated) in the afternoon. Remittent fevers are similar to intermittent fevers except the temperature does not return to normal at all until the patient becomes well (Figure 4-2).

When body temperature is abnormally low, the condition is called **hypothermia.** Death is a risk when the

Box 4-6 Nursing Interventions for the Patient with an Abnormal Body Temperature

- If temperature reading is abnormal, repeat measurement. If indicated, select another site.
- Remove or reduce the patient's external coverings.
- Keep patient's clothing and bed linens dry.
- Monitor patient's temperature at least every 4 hours or prn.
- Administer medication (usually acetaminophen) as ordered by the health care provider.
- Limit patient's physical activity. Increase frequency of rest periods.
- Increase or encourage oral fluid intake if not contraindicated (i.e., congestive heart failure [CHF]). If temperature is elevated, assess for additional related data suggesting systemic infection such as anorexia, headache, thirst, and chills.
- If temperature is above normal, further assess for possible site of localized infection such as pain or tenderness, purulent exudates, erythema, edema, and area of unusual warmth.
- If temperature continues to be elevated, encourage oral hygiene, because oral mucous membranes dry easily from dehydration.
- If patient's temperature is subnormal, cover patient with more blankets; close room doors or windows to eliminate drafts; encourage warm liquids; and remove wet clothes and replace with dry ones.

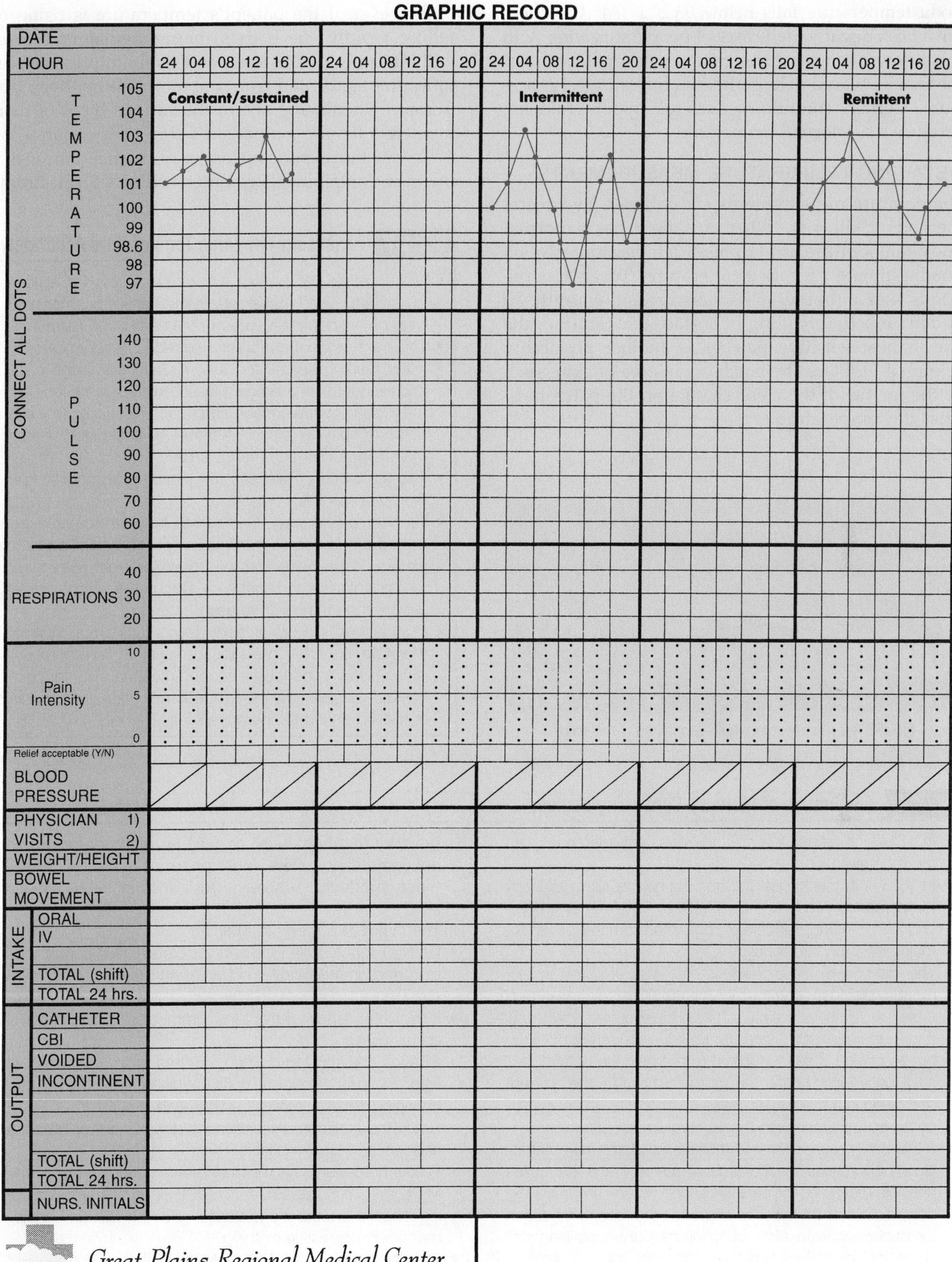

FIGURE 4-2 Temperature measurements recorded on a flow sheet showing types of fevers.

body temperature falls below 93.2° F (34° C). There have been documented cases of people surviving with much lower temperatures. Sometimes a patient is intentionally placed in hypothermia for a surgical procedure. Certain conditions, such as hypothyroidism, produce a subnormal temperature.

OBTAINING TEMPERATURE MEASUREMENTS

Temperature measurements are obtained by several methods (Skill 4-1). When a patient has a normal body temperature, a peripheral temperature gives a good estimate of core temperature. Touch the patient's skin and observe its moisture and warmth. To obtain an actual reading of surface temperature, the use of heat-sensitive patches is another possibility (Figure 4-3). Place the patch on an area of skin, such as the forehead; the color change on the patch indicates the temperature.

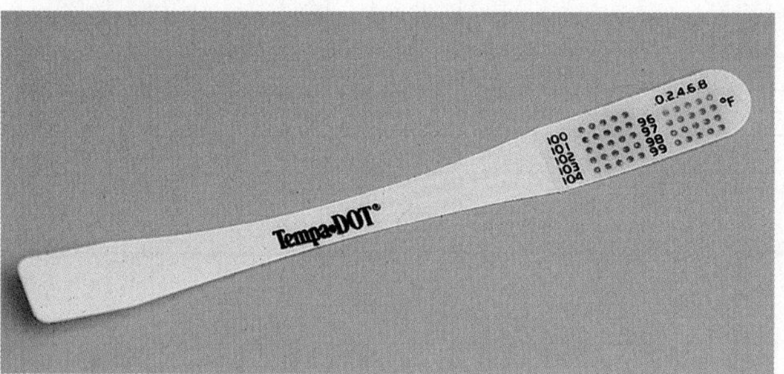

FIGURE 4-3 Disposable, single-use thermometer strip.

However, if the patient's temperature is rising or falling rapidly, the body's thermoregulatory system will affect peripheral sites, and temperatures can significantly lag behind true core temperature. Keep this in mind when using one of the various types of thermometers to assess a patient's core temperature (Box 4-7). Note that experts no longer recommend the use of mercury-containing thermometers (Box 4-8). Electronic

Box 4-7 Assessing Tympanic Temperature Accurately

- Make certain the patient has been indoors for at least 10 minutes. Also make certain the patient has not been lying on his or her ear, which could artificially warm it.
- The base of the thermometer provides battery power.
- If the reading seems too low, replace the probe cover and repeat the procedure. Make certain that the lens and the probe cover are clean and intact. Reassess the temperature, paying close attention to technique. Follow manufacturer's recommendations.
- The eject button releases the plastic probe cover from the tip of the thermometer.
- Be alert to temperature variations from ear to ear, especially if the temperature does not fit the patient's clinical picture. Sometimes you will obtain different readings in the patient's left and right ears. Document which ear was used for the temperature assessment.
- Fluctuations in normal body temperature are minimal; therefore, if there is a significant variation from normal, it is necessary to perform a second measurement for comparison. Ensure that the probe is not placed improperly or moved during temperature measurement.

Box 4-8 Elimination of Mercury-Containing Devices

- In 1714, Fahrenheit invented the constant reference point thermometer using mercury in glass.
- In 1868, Wunderlich established the normal range of body temperatures in humans as 97.25° to 99.5° F, using Fahrenheit's constant-reference-point thermometer. This remains the standard today.
- The mercury-in-glass thermometer was the only instrument available for use for more than 200 years. It was portable, accurate, and easy to use. However, we now know these thermometers are potentially dangerous if they break, posing a serious threat to not only the patient, but also the environment. One gram of mercury, the amount contained in a mercury-in-glass thermometer, is enough to contaminate a lake with the surface area of 20 acres.
- A technical report from the American Academy of Pediatrics (2001) addresses the hazards of mercury and discusses possible measures for pediatricians to reduce children's exposure. One of the chief findings was the recommendation for pediatricians to stop using all mercury-containing devices, including thermometers, and encourage parents to do the same. If the thermometer breaks, the mercury vaporizes and can be inhaled, causing toxicity. The statement calls for an end to the use of all mercury-containing thermometers. **Most health care facilities, clinics, and physicians' offices have discontinued the use of glass mercury thermometers, as well as mercury-calibrated sphygmomanometers. Most pharmacies no longer sell these products.** However, glass thermometers are still used in homes.

In the event of a mercury spill*:

- Do NOT touch spilled mercury droplets. If skin contact has occurred, immediately flush area with water for 15 minutes.
- If possible, remove patient from immediate environment of contamination.
- Change any clothing or linen that has been contaminated with mercury. Perform hand hygiene thoroughly after changing. Wash clothing before reuse.
- Notify the environmental services department or obtain a mercury spill kit, if available.
- Follow procedures for mercury removal as directed by the Material Safety Data Sheet (MSDS). Spills are removed using special absorbent materials, filtered vacuum equipment, and protective clothing.
- Promote exhaust ventilation to reduce concentration of mercury vapors.
- Follow agency guidelines for laundering clothing.
- Complete occurrence or incident report as directed by institution procedure.

*From Potter, P., and Perry, A. (2005). *Fundamentals of nursing* (6th ed.). St. Louis, Elsevier.

Skill 4-1 Measuring Body Temperature

Nursing Action *(Rationale)*

1. Perform hand hygiene. *(Reduces spread of microorganisms.)*
2. Assess for signs and symptoms of temperature alterations and for factors that influence body temperature. *(Enables the nurse to more accurately assess nature of variations.)*
3. Introduce self to patient. *(Decreases patient's anxiety.)*
4. Identify patient by identification band. *(Ensures correct patient for procedure.)*
5. Explain the procedure to patient: site of temperature reading and importance of maintaining proper position until reading is complete. *(Gains patient's cooperation.)*
6. Prepare for procedure:
   a. Assemble the thermometer, soft disposable tissues, lubricant (for rectal temperature only), pen and note pad, disposable gloves, plastic sleeve, or disposable probe cover. *(Promotes an efficiently completed procedure.)*
   b. Provide for patient privacy. *(Decreases anxiety level.)*
   c. Determine whether patient has consumed hot or cold beverages or food or has been smoking; if so, wait 20 to 30 minutes before measuring oral temperature. *(Ensures accuracy.)*
7. Obtaining an oral temperature reading with an electronic thermometer:
   a. Follow steps 1 through 6.
   b. Perform hand hygiene and don disposable gloves (optional). *(Reduces spread of microorganisms.)*
   c. Remove thermometer pack from charging unit. *(Adds maneuverability; battery power is available.)* Remove probe from storage well of recording unit. Grasp top of stem, being careful not to apply pressure to eject button. *(Ensures proper working order.)*
   d. Insert probe snugly into probe cover (see illustration)—red probe for rectal readings, blue probe for oral and axillary readings (see Figure 4-4). *(Using probe cover helps reduce spread of microorganisms.)*
   e. Inspect digital display. *(Ensures that unit is ready for use.)*
   f. Request patient to open the mouth, and gently insert probe into the posterior sublingual pocket (see illustration). Request patient to hold thermometer in place with lips closed. *(Ensures an accurate reading.)*
   g. Wait for audible signal. *(Indicates temperature reading is complete.)*
   h. Remove probe from patient's mouth and remove probe cover by pressing the eject button, directing probe cover into trash receptacle. *(Reduces spread of microorganisms.)*
   i. Provide for patient comfort.
   j. Read and write down reading from digital display before reinserting probe into holder. *(Ensures accurate recording.)*
   k. Perform hand hygiene. *(Reduces spread of microorganisms.)* Return electronic unit to charger. *(Maintains battery charge.)*
   l. Complete procedure by following step 12, a through d.
8. Measuring rectal temperature with an electronic thermometer. CAUTION: If you are not able to insert thermometer adequately into the rectum, remove thermometer and consider alternative method for obtaining temperature. Never force thermometer.
   a. Follow steps 1 through 6b.
   b. Don gloves. *(Maintains standard precautions.)*

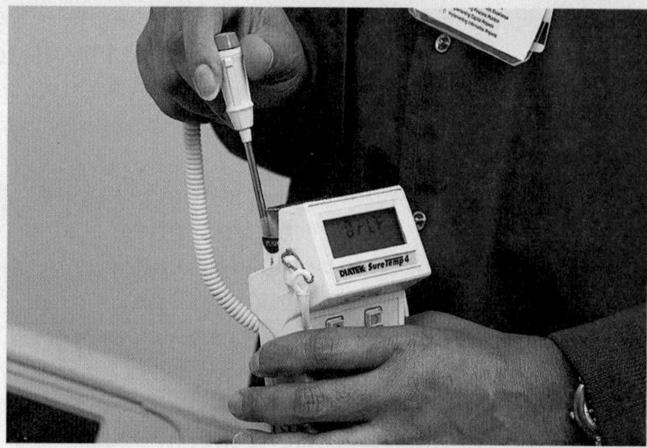

Step 7d

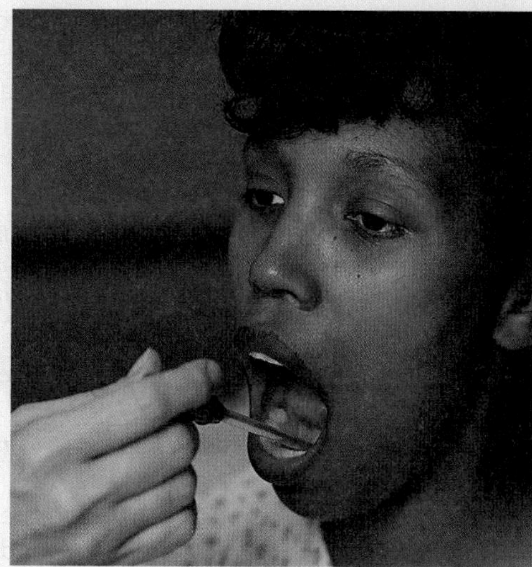

Step 7f

Continued

Skill 4-1 Measuring Body Temperature—cont'd

- **c.** Assist patient to the Sims' position with upper leg flexed. Move aside the bed linens to expose only the rectal area. *(Ensures correct thermometer placement and prevents unnecessary exposure of patient.)*
- **d.** Remove thermometer pack from charging unit. Make certain rectal (red) probe is attached to the unit, and slide disposable plastic cover over thermometer probe until it locks into place. *(Reduces spread of microorganisms.)*
- **e.** With thermometer in probe cover, lubricate 1 inch of tip. *(Eases insertion.)*
- **f.** For an adult, with patient in the Sims' position, gently spread buttocks and insert thermometer probe 1.5 inches into rectum (see illustration). Hold onto thermometer throughout procedure. *(Ensures safety.)*
- **g.** Hold electronic probe until audible signal occurs; only then read temperature on digital display (keep probe in place until signal occurs). *(Ensures accurate reading.)*
- **h.** Carefully remove probe from rectum; push eject button to remove probe cover and dispose into appropriate receptacle. *(Reduces spread of microorganisms.)*
- **i.** Return probe to storage unit, and later return the unit to its charging device. *(Prevents damage to the unit and ensures accurate working for the next assessment.)*
- **j.** Clean anal area of lubricant and possible feces. Remove and dispose of gloves and perform hand hygiene. *(Provides comfort and hygiene and reduces the spread of microorganisms.)*
- **k.** Assist patient to position of comfort. *(Restores self-esteem.)*
- **l.** Write down reading for later documentation. *(Ensures accurate recording.)*
- **m.** Complete procedure by following step 12, a through d.

9. Measuring axillary temperature with an electronic thermometer:

- **a.** Follow steps 1 through 6b.
- **b.** Don gloves. *(Maintains standard precautions.)*
- **c.** Assist patient to supine or sitting position. *(Provides easy access to axilla.)*
- **d.** Expose axilla; make certain the area is clean and dry. *(Ensures accurate reading.)*
- **e.** Prepare electronic thermometer following step 7, c through e.
- **f.** Insert probe into center of axilla; lower arm over thermometer, placing arm across patient's chest (see illustration). In an infant or young child, it is sometimes necessary to hold the arm against the child's side when using the axillary method. If infant is in a side-lying position, the lower axilla will record the higher temperature. *(Maintains proper positioning of temperature probe.)*
- **g.** Hold electronic probe until audible signal occurs. Reading will appear on digital display (see illustration). *(Probe must stay in place for accurate reading to occur.)*
- **h.** Remove probe from patient's axilla. Push eject button to remove probe cover and dispose into trash container. *(Reduces spread of microorganisms.)*
- **i.** Return electric probe to storage well of recording unit. *(Prevents damage to unit.)*
- **j.** Assist patient to regown and position for comfort. *(Restores a sense of well-being.)*

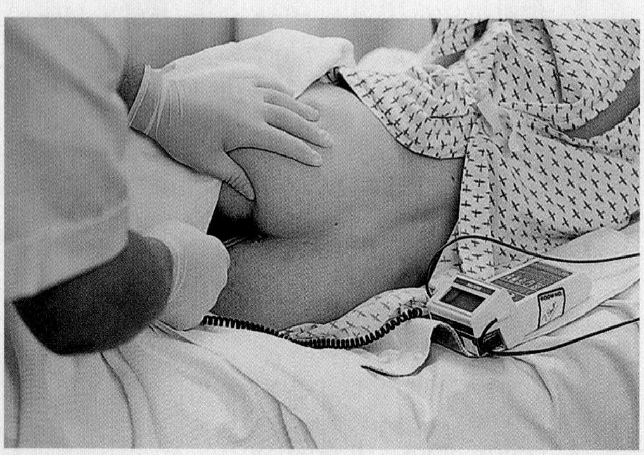

Step **8h**

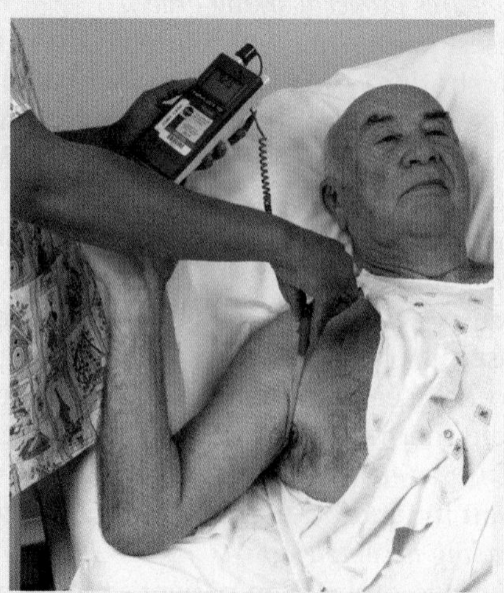

Step **9f**

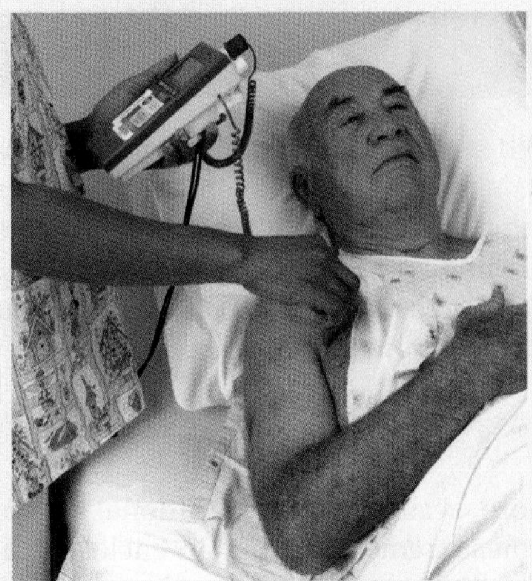
Step 9g

k. Remove and dispose of gloves in proper receptacle, and perform hand hygiene. *(Reduces spread of microorganisms.)*
l. Return thermometer to charger base. *(Maintains battery charge.)*
m. Write down reading for later documentation. *(Ensures accurate recording.)*
n. Complete procedure by following step 12, a through d.

10. Measuring tympanic temperature with an electronic thermometer.
   a. Follow steps 1 through 6a.
   b. Assist patient to a comfortable position with head turned toward the side, away from you. *(Ensures comfort and exposes auditory canal for accurate temperature reading.)*
   c. Remove thermometer handheld unit from charging base. *(Provides easy access to thermometer.)*
   d. Slide disposable plastic speculum cover over otoscope-like tip until it locks into place. *(Prepares the unit to measure temperature; the plastic speculum reduces spread of microorganisms.)*
   e. Follow manufacturer's instructions for tympanic probe positioning.
      (1) Gently tug ear pinna upward and back for an adult, down and back for a child *(because of age-related anatomic differences).*
      (2) Move thermometer gently in a figure-8 fashion. *(Ensures correct placement.)*
      (3) Fit ear probe snugly into canal. Do not allow further movement. *(Ensures correct reading.)*
      (4) Point digital readout toward you, following manufacturer's positioning recommendations. *(Steps i through iv ensure correct positioning of the probe with respect to ear canal; the ear tug straightens the external auditory canal, allowing maximum exposure of the tympanic membrane.)*
   f. Depress scan button on handheld unit and read assessment. Temperature reading appears on digital display.
   g. Carefully remove sensor from ear and push release button to eject plastic speculum cover; discard into proper receptacle. *(Reduces spread of microorganisms.)*
   h. Return handheld unit to charging base. *(Maintains battery charge.)*
   i. Assist patient to a comfortable position. *(Restores sense of well-being.)*
   j. Perform hand hygiene. Dispose of gloves, if worn, into proper receptacle. *(Reduces spread of microorganisms.)*
   k. Write down reading (for documentation later).
   l. Complete procedure by following step 12, a through d.

11. Measuring temporal artery temperature. (This skill can be delegated to assistive personnel who are knowledgeable in the procedure, but it is your responsibility to assess the significance of the findings.)
   a. Follow steps 1 through 6a.
   b. Ensure that forehead is dry. *(Decreases any chance of moisture interfering with temperature measurement.)*
   c. Place probe flush on patient's forehead. *(Prevents measuring ambient temperature by mistake.)*
   d. Press the scan button. *(Continuous scanning for the highest temperature will occur until you release the scan button.)*
   e. Keeping the probe flush on the skin, slowly brush the thermometer straight across forehead. *(Promotes accuracy in measurement.)*
   f. Keeping the scan button pressed, sweep the probe across the forehead and continue to just behind the earlobe.
   g. The thermometer makes a clicking sound when highest temperature is reached. Read and document temperature.
   h. Wipe probe with alcohol, or remove and dispose of probe cover.
   i. Complete procedure by following step 12, a through d.

12. Complete the procedure for body temperature measurement.
   a. Compare temperature findings with baseline and normal temperature range for patient's age-group. *(Comparison reveals presence of abnormalities.)*
   b. If temperature is abnormal, repeat procedure. If indicated, choose an alternate site or instrument. *(Second reading confirms initial findings of abnormal body temperature.)*

Continued

Skill 4-1 Measuring Body Temperature—cont'd

c. Record temperature on vital sign flow sheet, graphic flow sheet, or nurse's notes and report abnormal findings to nurse in charge or physician (see Figure 4-1 and Box 4-5). *(Recording promptly prevents omissions from the record. Abnormalities often necessitate immediate therapy.)* When recording an axillary temperature, write *Ax* above your documentation. When recording a rectal temperature, write *R* above the reading.

d. Do patient teaching (see patient teaching in Health Promotion box on p. 59).

thermometers (Figure 4-4) consist of a rechargeable battery-powered display unit, a thin wire cord, and a temperature-processing probe with a disposable cover. Separate probes are available for oral temperature measurement (blue tip) and rectal temperature measurement (red tip). Use only the specially designated electronic thermometer to obtain the **tympanic** (membranous "eardrum") temperature (Figure 4-5).

Tympanic thermometers have been available for 15 years and are now widely accepted. They are very likely more accurate than traditional thermometer, because measurement is from an enclosed cavity unaffected by the environmental temperatures. The tympanic membrane shares its blood supply with the hypothalamus, the body's temperature control center, and thus it is a good source for obtaining core-temperature readings. To obtain the reading, place the sensor probe on the tympanic thermometer in the external ear; the sensor measures infrared heat. These thermometers boast many advantages: They are easy to use and produce readings in a few seconds. They are suitable for patients of all ages, except infants, virtually eliminate the risk of cross-contamination, and are cost effective (see Skill 4-1). In contrast to rectal and oral measurement, they necessitate neither the exposure of the patient nor the patient's active participation. A switch on the thermometer provides oral and rectal equivalents.

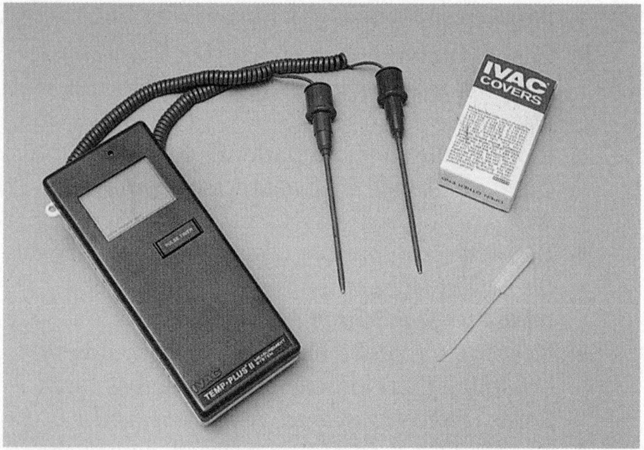

FIGURE 4-4 Electronic thermometer. Blue probe is for oral or axillary use. Red probe is for rectal use.

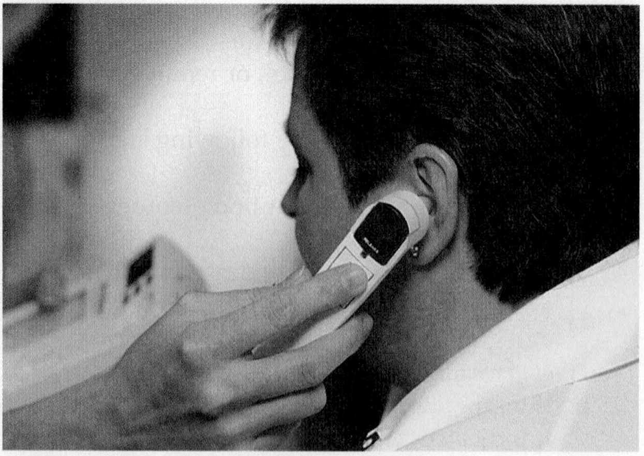

FIGURE 4-5 Tympanic thermometer with probe cover inserted into auditory canal.

One further way of measuring core temperature, the fairly new temporal artery method, provides a reliable, noninvasive measurement. It makes use of an infrared sensor that you brush across the patient's forehead, continuing posterior to the ear (see Skill 4-1). The handheld scanner then displays a measurement of the temperature of temporal artery cutaneous blood flow (Potter, 2006).

Your assessment of the patient will guide your choice of method to measure the temperature (Table 4-2). Do not attempt to obtain the oral temperature in the comatose or the disoriented patient, in small infants, or in patients with surgery fracture, because this method requires the patient's cooperation. Rectal measurements are contraindicated for patients with recent rectal surgery or certain conditions of the perineum. Axillary measurement is considered the least accurate method and is used less frequently since the advent of the tympanic membrane thermometer (see Skill 4-1). Be aware that rectal readings are normally 1° F higher, and axillary readings 1° F lower, than oral readings. When obtaining an oral or a tympanic reading, it is not usually necessary to provide privacy for the patient. Use of the temporal artery scanner is appropriate in virtually all situations. Diaphoresis does not interfere with the accuracy of the measurement as long as you brush the

Table 4-2 Selection of Sites for Temperature Measurement

ADVANTAGES	DISADVANTAGES AND LIMITATIONS
ORAL	
Most accessible site; comfortable for patient; necessitates no position change	Do not use for patients who could be injured by thermometer, who are unable to hold thermometer properly, or who might bite down on thermometer (glass thermometer); infants or small children; disoriented or unconscious patients; patients who have had oral surgery; patients with trauma to face or mouth; patients experiencing oral pain; patients who breathe only with mouth open; patients with history of convulsions; or patients experiencing a shaking chill.
RECTAL	
Argued to be more reliable when oral temperature cannot be obtained	Use sensitivity, because use is embarrassing. Do not use for patients after rectal surgery; patients who have a rectal disorder, such as tumor or hemorrhoids; or patients who cannot be positioned for proper thermometer placement, such as those in traction. There is a risk of body fluid exposure, and lubrication is required.
AXILLA	
Safe method because noninvasive	Least accurate
TYMPANIC	
Noninvasive, accurate, safe; provides core reading; lessens need to handle newborns, which aids in preventing heat loss	Excessive cerumen (earwax) has the possibility to interfere with accurate reading; continuous measurement of temperature is not possible; new disposable probe cover necessary for each patient, which raises the cost; patients must remove hearing aid in the ear that temperature is being measured
TEMPORAL ARTERY	
Provides core temperature; rapid, noninvasive method; tolerated well by children	Diaphoresis and airflow across the face may affect the accuracy; possible for any bandages or dressings on the face or head to prevent measurement with the device

scanner all the way across the forehead through to behind the ear.

AUSCULTATING USING THE STETHOSCOPE

Use a **stethoscope** (an instrument that is placed against the patient's chest or back to hear heart and lung sounds) (Figure 4-6) to measure the apical rate of the heart (see definitions of *apical* and *radial* in the following section on the pulse). The major parts of the stethoscope are the earpieces, the binaurals, the tubing, and the chestpiece.

Make sure the plastic or rubber earpieces fit snugly and comfortably in your ears. If the fit is proper, the binaurals will be angled and strong enough that the earpieces stay firmly in your ears without causing discomfort. To ensure the best reception of sound, the earpieces follow the contour of the ear canal, pointing toward your face when the stethoscope is in place.

The proper polyvinyl tubing is flexible and 12 to 18 inches (30 to 40 cm) long. Longer tubing decreases the transmission of sound waves. The tubing is thick-walled and moderately rigid to eliminate transmission of environmental noise and prevent the tubing from kinking, which distorts sound wave transmission. Some stethoscopes have single and some have dual tubes.

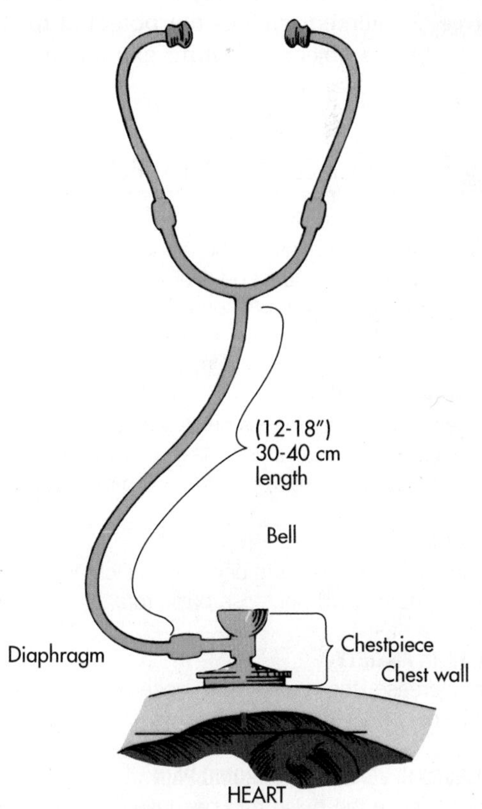

FIGURE 4-6 Parts of a stethoscope. Chestpiece must be placed firmly against the chest wall.

The chestpiece consists of a bell and a diaphragm. According to which you choose to use, rotate the bell or the diaphragm into proper position on the chestpiece so you are able to hear sounds through the stethoscope. To test, lightly tap to determine which side is functioning.

The diaphragm is the circular, flat-surfaced portion of the chestpiece covered with a thin plastic disk (see Figure 4-6). It transmits the high-pitched sounds created by the high-velocity movement of air and blood. You will **auscultate** (listen for sounds within the body to evaluate the condition of heart, lungs, pleura, intestines, or other organs or to detect fetal heart tones) bowel, lung, and heart sounds using the diaphragm. Position the diaphragm to make a tight seal against the patient's skin. Exert enough pressure to leave a temporary red ring on the patient's skin when the diaphragm is removed.

The bell is the bowl-shaped chestpiece, usually surrounded by a rubber ring (see Figure 4-6). The ring prevents the cold metal from chilling the patient's skin. The bell transmits low-pitched sounds created by the low-velocity movement of blood. You will auscultate heart and vascular sounds using the bell. Apply the bell lightly, resting the chestpiece on the skin. Compressing the bell against the skin reduces low-pitched sound amplification and creates a "diaphragm of skin."

When listening through the stethoscope, maintain a position that allows the tubing to extend straight and hang free. Movement creates the potential for tubing to rub or bump objects, creating extraneous sounds. Kinked tubing muffles sounds. When you are using the stethoscope, it is best for both you and the patient to remain quiet.

The stethoscope is a delicate instrument and requires proper care for optimal function. Remove the earpieces regularly and clean them of cerumen (earwax). Clean the bell and diaphragm of dust, lint, and body oils. Keep the tubing away from your body oils. Do not drape the stethoscope around your neck next to the skin. Cleaning the tubing or head with alcohol can dry and crack the material and is not recommended. Mild soap and water are preferred.

PULSE

THE BODY'S REGULATION OF PULSE

A **pulse** is a rhythmic beating or vibrating movement. In the body, it signifies the regular, recurrent expansion and contraction of an artery produced by the waves of pressure that are caused by the ejection of blood from the left ventricle of the heart as it contracts. Each pulse beat corresponds to a contraction of the heart. The adult pulse rate is normally between 60 and 100 beats per minute, with the approximate average being 80.

The condition of the heart and the patient's age, sex, emotional state, size, temperature, and amount of physical activity can influence the pulse rate. If the pulse is faster than 100 beats per minute, the adult patient has **tachycardia**; if it is slower than 60 beats per minute, the patient has **bradycardia**. Tachycardia has many potential causes: shock, hemorrhage leading to

Box 4-9 Factors Influencing Pulse Rates

AGE
The pulse rate decreases as the aging process progresses from infancy through adulthood. Pulse rate in the older adult is sometimes greater than 80 beats per minute because of weakened heart muscle or because of medication.

EXERCISE
Short-term exercise increases pulse rate. Long-term exercise strengthens heart muscle, resulting in a lower-than-normal rate at rest and a quicker return to resting rate after exercise.

FEVER, HEAT
Both increase the pulse rate because of increased metabolic rate. Hypothermia will decrease pulse rate.

ACUTE PAIN, ANXIETY
These increase the pulse rate because of sympathetic stimulation.

UNRELIEVED SEVERE PAIN, CHRONIC PAIN
These decrease the pulse rate because of parasympathetic stimulation.

MEDICATIONS
Various medications alter pulse rate. For example, digitalis decreases the pulse rate; atropine and epinephrine increase the pulse rate.

HEMORRHAGE
Loss of blood increases the pulse rate because of the sympathetic stimulation.

POSTURAL CHANGES
Lying down initially decreases the pulse rate. Standing or sitting increases the pulse rate.

METABOLISM
Certain diseases such as hyperthyroidism sometimes cause a chronic elevated pulse rate. Hypothyroidism sometimes causes a slowing of the pulse.

PULMONARY CONDITIONS
Pulmonary conditions increase pulse rate because these diseases cause poor oxygenation.

hypovolemia (an abnormally low circulating blood volume), exercise, fever, medication or substance abuse, and acute pain. Some drugs, such as epinephrine, also increase the pulse rate. One cause of bradycardia is unrelieved severe pain; pain stimulates the parasympathetic nervous system, which slows the heart rate. Some drugs, such as beta blockers, lower the heart rate. Resting in a supine position also has the potential to decrease the heart rate, as will the cardiac condition called *heart block* (Box 4-9).

If the amount of time between beats varies, there will be an irregular pulse or **dysrhythmia** (any disturbance or abnormality in a normal rhythmic pattern, specifically, irregularity in the normal rhythm of the heart). In the normal pulse, the amount of time between beats is even.

The volume of the pulse refers to the amount of blood pushing against the artery wall with each beat. A weak pulse is difficult to palpate; a bounding pulse is easily felt with light palpation. A pulse that you are unable to feel at all is imperceptible. Another means to communicate the volume of the pulse is by the use of numbers (Table 4-3). Follow agency policy when describing the pulse.

OBTAINING PULSE MEASUREMENTS

When taking the pulse, note the rate, the rhythm, and the volume, or strength, of the pulse. Palpate pulses using the pads of your index and middle fingers (Skill 4-2). Only apply slight pressure over the artery to avoid obliterating the pulse (by occluding blood flow). Assess pulses on both sides of the peripheral vascular system. Assess both radial pulses, for example, to compare the characteristics of each. In many disease states (e.g., thrombus [clot] formation, aberrant [abnormal] blood vessels, cervical rib syndrome, or aortic dissection), a pulse in one extremity will be unequal in strength or absent. It is acceptable to assess all symmetric pulses simultaneously except for the carotid pulse. Never measure both carotid pulses simultaneously because excessive pressure has potential to occlude blood supply to the brain. Do not reach across the patient's neck to count the carotid pulse (it is possible to occlude the patient's airway with the pressure of your arm). Measure the carotid pulse in the patient's neck on the side facing you.

It is possible to assess any artery for pulse rate, but the radial and carotid arteries are easily palpated peripheral pulse sites (Figure 4-7). People learning to

Table 4-3 Pulse Volume Variations

NUMBER	TYPE	DESCRIPTION
0	Absent pulse	None felt
1+	Thready pulse	Difficult to feel; not palpable when only slight pressure applied
2+	Weak pulse	Somewhat stronger than a thready pulse but not palpable when light pressure applied
3+	Normal pulse	Easily felt but not palpable when moderate pressure applied
4+	Bounding pulse	Feels full and springlike even under moderate pressure

Skill 4-2 Obtaining a Pulse Rate

Nursing Action *(Rationale)*

1. Perform hand hygiene. *(Decreases spread of microorganisms.)*
2. Introduce self to patient. *(Decreases patient's anxiety.)*
3. Identify patient by identification band. *(Verifies correct patient for procedure.)*
4. Explain procedure. *(Seeks cooperation and assistance from the patient and decreases patient's anxiety.)*
5. Prepare for procedure by doing the following:
   a. Assemble all necessary supplies, including a wristwatch with second hand. *(Organizes procedure.)*
   b. Provide privacy for the patient if necessary. *(Decreases patient's anxiety.)*
6. Implement procedure:
   Count pulse for 60 seconds.*
   a. Palpate pulse:
      (1) For **radial pulse,** lightly place tips of first and second fingers in groove formed along radial side of forearm, lateral to flexor tendon of wrist (see illustration). *(Pulse is relatively superficial and should not require deep palpation.)*
      (2) For **ulnar pulse,** place fingertips along ulnar side of forearm (see illustration). *(Palpated when arterial insufficiency to hand is expected or when nurse assesses effects radial occlusion might have on circulation to hand.)*

*It is the belief of the authors that a beginning student is unable to assess a pulse correctly in 15 or 30 seconds. A count of 60 seconds is necessary.

Continued

Skill 4-2 Obtaining a Pulse Rate—cont'd

(3) For **brachial pulse,** locate groove between biceps and triceps muscles above elbow at antecubital fossa. Place tips of first three fingers in muscle groove (see illustration). *(Artery runs along medial side of extended arm, requiring moderate palpation.)*

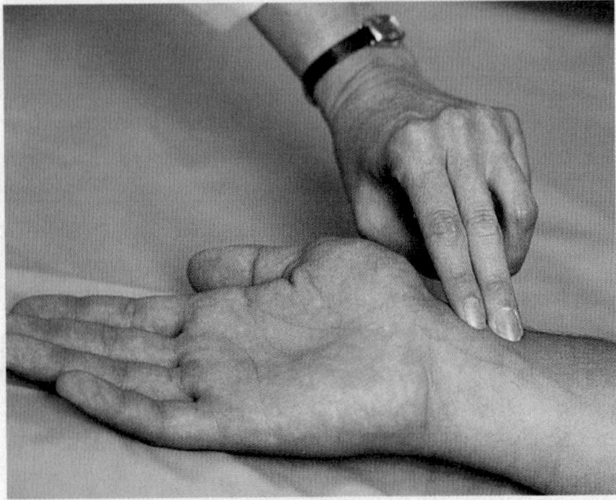

Step **6a(1)**

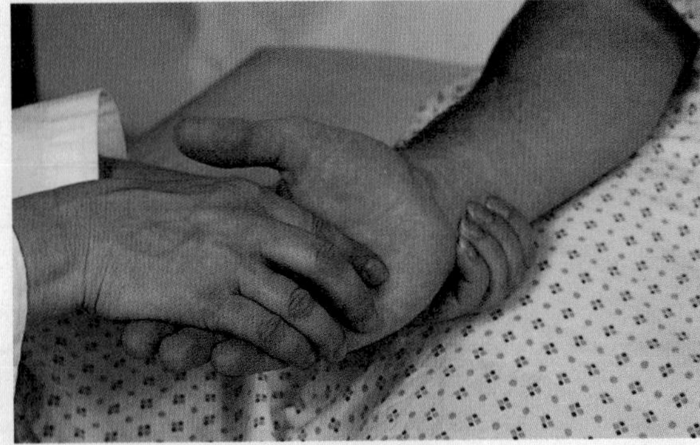

Step **6a(2)**

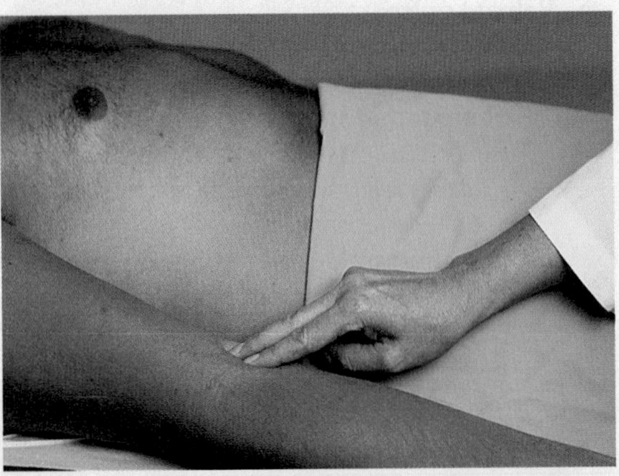

Step **6a(3)**

(4) For **femoral pulse,** with patient supine, place first three fingers over inguinal area below inguinal ligament, midway between pubic symphysis and anterosuperior iliac spine (see illustration). *(Supine position prevents flexion in groin area, which interferes with artery access.)*

(5) For **popliteal pulse,** instruct patient to slightly flex knee with foot resting on table or bed. Instruct patient to keep leg muscles relaxed. Palpate deeply into popliteal fossa with fingers of both hands placed just lateral to midline. It is also possible for patient to lie prone to achieve exposure of artery (see illustration). *(Flexion of knee and muscle relaxation improve accessibility of artery. Popliteal pulse is one of the more difficult pulses to palpate.)*

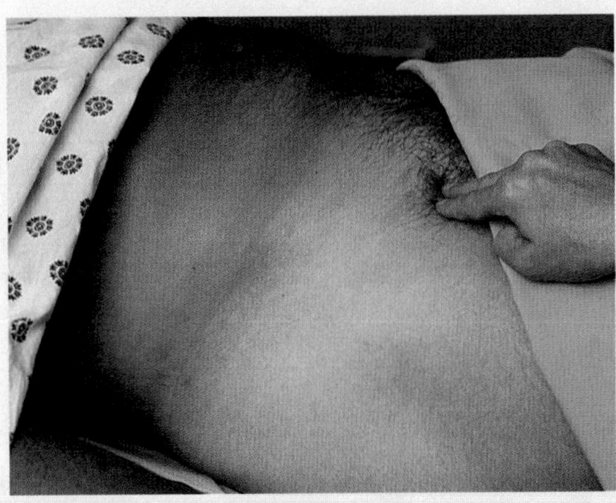

Step **6a(4)**

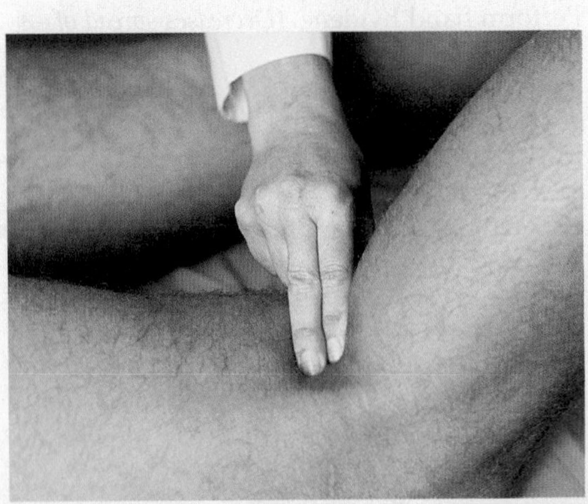

Step **6a(5)**

(6) For **dorsalis pedis pulse,** instruct patient to lie supine with feet relaxed. Gently place fingertips between great and first toes and slowly move them along groove between extensor tendons of great and first toes, until pulse is palpable (see illustration). *(Artery lies superficially and does not require deep palpation. Pulse is sometimes congenitally absent in healthy adults.)*

(7) For **posterior tibial pulse,** instruct patient to relax and slightly extend feet. Place fingertips behind and below medial malleolus (ankle bone) (see illustration). *(Artery is easily palpable with foot relaxed.)*

b. Determine strength of the pulse. Note thrust of vessel against fingertips. Strength equals volume of blood ejected against arterial wall with each heart contraction.

7. Write down radial pulse rate (for documentation later).
8. Perform hand hygiene. *(Reduces spread of microorganisms.)*
9. Document rate on graphic flow sheet (see Figure 4-1). *(Records procedure.)*
10. Follow up by reporting any abnormal pulse rates. *(Rate sometimes has to be reassessed.)*
11. Do patient teaching (see patient teaching in Health Promotion box on p. 58 and Skill 4-1).

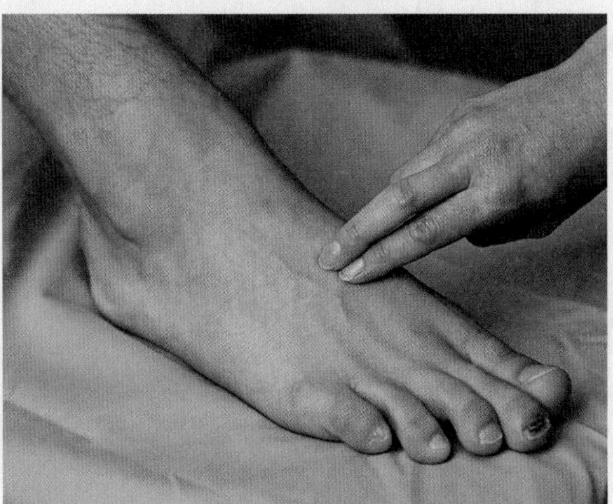

Step **6a(6)**

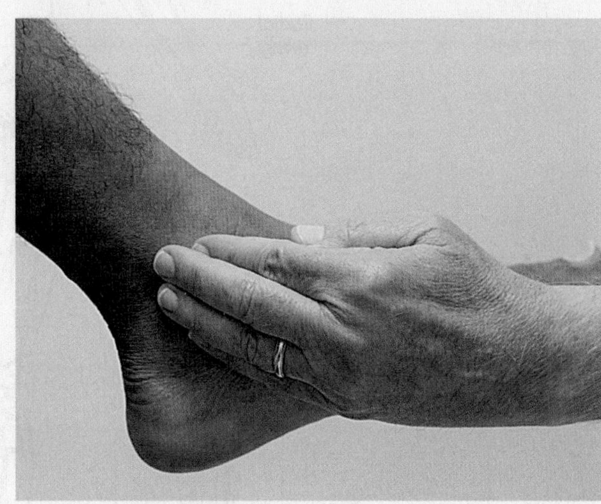

Step **6a(7)**

monitor their own heart rates (e.g., athletes) often use them. When a patient's condition suddenly deteriorates (Box 4-10), the carotid site is the best for finding a pulse quickly. The heart will continue delivering blood through the carotid artery to the brain as long as possible. When cardiac output declines significantly, peripheral pulses weaken and are difficult to palpate. (See Chapter 5 for further identification of the pulse sites.)

Obtain the radial pulse rate at the radial artery, which is located on the thumb side of the inner wrist. On initial assessment, palpate all major pulses and auscultate the apical rate. Major pulses include temporal, facial, carotid, brachial, radial, femoral, popliteal, and posterior tibial and dorsalis pedis (see Figure 4-7); the pulses provide both general and specific information. A pulse palpated at the dorsalis pedis, for example, indicates blood flow to the foot.

Auscultate the apical rate on all cardiac patients, as well as when the radial pulse is irregular or is difficult to palpate or when certain medications such as digoxin (Lanoxin) make this necessary (Skill 4-3). **Apical** refers to apex (the tip, the end, or the top of a structure) of the heart. The **apical pulse** represents the actual beating of the heart. Use the apical pulse site when taking the pulse rate of an infant. When you auscultate the apical rate, the "lubb-dupp" you hear represents one cardiac cycle, or heartbeat (Figures 4-8 and 4-9).

You will sometimes note a difference between the radial and apical rates. This is called a **pulse deficit.** To confirm a **pulse deficit,** one nurse listens to the apical rate, and a second nurse palpates the radial pulse at the same time, using the same watch for 1 full minute. There is a deficit when the radial rate is less than the apical rate. For example, an apical rate of 92 and a radial rate of 88 means there is a pulse deficit of 4. A pulse deficit signifies that the pumping action of the heart is faulty. This is often seen in atrial fibrillation.

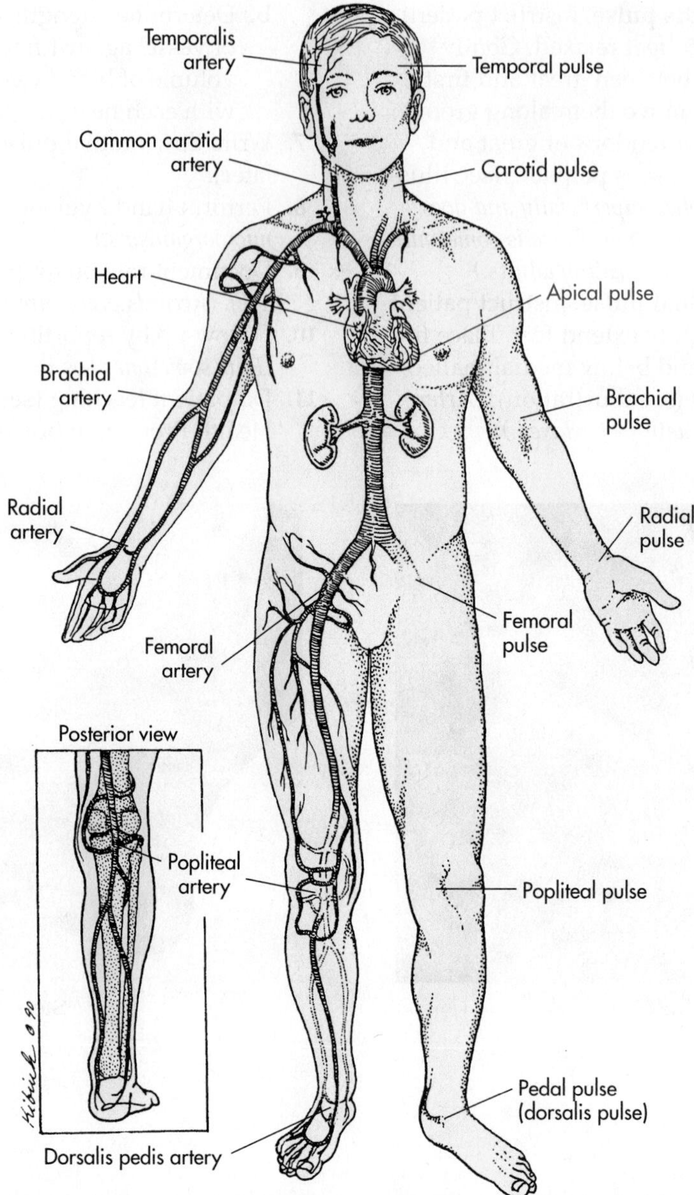

FIGURE 4-7 Pulse sites.

Box 4-10 Nursing Interventions for the Patient with an Abnormal Pulse

- If patient's pulse is weak or difficult to palpate, perform complete assessment of all peripheral pulses.
- Observe for symptoms associated with altered tissue perfusion, such as pallor or cyanosis of tissue distal to weak pulse and for coldness of extremity and any change in level of consciousness (LOC).
- Observe for factors associated with a decrease in cardiac output that results in diminished peripheral pulses such as hemorrhage, hypothermia, or heart muscle damage.
- If pulse is above normal, assess for related data such as pain, fear, anxiety, recent exercise, low blood pressure, elevated temperature, or inadequate oxygenation.
- Observe for symptoms such as dyspnea, fatigue, chest pain, orthopnea, syncope, cyanosis, or pallor of skin.
- If pulse is below normal, assess apical pulse and ascertain the presence of such factors as digoxin and antidysrhythmic medications. It is sometimes necessary to withhold medication pending the physician's evaluation of the situation.
- If the pulse is weak or irregular, assess apical pulse for a pulse deficit. Sometimes the physician orders an electrocardiogram or 24-hour heart monitor.
- When assessing for a pulse deficit, which sometimes indicates alteration in cardiac output, count the apical pulse while your colleague counts the radial pulse. Begin the assessment, counting out loud so you assess pulses simultaneously. The nurse with the watch should indicate when to begin counting, either by counting out loud or by another predetermined signal. This same nurse will indicate when to stop counting. If pulse count differs by more than two, a pulse deficit exists.

Skill 4-3 Obtaining an Apical Pulse Rate

Nursing Action *(Rationale)*

1. Perform hand hygiene. *(Reduces spread of microorganisms.)*
2. Introduce self to patient. *(Decreases patient's anxiety.)*
3. Identify patient by identification band. *(Ensures correct patient for procedure.)*
4. Explain procedure. *(Seeks cooperation and assistance from patient and decreases patient's anxiety.)*
5. Prepare for procedure by doing the following:
   a. Assembling all necessary supplies—stethoscope and watch with second hand. *(Organizes procedure.)*
   b. Providing privacy for patient if necessary. *(Decreases patient's anxiety.)*
6. Implement procedure:
   a. Clean earpiece and diaphragm of stethoscope with alcohol swab as necessary. *(Ensures instrument is clean and promotes auscultation.)*
   b. With patient in supine or sitting position, expose sternum and left side of chest. *(Exposes portion of chest wall for selection of auscultation site.)*
   c. Palpate angle of Louis, located just below suprasternal notch at point where horizontal ridge is felt along body of sternum. Place index finger just to right (patient's left) of sternum and palpate second intercostal space. Place next finger in intercostal space below, and proceed downward until fifth intercostal space is located. Move index finger horizontally along fifth intercostal space to left midclavicular line (see illustration). Palpate point of maximal impulse (PMI), also called the apical area. *(Use of anatomic landmarks allows correct placement of stethoscope over apex of heart. Position enhances ability to hear heart sounds clearly. PMI is over apex of heart.)*
   d. Place bell or diaphragm of stethoscope over PMI (apical area) (see illustration).
      (1) Count pulse rate for 60 seconds. *(Ensures accuracy.)*
      (2) Assist patient to dress. *(Provides for patient's comfort.)*
7. Write down pulse rate (for later documentation).
8. Perform hand hygiene. *(Reduces spread of microorganisms.)*
9. Document pulse rate on graphic flow sheet (e.g., P 83 ap) (see Figure 4-1).
10. Follow up by reporting an abnormal pulse rate (see Box 4-9).
11. Do patient teaching (see patient teaching in Health Promotion box on p. 58).

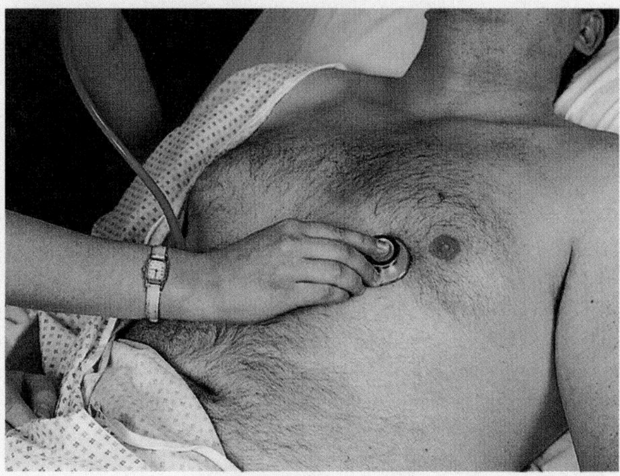

Step **6c, 6d**

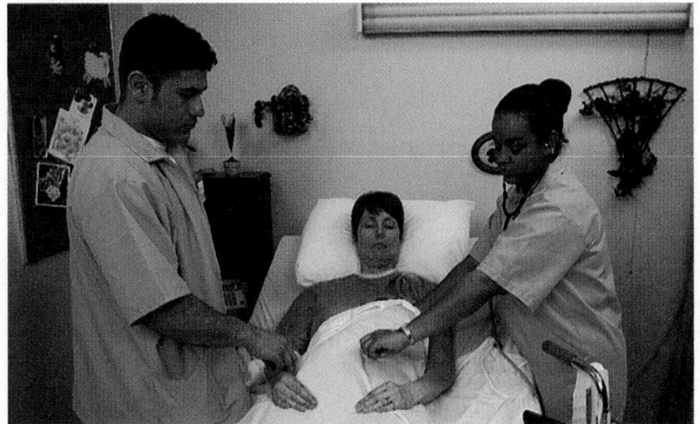

FIGURE 4-8 Taking an apical or radial pulse. One worker takes the apical pulse, and the other takes the radial pulse. NOTE: Two nurses are using the same watch.

RESPIRATION

RESPIRATORY FUNCTION

Respiration (the taking in of oxygen, its utilization in the tissues, and the giving off of carbon dioxide; the act of breathing, i.e., inhaling and exhaling) is both internal and external. Internal respiration refers to the exchange of gas at the tissue level caused by the process of cellular oxidation (any process in which the oxygen content of a compound is increased), as well as the gas exchange that occurs in the alveoli of the lungs. The breathing movements of the patient that you will observe are called *external respirations.* The cycle of external respirations has two parts: inspiration and expiration. **Inspiration** is inhaling air with oxygen into the lungs, and **expiration** is exhaling air with carbon diox-

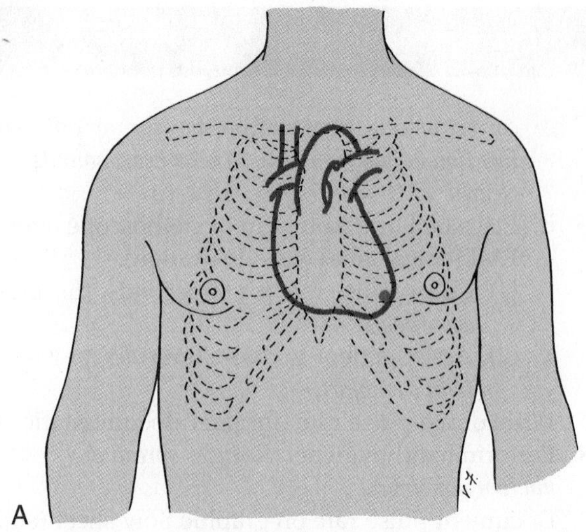

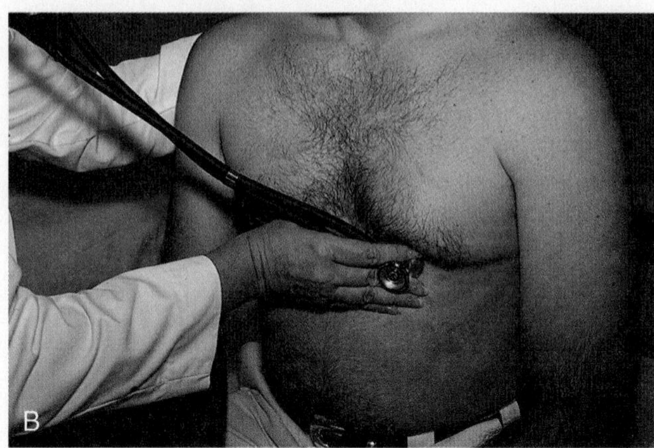

FIGURE 4-9 **A,** Point of maximum impulse is at fifth intercostal space. **B,** Assessing apical pulse.

ide out of the lungs. The rate of respiration is controlled by the medulla oblongata in the brain.

Any activity that increases metabolism (the aggregate of all chemical processes that take place in living organisms resulting in growth, generation of energy, elimination of wastes, and other bodily functions as they relate to the destruction of nutrients in the body after digestion) will increase the need for oxygen by the body and will increase respiratory rate.

The normal respiratory rate for an adult is between 12 and 20 respirations per minute (Boxes 4-11 and 4-12). The patient with a rapid respiratory rate has **tachypnea.** Exercise and fever increase respiratory rate. A slow respiratory rate, below 10 per minute, is

Box 4-11 Factors Influencing Respiration

DISEASE OR ILLNESS
Chronic lung disease (e.g., emphysema or bronchitis) alters the normal stimulus for ventilation. Lung tissue disease, reduced red blood cell levels, chest pain, kidney diseases, febrile disease, and diseases of the heart are a few of the conditions that alter the rate and the depth of respirations.

STRESS
An anxious or fearful patient will likely have increases in the rate and depth of respirations; as a result, it is possible for hyperventilation to occur.

FEVER
Hyperpyrexia (greatly elevated temperature) results in an abnormally rapid rate of breathing.

AGE
With growth from infancy to adulthood, the lungs' capacity increases and respiratory rate gradually declines. In older adults, lung capacity and depth of respirations decrease, and respiratory rate increases.

SEX
Men have a greater lung capacity than women.

BODY POSITION
In slumped or stooped positions, ventilation is often impaired, with a reduced depth of respirations. A straight, erect posture promotes full chest expansion. Lying flat should be avoided since full chest expansion is limited in this position.

MEDICATIONS
Narcotic analgesics depress the patient's ability to increase the volume of air inspired, and the rate of respirations is decreased. Other medications have the potential to increase or decrease the rate and depth of respirations and affect the rhythm. The rate and depth of respirations is increased with the use of amphetamines and cocaine. Conversely, bronchodilators cause dilation of the airways, causing the respiratory rate to decrease.

EXERCISE
Exercise increases the rate and the depth of respirations.

ACUTE PAIN
Pain increases the rate and the depth of respirations as a result of sympathetic stimulation; breathing becomes shallow.

SMOKING
Long-term smoking changes the lungs' airways, resulting in an increased respiratory rate.

BRAINSTEM INJURY
Injury to the brainstem impairs the respiratory center and inhibits respiratory rate and rhythm.

HEMOGLOBIN FUNCTION
Respiratory rate and depth are increased by conditions caused by decreased hemoglobin function. Examples include anemia, in which the blood's oxygen-carrying capacity is limited, and increased altitude, in which the amount of saturated hemoglobin is reduced.

Box 4-12 Nursing Interventions for the Patient with Abnormal Respirations

- Occasional periods of apnea are a symptom of underlying disease in the adult and must be reported to the physician or nurse in charge. Irregular respirations and short apneic spells of less than 20 seconds are normal in a newborn.
- Position of discomfort may cause patient to breathe more rapidly. Assess patients with difficulty breathing (dyspnea) such as those with heart failure or abdominal ascites or who are in late stages of pregnancy in the position of greatest comfort.
- Repositioning may increase the work of breathing, which will increase respiratory rate; allow for a period of rest.
- Respiratory rate less than 10 or more than 20 breaths per minute and shallow and slow respirations (hypoventilation) is likely to necessitate immediate intervention.
- See Chapter 42, for discussion of inspirometry.
- See Chapter 49, for discussion of pulse oximetry and assessment of adequate oxygenation.
- Observe for related factors such as obstructed airway or stertorous respirations.
- Observe for related signs and symptoms such as cyanotic nailbeds, lips, or mucous membranes; restlessness; irritability; confusion; dyspnea; shortness of breath; productive cough; and abnormal breath sounds.
- Consider possible effects of anesthesia or medications such as opioids.
- Assist patient to a supported sitting position (semi-Fowler's or full Fowler's, unless contraindicated).
- Provide oxygen as ordered by physician (see Chapter 20) if patient shows signs of respiratory distress.

known as **bradypnea.** The depth of respiration is determined by the amount of air taken in with inhalation. Normally, 500 mL of air is inspired with each breath. The diaphragm (a dome-shaped musculofibrous partition that separates the thoracic and abdominal cavities) aids respirations by moving down during inspiration and moving up during expiration. The proper rhythm of respiration is regular and uninterrupted. Occasional sighing is normal and allows all alveoli (plural for alveolus, an air cell of the lungs where gases are exchanged in respirations) to be aerated. Normal respirations are not audible except with the aid of a stethoscope.

ASSESSMENT OF RESPIRATION

In assessing respirations, note the rate, the depth, the quality, and the rhythm (Skill 4-4). Movement by the diaphragm and the intercostal muscles allows you to judge the depth of respirations. Shallow respirations make ventilation difficult to observe, and only a small amount of air is exchanged in the lungs. **Dyspnea** is breathing with difficulty. It is possible that the patient is laboring to get enough oxygen, with pursed lips, flared nostrils, and clavicular and costal retractions (the visible sinking-in of the soft tissues of the chest between and around the firmer tissues of the cartilaginous and body ribs, as occurs with increased inspiratory effort).

Also assess patterns of breathing (Figure 4-10). Apnea is a lack of spontaneous respirations. **Cheyne-Stokes respirations** are an abnormal pattern of respiration characterized by alternating periods of apnea and deep, rapid breathing. The periods of apnea increase as time goes on. Cheyne-Stokes respirations are noted in the critically or terminally ill patient. Hyperventilation is when the rate of ventilation exceeds normal metabolic requirements for exchange of respiratory gases, such as during emotional trauma. Volume and depth of respirations increase. Hypoventilation occurs when the rate of ventilation entering the lungs is insufficient for metabolic needs. Respiratory rate is below normal, and depth of ventilation is depressed. One situation in which hypoventilation is seen is after open cholecystectomy is performed, when deep breathing results in discomfort.

The best time to assess respirations is when counting a radial or an apical pulse. The patient will be unaware you are doing so and will not consciously alter respirations.

BLOOD PRESSURE

FACTORS DETERMINING BLOOD PRESSURE

The **blood pressure** is the pressure exerted by the circulating volume of blood on the arterial walls, the veins, and the chambers of the heart. Blood pressure is mea-

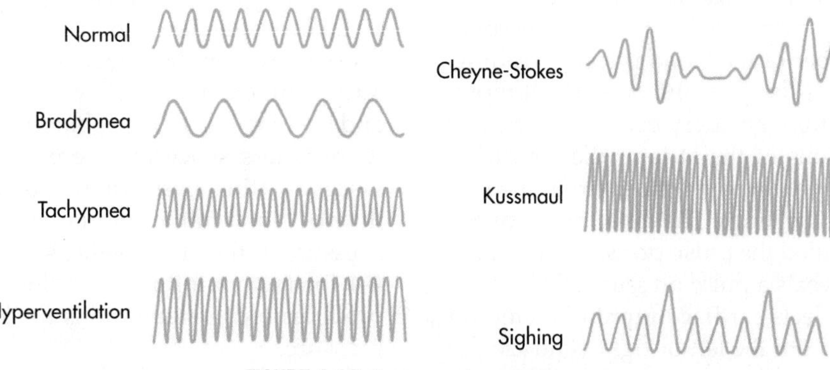

FIGURE 4-10 Patterns of respirations.

Skill 4-4 Obtaining a Respiratory Rate

Nursing Action *(Rationale)*

1. Perform hand hygiene. *(Reduces spread of microorganisms.)*
2. Introduce self to patient. *(Decreases patient's anxiety.)*
3. Identify patient by identification band. *(Verifies correct patient for procedure.)*
4. Explain procedure. *(Seeks cooperation and assistance from patient and decreases patient's anxiety.)*
5. Prepare for procedure:
   a. Assemble all necessary supplies, including a wristwatch with a second hand. *(Organizes procedure efficiently.)*
   b. Provide privacy for patient if necessary. *(Decreases patient's anxiety.)*
   c. If patient has been active, wait 5 to 10 minutes. *(Exercise increases respiratory rate and depth.)*
   d. Be certain patient is in a position of comfort, preferably sitting or lying supine with the head of the bed elevated 45 to 60 degrees, if patient can tolerate it. *(Discomfort causes the patient to breathe more rapidly. The erect, sitting position promotes full ventilation.)*
6. Implement procedure:
   a. Place fingertip as if to obtain a radial pulse (see illustration). Because patients sometimes unconsciously alter the respiratory rate when being observed, it is best to obtain the respiratory rate at the same time as the radial pulse reading.
   b. Observe respiratory rate for 60 seconds. *(Ensures accuracy.)* Count each rise of the chest wall. One inhalation and exhalation = one respiration.
   c. Provide for patient comfort. *(Promotes patient's self-esteem.)*
7. Write down rate (for documentation later).
8. Perform hand hygiene. *(Reduces spread of microorganisms.)*
9. Document the rate on the graphic flow sheet (see Figure 4-1).
10. Follow up by reporting any abnormal respiratory rates (see Box 4-11). *(Rate sometimes has to be reassessed.)*
11. Do patient teaching (see patient teaching in Health Promotion box on p. 58).

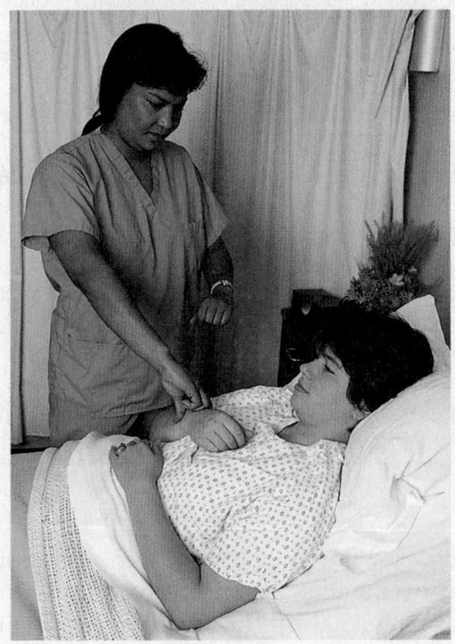

Step **6a**

sured in millimeters of mercury (mm Hg). Two pressures are actually elements of what we call *blood pressure.* The **systolic** pressure is the higher number and represents the ventricles contracting, forcing blood into the aorta and the pulmonary arteries. The occurrence of systole is indicated by the first sound heard on auscultation. The lower number of the blood pressure reading, the second pressure, is the **diastolic** pressure. It represents the pressure within the artery between beats, that is, between contractions of the atria or the ventricles, when blood enters the relaxed chambers from the systemic circulation and the lungs. The difference between the two readings is called the **pulse pressure.** A reading of 120/80 mm Hg reveals a pulse pressure of 40.

Blood pressure reflects **cardiac output** (the amount of blood discharged from the left or right ventricle per minute), the quality of the arteries, the blood volume, and blood viscosity. When blood is pumped by the heart into the arteries, the pressure within the arteries rises. The greater the amount of blood pumped by the heart, the greater the pressure.

Likewise, if the blood volume is increased, the pressure within the artery will increase. When the arteries' lumens (channels within the arteries) narrow and become less flexible, blood pressure rises because there is less space for the blood to enter. Increased viscosity (thickness) of the blood causes a slower flow of blood in the capillaries, which causes backup pressure in the larger vessels. See Box 4-13 and Table 4-4 for factors influencing blood pressure. Table 4-5 provides recommendations for a follow-up on blood pressure.

Box 4-13 Factors Influencing Blood Pressure

Normal blood pressure levels vary throughout life.

Age	*Blood Pressure (mm Hg)*
Newborn (3000 g [6.6 lb])	Mean 36-40
1 month	85/54
1 year	95/65
6 years	105/65
10-13 years	110/65
14-17 years	<120/75
18 years and up	<120/80

In children and adolescents, hypertension is defined as blood pressure that is, on repeated measurement, at the 95th percentile or greater, adjusted for age, height, and sex.

Anxiety, fear, pain, and emotional stress. May increase blood pressure because of increased heart rate and increased peripheral vascular resistance.

Medications. Can either lower or increase blood pressure depending on their pharmacologic action.

Hormones. Variations in blood pressure may be manifested as a person ages because of hormonal alterations. Pregnancy may cause mild to severe elevations in blood pressure.

Diurnal (happening daily). Variations may include a lower blood pressure in the morning, rising throughout the day, peaking in late afternoon or evening, and lowering at night; individual variations are significant.

Race. The rate of hypertension is higher in urban blacks than in European Americans. Hypertension-related deaths are also higher among blacks. The tendency for this population to have hypertension is believed to be genetically and environmentally related.

Sex. There is no clinically significant difference in blood pressure levels between boys and girls. After puberty, males tend to have higher blood pressure readings. After menopause, women tend to have higher levels of blood pressure than men of similar age.

Data from the National High Blood Pressure Education Program (NHBPEP) National Heart, Lung, and Blood Institute; National Institutes of Health, the seventh report of the Joint National Committee on Detection, Evaluation, and Treatment of High Blood Pressure. (2003) *JAMA,* 289(19):2560; and American Heart Association, "Am I at Risk?" April 1, 2009; accessed from http://www.americanheart.org/presenter.jhtml?identifier=2142. Accessed July 8, 2009.

Table 4-4 Classification of Blood Pressure for Adults Ages 18 and Over

CATEGORY	SYSTOLIC (mm Hg)*		DIASTOLIC (mm Hg)*
Normal	<120		<80
Prehypertension†	120-139	or	80-89
Hypertension	140 or higher	or	90 or higher

Data from the American Heart Association Recommendations on high blood pressure (2003), accessed March 24, 2009, from www.americanheart.org.
*Treatment based on highest category.
†Based on average of two or more readings taken at each of two or more visits after initial screening. Patient is not taking antihypertensive drugs and not acutely ill. When systolic and diastolic blood pressure fall into different categories, the higher category should be selected to classify the individual's blood pressure status. For example, 162/92 mm Hg should be classified as stage 2 hypertension.

Table 4-5 Recommendations for Blood Pressure Follow-Up

INITIAL BLOOD PRESSURE	FOLLOW-UP RECOMMENDED*
Normal	Recheck in 2 years
Prehypertension	Recheck in 1 year†
Stage 1 hypertension	Confirm within 2 months†
Stage 2 hypertension	Evaluate or refer to source of care within 1 month. For those with higher pressure (e.g., >180/110 mm Hg), evaluate and treat immediately or within 1 week, depending on clinical situation and presence of complications.

From Perry, A., & Potter, P. (2006). *Clinical nursing skills & techniques* (6th ed.). St. Louis: Elsevier.
*Modify the scheduling of follow-up according to reliable information about past blood pressure measurements, other cardiovascular risk factors, and target organ damage.
†Provide advice about lifestyle modifications.

The optimal blood pressure reading for a healthy middle-aged adult is less than 120/80 mm Hg. Values of 120-139/80-89 mm Hg are considered *prehypertensive.* **Hypertension** occurs when the elevated pressure is sustained above 140/90 mm Hg. The diagnosis of hypertension in adults is not made with only one random elevated reading. For this diagnosis, an average of 90 mm Hg or higher of two or more diastolic readings on at least two subsequent visits is necessary, or an average higher than 140 mm Hg of two or more systolic readings on at least two visits. Primary, or essential, hypertension is the most common form. The cause is unknown but is believed to be related to aging. Risk factors also contribute; consider their significance when doing patient teaching. These risk factors include family history of hypertension, obesity, smoking, heavy alcohol consumption, elevated blood cholesterol level, and continued exposure to stress.

A blood pressure below normal is **hypotension.** It is considered healthy to have a low blood pressure providing there are no ill effects, such as vertigo (dizziness) or syncope (fainting). **Orthostatic hypotension** (a drop of 25 mm Hg in systolic pressure and a drop of 10 mm Hg in diastolic pressure when a person moves from a lying to a sitting or from a sitting to a standing position) occurs when a person rises too quickly, usually from a supine position. The patient frequently feels lightheaded and unstable. Advise the patient to rise slowly from lying to sitting to standing, thus preventing blood volume from shifting suddenly (Box 4-14). Hypotension resulting from shock or massive hemorrhage is very serious and necessitates immedi-

Box 4-14 Measurement of Orthostatic Blood Pressure

Some patients, especially those who are older or taking certain medications, will experience a drop in blood pressure and/or an increase in pulse when changing from a lying to a sitting or from a sitting to a standing position.

Certain medications, including many antiseizure medications, antipsychotics, and antihypertensives, commonly cause orthostatic hypotension. Patients taking these medications often have a routine order to have orthostatic blood pressure readings taken.

1. Obtaining orthostatic blood pressure measurements requires critical thinking and ongoing nursing judgment; do not delegate this task.
2. Obtain supine patient's blood pressure in each arm. Select arm with highest systolic reading for subsequent measurements.
3. Leaving blood pressure cuff in place, assist patient to sitting position. After 1 to 3 minutes with patient in sitting position, obtain blood pressure. If orthostatic symptoms occur, such as dizziness, weakness, lightheadedness, feeling faint, or sudden pallor, terminate blood pressure measurement and assist patient to a supine position.
4. Leaving blood pressure cuff in place, assist patient to standing position and obtain blood pressure. If orthostatic symptoms occur (see above), terminate blood pressure measurement and assist patient to a supine position. In most cases, orthostatic hypotension will be detectable within 1 minute of standing.
5. Record patient's blood pressure in each position, for example, "140/80 supine, 132/72 sitting, 108/60 standing." Note any additional symptoms or complaints.
6. Report findings of orthostatic hypotension or orthostatic symptoms to physician or nurse in charge. Instruct patient to obtain assistance when getting out of bed if orthostatic hypotension is present or orthostatic symptoms occur.

ate medical intervention. See Table 4-6 for conditions causing alterations in blood pressure.

OBTAINING BLOOD PRESSURE MEASUREMENTS

Blood pressure readings are taken with a **sphygmomanometer** and a stethoscope. A sphygmomanometer (a device for measuring the arterial blood pressure) consists of an inflatable cuff and a gauge. The gauge is aneroid (use of mercury-calibrated manometers is no longer advised) (see Box 4-8) (Figures 4-11 and 4-12). Inflate the cuff around the patient's arm to compress the artery, which will occlude blood flow; then slowly deflate it, which will allow blood flow to resume (see the Evidence-Based Practice box). While you do this, listen at the brachial artery with the stethoscope to hear pulsating sounds. These are called **Korotkoff sounds.** The sounds go through five phases (Figure 4-13). When you hear the first sound, make a mental note of the point you see on the sphygmomanometer gauge, and note again the point at which the sound disappears. That first point is the systolic pressure, and the second is the diastolic pressure.

As you lower the pressure, the Korotkoff sounds sometimes seem to disappear temporarily. In this case, listen for a subtle difference in the quality of what you hear as the manometer approaches the diastolic reading. In patients with hypertension, the sounds usually heard over the brachial artery disappear as pressure is reduced and then reappear at a lower level. This temporary disappearance of sound is the auscultatory

Table 4-6 Conditions Causing Alterations in Blood Pressure

CONDITION	EFFECT	CAUSE
Hemorrhage	Lowers pressure	Decreased blood volume
Increased intracranial pressure	Raises pressure	Disturbance of cardiovascular control mechanisms in brainstem resulting from pressure exerted on the medulla oblongata
Acute pain	Raises pressure	Increased vasomotor tone and peripheral vascular resistance as a result of sympathetic stimulation
End-stage renal disease	Raises pressure	Increased blood volume resulting from increased retention of sodium and water; release of renin, a vasopressor that increases peripheral vascular resistance
Primary essential hypertension	Raises pressure	Increased peripheral vascular resistance resulting from progressive thickening of arterial walls
General anesthesia	Lowers pressure	Decreased vasomotor tone resulting from depression of vasomotor center in brainstem
Exercise	Raises pressure	Increased cardiac output
Postural change	Lowers pressure	Decreased blood volume as person moves from lying to sitting or standing position; normally, variations are minimal
Smoking	Raises pressure	Increased vasoconstriction

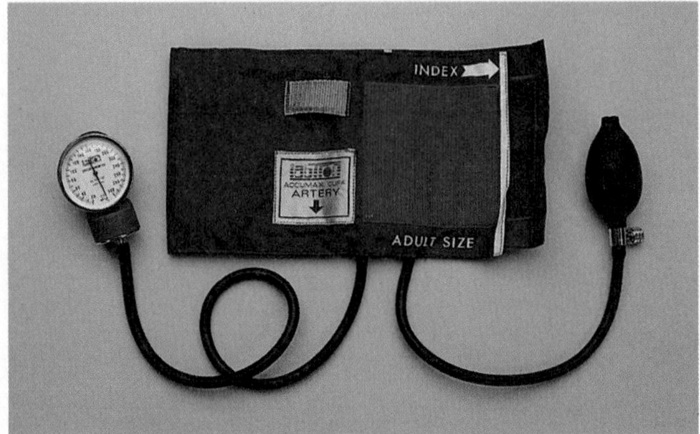

FIGURE 4-11 Aneroid manometer and cuff.

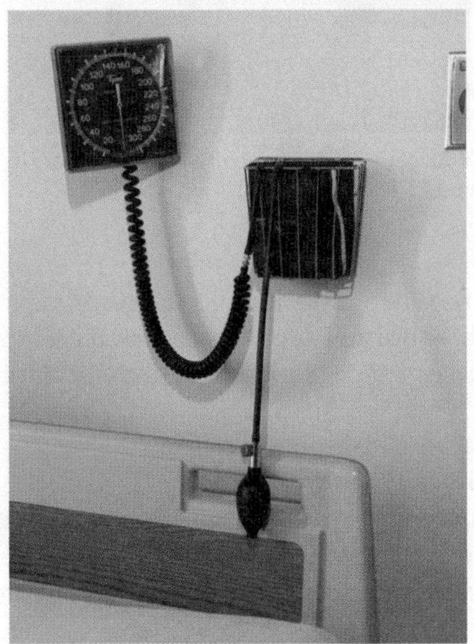

FIGURE 4-12 Wall-mounted aneroid sphygmomanometer.

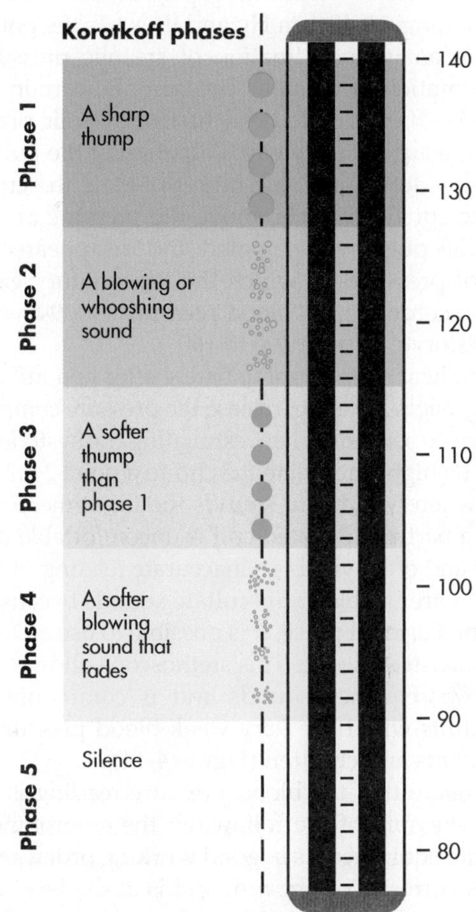

FIGURE 4-13 The sounds auscultated during blood pressure measurement can be differentiated into five Korotkoff phases. In this example, blood pressure is 140/90 mm Hg.

Evidence-Based Practice Forearm Versus Upper Arm Blood Pressure Measurements

Evidence Summary

Blood pressure measurement is an important factor when determining the diagnosis of hypertension and evaluating therapies. Because hypertension leads to serious complications, eliminating errors in measuring blood pressure is important. When the upper arm is not accessible or when the blood pressure (BP) cuff does not fit the patient's upper arm, the forearm has been used for BP measurement. In this research study BP measurements taken on the forearm and the upper arm were compared when patients were supine and when the head of the bed was elevated at 45 degrees. The researchers wanted to know if placement of the BP cuff affected systolic and diastolic BP. Two hundred twenty-one medical surgical inpatients had their BP measured at both arm locations in the supine and head-elevated positions. Researchers selected cuff size based on forearm and upper arm circumference. Results indicated a significant difference between upper arm and forearm blood pressures in both positions. Both systolic and diastolic blood pressure differed as much as 33 mm Hg.

Application to Nursing Practice

- A consistent approach to the placement of upper extremity blood pressure cuff allows accurate assessment of change in condition.
- Appropriate cuff size is essential for accurate measurement.
- You cannot substitute forearm BP measurements for upper arm blood pressure measurements.

Reference

Schell, K., et al. (2006). Clinical comparison of automatic noninvasive measurements of blood pressure in the forearm and upper arm with the client supine or with the head of the bed raised 45 degrees: a follow-up study, *American Journal of Critical Care,* 15(2):196.

From Potter, P.A. & Perry, A.G. (2009). *Fundamentals of nursing: concepts, process, and practice.* (7th ed.). St. Louis: Mosby.

gap. It typically occurs between the first and the second Korotkoff sounds. The gap in sound sometimes covers a range of 40 mm Hg and thus has the potential to cause an underestimation of systolic pressure or overestimation of diastolic pressure. Be certain to inflate the cuff enough to hear the true systolic pressure before the auscultatory gap. Palpation of the radial artery helps determine how high to inflate the cuff. Inflate the cuff 30 mm Hg above the pressure at which the radial pulse was palpated and disappeared. The range of pressures in which the auscultatory gap occurs is recorded (e.g., "blood pressure 190/94, with an auscultatory gap from 190 to 160").

If you hear sounds immediately after you inflate the cuff and begin listening, release the pressure completely and wait 60 seconds. Then, estimating the systolic pressure to be higher, reinflate the cuff to a point 30 mm Hg above where you heard sounds the first time. Reinflation of a partially deflated cuff is uncomfortable for the patient and often yields an inaccurate reading.

If you are unable to auscultate sounds because of a weakened arterial pulse, it is possible to use a Doppler ultrasonic stethoscope. This stethoscope allows you to hear low-frequency sounds and is commonly used with adults who have very weak blood pressure and with infants and children (Figure 4-14).

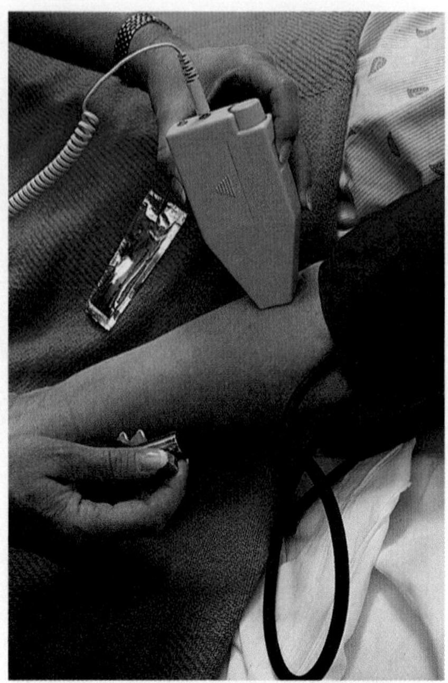

FIGURE 4-14 Doppler stethoscope over brachial artery to measure blood pressure.

To ensure that the blood pressure reading is accurate, make sure of the following: the environment is quiet, the equipment is in good working order, and the cuff fits correctly on the arm and is at the level of the heart. Have the gauge in plain view, not off to the side of the arm. Have the patient lying down or sitting up with both feet flat on the floor (legs not crossed) (Skill 4-5). See Box 4-15 for nursing interventions for the patient with abnormal blood pressure reading. See Box 4-16 for assessment of blood pressure in both arms.

Assessment of Blood Pressure in the Lower Extremities

Occasionally, dressings, casts, intravenous catheters, or other devices make the upper extremities inaccessible, so you will have to measure blood pressure in

Skill 4-5 Obtaining a Blood Pressure Reading

Nursing Action *(Rationale)*

1. Perform hand hygiene. *(Reduces spread of microorganisms.)*
2. Introduce self. *(Decreases patient's anxiety.)*
3. Identify patient by identification band. *(Verifies correct patient for procedure.)*
4. Explain procedure. *(Seeks cooperation and assistance from patient and decreases patient's anxiety.)*
5. Determine whether patient has ingested caffeine or has been smoking. *(If so, wait 30 minutes before assessment, since caffeine and smoking can cause false elevations.)*
6. Prepare for procedure:
   a. Assemble all necessary supplies, sphygmomanometer, and stethoscope. *(Organizes procedure efficiently.)* Determine the correct cuff size. *(An improper size will give an inaccurate reading.)* The cuff should be approximately 40% of the circumference of the extremity on which the cuff is to be used. *(A higher, inaccurate reading will be obtained if too small a cuff is used; a lower, inaccurate reading will be obtained if too large a cuff is used.)*
   b. Provide privacy. *(Decreases patient's anxiety.)*
   c. Request that patient assume sitting or lying position. Be certain room is quiet and warm. *(Maintains comfort.)*
   d. Determine site for blood pressure measurement. Do not apply cuff to arm when in the following situations *(applying the cuff would complicate these preexisting conditions)*:
      (1) Catheter is in antecubital fossa and fluids are infusing.
      (2) Arteriovenous shunt is in place.

(3) Breast or axillary surgery has been performed on that side.
(4) An arm or hand has been traumatized or is diseased.
(5) A lower arm cast or bulky bandage is in place.

7. Implement procedure:
   a. Apply cuff to bare arm with patient's palm facing upward. Do not hyperextend. The cuff is applied 1 to 2 inches above the antecubital space (see illustrations). The cuff is centered over the brachial artery. The patient's upper arm is held at the level of the heart, and the lower arm is rested on a firm surface. *(Ensures accuracy of procedure.)*
   b. Palpate radial artery (see illustration in Skill 4-2).
   c. Inflate cuff. Note the point on the manometer gauge when the radial pulse is obliterated. *(This is the approximate systolic pressure.)*
   d. Deflate the cuff. *(Deflating the cuff allows congestion to leave the arm, preventing a false-high reading.)* Rest arm for 1 minute.
   e. Palpate the brachial artery and place the bell or the diaphragm of the stethoscope over it.
   f. Reinflate cuff to 30 mm Hg above point at which radial artery was obliterated. *(Avoids the auscultatory gap.)* Estimating prevents false-low readings that will possibly result from the presence of this auscultatory gap (inaudible sounds below the systolic pressure). This phenomenon occurs in about 5% of adults and is prevalent in individuals with hypertension.
   g. Slowly deflate cuff. Cuff is deflated at a rate of 2 mm Hg per second. Note the point at which the pulse is heard. *(This is the systolic pressure.)* Note the point at which no pulse is heard. *(This is the diastolic pressure.)*
   h. When the Korotkoff sounds are no longer audible, continue to listen for another 10 to 20 mm Hg. *(Confirms blood pressure reading. Too-rapid deflation often causes a measurement error.)*
   i. Completely deflate and remove the cuff.
   j. Assist the patient to dress. *(Provides patient comfort.)*
8. Write down reading (for documentation later).
9. Perform hand hygiene. *(Reduces spread of microorganisms.)*
10. Document reading on graphic flow sheet (e.g., blood pressure 120/80 mm Hg) (see Figure 4-1).
11. Follow up by reporting abnormal readings immediately (see Box 4-16 for assessment of blood pressure in both arms, and Box 4-14 for assessment of orthostatic blood pressure). *(Reading sometimes has to be reassessed.)*
12. Do patient teaching (see patient teaching in Health Promotion box on p. 58).

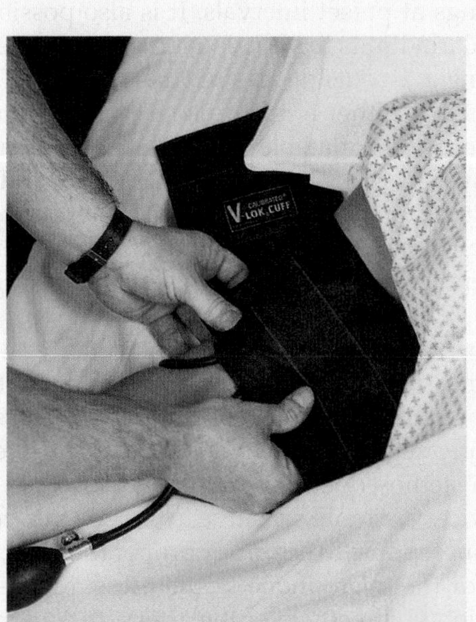

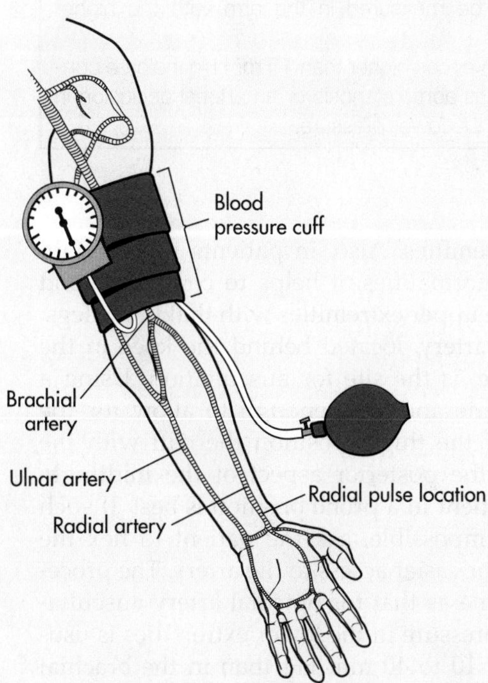

Step 7a Location of the brachial artery and placement of the cuff.

Box 4-15 Nursing Interventions for the Patient with Abnormal Blood Pressure Reading

- Repeat assessment, but first eliminate extraneous noise, such as television and conversation. Noise interferes with accuracy. Falsely elevated readings will be obtained if patient moves, talks, or coughs during blood pressure measurement.
- If you hear sounds immediately, release the pressure, wait 60 seconds, and estimate systolic pressure at higher reading. Reinflate cuff 30 mm Hg above the sound first heard. Reinflation of a partially deflated cuff is uncomfortable for the patient and often yields an inaccurate reading.
- Patient should be seated or lying in a quiet environment, free from temperature extremes, for at least 5 minutes before blood pressure is obtained. This is a good time to discuss with patient the benefits of exercise and weight control in reducing the risks for hypertension and coronary artery disease or lowering an existing blood pressure elevation.
- Electronic blood pressure cuff and machine must be matched by the manufacturer. Do not interchange blood pressure cuffs from machines of different manufacturers.
- Because blood pressure measurement can frighten children, this is a good time to prepare the child for the squeezing feeling of the inflated blood pressure cuff by saying, "This will feel like a tight hug for a minute," or "This will feel like a rubber band on your finger."
- If using an electronic blood pressure machine, tell the patient and family that these machines have audible alarm systems. Explain and allow the patient to hear sound. Inform patient that "the alarms do not always mean you have a problem, but also show that the machine needs attention."
- If an abnormal blood pressure reading is obtained, measure blood pressure on the other arm or on a lower extremity or use an ultrasonic Doppler instrument (see Figure 4-14).
- Ask another nurse to reassess readings.
- If blood pressure is above normal, observe for related symptoms such as headache (usually occipital), flushed face, and epistaxis (nosebleed). Older patients may notice fatigue.
- Be certain size of cuff is appropriate.
- Administer medications as ordered.
- Compare your current reading with the patient's baseline.
- If blood pressure is below normal, observe for symptoms such as weak, thready pulse; weakness; vertigo; confusion; pale, dusky, or cyanotic skin; or cool, mottled skin.
- Position patient in supine position and limit activity.
- Increase rate of intravenous fluid if infusing.

Box 4-16 Assessing Blood Pressure in Both Arms

- For the initial assessment, measure blood pressure in both arms, especially if the patient has heart disease or if the reading in the first arm is abnormal.
- Normally, a difference of 5 to 10 mm Hg exists between the arms. In subsequent assessments, the blood pressure should be measured in the arm with the higher pressure.
- Pressure differences higher than 10 mm Hg indicate conditions such as aortic stenosis or an arterial occlusion in the arm with the lower pressure.

the lower extremities. Also, in patients with certain circulatory abnormalities, it helps to compare blood pressure in the upper extremities with that in the legs. The popliteal artery, located behind the knee in the popliteal space, is the site for auscultation. Using a cuff that is wide and long enough to allow for the larger girth of the thigh, position the cuff with the bladder over the posterior aspect of the midthigh. Placing the patient in a prone position is best. If such a position is impossible, ask the patient to flex the knee slightly for easier access to the artery. The procedure is the same as that for brachial artery auscultation. Systolic pressure in the lower extremities is usually higher by 10 to 40 mm Hg than in the brachial artery, but the diastolic pressure is essentially the same (Figure 4-15, *A* and *B*).

Automatic Measurement Devices

There are many electronic devices that determine blood pressure automatically (Figures 4-16 and 4-17). On medical-surgical floors, in operating rooms, postanesthesia care units, intensive care units, and postpartum units (see Coordinated Care box), their use is now frequent.

Once the cuff is applied, it is possible to program the device to obtain and record blood pressure readings at preset intervals. It is also possible to program alarm limits to alert you if the blood pressure measurement is outside desired parameters. The system includes either a microphone or a pressure sensor built into the inflatable cuff. The microphone or acoustic system picks up Korotkoff sounds and registers diastolic and systolic readings. The pressure sensor or the ultrasonic system responds to the pressure waves generated by the movement of blood through the artery.

The advantages of automatic devices are the ease of use and efficiency when repeated or when frequent measurements are indicated. The automatic blood pressure cuff is also useful for home use if the patient or caregiver has hearing difficulties. The ability to use a stethoscope is not required. However, automatic devices are more sensitive to outside interference and are susceptible to error. For proper function, it is necessary for the microphone or the pressure sensor to be positioned directly over the artery. Patient movements, vibration, or outside noise have the potential to interfere with the microphone or the sensor signal. Most auto-

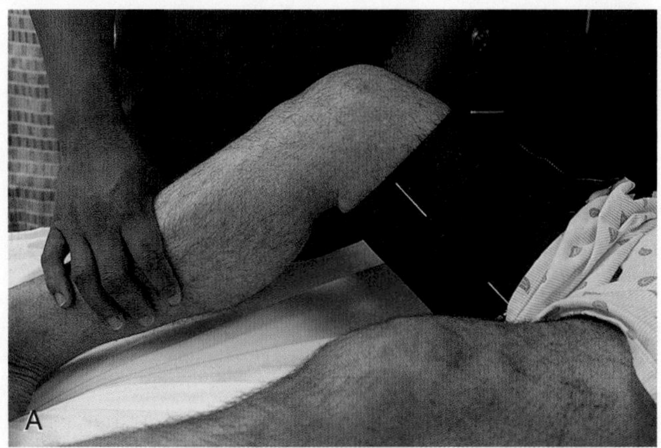

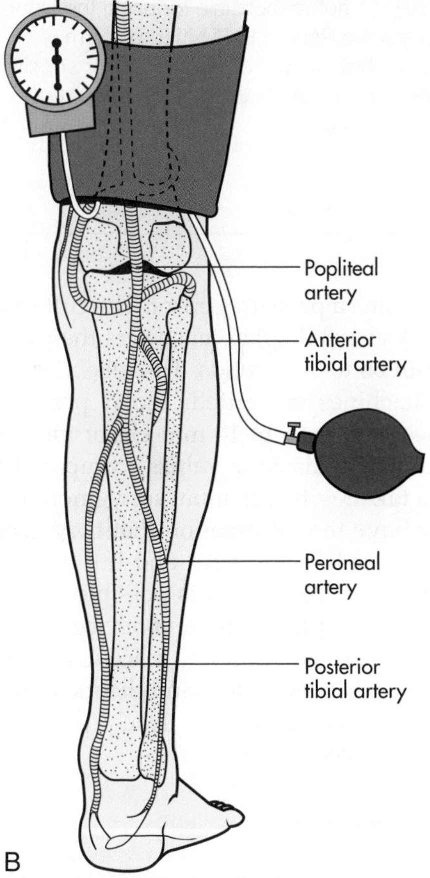

FIGURE 4-15 **A,** Lower-extremity blood pressure cuff positioned above popliteal artery at midthigh. **B,** Location of the popliteal artery and placement of the cuff.

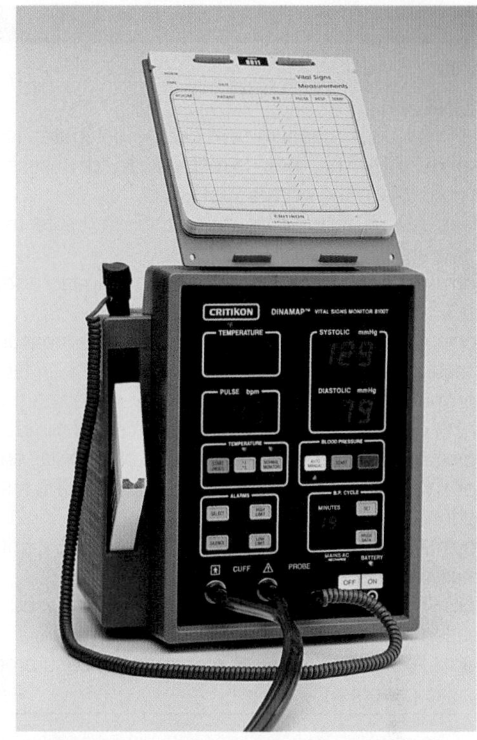

FIGURE 4-16 Monitor displays blood pressure reading.

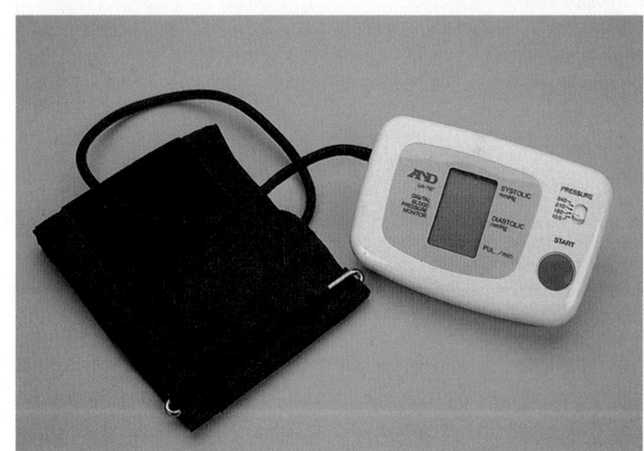

FIGURE 4-17 Electronic sphygmomanometer.

matic blood pressure devices are unable to process sounds or vibrations of low blood pressure (Box 4-17). In addition, the range of device sophistication sometimes makes it difficult to compare blood pressure measurements.

The use of automatic blood pressure devices permits assessment of blood pressure during interpersonal interactions. Nonetheless, avoid speaking to the patient for at least a minute before initiating a blood pressure recording. Talking to a patient when the blood pressure is being assessed increases readings 10% to 40%.

Self-Measurement

More people today measure their own blood pressure, thanks to improved technology in home monitoring devices and a greater interest in health promotion. Two of the more common types of devices the general public uses are portable home devices and stationary automated machines.

Coordinated Care

Supervision

VITAL SIGNS

The skill of vital signs measurement can be delegated to assistive personnel (AP). The nurse is responsible for assessing the effect of changes in the body's vital signs.

- Inform AP of appropriate route and device to measure temperature.
- Inform AP of specific factors related to patient that can falsely raise or lower temperature.
- Inform AP of the frequency of temperature measurement for select patient.
- Inform AP if there are any factors that will effect the positioning of a patient when measuring a rectal temperature.
- Inform AP of patient's history or risk of irregular pulse.
- Inform AP of frequency of pulse measurement for select patient.
- Inform AP of the proper positioning of the patient when measuring the apical pulse.
- Inform AP of patient history or risk for increased or decreased respiratory rate or irregular respirations.
- Inform AP of frequency of respiration measurement for specific patient.
- Inform AP if patient has alterations affecting the appropriate limb for blood pressure measurement.
- Inform AP of appropriate-size blood pressure cuff for designated extremity.
- Inform AP of frequency of blood pressure measurement for select patient.
- Inform AP before blood pressure measurement if the patient is at risk for experiencing orthostatic hypotension.
- Determine that AP is aware of the usual values of each vital sign for patient.
- Inform AP of abnormalities of each vital sign that should be reported and reconfirmed by the nurse.
- A nurse's aide (N/A), certified nursing assistant (CNA), and AP are not responsible for using the Doppler. This is a skill for the RN or LPN/LVN to perform.
- Explain which weight device to use for specific patient.
- Observe for patient's intolerance and report information back to the nurse.

Box 4-17 Patient Conditions that Make Use of Electronic Blood Pressure Measurements Inappropriate

Irregular heart rate
Peripheral vascular obstruction (e.g., clots, narrowed vessels)
Arrhythmias
Shivering
Seizures
Excessive tremors
Unable to cooperate to minimize arm motions
Older adults
Obese extremity

The portable home devices include the aneroid sphygmomanometer (see Figure 4-11) and electronic digital readout devices that do not require use of a stethoscope. The electronic devices inflate and deflate cuffs with the push of a button (see Figure 4-17). Although the electronic devices are often easier to manipulate, there are some disadvantages. They easily become inaccurate and require recalibration more than once a year. Because of their sensitivity, improper cuff placement or movement of the arm frequently causes electronic devices to give incorrect readings. A useful blood pressure device that overcomes these difficulties fits around the wrist, does not require a stethoscope, is easy to use, and is well adapted for home use. This device also inflates and deflates at the push of a button.

Stationary automated machines are often located in public places such as grocery stores, pharmacies, fitness clubs, banks, airports, and work sites. Users simply rest the arm within the machine's inflatable cuff, which contains a pressure sensor. The cuff fits over the clothing. A visual display tells users their blood pressure within 60 to 90 seconds. The reliability of the stationary machines is limited. Blood pressure values sometimes vary by 5 to 10 mm Hg or more (for both the systolic and diastolic values) compared with the pressures taken with a manual sphygmomanometer.

If they have the information that they need to perform the procedure correctly, and if they know when to seek medical attention, it is possible for consumers to learn to use self-measurement devices to their benefit. Advise patients of possible inaccuracies in the machines, help patients understand the meaning and implications of readings, and teach patients proper measurement techniques.

WEIGHT AND HEIGHT

With the initial measurement of vital signs, measure the patient's height (the vertical measurement of a structure, organ, or other object from bottom to top, when it is placed or projected in an upright position) and weight (the force exerted on a body by the gravity of the earth; normal weight depends on the frame of the individual). Height and weight determination is important: It helps assess normal growth and development, aids in proper drug dosage calculation, and is often used to assess the effectiveness of drug therapy, such as diuretics.

Never accept a stated height and weight. Only in cases of extreme illness is it acceptable to delay obtaining these valuable assessments. You will often weigh malnourished patients, patients who are undergoing diuretic therapy, and patients who have diseases that

Skill 4-6 Measuring Height and Weight

Nursing Action *(Rationale)*

1. Perform hand hygiene. *(Reduces spread of microorganisms.)*
2. Introduce self. *(Decreases patient's anxiety.)*
3. Identify patient by identification band. *(Verifies correct patient for procedure.)*
4. Explain procedure to patient. *(Gains cooperation and assistance and decreases patient's anxiety.)*
5. Prepare for procedure:
   a. Assemble supplies, including scale—standing, chair, or bed type. *(Organizes procedure efficiently.)*
   b. Provide privacy. *(Decreases patient's anxiety.)*
6. Implement procedure:
   a. Balance scale at zero. *(Ensures accurate reading.)*
   b. Place paper towel over base of scale where patient will stand, if patient is barefoot. *(Promotes medical asepsis.)*
   c. Have patient step onto scale. Patient should be weighed in same amount of clothing each time—preferably gown; slippers are optional. *(Promotes an accurate comparison.)*
   d. Measure height with patient standing upright, if patient can tolerate this. *(Promotes accurate measurement.)*
   e. Measure weight. *(Provides accurate measurement.)*
   f. Assist patient off scale by having patient step to side. *(Safer than stepping backward.)*
   g. Assist to bed or chair to provide for patient's comfort. *(Promotes patient's self-esteem.)*
7. Write down measurement (for documentation later.)
8. Perform hand hygiene. *(Reduces spread of microorganisms.)*
9. Document measurements (e.g., height: 64 inches, weight: 136 lb) (see Figure 4-1).
10. Follow up by reporting measurement. *(Reading often varies and will have to be reassessed.)*

increase fluid retention, such as heart, liver, and kidney disease.

OBTAINING WEIGHT MEASUREMENTS

Patients are weighed to give the physician information for prescribing medication dosages and to determine nutritional status and water balance. Because 1 liter (L) of fluid equals 1 kilogram (kg) (2.2 pounds [lb]), a weight change of 1 kg (2.2 lb) will often reflect a loss or gain of 1 L of body fluids. A significant loss of weight frequently points to an underlying disease.

Weigh the patient at the same time of day, on the same scale, and in the same type or amount of clothing to allow an objective comparison of subsequent weighings. An ideal time to weigh patients is at 6 AM, after voiding and before breakfast is served.

Calibrate the scale by setting the weight at zero and noting whether the balance beam registers in the middle of the mark. Be sure scales with a digital display read zero before each use.

There are standing, chair, and lift scales. Patients capable of bearing their own weight use a standing scale (Skill 4-6). Have the patient stand on the scale platform and remain still. Slowly adjust the scale weight on the balance beam until the tip of the beam registers in the middle of the mark. Digital scale readouts display weight in a matter of seconds.

Stretcher and chair scales are available for patients unable to bear weight (Figure 4-18). After being transferred to the scale, the patient is lifted above the bed by a hydraulic device, and the weight is measured on a balance beam or digital display. Caution must be used to promote patient safety when transferring patients to and from the scales.

To facilitate weighing very ill patients, portable bed scales are available in some agencies. A hydraulic device lifts the patient above the bed, and the weight is measured on a balance beam or digital display. To weigh a patient, position the scale next to the bed. Be sure to transfer the patient carefully to and from the scale platform.

OBTAINING HEIGHT MEASUREMENTS

For patients who are able to stand, ascertain height by using the metal rod attached to the back of the standing scale, which swings out and over the top of the head. It is also possible to use a measuring stick or tape attached vertically to the wall. Place paper towels on the scale platform or floor so that the patient's feet will remain clean. Ask the patient to remove his or her shoes, step onto the platform or against the wall, and stand erect, exercising good posture. Once you have obtained the measurement, help the patient to step off the scales by moving to the side and not backward, for safety reasons.

❖ NURSING PROCESS

The role of the licensed practical nurse or licensed vocational nurse (LPN/LVN) in the nursing process as stated is that the LPN/LVN will:

- Participate in planning care for patients based on patient needs

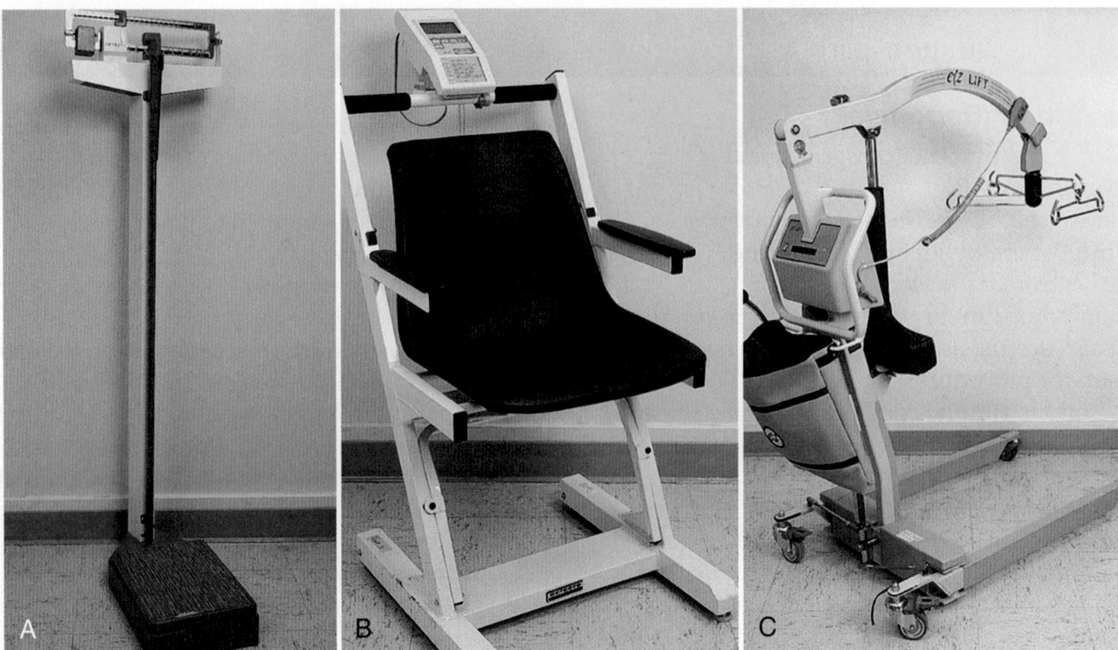

FIGURE 4-18 Types of scales. **A,** Standing scale. **B,** Chair scale. **C,** Lift scale.

- Review patient's plan of care and recommend revisions as needed
- Review and follow defined prioritization for patient care
- Use clinical pathways, care maps, or care plans to guide and review patient care

▪ Assessment

At initial contact with a patient, routinely obtain a baseline measurement of vital signs to provide a means for comparison with subsequent vital signs values. Your findings aid in determining whether it is necessary to assess specific body systems more thoroughly. For example, after assessing an abnormal respiratory rate, also auscultate lung sounds. In certain situations, you will limit your assessment of vital signs to measurement of a single vital sign for the purpose of reviewing a specific aspect of a patient's condition. For example, after administering an antihypertensive medication, measure the patient's blood pressure to evaluate the medication's effects. Part of your clinical judgment involves deciding which vital signs to assess and measure as well as when, and how frequently.

This assessment will include the following:

- Normal daily fluctuations
- Factors likely to interfere with accuracy of vital signs reading
- Medications that have potential to influence vital signs
- Factors that influence vital signs
- Conditions that precipitate fever, such as infections
- Previous baseline vital signs from patient's record. Baseline information provides basis for comparison and assists in assessment of current status.

▪ Nursing Diagnosis

Review all data gathered during assessment. Defining characteristics, when clustered, will reveal a diagnosis. The following are possible nursing diagnoses related to vital signs:

- Deficient fluid volume
- Hyperthermia
- Hypothermia
- Risk for imbalanced body temperature
- Impaired gas exchange

▪ Expected Outcomes and Planning

The appropriate focus for the plan of care is on those nursing interventions that will identify abnormalities and restore homeostasis (a relative constancy in the internal environment of the body; naturally maintained by adaptive responses that promote healthy survival).

A possible patient-centered goal is often "patient's vital signs will be within normal range"; or, for patients with chronic diseases that alter vital signs, such as chronic obstructive pulmonary disease (COPD), "baseline will be established."

Expected outcomes often include the following:

- Patient's vital signs are within normal range for age-group.
- Baseline is established for patients with chronic diseases such as COPD.

Implementation

The severity of an alteration in a vital sign will influence your priorities in the care of the patient.

What procedures the health care team uses to intervene and treat an abnormal vital sign depends on the cause, any adverse effects, and the strength and intensity of the abnormal vital signs as well as how long the abnormality persists. Direct interventions toward providing comfort to the patient, as well as to keeping complications to a minimum (see Boxes 4-6, 4-10, 4-12, and 4-15.)

Evaluation

Evaluate all nursing interventions by comparing the patient's actual responses to the outcome of the care plan. An example follows:

Outcome: Patient's blood pressure, pulse, respirations, and temperature are within normal range for age-group.

Evaluative measures: Assess vital signs on a regular basis, such as every 4 hours and after activity.

Get Ready for the NCLEX® Examination!

Key Points

- Vital signs include the physiologic parameters of temperature, pulse, respiration, and blood pressure.
- Vital signs are often measured as part of a complete physical examination or, more commonly, in a review of the patient's condition.
- Obtain vital signs whenever the patient's condition changes adversely.
- Knowledge of the factors influencing vital signs assists you in interpreting abnormal values.
- Vital signs measurements provide a basis for evaluating the patient's response to medical and nursing interventions.
- Approach the patient in a calm, caring manner while demonstrating proficiency in handling supplies needed for vital sign measurement.
- Vital signs are best measured when the patient is inactive (at rest) and the environment is controlled for comfort.
- Assess the presence and character of peripheral pulses to determine the adequacy of peripheral blood flow.
- A fever is one of the body's normal defense mechanisms.
- Temperatures are obtained by oral, rectal, axillary, and tympanic routes.
- The use of in-glass mercury thermometers and all mercury-containing devices for patient care is no longer advisable because of danger of mercury toxicity.
- Do not perform rectal temperature measurements on newborns, infants, or adults with rectal alterations.
- The tympanic route is the most accessible and acceptable site for measuring core body temperature.
- When assessing blood pressure, having the proper equipment is as important as using the correct technique.
- Most facilities have developed a fifth vital sign—pain control or comfort level. Pain has an observable effect on vital signs.
- Temperature, pulse, respiration, and blood pressure are interrelated; a change in one has potential to alter the others.
- Self-measurement of blood pressure is useful when it leads to detection of an elevated blood pressure in people previously unaware of a problem and in monitoring blood pressure in people already diagnosed with hypertension.
- There is no clinically significant difference in blood pressure levels between boys and girls. After puberty, males tend to have higher blood pressure readings. After menopause, women tend to have higher levels of blood pressure than men of similar age.
- The automatic blood pressure cuff is useful for home use if patient or caregiver has hearing difficulties.

Additional Learning Resources

Go to your Companion CD for an audio glossary, animations, video clips, and more.

evolve Be sure to visit the Evolve site at http://evolve.elsevier.com/Christensen/foundations/ for additional online resources.

Review Questions for the NCLEX® Examination

1. A 44-year-old patient is undergoing antibiotic therapy for pneumonia. His rectal temperature reading is 101.6° F. His oral temperature would be considered to be:
   1. 101.6° F (38.7° C).
   2. 100.6° F (38.1° C).
   3. 99.6° F (37.5° C).
   4. 97.6° F (36.4° C).

2. A 30-year-old patient develops a postpartum temperature that is elevated in the evening but returns to a normal reading in the morning. This has occurred for several days. This pattern of fever would be classified as:
   1. constant.
   2. intermittent.
   3. remittent.
   4. crisis.

3. A 66-year-old patient has a 10-year history of coronary artery disease. He is presently recovering from a myocardial infarction. For the most accurate assessment of pulse rate, the nurse obtains a(n):
   1. carotid pulse.
   2. radial pulse.
   3. apical pulse.
   4. brachial pulse.

4. A 16-year-old patient is admitted to the emergency department with an exacerbation of asthma. Her respirations are 40 per minute. After treatment, her rate returns to normal limits. Normal limits for the patient's respirations would be:
   1. 30 to 60.
   2. 12 to 20.
   3. 8 to 12.
   4. 24 to 30.

5. During a routine physical, a 48-year-old woman's blood pressure is noted at 180/90 mm Hg. She fears she is hypertensive. The nurse explains that the diagnosis of hypertension is made when there is a sustained elevated blood pressure of over:
   1. 160/100.
   2. 140/90.
   3. 130/70.
   4. 120/80.

6. A 65-year-old man has a history of emphysema resulting from 30 years of cigarette smoking. He frequently complains of dyspnea. Dyspnea is defined as:
   1. pallor.
   2. absence of retractions.
   3. cyanosis.
   4. difficulty breathing.

7. A 52-year-old woman complains of palpitations resulting from anxiety over her impending surgery. Her pulse rate is found to be 110 per minute. One possible description of her heart rate is:
   1. bradycardia.
   2. tachycardia.
   3. tachypnea.
   4. hypertension.

8. The nurse obtains a supine blood pressure reading of 130/64 mm Hg. One hour later, the nurse obtains a supine blood pressure reading of 134/62 mm Hg and a sitting blood pressure reading of 95/62 mm Hg. The nurse's immediate action is to:
   1. assist the patient to return to a supine position.
   2. obtain a blood pressure reading in the other arm.
   3. report the findings to the nurse in charge.
   4. question the patient about syncope.

9. The nurse is assessing a patient's blood pressure for the first time postoperatively. After inflating the cuff until the radial pulse is obliterated, the nurse:
   1. deflates the cuff slowly and waits 15 to 20 seconds before reinflating.
   2. deflates the cuff rapidly and waits 15 to 30 seconds before reinflating.
   3. deflates the cuff slowly and waits 1 minute before reinflating.
   4. deflates the cuff rapidly and waits 1 minute before reinflating.

10. The nurse has been assigned several patients. Which one of the following patients is most likely to have a higher-than-normal temperature?
    1. A depressed, apathetic patient
    2. A patient assessed with hemorrhage
    3. A patient who is recovering from surgery
    4. A patient experiencing strong emotions

11. A 16-year-old patient is admitted after a motorcycle accident. The nurse is assessing his pulse pressure. His blood pressure reading is 140/102 mm Hg. Which is the correct pulse pressure?
    1. 40
    2. 38
    3. 140
    4. 102

12. The nurse is preparing to assess a 2-day-old infant's pulse rate. Which site should be used?
    1. Scalp artery
    2. Femoral artery
    3. Apical site
    4. Radial site

13. Nurses often assess for the apical and radial pulses. Which statement is correct concerning the apical and radial pulse measurements?
    1. The apical pulse should be taken for 1 full minute and then the radial pulse for 1 full minute.
    2. The apical and radial pulse rates are lower when the temperature is elevated.
    3. The apical and radial pulses are taken at the same time for 30 seconds.
    4. The apical and radial pulses are taken at the same time for 60 seconds.

14. The physician has ordered an orthostatic blood pressure measurement. Which statement is correct concerning the orthostatic method of assessing blood pressure?
    1. The measurement is taken in the supine position, then sitting up, and then when the patient is standing.
    2. The measurement is taken first with the patient sitting up and then with the patient lying down.
    3. The nurse waits 5 minutes before assessing the blood pressure in the sitting position after assessing the blood pressure in the supine position.
    4. The nurse has the patient lie down for at least 10 minutes before performing the procedure.

15. The patient's oral temperature is 37° C. The nurse reports that the patient is:
    1. febrile.
    2. afebrile.
    3. hypotensive.
    4. hypertensive.

16. The nurse recalls that an important factor in the measurement of vital signs is that:

1. ranges of normal for vital signs are very narrow and apply to all patients.
2. the most significant aspect of measuring vital signs is their documentation.
3. environmental factors have an insignificant effect on the patient's vital signs.
4. all measuring equipment is chosen on the basis of the patient's conditions and characteristics.

17. The patient has been hospitalized after a severe head injury. The nurse recognizes that the patient's difficulty in maintaining a normal body temperature when there is no infection present is possibly the result of:

1. choosing the wrong time of day to obtain vital signs.
2. errors by the nurse in measuring temperature.
3. increased vasodilation of the superficial vessels contributing to excess heat losses.
4. the patient's head injury causing interference with the function of the hypothalamus.

18. A pulse deficit provides information about the heart's ability to adequately perfuse the body. A pulse deficit is:

1. the difference between the radial and the apical pulse rates.
2. the digital pressure felt when taking radial and ulnar pulses.
3. the amount of pressure felt when taking radial and ulnar pulses.
4. the difference between the systolic and the diastolic blood pressure readings.

19. The nurse finds that the patient's oral temperature is 98.8° F (37.1° C). The next nursing action is to:

1. administer an antiemetic drug.
2. offer the patient an additional blanket.
3. report that the patient is normal.
4. compare this with the patient's baseline.

20. To measure the patient's radial pulse rate, the nurse:

1. palpates a superficial artery at the medial side of the wrist.
2. places the binaurals directly and firmly into the ears.
3. compresses the bell of the stethoscope firmly over the heart.
4. locates the pulsation on the anterior part of the wrist lateral to the flexor tendon.

21. The assistive personnel report to you that the patient is feeling "funny." The nurse's first action would be to:

1. notify the physician.
2. obtain the patient's vital signs yourself.
3. delegate the assistant to retake the vital signs.
4. tell the assistant to keep assessing the patient and report any further complaints.

22. The nurse is taking vital signs measurements and notes that the patient has a strong radial pulse that diminishes in intensity and that there are interruptions in rhythm about every four to six beats. The immediate action is to:

1. report the findings to a physician.
2. measure a 60-second apical pulse.
3. connect the patient to a cardiac monitor.
4. obtain a 60-second apical-radial pulse.

23. When documenting a patient's blood pressure, the systolic pressure is recorded as the point at which the:

1. first Korotkoff sound appears.
2. second Korotkoff sound appears.
3. fourth Korotkoff sound appears.
4. fifth Korotkoff sound appears.

24. Which method of measuring temperature reveals core temperature?

1. Skin
2. Temporal
3. Oral
4. Axillary

25. The nurse is providing discharge teaching to a patient who has recently been diagnosed with a cardiac condition. In teaching this patient how to assess the radial pulse, the nurse will instruct him to palpate the:

1. radial artery.
2. carotid artery.
3. brachial artery.
4. femoral artery.

26. When teaching the patient about monitoring his own pulse, the nurse informs the patient that the pulse may be elevated by:

1. taking beta blockers.
2. fever.
3. sleeping.
4. standing up too quickly.

27. The nurse measures the blood pressure of an adult patient being seen in the clinic for complaints of an earache. The patient's blood pressure is 162/94 mm Hg, and he asks if he has hypertension. The nurse knows that the physician will diagnose hypertension when the patient:

1. has a blood pressure above normal range on the next clinic visit.
2. monitors his blood pressure at home and finds two more elevated readings.
3. has a blood pressure above normal range on two subsequent clinic visits.
4. complains of a constant headache.

28. The nurse begins to measure the blood pressure of an adult. The patient says that his doctor has instructed him to always use a large cuff. The nurse knows that the reason for this is that:
   1. a blood pressure cuff that is too small will give inaccurately high readings.
   2. a blood pressure cuff that is too small will likely injure the brachial artery.
   3. large cuffs are typically more accurate on adults than normal-size cuffs.
   4. normal-size cuffs should be used for pediatric patients.

29. The nurse notices the nursing assistant talking with patients as he uses an electronic cuff to measure their blood pressure. The nurse instructs the nursing assistant to avoid talking with patients while using an electronic cuff because while talking the blood pressure may elevate as much as:
   1. 5% to 35%.
   2. 10% to 40%.
   3. 20% to 50%.
   4. 30% to 60%.

30. The nurse is developing a care plan for a patient taking a diuretic to treat fluid retention. The nurse knows that weighing the patient on a daily basis will assist in monitoring the effectiveness of the medication since a weight loss of 1 kg indicates a fluid loss of:
   1. 1 L.
   2. 10 L.
   3. 100 L.
   4. 1000 L.

chapter 5

Physical Assessment

evolve

Barbara Lauritsen Christensen and Elaine Oden Kockrow

http://evolve.elsevier.com/Christensen/foundationsadult

Objectives

1. Discuss the difference between a sign and a symptom.
2. Compare and contrast the origins of disease.
3. List the four major risk categories for development of disease.
4. Discuss frequently noted signs and symptoms of disease conditions.
5. List the cardinal signs of inflammation and infection.
6. Describe the nursing responsibilities when assisting a physician with the physical examination.
7. List equipment and supplies necessary for the physical examination/assessment.
8. Explain the necessary skills for the physical examination/nursing assessment.
9. Discuss the nurse-patient interview.
10. List the basic essentials for a patient's health history.
11. Discuss the sequence of steps when performing a nursing assessment.
12. Discuss normal and abnormal assessment findings in the head-to-toe assessment.
13. Describe documentation of the physical examination/nursing assessment.
14. Explain ways to develop cultural sensitivity.

Key Terms

acute (p. 95)
assessment (p. 97)
auscultation (ăw-skŭl-TĀ-shŭn, p. 100)
borborygmi (bŏr-bō-RĬG-mē, p. 116)
bruits (BRŪ-ē, p. 110)
chronic (p. 95)
crackles (p. 112)
disease (p. 94)
drainage (p. 93)
dullness (p. 100)
edema (p. 95)
erythema (ĕr-ĕ-THĒ-mă, p. 95)
etiology (ē-tē-ŎL-ĕ-jē, p. 94)
exudate (ĔKS-ū-dāt, p. 93)
flatness (p. 100)
focused assessment (p. 106)
functional disease (p. 95)
infection (p. 95)
inflammation (p. 95)
inspection (p. 100)
level of consciousness (LOC) (p. 106)
neoplastic (nē-ō-PLĂS-tĭk, p. 94)
nursing health history (p. 101)
nursing physical assessment (p. 106)
objective data (p. 93)
organic disease (p. 95)
palpation (p. 100)
percussion (pŭr-KŬ-shŭn, p. 100)
pruritus (prū-RĪ-tŭs, p. 94)
purulent (PYŪ-rū-lĕnt, p. 95)
remission (p. 95)
signs (p. 93)
subjective data (p. 94)
symptoms (p. 93)
thrill (p. 110)
turgor (TŬR-gŏr, p. 109)
tympany (TĬM-pă-nē, p. 100)
wheezes (p. 112)

SIGNS AND SYMPTOMS

Signs are **objective data** as perceived by the examiner, in your case, what you see, hear, measure, or feel. More than one person is able to verify objective data by observation and measurement. Examples of signs are rashes, altered vital signs, abnormal lung or heart sounds, and visible drainage or exudate. **Drainage** refers to the passive or active removal of fluids from a body cavity, wound, or other source of discharge by one or more methods. Examples are the closed urinary drainage system or an open drainage system, such as from a Penrose drain. **Exudate** refers to fluid, cells, or other substances that are slowly exuded, or discharged, from cells or blood vessels through small pores or breaks in the cell membrane, usually as a result of inflammation or injury. Perspiration, pus, and serum are sometimes identified as exudates.

You will use your senses of sight, hearing, touch, and smell to gather these objective data or signs. Objective data also include laboratory findings, as well as diagnostic imaging and other diagnostic studies.

Symptoms are subjective indications of illness that the patient perceives. Examples of symptoms are pain, nausea, vertigo, pruritus, diplopia, numbness, and anxiety. You will be unaware of symptoms unless the patient describes the sensation. We refer to symptoms as **subjective data.**

In subjective data collection, the interviewer encourages a full description by the patient of the onset, the course, and the character of the problem and any factors that aggravate or alleviate it. Many signs accompany symptoms; for example, you will often see erythema and a rash when a patient complains of **pruritus** (itching). It is possible to objectively confirm some symptoms; for example, absence of response to a pinprick will confirm patient complaints of numbness of a body part.

DISEASE AND DIAGNOSIS

Disease, a pathologic condition of the body, is any disturbance of a structure or function of the body. A recognized set of signs and symptoms characterizes a given disease. How these signs and symptoms are clustered or grouped allows the health care provider to make a medical diagnosis. As a nurse, you will also rely on assessment of signs and symptoms, in this case to formulate a nursing diagnosis. Unlike the medical diagnosis, which deals with pathophysiologic factors and the cure of disease, the nursing diagnosis recognizes holistic needs of the patient that you will treat using nursing interventions. Some nursing interventions you will make independently. To accomplish others, you will depend on or collaborate with other members of the health care team.

ORIGINS OF DISEASE

Disease or illness originates from many causes; these are sometimes hereditary, and sometimes congenital, inflammatory, degenerative, infectious, deficiency, metabolic, neoplastic, traumatic, environmental, or some combination of these. For other diseases, no apparent cause is known. These illnesses, such as autoimmune diseases, are said to have an unknown **etiology,** or cause.

Hereditary diseases are transmitted genetically from parents to children. Some examples are cystic fibrosis, sickle cell anemia, color blindness, and hemophilia.

Congenital diseases appear at birth or shortly thereafter but are not caused by genetic abnormalities. These diseases result from some failure in development during the embryonic stage, or the first 2 months, of pregnancy. Contributing factors include inadequate oxygen, maternal infection, drugs, alcohol, malnutrition, and radiation. Both structural and functional defects occur. Examples include absence of limbs (structural) and blindness (functional).

Inflammatory diseases are those in which the body reacts with an inflammatory response to some causative agent. Microorganisms are the cause in many instances, such as with pharyngitis or bronchitis. Other inflammatory diseases, such as hay fever, are manifestations of an allergic reaction. Still others have an unknown cause.

Degenerative disease implies degeneration, often progressive, of some part of the body. It is possible that the aging process plays a role in these types of diseases. Osteoarthritis is a common example.

Infectious diseases result from the invasion of microorganisms into the body. Examples of infectious diseases include acquired immunodeficiency syndrome (AIDS), tuberculosis, measles, and pneumonia.

Deficiency diseases result from the lack of a specific nutrient. Nutrients are minerals, vitamins, proteins, fats, and carbohydrates. Scurvy is a deficiency disease resulting from a lack of vitamin C. Iron deficiency anemia sometimes results from a severe deficiency of iron in the diet.

Metabolic disease is caused by a dysfunction that results in a loss of metabolic control of homeostasis in the body. The dysfunction usually involves endocrine glands, which secrete hormones to regulate body processes. Diabetes mellitus results from the dysfunction of the pancreas. Other examples of metabolic disease are hypothyroidism and acromegaly, which involve the thyroid and pituitary glands.

Neoplastic disease is described as an abnormal growth of new tissues. The new growth is sometimes benign and sometimes malignant (cancerous). Malignant neoplasms are a serious threat to health, because of the rapid growth of the cells and their ability to invade and metastasize.

Traumatic conditions result from both physical and emotional trauma. Physical trauma, such as a motor vehicle accident, has the potential to result in traumatic brain injury (TBI). TBI frequently leaves the individual mentally and physically impaired. An individual who suffers emotional trauma, such as the loss of a loved one, sometimes becomes unable to manage the activities of daily living (ADLs) he or she participated in before the trauma.

Environmental diseases are a group of conditions that develop from exposure to a harmful substance in the environment. "Tight building syndrome" is an example of an environmental illness. The individual complains of headache, vertigo (dizziness), and respiratory infections. These signs and symptoms result from the fact that the well-built buildings of today do not allow circulation of fresh air and instead recycle air containing fumes and microorganisms. Radon gas and asbestos are other substances in the environment that potentially lead to disease.

Although many disease conditions have an unknown cause, many now consider a number of conditions to result from **autoimmune responses.** In an autoimmune response, the body develops immunoglobulins (antibodies) against its own tissues or body substances. Researchers are investigating the possible autoimmune nature of rheumatoid arthritis and ulcerative colitis.

RISK FACTORS FOR DEVELOPMENT OF DISEASE

A risk factor is any situation, habit, environmental condition, genetic predisposition, physiologic condition, or other variable that increases the vulnerability of an individual or group to illness or accident. Risk factors for the development of coronary artery disease, for example, include heredity, cigarette smoking, high blood levels of cholesterol, and stress. The presence of risk factors does not necessarily mean that a person will develop a disease condition, only that the chance of doing so is higher. You will assess the patient's risk factors and use them to help you formulate nursing diagnoses, because nursing diagnoses are made for the patient's potential, as well as actual, problems.

Risk factors fall into four major categories: genetic and physiologic, age, environment, and lifestyle (Box 5-1). Some, such as many environmental and lifestyle risk factors, are modifiable; others, such as age and family history, are not.

TERMS USED TO DESCRIBE DISEASE

Diseases are described in terms of duration. **Chronic** disease develops slowly and persists over a long period, often for a person's lifetime. Diabetes mellitus (inability of the body to use glucose) is an example of a chronic disease. Chronic disease is frequently further described as early, late, or terminal; another possibility is that it is in remission. **Remission** means there has been a partial or complete disappearance of clinical and subjective characteristics of the disease. Remission is sometimes spontaneous and sometimes a result of therapy.

In comparison, a disease described as **acute** begins abruptly with marked intensity of severe signs and symptoms and then often subsides after a period of treatment. An episode of appendicitis is considered acute.

Disease is also often described as being organic or functional. An **organic disease** results in a structural change in an organ that interferes with its functioning. Stroke is an organic disease of the brain. Manifestations of **functional disease** often appear to be those of organic disease, but careful examination fails to reveal evidence of structural or physiologic abnormalities. Many nervous and mental diseases are classified as functional.

FREQUENTLY NOTED SIGNS AND SYMPTOMS OF DISEASE

Although signs and symptoms of inflammation and infection are similar, it is important not to confuse the two. **Infection** is caused by an invasion of microorganisms, such as bacteria, viruses, fungi, or parasites, that produces tissue damage. **Inflammation** is a protective response of body tissues to irritation, injury, or invasion by disease-producing organisms. The cardinal signs of infection and inflammation include **erythema** (redness), **edema** (swelling), heat, pain, **purulent** drainage (pus), and loss of function (Table 5-1).

The inflammatory response is actually the body's defense against some causative agent. The erythema and heat are the result of increased blood flow to the

Box 5-1 Risk Factors for Disease

GENETIC AND PHYSIOLOGIC

- A family history of cancer increases the risk that an individual will develop cancer (genetic).
- Malnourishment predisposes an individual to illness (physiologic).

AGE

- Thinning skin in older adults makes this group more susceptible to skin trauma.
- Osteoporosis makes the older adult more prone to fractures, especially of the hip.

ENVIRONMENT

- Radon gas seeping from the earth into a basement increases the risk of cancer development.
- Asbestos in building structures increases the risk of cancer of the pleura (in lung).
- Air, water, and noise pollution increase the risk of illness.
- High crime rates and overcrowding also lead to stress that makes individuals more susceptible to disease.
- Within the family, conflicts or other problems have the potential to create stressors that put individual members or the family as a whole at increased risk of illness.
- Extremes of heat and cold have potential to damage or destroy body cells.

LIFESTYLE

- Smoking increases the risk of many diseases including oral (mouth) cancer; pharyngeal cancer; laryngeal cancer; lung cancer; renal cancer; esophageal cancer; pancreatic cancer; bladder cancer; uterine and cervical cancer; cardiovascular disease; and osteoporosis. Smoking is the most preventable cause of death in our society.
- Overeating or poor nutrition, insufficient rest and sleep, and poor personal hygiene also add to increased risk for illness for the individual.
- Other habits that place a person at risk for illness include alcohol and substance abuse.
- Sunbathing increases the risk of skin cancer.
- Any emotional stress has potential to be a risk factor if severe or prolonged or if the person is unable to adequately cope. In such a case, emotional stress increases the chance of illness. Events such as death, divorce, or pregnancy, as well as job-related stressors, are known to place the individual at risk.

Table 5-1 Frequently Noted Signs and Symptoms of Disease Conditions

TERM	DEFINITION
Anorexia	Lack of appetite resulting in the inability to eat. This symptom can occur in many disease conditions.
Asthenia	A condition of debility, loss of strength and energy, and depleted vitality.
Bradycardia	A circulatory condition in which the myocardium contracts steadily but at a rate of less than 60 contractions per minute.
Constipation	Difficulty in passing stools or an incomplete or infrequent passage of hard stools. There are many causes, both organic and functional.
Coughing	A sudden audible expulsion of air from the lungs. Coughing is an essential protective response that serves to clear the lungs, the bronchi, and the trachea of irritants and secretions and to prevent aspiration of foreign material into the lungs. It is a common sign of diseases of the larynx, the bronchi, and the lungs.
Cyanosis	Bluish discoloration of the skin and mucous membranes caused by an increase of deoxygenated hemoglobin in the blood.
Diaphoresis	The secretion of sweat, especially the profuse secretion associated with an elevated body temperature, physical exertion, exposure to heat, and mental or emotional stress.
Diarrhea	Frequent passage of loose, liquid stools; generally results from increased motility in the colon. This is usually a sign of an underlying disorder. The characteristics of the diarrhea give evidence as to the source. Dark black, tarry stools sometimes means there is bleeding in the intestines. Bright red blood in the feces indicates active bleeding from the lower portion of the intestinal tract.
Dyspnea	A shortness of breath or difficulty in breathing that is sometimes caused by certain heart and lung conditions, strenuous exercise, or anxiety.
Ecchymosis	Discoloration of an area of the skin or mucous membrane caused by the extravasation of blood into the subcutaneous tissues as a result of trauma to the underlying blood vessels or by fragility of the vessel walls (also called a *bruise*).
Edema	An abnormal accumulation of fluid in interstitial spaces. Some causes include overhydration, excess sodium intake, capillary hyperpermeability, and loss of serum albumin (a protein), which causes fluid to leave the vessels and collect in the interstitial space. Skin that is edematous will be taut and shiny. Pitting sometimes occurs when the skin is pressed; a small indentation will remain after the finger is removed.
Erythema	Redness or inflammation of the skin or mucous membranes that is the result of dilation and congestion of superficial capillaries; erythema is seen in a mild sunburn.
Fever	An abnormal elevation of the temperature of the body above 98.6° F (37° C) because of disease; also called *pyrexia*. It results from an imbalance between the elimination and production of heat. Infection and many different diseases often lead to febrile condition, or elevated temperature.
Fetid	Pertaining to something that has a foul, putrid, or offensive odor. Also called *malodorous*.
Inflammation	The protective response of the tissues of the body to irritation or injury.
Jaundice	Yellow tinge to the skin; often indicates obstruction in the flow of bile from the liver.
Lethargy	The state or quality of being indifferent, apathetic, or sluggish.
Nausea	A sensation often leading to the urge to vomit. Common causes include intense pain, gallbladder disease, inflammation of the stomach, paralytic ileus, and food poisoning.
Orthopnea	An abnormal condition in which a person has to sit or stand to breathe deeply or comfortably. Occurs in many disorders of the respiratory and cardiac systems.
Pain	An unpleasant sensation caused by noxious (extremely destructive or harmful) stimulation of the sensory nerve endings. It is a cardinal symptom of inflammation and is valuable in the diagnosis of many disorders and conditions. Pain has varied manifestations: mild or severe, chronic, acute, burning, dull or sharp, precisely or poorly localized, or referred.
Pallor	An unnatural paleness or absence of color in the skin; often results from a decrease in hemoglobin and erythrocytes (red blood cells).
Pruritus	A symptom of itching and an uncomfortable sensation leading to an urge to scratch. Some causes are allergy, infection, jaundice, elevated serum urea, and skin irritation.
Purulent drainage (pus)	A creamy, viscous, pale yellow or yellow-green fluid exudate that is the result of fluid remains of liquefied necrosis of tissues. Bacterial infection is the most common cause. The character of the pus, including its color, consistency, quantity, or odor, often has diagnostic significance.
Sallow	Pertaining to an unhealthy, yellow color; usually said of a complexion or skin.
Scleral icterus	The color of the sclera is yellow. This jaundice is due to coloring of the sclera with bilirubin that infiltrates all tissues of the body.
Tachycardia	An abnormal condition in which the heart contracts regularly but at a rate greater than 100 beats per minute. The heart rate accelerates in response to fever, exercise, or nervous excitement.
Tachypnea	An abnormally rapid rate of breathing seen in many disease conditions.
Vomit	To expel the contents of the stomach through the esophagus and out of the mouth. The quality of the vomitus often gives a clue to the underlying cause. "Coffee-ground" vomitus indicates bleeding in the stomach. The blood takes on a coffee-ground appearance because of the effect of the digestive juices. Vomiting of bright red blood is potentially a sign of gastric hemorrhage.

area. The damaged tissue releases chemical substances that cause the capillary walls to become more permeable. This enables white blood cells and plasma to move from the blood to the affected area. The white blood cells (neutrophils) digest microorganisms and cellular debris. This excess of fluid in the tissues, or edema, increases pressure on sensitive nerve endings, causing pain. Loss of function imposes a period of rest for the injured area. Purulent exudate is the accumulation of neutrophils, dead cells, bacteria, and other debris from the infectious process.

ASSESSMENT

A complete health **assessment** is an evaluation or appraisal of the patient's condition. The process involves the orderly collection of information concerning the patient's health status. It is performed by medical and nursing personnel and usually comprises taking a medical history and performing a physical examination. The data collected establish a baseline. This baseline allows the physician or the nurse to identify problems and plan care; in addition, ongoing assessments produce contrasting data that permit you to evaluate the effectiveness of care.

MEDICAL ASSESSMENT

When the health care provider conducts a physical examination, you will often be expected to carry out certain assistive functions. Preparing the examining room, assisting with equipment, preparing the patient, and collecting specimens are a few examples of responsibilities you need to be familiar with to facilitate the physical examination. There are both preexamination and postexamination responsibilities.

As you prepare the patient for the physical examination and assist with its performance, make sure to satisfy the following questions and requirements:

- Is an informed consent necessary? Has it been signed by the patient or next of kin? Has it been witnessed? Has it been dated?
- Have all test prerequisites been completed? Have vital signs been obtained? Has the patient's height and weight been determined? Is skin prep required? Has a urinalysis been ordered? A complete blood count (CBC)? Coagulation profile? Chest x-ray? Are all necessary supplies present (Box 5-2)?
- Has the patient voided? Is the patient wearing a hospital gown?
- Has the patient been adequately advised concerning the examination? Time? Place? Examiner? Sequence of events? Does the patient have any unanswered questions (Box 5-3)?
- Will the physical examination be performed in the patient's room? Is the working area cleared of unnecessary articles? Have the privacy curtains been pulled to provide patient privacy? Have visitors been asked to leave and shown where to wait? Has the door been closed? (Privacy is essential.)
- If an examination room is provided, how will the patient get to the room? Transfer by gurney? Transfer by wheelchair? By ambulating? Has the examining room been prepared? Are all necessary supplies and equipment arranged for easy access (Figure 5-1)?
- How much assistance will the patient need to safely climb onto and recline on the examining table? What position will the patient be required to

Box 5-2 Equipment and Supplies for Physical Examination and Assessment

- Cotton applicators
- Cytobrush
- Disposable pad
- Drapes
- Eye chart (e.g., Snellen chart)
- Flashlight and spotlight
- Forms (e.g., physical examination results, laboratory requisitions)
- Gloves (sterile and clean)
- Gown for patient
- Lubricant
- Ophthalmoscope
- Otoscope
- Papanicolaou (Pap) smear slides
- Paper towels
- Percussion hammer
- Safety pins
- Scale with height measurement rod
- Spatula
- Specimen containers and microscope slides
- Sphygmomanometer and cuff
- Stethoscope
- Swabs or sponge forceps
- Tape measure
- Thermometer
- Tissues
- Tongue depressor
- Tuning fork
- Vaginal speculum
- Wristwatch with second hand

Box 5-3 Psychological Preparation for a Physical Examination

Psychological preparation will often be your highest priority before the examination. Patients become embarrassed when required to answer sensitive questions about body functions or when certain body parts are exposed and examined. The possibility of the examiner finding something abnormal also creates anxiety. First tell the patient about the examination in general terms. Then, as each body system is examined, give a more detailed explanation. Use simple terms when describing steps of the examination because complicated terminology will perplex some patients and easily add to their fears.

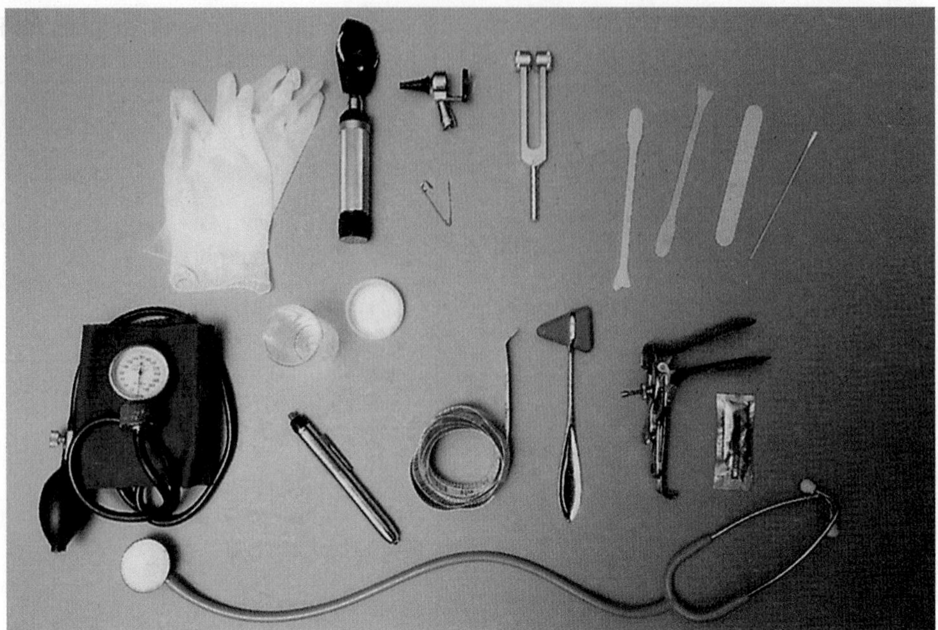

FIGURE 5-1 Equipment used during a physical examination *(clockwise from upper left)*: disposable gloves, ophthalmoscope, otoscope attachment, sterile safety pin, tuning fork, cervical spatulas, tongue depressor, cotton-tip swab, lubricant, vaginal speculum, reflex hammer, tape measure, penlight, specimen cup, sphygmomanometer, and stethoscope *(bottom)*.

assume during procedures (Table 5-2)? For perineal examination, has the patient been draped adequately to expose only the area being examined?

- Will you be required to remain in the examining room? It is recommended that you do not leave the patient alone. Most examiners appreciate a nurse in attendance; however, there are times when this is not necessary.
- Is the patient acquainted with the examiner? Are introductions necessary?
- Does the lighting require adjustment? Does the examiner expect you to provide instruments, supplies, and equipment as they are needed?
- Will specimens be obtained? How should they be labeled? Where should they be sent? How? (See Chapter 19.)
- How much attention and encouragement will the patient need during the examination?
- How much assistance will the patient need to assume a comfortable position following the examination? To cleanse himself or herself? To get dressed? To return to the room? To call for further assistance if needed?
- What signs and symptoms related to the procedure are you called on to make note of? Make these assessments at frequent intervals, and report results to the examiner.
- What information is required in the documentation of the procedure? Note vital signs, pertinent signs and symptoms, complaints of pain, anxiety level, and specimens obtained and sent to the laboratory. Report any abnormalities to the examiner.
- What other members of the health care team need to be informed of the procedure? Usually those who are directly responsible for the patient's care require notification.
- Does the examination room require attention? Was order maintained? Is there equipment that has to be disposed of or cleaned and returned to its proper location? It is always advisable to keep special examining rooms and equipment in readiness for the next patient.

Perform an assessment to determine the actual or potential (risk for) patient problems that will require nursing interventions for the safety and well-being of the patient. For example, if during the examination you observe that the patient has a need for oxygen (a basic human need), take steps to ensure placement of oxygen, positioning, deep breathing, and coughing to meet this need.

It is imperative that you perform accurate assessments because you, as the nurse, are the caregiver who is in constant contact with the patient. It is your role to monitor the patient, which permits you to discover developing complications and to evaluate medical treatments.

NURSING ASSESSMENT

Nursing assessment comprises the gathering, verifying, and communicating of data about the patient. The purpose of the assessment is to establish a baseline database about the patient's level of wellness, health practices, past illnesses, related experiences, and health care goals. The information contained in the database is the basis for an individualized plan of nursing care developed throughout the nursing process.

Data collected during this process includes the nursing health history, physical examination findings, re-

Table 5-2 **Positions for Examination**

POSITION	AREAS ASSESSED	RATIONALE	LIMITATIONS
Sitting	Head and neck, back, posterior thorax and lungs, anterior thorax and lungs, breasts, axillae, heart, vital signs, and upper extremities	Sitting upright provides full expansion of lungs and provides better visualization of symmetry of upper body parts.	Some physically weakened patients will be unable to sit. Use supine position with head of bed elevated instead.
Supine	Head and neck, anterior thorax and lungs, breasts, axillae, heart, abdomen, extremities, pulses	This is the most normally relaxed position. It provides easy access to pulse sites.	If patient becomes short of breath easily, consider raising head of bed.
Dorsal recumbent	Head and neck, anterior thorax and lungs, breasts, axillae, heart, abdomen	Position is used for abdominal assessment because it promotes relaxation of abdominal muscles.	Patients with painful disorders are more comfortable with knees flexed.
Lithotomy*	Female genitalia and genital tract	This position provides maximal exposure of genitalia and facilitates insertion of vaginal speculum.	Lithotomy position is embarrassing and uncomfortable, so keep time that patient spends in it to a minimum. Keep patient well draped.
Sims'	Rectum and vagina	Flexion of hip and knee improves exposure of rectal area.	Joint deformities may hinder patient's ability to bend hip and knee.
Prone	Musculoskeletal system	This position is used only to assess extension of hip joint.	Patients with respiratory difficulties tolerate this position poorly.
Lateral recumbent	Heart	This position aids in detecting murmurs.	Patients with respiratory difficulties tolerate this position poorly.
Knee-chest*	Rectum	This position provides maximum exposure of rectal area.	This position is embarrassing and uncomfortable.

*A patient with severe arthritis or other joint deformity may be unable to assume this position.

sults of laboratory and diagnostic tests, and information from health care team members and the patient's family or significant others. Obtain the health history while you initiate the nurse-patient relationship by interviewing the patient. You will use various techniques to progress through the interview (see Chapter 3). When assessing the patient, always pay special attention to areas about which the patient has expressed concern.

Once you have completed the interview, you will proceed to the physical assessment. Here you will call on your skills of inspection, palpation, auscultation, and percussion to collect physical examination data (Box 5-4). Laboratory and diagnostic tests validate findings from the history and physical examination and often lead to identification of problems not previously noted (Box 5-5).

Initiating the Nurse-Patient Relationship

Perhaps the most challenging patient interview you will ever have to conduct is the first one with every patient. For some patients, being interviewed by a nurse is a new experience. Your first task is thus to establish an effective nurse-patient relationship before proceeding to the nursing health history.

Box 5-4 Physical Assessment Techniques

INSPECTION

Visually inspect the patient's body and observe moods, including all responses and nonverbal behaviors. This **inspection,** or purposeful observation, is the technique you will use most frequently. It begins with your first contact with the patient and continues throughout the gathering of the nursing history. Use inspection to systematically collect data about significant behaviors or physical features. It is important to be accurate and thorough, using a systematic approach such as a head-to-toe assessment.

PALPATION

With **palpation,** you use the hands and sense of touch to gather data. Hands are highly sensitive to texture, temperature, and moisture and thus help determine the quality of an area. Use palpation to detect tenderness, temperature, texture, vibration, pulsations, masses, and other changes in structural integrity. Palpate each body part, usually according to a systematic assessment pattern. Palpation rules out or confirms suspicions raised during interview and inspection. Because touching has potential to elicit fear, embarrassment, pain, or other strong emotions, explain your actions and the reasons for them. In addition, instruct the patient to let you know whether palpation produces sensations of tenderness, pressure, or pain. The three palpation techniques are light, moderate, and deep. Light and moderate palpation are illustrated in Figures 5-11 and 5-12.

When using palpation, be sure your fingernails are short, and warm your hands before touching the patient. Social conversation during palpation is appropriate at times to distract the patient and help him or her relax. Use the pads of your fingers; place them flat against the patient's skin with slight pressure and gentle rotation of the area under examination. Your thumb and forefinger can be used to palpate muscle mass on arms and legs. Palpate pulses with the pads of your fingers. Someone who is not appropriately trained to perform palpation can cause internal injuries. When doing palpation, also observe the patient's facial expressions; if you see a grimace indicating pain, for instance, ask the patient to describe it.

AUSCULTATION

Auscultation is the process of listening to sounds produced by the body. Three systems produce sounds you will auscultate: the cardiovascular system, the respiratory system, and the gastrointestinal system. For auscultation of these systems, you will use a stethoscope, an instrument that amplifies sounds produced by internal organs. You will also use the technique of auscultation to detect the fetal heart sound.

To master the auscultation technique and gain experience at interpreting the sounds you hear, you will need repeated practice on both healthy and ill patients. Accurate assessment requires a quiet environment. Television, sounds from nasogastric suction, movement of bed linen, and conversation all have the ability to interfere with accurate auscultation. Try closing your eyes while listening to reduce visual distractions. Never rush auscultation. Take time to assess each area properly.

Place the diaphragm of the stethoscope gently over the patient's skin. If the area is hairy, dampening it sometimes decreases the sound of the hair rubbing against the diaphragm.

PERCUSSION

Percussion is use of the fingertips to tap the body's surface to produce vibration and sound. The sounds indicate the density of the underlying tissue and thus help you detect the location of body organs and structures. For example, percussion over a hollow organ such as the stomach produces a high-pitched, drumlike sound called **tympany.** Percussion over a dense organ such as the liver produces a low-pitched, thudlike sound called **dullness.** Percussion over a muscle produces a soft, high-pitched, flat sound called **flatness.** To perform percussion, place the palmar surface of one hand against the patient's body while tapping with the fingers of your other hand. Tap each area two or three times. Properly performed, percussion is not painful for the patient, but if it does cause discomfort, discontinue it and document the results. This assessment technique is the one you will use least frequently.

The first step in initiating the nurse-patient relationship is to introduce yourself, stating your name, your position, and the purposes of the interview. In the following Communication box, the nurse introduces herself, gives an estimate of the time needed for the assessment, and tells the patient the reason for the assessment. Indicating the length of time is important because it helps ensure cooperation. Do not consider the patient, even one in a hospital, a captive audience. Take steps to ensure that you do not use the patient's time inappropriately. In the example, the nurse also gives the patient an opportunity to ask questions. It is important to determine whether the patient has any pressing questions before beginning the more targeted part of the interview. By answering these questions, it is possible to meet some of the patient's immediate needs and help the patient feel more comfortable answering your questions. For example, sometimes a patient who is unsure of how the hospital bed operates will be distracted and think more about the bed than about your questions; this patient will be less likely to provide complete information for the database. Finally, note how the nurse asks whether it is acceptable

 Communication

Prior to Assessment

Nurse: Good morning, Mr. Carouthers. I'm Ms. Arrow, a student nurse. I'll be caring for you today. A portion of my nursing care is to conduct an assessment of you. My assessment will help me plan your nursing care. I will be including your temperature, pulse, respirations, blood pressure, heart rate, orientation, pain scale, lung sounds, O_2 saturations, abdominal sounds, arterial pulses, and skin color in my assessment. It will take me about 30 minutes. Do you have any questions? (pause) May I begin now? (pause) I will start with your vital signs.

Box 5-5 Common Laboratory and Diagnostic Tests

BLOOD ANALYSIS
Complete blood count (CBC), includes red blood cell (RBC), hemoglobin (Hgb), hematocrit, erythrocyte indices, platelets, white blood cell (WBC) with differential, and examination of peripheral blood cells
Electrolyte tests: sequential multiple analysis—6 (SMA-6), SMA-12
Arterial blood gas (ABG) analysis
Fasting blood sugar (FBS) test
Blood chemistry profile
Megaloblastic anemia profile
Prothrombin time (PT)
Partial thromboplastin time (PTT)
International normalized ratio (INR)

URINE ANALYSIS
Urinalysis (UA)
Urine culture and sensitivity test
24-hour urine collection for creatinine clearance, protein content

DIAGNOSTIC IMAGING EXAMINATIONS
Chest roentgenogram (chest x-ray [CXR])
Upper gastrointestinal (UGI) examination
Barium enema (BE) examination
Intravenous pyelogram (IVP)
Scans of the body, the head, the chest, the abdomen, the pelvis, and the bones

STOOL ANALYSIS
Guaiac tests (Hematest stools)
Ova and parasite tests
Culture and sensitivity
Clostridium difficile
Escherichia coli: O157:H7

SPUTUM ANALYSIS
Culture and sensitivity test
Acid-fast bacilli (AFB) test
Cytology tests

OTHER
Colonoscopy examinations
Endoscopy examinations
Electrocardiogram (ECG), echocardiogram, transesophageal echocardiogram
Stress test
Tuberculosis (TB) skin test

to conduct the interview at that time, thereby giving the patient a choice.

The next step in initiating the nurse-patient relationship is to communicate your trustworthiness and discretion to patients. Illnesses that cause people to seek help are often accompanied by anxiety, powerlessness, altered family processes, economic concerns, and changes in self-image. Patients are frequently asked to provide highly personal information about themselves and their families. Generally, people share such information only with family members or close friends. To be able to do so with you, it is crucial that the patient be comfortable that you will share this information only with caregivers who need it to provide proper care. Assure patients that information concerning past or present levels of wellness or family relationships is strictly confidential.

Finally, the nurse-patient relationship is enhanced by the professionalism and competence you convey. Your attitude of professionalism and your professional manner and appearance encourage a supportive therapeutic relationship with the patient that will enable you and the patient to communicate freely, thereby allowing identification of health care needs and goals.

The Interview

Conduct the interview in a relaxed, unhurried manner in a quiet, private, well-lighted setting. Convey feelings of compassion and concern and, at the same time, remain objective. It is essential that the patient feel that the information you are seeking is truly important to you; demonstrate an interest in the patient's state of wellness.

Determine by what name the patient wishes to be addressed, and then use that name during the interview. An accepting posture, in which you are sitting in a relaxed manner at eye level with the patient, is likely to enhance the interview. A pleasant facial expression will promote communication, and eye contact helps confirm to the patient that he or she has your full attention.

One way to enhance communication is by using nonjudgmental language. Statements such as, "Yes, I see," or "What happened next?" will encourage the patient to clarify without feeling threatened. Reflecting what the patient has said in your own words clarifies statements, as does summarizing and restating what the patient has said. Your approving nods and gestures facilitate the exchange of information. You must be responsive to the patient's condition at all times. It may be necessary to stop the interview to stabilize the patient's condition and ensure comfort and safety before proceeding. (Read more about interviewing in Chapter 3.)

NURSING HEALTH HISTORY

The **nursing health history** is the initial step in the assessment process. Data collected provide you with information about the patient's level of wellness, changes in life patterns, sociocultural role, and mental and emotional reactions to illness. The objective is to identify patterns of health and illness, risk factors for physical and behavioral health problems, deviations from normal, and available resources for adaptation to life's changes.

Biographic Data

In most facilities, the admitting department will obtain the biographic data; begin the interview by referring to this information. It generally includes data such as date of birth, sex, address, family members' names and addresses, marital status, religious preference and practices, occupation, source of health care, and insurance, Medicare, and Medicaid benefits. Verify this information with the patient to ensure that it is correct.

Reasons for Seeking Health Care

Ask why the patient has sought health care, because the information contained on the admission form sometimes differs considerably from the patient's subjective reason for seeking health care. This is often referred to as the **chief complaint.** Perhaps you will ask simply, "What is the reason for your admission?" This allows the patient not only to describe the reason for admission, but also to make her or his expectations known to you. To get the most information from the patient about health concerns, one possibility is to use the OPQRSTUV method (Box 5-6). Be sure to document this information in the patient's own words, using quotation marks. This will help remove the possibility of bias from later interpretation of the data.

It is also appropriate to elicit the patient's expectations of the health care providers. Determine whether patients expect to be "cured," or become "free of pain" or "able to care for self." This information assists in establishing the goals of nursing interventions, as well as in determining whether patients' expectations of themselves and the health care providers are realistic. In addition, such expectations provide you with information on patient perceptions about patterns of illness or changes in lifestyle.

Present Illness or Health Concerns

The data collected relate to the progression of the present illness from the onset to the current signs and symptoms. They must be detailed and comprehensive to allow you to plan appropriate interventions. By following the guidelines in Box 5-7, you have the ability to ensure that data collection is complete.

Health History

Information from the health history provides data on the patient's health care experiences. Determine whether the patient has ever been hospitalized or has undergone surgery. Also essential in planning nursing interventions are descriptions of allergies, including allergic reactions to food, drugs, or pollutants. If an allergy is present, note the specific reaction and treatment on the assessment form.

Box 5-6 History of Present Illness

When discussing the history of the present illness with your patient, make sure the patient describes his or her problems fully. To do this, ask the patient the following questions about each complaint:

Time of onset. When was the first date (the problem) happened? What time did it begin?

Type of onset. How did (the problem) start: Suddenly? Gradually?

Original source. What were you doing when you first experienced or noticed (the problem)? What seems to trigger it: Stress? Position? Certain activities? Arguments?

Characteristics. What is the problem like? If describing a discharge: Thick? Runny? Clear? Colored? If describing a psychological problem: Do the voices drown out other sounds? Whose voice does it sound like?

Severity. How bad is (the problem) when it is at its worst? Does it interfere with your normal activities? Does it force you to lie down, sit down, slow down?

Radiation. In the case of pain, does it travel down your back or arms, up your neck, or down your legs? What is the pain intensity on a scale of 0 to 10?

Time relationship. How often do you experience (the problem): Hourly? Daily? Weekly? Monthly? When do you usually experience it: Daytime? At night? In the early morning? Are you ever awakened by it? Does it ever occur before, during, or after meals? Does it occur seasonally?

Duration. How long does an episode last?

Course. Does (the problem) seem to be getting better, getting worse, or does it remain the same?

Associations. Does (the problem) lead to anything else? Is it accompanied by other signs and symptoms?

Source of relief. What relieves it: Changing diet? Changing position? Taking medications? Being active?

Source of aggravation. What makes it worse?

You can remember all these questions using the letters OPQRSTUV:

O Onset-Timing: onset, duration

P Precipitating-Provocative-Palliative
What causes it? What makes it better? What makes it worse?

Q Quality-Quantity: describe it: sharp, dull . . .
How does it feel, look, or sound, and how much of it is there? How often, when, how long

R Region-Radiation
Where is it? Does it spread?

S Severity scale
Does it interfere with activities? How does it rate on a severity scale of 0 to 10?

T Treatments
What helps? For how long?

U Understanding: What do you think is causing it? How does it affect you?

V Values: Goals of care; expectations

Box 5-7 Review of Systems

It is probable that you will not include questions pertaining to all the aspects of each system every time you take a nursing health history. Nevertheless, do include some questions regarding each system in every history. These essential areas are listed in bold type in the outline that follows. Whenever the patient gives positive responses to the first questions for that system, include questions about the more comprehensive and detailed areas relating to each system listed afterward. Keep in mind that these lists do not represent an exhaustive enumeration of questions; even more details are frequently required within an organ system, depending on the patient's problem.

A. **General constitutional symptoms:** Fever, chills, malaise, fatigability, night sweats; weight (average, preferred, present, change, appetite)

B. **Skin:** Rash or eruption, pruritus, pigmentation or texture change; diaphoresis (excessive sweating); abnormal nail or hair growth

C. **Skeletal:** Joint stiffness, pain, restriction of motion, edema, erythema, heat, bone deformity

D. **Head**
   1. General: Frequent or unusual headaches, vertigo (dizziness), syncope (fainting), severe head injuries
   2. Eyes: Visual acuity, blurring, diplopia (double vision), photophobia (abnormal sensitivity to light), scotomas (spots before the eyes), nystagmus (involuntary rhythmic movements of the eye), pain, recent change in appearance or vision, glaucoma, use of eyedrops or other eye medications, history of trauma or familial eye disease
   3. Ears: Hearing loss, pain, discharge, tinnitus, vertigo
   4. Nose: Sense of smell, frequency of colds, obstruction, epistaxis (nosebleed), postnasal discharge, sinus pain
   5. Mouth: Bleeding or edema of gums; recent tooth abscesses or extractions; soreness of tongue or buccal mucosa, ulcers; disturbance of taste; throat: hoarseness or change in voice; dysphagia (difficulty swallowing); frequent sore throats

E. **Endocrine:** Thyroid enlargement or tenderness, heat or cold intolerance, unexplained weight change, diabetes mellitus, polydipsia (excessive thirst), polyuria, changes in facial or body hair, increased hat and glove size, skin striae (streak or linear scar from rapidly developing tension in the skin)

F. **Reproduction**
   1. Males: Onset of puberty, erections, emissions, testicular pain, libido, infertility
   2. Females:
      a. Menses: Onset, regularity, duration of flow, dysmenorrhea (pain associated with menstruation), last period, intermenstrual discharge or bleeding, pruritus, date of last Papanicolaou (Pap) smear, age at menopause, libido, frequency of intercourse, sexual difficulties
      b. Pregnancies: Number, miscarriages, abortions, duration of pregnancy in each and any complication during any pregnancy or postpartum period; use of oral or other contraceptives
      c. Breasts: Pain, tenderness, discharge, lumps, mammograms; family history of breast cancer

G. **Respiratory:** Pain relating to respiration, dyspnea, cyanosis, crackles, wheezing, cough, sputum (character and quantity), hemoptysis (expectorating blood from respiratory tract), night sweats, exposure to tuberculosis (TB); date and result of last chest x-ray examination; dependence on supplemental oxygen

H. **Cardiac:** Chest pain or distress, precipitating causes, timing and duration, relieving factors, palpitations, dyspnea, orthopnea (number of pillows needed), edema, claudication (weakness of legs accompanied by cramplike pain), hypertension, previous myocardial infarction, heart failure, estimate of exercise tolerance, past electrocardiogram (ECG) or other cardiac tests; history of coronary artery bypass surgery, percutaneous transluminal coronary angioplasty, or percutaneous balloon valvuloplasty

I. **Hematologic:** Anemia, tendency to bruise or bleed easily, thromboses, thrombophlebitis, any known abnormality of blood cells, transfusions

J. **Lymph nodes:** Enlargement, tenderness, suppuration (to produce purulent material [pus])

K. **Gastrointestinal:** Appetite, digestion, intolerance for any type of foods, dysphagia (difficulty swallowing), heartburn, nausea, vomiting, hematemesis, regularity of bowels, constipation, diarrhea, change in stool color or contents (clay colored, tarry, fresh blood, mucus, undigested food), flatulence, hemorrhoids, hepatitis, jaundice, dark urine; history of ulcer, gallstones, polyps, tumor; previous x-ray examinations (where, when, findings)

L. **Genitourinary:** Dysuria, flank or suprapubic pain, urgency, frequency, nocturia, hematuria, polyuria, hesitancy, dribbling, loss in force of stream, passage of stone, edema of face, stress incontinence, hernias, sexually transmitted infection (inquire what kind and signs and symptoms, and list results of serologic test for syphilis [STS], if known)

M. **Neurologic:** Syncope (brief lapse in consciousness caused by transient cerebral hypoxia); history of stroke, seizures, weakness or paralysis, abnormalities of sensation or coordination, tremors, loss of memory; unusual frequency, distribution, or severity of headaches; serious head injury in past

N. **Psychiatric:** Depression, mood changes, difficulty concentrating, nervousness, tension, suicidal thoughts, irritability, sleep disturbances

Also use the health history to identify habits and lifestyle patterns. Use of alcohol, tobacco, illegal drugs, caffeine, herbal products, or over-the-counter drugs or prescription medications have potential to place the patient at risk for diseases involving the liver, the lungs, the heart, the nervous system, or thought processes. Note the type of habit, as well as the frequency and duration of use, to provide essential data. This is sometimes an uncomfortable area for both the patient and the nurse. To have a better chance of obtaining an accurate response, ask the patient, "How much alcohol do you drink?" rather than asking if the patient drinks alcohol.

Assess the patient's ability to perform ADLs. Patterns of sleep, exercise, and nutrition are important to assess when planning nursing interventions. Take care to correlate the patient's lifestyle patterns to how the nursing care plan will dictate these activities within a health care setting. If possible, see that variations in sleep, activity, and nutritional patterns are accommodated.

Family History

The purpose of the family history is to obtain data about immediate and blood relatives. This includes health or cause of death, as well as history of illnesses (e.g., diabetes mellitus, hypertension, heart disease, cancer). The objectives are to determine whether the patient is at risk for illnesses of a genetic or familial nature and to identify areas of health promotion and illness prevention. The family history also provides information about family structure, interaction, and function that are often useful in planning care. For example, a cohesive, supportive family is a possible resource in assisting a patient to adjust to an illness or disability; it is important in this case to incorporate the family into the plan of care. Conversely, if the patient's family is not supportive, it is often more therapeutic to refrain from involving them in care, particularly if the family history reveals that the patient is experiencing stress related to familial relationships.

Environmental History

The environmental history provides data about patients' home and work environments. The environmental history, for example, identifies exposure to pollutants that can affect health, high crime rates that prevent patients from walking around their neighborhoods, and resources available to assist patients in returning to the community.

Psychosocial and Cultural History

The psychosocial and cultural history includes data about the patient's primary language, cultural group, educational background, attention span, and developmental stage. It also provides information about the patient's and family's coping skills and support systems. It will help you identify potential or actual problems in dealing with the present illness and plan appropriate interventions. Make certain to identify major values, beliefs, and behaviors related to particular health concerns. Individualize assessments and interventions to the patient and family. Avoid making assumptions about cultural beliefs and behaviors without receiving validation from the patient (see Cultural Considerations box).

Review of Systems

The review of systems (ROS) is a systematic method for collecting data on all body systems (see Box 5-7). During the ROS, you will ask the patient about normal functioning of each system and any changes the patient has noted. Such changes are usually subjective data because they are described in terms of how the patient perceives them.

As you proceed through the nursing health history, record the data you obtain in a clear, concise manner using appropriate terminology. A clear, concise record is necessary because other health care professionals are likely to use the nursing health history when delivering health care. Figure 5-2 illustrates the correct way to record such information.

When you are determining the status of each body system, ask the patient specific questions relating to

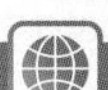 Cultural Considerations

Developing Cultural Sensitivity

Cultures are complex, integrated systems that include knowledge, skills, art, morals, law, customs, and any other acquired habits and capabilities of a group of people. Cultural beliefs and personal characteristics determine health behavior in individuals and families. More than half of all health problems are the result of behavior and lifestyle. If nursing's goal is to promote health while respecting individual value systems and lifestyles, it is imperative that culture-based behavior be understood.

The following are ways to develop cultural and ethnic sensitivity:

- Recognize that cultural and ethnic diversity exists.
- Demonstrate respect for people as unique individuals.
- Respect the unfamiliar.
- Identify and examine your own cultural and ethnic beliefs.
- Recognize that some cultural and ethnic groups have definitions of health and illness, as well as practices aimed at promoting health and curing illness, that will differ from your own.
- Interpret patients' signs and symptoms, and respond to them, in accordance with their cultural norms.
- Be willing to modify health care delivery in keeping with the patient's cultural background.
- Do not expect all members of one cultural group to behave in exactly the same manner.
- Appreciate that each person's cultural values are ingrained and therefore very difficult to change.

NURSING ADMISSION ASSESSMENT

Admitted: Ambulatory, Cart, Wheelchair, Arms, Ambulance

From: Office, ER, Surgery, Radiology, Recovery Room Transferred From: physician's office

Oriented to Room: Call Light, Side rails, TV, Phone, Safety/Smoking Policy: Yes ✓ No ____

Vital Signs: T 101² P 92 P 24 BP 160/92 HT 5'4" WT 190 Dentures upper/lower

Diet at home: 2 g sodium

Allergies: Drug penicillin Reaction hives

Other: none Organ Donor: Yes ____ No X

Reason for Admission Elevated temperature & fluid retention Signature E. Fletcher, LPN Date: 1/9/10 Time: 2010

EYES: Impaired vision, Blind, Cataract, Glaucoma, Contacts, Glasses, Prosthesis R. L.
Comments: cataract surgery (rt eye) 2008 OD

EARS, NOSE, THROAT: Hard of hearing, Deaf, Lesions, Hearing Aid, R, L., Tracheotomy
Comments:

RESPIRATORY: Pain, Dyspnea, Wheeze, Asthma, Sinusitis, COPD, Cough, Productive ____ Nonproductive X Oxygen needed, Smoker
Comments: c/o shortness of breath upon exertion crackles right base

CIRCULATION: Apical, Radial, Strong, Weak, Thready, Bounding, Regular, Palpitations, Chest pain, Numbness, Bruising, Edema, Hypertension, Hx MI, CHF, Pacer, Bypass Surgery
Comments: st" 4 pound weight gain in the last 3 days 3+ pitting edema bilaterally

ENDOCRINE: Thyroid, Diabetes
Comments: no problems

GI TRACT: Heartburn, Ulcers, Pain, Hernia, Dysphagia, Nausea, Vomiting, Loss of Appetite, Distention, Diverticulitis
Comments:

ELIMINATION: Last BM 2 days ago, Normal, Constipated, Diarrhea, Tarry, Bright red, Clay colored, Hemorrhoids, Involuntary, Use of laxatives, Yes/No enema, Yes/No, Ileostomy, Colostomy
Comments:

URINARY: Incontinence, Nocturia, Hematuria, Dysuria, Burning, Frequency, Urgency, Dribbling, infections, Cath: Yes/No
Comments:

NEUROLOGICAL: Convulsions, Paralysis, Syncope, Paresthesia, Dizziness, Coordination, Weakness, Headaches
Comments:

SKIN: Color pale Turgor poor Temp warm
Describe any Rashes, Lesions, Ecchymosis, Petechiae, Scars, Diabetic sores,
Comments: central abdominal scar

MUSCULOSKELETAL: Pain, Stiffness, Contractures, Deformities, Tremors, Backaches, Weight bearing, Amputation
Comments:

FEMALE REPRODUCTION: LMP EDC
Menopause, Breast pain, Breast tenderness, Vaginal discharge
Comments: post

PREVIOUS SURGERIES: herniorrhaphy ventral 2005; Rt eye Cataract surgery 2008

MEDS TAKEN AT HOME:

Med:	Dose:	Last Taken:
Cozaar	50 mg hour of sleep	Last PM
Coreg	12.5 mg BID	AM
Lasix	40 mgm qAM	AM
K-Lor	10 mEq BID	AM
Restoril	15 mg hour of sleep	Last PM

DISPOSAL OF MEDS:
Did not bring ✓
Pt. has ____ Family took home ____
Retained/taken to Pharmacy ____
Other:

Signature: Carolyn Oden RN
Time:

FIGURE 5-2 Nursing admission assessment.

the functioning of the system. For example, you will perhaps begin assessment of the respiratory system with the question, "Are you having any difficulty with your breathing?" Remember to be alert to the patient's comfort and well-being in the moment; thus, if the answer is "Yes," it is very possible that you will have to focus on airway, breathing, and circulation (ABCs) now, before continuing with questions. Once the patient's respiratory status is stable, continue the questioning with, "Please explain," or more specific questions, such as, "Do you have shortness of breath?" An ROS guide can be used to guarantee a complete interview.

The Communication box below shows an example of an interview using the OPQRSTUV technique. However, the ROS you carry out during the patient interview at the beginning of the physical assessment gives you much more information about the patient than what is contained merely in the words actually spoken. You will observe patient mobility and gain in-

Communication

Admission Assessment

Mr. Jacobi is admitted to the hospital with a diagnosis of possible peptic ulcer.

Nurse: Mr. Jacobi, can you tell me about your pain? What brings it on?

Patient: I get the pain several times a day after I eat. *(provocative) (timing)**

Nurse: What does it feel like?

Patient: It feels like burning. *(quality)*

Nurse: Where does the pain occur?

Patient: In my stomach. *(region)*

Nurse: How does the pain rate, on a scale of 0 to 10?

Patient: About an 8. *(severity)*

Nurse: How long have you had this pain?

Patient: It began about 6 months ago. *(timing)*

*See the description in Box 5-6 of the OPQRSTUV method of interviewing.

sight about the patient's intellect, level of orientation, and emotional and psychological state.

Assess the appropriateness of the patient's answers. By asking questions such as "Who are you?" "Why are you here?" "What is the date?" and "Where are you?" you determine the patient's **level of consciousness (LOC)** and level of orientation. Is the patient oriented to person, place, time, and purpose?

NURSING PHYSICAL ASSESSMENT

The physical examination you perform is sometimes also referred to as the **nursing physical assessment** or even just the nursing assessment. Nurses are most often the first to detect changes in the patient's condition. The skills of physical assessment provide you with powerful tools to detect subtle as well as obvious changes in a patient's health. The data you collect comprise the first step of the nursing process. Remember that the purpose of the nursing assessment is to determine the patient's state of health or illness. It is the initial step you use to form the nursing care plan, just as the physician performs a physical examination to determine the medical diagnosis and a proposed course of treatment. Many of the questions raised by the nurse in preparation to assist the physician are also a necessary part of the nursing physical assessment. Special considerations for assessing older adults are listed in the Life Span Considerations box.

Life Span Considerations

Older Adults

Assessment

- All systems will manifest changes to a greater or lesser extent with aging. An awareness of how aging affects an older adult helps sort out expected changes from pathologic processes. Adapt assessments to uncover problems and intervene effectively. All older adults do not show the physical signs of aging at the same rate.
- It is essential to allow adequate time for a thorough assessment. Several shorter sessions are likely to be better tolerated than one long session.
- During the assessment, monitor for signs of fatigue such as slumping, sighing, or irritability.
- For comfort during the assessment, do the following:
  - —Ensure privacy. If the older person has cognitive difficulty or wishes family member's assistance, allow it. Be careful that the family member does not dominate the conversation.
  - —Encourage the older person to void before the assessment.
  - —Conduct the assessment in a room where bathroom facilities are readily available.
  - —Verify that the temperature of the room is warm enough for the older person and free from drafts.
- Explain what you are doing in terms the older person can understand and avoid the use of medical jargon. Speak slowly and clearly so that the older person is able to hear what is being said and has the opportunity to process the information.
- Be patient and listen. Older people often take longer to reply, but it is important to allow them to complete ideas in their own words without interruption.
- Obtain objective and subjective data during the assessment.

When to Perform a Nursing Physical Assessment

The best time to assess the patient is as soon after admission as possible. In some facilities, policy dictates that the assessment be completed within 24 hours of admission. A registered nurse (RN) performs the initial baseline nursing assessment; however, the ongoing assessment is the responsibility of both the registered nurse and the licensed practical nurse or licensed vocational nurse (LPN/LVN).

The formal head-to-toe assessment is initially completed when the patient is admitted; however, portions of the assessment can be performed when you observe a change in the patient's condition. This is also referred to as a **focused assessment:** attention is concentrated or focused on a particular part of the body, where signs and symptoms are localized or most active, in order to determine their significance. Make a nursing assessment part of daily nursing care. By performing an assessment at the beginning of each shift, you can identify changes in the patient's condition, anticipate potential problems, communicate those changes to other medical personnel, and alter the nursing plan of care accordingly.

Where to Perform a Nursing Physical Assessment

Regardless of the setting—hospital, clinic, extended care facility, or the patient's home—it is important that the location for performing the nursing assessment be comfortable and safe for the patient. Ensure that an adjustable table or bed is available, and consider the patient's privacy. Be careful that the location is free of distracting sights, sounds, and odors. Keep the ambient temperature comfortable, because the patient's body will be exposed during the assessment. In most cases, the patient's own room works very well and is convenient for both you and the patient.

Methods of Performing a Nursing Physical Assessment

It is possible to organize the assessment in head-to-toe order or system by system. In either case, proceed systematically. By performing the assessment in the same manner each time, you have the ability to avoid inadvertently omitting a portion of the assessment. Box 5-8 is an example of a pocket guide to follow during the physical assessment; you will also find it useful when charting the assessment in your nursing notes.

If the patient expresses special concerns, or you observe any, it will often be best to perform a focused assessment of the system or area involved or a symptom analysis. However, if a complete physical assessment is necessary, it is usually best to assess any painful

Box 5-8 Physical Assessment Guide

1. Neurologic—Level of consciousness: alert, drowsy, lethargic, oriented ×1 (person), ×2 (person, place), ×3 (person, place, and time), ×4 (person, place, time, and purpose)
2. Integumentary—Skin condition, color, temperature, turgor, skin impairments, moist, dry
3. Cardiovascular—Apical pulse (strength and regularity), capillary refill (less than 3 sec) in upper and lower extremities, pedal pulses (1+ to 4+), pitting edema (1+ to 4+) (see Box 5-11), nonpitting edema, type of intravenous fluid with rate, site condition (without edema or erythema)
4. Respiratory—Posteriorly (lower lobes), anteriorly (upper lobes), right axilla (right middle lobe); auscultate for crackles, wheezes (sibilant and sonorous), pleural friction rub, respiration characteristics (tachypnea, orthopnea, dyspnea—resting or exertional); assess arterial oxygen saturation (Sao_2) via pulse oximeter; oxygen therapy with route (cannula, mask), and liters per minute of oxygen flow (e.g., O_2 2 L/min per nasal cannula)
5. Gastrointestinal—Diet, appetite, fluid intake; observe for distention; auscultate for presence of bowel sounds ×4 (active, hypoactive, hyperactive, absent by quadrants); palpate masses, tenderness, bowel movement with description, including colostomy or ileostomy stoma assessment, amount and consistency; nasogastric suction (color and amount)
6. Urinary—Urine amount, color, odor; presence of catheters (Foley, nephrostomy, suprapubic, ureteral); voiding; include ureterostomy stoma assessment
7. Mobility—Activity level: bed rest, chair, up ad lib; gait and level of tolerance; ambulation aides needed, such as walker, cane, or crutches

areas last. This will ensure better cooperation from the patient.

Performing the Nursing Physical Assessment

Items essential to the nurse's assessment are a penlight or flashlight, a stethoscope, a blood pressure cuff, a thermometer, gloves, gait belt, watch with second hand, scissors, black pen, and a tongue blade (see Figure 5-1 and Box 5-2). You will also make use of your senses of touch, smell, sight, and hearing. Always wash your hands before beginning the physical assessment. Follow the Centers for Disease Control and Prevention (CDC) (2002b) guidelines on standard precautions and hand hygiene guidelines.

Provide the patient the opportunity to empty his or her bladder before the examination. This makes the patient more comfortable and allows easier assessment of the bladder.

Obtain the patient's vital signs, including temperature, pulse, respirations, and blood pressure. Perform pain assessment to obtain the fifth vital sign (Box 5-9). The vital signs data you gather at the beginning of the assessment often provide clues to areas that warrant more critical evaluation. The beginning of the examination is also a good time to measure the patient's height and weight. For accuracy, measure height and weight yourself and then compare your results with the patient's stated height and weight. If there is a significant difference between these measurements, possible causes will have to be explored.

Box 5-9 Pain Assessment Scale

Use a pain rating scale to systematically assess pain intensity and manage pain. The most commonly used numerical scale is 0 to 10. Ask the patient to rate pain from 0 (no pain) to 10 (worst pain). Ratings of 3 to 5 are considered mild pain, ratings of 5 to 7 are considered moderate pain, and ratings greater than 7 are considered severe pain. Some agencies use a scale of 0 to 5. For children, use happy and sad faces to rate the pain. For clinical assessment, any of these scales is adequate and appropriate. However, it is important to always use the same scale with the same patient. See Figure 16-6 for sample pain intensity scales.

Head-to-Toe Assessment

When performing a head-to-toe assessment, begin with a neurologic assessment, and then assess the skin, the hair, the head, and the neck, including eyes, ears, nose, and mouth. Examine the chest, the back, the arms, the abdomen, the perineal area, the legs, and the feet in that order.

Note that the assessment does not stop after you have completed the head-to-toe assessment. It is a continuous process. Use the mnemonic *ABC, in and out, PS* for quick follow-up assessments (Box 5-10).

Neurologic. It is possible to integrate the neurologic assessment into the rest of the assessment. For instance, after taking the radial pulse, have the patient grasp your hands to test for equal grip. Always begin the neurologic assessment with the patient's level of consciousness and level of orientation.

Consciousness is awareness of one's thoughts and feelings and of the environment. The levels of consciousness (responsiveness) are generally described according to the behavior exhibited by the individual (Table 5-3).

It is critical to carefully assess the neurologic status of patients who have a head injury or signs or symptoms of a neurologic deficit from a neurologic disease (Jarvis, 2008). Neurologic assessment includes the following:

1. Level of consciousness: The earliest and most important factor in neurologic assessment is a change in the level of consciousness. Determine if the patient is oriented ×1 (person), ×2 (person and place), ×3 (person, place, and time), or ×4 (person, place, time, and purpose). Patients are

Box 5-10 How to Make Assessing Patients as Easy as ABC

Use a simple mnemonic to help you accurately check more patients in less time.

Take, for example, this scenario: You have just assisted a patient, Mr. Jonas, from his bed to a chair. Has this routine maneuver compromised his condition in any way? Are tubes and lines unimpeded? Is the patient comfortable in his new position?

To help you quickly answer these questions after transfers and periodically throughout your shift, we developed a handy mnemonic: **ABC, in and out, PS.** Use it for quick follow-up assessments after you complete the initial (and more thorough) assessment.

Here is what the letters and words in the mnemonic mean:

A = Airway. Is the airway compromised? Does Mr. Jonas's position have to be changed? It is not unusual for a weak, elderly, or very ill patient to slump or slide down in a bed or wheelchair, compromising the airway.

B = Breathing. Assess ease and rate. If Mr. Jonas is eupneic and the rate is normal, move on. If you detect problems, assess further.

C = Circulation. Check general color and quickly palpate extremities for tissue perfusion, assessing pulses and skin temperature.

In = What's going in? Check the identity and level of every solution Mr. Jonas is receiving by intravenous (IV) route or enterally. Look at drip rates and machine settings; check tubing (is anything taut or twisted?) and IV sites. Also check the rate of oxygen delivery and note if the oxygen delivery device is in place. To keep on track, start at each source (for example, the enteral feeding bag) and follow the tubes or lines to the insertion site on the patient's body, checking as you proceed.

Out = What's coming out? Is any drainage coming out of dressings? If so, is the color and amount appropriate? Check that chest tubes and urinary catheters are free from tension and kinks, and note the amount and characteristics of drainage. Again, to keep on track, start where the tube or drain exits Mr. Jonas's body and follow it to the collection receptacle.

P = Pain. Exactly how you will proceed depends on Mr. Jonas's condition and the results of your last in-depth pain assessment, but plan to check his comfort at every encounter. If he sits in the chair for a while, for instance, he will possibly become uncomfortable and want to go back to bed. Or perhaps he will become chilly and want another blanket.

S = Safety. Are side rails up as needed and are personal items and the call bell within easy reach? Are restraints (if used) properly applied? Is the bed or wheelchair locked and the area clutter free?

With this quick but complete approach, you can hit the essential points of assessment and easily pick up clues that signal a need for more assessment. And if all is well, you are reassured that your patient is stable, safe, and comfortable.

By Jacqueline Boyce Fitzpatrick, RN, MS, associate professor of nursing, State University of New York College of Agriculture and Technology, Morrisville; Marilyn Cary Shinners, RN, MS, nursing instructor, Samaritan Hospital School of Nursing, Troy, New York. From Fitzpatrick, J. (1996). How to make assessing as easy as ABC. *Nursing, 26*(8):51.

Table 5-3 Level of Consciousness (Responsiveness)

LEVEL	BEHAVIORS
Consciousness	Appropriate response (rate and quality) to external stimuli; oriented to time, place, person, and purpose
Confusion	Inappropriate response to stimuli and decreased attention span and memory; inappropriate reactions to simple commands
Lethargy (hypersomnia)	Drowsiness or increased sleep time; is able to be aroused; responds appropriately; possibly falls asleep again immediately
Delirium	Confusion, disorder perception, and decreased attention span; motor and sensory excitement; inappropriate reactions to stimuli; marked anxiety
Coma	Loss or lowering of consciousness
Stage I (stupor)	Arousable for short periods to verbal, visual, or painful stimuli; simple motor and verbal response to stimuli; slow responses; corneal and papillary reflexes sluggish; deep tendon and superficial reflexes unaffected; possible to obtain pathologic reflexes
Stage II (light coma)	Simple motor and verbal (moaning) response to painful stimuli; mass motor movement or flexion (avoidance) response
Stage III (deep coma)	Decerebrate posturing to painful stimuli (extension of body and limbs and pronation of arms)
Stage IV	Flaccid muscles; papillary reflex absent, apneic; on ventilator; superficial and some deep tendon reflexes present
Brain death	Presence of all of the following: Two electroencephalographic (EEG) tracings 24 hours apart indicate absence of brain waves; cerebral function absent for 24 hours; failure of cerebral perfusion; expert opinion rules out hypothermia or drug toxicity
Syncope	Temporary loss of consciousness (partial or complete) associated with increased rate of respiration, tachycardia, pallor, perspiration, and coolness of skin
Fugue state	Dysfunction of consciousness (hours or days) in which the individual carries on purposeful activity that he or she does not remember afterward
Amnesia	Memory loss over time or for specific subjects; individual affected responds appropriately to external stimuli

From Barkauskas, V., Baumann, L., & Darling-Fisher, C. (2006). *Health and physical assessment.* (4th ed.). St. Louis: Mosby.

alert if they have the ability to open their eyes spontaneously, if they are oriented to person, place, time and purpose, or if they are able to comply correctly to verbal clues (Jarvis, 2008).
2. Motor function: Ask the patient to move each extremity. Have the patient smile, frown, and lift the eyebrows.
3. Pupillary response: Check the pupils for size, equality, and shape. Use a penlight to shine into each pupil. Each pupil should constrict quickly (Jarvis, 2008). Pupils should be equal in size (3 to 7 mm in diameter). When assessing the pupils and the reaction is normal in all exams, record the letters PERRLA (pupils equal, round, reactive to light, and accommodation (Potter and Perry, 2009).

The third cranial nerve (cranial nerve III) runs parallel to the brainstem. The function of the oculomotor nerve is essential for eye movements (supplying extrinsic and intrinsic eye muscles). The intrinsic muscle affects the size and the equality of the pupils. A traumatic brain injury often results in increased intracranial pressure and edema of the brainstem with pressure on cranial nerve III, causing the ominous sign of a unilateral, dilated, and nonreactive pupil (Jarvis, 2008).

Other major areas of neurologic examination include the following:

1. Proprioception (pertaining to the sensations of body movements and awareness of posture) and cerebellar function
2. Deep tendon reflexes
3. Cranial nerve assessment (performed by the RN)

Vital signs. Vital signs are very important in assessment of the critically ill patient; however, pulse and blood pressure are not reliable indicators of central nervous system deficit. You will be able to note an increase in systolic blood pressure with widening pulse pressure, bradycardia, and an irregular breathing pattern (Cushing's triad) late in the course of the development of increased intracranial pressure (Jarvis, 2008).

Glasgow Coma Scale. The Glasgow Coma Scale (GCS) is a standardized, objective measurement of the level of consciousness. The scale has a numeric value. The scale is divided into three areas: eye opening, verbal response, and motor response. Assess each of the three areas separately, and give a number for the patient's correct response. Total the three numbers. A normal GCS demonstrating no brain trauma is 15. A score of 8 or less indicates severe brain injury (Jarvis, 2008).

Clues to areas of neurologic abnormality are sometimes evident during the patient's history, such as orientation, speech, and ability to interact with the examiner. Continue to evaluate the patient throughout the assessment process for a more accurate neurologic assessment.

Skin and hair. Observe the skin for color, temperature, moisture, texture, turgor, and evidence of injury or skin lesions. Normal skin tones vary with race, heredity, and sun exposure. Note the overall appearance, as well as the color in the sclera, the mucous membranes, the tongue, the lips, the nailbeds, and the palms and soles. A general uniformity of color from dark brown to light tan with pink or yellow overtones (depending on the patient's race) is normal. Changes in skin color that sometimes provide evidence of systemic disease include pallor, cyanosis, jaundice, erythema, and ecchymosis. The appearance of cyanotic (dusky blue) fingers, lips, or mucous membranes is abnormal in both light- and dark-skinned individuals. Jaundice in dark-skinned individuals sometimes appears as yellow staining in the sclera, the hard palate, and the palmar or plantar surfaces.

Normally the skin is warm, dry, and smooth, with good turgor. **Turgor** refers to the elasticity of the skin caused by the outward pressure of the cells and interstitial fluid (Figure 5-3). Dehydration results in *decreased* skin turgor and is manifested by lax skin that, when grasped and raised between two fingers, slowly returns to its previous position. Marked edema results in *increased* turgor, manifested by smooth, taut, shiny skin that cannot be grasped and raised.

Note any skin lesions or evidence of other skin impairments. Document their size, shape, color, pattern, location, and any presence of exudate.

Examine the hair over the entire body to determine the distribution, the quantity, and the quality. Hairless lower extremities sometimes signify an arterial disorder with reduced arterial blood flow. The hair is normally of a smooth texture and not oily or dry. A normal scalp is free of dandruff, lesions, and parasites. Wear gloves if you wish to inspect the hair and scalp. Abnormalities are sometimes related to external factors, such as the use of beauty products, and sometimes to internal factors, such as systemic or localized illnesses.

Head and neck. Assessment of the head includes the eyes, the ears, the nose, and the mouth. The neck assessment involves the arteries, the veins, and the lymph nodes. Facial expression and appearance are likely to be the first observations you make and often

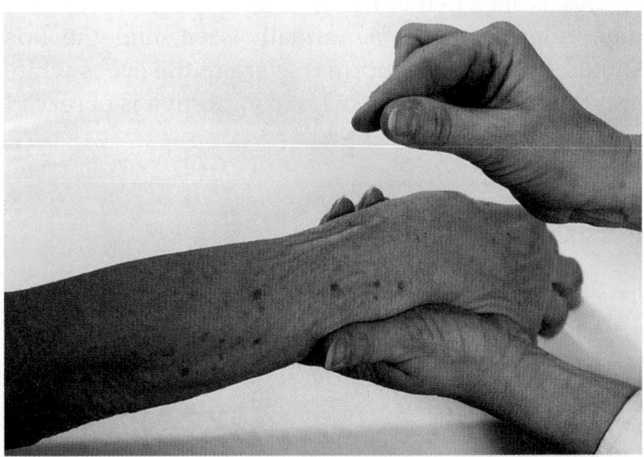

FIGURE 5-3 Assess skin turgor by first grasping fold of skin on back of patient's hand, sternum, forearm, or abdomen. Note ease and speed with which skin returns to place.

give clues to the emotional state of the patient. Note the symmetry of the face; normal facial movements are also symmetric and appropriate. The head is normally upright and still.

It is possible to make a gross assessment of range of motion (ROM) by having the patient move the head from side to side and in a nodding motion. The patient should be able to move the head comfortably through these motions. Using the pads of the fingers, palpate beneath the jaw and down each side of the neck to feel for enlarged lymph nodes. Although it is not abnormal to have an enlarged node, tenderness is not normal. Palpate the carotid arteries gently and one at a time (Figure 5-4). The normal carotid pulse is regular and palpable without a **thrill**, a vibrating sensation you perceive as you palpate along the artery.

Inspect for jugular venous distention. The jugular veins give information about activity on the right side of the heart. Specifically, they reflect filling pressure and volume changes. Distention results when ineffective pumping action of the right ventricle causes increased volume and pressure within the veins (Jarvis, 2008). Normally the veins will not be observable with the patient in a sitting position. Jugular venous distention is seen in venous hypertension or right-sided heart failure. It is possible to perform auscultation of the carotid artery by listening with the bell of the stethoscope. Normally, no bruits are audible. **Bruits** are abnormal "swishing" sounds heard over organs, glands, and arteries. A bruit results from an abnormality in an artery resulting from a narrow or partially occluded artery such as occurs in atherosclerosis (Jarvis, 2008).

Mouth and throat. Inspect the lips and the mucous membranes of the mouth with a tongue blade and penlight, assessing all surfaces of the oral cavity. Normal mucous membranes are moist, pink, and free of lesions. With dehydration, mucous membranes look dry. The lips should be smooth, moist, and free of cracking. The condition of the teeth and gums gives the nurse insight into the health habits of the patient. Breath odors often indicate disease; it is not normal for the breath to be foul, fruity, or musty.

Eyes. Note whether the eyes are symmetric. No exudate from the eyes is normally seen, and the lids should be open. The normal sclera of the eye is white and the conjunctiva pink. The conjunctiva is observed by gently depressing the lower lid. Periorbital edema (edema around the eye) is abnormal.

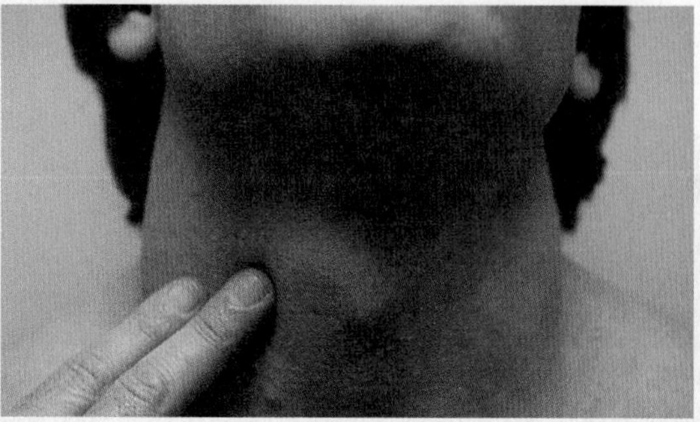

FIGURE 5-4 Palpation of carotid artery.

Assess both eyes individually. Also observe the eyes for pupillary reflex. Do this by darkening the room and using the penlight to shine light into the pupil. Have the light come from the side of the eye; shine the light across the eye, with the patient looking straight ahead at a focal point. The normal eye will show the pupil constricting when the light is applied. The pupil toward which the light is directed will normally constrict; this reaction is the direct papillary response to light. If normal, the other pupil will also constrict; this reaction is the consensual response to light. The rate and degree of constriction should be equal. A tip to recall this finding is to use the acronym PERRLA, which stands for *pupils equal, round, reactive to light, and accommodation.*

Ears. First note whether the ears are symmetric. By pulling gently back and up on the external ear to straighten, you will be better able to examine the ear canal with help from the penlight. With a child under age 3, pull the pinna back and down. Normally there is no pain associated with this movement. The ear canal is normally free of excess cerumen (earwax), blood, and any other discharge. During this assessment, note whether the patient is appropriately following commands, indicating an ability to hear.

Nose. The nose is usually symmetric, although variation in size is considered normal. To test for patency, press against one nostril and ask the patient to breathe. Air should flow through the nose. Assess both nostrils, observing for bleeding or drainage.

Chest, lungs, heart, and vascular system. Perform assessment of the chest and lungs with the patient in a sitting position. Inspect the chest for bilateral chest expansion, which is normally symmetric. Note the rate and depth of respirations. The normal rate for an adult is 12 to 20 breaths per minute. Normal breathing is quiet.

Tachypnea is a rapid rate of breathing at a rate greater than 24 breaths per minute. Tachypnea occurs in fever, fear, exercise, pneumonia, alkalosis, or respiratory insufficiency. Bradypnea refers to slow breathing of fewer than 10 breaths per minute. Bradypnea occurs in increased intracranial pressure, or depression of the respiratory center in the medulla oblongata owing to the action of opioids. Cheyne-Stokes respiration is an abnormal cycle of respirations that begins with slow, shallow respirations that become rapid. Respirations become slower and are followed by periods of apnea (20 seconds) before the cycle repeats itself. The most common causes of Cheyne-Stokes respiration are heart failure, opioid overdose, renal failure, meningitis, and severe head injury (Jarvis, 2008).

Note any sounds that are audible without the stethoscope; later you will auscultate them and determine their origin. Posture is often indicative of acute or chronic respiratory disease. The patient who is unable to lie supine or who must lean forward to breathe is showing signs of this distress. A large, rounded "barrel chest" is diagnostic for adults with pulmonary disease such as emphysema. Assess arterial oxygen saturation (Sao_2, the amount of oxygen bound to hemoglobin) via pulse oximetry, a noninvasive method of monitoring in which a sensor is attached to the person's finger or earlobe. An Sao_2 of 90% to 100% is needed to replenish O_2 in plasma.

Breasts. It is acceptable to examine the breasts during a lung assessment. Many patients also do so on a monthly basis. Teach breast self-exam to both male and female patients.

Lung sounds. Through auscultation, it is possible to obtain information about the functioning of the respiratory system and about the presence of any obstruction in the air passages. Most commonly, you will use the diaphragm of the stethoscope, which is designed to transmit the usually higher pitch of abnormal breath sounds.

It is preferable to auscultate lungs with the patient in a sitting position. Place the patient in a sitting position, leaning forward with arms across the lap. Instruct the patient to breathe through his or her mouth quietly and more deeply and slowly than in a usual respiration. Place the stethoscope firmly but not tightly on the skin, and listen for one full inspiratory-expiratory cycle at each point. Never listen with a stethoscope over clothing. Systematically auscultate the apices and the posterior, lateral, and anterior chest. Use a zigzag approach, comparing the findings at each point with the corresponding point on the opposite side (Figures 5-5 and 5-6).

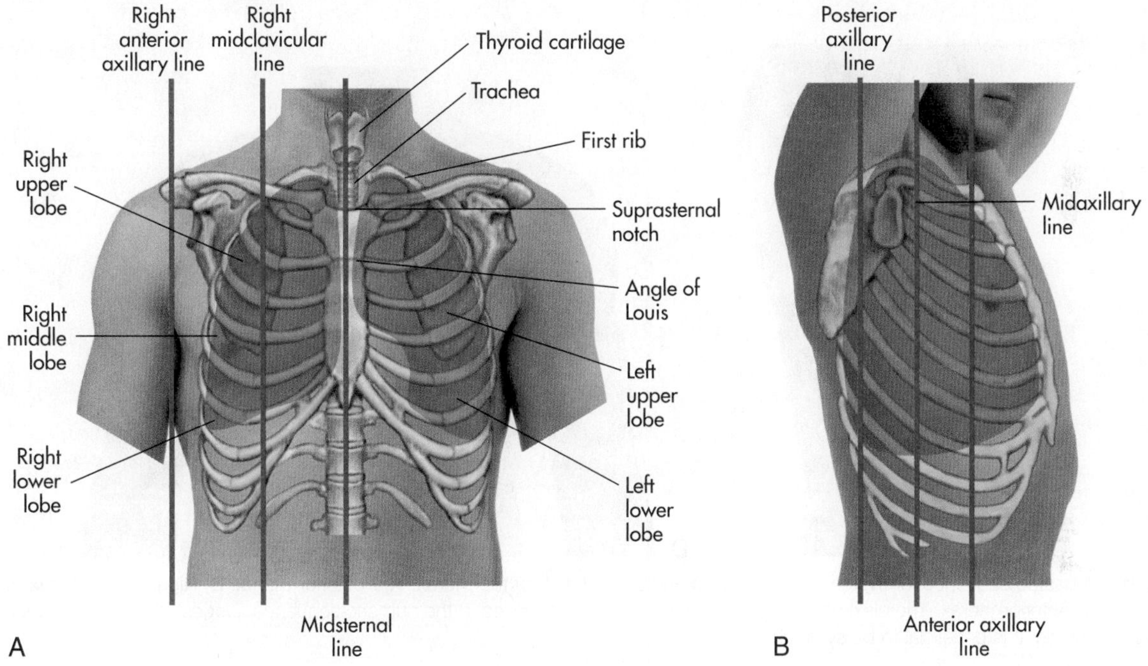

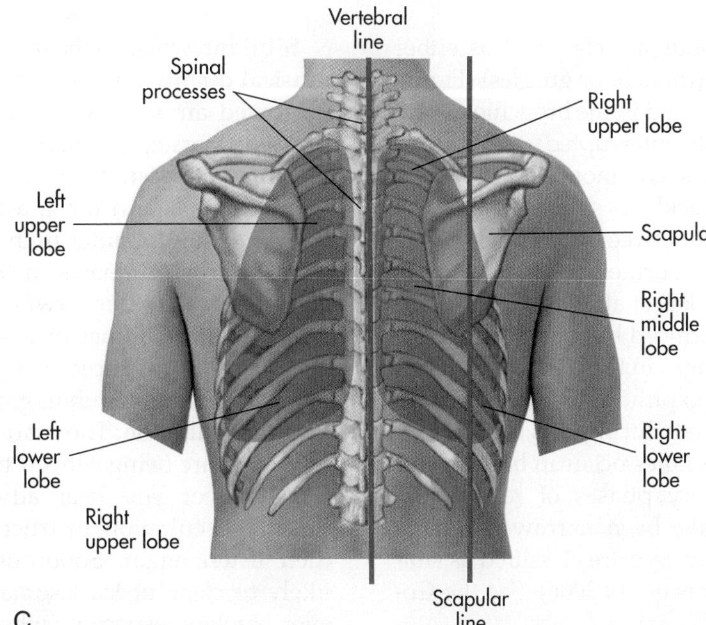

FIGURE 5-5 Thoracic landmarks. **A,** Anterior thorax. **B,** Right lateral thorax. **C,** Posterior thorax.

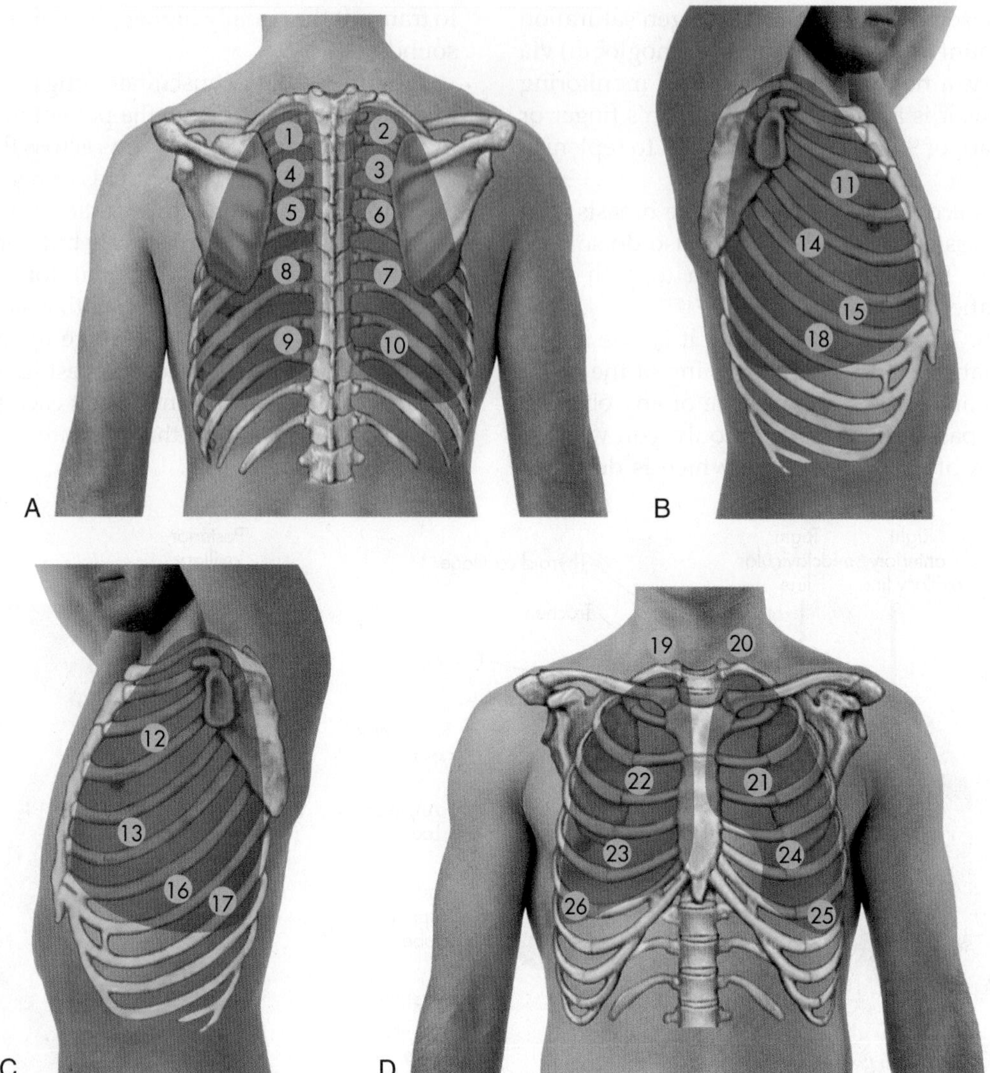

FIGURE 5-6 Suggested sequence for systematic percussion and auscultation of the thorax. **A,** Posterior thorax. **B,** Right lateral thorax. **C,** Left lateral thorax. **D,** Anterior thorax. The pleximeter finger or the stethoscope is moved in the numeric sequence suggested; however, other sequences are possible. It is beneficial to be systematic.

Adventitious breath sounds are classified as either crackles (rales) or wheezes (rhonchi or gurgles) (Figure 5-7). **Crackles,** produced by fluid in the bronchioles and the alveoli, are short, discrete, interrupted, crackling, or bubbling sounds that are most commonly heard during inspiration. The sound of crackles is similar to that produced by hairs being rolled between the fingers while close to the ear. Crackles are further described as fine, medium, or coarse (Barkauskas et al., 2006).

Wheezes are sounds produced by the movement of air through narrowed passages in the tracheobronchial tree. They predominate in expiration because bronchi are shortened and narrowed during this respiratory phase. However, they sometimes occur in both the inspiratory and the expiratory phases of respiration, suggesting that lumina have been narrowed during both respiratory phases. Wheezes are classified as sibilant or sonorous (Barkauskas et al., 2006). See the Coordinated Care box.

Sibilant wheezes have a high-pitched squeaking, musical quality and are produced by airflow through narrowed airways. **Sonorous** wheezes have a lower-pitched, coarser, gurgling, snoring quality and usually indicate the presence of mucus in the trachea and the large airways. **Stridor** is a high-pitched, inspiratory, crowing sound, louder in the neck than over the chest wall. Stridor originates in the larynx or the trachea, and indicates upper airway obstruction from edematous, inflamed tissues or a foreign body. **Pleural friction rubs** are produced by inflammation of the pleural sac; you will hear a rubbing, grating, or squeaky sound upon auscultation. The grating sounds as if two pieces of leather are being rubbed together.

Whenever you hear adventitious breath sounds during auscultation, instruct the patient to cough, and then listen again. Sonorous wheezes are the most likely to clear, at least somewhat, with cough. However, crackles, especially when patients are on bed rest,

Fine crackles: high-pitched, discrete, discontinuous crackling sounds heard during the end of inspiration; not cleared by a cough

Medium crackles: lower, more moist sound heard during the midstage of inspiration; not cleared by a cough

Coarse crackles: loud, bubbly noise heard during inspiration; not cleared by a cough

Rhonchi (sonorous wheeze): loud, low coarse sounds like a snore most often heard continuously during inspiration or expiration; coughing may clear sound (usually means mucus accumulation in trachea or large bronchi)

Wheeze (sibilant wheeze): musical noise sounding like a squeak; most often heard continuously during inspiration or expiration; usually louder during expiration

Pleural friction rub: dry, rubbing, or grating sound, usually caused by inflammation of pleural surfaces; heard during inspiration or expiration; loudest over lower lateral anterior surface

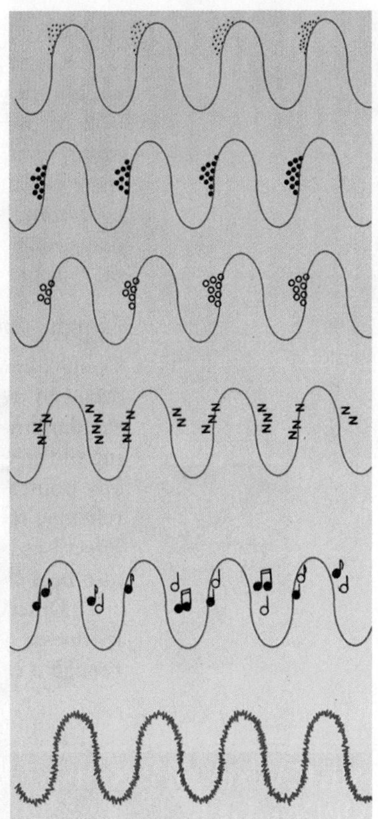

FIGURE 5-7 Adventitious breath sounds.

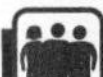 Coordinated Care

Leadership

ASSESSING LUNG SOUNDS

Assessment of the lung and thorax requires application of skills and knowledge unique to a nurse. For these skills, delegation is inappropriate. For patients with abnormal lung sounds, instruct assistive personnel (AP) to observe a patient's respirations and report any changes in rate and depth and to keep the head of the bed elevated for the patient to breathe.

sometimes also clear somewhat with cough. Document this finding with the breath sounds.

Spine. With the patient in a sitting position, note the curvature of the spine. Also assess the patient's posture when standing. Run your fingers down the patient's spine, which should be straight, assessing for the normal lumbosacral curve. Common postural abnormalities include lordosis, kyphosis, and scoliosis. Kyphosis, or humpback, is an exaggeration of the posterior curvature of the thoracic spine. Lordosis, or swayback, is an increased lumbar curvature. Scoliosis is a lateral spinal curvature. Check that the skin of the back is of normal color, temperature, and moisture.

Heart sounds. Heart sounds are auscultated with the stethoscope using both the bell and the diaphragm. The normal "lubb-dupp" sound of the heart is caused by the closure of the atrioventricular and the semilunar valves, respectively. The first normal heart sound, S_1, occurs with closure of the atrioventricular valves (AV) and thus signals the beginning of systole. S_1 is usually auscultated most clearly at the apex. The second normal heart sound, S_2, occurs with closure of the semilunar valves and signals the end of systole. S_2 is auscultated most clearly at the base (Jarvis, 2008). Extra heart sounds are S_3 and S_4. S_3, which sounds after S_2, is best heard at the apex. S_3 is sometimes normal in children, but is usually abnormal in adults. S_3 has a dull, soft sound and is sometimes an early sign of heart failure. S_4 is heard late in diastole when the atria contract. It is auscultated most clearly at the apex and is heard immediately before S_1. The sound is soft with a low pitch. S_4 is sometimes normal and sometimes pathologic; it is heard in patients with coronary artery disease after myocardial infarction (MI) or cardiomyopathy (Jarvis, 2008). With the patient in various positions (Figure 5-8), listen to the heart sounds for several cardiac cycles in each of the four points on the patient's chest (see Figure 5-6). Listen for the intensity of the sound, ranging from faint to strong. Also determine the regularity of the rhythm: regular, regularly irregular, or irregularly irregular. For patients with faint heart sounds, very irregular rhythms, very rapid heart rates, or noisy respirations, it helps to palpate the carotid or the radial pulses simultaneously with the auscultation of the heart sounds.

Peripheral vascular system. Arteries provide oxygen and nutrients to the tissues. You will assess the peripheral arteries by palpating peripheral arterial pulses. An

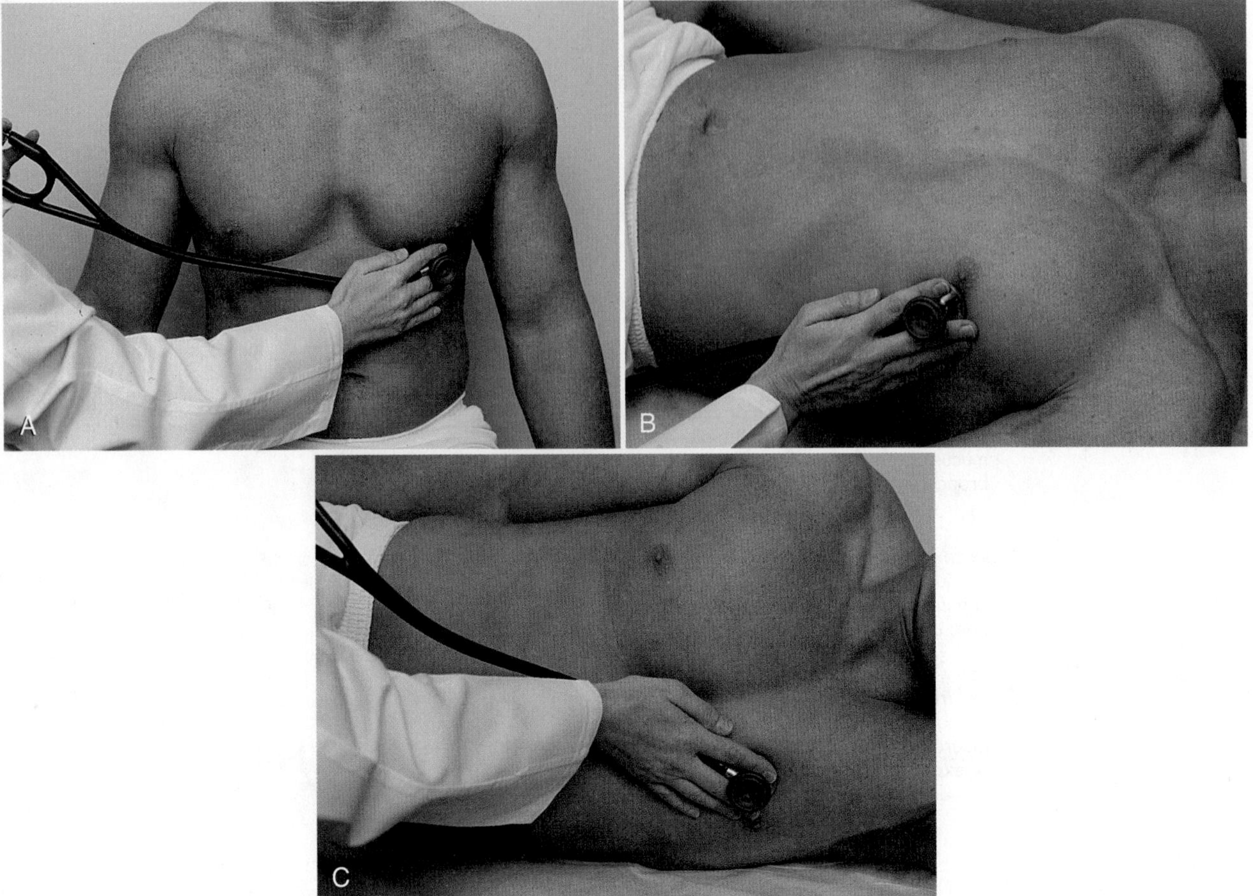

FIGURE 5-8 Sequence of patient positions for auscultation of heart sounds. **A,** Sitting up, leaning slightly forward. **B,** Supine. **C,** Left lateral recumbent.

arterial pulse is a pressure wave transmitted through the arterial system with each contraction of the heart. Peripheral pulses that you will be able to assess are radial, brachial, ulnar, femoral, popliteal, dorsalis pedis, and posterior tibial (Figure 5-9).

Using the pads of your fingertips, apply enough pressure at the pulse to gather information on the pulse rate, rhythm, and strength. Do not press so hard that the artery is occluded. If you encounter difficulty in locating the pulse, carefully move your fingers to slightly different positions in the area and vary the pressure you are exerting. Assess the pulse rate by counting the pulsation for 60 seconds. Check the rhythm for regularity. The strength of the pulse can by measured by using the following scale: 0 = absent, 1+ = thready, 2+ = weak, 3+ = normal, and 4+ = bounding. Follow agency policy when describing the pulse.

Begin with the most distal pulses to assess the arterial circulation at the farthest palpable point. Palpate the brachial pulse over the antecubital fossa (anterior surface of the elbow joint). Palpate the radial pulse by placing the pads of your first and second fingers on the palmar surface of the patient's relaxed and slightly flexed wrist medial to the radius bone. Palpate the femoral pulse midway between the anterosuperior iliac crest and the symphysis pubis, below and medial to the inguinal ligament. Palpate the popliteal pulse by pressing deeply into the dorsal aspect of the knee while the knee is slightly bent. Palpate the dorsalis pedis pulse by applying light touch between the first and second toes and slowly moving up the dorsum of the foot. The dorsalis pedis artery runs along the top of the foot in line with the groove between the extensor tendons of the great toe and the first toe. In adults over 45 years, occasionally the dorsalis pedis pulse is hard to find. Palpate the posterior tibial pulse slightly below and posterior to the medial malleolus of the ankle (Barkauskas et al., 2006).

Ischemia results if there is a decreased supply of oxygenated blood to the tissues; often this is caused by a narrowing of an artery. An embolism sometimes results in complete occlusion of an artery and death of tissue distal to the occlusion. Atherosclerosis has the potential to cause a partial occlusion of an artery and thus an insufficient delivery of oxygenated blood to the tissues. This sometimes results in a condition called claudication, which results in cramplike pains in the lower extremities, usually occurring after walking. The pain is caused by insufficient oxygen to the leg muscles (Jarvis, 2008).

Inspect the extremities for symmetry, color, and varicosities. They are normally symmetric and with-

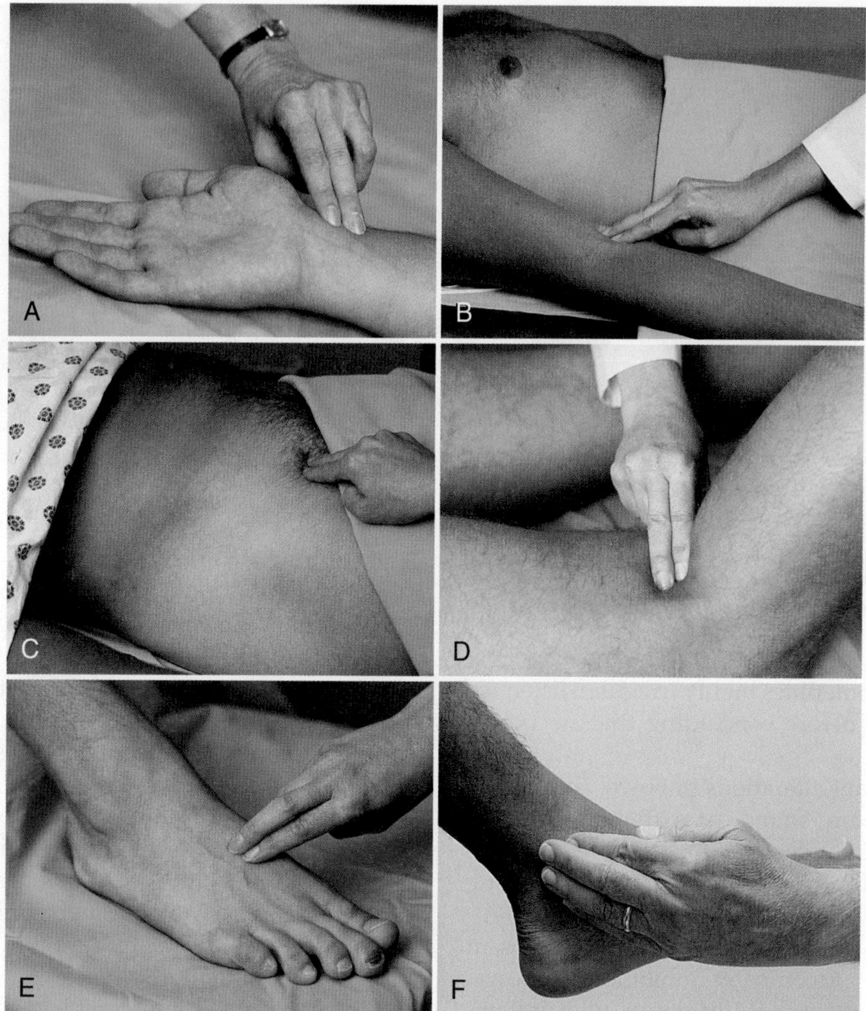

FIGURE 5-9 Palpation of arterial pulses. **A,** Radial. **B,** Brachial. **C,** Femoral. **D,** Popliteal. **E,** Dorsalis pedis. **F,** Posterior tibial.

out edema or discoloration. Palpate the hands and feet for temperature; normally, they are warm. Peripheral veins are normally fairly flat and barely visible.

Perform the capillary refill, or blanch, test by pressing firmly for 5 seconds on the fingernail or toenail and estimating the speed at which the blood returns (the tips of the fingers and toes can be used if the person has thick, unblanchable nailbeds). In a person with good cardiac function and distal perfusion, capillary refill usually takes less than 3 seconds. A capillary refill of more than 3 seconds is considered a sign of sluggish digital circulation, and a time of 5 seconds is considered abnormal. Poor cardiac function, dehydration, and peripheral vascular diseases are examples of disease processes that often cause delays in capillary refill.

Gastrointestinal system. During the remaining portion of the examination, the patient may remain in the supine position with knees elevated. During this portion of the assessment, be sure the patient is properly draped to decrease exposure of the pubic area and the breasts. Interview the patient regarding expelling of flatus, the latest bowel movement, and any complaints of nausea, vomiting, or altered appetite. After the interview, examine the abdomen. First inspect the abdomen for shape, contour, lesions, scars, lumps, or rashes. Normally, the abdomen's contour is even, and skin color is the same as that of the thorax. You will then auscultate for bowel sounds (Note: *before* palpating) by placing the diaphragm of the stethoscope over the divisions of the abdomen (Figure 5-10) and listening for the sounds of peristalsis (wavelike movements of the intestine). It is helpful, before you begin, to make sure the room is quiet: If the patient is on a nasogastric suction machine, or if a radio or television is on, turn them off. Light pressure on the stethoscope is sufficient to detect bowel sounds. Because peristalsis is continuous, you will normally hear sounds in all quadrants. Bowel sounds occur every 15 to 60 seconds and are classified as active, hyperactive, hypoactive, or absent. The normal rate of bowel sounds is 4 to 32 per minute.

Listen to bowel sounds for 1 minute in all quadrants to ensure you do not miss any sounds and to localize specific sounds. It is especially important to be thorough and take your time when evaluating for a silent abdomen (i.e., the absence of bowel sounds), which indicates the arrest of intestinal motility. Because peri-

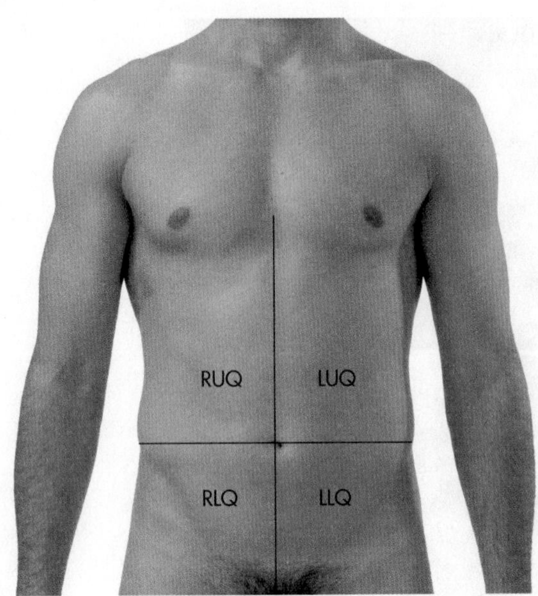

FIGURE 5-10 Anatomic divisions of the abdomen (quadrants).

staltic sounds are sometimes highly irregular, listen for at least 4 minutes before concluding that no bowel sounds are present.

The two significant alterations in bowel sounds are (1) the absence of any sound, or extremely soft and widely separated sounds, and (2) increased sounds with a characteristically high-pitched, loud, rushing sound (**borborygmi**):

- **Decreased bowel sounds.** Diminished or absent bowel sounds accompany inhibition of bowel motility. Decreased motility occurs with inflammation, gangrene, or paralytic ileus. Decreased peristalsis frequently accompanies peritonitis, electrolyte disturbances, the aftermath of surgical manipulation of the bowel, and late bowel obstruction. In addition, diminished bowel sounds are often correlated with lower lobe pneumonia.
- **Increased bowel sounds.** Loud, gurgling borborygmi often accompanies increased motility of the bowel, such as with diarrhea. Sounds of loud volume also are heard over areas of stenotic bowel. Sounds from an early bowel obstruction are high pitched. Frequently these are splashing sounds, similar to the emptying of a bottle into a hollow vessel. Fine, metallic, tinkling sounds are emitted as tiny gas bubbles break through the surface of intestinal juices. Common pathologic conditions associated with increased bowel sounds are gastroenteritis and subsiding ileus. Increased motility is sometimes caused by the use of a laxative, and sometimes by gastroenteritis.

Assessment of the abdomen for distention, firmness, and tenderness is also very important. After auscultating for bowel sounds, palpate the underlying structures. Palpation comes after auscultation because the manipulation has potential to stimulate intestinal activity and thus alter bowel sounds. Both

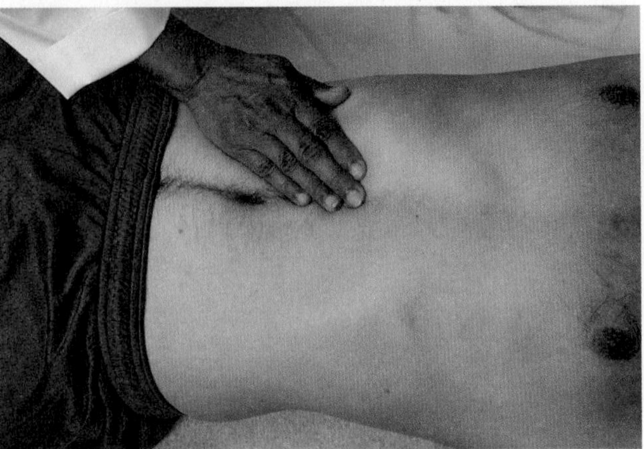

FIGURE 5-11 Light palpation of the abdomen to assess for distention, masses, or tenderness.

light and deep palpation are used. Beginning with light palpation, note texture, temperature, and moisture of the skin in all regions (Figure 5-11). Normal skin of the abdomen is smooth, dry, and warm. Light palpation will enable you to detect superficial lesions just below the skin. Advanced practice nurses will use deep palpation to detect tenderness or masses of the abdomen. In the upper right quadrant just below the rib cage, it will sometimes be possible to palpate the liver (Figure 5-12). If the liver is felt, it sometimes means that it is enlarged. The normal liver is smooth and nontender. The abdomen itself will normally be free of masses, and palpation will not be uncomfortable for the patient.

To ensure that the patient is relaxed during the palpation, be sure your hands are warm, and use conversation to distract the patient. Note the patient's face when you are palpating and check for grimacing. Sometimes the patient will also guard a tender area, which means he or she will tighten up abdominal muscles when the area is touched.

Use percussion on the abdomen to note the density of underlying tissue. Also percuss to locate the margins of internal organs. The normal abdomen has a

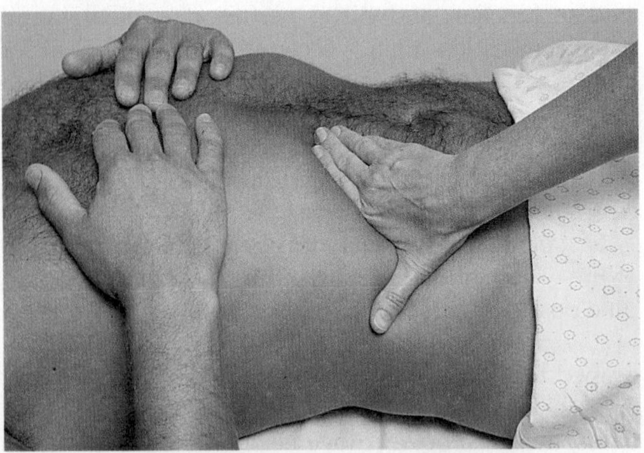

FIGURE 5-12 Palpation of the liver using moderate palpation.

tympanic (drumlike) sound, with dullness noted over the liver. A hollow sound heard over the stomach or intestines indicates flatus.

Genitourinary system. Nurses do not perform the vaginal examination with a speculum unless they have had advanced training. Assessment of the urinary system is performed using observation and palpation. It is most convenient for you to perform this inspection during the perineal care of the patient. Wear gloves when inspecting the labia for lesions. Inspect the pubic hair for lice, and note any vaginal discharge. Normal labia are pink, moist, and free of lesions. A normal white vaginal discharge known as leukorrhea is sometimes present.

Inspect the male genitalia for lesions and lice; look for discharge from the penis. Palpate the scrotum for lumps or hernias. If the male is uncircumcised, gently retract the foreskin to inspect for lesions on the glans penis.

While inspecting the genitalia on both males and females, palpate the femoral artery in that area (see Figure 5-9, *C*). Use palpation of the suprapubic area to determine distention.

Rectum. The rectal area is best examined with the patient in a Sims' position. Spread the buttocks to look for hemorrhoids or lesions. Normal skin around the anus is darker than surrounding skin. To further assess the intestinal system, explain the procedure for obtaining a stool specimen to the patient and leave a Hemoccult slide with the patient. The results of the test usually indicate whether gastrointestinal bleeding is present.

Legs and feet. The legs and feet are the final area of assessment. Palpate femoral, popliteal, dorsalis pedis, and posterior tibial as described earlier (see Figure 5-9, *C* to *F*). Assess the extremities for temperature. Cold extremities signal possible peripheral vascular disease with inadequate arterial perfusion. Observe the legs and feet, and palpate them for edema. **Edema** is an excessive accumulation of fluid in the interstitial spaces caused by leakage of fluid from veins and capillary beds. This occurs as a result of many disease processes, such as congestive heart failure, pathologic conditions of the kidneys, burns, lymphatic stasis, and trauma. Observe for edema in dependent parts of the body such as the feet, the legs, the scrotum, and the sacral area.

Pitting sometimes does and sometimes does not occur with edema. To check for pitting, press against a bony prominence for 5 seconds, and then lift your finger. Observe the skin for rebounding, and feel the area for the presence of an indentation. If the tissue rebounds immediately, the patient does not have pitting edema. An indentation indicates pitting edema, which is usually graded on a scale of 1 to 4 as follows (Box 5-11) (Barkauskas et al., 2006):

1+ Slight pitting; no visible change in the shape of the extremity; disappears rapidly

2+ Somewhat deeper pitting; no marked change in the shape of the extremity; disappears in 10 to 15 seconds

3+ Noticeably deep pitting; full and edematous extremity; sometimes lasts for more than 1 minute

4+ Very deep pitting; very edematous and distorted extremity; lasts as long as 2 to 5 minutes before return

If edema is not pitting, it cannot be given a grade on this scale. Edema without pitting often arises from arterial disease and arterial occlusion. Unilateral edema is likely due to occlusion of a major vein.

Check the color, motion, sensation, and temperature (CMST) of both feet. Normal skin color on the legs is similar to that of the rest of the body. Test for sensation by asking the patient to close his or her eyes; then touch the patient's toes and ask whether the patient feels it. Ask the patient if he or she has pain or decreased sensation in the lower extremities, which sometimes indicates peripheral neuropathy. Normally, both feet are equally warm and pedal pulses are present. Direct the patient to flex the knees and ankles to test for ROM, although you will make a better assessment of ROM by observing the patient's gait. Sometimes corns or bunions interfere with the patient's mobility. Varicosities (enlarged veins) are not normally present.

Box 5-11 Pitting Edema Scale

1+ Trace—a barely perceptible pit (2 mm)

2+ Mild—a deeper pit (4 mm), with fairly normal contours, that rebounds in 10 to 15 seconds

3+ Moderate—a deep pit (6 mm); lasts for 30 seconds to more than 1 minute

4+ Severe—an even deeper pit (8 mm), with severe edema that possibly lasts as long as 2 to 5 minutes before rebounding

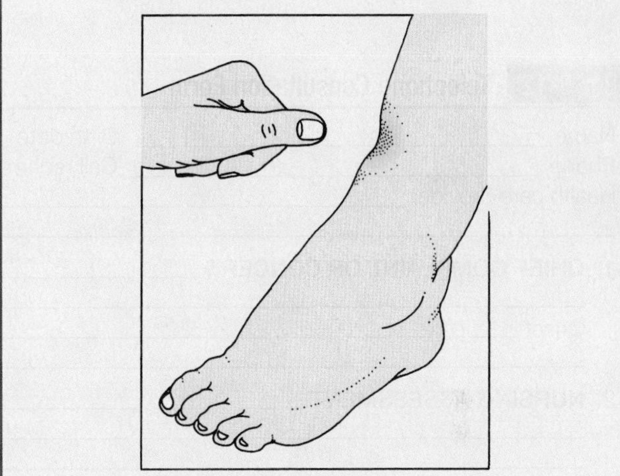

Documenting the Interview and the Assessment

Most institutions have a standardized form to follow when completing the patient history and the physical assessment. It serves as the baseline for evaluation of subsequent changes in the patient's condition, as well as decisions related to therapy (see Figure 5-2). Therefore it is important for the information to be objective, clear, complete, and concise.

Telephone Consultation

With the rapid changes taking place in health care today, nurses find themselves working in a variety of new settings. One example is in the area of telephone consultation, especially in the physician's office or clinic. When a patient calls with a health problem, the nurse is usually the person to whom he or she talks. If you take a call like this, sometimes you will dispense advice or instructions on the spot, and sometimes you will direct the patient to come in for a visit, see another health care provider, or seek care in the emergency department. Any interventions you make will be based on your assessment of the patient, despite the fact that

Box 5-12 Telephone Consultation Form

Name ______ Birth date ______ Date ______
Phone ______ Call received ______ AM ______ PM
Health care provider ______

1. **CHIEF COMPLAINT OR CONCERN** ______

Onset ______

2. **NURSING ASSESSMENT** ______

☐ Temperature ______	☐ Sore throat ______
☐ Rash ______	☐ Swollen glands ______
☐ Cough ______	☐ Earache ______
☐ Congestion ______	☐ Body aches ______
☐ Chest pain ______	☐ Abdominal pain ______
☐ Shortness of breath ______	☐ Nausea ______ ☐ Vomiting ______
☐ Sweating ______	☐ Diet ______
☐ Dizziness ______	☐ Appetite: Poor or good ______
☐ Indigestion ______	☐ Diarrhea ______
☐ Weakness ______	☐ Constipation ______
☐ Left arm or other pain ______	☐ Urination: Painful, frequent, or urgent ______

Health history ______

Medications ______

Allergies ______

L.M.P. ______ Birth control method ______
Immunizations; last tetanus ______

3. **NURSING INTERVENTIONS AND ADVICE** ______

DISPOSITIONS: ☐ 911 ☐ Appointment ______
☐ Advice ☐ ED ______
☐ Referral(s) ______

Instructions accepted Yes ☐ No ☐
Noncompliance warning Yes ☐
If S/S increase (or no improvement) call back for: ______
Nurse's signature ______

all the assessment data you will use comes directly from the patient. Will you always know the appropriate questions to ask? Several publications are currently available to use as a guideline to assist the nurse. Box 5-12 is an example of a telephone consultation form that is completed by the nurse and used by other health care personnel in caring for the patient. It is essential to follow Health Insurance Portability and Accountability Act (HIPAA) guidelines to protect the privacy of patient information.

Get Ready for the NCLEX® Examination!

Key Points

- The health care provider perceives signs by using the senses of sight, touch, smell, and hearing.
- The patient feels symptoms, sensations such as pruritus (itching), pain, and dizziness.
- Diseases originate from several different causes and are hereditary, congenital, traumatic, neoplastic, infectious, inflammatory, degenerative, deficiency, or environmental in nature.
- Risk factors for acquiring a disease include age, genetics, environment, and lifestyle variables.
- The universal signs of infection are erythema, edema, pain, heat, loss of function, and purulent, malodorous drainage.
- Some frequently noted signs and symptoms of disease are cyanosis, pallor, erythema, edema, nausea, vomiting, diarrhea, dyspnea, tachycardia, and fever.
- When a physician conducts a physical examination, the nurse is often requested to assist the examiner. The nurse has certain responsibilities, such as preparing the examining room, assisting with equipment, and preparing the patient.
- Results of laboratory evaluation of specimens such as urine and stool often add to the information about the patient.
- Optimally, a complete nursing physical assessment is performed as soon after admission as possible.
- Interviewing the patient initially serves to identify signs, symptoms, and areas of patient concern that the examination will seek to clarify.
- Properly performed, the physical assessment proceeds in an orderly fashion: head to toe or system by system.
- Perform assessment using specific skills of observation, palpation, percussion, and auscultation.
- Your role requires you to be familiar with normal assessments and thus able to identify abnormalities.
- Perform a physical assessment of each patient at the beginning of each nursing shift to determine actual or potential patient problems that will require medical or nursing interventions to promote the safety and well-being of the patient.

Additional Learning Resources

Go to your Companion CD for an audio glossary, animations, video clips, and more.

evolve Be sure to visit the Evolve site at http://evolve.elsevier.com/Christensen/foundations/ for additional online resources.

Review Questions for the NCLEX® Examination

1. The nurse has just gotten the patient in the chair after his bath. If using the mnemonic ABC, in and out, PS, what does the "P" indicate?

1. Purulent
2. Pus
3. Pain
4. Pallor

2. A 22-year-old patient has been admitted with acute bronchitis. When performing a lung assessment, the nurse is able to auscultate the lower lobes by listening to what location on the body?

1. Posteriorly
2. Anteriorly
3. Laterally
4. Superiorly

3. A 90-year-old patient is having difficulty answering the nurse's questions while completing the patient history. What will the nurse keep in mind about caring for older adults?

1. All older adults age at the same rate.
2. It is best to write down all of the questions and have the patient's family complete the information.
3. Sit down at eye level with the patient and allow a longer period to answer each question.
4. Talk more loudly and raise the pitch of the voice.

4. The patient has heart failure. When assessing her lower extremities, the nurse notices that a deep indentation remains for 30 seconds when the skin over the medial malleolus is pressed. The nurse documents this finding as:

1. nonpitting edema.
2. 2+ pedal pulses.
3. 3+ pitting edema.
4. 2+ pitting edema.

5. The nurse answers the patient's call light just after lunch. The patient complains of severe abdominal pain. What type of assessment should the nurse perform?

1. Head-to-toe assessment
2. Focused assessment
3. System-by-system assessment
4. Complete assessment

6. A 72-year-old man is admitted for chest pain. How would the nurse document the information the patient gives about his symptoms?
   1. Use the patient's own words in quotation marks.
   2. Briefly summarize what the patient says.
   3. Interpret the patient's comments using medical terminology.
   4. Use the information for the chief complaint from the admission sheet.

7. During the review of systems, the nurse questions the 88-year-old patient about her gastrointestinal system. The nurse will ask about what symptom?
   1. Wheezing
   2. Pyrosis (heartburn)
   3. Polyuria
   4. Dyspnea

8. The nurse has been assigned to care for a 62-year-old man. After introducing herself to the patient and explaining that she will be performing a nursing assessment, what is the first area to be assessed after taking vital signs?
   1. Assess for level of consciousness and orientation.
   2. Assess the skin.
   3. Listen to lung sounds.
   4. Check for pitting edema.

9. A 56-year-old woman has been admitted for dehydration after a prolonged period of diarrhea. Which finding do you expect to observe in this patient?
   1. Skin warm, moist, pink with good skin turgor
   2. Skin hot, dry, pale with decreased skin turgor
   3. Skin cool, dry, pink with increased skin turgor
   4. Skin cool, moist, pale with decreased skin turgor

10. The nurse is performing an initial nursing assessment on an 82-year-old woman. When palpating her carotid arteries a vibration is felt along the artery. This vibration is called a(n):
    1. palpation.
    2. thrill.
    3. bruit.
    4. aneurysm.

11. Which position is not used to assess the female genitalia?
    1. High Fowler's
    2. Dorsal recumbent
    3. Lithotomy
    4. Sims'

12. Which risk factor for cardiovascular disease can be modified?
    1. Age
    2. Race
    3. Diet
    4. Family history

13. An 82-year-old patient is admitted with respiratory difficulty. His respiratory rate is 36 breaths per minute, and he appears anxious. His chest x-ray film reveals right lower lobe pneumonia. The patient's respiratory rate of 36 breaths per minute is termed:
    1. sonorous.
    2. bradypnea.
    3. tachypnea.
    4. apnea.

14. The nurse auscultating breath sounds on a patient who has right lower lobe pneumonia detects adventitious breath sounds, which are a loud, bubbly noise heard during inspiration. These are called:
    1. coarse crackles.
    2. sonorous wheezes.
    3. pleural friction rub.
    4. sibilant wheezes.

15. The nurse assesses a 72-year-old patient who complains of a severe headache and vertigo. These data would be classified as:
    1. objective data.
    2. subjective data.

16. Which would be included in an assessment of the peripheral vascular system? *(Select all that apply.)*
    1. Assess the pulse rate by counting the pulsations for 60 seconds.
    2. Peripheral pulses that can be assessed include brachial, radial, ulnar, femoral, popliteal, dorsalis pedis, and posterior tibial.
    3. In a person with good cardiac function and distal perfusion, capillary refill should take less than 6 seconds.
    4. The strength of the pulse can be measured by using the following scale: 0, 1+, 2+, 3+ and 4+

17. The normal rate of bowel sounds is _____ per minute.
    1. 2 to 18
    2. 22 to 44
    3. 4 to 32
    4. 38 to 52

18. The main reason that auscultation precedes palpation of the abdomen is to:
    1. prevent distortion of vascular sounds.
    2. prevent distortion of bowel sounds.
    3. determine any areas of tenderness or pain.
    4. allow the patient to relax and be comfortable.

chapter 6

Nursing Process and Critical Thinking

evolve

Toni C. Wortham

http://evolve.elsevier.com/Christensen/foundationsadult

Objectives

1. Explain the use of each of the six phases of the nursing process.
2. List the elements of each of the six phases of the nursing process.
3. Describe the establishment of the database.
4. Discuss the steps used to formulate a nursing diagnosis.
5. Differentiate between types of health problems.
6. Describe the development of patient-centered outcomes.
7. Discuss the creation of nursing orders.
8. Explain the evaluation of a nursing care plan.
9. Demonstrate the nursing process by preparing a nursing care plan.
10. Explain North American Nursing Diagnosis Association International (NANDA-I), *Nursing Interventions Classification (NIC)*, and *Nursing Outcomes Classification (NOC)*.
11. Describe the use of clinical pathways in managed care.
12. Discuss critical thinking in nursing.
13. Define evidenced-based practice.

Key Terms

actual nursing diagnosis (ĂK-chū-ăl NŬRS-ĭng dī-ăg-NŌ-sĭs, p. 126)
assessment (p. 122)
biographic data (bī-ō-GRĂF-ĭk DĀ-tă, p. 123)
case management (kās MĂN-ĭj-mĕnt, p. 133)
clinical pathway (CLĬN-ĭ-căl PĂTH-wāy, p. 133)
collaborative problems (kŏ-LĂB-ŭr-ă-tĭv PRŎB-lĕmz, p. 126)
cue (kyū, p. 122)
database (p. 123)
defining characteristics (dē-FĪN-ĭng kăr-ăk-tŭr-ĬS-tĭks, p. 125)
diagnose (dī-ăg-NŌS, p. 123)
evaluation (ē-văl-yū-Ā-shŭn, p. 131)
goal (p. 127)
implementation (ĭm-plĕ-mĕn-TĀ-shŭn, p. 131)
managed care (p. 133)
medical diagnosis (MĔD-ĭ-kăl dī-ăg-NŌ-sĭs, p. 126)
NANDA-I (p. 124)
nursing diagnosis (p. 124)
nursing interventions (p. 129)
nursing process (p. 121)
nursing-sensitive patient outcomes (p. 132)
objective data (ŏb-JĔK-tĭv DĀ-tă, p. 122)
outcome (p. 127)
planning (p. 128)
problem (p. 123)
risk nursing diagnosis (p. 126)
standardized language (p. 132)
subjective data (sŭb-JĔK-tĭv DĀ-tă, p. 122)
syndrome nursing diagnosis (SĬN-drōm NŬRS-ĭng dī-ăg-NŌ-sĭs, p. 126)
variance (VĂR-ē-ăns, p. 133)
wellness nursing diagnosis (p. 126)

The definition of nursing has evolved as health care expectations have changed. In 1998, nursing was defined as "the diagnosis and treatment of human response to actual or potential health problems" (American Nurses Association [ANA], 1998). The current definition states, "Nursing is the protection, promotion, and optimization of health and abilities, prevention of illness and injury, alleviation of suffering through the diagnosis and treatment of human response, and advocacy in the care of individuals, families, communities, and populations" (ANA, 2003). This broader definition seeks to illustrate nursing's growth as a profession. The nursing process serves as the organizational framework for the practice of nursing.

The **nursing process** is a systematic method by which nurses plan and provide care for patients. This involves a problem-solving approach that enables you, as a nurse, to identify patient problems and potential problems. Once these problems are identified, you are then able to plan, deliver, and evaluate nursing care in an orderly, scientific manner. The nursing process consists of six dynamic and interrelated phases: assessment, diagnosis, outcome identification, planning, implementation, and evaluation (Figure 6-1). The *Nursing: Scope and Standards of Practice* of the American Nurses Association (ANA) outlines the steps of the nursing process (Box 6-1). (The LPN/LVN has a significant role in the nursing process, which is discussed later in the chapter.)

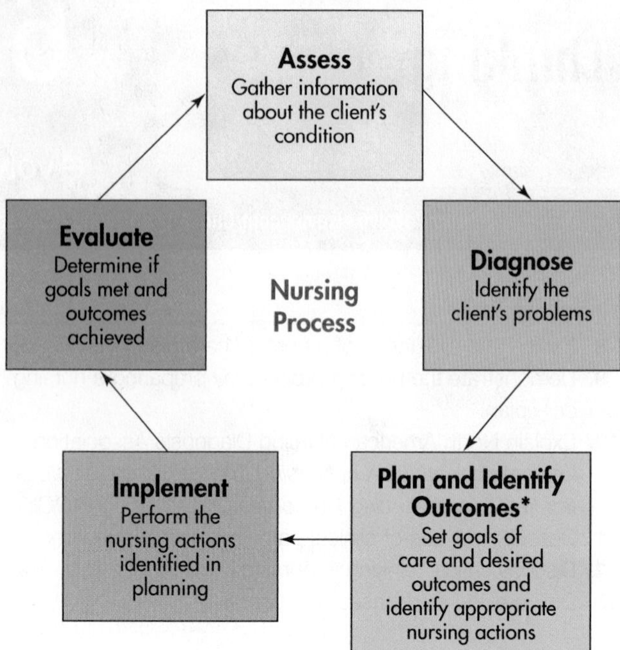

FIGURE 6-1 Relationships among the steps of the nursing process. *Note: Combined American Nurses Association (ANA) standards 3 and 4.

Box 6-1 American Nurses Association (ANA) Practice Standards

STANDARDS OF PRACTICE

Standard 1. *Assessment:* The nurse collects comprehensive data pertinent to the patient's health or the situation.

Standard 2. *Diagnosis:* The registered nurse analyzes the assessment data to determine the diagnoses or issues.

Standard 3. *Outcomes identification:* The registered nurse identifies expected outcomes for a plan individualized to the patient or situation.

Standard 4. *Planning:* The registered nurse develops a plan that prescribes strategies and alternatives to attain expected outcomes.

Standard 5. *Implementation:* The registered nurse implements the identified plan.

Standard 6. *Evaluation:* The registered nurse evaluates the patient's progress toward attainment of outcomes.

Reprinted with permission from American Nurses Association. (2004). *Nursing: scope and standards of practice*. Silver Spring, Md: Author.

ASSESSMENT DATA

The ANA defines **assessment** as "a systemic, dynamic process by which the nurse, through interaction with the client, significant others, and health care providers, collects and analyzes data about the client" (ANA, 2004). You gather information to identify the condition of the patient's health. You make assessments on first contact with a patient and continuously throughout patient care. The remaining phases of the nursing process depend on the accuracy and completeness of this initial data collection.

When the patient enters the health care system, the nurse begins the data collection. Depending on the status of the patient at the time of admission, you can perform either a complete assessment or a focused assessment.

A complete assessment involves a review and physical examination of all body systems (musculoskeletal, respiratory, gastrointestinal, etc.; see Chapter 5). This type of assessment also includes cognitive, psychosocial, emotional, cultural, and spiritual components and is appropriate for a patient who is stable and not in acute distress. Information about functional abilities, lifestyle, and developmental concerns is also important.

A focused assessment is advisable when the patient is critically ill, disoriented, or unable to respond. A focused assessment gathers information about a specific health problem. For example, if the patient reports abdominal distention, lack of appetite, and straining to have a bowel movement, one possible nursing diagnosis to suspect is constipation. To investigate further, you will then ask further questions about the intake of foods high in fiber, fluid intake, and amount of exercise.

Focused assessments are also performed continuously throughout nurse-patient contact. The nurse who monitors intake and output, skin turgor, and oral mucous membranes is performing a focused assessment for deficient fluid volume (Alfaro-LeFevre, 2009; Carpenito-Moyet, 2008a; Wilkinson & Ahern, 2009). The assessments made to determine progress toward the achievement of desired outcomes are also focused assessments.

TYPES OF DATA

When performing an assessment, you gather subjective and objective data. A **cue** is a synonym for significant data that usually demonstrate an unhealthy response (Wilkinson & Van Leuven, 2007). **Subjective data** are the verbal statements provided by the patient. Statements about nausea and descriptions of pain, fatigue, and anxiety are examples of subjective data. Other terms for subjective data are **symptoms** and **subjective cues.** Subjective data are hidden until shared by the subject, the patient.

Objective data are observable and measurable signs. One is able to record objective data. A camera records a rash, a skin lesion, or puffy eyes. A tape recorder gives evidence of crying or slurred speech. A thermometer records a temperature elevation. Other terms for objective data are **signs** and **objective cues.** See Table 6-1 for a comparison of subjective and objective data.

SOURCES OF DATA

Data are obtained from primary or secondary sources. The primary source of data is the patient. In most instances, the patient is considered to be the most accurate reporter. The alert and oriented patient is able to

Table 6-1 Comparison of Subjective and Objective Data

SUBJECTIVE DATA	OBJECTIVE DATA
"I feel nauseated."	50 mL green-tinged vomitus
"My chest hurts."	Blood pressure 100/60 mm Hg, pulse 100/min, respirations 32/min, patient holds fist over sternum
"I'm nervous."	Wringing hands, pacing in hall, pulse 112/min, respirations 28/min
"I'm tired."	Dark circles under eyes, yawning, catnaps during the day
"My foot hurts."	1″ × 2″ open lesion on left heel

provide information about past illnesses and surgeries and present signs, symptoms, and lifestyle.

When the patient is unable to supply information because of deterioration of mental status, age, or seriousness of illness, you will use secondary sources. Secondary sources include family members, significant others, medical records, diagnostic procedures, and nursing literature. Members of the patient's support system are often able to furnish information about the patient's past health status, current illness, allergies, and current medications.

Other health team professionals are also helpful secondary sources. Physicians, other nurses, dietitians, respiratory and physical therapists, and others frequently provide data about the patient. The nurse reviews nursing literature to determine what information may be needed. Nursing textbooks provide information about etiology (cause), pathophysiology, clinical manifestations, assessment, diagnostic tests, medical management, nursing interventions, patient teaching needs, and prognosis. This important information then guides further data collection.

METHODS OF DATA COLLECTION

Two basic methods are used to collect data. In the first method, you conduct an interview, the nursing health history, to obtain information about the patient's health history. You will commonly assess several common components in the course of the interview. Ask about **biographic data** to provide information about the facts or events in a person's life. Also request information about the reason the patient is seeking health care, a history of the present illness, the health history, and the family history. Because the environment in which the patient lives and works often plays a part in the patient's health status, you will often obtain an environmental history. A psychosocial history yields information about a combination of psychological and social factors. To gather information about the function of each body system, follow the nursing health history with a review of systems.

The second method of data collection is the performance of a physical examination. The physical examination is often guided by subjective data provided by the patient. For example, follow up on statements of pain by examining that part of the body. A head-to-toe format provides a systematic approach that helps avoid omitting important data (see Chapter 5).

When you have obtained the history and completed the physical examination with accuracy, you have the needed information to establish a **database** (a large store or bank of information). Analysis of the database leads to the identification of nursing diagnoses. In addition, it makes information available for the physician that assists in the medical management of the patient.

DATA CLUSTERING

After collecting and validating the data obtained from the health history, physical examination, and related diagnostic procedures, you will organize the data. By grouping related cues together, you perform data clustering. The clustering of related data helps to identify patterns that will assist with the identification of nursing diagnoses. Examples of appropriate data clustering and the related nursing diagnosis follow:

- "Thirst; dry skin; dry oral mucous membranes; increased body temperature; and decreased urine output" is a cue cluster that identifies *deficient fluid volume* as a nursing diagnosis (Alfaro-LeFevre, 2009; Carpenito-Moyet, 2008; NANDA-I, 2007; Wilkinson & Ahern, 2009).
- "Statements of inability to control symptoms of (specify problem), apathy, depression, and anxiety" is a cue cluster that potentially identifies the nursing diagnosis of *powerlessness* (Alfaro-LeFevre, 2009; Carpenito-Moyet, 2008, NANDA-I, 2007; Wilkinson & Ahern, 2009).

DIAGNOSIS

To **diagnose** is to identify the type and cause of a health condition. The American Nurses Association defines diagnosis as "a clinical judgment about the client's response to actual or potential health conditions or needs. The diagnosis provides the basis for determination of a plan of care to achieve expected outcomes" (ANA, 2004). The licensed practical nurse or licensed vocational nurse (LPN/LVN) and the registered nurse (RN) observe and collect data. Once the initial assessment has been completed, the data requires analysis. In most situations, the registered nurse is responsible for analyzing and interpreting data to identify health problems.

A **problem** is any health care condition that requires diagnostic, therapeutic, or educational actions. When the patient has a problem or a potential problem, cues are usually present that will help the nurse identify the area of concern.

Several guidelines help you identify the cues that have significance for nursing care. Consider any of the

Table 6-2 Determination of Significant Cues

PATIENT VALUES	NORM*	CONCLUSION
42-year-old man with blood pressure 165/92 mm Hg	Less than 120/80 mm Hg	High blood pressure
18-year-old patient with respirations of 32/min	16 to 22/min	Tachypnea
Small-frame woman with weight of 178 lb, height 5′ 1″	105 to 118 lb	Weight above accepted normal standard
22-month-old child not walking	12 months	Walking delayed
Male adult patient with hemoglobin of 8 g/dL	14 to 18 g/dL	Below normal limits
Female adult patient with hemoglobin of 12 g/dL	12 to 16 g/dL	Within normal limits
25-year-old patient with pulse of 120 beats/min	60 to 100 beats/min	Tachycardia
Newborn patient with pulse of 132 beats/min	130 to 150 beats/min	Within normal limits
Adult patient with thrombocyte count of 20,000/mm^2	150,000 to 400,000/mm^2	Thrombocytopenia

*Conclusion is based on the appropriate norm for the age and sex of the patient.

following to be important (Table 6-2): (1) deviations from population norms; (2) changes in the patient's usual health status; (3) developmental delays; (4) dysfunctional behavior; and (5) changes in usual behavior (Gordon, 1994).

NURSING DIAGNOSIS

A **nursing diagnosis** is a type of health problem that can be identified. In 1990, the North American Nursing Diagnosis Association (NANDA), now known as NANDA International **(NANDA-I)**, approved an official definition for nursing diagnosis that remains in current use. A nursing diagnosis is a "clinical judgment about individual, family, or community responses to actual or potential health problems/life processes. A nursing diagnosis provides the basis for selection of nursing interventions to achieve outcomes for which the nurse is accountable" (NANDA-I, 2009, p. 419). Nurses are legally permitted to identify and prescribe the primary interventions to treat or prevent problems that are nursing diagnoses. It is important for you to be aware of this important point. By definition, if the nurse is not able to prescribe the primary treatment, the problem is *not* a nursing diagnosis (Alfaro-LeFevre, 2009; Carpenito-Moyet, 2008).

You will perhaps notice that some of the nursing diagnoses approved for use do not conform to the NANDA-I definition. The explanation for this inconsistency is that many labels were added to the list before development of the 1990 NANDA definition. Ask your instructor for guidance, or use references that provide suggestions for appropriate label use in "author's notes" or "suggestions for use" (Alfaro-LeFevre, 2009; Carpenito-Moyet, 2008; Wilkinson & Ahern, 2009).

Components of a Nursing Diagnosis

Nursing research is ongoing in its identification of nursing diagnoses. When nurses submit nursing diagnoses, the following four components are addressed: (1) nursing diagnosis title or label; (2) definition of the title or label; (3) contributing, etiologic, or related factors; and (4) defining characteristics. The selection of an accurate nursing diagnosis depends on closely matching the elements in the patient situation with all four components of the nursing diagnosis. These four components are found in numerous nursing diagnosis handbooks, and each component is explained in the following discussion.

Title or Label

The problem that is identified after cue clustering and analysis is given a title or label. Frequently the name given to the problem is simply called the *nursing diagnosis.* In this chapter, we will use the terms *nursing diagnosis* and *nursing diagnostic label* to describe this component. The nursing diagnosis provides a concise name for the identified health problem. Lists of nursing diagnoses are often presented in alphabetical order. *Constipation, fatigue, hopelessness, powerlessness,* and *pain* are examples of nursing diagnostic labels.

Adjectives add meaning to the nursing diagnosis label by describing or modifying the label. Examples of adjectives are *imbalanced, ineffective, perceived, impaired,* and *excess.* The nursing diagnoses listed in the nursing care plans and nursing process sections of this book will follow the format used by NANDA-I in the original list (i.e., placing the noun first for easier location and identification in a list). When writing the nursing diagnosis, however, place the adjective *before* the noun modified. This provides a more natural word order and is less awkward. For example, *impaired physical mobility* is easier to say and understand than *mobility, impaired physical.*

Both international nursing groups and American nurses have challenged NANDA-I to simplify the language of nursing diagnoses. Although this is ongoing work, many labels have already undergone modification. *Altered comfort: pain* has been shortened to *acute pain* or *chronic pain.* Similarly, *alteration in bowel elimination: constipation* has been changed to *constipation.*

NANDA-I is currently using an organization structure for the diagnostic labels that is called Taxonomy II. New modifiers have been suggested as part of the organizational system. (See Table 6-3 for terms and their definitions.) The work of NANDA-I was never intended to be stagnant, so it is important for you to

Table 6-3 Descriptors for Taxonomy II

DESCRIPTOR OR MODIFIER	MEANING
Ability	Capacity to do or act
Anticipatory	To realize beforehand, to foresee
Balance	State of equilibrium
Compromised	Made vulnerable to threat
Decreased	Lessened; lesser in size, amount, or degree
Defensive	Used or intended to protect from a perceived threat
Deficient	Inadequate in amount, quality, or degree; not sufficient; incomplete
Delayed	Postponed, impeded, or retarded
Depleted	Emptied wholly or in part, exhausted of
Disabling	Making unable or unfit, incapacitating
Disorganized	Characterized by destruction of the systematic arrangement
Disproportionate	Not consistent with a standard
Disturbed	Agitated or interrupted, interfered with
Dysfunctional	Abnormal, incomplete functioning
Effective	Producing the intended or expected effect
Excessive	Characterized by an amount or quantity that is greater than necessary, desirable, or useful
Functional	Normal complete functioning
Imbalanced	State of disequilibrium
Impaired	Made worse, weakened, damaged, reduced, deteriorated
Inability	Incapacity to do or act
Increased	Greater in size, amount, or degree
Ineffective	Not producing the desired effect
Interrupted	Characterized by a break in continuity or uniformity
Low	Containing less than the norm
Organized	Formed into a systematic arrangement
Perceived	Having been brought into awareness of by means of the senses; characterized by assignment of meaning
Readiness for enhanced (for use with wellness diagnosis)	To make greater; to increase in quality, to attain something more desired (transition from a specific level of wellness to a higher level of wellness)
Situational	Related to particular circumstance(s)
Total	Complete, to the greatest extent or degree

Data from North American Nursing Diagnosis Association–International (NANDA-I). (2009). *Nursing diagnoses: definitions & classification 2009-2011*. Oxford, United Kingdom: Author.

monitor language changes and label additions every 2 years following the NANDA-I meetings. It is also possible to visit the NANDA-I website at www.nanda.org to keep current with the changes. Something new at NANDA-I is the periodic opportunity to vote on new diagnoses.

Definition

The definition presents a clear, precise description of the problem. This description helps identify the difference between similar nursing diagnoses. For example, if you need to select either *constipation* or *perceived constipation,* the following definitions will be helpful. Constipation is defined as "decrease in normal frequency of defecation accompanied by difficult or incomplete passage of stool and/or passage of excessively hard, dry stool" (NANDA-I, 2009, p. 102). Perceived constipation is defined as "self-diagnosis of constipation and abuse of laxatives, enemas, and/or suppositories to ensure a daily bowel movement" (p. 104). To increase the accuracy of your diagnosis selection, carefully study the definitions for nursing diagnoses in nursing diagnosis handbooks.

Contributing, Etiologic, and Related Factors and Risk Factors

Contributing, etiologic, and related factors are conditions that are often involved in the development of a problem and are also found in nursing diagnosis handbooks. These factors may become the focus for nursing interventions. Most authors also refer to the contributing factors as the "related to's." Contributing, etiologic, and related factors are written as the "related to" in actual nursing diagnoses statements. A contributing, etiologic, or related factor for the nursing diagnosis of anxiety is *a threat to or change in health status* (Carpenito-Moyet, 2008).

Risk factors are circumstances that increase the susceptibility of a patient to a problem. Prolonged immobility increases the risk for skin impairment and is a risk factor for the nursing diagnosis of impaired skin integrity. Risk factors are written as the "related to" in risk nursing diagnostic statements.

Defining Characteristics

Defining characteristics are the clinical cues, signs, and symptoms that furnish evidence that the problem exists. The cues, signs, and symptoms that were identified in the patient's assessment are written as the "manifested by" in the nursing diagnosis statement. Examples are presented in the following discussion that describes writing nursing diagnostic statements. Look for defining characteristics for each nursing diagnosis title or label in nursing diagnosis handbooks.

Writing Nursing Diagnosis Statements

There are four main types of nursing diagnoses: actual, risk, syndrome, and wellness. The following discussion provides descriptions of each type and furnishes guidelines for writing each type of nursing diagnosis statement.

Actual Nursing Diagnosis

NANDA-I describes an **actual nursing diagnosis** as the "human responses to health conditions/life processes that exist in an individual, family, or community. It is supported by defining characteristics (manifestations, signs, and symptoms) that cluster in patterns of related cues or inferences" (NANDA-I, 2009, p. 419). Cues obtained from a nursing assessment indicate that a problem exists. In an educational setting, the actual nursing diagnosis statement is usually represented by a three-part statement. In a clinical setting, you will sometimes see only the first two parts used. The three parts are written in the following order: (1) the nursing diagnosis label from the NANDA-I list; (2) the contributing, etiologic, or related factor; and (3) the specific cues, signs, and symptoms from the patient's assessment. Some authors describe this as the problem, etiology, signs and symptoms (PES) format (Alfaro-LeFevre, 2009; Wilkinson & Van Leuven, 2007). Connecting phrases are used to join the three parts of the statement. "Related to (r/t)" links the first and second parts of the statement. "Manifested by (m/b)" joins the second and third parts of the diagnostic statement. Note the italicized connecting words of an actual nursing diagnostic statement in the following example.

- Constipation *related to* insufficient fluid intake *manifested by* increased abdominal pressure, no bowel movement for 5 days, and straining with defecation.

Risk Nursing Diagnosis

NANDA-I describes a **risk nursing diagnosis** as the "human responses to health conditions/life processes that may develop in a vulnerable individual, family, or community. It is supported by risk factors that contribute to increased vulnerability" (NANDA-I, 2009, p. 419). The assessment indicates that risk factors are present that are known to contribute to the development of the problem. Risk nursing diagnoses are written as two-part statements: (1) the nursing diagnosis label from the NANDA-I list and (2) the risk factor(s). As in an actual nursing diagnosis, the two parts are connected by the words "related to." An example of a risk nursing diagnosis statement is as follows:

- Risk for impaired skin integrity related to physical immobilization

Note that there is no third part (manifested by) in this statement. If there were signs or symptoms, an actual problem would exist.

Syndrome Nursing Diagnosis

A **syndrome nursing diagnosis** is used when a cluster of actual or risk nursing diagnoses are predicted to be present in certain circumstances (Carpenito-Moyet, 2008; Wilkinson & Van Leuven, 2007). *Post-trauma syndrome, risk for disuse syndrome, impaired environmental interpretation syndrome, and relocation stress syndrome* are the current syndrome diagnoses. Because these diagnoses are so specific, the syndrome diagnoses are written as one-part statements.

Wellness Nursing Diagnosis

NANDA-I describes a **wellness nursing diagnosis** as "human responses to levels of wellness in an individual, family, or community" (NANDA-I, 2009). A wellness nursing diagnosis is written as a one-part statement. The words "readiness for enhanced" are used in a wellness nursing diagnosis (NANDA-I, 2009). An example of a wellness nursing diagnosis is *readiness for enhanced decision making* (NANDA-I, 2009).

OTHER TYPES OF HEALTH PROBLEMS

It is important to distinguish collaborative problems and medical diagnoses from nursing diagnoses. These two types of problems are defined and discussed separately.

Collaborative Problems

Collaborative problems are certain physiologic complications that nurses monitor to detect their onset or changes in the patient's status. You will manage collaborative problems using physician-prescribed and nursing-prescribed interventions to minimize the complications of the events (Carpenito-Moyet, 2008). Examples of collaborative problems for a diabetic patient are as follows:

- Potential complication: hypoglycemia (or PC: hypoglycemia)
- Potential complication: diabetic ketoacidosis or (PC: DKA)

Medical Diagnosis

A **medical diagnosis** is the identification of a disease or condition by a scientific evaluation of physical signs, symptoms, history, laboratory test, and procedures. The physician is licensed to make medical diagnoses. Examples of medical diagnoses are congestive heart failure, pneumonia, diabetes mellitus, and hepatitis B.

Differentiating Medical and Nursing Diagnoses

Students often have difficulty making a distinction between a medical and a nursing diagnosis. Physicians and advanced practice nurses diagnose diseases or disorders such as those listed earlier. These diseases or disorders are the result of changes in the structure or the function of an organ or body system. Diagnostic studies such as x-ray examinations and blood studies help to identify medical diagnoses. Although the patient is often able to recover from a medically diagnosed condition, the diagnosis itself does not change. The patient who recovers from a heart attack has a past history of a heart attack. The patient who was diagnosed with diabetes is likely to still have diabetes.

In the case of nursing diagnoses, the situation is different. Remember: Nursing diagnoses address *human responses* to health problems and life processes. As a nurse, in other words, you address the patient's concerns about the medical problem. Ask yourself, how is the patient responding to the diagnosis of cancer? You will have the opportunity to address feelings of anxiety, fear, anticipatory grieving, activity intolerance, nausea, and so on. These problems often change as you carry out interventions. Perhaps you will assist the patient who is concerned about dying with grief resolution, or perhaps teach the patient coping strategies. As you do so, their nursing diagnoses will change. The medical diagnosis of diabetes mellitus will not go away; however, it is hoped that the patient will no longer have the nursing diagnosis of *risk for ineffective therapeutic regimen management* once he or she has received education about his or her diabetes and is compliant with those instructions (Doenges & Moorhouse, 2008).

OUTCOMES IDENTIFICATION

The nurse develops expected outcomes for the established nursing diagnosis. The outcomes statement indicates the degree of wellness desired, expected, or possible for the patient to achieve. Alternative terms referring to this statement are a patient goal, a patient-centered goal, an objective, a behavioral objective, or a patient outcome. A patient outcome statement provides a description of the specific, measurable behavior (outcome criteria) that the patient will be able to exhibit in a given time frame following the interventions.

It is important to differentiate a goal statement and an outcome statement. A **goal** statement is a statement about the purpose to which an effort is directed. For example, perhaps you want to prevent constipation or promote activity. You then carry out activities to accomplish these goals. However, this type of goal statement does not describe the desired behavior that a patient is expected to demonstrate following nursing interventions. During the outcomes part of the nursing process, it is incorrect for you to write a goal statement of this type, because it indicates what you, *the nurse,* are meant to do rather than what *the patient* has to do. It is recommended that you use the term *desired patient outcome* because this term more clearly focuses on the change desired in the patient. *Outcome* is also the term used by the ANA. Once again: The desired patient **outcome** states the behaviors that the patient will be able to perform rather than what the nurse will do.

Desired patient outcome statements serve two functions. First, they guide the selection of nursing interventions. Nursing interventions are selected to promote the achievement of the desired outcome. Second, the outcome statement establishes the measuring standard that is used to evaluate the effectiveness of the nursing interventions. Therefore the outcome statement has to provide the specific details that can be used as the yardstick to judge progress or problem solution.

A well-written patient-centered goal or desired patient outcome statement does the following:

- Uses the word *patient* or a part of the patient as the subject of the statement
- Uses a measurable verb
- Is specific for the patient and the patient's problem
- Does not interfere with the medical plan of care
- Is realistic for the patient and the patient's problem
- Includes a time frame for patient reevaluation

Because the subject of the patient outcome statement is meant to be the patient or a part of the patient, the outcome statement should begin with the words, "The patient will" or "The patient's . . . will."

Measurable verbs indicate the precise behavior that you anticipate hearing or seeing. *Define, describe, list, walk, demonstrate,* and *verbalize* are examples of measurable verbs.

The properly written patient outcome statement is specific to the patient and the patient's medical problem. A patient who is in traction because of a bone fracture has mobility restrictions. An outcome statement indicating that all joints will be moved through full range of motion is not safe for this patient's problem.

The patient outcome statement also has to be realistic for the patient and the patient's medical problem. Although some 88-year-old patients are joggers, it is probably not reasonable to expect an 88-year-old patient to learn to jog.

A time frame is written into the patient outcome statement to provide a deadline for evaluation of the patient's progress. Nursing experience will increase your ability to predict realistic time frames.

Patient outcome statements indicate a reversal of the problem identified by the NANDA-I nursing diagnosis label, as shown in the following example:

Nursing Diagnosis	Goal/Outcome Statement
Impaired skin integrity related to prolonged immobility manifested by 2-inch–diameter ulcer on coccyx	Patient will have intact skin within 3 weeks. (NOTE: *intact skin* is a reversal of the *impaired skin*.)

There are two ways to approach writing patient outcome statements. The above example illustrates the simple reversal of the problem statement in a concise fashion. A second approach is to list the desired behavior in broader terms and then list exact criteria or standards. The following examples illustrate both methods. Note the use of "as evidenced by" that precedes the more exacting criterion:

- The patient will have one soft, formed bowel movement every day during hospitalization.
- The patient will improve mobility as evidenced by the ability to ambulate 200 feet by the third day following surgery.

PLANNING

During the **planning** phase of the nursing process, you establish priorities of care, select and convert nursing interventions into nursing orders, and communicate the plan of care using standardized languages or recognized terminology to document the plan. It is the nurse's responsibility to decide what it is possible to do to lessen or solve an actual problem or to prevent a risk problem from becoming an actual problem. The decision about what interventions will likely be effective is made during the planning phase.

PRIORITY SETTING

The nurse in today's busy health care facility is caring for many patients with complex problems and is challenged daily to use time and effort wisely. Priorities must be established to provide care for each patient.

Once you have developed a list of nursing diagnoses, you will be able to rank the problems in order of importance for the patient's life and health. A useful framework to guide the prioritization is Maslow's hierarchy of needs. This structure is based on the principle that it is necessary to meet lower-level needs before it is possible to satisfy higher-level needs. The physiologic needs are more vital than the safety and security needs, and the safety and security needs are more critical than the love and belonging needs. Review Maslow's hierarchy in Figure 6-2. Life-threatening and health-threatening problems are ranked before other types of problems. Actual problems will often be

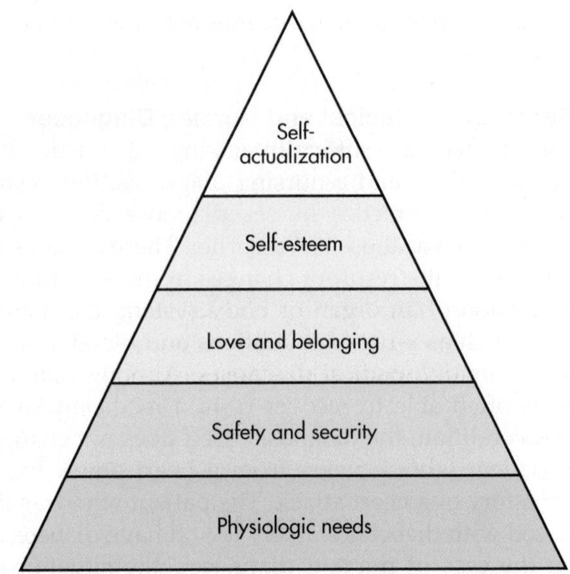

FIGURE 6-2 Maslow's hierarchy of needs. Physical needs include physiologic (personal hygiene, activity, sexuality) and homeostatic (vital functions [oxygenation], eating and drinking, sleep and rest, and elimination). Safety and security needs include safety and accident prevention, religion and philosophy, and feelings of well-being. Love and belonging needs are communication, affection, identity, modesty, companionship, and dependence. The self-esteem need is recognition, and the self-actualization need is a desire for self-fulfillment.

ranked before risk problems unless the risk problem, if it were to develop, would be life threatening. For example, *risk for ineffective airway clearance* might be prioritized higher than an actual problem of constipation. Alfaro-LeFevre (2009) suggests asking, "What problems need immediate attention and what could happen if I wait until later to attend to them?" The answer to these questions will help you prioritize care.

It is always best to consult patients about their prioritization of problems. Plans are more effective when the patient is involved in the process.

Time factors and severity of illness are important considerations when determining what problems to address initially. The patient who is admitted to the emergency department with a possible heart attack (myocardial infarction) is not ready at that time to hear dietary instructions to reduce cholesterol.

Priorities change as the patient progresses through hospitalization. As some problems are resolved, the approach to other problems opens up. The following example illustrates how the concerns of nursing change during one patient's hospital stay:

> A 28-year-old woman admitted for an abdominal hysterectomy may have the preoperative diagnosis of fear or anxiety. *Acute pain* is an important nursing diagnosis in the first few days following surgery. As the pain is controlled, *imbalanced nutrition: less than body requirements* and *risk for constipation* are managed. When the patient approaches discharge, teaching about wound care and activity restrictions becomes the focus for nursing diagnoses. Because of the loss of reproductive ability, self-es-

teem problems have to be confirmed or ruled out as possible nursing diagnoses for this patient. Note how the nursing diagnoses changed while the medical procedure did not.

SELECTING NURSING INTERVENTIONS

Nursing interventions are those activities that promote the achievement of the desired patient outcome. Interventions include activities that the nurse selects to resolve a nursing diagnosis, monitor for the development of a risk problem, or carry out physician orders. Nursing interventions are classified as physician prescribed or nurse prescribed.

Physician-prescribed interventions are those actions ordered by a physician for a nurse or other health care professional to perform (Carpenito-Moyet, 2008). It is important to remember that physicians' orders are not orders for nurses but are prescriptive instructions for patients (Carpenito-Moyet, 2008). Even though the physician has given the order, it is still necessary to use nursing judgment. You follow orders when administering medications, performing wound care, and ordering diagnostic tests. Assessing, teaching, and validating the safety of physician orders are important nursing responsibilities.

Nurse-prescribed interventions are any actions that a nurse is legally able to order or begin independently. Nurses write interventions for themselves or other nursing staff (Carpenito-Moyet, 2008). Examples of independent nursing interventions are providing a back massage, turning a patient every 2 hours, and monitoring for complications. When determining appropriate nursing interventions, the nurse should consider the contributing, etiologic, and related factors; risk factors; the patient-centered goal or desired patient outcome; and the nursing diagnosis label itself. Nursing interventions are focused on any or all of these areas.

Nursing interventions often are aimed at reducing or eliminating the causative factor. For example, for the nursing diagnosis *anxiety related to lack of knowledge about hospital procedures,* an appropriate nursing intervention is to teach the patient about typical routines and procedures. Providing information and reducing the lack of knowledge is likely to help reduce the fear of the unknown and thus reduce anxiety.

The patient outcome is also considered when selecting nursing interventions. For example, when the patient outcome statement says, "The patient will plan a week's menu for an 1800-calorie diabetic diet within 1 week's time," the interventions are selected to increase the patient's knowledge about planning for a diabetic diet.

The nursing diagnosis label itself may also direct the interventions. If the nursing diagnosis label is *acute pain,* interventions to relieve acute pain are selected.

A variety of sources list nursing interventions. Nursing textbooks, periodicals, and special "care plan" books are available in college bookstores and libraries. Some Internet sites are also helpful in choosing interventions. If your facility or school uses the *Nursing Interventions Classification (NIC),* that information provides another helpful source for nursing interventions and activities. (NIC is discussed later in this chapter.) Co-workers are a good source of ideas for interventions. Nursing conferences held to plan patient care often provide an environment for the development of creative approaches to patient care. With some frequency, patients also provide suggestions for interventions. If the patient states that a hot cup of coffee first thing in the morning stimulates a bowel movement, the wise nurse will include that intervention on the nursing care plan unless it is contraindicated.

WRITING NURSING ORDERS

Because nursing interventions offered in textbooks and care planning manuals are often broad, general statements that indicate an activity to be performed, it is often necessary to convert these nursing interventions to more specific instructional statements. For example, perhaps a text suggests the following general interventions:

- Increase dietary bulk
- Increase activity
- Encourage fluids

This information is helpful because it prescribes a direction for care, but the information provided is lacking in specific details. How will you carry out the interventions? How will dietary bulk be increased? How much and what types of foods are to be eaten? "How often," is another question left unanswered. How will fluids be increased? How much of what types of fluids should be included, and how often should the fluids be provided? For care planning purposes, it is necessary for you to be able to change the guiding general statement about the nursing intervention to a more specific statement. This detailed statement is called a *nursing order* and is necessary because the nurse who is writing the care plan is providing instructions for all caregivers. It is therefore essential that instructions be extremely clear and concise. Nursing orders have to be written to reduce the likelihood of misinterpretation. Details are provided to convey the intended meaning. Therefore nursing orders properly include the following:

- Date
- Signature of nurse responsible for the care plan
- Subject (who will be carrying out the activity)
- Action verb
- Qualifying details

In most cases, the subject of the nursing order is understood to be the nurse. When the nurse is not the subject, identify the person responsible for the action. Compare the following examples:

- Physical therapist will ambulate patient three times a day at 0900, 1400, and 1900.

- Ambulate the patient three times a day at 0900, 1400, and 1900, as tolerated.

The correctly written nursing order includes an action or command verb. These verbs tell what the caregiver should do. Examples of action or command verbs are *ambulate, offer, encourage, demonstrate, turn, teach,* and *monitor.*

A proper nursing order is specific for the problem, realistic for the patient, compatible with the medical plan of care, and based on scientific principles. The following examples illustrate appropriate conversion of general nursing interventions into specific nursing orders:

- Add four servings of fruits and vegetables of patient's choice to daily menu, one extra serving per meal and one snack.
- Ambulate patient 200 feet with the assistance of two personnel at 1000, 1500, and 2100.
- Offer water and juices up to 2000 mL per day according to the following schedule: 7 to 3 shift, 1200 mL; 3 to 11 shift, 600 mL; 11 to 7 shift, 200 mL.

COMMUNICATING THE NURSING CARE PLAN

After completing the initial assessment, analyzing the data, writing the nursing diagnoses, selecting outcomes, and selecting appropriate nursing interventions (which are then made more specific by nursing orders), it is the nurse's responsibility to communicate the detailed plan of care for the patient. The written nursing care plan is the tangible product of the nursing process (Table 6-4). (Refer to Chapter 7 for additional information on charting and documentation.)

Because the nursing staff is constantly changing (nurses work different shifts and have days off), it is important for continuity of patient care to have written guidelines. Continuity increases patient trust in the nursing staff and promotes outcome achievement.

Nursing care plans are sometimes prepared for each patient, sometimes standardized for a group of patients with common illnesses, and sometimes they are computerized. Individually prepared care plans are the most time consuming, but often provide care that is best matched to the specific patient's needs and situation. An individualized plan of care takes into consideration pertinent patient characteristics such as age, culture, and medical diagnosis.

Standardized nursing care plans are appropriate for patient populations with routine, expected care requirements. Women who have had a vaginal delivery or a cesarean delivery are ideal patient populations for standardized care plans. Many standardized care plans include blank spaces that the nurse fills in to individualize them to some degree.

Some computerized systems print an updated nursing care plan for each shift. The nurse reads the printout of the planned nursing interventions, performs the interventions, and documents them on the computerized care plan.

Linear Care Plans versus Concept Maps

Among nursing faculty, there is often a range of different expectations for the care planning process. Formats for the written nursing care plan vary from school to school. Components that are common in an educational setting are NANDA-I diagnostic labels, patient-centered goals and desired patient outcomes, and nursing interventions and orders.

Nursing faculty sometimes require you to submit the care plan in a 4- or 5-column format that is referred to as a *linear style.* With this system, it is often necessary to provide scientific principles to explain why the intervention is needed or how the intervention will work. You may be asked to provide reference page numbers to identify the source of the scientific principle.

Table 6-4 Nursing Care Plan Form

NURSING DIAGNOSIS	NURSING ORDER	SCIENTIFIC PRINCIPLE	EVALUATION
Acute pain r/t tissue trauma from broken fibula and tibia m/b grimaces, statements that right leg hurts, and elevated blood pressure 140/100 mm Hg **NEED DEPRIVED** Physical comfort **DESIRED OUTCOME** Patient will demonstrate improved comfort level as evidenced by relaxed facial expression, statements of pain relief, and return of vital signs to patient's normal range within 30 minutes of nursing interventions	1. Assess verbal and nonverbal indications of pain 2. Monitor blood pressure and pulse for increase over baseline value every 4 hr 3. Elevate right leg on two pillows at all times except meals 4. Offer back rub and position change when statements of pain are made	1. Fractures cause swelling and pressure on nerves. Patient pain report establishes need for intervention. 2. Pain increases heart rate and blood pressure. 3. Gravity helps reduce edema, which reduces pain. 4. Sensory nerve impulses from the skin "close the gate" and prevent pain transmission.	Outcome achieved Focus: Pain D = States pain in lower right leg. Blood pressure 140/100 mm Hg A = Right leg elevated on two pillows. Back rub given for 10 minutes R = States pain relieved. Blood pressure 132/88 mm Hg

A, Action; *D,* data; *m/b,* manifested by; *R,* response/evaluation; *r/t,* related to.

Other nursing faculty prefer the care plan to be represented as a concept map. A concept map, using different shapes and connecting lines to show relationships, provides a visual representation of the care plan (Berman et al., 2008). Perhaps, for instance, you will put the nursing diagnosis into a rectangular shape, interventions into a circle, and outcomes into a triangle. Follow the specific guidelines of the nursing program for topics to be included on a concept map and its organization.

IMPLEMENTATION

During the **implementation** phase of the nursing process, you and other members of the team put the established plan into action to promote outcome achievement. This is the fifth phase of the nursing process. The implementation phase includes ongoing activities of data collection, prioritization, performance of nursing interventions, and documentation (Alfaro-LeFevre, 2009).

In emergency situations, you will proceed directly from assessment of the problem to intervention. For example, for a patient whose respiratory or cardiac function has failed, initiate cardiopulmonary resuscitation.

Daily contact with the patient and the patient's family provides opportunities for additional data collection. Often, you will note increasing pain or fatigue, or changes from the patient's initial health status. As a result of this ongoing assessment, it is likely that you will have to alter priorities of care. As the patient's condition warrants, you will perhaps delay, cancel, or even accelerate certain activities.

Nursing interventions include both nurse-prescribed and physician-prescribed activities. (See the discussion of selecting nursing interventions in the Planning section earlier in this chapter.) Interventions that the nurse may perform include the following (Alfaro-LeFevre, 2009):

- Performing an activity for a patient
- Assisting the patient to perform an activity
- Teaching the patient or family about health maintenance
- Counseling the patient and family
- Monitoring for problems or complications
- Administering medications, and monitoring for therapeutic and nontherapeutic effects
- Referring the patient for care and follow-up activities

EVIDENCE-BASED PRACTICE

Today's nursing practice emphasizes the use of research to determine best practices, or the interventions or approaches to patient care that will have the best impact on patient outcomes. In contrast, professionals in the past used educational knowledge, consultation with peers and specialists, and their own experiences to make decisions about patient care and to select interventions. The modern clinician who uses evidence-based practices integrates his or her clinical experience with current research to help guide patient care decisions (Craven & Hirnle, 2007).

Nurses are now creating evidence-based guidelines using the results of research that are available in the form of systemic reviews. The Cochrane Database of Systematic Reviews, for example, is a full-text database that contains high-quality systematic reviews that have implications for nursing practice (Craven & Hirnle, 2007). With these tools, nurses write policies and procedures for their institutions.

DOCUMENTATION

Finally, remember that documentation is a vital component of the implementation phase. The written documentation of the nursing process is a legal record of what has transpired while the patient was in the health care facility. "If it was not charted, it was not done" remains a constant principle of nursing (see Chapter 7).

EVALUATION

Evaluation is a determination made about the extent to which the established outcomes have been achieved. You will take several steps to complete the evaluation phase: (1) Review the patient-centered goals or desired patient outcomes that were established earlier. These outcome statements present standards and criteria that are observable and measurable. (2) Reassess the patient to gather data indicating the patient's actual response to the nursing interventions. (3) Compare the actual outcome with the desired outcome and make a critical judgment about whether the patient-centered goal or desired patient outcome was achieved.

This critical judgment will lead you to make one of three conclusions or decisions: the outcome was achieved, the outcome was not achieved, or the outcome was partially achieved. Document the decision along with the basis for that decision, as in the following example:

Goal and Outcome Statement	Evaluation and Documentation
The patient will demonstrate self-administration of insulin using sterile technique and selecting correct site by 5/21/10.	5/21/10: Outcome achieved. Patient correctly administered regular insulin into upper thigh using sterile technique.

Typically, the plan of care undergoes changes during this phase of the nursing process. You will make modifications according to whether the outcome has been achieved, partially achieved, or not achieved. If the problem has been resolved, remove that problem from the current nursing care plan.

When the outcome has been partially achieved or not achieved, further analysis is needed. At this point, you review all phases of the nursing process. The following are examples of questions to ask yourself to ensure the accuracy of the nursing process:

- Was the assessment complete and accurate?
- Was the problem identified correctly?
- Was the desired patient outcome realistic and specific?
- Were the interventions realistic and did all personnel implement them consistently?
- Did new problems develop?
- Was adequate time allowed?

Once you have found answers to these questions, it is possible to modify the nursing care plan. You will intervene appropriately to correct any errors that have been identified, and will then refine the nursing care plan as needed.

STANDARDIZED LANGUAGES: NANDA-I, *NIC*, AND *NOC*

The importance of using standardized languages cannot be overemphasized. "A **standardized language** is one in which the terms are carefully defined and mean the same thing to all who use them" (Wilkinson & Van Leuven, 2007). When nurses use understandable, exact, consistent vocabulary, the benefits are numerous. Standardized nursing languages help accomplish the following (Wilkinson & Van Leuven, 2007):

- Improve communication by providing consistent terminology to describe clinical problems and treatments
- Support computerized patient records
- Improve testing of nursing interventions for effectiveness
- Define and expand nursing knowledge
- Facilitate research to improve patient care
- Demonstrate nursing's contribution to patient care
- Influence health policy decisions

NANDA-I, *Nursing Interventions Classification (NIC)*, and *Nursing Outcomes Classification (NOC)* are examples of standardized languages describing diagnoses, interventions, and outcomes, respectively, that are recognized by the ANA. (*NIC* and *NOC* are discussed in the following sections.) The groups behind NANDA-I, *NOC*, and *NIC* (NNN) are working together to demonstrate links between these three standardized languages and thus to improve communication both in the United States and internationally. An example of an NNN linkage is listed as follows (Johnson et al., 2006):

Nursing Diagnosis	Nursing Outcome	Nursing Intervention
Impaired physical mobility	Balance	Exercise therapy: muscle control

NURSING INTERVENTIONS CLASSIFICATION (NIC)

This standardized language, developed at the University of Iowa, encourages enhanced communication between nurses about nursing interventions. This system is useful to computer-based systems and describes nursing practice. The current *NIC* edition lists 542 interventions. Each *NIC* intervention has a label, a definition for that label, and a list of activities that can be used for that intervention. The title given to nursing interventions is concise. Examples of nursing interventions are *airway management; analgesic administration; teaching: prescribed diet;* and *therapeutic play.* Some *NIC* interventions are called *indirect interventions* because they occur away from the bedside but on behalf of the patient. Examples of indirect care interventions are *emergency cart checking, shift report, staff development,* and *supply management* (Bulechek et al., 2008).

The list of activities is very helpful to guide beginning nurses. The following example shows a NIC intervention and lists 3 of the 36 possible activities for the intervention (Bulechek et al, 2008). Note the definition given and the indicated number that can be retrieved by computer systems. These numbers "run in the background" and are not for memorization.

> ***NIC* intervention: 6540**
> **Infection control: (Minimizing the acquisition and transmission of infectious agents)**
> Activities:
> - Isolate persons exposed to communicable disease.
> - Wash hands before and after each patient-care activity.
> - Ensure appropriate wound care technique.

NURSING OUTCOMES CLASSIFICATION (NOC)

NOC, which measures the effects of nursing care, is the effort of a group of researchers working at the University of Iowa. These researchers have developed a standardized system with an organized structure to name and measure **nursing-sensitive patient outcomes.** Identifying outcomes that are responsive to nursing care is important work for nursing, especially in connection with efforts to contain costs and establish best practices (Moorhead et al., 2008). There are currently 385 outcomes with accompanying definitions, measurement standards, indicators, and references (Moorhead et al., 2008).

The *NOC* outcomes use brief phrases to describe the result of nursing care. Indicators are given as subheadings for each outcome. These indicators use a measurement scale to evaluate the degree of outcome attainment. An example of an *NOC* outcome with 1 of the possible 19 indicators follows. Note that it is possible to describe the outcome statement and indicator with selected key words from a patient outcome statement ("The patient will demonstrate beginning *grief resolution* as evidenced by the ability to *verbalize reality of loss* after nursing interventions"). Also note the coded nature of the outcome and indicators that will be used to enhance entry and retrieval of information from a computer database.

- Grief resolution (outcome 1304). Verbalizes reality of loss (indicator 130403). The scale used for this indicator measures from never demonstrated to consistently demonstrated (1-5 scale) (Moorhead et al., 2008).

Note that it is possible to use these measurement scales to establish a baseline assessment, and then apply the scale again during the evaluation phase. Some facilities use these indicators to plan for patient discharge. For example, if the patient does not achieve a 4 or 5 on a scale, then a referral is sometimes necessary.

ROLE OF THE LICENSED PRACTICAL NURSE OR LICENSED VOCATIONAL NURSE

The role of the LPN/LVN in the nursing process may vary from state to state and with different institutions. As a student practical and vocational nurse, you are responsible to review your state's nurse practice acts for guidance in determining your responsibility in your state or practice.

Often, the LPN/LVN is responsible for providing direct bedside nursing care. This direct care position allows you to closely observe, prioritize, intervene, and evaluate the care provided to and for the patient. See Box 6-2 for a summary of the role of the LPN/LVN in the nursing process.

Box 6-2 Role of the LPN/LVN in the Nursing Process

ASSESSMENT

- Observe and report significant cues to the nurse in charge or to the physician.

DIAGNOSIS

- Assist with the determination of accurate nursing diagnoses.
- Gather further data to confirm or eliminate problems.

OUTCOMES IDENTIFICATION AND PLANNING

- Assist with setting priorities.
- Suggest interventions.
- Assist with the development of realistic patient-centered goals and desired patient outcomes.

IMPLEMENTATION

- Assist with the establishment of priorities.
- Carry out physician and nursing orders.
- Evaluate the effectiveness of nursing activities.

EVALUATION

- Assist with reevaluation of the patient's health state after nursing interventions.
- Suggest alternative nursing interventions when necessary.

NURSING DIAGNOSES AND CLINICAL PATHWAYS

To practice in the changing world of health care today, you are called on to go beyond performing technical skills and providing direct patient care. Your responsibilities include working with outcomes, cost, resources, and other members of the health care team. As discussed in Chapter 1, **managed care** is a health care system that provides control over health care services for a specific group of individuals in attempts to control cost (Potter & Perry, 2007). A goal of managed care is to provide care to keep people healthy and avoid the higher cost of caring for an ill individual. A second goal of managed care is to standardize both diagnosis and treatment across the United States (Daniels et al., 2007). **Case management** refers to the assignment of a health care provider to a patient so that the care of that patient is overseen by one individual. The case manager advises nursing staff on specific nursing care issues, assists the patient and the patient's family in receiving required services, coordinates these services, and evaluates the adequacy of these services. The case manager focuses particularly on planning for patient discharge (Potter & Perry, 2007).

Case management usually depends on the use of clinical pathways, whose development was driven by the need to control costs. A **clinical pathway** is a multidisciplinary plan that schedules clinical interventions over an anticipated time frame for high-risk, high-volume, high-cost types of cases. Synonyms for clinical pathways are *critical pathways, multidisciplinary action plans, action plans,* and *care maps.* Institutions use representatives from disciplines such as nursing, medicine, pharmacy, social services, dietary therapy, and physical therapy to develop agency-specific multidisciplinary plans of care. Clinical pathways include such elements as diagnostic tests, treatments, activities, medications, consultations, education, daily outcomes, and discharge planning. Some systems allow for documentation onto the clinical path (Craven & Hirnle, 2007).

When a patient does not achieve the projected outcome, a **variance,** or exit, is said to have occurred. Variances and exits are examined by members of the multidisciplinary team to determine whether the failure to achieve the outcome was a problem with the system, the provider, or the patient (Craven & Hirnle, 2007). Variance analysis is then used to promote continuous quality improvement. Repetition of variances often leads the health care team to revise a clinical pathway.

The conventional nursing care plan has been eliminated in many facilities that use a managed care system. Alfaro-LeFevre (2009) states that the nursing process and care planning is still alive and well, just changed. Hospitals are still required to have a recorded plan of care. Sometimes, parts of the care plan are scattered. Perhaps the initial assessment is in the nursing admission notes, the outcomes and interventions on a clinical pathway, and the evaluation of outcome achievement in the daily nursing notes (Alfaro-LeFevre, 2009).

CRITICAL THINKING

Critical thinkers think with a purpose. They question information, conclusions, and points of view. Critical thinkers look beneath the surface. They are logical and fair in their thinking. The skills related to critical thinking are applied to reading, listening, and writing and across all subjects. Critical thinking is a complex process, and no single simple definition explains all aspects of critical thinking. Each author who writes about critical thinking has his or her own definition. Alfaro-LeFevre (2009) defines an element of critical thinking as "purposeful, informed, outcome-focused (results-oriented) thinking that requires careful identification of key problems, issues, and risks." The National League for Nursing (2000) defines critical thinking for nursing as "a discipline-specific, reflective reasoning process that guides a nurse in generating, implementing, and evaluating approaches for dealing with client care and professional concerns."

Why do nurses need to think critically? The answer lies in the nature of the nursing process. One of the first skills you learn as a nursing student is to take a temperature. How do you choose between obtaining tympanic (ear), oral, rectal, skin, or axillary measurements? Critical thinking will lead you through your decision making. One consideration is the need for accuracy in the results. Also, certain medical or surgical problems will perhaps interfere with the accuracy of the reading. If a patient has an ear infection, the results of a tympanic reading will not be accurate. You know to avoid using a rectal thermometer when the patient is recovering from hemorrhoid surgery. If the patient is likely to have a seizure, you do not take an oral reading with a glass thermometer; in fact, you will remember that experts now advise against using mercury-containing thermometers altogether. It is also necessary to take into consideration the condition of the site to be used. As you know, heavy perspiration often interferes with axillary temperature readings. Ask yourself whether the patient has ingested hot or cold beverages. These temperature extremes would interfere with the accuracy of an oral temperature reading.

As you can see from this example, it is crucial for nurses to not only be able to *perform skills* (the "doing" of nursing), but also to *think about* what he or she is doing. Nurses use a knowledge base (nursing science) to make decisions, generate new ideas, and solve problems. Nursing students add to their knowledge base by studying facts, principles, and theories. Knowledge of psychology, anatomy, physiology, pharmacology, and other related course work helps you gain the scientific knowledge base to think critically.

Critical thinkers have several characteristics in common. They use reason rather than prejudice, self-interest, or fear. Critical thinkers reflect or think about what is being learned. They look for relationships between concepts or ideas. Reflection is used to analyze and critique behaviors. Thus self-correction becomes a part of critical thinking. Critical thinkers realize that they do not know everything. Critical thinking also involves creative thinking. Creative thinking becomes necessary when traditional nursing approaches are not effective (Alfaro-LeFevre, 2009).

To help determine the difference between thinking and critical thinking, consider the following nonclinical situations:

- **Situation 1:** On the day before classes begin, the student is anxious about getting started and is unsure of her chances of success. She is thinking, "I hope I don't get lost. I hope the teachers are nice. I wonder if I will be able to pass the tests. Will I succeed?" On the day classes begin, she drives to school, finds a parking space, and enters the building to locate her classroom.
- **Situation 2:** On the day before classes begin, the student is anxious about getting started and is unsure of her chances of success. She is thinking, "I will drive to the school so I can judge how much time to allow for travel. I want to go early and locate my classroom today so I will have an easier time tomorrow. Maybe I can get some course materials early so I can organize my notebook."

Both of these situations describe individuals who are thinking. The student in situation 1 is experiencing a mental activity, but it is aimless and without purpose. The student in situation 2 has recognized the need to gain control and get organized. This student is beginning to think critically and with a purpose, which is to decrease the anxiety associated with her first day of class.

The following clinical situations provide examples of some aspects of critical thinking at the bedside:

- **Situation 1:** An infant was admitted to the hospital with an elevated temperature. According to hospital routine, the nursing staff took an oral thermometer reading and kept the thermometer in the infant's room to prevent cross-contamination. As the days went by, the infant continued to have an elevated temperature. Several tests were performed to identify the cause of the fever. One morning the nurse in charge realized that things just "didn't add up" with this infant. She was an experienced pediatric nurse. She observed that the infant did not look flushed, was eating well, and was not irritable as is often seen with sick infants. Taking all of these observations into consideration, she did not expect the infant to have an elevated temperature. This nurse obtained a different thermometer and took the infant's temperature. The temperature was normal. The first thermometer was defective. This experienced pediatric nurse used her knowledge base, questioned the original findings, and used logic and reason to save this infant from additional tests and hospitalization time.

- **Situation 2:** A diabetic patient was admitted to the hospital for a bladder infection. At the change of shift, the oncoming nurse entered the room to make an assessment. The nurse noted that the patient was unresponsive. How would the nurse use critical thinking to work out the problem? Using a scientific knowledge base, the nurse knew that he was probably facing one of two likely problems—hypoglycemia or hyperglycemia. However, first the nurse performed a quick "ABC" assessment and determined that the patient's airway was open, the patient was breathing, and the patient's heart was circulating blood. Then, since the patient was admitted with an infection, the nurse suspected that the patient was experiencing a rise in blood glucose levels, or hyperglycemia. He obtained a fingerstick blood sugar reading of 346. The nurse also noted that the patient's skin was warm, dry, and flushed. The patient's respirations were deep, and her breath smelled "fruity." The nurse quickly called the physician to report these findings and anticipated receiving orders to give the patient more insulin. Logic, a questioning attitude, and use of educational knowledge helped this nurse think critically.

Alfaro-LeFevre (2009) suggests that individuals become better critical thinkers by verbalizing their thoughts aloud. Anticipating questions, asking an expert, and asking *why* are all examples of other strategies to improve critical thinking. It often takes a while to become comfortable with these ideas, but doing so will help you gain insight into your thinking. Hearing others think aloud will help you learn how other people reason. Study to gain specific theoretical knowledge, and ask other people to evaluate their thinking. Alfaro-LeFevre (2009) recommends sharing mistakes and thus turning them into learning opportunities.

Get Ready for the NCLEX® Examination!

Key Points

- The nursing process consists of six interconnected phases: assessment, diagnosis, outcome identification, planning, implementation, and evaluation.
- A complete and valid assessment influences the remaining phases of the nursing process.
- The patient is the primary source of data; all others are secondary sources.
- The nurse prescribes the primary interventions to treat a nursing diagnosis.
- The nurse uses assessment data to develop the nursing diagnosis.
- The nurse projects end results that are measurable, desirable, and observable, during outcome identification.
- The nurse develops an individualized plan of care considering pertinent patient characteristics such as age, culture, medical diagnosis, and mutual interest.
- Nursing interventions are planned activities to promote outcome achievement.
- Evaluation is an ongoing component of each phase of the nursing process.
- During evaluation, the actual patient outcome is compared with the desired patient outcome, and a judgment is made about outcome achievement.
- The plan of care is changed according to evaluation and the resulting identification of needs.
- NANDA-I, *NIC,* and *NOC* continue to develop standardized nursing languages to aid communication and research.
- The LPN/LVN has a significant role in the nursing process.
- Managed care and case management systems have emerged in response to rising health care costs.
- A clinical pathway is a multidisciplinary plan that schedules clinical interventions over an anticipated time frame for specific types of patient health problems.
- Critical thinking has been defined by one source as purposeful, informed, outcome-focused thinking (Alfaro-LeFevre, 2009).
- Evidence-based practice provides the latest guidelines for client care based on best practices provided by research.

Additional Learning Resources

 Go to your Companion CD for an audio glossary, animations, video clips, and more.

evolve Be sure to visit the Evolve site at http://evolve.elsevier.com/Christensen/foundations/ for additional online resources.

Review Questions for the NCLEX® Examination

1. Which is a medical diagnosis?
   1. Acute pain
   2. Pneumonia
   3. Activity intolerance
   4. Ineffective airway clearance
2. Which nurse is demonstrating critical thinking?
   1. The nurse who follows a physician's order without question
   2. The nurse who admits a seriously ill patient to a room far from the nurses' station
   3. The nurse who checks the accuracy of an intravenous pump used to deliver medications
   4. The nurse who administers medications using the five "rights" of medication administration (right drug, right dose, right route, right time, and right patient)

3. The student who plans to use *Nursing Interventions Classification (NIC)* material will benefit from a list of:
   1. nursing interventions.
   2. nursing activities.
   3. nursing outcomes.
   4. nursing indicators.

4. A patient is admitted to a large teaching hospital with coronary artery disease and has a bypass graft performed to increase blood supply to his heart muscle. His wound continues to drain and, when he is discharged, home health nurses will visit to continue to care for him. The person responsible for coordinating the patient's discharge plans is probably the:
   1. RN team leader.
   2. social worker.
   3. case manager.
   4. physician.

5. Which diagnosis includes all appropriate components of an actual nursing diagnosis?
   1. Impaired gas exchange
   2. Potential complication: gastric bleeding related to gastric ulcer
   3. Fear related to separation from support system manifested by statements of being scared, pallor, and increased respirations
   4. Risk for falls related to confusion manifested by calling nurse by name of aunt

6. "Constipation related to the effects of analgesic medications on the bowel manifested by statements of straining to have a bowel movement and no bowel movement in 5 days" is an example of:
   1. an actual nursing diagnosis.
   2. a risk nursing diagnosis.
   3. a wellness nursing diagnosis.
   4. a medical diagnosis.

7. Based on Maslow's hierarchy of needs, which nursing diagnosis label has the highest priority?
   1. Risk for aspiration
   2. Deficient fluid volume
   3. Acute pain
   4. Stress urinary incontinence

8. Which patient outcome statement meets the necessary criteria?
   1. The patient will identify the types of foods to include in a high-fiber diet.
   2. The nurse will teach the patient about constipation prevention.
   3. The nurse will increase total fluids during hospitalization.
   4. The patient will have a soft, formed bowel movement on the third day after nursing interventions.

9. The patient is admitted to the hospital with an upper respiratory infection. The nurse writes the following nursing diagnosis: *Risk for deficient fluid volume related to refusal to drink fluids secondary to a sore throat.* Which is the best outcome statement for the patient?
   1. The nurse will offer 2000 mL of fluids per day during hospitalization.
   2. The patient will experience a less sore throat in 8 hours.
   3. The patient will maintain adequate hydration as evidenced by moist mucous membranes; elastic skin turgor; and voiding of clear, dilute urine.
   4. The nurse will maintain an intravenous infusion of fluids for the ordered length of time.

10. A woman who has had four children comes to the clinic. She tells the nurse that when she laughs or coughs she "wets her underwear." The nurse discusses with the patient exercises that are helpful to reduce this stress incontinence. The nurse teaches the patient to perform Kegel exercises 25 times a day with *four to six repetitions* each time. The italicized words indicate:
    1. the nursing process.
    2. a nursing diagnosis.
    3. an outcome statement.
    4. a nursing order.

11. A 14-year-old patient is admitted to the emergency department with a possible medical diagnosis of acute appendicitis. The nurse begins to perform an assessment by interviewing:
    1. the patient's parents.
    2. the patient.
    3. the physician.
    4. the admissions nurse.

12. A patient who describes his illness is providing:
    1. subjective data.
    2. objective data.
    3. overt data.
    4. signs of his illness.

13. Defining characteristics:
    1. are descriptions of the problem.
    2. tell how the nursing diagnosis is manifested.
    3. give a name to the cluster of signs and symptoms.
    4. list factors that contribute to the problem.

14. The main purpose of cue clustering is to:
    1. organize the data.
    2. assist in the formation of a nursing diagnosis.
    3. select appropriate nursing interventions.
    4. validate the completeness of the assessment.

15. Which nursing diagnostic label would be ranked first in priority?

1. Risk for ineffective airway clearance
2. Colonic constipation
3. Alteration in nutrition: less than body requirements
4. Total urinary incontinence

16. The phrases used to connect the parts of a nursing diagnosis are:

1. "related to" and "due to."
2. "due to" and "manifested by."
3. "related to" and "manifested by."
4. "due to" and "as evidenced by."

17. During the last phase of the nursing process, the nurse:

1. gathers data to use in planning care.
2. selects nursing interventions to achieve the desired outcomes.
3. compares the desired outcome with the actual outcome.
4. prioritizes nursing interventions.

18. A nursing diagnosis expresses:

1. the patient's needs according to Maslow's hierarchy.
2. the patient's disease process.
3. the required nursing intervention.
4. a conclusion about the patient's response to an illness.

19. The patient is experiencing severe respiratory distress that is related to his chronic obstructive pulmonary disease. Which source of information would the nurse use when performing a nursing history?

1. The patient
2. The patient and his wife
3. The physician
4. The medical record

20. The LPN/LVN has finished bathing a patient. The patient states that he is sick to his stomach and has refused his breakfast. What additional clinical evidence would support the nursing diagnosis of *nausea?*

1. Unwillingness to ambulate
2. Increased swallowing of saliva
3. Statements describing acid reflux
4. Decreased awareness of his environment

21. Which choice constitutes objective data?

1. "When I walk to the mailbox, I get very short of breath."
2. "My legs ache when I climb stairs."
3. 7-inch transverse abdominal incision
4. Statements of pain

22. A newborn has the nursing diagnosis of *risk for ineffective thermoregulation.* What is the most accurate outcome for this diagnosis?

1. Parents state that they will keep the infant's room warm.
2. Parents state that they will wrap their infant in two blankets.
3. Parents state that they will keep their infant's temperature between 97.5° F and 98.6° F.
4. Parents state that they will be sure that their infant wears something on her head at home.

23. The nurse notes skin breakdown on a patient's coccyx during a bath. This data will be used to write a nursing diagnosis statement as:

1. the nursing diagnosis.
2. the etiologic or related factor.
3. the defining characteristic.
4. not necessary for writing the statement.

24. Which example includes all appropriate components of a *risk for* nursing diagnosis?

1. Risk for activity intolerance
2. Risk for aspiration related to difficulty swallowing
3. Potential complication: hemorrhage
4. Risk for ineffective airway clearance manifested by wheezing

Chapter

7

Documentation

evolve

http://evolve.elsevier.com/Christensen/foundationsadult

Elaine Oden Kockrow

Objectives

1. List the five purposes for written patient records.
2. Describe the differences between traditional and problem-oriented medical records.
3. State important legal aspects of chart ownership, access, confidentiality, and patient care documentation.
4. Describe the purpose of and relationship between the Kardex and the nursing care plan.
5. Explain the relationship of the nursing care plan to care documentation and patient care reimbursement.
6. Describe the basic guidelines for and the mechanics of charting.
7. Describe the differences in documenting care using activities of daily living and physical assessment forms, narrative, SOAPE, and focus formats.
8. Discuss issues related to computerization in documentation.
9. Discuss long-term health care documentation.
10. Discuss home health care documentation.
11. Discuss documentation and clinical (critical) pathways.

Key Terms

auditors (p. 139)
chart (health care record) (p. 138)
charting (p. 138)
charting by exception (CBE) (p. 145)
database (DĂ-tă-bās, p. 142)
diagnosis-related groups (DRGs) (p. 139)
documenting (p. 138)
Kardex (or Rand) (p. 145)
narrative charting (p. 142)
nomenclature (p. 153)
nursing care plan (p. 145)
nursing notes (p. 139)
peer review (p. 139)
problem list (p. 142)
problem-oriented medical record (POMR) (p. 142)
quality assurance, assessment, and improvement (p. 139)
recording (p. 138)
SOAPE (SŌP, p. 144)
SOAPIER (SŌP-ē-ŭr, p. 142)
traditional (block) chart (p. 142)

The **chart (health care record)** has never been more important in the health care system than it is today; it is a legal record that is used to meet the many demands of the health, accreditation, medical insurance, and legal systems.

The process of adding written information to the chart is called **charting, recording,** or **documenting.** Documenting involves recording the interventions carried out to meet the patient's needs. It is essential when charting interventions to document the type of interventions, the time care was rendered, and the signature of the person providing care. Anything written or printed that is a record or proof of activities will, by definition, play a role in this process. Although there are many details to remember when documenting in the chart, the process is not difficult; however, it is often time consuming. Good documentation reflects the nursing process. Documentation is an integral part of the implementation phase of the nursing process (see Chapter 6) and is necessary for the evaluation of patient care, as well as for reimbursement for the cost of care provided.

It is essential for you to understand how to use medical records effectively and efficiently. This chapter covers the purposes for written records, the common types of records, the basic guidelines and rules for documentation, and legal concerns. The knowledge of these guidelines and the ability to chart completely, accurately, and legibly are requirements for licensure and employment as a nurse. See Table 7-1 and Chapter 6 for information on the nursing process and documentation.

PURPOSES OF PATIENT RECORDS

There are five basic purposes for accurate and complete written patient records: (1) written communication, (2) permanent record for accountability, (3) legal record of care, (4) teaching, and (5) research and data collection.

Table 7-1 Essential Elements of Documentation

NURSING PROCESS	OBSERVATION SOURCES	WHERE TO DOCUMENT
ASSESSMENT Physiologic status Functional status Knowledge Psychosocial well-being Family Safety	Patient and family interview History and physical examination Laboratory and radiology results Medication records Environment	Discharge and transfer forms Progress notes Flow sheets
DIAGNOSIS	Nursing judgment	Patient care plan Critical pathways Protocols Progress notes Patient problem lists Admission sheets
OUTCOMES IDENTIFICATION/PLANNING Outcome definition Defining care priorities Defining intervention strategy Activation of care plan	Patient care plan Critical pathways Projected length of stay Standards of care Admission assessment data Staff reports	Patient care plan Critical pathways Protocols Progress notes Patient problem lists
IMPLEMENTATION	Progress notes Patient rounds Direct patient care	Progress notes Critical pathways Protocols
EVALUATION	Patient and family interview Physical assessment Staff reports Progress notes Diagnostic test results Flow sheets	Patient care plan Critical pathways Progress notes Protocols Patient problem lists

The patient's chart provides a concise, accurate, and permanent record of past and current medical and nursing problems, plans for care, care given, and the patient's responses to various treatments. The record facilitates accurate communication and continuity of care among all members of the health care team. Recorded information is not as easily lost or altered as the spoken word. Proper charting covers all areas of patient needs and concerns: physical, emotional, psychological, social, and spiritual.

This permanent record is sometimes also used by various government and other agencies to evaluate the institution's patient care, to justify cost reimbursement for care provided, and to establish or review accreditation. Current regulations require chart audits (review of specific chart components for completion and appropriateness) by officially appointed **auditors** (people appointed to examine patients' charts and health records to assess quality of care). Auditors will look to see whether all ordered care was charted as given and whether responses to specific care plan items and treatments are noted. Institutions have medical and **peer review** systems (an appraisal by professional co-workers of equal status). Peer review appraises the manner in which an individual nurse conducts practice, education, or research. Institutions also have specific procedures to provide for **quality assurance, assessment, and improvement,** which is an audit in health care that evaluates services provided and the results achieved compared with accepted standards. Accurate and legible records are the only means institutions have to prove that they are providing care to meet the patient's needs and established standards.

Cost reimbursement rates by the government plans (Medicare, Medicaid) are based on **diagnosis-related groups (DRGs)** (a system that classifies patients by age, diagnosis, and surgical procedure, using 300 different categories to predict the use of hospital resources, including length of stay). Many private insurance companies now use similar illness categories when setting hospital payment rates. Institutions are reimbursed by insurance companies or government programs only for documented patient care. The payors carefully review the **nursing notes** (the form on the patient's chart on which nurses record their observations, the care given, and the patient's responses) when deciding whether the necessary and ordered care is being given or was given.

The patient chart or health record is a legal document; when necessary and appropriate, it is used in court proceedings. Although the physician or institution owns the original record, lawyers and courts are able to gain access to it; to protect those involved in inpatient care, therefore, it is important to chart in a very detailed manner.

Patient health records are also used for teaching. Students in the health care professions learn more quickly and easily if examples of good charting are shared. Individuals also learn from their mistakes and the mistakes of others.

There are many uses for patient records involving research and data collection in the health field. For example, the government periodically publishes data on certain diseases and the effectiveness of new treatments. In addition, the pressure to contain or limit health care costs has made data regarding the usual length of hospitalization and the cost of treatment for specific illnesses or surgeries important for governmental and other health insurance providers.

BASIC GUIDELINES FOR DOCUMENTATION

The quality and accuracy of the nursing notes is extremely important. They have a decisive impact on the success or failure of communication: sometimes they clearly and concisely convey the intended message; and sometimes, in contrast, they cause confusion and errors in communication and patient care. Correct choice of words as well as spelling, grammar, and punctuation, in addition to good penmanship and other writing skills, are critical. Make sure the information recorded in the chart is clear, concise, complete, and accurate.

The registered nurse (RN) has primary responsibility for each patient's initial admission nursing history, the physical assessment, and development of the care plan based on the nursing diagnoses identified. Contributions by all team members during this initial process and during later updating sessions are important.

The forms you will use to make these notes vary; follow your institution's policy. Each facility uses a combination of graphics, care flow sheets, and narrative or SOAPE notes (see description in later material) to document observations, care, and responses. Be sure to always correlate your notes with the medical orders, Kardex information, and the nursing care plan.

CHARTING RULES

See Box 7-1 for generally accepted documentation rules that provide consistency in documentation between health care providers and facilities. These rules also meet the standards expected by the individuals and the agencies using the charts.

LEGAL BASIS OF DOCUMENTATION

Accurate documentation is one of the best defenses in the event that legal claims associated with nursing care are made (see Chapter 2). To limit nursing liability, it is necessary that the nursing documentation

Box 7-1 Basic Rules for Documentation

- All sheets should have the correct patient name, date, and time if appropriate.
- Use only approved abbreviations and medical terms.
- Be timely, specific, accurate, and complete.
- Write legibly (print if handwriting is not legible).
- Follow rules of grammar and punctuation.
- Fill all spaces; leave no empty lines. Chart consecutively. Go line by line. Do not indent left margin.
- Chart after care is provided, not before.
- Chart as soon and as often as necessary.
- Chart only your own care, observations, and teaching; never chart for anyone else.
- Use direct quotes when appropriate.
- Be objective in charting—only what you hear, see, feel, smell.
- Describe each item as you see it—for example, "white metal ring with clear stone" (rather than "diamond ring"). Do not speculate, guess, or assume.
- Chart facts; avoid judgmental terms and placing blame.
- Write only what you observe—not opinions. Never use charting to accuse someone else.
- Sign each block of charting or entry with full legal name and title.
- When a patient leaves a unit (e.g., to go to x-ray, lab, or office), chart the time and the method of transportation on departure and return.
- Chart all ordered care as given or explain the deviation (NPO for lab, off unit, refused, etc.).
- Note patient response to treatments and response to analgesics or other special medications.
- Use only hard-pointed, permanent black ink pens; no erasures or correcting fluids are allowed on charts.
- If a charting error is made, draw one line through the faulty information, mark error, initial if required, and make the correct entry.
- When making a late entry, note it as a late entry and then proceed with your notation—for example, "Late entry ______________."
- Follow each institution's policies and procedures for charting.
- Avoid using generalized empty phrases such as "status unchanged" or "had good day."
- If you question an order, record that clarification was sought. For example, do not record "physician made error," but chart "Dr. Bradley was called to clarify order for __________."

NPO, Nothing by mouth status.

clearly indicates that individualized, goal-directed nursing care was provided to a patient based on the nursing assessment. The record has to describe exactly what happened to a patient. This is best achieved when you chart immediately after providing care. Even though nursing care may have been excellent, in a court of law "care not documented is care not provided." It is your responsibility to indicate all assessments, interventions, patient responses, instructions, and referrals in the medical record.

Cases of malpractice often involve one or more of four common forms of inadequate documentation: (1) not charting the correct time when events occurred, (2) failing to record verbal orders or failing to have them signed, (3) charting actions in advance to save time, and (4) documenting incorrect data. Table 7-2 provides guidelines for legally sound documentation.

COMMON MEDICAL ABBREVIATIONS AND TERMINOLOGY

You will not be able to effectively and efficiently use a health record until you have developed some understanding and knowledge of common abbreviations and medical terms. This information is also required for concise and accurate documentation of care. Most facilities have a published list of generally accepted

Table 7-2 Legal Guidelines for Documentation

GUIDELINES	RATIONALE	CORRECTIVE ACTION
Do not erase, apply correction fluid, or scratch out errors made while recording.	Charting becomes illegible: It may appear as if you were attempting to hide information or deface record.	Draw a single line through error, write the word error above it and sign your name or initials. Then record note correctly.
Do not write retaliatory or critical comments about patient or care by other health care professionals.	It is possible to use statements as evidence for unprofessional behavior or poor quality of care.	Enter only objective descriptions of patient's behavior; record patient comments as quotations.
Correct all errors promptly.	Errors in recording often lead to errors in treatment.	Avoid rushing to complete charting; be sure information is accurate.
Record all facts.	Record is required to be accurate and reliable.	Be certain entry is factual; do not speculate or guess.
Do not leave blank spaces in nursing notes.	It is possible for another person to insert additional or incorrect information in space.	Chart consecutively, line by line; if space is left, draw line horizontally through it and sign your name at end.
Record all entries legibly and in black ink.	Illegible entries are open to misinterpretation, which causes errors and lawsuits; ink is not subject to erasure; black ink is more legible when records are photocopied or transferred to microfilm.	Never erase entries or use correction fluid, and never use pencil.
If you question an order, record that clarification was sought.	Seeking clarification is correct action to take, since you are just as liable for prosecution as the physician is if you carry out an order you know to be improper; however, it is not professional to criticize another professional in the notes (see entry above).	Do not record "physician made error." Instead, chart that "Dr. Smith was called to clarify order for analgesic."
Chart only for yourself.	You are accountable for information you enter into chart.	Never chart for someone else (Exception: if caregiver has left unit for day and calls you with information that has to be documented, include the name of the source of information in the entry and include that information was provided via telephone.)
Avoid using generalized, empty phrases such as "status unchanged" or "had good day."	Specific information about patient's condition or case is sometimes accidentally deleted or overlooked if information is too generalized.	Use complete, concise descriptions of care.
Begin each entry with time of entry, and end with your signature and title.	This guideline ensures that correct sequence of events is recorded; signature documents who is accountable for care delivered.	Do not wait until end of shift to record important changes that occurred several hours earlier; be sure to sign each entry.
Keep your computer password for documentation to yourself.	Maintains security and confidentiality.	Once logged into the computer, do not leave the terminal unattended.

NURSE'S NOTES: 0800–1300 0 45 oriented x4, pain scale 0/10, hand & leg strength strong to
right, weak to left. Skin pink, warm & dry, turgor good, incision to Rt. anterior chest wall s̄
erythema or edema, Jackson-Pratt draining serosanguineous exudate. Apical pulse 78 and
regular, capillary refill <3 sec to hands and feet bilaterally, pedal pulses bilaterally found c̄
doppler, IV to L. hand infusing at 85 mL/hr, site s̄ edema or erythema –. morphine pCA for
pain control. Lung sounds clear bilaterally, O_2 sats 94%, O_2 @ 1L per NC, incentive spirometer
1250 mL, ADA diet 1/4 eaten, BS x4, unable to void, up c̄ assistance, unsteady gait, TPR Bp
98, 72, 20, 122/64, pain level on a 0/10 scale. ——— T. Fye SPN
Jackson-Pratt drained 20 mL serosanguineous exudate. Patient and family members taught
proper protocol to empty and record J.P. drain upon dismissal (1205) Voided 175 mL of clear
amber urine. ——— T. Fye SPN

N-135 11/10 Nurse's Record

FIGURE 7-1 Example of narrative charting.

medical abbreviations and the terms approved for use in charting. Be aware that the use of abbreviations when charting is often problematic. For example, is "BS" breath sounds, or bowel sounds, or blood sugar? (See Appendix A for commonly used abbreviations and Appendix B for the Joint Commission's list of abbreviations to avoid.)

METHODS OF RECORDING

The documentation system selected by a nursing service will optimally reflect the philosophy of the department and the way nursing care is implemented. Professionally executed charting proves what you have done and communicates the patient's status and progress. The nursing process shapes your approach to providing care, and in turn, effective documentation of the care you provide reflects the nursing process.

TRADITIONAL CHART

The **traditional (block) chart** is divided into sections or blocks. Emphasis is placed on specific sections, or sheets, of information. Typical sections are the following: admission sheet, physician's orders, progress notes, history and physical examination data, nurse's admission information, care plan and nursing notes, graphics, and laboratory and x-ray examination reports. The order, the content, and the number of the sections vary among institutions. Nurses use flow sheets, graphics, and **narrative charting** (recording of patient care in descriptive form) (see Figure 7-1) to chart observations, care, and responses. Narrative charting is often intimidating to students. Nursing notes in this form are easier to complete if you remember that the steps of the nursing process are followed and that the notes are supposed to include the same information as a SOAPE note (discussed later in this chapter). Narrative charting includes the data (subjective, objective, or both) about the basic patient need or problem, whether anyone has been contacted or consulted, care and treatments provided (implementation), and the patient's response to treatment (evaluation). Information obtained from the nurse's assessment of the patient is clustered (see Chapter 6) and organized in a head-to-toe manner. This type of charting is written in an abbreviated story form instead of in the outline style of the problem-oriented medical record (POMR) format described in the following section.

PROBLEM-ORIENTED MEDICAL RECORD

The **problem-oriented medical record (POMR)** is organized according to the scientific problem-solving system or method. The principal sections are database, problem list, care plan, and progress notes. The accumulated data, or **database,** from the history, the physical examination, and the diagnostic tests are used to identify and prioritize the health problems on the master medical and other problem list.

This **problem list** (Figure 7-2) of active, inactive, potential, and resolved problems serves as the index for chart documentation. Together, representatives of all the disciplines involved with the patient's care develop a care plan with nursing diagnosis for each problem Figure 7-3). All health care providers—physicians, nurses, social workers, and therapists—chart on the same progress notes using forms such as narrative notes, flow sheets, and discharge summaries to document patient progress. This is done to facilitate and enhance communication between care providers.

SOAPIER (SOAPE documentation) (Box 7-2) is an acronym for seven different aspects of charting. For notes on specific patient problems, only the necessary parts needed for completeness are used.

S—Subjective information is what the patient states or feels; only the patient can provide this information.

O—Objective information is what the nurse can measure or factually describe.

MASTER PROBLEM LIST				
Date	Problem	Resolved	Reviewed	Reactivate
7/4/10	#1 Deficient knowledge R/T preoperative and postoperative procedures.	7/6/10		
7/5/10	#2 Pain R/T incision.	7/6/10		
7/5/10	#3 Temperature elevation 2° due to bladder infection.			

Addressograph
000-123
Spaur, Phyllis - Room 348A
Female - 60
Dr. Pearson-Pompei

FIGURE 7-2 Master problem list.

Great Plains Regional Medical Center

000-123
Spaur, Phyllis - Room 348A
Female - 60
Dr. Pearson-Pompei

PATIENT CARE PLAN

Admitting Diagnosis: Cholelithiasis Operation: Cholecystectomy Surgery Date: 7/4/10
Additional Diagnosis: UTI Surgeon: Dr. Pearson-Pompei Adm. Date: 7/3/10 Dism. Date:

Nursing Diagnosis with Outcome	Start Date	Nursing Interventions	Date D/Cd	Init	Reassessment	Date D/Cd	Init
#1 Hyperthermia	7/4/10	Vital signs q̄ 4 and PRN		JC			
R/T UTI		Encourage fluids as tolerated					
M/B temperature		I & O, provide high calorie in					
> 101° (0)		between meal snacks. Assess comfort					
feeling flushed		Medicate for temperature > 102° (0)					
Skin		q̄ 4 PRN					
warm to touch							
Goal: maintain							
normal body							
temperature							
97.8–98° within							
24 hours							

INITIALS AND SIGNATURE *F. E. Frances Ellefson R.N.*

FIGURE 7-3 Patient care plan with nursing diagnosis.

A—Assessment refers to an analysis or potential diagnosis of the cause of the patient's problem or need.

P—Plan is the general statement of the plan of care to be given or action to be taken.

I—Intervention or implementation is the specific care given or action taken.

E—Evaluation is an appraisal of the response and effectiveness of the plan.

R—Revision includes the changes that may be made to the original plan of care.

Box 7-2 SOAPE and SOAPIER Documentation Formats

SOAPE	SOAPIER
Subjective	Subjective
Objective	Objective
Assessment	Assessment
Plan	Plan
Evaluation	Intervention
	Evaluation
	Revision

Last name: Spaur	First name: Phyllis	Attending Physician Dr. Pearson-Pompei	Room No. 348A	Hosp No. 000-123

Date	Notes Should Be Signed by Physician
7-5-10	0930 Problem #1 elevated temperature
	(Nursing diagnosis: hyperthermia)
	S Feels hot & flushed. Has burning on urination and heavy feeling over bladder area. c/o "some discomfort" in lt. flank
	O Temperature 101^2 (0) elevated from 99^8 @ 7:30 AM. Skin warm, flushed, dry. Urinating in 100-200 mL am'ts. Urine dark,
	amber and cloudy. Foley Cath. dc'd 7/4 @ 10 PM. Lungs clear.
	A Possible bladder infection secondary to Foley catheter.
	P Notify Dr. Pearson-Pompei of temperature elevation, dysuria and back discomfort. Assess for other signs of infection. To x-ray
	for chest evaluation. Begin oral antibiotics after catheterization and urine specimen to laboratory for C & S per Dr. Pearson-Pompei
	orders. Encourage increased oral fluids.
	E Urine to laboratory, x-ray of chest ordered, chest and breath sounds clear. Nonproductive cough. Taking fluids well. 10:30 PM
	urine less concentrated.

FIGURE 7-4 SOAPE charting progress notes.

SOAPE is the briefer adaptation of the charting format for the POMR. In this more compact form, the care given or action taken (intervention [I]) is included in the notations under planning. The needed plan revisions (R) are noted in the evaluation section after the evaluation of the response to treatment. Figure 7-4 shows the charting forms in the progress notes that are commonly used in the medical record.

FOCUS CHARTING FORMAT

In the **focus charting format** (Box 7-3), which was developed by nurses, a modified list of nursing diagnoses is used as an index for nursing documentation instead of problem lists. Note the similarity of this list to the problem list used for the POMR. Indeed, you will be able to use focus charting with both traditional and POMR charting.

Focus charting uses the nursing process and the more positive concept of the patient's needs rather than medical diagnoses and problems. The focus is sometimes a current patient concern or behavior, and sometimes a significant change in patient status or behavior or a significant event in the patient's therapy. A focus is not a medical diagnosis.

DARE is the acronym for four different aspects of charting using the focus format (see Box 7-3). Data (D) is both subjective and objective and is equivalent to the assessment step of the nursing process. Action (A) is a combination of planning and implementation. Response (R) of the patient is the same as evaluation of effectiveness. Some facilities include education or patient teaching (E). You do not need to use all the DARE steps each time you make notes on a particular focus (Figure 7-5).

Box 7-3 Focus Charting Format

Data
Action
Response and evaluation
Education and patient teaching

EXAMPLE OF FOCUS CHARTING

Date	Time	Focus		Data, Actions, Patient Response, and Education
7/5/10	8:20 AM	Hypotension	D	BP in left arm 90/60, patient's skin diaphoretic, patient responds to name
			A	Placed patient in Trendelenburg position, increased IV fluid rate to 100 mL/hr per protocol, called Dr. Arkin.
			R	Patient remains responsive, BP in left arm 94/68 3 min after increasing fluid S Wilson RN
7/5/10	4:20 PM	Pain	D	Twisting in bed, grimacing with movement, states "has sharp lower back pain"
			A	Administered morphine sulfate 10 mg IV in RVL
			R	Verbalized relief within 15 min, lying quietly. T. Newson, RN
			E	Instructed patient to move slowly when getting out of bed and to call for assistance when necessary

FIGURE 7-5 Focus charting nurse's notes.

CHARTING BY EXCEPTION

Some facilities require the narrative notes for each shift to include a minimum of three entries, as well as a flow sheet on which you will chart all the care you give or withhold. Behind this policy is the legally derived charting concept that "care is not given if care is not charted." It is true that all care has to be charted, but this is a time-consuming, detailed, and defensive manner of doing so.

To get around this problem, many hospitals now have a policy called **charting by exception (CBE).** You will chart complete physical assessments, observations, vital signs, intravenous (IV) site and rate, and other pertinent data at the beginning of each shift. During the shift, the only notes you will make will be for additional treatments done or planned treatments withheld, changes in patient condition, and new concerns. Make notations reflecting progress or revisions for all active nursing diagnoses on the nursing care plan.

With the CBE method of documentation, you will use more detailed flow sheets, which reduce the time needed to chart. One format often used is the problem, intervention, and evaluation (PIE) format. In that it is a problem-solving approach, PIE is similar to the SOAPE format; the main difference is that SOAPE charting originated from the medical model, whereas PIE charting arose from the nursing process. The SOAPE method of documentation is also oriented to the problems, interventions, and evaluations involved in nursing care. It was designed to provide an ongoing plan of nursing care with daily documentation. The care and assessment flow sheets consist of standardized assessment criteria and interventions. With this method, you will assess all areas and compare the results to normal standards. The PIE format may be written in several ways; use the format dictated by your agency's policy according to what area you are assigned. At each shift, evaluate each patient problem at least once, and if the problem remains unresolved, make sure it is continuously addressed until resolution is reached. After the patient problem is resolved, it is no longer covered by the daily documentation.

Sometimes you will use a variation of the PIE format that includes assessment (A) data before the PIE (APIE). This assessment data will include both subjective (S) and objective (O) data. This will assist you to follow the steps of the nursing process (Figure 7-6).

Date	Time	Progress notes
7/6/10	0900	A - Assessment: (s) states -"sharp shooting pain in epigastric region" (o) guarding abdomen and refuses lunch tray. States "I am nauseated."
	0915	P - Problem: Pain related to unknown cause
	0920	I - Intervention: Demerol 100 mg given IM in R ventral gluteal region
	1000	E - Evaluation: States "the pain is gone." *C. Sommers, LPN*

FIGURE 7-6 APIE documentation.

RECORD-KEEPING FORMS AND EXAMPLES

Different facilities use a variety of forms to make medical record documentation easy and quick, yet comprehensive. There are many forms that help eliminate the need to duplicate data repeatedly in the nursing notes. The forms present several types of information in a format more accessible than compilation of all progress notes. Most of the forms are self-explanatory as to the type of information required from the nurse (Figure 7-7). It is unnecessary to chart a narrative note each time you give a medication (see Chapter 23) or a bath (see Chapter 18) or assess vital signs (see Chapter 4).

The nursing **Kardex (or Rand)** system is a card system used to consolidate patient orders and care needs in a centralized, concise way. The cumulative care file or Rand is kept at the nursing station for quick reference. Card forms vary among institutions based on information required for care (Figure 7-8, p. 149).

The **nursing care plan** (preprinted guidelines used to care for patients with similar health problems) is developed to meet the nursing care needs of a patient. Sometimes you will see a standardized care plan for a certain condition or surgery; special needs and interventions are indicated so you are able to tailor care to the individual. This kind of plan, developed by nurses for nurses, is based on nursing assessment and nursing diagnosis. Standardized nursing care plans include the pertinent nursing diagnoses, goals, and plans for care and specific actions for care implementation and evaluation.

Incident Reports

You will fill out an **incident report** (any event not consistent with the routine operation of a health care unit or the routine care of a patient) (Figure 7-9, p. 150) or other hospital notification form when patient care is delivered that is not consistent with facility or national standards of expected care; for example, you neglect to give a medication or treatment or give an incorrect dose of a drug. Either of these events has the potential to cause injury. Incident reports are also filled out for any unusual event in a hospital (e.g., injuries to a patient, visitor, or hospital personnel). Many staff members are reluctant to fill out these forms, but this information helps the facility risk manager and unit

PHYSICAL ASSESSMENT (HEAD TO TOE)
TIME OF ASSESSMENT: ____________

	NOTES:
1. NEUROLOGIC: Level of consciousness	
Confused	
Oriented x 1. person 2. place 3. time 4. purpose	
PERRLA—Babinski: positive, negative	
Hand strength: strong, weak	
Leg movement: strong, weak	
2. INTEGUMENTARY	
Condition: moist or dry	
Temperature:	
Turgor	
Tenting	
Incision	
Location:	
Without erythema	
Exudate:	
Sutures/staples intact	
Sutures/staples not intact	
Open wound	
Hemovac: Color Amt	
Davol: Color Amt	
Jackson-Pratt: Color Amt	
Penrose: Color Amt	
Wound vac: Color Amt	
Dressing	
Clean & dry	
Needs changed	
3. CARDIOVASCULAR	
Apical pulse rate:	
Capillary refill <3 sec: Yes or No	
Pedal pulses (1-4+): L & R	
Pedal edema (1-4+): L & R	
Nonpitting edema	
IV	
Solution	
Peripheral	
Central line	
Rate:	
Site & condition:	
4. RESPIRATORY	
Anteriorly	
Posteriorly	
O_2 Saturation level: %	
Crackle	
Wheezes: sonorous or sibilant	
Pleural friction rub	

FIGURE 7-7 Nursing care record.

Dyspnea Tachypnea Orthopnea	
O_2 Therapy: type:	
Rate: Liters per:	
Incentive spirometer	
Inspiratory capacity: mL	
Chest tube to H_2O seal ____ cm	
Chest tube to H_2O seal and wall suction ____ mm Hg	
Color and amount ____ mm Hg	
5. GASTROINTESTINAL	
Appetite ____ Type of diet ____	
Dentures: yes or no	
Oral fluid intake:	
Bowel sounds *4:	
Active Hyper Hypo Absent	
Distention Tympanic Tenderness	
Flatulence	
BM #: Color: Consistency:	
Stoma pink & viable: Yes or No	
N/G	
Amt: mL	
Color of drainage	
Peg tube ____	
Site condition ____ Flush ____ Feeding ____	
Gastrostomy tube ____	
Site condition ____ Flush ____ Feeding ____	
Jejunostomy ____	
Site condition ____ Flush ____ Feeding ____	
6. URINARY	
Output amount: ____ hours of output ____	
Color:	
Odor:	
Catheter	
Type: Foley Ureterostomy	
Suprapubic Nephrostomy	
Urostomy	
CBI credit:	
True urine:	
7. MOBILITY	
Activity level:	
Bed rest. chair. up with assistance. walker.	
crutches. cane	
Up ad lib: yes or no	
Gait: unsteady or steady	
Level of tolerance:	
Traction: Kind: Weight:	

FIGURE 7-7, cont'd Nursing care record.

Continued

8. REPRODUCTIVE	
Prostate problems: yes no	
Hysterectomy: yes no	
Breast—monthly breast self-exam: yes no	
Mastectomy:	
___ Rt ___ Left ___ Appearance	
Vaginal drainage: yes no	
9. SENSORY	
Hard of hearing: yes no	
Hearing aid: yes no	
Glasses	
Contacts	

VITALS	VITALS	ADLs
TIME TAKEN: hrs	TIME TAKEN: hrs	BED BATH-TIME:
Temp:	Temp:	Supplies needed: 1 linen bag
Pulse:	Pulse:	2-3 towels
Respirations:	Respirations:	2-3 washcloths
Blood pressure:	Blood pressure:	4-5 disposable washcloths
How taken:	How taken:	Soap, shampoo, deodorant, comb
Level of pain:	Level of pain:	1 disposable garbage bag
NOTES:	NOTES:	Cotton swabs
		Orange stick/nail file
		Lip conditioner
		Toothbrush, toothettes, toothpaste
		Denture supplies
CHECK:	CHECK:	Other supplies need by pt:
Water filled & cool	Water filled & cool	
Bed straightened	Bed straightened	
Patient comfortable?	Patient comfortable?	LINEN CHANGE OF BED:
Patient requests:	Patient requests:	1 linen bag (if not doing @ bedtime)
		1 contour sheet
		1 flat sheet
		1 pull sheet
		Pillow case(s) - How many pillows?
		1 blanket
		1 bedspread
		Add'l supplies needed for pt:
__ ALL INFO CHARTED	__ ALL INFO CHARTED	__ ALL INFO CHARTED

FIGURE 7-7, cont'd Nursing care record.

managers prevent future problems through education and other corrective measures.

When filling out an incident report, give only objective, observed information. Do not admit liability or give unnecessary details. Do list date, time, care given the patient, and the name of the physician notified. When charting the incident in the patient's nursing notes, do not mention the incident report, because doing so makes it easier for an attorney to request that document for a court case (Table 7-3).

Twenty-Four-Hour Patient Care Records and Acuity Charting Forms

The nursing records are often consolidated into a system that accommodates a 24-hour period. A 24-hour record-keeping system helps eliminate unnecessary record-keeping forms. It is easier to obtain accurate assessment information and documentation of activities of daily living with 24-hour notations. In addition, 24-hour patient care records often use flow sheets and checklists to further enhance efficiency.

Date Activities
7/5 Bed rest
7/6 BRP
Dangle
Chair
w/Chair
Crutched
Walker
Ad. Lib.
Turn
7/7 Up with Assistance

Date Elimination
7/5 Catheter dc'd 7/6
Commode
Adult Diaper
Colostomy Old/New
Ileostomy Old/New
Hematest
Save Stools
Strain all Urine
Urostomy
7/5 Intake/Output
Ileo Conduit
Enema/Flush PRN
CBI

Date Supportive
Cradle/Footboard
Overhead Frame
TED Hose
Telemetry #
NG Tube
Tracheotomy
Traction
Oxygen
Siderails
Restraints
Egg Crate
7/5 IV's/Int. lock
Isolation
PCA Pump
Oral Suction
K-Pad

Date Wounds
Packing
Hemo drain
Drain
7/5 Incision
Suction
Solcotrans
7/5 T-Tube
Chest Tube

Date Hygiene
7/6 Bed Bath
7/7 Assist
Self Bath
Shower/Tub
Sitz
Towel Bath
Oral
Hair
Skin/Decubitus

Date	Diet
7/6	Clear liquids

Snacks	Beverages
	B Hot tea
	D Hot tea
	S Hot tea

Food Allergies: milk

LABORATORY and RADIOLOGY
7/5: Chest x-ray, ECG, CBC
7/7: Chest x-ray, UA/C&S

DATE	TREATMENTS	DISC.
	DAILY WEIGHT SCALE	
7/5	Incentive spirometer q 4 hr. while awake.	
7/5	Vital signs q 4hr.	
7/5	Turn, cough, and deep breath q 2 hr.	
7/5	Reinforce dressings PRN.	
7/6	Chg. abdominal dressings PRN.	
7/6	Record T-tube drainage.	

CONTACT (next of kin)
W.L. Spaur - husband
534-3974
Chaplain/Minister
G Timmons

BLUE DOT:

RECENT/PRESENT SURGERY:
Open Cholecystectomy 7/5/10

ADDITIONAL DIAGNOSIS:
UTI 7/7

Room:	Age:	Name:	Sex:	S(M)W.D.	Religion	Diagnosis:	Attending Physician:	Consulting Physician:
348A	60	Phyllis Spaur	Fe		Prot	Cholelithiasis & Cholecystitis	Dr. Pearson-Pompei	Dr. Jennifer Christensen

FIGURE 7-8 Nursing Kardex (or Rand) card.

Twenty-four hour patient care records provide the foundation for an acuity charting system. **Acuity charting** uses a score that rates each patient by severity of illness. By documenting and analyzing your interventions, you obtain an overall level of acuity for each patient. For example, perhaps an acuity system rates patients from 1 to 5 (1 is high, 5 is low). A patient returning from surgery with multisystem problems is an acuity level 1. On the same continuum, another patient awaiting discharge after a successful recovery from surgery is an acuity level 5. One benefit is the ability to determine efficient staffing patterns according to the acuity levels of the patients on a particular nursing unit. The patient-to-staff ratios depend on a composite gathering of data in regard to the 24-hour interventions necessary for implementing care.

Discharge Summary Forms

Much emphasis is placed on preparing a patient for a timely discharge from a health care institution. Ideally, discharge planning begins at admission and in some cases even before admission, as is necessary with same-day surgery admissions and childbirth. Nurses continue discharge planning as the patient's condition changes. It is best for patients and family to be involved in the discharge planning process.

A discharge summary form provides important information pertaining to the patient's continued health care after discharge. You will always provide to the patient or the family (or both) the reason for hospitalization, significant findings, the patient's status, and any specific teaching plan. Discharge summary forms (see Figure 11-5) make the summary concise and instructive. Often, the form includes a copy that you give to the patient, a family member, or a home health care nurse. Home health care agencies or extended nursing care facilities also benefit from receiving information on these summary forms and use it to provide better continuity of care.

DOCUMENTATION AND CLINICAL (CRITICAL) PATHWAYS

With the arrival of managed care, documentation tools that integrate the standards of care of multiple disciplines have been developed. Managed care is a systematic approach to care that provides a framework for the coordination of medical and nursing interventions.

GREAT PLAINS REGIONAL MEDICAL CENTER

Report of Medication, (Patient) Visitor Safety Variance

If no addressograph, write in name, age, sex, and chart number. For a visitor, please include address and telephone number.

Addressograph

To be completed by the person most closely involved or the person discovering the incident/occurrence.

PATIENT NAME: *John Jordan* AGE: *76* SEX: *male*

ADDRESS: *506 South Ash Street* *North Platte, NE 69101*

TYPE OF PATIENT: *X* Inpatient ____ Outpatient ____ Emergency
(check one) ____ Visitor ____ Employee

Date and time of variance: *4-9-10 0900*

Exact location of variance: *230A*

Description of variance: *Found patient lying on floor at foot of bed sts "I was having a liquid stool and I couldn't push the nurse's call light." Noted a large liquid stool on floor near patient. Side rails up X 2.*

What was the nature of the injury to the (patient) visitor, etc.: *4 cm. abrasion to left trochanteric area.*

Equipment or supplies involved: *none*

ID # & Present Location: *3001*

Why did variance occur? *patient too weak to push nurse's call light and an unsteady gait.*

Physician Notified? ____ yes *X* no when? *0915*

Signature *Carol Oden RN* Physician: *DR. J.H. CHRISTENSEN*

Witness *Patty Baker RN*

If the incident is related to patient care, this sheet must remain on inpatient medical record for 24 hours, after which it shall be taken to the Risk Management Department.

CONFIDENTIAL - NOT PART OF THE MEDICAL RECORD

FIGURE 7-9 Incident report.

Table 7-3 Examples of Incident Report Entries

PROPER ENTRY	INCORRECT ENTRY
6 PM Patient found on floor at foot of bed; able to respond to name when called. 2-cm abrasion noted across left forehead. Vital signs stable. Dr. Smith notified and arrived on floor at 6:15 PM. Placed patient on fall-prevention protocol.	Patient found on floor at foot of bed, probably fell on way to bathroom. Small abrasion over left forehead. Dr. Smith notified. Patient instructed to use call light when needing to go to bathroom.
Administered morphine sulfate 10 mg at 4 PM; 6 mg morphine sulfate ordered. Monitored vital signs q 15 minutes; called Dr. Jones; vital signs remain stable.	Administered 10 mg morphine sulfate at 4 PM without checking order before administering; 6 mg morphine sulfate ordered.
Needlestick to right index finger, caused minimal bleeding. Notified employee health department.	Needlestick to right index finger, likely due to needle left in bed linen after blood drawing. Notified employee health.

From Perry, A.G., & Potter, P.A.. (2005). *Clinical nursing skills and techniques* (6th ed.). St. Louis: Elsevier.

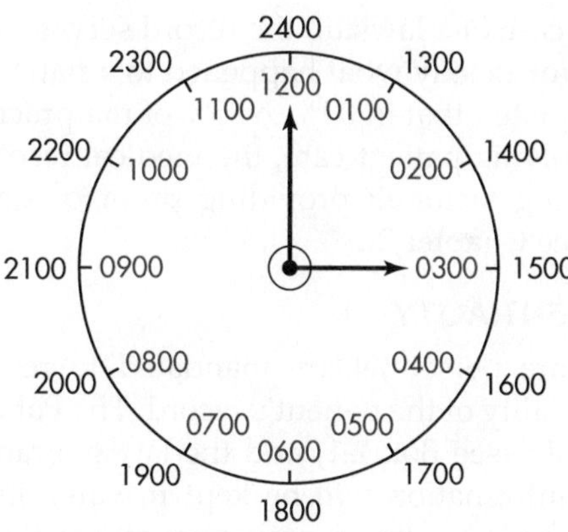

FIGURE 7-10 Military time clock.

These documentation tools are called **clinical (critical) pathways.** Clinical (critical) pathways allow staff from all disciplines to develop standardized, integrated care plans for a projected length of stay for patients of a specific case type. The case types that have clinical (critical) pathways are usually those that occur in high volume and are predictable. A clinical (critical) pathway for a total hip repair will recommend on a day-to-day basis the level of activity, pain control therapy, advancement in diet, and educational topics necessary for a normal patient's recovery.

The exact contents and format of these clinical (critical) pathways vary among institutions. The contents will include a care plan, interventions specific for each day of hospitalization, and a documentation tool. The clinical (critical) pathway replaces other nursing forms such as the nursing care plan.

You and other team members use the pathways both to monitor a patient's progress and as a documentation tool. CBE is frequently the method used with pathways. Staff members document only when anticipated interventions are not provided as projected.

Many agencies use military time, a 24-hour system that uses digit numbers to indicate morning, afternoon, and evening times (Figure 7-10).

HOME HEALTH CARE DOCUMENTATION

The home health care business continues to expand as growing numbers of older adults require an increasing use of home health care services. Medicare has specific guidelines for establishing eligibility for home health care reimbursement. In the fulfillment of these Medicare guidelines, documentation by home health care nurses has become a significant problem area: 50% of nursing time is spent in documentation (Box 7-4).

Documentation in the home health care system has different implications than in other areas of nursing. The primary difference is the nature of the home setting, which dictates that a narrower scope of people (e.g., patient, family, direct health care provider) witness the majority of care. Home health care requires that the entire health care team work closely together. It is necessary that the documentation of care is accurate and complete so that all members of the team are able to ascertain what care is rendered in the home. In addition, the documentation provides both the quality control and the justification for reimbursement from Medicare, Medicaid, or private insurance companies. Nurses have to document all their services for payment (e.g., direct skilled care, patient instructions, skilled observations, and evaluation visits). The nurse is the pivotal person in the documentation of the delivery of home health care.

Box 7-4 Home Care Forms for Documentation

The usual forms used to document home care include the following:

- Assessment form
- Referral source information and intake form
- Discipline-specific care plans
- Physician's plan of treatment
- Medication sheet
- Clinical progress notes
- Miscellaneous (conference notes, verbal order forms, telephone calls)
- Discharge summary
- Reports to third-party payers

Home health care documentation has unique problems because different health care providers have different uses for the medical record. Some parts of the record are needed in the home with the patient; other chart forms are needed in an office setting. Duplication of documentation is difficult to avoid; it is helpful for agency policies to indicate what forms you, as the home health nurse, will leave at your office versus what forms you take into the home. With the use of modems and laptop computers, it is possible for records to be available in multiple locations, which allows the multidisciplinary use of them that is often called for in home health care.

Delivery of home health care is changing along with other advancements in technology. You will often be able to communicate and even assess patient needs via modem linkages. The future continues to hold solutions for nursing care in the home via "distance learning." The changing mode of health care delivery also has an impact on documentation.

LONG-TERM HEALTH CARE DOCUMENTATION

An ever-increasing number of older adults require care in long-term health care facilities. Because many individuals will live in this setting for the rest of their lives, they are referred to as residents rather than patients. The acuity of residents' conditions, as well as the number of their disabilities, continues to escalate commensurate with their age. Nursing personnel often face challenges much different from those in the acute care setting. These differences establish a significantly different basis for nursing documentation.

Outside agencies are instrumental in determining the standards and policies for documentation in long-term health care. For example, the Omnibus Budget Reconciliation Act (OBRA) of 1987 instituted extremely significant Medicare and Medicaid requirements for long-term care provision and documentation. Among the requirements of OBRA are minimum data sets (MDS) and regulated standards for resident assessments, individualized care plans, and qualifications for health care providers (RNs and licensed practical nurses and licensed vocational nurses [LPN/LVNs]). In addition, the department of health in each state governs the frequency of the required written nursing entries in the records of residents in long-term care facilities.

Long-term care documentation supports a multidisciplinary approach in the assessment (referred to as the MDS) and the planning process (referred to as resident assessment protocols) of the residents. Often, long-term care agencies also have skilled care units where patients or residents stay when, in response to mandates for shorter hospital stays, they require increased levels of care and are not able to return directly to their usual residence after a hospital admission. Multidisciplinary communication among such health care providers as nurses, certified nurse assistants (CNAs), social workers, recreational therapists, and dietitians is essential in the regulated documentation process. The fiscal management of long-term care hinges on the justification of nursing care as demonstrated in sound documentation of the services rendered.

SPECIAL ISSUES IN DOCUMENTATION

RECORD OWNERSHIP AND ACCESS

The original health care record or chart is the property of the institution or the physician. On admission to the health care facility, the patient is usually asked to sign a form granting permission for appropriate people to have access to the record as necessary. Patients usually do not have immediate access to their full records. One exception is federal health care agencies, such as Veterans Administration (VA) hospitals.

Patients have gained access rights to their records in most states, but only if they follow the established policy of each facility. Usually a written request for chart access must be submitted, and institutions specify a period allowing the physician and the facility to review the record and give a response. Sometimes the institution requires that a staff member or physician be present while the individual looks through the chart to answer questions and to protect the integrity of the record.

Lawyers, with the patient's written permission, are given access to the chart. Courts have the legal right to obtain records for their review and use.

In the case of a lawsuit, the record serves as the description of exactly what happened to a patient. It has been estimated that in 80% to 85% of malpractice lawsuits involving patient care, the medical record is the determining factor in providing proof of significant events (see Chapter 2).

CONFIDENTIALITY

Health care personnel are mandated to respect the confidentiality of the patient's record. The Patient Care Partnership (see Box 1-1) and the law guarantee that medical information will be kept private, unless the information is needed in providing care or the patient gives permission for others to see it. The Health Insurance Portability and Accountability Act (HIPAA), an act of Congress passed in 1996, affords certain protections to persons covered by health care plans, including continuity of coverage when changing jobs, standards for electronic health care transactions, and primary safeguards for the privacy of individually identifiable patient information.

Ethical codes of practice also emphasize your obligation to preserve patients' privacy by holding patient information in highest confidentiality. Do not read a record, or allow others to do so, unless there is a clinical reason, and hold the information regarding the patient in confidence. Furthermore, trust is necessary for good nurse-patient relationships, and breaking confidences is a way to lose patient trust. If you break laws concerning confidentiality of the medical record, the possibility rises that you will face a lawsuit (see Chapter 2).

DOCUMENTATION BY COMPUTER

In many health care settings, **computer-based records** (electronic medical records) facilitate delivery of patient care and support the data analysis necessary for strategic planning. Computer-based records contain information that is identical to that found in traditional records, but they eliminate repetitive entries and allow more freedom of access to the database (Figure 7-11). In general, although they are expensive, computer documentation systems increase efficiency, consistency, and accuracy and decrease costs. Legibility is a further benefit they offer.

The scope of the use of computer systems for documentation in health care agencies varies depending on the agency. Most health care agencies have incorporated information systems for management of admissions, billing, and the communication of orders for diet, pharmacy, and diagnostic tests. Use of these systems allows departments within an institution to interact, and it provides a database for research and quality assurance. In addition, agency-wide computer information systems are more efficient because information entered in the system can be automatically transferred to other areas. Many agencies have incorporated soft-

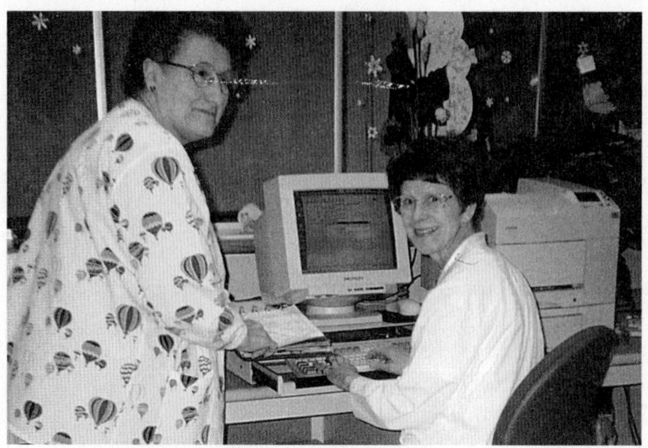

FIGURE 7-11 Nurses use computer for documentation.

ware for documentation of patient care. Systems often include options for generating individualized care plans, automated Kardex forms, and acuity levels, as well as providing a mechanism for recording ongoing assessment data (Figure 7-12).

Although some systems permit computer input only at the nurses' desk, bedside systems—including handheld systems—are becoming more common. Bedside charting systems, also referred to as point-of-care (POC) systems, often provide prompts for certain data to be entered, resulting in more accurate and complete record keeping. In addition, charting at the bedside saves time and allows current information to be immediately available to all who need it. Some systems automatically retrieve and record information from electronic devices (e.g., vital signs) and simultaneously enter the data in all relevant locations in the record, which cuts down on duplication of effort.

Electronic charting procedures vary by agency. Data are often recorded in flow-sheet format for easy storage and retrieval. Some agencies incorporate the use of free-text narratives in addition to standardized phrases, to allow specific and individualized documentation. The standard phrases indicate information such as nursing diagnoses, interventions, or outcomes classification systems. Assessment data, for instance, are entered by selecting from a list of preformulated choices. This means that the accuracy and pertinence of the data you enter depends on your familiarity with the language the system uses to name the nursing problems, the lists of data for assessment, and anything else that is entered by picking from a list.

These naming conventions, or **nomenclature** (a classified system of technical or scientific names and terminology), raise one of many concerns regarding computer-based documentation. The field of medical or nursing informatics (the study of information processing) is constantly evolving, which requires that software programs be updated on a regular basis to stay abreast of changes in terminology. In addition, there is a need to invest considerable time in training personnel, both in charting procedures and the terminology the system uses, as well as conducting ongoing refresher training. The agency-specific nature of the electronic record-keeping system is another problem. For one thing, because procedures and terminology are unique to the agency, newly hired personnel need to learn a new system even if they have already had considerable experience in the field. In addition, the software used by one agency often is incompatible with the software used by other agencies and providers. Thus instead of facilitating communication between institutions, the electronic records actually inhibit it.

Furthermore, although charting by computer is an efficient method of documentation, the security of the system raises legal and ethical issues. Confidentiality, access to information, and inappropriate alterations in patient records are areas of increasing concern. The network is protected by a firewall from illegitimate outside access. Some computer systems permit online access from remote sites, but this further complicates the task of keeping the system secure. To protect the patient's rights and keep the patient's record confidential, anyone who enters data into or consults a computerized record has to log on to the system using a secure password. Optimally, the institution will change passwords monthly to maintain security. Because your password is assigned only to you, anything you enter will automatically be credited to you as though you had signed it. Do not ever share your password with anyone. Make sure to log off the system before leaving the terminal to ensure that information about a patient does not remain on the monitor display for others to view.

It is also necessary to protect computer-generated printouts and prevent the indiscriminate duplication or distribution of information about patients. Most facilities using computer charting incorporate a system for logging and tracking computer printouts (Box 7-5), as well as having protocols for shredding the copies that are made.

The American Nurses Association's (ANA) Nursing Information and Data Set Evaluation Center (NIDSEC) has developed guidelines for nursing information systems. The standards provide a framework for evaluation of nomenclature, clinical content, storage and retrieval of data, and confidentiality and security components (ANA, 1997).

USE OF FAX MACHINES

Very limited amounts and types of information from a patient's record can be printed or faxed. Fax machines send written documents over telephone lines to quickly transmit data between hospitals and other facilities, such as doctors' offices. You are responsible for knowing

SHIFT ONGOING ASSESSMENT

Adult Review of Systems (Ongoing)

Pain

FLACC Pain Scale

Face: Frequent frown/clench jaw/quiver chin (2); pt unable to state pain according to pain scale, stated "I wouldn't know"
Legs: paraplegic activity—squirming/shifting back & forth/tense (1)
Cry: moans/whimpers/complains (1)
Consolability: reassure by touch/hug/distractible (1)
Total FLACC scale: 5, explained to her how to use her PCA pump, had her demonstrate back to me, nurse notified. Analgesic given

Cardiovascular

Apical pulse regular

Edema

Edema location: ankles and feet bilaterally; on a scale of 1-4, edema is 2+ pitting

Central Nervous

Alert; absence of fine motor skills; unable to move legs due to paralysis; hand grasp equal; very strong paraplegic

Ear-Eye-Nose-Throat

WNL Ear: External ears normal shape and appearance. No lesions or drainage. *WNL Eye:* Eyes bilaterally symmetrical. Eyebrows, lids, and lashes intact without deformities. Conjunctivae and cornea clear. Sclera white without redness. PERRLA. *WNL Nose:* Normal shape and appearance. No lesions or drainage. Normal breathing through nares. *Other comments:* lips cracked, applied Vaseline

GI

Abdomen: tender; very tender due to 2nd day post of sigmoid colostomy soft
Bowel sounds: absent

Colostomy

Clean, pink, stoma; beefy red with small amount of serosanguineous exudate; bag changed; applied first flange with bag per protocol, bleeding in PACU preventing application of bag to ostomy immediately post-op

GU Assessment (Ongoing)

Foley catheter catheter care performed 1030; Foley tubing taped to thigh; output of 100 mL urine: odor; sediment; color: dark yellow

Integumentary

Pink; warm; moist; skin turgor: good; <2 sec capillary refill is <2 seconds; bilaterally feet and hands. Other comments: central abdominal incision well approximated without erythema or edema. Third staple down is loose. Dressing change performed per sterile technique 0900. Small amount of serosanguineous exudate in dressing.

Musculoskeletal

Gait: nonambulatory. Resting in bed; other comments: paraplegic, bed to wheelchair

Intravascular Access (Ongoing)

Peripheral IV

Site 1 peripheral IV: left forearm per infusion pump; IV solution/rate: D5 1/2 NS running at 100 mL/hr; site without erythema or edema

Respiratory

Oxygen sats 92% on room air. WNL Respiratory: respirations are nonlabored. Breath sounds clear bilaterally. c/o pain with deep breathing

Pulses

Pedal pulse left: strong; pedal pulse right: strong; radial pulse right: strong; radial pulse left: strong

SHIFT ONGOING ASSESSMENT

Incisions/drsg/drains/chest tube

Dressing

Site 1 dressing: Lt knee clean, dry, and intact

Hemovac

Site 1 Hemovac: superior Lt knee sanguineous drainage

SHIFT ONGOING ASSESSMENT

q1h & q2h Shift Assessment

Pain

Pain scale: 3; *location:* Lt knee no complaints voiced; respirations even and unlabored; up in chair; eating noon meal with husband
IV site patent without erythema or edema; denies needs

FIGURE 7-12 Computerized reporting of ongoing data assessment.

Box 7-5 Guidelines for Safe Computer Documentation

- Do not share with another caregiver the password that you use to enter and sign off computer files. (NOTE: A good system requires frequent changes in personal passwords to prevent unauthorized people from accessing and tampering with records. Some facilities use fingerprint scanners instead of passwords.)
- After logging on, never leave the computer terminal unattended without first logging off.
- Follow the correct protocol for correcting errors. To correct an error after storage, mark the entry "mistaken entry," add the correct information, and date and initial the entry. If you record information in the wrong chart, write "mistaken entry—wrong chart," and sign off.
- Make sure that stored records have backup files—an important safety check. If you inadvertently delete part of the permanent records, type an explanation into the computer file with the date, the time, and your initials, and submit an explanation in writing to your manager.
- Do not leave information about a patient displayed on a monitor where others have the opportunity to see it.
- Follow the agency's confidentiality procedures for documenting sensitive information, such as a diagnosis of human immunodeficiency virus (HIV) infection.
- Printouts of computerized records also have to be protected. Shredding of printouts and keeping a log that accounts for every copy (whether electronic or printed) of a computerized file that you have generated from the system are ways to keep waste and creation of duplicate records to a minimum and protect the confidentiality of patients.

the policies and procedures of your employing institution for printing and faxing of patient information in order to avoid unauthorized release of information. According to Hebda and colleagues (2005), several steps are possible to protect the security of confidential patient information:

- Verifying the information that is permissible to fax
- Verifying the fax number that you are dialing
- Validating the source and destination of the fax before transmitting information
- Identifying yourself and the intended recipient by including a cover sheet, especially if the fax number is used by more than one person
- Using preprogrammed speed-dial keys to lessen the chance of dialing incorrect fax numbers
- Keeping fax machines in a secure area to maintain confidentiality
- Limiting use of the fax machine to designated personnel
- Logging fax transmissions electronically if the fax machine provides this capability

Get Ready for the NCLEX® Examination!

Key Points

- Documentation is part of the implementation phase of the nursing process and is used in evaluation.
- Use only approved abbreviations and medical terms when charting in a patient's record. Knowledge of the common abbreviations and terms is required.
- There are five purposes for written patient records. Records are (1) a means of written communication to facilitate continuity of care, (2) a permanent record for accountability purposes (audits, accreditation, and cost reimbursement), (3) a legal record, (4) used in teaching, and (5) used for research and data collection.
- Two common types of medical records or charts are the traditional (block) chart and the problem-oriented medical record (POMR).
- The POMR uses a master patient problem list as an index to the chart. These listed problems are usually medical diagnoses.
- SOAPIER is one format for charting in the POMR. The letters stand for subjective (S), objective (O), assessment (A), plan (P), implementation (I), evaluation (E), and revision (R).
- Two other common formats for charting nursing notes are narrative and focus. Focus charting includes data (D), action (A), response and evaluation (R), and education and patient teaching (E).
- It is essential for charting to be legible, clear, concise, accurate, and complete. These guidelines serve as a national standard for licensed nurses.
- The specific institution or unit will often have specific forms and charting formats; in addition, follow the general guidelines and rules for charting.
- Medical records are legal documents. The physician or institution owns the original record.
- Lawyers, courts, and patients are able to gain access to the record but only by following specified access procedures.
- The contents of a health record are confidential information protected by the law and the Patient Care Partnership.
- The nursing Kardex or Rand is a card-filing system used by nurses to condense all the orders and other care information needed quickly for each patient. It is kept at the nursing station for quick reference and is updated frequently.
- Computerized information systems provide information about a patient in an organized and easily accessible fashion.

- Clinical pathways allow staff from all disciplines to develop integrated care plans for a projected length of stay for patients of a specific case type.
- Many agencies use military time. This system uses four-digit numbers to indicate morning, afternoon, and evening times.
- A 24-hour record-keeping system helps eliminate unnecessary record-keeping forms.
- The acuity level determined by analyzing what nursing care is necessary allows patients to be rated in comparison to one another. Staffing patterns can then be determined by examining the acuity levels for the patients on a particular nursing unit.
- Nursing access to computer terminals and care documentation systems has the potential to save time and energy needed for patient care services. These systems are expensive but are a great benefit to the nurses able to use them.
- Fax machines are used to send written documents over telephone lines to quickly transmit data between hospitals and other facilities, such as doctors' offices.

Additional Learning Resources

Go to your Companion CD for an audio glossary, animations, video clips, and more.

evolve Be sure to visit the Evolve site at http://evolve.elsevier.com/Christensen/foundations/ for additional online resources.

Review Questions for the NCLEX® Examination

1. When documenting care and observations in a patient record:
   1. use of approved medical terms and abbreviations is permitted.
   2. use of any locally used abbreviations is permitted.
   3. to prevent errors, no abbreviations are permitted to be used.
   4. a nurse does not worry about the use of abbreviations.

2. Patient health care records are:
   1. confidential information and cannot be taken to court.
   2. owned by the patient, who has a right to see the data.
   3. not used by anyone else but the direct care providers.
   4. concise, legal records of all care given and responses.

3. When the POMR method is used for documentation:
   1. the problem list has only active and resolved problems.
   2. only the physician charts on the progress notes.
   3. the charting format is SOAPE or SOAPIER.
   4. focus or the DARE charting format is never used.

4. The nurse is using the SOAPE method to chart. In this method the *S* stands for:
   1. signs and symptoms that the nurse assesses.
   2. subjective information the patient states or feels.
   3. subjective information the nurse measures.
   4. solutions to problems the nurse identifies.

5. When charting, the nurse should:
   1. chart as soon and as often as necessary.
   2. remember to chart only basic care information.
   3. leave blank lines for others if asked.
   4. chart facts using judgmental terms if needed.

6. Understanding that health care personnel must respect the confidentiality of patients' records, the nurse:
   1. has an ethical prerogative to look at a friend's chart to see the diagnosis.
   2. knows that only the Patient's Bill of Rights advocates confidentiality.
   3. reads charts only for a professional reason.
   4. shares information from a chart to protect a friend.

7. The use of computers in the hospital by nurses:
   1. can save on charting time once nurses are comfortable using computers.
   2. is not considered important or efficient.
   3. can be done only on a shared terminal at the desk.
   4. lacks security measures to protect confidentiality.

8. When completing an incident report, the nurse is aware that it is necessary to:
   1. document in the chart that the incident report has been filed.
   2. have all parties involved sign the report.
   3. ask the supervising nurse to complete the incident report.
   4. document facts regarding the incident.

9. Which statement is correct about formats for documentation?
   1. Focus charting is a goal-oriented system.
   2. Clinical pathways are the most commonly used format now.
   3. Charting by exception documents those conditions, interventions, or outcomes outside the norm.
   4. Standardized care plans are not cost effective.

10. Which statement is a recommended guideline for charting?
    1. Pull a chart by the room number on the label.
    2. Include content that suggests a risk situation.
    3. Skip lines between charting entries.
    4. Have the patient's name and identification number on every sheet.

11. The 24-hour patient care record-keeping system is useful in:
    1. shortening the patient's hospital stay.
    2. keeping a more detailed account.
    3. ensuring the patient's privacy.
    4. consolidating the nursing record.

12. Acuity charting requires:
    1. staff to document their interventions.
    2. detailed assessment information.
    3. a patient's successful recovery from surgery.
    4. a discharge summary.

13. Which statement is a safe principle of computerized charting?
    1. A computer terminal may be left unattended during lunchtime.
    2. Each unit or department has its own password.
    3. There is no room for mistakes in computerized charting.
    4. Do not leave patient information displayed on the monitor.

14. Which accreditation agency specifies guidelines for documentation?
    1. The Joint Commission (TJC).
    2. American Nurses Association.
    3. National League of Nursing.
    4. American Academy of Colleges of Nursing.

15. The primary purpose of Title II of the Health Insurance Portability and Accountability Act (HIPAA) is to:
    1. ensure proper documentation in patient's medical records.
    2. maintain privacy and confidentiality of patient's health information.
    3. regulate the availability and range of group insurance plans.
    4. limit restrictions on insurance coverage based on preexisting conditions.

16. Which statement is correct about abbreviations?
    1. Every facility should have an approved abbreviations list.
    2. Creating abbreviations saves time for the reader.
    3. Abbreviating drug names and dosages helps reduce medication errors.
    4. Whiting out questionable abbreviations could make a jury think you're hiding something.

17. When comparing documentation for acute care in hospitals with documentation for long-term care, major differences are related to:
    1. the goal of the highest quality care at the lowest cost.
    2. using a multidisciplinary approach for assessment and planning.
    3. the prospective payment system determining the standards for reimbursement.
    4. increasing numbers of older adults and disabled people in the United States requiring long-term care.

18. The nurse documents in the patient record, "0830 patient appears to be in severe pain and refuses to ambulate. Blood pressure and pulse are elevated, physician notified, and analgesic administered as ordered with adequate relief. J. Doe RN." The most significant statement about the documentation would be that it is:
    1. inadequate because the pain is not described on a scale of 1 to 10.
    2. good because it shows immediate responsiveness to the problem.
    3. acceptable because it includes assessment, intervention, and evaluation.
    4. unacceptable because it is vague subjective data without supportive data.

19. The best description of narrative documentation is that it:
    1. organizes data by problem or diagnosis.
    2. describes occurrences in chronological order.
    3. includes objective data, subjective data, assessment, and plan.
    4. originated from the medical model.

20. In most states, patients can gain access to their medical records by:
    1. asking the nursing staff to allow them to view each entry in the record.
    2. submitting a written request to the facility to view the record.
    3. requesting the state board of health to allow access to the record.
    4. asking the staff for copies of their records.

21. Standards and policies regarding documentation in long-term care facilities is guided by:
    1. MDS.
    2. CBE.
    3. DARE.
    4. POMR.

22. The government reimburses agencies for health care costs incurred by Medicare and Medicaid recipients based on:
    1. thorough documentation by the nurse.
    2. submission of appropriate physician progress notes.
    3. clinical (critical) pathways.
    4. diagnosis-related groups.

chapter

8 Cultural and Ethnic Considerations

evolve

http://evolve.elsevier.com/Christensen/foundationsadult

Elaine Oden Kockrow and Relda T. Kelly

Objectives

1. Identify the importance of transcultural nursing.
2. Describe ways that culture affects the individual.
3. Explain how personal cultural beliefs and practices affect nurse-patient and nurse-nurse relationships.
4. Identify and discuss cultural variables that potentially influence health behaviors.
5. Explain how the nurse is able to use cultural data to help develop therapeutic relationships with the patient.
6. Discuss the use of the nursing process when caring for culturally diverse patients.
7. Discuss culturally sensitive communication with the older adult.

Key Terms

biomedical health belief system (p. 171)
cultural competence (KŬL-chŭr-ăl KŎM-pĕ-tĕns, p. 159)
culture (p. 158)
ethnicity (ĕth-NĬS-ĭ-tē, p. 161)
ethnic stereotype (p. 159)
ethnocentrism (ĕth-nō-SĔN-trĭz-ŭm, p. 159)
folk health belief system (p. 171)
holistic health belief system (p. 171)
mores (MŎR-āz, p. 159)
race (p. 161)
society (p. 158)
stereotype (STĔR-ē-ō-tīp, p. 159)
subculture (p. 158)
transcultural nursing (p. 160)

The United States has been described as a "melting pot" of people from many different countries. This description implies that people are so completely blended together that everyone shares the same values, beliefs, health practices, communication styles, and religion. A better description is to say our country is like a pot of vegetable soup—many different, but distinct, pieces are combined to form a rich assortment. This assortment makes up our **society** (a nation, community, or broad group of people who establish particular aims, beliefs, or standards of living and conduct). What's more, the "soup recipe" is no longer what is was, and as a result our societal "flavor" is changing. At the beginning of the twentieth century, the majority of immigrants to this country were of European ancestry. Today, according to the 2000 U.S. Census, 24.9% of the population is of African, Asian, Hispanic, American Indian, or some other ancestry (U.S. Census Bureau, 2000). It is estimated that the U.S. Muslim population numbers about 7 million and is growing steadily (e-Ethics, Park Ridge Center). Although these numbers do not specifically identify all cultural groups, they give us an idea of the diversity of the population.

CULTURE DEFINED

Culture is a set of learned values, beliefs, customs, and practices that are shared by a group and are passed from one generation to another. Because of the influx of diverse cultures, the United States is rapidly becoming multicultural and multilingual. Many immigrants have come from areas of the world devastated by wars, natural disasters, famine, and poverty. They have had little preparation or time to learn English or American culture before arriving. Many of these immigrant populations have formed subcultures in United States society.

There are often separate subcultures within a given group. A **subculture** shares many characteristics with the primary culture, but has characteristic patterns of behavior and ideals that distinguish it from the rest of a cultural group. Even among Americans who have lived here for several generations, these subcultures exist. For example, a person who grew up in the mountains of Appalachia will have very different cultural practices than a person from New York City. Understanding these variables and accepting each person as an individual is the first step in giving holistic care to patients.

Even though cultures often differ considerably from one another, they share certain basic characteristics. Box 8-1 identifies four common characteristics of all cultures.

All members of a culture will not exhibit the same behaviors. These variations within a cultural group occur because of individual differences. Examples of these differences are as follows:

- Age
- Religion
- Dialect or language spoken

Box 8-1 Common Characteristics of Cultures

- Culture is learned, beginning at birth, through language and socialization. Behaviors, values, attitudes, and beliefs are learned within the cultural family system.
- Culture is dynamic and ever-changing, but it remains stable. Language, traditions, and norms of customs may act as stabilizers for a culture.
- All members of the same cultural group share the patterns that are present in every culture. These include communication, means of economic and physical survival, transportation systems, family systems, social customs and mores, and religious systems. (**Mores** are accepted traditional customs, moral attitudes, or manners of a particular social group.)
- Culture is an adaptation to specific factors or conditions in a specific location, such as the availability of natural resources. When people are removed from that location, their customs continue even though they are no longer called for in the new setting.

- Gender identity and roles
- Socioeconomic background
- Geographic location of country of origin or current residence
- Amount and type of interaction between younger and older generations
- Degree to which values in current country are adopted

Because culture influences each person in various ways, you are ill advised to stereotype members of any cultural group. A **stereotype** is a generalized expectation about forms of behavior, an individual, or a group. An **ethnic stereotype** is a fixed concept of how all members of an ethnic group act or think. Stereotypes sometimes do and sometimes do not have any relationship to reality.

CULTURAL COMPETENCE AND TRANSCULTURAL NURSING

Most people look at the world from their own cultural viewpoint. They often believe that the beliefs and practices of their particular culture are best. This is called **ethnocentrism.** It is crucial for you to learn to value the beliefs of others and realize that practices of other cultures can be valuable in health care.

To give care to patients from many different cultures, you will be called on to develop **cultural competence.** This means that you are aware of your own cultural beliefs and practices and how they relate to those of others, which will be different. One way to identify these beliefs and practices is to do a self-assessment. This self-assessment is important. Your personal beliefs and practices influence, and sometimes put some limitations on, your ability to care for those from other cultures. Understanding your personal beliefs gives you an ability to respond to those from different cultures with openness, understanding, and acceptance of cultural differences between you.

You also need to accept that it is not possible to act the same with all patients and still give effective, individualized, holistic care. Sometimes nurses are so concerned about treating everyone the same that they ignore cultural differences. Rather than ignore the differences, think about including questions about cultural practices when using the nursing process. This information is critical and is important to include when you are developing a plan of care to meet patient needs. Box 8-2 gives some guidelines for cultural

Box 8-2 Cultural Assessment for Health Care

NURSING DATA COLLECTION (OBTAINED THROUGH INTERVIEW OR OBSERVATION)

- What language is used? If the patient does not commonly use English, how well does the patient understand English? Who does the patient depend on to translate information?
- What cultural practices have the potential to interfere with receiving health care?
  —Personal space practices
  —Modesty and privacy concerns
  —Difficulty with care being performed by members of the opposite sex
  —Differences in health care beliefs
  —Use of folk medicines or treatments
- What dietary practices have the potential to interfere with treatment for this illness?

INTERVIEW QUESTIONS

- Who will make decisions about your treatment?
  —Who is the person in your family that needs to be involved with health care decisions?
  —Are there members of your community who will be asked to help with making decisions about your care?
- Can you describe what is wrong?
- What do you think has caused your problem (illness, condition)?
- Why do you think this has happened at this time?
  —Why did it happen to you?
  —Why did it affect (body part)?
- How long have you had this problem?
  —Why did you come for help now?
- What do you think will help to clear up your problem?
- Who else do you think can help you?
  —Have you gone to this person for help?
  —What did the person do?
  —Did this treatment help?
- What results do you hope to get from your care?
- How will your illness affect your family?

Adapted from Potter, P.A., & Perry, A.G. (2009). *Fundamentals of nursing* (7th ed.). St. Louis: Mosby.

Evidence-Based Practice | **Cultural Beliefs and Rituals Surrounding Death**

Evidence Summary

Although culture and religion are important to people who are dying, as well as to their families, practices surrounding the death of a loved one vary among cultures and religions. Focus groups were used in this research study to find similarities and differences among cultural and religious beliefs, ceremonies, and rituals that surround death. Many cultures and religions use their beliefs to allow them to pray, talk, and remember their loved one. Rituals often accompany ceremonies and are used to delay death, ward off evil, ensure that the dying person is remembered, and help the family cope with the death. Respect for dying family members and protection of their souls were important for all of the participants in the study. Many practices that surround death are influenced by religion and culture. Those who are Hispanic and Latino often have rituals that are heavily influenced by Catholicism. African American and Caribbean participants identified the importance of faith, hope, and prayer, and similarities were found between Hindu and Buddhist beliefs about funeral arrangements, afterlife, family customs and Karma.

Application to Nursing Practice

- Be aware of religious and cultural preferences when helping patients and families prepare for death.
- Ask families about the rituals and ceremonies they use to help them cope with the death of a loved one.
- Allow patients and families the ability to participate in planning which rituals will be done at the patient's bedside.
- Be sensitive to cultural perceptions regarding organ donation, viewing the body, and preparing for burial.

Reference

Lobar SL and others: Cross-cultural beliefs, ceremonies, and rituals surrounding death of a loved one, *Pediatr Nurs* 32(1):44, 2006.

From Potter, P.A. & Perry, A.G. (2009). *Fundamentals of nursing: concepts, process, and practice.* (7th ed.). St. Louis: Mosby.

information that can be gathered when assessing the patient.

Because of the many variations in cultural and subcultural practices, it is a challenge to provide culturally appropriate nursing care in the twenty-first century. Understanding these variables and integrating your understanding into all aspects of nursing care is what we term **transcultural nursing.** Do your best to achieve a high level of transcultural nursing in day-to-day practices.

It is important to understand that people from different cultures have a variety of practices related to health care, treatment methods, and responses to illness and death (see the Evidence-Based Practice box). In many cases, these differences extend to practices related to childbirth and the ways people of different age-groups are cared for (Life Span Considerations for Older Adults box). In addition, cultural beliefs frequently affect diet and nutrition. Remember to assess areas that are potentially under the influence of cultural factors.

In addition to caring for people from various cultures, you will also find that many other health care providers come from different ethnic, cultural, and religious backgrounds than you or your patients. Some of these nurses have received their education in foreign countries and have moved to the United States for better opportunities. Others were born in this country but are part of a different cultural or racial group than you or other colleagues.

Learning about cultural differences that exist among you and your co-workers will improve your working relationships. Discuss these cultural practices with your co-workers. In much the same way this kind of openness will help you care for your patients, it will help you understand and accept differences among you and your colleagues. If conflicts arise, try to discuss and understand each other and your diverse cultural expectations. Resolving these conflicts is essential to providing good care to patients.

Life Span Considerations

Older Adults

Cultural Background

- Cultural background has an impact on family dynamics and plays an important role in determining the role and the status of the older person.
- Older adults form a unique cultural group based on shared historical experiences. Often there are fewer differences between two older individuals of diverse cultural backgrounds than between two people of the same culture but from different age-groups because of shifts in value systems that occurred over time.
- Some older adults are less tolerant of other cultures as a result of influences or experiences early in their lives. This raises the possibility of misunderstandings and distrust when the caregiver is of a cultural group different than the older person.
- Older people experiencing disturbed cognitive function resulting from Alzheimer's disease or other conditions sometimes speak without regard for the cultural sensitivity of others and thus make hurtful comments to caregivers and other people.
- Many older adults value home remedies and cultural practices regarding health care and will sometimes resist the attempts of caregivers to change even their harmful practices.
- Many older people find comfort in following religious practices that perhaps are not currently used by their religion. If these practices are not harmful, it is best to respect the older person's wishes.

RACE AND ETHNICITY

There are various reasons why a given individual demonstrates a given cultural practice. Perhaps the person is from a foreign country or a region of the

Table 8-1 Changes in Racially Designated and Hispanic Populations, 1990–2000

	1990		2000		
RACE AND HISPANIC OR LATINO	NUMBER	PERCENT OF TOTAL POPULATION	NUMBER	PERCENT OF TOTAL POPULATION	PERCENT CHANGE
Total population	248,709,873	100.0%	281,421,906	100.0%	+1.13%
White	199,686,070	80.3%	211,460,626	75.1%	−5.2%
Black or African American	29,986,060	12.1%	34,658,190	12.3%	+0.2%
American Indian or Alaska Native	1,959,234	0.8%	2,475,956	0.9%	+0.1%
Asian or Pacific Islander	7,273,662	2.9%	10,641,833	3.7%	+0.8%
Some other race	9,804,847	3.9%	15,359,073	5.5%	+1.6%
Two or more races	NA	NA	6,826,228	2.4%	NA
Hispanic or Latino (of any race)	22,354,059	9.0%	35,305,818	12.5%	+3.5%

From U.S. Bureau of the Census. (1990). Table DP-1: *General population and housing characteristics;* (2000). Table P3: *Race*, and Table P11: *Hispanic or Latino (total population)*. Available at http://factfinder.census.gov.

United States where that practice is common. Perhaps the person's practice is related to his or her **race** (a group of people who share biologic physical characteristics) and hereditary factors. Going beyond mere racial makeup, **ethnicity** refers to a group of people who share a common social and cultural heritage based on shared traditions, national origin, and physical and biologic characteristics. They often share social practices such as language, religion, dress, music, and food. Factors related to culture, race, and ethnicity often overlap, and many people combine a variety of practices related to several of these factors. It is important to understand that not everyone in a cultural, racial, or ethnic group will have identical practices. This is why it is important to treat each person in an individual, holistic manner.

ETHNIC AND RACIAL GROUPS IN THE UNITED STATES

As stated, the United States is home to people from many cultures. In addition, most people belong to one or more subcultures. Keep this overlap in mind, and do not make assumptions about a patient's beliefs or practices based on the person's name, skin color, or language.

We commonly make assumptions about the predominant cultures and subcultures in our country based on our own family or community. It is important to keep a larger view of our society to have a better understanding of our country. The 2000 census asked individuals to choose their racial origin from one of six categories: white, black or African-American, American Indian or Alaska Native, Asian, Native Hawaiian or other Pacific Islander, and other. Another category was provided indicating an origin in two or more races. In addition, individuals were asked to choose between two other categories: Hispanic or Latino and not Hispanic or Latino (U.S. Census Bureau, Census 2000).

Note the changes between the 1990 and the 2000 census results in these areas (Table 8-1). Significantly, the white population has decreased, whereas increases have occurred in almost all other racial groups. The largest increase has occurred in the Hispanic population, which rose from 9% to 12.5% of the population between 1990 and 2000. Predictions for the future indicate that this trend will continue and that the minority cultures will, in combination, make up a majority of the U.S. population by the middle of this century (U.S. Census Bureau, Census 2000).

One significant aspect of this diversity is the language we use to communicate. Many new immigrants from these diverse cultures do not speak English at all or have a limited grasp of the language. Often the younger members of the family are the ones who help the adults communicate with others outside of the cultural community. Adults will frequently bring a young child along as a translator when shopping or seeking health care.

CULTURALLY RELATED ASSESSMENTS

To care for patients from a different culture, it is important to be able to find out what the person believes. It is not reasonable to expect the patient to accept your care and health teaching if the patient does not believe that the practices will help him or her to recover (Figure 8-1).

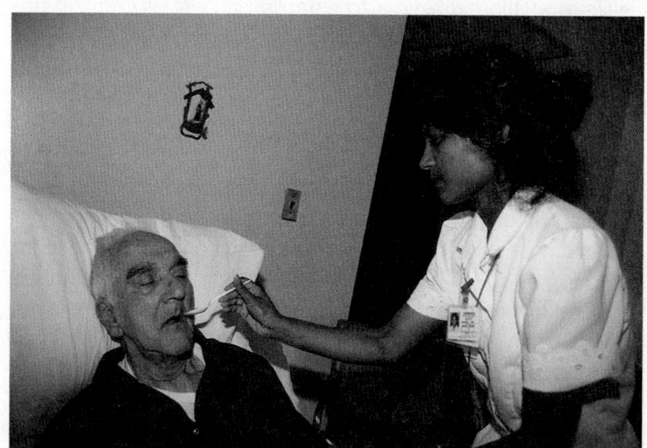

FIGURE 8-1 The nurse reaches past racial and cultural differences to assist the patient.

Later in this chapter, you will read brief examples of specific beliefs and practices of some cultures. It is hoped that these will be helpful when assessing your patients. However, remember that it is important to avoid stereotyping an individual according to common cultural practices. Perhaps the person accepts all of the practices within a culture or subculture, but perhaps he or she does not.

When you assess a patient, there are several areas to explore: communication, space, time, social organization, religious beliefs, health practices, and biologic variations.

COMMUNICATION

The most apparent communication variation is the language spoken. It is important to determine whether you and the patient can understand each other. For example, if you speak only English, and the patient speaks only Spanish, it will be next to impossible to explain even basic information. Remember that when a patient does not understand what you are saying, he or she will sometimes say yes or nod the head nonetheless, giving the mistaken impression of agreeing with you. Many people do this to avoid embarrassment or to be polite. Do not automatically assume the patient or his or her family understands.

Sometimes, the patient understands some English or you will speak some of the patient's language. If the patient has a poor grasp of English, it is possible that he or she will tire quickly when trying to understand what is being said. It is important to keep your questions or directions brief and simple. It is better to go back later and provide more information than to give long explanations. Sometimes, the patient's ability to read written English will be better than his or her speaking ability. In such cases, the patient will benefit from written explanations accompanied by pictures when possible.

One approach is to try to find an interpreter. Many health care facilities have employees on call to translate when there is a language barrier. Other times, family members are able to translate. Always remember that it is important that the patient understands essential information such as why care is being given and why medications are ordered. It is your responsibility to make every effort to provide this information to the patient. Using effective communication techniques will be beneficial as you care for patients from different cultures than your own (Box 8-3).

Even among English-speaking people, different cultural groups assign different meanings to the same words. For example, a person from the United Kingdom will probably say he is going to take the "lift." An American is not necessarily going to understand that he is referring to an elevator ride. Within the United States, the variety of regional accents further complicates the communication picture. People from different areas of the country (for example, people from the North and the South) often struggle to understand each other owing to the different accents or regional expressions they use. Some cultural or regional groups speak very rapidly, and this adds to the difficulty of understanding.

Other cultural patterns also play a role in communication. For example, in some cultural groups it is common for many family members to accompany a person to the health care setting. This tends to make communication difficult between nurse and patient, especially if large groups of family members are present. They sometimes all try to assist by answering at once. Or perhaps, when in the presence of strangers a person from another group only answers direct questions and thus appears rude or uncommunicative. Unfortunately, the appearance of rudeness is a common byproduct of a cross-cultural mismatch in communication. Sometimes, out of the mistaken belief that this

Box 8-3 Strategies for Communication with Patients from Different Cultures

- Take a little extra time to establish a level of comfort between you and the patient.
- Ask questions in an unhurried manner. Rephrase a question and ask it again if the answer seems inconsistent with other information the patient has provided.
- Observe the cultural differences in communication, and honor those differences. Use eye contact, touch, and seating arrangements that are comfortable for the patient.
- Ask patients about the meaning health and illness have for them, and their understanding of treatments and planned care. Investigate how the illness is likely to affect their life, relationships, and self-concept. Find out what patients consider to be the cause of their illness. Ask how patients prefer to manage their illness.
- To establish a therapeutic relationship, listen to the patient's perception of his or her needs, and respect the patient's perspective.
- Listen actively and attentively; try not to anticipate the patient's response.
- Talk to patients in an unhurried manner that considers social and cultural amenities.
- Give patients time to answer.
- Use validation techniques to verify that the patient understands. Remember that smiles and head nodding may indicate that the patient is trying to please you, not necessarily that you are understood.
- Sexual concerns may be difficult for patients to discuss. Having a nurse of the same sex may facilitate communication.
- Use alternative methods of communication, such as a foreign language phrase book, an interpreter, gestures, or pictures, for patients who do not speak English.
- Learn key phrases in languages that are commonly spoken in your community.

From Harkreader, H., Hogan, M.A., Thobaben, M. (2007). *Fundamentals of nursing: Caring and clinical judgment* (3rd ed.). Philadelphia: Saunders.

will help the hearer understand better, a person will speak more loudly to emphasize a point, In fact, it often has the opposite effect of the one desired: Members of some cultures will interpret the raised voice as rudeness or aggression and will shut out the sound altogether.

Consider, in contrast, the use of silence. Silence indicates many things to many cultures: a lack of understanding, stubbornness, apprehension, or discomfort; or agreement, disagreement, respect, or disdain. Among American Indian, Chinese, and Japanese cultures, silence is sometimes used to allow the listener to consider what the speaker has said before continuing. Members of other cultures, such as Russians, the French, and the Spanish, tend to become silent to indicate consensus between parties. In Asian cultures, people often use silence as a sign of respect, especially to elders (Cultural Considerations box). Mexicans will perhaps use silence when they disagree with a person of authority. In other cultures, the presence of silence creates discomfort, and people will make every attempt to fill gaps in conversation.

Nonverbal communication is usually expressed through body language. Some groups are more comfortable than others with touching or maintaining eye contact. Touch is particularly culturally related. In the United States, many people consider even casual touching inappropriate except among intimates. Recent immigrants from England and Germany are even less likely to touch each other in public, or allow casual touching by strangers. Spanish, French, Italian, Jewish, and South American individuals are likely to be much more comfortable about touching each other and being touched.

Cultural Considerations

Culturally Sensitive Communication

- Ask older adults how they like to be addressed. If in doubt, address them formally.
- Determine the patient's preferences for touch. For example, in the United States, Americans often greet each other with a firm handshake. However, many Native Americans see this as a sign of aggression, and touch outside the marriage is sometimes forbidden in older adults from the Middle East.
- Investigate the patient's preferences for silence. Generally, Eastern cultures value silence, whereas Western cultures are uncomfortable with silence.
- Be aware of the patient's beliefs about eye contact during conversation. Direct eye contact in European American cultures is a sign of honesty and truthfulness. However, eye contact with other groups, such as older Native Americans, is not allowed. Older Asian adults sometimes avoid eye contact with authority figures because this is considered disrespectful, and direct eye contact between the sexes in Middle Eastern cultures is sometimes forbidden except between spouses.

From Potter, P.A., & Perry, A.G. (2009). *Fundamentals of nursing* (7th ed.). St. Louis: Mosby. Data from Meiner, S.E., & Lueckenotte, A.G. (2006). *Gerontologic nursing* (3rd ed.). St. Louis: Mosby.

Eye contact also has significant cultural interpretations. Many people in the United States regard maintaining eye contact as an indication of openness, interest in others, attentiveness, and honesty. Lack of eye contact is thus interpreted as a sign of shyness, humility, guilt, embarrassment, rudeness, thoughtlessness, or dishonesty. Other cultures have various other reasons for not maintaining eye contact. Some Asian cultures and American Indians relate eye contact to impoliteness or an invasion of privacy. Certain East Indian cultures avoid eye contact with people of lower or higher socioeconomic classes. Among some Appalachian people, maintaining eye contact indicates hostility or aggressiveness.

Assessing the communication variables of a patient from another culture is important. Once you have made an assessment of cultural factors, you then have to respond appropriately. Make every effort to communicate with others at their personal level of comfort in order to establish good rapport. For example, if the patient is from a culture that avoids eye contact, try to look away when talking with the patient. If touch is unacceptable among casual acquaintances, avoid patting the shoulder or touching a hand when talking with the patient. Be sensitive to any difficulty a patient is having with the more intimate touching that inevitably accompanies many nursing interventions.

When you violate cultural beliefs and practices, it will likely interfere with establishing a therapeutic relationship with the patient and the patient's family. Do not expect to completely adjust your personal cultural practices, but make an effort to understand and accept the differences among practices in various cultures. It is important not to judge the patient's behavior according to your own personal practices.

SPACE

Cultural interpretation of space varies and is an important element of assessment. Cultures assign different comfort areas to personal space. Generally, in Western cultures, people in a casual or public setting are most comfortable when they can maintain 3 to 6 feet between them during a conversation (Giger & Davidhizar, 2008). Closer contact is reserved for more intimate relationships. Members of some cultures are accustomed to more close contact and sometimes inadvertently invade the space of a person from a Western culture. Occasionally the need for personal space also manifests itself in a desire to use a certain space. For example, perhaps a resident in a nursing home always wishes to sit in a particular chair or in a specific part of the room. Another resident chooses to sit at the same table for each meal. If someone changes any of these arrangements, either of these residents will possibly become upset.

Body movements are often culturally related. In the United States, certain gestures are generally understood by most longtime citizens. However, some commonly used gestures have the potential to offend someone from another culture. For example, forming a circle with the thumb and forefinger means "A-OK" in the United States. To someone from Brazil, this is an obscene gesture. Italian or Jewish people typically use more body movements to illustrate or emphasize what they are communicating than individuals from Asian cultures. As noted earlier, touch is used more commonly in some cultures than others.

TIME

The measurement of time and the rhythms of people's activities and interactions often have different meanings in various cultures. These different meanings have the potential to create some problems when you are caring for patients from other cultures. Our nursing practice emphasizes providing medications and treatments on a rigid schedule. The United States and many Northern European cultures generally give a high priority to being on time for appointments, and people typically expect everyone to follow this pattern. Japanese Americans also are generally prompt and adhere to fixed schedules, especially when meeting with a person they regard highly. However, people in many cultures feel that other concerns are more important. In Eastern cultures, including Chinese, East Indian Hindu, Filipino, and Korean, schedules and time are much more flexible concepts. Some Asians will spend a lot of time getting to know someone and will view abrupt endings to a conversation as rude. Mexican Americans may be late for an appointment because they focus more on a current activity and are less concerned about a previously planned meeting. According to Giger and Davidhizar (2008) this concept, known as "elasticity," implies that it is possible to recover future activities but not present ones. Perhaps you will find yourself getting angry when a patient is late for an appointment, fails to come at all, or does not follow therapeutic schedules, if you do not understand these cultural differences.

Perception of time or time orientation also varies among cultures. Many people in the United States tend to be future oriented. Present actions are taken based on a future outcome. An example is a person who takes medication to treat hypertension to prevent illness. Among members of other cultures, notably black, Hispanic, and American Indian, individuals tend to be more present oriented. Sometimes, like people described earlier who prolong a current encounter rather than rushing off to be on time for another one, a present-oriented person chooses to satisfy a current, more urgent need rather than prepare for a less immediate one that is some time away. A pregnant woman, for instance, will miss her own doctor's appointments to take care of her family; if her older child needs a ride to school, the mother will skip the appointment and drive the child. It is often difficult to encourage a patient with this belief system to follow through on treatment for a chronic illness. Such a patient will perhaps view the cost of a medication for hypertension to prevent future problems as an optional expense. Paying the rent or buying food for the family is a current need that takes precedence.

Timeliness varies among nursing professionals as well. Conflicts often arise when a colleague is always late for work. It is important to discuss the reasons for this, rather than to assume the person does not care about the job. If the habit is due to a cultural belief, the staff members involved need to develop a strategy to solve the problem accordingly.

SOCIAL ORGANIZATION

Cultural behavior is socially acquired, not genetically inherited. How we react to those who are members of other cultures reflects an internalized response that is part of our culture. Often, we are not aware of the strong impact these patterns of cultural behavior have each day in our lives. We may behave in a hostile manner toward a person of a particular ethnic group or a person with a different skin color merely because of an inner, culture-related belief. It is important to recognize these biases and to deal with them rationally. Understanding other cultures will help to overcome prejudices that have nothing to do with an individual. Each of us needs to accept the idea that our particular culture is not superior.

Self-concept is also influenced by culture and cultural identity. Individuals view themselves as part of a particular social group. They describe themselves in terms such as "African American" or "black," "Hispanic," "German American," "Irish Catholic," or "Texan." Clearly, these descriptions vary greatly. What is important is to understand how the person sees herself or himself. A good cultural assessment will take this self-description into account.

The varying social structures within a culture also have an impact on how individuals and families function. Some cultures are patriarchal, and the men (often the oldest) make most of the decisions. In a culture that is matriarchal, the women probably make the decisions about health care, provide the care, and discipline the children. It is important in a health care setting to determine with what sort of structure you are dealing. For example, a family in a patriarchal society will sometimes delay any decision making regarding health care for one of the family members until the oldest man in the family is consulted. Another family, in a matriarchal society, will expect the women to give care to a family member in the hospital.

The description of family may differ among cultures. See Box 9-2 for a description of some common family structures. Some of these structures are based on biologic relationships. Others are based on meeting basic needs for family by forming a group among unrelated individuals. Knowing the family structure will help you to better understand the patient. A common mistake is to assume that every family is a traditional nuclear family. In fact, this family structure is becoming increasingly rare. It is more important to know who the patient depends on for comfort and decision making and how the patient describes the family.

RELIGIOUS BELIEFS AND HEALTH CARE

In addition to families, other groups display cultural behaviors. Religious beliefs are frequently entwined with cultural beliefs. Some cultures expect all members to adhere to a particular religion. In these societies, religious and cultural beliefs are difficult to separate. In the United States, there are wide variations in religious practices (Box 8-4). In addition, as people from varying cultures intermarry, religious practices also become more varied.

Data for religious preferences are not collected by the U.S. Bureau of the Census, so there is no way of accurately determining the numbers of followers of the various religions in the United States. However, nursing care clearly is affected by patients' religious beliefs and practices, and it is important for you to be aware of and open to the wide range of such beliefs to ensure that you give care that is sensitive to the needs of individual patients.

Assessing family and social organization becomes increasingly more complicated as our society brings together more and more diverse cultures. It is not unusual for a family to be bicultural or biracial or to follow two different faith practices. Be constantly on guard against making assumptions about patients based on appearance, language, ethnic origin, names, or religious practices. Only by assessing the individual and her or his family on their own terms will you begin to understand the person.

Text continued on p. 170.

Box 8-4 Religious Beliefs and Practices Affecting Health Care in the United States

OBSERVANT JEWS (ORTHODOX JUDAISM AND SOME CONSERVATIVE GROUPS)

Birth: For observant Jews, babies are named by the father. Male children are named 8 days after birth, when ritual circumcision is done. A mohel performs the circumcision. Circumcision is often postponed if the infant is in poor health. Female babies are usually named during the reading of the holy Torah. Nurses need to be sensitive to the wishes of the parents when caring for babies who have not yet been named.

Care of women: A woman is considered to be in a ritual state of impurity whenever blood is coming from her uterus, such as during menstrual periods and after the birth of a child. During this time, her husband will not have physical contact with her. When this time is completed, she will bathe herself in a pool called a mikvah. Nurses need to be aware of this practice and be sensitive to the husband and wife because the husband will not touch his wife. He cannot assist her in moving in the bed, so the nurse will have to do this. An Orthodox Jewish man will not touch any woman other than his wife, daughters, and mother. Home health care workers need to be aware of these practices.

Dietary rules: (1) Kosher dietary laws include the following: no mixing of milk and meat at a meal; no consumption of food or any derivative thereof from animals not slaughtered in accordance with Jewish law; use of separate cooking utensils for meat and milk products; if for medical reasons a patient requires milk and meat products for a meal, the dairy foods should be served first, followed later by the meat. (2) During Yom Kippur (Day of Atonement), a 24-hour fast is required, but exceptions are made for those who cannot fast because of medical reasons or age. (3) During Passover, no leavened products are eaten. (4) Observant Jewish patients often wish to say prayers over the bread and wine before meals. Time and a quiet environment should be provided for this.

Sabbath: Observed from sunset Friday until sunset Saturday. Orthodox law prohibits riding in a car, smoking, turning lights on and off, handling money, and using television and telephone. Nurses need to be aware of this when caring for observant Jews at home and in the hospital. Have medical or surgical treatments postponed if possible.

Death: Judaism defines death as occurring when respiration and circulation are irreversibly stopped and no movement is apparent. (1) Euthanasia is strictly forbidden by Orthodox Jews, who advocate the strict use of life-support measures. (2) Before death, Jewish faith indicates that visiting of the person by family and friends is a religious duty. The Torah and Psalms are often read and prayers recited. A witness needs to be present when a person prays for health so that if death occurs God will protect the family and the spirit will be committed to God. Extraneous talking and conversation about death are not encouraged unless initiated by the patient or visitors. In Judaism, the belief is that people should have someone with them when the soul leaves the body; so allow family and friends to stay with patients. After death, the body is not to be left alone until burial, usually within 24 hours. (3) When death occurs, the body is to remain untouched for 8 to 30 minutes. Medical personnel are not to touch or wash the body; only an Orthodox person or the Jewish Burial Society is permitted to care for the body. Handling of a corpse on the Sabbath is forbidden to Jewish persons. If need be, the nursing staff is permitted to provide routine care of the body, wearing gloves. Water receptacles in the room have to be emptied, and the family often requests that mirrors be covered to symbolize that a death has occurred. (4) Orthodox Jews and some Conservative Jews do not approve of autopsies. If an autopsy is necessary, all body parts are required to remain with the body. (5) For Orthodox Jews, the body is required to be buried within 24 hours. No flowers are permitted. A fetus is required to be buried. (6) A 7-day mourning period is required by the immediate family. They stay at home except for Sabbath worship. (7) Make sure that organs or other body parts such as amputated limbs are made available for burial for Orthodox Jews, because they believe that all of the body must be returned to the earth.

Birth control and abortion: Artificial methods of birth control are not encouraged. Vasectomy is not allowed. Abortion is permitted only to save the mother's life.

Organ transplant: Donor organ transplants generally are not permitted by Orthodox Jews but with rabbinical consent are sometimes allowed.

Modified from Carson, V.B. (1989). *Spiritual dimensions of nursing practice*. Philadelphia: Saunders.

Continued

Box 8-4 Religious Beliefs and Practices Affecting Health Care in the United States—cont'd

OBSERVANT JEWS (ORTHODOX JUDAISM AND SOME CONSERVATIVE GROUPS)—cont'd

Shaving: The beard is regarded as a mark of piety among observant Jews. For very Orthodox Jews, shaving is never done with a razor but with scissors or an electric razor, because no blade is to contact the skin.

Head covering: Orthodox men wear skullcaps at all times, and women cover their hair after marriage. Some Orthodox women wear wigs as a mark of piety. Conservative Jews cover their heads only during acts of worship and prayer.

Prayer: Praying directly to God, including a prayer of confession, is required for Orthodox Jews. Provide quiet time for prayer.

REFORM JEWS

Birth: Reform Jews sometimes do and sometimes do not adhere to the practices described for Orthodox Jews. They favor ritual circumcision, but it is not imperative.

Care of women: Reform Jews do not observe the rules against touching.

Dietary rules: Reform Jews do not usually observe kosher dietary restrictions.

Sabbath: Usually worship in temples on Friday evenings. No strict rules.

Death: Advocate use of life support without heroic measures. Allow for cremation but suggest that ashes be buried in a Jewish cemetery.

Organ transplants: Donation or transplantation of organs is allowed with permission of a rabbi.

Head coverings: Variable; generally pray without wearing skullcaps (men) or head coverings (women).

ROMAN CATHOLIC

Birth: Because Roman Catholics believe that unbaptized children are cut off from heaven, infant baptism is mandatory. For newborns with a grave prognosis, stillborns, and all aborted fetuses (unless evidence of tissue necrosis and prolonged death are present), emergency baptism is required. The nurse calls a priest to perform the baptism unless the possibility exists that death will occur before the priest arrives. In that case, anyone is permitted to baptize by pouring warm water on the infant's head and saying, "I baptize you in the name of the Father, of the Son, and of the Holy Spirit." All information about the baptism is recorded on the chart, and the priest and family are notified.

Holy Eucharist: For patients and health care providers who are to receive communion, abstinence from solid food and alcohol is required for 15 minutes (if possible) before reception of the consecrated wafer. Medicine, water, and nonalcoholic drinks are permitted at any time. If a patient is in danger of death, the fasting requirement is waived because the reception of the Eucharist at this time is very important.

Anointing the sick: The priest uses oil to anoint the forehead and the hands and, if desired, the affected area. The rite is performed on any who are ill and desire it. People receiving the sacrament seek complete healing and strength to endure suffering. Before 1963, this sacrament was given only to people at time of imminent death, so the nurse must be sensitive to the meaning this has for the patient. If possible, the nurse calls a priest before the patient becomes unconscious but may also call when there is sudden death, because it is also possible to give the sacrament shortly after death. The nurse records on the care plan that this sacrament has been administered.

Dietary habits: Obligatory fasting is excused during hospitalization. However, if there are no health restrictions, some Catholics will still observe the following guidelines: (1) Anyone 14 years of age or older has to abstain from eating meat on Ash Wednesday and all Fridays during Lent. Some older Catholics still abstain from meat on all Fridays of the year. (2) In addition to abstinence from meat, people 21 to 59 years of age are required to limit themselves to one full meal and two light meals on Ash Wednesday and Good Friday. (3) Eastern Rite Catholics are stricter about fasting and fast more frequently than Western Rite Catholics, so it is important for the nurse to know if a patient is Eastern or Western.

Death: Each Roman Catholic is to participate in the anointing of the sick as well as the Eucharist and penance before death. The body is not to be shrouded until after these sacraments are performed. All body parts that retain human quality are required to be appropriately buried or cremated.

Birth control: Prohibited except for abstinence or natural family planning methods. Referral to a priest for questions about this is often of great help. Nurses teach the techniques of natural family planning if they are familiar with them; otherwise, make referral to the physician or to a support group of the Church that instructs couples in this method of birth control. Sterilization is prohibited unless there is an overriding medical reason.

Organ donation: Donation and transplantation of organs are acceptable as long as the donor is not harmed and is not deprived of life.

Religious objects: Rosary prayers are said using rosary beads. Medals bearing the images of saints, relics, statues, and scapulars are important objects that are often pinned to a hospital gown or pillow or kept at the bedside. Make sure extreme care is taken not to lose these objects, because they have special meaning to the patient.

EASTERN ORTHODOX

Birth: The child is required to be baptized within 40 days after birth. If sprinkling or immersion into water is not possible, baptism is performed by moving the baby in the air in the sign of the cross. It is obligatory for an ordained priest or a deacon to perform the ritual in this manner.

Holy Eucharist: The priest is notified if the patient desires this sacrament.

Anointing the sick: The priest conducts this in the hospital room.

Dietary habits: Fasting from meat and dairy products is required on Wednesdays and Fridays during Lent and on other holy days. Hospital patients are exempt if fasting is detrimental to health.

Special days: Christmas is celebrated on January 7 and New Year's on January 14. This is important to the care of a patient who is hospitalized on these days.

Death: Last rites are obligatory. This is handled by an ordained priest who is notified by the nurse while the patient is conscious. The Russian Orthodox Church does not encourage autopsy or organ donation. Euthanasia, even for the terminally ill, is discouraged, as is cremation.

Birth control: Birth control and abortion are not permitted.

Box 8-4 Religious Beliefs and Practices Affecting Health Care in the United States—cont'd

ASSEMBLIES OF GOD (PENTECOSTAL)

Baptism: Water baptism by complete immersion is practiced when an individual has received Jesus Christ as Savior and Lord based on Acts 2:38.

Holy Communion: Notify clergy if the patient desires to receive this sacrament.

Anointing the sick: Members believe in divine healing through prayer and the laying on of hands. Clergy is notified if patient or family desires this.

Dietary habits: Abstinence from alcohol, tobacco, and all illegal drugs is strongly encouraged.

Death: No special practices.

Other practices: Faith in God and in the health care providers is encouraged. Members pray for divine intervention in health matters. Encourage and allow patients time for prayer. Members sometimes "speak in tongues" during prayer.

BAPTIST (MORE THAN 27 DIFFERENT GROUPS IN THE UNITED STATES)

Baptism: Do not practice infant baptism.

Holy Communion: Notify clergy if the patient desires to receive this sacrament.

Dietary habits: Total abstinence from alcohol is expected.

Death: No general service is provided, but the clergy does minister through counseling, prayer, and Scripture as requested by the patient or family, and the patient is encouraged to believe in Jesus Christ as Savior and Lord.

Other practices: The Bible is held to be the word of God, so either allow quiet time for Scripture reading or offer to read to the patient.

CHRISTIAN CHURCH (DISCIPLES OF CHRIST)

Baptism: Do not practice infant baptism but have dedication service. Believers are baptized by immersion.

Holy Communion: Open communion is celebrated each Sunday and is a central part of worship services. Notify the clergy if the patient desires it; or sometimes the clergy member suggests it.

Death: No special practices.

Other practices: Church elders as well as clergy are appropriate to notify to assist with meeting the patient's spiritual needs.

CHURCH OF THE BRETHREN

Baptism: Do not practice infant baptism but have dedication service.

Holy Communion: Usually received within church, but clergy will give it in the hospital when requested.

Anointing the sick: Practiced for physical healing as well as spiritual uplift and held in high regard by the church. The clergy is notified if the patient or the family desires.

Death: The clergy is notified for counsel and prayer.

CHURCH OF THE NAZARENE

Baptism: Parents have the choice of baptism or dedication for their infant. Emphasis is on the believer's baptism, which is regarded as a symbol of the New Covenant in Jesus Christ.

Holy Communion: Pastor will administer if the patient wishes.

Dietary habits: The use of alcohol and tobacco is forbidden.

Death: Cremation is permitted, and stillborn term infants are buried.

Other practices: Believe in divine healing but not to the exclusion of medical treatment. Patients sometimes desire quiet time for prayer.

EPISCOPAL (ANGLICAN)

Baptism: Infant baptism is practiced and is considered urgent if the infant is critically ill. The priest is notified to administer the sacrament. Laypersons are permitted to baptize in an emergency.

Holy Communion: Notify the priest if the patient wishes to receive this sacrament.

Anointing the sick: Priest often administers this rite when death is imminent, but it is not considered mandatory.

Dietary habits: Some patients abstain from meat on Fridays. Others fast before receiving the Eucharist, but fasting is not mandatory.

Death: No special practices.

Other practices: Confession of sins to a priest is optional; if the patient desires this, the clergy should be notified.

LUTHERAN (10 DIFFERENT BRANCHES)

Baptism: Baptize only living infants any time, but usually 6 to 8 weeks after birth. Adults are also baptized, and modes of baptism, as appropriate, include sprinkling, pouring, or immersion.

Holy Communion: Notify the clergy if the patient desires this sacrament. Clergy sometimes also inquire about the patient's wishes.

Anointing the sick: Patients sometimes request an anointing and blessing from the minister when the prognosis is poor.

Death: A service of Commendation of the Dying is used at the patient's or family's request.

MENNONITE (12 DIFFERENT GROUPS)

Baptism: No infant baptism, but the child is sometimes dedicated if requested by the parents.

Holy Communion: Served twice a year, with foot washing as part of ceremony.

Dietary habits: Abstinence from alcohol is urged for all.

Death: Prayer is important at time of crisis, so contacting a minister is important.

Other practices: Women sometimes wear head coverings during hospitalization. Anointing with oil is administered in harmony with James 5:14 when requested.

METHODIST (MORE THAN 20 DIFFERENT GROUPS)

Baptism: Notify the clergy if the parent desires baptism for a sick infant.

Holy Communion: Notify the clergy if a patient requests it before surgery or another health crisis.

Anointing of the sick: If requested, the clergy will come to pray and sprinkle the patient with olive oil.

Death: Scripture reading and prayer are important at this time.

Other practices: Donation of one's body or part of the body at death is encouraged.

PRESBYTERIAN (10 DIFFERENT GROUPS)

Baptism: Infant baptism is practiced by pouring or sprinkling. Immersion is also practiced at times for adults.

Holy Communion: Given when appropriate and convenient, at the hospitalized patient's request.

Continued

Box 8-4 Religious Beliefs and Practices Affecting Health Care in the United States—cont'd

PRESBYTERIAN (10 DIFFERENT GROUPS)—cont'd

Death: Notify a local pastor or elder for prayer and Scripture reading if desired by the family or patient.

QUAKER (FRIENDS)

Baptism and Holy Communion: Friends have no creed; therefore a diversity of personal beliefs exists, one of which is that outward sacraments are usually not necessary because there is the ministry of the Spirit inwardly in such areas as baptism and communion. A few Friends baptize with water.

Death: Believe that the present life is part of God's kingdom and generally have no ceremony as a rite of passage from this life to the next. Ascertain the patient's personal beliefs and wishes, and then act on the patient's wishes.

Other practices: The name of the Quaker infant is recorded in official record books at the local meeting.

SALVATION ARMY

Baptism: No particular ceremony, but they do have an Infant Dedication ceremony.

Holy Communion: No particular ceremony.

Death: Notify the local officer in charge of the Army Corps for any soldier (member) who needs assistance.

Other practices: The Bible is seen as the only rule for one's faith; therefore make the Scriptures available to a patient. The Army has many of its own social welfare centers, with hospitals and homes where unwed mothers are cared for and outpatient services provided. No medical or surgical procedures are opposed, except for abortion on demand.

SEVENTH-DAY ADVENTIST

Baptism: No infant baptism is practiced, but have dedication services.

Holy Communion: Although this is not required of hospitalized patients, the clergy is notified if the patient desires.

Anointing of the sick: The clergy are contacted for prayer and anointing with oil.

Dietary habits: Because the body is viewed as the temple of the Holy Spirit, healthy living is essential. Therefore the use of alcohol, tobacco, coffee, and tea and the promiscuous (careless) use of drugs are prohibited. Some are vegetarians, and most avoid pork.

Special days: The Sabbath is observed on Saturday.

Death: No special procedures.

Other related practices: Use of hypnotism is opposed by some. People of homosexual or lesbian orientation are ministered to in the hope of "correction" of these practices, which are believed to be wrong. Make sure a Bible is always available for Scripture reading.

UNITED CHURCH OF CHRIST

Baptism: Practice infant and adult baptism. Three modes are used as appropriate: pouring, sprinkling, and immersion.

Holy Communion: Clergy is notified if the patient desires to receive this sacrament.

Death: If the patient desires counsel or prayer, notify the clergy.

ISLAM

Birth: A baby is bathed immediately after birth, before giving it to the mother. The father (or mother if the father is not available) then whispers the call to prayer in the child's ears so that the first sounds it hears are about the Muslim faith. Circumcision is culturally recommended before puberty. A baby born prematurely but at least 130 days of gestation is given the same treatment as any other infant.

Dietary habits: No pork or alcoholic beverages are allowed. All halal (permissible) meat must be blessed and killed in a special way. This is called zabihah (correctly slaughtered).

Death: Before death, family members ask to be present so that they can read the Koran and pray with the patient. An Imam will come if requested by the patient or family but is not required. Patients face Mecca and confess their sins and beg for forgiveness in the presence of their family. If the family is unavailable, any practicing Muslim is permitted to provide support to the patient. After death, Muslims prefer that the family wash, prepare, and place the body in a position facing Mecca. If necessary, health care providers are allowed to perform these procedures as long as they wear gloves. Burial is performed as soon as possible. Cremation is forbidden. Autopsy is also prohibited except for legal reasons, and then no body part is to be removed. Donation of body parts or organs is not allowed, because according to culturally developed law, people do not own their bodies.

Abortion and birth control: Abortion is forbidden, and many conservative Muslims do not encourage the use of contraceptives believing that is interferes with God's purpose. Others believe that it is best for a woman to have only as many children as her husband can afford. Contraception is permitted by Islamic law.

Personal devotions: At prayer time, washing is required, even by those who are sick. A patient on bed rest will sometimes require assistance with this task before prayer. Provision of privacy is important during prayer.

Religious objects: The Koran is not to be touched by anyone ritually unclean, and nothing is to be placed on top of it. Some Muslims wear taviz, a black string on which words of the Koran are attached. These should not be removed and must remain dry. Certain items of jewelry such as bangles may have religious significance; do not allow them to be removed unnecessarily.

Care of women: Because women are not allowed to sign consent forms or make a decision regarding family planning, it is mandatory for the husband to be present. Women are very modest and frequently wear clothes that cover all of the body. During a medical examination, it is necessary that the woman's modesty be respected as much as possible. Muslim women prefer female doctors. For 40 days after giving birth and also during menstruation, a woman is exempt from prayer because this is a time of cleansing for her.

AMERICAN MUSLIM MISSION

Baptism: No baptism is practiced.

Dietary habits: In addition to refusing pork, many will not eat foods traditional in black culture such as cornbread and collard greens.

Box 8-4 Religious Beliefs and Practices Affecting Health Care in the United States—cont'd

AMERICAN MUSLIM MISSION—cont'd

Death: The family is contacted before any care of the deceased is performed. There are special procedures for washing and shrouding the body.

Other practices: Quiet time is necessary to permit prayer. Members are encouraged to use black physicians for health care.

CHRISTIAN SCIENCE

Birth: Use physician or nurse-midwife during childbirth. No baptism ceremony.

Dietary habits: Because alcohol and tobacco are considered drugs, they are not used. Coffee and tea are often declined.

Death: Autopsy is usually declined unless required by law. Donation of organs is unlikely, but this is an individual decision.

Other practices: Do not normally seek medical care because they approach health care in a different, primarily spiritual, framework. They commonly use the services of a surgeon to set a bone but decline drugs and, in general, other medical or surgical procedures. Hypnotism and psychotherapy are also declined. Family planning is left to the family. They seek exemption from vaccinations but obey legal requirements. Report infectious diseases and obey public health quarantines. Nonmedical care facilities are maintained for those needing nursing assistance in the course of a healing. The Christian Science Journal lists available Christian Science nurses. When caring for a Christian Science believer, allow and encourage time for prayer and study. Patients often request that a Christian Science practitioner be notified to come.

JEHOVAH'S WITNESS

Baptism: No infant baptism is practiced. Baptism by complete immersion of adults is done as a symbol of dedication to Jehovah, because Jesus was baptized.

Dietary habits: Use of alcohol and tobacco is discouraged, because these harm the physical body.

Death: Autopsy is a private matter to be decided by the persons involved. Burial and cremation are acceptable.

Birth control and abortion: Use of birth control is a personal decision. Abortion is opposed based on Exodus 21:22-23.

Organ transplants: Use of organ transplant is a private decision; if used, it is required that the organ be cleansed with a nonblood solution.

Blood transfusions: Blood transfusions violate God's laws and are therefore not allowed. Patients do respect physicians and will accept alternatives to blood transfusions. These include the possible use of nonblood plasma expanders, careful surgical techniques to decrease blood loss, use of autologous transfusions, and autotransfusion through use of a heart-lung machine. Be sure to check unconscious patients for medical-alert cards or bracelets that state that the person does not want a transfusion. Because Jehovah's Witnesses are prepared to die rather than break God's law, you need to be sensitive to the spiritual as well as the physical needs of the patient.

THE CHURCH OF JESUS CHRIST OF LATTER-DAY SAINTS

Baptism: If a child over age 8 is very ill, whether baptized or unbaptized, call a member of the church's priesthood.

Holy Communion: Hospitalized patients often desire to have a member of the church priesthood administer this sacrament.

Anointing the sick: Mormons frequently are anointed and given a blessing before going to the hospital and after admission by laying on of hands.

Dietary habits: Abstinence from the use of tobacco; beverages with caffeine such as cola, coffee, and tea; alcohol and other substances considered injurious. Mormons eat meat but encourage the intake of fruits, grains, and herbs.

Death: Prefer burial of the body. Notify a church elder to assist the family. If need be, the elder will assist the funeral director in dressing the body in special clothes and will give other help as needed.

Birth control and abortion: Abortion is opposed except when the life of the mother is in danger. Only natural means of birth control are recommended. Artificial means are permitted when the health of the woman is at stake (including emotional health).

Personal care: Cleanliness is very important to Mormons. A sacred undergarment may be worn at all times by Mormons and is removed only in emergency situations.

Other practices: Allowing quiet time for prayer and the reading of the sacred writings is important. The church maintains a welfare system to assist those in need. Families are of great importance, so visiting is important to encourage.

UNITARIAN UNIVERSALIST ASSOCIATION

Baptism: No baptism.

Death: Cremation is often preferred rather than burial.

Other practices: Use of birth control is advocated as part of responsible parenting. Strong support for a woman's right to choice regarding abortion is maintained. Unitarian Universalists advocate donation of body parts for research and transplants.

UNIFICATION CHURCH

Baptism: No baptism.

Special days: Sunday mornings are used to honor Reverend and Mrs. Moon as the true parents, and members get up at 5 AM, bow before a picture of the Moons three times, and vow to do what is needed to help the reverend accomplish his mission on Earth.

Death: Believe that after death one's place of destiny will depend on his or her spirit's quality of life and goodness while on Earth. In the afterlife, one will have the same aspirations and feelings as before death. Hell is not a concern, because it will not be a place as heaven grows in size. People who leave the Unification Church are warned of the possibility that Satan will try to possess them.

Other practices: All marriages are required to be solemnized by Reverend Moon to be part of the perfect family and have salvation. The church supplies its faithful members with life's necessities. Members sometimes use occult practices to have spiritual and psychic experiences.

HEALTH PRACTICES

For many years, the belief popular in the United States was that modern biomedical health care is the best and only way to treat diseases. Today, many physicians and nurses still find it difficult to believe that any alternative therapies will be as effective as the biomedical methods that they have seen used for many years. Recently, however, a variety of alternative health services such as folk remedies, holistic therapies, and spiritual interventions have aroused attention even among the traditional medical community. Scientific research is being done in these areas to determine the effectiveness of these methods. Some are now being accepted more readily and are sometimes used concurrently with biomedical methods (see Chapter 17).

Several factors are driving this change in thinking about health care. Some of the long-established methods have become less effective, notably antibiotics used to treat infections. A number of folk remedies have been shown to be effective in treating certain diseases. More physicians with varied backgrounds and beliefs about health and illness now practice in the United States. As discussed earlier, our population continues to become more diverse. As new groups of people from other cultures arrive, they bring with them a variety of methods to deal with health issues (Figure 8-2). Many practices are benign but ineffective, and some are dangerous, but some are therapeutic and useful. It is important to allow a patient to follow practices that are in accordance with their cultural identity and personal beliefs when they are receiving health care in the traditional health care system, without allowing the effectiveness of either approach to be compromised.

The characteristics of four basic concepts of health beliefs are described in Table 8-2. For many years, Western cultures have almost universally used the biomedical method of treating illness and maintaining health. Folk medicine encompasses many different traditions in cultures around the world. It often includes native healers who use a variety of methods in treating disorders (Figure 8-3). At times, this belief system also incorporates religious practices and magic. Within this system, methods are used to manipulate the environment to improve health.

Do not assume that patients born in the United States accept the biomedical view of health care. Individuals in many subcultures of the United States practice folk medicine. These people will sometimes avoid seeking care from physicians, or will practice folk medicine while also receiving traditional care.

As our medical system becomes more open to considering a variety of alternative health care systems, you will be expected to understand the relationships between different views. Assessing the health practices of patients is an important part of achieving this understanding. If individual beliefs are discussed openly, the patient will probably be more willing to tell you about using other health care methods in addition to those directed by the doctor. Be aware that this information has to be shared with the doctor to prevent conflicts among treatments.

BIOLOGICAL VARIATIONS

Cultural groups are identified in a variety of ways. In some instances, the members share strong biologic characteristics. This is especially true if the cultural group is primarily made up of individuals from a particular race or geographic region. When assessing these individuals, include these characteristics. Some of the obvious ones are body structure, skin color, and hair color and texture. For example, you will probably expect a cultural group from the Scandinavian region to have many people with blonde hair and blue eyes. Asians are likely to have straight, coarse, dark hair. More important, in your practice, is a family history of diseases that are common within the ethnic group. Some diseases, such as sickle cell anemia, are more frequently found among those of African ancestry. Other diseases, such as diabetes, asthma, or heart disease, tend to be more prevalent among certain cultural groups. For example, even when diet and lifestyle are considered, diabetes occurs more frequently among American Indians.

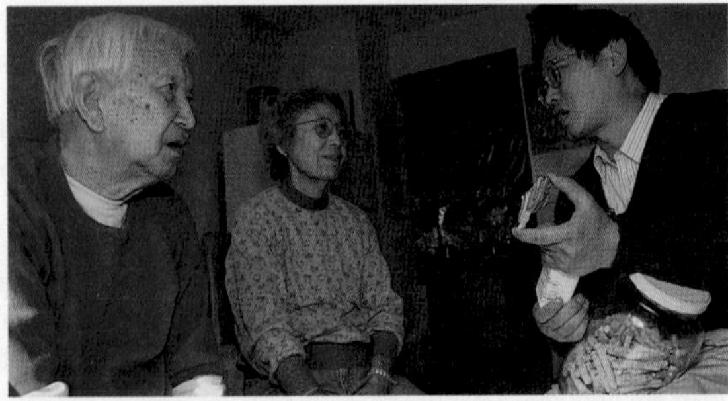

FIGURE 8-2 While providing information in a home care setting, a nurse compares traditional and Western remedies. Culture influences how people perceive health, illness, and pain. The nurse must take cultural variations into account to effectively communicate with patients and their families.

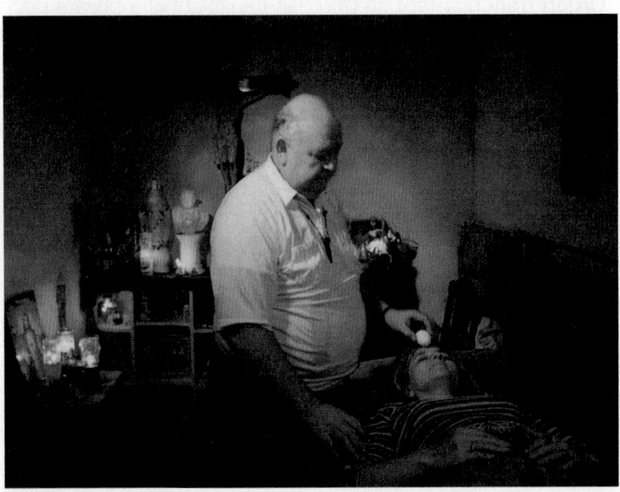

FIGURE 8-3 Within the Mexican-American folk medicine system, the *curandero* is the folk healer.

Table 8-2 Health Belief Systems

BELIEF SYSTEM	CHARACTERISTICS
Biomedical health belief system	Life is regulated by biomedical and physical processes. Life processes can be manipulated by human beings using mechanical interventions. Health is the absence of disease or signs and symptoms of disease. Disease is an alteration of the structure and function of the body. Disease has a specific cause, onset, course, and treatment. It is caused by trauma, pathogens, chemical imbalances, or failure of body parts. Treatment focuses on the use of physical and chemical interventions.
Folk health belief system	This is commonly referred to as "third-world" beliefs and practices. It is often called strange or weird by nurses and other health professionals who are unfamiliar with folk medicine beliefs. In most instances, these practices do not seem "strange or weird" once health care providers become acquainted with them. This system classifies illnesses or diseases as natural or unnatural. According to this belief system, natural events have to do with the world as God made it and as God intended it to be. Thus there is a certain amount of predictability for daily life. Unnatural events imply the exact opposite because they upset the harmony of nature. Thus unnatural events are those events that interrupt the plan intended by God and at their very worst represent the forces of evil and the machinations of the devil. They have no predictability and are beyond the control of ordinary mortals. Treatment is done by carrying out rituals, repentance, or giving in to the supernatural force's wishes.
Holistic health belief system	Religious experiences are based on cultural beliefs and may include such things as blessings from spiritual leaders, apparitions of dead relatives, and even miracle cures. Healing powers may also be ascribed to animate as well as on inanimate objects. Religion dictates social, moral, and dietary practices designed to assist an individual in maintaining a health balance as well as playing a vital role in illness prevention (e.g., burning of candles, rituals of redemption, and prayer). Baptism may be seen as a ritual of cleansing and dedication as well as prevention of evil. Anointing the sick may be seen as preparation for death and may also be performed as the hope of a miracle. Circumcision is also viewed as a religious practice. Treatment is designed to restore balance with physical, social, and metaphysical worlds. It may extend beyond treating the person to treating the environment to decrease pollution or prevent hunger, homelessness, etc.
Alternative or complementary belief system	In 1990, 34% of Americans (approximately 61 million people) used one or more nonmedical forms of therapy to treat an illness. Acupuncture, aromatic therapy, meditation, therapeutic touch, and a variety of other techniques prevail as feasible alternative therapies (see Chapter 17). Most of the individuals using an alternative therapy did so without informing their health care provider. Alternative therapies address the whole patient by viewing symptoms as the tip of the iceberg and as the body's means for communicating to the mind that something needs to be changed, removed, or added to one's life. The mind and body are seen as a whole unit.

Data from Giger, J.M., & Davidhizar, R.E. (2008). *Transcultural nursing: Assessment and intervention.* (5th ed.). St. Louis: Mosby.

Another important health consideration is the effect of culturally determined dietary practices. Many traditional foods are high in saturated fats, sodium, and sugar. If these foods are eaten frequently, they have the potential to affect patients' health as well as the health of their family members. In some cases, members of some cultural groups have dietary deficiencies caused by low intake of protein, complex carbohydrates, and fresh fruits and vegetables. When assessing the patient, include questions to determine whether the patient follows cultural dietary practices or eats a more general diet. Several diverse cultural groups (Chinese, Korean, Mexican, Puerto Rican, and Vietnamese) have beliefs that diseases and foods are classified as either "hot" or "cold." The diet is adjusted according to the perceived balance, and thus diseases are treated with the proper foods. This practice sometimes leads to a failure to meet basic nutritional needs and thus to dietary problems (see Chapter 21).

THE NURSING PROCESS AND CULTURAL FACTORS

When caring for patients, you will typically use the nursing process to develop a plan of care. Using the information you gather in your assessment, determine cultural behaviors, and then develop a plan of care accordingly.

Sometimes it is difficult to appropriately apply North American Nursing Diagnosis Association International (NANDA-I) nursing diagnoses to culturally diverse patients. People from other cultures often do not share the biomedical health belief system on which these diagnoses are based. It is unrealistic to use our system exclusively to classify their problems and needs. Unfortunately we sometimes end up labeling the patient's behavior as abnormal when it is actually quite normal in the person's own cultural context. The difficulties go even further, however. The goal of the nursing diagnosis system is to help change patients' behavior, but doing so by imposing biomedically-

Table 8-3 Nursing Diagnoses and Cultural Limitations

NURSING DIAGNOSIS	LIMITATIONS
Deficient knowledge	Patient decision-making and health-seeking behavior is directed by a different health belief system. Nurse also has knowledge deficit if care plan and nursing interventions are based solely on nurse's own health belief system.
Impaired verbal communication	Ability to understand each other is the problem—communication is not impaired. Patients sometimes seem unable to speak normally when they attempt to respond to someone speaking another language. Nonverbal communication between patient and nurse is likely to become more significant.
Ineffective health maintenance	Patient is very possibly following acceptable guidelines for health maintenance in his or her culture. Nurse expects person to change behavior to meet nurse's cultural view.
Noncompliance	Patient makes decisions based on health belief that is different. Concept of time possibly delays implementation. Religious beliefs sometimes affect adherence to biomedical treatment regimens. Perhaps others in the patient's cultural context counsel the patient to follow alternative health practices.

based health care beliefs and practices on them, without regard to their cultural identity, violates the basic tenets of nursing's patient-centered approach.

Certain nursing diagnoses are particularly problematic. Be careful about using nursing diagnoses such as deficient knowledge, impaired verbal communication, ineffective health maintenance, and noncompliance. Table 8-3 discusses limitations when using these nursing diagnoses.

To provide care and lessen the limitations of the NANDA-I nursing diagnoses, evaluate behavior from the perspective of the patient's culture. You, the health care system, or both may be required to change to accommodate, maintain, or reinforce patients' health beliefs and practices. Perhaps you will do this by reprioritizing nursing goals and changing procedures. It is important to find a compromise between your health beliefs and practices and those of the patient. The patient and her or his family are unlikely to accept any of the health teaching or treatments you attempt to provide if their own beliefs are not recognized. It is imperative to develop a mutually acceptable alliance with the patient. Remember that your ultimate goal is to assist the patient to achieve optimum health. One possible implication of this is that you will need to adjust many of the accepted nursing interventions to accommodate patients and their cultures.

Because of a patient's cultural background, therefore, you will sometimes modify how you perform an assessment or give care, or adapt the usual routines of your institution to the patient's needs. For instance, consider how to respect and accommodate cultural practices among Muslim patients. Allow Muslim women to keep the head, arms, and legs covered as much as possible. In addition, make every attempt to assign female staff members to care for Muslim women. Because Muslims pray several times each day, schedule care around these times to allow the patient privacy and the necessary leisure to pray. Be ready to consider similar accommodations to meet the needs of patients in other culturally dependent, special circumstances.

CULTURAL PRACTICES OF SPECIFIC GROUPS

As shown in Figure 8-4, Hispanics make up 24.3% of the population in western states of the United States and account for as much as 50% of the population in some counties. There are also subcultures within the Hispanic culture, and Hispanics' origins vary as well. According to the 2000 U.S. Census Bureau report, the largest Mexican populations are found in areas of California, Texas, Illinois, and Arizona. Puerto Ricans are concentrated in New York, Florida, New Jersey, and Pennsylvania. About two thirds of all Cubans in the United States live in Florida (U.S. Census Bureau, Census 2000). Although these groups share some common beliefs, they each have distinct practices. It is important to determine the place of origin when caring for a Hispanic patient.

Approximately 1.9 million American Indians among 10 tribes live in the United States (U.S. Census Bureau, Census 2000). American Indian populations were found in Arizona, Oklahoma, New Mexico, Alaska, California, North Carolina, South Dakota, New York, Montana, Washington, and Minnesota. Providing culturally appropriate nursing care is complicated by the fact that each nation or tribe of American Indians has its own language, religion, and belief system. Practices differ significantly among groups and among members of the same tribe. When the term "American Indian" is used, it is intended to refer to tribes residing within the continental United States.

It is impossible in the context of this chapter to give a complete picture of all cultural practices and beliefs for groups living in the United States. Table 8-4 gives examples of common cultural practices of prevalent groups in our culture. Always keep in mind the strong influence culture has on patients, colleagues, and you yourself. It is especially important to be aware of the community in which you practice. If you live in an area that is heavily populated by a culture that is unlike your own, it is your responsibility to learn as much as possible about the people and the culture.

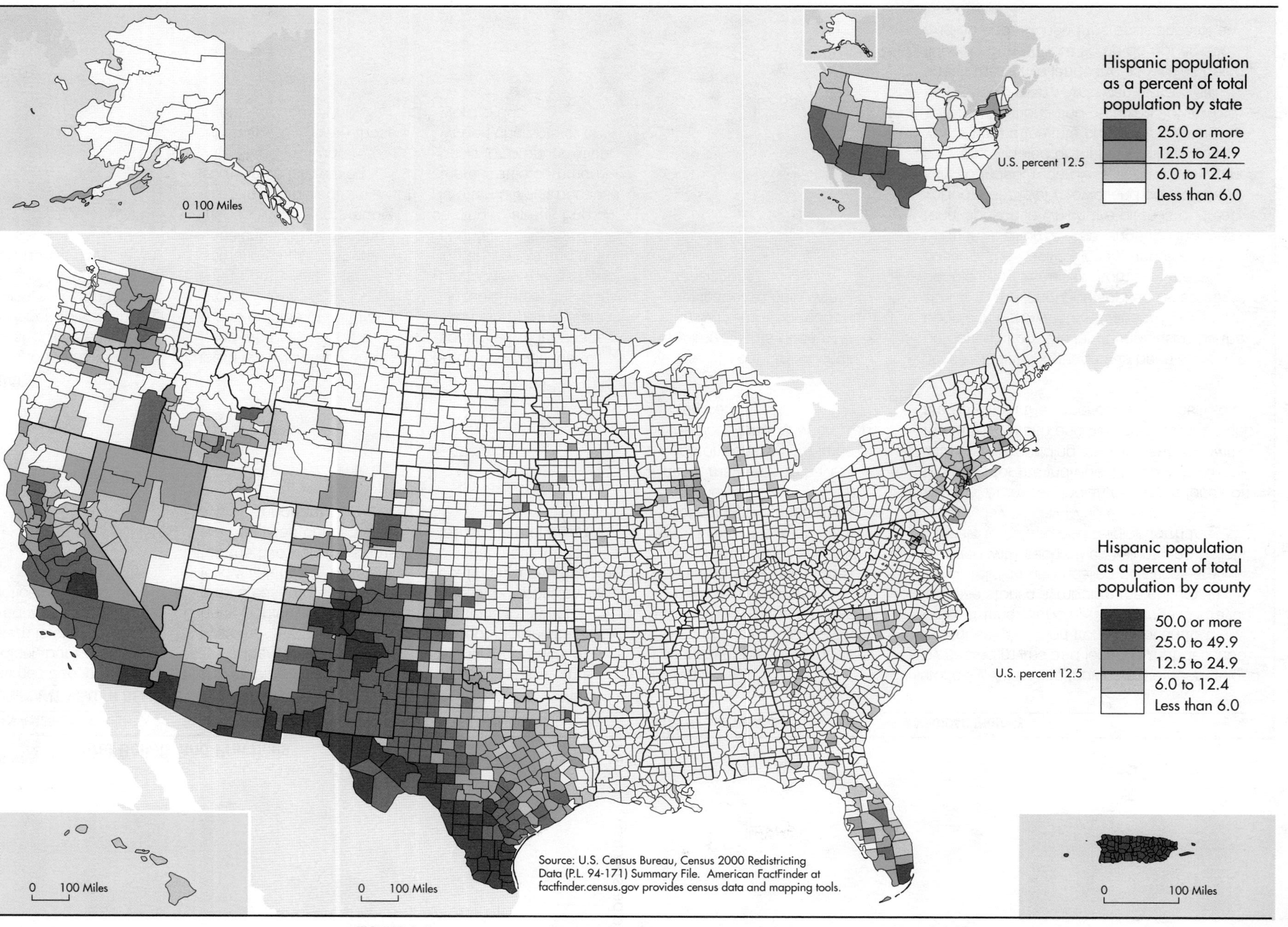

FIGURE 8-4 Hispanic percentage of the U.S. population according to Census 2000.

Table 8-4 Cultural Beliefs and Practices

MEXICAN AMERICANS	BLACKS (AFRICAN AMERICANS)	CHINESE AMERICANS	MUSLIM AMERICANS	AMERICAN INDIANS
PREDOMINANT HEALTH BELIEF SYSTEM				
Sometimes accept biomedical, but belief system is often heavily mixed with folk practices.	Highly diverse. Many adhere to biomedical system. Others, particularly from rural areas, more closely follow folk health beliefs. Often the two belief systems are practiced concurrently. Prayer is important.	Holistic belief system is primary influence. Will accept biomedical interventions for serious illness, but possibly will continue to practice traditional methods to reestablish natural balance.	Holistic. Essential to preserve modesty and privacy. Obligatory to keep body parts covered as much as possible. Use same-sex health care providers if at all possible. Always examine a female patient in presence of another female. Patient may wish to have doctor consult with Imam (religious leader) when planning care.	Historically, American Indians have been guided by sacred myths and legends that describe the tribes' evolution from inception to the present time. Supernatural beings portrayed in these stories symbolize the culture, in which religion and healing practices are blended with each other. Values and beliefs intrinsic to culture and religion form the Navajo day-to-day living experiences. Traditional American Indian concepts focus on the need for the individual to be in harmony with the surrounding environment and with the family. Health and religion cannot be separated within the American Indian culture.
LANGUAGE				
Spanish, often mixed with English. Children often are better able to speak English and sometimes translate for adults. Many adults never learn English.	English is understood and used when speaking with those outside of cultural group. Black English dialect is sometimes used when speaking with family and friends. Words commonly used in this dialect are sometimes intermixed with standard English when speaking with those in outside community.	Sometimes continue to speak native language even after many years in United States. It is possible to view this as honoring ancestors and native country. Learning to speak English is often difficult because there is little common basis for pronunciation, written characters, or word order.	Varies with country of origin. New immigrants often need family member or community leader to help with translations.	American Indian language has been shown to be derived from the languages used by the people in northwestern Canada. It is also similar to the language spoken by some people living in Alaska, some on the northern coast of the Pacific Ocean, and some in northern California. The language involves tonal speech in which the pitch is of great importance. Every vowel and consonant is fully sounded, regardless of how many times they are doubled or tripled within a word. Vowels are often interchanged, creating several variations and meanings of a word. Even today, many American Indians still speak the native language as well as being fluent in English, but some do not speak English and will need the assistance of an interpreter.

COMMUNICATION				
Sustained direct eye is contact considered rude, immodest, or dangerous. Women and children are susceptible to mal ojo (evil eye) and so avoid eye contact. Touch is used often. Touch has potential to neutralize mal ojo. Closeness and physical contact are valued in familiar situations. Modesty is highly valued, so it is possible that both men and women will be embarrassed when exposure of body is necessary.	Personal space comfort area tends to be close. Eye contact is sometimes uncomfortable, especially among older generation.	Maintaining eye contact is often considered ill mannered and disrespectful. Uncomfortable when face-to-face. Prefer to sit side-to-side or at right angles to carry on conversation. Touching is not usual during conversation—it is regarded as disrespectful or impolite. Touch possibly acceptable among same-sex acquaintances, but touching in public between opposite sexes is not acceptable.	Women do not usually shake hands with men. Women prefer to keep head, arms, and legs covered. Allow Imam to visit. Allow privacy to pray. Identify Muslim patients on chart and bracelet. Post signs to alert male staff members to avoid room with female Muslim patient.	Until recently, the Navajo language was unwritten. In World War II a special branch of the U.S. Marine Corps was developed for Navajos who served as Navajo code talkers. It has been estimated that this highly esteemed group saved millions of lives because the enemy was unable to understand the Navajo language or infiltrate the code. Instead of shaking hands, people of this culture will extend a hand and lightly touch the hand of the person they are greeting. Initially these people are silent and reserved, but once they become familiar, warm behavior is usually demonstrated. When introducing themselves by name, they give honor to ancestors by stating the clan and the location of their home area. They avoid eye contact, which is considered a sign of disrespect.
FAMILY ROLES				
Families sometimes expect to help care for patient. Male family members usually consulted before health care decisions are made. Only a wife permitted to give care to husband at home if genitalia are touched.	Women are primarily decision makers in family and are frequently head of the household. Extended family plays important role. Even when not related by blood, close ties exist. May refer to these people as "Aunt," "Uncle," "Grandmother," and include them in family decisions.	Loyalty and devotion to family is more important than individual feelings. Taking care of family members brings honor to family. Older children have authority over younger children in family. Decision making is organized in this way, and younger siblings must show respect and deference or it shames the family.	Decision-making unit is the family, not the individual. Husband will be consulted in any decisions about family. Imam often included in health-related decisions.	This culture is extremely family oriented, but it has a much broader meaning than just father, mother, and children. The biologic family is the center of social organizations and includes all members of the extended family. They are traditionally a matriarchal society. This means that when a couple marries, the husband makes his home with his wife's relatives and his family becomes one of several units that live in a group of adjacent hogans or other type of dwelling. Usually a male family member looked on as having the greatest amount of prestige will rise as leader for the extended family and provide necessary direction. However, in settling issues, all sides are listened to and the entire group determines the outcome. To be without relatives is to be really poor.

Continued

Table 8-4 Cultural Beliefs and Practices—cont'd

MEXICAN AMERICANS	BLACKS (AFRICAN AMERICANS)	CHINESE AMERICANS	MUSLIM AMERICANS	AMERICAN INDIANS
BIRTH RITES				
Inappropriate for husband to be present during birth. Father not expected to see wife or baby until both are cleaned and dressed. Female family members sometimes request to be present during labor and delivery.	Many folk customs potentially influence birth. Mother often supported through birth process by female family members. Breastfeeding is not readily accepted by new mothers or encouraged by older generations.	Fathers generally are not present in labor and delivery areas. Some mothers prefer acupuncture for birth rather than Western pain-control methods. Traditionally, mother does not see child for 12 to 24 hours.	Men are not present during labor and delivery. Some husbands wish to be present during the birth process. Women will seek a female physician. Pregnant women are exempt from fasting during Ramadan, the sacred ninth month during which Muslims fast from food and drink from dawn to dusk.	The tradition of massaging the newborn baby as a bonding experience between the mother and baby is still practiced. Assistance with ceremonies, particularly those associated with birth, is shared and has great importance. After delivery, the umbilical cord is taken from the newborn, dried, and buried near an object or place that symbolizes what the parents want for the child's future. The infant death rate remains disproportionately high for American Indians.
DEATH RITES				
Small children are shielded from the dying and death scene. Families take turns staying around the clock with the dying person. Grief sometimes is expressed by hyperkinetic or seizure type of behavior that serves to release emotions.	Extended family is very supportive during final illness. Family members will generally take turns staying with dying person. Some fear touching the body or being present when a person has died.	Often have aversion to death and anything concerning death. Donation of body parts is encouraged. Eldest son is responsible for all arrangements for the deceased. White, yellow, or black clothing is worn as sign of mourning.	Life is unique and precious; any intervention to hasten death is forbidden. Autopsy is acceptable with medical and legal need. It is important to allow family and Imam to follow Islamic practices to prepare body for funeral. Organ donations are permitted.	Assistance with ceremonies, particularly those associated with death, is shared and has great importance. People of this culture have a taboo against touching a dead person or any article associated with the deceased individual. Taboos associated with death in a hogan include the need to seal the entry and warn others to stay away; frequently the need to abandon or burn the hogan is observed.

DIETARY PRACTICES Lactose intolerance sometimes present. Rice, corn, and beans are good source of protein. Meats include beef, pork, poultry, and goat. Diet is high in fat because frying is common method of cooking. Fruits and vegetables that are native are included in diet. Sometimes there is an inadequacy in calcium, iron, vitamin A, folic acid, and vitamin C.	High incidence of lactose intolerance, so intake of milk and milk products is low. Many celebrations and rites revolve around food and feasting on traditional dishes (soul food). Traditional dishes such as collard greens, other leafy and yellow vegetables, legumes, beans, rice, and potatoes are high in nutritive value. Overall, the diet tends to be low in fiber, calcium, and potassium and high in fat. Dietary restrictions sometimes related to religious practices.	Diet is low in fat and sugar. Fat intake is limited because of cooking methods. Fish, pork, and poultry, as well as nuts, dried beans and tofu, are protein sources. Milk products are avoided because of lactose intolerance. Salt intake sometimes high as a result of eating preserved foods and seasoning with soy sauce. Rice is eaten with almost every meal.	Fasting during daylight hours is practiced during Ramadan. Medical condition often exempts person from fasting. Allow family to provide meals if allowed with treatment. Alcohol and drugs are forbidden. Make sure no pork products are included in foods.	Lack of food and food storage sometimes contribute to nutritional deficiencies. American Indians are believed to be at risk for tuberculosis, maternal and infant deaths, diabetes, and malnutrition. Lactose intolerance is extremely prevalent, affecting 79% of the American Indian population. One hypothesis suggests that some have a predisposition for diabetes that is seemingly triggered by changes in dietary practices and increasing obesity. Contemporary American Indian diet combines food indigenous to the areas with modern processed foods. Food practices are also influenced by tribal beliefs, practices, geographic area, and local availability of selected food. Foods preferred by many include meat and blue cornmeal. Milk is not a preferred food. The fat intake is primarily of saturated fats, and fiber intake is low. Commodity foods are supplied by the U.S. Department of Agriculture's food distribution program.

Get Ready for the NCLEX® Examination!

Key Points

- Transcultural nursing is practiced when the nurse consistently attempts to apply knowledge about culture to all aspects of care.
- To achieve cultural competence, you need an understanding of your own cultural beliefs and practices and an ability to perceive the health care setting from the patient's point of view. This understanding will help you to be more open and sensitive to the patient's cultural values.
- The impact of culture on behaviors, attitudes, and values depends on individual factors and varies among members of a specific cultural group.
- Beliefs and practices vary among as well as within cultures.
- Ethnocentrism can interfere with developing cultural competence. It is essential to be open to other cultures and value their beliefs as well as recognize that your own cultural beliefs are not necessarily superior to those of others.
- A preconceived idea that all members of a particular group possess the same attributes is known as stereotyping.
- Ethnic and racial stereotyping can lead to assumptions about an individual that are often inaccurate.
- Recognizing different health belief systems will assist you to develop a plan of care that incorporates varying beliefs.
- Nursing diagnoses are based on the biomedical health belief system and may have limitations when used to develop a plan of care for culturally diverse patients with different health beliefs.
- It is imperative to seek increased knowledge about cultural groups as transcultural nursing continues to be important in health care.

Additional Learning Resources

Go to your Companion CD for an audio glossary, animations, video clips, and more.

evolve Be sure to visit the Evolve site at http://evolve.elsevier.com/Christensen/foundations/ for additional online resources.

Review Questions for the NCLEX® Examination

1. The nurse works in a community with many Mexican-American families. The best way for her to learn about their culture would be to:
   1. eat at Mexican-American restaurants in the area.
   2. schedule a home visit with a Mexican-American family.
   3. conduct a library study or Internet search of information on the culture.
   4. observe cultural behaviors in a movie theater in the area.

2. The patient is admitted to the hospital complaining of diffuse symptoms such as nausea, vomiting, weight loss, headaches, insomnia, and chest pain, which she describes by saying, "My heart aches." Which intervention would be appropriate for this patient, whose cultural beliefs may differ from the nurse's beliefs about physical illness?
   1. Adhere to the philosophy, "I treat all my patients the same."
   2. Encourage the patient to describe her symptoms using only English.
   3. Contact an adviser who is familiar with the cultural beliefs of the patient.
   4. Allow the patient to continue taking herbal preparations while she is hospitalized.

3. A Muslim patient visiting the physician's office was told she will have to remove her clothes and put on an examination gown. The patient became upset and refused to do so. The nurse allows the patient to remain in her street clothes because she knows:
   1. the patient is embarrassed.
   2. as a Muslim, the patient must keep as much of her body covered as possible.
   3. the patient is being uncooperative.
   4. the patient cannot disrobe in front of another female.

4. The patient explains to the nurse that he became ill because the natural balance in his body was upset when he moved into a new apartment. He has been taking herbs and rearranging objects to change the environment. The nurse notes that the patient's health belief system is most likely:
   1. biomedical.
   2. folk.
   3. holistic.
   4. a combination of all three.

5. When the patient, a native of Mexico, comes to the clinic, she asks the nurse to allow her 10-year-old daughter to remain with her in the examining room. The nurse should:
   1. ask the child to leave to maintain privacy for the patient.
   2. explain to the patient that children are not allowed to stay in the examining room because of infection control.
   3. consider that the child may be there to serve as an interpreter for her mother.
   4. ignore the child.

6. The student nurse tells her instructor that she does not understand why a Chinese-American family is not grieving for their dying father. The instructor's response is based on knowing that the student nurse is:
   1. subculture oriented.
   2. stereotyping.
   3. ethnocentric.
   4. culturally racist.

7. The male nurse is assigned to care for a female Muslim patient. When the nurse enters the room to begin her care, the patient and her husband become upset. Her husband tells the nurse that he cannot care for his wife. This is probably because:
   1. the couple are prejudiced toward the nurse's race.
   2. the patient is a Muslim, so only women should be assigned to care for her.
   3. the nurse is not Muslim and therefore cannot care for the patient.
   4. the couple do not speak English.

8. A 25-year-old white nurse who was born and raised in the Midwest is typical of most native-born Americans because she believes that illness is generally caused by:
   1. fate and God's will.
   2. socioeconomic class.
   3. getting what you deserve.
   4. physiologic changes.

9. The nurse is planning to do a cultural assessment of a Chinese-American patient. It would be best if the nurse:
   1. sits facing the patient.
   2. touches the patient frequently to convey concern.
   3. positions the chair so that the nurse sits at a right angle to the patient.
   4. maintains good eye contact while asking questions.

10. A female nurse who is black is assigned to care for a new 86-year-old resident in a nursing home. When she enters his room, he makes several racially offensive remarks. What would be an appropriate response?
    1. Refuse to give care to the patient.
    2. Understand that he is possibly less tolerant of other races because of his own cultural experiences or he perhaps has disturbed cognitive functions.
    3. Become angry and retaliate by making racial statements directed at the patient.
    4. Tell her supervisor that she will not take care of any other white patients.

11. The nurse is assigned to care for a Muslim patient. When the nurse enters the room, he realizes that the patient is praying. The nurse should:
    1. stay in the room and wait until the patient is finished with his prayers.
    2. quietly leave the room and give the patient privacy to pray.
    3. interrupt the patient and tell him it is time for his care to be given.
    4. tell the patient that he cannot pray while he is in the hospital.

12. A Mexican American is pregnant with her second child. When the nurse is reviewing her diet, the patient states that she never drinks milk. The nurse knows that a cultural reason for this may be:
    1. the patient does not like the taste of milk.
    2. milk is forbidden in her cultural diet.
    3. lactose intolerance occurs often among Mexican Americans.
    4. the patient cannot afford to buy milk.

13. A 72-year-old black woman from Mississippi has been diagnosed with type 2 diabetes and hypertension. The student nurse tells the patient that her vegetables should be steamed and served plain. The patient responds, "But honey, I always cook my green beans with ham and salt and pepper. How can I eat them plain?" A culturally sensitive response might be:
    1. "I'm sorry, but you will just have to change your method of cooking."
    2. "I guess you will just have to give up eating green beans."
    3. "You must follow the physician's order if you want to get better."
    4. "Why don't you try cooking the beans with half as much ham and do not add salt?"

14. When caring for a patient who speaks a foreign language, it would be incorrect of the nurse to use impaired verbal communication as a nursing diagnosis because:
    1. an inability to understand each other is the problem, not impaired verbal communication.
    2. the patient is using a different health belief system that interferes with communication.
    3. the patient is perhaps following acceptable communication guidelines within his or her culture.
    4. the patient has deficient knowledge, not impaired verbal communication.

15. When the nurse is aware of her or his own cultural beliefs, the beliefs and practices of other cultures, and has the ability to interact effectively with individuals from other cultures, the nurse is said to be:
    1. stereotyping.
    2. ethnocentric.
    3. culturally aware.
    4. culturally competent.

16. Before implementation of any newly prescribed procedure, the nurse notices that the family of an older adult patient always consults the eldest son. The social organization of this family is most likely:
    1. Hispanic in origin.
    2. patriarchal.
    3. male dominated.
    4. traditional nuclear.

chapter

9 Life Span Development

evolve

http://evolve.elsevier.com/Christensen/foundationsadult

Elaine U. Polan

Objectives

1. Differentiate among the types of family patterns and their functions in society.
2. Describe different types of stresses that commonly affect today's families.
3. Describe the physical characteristics at each stage of the life cycle.
4. List the psychosocial changes at the different stages of development.
5. Discuss Erikson's stages of psychosocial development.
6. Describe Piaget's four stages of cognitive development.
7. Describe the cognitive changes occurring in the early childhood period.
8. Discuss the developmental tasks of the adolescent period.
9. List the developmental tasks for early adulthood.
10. Describe the developmental tasks for middle adulthood.
11. Define aging.
12. Discuss theories of aging.
13. Describe the normal age-related changes affecting the major body systems.
14. Discuss the effect of the aging process on personality, intelligence, learning, and memory.

Key Terms

adoptive family (p. 184)
ageism (p. 209)
autocratic family pattern (p. 184)
blended (reconstituted) family (p. 184)
cephalocaudal (sĕf-ă-lō-KŎ-dăl, p. 182)
chromosomes (KRŌ-mō-sōmz, p. 182)
cohabitation (p. 184)
conception (fertilization) (p. 181)
concrete operational phase (p. 199)
democratic family pattern (p. 184)
depression (p. 204)
development (p. 182)
disengagement stage (p. 185)
engagement or commitment stage (p. 185)
establishment stage (p. 185)
expectant stage (p. 185)
extended family (p. 183)
formal operational thought stage (p. 202)
foster family (p. 184)
growth (p. 182)
homosexual family (p. 184)
life expectancy (p. 180)
matriarchal family pattern (p. 184)
nuclear family (p. 183)
parenthood stage (p. 185)
patriarchal family pattern (p. 184)
preoperational thought stage (p. 194)
presbycusis (prĕz-bē-KYŪ-sĭs, p. 206)
presbyopia (prĕz-bē-Ō-pē-ă, p. 206)
proximodistal (prŏk-sĭ-mŏ-DĬS-tăl, p. 182)
schema (SKĒ-mă, p. 190)
school violence (p. 200)
senescence stage (sĕ-NĔS-ăns, p. 185)
sensorimotor stage (sĕn-sŏ-rē-MŌ-tŏr, p. 190)
single-parent family (p. 184)
social contract family (p. 184)
teratogen (tĕ-RĂ-tō-jĕn, p. 182)
zygote (ZĪ-gōt, p. 182)

As our nation develops, we are becoming consumed with health and well-being. Many improvements have contributed to better health and longer life. Better sanitation, medications, immunizations, exercise, and improved nutrition all help people stay healthy and live longer. Over the next decade, we expect to see an even greater proportion of the population grow older. Many factors have been identified as predictors of longevity, including health, happiness, avoidance of tobacco products, and job satisfaction. How long will you live? We are not in a position to predict the exact number, but we can estimate the number of years a person might live. This is known as life expectancy.

Life expectancy is the number of years an individual will probably live, based on the average for others with similar characteristics. Life expectancy in the United States in the beginning of the twentieth century was 47.3 years. This has increased over the past 100 years. Today, average life expectancy at birth in the United States is 77 years. Despite these changes, we still have plenty of room for improvement. There are currently 18 countries with populations of 1 million or more that have a life expectancy greater than that of the United States.

Within the United States, there are differences in life expectancy in different populations. For example, females outlive males by an average of 6 years. African-American females have a higher life expectancy today than white males. Other factors also influence life expectancy. Those with household incomes of greater than $25,000 live 3 to 7 years longer, depending on sex and race, than those in households with incomes of less than $10,000.

Infant mortality rate refers to the number of deaths before the first year of life. This number affects overall life expectancy statistics. The infant mortality rate for African Americans is more than double that for white infants. There is a great need for education and access to preventive health care for pregnant women of all ages and races.

Other factors also influence the life expectancy for different groups. According to *Healthy People 2010*, there are two goals for the population during the next 10 years: improving the length and quality of life and eliminating the health disparities and inequities in certain groups of the population. To motivate action toward change and progress, *Healthy People 2010* is organized around a list of 10 health indicators (Table 9-1).

HEALTH PROMOTION ACROSS THE LIFE SPAN

Development is a lifelong process that begins at **conception (fertilization)**, the beginning of pregnancy, and ends with death. There is continuity of development throughout the life span; middle adulthood and late adulthood have been recently recognized as having equal importance as the earlier stages of development. Experiences at one time of life affect future development. People are influenced by their genes, their families, and the world in which they live. The study of life span development is the study of how and why people change over time, as well as how and why they remain the same.

There are eight stages of life span development. These stages and their approximate ages are as follows:

- Infancy—birth to 1 year
- Toddler—1 to 3 years
- Preschool—3 to 5 years
- School age—6 to 12 years
- Adolescence—13 to 19 years
- Early adulthood—20 to 40 years
- Middle adulthood—40 to 65 years
- Late adulthood—65 years and over

Each stage of the life span is unique and has certain distinguishable features. The goal of studying the life span is to enable the student to better understand and relate to individuals at various stages of development. In particular, given the significant growth in the older population, it is incumbent on us to become more aware of the unique characteristics, needs, and problems of the older adult.

GROWTH AND DEVELOPMENT

An individual undergoes continuous changes throughout life to exist and function. These changes include the continuous replacement of cells, tissues, and fluids. Some changes are not physical in nature; they are

Table 9-1 ***Healthy People 2010*** **Health Indicators**

HEALTH INDICATORS	GOAL OF TAKING ACTION
Physical exercise	Increase bone and muscle strength
Overweight and obesity	Aid in weight control Enhance well-being
Tobacco use	Decrease risk for hypertension, hyperlipidemia, type II diabetes, heart disease, stroke, gallbladder disease, arthritis, cancer, sleep problems, and low self-esteem Decrease risk for heart disease, stroke, lung cancer, chronic lung disease, prematurity, spontaneous abortion, sudden infant death syndrome, and injuries caused by fires
Substance abuse	Decrease risk for child and spousal abuse, sexually transmitted diseases (HIV, hepatitis B or C), teen pregnancy, increased school failure rate, motor vehicle accidents, homelessness, and decreased worker productivity
Responsible sexual behavior	Prevent unplanned pregnancy, sexually transmitted diseases, and HIV/AIDS
Mental health	Provide mental health care, the lack of which potentially leads to depression; inability to maintain responsibilities as partner, parent, or worker; or suicide
Injury and violence	Reduce money spent for medical care, rehabilitation, loss of productivity and wages
Poor environmental quality	Decrease risk for premature births, respiratory illnesses, cancer
Immunization	Promote control of disease, elimination of infectious diseases, and prevention of illness and death
Access to health care	Provide health insurance coverage, primary care, routine medical checkups, and health supervision

From U.S. Department of Health and Human Services. (2000). *Healthy People 2010*. Washington, D.C.: U.S. Department of Health and Human Services.
AIDS, Acquired immunodeficiency syndrome; *HIV*, human immunodeficiency virus.

changes in cognition, communication, emotions, behavior, and feelings.

Growth refers to an increase in size of the whole or its parts. **Development** refers to function and the gradual process of change and differentiation, from simple to complex. Development proceeds as an orderly, sequential series of changes. Two directional terms important to understanding growth and development are *cephalocaudal* and *proximodistal*. **Cephalocaudal** is defined as growth and development that proceeds from the head toward the feet. The infant's head is large as compared with the rest of its body; gradually the body catches up. **Proximodistal** refers to growth and development that originates in the center and moves toward the outside. For example, the infant gains control of the shoulders before developing control of the hands and fingers.

The principles of growth and development may be summarized as follows:

- Growth and development proceed at a highly individualized rate that varies from person to person. Do not expect two people to react in the same manner to the same stimuli.
- Growth and development are continuous and interdependent processes characterized by spurts of growth and periods of rest.
- Growth and development proceed from the simple to the complex in a predictable sequence.
- Growth and development vary for specific structures at specific times. In other words, not all organs grow and develop at the same rate; for example, the ovaries in the female and the testes in the male do not mature until puberty.
- Growth and development are a total process that involves the whole person. The person grows physically, socially, mentally, and emotionally. Types of growth are interrelated.

PATTERNS OF GROWTH

Growth patterns appear to be genetically controlled. Nutrition, heredity, and environment play an important role in the patterns as well. The blueprint for all inherited traits is contained in the **chromosomes** (threadlike structures in the nucleus of a cell that function in the transmission of genetic information). At conception, the individual is endowed with a complex set of biologic potentials involving characteristics such as height; skin, hair, and eye color; and talents and interests, to name a few. Only identical twins have the same combinations of chromosomes (karyotype). The process of division, transmission, and mixing of chromosomes accounts for the variations in distinctive family traits or, in contrast, their continuity. This is discussed further in Chapter 25.

BEGINNINGS

Development begins with **conception**, or the union of the sperm and ovum, which combines the genetic material of both parents. Although environment plays a role, it is difficult to determine precisely what it is. Certainly, heredity and environment are interrelated, and their interaction results in the creation of a unique individual.

After fertilization, the **zygote** (the developing ovum from the time it is fertilized until, as a blastocyst, it is implanted in the uterus) contains 23 pairs of chromosomes, for a total of 46 chromosomes. One of each pair has been contributed by the mother and one by the father. The first question many parents ask following the birth of their baby is, Is it a boy or a girl? It is the sex chromosomes, one of the chromosome pairs, that determines the sex of the baby. The ovum always carries an X chromosome, whereas the sperm sometimes carries an X and sometimes a Y chromosome. The presence of a Y chromosome in the sperm that fertilizes the ovum means that the baby will be male.

$$\text{X ovum} + \text{Y sperm} = \text{XY (male)}$$
$$\text{X ovum} + \text{X sperm} = \text{XX (female)}$$

In addition to these sex characteristics, many other traits are potentially inherited. The transmission of certain abnormalities is genetically determined. Examples of such inherited disorders include Tay-Sachs disease, sickle cell disease, phenylketonuria, and spina bifida.

In some instances, environmental factors also play a role in contributing to certain diseases or defects in the unborn. A **teratogen** is a substance, agent, or process that interferes with normal prenatal development, causing the formation of one or more developmental abnormalities in the fetus. Drugs, alcohol, viruses, and cigarette smoke are just a few of the known harmful substances that are best avoided during pregnancy. It is estimated that a possible 5% to 25% of unfavorable outcomes in all pregnancies is attributable to smoking. It is also suggested that smoking increases the incidence of low-birth-weight babies.

Ethical Considerations

Genetic testing offers information to parents-to-be regarding the possibility that their offspring will inherit a genetic defect. Once parents are tested and know the results, they usually confront a difficult ethical decision and need support and counseling. Health professionals, who are in a position to advise these parents, face a dilemma. What is your opinion? Is it best to encourage them to undergo testing, or not?

THE FAMILY

The family is the basic unit of society. Families are composed of two or more individuals united by marriage, blood, adoption, emotional bonds, and social roles. The individuals of the family share emotional ties that usually persist over their entire lifetime (see Cultural Considerations box).

Cultural Considerations

Family and Culture

- Know the patient's family and kinship.
- Understand the values, the flow of authority, and decision-making patterns within the family.
- Understand different gender roles.
- Listen carefully to direct verbal and indirect nonverbal cultural cues.
- Be aware of common foods and eating rituals.
- Recognize that religious beliefs are likely to affect a person's response to health, illness, birth, and death.

Signs of several significant changes in American families are evident today. The factors that have contributed to the changed family are listed in Box 9-1. As a result of these influences, family roles and lifestyles have changed to meet society's needs.

TYPES OF FAMILIES

Regardless of the type of family, certain basic functions are inherent to the family unit. These basic functions include protection, nurturance, education, sustenance, and socialization. Ideally, unconditional affection, acceptance, and companionship are guaranteed to each family member. The family attempts to meet the individual's needs for growth and development, and in doing so it helps support personal fulfillment and strengthen each individual's self-esteem.

The family is the first socializing agent for teaching children society's expectations and limitations. As a part of that socialization, the family is responsible for ensuring that the child receives a formal education. The family is also responsible for instilling morals, values, and ideals into the children. These roles and functions of families are not necessarily stable or constant but are vulnerable to change. For example, the birth of a baby and the death of a family member make rearrangement of family roles and structures necessary. See Box 9-2 for types of families.

Nuclear Family

For a long time, the nuclear family was thought of as the so-called normal family. Today, the nuclear family is looked at as traditional without having an exclusive claim on normalcy. The **nuclear family** is a family unit consisting of parents and their biologic offspring. This family type had sex-based roles assigned to its members.

The modern-day nuclear family usually consists of a husband and wife with or without children living in an independent household setting. In the past, one parent, usually the man, was the breadwinner. Today these roles have been redefined in their structure and function. In many families, both parents work and share equally in the financial support and the roles and responsibilities of the family unit.

Extended Family

The **extended family** consists of the nuclear or traditional family and some additional family members all living in the same household: parents, their biologic children, grandparents, grandchildren, aunts, uncles,

Box 9-1 Changes Affecting Modern Families

- Economic changes—resulting in an increase in the number of women in the workforce
- The feminist movement
- More effective birth control
- Legalization of abortion
- Postponement of marriage, childbearing
- Increase in divorce rate

Box 9-2 Types of Families

NUCLEAR
- Consists of married man and woman and their children
- Lives in independent household

EXTENDED
- Consists of nuclear plus additional family members living in same household
- Provides a sharing of responsibilities

SINGLE-PARENT
- Occurs by divorce, death, separation, abandonment, or choice
- More common in recent years
- Typically, one adult performs roles of two people

BLENDED (RECONSTITUTED)
- Occurs when adults from previous marriage remarry and combine children within new household

SOCIAL CONTRACT AND COHABITATION
- Made up of man and woman living together without legal commitment but sharing roles and responsibilities

HOMOSEXUAL
- Involves homosexual partners living together with shared responsibilities

ADOPTIVE
- Consists of usually traditional nuclear-family members, husband, wife, and adoptive child

FOSTER
- Responsible for care, supervision, and nurturing of children in their charge

and other family members. A sharing of support, roles, and responsibilities is common to this family structure. This family type constitutes the basic family structure in many societies.

Single-Parent Family

The **single-parent family** exists today by choice or as the result of death, divorce, separation, or abandonment. More than 40% of single-parent families are the result of divorce. The head of the household is sometimes female and sometimes male. This type of family unit also results when an unwed parent lives alone or a single person decides to adopt a child. The single parent has the sole responsibility of carrying out the functions that are typically shared by two members.

Blended (Reconstituted) Family

The **blended (reconstituted) family** (also called the stepfamily) arises when adults remarry and bring together their children from previous marriages. This type of family potentially presents many types of stresses. Losses resulting from death or divorce sometimes cause both adults and children to be fearful of love and trust. A child's loyalties to an absent parent interfere at times with the formation of new ties to a stepparent, especially when the child goes back and forth between two households.

Social Contract Family and Cohabitation

The **social contract family** style is also referred to as **cohabitation.** It involves an unmarried couple living together and sharing roles and responsibilities.

Homosexual Family

The **homosexual family** is a family group composed around a same-sex couple. Homosexual adults form family units. Their members share bonds of emotional commitment and roles of child rearing. Many of these family structures consist of either natural children (from a heterosexual relationship) or adopted or foster children. Regardless of the specific family structure, all families share common parenting concerns and responsibilities.

Adoptive Family

The **adoptive family** is a family unit with adopted children. Each year, millions of couples increase their family size through adoption. Childless or infertile couples often are lonely and lack fulfillment and miss the joys of parenthood. The ordeal of adoption may be time consuming and anxiety provoking. The role of parenting can be both exciting and fulfilling for natural and adoptive families alike.

Foster Family

The **foster family** allows for the care, supervision, and nurturing of children whose parents are unable to care for them. The length of stay in the foster home is sometimes short and sometimes longer, and sometimes temporary; it depends on individual circumstances.

FAMILY PATTERNS

Family patterns refer to the way in which family members relate to each other. Examples of family patterns include autocratic, patriarchal, matriarchal, and democratic patterns. Several researchers have identified 12 qualities common to all functional families, listed in Box 9-3.

Autocratic Family Pattern

In the **autocratic family pattern,** the relationships are unequal. The parents attempt to control the children with strict, rigid rules and expectations. This family pattern is least open to outside influence.

Patriarchal Family Pattern

In the **patriarchal family pattern,** the adult male (or males of the family) usually assumes the dominant role. The adult male member functions in the work role, is responsible for control of finances, and makes most decisions.

Matriarchal Family Pattern

In the **matriarchal family pattern** (also known as the matrifocal family) the adult female (or females of the family) assumes primary dominance in areas of child care and homemaking, as well as financial decision making. In some families of this type, an older female relative provides child care so that the mother of the children is free to work outside of the home.

Democratic Family Pattern

In the **democratic family pattern,** the adult members function as equals. As is often true in other types of families, children are treated with respect and recog-

Box 9-3 Qualities of Functional Families

- Sense of commitment toward promoting the members' well-being
- Sense of appreciation and encouragement for tasks accomplished
- Directed effort toward spending quality time with individual members
- Sense of purpose that encourages progress during good or difficult times
- Sense of harmony between members of the family
- Effective communications between individuals
- Established values, rules, and beliefs
- Variety of different coping techniques to enhance functioning
- Use of effective problem-solving measures and the use of a variety of options
- Positive outlook
- Ability to be flexible and adapt to changes
- Use of varied resources to facilitate coping skills

nized as individuals. This style encourages joint decision making, and it recognizes and supports the uniqueness of each individual member. This family pattern favors negotiation, compromise, and growth.

STAGES OF FAMILY DEVELOPMENT

Engagement or Commitment Stage

The **engagement or commitment stage** begins when the couple acknowledges to themselves and others that they are considering marriage. At this time, opposition or support will be evident from friends and parents. There are wedding plans to be arranged. Housing, work, and furnishings are some of the items on the agenda requiring discussion and exploration.

Establishment Stage

The **establishment stage** extends from the wedding up until the birth of the first child. During this phase, one of the important tasks is the adjustment from the single, independent to the married, interdependent state. The challenges facing the newly married couple include learning to live with another person and together managing two-person decision making, conflict resolution, and communication. The relationship established with the couple's parents and families can enhance the cohesiveness or weaken the couple's ties. To the average young adult, marriage is an important, serious change that requires major adjustments. A good marriage does not just happen. It is something both parties have to work at and contribute to for success. Commitment, goals, and respect for each other all call for equal time and energy. Success at marriage satisfies Erikson's task of intimacy (see Table 9-2 on p. 187 and Psychosocial Development under Early Adulthood) and helps fulfill the individual's need for love and belonging (Figure 9-1).

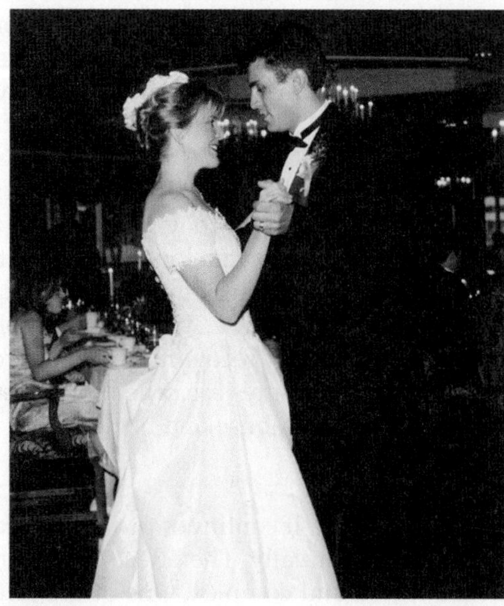

FIGURE 9-1 Establishment stage: the newly married couple.

Expectant Stage

The **expectant stage** begins with conception and continues through the pregnancy. One of the most important decisions of a person's life is that of starting a family. May people describe becoming parents as one of the most challenging, as well as most rewarding, roles in their lives. Pregnancy requires both physiologic and psychological adjustments. There are many important decisions to consider during pregnancy, including childbirth methods, continuation or modification of employment, child care, and feeding methods. The desired outcome of pregnancy is that a bond or attachment will be established between the parents and the new baby.

Ethical Considerations

When a woman is selected to be artificially inseminated for a fee to bear a child and then relinquishes the parenting rights to the baby's natural father, it is called *surrogacy*. What is your opinion regarding this practice, which has become more common in the United States?

Parenthood Stage

The **parenthood stage** begins at the birth or adoption of the first child. The transition to parenthood is a major event. Even couples with good preparation express a great deal of anxiety associated with the onset of this new role. One of the most frequently described problems is lack of time. There appears to be less free time, less sleep time, less time together, and less intimate sexual time. Compounding the lack of time is the stress of parenting and the self-doubt about ability and competency in this new role.

Disengagement Stage of Parenthood

The **disengagement stage** of parenthood is that period of family life when the grown children depart from the home. The role of parenting changes during this phase of the life cycle. The departure of children does not end the role of parenting. Even though grown children perhaps do not live with their parents, they usually continue to need emotional guidance and some financial support. Many grown children return to living at home for financial reasons. Regardless, during the disengagement stage, couples or the single parent need to redefine personal roles and structure time so that there is a sense of usefulness, accomplishment, and self-fulfillment.

Senescence Stage

The **senescence stage** is the last stage of the life cycle, which requires the individual to cope with a large range of changes. For the older adult, the family unit continues to be a major source of satisfaction and pleasure. Most older adults prefer to live independently. The greater life expectancy for women means that it is common for older women to outlive their spouses and continue life alone. Most older adults have regular contact with other family members. The grandparenting role requires new adaptations. This role requires a change in one's roles and sense of identity. In the past, grandparents often lived with their extended families because they had to, not necessarily because they wanted to. Grandparents of today are an independent breed. Grandparents want close, stable, emotionally satisfying family ties. Simultaneously, they tend to want an independent life, away from kin. They want to see and love their grandchildren but not be responsible for them.

CAUSES OF FAMILY STRESS

Various stressors affect the family unit. Chronic illness, abuse, and divorce are some of the most common factors. Stress, when it occurs, affects everyone, at all ages. Like adults, children often have feelings of stress. Stress in childhood results from either internal or external pressures or from a combination of both. At very early ages, stress sometimes results when the infant's needs are not met. Toddlers often perceive stress when they are separated from their mothers. School-age children sometimes feel stress from pressures in school or from parental expectations. Even social interactions at this stage have the potential to be somewhat difficult and stressful. Parents need to observe and listen to their children and be watchful for signs of stress (Box 9-4). It is essential that they be ready to help their children deal with their stress. One way to help is to anticipate what holds stress potential and to prepare children ahead of time. For example, if the child is starting a new school, it is a good idea for the parents to talk about it before the day of the event. Allow children to express their feelings. It is important for children to know that it is all right to have uneasy feelings. Children need to have someone validate their feelings. Talking about what is causing the child's uneasy feelings will help minimize the child's discomfort and help bring about possible solutions.

Chronic Illness

Chronic physical or emotional illness of the parent or the child affects all family members. Factors such as financial resources, family stability, and the adequacy of the support system determine an individual's ability to cope with a family member's chronic illness.

Box 9-4 Common Signs of Stress in Children

- Mood swings
- Acting-out behavior
- Change in eating or sleeping patterns
- Frequent stomachaches, headaches, or other unexplained somatic complaints
- Excessive clinging to parents
- Thumb-sucking
- Bed-wetting
- Return to behavior typical of an earlier stage of development

Working Mothers

Alternative family patterns are more common, and today's families often experience change and have to adjust to new circumstances. New family patterns have resulted in more women in the labor force. Working mothers are considered common today. Aside from the financial rewards, many feel that working mothers create a wider range of valid role models for young children. Many working mothers compensate for the time they are not with their child by establishing quality time during their limited at-home time. Some fathers are opting to assume primary child care responsibilities. Certainly, when both parents work outside the home, caregiving arrangements have to be considered. Child care is sometimes available; some of the various forms include in-home care by a relative or paid caregiver and out-of-home care in an organized or group setting. The federal government and most states have regulations controlling and regulating staff, size, and safety issues concerning daycare centers. In choosing a daycare center, look for the following: a balance of age-appropriate educational structure and an open environment, ample space with a variety of materials and activities, small class size with appropriate staff/child ratio, an environment that fosters active staff involvement, positive encouragement, and high-quality care in a safe environment.

Abuse

Abuse refers to physical, emotional, financial, verbal, sexual assault, or neglect. Each year, approximately 6 million women, children, and men are victims of physical abuse inflicted by parents, spouses, siblings, children, and other relatives. In many families, abuse is pervasive. A parent with ineffective coping skills will have difficulty maintaining family wellness and safety. Further, certain objective and measurable factors are related to family violence. They include financial strain, social isolation, low self-esteem, and previous history of abuse. The presence of several of these risk factors raises the risk that an individual will resort to abuse. The following are some common characteristics of parents who abuse their children: they were abused themselves as children; they are often loners; they are harsh, strict, and punitive; they have unreasonable expectations; and they are immature, lack self-control, and have low self-esteem. Early recognition, prompt reporting, and preventive measures are called for to help detect and end all forms of abuse and neglect.

Divorce

Divorce is widespread. It continues to affect more than 1 million children annually. The effects of divorce on children are varied and complex. One of the factors is the age of the child at the time of the divorce. Younger

Box 9-5 Tips for Divorcing Parents

- Encourage children to talk about their feelings.
- Do not use children as pawns or "go-betweens."
- Never speak negatively about ex-spouse in front of children.
- Seek professional help if children need additional support.

children often feel abandoned and feel they are no longer loved by both parents. Other factors that sometimes affect the child are the bitterness and conflict surrounding the divorce, the child's prior relationship with the absent parent, the effects of the divorce on the custodial parent, and the postdivorce relationship of the parents. Many children have reconciliation fantasies for extended periods after the divorce is finalized. Changes in one parent's status will create changes in emotional milieu, family role, finances, lifestyle, and often the home neighborhood (Box 9-5).

STAGES OF GROWTH AND DEVELOPMENT

The following sections of the text discuss development by age-group. It is necessary to take a look at a few aspects of development across a larger arc, however, in order to fully appreciate the scope of human growth and development.

PSYCHOSOCIAL DEVELOPMENT

Erik Erikson, an American psychoanalyst, viewed the life cycle as a series of developmental stages, each accompanied by a developmental task or challenge. Table 9-2 provides an overview of Erikson's stages of psychosocial development. Many of the subsections that follow include stage-appropriate characterization according to Erikson's framework.

COGNITIVE AND INTELLECTUAL DEVELOPMENT

Swiss theorist Jean Piaget's stages of cognitive development are outlined in Box 9-6.

COMMUNICATION AND LANGUAGE

Humans have an innate capacity to learn language. They are born with the mechanism and the capacity to develop speech and language skills. During infancy, the unique ability of the brain to sort out basic sounds and to extract from sentences the most meaningful elements becomes apparent. During early childhood, the brain's language-acquisition ability becomes even more sophisticated. Parents and other caregivers have an enormous potential to influence the infant's intellectual and language development. However, infants will not speak spontaneously. It rests with the environment to provide a means for them to acquire these skills. Speech requires intact physiologic functioning of (1) the respiratory system, (2) speech control centers in the cerebral cortex, and (3) the articulation and resonance structures of the mouth and nasal cavities. In addition, acquisition of language requires (1) an intact and discriminating auditory apparatus, (2) intelligence, (3) a need to communicate, and (4) stimulation. The rate of speech development varies from child to child and is directly related to neurologic competence and intellectual development. All children go through the same sequence of stages in language and speech development in early childhood unless abnormal conditions are present (Table 9-3).

Table 9-2 Erikson's Stages of Psychosocial Development

STAGE	APPROXIMATE AGE (YEARS)	DEVELOPMENTAL TASK	OUTCOMES
1. Infancy	Birth to 1	Basic trust vs. mistrust	Infants learn either to trust or to not trust that significant others will properly care for their basic needs, including nourishment, sucking, warmth, cleanliness, and physical contact.
2. Toddler	1 to 3	Autonomy vs. shame and doubt	Children learn either to be self-sufficient in many activities, including toileting, feeding, walking, and talking, or to doubt their own abilities.
3. Preschool	4 to 6	Initiative vs. guilt	Children want to undertake many adultlike activities, sometimes going beyond the limits set by parents and feeling guilty because of it.
4. School age	7 to 11	Industry vs. inferiority	Children eagerly learn to be competent and productive or feel inferior and unable to do any task well.
5. Adolescence	12 to 19	Identity vs. role confusion	Adolescents try to figure out "Who am I?" They establish sexual, ethnic, and career identities or are confused about what future roles to play.
6. Young adulthood	20 to 44	Intimacy vs. isolation	Young adults seek companionship and love with another person or become isolated from others.
7. Middle adulthood	45 to 65	Generativity vs. stagnation	Middle-aged adults are productive, performing meaningful work and raising a family, or become stagnant and inactive.
8. Late adulthood	65+	Ego integrity vs. despair	Older adults try to make sense out of their lives, either seeing life as meaningful and whole or despairing at goals never reached and questions never answered.

Box 9-6 Piaget's Stages of Cognitive Development

SENSORIMOTOR: BIRTH TO 2 YEARS
- Uses senses and motor abilities to understand the world and coordinates sensorimotor skills; this period begins with reflexes
- Develops schema
- Begins to interact with environment
- Learns that an object still exists when it is out of sight (object permanence) and begins to remember and imagine experiences (mental representation)
- Develops thinking and goal-directed behavior

PREOPERATIONAL THOUGHT: 2 TO 6 YEARS
- Develops egocentric thinking (understands the world from only one perspective—that of the self)
- Uses trial and error to discover new traits and characteristics
- Conceptualizes time in present terms only
- Uses symbols to represent objects
- Develops more logical, intuitive thinking
- Centers or focuses on a single aspect of an object, producing some distortion of reality
- Gains in imaginative ability
- Gradually begins to "de-center" (becomes less egocentric and understands other points of view)

CONCRETE OPERATIONAL THOUGHT: 7 TO 11 YEARS
- Understands and applies logical operations or principles to help interpret specific experiences or perceptions
- Has more realistic views; better understands other viewpoints
- Improves use of memory
- Focuses on more than one task; develops logical, socialized thoughts
- Recognizes cause-and-effect relationships
- Learns to identify behavior outcome
- Understands basic ideas of conversation, number classification, and other concrete ideas

FORMAL OPERATIONAL THOUGHT: 12+ YEARS
- Uses a systematic, scientific problem-solving approach
- Recognizes past, present, and future
- Is able to think about abstractions and hypothetic concepts and is able to move in thought "from the real to the possible"
- Becomes more interested in ethics, politics, and all social and moral issues as ability to take a broader and more theoretic approach to experience increases

Table 9-3 Normal Language and Speech Development during Early Childhood

AGE (YEARS)	NORMAL LANGUAGE DEVELOPMENT	NORMAL SPEECH DEVELOPMENT	INTELLIGIBILITY
1	Says two or three words with meaning Imitates sounds of animals	Omission of most final and some initial consonants Substitution of consonants "m," "w," "p," "b," "k," "g," "n," "t," "d," and "h" for more difficult sounds Use of unintelligible jargon peaks at age 18 months	Usually no more than 25% intelligible to unfamiliar listener
2	Uses two- or three-word phrases in context Has vocabulary of about 300 words and uses "I," "me," and "you"	Use of consonants "m," "w," "p," "b," "k," "g," "n," "t," "d," and "h" with vowels but inconsistently and with much substitution Omission of final consonants Articulation lags behind vocabulary	At age 2, 65% intelligible in context
3	Says four- or five-word sentences Has vocabulary of about 900 words Uses "who," "what," and "where" in asking questions Uses plurals, pronouns, and prepositions	Mastery of "b," "t," "d," "k," and "g"; "r" and "l" may still be unclear; omission or substitution for "w" Repetitions and hesitations common	At age 3, 70% to 80% clear
4 to 5	Has vocabulary of 1500 to 2100 words Able to use most grammatical forms correctly, such as past tense of verb with "yesterday" Uses complete sentences with nouns, verbs, prepositions, adjectives, adverbs, and conjunctions	Mastery of "f" and "v"; possible distortion of "r," "l," "s," "z," "sh," "ch," "y," and "th" Little or no omission of initial or last consonant	Speech is totally intelligible, although some are still imperfect
6-7	Has vocabulary of 3000 words Comprehends "if," "because," and "why"	Mastery of "r," "l," and "th"; possible continuing distortion of "s," "z," "sh," "ch," and "j" (usually mastered by 7.5 to 8 years of age)	Speech is totally intelligible

The basic sequence of language is as follows:

- *3 months—babbling.* When infants babble, they typically explore all the possible sounds they are able to make by enhancing the force of the air stream as it passes their vocal cords and by varying the positions of their tongue and mouth.
- *1 year—recognizes words.* Between ages 1 and 2, infants generally acquire the ability to produce holo phrases (one-word sentences that convey a complete message ["up"]). Infants learn to expand their holo phrases by attaching them back-to-back to other nouns or verbs. They thus form two-word sentences ("mommy milk," "daddy come"). Early speech is often referred to as telegraphic speech because, as in telegram messages, the articles, pronouns, prepositions, and conjunctions are omitted. In organizing and coding language, infants acquire an understanding of the most meaningful units of speech. No one teaches infants to use nouns and verbs first. They learn this sequence on their own.
- *Preschool—acquiring structure of native language.* The language explosion that occurs during the preschool years is most obvious in the growth of vocabulary, from 50 words at 18 months to 200 words at age 2 to between 8000 and 14,000 words at age 6. From ages 2 to 6, the average child learns between 6 and 10 words per day. Preschoolers have an outstanding ability to learn language. Most researchers regard early childhood as a crucial period for language learning.
- *6 years—able to speak and understand new words and sentences.* Even compared to the preschool years, language development from 6 years on is remarkable, albeit much more subtle, as children consciously come to understand more about the many ways language can be used. This understanding gives them greater control in their comprehension and use of language, and in turn, enhances the range of their cognitive powers generally.

A common rule of thumb about the evolution of early speech acquisition is that the number of words in an average response usually corresponds to the chronologic age of the child. For example, a 2-year-old might say, "Me do"; a 3-year-old might add a word, "Me do it"; and a 4-year-old might say, "Let me do it."

Girls advance more rapidly in language development than boys. Firstborn children develop language earlier than do later-born children, and children of multiple births (twins, triplets) develop language later than children of single births.

INFANCY: 1 TO 12 MONTHS

Physical Characteristics

An infant's physical development happens so rapidly that size, shape, and skills seem to change daily (see Chapter 27 for discussion of the newborn). Growth, which proceeds in a cephalocaudal and proximodistal sequence, is rapid during the first 6 months of life. The infant is expected to gain about 1.5 pounds per month until 5 months. The infant usually doubles his or her birth weight by 4 to 6 months. By the time the baby is 1 year of age, the birth weight has tripled (average weight is 21.5 pounds). Most of the weight gain in the first months of life is in the form of fat, which provides insulation and a source of nourishment to draw on if teething or other problems decrease food intake for a few days. After 8 months, weight gain includes more bone and muscle.

Height (length) increases by about 1 inch per month for the first 6 months. By 12 months of age, the infant's birth length has increased about 50%; the typical length is 30 inches (75 cm).

Vital Signs

Infants are subject to wide variations in body temperature related to activity levels and state of health. Apical rates slow down in infancy. At 2 months, the average apical rate is about 120 beats per minute. Count the apical pulse for a full minute, noting variations in rate, volume, and rhythm. Respiratory rates also decrease during infancy; these rates are related to activity level. Average resting respiratory rate for the 12-month-old is about 30 breaths per minute. Blood pressure readings will gradually increase to 90/60 mm Hg at 12 months.

Dentition

Teething begins at about 5 to 6 months of age. Signs of teething—irritability, edematous red gums, excessive drooling, and change in stooling—begin 3 to 4 weeks before the appearance of the tooth (Box 9-7). Dental decay can begin at any time after tooth development. Oral hygiene for the young infant consists of offering sips of clear water and wiping and massaging the infant's gums.

Advise parents to begin toothbrushing after the first teeth appear; this element of dental hygiene is important to continue throughout the life span. In areas without added fluoride in the water, recommend the use of fluoride toothpaste. To prevent bottle-mouth syndrome, instruct caregivers to avoid putting anything but water in the infant's night bottle. Sugar in milk, formula, or juice causes severe decay and de-

Box 9-7 Primary Dentition Schedule

6 months:	Teething begins with eruption of two lower central incisors
7 months:	Eruption of upper central incisors
9 months:	Eruption of upper lateral incisors
11 months:	Eruption of lower lateral incisors
12 months:	Approximately 6 to 8 teeth present
24 months:	Approximately 16 teeth present
30 months:	Completion of primary dentition—20 teeth present

struction of the tooth enamel. Also instruct all caregivers not to prop up the bottle and then leave the child alone with it, because this potentially leads to aspiration. Furthermore, holding the infant during feeding provides warmth, comfort, and bonding, all vital factors in providing a feeling of love and security.

Motor Development

At 2 months, the infant is able to hold the head up while in the prone position. By 4 months, the infant has the ability to hold the head up steadily to a 90-degree angle while in the prone position. At 6 months, most infants are able to balance the head quite well. By the end of the seventh month, infants have acquired the ability to sit up steadily without support.

Locomotion

Crawling, an early means of movement, is a motion made with the infant's abdomen touching the floor (Figure 9-2, *F*). A more advanced form of locomotion is creeping. The infant accomplishes this by resting the weight on the hands and knees. Infants sometimes crawl at 7 months and creep at about 9 months. Creeping appears after age 9 months in most children (Figure 9-2, *G*). Standing with support and walking follow at about 8 months to 15 months (Figure 9-2, *D*).

Psychosocial Development

Erikson defined the task of the infant as basic trust versus mistrust. The responsiveness of others to the needs of the infant helps establish the basis of trust. Infants obtain gratification when their basic needs are fulfilled. Infants whose needs are not met develop a sense of dissatisfaction or mistrust. (See Table 9-2 for an overview of Erikson's stages of psychosocial development.)

Cognitive and Intellectual Development

During this stage, the infant uses the senses to learn about self and environment. The infant learns by exploration of objects and events and by interaction. Piaget describes the infant as being in the sensorimotor stage of cognitive development.

In the **sensorimotor stage,** an infant's knowledge comes about primarily through sensory impressions and motor activities. Behavior is completely reflective. The infant develops an image or **schema** (an innate knowledge structure that allows a child to mentally organize ways to behave in the immediate environ-

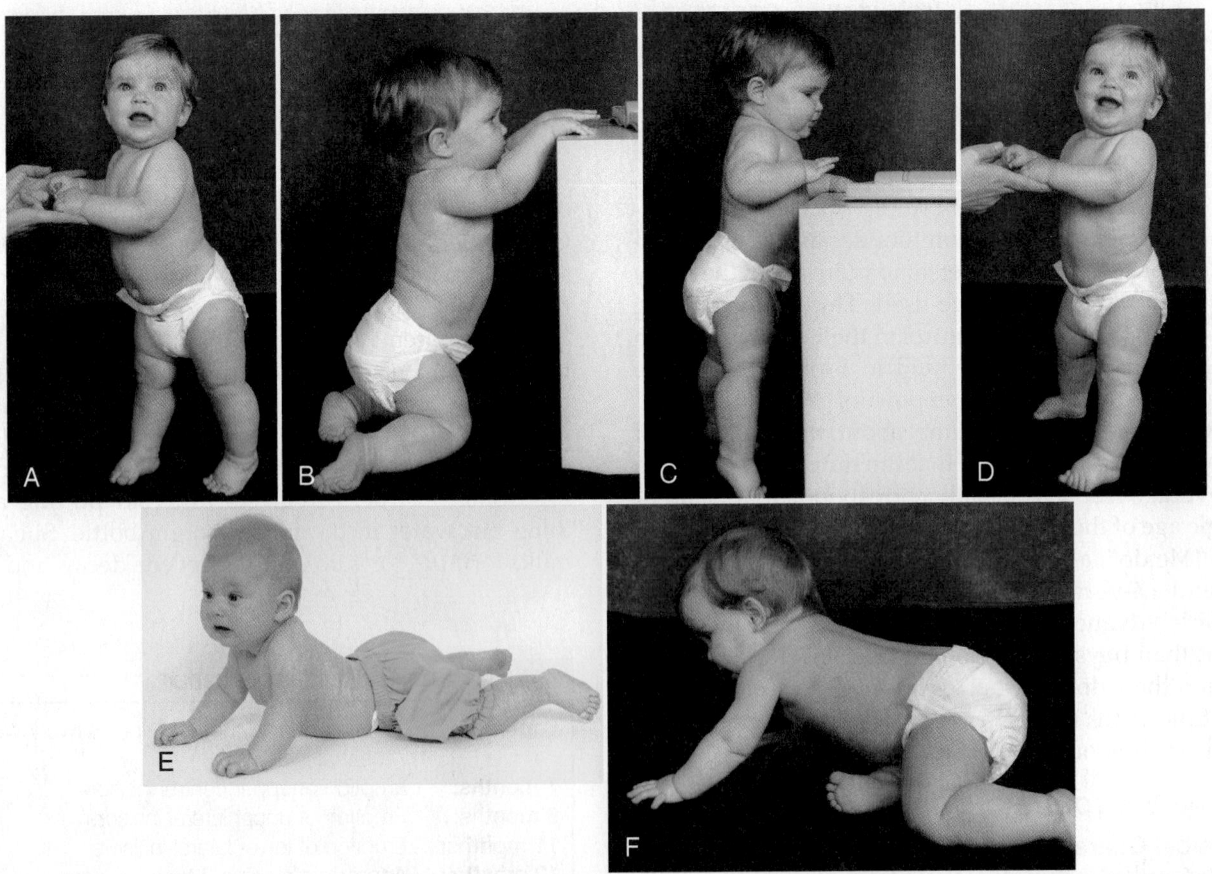

FIGURE 9-2 Development of locomotion. **A,** Infant bears full weight on feet by 7 months. **B,** Infant can maneuver from sitting to kneeling position. **C,** Infant can stand holding onto furniture at 9 months. **D,** While standing, infant takes deliberate step at 10 months. **E,** Infant crawls with abdomen on floor and pulls self forward, and then, **F,** creeps on hands and knees at 9 months. (Photos by Paul Vincent Kuntz, Texas Children's Hospital, Houston, Texas.)

ment) and assimilates and interprets the information. Infants learn by encountering and responding to stimulation from the environment. As the infant interacts with the environment, there are changes in mental structure and in development of thinking ability. During the first 1 to 4 months, the infant follows objects visually with the eyes and auditorily with the ears. By 4 months of age, infants become notably better at using both eyes together. This makes them more astute observers. From 4 to 8 months of age, the infant begins to recognize and imitate. Reaching and grasping are improved skills.

By age 3 months, most infants respond differently to the parents or primary caregiver than they do to other people. By age 4 months, many infants are able to identify the voices of the most familiar people in their lives. Smiling occurs in response to different people and events. At the sight of the parents or primary caregivers, the infant will smile and begin to vocalize.

Beginning at approximately 8 months of age, infants show anxiety when they are separated from their primary caregiver. There is shyness and a fear of strangers. The infant may cling and protest any separation from the primary caregiver(s). By age 9 months, most children will show alarm at the presence of a stranger. Parents and child develop a form of synchrony (happening at the same time; moving or operating at the same rate). It is thought that infants who develop a secure early attachment will later have the confidence to seek out future relationships. Studies on children ages 15 to 30 months who had good attachment relationships showed that they experienced a predictable behavior pattern following separation, known as separation anxiety.

Health Promotion

Nutrition

Both human breast milk and commercially prepared formula are options that meet the nutritional needs of the infant. Even though today's excellent infant formulas approximate human milk, breast milk is still almost always the best food for newborns. It has been called the "ultimate health food," because it offers so many benefits. However, infants who are fed with properly prepared formula and raised with love also grow up healthy and well adjusted. Breast milk or formula is the only food most babies need until they are about 4 to 6 months of age. Most experts agree that newborns should be fed when hungry. Early in life this may mean that babies are fed as often as every 2 hours. In the beginning, nursing mothers often start nursing for 10 to 15 minutes on each breast and then lengthen the feeding time as demanded by the infant. When the infant suckles more slowly or appears uninterested in either the breast or bottle, it is a good indication that he or she has had enough. Weighing the infant will help evaluate the success of either of the feeding methods. Signs of underfeeding include lack of satisfaction; cranky, fussy baby; little weight gain; and persistent wrinkling of the skin. Signs of overfeeding include vomiting after feeding and frequent watery stools. Full-term infants have enough stored iron to last for at least the first 5 to 6 months of age. After this time, iron supplements or food sources are options to replenish the diminishing supply. It is generally accepted that it is best to avoid certain foods in the first 6 months of life. Those foods include citrus fruits, egg whites, and wheat flour, all frequently identified as allergy-producing substances.

There is much controversy regarding the best time to introduce solid foods into the infant diet. Many physicians believe that very early introduction of solids leads to a variety of problems. Rather than deciding on when to introduce solid food, it is simpler to describe how to first introduce these foods into the infant diet. The rules for solid foods include the following:

- Introduce only one new food at a time, allowing several days between new foods.
- Introduce cereals first, fruits and vegetables next, and meats last.
- Avoid mixing foods to allow the infant to develop interest in different foods and tastes.

Never leave the infant alone while eating because infants choke easily on certain foods. Avoid giving older infants round, hard foods that are easily caught in the throat. Foods that have high potential to cause choking include popcorn, grapes, raisins, hot dogs, and chicken nuggets.

This often serves as an excellent time to look at the type of foods the whole family is eating. It is best to try to limit the amount of sodium, fats, and sugar in the family diet. Lifelong eating habits are largely established early on, in these toddler years. Offer the entire family plenty of fresh fruits, vegetables, lean meats, and whole grains.

In warmer weather, febrile conditions, prolonged vomiting, and diarrhea will place infants at higher risk for dehydration because of their small fluid volume. It is important for infants to receive adequate breast milk or bottle fed formula. Infants do not require additional fluids, especially water or juice, during the first 4 months of life. If an infant receives excessive intake of water, this can result in water intoxication, failure to thrive, and hyponatremia (Hockenberry & Wilson, 2007).

By age 8 to 9 months, most babies master eating mashed or junior foods. Self-feeding of finger foods allows the infant further opportunity for exploration. By 9 months of age, suggest introducing a training cup and beginning the process of weaning. This is usually a gradual process, with the cup substituted for one bottle at a time, usually starting with the lunchtime feeding.

Sleep, Play Activity, and Safety

Newborns and infants sleep 18 hours out of 24. These sleep periods usually consist of short, naplike periods. It is normal for the infant to be restless and make noises during these periods. Toward the end of the first 3 months, definite sleep patterns emerge, and nap and wake periods are clearly established. By the end of the first year, the infant will usually sleep 12 hours at night and take one nap during the day. Persistent crying during usual sleep or nap periods often signals discomfort or illness and calls for investigation.

A concern for parents of young infants is sudden infant death syndrome (SIDS). This disorder produces sudden, abrupt death with no identifiable warning signs. Formerly known as crib death, it appears to peak 2 to 3 months after birth. Steps to reduce the incidence of SIDS are outlined in the Safety Alert box.

Safety Alert!

Steps to Reduce the Incidence of SIDS

1. Back to sleep—place infants on their back to sleep.
2. Avoid exposure to cigarette smoke.
3. Avoid using soft bedding or pillows.
4. Keep room well ventilated.
5. Breastfeed if possible.
6. Maintain regular medical checkups for infants.

Play is important for learning. Play that captures the pleasures of using the senses and motor abilities is called sensorimotor play (Figure 9-3). Early play items include turning mobiles, mirrors, colorful shapes, and toys of different textures. As hand coordination improves, other items, such as rattles and shapes, become useful play objects. Toward the end of the first year, stacking items, blocks, and puzzles encourage developing motor skills. Music is useful to soothe the infant or to stimulate awareness of sounds and rhythms. Play style during infancy is described as solitary play. This means that the infant plays alone, not interacting with or needing other children to play. Allowing adequate freedom of movement helps enhance good development of muscles and bones. Young infants need room to stretch and kick. It is important to take care to prevent injury during this early stage of development. Do not push children to sit or walk before adequate muscle strength is achieved.

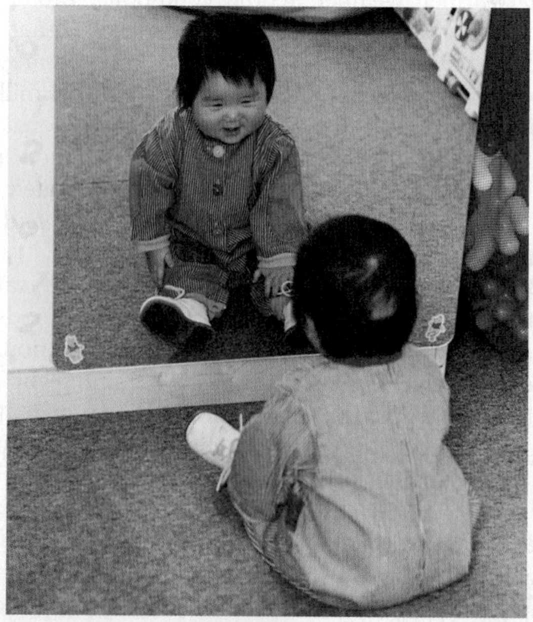

FIGURE 9-3 Nine-month-old infant enjoying own image in a mirror.

Accidents are the leading cause of injury and death in infants and young children. Safety precautions are essential to institute immediately at the birth of the child (Figure 9-4). The Safety Alert box lists safety rules for infants and young children.

Infancy is also a time of daily changes. Goals for the developmental tasks of infancy are shown in Box 9-8.

TODDLER: 1 TO 3 YEARS

Physical Characteristics

Rate of growth in the toddler years is slower than in infancy but follows the same general principles. It is orderly. It proceeds from head to foot, from the center outward, and from general to specific movements.

One of the most striking changes from infancy is the upright stance of the toddler. The chubby look of infancy is gone by 12 to 15 months. In the beginning of this stage, the toddler's body proportions result in a top-heavy appearance. By the end of this period, however, rapid growth of the extremities and slowed growth in the trunk produce a more proportionate body appearance (Figure 9-5). An exaggerated lumbar lordosis (convex lumbar curve) and protruding abdomen produce a potbelly appearance, which disappears as the abdominal muscles strengthen. By age 2.5 years,

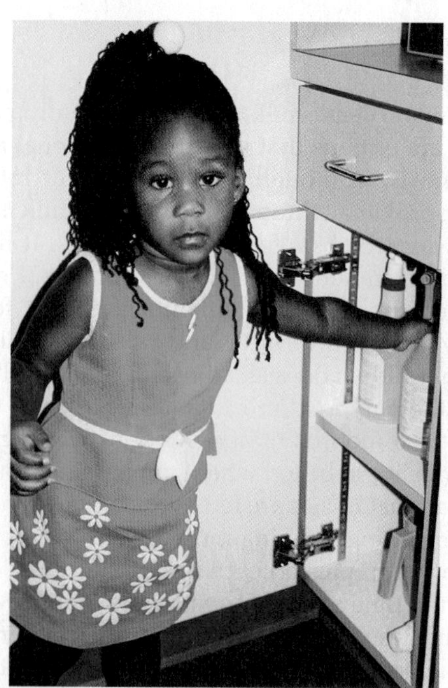

FIGURE 9-4 Children are most likely to ingest substances that are on their level, such as cleaning agents stored under sinks, rat poison, plants, or diaper pail deodorants.

Safety Alert!

Safety Rules for Infants and Young Children

- Never leave an unsupervised infant on an elevated surface.
- Never leave an infant unattended in a high chair, stroller, walker, or any other device.
- Secure stairways and exits.
- Keep crib sides up and set mattress at lowest setting.
- Never leave infants or young children unattended in a bath for even a few seconds.
- Keep windows locked and secured with child guards.
- Never use plastic bags or coverings on mattresses or near infant's playthings.
- Avoid the use of pillows with small infants.
- Infant cribs must meet U.S. Consumer Product Safety regulations to prevent strangulation between crib bars.
- Remove wires and dangling electric cords from the crawling child's reach. Cover outlets with protective caps.
- Inspect all toys carefully for long strings and small removable parts.
- Use pacifiers that have one-piece construction.
- Do not allow children to play with balloons.
- Avoid giving infants and young children hard candies, nuts, popcorn, and other foods that are easily aspirated.
- Lock all poisons and medicines out of infants' and young children's reach (see Figure 9-4).
- Avoid drinking hot fluids while holding an infant.
- Check temperature of foods and formula before feeding.
- Turn pot handles toward back of stove and remove burner knobs if within child's reach.
- Avoid smoking near infants and children to prevent burns and smoke inhalation.
- Keep infants and children away from hot surfaces, stoves, fireplaces, and barbecues.
- Use flame-retardant sleepwear.
- Never say that medication is candy to facilitate administration.
- Keep poison control hotline phone number accessible.
- Keep plants out of child's reach.
- Use plastic rather than glass eating and drinking utensils.
- Inspect toys and household items for sharp points.
- Inspect for chipped lead-based paint on surfaces painted before 1978 (production of lead paint for consumer use was banned in 1978).
- Keep knives and forks away from young children.
- Supervise infants and children playing around animals and pets.
- Teach children early about street dangers and supervise their play.
- Instruct children to never go anywhere with strangers.
- Teach young children the use of the telephone for emergencies.
- Instruct children that others should not touch their "private" body parts and to report happenings if they occur. Accept the child's story unless you can prove otherwise.
- Always use safety seats and restraints when transporting infants and young children.

Box 9-8 Developmental Tasks of Infancy

- Establishes trusting, meaningful relationships
- Recognizes primary caregiver
- Develops attachment behavior
- Learns to recognize objects
- Develops exploration skills
- Develops communication skills by beginning vocalization, developing nonverbal communication system, and imitating simple vocalizations
- Develops muscular control, eye-hand coordination, and object manipulation
- Develops mobility: crawling, creeping, cruising, walking
- Establishes patterns of living: eating, sleeping, elimination habits
- Begins to develop independent living skills: self-feeding, walking, undressing, communication of needs

all 20 deciduous teeth are present. Advise parents to begin routine dental examinations and toothbrushing during this period.

Vital Signs

During the toddler period, the pulse ranges from 90 to 120 beats per minute. Blood pressure averages 80 to 100 mm Hg systolic and 64 mm Hg diastolic. Body temperature ranges between 98° and 99° F (36.6° and 37.2° C). Respiration slows to 20 to 30 breaths per minute.

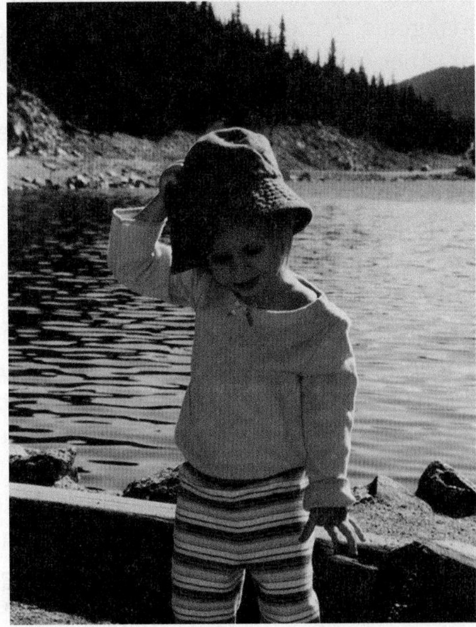

FIGURE 9-5 The toddler with proportionate body appearance.

Neuromuscular Development

Many gross motor skills emerge in this period, including walking, climbing stairs (2 years), and hopping (3 years). The toddler develops running, pulling, and holding-on-tight skills, exploring the world in ways previously impossible. This is also the time fine motor skills begin to be acquired, such as beginning to scribble (2 years) and copying a circle (3 years).

Toilet Training

Children do not reach the physiologic or psychological maturity necessary to begin toilet training until 18 to 24 months of age. Children need to reach maturity so they have neuromuscular control, the cognitive ability to understand what is expected of them, and the language skills to express their needs. Bowel control is achieved first. Bladder control begins at the same time but takes longer to achieve. Nighttime control is usually achieved after daytime control is established. Advise parents and caregivers to expect setbacks and accidents, particularly during times of stress or illness. Deemphasize accidents; never make the child feel inadequate. That is, praise success and ignore accidents. If praise is given for toileting successes and accidents are cleaned up without negativism, the toddler will gain a sense of self-control, inner goodness, and pride. However, if the toddler is punished and made to feel foolish, a sense of shame will develop. If the toddler is kept in diapers and given no opportunities to control the urges, a sense of doubt will be fostered. Feelings of shame and doubt are not healthy personality attributes.

Psychosocial Development

The toddler is an uninhibited, energetic little person, always seeking attention, approval, and achievement of personal goals. Sometimes the toddler is cuddly and loving; at other times, biting, hitting, or pinching prevails. The toddler only slowly realizes that everything desired cannot be had and that some behaviors annoy others. The toddler tries to be independent, yet becomes easily frightened and runs to the caregiver for protection, security, reassurance, and approval.

Erikson sees the toddler as struggling with autonomy (self-control) in opposition to shame and doubt. With newfound skills of independence, walking, talking, self-feeding, and beginning toilet training, the toddler is struggling to be independent. Characteristic of this search for autonomy is the toddler's use of the word "no," which gives a sense of control. The toddler possesses endless energy, yet often falls asleep almost while still in motion. As toddlers struggle for independence, you will frequently see possessiveness and a desire to have things go their way. Ritualistic behavior and repetitive rituals are self-consoling behaviors at this stage. Toddlers enjoy the same story, the same routine, and the same foods at each meal. Rituals decrease their anxiety by helping them know what to expect. When health care providers follow a hospitalized child's usual rituals, the toddler will feel safer and more secure in the strange environment.

Temper tantrums are common and are the result of frustration. A combination of wanting things "my way," the inability to communicate feelings, and the lack of impulse control are perhaps behind outbursts of temper. This type of negativism is best ignored unless the child or others are in danger of harm.

Toddlers need many experiences of being able to choose among alternatives (to play inside or outside, to wear green pants or red pants). However, advise caregivers to make use of questions and offer alternatives for children only in situations in which either choice will be acceptable. When a particular behavior is necessary (such as going to bed, holding hands to cross a street, letting go of another child's hair), it is better not to offer a choice. Erikson stressed that young children do not have the wisdom to know what behaviors are acceptable or unacceptable, healthy or unhealthy.

Discipline is a necessary means of teaching limit setting and impulse control. Basic principles of discipline are listed in Box 9-9. Toddlers seek attention, approval, and love as they struggle for independence.

Cognitive and Intellectual Development

The period from 12 to 24 months of age completes the last phase of sensorimotor development, in which the toddler's knowledge of the world comes about primarily through sensory impression and motor activities. The period of early childhood is the **preoperational thought stage**. (When the child focuses on the use of language as a tool to meet needs, the child has the emerging ability to think mentally.) The child uses trial and error to discover new traits and characteristics. According to Piaget, this stage extends from 2 to 7 years of age.

Toddlers are constantly absorbing new ideas, widening their cognitive world, and expanding memory. Activities can be connected to past events or memories. The toddler's concept of time is limited to the present. The child's thinking is egocentric at this stage. Toddlers are often demanding, wanting things to go their way.

Communication and Language

Cognitive and language development make it possible for toddlers to think about their actions and make their will known to their caregivers. "No!" and "Me!" (meaning "Let me do it myself") are oft-repeated holophrases of 2- and 3-year-olds.

Box 9-9 Basic Principles of Discipline

- Consistency: Apply rules uniformly
- Follow-through: Say and do what you mean
- Positive modeling: Practice role model–approved behavior
- Promptness: Administer any punishment in a nonhostile manner immediately after incident occurs
- Trust: Express trust in the child
- Prevention: Remove temptation
- Reinforcement: Offer positive reinforcement for acceptable behavior

During the toddler period, the child identifies objects by use. At 2.5 years of age, the toddler's vocabulary consists of about 450 words and two-word sentences consisting of a noun and verb, for example, "Me run." By 3.5 years of age, the child is able to answer questions and use brief sentences, and even recites television commercials. The 3-year-old's vocabulary is approximately 900 words. Strongly encourage parents to read to their toddlers. Being read to not only increases the child's vocabulary but provides a pleasant environment that enhances child-caregiver bonding.

Health Promotion

Nutrition

Good nutrition requires that the toddler's daily diet consist of one serving from the meat group; two or more servings of vegetables; and at least two servings of fruit, cereal, or breads. The MyPyramid guidelines (www.mypyramid.gov) should be followed. The child needs 24 ounces of milk per day. Too few solid foods can lead to iron deficiency. Most children are more likely to eat foods with which they are familiar; therefore gradual introduction of new foods is advisable. Bite-sized pieces, finger foods, and smaller portions are generally more acceptable. Idiosyncratic eating patterns are common at this stage. Toddlers need less food per unit of body weight than they did during infancy. A general guideline for serving size is 1 tablespoon of each solid food for each year of age. Parents need to be informed that during illness, brief periods of anorexia are usually not serious.

Sleep, Play Activity, and Safety

Toddlers expend a high level of energy in daily growth, play, and exploration. Adequate rest and sleep are essential for maintaining optimal wellness. The toddler requires 12 hours of sleep each night plus a daytime nap. Suggestions helpful in promoting healthy sleeping patterns include limiting stimulation before sleep time, using quiet-time activities before sleep, allowing a favorite bedtime toy, telling a specified number of stories, and establishing and maintaining bedtime rituals. Box 9-10 lists guidelines for bedtime preparation.

Play improves muscle coordination, balance, and muscle strength. The toddler's play style, described as

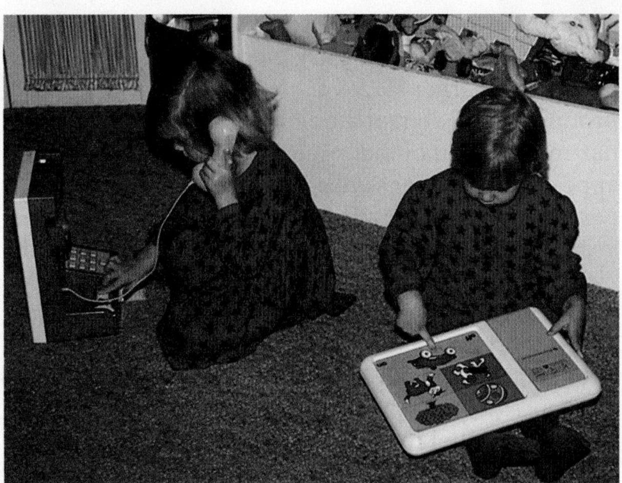

FIGURE 9-6 Parallel play.

parallel play (Figure 9-6), refers to the need that toddlers have to play alongside of, but not with, their peers. Unable to share and interact with their peers at this stage, they will play side by side with similar toys in similar ways, but they without interacting. Toddlers thrive on activities that keep them on the go. Running, jumping, and climbing help toddlers to develop bones and muscles. This age-group's natural curiosity about how things work encourages them to explore. Play groups help encourage the shy or reluctant child to participate and try new activities.

More than half of all childhood deaths are caused by accidents, many of which are motor vehicle accidents. About 90% of the accidents that occur in the home are believed to be preventable. Prevention methods must include both supervision and education.

The developmental tasks of toddlers are summarized in Box 9-11.

PRESCHOOL: 3 TO 5 YEARS

Physical Characteristics

Physical development during early childhood occurs on many fronts, with the most important—maturation of the nervous system and mastery of motor skills—being the least obvious; the most obvious are the striking changes in size and shape.

Box 9-10 Guidelines for Bedtime Preparation

- Reduce activity level before bedtime
- Establish a simple ritual (e.g., bathroom, story time, goodnight song)
- Make bedtime a pleasurable experience
- Familiarize child with routine nightly
- Reassure child that he or she is not alone
- Use a night-light
- Expect disruptions or setbacks during and after illness and stress or after stimulating activities

Box 9-11 Developmental Tasks of the Toddler

- Recognizes self as a separate person; tolerates separation from primary caregiver, expresses own ideas and needs
- Develops increased attention span
- Begins to develop communication skills
- Begins to develop self-control skills
- Masters toilet-training basics
- Achieves independent mobility
- Develops independent skills of daily living: feeding, dressing, toileting, and managing simple tasks

Growth during the preschool period tends to be slow and steady. The preschooler looks taller and thinner than at earlier stages as the toddler's lordosis and protuberant abdomen are left behind (as the abdominal muscles strengthen, the child loses the potbelly appearance). Average weight gain is less than 5 pounds per year. Linear growth is about 2 to 2.5 inches per year. Height of the 4-year-old is usually double the birth length. The gait of the preschooler becomes steadier. The preschooler is more capable of focusing and refining activities, and the body grows slimmer, stronger, and less top-heavy. Because of these developments, gross motor skills (large body movements such as running, climbing, jumping, and throwing) improve dramatically. Such tasks as tying shoelaces, cutting food with a knife and fork, and putting together a puzzle prove more difficult because of the preschooler's undeveloped fine motor skills (skills that involve small body movements); these are much harder for them to master than gross motor skills. It is important to encourage development of fine motor skills. The scribbling of the young child is comparable with the babbling of the infant. Both are ways to obtain practice with the means to later mastery of essential communication skills. Providing pencils, crayons, markers, and paper is as important as providing things to climb, things to throw, and places to run.

Vision in the younger preschooler is described as farsighted. Vision improves during this period, and most children achieve 20/30 visual accuracy by age 4. A yearly check of preschool children's vision is recommended. Sometimes ambylopia, a condition commonly known as lazy eye, is detected during a simple eye examination. Corrective measures such as patching the good eye usually strengthen the lazy eye and are necessary to prevent blindness. By age 6, the child begins to lose the deciduous teeth.

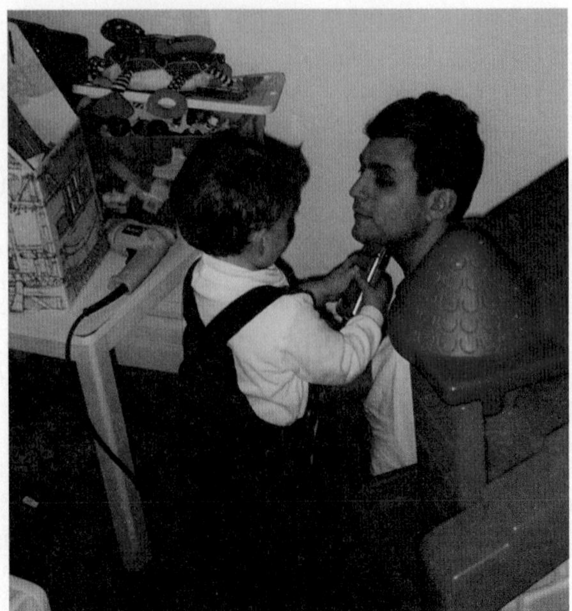

FIGURE 9-7 Trying out new roles.

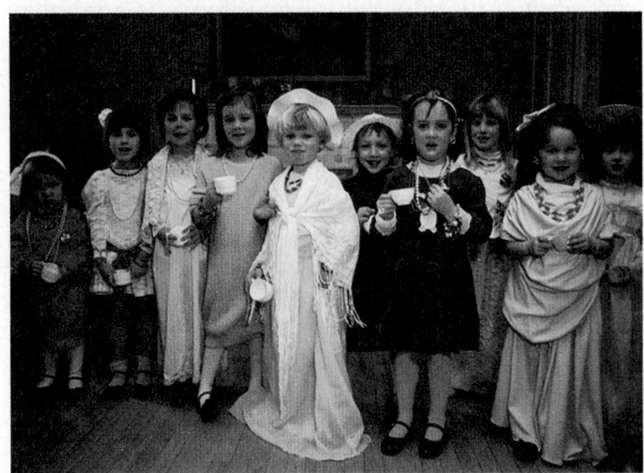

FIGURE 9-8 Young children enjoy dressing up.

Vital Signs

Heart rate for the preschooler ranges between 70 and 110 beats per minute. Respiratory rate slows down to about 23 breaths per minute at rest. Blood pressure averages 110/60 mm Hg. Temperature ranges from 97° to 99° F (36.1° to 37.2° C), depending on the method used for measurement.

Psychosocial Development

First the child learns to function independently, and subsequently to use imagination to creatively explore new experiences. Erikson describes the task of the preschooler in terms of initiative versus guilt. Preschoolers search for and create fantasies about the different kinds of people they would like to become. They pretend to be grown up and try out a variety of roles (Figures 9-7 and 9-8). During the preschool period, the child's superego (conscience) functions as a censor of behavior. The dilemma of the preschooler, according to Erikson, is to test his or her initiative without creating an overwhelming sense of guilt. Typical development of the preschooler includes gender identification. It is common at this time for the child to stereotype roles and to show marked interest in sexual differences. Strong sibling bonding is established (Figure 9-9).

Cognitive and Intellectual Development

According to Piaget, the preschool child is at the preoperational stage of cognitive development. Preschoolers use symbols to represent objects. They use trial and error to discover and adopt new traits and characteristics. Between ages 4 and 7 years, intuitive thinking develops and the child begins to think logically. Children in the preoperational stage see the world from their own viewpoint. They see things as absolutes, in terms of white and black. All things are to the preschool child either good or bad.

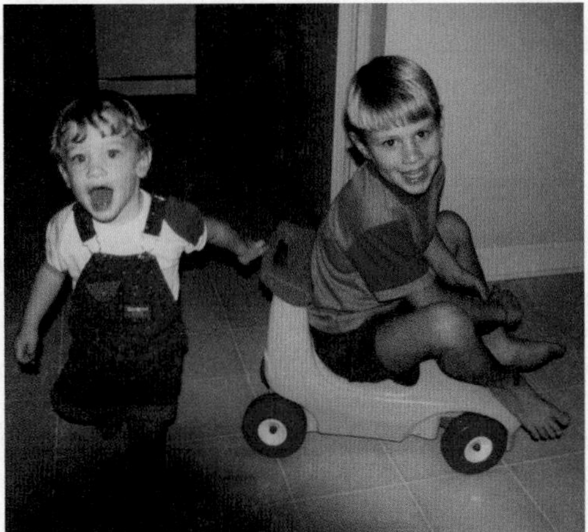

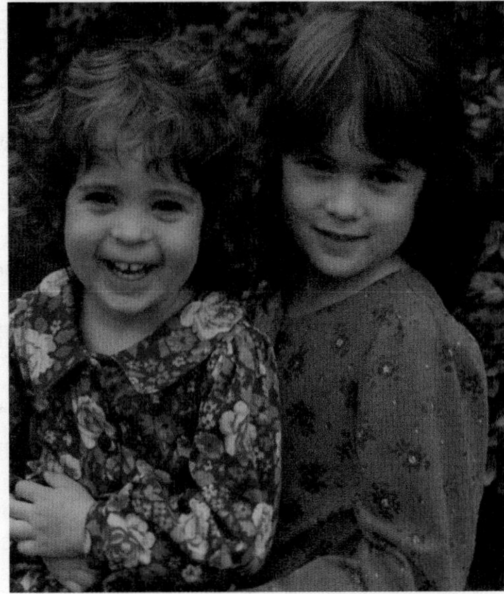

FIGURE 9-9 Siblings establishing a bond.

During the preschool stage, time is associated with weekly and seasonal events. Magical thoughts are typical of the child of this age, who believes that wishes have the power to make things happen. As a result the preschool child sometimes feels powerful—and responsible for events that occur. Believing that a wish has caused serious harm or even death to a loved one, the preschooler will at times feel guilty. The occasional "white lies" or untruths of this period usually reflect some of the child's fantasies. During this stage of development, the child needs trustworthy guidance to distinguish truth from fantasy. At this stage, the child is more vulnerable to certain fears, probably fallout from the typically vivid imagination. Excessive exposure to inappropriate television content and other media have potential to further distort reality testing. Common fears manifesting at this stage include fear of thunder, lightning, the dark, pain, abandonment, and monsters.

Communication and Language

By age 3 years, children are able to carry on a conversation. Pronunciation problems continue into the school years. Language becomes more adultlike. If the child is not talking by age 3 years, evaluation by a physician for possible hearing loss or other pathologic speech disturbances is necessary. Advise parents to continue to read to their child, because this helps expand language ability and comprehension and continues to foster positive child-caregiver relationships.

Health Promotion

Nutrition

Because body systems and muscles are still growing steadily, the preschool child continues to need high levels of protein. Dietary calcium and phosphorus are important to both toddlers and preschool children because of the increasing mineralization of their teeth and bones. Food habits, likes, dislikes, and appetites vary greatly from child to child. Some physicians recommend supplementary vitamins. Vitamins, like any other medication, are not intended and do not have the capacity to take the place of good eating habits (see Chapter 21).

Generally a weight increase of 20% or more is considered an indication of obesity. Most cultures hold strong views regarding obesity, resulting in emotional consequences for an obese child. Controlling weight is an important parental concern because it helps prevent serious health issues later in life. Overweight infants are more likely to become overweight later in life. It is possible that genetic factors predispose individuals to becoming obese. Children often adopt eating habits of parents. Make suggestions to parents of ways to help with their children's weight control: Model good eating behaviors, provide healthy food, and encourage physical activity.

Sleep, Play Activity, and Safety

Preschoolers often resist nap periods but still need 11 to 12 hours of sleep at night. Rest periods offered during the day enable children to reenergize and carry out the rest of their daily activities.

Play style for the preschool child becomes cooperative. The child begins to share, take turns, and interact with playmates (Figure 9-10). Preschoolers enjoy pretending to carry out activities such as cooking, shopping, and driving. Through dramatic play, the child tries on different roles and identifies with adult models. Not only is it fun for two or more children to cooperate in creating their own scenario, but it also helps their social development to try out social roles, express their fears and fantasies, and learn to cooperate. Experiences with imaginary playmates are not uncommon in this age-group. Children often feel a sense of control over what happens in their "imaginary world" and slowly learn to deal with reality through practice and experimentation.

Children during the preschool period are becoming more coordinated and want to begin participating in more organized games. By age 4 to 5, children learn to ride a bicycle with training wheels. They will need

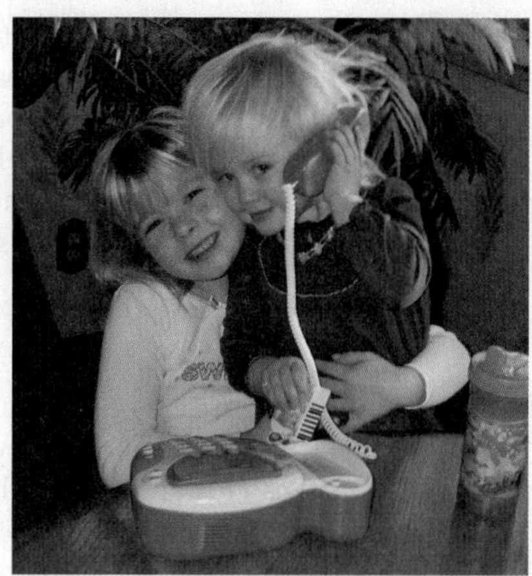
FIGURE 9-10 Playmates.

guidance because they have difficulty maneuvering their bicycle, and their judgment and awareness of safety issues is limited (see Safety Alert box for safety and injury prevention tips for preschool children). Swimming, skating, and dancing are activities that this age-group often begin to learn and enjoy. It is important for activities of this nature to be fun for the child. It is not beneficial or appropriate for children to be pressured to participate in activities that they do not like or enjoy. Also advise parents and caregivers to space activities so that children are not overstressed by having too many lessons, practices, or games.

Safety Alert!

Safety Tips and Injury Prevention for Preschool Children

- Use proper equipment that fits the child.
- Never leave children alone in pools of water. Teach children not to touch or go near pool drains.
- Inspect protective equipment, such as bicycle helmets, for potential hazards.
- Use protective sunscreen.

All the safety precautions described earlier apply to the preschool child as well as the infant and toddler (see the Safety Alert box). Instruct parents and caregivers to teach preschool children their full names, addresses, and telephone numbers. The child needs to know how to use the phone in case of an emergency.

Discipline and limit setting are needed and are as important to the child as are love and security. Necessary guidance includes offering alternative ways of expressing feelings and meeting needs (Box 9-12).

The preschool period is a time of learning to function independently and exploring the imagination. Box 9-13 shows the developmental tasks of preschoolers.

Box 9-12 Steps for Discipline and Limit Setting

- Define acceptable as opposed to unacceptable behaviors.
- Set limits: "I will not let you hurt anyone."
- Be consistent: keep the same rules, and enforce them reliably.
- Recognize escalating emotions and intervene: "I can see you're upset—let's go over there and sit down."
- Suggest "time out."
- Choose punishment that "fits" wrongdoing, and enact it in a timely way (and in a nonhostile manner).
- Praise and reinforce positive behavior: "I like the way you . . ."
- Always start over with a clean slate.
- Stay calm; avoid arguing.
- Avoid putdowns: "You're acting like a bad boy."
- Remember to listen to the child.

Box 9-13 Developmental Tasks of Preschoolers

- Develops stronger sense of self; is able to express own needs, ideas, and feelings; has capacity to postpone immediate gratification
- Attains greater attention span; listens more attentively
- Develops and refines gross motor skills and fine motor skills
- Recognizes sex identification
- Begins to work and play more cooperatively with others
- Improves communication skills
- Develops self-control skills; learns socially acceptable ways of expressing anger, frustration, and disappointment; obeys simple rules; develops self-awareness and sense of self-protection
- Seeks information, asks questions, learns values and beliefs of the family

SCHOOL AGE: 6 TO 12 YEARS

Physical Characteristics

During the school-age period, the growth pattern is usually gradual and subtle. The most obvious growth is in the long bones of the extremities and in the development of the facial bones. As a result of this bone growth, some children complain of "growing pains," particularly at night. Persistent pains call for evaluation by a physician to rule out any underlying pathologic condition. From ages 6 to 12, height and weight increase by about 2 inches and 4.5 to 6.5 pounds per year for both boys and girls.

Motor skills in boys and girls develop with some differences; boys often become stronger, and girls more graceful and accurate.

The child's posture becomes straighter. The causes of poor posture range from fatigue to emotional states or even minor skeletal defects. Ensure that school-age children are routinely screened for scoliosis (abnormal lateral curvature of the spine). Muscle mass and strength gradually increase, and the body loses the "baby fat" appearance of earlier childhood. Both gross motor and fine motor development continue to be refined during the school-age years.

Vision improves, and most children have 20/20 vision at this stage. Regular vision testing is advisable throughout the school years.

Vital Signs

Heart and respiratory rate steadily decrease, whereas blood pressure increases. Normal pulse rate is between 55 and 90 per minute, respiratory rate is 22 to 24 per minute, and blood pressure is 110/65 mm Hg.

Dentition

Permanent teeth develop rapidly. Regular dental checkups are recommended every 6 months throughout childhood.

Psychosocial Development

Entrance into school challenges the child and creates demands for new social and cognitive skills. The child becomes more independent and participates in a broader world of peers and new experiences. School-age children become increasingly aware of rules and socialization skills and expectations. The beginning abilities to compromise and compete are the challenges facing this age-group.

Erikson identified the task of the school-age years as industry versus inferiority. After the child realizes that "there is no workable future within the womb of his family," says Erikson, the school-age child "becomes ready to apply himself to given skills and tasks." Children develop their own goals and direct their efforts toward mastery of these goals. As children discover their talents and accomplishments, they gain self-confidence and a sense of purpose. During these years, the child learns to work and masters skills that produce satisfaction as the result of that work. Successful mastery of learning in school leads to strengthening and stabilizing the child's sense of self. According to Erikson, as children busily try to master the skills valued in their culture, they develop views of themselves as either competent or incompetent—as either industrious and productive or inferior and inadequate.

Input from the outside is a key factor in which direction the child's self-concept will take. If the environment inadequately supports a child's pursuits, the stage will perhaps be set for the development of feelings of inferiority and the lack of self-confidence. The good school setting is a pleasant, comfortable environment. Teachers and caregivers need to use praise, encouragement, and rewards to positively reinforce the school-age child's efforts. Teachers also have to be positive role models. School helps the child learn new routines and establish important social relationships (Figure 9-11).

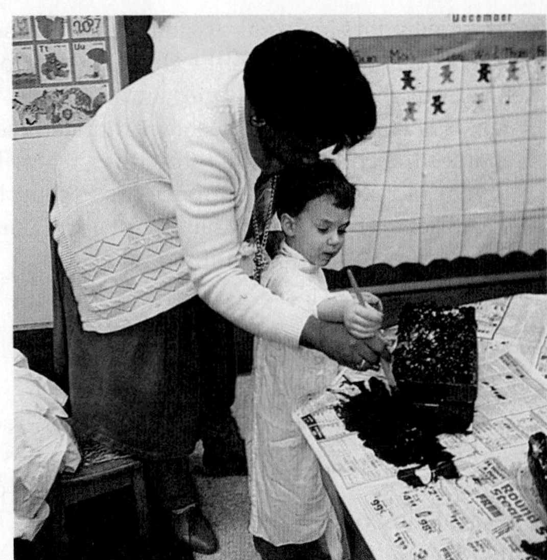

FIGURE 9-11 School represents an important change in a child's life, and teachers exert a significant influence on the child.

Cognitive and Intellectual Development

According to Piaget, children in the school years move into the **concrete operational phase**. During this phase, thoughts become increasingly logical and coherent, so that the child is able to classify, sort, and organize facts while still being incapable of generalizing or dealing with abstractions. Children have the capacity to think rationally about almost any specific and concrete perception. Between ages 7 and 11, children usually come to understand logical principles—again, as long as the principles can be applied to concrete, specific cases. They distinguish purpose from behavior and outcome and are able to focus on more than one aspect of a task. Children in this age-group have begun to develop logical socialized thought. They view the world more realistically than they did at younger ages, and they are capable of understanding the views of others. Movement is away from fantasy as the child realizes that a physical cause is behind an event. The child's developing cognitive skills serve as a motivator for learning how to work. A supportive learning environment will often enhance the child's approach to problem solving and helps lead to success.

The school-age child experiences gradual and subtle growth changes while learning new social and cognitive skills. Box 9-14 contains a list of the developmental tasks of the school-age child.

Communication and Language

Most 6-year-olds have a good command of sentence structure. The child's vocabulary has become more extensive and includes slang and swear words, which many children enjoy using for the effect they create. Fine motor development continues and, combined with growth in cognitive and communication skills,

Box 9-14 Developmental Tasks of the School-Age Child

- Develops a sense of belonging with family, peers
- Develops work habits; learns to organize, set, and reach goals, evaluate work, and accept criticism
- Learns competence in reading, writing, calculation, grammar, and communication
- Refines fine- and gross-motor coordination

produces refinements in written-language and musical abilities. By age 7, the hands of the child have become steadier. Printing becomes clearer and smaller. Between ages 8 and 10, the hand becomes more efficient, which enables the child to write rather than print. The 10- to 12-year-old child has the capacity to accomplish complex, intricate, fine-quality handcrafts and sometimes begins piano, violin, or guitar lessons.

Health Promotion

Nutrition

Total metabolic needs are largely determined by the energy expenditure of each individual child. The sedentary, quiet child who prefers fine motor activities requires fewer calories than the child who is more oriented to athletics or is more physically active. The recommended daily intake of food is listed at the MyPyramid website (see Chapter 21).

Building on toddler-age and preschool-age foundations, strong dietary habits and food preferences are laid down during the school-age period. Cultural influences, family habits, and peer pressure are all critical factors in how a child's food habits develop. Obesity during this period is closely correlated with obesity in adult years, and therefore it is necessary to maintain the child's weight within normal limits. In middle childhood, obese children are teased, picked on, and rejected. They know they are overweight, and they often hate themselves for it. Obese children usually have fewer friends than other children. The best way to get children to lose weight is to increase their physical activity. Indeed, inactivity is possibly as responsible for childhood obesity as overeating. Diets high in saturated fat increase a child's risk for high blood cholesterol, as well as earlier occurrence of heart disease unless steps are taken to lower these levels.

Sleep, Play Activity, and Safety

Fatigue, irritability, inattention, and poor learning are often signs of inadequate sleep. The 6-year-old needs about 12 hours of sleep at night. By 12 years of age, the child usually needs about 10 hours of sleep. Some children have frequent nightmares that disrupt their sleep. Stress, violence on television, and overtiredness all have the potential to contribute to a child's nightmares. Relaxation techniques such as quiet music, story time, and bathing often help the child relax before sleep.

School-age children need adequate exercise to enhance muscle development, coordination, balance, and strength. In addition, music, craft projects, board games, appropriate television, and video games are all enjoyed by the school-age child. Privacy and a place for their belongings are important at this age. The school-age child is often a willing worker and enjoys being paid for small jobs. Collection and hoarding of "treasures" among their belongings are a part of this stage of development.

Many children during the school years become involved with competitive or team sports (Figure 9-12). Children of this age show interest and loyalty to peers of the same sex. They learn to follow the rules of games. Some are able to benefit from team competitiveness and use it to motivate themselves to excel. Others shy away from competition and become disinterested or develop feelings of inadequacy and disappointment.

Accidents are still the leading cause of death in this age-group. Impulsiveness, poor judgment, curiosity, and incomplete control over motor coordination are some of the factors that increase the school-age child's risk of accidents.

Television often exerts a powerful influence on a child's development. One concern about television today is the increased amount of violence it portrays. Many believe that a good deal of available television content offers the child a potent model for aggressive behavior. Suggest ways for parents to help reduce the negative influence of television: (1) limit the amount of time children watch; (2) screen programs for content and age appropriateness; and (3) watch programs with children and discuss the content.

Preventing school violence is another critical issue these days. **School violence** is defined as anything that physically or psychologically injures schoolchildren or damages school property. Today there appears to be an increase in school violence in many locations. Two factors possibly contributing to this increase are an increased availability of weapons and a breakdown of communication. Experts agree that children need resources to help them deal with the daily stressors that they face. Many children today spend less time with

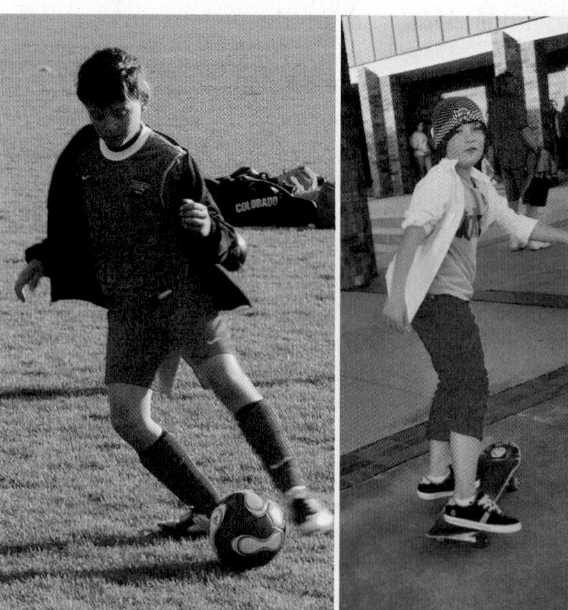

FIGURE 9-12 Activities engaged in by school-age children, such as soccer and skateboarding, vary according to the child's interest and opportunity.

parents and more time in front of a television and on the Internet watching or playing violent shows and games. Children need to feel comfortable discussing their feelings and concerns with parents and teachers, and to use these discussions to learn how to recognize if they are in danger or if others are exhibiting signs of troubled behavior. Encourage parents to ask questions about their child's feelings and their school activities on a daily basis. If children have difficulty talking to parents or answering their questions, advise parents to seek professional help. It is a key responsibility of parents to stay involved and be active participants in their child's daily affairs.

Children need to be taught constructive ways to handle their impulses; otherwise they are more likely to resort to unacceptable ways of channeling their feelings. One possibility is that they will look for revenge, which perhaps makes them feel in control and powerful. Although many children have access to weapons, most of them do not engage in violent behavior. However, we need to work to inhibit violent tendencies, and to look for ways to prevent the few who do act out their feelings in violent ways from causing harm to others (see Safety Alert box). The first step in preventing a tragedy is recognizing the behavioral tendencies that have the potential to lead to violence or other problem behavior. Give children the guidance and encouragement they need to recognize and report the signs of troubled behavior if they notice them in a friend or classmate without feeling that they have deceived the other person or let the other person down (Box 9-15).

Box 9-15 Common Signs of Troubled Childhood Behavior

- Problems getting along with peers
- Difficulty accepting authority and resistance to direction
- Outbursts of uncontrolled behavior
- Bullying tendencies
- Frequent victimizing or teasing
- Socially isolated
- Poor school performance
- Violence to pets or other living creatures
- Preoccupation with weapons
- Verbal expression of threatening behavior or revenge

Safety Alert!

Safety in Schools

- Secure weapons in homes.
- Develop a zero tolerance program with school officials.
- Work with a parent-teacher association (PTA) to make schools safe.
- Determine with school officials an emergency and security plan.
- Maintain open lines of communication between child and parent and school officials.

Gun safety is a must regardless of how one feels about guns. Gun enthusiasts, collectors, and law enforcement agents all are obliged to ensure the safety of others. Most children and many adults have a fascination with guns. Even when children and adults are taught gun safety, some will exhibit unsafe behavior when the opportunity arises. Even toy guns create the potential for dangerous situations. Parents and individuals with weapons in the home are under the obligation to take adequate steps to prevent accidents and injury from their weapons. Knowing how to handle a gun is not sufficient to protect the owner's family and others from injury. It is essential to remove ammunition from firearms and lock guns away securely and apart from ammunition, which is properly kept secured in another, separate locked area. In addition, and most importantly: teach children of all ages what to do if they find a gun (see Safety Alert box).

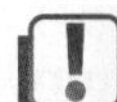

Safety Alert!

Gun Safety Rules

- Stop and **Do Not Touch** any gun, real or toy.
- Leave the area.
- Report to an adult.

ADOLESCENCE: 12 TO 19 YEARS

Physical Characteristics

The term *adolescence* covers the transition period from childhood to adulthood. Adolescence begins at puberty, and accompanying the pubertal changes are corresponding changes in the personality. *Puberty,* the period of life at which the ability to reproduce begins, entails the maturation of the reproductive system, including all the primary and secondary sexual developmental changes. Primary changes occur in the organs related to reproduction (ovaries, breasts, uterus, testes, and penis). Secondary sexual changes occur in other parts of the body (development of pubic and facial hair, voice changes, and fat deposits). Adolescence literally means "to grow into maturity" and is generally regarded as the psychological, social, and maturational process initiated by pubertal changes.

Adolescence is characterized as the second major period of rapid growth. Females grow 2 to 8 inches (5 to 20 cm), whereas males grow 4 to 12 inches (10 to 30 cm). During this adolescent period, females gain 15 to 55 pounds (7 to 25 kg), and males gain 15 to 65 pounds (7 to 30 kg). Whereas females develop more body fat, males develop more muscle tissue. After puberty, men average 50% muscle and 16% fat, whereas women average 40% muscle and 27% fat. Muscle strength and muscle mass increase in the male, causing the average male to have more muscle strength. Exercise facilitates the size, strength, and endurance of each adolescent.

In the female, menarche (the first menstrual period) signals the beginning of adolescence. In the male, sperm production signals the beginning of adolescence.

Body shapes are sex differentiated after puberty. Boys have broader shoulders, narrower hips, and larger limbs. Girls have larger breasts, a narrower waist, wider hips, and a lower center of gravity.

Both boys and girls experience voice changes. Girls' voices become fuller and richer because of the lengthening of their vocal cords. Boys' voices become lower and louder. The deeper male voice results from enlargement of the larynx (the Adam's apple) and lengthening of the vocal cords.

Sexual interests increase markedly in vigor and intensity and are usually focused on members of the opposite sex. New problems arise as adolescents find social disapproval and prohibitions arising in their own conscience conflicting with intense sexual drives.

Vital Signs

Average pulse rate is 70 beats per minute. Respiratory rate averages 20 breaths per minute. Blood pressure increases to 120/70 mm Hg.

Psychosocial Development

Exactly when adolescence begins is different in each individual. Some enter adolescence at an early age; others develop later. Regardless of the exact age of onset, we usually perceive the nearing of this stage by recognizing the onset of distinct behavioral changes. One mother remembers coming home from work one day to find her 11-year-old daughter tight-lipped about school and activities, no longer wanting her mother's opinion or listening ear. Her daughter was now spending most of her time at home in her room behind closed doors. A father takes delight in his son's musical talents and his band's energy and success, although the two do butt heads over the taste of their lyrics and the decibel level.

The period of adolescence is frequently described as difficult and involving a stormy search for oneself. Confronting every adolescent are a changing body, sexual demands, responsibilities, expectations, and questions about values and beliefs. The search for identity amid a world of social pressures creates a painful struggle. Erikson described the developmental task of adolescence as establishing a sense of identity. He proposed the conflict of identity versus role confusion as characteristic of adolescence. The search for a sense of identity, he believed, reaches crisis proportions at this time. Not only does the adolescent need to adjust to a sexually mature body, but also all previous conflicts (trust versus mistrust, autonomy versus doubt, initiative versus guilt, and industry versus inferiority) have to be resolved yet again in light of the newly sensuous self. The period of adolescence requires major reorganization of the personality, resolution of childhood insecurities, and acceptance of adult responsibilities. The value of peers is usually significant to the adolescent (Figure 9-13). Peers influence preferences of dress, speech, and leisure activities. The peer group is often the milieu to learn and test developing interpersonal skills. Many adolescents use conforming behavior to win praise and acceptance by peers. If handled properly, adolescence is often a great period of accomplishment and creativity (Box 9-16).

Cognitive Development

According to Piaget, an individual's cognitive function reaches maturity during adolescence. Piaget describes this stage as the **formal operational thought stage.** This is a higher process that permits abstract reasoning

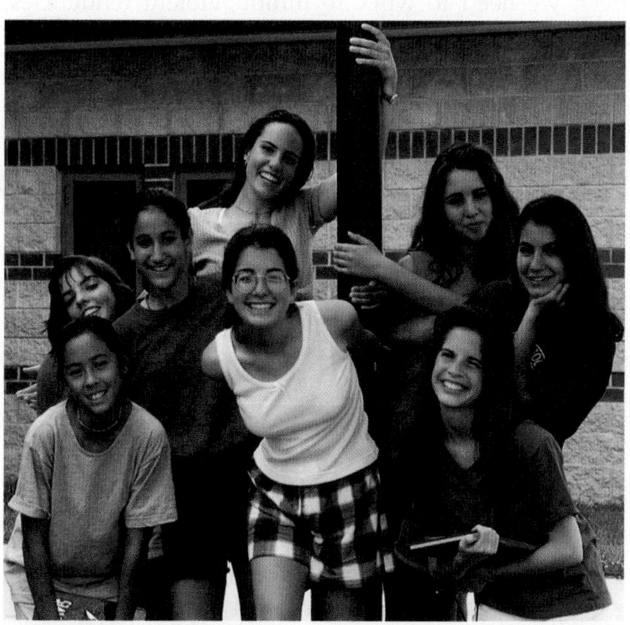

FIGURE 9-13 The peer group provides the adolescent with a sense of belonging.

Box 9-16 Parenting Tips during Adolescence

- Educate yourself and your adolescent
- Maintain open communication
- Choose your battles
- Set realistic expectations
- Set good examples for behavior
- Honor individuality
- Respect privacy
- Try to remember your own experiences during this stage
- Set appropriate rules and regulations
- Be consistent
- Stay involved—meet your child's friends and acquaintances
- Be active in school and after-school activities

and systematic, scientific problem solving. Adolescents become capable of reasoning and formal logic. At this time, it is possible that thoughts will be influenced more by logical principles than by personal perceptions and experiences. The adolescent thinks beyond the present. Without having to focus exclusively on the immediate situation, the adolescent is able to imagine the possible—a sequence of events that might occur, such as college and occupational possibilities; how things might change in the future, such as relationships with parents; and the possible consequences of actions they are considering, such as dropping out of school.

Moral Development

As children move through the stages of cognition and logical thinking, they also progress through stages of moral development. As with other developmental processes, moral development approaches or achieves adult levels during adolescence.

In some ways, adolescence is an uncomfortable in-between phase. Old principles are challenged, but new and independent values do not emerge immediately. As a consequence, young people find themselves searching for a moral code that will preserve their personal integrity and guide their behavior, especially in the face of strong pressure to violate the old values. They face many decisions involving moral dilemmas. They need to gradually internalize a set of principles that provide them with the resources to evaluate the demands of a situation and to plan a course of action consistent with their ideals.

Health Promotion

Nutrition

The rate of body growth and the adolescent's increased basal metabolic rate require an increase in the individual's caloric needs. At peak growth, females may need as much as 2600 calories per day and males as much as 3600 calories per day. Many factors affect the individual's dietary habits, including cultural background, family habits, work schedules, school, concern about weight gain, peer influence, and lack of knowledge concerning correct food choices. Protein needs are increased as a consequence of the rapid growth of this period. Advise them to obtain 12% to 16% of their total daily food intake from protein.

The adolescent diet is most likely to be deficient in calcium, iron, and zinc. There is a substantial increase in the need for these minerals during the period of rapid growth—calcium for skeletal growth; iron for expansion of muscle mass and blood volume, soft tissue growth, and the rapid growth demands of the expanding red cell mass; and zinc for the generation of both skeletal and muscle tissue. Adolescent boys have greater muscle mass, but adolescent girls have an additional iron loss from menstruation. Consequently, the need is probably equivalent in both sexes.

Increased amounts of milk are usually required to supplement an average diet to ensure an adequate calcium intake during this time.

The adolescent is advised to follow the guidelines at the MyPyramid website (see Chapter 21).

Sleep, Play Activity, and Safety

The adolescent needs to pace activities to allow for adequate rest. The adolescent often requires increased hours of sleep to restore energy levels. During puberty and adolescence, caution must be taken to prevent injuries related to exercise and sports. Injuries sometimes occur at this time in connection with the adolescent's growth spurt. Growth spurts cause the bones to grow more quickly than the muscles and tendons. This causes the muscles and tendons to become short and tight. This, combined with the general awkwardness of this stage, accounts for some of the frequent sports-related injuries. Teaching youngsters to do appropriate warm-up and stretching exercises before starting any strenuous sports can lessen the risk of injury (see sports-related safety tips in the Safety Alert box). Participating in organized sports at this age helps adolescents learn to work with others, meet challenges, and set personal goals. Parents have an opportunity to encourage children to exercise by setting an example and practicing good, healthy behaviors for themselves. Having parents involved on the sidelines supporting their adolescent's efforts potentially enhances self-esteem.

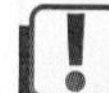
Safety Alert!

Sports-Related Safety Tips

- Use safety helmets.
- Use properly fitting equipment.
- Play on properly maintained surfaces.
- Perform warm-up exercises before sports practice.
- Avoid overuse.
- Insist on adequate supervision.
- Obtain proper training.
- Treat existing injuries and prevent reinjury.

Accident prevention is vitally important during this stage of development. The greatest number of deaths in this age-group is due to accidents. Driver's education, water safety training, education about safe sex practices, and drug education are necessary to inform adolescents of the risks and dangers inherent in these activities. The Safety Alert box lists safe sex practices that are crucial to emphasize early in adolescence, with special emphasis on abstinence.

Emotional Health

Adolescence is, as described earlier, a period of maturation covering the transition from childhood to adulthood (Box 9-17). In part as a result of the complexity of the tasks facing them, adolescents go through different moods that are common in this period. At times they

Safety Alert!

Guidelines for Practice of Safe Sex

- The safest sexual practice is abstinence.
- Be familiar with your sexual partners. Ask about their sexual lifestyle before you engage in sexual relations.
- Avoid engaging in sexual relations with intravenous drug users or with individuals who have had multiple sex partners.
- Use a latex condom as the best type of protection from infection.
- Condoms should be inspected for tears before use. Avoid lengthy storage and exposure to excessive heat.
- Fit the condom over the erect penis, leaving a small space at the end for the collection of semen.
- Hold the upper end of the condom when withdrawing from the vagina to prevent slippage.
- Avoid sexual relations with individuals who have genital lesions or unusual drainage.
- Be aware that there is an increased risk of human immunodeficiency virus infection with oral sexual practices. Anal intercourse requires additional education for safe practice.

Box 9-17 Developmental Tasks of the Adolescent

- Recognizes individuality
- Accepts strengths and weaknesses
- Develops own value system
- Assumes responsibility for own behavior
- Develops philosophy of life
- Adapts to somatic changes (changes affecting the body)
- Acquires skills necessary for adult living
- Refines social skills
- Develops independent living skills

are outgoing and gregarious and active participants in family matters. They will offer their opinions and seem to ignore others. There are also times when they are moody and loners who seem not to want any part of family activities. Such mood swings generally occur at this stage. It is important for families to recognize and distinguish normal moodiness from signs of depression in adolescents. **Depression** is defined as a mood disturbance characterized by feelings of sadness, despair, and hopelessness. People who are depressed are often unable to improve their condition without help from professional therapy. Teach parents, teachers, and health care workers to recognize the common signs of depression. It is crucial to have early detection and intervention when dealing with depression because this leads to higher success rates. Untreated depression can lead to suicide (Box 9-18). Advise parents to seek professional help if their child expresses feelings of marked depression. It is important to take all threats seriously, and imperative to be alert to sudden changes in behavior, such as a change from extreme sadness to manic behavior. This mood swing potentially signals a decision to carry out the person's suicide plan.

Box 9-18 Signs of Depression and Indicators of Suicide Risk

- Change in appetite
- Change in mood—sadness, hopelessness
- Inability to concentrate
- Loss of interest in activities
- Change in sleep habits (either always sleeping or unable to sleep)
- Talk of suicide
- Preoccupation with death or dying
- Giving away possessions

EARLY ADULTHOOD: 20 TO 40 YEARS

The transition to adulthood in the United States is marked by such events as taking on financial responsibilities, making career choices, beginning social relationships, entering marriage, and becoming a parent. All the challenges and accomplishments of the earlier developmental stages have helped prepare the individual for the responsibilities of adult maturity. Fantasies of what adulthood will entail usually give place to more realistic expectations and hopes.

Early adulthood, the period of optimal physical condition, is marked by momentous changes in lifestyle. Box 9-19 contains a list of the developmental tasks of early adulthood.

Physical Characteristics

The body during early adult years is at its optimal level of functioning. The typical young adult is a fine physical specimen. During the middle twenties, most body functions are fully developed, and muscular strength, energy, and endurance are now at their peak. At about age 50, declines in physical capabilities begin but usually so gradually that they are hardly noticed.

Physical appearance is always influenced by heredity, environment, and general state of wellness. Females usually reach their maximum height at about 16 to 17 years of age. Males sometimes continue to grow until 18 to 20 years of age. Between ages 30 and 45, height is stable, and then it begins to decline be-

Box 9-19 Developmental Tasks of Early Adulthood

- Achieves independence, both financial and social
- Maximizes personal worth and identity
- Develops meaningful and satisfying social relationships
- Assumes responsibilities and independent decision making
- Learns to balance personal needs and societal expectations
- Accepts self and others
- Distinguishes physical attraction from love and permanent commitment
- Decides on a marriage, career, and children

cause of settling of spinal disks. There is often an increase in fatty tissue, causing weight gain; a decrease in muscle strength; and a stabilization of reaction time. The senses are also at their sharpest during young adulthood. Visual acuity is keenest at about age 20 and does not begin to decline until about age 40. Both vision and hearing tend to diminish slightly in middle adulthood. Cardiac output, vital capacities, and organ reserves gradually decrease in middle adulthood.

Diet plays an important role, as it does throughout the developmental stages. Both heart disease and cancer are major concerns in the adult years. Proper diet and exercise often has a decisive impact on the control of heart disease, which is caused by increased cholesterol deposits occluding the walls of blood vessels. Likewise, low-fat, high-fiber, and low-cholesterol diets are recommended as preventive measures against cancers of the breast, the stomach, and the intestine. Other lifestyle habits such as the use of tobacco, drugs, and alcohol will also affect the adult's health status (see Health Promotion box).

In the past few decades, it has become more popular to pay attention to physical fitness, with benefit to general welfare. Regular, paced exercise increases heart and lung capacity, lowers blood pressure, helps control weight, enhances body function, and improves emotional health.

By adulthood, men and women have reached their sexual maturity. Sexual drive continues for both men and women throughout adulthood.

Psychosocial Development

About 95% of Americans marry at some point in their lives. Dual-career families have grown out of the economic realities of our times, as well as women's interest in pursuing careers. The feminist movement has resulted in many positive social changes. Both the home and the workplace demonstrate the effects of these changes and the dual-career lifestyle.

Another important option confronting this age-group is the decision to start a family (Figure 9-14). If procreation is the choice, a subsequent issue is how many children to have. Further thought is required regarding considerations such as financial means, safety,

Health Promotion

Recommendations for a Healthy Lifestyle

- Follow the guidelines at www.mypyramid.gov.
- Drink adequate fluids.
- Avoid smoking and drugs.
- Consume little or no alcohol.
- Maintain optimal weight.
- Participate in a scheduled program of daily exercise.
- Obtain adequate restorative sleep.
- Practice stress reduction.
- Enjoy leisure activities.

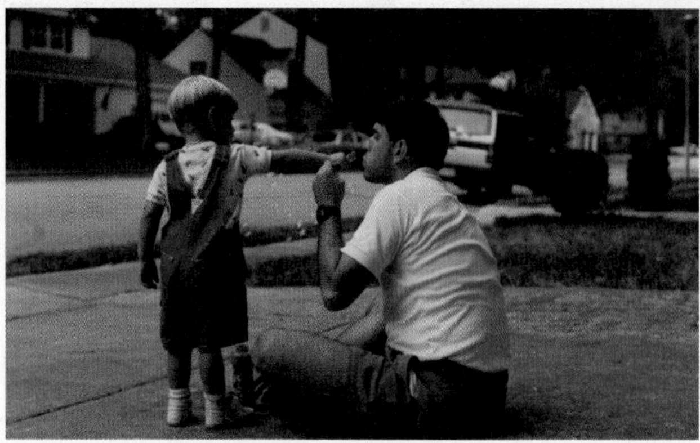

FIGURE 9-14 Father and child bonding.

family support, housing, the relationship to members of the extended family, and the roles and responsibilities of the nuclear family unit. It is important for young adults establishing a family today to have open communication about self-development, which includes issues of dual careers, child-rearing practices, and domestic duties within the home.

Family development and harmony are major goals for many young adults, both male and female. Although family size and structure have undergone dramatic changes in the past decades, concerns about individual members' health and safety continue to form a primary focus within the family as a unit. Family life is influenced by the characteristics of individual family members. Typically, healthy family adjustment is associated with the age of the individuals, job security, the family's and the individuals' places in the community, and healthy patterns of living (good nutrition, personal cleanliness, physical fitness). Therefore the physical and mental health of one family member affects all family members.

Erikson identified early intimacy versus isolation as the developmental task of adulthood. Intimacy is the ability to develop one's deepest hopes and concerns in connection to another person. One aspect of intimacy is the capacity to accept the closeness of another person. Intimacy leads to commitment, sharing, and compromise. The "virtue" that develops in young adulthood is the virtue of love, or the mutuality of devotion between partners who have chosen to share their lives. As young adults resolve conflicting demands of intimacy, competitiveness, and distance, they develop an ethical sense, which Erikson considers the mark of the adult. The opposite of intimacy, the distancing of oneself from intimate relationships, is the negative resolution of the task of this life stage and leads to isolation and self-absorption.

Cognitive Development

Piaget saw adulthood as actively developing the formal operational approach to learning and problem solving. He believed that the same cognitive operations apply throughout adulthood to a larger, more expansive list of experiences. Adults tend to think in an integrative way.

Health Promotion

Nutrition

Fewer total numbers of calories are needed compared to adolescence, because the adult has completed biophysical growth. Calories are needed to maintain body functioning for cell replacement and repair and for provision of energy. Calorie needs vary based on age, sex, size, physical activity, metabolism, and levels of stress.

Rest and Sleep

Most adults function well with 7 to 9 hours of restorative sleep. Adults do not commonly schedule daytime rest opportunities to prevent fatigue; however, they can increase their productivity by obtaining adequate rest during the day. Adequate rest is essential for the pregnant woman to ensure the health of both herself and her unborn baby.

Physical and Dental Examinations

Annual physical and dental examinations are recommended. For the male, a routine testicular examination and for the female annual Papanicolaou (Pap) smears are essential for early detection of cancer. Recommend monthly breast self-examinations for women older than age 20 and a baseline mammogram between ages 35 and 40. Beginning at age 40, advise men to obtain a yearly physical examination including a digital rectal examination, and beginning at age 50 including a prostate-specific antigen (PSA) study to screen for prostate cancer (see Chapters 50, 52, and 57). Schedule routine dental examinations for adults every 6 months. Eye examinations are necessary every 2 years unless otherwise indicated.

Safety

Accidents are the leading cause of disability and death in this age-group. Injuries commonly result from work, vehicle, and sports accidents, as well as from violence.

MIDDLE ADULTHOOD: 40 TO 65 YEARS

The middle adulthood period is arbitrarily designated as occurring between 40 and 65 years of age. Most individuals of this age-group enjoy a healthy body. Some changes result in a gradual shift of balance away from peak performance. The extent of these changes is directly related to diet, heredity, exercise, rest, mental outlook, stress, and disease.

Middle adulthood is characterized by shifts in responsibilities and physical adjustments. Box 9-20 contains a list of the developmental tasks of middle adulthood.

Box 9-20 Developmental Tasks of Middle Adulthood

- Balances goals and realities and redirects energies as necessary
- Extends caring and concern beyond immediate family (to neighborhood, community, society)
- Develops career and job satisfaction
- Adapts to physical changes
- Establishes new roles and relationships with spouse, children, grandchildren, and parents

Physical Characteristics

Bone mass decreases as skeletal growth cells are depleted. This bone loss leads to an increased risk of osteoporosis. Women lose calcium from bone tissue after menopause. Men also lose calcium from bones but at a more gradual rate than women, and their risk of osteoporosis is lower. Slight changes in height continue to occur as a result of the compression of the spinal vertebrae and the hardening of collagen fibers. A decrease in muscle fibers results in a reduction of muscle mass. Heredity, nutrition, and exercise patterns account for much of the individual variation commonly seen. Changes in muscle strength are perhaps related more to level of activity than to age. A redistribution of body weight leads to changes in body shape and contour. A decrease in basal metabolism and less activity often necessitates calorie reductions to prevent weight gain.

Basic neurologic functioning remains at a high level during this age period.

Noticeable changes in vision occur owing to **presbyopia** (defect in vision in advancing age involving loss of accommodation or the recession of the near point caused by loss of elasticity of crystalline lens and the ensuing change in close vision).

Other sensory changes may include **presbycusis** (a normal progressive, age-associated loss of hearing acuity, speech intelligibility, auditory threshold, and pitch). These changes usually begin around age 40 and occur more commonly in men than in women.

One of the most noticeable changes that occurs during this period is in the appearance of the individual's skin. There is a decrease in the elastic fibers and a slight loss of subcutaneous tissue, giving skin a looser, more wrinkled appearance. Hair color often changes with age with the onset of graying. Graying usually begins at the temples. Hair growth and distribution sometimes changes during the middle adult years. Scalp hair tends to become thinner.

There is a higher incidence of periodontal (gum) disease in the middle adult years. Preventive treatment programs including fluoride usage, regular flossing, and dental cleaning are important.

Hormonal changes include the woman's declining production of estrogen and progesterone. Menopause (female climacteric) is a gradual process that takes about 5 years to complete. A woman's perception of menopause is likely to be affected by her perceptions of her general health. During this process, the functions of the ovaries will diminish and eventually cease. Noticeable signs and symptoms of menopause typically include irregular menstrual periods, flow changes, excess fluid retention, breast tenderness, hot flashes—feeling "hot," flushing, and blushing—palpitations, night sweats, and irritability or mood swings. Some women have very few signs or symptoms related to menopause. Some women receive small doses of estrogen aimed at relieving the complications of decreased estrogen levels. Some suggest that hormone replacement therapy (HRT) offers a way to reduce osteoporosis and the risk of atherosclerosis and heart disease; however, HRT is also feared to increase the risk of stroke, endometrial cancer, and breast disease, as well as raise blood pressure. Therefore it is necessary to evaluate the risks versus the benefits of this treatment on an individual basis. The woman is able to continue to experience positive, satisfying sexuality and sexual responses throughout her middle adult years. With any fears of pregnancy now out of the picture, many women enjoy a period of enhanced sexuality.

Possible evidence of the male climacteric includes decreased libido (sex drive), loss of body hair, and delayed erection. Men do not lose the ability to reproduce during the middle adult years. Changes in male sexual function are often more related to psychological than physiologic occurrences. A man's actual capacity to function sexually often has more to do with self-perception and mental outlook and less with the changes he experiences in body appearance, including weight gain, hair loss, and decreased muscle strength. These changes cause some men to go through what is described as a "midlife crisis." During this time, many people may engage in extramarital affairs, often leading to divorce. Many men are unaffected by the physiologic and psychological occurrences of the climacteric.

Psychosocial Development

According to Erikson, the developmental task of middle age is generativity versus stagnation. This means accepting responsibility for and offering guidance to the next generation. Generativity encompasses productivity, continuity, and creativity (Figure 9-15). If this developmental task is not met, people become stagnant—inactive or lifeless. The middle adult years are a time for vocational, interpersonal, and personal fulfillment. The impulse to foster development of the young is not limited to guiding one's own children and does not cease with their maturation. Many middle-aged adults enjoyably express this desire through activities such as teaching and mentorship, a mutually fulfilling relationship that satisfies a younger protégé's need for guidance along with an older person's need for generativity. Resumption of education, career growth or changes, reentry into the workforce, and involvement with community activities create a multitude of possibilities for personal growth and satisfaction during the middle adult years.

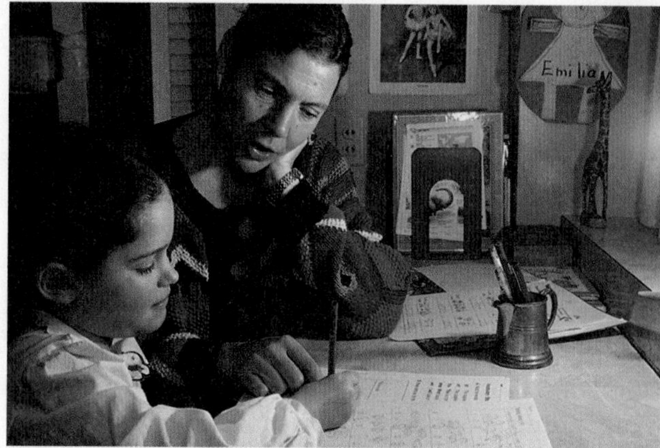

FIGURE 9-15 According to Erikson, generativity is the developmental task of middle adulthood. Nurturing and guiding the younger generation is a task people accomplish with their own children or with other children and adolescents in their family and community.

Family roles change during this stage. Children are sometimes present in the home, and sometimes not. For most caregivers, a significant change in their lives occurs with the end of daily, active responsibility for children. Relationships between spouses change, and the couple often has to regain familiarity with each other. For many, this offers the opportunity for new or renewed companionship. Survival of the marriage after children leave home possibly depends on the growth, the maturity, and the commitment of each partner. The majority of empty-nest women actually look forward to their emancipation from parenting duties, seeing it as an occasion to further develop their personal and social roles.

The role of grandparenting often begins at this developmental stage. Because it often does not have the constraints and responsibilities of child rearing, grandparenting becomes a rich and rewarding experience for many middle-aged adults. The past few decades have probably been the best time ever to be an American grandparent and to enjoy grandparenting as a joyful experience. Grandparents now have the longest, healthiest life spans ever recorded, the best social services, and the most independence. Many still hover just above the poverty line and some are below it; however, many grandparents are prosperous. Many of today's grandparents have lots of grandchildren to enjoy. Many American grandparents are not involved in the upbringing and disciplining of their grandchildren, preferring a "norm of noninterference." Grandparents often refrain from giving their grown children child-rearing instruction, even when they do not like something they see going on with their grandchildren. Most contemporary grandparents value their independence; many are unwilling to exchange their hard-won and long-awaited lifestyles for another round of the hard, often frustrating work of raising children.

On the other hand, most adults are not prepared for the increased responsibility of caring for aging parents. Economic stress and emotional pressure are both associated with the role reversal sometimes known as "parenting the parent." Studies have indicated that a midlife daughter is most likely to be involved in elder care with her parents and her husband's parents.

Health Promotion

Nutrition

Many adults slow down in their middle adult years; therefore, they need fewer calories than they did in their teens and twenties. The Centers for Disease Control and Prevention (CDC) reports that 65% of Americans over age 20 are overweight or obese, which is defined as being 20% over the desirable weight for one's sex, height, and body build. Inadequate calorie intake, or undernutrition, is also becoming more common. In some cases, this is due to poverty; however, in many cases it is a result of self-imposed dieting. A good diet with supplemental vitamins and minerals combined with regular exercise often helps lessen the effects of menopause.

Positive lifestyles with regular exercise are important to maintain healthy joints and bones. Activities that are stress reducing such as walking, swimming, golf, and tennis also have the potential to enhance calcium utilization. Premenopausal women need to obtain about 1,000 to 1,200 mg of dietary calcium per day. It is also important that the diet be rich in phosphorus and magnesium. A diet rich in green leafy vegetables, fresh fruits, whole-grain cereals or breads, and dairy products will help support healthy bones. A reduced intake of fat is recommended; most of it should come from unsaturated fats such as soy, sunflower, corn, or safflower oil. High blood levels of saturated fats and cholesterol contribute to atherosclerosis, coronary heart disease, and cancer.

Physical and Dental Examinations

The person in middle adulthood needs regular physical and dental examinations. Preventive American Cancer Society guidelines should be followed (see Chapter 57).

Sleep and Rest

The adult in this age-group sleeps less and experiences more nighttime awakenings than younger adults. In somewhat circular fashion, the subsequent need for additional daytime rest sometimes lessens the number of nighttime hours of sleep required.

LATE ADULTHOOD: 65 YEARS AND OLDER

Older adults represent a rapidly growing segment of the population, and it is important for us all to prepare for and understand the aging process (Box 9-21). There are many approaches to examining the experience of growing old. Aging is a normal condition of human existence and has been studied from sociologic, physiologic, and psychological perspectives. Throughout the life span, all these aspects of the human experience are interrelated. Gerontologists, who study the older adult and the aging process, note that many 70-year-olds today act and think as 50-year-olds did as recently as the 1960s.

The fact remains that everyone ages. The physiologic changes are not universal, however, or even necessarily inevitable, and the changes are often amenable to many interventions and treatments. An individual's adjustment to aging is a uniquely complex process. How an individual responds to the age-related changes

Box 9-21 Developmental Tasks of Late Adulthood

- Accepts own life
- Recognizes accomplishments
- Finds satisfaction with new roles, relationships, and leisure time
- Maximizes independence and maintains high level of involvement
- Accepts own mortality and prepares for death

Life Span Considerations

Older Adult

The Effects of Aging on Older Adults

- With increased emphasis on wellness and preventive care, today's older adults are living longer, healthier lives. However, longer life spans result in an increased presence of chronic and degenerative disorders.
- Each generation has its own central life tasks to complete. As life expectancy grows, more generations coexist, and the needs of one age-group sometimes come into conflict with those of others. This increases intergenerational stress and, typically, to alterations in family dynamics.
- Changes in roles and relationships present major developmental challenges to older adults.
- According to the U.S. Census Bureau, approximately 12% of the population is older than age 65. By 2030, this percentage will increase to 20%.*
- Health care needs of the aging population will place increased demands on the health care delivery system.
- The cost of providing care for the older adult population is a major societal concern. It is likely to have a significant impact on the amount and the type of health care coverage provided by insurance companies and the government.
- Older adults are a politically active group, and as their numbers increase they are having an impact on all aspects of society, including the entertainment, travel, and housing industries.
- Although some older adults are poor, as a group they generally have more income than younger individuals and therefore have a significant effect on the economy.

*Data from Ebersole, P., et al. (2008). *Toward healthy aging: Human needs and nursing response.* (7th ed.). St. Louis: Mosby.

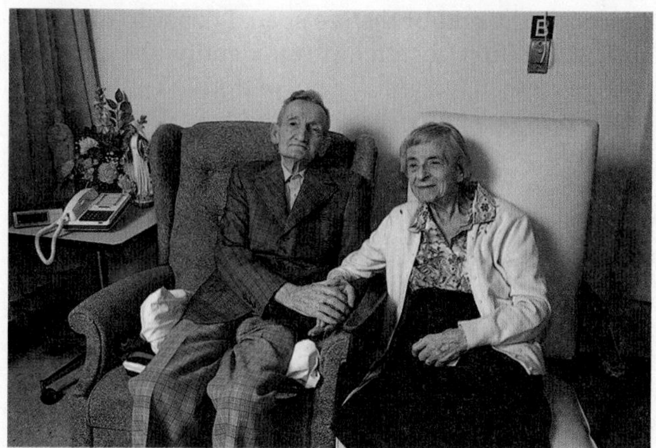

FIGURE 9-16 According to Erikson, generativity versus stagnation is the developmental task of older adulthood. A loving relationship with a spouse is an example of a positive influence during this stage of life.

visible in the mirror has much to do with the person's self-esteem. Successful aging depends on the individual's capacity to cope and ability to change. The process of aging affects the individual, the family, and society at large (see Life Span Considerations for Older Adults box).

The sociologically relevant issues of aging have to do with work, retirement, social security, and health care. As more and more people reach late adulthood, it is incumbent on society to recognize and value these individuals' knowledge, skills, and contributions. Preparations and planning for the future that are addressed and encouraged in the early adult years help prepare, support, and enhance adjustments once they are necessary. Implementation of flexible services and financial assistance programs helps people fulfill their goals.

The response to getting older is often also related to lifelong health habits, diet, and exercise patterns. Family, love, friendships, and intimate relationships are additional factors important to survival and well-being (Figures 9-16 and 9-17). These relationships are crucial to people's happiness whatever their age. Love relationships vary in intensity and meaning in adulthood. Early on, these relationships usually have an intense physical basis, which leads to intimacy, respect, and commitment. Although intense sexual drive decreases with age, sexual behavior remains an important part of many adult relationships.

Ageism

Ageism—a form of discrimination and prejudice against the older adult—is an unfortunate reality. Like racism and sexism, ageism works to prevent people from being as happy and productive as they otherwise have the ability to be. It is passed on from generation to generation by the process of socialization. Society today must relinquish old stereotypes about the older adult and learn to affirm the positive aspects of aging (Figure 9-18). It is a mistake to view aging only as a decline; it involves growth as well.

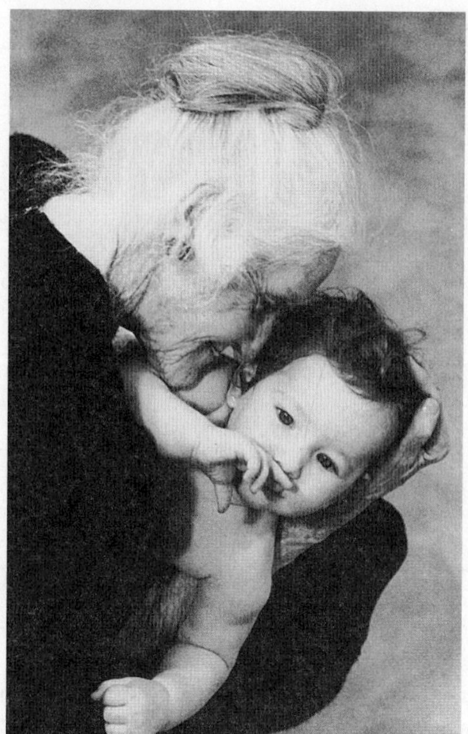

FIGURE 9-17 Beauty throughout the life span.

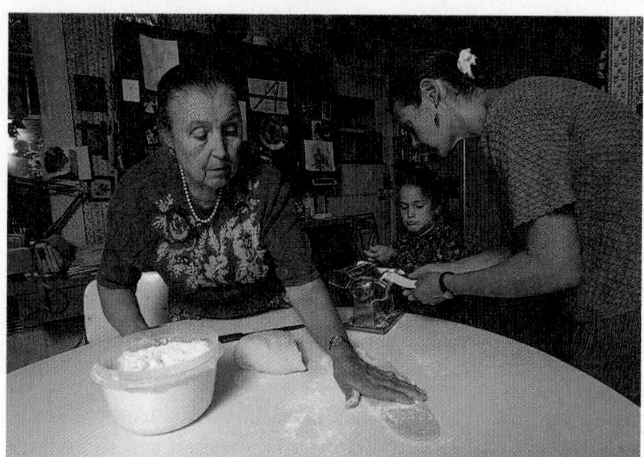

FIGURE 9-18 Three generations of Italian Americans make a pasta dinner together.

The purpose of this section is to refute the negative stereotypes, to present a realistically positive view of aging, and to help you identify the normal physical patterns of aging so you are able to identify deviations from the norm. Before reading this portion of the chapter, examine your personal beliefs about aging. Box 9-22 provides a brief list of true-false statements that will help you clarify your beliefs.

The number of older people has grown steadily over the past century. According to the U.S. Census Bureau (2007), 35.1 million persons, or about 12.4% of the population, are older than 65 years. By 2030, almost 72 million people will be 65 years or older (Ebersole et al., 2008).

Box 9-22 Your Beliefs on Aging

TRUE OR FALSE?

___ 1. All older people become senile.
___ 2. Most older people live in a nursing home or other institutional setting.
___ 3. Most older people are isolated from their families.
___ 4. Most older people have no interest in or capacity for sexual relationships.
___ 5. Older workers are less productive than younger workers.
___ 6. Intelligence declines in old age.
___ 7. Older people do better to cease exercising and just rest.
___ 8. Marked personality changes occur in the older person.
___ 9. Older people naturally become inflexible and demanding.
___ 10. Older people obtain less satisfaction from life.

Note: All of these statements are false.

Every year another group of adults reaches late adulthood. Who are these people? What are they like? To understand the older population, we must first consider what we mean by late adulthood. For our purposes, late adulthood will be defined as age 65 and older. We can further subdivide this state into "young older adult" (ages 65 to 74), "middle older adult" (ages 75 to 84), and "older older adult" (older than age 85). This population is constantly changing as new individuals enter the group and others leave through death. Each person has a unique personal history that reflects many influences. Box 9-23 lists keys to successful aging. The fastest growing segment of the U.S. population is the group aged 85 years and older.

Box 9-23 Keys to Successful Aging

- Practice pleasurable activities.
- View life as meaningful.
- Maintain a positive self-image.
- Accept responsibility for the past.
- Be optimistic.
- Remain motivated to maintain or expand intellectual capacity.
- Participate in a planned exercise program.

Biologic Theories of Aging

For centuries, humanity has been fascinated with the concept of aging. Many theories have attempted to define the causes of and to develop measures to halt or postpone the aging process. One of the earliest theories of aging, generated by Hippocrates, speculated that aging was an irreversible natural event caused by a decrease in body heat. Later, Galen supported this concept and **postulated** (claimed as real or true) that aging was a lifelong process rather than an event occurring at the end of the life span. Leonardo da Vinci, among the first to attempt to identify the physical changes associated with aging, performed autopsies to compare old men and young children. In the period after 1900, only a few scientists focused on aging as their main interest. Finally, in the past 30 years, we have begun to see a renewed interest in researching the causes of the aging process. Recent theories focus on the roles of autoimmunity, free radicals (compounds with an extra electron or protein), wear and tear, and biologic programming, among others. The only definitive conclusion we have at this time, however, is that aging is a slow, continuous, complex process that probably involves both intrinsic and extrinsic factors.

Autoimmunity Theory

The autoimmunity theory holds that with aging, the body becomes less able to recognize or tolerate the "self." As a result, the immune system produces antibodies that act against the self. This theory is supported by the increased accumulation of lymphocytes, plasma cells found in the tissues of normal, healthy, older people.

The primary organs of the immune system (thymus and bone marrow) are believed to be affected by the aging process. As we age, the thymus decreases in size and weight and becomes less able to produce T cells. The bone marrow stem cells also show reduced efficiency in performing certain functions. As immune system function decreases, the risk of developing infection and cancer increases (see Chapter 55).

Free Radical Theory

Free radicals are highly reactive cellular components derived from unstable atoms or molecules. Free radicals have a reduced cellular efficiency and cause cellular waste to accumulate. Some free radicals are produced by radiation, heat, and oxidation. The presence of free radicals possibly accelerates aging and results in the death of an organism. Lipofuscin is a pigmented material that accumulates in many organs as a part of aging. This accumulation interferes with the diffusion and transportation of essential metabolites and perhaps also contributes to the aging process.

Wear-and-Tear Theory

According to the wear-and-tear theory, age is not based on chronologic age but is determined by the amount of wear and tear we experience. Many believe that the structural and functional changes associated with growing old are accelerated by abuse of the body.

Biologic Programming Theory

Some theorists claim that there is a hereditary basis for aging, evidenced by the similarities in life expectancies in a particular family. Further evidence supporting the theory of biologic programming comes from in vitro cell studies. One early theory suggested that aging was a programmed genetic occurrence that was caused by specific aging genes (Darrach, 1992; Recer, 2000; Schlessinger, 2000). Another theory (Davidovic, 2003) cited aging as the result of progressive environmental damage to cells, interfering with normal cell functions. Aging has been attributed to the accumulation of lipofuscin, lipids, and fat. Changes in collagen structure and degenerative changes in elastin make tissues stiffer, less pliable, and less elastic and efficient.

Psychological Theories of Aging

Disengagement Theory

According to supporters of the disengagement theory of aging, a natural withdrawal, or disengagement, between the individual and society is best. This withdrawal is initiated either by the individual or by others in society. Adherents to this belief suggest that such withdrawal prevents older adults from experiencing frustration when they can no longer function adequately, while allowing a younger member of society to fulfill the now-empty role. They characterize this process as a normal, inevitable, universal process. Two major criticisms of the disengagement theory are as follows:

- It does not allow for the many active, functional older adults.
- The process is not seen in all cultural groups, and it is therefore not universal.

Activity Theory

According to this theory, the older person who is more active socially is more likely to adjust well to aging. Older adults with more social involvement have higher morale and better life satisfaction and personal adjustment. The number and the quality of the activities are important. If a person gives up activities or roles, advise them to find replacements. Meaningful activities involving close personal contact with others are extremely important. Activities of this nature reinforce our self-concept, which in turn is associated with a higher life satisfaction.

Continuity Theory

Supporters of this theory suggest that the critical factors in adjustment to old age are the coping abilities we developed previously and our ability to maintain our previous roles and activities. It is often useful to know and understand a person's personality type to predict their response to the aging process. People who were never highly involved will likely maintain the same mild level of involvement in old age. On the other hand, individuals who were highly involved and actively engaged with society need to remain active and involved with similar intensity. Supporters of the continuity theory contend that our adjustment to the aging process will be eased by maintaining roles and interests similar to those we developed earlier in life.

Physical Characteristics

Aging is a complex process that affects cells, tissues, and organs. Like growth and development, aging occurs at a highly individualized rate. There is a gradual reduction in the number and a change in the composition of aging cells. There is usually a slow increase in body weight until 45 to 50 years of age, and then a gradual decline begins. Body fat content and distribution differ in men and women. The accumulation of adipose tissue in females is typically found over the chest, the waist, the hips, and the thighs. Adipose tissue in the male is deposited mostly in the waist, the chest, and the lower abdomen.

Loss of height begins after age 50. Most of the noticeable decrease in trunk length is a result of the increase in spinal curvature caused by a slight thinning of the intervertebral disks. In addition to the shortening of the spine, certain abnormal postures and contours are noted. Kyphosis, an exaggeration of the thoracic curvature, may increase with aging. This sometimes leads to a barrel-chest appearance, which possibly affects the position of the diaphragm and reduces the effectiveness of inspiration. These and other postural changes have the potential to affect body posture, mobility, gait, and respiratory efficiency.

Common age-related changes specific to each body system are listed in Table 9-4, along with suggested nursing interventions to minimize the effect of these changes.

Psychosocial Development

Years of living and our successes, failures, strengths, weaknesses, and all the early experiences influence our emotional stability when we are older. Despite the physiologic changes associated with the aging process, it is most appropriate to view the older years as a time of satisfaction and pleasure. Many older adults choose to work after age 65. These activities provide interest, intellectual stimulation, and added income (Figure 9-19). Older people need to recognize their changing capabilities and begin a process of adjustment.

Erikson described the challenge of late adulthood as ego integrity versus a sense of despair. The task here is to evaluate one's life and accomplishments and find satisfaction and meaning in life. The process of reminiscing with others often serves to further validate the meaning and importance of the individual's life. Those who can feel that their lives have been well spent and are satisfied with their decisions and achievements have mastered this task of integrity. This allows the person to continue life with a sense of dignity and peacefulness. Adults who are dissatisfied with their accomplishments often experience conflict and despair. Dissatisfaction contributes to a feeling of restlessness and a sense of panic that time is "running

Table 9-4 Common Age-Related Changes

SYSTEM	NORMAL CHANGES	SUGGESTED NURSING INTERVENTIONS
MUSCULOSKELETAL SYSTEM		
Bones, muscles, joints, and connective tissue	Mineral salts move from bones to blood, making bones more porous; tendons, ligaments less elastic; increase in joint stiffness with less range of motion; varying degrees of increase of flexion at wrists, hips, knees, producing less joint mobility, agility, and endurance; thinning of vertebral disks	Maintain mobility. Encourage exercise (with physician's guidance). Encourage passive and active exercises. Avoid fatigue. Use assistive aids when indicated.
NERVOUS SYSTEM	Fewer, smaller neurons (nerve cells), slowed reaction time, decrease in tactile sensitivity, decrease in pain perception, altered motor coordination	Allow adequate time to complete activities. Be alert to danger of and prevent burning and chilling related to diminished sensitivity. Encourage position changes; inspect skin daily.
SPECIAL SENSES		
Taste and smell	Decline in taste and smell perception	Use smoke detectors. Serve attractive, colorful food.
Vision	Decreased tear production, increase in lens density; presbyopia (farsightedness; loss of elasticity of lens); yellowing of lens; slowing of accommodation (reaction to changes in light and distance); narrowing of visual field; decrease in depth perception	Encourage annual eye examinations. Use more diffuse lighting. Use bright colors (red, yellow). Place articles within visual field. Use night-lights.
Hearing	Presbycusis (increased difficulty hearing high-pitched sounds); increase in degenerative changes within ear structure; increase in buildup of wax production	Speak slowly, clearly. Face individual. Do not shout. Speak in lower tones. Control background noise. Encourage use of aids if available.
RESPIRATORY SYSTEM		
Ribcage	Increase in calcification of thorax; respiratory muscles weaken, producing diminished respiratory efficiency; maximum breathing capacity reduced; more susceptible to respiratory infection; easily fatigued	Allow for rest periods. Encourage coughing and deep breathing.
Lungs	Alveoli (air sacs) thinner, smaller, with decreased alveolar surface for gaseous exchange; decreased cough reflex action; decreased ciliary action, reduced maximum breathing capacity	Maintain adequate exercise and nutrition. Encourage regular physical examinations. Avoid overexertion and allow for rest between activities. Discourage smoking. Obtain streptococcal pneumonia (pneumococcal) vaccine.

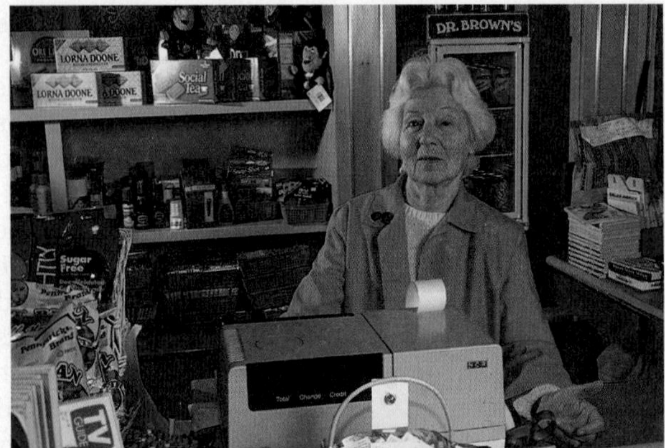

FIGURE 9-19 Many older people continue to work and learn after the traditional retirement age.

out." Often the individual feels the need for more time and a chance to do things over again differently.

Many other factors also affect the older adult's adjustment to this stage of life. Retirement is a major adjustment for the older adult. Health and financial resources are critical elements in determining our life satisfaction after retirement. Generally speaking, our society is relatively unprepared for the phenomenon known as retirement. Retirement creates many changes—some welcome, some not. Examples are changes in roles, self-esteem, support systems, life patterns, and leisure time. Retirement brings more time to spend as one wishes. Therefore individuals need to plan and discuss their hopes and expectations for the retirement period. Planning for retirement helps us identify activities that will be mean-

Table 9-4 **Common Age-Related Changes—cont'd**

SYSTEM	NORMAL CHANGES	SUGGESTED NURSING INTERVENTIONS
CARDIOVASCULAR SYSTEM	Fewer blood cells produced; loss of elasticity and narrowing of blood vessels, with an increase in blood pressure; valves thicker, more rigid; heart requires more time to return to resting state; decreased cardiac output	Encourage regular, paced exercise with adequate rest periods. Maintain low-fat, low-sodium diet. Obtain regular physician examinations.
INTEGUMENTARY SYSTEM		
Skin	Paler, thinner, irregularly pigmented; decrease in moisture; decrease in sweat and sebaceous gland activity; less elastic, more wrinkling; loss of subcutaneous fat; skin more fragile and prone to injury	Inspect skin for impairment or signs of pressure. Change position frequently. Wash with water and mild soap as needed. Rinse thoroughly and pat skin dry. Use lotions to replenish moisture. To maintain body warmth, provide adequate clothing.
REPRODUCTIVE SYSTEM		
Female	Fallopian tubes atrophy and shorten; ovaries smaller, thinner; uterus, cervix smaller; vagina less elastic, more alkaline, drier; reproductive capacity ceases	Suggest use of vaginal lubricants if indicated. Instruct person to have annual mammogram and vaginal examination with Papanicolaou test.
Male	Increased size of prostate; decreased testosterone levels; decreased circulation, and decreased rate and force of ejaculation	Instruct person to have annual prostate examination and prostate-specific antigen (PSA) test.
ENDOCRINE SYSTEM	Slowing of thyroid gland activity; decreased basal metabolic rate; decreased hormone production, affecting other systems	Recommend annual physical examination with thyroid function testing.
URINARY SYSTEM	Fewer cells in kidney, decreased renal blood flow; less effective filtration; decreased bladder elasticity and capacity; need to void more frequently	Observe for signs of urinary tract infections. Observe closely for adverse drug reactions. Observe male for signs of benign prostatic hypertrophy causing impairment of urinary flow.
HAIR	Increase in graying; balding and changes in thickness of hair occur; changes in distribution of body hair	
NAILS	More fragile, brittle; appear dull, opaque yellow or gray in color; toenails thicken	Have toenails trimmed by podiatrist as indicated.
GASTROINTESTINAL SYSTEM	Decreased saliva production; decreased chewing efficiency; decreased esophageal motility; total capacity of stomach reduced; decreased gastric enzyme secretion; liver smaller; less absorption of nutrients; slowing of peristalsis	Ensure adequate fluid intake. Encourage annual dental checkups. Offer five or six small daily meals, rather than three large ones. Assess for indigestion. Encourage regular toileting habits.

ingful and promote self-esteem and a sense of usefulness to both ourselves and society.

Family Roles

For many individuals, the older years become a time to explore their feelings about parenting and grandparenting. Grandparenting today, as discussed earlier, is often very different from the role of grandparenting three or four decades ago. Today's grandparent often works and remains highly active. For others, caring for grandchildren has become a full-time responsibility that leads to multiple stresses. Raising grandchildren has the potential to cause financial stress, cause a decrease in living space, and limit roles. Events affecting children such as divorce, abandonment, unemployment, death or illness, and incarceration are some of the factors that have contributed to the increased numbers of grandparents raising grandchildren on a full-time basis. Support groups, community resources, and other organizations are some of the resources to assist grandparents in their grandparenting roles.

During this stage, couples may need to adjust to increased time together, and often enjoy the increase in companionship and closeness. Maintaining old friendships and exploring ways to form new ones, along with continuing strong family ties, is a means to help soften the losses that are frequently experienced during this period.

The death of a spouse is traumatic at any age. In the older years, being widowed is more common for women than men. Children and a strong social network often play important roles in supporting the surviving spouse. The experience of being widowed goes beyond ending a partnership. Role changes, changes in lifestyle, and access to fewer financial resources are just some of the adjustments that are called for when a spouse dies. Some older people find remarriage as a solution to the challenge of being widowed and find the companionship, love, and security they seek.

Cognitive and Intellectual Development

Evidence suggests that older adults in good health and nurturing environments will have the capacity to maintain or increase their level of functioning, particularly in their areas of interest or specialization. Several factors are important to continued cognitive functioning: level of education, work roles, personality, health, lifestyle, and the relevancy or associated meaning of the tasks we are called on to perform. It is possible that some "practical" abilities will decline with age, whereas others remain stable or improve with age.

Memory

Some older adults notice some changes in memory. Such benign forgetfulness is far more common than the forgetfulness associated with Alzheimer's disease. As adults advance in years, there appears to be a greater loss of recent memory over remote memory. An older individual will perhaps forget what was served for breakfast 2 hours earlier and yet may remember in great detail the events of a wedding many decades ago. Older people are slower than younger people but often are more accurate in what they remember and do. Many people believe that this is deliberate: the older person is more willing to sacrifice speed for accuracy.

Health Promotion

Health promotion rests on the belief that individuals are able to have a strong influence on their health status. Environment, social patterns, diet, exercise, and personal habits are all factors that determine a person's state of health. It is imperative that health care workers clarify the common misconceptions about health and aging. It is essential to emphasize that people of all ages can benefit from living a healthy lifestyle, even in the later years (see Health Promotion box discussing the benefits of exercise).

Advise older adults to receive both pneumococcal and influenza vaccines yearly. Individuals who have compromised immune systems, who have a history of an allergy to eggs or egg products, or who have had a severe reaction to a previous vaccine should check with their physician before immunization.

> **Health Promotion**
>
> **Benefits of Exercise in the Older Adult**
>
> - Maintains or improves cardiovascular fitness
> - Prevents or reduces intensity of chronic diseases such as coronary artery disease, congestive heart failure, hypertension, osteoarthritis, osteoporosis, diabetes, obesity, and chronic obstructive lung disease
> - Prevents many falls and fractures
> - Improves muscle strength, flexibility, and balance
> - Enhances self-care abilities and promotes independent activities
> - Encourages social contact
> - Decreases anxiety, depression, and insomnia

Nutrition

Adequate nutrition plays a significant role in health maintenance and contributes to the older person's quality of life. Activities related to food and diet include transportation for food purchase, meal planning, and meal preparation. It often falls to family members to provide older individuals with assistance for these activities. Older adults need a diet of foods of higher quality and lower quantity that provide the basic necessary nutrients. Although caloric needs are highly individualized, older adults are in general less active and have more adipose tissue and less body mass, and therefore often need less daily caloric intake. Diets that are low in saturated fats and carbohydrates and high in fiber are usually recommended. Common threats to the adequacy of the older adult's diet are poor oral health, lack of appetite, food intolerances, and constipation. Proper nutritional assessment and counseling helps to identify problems and useful interventions. To ensure dietary compliance, take long-standing habits and cultural influences into consideration when introducing any dietary changes.

Various psychosocial factors also have the potential to affect the older person's diet. The choice of foods purchased and included in the diet sometimes comes down to economic factors. Loneliness also contributes to inadequate dietary intake for some people. If a person is not able to shop for and prepare meals, it is likely that his or her diet will become less than desirable. Another crucial component in the older person's diet is adequate fluid intake. Advise older adults to maintain a minimum daily intake of 1,500 mL/day. Often, an older person will avoid fluids out of a fear of incontinence and a lack of thirst.

Activity

Throughout the life span, evenly paced, satisfying exercise is crucial to general well-being. Exercise has benefits on cardiovascular functioning, lowering blood pressure while enhancing oxygen utilization, and maintaining joint mobility. It is misguided to exercise to the point of exhaustion; always recommend following up with a rest period to recuperate and restore the body to its maximum level of functioning (see the Health Promotion box for benefits of exercise).

Sleep

Older individuals require more rest but need less actual sleep. There is an increased incidence of accidents that occur during nighttime awakenings, and it is necessary to deal with safety concerns. Using night-lights and reducing excess furniture and clutter are some methods of decreasing the risk of nighttime injury. Sleep for the older person is often affected by medications, alcohol, caffeine, stress, and environmental noise and temperature.

Safety

Most accidents are preventable (see safety tips for older adults in Safety Alert box). The key to prevention is knowledge and recognition of and attention to the factors that contribute to the increased risk for accident or injury. Diminished sight, along with changes in posture or balance, sometimes expose the older person to the risk of falls. A single fall has the potential to produce an injury necessitating a long period of immobilization, thus diminishing the person's independence and self-esteem.

Safety Alert!

Safety Tips for the Older Adult

- Minimize clutter and excess furniture in rooms and hallways.
- Remove scatter rugs.
- Use hand rails on stairs.
- Install grab bars in showers and bathroom.
- Use night-lights.
- Get up slowly from a lying-flat position.
- Use caution in going from well-lighted areas to darkened areas or vice versa.
- If self-medicating, use dispensing aids to decrease the risk of error.
- Wear properly fitting shoes and clothing.
- Allow enough time—do not rush or hurry.

Get Ready for the NCLEX® Examination!

Key Points

- Development is a lifelong process that begins at conception and ends at death.
- All types of families serve similar basic functions: protection, nurturance, education, sustenance, and socialization of their members.
- Growth patterns suggest rapid growth during infancy, continued growth during toddler and preschool years, and slowed but steady growth during the school years, followed by a rapid surge of growth during puberty and adolescence.
- Erikson identified a central task that needs to be resolved at each stage of the life span: infancy, toddler, preschool, school age, adolescence, early adulthood, middle adulthood, and late adulthood.
- Piaget focused on the concept of cognitive development beginning in infancy and continuing throughout the childhood years.
- Accidental injuries are a major cause of death during infancy, childhood, and adolescence.
- Consistent discipline and supervision are needed throughout childhood.
- Peer relationships become significant at school age.
- Adolescence is the transitional period between childhood and adulthood.
- Adulthood is marked by significant events: career decisions, marriage, new social relationships, and financial concerns.
- Certain physical changes become evident during middle age, including graying of hair and vision changes.
- Menopause and hormonal changes characterize the reproductive changes of the middle-age female.
- Roles undergo change during middle adulthood, including nuclear family roles, relationships with grown children, grandparenting, and possibly career changes.
- Late adulthood is marked by a gradual slowing of the body's functioning.
- Several significant physical changes become evident in the older adult.
- Family changes and an increased awareness of one's mortality are common adjustments called for by the aging process.
- Life review and acceptance of one's strengths and weaknesses are necessary aspects of the aging process.
- Several theories attempt to explain aging; however, no one theory is universally accepted.
- Aging, like growth, is a highly individualized process.

Additional Learning Resources

Go to your Companion CD for an audio glossary, animations, video clips, and more.

evolve Be sure to visit the Evolve site at http://evolve.elsevier.com/Christensen/foundations/ for additional online resources.

Review Questions for the NCLEX® Examination

1. According to Piaget, thinking during the first few months is primarily based on:
   1. imitation.
   2. intuition.
   3. logical operations.
   4. reflex behavior.

2. The first socializing agent for the child is:

1. daycare.
2. family.
3. school.
4. play groups.

3. At 4 years of age, a child is working on Erikson's task of:

1. trust versus mistrust.
2. industry versus inferiority.
3. autonomy versus shame and doubt.
4. initiative versus guilt.

4. Which type of play is most common at ages 4 and 5?

1. Solitary
2. Parallel
3. Competitive
4. Make-believe

5. Growth during the school-age period:

1. occurs at a rate similar to that during infancy.
2. is slow and consistent.
3. is mainly in the body's upper region.
4. is more rapid than during the preschool period.

6. An 8-year-old loves to draw and do craft projects. Her need for praise and encouragement for her work efforts demonstrates her development of Erikson's task of:

1. autonomy.
2. initiative.
3. industry.
4. identity.

7. Peak physical strength and endurance occurs during:

1. adolescence.
2. early adulthood.
3. middle adulthood.
4. late adulthood.

8. Menopause usually occurs:

1. in the early 30s.
2. by age 40.
3. in the late 50s.
4. in the late 40s to early 50s.

9. In correcting the myths about aging, the nurse recognizes that healthy older adults:

1. have periods of confusion.
2. are likely to become senile.
3. have few or no sexual needs.
4. have a slower reaction time.

10. The principle that describes the direction of growth beginning at the head and moving to the lower extremities is called:

1. integrated.
2. proximodistal.
3. cephalocaudal.
4. differential.

11. The cognitive approach to understanding development is explained by ________ theory.

1. Maslow's
2. Piaget's
3. Erikson's
4. Skinner's

12. Following fertilization, the newly formed structure is known as a:

1. gene.
2. chromosome.
3. zygote.
4. germ cell.

13. According to Erikson, when the infant is cuddled, fed, and loved, the infant will develop:

1. autonomy.
2. trust.
3. industry.
4. identity.

14. The type of play typical of the preschool child is:

1. parallel play.
2. imaginary play.
3. organized, team play.
4. cognitive play.

15. According to Piaget, the child between 7 and 11 years of age is in the:

1. sensorimotor stage.
2. preoperational stage.
3. stage of concrete operation.
4. stage of formal operation.

16. In the female, the onset of the postpuberty period is marked by the onset of:

1. breast development.
2. appearance of pubic and axillary hair.
3. menarche.
4. mood changes.

17. The typical adolescent is likely to:

1. reject peer pressure.
2. try to be different from the crowd.
3. reject the advice of elders.
4. attempt to copy his or her peers.

18. According to Erikson, the task for the young adult is:

1. trust versus mistrust.
2. identity versus confusion.
3. generativity versus stagnation.
4. intimacy versus isolation.

19. Which are health-promoting behaviors the nurse will recommend? *(Select all that apply.)*

1. Regular medical checkups
2. Appropriate prescription use
3. Sedentary lifestyle
4. Eating low-cholesterol foods

20. Which segment of the population is currently the fastest growing?
    1. Baby boomers
    2. From 65 to 70 years of age
    3. From 71 to 80 years of age
    4. Older than 85 years of age

21. A 2-year-old's negative behavior is normal for her age. It is helping her to meet her need for:
    1. discipline.
    2. trust.
    3. independence.
    4. love.

22. The period of cognitive development when the child's knowledge comes about through sensory impressions is called:
    1. preoperational.
    2. sensorimotor.
    3. concrete operational.
    4. formal operational.

23. Growth during the school-age period can best be described as:
    1. irregular and slow.
    2. steady and slow.
    3. regular and fast.
    4. irregular and fast.

24. Typical behavior for toddlers includes:
    1. role modeling.
    2. ritualistic behavior.
    3. competitiveness.
    4. industry.

25. During early adulthood, individuals are physically:
    1. beginning to deteriorate.
    2. already slowing down.
    3. increasing lung capacity and muscle strength.
    4. fairly stable at optimal level of function.

26. To counteract the effect of aging, ____________ will help to increase the flow of ____________.
    1. rest; blood
    2. sleeping; oxygen
    3. exercise; oxygen
    4. carbohydrates; oxygen

27. Teach patients that influenza immunization:
    1. produces an immediate effect.
    2. is effective against all strains of influenza.
    3. has a lifelong effect.
    4. is contraindicated for use by people who are allergic to eggs or egg products.

28. Advise older adults in nutritional counseling to:
    1. eat more fats and proteins.
    2. eat a diet low in fiber and high in carbohydrates.
    3. eat a diet low in saturated fats and carbohydrates.
    4. rely on food supplements for all nutrient needs.

29. According to Erikson, the developmental tasks for older adults are:
    1. intimacy versus isolation
    2. generativity versus stagnation
    3. ego integrity versus despair
    4. initiative versus guilt

30. Which developmental skill is commonly accomplished by the fourth month of life?
    1. Sitting up unsupported
    2. Holding head up at 90-degree angle
    3. Creeping
    4. Transferring objects from one hand to the other

31. The introduction of solid foods to the infant should rely on:
    1. introducing several foods at once.
    2. limiting foods to those preferred by the family.
    3. introducing one new food at a time.
    4. mixing new foods together to conceal certain tastes.

32. Nighttime bottles should be avoided since milk and juice during the night lead to:
    1. dental caries.
    2. dental malocclusion.
    3. otitis media.
    4. lactose intolerance.

33. Preschool children need to be tested for amblyopia. This condition may lead to:
    1. blindness.
    2. deafness.
    3. muscle weakness.
    4. paralysis.

chapter 10

Loss, Grief, Dying, and Death

evolve

http://evolve.elsevier.com/Christensen/foundationsadult

Elaine Oden Kockrow and Barbara Lauritsen Christensen

Objectives

1. Explain the role of loss in the grief reaction.
2. Discuss how changes in the health care system have affected nursing interventions for the dying patient.
3. Describe the stages of dying.
4. Identify needs of the grieving patient and family.
5. Discuss principles of palliative care.
6. Recognize the five aspects of human functioning and how each interacts with the others during the grieving–dying process.
7. Identify unique physical signs and symptoms of the near-death patient.
8. Discuss nursing interventions for the dying patient.
9. Describe techniques in assisting the dying patient to say good-bye.
10. List nursing interventions that may facilitate grieving in special circumstances (perinatal, pediatric, older adult, and suicide).
11. Describe nursing responsibilities in care of the body after death.
12. Discuss approaches to facilitate the grieving process.
13. Explain concepts of euthanasia, do not resuscitate (DNR) orders, organ donations, fraudulent methods of treatment, and the Dying Person's Bill of Rights.
14. Discuss support for the grieving family.
15. Explain advance directives, which include the living will and the durable power of attorney.
16. Discuss complicated grieving.

Key Terms

advance directives (p. 234)
anticipatory grief (ăn-TĬS-ĭ-pă-TŌ-rē, p. 220)
autopsy (AW-tŏp-sē, p. 240)
bereavement (bĭ-RĒV-měnt, p. 220)
bereavement overload (p. 222)
complicated grieving (p. 224)
death (p. 218)
do not resuscitate (DNR) (p. 234)
durable power of attorney (p. 234)
dysfunctional grieving (p. 224)
euthanasia (yū-thĕ-NĀ-zhă, p. 233)
grief (p. 218)
grief therapy (p. 219)
grief work (p. 218)
inquest (p. 240)
living will (p. 234)
loss (p. 218)
maturational loss (măch-ŭ-RĀ-shŭn-ăl, p. 219)
morbidity (p. 220)
mortality (p. 219)
mortician (p. 241)
mourning (p. 220)
palliative care (PĂL-ē-ă-tĭv, p. 238)
postmortem care (p. 241)
situational loss (p. 219)
thanatology (thăn-ă-TŎL-ŏ-jē, p. 222)
unresolved grief (p. 222)

Life is a series of losses and gains. When any aspect of self becomes no longer available to a person, that person suffers a **loss**. Loss and **death** (cessation of life) are universal in the human experience, but they are unique events to the individual. Coping mechanisms determine a person's ability to face and accept loss. **Grief** is a pattern of physical and emotional responses to bereavement, separation, or loss. It is a natural response to loss. All losses have the possibility of triggering the grief process. The severity of the loss may vary, but the grief that accompanies it is real nonetheless.

Illness and hospitalization frequently cause loss, and nurses work with many patients who experience losses of different types. You help them understand and accept loss so that life can continue. The process of adapting to and mourning a loss is called **grief work**. After a loss, serious emotional, mental, and social problems may occur if a patient does not perform grief work.

Humans can anticipate death. This causes a variety of possible responses: anxiety, planning, denial, love, loneliness, achievement, or lack of achievement. Death affects dying patients and their families, significant others, friends, and caregivers. It can be an overwhelming experience. A person's style of dying reflects that person's style of living, and attitudes about death depend on a person's beliefs and emotional strengths.

Care of dying patients and their families can be one of the most challenging aspects of nursing care. Dying is the final stage of human growth and development; thus it is essential that you as a nurse be as knowledgeable about the process of dying as you are about the process of birth. Because health care usually emphasizes the cure of disease and the promotion of health, health care providers often perceive the death of a patient as a form of failure. Health care personnel caring for dying patients often withdraw from patients emotionally while providing adequate physical care.

When you deal with grieving families and dying patients, you will be confronted with your own **mortality** (the condition of being subject to death) and other distressing issues that accompany loss. It is possible that your subjective experience will influence the quality of the care you deliver. However, if you understand loss, the stages of the grief process, and the task of dying, you will find it easier to deliver quality care to those patients and families experiencing death.

CHANGES IN HEALTH CARE RELATED TO DYING AND DEATH

Before the 1950s, it was common for patients to die at home in their own beds with assistance only from their family. From the 1950s to the 1980s, the health care system became highly mechanized and dying occurred mostly in institutions, often with sophisticated equipment attached to the dying individual to prolong life. When diagnosis-related groups (DRGs) came into play by the early 1980s, the trend changed again. Today, in general, the only patients placed in hospital beds are those who are considered at risk for medical complications or who need hospital recovery time after surgery or special procedures. This type of bed is often used in the home as well. Many recuperating or terminally ill patients are discharged to home, a convalescent center, or a nursing home. Nurses providing care to the terminally ill patient in the home health care setting have felt the impact of this development. At home, these patients are now receiving intravenous infusions, including blood products, and other technical and mechanical assistance. Nurses in health care facilities and homes are the health care providers most often available to the grieving family during the crisis of death. These nurses are often licensed practical nurses (LPNs) or licensed vocational nurses (LVNs).

HISTORICAL OVERVIEW

Discussions of the dynamics surrounding grief, dying, and death are not new. In the 1960s, pioneers in death and dying theory such as Kübler-Ross and Glasser and Strauss produced works that stimulated the health care industry. Dying and death became topics of research and seminars. In the 1970s, hospices in the United States became recognized as health care delivery systems (see Chapter 40). **Grief therapy** (mental health treatment aimed at helping a patient deal with the pain of loss; a program that assists the bereaved to cope with a loss) was introduced in the 1980s when Bowlby and Worden added new insights to what was known about the needs and care of the dying patient.

Care providers have been learning to assist patients and families to exercise more control over their care. Individuals become involved by determining treatment options and choosing the setting, circumstances, and management of the dying process. Advance directives are being upheld as legal documents in courts of law, and terminal health care is shifting away from hospital settings. Because of developments such as these, nurses will continue to play a primary role in the care of the dying person at home and of the family experiencing loss.

LOSS

Not all losses are obvious or immediate. Obvious losses are such events as the death of a loved one, divorce, breakup of a relationship, or loss of a job. Not so obvious are the losses precipitated by illness, aging, and changing schools, jobs, or neighborhoods.

Some losses are actual and some perceived. An actual loss is easily identified, such as a woman who has a mastectomy. A perceived loss, such as the loss of confidence or when a woman who hopes to give birth to a female child delivers a male child instead, is less obvious. Perceived losses are easily overlooked or misunderstood, yet the associated process of grief follows the same sequence as with losses that are considered "real."

Another way to look at loss is to classify it as maturational, situational, or both. **Maturational loss** is a loss resulting from normal life transitions. Examples include the loss of childhood dreams, the loss felt by an adolescent when a romance fails, and the loss felt when leaving the family home for college or marriage and establishing a home of one's own. Later, as the individual ages, he or she experiences menopause and loss of hair, teeth, hearing, sight, and "youth." **Situational loss** is defined as a loss occurring suddenly in response to a specific external event, such as the sudden death of a loved one. Losing a job can lead to a loss of self-esteem. Such changes promote emotional growth and the development of coping skills. People use these skills later to cope with even more significant losses. Early experiences with loss can prepare the individual to deal with loss throughout the life cycle.

Each person experiences loss as it individually affects him or her. Each loss is followed by a time of grieving.

Personal loss is any significant loss that requires adaptation through the grieving process. When some-

Box 10-1 Factors Influencing the Experience of Loss

- Childhood experiences
- Significance assigned to the loss
- Physical and emotional state
- Accumulated loss experience
- View of loss as crisis
- Duration and timing
- Abruptness or suddenness
- Financial impact
- Availability of resources
- Cultural factors
- Personal attributes
- Relationship with the lost person or object

thing or someone can no longer be seen, felt, heard, known, or experienced, there is a sense of loss. The type of loss influences the degree of stress it causes. For example, the loss of an object might not generate the same stress as the loss of a significant other. On the other hand, individuals respond to loss differently. In general, people expect the death of a family member to cause more stress than the loss of a pet. However, for an older person living alone, it is very possible that the death of a pet that has been a constant companion will cause more emotional stress than that of a cousin who had not been seen in years.

Thus it is important for you as a nurse to recognize how highly individualized each person's interpretation of a loss is, whatever type of loss it may be. Loss is a complex phenomenon influenced by many factors (Box 10-1). It threatens self-concept, self-esteem, security, and sense of worth. It is important that you recognize the meaning of each loss to a patient and its impact on physical and psychological functioning.

GRIEF

Grief is the subjective response to actual or anticipated loss. It is a natural, normal, and universal part of human experience. **Bereavement** is defined as a common depressed reaction to the death of a loved one. **Mourning** (reaction activated by a person to assist in overcoming a great personal loss) refers to culturally defined patterns for the expression of grief. Mourning patterns include funerals, wakes, memorials, black dress, and defined time of social withdrawal.

Grief involves thought, feelings, and behaviors. There exist many examples of increased **morbidity** (an illness or an abnormal condition), both physical and mental, after significant losses. For example, there is an increase in the breakup of marriages and other significant relationships after the loss of a child or when one partner suffers a loss of a body part or function.

When allowed to operate normally, however, grief has a useful function. Grief is not an episode. It is a process, sometimes one that goes on forever (e.g., parents grieving for a child). On the other hand, the grieving process can lead to resolution of the hurt and the reestablishment of one's life. Still, the emotional pain involved in grief comes and goes with a person's life experiences. Many years after a loss, something reminds the person of it and the associated feelings return. The reminder might be an encounter with smells, places, foods, dates, holidays, clothing, or other people.

The grieving person may try a variety of strategies to cope. The following tasks facilitate the passage from grief to closure:

- Accepting the reality of the loss
- Experiencing the pain of grief
- Adjusting to an environment that no longer includes the lost person, object, or aspect of self
- Reinvesting emotional energy into new relationships

The successful completion of these tasks leads to healthy adjustment to loss. These tasks are not sequential. In fact, grieving people often work on all four tasks simultaneously, or place priority on only one or two. One of your roles is to assist patients and families in working through these tasks.

In the past, society discouraged the open display of grief. Unhappy children were told not to cry when playmates moved away, awkward adolescents were told not to be embarrassed about sudden growth spurts, and dying people were told to remain calm and dignified. Changes in attitudes, beliefs, and values have promoted more open expressions of grief. For example, nurses learn to seek support from peers and to express their concerns about dealing with terminally ill patients. Similarly, family members seek support from caregivers to express anger over loss. Grieving leads to new understandings that promote growth if a person is able to be open and obtains encouragement and adequate support from others.

Sometimes losses such as physical deformity or the death of close friends stimulate behaviors and feelings associated with the grieving process. These behaviors and feelings also occur when individuals face their own death. A patient who is dying is undergoing loss as well as the impact of the family's grief. Some patients feel that their family does not need any other problems and cannot cope with additional concerns. The dying patient in this situation sometimes depends extensively on the nurse, and identification of sources of support becomes a major task (Figure 10-1).

Loss, through death or otherwise, is somewhat easier to cope with if it is expected. Sometimes the diagnosis of terminal illness allows a period of **anticipatory grief** (to expect, await, or prepare oneself for the loss of a family member or significant other) when both the dying person and the mourners are able to cry together and enjoy their mutual affection. Having time for anticipation does not necessarily ease the pain of loss, because attachment is often strengthened during the period of anticipatory grief. However, sometimes the emotions expressed at this time make the loss less

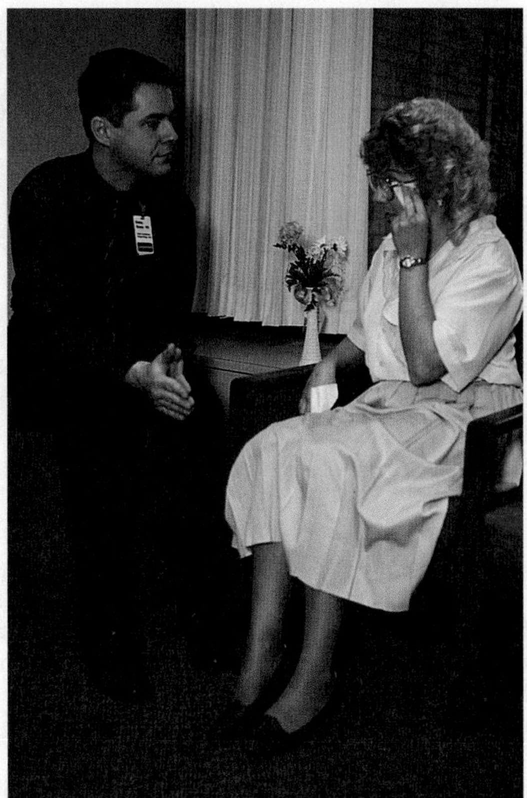

FIGURE 10-1 Nurses assist family members in finding resources to help with the grieving process.

conflicted than when such exchanges never occur. When individuals achieve an awareness of mortality, this maturity often leads them to anticipate eventual grief. They make a special effort to express affection and appreciation of their older adult relatives, even when there is no evidence of impending death.

The sudden death of someone who is not "supposed to" die (sometimes referred to as "out-of-sequence" death) is the most difficult grief to bear. The clearest example is the death of a child, especially one who has lived long enough to have a distinct personality and position in the family. If the death is a violent and sudden one, the loss is particularly devastating. Parents and siblings are often wracked by powerful and personal emotions of guilt, denial, and anger, as well as sorrow. One protective impulse is to blame someone—perhaps oneself for not having been more careful or more loving, perhaps a spouse, and perhaps even the dead child.

Blame and guilt, however, have the power to destroy a family just when family members need each other most. The Compassionate Friends, a national self-help support organization that assists families following the death of a child, finds that many married couples are driven apart by their separate reactions to the death. Perhaps one parent needs to talk about the death, whereas the other cannot bear to hear the child's name. Siblings suffer, too—partly because parents are so involved in their own grief that the surviving children are deprived of attention, and partly because a child's grief may follow a different course from that of adults. Denial and regression are common at first, with sorrow and acceptance coming much later than for adults. Each family member should make an effort to understand and accept the many possible individual forms and paces of mourning that may be exhibited by others. Children in particular need to know that all questions and feelings are acceptable.

SENSE OF PRESENCE

Individuals who have experienced a loss sometimes have a nonthreatening, comforting perception that the deceased is present. Such perceptions, known as *sense of presence*, vary from general feelings of the deceased's presence to having actual sensory experiences. Sometimes these sensory experiences manifest as dreams or conversations; sometimes they involve the senses and include visions, hallucinations, or the perception of voices, smells, or touch. A sense of presence is thought to be a form of searching behavior, a means of consciously or unconsciously denying the reality of the loss. Searching allows the individual to see the deceased as safe, comfortable, and at peace. Sense of presence is known to occur during the grief process and beyond (Harkreader, 2007).

GRIEF ATTACKS

The involuntary and unexpected reappearance of emotions and behaviors associated with grief is known as a *grief attack*. This phenomenon occurs in response to routine events and sometimes results in emotional outbursts. Sometimes exposure to experiences that were shared with the deceased, such as special music or places, is what generates a grief attack. In contrast, sometimes the trigger for these episodes is an unrelated event, such as a death depicted in a movie.

Although the sadness of a loss never disappears completely, emotions become more balanced over time. The individual finds that daily life goes on and emotional responses disrupt less, mostly during special times such as anniversaries and holidays (Harkreader, 2007).

NURSES' GRIEF

The universality of the loss experience often leads nurses who work with the terminally ill and the bereaved to develop a heightened empathy for their patients. Identifying with your patients and sharing the impact of loss is likely to help you prepare for the ultimate loss experience: death. On the other hand, your role in supporting grieving patients and families can become complicated when you are experiencing grief yourself, especially when working with dying patients. Never allow their grief to unduly influence your care of patients and families. Nurses who are not aware of their own grief issues have more difficulty relating to patients as unique individuals. Perhaps, for example, a dying patient reminds you of a beloved grandparent and you become too emotionally involved. There are other tasks and abilities that you will also find useful for working with dying patients: for example, coming to grips with and understanding the grief process, appreciating the experience of the dying patient, using effective listening skills, acknowledging personal limits, and knowing when there is a need to get away and take care of yourself. Recognizing the need to grieve will assist you in moving through this process.

If you experience multiple losses in the course of your work and fail to adequately process them, you run the risk of **bereavement overload** (before an initial loss is resolved, it is compounded by an additional loss). Frustration, anger, guilt, sadness, helplessness, anxiety, depression, and feelings of being overwhelmed are common. Self-care is critical to survival. As a nurse, you need to do for yourself what you do for your patients and their families. You need to mourn your losses (Box 10-2). Unrelieved grief and stress can lead to diminished well-being and inability to care for others (Figure 10-2). An ongoing personal support system is crucial if you are working in areas where a high number of deaths occur. Without opportunities for energy renewal and mutual support, you will not develop closure for each case. What happens when the stresses of the job exceed its rewards and you lack the support of peers, is burnout. (See Chapter 58 for further discussion of burnout.)

You, who are always giving, will eventually realize that receiving is also necessary if you want to be effective. Nursing is a job with increasingly high demands.

Box 10-2 Survival Strategies for Nurses

- Identify personal spiritual beliefs.
- Take regular breaks or time-outs from the patient care area, and consider rotating out of high-stress areas.
- Identify specific patients who are the most stressful so that stress can be anticipated.
- Trade off patients or ask for special assistance in working in stressful situations.
- Acknowledge physical needs as key factors in stress reduction.
- Integrate decompression routines into daily life (e.g., before leaving the work area and going home, take a moment to review the day and set it aside).
- Engage in life-affirming activities (e.g., spend time with lively, healthy children).
- View losses as an opportunity to reevaluate and grow.
- Avoid the "rescuer" or "savior" complex; recognize limits.
- Recognize the need for support and do not hesitate to ask for it.
- Say "I choose" rather than "I should."
- Develop the skills of setting limits and feeling okay about saying no.
- Laugh and play in the face of tragedy without guilt.
- Seek consultation on a regular basis.

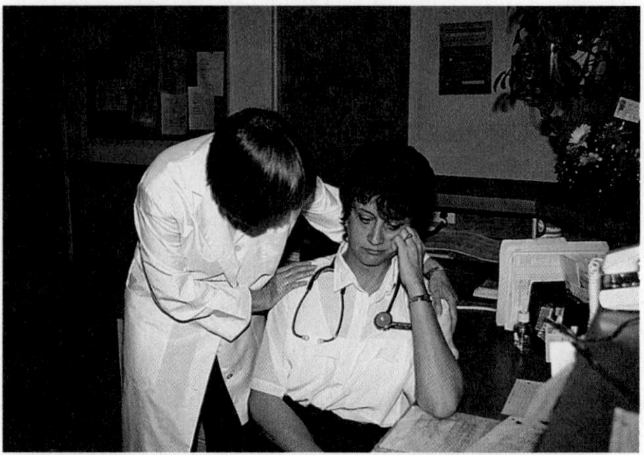

FIGURE 10-2 Nurses benefit from support of colleagues during their time of loss.

You need the ability to modify your role and acquire new ones that are compatible with new trends in health care delivery and permit ethical decision making about allocation of resources. An understanding of the impact work has on you will allow you to use problem-solving techniques to guide your choices and prevent dysfunctional responses to loss.

Being informed and up to date, practicing within the legal parameters of professional responsibilities, and using current trends in health care, you will be an expert in many fields, including the expertise of caring for the dying patient.

STAGES OF GRIEF AND DYING

There is no right or wrong way to grieve. The concepts and theories of grief are only tools for you to use to anticipate potential needs of patients and families and to plan interventions to help your patients understand their grief while trying to deal with it. It is a mistake, and possibly harmful, to expect patients to progress in some specific manner over a specified time. Your role as a nurse is to assess grieving behaviors, recognize the influence of grief on behavior, and provide empathic support.

Thanatology (the study of dying and death) has sparked much interest since the 1970s. See Box 10-3 for more information on theories of grief and mourning.

Table 10-1 describes some of the concepts of death and dying typically held by specific age-groups. With knowledge of these developmental stages, you will better understand a patient's responses to a life-threatening situation and the grief responses of individuals after a loss.

COMPLICATED GRIEF

Bereavement is a state of great risk physically, as well as emotionally and socially. For this reason, the importance of grief work cannot be overstated.

Various theorists have described behaviors indicative of unresolved grief. As the term indicates, **unresolved grief** signifies some disturbance of the normal

Box 10-3 Theories of Grief and Mourning

KÜBLER-ROSS'S STAGES OF DYING

A behavior-oriented theory that includes five stages:

- **Denial:** Individual acts as though nothing has happened and may refuse to believe or understand loss has occurred.
- **Anger:** Individual resists the loss and may strike out at everyone and everything.
- **Bargaining:** Individual postpones awareness of reality of the loss and may try to deal in a subtle or overt way as though the loss can be prevented.
- **Depression:** Individual feels overwhelmingly lonely and withdraws from interpersonal interaction.
- **Acceptance:** Individual accepts the loss and looks to the future.

BOWLBY'S PHASES OF MOURNING

A behavioral theory that includes four phases:

- **Numbing:** Individual describes phase as feeling "stunned" or "unreal." A period of intense emotion. Serves to protect the body from consequences of loss. Lasts from a few hours to a week or more.
- **Yearning and searching:** Arouses acute distress in most persons. A painful phase characterized by physical symptoms such as tightness in the chest and throat, shortness of breath, a feeling of weakness and lethargy, insomnia, and anorexia. Phase may last for months or years.
- **Disorganization and despair:** Individual endlessly examines how and why the loss occurred. Common time for person to express anger. Gradually phase gives way to an acceptance that loss is permanent.
- **Reorganization:** Individual begins to accept unaccustomed roles, acquires new skills, builds new relationships. Phase may last a year or more. Individual needs support to unlink self from the lost relationships.

WORDEN'S TASKS OF MOURNING

A behavioral theory that indicates four tasks:

- **Accept reality of loss:** There is always some period of disbelief and surprise over a loss. This task involves processes required to accept that the person or object is gone and will not return.
- **Work through pain and grief:** Emotional pain comes as a natural part of loss. Individuals who deny or shut off the pain prolong their grief.
- **Adjust to environment in which the deceased is missing:** Individual does not realize full impact of loss for at least 3 months. At this point, friends and associates stop calling, and the person is left prey to loneliness. Often, the individual must take on roles formerly filled by the deceased.
- **Emotionally relocate the deceased and move on with life:** Individual does not forget the deceased or give up the relationship with the deceased. The deceased, however, must take a new, less prominent, place in a person's emotional life. People dealing with this task fear they will forget their loved one.

From Perry, A.G., & Potter, P.A. (2005). *Clinical nursing skills and techniques* (6th ed.). St. Louis: Elsevier.

Table 10-1 Age-Related Influences on the Concept of Death

Age	Influences
Infancy to 5 years	• Does not understand concept of death • Infant's sense of separation forms basis for later understanding of loss and death • Believes death is reversible, a temporary departure, or sleep
5 to 9 years	• Understands that death is final • Believes own death can be avoided • Associates death with aggression or violence • Believes wishes or unrelated actions can be responsible for death
9 to 12 years	• Understands death as the inevitable end of life • Begins to understand own mortality • Concept of death expressed as interest in afterlife or as fear of death
12 to 18 years	• Fears a lingering death • May fantasize that death can be defied, acting out defiance through reckless behaviors (e.g., dangerous driving, substance abuse) • Seldom thinks about death, but views it in religious and philosophic terms • May seem to reach "adult" perception of death but be emotionally unable to accept it
18 to 45 years	• Has attitude toward death influenced by religious and cultural beliefs
45 to 65 years	• Accepts own mortality • Encounters death of parents and some peers • Experiences peaks of death anxiety • Death anxiety diminishes with emotional well-being
65+ years	• Fears prolonged illness • Encounters death of family members and peers • Sees death as having multiple meanings (e.g., freedom from pain, reunion with already deceased family members)

Box 10-4 Complicated Grief

When a person has difficulty progressing through the normal stages of grieving, bereavement becomes complicated. In these cases, bereavement appears to "go wrong" and loss never resolves. This threatens a person's relationship with others. Complicated grief includes four types:

- **Chronic grief:** Active acute mourning characterized by normal grief reactions that do not decrease but persist over long periods. Persons verbalize an inability to "get past" the grief.
- **Delayed grief:** Characterized by normal grief reactions that are suppressed or postponed. The survivor consciously or unconsciously avoids the pain of the loss. Active grieving is held back, only to resurface later, usually in response to a trivial loss or upset. For example, a wife only grieves a few weeks after the death of her spouse, only to become hysterical and sad a year later when she loses her car keys. The extreme sadness is a delayed response to the death of her husband.
- **Exaggerated grief:** Persons become overwhelmed by grief, and they cannot function. This is reflected in the form of severe phobias or self-destructive behaviors such as alcoholism, substance abuse, or suicide.
- **Masked grief:** Survivors are not aware that behaviors that interfere with normal functioning are a result of their loss. For example, a person who has lost a pet develops changes in sleeping or eating patterns.

DISENFRANCHISED GRIEF

Individuals experience grief when they experience a loss and they cannot openly acknowledge it, or when it is not socially accepted or publicly shared. Examples include the loss of a partner from acquired immunodeficiency syndrome (AIDS), the friend who becomes a drug addict, or a mother whose child dies in utero.

From Perry, A.G., Potter, P.A. (2005). *Clinical nursing skills and techniques* (6th ed.). St. Louis: Elsevier.

progression toward resolution. **Complicated grieving** (unresolved grief or complicated mourning; also called **dysfunctional grieving**) is a delayed or exaggerated response to a perceived, actual, or potential loss. Complicated grieving occurs when an individual (1) gets "stuck" in the grief process and becomes depressed; (2) is unable to express feelings; (3) cannot find anyone in his or her daily life who acts as the listener he or she needs; (4) suffers a loss that stirs up other, unresolved losses and causes him or her to explore long-standing feelings or emotional concerns; or (5) lacks the reassurance and support to trust the grief process and fails to believe that he or she can work through the loss. A surviving spouse who seeks additional support for many years after the loss of his or her significant other (Box 10-4) provides one example. The more signs, symptoms, and behaviors the mourner has, the stronger the likelihood of unresolved grief (Nursing Care Plan 10-1). It is important that you recognize these individuals and refer them for appropriate counseling or treatment (see Figure 10-1).

SUPPORTIVE CARE DURING THE DYING AND GRIEVING PROCESS

Assessment

To give compassionate nursing care and support to the family and the patient during the grieving and dying process, consider the five aspects of human functioning: physical, emotional, intellectual, sociocultural, and spiritual. Do an assessment in each area, using the nursing process, to fully understand the patient's needs and provide appropriate interventions.

Physical Assessment

While interviewing and observing the patient, assess such areas as sleeping patterns, body image, activities of daily living (ADLs), mobility, general health, medication use, and pain. Also address the basic needs of nutrition, elimination, oxygenation, activity, rest, sleep, and safety (Nursing Care Plan 10-2).

Interventions should target (1) energy conservation, (2) pain-reduction techniques, (3) comfort measures, (4) promotion of sleep and rest, and (5) increasing self-esteem through body image acceptance.

Emotional Assessment

Preparing for death is an endeavor filled with anxiety and fear for most people. Assess the patient's and the family's level of anxiety, guilt, anger, or acceptance. Major fears of the dying patient include fears of abandonment (fear of dying alone), loss of control, pain and discomfort, and the unknown.

Nurses intervene appropriately when they are able to accept the patient's and the family's feelings, whatever they may be. You can also offer encouragement and support and give the patient "permission to die" by assisting the patient in saying good-bye.

Intellectual Assessment

Intellectual assessment includes an evaluation of the patient's and the family's educational level, their knowledge and abilities, and the expectations they have in regard to how and when death will occur. Some aspects of functioning in the intellectual dimension are frequently altered during the dying process because of physiologic changes, medications, the patient's emotional state, or the disease process. By remaining alert to these changes, you will be able to avert problems if the patient's memory or sensations are decreased.

In most cases, you will direct interventions toward patient and family education and support. If you help

Nursing Care Plan 10-1 The Patient Experiencing Complicated Grieving (Unresolved Grief)

Ms. Stuart is 78 years old and is being admitted for weakness, complaints of chronic fatigue, anorexia, and weight loss. Her nursing history reveals that Ms. Stuart refuses to care for herself, has ceased participating in her church activities, and is unable to discuss the deceased without crying. The social history of Ms. Stuart reveals that her only child, a daughter, died unexpectedly at age 47. Her husband of 50 years died 1 year later. Ms. Stuart is accompanied by her grandchildren, who offer support and concern. The nursing assessment reveals that Ms. Stuart lacks resolution of previous grieving response and is experiencing bereavement overload.

NURSING GOAL–EXPECTED OUTCOME *Promote resolution of the grieving process*

Nursing Diagnosis	Patient Goals and Expected Outcomes	Nursing Interventions
Complicated grieving, related to bereavement overload secondary to death of daughter and husband manifested by refusing to care for self, abstaining from participation in church activities, the inability to discuss the deceased without crying, alterations in eating habits, and interference with performance of activities of daily living (ADLs)	Patient will establish new and meaningful relationships and interests. Patient will engage in constructive, meaningful lifestyle (precrisis level of functioning). Patient will relate realistically to both the pleasures and the disappointments of the lost relationships. Patient will participate in decision making and cooperate with recommended treatment within 2 weeks.	Establish trust and positive regard by creating an atmosphere of sharing. Offer privacy and security. Identify significance of multiple losses. Discuss ambivalence. Assess stage of grief and support patient's expressions of grief. Use active listening. Facilitate discussion of positive and negative aspects of loss. Provide opportunities for social interaction, especially with those who have coped with similar losses. Teach patient and significant others about the grieving process. Assure patient that feelings are normal. Expect patient to meet responsibilities and give positive reinforcement. Help patient identify ways to adapt lifestyle to accommodate loss. Explore ways to assist patient to make new emotional investments. If you become uncomfortable with your unresolved feelings of loss, contact another nurse to counsel the patient.

Critical Thinking Questions

1. Ms. Stuart is admitted to the medical unit for severe weakness, weight loss, and chronic depression. She is reluctant to get out of bed to dress and have meals. How could the nurse facilitate progression through the grieving process?
2. Ms. Stuart appears thin, with poor tissue turgor. How could the nurse and dietitian encourage improvement of her nutritional status?
3. The nursing assessment for Ms. Stuart revealed a flat affect, little verbalization, and poor personal hygiene. Which therapeutic nursing interventions would help achieve patient goals and expected outcomes?

keep everyone informed of procedures, changes in the patient's condition, and hospital policies, they can make more well-informed and satisfactory decisions.

Sociocultural Assessment

Your assessment of the patient's and the family's support systems is valuable. For one thing, it helps to ascertain whether family members want to assist in the patient's daily care. Not only does this lessen the family's sense of loss of control, but it also helps clarify what tasks the family will do and what will be done by nursing staff. If these needs and desires are not clear, distrust and hostility between family and nursing staff can result. Each family and each individual member in that family are unique in what they wish to do. Never assume that families want to deliver daily care. Many do, but others do not, and they need the opportunity to make that choice (Box 10-5).

Family members need support to get through the dying and death of their loved one. At the same time, it is good for them to provide support; encourage them to do so. Recognize the value of family members as resources and assist them in working with the dying person.

In the home, the family becomes closely involved in the patient's care (see Chapters 37 and 40). A terminal

 Nursing Care Plan 10-2 The Patient Facing Death

Ms. Barton is 68 years old and has been admitted to the hospital for weakness and debilitation caused by widespread metastatic cancer of the colon. She complains of pain and is anxious to return home. Both Ms. Barton and her family are aware of her terminal state. The nursing history identified that Ms. Barton (1) is unable to care for herself because of severe weakness; (2) has chronic pain; (3) has a decreased appetite; (4) appears anxious and wants to be home with her family; and (5) is grieving the loss of her health and expresses fears regarding her death.

NURSING GOALS *Control pain; prevent injury; ensure safety; provide for activities of daily living (ADLs), including adequate nutrition, hydration, and elimination; relieve anxiety; and facilitate the normal grieving process*

NURSING DIAGNOSIS *Chronic pain related to disease progression*

Patient Goals and Expected Outcomes	Nursing Interventions	Evaluation
Patient will verbalize moderate comfort and decreased pain while receiving analgesics and other comfort measures	Position patient comfortably; change position gradually and unhurriedly. Provide pain-relief measures patient prefers (e.g., relaxation therapy, diversion, and distraction). Give analgesics as ordered. Evaluate pain for intensity and quality. Know that pain is what patient says it is. Observe patient's freedom of movement. Request patient to rate pain on a scale of 1 to 10 and compare with baseline data. Use after nursing therapies are administered. Use combinations of analgesics or other therapies as patient's needs change. Provide frequent rest periods in a quiet environment. Time and pace nursing activities to conserve patient's energy. Minimize irritants through skin care, including daily baths, lubrication of skin, frequent repositioning, and dry, clean bed linens.	Patient states pain is relieved or decreased in intensity within 30 minutes to 1 hour after administration of medication 75% of the time.

NURSING DIAGNOSIS *Self-care deficit, bathing–hygiene, dressing, toileting, related to advanced disease*

Patient Goals and Expected Outcomes	Nursing Interventions	Evaluation
Patient will carry out ADLs at highest ability with nurse's assistance as necessary	Assist with ADLs but allow patient and family to assist when able. Provide sufficient time for ADLs. Include patient in determining care routine. Provide frequent oral care every 2 to 4 hours. Use soft toothbrushes or foam swabs for frequent mouth care. Apply a light film of petroleum jelly to lips and tongue. Remove crusts from eyelid margins and provide eye care. Reduce corneal drying with artificial tears. Protect skin from irritation and breakdown using absorbent pads and clean linen.	Patient indicates satisfaction with level of personal hygiene achieved.

Nursing Care Plan 10-2 The Patient Facing Death—cont'd

NURSING DIAGNOSIS *Imbalanced nutrition, less than body requirements related to disease progression*

Patient Goals and Expected Outcomes	Nursing Interventions	Evaluation
The patient will be able to consume 50% of her meals	Maintain and document food intake. Confer with dietitian to introduce kcal and protein and discuss patient's nutritional needs. Assist with frequent oral hygiene. Assist with environmental control (temperature, appearance, odors). Identify food preferences and provide the preferences as often as possible. Suggest that smaller portions may be more palatable. Allow home-cooked meals, as preferred by patient (gives family a chance to participate). Provide relief of thirst by using ice chips, sips of fluids, or moist cloth to lips.	Patient has maintained weight over 2 weeks or demonstrates weight gain weekly.

Critical Thinking Questions

1. Ms. Barton complains of severe bone pain and nausea. She appears cachexic and extremely weak. What are some nursing interventions to decrease Ms. Barton's symptoms?
2. Ms. Barton says, "I want to go home to die. I don't want to stay in the hospital. All I want to do is go home and be with my family." How can the hospice team most beneficially assist Ms. Barton?
3. When the nurse enters Ms. Barton's room to begin ADLs, she notes the patient's extreme fatigue and lethargy. What are some nursing interventions to conserve Ms. Barton's strength?

Box 10-5 Suggestions for Involving the Family in the Care of the Dying Patient

- The thanatologic philosophy dictates that family members be free to choose if and when they wish to be with the patient who is dying. No barrier because of "visitation hours" should be raised.
- Allow young children to visit a dying patient when the patient is able to communicate.
- Be willing to listen to family members' complaints about the patient's care and to their feelings about the patient.
- Help family members learn to interact with the dying person (e.g., using attentive listening, avoiding false reassurances, conducting conversations about normal family activities or problems).
- Allow family members to help with as much or as little care as they desire.
- When the family becomes fatigued with care activities, relieve them from their duties so that they can acquire needed rest and support. Refer them to resources for meals and lodging.
- Support the act of shared grieving among patient and family. Provide privacy when preferred. Do not discourage open expression of grief between family and patient.
- As the time of death approaches, assist family members to stay in communication with the dying patient through short visits, caring silence, touch, and telling the patient of their love for him or her.
- After death, assist the family with decision making, such as selection of a mortician, transportation of family members, and collection of the patient's belongings.

illness places heavy demands on social and financial resources. The emotional strain often disrupts normal communication channels. Sometimes the family becomes afraid to interact with the patient.

When families choose to take the patient home for care, be sure that they are well prepared before discharge for what they need to know. Arrange for hospice services to assist the family, if they are receptive; emphasize continuity of care and constant availability for when the patient is experiencing an emotional or physical crisis and needs ongoing support.

During the social assessment, it is necessary to learn who the patient considers to be the most supportive person in his or her life. It may be a friend, a co-worker, or a church member. Help this person to become a part of the patient's supportive network and be included in planning the patient's care. Encourage these social support people to become involved, and at the same time maintain and promote the patient's independence whenever possible.

Spiritual Assessment

Assess the spiritual dimension by gaining insight into the patient's philosophy of life and religious resources. Find out what significance the rituals of the particular faith group have for the patient in dealing with his or her death.

It is important to do the following:

- Assess your own feelings related to death and dying experiences.
- Suspend judgment and the tendency to interpret and analyze; instead, create an atmosphere of openness to discuss the patient's spiritual concerns.

Interventions in this area will come from clergy, friends, family, health care providers, and significant others. Supporting the patient's and the family's belief systems and values is important (see Chapter 8).

One aspect of this belief system is hope. Hope can take many forms. Your challenge is to assist the patient and the family to identify those hopes that are most important to them and that will help them to cope.

Hope can be considered a life force that is both multidimensional (taking many forms) and fluid. Hope is the common thread identified in all stages of grief. It is characterized by confidence, even though the hopeful individual does not necessarily expect to achieve a specific goal. Hope is not comprised in a single act but is a complex series of changing thoughts, feelings, and actions. Many sources report a significant relationship between the level of hope and the level of coping. In addition, the strength of religious connections and the performance of family role responsibilities are significantly related to the variables of hope and coping.

It is difficult to maintain hope during the dying process. As the patient's condition deteriorates, your challenge becomes one of assisting the patient and family in translating their hope for a cure into realistic hopes that are focused on short-term, achievable goals. These may be the hope for a comfortable and pain-free life or the desire to live long enough to participate in some important family event, such as the wedding of a child. A total lack of hope exhausts the human spirit. When hope is relinquished, death rapidly follows.

Shock and Denial

During the grieving process that follows a loss, your presence can help stabilize a grieving individual's feelings of confusion, shock, and denial. You can help by offering small amounts of information at a time, answering questions, and repeating information as

Box 10-6 Breaking Bad News

Generally, it is the physician who delivers unexpected bad news, but occasionally nurses must give families the news of a death. Accompany the physician who is approaching a family with unexpected or traumatic news, especially when it involves a death, and remain with the family after the physician leaves. When you have to deliver bad news, use the following guidelines:

- Determine the relationship of family members to whom you will be talking and their role in the patient's care and daily life. Be sensitive to cultural influences within family structure and roles. It is important to ascertain family dynamics so that the appropriate persons receive the information from a health professional.
- Plan words ahead, organize thoughts, and have all the facts and the answers to questions that can be predicted.
- Provide privacy, and establish rapport. If other team members have already developed such rapport, include them in the meeting with the family.
- Introduce personnel, and identify nurses in the care of the patient.
- Create an environment that allows time for the presentation of information and discussion of the meaning and consequences of the information. Turn off pager or cell phone, sit down, maintain eye contact, and listen attentively.
- Determine what the family already knows, and what the individuals want to know. Do not make assumptions about the extent of information or details desired by family members.
- Use language that is unambiguous; avoid medical terms and acronyms. Use basic terms to discuss medical situations and interventions. Present information at a level commensurate with the educational level of the participating family members. Use medical personnel as interpreters, if needed, rather than having a family member interpret facts and medical information to other family members.
- Assess nonverbal body language and indicators of emotional status.
- Continually assess and reassess family members' understanding of information being presented and discussed. State information repeatedly until it is heard and understood by families who are in shock or numb from the related events.
- Bring in clergy who can support and remain with families after the formal discussion of facts has concluded, if the family desires. Seek nursing supervisor assistance when needed to further assist family members as indicated (see Figure 10-1).
- Confirm that safe transportation is available when the family is ready to leave. Escort them out and up to the car in which they will drive away from the facility.
- A last measure of respect for the deceased person is conveyed when a staff member accompanies the family as they exit the place where a loved one has died.

From Harkreader, H., & Hogan, M. (2004). *Fundamentals of nursing: Caring and clinical judgment* (2nd ed.). St. Louis: Elsevier.

necessary. Remain with bereaved individuals who are experiencing shock, are stunned, or are showing signs of hostility. Also offer support to the grieving individual by allowing the individual to direct the discussion and by contacting appropriate supportive personnel, such as clergy (Harkreader, 2007). See Box 10-6 for tips on breaking bad news to the family or patient.

NURSING PROCESS *in Loss and Grief*

The role of the licensed practical nurse/licensed vocational nurse (LPN/LVN) in the nursing process as stated is that the LPN/LVN will:

- Participate in planning care for patients based on patient needs
- Review patient's plan of care and recommend revisions as needed
- Review and follow defined prioritization for patient care
- Use clinical pathways, care maps, or care plans to guide and review patient care

By completing assessment, diagnosis, planning, outcomes identification, implementation, and evaluation, you can develop a nursing care plan.

Assessment

Begin care of the grieving patient by collecting subjective and objective data about the meaning of loss to the patient and family or significant others. Interview the patient and family, observing their responses and behavior. Do not try to assess how the patient *should be* reacting but how the patient *is* reacting. Some behaviors or phases will occur in sequence. In contrast, some in the expected order will most likely be skipped or will recur. Many variables affect grief. Assessment of these variables gives the nurse a broad database by which to individualize care. When you provide care to patients from other backgrounds, perform assessment attentively and listen for clues to beliefs and practices regarding health and illness.

Interpretation of a loss varies greatly with a person's cultural and ethnic background. Many sources note that ethnicity is strongly related to attitudes toward life-sustaining treatments during terminal illness. The form the expression of grief takes generally is linked to cultural background and family practices. Culturally determined traditions often dictate how a family support system is to behave. For example, in the Western tradition, the grieving process is usually personal and private, with individuals showing emotional restraint. The ceremonies surrounding a person's death offer time and a means for grief resolution and reminiscing. In Eastern nations, respect for the dead is shown by loud wailing and physical demonstration of grief for a specified period. Despite these general tendencies, however, members of the same ethnocultural background often respond differently to loss and death.

Nursing Diagnosis

After thorough and thoughtful data collection, identify nursing diagnoses applicable to the patient's clinical situation. Formulate an individualized nursing diagnosis by noting and analyzing any clustering of patient or family behaviors, actual or potential losses, and data involving the loss (Box 10-7).

The mere presence of one or two defining characteristics is usually insufficient to make an accurate diagnosis. Be vigilant and do not overlook competing diagnoses. For example, if a patient who is dying manifests an increase in crying or tearfulness, displays of anger, and frequent nightmares, you will have to consider several possible nursing diagnoses, because these characteristics are common to more than one diagnosis. Among the choices are **acute pain, ineffective coping,** and **spiritual distress.** Until you examine all of the available data and inquire about the presence of other behaviors and symptoms, you will not be able to determine a correct diagnosis with any accuracy.

To be able to select appropriate interventions for the patient's care, it is also necessary to identify the relevant context, or the related factor. For example, dysfunctional grieving related to loss of physical function will necessitate different interventions than dysfunctional grieving related to the loss of a job.

For the patient who is seriously ill, it is possible for several nursing diagnoses to apply. It is impossible to address all of these complex problems simultaneously. On any given day or at any one time, two or three problem areas will demand your attention. These priorities will shift according to the patient's condition; rework them constantly.

Box 10-7 NANDA-I–Approved Nursing Diagnoses Related to Grieving

Grieving related to:
- Potential loss of significant other
- Potential loss of physiopsychosocial well-being

Complicated grieving related to:
- Actual or potential object loss
- Absence of anticipatory grieving
- Lack of resolution of previous grieving response
- Loss of significant other
- Thwarted grieving response to a loss

Imbalanced nutrition, less than body requirements related to:
- Depressed grief response

Interrupted family processes related to:
- Situational transition or crisis

Hopelessness related to:
- Failing or deteriorating physiologic condition

Spiritual distress (distress of the human spirit) related to:
- Separation from religious and cultural ties

Data from North American Nursing Diagnosis Association International (NANDA-I). (2009). *Nursing diagnoses: Definitions and classification 2009-2011*. Oxford, U.K.: Author.

In addition to making a diagnosis related directly to grief, it is likely that you will also diagnose other health problems common to grieving, such as anxiety or imbalanced nutrition, less than body requirements. In these situations, focus your interventions on supporting or resolving grief before attempting to solve the other problems. For example, if the patient continues to have loss of appetite related to severe anxiety, simply improving the nutritional value and variety of available foods will have little impact on nutritional status.

Expected Outcomes and Planning

Plan nursing interventions so as to meet the physiologic, emotional, developmental, and spiritual needs of the grieving patient. Draw on resources among the patient's friends and family, clergy, support groups, and legal consultants.

The plan of care focuses on achieving specific goals and outcomes that relate to the identified nursing diagnosis.

The following are examples of possible goals and outcomes:

Goal 1: Patient will actively participate in grief work.

Outcome: Patient expresses thoughts and feelings related to loss.

Goal 2: Patient will verbalize finding meaning in life.

Outcome: Patient verbalizes future goals and plans.

In developing a comprehensive plan to help patients deal with loss and grief, use other professionals within the health care team and in the greater community as resources. By suggesting consultation with other professionals or by providing resources, you contribute to the patient's well-being. Then incorporate use of these external resources into the plan of care. For instance, patients may have concerns about financial matters or the making or revising of a will; the best intervention for them will perhaps be referral to Legal Aid or to a private attorney. Also remember to treat each patient and family as unique, and recognize that their needs, fears, hopes, expectations, and concerns will change throughout the illness.

Implementation

Nursing care of the terminally ill patient is often demanding and stressful. It is important to recognize the value of family members as resources and assist them in working with the dying patient (see Box 10-5 and Patient Teaching box on the dying patient's family). Also consider any special needs of the older adult (see Life Span Considerations for Older Adults box).

A return to full functioning will not be an expected outcome for a terminally ill patient or even a person who experiences significant disability or other loss of function. However, you always have the goal of enabling the patient to return to optimal physical and emotional functioning. This does not mean that the patient and family will not experience sadness or other disturbing emotions, but that they will adapt and cope effectively with the stressors in their life. You can make use of a variety of techniques and interventions to assist patients to function optimally under severe stress; make effective decisions regarding their care; and cope with disappointment, frustration, and other emotions that are caused by their illness.

Patient Teaching

The Dying Patient and the Family

- Describe and demonstrate feeding techniques and selection of foods to facilitate ease of chewing and swallowing.
- Demonstrate bathing, mouth care, and other hygiene measures and allow family to perform return demonstration.
- Show video on simple transfer techniques to prevent injury to themselves and the patient; help family members practice.
- Teach family to recognize signs and symptoms to expect as the patient's condition worsens and provide information on whom to call in an emergency.
- Discuss ways to support the dying person and listen to needs and fears.
- Solicit questions from family and provide information as needed.
- Provide teaching, information, and encouragement in the use of creative outlets for expressing feelings and communicating with others. Encourage the use of tape-recorded messages, drawings, writings, imagery, music, and poetry. (This also assists patients and families in creating memories that can be very comforting later.)
- Inform patient and family of relaxation techniques.
- Observe the family and patient interacting using effective communication skills.

Evaluation

Refer to the goals and outcomes identified when planning care, and perform measures designed to evaluate the achievement of those goals.

Goal 1: Patient will actively participate in grief work.

Evaluative measures:

- Patient observed discussing loss with significant other.
- Patient demonstrates progress in dealing with stages of grief at his or her own pace.
- Patient participates in self-care, ADLs, and family conversations.

Goal 2: Patient will verbalize finding meaning in life.

Evaluative measures:

- Patient indicates to the health care team or family that he or she finds "peace" in meditation.
- Patient verbalizes goals and plans.
- Patient verbalizes progress in resolution of grief.

The patient expects individualization of care, including comfort, dignity, and cooperation, to maximize quality of life. The success of the evaluation depends partially on the bond you form with the patient. Unless the patient can fully trust you, the sharing of personal desires is not likely to occur. Once you establish rapport, you must be ever vigilant to avoid problems that threaten it.

Life Span Considerations

Older Adults

Dying and Death

- Many older adults have long-standing religious beliefs that are likely to influence their response to death and dying. Make sure spiritual counselors are available.
- Many older adults have come to accept death; others remain in earlier stages. Sometimes verbalization of the "wish to die" indicates acceptance and sometimes, depression.
- Some older adults feel free to discuss death; others avoid this topic. Encourage patients to discuss their feelings by giving permission and making yourself available to the bereaved.
- The older person may experience many losses that result in a grief response. These include loss of job, possessions, home, friends, spouse, and autonomy. The older adult often needs emotional support to cope with grief.
- Loss of a spouse in older adulthood is highly likely to result in a relocation. This increases the stress level of an already grieving older person and the risk of new health problems or an exacerbation of existing illness.
- Many older adults have instituted advance directives regarding their wishes in case of terminal illness.
- Older adults have the right to a dignified death.
- When caring for an older patient who is dying, it is important to prevent feelings of loneliness and abandonment as well as maintain the patient's self-esteem. This can be achieved by ensuring that attentive care is given: speak directly to the patient, ensure that pain control measures are effective, and keep the room environment pleasant.
- The older adult often feels a loss of control; therefore, it is important for the nurse to offer choices to the patient regarding care. Family members are often unaware that the dying older adult seeks their permission to die. Educate family members about this need and allow family members to be with the dying patient at any time.
- Comorbidity (more than one disease process) is common among older adults.
- Uncertainty of the prognosis of chronic illnesses can make treatment decisions difficult.
- Geriatric pharmacology and awareness of multiple drug interactions is vital.
- The most frequent symptoms experienced by the dying older adult are pain, respiratory distress, and confusion.
- Older adults often have experienced numerous losses, which affects their reactions to subsequent losses.

Data from Elkin M., Perry A., & Potter P. (2008). *Nursing interventions and clinical skills* (4th ed.). St. Louis: Mosby; and Ebersole, P., Hess. P., & Luggen, A. (2004). *Toward healthy aging: Human needs and nursing response* (6th ed.). St. Louis: Mosby.

The following are examples of questions that will validate the achievement of the nursing interventions:

- "Am I meeting your expectations while providing your care?"
- "Would you like me to assist you in a different manner?"
- "Do you have a specific request that I can use in your care at this time?"
- "Is there another problem that we are overlooking or that you feel is of higher priority?"
- "Are we dealing with your problems in a timely manner?"

Through communication and assessment, continue to evaluate whether the outcome criteria have been satisfied. Use this process to judge the extent to which the goals that were initially chosen have been accomplished. Often it will be easy to evaluate how well the patient's needs have been met, but harder to ascertain the same for the family.

SPECIAL SUPPORTIVE CARE

Often death occurs outside the realm of serious illness, injury, or aging. Perinatal, pediatric, suicidal, and older adult deaths are some examples that warrant special consideration.

PERINATAL DEATH

The death of a child is often viewed as one of the most devastating losses that can occur in a family. If the death of the child occurs before, during, or shortly after birth, it is called perinatal death.

Give special consideration to permitting the parents and family to grieve adequately. Loved ones have few or no memories about the child to hold onto, and "acting as though it never happened" places parents in jeopardy of living with unresolved grief. When possible, enable the parents to see, touch, and hold the infant, so that they can face the reality of the situation and resolve their grief. Listen attentively, and allow the parents to express their feelings over their loss. Refer to the baby as "your baby," "your son," or "your daughter," or use the given name, to reinforce that the baby was indeed a unique individual who was loved and will be missed. Support the usual cultural rituals after death for the baby, such as a funeral or memorial service.

Some agencies give a lock of the baby's hair, a blanket the baby was wrapped in, or an identification bracelet to the parents. In some cases, parents have refused these items, only to express a desire for these mementos later. Most agencies keep them and then gladly present the parents with these items in a small satin-covered box tied with a matching ribbon. A disposable camera may even be provided to the family. These same agencies acknowledge the first-year anniversary of the infant's death.

PEDIATRIC DEATH

Children faced with death need special nursing skills. Be aware of how children view or understand death, both their own and that of others. These children are usually aware that they are going to die. They often try to protect their parents. They need to be told the truth in language they can understand and be allowed to share fears, feelings, and opinions (see Life Span Considerations for Infants and Children box).

Most of all, children, like adults, need reassurance from their nurse, physician, and family that they will not suffer or be abandoned and left alone. A letter written by a 13-year-old boy who died of leukemia beautifully summarizes the needs of the dying child. This letter was written to the editor of a newspaper in the 1970s and published in a column written by Saul Kapel, M.D. (1974):

> I am a 13-year-old boy. I am dying. I write this to you who are and will become nurses and doctors in the hope that by sharing my feelings with you, you may someday be better able to help those who share my experience.
>
> But no one likes to talk about such things. In fact, no one likes to talk much at all. Doctoring and nursing must be advancing, but I wish it would hurry. The dying person is not yet seen as a person and thus cannot be communicated with as such. He is a symbol of what every human fears and what we each know. . . .
>
> But for me, fear is today and dying now. You slip in and out of my room, give me medication and check my blood pressure. Is it because you are insecure or just a human being that I sense your fright? Why are you afraid?
>
> I am the one who is dying. I know you feel insecure, don't know what to say, don't know what to do. But please believe me, if you care, you can't go wrong. Just admit that you care. This is really what we search for. We may ask for whys and wherefores, but we really don't want answers.

 Life Span Considerations

Infants and Children

A Child's Understanding of Death

A child's reaction to and understanding of death and dying depend on the developmental stage of the child and parental values and beliefs, culture, and religious orientation. The first way to help children to develop positive attitudes toward death is to counsel parents. Parents need to understand a child's age-specific understanding of death and the normal reactions of a child to death. Parents may use "small deaths"—of a pet, for example—to help children become familiar and comfortable with a loss.

When death occurs in a family, parents often try to shield children from the loss. They fear the child will not be able to cope with the grief. However, allowing children to feel emotions appropriate to events prepares them for more traumatic experiences later in life. The child's developmental level determines the proper amount and type of detailed information to discuss with the child.

When a child is dying, parents and siblings often feel considerable anger and resentment. The death of a child is usually seen as unfair. Some parents' inclination is to withhold information about the illness from the dying child. Even young children, however, often perceive that something is wrong with them because of the changes in behavior they see in parents. Work together with parents to plan their child's care, and determine the level of participation they desire. Do not attempt to assume a parental role or relinquish important nursing responsibilities. Parents and children need to know specifics about the plan of therapy and the normalcy of their reaction to the loss. It is common for friends and relatives to avoid contact with the dying child and family because of fear over the child's illness. Parents must decide whether they wish to maintain contact with significant others. Such a resource frequently proves valuable.

The following are basic guidelines to follow while providing care for a child who is dying or experiencing the death of a loved one:

- Allow young children to visit a dying parent or grandparent if all parties consent. (Some dying patients have strong feelings about possibly traumatizing children during this transition.)
- Ascertain the child's understanding and experience of death. There are developmental theories regarding children's concepts of death based on cognitive stage of development.
- Respect the family's wishes in how and what to tell children about serious illness, dying, and death. If the parents wish to be honest with the child, it is important to provide straightforward, yet caring explanations.
- Use of play therapy or drawing may help a child express his or her emotions, fears, and understanding about death.
- Answer parents' questions with specific details, taking into consideration the family's cultural background and knowledge level.
- Parents should be allowed to stay with the child at any time of day or night.
- Reassure parents that everything possible was done for the child.
- When possible, the topic of organ donation should be approached with the family before the death of the child. Many families appreciate this topic being brought to their attention because they would not think of it on their own. Many find it comforting to know they are able to help others.
- Make every effort to arrange for family members, especially parents, to be with the child at the time of death, if they wish to be present. For many, viewing the body is a sign of closure—an opportunity to finish their good-byes.
- Treat the family and child as a unit. Encourage parents to stay with the child and participate in care as much as desired or possible.
- Understand that decisions to end treatment can be more difficult when children are involved.

Data from Elkin, M., Perry, A., & Potter, P. (2008). *Nursing interventions and clinical skills* (4th ed.). St. Louis: Elsevier; and Hockenberry M., & Wilson D. (2003). *Wong's essentials of pediatric nursing* (7th ed.). St. Louis: Elsevier.

Don't run away. Wait. All I want to know is that there will be someone to hold my hand when I need it. I'm afraid. Death may be routine to you, but it is new to me. You may not see me as unique, but I've never died before. To me once is unique.

You whisper about my youth, but when one is dying, is he really so young anymore? I have lots I wish we could talk about. It really would not take much of your time, because you are in here quite a bit anyway.

If only we could be honest—both admit of our fears, touch one another. If you really care, would you lose so much of your professionalism if you even cried with me just person to person? Then it might not be so hard to die in a hospital with friends and relatives close by.

This essay heartrendingly describes the need of a child for honest and caring communication. Parents and loved ones have much difficulty in accepting the reality of a child's impending death. Death of a child is an "out-of-sequence" death and therefore is often more difficult to accept. Parents often harbor extreme guilt. They may express hostility and anger toward health care providers, God, or the world in general. Grandparents suffer a double grief—for themselves and for their son or daughter. Siblings also are extremely affected and need much support at this time. After a child's death, as well as during the dying process, survivors can often derive benefit from supportive group therapy.

SUICIDE

Survivors of a person who has committed suicide suffer grief in its many forms, in addition to profound guilt or shame. Sometimes they become obsessed with their failure to "see the signs." Rejection and lack of social and religious support is something survivors fear and, unfortunately, often experience. Suicide is usually not considered acceptable; many families of suicide victims are not given the same support from the church, community, or workplace as those whose loved ones have died from other causes. Because of the family's anger, fear, and shame, others do not reach out to help. However complicated, though, the grief of survivors is intense. As one mother said following the death of her son by suicide, "the loss of Leslie is so very great. I know my heart will ache forever." Survivors are at high risk for suicide themselves, and a grief counselor is frequently helpful.

GERONTOLOGIC DEATH

It is often assumed that older adults will display some understanding and acceptance of the death process. This is not always true. You must treat the older patient as an individual, and assess the patient's needs in the same way as you would those of any individual facing a terminal illness (see box on Life Span Considerations for Older Adults). It is important to include the older person in self-care and in decisions to undergo or refuse extensive therapeutic or resuscitative measures. Even when aggressive technologic options are rejected, patients still need intensive nursing interventions and pain-control measures. Sometimes families who suffer the loss of an older person accept the death, but they have to experience the grieving process nonetheless.

Factors influencing grief in older adults include the following:

- Physical changes that accompany aging
- Loss of employment
- Loss of social respect
- Loss of relationships
- Loss of self-care capabilities
- Fear of loss of control
- Sense of fulfillment and contributions made
- Personality traits
- Feelings of self-worth
- Degree to which functional ability is retained

SUDDEN OR UNEXPECTED DEATH

Sudden, unexpected, or violent death, such as through accident, homicide, or sudden illness (e.g., myocardial infarction), is also difficult to cope with. This family will also need support. Often there is preoccupation with the final hours or minutes before death. There is "unfinished business," such as things left unsaid or undone. There are usually guilt feelings: "If only I had not let him go to the party, he would still be alive." There is always the involvement of law authorities such as the police or coroner. Sometimes there is an obsessive need to understand or know why this has happened.

ISSUES RELATED TO DYING AND DEATH

EUTHANASIA

Euthanasia (Greek for "easy death") is sometimes active: a deliberate action taken with the purpose of shortening life to end suffering or to carry out the wishes of a terminally ill patient. There is also passive euthanasia: permitting the death of a patient by withholding treatment that might extend life, such as medication, life-support systems, or feeding tubes.

Although active euthanasia is highly controversial, most people are not in favor of preserving life in all cases. In a *New York Times*–CBS poll taken in 1990, 53% of the respondents said that health care providers should be allowed to assist an ill person in taking his or her own life. Technologies that can keep patients alive indefinitely after the brain has, for all practical purposes, stopped functioning are largely responsible for the change in attitudes over the past 25 years. Euthanasia raises thorny ethical questions for society and for patients and their families. There is a pressing need to define and monitor a problem that one health care provider who prefers to remain anonymous has called "so fundamental that it has moved beyond the boundaries of medicine."

DO NOT RESUSCITATE

It is proper for patients and families to retain control over decisions about withholding or withdrawing treatment. Death with dignity remains a concern for all. It is best for a **do not resuscitate (DNR)** decision to be a joint decision of the patient, the family, and the health care providers. Make sure the patient and family obtain an explanation of all facts regarding the patient's condition, as well as all treatment options. DNR means only not to resuscitate. It does not mean to withhold any other care, such as hygiene, nutrition, fluids, or medications. The physician writes a "no code" or "do not resuscitate" (DNR) order once a health care provider has documented in the progress notes the deterioration of the patient's condition and the decision by the physician and the patient not to administer cardiopulmonary resuscitation. Often the instructions regarding lifesaving treatment are written in the patient's living will or durable power of attorney. Check that the no-code or DNR order is written, not given verbally. Under optimal circumstances, the physician regularly reviews DNR orders in light of changes in the patient's condition. Be familiar with your institution's policies and procedures concerning DNR orders. Physicians can list all specifics of DNR orders as a follow-up to the patient's living will. In one situation, for example, a physician orders vasopressor and fluid management to maintain a patient's blood pressure but specifically prohibits chest compression or intubation for cardiac dysrhythmias or respiratory arrest. Thoroughly document in the patient's chart all DNR orders and the associated discussion with the patient and family.

ADVANCE DIRECTIVES

Advance directives are signed and witnessed documents providing specific instructions for health care treatment in the event that a person is unable to make these decisions personally at the time they are needed.

There are two basic types of advance directives: living wills and durable powers of attorney for health care. Many patients have instituted one or both.

The Patient Self-Determination Act (PSDA) (1991) requires health care institutions to provide written information to patients concerning the patient's rights under state law to make decisions, including the right to refuse treatment and formulate advance directives. It is especially important to understand patients' cultural beliefs and values when explaining advance directives. Regulatory mandates to benefit the public are based on the dominant value in American society of self-determination. This may be in conflict with a patient's cultural heritage.

Under the act, it must be documented in the patient's record whether the patient has signed an advance directive. The hospital is also required to ensure that state law is followed. The institution must provide education for the staff and the public concerning living wills and durable powers of attorney. For either type of advance directive to be enforceable, it is mandatory that the patient be legally incompetent or lack capacity to make decisions regarding health care treatment. The termination of legal competency is made by a judge, and the determination of decisional capacity is usually made by the physician and the family. Therefore, the advance directive is implemented within the context of the health care team and the health care institution. Be familiar with the institution's policies involving the act.

A **living will** is a written document that directs treatment in accordance with a patient's wishes in the event of a terminal illness or condition (Figure 10-3). Living wills are often difficult to interpret and are not clinically specific in unforeseen circumstances. Each state providing for living wills has its own requirements for executing them. Generally, the presence of two witnesses is required when the patient signs the document; neither may be a relative or physician. If health care workers follow the directions of the living will, they are immune from liability.

A **durable power of attorney** for health care designates an agent, surrogate, or proxy to make health care decisions on the patient's behalf based on the patient's wishes.

In addition to federal statutes, the ethical doctrine of autonomy ensures the patient the right to refuse medical treatment. This right was upheld in the *Bouvia v. Superior Court* case in 1986. That case allowed the discontinuation of the patient's tube feedings as per the patient's prior request. The courts have also upheld the right of a legally competent patient to refuse medical treatment based on religious beliefs. Jehovah's Witnesses, for example, accept medical treatment but refuse blood transfusions. In the absence of a truly compelling reason otherwise, the right to make such choices is protected. The U.S. Supreme Court stated in the *Cruzan v. Director Missouri Department of Health* case in 1990 that "we assume that the U.S. Constitution would grant a constitutionally protected competent person the right to refuse lifesaving hydration and nutrition." In cases involving the patient's right to refuse or withdraw medical treatment, the courts balance the patient's interest with the state's interest in protecting life, preserving medical ethics, preventing suicide, and protecting innocent third parties. Children are generally considered innocent third parties. Although the courts will not force adults to undergo treatment that is refused for religious reasons, they will grant an order allowing hospitals and physicians to treat children of Christian Scientists or Jehovah's Witnesses who have denied consent for treatment of their minor children.

When patients are legally incompetent and are unable to make health care decisions, the court steps in. Balancing the state's interest with that of the patient,

LIVING WILL DECLARATION OF

____

If I should lapse into a persistent vegetative state or have an incurable and irreversible condition that, without the administration of life-sustaining treatment, will, in the opinion of my attending physician, cause my death within a relatively short time and I am no longer able to make decisions regarding my medical treatment, I direct my attending physician, pursuant to the Rights of the Terminally Ill Act, to withhold or withdraw life-sustaining treatment that is not necessary for my comfort or to alleviate pain.

Declarant Signature

Signed this ________ day of ____________, 20 ___

Social Security Number: ________________ Date of Birth ____________

Address: ________________ Signature ________________

City/State: ________________

The declarant voluntarily signed this writing in my presence.

Signature of witness: ________________ Printed name/Date: ____________

Signature of witness: ________________ Printed name/Date: ____________

-OR-

NOTARY

The declarant voluntarily signed this document in my presence.

STATE OF NEBRASKA)
) SS.
COUNTY OF __________)

Notary Public

FIGURE 10-3 Example of a living will.

the court attempts to deliver a judgment representing what the patient would have chosen if competent. The Supreme Court held in the Cruzan case that states had the right to require "clear and convincing evidence" of a legally incompetent patient's prior wishes when making determinations to discontinue life-sustaining treatment. In that case, nutrition and hydration were recognized as life-sustaining medical treatment that could be withdrawn.

Every state now requires "clear and convincing" evidence of the patient's choice, but individual states differ as to what standard satisfies the requirement. In the absence of evidence indicating the patient's prior choice, most states allow treatment to be stopped based on other factors, including the best interest of the patient balanced with the state's interest (Box 10-8).

ORGAN DONATIONS

Legally competent people are free to donate their bodies or organs for medical use. Consent forms are available for this purpose. In many states, it is possible for adults to request organ donation by signing the back of their driver's license. State laws determine if a nurse is allowed to serve as a witness when individuals wish to give consent for the donation of organs, tissue, or the body. Be aware of the policies and procedures of your employing institution.

In most states (National Organ Transplantation Act, Public Law 98-507, 10-14, 1984), required request laws stipulate that at the time of a person's death, a qualified health care provider must ask family members to consider organ or tissue donation. Required request laws came about because of the shortage of suitable organs for transplantation.

The Uniform Anatomical Gifts Act addresses many problems of organ donation and stipulates that the physician who certifies death shall not be involved in removal or transplantation of the organs. The National Organ Transplantation Act, which governs this area of medical and nursing practice, prohibits selling or purchasing organs. Organ and tissue donations remain voluntary.

Donations can include the following:

Vital Organs	***Nonvital Tissues***
Kidney	Cornea
Heart	Long bones
Lung	Skin
Liver	Middle ear bones
Pancreas	

Vital organs are recovered after a patient is pronounced clinically dead or brain dead; circulatory and ventilatory support is maintained to perfuse the organs before removal.

RIGHTS OF DYING PATIENTS

Death with dignity is the goal in caring for the dying patient. The Dying Person's Bill of Rights (Box 10-9) is

Box 10-8 The Living Will and Durable Power of Attorney

- People who receive extraordinary measures to prolong life are often unconscious or mentally incompetent by the time these measures are put into effect. Therefore, it is only by deciding ahead of time what kind of care you want and communicating these decisions to others that you can ensure that you receive the extent of care that you want. This can be done through such documents as a living will and a medical durable power of attorney. If your state has adopted legislation for either or both documents, you should use the legally approved wording.
- Address the living will and give copies of it to your family physician, your attorney, and close family members. It specifies that if the time comes when you can no longer take part in decisions for your own future, this statement will stand as an expression of your wishes and directions while you are still of sound mind.
- You may, for example, direct that if a situation should arise in which there is no reasonable expectation of recovery from extreme physical or mental disability, you be allowed to die and not be kept alive by medications, artificial means, or "heroic measures." You may also, of course, use a living will to request such measures to keep you alive as long as possible. You may request pain-relieving medication, even though it may shorten your life. You may spell out specific provisions with regard to, for example, cardiac resuscitation, mechanical respiration, antibiotics, tube feeding, and permission to offer your organs as transplants to other people.
- Some "living will" legislation applies only to terminally ill patients—not to patients who are incapacitated by illness or injury but may live many years in severe pain, who are in a coma, or who are in some other greatly disabled state. Therefore it is advisable to draw up a durable power of attorney, an instrument that appoints another person (a health care surrogate) to make decisions in the event of your incompetence. A number of states have enacted statutes expressly for decisions about health care, known as a "medical durable power of attorney." In these states, filling out a form is all that is required; you do not have to consult an attorney.
- Depending on the statute, the agent you appoint (someone you trust and have confidence in) may give, withdraw, or withhold consent to specific medical or surgical measures; hire and fire medical personnel; gain access to your medical records; go to court to carry out your wishes; spend or withhold funds for treatment; and interpret your living will.

REMEMBER

- Both documents must be signed and dated before two witnesses who are not blood relatives and to whom you are not leaving property.
- For the durable power of attorney, you must have your signature notarized. If you choose more than one proxy for decision making on your behalf (a good idea in case your first choice is not available), give an order of priority (1, 2, 3).
- Give a copy to your physician to keep in your medical file, and be sure that the physician agrees with your wishes.
- Give copies to close relatives, friends, or both.
- Tell these people about your intentions now.
- Look over your living will once a year. Redate it and initial the new date to make it clear that your wishes are unchanged.

Box 10-9 The Dying Person's Bill of Rights

- I have the right to be treated as a living human being until I die.
- I have the right to maintain a sense of hopefulness, however changing its focus may be.
- I have the right to be cared for by those who can maintain a sense of hopefulness, however changing this might be.
- I have the right to express my feelings and emotions about my approaching death in my own way.
- I have the right to participate in decisions concerning my care.
- I have the right to expect continuing medical and nursing attention even though "cure" goals must be changed to "comfort" goals.
- I have the right not to die alone.
- I have the right to be free from pain.
- I have the right to have my questions answered honestly.
- I have the right not to be deceived.
- I have the right to have help from and for my family in accepting my death.
- I have the right to die in peace and dignity.
- I have the right to retain my individuality and not be judged for my decisions that may be contrary to beliefs of others.
- I have the right to discuss and enlarge my religious and/or spiritual experiences, whatever these may mean to others.
- I have the right to expect that the sanctity of the human body will be respected after death.
- I have the right to be cared for by caring, sensitive, knowledgeable people who will attempt to understand my needs and will be able to gain some satisfaction in helping me face my death.

From Barbus, A. (1975). The dying patient's bill of rights. *American Journal of Nursing, 75,* 99.

honored at hospitals and other health care agencies and is posted in prominent areas.

FRAUDULENT METHODS OF TREATMENT

Often the patient and family seek unconventional methods of treatment to prolong the patient's life. Such treatments may include special diets, enemas, unproven drugs, and machines or devices. You may be called on to help patients and families to sort out which treatments are real and which are fraudulent. Fraudulent treatments are those that are misrepresented, whether by concealment or nondisclosure of facts, for the purpose of inducing another to use them. View with suspicion any treatment that does not offer the patient informed consent after providing information regarding options, results, and approvals from federal agencies.

THE DYING PATIENT

COMMUNICATING WITH THE DYING PATIENT

You express respect for the patient, offer realistic hope, and impart appropriate reassurance and support when you use therapeutic communication. Supportive words without an accompanying supportive attitude will ring hollow and fail to provide comfort. Reassurance that is unrealistic or given merely to calm a patient will not work. Stating that "everything will be just fine" when this is untrue will only increase the patient's anxiety and violate his or her trust in you. It is far better to give reassurance in a limited way that is consistent with the facts.

Therapeutic communication also requires you to pay careful attention to what the patient expresses verbally and nonverbally. Always verify with the patient any interpretations or summaries of the patient's thoughts and feelings to make sure they are both accurate and effective.

If patients prefer not to communicate at a particular time, they need to know that you will accept and respect their wishes. Indicate your willingness to return at another time when the patient is feeling more comfortable. Be available to listen actively, nonjudgmentally, and with acceptance. Allow the patient to express emotions and feelings without fear.

Behavior that indicates you are listening to the patient is called "attending behavior." It includes appropriate eye contact, attentive body language, and verbal following. For a dying patient who is receiving numerous messages of rejection from other members of society, eye contact with you is especially important. Show your attentiveness in nonverbal as well as verbal ways. For instance, sit in a chair close to the patient's bed to reduce the physical distance and the emotional distance it implies. When appropriately used, touching is a highly effective means of communication. Later in the illness, when strength for or interest in verbal communication has dwindled, a patient will derive particular benefit from being touched. Holding a hand, patting an arm, gently wiping away a tear—all indicate attending behavior, as well as concern and care.

It is vitally important to remember that there is no way for you to "solve" the problem of dying. You can have a positive impact on the dying patient's feelings and fears, however. Communicate openly and sensitively with the patient. By doing so, you not only facilitate the expression of emotion, but also affirm that the patient is a living human being who has your support and compassion.

One of the most important tasks of the bedside nurse is to empower patients and families to participate in the final act of living. Communicate reassurance, confidence, and support for the vulnerable patient and family by sustaining your assessment practices, continuing to communicate, and providing skilled physical care. The seasoned hand of a skilled professional supporting and guiding the patient can change the journey through dying and death from a frightening process to one of peace and comfort.

Other resources to call on during management of the dying patient will be specific for each individual. Patients sometimes desire greater focus on spiritual needs; many request a visit by a clergyman or clergywoman or the performance of a religious ritual. Other patients seek answers in nutritional approaches, miracles, and other sources of hope, although these often come with a high price tag. Encourage nontraditional therapies if they give the patient hope and do no harm (see Chapter 17). Your primary role in the care of the dying patient is to explain realistic options without destroying hope. What makes the difference between the perceived success or failure of a dying experience is attitude: yours and your patient's.

ASSISTING THE PATIENT IN SAYING GOOD-BYE

One of the most difficult tasks a terminally ill patient faces is taking leave of loved ones. The patient who is aware of dying needs to say good-bye, whether in a verbal, nonverbal, concrete, or symbolic way. For their part, family members must also work through the process of acknowledging the impending parting. Good-byes help them move toward the completion of unfinished business with the patient that will otherwise complicate their transition through the grieving process. Your help in this area is important to both the dying person and the family (see Communication box).

First, provide a private, comfortable environment. Sometimes, emotional expression becomes overwhelming for the patient, the family, or both; offer to remain present or nearby to help reestablish equilibrium if necessary, or to ask a colleague to do so. There are various ways to assist patients in saying their good-byes such as role playing, letter writing, or making audio or video recordings. Help patients focus on what they want to say. One way to facilitate this is to ask them to talk to their loved ones as if they were going to be separated for a long time. Encourage them to express those feel-

Communication

Counseling a Family Member

Family member: I can't go back in that room. He just lies there and stares. I don't know what to do or say.

Nurse: Being near someone who is dying can be uncomfortable.

Family member: It makes me so sad to see him like that. Do you think he knows I'm there?

Nurse: It's very possible that he does. Would you like me to go in with you?

Family member: Yes, please. I wonder if he can hear me?

Nurse: It must be very difficult for you not to be certain that he is hearing you. If there is something you want to say to him, get close, take his hand, and speak directly to him. Most people in his condition can hear but are very weak and may not have the strength to respond.

Family member: I just feel like I am not able to do anything for him anymore.

Nurse: Just being there is letting him know that you care. That's something very important to any person.

Family member: I suppose you're right. I guess I'm ready to go in now.

Nurse: I'll be right here by your side.

ings and thoughts they would most want their loved ones to know in their absence. Help the dying person to formulate appropriate letters or tape recordings by asking, "What would you want to say to your 6-year-old when the child is 12?" Often dying patients become depressed because they do not have a purpose in life. Working on tasks such as poems, letters, and recordings affords patients feelings of control and productivity in their last days.

PALLIATIVE CARE

People who face life-threatening illnesses can take advantage of many medical and technologic advances to reverse the course of their disease or to prolong their lives. For patients with life-limiting illness, it becomes important that you find ways to help them approach their end of life. Such is the goal of **palliative care:** the prevention, relief, reduction, or soothing of symptoms of disease or disorders without effecting a cure. Palliative care allows patients to make more informed choices, achieve better alleviation of symptoms, and have more opportunity to work on issues of life closure. According to the World Health Organization (2003), when you deliver palliative care, you do the following:

- Provide relief from pain and other distressing symptoms
- Affirm life and regard dying as a normal process
- Neither hasten nor postpone death
- Integrate psychologic and spiritual aspects of patient care
- Offer a support system to help patients live as actively as possible until death
- Offer a support system to help families cope during the patient's illness and their own bereavement
- Enhance the quality of life

Palliative care is a philosophy of total care. It is appropriate to deliver palliative care at any time and to patients of any age, with any diagnosis. Although it has particular relevance to the care of the terminally ill, it is not just reserved to the last few months of life. The approach to care usually involves an interdisciplinary team of physicians, nurses, social workers, pastoral care professionals, physical and occupational therapists, and pharmacists. Massage therapists or music or art therapists who provide alternative therapies are also a part of the team at times. In the context of end of life, a palliative care approach ensures that a patient experiences a "good death," free of avoidable pain and suffering in accord with the patient's and family's wishes, and reasonably consistent with clinical, cultural, and ethical standards.

One of your most important tasks as a nurse providing palliative care is to establish a caring relationship with both patient and family. Furthermore, the symptom-control measures you provide are important to helping maintain the patient's dignity and self-esteem, prevent abandonment or isolation, and establish a comfortable and peaceful environment for death to occur (Box 10-10).

PHYSICAL CARE

You have an important responsibility in assisting patients to meet their physical needs. Providing adequate

Box 10-10 Long-Term Care Considerations

- Less physician involvement means nurses have an important role in assessing and managing pain and symptom control.
- Challenges include providing privacy and autonomy for the patient and family, involving the family as much as possible or desired, individualizing care, keeping family members informed of changes, and making the environment as homelike as possible.
- The goal of a nursing facility is to provide a caring environment for those who are dying. However, there are many facilities that sorely lack appropriate supportive care. Compassionate care allows family members to be present whenever they choose, day or night, and involves aggressive and appropriate symptom management.
- Nighttime is a time of least attention and a time of loneliness and pain. Night is also a time when people fear they will die alone and no one will know. If a friend or relative cannot stay with the patient, a mature sitter is an option. A volunteer from hospice might provide the same support. For those older adults who have developed a lifestyle around aloneness, solitude might be preferred. Be sensitive to the patient's preference.

Data from Perry, A.G., & Potter, P.A. (2005). *Clinical skills and techniques* (6th ed). St. Louis: Elsevier.

 Coordinated Care

Collaboration

CARING FOR THE DYING PATIENT

The task of supporting patients and families in grief should not be delegated to assistive personnel. A professional nurse has the responsibility for recognizing a patient's grief and knowing the appropriate communication and counseling strategies to use. Provide assistive personnel with information, assistance, and direction, including the following:

- Ask assistive personnel to inform you when the patient expresses behaviors of grief (e.g., crying, anger, loss of appetite).
- Encourage assistive personnel to conduct conversations with patients, but to inform you when patients express needs or concerns.
- Ask assistive personnel to inform you when family members arrive so you can meet with them and assess how they are coping.

A professional nurse is responsible for assessment of patients' symptoms and a determination of what symptoms can be independently managed and what symptoms require medical intervention. Certain symptom therapies can be delegated to assistive personnel such as positioning and environmental controls, hygiene approaches, and hydration. Therapies involving administration of opioids, anxiolytics, antidepressants, and so on, require a nurse's intervention. The nurse provides assistive personnel with instruction and assistance regarding the following:

- When to notify you if the patient's symptoms worsen or change in nature
- Potential adverse effects of pharmacologic agents and what to report to you
- The need to maintain communication with dying patients who still retain the sense of hearing

Care of the body after death can be delegated to assistive personnel. However, you should recognize that often family will expect to see you more than usual to provide support. Also, care after death can, in fact, begin before the actual death so that patients and families can preserve cultural practices. Check agency policy regarding which staff members are permitted to remove invasive tubes or lines. At the time of death, it may be best for you and assistive personnel to work together in preparing the body (see Skill 10-1).

- Inform other care providers of any preference the family might have because of cultural, religious, or ethnic beliefs that will influence the routine procedures of caring for the patient's body.
- Reinforce the importance of handling the body with respect.

Modified from Perry, A.G., & Potter, P.A. (2005). *Clinical nursing skills and techniques* (6th ed.). St. Louis: Elsevier.

nutrition and maintaining elimination patterns are priorities for the dying patient (see Chapter 40). Keep the patient clean, dry, well groomed, odor free, and comfortable; this decreases the chances of skin impairment and also provides the patient with feelings of self-esteem and self-worth (see Chapters 16 and 18). Sometimes you will be called on to provide care in a facility (see Coordinated Care box) and sometimes in the patient's home (see Home Care Considerations for the Dying Patient box).

Adjusting the environment to increase comfort and safety is paramount. Use side rails for safety and, when possible, to assist weak patients to adjust their own positions.

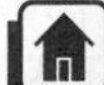 Home Care Considerations

The Dying Patient

- The trend is toward more people choosing to die at home.
- The family needs to know whom to call for help if symptom control is needed, what to do at the time of death, who must be notified, and how the body is to be transported.
- Knowledge of types of home care reimbursement is essential, including Medicare and Medicaid hospice benefits.
- Family members assume primary care responsibility, necessitating ongoing teaching and support. Educate family members about symptom management approaches and when to seek help.
- Volunteers may be needed to give family respite time.

Data from Elkin, M., Perry, A., & Potter, P. (2008). *Nursing interventions and clinical skills* (4th ed.). St. Louis: Mosby.

ASSESSMENTS AND INTERVENTIONS

Care of the dying patient has many facets. Of all the needs of the dying patient, the three most crucial are for love and affection, the control of pain, and the preservation of dignity and self-worth.

The patient near death continues to need meticulous nursing interventions. Because of the increased weakness and deterioration of the body, the patient's physical needs are important. However, one of your goals in end-of-life nursing goes beyond merely allaying the physical suffering of your patients to the greatest extent possible. Ideally, you will also help patients recognize and accept death as a reality of life so that they can undertake their last task in life with credit and dignity. Work to prevent the abandonment by family, friends, and caregivers that is so frequently a part of the dying patient's experience. It must be repeated: one of the worst fears of any individual is to be left to die alone.

Assess the patient for impending death. Although patients may appear comatose, unconscious, or unresponsive, this appearance is often a result of extreme fatigue, and you will find that patients are aware of activities occurring around them. Sometimes you will note that the patient becomes restless and picks or pulls at the bed linens. Remember that this is among the signs and symptoms of decreased oxygenation. Discoloration of arms and legs is a result of impaired circulation. Table 10-2 shows signs of approaching death as expressed in patient needs and the appropriate interventions.

Table 10-2 Needs and Interventions for the Patient near Death

PATIENT NEEDS	INTERVENTIONS
Discomfort	Provide thorough skin care including daily baths, lubrication of skin, and dry, clean bed linens to reduce irritants. Provide oral care at least every 2 to 4 hours. Use soft toothbrushes or foam swabs for frequent mouth care. Apply a light film of petroleum jelly to lips and tongue. Eye care removes crusts from eyelid margins. Artificial tears reduce corneal drying.
Fatigue	Help patient to identify values or desired tasks; then help patient to conserve energy for only those tasks. Promote frequent rest periods in a quiet environment. Time and pace nursing care activities.
Nausea	Administer antiemetics; provide oral care at least every 2 to 4 hours; offer clear liquid diet and ice chips; avoid liquids that increase stomach acidity such as coffee, milk, and juices with citric acid.
Constipation	Give preventive care, which is most effective: increase fluid intake; include bran, whole-grain products, and fresh vegetables in diet; and encourage exercise. Administer prophylactic stool softeners. Assess for fecal impaction.
Diarrhea	Confer with physician to change medication, or get order for antidiarrheal medication, if possible. Provide low-residue diet.
Urinary incontinence	Protect skin from irritation or breakdown. Indwelling urinary catheter or condom catheters may be used.
Inadequate nutrition	Serve smaller portions and bland foods, which may be more palatable. Allow home-cooked meals, which may be preferred by patient and gives the family a chance to participate.
Dehydration	Remove factors causing decreased intake; give antiemetics, and apply topical analgesics to oral lesions. Reduce discomfort from dehydration; give mouth care at least every 4 hours; and offer ice chips or moist cloth to lips.
Dyspnea, shortness of breath	Treat or control underlying cause. Maximize patient's oxygenation (e.g., position patient upright, provide supplemental oxygen, maintain a patent airway, and reduce anxiety or fever). Administer medications such as bronchodilators, inhaled steroids, or narcotics to suppress cough and ease breathing and apprehension.

From Perry, A.G., & Potter, P.A. (2009). *Fundamentals of nursing* (7th ed.). St. Louis: Elsevier.

You will observe changes in vital signs, including (1) slow, weak, and thready pulse; (2) lowered blood pressure; and (3) rapid, shallow, irregular, or abnormally slow respirations. Mouth breathing occurs, which leads to dry oral mucous membranes. The patient often has a detached look in the eyes. There is a diminished sensory and motor function in the lower extremities, progressing to the upper extremities. Touch sensation diminishes; pressure and pain sensations remain intact. As death becomes imminent, the pupils will become dilated and fixed, Cheyne-Stokes respirations will occur, the pulse will become increasingly weaker and more rapid, and the blood pressure will continue to fall. Peripheral circulation diminishes. The skin is cool and clammy; profuse diaphoresis may occur. If mucus collects in the patient's throat, you will hear noisy respirations. This sound is referred to as the **death rattle.** A period of peace may immediately precede the moment of death. The clinical signs of death are the following:

1. Unreceptivity and unresponsiveness
2. No movement or breathing
3. No reflexes
4. Flat encephalogram
5. Absence of apical pulse
6. Cessation of respirations

INQUEST

An **inquest** is a legal inquiry into the cause or the manner of a death. When a death is the result of an accident, for example, an inquest is held into the circumstances of the accident to determine any blame. The inquest is conducted under the jurisdiction of a coroner or medical examiner. A *coroner* is a public official, not necessarily a physician, appointed or elected to inquire into cause of death. A *medical examiner* is a physician and usually has advanced education in pathology or forensic medicine. Agency policy dictates who is responsible for reporting deaths to the coroner or medical examiner.

POSTMORTEM CARE

In most states, the physician is responsible for certifying a death in the medical record. The physician notes time of death and records a description of therapies or actions taken in the medical record. The physician may request permission from the family for the **autopsy** (examination performed after a person's death to confirm or determine the cause of death). Autopsies are required in circumstances of unusual death (e.g., violent trauma or unexpected death in the home).

Because of the therapeutic nurse-patient relationship, you may be the best person to care for the patient's body after death **(postmortem care)**. Keep in mind the need to care for the patient's body with dignity and sensitivity. Provide postmortem care as soon as possible after death to prevent tissue damage or disfigurement. If the family has requested organ donation, take immediate measures as appropriate. Know the state laws and the policies and procedures of your employing institution.

Prepare the body and the room to keep the stress of the experience to a minimum, after the patient has been pronounced dead by a physician or professional nurse and before the family views the body. Remove supplies and equipment from sight. Remove, clamp, or cut tubes remaining in the body to within 1 inch (2.5 cm) of the skin, and tape them in place. Care of tubes and specimens depends on agency policy, as well as whether an autopsy will be performed. Never, however, remove tubes, dressings, drains, and other equipment that is in place on or in the patient when an autopsy is to be performed. Clear away soiled linen and other clutter. Use spray deodorizer to help eliminate unpleasant odors.

Prepare the body by making it look as natural and comfortable as possible. Place the body in the supine position with arms at the sides, palms down or across the abdomen (but not one hand over the other); this helps the **mortician** (person trained in the care of the dead) better prepare it for interment. Discoloration of the face can result if blood is allowed to pool; to prevent this, place a small pillow or folded towel under the head. The eyelids usually remain closed if gently held down for a few seconds. If this does not occur, a moistened cotton ball will hold them in place. Insert the patient's dentures to maintain normal facial features. A rolled-up towel under the chin keeps the mouth closed (Skill 10-1). The Cultural Considerations box on care of the body after death presents culturally related attitudes to preparation of the body.

At the time of death, make notation of any valuables, such as watch, rings, or money, and secure these articles so that they may be delivered to the family according to agency policy. Documentation of all valuables and their disposition in the patient's medical record is required (Box 10-11).

Box 10-11 Documentation of End-of-Life Care

Documentation includes the following:

- Time of death and actions taken to prevent the death if applicable
- Who pronounced the death of the patient
- Any special preparation and type of donation, including time, staff, and company
- Who was called and who came to the hospital—donor organization, morgue, funeral home, chaplain, and individual family members making any decisions
- Personal articles left on the body and taped to skin or tubes left in
- Personal items given to the family—specific names and description of items
- Time of discharge and destination of the body
- Location of name tags on the body
- Special requests by the family
- Any other personal statements that might be needed to clarify the situation

Cultural Considerations

Care of the Body after Death

African Americans. Prefer having member of the health care team clean and prepare the loved one's body. Some consider organ donation a taboo, but may agree to an autopsy. In African-American families, cremation is usually not done. Organ donation is usually not done except for an immediate family need.

Chinese Americans. Some families will prefer to bathe the patient themselves. Often believe the body should remain intact; organ donation and autopsy are uncommon.

Filipino Americans. Some families may prefer to wash the body themselves and are likely to want time for all family members to say good-bye. May not permit organ donation or autopsy.

Hispanics or Latino Americans. Family members may help with care of the body and are likely to want to say good-bye. Organ donation and autopsy are uncommon.

Judaism. Dying person may want deathbed confessional, or other prayers. Usually oppose autopsies but may consider organ donation. Body must not be left unattended until burial. Family member may remain present while body is prepared by nursing staff for transport to morgue and then to funeral home.

Roman Catholicism. Dying person should receive sacraments of Penance and Anointing of the Sick within 30 days before death. Religion does not oppose autopsies or organ donation.

Islam (Muslim). When a person is close to death, he or she will recite the Islamic Creed with help from others. After death, close the person's eyes, close the mouth, and straighten arms and legs.

Hinduism. Dying person should be in a peaceful room if not a home. Person or someone else should recite the Gita. Family members prefer to wash the body.

Buddhism. An ordained monk or nun should be present to care for the dying person. When the person has died, cover the body with a cotton sheet. Do not touch or manipulate the body. Do NOT close the eyes or the mouth. No noise, talking, or crying is allowed.

Data from Mazanec P., & Tyler M.K. (2003). Cultural considerations in end-of-life care. *American Journal of Nursing, 103*(3), 50; and Giger J.N., & Davidhizar, R.E. (2008). *Transcultural nursing: Assessment and interventions.* (5th ed.). St. Louis: Mosby.

Skill 10-1 Care of the Body after Death

Nursing Action *(Rationale)*

1. Gather equipment. *(Organizes procedure.)*
   - Disposable gloves, gown, and other protective clothing
   - Plastic bag for hazardous waste disposal
   - Washbasin, washcloth, warm water, bath towel
   - Clean gown or disposable gown for body
   - Absorbent pads
   - Body bag or shroud kit (know agency policy)
   - Paper tape and gauze dressing
   - Suitable receptacle for patient's belongings and other items to be returned to family
   - Valuables envelope
   - Identification tags as required by agency policy
2. Wash hands. *(Reduces spread of microorganisms.)*
3. Don clean gloves. *(Protects nurse from contamination.)*
4. Close patient's eyes and mouth if needed. *(Provides a more normal appearance.)*
5. Remove all tubing and other devices from patient's body.* *(Makes patient look more peaceful.)*
6. Place patient in supine position. *(Allows access for procedures.)* Elevate the head. *(Prevents discoloration.)* Do not place one hand on top of the other. *(This can lead to discoloration.)*
7. Replace soiled dressings with clean ones. *(Prevents odor.)*
8. Bathe patient as necessary. *(Reduces odor.)*
9. Brush or comb hair. *(Gives more normal appearance.)*
10. Apply clean gown. *(Prepares body for viewing.)*
11. Care for valuables and personal belongings. *(For legal considerations.)* If wedding band is to remain on the deceased, secure ring to finger with a small strip of tape over ring. *(Prevents loss and protects jewelry.)*
12. Allow family to view body and remain in room. *(Provide emotional support if family wishes.)* A sheet or light blanket placed over the body with only the head and upper shoulders exposed will maintain dignity and respect for the deceased. Remove unneeded equipment from the room. Provide soft lighting and offer chairs. *(Demonstrates respect for significant others.)*
13. After the family has left the room, attach special label if patient had a contagious disease. *(Protects those who handle the body.)*
14. Close door to room. *(Prevents exposure to patients and visitors.)*
15. Await arrival of ambulance or transfer to morgue. *(Out of respect for patient.)* (Some agencies use a shroud to enclose the body before transfer to the morgue. See illustrations.)
16. Document procedure and disposition of patient's body, as well as belongings and valuables. *(For legal purposes.)*

*Some situations require that all tubing remain in the body (e.g., when an autopsy is scheduled). Know agency policy.

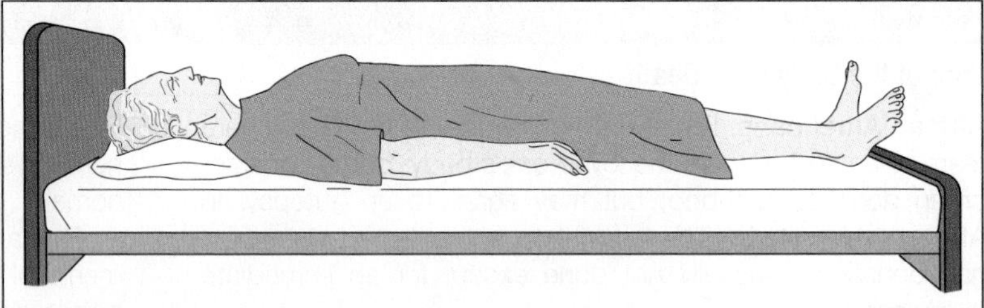

Step 15 A, Applying a shroud. The body is in the dorsal recumbent position. Arms are straight at the sides. There is a pillow under the head and shoulders.

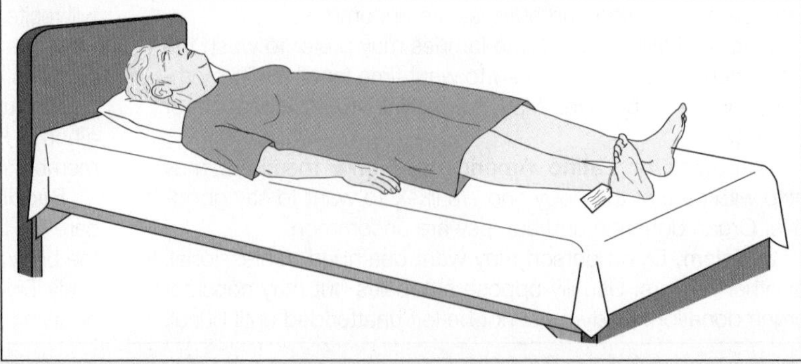

Step 15 B, Place the body on the shroud.

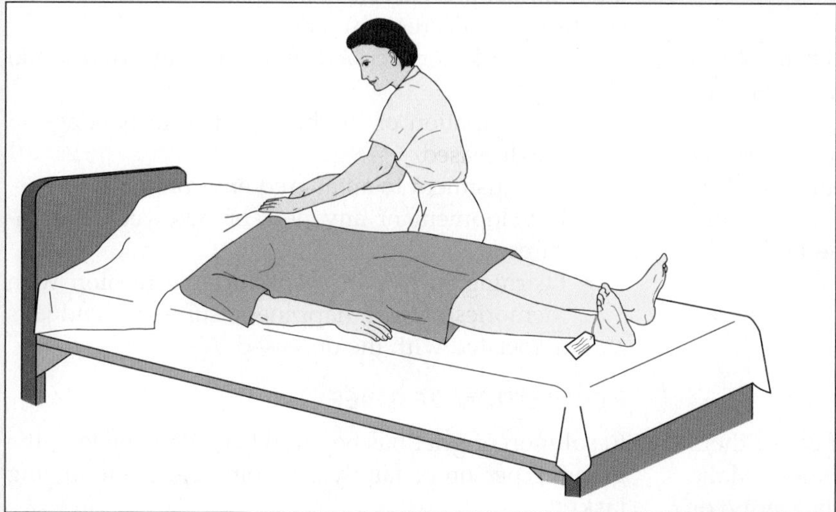

Step 15 **C,** Bring the top of the shroud down over the head.

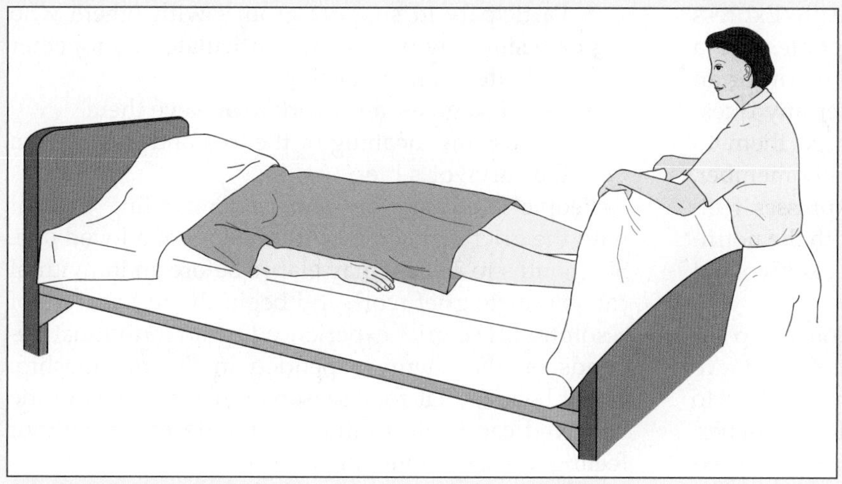

Step 15 **D,** Fold the bottom over the feet.

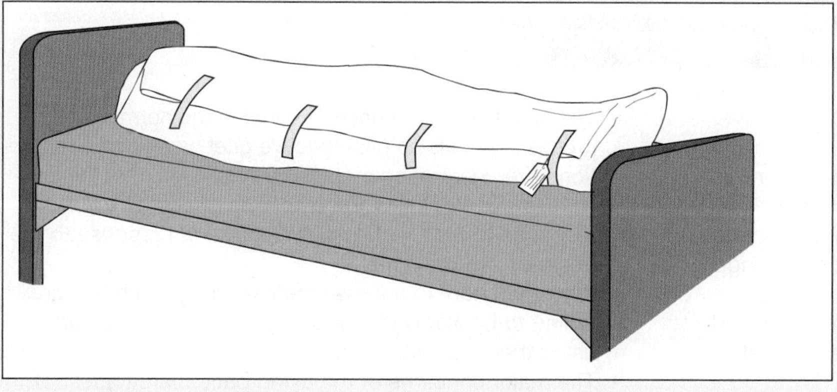

Step 15 **E,** Fold the sides over the body, tape or pin the sides together, and attach the identification tag.

Offer the family the opportunity to view the body. It is often helpful to suggest that this is an opportunity to say good-bye to their loved one, especially if they were not present at the time of death. If the family hesitates to view the body, let them think about it. If they decide not to view the body, accept their decision without judgment. If the family decides to view the body, assure them that they will not be alone. Offer to accompany them, and tell them that you would be glad to call on someone else to be present if they would like. Spend as much time as possible assisting the grieving family, and offer to contact other support services, such as social services and the spiritual adviser. (Many health care facilities now employ a full-time chaplain who may be summoned in the event of death.) The family now becomes the patient.

DOCUMENTATION

Document the care given to the dying patient objectively, completely, legibly, and accurately. As death approaches, make frequent documentation, and include the signs of impending death as they occur. Recording who was present at the time of the patient's death is important. Continue documentation until the last entry, which states where and to whom the body was transferred (see Box 10-11).

THE GRIEVING FAMILY

SUPPORT

Needs of the grieving family and significant others deserve your caring, compassionate attention. Make every attempt to contact someone—family, clergy, or friends—to be with the grieving survivor if he or she is alone at the time of the loved one's death. Express words that convey sympathy. If appropriate, use a spontaneous touch, such as a hand on the arm or an embrace, as a comforting gesture. Answer any questions the family may have, and encourage them to view, touch, and talk to the deceased family member. Remain nonjudgmental as the family expresses feelings of anger, guilt, or unfairness. Help with the notification of the mortician and any individuals involved in the procurement of donated organs.

Informing others can be a major emotional step for family members. Your presence and offer of assistance in this area is very supportive. Direct family members to support groups and other referral agencies (churches, therapists, social workers); such connections will expand the family's social network, as well as foster relatedness and decrease isolation.

Grief work is described as follows by Martocchio (1985):

- Emancipation of the bereaved from bondage to the deceased
- Readjustment to an altered environment
- Development of any new or renewed relationships
- Learning to live in a comfortable fashion with memories of hurt, happiness, suffering, and joys associated with the deceased

RESOLUTION OF GRIEF

Resolution of grief has begun when, after the loss, the grieving person or family can complete the following tasks:

- Have positive interactions with others
- Participate in support groups with others who are similarly bereaved to articulate loss together and offer companionship
- Establish goals, and work to achieve them
- Discuss the meaning of the loss and its effect on the survivor's life

People need support and understanding to deal with the grief that comes with the loss of a loved one. Six months to 2 years may elapse before an individual can complete grief work and begin the full process of resolution. The grief experienced by an individual depends on the energy expended in the relationship. Many believe that four seasons must pass before the bereaved can begin to think of the deceased without feeling intense emotional pain.

Get Ready for the NCLEX® Examination!

Key Points

- Care of the dying patient has moved from the home to hospitals and back again over the past 50 years.
- Dr. Elizabeth Kübler-Ross has been instrumental in identifying the five stages of death and dying: denial, anger, bargaining, depression, and acceptance.
- Losses occur throughout the life cycle, provide the individual experience with loss, and promote emotional growth and development of coping skills.
- The effect a loss will have on a person is individualized; duration, abruptness, extent, time required for treatment or replacement, or financial impact of the loss will all play a part.
- Grief is not an episode but a process, an active, not a passive, process. It takes work and emotional energy. The grief experienced by an individual depends on the energy expended in the relationship.
- When people do not do "grief work" following any significant loss, they are at risk for emotional, mental, and social problems.
- The grief theory demonstrates that in the normal grief process, there is an onset, active grief work, and a resolution or reorganization of the survivors' lives after the loss.
- Nurses experience all the emotions of grief not only in response to their own losses but also in response to the death of their patients.
- It is mandatory to assess whether family members are willing to be involved in a dying patient's care before using them as resources.
- The major concerns of the dying patient are (1) fear of abandonment (fear of dying alone), (2) fear of loss of control, (3) fear of pain and discomfort, and (4) fear of the unknown.
- Euthanasia is an ethical and legal issue faced by nurses. Active euthanasia is illegal in the United States.
- A do not resuscitate (DNR) order means only that. It does not mean to withhold hygiene, hydration, nutrition, or medications.
- Patients who decide ahead of time what kind of care they want and communicate these decisions to others do much to ensure that they receive the extent of care

that they desire. These communications, called advance directives, most often involve the living will and the durable power of attorney.

- The Dying Person's Bill of Rights speaks to the elements characteristic of dying with dignity.
- Assisting a dying patient in saying good-bye is an intervention nurses can initiate.
- The physical care requirements of the dying patient are primarily nursing interventions. Providing adequate nutrition, elimination, hygiene, safety, and comfort are nursing priorities.
- Continuing to speak to and include the patient in his or her care is essential, because as death approaches the dying patient becomes weaker. Patients may appear comatose yet be aware of activities around them.
- Signs of impending death are (1) slow, thready, and weaker pulse; (2) lowered blood pressure; (3) rapid, shallow, irregular, or abnormally slow respirations; and (4) mottling of lower extremities.
- Postmortem care is the care administered to the body after death. Follow procedures including cleansing, positioning, and labeling the body.

Additional Learning Resources

Go to your Companion CD for an audio glossary, animations, video clips, and more.

evolve Be sure to visit the Evolve site at http://evolve.elsevier.com/Christensen/foundations/ for additional online resources.

Review Questions for the NCLEX® Examination

1. During end-of-shift report, it is stated that an 86-year-old patient is dying as a result of end-stage renal disease. The nurse recalls that dying is considered:
   1. undesirable at any time.
   2. a failure for the nurse.
   3. impossible with modern medical devices.
   4. the final stage of human growth and development.

2. A nurse attempts to avoid caring for a 92-year-old patient who is dying of heart failure. If the nurse cannot avoid caring for this patient, she provides care but in a detached manner. This nurse is demonstrating:
   1. poor nursing care.
   2. grief reaction.
   3. withdrawal.
   4. bereavement.

3. A 65-year-old patient has been admitted with various physical complaints resulting from unresolved grief. During her morning care, she says, "It's been 6 months since Harry died. When is it going to get easier?" An appropriate answer by the nurse concerning grief work completion would be that grief work is completed:
   1. when the family returns to work, school, and social activities.
   2. after the funeral, wake, or memorial services.
   3. as soon as the bereaved can talk freely.
   4. on an individualized basis.

4. A 77-year-old patient has been admitted with pneumonia. Her husband asks the nurse about the living will. The nurse remembers that living wills:
   1. allow the courts to decide when care can be given.
   2. allow the individual to express his or her wishes regarding care.
   3. are legally binding in all states.
   4. allow health care workers to withhold fluids and medications.

5. The patient's daughter remained at the bedside of her dying mother throughout the night. When her mother died the following morning, the daughter cried out angrily at the nurse and the physician. The nurse's most appropriate action would be to:
   1. explain that everything possible was done for her mother.
   2. remain with the daughter and listen to what she is saying.
   3. leave the daughter in privacy and allow her to work through her grief.
   4. notify a clergyman and call other family members.

6. A newly licensed nurse is assigned to his first dying patient. The nurse would be best prepared to care for this patient if he:
   1. had completed a course dealing with death and dying.
   2. is able to control his own emotions about death.
   3. had experienced the death of a loved one.
   4. has resolved the matter of his own mortality.

7. A nurse is assigned to a patient who was recently diagnosed with a terminal illness. While the nurse was assisting her with morning care, the patient asked about organ donation. The most appropriate action would be to:
   1. assist her in obtaining the necessary information to make this decision.
   2. have the patient first discuss the subject with her family.
   3. suggest she delay making a decision at this time.
   4. contact the physician so consent can be obtained from the family.

8. A person experiences anticipatory grief when he:
   1. faces the possibility of losing a loved one.
   2. has placed the death of a loved one in perspective.
   3. displays grief responses after a loved one's death.
   4. has difficulty making decisions after a loved one's death.

9. The phases of bereavement:
   1. usually do not occur in order.
   2. are all present at the same time.
   3. occur before anticipatory grief.
   4. usually begin with reorganization.

10. When preparing a deceased patient for family viewing, the nurse:

1. covers the body with a warm blanket, if possible.
2. removes all equipment (tubes, drains, etc.) unless an autopsy has been ordered.
3. restricts family members from viewing a patient who has been disfigured.
4. covers the deceased patient's arms and hands.

11. Which is an appropriate therapeutic listening technique?

1. Saying, "I know just how you feel."
2. Saying, "Her death was for the best."
3. Never crying in front of family members
4. Talking slowly and encouraging family members to share their feelings

12. The nurse helps family members make difficult decisions by:

1. discussing autopsy and organ donation at the time of the loved one's death.
2. addressing one matter at a time, giving them adequate time to discuss each issue.
3. publicly discussing issues with other hospital staff.
4. addressing all of the issues at once.

13. Which phrase is most likely to help a grieving family member express himself or herself more easily?

1. "Tell me how you're feeling."
2. "I know just how you feel."
3. "Things will get better."
4. "Time heals all wounds."

14. If a bereaved family member has an unresolved issue with a deceased patient, the nurse should tell him:

1. that he is simply experiencing normal anticipatory grief.
2. that he missed his chance to make amends and now it is too late.
3. to verbalize his thoughts and feelings to his loved one.
4. not to worry, and explain that he is just going through the searching and yearning phase of bereavement.

15. For those who work with grief, death, and dying, it is essential to have constant vigilance over their:

1. patients.
2. own issues.
3. schedules.
4. colleagues.

16. Nurses care for all types of patients with various conditions, including those with a terminal illness. Which statement is true?

1. Death from terminal illness is sudden and unexpected.
2. Physicians know when death will occur.
3. An illness is terminal when there is no reasonable hope of recovery.
4. All severe injuries result in death.

17. Many forces influence living and dying. Which psychological force influences living and dying?

1. Hope and the will to live
2. Reincarnation and belief in the afterlife
3. Denial and anger
4. Bargaining and depression

18. There are many issues related to dying and death. One of the more controversial is euthanasia. Euthanasia is defined as:

1. a sudden or unexpected death.
2. the belief that the spirit or soul is reborn into another human body or another form of life.
3. an "easy death."
4. perinatal death.

19. Special considerations for children are necessary when dealing with death. Children between ages 5 and 7 years view death as:

1. temporary.
2. final.
3. something adults do.
4. going to sleep.

20. Following the death of a patient, the nurse leaves the room quickly and is found sobbing in the utility room. Which action is the most supportive?

1. Sending the nurse home for the rest of the shift
2. Reassigning the nurse to an area where it is unlikely a patient will die
3. Sitting with her and allowing her to express herself
4. Insisting that she perform postmortem care for the patient

21. The type of care that allows patients to make more informed choices, achieve better alleviation of symptoms, and have more opportunity to work on issues of like closure is:

1. acute care.
2. mourning care.
3. palliative care.
4. terminal care.

22. A factor that uniquely influences an older adult's grief response is:

1. cultural background.
2. socioeconomic resources.
3. sense of contribution in life.
4. support available from family members.

23. A healthy 25-year-old who sustained a head injury during a motor vehicle accident is in the emergency department. The patient has no brain activity and is on life support. The family has expressed an interest in organ donation. The nurse is aware that:

1. organ donations can only occur if the patient has given prior consent.
2. vital organs such as the heart and pancreas must be harvested while the patient remains on the ventilator.
3. brain death can be reversed, so the family should be informed to take more time in making their decision.
4. the attending physician will be present in the operating room during harvesting of the organs.

24. A bereaved widow of 3 months tells the nurse she has clearly smelled her deceased husband's aftershave scent as she sat in church recently. She questions if she might be "going crazy." The nurse can help her to understand she is experiencing:

1. intrusive memories.
2. dysfunctional or complicated grief.
3. sense of presence.
4. grief attacks.

25. When giving postmortem care, if the patient is in the supine position, it is best to place:

1. one hand on top of the other across the patient's abdomen.
2. one hand on top of the other across the patient's chest.
3. arms at the sides of the body with the palms facing down.
4. arms at the sides of the body with the palms facing up.

26. Following the diagnosis of a terminal illness, the nurse educates the patient and the family members about palliative care. The nurse explains that palliative care should be initiated:

1. as soon as possible after learning of the diagnosis of the terminal illness.
2. during the last 3 to 6 months of life.
3. during the last 3 to 6 weeks of life.
4. anytime following the diagnosis of the terminal illness.

27. The adult children of a dying patient, who is alert and oriented, disagree on the patient's choice of a do not resuscitate order. The children ask the opinion of the nurse, who has cared for this patient over an extended period. The nurse's best response is to:

1. encourage the children to speak with the physician regarding their concerns.
2. remind the children that this is the wish of their parent.
3. ask the patient to speak with the children regarding their concerns.
4. listen to the children's concerns and encourage them to talk to their parent.

chapter 11

Admission, Transfer, and Discharge

evolve

http://evolve.elsevier.com/Christensen/foundationsadult

Elaine Oden Kockrow and Barbara Lauritsen Christensen

Objectives

1. Identify guidelines for admission, transfer, and discharge of a patient.
2. Discuss the concepts of the Health Insurance Portability and Accountability Act (HIPAA).
3. Describe common patient reactions to hospitalization.
4. Identify nursing interventions for common patient reactions to hospitalization.
5. Discuss the nursing process and how it pertains to admitting, discharging, and transferring the patient.
6. Discuss the nurse's responsibilities in performing an admission.
7. Describe how the nurse prepares a patient for transfer to another unit or facility.
8. Discuss discharge planning.
9. Explain how the nurse prepares a patient for discharge.
10. Identify the nurse's role when a patient chooses to leave the hospital against medical advice.

Key Terms

admission (p. 248)
against medical advice (AMA) (p. 263)
continuity of care (p. 257)
discharge (p. 260)
discharge planning (p. 260)
disorientation (dĭs-ŏr-rē-ĕn-TĀ-shŭn, p. 248)
empathy (ĔM-pă-thē, p. 249)
health care facility (p. 248)
home health agency (p. 260)
separation anxiety (p. 248)
third-party payors (p. 257)
transfer (p. 257)

COMMON PATIENT REACTIONS TO HOSPITALIZATION

Admission (entry of a patient into the health care facility) to a hospital or other **health care facility** (any agency that provides health care) is an anxious time for patients and their families. The patient is usually very concerned about health problems or potential health problems and the potential outcome of treatment. Often the patient is having pain or other discomfort. The first contact with nurses and health care workers is important. It provides an opportunity to lessen anxiety and fears and initiate a positive attitude regarding the care to be received.

A way to significantly ease the patient's anxiety and promote cooperation and positive response to treatment is to follow admission routines that are efficient and show appropriate concern for the patient. Admission routines that the patient perceives as careless or excessively impersonal, in contrast, tend to heighten anxiety, reduce cooperation, impair response to treatment, and perhaps aggravate symptoms.

It is your responsibility to assist the patient in maintaining dignity and a sense of control and in becoming comfortable in the new environment of the health care facility. This environment differs from a patient's home and has new sights, sounds, and smells that may interfere with the patient's comfort.

Each person's reaction to hospitalization is unique; however, some common reactions are to be expected, such as fear of the unknown, loss of identity, **disorientation** (mental confusion characterized by inadequate or incorrect perception of place, time, and identity), **separation anxiety** (fears and apprehension caused by separation from familiar surroundings and significant people), and loneliness. These reactions are related to some of the needs described by Maslow (1954) (see Figure 1-5).

Fear of the unknown, which causes insecurity, is perhaps the most common reaction. This relates to the need Maslow calls *safety.* Explanations about hospital policies, information about medical orders and procedures, and simple, direct answers to common questions the patient or family often have help the person feel more comfortable and in control. Basic issues, if they remain mysterious, cause anxiety and insecurity: How do I work the bed? How do I call the nurse? How or when do I get some food? When can my family visit? What are they going to do to me next? You display caring and relieve some of this anxiety when you orient the patient and family to the room and explain how the equipment works.

During the admission process to a health care facility, many patients feel a loss of identity that reflects a need for esteem, love, and belonging. Recognition, as described by Maslow, is part of this need. Sometimes putting the identification (ID) band on the patient's wrist reduces the patient to feeling like the number and name on the ID rather than a person. Explain that this is a necessary procedure to provide a positive means of identification just in case medications, anesthesia, discomfort, and emotional reactions cause the patient to be disoriented or unresponsive.

It is important to learn new patients' names quickly. Address them by using Mr., Mrs., Ms., or Miss with the last name, and only use a first name at the patient's request. Using "honey," "dear," "Gramps," or "Grandma" is never appropriate.

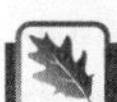

Life Span Considerations

Older Adults

Admission, Transfer, and Discharge

- The older adult admitted to the hospital today is likely to be seriously ill.
- In a normally alert and oriented older adult, medical conditions that necessitate hospitalization often result in some level of disorientation.
- Older adults, who often have some limitation of vision or hearing, are more likely to become agitated or fearful during hospitalization. Many experience relocation stress.
- Transfers, even within the hospital, tend to be confusing and upsetting to them.
- Hospitalized older adults frequently are concerned that they will be unable to return to their homes and will need institutional placement.
- Appropriate referrals for home nursing, therapy, homemaking, Meals on Wheels, or other services are essential for older adults.
- Older adult patients need you to converse with them slowly and clearly because hearing may be less acute. Face the patient to make lip-reading possible. Do not rush older patients; wait for the patient to answer you rather than letting family members answer.
- The change in environment and daily routine sometimes causes disorientation, loss of appetite, or reversal of sleeping-waking patterns. Anxiety about hospitalization has potential to interfere with memory.
- The stress of hospitalization will sometimes be serious for the older patient because of a reduction in adaptive capacity. Helplessness, lack of control, and dependency often emerge, although it is possible to restore some degree of personal control.
- When an older adult patient is transferred to a new facility, the relocation is also stressful. Ensure that significant support people are still accessible, the patient is thoroughly oriented to new surroundings, the patient is allowed to take along important memorabilia, and the patient has an opportunity to make decisions about care.

Separation anxiety and loneliness are reactions that reflect the needs Maslow identified as belongingness and love. We all know about separation anxiety in young children, but adults and the older adult often have this reaction as well. In children, it generally is expressed by crying; with adults, you will possibly note that they are either very quiet or very talkative; the older adult sometimes exhibits disorientation or depression.

The company of friends and loved ones is the best antidote to separation anxiety. Liberal visiting hours in health care facilities encourage family and friends to visit. Many hospitals now allow even small children to visit relatives, especially their own mother when she has had a new baby. Encourage parents to stay with their hospitalized child to prevent the anxiety separation from them causes. This also gives the child a feeling of security. In some facilities, pets are allowed to visit; pets even live in some nursing homes.

You have the ability to help reduce the severity of these common reactions to hospitalization with a warm, caring attitude and with courtesy and **empathy** (ability to recognize and to some extent share the emotions and state of mind of another and to understand the meaning and significance of that person's behavior). To help them adapt, treat patients with respect; maintain their dignity; involve them in the plan of care; and whenever possible, adjust hospital routine to meet their desires. Special considerations for the older adult are listed in the Life Span Considerations for Older Adults box.

ROLE OF THE ADMITTING CLERK OR SECRETARY

One of the many roles of the admitting clerk or secretary includes obtaining important identifying information from the patient. To maintain the patient's safety and legal rights, it is important to obtain this information in a private manner. If the patient is non–English speaking or has extensive hearing impairment, it is best for the clerk or secretary to contact an interpreter to ensure that accurate information is obtained during the admission procedure. In the event that there is no admitting clerk or secretary on duty, it is possible that these admission responsibilities will become the responsibility of the nurse who will be caring for the patient (Perry & Potter, 2006).

After obtaining identifying information, place the ID band on the patient's wrist. Before performing therapies or procedures, health care personnel will check the ID band to verify the patient's full legal name, the birth date, the patient's facility identification number, and the name of the admitting physician. An additional, usually red band is also applied to alert personnel to patient allergies. If the patient is unconscious at the time of admission, it is not possible to make proper identification until a family member or legal guardian is present. If the patient is the victim of a crime, some agencies' policy will provide guidelines for their ID to be anonymous (Perry & Potter, 2006).

Both The Joint Commission and Medicare and Medicaid Services require that all hospitals present a consent form for general treatment and the Patient's Bill of Rights to the patient or the patient's legal guardian at the time of admission. Doing so is the responsibility of the admitting clerk or secretary. All health care facilities also have other policies and procedures that further inform the patient of his or her rights and of the nurse's responsibilities in ensuring these rights are honored (Perry & Potter, 2006).

Additional important topics to address at the time of admission are the Patient Self-Determination Act of 1991, and the Health Insurance Portability and Accountability Act (HIPAA). As directed by the Patient Self-Determination Act, patients being admitted to a Medicare- and Medicaid-recipient facility are required to be made aware of their right to accept or refuse medical treatment and to receive information on advance directives. It is mandatory to refer the patient to the appropriate resource if he or she wishes to further discuss advance directives or complete an advance directive document (Perry & Potter, 2006).

HIPAA is a federal mandate that ensures the privacy of the patient's protected health information (PHI). Patient's are informed of their privacy rights regarding their PHI upon admission, and are usually given a written form that explains how the facility will protect these rights. HIPAA also requires that facilities only use or disclose PHI for the purpose of treating the patient or for the purpose of payment for services. Any other uses of PHI require authorization by the patient. In addition, HIPAA requires that only those health care providers directly involved in the care of the patient are given information, and only on a need-to-know basis. In other words, the least amount of PHI necessary to provide care is disclosed to the fewest people necessary. Under HIPAA, patients have the right to gain access to their records, request amendments to their PHI, or request restrictions in the use of their PHI. Patients also have the right to request a record of all PHI disclosures. They are permitted to request PHI to be sent to an alternate address or phone number than what was listed at the time of admission. It is important for all health care personnel to be familiar with their facility's policies and procedures relating to HIPAA guidelines (Perry & Potter, 2006).

CULTURAL CONSIDERATIONS FOR THE HOSPITALIZED PATIENT

If the patient does not speak English and is not accompanied by a bilingual family member, contact the appropriate resource (usually the social services department) to secure an interpreter. (See Chapter 8 for in-depth discussion of cultural issues in health care.)

The following are guidelines for communicating with patients from various cultures during the admission, discharge, and transfer procedures (see Cultural Considerations box):

- Respect the patient as an individual. Avoid judging patients' intellectual abilities on the basis of how they use language.

Cultural Considerations

Admission, Transfer, and Discharge

- Observe interactions between the patient and family members. Some families prefer to make decisions as a unit (family decision making); others will perhaps look to either the authority figure within the family or to the eldest member for decision making (Perry & Potter, 2006).
- Some Haitian-American patients are more likely to feel they are receiving effective treatment when a nurse is seen. In Haiti, a nurse is given more authority and status than a physician, and the patient tends to be more cooperative with directions given by a nurse. When nursing measures are being implemented (e.g., taking the patient's blood pressure), tell the patient verbally what you are doing and that it is for the patient's benefit. Nursing actions are seen as caring and helpful.
- Many Haitians believe that leaves have a special significance in healing. You will sometimes find leaves in the clothes and on various parts of the body. Leaves are thought to have mystical power related to regaining or keeping health.
- Some Haitian-Americans associate wheelchairs with being sick. Therefore, the patient who is allowed to walk out of the hospital at discharge is more likely to feel that care has been effective.
- It is possible that a poor patient and a wealthy patient with Haitian background, although from the same country, will find it very distasteful to share the same room in the hospital.
- According to traditional Japanese belief, contact with blood, skin disease, and corpses causes illness. Some Japanese also believe improper care of the body, including poor diet and lack of sleep, causes illness.
- Be aware when caring for Orthodox Jewish patients that the use of electronic equipment is avoided during the Sabbath, which is from sundown Friday to sundown Saturday. Sometimes it will be necessary to find alternatives to the use of call lights and telephones for these patients (Perry & Potter, 2006).
- Remember that just because two patients are black does not mean they will share common interests; sometimes they will find not even find each other suitable for sharing a hospital room.
- Most Appalachians (found chiefly in the Eastern and some Southern states) intertwine both religion and culture; therefore, in the interests of cultural sensitivity, include the assessment of the patient's religious beliefs on admission to the health care system. Because some Appalachians tend to be fundamental and fatalistic in their religious beliefs, it is essential to consider this belief an influencing variable.
- Chinese-Americans believe the number 4 is unlucky because it sounds like the Chinese word for death. If possible, do not assign 4 as a room number.

- Avoid treating these patients differently from other patients, because "special" treatment may be interpreted as patronizing.
- Do not assume patients are angry, aggressive, or hostile if they speak more loudly or emotionally than most other patients.
- Use titles such as "Mr." or "Ms."
- Never attempt to use ethnic dialects with patients. This could be interpreted as making fun of patients or as condescension.
- Avoid trying to impress patients by saying you have friends of the same racial background.
- Be attentive to the patient's nonverbal communication. This often helps clarify seemingly confusing verbal communication.
- If you do not understand what a patient is saying, ask for clarification. Do not let embarrassment at not understanding raise the risks posed by misinformation.

ADMITTING A PATIENT

The admission procedure generally begins in the admitting department. Here the admissions staff gather information to start the patient's record. This information usually includes name, address, telephone number, age, birth date, Social Security number, next of kin, insurance company and policy number, place of employment, physician's name, and reason for this admission and for previous admissions. This information is primarily used in the business office for billing purposes. The ID band is prepared with the patient's name, age, admitting number, physician's name, and room number. The admitting clerk usually puts the band on the patient's wrist. The unit where the patient is assigned for care is notified, and the patient is escorted to the room.

Admitting departments will usually have the patient sign consent for treatment before transfer to the nursing unit.

Some hospitals have telephone admitting. The day before a planned admission, a clerk from the admitting office calls the patient at home and gathers all the information needed to begin the records. Instructions are given regarding time to arrive at the hospital, items to bring to the hospital, and things that it is better not to bring to the hospital (e.g., jewelry and large sums of money). When the patient arrives the next day, the records and ID band need only have the room number put on them.

People brought to the emergency department are sometimes admitted directly to a patient care room or a special care unit (SCU), intensive care unit (ICU), coronary care unit (CCU), or burn unit. In these situations, a family member, usually the next of kin, goes to the admitting office to provide the necessary information.

When the unit staff is notified that a new patient is en route, they will make the room ready. A room that is neat and clean, of appropriate temperature, with lighting and personal care items in place, makes the patient feel expected and welcome. In contrast, a room that is not prepared will most likely make the patient feel unexpected or that the arrival is inconvenient to the nurse. This makes a poor first impression and impedes the development of a therapeutic nurse-patient relationship.

If special equipment will be required by the new patient, such as oxygen or traction, have it in place and ready when the patient arrives. A patient arriving on a stretcher will need the bed in the high position; the low bed position is best for a patient arriving by wheelchair or walking.

Greeting the patient by name and making the patient feel welcome is one of the most important aspects of the admission procedure. Be careful to call the patient by his or her surname if the patient is an adult, unless otherwise directed. Introduce yourself by name and title (e.g., Miss Rodriguez, SPN, or Mr. Smith, LVN). A person who is warmly welcomed will be more at ease in this new environment.

It is important to remember that patients do not get ill and require hospitalization at your convenience. The patient's admission to the unit may occur at any time. Regardless of the time or the activity occurring on the nursing unit, be courteous to, interested in, and receptive of the new patient. The new patient needs to be given an orientation to the unit and the room (Box 11-1).

Also explain the hospital routine. Knowing when meals are served, when family and friends are allowed to visit, when laboratory tests or diagnostic imaging evaluations are scheduled, when the physician usually makes rounds, and the policy on side rails will give the patient a sense of security and lessen anxiety. Many hospitals have booklets for the patient explaining these routine activities; these serve as reminders of your explanations. Some booklets include information about the availability of various social services, religious services, and facilities such as cafeteria, library, and gift shop. Use the opportunity for patient teaching (Patient Teaching box).

Box 11-1 Patient Room Orientation

Orientation should include the following:
- The relationship of the room to the nurses' station
- The location of lounge areas
- The location of shower and bathroom facilities
- How to call the nurse from the bed and the bathroom
- How to use the intercom system
- How to adjust the bed and the lights
- How to operate the television
- How to operate the telephone and the radio
- Explanation of policies applicable to the patient

Patient Teaching

Patient Admission to the Health Care Facility

- Some teaching occurs during the admission process. The nurse provides information regarding physical assessment findings, planned diagnostic procedures, or hospital routines. A formal teaching plan will not begin until assessment is completed and a care plan is developed.
- In an emergency situation, instruct family members on the rationale for any procedures and routines to expect in the patient's care.
- Teaching begins early in a patient's hospitalization. Introduce instruction when the patient is able to be attentive and learn from the information. This is sometimes difficult in an acute care setting. Keep information specific and focus on topics such as nature of the patient's illness, medications needed for treatment, and use of equipment in self-care (e.g., dressing, ambulatory devices).
- Explain shift times and shift changes to the patient.
- Consider how hospitalization influences an adult patient's occupational status. Will the illness seriously delay work that the patient is assigned to complete? Will there be a considerable delay before the patient can return to work?
- Confirm the patient's understanding of transfer and procedures through discussion and questions. Explain the reason for the transfer, the time it is to occur, and what procedures are planned.
- Be prepared to repeat information and instructions to the patient and significant others during the transfer of a patient, since transfers often elicit feelings of anxiety.
- Before the patient leaves the agency, provide for return demonstration of any skills taught.
- Patients who have short stays in health care agencies often do not receive teaching until day of discharge.
- It is not always possible to anticipate some prescriptions. The day of discharge is sometimes the only opportunity to teach patient about medications. Some agencies have brochures or cards that provide specific information about individual medications (see Figure 11-4).
- Obtain the help of social workers or discharge planners to ensure the transfer of a patient to a long-term care facility is appropriate in meeting the patient's physical and mental needs.

The admitting procedure on the patient care unit is much more extensive than that in the admitting department (Skill 11-1). Check the ID band and verify the information with the patient. Make an assessment of immediate needs such as pain, shortness of breath, or severe anxiety, and report the results. If there is another patient in the room, introduce the two patients.

Have the patient give jewelry, money, and medications to the family to take home. If no family member is present, see that valuables are put in the hospital safe. Carefully follow the hospital policy for patient

Skill 11-1 Admitting a Patient

Nursing Action *(Rationale)*

1. Wash hands. *(Reduces spread of microorganisms.)*
2. Prepare the room before the patient arrives: care items in place; bed at proper height and open; light on. *(This makes patient feel expected and welcome.)*
3. Courteously greet the patient and family. Introduce yourself. Project interest and concern. Introduce roommate. *(The patient and family are more at ease when they know the people around them.)*
4. Check the ID band and verify its accuracy. *(Ensures identification before tests or surgery are performed or medication is given. In long-term care facilities, the residents do not wear ID bands. A picture of the resident is used for identification purposes.)*
5. Assess immediate needs. *(Establishes trust when needs are recognized and met.)*
6. Orient the patient to the unit, the lounge, and the nurses' station. *(Promotes safety.)*
7. Orient the patient to the room. Explain the use of equipment, call system, bed, telephone, and television. *(Allows the patient some control over the environment and promotes safety.)*
8. Explain hospital routines, such as visiting hours, meal times, and morning wake-up. *(Decreases fear of unknown and gives a feeling of security.)*
9. Provide privacy if the patient desires. Family members are sometimes asked to leave the room. Admission of an infant or small child requires emotional support for both child and parents. Parents are generally encouraged to stay with their child to prevent separation anxiety. The most reliable source of admission information is the parent. Assist the patient to undress if necessary. *(Helps maintain dignity and shows respect for the patient. Helping the patient undress prevents fatigue and falls. Provides opportunity to assess range of motion and the skin.)*
10. Follow hospital policy for care of valuables, clothing, and medications. *(Helps prevent loss of valuables, clothing, or medications, which is disturbing to the patient and family and potentially results in legal problems.)*

11. Obtain the patient's health history and do the initial nursing assessment. *(Provides a basis for individualized care.)* When a patient is admitted in critical condition, only the most pertinent information need be collected immediately. The remaining information will be obtained at a later time. Young children are very curious about what is happening to them and the environment around them. Encourage the child to use equipment on dolls to help reduce anxieties. Encourage children to express how they feel. It is generally best to perform invasive procedures (e.g., obtaining blood specimens, starting intravenous lines) in a treatment room. *(Enables the child to perceive his or her room as a safe area.)*
12. Provide for safety: bed in low position, side rails up, call light within easy reach. *(Promotes patient safety.)*
13. Begin care as ordered by the physician. *(The patient and family will develop a positive attitude about the institution when care is started immediately.)*
14. Invite family back into the room if they left earlier. *(Decreases family anxiety when they observe the patient is settled.)*
15. Wash hands. *(Reduces spread of microorganisms.)*
16. Record the information on the patient's chart according to agency policy. *(Provides information that can also be used by other health professionals. It is the beginning of the permanent record.)*
17. Allow patient and family time alone together, if desired. *(Admission procedure is often stressful and fatiguing. Allows time for decision making.)*
18. Do patient teaching (see Patient Teaching box).

valuables. Losing a patient's valuables incurs serious legal implications for both you and the hospital. Document disposition of valuables on the medical record. In an Alzheimer's unit of a long-term care facility or in a mental health unit, the facility does assume some responsibility for patient belongings, because the patient is not competent to do so. In this case, the careful listing and description of the patient's property become even more important. Hospitals will in some cases be required to reimburse this patient for lost items. In these units, patients generally are not allowed to keep any jewelry (other than a wedding ring) or any money at the bedside. Some facilities require all medications brought in by the patient to be sent to the pharmacy to be identified. These same medications are then returned to the patient upon dismissal. Be sure to document all of these in the patient's record.

The patient is usually asked to put on pajamas or a hospital gown. Sometimes you will have to help the patient change clothes. If this help is not needed, provide the patient a few minutes of privacy to change. Make an inventory of clothing along with other personal items the patient uses, such as glasses, contacts, dentures, prostheses, crutches, hearing aids, wigs, or Bible. Also record any jewelry or money that will be kept in the patient's room. Figure 11-1 is of a sample clothing and valuables inventory checklist.

Once the patient is established in his or her room, take the health history and do the initial nursing assessment (Coordinated Care box). The health history generally includes the reason for admission; signs and symptoms the patient is experiencing; past illnesses, surgical procedures, and hospitalizations; medications (both prescription and nonprescription); allergies (food, medications, other); eating habits; urinary and bowel patterns; sleep routine; and activity and exercise habits

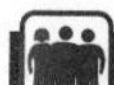

Coordinated Care

Delegation

ASSESSMENT AND DATA COLLECTION

The Joint Commission (TJC) requires each patient to have an admission assessment prepared by a registered nurse (RN) (TJC, 2003). The RN is then allowed to delegate aspects of data collection, for example, to the licensed practical nurse or licensed vocational nurse (LPN/LVN).

Data from The Joint Commission. (2003). *Comprehensive accreditation manual for hospitals: The official handbook (CAMH).* Oak Brook Terrace, Ill.: Author.

and routine. Other information to be included in a history is the language spoken (and languages understood), family members or significant others, home situation, interests, abilities, activities of daily living, and occupation.

The initial assessment properly includes level of consciousness, vital signs, height, weight, breath sounds, bowel sounds, range of motion, condition of skin, vision, and hearing. Figure 11-2 is an example of a record used to collect this information. Figure 11-3 shows a typical medication record to keep track of the medications a patient is taking upon admission and during the course of this hospitalization.

Prioritize the patient's needs. Each facility is required to set a time frame for completion of the admission procedure.

The physician is notified when the patient has been admitted. If no orders have been received yet, the physician will give orders at this time.

Skill 11-1 identifies the general steps to follow in admitting a patient. Specific hospital policies and the patient's condition may necessitate some alterations to these steps. See Box 11-2 for managing emergency admissions.

CLOTHING LIST		
[ ] Clothing- [ ] Belt [ ] Blouse [ ] Boots [ ] Bra [ ] Coat/jacket [ ] Dress/skirt [ ] Hat/cap/gloves	[ ] Hose/socks [ ] Jeans/slacks [ ] Luggage [ ] Nightgown/pajamas [ ] Robe [ ] Shirt [ ] Shoes [ ] Shorts [ ] Slip	[ ] Slippers [ ] Sweat pants [ ] Sweat shirt [ ] Sweater [ ] Tie [ ] Underwear [ ] Other clothing- [ ] Clothing sent with family [ ] No clothing items
[ ] Personal items- [ ] Bible/book [ ] Crutches [ ] Curling iron [ ] Hair dryer [ ] Upper dentures [ ] Lower dentures [ ] Partial dentures [ ] Right hearing aid [ ] Left hearing aid	[ ] Prosthesis [ ] Radio/tape player [ ] Razor [ ] Toothbrush [ ] Walker [ ] Other personal items-	[ ] Personal items sent with family- [ ] All personal items sent with family [ ] No personal items
[ ] Valuables- [ ] Bracelet- [ ] Earrings- [ ] Glasses/case- [ ] Contacts [ ] Medals/rosary [ ] Money-	[ ] Necklace- [ ] Purse [ ] Rings- [ ] Wallet [ ] Wrist watch- [ ] Other valuables-	[ ] Valuables sent with family- [ ] All valuables sent with family [ ] Valuables sent to safe (receipt on chart) [ ] Valuables in Same Day Surgery locker number-

I take full responsibility for retaining in my possession the items/clothing listed above and any others brought to me while I am a patient at Great Plains Regional Medical Center.

Admission signatures completed at time of admission		Discharge signatures completed at time of discharge	
Patient/Family:	Date/Time:	Patient/Family:	Date/Time:
Staff 1: Staff 2:	Date/Time:	Nurse:	Date/Time:

FIGURE 11-1 Example of a clothing and personal belongings list.

Box 11-2 Managing Emergency Admissions

- For the patient admitted through the emergency department (ED), immediate treatment takes priority over routine admission procedures. After ED treatment, the patient arrives on the nursing unit with a temporary ID bracelet, a physician's order sheet, and a record of treatment. Read this record and confer with the nurse who cared for the patient in the ED to gain insight and to ensure continuity of care.
- Next, record any ongoing treatment, such as an intravenous infusion, in the nursing notes. Obtain and record the patient's vital signs, and follow the physician's orders for treatment. If the patient is conscious and not in great distress, explain any treatment orders. If family members accompany the patient, ask them to wait in the lounge while you assess the patient and begin treatment. Permit them to visit the patient after the patient is settled in his or her room. When the patient's condition allows, proceed with routine admission procedures.

NURSING ADMISSION STATEMENT

Admitted: Ambulatory, Cart, Wheelchair, Arms, Ambulance

From: Office, ER, Surgery, Radiology, Recovery Room Transferred From: ________

Oriented to Room: Call Light, Side Rails, TV, Phone, Safety/Smoking Policy: Yes ____ No ____

Vital Signs: T ____ P ____ R ____ BP ____ HT ____ WT ____ Dentures ____

Diet at Home ________

Allergies: Drug ________ Reaction

Other ________ Organ Donor: Yes ____ No ____

Reason for Admission ________ Signature ________

Date: ________ Time: ________

EYES: Impaired Vision, Blind, Cataract, Glaucoma, Contacts, Glasses, Prosthesis R.L.
Comments: ________

EARS, NOSE, THROAT: Hard of hearing, Deaf, Lesions, Hearing Aid, R.L., Tracheotomy
Comments: ________

RESPIRATORY: Pain, Dyspnea, Wheeze, Asthma, Sinusitis, COPD, Cough,
Productive ____ Nonproductive ____
Oxygen needed, Smoker
Comments: ________

CIRCULATION: Apical, Radial, Strong, Weak, Thready, Bounding, Regular, Palpitations, Chest pain, Numbness, Bruising, Edema, Hypertension, Hx MI, CHF, Pacer, Bypass Surgery
Comments: ________

ENDOCRINE: Thyroid, Diabetes
Comments: ________

GI TRACT: Heartburn, Ulcers, Pain, Hernia, Dysphagia, Nausea, Vomiting, Loss of Appetite, Distention, Diverticulitis
Comments: ________

ELIMINATION: Last BM ____ Normal, Constipated, Diarrhea, Tarry, Bright red, Clay colored, Hemorrhoids, Involuntary, Use of laxatives, Yes/No Enema, Yes/No Ileostomy, Colostomy
Comments: ________

URINARY: Incontinence, Nocturia, Hematuria, Dysuria, Burning, Frequency, Urgency, Dribbling, Infections, Cath: Yes/No
Comments: ________

NEUROLOGICAL: Convulsions, Paralysis, Syncope, Paresthesia, Dizziness, Coordination, Weakness, Headaches
Comments: ________

SKIN: Color ____ Turgor ____ Temp ____
Describe any rashes, Lesions, Ecchymosis, Petechiae, Scars, Diabetic sores
Comments: ________

MUSCULOSKELETAL: Pain, Stiffness, Contractures, Deformities, Tremors, Backaches, Weight bearing, Amputation
Comments: ________

FEMALE REPRODUCTION: MP ____ EDC ____
Menopause, Breast pain, Breast tenderness, Vaginal discharge
Comments: ________

PREVIOUS SURGERIES:

MEDS TAKEN AT HOME:

Med:	Dose:	Last Taken:

DISPOSAL OF MEDS:
Did not bring ____
Pt. has ____ Family took home ____
Retained/taken to Pharmacy ____
Other: ____
Signature: ____
Time: ____

N-37 (Rev. 6/98)

FIGURE 11-2 Nursing admission assessment form.

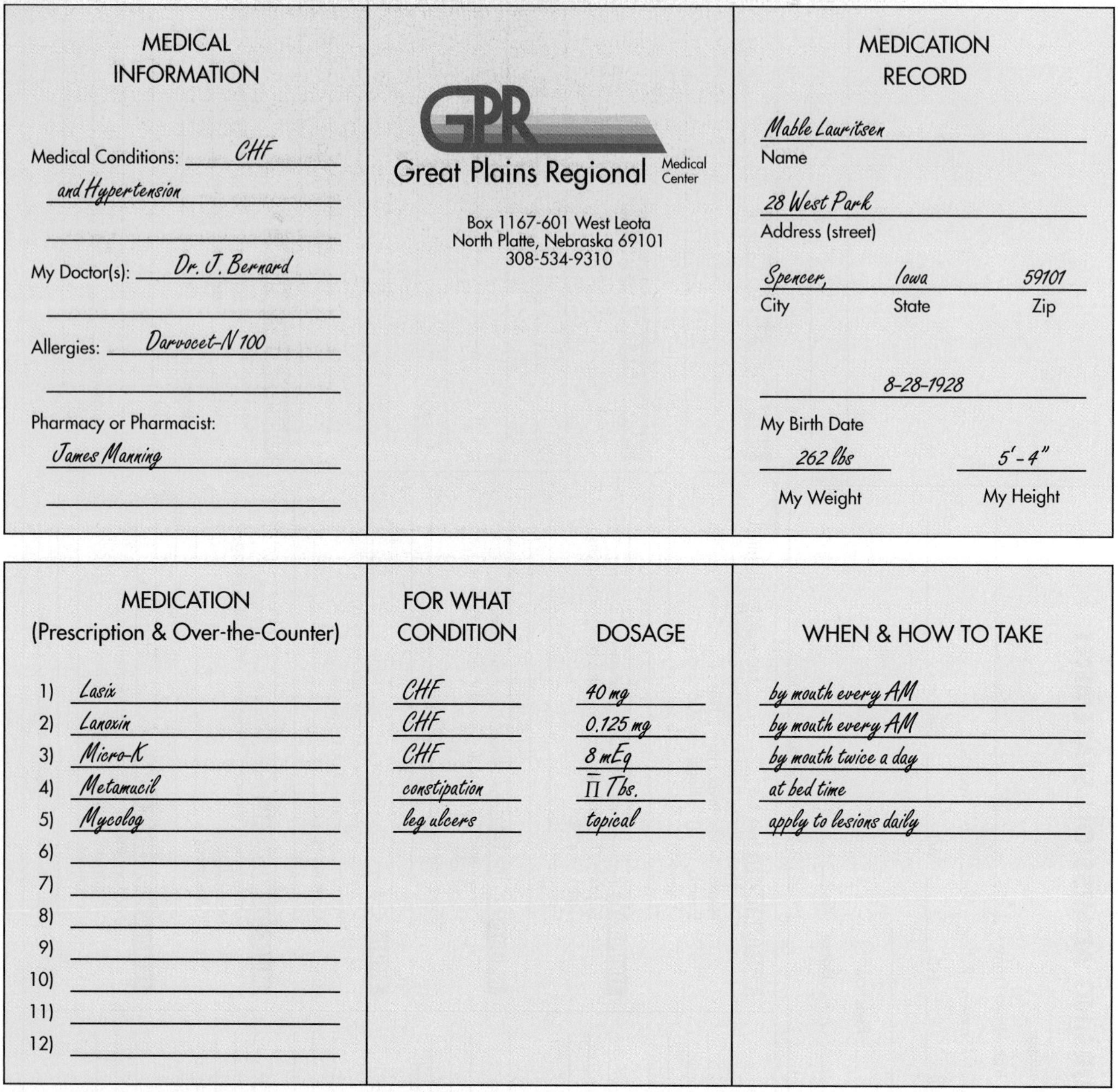

MEDICAL INFORMATION		MEDICATION RECORD
Medical Conditions: CHF and Hypertension	GPR Great Plains Regional Medical Center	Mable Lauritsen Name
My Doctor(s): Dr. J. Bernard	Box 1167-601 West Leota North Platte, Nebraska 69101 308-534-9310	28 West Park Address (street)
Allergies: Darvocet-N 100		Spencer, (City) Iowa (State) 59101 (Zip)
Pharmacy or Pharmacist: James Manning		8-28-1928 My Birth Date
		262 lbs (My Weight) 5'-4" (My Height)

	MEDICATION (Prescription & Over-the-Counter)	FOR WHAT CONDITION	DOSAGE	WHEN & HOW TO TAKE
1)	Lasix	CHF	40 mg	by mouth every AM
2)	Lanoxin	CHF	0.125 mg	by mouth every AM
3)	Micro-K	CHF	8 mEq	by mouth twice a day
4)	Metamucil	constipation	$\overline{\text{II}}$ Tbs.	at bed time
5)	Mycolog	leg ulcers	topical	apply to lesions daily
6)				
7)				
8)				
9)				
10)				
11)				
12)				

FIGURE 11-3 Example of a patient's medication record.

❖ NURSING PROCESS *for Patient Admission*

The role of the licensed practical nurse or licensed vocational nurse (LPN/LVN) in the nursing process as stated is that the LPN/LVN will:

- Participate in planning care for patients based on patient needs
- Review patient's plan of care and recommend revisions as necessary
- Review and follow defined prioritization for patient care
- Use clinical pathways, care maps, or care plans to guide and review patient care

■ Assessment

Assessment of the patient begins at admission. Collect both subjective and objective data. Most facilities have a patient database form to assist in organizing these data (see Figures 11-2 and 11-3).

■ Nursing Diagnosis

The following nursing diagnoses for the patient being admitted are likely to emerge upon clustering of defining characteristics from the assessment data:

- Anxiety
- Risk for injury

Expected Outcomes and Planning

Planning involves the development of patient-oriented goals based on the nursing diagnosis formed.

Goal 1: Patient will be prepared to anticipate treatment and procedures during hospitalization.

Goal 2: Patient will not suffer accidental injury.

Implementation

Nursing interventions include the following:

- Orient or acquaint the patient to the hospital to put the patient at ease.
- Identify risk behaviors or limitations to assist the staff in making the environment safe (see Skill 11-1).
- Confirm through discussion and questions that the patient understands the diagnostic tests and procedures.
- Monitor the patient's ability to ambulate alone.
- Monitor the patient's ability to operate the hospital bed, the call light, and the emergency button.

Evaluation

Goal 1: Patient demonstrates understanding of procedure (specify).

Goal 2: Patient has remained injury free.

TRANSFERRING A PATIENT

The changing condition of a patient, whether in the direction of improvement or becoming more critical, frequently necessitates **transfer** (moving a patient from one unit to another [intraagency transfer] or moving a patient from one health care facility to another [interagency transfer]). Transfers are sometimes to another unit in the hospital and sometimes to another health care institution, such as a nursing home or rehabilitation hospital (Box 11-3, Figure 11-4).

Often a patient whose condition becomes critical will be moved to special care areas, such as the ICU or the CCU. A patient whose condition improves is likely to be moved from a special care area to a general care area or a step-down unit. Other patients will be transferred to a nursing home for continued care at a lower cost. Transfers may also be done at the patient's request; for example, some patients wish to have a private room or a quieter room.

The patient transfer requires thorough preparation and careful documentation. Preparation includes an explanation of the transfer to the patient and family, discussion of the patient's condition and plan of care with the staff of the receiving unit or facility, and arrangements for transportation, if necessary. Documentation of the patient's condition before and during transfer and adequate communication among nursing staff ensures **continuity of care** (continuing of established patient care from one setting to another) and provides legal protection for the transferring facility and its staff.

Box 11-3 Nursing Home Considerations

Admission to a nursing home sometimes occurs as a transfer from the hospital (see Skill 11-2) and sometimes as a direct admission. Do a health history and initial nursing assessment to determine the patient's condition. Encourage the patient to bring clothing and other personal items such as pictures; even personal furniture may be brought to place in the room to give a feeling of familiarity (see Chapters 33, 38, and 39). It is important to follow agency policies and requirements of **third-party payors** (entities [people or elements] other than the giver or receiver of service responsible for payment, e.g., Medicare or insurance company) so that benefits will not be lost. Discharge from a nursing home is essentially the same as discharge from a hospital. There will be more personal belongings to gather and pack.

Transfer combines admission and discharge. The patient is discharged from one unit and received on the new unit, much like an admission. A physician's order is often needed to begin the transfer process. Skill 11-2 gives general steps to follow when transferring a patient. Box 11-4 lists special considerations for transferring patients.

❖ NURSING PROCESS *for Patient Transfer*

Assessment

Assess the following: reason for patient transfer, the patient's physical condition, the patient's level of understanding regarding the purpose of the transfer, and the method of transfer.

Nursing Diagnosis

The following nursing diagnoses for patients requiring a transfer are likely to emerge upon clustering of defining characteristics from assessment data:

- Anxiety
- Risk for injury

Expected Outcomes and Planning

Transfer planning involves the development of patient-oriented goals based on the nursing diagnosis formed.

Goal 1: Patient will remain stable during transfer.

Goal 2: Patient will incur no injury during transport procedures.

Implementation

Nursing interventions include the following:

- Explain to patient and family the reason for the transfer, when it is to occur, and what procedures are planned.
- Encourage questions (see Skill 11-2).

Patient Transfer Form

Patient Transfer Form	Date: 1-31-10	Medical record No.: 432-612-1111
Patient's name: Nels Lauritsen Phone # 262-1349	Diet on transfer: Low sodium	Date of transfer: 1-31-10
Address: 28 West Park, Spenser, Iowa	Attending physician at time of transfer: Dr. J. H. Christensen	

Diagnosis:
Primary: myocardial infarction
Secondary: congestive heart failure
All other conditions: ______ Allergies: penicillin

Current medications: (date and time last dose)

Bumex 1 mg po daily
Lanoxin 0.25 mg po daily
Colace tabs po H.S.
Slow-K 10 mEq po B.I.D.
Procardia XL 30 mg po B.I.D.
Nitrostat 6.5 mg po daily

Nursing evaluation

a. Speech	☒ Normal	☐ Impaired	☐ Unable to speak	
b. Hearing	☐ Normal	☒ Impaired	☐ Deaf	
c. Sight	☐ Normal	☒ Impaired	☐ Blind	
d. Mental status	☒ Always alert	☐ Occasionally confused	☐ Always confused	
e. Feeding	☒ Independent	☐ Help with feeding	☐ Cannot feed self	
f. Dressing	☒ Independent	☐ Help with dressing	☐ Cannot dress self	
g. Elimination	☐ Independent	☒ Help to bathroom	☐ Bedpan or urinal required	☐ Incontinent
h. Bathing	☒ Independent	☒ Help with bathing	☐ Bed bath with help	☐ Bed bath
i. Ambulatory status	☐ Independent	☒ Walks with assistance	☐ Help from bed to chair	☐ Bed bound

Appliances or support: walker, up c̄ assistance

Physical activity: ______

Nursing assessment and other pertinent information: grieving the loss of wife 2 months ago, alert and oriented ×3, crackles in right apex, last BM this AM - brown semiformed stool, last set of vitals = 97°-80-22 100/60. Abdomen soft and nondistended, pedal pulse +2 bilaterally

Nurse's signature: Barbara J. Christensen Title: RN MS Date: 1-31-10

FIGURE 11-4 Example of a patient transfer form.

Box 11-4 Special Considerations for Transferring Patients

- Arrange transportation by ambulance with social services department, if the patient requires it, for transfer to another facility. Ensure that the necessary equipment is assembled to provide care during transport.
- Be especially careful that all documentation is complete when the patient is being transferred to another facility. (A communication breakdown carries high potential to interfere with the patient's chance for recovery.)
- If the patient is being transferred to a different facility, make sure that all of the appropriate patient care measures have been performed: suctioning of airway, administering prescribed medication, changing soiled dressings, bathing an incontinent patient, and emptying collection devices.

Skill 11-2 Transferring a Patient

Nursing Action *(Rationale)*

1. Wash hands. *(Reduces spread of microorganisms.)*
2. Check physician's order for transfer. *(Verifies if and when a patient is to be transferred.)*
3. Inform patient and family of the transfer. *(Reduces the fear of the unknown and strengthens the nurse-patient relationship.)*
4. Notify the receiving unit of the transfer and when to expect the patient. *(Allows preparation time to best welcome the new patient and begin care in a courteous, thoughtful, and unhurried manner.)*
5. Gather all the patient's belongings and necessary care items to accompany the patient. *(Builds trust and prevents loss of items.)*
6. Assist in transferring the patient, usually by stretcher or wheelchair. *(Ensures patient safety. The patient's condition will determine mode of transportation.)*
7. Introduce patient and family to nurses on new unit and to roommate. *(Establishes the beginning of new therapeutic nurse-patient relationship and gives a sense of belonging.)*
8. Provide a brief summary of medical diagnosis, treatment care plan, and medications. Review medical orders with nurse assuming care. If transfer is to another facility, complete an interagency transfer form. *(Gives personnel on the receiving unit pertinent information for continuing care. Reviewing records together prevents errors.)*
9. Explain equipment, policies, and procedures that are different on the new unit. *(Gives the patient some control and reduces anxiety.)*
10. Wash hands. *(Reduces spread of microorganisms.)*
11. Record condition of patient and means of transfer. The nurse on the new unit will also record an assessment of the patient's condition on arrival. *(Properly executed, the patient's medical record will reflect all care given and the patient's response to that care while in the hospital.)*
12. Notify other hospital departments, such as diagnostic imaging, laboratory, switchboard, dietary, and business offices, of the transfer. *(Keeps records current and prevents errors.)*
13. An interagency transfer is usually made by air or ground ambulance or by private car. Make sure the patient is dressed or covered appropriately for environmental comfort. If oxygen is required, a small transport tank is usually used. A nurse generally accompanies a critically ill patient who is being transferred. *(Promotes continuity of care.)*
14. Infants are generally transported in an isolette that is later returned to the sending health care facility. Parents usually accompany their child during transfer unless the transfer is by air ambulance. In this case, the parents will generally follow in family transportation. *(Promotes continuity of care.)*
15. Do patient teaching (see Patient Teaching box on p. 252). See Box 11-4 for special considerations for patient transfer.

- Confirm the patient understands the transfer and procedures through discussion and questions.
- Inspect the patient's positioning in or on transport vehicle.
- During final assessment, compare present data with previous findings.

Evaluation

Goal 1: Patient's vital signs are within normal limits.

Goal 2: Patient states medication for pain remains effective (e.g., pain is 3 on a scale of 1 to 10).

Goal 3: Patient is secured into wheelchair or gurney and remains injury free.

DISCHARGING A PATIENT

DISCHARGE PLANNING

Most patients, especially those who are at risk, benefit from the process of discharge planning. **Discharge planning** is defined as the systematic process of planning for patient care after discharge from the hospital.

Although **discharge** from a health care facility is usually considered routine, effective discharge requires careful planning and continuing assessment of the patient's needs during his or her hospitalization. Ideally, discharge planning begins shortly after admission. Discharge planning has several purposes: to teach the patient and the family about the patient's illness and its effect on his or her lifestyle; to provide instructions for home care; to communicate dietary or activity instructions; and to explain the purpose, adverse effects, and scheduling of medication treatment. It can also include arranging for transportation; follow-up care, if necessary; and coordination of outpatient or home health care services.

Good discharge planning involves the patient from the beginning, uses the strengths of the patient in planning, provides resources to meet the patient's limitations, and is focused on improving the patient's long-term outcomes.

The Joint Commission (TJC) (2008) requires the following instruction before patients leave health care facilities:

- Safe and effective use of medications and medical equipment
- Instruction on nutrition and modified diets
- Rehabilitation techniques to support adaptation to and/or functional independence in the environment
- Access to available community resources as needed
- When and how to obtain further treatment
- The patient's and family's responsibilities in the patient's ongoing health care needs and the knowledge and skills needed to carry out those responsibilities
- Maintenance of good standards for personal hygiene and grooming

It is also necessary to identify risk factors. Risk factors for discharge planning include the following:

- Older adult age-group
- Multisystem disease process
- Major surgical procedure
- Chronic or terminal illness

Discharge planning is a multidisciplinary process involving participation by all members of the health care team, the patient, and the patient's family. Many larger hospitals have discharge planners or coordinators. Considered part of the health care team, these people orchestrate the discharge planning. This is especially important when the patient is considered at risk. More often, however, the staff or the head nurse is responsible for discharge planning. With the assistance of social workers or community-based nurses, the staff identifies and anticipates patient needs after discharge from the hospital and formulates a plan for meeting those needs (see Box 11-5, Home Care Considerations box, and Figure 11-5).

Another approach to discharge planning is to perform transitional care using transition specialists. This role was developed to facilitate the transition from hospital (where discharge planning is initiated) to recovery (in the home). The transition specialist begins discharge planning and usually makes a home visit before the patient is discharged. Following discharge to the home, this specialist is available to the patient and family. This type of transitional care and coordination is cost effective and has improved the quality of care.

Communication among the patient, the family, and health care agencies is essential for effective discharge planning. The nurse establishes a dialogue between these various people and coordinates the discharge plan before the patient leaves the hospital. Any necessary referrals to other agencies are initiated before the patient is discharged. The nurse, if there is no discharge planner available, is responsible for coordinating such referrals, including signed physician's orders for specific care, treatments, or medications, to enable the patient to obtain reimbursement from third-party payors.

A discharge summary is part of the discharge plan. This summary includes the patient's learning needs, how well they have been met, the patient teaching completed, short- and long-term goals of care, referrals made, and coordinated care plan to be implemented after discharge.

Home Care Considerations

The Discharged Patient

- A patient requiring care at home is often referred to a **home health agency** (an organization that provides health care in the home) (see Chapter 37). Typical services include skilled nursing care or simply assistance with activities of daily living. A physician's order is necessary for these services to be reimbursable from insurance or Medicare and Medicaid. A health history and initial assessment are performed, just as in the hospital.
- Home care patients will either be transferred for a few hours to a clinic or outpatient services facility for diagnostic tests or treatments, or transferred and admitted to the hospital or nursing home.
- Discharge from a home health agency involves the same kind of teaching as discharge from the hospital. You are responsible to ascertain whether the patient or family is able to provide any care still needed. Gather any equipment and supplies to be returned from the patient's home to the agency.
- Assess availability and skill of the primary caregiver (e.g., spouse or neighbor); assess time available, ability, willingness, emotional and physical stamina, and knowledge.
- Perform the following assessments of immediate family members: attitude; ability to adjust to demands of patient care; impact of care demands on their lives, including noise levels and preparations of special diets; and impact of potential ongoing nature of the patient's needs. Family members who are not properly prepared for their role as caregivers are more likely to be overwhelmed by the patient's needs, which raises the risk of neglect or otherwise avoidable hospital readmissions.
- Assess additional resources, including friends or neighbors who are available to help.
- Evaluate emergency preparations: for example, call bell or phone is set up within patient's reach, and appropriate protocol is written out.

Box 11-5 Discharge Teaching Goals

Discharge teaching goals should aim to ensure that the patient does the following:

- Understands his or her illness
- Complies with his or her medication therapy
- Carefully follows his or her diet
- Manages his or her activity level
- Understands his or her treatments
- Recognizes his or her need for rest
- Knows about possible complications
- Knows when to seek follow-up care

Be certain that the discharge teaching includes the patient's family or other caregivers to ensure that the patient receives proper care at home.

DISMISSAL INSTRUCTION SHEET

Name *Marjorie Oden* Allergies *NKA*

1. Diet: Regular ____ Soft *X* Liquid ____ Special instructions: ____

2. Activity: Walking *X* Rest *X* Lifting *10 lb.* Driving *no*
   Work ____ Other ____
3. Bowels: *Laxative of choice*
4. Bathing: Shower *X* Tub *no* Sponge *—*
5. Wound care: Incision care ____
   Dressing change ____
   Special instructions ____
6. Tubes, drains, heplock, appliances: Special instructions *Leave Steri-Strips in place on abdomen until physician's visit*

   Saline lock patient instruction sheet given: yes ____ NA *X* Prescriptions sent: yes *X* NA ____
   Physician's instruction sheet given: yes *X* NA ____ Home med sent: yes *X* NA ____
7. Medications:

Drug	Dose	Frequency	Route	Special Instructions
Koflex	*250 mg*	*three times daily*	*by mouth*	*Take with food or milk*
Tylenol ES	*tabs 2*	*every 4 hr*	*by mouth*	*As needed for pain control*
Colace	*caps 2*	*daily*	*by mouth*	*At hours of sleep*
Halcion	*0.125 mg*	*daily*	*by mouth*	*As needed for sleep*

8. Other instructions: *Call physician if any redness, pain, or swelling of incision or temperature greater than 100° F*

9. Office visit: Call for an appointment on *5-9-10 at 2 PM* (date)
   Doctor *A. Yocum* Address *1402 Iowa Avenue* Phone number *308-2890*

Please bring this instruction sheet to your first appointment with your doctor.

Instructions received and understood,
Patient or responsible party *Marjorie Oden* Signature ____ Relationship ____
Nurse signature *Elaine Kockrow R.N.* Date *5-2-10*

Great Plains Regional Medical Center

BOX 1167 • 601 WEST LEOTA STREET • NORTH PLATTE, NEBRASKA 69103 • 308-534-9310

Label

FIGURE 11-5 Example of a dismissal instruction sheet.

REFERRALS FOR HEALTH CARE SERVICES

Often a patient who is discharged will require the further services of various disciplines (departments) within a hospital, such as dietary, social work, or physical therapy. The nurse is often the first to recognize the patient's needs. It is important to remember the specialized skills and knowledge of other health professionals. They are often in a position to give a patient services that you, as a nurse, are not able to offer. Make referrals as soon as possible after the patient's need is identified. In many agencies, a physician's order is needed for a referral, especially when specific therapies are planned (e.g., physical therapy) (see Health Promotion box).

THE DISCHARGE PROCESS

Many hospitals have a form with written instructions and teaching documentation for the patient to sign acknowledging understanding of the instructions. These instructions serve as a guide for the patient to use at home (see Figure 11-5). Skill 11-3 outlines the steps for discharging a patient. Box 11-6 discusses what to do if

Health Promotion

Referrals and Discharge Planning

The following list summarizes the role that various health disciplines play in referrals during discharge planning.

DIETITIAN
- Provides proper nutrient and food source requirements in patients' diets
- Instructs patients on meal planning and diet restrictions

SOCIAL WORKER
- Provides counseling for major life crises such as terminal illness and family problems
- Assists in finding community resources such as equipment for home health care or an agency that will accept patients after discharge from a hospital
- Assists in finding financial resources to cover medical costs

PHYSICAL THERAPIST
- Assists in the examination and treatment of physically disabled or handicapped people
- Assists in rehabilitating patients and restoring musculoskeletal function to a patient's greatest potential

OCCUPATIONAL THERAPIST
- Teaches patients to adapt to physical handicaps by learning new vocational skills or activities of daily living

SPEECH THERAPIST
- Assists patients with disorders affecting normal oral communication

CLINICAL NURSE SPECIALIST
- Consults with nursing staff on appropriate nursing interventions for complex nursing diagnoses
- Provides instruction to patients and family members who will assume patient care

HOME HEALTH CARE NURSE
- Provides follow-up discharge visits to a patient's home for the delivery of nursing services

Skill 11-3 Discharging a Patient

Nursing Action *(Rationale)*

1. Wash hands. *(Reduces spread of microorganisms.)*
2. Make certain there is a written discharge order. *(Verifies physician's decision regarding time for the patient to be discharged.)*
3. Contact agency's business office to determine if final payment of bill has been made. Arrange for patient and family to visit office. *(Source of concern for many patients is whether agency has accepted insurance or other payment forms.)*
4. If no discharge order has been written, have patient sign against medical advice (AMA) form (see Figure 11-6). *(Generally patients cannot be held against their wishes.)* The patient's signature acknowledges full responsibility for what happens after the patient leaves. Make sure the physician is notified.
5. Notify the family or the person who will be transporting the patient home. *(Prevents delay in discharge.)*
6. Verify that the patient and the family understand the instructions for care (medications, special diet, exercise). *(Ensures appropriate home care.)*
7. Gather equipment, supplies, and prescriptions that the patient is to take home. *(Provides service patient and family are unable to perform for themselves.)*
8. Check to see that business office has given a release. *(Prevents undue waiting by the patient when leaving.)*
9. Assist the patient in dressing and packing items to go home. *(Conserves patient's strength.)*
10. Check clothing and valuables list made on admission according to policy. *(Prevents patient from leaving personal items at facility.)*
11. a. Transfer the patient and his or her belongings via wheelchair to the vehicle outside (see illustration).
    b. Many patients are discharged via gurney (see illustration).

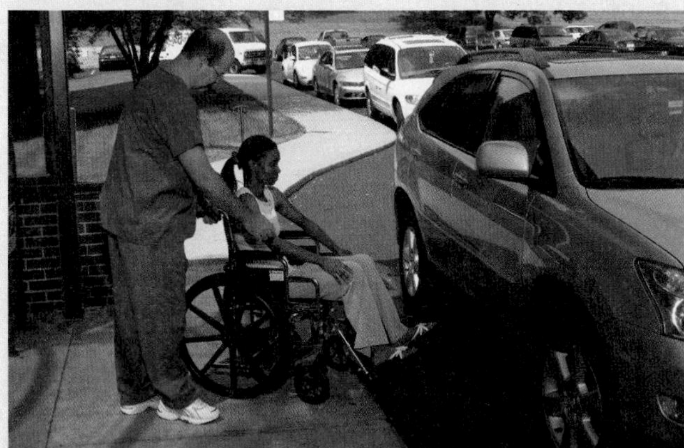

Step **11a**

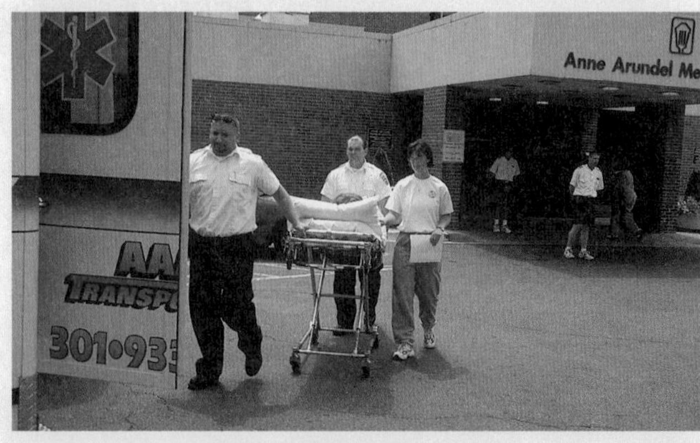

Step **11b**

c. Assist patient into the vehicle. Help family place personal belongings into car. As with all procedures, use good communication skills and wish the patient well as he or she leaves the facility. *(Provides patient safety and complies with policy of most health care facilities. Agency's liability ends once patient is safely in vehicle.)*

12. Wash hands. *(Reduces spread of microorganisms.)*

13. Chart entire discharge procedure. *(Completes the record. Legally this is important and helps to prevent problems in the future.)* Document the following:
    - Teaching
    - Patient's condition
    - Method of discharge

14. When the patient is a child, the parents must be included in all aspects of teaching and in the entire discharge procedure. Some hospitals have a special form to be signed by the person legally responsible for taking the child away from the facility.

a patient decides to leave the hospital against medical advice (Figure 11-6).

❖ NURSING PROCESS *for Patient Discharge*

■ Assessment

Every hospitalized patient requires discharge planning, which is initiated on admission. There are conditions, however, that place a patient at greater risk for being unable to meet continuing health care needs after discharge. Make sure to note the following risk factors, if present:

- Older adult age-group
- Multisystem disease process
- Major surgical procedure
- Chronic or terminal illness
- Emotional or mental instability

Assess the patient's and family's needs for health teaching and collaborate with physicians and staff in other disciplines to assess any needs for referral.

Box 11-6 Discharge Against Medical Advice

Occasionally, the patient or the patient's family may demand discharge **against medical advice (AMA)** (when a patient leaves a health care facility without a physician's order for discharge). If this occurs, notify the physician immediately. If the physician fails to convince the patient to remain in the facility, the physician will ask the patient to sign an AMA form (see Figure 11-6) releasing the facility from legal responsibility for any medical problems the patient experiences after discharge.

If the physician is not available, discuss the discharge form with the patient and obtain the patient's signature. If the patient refuses to sign the AMA form, do not detain the patient. Doing so is a violation of the patient's legal rights.* After the patient leaves, document the incident thoroughly in your notes and notify the physician.

*It is not permitted to forcibly detain a rational adult patient who will not sign the form. Only if a court order was issued for the admission, as in some cases of mental illness, is it possible to forcibly detain a patient. It is possible to file a lawsuit for false imprisonment against the hospital and/or personnel for keeping patients against their wishes. It is important to document the refusal to sign the form and the information given about the risks of leaving in the patient's chart.

STATEMENT OF PATIENT LEAVING HOSPITAL AGAINST ADVICE

This is to certify that I am leaving ______________________ Hospital at my own insistence and against the advice of the hospital authorities and my attending physician. I have been informed by them of the dangers of my leaving the hospital at this time. I release the hospital, its employees and officers, and my attending physician from all liability for any adverse results caused by my leaving the hospital prematurely.

Signed ______________________

I agree to hold harmless the ______________________ Hospital, its employees and officers, and the attending physician from all liability, with reference to the discharge of the patient named above.

____
(Husband, wife, parent, etc.)

Date ______________________

Witness ______________________

FIGURE 11-6 Example of form used when a patient leaves the hospital against medical advice.

Nursing Diagnosis

The following nursing diagnoses for the patient needing discharge may emerge upon clustering of defining characteristics from assessment data:

- Impaired home maintenance
- Self-care deficit, bathing/hygiene

Expected Outcomes and Planning

Planning involves the development of patient-oriented goals based on nursing diagnoses.

Goal 1: Patient or family member will be able to care for individual needs.

Goal 2: Health care resources will be available at home.

Implementation

On the day of discharge, nursing interventions include the following:

- All equipment, supplies, and prescriptions that the patient is to take home are gathered.
- The nurse verifies that the patient and the caregiver understand the instructions for care.
- Have patient or family member perform any treatments to be continued in the home (return demonstration).
- Home health nurse will inspect home environment to assess for obstacles or risks.

Evaluation

Goal 1: Home health agency has been notified of patient's needs on arrival at home.

Goal 2: Home health agency's initial visit is completed before discharge or soon thereafter.

Get Ready for the NCLEX® Examination!

Key Points

- Admission into a hospital begins with making certain that the patient is knowledgeable about routine procedures and activities that will occur during the hospital stay.
- The Patient Self-Determination Act requires all Medicare- and Medicaid-recipient hospitals to provide patients with information about their right to accept or reject medical treatment.
- The patient has the right to be treated with dignity, courtesy, and respect.
- The nurse's attitude often influences the patient's feelings about the care received.
- Common reactions to hospitalization are fear of the unknown, loss of identity, disorientation, separation anxiety, and loneliness.
- An adult patient should always be addressed as Miss, Ms., Mrs., or Mr. (last name), unless the patient grants permission to do otherwise.
- Transfers may be intraagency (patient is discharged from one unit and received on the new unit, much like an admission).
- Transfers may also be interagency (patient leaving one health care facility to enter another health care facility).
- Coordination is the key to the efficient and safe transfer of a patient.
- Discharge planning begins when a patient is admitted to a hospital.
- A medical condition will sometimes place a patient at risk for needing more thorough discharge planning.
- Nurses will find it necessary to involve other health care providers in discharge planning when the expertise of those providers is needed to help plan or provide ongoing care.
- Although discharge from a health care facility is usually considered routine, effective discharge requires careful planning and continuing assessment of patients' needs during their hospitalization.
- Every patient in the hospital requires discharge planning.
- Successful discharge planning is a centralized, coordinated, multidisciplinary process that ensures the patient has a plan for continuing care after leaving the hospital.
- The ultimate goal of discharge planning is to give patients and families the knowledge, skills, and resources needed to assume self-care or patient care after discharge.
- When the patient is leaving without a physician's discharge order, it is necessary to have the appropriate forms (AMA) signed and the physician notified.
- Generally, it is not permitted to keep a person in a health care facility against his or her will.

Additional Learning Resources

Go to your Companion CD for an audio glossary, animations, video clips, and more.

evolve Be sure to visit the Evolve site at http://evolve.elsevier.com/Christensen/foundations/ for additional online resources.

Review Questions for the NCLEX® Examination

1. During the registration process, the admission clerk is responsible for:
    1. informing the patient of the Patient's Bill of Rights.
    2. obtaining a list of patient allergies.
    3. informing the patient of current physician's orders.
    4. ensuring the patient has an allergy band.

2. A 36-year-old schoolteacher is admitted for observation and various diagnostic tests. The initial nursing action in her admission process is to:
    1. introduce self and roommates.
    2. measure vital signs.
    3. help her get undressed and into bed.
    4. notify the physician.

3. A 90-year-old great-grandfather has been hospitalized with pneumonia. It is necessary to reorient him to his surroundings periodically. The nurse assisting him with his morning care remembers that to call an older male patient "Gramps" is:
   1. just fine if he has grandchildren.
   2. acceptable if you cannot remember his name.
   3. acceptable if you feel comfortable calling him "Gramps."
   4. never appropriate.

4. A patient has been transferred out of the ICU to a medical unit. A nurse has been assigned to complete the transfer. This type of transfer is called a(n):
   1. patient-initiated transfer.
   2. interagency transfer.
   3. business office transfer.
   4. intraagency transfer.

5. A 52-year-old patient is being transferred to the surgical unit from the recovery room following extensive surgery as the result of trauma from an automobile accident. The nurse assigned to complete his care remembers that when admitting, transferring, or discharging a patient:
   1. the patient is a human being deserving dignity, courtesy, and respect.
   2. the patient is ill and unable to make decisions or give accurate information.
   3. the nurse knows best and should tell the patient what to do.
   4. families get in the way and should be encouraged not to get involved in the patient's care.

6. A 45-year-old patient has been recently diagnosed and hospitalized for type 1 diabetes mellitus. The multidisciplinary health care team has been preparing her for dismissal. The purpose of discharge planning is to:
   1. make certain the patient takes her medication as prescribed.
   2. provide medical treatment.
   3. provide ongoing patient education.
   4. ensure continuity of care.

7. An 84-year-old patient has been hospitalized for 6 days with a diagnosis of a stroke. The nurse knows planning for the patient's dismissal should begin:
   1. when his condition has stabilized.
   2. on his admission to the hospital.
   3. when he begins to ask questions.
   4. when his family asks for information.

8. A patient is determined to leave the hospital. His physician is not aware of his intent, nor is it in his best interest to be discharged at this time. When a patient chooses to leave a health care facility without a physician's written order, the nurse should:
   1. call the family so they can expect the patient at home.
   2. allow the patient to leave because no one can be held against his or her will.
   3. call security because there must be a physician's order before a patient may leave.
   4. explain the risks of leaving and request that the patient sign a paper accepting responsibility for problems that may occur.

9. The nurse is admitting a patient to the nursing unit. The nurse's first action is to:
   1. greet the patient by name.
   2. ask the patient his or her name.
   3. tell the patient everything will be all right.
   4. introduce the roommate.

10. The patient is being discharged. The nurse should:
    1. tell the patient everything will be all right.
    2. encourage the patient not to worry.
    3. wish the patient well.
    4. introduce the patient to the office staff.

11. A patient is being admitted to the hospital for stabilization of her heart condition. Before arriving on the nursing unit, the admissions department will:
    1. have the patient sign consent for treatment.
    2. itemize the patient's belongings.
    3. measure the patient's vital signs.
    4. review the physician's orders.

12. When a patient arrives on the nursing unit, the LPN is probably responsible for:
    1. admission charting.
    2. admission interview.
    3. formulating nursing diagnoses.
    4. obtaining vital signs.

13. Nursing documentation at discharge should include a:
    1. summary account of the hospital stay.
    2. account of all financial obligations.
    3. method of discharge.
    4. summary of personnel who cared for the patient.

14. The services of a transition specialist for patient discharge often leads to an increase in:
    1. insurance reimbursement rates for facilities.
    2. continuity of care from hospital to home.
    3. completion of hospital documentation requirements.
    4. readmitting of patients to hospitals.

chapter

12 Medical-Surgical Asepsis and Infection Prevention and Control

evolve

http://evolve.elsevier.com/Christensen/foundationsadult

Elaine Oden Kockrow

Objectives

1. Explain the difference between medical and surgical asepsis.
2. Discuss the events in the inflammatory response.
3. Describe the signs and symptoms of a localized infection and those of a systemic infection.
4. Explain how each element of the chain of infection contributes to infection.
5. List five major classifications of pathogens.
6. Differentiate between *Staphylococcus aureus* and *Staphylococcus epidermidis* in terms of virulence.
7. Discuss nursing interventions used to interrupt the sequence in the infection process.
8. Identify the body's normal defenses against infections.
9. Discuss examples of how to prevent infection for each element in the chain of infection.
10. Demonstrate the proper procedure for hand hygiene.
11. Discuss standard precautions, explaining their rationale.
12. Demonstrate technique for gowning and gloving.
13. Identify principles of surgical asepsis.
14. Correctly don and remove surgical mask, sterile gown, and sterile gloves.
15. Explain closed gloving.
16. Discuss infection prevention and control measures for the home.
17. Describe the accepted techniques of preparation for disinfection and sterilization.
18. Discuss patient teaching for infection prevention and control as an element of health promotion.

Key Terms

antiseptic (ăn-tĭ-SĔP-tĭk, p. 268)
asepsis (ā-SĔP-sĭs, p. 267)
carrier (KĂR-ē-ŭr, p. 271)
Centers for Disease Control and Prevention (CDC) (SĔN-tĕrz fŏr dĭ-ZĒZ kŏn-TRŌL ănd prē-VĔN-shŭn, p. 276)
contamination (kŏn-tăm-ĭ-NĀ-shŭn, p. 272)
disinfection (dĭs-ĭn-FĔK-shŭn, p. 268)
double bagging (DŬB-ĕl BĂG-ĭng, p. 284)
endogenous (ĕn-DŎJ-ĕn-ŭs, p. 275)
exogenous (ĕks-ŎJ-ĕn-ŭs, p. 275)
fomite (FŌ-mīt, p. 272)
health care–associated infection (hĕlth-kār ă-SŌ-sē-ā-tĭd ĭn-FĔK-shŭn, p. 274)
host (HŌST, p. 273)
infection prevention and control (ĭn-FĔK-shŭn prē-VĔN-shŭn, p. 267)
medical asepsis (MĔD-ĭ-kăl ā-SĔP-sĭs, p. 267)
microorganisms (mī-krō-ŎR-găn-ĭz-ĕmz, p. 266)
reservoir (RĔZ-ŭr-vwăhr, p. 271)
spore (spōr, p. 268)
standard precautions (STĂN-dŭrd prē-KĂW-shŭnz, p. 276)
sterilization (stĕr-ĭ-lĭ-ZĀ-shŭn, p. 302)
surgical asepsis (SŬR-jĭ-kăl ā-SĔP-sĭs, p. 267)
vector (VĔK-tŭr, pp. 271, 272)
vehicle (VĒ-ĭ-kĕl, p. 272)
virulent (VĬR-ū-lĕnt, p. 275)

With research and the discovery that microorganisms cause infection came the realization that, to prevent illness or disease, it is necessary to somehow inhibit or stop their growth and reproduction. The method of aseptic technique initiated by Joseph Lister (1827–1912) helped reduce morbidity and mortality from surgery and wound care. Lister is known as the father of aseptic technique, although many scientists, researchers, and physicians contributed to its development.

These methods are still used in health care today. It is imperative in today's health care environment that nurses practice effective infection prevention and control measures, not only for the purpose of protecting patients from drug-resistant microorganisms and occupational exposure, but also to keep health care delivery costs down.

ASEPSIS

The increase of transmissible infections, not only in health care institutions but also in the home, is an issue of great societal concern. **Microorganisms** (any tiny, usually microscopic, entity capable of carrying on living processes) are naturally present on and in the human body, as well as in the environment. Many of these microorganisms are harmless (nonpathogenic) and in most individuals do not produce disease. Some are even helpful. However, if an individual is highly susceptible to infection, it is possible for the nonpathogenic microorganisms to be dangerous. There are also known microorganisms (pathogens) that do cause specific diseases or infections.

Any patient entering a health care facility is at a greater risk of developing an infection because of lowered resistance, increased exposure to numbers and types of disease-causing organisms, or the need for an invasive procedure. Your knowledge of infection, the application of infection prevention and control principles, and use of common sense help protect patients from infection. In whatever action you perform as a nurse, be sure that infection prevention and control is part of your routine. Infection prevention and control consists of the implementation of policies and procedures in hospitals and other health care facilities to minimize the spread of health care–associated or community-acquired infections to patients and other staff members. In many situations, you will be exposed to pathogenic microorganisms. For your own protection as well as that of others, learn to prevent the spread of infection by using both routine and specialized practices of cleanliness and disinfection. These techniques aid in accomplishing asepsis (absence of pathogenic microorganisms). Asepsis is divided into the following two categories:

1. Medical asepsis consists of techniques that inhibit the growth and spread of pathogenic microorganisms. Medical asepsis is also known as **clean technique** and is used in many daily activities, such as hand hygiene and changing patients' bed linen. You follow principles of medical asepsis in the home, for instance, with the common practice of washing your hands before preparing food.
2. Surgical asepsis destroys all microorganisms and their **spores** (the reproductive cell of some microorganisms, such as fungi or protozoa). Surgical asepsis is known as sterile technique and is used in specialized areas or skills, such as care of surgical wounds, urinary catheter insertion, invasive procedures, and surgery.

INFECTION

For a microorganism to be transported and be effective in continuing contamination, it follows a definite cycle or chain of events. The following six elements are necessary for infection to occur (Figure 12-1):

1. The infectious agent—a pathogen
2. Reservoir—where the pathogen can grow
3. Exit route from reservoir
4. Method or vehicle of transportation, such as exudate, feces, air droplets, hands, and needles
5. Entrance through skin, mucous lining, or mouth
6. Host—another person or animal

To prevent the spread of a microorganism, the cycle must be interrupted. Through daily practices of medical asepsis, this is possible. These practices help to inhibit (to stop or slow a process) the growth and reduce the number of microorganisms.

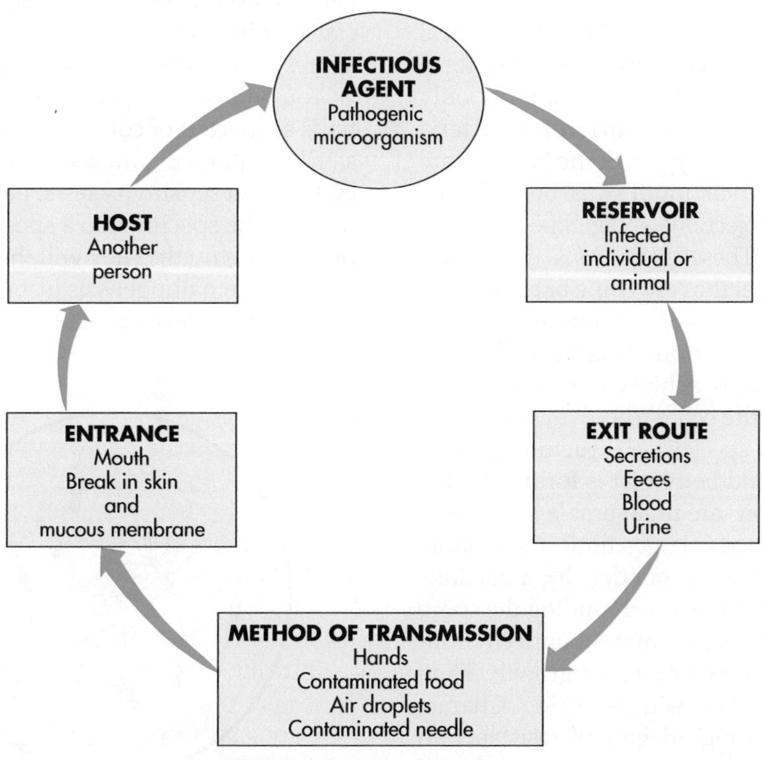

FIGURE 12-1 The chain of infection.

INFECTIOUS AGENT

Pathogenic microorganisms are infectious agents. These pathogens vary among bacteria, viruses, yeasts, fungi, and protozoa. All these microorganisms require food for growth and a suitable environment in which to live. Unwashed hands, wound dressings, soiled linen, and decaying teeth provide ideal areas for pathogenic growth. The strength of the microorganism, the number of microorganisms present, the effectiveness of a person's immune system, and the length of exposure to the microorganisms determine a pathogen's ability to produce disease. You as a nurse have a duty to provide a safe environment for a patient. In large part, you accomplish this by performing hand hygiene, donning gloves, disinfection (the use of a chemical that can be applied to objects to destroy microorganisms), using an antiseptic (a substance that tends to inhibit the growth and reproduction of microorganisms—may be used on humans), and sterilizing.

Bacteria

Bacteria have many different characteristics. In addition to their three basic shapes—round, oblong, and spiral—there are many variations. Some are elongated or have pointed ends, and some are flattened on one side. Some are shaped like commas, and others appear square. Spirilla are often tightly coiled, like a corkscrew. During cell division, some bacteria remain together to form pairs, whereas others will perhaps form long chains. All these alternative details are part of how we are able to identify specific kinds of bacteria.

Bacteria also frequently have different chemical compositions, require different nutrients, and form different waste products. **Aerobic** bacteria grow only in the presence of oxygen, whereas **anaerobic** bacteria grow only in the absence of oxygen. Some bacteria are capable of movement. Their motility is possible because of fine, hairlike projections—flagella—that arise from the bacterial cell. These projections move in a wavelike fashion to propel the cell. Some bacteria have only one flagellum attached to one end of the cell, and others have many flagella surrounding the cell. Locomotion of the spirochete is achieved by a wiggling motion involving the entire cell body.

Some bacteria form a specialized structure called a spore. The spore is a round body that is formed by the bacterium when conditions are unfavorable for growth of the bacterium. The spore enlarges until it is as large as the bacterial cell and is surrounded by a capsule. Eventually the portion of the cell surrounding the spore disintegrates. The spore remains dormant until environmental conditions become favorable for growth. Then the spore germinates and begins reproducing. Characteristically, spores have a high degree of resistance to heat and disinfectants. They are impervious (unable to be affected) to the usual laboratory staining methods.

Some bacteria have the ability to form capsules about the cell wall. These mucilaginous (thick, sticky, slimy substance) envelopes seem to form when the bacterial environment is unfavorable; it is believed that the formation may be a defensive mechanism to protect the bacteria. The composition of the capsules varies with the species of bacteria. However, they are possibly composed of protein or fat substances, and some will probably contain nitrogen and phosphorus. As with spores, staining in the laboratory usually requires special procedures. Capsule formation also contributes to the development of multidrug resistance. When capsules are present, antibiotic therapy is sometimes ineffective because the capsule prevents the drug from reaching the bacteria within the capsule.

Knowing the type of organism is important to the treatment of the patient. With many diseases, proper diagnosis and treatment are not possible until the specific microorganism causing the illness has been identified. Specially trained laboratory personnel perform this identification. In some instances, they examine a specimen before staining it, but this is usually less satisfactory. Most bacteria are not visible without a special staining process, in which a dye is applied to a specially prepared glass slide containing a small amount of the material to be examined. It is possible to identify most bacteria by this simple process; however, other bacteria require additional staining. Depending on whether it is possible to remove a color by using a solvent or the color is retained after the use of the solvent, the organism is identified as being gram positive or gram negative. Some bacteria are known as acid-fast bacteria, depending on the staining process. Special staining is required for bacteria that have flagella, spores, or capsules (Figure 12-2).

You will collect specimens of body fluids and secretions suspected of containing pathogenic organisms in sterile containers and send them to the laboratory for culture and sensitivity tests. Laboratory personnel will transfer the specimen to a special culture medium that promotes growth. They will then study the culture and identify the pathogens as just described. The results of the sensitivity tests assist the practitioner in determin-

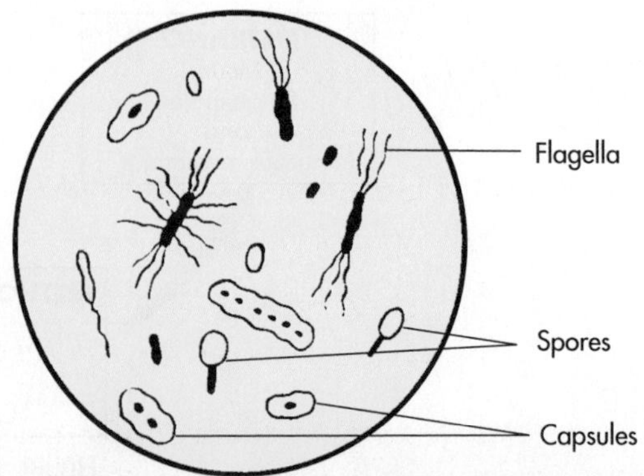

FIGURE 12-2 Flagella, spores, and capsules.

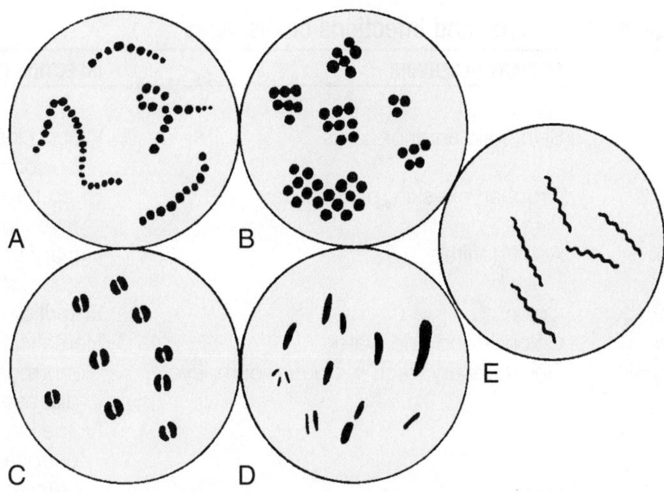

FIGURE 12-3 Some common disease-producing bacteria. **A,** Streptococci. **B,** Staphylococci. **C,** Diplococci. **D,** Bacilli. **E,** Spirilla.

ing which antimicrobial agent will effectively inhibit the pathogens' growth. The practitioner then orders appropriate antimicrobial agents on the basis of these tests, which typically take 48 to 72 hours to complete. Different organisms require different antibiotics to be destroyed.

Bacterial infections are transmitted from person to person by direct contact, by inhalation of droplet nuclei, and by indirect contact with articles contaminated with the pathogen. Some are also transmitted through the ingestion of contaminated food and drink (Figure 12-3).

The *Streptococcus* bacterium is responsible for more diseases than any other organism, but methicillin-resistant *Staphylococcus aureus* (MRSA) is growing in number and is responsible for a number of serious and sometimes fatal infections, such as necrotizing MRSA pneumonia. The incidence of MRSA has been estimated to be 3.95 cases per 1000 patient discharges (Kuehnert et al., 2005). Some strains produce serious or even fatal diseases; other strains produce disease only under special conditions; and some strains are nonpathogenic (Table 12-1). The β-hemolytic group of streptococci is responsible for 4.1 to 7.2 cases per 100,000 people. Some of the diseases caused by this group are extremely serious, sometimes fatal.

Rocky Mountain spotted fever has been found in almost every area of the United States, and its prevalence seems to be increasing. It is transmitted to humans through the bite of an infected tick. Several varieties of ticks carry the disease. The ticks live on many different kinds of animals found in rural and wooded areas. They are also able to live on common house pets such as cats and dogs. People working in areas where ticks are known to be abundant are more likely to become infected. The tick attaches itself to the skin, and the longer it remains attached, the more likely the person is to become infected. In removing the tick from the skin, it is essential to take great care not to crush or squeeze it.

Anthrax

The spore-forming bacterium *Bacillus anthracis* causes the acute infectious disease of anthrax. Anthrax infection occurs in three forms:

- Cutaneous (skin) (Figure 12-4)
- Inhalation
- Gastrointestinal

Anthrax occurs more commonly in animals, but it also has the ability to infect humans. It is seen more often in agricultural regions of South and Central America, southern and eastern Europe, Asia, Africa, the Caribbean, and the Middle East, where it is found in animals. It rarely occurs in domesticated animals in the United States.

B. anthracis spores are able to live in the soil for many years. Casual contact from person to person does not spread anthrax, nor does sharing an office; the infection is not transmitted by coughing or sneezing. In cases of intentional exposure, as in a bioterrorist release, the

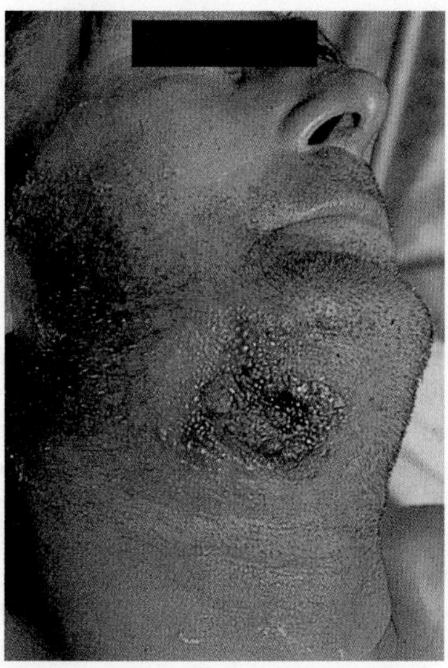

FIGURE 12-4 Cutaneous anthrax infection.

Table 12-1 Common Pathogens, Reservoirs, and Infections or Diseases

ORGANISM	PRIMARY RESERVOIR	INFECTION OR DISEASE
BACTERIA		
Staphylococcus aureus	Skin, hair, anterior nares	Wound infection, pneumonia, food poisoning
β-Hemolytic group A streptococci	Oropharynx, skin, perineal care	Strep throat, rheumatic fever, scarlet fever, impetigo
β-Hemolytic group B streptococci	Adult genitals	Urinary tract infection, wound infection, neonatal sepsis
Escherichia coli	Colon	Enteritis
E. coli serotype O157:H7	Colon—food and water	Hemolytic-uremic syndrome (HUS)
Neisseria gonorrhoeae	Genitourinary tract, rectum, mouth, eye	Gonorrhea, pelvic inflammatory disease, conjunctivitis
Staphylococcus epidermidis	Skin	IV line infection, bacteremia, endocarditis
Tubercle bacillus *(Mycobacterium tuberculosis)*	Lungs	Tuberculosis infection Tuberculosis disease
Bacillus anthracis	Infected animals or their products; bio-terrorist release	Cutaneous anthrax Inhalation anthrax Gastrointestinal anthrax
Rickettsia rickettsii	Wood tick	Rocky Mountain spotted fever
VIRUSES		
Herpes simplex virus I and II	Lesions of the mouth, skin, adult genitals	Cold sores, sexually transmitted infections
Hepatitis A and E	Food or water, feces	Hepatitis A and E
Hepatitis B, C, D, and G	Blood, body fluids, and excretions	Hepatitis B
Human immunodeficiency virus (HIV)	Blood, semen, vaginal secretions, breast milk	HIV-positive status, HIV infection
Varicella-zoster virus	Vesicle fluid, respiratory tract infections	HIV disease Varicella (chickenpox) primary infection, herpes zoster (shingles) reactivation
FUNGI		
Pneumocystis jiroveci (carinii)	Intestinal tract, genitourinary tract, respiratory tract, and circulatory system of humans and animals	Pneumonia referred to as an opportunistic infection in acquired immunodeficiency syndrome (AIDS)
Candida albicans	Mouth, skin, colon, genital tract	Thrush, dermatitis, sexually transmitted diseases
Cryptococcus	Bird feces	Pneumonia-like illness, meningoencephalitis
PROTOZOA		
Plasmodium falciparum	Mosquito	Malaria
Entamoeba histolytica	Intestinal tract (specifically the large intestine)	Diarrhea, colitis

IV, Intravenous.

most likely routes of infection are breathing in the spores or spore contact with skin. *B. anthracis* is considered by the Centers for Disease Control and Prevention (2006a) to be one of a number of potential agents for use in biological terrorism (see Chapter 24).

Anthrax infection is diagnosed when *B. anthracis* is detected in blood, skin lesions, or respiratory secretions by means of a laboratory culture or by measuring specific antibodies in the blood of infected people.

Treatment consists of antibiotics such as ciprofloxacin (Cipro) or doxycycline (Vibramycin). There is a vaccine to prevent anthrax infection. Vaccination is recommended for those at high risk of exposure, such as laboratory scientists handling the bacterium or members of the armed forces. If left untreated, anthrax can be fatal.

Viruses

Viruses are the smallest known agents to cause disease. They are not complete cells but are composed of either RNA or DNA. They consist of a protein coat around a nucleic acid core and depend on the metabolic processes of the cell they enter. Before 1900, scientists discovered that certain agents, unlike bacteria, have the ability to pass through a laboratory filter. In addition, they were unable to observe these tiny bodies with the ordinary microscope. In 1898, Martinus W. Beijerinck called these small bodies *viruses,* and they became known as *filterable viruses.*

For years, scientists knew little about viruses, even though they were able to observe their effect on humans and animals. In 1941, the electron microscope became available. With this advancement, the science of virology was born and a whole new era in the study of human disease was opened. In addition, the development of other tools and techniques has resulted in rapid advances in the study of viruses: the use of certain dyes that become luminous when exposed to ultraviolet light (fluorescent microscopy), tissue culture methods, ultracentrifuge, cytochemistry, and the development of other technical laboratory aids.

Viruses gain entrance to the body through various portals: the respiratory tract, the gastrointestinal tract, or broken skin resulting from an animal bite. Sometimes the virus is injected by a mosquito or hypodermic needle. Viruses are selective in the type of body cells they attack, but once they have found cells for which they have an affinity, they enter the cell and reproduce rapidly. As they multiply, they interrupt the cell activities and use the cell material to produce new virus material.

Viral infections are usually self-limiting. They run a given course, and recovery usually occurs. One exception is rabies, which is almost always fatal. Another exception is acquired immunodeficiency syndrome (AIDS). As the human immunodeficiency virus (HIV) reproduces and the immune system continues to be stressed to the point where it can no longer fight off even the most common infection, the patient then receives the diagnosis of AIDS. Other viral diseases have the capacity to cause death if complications occur or if they attack extremely weak, elderly, or debilitated people. The common cold is caused by a virus; the typical aching feeling, fever, and chilling sensations it entails are usually relieved by staying in bed and taking certain over-the-counter remedies. No medicine will cure the cold; medicine only relieves the discomfort. Antibiotics do not alter the course of the vast majority of viral diseases.

Viruses are classified in various ways, either according to the human diseases they cause or by the characteristics of a specific group. In the latter classification system, each subgroup will often have many types or strains (see Table 12-1).

Fungi

Fungal (mycotic) infections are among the most common diseases found in humans. Fungi are among the most plentiful forms of life. They belong to the plant kingdom, and although many of them are harmless, some are responsible for infections. Fungus types that are familiar to everyone include the fuzzy black, green, or white growth on stale bread, decayed fruit, or damp clothing. Mycotic infections are diseases caused by yeasts and molds. Some are superficial, involving the skin and the mucous membranes. Most frequently, the infections involve the external layers of the skin, the hair, and the nails and are commonly referred to as ringworm (dermatomycosis). In children, the most frequent site affected is the scalp. The condition is considered infectious, and often the child is not permitted to attend school until the infection has been cured. Other common sites include men's beards (barber's itch), the feet (athlete's foot), and around the nails. Domestic pets sometimes have ringworm infection and are frequently the source of infection for humans (see Table 12-1).

Fungi also invade the deeper tissues of the body at times. Most of these infections produce no signs or symptoms; however, some become serious and potentially fatal, especially in a patient who is severely immunocompromised. Those most common in the United States are coccidioidomycosis (valley fever) and histoplasmosis (a systemic fungal respiratory disease).

Protozoa

The protozoa are single-celled animals; in some form, they exist everywhere in nature. Some of the parasitic forms of protozoa are found in the intestinal tract, the genitourinary tract, the respiratory tract, and the circulatory system of humans and other animals. The disease-producing protozoa are responsible for malaria, amebic dysentery, and African sleeping sickness (see Table 12-1).

RESERVOIR

To thrive, organisms require food and a proper atmosphere. Characteristics of an environment that supports organism growth include food, oxygen, water, temperature, pH, and light. Any natural habitat of a microorganism that promotes growth and reproduction is a **reservoir.** Many areas of the body typically host a variety of microorganisms, but the presence of these microorganisms does not always cause illness. Examples of reservoirs are soiled or wet dressings and hospital equipment such as a bedside stand, an overbed table, suction equipment, or urinary drainage bags.

A **carrier,** or **vector,** is a person or animal who does not become ill but harbors and spreads an organism, causing disease in others.

Among your functions as a nurse is to prevent known carriers from coming into contact with the patient, change wet or soiled dressings, clean hospital equipment, change suction canisters routinely, and use medical asepsis when handling urinary drainage bags (Box 12-1).

EXIT ROUTE

A microorganism does not have the capacity to cause disease in another host without finding a point of escape from the reservoir. Exit routes in humans are the

Box 12-1 Measures to Reduce Reservoirs of Infection

BATHING
- Use soap and water to remove drainage, dried secretions, excess perspiration, or sediment from disinfectants.

DRESSING CHANGES
- Change wet or soiled dressings.

CONTAMINATED ARTICLES
- Place used tissues, soiled dressings, and soiled linen in moisture-resistant bags for proper disposal. Place pourable, drippable, or squeezable dressings in biohazard bags.

CONTAMINATED NEEDLES AND SHARPS
- Place syringes, uncapped hypodermic needles, and sharps such as scalpels in moisture-resistant, puncture-proof containers. Keep these in patients' rooms or treatment areas so that it is not necessary to carry exposed, contaminated equipment any distance.
- Do not recap needles or attempt to break them.

BEDSIDE UNIT
- Keep table surfaces clean and dry.

BOTTLED SOLUTIONS
- Do not leave bottled solutions open for prolonged periods.
- Keep solutions tightly capped.
- Date bottles when opened.
- Use only as directed by the manufacturer.

SURGICAL WOUNDS
- Maintain the patency of drainage tubes and collection bags to prevent accumulation of serous fluid under the skin surface.

DRAINAGE BOTTLES AND BAGS
- Empty and dispose of drainage suction canisters according to agency policy.
- Empty all drainage systems on each shift unless otherwise ordered by a physician.*
- Never raise a drainage system (e.g., urinary drainage bag) above the level of the site being drained unless it is clamped off.

*Closed, water-sealed chest drainage system receptacles are never emptied, only replaced if necessary, per hospital protocol.

gastrointestinal, respiratory, and genitourinary systems; tissue; blood; and wounds.

By performing hand hygiene, you have the capacity to prevent the spread of microorganisms, or cross-contamination. Also teach the patient to cover the nose and mouth when coughing or sneezing.

METHOD OF TRANSMISSION

A contaminated **vehicle** is the means by which microorganisms are carried about and transported to the next host, once they have left the reservoir. **Contamination** means a condition of being soiled, stained, touched by, or otherwise exposed to harmful agents; an example is the entry of infectious or toxic materials into a previously clean or sterile environment, making an object potentially unsafe for use. If the vehicle is a living carrier, it is called a **vector.** If the vehicle is an inanimate (nonliving) object, it is called a **fomite.** Some of the many common fomites are computers (many people touch the computer throughout the day), medical records and charts, stethoscopes, thermometers, bandage scissors, used tissues, drinking glasses, needles, and soiled dressings.

Transmission by this kind of common contact with a fomite or vector is known as the indirect method of transmission. Transmission through direct contact is also possible, such as when you use poor hand hygiene technique and then turn or bathe a patient.

Air currents easily carry microorganisms. When you make a bed, therefore, do not shake the linens. Use a dampened or treated cloth when dusting to prevent circulation of dust particles.

The floor is the dirtiest area in any building. Discard anything dropped onto it, such as soiled linens and other supplies. Feet and furniture are the only items that belong on the floor.

Because so many factors can promote the spread of infection to a patient, it is essential for all hospital personnel providing direct care (physical therapists and physicians, as well as nurses) and those performing diagnostic and support services (laboratory technicians, respiratory therapists, dietary workers) to follow infection prevention and control practices to prevent or minimize the spread of infection.

ENTRANCE OF MICROORGANISMS

Once the microorganism has exited the reservoir and has been transmitted to a susceptible host, it has to find a way to enter. When the host's defense mechanisms are reduced (see the next section), the microorganism has a greater chance to enter. If the patient's skin is punctured with a contaminated needle, microorganisms are able to enter and be absorbed into the bloodstream. Incorrect handling of a wound dressing allows microorganisms to enter the open wound and cause an infection.

Many of the entrance and exit routes microorganisms take are the same, and methods used to prevent or control both processes are also similar. The skin is the first line of defense; keep it intact, lubricated, and clean. Closely observe areas of possible skin impairment, and treat them accordingly (see Chapter 18).

Accidental needlesticks are a hazard for all health personnel. Report them immediately so that it is possible to start prophylactic measures. Available and appropriate waste containers are essential for safe disposal of sharp instruments. Never recap needles.

Improper care of Foley catheter or other drainage apparatus often provides an entrance for microorganisms and allows the infectious process to continue.

Ensure that tubes remain connected and intact. Take care when turning, positioning, or transferring a patient to prevent tubes from becoming tangled or pulling apart.

Correct cleansing of wounds will prevent the entrance of microorganisms. To accomplish this, clean away from the wound, wear sterile gloves, and use an antiseptic agent. Wear gloves when handling soiled dressings, and place the dressings in the appropriate container for disposal.

HOST

A **host** is an organism in which another, usually parasitic, organism is nourished and harbored.

Susceptibility to an infection is defined by the amount of resistance shown to the pathogen. Microorganisms are constantly in contact with people, but an infection will not develop unless a person is susceptible to the microorganism's strength and numbers. As the pathogen's strength and numbers increase, the person becomes more susceptible. Factors that affect a person's immunologic defense mechanisms are described in Box 12-2.

Immunizations have proven effective in reducing susceptibility to infectious disease. These are given before a person has been exposed to a disease (to provide protection before contact) or after exposure (if the person's history indicates possible contact with an infectious microorganism). Table 12-2 on p. 274 lists the normal defense mechanisms against infection.

Be a role model and keep up to date with your own immunizations, as well as teaching your patients and other caregivers to do so.

INFECTIOUS PROCESS

When you understand the chain of infection, you gain the ability to intervene to prevent infections from developing. When the patient acquires an infection, there are signs and symptoms you will be able to observe, and appropriate actions to take to prevent its spread. Infections follow a progressive course (Box 12-3). The severity of the patient's illness depends on the extent of the infection, the virulence (disease-causing power) of the microorganisms, and the susceptibility of the host.

Box 12-2 Factors Affecting Immunologic Defense Mechanisms

- Increasing age and extreme youth
- Stress
- Nutritional status
- Hereditary factors
- Disease processes
- Environmental factors
- Medical therapy
- Chemotherapy
- Radiation
- Lifestyle
- Occupation
- Diagnostic procedures
- Travel history
- Trauma

Box 12-3 Stages of an Infectious Process (Localized or Systemic)

INCUBATION PERIOD

Interval between entrance of pathogen into body and appearance of first symptoms (e.g., chickenpox, 1 to 3 weeks; common cold, 1 to 2 days; influenza, 1 to 3 days; mumps, 12 to 26 days)

PRODROMAL STAGE

Interval from onset of nonspecific signs and symptoms (malaise, low-grade fever, fatigue) to more specific symptoms (during this time, microorganisms grow and multiply, and patient is more capable of spreading disease to others). For example, herpes simplex begins with itching and tingling at the site during the prodromal stage, before the lesion appears.

ILLNESS STAGE

Interval when patient manifests signs and symptoms specific to type of infection (e.g., common cold manifested by sore throat, sinus congestion, rhinitis; mumps manifested by earache, high fever, parotid and salivary gland swelling)

CONVALESCENCE

Interval when acute symptoms of infection disappear (length of recovery depends on severity of infection and patient's general state of health; recovery takes from several days to months)

If infection is **localized** (e.g., a superficial wound infection), proper care controls the spread and minimizes the illness. The patient usually experiences localized symptoms such as pain and tenderness at the wound site. An infection that affects the entire body instead of just a single organ or part is **systemic** and has potential to become fatal.

The course of an infection influences the level of nursing care you will provide. You are responsible for properly administering antimicrobial agents and monitoring the response to drug therapy. Supportive therapy includes providing adequate nutrition and rest to bolster the body's defense against the infectious process. The complexity of care further depends on body systems affected by the infection.

Regardless of whether infection is localized or systemic, you play a critical role in minimizing its spread. For example, the organism causing a simple wound infection will often spread to involve an incisional wound site if you use improper technique during the dressing change. If you have a break in your own skin, it is also possible for you to acquire infections from patients if your technique for controlling infection transmission is inadequate.

INFLAMMATORY RESPONSE

The body's response to injury or infection at the cellular level is inflammation. Inflammation is a protective vascular reaction that delivers fluid, blood products,

Table 12-2 Normal Defense Mechanisms Against Infection

DEFENSE MECHANISMS	ACTION	FACTORS THAT MAY ALTER DISEASE
SKIN		
Intact multilayered surface (body's first line of defense against infection)	Provides barrier to microorganisms	Cuts, abrasions, puncture wounds, areas of maceration
Shedding of outer layer of skin cells	Removes organisms that adhere to skin's outer layers	Failure to bathe regularly
Sebum	Contains fatty acid that kills some bacteria	Excessive bathing
MOUTH		
Intact multilayered mucosa	Provides mechanical barrier to microorganisms	Lacerations, trauma, extracted teeth
Saliva	Washes away particles containing microorganisms Contains microbial inhibitors (e.g., lysozyme)	Poor oral hygiene, dehydration
Eye tearing and blinking	Provides mechanisms to reduce entry (blinking) or to assist in washing away (tearing) particles containing pathogens, thus reducing number (dose) of organisms	Injury, exposure—splash or splatter of blood or other potentially infectious material into the eye
RESPIRATORY TRACT		
Cilia lining upper airway coated by mucus	Trap inhaled microbes and sweep them outward in mucus to be expectorated or swallowed Engulf and destroy microorganisms that reach lungs' alveoli	Smoking, high concentration of oxygen and carbon dioxide, decreased humidity, cold air Smoking
URINARY TRACT		
Flushing action of urine flow	Washes away microorganisms on lining of bladder and urethra	Obstruction to normal flow by urinary catheter placement, obstruction from growth or tumor, delayed micturition Introduction of urinary catheter, continual movement of catheter in urethra
GASTROINTESTINAL TRACT		
Acidity of gastric secretions	Chemically destroys microorganisms incapable of surviving low pH	Use of antacids
Rapid peristalsis in small intestine	Prevents retention of bacterial contents	Delayed motility resulting from impaction of fecal contents in large bowel or mechanical obstruction by masses
VAGINA		
At puberty, normal flora cause vaginal secretions to achieve low pH	Inhibit growth of many microorganisms	Antibiotics, excessive douching, and oral contraceptives disrupting normal flora

and nutrients to interstitial tissues in the area of an injury. The process neutralizes and eliminates pathogens or necrotic (dead) tissues and establishes a means of repairing body cells and tissues. Signs of inflammation frequently include edema (swelling), rubor (redness), heat, pain or tenderness, and loss of function in the affected body part. When inflammation becomes systemic, other signs and symptoms develop, including fever, leukocytosis, malaise, anorexia, nausea, vomiting, and lymph node enlargement.

The inflammatory response is triggered by physical agents, chemical agents, or microorganisms. Mechanical trauma, temperature extremes, and radiation are examples of physical agents. Chemical agents include external and internal irritants such as harsh poisons or gastric acid. Microorganisms trigger this response as well, as previously discussed. The inflammatory response sometimes occurs in the absence of an infectious process.

HEALTH CARE–ASSOCIATED INFECTIONS

More than 40 million people are admitted to hospitals each year, and as many as 10% of them acquire a **health care–associated infection** (HAI) while there. Criteria for HAIs require that the infection manifests at least 48 hours after hospitalization or contact with another health agency. These infections pose a far-reaching and serious problem. Hospitals harbor microorganisms that are often highly **virulent** (of or pertaining to a highly pathogenic or rapidly progressive condition), making them more likely places to acquire an infection. The patient's immune system will probably already be weakened from disease or therapy, which makes the patient more susceptible to pathogens. HAIs not only necessitate longer hospital stays for the patient but also increase costs for both the patient and the hospital.

An **exogenous** (growing outside the body) infection is caused by microorganisms from another person. An **endogenous** (growing within the body) infection is caused by the patient's own normal microorganisms, which become altered and overgrow or are transferred from one body site to another (e.g., microorganisms in fecal material are transferred to skin by hands and infect a wound).

HAIs are most commonly transmitted by direct contact between health care personnel and patients or from patient to patient. For this reason, it is crucial to place a strong emphasis on sanitary procedures, such as hand hygiene and environmental cleaning.

You are responsible for providing the patient with a clean and safe environment. Your conscientiousness and accuracy in performing clean and aseptic procedures increase the effectiveness of infection prevention and control. To decrease the occurrence or duration of HAIs, many agencies have an infection prevention and control department, which investigates and establishes policies to ensure that all personnel maintain aseptic techniques while performing a procedure on a patient. These procedures include clean technique, which is used in all areas, and sterile technique, which is used in specialized areas.

HAIs significantly increase health care costs. Extended lengths of stay in health care institutions increase disability, and prolonged recovery times add to the expenses the patient has to bear, as well as the health care institution and the funding bodies (Medicare and Medicaid). Beginning in the fall of 2008, Centers for Medicare and Medicaid Services (CMMS) no longer reimburse hospitals for catheter-associated urinary tract infections (UTIs) and bloodstream infections. In coming years, surgical site infections and ventilator-associated infections will also cease to be reimbursed. Often costs for HAIs are not reimbursed; as a result, prevention carries financial benefit.

INFECTION PREVENTION AND CONTROL TEAM

Infection prevention and control is a valuable discipline in the health care arena. The Occupational Safety and Health Administration (OSHA), The Joint Commission risk management, and hospital administration place an ever-increasing emphasis on infection prevention and control. Administratively, infection preventionists and other members of the infection prevention and control team function within the hospital via the infection prevention and control committee.

INFECTION PREVENTIONIST

Many agencies employ nurses who are specially trained in infection prevention and control. They are responsible for advising hospital personnel on the development and implementation of safe patient care delivery practices and for monitoring infection outbreaks within the health care agency. Duties of an infection preventionist include:

- Providing staff education on infection prevention and control.
- Reviewing and revising infection prevention and control policies and procedures to ensure they are in compliance with local, state, and federal regulations as well as with certification agencies such as CMMS and The Joint Commission.
- Reviewing patients' medical records and laboratory reports and recommending appropriate transmission-based isolation procedures.
- Screening patient records for community-acquired infections (those that are acquired outside of the health care setting). These infections often are distinguished from health care–associated infections by the type of organisms that affect patients who are recovering from a disease or injury.
- Consulting with occupational health departments concerning recommendations to prevent and control the spread of infection among health care personnel, such as tuberculosis testing.
- Compiling data and analyzing the results regarding the epidemiology of health care–associated (or health care–acquired) infections.
- Notifying the local public health department of incidences of communicable diseases.
- Conferring with various hospital departments to investigate unusual events or clusters of infection.
- Educating patients and families in the prevention and control of infection.
- Identifying infection control problems with medical or patient equipment.
- Assessing microorganism sensitivity to antibiotics in use and reminding medical staff of resistance demonstrated by sensitivity examination.

An infection preventionist is a valuable resource in the prevention and control of HAIs.

OCCUPATIONAL HEALTH SERVICE

The occupational health service plays an important role in the prevention or the control of an infection in a health care setting by taking measures to protect the health care worker and patients from certain infections.

When any needlestick occurs, it is essential to report it immediately. Hepatitis B, or serum hepatitis, is the infection most commonly transmitted by contaminated needles. Health care agencies require workers who have had a needlestick to complete an injury report and seek appropriate treatment (Box 12-4).

Many agencies mandate all workers and students to obtain titers as proof of immunity against varicella, measles, mumps, and rubella. Titers are lab tests that measure the amount of an antibody in the bloodstream. If the amount of the antibody is not high enough, the institution will often require personnel to receive a vaccination or be revaccinated to prevent the disease.

Box 12-4 Vaccination and Follow-up Care

HEPATITIS B

1. Federal law requires that health care employers make available the hepatitis B vaccine and vaccination series to all employees who have occupational exposure. If an employee declines the vaccine, the employee is required to sign a declination form. Evaluation and follow-up care will be available to all employees who have been exposed.
2. Hepatitis B vaccinations will be made available to employees within 10 working days of assignment; this means before the employee starts to provide patient care and after the employee receives education and training about the vaccine.
3. A blood test (titer) is offered in some facilities 1 to 2 months after completing the 3-dose vaccine series (check the health care facility or agency policy).
4. The vaccine is offered at no cost to employees. Vaccine does not require any boosters.
5. After exposure, no treatment is needed if there is a positive blood titer on file. If no positive titer is on file, it is mandatory to follow the CDC guidelines.

HEPATITIS C (HCV)

1. If the source patient tests positive for HCV, the employee will receive a baseline test.
2. At 4 weeks after exposure, the employee is to be offered a HCV-RNA test to determine if the employee contracted HCV.
3. If positive, the employee is started on treatment. (There is no prophylactic treatment for HCV after exposure.)
4. Early treatment for infection has the potential to prevent chronic infections.

HUMAN IMMUNODEFICIENCY VIRUS (HIV)

1. If the patient tests positive for HIV infection, a viral load study is performed to determine the amount of virus present in the blood.
2. If the exposure meets the CDC criteria for HIV prophylactic treatment, or postexposure prophylaxis (PEP), it is optimally started as soon as possible, preferably within 2 hours after the exposure (CDC, 2005b). All medical evaluations and procedures, including the vaccine and vaccination series and evaluation after exposure (prophylaxis), are made available at no cost to at-risk employees. A confidential written medical evaluation will be available to employees with exposure incidents.

From Centers for Disease Control and Prevention, www.cdc.gov. and Occupational Safety and Health Administration, www.osha.gov (2005). *Occupational Safety and Health Act of 2001*.

STANDARD PRECAUTIONS

With the increased awareness of contamination from bloodborne pathogens (e.g., hepatitis B virus, HIV) came the realization that definite precautions are necessary to prevent infections.

The **Centers for Disease Control and Prevention (CDC),** part of the U.S. Department of Health and Human Services, provides facilities and services for investigation, prevention, and control of disease. The CDC has conducted studies on health care workers with documented skin or mucous membrane exposure to blood or body fluids of infected patients (Siegel et al., 2007). The studies show that infection resulted when health care workers did not use protective measures.

It is difficult to accurately identify all patients infected with bloodborne pathogens. In the past, the CDC recommended that health care workers use "universal blood and body fluid precautions," or "universal precautions," and body substance isolation when caring for all patients. These two sets of precautions have now been incorporated into one standard set of guidelines, called **standard precautions** (Box 12-5).

The increased incidence of tuberculosis (TB) has led to a heightened stress, along with these precautions, on wearing the particulate respirator mask (Figure 12-5) to protect against airborne pathogens.

The CDC guidelines for isolation precautions in hospitals, revised in 2007, have been adopted by many health care facilities (Siegel et al., 2007). The goal of these guidelines is to interrupt the chain of infection and reduce transmission of bloodborne pathogens and other potentially infectious materials from moist body substances. They apply to (1) blood; (2) all body fluids,

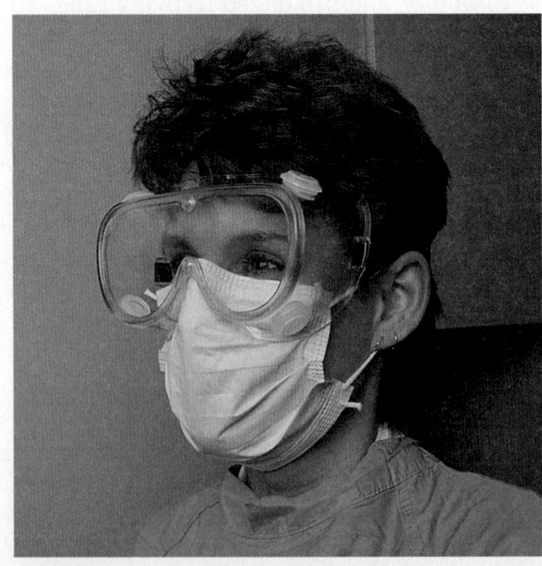

FIGURE 12-5 Nurse wearing protective goggles and mask.

Box 12-5 Standard Precautions

HAND HYGIENE

- Hand hygiene is considered of utmost importance when practicing standard precautions. Hands are to be washed before patient care and after touching blood, body fluids, secretions, excretions, and contaminated items, regardless of whether gloves are worn. Perform hand hygiene immediately after gloves are removed, between patient contacts, and when otherwise indicated to prevent transfer of microorganisms to other patients or environments. It may be necessary to wash hands between tasks and procedures on the same patient to prevent cross-contamination of different body sites.
- Use approved soaps and alcohol-based hand sanitizers and lotions.

GLOVES

- Wear clean, unsterile gloves when the potential for touching blood, body fluids, secretions, excretions, and contaminated items exists. Put on clean gloves just before touching mucous membranes and nonintact skin. Change gloves between tasks and procedures on the same patient after contact with material that possibly contains a high concentration of microorganisms. Remove gloves promptly after use, before touching noncontaminated items and environmental surfaces. Perform hand hygiene immediately after removing gloves to prevent transfer of microorganisms to other patients or environment.

MASK, EYE PROTECTION, FACE SHIELD

- Wear a mask and eye protection or a face shield to protect mucous membranes of the eyes, the nose, and the mouth during procedures and patient care activities that are likely to generate splashes or sprays of blood, body fluids, secretions, and excretions.

GOWN

- Wear a fluid-resistant gown (a clean, unsterile gown is adequate) to protect skin and prevent soiling of clothing during procedures and patient care activities that are likely to generate splashes or sprays of blood, body fluids, secretions, or excretions or cause soiling of clothing. Select a gown that is appropriate for the activity and amount of fluid likely to be encountered. Remove the soiled gown as promptly as possible and perform hand hygiene to prevent transfer of microorganisms to other patients or environments.

MISCELLANEOUS GUIDELINES

- Place used sharps, such as needles or scalpels, in a designated sharps disposal container.
- Do not purposefully bend, break, or recap needles.
- Place disposable wastes and articles contaminated with blood or large amounts of body fluids in a biowaste container for a trash pickup.
- Clean up spills of blood or body fluids per hospital protocol (i.e., blood spill kit).
- Place all soiled linen in a laundry bag. Do not overfill the bag, to prevent contamination of the environment.
- For patients with diarrhea: Strongly recommend soap and water for hand hygiene.
- For patients who are coughing: Wear a face mask if within 3 feet of patient and teach patient about respiratory hygiene.
- Use mouthpieces, resuscitator bags, or other ventilation devices if resuscitation is needed.
- Health care workers: If you have exudative (draining) lesions, refrain from all direct patient care and from handling patient care equipment until wound is healed.
- Handle laboratory specimens from all patients as if they are infectious (refer to agency manual).
- Use private rooms for patients with communicable diseases subject to airborne transmission or patients who soil their environment uncontrollably with body substances. For certain diseases (e.g., meningococcal meningitis), personnel and family entering the patient's room are to wear masks. This is true for the first 24 hours until antibiotics have been started, then is no longer required per the CDC. Roommates who are immune to the patient's disease or who are currently infected with the same disease are permitted to share rooms (institutional policy may vary on this specific procedure).

From Siegel, J.D., et al. (2007). *Guideline for isolation precautions: Preventing transmission of infectious agents in healthcare settings*. Retrieved from www.cdc.gov/ncidod/dhqp/pdf/isolation2007.pdf.

secretions, and excretions except sweat, regardless of whether or not they contain visible blood; (3) nonintact skin; and (4) mucous membranes. Standard precautions are designed to reduce the risk of transmission of microorganisms from both recognized and unrecognized sources of infections.

These precautions promote hand hygiene and use of gloves, masks, eye protection, and gowns when appropriate for patient contact.

HAND HYGIENE

Hand hygiene is the single most important and basic preventive technique for interrupting the infectious process. Box 12-6 indicates when it is essential to initiate hand hygiene.

Box 12-6 Hand Hygiene Is Essential

- When hands are visibly soiled
- Before and after caring for a patient
- After contact with organic material, such as feces, wound drainage, and mucus
- In preparation for an invasive procedure, such as suctioning, catheterization, or injections
- Before changing a dressing or having contact with open wounds
- Before preparing and administering medications
- After removing disposable gloves or handling contaminated equipment
- Before and after using the toilet
- Before and after eating
- At the beginning and end of the shift

Performing hand hygiene (Skill 12-1) will provide the necessary protection before you care for a patient. To effectively clean hands soiled with dirt or organic matter, or if you have handled a contaminated article, soap or detergents that contain antiseptic and water are required. The standard is to wash for 15 to 30 seconds using hospital approved soap, running hands under warm water (both cold and very hot water increase the risk of drying and chapping the skin). Box 12-7 contains an overview of the CDC hand hygiene guidelines, and Box 12-8 addresses the use of alcohol-based waterless antiseptics for hand hygiene. All forms of health care–associated infections can result from improper hand hygiene and use of contaminated equipment.

The CDC has pointed out the need for the health care worker in contact with patients to remove all artificial fingernails to maintain infection control principles (see Evidence-Based Practice box).

Skill 12-1 Performing Hand Hygiene Using Soap and Water

Nursing Action *(Rationale)*

1. Inspect hands, observing for visible soiling, breaks, or cuts in the skin and cuticles. *(Poor personal hygiene and an open area of the skin provide areas in which microorganisms are able to grow.)*
2. Determine amount of contaminant of hands. *(Determines the type of hand hygiene needed.)*
3. Assess areas around the skin that are contaminated. *(Prevents contamination of hands during and after hand hygiene procedure.)*
4. Remove jewelry (except plain wedding band), and push watch and long sleeves above wrist. *(Microorganisms collect in jewelry and watch bands; removing jewelry makes it easier to wash all areas of hands and wrists.)*
5. Adjust the water to appropriate temperature and force. *(Water that is too hot or too cold can chap skin, and too much force will cause splashing and spread microorganisms to other areas, especially your clothing.)*
6. Wet hands and wrists under the running water, always keeping hands lower than elbows. *(Hands are the most contaminated part of the upper extremities; water should flow from the wrists [least contaminated area] over the hands, and then down the drain.)*
7. Lather hands with liquid soap (about 1 teaspoon). *(Soap lather emulsifies fat and aids in cleansing.)*
8. Wash hands thoroughly using a firm, circular motion and friction on back of hands, palms, and wrists. Wash each finger individually, paying special attention to areas between fingers and knuckles by interlacing fingers and thumbs and moving hands back and forth, causing friction (see illustration). *(Helps to loosen soil and microorganisms, both resident [normally present] and transient [acquired from contamination].)*
9. Wash for 15 to 30 seconds, rinse thoroughly, relather, and wash another minute, using continuous friction. *(Rinsing removes the loosened microorganisms, and relathering ensures more thorough cleaning. The greater the contamination, the more need for longer washing.)*

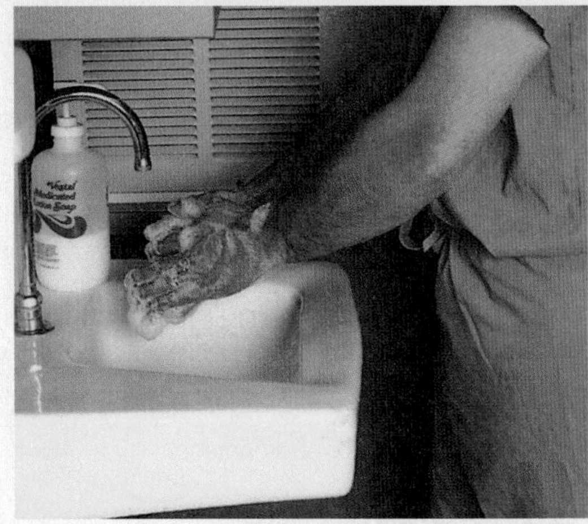

Step 8

10. Rinse wrists and hands completely, again keeping hands lower than elbows (see illustration). *(Water should run from cleaner area [the wrists] over the hands, and then down the drain, rinsing the dirt and microorganisms away.)*
11. Clean fingernails carefully under running water, using fingernails of other hand or blunt end of an orange stick. *(Reduces chance of microorganisms remaining under nails.)*

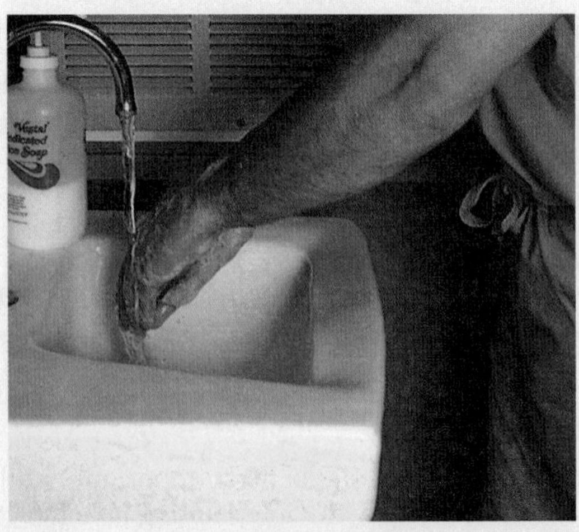

Step 10

12. Dry hands thoroughly with paper towels. Start by patting at fingertips, then hands, and then wrists and forearms. *(Prevents chapping. Drying should progress from clean to less clean, and the cleanest areas are now your fingers and hands.)*
13. Turn off faucets using a dry paper towel. *(Keeps clean hands from touching contaminated handles.)*
14. Use hospital-approved hand lotion if desired. *(Keeps skin soft and lubricated so it will not crack easily.)*
15. Inspect hands and nails for cleanliness. *(Ensures cleanliness of hands and nails.)*
16. If hands are not visibly soiled, use an alcohol-based waterless antiseptic for routine decontamination of hands in all clinical situations, unless you are caring for a patient with *Clostridium difficile* or *Candida* infection. The spores are impervious (incapable of being affected) to alcohol, so soap and water must be used in this instance. (See illustrations; also see Box 12-8).
17. Provide patient teaching (see Patient Teaching box on infection prevention and control).
18. Explain to the patient the importance of hand hygiene. *(Helps the patient understand that hand hygiene slows down the spread of infection.)*
19. If contamination continues, it is necessary to reassess technique.

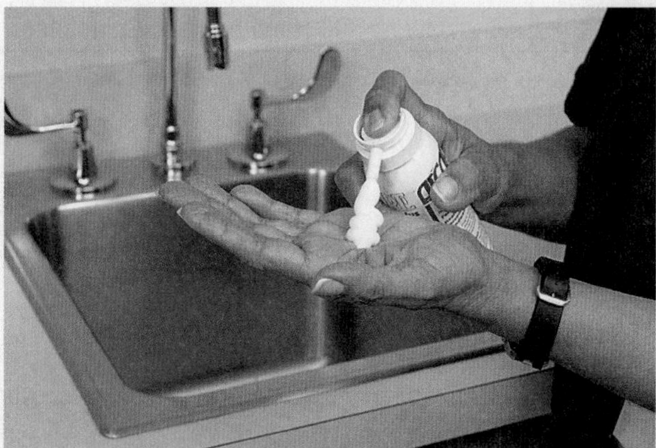

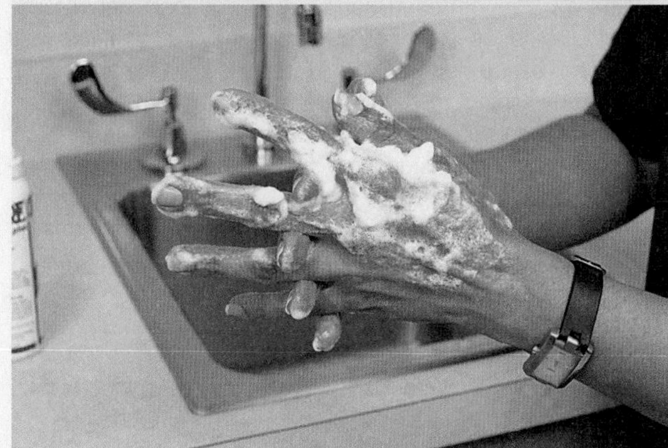

Step **16**

Evidence-Based Practice: Pathogens and Artificial Fingernails

Evidence Summary

Female health care workers (HCWs) frequently have artificial or manicured nails. Researchers posed the question as to whether bacteria reside in higher than normal numbers on artificial nail material.

In three separate studies the identity and quantity of microbial flora from HCWs wearing artificial nails were compared with those from HCWs with normal nails. In both studies, nail surfaces were swabbed and subungual (area under nails) debris was collected to obtain material for culture. In the first study, 12 HCWs who did not normally wear artificial nails wore polished artificial nails on their nondominant hand for 15 days. Identity and quantity of microflora were compared between the artificial nails and the polished normal nails of the other hand. Potential pathogens were isolated from more samples obtained from artificial nails than normal nails. Colonization of artificial nails increased over time. More organisms were found on the surface of artificial nails than normal nails.

In the second study the flora of the nails of 30 HCWs who wore permanent acrylic artificial nails were compared with that of HCWs who did not wear artificial nails. HCWs wearing artificial nails were more likely to have a pathogen isolated than the other group.

In this study, artificial nails were more likely to harbor pathogens, especially gram-negative bacilli and yeasts, than normal nails. The longer artificial nails were worn, the more likely that a pathogen was isolated.

The third study examined an outbreak of *Pseudomonas aeruginosa* in a neonatal intensive care unit. This outbreak was attributed to two nurses. One nurse had long artificial nails, and another nurse had long natural nails. Both nurses carried on their hands the implicated strain of *P. aeruginosa.* The investigation found that the neonates were more likely to have been cared for by the two nurses during the exposure period. This indicated that the artificial and long natural nails may have contributed to causing this outbreak.

Application to Nursing Practice

- Nurses should not wear artificial nails or extenders when performing patient care (CDC, 2002).
- Natural nails should be kept well manicured at ¼ inch long and free of nail gels and acrylic products.

Reference

Boyce, J.M., & Pittet, D. (2002). *HICPAC/SHEA/APIC/IDSA Hand Hygiene Task Force and the CDC Healthcare Control Practices Advisory Committee draft guidelines for hand hygiene in healthcare settings.*

From Potter, P.A., & Perry, A.G. (2009). *Fundamentals of nursing: Concepts, process, and practice.* (7th ed.). St. Louis: Mosby.

Box 12-7 Overview of CDC Hand Hygiene Guidelines

The Centers for Disease Control and Prevention (CDC) makes recommendations for hand hygiene in health care settings. Hand hygiene is a term that applies to handwashing, use of an antiseptic hand rub, or surgical hand antisepsis. Evidence suggests that hand antisepsis, the cleansing of hands with an antiseptic hand rub, is more effective in reducing health care–associated infections than plain handwashing.

FOLLOW THESE GUIDELINES IN THE CARE OF ALL PATIENTS

- Continue practice of washing hands with either a nonantimicrobial or an antimicrobial soap and water whenever hands are visibly soiled.
- Use an alcohol-based hand rub to routinely decontaminate the hands in the following clinical situations: (NOTE: If alcohol-based hand rubs are not available, the alternative is handwashing.) (See Skill 12-1, Step 16.)
  - —Before and after patient contact
  - —Before donning sterile gloves when inserting central intravascular catheters
  - —Before performing nonsurgical invasive procedures (e.g., urinary catheter insertion, nasotracheal suctioning)
  - —After contact with body fluids or excretions, mucous membranes, nonintact skin, and wound dressings
  - —If moving from a contaminated body site (rectal area or mouth) to a clean body site (surgical wound, urinary meatus) during patient care
  - —After contact with inanimate objects (including medical equipment) in the immediate vicinity of the patient
  - —After removing gloves
- Before eating and after using a restroom, wash hands with soap (nonantimicrobial or antimicrobial) and water.
- Antimicrobial-impregnated wipes (i.e., towelettes) are not a substitute for using an alcohol-based hand rub or antimicrobial soap.
- If exposure to *Bacillus anthracis* is suspected or proven, wash hands with soap (nonantimicrobial or antimicrobial) and water. The physical action of washing and rinsing hands is recommended because alcohols, chlorhexidine, iodophors, and other antiseptic agents have poor activity against spores.

FOLLOW THESE GUIDELINES FOR SURGICAL HAND ANTISEPSIS (see Skill 12-6)

- Surgical hand antisepsis reduces the resident microbial count on the hands to a minimum.
  - —The CDC recommends using an antimicrobial soap to scrub hands and forearms for the length of time recommended by the manufacturer. Refer to agency policy for time required.
  - —When using an alcohol-based surgical hand-scrub product with persistent activity, follow the manufacturer's instructions. Before applying the alcohol solution, prewash hands and forearms with a nonantimicrobial soap, and dry hands and forearms completely. After application of the alcohol-based product as recommended, allow hands and forearms to dry thoroughly before donning sterile gloves.

GENERAL RECOMMENDATIONS FOR HAND HYGIENE

- Use hospital-approved hand lotions or creams to minimize the occurrence of irritant contact dermatitis associated with hand antisepsis or handwashing.
- Do not wear artificial fingernails or extenders when having direct contact with clients at high risk (e.g., those in intensive care units or operating rooms).
- Keep natural nail tips less than ¼ inch long.
- Wear gloves when contact with blood or other potentially infectious materials, mucous membranes, and nonintact skin could occur.
- Remove gloves after caring for a patient. Do not wear the same pair of gloves for the care of more than one patient, and do not wash gloves between uses with different patients.
- Change gloves during patient care if moving from a contaminated body site to a clean body site.

Modified from Boyce, J.M., & Pittet, D. (2002). *HICPAC/SHEA/APIC/IDSA Hand Hygiene Task Force and the CDC Healthcare Control Practices Advisory Committee draft guidelines for hand hygiene in healthcare settings.*

Box 12-8 Using an Alcohol-Based Waterless Antiseptic for Routine Hand Hygiene

The Centers for Disease Control and Prevention (CDC) (2002) recommends the use of alcohol-based waterless antiseptics to improve hand hygiene practices, protect health care workers' hands, and reduce transmission of pathogens to patients and personnel in health care settings. Alcohols have excellent germicidal activity and are more effective than either plain soap or antimicrobial soap and water. Emollients are added to alcohol-based antiseptics to prevent drying the skin.

If hands are not visibly soiled, use an alcohol-based waterless antiseptic for routine decontamination of hands in most clinical situations.

1. Apply an ample amount of product to palm of one hand. *(Enough product is needed to thoroughly cover the hands.)*
2. Rub hands together, covering all surfaces of hands and fingers with antiseptic.
3. Rub hands together for several seconds until alcohol is dry. Allow hands to dry before applying gloves. If an adequate volume is used, it will take 15 to 25 seconds for hands to dry. *(Drying ensures full antiseptic effect.)*
4. If hands are dry or chapped, a small amount of lotion or barrier cream can be applied. *(Use the hospital-provided container of lotion because other lotions will possibly interfere with antimicrobial action or disintegrate gloves.)*

Data from Boyce, J.M., & Pittet, D. (2002). *HICPAC/SHEA/APIC/IDSA Hand Hygiene Task Force and the CDC Healthcare Control Practices Advisory Committee draft guidelines for hand hygiene in healthcare settings.*

NOTE: Hand gels are not recommended if caring for a patient with *Clostridium difficile (C. diff)* diarrhea or *Candida* infections. The spores are impervious to the alcohol.

In addition to hand hygiene, there are other actions to take to reduce the chance of transmitting microorganisms. Teach patients and visitors about appropriate times for hand hygiene (see Patient Teaching box on infection prevention and control). Provide patients with their own set of personal care articles, such as bedpan, urinal, bath basin, water pitcher, and drinking glass, to prevent cross-contamination. Since microorganisms are also transmitted by indirect contact with contaminated equipment and soiled linen, place these articles in special waste containers or laundry bags and keep them away from your uniform.

The risk of transmitting health care–acquired infections or infectious disease among patients is high when standard precautions are not followed. Stay informed about patients who have a known source of infection, and alert other health care workers. By following recommendations for infection prevention and control practices, you and other health care workers will be protected from exposure and will lessen the risk of the patient acquiring a health care–associated infection.

GLOVING

Nurses and other health care personnel don gloves if there is any possibility of contact with infectious material. The CDC (Boyce & Pittet, 2002) gives the following advice regarding gloves:

- Wear gloves only once, and then place them into the appropriate waste containers for safe disposal.
- If you have not completed the patient's care but have come into contact with infectious material, change the gloves before continuing the patient's care.
- There is the risk of perforating the gloves during use, so perform hand hygiene after removing the gloves (Skill 12-2).

Family members need to understand the importance of using gloves. Explain that gloves become contaminated if they touch infected material or a contaminated object (see Patient Teaching box on gloving technique).

Latex Allergy

Latex allergy causes an individual to have a reaction to certain proteins found in natural rubber latex, a product manufactured from a milky fluid derived from the rubber tree found in Africa and Southeast Asia. The latex proteins are able to enter the body through the skin and mucous membranes, intravascularly, and by inhalation. Suspect the presence of latex allergy and obtain an evaluation by a physician when anyone, patient or health care worker, develops red, watery, itchy eyes; sinus or nasal tachycardia; and hypotension after exposure to latex. Anaphylaxis, a potentially life-threatening condition, sometimes occurs.

More than 20,000 medical products contain latex. Synthetic versions of many products are available. Even though an individual product is "latex free," an environment is "latex safe" only when all items of latex that have potential to come in contact with the allergic individual are removed (Box 12-9).

Be alert to the possibility of other health care personnel or the patient being allergic to the latex gloves. Reactions vary from contact dermatitis to anaphylactic shock (see Chapter 24). When wearing latex gloves, ask patients if they have a known allergy to latex products before touching them. If they do, use nonlatex gloves. Make sure the fact is posted and passed along to all caregivers.

Patient Teaching

Infection Prevention and Control

- Teach the patient about the infection process, especially how an infection is transmitted, and stress the importance of interrupting the process. Use a simple diagram to illustrate this (see Figure 12-1). Teaching caregivers is extremely important as well.
- Use an example for each step that is familiar to the patient.
- Provide a simple explanation of clean as opposed to contaminated items.
- Although hand hygiene is a basic aseptic technique, stress when and how the procedure should be performed to be effective in preventing infection. Demonstrate hand hygiene within sight of the patient whenever possible.
- Instruct patient about signs and symptoms of wound infection.
- Teach the applications of aseptic principles to self-care activities such as wound care and medication administration.
- When isolation apparel (such as mask, gown, or gloves) is to be used, demonstrate the procedures for the patient and visitors.
- Instruct patient to place contaminated dressings and other disposable items containing infectious body fluids in leak-resistant bag. Place needles in bleach bottles with the cap taped or glued on, or place in a sharps container and take to local hospital for disposal.
- Always allow a question-and-answer session for the patient (some patients will need special assistance in understanding the precautions).

Patient Teaching

Gloving Technique

- Make certain the patient knows you are isolating the microorganism and not the patient.
- Some patients will need special assistance in understanding the precautions.
- Demonstrate to the patient how to don gloves.

Skill 12-2 Gloving

Nursing Action *(Rationale)*

Donning Gloves

1. Remove gloves from dispenser. *(Keeps gloves handy and ready for use.)*
2. Inspect gloves for perforations. *(Prevents pathogenic microorganisms from entering through perforation in gloves.)*
3. Don gloves when ready to begin patient care. Wearing gloves with a gown does not necessitate any special technique for putting them on; wear them pulled over cuffs of gown. *(Ensures full coverage of your wrists.)*
4. Change gloves after direct handling of infectious material such as wound drainage. *(Prevents cross-contamination.)*
5. Do not touch side rails, tables, or bed stands with contaminated gloves. *(Prevents spread of microorganisms throughout environment.)*

Removing Gloves

6. Remove first glove by grasping outer surface at palm with other gloved hand and pulling glove inside out and off (see illustration). Place this glove in the hand that is still gloved. *(Prevents you from touching own skin with contaminated glove.)*
7. Remove second glove by placing finger under cuff and turning glove inside out and over other glove (see illustration). Drop gloves into waste container. *(Prevents you from touching contaminated glove. Wraps contamination inside gloves to help protect others.)*
8. Perform hand hygiene. *(Helps prevent cross-contamination.)*
9. Provide patient teaching (see Patient Teaching box on gloving technique).
10. If contamination continues, it is necessary to reassess technique.

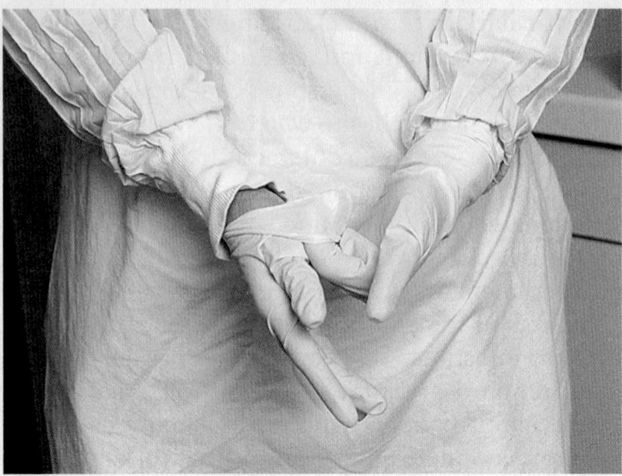
Step 6

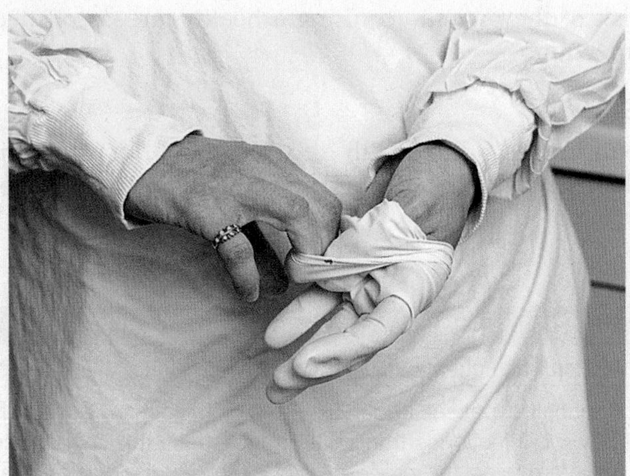
Step 7

Box 12-9 Preventing Latex Allergy

The American Nurses Association (ANA) provides the following suggestions for nurses to avoid becoming latex allergic:

1. Whenever possible, wear powder-free gloves (they are lower in protein allergens).
2. Wear gloves that are appropriate for the task (e.g., avoid use for cleaning).
3. Wash with a pH-balanced soap immediately after removing gloves.
4. Apply only non–oil-based hand care products (oil-based products break down latex).
5. If a reaction or dermatitis occurs, report to employee health and/or seek medical treatment immediately.

GOWNING

The use of a gown while administering care to a patient in isolation is important primarily to protect your clothing from being soiled. The gown also provides protection against infectious microorganisms possibly given off by the patient. It is recommended that you discard your gown when leaving the patient's room rather than reuse it. This aids in preventing the spread of pathogens to other patients or personnel. This procedure also applies to visitors.

Another rationale for use of a gown is protection of a patient whose immune system is inadequate. In this situation, health care personnel and visitors wear a sterile gown to prevent the transfer of pathogens from themselves to the patient.

There are several types of isolation. Some necessitate wearing a gown, whereas others do not. Donning an isolation gown is indicated when caring for patients with diseases characterized by heavy drainage or exudate, infectious and acute diarrhea, other gastrointestinal disorders, respiratory disorders, skin wounds or burns, and urinary disorders.

Isolation gowns open at the back and have ties at the neck and the waist. This keeps the gown securely closed, protecting the back as well as the front of your uniform. It is necessary that the gown be long enough to cover your uniform and, for added protection, have long sleeves with cuffs.

To don gowns correctly, follow the procedure listed in Skill 12-3.

Skill 12-3 Gowning for Isolation

Nursing Action *(Rationale)*

1. Remove your watch and push up long sleeves, if you have them. *(Ensures that uniform sleeve is under gown sleeve for protection.)*
2. Place your watch on a paper towel or in a see-through plastic bag before taking vital signs. *(Prevents cross-contamination.)*
3. Perform hand hygiene. *(Reduces spread of microorganisms.)*
4. Don gown and tie it securely at neck and waist (see illustrations). *(Provides protective covering of the entire uniform.)*
5. Remove gown after providing necessary patient care (see illustration). *(Has protected the nurse.)*

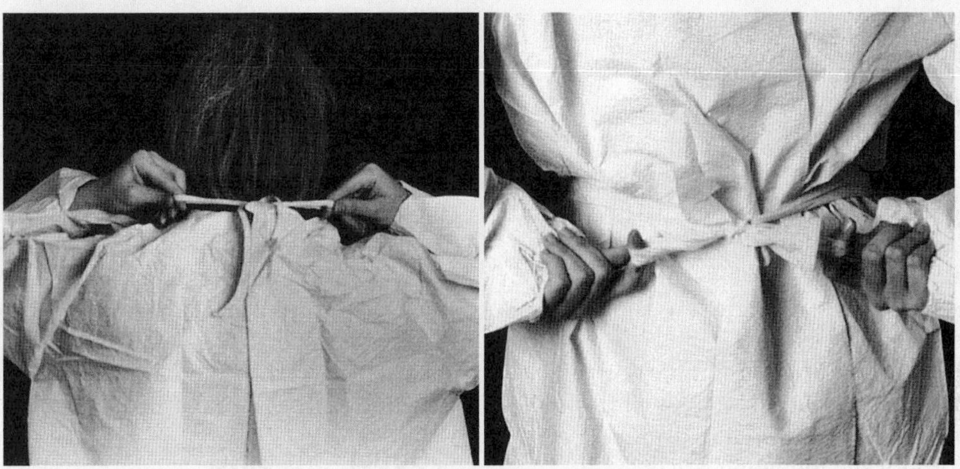

Step 4

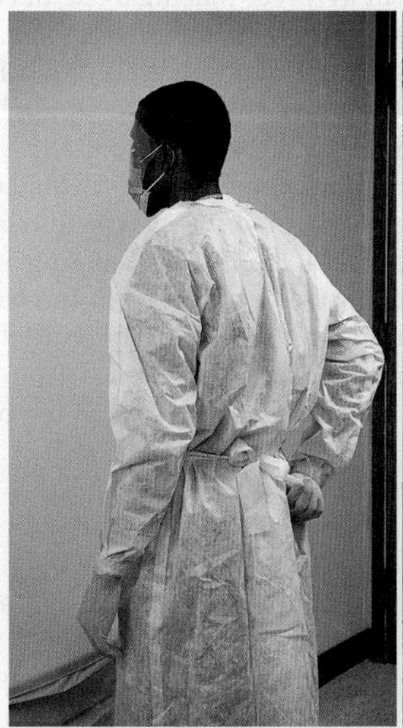

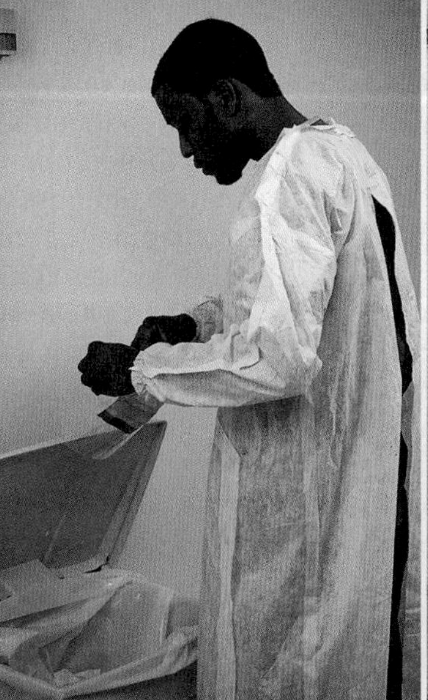

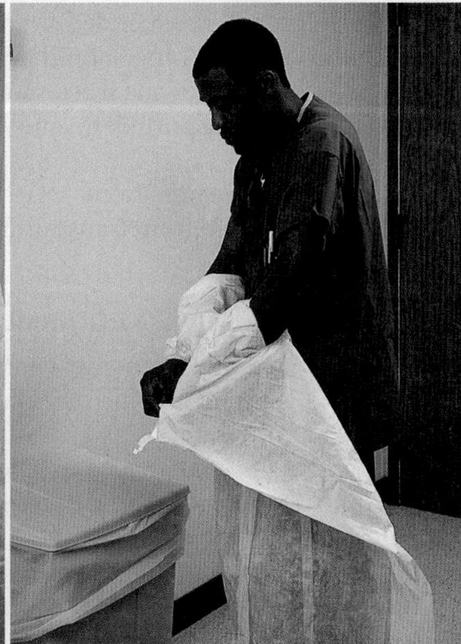

Step 5

Continued

Skill 12-3 Gowning for Isolation—cont'd

6. Discard soiled gown appropriately (see illustration). *(Prevents contamination.)*
7. Perform hand hygiene. *(Prevents spread of microorganisms.)*
8. Record use of gown in isolation procedure if agency's policy so dictates. *(Provides proof that appropriate procedure was followed.)* Some agencies charge a daily rate for isolation precautions. This is noted on a daily basis in the patient's record. Therefore repeated notations throughout the 24 hours are not necessary.
9. Provide patient teaching (see Patient Teaching box on infection prevention and control).
10. If contamination continues, it is necessary to reassess technique.

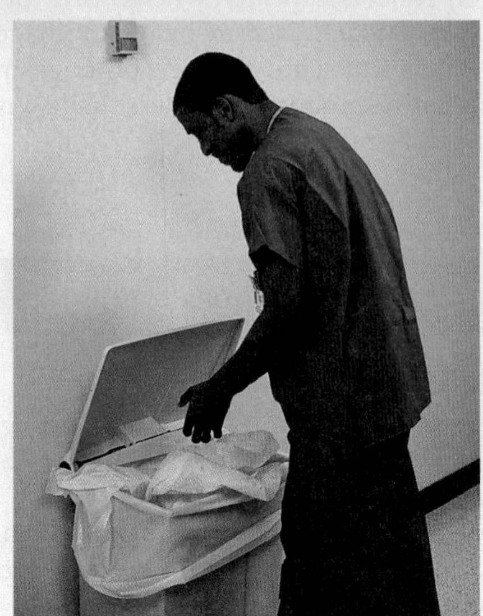
Step 6

MASK AND PROTECTIVE EYEWEAR

When a mask is correctly applied, it will fit snugly below your chin and securely over your nose and mouth, and the top edge will fit below your eyeglasses, if you wear them. (This prevents fogging of your glasses.) Masks are available with eyeshields like glasses to cover your eyes (or glasses). Goggles are another possible way to protect your eyes (see Figure 12-5). Change your mask at least every 20 to 30 minutes or if it becomes moist. Do not reuse a mask or allow it to dangle around your neck and then reuse it (Skill 12-4).

A mask is worn for the following reasons:

- To protect the wearer from inhaling microorganisms that travel on airborne droplets for short distances or that remain suspended in the air for longer periods, or if splashing should occur
- To prevent inhaling pathogens if resistance is reduced or if being transported to another area (patient wears mask)
- To discourage the wearer from touching the mouth, nose, or eyes and from transmitting infectious material

DISPOSING OF CONTAMINATED EQUIPMENT

Health care facilities generate immense quantities of contaminated materials, some of which are disposable and some of which are reusable. It is essential to design and implement an effective mechanism to handle this material within the facility. The disposal of contaminated materials also comes under the review of the infection preventionist and the infection prevention and control committee. Until the biowaste is removed from the property by the waste hauler, use of specially labeled (usually red) bagging is required for its removal from the nursing unit and storage in the medical waste storage area. A major risk to personnel is in the disposal of sharps (needles, blades), which are often contaminated by blood. When left in linens or in dressings, these have the potential to injure workers cleaning patient or resident care areas and examination rooms. To prevent this problem, it is necessary to provide all patient and resident care areas where sharps are ever used with puncture-proof containers into which health care workers place used disposable needles, syringes, and other sharps.

DOUBLE BAGGING

The CDC recommends **double bagging** (an infection control practice that involves placing a bag of contaminated items into another, clean bag that is held outside an isolation room by other personnel) when it is impossible to keep the outer surface of a single bag free from contamination. Label or color code the second bag to alert nursing personnel and to prevent contamination of housekeeping personnel who will handle the contaminated material. Use double bagging if necessary for safe removal of any article from the room.

The CDC recommends the following guidelines for handling isolation linen:

- Place soiled linen in a laundry bag in the patient's room.
- Treat all linen as though it is infectious.
- Linen requires less handling if it is placed in a bag that is soluble in hot water; however, it is often necessary to double bag such a bag because it punctures or tears easily.

Note that double bagging is no longer recommended as a universal practice, unless a cloth bag is being placed in a plastic bag. In most cases, a single bag is

Skill 12-4 Donning a Mask

Nursing Action *(Rationale)*

1. Remove mask from container. *(Mask is readily available for use.)*
2. Don mask when ready to begin patient care by covering your nose, mouth, and eyes (or glasses) with the device. Wear a mask with a protective eyeshield when there is risk of splashing. Secure mask in place with elastic band or by tying the strings behind your head (see illustration). *(Provides protection from microorganisms.)*
3. Wear mask until it becomes moist, but no longer than 20 to 30 minutes. *(Moisture renders a mask ineffective.)*
4. Make certain patient feels comfortable and accepted. *(Contributes to patient's well-being.)*
5. Remove mask by untying the strings or moving the elastic. Make certain not to touch contaminated area (see illustration). *(Prevents your coming into contact with contaminated mask.)*
6. Dispose of soiled mask in appropriate container. *(Protects other health care workers.)*
7. Wash hands thoroughly. *(Removes microorganisms.)*
8. Record use of mask during patient care (some agencies require documentation of specific barriers used). *(Provides proof of wearing mask for protection of patient and nurse.)*
9. If contamination continues, it is necessary to reassess technique.
10. Provide patient teaching (see Patient Teaching box on infection prevention and control).

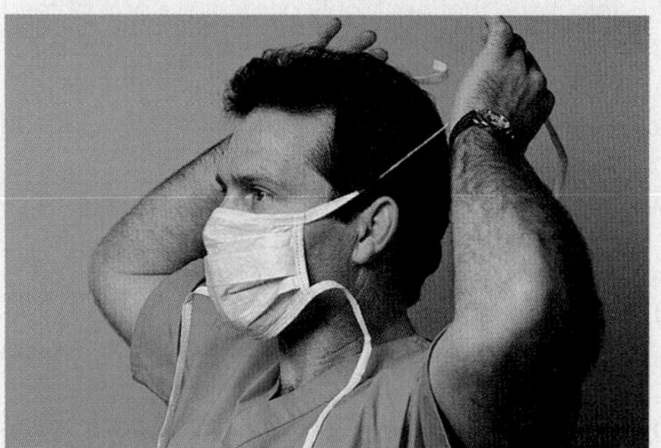

Step **2**

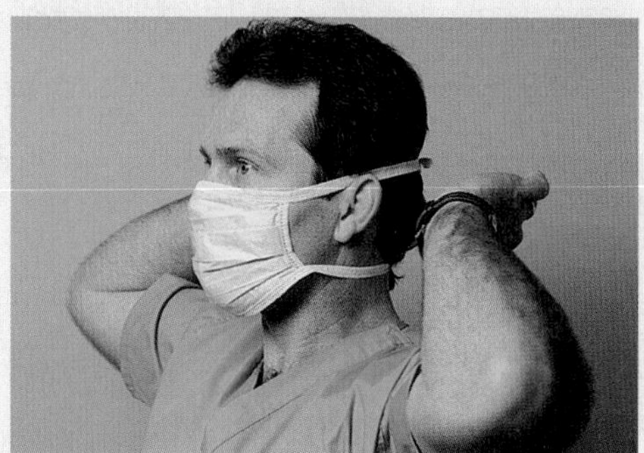

Step **5**

adequate if it is possible to place the contaminated articles in the bag without contamination of the outside of the bag.

ISOLATION TECHNIQUE

The CDC issued isolation guidelines, in addition to standard precautions, that contain two tiers of approach (Siegel et al., 2007). The first contains precautions designed to care for all patients in health care facilities regardless of their diagnosis or presumed infectiousness. This first tier is called **standard precautions.**

The second tier condenses the disease-specific and categories approach to isolation into new transmission categories: airborne, droplet, and contact precautions. These precautions are designed for specific patients with highly transmissible pathogens (Box 12-10, Figures 12-6 through 12-8).

The type of isolation techniques followed for a given patient will depend on how transmissible the pathogen in question is. Follow some basic principles regardless of which technique is used:

- Perform thorough hand hygiene before entering and after leaving a patient's room.
- Use your understanding of the disease process and the method of transmission of the infectious microorganism to help determine which protective barriers to use.
- Dispose of contaminated equipment and articles in a safe and effective manner to prevent transmission of pathogens to other individuals.
- If the patient is to be transported to other areas in the agency (away from the isolation room), take necessary measures to protect those who will potentially be exposed. Transport the patient in accordance with hospital protocol.

Environmental barriers keep pathogens in a confined area. Examples of such barriers are a private or isolation room, closed door, protective gown, mask, goggles, and gloves.

Place the patient with an infectious disease in a private or isolation room equipped with the appropriate hand hygiene and toilet facilities. Private rooms used for airborne illness isolation have negative-pressure airflow that prevents infectious particulates from flowing out of the closed environment. Special rooms with positive-pressure airflow are also used for highly susceptible patients such as transplant recipients. In this

Box 12-10 Types of Precautions and Patients Requiring Those Precautions

STANDARD PRECAUTIONS (TIER 1)

Use standard precautions for the care of all patients. This general mandate is necessary because it is sometimes not known if the patient is colonized or infected with certain pathogenic microorganisms. Barrier precautions reduce the need to handle sharps.

TRANSMISSION PRECAUTIONS (TIER 2)

Airborne Precautions (see Figure 12-6)

In addition to standard precautions, use airborne precautions for patients known or suspected to have serious illnesses transmitted by airborne droplet nuclei. Examples of such illnesses include the following:

- Measles
- Varicella (including disseminated zoster)
- Tuberculosis

Droplet Precautions (see Figure 12-7)

In addition to standard precautions, use droplet precautions for patients known or suspected to have serious illness transmitted by large particle droplets. Examples of such illnesses include the following:

- Invasive *Haemophilus influenzae*, including meningitis, pneumonia, epiglottitis, and sepsis
- Invasive *Neisseria meningitidis* disease, including meningitis, pneumonia, and sepsis

Examples of other serious bacterial respiratory infections spread by droplet transmission include the following:

- Diphtheria (pharyngeal)
- *Mycoplasma* pneumonia
- Pertussis
- Pneumonic plague
- Streptococcal pharyngitis, pneumonia, and scarlet fever in infants and young children

Examples of serious viral infections spread by droplet transmission include the following:

- Adenovirus
- Influenza
- Mumps
- Parvovirus B19
- Rubella
- Tuberculosis caused by *Mycobacterium tuberculosis*

Tuberculosis (TB) Isolation

- TB isolation should be practiced for all patients with known or suspected TB. (Suspected TB is defined by agency policy and generally means any patient with a positive acid-fast bacillus (AFB) smear, with a cavitating lesion seen on chest x-ray study, or identified as high risk by a screening tool.)
- Isolation is mandatory in a single-patient room designated as negative-pressure airflow and having at least 6 to 12 air exchanges per hour. It is necessary to vent room air to the outside and, to maintain negative pressure, to close the door.
- It is obligatory for health care workers to wear an N-95 or higher particulate respirator mask when entering an AFB isolation room (check agency's policy for type of mask).
- It is obligatory for health care workers to be fit-tested* before using a respirator for the first time. This ensures that the type and the size of the respirator is appropriate for the individual.
- It is obligatory for health care workers to fit-check† the respirator's fit before each use.
- Respirator is permitted to be reused and stored according to manufacturer's recommendations and agency policy.

Contact Precautions (see Figure 12-8)

In addition to standard precautions, use contact precautions for patients known or suspected to have serious illnesses easily transmitted by direct patient contact or by contact with items in the patient's environment. Examples of such illnesses include the following:

- Gastrointestinal, respiratory, skin, or wound infections or colonization with multidrug-resistant bacteria judged by the infection prevention and control committee, and current state, regional, and national recommendations, to be of special clinical and epidemiologic significance
- Enteric infections with a low infectious dose or prolonged environmental survival, including the following:
  a. *Clostridium difficile*
  b. Diapered or incontinent patients with the following:
    1. *Escherichia coli* O157:H7
    2. *Shigella*
    3. Hepatitis A
    4. Rotavirus
- Respiratory syncytial virus, parainfluenza virus, and enteroviral infections in infants and young children
- Skin infections that are highly contagious or that tend to occur on dry skin, including the following:
  a. Diphtheria (cutaneous)
  b. Herpes simplex virus (neonatal or mucocutaneous)
  c. Impetigo
  d. Major (noncontaminated) abscesses, cellulitis, or decubitus ulcers
  e. Pediculosis
  f. Scabies
  g. Staphylococcal furunculosis in infants and young children
  h. Methicillin-resistant *Staphylococcus aureus* (MRSA)
  i. Vancomycin-resistant enterococci (VRE)
  j. Extended-spectrum beta-lactamase (ESBL) (Necessitates 9 months of contact precautions. This enzyme attaches to the cell wall of *E. coli* and some *Klebsiella* organisms, which in turn makes the organisms multidrug-resistant. Once treatment is completed, the enzyme is still found in the feces for up to 9 months.)
  k. Zoster (disseminated or in the immunocompromised host)
  l. Viral or hemorrhagic conjunctivitis
  m. Viral hemorrhagic infections (Ebola, Lassa, or Marburg)

Immunocompromised Patients

Immunocompromised patients vary in their susceptibility to health care–associated infections depending on the severity and the duration of immunosuppression. They are generally at increased risk for bacterial, fungal, parasitic, and viral infections from both endogenous and exogenous sources. In general, the use of standard precautions for all patients and transmission-based precautions for specified patients reduces the acquisition by these patients of institutionally acquired organisms from other patients and environments. Leukopenic patients will sometimes require additional protective measures, other than standard precautions. In such instances, the physician or infection preventionist instructs nursing staff as to the necessary protective measures (e.g., masks, private room). They place an isolation sign on the door, which lists the additional protective measures that staff and visitors are required to follow for the safety of the patient.

Monitoring of Isolation

Transmission-based isolation practices are monitored on an ongoing basis by the infection preventionist.

*Fit-test: Procedure to determine adequate fit of respirator, usually by qualitative measure (wearers are exposed to a concentrated saccharin solution and asked if they can detect taste while wearing respirator).

†Fit-check: Procedure in which worker uses negative pressure to see if mask is properly sealed to face.

AIRBORNE PRECAUTIONS

(in addition to standard precautions)

VISITORS: Report to nurse before entering.

Use Airborne Precautions as recommended for patients known or suspected to be infected with infectious agents transmitted person-to-person by the airborne route (e.g., *M. tuberculosis*, measles, chickenpox, disseminated herpes zoster).

Patient placement

Place patients in an **AIIR** (Airborne Infection Isolation Room).
Monitor air pressure daily with visual indicators (e.g., flutter strips).

Keep door closed when not required for entry and exit.

In ambulatory settings instruct patients with a known or suspected airborne infection to wear a surgical mask and observe Respiratory Hygiene/Cough Etiquette. Once in an AIIR, the mask may be removed.

Patient transport

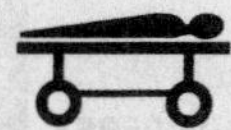

Limit transport and movement of patients to **medically-necessary purposes.**

If transport or movement outside an AIIR is necessary, instruct patients to **wear a surgical mask**, if possible, and observe Respiratory Hygiene/Cough Etiquette.

Hand Hygiene

Hand Hygiene according to standard precautions.

Personal Protective Equipment (PPE)

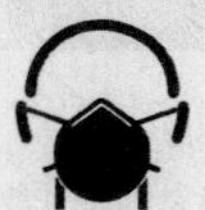

Wear a fit-tested NIOSH-approved **N-95** or higher level respirator for respiratory protection when entering the room of a patient when the following diseases are suspected or confirmed: Listed on back.

APR

FIGURE 12-6 Airborne Precautions.

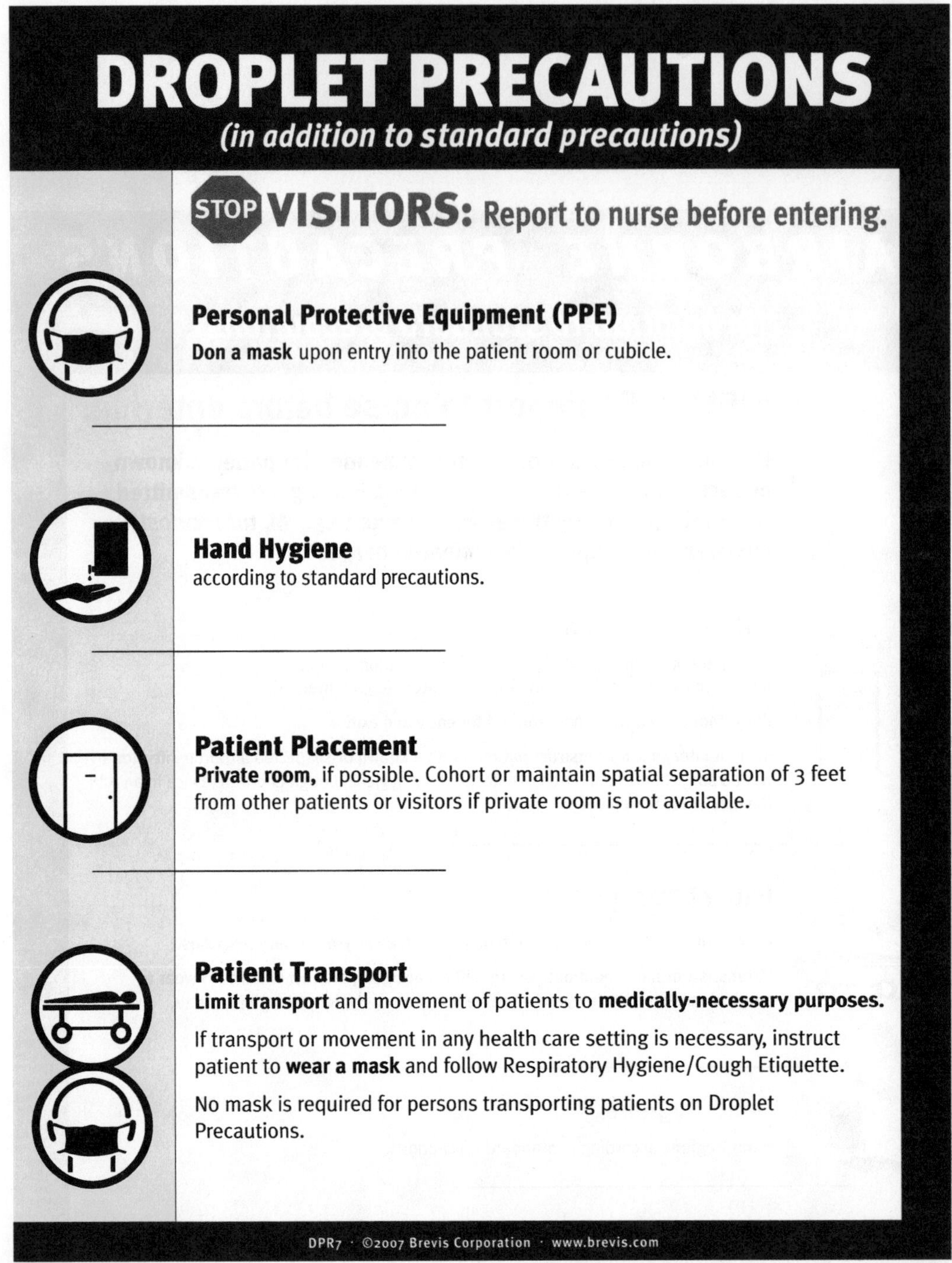

FIGURE 12-7 Droplet Precautions.

case, no organisms are able to enter the room. The routine care of a patient in isolation follows from the same hygienic principles as the care given to all patients. Remember that all articles that come into contact with the patient are contaminated, and handle them appropriately to maintain asepsis. Dedicated equipment for assessing vital signs remains in the room if possible. Otherwise it is mandatory to safely disinfect the equipment when you remove it from the room.

It is important in the care of the patient to consider the psychological or emotional deprivation that will possibly result from transmission-based isolation precautions. The patient is forced into solitude and deprived of normal social contacts. Proper care of the patient will make him or her feel wanted and cared for like all other patients. Spend extra time with the patient, keep the room clean and pleasant, and teach the patient the rationale for the precautions. The patient's emotional state has the potential to interfere with recovery, so make every effort to keep feelings of psychological and physical isolation to a minimum. Make sure the patient and significant others have an under-

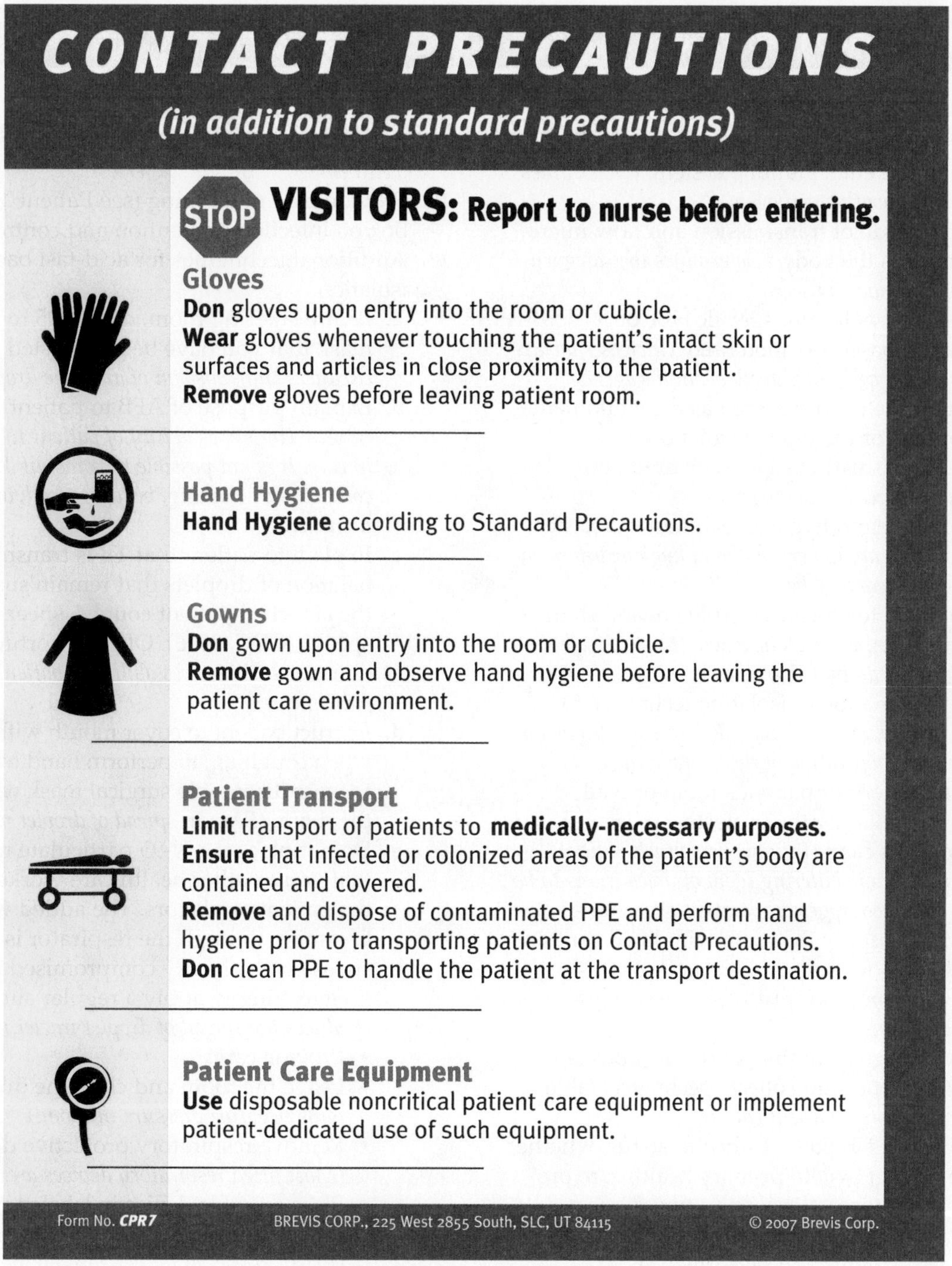

CONTACT PRECAUTIONS
(in addition to standard precautions)

STOP **VISITORS: Report to nurse before entering.**

Gloves
Don gloves upon entry into the room or cubicle.
Wear gloves whenever touching the patient's intact skin or surfaces and articles in close proximity to the patient.
Remove gloves before leaving patient room.

Hand Hygiene
Hand Hygiene according to Standard Precautions.

Gowns
Don gown upon entry into the room or cubicle.
Remove gown and observe hand hygiene before leaving the patient care environment.

Patient Transport
Limit transport of patients to **medically-necessary purposes.**
Ensure that infected or colonized areas of the patient's body are contained and covered.
Remove and dispose of contaminated PPE and perform hand hygiene prior to transporting patients on Contact Precautions.
Don clean PPE to handle the patient at the transport destination.

Patient Care Equipment
Use disposable noncritical patient care equipment or implement patient-dedicated use of such equipment.

Form No. CPR7 BREVIS CORP., 225 West 2855 South, SLC, UT 84115

FIGURE 12-8 Contact Precautions.

standing of the patient's disease and know the importance of following the precautions. Teach family and visitors how to wear isolation apparel, and ensure that the procedure is followed (Skill 12-5).

PULMONARY TUBERCULOSIS (TB) PRECAUTIONS

The dramatic upsurge in the incidence of pulmonary TB, in some cases involving multidrug-resistant strains of the microorganism, has increased concern regarding health care–associated transmission. Guidelines for preventing pulmonary TB in health care settings stress the importance of early identification and treatment of people with known or suspected TB and proper isolation in the health care setting. Suspect the presence of pulmonary TB in any patient with respiratory symptoms lasting longer than 3 weeks. Good assessment skills hasten the possibility of a diagnosis, which is essential, because the risk of exposure is greatest before a diagnosis is made and isolation precautions are implemented. Suspicious symptoms include fatigue, unexplained weight loss, dyspnea, fever, night

Skill 12-5 Isolation Technique

Nursing Action *(Rationale)*

1. Determine causative microorganism and effectiveness of patient's immune system. *(Determines virulence of causative pathogen.)*
2. Recognize mode of transmission and how microorganism exits the body. *(Determines the category or type of isolation to use.)*
3. Follow agency policy for specific type of transmission-based isolation used. *(Increases awareness of isolation categories available in the agency.)*
4. Ensure that the environment has the equipment and supplies for the type of isolation:
   a. Private or isolation room with anteroom. *(Reduces spread of pathogens.)*
   b. Adequate hand hygiene facilities. *(All workers and visitors are to perform hand hygiene before entering and leaving the area.)*
   c. Containers for trash, soiled linen, and sharp instruments, such as needles. *(Ensures safe disposal of contaminated articles.)*
5. Provide explanation of isolation technique to patient, family, and visitors. *(Relieves apprehension and promotes cooperation of those involved.)*
6. Post sign on door of patient's room or wall outside room stating the protective measures in use for patient care. *(Informs personnel, patient, family, and visitors entering room of precautions to be followed and encourages cooperation.)*
7. Be certain to supply the room with lined containers designated for soiled linens and for trash. *(Prevents transmission of pathogens from seepage through container.)*
8. Assess vital signs, administer medications, administer hygiene, and collect specimens (Table 12-3). *(Administers patient care.)*
9. Report changes in patient's health status, whether positive or negative, to primary health care provider or supervisor. *(Ensures continued care and helps determine patient progress.)*
10. Record assessments and performance of transmission-based isolation precautions. *(Provides proof of appropriate patient care.)* Document per agency policy.
11. Determine patient's understanding of activities in room. *(Increases patient's comfort and feeling of well-being.)*
12. Provide patient teaching (see Patient Teaching box on infection prevention and control).
13. Additional techniques for acid-fast bacillus (AFB) isolation:
    a. Before entering room, don N-95 respirator mask that you have been fit-tested for. *(Reduces transmission of airborne droplet nuclei.)*
    b. Explain purpose of AFB to patient, family, and others. *(Improves ability of patient to participate in care. It is not possible to transmit TB through contact with clothing, bedding, food, or eating utensils.)*
    c. Explain to patient that TB is transmitted by inhalation of droplets that remain suspended in the air when patient coughs, sneezes, or speaks (CDC, 2006). Offer opportunity for questions. *(Improves ability of patient to participate in care.)*
    d. Instruct patient to cover mouth with tissue when coughing, to perform hand hygiene, and to wear disposable surgical mask when leaving the room. *(Reduces spread of droplet nuclei.)*
    e. Do not place the N-95 particulate respirator that you or other health care workers wear on the patient or visitors. The added work of breathing through the respirator is an added stress on an already compromised pulmonary system. Simply apply a regular surgical mask. *(Reduces the spread of droplet nuclei.)*
       - Provide care.
       - Leave the room and close the door. *(Maintains negative pressure in room.)*
       - Remove respiratory protective device last. *(Most fitted respiratory devices are reusable.)*
       - Place reusable device in labeled paper bag for storage, being careful not to crush device. *(Plastic bags seal in moisture.)* (Check agency policy for number of times it can be reused.)
       - Record assessments and performance of patient care. *(Promotes continuity of care.)*

sweats, and hemoptysis (a cough that can be productive of blood). Isolation for patients with known or suspected TB includes a negative-pressure isolation room (see Box 12-10). Such rooms have negative pressure in relation to surrounding areas in the facility so that room air is exhausted directly to the outside, or through special high-efficiency particulate air (HEPA) filters if recirculation is unavoidable. High-hazard procedures on patients with suspected or confirmed infectious TB must be performed in negative-pressure rooms.

OSHA and CDC guidelines require health care workers who care for active or suspected TB patients to wear HEPA respirators (Jensen et al., 2005; United States Department of Labor, 2009). The respirators have the capacity to filter particles smaller than 5 μm in size with a filter efficiency of 95% or higher. It is mandatory to fit-test the masks of health care employ-

Table 12-3 Specimen Collection Techniques for the Patient in Isolation

AMOUNT NEEDED*	COLLECTION DEVICE*	SPECIMEN COLLECTION AND TRANSFER
WOUND (CULTURE) SPECIMEN		
As much as possible (after cleaning surface of skin or wound bed to remove flora or debris)	Sterile cotton-tipped swab or syringe	Clean site with sterile water or saline before wound specimen collection. Don gloves and place clean test tube or culturette tube on clean paper towel. After swabbing center of wound site, grasp collection tube by holding it with paper towel. Carefully insert swab without touching outside of tube. After removing gloves, washing hands, and securing tube's top, transfer labeled tube into bag for transport to laboratory. Document that procedure was performed.
BLOOD (CULTURE) SPECIMEN		
This specimen is usually obtained by the laboratory technician. 10 mL per culture bottle, from two different venipuncture sites (volume may differ based on collection containers and age of patient)	Syringes, needles, and culture media bottles	Don gloves and perform venipuncture per hospital protocol at two different sites to decrease likelihood of both specimens being contaminated by skin flora. Inject 10 mL of blood into each bottle. Remove gloves and wash hands. Secure tops of bottles, label specimens, complete requisition, and send to laboratory. Document that procedure was performed.
STOOL (CULTURE) SPECIMEN		
Small amount, approximately size of a walnut	Clean specimen cup with seal top (not necessary to be sterile) and sterile tongue blade	Don gloves and place cup on clean paper towel in patient's bathroom. Using tongue blade, collect needed amount of feces from bedpan, not the toilet. Transfer feces to specimen cup without touching cup's outside surface; cover with lid provided. Remove gloves, wash hands, and place seal on cup. Repeat handwashing. Transfer specimen cup into clean bag for transport to laboratory after ensuring cup is correctly labeled. Document procedure was performed.
URINE (CULTURE) SPECIMEN		
5-15 mL for adults	Syringe and sterile cup	Don gloves and place cup or tube on clean towel in patient's bathroom. Use alcohol swab pad, syringe, and needle to collect specimen if patient has Foley catheter. (All Foley catheters are equipped with needleless ports, which have to be cleaned per manufacturer's guidelines; alcohol swabs are not sufficient.) Otherwise, have patient follow procedure to obtain clean-voided specimen (see Chapter 19). Transfer urine into sterile container by injecting urine from syringe or pouring it from container. Secure top of labeled container, remove gloves, and wash hands. Transfer labeled specimen into clean bag for transport to laboratory, after ensuring container is labeled correctly. Document procedure was completed.

From Pagana, K.D., & Pagana, T.J. (2005). *Mosby's diagnostic and laboratory test reference* (7th ed.). St. Louis: Mosby.
*Agency policies may differ on type of container. Ensure that all specimen containers used have the biohazard symbol on the outside, amount of specimen required, and are bagged for transport to a laboratory.

ees who work in the rooms of TB patients in a reliable way to obtain a face-seal leakage of 10% or less. Under National Institute for Occupational Safety and Health (NIOSH) criteria, the minimally acceptable level of respiratory protection for TB is the N-95 respirator (see Skill 12-5). Training in the wearing and storage of the respirator is required for hospital staff. OSHA also requires employers to provide training concerning transmission of TB, especially in areas where risk of exposure is high, such as in bronchoscopy procedural areas. Other requirements include annual TB skin testing for health care workers and appropriate follow-up when a previously negative skin test becomes positive.

SURGICAL ASEPSIS

Surgical asepsis, or sterile technique, requires that you use different precautions from those of medical asepsis. **Surgical asepsis** consists of maintaining the absence of all microorganisms, including pathogens and spores, from an object. It is essential that you understand that the slightest break in technique, when you are working with a sterile field or with sterile equipment, results in contamination. Practice surgical asepsis (e.g., when filling a syringe or changing a dressing on a wound) to keep microorganisms away from an area.

Although surgical asepsis is practiced in the operating room, the labor and delivery area, and major diagnostic or procedure areas, you will also sometimes use surgical aseptic techniques at the patient's bedside. This includes, for example, when you insert IVs or urinary catheters, suction the tracheobronchial airway, and reapply sterile dressings. In an operating room, follow a series of steps to maintain sterile techniques, including donning a mask, protective eyewear, and a cap; performing surgical hand hygiene; and donning a sterile gown and gloves. In contrast, when you are changing a dressing at a patient's bed-

Box 12-11 Principles of Sterile Technique

1. **A sterile object remains sterile only when touched exclusively by other sterile objects.** (This principle guides your placement of sterile objects and how you handle them.)
   a. Sterile touching sterile remains sterile; for example, wear sterile gloves and use sterile forceps to handle objects on a sterile field.
   b. Sterile touching clean becomes contaminated; for example, if the tip of a syringe or other sterile object touches the surface of a clean disposable glove, the object is contaminated.
   c. Sterile touching contaminated becomes contaminated; for example, when you touch a sterile object with an ungloved hand, the object is contaminated.
   d. Sterile touching questionable is contaminated; for example, when you find a tear or break in the covering of a sterile object, discard the object regardless of whether it appears untouched or not.
2. **Place only sterile objects on a sterile field.** Properly sterilize all items before use. It is essential to keep the package or container holding a sterile object intact and dry. A package that is torn, punctured, wet, or open is unsterile.
3. **A sterile object or field out of the range of vision or an object held below a person's waist is contaminated.** Never turn your back on a sterile tray or leave it unattended. It is possible for contamination to occur accidentally from a dangling piece of clothing, falling hair, or an unknowing patient touching a sterile object. Consider any object below waist level contaminated since you are not able to keep it in constant view. Keep sterile objects in front of you with your hands as close together as possible.
4. **A sterile object or field becomes contaminated by prolonged exposure to air.** Avoid activities that potentially create air currents, such as excessive movements or rearranging linen after a sterile object or field becomes exposed. When opening sterile packages, it is important to keep to a minimum the number of people walking into the area. Microorganisms also travel by droplets through the air. Make sure no one talks, laughs, sneezes, or coughs over a sterile field or when gathering and using sterile equipment. Never perform sterile procedures if you have a cold or other respiratory ailment unless you are wearing a specialized mask. Microorganisms have the potential to travel through the air and fall on sterile items or fields if you reach over the work area. When opening sterile packages, hold the item or piece of equipment as close as possible to the sterile field without touching the sterile surface. Keeping movement and rearranging of sterile items to a minimum also reduces contamination by air transmission.
5. **When a sterile surface comes in contact with a wet, contaminated surface, the sterile object or field becomes contaminated.** Moisture seeping through a sterile package's protective covering permits microorganisms to travel to the sterile object. When stored sterile packages become wet, discard the objects immediately or send the equipment for resterilization. When working with a sterile field or tray, you will sometimes have to pour sterile solutions. Any spill is a possible source of contamination unless the object or field rests on a sterile surface impervious to moisture. For example, urinary catheterization trays contain sterile supplies that rest in a sterile, plastic container. Any sterile solutions spilled within the container will not contaminate the catheter or other objects. In contrast, if you place a piece of sterile gauze in its wrapper on a patient's bedside table and the table surface is wet, consider the gauze to be contaminated.
6. **Fluid flows in the direction of gravity.** A sterile object becomes contaminated if gravity causes a contaminated liquid to flow over the object's surface. To prevent contamination during a surgical hand scrub, raise and hold your hands above your elbows. This allows water to flow downward without contaminating your hands and fingers. The principle of water flow by gravity is also the reason for drying in a sequence from fingers to elbows, with hands held up, after the scrub (see Skill 12-6).
7. **Consider the edges of a sterile field or container to be contaminated.** Frequently, you will place sterile objects on a sterile towel or drape. Because the edge of the drape touches an unsterile surface, such as a table or bed linen, it is necessary to consider a 1-inch (2.5-cm) border around the drape to be contaminated. The edges of sterile containers become exposed to air after they are open and are thus contaminated. After you remove a sterile needle from its protective cap or after removing a forceps from a container, do not allow the objects to touch the container's edge. The lip of an opened bottle of solution also becomes contaminated after it is exposed to air. When pouring a sterile liquid, first pour a small amount of solution and discard it. The solution thus washes away microorganisms on the bottle lip. Then pour a second time on the same side to fill a container with the desired amount of solution.

side, you will often only perform hand hygiene and don sterile gloves.

Because surgical asepsis requires exact techniques, you will need the patient's cooperation. For this reason, prepare the patient before any procedure. Certain patients fear moving or touching objects during a sterile procedure, whereas others will even try to assist. Explain how a procedure is to be performed and instruct the patient how to avoid contaminating sterile items, including the following measures:

- Try not to make sudden movements of body parts covered by sterile drapes
- Refrain from touching sterile supplies, drapes, or the nurse's gloves and gown
- Avoid coughing, sneezing, or talking over a sterile area

PRINCIPLES OF STERILE TECHNIQUE

When beginning a surgically aseptic procedure, follow the principles listed in Box 12-11 to ensure maintenance of asepsis. Failure to follow each principle conscientiously endangers patients, placing them at risk for infection.

Assemble all the equipment necessary for a sterile procedure before the procedure begins. By doing so, you avoid the need to leave a sterile area unattended because some equipment is missing. Have a few extra supplies available in case objects accidentally become contaminated. If an object becomes contaminated during the procedure, discard it immediately.

SURGICAL HAND SCRUB

In the operating room setting, effective handwashing or use of select surgical hand rub to achieve surgical hand hygiene is imperative. To reduce patients' risk of postoperative infection, use an antimicrobial preparation for hand hygiene as an integral part of the presurgical scrubbing procedure for operating room personnel. Although it is not possible to sterilize the skin, it is possible to greatly reduce the number of microorganisms by chemical, physical, and mechanical means.

The surgical hand scrub (Skill 12-6) is the traditional method for surgical asepsis. Through the use of an antimicrobial agent and sterile brushes, the surgical hand scrub removes debris and transient microorganisms from the nails, the hands, and the forearms; reduces the resident microbial count to a minimum; and inhibits rapid or rebound growth of microorganisms. New evidence suggests that a brushless technique with an agent containing at least 60% alcohol, with or without water, has the same microbial efficacy and provides an alternative to the traditional hand scrub

Skill 12-6 Surgical Hand Hygiene

Nursing Action *(Rationale)*

1. Inspect hands for presence of abrasions, cuts, or open lesions. *(These conditions increase likelihood of more microorganisms residing on skin surfaces.)*
2. Apply surgical shoe covers, cap or hood, face mask, and protective eyewear. *(Mask prevents escape into air of microorganisms that can contaminate hands. Other protective wear prevents exposure to blood and body fluid splashes during the procedure.)*
3. Perform surgical hand hygiene (traditional method):
   - **a.** Turn on water using knee or foot controls and adjust to comfortable temperature.
   - **b.** Wet hands and arms under running lukewarm water and lather with detergent to 5 cm (2 inches) above elbows. (Keep hands above elbows at all times.) *(Hands become cleanest part of upper extremity. Keeping hands elevated allows water to flow from least to most contaminated areas, since water runs by gravity from fingertips to elbows. Washing a wide area reduces risk of contaminating gown that you will don later.)*
   - **c.** Rinse hands and arms thoroughly under running water. **REMEMBER TO KEEP HANDS ABOVE ELBOWS.** *(Rinsing removes transient microorganisms from fingers, hands, and forearms.)*
   - **d.** Under running water, clean under nails of both hands with nail pick. Discard after use (see illustration). *(Removes dirt and organic material that harbor large numbers of microorganisms.)*
   - **e.** **(1)** Wet clean sponge and apply antimicrobial detergent. Scrub nails of one hand with 15 strokes. Holding sponge perpendicular to hand (see illustration) scrub palm, each side of thumb and fingers, and posterior side of hand with 10 strokes each.

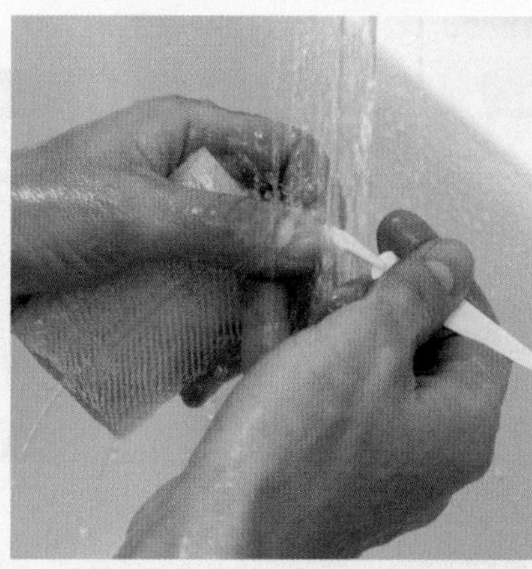

Step **3d**

Continued

Skill 12-6 Surgical Hand Hygiene—cont'd

(2) Mentally divide your arm into thirds, and scrub each third 10 times (see illustration). Entire scrub should last 5 to 10 minutes. Rinse sponge and repeat sequence for other arm. It is permitted to substitute with a two-sponge method. Check agency policy. *(Friction loosens resident bacteria that adhere to skin surfaces. Ensures coverage of all surfaces. Scrubbing is performed from cleanest area [hands] to marginal area [upper arms.])*

f. Discard sponge and rinse hands and arms thoroughly (see illustration). Turn off water with foot or knee control and back into room entrance with hands elevated in front of and away from the body. *(After touching skin, consider sponge contaminated. Rinsing removes resident bacteria. Prevents accidental contamination.)*

g. (1) Walk up to sterile tray and lean forward slightly to pick up a sterile towel (see illustration).

(2) Dry one hand thoroughly, moving in sequence from fingers to elbow. Dry in a rotating motion. Dry from cleanest to least clean area (see illustration). *(Drying prevents chapping and facilitates donning of gloves. Leaning forward prevents accidental contact of arms with scrub attire.)*

h. Repeat drying method for other hand by carefully reversing towel or using a new sterile towel. *(Prevents accidental contamination.)*

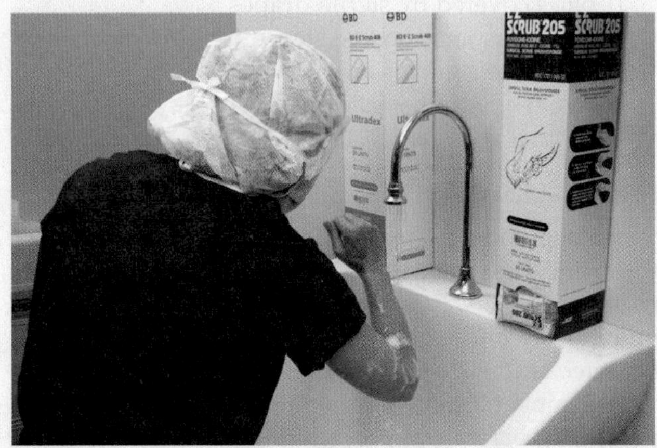

Step **3f**

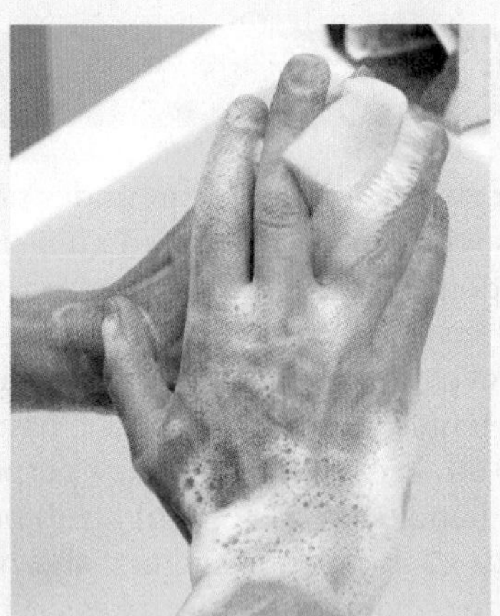
Step **3e(1)**

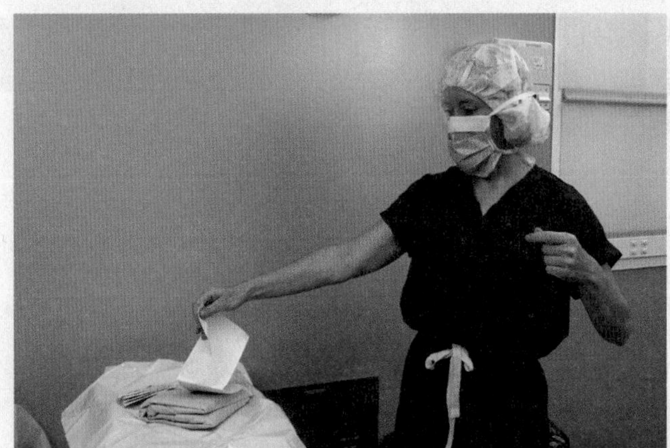
Step **3g(1)**

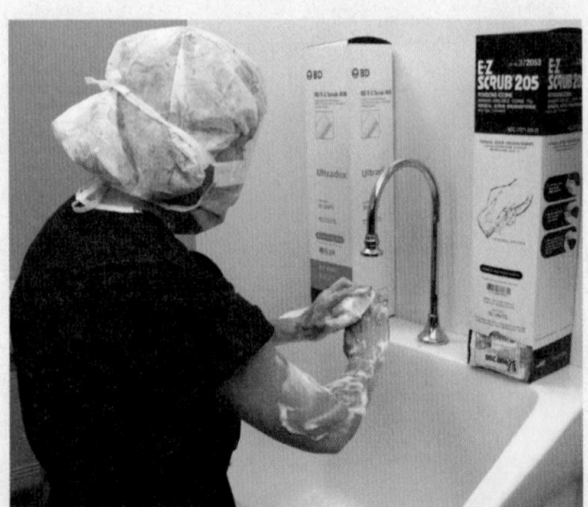

Step **3e(2)**

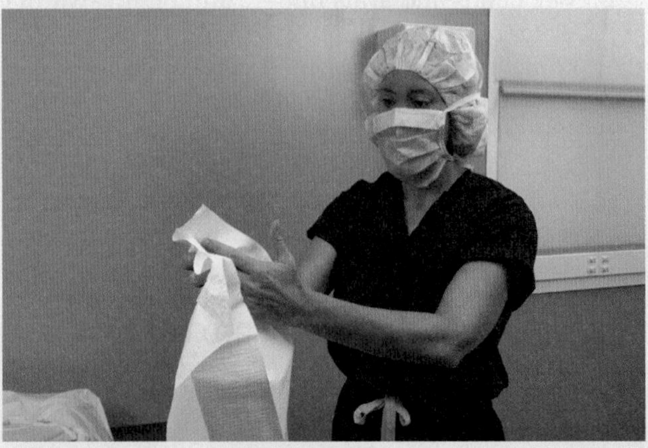
Step **3g(2)**

i. Discard towel. *(Prevents accidental contamination.)*
j. Proceed with sterile gowning.

4. Alternate method of surgical hand hygiene using alcohol-based antiseptic:
   a. Wash hands with soap and water for 15 to 30 seconds to remove soil. *(Removes dirt and organic material that harbor large numbers of microorganisms.)*
   b. Under running water, clean under nails of both hands with nail pick. Discard after use and dry hands with a paper towel. *(Removes dirt and organic material that harbor large numbers of microorganisms.)*
   c. Apply enough alcohol-based waterless antiseptic to one palm to cover both hands thoroughly. Spread the antiseptic over all surfaces of the hands and the fingernails. Follow product instructions for length of time to rub over hand surfaces. Allow to air-dry. *(Ensures coverage of all surfaces. Air-drying ensures complete antisepsis.)*
   d. Repeat the process and allow hands to air-dry before applying sterile gloves.

with a brush. Both hand antiseptic methods are currently used in operating room settings. Skill 12-6 addresses both techniques.

Surgical personnel wear surgical attire (i.e., scrubs) in the operating room to reduce the chance for contamination from themselves to patients and vice versa. Fingernails should be short, clean, and healthy. If you wear polish, make sure it is not chipped and not older than 4 days. Do not wear artificial nails. Artificial nails tend to harbor gram-negative microorganisms and fungus. Remove all rings, watches, and bracelets before the surgical scrub.

The Association of Perioperative Registered Nurses (AORN) (2005) has a revised set policies and procedures; also refer to agency policy on surgical hand hygiene (see Chapter 42).

MANAGING STERILE PACKAGES

Sterile items such as syringes, gauze dressings, and catheters are packaged in paper or plastic containers that are impervious (unable to be penetrated) to microorganisms as long as they are dry and intact. Some institutions wrap reusable supplies in a double thickness of linen or muslin. Paper packages are permeable to steam and thus allow for steam autoclaving. A disadvantage of paper wrappers is that they tear or puncture relatively easily. Place sterile items in clean, enclosed storage cabinets, and never keep them in the same room as dirty equipment.

Sterile supplies have dated labels or chemical tapes that indicate the date when the sterilization expires. The tapes change color during the sterilization process. Failure of the tapes to change color means the item is not sterile. Never use or allow use of a sterile item or piece of equipment after the expiration date. Some agencies use the "event-related" contamination rule. If the integrity of the sterile package is questionable (i.e., wet, torn, discolored), the item is not used. If you find moisture after opening a sterile tray, either discard the item or return it to the institution's supply area for resterilization.

Before opening a sterile item, perform thorough hand hygiene. Assemble the supplies at the work area, such as the bedside table or in the treatment room, before opening packages. A bedside table or countertop provides a large, clean working area for opening items. Make sure the work area is above your waist level. Do not open sterile supplies in a confined space where it is possible for a dirty object to fall on or strike them.

It is possible to open sterile packaged items without contaminating the contents even when you are not wearing sterile gloves. Commercially packaged items are usually designed so that you only have to tear away or separate the paper or plastic cover. Hold the item in one hand while pulling the wrapper with the other (Figure 12-9, *A*). Take care afterwards to keep the inner contents sterile before use. When opening items packed in linen and some commercially prepackaged items, use the steps described in Box 12-12 and illustrated in Figure 12-9, *B* through *E*, and Figure 12-10.

PREPARING A STERILE FIELD

When performing sterile procedures, you need a sterile work area that provides room for handling and placing of sterile items. A sterile field is an area that is free of microorganisms and is prepared to receive sterile items. Prepare the field by using the inner surface of a sterile wrapper as the work surface or by using a sterile drape (Skill 12-7).

Sometimes you will choose to wear sterile gloves while preparing items on the field. You are then able to touch the entire drape, but an assistant will have to open and pass sterile items to you. Do not allow your gloves to touch the outside wrappers of sterile items.

POURING STERILE SOLUTIONS

Often you will be called on to pour sterile solutions into sterile containers. A bottle containing a sterile solution is sterile on the inside and contaminated on the outside. The bottle's neck is also contaminated, but the inside of the bottle cap is sterile. After opening a cap or lid, hold it in your hand or place it, sterile side (inside) up, on a clean surface. This means that you can see the inside of the lid as it rests on the table surface. Never allow a bottle cap or lid to rest sterile side down on a

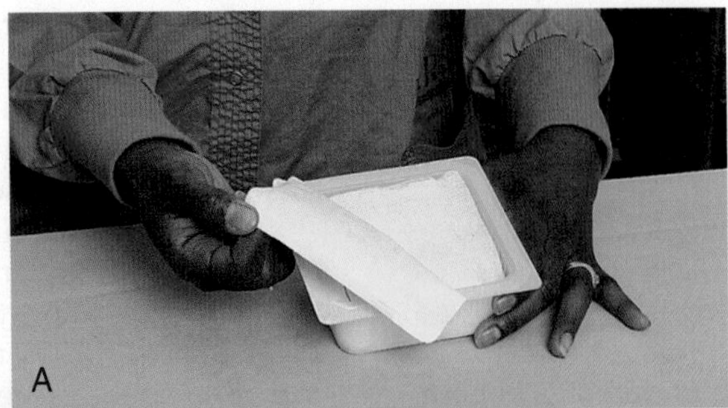

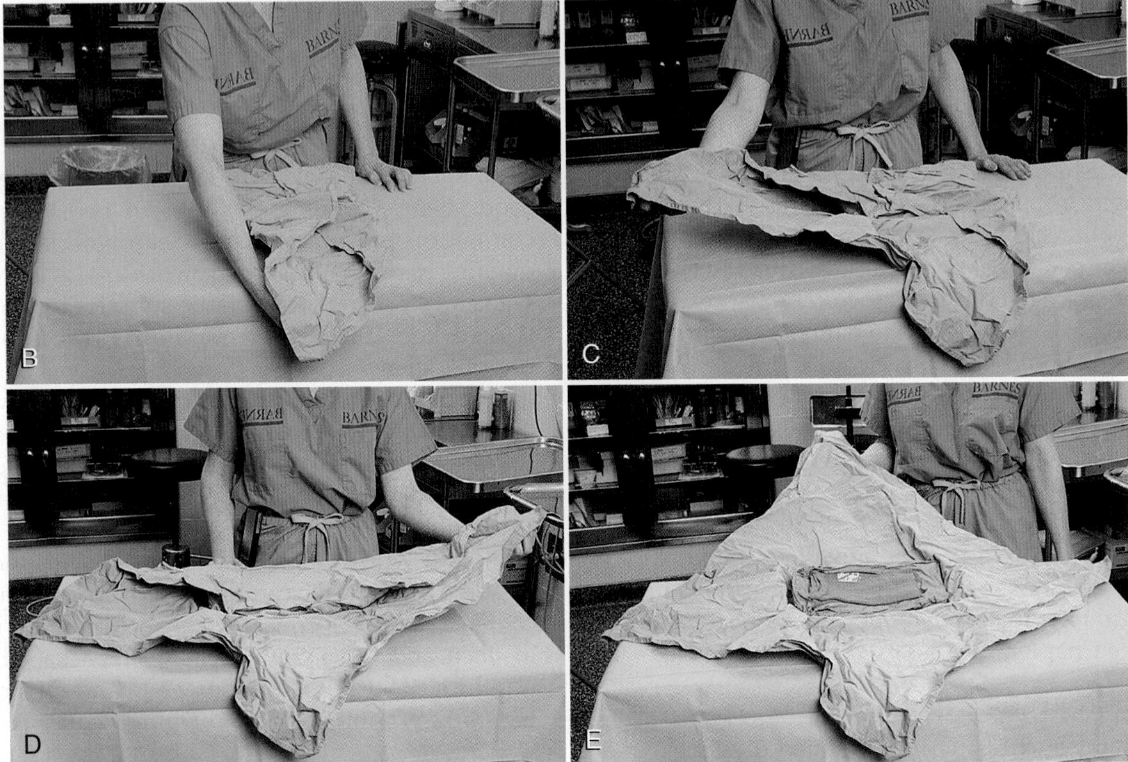

FIGURE 12-9 **A,** When opening a commercially packaged sterile item, tear the wrapper away from your body. **B,** When opening sterile packaged items on a flat surface, open the top flap away from your body. **C,** Keep your arm out, away from the sterile field, while opening the side flap. **D,** Opening the second side flap. **E,** Opening the back flap.

Box 12-12 Opening Sterile Packages

1. Perform hand hygiene.
2. Place the item flat in the center of the work surface.
3. Remove the tape or seal indicating the sterilization date.
4. Grasp the outer surface of the tip of the outermost flap.
5. Open the outer flap away from your body, keeping your arm outstretched and away from the sterile field.
6. Grasp the outside surface of the first side flap.
7. Open the side flap, allowing it to lie flat on the table surface. Keep your arm to the side and not over the sterile surface. Do not allow flaps to spring back over the sterile contents.
8. Grasp the outside surface of the second side flap and allow it to lie flat on the table surface.
9. Grasp the outer surface of the last and innermost flap.
10. Stand away from the sterile package and pull the flap back, allowing it to fall flat on the surface.
11. Use the inner surface of the package cover (except for the 1-inch border around the edges) as a sterile field to handle this or additional sterile items (see Figure 12-10). Grasp the 1-inch border to maneuver the entire field on the table surface.
12. When opening a small, sterile item, hold it in your hand so that you can pass it to a person wearing sterile gloves or transfer it to a sterile field. Hold the package in your nondominant hand while you open the top flap and pull it away from you. Using your dominant hand, carefully open the side and top flaps away from the enclosed sterile item in the same order in the earlier steps (see Figure 12-9).

Skill 12-7 Preparing a Sterile Field

Nursing Action *(Rationale)*

1. Prepare sterile field just before planned procedure. *(Prevents exposure of sterile field and supplies to air contamination.)* Make sure to use supplies immediately.
2. Select clean work surface that is above waist level. *(Consider sterile objects held below waist contaminated.)*
3. Assemble necessary equipment. *(Preparing equipment in advance prevents breaks in technique.)*
   - Sterile drape
   - Assorted sterile supplies
4. Check dates, labels, and condition of package for sterility of equipment. *(Consider equipment stored beyond expiration date, or a package that is damaged, unsterile.)*
5. Wash hands thoroughly. *(Prevents spread of microorganisms.)*
6. Place pack containing sterile drape on work surface and open (see Figure 12-9). *(Ensures sterility of packaged drape.)*
7. With fingertips of one hand, pick up folded top edge of sterile drape. *(Up to the 1-inch border around drape is unsterile and permitted to be touched.)*
8. Gently lift drape up from its outer cover and let it unfold by itself without touching any object. Discard outer cover with your other hand. *(If sterile object touches any unsterile object, it becomes contaminated.)*
9. With other hand, grasp adjacent corner of drape and hold the entire edge straight up and away from your body. Now, properly place drape while using two hands and making sure to keep the drape away from unsterile surfaces. *(Prevents contamination.)*
   a. Holding drape, first position the bottom half over intended work surface. *(Prevents you from reaching over sterile field.)*
   b. Allow top half of drape to be placed over work surface last. *(Creates a flat, sterile work surface.)*
10. Perform procedure using sterile technique. *(Prevents contamination.)*

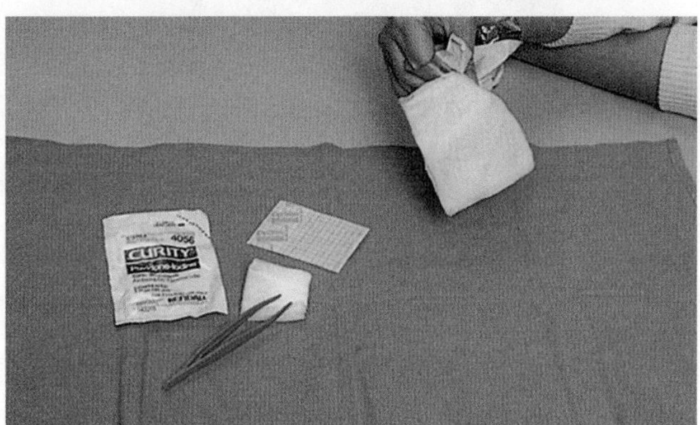

FIGURE 12-10 Placing items on a sterile field.

sterile surface because the cap's outer edge is unsterile and will contaminate the surface. Likewise, placing a sterile cap down on an unsterile surface increases the chances of the inside of the cap becoming contaminated.

Hold the bottle with its label in the palm of your hand to prevent the solution from wetting the label and causing it to fade. Before pouring the solution into the container, "lip" the bottle by pouring a small amount (1 to 2 mL) into a disposable cup or plastic-lined waste receptacle, and discarding it. The poured solution cleans the lip of the bottle. Keep the edge of the bottle from touching from the edge or the inside of the receiving container, which is unsterile.

Pour any solution slowly to avoid splashing the underlying drape or field. Never hold the bottle so high above the recipient container that even, slow pouring will cause splashing. Hold the bottle outside the edge of the sterile field (Figure 12-11).

DONNING A STERILE GOWN

It is necessary to don a sterile gown (Skill 12-8) before working in the operating room, as well as before assisting with certain sterile procedures or working in special treatment areas. The sterile gown decreases the risk of contaminating sterile objects when you handle them. In addition, the sterile gown prevents contami-

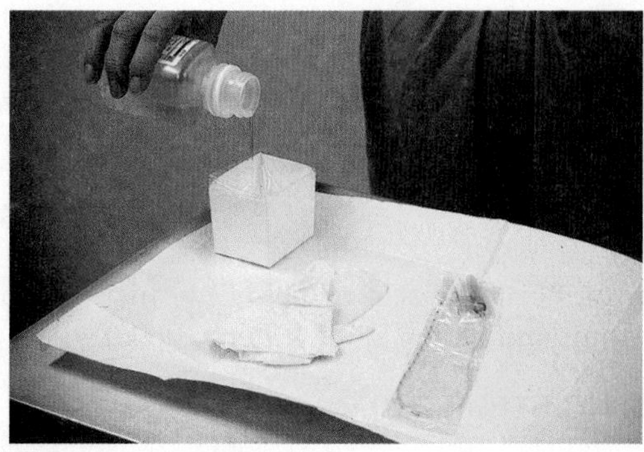

FIGURE 12-11 Place receptacle into which you pour fluids near edge of sterile table to prevent the need for reaching over sterile field to pour.

Skill 12-8 Donning a Sterile Gown

Nursing Action *(Rationale)*

1. Don surgical cap, shoe covers, protective eyewear, and mask, and then perform surgical hand hygiene. *(Prevents contamination of the surgical field as well as protects the nurse from blood and body fluid exposure.)*
2. Ask the circulating nurse to open the sterile gown package and the sterile glove package. *(Prevents you from contaminating your own hands following the surgical handwash since the outer wraps are not sterile.)*
3. Don the gown.
   a. If available, the scrub nurse will assist by pulling the gown over your extended hands and arms. If there is no assistance from a scrub nurse:
      (1) Pick up the gown touching only the inner surface below the neck. *(Touching the outer, sterile surface causes the gown to become contaminated since your hands are not yet gloved and thus unsterile.)*
      (2) Maintain constant control of the folded layers of the gown. *(Prevents the gown from brushing against unsterile surfaces.)*
      (3) While holding the gown at arm's length, allow the gown to unfold from top to bottom. Be sure that the gown does not touch the floor (see illustration). *(Prevents contamination.)*
      (4) While holding the inside of the gown near the shoulders and below the neckband, slide hands and arms into the sleeves with your fingers stopping at the end of the cuffs (see illustration). *(The fingers remain inside the sleeves in order to don the sterile gloves by means of closed gloving.)*
      (5) Ask another staff member to grasp the cord that is attached to the ties of the gown in order to draw the ties around to the back with the gown overlapping itself. The staff member should now tie the gown, avoiding touching any part of the gown except the ties. *(Do not allow the front or the sides of the gown to be touched by the staff member since these areas are sterile.)*

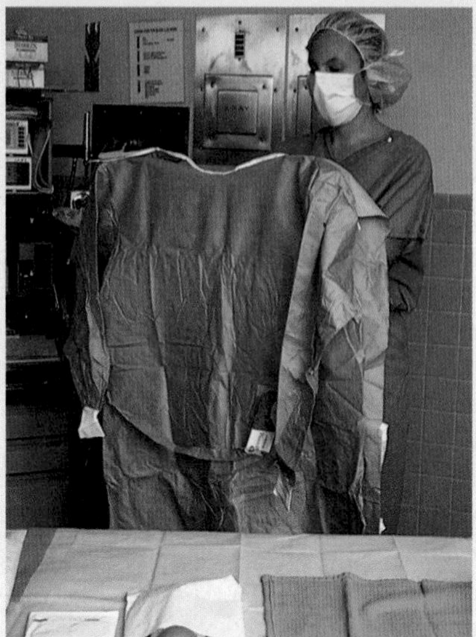
Step **3a(3)**

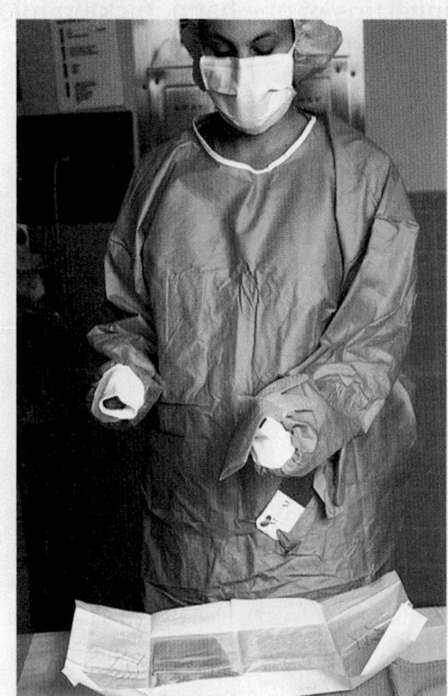
Step **3a(4)**

nation of sterile objects or fields by microorganisms shed from your skin (Potter & Perry, 2006).

DONNING STERILE GLOVES

Sterile gloves are an additional barrier to bacterial transfer. There are two methods of donning gloves: open (Skill 12-9) and closed (Figure 12-12). Nurses who work on general nursing divisions use open gloving before procedures such as dressing changes or urinary catheter insertions. Use the closed gloving method when donning a sterile gown before procedures in the operating room and special treatment areas.

Make sure to select the proper glove size. It is necessary for the glove to be snug enough for you to pick things up easily, and yet not so tightly stretched that it tears easily.

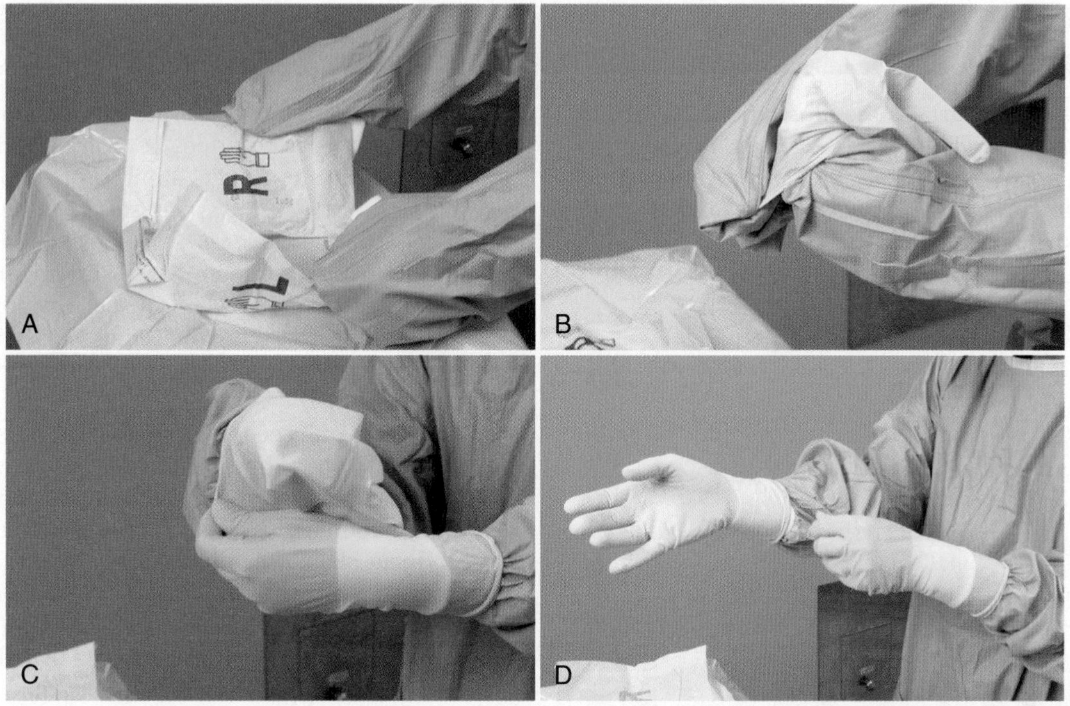

FIGURE 12-12 Closed gloving. **A,** Open glove package. **B,** Grasp back of dominant hand's glove cuff with nondominant hand and stretch over end of dominant hand's sleeve. **C,** Glove nondominant hand in same manner. **D,** Use gloved dominant hand to pull on glove, keeping nondominant hand inside sleeve until it emerges into glove.

Skill 12-9 Performing Open Sterile Gloving

Nursing Action *(Rationale)*

1. Have package of properly sized sterile gloves at treatment area. *(Facilitates procedure.)*
2. Perform thorough hand hygiene. *(Removes bacteria from skin surfaces.)*
3. Remove outer glove package wrapper by carefully separating and peeling apart sides (see illustration). *(Prevents inner glove package from accidentally opening and touching contaminated objects.)*
4. Grasping inner side of package, lay package on clean, flat surface just above waist level. Open package, keeping gloves on wrapper's inside surface (see illustration). *(Inner surface of glove package is sterile. Sterile objects held below the waist are considered contaminated.)*
5. Identify right and left gloves. Each glove will have cuff approximately 2 inches (5 cm) deep. *(Proper identification of gloves prevents contamination by improper fit.)*
6. Glove dominant hand first. With thumb and first two fingers of nondominant hand, grasp edge of cuff of glove for dominant hand. Touch only

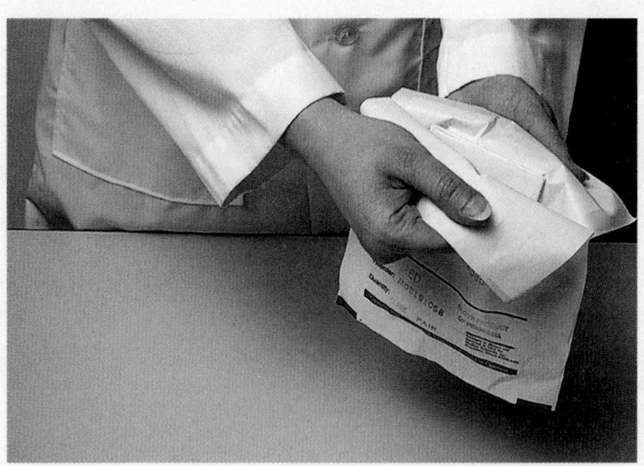

Step **3**

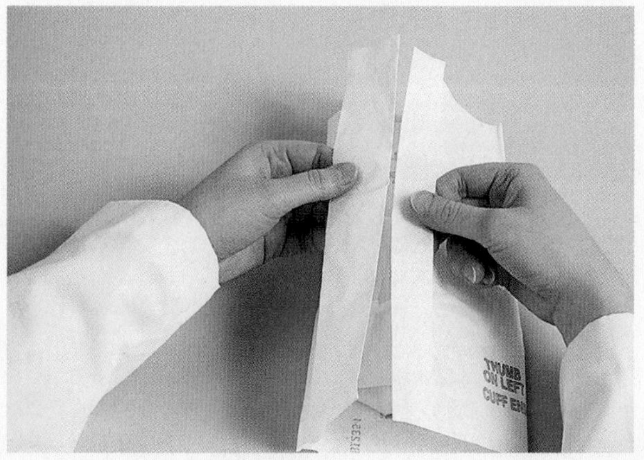

Step **4**

Continued

Skill 12-9 Performing Open Sterile Gloving—cont'd

glove's inside surface (see illustration). *(Gloving of dominant hand first improves dexterity. Touching inside surface is permitted since inner edge of cuff will lie against skin. If glove's outer surface touches hand or wrist, it is contaminated.)*

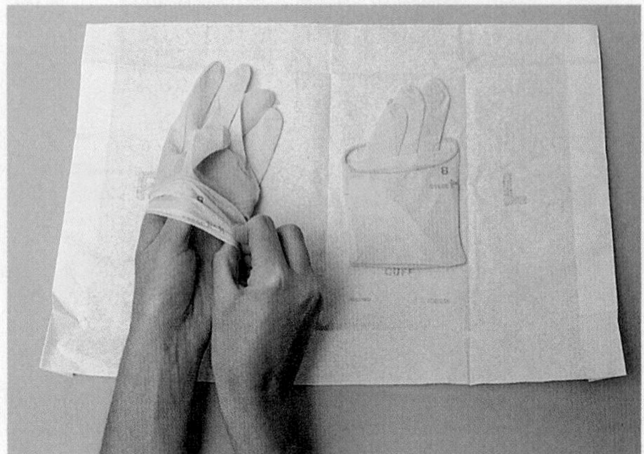

Step **6**

7. Carefully pull glove over dominant hand, leaving cuff; make sure cuff does not roll up wrist. Make sure thumb and fingers are in proper spaces (see illustration). *(If glove's outer surface touches hand or wrist, it is contaminated.)*
8. With gloved, dominant hand, slip fingers underneath second glove's cuff in such fashion that the cuff will protect the gloved fingers (see illustration). *(Sterile touching sterile prevents glove contamination.)*
9. Carefully pull second glove over nondominant hand. Do not allow fingers and thumb of gloved, dominant hand to touch any part of exposed nondominant hand. Keep thumb of dominant hand abducted back (see illustration). *(Contact of gloved hand with exposed hand results in contamination.)*
10. After second glove is on, interlock hands. *Be sure to touch only sterile sides.* The cuffs usually fall down after application (see illustration). *(Ensures smooth fit over fingers.)*

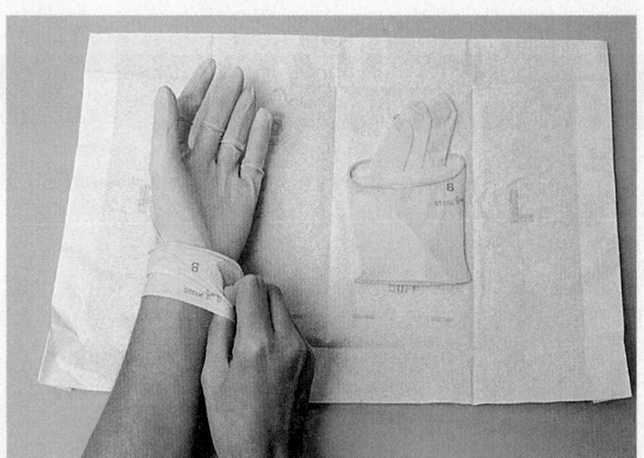

Step **7**

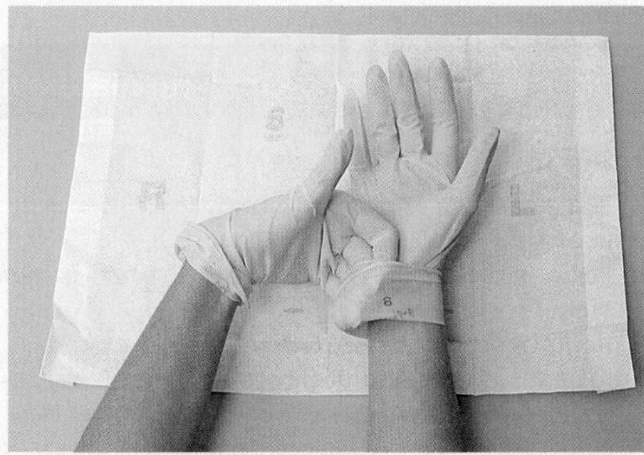

Step **9**

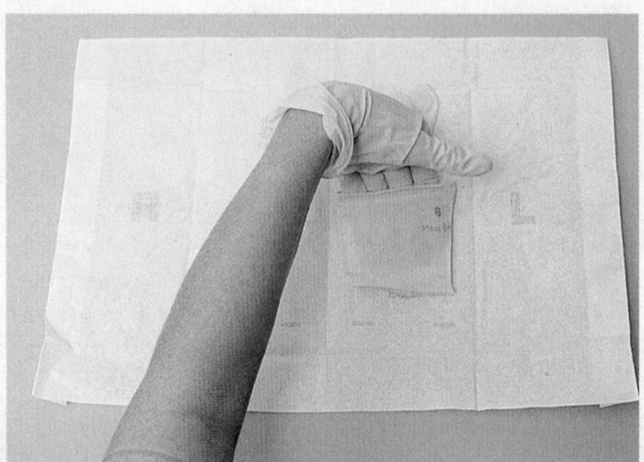

Step **8**

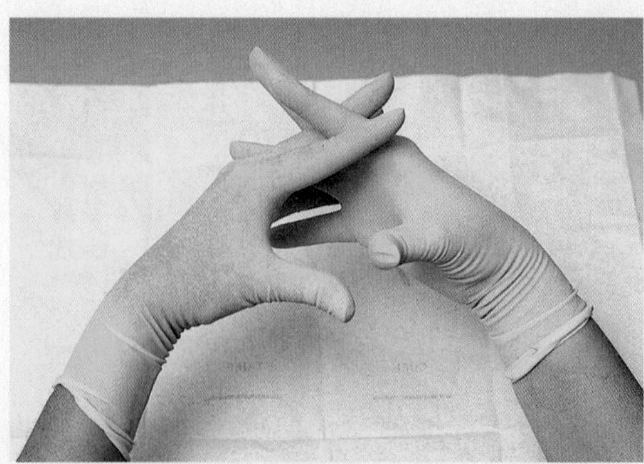

Step **10**

Glove Removal and Disposal

11. Grasp outside of one cuff with other gloved hand; avoid touching wrist (see illustration). *(Minimizes contamination of underlying skin.)*
12. Pull glove off, turning it inside out (see illustration). Discard in receptacle. *(The outside of glove does not touch skin surface.)*

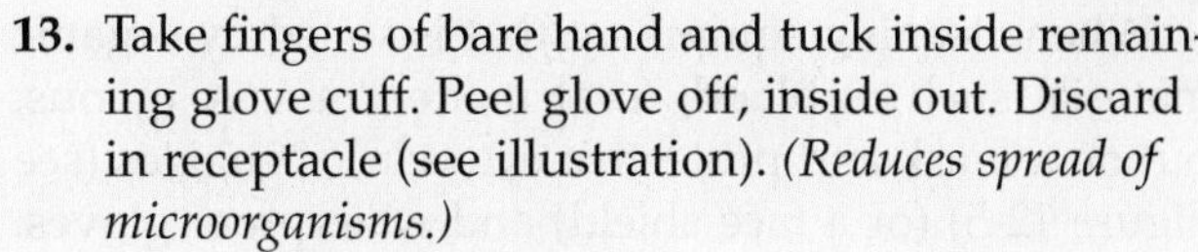

13. Take fingers of bare hand and tuck inside remaining glove cuff. Peel glove off, inside out. Discard in receptacle (see illustration). *(Reduces spread of microorganisms.)*

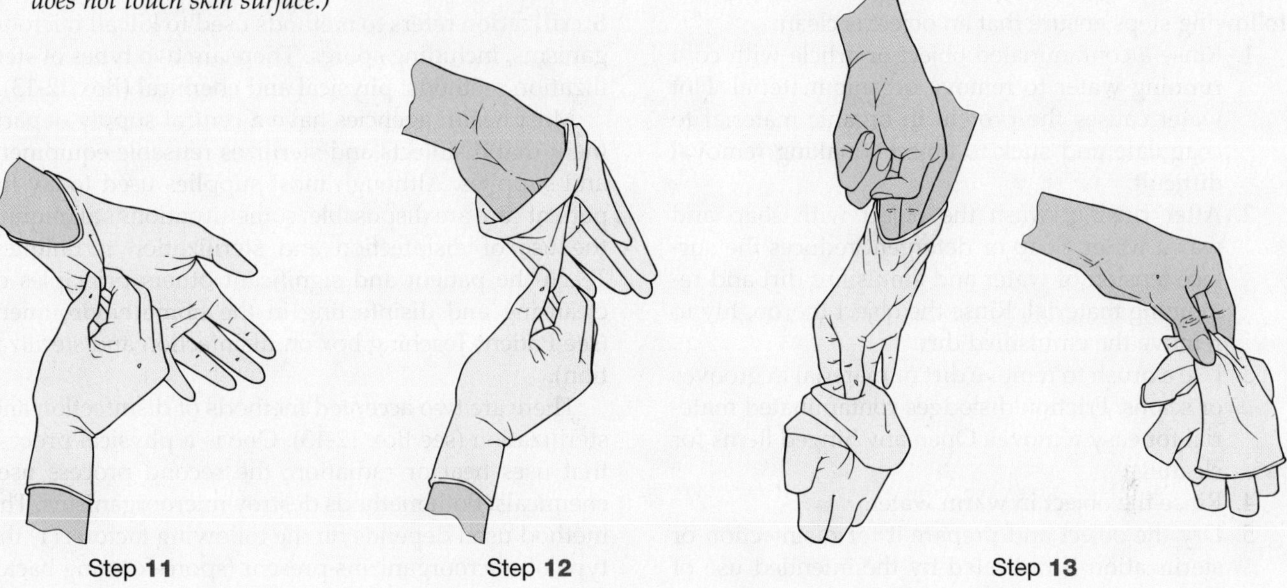

Closed Gloving

Closed gloving is practiced when the nurse wears a sterile gown. To perform the closed gloving procedure, keep your hands covered with the gown sleeves as you open the inner sterile glove package. As with open gloving, you will glove the dominant hand first. With your nondominant hand inside the gown cuff, pick up the glove for your dominant hand by grasping the folded cuff through the gown material. Extend your dominant forearm palm up and place the palm of the glove against the palm of your dominant hand. Glove fingers will point toward elbow.

Grasp the back of the glove cuff with your nondominant hand, still through the gown material, and turn the glove cuff over the end of your dominant hand and the gown cuff (Figure 12-12, *B*). Grasp the top of the glove and the underlying gown sleeve with your covered, nondominant hand. Carefully extend fingers of your dominant hand into the glove, making sure the glove's cuff covers the gown's cuff. Then go on to glove your second, nondominant hand in the same manner, reversing hands (Figure 12-12, *C*). Use your gloved, dominant hand to pull on the nondominant hand's glove, once again keeping your hand inside the gown sleeve (Figure 12-12, *D*) until you are able to extend it out of the sleeve and directly into the glove.

By the use of this closed gloving procedure, you maintain the sterile barrier and prevent contamination. You are now ready to assist with sterile materials and instruments such as those called for during surgery or treatments such as wound debridement.

CLEANING, DISINFECTION, AND STERILIZATION

Pathogenic microorganisms are present on most articles in the home and public areas, including health care agencies. By following basic clean or aseptic technique, you are able to interrupt the spread of infection. Antiseptics are a means to inhibit the growth of microorganisms, although killing them this way is not possible. Antiseptics are also referred to as **bacteriostatic** solutions. *Bacterio* means "microorganism" and *static* means "referring to that which cannot move or grow." Use of antiseptics on human tissue is acceptable and is often performed before surgery, during wound care, for mouth care, and for washing hands.

CLEANING

Cleaning is the removal of foreign materials, such as soil and organic material, from objects. Generally, cleaning involves use of water and mechanical action with or without detergents.

When an object comes in contact with infectious or potentially infectious material, the object is contaminated. If the object is disposable, it is usually discarded unless formal policies and procedures are in place for reprocessing the object. It is necessary to thoroughly clean reusable objects and then either disinfect or sterilize them before reuse.

When cleaning equipment that is soiled by organic material such as blood, fecal matter, mucus, or pus, put on a mask and protective eyewear or goggles (see Figure 12-5) (or a face shield) and waterproof gloves. These barriers provide protection from infectious organisms (as discussed earlier). You will need a stiff-bristled brush and detergent or soap for cleaning. The following steps ensure that an object is clean:

1. Rinse a contaminated object or article with cold running water to remove organic material. Hot water causes the protein in organic material to coagulate and stick to objects, making removal difficult.
2. After rinsing, wash the object with soap and warm water. Soap or detergent reduces the surface tension of water and emulsifies dirt and remaining material. Rinse the object thoroughly to remove the emulsified dirt.
3. Use a brush to remove dirt or material in grooves or seams. Friction dislodges contaminated material for easy removal. Open any hinged items for cleaning.
4. Rinse the object in warm water.
5. Dry the object and prepare it for disinfection or sterilization if indicated by the intended use of the item.
6. Consider the brush, the gloves, and the sink in which the equipment is cleaned contaminated and make sure it is cleaned and dried per hospital protocol.

DISINFECTION

Disinfection is used to destroy microorganisms. However, it does not destroy spores. The solutions used are called **disinfectants**, or possibly **bactericidal solutions** (the suffix *-cidal* is derived from a Latin word meaning "to kill"). These solutions are too strong for human skin to tolerate and are used only on inanimate objects. If a disinfectant solution comes in contact with human tissue, the tissue will feel "slippery." This is the first step of tissue breakdown. When using a disinfectant solution, use clean gloves to protect your skin (Skill 12-10).

STERILIZATION

Sterilization refers to methods used to kill all microorganisms, including spores. There are two types of sterilization methods: physical and chemical (Box 12-13).

Most health agencies have a central supply department that disinfects and sterilizes reusable equipment and supplies. Although most supplies used today for patient care are disposable, some situations still require the use of disinfection and sterilization techniques. Teach the patient and significant others principles of cleansing and disinfecting in the home environment (see Patient Teaching box on disinfection and sterilization).

There are two accepted methods of disinfection and sterilization (see Box 12-13). One is a physical process that uses heat or radiation; the second process uses chemicals. Both methods destroy microorganisms. The method used depends on the following factors: (1) the type of microorganisms present (spore-forming bacteria are resistant to destruction); (2) how many microorganisms are present (it takes longer to kill a large number); and (3) the type of article in need of cleansing (some materials are so sensitive that heat or certain chemicals destroy them). Other determinants of the sterilization method used are (1) the intended use for the article (surgery, for instance, requires that all organisms be destroyed, whereas medical asepsis requires removal of pathogens only), and (2) the methods of sterilization available.

Chemicals used effectively in sterilization and disinfection are iodine, alcohol, and chlorine bleach com-

Skill 12-10 Preparing for Disinfection and Sterilization

Nursing Action *(Rationale)*

1. Prepare equipment and supplies. *(Ensures organization of procedure.)*
   - Disinfectant to use for cleansing. *(Aids in appropriate care of equipment and reusable supplies.)*
   - Method of sterilization. *(Ensures that appropriate method is used.)*
   - Gloves. *(Protects you from contamination.)*
   - Running water. *(Aids in cleansing and rinsing of articles.)*
   - Scrub brush. *(Aids in cleansing grooves.)*
   - Cloth wrapper. *(Provides the means for wrapping articles requiring sterilization.)*
2. Don gloves. *(Protects you from contamination.)*
3. Rinse article under cool running water. *(Emulsifies or softens soil for removal.)*
4. Wash article with detergent. *(Emulsifies or softens dirt for easy removal.)*
5. Use scrub brush to remove material in grooves. *(Friction loosens material in corners and grooves.)*
6. Dry article thoroughly. *(Prevents the growth of microorganisms.)*
7. Prepare article for sterilization by wrapping it in cloth wrapper. *(Promotes appropriate sterilization of the article.)*
8. Clean work area and put in order. *(Prevents the spread of microorganisms.)*
9. Perform patient teaching (see Patient Teaching box on disinfection and sterilization at home).

Box 12-13 Methods of Disinfection and Sterilization

PHYSICAL METHOD

1. Steam under pressure, or moist heat, is the most practical and dependable method for destruction of all microorganisms. This process is called sterilization. Examples of sterilization equipment are the autoclave, which is used in hospitals and other agencies, and the pressure cooker, which is used in a home environment.
2. Boiling water is the best method for home use and is the least expensive. However, this technique will not destroy bacterial spores and some viruses. It is necessary to boil the article for a minimum of 15 to 20 minutes for disinfection.
3. Radiation is used to sterilize pharmaceutical goods, foods, and heat-sensitive items. It is extremely effective on articles that are difficult to sterilize by other methods.
4. Dry heat is a method used for disinfecting articles that are destroyed by moisture. Health agencies seldom use this method, but in the home an article can be disinfected by being placed in the oven for 2 hours at 320° F or for 45 minutes at 350° F.

CHEMICAL PROCESS

1. Gas (ethylene oxide) is used for sterilization. It destroys spores formed by bacteria.
2. Chemical solutions are often used to disinfect instruments because they are effective in destroying microorganisms. One way to store clinical thermometers is in a chemical solution, and some articles are soaked in a solution to prepare them for another, more definitive method of disinfection or sterilization.

Patient Teaching

Disinfection and Sterilization at Home

- Teach the patient about using an oven or a pressure cooker for sterilization.
- Teach the patient that microwaves are widely used.
- Teach the patient that exposure to sunlight is helpful.
- Teach the patient about destroying microorganisms by boiling contaminated articles.

pounds. Chlorine bleach is useful for household disinfecting and in disinfection of water, but it is important never to mix it with ammonia because of the resulting emission of toxic fumes. Chlorine bleach has a tendency to corrode some metals. Iodine is a good bactericidal agent (i.e., it kills bacteria but not spores). Iodine leaves behind stains and is not used as widely as it once was.

Meticulous physical cleaning is required to precede both high-level disinfection and sterilization. Visible pieces of contamination (tissue, blood) will prevent disinfection or sterilization from occurring. Expect high-level disinfection and sterilization to destroy vegetative (those substances of or pertaining to the plant kingdom) microorganisms, most fungal spores, tubercle bacilli, and some viruses (see Skill 12-10).

PATIENT TEACHING FOR INFECTION PREVENTION AND CONTROL

Patients and families often have to learn to use infection prevention and control practices at home. Aseptic technique becomes almost second nature to the nurse, who practices it daily. However, the patient is less aware of the factors that promote the spread of infection or of the ways to prevent its transmission. You will be obliged to educate patients about the nature of infection and the techniques to use in planning or controlling its spread (Patient Teaching [p. 281], Life Span Considerations for Older Adults, and Cultural Considerations [p. 304] boxes regarding infection control).

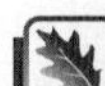

Life Span Considerations

Older Adults

Infection Prevention and Control

- The older adult experiences an alteration in integrity of the oral mucosa. Promote careful oral hygiene and stress regular dental care.
- The older adult experiences a decrease in the production of digestive acid. Teach the older patient to carefully wash hands before food preparation, to adequately cook foods, and to refrigerate unused portions promptly.
- The dermal and epidermal skin layers of the older adult become thinner, and elasticity is decreased. Turn the bedridden patient frequently, and carefully observe the skin for impairment.
- The older adult experiences urethral stricture, neurogenic bladder, and prostatic enlargement. In the older patient with an indwelling Foley catheter, assess for adequate drainage and maintain cleanliness of the urethra and the perineal area.
- Older adults experience a decrease in ribcage movement during inspiration. In caring for older adults postoperatively, elevate the head of the bed (if indicated) and encourage the patient to cough and breathe deeply and to get out of bed as soon as possible to prevent postoperative complications such as hypostatic pneumonia.

INFECTION PREVENTION AND CONTROL FOR HOME AND HOSPICE SETTINGS

Patients are now commonly discharged from acute care to home care sooner than in the past. Thus they often require care from home health personnel. Infections that develop within 30 days after discharge, such as a wound infection at an operative site, are at times an outcome of hospitalization, and the hospital infection preventionist needs to receive a report of them. As more patients elect to die at home, care for the dying will make similar care and reporting measures necessary in more cases. The epidemiologic (pertaining to the study of the occurrence, distribution, and causes of disease in humankind) basis of infections developing in homes is sometimes of a

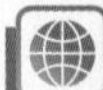

Cultural Considerations

Infection Prevention and Control

- Cultural heritage affects all dimensions of health. It is vital to consider cultural background when teaching patients measures related to infection prevention and control.
- The way that culture influences behaviors, attitudes, and values depends on many factors and thus is often not the same for individual members of a cultural group.
- Clean water is a difficult commodity for the Alaskan Eskimo to obtain reliably. In some villages on the ocean, it is necessary to bring in drinking water as ice from several miles upriver. In this process, the chunks of ice destined for human consumption are often handled by many people and must then be melted, boiled, and cooled.
- Japanese Americans believe that disease is caused by contact with polluting agents such as blood, corpses, and skin diseases, which accounts for their emphasis on cleanliness.
- The germ theory can be confusing to Vietnamese individuals, who have no knowledge of this concept. Many patients with animistic beliefs (a belief in the existence of spirits and demons) have a supernatural or spirit world disease-cause manner of thinking. In an effort to move the patient's understanding into the scientific or natural world, germs are presented as the cause of disease because they are part of the Western world. For all practical purposes, however, germs are not visible and are far less real to the individual with animistic beliefs than the spirits and demons that the patient knows are able to cause trouble.
- Jewish people have incorporated certain everyday habits into laws of observance. Usually these represent good hygiene or have been proven to be medically sound practices. For example, they wash hands on awakening from sleep, after elimination of bodily wastes, after hair cutting, after touching a vermin (insects and small animals such as rats or weasels), after being close to a dead body, and before eating or drinking.
- The Cajun people believe in faith healing and are less likely to take preventive health measures.

community-wide nature. Thus the patient may develop influenza, an enteric infection, or a streptococcal pharyngitis as it passes through the community.

As home care and hospice programs continue to expand, questions about infection prevention and control in these settings are emerging. The reliability of hospital infection rates depends directly on accurate attribution of the source of infection. Such accuracy tends to be problematic when rapid hospital discharges leave unclear the source of an infection. Hospitalized patients need to receive education and instruction at discharge about reporting to appropriate personnel the occurrence of any signs and symptoms of infection such as pain, erythema (redness), edema (swelling), drainage or exudate, and fever (Health Promotion box).

❖ NURSING PROCESS

The role of the licensed practical nurse/licensed vocational nurse (LPN/LVN) in the nursing process as stated is that the LPN/LVN will:

- Participate in planning care for patients based on patient needs

Health Promotion

Prevention of Infection in the Home Setting

The basic principles of hygiene are important to prevent the spread of infection in the home setting: bathing; not sharing personal articles such as combs, toothbrushes, razors, and washcloths; and covering one's mouth when coughing and sneezing. Patient education as to the risk of spreading hospital-acquired organisms to family or friends is very important, especially when family members will be assisting at home in changing dressings, intravenous infusions, or incontinent patients' diapers.

Other principles include the following:

- **Hand hygiene.** Wash hands after using the bathroom, after contact with any secretions, before eating, and before and after patient care. Use warm water, soap, and friction for 15 to 30 seconds, and dry hands thoroughly.
- **Food preparation.** Do not have any person with an infectious gastrointestinal disease prepare food until symptoms resolve. Do not thaw and then refreeze foods. Make sure to store cooked foods immediately in clean containers in the refrigerator. Wash hands before food preparation. Using a dishwasher or washing dishes in hot soapy water decreases the risk of contamination.
- **Tube feedings.** Prepare enough formula for only 8 hours (commercially prepared) or 4 hours (home prepared). Contaminated enteral feeding will sometimes cause salmonella or stapylococcal infections. Cleanse or replace feeding bag and tubing per manufacturer's recommendations.
- **Linens.** Wash linens that are contaminated with blood or body fluids separately in hot, soapy water using 1 cup of bleach per load, and dry them in a dryer on the hot cycle.
- **Waste containers.** Keep waste containers available in the patient contact area for the disposal of dressings, diapers, tissues, and other disposable items. Place a sturdy bag inside the waste container to prevent spilling and leakage. Flush body fluids such as urine, vomitus, feces, and blood down the toilet.
- **Body fluid spills.** Clean up any accidental body fluid spill as soon as possible, while wearing gloves. To disinfect, spray a solution of 1 cup of bleach diluted with 10 cups of water over the spill, and clean up with paper towels. Then place the paper towels in the plastic-lined waste container.

- Review patient's plan of care and recommend revisions as needed
- Review and follow defined prioritization for patient care
- Use clinical pathways, care maps, or care plans to guide and review patient care

Assessment

By evaluating signs and symptoms revealed during assessment, you are able to determine whether a patient's clinical condition indicates a risk for infection. Early recognition of infection will help you in making a correct nursing diagnosis and thus establishing an appropriate treatment plan. Also consider how well the patient is adjusting to the disease and what, if any, are the needs for resources to assist in the management of health problems. Including the patient's family is also important: How does the infection affect them?

Assess laboratory data as soon as available. Laboratory values such as increased white blood cell count or a positive blood culture often indicate infection. When assessing laboratory data, consider the age of the patient. For example, in the older adult, smaller amounts of bacteria such as *Salmonella* have potential to cause gastrointestinal infections because of the decrease in bactericidal gastric acids and deterioration of the mucosal layer of the stomach.

Sometimes positive laboratory results indicate the patient's risk for infection and the need to use barrier precautions or isolation. In this case, consult the infection preventionist or refer to the facility's infection prevention and control policy manual.

Nursing Diagnosis

The selection of a nursing diagnosis is based on data collected during assessment. Possible nursing diagnoses for patients susceptible to or affected by an infection include the following:

- Impaired tissue integrity
- Risk for infection (Nursing Care Plan 12-1)
- Social isolation

Expected Outcomes and Planning

The plan of care focuses on achieving specific goals and outcomes related to the nursing diagnoses chosen. Interventions are determined with the aid of the patient, the family, the physician, and other members of the health care team. These goals and outcomes possibly include the following:

Goal 1: Transmission of infectious organism is prevented.

Outcome: Patient does not experience onset of health care–associated infection.

Goal 2: Progress of infection is controlled or decreased.

Outcome: Inflammation or signs and symptoms over an involved site decrease in 5 days.

Implementation

Your role is to prevent the onset and spread of infection and promote measures for treatment. By recognizing and assessing a patient's risk factors and implementing appropriate measures, you have the capacity to reduce the risk of infections. Appropriate measures to include are good hand hygiene techniques and the proper use of sterile supplies and barrier protection. If

Nursing Care Plan 12-1 The Patient with an Infection

This care plan has been adopted for the patient who is at risk for infection. Mr. Russell is a 68-year-old male in the nursing unit for 8-hour postop care after bowel resection. He has intravenous fluids infusing and a urethral catheter in place.

NURSING DIAGNOSIS ***Risk for infection, related to presence of abdominal incision, intravenous devices, age, presence of indwelling urinary catheter***

Patient Goals and Expected Outcomes	Nursing Intervention	Evaluation
Patient remains free of infection as evidenced by normal vital signs and absence of purulent drainage from abdominal incision, tubes, and catheter	Assess for presence or existence of risk factors such as abdominal incision, indwelling catheter, and venous or arterial devices Monitor white blood count (WBC) Monitor the following for signs and symptoms of infection: Erythema (redness) Edema (swelling) Increased pain Purulent exudates (drainage) at incision, exit sites of IV, Foley catheter Elevated temperature Color of respiratory secretions Appearance of urine	Patient demonstrates understanding of necessary precautions to prevent infection Patient remains free of infection

Continued

Nursing Care Plan 12-1 The Patient with an Infection—cont'd

Patient Goals and Expected Outcomes	Nursing Intervention	Evaluation
Patient remains free of infection as evidenced by normal vital signs and absence of purulent drainage from abdominal incision, tubes, and catheter—cont'd	Assess nutritional status Perform asepsis for wound care, catheter care, and IV access management Maintain hand hygiene before patient contact and between procedures with patient Encourage diet and fluid intake (contact dietitian as necessary) Encourage coughing and deep breathing; consider use of incentive spirometer Teach patient and family how to perform hand hygiene correctly	

Critical Thinking Questions

1. Mr. Russell has a peripheral IV infusing and complains of discomfort at the site of insertion. What should the nurse do?
2. Mr. Russell has a urinary catheter connected to continuous drainage. He complains of burning at the site of insertion and the nurse notes dark, concentrated urine in the tubing. What should the nurse do next?
3. The nurse notes on the sheet of laboratory results for the patient that his WBC count is 10,000/mm^3. Why is this a concern, and what is recommended as a precautionary measure?

the patient does develop an infection, you will want to continue these interventions to ensure that health care personnel and other patients are not exposed to the pathogenic organism.

Evaluation

The success of the nurse who practices infection prevention and control techniques is measured according to the extent to which the goals are achieved for reducing or preventing infection. Evaluation is by nature ongoing because a patient's condition can change at any time. You are then in a position to decide to continue nursing interventions, revise them as necessary, or determine that the problem has been resolved. This will be accomplished by referring to the goals and outcomes identified when planning care.

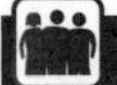

Coordinated Care

Delegation

INFECTION PREVENTION AND CONTROL

Hand hygiene or antisepsis involves a set of basic procedures that all caregivers are obliged to perform correctly. If you observe other caregivers or family caregivers cleanse their hands incorrectly, reinforce the importance of the correct technique and procedural steps.

Observe the consistency and thoroughness of staff in washing or disinfecting hands.

Applying disposable gloves is a basic procedure that should be performed correctly by assistive personnel (AP). If you observe AP failing to use gloves when necessary, reinforce the importance of the procedure.

It is acceptable to delegate to AP basic care procedures (e.g., bathing and feeding) that are performed under transmission-based isolation precautions. You are responsible for assessing whether it is more effective to provide direct care or delegate care activities, depending on the patient's clinical status. Procedures such as medication administration and care of intravenous (IV) lines require the application of critical thinking knowledge unique to the nurse.

Clarify for the AP the type of isolation precautions to use (see Figures 12-6 through 12-8).

It is acceptable to delegate to AP basic care procedures (e.g., bathing and feeding) that are performed under airborne infection isolation (see Skill 12-5). You are responsible for assessing whether it is more effective to provide direct care or delegate care activities, depending on the patient's clinical status. Procedures such as medication administration and care of IV lines require the critical thinking and knowledge application unique to the nurse.

Clarify for AP special precautions in use of a fitted respirator mask.

Nurses generally perform procedures requiring sterile technique and do not delegate them to AP. In some settings, AP (surgical technicians) are specifically trained to perform sterile technique under the supervision of a nurse. Check agency policy. The AP can help you in the circulating nurse role by opening sterile supplies (see Box 12-11), setting up a sterile field (see Skill 12-7), and running errands under your direction.

Goal 1: Transmission of infectious organisms is controlled.

Evaluative measures: Assess patient's temperature; observe wound sites for erythema, edema, tenderness, or exudate.

Goal 2: Progression of infection is controlled or decreased.

Evaluative measures: Inspect size of inflamed area over consecutive intervals; gently palpate involved site to note reduction in tenderness.

See the Coordinated Care box for infection prevention and control procedures.

Get Ready for the NCLEX® Examination!

Key Points

- The mucous membranes of the respiratory, gastrointestinal, and genitourinary tracts provide primary defense against pathogenic microorganisms, as does intact skin.
- An infection has potential to develop as long as the six elements composing the infectious chain are uninterrupted.
- A microorganism's virulence depends on its ability to resist attack by the body's normal defenses.
- Age, poor nutrition, stress, inherited conditions, chronic disease, and treatments or conditions that compromise the immune system increase susceptibility to infection.
- The signs of local inflammation and infection are similar, but it is possible for the inflammatory response to occur in the absence of an infectious process.
- Surgical asepsis requires more stringent techniques than medical asepsis and is directed toward eliminating all microorganisms and their spores.
- Contamination of a sterile object or field occurs when it comes into contact with a wet surface that contains microorganisms or when it is exposed to airborne microorganisms.
- The CDC recommends that health care workers consider all patients as infectious and to use standard precautions to reduce the risk of exposure to blood and body fluids.
- Following aseptic principles is the key to a nurse's success in preventing patients from acquiring infection.
- Do not take an article (e.g., sphygmomanometer or blood pressure cuff) into an isolation room if the article is to be used by another patient.
- Lack of proper hand hygiene is the main cause of the spread of infections.
- An infection preventionist monitors the incidence of infections within an institution and provides educational and consultative services to maintain aseptic practices to staff, patients, and their caregivers.
- Isolation transmission-based precautions are used to prevent personnel and patients from acquiring infections and prevent transmission of microorganisms to other persons.
- Wearing gloves, gowns, and masks in combination with eye protection devices such as goggles or glasses with solid side shields is mandatory when contact with blood or potentially infectious material is possible or whenever splashing or spraying of blood or potentially infectious material is possible.
- The restricted environment subjects a patient in transmission-based isolation to psychological and emotional deprivation.
- Standard precautions are used to prevent the spread of organisms present in blood, all other body fluids, nonintact skin, and mucous membranes.
- Standard precautions are used with all patients since it is often unknown which patients have an infection. This includes the use of barrier protection when appropriate.
- If the skin is broken or if you perform an invasive procedure into a body cavity normally free of microorganisms, surgical aseptic practices are followed.
- The major sites for health care–associated infections include the urinary and respiratory tracts, the bloodstream, and surgical or traumatic wounds.
- You need to be a role model and keep up to date with your own immunizations, as well as teaching your patients to do so.
- Proper cleansing requires mechanical removal of all foreign materials from an object or area.
- Cultural influences play a major role in patient education and follow-up care.

Additional Learning Resources

Go to your Companion CD for an audio glossary, animations, video clips, and more.

evolve Be sure to visit the Evolve site at http://evolve.elsevier.com/Christensen/foundations/ for additional online resources.

Review Questions for the NCLEX® Examination

1. A 24-year-old was admitted to a medical unit with the diagnosis of hepatitis A and placed in contact isolation. The purpose of this is to:
   1. prevent transmission of infectious microorganisms.
   2. control the environment of the patient.
   3. protect the patient from infectious microorganisms.
   4. protect only the family.

2. The nurse is working in a clinical medical area with a census of 15. Each patient has a different illness. The most important skill the nurse can use to protect each patient from health care–associated infections is:
   1. wearing a gown.
   2. placing each patient in isolation.
   3. hand hygiene.
   4. wearing gloves.

3. The nurse caring for the patient in isolation wears latex gloves. Which is an important consideration?
   1. First assess the patient for potential latex allergy.
   2. Vinyl gloves actually provide higher barrier protection than latex.
   3. The cost of latex gloves is significantly higher than that of synthetic gloves.
   4. Latex gloves are so reliable as barriers that hand hygiene is not required.

4. The nurse notes that the patient understands proper technique for hand hygiene when the patient states:
   1. "The water I wash my hands with should be as hot as I can tolerate to kill all of the germs on my skin."
   2. "If there isn't time to completely wash my hands, it will be all right to rinse them quickly in warm water."
   3. "After washing my hands with soap for at least 15 seconds, I will rinse them thoroughly under running water."
   4. "I will put soap into a basin of warm water, lather my hands for 15 seconds, and then rinse them in the basin."

5. Identification of the chain of infection allows health care providers to:
   1. test patients for resistance to communicable diseases.
   2. request more money for building isolation hospitals.
   3. work with the physician to identify the most appropriate antibiotic.
   4. determine points at which the infection can be stopped or prevented.

6. A patient in isolation is experiencing signs of social deprivation. Which intervention by the nurse is appropriate?
   1. Allow visitors to remove masks while in the patient's room.
   2. Leave the door of the negative-pressure room open slightly.
   3. Remind the patient that the isolation is for his or her own benefit.
   4. Set specific times when the nurse will return to the patient's room.

7. A 45-year-old man was admitted to the hospital with cellulitis of the right foot. Three days later, he developed bacterial pneumonia. This type of bacterial infection is classified as:
   1. acute primary.
   2. health care–associated.
   3. interstitial.
   4. mycoplasmic.

8. Which statement is true of sterile technique?
   1. Sterilization is the practice that helps confine or reduce the number of microorganisms.
   2. When an item has been disinfected, it is to be considered sterile.
   3. Recently opened wrappers are considered sterile to within 1 inch of their edges.
   4. Surgical asepsis and clean technique are the same.

9. Because sterile technique is used in many procedures of patient care, it is important for the nurse to remember to hold sterile objects:
   1. close to shoulder level.
   2. just below waist level.
   3. anywhere as long as they are handled with sterile gloves.
   4. above waist level.

10. Although surgical asepsis is practiced in the operating room and in other specialty areas, the nurse will at times also use surgical aseptic technique at the patient's bedside. For which procedure will the nurse employ surgical asepsis?
    1. Inserting an IV
    2. Performing perineal care
    3. Performing oral care
    4. Obtaining a sputum specimen

11. The nurse is performing a surgical hand scrub. During a surgical hand scrub, the hands are held:
    1. above the elbows.
    2. with the fingers pointing downward.
    3. whichever way is convenient.
    4. just below the waist.

12. To practice strict surgical asepsis, the nurse will:
    1. adhere to principles of sterile technique.
    2. perform routine environmental cleaning.
    3. disinfect surfaces that come into contact with body fluids.
    4. maintain proper hand hygiene before and after patient care.

13. When donning sterile gloves, the nurse will:
    1. touch only the inside surface of the first glove while pulling it onto the hand.
    2. place the fingers of the dominant hand into the outside cuff of the first glove.
    3. let the cuff of the glove roll up over the hand as it is being pulled onto the hand.
    4. begin the procedure by pulling the first glove upward and over the nondominant hand.

14. To remove gloves at the end of a procedure, the nurse will:
    1. pull each finger from each of the gloves first, then roll the glove back over the hand.
    2. remove the glove from the nondominant hand by reaching inside the glove and pulling it off.
    3. remove one glove, then use the bare fingers to push the remaining glove off from inside the cuff.
    4. hold both gloved hands under running water and roll the gloves down to keep microorganisms contained.

15. Which is a principle of surgical asepsis?
    1. Any sterilized item is considered unsterile once it is allowed to fall below knee height.
    2. Sterile fields and sterilized items are no longer sterile if they contact a clean surface.
    3. A person not wearing sterile garments can come no closer to a sterile field than 3 feet.
    4. The front and back of a sterile gown being worn are considered sterile from shoulders to knees.

16. A patient isolated for pulmonary tuberculosis seems to be angry, but the nurse knows this is a normal response to isolation. The best intervention would be to:
    1. provide a dark, quiet room to calm the patient.
    2. explain isolation procedures and provide meaningful stimulation.
    3. reduce the level of precautions to keep the patient from becoming angry.
    4. limit family and other caregiver visits to reduce the risk of spreading the infection.

17. After administering care to a patient, the nurse needs to remove a tray of soiled instruments from the room and "bag" the materials. Some of the items are metal, whereas others are made of plastic. The nurse knows that:
    1. it is acceptable to place everything into one bag as long as it is labeled properly.
    2. it is necessary to bag the metal items and send them for autoclaving, and acceptable to dispose of the plastic items.
    3. it is necessary to separate the items: plastic goes into one bag for gas sterilization, and metal into another to be autoclaved.
    4. the type of bag doesn't matter as long as it is labeled "isolation."

18. The nurse is assisting the physician with an irrigation of a draining abdominal wound by preparing the sterile tray. It is necessary to maintain sterility of the tray at all times. During the process the nurse will:
    1. use sterile forceps while reaching across it to move the contents around.
    2. wear clean gloves to handle the contents of the tray.
    3. allow the open tray to stand unattended for 20 minutes, then cover it with a towel.
    4. put on sterile gloves to handle the contents of the tray.

19. The nurse is assigned to represent the unit on the infection prevention and control committee. The committee is discussing the CDC's hand hygiene recommendations for implementation in the hospital. Which statement demonstrates an understanding of the CDC's recommendation?
    1. Health care providers will wear gloves at all times when providing patient care.
    2. Disinfecting hands following glove removal is not necessary.
    3. Alcohol-based hand cleaner is effective on hands that are not visibly soiled with blood and body fluids.
    4. It is necessary to remove waterless alcohol-based hand cleaner with paper towels to remove pathogens from hands.

20. The nurse just completed a sterile dressing change on a patient's postoperative incision, and is preparing to measure the patient's vital signs. In regard to the gloves worn during application of the sterile dressing, the nurse should:
    1. leave the gloves on, since they are sterile, and measure the vital signs.
    2. remove the gloves, and perform hand hygiene before measuring the vital signs.
    3. remove the gloves, and leave the room to perform hand hygiene.
    4. remove the gloves, measure the vital signs, and then perform hand hygiene.

21. The nurse will wear a gown during care of an infected wound for any patient in this type of isolation:
    1. airborne precautions.
    2. droplet precautions.
    3. contact precautions.
    4. TB precautions.

22. The nurse is preparing to change the tracheostomy ties on a patient. Which precaution would necessitate wearing a mask?
    1. Airborne precautions
    2. Droplet precautions
    3. Contact precautions
    4. Standard precautions

23. The nurse is preparing to open the outer sterile wrap of a Foley (indwelling catheter) tray. Which flap of the wrap (in which direction) should be opened first?
    1. The flap that opens away from the nurse
    2. The flap that opens to the left
    3. The flap that opens to the right
    4. The flap that opens toward the nurse

24. The patient asks the nurse how his skin will be sterilized before his surgery. The nurse's best response is:
    1. "We will use alcohol to sterilize your skin."
    2. "It is not possible to sterilize skin, but we will use an antimicrobial solution to eliminate most microorganisms."
    3. "There are a series of steps used in sterilizing your skin in order to prevent you from getting an infection."
    4. "We will use Betadine solution to sterilize your skin."

chapter

13 Surgical Wound Care

evolve

http://evolve.elsevier.com/Christensen/foundationsadult

Elaine Oden Kockrow

Objectives

1. Discuss the body's response during each stage of wound healing.
2. Discuss the role of nutrition in wound healing.
3. Identify common complications of wound healing
4. Differentiate between healing by primary and secondary intention.
5. Discuss the classification of wounds according to the Centers for Disease Control and Prevention.
6. Discuss the factors that impair wound healing and the interventions for each type of wound.
7. Explain procedure for applying dry dressings: wet-to-dry dressings.
8. Discuss dehiscence and evisceration and the nursing care they involve.
9. Identify the procedure for removing sutures and staples.
10. Discuss care of the patient with a wound drainage system: Hemovac or Davol suction, T-tube drainage.
11. Identify procedure for performing sterile wound irrigation.
12. Identify the nursing interventions for the patient with vacuum-assisted closure (VAC) of a wound.
13. Describe the purposes of and precautions taken when applying bandages and binders.
14. List nursing diagnoses associated with wound care.

Key Terms

bandage (p. 333)
binder (p. 334)
dehiscence (dē-HĬS-ĕns, p. 338)
drainage (p. 325)
evisceration (ē-vĭs-ŭr-Ā-shŭn, p. 338)
exudate (ĔKS-ū-dāt, p. 311)
granulation (grăn-ū-LĀ-shŭn, p. 311)
incision (ĭn-SĬZH-ŭn, p. 310)
infectious process (p. 314)
inflammatory response (p. 314)
irrigation (p. 321)
primary intention (p. 311)
puncture (p. 310)
purulent (PYŪ-rū-lĕnt, p. 311)
sanguineous (săng-GWĬN-ē-ŭs, p. 314)
secondary intention (p. 311)
serosanguineous (SĒR-ō-săng-GWĬN-ē-ŭs, p. 314)
serous (SĒR-ŭs, p. 314)
T-tube (p. 329)
tertiary intention (TŬR-shē-ăr-ē, p. 311)
vacuum-assisted closure (p. 330)
wound (p. 310)

The term **wound** refers to any injury to the body's tissues involving a break in the skin. Injury results in either an open or closed wound; whether the injury is intentional or unintentional does not make any difference in its classification or treatment. Promoting wound healing is the nursing focus during the postsurgical recovery phase. Various stresses affect a wound's ability to repair itself. Stress and strain (nausea, vomiting, abdominal distention, coughing, respiratory efforts) place tension against a surgical incision, especially an abdominal incision. During this phase, the abdominal muscles contract and cause intraabdominal pressure; if the incisional area is weak, dehiscence is possible. As the postoperative period lengthens, patient-related factors influence wound healing: age, nutritional status, physical condition, preexisting health problems (e.g., diabetes), and medication habits. Other factors that have the capacity to affect wound healing include preoperative skin preparation, type of surgical procedure, environment within the surgical suite, and postoperative wound care.

WOUND CLASSIFICATION

Wound classifications derive from their cause, the severity of injury, the amount of contamination, or the skin's integrity. It is vitally important to understand the causative factors of a wound to determine the proper treatment plan. Obtain a complete history, including what caused the wound and any underlying disease process.

In planned surgery, the practitioner makes a wound by **incision** (a cut produced surgically by a sharp instrument creating an opening into an organ or space in the body) or **puncture** (stab wound for a drainage system); the surgical wound is usually closed or managed (e.g., a drain inserted, a stoma created) in the final stage of the procedure. By contrast, in traumatic injury (e.g., from a knife stabbing) and unplanned or emergency surgeries, the practitioner brings wound edges together to aid healing. Unless a "dirty surgery" is performed (e.g., a perforated bowel, ruptured appendix), a surgical incision is cleaner and easier to repair than a traumatic wound.

The Centers for Disease Control (CDC, 1985) classify wounds according to the amount of contamination involved: clean, clean-contaminated, contaminated, and dirty or infected. A clean wound is an uninfected surgical wound; the chance of an infection occurring postoperatively is less than 5%. A surgical incision made into the respiratory, the gastrointestinal (GI), or the genitourinary tract after special presurgical preparation is called a clean-contaminated wound. The likelihood that an infection will occur postoperatively in a clean-contaminated wound is between 3% and 11%. A contaminated wound results from the presence of GI products (e.g., feces with *Escherichia coli* in the colon); from an acute, nonpurulent inflammation (e.g., inflamed appendix); or when aseptic technique is broken during surgery (e.g., scalpel is reused after incising a contaminated area). A wound infection occurs 10% to 17% of the time from a contaminated wound. Dirty or infected wounds have a 27% chance of causing a wound infection. Wounds in this category (e.g., gangrenous toe) are infected before surgery.

WOUND HEALING

The healing process begins immediately after an injury and sometimes continues for a year or longer. Although the healing process follows the same pattern, the type of wound and tissue, the wound's severity, and the overall condition of the patient influence the overall process. Wound healing follows four phases: hemostasis, inflammatory phase, reconstruction, and maturation.

PHASES OF WOUND HEALING

Hemostasis (termination of bleeding) begins as soon as the injury occurs. As blood platelets adhere to the walls of the injured vessel, a clot begins to form. Fibrin in the clot begins to hold the wound together, and bleeding subsides.

During the inflammatory phase, there is an initial increase in the flow of blood elements (antibodies, electrolytes, plasma proteins) and water out of the blood vessel into the vascular space. This process causes the cardinal signs and symptoms of inflammation: erythema (redness), heat, edema (swelling), pain, and tissue dysfunction. Leukocytes appear and begin to engulf bacteria, fungi, viruses, and toxic proteins. If an infection is not present, the number of leukocytes decreases. During the inflammatory phase, cells in the injured tissue migrate, divide, and form new cells. Slowly, blood clots dissolve and the wound fills; the sides of the wound usually meet in 24 to 48 hours. As the inflammatory phase ends, new cells and capillaries fill in the wound from the underlying tissue to the skin surface. This process seals the wound and protects it from contamination.

Collagen formation occurs during the reconstruction phase. This phase begins on the third or fourth day after injury and lasts for 2 to 3 weeks. Fibroblasts produce collagen, a gluelike protein substance that adds tensile strength to the wound and the tissue. Collagen formation increases rapidly between postoperative days 5 and 25. During this phase, the wound takes on the appearance of an irregular, raised, purplish, immature scar. During this time, encourage the patient to consume foods rich in protein and vitamins A and C, which assist in wound repair. If a patient is not well nourished, the physician sometimes orders nutrient supplements. Wound dehiscence most frequently occurs during the reconstruction phase.

Approximately 3 weeks after surgery, fibroblasts begin to exit the wound. The wound continues to gain strength, although healed wounds rarely return to the strength the tissue had before surgery. Although tissue heals at varying speeds, internal wounds (stomach, colon) regain strength faster than skin wounds. Occasionally a keloid, which is an overgrowth of collagenous scar tissue at the site of a wound, will form during this maturation phase. The keloid's color ranges from red to pink to white. This new tissue is elevated, rounded, and firm. African-Americans, dark-complexioned whites, and young women have the highest incidence of keloid formation. Therapy sometimes worsens the condition; only skilled professionals are qualified to perform it.

PROCESS OF WOUND HEALING

The process of wound healing occurs by primary intention (primary union), secondary intention (granulation), or tertiary (third) intention (Figure 13-1). Wounds in which skin edges are close together and little tissue is lost, such as those made surgically, heal by **primary intention;** minimal scarring results. Primary intention healing begins during the inflammatory phase of healing; in surgery this is usually during closure of the wound.

Healing by **secondary intention,** when a wound must granulate during healing, occurs when skin edges are not close together (approximated) or when pus has formed. Some wounds develop a **purulent** (producing or containing pus) **exudate** (fluid, cells, or other substances that have been slowly exuded, or discharged, from cells or blood through small pores or breaks in cell membranes) when injured or diseased tissue dies. In this case, the surgeon provides a means for its release through a drainage system or by packing the wound with gauze. Slowly the necrotized tissue decomposes and escapes, and the cavity begins to fill with **granulation** tissue, or soft, pink, fleshy projections consisting of capillaries surrounded by fibrous collagen. The amount of granulation tissue required to fill the wound depends on the wound's size; scarring is greater in a large wound.

In healing by **tertiary intention** (delayed primary intention), the practitioner leaves a contaminated wound

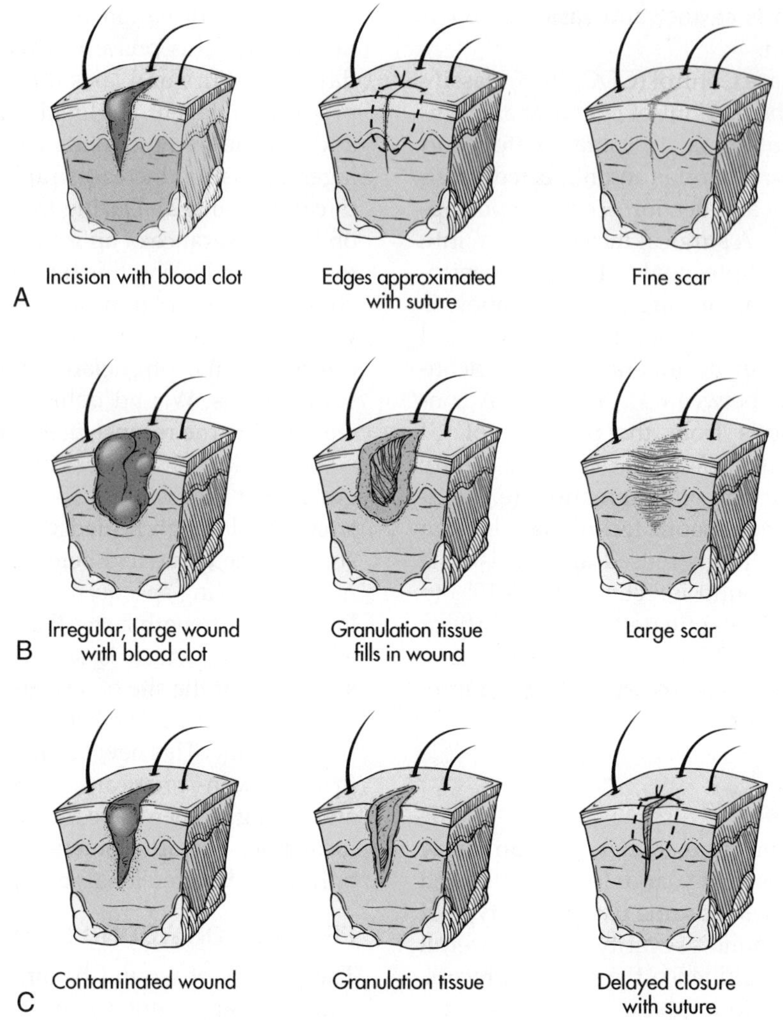

FIGURE 13-1 Types of wound healing. **A,** Primary intention. **B,** Secondary intention. **C,** Tertiary intention.

open and closes it later, after the infection is controlled, by suturing two layers of granulation tissue together in the wound. It also occurs when a primary wound becomes infected, is opened, is allowed to granulate, and is then sutured. Tertiary intention healing results in a larger and deeper scar than healing by primary or secondary intention.

These stages provide a model for acute (as opposed to chronic) wound healing. An important concept in wound healing is that the stages of wound healing, although progressive, do not necessarily occur in a linear (strictly sequential) fashion. Some normally healing wounds are in all three stages of wound healing simultaneously.

FACTORS THAT AFFECT WOUND HEALING

To promote healing, closely monitor fluid and nutritional needs (i.e., proteins, carbohydrates, fats, vitamins) of the patient. If the patient is not able to tolerate food or fluids, provision of total parenteral nutrition or nasogastric feedings is a possibility. Because patients are often unable to tolerate large meals or solid foods, dietary services will provide small frequent feedings. Offer fluids, when tolerated, on an hourly basis. Unless there are contraindications, encourage an intake of 2000 to 2400 mL in 24 hours. As the patient progresses from clear to full liquids, provide fluids the patient enjoys. Until the patient's hydration level is stable (usually 24 to 72 hours), monitor the patient's intake and output (I&O).

Assist the patient to achieve a balance between rest as a means to facilitate healing and activity to decrease venous stasis. When the patient is confined to bed, encourage him or her to move one body section at a time—head, chest, hips, legs. To sit up, the patient should roll to the side and, using the elbow as a lever, push to a sitting position; this reduces the stress placed on the incision. If coughing occurs, apply a pillow, rolled bath blanket, or the palms of the hands to the incisional area to lessen intraabdominal pressure; this technique is called *splinting*. It is sometimes necessary to limit visitors if the patient tires too easily.

Preexisting conditions, such as heart murmurs, and chronic diseases (arthritis, diabetes mellitus, hypertension) add stress to the recovering body and necessitate ongoing monitoring (Table 13-1).

Table 13-1 **Factors that Impair Wound Healing**

PHYSIOLOGICAL EFFECTS	INTERVENTIONS
AGE	
Aging alters all phases of wound healing. Vascular changes impair circulation to wound site. Reduced liver function alters synthesis of clotting factors. Inflammatory response is slowed. Formation of antibodies and lymphocytes is reduced. Collagen tissue is less pliable. Scar tissue is less elastic.	Instruct patient on safety precautions to prevent injuries. Be prepared to provide wound care for longer period. Teach home caregivers wound care techniques (see Patient Teaching box on p. 339).
MALNUTRITION	
All phases of wound healing are impaired. Stress from burns or severe trauma increases nutritional requirements.	Provide balanced diet rich in protein, carbohydrates, lipids, vitamins A and C, minerals (e.g., zinc, copper), and B vitamins. Provide adequate amounts of calories and fluids.
OBESITY	
Fatty tissue lacks adequate blood supply to resist bacterial infection and deliver nutrients and cellular elements.	Observe obese patient for signs of wound infection, dehiscence, and evisceration.
IMPAIRED OXYGENATION	
Low arterial oxygen tension alters synthesis of collagen and formation of epithelial cells. If local circulating blood flow is poor, tissues fail to receive needed oxygen. Decreased hemoglobin (anemia) reduces arterial oxygen levels in capillaries and interferes with tissue repair.	Provide diet adequate in iron, vitamin B, and folic acid. Monitor hematocrit and hemoglobin levels of patients with wounds.
SMOKING	
Smoking reduces amount of functional hemoglobin in blood, thus decreasing tissue oxygenation. Smoking sometimes increases platelet aggregation and causes hypercoagulability. Smoking interferes with normal cellular mechanisms that promote release of oxygen to tissues.	Discourage patient from smoking by explaining its effects on wound healing.
DRUGS	
Steroids reduce inflammatory response. Antiinflammatory drugs suppress protein synthesis, wound contraction, epithelialization, and inflammation. Prolonged antibiotic use increases risk of superinfection. Chemotherapeutic drugs often depress bone marrow function, number of leukocytes, and inflammatory response.	Carefully observe patient; signs of inflammation are not always obvious. Vitamin A has the capacity to counteract effects of steroids.
DIABETES MELLITUS	
Chronic disease causes small blood vessel disease that impairs tissue perfusion. Diabetes causes hemoglobin to have greater affinity for oxygen, so it fails to release oxygen to tissues. Hyperglycemia alters ability of leukocytes to perform phagocytosis and also supports overgrowth of fungal and yeast infections.	Instruct patient to take preventive measures to avoid cuts or breaks in skin. Provide preventive foot care. Control blood sugar to reduce the physiologic changes associated with diabetes.
RADIATION	
Fibrosis and vascular scarring eventually develop in irradiated skin layers. Tissues become fragile and poorly oxygenated.	Closely observe patients who have had surgery for wound complications.
WOUND STRESS	
Vomiting, abdominal distention, and respiratory effort sometimes stress suture line and potentially disrupt wound layer. Sudden, unexpected tension on incision inhibits formation of endothelial cell and collagen networks.	Control nausea with ordered antiemetics. Keep nasogastric tubes patent and draining to prevent accumulation of secretions. Instruct patient to splint abdominal wound during coughing.

SURGICAL WOUND

The selection of the site for the surgical wound is based on the tissue and the organ(s) involved, the nature of the injury or disease process, the presence of inflammation or infection, and the strength of the site. If a surgical procedure calls for a drainage system, the positioning of the drain will also influence the placement of the incision. The surgeon's goal is to enter the cavity involved and repair the injured or diseased area, as quickly and with the least trauma possible. To facilitate the surgery, patients are often placed in positions that add stress to the tissue. Pain after surgery thus results at times from strained muscles and ligaments, as well as from the surgical process.

Many options are available to the surgeon for closing the surgical incision. Common closures are sutures, staples, Steri-Strips, butterfly strips, and transparent sprays and films. A binder or bandage helps support the incision or secure dressings and makes use of adhesive materials unnecessary. Inspect dressings every 2 to 4 hours for the first 24 hours. The day of surgery, most wounds produce either sanguineous (composed of or pertaining to blood) or serosanguineous (thin and red, composed of serum and blood) exudate. Later, as the exudate subsides, it becomes serous (thin and watery, composed of the serum portion of blood) (Table 13-2). Because pressure to wounds retards bleeding, you will usually keep surgical wounds covered with a gauze dressing. To prevent hemorrhaging from going undetected, it is imperative that you inspect both the dressing or incisional area and the area under the patient. Exudate follows the flow of gravity; therefore, depending on the contour of the body, the dressing will sometimes remain dry even though blood or exudate is flowing away, under the body.

The extent of the inflammatory response (a tissue reaction to injury) depends on the level of injury inflicted, the size of the area involved, and the physical condition of the patient. Gradually, fluid from the cells and leukocytes collect along the vessel walls, and fibrin walls off the injury and provides a matrix along which new cells will form. Leukocytes perform one of their important functions, phagocytosis (a process by which certain cells engulf and dispose of microorganisms and cell debris), by surrounding, engulfing, and digesting exudate from the injured cell. The leukocyte becomes the body's vacuum cleaner by removing its debris. Evidence of leukocyte action is given through changes in the white blood cell (WBC) count. An infectious process (a condition caused by the invasion of the body by pathogenic microorganisms) is usually evidenced by an elevated WBC count.

Table 13-2 Types of Wound Drainage

TYPE	APPEARANCE
A. Serous	Clear, watery plasma
B. Purulent	Thick, yellow, green, tan, or brown
C. Serosanguineous	Pale, red, watery: mixture of serous and sanguineous
D. Sanguineous	Bright red: indicates active bleeding

From Elkin, M.K., Perry, A.G., & Potter, P.A. (2007). *Nursing interventions and clinical skills.* (4th ed.). St. Louis: Mosby.

STANDARD STEPS IN WOUND CARE

All nursing skills include by necessity certain basic steps for the safety and well-being of the patient and the nurse. To save space and minimize repetition, instructions for these steps are not included in the description of each skill unless it is necessary to clarify their application for that skill in particular. Keep the following essential steps in mind and remember to follow them with exactness to deliver appropriate and responsible nursing interventions. As usual for the skills described in this text, the rationale for each step follows each instruction in parentheses.

Before performing the skill:

1. Refer to the medical record, care plan, or Kardex for special interventions. *(Provides basis for care. Many nursing interventions require a physician's order. Verification is ensured when you review the medical record.)*
2. Introduce yourself; include your name and title or role. *(Decreases patient anxiety.)*
3. Identify patient by checking armband and requesting patient to state his or her name. *(Identifies correct patient for procedure.)*
4. Explain the procedure and the reason it is to be done in terms the patient is able to understand,

and give patient time to ask questions. Advise patient of any potential unpleasantness that will be experienced. *(Seeks cooperation, decreases patient's anxiety, and prepares patient. Also helps determine if procedure is still appropriate.)*

5. Assess need for and provide patient teaching during procedure. *(Promotes patient's independence.)*
6. Assess patient. Each skill has an assessment section that includes specific data. *(Provides baseline information for later comparisons.)*
7. Perform hand hygiene and don clean gloves according to agency policy and guidelines from the CDC and the Occupational Safety and Health Administration (OSHA) (see Chapter 12). *(Reduces the spread of microorganisms.)*
8. Assemble equipment and complete necessary charges. *(Organizes procedure. Some equipment is reusable and is kept at the bedside. Some of the equipment is disposable and charged to the patient as used. Know agency policy. Specific equipment is listed for each skill.)*
9. Prepare patient for intervention:
   a. Close door or pull privacy curtain. *(Provides privacy and promotes patient's comfort.)*
   b. Raise bed to comfortable working height; lower side rail on side nearest you. *(Promotes proper body mechanics by minimizing muscle strain on caregivers and preventing injury and fatigue.)*
   c. Position and drape patient as necessary. *(Respect for privacy is basic for preserving human dignity. Patients have the right to privacy. Specific positions are included in each skill.)*

During the skill:

10. Promote patient involvement as possible. *(Participation encourages patient motivation and cooperation.)*
11. Assess patient's tolerance, being alert for signs and symptoms of discomfort and fatigue. Inability to tolerate a procedure is described in the nursing notes. *(Patient's ability to tolerate interventions varies depending on severity of illness and disability. Nurses need to use judgment in providing the opportunity for rest and comfort measures.)*

Completion of procedure:

12. Assist patient to a position of comfort and place needed items within easy reach. Be certain patient has a means to call for assistance and knows how to use it. *(Promotes safety—patients who attempt to reach items not close by risk falling or injury.)*
13. Raise the side rails and lower the bed to the lowest position. *(This reduces the risk of patients getting out of bed unattended. According to your best nursing judgment, allow alert, cooperative patients to have their side rails down during daytime hours without the risk of injury.)*
14. Remove gloves (see Skill 13-3, step 6) and all protective barriers, such as gown, goggles, and masks if worn. Store or remove and dispose of soiled supplies and equipment according to agency policy and guidelines from the CDC and OSHA (see Chapter 12). *(Reduces spread of microorganisms, cleans environment, and enhances patient comfort.)*
15. Perform hand hygiene after patient contact and after removing gloves. *(Wearing gloves does not eliminate the need to wash hands. Hand hygiene is the single most important technique in prevention and control of the spread of microorganisms; see Chapter 12.)*
16. Document patient's response, expected or unexpected outcomes, and patient teaching. *(Timely and proper documentation records patient progress and promotes continuity of care. Recording also fulfills legal responsibility of nurse.)* Specific notes for documentation are included in each skill.
17. Report any unexpected outcomes. *(Additional therapies may be necessary.)* Specific notes for reporting are included in each skill.

CARE OF THE INCISION

Surgical wounds, because they are created under aseptic conditions, generally heal well and quickly. For psychological reasons and to prevent trauma until epithelialization occurs, as well as to keep bleeding and exposure to bacteria to a minimum, the wound is usually covered at least initially by a dressing. Dressings over closed wounds are usually removed by the third day. Some surgeons remove dressings the first postoperative day if no drains are present.

Incision coverings take the form of gauze, semiocclusive, or occlusive dressings (Figure 13-2). Gauze dressings permit air to reach the wound; semiocclusive dressings permit oxygen but not air impurities to pass; and occlusive dressings permit neither air nor oxygen to pass. Occlusive and semiocclusive dressings are thought to promote healing by keeping wounds moist (yet sterile) so epithelial cells are able to slide more easily over the surface of the wound during epithelialization. Sometimes you will use tape, and sometimes ties or bandages and cloth binders, to secure a dressing over a wound site. The choice of anchoring depends on the wound size, the location, the presence of drainage, the frequency of dressing changes, and the patient's level of activity. Montgomery straps, which remain in place around the wound while permitting the dressing over the wound to be changed, are one possibility; they reduce the need for frequent removal and reapplication of tape, which can cause considerable skin irritation (Box 13-1). If an occlusive dressing is used, place tape strips on all sides of the dressing. Otherwise place the tape strips several inches apart to make the wound accessible to atmospheric oxygen.

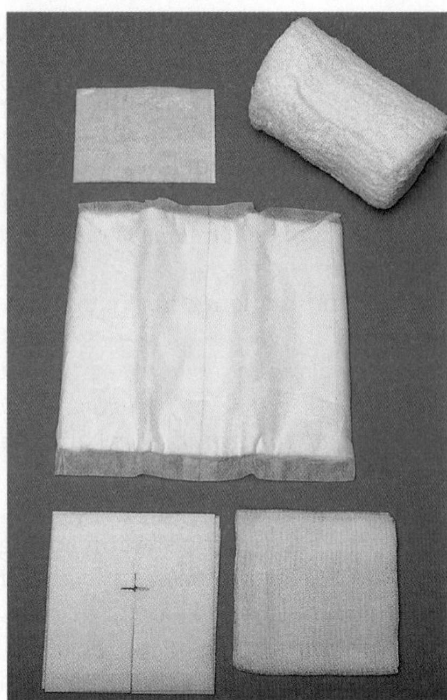

FIGURE 13-2 Types of dressings. Top to bottom: Telfa, rolled gauze, ABD, flat gauze 4 × 4, and drain dressing.

Box 13-1 How to Make Montgomery Straps

Using Montgomery straps to secure dressings helps prevent tape irritation of skin when dressings require frequent changing (see the figure for step 14 in Skill 13-1). If ready-made Montgomery straps are not available, follow these steps to make your own:

1. Cut four to six strips of 2- to 3-inch–wide (5 to 7.6 cm) hypoallergenic tape of sufficient length to allow the tape to extend about 6 inches beyond the wound on each side. (The length of the tape depends on the patient's size and the type and amount of dressing.)
2. Fold each strip 2 to 3 inches back on itself (sticky sides together) to form a nonadhesive tab. Then cut a small hole in the folded tab's center, close to its top edge. Make as many pairs of straps as you will need to snugly secure the dressing.
3. Clean the patient's skin to prevent irritation. After the skin dries, apply skin protectant. Then apply the sticky side of each tape to a skin barrier sheet composed of opaque hydrocolloidal or nonhydrocolloidal materials, and apply the sheet directly to the skin near the dressing. Thread a separate piece of gauze tie, umbilical tape, or twill tape (about 12 inches [30.5 cm]) through each pair of holes in the straps, and fasten each tie as you would a shoelace. Do not stress the surrounding skin by securing the ties too tightly.
4. Repeat this procedure according to the number of Montgomery straps needed.
5. Replace Montgomery straps whenever they become soiled (every 2 to 3 days). If skin maceration occurs, place new tape about 1 inch (2.5 cm) away from any irritation. See Skill 13-1, step 14.

Adapted from Springhouse. (2001). *Handbook of nursing procedures*. Philadelphia: Lippincott Williams & Wilkins.

There is a trend either to leave sutured, clean wounds not dressed after surgery or to use loose dressings. These methods allow atmospheric oxygen to circulate above the wound, aiding in the healing process. In many cases, if a dressing has been used for closed wounds, it is removed within 24 hours postoperatively to allow air circulation. Within 24 hours, enough fibrin has usually been produced at the wound site to stop the entry of microorganisms. Refer to agency policy and the physician's or the surgeon's preference. Often the physician or surgeon does the initial dressing change.

A dry dressing (as opposed to wet-to-dry, or semiocclusive or occlusive dressings) is often the choice for management of a wound with little exudate or drainage such as abrasions and nondraining postoperative incisions. In addition to keeping initial bleeding to a minimum, the dressing protects the wound from injury, prevents introduction of bacteria, reduces discomfort, and speeds healing. A dry dressing also prevents deeper tissues from drying out by keeping the wound surface moist (go to woundsource.com on the Internet for a helpful resource). The dry dressing does not debride the wound and is not the proper selection for wounds requiring debridement. If a dry dressing adheres to a wound, moisten the dressing with sterile normal saline or sterile water before removing the gauze. Moistening the dressing in this manner decreases the adherence of the dressing to the wound and reduces the risk of further trauma to the wound (Skill 13-1).

Because removal of dressings can be painful, it frequently helps to give an analgesic at least 30 minutes before exposing a wound. If underlying drains are present, take care not to accidentally remove or displace them when you remove dressings.

Follow sterile technique whenever handling the wound or the dressing (see Chapter 12 for principles of sterile technique). Asepsis not only protects you from wound drainage, but also decreases the introduction of **pathogenic** (any microorganism capable of producing disease) organisms into the wound (Figure 13-3). Using

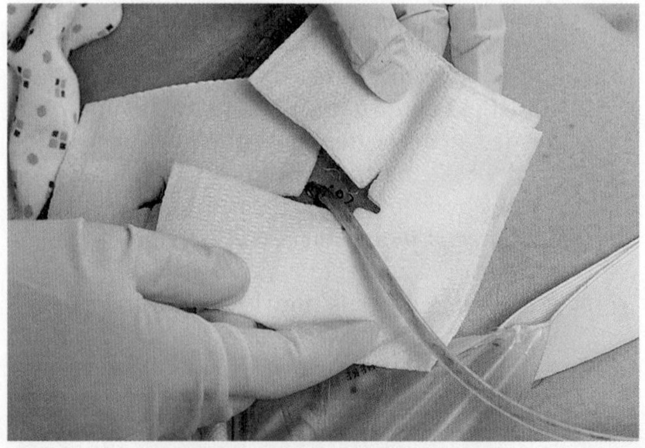

FIGURE 13-3 Applying a drain dressing.

Skill 13-1 Changing a Sterile Dry Dressing

Nursing Action *(Rationale)*

1. See standard steps in wound care 1 to 9, pp. 314 to 315.
2. Assemble equipment:
   - Clean gloves
   - Sterile gloves
   - Refuse container
   - Dressing set
   - Sterile normal saline (if indicated)
   - Antiseptic swabs
   - Ointment, if ordered
   - Sterile 4 × 4 gauze squares
   - Nonadherent dressing
   - Fluff or loose gauze
   - Sterile abdominal pads
   - Barrier drape (optional)
   - Tape (e.g., paper or micropore), Montgomery straps (see Box 13-1), or binder
   - Adhesive remover (optional)
   - Protective apparel (gown, goggles, mask [optional])
   - Disposable measuring device to accurately assess wound size and amount of drainage
3. Place refuse container in convenient location away from sterile field. *(Prevents need to reach across sterile field and thus prevents contamination.)*
4. Set up sterile field. *(Maintains asepsis during procedure and organizes approach to procedure.)*
   a. Open sterile dressings.
   b. Use barrier drape as needed.
   c. Open sterile gloves.
   d. Open dressing set, if needed.
   e. Prepare antiseptic swabs.
5. Loosen tape by gently removing toward incision and gently using thumb to retract skin away from tape (countertraction). *(Minimizes tissue trauma and decreases patient discomfort.)*
6. Don clean gloves and remove dressing and discard. If drains are present, remove dressings one layer at a time. *(Prevents accidental removal of drain.)*
7. Assess status of wound and wound drainage. *(Provides evaluation of healing process and collection of data for accurate documentation.)*
8. Remove gloves; discard. Wash hands and don sterile gloves. *(Prevents spread of microorganisms and maintains surgical asepsis.)*
9. Cleanse wound and surrounding area with antiseptic swab, starting from incision and moving outward, using one stroke per swab (see illustration). Discard swabs. *(Aids in removing bacteria from wound areas. Prevents contaminating previously cleaned area.)*

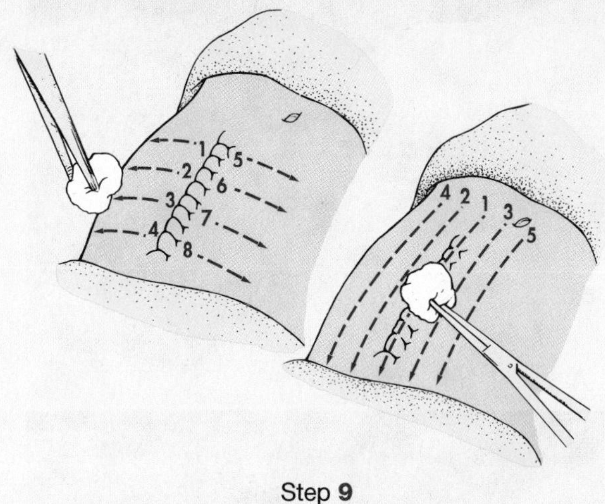

Step 9

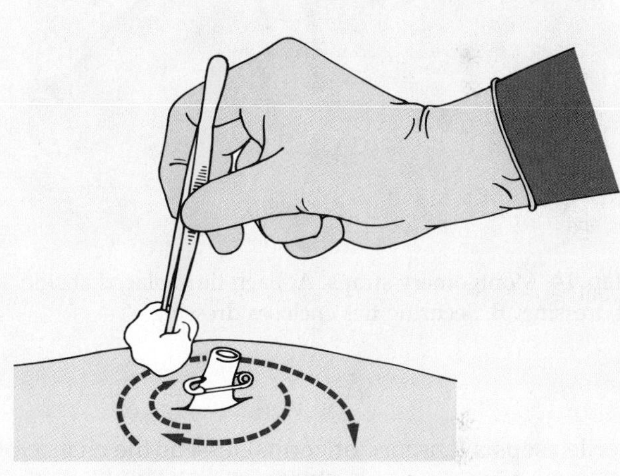

Step 11

10. Use sterile gauze to dry in same manner, or allow antiseptic to air-dry. *(Drying reduces excess moisture that could eventually harbor microorganisms.)*
11. Cleanse drain site if applicable (see illustration). *(Helps to remove bacteria or prevent bacteria from entering wound area.)*
12. Apply antibiotic ointment, if ordered, using same techniques as for cleansing. *(Helps reduce growth of microorganisms.)*
13. Cover wound with appropriately sized dry sterile dressing and use drain dressing, if applicable (see Figure 13-3). *(Protects wound and skin around drain site from skin impairment.)*
14. Secure dressing with tape, Montgomery straps (see illustration), or binder. Some facilities use a Skin Prep at tape sites to protect skin from irritation. Consider use of Montgomery straps when dressings require frequent changing to prevent tape irritation of skin (see Box 13-1). *(Supports*

Continued

Skill 13-1 Changing a Sterile Dry Dressing—cont'd

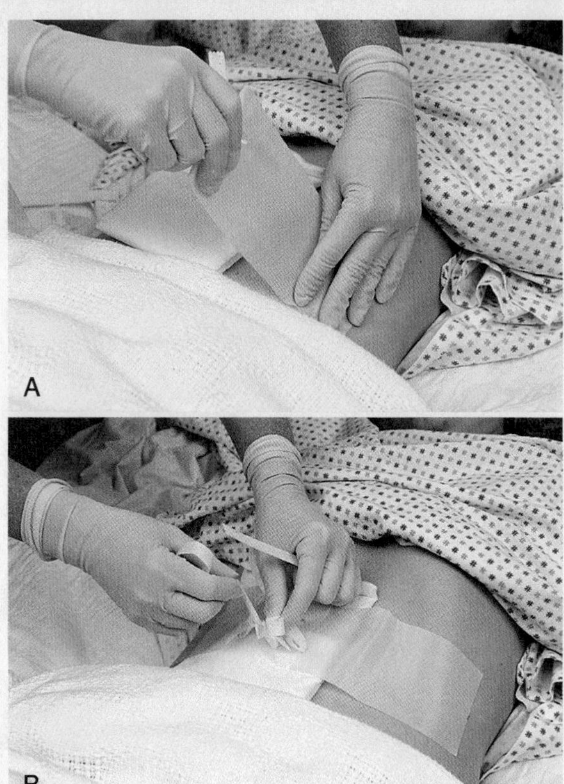

Step **14** Montgomery straps. **A,** Each tie is placed at side of dressing. **B,** Securing ties encloses dressing.

wound and ensures placement and stability of dressings.)

15. See standard steps in wound care 10 to 17, p. 315.
16. Document: *(Records patient's progress and therapy provided.)*
    - Location
    - Status of wound
    - Description of exudate or drainage (see Table 13-2)
    - Dressings applied
    - Any changes
    - Patient's response to procedure
    - Patient teaching (see Patient Teaching box on p. 339)
17. Report to physician any unexpected appearance of wound or drainage or accidental removal of drain within an hour. *(Unless patient shows evidence of wound dehiscence, notification of physician of unexpected findings within an hour is adequate.)*

sterile **asepsis** (absence of germs) lessens the chance of the patient acquiring a health care–associated infection (Box 13-2). Employ standard precautions (see Chapter 12) when handling body secretions. Good hand hygiene technique and the use of sterile aseptic procedures are essential when providing surgical wound care. Wear a gown, mask, and protective goggles if you anticipate soiling or splashing of wound exudate.

Box 13-2 Health Care–Associated Wound Infections

- Health care–associated infections are a continual threat to patients, especially the postsurgical patient.
- Virulence of the bacterial contamination and resistance of the patient are two major factors in determining whether a wound becomes infected.
- Because wound infections usually have an incubation period of 4 to 6 days, some patients are discharged before problems are noted.
- Patient teaching includes ongoing observations to determine if medical treatment is required.
- Exudate and drainage are a sign of healing, but accurate assessments will sometimes provide signals of potential complications of wound healing.

WET-TO-DRY DRESSING

The primary purpose of wet-to-dry dressing (Skill 13-2) is to mechanically debride a wound. The moistened contact layer of the dressing increases the absorptive ability of the dressing to collect exudate and wound debris. As the dressing dries, it adheres to the wound and, when the dressing is removed, debrides it. These dressings are most appropriate for wounds that do not have significant amounts of ischemic or necrotic tissue or large amounts of drainage or exudate. Take care not to apply a dressing so wet that it remains wet continuously. A too-wet dressing has the potential to cause tissue maceration and bacterial growth.

Commonly used wetting agents include normal saline and lactated Ringer's solution, isotonic solutions that aid in mechanical debridement. Acetic acid is effective against *Pseudomonas aeruginosa* but is toxic to fibroblasts in standard dilutions. Sodium hypochlorite solution (Dakin's) is sometimes used to facilitate debridement in a wound with necrotic debris and is an effective deodorizing solution. Povidone-iodine, usually one-quarter to one-half strength, is a rapid-acting antimicrobial agent for cleansing intact skin. In wounds,

Skill 13-2 Changing a Wet-to-Dry Dressing

Nursing Action *(Rationale)*

1. See standard steps in wound care 1 to 9, pp. 314 to 315.
2. Assemble equipment:
   - Barrier drape
   - Sterile dressing
   - Gauze
   - Sterile basin
   - Sterile solution
   - Antiseptic swabs
   - Instrument set, if needed
   - Clean gloves
   - Sterile gloves
   - Refuse container
   - Tape or Montgomery straps
   - Waterproof pad
3. Place waterproof pad appropriately. *(Prevents soiling of bed or linens.)*
4. Place refuse container appropriately. *(Prevents need to reach across sterile field and thus prevents contamination.)*
5. Set up sterile field. *(Maintains sterile technique during procedure and organizes approach to procedure.)*
   a. Open barrier drape.
   b. Add sterile dressing and gauze.
   c. Add sterile basin.
   d. Pour sterile solution into basin.
   e. Add instrument set, if needed.
   f. Add antiseptic swabs.
6. Loosen tape by gently removing toward incision and, using thumb, gently retracting the skin away from tape (countertraction). *(Minimizes tissue trauma. Decreases patient discomfort.)*
7. Don clean gloves. Remove dressing and discard. Do not moisten dressings to remove, because this will interfere with the debriding process. To be considerate of patient, provide analgesic medication at least 20 to 30 minutes before the procedure. *(Protects you from microorganisms. Prevents contamination of wound from soiled dressing and promotes patient comfort.)*
8. Assess status of wound and wound exudate or drainage on dressing (see Table 13-2). *(Provides evaluation of healing process and collection of data for accurate documentation.)*
9. Remove gloves; discard. Perform hand hygiene and don sterile gloves. *(Reduces spread of microorganisms and maintains surgical asepsis.)*
10. Cleanse wound and surrounding area with antiseptic swab, starting from incision and moving outward, using one stroke per swab. Discard swabs. *(Removes old drainage and bacteria from skin area.)*
11. Place gauze into basin. *(Wets gauze with solution.)*
12. Wring excess solution from dressing, leaving it slightly moist. *(Prevents growth of bacteria caused by dressing that is too wet.)*
13. Apply moist gauze dressing as a single layer directly onto wound surface. If wound is deep, gently pack gauze into wound with forceps until all wound surfaces are in contact with moist gauze (see illustration). *(Allows solution to come into contact with wound, which makes it effective. Moist gauze absorbs drainage and adheres to debris.)*
14. Apply dry dressing over wet gauze. *(Pulls moisture from the wound and allows for absorption of excess moisture.)*

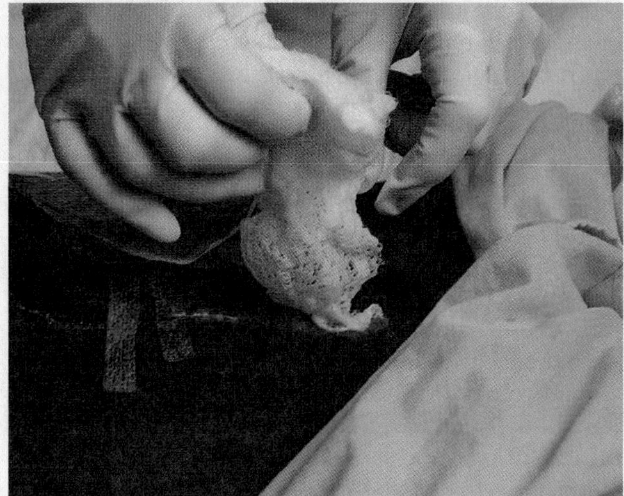

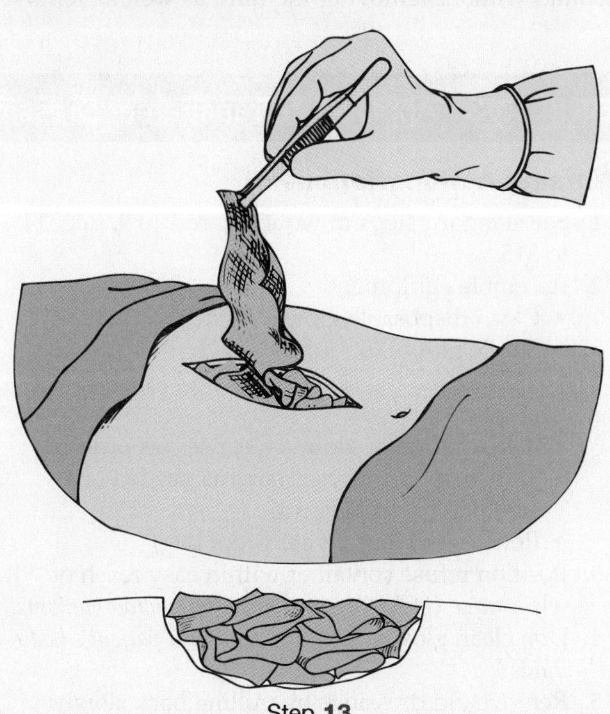

Step 13

Continued

Skill 13-2 Changing a Wet-to-Dry Dressing—cont'd

15. Cover with additional dressing as needed. *(Protects wound from bacteria.)*
16. Secure with tape or Montgomery straps. *(Secures dressings in place.)*
17. See standard steps in wound care 10 to 17, p. 315.
18. Document: *(Documents patient's progress and therapy provided.)*
    - Wound status
    - Description of exudate or drainage (see Table 13-2)
    - Dressings applied
    - Patient's response to procedure
    - Patient teaching (see Patient Teaching box on p. 339)
19. Discuss change in dressing procedure with physician as wound surface becomes clean and granulation tissue is evident. *(Promotes anticipated wound healing.)*
20. Be aware this type of dressing is not so widely used (see Evidence-Based Practice box on p. 333)

the solution is toxic to fibroblasts and has questionable efficacy in infected wounds. Other antibiotic solutions may be ordered, although their use is controversial. Wetting solutions should be discarded 24 hours after opening and replaced with fresh solution because they can harbor microorganism growth.

TRANSPARENT DRESSINGS

Another type of dressing is a thin, self-adhesive transparent film (e.g., Op-site or Tegaderm) that belongs in the semiocclusive or occlusive categories. A synthetic permeable (capable of allowing the passage of fluids or substances in solution) membrane, it acts as a temporary second skin. It has several advantages. It adheres to undamaged skin to contain exudate and minimize wound contamination. It also serves as a barrier to external fluids and bacteria yet still allows the wound to breathe. It promotes a moist environment that speeds epithelial cell growth. You will be able to assess the wound without removing the film, as well as remove the film without damaging underlying tissues. Transparent dressings are available with and without adhesive borders. It is acceptable for them to stay in place up to 7 days, if complete occlusion is maintained.

For best results, use these dressings on clean, debrided wounds that are not actively bleeding. The film is ideal for small, superficial wounds and as a dressing over an intravenous catheter site. Apply it so no wrinkles form, but do not stretch it over the skin. Another option in some cases is to use it over another, smaller dressing (e.g., Telfa) cut to fit the area of the wound. Impregnated gauzes are more popular. It is possible to apply topical medications over nonadhesive transparent dressings without disturbing the dressing. Nonadhesive transparent dressings will fall off as the wound heals. If the dressing does stick to the wound and removal is necessary, moisten with normal saline. With physician approval, the patient is permitted to shower or bathe with the dressing in place.

See Skill 13-3 for applying a transparent dressing.

Skill 13-3 Applying a Transparent Dressing

Nursing Action *(Rationale)*

1. See standard steps in wound care 1 to 9, pp. 314 to 315.
2. Assemble equipment:
    - Clean disposable gloves
    - Sterile gloves (optional)
    - Sterile dressing set (scissors and forceps; optional)
    - Sterile saline or wound cleanser (as ordered)
    - Transparent dressings (size as needed and sterile 2 × 2 gauze pad)
    - Refuse container (waterproof bag)
3. Position refuse container within easy reach of work area. *(Helps prevent spread of microorganisms.)*
4. Don clean gloves. *(Protects you from patient's body fluids.)*
5. Remove old dressings by pulling back slowly across dressing in direction of hair growth and toward the center. *(Reduces excoriation, pain, and irritation of skin after dressing removal.)*
6. Remove disposable gloves by pulling them inside out over soiled dressings, and dispose of them in refuse container (see illustration). *(Provides containment of soiled dressings and prevents contact of your hands with drainage.)*
7. Inspect wound for color, odor, and drainage or exudates. Measure if indicated. *(Appearance indicates status of wound healing.)*
8. Clean area gently, swabbing toward area of most exudate, or spray with cleanser—know agency policy and physician's order. *(Reduces transmission of microorganisms from contaminated area to cleaner site.)*
9. Reapply sterile or clean gloves as indicated. *(Prevents risk of exposure to body fluids if present.)*

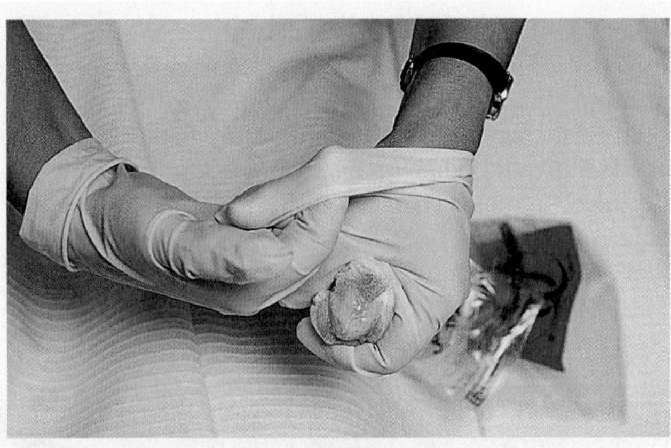

Step 6

10. Dry skin around wound thoroughly with sterile gauze. Make sure skin surface is dry. *(Transparent dressings with adhesive backing will not adhere to damp surface.)*
11. Apply transparent dressing according to manufacturer's direction.
    a. Remove paper backing, taking care not to allow adhesive areas to touch each other (see illustration). *(Often results in wrinkles and becomes impossible to use.)* NOTE: Chevrons of tape (wrapped around the needle head) are no longer widely used, because the tape is not sterile and may cause infection.
    b. Place film smoothly over wound without stretching (see illustration).

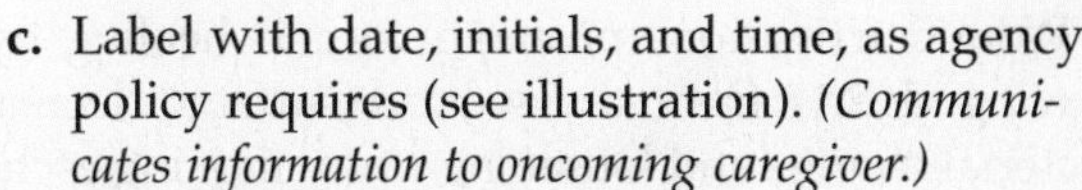

    c. Label with date, initials, and time, as agency policy requires (see illustration). *(Communicates information to oncoming caregiver.)*
12. Remove gloves, discard them in refuse container, and wash hands. *(Prevents transmission of microorganisms.)*
13. See standard steps in wound care 10 to 17, p. 315.
14. Document: *(Records care given and progress of wound.)*
    - Wound status
    - Description of exudate or drainage
    - Dressing applied
    - Patient's response to procedure
    - Patient teaching
15. Report any unexpected appearance of the wound or exudates. *(Further treatment may be necessary.)*

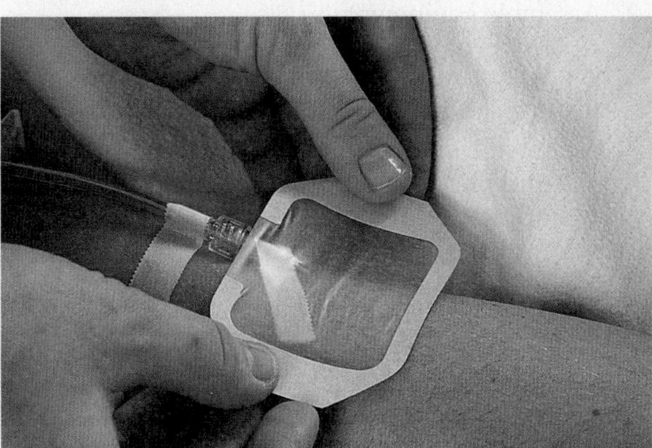

Step 11b

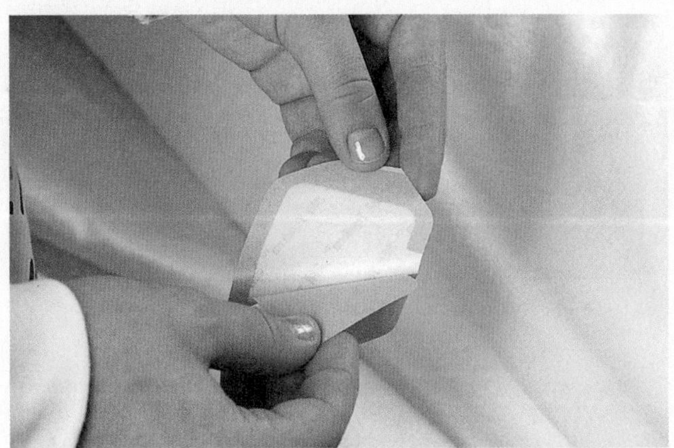

Step 11a

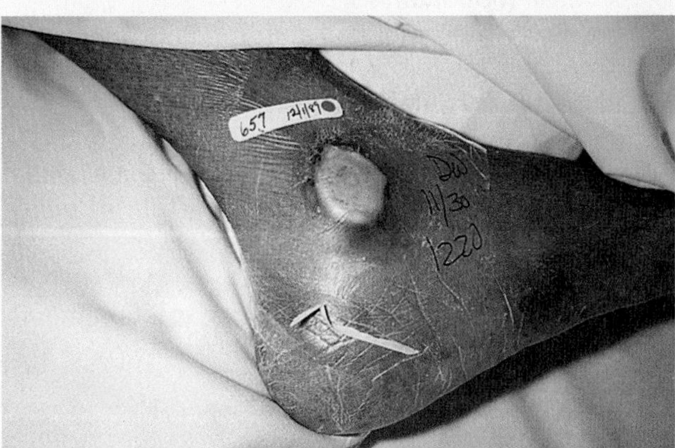

Step 11c

IRRIGATIONS

Irrigation is gentle washing of an area with a stream of solution delivered through an irrigating syringe. Use this nursing intervention for wounds on any part of the torso or the extremities. In addition to cleansing an area, you have the ability to introduce prescribed medications in solution form. Principles of basic wound irrigation include the following:

1. Cleanse in a direction from the least contaminated area to the most contaminated.
2. When irrigating, make sure all the solution flows from the least contaminated to the most contaminated area.

Wound irrigations promote wound healing by removing debris from the wound surface, decreasing bacterial counts, and loosening and removing eschar (a black, leathery crust). Solutions used for irrigations include warm water, saline, and mild detergents. Nonsurgical indications include management of pressure ulcers (see Chapter 18). Meticulous hand hygiene and proper infection control procedure before and after removing soiled dressings, coupled with proper irrigation procedures, limit the risk of health care–associated infection. Perform basic wound cleansing by applying antiseptic solutions with sterile gauze or by irrigation. Skin cleansing in the area of the suture line or the drain site is indicated when an excessive amount of drainage occurs. The presence of wound exudate is an expected stage of epithelial cell growth.

When performing an irrigation (Skill 13-4), make sure to provide for patient comfort: an irrigation has

Skill 13-4 Performing a Sterile Irrigation

Nursing Action *(Rationale)*

1. See standard steps in wound care 1 to 9, pp. 314 to 315.
2. Assemble equipment:
   - Refuse container
   - Clean gloves
   - Sterile gloves
   - Dressing set
   - Antiseptic swabs
   - Sterile basin
   - Warmed, sterile irrigation solution (200 to 1000 mL)
   - Irrigation syringe, Waterpik, or spray bottle or soft catheter for deep wounds
   - Clean basin
   - Waterproof pad
   - Sterile dressings
   - Gown and goggles (optional)
   - Tape, gauze, and elastic bandage, if appropriate
   - Mask (optional)
3. Position waterproof pad appropriately. *(Protects patient and bed linens from contaminated fluids.)*
4. Place refuse container in convenient location away from sterile field. *(Prevents need to reach across sterile field and thus prevents contamination.)*
5. Set up sterile field. *(Maintains asepsis during procedure and organizes approach to procedure.)*
   a. Set up sterile basin.
   b. Add sterile, warmed irrigation solution to basin.
   c. Add antiseptic swabs.
   d. Open sterile gloves.
   e. Add dressing set (optional).
   f. Add sterile syringe and catheter if necessary.
   g. Add disposable measuring device.
6. Don gown and goggles if you anticipate splashing. *(Protects you from splashes.)*
7. Don clean gloves and remove dressing. Discard dressing in refuse container. *(Protects you from pathogens and prevents wound contamination from soiled dressing.)*
8. Remove gloves, discard into proper receptacle, and wash hands. *(Reduces transmission of microorganisms.)*
9. Assess status of wound and exudate or drainage on dressing (see Table 13-2). *(Provides evaluation of healing process and collection of data for accurate documentation.)*
10. Place collection basin appropriately (see illustration). *(Collects contaminated solution.)*
11. Perform hand hygiene and don sterile gloves. *(Maintains asepsis.)*
12. Cleanse area around wound with antiseptic swabs. *(Removes bacteria and drainage.)*
13. Fill irrigating syringe with solution. Attach soft catheter if irrigating a deep wound with small opening. *(Allows for direct flow of solution into wound.)* Use a 19-gauge needle (or angiocath) with a 35-mL syringe to clean most pressure ulcers, especially deep ulcers (see illustration).
14. Instill solution gently into wound, holding syringe approximately 1 inch above wound. If using catheter, gently insert into wound opening until slight resistance is met, pull back, and

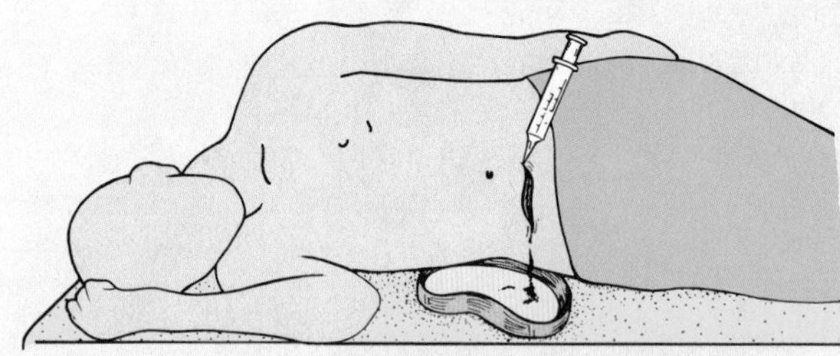

Step **10**

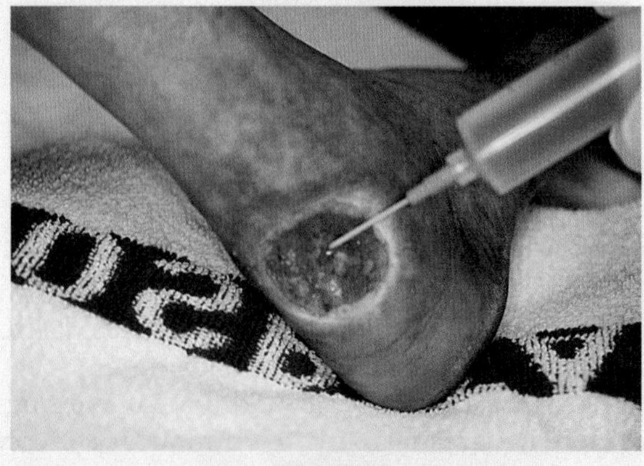

Step **13**

gently instill solution. *(Minimizes tissue trauma, irritation, and bleeding.)* In some instances, it is possible to replace the needle with a Waterpik. Refer to physician's orders or facility policies.

15. Allow solution to flow from clean area of wound to dirty area. *(Prevents contamination of clean tissue by exudate.)*
16. Pinch off catheter during withdrawal from wound. *(Avoids aspiration of contaminating fluid into syringe.)*
17. Refill syringe and continue irrigation until solution returns clear. *(Thoroughly cleanses wound.)*
18. Blot wound edges with sterile gauze. *(Prevents tissue damage from excess moisture.)*
19. Dress wound again, if applicable. *(Protects wound from injury and microorganisms and provides for patient comfort.)*
20. See standard steps in wound care 10 to 17, p. 315.
21. Document: *(Records care given and progress of wound.)*
    - Status of wound
    - Performance of wound irrigation
    - Solution used
    - Character of exudate and drainage
    - Patient's response to procedure
    - Patient teaching (see Patient Teaching box on p. 339)
22. Report immediately to attending physician any evidence of fresh bleeding, sharp increase in pain, retention of irrigant, or signs of shock. *(These are signs of tissue damage and fistula or sinus tract development. Shock phenomena sometimes indicate internal bleeding or tissue damage.)*

potential to cause pain. Patients will often need to be medicated before you perform the procedure. Gentleness is important in performing any type of irrigation to prevent tissue damage and pain.

Use sterile technique or clean technique for wound cleansing and irrigation. Introduce the cleansing solution directly into the wound with a syringe, syringe and catheter, shower, or whirlpool. When using a syringe (Waterpiks are available in some facilities), keep the tip 1 inch (2.5 cm) above the wound or area you are cleansing. This prevents contamination of the syringe. Careful attention to placement of the syringe also prevents unsafe pressure of the flowing solution. Make sure that the flow of irrigant moves from the area being cleansed to an area that is both distal to and lower than the wound area. In wound care, the area being cleansed is considered clean and the surrounding skin surfaces are considered contaminated without respect to whether the wound is infected. Within the wound, direct the flow from healthy tissue toward infected tissue. If the patient has a deep wound with a narrow opening, attach a soft catheter to the syringe to maintain sterile technique while permitting the fluid to enter the wound. To prevent fluid being retained in the wound, position the patient on his or her side to encourage the irrigant to flow away from the wound. With small wounds, it is often helpful to use a 35-mL syringe with a 19-gauge needle attached to obtain optimal pressure for cleansing with minimal risk of tissue injury.

Ambulatory or home patients are sometimes able to avail themselves of a handheld shower for wound cleansing, holding the shower spray approximately 12 inches from the wound. If the force of the spray results in too much pressure for comfort, suggest that the patient tie a clean washcloth around the shower head to disperse the force. An alternative means of irrigating wounds in acute care areas is the shower table, frequently used for cleansing in burn and trauma wound care units. For patients who require cleansing but cannot tolerate the aforementioned methods, the whirlpool is useful. Physical therapists often perform or assist with performing the whirlpool procedure, and then help apply dressings.

COMPLICATIONS OF WOUND HEALING

Impaired wound healing, regardless of the cause, requires accurate observation and ongoing interventions. Because wound complications are potentially life threatening, it is vital throughout the patient's recovery phase to monitor signs and symptoms and assess their severity (Table 13-3).

Wound bleeding potentially indicates a slipped suture, dislodged clot, coagulation problem, or trauma to

Table 13-3 Terms Associated with Wound Complications

TERM	DEFINITION
Abscess	Cavity containing pus and surrounded by inflamed tissue, formed as a result of suppuration in a localized infection
Adhesion	Band of scar tissue that binds together two anatomical surfaces normally separated; most commonly found in the abdomen
Cellulitis	Infection of the skin characterized by heat, pain, erythema, and edema
Dehiscence	Separation of a surgical incision or rupture of a wound closure
Evisceration	Protrusion of an internal organ through a wound or surgical incision
Extravasation	Passage or escape into the tissues; usually of blood, serum, or lymph
Hematoma	Collection of extravasated blood trapped in the tissues or in an organ resulting from incomplete hemostasis after surgery or injury

Box 13-3 Responding to Wound Evisceration

If a patient's wound eviscerates, you will need to respond swiftly and accurately, as outlined here:

1. Stay calm. Projecting a calm and confident manner will help keep the patient and the family calm as well.
2. Ask a colleague to obtain supplies and to notify a physician while you stay with the patient.
3. Raise the gatch near the foot of the bed and help the patient into a low Fowler's position with the knees slightly flexed. This position will ease pressure on the wound, prevent further tearing of the wound edges, and reduce the risk of further evisceration.
4. Cover the protruding organ(s) with a sterile dressing moistened with sterile normal saline solution to help prevent wound contamination and keep the abdominal contents moist. If no sterile dressing is available, use clean towels or dressings.
5. Monitor the patient closely and assess vital signs and pulse oximetry readings. Frequent monitoring will help detect impending shock.
6. Establish intravenous access to provide fluids and prepare the patient for surgery as ordered. The patient will most likely need surgery to repair the wound and will not be permitted oral intake.
7. Continue to provide emotional support to patient and family. Wound evisceration can be extremely frightening. A calm, supportive approach helps the patient through this emergency.

Adapted from Harkreader, H., Hogan, M.A., & Thobaben, M. (2007). *Fundamentals of nursing*. (3rd ed.). Philadelphia: Saunders.

blood vessels or tissue. To help detect increased drainage and color changes, inspect the wound and dressing. If hemorrhage results internally, the dressing will sometimes remain dry while the abdominal cavity collects blood. Consider whether the patient is hemorrhaging if you observe the following: increased thirst; restlessness; rapid, thready pulse; decreased blood pressure; decreased urinary output; and cool, clammy skin. By monitoring vital signs, intake and output (I&O), skin condition, wound site, and overall patient response, you facilitate the timely identification of hemorrhage and hypovolemic shock. Internal abdominal bleeding, if allowed to continue, causes the abdomen to become rigid and distended. If hemorrhage is not detected and stopped, hypovolemic shock will possibly cause the circulatory system to collapse, causing death.

When wound layers separate, resulting in dehiscence, some patients will tell you that something has given way (see Chapter 42). Sometimes this feeling is brought on by periods of sneezing, coughing, or vomiting. Evidence of serosanguineous drainage on the dressing is an important sign to assess. Dehiscence is sometimes preceded by serosanguineous drainage. If the wound is not covered and dehiscence occurs, have the patient remain in bed and receive nothing by mouth (NPO); tell the patient not to cough, place a warm, moist sterile dressing over the area until the physician evaluates the site, and provide reassurance. When a skin suture breaks and dehiscence occurs, you will often be able to close the wound effectively using Steri-Strips or a butterfly strip. Dehiscence most frequently occurs between the fifth and twelfth postoperative days. Because most patients have been dismissed from the hospital by day 12, include in patient teaching how to recognize dehiscence and what care to provide.

If an evisceration (when internal organs protrude through opened incision) follows the dehiscence, the patient is to remain in bed in a low Fowler's position, with the knees flexed to reduce pressure on the wound. Keep the patient on NPO status, and cover the wound and contents with warm, sterile saline dressings. Notify the surgeon immediately (Box 13-3).

Wound infection, or wound sepsis, results when the wound becomes contaminated. The CDC label a wound infected when it contains purulent (pus) drainage. A patient with an infected wound displays a fever, tenderness and pain at the wound site, edema, and an elevated WBC count. Purulent drainage has an odor and is brown, yellow, or green, depending on the pathogen. Culture of the exudate from an infected wound confirms the presence of the pathogenic organism, and it is then possible to order the appropriate medical therapy (see Chapter 19).

STAPLE AND SUTURE REMOVAL

Institutional policy determines whether only the physician or the physician and the nurse may remove sutures and staples. Always obtain the physician's written order before implementing either skill. The time of removal is based on the stage of incisional healing and the extent of surgery.

Sutures and staples are generally removed in 7 to 10 days after surgery, or sooner, if healing is adequate. Sometimes one suture or staple comes out at a time, and sometimes removal is in two phases: First, every other suture or staple is removed and replaced with a Steri-Strip, and the same sequence occurs with the remainder in the second phase. The physician determines the timing and method and orders the removal.

Sutures are threads of wire or other material (silk, steel, cotton, linen, nylon, or Dacron) used to sew body tissues together. Sutures are placed within tissue layers in deep wounds and superficially as the final means for wound closure. The deeper sutures are usually made of an absorbable material that disappears in several days. There are many kinds of sutures: inter-

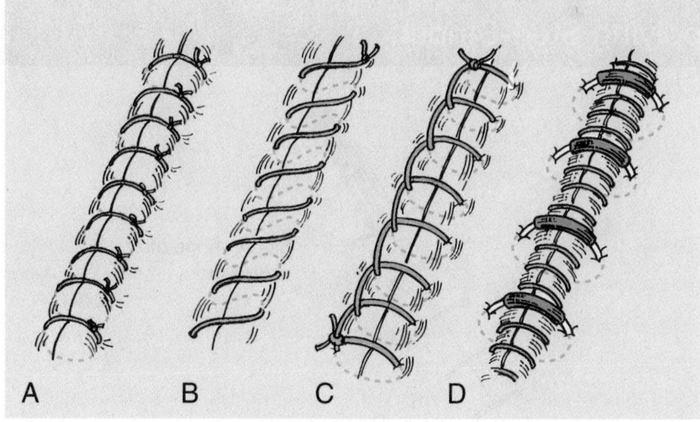

FIGURE 13-4 Sutures. **A,** Interrupted, or separate, sutures. **B,** Continuous suture. **C,** Blanket continuous suture. **D,** Retention suture covered with rubber tubing to provide greater strength.

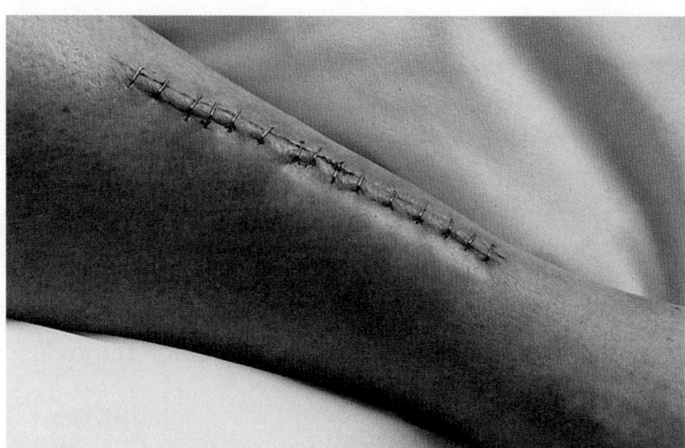

FIGURE 13-5 Wound closure with staples.

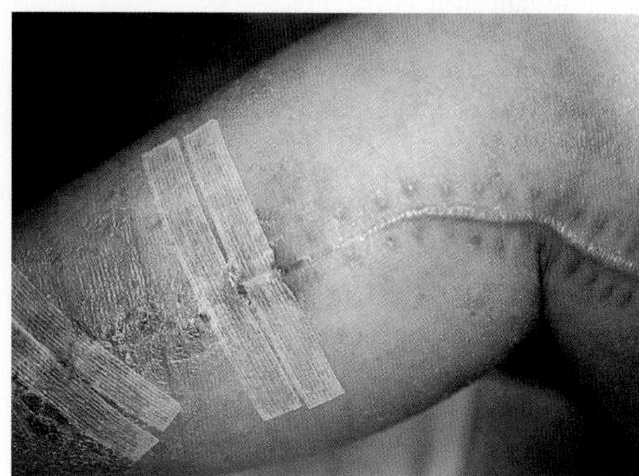

FIGURE 13-6 Steri-Strips placed over incision for closure.

rupted or separate sutures, continuous sutures, blanket sutures, or retention sutures covered with rubber tubing to provide greater strength (used primarily in obese patients who have had abdominal surgery). The cosmetic result of these latter sutures is often not as desirable as that obtained with finer suture material (Figure 13-4).

Staples are made of stainless steel wire, are quick to use, and provide ample strength. They are popular for skin closure of abdominal incisions and orthopedic surgery when appearance of the incision is not critical (Figure 13-5). The time of removal is based on the stage of incisional healing and the extent of surgery. Sutures and staples are generally removed within 7 to 10 days after surgery if healing is adequate. Retention sutures are left in place longer (14 days or more). Leaving sutures in too long makes removal more difficult and increases the risk of infection. Removal of staples requires a sterile staple extractor and maintenance of aseptic technique (Skill 13-5).

Routinely, you will remove every other suture or staple first and replace each with a Steri-Strip (Figure 13-6) and, if the incision remains securely closed, you will remove the rest by the same process. If any sign of suture line separation is evident during the removal process, leave the remaining sutures in place, document a description, and report it to the physician. In some cases, these sutures are left in place and removed several days to a week later.

The patient's history of wound healing, the site of the wound, the tissues involved, and the purpose of the sutures determine the selection of the suture material. For example, a patient with repeated abdominal surgeries will often require wire sutures for greater strength to promote wound closure.

EXUDATE AND DRAINAGE

Exudate is fluid, cells, or other substances that have slowly exuded or discharged from cells or blood vessels through small pores or breaks in cell membrane. Drainage is the removal of fluids from a body cavity, wound, or other source of discharge by one or more methods; it may occur passively on its own or with mechanical assistance (see the following section on drainage systems).

Exudate and drainage are described as serous, sanguineous, or serosanguineous. Serous exudate or drainage is a clear, watery fluid that has been separated from its solid elements (e.g., the exudate from a blister). Serous fluid has the characteristics of serum.

Skill 13-5 Removing Staples or Sutures (Applying Steri-Strips)

Nursing Action *(Rationale)*

1. Refer to standard steps in wound care 1 to 9, pp. 314 to 315.
2. Assemble equipment:
   - Refuse container
   - Clean gloves
   - Sterile gloves (optional)
   - Sterile sutures or staple removal set
   - Antiseptic swabs
   - Appropriate sterile dressings, including butterfly or adhesive Steri-Strips
   - Compound benzoin tincture or other skin protectant such as Skin Prep
3. Place refuse container in convenient location away from sterile field. *(Prevents need to reach across sterile field and thus prevents contamination.)*
4. Set up sterile field. *(Maintains asepsis during procedure and organizes approach to procedure.)*
   a. Open suture or staple set.
   b. Open sterile dressings (use sterile barrier if necessary for sterile field).
5. Remove dressing and soiled gloves. Discard into plastic refuse bag. (Use bag as needed for additional refuse.) *(Protects you from microorganisms and prevents contamination from soiled dressing.)*
6. Assess status of wound and drainage on dressing. *(Allows determination of alterations in healing process and collection of data for accurate documentation.)*
7. Perform hand hygiene and don sterile gloves. *(Allows you to handle sterile equipment.)*
8. Cleanse area with antiseptic swabs, starting from incision outward, using one stroke per swab. *(Removes bacteria from wound area.)*

Staple Removal

9. Prepare patient for pulling sensation and site tenderness during removal. Place staple remover under staple while slowly closing the ends of the staple remover together. Squeeze the center of the staple with the tips, freeing the staple from the skin (see illustration). *(Prevents putting excess pressure on suture line and secures removal of each staple.)*
10. Release handles and discard staple in refuse container. *(Prevents contamination of sterile field with used staple.)*
11. Repeat steps 9 and 10 until all staples have been removed. *(Permits complete removal of all staples.)* Every other staple may be removed and Steri-Strips applied, or two or three staples removed at a time and Steri-Strips applied until all staples have been removed and Steri-Strips applied.
12. Count number of staples removed. *(Provides count for documentation.)*

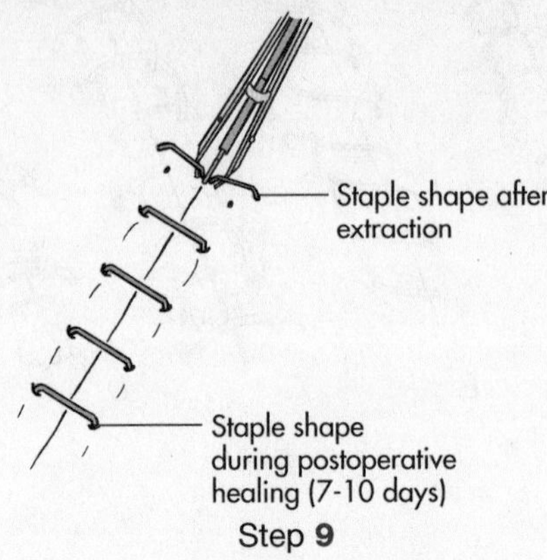

Step 9

Special Considerations for Suture and Staple Removal:

- Wire sutures are removed by physician.
- Limit amount of dressing supplies because either a light dressing or no dressing will be needed after suture or staple removal.
- Notify physician immediately if inadequate wound healing is noted; discontinue removal of staples.
- It is common to see wounds closed with Steri-Strips, or sterile tape applied along both sides of a wound to keep the edges approximated and closed (see Figure 13-6).

Interventions to Follow When Applying Steri-Strips:

a. Gently cleanse suture line with antiseptic swab. *(Removes as much surface bacteria as possible.)*
b. Carefully inspect the incision. *(Ensures that all sutures have been removed.)*
c. Apply tincture of benzoin to the skin on each side of suture line over an area 1.5 to 2 inches (4 to 5 cm) wide, and allow to dry a few minutes until tacky. *(Makes Steri-Strips adhere more securely.)*
d. When skin is dry, cut Steri-Strips to allow strips to extend 1.5 to 2 inches (4 to 5 cm) on each side of the incision. Some physicians request the strips be placed side by side, whereas others request they be spaced evenly and appropriately apart (see Figure 13-6).
e. Instruct patient to take showers rather than soak in bathtub according to physician's preference. Steri-Strips are not removed and are allowed to loosen and peel off gradually.
f. On removal of sutures, many physicians request that only one to three sutures be removed at a time, and Steri-Strips applied in their place. This action is repeated until all sutures are removed and Steri-Strips applied.

13. Assess healing status of wound. *(Determines need for butterfly or Steri-Strip skin closures.)*
14. Cleanse area with antiseptic swabs. *(Decreases the risk of infection.)*

Removal of Interrupted Sutures (see Figure 13-4, *A*)

15. Each suture has a knot. Each interrupted suture is secured with its own knot. Knots are lined up on the same side of incision.
16. Grasp and elevate knotted end of suture with hemostat or forceps. *(Exposes the knot and ensures removal of suture and maintains skin integrity.)*
17. Snip suture at skin level on opposite side, proximal to knot (see illustration). *(Releases suture.)*
18. Gently remove entire suture with forceps and discard on sterile gauze. *(Prevents contaminating sterile field with used materials.)*
19. Repeat steps 16 to 18 until all sutures have been removed. *(Ensures removal of all sutures.)*

Removal of Continuous Sutures (see Figure 13-4, *B*)

20. To remove continuous sutures:
    - **a.** Snip suture close to skin surface at end distal to knot.
    - **b.** Snip second suture on same side.
    - **c.** Grasp knot and gently pull with continuous smooth action, removing suture from beneath the skin. Place suture on gauze.
    - **d.** Grasp and lift next suture, and snip with tip of scissors close to skin.
    - **e.** Grasp suture and gently remove loop of suture. Never pull the contaminated stitch through tissue.
    - **f.** Repeat these steps until the end knot is reached. Cut the last one and remove it by grasping and pulling the knot.

Removal of Blanket Continuous Suture (see Figure 13-4, *C*)

21. To remove blanket continuous sutures:
    - **a.** Cut the suture opposite the looped blanket edge.
    - **b.** Remove each suture by grasping at the looped end.
22. Apply sterile dressing or leave open to air as ordered. (Dressing is often needed only if patient's clothing will irritate wound area.) *(Protects wound and facilitates healing process.)*
23. Refer to standard steps in wound care 10 to 17, p. 315.
24. Document: *(Records care given and progress of wound.)*
    - Number of staples or sutures removed
    - Condition of staple or suture line
    - Patient's response
    - Dressings applied, if necessary
    - Patient teaching (see Patient Teaching box on p. 339)

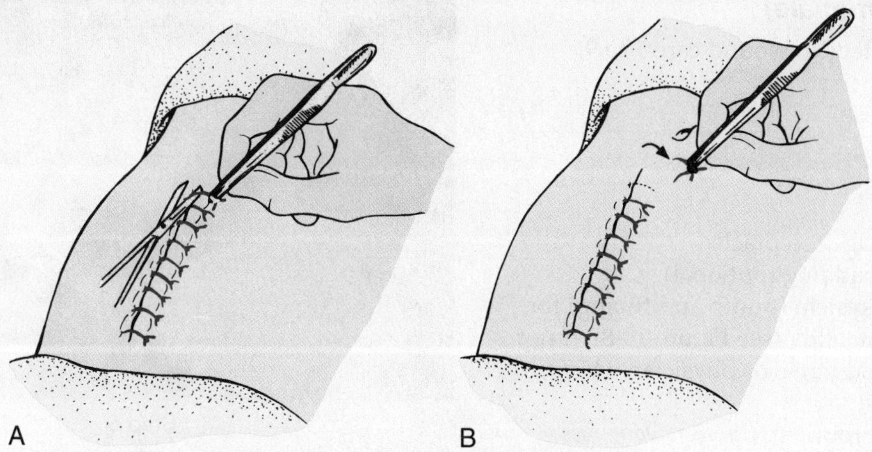

Step 17 **A,** Cut the suture as close to the skin as possible, away from the knot. **B,** Remove the suture; never pull the contaminated stitch through tissue.

Serum is the clear, thin, sticky fluid portion of blood that remains after coagulation. In contrast, sanguineous exudate or drainage is fluid that contains blood. Thus serosanguineous exudate or drainage is thin and red (usually described as pink), because it is composed of both serum and blood. If the tissue is infected, exudate or drainage is likely to be purulent or brown-green. Exudate or drainage from specific organs will have its own particular color (e.g., bile from the liver and gallbladder is green or green-brown).

The type and the amount of exudate or drainage produced depend on the tissue and organs involved. Treat exudate or drainage in quantities greater than 300 mL in the first 24 hours as abnormal, and report it immediately. When patients first ambulate, a slight increase of exudate or drainage sometimes occurs. If sanguineous exudate or drainage continues, it is possible that small blood vessels are oozing.

Not all surgical wounds drain. If exudate or drainage does occur, accurate assessments are vital. The following exudate and drainage characteristics are important to note and chart: color, amount, consistency (thick or thin), and odor. If the exudate or drainage has a pungent or strong odor, infection is likely. Perform a wound culture (see Chapter 19). Exudate will most likely be contained either in a drainage system or on a dressing. If a dressing is used, you will be able to monitor the amount of exudate or drainage (such as from a Penrose drain) by weighing the soiled dressing (1 g of exudate or drainage equals 1 mL), by circling and dating the drainage area and comparing the circled area to later observations, or by reporting the number and the type of dressings used and saturated over what interval. Until the surgeon orders a dressing change, never remove the soiled dressings, only reinforce them.

DRAINAGE SYSTEMS

Frequently, surgical procedures are performed to remove or repair organs that lie within the body (e.g., gallbladder removal). In these cases, a mechanism is needed to assist gravity in removing exudate from the cavity. If a gastrectomy is performed using an upper abdominal midline incision, fluid will collect and remain at the surgical site. To facilitate drainage, the surgeon makes a secondary incision, or stab wound, close to the surgical incision. The site for the stab wound is planned deliberately. It is the intent of the surgeon to drain exudate away from the incision, not toward it. If the exudate enters the surgical incision, contamination and infection are likely to follow.

Several methods are available to facilitate the flow of exudate away from the wound site. **Closed drainage** is a system of tubing and other apparatus attached to the body to remove fluid in an airtight circuit that prevents environmental contaminants from entering the wound or cavity. **Open drainage** passes through an open-ended tube into a receptacle or out onto the dressing. **Suction drainage** uses a pump or other mechanical device to help extract a fluid (Skill 13-6).

Gentle suction is needed in some surgeries to help gravity move the exudate. A drainage system is chosen to fit the area to be drained and according to the type of exudate and amount of drainage expected. A rubber or plastic drain is sometimes used to remove exudate from the wound and deposit it out through the skin onto a dressing (open drainage system), or sometimes is positioned through the surgical incision or stab

Skill 13-6 Maintaining Hemovac or Davol Suction and T-Tube Drainage

Nursing Action *(Rationale)*

1. Refer to standard steps in wound care 1 to 9, pp. 314 to 315.
2. Assemble equipment:
   - Clean gloves
   - Alcohol pads
   - Swabs
   - Calibrated drainage receptacle
   - Moisture-proof padding (optional)
3. Examine drainage system (pump and tubing) for seal, patency, and stability (see Figure 13-8). If not working, notify head nurse or physician. *(Maintains efficiency of system.)*
4. Don goggles, if appropriate. *(Protects your eyes from contaminants.)*
5. Remove Hemovac or Davol plug labeled "pouring spout." *(Permits accurate measuring of drainage.)*
   a. Empty drainage into measuring device.
   b. When emptying Hemovac, compress device by pushing top and bottom together with your hands.
6. Hold pump of Hemovac tightly compressed and reinsert plug to reestablish closed drainage system (see illustration). When caring for a Davol, reestablish suction by pumping bulb until balloon is completely inflated. Recap drainage port. For both Hemovac and Davol, keep plug out of drainage stream—hold the plug by stem. *(Maintains unit sterility.)*

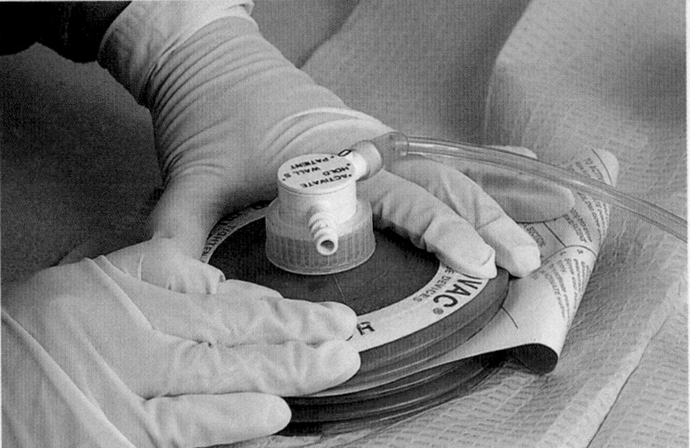

Step 6

7. Observe the drainage for color, consistency, and odor. *(Provides basis for documentation.)*
8. Measure and record amount of drainage; rinse measuring container. *(Provides basis for documentation.)*
9. Position drainage system on bed, and secure system. *(Maintains efficiency of system.)*
10. Dispose of drainage and rinse container. Remove gloves and wash hands. *(Reduces spread of microorganisms.)*

11. If specimen is ordered, send to laboratory. (If dressing change is necessary, do it at this time.) *(Provides continuity of care.)*
12. Observe Davol or Hemovac every 2 to 4 hours. *(Ascertains integrity of suction.)* Measure drainage every 8 hours or as ordered. *(Recording an accurate output of drainage is necessary so the physician is able to determine any change in the amount or the character of wound drainage.)*
13. Refer to standard steps in wound care 10 to 17, p. 315.
14. Document: *(Records care given and progress of wound.)*
    - Time of procedure
    - Amount of drainage
    - Characteristics of drainage
    - Patient response
    - Suction reestablished
    - Patient teaching (see Patient Teaching box on p. 339)
15. Report any abnormal characteristics of drainage (see Table 13-2).

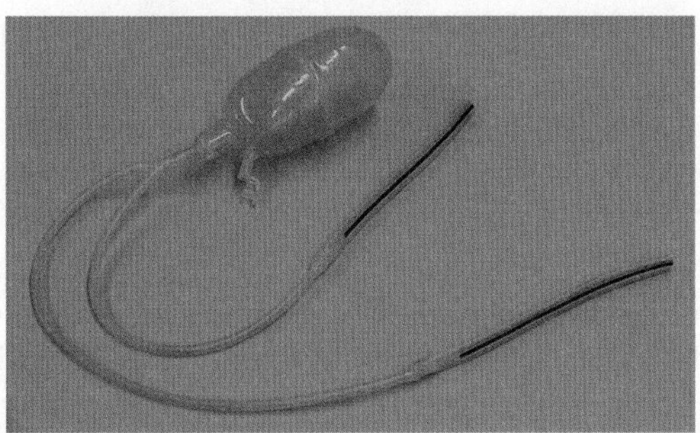

FIGURE 13-7 Jackson-Pratt drains have wide, flat areas that have to be brought through the stab wound with great force.

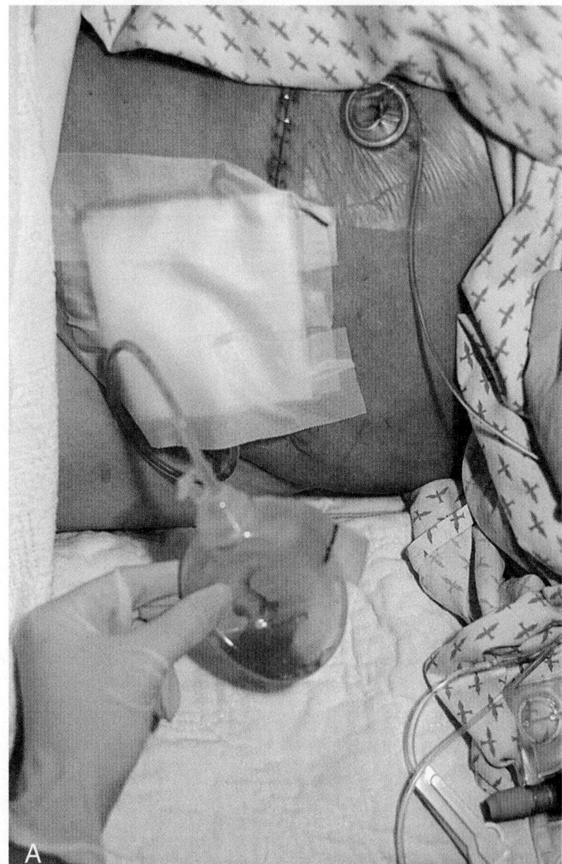

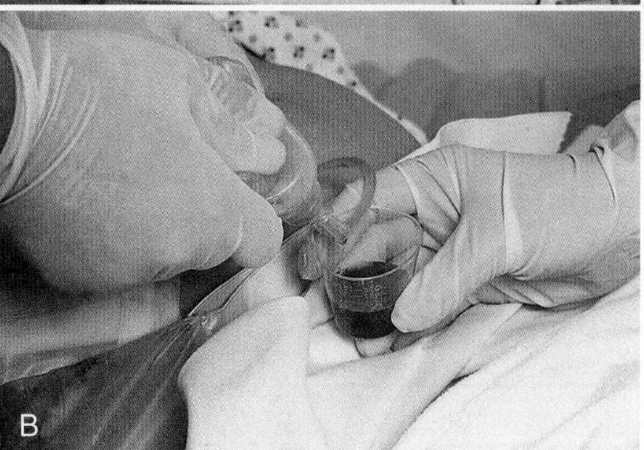

FIGURE 13-8 Jackson-Pratt drainage device. **A,** drainage tubes and reservoir. **B,** Emptying drainage reservoir.

wound. The Penrose drain commonly serves this purpose. When it is inserted, a sterile safety pin is placed through the drain to keep it from sliding into the wound. When the surgeon wants a gentle vacuum, it is possible to use a closed drainage system. The portable vacuum container (e.g., Hemovac, RediVac) is an expandable unit that is connected by tubes to the drainage site (see Skill 13-6). As the unit creates gentle suction, exudate collects in the drainage receptacle. The Jackson-Pratt and Davol evacuators are other types of closed drainage systems that use a bulb to provide the needed vacuum (Figures 13-7 and 13-8).

A drainage system requires close monitoring. In addition to noting the color, the consistency, and the amount of drainage, it is important to check the tube's patency. Do not allow a tube to become kinked or occluded; if blood clots or exudate have slowed drainage, record this and report it.

T-Tube Drainage System

After surgical removal of the gallbladder (an open cholecystectomy), the bile duct is often inflamed and edematous. The physician will frequently insert a drainage tube into the duct to maintain a free flow of bile until edema subsides. This tube is called a T-tube. The long end of the T-tube exits through the abdominal incision or through a separate surgical wound (Figure 13-9). The tube drains by gravity into a closed drainage system. The collection bag is emptied and measured every shift or as necessary (Box 13-4).

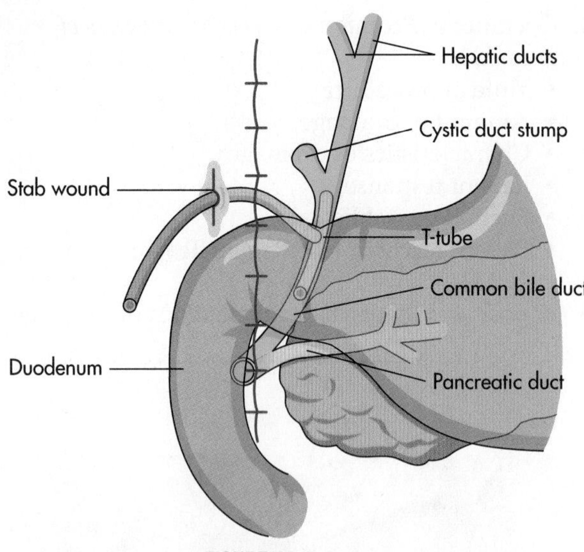

FIGURE 13-9 T-Tube.

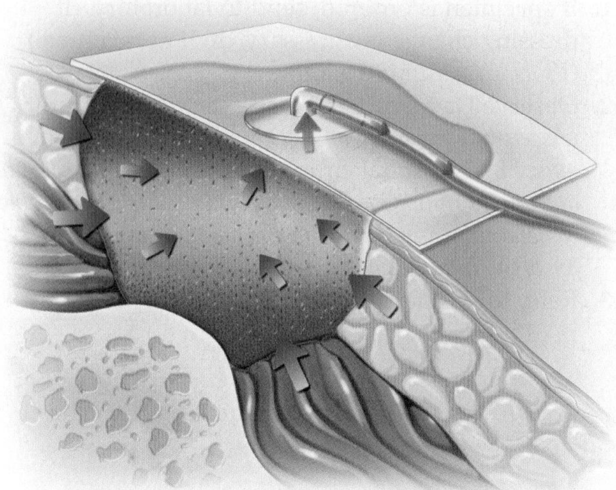

FIGURE 13-10 Wound VAC system uses negative pressure to remove fluid from area surrounding the wound, reducing edema and improving circulation to the area.

Box 13-4 Care of the T-Tube Drainage System

Nursing interventions for the patient with bile drainage include the following:

- Include specific measures or techniques for dressing change in the nursing care plan to provide continuity of care.
- Assess the patency of the drainage tube frequently, preventing twists or kinks to ensure appropriate, continuous drainage.
- Keep the collection receptacle below the level of the wound or common bile duct to ensure appropriate drainage.
- Keep the receptacle compressed, and frequently monitor it to maintain a vacuum. (Many T-tube drainage systems use drainage by gravity only.)
- Protect the skin surrounding the wound from bile drainage to prevent tissue damage.
- Assess excessive bile leakage from the wound, because it may indicate occlusion of drainage tube.
- Assess for normal bile drainage: amount varies from 250 to 500 mL/24 hours, with color normally greenish brown, thick, and slightly blood tinged in the first 24 hours.
- Consider the use of Montgomery straps when the dressing requires frequent changing, to prevent tape from impairing skin integrity (see Box 13-1 and Skill 13-1, step 14).
- Assess the need for patient teaching during the dressing change and wound care.
- Secure the vacuum unit to the patient's gown with a safety pin, avoiding tension on the tubing.
- Record the amount of drainage on the intake and output sheet to provide an accurate intake and output record.

Wound Vacuum-Assisted Closure

The wound **vacuum-assisted closure** (wound VAC) is a device that assists in wound closure by applying localized negative pressure to draw the edges of a wound together. VAC accelerates wound healing by promoting the formation of granulation tissue, collagen, fibroblasts, and inflammatory cells in order to completely close or improve the condition of a wound in preparation for a skin graft. The use of negative pressure removes fluid from the area surrounding the wound, thus reducing local or peripheral edema and improving circulation to the area (Figure 13-10). In addition, after 3 or 4 days of therapy, bacterial counts in the wound drop.

Wound VAC is used to treat both acute wounds (such as traumatic wounds, flaps, and grafts) and chronic wounds. The schedule for changing wound VAC dressings varies. An infected wound sometimes calls for a dressing change every 24 hours, whereas dressing changes three times a week suffice for a clean wound. As the wound heals, the wound base becomes redder and granulation tissue lines its surface. The wound has a stippled or granulated appearance. Last, the surface area of the wound changes size, either increasing or decreasing depending on wound location and the amount of drainage removed by the wound VAC system. As the wound heals, paler areas in the wound often develop. This indicates an increase in fibrous tissue. The wound will have to be assessed for location, appearance, and size. This will provide information regarding status of wound healing, presence of complications, and the proper type of supplies and assistance needed to apply the new transparent dressing (Skill 13-7).

You will want to assess the patient's comfort level using a scale of 0 to 10. This will determine effectiveness of comfort control measures before, during, and after dressing change. Assess the patient's knowledge of the purpose of the dressing change because this will determine the level of support and explanation required. Keep your focus on the expected outcomes of preventing infection, promoting healing, control of pain, and patient and family education.

Skill 13-7 Wound Vacuum-Assisted Closure

Nursing Action *(Rationale)*

1. See standard steps in wound care 1 to 9, pp. 314 to 315.
2. Assemble equipment (see illustration):
   - VAC system (requires physician's order)
   - VAC foam dressing
   - Tubing for connection between VAC system and VAC dressing
   - Gloves, clean and sterile
   - Scissors (sterile)
   - Skin Prep or skin barrier
   - Moist washcloth
   - Plastic or waterproof refuse bag
   - Linen bag
3. Position patient comfortably, and drape to expose only wound site. Instruct patient not to touch wound or sterile supplies. *(Maintaining patient comfort assists in completing skill smoothly. Draping provides access to wound while keeping unnecessary exposure to a minimum.)*
4. Place disposable waterproof bag within reach of work area with top folded to make a cuff. *(Facilitates safe disposal of soiled dressings.)*
5. When VAC system is in place, begin by pushing therapy on-off button. *(Deactivates therapy and allows for proper drainage of fluid in drainage tubing.)*
   - Keeping tube connected to VAC system, disconnect tubes from each other to drain fluids into canister.
   - Before lowering, tighten clamp on canister tube.
6. With dressing tube unclamped, introduce 10 to 30 mL of normal saline, if ordered, into tubing to soak underneath foam. *(Facilitates loosening of foam when tissue adheres to foam.)*
7. Gently stretch transparent film horizontally, and slowly pull up from the skin. *(Reduces stress on suture line or wound edges and reduces irritation and discomfort.)*
8. Remove old VAC system dressing, observing appearance and drainage on dressing. Use caution to prevent tension on any drains that are present. Discard dressing and remove gloves. Perform hand hygiene. *(Determines dressings needed for replacement. Prevents accidental removal of drains that are sometimes sutured in place and sometimes not.)*
9. Apply sterile or clean gloves. Irrigate the wound (see Skill 13-4) with normal saline or other solution ordered by the physician. Gently blot to dry. (If this is a new surgical wound, sterile technique will possibly be ordered. Chronic wounds often require clean technique.) *(Irrigation removes wound debris.)*
10. Measure wound as ordered: at baseline, at first dressing change, weekly, and at discharge from therapy. Remove and discard gloves. (Wound cultures are sometimes ordered on a routine basis. However, when drainage looks purulent, there is change in amount or color, or drainage has a foul odor, obtain wound cultures even when they are not scheduled for that particular dressing change.) *(Objectively documents wound healing process in response to negative pressure, wound therapy.)*
11. Depending on the type of wound, apply sterile gloves or new clean gloves. *(Fresh sterile wounds*

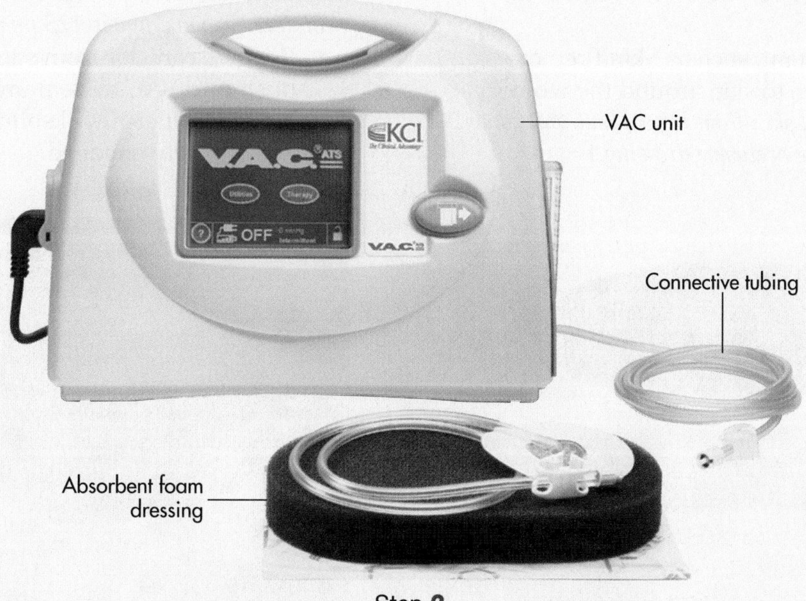

Step **2**

Continued

Skill 13-7 Wound Vacuum-Assisted Closure—cont'd

require sterile gloves. Chronic wounds often require clean technique.) Do not use the same gloves worn to remove old dressing. *(Cross-contamination is a possible result.)*

12. Prepare VAC foam.
    a. Select appropriate foam (see illustration).
    b. Using sterile scissors, cut foam to wound size. Proper size of foam dressing helps maintain negative pressure to entire wound. It is essential to cut dressing to fit the size and shape of the wound, including tunnels and undermined areas. (Patients sometimes experience more pain with the black foam because of excessive wound contraction. For this reason you will perhaps have to switch to the PVA soft foam.) *(Black polyurethane [PU] foam has larger pores and is most effective in stimulating granulation tissue and wound contraction. White polyvinyl alcohol [PVA] soft foam is denser, with smaller pores; use it when the growth of granulation tissue has to be restricted.)*
13. Gently place foam in wound, making sure that the foam is in contact with entire wound base, margins, and tunneled and undermined areas. *(Maintains negative pressure to entire wound. Edges of the foam dressing have to be in direct contact with the patient's skin.)*
14. Apply wrinkle-free transparent dressing over foam and secure tubing to the unit (see illustrations). (For deep wounds, regularly reposition tubing to minimize pressure on wound edges. In addition, it is important to frequently reposition patients with restricted mobility or sensation so that they do not lie on the tubing and cause further impairment of skin integrity.) *(Connects the negative pressure from the VAC system to the wound foam.)*
15. Apply skin protectant, such as Skin Prep or Stomahesive water, to skin around the wound. *(Protects periwound skin from injury that will sometimes result from the occlusive dressing.)*

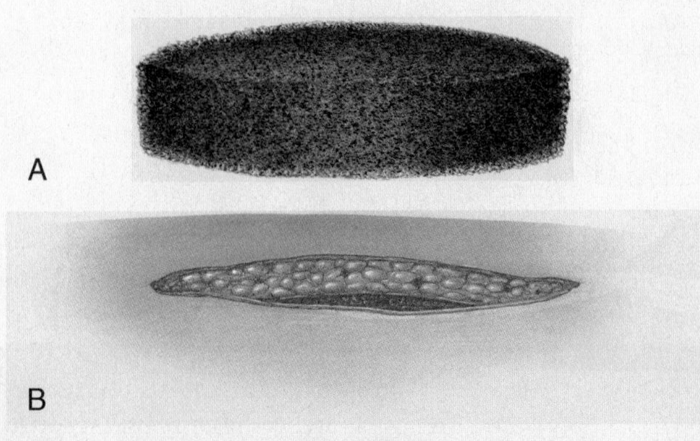

Step **12a**

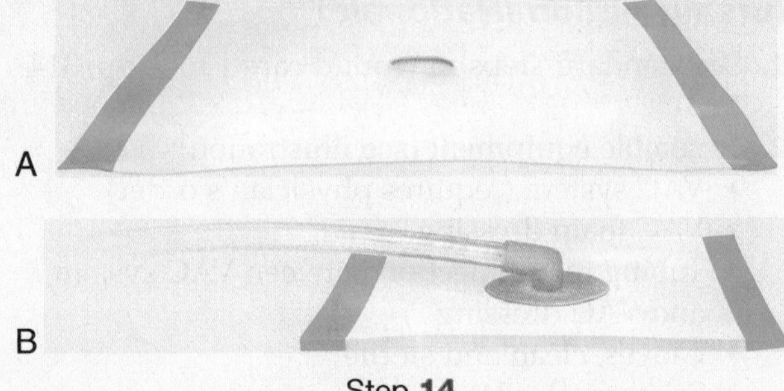

Step **14**

16. Apply wound VAC dressing. *(Ensures that the wound is properly covered and a negative pressure seal can be achieved.)* (Box 13-5)
    a. Cover with VAC foam, keeping margin of 1 to 2 inches (3 to 5 cm) of surrounding healthy tissue. Apply wrinkle-free transparent dressing. *(Excessive tension has potential to compress foam dressing and impede wound healing. Excessive tension also produces a shear force on periwound area.)*
    b. Secure tubing to transparent film, aligning drainage holes to ensure an occlusive seal. **Do not apply tension to drape and tubing.**
17. Secure tubing several inches away from the dressing. *(Prevents pull on the primary dressing, which can cause leaks in the negative pressure system.)*
18. Once wound is completely covered (see illustration), connect the tubing from the dressing to the tubing from the canister and the VAC system. *(Administration of intermittent or continuous negative pressure between 5 mm Hg and 200 mm Hg is acceptable, according to physician's order and patient comfort. The average is 125 mm Hg.)*
    a. Remove canister from sterile packaging, and push into VAC system until a click is heard. NOTE: An alarm will sound if the canister is not properly engaged.

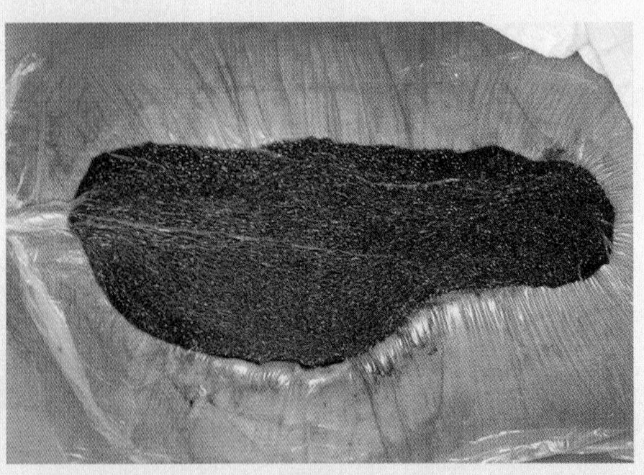
Step **18**

b. Connect the dressing tubing to the canister tubing. Make sure both clamps are open.
c. Place VAC system on a level surface, or hang from the foot of the bed. NOTE: The VAC system will alarm and deactivate therapy if the unit is tilted beyond 45 degrees.
d. Press green-lit power button, and set pressure as ordered.

19. Discard old dressing materials, remove gloves, and perform hand hygiene. *(Reduces transmission of microorganisms.)*
20. Inspect wound VAC system to verify that negative pressure is achieved. *(Negative pressure is achieved when an airtight seal is achieved.)* (see Box 13-5)
    a. Verify that display screen reads "THERAPY ON."
    b. Be sure clamps are open and tubing is patent.
    c. Identify air leaks by listening with stethoscope or by moving hand around edges of wound while applying light pressure.
    d. If a leak is present, use strips of transparent film to patch the edges of the wound.
21. Refer to standard steps in wound care 10 to 17, p. 315.
22. Document:
    - Appearance of wound color; characteristics of any drainage. Compare wound with baseline wound assessment.
    - Presence of wound healing augmentation such as wound VAC.
    - Response to dressing change.
    - Record date and time of dressing change on new dressing.
23. Report immediately to the physician:
    - Bright, brick-red bleeding
    - Evidence of poor wound healing
    - Evisceration
    - Dehiscence
    - Possible wound infection *(These signs are abnormal and necessitate immediate interventions.)*

Evidence-Based Practice — Moisture-Associated Skin Damage from Dressings

Evidence Summary

Wound management and wound healing are critical to patients at risk for pressure ulcers and those with pressure ulcers or with other chronic wounds. Advances in wound care show the benefit of a moist wound environment and the accepted practice of moist wound healing. However, a moist wound environment may damage the wound edges (periwound skin). This damage is maceration; the tissues of the periwound skin soften, and the connective fibers are damaged. This condition is also classified as moisture-associated skin damage (MASD). This study reviewed the existing literature to evaluate the effect of moist wound healing on the periwound skin. Although further research is needed to identify and evaluate the best strategy for managing existing periwound maceration, there are some clinical applications that may help prevent or manage MASD.

Application to Nursing Practice

- Use of a skin protectant (no-sting film barrier, petrolatum- or zinc-based protectant) helps to prevent periwound skin maceration.
- Dressing selection needs to be individualized to the type of wound and wound-healing goals.
- Topical preparations such as BCT ointment (Xenaderm) help manage periwound MASD.
- Use of negative-pressure wound therapy (NPWT) may reduce the risk of periwound maceration by reducing local edema and exudates in the periwound tissue. (See Skill 13-7.)

Reference

Gray, M., & Weir, D. (2007). Prevention and treatment of moisture-associated skin damage (maceration) in the periwound skin, *Journal of Wound, Ostomy, and Continence Nursing, 34*(2):153.

From Potter, P.A., & Perry, A.G. (2009). *Fundamentals of nursing: concepts, process, and practice.* (7th ed.). St. Louis: Mosby.

Box 13-5 Maintaining an Airtight Seal

To avoid wound desiccation (to cause to dry up), it is essential that the wound stay sealed once therapy is initiated. Problem seal areas include wounds around joints and near the sacrum. The following tips may assist you to create and maintain an airtight seal:

- Shave hair around wound.
- Cut transparent film to extend 1 to 2 inches (3 to 5 cm) beyond wound parameter.
- Prevent wrinkles in transparent film.
- Use multiple small strips of transparent film to hold dressing in place before covering dressing with large piece of transparent film.
- Avoid use of adhesive remover because it leaves a residue that hinders film adherence.

Adapted from Elkin, M., Perry, A.G., & Potter, P.A. (2007). *Nursing interventions and clinical skills.* (4th ed.). St. Louis: Mosby.

BANDAGES AND BINDERS

A **bandage** is a strip or roll of cloth or other material that can be wound around a part of the body in a variety of ways for multiple purposes. Bandages are available in rolls of various widths and materials, including gauze, elasticized knit, elastic webbing, flannel, and muslin. Gauze bandages are lightweight and inexpensive, mold easily around contours of the body, and permit air circulation that helps prevent skin maceration (the softening and breaking down of skin from prolonged exposure to moisture) (see Evidence-Based Practice box). Elastic bandages conform well to body parts but also can be used to exert pressure over a body part. Flannel and muslin bandages are thicker than gauze and thus stronger for supporting or applying pressure. A flannel bandage also insulates to provide warmth.

A **binder** is a bandage that is made of large pieces of material to fit a specific body part, for example, an abdominal binder or a breast binder. Most binders are made of elastic, cotton, muslin, or flannel.

Correctly applied bandages and binders do not cause injury to underlying and nearby body parts or create discomfort for the patient (Skills 13-8 and 13-9, Table 13-4). For example, a chest binder must not be so tight as to restrict chest wall expansion. Before a bandage or binder is applied, your nursing responsibilities include the following (see Coordinated Care box):

- Inspecting the skin for abrasions, edema, discoloration, or exposed wound edges
- Covering exposed wounds or open abrasions with sterile dressings
- Assessing the condition of underlying dressings and changing them if soiled

Text continued on p. 337

Skill 13-8 Applying a Bandage

Nursing Action *(Rationale)*

1. Refer to standard steps in wound care 1 to 9, pp. 314 to 315.
2. Assemble equipment:
   - Correct width and number of bandages
   - Safety pins, fasteners, and/or tape
   - Gloves, if wound drainage is present
3. Ensure that skin and dressing are clean and dry. *(Allows bandages to be applied to clean, dry areas to prevent further impaired skin integrity.)*
4. Separate any adjacent skin surfaces. *(Prevents irritation and impairment of skin integrity.)*
5. Align part to be bandaged, providing slight flexion as appropriate and not contraindicated. *(Promotes comfort and functional use.)*
6. Apply bandage from distal to proximal part. *(Encourages return of venous blood flow to heart.)*
7. Apply bandage with even distribution of pressure. *(Maintains uniform bandage tension, prevents impairment of circulation.)*
   a. For the circular bandage, see Table 13-4.
   b. For the spiral bandage, see Table 13-4.
   c. For the spiral-reverse bandage, see Table 13-4.
   d. For the recurrent (stump) bandage, see Table 13-4.
   e. For the figure-of-8 bandage, see Table 13-4.
   f. Secure first bandage before applying additional rolls. Apply additional rolls without leaving any uncovered areas. *(Prevents wrinkling or loose ends.)*
8. Assess tension of bandage and circulation of extremity. *(Ensures that bandage is applied appropriately.)*
9. Refer to standard steps in wound care 10 to 17, p. 315.

Skill 13-9 Applying a Binder, Arm Sling, and T-Binder

Nursing Action *(Rationale)*

1. Refer to standard steps in wound care 1 to 9, pp. 314 to 315.
2. Assemble equipment:
   - Binder
   - Safety pins
   - Washcloth
   - Towel
   - Soap
   - Water
   - Cotton or gauze pad
   - Pain medication, if indicated
   - Dressing, as necessary
3. Change dressing if appropriate; cleanse skin if needed. *(Prepares underlying skin surfaces for binder application.)*
4. Separate skin surfaces or pad bony prominences. *(Protects skin surfaces from contact, preventing irritation and impairment of skin integrity.)*
5. Apply binder.
   a. Triangular binder (sling)
      (1) Have patient flex arm at approximately 80-degree angle, depending on purpose of binder. *(Allows proper angle for application.)*
      (2) Place end of triangular binder over shoulder of the uninjured side, anterior to posterior (see illustration). *(Places point of triangle under patient's elbow of injured arm.)*
      (3) Grasp other end of binder and bring it up and over injured arm to shoulder of injured arm. *(Supports the impaired arm.)*
      (4) Use square knot to tie two ends together at lateral area of neck on uninjured side. *(Prevents slippage to knot. Prevents wear on bony prominences.)*
      (5) Support wrist well with binder; do not allow it to extend over end of binder.

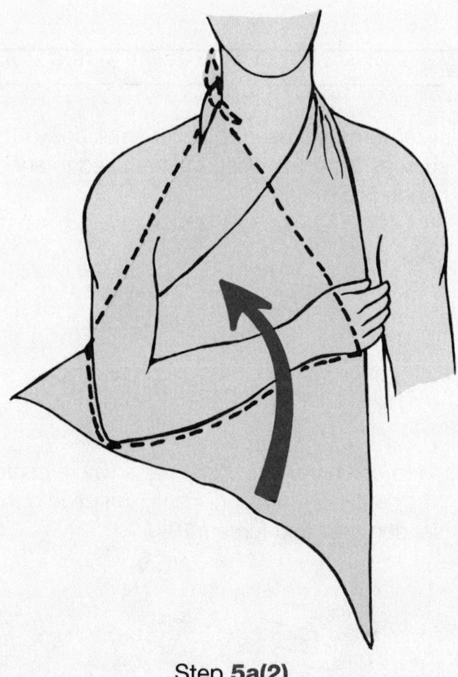
Step **5a(2)**

(Maintains body alignment. Prevents circulation impairment.)

(6) Fold third triangle end neatly around elbow and secure with safety pins. *(Secures binder. Prevents arm from slipping out.)*

b. T-binder (see illustration)

(1) Using appropriate binder, place the waistband smoothly under patient's waist; patient should be positioned lying supine; tail(s) should be under patient. *(Allows use of appropriate binder; single tail for female patients and two tails for male patients.)*

(2) Secure two ends of waistband together with safety pin. *(Allows securing at the waist.)*

(3) Single tail—bring the tail up between legs to secure dressing in place. Two tails—bring tails up one on each side of penis or large dressing. *(Secures dressing, pad, or other item without causing pressure on the genitalia.)*

(4) Bring tails under and over waistband; secure with safety pins.

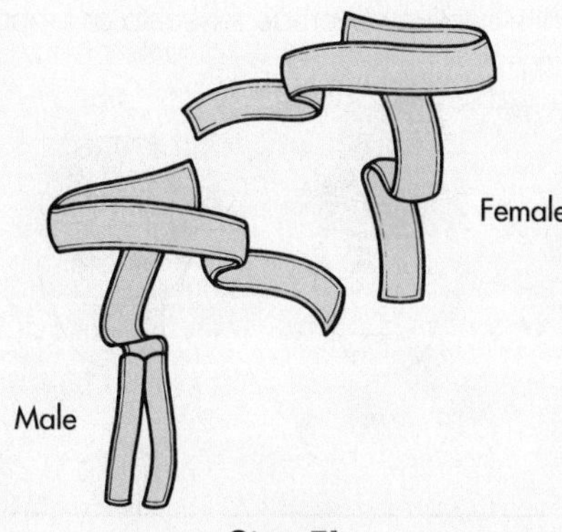

Step **5b**

c. Elastic abdominal binder (see illustration)

(1) Center binder smoothly under appropriate part of patient. *(Promotes effectiveness of binder.)*

(2) Close binder: Pull one end of binder over center of patient's abdomen while maintaining tension on that end of binder; pull opposite end of binder over center and secure with Velcro closure tabs, metal fasteners, or horizontally placed safety pins. *(Provides continuous wound support and comfort.)*

(3) Observe patient's respiratory status. *(Abdominal binders that are too tight will often interfere with respirations.)*

d. For postsurgical application of Scultetus abdominal binders, proceed upward from bottom (except for a patient after cesarean delivery) to minimize pull on the suture line (see illustration).

6. Note comfort level of patient. Smooth out binder to prevent wrinkles. Adjust binder as necessary. *(Promotes comfort and chest expansion.)*

7. Refer to standard steps in wound care 10 to 17, p. 315.

8. Document:
- Time of application
- Type of binder
- Patient's response
- Patient teaching (see Patient Teaching box on p. 339)

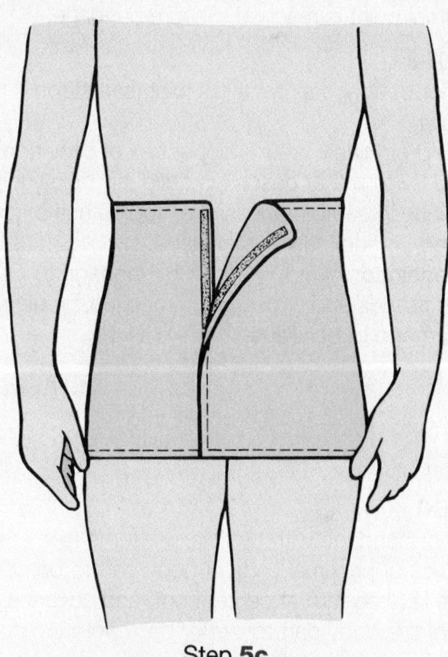
Step **5c**

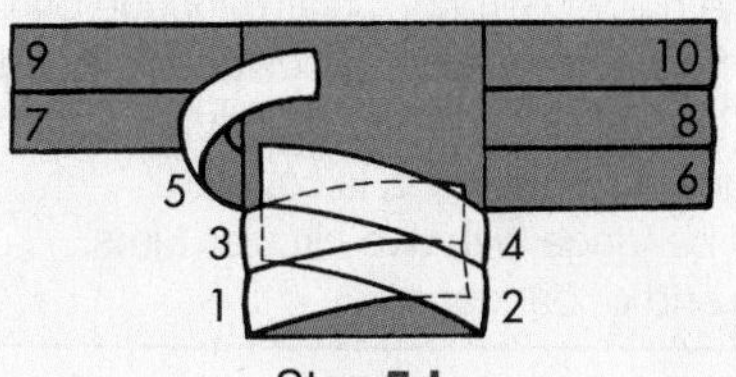

Step **5d**

Table 13-4 Basic Bandage Turns

BASIC BANDAGE TURNS	USE
CIRCULAR 1. Unroll 3 to 4 inches of bandage from back of roll. 2. Place flat bandage surface on anterior surface of portion of body to be covered and hold end in place with thumb of nondominant hand. 3. Continue rolling bandage around same area until two overlapping layers of bandage cover part. Remove excess bandage roll. 4. Secure end of bandage with safety pin or clip if it is attached to end of bandage. If end of bandage has raw edge, fold 0.5 to 1 inch under before securing bandage. Gauze bandage is possible to secure with strip of adhesive tape.	Circular turns are used to cover small body regions such as a digit or wrist and are used to anchor bandaging materials. 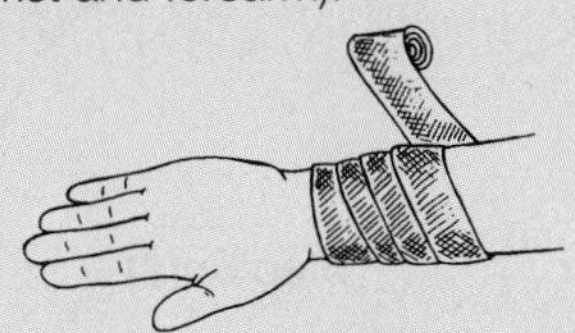
SPIRAL 1. Anchor bandage at distal end of body part with two circular turns (note steps 1 through 3, Circular). 2. Advance bandage on ascending angle, overlapping each preceding turn by half to two-thirds the width of bandage roll until proximal border of area is covered. 3. Secure end of bandage.	Used to cover cylindric body parts where contour of part does not vary significantly in size (e.g., slender wrist and forearm). 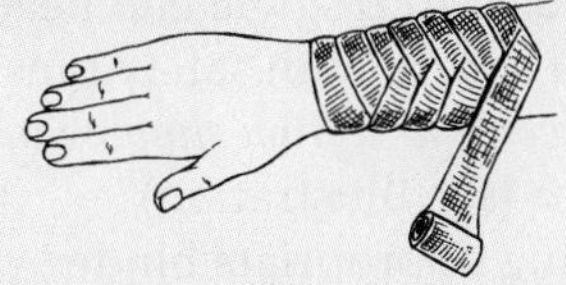
SPIRAL-REVERSE 1. Anchor bandage at distal border of area to be covered (use one to three circular turns). 2. Advance bandage on ascending angle of approximately 30 degrees. 3. Halfway through each turn fold bandage toward you and continue around part in downward stroke. 4. Continue advancing bandage as in steps 2 and 3 until desired proximal point is reached. Secure bandage.	Used to cover inverted cone-shaped body parts such as calf or thigh.
FIGURE-OF-8 1. Anchor bandage at center of joint (see steps 1 through 3, Circular). 2. Ascend obliquely around upper half of circular turn above joint followed by turn that descends obliquely below joint. 3. Continue in same manner, overlapping half of previous turn until desired immobilization is attained. 4. Be certain to cover the joint with bandage to prevent fluid shift to those tissues and subsequent impaired circulation. 5. Secure end of bandage.	Used to cover joints and provide immobilization. Outer surface of fabric is against skin during ascending application of bandage. Each reverse turn places alternate side of bandage toward skin. 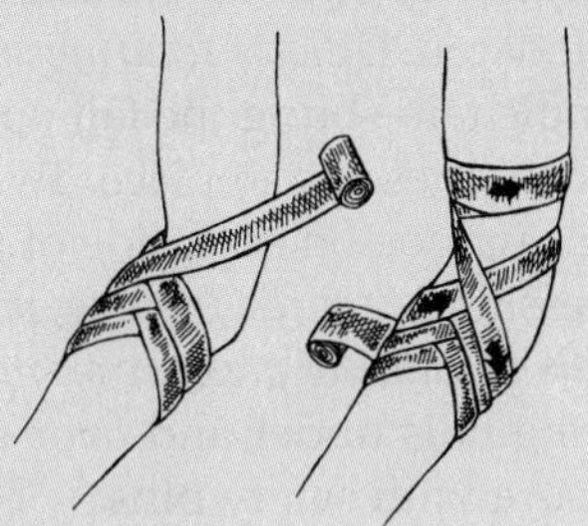
RECURRENT 1. Anchor bandage with two circular turns (see steps 1 through 3, Circular) at proximal ends of body part to be covered. 2. Make reverse turn at center front, and advance fabric over distal end of the body part to center back, forming covering perpendicular to first circular turns. 3. Make reverse turn at back and bring bandage forward, overlapping one half of perpendicular bandage on one side. Make reverse turn at front and overlap opposite side of center, continuing on to back. Repeat these steps, overlapping each previous strip of bandage until entire area is covered. 4. Anchor bandage with two circular turns. 5. Secure end of bandage.	Provides caplike coverage for scalp or amputation stump. 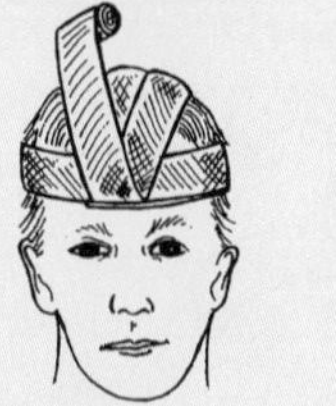 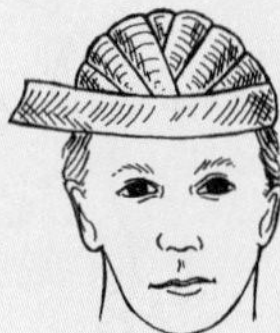

 Coordinated Care

Delegation

DRESSING CHANGES

Check institutional policy and the state's nurse practice act regarding which wound care interventions can be delegated to assistive personnel (AP). In some states, aspects of wound care such as dressing change are permitted to be delegated. Possibly this will include the changing of dry dressings using clean technique for chronic wounds. In this situation, instruct staff on what to report when a wound is cleansed. It is also necessary for AP to know how to use clean technique so as to avoid cross-contamination. All wound assessment—the care of acute new wounds and those that require sterile technique for dressing changes—generally remains within the domain of professional nursing practice. The assessment of the wound requires the critical thinking and knowledge application unique to a nurse even when the dressing change is delegated to others.

It is acceptable to delegate the skill of applying a transparent dressing to an AP.

Assessment of wound drainage and maintenance of drains and the drainage system require the critical thinking and knowledge application unique to a nurse. However, delegation to an AP is often appropriate for emptying a closed drainage container, measuring the amount of drainage, and reporting the amount on the patient's intake and output (I&O) record.

The skill of suture removal requires the critical thinking and knowledge application unique to the nurse. For this skill, delegation is inappropriate.

It is acceptable to delegate the skills of applying a binder (abdominal or breast) to AP. However, it is the responsibility of the nurse to assess the patient's ability to breathe deeply, cough effectively, and move independently before and after binder application. The nurse is also responsible for assessing the patient's skin for irritation or abrasion, the underlying wound, and patient's level of comfort.

The skill of applying the wound vacuum-assisted closure (VAC) is inappropriate to delegate owing to the unique knowledge necessary for application.

- Assessing the skin of underlying body parts and parts that will be distal to the bandage for signs of circulatory impairment (coolness, pallor or cyanosis, diminished or absent pulses, numbness, and tingling) to provide a means for comparing changes in circulation after bandage application

After a bandage is applied, you will assess, document, and immediately report changes in circulation, skin integrity, comfort level, and body function, such as ventilation or movement. If you apply a bandage, it is acceptable for you also to loosen or readjust it as necessary. Obtain a physician's order before loosening or removing a bandage the physician applied. Explain to the patient that any bandage or binder will by definition feel relatively firm or tight. Assess any bandage carefully to be sure it is properly applied and is providing therapeutic benefit, and replace soiled bandages. Like a damp dressing, a bandage or binder is a potential harbor for microorganisms (Box 13-6).

Box 13-6 Guidelines for Applying a Bandage or Binder

1. Position body part to be bandaged in comfortable position of normal anatomical alignment. Bandages cause restriction in movement. Immobilization in position of normal functioning reduces risks of deformity or injury.
2. Prevent friction between and against skin surfaces by applying gauze or cotton padding. Skin surfaces in contact with each other (e.g., between toes, under breasts) will likely rub against each other and cause abrasion or chafing. Bandages over body prominences will often rub against skin and cause impairment of skin integrity.
3. Apply bandages securely to prevent slippage during movement. Friction between bandage and skin can cause impairment of skin integrity.
4. When bandaging extremities, apply bandage first at the distal end and progress toward the trunk (heart).
5. Gradual application of pressure from the distal toward the proximal portion of the extremity promotes venous return and keeps the risk of edema or circulatory impairment to a minimum.
6. Apply bandages firmly, with equal tension exerted over each turn or layer. Avoid excess overlapping of bandage layers. (Approximately one third to one half of previous layer should be covered by successive layers.) Proper application prevents unequal pressure distribution over bandaged body part. Localized pressure causes circulatory impairment.
7. Position pins, knots, or ties away from wound or sensitive skin areas. These materials potentially exert localized pressure and cause irritation.
8. Remove and reapply an elastic bandage at least once every 8 hours unless otherwise directed by physician.
9. Remove elastic bandage whenever necessary to readjust wrinkles, looseness, or tightness; because of patient discomfort; or when you note signs and symptoms of nerve or vascular impairment.
10. Apply bandages to the lower extremities before the patient sits or stands (i.e., with patient lying down).
11. Use increasingly wider bandages as size of area to be covered increases.
12. Use adhesive tape rather than loose clips or pins to fasten bandages on small child or infant. Safety pins are more effective than clips and do not fall out of bandage. Many facilities prefer tape for safety and maintenance of skin integrity.
13. Patients with tubes or drains who have binders will require frequent assessment to ensure patency of tubes for drainage.

NURSING PROCESS

The role of the licensed practical nurse/licensed vocational nurse (LPN/LVN) in the nursing process as stated is that the LPN/LVN will:

- Participate in planning care for patients based on patient needs
- Review patient's plan of care and recommend revisions as needed
- Review and follow defined prioritization for patient care
- Use clinical pathways, care maps, or care plans to guide and review patient care

Assessment

Note whether wound edges are closed. Assessment will consist of location, size or dimensions, exudates, wound bed or edges, tunnel or undermining, periwound characteristics, pain, signs and symptoms of infection. A surgical incision will properly have clean, well-approximated edges. Crusts often form along the wound edges from exudate. A puncture wound is usually a small, circular wound with the edges coming together toward the center. If a wound is open, separate the wound edges and inspect the condition of underlying tissue such as adipose and connective tissue. Also look for complications such as **dehiscence** (separation of surgical incision or rupture of wound closure, typically an abdominal incision) and **evisceration** (the protrusion of an internal organ through a wound or surgical incision, especially in the abdominal wall). The outer edges of a wound normally appear inflamed for the first 2 to 3 days, but this slowly disappears. Within 7 to 10 days, a normally healing wound fills with epithelial cells, and edges close. If infection develops, the wound edges become brightly erythematous and edematous.

If a closed wound is covered by a dressing, observe the dressing but do not change it until an order is issued. If a dressing becomes saturated with exudate before the order is given, reinforce the dressing over the incisional area by placing sterile gauze on top of the original dressing and anchoring it securely. Record and report any dressing that is reinforced. Observe the amount of exudate observed and document the dressings applied.

Nursing Diagnosis

After completing an assessment of the patient's wound, you will identify nursing diagnoses that will direct supportive and preventive care. Existence of a wound clearly indicates the following nursing diagnosis:

- Impaired skin integrity

This nursing diagnosis will lead you to initiate interventions that promote the healing process.

Some patients will be at risk for poor wound healing because of preexisting conditions that impair healing (see Table 13-1). Thus, even though the patient's wound appears normal, it is important that you identify nursing diagnoses that direct nursing interventions toward support of wound repair, such as the following:

- Imbalanced nutrition: more than body requirements
- Imbalanced nutrition: less than body requirements
- Ineffective tissue perfusion (specify type)

The nature of a wound can cause problems unrelated to wound healing. Pain and impaired mobility can affect a patient's eventual recovery. For example, a large abdominal incision can cause enough pain to interfere with the patient's ability to turn in bed effectively (Box 13-7).

Expected Outcomes and Planning

You will establish a plan of care based on the patient's health care needs. These needs are identified during the assessment phase of the nursing process. Next you form the nursing diagnostic statement and devise the plan of care. Consider the patient's plan of care for discharge because patients are discharged earlier than in the past (Home Care Considerations box). Incorporate patient and family teaching into the patient's plan of care (Patient Teaching box). Consider special needs of the older adult when performing wound care (Cultural Considerations and Life Span Considerations for Older Adults boxes).

Box 13-7 Nursing Diagnoses Related to Wound Healing

- Ineffective breathing pattern, related to:
  —Pain secondary to abdominal or thoracic incision
- Risk for infection, related to:
  —Malnutrition
  —Tissue loss and increased environmental exposure
- Impaired physical mobility, related to:
  —Pain of surgical wound or site of surgery (e.g., joint replacement)
- Imbalanced nutrition: less than body requirements, related to:
  —Inability to ingest or tolerate food
- Acute pain, related to:
  —Surgical incision
- Situational low self-esteem, related to:
  —Perception of scars
  —Perception of surgical drains
  —Reaction to surgically removed body part
- Impaired skin integrity, related to:
  —Surgical incision
  —Pressure
  —Chemical injury
  —Secretions and excretions
- Risk for impaired skin integrity, related to:
  —Physical immobilization
  —Exposure to secretions

Home Care Considerations

Wound Care

- Demonstrate wound care and provide time for return demonstration.
- Explain need for specialized supplies such as irrigating solutions and dressings and need to maintain sterile asepsis when performing care.
- Instruct as to where and how to obtain additional supplies.
- Instruct about signs of improper wound healing and wound infections.
- Explain why wound is being allowed to heal by secondary intention.
- Assess understanding of need for the methods of wound care.
- Instruct primary caregiver and patient in how to maintain clean technique when changing dressings. Wear clean gloves, and perform hand hygiene after procedure. Use of clean dressings is permitted in the home environment.
- Make certain patient knows when and what signs and symptoms to report to physician or primary caregiver.
- Assess extent of wound or incision in relation to patient's level of activity to determine type of dressing that will achieve desired purpose.
- Assess area where procedure will be performed for adequate lighting and running water. Determine whether there is table or cabinet on which sterile supplies may be placed with reasonable security.
- Bedroom or bathroom is usually ideal for procedure.
- Cleansing wound in the shower is acceptable if approved by physician.
- If drainage system is present, explain how system operates.
- Explain importance of drainage system.
- Demonstrate procedure for emptying the drainage chamber and how to reseal it without contaminating unit.
- Make sure the drain is protected from the disoriented patient, who may pull it out.
- Teach proper application of binder.
- Teach proper care of binder.

Patient Teaching

Wound Care

- Assist patient to accept the surgical wound by stating the progress of the wound and how healing is occurring.
- Teach importance of early ambulation after surgery.
- Teach importance of a nutritious diet in wound healing.
- Explain that dressings will perhaps be required at home and how to purchase what will be needed. Inform of home health services if needed or per physician's order.
- Wounds out of patient's reach and vision necessitate assistance by a family member or other caregiver.
- Explain expected wound appearance, what should be reported, and risks of improper wound care.
- After demonstrating wound care, allow the patient or the family member to perform wound care with supervision.
- Teach the importance of keeping dressings, sutures, and staples dry and clean.
- Explain the importance of washing hands before and after dressing changes.
- Teach signs and symptoms of infection.
- Instruct the patient to notify the physician if signs of wound infection appear.
- Follow physician's instructions for limiting activity.
- Provide written instructions in addition to verbal ones.
- Allow time for patient's questions.
- If drainage system is present:
  - —Explain purpose of drainage system.
  - —Explain importance of measuring output.
  - —Instruct to keep Hemovac or Davol tubing clipped or pinned to gown to prevent accidental dislodgement.
  - —Teach what to do if the drain accidentally comes out.
- If binder is present, teach function of the binder.
- Teach to report if binder is loose or causing pain or discomfort.
- Teach to report any breathing restrictions if binder is too tight.

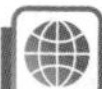

Cultural Considerations

Wound Care

Detecting cyanosis and other changes in skin color in patients is an important clinical skill. However, this detection can become a challenge in dark-skinned patients. Cyanosis is defined as a slightly blue-gray slatelike or dark purple discoloration of the skin due to a reduction of at least 5 g of hemoglobin in arterial blood. Color differentiation of cyanosis varies according to skin pigmentation. In dark-skinned patients, you need to know the individual's baseline skin tone. Do not confuse the normal hyperpigmentation of Mongolian spots that are seen on the sacrum of African-American, Native American, and Asian-American patients as cyanosis. Observe the patient's skin in daylight without glare.

Keep in mind the following points:

- Cyanosis is difficult but possible to detect in a dark-skinned patient.
- You need to be aware of situations that produce changes in skin tone.
- Examine body sites with the least melanin (mucous membranes) for underlying color identification.
- The pigmented skin should be assessed for specific color changes in skin tone.

Life Span Considerations

Older Adults

Wound Care

- Assess ability of the older adult to perform self-care, to reach the wound, and to manipulate the wound dressings.
- The skin of older adults is fragile and sometimes does not tolerate adhesives. It is necessary to avoid frequent dressing changes. Use paper tape.
- Decrease extraneous noises as much as possible to alleviate or prevent patient anxiety.
- Increase time allowed for the skills and allow time for repetition of teaching.
- Slow the pace.
- Give small amounts of information at a time.
- Older patients learn better by doing and using multiple senses than by reading instructions.
- The increased fragility of the skin of the older adult will sometimes contraindicate the use of a binder. Assess skin thoroughly before any binder application.
- Observe underlying skin of the older adult more frequently.
- Patient needs two binders since binders are washable and must be "line dried." Thus the patient has one to wear while the other is being washed and dried.
- Older adults often need reassurance about the suture removal procedure. Assess mental status for comprehension of the procedure.
- Older skin is frequently at higher risk for dehiscence after sutures are removed.
- Be aware that patients will need additional fluid intake to prevent dehydration.
- It will sometimes be necessary to take certain measures to prevent a confused patient from pulling out the drain.
- Compensate for any auditory, visual, or cognitive impairment the patient has when performing a dressing change.
- A decrease in sensory receptors causes decrease in pain sensation.

Goals such as the following are developed for the patient based on the nursing diagnosis.

Goal 1: Patient's wound heals without complications.

Goal 2: Patient has minimal pain.

Expected outcomes are based on the goals of care:

Outcome 1: Patient's wound is free of infection; drainage begins to diminish in amount.

Outcome 2: Patient reports minimal discomfort.

■ Implementation

While performing wound care, you will observe the wound for signs and symptoms of infection. Make certain sterile technique is used when gloving, handling sterile equipment and dressings, performing procedures that involve care of the open wound, and caring for wound drainage systems. Documentation of wound care is required to include the appearance of the wound, presence of drains and drainage or exudate, medication or solutions used in wound care, type of dressings applied, and patient response to the procedure. Report any variation from normal healing. Include specific interventions or techniques of dressing changes in the nursing care plan to provide continuity of care.

■ Evaluation

Evaluate wound healing with each dressing change, after application of heat and cold therapies, after wound irrigation, and after stress to the wound site.

Determine whether expected outcomes have been met. The following evaluative measures are possible to take: Assess condition of the wound, ask whether patient notes discomfort during procedure, and inspect condition of dressings at least every shift. Note the following examples:

Goal 1: Patient's wound heals without complications.

Evaluative measure: Assess the wound and dressing for odor, exudate, separation, color, and edema.

Goal 2: Patient has minimal pain; rates pain at 3 on a scale of 1 to 10.

Evaluative measures: Compare dosage and frequency of pain medication delivered over recovery period. Request patient to rate pain on a scale of 0 to 10, with 10 being the most pain and 0 being no pain.

Get Ready for the NCLEX® Examination!

Key Points

- Wounds are described as open or closed. Care of the open wound is determined by the extent of the wound.
- It is essential to maintain sterile technique when providing care for an open wound.
- Size, description of appearance, amount and type of exudate, presence of drains, integrity of wound closures, and pain level are included in a proper wound assessment.
- The wet-to-dry dressing can be used to mechanically debride a wound of necrotic tissue or wound exudate.
- Do not moisten the wet-to-dry dressing before removing it since this defeats the goal of debriding the wound.
- Wound drains remove secretions within tissue layers to promote wound closure.

- A drainage system requires close monitoring. In addition to noting color, consistency, and amount of drainage, checking the tube patency is important.
- After a bandage or binder is applied, you will assess, document, and immediately report changes in circulation, skin integrity, comfort level, and body function, such as ventilation or mobility.
- Remove dressings gently to prevent further injury to the wound. Dispose of used dressings appropriately to prevent cross-contamination.
- The type of suture securing a wound influences the method of suture removal.
- Wound care involves cleaning wounds, changing dressings, maintaining drains, irrigating, inserting packing, applying heat and cold treatments (see Chapter 20), and/or applying bandages and binders.
- Major types of wound exudate are serous, purulent, and sanguineous. The main complications of wound healing are hemorrhage, infection, dehiscence, and evisceration.
- Major nursing responsibilities related to wound care include preventing infection, preventing further tissue damage, preventing hemorrhage, promoting healing, and preventing skin excoriation around draining wounds.
- Wound assessment requires a description of the appearance of the wound base, the wound's size, the presence of exudates, and the periwound skin condition.
- When cleansing wounds or drain sites, clean from the least to the most contaminated area, away from the wound edges.
- Physical stress from vomiting, coughing, or sudden muscular contraction have potential to cause separation of wound edges or dehiscence.
- Apply bandages and binders in a manner that does not impair circulation or irritate the skin.

Additional Learning Resources

Go to your Companion CD for an audio glossary, animations, video clips, and more.

evolve Be sure to visit the Evolve site at http://evolve.elsevier.com/Christensen/foundations/ for additional online resources.

Review Questions for the NCLEX® Examination

1. The patient has just returned from the postanesthesia care (PAC) unit. During report, the nurse is told that the patient has a Penrose drain in the left lower quadrant (LLQ). The purpose of a Penrose drain is:
   1. to instill solution for wound irrigation.
   2. to prevent blockage of a passageway.
   3. to drain the wound area by suction.
   4. to drain the wound area by gravity.

2. Which nursing intervention would be appropriate should the patient's abdominal wound eviscerate?
   1. Place her in high Fowler's position.
   2. Give her fluids to prevent shock.
   3. Replace dressings with sterile fluffy pads.
   4. Apply warm, moist sterile dressings.

3. The nurse prepares to irrigate a patient's wound. The primary reason for performing this procedure is to:
   1. remove debris from the wound.
   2. decrease scar formation.
   3. improve circulation from the wound.
   4. decrease irritation from wound drainage.

4. What is the best indicator that a wound has become infected?
   1. Palpation of the wound reveals excess fluid under its edges.
   2. Wound cultures are positive.
   3. Purulent drainage is coming from the wound area.
   4. The wound has a distinct odor.

5. Which nursing entry is the most complete in its description of a wound?
   1. Wound appears to be healing well, dressing dry and intact
   2. Wound well approximated with minimal drainage
   3. Drainage size of quarter; wound pink; 4×4 applied
   4. Incisional edges approximated without erythema or exudate; two 4×4s applied

6. A patient has peripheral edema that causes the left calf of the leg to swell. Which is the most appropriate technique for applying a bandage around the affected extremity?
   1. Increase tension with each successive turn when applying the bandage.
   2. Place clips and tape over the area with the most swelling to prevent slippage.
   3. Assess the skin integrity carefully before reapplying each new bandage.
   4. Encourage peripheral blood flow by beginning bandaging at the proximal end and working to the distal area.

7. Which statement is correct in regard to the use of an abdominal binder?
   1. It replaces the need for underlying dressings.
   2. It should be kept loose for patient comfort.
   3. The patient has to be sitting or standing when it is applied.
   4. The patient must have adequate ventilatory capacity.

8. The first step in packing a wound is to:
   1. assess its size, shape, and depth.
   2. prepare a sterile field.
   3. select gauze packing material.
   4. irrigate the wound.

9. The correct procedure for the wet-to-dry dressing method is to:
   1. place dry gauze into the wound and remove it when it is wet.
   2. medicate the patient for pain after you change the dressing.
   3. complete this type of dressing change just once a day.
   4. place moist gauze into the wound and remove it when it is dry.

10. Serous drainage from a wound is described as:

1. fresh bleeding.
2. thick and yellow.
3. clear, watery plasma.
4. beige to brown and foul smelling.

11. A binder placed around a surgical patient with a new abdominal wound is indicated for:

1. collection of wound drainage.
2. reduction of abdominal swelling.
3. reduction of stress on the abdominal incision.
4. stimulation of peristalsis from direct pressure.

12. The purpose of a wet-to-dry dressing is:

1. debridement.
2. cooling.
3. comfort.
4. antiinfection.

13. A surgical wound infection can be reduced by:

1. adhering to the principles of hand hygiene.
2. cleansing the incision from the least contaminated to the most contaminated area.
3. leaving the incision open to the air.
4. changing the dressing using sterile technique.

14. When changing a patient's dressing, which nursing action is correct?

1. Enclose the soiled dressing within a latex glove.
2. Clean the wound in circles toward the incision.
3. Free the tape by pulling it away from the incision.
4. Remove the soiled dressing with sterile gloves.

15. When emptying the drainage in a Hemovac reservoir, which nursing action is essential for reestablishing the negative pressure within this drainage device?

1. Fill the reservoir with sterile normal saline.
2. Secure the reservoir to the skin near the wound.
3. Compress the reservoir and close the vent.
4. Open the vent, allowing the reservoir to fill with air.

16. Which patient is more at risk for wound dehiscence?

1. The patient who smokes
2. The obese patient
3. The patient with a history of peripheral vascular disease
4. The immunocompromised patient

17. Which wound drain is classified as providing gravity-assisted drainage?

1. Jackson-Pratt
2. Hemovac
3. Penrose
4. Wound VAC system

18. The physician has ordered all sutures on an abdominal hysterectomy patient be removed on the tenth postoperative day, and Steri-Strips applied. During suture removal, the nurse notices the incision edges are slightly separating. The nurse's best action is to:

1. continue removing the sutures and apply the Steri-Strips.
2. stop the suture removal and contact the physician immediately.
3. continue removing the sutures and applying the Steri-Strips, then cover the incision with a dry sterile dressing.
4. stop the suture removal, apply Steri-Strips where sutures have already been removed and notify the physician.

19. When providing care to a patient with a Hemovac drain, the nurse should:

1. record the appearance of the drainage in the nursing progress notes and include the amount in the intake and output calculations.
2. clamp the tubing during patient ambulation and activity in order to prevent excess drainage during these times.
3. empty the bulb drainage receptacle when it is one fourth full.
4. pin the bulb above the insertion site to assist in proper drainage of exudate.

20. During assessment of a patient following abdominal surgery, the nurse suspects internal hemorrhaging based on which finding?

1. The dressing is saturated with bright red sanguineous drainage, and the patient has an increased urinary output.
2. The dressing is dry and intact, and the patient's blood pressure has decreased and pulse and respirations have increased.
3. The dressing is saturated with serosanguineous drainage, and the patient is diaphoretic with a decrease in pulse and respirations.
4. The dressing is dry and intact, and the patient complains of shortness of breath and has an elevated temperature.

chapter 14

Safety

evolve

Elaine Oden Kockrow and Barbara Lauritsen Christensen

http://evolve.elsevier.com/Christensen/foundationsadult

Objectives

1. Discuss necessary modifications of the hospital environment for the left-handed patient.
2. Relate OSHA's guidelines for violence protection programs to the workplace.
3. Summarize safety precautions whose implementation helps prevent falls.
4. Relate specific safety considerations to the developmental age and needs of individuals across the life span.
5. Identify nursing interventions that are appropriate for individuals across the life span to ensure a safe environment.
6. Discuss safety concerns in the health care environment.
7. Describe safe and appropriate methods for the application of safety reminder devices.
8. Discuss nursing interventions that are specific to the patient requiring a safety reminder device.
9. Cite the steps to be followed in the event of a fire.
10. Discuss the role of the nurse in disaster planning.
11. Describe nursing interventions in the event of accidental poisoning.
12. Detail measures to create a restraint-free environment.
13. Discuss high-risk syndromes of bioterrorism.
14. Discuss terrorism.

Key Terms

bioterrorism (p. 363)
Centers for Disease Control and Prevention (CDC) (SĔN-tĕrz fŏr dĭ-ZĒZ kŏn-TRŌL ănd prē-VĔN-shŭn, p. 357)
codes (p. 362)
disaster manual (p. 362)
disaster situation (p. 361)
endemic (ĕn-DĔM-ĭk, p. 364)
epidemic (ĕp-ĭ-DĔM-ĭk, p. 364)
Hazard Communication Act (p. 357)
Occupational Safety and Health Administration (OSHA) (p. 357)
PASS (p. 359)
poisoning (p. 360)
RACE (p. 359)
safety reminder device (SRD) (p. 346)
sentinel event (SĔN-tĭ-nĕl, p. 343)
terrorism (p. 362)

The need for a safe environment applies to all of us, all of the time. A focus on the immediate environment raises certain concerns, and the local and national environment in which one lives and works brings others to the fore. Such issues as water and air pollution, disposal of waste and toxic materials, safety on the highways, protecting endangered species, and preserving forests illustrate general concerns about environmental safety.

SAFETY IN THE HOSPITAL OR HEALTH CARE ENVIRONMENT

Traditionally, the patient's overall safety in the hospital or other health care environment has been a primary concern of nursing. Today the focus on a safe environment has expanded as we have come to recognize and identify potential hazards and threats faced by hospital personnel, patients, and visitors (Box 14-1).

A safe environment implies freedom from injury with focus on helping to prevent falls, electrical injuries, fires, burns, and poisoning. Your role requires you to be alert to potential safety problems, including workplace violence, and to know how to report and respond when safety is threatened.

Providing and maintaining a safe environment involves the patient, visitors, and members of the health care team. Both protection and education are primary nursing responsibilities, and you will be directly and actively involved in ensuring a safe health care environment. Checking to see that the call light or signal system is working and accessible is an example of how you help maintain a safe environment.

Each year The Joint Commission releases national patient safety goals for health care facilities. These goals are based on evidenced-based practices developed from a review of national databases and assist facilities in maintaining patient safety. A component of these goals includes the identification of sentinel events. The Joint Commission defines a **sentinel event** as "any unexpected occurrence involving death or serious physical or psychological injury, or the risk thereof." The reporting of certain sentinel events to The Joint Commission is required, including a thorough review of the event as well as the plan for improvements that will prevent the

Box 14-1 Precautions to Promote Safety

- Orient patient to the environment to provide familiarity.
- Place bedside table and overbed table within reach. Ensure that frequently used items, such as the telephone, eyeglasses, or other personal belongings, are easily accessible.
- Assist patients when they get out of bed if they have had surgery, received narcotics for analgesia, or been in bed for an extended period.
- Keep environment free of litter because such items as books, magazines, and shoes will sometimes cause the patient to trip and fall.
- Follow facility policies regarding the use of side rails.
- Keep adjustable beds in the low position except when giving care.
- If bed is equipped with an alarm, turn on for the restless, disoriented patient.
- Lock wheels on beds, wheelchairs, and gurneys.
- Encourage patients to wear slippers or shoes with low heels when ambulating. Recommend terrycloth slippers with rubber, skid-resistant soles; advise against loose, poorly fitting soft shoes.
- Wipe or mop up spilled liquids promptly. Personnel and patients all need to be alert to signs warning of wet or slippery floors.
- Encourage the use of hand rails in the bathrooms and halls.
- Provide adequate lighting.
- Demonstrate the proper use of emergency call buttons or cords.
- Instruct patient to use the call bell for assistance.
- Some institutions have adopted "fall precaution" policies in which every patient is evaluated on admission to determine his or her degree of likelihood for a potential fall (see Figure 14-1).

event from occurring again. Examples of sentinel events include medication errors and errors in procedures and treatments that led to death of an individual, and inappropriate application of safety reminder devices (SRDs) (formerly referred to as **restraints**).

FALLS

Falls are a common problem. Be alert to patients who are likely to fall. It is important to perform a fall risk assessment upon admission to the unit and whenever there has been a significant change in the patient's condition. The majority of patient falls occur during transfer either to a bedside commode or to a wheelchair. Patient falls are a major safety consideration for *all* institutions (see Coordinated Care box). The very young and older adults are not the only individuals at risk in the health care environment. Individuals who become ill or who are injured are also at risk. An

 **Coordinated Care**

Delegation

PATIENT SAFETY AND FALL PREVENTION

Preventing falls is the responsibility of all caregivers, including assistive personnel (AP). However, assessment for risk of fall or injury requires the critical thinking and knowledge application unique to the nurse and is not delegated. When delegating safety measures, stress the importance of the following:

- The patient's mobility limitations and any specific measures to minimize risks
- Environmental safety precautions (e.g., bed locked and in low position, call bell and personal items within reach, clear pathway, nonskid footwear)
- What to do when a patient starts to fall while being assisted with ambulation (i.e., ease patient into a sitting position in a chair or on the floor, and alert the nurse)

It is acceptable to delegate monitoring patient behavior for risk of injury, and promoting a safe environment is a responsibility of AP as well as of nursing staff. However, assessment of a patient's behaviors and decisions about less restrictive interventions require the critical thinking and knowledge application unique to the nurse.

It is acceptable to delegate application of safety reminder devices (SRDs) to AP. However, assessment of when SRDs are needed and the appropriate type to use requires the critical thinking and knowledge application unique to the nurse and is not delegated. Stress the importance of the following:

- Correct placement of the SRD
- Observing for constriction of circulation, skin integrity, and adequate breathing
- When and how to change position and provide range-of-motion exercises, skin care, toileting, and opportunities for socialization

It is acceptable to delegate care of the patient receiving radiation therapy to AP. Stress the importance of the following:

- Patient's activity limitations
- Safety regulations (e.g., use of dosimeter, time and distance limits)
- Use of protective equipment (shields, gloves)
- Visitor restrictions (no one younger than 18 years of age or who is or may be pregnant)
- Care and handling of patient care–related items and substances (e.g., linen, trash, dietary tray, specimens, urine, feces)

It is acceptable to delegate setting up seizure precautions and protection for patients at risk for seizures to AP. Stress the importance of protection from falls, avoiding attempts to restrain, and not placing anything in the patient's mouth. Interventions for a patient experiencing a seizure are not to be delegated. Assessment of the patient's airway patency, breathing, and circulatory status require the critical thinking and knowledge application unique to the nurse and are not permitted to be delegated. See Chapter 54 for further care of the patient with seizures.

unfamiliar environment and the various symptoms and signs associated with the patient's diagnosis often place an individual at risk. The use of anesthesia, sedatives, or narcotics increases the risk of falling, as does an unstable gait or a problem with balance. Various safety precautions can be taken to prevent falls (Figure 14-1).

Gait belts are another way to help patients ambulate safely. A gait belt is a leather or canvas (or other very strong material) belt that encircles the patient's waist (some belts have handles attached for you to grasp) while the patient ambulates. Correct technique in the use of the gait belt is as follows:

1. Apply gait belt securely around the patient's waist.
2. Walk to the side of patient, with one arm around patient's waist and one hand on belt. Unless the patient has a tendency to lean toward one particular side, walk on the patient's weaker side so that you are able to give assistance if the patient starts to fall. See the illustration for Skill 14-1, Step 6d(1).
3. Have patient support self by leaning on or holding your arm.
4. Walk with your closest leg just behind the patient's knee.
5. Walk with your knees and hips flexed.
6. If patient is weak:
   - Walk alongside bed or heavy furniture.
   - Use hand rail in hallway, if available.
   - Encourage patient to use furniture or rails for support.
7. Following ambulation, loosen or remove the gait belt.
8. Document procedure.

INFANTS AND CHILDREN

Ensuring the safety of the environment of infants and children requires protecting the child and educating the parents to do so as well. Anticipate potential injuries and individualize your care and teaching. Accidents involving children are largely preventable, but parents and caregivers need to be aware of specific dangers at each stage of growth and development. Growth and the acquisition of new motor skills place the child at great risk for injury. See Chapters 29 through 32 for a more detailed discussion.

There are many dangers in a child's environment. All household cleaning items are potentially poisonous when ingested, and it is mandatory to keep them out of children's reach. Keep in mind that most children younger than 6 years of age are not able to read labels on cleaning materials or medication containers. Young infants in the oral stage of development put al-

Instructions:
Results of this assessment may be used as a guideline to define "fall-prone" patients. Any patient scored as 15 or greater is considered fall prone. Patients should be reassessed as their condition changes or deteriorates.

	Date	Date	Date
History of seizures or fainting (10)			
Older than age 70 (3)			
Recent falls (10)			
Language barrier, loss of hearing (1)			
Confused or disoriented (10)			
History of drug/alcohol abuse (3)			
Receiving multiple medications (such as tranquilizers, narcotics, sleepers) (5)			
New disability (amputee, new CVA, leg cast) (7)			
Neurologic problems (change of levels of consciousness, balance, gait, weakness) (3)			
Cardiovascular problems (BP variations, lightheadedness) (3)			
Overly independent attitude of patient and/or family (4)			
Poor eyesight (uncorrected) (3)			
Urinary/bowel urgency (history of incontinence, use of diuretics and/or laxatives) (5)			
Total			
Patient placed on Blue Dot System (date)			
Ambularm initiated (date)			

Signature ______________________ Date __________

Signature ______________________ Date __________

Signature ______________________ Date __________

FIGURE 14-1 Fall-prone patient assessment guide.

most anything into their mouths. As infants learn to crawl, electrical sockets and cords also become a danger. Protect toddlers and young children from burns by turning pot handles on a stove away from the child's reach. Carefully monitor the temperature of bath water. See that no infant, toddler, or preschool child is ever left unattended in a bathtub or pool of water, even for a moment. Protect infants and toddlers from falling out of bed; keep side rails up at all times. When giving care, always place your hand on the infant or toddler if you turn, for instance, to obtain supplies. See Chapters 29 through 32 for a more detailed discussion.

OLDER ADULTS

Changes associated with aging significantly affect the ability of older adults to protect themselves from injury (Life Span Considerations for Older Adults box). For example, unsteadiness in gait typically leads to falls. Age-related eye changes sometimes affect the ability to see the height of stairs. Vertigo (dizziness) is often related to chronic disease conditions and to side effects of some medications. Encourage the use of eyeglasses, hearing aids, and assistive devices such as canes in patients with deficits.

Make certain to assist frail or disoriented older patients to drink hot liquids such as soups, coffee, or tea. People in this age-group are more vulnerable to burns from spilled hot liquids, as well as from heating pads and electric blankets. For safety, change or correctly position long, loose clothing and straps from safety reminder devices that might cause tripping.

SAFETY REMINDER DEVICES

A **safety reminder device (SRD)** is defined as any of the numerous devices used to immobilize a patient or part of the patient's body, such as arms or hands. The most common type of SRD is the soft restraint, often referred to as a **Posey** after the company that manufactures this type of restraint.

You will use SRDs for various reasons, primarily for considerations of patient safety. Sometimes an SRD serves to safeguard the continuity of treatment (e.g., the wrist SRD prevents patients from removing intravenous lines, feeding tubes, or drainage tubes). Certain patient populations, such as the older adult and the disoriented patient, are more likely to need SRDs. Their use prevents the disoriented patient from wandering and prevents or reduces the risk of the patient falling from a bed, chair, or wheelchair (Figures 14-2

Life Span Considerations

Older Adults

Safety

Physiologic changes in aging increase the need for safety precautions:

- Changes in vision, including altered depth perception, increased sensitivity to glare, and decreased visual acuity in dim light, increase the risk of falls owing to misperception of visual cues.
- Changes in hearing, including varying degrees of deafness and tinnitus (ringing in the ears), increase the risk of injury from hazards in the environment, since certain warnings that are commonly detected by auditory cues, such as motor vehicle horns, alarms, or even spoken warnings, go unheard.
- Prevent sensory overload in older adults since both reflexes and the ability to respond to multiple stimuli slow with aging.
- Changes in muscle strength and joint function resulting in slowed reaction time, altered gait, and altered sense of balance make it more likely that stumbling will result in a fall.
- Changes in the cardiovascular system such as anemia, orthostatic hypotension, and heart block increase the risk of syncope, which increases the risk of falls.
- Changes in the peripheral vascular system sometimes result in loss of sensitivity to heat, cold, or foreign objects, which increases the risk of tissue damage resulting from burns, frostbite, and pressure.
- Older adults take many medications that increase the need for safety precautions. For example, sedatives, hypnotics, and tranquilizers affect reaction time and increase the risk of injury. Antihypertensives, diuretics, and antihistamines increase the risk of orthostatic hypotension (a drop of 25 mm Hg in systolic pressure and 10 mm Hg in diastolic pressure), which increases the risk of falls.
- Keep to a minimum the use of safety reminder devices (SRDs) with older adults and, when necessary, the amount of any restraint used. SRDs reduce mobility and result in a loss of strength that can increase the risk of falls or injury.
- Accidental poisoning is a significant problem in older adults. Visual changes raise the potential for misreading of labels on medication or other package labels and lead to overdose or other errors in administration. Medication organizers or dispensers are available for purchase at any drugstore at reasonable cost. They need only to be filled once a week (or once a day) and the medications taken at specific times during the day. In addition, many older adults do not consider over-the-counter medications to be "real" medicine, so they take them freely and fail to mention them when questioned regarding drug use. Many over-the-counter medications increase the risk of injury to the older adult by potentiating or interfering with the effects of prescription drugs.

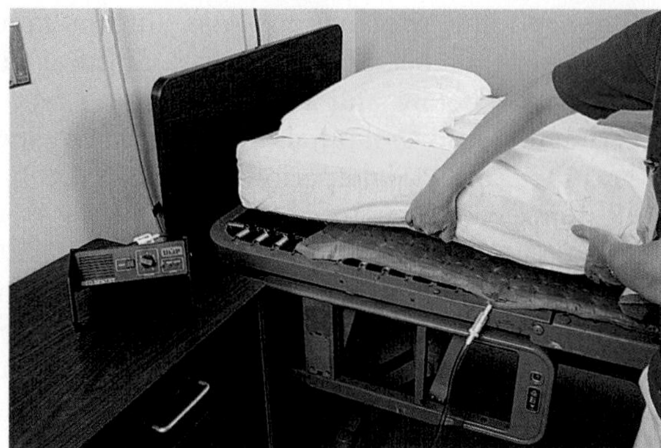

FIGURE 14-2 Weight-sensitive alarm.

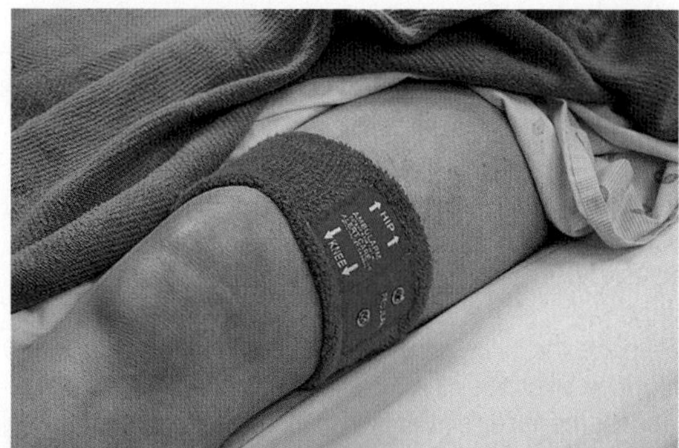

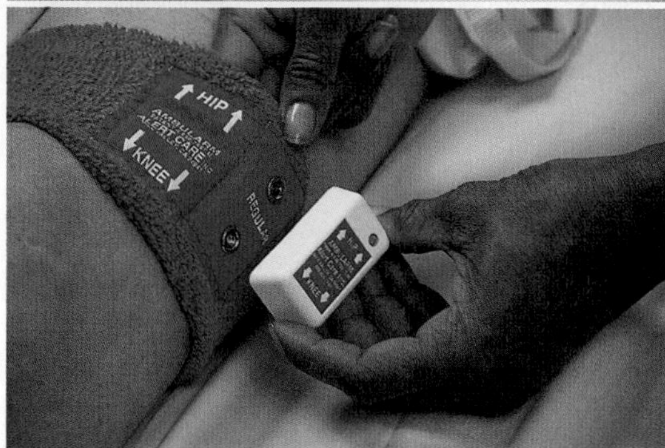

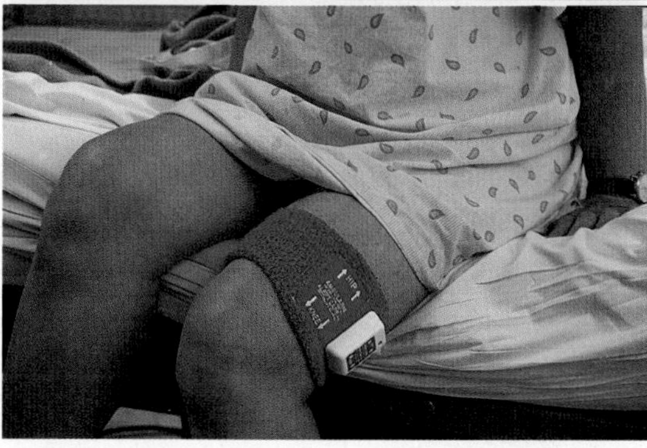

FIGURE 14-3 Using monitoring devices as an alternative to restraints. Measure correctly to determine correct size for the Ambularm, because the band that is too loose will sometimes slip off and a band that is too tight will sometimes interfere with circulation or cause skin irritation. The use of the Ambularm is contraindicated in the presence of impaired circulation, edema (swelling), skin irritation, or impairment of skin integrity (breaks in the skin such as skin tears or ulcers).

and 14-3). In some instances, you will have to restrict an aggressive patient's movements to protect other patients and staff from harm.

The use of SRDs also tends to result in increased restlessness, disorientation, agitation, anxiety, and a feeling of powerlessness. It contributes to patient immobility and associated problems with immobility such as dehydration, health care–associated infection, and incontinence. The resulting disuse of body parts has the potential to increase disability and lead to further patient weakness and unsteadiness. Patients often pull against the SRDs, causing skin and circulation problems.

Therefore, although SRDs have been used with some 7% to 10% of the hospital population in North America, this practice is rapidly decreasing in popularity. Today, ethical and legal issues surround their use. The focus today is on attempting alternative strategies before turning to the use of SRDs (Box 14-2). By assessing individual patient needs, characteristics of the environment, and organizational change, you will

Box 14-2 Designing a Restraint-Free Environment

Care of the patient who may be prone to threats to safety and security requires a creative, systematic, and attentive approach. A wide variety of electronic devices have been developed to alert staff to a patient's need for assistance. A weight-sensitive alarm can be placed under a patient in bed or in a chair. When the patient tries to get up an alarm sounds (see Figure 14-2). An Ambularm is a monitoring device that fits around the patient's leg directly above the knee (see Figure 14-3, *A* and *B*). When the patient swings a leg over the side of the bed, an alarm sounds from a battery that snaps to the leg band (see Figure 14-3, *C*).

To design a restraint-free environment:

- Orient patient and family to surroundings; explain all procedures and treatments.
- Encourage family and friends to stay, or use sitters for patients who need supervision.
- Assign confused or disoriented patients to rooms near the nurses' station. Observe these patients frequently.
- Provide appropriate visual and auditory stimuli (e.g., family pictures, clocks, radio).
- Eliminate bothersome treatments as soon as possible. For example, discontinue tube feedings and begin oral feedings as quickly as the patient's condition allows.
- Use relaxation techniques (e.g., massage).
- Institute exercise and ambulation schedules as the patient's condition allows.
- Maintain toileting routines.
- Consult with physical and occupational therapists to enhance patient's abilities to carry out activities of daily living.
- Evaluate all medications patient is receiving to determine if the medication is having the desired therapeutic effect.
- Conduct ongoing assessment and evaluation of patient's care and patient's ongoing response to care.

often be able to plan interventions that permit you to reduce your reliance on SRDs. In any case, make sure that patient safety and the safety of others is your primary motive to apply an SRD.

Most health care facilities have specific policies and procedures related to the use of SRDs (see Box 14-3 and Skill 14-1), and most require a specific order from a physician. Some agencies require that a physician order for SRDs be renewed every 24 hours. Be familiar with your facility's policies for SRD use. Use them judiciously and with kindness. Explain to the patient the need for the devices even if the patient does not seem to understand the explanation. Also inform family members about the need for SRDs (see Cultural Considerations box below and Patient Teaching box on p. 354). Include information about the specific device used and the approximate period for use. If you have any questions, consult your supervisor.

Documentation about the need for the SRDs, the type of device used, and the patient's response is crucial (Figure 14-4). Perform a comprehensive assessment focusing on the patient's behavior, activity, and skin condition. Note all nursing interventions, including patient and family teaching about the SRDs.

Text continued on p. 354

Box 14-3 Nursing Home Variations for Safety Reminder Devices

Legislation has greatly affected the use of SRDs in the long-term care facility. Under the Omnibus Budget Reconciliation Act (OBRA) of 1987, residents' rights are specifically addressed in terms of SRDs. This act, effective October 1, 1990, mandates specific guidelines and prohibits routine use of SRDs in nursing homes. The act regulates the use of extremity SRDs, hand mitts, safety vests, and wheelchair safety bars. SRDs may be used only to ensure the physical safety of the resident or other residents. There must be a written order by the physician detailing the duration and circumstances under which the SRDs are to be used.

OBRA states the following as acceptable reasons for the use of physical restraints:

- All other interventions have been attempted before the use of restraints.
- Other disciplines have been consulted for their assistance.
- Supporting documentation has been completed.

ESSENTIALS OF SRD DOCUMENTATION

- Reason for the physical restraint
- Explanation given to patient and family
- Date and time of the patient's response to treatment
- Duration
- Frequency of observation and patient's response
- Safety
  - —Release the physical restraint at least every 2 hours
  - —Routine exercise of extremities
  - —Assessment for circulation and skin integrity
- Assessment for continued need for the physical restraint
- Patient outcome

Cultural Considerations

Safety in Health Care Settings

- Cultural heritage affects all dimensions of health; it is vital that you consider cultural background when planning for patient safety.
- The way that culture influences behaviors, attitudes, and values depends on many factors and thus may not be the same for individual members of a cultural group.
- Before assessing the cultural background of a patient, assess the influence of your own culture.
- Adapt the planning and implementation of nursing interventions for safety as much as possible to a patient's cultural background.
- Evaluate your own attitudes and emotions toward providing nursing interventions for safety to patients from diverse sociocultural backgrounds.
- Patients from western Europe and the British Isles sometimes seems aloof and distant in terms of space. It is often very difficult for them to have an outsider in their home who is suggesting changes with regard to their personal belongings, even though the purpose is to reduce physical hazards.
- It is particularly difficult to determine a patient's attitude toward his or her home when another language is spoken. Use an interpreter or engage the patient's family to interpret if available. Attentiveness to the patient's nonverbal communication becomes extremely important as you assess the home.
- Another culturally sensitive issue is the patient's sense of environmental control. Be aware of health beliefs and practices that will affect the outcome of interventions. For example, reliance on family and religious organizations, as opposed to community resources, is likely to affect compliance with nursing interventions and referrals.

Skill 14-1 Applying Safety Reminder Devices

Nursing Action *(Rationale)*

1. Refer to medical record, care plan, and Kardex. Review agency policy. *(Provides basis of care; a physician's order is required before safety reminder devices [SRDs] are applied.)*
2. Perform hand hygiene. *(Reduces spread of microorganisms.)*
3. Introduce self. *(Decreases patient's anxiety.)*
4. Identify patient. *(Identifies correct patient for procedure.)*
5. Procedure:
   a. Explain procedure. *(Enlists cooperation or assistance from patient and family and decreases anxiety.)*
   b. Prepare for procedure by providing privacy and assembling necessary supplies. *(Organizes procedure and decreases patient's anxiety.)*
   c. Assess patient for need for SRD (a comprehensive nursing assessment of the patient's potential for injury and treatment in relation to the need for an SRD is crucial before applying SRD). *(Restraining a patient without a physician's order or without reasonable cause incurs risk of charges of false imprisonment. Some facilities have specific requirements for SRD use in certain situations [e.g., the presence of an endotracheal tube].)*
6. Apply appropriate type of SRD:
   a. **Wrist or ankle (extremity) SRD** designed to immobilize one or more extremities
      (1) If using Kerlix gauze, make a clove hitch by forming a figure-of-8 and picking up the loops. *(The clove hitch does not tighten when pulled.)*
      (2) Place gauze or padding around the extremity. *(Decreases risk of injury to underlying skin.)*
      (3) Slip the wrist(s) or ankle(s) through loops directly over the padding—if using a commercially made SRD, wrap the padded portion of the device around affected extremity, thread tie through slit in device, and fasten to second tie with a secure knot (see illustration). *(Decreases risk of injury to underlying skin.)*

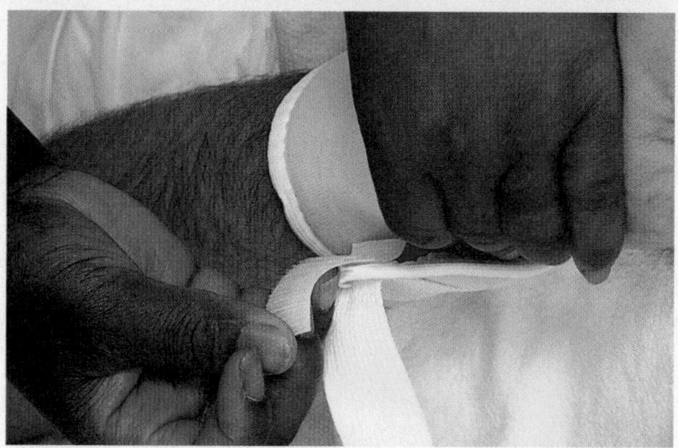

Step **6a(3)**

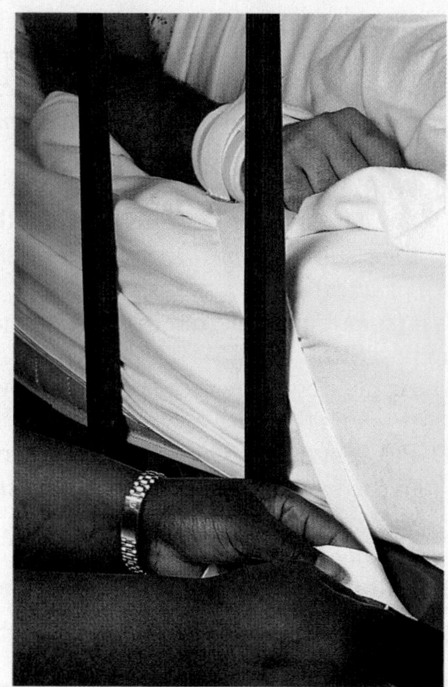

Step **6a(4)**

      (4) Secure ends of ties to the movable portion of the bed frame that moves with the patient when the bed is adjusted, NOT TO SIDE RAILS (see illustration). *(If side rails are lowered with the SRD attached, injury is possible result.)*
      (5) Leave as much slack as possible (1 to 2 inches). *(Provides for movement.)*
      (6) Palpate pulses below the SRD. *(Ensures that the device is not so tight as to occlude circulation.)*

Continued

Skill 14-1 Applying Safety Reminder Devices—cont'd

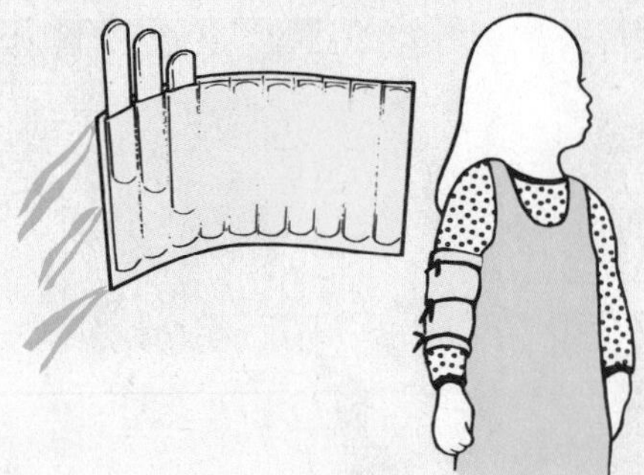

Step **6b(1)**

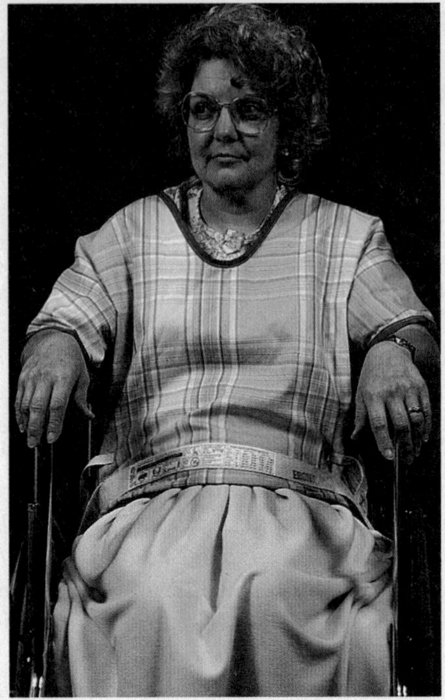

Step **6c(2)**

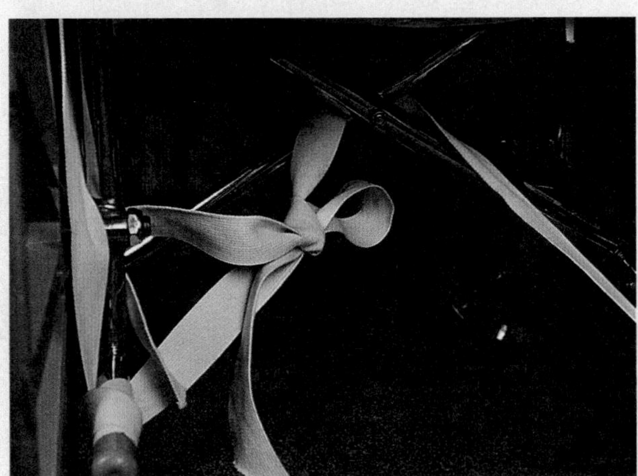

Step **6c(4)**

b. Elbow SRD

(1) Place SRD (a piece of fabric with slots for the insertion of tongue blades to keep the elbow straight) over the elbow or elbows (see illustration). *(Elbow SRDs are often used with children to prevent elbow flexion so they cannot disturb tubes, catheters, and dressings.)*

(2) Wrap SRD(s) snugly, tying them at the top. For small infants, tie or pin SRDs to their shirts. *(Tying or pinning the restraint to the infant's shirt ensures a secure fit.)*

c. Vest (sometimes referred to as a wrap jacket or chest SRD)

(1) Apply device over the patient's gown. *(Protects the skin.)*

(2) Put vest on patient with V-shaped opening in the front (see illustration). *(If vest is on backward and patient becomes restless, choking is possible result.)*

(3) Pull tie at end of vest flap across the chest and slip tie through slit on opposite side of vest.

(4) Wrap the other end of the flap across patient and tie the straps to frame of bed or behind wheelchair. *(Helps secure vest SRD to the patient.)* Use the quick-release knot (see illustration). *(A tight restraint potentially causes constriction and impedes circulation. Assessing for constriction prevents neurovascular injury.)*

(5) With a proper fit, there is room for a fist in the space between the vest and the patient. *(This determines that the vest is not too tight.)*

d. Gait or safety reminder belts

(1) Apply belt over the patient's gown (see illustration). *(Protects the skin.)*

(2) If patient is ambulating, place belt around the patient's waist. The belt usually has a buckle to secure the belt in place. *(Provides a snug fit and prevents slipping.)*

(3) If the belt does not have a buckle, use a slip knot. *(Allows for quick removal in case of emergency.)*

7. Use a quick-release knot rather than a regular knot to secure the safety reminder device to bed frame (see illustration). *(A quick-release knot is quick to undo in an emergency.)*

8. Secure SRDs so that the patient cannot untie them. *(Prevents patient injury.)*

9. Apply SRD with gentleness and compassion.

10. Perform hand hygiene. *(Reduces spread of microorganisms.)*

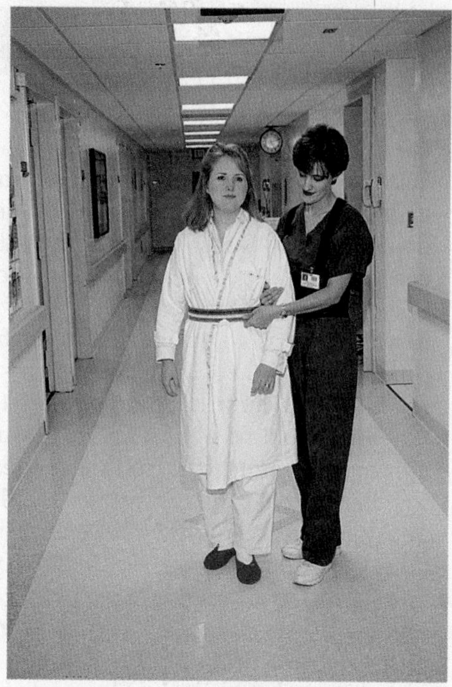

Step **6d(1)**

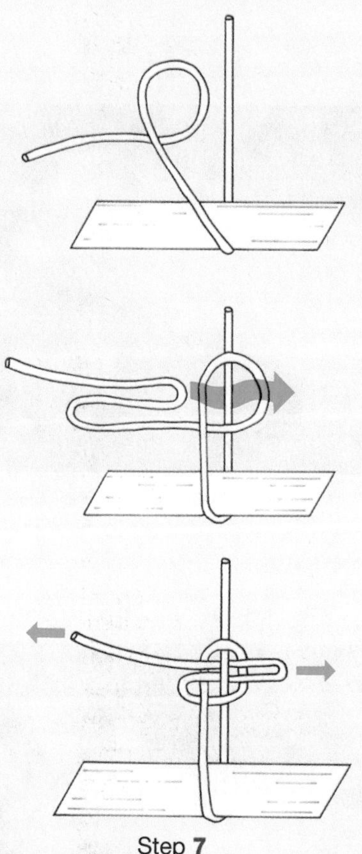

Step **7**

11. Document procedure. *(Notes procedure and patient's response.)*
    - Reason(s) SRD needed
    - If appropriate, the notification of the physician and time order obtained
    - The time and type of SRD applied
    - The ongoing assessment and monitoring of the patient's skin, extremity circulation, and mental status
    - The response(s) of the patient
    - The periodic removal of the SRD and any skin care performed
    - If SRD removed, note time and follow-up assessments
    - If reapplication is needed, note reasons, time, and patient assessment
    - A flow sheet is an excellent tool for this documentation (see Figure 14-4)
12. Follow-up
    a. Monitor for skin impairment. *(Excessive pressure potentially leads to loss of skin integrity.)*
    b. With the use of extremity SRD, assess extremity distal to SRD every 30 minutes or more often according to agency policy. *(Identifies any problems or need to remove or adjust SRD.)*
        (1) Remove SRD on one extremity at a time at least every 2 hours (know agency policy) for 5 minutes. *(Allows supervised movement of extremity, enhances circulation, and reduces apprehension.)*
    c. Monitor position of SRD, circulation, skin condition, and mental status frequently. *(Ensures patient safety.)* Remove SRD when no longer needed.
    d. With the use of vest SRD, monitor respiratory status. *(Respiratory distress is possible if there is restriction from the vest.)*
    e. Do NOT leave the patient unattended during temporary removal of SRD. *(An unattended patient is at risk for injury.)* Do take advantage of removal to change patient's position and inspect skin.
    f. Gently massage the skin beneath SRD—apply lotion or powder if desired. *(A gentle massage of the skin increases circulation to area.)*
    g. Change SRD when soiled or wet. *(Reduces risk of skin impairment and infection.)*
    h. Assess frequently for tangled ties or pressure points from knots; adjust SRD device(s) as needed. *(Excess pressure leads to loss of skin integrity and impaired circulation.)*
13. Evaluation
    a. The SRD is adequate and appropriate for the individual patient's condition. *(Prevents interruption of treatment or therapy; prevents patient from falling from bed, chair, or wheelchair, and possibly from harming others.)*

Continued

Skill 14-1 Applying Safety Reminder Devices—cont'd

b. SRDs are correctly applied. *(Correct application prevents injury to the patient or to others.)*
c. Quick-release knots are easily released. *(Ensures quick access to the patient in case of an emergency.)*
d. Related problems (e.g., of the skin or of the musculoskeletal system) are identified. *(Complications are prevented by performing timely interventions.)*

14. Provide patient teaching (see Patient Teaching box on safety promotion).
15. Pediatric considerations
    - When it is necessary to restrain a child for a procedure, it is best that the person applying the restraint not be the child's parent or guardian.
    - A mummy restraint is a safe, efficient, short-term method to restrain a small child or infant for examination or treatment.
        a. Open a blanket, and fold one corner toward the center. Place the infant on the blanket with shoulders at the fold and feet toward the opposite corner (see illustration).
        b. With infant's right arm straight down against body, pull the right side of the blanket firmly across the right shoulder and chest, and secure beneath the left side of body (see illustration).
        c. Place the left arm straight against the body, bring the left side of the blanket across the shoulder and chest, and lock beneath the infant's body on the right side (see illustration).
        d. Align the infant's legs, pull the corner of the blanket near the feet up toward the body, and tuck snugly in place or fasten securely with safety pins (see illustration).
    - Remain with the infant while restrained, and remove the restraint immediately after treatment is complete. If restraint is required for an extended period, remove it at least every 2 hours and perform range-of-motion exercises on all extremities.

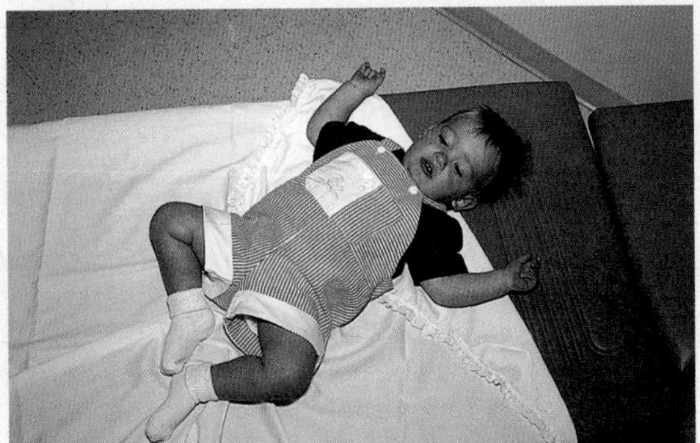
Step **15a**

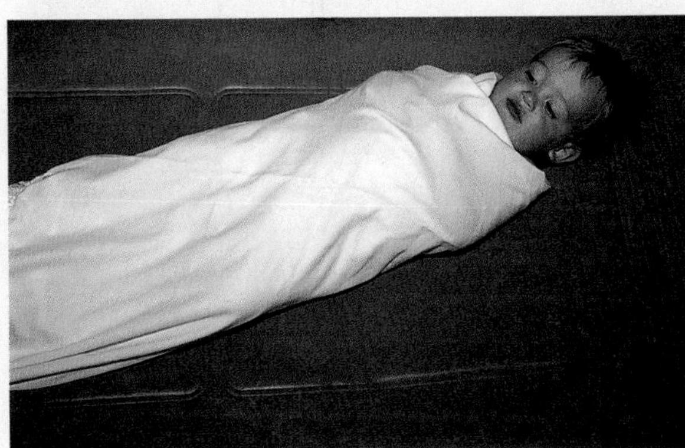
Step **15c**

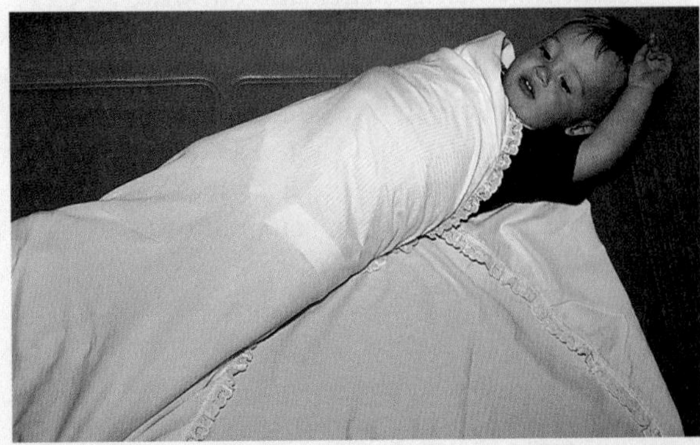
Step **15b**

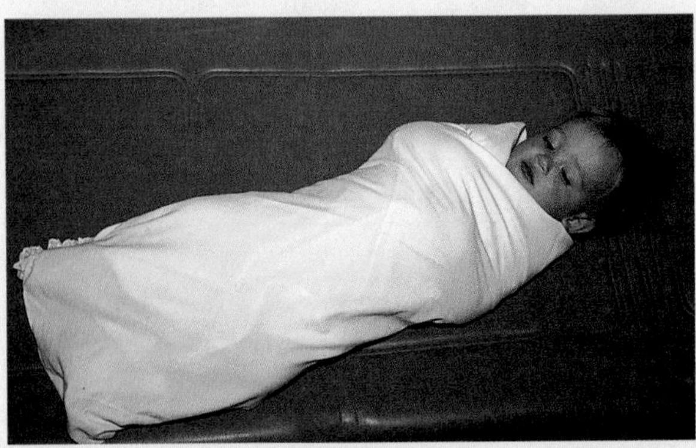
Step **15d**

Restraint Application Date ____________ Time Restraints Applied ____________ Patient Name ____________

Physician Order Date and Time ____________ Medical Record # ____________

Type of Restraint ____________ Length of Time Physician Ordered Restraint ____________

Date												
Hour of Day												
I. Patient Assessment												
A. Circulation												
P 5 Pink B 5 Blanches												
B. Skin Condition												
R 5 Red B 5 Blistered												
E 5 Edema N 5 Normal												
SB 5 Skin Broken												
C. Respiratory Status												
N 5 Normal L 5 Labored												
S 5 Shallow												
CS 5 Cheyne-Stokes												
II. Restraint Released												
Extremity Exercised												
R/R 5 Restraint Released												
E 5 Exercised												
III. Water/Food Offered												
T 5 Taken												
Re 5 Refused												
IV. Toileting Offered												
V 5 Voided												
BM 5 Bowel Movement												
Re 5 Refused												
C 5 Catheter												
V. Personal Hygiene Offered												
D 5 Dental												
B 5 Bath												
S 5 Shower												
P 5 Partial												
Re 5 Refused												
INITIALS												
SIGNATURE												

FIGURE 14-4 Safety reminder device (restraint) protocol charting record.

Patient Teaching

Safety Promotion

- Teach primary caregiver the dangers associated with restraining a patient with history of seizures and how to modify environment for patient's protection.
- Instruct primary caregiver how to correctly restrain a patient who is nauseated and vomiting.
- Instruct primary caregiver how to routinely change patient's position and use passive range of motion.
- Explain to the patient and members of the family why safety reminder devices (SRDs) are necessary.
- Provide information about the type of SRD to be used and the approximate time frame for use.
- Inform patient and family that patient will still receive comfort measures such as repositioning and limb exercises.
- Inform patients and parents about potential sources of poisoning found in the home and appropriate safety precautions (see Box 14-10).
- Inform patients and parents about poison control centers. Provide number of closest center or instruct to call 9-1-1.
- Teach basic interventions to follow in the case of a poisoning.
- See that safety items such as stickers with poison center information are available.
- Teach parents and caregivers not to try home remedies. When ingestion of a dangerous substance is suspected, it is necessary to seek appropriate medical intervention immediately (see Cultural Considerations box).
- Removal of poisonous and toxic substances does not take the place of education as a means to prevent accidental poisoning.
- Instruct family to place bedside tables and overbed tables close to the patient.
- Encourage the patient to rise from the bed or chair slowly to prevent vertigo (dizziness) resulting from postural hypotension.
- Advise the family to remove clutter from bedside tables, hallways, bathrooms, and grooming areas.
- Encourage family to mount grab bars around toilets and showers; instruct the patient how to use them.
- Recommend that rugs and carpets be securely attached to floors and stairs.
- Recommend that bath mats and nonskid strips be attached to bathtubs and the floors of shower stalls.
- Recommend that electrical cords be secured against baseboards so that the patient will not trip over them easily.
- Ensure that the call bell is within easy reach of the hospitalized patient, and show patient the location of emergency call bells in bathrooms. (It is essential to respond to call lights quickly, especially for patients needing assistance to the bathroom.)
- See that wheelchairs remain locked when transporting a patient from bed to wheelchair or back to bed.
- Instruct caregivers to check that side rails are up and safety straps secured around the patient who is on a gurney (stretcher) (see Coordinated Care box).
- Use the fire drill procedure as an opportunity to talk about fire safety.

Box 14-4 Levels of Latex Sensitivity

- *Contact dermatitis:* A nonallergic response characterized by skin redness and itching.
- *Type IV hypersensitivity:* Cell-mediated allergic reaction to chemicals used in latex processing. Delayed reaction—including redness, itching, and hives—up to 48 hours is possible. Localized swelling, red and itchy or runny eyes and nose, and coughing often develop.
- *Type I hypersensitivity:* A true latex allergy that is possibly life threatening. Reactions are likely based on type of latex protein and degree of individual sensitivity, including local and systemic. Symptoms include hives, generalized edema, itching, rash, wheezing, bronchospasm, difficulty breathing, laryngeal edema, diarrhea, nausea, hypotension, tachycardia, and respiratory or cardiac arrest.

LATEX SENSITIVITY

All patients need to be questioned regarding allergies, and it is imperative that they be specifically asked about latex allergies. A latex allergy can precipitate a respiratory arrest, which is a life-threatening event (Box 14-4). This potential reaction must be kept in mind at all times. Do not wear, or permit others to wear, latex gloves when caring for patients with latex allergies. For individuals at high risk or with suspected sensitivity to latex, it is important to use exclusively latex-free products, including gloves, and to inspect the contents of all patient care supply kits for items that contain latex. Institutions have latex-free procedure kits available for use.

LEFT-HANDED PATIENT

The left-handed patient presents a unique challenge to the health care team, especially to the nurse. The typical hospital room environment is set up to accommodate the right-handed patient (see Chapter 18, Figure 18-1). Seldom, if ever, is the patient asked, "Which hand do you use the most?" or "Which hand do you write with?" Patients will struggle and strain to cope by contorting (twisting) the body, which creates a "risk for injury" situation. Be perceptive, and document in the patient's record the fact that the patient is left-handed (Box 14-5).

ELECTRICAL HAZARDS

Much of the equipment used in health care settings is electrical and requires good maintenance. Use properly grounded and functional electrical equipment to decrease the risk of electrical injury and fire. Teach patients and family how to reduce their risk of electrical injury in the home (e.g., discuss prevention of electri-

Box 14-5 Safety Features for the Left-Handed Patient

- During personal hygiene, place all bathing articles at the patient's left.
- As back care is performed, allow patient to turn to the right side, because the left arm and hand will be stronger to assist in turning over.
- Place the drainage receptacle for the indwelling catheter to patient's left.
- Arrange meal trays by placing all liquids on the left side of the trays.
- When assisting the left-handed patient to ambulate, walk to the patient's left side.
- Use the patient's right hand and arm for intravenous therapy and injections whenever possible.
- Allow more time for the patient to master skills during patient teaching if you are right-handed. The left-handed patient has to translate your hand movements to the opposite hand.
- If you are left-handed, consider the problems that right-handed patients will have with your instructions. Unlike left-handers, right-handers are not accustomed to making modifications according to "handedness."
- Adjust the patient's environment by placing bed stand, table, chair or commode, and call light to the patient's left.

cal shock, avoidance of use of electrical appliances near water source, methods of grounding appliances, avoidance of operating unfamiliar equipment).

RADIATION

Radiation presents a health hazard, if used incorrectly, in health care settings and the community. Radiation and radioactive materials are used in the diagnosis and treatment of patients. Hospitals have strict guidelines on the care of patients who are receiving radiation and on the handling of radioactive materials. Be familiar with established agency protocols. To reduce your exposure to radiation, limit time spent near the source, keep as great a distance from the source as possible, and use shielding devices such as lead aprons. Staff members working near radiation on a routine basis are required to wear devices that track their cumulative exposure to radiation. Following collection and processing of these devices, those staff members whose radiation exposure readings fall above a set limit are frequently assigned to an alternative work area away from radiation exposure. Follow-up medical attention is often mandated for them, as well.

The community is put at risk for radiation exposure if radioactive waste products are disposed of or transported incorrectly. Community health agencies, the Environmental Protection Agency (EPA), the Nuclear Regulatory Commission (NRC), the Department of Energy (DOE), and the Department of Transportation (DOT) have established specific, strict guidelines for the disposal of radioactive waste (EPA, 2008). If a radioactive leak occurs, these agencies institute measures to

Box 14-6 Mercury Spill Cleanup Procedure

In the event of a mercury spill, follow these steps while waiting for trained personnel to arrive:

1. Evacuate the room except for a housekeeping crew (if available).
2. Ventilate the area. Close interior doors and open any outside windows.
3. DO NOT VACUUM THE SPILL.

After the mercury has been recovered:

4. Mop the floor with a mercury-specific cleanser (see agency policy).
5. Dispose of collected mercury according to local environmental safety regulations.

prevent exposure of surrounding neighborhoods, to clean up radioactive leaks as quickly as possible, and to ensure that anyone injured receives prompt medical care.

MERCURY SPILL

It is important for you to know who to contact when exposure to a hazardous chemical such as mercury occurs in the health care setting. Exposures in a health care facility include broken thermometers or sphygmomanometers, although these devices are no longer allowed in most health care delivery facilities. Mercury enters the body through inhalation and absorption through the skin. Exposures that occur in a hospital setting are usually brief but still have the potential to affect the brain or kidney. However, full recovery is likely to occur once the body cleans itself of the contamination. Box 14-6 summarizes steps to take in the event of a mercury spill. Though it is not likely to occur in the health care setting, it is important to be aware of the facility's policy for proper cleanup of a mercury spill.

WORKPLACE SAFETY

The hospital environment is a source of potential safety hazards to health care workers. Of significant impact is the threat of workplace violence (Box 14-7). In addition, various biologic, chemical, radiologic, and physical hazards are present. The increased use of lasers in the health care setting requires specific safety precautions because a laser has the potential to cause skin and eye injury, as well as start a fire, if used improperly. Therefore, make sure to provide protection for the eyes of the patient and the staff working with the laser. Personnel involved with laser-based procedures wear specially designed eyewear. Because a laser beam generates an enormous amount of energy, it is possible for dry combustibles in the surgical field to accidentally ignite, posing a threat to the patient and staff. Make sure that water and a halon fire extinguisher are readily available. In order to prevent injury

Box 14-7 Workplace Violence

According to the Occupational Safety and Health Administration (OSHA), more assaults occur in health care settings than in other industries. Violence does not always involve physical injury; it also includes any intense extreme behavior used to frighten, intimidate, threaten, or injure a person or damage or destroy property. The behavior is sometimes physical, sometimes verbal, and sometimes even nonverbal, such as a gesture. Legally, if by either threat or gesture someone causes you to fear being struck, an assault has occurred. Any unwelcomed physical contact from another person is battery. In other words, one does not have to be physically "hurt" to get protection under the law.

According to information from the Bureau of Labor Statistics (BLS) available at www.bls.gov, 69 homicides occurred in the health care setting from 1996 to 2000. However, most workplace violence, including in the health care setting, results in nonfatal injuries. Of nonfatal injuries incurred while on the job in health care and social services in the year 2000, 48% were attributed to assault. The health care workers most commonly victimized by on-the-job assault were nurses, orderlies, and attendants.

Unfortunately, these statistics do not provide the full picture, and as many as half of workplace violence incidents are not reported. Sometimes nurses do not report a violent incident because they are unsure what constitutes violence, do not know of the requirement to report the incident, or do not know whom to inform; sometimes they do not file a report because the injuries do not require emergency treatment or time off from work.

Risk factors for work-related assaults in health care agencies include the following:

- On-site presence of handguns in the possession of patients, families, friends, and co-workers
- Patients who are hospitalized and under police custody at the same time (people arrested or convicted of crimes)
- On-site presence of acutely disturbed and violent people seeking health care
- On-site presence of mentally ill people who do not take medicine, do not receive follow-up care, and are not hospitalized unless they are an immediate threat to themselves or others
- On-site presence of upset, agitated, and disturbed family members and visitors
- Long emergency department waits that increase a person's agitation and frustration
- On-site agency pharmacies that are a source of drugs and therefore a target for robberies
- Gang members and substance abusers having access to agencies as patients or visitors
- Staff being alone with patients during care or transport to other agency areas during examination or treatment
- Low staffing levels during meals, during emergencies, and at night
- Poorly lighted parking areas or distant parking areas
- Lack of staff training in recognizing and managing potentially violent situations

OSHA (2008) provides guidelines for violence prevention programs with a goal of eliminating or reducing employee exposure to situations that have potential to cause death or injury. The worksite is analyzed for hazards. Prevention strategies are developed and implemented. Also, employees are required to receive safety and health training per facility protocol. Your responsibilities in violence prevention programs include the following:

- Understand and follow the workplace violence prevention program
- Understand and follow safety and security measures
- Voice safety and security concerns
- Report violent incidents promptly and accurately
- Serve on health and safety committees that review incidents of workplace violence
- Take part in training programs that focus on recognizing and managing agitation, assaultive behavior, and criminal intent

Practice the following safety measures when dealing with agitated or aggressive people:

- Stand away from the person. Judge the length of the person's arms and legs. Stand far enough away that the person will not be able to hit or kick you.
- Position yourself close to the door. Do not allow yourself to become trapped in the room.
- Note the location of panic buttons, call bells, alarms, closed-circuit monitors, and other security devices.
- If you wear your ID badge around your neck, make sure it will break away if pulled.
- Keep your hands free.
- Stay calm. Talk to the person in a calm manner. Do not raise your voice or argue, scold, or interrupt the person.
- Do not touch the person.
- Tell the person that you will get the supervisor to speak to the person.
- Leave the room as soon as you are able. Make sure the person is safe.
- Notify the supervisor or security officer of the situation.
- Complete an incident report according to agency policy.

From Occupational Safety and Health Administration (OSHA). Available at www.osha.gov. National Institute for Safety and Health (NIOSH) Bureau of Labor Statistics (BLS). Available at www.bls.gov/data/#injuries. Accessed October, 2008.

to patients, staff, and equipment, it is imperative to have sufficient and appropriate fire extinguishers in magnetic resonance imaging (MRI) areas.

Hospital workers are also exposed to blood and body fluids, contaminated needles, radiation, and vaccine-preventable diseases such as rubella and hepatitis B. Immunization programs help protect hospital personnel and, in turn, patients at risk of being infected by hospital personnel. For example, the Centers for Disease Control and Prevention (1999, 2001) highly recommend the hepatitis B vaccine for employees who work in high-risk areas. Any employee who refuses the vaccine is required to sign a refusal form but is allowed to request vaccination at a later date. Some schools of nursing also require that students have the hepatitis B vaccine before beginning their clinical experiences. Newer intravenous tubing and accessories are now available that do not require needles, thus reducing the risk of needlesticks. It is possible to further reduce needlesticks by following the "do not recap" procedure and properly disposing of needles after use. A stray needle lying in bed linens or carelessly thrown into a wastebasket is a prime source of exposure to bloodborne pathogens. There are commercial devices available to help with the so-called scoop technique, a one-handed method of more safely recapping, in cases of real need. Hepatitis types B and C are the infections most commonly transmitted by contaminated needles.

The National Institute for Occupational Safety and Health (NIOSH) focuses on safety and issues related to health. Identifying risks associated with the preparation of certain drugs and looking at ways to control exposure during preparation and administration is just one example of how this group works to ensure a safe health care environment for health care workers. The Hazard Communication Act of the Occupational Safety and Health Administration (OSHA) (a federal organization that provides guidelines to help reduce safety hazards in the workplace) requires hospitals to inform employees about the presence of or potential for harmful exposures and how to reduce the risk of exposure. The Centers for Disease Control and Prevention (CDC) (a federal agency that provides facilities and services for the investigation, identification, prevention, and control of disease) also provide guidelines for working with infectious patients (e.g., standard precautions) (see Chapter 12). Request information and follow recommended guidelines for reducing your exposure to the variety of hazards present in the hospital environment.

FIRE SAFETY

Both the home and the health care facility are at risk for fires. Fires in the health care facility are often related to smoking in bed or faulty electrical equipment. According to some statistics, more than 8100 hospital fires and over 4300 nursing home fires occur each year, but these have been reduced by *No Smoking* laws.

An established fire safety program is mandatory for all health care facilities (Box 14-8). Most facilities have a

Box 14-8 Fire Safety Interventions and Safe Evacuation of Patients

ACTION *(RATIONALE)*

1. Follow facility fire plan in the event of a fire. *(Fire plan outlines procedures to follow.)*
   a. Ascertain patient's age, sensory impairments, level of mobility, ability to comprehend instructions, and overall need for protection. *(Protects and assists patient in interpreting environmental stimuli relevant to safety.)*
   b. If indicated, assess patients for type of evacuation assistance needed. *(Move individuals at risk for injury to a safer area.)*
   c. Provide clear explanations to patients and visitors in a calm manner. *(Anxiety hinders understanding of situation and ability to follow instructions.)*
   d. Assist with evacuations if needed:
      (1) Usually patients are moved horizontally (e.g., out of rooms, across halls, and through the next set of fire doors). *(The fire and its potential for spreading often necessitate movement to a safer area. Some agencies have fire doors that are normally held open by magnets and close automatically when a fire alarms sounds. It is important to keep equipment away from these doors.)*
      (2) If smoke or fire prevents you from moving patients across the hall, proceed vertically down to a lower level. **Never use elevators as an exit route. A fire will spread very quickly up through the elevator shaft.**
      (3) If a patient cannot walk or be moved by bed, stretcher, or wheelchair from the fire area, it is often necessary to carry the patient. *(Use the carrying method that is safe for both you and the patient; fire department personnel will help with the evacuation.)*
      (4) Infant and child removal
         (a) Place a blanket or sheet on floor.
         (b) Place two infants in each bassinet, using diapers or small blankets for padding.
         (c) Place the bassinet in the middle of the blanket.
         (d) Use the baby vest if available or fold the blanket over one end, fold the corners in, then roll the sides in to form a pocket.
         (e) Grasp the folded corners of the blanket and pull the infants to safety. Two people (or, if necessary, one person) are able to drag eight babies to the prescribed area.
         (f) Alternatively, place as many children as possible in one crib and pull the crib to the prescribed area.
      (5) Universal carry
         The universal carry is a method of removing a patient from a bed to the floor. It is a quick and effective method for removing a patient who is in immediate danger. This carry can be used by anyone, regardless of patient size.
         (a) Spread a blanket, sheet, or bedspread on the floor alongside the bed, placing one third of it under the bed and leaving about 8 inches to extend beyond the patient's head.
         (b) Grasp the patient's ankles, and move the patient's legs until they fall at the knee over the edge of the bed.
         (c) Grasp each shoulder, slowing pulling the patient to a sitting position.
         (d) From the back, encircle the patient with your arms, place your arms under the patient's armpits, and lock your hands over the patient's chest.

Continued

Box 14-8 Fire Safety Interventions and Safe Evacuation of Patients—cont'd

(e) Slide the patient slowly to the edge of the bed, and lower the patient to the blanket. If the bed is high, instruct the patient to slide down one of your legs.
(f) Taking care to protect the patient's head, gently lower the head and upper torso to the blanket and wrap the blanket around the patient.
(g) At the patient's head, grip the blanket with both hands, one above each shoulder, holding the patient's head firmly in the 8 inches of blanket. Do not let the patient's head snap back.
(h) Lift the patient to a half-sitting position, and pull the blanketed patient to safety.

(6) Blanket drag
If vertical or downward evacuation by an interior stairway is necessary, in many cases one person can handle a helpless patient by using the blanket drag.
(a) Double a blanket lengthwise, and place it on the floor parallel and next to the bed, leaving 8 inches to extend above the patient's head.
(b) Using cradle drop, kneel drop, universal carry, or other suitable means, remove the patient from the bed to the folded blanket on the floor alongside the bed.
(c) Grasp the blanket above the patient's head and pull to the stairway; start down the stairs with patient coming headfirst onto the stairway.
(d) Position yourself one, two, or three steps lower than the patient, depending on your height and the patient's height. The patient's lower body inclines upward.
(e) Place your arms under the patient's arms, and clasp your hands over the patient's chest.
(f) Back slowly down the stairs, constantly maintaining close contact with the patient, keeping one leg against the patient's back.

(7) When considering the two-person swing, as well as all evacuation methods, take into consideration the patient's size and weight.
(a) Two staff members grasp each others' forearms to form a seat for the patient to sit in (see Figure 14-5, *A*).
(b) Other personnel lift the patient into the seat formed in step (7)(a) and removed from area (see Figure 14-5, *B*).

2. Follow-up
   a. Listen to the "All clear" announcement after a drill or follow specific instructions from the fire department or supervisor regarding the return of patients. ("This area is safe for patients and staff.")
   b. Reduce the potential for fire-related injuries by doing the following:
      (1) Follow and enforce the smoking policy. Most facilities have adopted a *No Smoking* policy to promote a smoke-free environment for patients and employees.
      (2) Know the location of fire alarm boxes and type of fire extinguishers available.
      (3) Know the location of the fire exits.
      (4) Be familiar with the hospital fire safety program and protocols for evacuation.
      (5) Keep hallways free of unnecessary supplies, furniture, and other obstacles.
      (6) Check to see that electrical equipment is operating safely. *(Planning saves valuable time and improves overall performance.)*
   c. Participate, when possible, in fire drills. Fire safety education programs are necessary to meet the requirements of accrediting agencies, such as The Joint Commission. *(Learning experiences are provided through participation in fire drills and formal critiques of the activity.)*
3. Evaluation
   a. The immediate environment of the patient is safe from potential fire hazards. *(Fire safety practices help prevent fires.)*
   b. In the event of a fire, established protocols are followed. *(The emergency will be handled rapidly and appropriately.)*

Box 14-9 Fire Prevention Guidelines for Nurses

- Keep the phone number for reporting fires visible on the telephone at all times.
- Know the agency's fire drill and evacuation plan.
- Know the location of all fire alarms, exits, and fire extinguishers.
- Use the mnemonic *RACE* to set priorities in case of fire:
  R—Rescue and remove all patients in immediate danger.
  A—Activate the alarm. Always do this before attempting to extinguish even a minor fire.
  C—Confine the fire by closing doors and windows and turning off all oxygen and electrical equipment.
  E—Extinguish the fire using an extinguisher.
- Memorize the mnemonic *PASS* to operate the fire extinguisher:
  P—Pull the pin to unlock the handle.
  A—Aim low at the base of the fire.
  S—Squeeze the handle.
  S—Sweep the unit from side to side (see Figure 14-6).

safety committee that is actively involved in establishing and monitoring prevention and fire education programs. Fire prevention includes good housekeeping, maintenance, and employee discipline (Box 14-9).

Housekeeping responsibilities include eliminating all unnecessary combustible material; and maintenance responsibilities include ensuring the proper functioning of fire protection devices, such as alarms, extinguishers, and sprinklers. It is mandatory to identify, light, and unlock exits. Cooking and laundry equipment, filters, and air ducts are to be kept free of lint and grease. It is obligatory to inspect and maintain all mechanical and electrical equipment regularly to keep fire hazards to a minimum.

All employees need to know the telephone number and procedure for reporting a fire, as well as the location of the nearest alarms and firefighting equipment. Additionally, it is crucial that health care workers

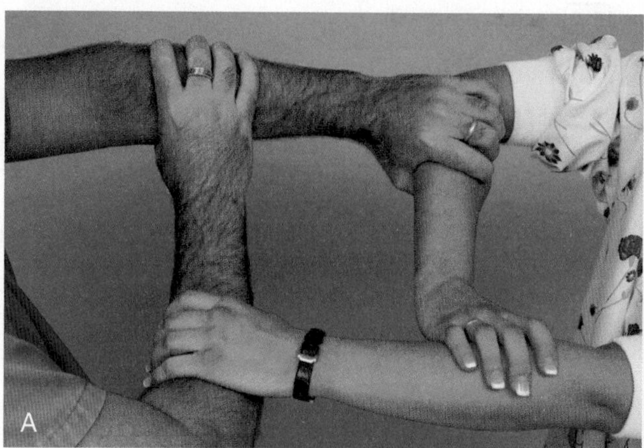
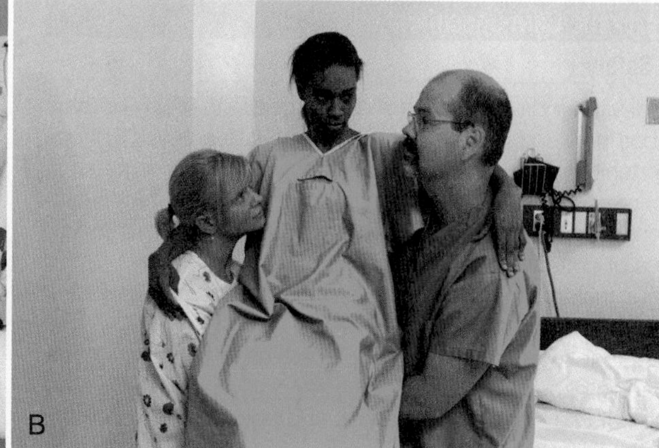

FIGURE 14-5 The two-person evacuation carry. **A,** Hands positioned to form two-person evacuation swing. **B,** Patient is seated firmly on swing and holds nurses by shoulders for emergency evacuation.

know their roles in the overall hospital evacuation plan (Figure 14-5). Checking for fire hazards on an ongoing basis is a must.

An important element in any fire safety program is an understanding of what type of fire extinguisher to use on different types of fires. Use the appropriate fire extinguisher for each type of fire:

- Paper, wood, and cloth fires require a type A fire extinguisher.
- Flammable liquid fires, such as those caused by grease and anesthetics, require a type B fire extinguisher.
- Electrical fires require a type C fire extinguisher.
- Fire extinguishers marked ABC are acceptable for use on any type of fire.

Knowing which type of extinguisher is on the unit before a fire occurs is vital. Most fire safety programs afford health care workers the opportunity to handle the different types of fire extinguishers.

Certain areas of the health care facility require additional fire safety programs and precautions. For example, fires and smoke inhalation are potential problems associated with the use of lasers in surgery and with oxygen therapy. Other common ignition sources in the operating area are electric cautery equipment and high-intensity light cords. In the event of a fire, patients on life-support systems will possibly need manual respiratory support with an ambu bag.

By remembering the formula RACE (**R**escue patients, sound the **A**larm, **C**onfine the fire, and **E**xtinguish or **E**vacuate), you will be prepared when safety is threatened by fire. In the event of fire, rescue patients in *immediate* danger, and then follow the facility's procedure for activating the fire alarm and reporting the location and extent of the fire. Then take measures to contain or extinguish the fire if there is no immediate threat to safety. These measures include closing doors and windows, turning off oxygen and electrical equipment, and using the appropriate fire extinguisher (Figure 14-6). The mnemonic PASS will help you remember how to operate the fire extinguisher.

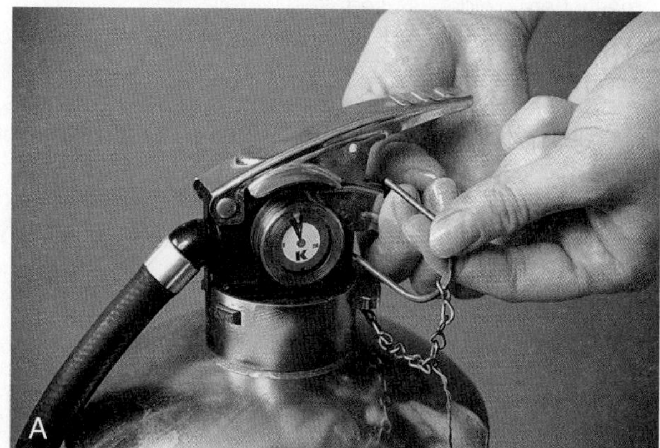
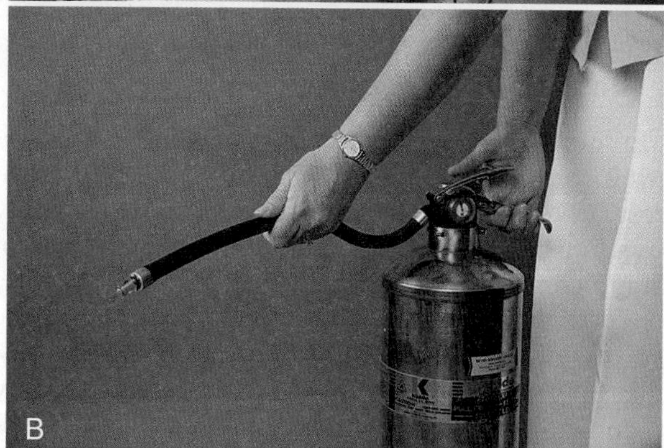
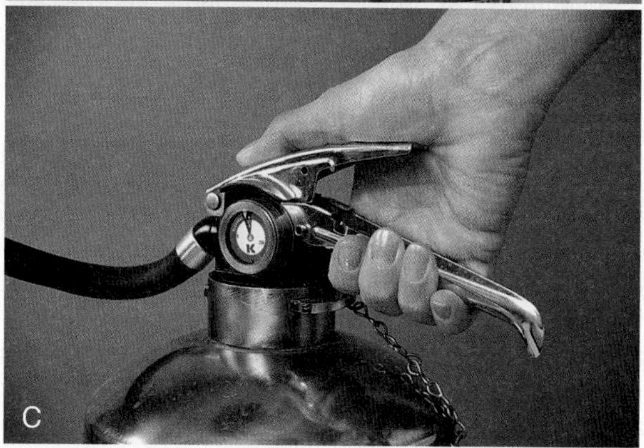

FIGURE 14-6 Operating a fire extinguisher. **A,** Pull the pin. **B,** Aim at the base of the fire. **C,** Squeeze the handles. Sweep from side to side to coat the area evenly.

Home Care Considerations

Fire Safety

- Today, as more patients are discharged with follow-up care to be provided in the home, the nurse has an excellent opportunity to evaluate fire safety practices in the home environment. Patients who are elderly or who have mobility limitations will often need your assistance to achieve an environment free of potential fire hazards.
- Give instructions about the proper use of monitoring or therapy equipment used.
- See that several electrical circuits are used to prevent overloading of any single one.
- Do not use electrical appliances and equipment near sinks, bathtubs, or showers.
- Review smoking practices, and give instructions to not smoke in bed or when sleepy.
- Do not permit smoking by the patient, family, or visitors in areas where oxygen is used.
- Advise against the use of electrical appliances (e.g., electric razors) around oxygen.
- Encourage the installation of fire alarms, smoke detectors, and carbon monoxide detectors, as well as the purchase of a portable fire extinguisher.
- Have the family plan fire escape routes from each room and practice exit drills. Establish a place to meet outside to verify that everyone is safe.
- Teach *stop*, *drop*, and *roll* to extinguish fire on clothing.
- Do not place electrical cords under carpeting.
- Allow only certified electricians to work on wiring.
- Avoid using candles for light or heat, and never leave a burning candle unattended.

Patient Teaching

The Non-Use of Ipecac at Home

According to the National Capital Poison Center in 2009:

- The American Academy of Pediatrics and the American Association of Poison Control Centers recommend that ipecac syrup not be kept in homes for available use.
- The U.S. Food and Drug Administration (FDA) is considering making ipecac syrup available to the public by prescription only.
- Most pharmacies no longer carry ipecac syrup.
- The first action recommended in the event of ingestion of a poison is to call the local poison control center at 1-800-222-1222.

From National Poison Control Center. (n.d.). *Ipecac syrup.* Available at www.poison.org/prepared/ipecac.asp. Accessed April, 2009.

Enforcing the facility's smoking policy and monitoring for potential electrical hazards help prevent fires. For example, never use or allow to be used any frayed or broken electrical cords or a faulty piece of equipment. Notify the maintenance department of any defects in the equipment. Report any shocks felt while using equipment. Monitor *No Smoking* rules carefully, especially near patients receiving oxygen. The safety of patients and caregivers depends on the staff's knowledge of fire prevention guidelines and fire procedures (see Home Care Considerations box).

ACCIDENTAL POISONING

Poisoning (the condition or physical state produced by the ingestion, injection, inhalation, or exposure of a poisonous [toxic] substance) is one of the major causes of death in children under 5 years of age. Wong and others (2006) note that there are more than 500 toxic substances in the average home. Although legislation passed in the early 1970s required the use of child safety packaging for certain substances, a significant number of accidental poisonings continue to occur. Specific antidotes and treatments are now available for all types of poisons. Note that syrup of ipecac is no longer recommended for use (see Patient Teaching box on non-use of ipecac).

The older adult is also at risk. Changes associated with aging interfere with the individual's ability to absorb and excrete drugs. Some older adults share drugs with friends or limit their medications because of the expense. Changes in eyesight sometimes lead to an accidental ingestion. If elderly patients have any memory impairment, they are liable to forget when they last took either prescribed or over-the-counter medication.

Hospitalized patients and those in other types of health care facilities are at risk for accidental poisoning because of the many poisonous substances in the environment. Make sure cleaning solutions and disinfectants are properly labeled and stored. To prevent poisoning, remove toxic agents from areas where accidental poisoning is possible. Do not remove toxic or poisonous substances from their original containers because incorrect labeling is one of the likely results, and never use substances from unmarked containers. Label poisonous substances conspicuously, and store them appropriately immediately after use.

Drugs, of course, are potentially hazardous if prepared or administered inappropriately. Human carelessness causes errors of both types. Always follow drug administration procedures (see Chapter 23). Make sure to attend staff inservice programs that present new drugs or provide updated information on frequently used drugs.

Poison control centers are valuable sources of information when poisoning occurs or is suspected. Keep the number of the closest poison control center clearly posted. Information received from the center helps both in treatment and referral. Most health care facilities also have posted instructions about how to handle poisoning cases (Box 14-10). Make sure you know where these are located (see Chapter 24).

Box 14-10 Accidental Poisoning Interventions

ACTION *(RATIONALE)*

1. When a poisoning occurs:
   a. Obtain an accurate history. *(Identifies possible antidote[s] and method of treatment needed.)*
      (1) Identify the route (e.g., injected, ingested, inhaled), type, and amount of poisonous substance(s) received.
      (2) Determine how long ago the poisoning happened.
      (3) Obtain a history of allergies, prescribed medications, medical problems, and general state of physical and mental health.
   b. Assess for changes in mental status and the presence of motor and sensory deficits. *(Incomplete data possibly results in incorrect identification of patient's health needs.)*
   c. Notify the poison control center and follow facility protocols (see Patient Teaching box on non-use of ipecac). *(Treatment guidelines will be furnished.)*
   d. Do not induce vomiting if poisoning is related to the following substances: household cleaners, lye, furniture polish, grease, or petroleum products. *(Vomiting increases risk of internal burns.)*
   e. Do not induce vomiting in an unconscious individual. *(Vomiting increases danger of aspiration.)*
2. Perform hand hygiene. *(Reduces spread of microorganisms.)*
3. Document procedure. *(Note procedure and patient's response.)*
4. Follow-up
   a. Continue to monitor vital signs and response to treatment. *(Ongoing assessment is a part of the treatment.)*
   b. Reduce the potential for accidental poisoning by doing the following:
      (1) Be aware of potentially poisonous substances (e.g., drugs, plants, and cleaning solutions).
      (2) Inform patients and families about how to handle a poisoning emergency.
      (3) Ensure that poisonous substances are labeled, locked, and out of the reach of children. *(It is possible to greatly reduce the risk of accidental poisoning. Quick and appropriate action will often decrease the effects of the poisoning.)*
   c. Know where emergency instructions are located. *(Procedures and guidelines for handling the emergency are outlined.)*
   d. Know the number of the poison control center (National Poison Control Center: 1-800-222-1222; www.poison.org) or call 9-1-1 and be prepared to provide information about the poison. *(The poison control center will provide information needed to treat the patient, and all dispatchers will offer referral assistance.)*
   e. The immediate environment is safe from potential poisoning hazards when poisonous substances are labeled, locked, and properly stored. *(Safety practices reduce the risk of accidental poisoning.)*

SPECIAL CONCERNS

- Always follow drug administration policies and procedures. Have your dosage calculations checked, especially if a mixed or prepared drug is to be infused.
- Keep informed of new medications and recommended dosages.
- Properly label and store cleaning solutions and disinfectants.
- Never use substances from unmarked containers.

DISASTER PLANNING

Disaster planning, or emergency preparedness, enables rescuers to respond effectively and efficiently when confronted with a disaster situation. A **disaster situation** is an uncontrollable, unexpected, psychologically shocking event that is unique and likely to have a significant impact on a variety of health care facilities. Examples of natural threats to safety are earthquakes, hurricanes, floods, and tornados. Bombings, arson, riots, and hostage taking represent acts of violence carried out by people and will not always affect a facility's day-to-day operations.

Factors that affect disaster response include the time of the day; the scope and duration of the triggering event; readiness of the health care facility, personnel, and equipment; preparations for appropriate procedures; and the extent to which the various community agencies and institutions collaborate with one another. Health care facilities are expected to receive victims and survivors and to assist rescuers.

Disasters are referred to as external or internal. The external disaster originates outside the health care facility and results in an influx of casualties brought to the facility (e.g., an explosion in a chemical plant, an airplane crash, a train accident). The emergency department is the main focus of activity. Typically, there is no immediate safety threat to staff, patients, or hospital property.

The internal disaster represents an extraordinary situation that is brought about by events within the health care facility. In many cases, the organization's ability to function normally is threatened. An internal disaster has the ability to threaten the safety of patients, visitors, staff, and facility property.

Disaster planning consists of putting appropriate measures into place to ensure that health care facilities and personnel have the capacity to manage a disaster effectively (Boxes 14-11 and 14-12). Most state and federal regulators require disaster drills to be conducted on a routine basis to prepare health care facilities and personnel to meet their responsibilities effectively. It is

Box 14-11 Disaster Planning Interventions

ACTION *(RATIONALE)*

1. **Planning**
   a. Review facility disaster plan frequently to update knowledge. The development of the disaster-preparedness plan is an evolving and ongoing process. The purpose of disaster-preparedness planning is to prepare the facility and health care workers for both external and internal disasters. *(Information helps health care workers anticipate their roles in the event of a disaster.)*
   b. Know your own particular responsibilities in a disaster emergency. *(Valuable time is saved and overall performance improved.)*
   c. Participate, when possible, in disaster drills. Learning experiences are provided through disaster drills and formal critiques of the responses. *(Drills are helpful in evaluating the overall safety program and are required by accrediting agencies.)*
   d. Participation in a crisis support group is desirable if directly involved in a disaster or a disaster response. Individuals often experience some level of emotional or critical incident stress. *(Crisis support teams or groups encourage staff to share thoughts and feelings related to the experience [debriefing].)*
2. **Follow facility disaster plan in the event of a disaster.** *(Disaster plan outlines procedures to follow and is most effective when personnel respond appropriately.)*
   a. Identify the type of disaster emergency by recognizing the code that is used to announce it. *(Unfamiliarity with the codes tends to result in loss of valuable time and injury to patients or personnel.)*
   b. Identify each patient's age, sensory impairments, level of mobility, ability to comprehend instructions, and overall need for protection. *(Helps you to protect and assist patients in interpreting environmental stimuli relevant to safety.)*
   c. If indicated, assess patients for possible discharge or transfer. Protection of inpatients, as well as casualties from a disaster, is a top priority. *(It is possible that space will be needed for disaster victims.)*
   d. Provide clear explanations to patients and visitors in a calm manner. *(The amount of information patients and families have about the situation [drill, disaster event] will affect their ability to cooperate and participate in any planned or unplanned activity.)*
   e. If a disaster occurs when you are off duty, follow your facility protocols for reporting in (i.e., some facilities require you to report for duty at your regularly scheduled times, whereas others require you to contact your manager for instruction). Community agencies and resources are incorporated into the overall plan. *(Additional personnel [e.g., student nurses and clinical faculty] will in some cases assist with inpatient care to free staff for more critical disaster victims.)*
   f. If an internal disaster occurs, assist with planned evacuations as needed. *(Some disasters necessitate moving patients to a safer area.)*
   g. Listen for the "All clear" announcement after a disaster drill. *(This indicates that the drill is over.)*
3. **Evaluation.** Compare actual outcomes and performances with disaster-preparedness plan (usually a critique session is held). *(Evaluation allows facility to examine whether plan accomplished goals and objectives; permits necessary changes to be made.)*

Box 14-12 Variations for Disaster Planning: The Nursing Home

Nursing home residents will also sometimes require evacuation and relocation in the case of an internal disaster. The successful nursing home disaster-preparedness plan, like those for hospitals, outlines the sequence of events to be followed:

- Residents will require some type of identification (picture ID or identification bracelet, such as those used in the memory support unit for patients diagnosed with Alzheimer's disease (AD).
- At the designated triage site, nurses will decide where residents will go.
- Residents will sometimes require admission to a hospital or other building, such as a school or church, for temporary shelter and care.
- It is necessary that the disaster plan include instructions and guidelines for what is to be done after the relocation is completed.
- Notification of families and physicians is critical.
- A log is kept to document events. List the name of the patient, who and how transported, and where patient was sent so family and physicians are aware of his or her location and transfers as they occur.

essential that personnel be familiar with the location and the contents of the facility's **disaster manual** (sometimes called the Emergency Operations Plan or Emergency Management Plan). This manual specifies chain of command, callback procedures, assignment procedure, departmental responsibilities, patient evacuation procedure and routes, procedures for the receipt and management of casualties, and policies related to the overall management of supplies and equipment.

Make sure you know the various **codes** (a system of notification to be transmitted rapidly) used by your health care facility to alert personnel to the various emergencies affecting the facility.

TERRORISM

Terrorism, or the possibility of a terrorist attack, has recently emerged as an environmental health threat. **Terrorism** is a violent or dangerous act used to intimidate or coerce a person or government to further a political or social agenda. Before 1990 and the Gulf War, the possibility of the United States coming under attack from terrorist groups using biological, chemical, or nuclear weapons seemed remote. After the terrorist attacks on the World Trade Center in New York City and the Pentagon on September 11, 2001, the government implemented the Homeland Security Act of 2002. Its purpose was to have a single agency to oversee the development of a comprehensive approach to a large domestic incident. The Department of Homeland Security is primarily concerned with preventing and managing potential attacks by an individual or small group on one of our cities, a large sporting event, or a unit of our military forces.

BIOTERRORISM

Bioterrorism is the use of biological agents to create fear and threat. It is crucial for health care facilities to be prepared to treat mass casualties from such an attack. A facility's emergency management plan provides details on how to respond to a terrorist attack, for example, determining the agent used, determining the time and location of the attack and the affected population, obtaining and delivering supplies, and providing treatment. Education and training is required to prepare nurses to respond to an attack by taking the necessary steps to initiate an agency's emergency management plan.

Bioterrorist Attacks

Although the only bioterrorist attack to date was the anthrax attack shortly after September 11, 2001, the threat is very real. Be prepared to make accurate and timely assessments in any type of setting. If an attack occurs, it will most likely involve the use of biological agents such as anthrax, botulism, smallpox, or bubonic plague. A bioterrorist attack will most likely resemble a natural outbreak initially, but sometimes the microorganisms used will be modified to obtain increased virulence or will have resistance to antibiotics or vaccines. Biological attacks will sometimes be **overt** (announced) and sometimes **covert** (unannounced). In the case of an overt attack, rapid assessment of its real scope is necessary, followed by an appropriate response. Covert attacks become obvious only after victims seek medical care, that is, after the incubation period has passed and clinical signs begin to appear. In both cases, it is essential for you to recognize and understand how to manage high-risk syndromes (groups of signs and symptoms resulting from a common cause or appearing together to present a clinical picture of a disease) (Box 14-13). Acutely ill patients representing the earliest cases after a covert attack will

Box 14-13 High-Risk Syndromes

1. **Anthrax** (acute infectious disease caused by *Bacillus anthracis*, a spore-forming, gram-positive bacillus). Humans become infected through skin contact, ingestion, or inhalation. Person-to-person transmission of inhalational disease does not occur. Direct exposure to vesicle secretions of skin anthrax potentially results in secondary cutaneous infection.
   Clinical Features: Pulmonary: flulike symptoms, possible brief interim improvement, within 2 to 4 days there is abrupt onset of respiratory failure and hemodynamic collapse. Gram-positive bacilli on blood culture tests. *Cutaneous*: local skin involvement, common on head, forearms, and hands; localized itching followed by a papular lesion that becomes vesicular and within 2 to 6 days becomes a depressed black eschar. *Gastrointestinal:* abdominal pain, nausea, vomiting, and fever after eating contaminated food (usually meat); bloody diarrhea, hematemesis; gram-positive bacilli on blood culture. Symptoms begin within 1 day to 8 weeks (average 5 days) depending on route of exposure and amount of agent.
2. **Botulism** (caused by *Clostridium botulinum*, an anaerobic gram-positive bacillus that produces a potent neurotoxin). Foodborne botulism is the most common form. An airborne form of botulism also occurs.
   Clinical Features: Foodborne botulism causes abdominal cramping, diarrhea, and other gastrointestinal symptoms. Both foodborne and inhalation botulism cause the following: responsive patient with absence of fever; drooping eyelids, weakened jaw clench, difficulty swallowing or speaking; blurred vision and double vision; symmetric paralysis of arms first, followed by respiratory muscles, then legs; respiratory dysfunction from respiratory muscle paralysis; **no sensory deficits.** Neurologic symptoms begin 12 to 36 hours after ingestion of foodborne botulism and 24 to 72 hours after inhalation of the airborne form. The disease is not transmitted from person to person.
3. **Plague** (an acute bacterial disease caused by the gram-negative bacillus *Yersinia pestis*). A bioterrorism-related outbreak is likely to be airborne.
   Clinical Features: Fever, cough, chest pain, hemoptysis, mucopurulent or watery sputum with gram-negative rods in a Gram stain test. X-ray film shows bronchopneumonia. Person-to-person transmission is possible via large aerosol droplets. Symptoms usually appear within 1 to 3 days.
4. **Smallpox** (an acute viral illness caused by the variola virus). Disease has the potential to cause severe morbidity in a nonimmune population. Transmission via the airborne route is possible. A single case of smallpox is a public health emergency.
   Clinical Features: Symptoms similar to other acute viral illnesses, such as the flu. Skin lesions appear, quickly progressing from macules to papules to vesicles. Other symptoms include 2 to 4 days of fever and myalgia; rash most prominent on face and extremities (including palms and soles); rash scabs over in 1 to 2 weeks. Smallpox is transmitted by large and small respiratory droplets. Patient-to-patient transmission is likely from airborne and droplet exposure, and by contact with skin lesions or secretions. Symptoms begin in 7 to 17 days (average 12 days).

Adapted from Potter P.A., & Perry, A.G. (2007). *Basic nursing: essentials for practice* (6th ed.). St. Louis: Mosby.

usually seek care in emergency departments. Less ill patients, or those at the onset stage of an illness, sometimes seek care in primary care settings or try to manage the signs and symptoms on their own.

There are basic epidemiologic (the distribution and determinants of health-related states and events in populations) principles to assess whether a patient's presentation of symptoms is typical of an endemic (the expected or normal incidence native to or occurring naturally to a specific area or environment) disease or is an unusual event that calls for investigation. Consider the possibility of a bioterrorism-related outbreak when you observe trends or events such as the following:

- A rapidly increasing incidence of a disease (e.g., within hours or days) in a normally healthy population
- An unusual increase in the number of people seeking care, especially with fever or respiratory or gastrointestinal complaints
- An epidemic disease, or a disease that emerges rapidly at an uncharacteristic time or in an unusual pattern
- Lower incidence among patients who had been indoors, in areas with filtered or closed ventilation, compared with people who had been outdoors
- Clusters of patients arriving from a single locale
- Large numbers of rapidly fatal cases
- Any patient who develops a disease that is relatively uncommon and has bioterrorism potential

It is essential that you have the ability to recognize a casualty of a biological attack and to carry out your roles and responsibilities quickly and efficiently. Timely communication is critical for alerting both the medical and general community at large to a bioterrorist attack. Health care agencies' emergency plans will outline the departments to contact in the event of an attack and who is responsible for reporting the suspected occurrence to the local public health authorities.

Infection prevention and control practices are critical in the event of a biological attack. Manage all patients with suspected or confirmed bioterrorism-related illnesses using standard precautions (see Chapter 12). For certain diseases, such as smallpox or pneumonic plague, airborne and contact isolation precautions will be needed. Although a number of infections associated with biological agents are not transmissible from patient to patient, in general make sure to limit the transport and movement of patients to what is essential for treatment and care. Also ensure that you and other staff are utilizing all safety precautions to protect yourselves as well as those in the immediate surroundings.

TERRORISM BY NUCLEAR EXPOSURE

One example of how the threat of nuclear terrorism will possibly manifest is an attack on a domestic nuclear weapon facility. Another is the use of a so-called "dirty bomb," which is a radiation-dispersal device that couples nuclear waste with a conventional bomb.

A patient is contaminated by radiation from a source on the body or the clothing, from ingesting it, or by absorbing it through a skin opening. The effects on the patient are determined by the amount of radiation absorbed (absorbed radiation is measured by the gray [Gy], equal to 100 rads). When less than 0.75 Gy is absorbed, patients usually do not have any symptoms. Patients who absorb 8 Gy will usually die, and an absorption of 30 Gy is always fatal.

The patient who absorbs more than 0.75 Gy is at risk for developing acute radiation syndrome; the severity and nature of symptoms will vary, depending on the amount of radiation absorbed:

- **Hematopoietic:** Deficiency of white blood cells and platelets, which leads to bleeding, anemia, infections, impaired wound healing, and immunodeficiency
- **Gastrointestinal:** Loss of mucosal barrier and cells lining the intestine, which results in fluid and electrolyte loss, vomiting, hematemesis, diarrhea, melena, loss of normal flora, and sepsis
- **Cerebrovascular and central nervous systems:** Cerebral edema, hyperpyrexia, hypotension, confusion, and disorientation
- **Skin:** Loss of epidermis and possibly the dermis

During the prodromal phase immediately following exposure, signs and symptoms in more than one of these areas typically appear. The latent phase, when all symptoms generally disappear for a few days to a few weeks, follows in a day or two. Then, in the illness phase, the signs and symptoms reappear and intensify. Following this peak, the patient will either begin to recover or will die. Death typically occurs from infection or other complications.

OSHA requires that hospitals have an emergency plan for treating patients contaminated with radioactive substances. A decontamination unit is set up near the emergency department.

CHEMICAL TERRORISM

The following are several types of agents it is possible to use in chemical terrorism.

- **Pulmonary agents:** Include the gases chlorine (Cl), phosgene, ammonia, and hydrochloric acid. These agents cause shortness of breath, chest tightness, and wheezing and, in some cases, pulmonary edema. Symptoms sometimes take up to 2 to 24 hours to appear. Fluid in the lungs leads to hypovolemia and hypotension. Patients often require mechanical ventilation and supportive care.
- **Incapacitating agents:** Include 3-quinuclidinyl benzilate, a glycolate anticholinergic compound typically known by its NATO code BZ and agent 15 (an Iraqi version of BZ). These agents impair rather than kill or seriously injure victims. The effects include decreased organ function, hyperthermia, hallucinations, altered perceptions, and erratic behavior.

- **Cyanide agents:** Hydrogen cyanide is one example; these agents form cyanide when metabolized and are either ingested or inhaled. A patient in severe respiratory distress without cyanosis has probably been exposed to cyanide. Cyanide has a pungent odor similar to bitter almonds or peaches. When an individual is exposed to a high concentration, death will occur within 5 to 10 minutes.
- **Nerve agents:** Taubin, sarin, soman, and V-agents are some of the most toxic nerve agents and they cause death in a matter of minutes. Symptoms include increased saliva production, chest pressure, rhinorrhea, vomiting, muscle weakness, incontinence, and convulsions. Symptoms will usually appear up to 10 hours following exposure to a low concentration.
- **Vesicant agents:** Sulfur mustard (H), distilled mustard (HD), nitrogen mustard (HN 1, 3), mustargen (HN 2), lewisite (L), and phosgene oxime (OX) are in this group. Vesicants are more lethal than pulmonary agents and cyanide agents because they sometimes remain in the environment for weeks, which results in a continuing source of exposure. Sulfur mustard smells like mustard or garlic, whereas another agent smells like geraniums, and yet another has a peppery smell. Vesicants affect the skin, the eyes, and the airway, and large doses damage the bone marrow. These agents have the capacity to cause the formation of vesicles that progress to severe tissue necrosis and sloughing. Symptoms of sulfur mustard exposure appear in 4 to 8 hours, but cellular damage occurs in 2 minutes with agents like lewisite and phosgene.

NURSING PROCESS *for Patient Safety*

The role of the licensed practical nurse/licensed vocational nurse (LPN/LVN) in the nursing process as stated is that the LPN/LVN will:

- Participate in planning care for patients based on patient needs
- Review patient's plan of care and recommend revisions as needed
- Review and follow defined prioritization for patient care
- Use clinical pathways, care maps, or care plans to guide and review patient care

Assessment

Using the nursing process, you can reduce the risk of injury to patients and staff. Seek to determine which patients are at risk for injury as soon as possible. Identify actual and potential threats to the patient's safety, the effect of the underlying illness on the patient's safety, and the risks for the patient's developmental stage. Specific interventions help ensure a safe environment. If safety is threatened, follow established guidelines to resolve the situation (Nursing Care Plan 14-1).

Nursing Diagnosis

Identification of defining characteristics from the data direct your efforts to identify appropriate nursing diagnoses. Include specific causes of a patient's safety risk among the nursing diagnoses so you are able to individualize nursing care. For example, a patient with an unsteady gait will be at risk for falling or injury. Nursing diagnoses related to patient safety could include the following:

- Risk for falls
- Impaired physical mobility
- Risk for injury

Expected Outcomes and Planning

In the plan of care, identify nursing interventions that prevent threats to safety and meet safety needs. Perform planning and goal setting with the patient, the family, and other members of the health care team. Goals and priorities are based on the risk to patient safety and health promotion. The overall goal for a patient with a threat to safety is remaining free from injury (see Nursing Care Plan 14-1).

Implementation

Nursing interventions are designed to promote the safety of the patient in the home as well as the health care setting. These interventions include health promotions, developmental considerations, environmental protection, and education of family members or patient caregivers (see Nursing Care Plan 14-1).

Evaluation

Evaluate nursing interventions for reducing threats to safety by comparing the patient's response to the expected outcomes for each goal of care. Assess patient for signs and symptoms of injury and assess the environment for physical hazards continually throughout hospitalization. Remove the hazards and modify the environment as necessary.

Observe for correct application of SRDs. Observe skin, monitor pulses, assess the restrained body part every 30 minutes, and release the restrained body part every 2 hours. Continuously monitor for complications of immobility.

Nursing Care Plan 14-1 Patient Safety

This care plan has been adapted for the patient who is at risk for injury and has been determined to need an SRD.

NURSING DIAGNOSIS ***Risk for injury, related to disease process, weakness, lack of mental acuity, medications, or age***

Patient Goals and Expected Outcomes	Nursing Interventions	Evaluation
Patient or caregiver will demonstrate knowledge and understanding of potential hazards and will practice preventive measures or will be protected from injury as necessary during hospitalization	Assess the following: (1) Patient's mental, visual, and auditory acuity (fall assessment, see Figure 14-1) (2) Patient's level of consciousness (3) Patient's ability to perform activities of daily living (ADLs), exercise, and ambulation. Consult with family on options other than restraints. Prevent clutter; wipe up spills; provide adequate lighting. Orient patient to surroundings and assess effectiveness of reality orientation. Maintain side rails and bed alarm. Maintain bed in low position when care is not being given. Place patient in room close to nurses' station. Assist patient with ADLs as needed. Obtain medication history and administer medications according to agency policy. Document nursing interventions for medications and monitor side effects. Use SRDs as per protocol. Assess respiratory status every 2 hours if the chest SRD is used. Offer fluids every 2 hours while awake unless contraindicated. Offer use of commode, bedpan, or urinal every 2 hours while awake. Release SRDs and exercise extremities according to agency policy, and assess extremities for alteration in peripheral tissue perfusion by testing capillary refill (blanch response); palpating radial and pedal pulses; assessing for edema, pallor, cyanosis, and coldness of extremities; and eliciting description of extremity sensations from patient (paresthesia). Document type of SRD used, including patient response and patient and family teaching about need for SRD. Review use of SRD at least every 24 hours, with the goal of discontinuing the SRD at the earliest possible time.	Patient demonstrates understanding of potential health hazards. Patient practices injury prevention for self. Patient remains injury free.

Critical Thinking Questions

1. The nurse walking down the hall hears a patient calling out for help. The nurse assesses the situation and realizes that the patient does not remember how to use the call light. What factors possibly contribute to the patient's inability to remember, and how should the nurse teach the patient to use the call bell?
2. The nurse enters the patient's room to answer the call bell and sees the patient frantically pointing to the trash can next to the bed. The nurse smells smoke and sees small flames. What is possible to help prevent fires, and what should the nurse do in this situation?

Get Ready for the NCLEX® Examination!

Key Points

- Discuss safety measures for coping with violence in the workplace.
- Preventing falls, electrical injuries, fires, burns, and accidental poisoning is key to maintaining a safe environment.
- Left-handed patients need special considerations to cope in a right-handed hospital environment.
- Infants, young children, older adults, and the ill or injured patient are at risk for falling.
- Proper patient orientation includes information about the use of the call light and bed controls. Place frequently used items within reach of patients.
- Question all patients regarding allergies. It is imperative to ask specifically about food and latex allergies.
- Keep adjustable beds in the low position except when care is given.
- Gait belts are an added safety feature to use when assisting patients to ambulate.
- Consider designing a restraint-free environment before applying an SRD.
- Make sure your priority is patient safety or the safety of others when applying an SRD.
- SRD use has the potential to result in increased restlessness, disorientation, agitation, anxiety, and feelings of powerlessness.
- Once SRDs are applied to a patient, it is mandatory to document the position of the device, circulation, physical and mental status, and ongoing need for the device.
- When extremity SRDs are applied, place gauze or padding around the extremity and secure the ends of the ties to the bed frame, not to the side rails.
- Remove SRDs at least every 2 hours and assess the skin. Do not leave the patient unattended during this time.
- Know agency policy and procedures regarding SRD use and documentation.
- Electrical accidents are often prevented by reporting frayed or broken electrical cords or any shocks felt when using equipment.
- It is possible to reduce fire-related injuries by knowing the location of exits, fire alarm boxes, and fire extinguishers.
- By remembering the formula RACE (**R**escue patients, sound the **A**larm, **C**onfine the fire, and **E**xtinguish or **E**vacuate), you will be prepared when safety is threatened by a fire.
- Participation in fire and disaster drills helps staff become familiar with established protocols.
- Poison control centers are valuable sources of information when poisoning is suspected or has occurred.
- A terrorist attack is a potential environmental health threat.
- Bioterrorism, or the use of biological agents to create fear and threat, is the most likely form a terrorist attack will take.
- Several national organizations, including OSHA, NIOSH, and the CDC, provide guidelines that help reduce safety hazards in the workplace.

Additional Learning Resources

 Go to your Companion CD for an audio glossary, animations, video clips, and more.

evolve Be sure to visit the Evolve site at http://evolve.elsevier.com/Christensen/foundations/ for additional online resources.

Review Questions for the NCLEX® Examination

1. On the transfer sheet of a patient admitted to a health care facility is the order "restrain prn." SRDs are used in the hospital setting to prevent patient injury. Which statement is correct?

1. SRDs often decrease anxiety because the patient feels safer.
2. All older adult patients need some type of SRD at night.
3. Allow as much freedom of movement as possible when applying SRDs.
4. When using soft SRDs to prevent injury from falling out of bed, tie them to the side rail.

2. In the situation of question 1, what is an appropriate goal (expected outcome) for the patient requiring a physical restraint?

1. Patient will remain free of injury.
2. Patient will allow SRDs to be used.
3. Nurse will check SRD every 30 minutes.
4. Use least restrictive form of SRD possible.

3. Documentation related to use of an SRD is required to include:

1. the nurse's feelings about having used the SRD.
2. the specific type of SRD used.
3. confirmation of a prn order for use of the SRD.
4. evidence that the patient was assessed every 8 hours.

4. When caring for the patient who requires the use of an SRD, the nurse remembers that an appropriate nursing intervention when caring for a patient who needs an SRD is to:

1. monitor the skin for signs of impairment.
2. remove the SRD once every 24 hours.
3. secure the ends of the ties to the side rails.
4. ensure that the SRD is in place at all times.

5. The nurse discovers smoke in a soiled utility room and remembers that the initial step taken to protect the patient in the event of a fire is to:

1. notify the fire department.
2. disconnect the oxygen supply.
3. use any extinguisher on the fire.
4. remove the patient from the area.

6. The patient who requires the use of an extremity SRD has an edematous extremity. The most appropriate nursing action is to:
   1. elevate the involved extremity.
   2. increase the padding around the extremity.
   3. notify the physician for a different type of SRD.
   4. remove the SRD and watch the patient more closely.

7. A type C fire extinguisher is required for which of the following types of fire?
   1. Paper
   2. Cloth
   3. Grease
   4. Electrical

8. When assessing a patient's knowledge of the fire safety precautions, which action indicates the need for further fire safety instruction?
   1. Fire exits and corridors are kept clear.
   2. A *No Smoking* sign is posted when oxygen is in use.
   3. A heating pad cord is taped when a frayed area is noted.
   4. Facility smoking policies are a part of the admission procedure.

9. Which factor places a child at greatest risk for specific types of injuries?
   1. Sex of the child
   2. Overall health
   3. Educational level
   4. Developmental level

10. During the 7 AM to 3 PM shift on the adult surgical unit, the code is announced for an external disaster emergency. Which event best represents this type of situation?
    1. A school bus accident
    2. A bomb threat in the mail room
    3. A hostage-taking event in the emergency department
    4. An electrical fire in the maintenance department

11. Vomiting is most likely to be induced if poisoning is related to the ingestion of which substance(s)?
    1. Lye
    2. Petroleum products
    3. Household cleaners
    4. Salicylates, such as aspirin

12. A 63-year-old patient is brought to the emergency department for treatment of an accidental poisoning. The first step in the treatment is to:
    1. induce vomiting.
    2. assess the patient.
    3. place the patient in an upright position.
    4. notify the poison control center.

13. Which is the greatest safety issue for caregivers of older adults?
    1. Accidental poisoning
    2. Electrical shock
    3. Accidental falls
    4. Thermal burns

14. A potential environmental health threat is the possibility of:
    1. bioterrorism.
    2. noise pollution.
    3. water pollution.
    4. air pollution.

15. In the event of a mercury spill, which statement is true?
    1. It is acceptable to clean the mercury spill with alcohol and ordinary cleaning cloths.
    2. Close all windows and doors to prevent the mercury spill from spreading out of the area.
    3. Do not vacuum the spill.
    4. Place the recovered mercury in a plastic bag and close tightly.

chapter

15

Body Mechanics and Patient Mobility

evolve

Elaine Oden Kockrow

http://evolve.elsevier.com/Christensen/foundationsadult

Objectives

1. State the principles of body mechanics.
2. Explain the rationale for using appropriate body mechanics.
3. Discuss considerations related to mobility for older adults.
4. Discuss the complications of immobility.
5. Demonstrate the use of assistive devices for proper positioning.
6. State the nursing interventions used to prevent complications of immobility.
7. Demonstrate placement of patient in Fowler's, supine (dorsal), Sims', side-lying, prone, dorsal recumbent, and lithotomy positions.
8. State the assessment for the patient's neurovascular status, including the phenomenon of compartment syndrome.
9. Describe range-of-motion exercises and their purpose.
10. Demonstrate joint range-of-motion exercises.
11. Identify complications caused by inactivity.
12. Relate appropriate body mechanics to the techniques for turning, moving, lifting, and carrying the patient.
13. Discuss use of the continuous passive motion machines.
14. Discuss the nursing process for patient mobility.

Key Terms

abduction (ăb-DŬK-shŭn, p. 379)
adduction (ă-DŬK-shŭn, p. 379)
alignment (ă-LĪN-mĕnt, p. 371)
base of support (p. 371)
body mechanics (p. 370)
compartment syndrome (p. 377)
contracture (kŏn-TRĂK-chŭr, p. 382)
dorsal (supine) (DŎR-săl, sū-PĪN, p. 373)
dorsal recumbent (DŎR-săl rē-KŬM-bĕnt, p. 373)
dorsiflexion (dŏr-sĭ-FLĔK-shŭn, p. 381)
extension (p. 379)
flexion (p. 379)
Fowler's (p. 373)
genupectoral (jĕ-nyū-PĔK-tŏr-ăl, p. 374)
hyperextension (hī-pŭr-ĕk-STĔN-shŭn, pp. 372, 379)
immobility (p. 375)
joint (p. 379)
lithotomy (lĭ-THŎT-ŏ-mē, p. 375)
mobility (p. 375)
orthopneic (ŏr-thŏp-NĒ-ĭk, p. 374)
physical disuse syndrome (p. 379)
pronation (prō-NĀ-shŭn, p. 380)
prone (p. 374)
range-of-motion (ROM) (p. 379)
semi-Fowler's (p. 373)
Sims' (p. 374)
supination (sū-pĭ-NĀ-shŭn, p. 380)
Trendelenburg (Trĕn-DĔL-ĕn-bŭrg, p. 375)

Studies of Workers' Compensation claims show that nursing personnel have the highest claim rates of workers in any occupation or industry. Patient-handling tasks, such as lifting, transferring, and repositioning, are the primary causes of musculoskeletal disorder (MSD) among nurses. These tasks, which you typically perform manually without the use of assistive devices, are so much a part of your nursing routine that you hardly ever consider them. There is always the need to transfer patients: from bed to wheelchair, from wheelchair to toilet, from wheelchair to bathtub—and back again. They need you to raise them, lower them, reposition them, and even lift them off the floor. Patients are sometimes able to assist with these maneuvers and sometimes not; some of them will be cooperative and some combative; and quite a few will be obese.

Injuries are most likely when you are performing a task that requires you to exert yourself forcefully, perform repetitive movements, or maintain an awkward or static posture. The most serious injuries occur when you twist and lift at the same time or move a patient without help from other personnel or an assistive device.

Mechanical lifting devices and assistive patient-handling equipment such as roller boards, sliders, friction-reduction pads, transfer chairs, and gait belts work by taking on the energy and force that would otherwise be imposed upon you during the lifting, transferring, or repositioning of a patient. Regular use of lifts and other assistive devices reduces your risk of injury (see Evidence-Based Practice box).

Safe patient transfer requires adequate staffing, the right mix of personnel, and appropriate, readily available, well-maintained patient-lifting equipment.

Evidence-Based Practice — Evaluation of Devices for Transferring Patients

Evidence Summary

This study compared seven lateral transfer devices with the traditional drawsheet method in a variety of acute care nursing units. Caregivers, who were mostly nurses, were given surveys after they used a transfer device to rank the device's comfort, ease of use, perceived injury risk, time efficiency, and patient safety. Caregivers rated the air-assisted devices higher than all the other devices when performing a lateral transfer, and the traditional drawsheet method performed poorly when compared with the other devices.

Application to Nursing Practice

- Health care agencies need to provide devices to reduce the risk of injury associated with lateral transfers.
- Nurses need to stop using the traditional drawsheet method when transferring patients.
- Use assistive devices, preferably air-assisted devices, when performing lateral transfers.
- New devices to transfer patients are being developed; take an active role in the evaluation of these devices whenever possible.

Reference

Baptiste, A., Boda, S.V., Nelson, A.L., et al. (2006). Friction-reducing devices for lateral patient transfers, *AAOHN Journal,* 54(4):173.

From Potter, P.A., & Perry, A.G. (2009). *Fundamentals of nursing: concepts, process, and practice.* (7th ed.). St. Louis: Mosby.

Life Span Considerations

Older Adults

Mobility

- The skin of older adults is more fragile and susceptible to injury. When moving or transferring older adults, it is essential to avoid pulling them across bed linens because this has potential to cause shearing or tearing of the skin.
- Always support older adults under the joints when moving them in bed. Lifting in any other manner increases the stress on the joint and causes increased pain, particularly if there is some degenerative joint disease. Explain each step in simple language, and avoid jerky, sudden movements.
- Aging tends to result in loss of flexibility and joint mobility. This often interferes with normal transfer techniques and necessitates modifications to protect patient and nurse.
- Weakness and hypotension are common signs and symptoms noted in an older adult on bed rest. Proceed slowly and cautiously when helping a patient ambulate for the first time after prolonged immobility. While facilitating independence and proper utilization of patient's body mechanics, use assistive devices such as canes, walkers, and trapeze bars. Provide adequate help to ensure patient safety when moving from a lying to a sitting position and from a sitting to a standing position.
- Older adults who have many diseases or have undergone prolonged bed rest have greater risk for hypotension with postural change (orthostatic hypotension).
- Patients using medications to reduce blood pressure are at greater risk for orthostatic hypotension.
- Older adults, particularly those with altered sensory perception, sometimes become fearful when hydraulic lifts are used for transfers. Provide eyeglasses and basic instructions.
- There are limited positioning alternatives for the older adult who has arthritis, neuropathies, or other restrictive conditions.
- Discourage older adult patients from sitting for prolonged periods of time without stretching and moving. Lack of movement presents a risk for contractures of joints.
- Ensuring good body alignment when the patient is sitting is a way to prevent joint and muscle stress.
- Provide patient teaching that includes using strong joints and large muscle groups for activities that require extra strength in order to prevent strain and pain in joints.
- For older adult patients with osteoporosis, encourage appropriate exercise programs that will prevent fractures and reduce bone loss.
- Encourage exercise programs for those older adults who do not participate in regular exercise. Ensure that patients consult with their health care provider before beginning any exercise program.
- Special adjustments to an exercise program are often necessary to prevent any problems for those older adults in advanced age.
- Older adults who are not able to participate in a structured exercise program are frequently able to achieve improved circulation and joint mobility by stretching and by exaggerating normal movements.

Data from Potter, P.A., & Perry, A.G. (2009). *Fundamentals of nursing: concepts, process, and practice.* (7th ed.). St. Louis: Mosby.

Equally important is the use of appropriate body mechanics or movements that protect your large muscle groups from injury and provide safety for patients when you are helping them to ambulate. Take special care with older adults (see Life Span Considerations for Older Adults box regarding mobility). Assistive devices such as splints, crutches, braces, canes, gait belts, and walkers are available to aid in promoting patient activity. Also important is the need to teach the patient appropriate positioning for home care, and to help a family member to learn how to assist the patient at home.

USING APPROPRIATE BODY MECHANICS

Understanding **body mechanics** (the field of physiology that studies muscular actions and the functions of muscles in maintaining the posture of the body) includes knowing how we use certain muscle groups. You use body mechanics daily in making beds, assist-

Table 15-1 Body Mechanics for Health Care Workers

ACTION	RATIONALE
When planning to move a patient, arrange for adequate help. Use mechanical aids if help is unavailable.	Two workers lifting together divide the workload by 50%.
Encourage patient to assist as much as possible.	This promotes patient's abilities and strength while keeping workload to a minimum.
Keep back, neck, pelvis, and feet aligned. Avoid twisting.	Twisting increases risk of injury.
Flex knees; keep feet slightly apart.	A broad base of support increases stability.
Position yourself close to patient (or object being lifted).	The force is minimized: 10 pounds at waist height close to the body is equal to 100 pounds at arm's length.
Use arms and legs (not back).	The leg muscles are stronger, larger muscles capable of greater work without injury.
Slide patient toward yourself using a pull sheet.	Sliding requires less effort than lifting. Pull sheet keeps to a minimum any shearing forces, which can damage patient's skin.
Set (tighten) abdominal and gluteal muscles in preparation for move.	Preparing muscles for the load limits strain to the least possible level.*
Person with the heaviest load coordinates efforts of team involved by counting to 3.	Simultaneous lifting keeps the load for any one lifter to a minimum.

*Back injuries are still the most common occupational injury among nurses.

ing the patient to walk, carrying supplies and equipment, lifting, providing patient care, and carrying out other procedures.

It is essential to look after the musculoskeletal system to prevent injury to yourself and the patient. Learn self-protection (Table 15-1), and teach the patient to protect himself or herself. Practice the appropriate use of body mechanics consistently in your work and in your personal life. Maintaining appropriate body alignment is the key factor in proper body mechanics. The term **alignment** refers to the relationship of various body parts to each other. Alignment helps balance and helps coordinate movements smoothly and effectively.

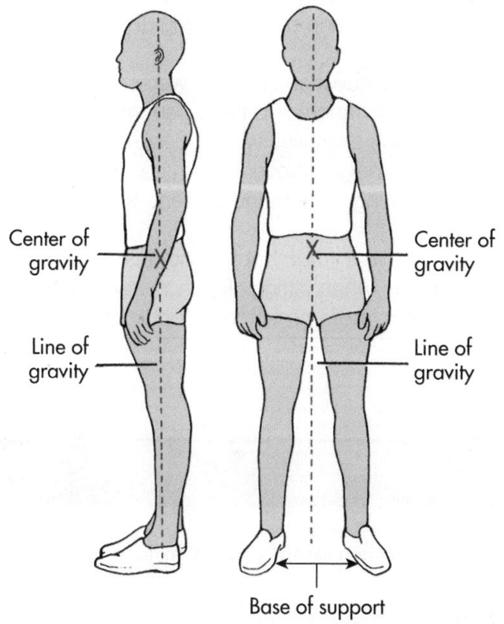

FIGURE 15-1 Good position for body mechanics: chin is high and parallel to the floor, abdomen is tightened (internal girdle) in and up with gluteal muscles tucked in, and feet are spread apart for a broad base of support.

Maintain a wide **base of support** (a stance with feet slightly apart) when standing. This helps provide better stability. Keep the base (distance between your feet) about 1.5 times the length of your shoes (Figure 15-1). When you are more stable, you are less likely to become overbalanced while carrying out an activity such as assisting the patient in and out of bed or ambulating in the room.

Skeletal muscles and the nervous system maintain equilibrium, or balance, which facilitates appropriate body alignment when lifting, bending, moving, and doing other activities. Bending your knees and hips before attempting these activities protects your back from the stress and potential injury inherent in the physical work of nursing. When stooping, flex or bend your hips and knees and maintain appropriate body alignment (i.e., keep your back straight). Avoid bending from the waist because this will, in time, strain the lower back (Figure 15-2). Work at a height or level that is comfortable and easy for you; this will help prevent undue stress and strain on your back muscles. One

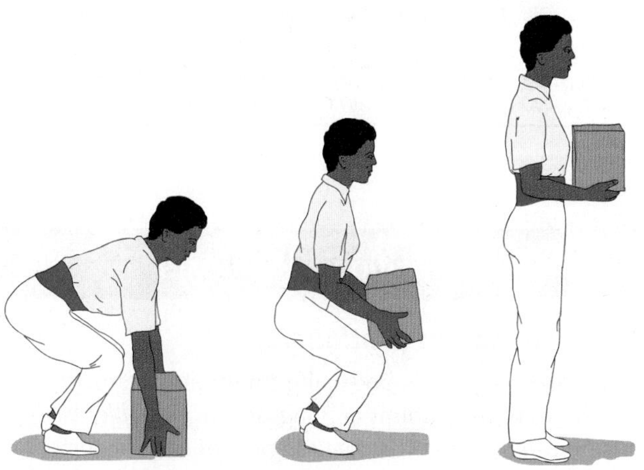

FIGURE 15-2 Picking up a box using good body mechanics. Box is carried close to the nurse's body and base of support.

way to accomplish this is by adjusting the height of the bed to a level appropriate for your height.

Using large muscle groups (such as arm and shoulder muscles, hips, and thigh muscles), helps in performing a bigger workload more safely. The more muscle groups you use, the more evenly you distribute the workload. If you widen your base of support in the direction of movement, you require less effort to carry out an activity. To avoid twisting your spine, stand directly in front of the person or object you are working with.

There are many other ways to protect both you and the patient from injury: Carry objects close to the midline of your body (see Figure 15-2), avoid reaching too far, avoid lifting when other means of movement are available (such as sliding, rolling, pushing, or pulling), use devices instead of or in combination with lifting, and use alternating periods of rest and activity. Know the maximum weight that is safe to carry. If you weigh 130 pounds, do not try to lift an immobilized 100-pound patient on your own. Although it is possible that you will be able to do it, there is a risk of injury to both you and the patient.

Assess your own abilities and limitations and that of your partner, if working in pairs. For example, note whether an individual has a bad knee, a trick knee, an old fractured ankle with limited motion, or a history of back injury (Box 15-1).

Box 15-1 Correct Use of Body Mechanics

Actions to promote proper body mechanics *(with rationale)*:

- Position feet 6 to 8 inches apart. *(Provides adequate base of support.)*
- Align and balance weight on both feet. *(Distributes weight evenly.)*
- Flex knees slightly. *(Prevents* **hyperextension** *[extreme or abnormal stretching].)*
- Tilt pelvis forward by pulling buttocks inward so gluteal muscles are contracted in and down. *(Helps straighten the lumbar curve of the spine, increasing power and reducing strain.)*
- Contract abdominal muscles in and up. *(Provides support and reduces muscle strain.)*
- Hold chest up. *(Allows adequate lung expansion.)*
- Keep head erect. *(Helps maintain appropriate alignment of the spine.)*
- Use appropriate body mechanics in all activities: standing, sitting, bending, and lifting. *(Produces most efficient body movement.)*
- Face your work area. *(Prevents unnecessary twisting.)*
- Push, slide, or pull heavy objects. *(Places less strain on body than lifting does.)*
- Lift twice—first mentally, and then physically. *(Helps determine if assistance is needed.)*
- Do not lift objects higher than chest level. Do not reach above your shoulders. *(It is much safer to use a step stool to reach an object higher than chest level.)*

POSITIONING PATIENTS

You and allied staff are called on daily to position patients. There are many positions to prevent patients from developing complications (Skill 15-1, Patient Teaching box on mobility). Inappropriate positioning poses the risk of causing permanent disability.

Patient Teaching

Mobility

- Instruct the family on proper mobility techniques if the patient is unable to understand teaching for reasons such as impaired cognition.
- Teach patient ways to assist with positioning.
- Provide opportunity for return demonstration.
- Teach patient and family signs and symptoms of skin impairment and contractures.
- Teach patient to avoid prolonged sitting. Frequent stretching decreases joint and muscle contractures.
- Teach importance of maintaining skin integrity.
- Explain importance of proper body alignment.
- Explain importance of rising slowly from lying to sitting, from sitting to standing, and after stooping. (Prevents orthostatic hypotension.)
- Provide time for questions and answers.
- Emphasize importance of patient performing active range-of-motion (ROM) exercises when possible.
- If the patient's height prevents the feet from touching the floor when sitting, teach the patient to rest them on a footstool.
- In order to prevent thrombophlebitis, teach patients not to cross their legs when sitting. Teach those at increased risk the signs and symptoms of thrombophlebitis, as well.

Skill 15-1 Positioning Patients

Nursing Action *(Rationale)*

1. Assess patient's body alignment and comfort level while patient is lying down. *(Provides baseline data concerning body alignment and comfort level. Helps determine ways to improve position and alignment.)*
2. Assemble equipment and supplies. *(Organizes procedure.)*
   - Pillows
   - Footboard
   - Trochanter roll
   - Sandbags

- Hand rolls
- Safety reminder devices
- Side rails

3. Request assistance as needed. *(Provides for safety.)*
4. Introduce self. *(Decreases patient's anxiety.)*
5. Identify patient. *(Ensures procedure is performed with correct patient.)*
6. Explain procedure. *(Enlists cooperation from patient and decreases patient anxiety.)*
7. Wash hands. Wear gloves as necessary according to agency policy and guidelines from the Centers for Disease Control and Prevention (CDC) and Occupational Safety and Health Administration (OSHA). *(Reduces spread of microorganisms.)*
8. Prepare patient. *(Prepares for procedure.)*
   - **a.** Close door or pull curtain. *(Provides privacy.)*
   - **b.** Raise level of bed to comfortable working height. *(Promotes good body mechanics in the nurse and safety for the patient.)*
   - **c.** Remove pillows and devices used in previous position. *(Makes access to patient easier.)*
   - **d.** Put bed in flat position or as low as patient can tolerate, and lower side rail closest to you. *(Facilitates procedure.)*
9. Position patient.
   - **a.** **Dorsal (supine)** position (lying flat on the back) (see illustration):
     - **(1)** Place patient on back with head of bed flat. *(Necessary for placing patient in supine position.)*
     - **(2)** Place small rolled towel under lumbar area of back. *(Provides support for lumbar spine.)*
     - **(3)** Place pillow under upper shoulder, neck, and head. *(Maintains correct alignment and prevents flexion contractures of cervical lumbar spine.)*
     - **(4)** Place trochanter rolls or sandbags parallel to lateral surface of thighs. *(Reduces external rotation of hip.)*
     - **(5)** Place small pillow or roll under ankle to elevate heels. *(Reduces pressure on heels, helping to prevent skin impairment.)*
     - **(6)** Support feet in dorsiflexion with firm pillow, footboard, or high-top sneakers. *(Prevents footdrop.)*
     - **(7)** Place pillows under pronated forearms, keeping upper arms parallel to patient's body (see illustration). *(Reduces internal rotation of shoulder and prevents extension of elbows. Maintains correct body alignment.)*
     - **(8)** Place hand rolls in patient's hands. *(Reduces extension of fingers and abduction of thumb.)*
   - **b.** **Dorsal recumbent** position (supine position with patient lying on back, head, and shoulder with extremities moderately flexed; legs are sometimes extended):
     - **(1)** Move patient and mattress to head of bed. *(Ensures appropriate body alignment.)*
     - **(2)** Turn patient onto back. *(Appropriately positions patient.)*
     - **(3)** Assist patient to raise legs, bend knees, and allow legs to relax. *(Puts patient in dorsal recumbent position.)*
     - **(4)** Replace pillow. Patient will sometimes need a small lumbar pillow. *(Provides comfort.)*
   - **c.** **Fowler's** position (posture assumed by patient when head of bed is raised 45 to 60 degrees) (see illustration).
     - **(1)** Move patient and mattress to head of bed. *(Ensures appropriate body alignment.)*
     - **(2)** Raise head of bed to 45 to 60 degrees. *(Positions patient appropriately.)*
     - **(3)** Replace pillow. *(Provides comfort, maintains proper body alignment, and ensures skin integrity.)*
     - **(4)** Use footboard. *(Prevents patient from slipping down in bed.)*
     - **(5)** Use pillows to support arms and hands. *(Provides comfort and maintains correct alignment.)*
     - **(6)** Place small pillow or roll under ankles. *(Reduces risk of skin impairment over heels.)*
   - **d.** **Semi-Fowler's** position (posture assumed by patient when head of bed is raised approximately 30 degrees).
     - **(1)** Move patient and mattress to head of bed. *(Ensures appropriate body alignment.)*
     - **(2)** Raise head of bed to about 30 degrees. *(Positions patient appropriately.)*

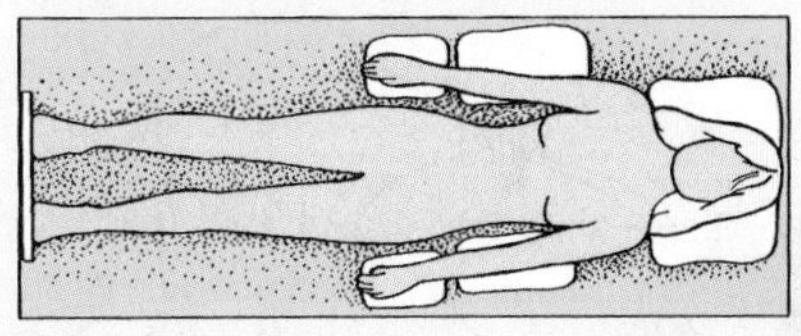

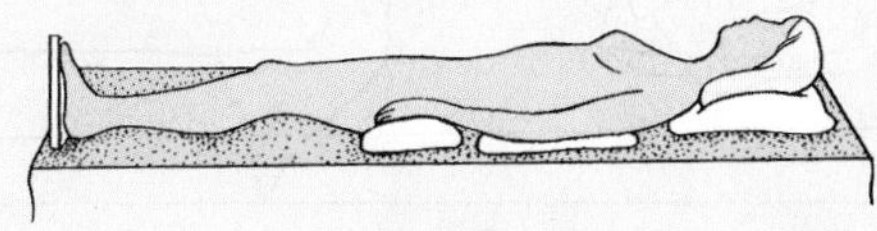

Step **9a**

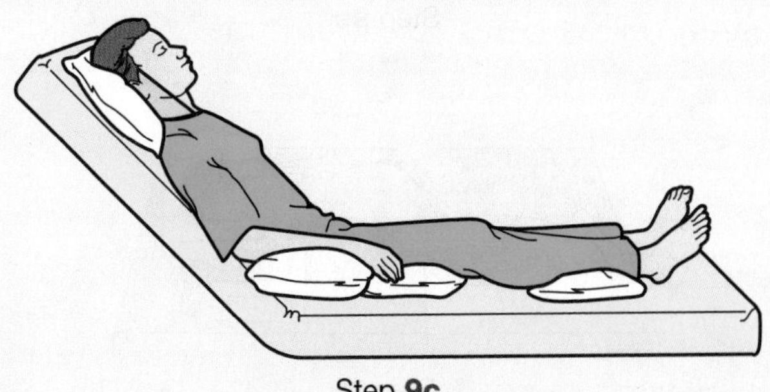

Step **9c**

Continued

Skill 15-1 Positioning Patients—cont'd

(3) Replace pillow. *(Provides patient comfort.)* See suggestions in Step 9c for positioning of pillows.

e. **Orthopneic** position (the posture assumed by the patient sitting up in bed at 90-degree angle, or sometimes resting in forward tilt while supported by pillow on overbed table) (see illustration). Often used for the patient with a cardiac or respiratory condition.

(1) Elevate head of bed to 90 degrees. *(Facilitates positioning.)* Patient will sometimes sit on side of bed with legs dangling or propped on a chair.

(2) Place pillow between patient's back and mattress. *(Provides back support.)*

(3) Place pillow on overbed table and assist patient to lean over, placing head on pillow. *(Facilitates ease of breathing. Women are more comfortable with arms on pillow and head on arms.)*

f. **Sims'** position (position in which patient lies on side with knee and thigh drawn upward toward chest) (see illustration). The left Sims' position is appropriate positioning for the enema procedure and administering a rectal suppository.

(1) Place patient in supine position. *(Prepares patient for position.)*

(2) Position patient in lateral position, lying partially on the abdomen. *(Patient is rolled only partially on abdomen.)*

(3) Draw knee and thigh up near abdomen and support with pillows. *(Positions patient appropriately.)*

(4) Place patient's lower arm along the back. *(Provides appropriate body alignment.)*

(5) Bring upper arm up, flex elbow, and support with pillow. *(Provides comfort and decreases strain on joints.)*

(6) Allow patient to lean forward to rest on chest. *(Provides maximum comfort.)*

g. **Prone** position (lying face down in horizontal position) (see illustration).

(1) Assist patient onto abdomen with face to one side. *(Facilitates positioning.)*

(2) Flex arms toward the head. *(Provides appropriate body alignment.)*

(3) Position pillows for comfort. Place a pillow under lower leg to release any "pull" on the lower back, or place a pillow under the head as shown (or both). *(Increases comfort and maintains proper body alignment.)*

h. Knee-chest **(genupectoral)** position; patient kneels so that weight of body is supported by knees and chest, with abdomen raised, head turned to one side, and arms flexed (see illustration).

(1) Turn patient onto abdomen. *(Facilitates positioning.)*

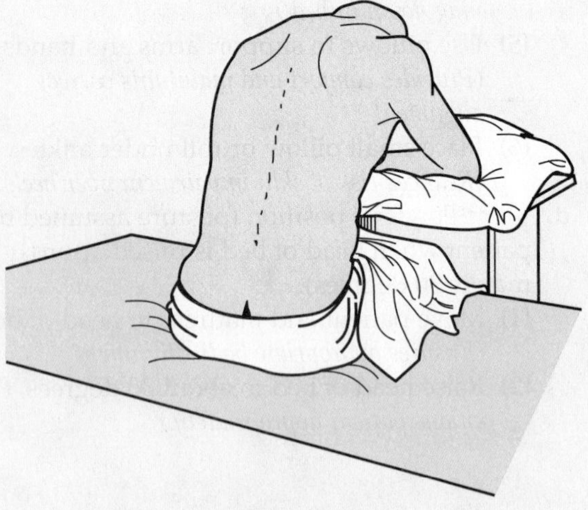

Step **9e**

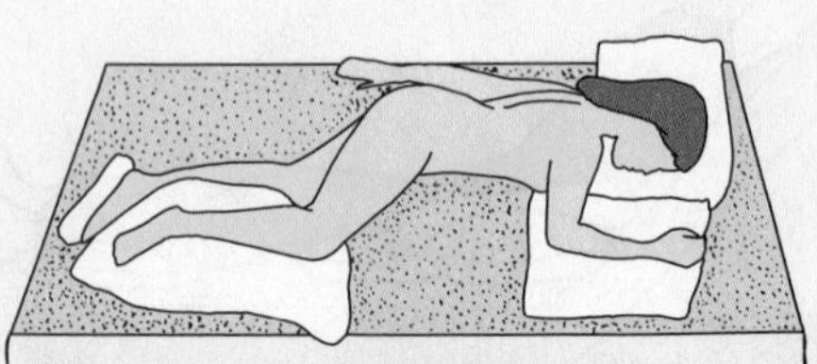

Step **9f**

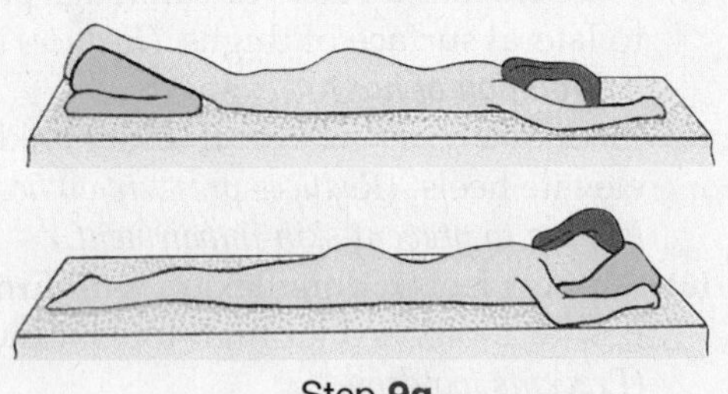

Step **9g**

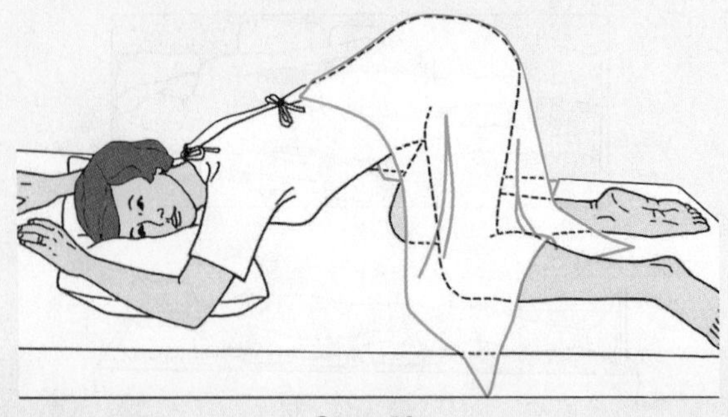

Step **9h**

(2) Assist patient into kneeling position; arms and head will rest on pillow while upper chest rests on bed. *(Allows for as much comfort as possible in this position.)*

i. **Lithotomy** position; patient lies supine with hips and knees flexed and thighs abducted and rotated externally (sometimes feet are positioned in stirrups) (see illustration).

(1) Position patient to lie supine (lying on the back). *(Facilitates positioning.)*

(2) Request patient to slide buttocks to edge of examining table. *(Facilitates positioning.)*

(3) Lift both legs; have patient bend knees and place feet in stirrups. *(Positions patient appropriately.)*

(4) Drape patient. *(Provides privacy.)*

(5) Provide small lumbar pillow if desired. *(Provides comfort. Pillow under head also provides comfort.)*

j. **Trendelenburg** position (patient's head is low and the body and legs are on inclined plane) (see illustration). This is no longer widely used.

(1) Place patient's head lower than body with body and legs elevated and on an incline. Foot of bed is sometimes elevated on blocks. (Not used if patient has a head injury.) Trendelenburg position is not usually used to treat shock because of pressure it causes on diaphragm by organs in the abdomen.

k. Lateral position (see Chapter 18).

10. Assess patient for the following: *(Provides follow-up with appropriate nursing interventions.)*
    - Proper body alignment. Small children often need to be propped with pillows to help them maintain a position.
    - Comfort. Performing a back massage after turning from one position to another helps prevent impaired skin integrity.
    - Skin integrity. Skin of older adults is often thin and nonelastic and needs special care to prevent tearing and further impaired skin integrity.
    - Breathing. Additional support is necessary in some positions if patient finds it difficult to maintain ease of respiratory effort.
    - Tolerance of position. Provides ongoing observations regarding patient's activity tolerance and indicates complications of immobility.
    - Repositioning. Reposition debilitated, unconscious, or paralyzed patients at least every 2 hours.

11. Perform hand hygiene. *(Reduces spread of microorganisms.)*

12. Document. *(Records procedure, patient's response, and effectiveness of nursing interventions.)*
    - Procedure
    - Observations (e.g., skin condition, joint movement, patient's ability to assist with positioning)
    - Patient teaching (see Patient Teaching and Home Care Considerations boxes).

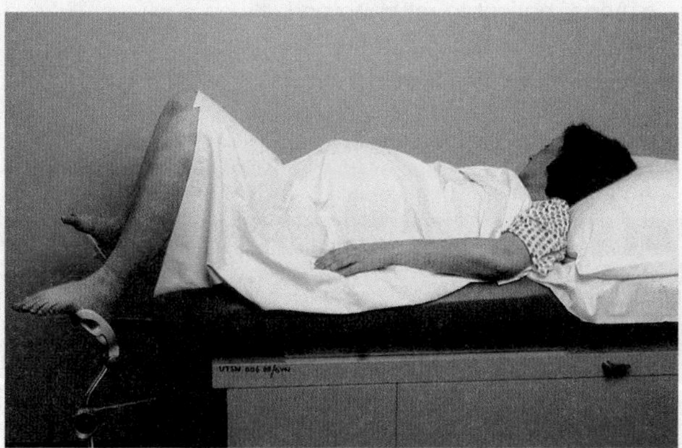

Step 9i

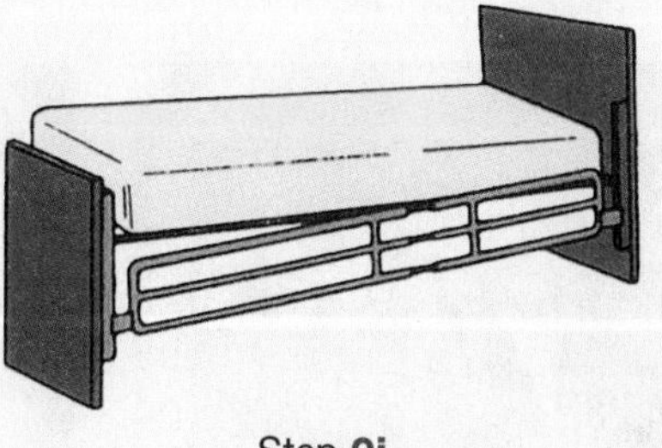

Step 9j

MOBILITY VERSUS IMMOBILITY

Mobility is a person's ability to move around freely in his or her environment. Moving about serves many purposes, including expressing emotion, self-defense, attaining basic needs, performing recreational activities, and completing activities of daily living (ADLs), those activities of physical self-care such as bathing, dressing, and eating. In addition, mobility is fundamental to maintaining the body's normal physiologic activities. To maintain normal physical mobility, it is necessary for the body's nervous, muscular, and skeletal systems to be intact, functioning, and used regularly. Although we all welcome a rare day to lie in bed and rest, the person who is **immobile** (experiencing **immobility**, the inability to move around freely) is predisposed to developing a wide variety of complications (Box 15-2).

Many types of health problems potentially lead to a decline in a patient's mobility. Patients with certain illnesses, injuries, or surgeries will sometimes experience a period of immobilization as a result of changes

Box 15-2 Complications of Immobility and Preventive Measures

COMPLICATIONS

- Muscle and bone atrophy
- Contractures
- Pressure ulcer
- Constipation
- Urinary tract infection
- Disuse osteoporosis—fractures occur easily
- Renal calculi (kidney stones)
- Hypostatic pneumonia
- Pulmonary embolism
- Postural hypotension
- Anorexia
- Insomnia
- Asthenia (muscular weakness)
- Disorientation
- Thrombophlebitis (blood clot with accompanying inflammation of the involved vein, usually of the lower extremity)

INTERVENTIONS

- Reposition at least every 2 hours
- Ensure adequate intake—encourage fluids
- Encourage a well-balanced diet
- Prevent deformities (e.g., footboard or other measures to prevent footdrop)
- Handle and transfer patients carefully; maintain proper body alignment
- Position lower extremities properly (a pillow or wedge between the legs, never under knees)
- Early ambulation
- Antiembolism measures (thromboembolic deterrent [TED] hose or decompression boots)
- Progressive ambulation
  —Roll up head of bed
  —Dangle over side of bed
  —Stand
  —Take a few steps
  —Sit in the chair
  —Up to bathroom
  —Up and about the room
  —Up and out in the hallway
  —Up as desired

DURING AMBULATION

1. Observe the patient closely
2. Encourage the patient to do the following:
   - Take slow, deep breaths
   - Keep eyes open and look straight ahead
   - Keep head up

   (These measures will aid in preventing vertigo, syncope, weakness, and nausea and vomiting.)
3. If the patient starts to fall, do not attempt to prevent the fall. Ease the patient to the floor. This allows you to break the fall, control its direction, and also protect the patient's head. Follow these steps when assisting a patient's fall:
   - Stand with your feet apart. Keep your back straight.
   - Bring the patient close to your body as quickly as possible. Use the gait belt if one is worn. If not, wrap your arms around the patient's waist. Move your leg so the patient's buttocks rest on it. Move the leg near the patient (see illustration).
   - Lower the patient to the floor by letting the patient slide down your leg. Bend at your hips and knees as you lower the patient (see illustration). *(The gravitational pull will enable the patient to be lowered to the floor with a minimal amount of strain to your musculoskeletal system.)*
   - Call for assistance.
   - Assist patient to return to bed.
   - Report and document the following:
     —How the fall occurred
     —How far the patient walked
     —How activity was tolerated before the fall

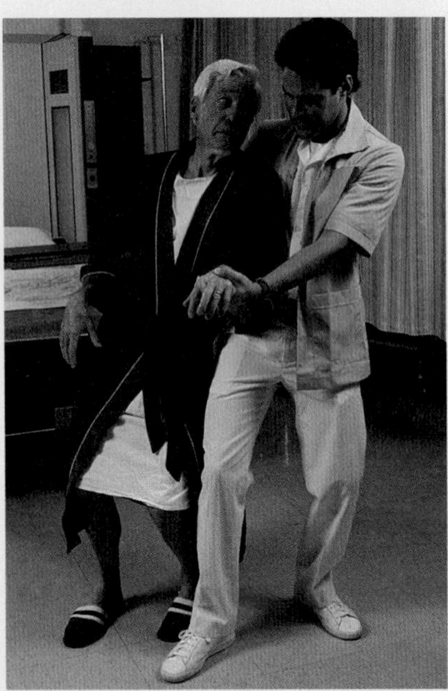

May support the falling patient under the arms as shown.

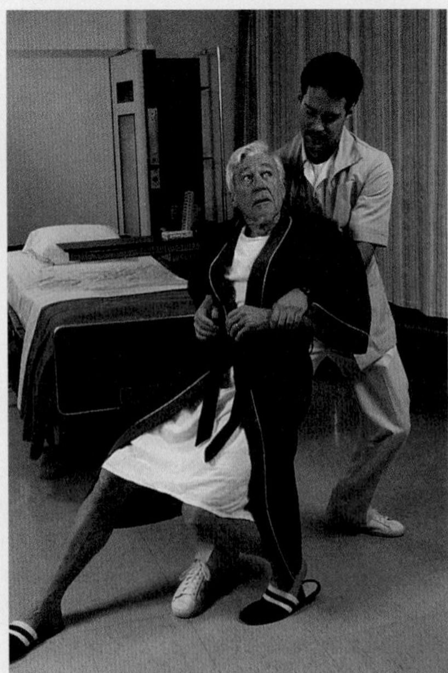

The patient's buttocks rest on your leg.

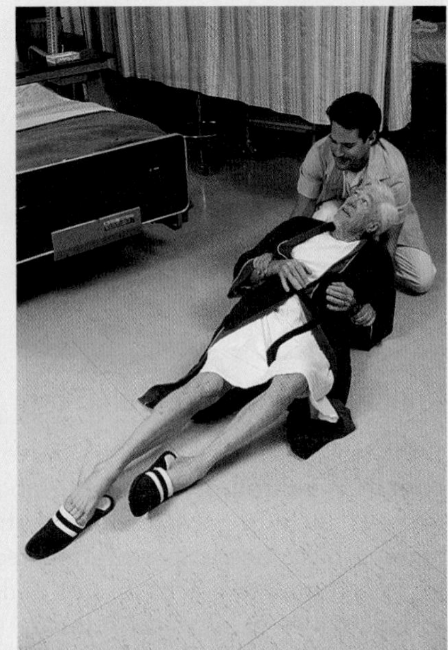

Slide the patient down your leg to the floor.

Box 15-2 Complications of Immobility and Preventive Measures—cont'd

—Any complaints before the fall
—The amount of assistance needed by the patient while walking
- Complete an incident report, if required. *(Know agency policy.)*

4. On a daily basis encourage the following:
   - Deep breathing and coughing exercises (spirometry)
   - Careful use of medications
5. Be certain to provide the following:
   - Suitable diversion
   - Meticulous skin care
   - Range-of-motion exercises
   - Reality therapy

Table 15-2 Assistive Devices for Proper Positioning

DEVICE	REASON FOR USE
Pillow	Provides support of body or extremity; elevates body part; splints incisional area to reduce postoperative pain during activity or coughing and deep breathing
Foot boots	Maintains feet in dorsiflexion
Trochanter roll (see Figure 15-3)	Prevents external rotation of legs when patient is in supine position; possible to make with a bath blanket
Sandbag	Provides support and shape to body contours; immobilizes extremity; maintains specific body alignment
Hand roll (see Figure 15-4)	Maintains thumb slightly adducted and in opposition to fingers; maintains fingers in slightly flexed position
Hand-wrist splint	Individually molded for patient to maintain proper alignment of thumb; slightly adducted in opposition to fingers; maintains wrist in slight dorsiflexion
Trapeze bar (see Figure 15-5)	Enables patient to raise trunk from bed; enables patient to transfer from bed to wheelchair; allows patient to perform exercises that strengthen upper arms
Side rail	Helps weak patient to roll from side to side or to sit up in bed
Bed board	Provides additional support to mattress and improves vertebral alignment
Wedge pillow	Also called *abductor pillow* (triangular pillow made of heavy foam); used to maintain the legs in abduction following total hip replacement surgery

Modified from Potter, P.A., & Perry, A.G. (2007). *Basic nursing: essentials for practice.* (6th ed.). St. Louis: Mosby.

in medical and physical status. In some cases, immobilization is also used therapeutically to limit the movement of the whole body or a body part, and some patients will be under ambulation restrictions.

Interventions to prevent complications of immobility are varied, and many do not require a physician's order (see Box 15-2).

There are various assistive devices to use to maintain correct body positioning and to help prevent complications that commonly arise when a patient needs prolonged bed rest (Table 15-2). Several of the devices are especially useful when caring for patients who have a loss of sensation, mobility, or consciousness (Figures 15-3 through 15-5).

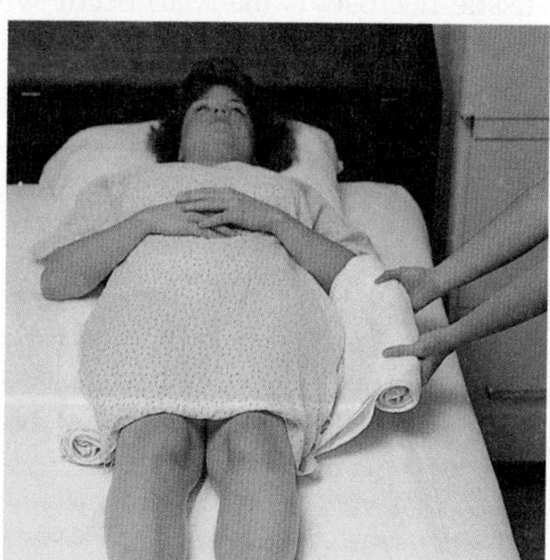

FIGURE 15-3 Trochanter roll.

NEUROVASCULAR FUNCTION

Your major responsibility is frequent monitoring of neurovascular function, or circulation, movement, and sensation (CMS) assessment. Check for skin color, temperature, movement, sensation, pulses, capillary refill, and pain. Always compare the affected limb with the unaffected one (Table 15-3).

This assessment is especially important when compression from external devices, such as casts and bulky dressings, creates the risk of compartment syndrome,

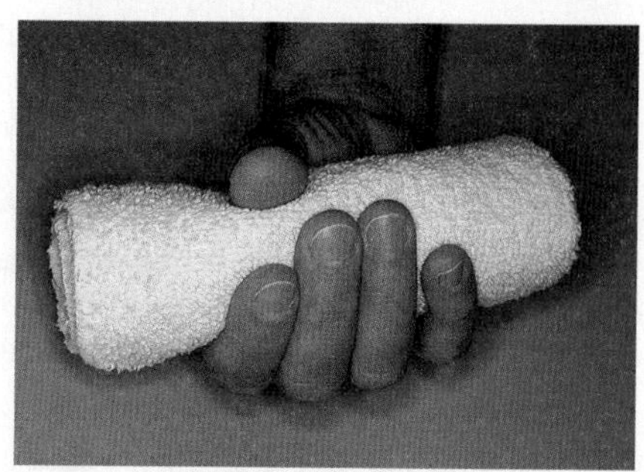

FIGURE 15-4 Hand roll.

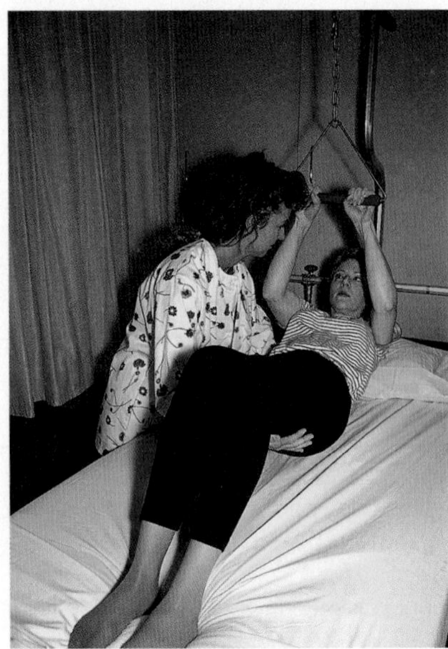

FIGURE 15-5 Patient using a trapeze bar.

which has the potential to cause extensive tissue damage. This phenomenon occurs in the extremities, especially the legs, where a sheath of inelastic fascia partitions blood vessel, nerve, and muscle tissue. Normally, the pressure in this compartment is less than capillary pressure. However, compression created by external pressure or the accumulation of excessive tissue fluid from severe burns, insect bites, or infiltration of intravenous fluids will increase compartmental pressure and in some cases lead to compartment syndrome. Ischemic tissue necrosis is likely to occur within 4 to 8 hours unless this pressure is relieved and compartment syndrome reversed.

Increased pain on passive motion when compared with active motion, or loss of sensation in the web space between the great and second toes (or between the thumb and the second finger), indicates the early stage of compartment syndrome. When the patient is in late-stage compartment syndrome and damage is not reversible, the patient will typically demonstrate signs referred to as the *six Ps*:

- Pain, not relieved
- Paresthesias
- Pallor
- Pulse absent (pulselessness)
- Paralysis
- Palpated tense tissue

Do not wait until these signs and symptoms are present. The earlier compartment syndrome is treated, the better the prognosis is. Compartment syndrome sometimes necessitates amputation of the limb when the neurovascular compromise is not promptly assessed and managed. Notify the physician immediately of signs of compartment syndrome.

PERFORMING RANGE-OF-MOTION EXERCISES

Regardless of whether the causes of immobility are permanent or temporary, the immobilized patient needs some type of exercise to prevent excessive muscle atrophy and joint contracture. You and allied staff, or members of the physical therapy department, will help the patient confined to bed for long periods to

Table 15-3 Assessing Neurovascular Status

CHARACTERISTIC	ASSESSMENT TECHNIQUE	NORMAL FINDINGS
Skin color	Inspect the area distal to the injury.	No change in pigmentation compared with other parts of the body
Skin temperature	Palpate the area distal to the injury (the dorsum of the hands is most sensitive to temperature).	The skin is warm
Movement	Ask the patient to move the affected area or the area distal to the injury (active motion).	The patient is able to move without discomfort
	Move the area distal to the injury (passive motion).	No difference in comfort compared with active movement
Sensation	Ask the patient if numbness or tingling is present (paresthesia).	No numbness or tingling; no difference in sensation in the affected and unaffected extremities
	Palpate with a safety pin or paper clip, especially the web space between the first and second toes or the web space between the thumb and the forefinger.	Loss of sensation in these areas indicates peroneal nerve or median nerve damage
Pulses	Palpate the pulses distal to the injury.	Pulses are strong and easily palpated; no difference in the affected and unaffected extremities
Capillary refill	Press the nail beds distal to the injury until blanching occurs (or until the skin near the nail blanches, if nails are thick and brittle).	Blood returns (return to usual color) within 3 seconds (5 seconds for older adult patients)
Pain	Ask the patient about the location, the nature, and the frequency of pain.	Pain is usually localized and is often described as stabbing or throbbing

From Ignatavicius, D.D., & Workman, M.L. (Eds.). (2006). *Medical-surgical nursing: critical thinking for collaborative care.* (6th ed.). Philadelphia: Saunders.

perform range-of-motion (ROM) (any body action involving the muscles and joints in natural directional movements) exercises. **Passive** ROM exercise is performed by caregivers and **active** ROM by patients. You will move, or assist the patient to move, the designated joint (any one of the connections between bones) to the point of resistance or pain, using care to avoid injury. Gradually increase the ROM with subsequent exercises as tolerated (Table 15-4, Skill 15-2).

Some patients who are weak or partially paralyzed will be able to move a limb partially through ROM. Then you will help the patient finish the full ROM. This is referred to as **passive assisted** ROM. Another form of ROM exercise is referred to as **active assisted** ROM, in which the patient uses the strong arm to exercise the weaker or paralyzed arm. Always encourage the patient to be as independent as possible.

Assess patients for their level of mobility. The patient who is able to move about freely will independently perform ADLs and active ROM exercises. If the patient is partially immobile and unable to move about freely (paraplegic, quadriplegic), you or allied staff will use a mechanical device to assist the patient with passive ROM exercises.

Encourage and assess active ROM every day (see Life Span Considerations for Older Adults box on p. 382). The total amount of activity required to prevent physical disuse syndrome (a state in which an individual is at risk for deterioration of body systems as the result of prescribed or unavoidable inactivity) is

Text continued on p. 382

Table 15-4 Joint Range-of-Motion Exercises

BODY PART	TYPE OF JOINT	TYPE OF MOVEMENT
Neck and cervical spine	Pivotal	**Flexion:**[1] bring chin to rest on chest. **Extension:**[2] return head to erect position. **Hyperextension:**[3] bend head back as far as possible. Use caution with older adults.
		Lateral flexion: tilt head as far as possible toward each shoulder.
		Rotation: turn head as far as possible to right and left.
Shoulder	Ball and socket	Flexion: raise arm from side position forward to position above head. Extension: return arm to position at side of body. Hyperextension: move arm behind body, keeping elbow straight.
Shoulder—cont'd	Ball and socket—cont'd	**Abduction:**[4] raise arm to side to position above head with palm away from head. **Adduction:**[5] lower arm sideways and across body as far as possible.
		Internal rotation: with elbow flexed, rotate shoulder by moving arm until thumb is turned inward and toward back. External rotation: with elbow flexed, move arm until thumb is upward and lateral to head.
		Circumduction: move arm in full circle. (Circumduction is combination of all movements of ball-and-socket joint.)

Modified from Potter, P.A., & Perry, A.G. (2007). *Basic nursing: essentials for practice.* (6th ed.). St. Louis: Mosby.

[1]*Flexion:* movement of certain joints that decreases angle between two adjoining bones.

[2]*Extension:* movement of certain joints that increases angle between two adjoining bones.

[3]*Hyperextension:* extreme or abnormal extension.

[4]*Abduction:* movement of limb away from body.

[5]*Adduction:* movement of limb toward axis of body.

Continued

Table 15-4 Joint Range-of-Motion Exercises—cont'd

BODY PART	TYPE OF JOINT	TYPE OF MOVEMENT
Elbow	Hinge 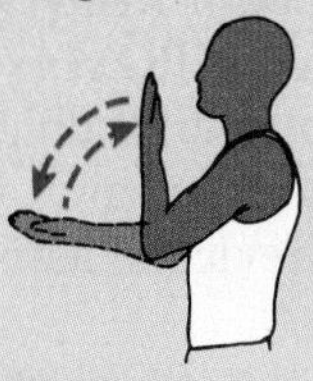	Flexion: bend elbow so that lower arm moves toward its shoulder joint and hand is level with shoulder. Extension: straighten elbow by lowering hand. Hyperextension: bend lower arm back as far as possible.
Forearm	Pivotal 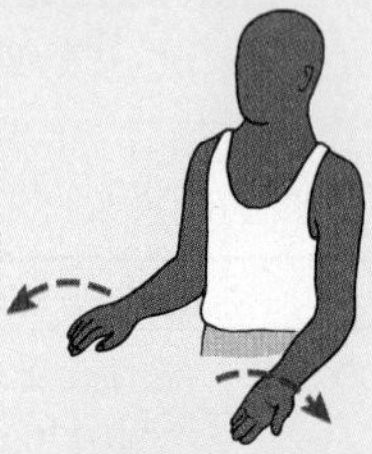	**Supination:**[6] turn lower arm and hand so that palm is up. **Pronation:**[7] turn lower arm so that palm is down.
Wrist	Condyloid 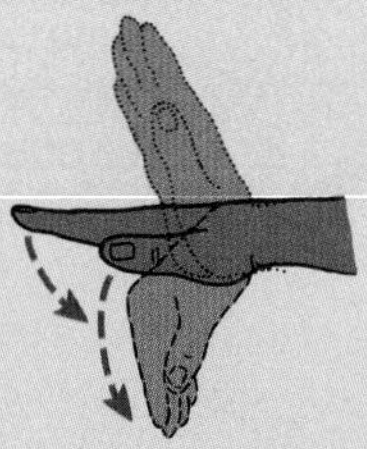	Flexion: move palm toward inner aspect of forearm. Extension: move fingers so that fingers, hands, and forearm are in same plane, in a straight line. Hyperextension: bring dorsal surface of hand back as far as possible.
	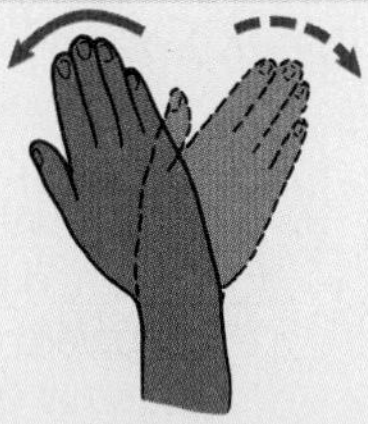	Radial flexion: bend wrist medially toward thumb. Ulnar flexion: bend wrist laterally toward fifth finger.
Fingers	Condyloid hinge 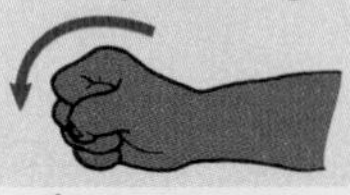	Flexion: make fist. Extension: straighten fingers.
	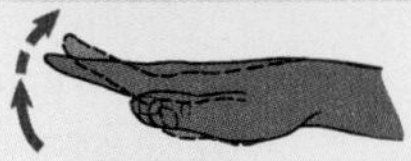	Hyperextension: bend fingers back as far as possible.
	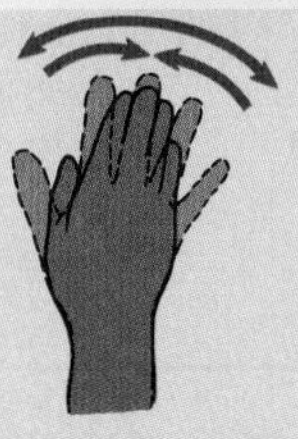	Abduction: spread fingers apart. Adduction: bring fingers together.
Thumb	Saddle 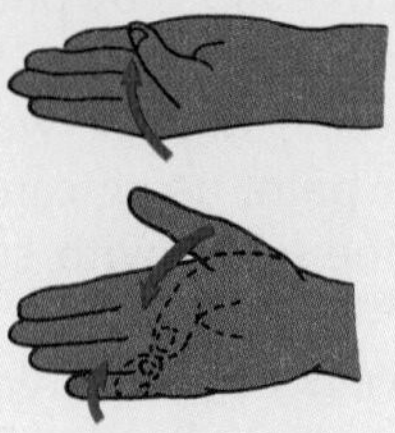	Flexion: move thumb across palmar surface of hand. Extension: move thumb straight away from hand. Abduction: extend thumb laterally (usually done when placing fingers in abduction and adduction). Adduction: move thumb back toward hand. Opposition: touch thumb to each finger of same hand.
Hip	Ball and socket 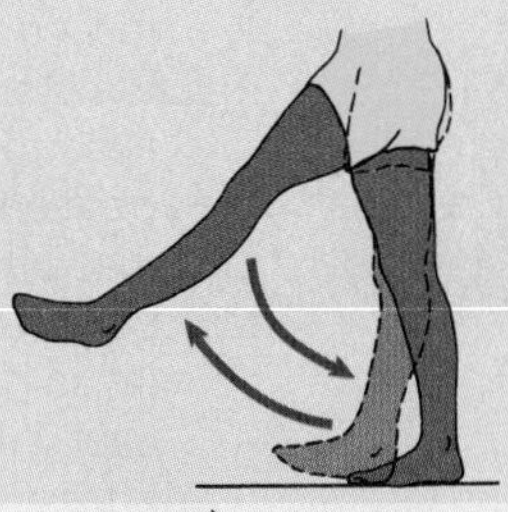	Flexion: move leg forward and up with knee in extension. Extension: move leg back beside other leg while knee joint remains in extension.
	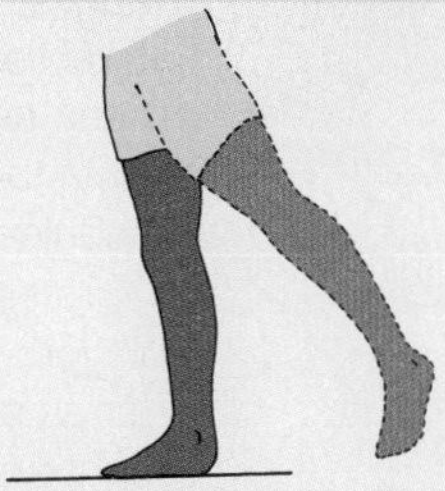	Hyperextension: move leg behind body.
	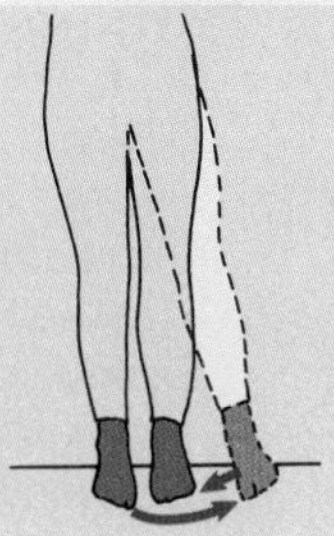	Abduction: move leg laterally away from body. Adduction: move leg back toward medial position and beyond if possible.
	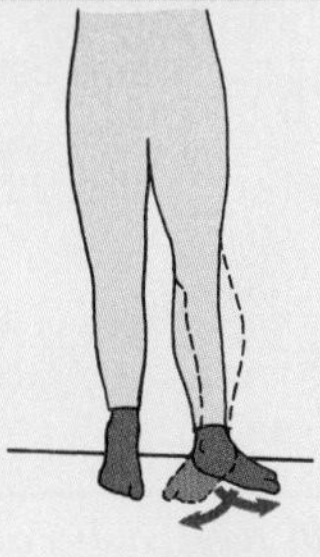	Internal rotation: turn foot and leg toward other leg. External rotation: turn foot and leg away from other leg.

[6]*Supination:* kind of rotation that allows palm of hand to turn up.
[7]*Pronation:* palm of hand turned down.

Table 15-4 Joint Range-of-Motion Exercises—cont'd

BODY PART	TYPE OF JOINT	TYPE OF MOVEMENT	BODY PART	TYPE OF JOINT	TYPE OF MOVEMENT
Hip—cont'd	Ball and socket—cont'd	Circumduction: move leg in circle.	Foot	Gliding	Inversion: turn sole of foot medially. Eversion: turn sole of foot laterally.
Knee	Hinge	Flexion: bring heel back toward back of thigh. Extension: return heel to floor.	Toes	Condyloid hinge	Flexion: curl toes downward. Extension: straighten toes.
Ankle	Hinge	**Dorsiflexion:**[8] move foot so that toes are pointed upward. Plantar flexion: move foot so that toes are pointed downward.			Abduction: spread toes apart. Adduction: bring toes together.

[8]*Dorsiflexion:* to bend or flex backward.

Skill 15-2 Performing Range-of-Motion Exercises

Nursing Action *(Rationale)*

1. Refer to medical record, care plan, or Kardex for special interventions. *(Provides basis for care.)*
2. Assemble equipment. *(Organizes procedure.)*
   - Clean gloves, if necessary (see step 6)
3. Introduce self. *(Decreases patient's anxiety.)*
4. Identify patient. *(Ensures procedure is performed with correct patient.)*
5. Explain procedure. *(Enlists cooperation and decreases patient's anxiety.)*
6. Perform hand hygiene and don clean gloves according to agency policy and guidelines from CDC and OSHA. *(Reduces spread of microorganisms.)*
7. Prepare patient for intervention:
   a. Close door to room or pull curtain. *(Provides privacy.)*
   b. Drape for procedure if appropriate. *(Prevents unnecessary exposure of patient.)*
   c. Raise bed to comfortable working level. *(Promotes good body mechanics in the nurse and safety for the patient.)*
   d. Assist patient to a comfortable position, either sitting or lying down. *(Ensures patient's comfort.)*
   e. Medicate patient as needed. *(Promotes patient comfort.)*
8. Support the body part above (proximal to) and below (distal to) the joint by cradling the extremity or by using cupped hand to support the joint being exercised (see illustration). *(Protects the weaker joints and muscles.)*
9. Begin by doing exercises in normal sequence (see Table 15-4. Repeat each full sequence 5 times during the exercise period. *(It is easiest to perform exercises in head-to-toe manner.)* Discontinue exercise if patient complains of pain or if there is resistance or muscle spasm.

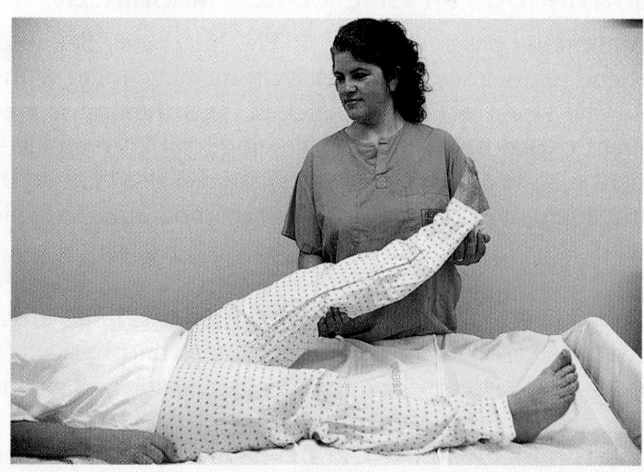

Step 8

Continued

Skill 15-2 Performing Range-of-Motion Exercises—cont'd

10. Assist patient by putting each joint through full range of motion (see Table 15-4). *(Provides baseline for joint movement.)*
11. Position patient for comfort. To prevent contracture (an abnormal shortening of a muscle), do not allow patients with joint pain to remain continuously in position of comfort; it is necessary to exercise joints routinely. *(Immobility contributes to contractures.)* Periodically provide back massage. *(Provides comfort.)*
12. Adjust bed linen. *(Provides comfort and privacy.)*
13. Remove and dispose of gloves and wash hands. *(Reduces spread of microorganisms.)*
14. Document the following: *(Records procedure and patient's response.)*
    - Joints exercised
    - Presence of edema or pressure areas
    - Any discomfort resulting from the exercises
    - Any limitations of ROM
    - Patient's tolerance of the exercises
    - Patient teaching (see Patient Teaching box on p. 372 and Home Care Considerations box on p. 391)

Life Span Considerations

Older Adults

Range-of-Motion Exercises

- Some older adults who have chronic illnesses will need you to break range-of-motion (ROM) exercises into two or more sessions to control fatigue.
- Inadequate intake of calcium or exposure to sunlight increases older adults' risk of bone loss and increases the need for ROM and weight-bearing exercise.
- Older people who fear falling often display reluctance to move from bed to chair. Encouragement, reassurance, and assistance from family members and caregivers decrease anxiety.
- Older adult patients who are depressed often prefer to stay in bed, especially when they were accustomed to being very independent and active and are now needing assistance.
- Many older adults with arthritis require additional time in the morning before resuming activities.
- Even without arthritis, older adults often need more time in the morning to resume activity.

only about 2 hours for every 24-hour period. Schedule this activity throughout the day to prevent the patient from remaining inactive for long periods.

CONTINUOUS PASSIVE MOTION MACHINES

Continuous passive motion (CPM) machines flex and extend joints in order to passively mobilize them without the strain of active exercises. This therapy is frequently used immediately following total knee replacement surgery (knee arthroplasty) but can also be used in outpatient or home physical therapy programs. The initial postoperative setting for a knee arthroplasty is usually 2 cycles per minute, with between 20 and 30 degrees of flexion and full extension. However, it is imperative that the CPM machine be set according to the physician's orders for the degree and the speed of flexion and extension for each individual patient (Elkin et al., 2007).

It is possible to use CPM machines on joints other than the knee, including the hip, the shoulder, and the ankle. Mobilizing the joint prevents complications, such as joint contracture, atrophy of surrounding muscles, and thromboembolism. When using a CPM machine, consider the following (Elkin et al., 2007):

- It will sometimes be necessary for older adults requiring CPM therapy following discharge to enter a rehabilitation facility or have home care, because the equipment is not easy to manipulate.
- Older adults with fragile skin are at a high risk of skin impairment from pressure of the CPM machine. Closely monitor pressure point areas such as the heel.
- Physical therapy is frequently used in addition to the CPM therapy.
- If the patient is using the CPM at home, ensure that the patient and family members assisting with care are given instructions on how to use the CPM machine, prescribed settings, and parameters for contacting the physician.
- The goals of CPM therapy are to increase or maintain physical mobility by improving joint range of motion and to prevent skin breakdown at pressure points.
- It is acceptable to delegate care of the patient during CPM therapy to assistive personnel, but assessment of the patient must not be delegated to assistive personnel. Assessment remains a nursing responsibility.

MOVING THE PATIENT

You will often be required to assist in moving the patient. Moving includes lifting the patient up in bed, to the side of bed, to the tub, and into a car (Skill 15-3), turning and dangling the patient and assisting the patient in and out of the bed for ambulation. Sometimes you will use mechanical equipment for lifting patients, such as the hydraulic lift, roller board, and gurney lift. Remember to lift twice—first mentally and then

Text continued on p. 387

Skill 15-3 Moving the Patient

Nursing Action *(Rationale)*

1. Refer to the medical record, care plan, or Kardex for special interventions. *(Provides basis for care.)*
2. Assemble equipment. *(Organizes procedure.)*
   - Hospital bed
   - Chair
   - Side rails
   - Patient's slippers
   - Cotton blanket
   - Pillows
   - Extra personnel
   - Lifting devices (see Skill 15-4)
3. Introduce self. *(Decreases patient's anxiety.)*
4. Identify patient. *(Ensures procedure is performed with correct patient.)*
5. Explain procedure. *(Enlists cooperation and assistance from patient and decreases patient's anxiety.)*
6. Wash hands. *(Reduces spread of microorganisms.)*
7. Prepare patient for interventions.
   a. Close door or pull curtain. *(Provides privacy.)*
   b. Adjust bed level for safe working height. *(Promotes good body mechanics in the nurse and safety for the patient.)*
   c. Medicate patient as needed. *(Promotes patient comfort.)*
8. Arrange for assistance as necessary. *(Provides for safety.)*
9. Lift and move patient up in bed (sometimes requires one nurse and sometimes more):
   a. Place patient supine with head flat. *(Creates less resistance on flat surface.)*
   b. Face the patient and establish your base of support. *(Protects your back.)*
   c. Place one arm under patient's axilla if at all possible; place opposite arm under shoulder and neck. *(Supports patient.)*
   d. Ask patient to flex knees and push up with flat of feet, not heels, on count of 3 while you assist. *(Protects your back and promotes patient's mobility.)*
   e. If more than one of you are working together, position yourselves on opposite sides of the patient's bed facing each other and support patient's back with one arm each, with the second arm under shoulder and neck. *(Protects nurses and provides patient safety.)*
   f. On count of 3, both of you perform maneuver to move patient up to head of bed. *(Coordinates move.)*
   g. Another way to accomplish this is to use a pull sheet, made with a small sheet folded in half or a bath blanket folded to fit under the patient.
      (1) Roll patient first to one side and then the other, placing pull sheet underneath patient from shoulders to thighs. *(Facilitates the position change.)*
      (2) Flex your knees and face your body in the direction of the move. The foot farthest away from the bed faces forward for broader base of support (see illustration).
      (3) With one nurse on each side of patient, grasp pull sheet firmly with hands near patient's upper arms and hips, rolling the sheet material until your hands are close to the patient. *(The closer you are to the patient, the less you need to raise the patient up to clear the bed during the move.)*
      (4) Instruct patient to rest arms over body and to lift head on the count of 3; at the same time, pull the sheet to move the patient up to head of bed (see illustration).

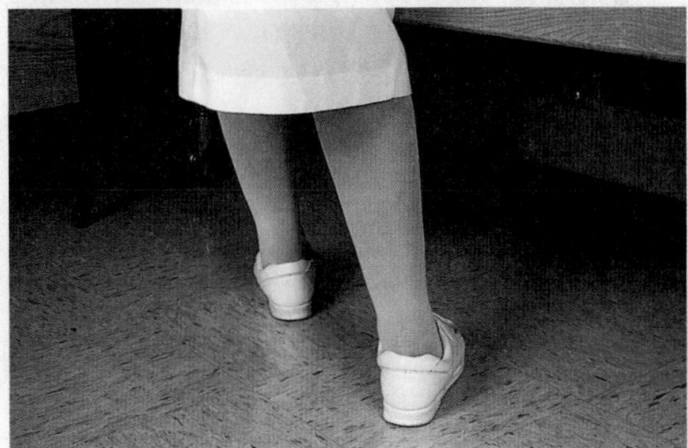

Step **9g(2)**

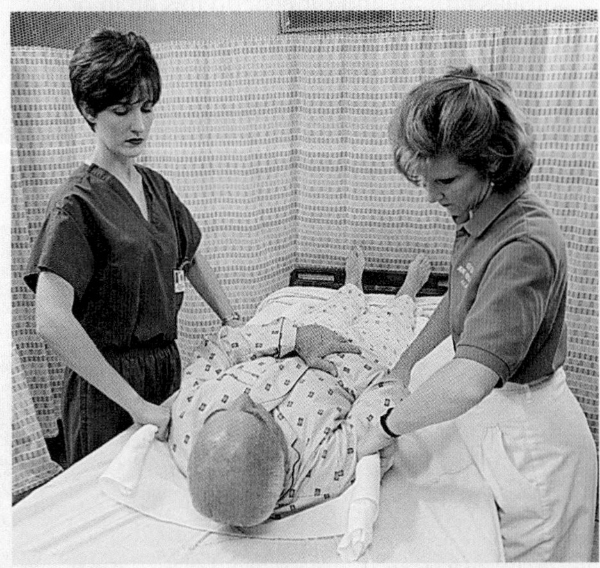

Step **9g(4)** A lift sheet is used to move the patient up in bed. The lift sheet extends from the patient's head to above the knees. The lift sheet is rolled close to the patient and held near the shoulders and buttocks.

Continued

Skill 15-3 Moving the Patient—cont'd

10. Turning the patient:
    a. Stand with your feet slightly apart and flex your knees. *(Provides base of support.)*
    b. Place one arm under patient's neck and shoulders and other arm under waist. *(Provides patient's safety and support.)*
    c. Move patient toward you, bracing your knee on bed for leverage. *(Reduces strain on your back.)*
    d. Turn patient on side facing raised side rail, toward you. *(Prevents patient from falling out of bed.)*
    e. Flex one of patient's legs over the other. Place pad or pillow between legs. *(Reduces pressure on lower leg.)*
    f. Align patient's shoulders; place pillow under head. *(Ensures proper body alignment.)*
    g. Support patient's back with pillows as necessary. A "tuck back" pillow is made by folding pillow lengthwise. Tuck smooth area slightly under patient's back. *(Helps keep patient in position.)*
11. Dangling patient:
    a. Assess pulse and respirations. *(Provides baseline for assessing patient's response to dangling.)*
    b. Move patient to side of bed toward you. *(Makes it easier for patient to sit up. Request patient do by self if possible.)*
    c. Lower bed to lowest position. *(Provides patient safety when getting up.)*
    d. Raise head of bed. *(It is easier for patient to swing around to sitting position.)*
    e. Support patient's shoulders and help to swing legs around and off bed; do this all in one motion by simply pivoting patient. Make sure patient's feet touch floor (see illustration). *(Prevents strain on patient, especially if patient has an incision.)*

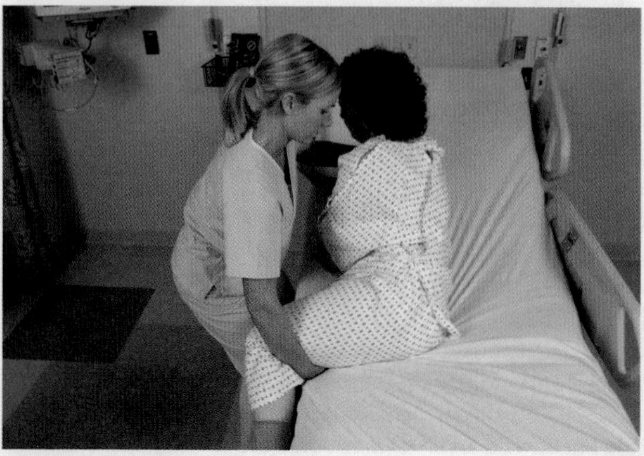

Step **11e**

    f. Another way to accomplish this is by rolling the patient onto his or her side before sitting the patient up. *(Decreases the amount you need to lift, since the patient's body weight actually helps the patient to sit upright.)* Then simply stoop; and as you stand you move and bring the patient along with you. *(This causes less back strain for you, and the patient does not feel pulled on.)*
    g. Help patient don slippers; cover legs. *(Prevents patient from becoming chilled.)* For safety, have patient don slippers while in bed.
    h. Assess patient's pulse and respirations. *(Determines patient's response to procedure.)*
12. Log-rolling the patient (back, neck, or head conditions sometimes necessitate log-rolling following injury or surgery):
    a. Enlist the help of at least one additional person. *(Ensures patient safety.)*
    b. Lower the head of the bed as much as the patient can tolerate. *(Maintains alignment of the spinal column.)*
    c. Place a pillow between the patient's legs. Use of a pull sheet placed between shoulders and knees facilitates turning (see Step 9g[1]). *(Maintains position of the lower extremities.)*
    d. Extend the patient's arm over the patient's head unless shoulder movement is restricted. *(Prevents rolling over it during the turn.)* If shoulder movement is restricted, keep the arm in extension next to the body.
    e. With both nurses on the same side of the bed, one of you places one hand on the patient's shoulder and the other on the hip while the other of you places one hand to support the patient's back and the other behind the knee. If you use a pull sheet, space your hands in such a way to provide even support for the length of the rolled sheet and to distribute weight evenly (see illustrations).
    f. On count of 3, turn the patient with a continuous, smooth, and coordinated effort. *(Maintains body in alignment, preventing stress on any part of the body.)*
    g. Support the patient with pillows as previously discussed (see Step 10g). *(Promotes patient comfort.)*
13. Transferring the patient from bed to straight chair or wheelchair:
    a. Lower bed to lowest position. *(Provides patient safety when getting up.)*
    b. Raise head of bed. *(Makes it easier for patient to swing around to sitting position.)*
    c. Support patient's shoulders and help swing legs around and off bed; perform all in one

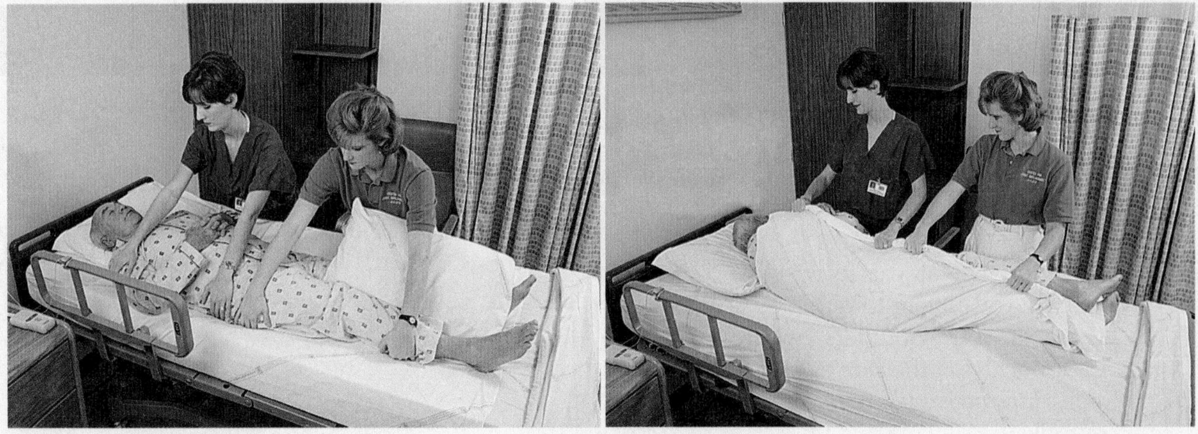

Step **12e**

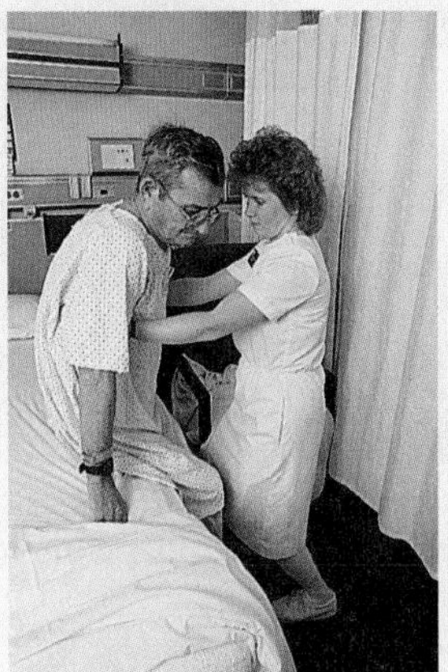

Step **13c**

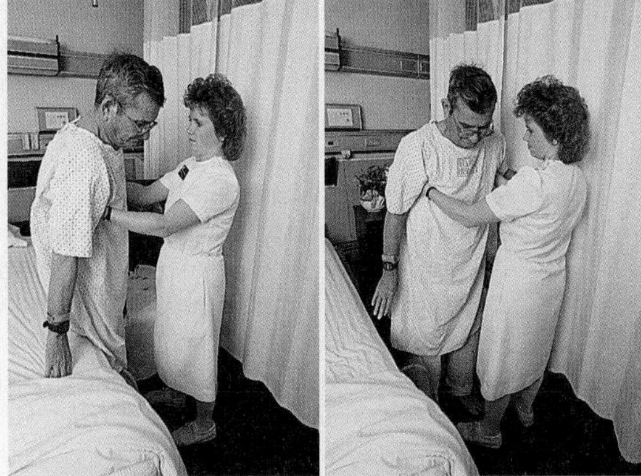

Step **13f**

motion (see illustration). *(Prevents strain on patient, especially if patient has incision.)*

d. Help patient don robe and slippers (or do this before beginning procedure). *(Prevents chilling.)*

e. Have chair positioned beside bed with seat facing foot of bed. *(Provides easy access to chair.)*
   (1) Place wheelchair at right angle to bed and lock wheels after bed is lowered. *(Provides safety.)*
   (2) Place straight chair against wall, or have another nurse hold the chair. *(Provides safety.)*

f. Stand in front of patient and place your hands at patient's waist level or below, and allow patient to use his or her arms and shoulder muscles to push down on the mattress to facilitate the move (see illustrations). *(Prepares the patient for movement to chair.)*

g. Assist patient to stand and swing around with back toward seat of chair. Keep your strong side toward the chair. *(Provides safety.)*

h. Help patient to sit down as you bend your knees to assist process (see illustration). *(Prevents patient from slipping and falling. If patient begins to fall, prevent patient injury by holding patient and allowing patient to sit down gently on floor*; see Box 15-2, step 3.)

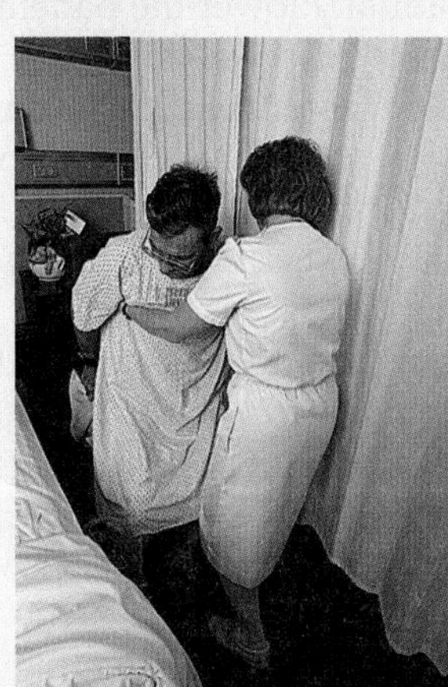

Step **13h**

i. Apply blanket to legs. *(Provides extra warmth.)*

j. If transfer belt is used, apply after patient is sitting on side of bed and follow these guidelines:
   (1) Stand in front of the patient. *(Permits excellent view of patient.)*
   (2) Have the patient hold on to the mattress, or ask the patient to place his or her fists

Continued

Skill 15-3 Moving the Patient—cont'd

on the bed by the thighs. *(Any assistance from the patient minimizes strain on you.)*

(3) Make sure the patient's feet are flat on the floor. *(Provides balance and stability for patient.)*

(4) Have the patient lean forward.

(5) Instruct the patient to place his or her hands on your shoulders, not around your neck or at the side as shown. *(Arms around the neck could result in neck injury to nurse.)*

(6) Grasp the transfer belt at each side. *(Offers stability of patient for the nurse.)*

(7) Brace your knees against the patient's knees. Block the patient's feet with your feet (see illustration). *(Provides safety and prevents patient's foot from slipping.)*

(8) Ask the patient to push down on the mattress and to stand on the count of 3. Pull the patient into a standing position as you straighten your knees (see illustration). *(Provides for less strain on your back.)*

(9) Pivot the patient so he or she is able to grasp the far arm of the chair. Back of the legs will be touching the chair. *(Enables patient to assist in the transfer.)*

(10) Continue to turn the patient until the other arm rest is grasped.

(11) Gradually lower the patient into the chair as you bend your hips and knees. The patient assists if able by leaning forward and bending his or her elbows and knees. *(Encourages patient to assist in transfer and increases muscle strength and a sense of control.)*

(12) Make sure buttocks are to the back of the chair. *(Ensures patient safety.)*

(13) Cover patient's lap and legs. *(Promotes patient's comfort and privacy.)*

14. Transferring from bed to stretcher or gurney back to bed:

a. Position bed flat and raise to the same height as stretcher or gurney. Lower side rails. *(Facilitates procedure.)*

b. Cover patient with top sheet or blanket and remove linens without exposing patient. *(Provides privacy.)*

c. Assess for intravenous (IV) line, Foley catheter, tubes, or surgical drains, and position them to avoid tension during the transfer. *(Prevents accidental tension and possible removal of tubes.)*

d. Position the gurney as close to the bed as possible, and lock the wheels of the bed and

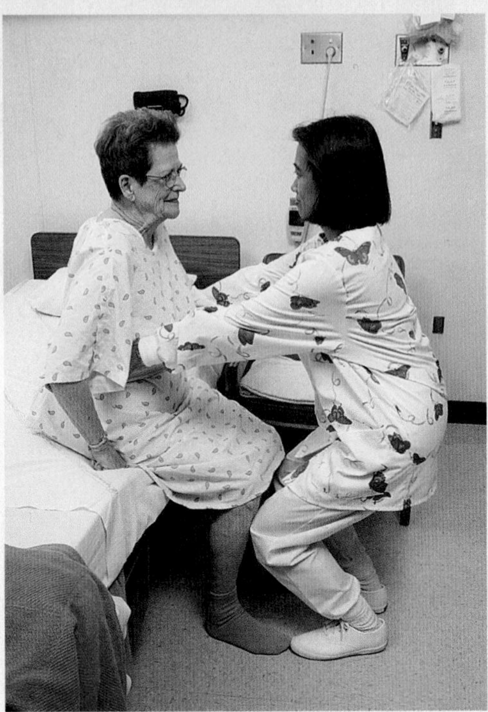

Step 13j(7) Prevent the patient from sliding or falling by bracing the patient's knees and feet with your own knees and feet.

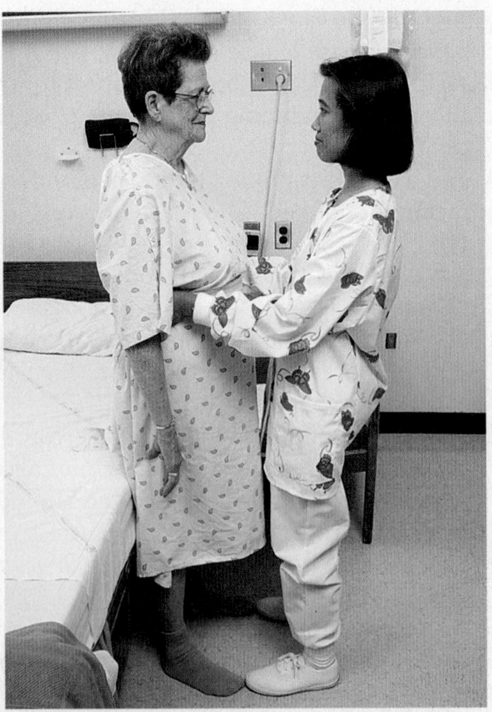

Step 13j(8) The patient is pulled up to a standing position and supported by holding the transfer belt and blocking the patient's knees and feet.

gurney (with side rails lowered). *(Ensures patient's safety.)*

e. When patient is able to assist, stand near side of gurney and instruct patient to move feet, then buttocks, and finally upper body to the gurney, bringing blanket along. Be certain patient's body is centered on the gurney. *(Promotes safety and security.)*

f. When patient is unable to assist, place a folded sheet or bath blanket under the patient so that it supports patient's head and extends to midthighs. Roll the sheet or bath blanket close to the patient's body. Assist patient to cross arms over chest. Two nurses reach over the bed to patient and two more nurses stand as close to the gurney as possible. A fifth nurse stands at the foot to transfer the feet (see illustration). Using a coordinating count of 3, all five nurses lift the patient to the edge of the bed. With another effort, lift the patient from edge of bed to gurney (see illustration). Roller devices are available in some facilities to facilitate this transfer.

15. Perform hand hygiene. *(Reduces spread of microorganisms.)*

16. Assess patient for appropriate body alignment after move. When repositioning, always assess previously dependent skin surfaces (pressure areas). Position pillows for comfort. Do not overtire patient during ambulation. As in all transfers, make certain call device is in easy reach. *(Evaluates, determines, and promotes patient safety and comfort.)*

17. Document procedure. *(Notes procedure and patient's response.)*
    - Patient's response
    - Expected and unexpected outcomes
    - Patient teaching (see Patient Teaching box on p. 372 and Home Care Considerations box on p. 391)

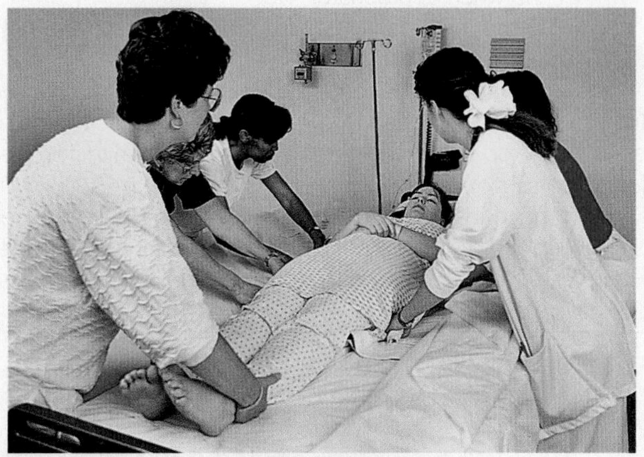

Step **14f**

physically—to be certain you have sufficient assistance. Sometimes providing assistance will make the patient more dependent and less inclined to move on to self-care. Assess the patient's ability to assist with moving. Patients are often reluctant to move if it will cause more pain for them. Administer medication to the patient before activities that you anticipate will fall in this category (Box 15-3 and Coordinated Care box).

Box 15-3 Long-Term Care Considerations for Mobility

- Patients who have maintained bed rest for a long time sometimes revert back to a favorite position. Frequently assess these patients, and turn more often as needed.
- Use lift (draw) sheet as often as possible to prevent placing shearing force on fragile skin.
- Allow patient to assist with moving and positioning whenever possible to promote independence.
- Perform safety and maintenance checks of ambulation devices on a routine basis.
- Perform periodic assessments to ensure that the patient is using ambulation device properly.
- Consult physical therapist for additional assistance or exercises and to ascertain patient's response to exercise program.
- Group activities (e.g., simple games, walking, tossing a ball in a large circle) are useful in maintaining ROM.

USING THE LIFT FOR MOVING PATIENTS

Mechanical devices, such as the hydraulic lift used with a Hoyer sling (Figure 15-6), are useful for moving patients safely, protecting the nurse's back, and full-weight lifting of patients who cannot assist. Follow agency policy for use of the lift (Skill 15-4).

NURSING PROCESS *for Patient Mobility*

The role of the licensed practical nurse/licensed vocational nurse (LPN/LVN) in the nursing process as stated is that the LPN/LVN will:

- Participate in planning care for patients based on patient needs
- Review patient's plan of care and recommend revisions as needed
- Review and follow defined prioritization for patient care
- Use clinical pathways, care maps, or care plans to guide and review patient care

Assessment

Assessment focuses on ROM, muscle strength, activity tolerance, gait, and posture. Observation during ADLs enables you to estimate the patient's fatigability, muscle strength, and ROM. Further assessment helps determine the type of assistance the patient re-

Delegation

MOBILITY

The following information is needed when delegating the skill of position changes to minimize orthostatic hypotension to assistive personnel (AP):

- Have patient wear shoes with a nonslip surface during transfer or ambulation.
- Make slow, gradual position changes.
- Help patient sit in chair or return to bed if patient has symptoms of orthostatic hypotension.
- When assisting with ambulation:
  —Do not try to hold patients if they become dizzy or faint. Ease them into a sitting position in a chair or onto the floor.
  —Use assistive devices such as walkers, crutches, or cane when appropriate.
  —Be sure the area is free of clutter, wet areas, and rugs that may slide.

It is acceptable to delegate the skills of safe and effective transfer from bed to chair to AP who have successfully demonstrated good body mechanics and safe transfer techniques for patients involved.

Teaching patients how to use assistive devices requires critical thinking and knowledge application unique to a nurse. However, AP are able to assist ambulatory patients with assistive devices.

- Have patient wear shoes with a nonskid surface during ambulation.
- Be sure the area is free of clutter, wet areas, and rugs that may slide or buckle.
- Make sure AP know how to use an IV pole to assist in ambulation for patients with continuous IV therapy.
- Make sure patient uses the correct gait and weight bearing during ambulation.
- Ease patient to a sitting position in a chair or on the floor if he or she becomes dizzy or faint.
- Alert the nurse if patient becomes dizzy or lightheaded or suffers a fall.

It is acceptable to delegate the skill of performing ROM exercises to AP. Patients with spinal cord or orthopedic trauma or surgery usually require exercise by nurses or physical therapists. When delegating this skill, instruct AP to perform exercises slowly and provide adequate support to the joint being exercised. In addition, remind AP not to exercise joints beyond the point of resistance or to the point of fatigue or pain. In addition, if muscle spasms occur, stop exercise until the spasms have subsided.

It is acceptable to delegate the skill of safe and effective transfer using a Hoyer lift to AP who have demonstrated ability to use good body mechanics and safe transfer techniques, as well as equipment (Hoyer lift).

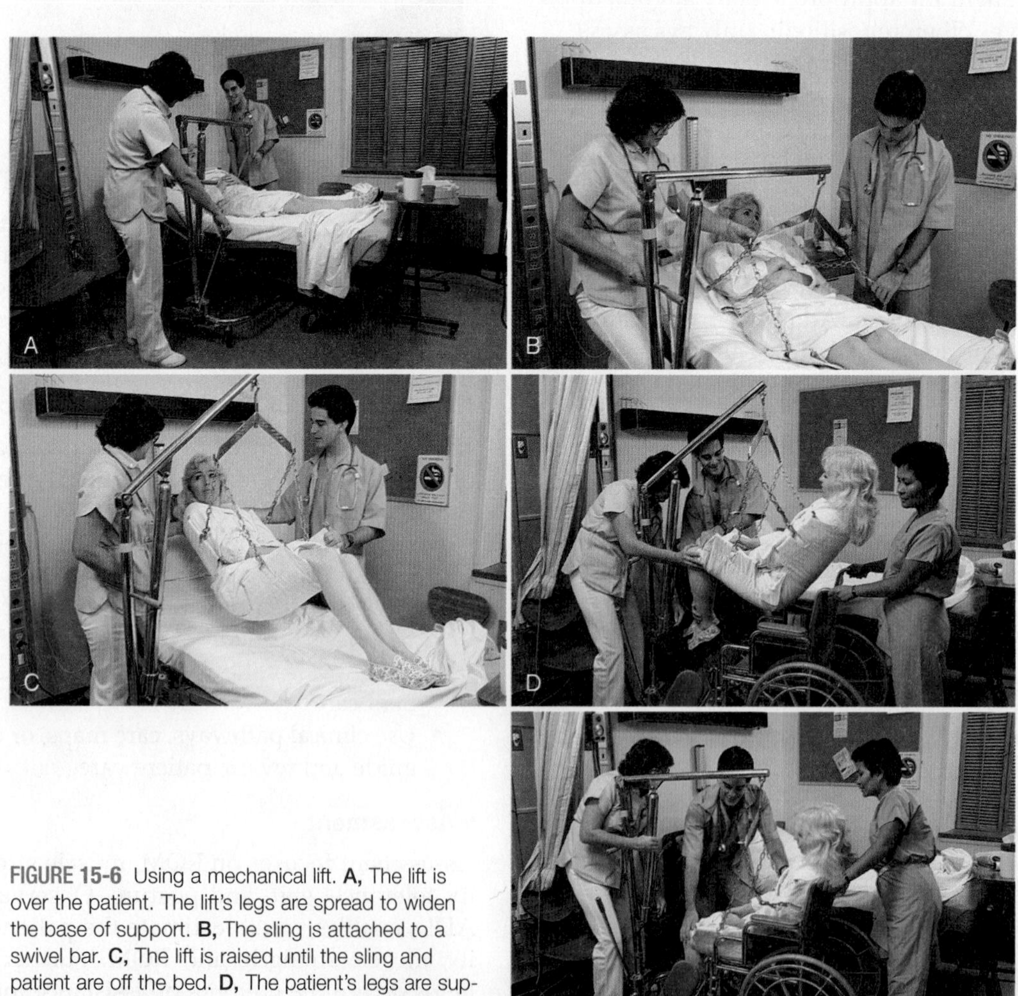

FIGURE 15-6 Using a mechanical lift. **A,** The lift is over the patient. The lift's legs are spread to widen the base of support. **B,** The sling is attached to a swivel bar. **C,** The lift is raised until the sling and patient are off the bed. **D,** The patient's legs are supported as the patient and lift are moved away from the bed. **E,** The patient is guided into a chair.

Skill 15-4 Using Lifts for Moving Patients

Nursing Action *(Rationale)*

1. Refer to medical record, care plan, or Kardex for special interventions. *(Provides basis for care.)* Read manual for direction.
2. Assemble equipment:
   - Hoyer lift frame (see Figure 15-6)
   - Seat sling attachment (may be one piece or two)
   - Two cotton bath blankets
3. Introduce self. *(Decreases patient's anxiety.)*
4. Identify patient. *(Ensures procedure is performed with correct patient.)*
5. Explain procedure. *(Enlists cooperation and assistance from patient and decreases patient's anxiety.)*
6. Perform hand hygiene. *(Reduces spread of microorganisms.)*
7. Prepare patient for interventions.
   a. Close door or pull curtains. *(Provides privacy.)*
   b. Adjust bed level to working height (even with level of arm of chair [of lift] if chair is not removable or level with seat if chair is removable.) *(Promotes safety.)*
   c. Medicate patient as needed. *(Promotes patient comfort.)*
   d. Place cotton bath blanket over chair for patient's comfort.
   e. Cover patient with remaining bath blanket.
8. Secure adequate number of personnel. *(Provides necessary assistance and patient safety.)*
9. Place chair near bed. *(Prepares seat for patient.)*
10. Appropriately place canvas seat under patient; support head and neck. *(Helps in lifting safely.)*
11. Slide horseshoe-shaped bar under bed on one side. *(Places lift close to bed.)*
12. Lower horizontal bar to level of sling by releasing hydraulic valve, and lock valve. *(Places lift close to patient.)*
13. Fasten hooks on chain to openings in sling. *(Attaches lift to sling seat.)*
14. Raise head of bed. *(Places patient in sitting position.)*
15. Fold patient's arms over chest. *(Prevents patient injury.)*
16. Pump lift handle until patient is raised off bed. *(Ensures patient safety during lifting.)*
17. With steering handle, pull lift off bed and down to chair. *(Places patient safely in chair provided.)*
18. Release valve slowly to lift and lower patient toward chair. *(Appropriately places patient in chair.)*
19. Close off valve and release straps. *(Prevents patient injury from boom.)*
20. Remove straps and hydraulic lift. *(Provides safety and comfort.)*
21. Wash hands. *(Reduces spread of microorganisms.)*
22. Document procedure. *(Note procedure and patient's response.)*
   - Evaluate body alignment to help prevent skin impairment.
   - Evaluate patient's response to movement to help determine patient's mobility potential.
23. Perform patient teaching (see Patient Teaching and Home Care Considerations boxes).

quires to change position or transfer from bed to chair, or to toilet, tub, or car. These assessments will give you an understanding of the patient's overall level of mobility and coordination (see Cultural Considerations box).

Nursing Diagnosis

Assessment enables you to cluster relevant data and develop actual or potential (risk) nursing diagnoses related to the patient's needs. State the nursing diagnoses along with the probable cause "related to (r/t)." Identification of the cause of the problem further individualizes the care plan and leads to selection of appropriate care.

Example: Impaired physical mobility r/t activity intolerance secondary to (2 degrees) left shoulder pain.

Expected Outcomes and Planning

Set goals and expected outcomes with the patient to direct interventions. Individualize care planning to the patient, taking into consideration the patient's most immediate needs. These goals are based on the nursing diagnosis formulated.

Goal: Patient will demonstrate increased activity tolerance.

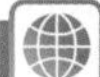
Cultural Considerations

Promotion of Patient Mobility

- Assess and listen carefully to patient's expressions of health and illness beliefs and practices.
- Be aware of the patient's personal space; seek permission before intruding in the patient's territory.
- The nursing process enables you to provide individualized care; adapt it so you are able to provide culturally sensitive care.
- When speaking with a patient (or family member) who does not understand English, many people try to compensate for the lack of understanding by speaking more loudly. Speaking slowly, distinctly, and in a normal volume is more effective (see Chapter 8).

Expected outcomes: Patient dangles legs or sits without vertigo, weakness, or orthostatic hypotension for 5 minutes with assistance.

▪ Implementation

Individualize nursing interventions according to the level of risk to the patient. You, the patient, and other members of the health care team work together to determine the most effective interventions (Nursing Care Plan 15-1). While implementing the established goals, also assess the patient's readiness to learn and teach appropriate body mechanics (see Home Care Considerations box on mobility).

You will be aware of the patient's motor deficits, ability to aid in transfer, and body weight. As a rule of thumb, never attempt to lift more than 35% of your own body weight, and always get assistance if in doubt about your ability to transfer a patient.

In recent years, the rate of injuries in occupational settings has increased dramatically. Half of all back pain is associated with manual lifting tasks. The most common back injury is strain on the lumbar muscles, which include the muscles around the lumbar vertebrae. Injury to these areas affects the ability to bend forward, backward, and side to side. The ability to rotate the hips and lower back is also decreased. To protect the patient and the nurse, it is essential to learn and master proper body mechanics.

Many special problems are to be considered in transfer. Many patients who have been immobile for several days or longer will be weak or complain of vertigo (dizziness) and sometimes develop orthostatic hypotension (a drop in blood pressure) when transferred. A patient with neurologic deficits will perhaps have paresis (muscle weakness) or paralysis unilaterally or bilaterally, which will complicate safe transfer. A flaccid arm will easily sustain injury during transfer if unsupported. Be creative when necessary when transferring trauma patients. As a general rule, use a transfer belt and obtain assistance for mobilization of such patients.

▪ Evaluation

Evaluates the success of interventions by comparing the patient's response to the outcome established for each nursing goal, such as the following:

1. Ask patient to rate fatigue on a scale of 1 to 10 (determines need for additional pain control).

Nursing Care Plan 15-1 The Patient with Activity Intolerance

Mr. Davis, a 56-year-old patient hospitalized with multiple orthopedic traumas, reports pain in his left shoulder during movement. He reports difficulty extending his shoulder joint in carrying out activities of daily living. You observe that he limits motion in his left arm. Range of motion (ROM) is reduced 30 degrees during abduction of arm.

NURSING DIAGNOSIS ***Impaired bed mobility, related to (r/t) left shoulder pain manifested by (m/b) limited mobility of left arm, c/o (complaints of) pain and favoring left arm***

Patient Goals and Expected Outcomes	Nursing Interventions	Evaluation
Patient will gain optimal ROM of left shoulder within 4 months Patient will perform self-care activities using left arm within 2 days Patient will report decreased pain Patient will increase ROM in upper extremity joints by 20 degrees Patient will follow a regular exercise program by discharge	Offer analgesic 30 minutes before ROM exercises (peak action of analgesic will occur as patient begins exercises). Schedule active ROM exercises between meals and hygiene activities (promotes frequent exercise to affected joints and reduces risk of contracture development). Teach patient specific ROM exercises for left shoulder and arm. (Teaching provides the patient with opportunity and knowledge to maintain and increase ROM.) (See Patient Teaching and Home Care Considerations boxes on mobility.)	Ask patient to report changes in perception of left shoulder pain, using a scale of 1 to 10. Observe patient while doing ROM exercises in upper extremities and while doing self-care.

Critical Thinking Questions

1. The nurse is in the process of transferring Mr. Davis from his bed to a chair using a mechanical lift. The nurse has prepared the chair and placed it near the bed. The nurse turns Mr. Davis to his side, places the sling under Mr. Davis to ensure adequate support of his head, returns Mr. Davis to his back, and slowly begins to lift him from his bed. What has the nurse forgotten to do, and why is it important?
2. The patient has a trapeze bar across the bed, trochanter rolls, and a footboard. Explain the rationale for using each of these devices to maintain proper body alignment.

2. Note patient's behavioral response to transfer (reveals level of motivation and self-care potential).

To evaluate the patient's perception of the interventions, first it is necessary to have knowledge of the patient's expectations concerning joint mobility, posture, or body alignment. What is acceptable or anticipated on your part will sometimes be vastly different from what the patient and family members anticipate or are able to accept.

Home Care Considerations

Mobility

- Instruct family or caregiver in the rationale for slow, gradual position changes.
- Instruct family or caregiver in the use of a gait belt and correct body mechanics for transfer of patient.
- Instruct family or caregiver to not attempt ambulation if patient complains of dizziness or lightheadedness.
- Transfer ability at home is greatly enhanced by prior teaching of family, assessment of home for safety risks and functionality, and provision of applicable aids.
- Have family practice transfer in hospital and achieve success before taking patient home.
- Alternatively, have the patient who lives alone practice activities because they will be used at home to manage the toileting and showering. Teach patients to transfer to armchairs for ease of rising and sitting.
- Make sure the home is free of risks (i.e., throw rugs, electric cords, slippery floors). If wheelchair is used, see that access is possible through all doors, and that space for transfer is available in bedroom and bathroom.
- Make sure arrangements are made for a home health nurse or support person to continue to assist the family at home.
- Instruct patient in how to use the ambulation aids on various terrains (e.g., carpet, stairs, rough ground, inclines).
- Instruct patient in how to maneuver around obstacles such as doors and how to use the aid when transferring, such as to and from a chair, toilet, tub, and car.
- Attach a "saddle bag" to patient's walker to carry objects; caution patient not to overfill to prevent forward tipping of walker.
- Assess family member or primary caregiver's ability, availability, and motivation to assist patient with exercises that patient is unable to perform independently.
- Assist family or primary caregiver to arrange home environment to promote exercise program (e.g., space allocation, lighting, temperature, safety precautions).
- Teach family members about body mechanics.
- In the absence of a hospital bed and equipment, creative adaptation will be required.
- Consider the need for a bed that places the bedridden patient at caregiver's waist level.
- Teach caregivers to change patient's position every 1 to 2 hours, if possible, to maintain musculoskeletal alignment, and to reduce pressure on bony prominences. Develop and post a realistic turning schedule.

Get Ready for the NCLEX® Examination!

Key Points

- It is essential to protect the musculoskeletal system to prevent injury to both patient and nurse.
- You need less effort to carry out an activity if you widen your base of support in the direction of movement.
- Practice appropriate body mechanics consistently.
- Maintaining correct body alignment is the key to proper body mechanics.
- Correct body alignment promotes balance and helps coordinate movements.
- Permanent disability can occur from inappropriate positioning.
- Proper positioning permits activity, enhances comfort, and prepares patients for procedures.
- Immobility sometimes results from illness or trauma, and sometimes it is prescribed for therapeutic reasons. Whatever the reason, immobility poses the risk of serious complications. Interventions to avoid these complications are possible.
- You will perform range-of-motion exercises to promote circulation, prevent contractures, and provide joint mobility.
- When turning, moving, lifting, or carrying a patient, secure adequate assistance to reduce strain and prevent injury to both you and the patient. Perform procedure safely and properly, facilitating patient's independence, and teach patient and others safety in moving.
- Mechanical devices such as a hydraulic lift, roller board, and gurney lift are used for moving patients safely.
- Use the nursing process to provide care for patients who are at risk for or are experiencing activity intolerance and impaired mobility.

Additional Learning Resources

Go to your companion CD for an audio glossary, animations, video clips, and more.

evolve Be sure to visit the Evolve site at http://evolve.elsevier.com/Christensen/foundations/ for additional online resources.

Review Questions for the NCLEX® Examination

1. The nurse is assigned to care for an 82-year-old patient who weighs 252 pounds and is a bilateral below-the-knee amputee. The safest method to transfer this patient from bed to chair would be:
   1. log-rolling.
   2. using two nurses to lift.
   3. a hydraulic lift with a Hoyer sling.
   4. a gurney lift.

2. The nurse helps ambulate an 84-year-old patient who has peripheral vascular disease that caused a severe stasis ulcer. The patient becomes very weak, complains of feeling faint, and begins to fall. The most appropriate action to prevent injury to the patient would be to:
   1. support her while falling and allow her to sit on the floor.
   2. carefully attempt to return her to her room.
   3. tell her to hold onto the wall and that you will get more assistance.
   4. ask her to take deep breaths and look straight ahead.

3. A 56-year-old patient had an open cholecystectomy. The nurse is going to dangle the patient before ambulation. After sitting him on the edge of the bed, which nursing intervention should the nurse perform before proceeding with the ambulation?
   1. Assess his temperature.
   2. Assess his pulse and respirations.
   3. Perform an oximetry check.
   4. Remove antiembolism stockings.

4. The patient accidentally knocks the emesis basin to the floor. When picking up the emesis basin, the nurse will use proper body mechanics to:
   1. lower his or her body by flexing the knees and bending the hips.
   2. bend from the waist and hips.
   3. flex the knees and bend at the waist.
   4. keep his or her legs straight and flex the waist.

5. A 72-year-old patient with a stroke has slid to the foot of the bed. To use appropriate body mechanics, the nurse maintains a wide base of support and faces the patient in the direction of movement, thus allowing the nurse to:
   1. use the back muscles.
   2. use the large muscles across the scapula.
   3. exert less physical effort.
   4. use the gluteal muscles.

6. An 82-year-old patient has had a right total hip replacement. On the first postoperative day, the nurse repositions the patient to her left side, placing a pillow between her legs and another to her back. The nurse assesses the proper placement of the patient's body to evaluate:
   1. base of support.
   2. body alignment.
   3. head and chin tilt.
   4. gluteal pressure.

7. It is the patient's first night after an abdominal hysterectomy. She has not voided for 9 hours, and the nurse is to insert a 16-F Foley catheter into her bladder. The preferred position is:
   1. dorsal recumbent.
   2. lithotomy.
   3. Sims'.
   4. prone.

8. The nurse is assigned to care for a 64-year-old patient who was admitted for exacerbation of chronic obstructive pulmonary disease and pneumonia. He has dyspnea and is unable to rest in a supine position. The nurse elevates the head of the bed to 90 degrees, places a pillow on the overbed table, and assists the patient to lean forward, placing his head on the pillow. This position is called:
   1. semi-Fowler's.
   2. dorsal.
   3. Sims'.
   4. orthopneic.

9. The nurse explains to the patient that the log-rolling technique will be used to help the patient change position by stating:
   1. "Log-rolling will help you keep your hips slightly flexed toward your chest."
   2. "By having you dangle your legs at the bedside, you will be more comfortable."
   3. "Because of your injury, it is extremely important that the head of your bed remain up at all times."
   4. "It is important to keep your neck and spine in straight alignment while we help you move onto your side."

10. The nurse and an assistant are to move a dependent patient from the supine to the lateral position and will:
    1. move the patient to the center of the bed first.
    2. ensure that the upper arm and leg are supported with pillows.
    3. place a firm pillow at the abdomen and chest for additional support.
    4. turn the patient's shoulders to one side and hips toward the other side.

11. An older adult patient has been lying in the supine position for 3 hours and tells the nurse that she is too uncomfortable to move right now. The nurse will:
    1. express concern that she is uncomfortable and promise to come back later.
    2. assess the patient's need for pain medication before helping her change position.
    3. explain to the patient that if she doesn't move now, she will develop pneumonia.
    4. find another nurse to help move the patient to the lateral position immediately.

12. A principle of good body mechanics includes:
    1. keeping the knees in a locked position.
    2. maintaining a wide base of support and bending at the knees.
    3. bending at the waist to maintain one's balance.
    4. holding objects away from the body for improved leverage.

13. A patient becomes faint while sitting on the side of the bed. To prevent injury to the patient, the nurse will:

1. call for assistance.
2. lay patient straight back and support head.
3. allow patient to lower head to rest on your abdomen.
4. find an emesis basin as patient will probably vomit.

14. A patient has been immobilized for 5 days because of extensive abdominal surgery. When getting this patient out of bed for the first time, a nursing diagnosis related to the safety of the patient would be:

1. pain.
2. impaired skin integrity.
3. altered tissue perfusion.
4. risk for activity intolerance.

15. Which assistive device allows the patient to pull with the upper extremities to raise his trunk off the bed, to assist in transfer from bed to wheelchair, or to perform upper arm exercises?

1. Trapeze bar
2. Trochanter roll
3. Hand rolls
4. Footboard

16. In which position is the patient lying face down or chest down?

1. Supine
2. Lateral
3. Prone
4. Fowler's

17. A necessary safety precaution when helping a patient to ambulate is to:

1. have family members present.
2. have patient wear well-fitting rubber-soled shoes or slippers.
3. have at least two people present to assist the patient.
4. be sure no pain medication was given for at least 3 hours before ambulation.

18. Active and passive ROM exercises benefit the patient by preventing:

1. contractures.
2. arthritis.
3. muscle strain.
4. atrophy of surrounding tissue.

19. A footboard can prevent footdrop, also known as:

1. plantar flexion of the foot.
2. dorsiflexion of the foot.
3. ankle extension.
4. ankle hyperextension.

20. When using a drawsheet to assist in moving a patient up in bed, ask the patient to:

1. bend knees to assist in moving.
2. keep hands at sides.
3. raise arms above the head.
4. maintain straight body position.

chapter 16

Pain Management, Comfort, Rest, and Sleep

evolve

http://evolve.elsevier.com/Christensen/foundationsadult

Barbara Lauritsen Christensen

Objectives

1. Define the key terms as listed.
2. List 10 possible causes of discomfort.
3. Discuss McCaffery's description of pain.
4. Describe the use of gate control theory to guide selection of nursing interventions for pain relief.
5. Identify subjective and objective data in pain assessment.
6. Discuss the concept of pain assessment as the fifth vital sign.
7. Discuss the synergistic impact of fatigue, sleep disturbance, and depression on the perception of pain.
8. Analyze several scales used to identify intensity of pain.
9. Discuss pain mechanisms affected by each analgesic group.
10. Discuss the responsibilities of the nurse in controlling pain.
11. List several methods for pain control.
12. Identify nursing interventions to control painful stimuli in the patient's environment.
13. Discuss the differences and similarities between sleep and rest.
14. Outline nursing interventions that promote rest and sleep.
15. Discuss the sleep cycle, differentiating between non–rapid eye movement (NREM) and rapid eye movement (REM) sleep.
16. List six signs and symptoms of sleep deprivation.
17. Identify two nursing diagnoses related to sleep problems.

Key Terms

acute pain (ă-KYŪT pān, p. 396)
chronic pain (KRŎN-ĭk pān, p. 396)
endorphins (ĕn-DŎR-fĭnz, p. 396)
gate control theory (GĀT kŏn-trōl THĒ-ŏ-rē, p. 396)
non–rapid eye movement (NREM) (NŎN-răp-ĭd Ī mūv-mĕnt, p. 410)
noxious (NŎK-shŭs, p. 395)
patient-controlled analgesia (PCA) (PĀ-shĕnt kŏn-TRŌLD ăn-ăl-JĒ-zē-ă, p. 402)
rapid eye movement (REM) (RĂP-ĭd Ī mūv-mĕnt, p. 410)
referred pain (rē-FŬRD pān, p. 396)
synergistic (sĭn-ŭr-JĬS-tĭk, p. 396)
transcutaneous electric nerve stimulation (TENS) (trăns-kyū-TĀ-nē-ŭs ē-LĔK-trĭk NŬRV stĭm-ū-LĀ-shŭn, p. 398)
visual analog scale (VĬZH-ū-ăl ĂN-ă-lŏg skāl, p. 406)

One of your greatest challenges as a nurse is to provide comfort to the patient. To comfort means to give strength and hope, to cheer, and to ease the grief, pain, or trouble of another. Promoting physical and psychological comfort is a vital aspect of your role as a nurse.

Many factors contribute to a patient's lack of comfort, which manifests in many forms, including the following:

- Anxiety
- Constipation
- Constricting edema
- Depression
- Diaphoresis
- Diarrhea
- Distention
- Dry mouth
- Dyspnea
- Fatigue
- Fear
- Flatus
- Grief
- Headache
- Hopelessness
- Hyperthermia
- Hypothermia
- Hypoxia
- Incontinence
- Muscle cramping
- Nausea
- Pain
- Powerlessness
- Pruritus
- Sadness
- Singultus
- Thirst
- Urinary retention
- Vomiting

It is important to explore the patient's concept of what constitutes comfort. By actively listening to the patient, you will be better prepared to plan nursing interventions. When you know the possible elements of patient discomfort, you will recognize discomfort signals even when the patient is not able to verbalize, as in the case of a patient who is aphasic or one who is semicomatose. Be diligent in your efforts and pursue all the methods within your power to relieve patients' discomfort. If interventions are not successful, seek out and apply alternative interventions.

Regardless of age, patients typically receive comfort and a sense of well-being from gentle touch and eye contact (Figure 16-1).

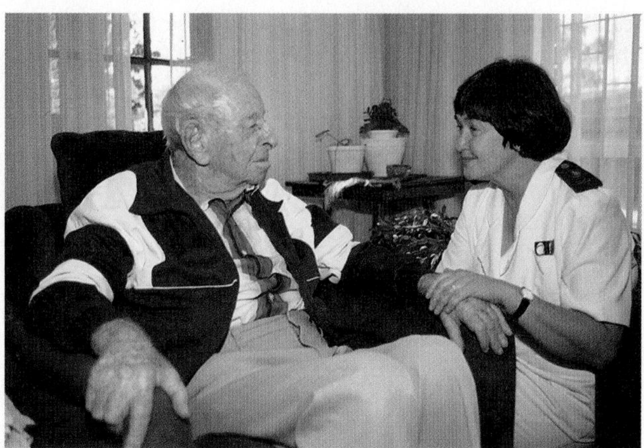

FIGURE 16-1 Eye contact and gentle touch promote comfort and well-being.

PAIN

NATURE OF PAIN

Pain is a complex, abstract, personal subjective experience. It is an unpleasant sensation caused by **noxious** (injurious to physical health) stimulation of the sensory nerve endings. It serves as a warning to the body because it often occurs where there is actual or potential tissue damage. Pain is often a cardinal symptom of inflammation and is valuable in the diagnosis of many disorders and conditions. Pain is also possible when there is no tissue damage, such as the pain of grief at the death of a loved one or the pain of migraine headaches. Pain causes fatigue and decreases the patient's ability to cope physically, emotionally, and mentally. Pain has the potential to be totally debilitating and is the most common reason that patients seek out a health care provider (Elkin et al., 2007).

Pain is subjective; the interpretation and significance of pain depend on an individual's learned experiences and involve psychosocial and cultural factors. The defining characteristic of pain is the verbal or nonverbal communication by the patient of the presence of pain (Box 16-1). McCaffery and Pasero's description of pain is a practical one: "Pain is whatever the experiencing person says it is, existing whenever he says it does" (McCaffery & Pasero, 2003). According to McCaffery and Pasero's description, you are obliged to believe every patient who says he or she has pain.

Only the person with pain, and not the health professional, is the expert about that pain: its onset, duration, location, intensity, quality, and pattern, as well as the degree of pain relief obtained from therapy. The patient often does not recognize that health professionals are not able to tell how much pain the patient is experiencing. Assist the patient to recognize his or her expertise about the pain and to use that expertise in partnership with health professionals to obtain better pain management. Empowering the patient to be an active partner in reporting information about the pain is an important nursing therapy.

A patient with pain does not always know how to report the pain to health professionals. You have an important role in helping the patient by conducting nursing pain assessments.

Box 16-1 Behavioral Characteristics of Patients in Pain

The patient with pain exhibits the following behaviors:

- Is self-protective; guards the painful area—places hands over the area
- Has narrowed focus: cannot think of anything but the pain, has reduced attention span
- Withdraws from social contact, avoids conversation or social contacts
- Has impaired thought processes
- Demonstrates distraction behavior, which includes moaning, rocking, crying, pacing, restlessness, or seeking out other people or activities
- Presents facial mask of pain: eyes that appear dull or lusterless, fixed or scattered facial movements, grimacing, teeth clenching, lip biting, or jaw tightening
- Experiences alterations in muscle tone, ranging from lassitude to rigidity
- Exhibits diaphoresis, changes in blood pressure and pulse rate, pupillary dilation, and increased or decreased rate of respiration
- Sometimes demonstrates no outward expression of pain. *Remember that lack of pain expression does not mean lack of pain. There is no specific "picture" of a patient in pain.*

DEFINITIONS OF PAIN

The most widely accepted definition of pain, adopted by the International Association for the Study of Pain (IASP) and the American Pain Society (APS), is as follows: "Pain is an unpleasant sensory and emotional experience associated with actual or potential tissue damage, or described in terms of such damage" (McCaffery & Pasero, 2003). This definition presents pain as a phenomenon with multiple components that makes an impact on a person's psychosocial and physical functioning. It acknowledges the complexity of the pain experience. Pain is not determined by tissue damage alone. In fact, no predictable relationship exists between identifiable tissue injury and the sensation of pain. For example, a patient's description of pain may be disproportionate to the evidence of tissue damage. In times of high stress and trauma, patients will sometimes describe pain as less severe than you expect it to be, whereas patients with chronic nonmalignant pain often describe pain for which little or no tissue damage can be found. The latter is possibly due to abnormalities in the neural processing of stimuli. The inability to identify tissue damage sufficient to explain the pain is not proof that the pain is of psychological origin.

TYPES OF PAIN

There are many types of pain: mild and severe; chronic and acute; intermittent and intractable (constant); burning, dull, and sharp; precisely and poorly localized; and referred. Referred pain is felt at a site other than the injured or diseased organ or part of the body. An example of referred pain is the pain of coronary artery insufficiency that will in some cases be felt in the left shoulder or arm, or the jaw.

Acute pain is intense and of short duration, usually lasting less than 6 months. Generally, acute pain provides a warning to the individual of actual or potential tissue damage. It creates an autonomic response that originates within the sympathetic nervous system, flooding the body with epinephrine and commonly referred to as the **fight-or-flight response.** Anxiety is usually associated with the pain. Because the pain is of short duration, physicians are likely to prescribe opioids and other analgesics.

Chronic pain is generally characterized as pain lasting longer than 6 months. Sometimes the pain is continuous and sometimes intermittent, and is at times as intense as acute pain. Chronic pain does not serve as a warning of tissue damage in process, but rather signals the fact of its having occurred. In rheumatoid arthritis, for example, joint pain will often continue when the disease process is no longer active because of the structural damage that has already occurred in the joint. The reason for some forms of chronic pain sometimes remains unknown. Because of the prolonged time involved in chronic pain, the patient often develops chronic low self-esteem, change in social identity, changes in role and social interaction, fatigue, sleep disturbance, and depression.

It is possible that fatigue, sleep disturbance, and depression act in a type of synergistic (the action of two or more substances or organs to achieve an effect of which each is individually incapable) relationship. The combination of fatigue, sleep disturbance, and depression has the potential to markedly change a person's perception of pain. Depression is associated with sleep disturbance, which in turn increases the intensity of the fatigue. The patient's world becomes smaller and smaller, in the worst case spiraling inward to restrict itself to just the patient's own body and mind. As the focus narrows more and more, it entraps the individual in a vicious cycle, making the pain difficult to treat. Pain-related disability, such as inability to perform activities of daily living, contributes to low self-esteem and social problems. Because depression is common in patients with chronic pain, always screen for suicidal ideation and report to a registered nurse (RN) for psychiatric evaluation referral (Siedlecki, 2004).

Because of the general differences between acute and chronic pain, some aspects of nursing interventions for these conditions will often differ. Keep in mind that the patient's perception of pain, whether acute or chronic, is real, and use appropriate measures to relieve that pain.

THEORIES OF PAIN TRANSMISSION

GATE CONTROL THEORY

The gate control theory of pain, proposed by Melzack (1983), suggests that pain impulses are regulated and even blocked by gating mechanisms located along the central nervous system (CNS). The proposed location of the gates is in the dorsal horn of the spinal cord. Pain and other sensations of the skin and muscles travel the same pathways through the large nerves in the spinal cord. If other cutaneous stimuli besides pain are transmitted, the "gate" through which the pain impulse must travel is temporarily blocked by the stimuli. The brain does not have the capacity to acknowledge the pain while it is interpreting the other stimuli. When gates are open, pain impulses flow freely (Figure 16-2). When gates are closed, pain impulses become blocked. Partial openings sometimes occur. A bombardment of sensory impulses, such as those from the pressure of a back rub, the heat of a warm compress, or the cold from ice applications, will close the gates to painful stimuli. It is possible with some patients to distract them from pain by removing the sensation of pain from their center of attention. Auditory or visual stimuli will often distract patients and help make pain more tolerable.

Gating mechanisms are also subject to alteration by thoughts, feelings, and memories. The cerebral cortex and the thalamus have the capacity to influence whether pain impulses reach a person's conscious awareness. There is conscious control over how pain is perceived, and this helps explain the various ways people react and adjust to pain.

ENDORPHINS

The body produces morphinelike substances called endorphins (potent polypeptides composed of many amino acids found in the pituitary gland and other areas of the CNS). Stress and pain activate endorphins. Analgesia results when certain endorphins attach to opioid receptor sites in the brain and prevent the release of neurotransmitters, thereby inhibiting the transmission of pain impulses. People who have less pain than others from a similar injury have higher endorphin levels. Pain relief measures, such as transcutaneous electric nerve stimulation (TENS), acupuncture, and placebos, are believed to cause the release of endorphins.

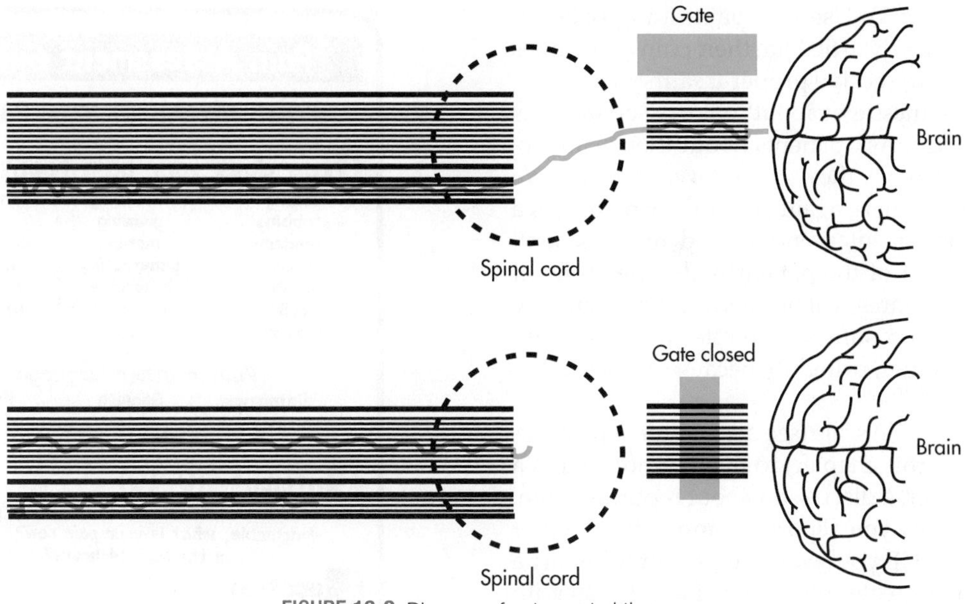

FIGURE 16-2 Diagram of gate control theory.

CONTROLLING PAIN

REQUIREMENTS OF THE JOINT COMMISSION FOR PAIN CONTROL

Assessing and managing pain has long been a major nursing responsibility. In the 1992 Standards Manual issued by The Joint Commission (TJC) (McCaffery & Pasero, 2003), effective pain management was stated as one of the rights of a dying patient. In 1994 TJC broadened this statement to cover all patients, stating, "The management of pain is appropriate for all patients, not just dying patients" (McCaffery & Pasero, 2003). TJC accreditation visits began to include a focus on what institutions were doing about pain management.

In 1997, under a grant from the Robert Wood Johnson Foundation, TJC began working collaboratively with institutions to create standards for pain assessment and treatment, with plans to conduct national quality improvement programs to help health care facilities meet these standards (McCaffery & Pasero, 2003). TJC now requires accredited facilities and organizations to develop policies and procedures that formalize this obligation (TJC, 2006).

The Joint Commission Standards

Under the new TJC standards, health care providers are expected to be knowledgeable about pain assessment and management, and facilities are expected to develop policies and procedures supporting the appropriate use of analgesics and other pain control therapies. Here are some key concepts (Acello, 2000):

- Patients have the right to appropriate assessment.
- Patients will be treated for pain or referred for treatment.
- Pain is to be assessed and regularly reassessed.
- Patients will be taught the importance of effective pain management.
- Patients will be taught that pain management is part of treatment.
- Patients will be involved in making care decisions.
- Routine and prn analgesics are to be administered as ordered.
- Discharge planning and teaching will include continuing care based on the patient's needs at the time of discharge, including the need for pain management.

MAKING PAIN THE FIFTH VITAL SIGN

One simple strategy to increase accountability for pain control is for an institution to make pain intensity ratings a routine part of assessment and documentation of vital signs. This suggestion comes from the American Pain Society (APS) and has been implemented in many hospitals, often simply by including pain on the vital sign record (APS, 1995; McCaffery & Pasero, 2003). This makes any presence of pain visible and raises awareness of the problem of unmanaged pain. Thanks to the work of pain and palliative care associations, more attention is being paid to pain management, and many institutions have included pain assessment as a vital sign.

When pain is assessed with the same zeal as are other vital signs, there is a much better chance of its being treated properly. Vital signs are monitored to detect changes or trends that signal a need for further assessment, diagnosis, and treatment. So it is with pain. Making pain a vital sign—along with pulse, temperature, blood pressure, and respiration—will ensure that you monitor pain on a regular basis (see

Chapter 4, Figure 4-1). Use of a pain-rating scale allows patients to clearly articulate their pain and makes them more likely to receive proper treatment.

The essential message about pain assessment is easy to summarize: Ask patients about their pain, accept and respect what they say, intervene to relieve their pain, and ask them again about their pain. It is a circle of assessment, intervention, and reassessment. Without assessment of the patient with pain, none of the pain relief measures will be useful. Approximately half the people who suffer moderate to severe pain will continue to suffer, primarily because nurses fail to assess pain.

Comparing the pain scale (see discussion of pain rating scales later in this chapter) to the thermometer is a helpful way to open a discussion about reporting pain. Explain that just as you report a temperature higher than 100° F (37.8° C), you want the patient to report a pain rating of 4 or greater on a scale of 0 to 10. As with temperature, the higher the pain score, the more concern and urgency are warranted (Figure 16-3). Help patients to understand that delaying analgesia until pain is severe has no benefits (McCaffery, 2002b).

Unrelieved pain has harmful physical effects, such as increased oxygen demand, respiratory dysfunction, decreased gastrointestinal motility, confusion, and depressed immune response. Possible emotional consequences of unrelieved pain include anxiety, depression, irritability, and an inability to enjoy life. Neglected pain erodes a patient's trust in the health care system and possibly leads to setbacks and increased costs in treatment. Conversely, appropriate pain management will typically bring about quicker recoveries, shorter hospital stays, fewer readmissions, and improved quality of life (Mayer et al., 2001).

Pain Assessment Guide

Tell Me About Your Pain

H ow does your pain feel?

aching	throbbing	shooting
stabbing	gnawing	sharp
tender	burning	exhausting
tiring	penetrating	nagging
numb	miserable	unbearable
dull	radiating	squeezing
crampy	deep	pressure

Pain in other languages

Vietnamese	Spanish	French
dau	dolor	douleur

I ntensity (0-10)

If 0 is no pain and 10 is the worst pain imaginable, what is your pain now?
... in the last 24 hours?

L ocation

Where is your pain?

D uration

Is the pain always there?
Does the pain come and go? (Breakthrough Pain)
Do you have both types of pain?

A ggravating and Alleviating Factors

What makes the pain better?
What makes the pain worse?

How does pain affect

sleep	energy	relationships
appetite	activity	mood

Are you experiencing any other symptoms?

nausea/vomiting	itching	urinary retention
constipation	sleepiness/confusion	weakness

Things to check

vital signs, past medication history, knowledge of pain, and use of non-invasive techniques

FIGURE 16-3 Pain assessment guide.

NONINVASIVE PAIN RELIEF TECHNIQUES

Pain is most effectively controlled through a combination of noninvasive pain relief measures and pharmacologic therapy. The purpose of noninvasive pain relief techniques, which are sometimes of help even when used alone, is to decrease the patient's perception of pain as well as improve the patient's sense of control. Useful noninvasive approaches include cutaneous stimulation (heat, cold, massage, and TENS), the removal of painful stimuli, distraction, relaxation, guided imagery, meditation, hypnosis, and biofeedback (Table 16-1). In guided imagery, the patient is encouraged to concentrate on an image that helps relieve pain or discomfort. For the best results, help the patient choose a scene that holds especially pleasant memories. Ask the patient where he or she feels the most relaxed, such as at a lake, in a forest, or in a meadow, then encourage the patient to use sensory memories to bring the image to life.

Whether the gate control theory explains why these techniques are successful, or whether they work by decreasing anxiety, they undoubtedly have many advantages for pain control. Most are inexpensive and easy to perform, have low risk and few side effects, and frequently do not require a physician's order. Probably the greatest advantage of these techniques is patients' ability to have some control over the treatment of their pain. Sometimes merely having options to choose from provides comfort to the patient. Although not everyone will react successfully to these pain relief measures, it is worthwhile to attempt any of them before advancing to more invasive techniques.

Transcutaneous Electric Nerve Stimulation (TENS)

A special pain relief system, **transcutaneous electric nerve stimulation (TENS),** uses a pocket-sized,

Table 16-1 **Nonpharmacologic Interventions for Pain***

INTERVENTIONS	COMMENTS
PHYSICAL	
Progressive muscle relaxation	Reduces mild to moderate pain. Requires 3 to 5 minutes of staff time for instruction.
Massage	Effective for reduction of mild to moderate discomfort. May be firm, gentle, or light stroking of the body part involved or the opposite extremity. Requires 3 to 10 minutes of staff time.
Transcutaneous electric nerve stimulation (TENS)	Effective in reducing mild to moderate pain by stimulating the skin with mild electric current. Electrodes are placed over or near the site of pain. Requires special equipment. Requires physician order.
Heat or cold application	Selection of heat versus cold varies with the situation. Moist heat relieves stiffness of arthritis and relaxes muscles. Cold applications reduce acute pain associated with inflammation from arthritis or from acute injury. Requires physician order.
PSYCHOLOGICAL AND COGNITIVE	
Music	Simple relaxation. Best taught preoperatively. Both patient-preferred and "easy-listening" music effective for mild to moderate pain.
Biofeedback	Reduces mild to moderate pain and operative site muscle tension. Requires patient to have high level of cognitive function. Requires skilled personnel and special equipment.
Imagery	Reduces mild to moderate pain. Requires skilled personnel.
Education	Effective for reduction of all types of pain. Should include sensory and procedural information and instruction aimed at reducing activity-related pain. Requires 5 to 15 minutes of staff time.

From Elkin, M.K., Perry, A.G., & Potter, P.A. (2007). *Nursing interventions and clinical skills.* (4th ed.). St. Louis: Mosby.
*Should be used with analgesic medication.

battery-operated device that provides a continuous, mild electric current to the skin via electrodes that are attached to a stimulator by flexible wires. The electric current is adjustable. As with other forms of cutaneous stimulation, it is thought that TENS works by stimulating large nerve fibers to "close the gate" in the spinal cord, thus blocking transmission of pain impulses. In addition, TENS is hypothesized to stimulate endorphin production.

TENS is typically used for patients suffering postoperative or chronic pain. Generally, you will place the electrodes on or near the painful site. Be alert to the possibility of a TENS unit interfering with the function of a cardiac pacemaker device.

INVASIVE PAIN RELIEF TECHNIQUES

Invasive means anything that enters the body. Examples of invasive techniques are nerve blocks, epidural analgesics, neurosurgical procedures, and acupuncture. Certain invasive techniques offer relief for many patients with pain. However, careful patient selection and proper technique are essential because the costs and risks are potentially high.

MEDICATION FOR PAIN MANAGEMENT

Analgesics often provide patients effective pain relief. Nurses and physicians frequently have misconceptions about the dangers and effects of analgesics. They often undertreat patients and even administer less medication than is ordered because of (1) misunderstandings or insufficient knowledge of pharmacologic principles, (2) concerns about addiction, and (3) anxiety over administering too large a dose of an opioid analgesic. Because of such uncertainties, the patient's pain is only reduced, not relieved. Make sure you understand the medications available for pain relief and their effects.

Nonopioids

Acetaminophen and nonsteroidal antiinflammatory drugs (NSAIDs)—the nonopioid analgesics—are the most widely available and frequently used analgesic group. Acetaminophen may block pain impulses peripherally that occur in response to inhibition of prostaglandin synthesis, primarily in the CNS. Nonopioids are used primarily for mild to moderate pain but are sometimes also used to relieve certain types of severe pain. Some NSAIDs are available without a prescription, such as aspirin, ibuprofen (Advil, Nuprin, Motrin), and naproxen sodium (Aleve). Aspirin blocks pain impulses in the CNS and reduces inflammation.

Remember that the maximum recommended dosage of acetaminophen is 4,000 mg (4 g) in 24 hours. Its toxic side effect, a basic consideration in all analgesic regimens, is hepatotoxicity. Patient responses to NSAIDs vary, so if one is ineffective, try another. Their mechanisms of action appear to be different enough to warrant changing NSAIDs until the best one for the patient is identified. All NSAIDs pose the risk of gastrointestinal (GI) bleeding.

Opioids

Opioids such as morphine, meperidine (Demerol), hydromorphone (Dilaudid), and fentanyl (Actiq, Duragesic) act on higher centers of the brain to modify perception and reaction to pain. Opioids decrease the perception of pain by binding to pain receptor sites in the CNS. The term *opioids* is now preferred over *narcotics* because of the association with illegal substance abuse (Elkin et al., 2007).

Opioid analgesics are the cornerstone for managing moderate to severe acute pain. Morphine is the standard agent for opioid therapy, but other opiates, such as hydromorphone HCl, levorphanol, oxycodone, and fentanyl are ordered as substitutes if the patient has an unusual reaction or allergy to morphine. Morphine is a highly effective drug; however, its use in the presence of compromised renal function must be monitored carefully.

The danger of morphine and other opioid analgesics is their potential to cause depression of vital nervous system functions. Most significantly, opiates cause respiratory depression by depressing the respiratory center within the brainstem. Based on studies of intravenous (IV), and epidural administration routes for opioids, the likelihood of clinically significant opioid-induced respiratory depression is less than 1%. Clinically significant respiratory depression occurs less often when administering opioids by the epidural route (0.07% to 0.4%) or by IV patient-controlled analgesia (0.1% to 0.23%) than when the intramuscular (IM) route is used (0.9%) (McCaffery, 2002b).

There are numerous opiate analgesics now on the market. Two new extended-release morphine tablets, Avinza and Kadian, provide 24-hour pain relief with once-daily administration. These medications are replacing the older MS Contin, which provides only 12 hours of pain relief. A new combination medication, Combunox, which contains 5 mg of oxycodone and 400 mg of ibuprofen, is now often prescribed for pain relief. Administration of the combined medication is limited by the maximum daily dosage of 3.2 g of ibuprofen (D'Arcy, 2006).

Because of its potential for inducing seizures, meperidine (Demerol) is no longer the drug of choice for pain management. The active metabolite in meperidine, normeperidine, is a CNS stimulant and sometimes produces irritability, tremors, muscle twitching, jerking, agitation, and seizures. Because normeperidine is eliminated by the kidneys, do not use it in patients with decreased renal function. It is a particularly poor choice in the older adult and patients with sickle cell disease because most have some degree of renal insufficiency. Repeated administration increases the risk of accumulation of normeperidine, so meperidine is not generally prescribed for patients requiring long-term opioid treatment, such as those with cancer or chronic nonmalignant pain. The effects of normeperidine have been observed even in young, otherwise healthy patients given sufficiently high doses of meperidine postoperatively.

Meperidine administration is contraindicated in patients receiving monoamine oxidase (MAO) inhibitors and in patients with untreated hypothyroidism, Addison's disease, benign prostatic hypertrophy, or urethral stricture. Meperidine is more likely than other opioid drugs to cause delirium in postoperative patients of all ages, especially if given epidurally or intravenously. By any route of administration, the logic of using meperidine for any type of pain management is questionable. There are opioid choices that are clearly safer (see Life Span Considerations for Older Adults box on pain control).

Tolerance and Addiction

Opioid tolerance and physiologic dependence are unusual with short-term postoperative use, and psychological dependence and addiction are extremely unlikely after taking opiates for acute pain. Studies conducted over 20 years have uniformly shown that the likelihood of addiction occurring as a result of taking opioids for pain relief, even over a long period, is rare—probably less than 1%. Often the term ***addiction*** is inappropriately applied to a patient, and the label becomes a barrier to pain relief for that person.

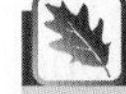

Life Span Considerations

Older Adults

Pain Control

- The effects of aging on the pain process are sometimes compounded in an older adult who has a chronic illness that affects the nervous system.
- An older person who is well instructed in use of pain measurement tools and without diseases affecting the nervous system (e.g., diabetes) tends to report pain intensity similar to a younger person.
- The risk for gastric and renal toxicity from nonsteroidal anti-inflammatory drugs (NSAIDs) is increased in older adults.
- Changes in peripheral vascular function and skin as well as decreased transmission of pain impulses place the older adult at risk for being unable to sense pain.
- Older age is associated with chronic health problems, increased risk for musculoskeletal pain, depression, and limitations in activities of daily living.
- Increased pain intensity has been noted in older individuals, particularly when adequate treatment is not provided for chronic and recurrent pain.
- Treatment of pain in the older adult is as likely to be successful as that in a younger person.
- Meperidine (Demerol) is a particularly poor choice for pain control in the older adult in that it is not to be used in patients with decreased renal function. Older adult patients often have some degree of renal insufficiency.
- Older adults sometimes become susceptible to side effects of opioids because of changes in serum proteins and liver and renal function, and a reduction in cardiac output.

Physical tolerance and physical dependence do occur in many patients after 1 to 4 weeks of regular opioid administration. Recognize that these effects are expected with long-term opioid treatment, but do not confuse them with addiction (McCaffery, 2002b).

A helpful rule is that relief of severe pain requires a greater amount of analgesic; remembering this helps overcome any fear of overtreating patients' pain. Dosages at the upper end of normally prescribed ranges are usually safe. If you administer a low dose and it proves ineffective, the patient will have to suffer until the required time interval has passed for another dose to be given.

Preventing and Managing Opioid-Induced Constipation

Opioids often delay gastric emptying, slow bowel motility, and decrease peristalsis. They also tend to reduce secretions from the colonic mucosa. The result is slow-moving, hard stool that is difficult to pass. At its worst, gastrointestinal dysfunction can result in ileus, fecal impaction, and obstruction.

Constipation is the most common side effect of opioids and the only one for which individuals do not develop tolerance. Thus it necessitates a preventive approach, regular assessment, and aggressive management. Factors contributing to constipation in patients taking opioids include advanced age, immobility, abdominal disease, and concurrent medications. Typically, you will direct patients placed on opioid analgesics to take a stool softener with a mild peristaltic stimulant, such as Senokot-S, and to continue regular use as long as the opioid regimen lasts.

Instruct the patient in proper diet, fluids, and exercise and provide for the patient's privacy and convenience. Keep in mind, however, that these aspects of bowel management are important but usually insufficient on their own to prevent opioid-induced constipation. Bulk laxatives, natural roughage, and large amounts of fluid are sometimes unpalatable and ineffective. In addition, if fluid intake is inadequate, bulk laxatives, such as psyllium (Metamucil), sometimes cause fecal impaction and obstruction. Stool softeners alone are inadequate.

Pain Mechanisms Affected by Each Analgesic Group

It is useful and clinically relevant to distinguish among analgesics that relieve pain by different mechanisms. Because different analgesics relieve pain in different ways, it is sometimes logical to combine analgesics from different groups to relieve one specific type of pain or to relieve different types of pain occurring in the same patient.

Following is a brief description of selected mechanisms of action thought to be unique to each analgesic group.

- **Nonopioids** (acetylsalicylic acid [aspirin], acetaminophen, and NSAIDs). The analgesia produced by acetaminophen (Tylenol) appears to be related to the inhibition of prostaglandins that may serve as mediators of pain and fever, primarily in the CNS but may also block pain impulses peripherally. Aspirin blocks pain impulses in the CNS and reduces inflammation by inhibition of prostaglandin synthesis. NSAIDs such as tramadol (Ultram), ibuprofen (Motrin), naproxen (Naprosyn), ketorolac tromethamine (Toradol), and celecoxib (Celebrex) also work in the CNS, but their better-characterized actions are peripheral (at the site of injury), where they are thought to exert analgesic effects through the inhibition of prostaglandin production. Prostaglandin is an inflammatory mediator, released when cells are damaged, that sensitizes nerves that carry information about pain. By inhibiting prostaglandin release, these drugs diminish transmission of pain stimuli.
- **Opioids.** Opioids probably relieve pain mainly by action in the CNS, binding to opioid receptor sites in the brain and the spinal cord. There are multiple opioid receptor sites. When a drug binds to any of these sites, pain relief occurs. When a drug attaches to these opioid receptor sites as an antagonist, pain relief and other effects are blocked. A well-known opioid antagonist is naloxone (Narcan), which antagonizes (blocks or reverses) the action of all opioids.
- **Adjuvant analgesics.** It is not possible to identify any one mechanism of action for pain relief for this analgesic group. This group is composed of diverse classes of drugs that relieve pain by a variety of mechanisms, many of which are not understood. For example, certain antidepressants appear to relieve pain by blocking the reuptake of serotonin, resulting in the presence of greater amounts of serotonin. Orally formulated local anesthetics such as mexiletine (Mexitil) and certain anticonvulsants such as carbamazepine (Tegretol) are sodium channel blocking agents, and this is perhaps part of the mechanism underlying their ability to relieve certain types of pain. Neuropathic pain is difficult to treat. Gabapentin (Neurontin), an anticonvulsant, binds to the neocortex and is used in the treatment of chronic neuropathic pain. Duloxetine (Cymbalta), an antidepressant, is used for control of the pain associated with diabetic neuropathy, as is pregabaline (Lyrica), an anticonvulsant.

Administration Routes for Analgesics

Learn the most effective analgesic and means of administration for the patient's specific need. It takes skill to determine the most effective method of administration.

The IV route is best for administration of opioid analgesics after major surgery. The most appropriate opioids for pain relief for rapidly escalating, severe pain include morphine, hydromorphone, and fentanyl. For rapid onset of analgesia to treat escalating pain, give these drugs by the IV route. They are suitable for bolus administration and continuous infusion, including patient-controlled analgesia (PCA). The ability to obtain a dose when it is needed places the patient in control and eliminates the wait for medication to be given.

IM administration of opioids is associated with wide fluctuations in absorption, including delayed absorption in postoperative patients, making it an ineffective and potentially dangerous method of managing pain. Furthermore, repeated IM injections are often painful and traumatic, deterring patients from requesting medications for relief of pain; they also have the potential to cause fibrosis of muscle and soft tissue and sterile abscesses. In general, therefore, avoid the IM route, especially repeated IM administration.

The oral route is often the optimal route, especially for chronic pain treatment, because of its convenience, its flexibility, and the relatively steady blood levels produced. However, the IV route is usually necessary when a quick onset of analgesia is desired or when the patient is unable to take oral medication. When the pain is under control, the regimen will then be changed to give the analgesic orally. Oral administration is convenient and inexpensive. Its use is appropriate as soon as the patient can tolerate oral intake and is the mainstay of pain management for ambulatory surgical patients.

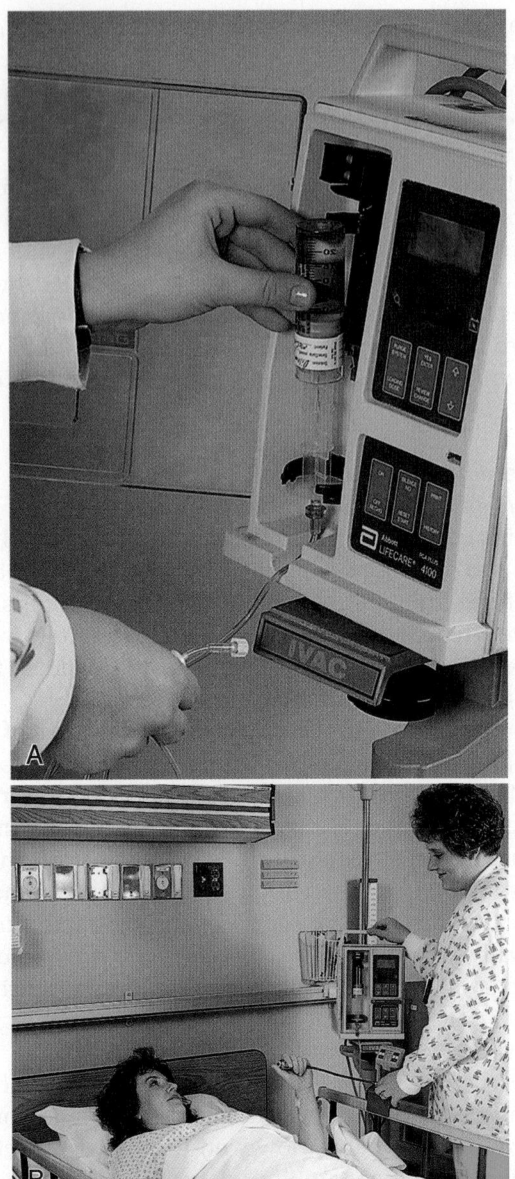

FIGURE 16-4 **A,** PCA pump with syringe chamber. **B,** Patient learns to use PCA pump.

Patient-Controlled Analgesia

A drug delivery system called **patient-controlled analgesia (PCA)** allows patients to self-administer analgesics whenever needed. The PCA is a portable, computerized pump with a chamber for a syringe (Figure 16-4). The pump delivers a small, preset dose of IV medication, usually morphine, meperidine, hydromorphone, or fentanyl. To receive a dose, the patient pushes a button on a cord attached to the pump. A timer prevents the system from delivering more than a specified number of doses every hour, to prevent overdose. Each dose may be as small as 1 mL or 1 mg of morphine every 6 to 12 minutes. It has a locked safety system that prevents tampering.

PCA is based on the idea that only the patient can feel the pain and only the patient knows how much analgesic will relieve it. By allowing patients to determine the need for doses, PCA addresses the significant variations in analgesic requirements between individuals.

Analgesia is more effective when the patient, rather than the nurse or the physician, is in control. PCA is similar to responsive prn dosing in that it requires patients to recognize that they are experiencing pain and request analgesia (e.g., by pressing a button on a pump to deliver a PCA bolus). The difference between prn and PCA is that with PCA, the patient rather than a nurse administers the analgesic, so the delay in waiting for a nurse's response to the request for analgesia is eliminated. Just as with effective prn administration, remind patients to "stay on top of pain" to maintain a steady analgesic level and self-administer a dose before pain is severe and out of control.

PCA has been used to manage all types of acute pain, although less often for cancer pain because most cancer pain is manageable with orally administered opioids. To be a candidate for PCA, a patient is

Patient Teaching

Preparation for Patient-Controlled Analgesia

- Teach the use of patient-controlled analgesia (PCA) before surgery so that patients will know how to use it after awakening from anesthesia. (Confused and unresponsive patients, patients with neurologic disease, patients with impaired renal or pulmonary function, and those unable to press the delivery button are not candidates for PCA.)
- Instruct patients on the purpose of PCA, operating instructions, lockout intervals, expected pain relief, precautions, and potential side effects, emphasizing that the patient controls medication delivery.
- Explain that the pump prevents overdose.
- Tell family members and friends not to operate the PCA device for the patient.
- Have the patient demonstrate use of the PCA delivery button.

required to be alert, oriented, and able to follow simple directions. Patient preparation and teaching is critical to the safe and effective use of PCA (see Patient Teaching box).

Older adult patients and those with respiratory compromise or hypovolemia are typically at high risk for respiratory complications with IV opioids of any type. They and patients with significant impairment of renal or hepatic function will most likely be determined unsuitable candidates to use PCA.

If someone other than the patient pushes the button on a PCA pump, even at the patient's request, it is termed *PCA by proxy.* Proxy administration of opioids leads to possible oversedation and opioid toxicity. PCA is for patient use only and nurses, patients, and visitors need to be reminded not to push the button.

Although patients with pain often self-administer their oral analgesics, the term PCA is applied usually when administering opioids by the IV and epidural routes. Typically, a special infusion pump is used to deliver PCA by these routes. In this context, PCA refers to the bolus dose the patient controls when pressing a button on or attached to the pump. PCA is delivered by one of two modes: PCA bolus doses with a continuous infusion (also called a basal rate) or PCA bolus doses alone.

It is your responsibility to assess the IV site and the PCA drug delivery system for proper functioning and correct drug dosing. Also assess the patient for signs of oversedation and respiratory depression. Document the amount of opioid used as well as any waste of the medication (Potter & Perry, 2009).

Epidural Analgesia

Another method of delivery of analgesia is the insertion of an epidural catheter and the infusion of opiates into the epidural space. Containing blood vessels, fat, and nerves, the epidural space is a "potential" space (there is no free-flowing fluid in it) between the walls of the vertebral canal and the dura mater of the spinal cord. It surrounds the spinal meninges and extends from the foramen magnum to the sacral hiatus. The epidural medication diffuses slowly from the epidural space across the dura and arachnoid membranes into the cerebrospinal fluid (Figure 16-5). Epidural administration of opioids brings the drug close to the action site (opioid receptors); therefore, as compared with systemic administration, relatively small doses are effective. Because of the vasculature in the epidural space, the drug is also absorbed systemically. There are three methods of administering epidural analgesia: by bolus doses, continuous infusion, and patient-controlled epidural analgesia (PCEA).

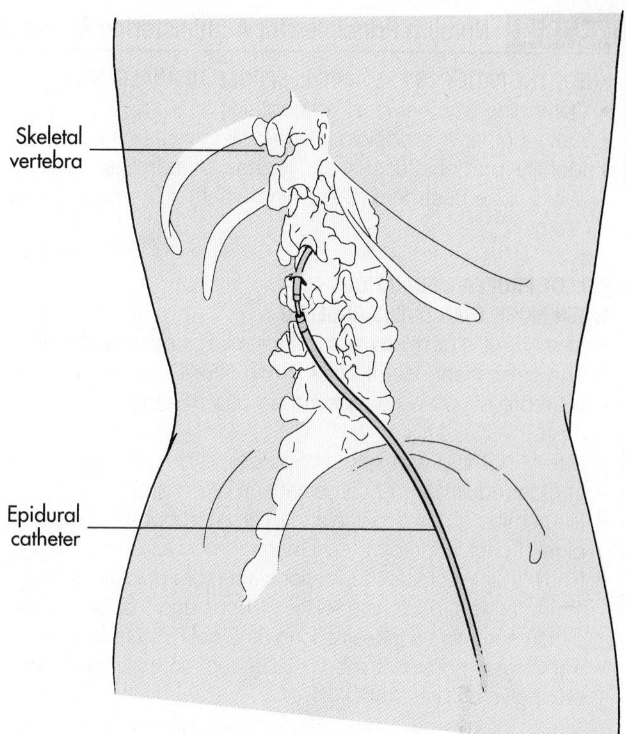

FIGURE 16-5 Epidural catheter.

Drugs used for epidural analgesia are morphine, fentanyl, and hydromorphone. The epidural opioids also have side effects: urinary retention, postural hypotension, pruritus, nausea, vomiting, and respiratory depression. Monitor respiratory rate carefully every 15 minutes during infusion. The epidural route of administration is an appropriate first-line route for moderate to severe acute pain expected to last for at least 24 hours. An abundance of research over the past two decades has demonstrated superior pain relief and improved functional outcomes after major surgery in patients who receive epidural analgesia, compared with patients receiving traditional postoperative pain management, such as IV PCA (Pasero, 2003). Epidural

Box 16-2 Nursing Principles for Administering Analgesics

KNOW THE PATIENT'S PREVIOUS RESPONSE TO ANALGESICS

- Determine whether relief was obtained.
- Ask whether a nonopioid was as effective as an opioid.
- Identify previous doses and routes of administration to avoid undertreatment. Determine whether the patient has allergies.

SELECT PROPER MEDICATIONS WHEN MORE THAN ONE IS ORDERED

- Use NSAIDs or milder opioids for mild to moderate pain.
- The concurrent use of opioids and NSAIDs often provides far more effective analgesia than use of either drug class alone.
- Use of NSAIDs can help reduce opioid side effects.
- In older adults, avoid combinations of opioids.
- Remember that morphine and hydromorphone are the opioids of choice for long-term management of severe pain.
- Know that injectable medications act more quickly, often relieving severe, acute pain within 1 hour, and that oral medication sometimes takes as long as 2 hours to take effect.
- For longer, more sustained relief in connection with chronic pain, give an oral drug.

KNOW THE OPTIMAL DOSAGE

- Remember that doses at the upper end of normal are generally needed for severe pain.
- Adjust doses, as appropriate, for children and older patients.
- Dosage typically requires adjustment over time.
- Know the comparative potencies of analgesics (refer to drug manual or pharmacy) in oral and injectable forms.

ASSESS THE RIGHT TIME AND INTERVAL FOR ADMINISTRATION

- Use an appropriate pain scale for more accurate pain assessment.
- Administer analgesics as soon as pain occurs and before it increases in severity.
- Do not give analgesics only on "as needed" schedules. An around-the-clock administration schedule is best.
- Give analgesics before pain-producing procedures or activities.
- Know the average duration of action for a drug, and time the administration so that the peak effect occurs when the pain is most intense.

CHOOSE THE RIGHT ROUTE

- Intravenous and oral routes are preferred.
- Intramuscular and subcutaneous administration are best avoided, because these routes are frequently painful and absorption is not reliable. Intramuscular injections have the potential to cause fibrosis of muscle and soft tissue and sterile abscesses.

From Potter, P.A., & Perry, A.G. (2007). *Basic nursing: essentials for practice.* (6th ed.). St. Louis: Mosby.

analgesia is beneficial for controlling acute pain during labor and for relieving chronic pain, such as that seen in patients with advanced cancer (Elkin et al., 2007) (Box 16-2).

The insertion and maintenance of the epidural catheter for the infusion are invasive techniques that are the responsibility of the anesthetist or the anesthesiologist. Nursing staff members are responsible for monitoring the patient's level of consciousness, pain intensity, respiratory rate, and the infusion rate and volume on the pump. Also examine the dressing site for signs of infection or leakage of medication around the catheter (Table 16-2).

RESPONSIBILITY OF THE NURSE IN PAIN CONTROL

The founding principle of effective pain management is Meinhart and McCaffery's statement that "the failure to treat pain is inhumane and constitutes professional negligence" (Meinhart & McCaffery, 1983). Every patient has the right to be free of pain; it is the nurse's responsibility to do everything possible to alleviate the patient's pain.

Assist the patient in pain relief by telling the patient, "I believe that you are in pain, and I will assist you in whatever way I can to reduce or relieve your pain." This reduces the patient's anxiety level. Do not make the patient expend energy convincing you that the pain is real. Begin pain intervention as soon as the patient states that she or he is in pain.

Encourage the patient to be an active participant by telling you when pain occurs. Also assess the patient for nonverbal expressions of pain. If any pain-producing procedure is scheduled, such as ambulating, coughing, or a dressing change, give an analgesic beforehand. Administer the drug so that its peak effect is reached during the patient's most active time.

Probably no other area of nursing involves patient advocacy to the same extent as pain control. In all nursing fields, the nurse advocates for the patient by clarifying concerns, answering questions, supplying all the information the patient needs to make decisions about care, and supporting the patient's decisions. Effective patient advocacy requires time, patience, and courage. Good listening skills are essential. Ask the patient how he or she is, and attentively wait to hear the answer.

At times you may be the only person who "advocates" or believes that the patient has pain. This will probably be a disconcerting experience for you, one that requires patience and energy. Advocacy is critical if you are to be effective in pain management.

The ultimate goal of pain management is to provide pain relief and enable the patient to carry on with activities of daily living in as comfortable a manner as possible. If pain is to be prevented or managed well, it

Table 16-2 Nursing Interventions for Patients with Epidural Infusions

GOAL	ACTIONS
Prevent catheter displacement	Secure catheter (if not connected to implanted reservoir) carefully to outside skin.
Maintain catheter function	Check external dressing around catheter site for dampness or discharge. (Leak of cerebrospinal fluid may develop.) Use transparent dressing to secure catheter and to aid inspection. Inspect catheter for breaks.
Prevent infection	Use strict aseptic technique when caring for catheter. Do not routinely change dressing over site. Change infusion tubing every 24 hours. (RN)
Monitor for respiratory depression	Monitor vital signs, especially respirations, per policy. Use pulse oximetry and apnea monitoring as appropriate.
Prevent undesirable complications	Assess for pruritus (itching) and nausea and vomiting. Administer antiemetics as ordered.
Maintain urinary and bowel function	Monitor intake and output. Assess for bladder and bowel distention. Assess for discomfort, frequency, and urgency.

From Potter, P.A., & Perry, A.G. (2009). *Fundamentals of nursing: concepts, process, and practice.* (7th ed.). St. Louis: Mosby.
RN, Registered nurse.

 Home Care Considerations

Pain Management in the Home

- Current practice features recognition of the need to include the patient and family in planning and implementing effective pain management strategies.
- With so much care being given in clinics, physicians' offices, and patients' homes rather than in hospitals, the need for well-informed patients and families has become even more important.
- Explain the pain management program that is likely to be used in the patient's home.
- Discuss and have the patient practice pain management techniques to use in the home.
- Home health and hospice patients are assessed for pain at every visit. Instruct patients to notify a home health or hospice nurse at any time of unrelieved pain.

is imperative that physicians, nurses, and others caring for the patient understand the pain management plan. Assessment of the patient's pain is ongoing and is documented with each assessment and reassessment. There is increasing emphasis on combining psychosocial and drug approaches in the pain treatment plan (see Home Care Considerations box).

Pain management is a challenge that every nurse must face, regardless of the practice setting. In fact, the nurse's role in pain management is probably more important than that of any other member of the health care team (see Nursing Care Plan 16-1).

NURSING ASSESSMENT OF PAIN

Collection of Subjective Data

Because pain is a subjective experience, it is vital that you become a well-versed and competent practitioner of the art of pain assessment. Obtaining accurate information from the patient concerning the pain, including characteristics and description of the pain, is critical. Characteristics worth noting include the site, the severity, the duration, and the location of pain. When documenting the presence of pain, describe the specific location and intensity. Charting "patient complains of pain" provides no useful information. It is necessary to ask the patient what relieves the pain, what actions cause the pain to be worse, and what does not relieve the pain. Sociocultural information is worthwhile to obtain; for instance, identify usual coping mechanisms and the patient's, the family's, and friends' expectations of appropriate behavior when in pain (see Cultural Considerations box). If medications are taken for relief of pain, the name, the dosage, the frequency, and the effect of the drugs must be determined.

Be sensitive to the patient's condition. Obviously, it is appropriate to ask only a few key questions at any given time of patients who are critically ill or in excruciating pain; do not subject them to a long list of questions. Project your interest and concern for the patient so that he or she will openly discuss the pain.

Try to have patients use their own words to describe the pain, because the terms they use will often provide clues about the etiology of the pain. For example, patients who experience chest pain during a myocardial infarction frequently describe the pain as a pressure or as if someone were squeezing the chest.

There has been interest recently in developing tools specifically for assessment of pain. Nurses are frequently faced with difficulties in assessing pain. A pain scale will help with this assessment; it allows the patient to rate the pain and you to measure its intensity.

Nursing Care Plan 16-1 The Patient with Chronic Pain

Mr. Jaccoud is a 45-year-old patient with a 15-year history of severe, crippling rheumatoid arthritis. He has had numerous joint replacements, has had a weight loss of 40 pounds in the past year, and has developed corneal ulcers from the presence of Sjögren syndrome. He is in constant chronic pain and has limited mobility. He states that he has difficulty accomplishing activities of daily living (ADLs).

NURSING DIAGNOSIS ***Chronic pain, related to joint and muscle inflammation and degeneration manifested by complaints of pain, anorexia, narrow focus of interest, fatigue, guarded movement, changes in sleep pattern, and social withdrawal***

Patient Goals and Expected Outcomes	Nursing Interventions	Evaluation
Patient or family (or both) will verbalize a reduction in anxiety and pain when using relaxation, massage, cutaneous stimulation, and analgesics within 1 hour after initiation of pain relief measures	Encourage patient to report pain or discomfort location, intensity, duration using the pain scale. Teach relaxation exercises. Perform massage to relieve pain and to enhance communication. Administer analgesics and apply cold or heat applications as ordered. Maintain transcutaneous electric nerve stimulation (TENS) as ordered. Encourage relaxation by teaching use of guided imagery.	Patient indicates improved pain relief within 1 hour of implementation of pain management techniques. Patient reports pain level reduced to 4 on a scale of 0 to 10.

NURSING DIAGNOSIS ***Chronic low self-esteem, related to inability to work and carry out ADLs, and with body image changes, manifested by preoccupation with body changes, verbalization of powerlessness, expressions of guilt, and self-negating verbalizations***

Patient Goals and Expected Outcomes	Nursing Interventions	Evaluation
Patient will verbalize understanding of changes in body image caused by disease process and will begin to exhibit increased confidence in dealing with self-esteem within 1 week	Encourage verbalization about fears and anxiety; listen attentively. Deal with behavioral changes, denial, powerlessness, anxiety, and dependence. Be supportive in setting goals. Encourage independence, and give praise for tasks accomplished. Modify environment, and allow time for patient to accomplish goals.	Patient states improved feeling of self-esteem within 1 week of implementation of techniques outlined.

Critical Thinking Questions

1. During the morning ADLs, Mr. Jaccoud states, "I feel so useless. I can't even place the urinal for myself." What would be the nurse's most therapeutic response?
2. What would be the most useful nursing intervention to achieve the goal of reduced pain during Mr. Jaccoud's assisted ambulation?
3. Which comfort measures could the nurse perform to ensure that Mr. Jaccoud has several hours of restorative sleep?
4. Mr. Jaccoud complains of his eyes burning and feeling dry and the lights annoying him. What measures are most likely to help relieve his symptoms?

Pain Rating Scales

Visual analog scales and numerical scales are commonly used to qualify the intensity of the pain experience (Figure 16-6).

With the **visual analog scale,** the patient marks a spot on a horizontal line to indicate pain intensity (intensity increases as the line moves from left to right). The most frequently used numerical scale is 0 to 10; the patient chooses the correct pain rating, with 0 being no pain and 10 being the worst pain imaginable. A visual scale with numerical ratings combines both, providing a description and facial expressions with assigned numbers from numbers 0 to 10 (see Figure 30-8). For clinical assessment, any of these scales is adequate and appropriate. It is important to always use the same scale with the same patient. All personnel in a given health care setting also need to use the same scale.

A good pain scale is easy to use and not time consuming. If a patient is able to read and understand a scale easily, the description of pain will be more accurate. If the patient wears a hearing aid or glasses, be sure they are worn when the patient is answering pain assessment questions or marking a pain scale. Several pain scales have been developed to assess pain in chil-

Cultural Considerations

Pain Management

- The primary strategy for working with a patient in pain from a different culture is to establish a relationship by listening, showing respect, and allowing the patient to help develop and choose treatment options.
- To further increase your cultural sensitivity, cultivate rapport with your patient and the patient's family, maintain an open attitude, and remain flexible.
- Understanding cultural background and personal characteristics will help you more accurately assess pain and its meaning to patients.
- In some instances, you will not be from a comparable culture or religion; therefore, the key is to assess the patient's needs, ways, and customs as thoroughly and sensitively as possible.
- You will perhaps not understand some non-Western pain remedies, so it is important that the patient feels free to ask for what is needed.
- It is important to respect the patient's attitudes and beliefs about pain, as well as preferred treatment options, even if these conflict with your beliefs about pain treatment.
- During the assessment process, explore how the patient feels about combining therapies so that the patient is made familiar with a range of pain treatment options.
- Many Latino men believe that men are supposed to endure pain without complaining and that alleviating it would be "unmanly" and demeaning in the eyes of their children.
- Many Chinese people avoid eye contact, making pain assessment more difficult.
- Italian, Jewish, African-American, and Spanish-speaking people often smile readily and use facial expressions and gestures to communicate pain or displeasure.
- Irish, English, and northern European people tend to show fewer facial expressions and are less responsive, especially to strangers such as professional caregivers.

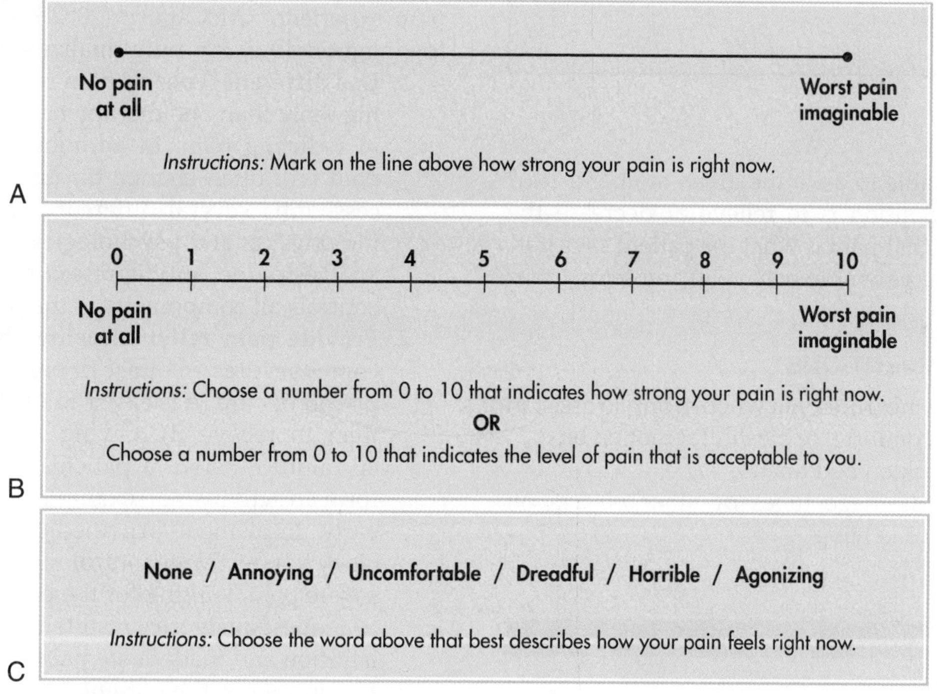

FIGURE 16-6 Sample pain scales. **A,** Visual analog. **B,** Numerical. **C,** Verbal descriptive.

dren. Wong and Baker developed the FACES pain rating scale (see Figure 30-8). Most patients require a pain level of 4 or less to function well.

Collection of Objective Data

Carefully observe the patient. Possible objective signs are tachycardia, increased rate and depth of respirations, diaphoresis, increased systolic or diastolic blood pressure, pallor, dilated pupils, and increased muscle tension. Some patients complain of nausea or weakness (Box 16-3). Other patients have a subjective complaint of pain with no observable objective signs.

If the pain is chronic or less severe, the physiologic changes are likely to be less prominent. You will sometimes notice changes in facial expressions, such as frowning or gritting teeth. Some people clench their fists and withdraw when in pain. Others will complain bitterly, cry, moan, toss about in bed, assume a fetal position, or clutch at the affected body part. Still others will pace, if they have energy to do so. Some patients in pain want someone in constant attendance, whereas others want to be left alone.

Be unbiased and nonjudgmental when gathering objective data; consider that the patient is doing the

Box 16-3 Objective Signs of Pain

PHYSIOLOGIC SIGNS

Pulse: increased rate
Respirations: increased depth and frequency
Blood pressure: increased systolic and diastolic
The body seeks equilibrium. In an hour or less, vital signs usually return to what they were previously, even if the patient is still in severe pain. Continuous severe pain will in some cases cause vital signs to increase again from time to time, but they rarely remain elevated.
Diaphoresis, pallor
Dilated pupils
Muscle tension (face, body)
Nausea and vomiting (if pain is severe)

BEHAVIORAL SIGNS

Rigid body position
Restlessness
Frowning
Grimacing
Clenched teeth
Clenched fists
Crying
Moaning

best he or she is able to do at the given moment. Your immediate intervention is to relieve or decrease the pain. Remember that pain is what the patient says it is. Do not expect the patient to behave in any set manner when in pain.

NURSING INTERVENTIONS

The following are measures you will perform to assist in pain control and comfort (see Health Promotion box):

- Tighten wrinkled bed linens
- Reposition drainage tubes or other objects on which patient is lying
- Place warm bath blankets if the patient is cold
- Loosen constricting bandages
- Change moist dressings
- Check tape to prevent pulling on skin
- Position patient in anatomic alignment
- Check temperature of hot and cold applications, including bath water
- Lift—do not pull—patient up in bed; handle gently
- Position patient correctly on bedpan
- Avoid exposing skin or mucous membranes to irritants (e.g., diarrheal stool or wound drainage)
- Prevent urinary retention by ensuring patency of Foley catheter
- Prevent constipation by encouraging appropriate fluid intake, diet, and exercise and administering prescribed stool softeners

Health Promotion

Promoting Comfort

- Measures that promote a sense of well-being to minimize or avoid discomfort include warm baths, thorough personal hygiene, and adequate rest.
- Pain has the potential to disable and immobilize a person enough to impair the ability to perform self-care activities. This results in social isolation, depression, and changes in self-concept. Help patients and families learn to discuss their feelings about the loss of function, and to find ways to cope with pain and the lifestyle it imposes.
- When a patient has chronic, disabling pain, instruct family members on proper positioning techniques and methods of assisting the patient with ambulation.
- A number of nonpharmacologic or complementary therapies are used for pain relief, including massage, guided imagery, music, biofeedback, meditation, hypnosis, exercise, therapeutic touch, acupuncture, and relaxation techniques.

Guidelines for Individualizing Pain Therapy

In providing pain relief measures, it is important for you to choose therapies suited to the patient's unique pain experience. McCaffery (2002b) suggests the following guidelines for individualizing pain therapy:

1. **Use different types of pain relief measures.** Using more than one therapy has an additive effect in reducing pain. In addition, the character of pain will often change throughout the day, necessitating several different therapies. Combining physical and psychological approaches (e.g., analgesics or antidepressants and relaxation) controls all components of the pain experience.
2. **Provide pain relief measures before pain becomes severe.** An ounce of prevention is worth a pound of cure (it is easier to prevent severe pain than to relieve it). Giving an analgesic 30 to 40 minutes before a patient must walk or perform an activity is an example of controlling pain early. Implement prn medications around the clock to effectively control moderately severe to severe pain. Waiting for the patient or the family to request analgesics results in delays in administration and inadequate pain control.
3. **Use measures the patient believes are effective.** The patient is the expert on the pain and will likely have realistic ideas about what measures to use (e.g., rubbing lotion on an edematous finger) and when to use them.
4. **Consider the patient's ability or willingness to participate in pain relief measures.** Some patients are not able to actively assist with pain therapy because of fatigue, sedation, or altered levels of consciousness. However, there are variations of pain relief measures that require little effort, such as relaxation exercises in bed or listening to music as a distraction. You will not relieve pain by forcing an unwilling patient to participate in therapy. The depressed patient with chronic pain has little motivation to participate.

5. **Choose pain relief measures appropriate to the severity of the pain as reflected by the patient's behavior.** It would be poor judgment to administer a potent opioid to a patient who is displaying only mild pain. Carefully assess what the patient says before choosing pain therapy. Some patients acquire relief from severe pain after using only mild analgesics. Only the patient can determine the degree of effectiveness of a therapy.
6. **If a therapy is ineffective at first, encourage the patient to try it again before abandoning it.** Often anxiety or doubt prevents patients from gaining relief from therapy. Some approaches, such as distraction, require practice. Some measures that seem ineffective merely require adjustment to become effective. For example, try increasing the dosage of an analgesic if severe pain is initially unrelieved. Be persistent and understanding in helping the patient learn to use measures that do not afford immediate relief.
7. **Keep an open mind about what has potential to relieve pain.** New ways are sometimes found to control pain. There is much to be learned about the pain experience. Rejecting a patient's unconventional therapies will lead to mistrust. It is, however, your responsibility to monitor therapies to ensure the patient's safety and well-being.
8. **Keep trying.** It is easy to become frustrated when efforts at pain relief fail. It is important not to abandon the patient when pain persists. Some patients in severe chronic pain who are ignored choose suicide as an alternative. If the patient gains no relief, reassess the situation and consider whether alternative therapies are needed.
9. **Protect the patient.** Pain therapy that causes more distress than the pain itself is misguided and inappropriate. Always observe the response to therapy. Any pain relief measure poses a risk of side effects, such as fatigue, anxiety, or additional pain. Your aim is to relieve pain without disabling the patient mentally, emotionally, or physically. It is important to maintain safety of the patient and environment.

SLEEP AND REST

A patient at rest feels mentally relaxed, free from worry, and physically calm. A patient at rest is free from physical or mental exertion. Everyone has their own method of obtaining rest and is usually able to adjust to new environments or conditions affecting the ability to rest.

You will probably care for patients for whom bed rest has been prescribed. This treatment confines patients to bed to decrease physical or psychological demands on the body. Bed rest does not necessarily mean a patient is resting. Emotional or metabolic stressors naturally cause the patient to be restless.

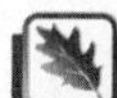

Life Span Considerations

Older Adults

Sleep

- Older adults require about the same amount of sleep as younger people but are more likely to achieve it in separate episodes; they take more naps and get less sleep at night.
- The sleep of an older adult is less deep. This increases the risk of early awakening and complaints of sleep disturbance.
- Sleep is likely to be disturbed in older adults with chronic health problems such as arthritis, heart failure, and chronic obstructive pulmonary disease. Adequate pain control and positioning facilitate breathing and help promote rest and sleep.
- Older adults often take medications such as diuretics and theophylline that are likely to disturb sleep. Carefully assess time of administration and the effect on sleep and modify when possible.
- Insufficient sleep may lead to memory and personality changes in older adults.
- Include nonpharmacologic comfort measures among nursing interventions to promote rest and sleep.

Sleep is a state of rest that occurs for a sustained period. The reduced consciousness during sleep provides time for repair and recovery of body systems for the next period of wakefulness. The theory that sleep is associated with healing suggests that achieving optimum sleep quality is important for patients' recovery. Sleep restores a person's energy and feeling of well-being.

Hospital or other health care facility routines are quick to disrupt the rest and sleep habits of the patient (Box 16-4). The extent of the change depends on the gravity of the illness, as well as the environment in which the patient is placed. It is important to remain aware of the patient's need for rest. Without it, the patient becomes fatigued and irritable and has a decreased ability to cope with stressors (see Life Span Considerations for Older Adults box on sleep).

PHYSIOLOGY OF SLEEP

Sleep is a cyclic physiologic process that alternates with longer periods of wakefulness. The sleep-wake cycle influences and regulates body functions and behavioral responses.

People experience cyclic rhythms as part of their everyday life. The most familiar rhythm is the 24-hour day-night cycle known as the diurnal or circadian rhythm. All circadian rhythms, including the sleep-wake cycle, are affected by light and temperature and external factors such as social activities and environmental stressors. All of us have a biologic clock that synchronizes our sleep cycles. Some people are able to fall asleep at 8 PM, whereas others go to bed at midnight or early in the morning. Different people also function best at different times of the day.

Box 16-4 Factors Affecting Sleep

PHYSICAL ILLNESS
- Pain and physical discomfort result in difficulty falling or staying asleep.
- Chronic pain sometimes has a circadian rhythm including increasing intensity at night, thus disrupting sleep.
- Illness frequently forces patients to sleep in positions to which they are unaccustomed.
- Respiratory diseases interfere with the rhythm of breathing and sometimes oblige a person to assume a certain position to be able to breathe easily. Both factors can disturb sleep.
- Patients with heart disease are often afraid to go to sleep at night.
- Hypertension causes early morning awakening and fatigue.
- Nocturia and "restless legs syndrome" disrupt sleep, causing patients to awaken and have trouble falling back to sleep during the night.
- Conditions that increase intracranial pressure or alter central nervous system physiology alter sleep patterns and sometimes cause excessive daytime sleeping.

ANXIETY AND DEPRESSION
- As anxiety and depression increase, so does lack of sleep; as sleep decreases, anxiety and depression increase.
- The bereaved often experience sleep problems related to fear of intruders, loneliness, and the dreams or nightmares that occur involving the lost loved one.

DRUGS AND SUBSTANCES
- Various drugs and substances affect the pattern and the quality of sleep.
- Hypnotics interfere with reaching deeper sleep stages, provide only temporary (1-week) increase in quality of sleep, and eventually cause "hangover" feeling during the day. Hypnotics often worsen sleep apnea in older adults.
- Older adults often take several drugs, the combined effects of which disrupt sleep.
- L-tryptophan, a protein found in foods such as milk, cheese, and meats, frequently helps induce sleep.

LIFESTYLE
- Daily routines such as work shifts influence sleep patterns; changing them, as with rotating shifts, disrupts these patterns. Only after several weeks of working a night shift does a person's biologic clock adjust.
- Performing unaccustomed heavy work, late-night social activities, and changing evening mealtimes are activities that can disrupt sleep.

SLEEP PATTERNS
- Sleep patterns include starting time and duration of sleep. The most significant cause of daytime sleepiness is inadequate or abnormal sleep at night.
- Everyone has an increased sleep tendency from 2 AM to 7 AM.
- When sleep patterns are disrupted, the natural tendency to be sleeping at certain times increases.
- Sleep patterns influence succeeding attempts to fall asleep because of changes in circadian rhythm. Sleeping 1 hour later results in falling asleep 1 hour later the next night.

STRESS
- Stress resulting from personal problems or situational crises causes tension and at times will cause a person to try too hard to fall asleep, to awaken frequently, or to oversleep.
- Stress causes release of corticosteroids and adrenalin, which leads to catabolism and sleeplessness.
- Patients with advanced cancer or chronic illness often are afraid to go to sleep for fear they might die.
- Older patients experience losses such as retirement or death of a loved one. The stress of these losses will sometimes cause older adults to suffer delays in falling asleep, earlier REM sleep, frequent awakening, increased total bedtime, and feelings of sleeping poorly.

ENVIRONMENT
- Environmental factors influence the ability to fall and remain asleep. Significant factors include ventilation, lighting, type of bed, sound level, and the presence or absence of a bed partner.
- In hospitals, unfamiliar noises and higher noise levels such as that created by wall suction, opening packages, ringing alarms, and flushing toilets have the capacity to cause sleep deprivation.
- Intensive care units are sources of high noise levels.

EXERCISE AND FATIGUE
- Exercise and fatigue in moderation usually facilitate restful sleep, but excess fatigue from exhausting or stressful work typically make falling asleep difficult.
- Exercise 2 hours before bedtime allows the body to cool down and promotes relaxation.

NUTRITION
- Weight gain causes longer sleep periods with fewer interruptions and later awakening.
- Weight loss sometimes causes reduction in total time spent asleep along with broken sleep and earlier awakening.

The biologic rhythm of sleep frequently becomes synchronized with other body functions. Normal variations in body temperature, for example, correlate with sleep patterns. When the sleep-wake cycle is disrupted (e.g., by working rotating shifts), other physiologic functions typically change as well. For example, a person will sometimes experience a decreased appetite and lose weight. Failure to maintain one's usual sleep-wake cycle is likely to adversely affect a person's overall health (Potter & Perry, 2009).

SLEEP CYCLE

Sleep involves two phases: **rapid eye movement (REM)** and **non–rapid eye movement (NREM)** (Box 16-5). NREM sleep is further divided into four stages through which a sleeper progresses during a typical sleeping cycle. The sleeping stages are highly individualized (Figure 16-7).

Normally an adult's routine sleep pattern begins with a presleep period during which the person is

Box 16-5 Stages of Sleep

NON–RAPID EYE MOVEMENT (NREM) SLEEP

Stage 1

Lightest level of sleep
Lasts a few minutes
Decreased physiologic activity beginning with a gradual fall in vital signs and metabolism
Person easily aroused by sensory stimuli such as noise
If person awakes, feels as though daydreaming has occurred
Reduction in autonomic activities (e.g., heart rate)

Stage 2

Period of sound sleep
Relaxation progresses
Arousal still easy
Lasts 10 to 20 minutes
Body functions still slowing

Stage 3

Initial stages of deep sleep
Sleeper difficult to arouse and rarely moves
Muscles completely relaxed
Vital signs decline but remain regular
Lasts 15 to 30 minutes
Hormonal response includes secretion of growth hormone

Stage 4

Deepest stage of sleep
Very difficult to arouse sleeper
If sleep loss has occurred, sleeper will spend most of night in this stage
Restores and rests the body
Vital signs significantly lower than during waking hours
Lasts approximately 15 to 30 minutes
Possible sleepwalking and enuresis
Hormonal response continues

RAPID EYE MOVEMENT (REM) SLEEP

Stage of vivid, full-color dreaming (less vivid dreaming sometimes occurs in other stages)
First occurs approximately 90 minutes after sleep has begun, thereafter occurs at end of each NREM cycle
Typified by autonomic response of rapidly moving eyes, fluctuating heart and respiratory rates, and increased or fluctuating blood pressure
Loss of skeletal muscle tone
Responsible for mental restoration
Stage in which sleeper is most difficult to arouse
Duration increasing with each cycle and averaging 20 minutes

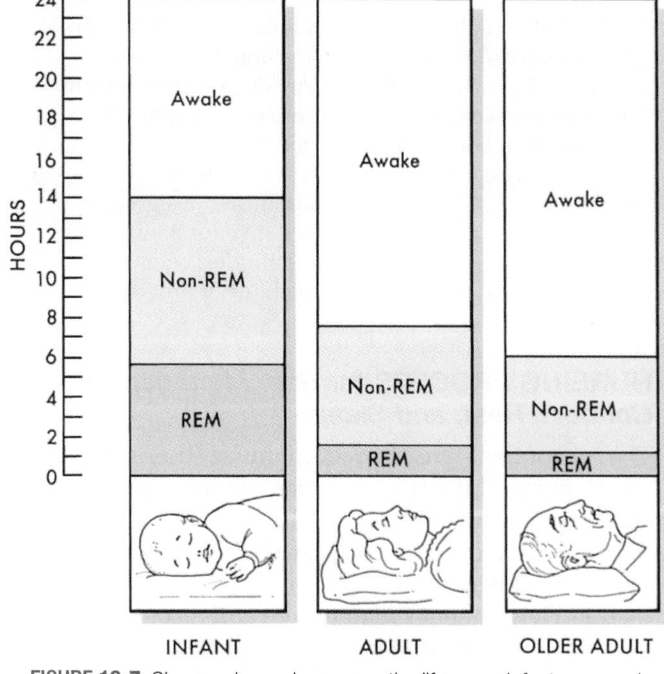

FIGURE 16-7 Sleep-wake cycles across the life span. Infants: approximately 40% of total sleep time is REM. Adults: 20% of total sleep time is REM. Older adults: total sleep time is slightly reduced; REM remains 20% of total.

aware only of a gradually developing drowsiness. This period normally lasts 10 to 30 minutes, but if a person has difficulty falling asleep, it will possibly last an hour or longer.

As adults fall asleep, they progress through the four stages of NREM sleep. At the end of the fourth stage, they come out of a deep sleep, go back to stage 2, and then enter a period of REM. A person reaches REM sleep in about 90 minutes (average). Each person differs, but a typical night's sleep consists of four to six such cycles.

Dreams occur during both the NREM and REM stages. The dream of REM sleep is believed to be functionally important, more vivid, and elaborate, allowing a person to clarify emotions and prepare the mind for events of the next day.

NREM sleep is necessary for body tissue restoration and healthy cardiac function (McCance & Huether, 2006; Potter & Perry, 2009). A person's biologic functions slow during NREM sleep. For example, a healthy adult has a heart rate of 70 to 80 beats per minute during the day; however, during sleep the heart beats at 60 beats per minute or less. Respirations and blood pressure are also decreased during sleep. It is very difficult to arouse the sleeper in REM sleep.

REM sleep is important for brain and cognitive restoration (Buysee, 2005). During REM sleep there are changes in cerebral blood flow and increases in cortical activity, oxygen consumption, and epinephrine release, which are beneficial to memory storage and learning (McCance & Huether, 2006).

SLEEP DEPRIVATION

Sleep deprivation is a problem many patients experience as a result of hospitalization. Sleep deprivation involves decreases in the amount, the quality, and the consistency of sleep. When sleep is interrupted or fragmented, changes in the normal sequence of sleep stages occur, and cycles are not completed. Gradually a cumulative deprivation develops.

Safety Alert!

Daytime Sleepiness

- Safety precautions are important for patients and residents who awaken during the night to use the bathroom and for those with excessive daytime sleepiness.
- Set beds lower to the floor to lessen the chance of the patient or resident falling when first standing.
- Some patients and residents who experience daytime sleepiness fall asleep while sitting up in a chair or wheelchair. Position the person so he or she will not fall out of the chair while sleeping.

Patients experience a variety of physiologic and psychological signs and symptoms. Possible physiologic signs and symptoms include hand tremors, decreased reflexes, slowed response time, reduction in word memory, decreased reasoning and judgment, and cardiac dysrhythmias. Possible psychological signs and symptoms include mood swings, disorientation, irritability, decreased motivation, fatigue, sleepiness, and hyperexcitability.

PROMOTING REST AND SLEEP

Determine the patient's usual rest and sleep patterns, decide whether they are sufficient, and note why the patient is not getting sufficient rest. Work with the patient and the family to develop a plan to provide for more rest. A typical plan includes limiting interruptions during the night for vital sign checks and other procedures, providing a quiet environment with a comfortable room temperature, limiting the number of visitors and the duration of visits, and carrying out all procedures within a given time frame (see Coordinated Care box).

In preparing the patient for sleep, wash the patient's back if the patient is on bed rest, gently massage it, change the linens, make certain the patient is warm enough, offer an uncaffeinated beverage such as milk (if allowed), change soiled dressings, and have the patient void.

Decrease environmental stimuli by dimming the lights and decreasing the noise level. Direct the patient to assume a comfortable position and assist if needed. A night-light is a necessity for promotion of safety in the older adult. Administer a sleeping medication or analgesic as ordered if the patient cannot sleep (see Box 16-4).

Coordinated Care

Supervision

PROMOTING SLEEP

- Encourage nursing assistants to provide a quiet, undisturbed environment for patients or residents that causes the least interference with sleep.
- Instruct the nursing assistant to provide comfort measures such as toileting, a back rub, and a comfortable bed to help the patient or resident prepare for sleep.
- Communicate to the nursing assistant that it is essential to keep excessive noise from conversation or equipment to a minimum because this will easily disturb residents or patients who are already having difficulty sleeping.

Nursing diagnoses and interventions for the patient with sleep disturbance include but are not limited to the following:

Nursing Diagnoses	Nursing Interventions
Disturbed sleep pattern, related to illness and psychological stress manifested by change in behavior, increased irritability, listlessness, and verbal complaints of not feeling well rested	Encourage patient to ambulate in the early evening, if permitted. Provide glass of milk 30 minutes before bedtime unless contraindicated. Perform all necessary procedures before 9 PM to ensure uninterrupted sleep. Massage back, freshen linens, reduce noise, and dim lights. Administer hypnotic as ordered.
Disturbed thought processes, related to sleep deprivation manifested by slower reaction time, altered attention span, and disorientation	Maintain periods of uninterrupted rest. Provide safe environment. Close door to patient room. Orient to reality. Administer analgesic or sedative (or both) about 30 minutes before bedtime, if ordered.

NURSING PROCESS *for Pain Management, Comfort, Rest, and Sleep*

The role of the licensed practical nurse/licensed vocational nurse (LPN/LVN) in the nursing process as stated is that the LPN/LVN will:

- Participate in planning care for patients based on patient needs
- Review patient's plan of care and recommend revisions as needed
- Review and follow defined prioritization for patient care
- Use clinical pathways, care maps, or care plans to guide and review patient care

Assessment

Pain assessment is one of the most frequent and difficult activities a nurse performs. It is crucial to assess the pain experience from the patient's perspective. Make sure patients are aware that informed reporting of pain is valuable and necessary if the health care team is to manage pain effectively.

Terminology

Specific terms are used when assessing pain. **Onset** indicates when the pain began. **Duration** is how long the pain lasts from the onset until it is resolved. Pain is also classified by location. To determine pain location, use a drawing of the body and have the patient mark all the areas where pain is felt. Another method is to ask the patient to point to the places where pain is felt, and you then document those places either on a body outline or descriptively in the medical record and on the care plan. Remind the patient to report new pain sites, because they may signal complications.

Severity indicates whether the pain is mild, moderate, or intense in nature. Sample pain scales are useful to assist you in assessing pain (see Figures 16-3 and 16-6). Terms the patient uses to describe the pain such as **sharp, stabbing, dull,** or **throbbing** provide more information.

Many patients experiencing acute pain will exhibit a rise in pulse rate and blood pressure, diaphoresis, and dilated pupils.

■ Nursing Diagnosis

An accurate nursing diagnosis of the patient with pain will enable you to effectively plan and implement relief measures. The following nursing diagnoses are directly associated with the care of patients with pain:

- Acute pain
- Chronic pain

Other possible nursing diagnoses that are appropriate when pain affects other aspects of a patient's life include the following (NANDA-I, 2007, 2009):

- Activity intolerance
- Anxiety
- Disturbed body image
- Caregiver role strain
- Constipation
- Ineffective coping
- Disabled family coping
- Risk for disuse syndrome
- Interrupted family processes
- Fatigue
- Fear
- Anticipatory grieving
- Dysfunctional grieving
- Hopelessness
- Deficient knowledge (specify)
- Impaired physical mobility
- Imbalanced nutrition: less/more than body requirements
- Powerlessness
- Ineffective role performance
- Bathing/hygiene self-care deficit
- Toileting self-care deficit
- Sexual dysfunction
- Sleep deprivation
- Disturbed sleep pattern
- Impaired social interaction
- Social isolation
- Disturbed thought processes

The extensiveness of the list alerts you to the numerous problems that may develop because of pain.

■ Expected Outcomes and Planning

When participating in the development of the plan of care, you will establish priorities based on the patient's level of pain and its effect on the patient's condition. You and the patient set realistic expectations for pain relief and discuss the degree of pain relief to expect. Typical patient-centered goals and outcomes include the following:

Goal 1: Patient attains a sense of well-being and improved comfort within 1 hour.

Outcome: Patient nonverbally (facial expression, tone of voice) demonstrates improved relief from pain within 1 hour.

Goal 2: Patient regains ability to perform self-care independently within 24 hours.

Outcome: Patient bathes and grooms self without hesitancy or restriction within 24 hours.

■ Implementation

It is important to establish a trusting nurse-patient relationship so the patient believes that relief measures will be beneficial. You help accomplish this best when you see the patient in a holistic manner, listen attentively to concerns, attend promptly to patient needs, and respect any response to pain. In a successful nurse-patient relationship, the nurse understands that the patient is the one who knows more about the patient's pain and its relief.

You will probably teach various measures to help the patient and the family deal with pain. Comfort measures sometimes avert the need for analgesics. Some measures are appropriate positioning and alignment in bed, washing and massaging the back, and ambulation unless contraindicated.

Try teaching distraction and relaxation techniques to the patient. Sometimes distraction and relaxation do not help control the patient's pain, so it is necessary to use analgesic medications.

Nursing interventions that promote the establishment of an effective relationship with the person who is experiencing pain and with the family should include the following:

- **Believe the patient.** The patient needs to be able to trust you to believe in the pain's existence. Convey this message verbally to the patient by saying, "I know you are in pain." Sometimes you will have to help the family believe the patient.
- **Clarify responsibilities in pain relief.** Discuss what you are going to do and what the patient and the family are expected to do.
- **Respect the patient's response to pain.** Accept the right of the patient to respond to the pain in

the necessary manner. The family also needs help in this area. Sometimes the patient will need help to accept the response to the pain, if the behavior is less than is expected by the patient and family.

- **Confer with the patient.** Encourage the patient to use coping techniques that have been effective in the past. Assist the patient and the family to use personal resources more effectively. Help the patient and the family to participate actively in setting goals for pain relief.
- **Explore the pain with the patient.** Find out what the pain means to the person enduring it and to the family.
- **Be with the patient often.** Act as a buffer for the patient and the family during difficult times. Your physical presence will reassure or distract the patient at times and offer variety at others, thus relieving the pain (McCaffery & Pasero, 2003).

Evaluation

Effective communication between you and the patient is essential in achieving pain control. Continuous evaluation allows you to determine whether new or revised therapies are required. Refer to the goals and outcomes identified when planning care, and perform evaluative measures to determine whether the goals have been reached. Examples of goals and evaluative measures include the following:

Goal 1: Patient obtains a sense of well-being and improved pain relief within 1 hour.

Evaluative measure: Ask the patient to rate the pain on a scale of 0 to 10, 10 being the most severe. Observe the patient's facial expressions and body movement, noting whether there is freedom of movement.

Goal 2: Patient regains ability to perform self-care independently within 24 hours.

Evaluative measure: Observe patient performing activities of daily living.

Get Ready for the NCLEX® Examination!

Key Points

- McCaffery has a realistic description of pain: "Pain is whatever the experiencing person says it is, existing whenever he says it does."
- Pain is largely a subjective experience.
- Pain is often a protective mechanism that warns of tissue injury.
- A nurse's bias and misconception of pain potentially results in ineffective control of the patient's pain.
- Pain scales are used to objectively evaluate pain intensity and the effectiveness of pain therapies.
- Making pain the fifth vital sign will ensure that pain is monitored on a regular basis.
- Individualize pain therapy by working closely with the patient, using assessment findings, and trying a variety of therapies.
- Patient-controlled analgesic devices and epidural analgesia give pain control with low risk of overdose.
- Nursing implications for administering epidural analgesia include closely monitoring for respiratory depression.
- Appropriate pain management has the potential to bring about quicker recoveries, shorter hospital stays, fewer readmissions, and improved quality of life.
- Constipation is the most common opioid side effect and the only one for which the individual does not develop tolerance.
- Fatigue, sleep disturbance, and depression act in a type of synergistic relationship that can markedly change one's perception of pain.
- The circadian rhythm is the 24-hour, day-night cycle known also as the diurnal rhythm.

Additional Learning Resources

Go to your Companion CD for an audio glossary, animations, video clips, and more.

evolve Be sure to visit the Evolve site at http://evolve.elsevier.com/Christensen/foundations/ for additional online resources.

Review Questions for the NCLEX® Examination

1. Following surgery for a total knee replacement, a patient was given an epidural catheter for fentanyl epidural analgesia. An important nursing intervention is to:

1. administer additional analgesic medications prn.
2. change the epidural dressing every shift.
3. assess respiratory rate carefully.
4. encourage unassisted ambulation.

2. A 52-year-old patient admitted for deep-vein thrombosis of the left internal iliac vein complains of excruciating pain in his left leg. The most appropriate nursing response is to reassure him by stating:

1. "Pain is what you say it is; I will assist you in whatever way I can."
2. "Your pain is an unpleasant sensation caused by inflammation of the vein and difficult to control."
3. "Your pain is one of the cardinal signs of inflammation."
4. "I know you are in pain, but it is important that we guard against possible addiction to opioids."

3. A 63-year-old patient is first-day postoperative after a lower anterior bowel resection. A common central nervous system analgesic often prescribed for control pain is:

1. aspirin.
2. acetaminophen (Tylenol).
3. morphine.
4. ibuprofen (Motrin).

4. A drug delivery system to control pain via a portable computerized pump with a chamber for a syringe is called:
   1. patient-controlled analgesia.
   2. transcutaneous electric nerve stimulation.
   3. a venous access device.
   4. a placebo.

5. The gate control theory of pain suggests that:
   1. the body contains a natural supply of a morphinelike substance called endorphins.
   2. there are specific nerve fibers that transmit pain impulses to the brain.
   3. pain impulses are regulated or even blocked by mechanisms located along the central nervous system.
   4. pain is a manifestation of an intricate chain of electrochemical events.

6. A patient admitted with severe cellulitis of the left breast states, "I have a severe burning pain, and it feels like my breast is on fire." She rates her pain as 7 on the 0-to-10 pain assessment scale. This collection of data by the nurse in assessing the patient's pain would be:
   1. deductive.
   2. speculative.
   3. objective.
   4. subjective.

7. The nurse listens attentively while the patient describes her angina pectoris pain as radiating down her left inner arm to the little finger and upward to the jaw and the shoulder. This type of pain is called:
   1. precisely localized.
   2. referred.
   3. intermittent.
   4. chronic.

8. The nurse is assessing the patient's description of his back pain. He states that it is "immobilizing, intense, and on a scale of 0 to 10, it is an 8." The pain assessment scale the patient is using is called:
   1. visual analog.
   2. categorical.
   3. functional.
   4. numerical.

9. People who have less pain than others from a similar injury have a:
   1. higher level of endorphins.
   2. lower level of endorphins.

10. Research shows nurses treating pain have a tendency to:
    1. overtreat.
    2. undertreat.

11. A patient was admitted to the orthopedic section for acute back pain. The physician chose to use cutaneous stimulation management, in which the analgesic effects are achieved by closing the gate to pain impulses and release of endorphins. An example of this pain control method is:
    1. epidural analgesia.
    2. transcutaneous electric nerve stimulation (TENS).
    3. NSAIDs.
    4. patient-controlled analgesia.

12. Unrelieved pain is:
    1. to be expected after major surgery.
    2. to be expected in a person with cancer.
    3. dangerous and can lead to many physical and psychological complications.
    4. an annoying sensation, but it is not as important as other physical care needs.

13. An important nursing responsibility related to pain is to:
    1. leave the patient alone to rest.
    2. help the patient appear to not be in pain.
    3. believe what the patient says about pain.
    4. assume responsibility for eliminating the patient's pain.

14. A nurse believes that patients with the same type of tissue injury will have the same amount of pain. This statement reflects:
    1. a belief that will contribute to appropriate pain management.
    2. a belief that will have no effect on the type of care provided to people in pain.
    3. an accurate statement about pain mechanisms and an expected goal of pain therapy.
    4. the nurse's lack of knowledge about pain mechanisms and is likely to contribute to poor pain management.

15. Research indicates that the risk of clinically significant opioid-induced respiratory depression is:
    1. less than 1%.
    2. 5%.
    3. 20%.
    4. 30%.

16. Which route is most appropriate for treating rapidly escalating severe pain?
    1. Oral
    2. IM
    3. IV
    4. Transdermal

17. Which opioid is no longer a drug of choice for managing pain because of its toxic complications, such as causing seizures?
    1. Codeine
    2. Morphine
    3. Meperidine
    4. Fentanyl

18. Which are reasons that the patient-controlled analgesia (PCA) pumps are frequently used for postoperative pain management? *(Select all that apply.)*
    1. PCAs increase patient satisfaction.
    2. PCAs decrease the frequency of patient complaints.
    3. PCAs control the patient's use of opioids and reduce the chance of addiction.
    4. PCAs encourage the use of pain analgesic before the patient experiences severe pain.

chapter

17

Complementary and Alternative Therapies

evolve

http://evolve.elsevier.com/Christensen/foundationsadult

Elaine Oden Kockrow and Barbara Lauritsen Christensen

Objectives

1. Differentiate between complementary and alternative therapies.
2. Describe the practice of holistic nursing.
3. Describe how herbs differ from pharmaceuticals.
4. Explain why a good health history is important for a patient using complementary and alternative therapies.
5. Explain the scope of practice of chiropractic therapy.
6. Describe the principles behind acupuncture and acupressure.
7. Discuss animal-assisted therapy.
8. Explain the difference between acupuncture and acupressure.
9. List three conditions whose presence sometimes contraindicates use of therapeutic massage.
10. Explain how essential oils may be used to provide aromatherapy.
11. Discuss the therapeutic results of yoga.
12. Explain the theory behind reflexology.
13. Describe the purpose and principles of biofeedback.
14. Describe the possible benefits of magnetic therapy.
15. Describe safe and unsafe herbal therapies.
16. Discuss the health benefits of t'ai chi.

Key Terms

acupressure (ĂK-yū-prĕsh-ŭr, p. 424)
acupuncture (ĂK-yū-pŭnk-chŭr, p. 423)
allopathic medicine (ăl-ō-PĂTH-ĭk MĔ-dĭ-sĭn, p. 416)
alternative therapies (p. 416)
aromatherapy (p. 424)
biofeedback (p. 429)
chiropractic therapy (kī-rō-PRĂK-tĭk, p. 423)
complementary therapies (p. 416)
herbal therapy (p. 418)
holistic nursing (hō-LĬS-tĭk NŬRS-ĭng, p. 417)
imagery (p. 426)
meridians (mĕ-RĬD-ē-ănz, p. 423)
pharmaceuticals (făhr-mă-SŪ-tĭ-kălz, p. 418)
Qi (CHĒ, p. 423)
reflexology (p. 424)
relaxation (p. 426)
t'ai chi *or* Taiji (tī JĒ, p. 428)
therapeutic massage (p. 424)
yoga (p. 428)

A greatly increased number of patients are turning to complementary and alternative therapies to help restore or maintain health. This chapter discusses several types of these nontraditional or unconventional therapies, which are frequently referred to as either complementary or alternative medicine (CAM) therapies.

Complementary therapies are therapies used in addition to conventional treatment recommended by a person's health care provider. As the name implies, complementary therapies do not substitute for but rather complement the conventional treatment. Complementary therapies include exercise, massage (Figure 17-1), reflexology, prayer, biofeedback, creative therapies (art, music, or dance therapy), guided imagery, acupuncture, relaxation strategies, chiropractic therapy, therapeutic touch, and herbalism.

Alternative therapies, on the other hand, often include the same interventions as complementary therapies, but frequently become the primary treatment modality that replaces **allopathic medicine** (traditional or conventional Western medicine).

The number of patients seeking unconventional treatments has risen considerably. Between one third and one half of the population of the United States uses one or more forms of CAM (CDC, 2004). In large part, this popularity is due to (1) the perception that the treatments offered by the medical profession do not provide relief for a variety of common illnesses; (2) the increasing interest of patients in becoming more educated about their health and the need to take a more active role in their treatment; (3) the increased number of articles in journals such as *Annals of Behavioral Medicine, Alternative Therapies in Health and Medicine,* and *Journal of Alternative and Complementary Medicine,* as well as coverage of CAM therapies in respected general medical journals; (4) programs seen on television; and (5) the attraction to a holistic approach to health care that incorporates the mind, the body, and the spirit.

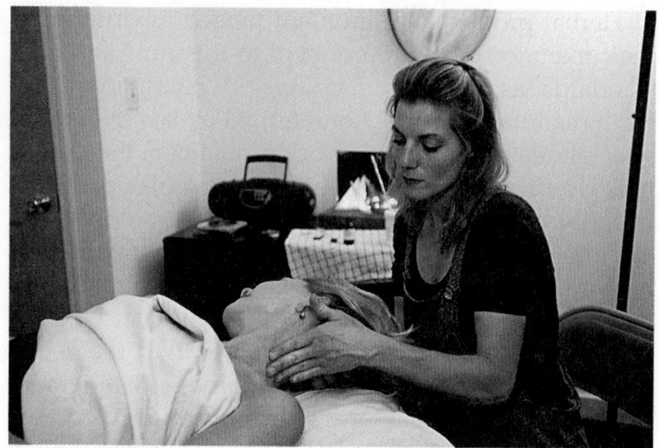

FIGURE 17-1 Massage therapy is used to relieve tension.

People also tend to turn to alternative therapies because they believe them to be less invasive and gentler than allopathic or traditional medicine and perceive them to incorporate a more holistic approach. Prevention is fundamental to most of the CAM therapies. They are not usually used as an immediate cure for an illness or acute injury but provide an ongoing method of maintaining maximum health. Practitioners often recommend lifestyle changes and encourage patients to follow health practices on a daily basis, thereby improving their overall health. Some practitioners incorporate therapies from a variety of treatments to provide holistic care for the patient (Box 17-1).

In contrast, the strength of allopathic medicine is its effectiveness in treating certain physical ailments (e.g., bacterial infections, structural abnormalities, acute emergencies). In general, it focuses less on preventing disease, decreasing stress-induced illnesses, managing chronic disease, and caring for the emotional and spiritual needs of individuals.

Both complementary and alternative therapies vary in the degree to which they are compatible with allopathic or conventional medicine. Many of the complementary therapies, such as acupuncture, make use of diagnostic and therapeutic methods specific to their field, whereas others, such as guided imagery, are essentially adjunctive in nature. For example, chiropractic practitioners frequently use diagnostic terminology and methods similar to those used by allopathic or conventional practitioners. They base interventions on conventional pathophysiology, anatomy, and kinesiology but at the same time explore mind-body connections that they believe drive the physiologic condition. Some alternative therapies, on the other hand, are not supported by scientific data, and some conflict with or even contradict traditional, scientifically-based medical practices.

Some patients will seek to make use of CAM therapies in conjunction with traditional medicine. However, others will choose to make the alternative health care provider the main source of health care. In any case, patients are often hesitant to talk to an allopathic health care provider about any treatment they are receiving other than that prescribed by a medical doctor. It is estimated that almost half of all health care consumers in the United States take some form of herbal or natural product supplement alone or in combination with conventional medicines but rarely report this practice to their health care providers.

Box 17-1 Holistic Nursing

Holistic nursing addresses and treats the mind-body-spirit of the patient. Nurses use holistic nursing interventions such as relaxation therapy, guided imagery, music therapy, simple touch, massage, and prayer. Such interventions affect the whole person (mind-body-spirit) and are effective, economical, noninvasive, nonpharmacologic complements to medical care. Holistic interventions can be used to augment standard treatments, to replace interventions that are ineffective or debilitating, and to promote or maintain health. The American Holistic Nursing Association (2007) maintains standards of holistic nursing practice, which define and establish the scope of holistic practice and describe the level of care expected from a holistic nurse.

- Nurses who provide holistic care need to recognize that prayer is a valued and frequently used coping strategy for many patients, especially cancer patients.
- One means at your disposal to help patients cope is to recognize and facilitate patients' use of prayer.
- Patients are likely to pray at times of symptom distress and emotional distress, and during diagnostic and therapeutic processes. At such times, your help is valuable in fostering conditions and an environment conducive to prayer.
- Although there are commonalities in prayer experiences, typically prayer is unique to the individual. Therefore, you will be called on to design nursing strategies for facilitating prayer with sensitivity to the uniqueness of each patient.
- You contribute to the patient's opportunity for prayer by helping the patient relax, offering spiritual reading material, placing the patient with a view of nature, offering a notebook for journaling, and safeguarding the patient's privacy by preventing unnecessary intrusion into the room during this time.

It is important, however, to gain as clear a picture as possible of all efforts a patient is making to improve or maintain health. Although many alternative therapies do not interfere with those therapies prescribed by a physician, some pose the risk of serious interactions. When obtaining a health history from a patient, carefully assess the patient's use of any other therapies that may interact with traditional medical care (Potter & Perry, 2009). Project an open, nonjudgmental attitude when obtaining a health history so that the patient feels comfortable in providing all information about any therapies he or she is currently receiving.

Insurance coverage is becoming more common for several of these treatments. Many policies cover chiropractic treatments and massage therapy if ordered by a health care provider. Acupuncture is also covered under some policies. Insurance companies are beginning to see the value of preventive measures, as well as treatment for acute injury or illness. From a risk management perspective, many of the alternative therapies are attractive since they work to maintain health, as well as restore it.

The Office of Alternative Medicine (now the National Center for Complementary and Alternative Medicine) was established in 1992 as part of the National Institutes of Health. The goals of this office are to facilitate the evaluation of alternative medical treatment, specifically acting as a clearinghouse to distribute information to the public, the media, and professionals and supporting, coordinating, and conducting research and research training in the area of alternative medicine.

HERBAL THERAPY

The use of **herbal therapy** as medical treatment goes back thousands of years. Neanderthal gravesites have been found that have the remains of plants surrounding the body. Herbalists were consulted by and worked in conjunction with medical physicians until the 1930s, when the last accredited herbal schools closed. In the meantime, the number of **pharmaceuticals**, or drugs, was increasing and their use becoming commonplace. Still, many of those drugs, as well as medications in use today, had their origins in herbs. An example is digitalis, which comes from the finger-shaped foxglove herb. Used in the treatment of heart failure, it is commonly prescribed by health care providers. Recently there has been an increased interest among the general population in the use of herbs and natural supplements to treat illness and maintain health.

Herbs differ from pharmaceuticals—even those that are plant based—in several ways. An herbal preparation usually uses an unpurified extract of the whole plant. One herb may be used for a variety of purposes and is usually gentler than pharmaceuticals. Pharmaceuticals that are derived from herbs include only the active part, and the rest of the plant is separated out and discarded; thus the pharmaceutical is likely to both be more potent and incur more adverse effects. There are several herbal medicine handbooks and websites that list adverse effects for each herbal preparation.

Because herbal medicines have not undergone the same rigorous research as have pharmaceuticals, the majority have not received approval in the United States for use as drugs. For this reason many herbal medicines are sold as foods or food supplements in health food stores and through private companies. The Dietary Supplement Health and Education Act passed in 1994 now allows for herbs to be sold as dietary supplements as long as there are no health claims written on their labels.

Herbal products are thus not treated as drugs, and their manufacturers are not held to the same stringent standards as are manufacturers of pharmaceuticals. Herb manufacturers are not required by law to demonstrate the safety, the efficacy, or the quality of their products. Herb manufacture remains unregulated and is likely to continue to be so in the current political and economic climate. Some manufacturers voluntarily adhere to so-called good manufacturing practices and make every effort to produce a quality product; others do not. However, nothing guarantees that the active chemical constituents in an herbal product will remain constant from manufacturer to manufacturer. Chemical analysis of samples labeled as the same herbal product, but purchased from various suppliers or outlets, has revealed wide variations in potency, quality, and chemical content. Unlike for prescription drugs, no standardized dosages have been established for most herbs, and few manufacturers produce the standardized preparations of predictable and consistent strength that make an herbal regimen possible to follow.

Herbal therapy is based on a different philosophy than conventional drug therapy. The goal of herbal therapy is to restore balance within the individual by facilitating the person's self-healing capacity. Drug therapy, on the other hand, is aimed at the treatment of specific diseases or symptoms. Herbal therapy is also prescribed on an individual basis, with unique herbal concoctions tailored for each person.

Many herbs are potentially toxic if used incorrectly. For example, some herbs are safe and effective when used topically in the amount specified, but are highly toxic if taken internally. Many of the toxic effects of herbs have yet to be determined, both because of insufficient research and because no law requires that adverse effects from herbal products be reported (Table 17-1).

With these cautions in mind, also remember that many herbs may produce beneficial effects when used as directed. Research continues to confirm the efficacy of many popular herbs, echinacea and ginkgo being only two of many examples.

There is much confusion and misinformation regarding herbal medicine. Herbal medicine has yet to be subjected to the same level of scientific scrutiny as traditional medical treatments. As a result, it has not yet gained wide acceptance by mainstream medicine. Because herb use is not widely accepted or understood by mainstream medical caregivers, patients often do not disclose their use of herbs to their health care provider. Many use prescription drugs concurrently with herbal remedies and face possible health risks as a result of adverse interactions. A well-informed, nonjudgmental care provider is most likely to inspire the patient's trust and gain not only a more accurate picture of the patient's herb use but also an opportunity to provide valuable information about herb safety issues (see Patient Teaching box).

Table 17-1 Commonly Used Herbs

HERB	USES	CONSIDERATIONS
Asian ginseng (*Panax ginseng*)	Improves overall health and well-being Atherosclerosis, bleeding disorders, colitis, diabetes, depressant cancer	Do not use if pregnant or breastfeeding. Do not use in the presence of cardiovascular disease, hypertension, diabetes, or concurrent therapy. Avoid use if taking anticoagulants because it can prolong clotting. Avoid taking with CNS stimulants, estrogen, furosemide, ibuprofen, caffeine, or drugs metabolized by CYP3H4. Drug interactions are possible with agents that inhibit monoamine oxidase (phenelzine, St. John's wort, selegiline).
Aloe vera (*Aloe ferox, A. barbadensis*)	Burns, skin irritation Has laxative properties	Internal use produces a cathartic action and has resulted in painful cramps, electrolyte imbalance, hemorrhagic diarrhea, and kidney damage. Drug interactions exist with antidysrhythmics, cardiac glycosides (like digoxin), antidiabetics, beta blockers, steroids, diuretics, and disulfiram. Herb interactions exist with licorice.
Cayenne (*Capsicum* sp.)	General cardiovascular health, reduces cholesterol level; topical application produces analgesia, controls bleeding	Topical application as a counterirritant produces a "heat" sensation. Repeated applications produce analgesia resulting from neuronal depletion of substance P (a mediator of pain transmission between peripheral nerves and spinal cord). Burning and pruritus diminish with continued use. Drug interactions exist with ACE inhibitors, heparin, ASA, disulfiram, and theophylline. Herb interactions exist with feverfew, garlic, ginger, and ginseng.
Comfrey (*Symphytum officinale*)	Cell proliferent, stimulates quick healing of strains and slow-healing wounds (for external use only)	When used internally, comfrey is potentially harmful: there are reports of liver toxicity. Some preparations contain significant levels of alcohol; use with caution. Monitor patients for abdominal distention, nausea, abdominal pain, and elevated liver function test results. Limit use to 4 to 6 weeks per year to prevent exposure to large amounts of toxic alkaloids.
Echinacea (*Echinacea purpurea, E. angustifolia, E. pallida*)	Stimulates immune function; excellent blood cleanser; upper respiratory infections; wound healing	Activity shown against influenza, herpes, and *Candida* infections. Adverse reactions include fever, taste disturbance, gastrointestinal disturbances, nausea and vomiting, diuresis, photosensitivity. Avoid use in patients with ragweed allergies. Prolonged use potentially leads to overstimulation of the immune system and possible immune suppression. Drug interactions are possible with amprenavir, protease inhibitors, disufiram, metronidazole, immunosuppressants, cyclosporine and methotrexate, prednisone, alcohol, warfarin, digoxin, contraceptives, SSRIs, MAOIs.
Evening primrose oil (*Oenothera biennis*)	Premenstrual syndrome, attention-deficit hyperactivity disorder, cardiovascular problems, hot flashes, mastalgia	Use of the oil will occasionally unmask previously undiagnosed epilepsy, especially when taken with a drug that treats depression or schizophrenia. Take drug with food to decrease adverse gastrointestinal reaction. Use is contraindicated for those with an allergy to evening primrose oil and those who are pregnant or breastfeeding. Do not use if you have history of epilepsy or are taking a tricyclic antidepressant, phenothiazine, or another drug that lowers the seizure threshold.
Ginger (*Zingiber officinale*)	Nausea, vomiting, motion sickness, appetite improvement, impotence, liver toxicity, burns	Overdose possibly produces CNS depression and dysrhythmias. Ginger sometimes enhances the effect of anticoagulants. Do not take large doses if pregnant, because the teratogenic potential is largely unstudied. No consensus exists regarding dosage or monitoring. Drug interactions are possible with antacids, histamine H_2 receptor blockers, proton pump inhibitors, anticoagulants, barbiturates, disulfiram, and metronidazole.
Ginkgo, Maidenhair tree (*Ginkgo biloba*)	Improves memory, increases circulation to the extremities and the brain	Studies have shown that ginkgo produces arterial and venous vasoactive changes that increase tissue perfusion and cerebral blood flow. Adverse reactions include dizziness, headache, subarachnoid and subdural hemorrhage, and cardiac insufficiency. There have been reports of seizures in children and bleeding complications. Potential drug interactions exist with antiplatelet therapy, anticoagulants, anticonvulsants, buproprion, tricyclic antidepressants, disufiram, metronidazole, MAOIs, SSRIs, and trazodone. Herb interactions include garlic.

ACE, Angiotensin-converting enzyme; *ASA,* acetylsalicylic acid (aspirin); *CNS,* central nervous system; *MAOI,* monoamine oxidase inhibitor; *SSRI,* selective serotonin reuptake inhibitor.

Continued

Table 17-1 Commonly Used Herbs—cont'd

HERB	USES	CONSIDERATIONS
Goldenseal (*Hydrastis canadensis*)	Antibiotic and antiseptic, especially effective on mucous membranes, urinary tract infection, diarrhea, and hemorrhoids Digestive aid and expectorant	Possibly reduces effect of anticoagulants. Increases hypoglycemic effects in patients using insulin. Possibly reduces or enhances hypotensive effect of antihypertensives. Possibly interferes or enhances cardiac effects of beta blockers, calcium channel blockers, and digoxin. Possibly enhances sedative effects of CNS depressants. Possibly enhances sedative effects of alcohol. Do not give to children.
Kava (Kava-kava) (*Piper methysticum*)	Anxiety, stress, and restlessness, insomnia, wound healing	Kava does not appear to cause physiologic dependence. Expect enhanced sedative effects if combined with other CNS depressants (alcohol, benzodiazepines, and opioid analgesics). Heavy use sometimes causes nutritional deficiencies, skin dermopathy, blood dyscrasias, pulmonary hypertension, cirrhosis, liver failure, hepatitis, and dopamine antagonism. It is generally well tolerated except in high doses or with long-term use. Do not use when using alcohol, and during pregnancy and breastfeeding, and do not use in children younger than 12 years of age. Drug interactions may exist with antiplatelet medications, MAOIs, drugs metabolized in cytochrome P-450 system, hepatotoxic drugs, L-dopa.
Lavender (*Lavandula officinalis*)	Antiseptic, antidepressant, sedative Relaxation, minor cuts, psoriasis, fragrance	Used for its calming mild sedative effect. Add to warm bath water if desired to aid in relaxation. Orally it is sometimes used as a tea to calm a "nervous stomach." Monitor patient closely for oversedation because it will possibly potentiate other sedative drugs. Possibly potentiates CNS depressant effects of alcohol. Avoid use if pregnant or breastfeeding. Some patients are allergic to lavender-containing perfumes. Do not confuse with true lavender oil or lavandin or spiked lavender oil. The latter two contain high enough levels of camphor to elicit neurotoxicity. Excessive inhalation of the oil sometimes leads to vertigo, nausea, and syncope. Tell patients to avoid hazardous activities until full effects are known.
St. John's wort (*Hypericum perforatum*)	Mild to moderate depression, anxiety, viral infection, insomnia, premenstrual syndrome, topical myalgia, inflammation	There are numerous case reports and clinical trials evaluating the efficacy and safety of St. John's wort. Most trials contain design flaws, but overall results suggest that St. John's wort is sometimes beneficial for mild to moderate depression. Adverse reactions are uncommon but include photosensitivity, constipation, vertigo, dry mouth, restlessness, and sleep disturbance. Avoid concurrent use with MAOIs, alcoholic beverages, opioids, prescription antidepressants, sympathomimetics, and foods such as chocolate, aged cheeses, and beer. Do not use if pregnant or breastfeeding. Do not use in children. Drug interactions include amiodarone, amitriptyline, chemotherapy drugs, cyclosporine, digoxin, drugs metabolized in cytochrome P-450 system, contraceptives (oral), protease inhibitors, theophylline and warfarin, SSRIs, reserpine, and nonnucleoside reverse transcriptase inhibitors.
Tea tree oil (*Melaleuca alternifolia*)	Skin irritations, acne, athlete's foot Topical antiseptic, antifungal inhalation for respiratory disorders	Do not take in combination with drugs that affect histamine release. Do not apply to dry skin, cracked or broken skin, open wounds, or areas affected by rash that is not fungal. Do not use internally because of systemic toxicity. Use externally only after dilution, especially for patients with sensitive skin. Do not use around nose, eyes, and mouth because it sometimes causes burns or pruritus in tender areas. Use the pure oil only with close supervision by a health care provider.
Valerian (*Valeriana officinalis*)	Insomnia, hyperactivity, stress, anxiety	Causes addictive effects in some patients taking barbiturates. Possibly potentiates sedative effects of catnip, hops, kona, and passionflower. Possibly potentiates the sedative effects of alcohol. Do not use if pregnant or breastfeeding. Evidence of toxicity includes difficulty walking, hypothermia, or increased muscle relaxation. Possible adverse reactions include hepatotoxic withdrawal.

Patient Teaching

Using Complementary and Alternative Therapies

- Use herbal preparations according to package or health care provider direction.
- When taking ginkgo, keep seeds out of children's reach because of the potential risk of seizures with ingestion.
- Consult your health care provider before starting a yoga program because some yoga postures are stressful to people with certain health problems (muscle injury is possible if the positions are not done correctly or if the body is forced into certain positions).
- Yoga is a complementary therapy, not a cure for disease. Patient will need to continue any conventional medical treatments he or she is currently following.
- When practicing yoga, try different positions cautiously; few people are able to do all the movements in the beginning. Yoga requires regular practice to be effective.
- Inform your primary care provider of any drugs you use, including herbal remedies, so that all agents—whether "nutraceutical" or pharmaceutical—will be considered in the plan of care.
- Stop taking the herb and notify your primary care provider if adverse effects or side effects occur.
- Avoid using combinations of herbs.
- "Natural" does not mean safe.
- Seek objective and scientifically based sources of information. Use caution when evaluating the claims made by herb manufacturers.
- Use only products that are standardized and known to contain a specific amount of active ingredients.
- Select herbal products carefully, buying only those that list the following information on the package: herb's common and scientific names, name and address of the manufacturer, batch or lot number, expiration date, dosage and administration guidelines, potential side effects, and details of how quality is ensured.
- Avoid using herbs and spices for at least 2 weeks before any surgery.
- Bear in mind that patients who self-prescribe medications will possibly have serious underlying physiologic or psychological conditions that require attention. Teach patient to devise health regimen that best suits his or her needs—whether or not herbs are used.
- Herb-drug interactions do occur, as well as herb-herb interactions, and they pose serious risks; therefore, it is best to let the primary care provider determine the safety of combining herbs and drugs.
- Purchase herbal products that have been standardized, that is, products for which the effects are known for a given dosage and for which the manufacturer ensures consistency from batch to batch.
- Buy from reputable sources. Ask the primary health care provider for assistance in determining where to purchase herbs.
- Avoid herbs during pregnancy and lactation or when attempting to become pregnant.
- Neither the safety nor the efficacy of herbs has been conclusively documented in scientific literature.
- It is in the patient's best interest to undergo a complete medical evaluation before self-medicating with supplements—whether to treat specific symptoms of an illness or as a preventive measure.
- Do not use herbs in larger-than-recommended dosages or for more than several weeks (unless approved by the health care provider).
- Do not give infants, children, and older adults herbal treatments without professional supervision.
- Postpone reflexology treatment if patient's feet have cuts, boils, bruises, or other injuries.
- Check with your health care provider before trying reflexology if patient has diabetes, peripheral vascular disease, or other vascular problems in the legs, such as thrombosis or phlebitis.
- Many people who claim to perform reflexology actually are performing a simple foot massage; advise patient to make sure the therapist has been trained in reflexology.
- Keep all herbs out of the reach of children and pets.

Reduced insurance coverage, constraints on access to care, and increased costs of prescriptions and services are the norm in today's health care climate. People are living longer, and chronic diseases (arthritis, diabetes, cancer, Alzheimer's, human immunodeficiency virus and acquired immunodeficiency syndrome [HIV/AIDS]) are on the rise. Conventional prescription drugs used to treat these conditions are often expensive, and because at least a portion of the cost is often not reimbursed by insurance carriers, consumers are paying more out of pocket for them. People are becoming increasingly interested in preventive strategies and holistic approaches to health, such as eating a nutritionally sound diet, maintaining fitness, and reducing stress. Interest in natural treatments and products continues to grow. Americans spent $3.24 billion on herbs in 1997 and $4.3 billion in 2000. The amount continues to increase.

As a nurse, you help patients make educated decisions about their health; there is no reason for this to exclude the use of herbs. Of particular concern is the fact that most patients receive information about herbs from the media and the Internet, sources whose claims do not always coincide with results of clinical studies. Teach patients that before taking any herbal product, it is best to review it with a health care professional, pharmacist, or certified herbalist.

Treatment is provided in a variety of ways. It is possible to take dried herbs orally in capsule or tablet form. Tinctures are made by placing herbs in alcohol or vinegar and allowed to sit until the liquid absorbs the properties of the herb. The liquid is then strained and used. Teas made of an infusion of herbs and hot water are drunk, or a moist compress is made from the tea and applied to the affected area. Topical application of herbs is also possible by making a salve or ointment (Table 17-2).

Thousands of herbs are available. Table 17-1 lists some of the most common herbs and their uses. Remind patients to take care to only use herbs from a reliable source. Before using any fresh herbs, it is best to obtain exact identification from a trained professional. Always know exactly what the herb is and what its actions are before using any herb.

Many herbs interact with various medications. For example, the combination of valerian and barbiturates will probably cause excessive sedation. Ginseng is likely to interfere with the actions of digoxin. Advise against taking St. John's wort concurrently with antidepressant medications. Screen patients carefully in regard to herbal use and possible interactions with other medications.

Table 17-2 Common Essential Oils and Their Uses

ESSENTIAL OIL	USE	CONSIDERATIONS
Chamomile	Pain, gastric intestinal spasms, stress, insomnia	Theoretic potential exists for decreased absorption of certain antispasmodic medications. Excessive anticoagulation possible when used with other anticoagulants. Avoid use in pregnancy because of potential abortifacient and teratogenic effects. Instruct patients with atopic eczema to avoid use because of potential allergic reactions.
Eucalyptus	Respiratory problems	Sometimes causes nausea, vomiting, diarrhea, and asthmalike attacks. Possibly enhances the effects of hypoglycemics. The oil has potential to affect any drug that the liver metabolizes, so monitor these patients for effect and toxic reaction. Decreases blood glucose levels—monitor patients for effect. Do not use with herbs that cause hypoglycemia such as basil, glucomannan, or Queen Anne's lace. When applied to an infant's or child's face, sometimes causes severe bronchial spasm. Do not use if pregnant, or breastfeeding, or if you have liver disease or intestinal tract inflammation.
Lavender	Insomnia, stress, depression	Possibly causes CNS depression, confusion, vertigo, syncope, drowsiness, headache, neurotoxicity, hypotension, nausea, vomiting, constipation, and respiratory depression. Possibly potentiates the effects of sedative drugs, so monitor patient closely for oversedation. Possibly potentiates CNS depressant effects of alcohol, so avoid use. Massaging with diluted oil is unlikely to be toxic. Do not use if pregnant or breastfeeding. Do not confuse true lavender oil with lavandin or spike lavender oil; the latter two contain high enough levels of camphor to elicit neurotoxicity.
Lemon	Colds and flu, mental stimulation Diuretic, antiinflammatory	Avoid oral ingestion of expressed oil if pregnant or breastfeeding. Do not use if hypersensitive to members of the citrus family. Skin reactions of photodermatotoxicity from expressed oil are possible. Herb-drug interactions have been reported.
Peppermint	Acne, stomach upset General stimulant	Patients with gastroesophageal reflux disease should avoid because peppermint sometimes exacerbates it. Do not use peppermint teas and mentholated ointment with infants and small children. Menthol sometimes causes sensitization and allergic reactions. Advise patients not to apply to broken skin. Internal use of peppermint other than for flavoring is not recommended.
Rosemary	Internally: Mental stimulant; use for stress, circulatory problems Externally: myalgias, neuralgia, pruritus, migraines	Promotes menstrual flow, induces abortions (do not use if pregnant); and relieves headache, liver, and gallbladder complaints and blood pressure problems. In high doses sometimes causes seizures. Asthma from repeated occupational exposure is possible. Also sometimes causes contact dermatitis and photodermatosensitivity. Encourage patients to take precautions and use sunscreen. Avoid use with herbal products containing alcohol. Do not use with pregnant or breastfeeding patients, children, or patients with seizure disorders. Bronchospasm and glottal spasm have been reported in children.
Tea tree	Antiseptic Skin irritations, viral illness, respiratory infection	Topical applications have not shown to be toxic, but ingesting the oil will possibly produce CNS depression and gastrointestinal irritation. Its antimicrobial activity has been well documented, but only anecdotal evidence exists for its efficacy in treating skin maladies. Advise patients of various product concentrations. It is probably best for those with propensity for contact dermatitis to avoid the use of tea tree oil.

CNS, Central nervous system.

CHIROPRACTIC THERAPY

Chiropractic therapy has been in existence since the late 1800s. Doctors of chiropractic medicine undergo extensive training in manipulation of the musculoskeletal system. Although chiropractic therapy has been severely criticized, it is currently considered an acceptable treatment for certain disorders, including back pain and headaches. Many insurance companies provide coverage for chiropractic therapy care.

This form of therapy is based on a holistic belief in the body's capacity to take care of itself. The chiropractic doctor adjusts the joints of the body by gentle manipulation to put an area of disturbed structural integrity, usually the vertebrae, back in proper alignment. When properly performed, this treatment does not cause pain to the patient. Often, patients seek treatment from a medical physician for an acute injury or illness, and use chiropractic care on a routine basis. If there is acute distress, visits are sometimes recommended several times a week or daily, but monthly visits to keep the patient at a maximum level of health are typical.

The chiropractor often uses radiographs to assist with diagnosis. A doctor of chiropractic medicine does not prescribe medications as part of the treatment. Other treatments, such as hot and cold packs, are sometimes used during the course of chiropractic treatment. The chiropractor will often consider lifestyle changes to help keep the patient functioning well without recurrence of the injury. A variety of suggested exercises often plays a role in treatment.

LIMITATIONS OF CHIROPRACTIC THERAPY

It is unwise to treat certain diseases or joint conditions with manipulation. Contraindications for chiropractic therapy include acute myelopathy, fractures, dislocations, rheumatoid arthritis, and osteoporosis. If a malignancy is suspected or determined through diagnostic testing, see that the patient is referred to a health care provider for further evaluation and treatment. Bone and joint infections also require pharmaceutical or surgical intervention. Care is required not to compromise the structural integrity of the bone, which is possible if excessive force is used.

ACUPUNCTURE AND ACUPRESSURE

Acupuncture and acupressure are therapies that are based on the belief that there is a form of energy or Qi (life force) that flows through the body along meridians (channels of energy). These meridians, or channels, can become blocked, thus causing illness or discomfort. Therapy involves stimulating the channels at specific points to open them and allow the Qi to flow freely. Pain is understood to result primarily from stagnant or blocked Qi, and opening up the dam in the flow of energy through a meridian relieves the pain.

Acupuncture is a method of stimulating certain points (acupoints) on the body by the insertion of special needles to modify the perception of pain, normalize physiologic functions, or treat or prevent disease. Fine needles inserted at specific points serve to open the meridians. These needles are sterile and extremely thin, much smaller than the needles used for insulin injection; each one is for one-time use only. The practitioner will usually insert the needles only a few millimeters. When all the needles are in place, the needles are stimulated manually, electrically, or with heat (Figure 17-2). After the needles have been in place for about 20 minutes, the practitioner removes and discards them. There is usually little discomfort while the needles are inserted, and most patients state that they feel no distress at all.

Acupuncture is the primary treatment modality used by physicians of Chinese medicine. Many allopathic or conventional Western physicians and health care professionals are also being trained and certified in acupuncture. Many states now have regulations and licensure requirements to practice as an acupuncturist.

The most common problems for which acupuncture is used include low back pain, myofascial pain, simple and migraine headaches, sciatica, shoulder pain, tennis elbow, osteoarthritis, whiplash, and musculoskeletal

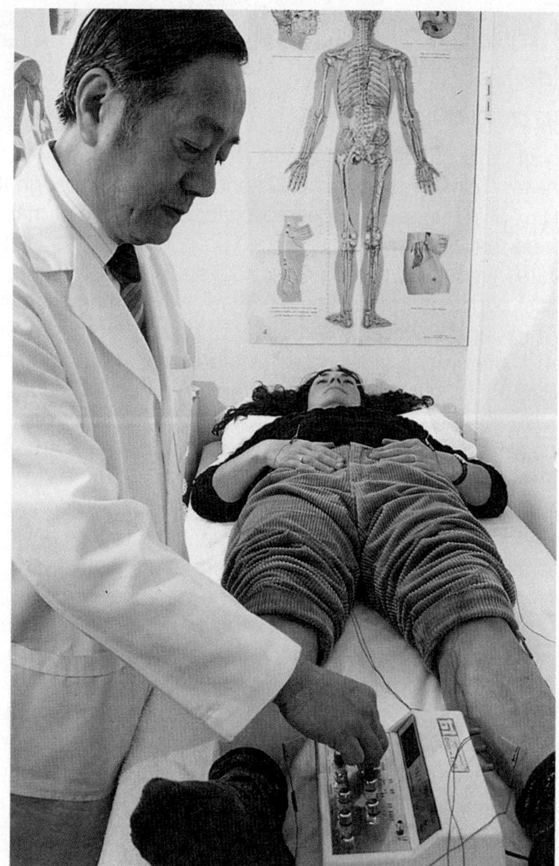

FIGURE 17-2 Acupuncture uses fine needles inserted at specific points to open the meridians.

sprains. Other problems that have been successfully treated include sinusitis, gastrointestinal disorders, bladder leakage, premenstrual symptoms, neurologic disorders, chronic pulmonary disease (including asthma), hypertension, smoking and other addictions, and clinical depression.

Acupressure uses gentle pressure at similar points on the body. Pressure is sometimes applied with a finger and sometimes with a small, blunt object. Acupressure is used primarily for prevention and relief of symptoms of muscle tension. The healing touch of acupressure reduces tension, increases circulation, and enables the body to relax deeply. By relieving stress, acupressure increases resistance to disease and promotes wellness. Acupressure is beneficial in situations of discomfort and promotes the ability to rest or sleep.

Acupuncture and acupressure usually require several treatments to achieve the desired results. These methods are properly performed only by a professional with appropriate training.

THERAPEUTIC MASSAGE

Nurses have long used massage to relax patients and help prevent impairment of skin integrity in the patient confined to bed. The effects are both physical and psychological (see Life Span Considerations for Older Adults box on touch). **Therapeutic massage** is massage performed by trained professionals to manipulate the soft tissues of the body and assist with healing (Nursing Care Plan 17-1). There are various types of massage designed to heal or prevent injury. Some massage is relaxing and other forms are energizing.

Obtain a general health profile before the first massage. With some conditions, massage is contraindicated. A patient with phlebitis or thrombosis needs to avoid massage of the affected extremity. Infectious skin diseases are also conditions where massage is contraindicated.

The massage is conducted in a warm, relaxing atmosphere (see Figure 17-1). A session will last approximately an hour. A whole-body massage is sometimes done, with extra attention being given to the affected area. Oils or lotions are often used during the massage. Make sure the patient is checked for allergies before their use.

 Life Span Considerations

Older Adults

Focus on Touch

- Touch is a primal need, as necessary as food, growth, or shelter. Think of touch as a nutrient transmitted through the skin. "Skin hunger" has been described as a form of malnutrition that has reached epidemic proportions in the United States, especially among older adults.
- Older adults need touch as much as or more than any other age-group. However, skin hunger or poverty of touch is often acute among older adults. It is an unfortunate irony that older adults often have fewer family members or friends to touch them just at the time when there is greatest need to use simple touch to enhance communication or when other senses are sometimes reduced in acuity.
- Simple touch helps older adult patients feel more connected to and accepted by those around them and to their environment. Self-esteem and sense of worth are enhanced.
- A nurse who reacts adversely to the skin changes of older adults will perhaps find it difficult to touch an older patient. Such reluctance goes on to communicate a negative message to the older adult.
- A truly holistic nursing approach to the care of older adults also includes the caregivers, who often experience poor health or have neglected their own health, find themselves challenged by their own psychosocial issues as they relate to the caregiving experience, feel the effects of multiple stressors, or feel spiritual distress.

Adapted from Potter, P.A., & Perry, A.G. (2009). *Fundamentals of nursing: concepts, process, and practice.* (7th ed.). St. Louis: Mosby.

AROMATHERAPY

Aromatherapy uses pure essential oils, produced from plants, to provide health benefits. The oils are formulated for inhalation or are applied topically. Sometimes the scent is dispersed into the air through the use of candles or oil dispersers. Aromatic oils are often used during massage. Bathing provides a good modality for aromatherapy when oil is added to the water. Occasionally, essential oils will be taken orally in small amounts but only when prescribed by a qualified practitioner.

Many scents are put to use for their psychological effects. Different scents are thought to invoke different responses in the body as well. Nurses know that certain odors in a clinical setting have the potential to cause nausea or vomiting. Aromatherapy works on similar principles. Specific scents are thought to relax or stimulate, improve digestion, increase hormone production, and improve circulation or memory. Table 17-2 presents some common essences and their uses.

Asthmatic patients will sometimes develop exaggerated symptoms from certain aromatic essence. Do not use essential oils on the skin of a patient with atopic eczema.

REFLEXOLOGY

In **reflexology** it is thought that it is possible to exert an effect on the entire body by applying pressure to specific areas on the feet. Reflexology is based on the premise that there are zones and reflexes in different parts of the foot that correspond one-to-one to each part, gland, and organ of the body. The manipulation of specific reflexes removes stress, enabling the release of disharmonies by a physiologic change in the body.

Nursing Care Plan 17-1 The Patient Using Complementary and Alternative Therapies

Ms. Lowe, 40 years old, has undergone an abdominal hysterectomy and is second-day postoperative. The nurse finds her awake at midnight. She voices concern about how long she will be in the hospital because she has four children, ages 4 to 15 years, at home and she is worried how well her family is managing without her. She also states that she has abdominal pain at the incision site that she rates at 5 on a scale of 0 to 10. Her vital signs are normal. Tylox, 1 or 2 capsules every 4 hours prn for pain, is ordered, but she does not want to take any more drugs. She wonders if there is anything else she can do to decrease her anxiety and pain.

NURSING DIAGNOSIS ***Anxiety, level 2, related to hospitalization. Pain, acute, related to surgical procedures.***

Patient Goals and Expected Outcomes	Nursing Interventions	Evaluation
Patient will state that anxiety is reduced to an acceptable level Patient will state that pain is 1 to 2 on a scale of 0 to 10	Explain the procedure for therapeutic massage. Position the patient comfortably. Reduce noise, lighting, and distractions. The nurse performs therapeutic massage. Make patient comfortable after procedure by proper positioning, freshening linens, darkening the room, and providing a quiet environment.	Patient states that feelings of anxiety are reduced and pain is now 2 on a scale of 0 to 10.

Critical Thinking Questions

1. Ms. Lowe complains of feeling fatigued and tense. List some nonpharmacologic methods of bringing about a state of physical and mental tranquility that may be helpful. Why might each of these methods be helpful for Ms. Lowe?
2. Ms. Lowe turns on her light and is crying. She complains of feeling helpless and inadequate to assume responsibility for her children and husband when she is discharged. What are some therapeutic interventions that will promote her feelings of stability and validation of her anxiety?

With stress removed and circulation improved, the body is allowed to return to a state of homeostasis.

Reflexology demonstrates the following four main benefits:

1. Relaxes the body and removes stress
2. Enhances the circulation
3. Assists the body to normalize metabolism naturally
4. Complements all other healing modalities

When the reflexes are stimulated, the body's natural electric energy works along the nervous system pathways and meridian lines to clear any blockages along those lines and in the corresponding zones. A treatment seems to break up deposits (felt as a sandy or gritty area under the skin) that interfere with this natural flow of the body's energy. Reflexologists do not diagnose medical conditions.

Novey (2000) states the following:

> Foot reflexology stands the test of patient acceptance as a valid means of making one feel good, relaxing, and functioning better than he otherwise would. As such foot reflexology qualifies as an important adjunct for health care. . . . There are 7200 nerve endings in each foot. Perhaps this fact, more than any other, explains why one feels so much better when our feet are treated. Nerve endings in the feet have extensive interconnections through the spinal cord and brain with all areas of the body. Surely the feet are a gold mine of opportunity to release tension and enhance health.

Place the patient in a comfortable position for treatment, either lying or sitting. Expose the feet so that the practitioner is able to perform specific massage movements and techniques on the feet. Treatments typically last up to 1 hour. Most people find treatments to be very relaxing.

Reflexologists believe that treatment has the capacity to interfere with other medical or alternative treatment; therefore, it is important that the patient informs the practitioner of any other treatments being received. Performance of reflexology on everyone is acceptable, from the newborn to the older adult. It is used both for a general "tune-up" and in a very sick body. Its use is appropriate throughout pregnancy care and presurgically and postsurgically. In all cases, use common sense in selecting this therapy.

WARNINGS, CONTRAINDICATIONS, AND PRECAUTIONS

Use lighter pressure on the corresponding reflex areas when heart problems, blood problems, high blood pressure, epilepsy, or diabetes are present. In diabetic patients using artificial insulin, overstimulation of the corresponding reflexes will possibly cause the pancreas to start producing insulin again and thus lead to a higher level of insulin than expected.

MAGNET THERAPY

Magnets have been used for thousands of years in healing and to improve overall health. Natural lodestones were found and are the earliest form of magnets known. Currently, a variety of companies produce magnets for use on various parts of the body. Magnets are sometimes used intermittently and sometimes worn all the time.

Magnets are used to increase circulation, increase energy, and decrease pain. Although it is not known exactly how magnets work, they are thought to increase circulation to the affected area and promote healing, as well as stimulate acupuncture points. Common physiologic responses resulting from magnetic field exposures include the following actions: (1) vasodilation; (2) analgesic action; (3) antiinflammatory action; (4) spasmolytic (arresting spasms) activity; (5) acceleration of healing; and (6) antiedema activity. The magnet is placed over the affected area and held in place by jewelry, cloth wraps, or tape. Magnet insoles are available to place in shoes.

Contraindications include pregnancy and the presence of pacemakers, insulin delivery systems, cochlear implants, and defibrillators, and concurrent use of an electric blanket or heating pad. Magnets are also not to be used with patients with myasthenia gravis because muscle weakness will possibly be aggravated because of the magnet's strong action on relaxing muscles. Other conditions in which magnets are contraindicated include hyperthyroidism and adrenal gland, hypothalamic, and pituitary dysfunction.

IMAGERY

Imagery or visualization techniques use the conscious mind to create mental images to evoke physical changes in the body, create a sense of improved well-being, and enhance self-awareness. Frequently imagery is combined with some form of relaxation training to facilitate the effect of the relaxation technique. Imagery is sometimes self-directed, and the individual creates his or her own mental images; and sometimes the process is guided, and a practitioner leads the individual through a particular scenario. Here is a sample scenario of guided imagery with you as the guide: First direct the patient to begin slow abdominal breathing while focusing on the rhythm of breathing. Then instruct the patient to visualize ocean waves coming to shore with each inspiration, and receding with each expiration. Next instruct the patient to take notice of the smells, the sounds, and the temperatures that he or she is experiencing. As the imagery session progresses, perhaps you will instruct the patient to visualize warmth entering the body during inspiration and tension leaving the body during expiration. Work along these lines, but individualize imagery scenarios for each patient, or leave them to the patient to develop.

Imagery has the power to evoke significant psychophysiologic responses such as alterations in immune function. Many imagery techniques involve visual imagery, but they also include the auditory, proprioceptive, gustatory, and olfactory senses at times. For example, visualize slicing a lemon in half and squeezing the lemon juice under your tongue. You've probably already noticed that this visualization produces increased salivation as effectively as the actual event. We typically respond to our environment according to the way we perceive it. But just as you responded physiologically (salivating) to something that didn't "really" happen (the lemon slicing and juice tasting), you have the power to regulate your response to an environmental stimulus by appropriately regulating your expectations and perception of it—through imagery and active visualization.

Imagery has applications in a number of patient populations. Imagery has been used to visualize the destruction of cancer cells by cells of the immune system, to control or relieve pain, and to achieve calmness and serenity. It has also been used in the treatment of chronic conditions such as asthma, hypertension, functional urinary disorders, menstrual and premenstrual syndromes, gastrointestinal disorders such as irritable bowel syndrome and ulcerative colitis, and rheumatoid arthritis (Potter & Perry, 2009).

RELAXATION THERAPY

Relaxation is the state of a generalized decrease in cognitive, physiologic, or behavioral arousal. Relaxation is also defined as the act or process of arousal reduction. The process of relaxation elongates the muscle fibers and reduces the neural impulses sent to the brain, and thus decreases the activity of the brain and other body systems. The relaxation response is characterized by decreased heart and respiratory rates, blood pressure, and oxygen consumption and increased alpha brain activity and peripheral skin temperature. The relaxation response can be obtained through a variety of techniques that incorporate a repetitive mental focus and the adoption of a calm, peaceful attitude. Teaching strategies for relaxation exercises are listed in Box 17-2.

Relaxation training involves developing cognitive skills that help people reduce the negative ways in which they respond to situations and their environment. The cognitive skills include **focusing** (the ability to identify, differentiate, maintain attention on, and return attention to simple stimuli for an extended period), **passivity** (the ability to stop unnecessary goal-directed and analytic activity), and **receptivity** (the

Box 17-2 Relaxation Strategies

RHYTHMIC BREATHING*

1. Provide a quiet environment.
2. Help the patient get comfortable by elevating the legs with the knees bent (relaxing the leg, back, and abdominal muscles).
3. Instruct the patient to close eyes and to breathe in and out slowly, saying rhythmically, "Breathe in, 2, 3, 4; breathe out, 2, 3, 4."
4. Once rhythmic breathing is established, instruct patient to listen to your voice, and with a low and steady voice, instruct patient to do the following:
   a. Breathe in and out slowly and deeply.
   b. Try to breathe from the abdomen.
   c. Feel more relaxed with each exhalation.
   d. Try to identify your own special feeling of relaxation (e.g., light and weightless or very heavy).
   e. While you are breathing, let your imagination take you to a place you remember as peaceful and pleasant; look around, listen to the sounds, feel the air, notice the smells.
   f. When you are ready to end this relaxation exercise, count silently from 1 to 3; on 1, move your lower body; on 2, move your upper body; on 3, breathe in deeply, open your eyes, and while breathing out slowly, say silently, "I am relaxed and alert." Stretch as if just waking up.

PROGRESSIVE RELAXATION

1. Follow steps 1, 2, and 3 of rhythmic breathing.
2. Once patient is breathing slowly and comfortably, instruct patient to tighten and relax an ordered succession of muscle groups, tensing them and then relaxing them, leaving each part feeling relaxed.
3. Instruct patient to begin by tensing and then relaxing the calves, then the knees, and so on.

RELAXATION BY SENSORY PACING

1. Follow steps 1 and 2 of rhythmic breathing.
2. Instruct patient to slowly repeat and finish either in a low voice or to self each of the following sentences:
   a. "Now I am aware of seeing . . ."
   b. "Now I am aware of feeling . . ."
   c. "Now I am aware of hearing . . ."
3. Instruct patient to repeat and complete each sentence four times, then three times, then twice, and finally once.

4. Instruct patient to allow the eyes to close when they feel heavy.

RELAXATION BY COLOR EXCHANGE

1. Follow steps 1, 2, and 3 of rhythmic breathing.
2. Instruct patient to notice any tension, tightness, aches, or pains in the body and to give that sensation the first color that comes to mind.
3. Instruct patient to breathe in pure white light from the universe and send the light to the tense or painful place in the body, letting the white light surround the color of the discomfort.
4. Instruct patient to exhale the color of the discomfort and let the white light take its place.
5. Instruct patient to continue breathing in the white light and exhaling the color of the discomfort, allowing the white light to fill the entire body and bring about a sense of peace, well-being, and energy.

MODIFIED AUTOGENIC RELAXATION

1. Follow steps 1, 2, and 3 of rhythmic breathing.
2. Instruct patient to repeat each of the following phrases to self four times, saying the first part of the phrase while breathing in for 2 to 3 seconds, then holding the breath for 2 to 3 seconds, and then saying the last part of the phrase while breathing out for 2 to 3 seconds.

Breathing In	***Breathing Out***
I am	relaxed.
My arms and legs	are heavy and warm.
My heartbeat	is calm and regular.
My breathing	is free and easy.
My abdomen	is loose and warm.
My forehead	is cool.
My mind	is quiet and still.

RELAXING WITH MUSIC

1. Provide patient with a tape recorder and headset.
2. Ask patient to select a favorite cassette of slow, quiet music.
3. Instruct patient to get into a comfortable position (either sitting or lying down but with arms and legs uncrossed) and to close eyes and listen to the music through the headset.
4. Instruct patient to imagine floating or drifting with the music while listening.

Data from Potter, P.A., & Perry, A.G. (2009). *Fundamentals of nursing: concepts, process, and practice.* (7th ed.). St. Louis: Mosby.
*In conditioning a relaxation response, a "signal breath" involving deep inhalation through the nose and forceful exhalation through the mouth is the key. The signal breath precedes and follows each run through the exercise.

ability to tolerate and accept experiences that are sometimes uncertain, unfamiliar, or paradoxic). In addition, the individual performs cognitive restructuring during which he or she replaces negative thoughts with positive ones. The long-term goal of relaxation therapy is for the person to continually monitor the self for indicators of tension and to consciously let go and release the tension contained in various body parts (Potter & Perry, 2009).

ANIMAL-ASSISTED THERAPY

As early as 1792, animals were used therapeutically in England at York Retreat, where psychiatric patients cared for rabbits and poultry. It was 1944 before animals were used in a therapeutic setting in the United States.

In animal-assisted therapy (AAT), a trained handler and animal pair work one-on-one with a patient toward explicit short- and long-term goals.

Currently AAT is used as a complementary therapy for people in both acute and long-term care settings. Dogs are most often used in AAT. Cats are less predictable, and many people are allergic to cat dander. Regular or miniature horses may also be used. AAT has many applications including overcoming physical limitations, improving mood, lowering blood pressure, and improving socialization skills and self-esteem.

YOGA

The word *yoga* means "yoke," or union of the personal self with the divine source. Yoga is a healing system of therapy and practice. It is a combination of breathing exercises, physical postures, and meditation that has been practiced for over 5000 years. Yoga has emerged as a therapeutic treatment and is now being recognized by Western medical practice. As scientific research points more and more to the integration of the whole person in healing disease, the medical community is no longer in a position to ignore the efficacy of yoga's body-mind connection.

With consistent and earnest practice, change and personal transformation take place on numerous levels. Typically, these changes include improved health and energy, reduced stress, feelings of well-being, and the healing of disease. What perhaps started as a search for increased flexibility and stress reduction slowly enlarges to a greater understanding of the self, emotional growth, and spiritual awakening.

There are a number of different systems of yoga. Hatha yoga is the most familiar type in the United States. However, all systems recognize the validity of certain basic principles, including control of the body through correct posture and breathing, control of the emotions and the mind, and meditation and contemplation (Figure 17-3).

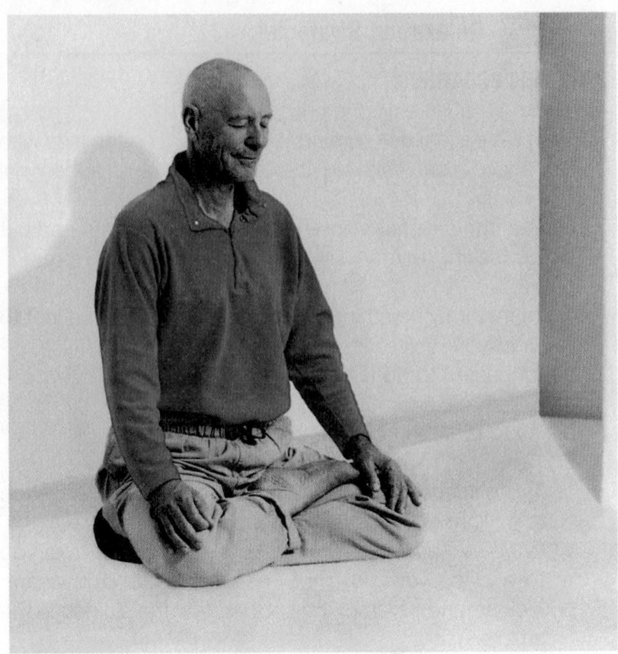

FIGURE 17-3 Yoga is useful to achieve control of the body through correct posture and breathing, control of the emotions and the mind, and meditation and contemplation.

A regular practice of yoga offers the potential to tone the muscles that balance all parts of the body, including internal organs, heart, lungs, glands, and nerves. It increases flexibility of the spine and therefore is good for treating chronic back problems. It is beneficial for the nervous system, promoting deep relaxation and reduction of stress. Everyone has the capacity to practice yoga—children, athletes, and other adults, indeed anyone who seeks a stronger, more supple body.

The origins of yoga go back to the *Vedas*, the oldest written record of Indian culture. Inscribed within the hymns and rituals of this 3000-year-old text is the earliest written reference to yogic activities.

In the sixth chapter of the *Bhagavad Gita*, Sri Krishna explains the meaning of yoga (Black & Hawks, 2009):

> When his mind, intellect and self are under control, freed from restless desire, so that they rest in the spirit within, a man becomes a Yukta—one in communion with God. A lamp does not flicker in a place where no winds blow; so it is with a yogi, who controls his mind, intellect, and self, being absorbed in the spirit within him. When the restlessness of the mind, intellect, and self is stilled through the practice of Yoga, the yogi by the grace of the Spirit within himself finds fulfillment. Then he knows the joy eternal, which is beyond the pale of the senses, which his reason cannot grasp. He abides in this reality and moves not therefrom. He has found the treasure above all others. There is nothing higher than this. He, who has achieved it, shall not be moved by the greatest sorrow. This is the real meaning of Yoga—a deliverance from contact with pain and sorrow.

T'AI CHI/TAIJI

T'ai chi—or Taiji, using the world-standard pinyin romanization scheme for Chinese words—was originally developed as a martial art in seventeenth-century China. Origins of the art are debated by proponents of various styles, but nearly all agree that the art was a fusion of existing martial arts practices with Daoist philosophical concepts, traditional Chinese medicine, and Ch'i Kung *(qigong)* theory and practice. The meaning of Taiji (Figure 17-4) is described by Y. Yang (2008):

> The word taiji (太极) is an ancient Daoist philosophical term symbolizing the interaction of yin and yang, which are opposite manifestations of the same forces in nature. The dynamic interaction of yin and yang, underlying the relation and changing nature of all things, is epitomized in the famous "Taiji Diagram."

It is helpful to think of yin and yang as complementary opposites—each necessarily relies upon, and gives

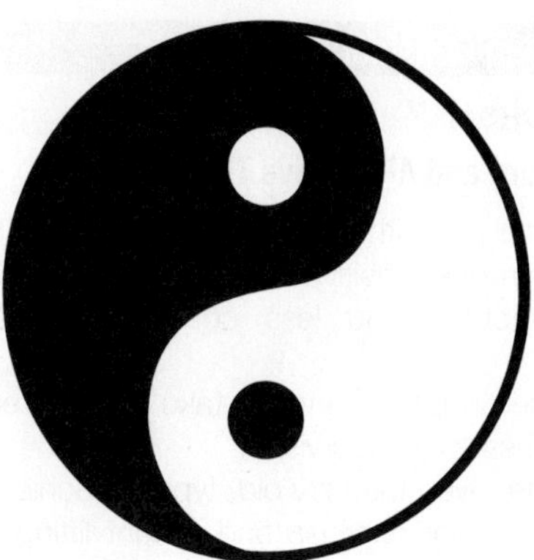

FIGURE 17-4 The Taiji diagram.

birth to, the other. For example, a fundamental theory of Taijiquan is that hardness comes from softness and quickness comes from slowness. In Taiji practice, emphasis is placed on relaxing the body and calming and focusing the mind. Taiji form movement is performed slowly, accentuating the intention, mechanics, accuracy, and precision of the motion. By practicing in accordance with Taiji principles of softness and slowness, the practitioner will paradoxically begin to experience a quality of hardness and strength and efficiency of movement that are significantly different from that of ordinary natural ability (Yang et al., 2008).

The Taiji training system includes form movement, static and dynamic qigong exercises, and two-person balance and reaction training called "push-hands." Form movement is typically performed slowly with relaxed body and calm and focused mind, and is thus referred to as a "moving meditation." Static standing and sitting meditation exercises are practiced as fundamental qigong exercises. Lying down meditation is another qigong practice that is an effective relaxation and stretching exercise. In its complete form, Taiji is a holistic art that emphasizes mind-body integration, physical and mental balance, and spiritual development. Practice of the art is direct exercise of central and peripheral nervous system function.

Taiji practice was originally intended to improve the variables of fundamental skills including balance, strength, flexibility, coordination, agility, reaction time, sensitivity or awareness, and confidence. Although essential for self-defense, these variables are at the same time fundamentally health issues. Because the intensity (e.g., range of motion and height of stance) of any Taiji form sequence is easily varied to suit the practitioner's physical capabilities, people of all physical abilities are able to practice Taiji, and it is especially well suited as a low- to medium-intensity exercise for older adults. Those unable to learn or perform movements do well to begin with the static qigong exercises.

Other health benefits of Taiji practice have long been recognized in China and are receiving increasing attention in the West. A search of the Medline biomedical bibliographic information source yields more than 100 papers discussing Taiji published in Western medical journals over the past 10 years. Health benefits documented in these studies include significant improvements in balance, leg strength, cardiorespiratory function, range of motion and treatment of arthritic symptoms, self-efficacy, sleep quality, prevention of osteoporosis, and immune function. Other health benefits, not yet studied in the West but known in China, include improvements in bowel function, general strengthening of the immune system, and improvements in cognitive function (attention, concentration, learning, and memory) (Yang et al., 2008).

BIOFEEDBACK

Biofeedback is a noninvasive method of determining a patient's neuromuscular and autonomic nervous system response by measuring body functions such as blood pressure, pulse, muscle tension, and skin temperature with the use of electronic or electromechanical equipment. These responses are conveyed to the patient through auditory, visual, physical, and/or physiologic signals. The goal of biofeedback is for patients to become aware of their responses, and in conjunction with relaxation techniques, to be able to control their response (Rakel & Faass, 2006). The immediate feedback gives the patient the ability to implement relaxation techniques and determine which are effective. In addition, the patient becomes more aware of physiologic functions and how thoughts and feelings influence physiologic responses. The end result is that the patient will be able to recognize physiologic responses and control these responses with relaxation techniques without the use of electronic equipment (Potter & Perry, 2009).

CLINICAL APPLICATIONS OF BIOFEEDBACK

In addition to reducing the stress response, biofeedback has been found to be beneficial in the treatment of disorders such as migraine headaches, pain, and both urinary tract and gastrointestinal tract disorders. As with any behavioral modification program, the commitment of the patient to the program determines how successful the outcome will be (Potter & Perry, 2009).

LIMITATIONS OF BIOFEEDBACK

Though biofeedback is considered noninvasive, precautions with the therapy are necessary in connection with repressed emotions or feelings that may surface during the relaxation and/or biofeedback sessions. It is important for the practitioner to be aware of these precautions so that proper psychological support is available at the time of the sessions or proper referral is made (Potter & Perry, 2009).

INTEGRATIVE MEDICINE AND THE NURSING ROLE

The interest in CAM therapies has increased significantly in the past 20 years. The majority of people using and seeking information about CAM are well educated and have a strong desire to actively participate in the decision making about their health care. This increased interest comes not only from health care consumers but also from allopathic physicians who have increasing concerns that current Western medicine is not meeting the needs of their patients. Many allopathic health care providers do not refer their patients for CAM because they are not familiar with the therapies and have had little, if any, education and training in complementary and alternative medicine. Many physicians have reservations about CAM because its modalities have not been appropriately tested in clinical trials with strict controls for the other factors that have the capacity to influence the outcomes. Many studies related to CAM have involved small numbers of subjects and were not well controlled. More research is needed to establish evidence-based practice and to validate the effectiveness of CAM therapies (Potter & Perry, 2009).

In North America and the United Kingdom, many professional groups are exploring the use of CAM and facilitating and monitoring research in this area. Proposals put forth by several of these groups include assessing the need of the public for CAM therapies, incorporating CAM educational components into the curriculum from all health care programs, providing appropriate information to the public, and encouraging and facilitating communication between CAM practitioners from various backgrounds and geographic locations. If CAM therapies are to be accepted and integrated into the Western medical approach, they will have to be subjected to more rigorous research—an undertaking that will perhaps worry some practitioners, but will also serve to refine and improve the therapies. The benefits of this integrative approach will become apparent to all health care providers, in fact: therapies that encourage patients to actively participate in preventing illness or managing chronic illness, and less passive reliance solely on surgery or drugs.

Integrative medicine, a health care strategy that is gaining popularity, involves an interdisciplinary, multiple-practitioner treatment group that a patient consults as a cooperative entity, instead of seeking care from one type of practitioner at a time. Patients have the option to choose the kind of practitioner they think would benefit their particular health problem, and the practitioners of different types and specialties also refer to and consult amongst each other. This represents a pluralistic and truly complementary health care system in which both alternative and allopathic practitioners work side by side to improve the well-being of their patients. Although this is not reality in the majority of settings, this approach of open communication and practice between allopathic and alternative practitioners has great potential to benefit a large number of patients (see Life Span Considerations for Older Adults box on complementary and alternative therapies). Patients likely to benefit from these groups are those who have chronic health problems that have historically been difficult to treat using traditional allopathic medicine, such as fibromyalgia or chronic fatigue syndrome.

Life Span Considerations

Older Adults

Complementary and Alternative Therapy

- Use essential oils with caution in older adults. These patients are usually more sensitive to essential oils and thus require smaller amounts and less concentrated forms of the essence.
- Advise older adult patients to take herbal treatments only under professional supervision.
- Older adults, even the very old, typically achieve positive results from regular exercise and weight lifting, including increased physical strength and flexibility and improved mental status in areas such as memory and depression. However, it is necessary to adapt the exercise regimen to each patient's physical condition.
- When using massage therapy, a lighter pressure will be necessary; possibly, other modifications for body status of an older adult patient will be also needed.
- Magnet therapy will interfere with pacemaker functions.

The integrative medicine approach is consistent with the holistic approach nurses are taught to practice. Nurses have the potential for becoming essential participants in this type of health care model. Many nurses already practice forms of CAM by offering relaxation, imagery, and massage to their patients. You will need a good knowledge of CAM therapies to make appropriate recommendations to allopathic primary care providers about potentially useful therapies. Be prepared to provide advice to patients regarding when to seek conventional therapy and when CAM therapy is appropriate (see Patient Teaching box). For example, if a patient complains of right lower abdominal pain, nausea, and vomiting, you will suspect appendicitis and recommend assessment by an allopathic physician. However, if the patient has a chronic gastrointestinal disorder and has been diagnosed with irritable bowel syndrome, it is possible that the patient will benefit from relaxation and herbal therapy. Be aware of your state nurse practice act with regard to complementary therapies and practice accordingly within the scope of these laws.

Nurses work closely with their patients and are in the unique position of becoming familiar with the patient's religious and cultural viewpoints (see Cultural Considerations box) and existential issues. You are in a good position to determine which CAM therapies are most appropriately aligned with these beliefs and offer recommendations accordingly.

Increased awareness of alternative and complementary therapies means that many patients will come to

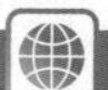

Cultural Considerations

Providing Culturally Appropriate Complementary and Alternative Therapy

- Avoid using the term "alternative therapy"; it is quite possible that patients will not consider what they are doing to be alternative at all. For some Chinese Americans, for instance, treatments such as acupuncture and use of herbal preparations are grounded in their culture and passed down from generation to generation. If anything, they are likely to consider what you are offering in the way of Western medicine to be alternative.
- Regardless of your faith in another type of care, you need to be sensitive to cultural differences (ethnic, racial, gender, etc.) and question the patient appropriately and then support the patient's choices as needed.
- Members of some cultures will often have more faith in an alternative practitioner than a traditional doctor. Respect the patient's beliefs and explore ways to combine therapies when there are no contraindications.
- Demonstrate your respect for the cultural differences by honoring the patient's culturally based health beliefs.
- Ask permission before touching the patient; ask the meaning of touch and the body areas considered touchable. Acceptable touch varies from culture to culture.
- To provide culturally appropriate and competent alternative and complementary therapies, it is important to remember that each individual is culturally unique and as such is a product of a mix of past experiences, cultural beliefs, and cultural norms.
- Acupuncture originated in China approximately 4000 to 5000 years ago, but very little acupuncture was performed in the United States outside of Chinese immigrant communities until the 1970s.
- Yoga began in India more than 6000 years ago.

See Chapter 8 for further discussion of cultural considerations.

you already having had experience with or open to investigating these therapies. Patients tend to be more receptive to holistic interventions and will often seek your guidance in exploring various options when making choices concerning their health care (Potter & Perry, 2009). Therefore it is important for you to be knowledgeable about the multiple CAM therapies available and the use of these therapies by your patients. It is also important for you to keep abreast of the current research being done in this area to provide accurate information, not only to patients but also to other health care professionals.

Get Ready for the NCLEX® Examination!

Key Points

- Complementary and alternative therapies are used to restore or maintain health.
- Patients tend to think of CAM therapies as gentler and less invasive than traditional medical treatments.
- Patients are often hesitant to tell a health care provider about CAM therapies they are using.
- Herbs used for treatment are formulated in many ways for consumption and use: as dried herbs in capsules or tablets, tinctures, teas, compresses, salves, or ointments.
- Some herbs sometimes interfere with medications. A thorough health history is important.
- Chiropractic treatment achieves its effects through manipulation of the musculoskeletal system. Gentle manipulation puts the vertebrae in proper alignment.
- Acupuncture and acupressure are done by applying needles or pressure to specific points on the body. The points correspond to meridians that flow through the body.
- In its complete form, t'ai chi (Taiji) is a holistic art that emphasizes mind-body integration, physical and mental balance, and spiritual development.
- Therapeutic massage is used to promote healing and prevent injury. Contraindications include a history of phlebitis or thrombosis of the extremities.
- Aromatherapy uses essential oils to provide health benefits. Inhalation is the most common method of using the oils.
- Pressure to the feet in the form of massage is done in reflexology.
- Reflexology is a focused pressure technique; it is based on the premise that zones or reflex areas exist in the feet that correspond to all organs, glands, and systems of the body.
- Magnet therapy is thought to improve circulation to a specific area, promote healing, increase energy, and decrease pain.
- Regular practice of yoga potentially tones the muscles that balance all parts of the body, including internal organs, heart, lungs, glands, and nerves, and control the emotions and mind.
- Although some CAM therapies have been researched and published in professional journals, others lack scientific proof. However, those that lack scientific proof need not be discarded since many patients report positive outcomes from these therapies.

Additional Resources

Go to your Companion CD for an audio glossary, animations, video clips, and more.

evolve Be sure to visit the Evolve site at http://evolve.elsevier.com/Christensen/foundations/ for additional online resources.

Review Questions for the NCLEX® Examination

1. In selecting alternative therapies, acupressure may be most effective with which patient?
   1. Restless, anxious patient
   2. Patient with ulcerative colitis
   3. Pregnant woman
   4. Psychiatric patient

2. The nurse's presentation on alternative therapies for a community group states that herbal therapies are:
   1. approved by the U.S. Food and Drug Administration under the Food, Drug, and Cosmetic Act.
   2. sold as medicines in most stores because they lack major side effects.
   3. allowed to be packaged as dietary supplements if they are without health claims.
   4. consistent in their standards for concentrations of major ingredients and additives.

3. A patient asks about different herbal therapies that may promote physical endurance and reduce stress. On which would the nurse provide information?
   1. Ginseng
   2. Ginger
   3. Echinacea
   4. Chamomile

4. When assessing a patient's use of alternative therapies, the nurse asks:
   1. "What herbal supplements have you taken?"
   2. "Have you ever used relaxation therapy?"
   3. "What types of activities or remedies do you use when you do not feel well?"
   4. "Do you use holistic treatments?"

5. Which statement is correct regarding complementary and alternative medicine?
   1. One third to one half of the U.S. population uses one or more forms of alternative therapy.
   2. Decreasing amounts of insurance coverage are available to meet the needs of alternative therapies.
   3. Discussion of alternative therapies is still not provided in traditional medical journals.
   4. Integration of alternative therapies is regulated by state and national agencies.

6. A benefit that the patient can gain from relaxation therapy is a decrease in:
   1. receptivity.
   2. peripheral skin temperature.
   3. oxygen consumption.
   4. alpha brain activity.

7. Which factor makes accurate administration of precise dosages of herbs difficult?
   1. Multiple clinical trials are under way
   2. Availability in many different forms
   3. Infrequent usage by consumers
   4. Excessive standardization by international organizations

8. Which instruction should be included when teaching a patient about safe herbal product usage?
   1. "Combine several herbs to maximize the benefits."
   2. "Believe all claims made by the manufacturer."
   3. "Continue using herbs if side effects develop because they will diminish."
   4. "Inform your primary care provider of all herbal products you use."

9. A method of stimulating certain points on the body by the insertion of special needles to modify the perception of pain, normalize physiologic functions, or treat or prevent disease is known as:
   1. acupressure.
   2. magnet therapy.
   3. acupuncture.
   4. chiropractic therapy.

10. Patient teaching about herbal therapies should address which statement?
    1. Inform the primary care provider of any drugs being used, including herbal remedies.
    2. Active ingredients per dose are always the same among different brands of the same herb.
    3. There are numerous clinical trials on the benefits and side effects of herbs, enabling clinicians to be well informed in recommending an herb or cautioning against it.
    4. Taking herbs does not require cautious use and results in few side effects.

11. Which is a contraindication for the use of reflexology?
    1. Taking chemotherapy for cancer
    2. General "tune-up"
    3. Pregnancy, presurgical status, and postsurgical status
    4. Presence of heart problems, blood pressure problems, epilepsy, or diabetes

12. Many complementary therapies, such as acupuncture, use diagnostic and therapeutic methods specific to their field, whereas others, such as ___________, are more easily learned and applied.
    1. massage therapy
    2. Chinese medicine
    3. shamanism
    4. breathwork and imagery

13. What does holistic nursing address and treat?
    1. Mind, body, and spirit of the patient.
    2. Disease, spirit, and family.
    3. Desires and emotion of the patient.
    4. Muscles, nerves, and spinal disorders.

14. One of the principles of complementary and alternative medicine (CAM) therapies is that the individual becomes:
    1. actively involved in the treatment.
    2. a total believer in what is being taught.
    3. submissive to the practitioner.
    4. less competent in his or her own care.

15. The herb comfrey is sometimes used by patients for its wound healing properties. It is important that the nurse inform the patient that this herb:
    1. should be taken internally.
    2. may cause cancer.
    3. can only be used externally.
    4. is a known antiseptic.

16. Patients with certain medical diagnoses should avoid chiropractic treatment. These diagnoses include:
    1. joint subluxation
    2. vertigo
    3. osteoporosis
    4. hypertension

17. Imagery is used to:
    1. gain relief for skin diseases.
    2. control and relieve pain.
    3. treat cardiac dysrhythmias.
    4. gain relief from alcohol addiction.

18. A patient tells the nurse that he takes the herb St. John's wort for mild depression. It is important that the nurse inform the patient that he should avoid consuming:
    1. foods high in salt or sodium.
    2. milk products.
    3. anything containing barley, such as beer.
    4. aged cheese and red wine.

Chapter

18 Hygiene and Care of the Patient's Environment

evolve

http://evolve.elsevier.com/Christensen/foundationsadult

Elaine Oden Kockrow

Objectives

1. Discuss the therapeutic hospital room environment.
2. Describe personal hygienic practices.
3. Discuss variations of the bath procedure determined by a patient's condition and physician's orders.
4. Describe the procedure for a bed bath.
5. Identify nursing interventions for the prevention and treatment of pressure ulcers.
6. Describe the procedures for oral hygiene, shaving, hair care, nail care, and eye, ear, and nose care.
7. Outline the procedure for a back rub.
8. Summarize the procedure for perineal care to a male patient and a female patient.
9. Discuss the procedures for skin care.
10. Describe the procedure for making an unoccupied bed.
11. Describe the procedure for making an occupied bed.
12. Discuss assisting a patient in the use of the bedpan, the urinal, and the bedside commode.

Key Terms

axilla (ăk-SĬL-ă, p. 442)
bedpan (BĔD-păn, p. 465)
canthus (KĂN-thŭs, p. 442)
cerumen (sĕ-RŪ-mĕn, p. 461)
chux (chŭks, p. 465)
circumorbital (sŭr-kŭm-ŎR-bĭ-tăl, p. 460)
dentures (DĔN-chŭrs, p. 452)
febrile (p. 440)
hygiene (HĪ-gēn, p. 434)
labia majora (LĀ-bē-ă mă-JŎR-ă, p. 459)
labia minora (LĀ-bē-ă mĭ-NŎR-ă, p. 459)
medical asepsis (ā-SĔP-sĭs, p. 434)
oral hygiene (ŎR-ăl HĪ-gēn, p. 450)
pathogenic (păth-ō-GĔN-ĭk, p. 436)
perineal care (pĕr-ĭ-NĒ-ăl, p. 457)
personal hygiene (PŬR-sŭn-ăl HĪ-gēn, p. 434)
prone (prōn, p. 443)
range of motion (ROM) (rānj ŏv MŌ-shŭn, p. 441)
Sims' position (SĬMZ pŏ-zĭ-shŭn, p. 443)
supine (SŪ-pīn [noun], sū-PĪN [adjective] p. 443)
syncope (SĬN-kō-pē, p. 439)
umbilicus (ŭm-BĬL-ĭ-kŭs, p. 442)
urinal (Ū-rĭn-ăl, p. 466)
vertigo (VŬR-tĭ-gō, p. 439)

Hygiene (the science of health) includes care of not only the skin but also the hair, the hands, the feet, the eyes, the ears, the nose, the mouth, the back, and the perineum. This chapter discusses the bath, components of the bath, bedmaking, and assisting the patient in the use of the bedpan, the urinal, and the bedside commode. Many factors influence the practice of an individual's personal hygiene (Box 18-1 and Cultural Considerations box).

When providing the patient's hygiene needs, you have an opportunity to observe the patient's ability to perform self-care. During the bath, you will note the patient's physical and emotional state, as well as assess all body systems. Because the bath, especially the bed bath, involves close contact with the patient, it offers an opportunity to use your communication skills to enhance the therapeutic relationship and learn about the emotional needs of the patient.

Patients often find themselves in a dependent role and need you to assist them in carrying out **personal hygiene** (the self-care measures people use to maintain their health). While carrying out your responsibilities in this area, preserve the patient's well-being, encourage as much of the patient's independence as possible, and respect the patient's privacy.

At times you will need to teach health promotion practices, and the performance of hygienic care provides an excellent opportunity for this. Project an attitude of acceptance when caring for a patient whose hygiene is obviously poor.

The different types of hygienic care are usually performed at certain times throughout the day. These times depend on various factors involving your organization and the way it schedules care (Box 18-2). Sometimes it will be most convenient to schedule hygiene measures to be performed at the same time as other care measures.

Your own conscientious practice of personal hygiene is essential (Box 18-3). Nurses are role models and teach by example. Hygienic practices promote **medical asepsis,** also known as clean technique. This is a technique that inhibits the growth and spread of

Box 18-1 Factors that Influence a Patient's Personal Hygiene

- *Social practices.* Social groups, family customs, age, friends, and work groups all influence practices of personal hygiene.
- *Body image.* Body image is a person's subjective concept of physical appearance. This body image affects the manner in which hygiene is maintained. You will need to provide education to the unclean patient about the importance of hygiene. However, be careful not to convey feelings of disapproval when caring for the patient whose hygiene practices differ from your own.
- *Socioeconomic status.* The patient's economic resources will often influence the type or extent of hygienic practices used.
- *Knowledge.* Knowledge alone is not enough. It is also essential to encourage the patient to maintain self-care. Often, learning about an illness or condition encourages patients to improve hygienic practices. For example, teaching the patient with diabetes the importance of foot care helps prevent infections. It is important to maintain a nonjudgmental attitude while providing hygiene for the patient.
- *Personal preference.* Individual patients will have individual desires and choices as to when to bathe, shave, and shampoo. Patients choose different shampoos, deodorants, and toothpastes according to personal needs or selections. Do not try to change the patient's preferences unless the patient's health is affected.
- *Physical condition.* Patients in the late stages of terminal illness or those who have undergone surgery often lack the physical energy or dexterity to perform personal hygiene. Some disease conditions will exhaust or incapacitate patients, thereby requiring you to perform all aspects of hygiene. Other disease conditions, such as serious cardiac or pulmonary problems, cause severe activity intolerance.
- *Cultural variables.* Patients from diverse cultural backgrounds follow different self-care practices. For example, in North America people take daily baths (tub or shower), but in many European countries it is not unusual to bathe completely only once a week. Avoid being judgmental when caring for patients with different hygienic practices (see Cultural Considerations box).

Cultural Considerations

Personal Hygiene

- Touching or lack of touch has cultural significance and symbolism and is a learned behavior. Cultural uses of touch vary. Although the rules of touch are typically unspoken and unwritten, they are usually visible to the observer. Stay within the rules of touch that are culturally prescribed.
- Chinese-Americans will sometimes view tasks associated with closeness and touch as offensive. Vietnamese-Americans are likely to feel very uneasy during a back rub. Ask patients what will make them most comfortable during a bath.
- It is essential that you use touch with discernment and avoid forcing touch on anyone. A momentary and seemingly incidental touch has the capacity to establish a positive, temporary bond between strangers, making them more compliant, helpful, positive, and giving.
- The astute nurse is mindful of the patient's reaction to touch and avoids being perceived as intrusive.
- Also consider the individual patient's beliefs, values, and habits.
- Individual preferences usually do not affect health in any significant manner and usually fit without problem into the plan of care.
- One culture that considers personal hygiene to be extremely important is that of the East Indian Hindus. A daily bath is part of their religious duty. Bathing after a meal is believed by some Hindus to be injurious. Likewise, a bath that is too hot has the potential to injure the eyes. Hot water may be added to cold water, but cold water is not to be added to hot water when one is preparing a bath. Once a bath is completed, the individual carefully dries the body thoroughly with a towel.

Box 18-2 Hygiene Care Schedule

- *Early morning care.* Nursing personnel on the night shift provide basic hygiene to patients getting ready for breakfast, scheduled tests, or early morning surgery; "AM care" includes offering a bedpan or urinal if the patient is not ambulatory, washing the patient's hands and face, and assisting with oral care.
- *Morning care, or after-breakfast care.* This care is performed after breakfast. Offer a bedpan or urinal to patients confined to bed; provide a bath or shower; provide oral, foot, nail, and hair care; give a back rub; change the patient's gown or pajamas; change the bed linens; and straighten the patient's bedside unit and room. This is often referred to as complete AM care.
- *Afternoon care.* Because hospitalized patients often undergo many exhausting diagnostic tests or procedures in the morning, they tend to greatly appreciate afternoon care. Afternoon hygienic care includes washing the hands and face, assisting with oral care, offering a bedpan or urinal, and straightening bed linen.
- *Evening care, or hour-before-sleep (HS) care.* Before bedtime, offer personal hygienic care that helps a patient relax to promote sleep; "PM care," sometimes referred to as HS care, typically includes changing soiled bed linens, gowns, or pajamas; assisting the patient in washing the face, hands, and back; providing oral hygiene; giving a back massage; and offering the bedpan or urinal to nonambulatory patients.

Box 18-3 Personal Hygiene for Nurses

- Take a daily bath or shower.
- Use a strong, odorless, and effective deodorant every day.
- Wear clean undergarments every day.
- Wear a clean uniform every day.
- Shampoo hair as often as necessary to maintain cleanliness.
- Keep hair off the collar or at least pulled back away from the face and in a contained hairstyle. Wear barrettes and bows that blend in with your hair.
- Wear white cotton socks or hose that are nylon, white, and free from defects; launder following each wearing.
- Wear white, comfortable shoes; keep clean and polished. Launder shoestrings on a regular basis.
- Keep fingernails short, clean, and well manicured. Wear clear or pale pink polish, if any (never have chipped polish). No acrylic nails! Pathogens get trapped underneath acrylic nails and have the potential to cause serious infections, especially in newborns.
- Wear makeup only in moderation.
- Wear only an engagement ring or wedding ring (or both). In departments such as the operating and delivery rooms, rings are not worn at all.
- Wear only small, unobtrusive earrings; wear only one pair. Large or dangling earrings are not recommended, nor are numerous rings. These are considered hazardous in departments such as pediatrics and some mental health areas.
- Use only a very light cologne, perfume, or aftershave (strong odors are objectionable to patients).
- Wear white-only T-shirts under uniform tops.
- Wear the standard departmental uniform. Jeans, sport slacks, blouses, and shirts are not recommended.
- Keep beards and mustaches clean, short, and well trimmed.
- Use breath mints; the smell of coffee or nicotine is often offensive to patients.

pathogenic (disease-producing) microorganisms (see Chapter 12).

PATIENT'S ROOM ENVIRONMENT

Patients with severe illnesses are often restricted to prolonged bed rest. Many patients with limitations such as traction, casts, or monitoring equipment are not allowed to leave their rooms. Patients with chronic disabilities and those in long-term care facilities are often confined to their rooms for long periods. Keep rooms comfortable and safe (Figure 18-1). By controlling factors such as room temperature, ventilation, noise, and odors, you create a more therapeutic environment. Keeping the room clean, neat, and orderly contributes to a sense of well-being.

MAINTAINING COMFORT

Consider the patient's age, severity of illness, and activity tolerance to best maintain patient comfort. The recommended room temperature is 68° to 74° F (20° to 23° C). Infants, older adults (see Life Span Considerations for Older Adults box), and the acutely ill are likely to need warmer temperatures. Physically active patients tend to be more comfortable in a cooler environment.

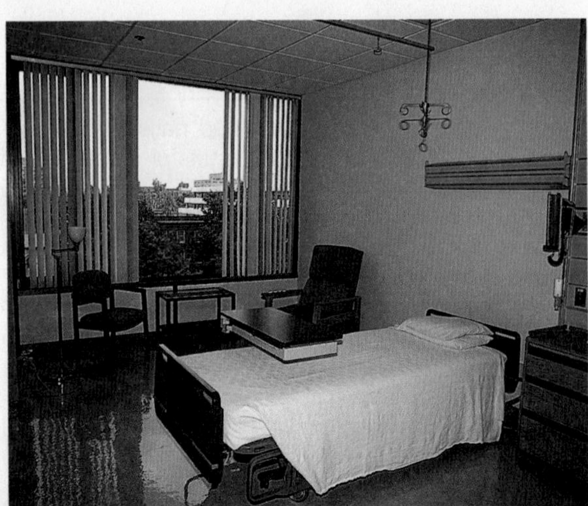

FIGURE 18-1 A typical hospital room.

Good ventilation is necessary to keep stale air and odors from lingering in the room. Take care to protect the patient from drafts.

Be conscientious about emptying and rinsing bedpans and urinals promptly after use. Do not allow visitors to smoke in patients' rooms. (Almost all health care facilities have instituted a no-smoking policy.)

Noises are unpleasant intrusions. Ill patients are more sensitive to the noises commonly heard within the hospital environment. Work with other hospital personnel to monitor the noise level that results from the moving of metal equipment on and off the elevator, TVs and radios, telephones ringing, loud talking, and laughter at the nurses' station. Manage equipment properly, answer phones immediately, and control voice volume. Ask patients to keep TVs and radios turned down.

Proper lighting is necessary for the safety of both you and the patient. Reduce lighting levels to encourage sleep, and brighten the room for stimulation. Adjust the lighting by closing or opening the drapes, adjusting overbed and floor lights, or by opening or closing room doors.

The patient is obliged to direct all energy toward recovery. Do everything within your power, therefore, to control stimuli within the patient's personal environment. This will promote a sense of security and enhance the patient's ability to gain needed rest and sleep (see Chapter 16).

ROOM EQUIPMENT

The usual hospital room contains certain basic furniture: bedside stand, bed, overbed table, chairs, and

 Life Span Considerations

Older Adults

Hygiene Practices

- Older individuals are more likely to become chilled during bathing or when left uncovered. Maintain a warmer room temperature than for younger people, and keep drafts to a minimum.
- Drape older adults properly during care to prevent chilling and provide for modesty.
- Older adults with limited mobility will need assistance in perineal care. Using a side-lying position increases the patient's comfort and provides the nurse with opportunity to provide perineal care and inspect surrounding skin.
- Impaired circulation or neurologic changes sometimes decrease the older person's ability to sense temperature changes in water, so use caution to prevent burns during tub or shower bathing.
- Too-frequent bathing and use of detergent soaps has harmful effects on the skin of most older adults. Base type and frequency of baths and choice of soap on individual needs.
- Rehydrate patient's skin with lotions and fluids.
- Immobility, incontinence, and poor nutrition increase the risk of skin impairment in older adults. Adequate diet, frequent change of position, use of pressure-reducing devices, regular toileting, and prompt cleansing of the skin after incontinence reduce the risks.
- Older adults with urinary incontinence need meticulous skin care to reduce skin irritation from urine and feces.
- The aging process contributes to changes in voiding and defecating. Often, the aging patient will require immediate response to a request for the bedpan or urinal or a trip to the toilet.
- Incontinence of urine or stool is NOT an expected result of the aging process.
- Decreased production of saliva in aging necessitates more frequent oral hygiene. Good cleaning of the oral cavity and teeth or dentures helps reduce the alteration in taste common with aging.
- Good oral hygiene practices help older adults preserve their ability to eat. Patients with diabetes need to visit the dentist a minimum of every 6 months. It is best for older adults, especially those at risk for oral problems, to avoid spicy, coarse, acidic, and sugary foods, which tend to cause dental caries.
- Treat older adults with respect. Keep grooming, including hair care and use of cosmetics, age appropriate.
- Because of normal changes in the nails and an increased incidence of circulatory problems or diabetes mellitus, older individuals are more likely to require special foot care.
- Changes in aging skin include thinning of epidermis and subcutaneous fat and dryness because of decreased activity of oil and sweat glands. These changes become visible in the feet. In addition, nails become opaque, tough, scaly, brittle, and hypertrophied.
- A lifetime of limited exercise often results in laxity of foot ligaments and musculature and leads to instability and impaired mobility.
- Common foot problems of older adults include heel pain caused by tearing of plantar fascia and foot musculature, metatarsalgia (pain beneath metatarsal head), hammertoes and claw toes, corns and calluses, pathologic nail conditions (e.g., ingrown toenails, fungal infections), arthritis, and neuropathies that cause diminished sensation in the foot.
- Older persons are also more vulnerable to bunions because feet tend to spread with aging.
- Usually the facial hair of the older adult does not grow quickly, and thus a shave is not necessarily a must every day.
- Older adults have fragile skin and require more protection. Be sure bed linens are clean, dry, and free of wrinkles.
- Encourage older adults to spend as much time out of bed as possible.
- Use drawsheets and waterproof pads with caution. Accumulation of moisture creates a risk for skin maceration and impairment.

lights (see Figure 18-1). In addition, the standard hospital room will have either a closet or drawer space.

The bedside stand serves to store the patient's personal articles and hygienic equipment such as towels, the emesis and bath basins, toothpaste and toothbrush, and comb and brush. The telephone, the drinking glass, and the water pitcher are ordinarily kept on the patient's bedside stand.

The overbed table is on wheels and is adjustable to various heights over the bed or a chair. Usually there is a storage area under the tabletop. This tabletop is ideal to use for your working space when you perform procedures. It also serves as a surface for meal trays, toileting items needed during hygienic care, and other objects frequently used by the patient.

Chairs are a necessity in the hospital room. Both straight chairs and lounge chairs are typical. Both the patient and visitors will make use of the lounge chair. Straight chairs are more maneuverable than lounge chairs. They are also more convenient when temporarily transferring the patient from the bed, such as during bedmaking. Relatives sitting with the patient are apt to use recliner chairs.

Lights in each patient's room provide comfort, safety, and ease. A call light is available at each bedside. The call signal indicates that a patient needs assistance. Many facilities are designed so that the call light from a patient's bathroom will flash off and on, perhaps many times, denoting a call of a more serious nature, in contrast to the bedside call light, which does not flash. Respond as soon as possible when a patient indicates a need for assistance.

Seriously ill patients often remain in bed for a long time, and the bed is the piece of equipment used most by a patient. Therefore hospital beds are designed for comfort, safety, and their capacity to accommodate position changes (Table 18-1). The standard hospital bed has a firm water-repellent mattress on a metal frame that is raised and lowered horizontally as needed. An even surface provides for the greatest comfort. Handles

Table 18-1 Bed Positions

POSITION	DESCRIPTION	USES
Fowler's	Head of bed raised to angle of 45 degrees or more; semisitting position	Preferred while patient eats; used during nasogastric tube insertion and nasotracheal suction; promotes lung expansion
Semi-Fowler's	Head of bed raised approximately 30 degrees; incline less than Fowler's position	Promotes lung expansion
Trendelenburg's	Entire bed tilted downward toward head of bed	For postural drainage; facilitates venous return in patients with poor peripheral perfusion
Reverse Trendelenburg's	Entire bed frame tilted downward toward foot of bed	Used infrequently; promotes gastric emptying and prevents esophageal reflux
Flat	Entire bed frame parallel with floor	For patients with vertebral injuries and in cervical traction; used for hypotensive patients; generally preferred by patients for sleeping

From Potter, P.A., & Perry, A.G. (2007). *Basic nursing: a critical thinking approach.* (6th ed.). St. Louis: Mosby.

on the sides serve to help removal or turning of the mattress.

Different bed positions are used to promote lung expansion, postural drainage, and other interventions. Most beds are powered by electricity, but some are operated manually. These beds are convenient to raise while you are working at the bedside and then lower when the patient is being transferred or when you leave the patient's room. The bed is also constructed so that you are able to raise and lower the head and the foot independently. In most cases, the controls are conveniently situated on the side of the bed. However, some beds are designed with the controls in the side rail, at the foot of the bed, or as part of the bedside stand. Teach the patient the proper use of the controls, and caution the patient to leave the bed at its lowest level to prevent injuries from falls.

Hospital beds have a number of safety features. Locks on the wheels prevent unwanted movement. Side rails (adjustable metal frames that you raise and lower by pushing or pulling a knob) are located on both sides of the bed. These side rails protect patients from falling, aid patients in positioning themselves, and provide upper extremity support as the patient gets out of bed. Never leave the bedside of a patient in bed if the side rail is lowered. Another safety feature is the special removable headboard on most beds. This is important when the medical team needs easy access to the patient's head during cardiopulmonary resuscitation.

BATHING

The extent of the patient's bath and methods used for bathing depend on the patient's capabilities, the degree of hygiene required, and the physician's order, as in the case of therapeutic baths. The types of therapeutic baths are outlined in the following sections. Some hygiene skills are acceptable to delegate to assistive personnel (see Coordinated Care box on bathing and other hygienic care measures).

SITZ BATH

This bath cleanses and aids in reducing inflammation of the perineal and anal areas of the patient who has undergone rectal or vaginal surgery or childbirth. Discomfort from hemorrhoids or fissures is also relieved by a sitz bath.

The appliance for the sitz bath is shown in Figure 18-2. Depending on the patient's diagnosis and the physician's order, the desired results are possible to obtain from a tub bath. However, the tub is the least desirable method because heat is also applied to the legs, thus reducing the effects on the pelvic region.

 Coordinated Care

Delegation

HYGIENE CARE MEASURES

Bathing

Skills of bathing are often delegated to assistive personnel (AP); however, skin and range-of-motion (ROM) assessment require the critical thinking and knowledge application unique to the nurse.

- Instruct the AP in what type of bath (complete, partial assist, tub, shower) is appropriate to the patient's diagnosis and needs.
- Remind the AP to notify you of any skin integrity problems so you can inspect areas of impairment or potential impairment.
- Remind the AP to use an organized approach and reassuring tone of voice so the patient feels safe and comfortable during bathing.
- Instruct the AP to encourage the patient to report any concerns or discomfort during the bath.
- Instruct the AP to encourage as much independence in the patient's self-care skills as appropriate and to provide positive feedback.

Oral Care

Skills of oral care, toothbrushing, and denture care are appropriate to delegate to AP, but the patient's gag reflex should be assessed first.

- Instruct the AP the proper way to position patient if patient is unconscious or debilitated.
- Remind the AP to report any changes in oral mucosa.
- Review with the AP the use of oral suction for cleansing oral secretions, if the patient is likely to require it.

Hair Care and Showering

The skills of shampooing and shaving are appropriate to delegate to AP unless the patient has a trauma or injury of the cervical spine.

- Instruct the AP how to properly position individual patients and any special products whose use is indicated.
- Make sure the AP knows how to correctly use medicated shampoos for lice or other conditions and the appropriate steps to prevent transmission to other patients.
- Remind the AP to report how the patient tolerated the procedure and any changes that indicate possible inflammation or injury.

Hand, Foot, and Nail Care

The skill of care of the fingernails and foot care for nondiabetic patients and patients without any circulatory compromise is appropriate to delegate to AP.

- Instruct AP in the proper way to use nail files and clippers (check agency policy on whether AP is permitted to use nail clipper on patients).
- Caution AP to use warm water.
- Remind AP to report any changes that indicate possible inflammation or injury.

Bedmaking

Bedmaking is usually delegated to AP.

- Instruct AP on whether an unoccupied or occupied bed is to be made.
- Review with AP the safety precautions or activity restrictions for patient; stress the use of side rails and the call system in the event that staff assistance is needed.
- Tell AP what to do if wound drainage, dressing material, drainage tubes, or IV tubing becomes dislodged or is found in the linen.
- Instruct AP on what to do if the patient becomes fatigued.

Care of the Incontinent Patient

The skill of providing care for incontinent patients is appropriate to delegate to AP. The following measures are all particularly important when assisting the incontinent patient:

- Caution AP to be aware of the patient's dignity and self-esteem needs and to take measures to prevent violating these needs.
- Ensure that AP know standard precautions guidelines related to handling of body fluids.
- Be sure AP report information to you such as abdominal pain, increased episodes of incontinence, changes in appearance of urine or stool, and evidence of skin breakdown.
- The supervisory nurse is responsible for ensuring that all older adult patients are given adequate privacy for elimination and that cultural modesty standards are observed.

Maintain a water temperature of 110° F (about 43° C) if the purpose is to apply heat to the affected area. If the purpose is to promote healing or to produce relaxation, use a water temperature of about 98° to 102° F (34° to 39° C). Remember to prevent chilling by covering the patient's legs with a bath blanket and the shoulders with a towel. Place a towel behind the patient's back for comfort.

Optimally, the sitz bath lasts from 20 to 30 minutes; it is usually ordered three times daily. If the patient has reading material, the time will seem to pass more quickly.

Observe the patient for signs and symptoms of weakness, such as rapid, weak pulse; tachypnea; and vertigo (dizziness) or syncope (fainting). Never leave the patient alone unless you are sure the patient is safe; then a call signal should be placed within easy reach. Instruct the patient to stay out of drafts and to rest after a sitz bath.

COOL WATER TUB BATH

The cool water tub bath is an option to relieve tension or lower body temperature. It is necessary to institute measures to prevent the patient from chilling. The water temperature is tepid, not cold—98.6° F (37° C).

WARM WATER TUB BATH

You will give the warm water tub bath chiefly to reduce muscle tension. The recommended water temperature is 109.4° F (43° C).

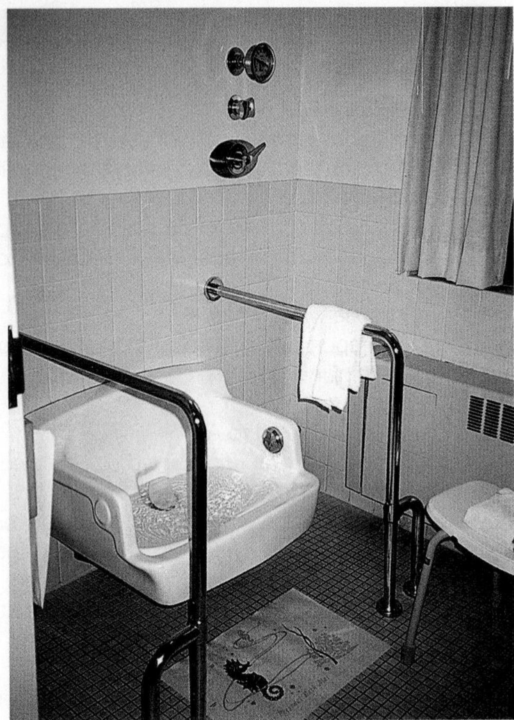

FIGURE 18-2 The sitz bath.

HOT WATER TUB BATH

The hot water tub bath helps relieve muscle soreness and muscle spasms. This procedure is not recommended for children. The proper water temperature for adults is 113° to 115° F (45° to 46° C). Keep in mind the danger of burns, and take precautions to prevent them. You will not use this bath for patients with neurologic disorders or circulatory impairment because of the risk of causing burns.

OTHER BATHS

A complete bed bath is for patients who are totally dependent and require total assistance (Skill 18-1). The seriously or critically ill patient will sometimes need a towel bath. As the patient's condition improves, only partial assistance becomes necessary. Assist the patient to bathe those body parts that are inaccessible to the patient.

If the patient's condition warrants it and ambulation has been ordered, the patient is often allowed to take a tub bath or shower.

A tepid sponge bath is administered to reduce the elevated temperature of patients who are **febrile** (condition characterized by an elevated body temperature).

A medicated bath is sometimes ordered. This bath is likely to include agents such as oatmeal, cornstarch, Burow's solution, and soda bicarbonate (alkaline bath). The medicated bath helps reduce tension, relax the patient, and relieve the pruritus caused by certain skin disorders.

When bathing patients who have dementia, you will probably find it necessary to adjust your style of interaction (Box 18-4).

Text continued on p. 448

Box 18-4 Bathing Patients Who Have Dementia

You will sometimes be required to adjust your style of interaction.

- When caregivers maintain a more relaxed demeanor and smile frequently while bathing patients with dementia, the patients demonstrate greater degrees of calmness and cooperation. Use language appropriate to the patient's level of comprehension, and try to determine which words and phrases the patients uses in reference to bathing—some say "washing up" rather than "having a bath," for example. Explain what you intend to do. If the patient complains of pain or discomfort, apologize and try to determine and address the cause: For example, "I'm sorry that I hurt you. I won't scrub as hard. Is that better?" Offer reassurance frequently, such as, "You are doing really well; we'll be finished soon," or "As soon as we're finished, I'm going to wrap you in a warm towel and put some of the lotion that you like on your skin."
- Use distraction and negotiation instead of demands.
  —Minimize noise in the bathing area.
  —Be sure bathing environment is warm.
  —Set priorities as to which body parts need bathing and which can be "skipped."
  —Use as few staff as possible.
  —If patient fears water, colored water or bubble bath may help.
- Reward patient after bathing.
  —Praise and rewards have to be realistic.

Skill 18-1 Bathing the Patient and Administering a Back Rub

Nursing Action *(Rationale)*

1. Refer to medical record, care plan, or Kardex for special interventions. *(Provides basis for care.)*
2. Assemble the necessary supplies. *(Organizes procedure.)*
   - Bath towels (2)
   - Washcloths (2)
   - Washbasin
   - Soap and soap dish
   - Bath blanket
   - Gown or patient's own pajamas or nightgown
   - Hygiene articles, such as lotion, powder, and deodorant
   - Laundry bag or hamper
   - Disposable gloves
   - Drapes

3. Introduce self. *(Decreases patient's anxiety.)*
4. Identify patient. *(Ensures procedure is performed with correct patient.)*
5. Explain procedure to patient. *(Enlists cooperation and decreases anxiety.)*
6. Perform hand hygiene and, as appropriate, don clean gloves. Know agency policy and guidelines from the Centers for Disease Control and Prevention (CDC) and Occupational Safety and Health Administration (OSHA). *(Reduces spread of microorganisms.)*
7. Prepare patient for intervention.
   a. Close door or pull curtain. *(Provides privacy.)*
   b. Drape for procedure as appropriate. *(Prevents unnecessary exposure.)*
   c. Suggest use of bedpan, urinal, or bathroom. *(Prevents interruptions during procedure and provides for patient's comfort.)*
   d. Arrange supplies. *(Provides convenient access to equipment.)*
   e. Adjust room temperature. *(Prevents patient from chilling.)*
   f. Raise bed to comfortable working position. *(Promotes proper body mechanics.)*
8. Bed bath.
   a. Lower side rail; position patient on side of bed closest to you. *(Ensures proper body mechanics.)*
   b. Loosen top linens from the foot of the bed; place bath blanket over the top linens. Ask patient to hold bath blanket while you remove top linens. If patient is unable, you will have to hold bath blanket in place while removing linens. *(Provides warmth and privacy.)*
   c. Place soiled laundry in laundry bag—do not touch uniform with soiled laundry. *(Reduces spread of microorganisms.)*
   d. Assist patient with oral hygiene. *(Prevents mouth diseases, improves self-image, and improves appetite.)* If patient is unable, perform procedure yourself (see Skill 18-2).
   e. Remove patient's gown, all undergarments, and jewelry. *(Facilitates a more effective bed bath.)* If an extremity is injured or has reduced mobility, begin removal of the gown from the unaffected side. If the patient has an intravenous (IV) tube, remove gown from the arm without IV first, then lower IV container or remove tubing from pump and slide gown covering down over the affected arm, and over tubing and container. Rehang IV container and check flow rate or reset pump (see illustration). Do not disconnect tubing. *(Undressing the unaffected side first makes it easier to manipulate gown over body part with reduced range of motion [ROM]*

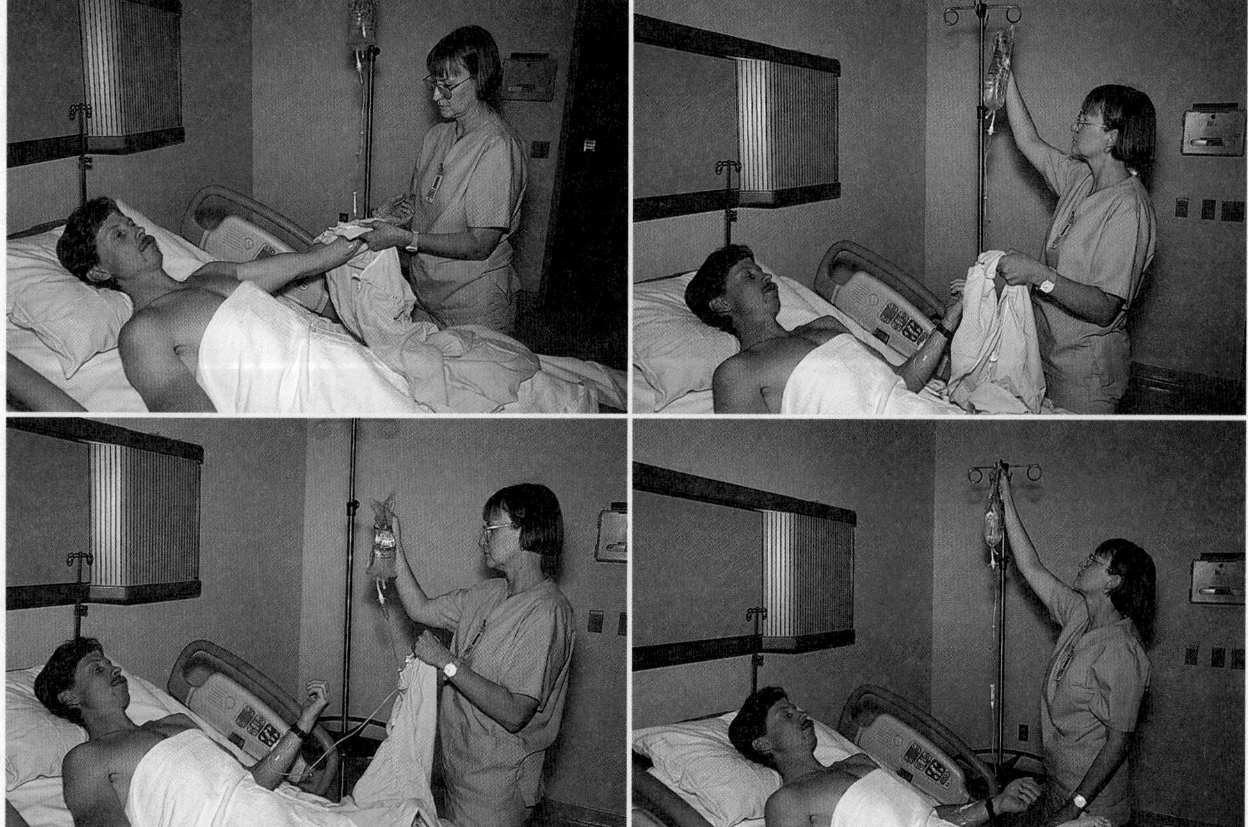

Step 8e

Continued

Skill 18-1 Bathing the Patient and Administering a Back Rub—cont'd

[normal movement that any given joint is capable of making].)

f. Raise side rail and fill washbasin two thirds full with water at 110° to 115° F (43° to 46° C). To prevent spillage, do not overfill basin. *(Maintains patient's safety.)*

g. Remove pillow and raise head of bed to semi-Fowler's position if patient is able to tolerate it. *(The patient's face, ears, and neck are more accessible for cleansing. Patients with breathing difficulties require a pillow or elevation of head of bed during bath.)*

h. Form mitt with bath cloth around your hand (see illustration); dip mitt and hand into bath water. Squeeze out excess water. *(Facilitates handling of bath cloth and prevents corners from brushing against patient. Do not place soap in bath water—too many suds will prevent adequate rinsing.)*

i. Wash around patient's eyes, using a different portion of washcloth for each eye. Cleanse from inner to outer **canthus** (corner of eye) (see illustration). Dry gently. *(Prevents irritation, spread of infection, and injury.)*

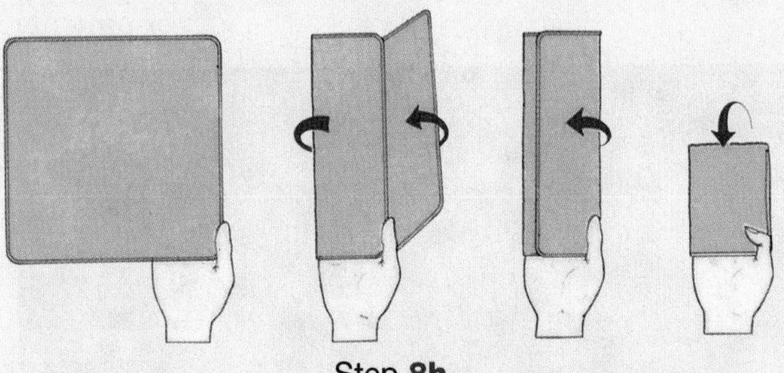

Step **8h**

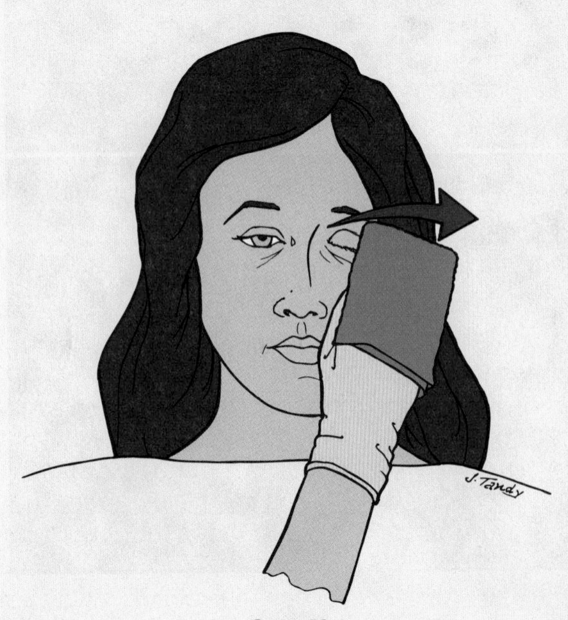

Step **8i**

j. Rinse bath cloth (then continue to use as mitt) and finish washing face. (Ask patient about using soap on face because some patients, especially female patients, do not use soap on face.) Now wash ears and neck. Cleanse pinna (the projecting part of the external ear) with cotton-tipped applicators. *(Rinsing cloth well will help reduce any skin irritation from the soap. Do not place soap in washbasin to keep rinse water from getting soapy.)*

k. Expose arm farthest from you. Place towel lengthwise under patient's arm. Place washbasin on towel, and place patient's hand in basin of water. Bathe arms using long, firm strokes; a firm stroke rather than a light stroke prevents tickling the patient. Supporting arm, raise it above patient's head to bathe the **axilla** (the underarm area or armpit). Rinse and dry well. In most cases, provide nail care at this time (see next step), although if desired it is possible to do separately (see Skill 18-3). Apply deodorant if desired. *(Beginning on far side prevents reaching over clean area; long, firm strokes stimulate circulation. Raising arm promotes ROM, as well as exposes axilla. Deodorant controls body odor. Axilla is bathed last because it is considered less clean than arm.)*

l. When doing nail care, allow patient's hand to soak for 3 to 5 minutes; push back cuticles gently with washcloth. Clean under nails and file smoothly as needed. Dry thoroughly. *(Enhances feeling of self-worth and decreases spread of infection. Soaking softens cuticles and loosens debris under nails.)*

m. Bathe arm closest to you. Follow steps k and l.

n. Cover patient's chest with bath towel; fold bath blanket down to waist and wash chest with circular motion. Be certain to cleanse and dry well in skinfolds and under breasts. *(Using circular motion while bathing chest prevents injury to delicate breast tissue. Covering chest with towel prevents unnecessary exposure. Cleansing well in skinfolds and under breasts maintains skin integrity.)* Continue to observe the condition of the patient's skin, degree of mobility, and behavior, and encourage the patient to verbalize concerns.

o. Fold bath blanket down to pubic area, keeping chest covered with dry towel. Wash abdomen, including **umbilicus** (the depressed point in the middle of the abdomen) (wash umbilicus using cotton-tipped applicators), and skinfolds. Dry thoroughly. *(Main-*

tains privacy. Prevents unnecessary exposure and prevents skin impairment.)

p. Raise side rail; empty basin into hopper or stool. *(Flushes microorganisms down the stool and does not contaminate sink.)*

q. Rinse basin and washcloth. Refill basin two thirds full with water at 110° to 115° F (43° to 46° C.) *(Promotes patient's safety and comfort.)*

r. Expose leg farthest away from you, keeping **perineum** (the genital area) covered. Place bath towel lengthwise on bed under patient's leg. Place washbasin on towel, and place patient's foot in basin (see illustration). (Patients with diabetes mellitus require special foot care.) Make certain to support patient's leg properly; flex knee and grasp heel. If patient is unable to place foot in washbasin, wash leg and foot with mitted washcloth. *(Beginning on the far side prevents reaching over clean area; bath towel prevents wetting bottom linens; supporting patient's leg properly prevents injury.)*

s. Using long, firm strokes, bathe leg. *(Promotes circulation.)* However, note that it is contraindicated to bathe the lower extremities of patients with history of deep-vein thrombosis (DVT) or hypercoagulation disorders with long firm strokes; use circular, gentle strokes for these patients. After soaking, do nail care (may be done at a separate time) (see Skill 18-3). If skin is dry, apply lotion if desired. Do not massage legs: **Never massage lower extremities.** *(Prevents possible embolus [a moving blood clot].)*

t. Bathe leg and foot closest to you as in steps r and s.

u. Raise side rail. Make sure patient is covered with bath blanket. Be certain to expose only those body parts being bathed. Change water (see steps p and q). *(Provides clean water and promotes good hygiene.)* Lower side rail. If patient tolerates, position **prone** (lying face-down) or in **Sims' position** (side-lying position). Place towel lengthwise on bed along back. Wash and dry back from neckline down to buttocks (see illustration). If patient tolerates a massage action, do so while washing back. *(Promotes circulation, thus preventing skin impairment, and promotes relaxation.)*

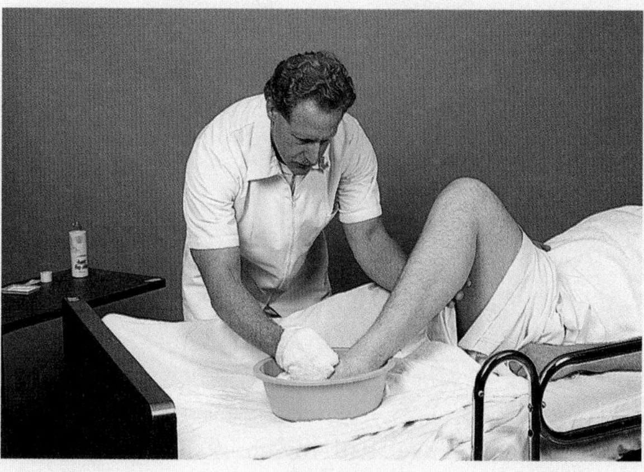

Step **8r**

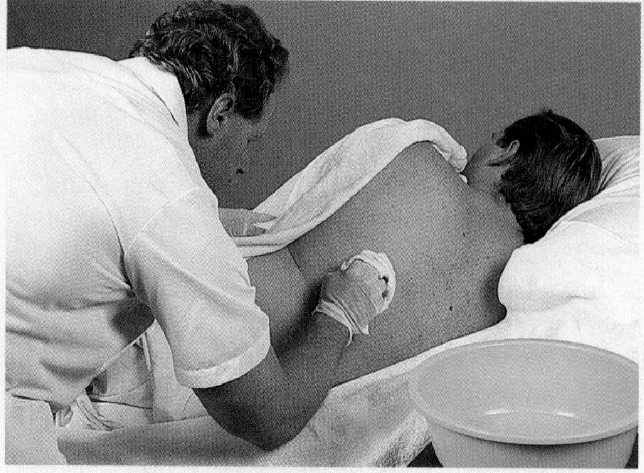

Step **8u**

v. Reposition patient **supine** (lying face-up). Provide basin of water, soap, washcloth, and towel, and instruct patient to cleanse perineal area. (Give patient privacy to do this.) If patient is unable to finish bath, don new gloves and complete this aspect of patient care (see Skill 18-4). *(Completes the bath procedure, decreases infection, and prevents skin impairment.)*

w. Make certain patient is covered with blankets. *(Prevents chilling.)* Raise side rail. *(Promotes safety.)* Empty, wash, and rinse basin. Replace basin in bedside stand. Place washcloth in laundry bag for soiled linen. *(Practice of medical asepsis reduces spread of microorganisms.)*

x. Position patient in Sims' or prone position close to you. Place towel lengthwise along patient's back. Give back rub (see step 14). *(Facilitates back care; provides comfort and promotes skin integrity.)* Never massage reddened areas. *(Potentially causes further skin breakdown.)*

y. Assist patient into clean gown. If ordered, assist patient to ambulate to chair; place towel over shoulders, and comb hair. *(Promotes positive self-image.)*

Women sometimes wish to apply makeup at this time. While patient is in chair, make unoccupied bed (see Skill 18-5). If patient is not ambulatory, you will have to make the occupied bed (see Skill 18-5). *(Maintains clean environment.)*

z. Place all soiled linen into laundry bag. Make certain all bath equipment is clean and put it

Continued

Skill 18-1 Bathing the Patient and Administering a Back Rub—cont'd

away as necessary. *(Reduces spread of microorganisms.)*

aa. Place call light, overbed table, nightstand, and telephone within easy reach. *(Promotes safety.)*

bb. Position patient for comfort, and provide warmth. *(Promotes patient's well-being.)*

cc. Remove gloves, if wearing any; discard them in proper receptacle, and perform hand hygiene. *(Reduces spread of microorganisms.)* Maintain a neat, clean work area.

9. The partial bed bath differs from the bed bath only in that the patient does not need assistance bathing many anatomic regions. Help by bathing those areas that the patient cannot reach. All steps of the bath are followed, and the same considerations prevail. Place supplies within easy reach. Change water as noted in the bed bath procedure, and give back care, skin care, nail care, and hair care. A partial bath, in which face, neck, axilla, and perineum are washed, is practiced in some agencies.

10. Towel bath.
   a. Follow steps 1 and 3 to 7.
   b. Assemble supplies. *(Organizes procedure.)*
      - Concentrate or solution (e.g., Septi-Soft)
      - Measuring device, such as plastic medication cup or liter-calibrated container
      - Towel–bath towel (3 × 7.5 ft)
      - Large plastic bag
      - Bath towel
      - Washcloths (2)
      - Bath blankets (3)
      - Disposable gloves
      - Linens for bedmaking
      - Clean gown
      - Articles for personal hygiene—comb, toothbrush, lotion, toothpaste, and mouthwash
   c. Prepare patient. *(Ensures that bath towel will be warm enough for patient's comfort, as well as for effective towel bath. It is necessary to ready the patient before the bath towel is prepared—the temperature cools down quickly.)*
      (1) Remove patient's clothing and excess bedding (top linens, bedspread). Place patient on bath blanket, and cover patient with bath blanket. *(Provides privacy and prevents unnecessary exposure of patient; provides for patient warmth.)*
      (2) Cover with plastic any surgical dressings, casts, or areas that are not to be gotten wet. *(Maintains integrity of dressing or cast.)*
      (3) Fanfold a clean bath blanket at foot of the bed. *(Provides easy access to clean blankets.)*
      (4) Position patient supine with legs partially separated and arms loosely at sides. *(Facilitates the towel bath.)*
   d. Prepare towel. *(Prevents unnecessary cleanups and promotes effective procedure.)*
      (1) Fold towel in half, top to bottom; fold in half again, top to bottom; fold in half again, side to side. Then roll towel–bath towel with bath towel and washcloths inside, beginning with folded edge (see illustration).
      (2) Place rolled-up towel–bath towel (with bath towel and washcloths inside) in plastic bag with selvage edges toward open end of bag.
      (3) Draw 2000 mL of water at 115° to 120° F (46° to 49° C) into plastic pitcher. If the towel is not warm, saunalike effect will not be produced and the patient will chill. Measure 30 mL of concentrate with a pump (a single stroke measures 30 mL). Mix 2000 mL of water and Septi-Soft.
      (4) Pour mixture over towel in plastic bag (see illustration).
      (5) Knead the solution quickly into towel; position plastic bag with open end in sink and squeeze out excess water, giving added wringing twist to selvage edges of towel.

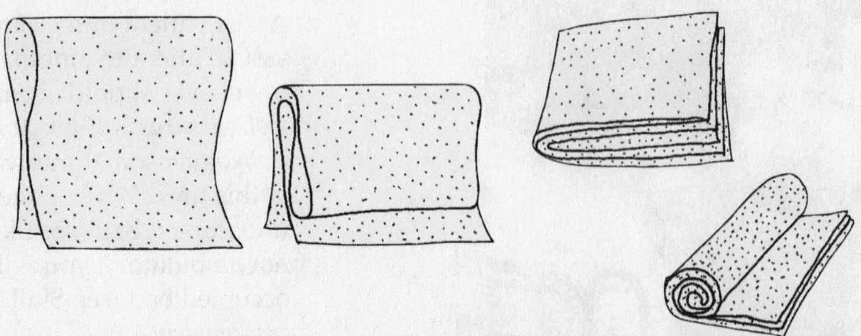

Step **10d(1)** NOTE: Bath towel and washcloth are inside the towel–bath towel.

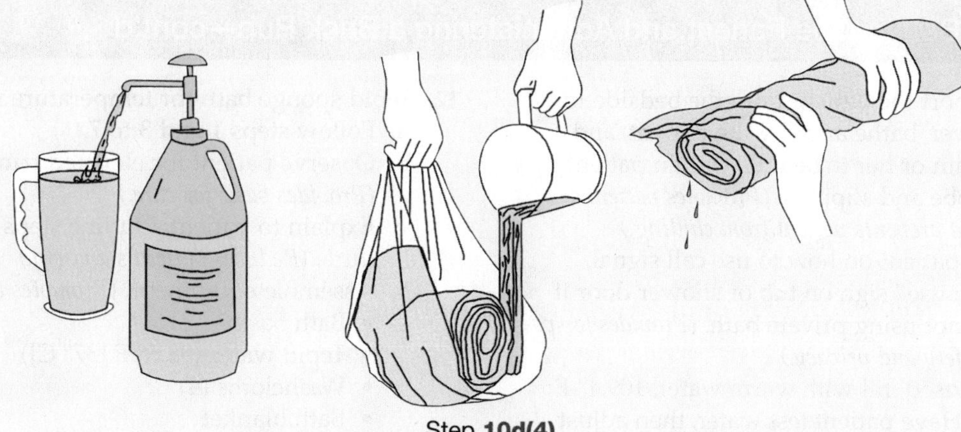
Step 10d(4)

e. Bathe patient using the following procedure. *(Promotes effective towel bath, provides warmth, and keeps bed dry, avoiding chilling the patient.)*

(1) Fold bath blanket down to waist. Remove warm, moist towel from plastic bag and place on patient's right or left chest with open edges up and outward. Unroll towel across chest.

(2) Open towel to cover entire body while removing top bath blanket. Tuck towel–bath towel in and around body (leave bath towel and washcloths in plastic bag to keep warm) (see illustration).

(3) Begin bathing at feet, using gentle, massaging motion. Employ clean section of towel for each part of body as you move toward patient's head.

(4) Fold lower part of towel upward away from feet as bathing continues. If you have an assistant, the bath is given more effectively.

(5) Continue to draw clean bath blanket upward and place over patient as you move upward. Leave 3 inches of exposed skin between towel and bath blanket. Skin will dry in 2 or 3 seconds. If towel bath is given properly, the patient will be refreshed and relaxed.

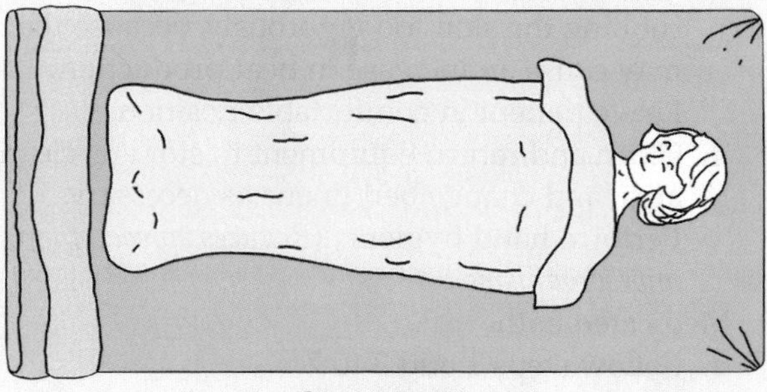
Step 10e(2)

(6) Wash face, neck, and ears with one of the prepared washcloths.

(7) Turn patient onto side.

(8) Use prepared bath towel for back care. (Give back rub—see step 14)

(9) Use second washcloth for perineal care (don disposable gloves). Sometimes you will need a basin of warm water, soap, washcloth, towel, and gloves to perform perineal care (see Skill 18-4).

(10) When bath is completed, remove towel and place with soiled linens in plastic laundry bag. *(Promotes medical asepsis.)*

(11) If top bath blanket is not soiled, fold for reuse later.

f. Make occupied bed. *(Provides comfort and promotes practices of medical asepsis)* (see Skill 18-5).

11. Tub bath or shower.

a. Follow steps 1 and 3 to 7.

b. Determine whether activity is allowed; consult with registered nurse (RN) in charge, if necessary.

c. Make certain tub or shower appliance is clean. See agency policy. Place nonskid mat on tub or shower floor and disposable mat outside of tub or shower. *(Promotes patient's safety. Conditions placing patients at risk for falls in the bathtub include neurologic impairment, arthritis, and poor balance.)*

d. Assemble all items necessary for bathing. *(Prevents unnecessary interruptions.)*

- Towel
- Washcloth
- Soap
- Deodorant
- Lotion
- Clean gown or patient's own pajamas or nightgown

e. Assist patient to tub or shower. Shower chairs are available in most facilities so you are able

Continued

Skill 18-1 Bathing the Patient and Administering a Back Rub—cont'd

to transport the patient from the bedside to the shower, bathe and dry the patient, and return him or her to bed. Be certain patient wears robe and slippers. *(Promotes patient's safety and prevents patient from chilling.)*

f. Instruct patient on how to use call signal. Place "in use" sign on tub or shower door if you are not using private bath. *(Provides for patient's safety and privacy.)*

g. If tub is used, fill with warm water, 109.4° F (43° C). Have patient test water, then adjust temperature. Instruct patient on use of faucets—which is hot and which is cold. If shower is used, turn water on and adjust temperature. *(Prevents accidental burns and promotes safety.)*

h. Caution patient to use safety bars. Discourage use of bath oil in water. It is essential to maintain safety at all times. Check on patient every 5 minutes (q5min). Do not allow to remain in tub more than 20 minutes. *(Maintains patient's safety and prevents vertigo and syncope.)*

i. Return when patient signals. Make an unoccupied bed while the patient bathes unless patient condition is such that you are required to remain with the patient. Return to the tub or shower room and offer to wash the patient's back. Knock before entering. *(Provides privacy and promotes comfort.)*

j. Assist patient out of tub and with drying. Observe the patient for signs and symptoms of weakness, which are rapid pulse, paleness, diaphoresis, unsteady gait, tachypnea, vertigo, and syncope. If patient complains of weakness, vertigo, or syncope, drain tub before patient gets out and place towel over patient's shoulders. *(Prevents falls and promotes comfort.)*

k. Assist patient into clean gown, robe, and slippers. Accompany to room, position for comfort, and give back rub (see step 14). *(Maintains warmth and safety.)*

l. Make unoccupied bed if patient can tolerate sitting in chair, if you did not do so earlier. Perform back, hair, nail, and skin care. *(Maintains clean environment to promote positive self-image and medical asepsis, and promotes patient's well-being.)*

m. Return to shower or tub. Clean according to agency policy. Place all soiled linens in laundry bag and return all articles to patient's bedside. *(Promotes orderly environment and reduces spread of microorganisms.)*

n. Perform hand hygiene. *(Reduces spread of microorganisms.)*

12. Tepid sponge bath for temperature reduction.

a. Follow steps 1 and 3 to 7.

b. Observe patient for elevated temperature. *(Provides basis for care.)*

c. Explain to patient: Outline steps of the procedure. *(Reduces patient's anxiety.)*

d. Assemble equipment. *(Promotes organization.)*
- Bath basin
- Tepid water (98.6° F [37° C])
- Washcloths (4)
- Bath blanket
- Patient thermometer

e. Cover patient with bath blanket, remove gown, and close windows and doors. *(Prevents chilling and provides privacy.)*

f. Test water temperature. Place washcloths in water, then apply wet cloths to each axilla and groin (the depressed area between the thigh and trunk). If patient is in tub, allow to stay in water for 20 to 30 minutes. *(Promotes cooler temperature and allows for more effective heat loss because blood vessels are close to the surface of the body in the axilla and the groin.)*

g. Gently sponge an extremity for about 5 minutes. If patient is in tub, gently sponge water over upper torso, chest, and back. *(Prevents sudden drop in body temperature.)*

h. Continue sponge bath to other extremities, back, and buttocks for 3 to 5 minutes each. Determine temperature and pulse q15min. *(Minimizes risk of patient chilling.)*

i. Change water and reapply freshly moistened washcloths to axilla and groin as necessary. *(Maintains tepid water temperature and continues to promote cooling.)*

j. Continue with sponge bath until body temperature falls to slightly above normal. Keep body parts that are not being sponged covered. Discontinue procedure according to agency policy. *(Prevents body temperature from falling below normal; body temperature will continue to drop.)*

k. Dry patient thoroughly and cover with light blanket or sheet. *(Prevents chilling.)* Avoid rubbing the skin too vigorously, because that may cause an increase in heat production. Leave patient in comfortable position.

l. Clean and return equipment to storage, clean area, and change bed linens as necessary. Perform hand hygiene. *(Reduces spread of microorganisms.)*

13. Medicated bath.

a. Follow steps 1 and 3 to 7.

b. Prepare tub bath (see steps 11c, f, g). *(Promotes orderly procedure.)*

c. Add agent as ordered by physician. *(Follows physician's orders.)*
d. Don gloves as necessary.
e. Assist patient to tub. *(Maintains patient's safety.)*
f. Allow patient to remain in tub for required time. *(Promotes effective procedure.)*
g. Assist patient out of tub. *(Maintains patient's safety.)*
h. Gently pat dry. (Allows medication to remain on patient's skin.) Teach patient not to scratch lesions. *(Avoids further irritation and prevents infection.)*
i. Assist patient into gown or pajamas. *(Prevents patient from chilling.)*
j. Assist patient to return to bed, and position for comfort. *(Allows patient to rest and relax. Promotes well-being.)*
k. Remove and dispose of gloves and perform hand hygiene. *(Reduces the spread of microorganisms.)*

14. Back rub.
    a. Prepare supplies. (*Organizes procedure.*)
        - Bath blanket (optional)
        - Bath towel
        - Skin lotion, powder. If powder is used, apply sparingly. *(Lotion lubricates skin, whereas powder will absorb body moisture and clump, which could result in skin irritation.)*
    b. Follow steps 1 and 3 to 7 and provide quiet environment.
    c. Lower side rail. Position patient with back toward you. Cover patient so that only parts to massage are exposed. *(Prevents unnecessary exposure.)*
    d. Warm hands if necessary. Warm lotion by holding some in hands. Explain that lotion often feels cool. *(Enhances relaxation.)*
    e. Begin massage by starting in sacral area using circular motions (see illustration). Stroke upward to shoulders. Massaging over bony prominences is no longer recommended. Massage may result in decreased blood flow and tissue damage in some patients.

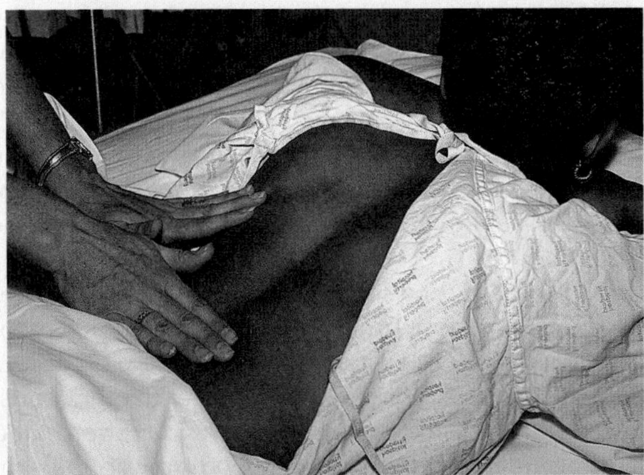
Step 14e

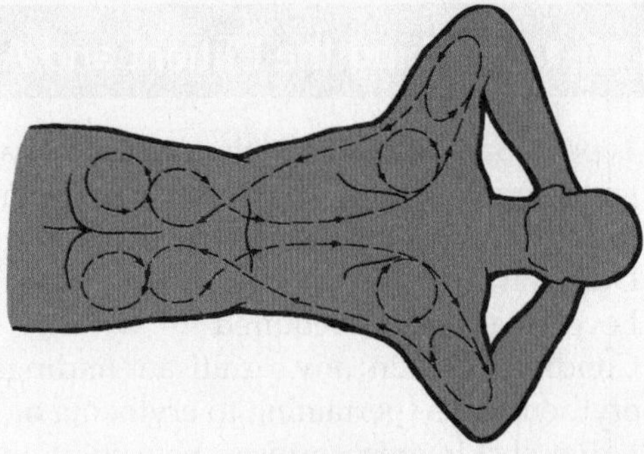
Step 14f

    f. Use firm, smooth strokes to massage over scapulae. Continue to upper arms with one smooth stroke and down along side of back to iliac crest (see illustration). Do not break contact with patient's skin. Complete massage in 3 to 5 minutes. *(A firm, gentle pressure provides relaxation. Using firm pressure prevents tickling the patient. Continuous contact with skin surface is soothing and stimulates circulation.)*
    g. Gently but firmly knead skin by grasping area between thumb and fingers. Work across each shoulder and around nape of neck. Continue downward along each side to sacrum. *(Kneading increases circulation; motion is soothing and relieving.)*
    h. With long, smooth strokes, end massage, remove excess lubricant from patient's back with towel, and retie gown. *(These strokes are relaxing and the most soothing of all massage movements.)* Position for comfort. Lower bed and raise side rail as needed and place call button within easy reach. *(Promotes patient's safety. Excess lotion often irritates skin. Comfortable position enhances the back rub's effect.)*
    i. Place soiled laundry in proper receptacle, and perform hand hygiene. *(Reduces spread of microorganisms.)*

15. Assess patient. *(Determines patient's ability to perform self-care and level of assistance required from you.)*
    - Tolerance of activity
    - Level of discomfort
    - Cognitive ability
    - Musculoskeletal function; extent of joint ROM
    - Risk for skin impairment (e.g., presence of paralysis or large casts or traction, or those patients who are weakened and disabled)
    - Knowledge of importance of skin hygiene
    - Vital signs *(Helps detect an unexpected outcome of an elevation in heart rate and systolic blood pressure.)*

16. Document. *(Timely documentation maintains accuracy of patient's record; condition of skin documents response to therapy [e.g., turning and positioning].)*

Continued

Skill 18-1 Bathing the Patient and Administering a Back Rub—cont'd

- Type of bath (e.g., sitz bath, medicated bath, or tepid sponge bath), water temperature, and solution used, when appropriate
- Duration of treatment
- Level of assistance required
- Condition of skin; any significant findings (e.g., erythematous [pertaining to erythema or redness] skin areas, bruises, nevi, joint or muscle pain, or exudate)
- Vital signs if applicable (e.g., sponge bath for temperature reduction)
- Patient's response
- Patient teaching (see Patient Teaching box)

17. Report alterations in skin integrity to nurse in charge or physician. *(Special medical treatment is sometimes necessary.)*

BACK CARE AND BACK RUB

You will typically administer the back rub after the patient's bath. Offer this opportunity to the patient, because it promotes relaxation, relieves muscular tension, and stimulates circulation. To give an effective back rub, massage for 3 to 5 minutes (see Skill 18-1). During the back rub, observe the skin for abnormalities. Monitor pulse and blood pressure of those patients with a history of hypertension or dysrhythmias. The back rub is contraindicated if the patient has such conditions as fractures of the ribs or vertebral column, burns, pulmonary embolism, or open wounds.

COMPONENTS OF THE PATIENT'S HYGIENE

CARE OF THE SKIN

When a person's physical condition changes, the skin often reflects this by alterations in color, thickness, texture, turgor, temperature, and hydration. As long as the skin remains intact and healthy, its physiologic function remains optimal.

Data Collection

Determine the condition of the patient's skin by observing its color, texture, thickness, turgor, temperature, and hydration. Be certain to use ample lighting. Natural or halogen lighting is suggested, but sunlight is preferred for assessing a patient who has dark skin. Normal skin has the following characteristics:

- Intact without abrasions
- Warm and moist
- Localized changes in texture across surface
- Good turgor (elastic and firm); generally smooth and soft
- Skin color variations from body part to body part

Pressure Ulcers

The nursing diagnosis of *impaired skin integrity,* either *actual* or *risk for,* will apply to every patient with whom you have contact. Prevention and treatment of skin impairment is usually one of your responsibilities. Prevention is the ultimate goal, but when this is not possible, good nursing interventions can result in (1) optimal healing of the impaired skin without complications, (2) a decrease in the patient's discomfort, (3) a decrease in length of hospitalization, and (4) a decrease in the cost of ongoing care.

Approximately 2.5 million hospitalized patients develop pressure ulcers each year despite national guidelines regarding their prevention and treatment. Of these 2.5 million patients, 60,000 die from complications, and the financial cost incurred from treating patients with pressure ulcers is estimated at $11 billion each year (Ayello & Lyder, 2007).

To encourage acute care facilities to become more aggressive in the prevention of pressure ulcer development, as of October 2008 the Centers for Medicare and Medicaid stopped covering the costs of treating pressure ulcers that developed during the patient's hospitalization. The goal is to prevent patients from experiencing the pain, loss of function, complications such as infection, prolonged hospital stays, and the increased costs associated with the development of pressure ulcers (Ayello & Lyder, 2007).

Pressure ulcers occur when there is sufficient pressure on the skin to cause the blood vessels in an area to collapse. The flow of blood and fluid to the cells is impaired, resulting in ischemia, or lack of oxygen and nutrients, to the cells. When the external pressure against the skin is greater than the pressure in the capillary bed (network of capillaries), blood flow decreases to the adjacent tissue. If the pressure continues without relief for more than 2 hours, cells in the involved layers of skin tend to undergo necrosis (death of tissue). Pressure is usually most severe over bony prominences (e.g., sacrum, ischial tuberosities, trochanteric areas of the hips, heels, and malleoli of the ankles).

In addition to unrelieved pressure, two mechanical factors play a common role in the development of pressure ulcers. The first is **shearing force.** This occurs when the tissue layers of skin slide on each other, causing subcutaneous blood vessels to kink or stretch and resulting in an interruption of blood flow to the skin (Figure 18-3).

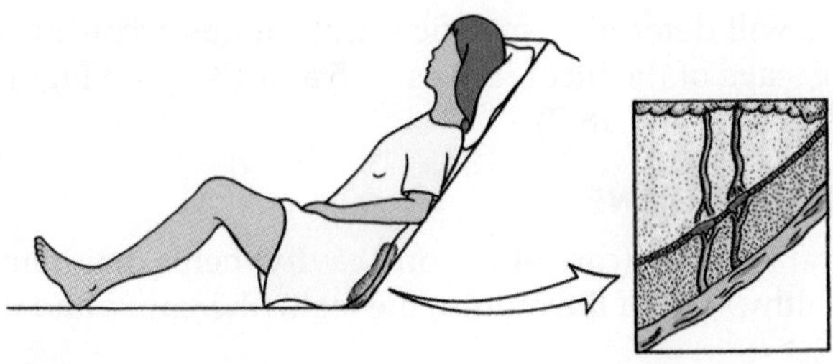

FIGURE 18-3 Diagram of shearing force exerted against sacral area.

The second mechanical factor is **friction.** The rubbing of skin against another surface produces friction, which may remove layers of tissue. Examples of when this might occur are (1) moving the patient in bed by sliding him or her across the bed linen, (2) improperly lifting the patient, and (3) improperly placing the bedpan.

The appearance of pressure ulcers is a major manifestation of impaired skin integrity. A patient who stays in one position without relief of pressure, especially over bony prominences, is at risk to develop a pressure sore. Patients especially at risk are chronically ill, debilitated, older, disabled, incontinent, and those with spinal cord injuries, limited mobility, or poor overall nutrition.

Those who are incontinent are at risk because continual contact of the skin with urine and feces often causes chemical irritation, which frequently leads to impaired skin integrity. Nutritional factors play a role both for those who are overweight and those who are underweight. Obesity increases the risk because fat tissue has less vascularity and resilience, and the added bulk and weight increase the pressure on bony prominences. Underweight increases the risk because of a lack of cushion over the bones and muscles. In addition, any condition that results in a decreased supply of oxygen and nutrients to the cells, such as anemia, atherosclerosis, or edema (swelling), increases the risk of skin impairment because the cells are not adequately nourished.

Patients who are at increased risk for any reason will need careful, ongoing assessment and a plan of care aimed at preventing skin impairment (see Coordinated Care box on skin care).

Definition and Staging

The definition of a pressure ulcer was revised by the National Pressure Ulcer Advisory Panel (NPUAP) in 2007, when the staging system of pressure ulcers was expanded from four to six categories. The NPUAP defines a pressure ulcer as a localized injury to the skin or underlying tissue, usually over a bony prominence, caused by pressure with shear or friction. The following sections describe the revised stages of pressure ulcer development (NPUAP, 2007).

Suspected deep tissue injury. During this stage, the wound appears as a localized purple or maroon area of discolored, intact skin or a blood-filled blister. This is caused by underlying soft tissue damage from pressure and/or shear. Characteristics of the area range from painful, firm, mushy, boggy, or warm, to cool compared to adjacent tissue. In patients with dark skin tones, deep tissue injury is sometimes difficult to detect but often starts with a thin blister over a dark wound bed. The wound sometimes becomes covered with thin eschar. Even with prompt treatment, some

 Coordinated Care

Collaboration

SKIN CARE

Assessment for the presence of skin impairment is a nursing responsibility and is not to be delegated to assistive personnel (AP). However, it is important to instruct AP to report the following to the nurse:

- Any changes in the patient's skin immediately
- Patient's exposure to body fluids (e.g., urine, feces, wound drainage, gastric secretions)

Instruct AP on the following assessment procedure:

1. Obtain appropriate equipment (check agency policy).
   a. Skin assessment documentation record
2. Observe pressure points. Compression of these areas for prolonged periods of time by bony prominences or external sources has the potential to cause tissue ischemia and cell death.
   a. Bony prominences—heels, ankles, knees, sacral area, ischial area, spinal area, shoulders, and elbows
   b. Cast edges, area next to nasogastric tubes, drainage tubes, and oxygen tubing
3. When reddened areas are found, gently press the area with a gloved finger to assess the capacity of the tissue to blanch. Reactive hyperemia occurs when a reddened area blanches upon palpation. If the area does not blanch, suspect tissue injury.
4. Check perineal area for signs of reddened, irritated skin. Perineal skin is at high risk for skin impairment in the patient with fecal and/or urinary incontinence.
5. Observe underlying skin areas where tape, tubing, casts, or splints are in contact with skin.
6. Note previous areas of skin impairment, check for any breaks in the skin integrity, and note any nonblanching erythema in this area. Areas of previous skin impairment do not heal to the same strength as intact noninjured skin; therefore, these areas are at higher risk of skin impairment.
7. Determine if potential or actual skin impairment is present and institute impairment–appropriate preventive or treatment protocols.
8. Record appearance of skin under pressure.
9. Record what preventive or treatment protocols were initiated.

Adapted from Potter, P.A., & Perry, A.G. (2009). *Fundamentals of nursing: concepts, process, and practice.* (7th ed.). St. Louis: Mosby.

wounds evolve rapidly, exposing additional layers of tissue.

Stage I. A stage I pressure ulcer is a localized area of skin—typically over a bony prominence—that is intact with nonblanchable redness. Darker-toned skin will perhaps not have visible blanching, but its color is likely to differ from the surrounding area. The wound characteristics vary: You will see areas that are painful, firm, soft, warm, or cool compared to adjacent tissue. This stage is typically difficult to detect in patients with dark skin tones.

Stage II. A stage II pressure ulcer involves partial-thickness loss of dermis. It appears as a shallow, open ulcer, usually shiny or dry, with a red-pink wound bed without slough or bruising. (Bruising raises the suspicion of deep tissue injury.) Some stage II ulcers manifest as intact or open (ruptured) serum-filled blisters. Do not use the term stage II to describe skin tears, tape burns, perineal dermatitis, maceration, or excoriation.

Stage III. A stage III pressure ulcer involves full-thickness tissue loss in which subcutaneous fat is sometimes visible, but bone, tendon, and muscle are not exposed. If slough is present, it does not obscure the depth of tissue loss. Possible features are undermining and tunneling. The depth of a stage III pressure ulcer varies depending on its anatomic location. On the bridge of the nose, the ear, the occiput, and the malleolus, which lack subcutaneous tissue, these ulcers are shallow. Extremely deep stage III pressure ulcers do develop in areas where there are significant layers of deep adipose tissue.

Stage IV. A stage IV pressure ulcer involves full-thickness tissue loss with exposed bone, tendon, or muscle. Sometimes slough or eschar is present on some parts of the wound bed. The ulcer often includes undermining or tunneling. As with stage III pressure ulcers, stage IV pressure ulcers vary in depth depending on their location. Because these ulcers extend into muscle and supporting structures, the patient is at risk for osteomyelitis.

Unstageable. An unstageable pressure ulcer involves full-thickness tissue loss, a wound base covered by slough (yellow, tan, gray, green, or brown), and/or eschar in the wound bed that will usually be tan, brown, or black. It is not possible to determine the true depth and stage of the ulcer until the base of the wound has been exposed. Stable eschar on the heels provides a natural biologic cover: Do not remove it.

Interventions

Nursing interventions for patients with pressure ulcers include ongoing assessment and evaluation of improvement. Assessment data include the size and the depth of the ulcer (Figure 18-4), the amount and the color of any exudate, the presence of pain or odor, and the color of the exposed tissue. Healing is a long-term process; therefore, make sure the plan of care is consistent over time and evaluate it for effectiveness. You will determine specific interventions according to the stage of the ulcer (Boxes 18-5 and 18-6, and Figures 18-5, 18-6, and 18-7).

ORAL HYGIENE

Oral hygiene (care of the oral cavity) helps maintain a healthy state of the mouth, the teeth, the gums, and the

Box 18-5 General Guidelines for Care of Pressure Ulcers

- Practice surgical asepsis when caring for the pressure ulcer to prevent a secondary infection. **Sterile** (free of all living microorganisms) technique includes the use of sterile dressings, sterile gloves, and sterile irrigating solution.
- Never massage reddened areas (risks causing further skin breakdown). Massage over bony prominences is no longer recommended. *(Massage results in decreased blood flow and tissue damage in some patients.)*
- Nutritional support, which promotes healthy tissue repair, is likely to be as important as local wound care for the patient.
- Observe the patient's hydration. If it is inadequate or if signs of dehydration (decreased skin turgor and recessed eyes) are present, carefully observe the patient's intake and output (I&O) and monitor fluid replacement therapy as ordered.
- Turn patients who are on complete bed rest every 2 hours. It is important to avoid the full lateral position, which results in direct pressure on the trochanteric region. It is preferable to use the 30-degree lateral-incline position (see Box 18-6).
- Reposition chair-bound patients every hour. If the chair-bound patient is able to shift his or her weight, teach him or her to do so every 15 minutes.
- Place patients who are at risk for skin impairment on a pressure-relieving mattress or chair cushion. These pressure-reducing devices are preferred over the use of sheepskin heel protectors. Placing a rolled bath blanket under the distal extremity to raise the heel off the bed (see Figures 18-6 and 18-7) is a much preferred method because this device relieves pressure on the heel completely. Doughnut types of cushions are not advisable because they sometimes cause a congestion of blood to the area, resulting in edema and decreased blood flow to the area.
- Other pressure-relieving devices to try are therapeutic beds and mattresses. Examples of pressure-relieving beds are the low-air-loss bed (KinAir) and the oscillating support surface bed (RotoRest), both produced by Kinetic Concepts, and the Clinitron bed produced by Support Systems International. Examples of the therapeutic mattress are the Roho, produced by Roho, and the First Step, produced by Kinetic Concepts. In addition, there are the alternating air mattress and the water mattress.
- Many kinds of topical agents to facilitate healing are available to apply to the wound and edges of the wound. Take care to evaluate the effectiveness of any product used on the ulcer. Use with caution any products that have the capacity to damage fragile skin and prevent epithelialization (formation of new cells), such as hydrogen peroxide or alcohol.

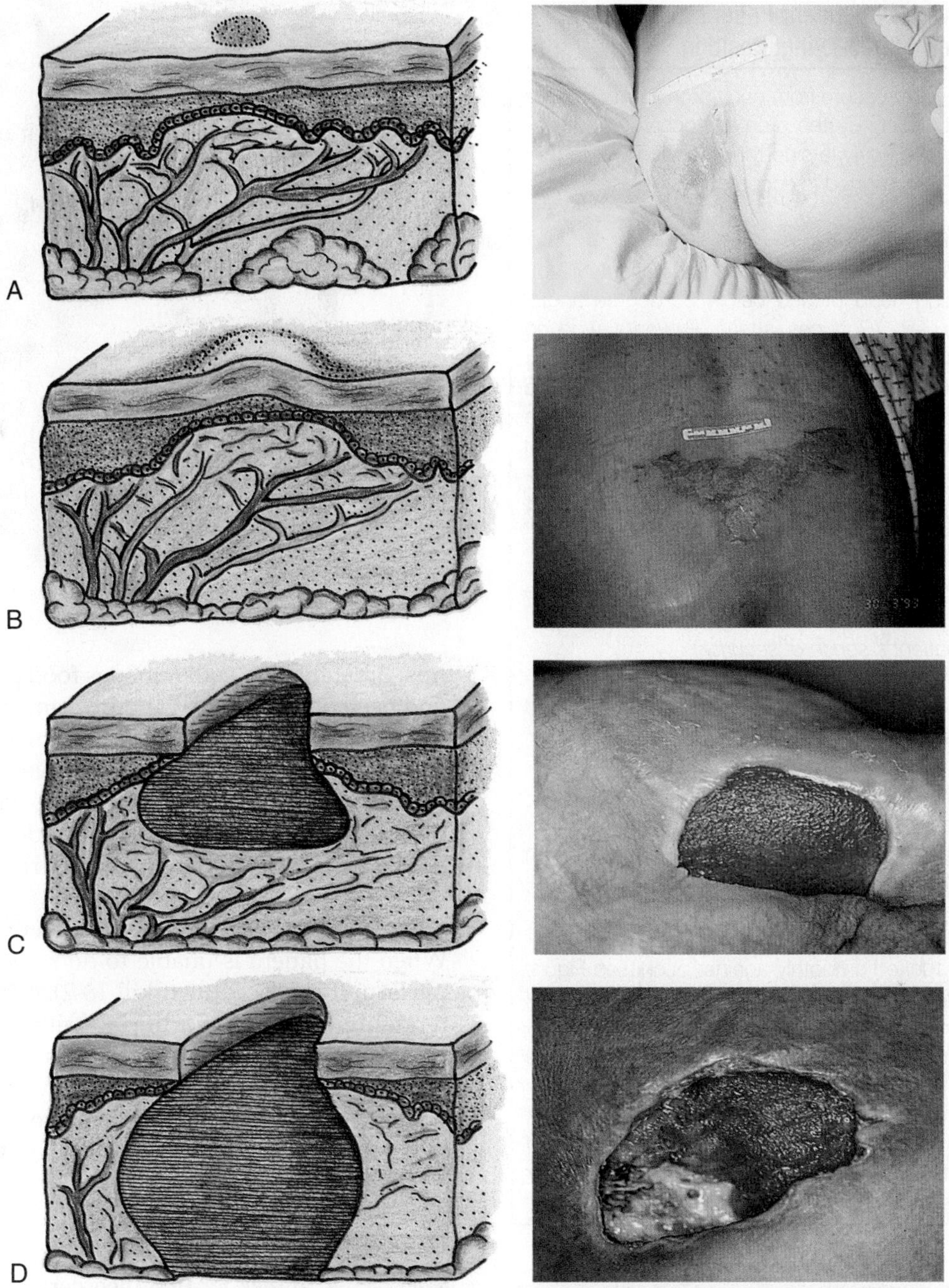

FIGURE 18-4 Pressure ulcers. **A,** Stage I pressure ulcer. **B,** Stage II pressure ulcer. **C,** Stage III pressure ulcer. **D,** Stage IV pressure ulcer.

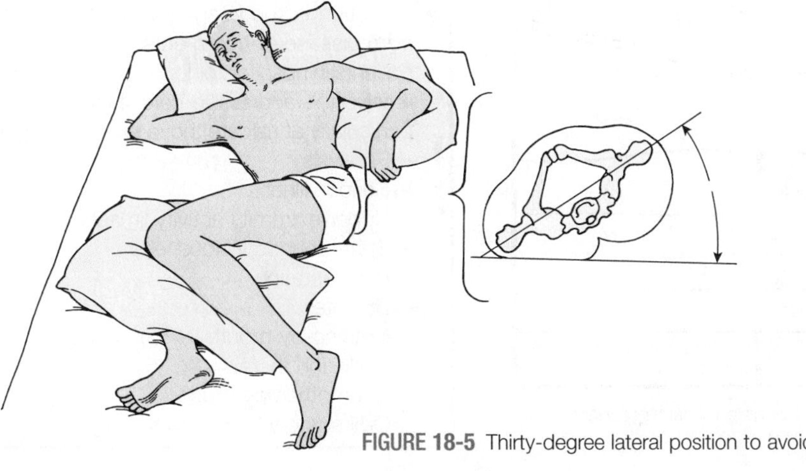

FIGURE 18-5 Thirty-degree lateral position to avoid pressure points.

Box 18-6 Moving Dependent Patient to 30-Degree Lateral (Side-Lying) Position

This move removes pressure from bony prominences of the entire back, but especially the greater trochanters. (If patient is able to move freely, a side-lying position with upper and lower shoulders aligned is acceptable.)

PROCEDURE *(Rationale)*

1. Lower the head of the bed as much as patient will tolerate, keeping head of bed below 30-degree angle. Lower side rail. *(Reduces shear. Prevents working against gravity.)*
2. Using a pull sheet, move patient to the side of the bed opposite the one toward which the patient will be turned. Raise side rail. Go to opposite side of the bed and lower side rail. *(Ensures that patient will be in center of the bed when turned.)*
3. Assist patient to raise arm nearest you above head, adjusting pillow if needed.
4. Grasp patient's shoulder and hip, and assist patient to roll toward you onto side. *(Turning patient toward you promotes patient's sense of security.)*
5. Flex both of the patient's knees after the turn, and support upper leg from knee to foot using a pillow or folded blanket. *(Keeps spine in good alignment.)*
6. Ease lower shoulder forward, and bring upper shoulder back slightly. Assess patient's comfort. *(Prevents excessive pressure directly on shoulder.)*
7. Support upper arm with pillows so that arm is level with shoulder. *(Improves respiratory effort by reducing pressure on chest to a minimum.)*
8. Optional: Place pillow behind and under patient's back so that it is tucked smoothly against back (see Figure 18-5). *(Provides support and prevents patient from rolling onto back.)*
9. Make certain patient's back is straight without evidence of twisting. Adjust as needed for comfort.
10. Pressure points to assess include the ear, the shoulder, the anterior iliac spine, the trochanter, the lateral side of the knee, the malleolus, and the foot. *(Prevents further skin impairment.)*

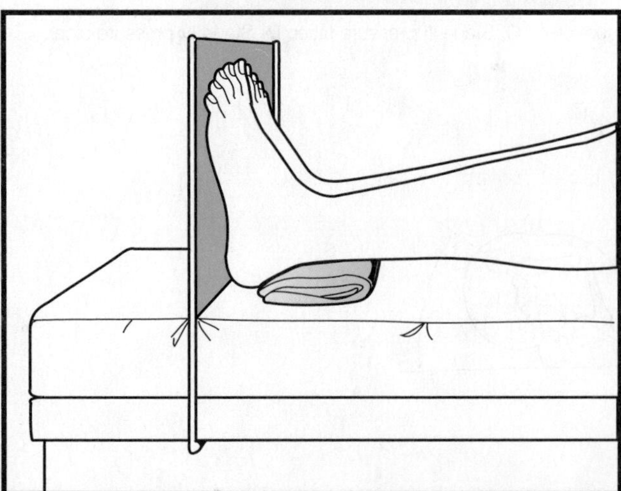

FIGURE 18-6 Using a rolled bath blanket as a pressure-reducing device.

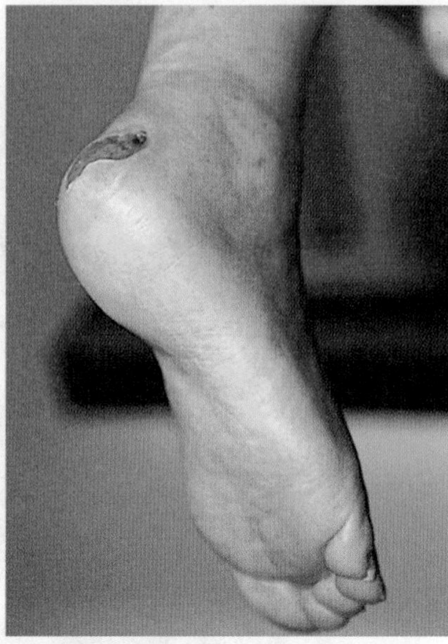

FIGURE 18-7 Pressure ulcer on heel.

lips. Brushing the teeth removes food particles, plaque, and bacteria; massages the gums; and relieves discomfort resulting from unpleasant odors and tastes. Complete oral hygiene gives a sense of well-being and thus can stimulate appetite. Proper care will prevent oral disease such as gingivitis or periodontitis and tooth destruction. Certain patients are at risk for oral disorders (Box 18-7).

Have patients brush their own teeth when possible. When the patient is unable to do so, you will need to perform this procedure (Skill 18-2).

Dentures (a set of artificial teeth not permanently fixed or implanted) are the patient's personal property; handle them with care, because they can be easily broken. Use an enclosed, labeled cup to soak dentures or to store them when they are not being worn (e.g., dur-

Box 18-7 Conditions that Place Patients at Risk for Oral Disorders

- Lack of knowledge about oral hygiene
- Inability to perform oral care
- Alteration in the integrity of teeth and mucosa resulting from disease or treatments
- Patients in hospitals or long-term care facilities often do not receive the aggressive care they need. Patients who are particularly at risk are those experiencing the following:
  —Paralysis
  —Serious illness
  —Upper-extremity activity limitations
  —State of unconsciousness
  —Disorientation
  —Diabetes
  —Nothing-by-mouth (NPO) status
  —Radiation therapy
  —Chemotherapy drugs
  —Oral surgery

Skill 18-2 Administering Oral Hygiene

Nursing Action *(Rationale)*

1. Refer to medical record, care plan, or Kardex for special interventions. *(Provides for basis of care.)*
2. Assemble supplies. *(Organizes procedure.)*
   a. For oral care.
      - Cleansing solution, such as diluted hydrogen peroxide, toothpaste, normal saline, soda solution, or mouthwash
      - Toothette, soft-bristled toothbrush, or tongue blade wrapped with gauze
      - Towel
      - Emesis basin
      - Disposable gloves
      - Flashlight
      - Dental floss (optional)
   b. For denture care.
      - Soft-bristled toothbrush
      - Denture brush
      - Emesis basin or sink
      - Cleansing agent
      - Water glass
      - Washcloth
      - 4 × 4 gauze
      - Denture cup
      - Disposable gloves
3. Introduce self. *(Decreases patient's anxiety.)*
4. Identify patient. *(Ensures procedure is performed with correct patient.)*
5. Explain procedure to patient. *(Enlists cooperation and decreases patient's anxiety.)*
6. Assess patient for the following, wearing gloves: *(Determines special needs and level of assistance required from nurse.)*
   - Integrity of lips, teeth, buccal mucosa, gums, palate, and tongue
   - Risk of dehydration (nothing-by-mouth [NPO] status)
   - Presence of nasogastric or oxygen (O_2) tubes
   - Chemotherapeutic drugs or radiation therapy to head and neck
   - Presence of artificial airway
   - Oral surgery; trauma to mouth
   - Aging
   - Diabetes mellitus
   - Ability to perform own oral care (independence is to be encouraged)
7. Perform hand hygiene and don clean gloves according to agency policy and guidelines from the CDC and OSHA. *(Reduces spread of microorganisms.)*
8. Prepare patient for intervention.
   a. Close door or pull privacy curtain. *(Provides privacy.)*
   b. Raise bed to comfortable working position. *(Promotes proper body mechanics.)*
   c. Arrange supplies. *(Provides convenient access to equipment.)*
   d. If patient tolerates the activity, provide supplies in the bathroom and allow patient privacy.
   e. If patient is on bed rest but tolerates the activity while remaining in bed—arrange overbed table in front of patient; provide supplies, and allow patient privacy. *(Patient involvement with procedure keeps anxiety to a minimum.)*
   f. If you are performing the procedure with an unconscious patient, position patient's head to the side toward you (dependent side if possible) and close to you (see step 9a). *(Proper positioning of head will prevent aspiration.)*
9. Oral care.
   a. Place towel under patient's face and emesis basin under patient's chin (see illustration). *(Facilitates procedure and prevents soiling of bed.)*
   b. Carefully separate patient's jaws. (*Protects your fingers.)*
   c. Cleanse mouth using brush, tongue blade, or Toothette moistened with cleansing agent. Clean inner and outer tooth surfaces (see illustration). Swab roof of mouth and inside

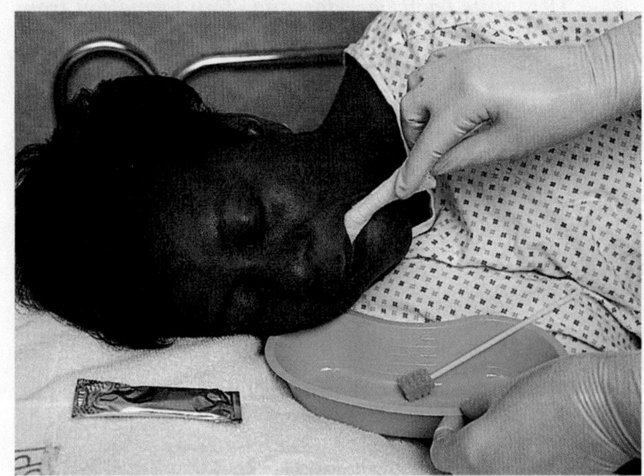

Step **9a**

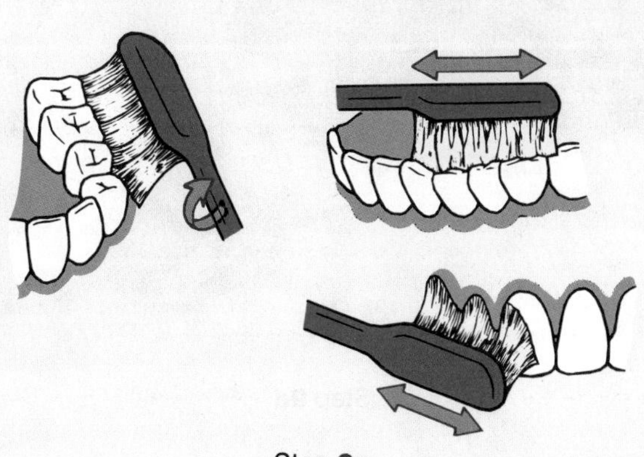

Step **9c**

Continued

Skill 18-2 Administering Oral Hygiene—cont'd

cheeks. Use flashlight for better visualization of oral cavity. Gently swab tongue. Rinse and repeat. Rinse several times. *(Removes food particles, secretions, and dried exudate. Moistens mucosa; leaves mouth fresh.)*

d. Apply lubricant to lips (see illustration). *(Provides moisture to prevent drying and cracking [cheilosis].)*

10. Cleaning dentures.

a. Fill emesis basin half full of tepid water. *(Acts as a cushion for the dentures if accidentally dropped, preventing damage to dentures. Temperature extremes will harm dentures.)*

b. Ask patient to remove dentures and place in emesis basin. If patient is unable to remove own dentures, break suction that holds upper denture in place by using thumb and finger. With gauze, apply gentle downward tug and carefully remove from patient's mouth. *(Gauze prevents slipping while handling dentures.)* Next remove lower denture by carefully lifting up and turning sideways. Remove and place in emesis basin.

c. Cleanse biting surfaces. Cleanse outer and inner tooth surfaces (see illustration). Be certain to cleanse lower surface of dentures. *(Prevents bacteria, odor, and stain formation from lodged food particles.)*

d. Rinse dentures thoroughly with tepid water. *(Warm water is more effective than cold water.)*

e. Before replacing dentures in patient's mouth or after storing dentures properly, gently brush patient's gums, tongue, and inside of cheeks and rinse thoroughly. *(Cleansing of the oral cavity is also necessary to promote healthy gums and mucosa.)*

f. Replace dentures either in patient's mouth or in container of solution placed in safe place. *(Dentures may become brittle and warped if not kept moist. Dentures are costly and must be handled with care.)*

g. When reinserting the dentures, replace the upper denture first if patient has both dentures. Apply gentle pressure to reestablish the suction. Moisten dentures for easier insertion. Make certain dentures are comfortably situated in patient's mouth before leaving the bedside. *(Promotes comfort.)*

11. Dispose of gloves in proper receptacle. Clean and store supplies. Perform hand hygiene. *(Reduces spread of microorganisms.)*

12. Position patient for comfort, raise side rail, and lower bed. *(Promotes comfort and safety.)*

13. Assess for patient comfort. *(Helps determine whether dentures are fitting properly.)*

14. Document. *(Timely documentation maintains accuracy of patient's record and communicates interventions given.)*

- Procedure
- Pertinent observations (bleeding gums, dry mucosa, ulcerations, or crust on tongue)
- Most facilities have flow sheets for documenting activities of daily living (ADLs), but also note condition of oral cavity in nursing notes
- Patient teaching (see Patient Teaching box)

15. Report bleeding or presence of lesions to nurse in charge or physician. *(Bleeding indicates possibility of serious systemic problems. Certain oral lesions are potentially cancerous.)*

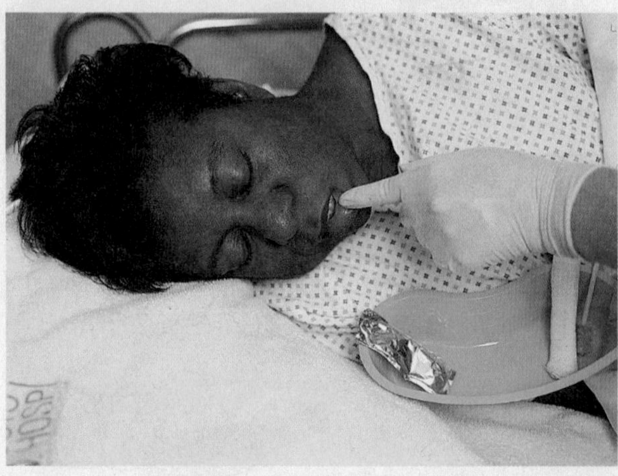

Step **9d**

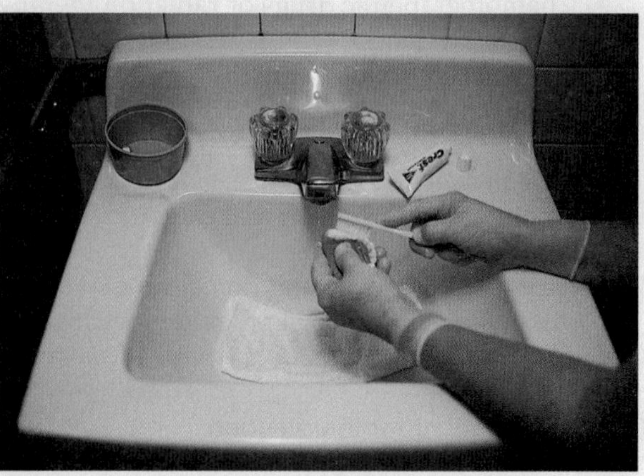

Step **10c**

ing surgery or a diagnostic procedure). Patients who return from surgery or a diagnostic test usually prefer to have their dentures reinserted as quickly as possible. Many people find the change in appearance that results when dentures are removed to be embarrassing.

Most patients prefer to clean their dentures themselves; encourage them to do so as often as for natural teeth to prevent infection and irritation. However, when it becomes necessary for you to assist with denture care, always consider the patient's preference of cleanser and soaking (see Skill 18-2).

Provide oral care on a regular basis; frequency of hygiene measures will depend on the condition of the patient's mouth. The beneficial outcomes of oral hygiene will probably not be seen for several days. Repeated cleansing is often needed to remove tenacious, dried exudate of the tongue and to restore the mucosa's hydration to normal.

HAIR CARE

Proper hair care is important to the patient's self-image. Combing, brushing, and shampooing are basic hygiene measures needed by all patients. Illness or disability will often prevent patients from performing their own daily hair care. A bedfast patient's hair soon becomes tangled. It is important to remember that most patients are aware of their appearance at all times. Therefore perform good hair care routinely, at least daily, to meet the hygiene needs of the patient. If the patient is not able to carry out this part of self-care, you will be required to give assistance. If the patient is able to take a shower or tub bath, you can easily shampoo the hair. One option is to use a portable chair in the shower, and another is to place a chair in front of a sink.

For the helpless, bedfast patient, it will be necessary to perform the shampoo with the patient in bed. Check whether a physician's order is necessary. Most facilities have portable blow-dryers and curling irons available, as well as shampoo boards (Skill 18-3). Dry shampoos are available in most facilities, but their effectiveness is questionable.

SHAVING THE PATIENT

Many patients prefer to shave at the time of bathing. Remember that those patients who have a bleeding disorder or who are taking **anticoagulants** (medications that increase the tendency to bleed) need to use electric razors. Do not allow a disoriented or depressed patient to use a razor with a blade, to prevent accidental or self-inflicted injury. A patient's beard, mustache, or sideburns are never removed without written consent, except for emergency purposes.

You will need to shave the patient when he is unable to, for instance, because he is too ill or has an arm immobilized in traction or a cast (see Skill 18-3).

Skill 18-3 Care of the Hair, Nails, and Feet

Nursing Action *(Rationale)*

1. Refer to medical record, care plan, or Kardex for special interventions. *(Provides basis for care.)*
2. Assemble supplies. *(Organizes procedure.)*
   a. Bed shampoo.
      - Bath towels (2)
      - Washcloth or hand towel
      - Water pitcher
      - Shampoo
      - Shampoo board
      - Wash basin
      - Bath blanket
      - Comb and brush
      - Hair dryer and curling iron (optional)

   b. Shaving.
      - Razor with sharp blade
      - Shaving cream or soap and brush
      - Bath towel
      - Face towel
      - Washcloth
      - Bath blanket
      - Basin with hot water, 115° F (46° C), or as patient prefers
      - Aftershave lotion or powder
      - Mirror

   c. Nail and foot care.
      - Wash basin
      - Emesis basin
      - Washcloth
      - Hand towel
      - Nail clippers, emery board, and orange-wood stick
      - Lotion
      - Disposable bath mat
      - Disposable gloves (optional)
3. Introduce self. *(Decreases patient's anxiety.)*
4. Identify patient. *(Ensures procedure is performed with correct patient.)*
5. Explain procedure. *(Enlists cooperation and reduces patient's anxiety.)*
6. Assess patient for the following: *(Determines special interventions necessary.)*
   - Contraindications to shampooing, shaving, or nail care. *(In some facilities only registered nurses [RNs] are permitted to trim the toenails of a diabetic patient. Follow agency policy.)*

Continued

Skill 18-3 Care of the Hair, Nails, and Feet—cont'd

- Restrictions to positioning.
- Condition of scalp, hair, nails, and feet; color and temperature of toes, feet, and fingers.
- Ability to care for own hair, nails, and feet. *(Encourages independence.)*
- Knowledge of foot and nail care practices.

7. Perform hand hygiene and don clean gloves according to agency policy and guidelines from the CDC and OSHA. *(Reduces spread of microorganisms.)*
8. Prepare patient for intervention. *(Readies patient for procedure.)*
   a. Close door or pull privacy curtain. *(Provides privacy.)*
   b. Raise bed to a comfortable working height. *(Promotes proper body mechanics.)*
   c. Arrange supplies at bedside or, if patient is able to perform procedure, have supplies available in the bathroom and offer assistance as needed. *(Patient's involvement with procedure reduces anxiety to a minimum.)*
9. Bed shampoo.
   a. Position patient close to one side of bed. Place shampoo board under patient's head and washbasin at end of spout (see illustration). Make sure spout extends over edge of mattress. *(Prevents wetting of bed linens.)*
   b. Position rolled-up bath towel under patient's neck. *(Reduces discomfort.)* Certain conditions such as cervical neck injuries, open incisions, or tracheostomy place the patient at risk for injury, in which case, a modified position is used.
   c. Brush and comb patient's hair. If hair is matted with blood, hydrogen peroxide is effective as a cleansing agent. *(Removes tangles and loosens dried secretions.)*

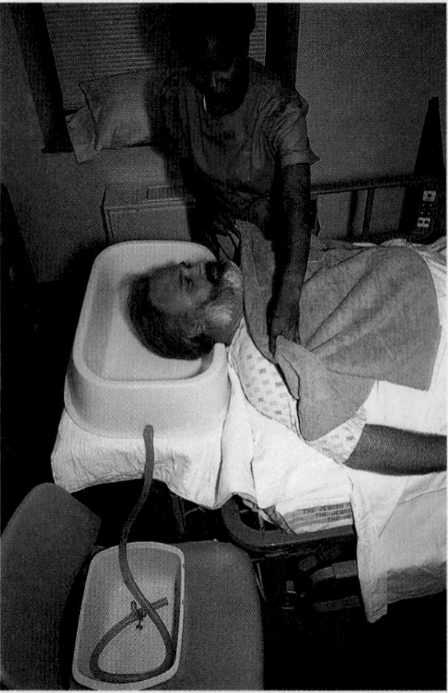

Step **9a**

   d. Obtain water in pitcher at about 110° F (43° C). *(Prevents burns.)*
   e. If patient is able, instruct patient to hold washcloth over eyes. Completely wet hair and apply small amount of shampoo. *(Prevents water and shampoo from getting into eyes.)*
   f. Massage scalp with pads of fingertips, not nails. Shampoo hairline, back of neck (lift head slightly), and sides of hair. *(Ensures thorough cleansing and increases scalp circulation. Use of pads of fingertips prevents injury to scalp.)*
   g. Rinse thoroughly and apply more shampoo, repeating steps e and f. Rinse, and repeat rinsing until hair is free of shampoo. *(Prevents scalp irritation.)*
   h. Wrap dry towel around patient's head. Dry patient's face, neck, and shoulders. Dry hair and scalp using second towel. *(Prevents patient from chilling.)*
   i. Comb hair and dry with hair dryer as quickly as possible. *(Prevents patient from chilling.)*
   j. Complete styling hair and position patient for comfort. *(Promotes sense of well-being.)*
10. Shaving the patient.
   a. Assist patient to sitting position if patient is able. *(Simulates the natural position.)*
   b. Observe face and neck for lesions, moles, or birthmarks. *(Cutting poses risk to cause infection, bleeding, or irritation.)*
   c. Use shaving cream or soap. *(Lathering will soften beard and facilitate shave.)*
   d. Shave in direction hair grows. Use short strokes. Start with upper face and lips, and then extend to neck. If patient is able, it will help if he hyperextends (tilts backward) his head to help shave curved areas. *(Provides for closer shave without irritation.)*
   e. Pull skin taut with nondominant hand above or below the area being shaved (see illustration). *(Promotes uniform shaving.)*
   f. Rinse razor after each stroke. *(Keeps cutting edge clean.)*
   g. Rinse and dry face. *(Removes remnants of lather and shaved hair.)*
   h. If patient desires, apply lotion or cologne. *(Causes cooling sensation that feels refreshing.)*
   i. Dispose of blades in sharps container. *(Protects others from accidental injury.)*
11. Hand and foot care.
   a. Position patient in chair. If possible, place disposable mat under patient's feet. *(Protects bare feet from floor.)*

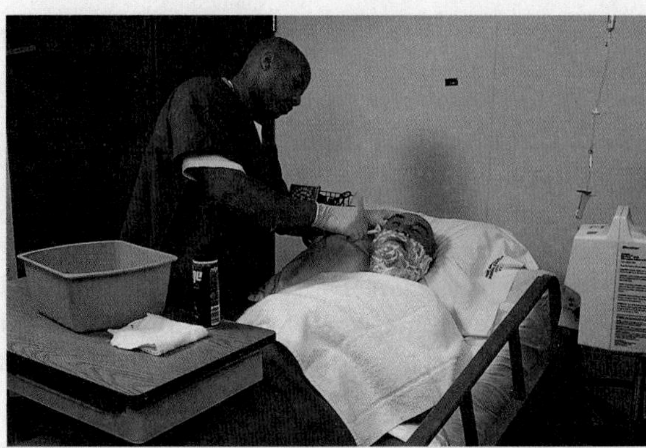

Step **10e**

b. Fill basin with warm water and test temperature. Place basin on disposable mat and assist patient to place feet into basin. **(Do not soak hands and feet of a diabetic patient; soaking increases risk of infection.)** Allow to soak 10 to 20 minutes. Rewarm water as necessary. *(Soaking in warm water will soften nails and ensure easy manipulation of cuticles. Keeping water warm prevents chilling the patient.)*

c. Place overbed table in low position in front of patient. Fill emesis basin with warm water and test water temperature. Place basin on table, and place patient's fingers in basin. Allow fingernails to soak 10 to 20 minutes. Rewarm water as necessary. *(Soaking loosens foreign particles under nails and ensures easy manipulation of cuticles. Keeping water warm prevents chilling the patient.)*

d. Using orangewood stick, gently clean under fingernails. *(Orangewood stick removes debris under nails that harbors microorganisms.)* With clippers, trim nails straight across and even with tip of fingers. With emery board, shape fingernails. Push cuticles back gently with washcloth or orangewood stick. *(Prevents injury to delicate nailbeds.)*

e. Don gloves, and with washcloth scrub areas of feet that are calloused. *(Reduces spread of microorganisms. Scrubbing after soaking helps remove dead skin layers.)*

f. Trim and clean toenails following step d instructions.

g. Apply lotion or cream to hands and feet. Return patient to bed and position for comfort. Dry fingers and toes thoroughly to impede fungal growth and prevent maceration (a softening and breaking down of tissue resulting from prolonged exposure to moisture). *(Creams and lotions lubricate dry skin.)*

h. On completion of procedure, observe the nails and the surrounding tissue for condition of skin and any remaining rough edges.

i. If the patient's nails are extremely hard or if the patient is unable to perform personal nail care, have a podiatrist (a person trained in the treatment of nail and foot problems) provide nail care.

12. Dispose of gloves in proper receptacle. Clean and store supplies. Place soiled laundry in hamper. Perform hand hygiene. *(Reduces spread of microorganisms.)*

13. Assess for patient's comfort, lower bed level, raise side rails, and place call button within easy reach. *(Promotes safety.)*

14. Document. *(Timely recording maintains accuracy of patient's record and communicates interventions given.)*
- Procedure
- Pertinent observations (e.g., breaks in the skin, inflammation, or ulcerations)
- Most facilities have flow sheets for ADLs; shaving and nail and foot care are usually not recorded in nursing notes; know agency policy
- Patient teaching (see Patient Teaching and Home Care Considerations boxes)

15. Report abnormal findings (breaks in the skin or ulcerations) to nurse in charge or physician. *(Additional interventions are sometimes required.)*

HAND, FOOT, AND NAIL CARE

Hands and feet often require special attention to prevent infection, odors, and injury. Problems arise from abuse or poor care of the hands and feet, for example, biting the nails or wearing ill-fitting shoes.

Assessment of the feet involves a thorough examination of all skin surfaces. Carefully assess the area between the toes. Observe patients with diabetes mellitus or peripheral vascular disease for adequate circulation to the feet. The elderly are also at risk for foot disorders because of poor vision or decreased mobility. Consider whether a podiatry consult is in order; consult the physician.

Administer care of the hands and feet during the morning bath, or at another time if desired (see Skill 18-3).

PERINEAL CARE

Perineal care (pericare, or care of the genitalia) is part of the complete bed bath. Those patients most in need of scrupulous pericare are those at risk for acquiring an infection, for example, patients with indwelling catheters, patients recovering from rectal or genital surgery, or postpartum patients. If patients are able to do their own pericare, allow them to do so. Never allow embarrassment to cause you to overlook this nursing intervention. A professional, dignified attitude helps diminish embarrassment and put patients at ease. Catheter care is done at least two times daily on all patients with indwelling catheters unless otherwise ordered by the physician.

Be alert for signs of vaginal or urethral exudate (discharge), skin impairment, unpleasant odors, complaints of burning during urination, or localized tenderness or pain of the perineum. Also observe for skin impairment in the perineal area, especially in those patients with urinary or fecal incontinence, rectal and perineal surgical dressings, and indwelling urinary catheters (Skill 18-4).

Perineal Care for the Patient with an Indwelling Catheter

Catheter care is to be performed twice daily on all patients with indwelling catheters unless otherwise ordered by the physician. Daily catheter care includes cleansing of the meatal-catheter junction with a mild soap and water and sometimes application of a water-

Skill 18-4 Perineal Care: Male and Female and the Catheterized Patient

Nursing Action *(Rationale)*

1. Refer to medical record, care plan, or Kardex for special interventions. *(Provides basis for care.)*
2. Assemble supplies. *(Organizes procedure.)*
   a. Perineal care.
      - Mild soap
      - Washbasin and warm water
      - Washcloths (2)
      - Bath towel
      - Bath blanket
      - Bedpan
      - Toilet tissue
      - Disposable gloves
      - Solution bottle
      - Waterproof pad
   b. Additional supplies for the catheterized patient.
      - Betadine (or ointment of physician's or agency's choice)
      - Sterile package of cotton-tipped applicators
3. Introduce self. *(Reduces patient's anxiety.)*
4. Identify patient. *(Ensures procedure is performed with correct patient.)*
5. Explain procedure. *(Enlists cooperation and reduces patient's anxiety.)*
6. Assess patient for the following, wearing gloves: *(Determines whether additional interventions are necessary.)*
   - Accumulated secretions
   - Surgical incision
   - Lesions
   - Ability to perform self-care
   - Extent of care required by patient
   - Knowledge of importance of perineal care
7. Remove and dispose of soiled gloves and perform hand hygiene and don clean gloves according to agency policy and guidelines from the CDC and OSHA. *(Reduces spread of microorganisms.)*
8. Prepare patient for interventions. *(Readies patient for procedure.)* Allow postpartum patients to perform this procedure by themselves while sitting on the stool, using a pericare squeeze bottle. Patients allowed tub or shower baths will do this by themselves. Make certain supplies are close by. *(Patient's involvement with procedure reduces anxiety.)*
   a. Close door or pull privacy curtain. *(Provides privacy.)*
   b. Raise bed to comfortable working height and lower side rail. *(Promotes proper body mechanics.)*
   c. Arrange supplies at bedside. *(Facilitates procedure.)*
   d. Assist patient to desired position in bed: dorsal recumbent for female or supine for male. *(Facilitates procedure.)*
   e. Drape for procedure. *(Reduces patient's embarrassment.)*
   f. When perineal care is given other than routinely during the bath, you will need to fill the perineal bottle (peribottle) with cleansing solution and position the patient in bed on the bedpan.
9. Female perineal care.
   a. Raise side rail and fill basin two thirds full of water at 105° to 109° F (41° to 43° C). *(Promotes patient safety. Filling basin only two thirds full prevents unnecessary splashing.)*
   b. Position waterproof pad or towel under patient's buttocks with patient lying in the dorsal recumbent position in bed. Drape patient with bath blanket placed in the shape of a diamond. There will be one corner under the patient's chin; one corner on each side of the patient, with the bath blanket wrapped around each foot and leg; and the last corner will be between the patient's legs. This corner can be lifted to expose the patient's perineum (see illustration). *(Draping in this manner keeps exposure to a minimum, decreasing the patient's anxiety.)*
   c. Using a disposable washcloth wrapped around one hand, wash and dry patient's upper thighs. *(Surrounding skin surfaces need cleansing also.)*

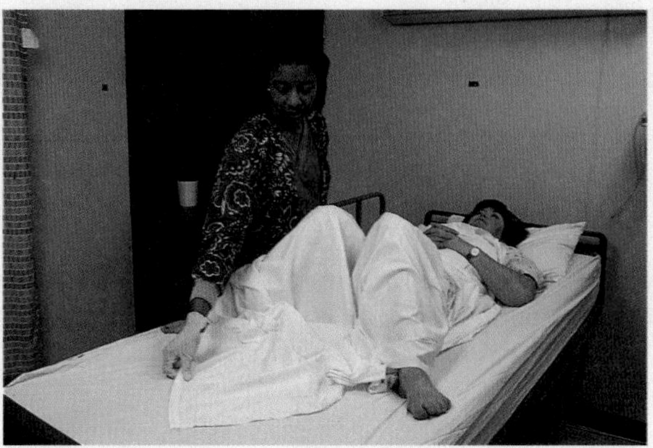

Step **9b**

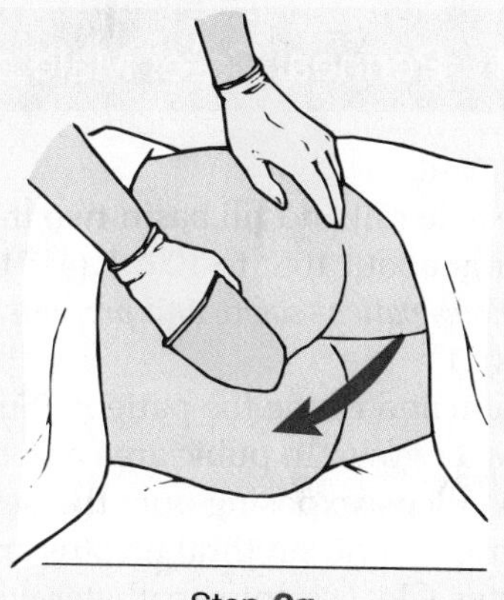

Step **9g**

d. Wash both labia majora (larger fold or lip) and labia minora (smaller fold or lip). Wash carefully in skinfolds. Cleanse in direction anterior to posterior. Use separate corner of washcloth for each skinfold. *(Prevents microorganisms around the anus from entering the meatus or vagina.)*

e. Separate labia to expose the urinary meatus (opening) and the vaginal orifice. Wash downward toward rectum with smooth strokes (see illustration). Use separate corner of washcloth for each smooth stroke. *(Reduces spread of microorganisms.)*

f. Cleanse, rinse, and dry thoroughly. *(Retained moisture harbors microorganisms.)* If patient is on bedpan and peribottle is used, direct flow of cleansing solution down over perineal area and dry thoroughly.

g. Assist patient to side-lying position and cleanse rectal area with toilet tissue, if necessary. Wash area by cleansing from perineal area toward anus (see illustration). You will often need several washcloths. Many facilities have disposable wipes. If so, use them. Wash, rinse, and dry thoroughly. *(Reduces spread of microorganisms and risk of skin impairment.)*

10. Male perineal care.

a. Raise side rail and fill basin two thirds full of water at about 105° to 109° F (41° to 43° C.) *(Promotes patient safety and prevents unnecessary spillage.)*

b. Gently grasp shaft of penis. Retract foreskin of uncircumcised patient. *(Secretions collect under foreskin.)*

c. Wash tip of penis with circular motion (see illustration).

d. Cleanse from meatus outward (see illustration). *(Prevents microorganisms from entering urethra.)* Two washcloths are often necessary. Wash, rinse, and dry gently.

e. Replace foreskin, and wash shaft of penis with a firm but gentle downward stroke. Replace the foreskin of the uncircumcised male patient after thorough cleansing. *(Prevents edema and discomfort.)*

f. Rinse and dry thoroughly. *(Retained moisture harbors microorganisms.)*

g. Cleanse scrotum gently. Cleanse carefully in underlying skinfolds. Rinse and dry gently. *(Pressure on scrotal tissue is often very painful.)*

h. Assist patient to a side-lying position. *(Facilitates procedure.)* Cleanse anal area. Follow step 9f of female perineal care.

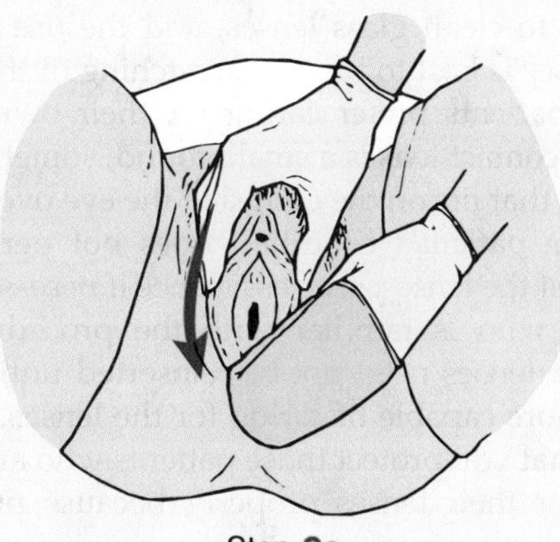

Step **9e**

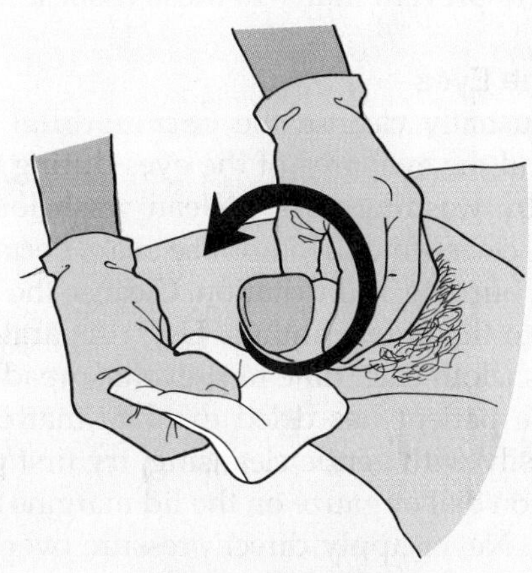

Steps **10c, 10d**

Continued

Skill 18-4 Perineal Care: Male and Female and the Catheterized Patient—cont'd

11. Catheter care.
    a. Raise side rail and fill basin two thirds full of water at about 105° to 109° F (41° to 43° C). *(Promotes patient safety and prevents unnecessary spillage.)*
    b. Position and drape the patient. (Supine position with gown to pubic area and bath blanket up over legs, exposing only the perineum.)
    c. Cleanse around urethral meatus and adjacent catheter. Cleanse entire catheter with soap and water. *(Reduces risk of urinary tract infections.)*
    d. Repeat cleansing to remove all exudate from meatus and catheter. *(Exudates are often irritating and serve as medium for infectious organisms.)*
    e. If ointment is ordered, open package of sterile cotton-tipped applicators. Do not touch cotton tip. Apply ointment to applicator. Do not touch wrapper to cotton tip. *(Maintains sterility.)*
    f. Apply ointment to junction of catheter and urethral meatus. *(Reduces irritation and reduces spread of microorganisms.)*
12. Remove gloves. Clean and store equipment. Dispose of contaminated supplies in proper receptacle. Perform hand hygiene. *(Reduces spread of microorganisms.)*
13. Position patient for comfort. *(Promotes relaxation.)*
14. Document. *(Timely recording maintains accuracy of patient's record and communicates interventions given.)*
    - Procedure
    - Pertinent observations such as the following:
      —Character and amount of discharge and odor if present
      —Condition of genitalia (erythema, edema, or discomfort)
    - Patient's ability to perform own care
    - Patient teaching (see Patient Teaching and Home Care Considerations boxes)
15. Report abnormal findings to nurse in charge or physician. *(Additional interventions are sometimes required.)*

soluble microbicidal ointment (Betadine or Neosporin are often ordered) (see Skill 18-4).

EYE, EAR, AND NOSE CARE

Special attention is given to cleansing the eyes, the ears, and the nose during the patient's bath. You often have the responsibility of assisting patients in the care of eyeglasses, contact lenses, or artificial eyes. For patients who wear eyeglasses, contact lenses, artificial eyes, or hearing aids, assess the patient's knowledge and methods used to care for the aids, as well as any problems caused by the aids. Patients who cannot grasp small objects, have limited mobility in the upper extremities, have reduced vision, or are seriously fatigued will require your assistance.

The eyes, ears, and nose are sensitive; therefore take extra care to prevent injury to these tissues.

Care of the Eyes

You will usually cleanse the **circumorbital** (circular area around the eye) area of the eyes during the bath, typically by washing with a clean washcloth moistened with clear water. Do not use soap, because it often causes burning and irritation. Cleanse the eye from the inner to the outer canthus. Use a separate section of the washcloth each time to prevent spread of infection. If the patient has dried exudate that is not removed easily with gentle cleansing, try first placing a damp cotton ball or gauze on the lid margins to loosen secretions. Never apply direct pressure over the eyeball; doing so has potential to cause serious injury. Remove any exudate from the eyes carefully and as often as necessary to keep the eye clean.

The eyes are well protected with eyelashes, tearing, and a split-second blink reflex and usually do not require special care. However, the unconscious patient is likely to need frequent special eye care. Secretions often collect along the margins of the lid and the inner canthus when the blink reflex is absent or when the eyes do not completely close.

Many patients wear eyeglasses. They represent a large financial investment. Therefore use care when cleaning glasses, and protect them from breakage or other damage when not worn.

Store eyeglasses in the case and place them in the drawer of the bedside stand when not in use to prevent accidental damage. Plastic lenses require special cleansing solutions and drying tissues. Warm water is adequate to clean glass lenses, and the use of a soft cloth to dry is best to prevent scratching of the lenses.

Most patients prefer caring for their own contact lenses. A contact lens is a small, round, sometimes colored disk that fits on the cornea of the eye over the pupil. If the patient's condition does not permit self-removal of the lenses, seek assistance if necessary from someone who is familiar with the procedure (Box 18-8). The lenses need not be reinserted until the patient is more capable of caring for the lenses. It is important that you protect those patients who are unable to care for their lenses properly, because prolonged

Box 18-8 Contact Lens Removal and Care

SOFT LENSES
- Wear gloves if exudate is suspected or present.
- If possible, have patient look straight ahead. Retract lower eyelid, and expose lower edge of lens.
- Using pad of index finger, slide lens off cornea to white of eye.
- Pull upper eyelid down gently with thumb of other hand, and compress lens slightly between thumb and index finger.
- Gently pinch lens, and lift out without allowing edges to stick together.
- If lens edges stick together, place lens in palm and soak thoroughly with sterile saline.
- Place lens in storage case.
- Follow recommended procedure for cleansing and disinfecting.

RIGID LENSES
- Wear gloves if exudate is suspected or present.
- Be sure lens is positioned directly over cornea. If it is not, have patient close eyelids. Place index and middle fingers of one hand beside the lens, and gently but firmly massage lens back over cornea.
- Place index finger on outer corner of patient's eye, and draw skin gently back toward ear.
- Ask patient to blink. Do not release pressure on lids until blink is completed.
- If lens fails to pop out, gently retract eyelid beyond edges of lens. Press lower eyelid gently against lower edge of lens.
- If patient is unable to assist, use a specially designed suction cup. Place cup on center of lens, and while applying suction, gently remove lens off patient's cornea.
- Place lens in storage case.
- Follow manufacturer's recommended procedure for cleansing and disinfecting.

wearing of contact lenses is likely to cause serious damage to the cornea. A large variety of products are available for lens care.

Care of the Ears

You will cleanse the ears during the bed bath. A clean corner of a moistened washcloth rotated gently into the ear canal works best for cleaning. Also, a cotton-tipped applicator is useful for cleansing the pinna. Teach patients never to use bobby pins, toothpicks, or cotton-tipped applicators to clean the internal auditory canal. These objects easily damage the tympanic membrane (eardrum) or cause **cerumen** (wax) to become impacted in the canal.

Hearing Aids

Hearing loss is a common health problem. The ability to hear enables patients to communicate and react appropriately to stimuli in their environment. The care of the hearing aid involves routine cleanings, battery care, and proper insertion technique. Assess the patient's knowledge of and routines for cleaning and caring for the hearing aid. Determine whether the patient hears clearly with the use of the aid by talking slowly and clearly in a normal voice tone. Have the patient suggest any additional tips for care of the hearing aid. When not in use, see that the hearing aid is stored where it will not become damaged. Take care to turn off the hearing aid when not in use to prolong the life of the battery. Clean the outside of the hearing aid with a dry, soft cloth (see Coordinated Care box on care of the hearing aid and Figure 18-8).

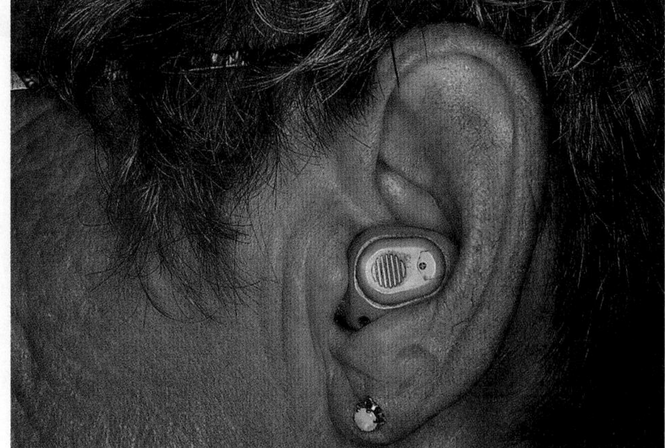

FIGURE 18-8 Hearing aid.

Care of the Nose

The patient is usually able to remove secretions from the nose by gently blowing into a soft tissue. This is often the only daily hygiene necessary. Teach the patient that harsh blowing causes pressure capable of injuring the tympanic membrane (eardrum), the nasal mucosa, and even sensitive eye structures. If the patient is not able to clean the nose, give assistance, using a saline-moistened washcloth or cotton-tipped applicator. Never insert the applicator beyond the cotton tip. If nasal secretions are excessive, suctioning will sometimes be necessary. When the patient receives oxygen per nasal cannula or has a nasogastric tube, cleanse the nares every 8 hours with a cotton-tipped applicator moistened with saline. Because secretions are more likely to collect and dry around the tube, you will also need to gently cleanse the tube with water and a mild soap.

BEDMAKING

You will usually make the patient's bed in the morning after the bath. When possible, make the bed while it is not occupied: when the patient is in the tub, showering, or out of the room for a diagnostic examination or procedure. When the patient is unable to be out of bed, you will make an occupied bed (Skill 18-5).

Always keep the patient's safety foremost in your mind. Comfort and privacy are also important. Re-

Text continued on p. 465

 Coordinated Care

Delegation

CARE OF THE HEARING AID

The skill of caring for a hearing aid is appropriate to delegate to assistive personnel.

- Confirm that patient knows proper way to care for prosthetic device.
- Clarify communication tips to use for individual patient while aid is being cleaned.
- Have care provider report presence of any drainage to registered nurse (RN).
- The small size of hearing aids (see Figure 18-8) frequently makes it difficult for older adults to handle and manipulate the devices. Have patients with this difficulty contact their hearing aid specialist for assistance. Family members are often able to assist with care of device.
- High-pitched signals associated with consonants *f, p, t, k, ch, sh*, and *st* are more difficult to hear clearly as people age.
- Inappropriate responses to questions or situations, inattentiveness, difficulty following instructions, and monopolization of conversation is often a red flag for some hearing loss the patient has that calls for evaluation. Make sure that you and family members remain alert to this possibility, instead of incorrectly assuming that the patient is confused.
- Be alert for patient assessment findings that indicate some possible depression. Hearing loss in association with depression is common, and correction of hearing loss actually resolves depression in some patients.
- Age-related hearing loss, presbycusis, is common. Patients and their families often compensate adequately for this auditory change by speaking slowly and clearly. Not all patients with this type of hearing loss require a hearing aid.
- Advise restricting initial use of a hearing aid to quiet situations in the home. Patients need to adjust gradually to voices and household sounds.
- Avoid exposure of aid to extreme heat or cold. Do not leave in its case near stove, heater, or sunny window. Do not use with hair dryer on hot settings or with sunlamp.
- Remove aid for bathing and when at hair stylist.
- Hair spray tends to clog hearing aid.
- Because of the typically high number of hearing aids in long-term care facilities, patients and their families need to clearly mark the hearing aid.
- Always store the hearing aid in the patient's bedside table.
- Instruct family to buy an extra battery to keep in patient's bedside table, whenever possible.
- Instruct patients not to remove their aids in common rooms of the facility (e.g., sunroom, recreation areas).

Skill 18-5 Bedmaking

Nursing Action *(Rationale)*

1. Refer to medical record, care plan, or Kardex to determine potential for orders or specific precautions for mobility and positioning. *(Provides basis for care.)*
2. Assemble supplies. *(Organizes procedure.)*
    - Laundry bag
    - Mattress pad (optional)
    - Bottom sheet—many facilities use the contour or fitted sheet
    - Protective drawsheet (optional)
    - Linen drawsheet
    - Top sheet, flat
    - Blanket
    - Spread
    - Chux (waterproof disposable underpad) or bath blanket (or both) (2)
    - Pillowcase(s)
    - Bedside chair or table
    - Disposable gloves (optional)
3. Introduce self. *(Reduces patient's anxiety.)*
4. Identify patient. *(Ensures procedure is performed with correct patient.)*
5. Explain procedure. *(Enlists cooperation and reduces patient's anxiety.)*
6. Perform hand hygiene and don gloves according to agency policy and guidelines from the CDC and OSHA. *(Reduces spread of microorganisms.)*
7. Prepare patient. *(Readies patient for procedure.)*
    a. Close door or pull privacy curtain. *(Provides privacy.)*
    b. Raise bed to appropriate height and lower side rail on the side closest to you. *(Promotes proper body mechanics.)*
    c. Lower head of bed (HOB) if patient tolerates it. *(Patient with a respiratory disorder will frequently not be able to tolerate lying flat. The use of contour sheets makes it easier to make hospital beds with the HOB elevated.)*
    d. Assess patient's tolerance of procedure. Be alert for signs of discomfort and fatigue. *(Use judgment in providing the opportunity for rest and comfort measures.)*
8. Occupied bed.
    a. Remove spread and blanket separately and, if soiled, place in laundry bag. If linens will be reused, fold neatly and place over back of chair. (Keep linens away from uniform.) Do not fan or shake linens. *(Reduces spread of microorganisms.)*

b. Place bath blanket over patient on top of sheet.
c. Request patient to hold onto bath blanket while you remove top sheet by drawing sheet out from under bath blanket at foot of bed. If patient is unable to assist, you will need to hold bath blanket in place while removing sheet. *(Prevents unnecessary exposure of patient.)*
d. Place soiled sheet in laundry bag. *(Reduces spread of microorganisms.)*
e. With assistance from co-worker, slide mattress to top of bed. *(If mattress has shifted to foot of bed, it will be difficult to tuck in linens.)*
f. Position patient to far side of bed with the back toward you. Assure patient that he or she will not fall out of bed. Adjust pillow for comfort. Be sure side rail is up. *(Provides for patient's safety.)*
g. Beginning at head and moving toward foot, loosen bottom linens. Fanfold linen drawsheet, protective drawsheet, and bottom sheet, tucking edges of linens under patient. *(Provides maximum work space.)*
h. Apply clean linens to bed by first placing mattress pad (if used). Fold lengthwise, making sure crease is in center of bed. Likewise, unfold bottom sheet and place over mattress pad. Place hem of bottom sheet (if flat sheet is used) with rough edge down and just even with bottom edge of mattress (see illustration of step 9g). *(Keeps energy and time you need for bedmaking to a minimum. Rough edge of hem away from patient prevents skin impairment to patient's heels.)*
i. Miter corners (if flat sheet) at head of bed (see illustration). Continue to tuck in sheet along side toward front, keeping linens smooth. *(Prevents linens from becoming easily loosened.)*
j. Reach under patient to pull out protective drawsheet (if used), and smooth out over clean bottom sheet. Tuck in. Unfold linen drawsheet and place center fold along middle of bed, smooth out over protective drawsheet, and tuck in. Tuck in folded linens in center of bed so they are under patient's buttocks and torso (see illustration).
k. Keep palms down as linens are tucked under mattress. *(Provides for patient's comfort.)*
l. Raise side rail and assist patient to roll slowly toward you over folds of linen. Go to opposite side of bed and lower side rail. *(Maintains patient's safety.)*
m. Loosen edges of all soiled linens. Remove by folding into a bundle (see illustration), and place in laundry bag. *(Reduces spread of microorganisms.)*
n. Spread clean linens, including protective drawsheet, out over mattress and smooth out wrinkles. Assist patient to supine position and position pillow for comfort. *(Maintains patient's comfort.)*
o. Miter top corner of bottom sheet, pulling sheet taut (see illustration). Tuck bottom sheet under mattress all the way to foot of bed. *(Maintains smooth linens. Avoid lifting mattress too far. Ensures tight fit.)*
p. Smooth out drawsheets. Pulling sheet taut, tuck in protective drawsheet and then tuck in linen drawsheet, first in center, then top, and bottom last. *(Ensures tight fit.)*

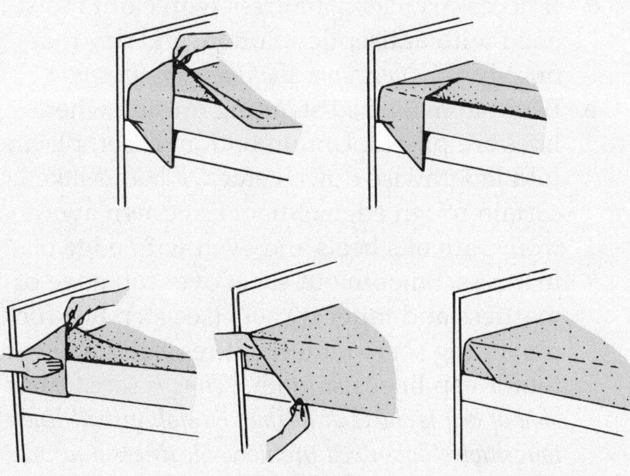

Step 8i

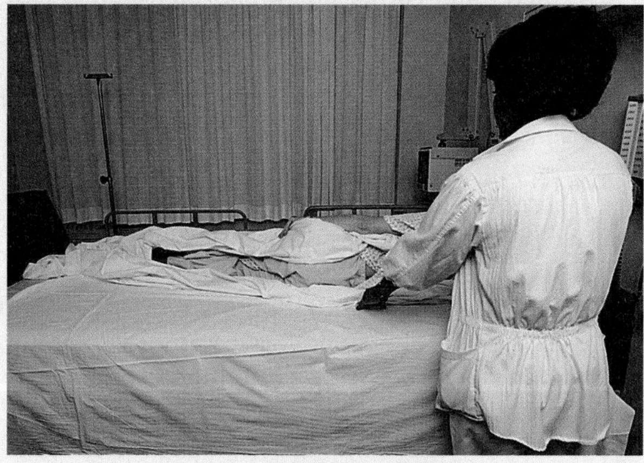

Step 8j

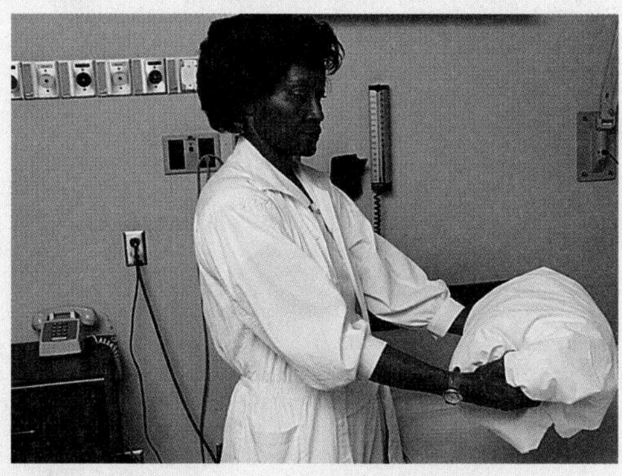

Step 8m

Continued

Skill 18-5 Bedmaking—cont'd

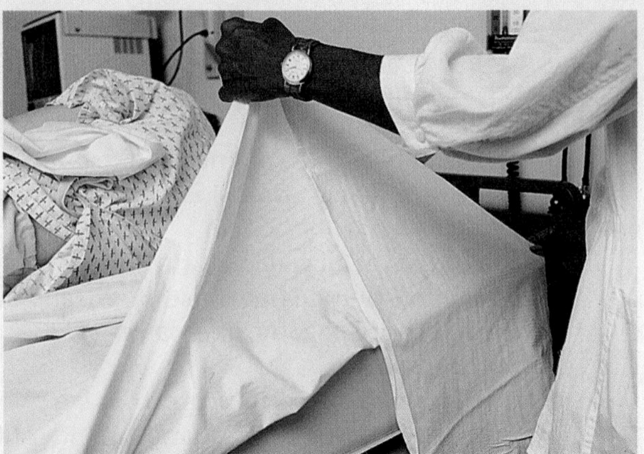
Step 8o

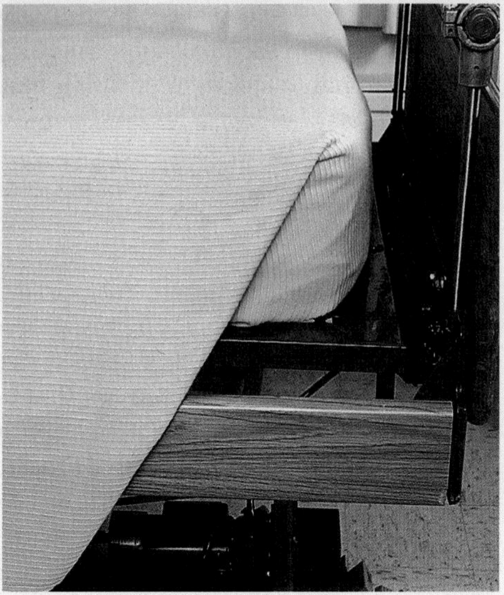
Step 8r

q. Place top sheet over bath blanket that is over patient. Request patient to hold top sheet while you remove bath blanket (see illustration). Place blanket in laundry bag. (Make sure center fold of sheet is in center of bed.) If blanket is used, place over sheet and place spread over blanket. Form cuff with top linens under patient's chin. *(Provides for patient's comfort and warmth.)*

r. Tuck in all linens at foot of bed, making modified miter corner (see illustration). Raise side rail and make opposite side of bed. Remember to allow for toe pleat. Make toe pleat by placing fold either lengthwise down center of bed or across foot of bed. *(Prevents unnecessary pressure on patient's feet, possibly causing footdrop.)*

s. Change pillowcase. Grasp closed end of pillowcase, turning case inside out over hand. Now grasp one end of pillow with your hand in the case and smooth out wrinkles, making sure pillow corners fit into pillowcase corners. *(Never place pillow on top of patient while changing its cover.)* As pillow is removed from under patient, support neck muscles. *(Prevents injury.)* Never hold pillow under your chin. *(Reduces spread of microorganisms.)*

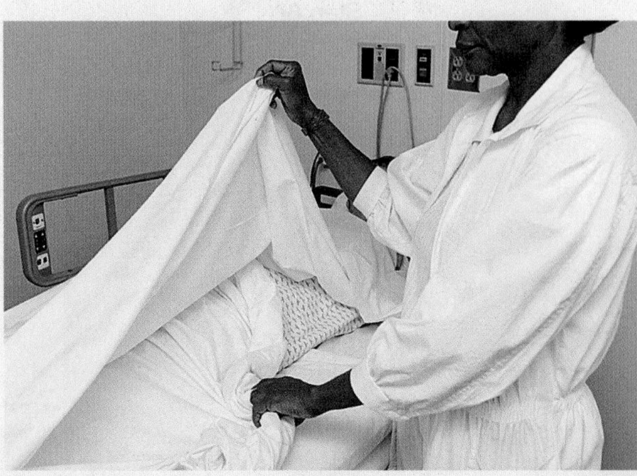
Step 8q

9. Unoccupied bed.
   a. Starting at head of bed, loosen linens all the way to foot. Go to opposite side of bed, loosen linens, roll all linens up in ball (see illustration of step 8m), and place in soiled laundry bag. Do not permit linens to come in contact with uniform. Do not shake or fan linens. Wash hands after handling soiled linens. Perform hand hygiene. *(Reduces spread of microorganisms.)*
   b. If blanket and spread are to be reused, fold neatly and place over back of chair. Remove soiled pillowcase.
   c. Slide mattress to head of bed. *(It is easier to tuck in linens.)*
   d. If necessary, clean mattress with cloth moistened with antiseptic solution, and dry thoroughly. *(Reduces spread of microorganisms.)*
   e. Begin to make bed standing on side where lines are placed. Unfold bottom sheet, placing fold lengthwise down center of bed. Make certain rough edge of hem lies down away from patient's heels and even with edge of mattress. Smooth out sheet over top edge of mattress and miter corners (see step 8i). Tuck remaining sheet under mattress all the way to foot. Keep linens smooth. *(Time is saved if one side of bed is made at a time. Fanfolding all linen lengthwise down bed promotes neatness and prevents wrinkling.)*

f. Place drawsheet on bed so that center fold lies down middle of bed. If protective drawsheet is to be used, place it on first. Smooth out over mattress and tuck in. *(Prevents loosening and wrinkling.)* Keep palms down. *(Prevents stones in wedding rings from catching in bed springs.)*

g. Place top sheet over bed and smooth out. Place blanket over top sheet. Smooth out. Place spread over blanket and smooth out. Make cuff with top linens (see illustration). *(Provides for patient's comfort.)*

h. Allow for toe pleat. Make modified mitered corner by not tucking tip of sheet under mattress. *(Provides for patient comfort.)*

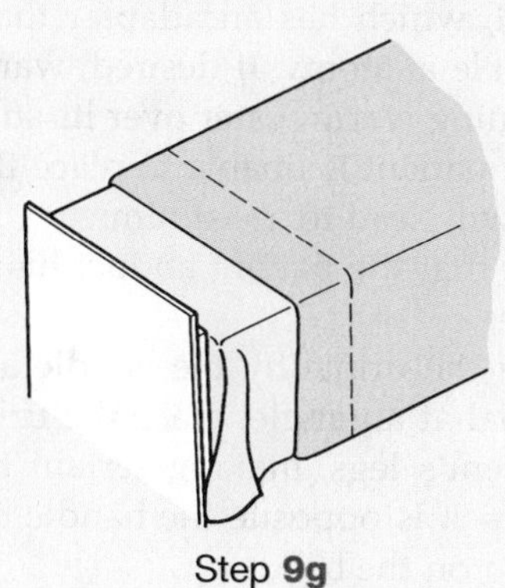

Step **9g**

i. Move to opposite side of bed and complete making bed as described in steps 9e to 9h. *(Saves your time and energy.)* Pull linens tight and keep taut as linens are tucked in.

j. Put on clean pillowcase (see step 8s). Place pillow at head of bed and position for comfort. Place call light within easy reach and lower bed level. *(Promotes patient's safety.)*

k. If patient is to return to bed, fanfold top linens down to foot of bed. Make sure cuff at top of linens is easily accessible to patient. *(It is easier for patient to return to bed.)*

10. Arrange personal items on bed table or bedside stand and place within patient's easy reach. *(Promotes patient's safety.)*

11. Leave area neat and clean. *(Promotes patient's sense of well-being.)*

12. Place all soiled linens in proper receptacle. Perform hand hygiene. *(Reduces spread of microorganisms.)*

13. Assist patient to bed, and position for comfort. *(Promotes patient's safety and comfort.)*

14. Documentation.
- Bedmaking does not have to be recorded.
- Record patient's vital signs, signs, and symptoms only if there are changes.

15. Report any abnormal findings to nurse in charge or physician.

member to use side rails, to keep the call light within easy reach, and to maintain the bed in the proper position: high position while working at the bedside, and low position when work is completed, to protect the patient from accidental falls.

It is your responsibility to keep the bed as clean and comfortable as possible. This is likely to require frequent inspections to make certain bedding is clean, dry, and wrinkle free. Check the linens for food particles after meals and for urine incontinence or involuntary stool. If linens are soiled with urine, feces, blood, or emesis, change them. Use **chux** (waterproof pads) with caution. Accumulation of moisture creates a risk for skin maceration and impairment.

Follow basic principles of medical asepsis (Box 18-9).

Use proper body mechanics while making the bed; for example, raise the bed to a working level to avoid bending down or stretching. Also apply the principles of body mechanics while turning and repositioning the patient.

There are two ways to make an unoccupied bed: open or closed. In the open bed, the top linens are fanfolded toward the foot of the bed to allow the patient to return to bed more easily. A closed bed is prepared following a patient's dismissal or transfer, or when the patient dies, before another patient is admitted. Housekeeping personnel clean the mattress and bed and apply fresh linens (see Skill 18-5).

Box 18-9 Principles of Medical Asepsis for Bedmaking

- Keep soiled linens away from uniform.
- Place soiled linens in hamper or plastic bag.
- Never fan linens in the air. *(This causes air currents, which spread microorganisms.)*
- Never place soiled linens on the floor. If clean linens touch the floor, place in laundry hamper immediately.
- Remove all unnecessary equipment and maintain a neat work area.

The postoperative bed is a form of the open bed. The top sheet and the spread are not mitered or tucked in at the corners. The top linens are usually fanfolded lengthwise or crosswise at the foot of the patient's bed. Arrange the top bed linens in such a way that they allow easy transfer of the surgical patient from the gurney to the bed. A complete linen change is done if the patient is returning from surgery (Figure 18-9).

ASSISTING THE PATIENT WITH ELIMINATION

A patient who is unable to get up to the bathroom for the purpose of **urination** (the act of emptying the urinary bladder) or of **defecation** (the act of eliminating feces) will use a **bedpan** (device for receiving feces or

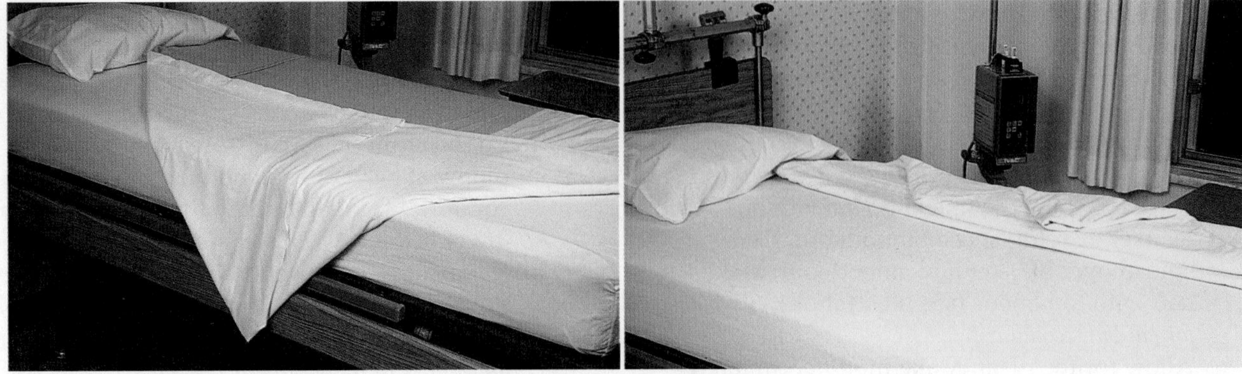

FIGURE 18-9 The postoperative bed.

urine from either male or female patients confined to bed) or urinal (a device for collecting urine from male patients; urinals for female patients are also available). Using a bedpan or urinal is a private and personal procedure. Make sure to afford the patient as much privacy as his or her condition allows.

Offer the bedpan or urinal frequently, because patients risk accidentally soiling bedclothes if their elimination needs are not met. It is not unusual for a patient to procrastinate using a bedpan because it is uncomfortable and embarrassing. Patients will sometimes try to get to the bathroom unassisted even if their condition prohibits ambulation. Remind patients of the possibility of accidents or falls (Box 18-10).

Report and record in the nursing notes any abnormalities in urine or stool (Box 18-11). Flow sheets are usually provided for documentation of normal voidings and stools.

Bedpans are made of metal or plastic. There are two types of bedpans. One type has a high back. The second type is flat and smaller and is called a fracture pan (Figure 18-10, *A*).

A urinal is made of metal or plastic. There are two types of urinals. One type serves the male patient for voiding (see Figure 18-10, *B*). The other type is called a **female urinal,** which has an adapter that accommodates the female anatomy. If desired, warm the metal urinal by running warm water over its surface.

If the male patient is unable to place the urinal for himself, you will need to assist him:

1. Request that the patient abduct his legs a slight distance.
2. Holding the urinal by the handle and directing the urinal at an angle, place the urinal between the patient's legs, making certain the long, flat side, which is opposite the handle of the urinal, is resting on the bed.
3. Gently raising the penis, place it fully within the urinal.

Empty the bedpan and the urinal immediately after use, and cleanse and store it properly. If the patient's intake and output are being monitored, measure urine and record result. Estimate liquid stool on the appro-

Box 18-10 Assisting the Patient with Elimination

- Allow the patient enough time for elimination. Ignoring the urge to defecate or urinate or not taking time to eliminate completely is a common cause of constipation or urine retention.
- It is essential to be prompt when called to assist the patient to the bathroom or onto the bedpan or bedside commode.
- When the patient shares a room with another patient, be certain to curtain off the patient's area. This enables the patient to relax, knowing that interruptions will not occur.
- Close the bathroom door. If it is necessary to remain nearby, stand outside door or curtain.
- For those patients unable to assume the normal squatting position, there are stool risers, which call for less effort to sit or stand.

Box 18-11 Characteristics of Normal Urine and Normal Stool

NORMAL URINE

- Ranges from a pale, straw color to amber (depends on the concentration)
- Is transparent at the time of voiding
- Has a characteristic odor: faintly aromatic
- Yields negative results when tested for protein, glucose, ketone bodies, red blood cells, white blood cells, and bacteria

NORMAL STOOL

- Brown
- Odor is affected by food types
- Has soft, formed consistency
- Frequency ranges from once a day to two or three times a week
- Resembles the shape of the rectum
- Contains undigested food, dead bacteria, fat, bile pigment, living cells, intestinal mucosa, and water

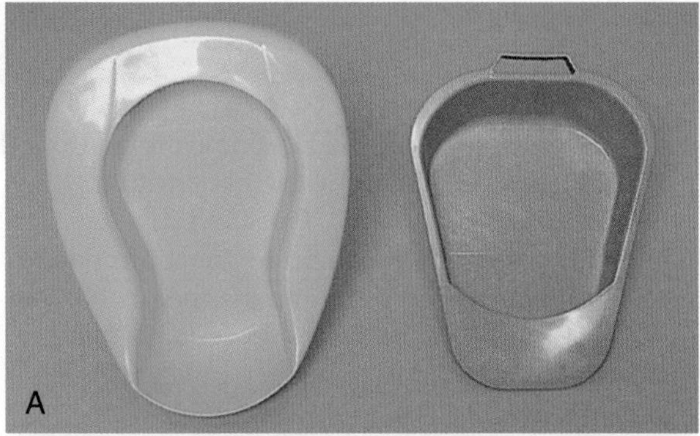

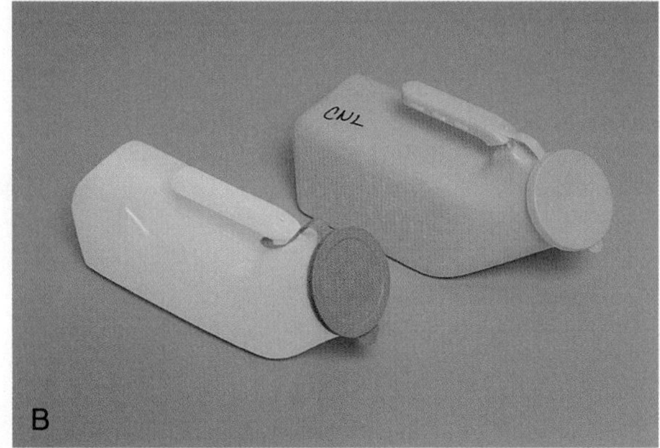

FIGURE 18-10 Selected equipment and supplies for elimination. **A,** Regular bedpan (left) and fracture pan (right). **B,** Male urinals.

priate form according to the agency's policy. See Skill 18-6 for positioning the bedpan.

Another option for elimination, instead of the bedpan or the urinal, is the bedside commode (Figure 18-11). It is useful at night and for the patient who is not able to ambulate as far as the bathroom easily.

Care of the Incontinent Patient

Incontinence is a very common problem, especially among older adults. Regardless of the cause, incontinence is psychologically distressing and socially disruptive.

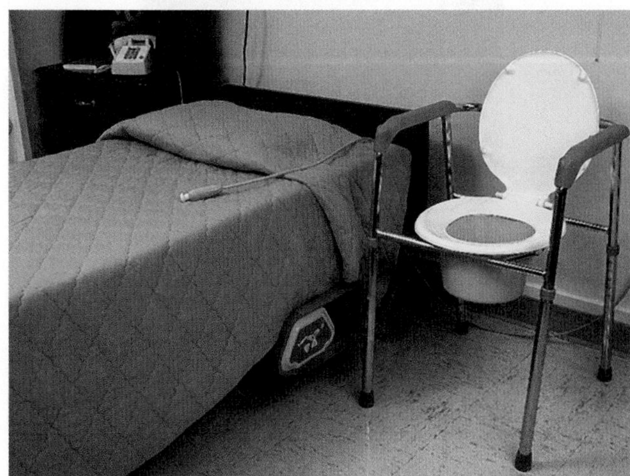

FIGURE 18-11 The bedside commode has a toilet seat with a container underneath. The container slides out from under the toilet seat for emptying and cleaning.

Urinary incontinence occurs because pressure in the bladder is too great, because the sphincters are weak, or because the innervation has been compromised as a result of illness or injury. Collaborate with other members of the health care team to assess the cause and the extent of incontinence and to assist in managing the problem. The physical therapist, for example, is prepared to assess the extent of musculoskeletal involvement and determine methods of treatment.

Incontinence sometimes involves a small leakage of urine occurring when a person laughs, coughs, or lifts something heavy. Teach the patient exercises to strengthen muscles around the external sphincters to help manage this type of incontinence. Pelvic floor exercises (Kegel exercises) involve tightening the ring of muscle around the vagina and anus and holding the muscle contraction for several seconds. Have the patient do this a minimum of 10 times, three times a day.

Alert patients need an incontinence product that is discreet and promotes self-care. Some incontinence products are designed for small amounts of leakage. Persistent urge, stress, or overflow incontinence will most likely necessitate referral for urologic evaluation.

Incontinence characterized by urine or fecal flow at unpredictable times necessitates the use of disposable adult undergarments or underpads as the primary means of management. Urine and feces are very irritating to the skin. Skin that is continually exposed quickly becomes inflamed and irritated. Cleanse the skin thoroughly after each episode of incontinence with warm soapy water and dry it thoroughly to help prevent skin impairment.

When urinary incontinence results from decreased perception of bladder fullness or impaired voluntary motor control, bladder training is often helpful.

❖ NURSING PROCESS *for Hygiene*

The role of the licensed practical nurse/licensed vocational nurse (LPN/LVN) in the nursing process as stated is that the LPN/LVN will:

- Participate in planning care for patients based on patient needs
- Review patient's plan of care and recommend revisions as needed
- Review and follow defined prioritization for patient care
- Use clinical pathways, care maps, or care plans to guide and review patient care

■ Assessment

Nursing assessment is an ongoing process. First it will always be necessary to determine whether the patient is able to tolerate hygienic procedures, which can be exhausting. Also observe the patient's physical condi-

Skill 18-6 Positioning the Bedpan

Nursing Action *(Rationale)*

1. Refer to medical record, care plan, or Kardex. *(Provides basis for care.)*
2. Assess patient's needs. *(Allows nurse to note any potential problems with patient's environment.)*
3. Assemble supplies according to patient's needs (see Figure 18-10). *(Organizes procedure.)*
4. Introduce self. *(Reduces patient's anxiety.)*
5. Identify patient. *(Ensures procedure is performed with correct patient.)*
6. Explain procedure. *(Enlists cooperation and reduces patient's anxiety.)*
7. Prepare patient. *(Facilitates procedure.)*
   a. Close door/pull privacy curtain. *(Elimination is a very personal function and is greatly facilitated by providing privacy.)*
   b. Arrange supplies close to the bedside. *(Provides easy access to supplies.)*
   c. Place protective pad under patient's buttocks, if necessary. *(Protects linens from soiling.)*
8. Perform hand hygiene and don clean gloves according to agency policy and guidelines from the CDC and OSHA. *(Reduces spread of microorganisms.)*
9. Warm metal bedpan under running warm water. *(Provides for patient's comfort.)*
10. When patient is able to assist self onto bedpan, nurse will position patient in supine position with knees flexed and bottom of feet flat on bed surface. As patient raises hips, nurse supports patient's lower back with her arm and positions bedpan under patient. When patient has finished with elimination, nurse removes bedpan in same manner. *(Allows for some measure of independence.)*
11. For patient unable to assist self on bedpan.
    a. Turn patient away from nurse toward opposite side rail, moving linens out of way. *(Provides for patient safety and maintains clean linens.)*
    b. Fit bedpan to patient's buttocks (see illustration). *(Prevents injury to patient's skin.)*
    c. Assist patient to turn over onto bedpan while nurse secures bedpan (see illustration). *(Allows nurse to use appropriate body mechanics.)*
    d. Raise head of bed 30 degrees. *(Promotes patient's comfort.)*
    e. Place toilet tissue and call light within easy reach. *(Provides for patient's convenience and promotes certain measure of independence.)*
12. For those patients who can be out of bed but are unable to ambulate far, there is the bedside commode (see Figure 18-11). Some are equipped with wheels, which allow the patient to be moved to the bathroom. *(Provides privacy.)*
13. When transferring a patient to the commode, assist the patient in the same manner as if assisting to a chair. *(Maintains proper body mechanics.)*
14. Document according to agency policy: *(Verifies patient's care.)*
    - Amount
    - Color
    - Consistency
    - Abnormal findings such as blood
15. Report unusual findings. *(Further interventions may be necessary.)*

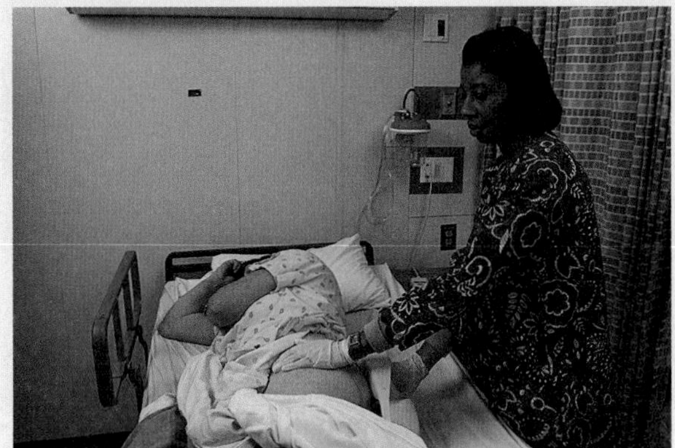

Step **11b**

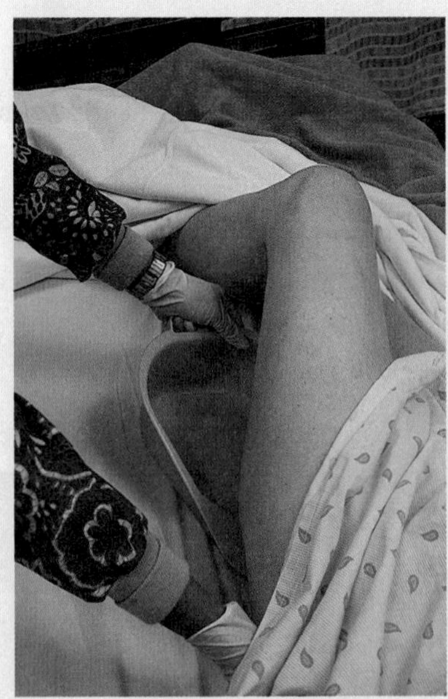

Step **11c**

tion and the integrity of the patient's skin, oral cavity, and sensory organs. Explore any developmental factors influencing the patient's hygiene needs. Note the patient's self-care ability and hygiene practices. Determine the patient's cultural preferences, as well.

Nursing Diagnosis

Nursing assessment helps identify the patient's need for and ability to maintain personal hygiene. You will then base interventions on the identified nursing diagnosis. Nursing diagnoses will possibly include the following:

- Impaired oral mucous membranes
- Impaired physical mobility
- Impaired skin integrity (Nursing Care Plan 18-1)
- Self-care deficit: bathing/hygiene
- Self-care deficit: dressing/grooming

Expected Outcomes and Planning

Considering the patient's preferences before planning is important. The hygiene measures that the patient desires or requires will determine the supplies and equipment that you will prepare. In some cases, you will also have to schedule hygiene measures around laboratory tests and diagnostic procedures, and involve the family in planning and adapting approaches for home care, as well as in hygiene instruction. Be aware of community resources that will be of assistance to meet the patient's needs.

Focus the interventions you administer on specific goals and outcomes that pertain to the identified nursing diagnoses, such as the following:

Goal: Patient's skin integrity remains intact.

Outcome: Patient's skin remains pink, warm, and with good turgor.

Nursing Care Plan 18-1 Skin Care

Mr. Payton is a 48-year-old patient immobilized because of trauma to the spinal cord. He has periods of diaphoresis. He has had liquid diarrhea for the past 48 hours. The skin on Mr. Payton's back, sacral regions, and buttocks is dry and intact, with a 2-cm area of erythema around the sacrum.

NURSING DIAGNOSIS ***Impaired skin integrity, related to immobilization and secretions***

Patient Goals and Expected Outcomes	Nursing Interventions	Evaluation
Skin will remain intact during hospitalization Skin will remain free of pressure Skin will have reduced or absent secretions Skin will be dry, warm, and smooth	Provide perineal care after each diarrheal episode. Change linen after diaphoresis or diarrheal episode. Apply lotion to areas that will easily become dried and chapped. Monitor length of time any areas of erythema persist. Determine turning interval (e.g., 2 hours). Place oscillating air mattress on patient's bed. Do not massage erythemic (reddened) area or bony prominences. Reassess skin area daily. Assess for history of preexisting chronic diseases (diabetes, malignancy, acquired immunodeficiency syndrome [AIDS], peripheral and/or cardiovascular conditions). Assess surface that patient spends majority of time on (mattress for bedridden patient, cushion for wheelchairs). Specifically assess skin over bony prominences (sacrum, trochanters, scapulae, elbows, heels, inner and outer malleoli, inner and outer knees, back of head).	Observe and time the duration of erythemic area after each position change; palpate underlying and adjacent tissues after each position change.

Critical Thinking Questions

1. Mr. Payton has a poor appetite and his chemistry profile reveals low protein, low albumin, and low anion gap (A/G) ratio. Explain why poor nutrition predisposes to impairment of skin integrity and poor tissue healing.
2. With Mr. Payton's history of diarrhea, explain the possible complication that could evolve if the dry, intact skin develops an open lesion.

Goal: Impairment is minimal if present.
Outcome: No further skin impairment, as noted by pink granulation tissues around pressure ulcer edges.

■ Implementation

Nursing interventions that promote the patient's personal hygiene include bedmaking, bathing, and care of hair, eyes, ears, nose, nails, and skin.

Providing hygiene is a basic part of a patient's care. Learn and use care practices that help alleviate the patient's anxiety and promote comfort and relaxation while you are performing each hygiene measure. For example, while giving a patient a bath and changing a gown, use a gentle approach in turning and repositioning. Using a soft, gentle voice while conversing with the patient helps relieve any fears or concerns. For patients suffering symptoms such as pain or nausea, administering symptom relief before hygiene procedures will better prepare the patient.

You are in a unique position to assess the patient's readiness to learn and to teach health promotion practices whenever possible (see Patient Teaching and Home Care Considerations boxes). This includes educating

 Patient Teaching

Hygiene

GENERAL PRINCIPLES

- Initiate patient teaching at the beginning of the hygienic procedure, and continue throughout the duration of the intervention.
- Teach and encourage independence no matter how minimal it seems to be (e.g., washing the face and perineal area, brushing teeth, combing hair).
- Explain steps of procedure in which patient will be participating.

TEACHING POINTS

- Teach elderly and other patients with reduced sensation how to assess temperature of the bath water (e.g., bath thermometer).
- Teach how to inspect surfaces between skinfolds for signs of irritation or impairment (breakdown) (e.g., erythema, scalding).
- Teach proper cleansing of the perineum (e.g., female patients—cleansing from front to back; uncircumcised males—retracting foreskin to adequately cleanse underneath).
- Teach patients who have a trapeze bar on their bed how to lift themselves on and off the bedpan.
- Teach patient importance of washing hands before and after performing catheter care.
- If patient achieves relaxation from back rub, teach family members how to perform procedure.
- Stress importance of consistent use of sunscreen with a protective factor of at least 15 and avoidance of unnecessary sun exposure.
- Teach methods to prevent tooth decay (e.g., reduce intake of carbohydrates between meals [sweet snacks], brush within 30 minutes of eating sweets, rinse mouth thoroughly with water or eat acid-containing fruit such as an apple, use fluoridated water).
- Teach how to prevent or heal dry lips by applying lip ointment or lubricant and avoiding licking the lips.
- Teach the proper storage methods for dentures. Stress techniques of cleaning that avoid damage to dentures (e.g., use brush with soft bristles; carry dentures in a container; hold dentures with cloth to avoid dropping).
- Teach patient to remove dentures at bedtime to give gums a rest, and to store dentures in solution to prevent drying and warping.
- Teach signs and symptoms of oral infection or irritation (e.g., erythematous or whitened areas, bleeding, lesions).
- Advise patient to brush teeth at least four times daily and to rinse well after brushing.
- Teach diabetic patients to visit their dentist every 3 to 4 months and to handle tissues gently. *(Diabetes depresses the immune system and decreases circulation to the mucosa.)*
- Teach proper hair care—regular shampooing, not to use chemicals and hot combs for straightening hair. *(May result in scalp burns, hair loss, or allergic reaction.)*
- Teach primary caregiver safety precautions for shaving, especially if patient is receiving anticoagulant therapy, and the technique to follow in the event a patient is accidentally nicked.
- Teach proper foot care:
  —Wash and soak feet daily using lukewarm water; thoroughly pat feet dry and dry well between toes. It is not recommended to soak the feet of a diabetic patient or a patient with peripheral vascular disease. This potentially leads to maceration (excessive softening of the skin) and infection.
  —File nails, never clip them.
  —Caution against self-treating corns or calluses. Consult a physician or podiatrist.
  —If needed, apply a mild foot powder.
  —Inspect feet daily.
  —Wear clean socks or stockings daily (change twice a day if feet perspire).
  —Do not walk barefoot.
  —Wear properly fitting shoes.
  —Wash and dry minor cuts immediately. Use only mild antiseptic (e.g., Neosporin ointment).
- Teach when cleansing the eye to go from the inner corner or canthus to the outer corner or canthus.
- Teach to never insert hairpins, toothpicks, or cotton-tipped applicators into the ear canal. If necessary, consult a physician.
- Teach about skin care:
  —Teach process of wound healing and expected wound appearance.
  —Teach signs and symptoms of pressure ulcers to report to health care team.
  —Teach prevention guidelines to halt further breakdown.
  —Teach importance of good nutrition and adequate fluid intake.

 Home Care Considerations

Hygienic Care

BATHING

- Include family members in discussion about patient's hygienic care, before discharge if possible.
- Set up equipment according to established routine.
- Advise installing grab bars around tub, carpeting bathroom floor, and using a portable shower seat for safety.
- The three types of baths for the homebound patient are the complete bed bath; the abbreviated bed bath, during which only the parts of the patient's body are washed whose neglect will potentially cause illness, odor, or discomfort; and the partial bath, which takes place at the sink, in the tub, or in the shower.
- The kind of bath chosen depends on assessment of the home, availability of running water, and condition of the bathing facilities.
- If beds do not have side rails, positioning is possible with pillows or by placing bed against the wall.
- Never leave bathing patient unattended. Adhesive strips on bottom of tub or shower, handrails, chairs, or stools in tub or shower will further protect patient.
- Follow patient's usual bathing and skin care routines.
- Assess patient to see whether there is need for a home health aide or other assistance after discharge.

SKIN CARE

- Assess perineum at every visit because of risk for infection and skin breakdown.
- Make sure to protect patient from falling off bed during back rub.
- The 30-degree lateral position or the prone position are sometimes useful at night to prolong the time needed between position changes, resulting in less sleep disruption for the patient and the caregiver.
- Identify community resources such as neighbors and relatives for assistance should patient need help with position changes, including after a fall.
- Customize pressure-relief maneuvers for the independent patient. Some individuals find it useful to use a watch with timer, mark even or odd hours, and use television commercials as guidelines to remember when to complete pressure-relief techniques.
- Identify clean storage area for dressing supplies.
- Determine availability of required supplies.
- Discuss need for home pressure-relief surface or bed.
- Identify adaptive equipment needed to care for patient at home, such as stool risers.

ORAL CARE

- Assess state of dental health of patient and family members and attitudes toward oral hygiene.
- Family members need instruction in oral care so that family understands how to protect the patient from aspirating while ensuring thorough cleansing of the oral cavity.
- Irrigate oral cavity with a bulb syringe; if unavailable, a gravy baster is acceptable to use as a substitute. A large syringe is another possibility.
- Cleanse mouth at least twice a day. If patient breathes through mouth, wrap gauze or soft linen around a tongue blade, moisten, and use every 1 to 2 hours to keep mouth moist and fresh.
- On regular visits, assess for signs and symptoms of infection or irritation, including erythematous, bleeding lesions of the gums.
- Provide special care to patients undergoing head and neck radiation because the gums will usually be dry and edematous and will likely interfere with proper denture fit.

HAIR CARE

- Assess temperature of the room, availability of water, and the most satisfactory position of the patient for the procedure.
- Provide extra protection from wetness for patients with casts.
- Obtain dry shampoo preparations when a wet shampoo is contraindicated.
- Construct a trough by arranging a plastic shower curtain or tablecloth under the patient's head and then tapering the cloth to form a narrow end that can drain into a container or basin next to the patient's bed.
- In the home setting, you will need to find ways the patient can shampoo the hair without causing injury. Some patients with a long leg cast will need to wash the hair at a sink until it is safe to shower or until the cast is removed and resumption of tub baths is permitted.
- Caution patients about using chemicals and hot combs for straightening hair. Such practices often cause considerable damage to the hair. Misuse results in possible scalp burns, hair loss, and allergic reactions that cause severe skin rashes, urticaria, and conjunctivitis.

SHAVING

- Provide adequate towels around patient's neck to help prevent spilling shaving cream or water on chest or bed.
- Provide adequate lighting for the procedure.
- Perform procedure in comfortable setting, such as bathroom or bedroom.
- Usually the facial hair of the older patient does not grow quickly, and thus a shave may not be necessary every day.
- If patient is on anticoagulant therapy, use an electric razor.

NAILS AND FEET

- Alternative therapies: moleskin applied to areas on feet that are under friction is less likely to cause local pressure than corn pads; spot adhesive bandages guard corns against friction but do not have padding to protect against pressure; wrapping small pieces of lamb's wool around toes reduces irritation of soft corns between toes.
- Assess use of patient's bathroom sink for soaking patient's hands, and tub for soaking patient's feet.
- Financial constraints are often responsible for patients wearing poorly fitted shoes, which can cause foot problems.

BEDMAKING

- Assess primary caregiver's ability and willingness to maintain a clean environment for the patient.
- Assess home laundry facilities to plan with the primary caregiver the most reasonable frequency with which linens will be laundered.
- Assess amount of linens in the home to establish with the primary caregiver the number of changes of sheets that it is possible to reserve for the patient's use.

patients on proper hygiene techniques and connecting patients with the community resources necessary to enable them to perform hygienic care. The greater the risk for hygiene problems the patient is at, the greater the patient's need to understand these risks, know the implications, and have the necessary information to make choices about when and how hygiene is performed.

Be mindful of the patient's independence and privacy and foster the patient's physical well-being.

Evaluation

Assess the success of the nursing interventions on completion of the hygienic measures. Reassess the condition of the patient's skin, nails, oral cavity, and sensory organs. Determine if the patient's comfort level has improved. Ask the patient to demonstrate hygiene self-care skills, and ask the patient if his or her expectations are being met.

Always be prepared to revise the care plan based on the evaluation. Systematic evaluation requires you to determine whether expected outcomes have been met. Refer to the identified goals and outcomes when planning interventions.

Goal: Patient's skin integrity remains intact.

Evaluative measure: Assess for pink skin, warm, moist, without abrasions, and with immediate color return on blanching.

Goal: Patient's skin impairment, if any, remains minimal.

Evaluative measure: Measure skin impairment, assess for granulation tissue, and note absence of necrotic tissue.

Get Ready for the NCLEX® Examination!

Key Points

- Hygiene is a personal matter; it is important to consider all factors influencing the personal hygiene routine.
- Make sure the patient's room is comfortable, safe, and large enough to allow the patient and visitors to move around freely.
- Assume the responsibility for providing the daily hygienic needs of patients if they are unable to care for themselves adequately.
- Providing hygienic care gives you the opportunity to assess all external body surfaces and the patient's emotional state.
- Assisting or providing the patient with daily hygienic needs allows you to use teaching and communication skills to develop a meaningful relationship with the patient.
- Consider the patient's personal preferences as you plan the daily hygienic care.
- Be sure to maintain the patient's privacy and comfort when providing daily care.
- Various sociocultural, economic, and developmental factors influence patients' hygiene practices.
- During assessment of the skin, observe the characteristics most influenced by hygienic measures.
- Patients who are immobilized, who are poorly nourished, and who have reduced sensation are at risk for impaired skin integrity.
- External pressure, shearing force, moisture, impaired peripheral circulation, edema, and obesity contribute to the development of pressure ulcers.
- When the external pressure against the skin is greater than the pressure in the capillary bed, blood flow decreases to the adjacent tissues.
- Pressure ulcers tend to occur initially in the superficial layers of the skin.
- Meticulous assessment of the skin and underlying tissue and identification of risk factors are important in preventing the circumstances favorable to development of pressure ulcers.
- Preventive skin care is aimed at controlling external pressure on bony prominences and keeping the skin clean, well lubricated, hydrated, and free of excess moisture.
- Proper positioning reduces the effects of pressure and guards against shearing force.
- Cleansing and topical agents used to treat pressure ulcers vary according to the stage of the ulcer.
- Wear gloves during hygienic care when there is risk of contacting body fluids.
- Techniques used during tepid sponging are designed to minimize the risk of a patient becoming chilled.
- Patients with diabetes mellitus require special consideration when you provide nail and foot care.
- When administering oral care to unconscious patients, take measures to prevent aspiration.
- The evaluation of hygienic care is based on the patient's expression of a sense of relaxation and well-being and an understanding of personal hygienic techniques.

Additional Resources

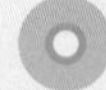
Go to your Companion CD for an audio glossary, animations, video clips, and more.

evolve Be sure to visit the Evolve site at http://evolve.elsevier.com/Christensen/foundations/ for additional online resources.

Review Questions for the NCLEX® Examination

1. When preparing for patient care, a student nurse learns that microorganisms are spread by:
   1. fresh air and sunshine.
   2. carrying linens away from one's uniform.
   3. placing soiled linens on the floor.
   4. using a common handwashing station.

2. During the bed bath, the patient is covered with a bath blanket:

1. to prevent skin impairment.
2. for cosmetic purposes.
3. to prevent the spread of microorganisms.
4. to prevent chilling.

3. A patient with severe, crippling rheumatoid arthritis is confined to bed for extended periods. An erythematous and edematous area over the coccyx that has potential to become an open lesion is noted. This is referred to as:

1. an inflammatory ulcer.
2. a pressure ulcer.
3. a stasis ulcer.
4. the inner canthus.

4. A 64-year-old patient with terminal cancer is too weak to perform her own perineal care. The student nurse will include bathing which areas as part of perineal care?

1. Back and buttocks
2. Eyes, ears, and nose
3. Upper torso and thighs
4. Upper thighs, genitalia, and anal area

5. Which patient would be at greatest risk for skin impairment?

1. Child on bed rest
2. Infant with cool skin temperature
3. Young man with diarrhea
4. A 60-year-old in a body cast

6. A 52-year-old patient is in her second postoperative day after an abdominal hysterectomy. The nurse plans to give the patient a bed bath. When caring for the patient's face, the nurse will:

1. use only water.
2. ask the patient her preference.
3. use soap in all areas except the eyes.
4. use a cleansing cream.

7. When bathing a 12-year-old patient with a leg cast, the nurse is aware that proper eye care would be:

1. to wash from the outer canthus to inner canthus.
2. to cleanse dried exudate with hot water.
3. to avoid drying circumorbital area after washing.
4. to use a different section of washcloth for each eye.

8. A patient with heart failure is stabilizing well and states that he would enjoy a tub bath. The nurse assists the patient with filling the bathtub. The correct water temperature is:

1. 109.4° F.
2. 110° to 115° F.
3. 98° to 100° F.
4. 85° to 98° C.

9. An 11-month-old infant is admitted with a tympanic temperature of 105° F. The physician orders a tepid sponge bath. The purpose of the tepid sponge bath is to:

1. reduce temperature in febrile patients.
2. cleanse the patient's groin and axillary areas.
3. stimulate circulation to the skin.
4. calm and relax the patient.

10. An 80-year-old uncircumcised man is in the first postoperative day after a transurethral prostatectomy. When administering perineal care, the nurse will:

1. retract the foreskin, cleanse the penis, and allow the foreskin to return to its former position.
2. sprinkle powder under the foreskin to facilitate retraction.
3. leave the foreskin slightly damp to allow retraction to its former state.
4. retract the foreskin, cleanse the penis, and return the foreskin with a gentle forward motion.

11. A 50-year-old patient was discharged home with a Foley catheter. The student nurse instructs the patient in the proper procedure for cleansing the female perineal area by teaching her to:

1. cleanse the area in circular motions around the rectum.
2. cleanse from the rectum toward the pubis.
3. cleanse from the pubis toward the rectum.
4. cleanse in circular motions around the vaginal area.

12. Which patient is most at risk for complications of the feet?

1. A young man in a career that requires standing
2. A disoriented, older adult man
3. A 60-year-old person with diabetes mellitus
4. A 62-year-old patient with total hip replacement

13. An 82-year-old patient is unconscious and requires meticulous oral hygiene. The optimal position for providing oral hygiene to the patient is ________ to prevent choking.

1. high Fowler's position
2. high Fowler's position with head hyperextended
3. supine with the head lowered
4. side-lying with head facing to the side

14. A 72-year-old patient has diffuse pancreatitis. The nurse will cleanse her ears while giving her a soothing bed bath. Which intervention for cleansing her ears is correct?

1. Cleansing the outer ear with the washcloth during the bath
2. Retracting the outer ear downward to loosen visible cerumen
3. Irrigating to remove tenacious cerumen
4. Using cotton-tipped applicators to remove cerumen

15. The student nurse has completed her educational instructions on the correct procedures for bedmaking. Which intervention is correct for bedmaking?

1. Preparing a closed bed for receiving postoperative patients
2. Shaking soiled linen before placement in the hamper
3. Mitering the corners of the bottom fitted sheet
4. Washing hands thoroughly after handling soiled linen

16. A retired dentist has been admitted to the hospital for thrombophlebitis of his left leg. Which stroke will you use when finishing his back rub?
    1. Long, firm strokes across the width of the back
    2. Light strokes while moving up the back in a circular motion
    3. Long, smooth strokes along the length of the back
    4. Circular motion upward from buttocks to shoulder

17. An 82-year-old patient is in his first postoperative day after lysis of adhesions. As part of his morning care, the nurse will remove and cleanse his dentures. Which of the following techniques is correct?
    1. Work over an open sink convenient to the water faucet.
    2. Rinse dentures thoroughly with hot water.
    3. Brush dentures with a soft toothbrush.
    4. Hold dentures securely in the palm of the hand.

18. The nurse will position the patient in the 30-degree lateral position to prevent pressure ulcers over the:
    1. spinous processes.
    2. ischial tuberosities.
    3. greater trochanters.
    4. occipital prominence.

19. Stage III pressure ulcers are identified as:
    1. nonblanchable reddened areas where the skin is intact.
    2. full-thickness skin loss extending to but not through the fascia.
    3. extensive destruction of skin and muscle with possible sinus tracts.
    4. areas of full-thickness skin loss with possible extension to the bone.

20. The patient has been changing a dressing on a pressure ulcer for several days and is now being seen in the physician's office. The patient states, "There is a lot of pink tissue at the base of the ulcer." The nurse expects this is due to:
    1. improper dressing technique and probable infection.
    2. presence of a layer of eschar that has to be removed.
    3. development of a fungal overgrowth interfering with healing.
    4. the normal process of healing with healthy granulation tissue.

21. In addition to bathing, which intervention is likely to best promote patient comfort?
    1. Books or tapes
    2. Back rub
    3. Snacks
    4. Postural drainage

22. Patients will experience conditions that threaten the integrity of oral mucosa; therefore:
    1. less oral hygiene is needed.
    2. more frequent mouth care is needed.
    3. no mouth care is to be performed.
    4. no antiinfective agents are to be used.

23. The goal of meticulous foot care for patients is to:
    1. prevent injury to the toes and feet.
    2. provide routine cleaning of the feet and nails.
    3. monitor the healing process of foot ulcers.
    4. determine if the patient's shoes are the proper size.

24. When providing hygiene to the older adult, it is important to remember that the older adult's skin is:
    1. fragile with decreased elasticity.
    2. fragile with increased elasticity.
    3. fragile with increased circulation.
    4. fragile with increased muscle mass.

25. Which tissues are most vulnerable to pressure?
    1. Skin and cartilage
    2. Skin and muscle tissue
    3. Skin and subcutaneous tissue
    4. Muscle and subcutaneous tissue

26. Which statement about moisture is correct?
    1. Topical moisture barriers protect the skin from breakdown and impairment.
    2. Evidence indicates that topical moisture barriers cause skin rashes.
    3. Excess moisture promotes wound healing and prevents skin impairment.
    4. Dry skin is resistant to breakdown.

27. The color of eschar is:
    1. pink or red.
    2. pale, almost white.
    3. tan, brown, or black.
    4. yellow, gray, or green.

28. When assessing the skin of a patient with dark skin, it is best to have which source of light?
    1. Halogen
    2. Fluorescent
    3. Soft
    4. Sunlight

29. Staging a pressure ulcer is not possible if:
    1. the ulcer is full thickness and the wound bed is covered with brown eschar.
    2. skin is intact with a blood-filled blister present that is cool to the touch.
    3. bone is exposed with yellow slough present in parts of the wound bed.
    4. subcutaneous fat is visible, along with tissue undermining.

Chapter 19

Specimen Collection and Diagnostic Examination

Elaine Oden Kockrow

evolve

http://evolve.elsevier.com/Christensen/foundationsadult

Objectives

1. Explain the rationales for collection of each specimen listed.
2. Discuss guidelines for specimen collection.
3. Describe the role of the nurse in procedures for specimen collection.
4. Discuss patient teaching for diagnostic testing.
5. State appropriate labeling for a collected specimen.
6. List the proper steps for teaching blood glucose self-monitoring.
7. Discuss the procedure for obtaining stool specimens.
8. State the correct procedures for collecting a sputum specimen.
9. List the proper steps when obtaining urine specimens.
10. List the nursing responsibilities for a glucose tolerance test.
11. Identify procedure for performing a phlebotomy.
12. Identify procedure for performing an electrocardiogram.
13. Describe the necessary documentation of the patient's condition before, during, and after a laboratory or diagnostic test.
14. Discuss nursing interventions necessary to properly prepare a patient who is to have a diagnostic examination.
15. List the diagnostic tests for which it is a nursing responsibility to determine whether the patient is allergic to iodine.

Key Terms

culture (p. 502)
cytology (sī-TŎL-ŏ-jē, p. 502)
electrocardiogram (ECG) (ĕ-lĕk-trō-KĂR-dē-ō-grăm, p. 514)
expectorate (ĕks-PĔK-tŏ-rāt, p. 502)
fixative (p. 488)
Hemoccult (HĒ-mō-kŭlt, p. 499)
midstream urine specimen (p. 494)
occult (ŏ-KŬLT, p. 499)
residual urine (p. 494)
sensitivity (p. 502)
specimen (p. 494)
tourniquet (TŪR-nĭ-kĕt, p. 509)
Vacutainer (p. 507)
venipuncture (VĔN-ĭ-pŭnk-chŭr, p. 507)

DIAGNOSTIC EXAMINATION

Diagnostic examination is performed by a physician sometimes at the patient's bedside and sometimes in a specially equipped room for therapeutic or diagnostic purposes. As a nurse, you are responsible for assessing the patient's knowledge of and preparing the patient for the procedure, assisting the physician with the procedure, and caring for the patient after tests are completed. Your knowledge and organization of the diagnostic procedure can be the key to success.

Patients have fundamental rights and protections while they are receiving care. One of the most important rights is informed consent, which requires that a patient (or a responsible family member if the patient is legally incompetent) fully understands what will be done during a test, surgery, or any medical procedure and understands its risks and implications *before* legally consenting to it.

Explaining a procedure, how it will be performed, and its potential benefits and risks is primarily the physician's responsibility. You will typically reinforce the physician's explanation and confirm that the patient comprehends it. Written consent is not always necessary for individual tests; informed verbal consent is adequate in many cases. The patient retains the legal right to withdraw consent—verbal or written—at any time and for any reason and to refuse care or treatment.

Anticipate the needs of the physician and have the proper supplies ready. Assist the patient through the procedure. It is especially important to keep the patient adequately informed of procedural details that have potential to cause discomfort. Many procedures cause moderate discomfort. Patients tend to tolerate the procedures better if a well-informed nurse stays at the bedside and describes each step and possible reactions.

Take special care with older adults during specimen collection and diagnostic examination (see Life Span Considerations for Older Adults box). Be aware that sociocultural variations often affect a patient's re-

Life Span Considerations

Older Adults

Specimen Collection and Diagnostic Tests

- Owing to a decrease in the agility required to collect a midstream specimen, catheterization of the older person is sometimes necessary. It is important to explain the purpose of the procedure and provide privacy during specimen collection.
- Older adults are prone to reduced drug clearance from decreased renal function or decreased hepatic function. Therefore monitor effects of narcotics and hypnotics that have the potential to interfere with breathing.
- Decreased peripheral circulation sometimes makes it difficult to collect a specimen for blood glucose determination. Try wrapping the hand in a warm, moist washcloth for a few minutes to facilitate the procedure.
- Changes in blood vessels make venipuncture more difficult in many older adults. Repeated sticks to obtain blood samples pose the risk of causing mental and physical trauma to the older adult.
- Collect stool specimens from older adults by using a bedpan or specimen pan in the toilet or commode. At home, collect stool by supporting a large piece of waxed paper or clear plastic under the toilet seat.
- Collection of sputum is often difficult because of poor cough capacity in older adults. It is sometimes necessary for a respiratory therapist to collect the specimen.
- Collection of wound drainage is often painful. Provide adequate analgesics to older adults before this is performed.
- Assessment of certain specimens involves comparing results to a color chart. Older adults often have difficulty reading the color chart.
- Many older adults will need a written reminder placed on the bathroom mirror to collect all urine samples.
- When obtaining a specimen by doing a venipuncture, remember that some older adults do not need a tourniquet for this procedure.
- Older adults have fragile veins that are easily traumatized during venipuncture.
- If multiple procedures are necessary, schedule adequate rest time between tests.
- Postprocedural restlessness in the older adult possibly indicates hypoxemia or pain. Assess the patient thoroughly for the cause.
- The older adult patient is typically taking multiple medications. Keep in mind that alterations in administration schedules will sometimes be necessary because of nothing-by-mouth (NPO) status for diagnostic tests.
- In the older adult, slight variations in vital signs or in behavior often indicate impending problems; therefore, skilled observations are critical.
- Be aware that NPO status in the older adult patient will possibly result in dehydration.
- Many older adults will have difficulty assuming various positions needed for specimen collection. Give assistance before and during procedure.
- If the patient is confused, an assistant is sometimes necessary to hold the patient's hand.
- Assess skin integrity of patient after lying on examining table. Older adults are at greater risk for skin impairment.
- Older adults will often need additional clothing, slippers, and extra blankets to keep them warm in waiting rooms and examination room.

Cultural Considerations

Diagnostic Testing

- If the patient's language skills inhibit communication, seek assistance from interpreters, word signs, or charts.
- A patient who is modest and self-conscious about the body will need psychological preparation before some procedures and tests.
- In almost all cases, you will be able to avoid cultural conflicts by communicating to the patient your respect for ethnicity and individuality. To accomplish this, you will sometimes find it useful to adapt your approach to the patient.
- Chinese-Americans will sometimes fear medical institutions because of language barriers and unfamiliarity with institutions or because of inadequate understanding of illness and treatment regimen. As a result, some Chinese-Americans will not comply with medical treatments. Many diagnostic tests, such as amniocentesis, glucose tolerance testing, ultrasonography, or drawing blood, are often perceived as being dangerous and unnecessary.
- Some Vietnamese-American patients believe that it is not possible to replace any body tissue or fluid that is removed, and that once it is removed, the body will continue to suffer the loss, not only in this life but also in the next life.
- Drawing blood for diagnostic purposes has the potential to cause a crisis for a Vietnamese-American patient. Some patients complain, although often not to the health care worker, of feeling weak and tired for varying periods—as long as months in some cases—following the procedure.
- Be sensitive that diverse age-groups and sociocultural groups typically use different words to describe urine and stool.

sponse and willingness to participate in various diagnostic procedures (see Cultural Considerations box).

When there are questions about diagnostic examination, consult the agency's procedural manual or the designated department involved.

It is essential to maintain confidentiality when disclosing results from testing and diagnostic procedures. Health care agencies are required to have and strictly follow policies regarding confidentiality of these records.

PREPARING THE PATIENT FOR DIAGNOSTIC EXAMINATIONS

Be prepared to answer any questions the patient has and to clarify the requirements for the examination. Be sure the patient knows if nothing is permitted to be taken by mouth (NPO) after midnight and if breakfast will be held until the examination is completed. The patient needs to know if a special room or if certain equipment is required for the test, as well as if any medications are needed before or during the test. An informed patient will be more cooperative during any test (Skill 19-1 and Patient Teaching box). You are responsible to know guidelines for and dangers of diagnostic examinations (Boxes 19-1 and 19-2, Table 19-1).

Text continued on p. 493

Skill 19-1 Preparing Patient for Diagnostic Examination

Nursing Action *(Rationale)*

1. Refer to medical record, care plan, or Kardex. *(Provides basis for care.)*
2. Ensure that informed consent has been obtained when necessary. Most invasive diagnostic tests require a signed informed consent form. The physician is ultimately responsible for disclosure, but you also need to be aware of agency policies regarding consent forms and ensure that informed consent is obtained before procedure. *(Ensures that legal implications of diagnostic procedures are taken into consideration.)*
3. Assemble equipment and supplies. *(Organizes procedure.)*
4. Introduce self. *(Decreases patient's anxiety.)*
5. Identify patient. *(Ensures procedure is performed with correct patient.)*
6. Explain procedure. Assess patient's understanding of procedure and purpose. If dye is to be used, assess patient for allergies (see Box 19-2). *(Promotes understanding and cooperation. Data help you set guidelines for teaching plan.)*
7. Prepare patient for procedure. *(Facilitates procedure.)*
   a. Transfer to examining room. Maintain safety precautions. *(Facilitates procedure—some facilities have special examination rooms, but many times a procedure is performed at the bedside.)*
   b. Close door and pull curtains. *(Provides privacy.)*
   c. Raise bed or arrange examination table to convenient height. *(Promotes proper body mechanics.)*
   d. Drape for procedure, if necessary. *(Prevents unnecessary exposure of patient.)* (See Table 19-1.)
8. Perform hand hygiene and don clean gloves according to agency policy and guidelines from the CDC and OSHA. *(Reduces spread of microorganisms.)*
9. Assist physician with procedure. *(Provides help to the physician while providing support to patient.)*
10. Answer patient's questions. *(Provides for patient's security and emotional support.)*
11. Deliver specimen to laboratory promptly. Label specimen according to agency policy (see Box 19-5): patient's name, age, room number, physician, date and time, type of specimen, and collector's initials. The CDC (2005b) and OSHA (2001a, 2001b) recommend inserting specimen (in container) into another plastic bag for transport to laboratory (see illustration). *(Prevents loss and potential delays in obtaining results. Outer plastic bag further prevents contamination from specimen.)*
12. Document procedure. *(Communicates performed procedure and patient's response.)*
    - Type of procedure
    - Time
    - Specimen obtained
    - Sent to laboratory with requisition
    - Patient's response
    - Patient teaching (see Patient Teaching box)

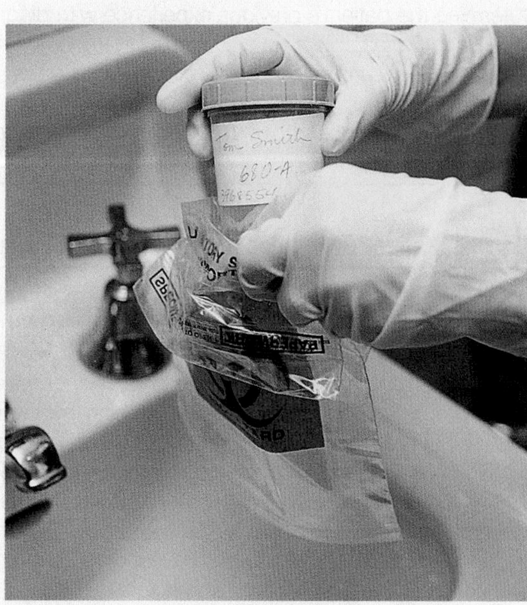

Step 11

 Patient Teaching

Specimen Collection and Diagnostic Tests

- Explain importance of collecting specimens on time and in the correct amount.
- Explain importance of specimen collection (why it is performed).
- Explain appropriate hand hygiene and to perform it before and after specimen collection.
- Explain proper procedure for obtaining each specimen and preparing for each diagnostic examination.
- Some specimen collection is not completed before dismissal. Make certain patient understands how to complete the collection.
- If dietary restrictions are required, explain importance of adhering to direction. EXAMPLE: A meat-free diet is often ordered before a stool specimen for occult blood.
- Explain results of test when applicable. EXAMPLE: Complete blood count.
- Request patient to perform return demonstration of obtaining a specimen. EXAMPLE: Skin puncture for measuring blood glucose level.
- Explain normal laboratory values when appropriate. EXAMPLE: Blood glucose levels desired.
- Explain when to notify physician. EXAMPLE: Elevated blood glucose level.
- Advise patient to perform oral hygiene after sputum collection as a comfort measure.
- Explain the importance of drinking fluids to decrease thickness of mucus; helpful before sputum collection.
- Ensure that patient understands the importance of obtaining an uncontaminated specimen.
- Allow time for patient questions, and provide answers.
- Instruct patient to check with physician about taking, or readjusting the time schedule for, prescribed medications on the day of the test or examination.

Box 19-1 General Guidelines for Diagnostic Examination

- Know the patient's baseline vital signs. Some diagnostic tests are invasive procedures and have associated complications. *(Changes from baseline vital signs provide early physiologic data about potential complications.)*
- Know the patient's level of education. Diagnostic tests require you to teach the patient about the test. *(Knowing the patient's educational background enables you to develop an individualized teaching plan.)*
- Determine the patient's awareness of actual or potential medical diagnoses. *(Provides you with data about the patient's knowledge and perception of medical diagnoses.)*
- Perform a thorough nursing assessment, including assessment of the patient's cultural background. *(Reveals abnormal findings, which can indicate or contraindicate a diagnostic test.)*
- Determine the patient's previous experience with diagnostic testing. *(Patients who have had smooth, uncomplicated diagnostic tests are usually less anxious about a test. If a patient has had a complication from a diagnostic test, it is possible that the patient will require more preprocedure education and support.)*
- Most agencies adhere to standard precautions—know your agency's policy. *(Some institutions have policies that require all specimen containers of body substances to be placed in small plastic bags for transportation to various laboratories. Attach requisitions to specimen container.)*
- Know normal values of the test being performed and causes of deviations from these normal values. (Be aware that some deviations from normal values occur as a result of medications or dietary intake.) *(Allows you to notify physician of end results in a timely manner.)*
- Refer to the policy manual for the institution's instructions for collection of each specimen during diagnostic examinations (see Table 19-1).
- Many factors have the potential to contribute to dysrhythmias in association with diagnostic exams, including medications such as digitalis and quinidine, hypertrophy of cardiac muscle, alcohol, thyroid dysfunction, coffee, tea, tobacco, electrolyte imbalances, edema, acid-base imbalances, and myocardial ischemia. *(Patients with dysrhythmias are at risk for cardiac arrest. Be familiar with crash cart location and knowledgeable about emergency equipment, medications, and cardiopulmonary resuscitation [CPR].)*

Box 19-2 Patient Evaluation for Iodine Dye Allergies

- Many types of contrast media are used in radiographic studies, for example, organic iodines and iodized oils.
- Possible allergic reactions to iodinated dye vary from mild flushing, itching, and urticaria to severe, life-threatening **anaphylaxis** (an exaggerated life-threatening hypersensitivity reaction to a previous encountered antigen; evidenced by respiratory distress, drop in blood pressure, or shock). In the unusual event of anaphylaxis, treatment consists of administration of drugs such as diphenhydramine (Benadryl), steroids, and epinephrine. Always have oxygen and endotracheal equipment on hand for immediate use.
- Always assess the patient for allergies to the iodine dye before its administration. Inform the radiologist if an allergy is suspected. The radiologist is likely to prescribe a Benadryl and steroid preparation to be administered before testing. Usually, hypoallergenic contrast media will be used during the test.*
- After the x-ray procedure, evaluate patient for delayed reaction to dye (dyspnea, rashes, tachycardia, hives). This usually occurs within 2 to 6 hours after the test. Treat with antihistamines or steroids, according to physician's order.
- Iodine is absorbed systemically, and it is necessary to consider all body secretions, especially urine, to be radioactive. You will usually keep the patient in a private room with its own bathroom. Check with your agency policy for specific guidelines.

*The American College of Radiology recommends that patients who have a prior documented contrast reaction be given a different contrast agent in combination with a premedication regimen if it is not possible to avoid using a contrast medium.

Table 19-1 Nursing Interventions for Diagnostic Examinations

PREEXAMINATION	POSTEXAMINATION
ABDOMINAL SCAN*	
Prepare requisition form. Explain procedure. Obtain informed consent, if required by institution. Assess lab results for kidney function. Instruct patient to be NPO for 4 hours before examination, if contrast medium is to be used. Assess patient for allergies to dye or shellfish—it is possible to do the abdominal scan with or without the dye. Assess patient for claustrophobia. Patients who are mildly claustrophobic often benefit from premedication with antianxiety drugs. Some patients will experience mild nausea from the contrast medium; provide emesis basin. Advise patients that a salty taste, flushing, and warmth during the dye injection are possible.	Evaluate patient for delayed reaction to dye (see Box 19-2). Encourage oral intake of fluids. Report results. Diarrhea is possible.
AMNIOCENTESIS	
Explain procedure. Encourage verbalization of concerns. Obtain written consent from patient and her spouse. Monitor fetal heart tones. No fluid or food restrictions. Monitor mother's blood pressure. Follow instructions regarding emptying the bladder, which depend on gestational age. Before 20 weeks of gestation, it is necessary to keep the bladder full to support the uterus. After 20 weeks, the bladder is typically emptied to minimize the chance of puncture. NOTE: The location of the placenta is determined by ultrasound before the study to permit selection of a site that will help prevent placental puncture.	Monitor fetal heart tones. If patient complains of vertigo or nausea, allow her to rest on her left side for several minutes before leaving examination room; assess mother's vital signs. If patient has any fluid loss or temperature elevation, abdominal pain or cramping, or fetal hyperactivity or unusual fetal lethargy, instruct her to notify her physician. Inform patient to contact her physician to obtain results (usually after 2 weeks). For women who have Rh-negative blood, administer RhoGAM because of the risk of immunization from the fetal blood. Observe puncture site for bleeding.
ARTERIOGRAPHY	
Explain procedure. Obtain written consent. Inform patient of a possible warm flushing feeling when dye is injected. Assess allergies to dye. Assess if patient has been taking anticoagulants. Keep patient NPO for 2 to 8 hours. Mark site of peripheral pulses with a pen (this will permit assessment after the procedure). If patient does not have peripheral pulse, document this so that arterial occlusion will not be suspected after the procedure. Administer medications as ordered. Ensure that the appropriate coagulation studies have been done and are within normal range. For cerebral angiograms, perform baseline neurologic assessment to compare subsequent assessments. Remove and safely store all dental prostheses and all valuables before study. Instruct patient to void before study. Inform the patient that bladder distention will possibly cause some discomfort during study.	Keep patient on bed rest for 8 hours. Monitor vital signs and observe for bleeding at puncture site. Assess peripheral arterial pulse at premarked site. If cerebral arteriograph has been done, perform neurologic assessment. Maintain pressure at the puncture site. Perform neurovascular assessment on patient's lower extremities; compare the involved extremity with the uninvolved extremity. Administer analgesic as indicated; notify physician if patient has severe, continuous pain. Have patient drink fluids to prevent dehydration. Evaluate patient for delayed allergic reaction to the dye (see Box 19-2). Notify physician if patient has continuous, severe pain.

NPO, Nothing by mouth or on nothing-by-mouth status.
*Showing a picture of the x-ray machine (used for scans and MRI) and encouraging the patient to verbalize concerns regarding claustrophobia will help reduce anxiety. Most patients who are mildly claustrophobic are able to tolerate these studies after appropriate premedication with antianxiety medications. Most of these tests require lying still on a hard table and peripheral venipuncture, which sometimes cause mild discomfort. Mild nausea is a common sensation when contrast dye is used. Have an emesis basin readily available. Some patients will experience a salty taste, flushing, and warmth during the dye injection. Encourage patients who receive dye injections to increase their fluid intake, because the dye is excreted by the kidneys and causes diuresis. Assure patients that they will be draped sufficiently so as to prevent unnecessary exposure.

Continued

Table 19-1 Nursing Interventions for Diagnostic Examinations—cont'd

PREEXAMINATION	POSTEXAMINATION
BARIUM ENEMA	
Prepare requisition form. Explain procedure. Provide needed emotional support. Instruct patient to be NPO after midnight (some facilities allow liquids for breakfast). Assist patient with bowel preparation, which varies among institutions. (In elderly patients, this preparation is sometimes exhausting and even causes severe dehydration in some.) *A typical day before preparation:* Clear liquid for lunch and supper (no dairy products). Have patient drink one glass of water or clear liquid every hour for 8 to 10 hours. Administer a cathartic at 2 PM. Administer three Dulcolax tablets at 7 PM. Keep patient NPO after midnight. *Day of examination:* Keep patient NPO. Administer a suppository or cleansing enema at 6 AM. Pediatric patients will have specific bowel preparations. Patients with an ileostomy or colostomy will have special preparations. Determine if the bowel is adequately cleansed. When fecal return is similar to clear water, preparation is adequate; if large, solid fecal waste is still being evacuated, preparation is inadequate. Notify radiologist, who in some cases will want to extend bowel preparation. Suggest the patient take some reading material to the radiology department to occupy time while expelling barium.	Allow patient to resume regular diet as soon as examination is completed. Encourage fluid intake. Monitor stools; barium sometimes causes constipation. Apply a local anesthetic ointment to the anal area after examination to relieve anal discomfort as per physician's order. Suggest to patient that a warm bath is often soothing. Administer milk of magnesia, 2 oz, after examination as per hospital protocol. Allow time for rest. Be aware of dehydration and electrolyte abnormalities. Inform patient the stools will be white; when all the barium is expelled, the stool will return to normal color.
BARIUM SWALLOW	
Prepare requisition form. Obtain consent if required by institution or agency. Explain procedure. Instruct patient to be NPO for at least 8 hours (usually NPO after midnight). Assess patient's ability to swallow (if patient tends to aspirate, inform the radiologist). Accompany hospitalized patient to x-ray department if vital signs are not stable and the test is to be performed.	Inform the patient of the need to evacuate all the barium. Advise patient that at first the stools are white, but will return to normal color when evacuation is completed. NOTE: Laxatives are sometimes ordered to facilitate evacuation of barium.
BLOOD CHEMISTRIES	
Prepare requisition form. Instruct patient to be NPO (as indicated). Water is permitted. Explain procedure. Prohibit smoking as per agency policy. Prohibit alcohol intake for 24 hours before test. Indicate to patient that dietary intake at least 2 weeks before testing will affect results.	Observe site for bleeding. Apply pressure as indicated. Be certain patient's meal is served after test is completed. Report results. Instruct patients with high levels regarding a low-cholesterol diet, exercise, and appropriate body weight.
BODY SCAN*	
Prepare requisition form. Explain procedure. See specific anatomical locations for particular interventions.	See specific anatomical locations for particular interventions.

NPO, Nothing by mouth or on nothing-by-mouth status.

*Showing a picture of the x-ray machine (used for scans and MRI) and encouraging the patient to verbalize concerns regarding claustrophobia will help reduce anxiety. Most patients who are mildly claustrophobic are able to tolerate these studies after appropriate premedication with antianxiety medications. Most of these tests require lying still on a hard table and peripheral venipuncture, which sometimes cause mild discomfort. Mild nausea is a common sensation when contrast dye is used. Have an emesis basin readily available. Some patients will experience a salty taste, flushing, and warmth during the dye injection. Encourage patients who receive dye injections to increase their fluid intake, because the dye is excreted by the kidneys and causes diuresis. Assure patients that they will be draped sufficiently so as to prevent unnecessary exposure.

Table 19-1 Nursing Interventions for Diagnostic Examinations—cont'd

PREEXAMINATION	POSTEXAMINATION
BONE MARROW ASPIRATION	
Prepare requisition form. Explain procedure. Assess coagulation studies and inform physician of any abnormalities. Obtain written consent. Advise patient that the procedure will be painful but only briefly. Assist in obtaining specimens. Provide needed emotional support. Obtain order for sedative, as necessary. Remind patient to remain very still throughout procedure. 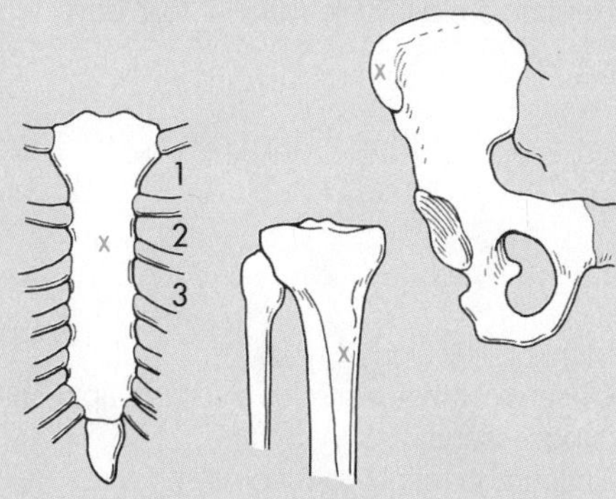 Bone marrow is located in spongy bone. The posterior superior iliac crest is the most commonly used area for bone marrow aspirations.	Apply pressure to puncture site. Apply adhesive dressing. Observe the puncture site for bleeding. Monitor patient for signs and symptoms of shock (e.g., increased pulse rate, decreased blood pressure) and for pain. Allow patient to resume normal activity 30 to 60 minutes after examination. Some patients need mild analgesics for tenderness at the puncture site for several days after this procedure. Instruct patient to notify physician if any tenderness persists or erythema occurs, because these indicate possible infection.
BONE SCAN*	
Prepare requisition form. Explain procedure. Instruct patient to remove jewelry and any metal objects. Encourage patient to drink several glasses of water. Tell the patient the injection causes slight discomfort. No fasting or sedation is required. Have patient void before examination. Assure patients that they will not be exposed to large amounts of radioactivity because only tracer doses of the isotope are used. Tell the patient the injection causes slight discomfort; no fasting or sedation is required.	Because only tracer doses of radioisotopes are used, no precautions need to be taken to prevent radioactive exposure to other personnel or family members. Observe injection site for erythema or edema; if hematoma forms, apply warm soaks to the area to relieve pain. Assure patient that the radioactive substance is usually excreted from the body within 6 to 24 hours. (To assess for allergic reaction, see Box 19-2.) Encourage fluid intake.
BRAIN SCAN*	
Explain procedure. Obtain informed consent. Keep patient NPO for 4 hours before examination if contrast dye is to be used. Instruct patient not to wear wig, hairpins, clips, or partial denture plates. Observe patient for iodine allergies. If ordered, give sedation. Inform patients that they will hear a clicking noise as the scanner moves.	Assess patient for iodine allergies (see Box 19-2). Encourage fluid intake. Report results.
BRONCHOSCOPY	
Prepare requisition form. Explain procedure. Obtain informed consent before patient is premedicated. Instruct patient to be NPO after midnight (4 to 8 hours). Administer preoperative medication as ordered.	Do not allow patient to eat or drink after procedure until no effects of anesthesia remain and gag reflex has returned (usually about 2 hours). Observe any sputum for blood; small amounts are normal.

Continued

Table 19-1 Nursing Interventions for Diagnostic Examinations—cont'd

PREEXAMINATION	POSTEXAMINATION
BRONCHOSCOPY—cont'd	
Remove and safely store contact lenses, dentures, and glasses. Reassure patients that they will be able to breathe during procedure. Instruct patient to perform good mouth care to minimize risk of introducing bacteria into the lungs during procedure. Instruct patient not to swallow the local anesthetic sprayed into the throat. Provide a basin for expectoration of the lidocaine. 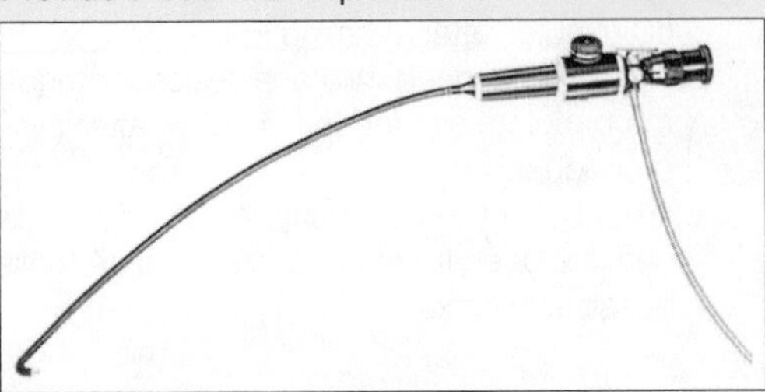 Flexible fiberoptic bronchoscope.	Monitor vital signs frequently. Fever is normal within the first 24 hours after bronchoscopy. Observe for impaired respirations. Observe closely until no effects of anesthesia remain. If patient complains of sore throat, provide warm saline gargles and lozenges as desired. If a tumor is suspected, collect a postbronchoscopy sputum sample for cytology determination. Inform patient to report bronchospasms or laryngospasms immediately. Reports are available within 2 to 7 days.
CARDIAC CATHETERIZATION	
Explain procedure. Obtain written consent. Provide needed emotional support. Instruct patient to be NPO for 4 to 8 hours. Determine if patient has any dye allergies (see Box 19-2). Administer preexamination medications as ordered. Prepare catheter insertion site by shaving and prepping the skin. Mark the site of the patient's peripheral pulses with a pen to facilitate postprocedure assessment. Instruct patient to void before going to the catheterization laboratory. Remove and safely store all valuables and dental prostheses. Obtain IV access for delivery of IV fluids and cardiac drugs, if necessary.	Monitor vital signs. Observe catheter site for bleeding; apply pressure as necessary. Encourage rest (4 to 8 hours). Encourage fluids; monitor urinary output. Keep affected extremity extended and immobilized to decrease bleeding. Assess the patient's pulses in both extremities. Compare pulses with preprocedure marking and assessments. Instruct the patient that the tests will be reviewed by the cardiologist and the results will be available in 1 or 2 days. Perform serial neurovascular assessment on the patient's involved extremity; compare with uninvolved extremity. Instruct the patient to report any sign of numbness, tingling, pain, or loss of function in the involved extremity immediately.
CHEST X-RAY	
Prepare requisition form. Explain procedure—no fasting required. Be certain there are no snaps or pins on gown and that the patient is not wearing a bra. Instruct the patient to remove all metal objects (necklaces, pins). Tell patients that they will be asked to take a deep breath and to hold it while the x-ray films are taken.	Report results. NOTE: No special care is required following the procedure.
COLONOSCOPY	
Prepare requisition form. Explain procedure. Obtain written consent. Assist with the bowel preparation.	Observe for abdominal pain, tenderness, and bleeding—gas pains from air in the bowel. Examine stools for gross blood. Offer normal diet if no bowel perforation exists.

IV, Intravenous; *NPO,* nothing by mouth or on nothing-by-mouth status.
*Showing a picture of the x-ray machine (used for scans and MRI) and encouraging the patient to verbalize concerns regarding claustrophobia will help reduce anxiety. Most patients who are mildly claustrophobic are able to tolerate these studies after appropriate premedication with antianxiety medications. Most of these tests require lying still on a hard table and peripheral venipuncture, which sometimes cause mild discomfort. Mild nausea is a common sensation when contrast dye is used. Have an emesis basin readily available. Some patients will experience a salty taste, flushing, and warmth during the dye injection. Encourage patients who receive dye injections to increase their fluid intake, because the dye is excreted by the kidneys and causes diuresis. Assure patients that they will be draped sufficiently so as to prevent unnecessary exposure.

Table 19-1 Nursing Interventions for Diagnostic Examinations—cont'd

PREEXAMINATION	POSTEXAMINATION
COLONOSCOPY—cont'd	
One type is the 2-day bowel preparation: clear liquids for 2 days along with a strong cathartic; on the day of examination an enema is given. The 1-day preparation uses a glycol bowel preparation. The patient drinks a gallon of GoLYTELY; enemas are usually not needed. (The entire gallon should be consumed within 4 hours.) Avoid oral bowel preparation in patients with upper gastrointestinal obstruction, suspected acute diverticulitis, or recent bowel surgery. Assure patients that they will be appropriately draped to prevent unnecessary embarrassment. Administer appropriate preendoscopy sedation as ordered. Record results from cathartics and enemas. Determine if the bowel is adequately cleansed. When fecal return is similar to clear water, preparation is adequate; if large, solid fecal waste is still being evacuated, preparation is inadequate. Notify physician who will be performing the colonoscopy, who will in some cases want to extend the bowel preparation.	Suggest a warm bath for relaxation. Allow time for rest. Take precautions until no medication effects remain. Assess patient's vital signs. Watch for decrease in blood pressure with an increase in pulse rate as an indication of hemorrhage. Notify physician if patient develops increased pain or significant gastrointestinal bleeding. Examine abdomen for evidence of colon perforation (abdominal distention and tenderness). Encourage patient to drink a lot of fluids when intake is allowed. This will make up for the dehydration from the bowel preparation.
COMPLETE BLOOD CELL (CBC) COUNT (see Skill 19-13)	
Prepare requisition form, if required by institution. Explain procedure.	Observe site for bleeding. Report results.
COMPUTED TOMOGRAPHY (CT)*	
Explain procedure. Obtain informed consent if required. Assess for allergies to iodine (see Box 19-2). Inform patient that it is necessary to remove wigs, hairpins or clips, and partial denture plates if scan will include head. Maintain NPO status 4 hours before oral contrast medium is administered, except in emergencies. See specific anatomical locations for particular interventions.	Encourage patient to drink fluids to prevent renal complications and to promote excretion of dye. See specific anatomical locations for particular interventions. 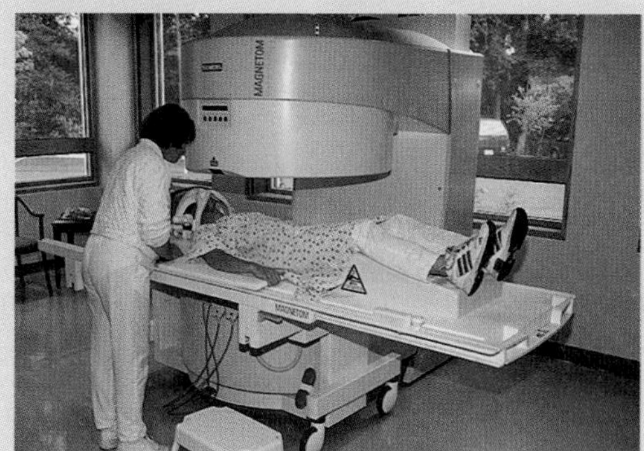 CT scan.
CYSTOSCOPY	
Explain procedure. Instruct patient to lie still during the procedure. Obtain written consent. Administer enemas as ordered, and record results. If patient will be under local anesthesia, liquid breakfast is sometimes allowed. If patient will be under general anesthesia, keep patient NPO after midnight on day of test. Administer preprocedure medications as ordered. Insert a Foley catheter if ordered (see Chapter 20).	Assess patient's ability to void for at least 24 hours after procedure—urinary retention sometimes occurs secondary to edema caused by instrumentation. Record urine color; if bright red, report to physician. Suggest warm sitz baths for relaxation. Encourage fluid intake to maintain a constant flow of urine. Observe vital signs; watch for decrease in blood pressure and increase in pulse, which indicate possible hemorrhage. Observe for hemorrhage and for sepsis. Administer antibiotic as ordered.

Continued

Table 19-1 Nursing Interventions for Diagnostic Examinations—cont'd

PREEXAMINATION	POSTEXAMINATION
CYSTOSCOPY—cont'd	Instruct patient not to walk or stand alone immediately after legs have been removed from stirrups. The orthostatic hypotension that sometimes results from standing erect has the potential to cause vertigo or syncope. Mild analgesics will sometimes be ordered for back pain, bladder spasms, and burning on urination. Antibiotics are occasionally ordered 1 day before and 3 days following. Encourage patient to prevent constipation. (Increases in intraabdominal pressure have the capacity to initiate severe lower urologic bleeding.) A postprocedure irrigation is sometimes ordered. If catheter remains in, provide catheter care instructions.
ECHOCARDIOGRAM Prepare requisition form, including pertinent patient history. Explain procedure; it is a painless study. Answer questions. NOTE: This procedure usually takes 45 minutes.	Remove the gel from the patient's chest wall with a tissue. Inform patient that the results will be available in a few hours after the physician has interpreted the study.
ELECTROCARDIOGRAM (ECG) (see Skill 19-14) Prepare requisition form. Include all medications the patient is taking. Explain procedure. No food or fluid restriction is necessary. Expose only the patient's chest and arms. Keep the abdomen and the thighs adequately covered. Assure the patient that the flow of electric current is from the patient; patient will not feel anything during this procedure.	Remove electrodes and gel from patient's skin with a tissue. If patient experiences chest pain during the study, indicate this on the ECG strip or request slip (it is possible that the pain will correlate to a dysrhythmia on the ECG tracing).
ELECTROENCEPHALOGRAM (EEG) Prepare requisition form. Explain procedure. Make sure hair is clean; administer shampoo as necessary; do not use any oils, sprays, or lotions. Confer with physician regarding the need to discontinue any medications before examination. Do not administer sedatives or hypnotics, unless ordered. Encourage food intake, but eliminate coffee, tea, and colas. Explain need to patient of remaining still during test—even blinking will create interference. Instruct patient if sleeping time is to be shortened the night before the test.	Assist the patient to remove the electrode paste with acetone or witch hazel. Shampoo hair. Ensure safety precautions until no effects of the sedatives remain; keep side rails up. Instruct the patient who has had a sleep EEG not to drive home alone.
ENDOSCOPY AND GASTROSCOPY Prepare requisition form. Administer preexamination medication, if ordered. Explain procedure. Obtain written consent before administering medication. Keep patient NPO after midnight. Provide emotional support. Remove and safely store patient's dentures and eyewear.	Perform oral hygiene measures. If an anesthetic has been sprayed on the throat, do not allow the patient to eat or drink until the gag reflex returns (2 to 4 hours). Ask patient to open mouth, and hold tongue down with tongue blade. Touch back of pharynx on each side with applicator stick.

NPO, Nothing by mouth or on nothing-by-mouth status.

Table 19-1 Nursing Interventions for Diagnostic Examinations—cont'd

PREEXAMINATION	POSTEXAMINATION
ENDOSCOPY AND GASTROSCOPY—cont'd	
Perform oral hygiene measures, because the tube will pass through the mouth. Reassure the patient that the procedure is not painful. Most patients are given conscious sedation, which is the administration of central nervous system depressant drugs and/or analgesics to supplement topical, local, or regional anesthesia during surgical or diagnostic procedures. It is most often used to supplement analgesia, relieve anxiety, and/or to provide amnesia for the event. Consciousness is depressed, and some patients will fall asleep but are not unconscious. Patients "wake up" in 20 to 30 minutes with no memory and no sense of time having passed. If the patient's throat is to be sprayed with an anesthetic, caution patient that he or she will not be able to speak during the examination, but respiration will not be affected. Check the patient for gag reflux. Instruct the patient not to bite down on the endoscope. 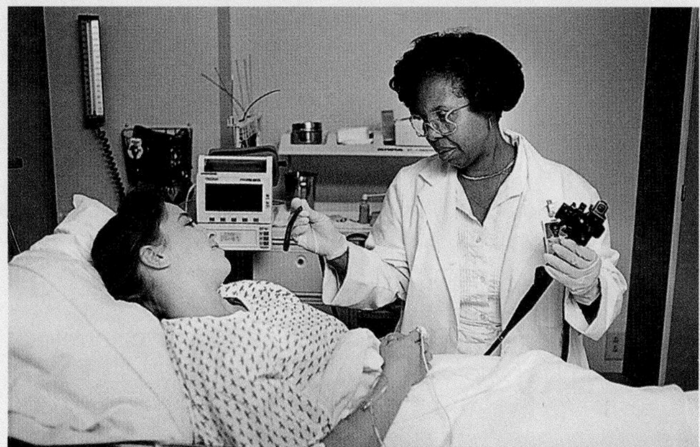 Assisting with endoscopy.	If conscious sedation has been administered, monitor patient carefully because oversedation or adverse patient response to sedation has the potential to result in life-threatening complications such as hypotension, loss of airway reflexes, inability to maintain patent airway, hypoventilation, and apnea. Explain that drinking cool fluids and gargling will help relieve some soreness. Observe the patient for bleeding, fever, abdominal pain, dysphagia, and dyspnea. Notify physician immediately if these occur. Monitor vital signs. Observe safety precautions until no effects of the sedatives remain. Inform patient that it is normal to have some bloating, belching, and flatulence after the procedure. 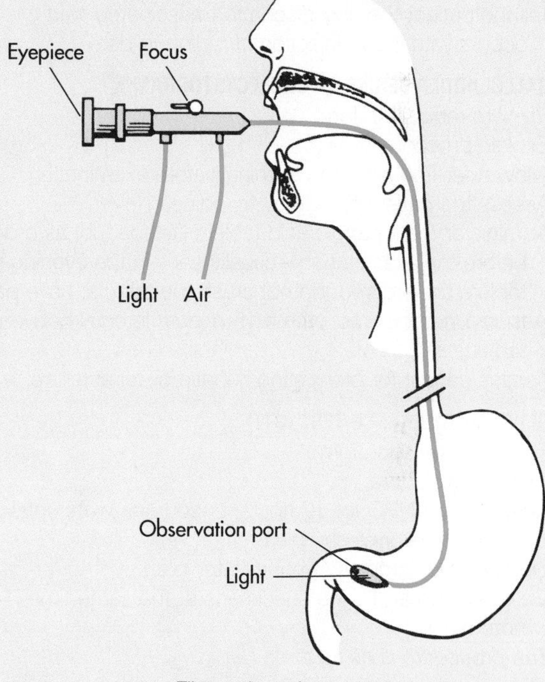 Fiberoptic endoscope.
EXERCISE TOLERANCE TEST (TREADMILL)	
Explain procedure. Keep patient NPO for 4 hours before the test, except for water, unless medications are otherwise ordered. Never hold heart medications. Instruct patient not to smoke. Instruct patient to wear suitable clothing—slippers are not acceptable. Inform patient about the risks of the test, and obtain informed consent. Inform patient of any medications it is necessary to discontinue before testing. Record patient's vital signs for baseline values. Apply and secure appropriate electrodes. Obtain a pretest ECG.	Resume diet as usual. Resume medication regimen. Have patient rest supine for several hours after examination. Instruct patient not to shower immediately after examination. Monitor and record vital signs until recordings and values return to pretest levels. Remove electrodes and paste or gel from patient's skin.

Continued

Table 19-1 Nursing Interventions for Diagnostic Examinations—cont'd

PREEXAMINATION	POSTEXAMINATION
FEMORAL ANGIOGRAM (see Arteriography)	
Provide emotional support. Observe patient for allergies to iodine dye (see Box 19-2). Obtain written consent. Keep patient NPO after midnight.	Observe catheter insertion site for inflammation, hemorrhage, or hematoma at the site, or absence of peripheral pulses. Observe the involved extremity for numbness, tingling, pain, or loss of function. Monitor vital signs. Apply cold compresses to the puncture site as needed to reduce discomfort and edema. If patient complains of continuous, severe pain, notify physician.
GALLBLADDER NUCLEAR SCANNING (this has largely replaced the gallbladder series)	
Explain procedure. Assure patients that they will not be exposed to large amounts of radiation. Instruct patient to fast at least 2 hours before the test. This fasting is preferred, but not mandatory. Tell the patient the only discomfort associated with this procedure occurs with the IV injection of radionuclide.	Obtain a meal for the patient if indicated.
GALLBLADDER SERIES OR CHOLECYSTOGRAM	
Prepare requisition form. Explain procedure. Allow a fat-free meal the evening before examination. Assess the patient for allergy to iodine. Administer the iopanoic acid tablets (Telepaque) as ordered the day before the examination—usually early in the evening (a number of tablets are ordered; do not crush the tablets; have patient take them one at a time, with a 15-minute interval between each tablet). Assess patient for preexisting hepatic or renal failure.	Monitor patient for side effects to the tablets, such as nausea, vomiting, diarrhea, abdominal pain, rash, and anaphylaxis. (If diarrhea develops before the examination, it is possible that the radiopaque dye will not be absorbed, resulting in nonvisualization of the gallbladder.) Resume usual diet as soon as series is completed. There is no other postprocedure care.
GLUCOSE TOLERANCE TEST (GTT)	
Prepare requisition form. Explain procedure. Keep patient NPO for 12 hours; encourage water intake so patient can provide urine samples. Obtain urine samples at hourly intervals.† Collect blood and urine specimens at the same time (1 hr, 3 hr) and note times.† *The procedure is as follows:* Make certain the patient empties the bladder; 30 minutes later obtain a fasting urinalysis (UA). Laboratory assistant will administer 75 g of dextrose orally. Collect urine specimen at ½ hour, 1 hour, 2 hours, 3 hours, and 4 hours after dextrose is given, depending on the physician's orders.† Educate patient about the importance of having adequate food intake with adequate carbohydrates (150 g) for at least 3 days before the test. Instruct patient to discontinue drugs, including tobacco, that have potential to interfere with test results. Consult physician. If necessary, give patient written instructions concerning the test requirements. Obtain patient's weight to determine the appropriate loading dose.	Mark on the tube the times specimens are collected. Send all specimens promptly to the laboratory. Observe venipuncture site for bleeding; apply pressure as necessary. Make certain patient receives meal when test is completed. Report results. An elevated blood glucose level at the 2-hour point usually indicates some disorder of carbohydrate metabolism; depending on how elevated the blood glucose level is, glucose will possibly be present in the urine. Administer insulin or oral hypoglycemic, if ordered.

GI, Gastrointestinal; *IV,* intravenous; *NPO,* nothing by mouth or on nothing-by-mouth status.
†Specific collection times depend on physician's orders.

Table 19-1 Nursing Interventions for Diagnostic Examinations—cont'd

PREEXAMINATION	POSTEXAMINATION
HEMATEST OF STOOLS (GUAIAC)—HEMOCCULT SLIDE TEST (see Skill 19-7)	
Explain procedure. Assist patient in obtaining specimens. There are many options for type of procedural materials (cards, tissue wipes, test paper). Tests are often permitted to be done at home with cards (Hemoccult) and mailed when collected. Inform patient of the need for multiple specimens obtained on separate days to increase test accuracy. Document specimens as sent to laboratory. Instruct patient not to eat red meat for at least 3 days before the test. Instruct patient not to mix urine with the stool specimen. Some laboratories recommend a high-residue diet to increase abrasive effect of stool. Note on laboratory slip any anticoagulants or medications the patient is taking. Be gentle when obtaining stool by digital rectal examination. Traumatic digital examination can cause a false-positive result, especially in patients with prior anorectal disease such as hemorrhoids.	No specific follow-up care. Read results and inform patient. If test results are positive, ascertain whether the patient violated any of the preparation recommendations.
INTRAVENOUS PYELOGRAM (IVP) OR INTRAVENOUS UROGRAPHY (IUG)	
Prepare requisition form. Be certain IVP is done before any barium studies. Explain procedure. Check for allergies to iodine and shellfish (the intravenous dye contains iodine). Administer cathartics or laxatives as ordered (children and infants are not given cathartics or laxatives). Keep patient NPO after midnight (if an IV solution is infusing, ask if physician wishes to decrease IV to keep-open rate to prevent hydration; for an IVP, fluid restriction is necessary for the dye to be taken up by the kidneys). Some institutions prefer abstinence from solid food for 8 hours before testing; some allow a clear liquid breakfast on test day. Assess the patient's blood urea nitrogen (BUN) and creatinine levels. (Renal function that is already abnormal sometimes deteriorates further as a result of the dye injection.) Give patient an enema or suppository on the morning of study, if ordered. NOTE: Indicate specific fasting times for older adult and debilitated patients.	Observe for anaphylaxis (respiratory distress, shock, and drop in blood pressure) (see Box 19-2). Allow patient normal diet. Encourage fluid intake to help eliminate any dye left in body and counteract any fluid depletion. Encourage patient to ambulate with assistance unless contraindicated. Some patients will be weak because of fasting and catharsis necessary for test preparation. Assess urinary output (a decreased output indicates possible renal failure).
KIDNEY, URETER, AND BLADDER X-RAY STUDY (KUB, Flat Plate of the Abdomen)	
Prepare requisition form. Explain procedure; no GI contrast media will be used. No fasting or sedation is required. Schedule this study before any barium studies. Ensure all radiopaque clothing has been removed.	No specific follow-up. Report results. Schedule IVP or gastrointestinal studies after completion of the KUB.
LIVER BIOPSY	
Explain procedure. Obtain written consent. Assess blood coagulation profile; essential that it is normal. Keep patient NPO after midnight before examination. Assist physician. Send specimens to laboratory promptly.	Keep patient on bed rest for 24 hours. Keep patient on right side for about 1 to 2 hours. (In this position, the liver capsule is compressed against the chest wall, thereby decreasing the risk of hemorrhage or bile leak.) Observe for hemorrhage. Apply pressure dressing.

Continued

Table 19-1 Nursing Interventions for Diagnostic Examinations—cont'd

PREEXAMINATION	POSTEXAMINATION
LIVER BIOPSY—cont'd	
Have specimen placed in proper **fixative** (any substance used to preserve gross or histologic specimens of tissue for later examination); usually 10% formalin is used, but confirm with the laboratory or the pathologist. If the liver specimen is for detection of lymphoma, saline solution is used. Administer any sedative medications as ordered.	Monitor vital signs frequently for evidence of hemorrhage (i.e., increased pulse and decreased blood pressure) and for peritonitis (increased temperature). Observe biopsy site. Tell patient to avoid coughing or straining, which tend to increase intraabdominal pressure. Instruct patient to avoid strenuous activities and heavy lifting for 1 to 2 weeks. Evaluate the rate, rhythm, and depth of respirations. Assess breath sounds. Report chest pain and signs of dyspnea, cyanosis, and restlessness (indicate possible pneumothorax).
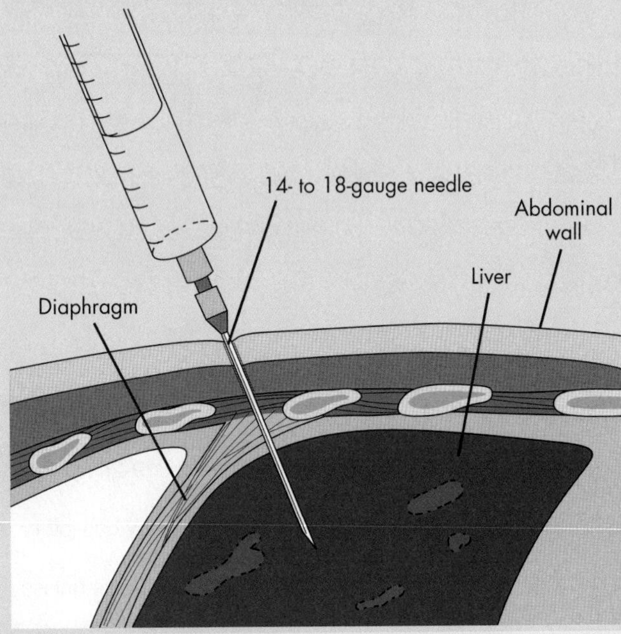	Liver biopsy. Percutaneous liver biopsy requires the patient's cooperation. The patient has to be able to lie quietly and hold his or her breath after exhaling.
LUMBAR PUNCTURE (Spinal Tap)	
Explain procedure. Obtain written consent. Have patient empty bladder and bowel. Provide necessary equipment. Assist patient to assume appropriate position. Hold manometer straight, if requested. Label and number specimens. Perform baseline neurologic assessment of the legs by assessing patient's strength, sensation, and movement. No fasting or sedation is required. Explain to patient that it is necessary to lie very still throughout procedure (movement has potential to cause injury). Encourage patient to relax and take deep, slow breaths with mouth open.	Apply digital pressure and an adhesive dressing to the puncture site. Notify physician if any unusual findings from puncture site occur. Report results. Place patient in the prone position with a pillow under the abdomen to increase intraabdominal pressure, which will indirectly increase the pressure in the tissues surrounding the spinal cord. This retards continued cerebrospinal fluid (CSF) flow from the spinal canal. Encourage fluids (using a drinking straw so patient can keep head flat). Usually the patient is kept in the reclining position for up to 12 hours to prevent discomfort from potential postpuncture spinal headache. Allow patient to turn from side to side as long as head is not raised. Label and number specimen containers appropriately and take to laboratory immediately (refrigeration will alter test results). A delay between collection time and testing has the capacity to invalidate results, especially cell counts. Instruct patient to report any abnormalities such as numbness and tingling in the legs. Assess patient for numbness, tingling, and movement of the extremities; pain at the injection site; drainage of blood or CSF at the injection site; and the ability to void. Notify physician of any unusual findings.

NPO, Nothing by mouth or on nothing-by-mouth status.

Table 19-1 Nursing Interventions for Diagnostic Examinations—cont'd

PREEXAMINATION	POSTEXAMINATION
LUMBAR PUNCTURE (Spinal Tap)—cont'd	
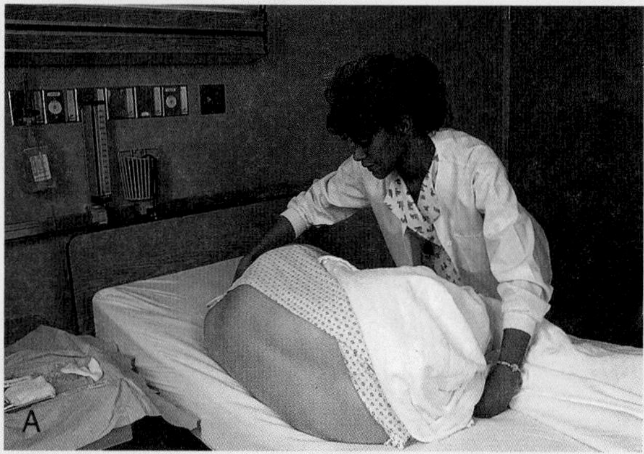 Position of patient **(A)** and needle insertion **(B)** for the lumbar puncture.	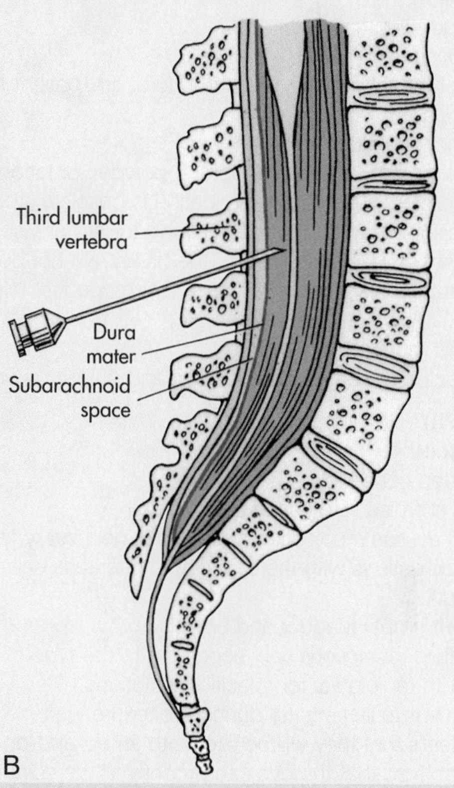
LUNG SCAN*	
Prepare requisition form. Obtain informed consent if required by institution. Explain procedure. Observe the patient for allergies to iodine (see Box 19-2). Keep patient NPO for 4 hours before test if contrast medium is administered. Have a recent chest x-ray film available. Remove jewelry around the chest area.	Apply pressure to venipuncture site. Encourage fluid intake. No radiation precautions are necessary. Encourage patients who received dye injection to increase fluid intake because the dye causes diuresis.
MAGNETIC RESONANCE IMAGING (MRI, Nuclear Magnetic Resonance Imaging [NMRI])*	
Prepare requisition form. Explain procedure. Obtain informed consent. Assess the patient for any contraindications to testing (e.g., aneurysm clips, plates). Instruct patient to remove all metal objects: dentures, partial dentures, jewelry, hairpins, and belts; provide safe storage. Inform patient of the need to remain motionless. Have patient empty bladder for comfort. Encourage adults to read or talk to child in scanning room. Some patients experience claustrophobia; antianxiety medications are often helpful. Explain that during the procedure, patient will hear a thumping sound. (Earplugs are available if the patient wishes to use them.) There are no food or fluid restrictions.	No postprocedure care is necessary. Report results. Patient is permitted to drive without assistance. 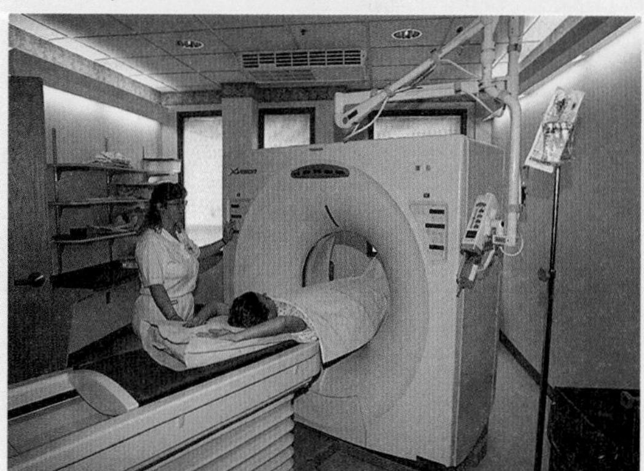 Assisting with MRI.

*Showing a picture of the x-ray machine (used for scans and MRI) and encouraging the patient to verbalize concerns regarding claustrophobia will help reduce anxiety. Most patients who are mildly claustrophobic are able to tolerate these studies after appropriate premedication with antianxiety medications. Most of these tests require lying still on a hard table and peripheral venipuncture, which sometimes cause mild discomfort. Mild nausea is a common sensation when contrast dye is used. Have an emesis basin readily available. Some patients will experience a salty taste, flushing, and warmth during the dye injection. Encourage patients who receive dye injections to increase their fluid intake, because the dye is excreted by the kidneys and causes diuresis. Assure patients that they will be draped sufficiently so as to prevent unnecessary exposure.

Continued

Table 19-1 Nursing Interventions for Diagnostic Examinations—cont'd

PREEXAMINATION	POSTEXAMINATION
MAMMOGRAPHY	
Prepare requisition form. Explain procedure. If patient is embarrassed by the procedure, ask patient to verbalize her feelings. Provide emotional support. Instruct patient not to wear deodorant, powder, or lotion. Some discomfort during the examination is possible (from breast compression). This compression allows for better visualization of the breast tissue. Assure patient the breast will not be harmed. If the patient has very tender breasts, this procedure is potentially painful. No fasting is required. Patient should disrobe above the waist and put on gown.	Explain how to obtain test results. Instruct patient on breast self-examination.
MYELOGRAPHY	
Explain procedure. Obtain written consent. Assess for allergies to dye and shellfish. Obtain and assess medication history. (It is necessary to avoid some medications with the capacity to decrease seizure threshold.) Have patient empty bladder and bowel. Food and fluid restrictions vary according to the type of dye used. Check with radiologist for specific restrictions. Instruct patient to lie very still during procedure. Inform patients that they will be tilted into an up-and-down position on the table so that the dye can properly fill the spinal canal and provide adequate visualization in the desired area.	If necessary, assist with proper positioning, as prescribed by the physician. Usually, you will place the patient on bed rest for several hours. The head position varies with the dye used. (EXAMPLES: Elevate the head after using oil-based and water-soluble agents. After an air-contrast study, position the head lower than the rest of the body.) Observe the patient for fever, stiff neck, occipital headache, or photophobia, which are signs and symptoms of meningeal irritation. Monitor vital signs. Monitor ability to void. Encourage fluids so patient does not get dehydrated; dehydration will result in a severe headache. Observe for seizure activity, which some types of dye potentially cause.
PARACENTESIS	
Explain procedure. Obtain written consent. Provide emotional support. Obtain equipment. Assist physician. No fasting or sedation is necessary. Have patient urinate before the test (helps prevent accidental bladder trauma). Measure abdominal girth. Obtain patient's weight. Obtain baseline vital signs. Although local anesthetics eliminate pain at insertion site, tell patients that they will feel a pressurelike pain as the needle is inserted.	Observe for syncope. Monitor vital signs. Encourage a period of rest after examination. Send specimen to laboratory for examination, if requested. (It is necessary to perform all laboratory tests immediately to ensure accurate results. Label all specimen containers appropriately.) Observe puncture site for bleeding, continued drainage, or signs of inflammation. Measure abdominal girth and weight of the patient and compare with baseline values. Observe for signs of hypotension if a large volume of fluid was removed. Record any recent antibiotic therapy on requisition slip. Monitor serum protein and electrolyte levels, especially sodium (protein content of ascitic fluid is high).

IV, Intravenous.

Table 19-1 Nursing Interventions for Diagnostic Examinations—cont'd

PREEXAMINATION	POSTEXAMINATION
PARACENTESIS—cont'd 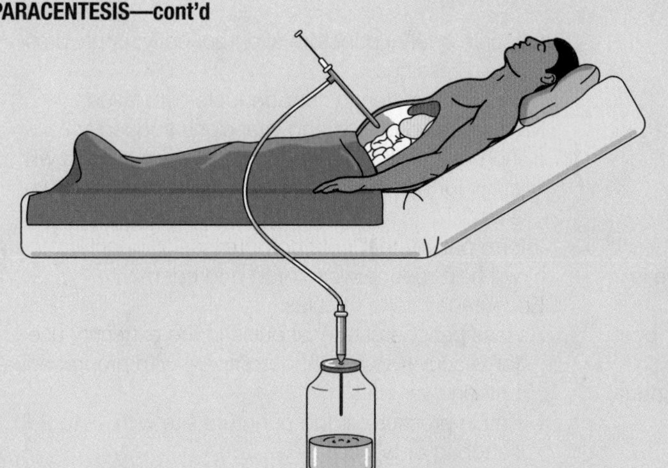 Paracentesis. A catheter is placed through the skin and the abdominal muscle wall into the peritoneal cavity containing free fluid.	Occasionally, fluid will continue to leak from the needle tract. It is possible to stop this with a suture. If unsuccessful, apply a collection bag to the skin to allow for measurement of volume of fluid and treatment of fluid loss.
POSITRON EMISSION TOMOGRAPHY (PET) Prepare requisition form. Obtain informed consent. Instruct patient not to have alcohol, caffeine, tobacco, or sedatives or tranquilizers for 24 hours before examination; no other restrictions are necessary. Have patient empty bladder before examination. Explain procedure (because many patients have not heard of this study, they are often anxious and require emotional support). Excessive anxiety has the capacity to affect brain function evaluation. Inform patients that two IV lines will probably be inserted, one for infusion of the isotope and the other for serial blood samples. Instruct diabetic patients to take their pretest dose of insulin at a meal 3 to 4 hours before the test. High glucose levels will potentially throw off accuracy and results of PET scans. Inform patient that the only discomfort associated with this study is the insertion of the two IV lines.	Instruct patient to change position slowly from lying to standing to prevent postural hypotension. Encourage patient to drink fluids and urinate frequently to aid in removal of the radioisotope from the bladder. Report results.
PROCTOSCOPY AND SIGMOIDOSCOPY Prepare requisition form. Explain procedure. Provide emotional support. Obtain written consent. Allow patient a light breakfast on day of examination. Administer enemas as ordered and record results. In most cases, two Fleet enemas are sufficient. Ensure patient is properly draped to prevent unnecessary embarrassment. Inform patients that they will feel discomfort and the urge to defecate as the scope is inserted. 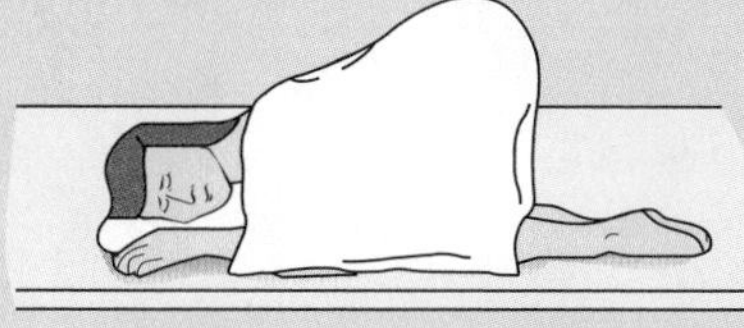 Position for proctoscopy.	Observe the patient for fever, rectal bleeding, abdominal distention, unusual complaints of pain, and increased tenderness. Inform patient that because air has been insufflated into the bowel during the procedure, he or she may have flatulence or gas pains. Ambulation often helps. If biopsies have been taken, slight rectal bleeding is possible. Instruct patient to report increasing abdominal pain (indicates possible bowel perforation). Fever and chills are further indications of a possible bowel perforation. Inform patient that frequent bloody bowel movements possibly indicates poor hemostasis if biopsy or polypectomy was performed. Observe for abdominal bloating and inability to pass flatus, which indicates possible colon obstruction, if a neoplasm was identified.

Continued

Table 19-1 Nursing Interventions for Diagnostic Examinations—cont'd

PREEXAMINATION	POSTEXAMINATION
RENAL ANGIOGRAPHY	
Explain procedure. Answer questions. Obtain written consent. Determine if patient has been taking anticoagulants. Assess patient for allergy to iodine dye (see Box 19-2). Keep patient NPO at least 2 to 8 hours before testing. Administer cathartics as ordered. Administer preprocedure medications. Inform patient of a possible warm flushing feeling as the dye is injected. Mark the site of the peripheral pulses with a pen (allows for postprocedure assessment). If no peripheral pulses are present, document this so that arterial occlusion will not be suspected on the postprocedure assessment. Ensure that the appropriate coagulation studies have been performed and are normal. Remove and safely store all valuables and dental prostheses. Have patient void (the dye sometimes acts as a diuretic). Inform patient that bladder distention sometimes causes some discomfort during the study.	Observe arterial puncture site frequently; apply pressure dressings. Monitor the extremity for adequate circulation. Monitor pedal pulses and vital signs frequently. Keep patient on bed rest for about 8 hours (this will allow for complete sealing of the arterial puncture site). Inform patient that cold compresses to puncture site will help reduce discomfort and edema. Encourage intake of fluids. Assess peripheral arterial pulse in the extremity used for vascular access and compare with preprocedure baseline values. Maintain pressure at the puncture site with 1- to 2-lb sandbag or IV bag. Assess extremities for signs of reduction in blood supply (i.e., absence of pulses, numbness, pallor, tingling pain, loss of sensory or motor function). Note and compare the color and temperature of the involved extremity with the uninvolved extremity. Notify physician if there is severe, continuous pain. Encourage fluids to prevent dehydration caused by diuretic action of the dye. Evaluate for delayed reaction to dye. Administer mild analgesics for minor discomfort at arterial puncture site.
THORACENTESIS	
Explain procedure. Obtain written consent. Obtain equipment. Assist patient to assume the appropriate position (usually sitting). Offer emotional support. No fasting or sedation is necessary. Inform patient to keep movement or coughing to a minimum to prevent the needle causing damage to the lung or the pleura during procedure. Administer cough suppressant if patient has troublesome cough. An x-ray film or ultrasound scan is often used to assist in location of the fluid. Fluoroscopy may also be used. Inform patients that although local anesthetics eliminate pain at the insertion site, a pressurelike pain is possible when the pleura is entered and the fluid is removed. 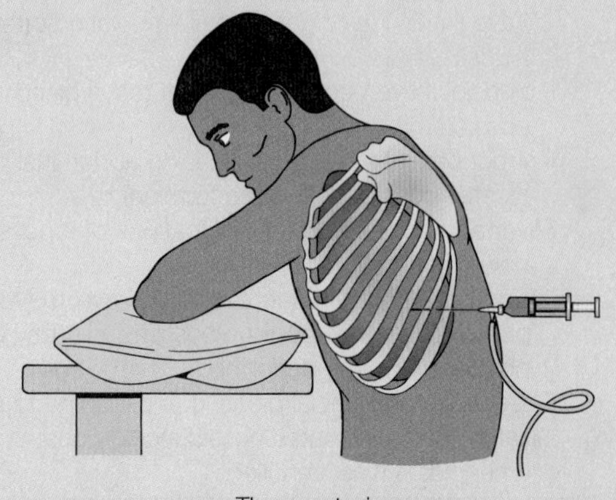 Thoracentesis.	Monitor vital signs. Monitor patient for coughing or for hemoptysis—indicates possible trauma to the lung. If no complaints of dyspnea, resume normal activity in an hour. Place small dressing over needle site. Usually, you will turn patient on the unaffected side for 1 hour to allow the puncture site to seal. Label specimen containers appropriately and send promptly to the laboratory. Obtain chest x-ray film, if ordered, to assess for pneumothorax. Assess patient for signs and symptoms of subcutaneous emphysema, or infection (e.g., tachypnea, dyspnea, diminished breath sounds, anxiety, restlessness, fever). Assess patient's lungs for diminished breath sounds, which are a sign of possible pneumothorax.

IV, Intravenous; *NPO,* nothing by mouth or on nothing-by-mouth status.

Table 19-1 Nursing Interventions for Diagnostic Examinations—cont'd

PREEXAMINATION	POSTEXAMINATION
ULTRASOUND OR SONOGRAM*	
Prepare requisition form. Explain procedure. If a pelvic sonogram is ordered, the patient needs a full bladder. If a gallbladder sonogram is ordered, keep patient NPO. Obtain a signed consent form, if required. No fasting or sedation is needed.	Because this procedure is noninvasive, no specific follow-up care is needed. Resume usual diet after examination. Remove the lubricant from the patient's skin. Encourage voiding.
UPPER GASTROINTESTINAL SERIES	
Prepare requisition form. Explain procedure and answer questions. Offer emotional support—the test will not cause discomfort. Keep patient NPO for at least 8 hours before examination. Advise patients of potential discomfort from lying on the hard table and possible sensation of bloating or nausea during the test.	Permit patient to eat as soon as series is completed, unless contraindicated. Encourage intake of fluids. Administer milk of magnesia, 2 oz, or per hospital protocol. Inform patient that if Gastrografin is used for contrast, significant diarrhea is possible. Monitor stools to make certain all of the barium has been eliminated. The stools will usually return to normal color after complete expulsion of the barium, which sometimes takes as long as a day and a half.
URINALYSIS (UA)	
Prepare requisition form. Explain purpose and specific method of urine collection. Wash perineal area, if soiled. If patient is menstruating, note this on requisition form. Use midstream urine collection guidelines (see Skill 19-2).	Report results. Take specimen to laboratory promptly. If not processed immediately, refrigerate specimen. If 24-hour urine is requested, refrigerate specimen or preserve with formalin when collected. It is necessary to perform examination for casts on fresh urine specimens.

*Showing a picture of the x-ray machine (used for scans and MRI) and encouraging the patient to verbalize concerns regarding claustrophobia will help reduce anxiety. Most patients who are mildly claustrophobic are able to tolerate these studies after appropriate premedication with antianxiety medications. Most of these tests require lying still on a hard table and peripheral venipuncture, which sometimes cause mild discomfort. Mild nausea is a common sensation when contrast dye is used. Have an emesis basin readily available. Some patients will experience a salty taste, flushing, and warmth during the dye injection. Encourage patients who receive dye injections to increase their fluid intake, because the dye is excreted by the kidneys and causes diuresis. Assure patients that they will be draped sufficiently so as to prevent unnecessary exposure.

SPECIMEN COLLECTION

All patients admitted to a health care facility will experience at least one laboratory specimen collection during their hospitalization. You are often responsible for collecting specimens of body secretions and excretions. Laboratory examination of specimens of urine, stool, sputum, blood, and wound drainage provides important information about body functioning and contributes to the assessment of health status. Laboratory test results often facilitate the diagnosis of health care problems, provide information about the stage and activity of a disease process, and measure the response to therapy.

Patients often experience embarrassment or discomfort when giving a sample of body excretions or secretions. Most people believe excretions should be handled discreetly; therefore, it is important to provide the patient with as much comfort and privacy as possible. Anxiety is also provoked by the invasive nature of some collection procedures, as is the fear of what the test results will be. Patients given a clear explanation about the purpose of the specimen and how it is to be obtained will be more cooperative in its collection. With proper instruction, many patients are able to obtain their own specimens of urine, stool, and sputum, thus avoiding embarrassment. Often the success of specimen collection depends on cooperation.

GUIDELINES FOR SPECIMEN COLLECTION

Laboratory tests are often expensive. Help prevent unnecessary costs by using the correct procedures for obtaining and processing specimens (Box 19-3). When there are questions about laboratory tests, consult the agency's procedure manual or call the laboratory.

It is your responsibility to notify the physician when laboratory and diagnostic studies deviate from the norm and intervention is necessary. Each health care facility has its own policy and procedure manuals. These manuals contain routine orders for each diagnostic test. The manuals are a valuable resource that

Box 19-3 Preventing Inaccuracy in Examination and Test Procedures

There are many factors that have the capacity to interfere with examinations and tests and that will potentially alter the accuracy of or even nullify their results:

- Drug interactions
- Insufficient bowel cleansing
- Failure to maintain fasting requirements
- Inadequate diet preparation
- Test requisition not complete, or absent
- Specimen not delivered on schedule
- Inappropriate specimen amount
- Contamination of sterile specimen
- Absence of required informed consent

prevents you from overlooking critical patient preparation information or the need to take action or notify the physician of results.

Remembering the meaning of root words, prefixes, and suffixes will help you learn to identify many confusing test names. Knowing the following suffixes is typically useful:

-ography Procedure in which an image is produced (e.g., mammography)

-ogram Actual image or results of a test (e.g., mammogram)

-oscopy Procedure in which body structures are visualized (e.g., colonoscopy)

-centesis Procedure involving puncture of a body cavity (e.g., thoracentesis)

Box 19-4 lists general guidelines for specimen collection.

COLLECTING A MIDSTREAM URINE SPECIMEN

There are several methods for collecting a urine **specimen** (a small sample of something, intended to show the nature of the whole) for urinalysis, one of the most commonly ordered diagnostic tests. Typically, several tests are ordered on one sample of urine, including determination of pH, protein, glucose, ketones, blood, and specific gravity. In addition, a urine specimen is sometimes ordered for culture and sensitivity, to diagnose and treat urinary tract infections. Your responsibilities are to collect and label the urine sample, to ensure its safe delivery to the laboratory, and to assess the results. You will also explain the collection procedure to the patient. If appropriate, notify the physician of the results.

It is necessary that the patient is aware of the upcoming test and knows to contact you before the next voiding. Instruct the patient to drink extra water to assist voiding, to not put toilet tissue in container, and to not allow fecal matter to come in contact with the urine specimen. A **midstream urine specimen** is urine collected after voiding is initiated (midstream) and before voiding is completed (Skill 19-2). This is the cleanest part of the voided specimen.

Box 19-4 General Guidelines for Specimen Collections

- Consider the patient's need and ability to participate in specimen collection procedures.
- Recognize that collection of a specimen sometimes provokes anxiety, embarrassment, or discomfort.
- Provide support for patients who are fearful about the results of a specimen examination.
- Recognize that children require a clear explanation of procedures and often benefit from the support of parents or family members.
- Obtain specimens in accordance with specific prerequisite conditions (e.g., fasting, nothing-by-mouth [NPO] status) as required.
- Wear gloves when collecting specimens of blood or other body fluids because it is not possible to identify everyone infected with human immunodeficiency virus (HIV) or other pathogens such as hepatitis B. (These standard precautions are advocated by the CDC [2005b] and OSHA [2001a, 2001b].)
- Perform hand hygiene and similarly cleanse other skin surfaces immediately and thoroughly if contaminated with blood or body fluids; wash hands immediately after removing gloves.
- Collect specimens in designated containers, at the correct time, in the appropriate amount.
- Properly label all specimens with the patient's identification; complete laboratory requisition form as necessary (see Box 19-5).
- Most specimens are transported to the laboratory in a separate outer plastic bag (see illustration for Skill 19-1, step 11).
- Deliver specimens to the laboratory within the recommended time, or ensure that they are stored properly for later transport.
- Use aseptic technique in all collections to prevent contamination, which has the potential to cause inaccurate test results.
- Transport specimens under special conditions (e.g., iced specimens or special containers with preservatives) as required.

COLLECTING A STERILE URINE SPECIMEN

To obtain a sterile urine specimen, either insert a straight catheter into the urinary bladder and remove urine, or obtain a specimen from the port of an indwelling catheter using sterile technique. Never use urine from a dependent drainage bag for a specimen because it is not fresh and will not provide accurate test results. It is possible to measure **residual urine** (urine left in the bladder after voiding) at the time of catheterization.

The patient voids, and catheterization is performed within 10 minutes. More than 50 mL of urine remaining in the bladder is considered residual urine; the patient will sometimes require insertion of an indwelling catheter.

Prepare the patient by explaining which type of urine specimen will be collected. It is important to relieve any anxiety by assuring the patient that there will

Skill 19-2 Collecting a Midstream Urine Specimen

Nursing Action *(Rationale)*

1. Refer to medical record, care plan, or Kardex. *(Provides basis for care.)*
2. Assemble supplies (see illustration). *(Organizes procedure.)*
   - Collecting kit
     —Sterile cotton balls or swabs
     —Antiseptic wipes
     —Sterile specimen container with label
   - Disposable gloves
   - Requisition slip
3. Introduce self. *(Decreases patient's anxiety.)*
4. Identify patient. *(Ensures procedure is performed with correct patient.)*
5. Explain procedure. Assess patient's understanding of procedure. *(Decreases patient's anxiety, promotes patient's cooperation, and ensures accuracy.)*
6. Prepare patient for procedure. *(Facilitates procedure.)*
   a. Close door and pull curtain. *(Provides privacy.)*
   b. Varying degrees of assistance will be required by patients who are seriously ill, have difficulty standing, or are disoriented. Some patients will need assistance in the bathroom, whereas others require a bedpan or urinal in bed. Older patients typically have difficulty in maintaining balance and raising or lowering toilet seats.
7. Perform hand hygiene and don clean gloves according to agency policy and guidelines from the CDC and OSHA. *(Reduces spread of microorganisms.)*

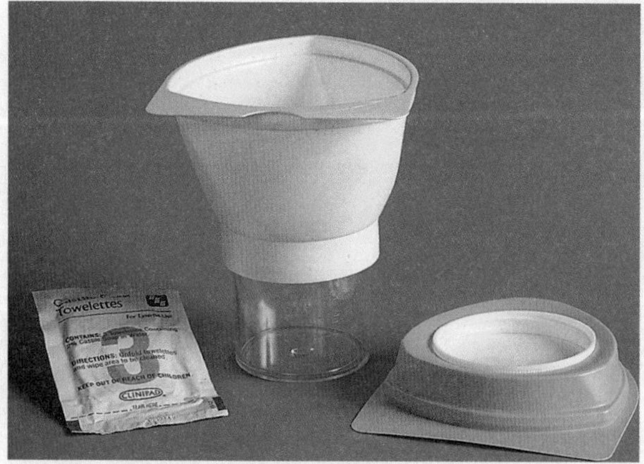

Step 2

8. If patient is able, allow patient to cleanse perineum in anterior-to-posterior direction with the antiseptic wipes. Separate the labia well on a female patient. Retract foreskin on an uncircumcised male. Use each cotton ball that is saturated with antiseptic solution one time only. If patient is unable to cleanse area, don gloves and assist with the procedure. *(Provides a cleaner specimen and prevents organisms at or near the meatus from being washed into the specimen. Cleansing from anterior to posterior aspect prevents microorganisms from the anus entering through the urinary meatus.)*
9. Guide female patients to straddle bedpan or toilet, if possible, to allow for labial spreading and keeping the labia separated while voiding. Request that patient (1) begin by voiding about 30 mL into the toilet seat collector, and then place the sterile specimen container, making sure the sides of the labia of the female do not touch it or each other; (2) without stopping flow, void a small amount into specimen cup; (3) remove cup and, without stopping flow, finish voiding into toilet seat collector. *(Collects midstream urine specimen appropriately. The first 30 mL, containing the organisms washed away from the meatus, is discarded.)*
10. Secure lid on container. *(Prevents spillage and contamination.)*
11. Remove gloves, discard in proper receptacle, and wash hands. *(Reduces spread of microorganisms.)*
12. Cleanse and return toilet seat collector, or empty and flush bedpan or urinal. *(Prepares equipment for next use.)*
13. Label specimen appropriately. Place in plastic bag for transport to laboratory (see illustration for Skill 19-1, step 11). *(Ensures proper identification of specimen; ensures accurate results; prevents loss and potential delays in obtaining results.)* Follow agency policy. (See Box 19-5.)
14. Ensure prompt delivery to laboratory with proper requisition slip (many facilities mandate within 1 hour). *(Ensures a fresh specimen for testing and prevents loss of specimen.)*
15. Document procedure. *(Provides communication of procedure and patient's response.)*
   - Time
   - Type of specimen collected
   - Sent to laboratory with requisition
   - Patient's response (if appropriate)
   - Patient teaching (see Patient Teaching box)

be no discomfort if the patient remains relaxed, only a sensation of mild pressure as the catheter is inserted and nothing when urine is collected from the catheter port. See Chapter 20 and Skill 20-12 for insertion of sterile urinary catheter.

If a urinary catheter is already in place, you have the option of obtaining a sterile urine specimen from the port of the urinary drainage system. When this approach is carried out, the sterility of the urinary drainage system is not compromised (Skill 19-3).

COLLECTING A 24-HOUR URINE SPECIMEN

Tests of renal function and urine composition, such as measurements of levels of adrenocortical steroids, hormones, protein, and creatinine clearance, necessitate a 24-hour collection of urine. Carefully follow the proce-

Skill 19-3 Collecting a Sterile Urine Specimen via Catheter Port

Nursing Action *(Rationale)*

1. Refer to medical record, care plan, or Kardex. *(Provides basis for care.)*
2. Assemble supplies. *(Organizes procedure.)*
   - Disposable gloves
   - Sterile specimen container with label
   - Clamp or rubber band
   - Sterile syringe and needle
   - Alcohol prep
   - Requisition slip
3. Introduce self. *(Decreases patient's anxiety.)*
4. Identify patient. *(Ensures procedure is performed with correct patient.)*
5. Explain procedure. *(Promotes cooperation and decreases patient's anxiety.)*
6. Perform hand hygiene and don clean gloves. *(Reduces spread of microorganisms.)*
7. Catheter port collection:
   a. Clamp just below catheter port for about 30 minutes (see illustration). *(Allows for urine to collect for removal.)*
   b. Return in 30 minutes; clean port with alcohol prep. *(Prevents needle puncture form causing contamination.)*
   c. Insert needle into port at 30-degree angle and withdraw 5 to 10 mL of urine for a specimen (see illustration). *(Inserting needle at an angle prevents puncturing opposite side of tubing. Provides for specimen.)*
   d. Place urine in sterile specimen cup. *(Keeps specimen sterile.)*
   e. Unclamp catheter. *(Allows continuous urine flow to resume.)*
   f. Label specimen and place in plastic bag for transport to laboratory (see illustration for Skill 19-1, step 11 and Box 19-5) and send to laboratory with requisition. *(Ensures proper identification of specimen; ensures accurate results; prevents loss and potential delays in obtaining results.)*
8. Remove gloves; dispose of them in proper receptacle, and wash hands. *(Reduces spread of microorganisms.)*
9. Document procedure and observations (see Skill 19-2, step 15). *(Records procedure and patient's response.)*

Step **7a**

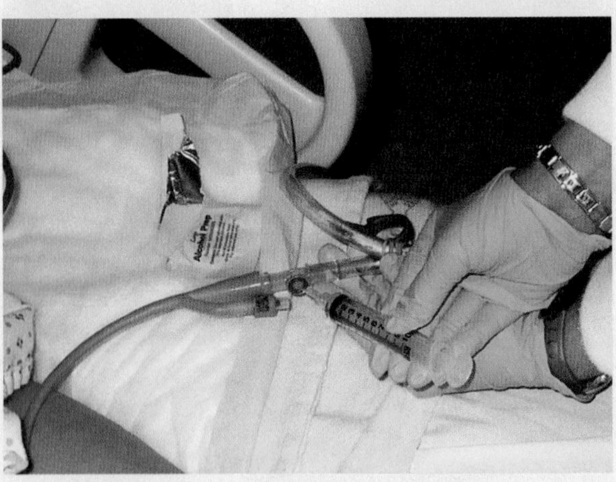

Step **7c**

dure for ensuring accurate performance of the test. Some tests require collecting the entire volume of urine from a 24-hour period (Skill 19-4). If urine is accidentally discarded or contaminated or the patient is incontinent, you will have to contact the physician for an order for an indwelling catheter.

MEASURING BLOOD GLUCOSE LEVELS

Using a meter to measure the blood glucose of a patient with diabetes provides more meaningful data than testing urine for the presence of glucose. The patient easily performs skin puncture at home, obtaining more accurate information than from the urine glucose or acetone determination test (Skill 19-5).

COLLECTING A STOOL SPECIMEN

Stool specimens are collected and examined for a variety of reasons, including the following: to determine the presence of infection, bleeding, or hemorrhage; to observe amount, color, consistency, and presence of fats; and to identify parasites, ova, and bacteria. Collect the feces, label the specimen appropriately, and send the specimen and the laboratory request to the laboratory. It is necessary to take stool to be examined for parasites immediately to the laboratory in order for parasites to be examined under the microscope while alive. It is also possible to collect a stool specimen from a colostomy or an ileostomy.

Inform the patient that a stool specimen is needed; then it is essential to carry out collection in a manner that will not cause stress or make the patient feel hurried or embarrassed. Arrange supplies if patient will collect the stool. When a stool specimen is to be obtained, place the specimen hat toward the back of the toilet, commode, or bedpan. When a urine specimen is to be obtained, place the specimen hat toward the front (Figure 19-1). You need to understand why the stool specimen is being collected to correctly choose the ap-

Skill 19-4 Collecting a 24-Hour Urine Specimen

Nursing Action *(Rationale)*

1. Refer to medical record, care plan, or Kardex. *(Provides basis for care.)*
2. Assemble supplies and equipment. *(Organizes procedure.)*
   - Specimen hat for bedpan, commode, or toilet; or urinal
   - Specimen container including preservative of agency's choice, and label
   - Gloves
   - Requisition
3. Introduce self. *(Decreases patient's anxiety.)*
4. Identify patient. *(Ensures procedure is performed with correct patient.)*
5. Explain procedure. *(Promotes cooperation and decreases anxiety.)*
   a. Stress importance of collecting all urine for a 24-hour period. *(Ensures a valid 24-hour kidney function test.)*
   b. Instruct patient not to allow tissue or fecal material to touch specimen or enter container. *(Contaminates specimen.)*
6. Post signs on patient's door, on bathroom door, and near patient's bed. *(Alerts staff and reminds patient to save all urine.)*
7. Wash hands and don gloves according to agency policy and guidelines from the CDC and OSHA each time a specimen is collected and transferred to the large collection container. *(Reduces spread of microorganisms.)*
8. Have patient void just before the 24-hour specimen collection is to begin; discard this voiding. *(This voiding has been formed in urinary system before the study began.)*
9. Place labeled container on ice if required. (Some agencies require refrigeration of all specimens. Others advocate that the urine container be placed on ice. For some collection procedures, such as the creatinine clearance test, refrigeration is not always necessary.) *(Keeps the specimen cool, which decreases decomposition and odor.)*
10. Save all urine for the 24-hour period; place each voided specimen into the larger container with preservative. *(It is essential to save all urine; otherwise results will be altered.)*
11. Instruct patient to void a few minutes before end of 24 hours; this urine is part of the 24-hour specimen. *(This will empty bladder before the end of testing.)*
12. Send specimen to laboratory promptly; be certain label includes date and time specimen started (see Box 19-5). If more than one container is necessary, make certain both are labeled and numbered. If patient is menstruating, be certain to note this on the requisition slip. *(Ensures proper identification of specimen; ensures accurate results; prevents loss and potential delays in obtaining results.)*
13. Document procedure and observations (see Skill 19-2, step 15). *(Communicates with others the patient care administered.)*
14. Perform patient teaching. (See Patient Teaching box.)

Skill 19-5 Measuring Blood Glucose Levels

Nursing Action *(Rationale)*

1. Refer to medical record, care plan, or Kardex. *(Provides basis for care.)*
2. Assemble supplies. *(Organizes procedure.)*
   - Lancet
   - Automatic lancing device
   - Alcohol swabs or cotton balls; or soap and water (see step 10)
   - Vial of test strips
   - Meter to measure glucose
3. Introduce self. *(Decreases patient's anxiety.)*
4. Identify patient. *(Ensures procedure is performed with correct patient.)*
5. Explain procedure to patient. *(Promotes cooperation and decreases patient's anxiety.)*
6. Wash hands and don gloves according to agency policy and guidelines from the CDC and OSHA. *(Reduces spread of microorganisms.)*
7. Remove cap from lancet using sterile technique. *(Maintains sterility of point.)*
8. Place lancet into automatic lancing device according to instructions in operating manual. *(Allows proper puncture of skin.)*
9. Select site on side of any fingertip (use heel for infant.) *(The side of the finger is less responsive to pain from puncture than other sites.)*
10. Wipe selected site with alcohol swab and discard swab. *(Prepares site. Some manuals now say wash hands with soap and water—no alcohol because it alters the test strip and dries the skin.)*
11. Ask patient to hold arm at side 30 seconds. *(Increases blood flow to site and allows site to dry.)*
12. Gently squeeze fingertip with thumb of same hand. *(Increases blood supply to site.)*
13. Hold lancing device. *(Provides easy access to device.)*
14. Place trigger platform of lancing device on side of finger and press (see illustration). *(Activates lancing mechanism.)*
15. Squeeze finger with downward motion; wipe off first drop of blood that appears and continue squeezing. *(Produces enough blood to cover test pad on test strip; producing and wiping first drop removes surface contaminants.)*
16. While holding strip level, touch new drop of blood on finger to test pad. Do not allow finger (skin) to touch the test pad (see illustration). *(Causes blood to cover test pad without smearing and prevents altering test results.)*
17. Begin recommended timing. After 60 seconds, blot blood off test strip, place reagent strip into appropriate site on meter, and wait for numeric readout. *(Ensures test accuracy.)*
18. Remove lancet from device and discard. *(Prevents accidental needlestick injury.)*
19. Remove gloves, discard, and wash hands. *(Reduces spread of microorganisms.)*
20. Document procedure and observations (see Skill 19-2, step 15). *(Communicates patient care administered.)*
21. Perform patient teaching. (See Patient Teaching box.)

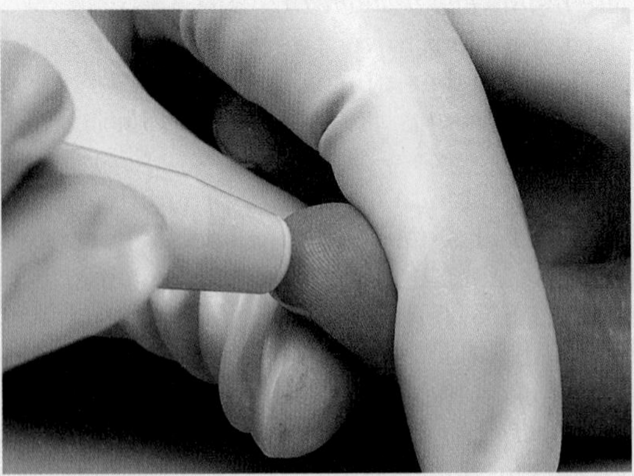

Step **14**

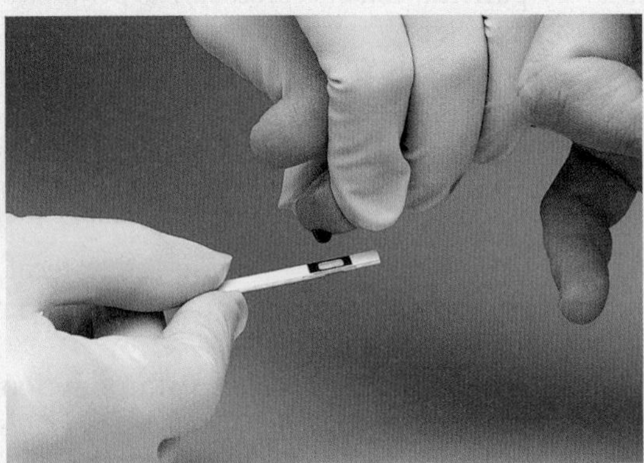

Step **16**

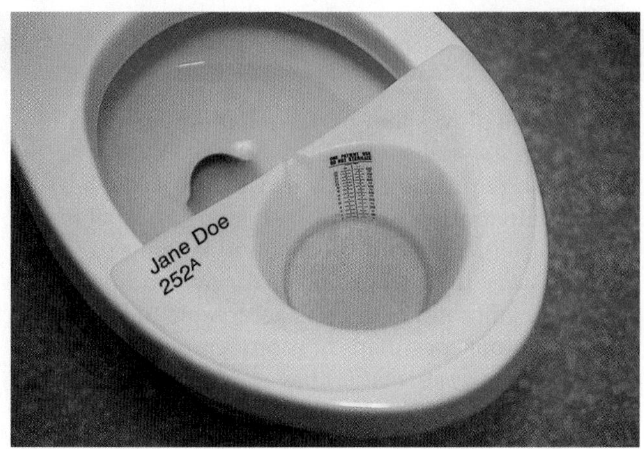

FIGURE 19-1 Specimen "hat."

propriate supplies. If stool specimen is for ova and parasites (O&P), obtain an appropriate container with special solution (Skill 19-6).

DETERMINING THE PRESENCE OF OCCULT BLOOD IN STOOL (GUAIAC)

The presence of blood in body waste is abnormal. Blood in the stool may be bright red, which indicates that the blood is fresh and that the site of bleeding is in the lower gastrointestinal (GI) tract. In contrast, black, tarry feces indicate the presence of old blood and that the site of bleeding is higher in the GI tract. When blood is present in the stool but you are not able to see it without the use of a microscope, it is referred to as **occult** (hidden). A **Hemoccult** test detects occult blood in feces (Skill 19-7).

Instruct the patient on how many stool specimens are ordered by the physician and how to collect a stool specimen. Then label the Hemoccult card appropriately (Box 19-5) and send it to the laboratory. Some facilities permit nursing staff to perform reagent testing without sending the Hemoccult card to the laboratory.

Box 19-5 Correct Labeling Information

- Patient's full name (last name, first name, and middle name or initial)
- Patient's identification number, bed number, room number, and medical record number
- Patient's age, sex (male or female)
- Physician's name
- Date and time of specimen collection
- Collector's name or initials
- Blood test ordered

Skill 19-6 Collecting a Stool Specimen

Nursing Action *(Rationale)*

1. Refer to medical record, care plan, or Kardex. *(Provides basis for care.)*
2. Assemble supplies. *(Organizes procedure.)*
   - Stool specimen cup or container
   - Gloves
   - Bedpan, specimen device, or commode
   - Tongue depressor
   - Label
   - Laboratory requisition
3. Introduce self. *(Decreases patient's anxiety.)*
4. Identify patient. *(Ensures procedure is performed with correct patient.)*
5. Explain procedure to patient; make certain patient understands what is expected. *(Promotes cooperation and decreases anxiety.)*
6. Wash hands and don gloves according to agency policy and guidelines from the CDC and OSHA. *(Prevents transmission of microorganisms.)*
7. Assist patient to bathroom when necessary. *(Provides patient safety.)*

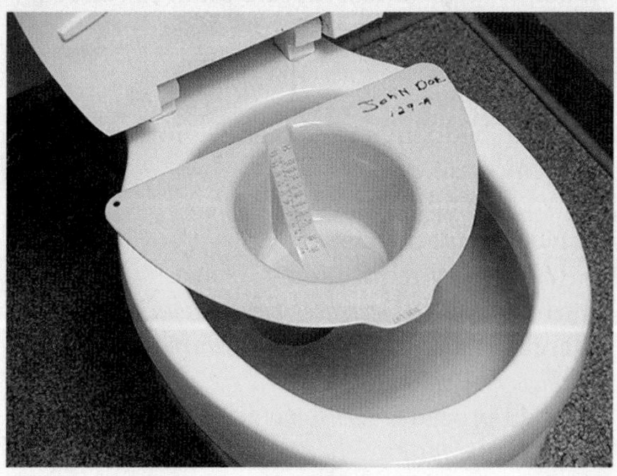

Step 8

8. Request patient to defecate into commode, specimen device, or bedpan, preventing urine from entering specimen (see illustration). *(Prevents contamination of specimen.)*
9. Transfer stool to specimen cup with use of a tongue blade, and close the lid securely (see illustration). *(Protects specimen.)*

Continued

Skill 19-6 Collecting a Stool Specimen—cont'd

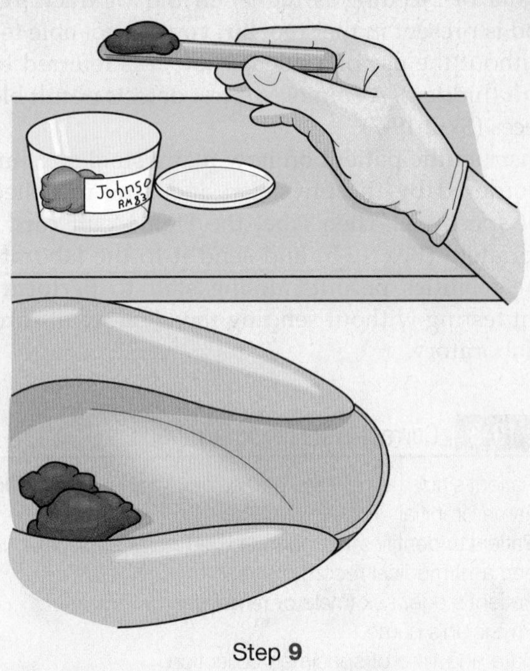

Step 9

10. Remove gloves and perform hand hygiene. *(Reduces spread of microorganisms.)*
11. Attach requisition slip, enclose in a plastic bag (see illustration for Skill 19-1, step 11), label (see Box 19-5), and send specimen to laboratory (it is necessary to take specimens for ova and parasites to the laboratory stat; it is acceptable to keep other stool specimens at room temperature). *(Ensures proper identification of specimen; ensures accurate results; prevents loss and potential delays in obtaining results.)*
12. Assist patient to bed. *(Provides for patient safety and comfort.)*
13. Document procedure and observations (see Skill 19-2, step 15). *(Communicates care administered.)*
14. Perform patient teaching. (See Patient Teaching box.)

Skill 19-7 Determining the Presence of Occult Blood in Stool

Nursing Action *(Rationale)*

1. Refer to medical record, care plan, or Kardex. *(Provides basis for care.)*
2. Assemble supplies. *(Organizes procedure.)*
   - Clean gloves
   - Clean bedpan or specimen device for commode
   - Hemoccult card
   - Wooden applicator
   - Hemoccult developer
   - Laboratory requisition
3. Introduce self. *(Decreases patient's anxiety.)*
4. Identify patient. *(Ensures procedure is performed with correct patient.)*
5. Explain procedure. *(Promotes cooperation and decreases patient's anxiety.)*
6. Perform hand hygiene and don gloves according to agency policy and guidelines from the CDC and OSHA. *(Reduces spread of microorganisms.)*
7. Collect stool specimen. (See Skill 19-6, steps 7 and 8.) *(Provides stool for Hemoccult.)*
8. Follow steps on Hemoccult slide test:
   a. Open flap (see illustration). *(Begins test.)*
   b. With tongue blade, smear very small amount of stool in first box (A). *(Prepares slide.)*
   c. With tongue blade, smear very small amount from another part of stool and transfer to box B. *(Prepares second slide.)*

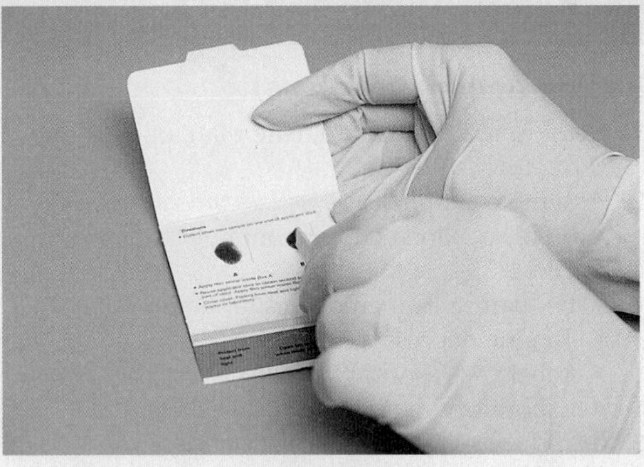

Step 8a

   d. Close card and label, if you have not already done so (see Box 19-5). *(Ensures accurate identification of specimen. It is advisable to label card before gathering specimen to prevent contamination.)*
   e. Enclose specimen in plastic bag and send to laboratory with requisition slip. *(Ensures proper identification.)*
   f. If testing is to be performed on the nursing unit, wait 3 to 5 minutes. Turn the card over and open the back of the slide. Place two

drops of developer over each smear. Read results within 60 seconds. Any trace of blue on or at the edge of the smear signifies a positive result for occult blood. Place one drop of developer on the quality control area. Read results within 10 seconds, according to manufacturer's directions. Document results of occult blood in stool and results of quality control area.

9. Remove gloves, discard, and perform hand hygiene. *(Reduces spread of microorganisms.)*
10. Document procedure and observations (see Skill 19-2, step 15). *(Communicates collection of stool specimen.)*
11. Perform patient teaching. (See Patient Teaching box.)

DETERMINING THE PRESENCE OF OCCULT BLOOD IN GASTRIC SECRETIONS OR EMESIS (GASTROCCULT TEST)

This test serves to determine bleeding in the esophagus, the stomach, the small intestine, or the large intestine. The test confirms the suspected presence of blood when there is red or black coloration of gastric contents, or coffee-grounds appearance of gastric contents in emesis or the product of nasogastric (NG) suction (Skill 19-8; see Chapter 20 for insertion of nasogastric tube).

COLLECTING A SPUTUM SPECIMEN

Sputum is secretion from the lungs. It contains mucus, cellular debris, microorganisms, or some combination of these, and it sometimes contains blood or pus. It is necessary to obtain a sputum specimen from deep in the bronchial tree. Expectoration of throat and mouth secretions is not to be used as a sputum specimen because saliva with food particles will not give desired results. Early morning is the best time to collect a sputum specimen because the patient has not yet cleared

Skill 19-8 Collecting Gastric Secretions or Emesis Specimen

Nursing Action *(Rationale)*

1. Refer to medical record, care plan, or Kardex. *(Provides basis for care.)*
2. Assemble supplies. *(Organizes procedure.)*
   - Gloves
   - Facial tissues
   - Emesis basin
   - Wooden applicator
   - 60-mL bulb syringe or catheter-tip syringe
   - Gastroccult test
   - Cardboard slide
   - Gastroccult developing solution
3. Introduce self. *(Decreases patient's anxiety.)*
4. Identify patient. *(Ensures procedure is performed with correct patient.)*
5. Explain procedure. *(Promotes cooperation and decreases patient's anxiety.)*
6. Perform hand hygiene and don gloves according to agency policy and guidelines from the CDC and OSHA. *(Prevents transmission of microorganisms.)*
7. To obtain specimen of gastric contents using nasogastric (NG) or nasoenteral tube, position patient in high Fowler's position in bed or chair. *(Keeps risk of aspiration of gastric contents to a minimum. Position relieves pressure on abdominal organs. If patient is nauseated, flat position in bed or one in which the patient is not able to sit straight sometimes causes abdominal discomfort.)*
8. Verify NG tube placement (see Chapter 20). *(Ensures aspiration of gastric contents.)*
9. Collect gastric contents via NG tube or nasoenteral tube (see Chapter 20). *(Only a small amount of specimen is needed for pH and occult blood testing.)*
   a. Disconnect tube from suction or gravity drainage.
   b. Attach bulb syringe or catheter-tip syringe.
   c. Aspirate 5 to 10 mL.
   d. Obtain sample of emesis with a 3-mL syringe or wooden applicator.
   e. Using applicator or syringe, apply 1 drop of gastric sample to test area of Gastroccult blood test slide. *(Sample must cover test paper for test reaction to occur.)*
   f. Apply two drops of commercial developer solution over sample and one drop between positive and negative performance monitors (see illustration).
   g. After 60 seconds, compare color of gastric sample with that of performance monitors. *(Positive performance monitor turns blue in 30 seconds and negative monitors remain white or beige. If sample turns blue, test is positive for occult blood. If sample turns green, test is negative.)*
   h. Verify that performance monitor turns blue or green in 30 seconds. *(Indicates slide is working properly.)*

Continued

Skill 19-8 Collecting Gastric Secretions or Emesis Specimen—cont'd

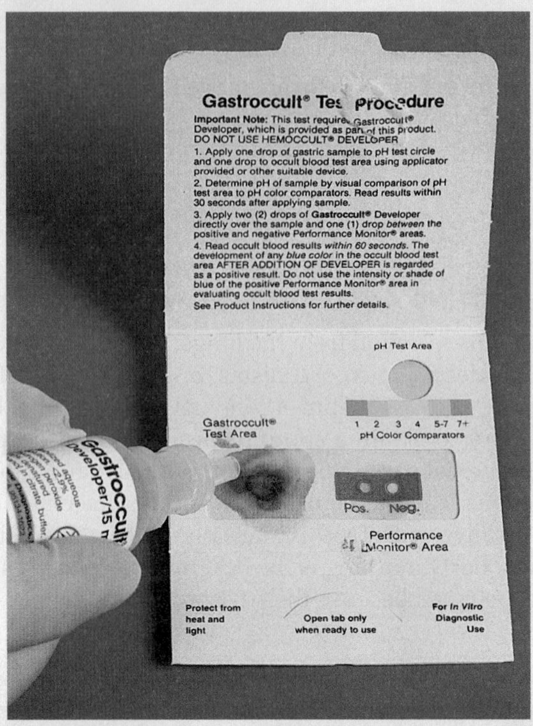

Step **9f**

10. Close card and label, if you have not already done so (see Box 19-5). *(Ensures accurate identification of specimen. It is advisable to label card before obtaining specimen to prevent contamination.)*
11. Enclose specimen in plastic bag and send to laboratory with requisition slip (see illustration for Skill 19-1, step 11). *(Ensures proper identification.)*
12. Reconnect NG tube to drainage system, suction, or clamp as ordered. *(NG tube serves to decompress abdomen by promoting drainage. Clamping is sometimes ordered to determine tolerance to stomach filling.)*
13. Dispose of equipment, remove gloves, and wash hands. *(Reduces spread of microorganisms.)*
14. Document procedure and observations. *(Communicates collection of specimen and completion of test.)*
15. Perform patient teaching. (See Patient Teaching box.)

the respiratory passages. Many tests are possible to perform on sputum, such as **culture** (a laboratory test involving cultivation of microorganisms or cells in a special growth medium) and **sensitivity** (a laboratory method of determining the effectiveness of antibiotics, usually performed in conjunction with culture), cytologic analysis or **cytology** (the study of cells, including their formation, origin, structure, function, biochemical activities, and pathology) examination, and test for acid-fast bacillus (the organism responsible for tuberculosis of the lung).

Collecting a Sputum Specimen by Suction

Some patients are not able to **expectorate** (eject mucus, sputum, or fluids from trachea and lungs by coughing or spitting) a specimen, and nasotracheal suctioning is required to obtain a sputum specimen. Suctioning sometimes provokes coughing, which has potential to induce vomiting and constriction of pharyngeal, laryngeal, or bronchial muscles. Suctioning also causes direct stimulation of vagal nerve fibers in some cases, resulting in cardiac dysrhythmias and increased intracranial pressure (Skill 19-9).

Closed-method collection containers protect you from contamination from body fluids. Explain the procedure and prepare the patient for the test. Instruct the patient the night before the test to drink extra fluids, because this will help loosen secretions and make it easier for the patient to expectorate for the specimen. Instruct the patient that it is not possible to use saliva as a specimen. Saliva is clear, whereas sputum is thick, colored, and tenacious (sticky) (Skill 19-10).

OBTAINING A WOUND CULTURE

If you detect purulent or suspicious-looking exudates or drainage, the physician will probably order a wound culture. Never collect a wound culture sample from old drainage because resident colonies of bacteria grow in exudate. It is necessary to obtain the specimen from inside the wound. Aerobic organisms grow in superficial wounds exposed to the air, and anaerobic organisms tend to grow within body cavities. To collect an aerobic specimen, insert a sterile swab from the culturette tube (Figure 19-2 on p. 505) into wound secretions, return the swab to the culturette tube, cap the tube, and crush the inner ampule so that the medium for organism growth coats the swab tip (Figure 19-3 on p. 505). Immediately send the labeled specimen to the laboratory with a requisition slip. To collect an anaerobic specimen deep in a body cavity, use a sterile syringe tip to aspirate visible drainage from the inner wound, expel any air from the syringe, and inject the syringe contents into a special vacuum container with culture medium. In some institutions, you will place a cork over the needle to prevent entrance of air, and then send the syringe to the laboratory with a requisition slip.

Skill 19-9 Collecting a Sputum Specimen by Suction

Nursing Action *(Rationale)*

1. Refer to medical record, care plan, or Kardex. *(Provides basis for care.)*
2. Assemble supplies. *(Organizes procedure.)*
   - Suction device (wall or portable)
   - Sterile suction catheter (size 14, 16, or 18) *(Use of too large a catheter causes trauma to nasal mucosa.)*
   - Sterile gloves
   - Sterile saline or container
   - In-line specimen container (sputum trap)
   - Oxygen therapy equipment, if indicated
   - Protective eyewear, if required (to protect eyes from sputum drops/particles)
3. Introduce self. *(Decreases patient anxiety.)*
4. Identify patient. *(Ensures procedure is performed with correct patient.)*
5. Explain procedure. Encourage patient to breathe normally to prevent hyperventilation. *(Promotes cooperation and decreases patient's anxiety.)*
6. Assess patient.
   - Determine when patient last ate a meal. *(It is best to obtain the specimen 1 to 2 hours after a meal or 1 hour before to keep gagging, which can cause vomiting and aspiration, to a minimum.)*
   - Respiratory status: rate, depth, pattern, lung sounds, and color. *(Changes in respirations indicate the possible presence of secretions in the tracheobronchial tree and potential need for supplementary oxygen.)*
   - Anxiety level. *(The procedure is usually contraindicated if patient is not able to cooperate or remain still during procedure.)*
7. Arrange equipment and prepare necessary charges. *(Facilitates procedure and facilitates proper billing.)*
8. Position patient for procedure.
   a. Close door or pull curtains. *(Provides privacy.)*
   b. The higher semi-Fowler's position is recommended. *(Promotes full lung expansion and facilitates ability to cough.)*
   c. Prepare suction machine or device and make certain it is functioning properly. *(Adequate amount of suction is necessary to aspirate sputum.)*
   d. Drape patient as necessary. *(Prevents unnecessary exposure.)*
   e. Adjust bed to appropriate height, and lower side rail. *(Promotes proper body mechanics and facilitates procedure.)*
9. Perform hand hygiene. *(Reduces spread of microorganisms.)*
10. Connect suction tube to adapter on sputum trap. *(Facilitates procedure.)*
11. Apply sterile glove to dominant hand. *(Allows handling of suction catheter without introducing microorganisms into the tracheobronchial tree—a sterile body cavity.)*
12. Preoxygenate the patient for 1 minute with 100% oxygen, if available. (Use caution if patient has chronic obstructive pulmonary disease [COPD] because 100% oxygen has the capacity to depress respiratory effort.)
13. Using gloved hand, connect sterile suction catheter rubber tubing on sputum trap. *(Aspirated sputum will go directly to trap instead of to suction tubing.)*
14. Gently insert tip of suction catheter prelubricated with sterile water through nasopharynx, endotracheal tube, or tracheostomy without applying suction (see illustration). *(Keeps trauma to airway as catheter is inserted to a minimum. Lubrication allows for easier insertion.)*
15. Warn patient to expect to cough and gently and quickly advance catheter into trachea. *(Triggers cough reflex.)*
16. As patient coughs, apply suction for 5 to 10 seconds, collecting 2 to 10 mL of sputum. *(Suctioning longer than 10 seconds risks causing hypoxia and mucosal damage.)*
17. Release suction and remove catheter, and then turn off suction. *(Releasing suction prevents unnecessary trauma to mucosa as the catheter is withdrawn.)*
18. Detach catheter from specimen trap, and dispose of catheter into appropriate receptacle. Connect rubber tubing on sputum trap to plastic adapter (see illustration). *(Aids in keeping specimen intact.)*
19. If any sputum is present on outside of container, wash it off with disinfectant. *(Prevents spread of infection to persons handling specimen.)*
20. Offer patient tissues after suctioning. Dispose of tissues in emesis basin or trash container. Remove

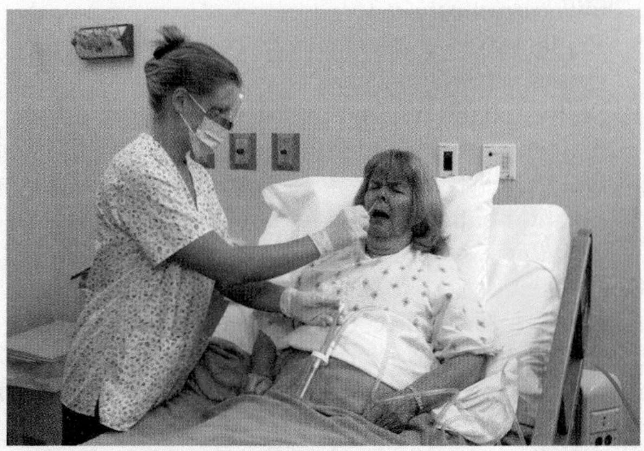

Step 14

Continued

Skill 19-9 Collecting a Sputum Specimen by Suction—cont'd

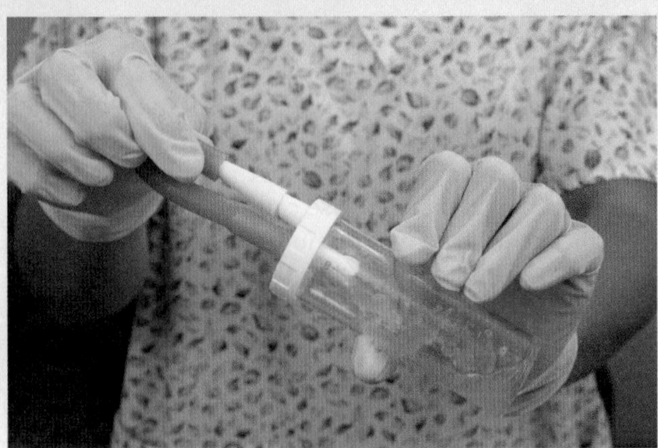

Step **18**

and dispose of gloves. *(Reduces spread of microorganisms.)*

21. Securely attach properly completed identification label and laboratory requisition to side of specimen container (not the lid). *(Ensures proper identification of specimen; ensures accurate results; prevents loss and potential delays in obtaining results)*
22. Enclose specimen in a plastic bag (see illustration for Skill 19-1, step 11). Send specimen immediately to laboratory. *(Bacteria multiply quickly. Prompt analysis of specimen is necessary for accurate results.)*
23. Offer patient mouth care, and assist to a comfortable position and place needed items within easy reach. *(Ensures patient's comfort and well-being.)*
24. Raise side rail and lower bed to lowest position. *(Ensures patient's safety.)*
25. Store, remove, or dispose of supplies and equipment as appropriate. *(Ensures equipment is available for next use.)*
26. Document procedure. *(Provides communication that procedure was carried out and patient's response.)*
    - Method used to obtain specimen
    - Date and time collected
    - Type of test ordered and how specimen was transported to the laboratory
    - Characteristics of sputum specimen
    - Patient's oxygenation and respiratory status
27. Perform patient teaching. (See Patient Teaching box.)

Skill 19-10 Collecting a Sputum Specimen by Expectoration

Nursing Action *(Rationale)*

1. Refer to medical record, care plan, or Kardex. *(Provides basis for care.)*
2. Assemble supplies. *(Organizes procedure.)*
    - Sterile sputum collector
    - Tissues
    - Label for specimen
    - Laboratory requisition
    - Gloves
3. Introduce self. *(Decreases patient's anxiety.)*
4. Identify patient. *(Ensures procedure is performed with correct patient.)*
5. Explain procedure. *(Promotes cooperation and decreases patient's anxiety.)*
6. Perform hand hygiene and don gloves according to agency policy and guidelines from the CDC and OSHA. *(Prevents transmission of microorganisms.)*
7. Position patient in Fowler's position. *(Helps with coughing.)*
8. Instruct patient to take three breaths and force cough into sterile container (see illustration). *(Helps patient expectorate mucus.)* (Be prepared to obtain the specimen by nasotracheal suctioning if patient is not able to cough.)
9. Label specimen container (see Box 19-5). *Ensures proper identification of specimen; ensures accurate results; prevents loss and potential delays in obtaining results.)*
10. Enclose specimen in plastic bag and attach laboratory requisition. Immediately send specimen to laboratory. If any sputum is present on outside of container, wash it off with disinfectant. *(Ensures specimen is sent to the laboratory. Bacteria multiply quickly. Prompt analysis of specimens is necessary for*

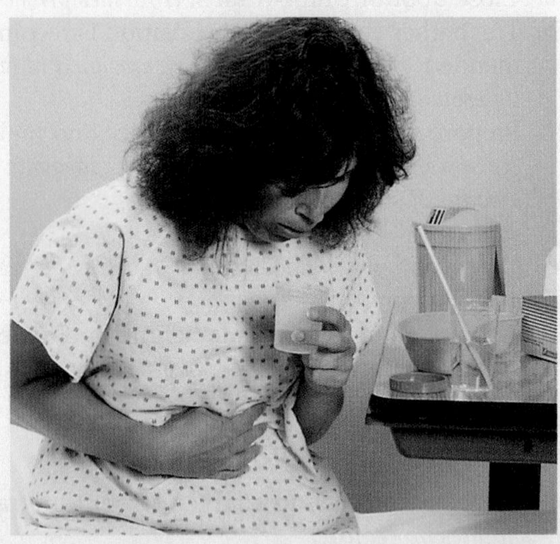

Step **8**

accurate results. Removing sputum from outside of container prevents spread of infection to anyone handling specimen.)

11. Remove gloves, discard, and perform hand hygiene. *(Reduces spread of microorganisms.)*
12. Document procedure and observations (see Skill 19-2, step 15). *(Communicates care administered.)*
13. Perform patient teaching. (See Patient Teaching box.)

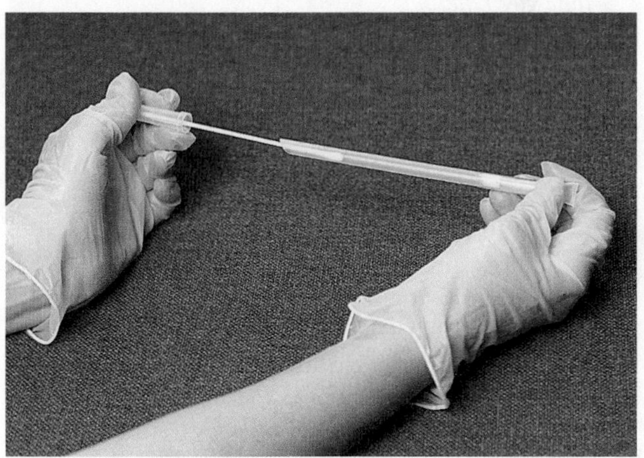

FIGURE 19-2 Wound culture tube.

Assess the patient for fever, chills, malaise, and elevated white blood cell count, which indicate a possible systemic infection. It is not possible to confirm or accurately treat infection without results from a wound culture.

Also assess the severity of pain at the wound site using a pain scale such as a scale of 0 to 10. If a patient requires an analgesic before a dressing change, it is ideal to give this medication 30 minutes before dressing change so it reaches peak effect when you perform the procedure.

Make sure you determine when the dressing change is scheduled, because you will likely obtain a wound culture as part of this procedure (see Chapter 13).

COLLECTING SPECIMENS FROM THE NOSE AND THROAT

When a patient has signs and symptoms of upper respiratory or sinus infection, a nose or throat culture is a simple diagnostic tool often used to determine the nature of the patient's problem. A nose culture is also now done for methicillin-resistant *Staphylococcus aureus* (MRSA). The laboratory staff places the specimen on a culture medium to determine if pathogenic microorganisms will grow. Regardless of what body fluids are cultured, certain principles apply. It is necessary to draw cultures before antibiotic therapy is started because the antibiotics have the capacity to interrupt the organism's growth in the laboratory. If the patient is receiving antibiotics, notify the laboratory and communicate specifically what antibiotics the patient is receiving.

Collection of a nose and throat specimen sometimes causes the patient discomfort owing to heightened sensitivity of the mucosal membranes; the same goes for collection of a throat culture. Collection of a throat culture often causes gagging, so it is important to collect a throat culture before mealtime or at least 1 hour after eating to lessen the chance of inducing vomiting. Make sure the patient clearly understands how each specimen is to be collected to keep anxiety and discomfort to a minimum (Skills 19-11 and 19-12).

When collecting nose and throat specimens, do the following:

- Assess the condition of and drainage from nasal mucosa and sinuses. *(Reveals physical signs that indicate possible infection or allergic irritation.)*
- Determine if patient has experienced postnasal drip, sinus headache or tenderness, nasal congestion, or sore throat. *(Further clarifies nature of problem.)*
- Assess the condition of posterior pharynx (see Chapter 5).
- Assess for systemic indications of infection, including fever, chills, and malaise.

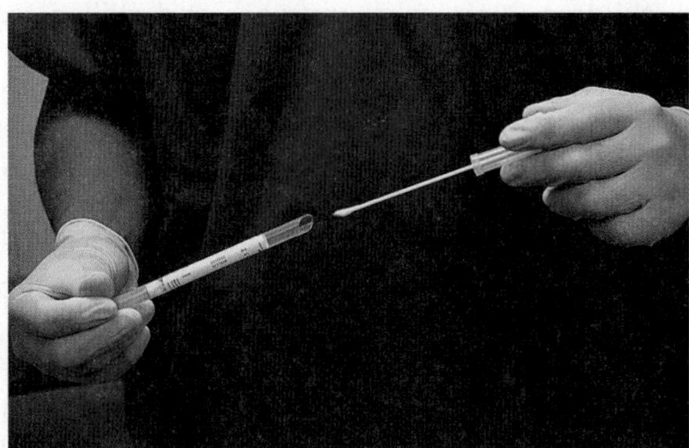

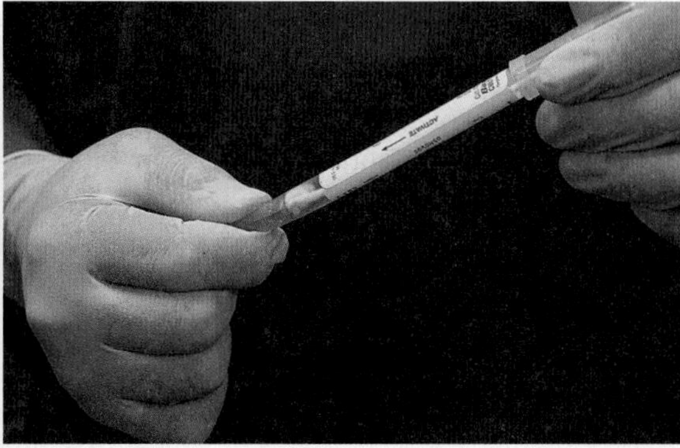

FIGURE 19-3 Aerobic culture tube.

Skill 19-11 Obtaining a Throat Specimen

Nursing Action *(Rationale)*

1. Refer to medical record, care plan, or Kardex. *(Provides basis of care.)*
2. Assemble supplies. *(Organizes procedure.)*
   - Disposable gloves
   - Two sterile swabs in sterile culture tubes (flexible wire swab with cotton tip often used for nose culture)
   - Nasal speculum (optional)
   - Tongue blades
   - Penlight
   - Emesis basin or clean container (optional)
   - Facial tissues
   - 2 × 2 gauze
   - Label (completed)
   - Laboratory requisition
3. Introduce self. *(Decreases patient anxiety.)*
4. Identify patient. *(Ensures procedure is performed with correct patient.)*
5. Explain procedure to patient; make certain patient understands what is expected. *(Promotes cooperation and decreases anxiety.)*
6. Perform hand hygiene and don gloves according to agency's policy and guidelines from the CDC and OSHA. *(Prevents transmission of microorganisms.)*
7. Instruct patient to tilt head backward. For patients in bed, place pillow behind shoulders. *(Facilitates visualization of pharynx.)*
8. Ask patient to open mouth and say "ah." *(Permits exposure of pharynx, relaxes throat muscles, and minimizes gag reflex.)*
9. Have swab stick ready for use. Consider loosening top so swab can be removed easily. *(Most commercially prepared tubes have a top that fits securely over end of swab, which allows you to touch outer top without contaminating swab stick.)*
10. If pharynx is not visualized, depress tongue with tongue blade and note inflamed areas of pharynx or tonsils. Depress anterior third of tongue only (illuminate with penlight as needed). *(It is necessary to visualize area to be swabbed. Placement of tongue blade along back of tongue is more likely to initiate gag reflex.)*
11. Insert swab without touching lips, teeth, tongue, or cheeks. *(Touching lips or oral mucosal structures potentially contaminates swab with resident bacteria.)*
12. Gently but quickly swab tonsillar area from side to side, making contact with inflamed or purulent sites. *(These areas contain the most microorganisms.)*
13. Carefully withdraw swab without striking oral structures. Immediately place swab in culture tube, cover using a 2 × 2 gauze, cover end of the tube, and crush ampule at bottom of tube. Push tip of swab into liquid medium. *(Retains microorganisms within culture tube. Placing tip in culture medium maintains life of bacteria for testing.)*
14. Securely attach properly completed label and requisition slip to side of specimen container (not lid). *(Ensures proper identification of specimen; ensures accurate results; prevents loss and potential delays in obtaining results.)*
15. Enclose in a plastic bag (see illustration for Skill 19-1, step 11). *(Complies with guidelines from the CDC and OSHA.)*
16. Send specimen immediately to laboratory or refrigerate. *(Leaving specimen at room temperature permits bacterial content to increase.)*
17. Discard gloves and perform hand hygiene. *(Prevents spread of microorganisms.)*
18. Document. *(Ensures procedure was completed.)*
    - Date and time collected
    - Type of specimen
    - Fact that specimen sent to laboratory with requisition slip
    - Patient response (if appropriate)
19. Perform patient teaching. (See Patient Teaching box.)

COLLECTING A BLOOD SPECIMEN (VENIPUNCTURE) AND BLOOD FOR CULTURE

Veins are a major source of blood for laboratory testing, as well as routes for intravenous (IV) fluids or blood replacement; therefore, maintaining their integrity is essential. Make sure to acquire and maintain skill in venipuncture to prevent unnecessary injury to veins.

Regardless of the method used to obtain a blood specimen, anticipate anxiety on the patient's part. The procedure is sometimes painful, and often just the appearance of the needle is frightening, especially to children. Your calm approach and skilled technique help limit anxiety.

Blood tests, one of the most commonly used diagnostic aids in the care and evaluation of patients, typically yield valuable information about nutritional, hematologic, metabolic, immune, and biochemical status. Tests allow physicians and other health care providers to screen patients carefully for early signs of physical alterations, plot the course of existing disease, and monitor responses to therapies.

You will often be responsible for collecting blood specimens; however, many institutions have specially

Skill 19-12 Obtaining a Nose Culture

Nursing Action *(Rationale)*

1 to 6. Refer to steps 1 to 6 of Skill 19-11.

7. Ask patient to blow nose, and then check nostrils for patency with penlight. Select nostril with greatest patency. *(Clears nasal passage of mucus that contains resident bacteria.)*

8. Ask patient to tilt head back. Patients in bed should have a pillow behind the shoulders.

9. Gently insert nasal speculum in one nostril (optional). Carefully pass swab into nostril until it reaches portion of mucosa that is inflamed or contains exudate. Rotate swab quickly. NOTE: If nasopharyngeal culture is to be obtained, use a special swab on a flexible wire that is possible to flex downward to reach nasopharynx. *(It is necessary that swab remain sterile until it reaches area to be cultured. Rotating swab covers all surfaces where exudate is present.)*

10. With dominant hand, remove swab without touching sides of speculum or nasal canal. *(Prevents contamination by resident bacteria.)*

11. With nondominant hand, carefully remove nasal speculum (if used), and place in basin. Offer patient facial tissue. *(Removing speculum carefully prevents trauma to nasal mucosa; offering patient facial tissue provides comfort.)*

12. Immediately place swab in culture tube. *(Prevents contamination of specimen.)*

13. Cover end of tube with 2 × 2 gauze, then crush ampule at bottom of tube to release culture medium. Push tip of swab into liquid medium. *(Placing tip in culture medium maintains life of bacteria for testing.)*

14. Place top on tube securely. *(Prevents spillage of specimen.)*

15. Discard supplies into trash. *(Prevents transmission of microorganisms.)*

16. Send to laboratory with completed requisition and attached label not attached to the lid of the container (see Box 19-5). Enclose in a plastic bag. *(Ensures proper identification of specimen; ensures accurate results; prevents loss and potential delays in obtaining results.)*

17. Remove and discard gloves, perform hand hygiene. *(Reduces spread of microorganisms.)*

18. Document procedure. *(Ensures procedure was completed.)*

19. Perform patient teaching. (See Patient Teaching box.)

trained technicians whose sole responsibility is to draw blood. Be familiar with your institution's policies and procedures and your state's nurse practice act regarding guidelines for drawing blood samples.

Venipuncture, the most common method, involves inserting a hollow-bore needle into the lumen of a large vein to obtain a specimen. In some cases, you will use a needle and syringe, and in others, a special **Vacutainer** tube that allows the drawing of multiple blood samples.

Assess the patient for special conditions that will have an impact on the test procedure or results. With some tests, certain preparations are necessary to obtain accurate measurements, such as that the patient be on NPO status. A variety of factors put the patient at risk when undergoing venipuncture, including anticoagulant therapy, low platelet count, bleeding disorders, presence of arteriovenous shunt or fistula, and having had breast or axillary surgery performed on that side. Abnormal clotting abilities, medications, and compromised circulation tend to impair blood flow. Assess the patient's ability to cooperate with the procedure; some patients will need assistance from another health care team member, for instance, when the procedure appears threatening to patient.

A physician's order is required for tests. Before collecting the specimen, review the order and make sure you will be drawing the correct specimens and amount for all the tests to be performed, so you will not have to draw multiple samples.

Older adults have fragile veins that are easily traumatized during venipuncture. Sometimes, application of a warm compress will help obtain samples. Using a small-bore catheter is another helpful strategy.

In the home care setting, you will often find it helpful to use a blood pressure cuff, rather than a tourniquet, when performing the venipuncture. Instruct patient to notify you or the physician if persistent or recurrent bleeding or expanding hematoma occurs at venipuncture site.

Children are often afraid of needles and the loss of blood. Explain what you are going to do. Explain that they have a lot of blood and that their bodies constantly make blood. Ask a parent or another staff member to hold and comfort the child. Use toys or books to distract the child. Keep the needle out of the child's sight for as long as possible. Perform the venipuncture and collect the blood quickly. Once you have finished, placing an adhesive bandage over the site is comforting. It reassures the child that blood will not leak from the body.

The bloodborne pathogens standard of the Occupational Safety and Health Administration (OSHA) requires that "Each employer having an employee(s) with occupational exposure . . . shall establish a written Exposure Control Plan designed to eliminate or minimize employee exposure." (OSHA, 1991) As a result, phlebotomy equipment includes needle safety devices. Using standard precautions and appropriate personal protective equipment helps to protect skin and mucous membranes from contact with blood; however, most barriers are easily penetrated by needles. New safety devices and features protect health care workers as follows:

- Provide a barrier between the hands and the needle after use
- Allow or require the worker's hands to remain behind the needle at all times
- Are an integral part of the device and not an accessory
- Are simple to operate and require little training to use effectively

A less invasive method of collecting a blood specimen is called a capillary puncture. It is commonly used to collect blood specimens from newborns and for glucose monitoring in all patients. The procedure is usually performed by puncturing a vascular area on a finger, toe, or heel with a lancet, although sometimes a sterile needle is used instead.

Regardless of the type of safety device in use, never recap needles and always carefully discard them in puncture-resistant containers close to the patient (Figure 19-4). A major significant exposure occurs when a deep puncture is caused by a needle that has been used to collect blood. Report all needlestick injuries. All needlestick injuries are not preventable; however, the use of needles with safety features has substantially decreased the risk of exposure to bloodborne pathogens for health care workers (Davenport & Myers, 2009; Centers for Disease Control and Prevention [CDC], 2005b; Occupational Safety and Health Administration [OSHA], 2001a, 2001b).

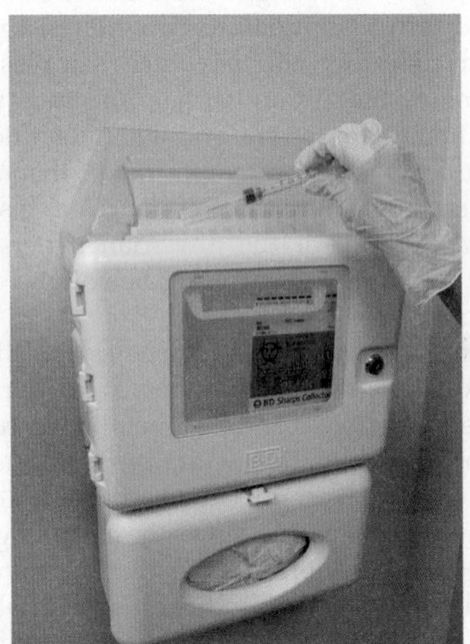
FIGURE 19-4 Safety container for used needles and other sharps.

Blood culture, a specific blood test used to detect the presence of bacteria in the blood (bacteremia), requires a special phlebotomy technique. Draw specimens for culture when the symptoms of fever and chills that often accompany bacteremia are present. It is important to draw at least two culture specimens from two different sites. The diagnosis of bacteremia is confirmed when both cultures grow an infecting agent. If only one culture produces bacteria, the assumption is that the bacteria were skin contaminants rather than the infecting agent. Because culture specimens obtained through an IV catheter are frequently contaminated, do not perform tests using them unless catheter sepsis is suspected. Blood culture specimens are always drawn before antibiotic therapy is started because the antibiotic usually interferes with the organism's growth in the laboratory.

Collection Methods

Several collection methods are available. Using a syringe and attached needle is one method. Another is the use of a Vacutainer. With the syringe method, you will draw the blood into the barrel by pulling back on the plunger. After the blood is collected, transfer it to a test tube.

The Vacutainer system has a needle, a holder for the needle and tube, as well as one or more evacuated tubes with rubber stopper complete the apparatus (Figure 19-5, *A*). In evacuated tubes, air is removed, creating a vacuum. When a vein is punctured, blood flows into the tube (Figure 19-5, *B*). After a tube fills, you will remove it from the holder and attach a new one without withdrawing the needle from the vein. The Vacutainer system thus allows the collection of many blood specimens with one venipuncture.

Collection Tubes

Types of Collection Tubes

Blood collection tubes come in different sizes. The blood tests ordered determine the amount of blood needed.

Also, some tests require additives, chemicals that are added to the collection tube and mixed with the blood. The chemicals preserve the blood until testing. In the Vacutainer system, the tubes contain the necessary additives. The rubber stoppers are color coded. Red, lavender, blue, green, gray, and yellow are common colors. The color coding signals the type of additive, the amount of blood to collect, and the recommended blood tests to perform on the sample. Color coding sometimes varies; always follow your agency's

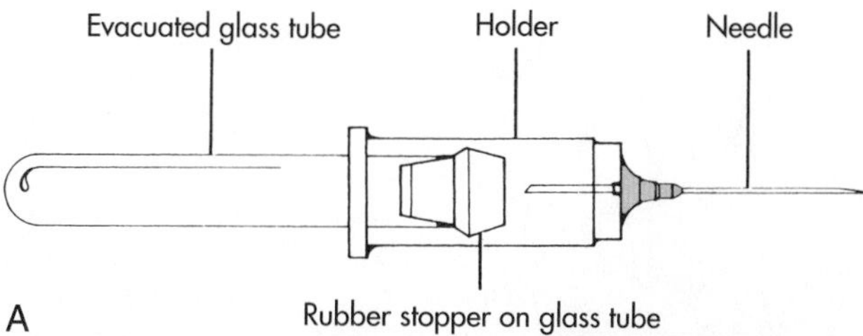

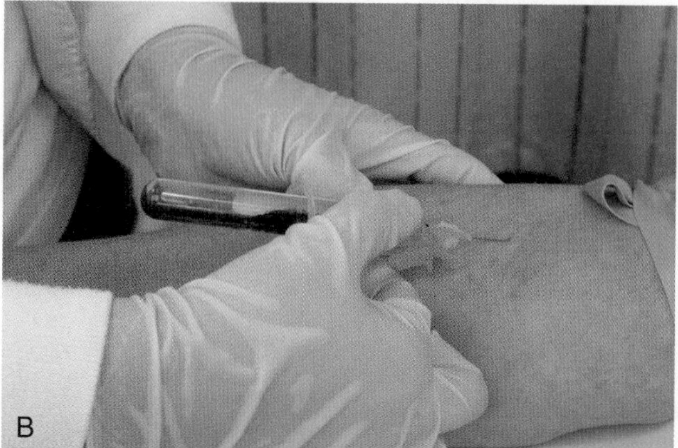

FIGURE 19-5 **A,** Parts of the Vacutainer. **B,** Blood collects in a Vacutainer tube.

procedures. Check the Vacutainer tube guide (Figure 19-6) when selecting tubes for blood tests.

After selecting the collection tubes, place them in order of use. The order is important to prevent tube contamination. Different tubes have different additives. Make sure you do not inadvertently transfer the additive from one tube to another by using the wrong order. Follow agency policy for the order in which to collect blood specimens.

Labeling Collection Tubes

After you have completed the collection and before sending the blood specimens to the laboratory, label the collection tube with the patient's identifying information (Figure 19-7). Labeling is necessary to make sure that the right tests are done for the right patient. When wrong test results are reported for the patient, the wrong treatment will be given and the patient is at risk for serious harm. See Box 19-5 for a patient's identifying information.

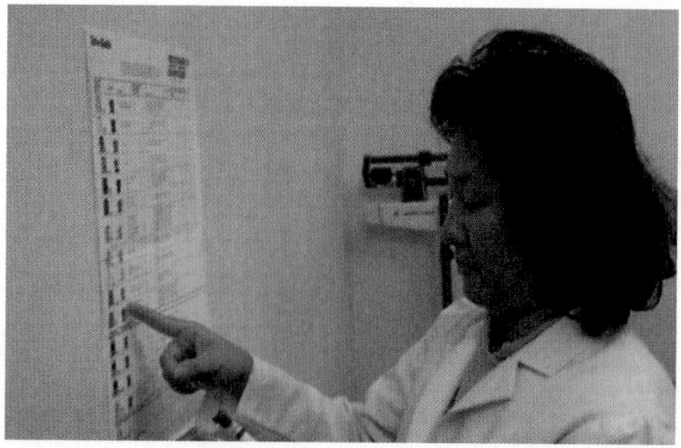

FIGURE 19-6 Vacutainer tube guide.

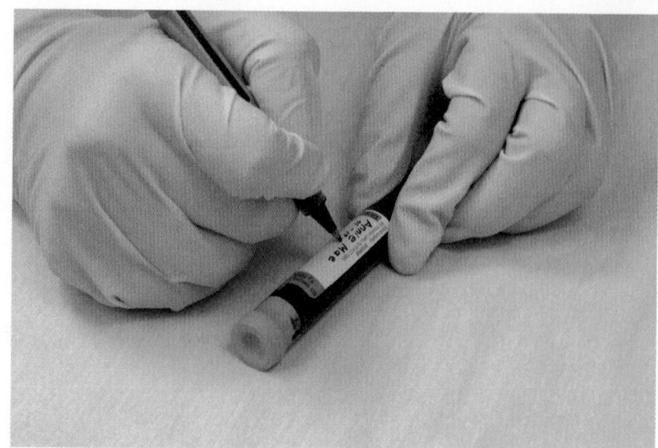

FIGURE 19-7 Labeling the blood tube.

Selecting a Venipuncture Site

The basilic and cephalic veins in the antecubital space are the most common venipuncture sites (Figure 19-8). These veins are large and near the skin surface. Hand veins offer alternative sites.

Before selecting the vein, select the arm to be used. Avoid using the arm on the side of a mastectomy or on the side of a paralysis. If the patient has an IV line, do not use that arm. Do not use the arm with an access site for hemodialysis. Confer with other staff members or laboratory personnel when in doubt.

Assess the arm you will use for skin impairment or hematomas. Do not use if these are present.

To begin the vein selection process, apply a tourniquet (Figure 19-9, *A*). A **tourniquet** is a constricting device traditionally applied to control bleeding. This device is applied above the bleeding site. It prevents arterial blood flow to the part below the tourniquet and prevents venous blood from returning to the heart. The veins fill with blood and distend, which makes them firmer and easier to see and feel, thus making the tourniquet useful for venipuncture (Figure 19-9, *B*).

Remove the tourniquet after collecting the blood specimen, before withdrawing the needle from the vein. To apply the tourniquet, place it 3 or 4 inches above the elbow. Cross one end tightly over the other, then tuck the upper end under band to form a half bow (see Figure 19-9, *A*). This will allow for quick release.

When used for blood draws, tourniquets serve to prevent venous blood flow—not arterial blood flow. Make sure the tourniquet is tight enough that the veins distend; however, the radial pulse should be palpable.

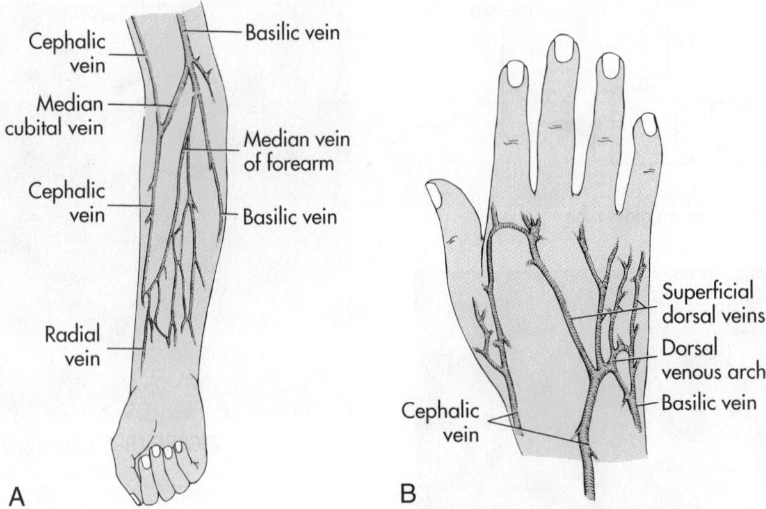

FIGURE 19-8 Selecting a venipuncture site. **A,** Inner arm. **B,** Dorsal surface of hand.

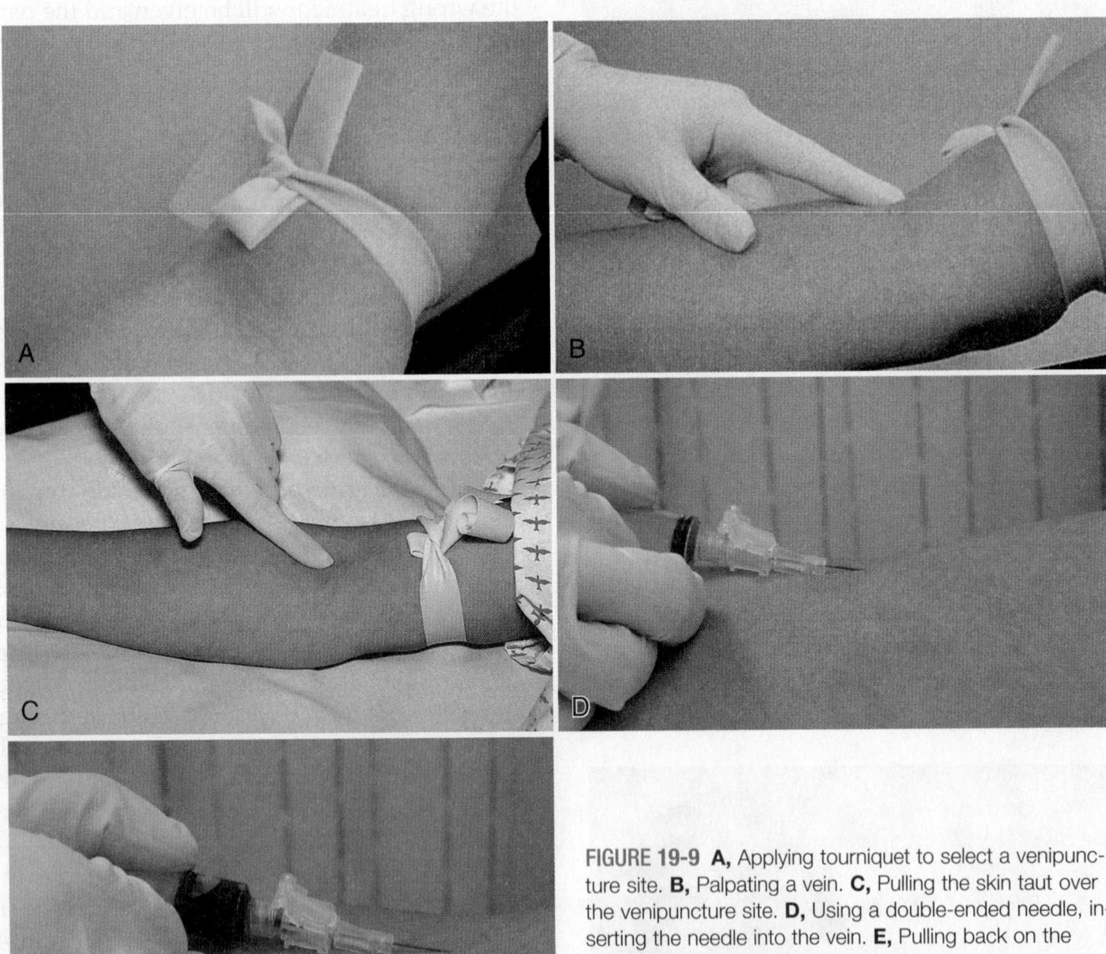

FIGURE 19-9 **A,** Applying tourniquet to select a venipuncture site. **B,** Palpating a vein. **C,** Pulling the skin taut over the venipuncture site. **D,** Using a double-ended needle, inserting the needle into the vein. **E,** Pulling back on the plunger to withdraw blood; note safety feature.

If the radial pulse is not detected, release and reapply the tourniquet. Assess for radial pulse. Leave the tourniquet in place for no longer than 1 minute.

To select a vein in the antecubital space, apply a tourniquet 3 to 4 inches above the elbow. Then ask the patient to open and close the fist. With the fist closed, look and feel for a vein. Look for a straight vein. A good vein for venipuncture feels full and firm, and it is elastic and springs back after palpating (see Figure 19-9, *B*). Avoid using veins with the following characteristics:

- Small and narrow—they are usually fragile.
- Weak—weak veins are soft and do not rebound.
- Sclerosed—sclerosed veins are hard and rigid.
- Easy to roll—the vein rolls when palpated.

Perform the venipuncture (Skill 19-13).

See Home Care Considerations box on p. 515 and Coordinated Care box on p. 516.

Skill 19-13 Performing the Venipuncture

Nursing Action *(Rationale)*

1. Refer to medical record, care plan, or Kardex. *(A physician's order is necessary.)*
2. Assemble supplies. *(Organizes procedure.)*
   - Alcohol or antiseptic swab (check agency policy for specific antiseptic solution)
   - Disposable gloves
   - Small pillow or folded towel
   - Rubber tourniquet
   - Sterile 2 × 2 gauze pads
   - Bandage or adhesive tape
   - Appropriate blood tubes, culture bottles
   - Identification labels
   - Laboratory requisition
   - Plastic bag for delivery of specimen to laboratory (or container as specified by agency)

   a. Syringe method.
      (1) Sterile needles (20- to 21-gauge for adults, 23- to 25-gauge for children, 23- to 25-gauge butterfly for older adults)
      (2) Sterile syringe of appropriate size

   b. Vacuum tube method.
      (1) Vacuum tube with needle holder
      (2) Sterile double-ended needles (20- to 21-gauge for adults, 23- to 25-gauge for children)
3. Introduce self. *(Decreases patient's anxiety.)*
4. Identify patient. *(Ensures procedure is performed with correct patient.)*
5. Explain procedure, including the reason it is being done. *(Promotes patient's cooperation and decreases patient anxiety.)*
6. Assess patient. *(Determines if test is still appropriate.)*
7. Arrange equipment and complete necessary charges. *(Facilitates procedure and facilitates proper billing.)*
8. Prepare patient for procedure.

   a. Close door or pull curtain. *(Provides privacy.)*

   b. Assist patient into supine or semi-Fowler's position with arms extended to form straight line from shoulders to wrists. Place small pillow or towel under upper arms. *(Helps stabilize extremity. Supported position in bed reduces chance of injury to patient if fainting occurs.)*

   c. Adjust bed to appropriate height, and lower nearest side rail. *(Promotes proper body mechanics and facilitates procedure.)*

   d. Drape patient. *(Prevents unnecessary exposure.)*
9. Perform hand hygiene and don gloves according to agency policy and guidelines from the CDC and OSHA. *(Reduces your exposure to bloodborne pathogens.)*
10. Apply tourniquet 3 to 4 inches above puncture site (see Figure 19-9, *A*). *(Causes vein to distend for easier visibility.)*
11. Palpate distal pulse. If pulse is not palpable, reapply tourniquet more loosely. *(If too tight, tourniquet will impede arterial blood flow.)*
12. Keep tourniquet on patient no longer than 1 to 2 minutes. If tourniquet is left on arm too long, remove and assess other extremity, or wait 60 seconds before applying. *(Prolonged time has potential to alter test results and cause pain and venous stasis.)*
13. Ask patient to open and close fist several times, finally leaving fist clenched. Avoid vigorous opening and closing of fist, which sometimes causes erroneous laboratory results. *(Facilitates distention of veins by forcing blood up from distal veins.)*
14. Quickly inspect extremity for best venipuncture site, looking for straight, prominent vein without swelling or hematoma. *(Straight and intact veins are easiest to puncture.)*
15. Palpate selected vein with fingers. Note if vein is firm and rebounds when palpated or if vein feels rigid and cordlike and rolls when palpated (see Figure 19-9, *B*). *(Patent, healthy vein is elastic and rebounds on palpation. Thrombosed vein is rigid, rolls easily, and is difficult to puncture.)*
16. Select venipuncture site (see Figure 19-9). *(Prevents discomfort to patient and inaccurate test results.)*

Continued

Skill 19-13 Performing the Venipuncture—cont'd

17. Obtain blood sample.
    a. Syringe method.
        (1) Use syringe with appropriate needle securely attached. *(Ensures needle will not dislodge from syringe during venipuncture.)*
        (2) Cleanse venipuncture site with alcohol swab, moving in circular motion outward from site for approximately 2 inches (5 cm). Allow to dry. *(Antimicrobial agent cleans skin surface of resident bacteria so organisms do not enter puncture site. Allowing alcohol to dry reduces "sting" of venipuncture.)*
        (3) Remove needle cover and inform patient that a "stick" lasting only a few seconds will be felt. *(Patient has better control over anxiety when prepared for what to expect.)*
        (4) Place thumb or forefinger of nondominant hand 1 inch (2.5 cm) below site, and pull skin taut (see Figure 19-9, C). *(Stabilizes vein and prevents rolling during needle insertion.)*
        (5) Hold syringe and needle at 15- to 30-degree angle from patient's arm with bevel up (see Figure 19-9, *D*). *(Reduces chance of penetrating both sides of vein during insertion. Keeping bevel up reduces vein trauma.)*
        (6) Slowly insert needle into vein (see Figure 19-9, *D*). *(Reduces chance of penetrating both sides of vein during insertion.)*
        (7) Hold syringe securely and pull back gently on plunger (see Figure 19-9, *E*). *(Holding syringe securely prevents needle from advancing. Pulling on plunger creates vacuum needed to draw blood into syringe.)*
        (8) Look for blood return. *(If blood flow fails to appear, needle is not well seated in vein; withdraw needle and prepare for a second attempt.)* NOTE: No more than two attempts should be made by a single nurse in the same session (Infusion Nurses Society, 2006).
        (9) Obtain desired amount of blood, keeping needle stabilized. *(Test results are more accurate when required amount of blood is obtained. Some tests are not possible to perform without minimum blood requirement. Movement of needle increases discomfort.)*
        (10) After specimen is obtained, release tourniquet (see illustration). *(Reduces bleeding at site when needle is withdrawn.)*
        (11) Apply 2 × 2 gauze pad or alcohol swab over puncture site without applying pressure, and quickly but carefully withdraw needle from vein; apply pressure with gauze following removal of needle (see illustration). *(Pressure over needle causes discomfort. Careful removal of needle keeps discomfort and vein trauma to a minimum.)*
        (12) Carefully transfer blood from syringe into vacuum tube.
        (13) Without recapping, discard needle in proper receptacle. *(Reduces risk of needlestick injury.)*
        (14) Remove and discard gloves; wash hands. *(Reduces spread of microorganisms.)*
    b. Vacuum tube method.
        (1) Attach double-ended needle to vacuum tube or Vacutainer (see illustration). *(Long end of needle is used to puncture vein. Short end fits into blood tube.)*
        (2) Have proper blood specimen tube resting inside vacuum tube, but do not push onto needle and puncture rubber stopper. *(Causes loss of tube's vacuum.)*

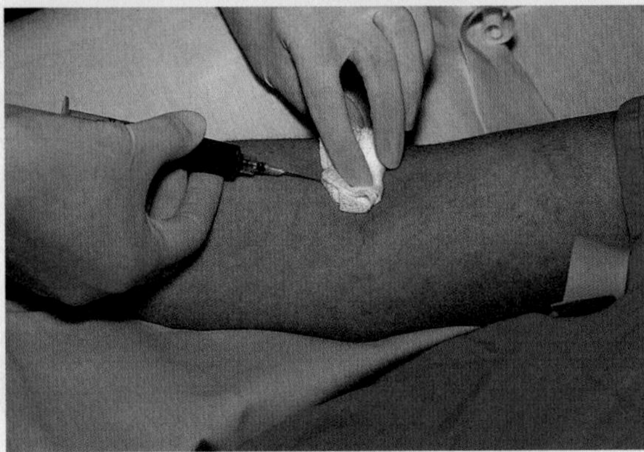

Step **17a(10)**

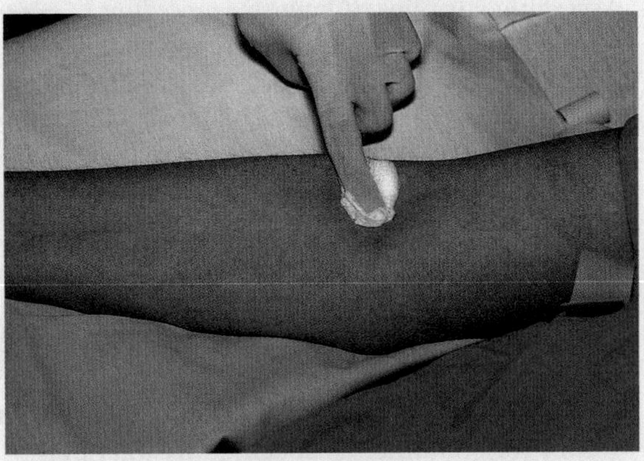

Step **17a(11)**

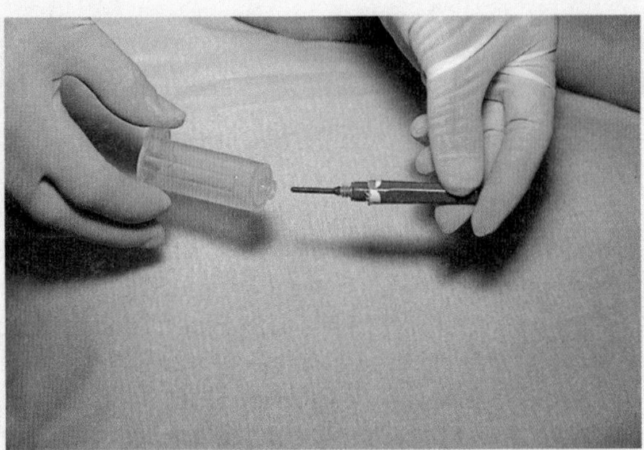

Step **17b(1)**

(3) Cleanse venipuncture site with alcohol swab, moving in circular motion outward from site for approximately 2 inches (5 cm). *(Cleans skin surface of resident bacteria so that organisms do not enter through puncture site.)*

(4) Remove needle cover and inform patient that a "stick" lasting only a few seconds will be felt. *(Patient has better control over anxiety when prepared for what to expect.)*

(5) Place thumb or forefinger of nondominant hand 1 inch (2.5 cm) below site and pull skin taut. Stretch skin down until vein is stabilized. *(Stabilizes vein and prevents rolling during needle insertion.)*

(6) Hold vacuum tube at 15- to 30-degree angle from arm with bevel up (see illustration). *(Reduces chance of penetrating both sides of vein during insertion. Keeping bevel up causes less trauma to vein.)*

(7) Slowly insert needle into vein (see Figure 19-9, *D*). *(Reduces chance of penetrating both sides of vein during insertion.)*

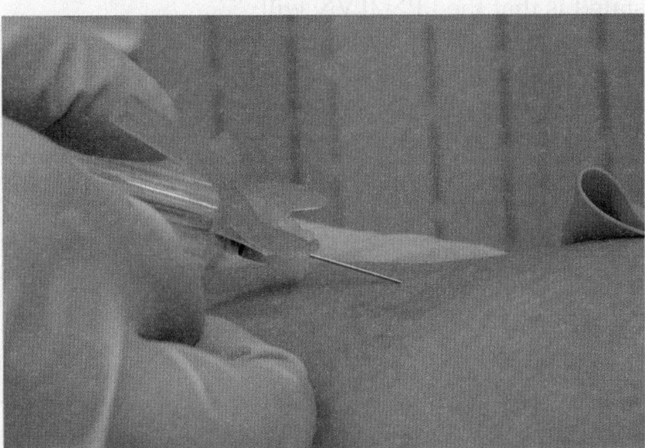

Step **17b(6)**

(8) Grasp vacuum tube securely so you do not move it and advance needle in vein, and advance specimen tube into needle of holder. *(Pushing needle through stopper breaks vacuum and causes blood to flow into tube. If needle in vein advances, it is possible to puncture vein on other side.)*

(9) Note flow of blood into tube (normally fairly rapid). *(Failure of blood to appear indicates that vacuum in tube is lost or needle is not well seated in vein.)*

(10) After specimen tube is filled, grasp vacuum tube firmly and remove tube without allowing needle in vein to move in or out. Insert additional specimen tubes as needed, as described in Step 8. *(Prevents needle from advancing or dislodging. It is necessary to fill tube completely to keep additives in certain tubes in proper proportion to blood volume of tube. Invert tubes with additives as soon as possible to mix.)*

(11) While last tube is filling, release tourniquet. *(Reduces bleeding at site when needle is withdrawn.)*

(12) Apply 2 × 2 gauze pad over puncture site without applying pressure, and quickly but carefully withdraw needle from vein. *(Pressure over needle causes discomfort. Careful removal of needle keeps discomfort and vein trauma to a minimum.)*

(13) Remove and discard gloves; perform hand hygiene. *(Reduces spread of microorganisms.)*

18. For blood obtained by syringe, transfer specimen to tubes.

a. Using one-handed technique, insert syringe needle through stopper of blood tube and allow vacuum to fill tube. Do not force blood into tube. *(Forcing blood into tube has the potential to cause hemolysis of red blood cells and invalidates test with tubes containing anticoagulants or additives. OSHA recommends one-handed technique to help prevent needlestick injury.)*

b. Alternative method is to remove needle from syringe and stopper from each test tube. Gently inject required amount of blood into each tube. Reapply stopper. *(Blood injected too quickly will sometimes cause frothing or hemolysis of red blood cells. Stopper maintains sterility of specimen.)*

19. When obtaining blood for culture.

a. Cleanse venipuncture sites with povidone-iodine or appropriate antiseptic. Allow to dry. *(Antimicrobial agent cleans skin surface so organisms do not enter puncture site or contaminate culture.)*

Continued

Skill 19-13 Performing the Venipuncture—cont'd

b. Clean bottle tops of vacuum tubes or culture bottles with appropriate antiseptic (check agency policy). *(Ensures specimen is sterile.)*
c. Collect 10 to 15 mL of venous blood by venipuncture from each venipuncture site. *(It is necessary to obtain cultures from two sites.)*
d. Discard needle on syringe; replace with new sterile needle before injecting blood sample into culture bottles. *(Maintains sterile technique and prevents contamination of specimen.)*
e. If both aerobic and anaerobic cultures are needed, inoculate anaerobic first. *(Anaerobic organisms often take longer to grow.)*
f. Mix medium gently after inoculation. *(Mixes medium and blood.)*
g. After venipuncture, apply 2 × 2 gauze pad over puncture site without applying pressure, and quickly but carefully withdraw needle from vein. *(Pressure over needle causes discomfort. Careful removal of needle keeps discomfort and vein trauma to a minimum.)*

20. For blood tubes containing additives, gently rotate back and forth 8 to 10 times. *(It is necessary to mix additives with blood to prevent clotting. Shaking has potential to cause hemolysis of red blood cells, producing inaccurate test results.)*
21. Inspect puncture site for bleeding and apply adhesive tape with gauze. *(Keeps puncture site clean and controls any final oozing.)*
22. Check tubes for any sign of external contamination with blood. Decontaminate with alcohol if necessary. Remove and discard gloves; wash hands. *(Prevents cross-contamination. Reduces risk of exposure to pathogens present in blood.)*
23. Securely attach properly completed identification label to each tube, affix proper requisition, and transfer to laboratory promptly. *(Ensures proper identification of specimen; ensures accurate results; prevents loss and potential delays in obtaining results.)*
24. Remove and appropriately discard gloves. Perform hand hygiene. *(Prevents the spread of microorganisms.)*
25. Assist patient to a comfortable position and place needed items within easy reach. *(Ensures patient's comfort and well-being.)*
26. Raise side rail and lower bed to lowest position. *(Promotes patient safety.)*
27. Store, remove, or dispose of supplies and equipment as appropriate. *(Ensures equipment is available for next use.)*
28. Document procedure.
    - Time
    - Test performed
    - Patient's response
    - Any adverse findings (e.g., hematoma, prolonged bleeding, unusual pain)

ELECTROCARDIOGRAM

Electrocardiograms are often done by technicians specifically trained for this test. The **electrocardiogram (ECG)** (sometimes called an EKG) is a graphic representation of electrical impulses generated by the heart during a cardiac cycle; it identifies abnormalities that interfere with electrical conduction through cardiac tissue. This procedure is usually done at the patient's bedside, but sometimes it is done in a specially equipped laboratory.

Assess the patient for knowledge level of the procedure; ability to understand and follow directions (this procedure requires patient to follow directions closely and assume proper positioning); ability to assume proper position; and vital signs (baseline) for comparison with postprocedure vital signs.

If the patient has large amounts of hair, you will sometimes have to clip or shave it at the placement site. This will promote adherence of the leads (electrodes) to the chest and on the extremity. Skill 19-14 describes how the ECG is performed.

❖ NURSING PROCESS *for Specimen Collection and Diagnostic Examination*

The role of the licensed practical nurse/licensed vocational nurse (LPN/LVN) in the nursing process as stated is that the LPN/LVN will:

- Participate in planning care for patients based on patient needs
- Review patient's plan of care and recommend revisions as needed
- Review and follow defined prioritization for patient care
- Use clinical pathways, care maps, or care plans to guide and review patient care

■ Assessment

You will need to do the following:

- Assess patient's knowledge of procedure to determine level of health teaching required.
- Observe verbal and nonverbal behavior to determine patient's anxiety.

Text continued on p. 518

 Home Care Considerations

Specimen Collection and Diagnostic Examination

URINE SPECIMEN

- It is best to collect urine specimens for culture and sensitivity in the laboratory setting rather than at home owing to the increased chance of bacterial growth because of the delay in testing. If a specimen is collected at home, the patient will have to refrigerate the specimen until time of transport to the laboratory and keep the specimen on ice during transport.
- When purchasing urine testing kits, the patient needs to know that all supplies except for the specimen container are usually supplied.
- Urine testing at home is typically performed with reagent strips.

STOOL SPECIMEN

- Frequently, patients are instructed to obtain stool specimens at home and then bring the specimen to the laboratory setting or physician's office.
- If obtaining a stool specimen for occult blood testing, the client is asked to prepare the slide at home and return the slide to the laboratory or physician's office for testing.
- Instruct the patient obtaining a stool specimen at home to avoid specimen contact with any solutions that clean, disinfect, or deodorize the toilet bowl.
- Older adults will often need assistance with the collection of stool specimens.

SPUTUM SPECIMEN

- Instruct patients obtaining sputum specimens at home on proper specimen collection and the importance of returning the specimen to the lab in a timely manner.

WOUND DRAINAGE

- Teach proper technique for obtaining a wound specimen (e.g., hand hygiene) if obtaining the specimen in the patient's home.

VENIPUNCTURE

- Since there is often no tourniquet available in the home setting, use a blood pressure cuff before venipuncture.

BLOOD GLUCOSE TESTING

- Encourage patients to attend a diabetic support group.
- Various glucose meters are available for home use.

OTHER SPECIMENS AND EXAMINATIONS

- Driving is restricted for 24 hours following procedures requiring conscious sedation.
- Instruct the patient not to make any legal decisions for 24 hours following procedures requiring conscious sedation.

Postprocedural Considerations

Following an intravenous pyelogram (IVP), discharge instructions typically include the following:

- To wash out the contrast medium via the kidneys, drink at least 24 ounces of water if not contraindicated.
- Delayed allergic reaction from the contrast medium is possible as much as 24 hours postprocedure. Instruct patients to call the primary physician. If the reaction is an emergency, the patient is to go immediately to the emergency department rather than contacting the primary physician.
- Provide the patient with written instructions upon discharge following a lumbar puncture. Instructions include directing the patient to get immediate medical attention if a severe headache or change in level of consciousness occurs following the procedure.
- Following a paracentesis, instruct the patient to contact the physician if he or she becomes febrile, or experiences pain, swelling, or discharge from the puncture site. Instruct male patients to contact the physician if they experience scrotal edema.
- Give patients who have undergone a thoracentesis written instructions that include signs and symptoms of complications related to perforation of the spleen or liver. Inform them that sometimes these signs and symptoms will not occur for several days following the procedure.

Following Bronchoscopy

- Instruct patients experiencing fever, chest pain or discomfort, and/or respiratory symptoms such as dyspnea, wheezing, or hemoptysis to contact the physician or seek medical attention immediately.
- Instruct patients that throat discomfort is common and is often relieved with throat lozenges.

Following Endoscopy

- Hoarseness and sore throat sometimes occur following the procedure; as long as the gag reflex has returned, encourage the patient to seek relief with throat lozenges or ice chips.
- Following a lower GI tract endoscopy, recommend a warm tub bath to ease any rectal discomfort.

Following Cardiac Catheterization

- Instruct the patient to contact the physician or seek immediate medical attention if any of the following occurs:
  —Bleeding from the puncture site (apply pressure).
  —Formation or an increase in size of any knots or lumps under the skin at the puncture site.
  —Increase in bruising at the puncture site or movement of bruising down the extremity with the puncture site.
  —Change or an increase in pain at the puncture site or in the extremity with the puncture site, or if the extremity becomes pale and/or cool to touch.
  —Swelling, redness, and/or warmth at the puncture site or in the extremity of the puncture site.

Adapted from Perry, A.G., & Potter, P.A. (2006). *Clinical nursing skills and techniques.* (6th ed.). St. Louis: Mosby.

 Coordinated Care

Collaboration

SPECIMEN COLLECTION

- The collection of urine specimens may be performed by assistive personnel (AP) who are familiar with aseptic and sterile technique. Inform the AP of when to collect a specimen and proper transport of the specimen. Direct the AP to notify you immediately if appearance of urine specimen is abnormal (e.g., presence of blood, cloudiness, or excess sediments).
- The collection of stool and emesis for testing is appropriate for AP to perform. The skills of assessing the significance of test results require the critical thinking and knowledge application unique to a nurse. Delegation of the analysis of test results is inappropriate. Direct the AP to notify you immediately if results are positive so you know to repeat the testing.
- The skills used to obtain and test gastric secretions from an NG or nasoenteral tube require the critical thinking and knowledge application unique to a nurse. Delegation of these procedures is inappropriate.
- Obtaining and testing the blood glucose level after skin puncture is appropriate to delegate to an AP who has been certified to perform the procedure. It is necessary to assess the patient to determine whether his or her need for glucose monitoring is appropriate for delegation. If the patient's condition changes frequently, do not delegate this procedure to AP.
- Phlebotomy staff and registered nurses (RNs) are permitted to obtain venipuncture samples. RNs who draw blood samples are usually certified by the agency that employs them. However, check agency policy to determine who is permitted to perform blood drawing.
- The skills used to obtain throat, nasal, and nasopharyngeal cultures require the critical thinking and knowledge application unique to a nurse. Delegation of these procedures is inappropriate.
- Collection of expectorated sputum specimens is appropriate to delegate to AP. The skills used to collect a sputum specimen using sterile suction require the critical thinking and knowledge application unique to a nurse. Delegation of this procedure is inappropriate.
- Obtaining a wound culture requires the critical thinking and knowledge application unique to a nurse. Delegation of this procedure is inappropriate.
- AP are permitted to transport stable patients to the testing department. Monitoring vital signs following the procedures is possible to delegate to an AP, but assessment is not. Monitoring during intravenous conscious sedation (IVCS) requires the critical thinking and knowledge application unique to a nurse. Delegation is inappropriate.
- Diagnostic studies requiring the use of a contrast medium subject patients to potentially life-threatening complications. Direct the AP to notify you immediately of any complications (e.g., allergic reactions, bleeding, respiratory distress, or coughing up blood).
- ECGs are often performed by technicians specifically trained for this test. Nurses with advanced training often monitor patient ECG patterns continuously in an intensive care setting, in the emergency department, or on units where telemetry is used. It is acceptable for AP to monitor the vital signs of stable patients. APs need to immediately notify you of chest pain or altered vital signs.

Skill 19-14 Performing an Electrocardiogram (ECG)

Nursing Action *(Rationale)*

1. Refer to medical record, care plan, or Kardex. *(Provides basis for care.)*
2. Assemble supplies. *(Organizes procedure.)*
   - ECG machine
   - Electropaste (gel)
   - ECG leads or electrodes
   - Alcohol wipes
   - Razor or clippers
   - Clean gloves (optional)
3. Introduce self. *(Decreases patient's anxiety.)*
4. Identify patient. *(Ensures procedure is performed with correct patient.)*
5. Explain procedure. Include the reason it is being done in terms the patient is able to understand. *(Promotes cooperation and decreases patient's anxiety; ensures accuracy.)*
6. Assess patient for chest pain, pulse, and respirations. *(Enables you to determine if test is still appropriate.)*
7. Arrange equipment and complete necessary charges. *(Facilitates procedure and proper billing.)*
8. Prepare patient for procedure.
   a. Close door or pull curtains. *(Provides privacy.)*
   b. Usually supine is the preferred position. Arrange for patient's comfort. *(Promotes accuracy of test.)*
   c. Drape patient as necessary. *(Prevents unnecessary embarrassment.)*
   d. Adjust bed to appropriate height, and lower the nearest side rail. *(Promotes proper body mechanics and facilitates procedure.)*
   e. Perform hand hygiene and don gloves according to agency's policy and guidelines from the CDC and OSHA. *(Reduces spread of microorganisms.)*

10. Perform ECG.
    a. Cleanse and prepare skin (shave or clip hair, as necessary after obtaining consent); wipe skin with alcohol. *(Promotes adherence of leads [electrodes] to chest or extremity.)*
    b. Apply electrode paste and attach leads (see illustration). *(Position of leads promotes proper display of ECG on paper.)* For 12-lead ECG:
        (1) Chest (precordial leads) (see illustration)
        - V_1—Fourth intercostal space (ICS) at right sternal border
        - V_2—Fourth ICS at left sternal border
        - V_3—Midway between V_2 and V_4
        - V_4—Fifth ICS at midclavicular line
        - V_5—Left anterior axillary line at level of V_4 horizontally
        - V_6—Left midaxillary line at level of V_4 horizontally

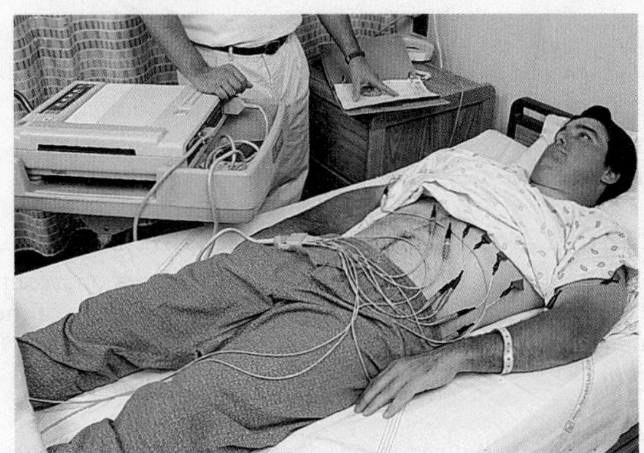

Step **10b**

        (2) Extremities—one at lower portion of each extremity:
        - $_aV_R$—Right wrist
        - $_aV_L$—Left wrist
        - $_aV_F$—Left ankle
    c. Obtain tracing (12-lead ECG is possible to obtain without removing precordial leads). *(Transfers electrocardiac conduction on ECG tracing paper for subsequent analysis by cardiologist.)*
    d. Disconnect leads; wipe excess electrode paste from chest. *(Promotes comfort and hygiene.)*
    e. Remove gloves, discard in proper receptacle, and perform hand hygiene. *(Reduces spread of microorganisms.)*
    f. Deliver ECG tracing to appropriate laboratory or nursing unit promptly. *(Provides for review of ECG by cardiologist.)*
11. Assist patient to a comfortable position and place needed items within easy reach. *(Ensures patient's comfort and well-being.)*
12. Raise side rail and lower bed to lowest position. *(Ensures patient's safety.)*
13. Store, remove, or dispose of supplies and equipment as appropriate. *(Ensures equipment is available for next use.)*
14. Document procedure. *(Provides communication that the procedure was carried out and patient's response.)*
    - Time
    - Test performed
    - Patient's response
    - Patient teaching (as appropriate)

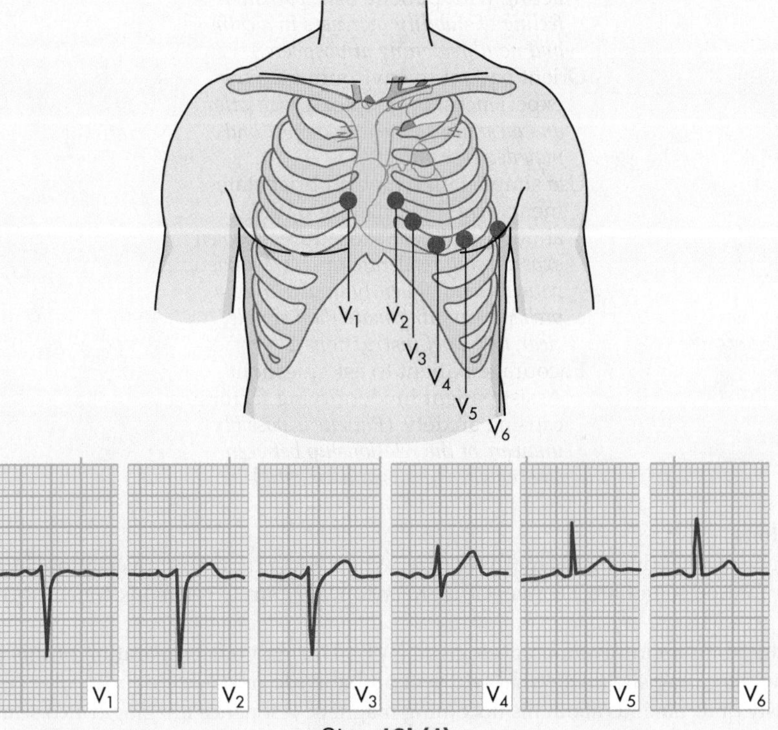

Step **10b(1)**

- Assess patient's ability to understand and follow directions.
- Assess patient's ability to assume position required for procedure and ability to remain in that position.
- Assess whether patient is allergic to antiseptics or anesthetic solutions or any of the dyes that will possibly be used.
- Assess patient's need for preprocedure analgesic administration.

Nursing Diagnosis

With an astute assessment, you will be able to determine the nursing problems and formulate the necessary nursing diagnoses. Nursing diagnoses are likely to include the following:

- Anxiety, related to the manner in which a specimen is obtained or a procedure is performed. Fear of the possible test results is often a factor (Nursing Care Plan 19-1).
- Deficient knowledge, related to the purpose of the collection or examination and the manner in which the specimen is collected or the test is performed.
- Risk for infection, related to the patient's skin or tissue impairment (broken during a diagnostic procedure).
- Acute pain, related to invasive diagnostic test (when some type of instrument is inserted into a part of the body).

Nursing diagnoses related to optimum oxygenation during diagnostic procedures involving the airway include the following:

- Impaired gas exchange
- Ineffective breathing pattern
- Risk for aspiration

Nursing Care Plan 19-1 Specimen Collection or Diagnostic Examination

This care plan has been adapted for the patient who is at risk for anxiety due to diagnostic tests and examinations.

NURSING DIAGNOSIS ***Risk for anxiety, related to intrusive diagnostic tests and procedures***

Patient Goals and Expected Outcomes	Nursing Interventions and Rationale	Evaluation
Patient describes a reduction in the level of anxiety experienced	Acknowledge awareness of patient's anxiety. *(Acknowledgment of the patient's feelings validates the feelings and communicates acceptance of these feelings.)* Stay with the patient if this appears necessary. *(The presence of a trusted person is often helpful.)* Maintain a calm manner while interacting with patient. *(The patient's feeling of stability increases in a calm and nonthreatening atmosphere.)* Orient patient to environment, new experiences, or people. *(Orientation and awareness promote comfort and may decrease anxiety.)* Use simple language and brief statements when instructing patient about diagnostic procedures. *(When experiencing moderate to severe anxiety, patients are frequently unable to comprehend anything more than simple, clear, and brief instructions.)* Encourage patient to ask questions. Assist patient in identifying factors causing anxiety. *(Patient is possibly unaware of the relationship between emotional concerns and anxiety.)*	Patient states fewer feelings of anxiety. Patient states an understanding of the upcoming examination.

Critical Thinking Questions

1. The patient has been very quiet during his morning care. When you attempt a conversation, he is obviously not interested. What is a way for you to initiate a conversation to encourage him to relate his concerns over his upcoming bronchoscopy?
2. Your patient is scheduled for an intravenous pyelogram (IVP). During your preparation of this patient, he remarks he once had a reaction while eating shellfish. What will you probably do next?
3. The patient is obviously quite anxious about his upcoming magnetic resonance imaging (MRI) scan. He breaks out in a cold sweat and is breathing rapidly, and when assessing his pulse, you note tachycardia. How will you respond to this patient?

- Ineffective airway clearance, related to collection of sputum specimen by sneezing and coughing or related to collection of sputum specimen by suctioning

Expected Outcomes and Planning

Identify goals and outcomes of care, and set priorities for the plan of care that most likely will result in goal achievement. Expected outcomes focus on the collection of an uncontaminated specimen by you or the patient and the patient understanding the purpose of the examination requiring the specimen.

All Specimens

- Patient explains procedure for specimen collection before collection is attempted.
- Patient explains purpose of specimen analysis before collection is attempted.
- Patient verbalizes lack of fear of specimen collection and test results.

24-Hour Urine Collection

- All of patient urine voided during time period is saved.

Urine and Stool Specimens

- Patient specimen is free of contaminants, such as urine or toilet tissue in stool or toilet tissue in urine.

Sputum Specimen Obtained by Suction

- Patient maintains adequate oxygenation throughout procedure.

Wound Drainage Specimen

- Specimen is free of contaminants from skin.

Contrast Media Studies

- Patient explains the purpose and basic steps of the procedure before it begins.
- Patient assumes the correct position and remains still during the procedure.
- Patient does not experience postprocedure complications, such as flushing, pruritus, and urticaria; respiratory depression or decreased cardiovascular function; diminished or absent peripheral pulses; hypotension and tachycardia; or decreased or absent urinary output.

Nuclear Imaging Studies (Scans)

- Patient expresses fears and anxieties related to testing and results.
- Patient does not experience postprocedure complications such as hematoma, erythema, or edema at injection site.

Implementation

Implementation includes performing those preexamination and postexamination responsibilities that will assist a patient to reach a maximum state of health (see Table 19-1).

If patient is discharged home, teach home care instructions (see Home Care Considerations box).

Evaluation

Evaluation involves observing for a patient's response to determine whether goals and outcomes have been met.

1. Ask patient to state purpose and explain steps of the procedure before it is started.
2. Ask if patient has questions or concerns about the procedure before it begins and later about test results. Assess nonverbal behaviors of anxiety before, during, and after procedure.
3. Ask patient to demonstrate body position required for procedure. Assess patient's body position throughout procedure and assist to maintain position as necessary.
4. Ask patient to describe level of comfort during and after procedure.
5. Assess patient's respiratory status (rate, rhythm, and depth of respirations; symmetry of chest movement) during and after abdominal paracentesis, thoracentesis, and bronchoscopy.
6. Compare patient's heart rate and blood pressure during and after procedure to preprocedure baseline. (Check hospital policy; sometimes as often as every 15 minutes, typically lasts 2 hours.)
7. Inspect dressing over puncture site for drainage every hour after the procedure until patient's condition is stable.
8. Assess patient for postprocedure complications.
   a. Assess patient for a decrease in blood pressure and tachycardia (could signify hemorrhage or allergic reaction to dye [see Box 19-2]).
   b. Assess patient for flushing, itching, and urticaria (could signify allergic reaction to dye [see Box 19-2]).
   c. Assess patient's respiratory status for sudden, severe shortness of breath (signifies possible laryngospasm and bronchospasm).
   d. Assess patient for abdominal pain, fever, and bleeding (signifies possible perforation of abdominal structures).
   e. Assess patient for low oxygen saturation; rate and depth of respirations; cyanosis or mottled skin; hypotension; changes in heart rate or rhythm (usually bradycardia); decreased or nonpalpable peripheral pulses; decreased or absent reflexes; and changes in level of consciousness related to conscious sedation.
9. Ask patient to describe postprocedure positioning and activity restriction for lumbar puncture, liver biopsy, and thoracentesis.

Get Ready for the NCLEX® Examination!

Key Points

- Laboratory examinations of specimens of urine, stool, sputum, blood, and wound drainage provide important information about body functioning and contribute to the assessment of health status.
- Patients who are given a clear explanation about the purpose of the specimen and how it is obtained will be more cooperative in its collection.
- Prepare properly to ensure that the patient is ready for the test and to prevent prolonging the hospital stay because of inadequate test preparations.
- Most people believe that it is best for excretions to be handled discreetly; therefore, it is important to provide the patient with as much comfort and privacy as possible.
- Health care professionals are obliged to take into consideration the patient's age and socioeconomic, cultural, and educational background when discussing and collecting laboratory specimens.
- Wear gloves when collecting specimens of blood or other body fluids to prevent spread of human immunodeficiency virus (HIV), hepatitis B, and other pathogens.
- Collect specimens in proper containers at the correct time and in the appropriate amount.
- Label all specimens properly with the patient's identification, and complete laboratory requisition as necessary.
- Most invasive diagnostic tests require a signed informed consent.
- Wound cultures serve to identify aerobic and anaerobic organisms.
- Some diagnostic tests are possible to perform at the patient's bedside; your responsibility in this case includes caring for the patient and assisting the physician.
- Following diagnostic testing, provide care and teach the patient what to expect, including the outcomes or side effects of the test.

Additional Resources

Go to your Companion CD for an audio glossary, animations, video clips, and more.

evolve Be sure to visit the Evolve site at http://evolve.elsevier.com/Christensen/foundations/ for additional online resources.

Review Questions for the NCLEX® Examination

1. A 64-year-old patient who is newly diagnosed with diabetes mellitus has been learning how to perform her own blood glucose monitoring. The nurse is aware that having the patient hold her arm at her side for 30 seconds before obtaining a blood sample to measure glucose will:

1. increase blood to the site.
2. provide easy access to device.
3. prepare the site.
4. prevent needle puncture of the nurse.

2. A sputum specimen has been ordered for a 75-year-old patient admitted with possible pneumonia of the right lower lobe. The patient is not able to cough. For patients who cannot expectorate sputum from deep in the bronchial tree, it is necessary to collect the specimen by:

1. pharyngeal suctioning.
2. nasotracheal suctioning.
3. oropharyngeal suctioning.
4. percussion and vibration.

3. The physician has ordered a stool specimen for blood that it is not possible to see with the naked eye. This examination is for:

1. profuse bleeding.
2. gross blood.
3. melena.
4. occult blood.

4. A 46-year-old patient is seen by the physician for recurrent symptoms of cystitis. He is to have a urine culture and sensitivity determination and a 24-hour urine collection for laboratory analysis. A urine culture study is required to:

1. identify the causative organisms.
2. determine the presence of malignant cells.
3. analyze the elements present in the urine.
4. localize the site of the inflammatory process.

5. To obtain a 24-hour urine specimen, which instruction should be given to the patient?

1. Collect each voiding in separate containers for the next 24 hours.
2. Discard the first voided specimen and then collect the total volume of each voiding for 24 hours.
3. For the next 24 hours, retain a 30-mL specimen of each voiding after recording the amount voided.
4. Keep a record of the time and the amount of each voiding for 24 hours.

6. A 72-year-old patient has an indwelling urinary catheter. A sterile urine specimen has been ordered for a culture and sensitivity. The nurse will obtain the sterile specimen by:

1. obtaining 60 mL of urine from the collection bag.
2. removing the present catheter, having the patient void, and then recatheterizing.
3. disconnecting the tubing from the catheter and draining 2 mL of urine.
4. aspirating 10 mL of urine with a sterile syringe from the tubing port.

7. A patient performing a fingerstick for blood glucose determination asks why the side of the fingertip is advised as the preferred site. The nurse knows that it is because:

1. the blood supply is greater in this area.
2. it is easier for the self-determination method.
3. the side of the finger is less responsive to pain than other sites.
4. it leaves more room for other site selection.

8. An important preexamination nursing intervention for the patient undergoing an invasive diagnostic examination is:

1. a cleansing bath with Hibiclens.
2. obtaining the informed consent.
3. encouraging the patient to drink several glasses of water.
4. instructing the patient not to wear deodorant, powder, or lotion.

9. A patient is scheduled for an upper GI series and a barium enema. The nurse explains that because of the procedure for an upper GI study and barium enema, the patient can expect to:

1. be NPO after midnight and have a series of enemas.
2. have coffee and toast the morning of the test.
3. take radiographic dye tablets.
4. have a needle inserted into the liver.

10. The physician has ordered a urine sample to be collected. The nurse will have to:

1. verify whether this is to be a sterile sample.
2. instruct the patient to save all urine for the next 24 hours.
3. choose a 20-mL syringe to aspirate urine from the catheter bag.
4. request that the patient use the bedpan for collection of the sample.

11. Before obtaining a blood sample, the nurse will first:

1. verify the patient identification.
2. ask the patient which arm is best to use.
3. reassure the patient that the procedure will not be painful.
4. clean the patient's skin thoroughly according to agency protocol.

12. On evaluation of the patient after a venipuncture, the nurse notes which occurrence as an unexpected outcome?

1. Patient's heart rate is 80 and regular
2. Soft lump is noted under the skin at the venipuncture site
3. Patient complains of a stinging sensation after the needle is removed
4. Small amount of blood is noted on the skin over the venipuncture site

13. The patient tells the nurse, "I have a very hard time getting a drop of blood from my finger for the blood sugar test." The nurse will:

1. ask the physician to order a different type of blood glucose monitoring system.
2. suggest that the patient use warm water on the finger just before using the blood lancet.
3. instruct the patient to use the same puncture site several times in a row for best results.
4. remind the patient that it is acceptable to skip blood glucose monitoring once in a while.

14. The nurse notes that the patient does not require further teaching regarding home use of stool testing for occult blood when the patient states:

1. "It is best if I can get two separate samples from the same stool."
2. "I need to apply a very thick smear of stool onto the guaiac slide."
3. "There is an electronic meter or blood sample required for this test."
4. "If the paper turns white after the stool is on it, I need to call my doctor."

15. The nurse has just completed attaching the leads for an electrocardiogram. The next step is to:

1. perform hand hygiene and don clean gloves.
2. position the patient lying supine.
3. obtain the tracing.
4. raise the side rail and lower bed to lowest position.

16. When obtaining a midstream urine specimen from a female patient, which instructions will be most important to tell the patient?

1. Start voiding directly into the sterile cup.
2. Discard the last of the stream of urine into the stool.
3. Wash hands before obtaining specimen.
4. Wipe from front to back when cleansing the urethral area.

17. Which nursing action is essential before a chest x-ray film is obtained?

1. Make certain the patient doesn't eat or drink.
2. Remove the patient's metal necklace.
3. Have the patient swallow contrast medium.
4. Administer a dose of medication for pain relief.

18. A nursing student asks the nurse to explain the difference in testing between a midstream urine specimen and a urinalysis. The nurse explains that the midstream specimen is commonly used to perform a test for:

1. culture and sensitivity of the urine specimen.
2. measuring the specific gravity of the urine.
3. determining the presence of glucose and ketones in the urine.
4. checking the urine for the presence of white blood cells (WBCs) and red blood cells (RBCs).

19. During the collection of a 24-hour urine specimen, it is important for the nurse to maintain the integrity of the urine by use of a chemical preservative or by:

1. discarding every other specimen collected.
2. ensuring the patient voids every 1 to 2 hours.
3. sending specimens to the lab every 2 to 3 hours.
4. keeping the specimen container chilled during the entire 24 hours.

20. When assessing a patient's urine sample, what will the nurse consider an abnormal finding?

1. Clear, amber color
2. Some sediment and a few mucus flecks
3. Blood
4. A slight aromatic odor

21. In order to obtain sputum rather than saliva for a sputum specimen, the nurse knows that the best time to collect the specimen is:

1. following episodes of coughing.
2. in the morning upon awakening.
3. immediately following respiratory treatments.
4. prior to initiating oxygen therapy.

22. Because of loss of subcutaneous tissue and skin elasticity in the older adult, which step of the venipuncture procedure will the nurse sometimes eliminate?

1. Application of the tourniquet before venipuncture
2. Applying pressure to the venipuncture site following the procedure
3. Cleansing of the intended venipuncture site with a topical antiseptic
4. Placement of a small dressing to the venipuncture site following the procedure

23. When obtaining a residual urine specimen, it is important to catheterize the patient after the patient voids within:

1. 10 minutes.
2. 30 minutes.
3. 50 minutes.
4. 90 minutes.

chapter 20

Selected Nursing Skills

Elaine Oden Kockrow

evolve

http://evolve.elsevier.com/Christensen/foundationsadult

Objectives

1. Describe the procedures for irrigating the eye and the ear.
2. Discuss heat and cold therapy and procedures.
3. Summarize the nurse's responsibilities for the patient receiving intravenous therapy and procedures.
4. Explain the nurse's responsibility when administering blood transfusion therapy.
5. Discuss complications of intravenous therapy.
6. Describe the complications of blood therapy.
7. Discuss nursing interventions and procedures for the patient receiving oxygen.
8. Develop nursing diagnoses for the patient receiving oxygen therapy.
9. Discuss care of (procedures for) a patient with a tracheostomy.
10. Differentiate among oropharyngeal, nasopharyngeal, and nasotracheal suctioning.
11. Discuss management of the patient with an indwelling catheter or urinary diversion:
    - Male catheterization
    - Female catheterization
    - Discontinuing an indwelling catheter
    - Catheter irrigation
    - Care of the urinary diversion
12. Identify the procedures for promoting bowel elimination:
    - Administering an enema
    - Inserting a rectal tube
    - Removing a fecal impaction
13. Describe nursing care required to maintain structure and function of a bowel diversion.
14. Explain nursing interventions for the patient with nasogastric intubation.
15. Discuss gastric and intestinal suctioning care.
16. Describe the procedure for nasogastric tube removal.
17. Explain the procedure for external and internal vaginal irrigation (douche).
18. Discuss the procedure for nasal irrigation.

Key Terms

bladder training (p. 582)
catheterization (kă-thĕ-tŭr-ĭ-ZĀ-shŭn, p. 569)
chevron (SHĔV-rŏn, p. 550)
compress (KŎM-prĕs, p. 532)
defecation (dĕf-ĕ-KĀ-shŭn, p. 589)
enema (p. 592)
feces (FĒ-sēz, p. 589)
flatulence (FLĂCH-yū-lĕns, p. 592)
impaction (ĭm-PĂK-shŭn, p. 592)
incontinence (ĭn-KŎN-tĭ-nĕns, p. 580)
induration (ĭn-dū-RĀ-shŭn, p. 545)
infiltration (ĭn-fĭl-TRĀ-shŭn, p. 545)
intravenous (IV) (ĭn-tră-VĒ-nŭs, p. 536)
irrigations (p. 525)
lumen (LŪ-mĕn, p. 531)
nasal cannula (KĂN-yū-lă, p. 557)
nasogastric (NG) tube (nā-zō-GĂS-trĭk, p. 583)
patency (PĂ-tĕn-sē, p. 545)
peripheral (pĕ-RĬF-ŭr-ăl, p. 536)
sensory deprivation (dĕp-rĭ-VĀ-shŭn, p. 564)
tracheostomy (trā-kē-ŎS-tō-mē, p. 560)
urinary catheter (KĂ-thĕ-tŭr, p. 569)
vasoconstriction (vā-zō-kŏn-STRĬK-shŭn, p. 531)
vasodilation (vā-zō-dī-LĀ-shŭn, p. 531)
venipuncture (VĔN-ĭ-pŭnk-chŭr, p. 536)

The implementation of nursing interventions calls for specific skills. To develop proficiency in these skills, you will need both knowledge and practice. Knowing the rationale for the action, as well as having the ability to adapt creatively and seek the assistance of others during its performance, improves the quality of nursing interventions. Thus nurses use knowledge, experience, and interaction to determine appropriate nursing interventions for each specific patient care situation.

STANDARD STEPS IN SELECTED SKILLS

To ensure the safety of both you and the patient, it is necessary to follow specific steps when performing nursing skills (Perry & Potter, 2009). To save space and minimize repetition in this chapter, the bulk of which is comprised of skills boxes, steps that are common to them all are presented here and not individually, unless there is a need to clarify their application in a particular context. Remember that these steps are essential: follow them with exactness to deliver appropriate and responsible nursing interventions. The skills boxes refer to them as *standard steps*.

Before the skill:

1. Refer to medical record, care plan, or Kardex for special interventions. *(Provides basis for care. Many nursing interventions require a physician's order. Verification is ensured when you review medical record.)*
2. Introduce yourself; include your name and title or role. *(Decreases patient anxiety.)*
3. Identify patient by checking armband and requesting patient to state his or her name. *(Ensures procedure is performed with correct patient.)*
4. Explain the procedure and the reason it is to be done in terms the patient is able to understand, and give patient time to ask questions. Advise patient of any unpleasantness that is likely or possible to be involved. *(Promotes cooperation, decreases patient's anxiety, and prepares patient. Also helps determine if procedure is still appropriate.)*
5. Assess need for and provide patient teaching during procedure. *(Promotes patient's independence.)*
6. Assess patient. Each skill box has an assessment section that includes specific data. *(Provides baseline information for later comparisons.)*
7. Perform hand hygiene and don clean gloves according to agency policy and guidelines from the Centers for Disease Control and Prevention (CDC) and Occupational Safety and Health Administration (OSHA) (Boyce & Pittet, 2002) (see Chapter 12). *(Reduces the spread of microorganisms.)*
8. Assemble equipment, and complete necessary charges. *(Organizes procedure. Some equipment is reusable and is kept at the bedside. Some of the equipment is disposable and charged to the patient when used. Know agency policy. Each skill box lists the specific equipment required.)*
9. Prepare patient for intervention:
   a. Close door or pull privacy curtain. *(Provides privacy and promotes patient comfort.)*
   b. Raise bed to comfortable working height, and lower side rail on side nearest you. *(Promotes proper body mechanics by keeping muscle strain on caregivers to a minimum and preventing injury and fatigue.)*
   c. Position and drape patient as necessary. *(Respect for privacy is fundamental to preserving human dignity. Patients have the right to privacy. Specific positions are included in each skill.)*

During the skill:

10. Promote patient involvement as possible. *(Participation encourages patient's buy-in and cooperation.)*
11. Assess patient's tolerance, being alert for signs and symptoms of discomfort and fatigue. Describe any inability to tolerate a procedure in your nursing notes. *(Patient's ability to tolerate interventions varies depending on severity of illness and disability. It is necessary to use judgment in providing the opportunity for rest and comfort measures.)*

Completion of procedure:

12. Assist patient to a position of comfort, and place needed items within easy reach. Be certain patient has a means to call for assistance and knows how to use it. *(Promotes safety—otherwise patients often attempt to reach items and risk falling or injury.)*
13. Raise the side rails, and lower the bed to the lowest position. *(This keeps to a minimum the risk of patients getting out of bed unattended. Use your judgment to safely allow alert, cooperative patients to have their side rails down during daytime hours without the risk of injury.)*
14. Remove gloves (see illustration) and all protective barriers you are wearing, such as gown, goggles, and masks. Store or remove and dispose of soiled supplies and equipment according to agency policy and guidelines from the CDC and OSHA (see Chapter 12). *(Reduces spread*

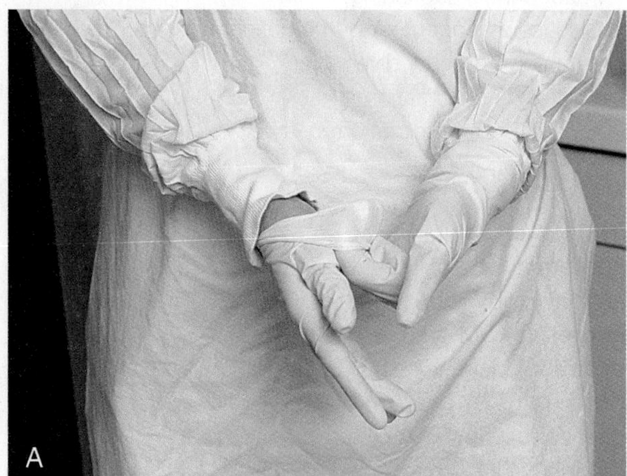

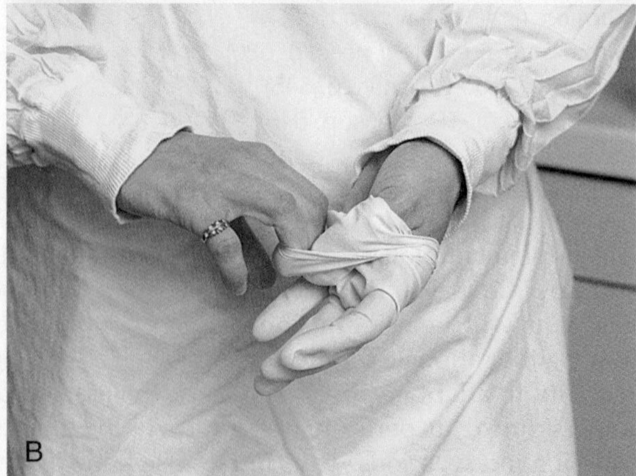

Step 14 Removing disposable gloves. **A,** Nurse places gloved finger inside cuff to pull first glove off hand. **B,** Second glove is removed as nurse slides fingers inside glove cuff and pulls.

of microorganisms, maintains cleanliness of environment, and enhances patient comfort.)

15. Perform hand hygiene after patient contact and after removing gloves. *(Wearing gloves does not eliminate the need to perform hand hygiene. Hand hygiene is the single most important technique in preventing and controlling the spread of microorganisms.)*
16. Document patient's response, expected or unexpected outcomes, and patient teaching. *(Timely and quality documentation records patient progress and promotes continuity of care. Recording also fulfills your legal responsibility.)* Specific areas of documentation are indicated in each skill box.
17. Report any unexpected outcomes. *(Additional therapies will sometimes be necessary.)* Specific notes for reporting are included in each skill.

SKILLS FOR SENSORY DISORDERS

IRRIGATIONS

Eye Irrigations

You will usually perform **irrigations** (a gentle washing of an area with a stream of solution delivered through a syringe) of the eye to relieve local inflammation of the conjunctiva, apply antiseptic solution, or flush out exudate or caustic or irritating solutions. In most cases, use warm normal saline and a small syringe or eyedropper to instill a few hundred milliliters of solution. Always perform irrigation in a direction from the inner to the outer canthus to lessen the chances of contaminants being absorbed through the nasolacrimal duct (Skill 20-1 and Patient Teaching box on eye care). Performing eye irrigation requires the skill and knowledge unique to a nurse. Delegation is inappropriate. Never allow the syringe tip to touch the eye. When caustic chemicals enter the eye, make sure to gently flush the eye continuously for at least 15 minutes with tap water to prevent burning of the cornea, and then refer the patient immediately to a physician.

Patient Teaching

Eye Care

- Use a calm, confident, soft voice when talking with patient, and reinforce the importance of the procedure. For example, "You're doing great; just relax; that's it, we need to flush this out of your eye as completely as possible to lessen the chance on an eye injury."
- Remove contact lenses if possible before beginning an irrigation or applying a compress.
- Reassure patient that eye can be closed periodically and that no object will touch eye.
- Request patient to report any pain or foreign body sensation in the eye after irrigation, as well as any excessive tearing or photophobia.
- Request patient to close the eye and avoid movement and report to you or physician at once if any symptoms occur.
- If a patient is in need of continuing eye irrigations at home but is unable to perform them, teach a responsible family member or caregiver.
- If the patient's field of vision is limited, the home environment should be assessed, and special safety precautions should be taken.

Skill 20-1 Eye Irrigation

Nursing Action *(Rationale)*

1. Refer to standard steps 1 to 9.
2. Assemble equipment:
   - Moisture-proof towel or pad
   - Aseptic or small bulb syringe or plastic squeeze bottle
   - Clean gloves (mask and protective eyewear are optional)
   - Warm irrigation solution as prescribed (volume depends on purpose; 200 to 500 mL) *(Using solutions at body temperature prevent adverse reactions.)*
   - Sterile basin for solution
   - Curved emesis basin
   - Gauze
   - Cotton-tipped applicators
   - Cotton balls
3. Assess condition of both eyes. *(Provides baseline data to help determine change after irrigation.)*
4. Place patient lying toward side to be irrigated. *(Prevents solution from flowing into other eye.)*
5. Place towel under patient's head. *(Prevents soiling of bed linens.)*
6. Use a plastic squeeze bottle unless very large amounts of solutions are needed. Sometimes a medicine dropper is sufficient. *(Depends on purpose of the irrigation.)*
7. Don gloves. *(Reduces spread of microorganisms.)*
8. Place an emesis basin at side of face. *(Collects irrigating solution.)*
9. Pour a small amount of irrigating solution into sterile basin (see Chapter 12).
10. Using the thumb and index finger of the nondominant hand, separate the patient's eyelids. Retraction keeps blinking to a minimum and allows irrigation of conjunctiva. *(Exposes eyeball and facilitates procedure.)* Never rest fingers on the eyeball but on the bone structure above and below the eye. *(Prevents placing direct pressure on the eyeball.)* If desired, wrap a piece of gauze around your gloved index finger to raise upper lid. *(For better cleaning if heavy discharge is present.)*

Continued

Skill 20-1 Eye Irrigation—cont'd

11. Gently direct the irrigating solution along the conjunctiva from the inner to the outer canthus (see illustration). *(Follows the normal directional flow of tears.)* Sometimes only a cotton ball or folded gauze square saturated with the irrigating solution is used (depends on condition of the eye and physician's order).
12. Avoid directing a forceful stream onto the eyeball. *(Reduces spread of microorganisms; also, a more forceful irrigation risks damage to the delicate eye structure.)*
13. Avoid touching any parts of the eye with irrigation equipment. *(Prevents any trauma to the eye structure.)*
14. Gently dry the eyelids with cotton balls. *(Avoids force that could damage the eye structure.)*
15. Refer to standard steps 10 to 17.
16. Document: *(Verifies performance of procedure and ensures continuity of care.)*
    - Duration
    - Type of solution
    - Amount of solution
    - Characteristics of drainage
    - Assessment before and after procedure
    - Patient's response
    - Patient teaching (see Patient Teaching box on eye care)

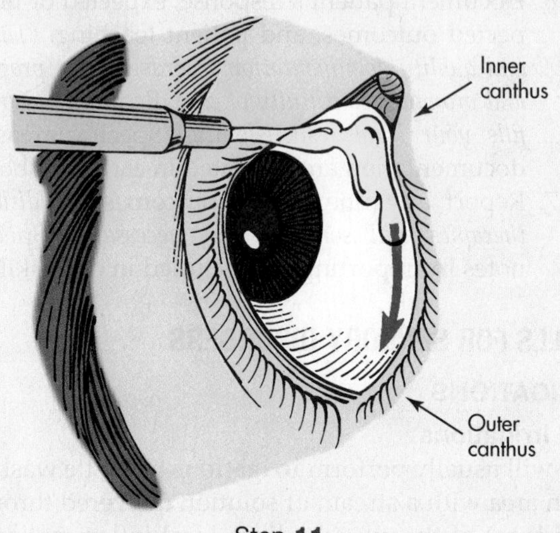

Step **11**

In the home, it is possible for a family member or the patient to perform eye irrigation with an eye cup. These cups are made of plastic or glass and are available in most drugstores. Instruct the patient about proper cleaning of the cup between uses and of the need to check for chips in the glass.

A copious irrigation of the eye is possible with the use of intravenous (IV) tubing and bag connected to a Morgan therapeutic lens. Connected to irrigation tubing, a Morgan lens permits continuous lavage and delivers medication to the eye. Use an adapter to connect the lens to the IV tubing and the solution container. Begin the irrigation at the prescribed flow rate. To insert the device, ask the patient to look down as you insert the lens under the upper eyelid. Then have the patient look up as you retract and release the lower eyelid over the lens.

Skill 20-2 provides directions on applying a warm, moist eye compress.

Ear Irrigations

Use a small syringe and solution at body temperature to cleanse a patient's external auditory canal of excess cerumen or exudate from a lesion or inflamed area. The use of solution at body temperature prevents discomfort and severe vertigo. Avoid irritating the canal's sensitive skin lining by not pulling the auricle excessively or introducing the tip of the irrigating syringe into the canal. Never occlude the auditory canal with the syringe tip because introducing fluid under pressure risks rupturing the tympanic membrane. A slow, gentle irrigation works best (Skill 20-3 and Patient Teaching box on ear care on p. 529). This procedure is contraindicated when a vegetable foreign body (such as a bean) obstructs the auditory canal. These foreign bodies attract and absorb moisture and will swell, causing intense pain and complicating removal of the object. This procedure is also contraindicated if the patient has a cold, an elevated temperature, an ear infection, or an injured or ruptured tympanic membrane. Performing ear irrigation on the external ear requires the skill and knowledge unique to a nurse. Delegation is not appropriate.

Nasal Irrigations

Irrigation of the nasal passages is performed for several reasons. It soothes inflamed mucous membranes and washes away dried mucus, secretions, and, it is hoped, any foreign matter present. If untreated, these dried, crusted deposits pose a risk of obstructing sinus drainage and airflow through the nares and causing headache, unpleasant odors, and infection to develop. The irrigation is possible to accomplish with use of a specially designed, sometimes electronic, device or with a bulb syringe. The skill of irrigating the nares is acceptable to delegate to assistive personnel. Check agency policy. If the irrigation is also to provide a means of administering medications, then delegation is inappropriate.

Skill 20-2 Warm, Moist Eye Compresses

Nursing Action *(Rationale)*

1. Refer to standard steps 1 to 9.
2. Assemble equipment (use separate equipment for bilateral eye infections):
   - Towels and/or waterproof pad
   - Sterile gloves, one pair for each eye treated
   - Basin of hot water
   - Prescribed solution, usually sterile water or normal saline solution
   - Sterile basin for sterile solution
   - Sterile 4 × 4 gauze pads
   - Sterile petroleum jelly or ophthalmic ointment, eyepatch if ordered (often used on skin around the eyes) *(Protects the skin.)*
3. Assess condition of both eyes. *(Provides baseline data to determine change after therapy.)*
4. Assist patient to a comfortable position. When applying hot compresses, have the patient sit, if possible. Support patient's head with a pillow and turn patient's head slightly to the unaffected side. *(This position helps hold the compress in place.)*
5. Place the towel or waterproof pad under patient's head. *(Protects bed linens.)*
6. Use sterile technique when infection or ulceration is present; clean technique is acceptable for allergic reactions. *(Reduces transmission of microorganisms.)*
7. Change gloves, dispose of in proper receptacle, and perform hand hygiene before treating each eye. *(Prevents transmission of microorganisms from one eye to the other.)*
8. Do not allow temperature of compresses to exceed 120° F (49° C). Heat solution by placing the uncapped bottle of solution in a basin of hot water. Pour the warmed solution into a sterile bowl, filling it halfway. Place sterile gauze pads in the bowl. *(Temperatures exceeding 120° F [49° C] will burn the delicate eye structures and the surrounding skin.)*
9. Take two 4 × 4 gauze pads from the basin. Squeeze out excess moisture. *(Prevents excess moisture from dribbling over the patient.)*
10. Instruct the patient to close the eyes. Gently apply the pads—one on top of the other—to the affected eye. Do not exert pressure on eyelids. If the patient complains that the compress is too hot, remove it immediately. *(Promotes patient's safety and prevents skin damage.)*
11. Change compress every few minutes, as necessary, for the prescribed length of time—usually 10 to 20 minutes. *(Maintains consistent temperature for the duration of therapy.)*
12. If sterility is not necessary, it is possible to apply moist heat by means of a clean washcloth. *(Clean technique is sufficient if infection is not present.)*
13. After removing each compress, assess the periorbital skin for signs that the compress solution is too hot. *(Maintains patient's safety.)*
14. Cleanse patient's eye and dry area with the remaining gauze pads. *(Promotes patient comfort.)*
15. If ordered, apply petroleum jelly or ophthalmic ointment, or eyepatch. *(Promotes healing.)*
16. Refer to standard steps 10 to 17.
17. Document: *(Verifies performance of procedure and ensures continuity of care.)*
    - Type of compress
    - Temperature of solution
    - Duration of application
    - Assessment of eyes before and after treatment
    - Application of ointment or dressing
    - Patient's response
    - Patient teaching (see Patient Teaching box on eye care)

Skill 20-3 Ear Irrigation

Nursing Action *(Rationale)*

1. Refer to to standard steps 1 to 9.
2. Assemble equipment:
   - Clean gloves (mask and protective eyewear are optional)
   - Curved emesis basin
   - Towel or moisture-proof pad
   - Cotton-tipped applicator
   - Otoscope
   - Warm irrigating solution prescribed (volume depends on purpose) *(Using solution at body temperature prevents adverse reaction.)*
   - Sterile basin for solution
   - Asepto or small-bulb syringe
   - Cotton balls
3. Advise patient of possible sensations involved: vertigo, fullness, and warmth.

Continued

Skill 20-3 Ear Irrigation—cont'd

4. Assess condition of external ear structures and canal for erythema, edema, and exudate.
5. Assist patient to either a side-lying or sitting position with head tilted toward affected ear, and position emesis basin under ear (patient sometimes helps hold basin) (see illustration). *(Irrigating solution will flow from auditory canal into the basin.)*
6. Place towel under patient's shoulder just under ear and emesis basin. *(Prevents soiling of bed linens.)*
7. Inspect auditory canal for any accumulation of cerumen or debris. Remove what you can see with the naked eye or the otoscope using cotton or the applicator and solution (do not force cerumen into the canal). *(Cleanses the canal for irrigation.)*
8. Assess irrigation solution for proper temperature (body temperature: 98.6° F [37° C]). Test temperature of solution by sprinkling a few drops of solution on your inner wrist. Fill bulb syringe with appropriate volume. *(Irrigating solution at body temperature keeps vertigo and discomfort to a minimum.)*
9. Straighten auditory canal for introduction of solution. In infants, pull auricle (or pinna) down and back. In adults, pull auricle up and back. *(Facilitates entrance and flow of irrigating solution.)*
10. With tip of syringe just above canal, irrigate gently by creating steady flow of solution against roof of canal. Do not occlude canal with tip of syringe (see illustration). *(Occlusion of canal with syringe causes pressure against tympanic membrane during irrigation. Flow of solution drains safely out of the canal while loosening debris.)*
11. Continue irrigation until all debris has been removed or all solution has been used. Reassess auditory canal with otoscope. *(Helps assess whether purpose of irrigation has been accomplished: to cleanse canal, instill antiseptic, or provide local heat.)*

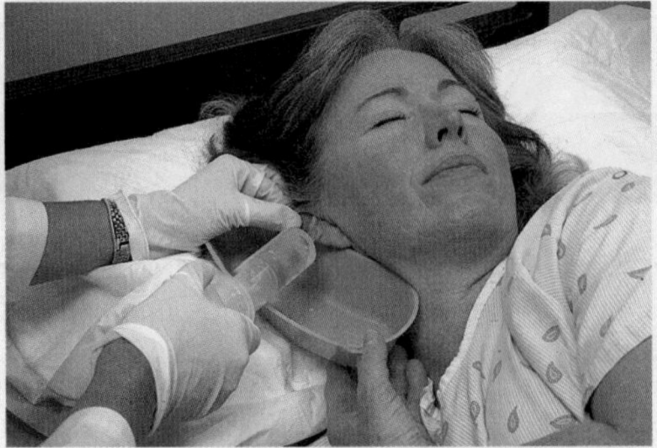

Step 5

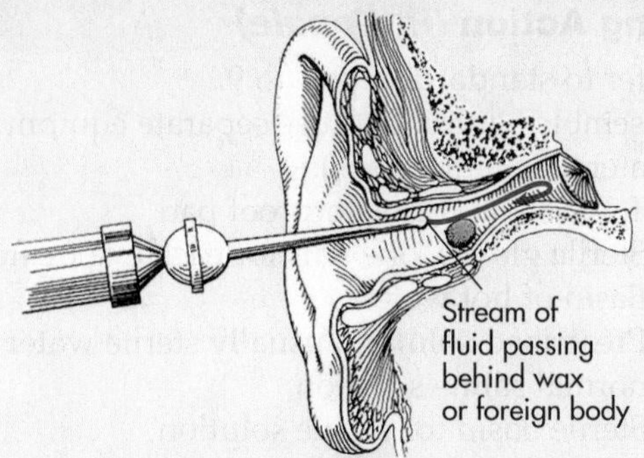

Step 10 Note that the irrigating tip is not occluding the ear canal and therefore allows drainage to occur.

12. Assess patient for vertigo or nausea. Onset of symptoms sometimes makes it necessary to pause the procedure temporarily. *(Irritation of the ear canal from irrigant sometimes causes vertigo and nausea.)*
13. Dry off auricle and apply cotton ball loosely to auditory meatus. *(Promotes comfort. Cotton ball collects excessive drainage.)*
14. Position patient on side of affected ear for 10 minutes. *(Allows solution remaining in auditory canal to drain.)*
15. Refer to standard steps 10 to 17.
16. Return to patient to assess character and amount of drainage and determine patient's level of comfort. *(Enables you to identify patient's tolerance of procedure.)*
17. Document: *(Verifies performance of procedure and ensures continuity of care.)*
    - Type, temperature, and volume of solution used
    - Character of exudate
    - Assessment of the ear canal before and after irrigation
    - Patient's response to irrigation
    - Patient teaching (see Patient Teaching box on ear care)
18. Ten minutes after irrigation, return to patient to remove cotton ball and reassess exudate. Permit patient to resume normal level of activity. *(Increase in exudate or onset of pain indicates possible injury to tympanic membrane.)*

 Patient Teaching

Ear Care

- Talk in a confident, calm voice to help patient relax. As the irrigation begins say, "Now you are going to feel the warm water. I am going to be very careful to do this gently. If you feel any discomfort at all, let me know."
- Advise patient not to make any sudden moves, to prevent trauma to the ear during irrigation.
- Older adults often require ongoing ear care for cerumen removal. Use of a softening agent such as slightly warmed mineral oil (0.5 to 1 mL), twice daily for several days before irrigation, is helpful.
- Older adults with large amounts of ear canal hair, those with a benign growth that narrows the ear canal, and those who habitually wear hearing aids are a higher risk for cerumen impaction.
- Instruct patient to clean ears with a damp washcloth wrapped around a finger. Do not use a cotton-tipped applicator (has potential to rupture eardrum).
- If patient uses a wax softener, instruct that these are softening products only and will not remove a cerumen impaction.
- Instruct patient to report the following signs and symptoms (which indicate a severe cerumen impaction) to the physician right away:
  —Decrease in hearing
  —Pain
  —Tinnitus (ringing in the ear)
  —Crackling noise in the ear

Patients with acute or chronic nasal conditions, including rhinitis, Sjögren's syndrome, or sinusitis, and patients who inhale allergens (e.g., coal dust) and toxins (e.g., paint fumes, sawdust, pesticides) often derive benefits from nasal irrigations. Sometimes the physician will order nasal irrigations after certain nasal surgeries to enhance healing by removing debris and stimulating repair of the mucosal membranes.

Advanced destruction of the sinuses, foreign bodies in the nasal passages (which it is possible to drive further in by irrigating), and frequent nosebleeds are contraindications to nasal irrigation. However, some physicians will order a nasal irrigation for these patients anyway, because they sometimes benefit in spite of the contraindications (Skill 20-4).

SKILLS FOR HEAT AND COLD THERAPY

Patients who have experienced injury to some part of the body often benefit from the application of heat and/or cold therapy. It is your responsibility to ensure patient safety during this therapy. Make sure you know how to operate equipment, assess the skin integrity of the body part, and verify the patient's ability to perceive temperature variations. Also ensure that the physician's order for the therapy is being implemented and be knowledgeable of how the body

Skill 20-4 Performing a Nasal Irrigation

Nursing Action *(Rationale)*

1. Refer to standard steps 1 to 9.
2. Assemble equipment and supplies: *(Organizes procedure.)*
   - Irrigating device (kits are available at most pharmacies)
   - Bulb syringe or oral irrigation device such as a Waterpik
   - Rigid or flexible disposable irrigation tip (for one patient's use only)
   - Plastic sheet
   - Apron or towels
   - Facial tissues
   - Bath basin or sink
   - Gloves
   - Hypertonic saline solution (500 to 1000 mL)
3. Describe sensations patient is likely to experience (e.g., feelings of fullness in the sinuses, warmth, and wetness). *(Relieves patient's anxiety.)*
4. Assess patient's comfort level and any nasal discharge. *(Provides baseline for assessment postprocedure.)*
5. Don gloves, and if used for assessment, remove, dispose of appropriately, and perform hand hygiene. *(Prevents spread of microorganisms.)*
6. Assemble and prepare equipment:
   - Warm saline solution (105° F [40.5° C]). *(Unlike a cold solution, a warm solution is comfortable and promotes healing.)*
   - If using an electrical device, plug instrument into an outlet near the patient. *(Facilitates procedure.)* Run about 240 mL of the saline solution through the tubing. *(Rinses any residual solution from the tubing and warms the tubing.)*
   - If using a bulb syringe, draw some warmed irrigant into the bulb and then expel. *(Rinses any residual solution from previous irrigation and warms the bulb.)*
7. Don disposable gloves. *(Reduces spread of microorganisms.)*
8. Have patient sit comfortably near the equipment in a position that allows the irrigation device tip to enter the nose without obstructing the return flow of irrigant. Assist patient to sit upright with the head bent forward over the collecting receptacle (basin or sink) and with the chest well flexed. The nose and the ear should be on the same plane vertically. *(The patient is less likely to breathe in the solution when holding the head in this position. This position will also keep solution from entering the eustachian*

Continued

Skill 20-4 Performing a Nasal Irrigation—cont'd

tube, which will now lie above the level of the solution stream.) Provide towels to collect any excess moisture. *(Helps keep patient dry and provides comfort.)*

9. Instruct patient to keep the mouth open and to breathe rhythmically during the procedure. *(This causes the soft palate to seal the throat, allowing the irrigant to flow out the other nostril and bring any discharge with it.)*
10. Instruct patient to neither speak nor swallow during the procedure. *(This prevents forcing any infectious material into the eustachian tube and/or sinuses.)*
11. If the patient reports the need to sneeze or cough, remove the irrigating device tip from the patient's nares. *(Helps prevent injury to the nasal mucosa.)*
12. Perform procedure.
    a. If using a commercial kit, follow directions on package.
    b. **Using an electrical irrigating device:** Insert the tip about ½ to 1 inch (1 to 3 cm) into the patient's nostril and turn on the irrigating device. Begin with a low-pressure setting, increasing pressure as needed. *(Obtains a gentle stream of irrigant, which helps prevent forcing material from the nose into the sinuses or eustachian tube, which poses risk of causing infection.)* Insert the irrigation tip far enough into the patient's nostril to ensure that the irrigating solution cleans the nasal membranes before draining out. Irrigate both nostrils.
    c. **Using a bulb syringe:**
        (1) Fill bulb with warm saline solution and insert tip about ½ to 1 inch (1 to 3 cm) into the patient's nostril. *(Prepares for effective procedure.)*
        (2) Squeeze bulb until a gentle stream of warm solution washes through the nose. Avoid forceful squeezing. Alternate nostrils until the return solution is clear. *(A gentle squeeze helps prevent forcing debris from the nasal passages up into the sinuses or eustachian tube, which poses risk of causing infection.)*
13. Inspect return solution for: *(Indicates possible infection that is necessary to report to physician.)*
    - Color
    - Viscosity
    - Volume
    - Blood
    - Necrotic material
14. Request that the patient wait a few minutes after the procedure before blowing excess fluid from the nostrils. Expect fluid to drain from the patient's nose for a brief time after the procedure and before the nose is blown. *(Allows for more thorough cleansing of mucous membranes.)* Instruct patient to blow gently from both nostrils at once. *(Prevents fluid or pressure buildup in the sinuses and helps loosen and expel any crusted secretions and mucus.)* Provide tissues. *(Helps contain secretions.)*
15. Clean irrigating equipment with soap and water, and then disinfect it according to agency policy. *(Prevents spread of microorganisms.)* Rinse, dry, and properly store equipment. *(Readies supplies for next procedure.)*
16. Refer to standard steps 10 to 17.
17. Document: *(Verifies performance of procedure and ensures continuity of care.)*
    - Time
    - Duration of procedure
    - Type of solution used (formula of ingredients used)
    - Amount and temperature of solution used
    - Appearance of returns
    - Assessment of patient's comfort level and breathing ease before and after procedure
    - Patient teaching. *(Ensures continuity of care.)* To teach irrigations at home, include the following points:
      —How to prepare saline solution:
        (1) Fill a clean 1-L plastic bottle with bottled or distilled water (4 cups + 1 oz = 1 L).
        (2) Add 1 teaspoon of noniodized salt. Some physicians order 1 teaspoon of soda also.
      —How to disinfect used devices at home:
        (1) Rinse well to remove debris. Follow cleaning directions that accompany electrical device or equipment (other than the bulb syringe).
        (2) How to hold the head for optimal safety, comfort, and effectiveness. *(Facilitates smooth progression of procedure.)*

responds to local applications of heat or cold (Potter & Perry, 2009).

Even though the skin's normal surface temperature is 93.2° F (34° C), the body's temperature receptors adapt well to temperatures in the wide range between 113° F (45° C) and 59° F (15° C). Typically, patients exposed to temperatures beyond 113° F (45° C) experience pain and burning, and exposure to temperatures below 59° F (15° C) causes numbness followed by pain. This wide range of adaptability, along with decreased sensitivity to temperature extremes, creates the risk of injury. Initially patients are able to sense

Table 20-1 **Factors in Preventing Injury from Heat and Cold Applications**

FACTOR	RATIONALE
Very young patients or older adult patients	Thinner skin layers in children and older adults increase risk of burns. Older patients have reduced sensitivity to pain.
Open wounds, skin impairment, stomas	Subcutaneous and visceral tissues are more sensitive to temperature variations. They also contain no temperature receptors and fewer pain receptors.
Areas of edema or scar formation	Reduced sensation to temperature stimuli occurs because of thickening of skin layers from fluid buildup or scar formation.
Peripheral vascular disease (e.g., diabetes, arteriosclerosis)	Body's extremities are less sensitive to temperature and pain stimuli because of circulatory impairment and local tissue injury. Cold application further compromises blood flow.
Disorientation or unconsciousness	Reduced perception of temperature extremes occurs.
Spinal cord injury	Alterations in nerve pathways prevent reception of sensory or painful stimuli.
Abscessed tooth or appendix	Infection is highly localized. Application of heat potentially causes rupture with spread of microorganisms systemically.

From Potter, P.A., & Perry, A.G. (2009). *Fundamentals of nursing: concepts, process, and practice.* (7th ed.). St. Louis: Mosby.

temperature changes, but within a short time, the patient's skin adapts to the temperature and the patient no longer feels the change. Therefore, it is imperative to identify those patients at greatest risk for developing injuries related to heat and cold applications (Table 20-1 and Life Span Considerations for Older Adults box on cold applications) (Potter & Perry, 2009).

LOCAL EFFECTS OF HEAT AND COLD

Heat produces vasodilation, whereas cold produces vasoconstriction. The physician considers these factors when choosing the proper therapy based on the needs of the patient.

Effects of Heat Application

Vasodilation causes the **lumen** (hollow channel within a tube) of blood vessels to dilate, increasing blood flow to that area of the body. However, if heat applications are applied to an area of the body for more than 1 hour, a heat-conserving mechanism sets in: vessels begin to constrict, decreasing blood flow to that area. In addition, heat application for more than 1 hour sometimes causes damage to epithelial cells, erythema, tenderness, and blistering. Therefore, it is important to apply heat for proper intervals in order to increase its therapeutic effects and help prevent complications (Potter & Perry, 2009).

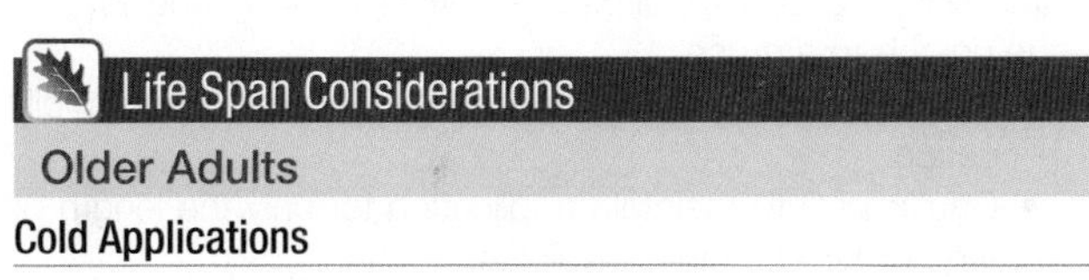

Life Span Considerations

Older Adults

Cold Applications

- Older adults are more sensitive to cold.
- Remain with the patient for the first 5 minutes of treatment to assess subjective response.
- Consider shortening duration of therapy.
- Assess skin every 2 to 3 minutes after first 10 minutes of therapy.
- Older adults frequently require more covering for warmth.

Effects of Cold Application

Exposure of the skin to cold results in **vasoconstriction** (the lumen of the blood vessel narrows). The term *tissue ischemia* (decreased blood supply to a body part or organ; often accompanied by pain and organ dysfunction) refers to tissue cells that are lacking in sufficient blood flow and nutrients. When the skin is exposed to cold, it initially becomes erythematous or reddened. This is generally followed by the skin taking on a mottled appearance (bluish purple discoloration), as well as a burning pain. If exposure to extreme cold continues for an extensive period, the skin will actually freeze (Potter & Perry, 2009).

ASSESSMENT

To prevent further injury, assess the patient for any signs of impairment in skin integrity and assess the patient's general condition for any indications of possible intolerance to heat or cold before applying either therapy. This assessment also enables you to determine the effectiveness of therapy and identify any complications following applications. It is also possible to assess the patient's ability to distinguish heat and cold temperature variations by observing the reaction to light touch or pinprick (Box 20-1 and Coordinated Care box on heat and cold therapy).

Also assess the patient for any contraindications to the use of either heat or cold therapy. Contraindications to heat therapy include any bleeding, since vasodilation caused by heat will increase bleeding; inflammation, which will sometimes worsen with heat; and cardiovascular problems, since heat has the potential to cause considerable vasodilation and thus interrupt blood flow to vital organs.

Cold therapy is contraindicated in several conditions. Do not use cold applications if edema has already occurred, since cold will decrease circulation to the area and prevent absorption of the interstitial fluid that has accumulated. Additional contraindications include impaired circulation, since cold reduces blood

Box 20-1 Factors Influencing Heat and Cold Tolerance

The body's response to heat and cold applications depends on the following factors:

- **Duration of treatment.** Short exposure to temperature extremes is better tolerated than lengthy exposure.
- **Body part.** Certain areas of the skin are more sensitive to temperature variations. These include the neck, the inner aspect of the wrist and forearm, and the perineal region. The foot and the palm of the hand are less sensitive.
- **Damage to body surface.** Exposed skin layers are more sensitive to temperature variations.
- **Prior skin temperature.** The body responds best to minor temperature adjustments. If a body part is cool and a hot stimulus touches the skin, the response is greater than if the stimulus is warm. (A gradual change in temperature is preferred.)
- **Body surface area.** People have less tolerance to temperature changes when a large area of the body is exposed to heat or cold.
- **Age and physical condition.** Tolerance to temperature variations changes with age. Patients who are very young and older adults are most sensitive to the heat and cold. If a patient's physical condition reduces the reception of sensory stimuli, tolerance to temperature extremes is high, but the risk of injury is also high.

From Potter, P.A., & Perry, A.G. (2007). *Basic nursing: essentials for practice.* (6th ed.). St. Louis: Mosby.

supply further, and shivering. Cold will likely increase shivering, resulting in a significant increase in body temperature (Potter & Perry, 2009).

It is essential to frequently observe patients with heat or cold applications who have an altered level of consciousness or are disoriented, since these patients are at an increased risk of complications from either type of application. You are also responsible for ensuring that equipment being used for heat and cold applications is in proper working order. Monitor fluid-containing equipment for any leaks. Monitor electrical equipment for any damaged cords or wires. Also check for even distribution of temperature of the equipment (Potter & Perry, 2009). Uneven temperature distribution suggests that the equipment is not functioning properly.

PATIENT SAFETY

Before the application of heat or cold therapy, instruct the patient on the purpose of therapy, the signs and symptoms of complications from therapy, and safety measures to prevent injury from therapy (Potter & Perry, 2009) (Box 20-2).

PHYSICIAN'S ORDER

A physician's order indicating the area, the frequency, and the intended duration is necessary for the application of heat or cold therapy. Sometimes the physician will order a specific temperature; in other cases, you will follow your facility's policy for temperatures of applications (Potter & Perry, 2009) (Table 20-2).

MOIST OR DRY APPLICATIONS

The physician will order either moist or dry applications. Determining factors for which application is appropriate include the type of injury, the type of wound, the area of the body affected, and whether any drainage or inflammation is present.

HOT, MOIST COMPRESSES

If a wound is open, it is necessary to use sterile compresses. A **compress** consists of gauze that is moistened with a prescribed warm solution. Sterile hot, moist compresses increase circulation to the affected area, decrease edema, and consolidate any purulent exudates, among other beneficial effects. Somewhat different from a compress, a hot pack is a large piece of cloth that is used on larger areas of the body.

Coordinated Care

Delegation

HEAT AND COLD THERAPY

Application of moist heat is acceptable to delegate to assistive personnel (AP). The skill of dry heat application and the necessary assessment and evaluation of the condition of the patient's skin requires critical thinking and application of knowledge unique to a nurse.

- Caution AP to maintain proper temperature of the application.
- Caution AP to maintain application for only the length of time ordered by the physician.
- Caution AP to check patient's skin for excessive redness and pain during application and to report any such adverse reactions to you.
- Ask AP to report to you when the treatment is complete so that you have the opportunity to evaluate the patient's response.

The application of cold therapy to intact skin is acceptable to delegate to assistive personnel. The skill of cold application and the necessary assessment and evaluation of the condition of the patient's skin requires the critical thinking and knowledge unique to a nurse.

- Caution AP to maintain proper temperature of the application.
- Caution AP to maintain application for only the length of time ordered by the physician.
- Caution AP to check patient's skin for excessive redness or pain and immediately report such adverse reactions to you.
- Ask AP to report to you when the treatment is complete so that you have the opportunity to evaluate the patient's response.

Box 20-2 Safety Measures When Applying Heat or Cold Therapy

- Explain to the patient sensations to be felt during the procedure. The treatment is meant to feel warm, but have the patient notify you if it feels uncomfortably so; in this case, discontinue the treatment.
- Instruct the patient to report changes in sensation or discomfort immediately.
- Provide a timer, clock, or watch so that the patient is able to help time the application.
- Keep the call light within the patient's reach.
- Refer to the agency's policy and procedure manual for safe temperatures.
- Do not allow the patient to adjust temperature settings (see Table 20-2).
- Do not allow the patient to move the material used for application of heat or cold or place hands on the wound site.
- Do not place the patient in a position that prevents movement away from the temperature source.
- Do not leave unattended a patient who is unable to sense temperature changes or move from the temperature source.
- Never use microwave ovens to heat compresses because the temperature achieved is often erratic and imprecise, and burns result easily.
- Never use pins to secure aquathermia or electric heating pad. Shock may occur.
- Never use pins to secure a chemical pack because it will leak and cause a burn.
- If bleeding, erythema, underlying inflammation, or elevated body temperature occurs, do not apply heat because it will only aggravate the problem.
- Use sterile supplies if there is an open wound.
- Patients with cardiac difficulty will sometimes develop hypotension, so be alert for vertigo and syncope and monitor blood pressure.

Modified from Potter, P.A., & Perry, A.G. (2009). *Fundamentals of nursing: concepts, process, and practice.* (7th ed.). St. Louis: Mosby.

Table 20-2 Temperature Ranges for Hot and Cold Applications

TEMPERATURE	FAHRENHEIT RANGE	CENTIGRADE RANGE
Very hot	105° to 115° F	41° to 46° C
Hot	98° to 105° F	37° to 41° C
Warm	93° to 98° F	34° to 37° C
Tepid	80° to 93° F	26° to 34° C
Cool	65° to 80° F	18° to 26° C
Cold	50° to 65° F	10° to 18° C

To maintain the temperature of a compress, it is necessary to either change the compress frequently or wrap the compress in an aquathermia pad, waterproof heating pad, a piece of plastic, or a dry towel. Remember that moist heat is a better conductor of heat than dry heat; therefore, maintain lower temperature settings for moist heat than for dry heat applications. In addition, keep the patient warm by keeping the room free from drafts or covering the patient with a light blanket, since moist heat will cause evaporation of heat from the skin as a result of the vasodilation (Potter & Perry, 2009) (Skill 20-5 and Home Care Considerations box on cold applications).

WARM SOAKS

Soaks involve immersing a body part in a warm solution or wrapping a body part in dressings that have been saturated with a warm solution. The benefits of soaks include increased circulation to the affected area, reduction of edema, wound debridement, muscle relaxation, and ability to apply medicated solution to large areas. Another method of accomplishing this is the whirlpool treatment (Figure 20-1).

To administer a soak, warm the solution to a temperature of 105° to 110° F (40.5° to 43° C). Then, taking care to maintain patient comfort, immerse the affected body part in the solution. Place waterproof pads under

 Home Care Considerations

Cold Applications

- Keeping gel packs in the freezer at home makes cold treatments easy.
- Teach patients never to use on skin any cold packs used in freezer chests for food or beverages.
- Suggest using a bucket filled with ice and water to immerse foot, hand, or elbow. Use a bath thermometer to test temperature.
- Freeze water in a plastic foam cup, and use it to treat a sprain or strain. Peel off the rim of the cup to or below the level of the ice, and apply ice in a circular motion.
- A bag of frozen vegetables conforms readily to a body part needing cold therapy for a brief time.
- Put ice and water in a zipper-locked bag to quickly make an ice bag for home use.

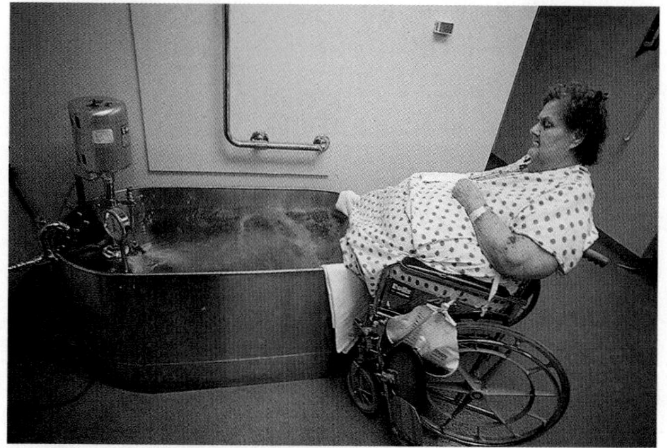

FIGURE 20-1 Whirlpool moist heat therapy. Note the towel placed over the edge of the tub beneath the patient's legs to prevent injury and promote comfort.

Skill 20-5 Applying a Hot, Moist Compress to an Open Wound

Nursing Action *(Rationale)*

1. Refer to standard steps 1 to 9.
2. Assemble equipment:
   - Waterproof pad
   - Prescribed solution warmed to appropriate temperature, approximately 110° to 115° F (43° to 46° C)
   - Sterile container for solution
   - Sterile gauze dressings
   - Commercially prepared compresses (optional)
   - Aquathermia or heating pad (optional)
   - Disposable gloves
   - Sterile gloves
   - Petroleum jelly (optional)
   - Sterile cotton swabs
   - Tape or ties
   - Dry bath towel
   - Bath thermometer
   - Bath blanket
3. Describe sensations to be felt (e.g., feeling of warmth and wetness). Explain precautions to prevent burning. *(Promotes cooperation, decreases patient's anxiety, and prepares patient.)*
4. Assess condition of exposed skin and wound on which compress is to be applied (see illustration). *(Provides baseline for determination of changes in skin during heat application. Very thin or impaired skin is more susceptible to injury from heat.)*
5. Place waterproof pad under area to be treated. *(Protects bed linens.)*
6. Assemble equipment. Pour warmed solution into sterile container. (If using portable heating source, keep solution warm. It is acceptable to leave commercially prepared compresses under infrared lamp until just before use.) Open sterile packages and drop gauze into container to immerse in solution. Set aquathermia pad (if used) to correct temperature and assess fluid level of unit. *(It is necessary for compresses to retain warmth for therapeutic benefit.)*

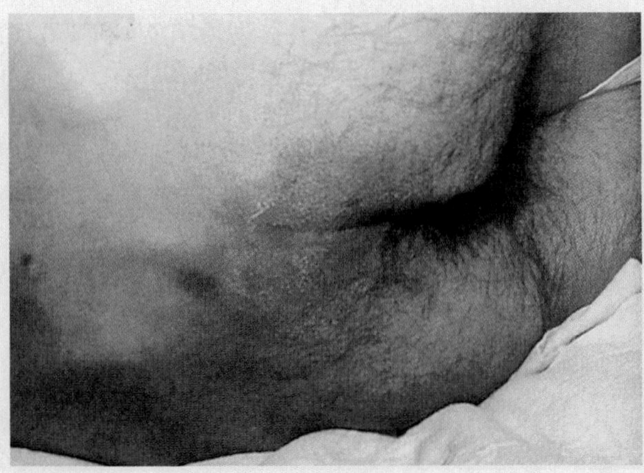

Step 4

7. Don disposable gloves. Remove any existing dressings covering wound. Dispose of gloves and dressings in proper receptacle. *(Reduces spread of microorganisms.)*
8. Apply sterile gloves. *(Allows you to manipulate sterile dressing and touch open wound.)*
9. Apply sterile petroleum jelly (optional) with cotton swab to skin around wound. Do not apply jelly on impaired skin. *(Protects skin from possible burns and maceration.)*
10. Pick up one layer of immersed gauze and squeeze out excess water. *(Excess moisture macerates skin and increases risk of burns and infections.)*
11. Apply gauze lightly to open wound. Observe response and ask whether patient feels discomfort. In a few seconds, lift edge of gauze to assess for erythema. *(Enables you to determine appropriate temperature; prevents burns.)*
12. If patient tolerates compress, pack gauze snugly against wound. Be certain all wound surfaces are covered by hot compress. *(Prevents rapid cooling from underlying air currents.)*
13. Wrap or cover moist compress with dry bath towel. If necessary, pin or tie in place. *(Insulates compress to prevent heat loss.)*
14. Change hot compress frequently as ordered. *(Prevents cooling and maintains therapeutic benefit of compress.)*
15. Apply aquathermia or waterproof heating pad over compress (optional). Keep it in place for desired duration of application (20 to 30 minutes). *(Promotes consistent temperature of compress. Local application of heat for more than 60 minutes often results in vasoconstriction. Removing hot compress after 30 minutes and reapplying in 15 minutes, if desired, maintains vasodilation and positive therapeutic effects.)*
16. Assess patient periodically for discomfort or burning sensation. Observe area of skin not covered by compress. *(Continued exposure to heat poses risk of burns to skin.)*
17. Remove pad, towel, and compress in 30 minutes. Again assess wound and condition of skin. *(Continued exposure to moisture will macerate skin. Prevents injury.)*
18. Apply dry, sterile dressing as ordered. *(Prevents entrance of microorganisms into wound site.)*
19. Refer to standard steps 10 to 17.
20. Ask patient if an unusual burning sensation is noticed that was not felt before. *(It is often difficult*

to determine the presence of a burn merely by color changes, if wound is inflamed or exudate is present.)

21. Document: *(Verifies performance of procedure and ensures continuity of care.)*
    - Type of application
    - Location and duration of application
    - Temperature of application
    - Condition of wound and skin
    - Patient response to therapy. *(Burn or other change will probably make future therapies necessary.)*

See Chapter 13 for additional wound care techniques.

the soak, and cover the container with towels or waterproof pads to keep heat loss to a minimum. The solution usually retains the desired temperature for approximately 10 minutes. As the temperature cools, it will be necessary to add heated solution to maintain a constant temperature; it is important to elevate the body part from the water while adding the heated solution. Upon completion of the soak, dry the body part completely to prevent tissue maceration (Potter & Perry, 2009).

PARAFFIN BATHS

A paraffin bath consists of a mixture of heated paraffin wax and mineral oil (1 part oil to 5 parts paraffin). Patients with painful arthritis or other joint discomforts of the hands and feet benefit most from these baths. In many institutions, only physical therapists administer the applications. Patients often heat paraffin baths at home in double boilers. Containers and appliances are now available for home use. Instruct patients to have the bath temperature at 128° to 130° F (53.3° to 54.5° C).

AQUATHERMIA (WATER-FLOW) PADS (K-PADS)

In health care institutions, the aquathermia pad—also known as a water-flow pad or K-pad (Figure 20-2)—is used as a source of moist or dry heat application in lieu of conventional heating pads. Aquathermia pads are safer than heating pads since a precise temperature is set by inserting a plastic key into the temperature regulator, or preset by the facilities central supply department. In addition, the pad is waterproof and works by circulating distilled water through the internal channels of the pad via hoses connected to an electrical unit that houses a heating element and motor.

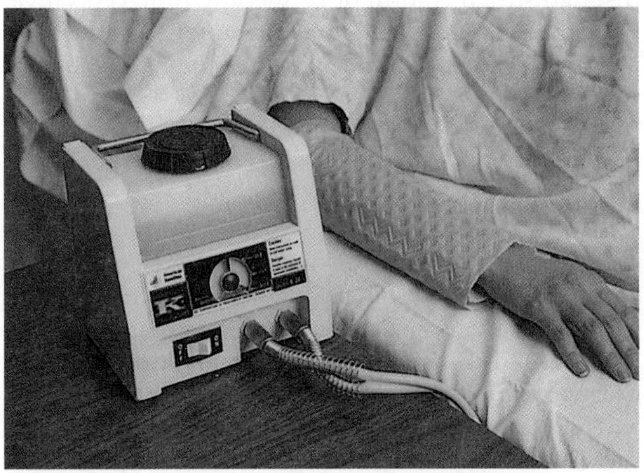
FIGURE 20-2 Aquathermia pad.

The recommended temperature setting for the aquathermia pad is between 105° and 110° F (40.5° and 43° C). To ensure proper functioning and safety of the unit and even distribution of water circulation, make sure the tubing is kept even with the unit and is secured in place. As the water reservoir runs low, fill the unit with distilled water rather than tap water to prevent mineral deposits from forming in the unit. Patients who benefit from the aquathermia pad include those with muscle strains, mild inflammation, and edema.

Place a thin towel or pillowcase next to the patient's skin so that the pad is not in direct contact with the patient. Secure the pad with tape, ties, or gauze rolls. Never secure aquathermia pads with safety pins, since this sometimes causes the heated water to leak. In addition, do not allow patients to lie on the pad, since this prevents even heat distribution. Applications typically last for 20 to 30 minutes. Assess the skin periodically during the application for any signs of burning. In the case of conditions such as thrombophlebitis, some physicians order the application on for 1 hour and off for 3 hours (Potter & Perry, 2009).

COMMERCIAL HOT PACKS

Warm, dry heat applications are possible with the use of commercially available disposable hot packs. Release of heat occurs when the chemicals contained in the pack are mixed by squeezing, kneading, or sticking the pack, according to package directions. Also follow instructions regarding the recommended time for applications.

Hot-water bottles are not recommended in acute care facilities. If they are used in the home setting, it is essential to practice extreme caution to prevent burns.

ELECTRIC HEATING PADS

Heating pads, frequently used in the home setting, are a conventional method of heat application. Heating pads contain an electrical coil surrounded by a waterproof pad covered by cotton or flannel fabric. The temperature regulation for these units is limited to the choice of low, medium, and high settings instead of exact temperatures. Safety precautions include avoiding the following: lying on the pad, using the high setting, and securing the pad with a safety pin (which poses the risk of causing electrical shock). Heating pads are not recommended in acute care facilities (Potter & Perry, 2009).

COLD, MOIST, AND DRY COMPRESSES

Cold compresses are either clean or sterile. Apply them for 20 minutes at 59° F (15° C). You will typically use cold compresses to treat inflammation and prevent edema; the procedure for application is the same as for warm compresses (see Skill 20-5).

Commercially prepared disposable cold packs work like disposable hot packs. They are packaged in various sizes and shapes and permit dry cold application. You are responsible for assessing the patient for signs of complications from cold therapy, including erythema, burning, numbness, mottling, extreme paleness, and cyanosis (blue discoloration of the skin). Teach the patient that there is a normal progression of sensation change during cold therapy: first cold, then pain relief followed by burning skin pain, and finally numbness. If the skin is uncovered or if the application has not been covered, apply towels (sterile towels over an injured area) and then apply cold application to the skin (Figure 20-3). To prevent frostnip, remove the cold pack or compress when the area feels numb.

ICE BAGS OR COLLARS

Ice bags or collars serve to reduce edema formation and bleeding and provide an anesthetic effect to areas of injury. Ice bags and collars are ideal methods of application to treat areas of localized hemorrhage and hematoma formation as well as for patients who have undergone dental surgery and those with muscle strain. Implement the following measures when using these devices: (1) Ensure there are no defects with the device by filling it with water to check for leaks. (2) Fill devices to a maximum of two thirds full of crushed ice so that the application will mold well to the body part and not be too heavy on the area. (3) Eliminate excess air from the device before securing the cap. Conduction of cold is interrupted by excess air in the device. (4) Dry excess moisture from the device and cover with flannel material, a towel, or a pillowcase. (5) Apply the ice pack or collar for 30 minutes and remove it after 1 hour (Potter & Perry, 2009).

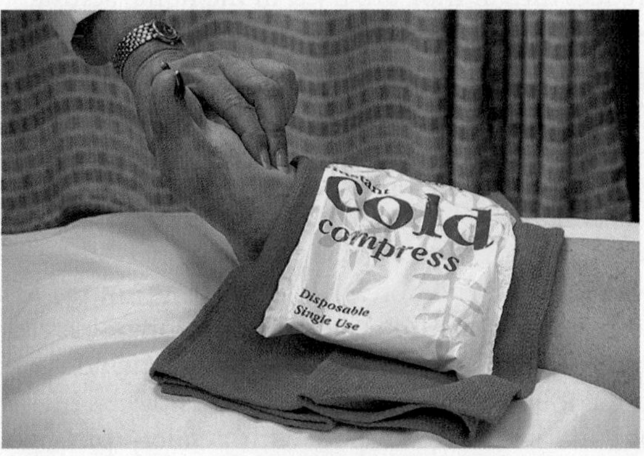

FIGURE 20-3 Commercial cold pack used for therapy.

SKILLS FOR ADMINISTERING PARENTERAL FLUIDS

Healing is directly associated with well-nourished body cells. In the absence of adequate electrolytes and nutrients, healing is hindered. For surgical patients, a patent **intravenous (IV)** site is maintained for the administration of nutrients, fluids, medications, and blood. The main goal of fluid IV administration is to correct or prevent fluid and electrolyte imbalances. Poor tissue absorption, inadequate gastrointestinal (GI) tract function, and the need for maintaining medications at optimum levels are indicators for IV therapy. IV therapy continues postoperatively until the patient tolerates fluids and oral nutrients. Also, medications delivered by IV route are absorbed much faster.

Observe the following three guidelines when monitoring IV therapy: (1) monitor the solution drip rate and maintain the infusion rate ordered, (2) infuse the amount of prescribed solution, and (3) maintain the patency of the IV **catheter** (a flexible tube that is possible to insert into a vessel or cavity of the body to withdraw or instill fluids). It is best to monitor the site every 1 to 2 hours, and assess the IV line at least every 4 hours.

INTRAVENOUS THERAPY AND VENIPUNCTURE

The most common method of drawing a blood sample involves inserting a hollow-bore needle into the lumen of a large vein. Peripheral IV therapy is the administration of fluid, electrolytes, nutrients or medications through an over-the-needle catheter or needle inserted into a vein in the arm. Fluid therapy is initiated by inserting the needle or cannula into a vein and connecting it to tubing through which the fluid is administered. During **peripheral** (pertaining to the outside surface, or surrounding area of an organ or other structure or fluid of vision) therapy, record the patient's intake and output (I&O). The term *peripheral* distinguishes this form of IV therapy from central venous therapy. Central venous therapy is administered through a catheter in the subclavian vein, the jugular vein, the vena cava, or the right atrium.

Each state nurse practice act determines the legal guidelines, and agency policies further define the qualifications of nurses allowed to administer IV medications or fluids, blood, or blood products (see Coordinated Care box on intravenous therapy). Only nurses who have been specially trained and who meet the legal qualifications and agency guidelines are involved in IV administration. Not all nurses are expected or required to administer IV therapy.

There are several steps to performing a **venipuncture** (insertion of a needle into a vein for the purpose of drawing a venous blood specimen) (Skill 20-6 and Figures 20-4 and 20-5). Before the procedure, assemble and

Text continued on p. 541

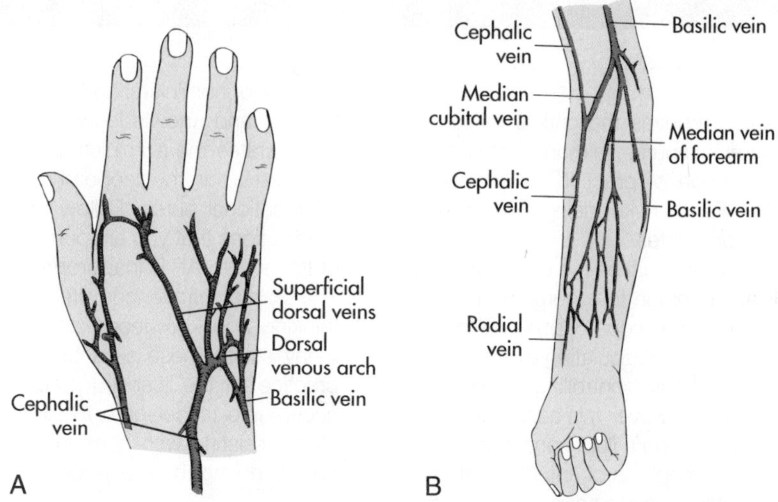

FIGURE 20-4 Common intravenous sites. **A,** Dorsal surface of the hand. **B,** Inner arm.

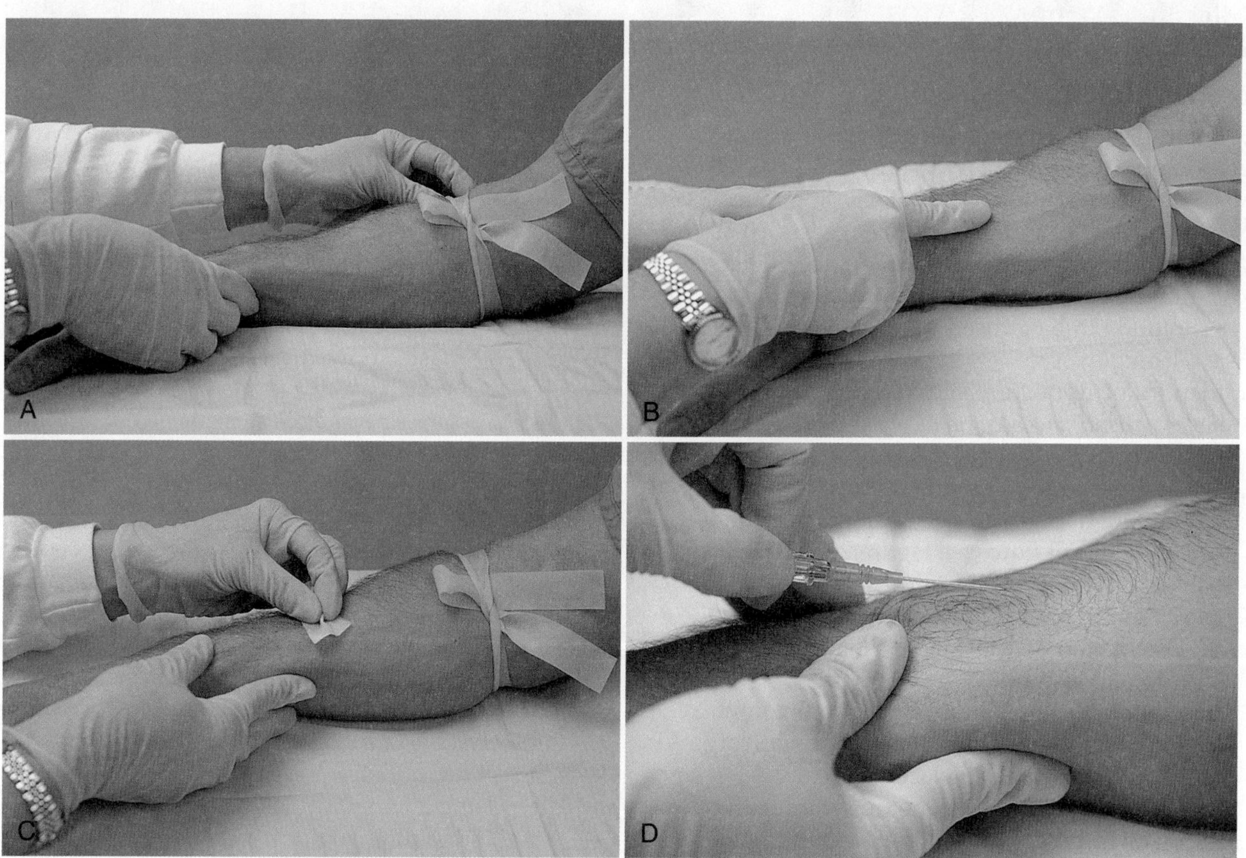

FIGURE 20-5 **A,** Apply tourniquet. **B,** Select intravenous site. **C,** Cleanse site for venipuncture. **D,** Pull skin taut as catheter is inserted.

 Coordinated Care

Collaboration

INTRAVENOUS THERAPY

- The skill of basic IV insertion requires the critical thinking knowledge application unique to a nurse. In many states this skill is included within the scope of practice for licensed practical (vocational) nurses. For this skill, delegation to assistive personnel (AP) is inappropriate.
- The skill of regulating IV flow rates requires the critical thinking and knowledge application unique to a nurse. In many states this skill is included within the scope of practice for licensed practical (vocational) nurses. Calculating and adjusting flow rates on gravity or electronic controlling devices is inappropriate for AP to perform. However, it is acceptable to delegate AP to inform the nurse when a fluid container is almost empty, when the patient complains of any discomfort, and when an electronic controlling device sounds an alarm.
- The skill of administering IV medications requires the critical thinking and knowledge application unique to a nurse. In many states the administration of certain IV medications is included within the scope of practice for a licensed practical or vocational nurse. Follow agency policy for the specific medications that you are permitted to administer. Delegation of this skill to AP is inappropriate.
- The skills of intravenous site maintenance require the critical thinking and knowledge application unique to a nurse. In many states these skills are included within the scope of practice for the licensed practical or vocational nurse. It is acceptable to delegate to AP the tasks of collecting supplies, assisting with comfort measures, and distracting the patient during the procedure.

Skill 20-6 Initiating Intravenous Therapy

Nursing Action *(Rationale)*

1. Refer to standard steps 1 to 9.
2. Assemble equipment:
   - Intravenous infusion tray, including tourniquet, alcohol swab or special agent such as povidone-iodine (Betadine), angiocatheter, tubing, adhesive tape, and dressing
   - Solution to be infused
   - Clean gloves
3. Identify venipuncture sites (see Figure 20-4). *(Promotes patient movement and comfort and locating adequate vein for infusion.)*
4. Apply tourniquet. Properly applied, tourniquet is tight enough to impede venous return but not occlude arterial flow (see Figure 20-5, *A*). *(Facilitates observation and puncture of distended veins.)*
5. Select venipuncture site (see Figure 20-5, *B*).
   a. Use the most distal site in the nondominant arm, if possible.
   b. Avoid areas that are painful to palpation.
   c. In the nondominant arm, select a vein large enough for catheter placement.
   d. Choose a site that will not interfere with planned procedures or the patient's activities of daily living.
      (1) Palpate the vein by pressing downward and noting the resistant, soft, bouncy feeling as pressure is released. Always use the same finger to palpate. *(Use of the same finger helps you develop a sensitivity to better assess the vein condition.)*
      (2) Promote venous distention by instructing the patient to open and close the fist several times, lowering the patient's arm, and rubbing or stroking the patient's arm.
      (3) Avoid sites distal to previous venipuncture sites, hardened cordlike veins, infiltrated sites or phlebotic (enlarged) vessels, and bruised areas. *(Such sites tend to cause infiltration of new IV lines and excessive vessel damage.)*
      (4) Avoid vessels in an extremity with compromised circulation such as in cases of mastectomy, dialysis graft, or paralysis. *(Venous alterations increase risk of complications such as infiltration.)*
6. Cleanse site with alcohol swab or special agent, using friction (see Figure 20-5, *C*). Cleanse in clean-to-dirty direction starting at selected insertion site and working outward, creating concentric circles. Use alcohol first, then chlorhexadine or Betadine. Allow to dry. *(Removes microorganisms from puncture site.)*
7. Stretch skin taut, and stabilize vein with nondominant hand (see Figure 20-5, *D*). *(Prevents vein from moving during procedure.)*
8. Insert the catheter:
   a. Using an angiocatheter:
      (1) Holding angiocatheter bevel up, pierce skin above and slightly to side of vein at 30-degree angle (see Figure 20-5, *D*). *(Allows needle to enter smoothly through skin and approach vein wall.)*
      (2) Lower angle to 10 degrees and enter vein wall. Slight resistance and "pop" accompany entry into vein. *(Reduces risk of going completely through vein and ensures placement within vein.)*
      (3) Follow vein lumen with tip of needle to ensure placement within vein, watching

for blood return through angiocatheter backflow chamber. *(Confirms placement within vein.)*

(4) Release tourniquet. *(Decreases potential for vein rupture.)*

(5) Holding guide needle in place, gently thread plastic catheter off needle and into vein. *(Prevents needle going through catheter and vein. Prevents catheter from being dislodged by slight movement.)*

(6) Applying gentle pressure over catheter in vein, remove guide needle.

b. Using a needleless over-the-needle catheter (ONC) with safety device:

(1) Insert ONC (see illustrations) with bevel up at 10- to 30-degree angle slightly distal to actual site of venipuncture in the direction of the vein. *(The Needle Stick Safety and Prevention Act effective April 2001 requires use of needle safety devices [CDC, 2002].)*

(2) Look for blood return in the flashback chamber on ONC indicating the needle has entered the vein (see illustrations for 8b[2], *A*). Advance catheter ¼ inch into vein and loosen stylet. Advance catheter over the needle into vein until head rests at venipuncture site (see illustrations for 8b[2], *B*). Do not reinsert the stylet once it is loosened. Advance safety device by using push-tab to thread catheter.

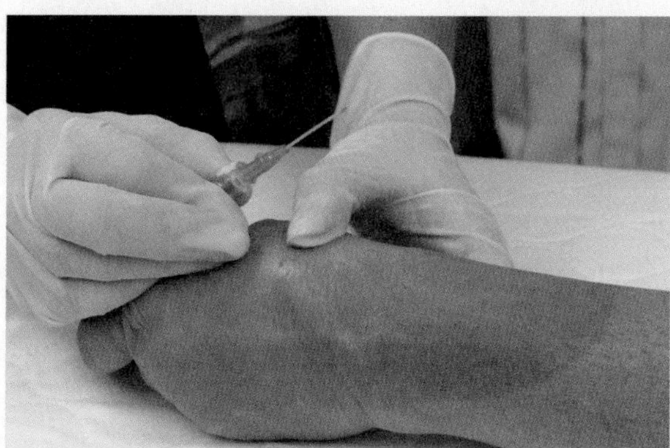

Step **8b(1)** **A,** Stabilize vein below insertion site with skin taut.

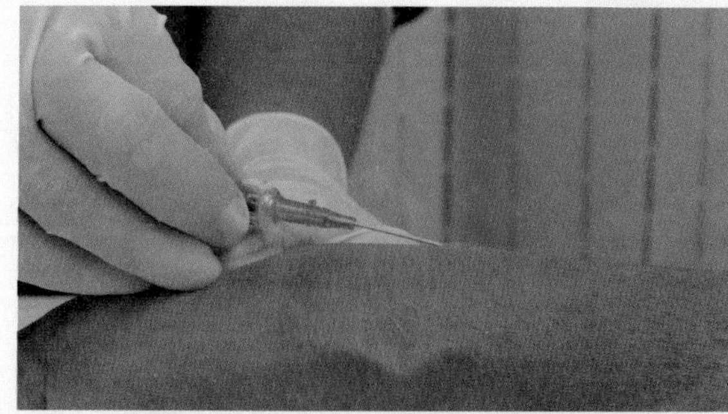

Step **8b(1)** **B,** Puncture skin with catheter at 10- to 30-degree angle. Catheter enters vein.

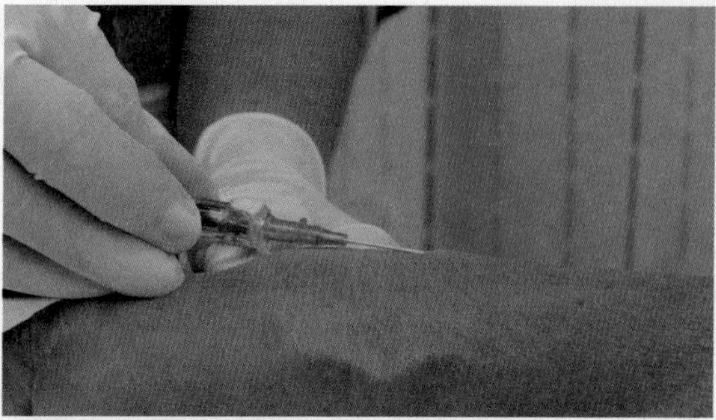

Step **8b(2)** **A,** Blood return in flashback chamber, catheter lowered flush with skin.

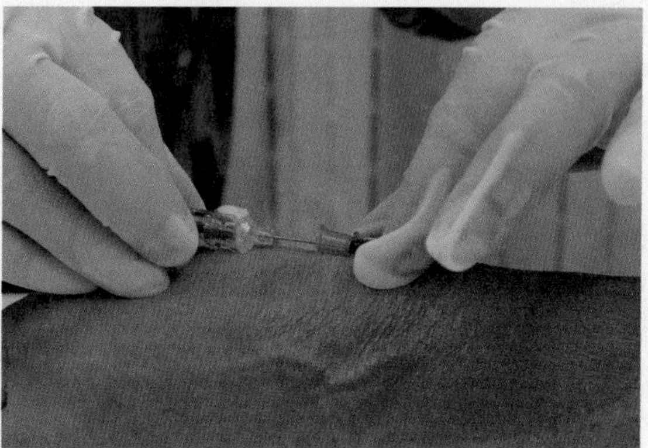

Step **8b(2)** **B,** Advance catheter into vein; use safety device push-tab.

(Increased venous pressure from tourniquet increases backflow of blood into catheter or tubing. Lowering the angle and advancing the cannula slightly allows for full penetration of the vein wall, placement of the catheter within the vein's inner lumen, and easy advancement of catheter off stylet. Threading catheter up to hub reduces the risk of introducing infectious organisms along the catheter length. Reinserting the stylet has potential to cause damage to the catheter and/or formation of a catheter embolus.)

(3) Stabilize the catheter. Apply gentle but firm pressure with the index finger of nondominant hand 1¼ inches (3 cm) above insertion site (see illustration 8b[3], *A*). Release tourniquet with dominant hand and retract stylet from ONC (see illustration 8b[3], *B*). Do not recap the stylet. For safety, slide the catheter off the stylet while gliding the protective guard over the stylet. A click indicates the device is locked. *(Permits venous flow, reduces backflow of blood, and prevents accidental withdrawal or dislodgment.)*

9. Attach sterile connection end of primed tubing to catheter hub. *(Helps prevent backflow, connects fluid source to venous access, and maintains sterility of system.)*

Continued

Skill 20-6 Initiating Intravenous Therapy—cont'd

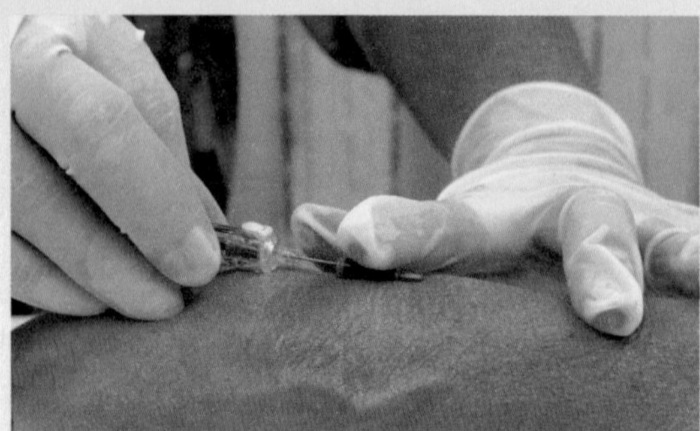

Step 8b(3) A, Apply gentle but firm pressure with index finger 1¼ inches (3 cm) above insertion site.

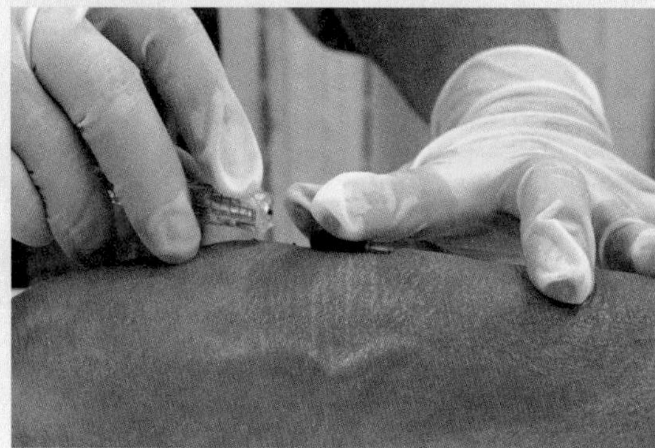

Step 8b(3) B, Release tourniquet from ONC.

10. Stabilizing insertion site, slowly open flow valve to begin intravenous infusion. *(Keeps catheter in place, initiates infusion, and helps prevent clotting of blood in catheter.)*
11. Following agency policy, secure and dress site with tape, medications, and dressings (see illustrations). *(Prevents unintentional dislodging of catheter from vein and prevents infection.)*
12. Label site and tubing according to agency policy. *(Serves as reminder to change site and tubing.)*
13. Adjust fluid flow rate according to accurate drop-rate calculations (see Chapter 23). *(Provides fluid therapy according to medical order.)*
14. Refer to standard steps 10 to 17.
15. Document (some agencies have a special form to record IV therapy):
    - Type of fluid
    - Injection site
    - Number of attempts made
    - Flow rate
    - Size and type of catheter or needle
    - Patient's response
    - Patient teaching (see Patient Teaching box and Life Span Considerations for Older Adults box on intravenous therapy)
16. Immediately report to physician any adverse conditions or reactions such as pulmonary congestion, shock, or thrombophlebitis.

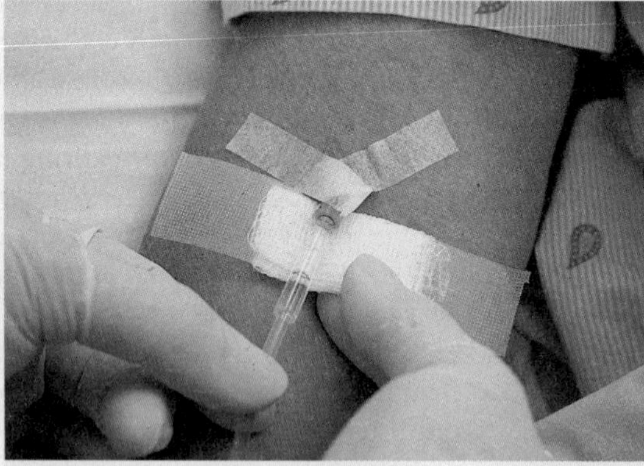

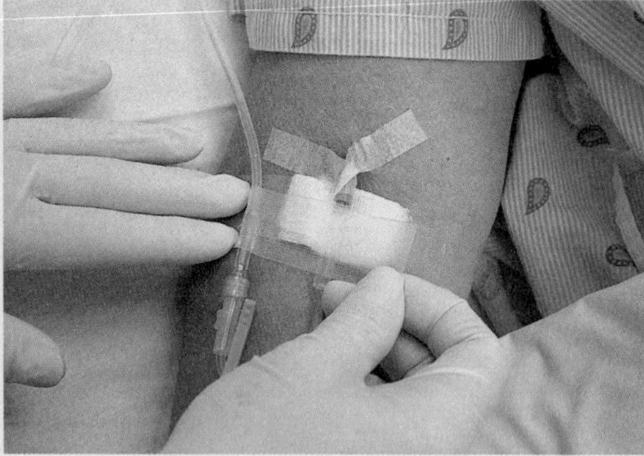

Step 11 A, Gauze dressing is used to secure IV site.

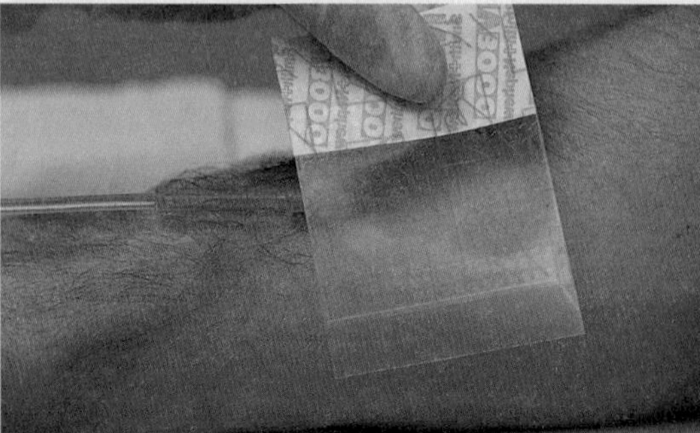

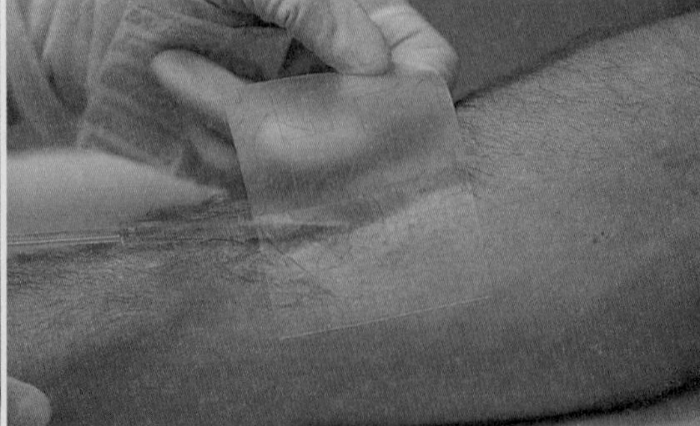

Step 11 B, Transparent dressing is used to secure IV site.

ready the equipment. Then assess the patient's veins, select and cleanse a puncture site, perform the venipuncture, and begin and secure the infusion. Teach the patient about the signs and symptoms of problems and ways to perform activities while receiving IV therapy (see Patient Teaching and Life Span Considerations for Older Adults boxes on intravenous therapy). Because a venipuncture is invasive and the pierced skin is no longer a barrier to microorganisms, it is necessary to follow strict aseptic principles when performing this procedure. Inspect equipment packaging for breakage of sterile seals, and be sure to use it before the expiration dates marked on the packaging barriers. Do not use equipment with damaged outer packaging.

Select the tubing based on the needs of the patient and the type of infusion to be initiated. When preparing to hang an infusion, remove the tubing's sterile packaging and inspect it for kinks. Also make sure that the flow valve is functional. Close the valve, and place the tubing within easy reach (Figure 20-6, *A*). Remove the correct fluid bag from its sterile packaging and invert it to allow easy access to the tubing insertion port. Remove the insertion port cover (see Figure 20-6, *B*), remove the tubing spike end cover, and insert the

Patient Teaching

Intravenous Therapy

- If intravenous (IV) apparatus is positional, instruct how to properly position arm to maintain flow.
- Instruct patient to wear clothes with wide sleeves.
- Instruct about signs and symptoms of infiltration, phlebitis, and inflammation, such as redness, swelling, or discomfort at site.
- Instruct to inform you if flow slows or stops or blood is seen in the tubing.
- Instruct how to ambulate with IV pole or stand.
- Instruct about procedures of IV therapy, including sterile technique while manipulating syringes and other supplies.
- Teach potential problems with infusion and appropriate reaction to problems.
- Teach to apply pressure with sterile gauze if needle falls out and, if patient is on anticoagulant therapy, to tape several pieces of sterile gauze in place for at least 20 minutes or until bleeding stops.
- Teach that it is best to take tub bath to wash up, but not to let IV tubing touch water and to unplug pump first if one is used. If showering is mandatory, the patient will have to insert hand and forearm into a plastic bag and tape the bag in place to ensure that IV site is completely covered, so as not to get it wet.
- Teach the importance of not changing the flow rate, not lying on the tubing, and not allowing the tubing to kink.
- Demonstrate care of the IV site while performing hygiene measures.
- Teach the need for IV fluid container to be above the insertion site.

Life Span Considerations

Older Adults

Intravenous Therapy

- Changes in cardiac and renal function related to the aging process or chronic conditions create the need for extreme accuracy in flow control and thus make use electronic infusion devices necessary (see Chapter 23).
- Fragility of veins in the older adult patient increases risk of infiltration. The infusion device sometimes continues to infuse fluid into sites where infiltration is occurring. Monitor infusion site carefully and frequently.
- Fragile skin requires the use of nonporous tapes and skin protectant solutions.
- Older adults are more prone to fluid imbalances and require careful monitoring of all infusions, (e.g., fluid volume overload).
- Visual and hearing deficits pose challenges to patient education. Face the patient while speaking clearly and calmly.
- Short-term memory loss, depression, and confusion sometimes lead patients to remove the IV catheter or change their attitude or decisions about care.
- Because of fragility of veins, use extra care in injecting bolus of medications.
- If the patient is not able to tolerate the volume of 1 unit of whole blood or red blood cells to be infused in 4 hours, request the blood bank to split the unit into two bags, and leave the second bag under the appropriate refrigeration during the infusion of the first.
- If accurate rate control with an electronic infusion device is required, check agency policy for information about use of specific brand for blood infusor.
- In older adults, use the smallest-gauge catheter or needle possible (e.g., 24- to 26-gauge). This is less traumatizing to the vein and allows better blood flow to provide increased hemodilution of the IV fluids or medications. Use this gauge for hourly flow rates of 75 to 100 mL/hour.
- Avoid the back of the older adult's hand or the dominant arm for venipuncture, because these sites greatly interfere with the older adult's independence.
- If the older adult has fragile skin and veins, use minimal tourniquet pressure.
- When the older adult has lost subcutaneous tissue, the veins lose stability and will roll away from the needle. To stabilize the vein, apply traction to the skin below the projected insertion site.
- Using an angle of 5 to 15 degrees on insertion is helpful, because the older adult's veins are more superficial.
- In the older person with fragile skin, prevent skin tears by keeping the amount of tape used to a minimum.

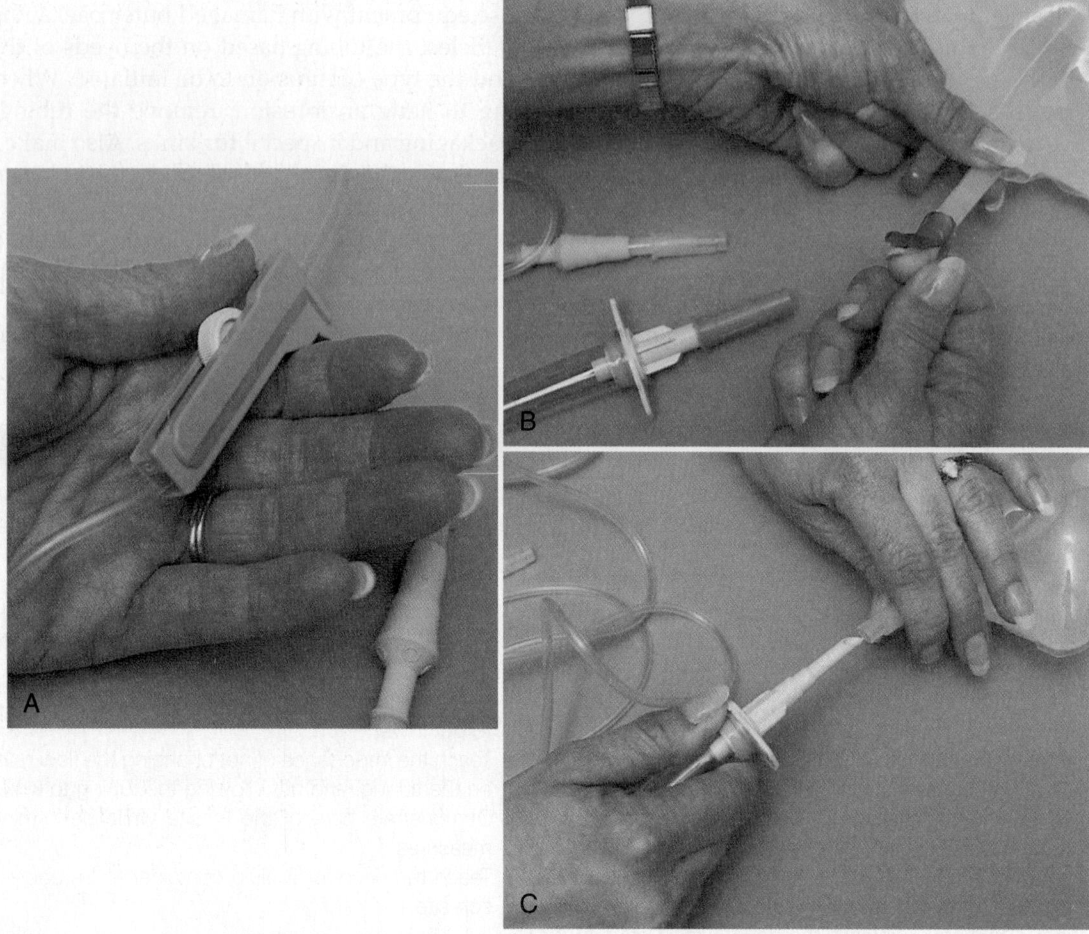

FIGURE 20-6 **A,** Close valve. **B,** Remove insertion port cover. **C,** Insert spike.

spike into the port until the plastic diaphragm covering the port is pierced (see Figure 20-6, C). Then hold the fluid bag upright and gently squeeze the tubing drip chamber to partially (one third to one half) fill it with fluid. Slowly open the flow valve to permit the flow of the solution down the tubing. This priming (filling of the tubing with solution) prevents air from being forced through the tubing into the patient's circulatory system, creating an air embolus. Also invert injection ports to fill with fluid during priming. Remember to select the venipuncture needle and catheter according to the solution to be infused and the size and condition of the patient's veins. Choose a catheter that is smaller than the vein, yet large enough for the solution to flow through it without clogging. A 20-, 21-, or 22-gauge catheter is acceptable for an adult. However, if blood is to be administered, use one with a larger lumen (18- or 20-gauge). The Infusion Nurses Society (INS) (2006) supports the position that it is acceptable to administer both blood components and whole blood via an 18- or 20-gauge catheter if the infusion is given rapidly to prevent hemolysis of the red blood cells or destruction of the components. However, if it is a slow infusion, use of a 22- to 24-gauge catheter is acceptable. Often the smaller-gauge needles will be the only possibility for giving volume expanders and blood components to a hemorrhaging patient displaying signs of shock.

Plastic IV catheters are flexible and have blunt tips that reduce infiltration and allow the patient to move more than the metal needles used in the past. These plastic catheters, called over-the-needle (ONC) or needleless catheters, have a metal needle, or stylet, inside them that you use to pierce the skin and guide the catheter into the vein. You then thread the catheter over the needle and into the vein, and remove the metal guide needle (see Skill 20-6 and Box 20-3).

Central Venous Access Devices

Central venous access devices (CVADs) were developed to address the difficulties faced by patients requiring repeated access to their venous system for the purpose of long-term IV therapy, blood sample collection, medication or blood administration, and fluid or nutrition administration. CVADs provide safer access to the venous system and avoid the dangers of multiple venipunctures, such as vein sclerosis (hardening), bruising, infection, and pain.

Various catheters and ports are used for patients requiring long-term IV therapy; therefore, it is important

Box 20-3 Special Considerations for Patients Receiving Intravenous Therapy

- Very young and older adult patients have fragile veins; avoid using sites that are easily moved or bumped. The most common intravenous (IV) site for infants is a scalp vein; sites in the foot are also used for pediatric patients.
- Obese patients present problems for venipuncture because of difficulty in locating superficial veins.
- Avoid using any extremity with circulatory or neurologic impairment, or the dominant extremity, whenever possible.
- When you anticipate the need to administer blood or blood components or the patient is preoperative, use a large-gauge (18 or 19 F) catheter for infusion of more **viscous** (state of being sticky or gummy) solutions.
- Critically ill patients at all stages of life require more frequent assessment to monitor status of therapy.
- When solution has less than 100 mL remaining, have new solution at patient's bedside and slow the flow rate before the end of your shift. This reduces risk of solution emptying during change-of-shift report.
- Institutions that do not use IV over-the-needle safety devices, which make disposal error free, sometimes have policies for using a "one-handed" technique to recap IV stylets. The Occupational Safety and Health Administration (OSHA) allows the one-handed technique. Lay the cap on a flat surface and, using one hand only, slide the needle into the cap.
- In patients with fragile or engorged veins (patients with congestive heart failure or those receiving anticoagulants), avoid using tourniquets. Have another nurse apply light hand pressure instead, and release it as soon as the catheter has punctured the vein wall. This will decrease the chance of excessive vein wall tearing and hematoma formation.
- Use a direct approach for large, easily seen veins: use the catheter to puncture the skin and the vein wall simultaneously.
- Use an indirect approach for small, fragile, or deeper veins: use the catheter to puncture the skin, relocate the vein, and then use the catheter to puncture the vein wall.
- If venipuncture is unsuccessful and you are obliged to make a second attempt, always obtain a new catheter first. Never reinsert the stylet into the catheter because this has potential to cause damage to the catheter and/or formation of a catheter embolism.
- Encourage patient to ask questions, and provide honest, forthright answers in a calm, reassuring manner. Tell patient, "The stick will hurt a little bit but will be less painful if you can hold very still. It's okay to move your other arm."
- After all preparation is complete and immediately before puncturing the skin, say, "It's going to be a big stick now," then proceed immediately to insert the catheter. Keep reminding the patient to take slow, deep breaths, especially if you have difficulty entering the vein. Distract the patient by talking about other subjects.
- Never make more than three attempts at inserting an IV yourself (most facilities' policies state no more than two). Know agency policy.

for you to be familiar with the devices. The three categories of CVADs are tunneled central venous catheters (CVCs), percutaneous CVCs, and implanted infusion ports. Common brand names for the various catheters, such as Hickman, Groshong, Raaf, and Port-a-Cath, do not indicate the type of catheter.

Percutaneous CVC insertion is possible to perform at the bedside, whereas tunneled CVCs are inserted under local or general anesthetic in the operating room. Both are inserted into a large vein. The percutaneous CVC is usually placed directly into the internal or the external jugular or the superior vena cava vein. The tunneled CVC is tunneled through the subcutaneous tissue (Figure 20-7), which creates a space between the catheter and the vein that allows the catheter to stay in place for an indefinite period; then it is advanced into the subclavian vein and into the superior vena cava (Figure 20-8). The percutaneous CVC is possible to insert through the cephalic or basilic veins in the arm and is then advanced into the superior vena cava. The ad-

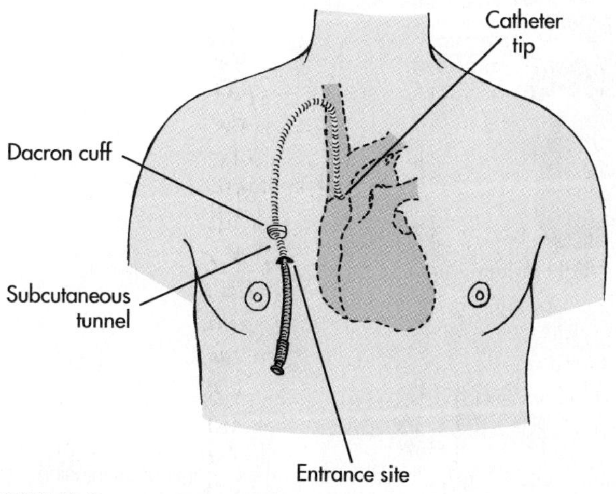

FIGURE 20-7 Small-gauge tunneled catheter in its place, threaded into superior vena cava.

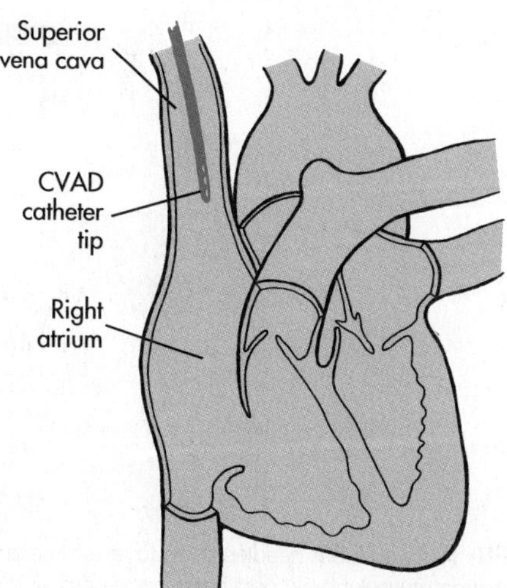

FIGURE 20-8 Catheter tip from CVAD lies in superior vena cava.

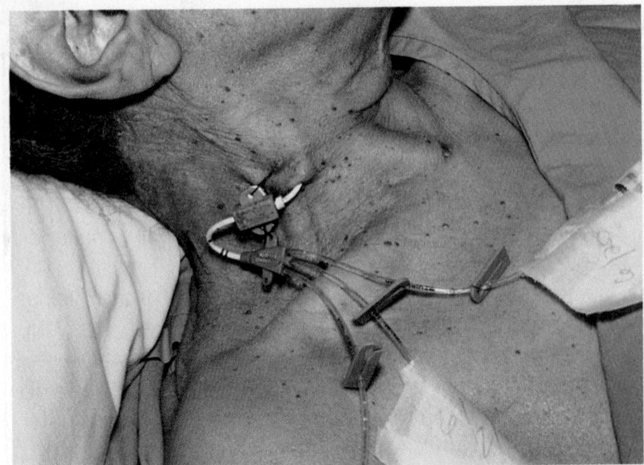

FIGURE 20-9 Triple lumen CVAD placed in jugular vein.

vantage of both types of CVC, which are placed into a large central vessel rather than a peripheral vessel, is that they produce less chance of irritation and inflammation of the vessel or vessel sclerosis.

CVCs are used to (1) administer various fluids, including chemotherapy and parenteral nutrition, (2) obtain blood samples, and (3) perform hemodialysis. Depending on the type of catheter, the device will have single, double, or triple lumens and is left in place according to the manufacturer's guidelines (Figure 20-9).

Implanted infusion ports are CVCs that are surgically implanted under local anesthesia into the subcutaneous tissue in the area of the intraclavicular fossa. The catheter is inserted into a large vessel, as with the other CVCs, and threaded into the superior vena cava (Figure 20-10, *A*). The four parts that make up the im-

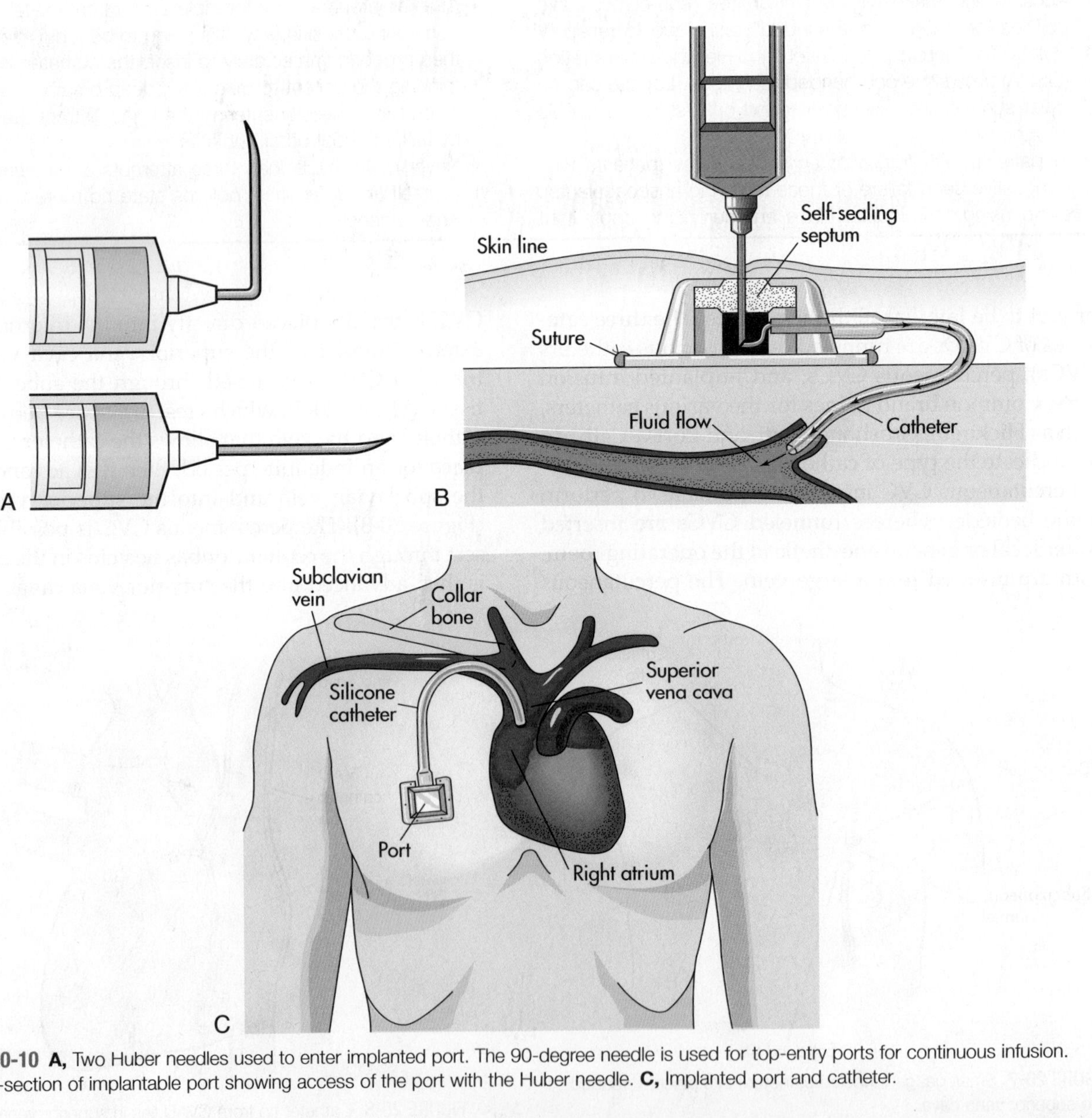

FIGURE 20-10 A, Two Huber needles used to enter implanted port. The 90-degree needle is used for top-entry ports for continuous infusion. **B,** Cross-section of implantable port showing access of the port with the Huber needle. **C,** Implanted port and catheter.

planted infusion port are the body of the port, the central septum and the reservoir, and the central line catheter (Figure 20-10, *B*). One of the advantages of the implanted infusion port is that while it is not in use, there are no external catheters to care for. The port placement is possible to palpate and is accessed with a either a 90-degree angle or straight Huber needle directly through the skin (Figure 20-10, *C*); it is necessary to heparinize the port every 4 weeks. Implanted infusion ports are used for the same purposes as all other CVCs.

You and your patients need to be aware that the two most common complications of CVCs are infection and occlusion of the catheter cannula. It is usually possible to prevent these complications by caring for the devices properly. Teach patients how to care for their devices in the home setting so that they are able to start and discontinue infusions and heparinize their devices independently. While in the home setting, patients will need to perform dressing changes to their CVCs using clean technique (Perry & Potter, 2009).

Peripherally Inserted Central Catheters (PICCs)

PICCs are an alternative to CVCs for patients requiring IV access beyond the length of time that peripheral IVs can be maintained. PICCs enter the central venous system, usually the subclavian vein, via the larger cephalic or basilic veins in the upper arm. Specially trained registered nurses (if the state nurse practice act permits) and physicians insert PICCs, which are possible to leave in place for extended periods as long as there are no problems with the device or complications.

Refer to your facility's policy and procedure manual for proper care of PICC lines. The advantages of PICCs are that they pose less risk of pneumothorax, hemothorax, and air embolisms than CVCs, are less expensive to maintain than CVCs, and pose less risk of phlebitis and infiltration than peripheral lines. The risks involved with PICCs include clotting, leaking from the catheter, migration of the catheter, infection, and catheter breakage.

PICCs will have a single or a double lumen; the PICCs range in lumen size from 16- to 24-gauge, and in length from 40 to 65 cm (16 to 26 inches). PICCs are typically used for therapy that is going to last from 7 days to 3 months, most commonly consisting of administration of IV fluids and medications, parenteral nutrition, and blood or blood products (Perry & Potter, 2009).

Intravenous Monitoring

You will select the IV site according to its capacity to accommodate the intended solution. Most insertion sites are located in the hand or the arm. A central vein, such as the subclavian vein, is used to deliver large amounts of fluids or concentrated solutions directly into the bloodstream.

Assessment of the IV site centers on the **patency** (a condition of being open and unblocked) of the system. Establish a routine for assessing the IV site, beginning at the solution container and ending at the site. Check the flow rate against the physician's order. Assess tubing for kinks or obstructions, and check the position of the patient's hand or arm. If the extremity is flexed, it is possible for the vein to become occluded. Remind patients to keep extremities extended. Inspect and palpate the site for edema, erythema, **induration** (hardness), heat, and discomfort. A burning sensation often means the solution is irritating the vein; slow the infusion rate and continue monitoring. Compare the hand or arm with the opposite hand or arm if the site seems edematous. Edema often indicates that infiltration has occurred.

If the patient is dehydrated, in shock, or critically ill, a slow infusion rate does not provide the cardiovascular system with enough fluid. By contrast, an infusion rate that is too rapid will potentially place too much fluid into the circulation and overload the cardiovascular, neurologic, and urinary systems. Fluid overload is sometimes fatal. Signs and symptoms associated with fluid overload include dyspnea; a rapid, weak pulse; cough; disorientation; increased or decreased blood pressure; crackles; pitting edema; weight gain; and decreased urine output. If you suspect that an overload has occurred, immediately slow the infusion rate and contact the charge nurse. Assess the volume infused by both the bag contents and the pump readout to ensure pump accuracy.

Infiltration

If you detect edema, first loosen the tape over the insertion site. Edema that does not subside generally indicates that the catheter is out of the vein and **infiltration** (presence of intravenous fluids within the subcutaneous space surrounding a venipuncture site) has occurred. Discomfort or dysfunction are other possible indications that the solution has infiltrated. In patients who have good skin turgor, the drip rate will decrease when there is an infiltration. When palpating the site, you will find that an infiltrated area feels cool, and the skin will often have a blanched appearance. If fluid seeps into the tissue and you confirm that infiltration has occurred, discontinue the infusion and use another site to continue therapy, preferably in the opposite extremity. Monitor the site of the infiltration; usually fluid resorbs within 24 hours. Do not apply warm compresses to infiltrations caused by blood and **vesicants** (drugs capable of causing tissue necrosis when extravasated [the inadvertent infiltration of intravenous fluids or medication into the subcutaneous tissue surrounding the infusion site]). Document the degree of infiltration (Table 20-3) and nursing interventions you perform. Follow your agency's policy on care to be provided.

Table 20-3 Infiltration Scale

GRADE	CLINICAL CRITERIA
0	No symptoms
1	Skin blanched Edema less than 1 inch in any direction Cool to touch With or without pain
2	Skin blanched Edema 1 to 6 inches in any direction Cool to touch With or without pain
3	Skin blanched, translucent Gross edema greater than 6 inches in any direction Cool to touch Mild to moderate pain Possible numbness
4	Skin blanched, translucent Gross edema greater than 6 inches in any direction Deep pitting tissue edema Circulatory impairment Moderate to severe pain Infiltration of any amount of blood product, irritant, or vesicant

From Infusion Nurses Society. (2006). Infusion nursing standards of practice. *J Intraven Nurs, 29*(1S), S60; and Potter, P.A., & Perry, A.G. (2009). *Fundamentals of nursing: concepts, process, and practice.* (7th ed.). St. Louis: Mosby.

Phlebitis

Phlebitis results from mechanical irritation (the needle moves inside the vein, injuring the vessel), the low pH of some IV solutions, and highly concentrated additives. Erythema, warmth, edema, and discomfort are classic signs of phlebitis (Table 20-4). Discontinue the IV and restart it in a different site, preferably in the opposite extremity with new IV tubing and fluids. Reducing injurious agents, maintaining sterile technique when beginning an IV, and using in-line filters decrease the incidence of vein irritation and trauma. Applying warm compresses to the inflamed area lessens discomfort.

Table 20-4 Phlebitis Scale

GRADE	CLINICAL CRITERIA
0	No clinical symptoms
1	Erythema at access site with or without pain
2	Pain at access site with erythema and/or edema
3	Pain at access site with erythema and/or edema Streak formation Palpable venous cord
4	Pain at access site with erythema and/or edema Streak formation Palpable venous cord greater than 1 inch in length Purulent drainage

From Infusion Nurses Society. (2006). Infusion nursing standards of practice. *J Intraven Nurs, 29*(1S), S59; and Potter, P.A., & Perry, A.G. (2009). *Fundamentals of nursing: concepts, process, and practice.* (7th ed.). St. Louis: Mosby.

Septicemia

Using sterile technique reduces the potential for introduction of pathogenic organisms through IV therapy. If a systemic infection does occur from pathogens introduced into the bloodstream, septicemia (blood poisoning) results. Signs and symptoms include a fever, chills, **prostration** (condition of extreme exhaustion), pain, headache, nausea, and vomiting. If this occurs, retain previously used IV catheters for possible culture (follow your agency's policy) and notify physician. The physician will order vigorous initiation of antibiotic therapy if blood cultures verify a septicemic condition. Document nursing interventions as stated in agency policy and procedure.

BLOOD TRANSFUSION THERAPY

Blood component transfusion therapy is most commonly used to replace blood loss. The fear of human immunodeficiency virus (HIV) infection has led some patients to refuse blood products. Testing procedures used by the American Red Cross to detect HIV have dramatically reduced the incidence of its transmission by means of blood products. Plasma expanders (Plasmanate, Dextran) are possible to use for patients who refuse blood transfusions because of personal or religious beliefs.

Individuals who have concerns about receiving another person's blood are permitted to store their own blood with the American Red Cross before anticipated surgery for infusion during their hospitalization. Autologous blood transfusion (a process of collecting a patient's blood and infusing it intravenously to the patient) using blood lost during surgery or after traumatic injury is also used in some facilities. One apparatus used for this procedure is the Atrium autotransfusion system. It is used during cardiac thoracic surgery or after traumatic chest injury. Using suction provided by the chest drainage device, the blood is collected in a special bag. The blood is best administered immediately or not more than 6 hours after initial collection. Before any autologous blood transfusion system is used, make certain of facility policy and protocols for handling and transfusing blood and administering anticoagulants. Other systems are available for continuous blood recovery and infusion during surgical procedures.

Initiating a Blood Transfusion

You are responsible for assessing and monitoring the patient before, during, and after the transfusion (see Coordinated Care box on blood transfusions). After an informed consent has been signed, initiate a primary IV infusion of 0.9% or sometimes 0.45% normal saline, and follow the established protocol for obtaining the

Coordinated Care

Collaboration

BLOOD TRANSFUSIONS

- The skill of transfusing blood products requires the critical thinking and knowledge application unique to a nurse. In some states, the administration of blood and blood components is included within the scope of practice for the LPN/LVN. Follow agency policy.
- Acceptable delegation to assistive personnel includes obtaining vital signs, collecting equipment, transporting units from the blood bank, and instituting patient's comfort measures. However, the primary responsibility for donor and recipient identification, infusing the unit within the required time, and assessing outcomes remains with the nurse transfusionist. (It is generally a registered nurse's responsibility.)

blood, double-checking the compatibility of the blood with the patient's blood, and identifying the patient. Take and record baseline vital signs. Then prime the special blood filter administration tubing and piggyback it into the primary infusion line (Figure 20-11). Remaining with the patient while slowly infusing the first 50 mL of blood allows you to assess the patient's response and monitor vital signs. Transfusion reactions are possible at any time during or even after a blood transfusion. However, the reactions usually occur within the first 15 minutes. Make sure you know the symptoms of a blood transfusion reaction and the nursing interventions to initiate for them.

In order to alleviate the patient's concerns over blood transfusions, it is important to provide information regarding alternatives, advantages, and risks of transfusions, as well as measures that are implemented to ensure a safe blood supply. Inform the patient that no guarantee is possible that transfusions will be entirely risk free (Elkin et al., 2007).

Blood typing and crossmatching of the Rh factor is performed before administration of blood products in order to ensure the donor and recipient's blood are as compatible as possible. In order to prevent transfusion reactions, it is imperative to carry out the verification process correctly. Verification before infusion of blood products consists of confirming the correct patient, blood product and product type, and crossmatching (Elkin et al., 2007).

Inspect blood product for signs of leakage or unusual appearance, including bubbles or purplish color. Report these signs immediately (the presence of contamination is possible), and return the blood product to the laboratory or blood bank.

Protocol for initiating a blood product transfusion includes remaining with the patient for the first 15 to 20 minutes of the transfusion to monitor for reactions, beginning the transfusion at a slow rate per agency policy, taking vital signs frequently per agency policy, and monitoring the patient for any complaints of discomfort that indicate a possible reaction (Potter & Perry, 2009).

The medical order specifies the rate of infusion. Ideally, each unit of blood will infuse within 2 to 4 hours. The risk of blood cell damage and infection increases after that time. Remember that blood is permitted to be out of the blood bank no longer than 4 hours. It is essential to follow the protocol regarding discarding

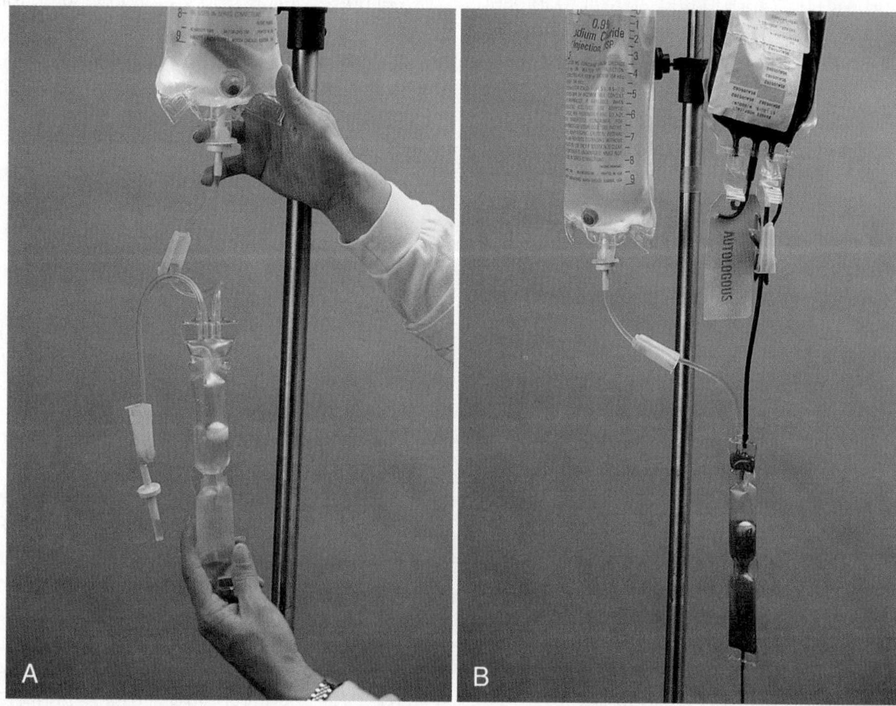

FIGURE 20-11 **A,** Opened blood administration set and tubing primed with normal saline 0.9%. Note that the filter is completely filled with the saline. **B,** Attached blood product to the normal saline 0.9%. Note that the clamp is closed on the saline and the clamp is opened above the filter to the blood product.

or returning of the container to the blood bank whenever a unit of blood is infused. In addition, use fresh (not reused) tubing for the primary tubing to administer each new unit of blood, piggybacking it into the primary IV line; and flush the tubing with normal saline before another unit of blood is infused so that the blood from both units is not mixed within the tubing. (Always refer to agency policy for specific instructions on tubing changes for blood products.) This prevents clotting within the tubing and keeps blood from mixing from unit to unit.

Blood Transfusion Reactions

Infusing blood that is not compatible with the patient's blood type leads to a reaction. A transfusion reaction is an emergency. Close monitoring is therefore crucial in assessing the patient's tolerance to the infusing blood. Patients experiencing transfusion reactions frequently say they are "not feeling right" or have a sense of impending doom. They sometimes have chills, fever, low back pain, pruritus (itching), hypotension, nausea and vomiting, decreased urine output, back pain, chest pain, and dyspnea. If the patient is unconscious, closely assess vital signs, urine output, and skin appearance. If you suspect a transfusion reaction, stop the transfusion. Keep the vein open with 0.9% sodium chloride (NaCl) solution, and notify the physician and the blood bank. Send the tubing and the blood to the lab for examination. Monitor the patient's vital signs and urine output every 15 minutes. Because a transfusion reaction tends to be frightening, reassure and support the patient.

If the patient is experiencing a hemolytic reaction, transfused blood is incompatible with the patient's blood type, and death is possible. Although a reaction normally occurs within the first 15 minutes, it is possible at any time during the infusion process. If the reaction is severe, the patient will possibly go into shock and die. Other types of blood transfusion reactions are nonhemolytic, allergic, and anaphylactic reactions. Another type of transfusion reaction is the delayed reaction, which occurs days to weeks later. Each type of reaction is caused by the incompatibility of a component within the unit of blood with the patient's blood.

After any blood transfusion reaction, return the remaining blood to the blood bank for analysis. Comply with your agency's policies for monitoring blood transfusions and reactions (Box 20-4).

Maintaining an Intravenous Site

Complications sometimes occur with peripheral intravenous (IV) infusions, typically in relation to the infusion or the catheter. Infiltration of the site, phlebitis of the vessel, and local or systemic infections are possible. Appropriate management of IV sites will prevent or keep these complications to a minimum (Skill 20-7) (Potter & Perry, 2009).

Text continued on p. 555

Box 20-4 Blood Transfusion Precautions

- In the event of a blood transfusion reaction, hang a new bag of normal saline with new tubing and allow it to infuse slowly. This prevents any more of the transfusing blood to enter the patient (even from the tubing) and keeps the vein open.
- Make sure IV catheters for blood transfusions are of appropriate size, keeping in mind the size of the vessel.
- One unit of blood is released at a time from the blood bank. Verification of each unit by two nursing staff members is required, along with some form of patient identification.
- Completely prime blood transfusion filters with saline to prevent collection of debris in a partially primed filter. Saline will reduce the viscosity of red blood cells by diluting them and thus flush blood from the tubing (see Figure 20-11, *A*).
- A transfusion reaction produces a hemolytic reaction that causes red blood cells to appear in the urine. Therefore it is important that the patient voids or catheter drainage devices be emptied before the transfusion is started so that if a reaction occurs, a fresh urine sample is available to test for red blood cells.
- A registered nurse (RN) regulates the flow rate so that only 10 to 24 mL of product infuses during the first 15 minutes, and the RN remains with the patient during this time (see Figure 20-11, *B*). If a reaction occurs, only a small amount of incompatible blood product will have been administered to the patient at this slow rate.
- An alteration in the vital signs from the baseline indicates the possibility that a transfusion reaction has occurred.
- An RN is required to hang the blood, but a licensed practical nurse or licensed vocational nurse (LPN/LVN) is permitted to verify type with the RN. The RN is required to sit with the patient for the first 15 to 30 minutes of transfusion.
- If you believe that a transfusion reaction is occurring, implement the following steps:
  1. Stop the transfusion **immediately.**
  2. Piggyback 0.9% normal saline directly into the vein with new tubing in order to prevent any more incompatible blood from being infused into the patient.
  3. Notify the physician immediately after stopping the transfusion.
  4. Monitor the patient's signs and symptoms of reaction continuously, and measure the vital signs every 5 minutes.
  5. Anticipate the physician's order of emergency drugs such as antihistamines, vasopressors, IV fluids, and steroids to counteract and treat the reaction.
  6. The development of cardiac and respiratory arrest is possible, so prepare to perform CPR if necessary.
  7. Collect a urine specimen and send it to the lab to assess for red blood cells from a hemolytic reaction.
  8. Do not discard the blood container, the tubing, the labels, or the transfusion record. These items will have to be sent to the laboratory.
  9. Document everything that occurred during the transfusion reaction.

Skill 20-7 Maintaining an Intravenous Site

Nursing Action *(Rationale)*

Changing a Peripheral Intravenous (IV) Dressing

1. Refer to standard steps 1 to 9.
2. Assemble equipment:
   - Clean gloves
   - Antiseptic swabs, alcohol, povidone-iodine, chlorhexidine
   - Skin protectant solution
   - Adhesive remover (optional)
   - Strips of sterile, precut tape (or 36-inch roll of tape)
   - Transparent dressing or sterile 2 × 2 gauze pads and tape
   - Arm board, hand board, or housing device (optional)
3. Assessment:
   - **a.** Determine when the dressing was last changed by checking the dressing label. *(This labeling provides instant identification for assessing and determining status of the site.)*
   - **b.** Observe present dressing for moisture and occlusiveness. Determine if moisture is from leakage from the puncture site or from an external source. *(Change soiled dressing immediately.)*
   - **c.** Observe IV system for proper functioning or complications (tubing or catheter kinks).
   - **d.** Palpate the catheter site through the intact dressing to elicit any complaints of tenderness, pain, or burning. *(Signs indicative of phlebitis.)*
   - **e.** Inspect exposed catheter site for edema, erythema, drainage, or blanching. *(Signs indicative of phlebitis or infiltration.)*
   - **f.** Monitor body temperature.
   - **g.** Determine patient's understanding of the need for continued IV infusion.
4. Remove any overlying tape. Then remove transparent membrane dressing by picking up one corner and pulling the side laterally while holding catheter hub (see illustration). Repeat for other side. *(Technique keeps discomfort during removal to a minimum.)*

   Or

   Remove gauze dressing and tape from old dressing one layer at a time by pulling toward the insertion site. Leave tape securing catheter to skin. Check agency procedure. *(If catheter moves during dressing change, there is potential for it to accidentally dislodge and puncture blood vessel.)*
5. Observe insertion site for redness, erythema, edema, exudate, pallor, or pain. If present, discontinue infusion. *(Signs indicative of phlebitis or infiltration.)*

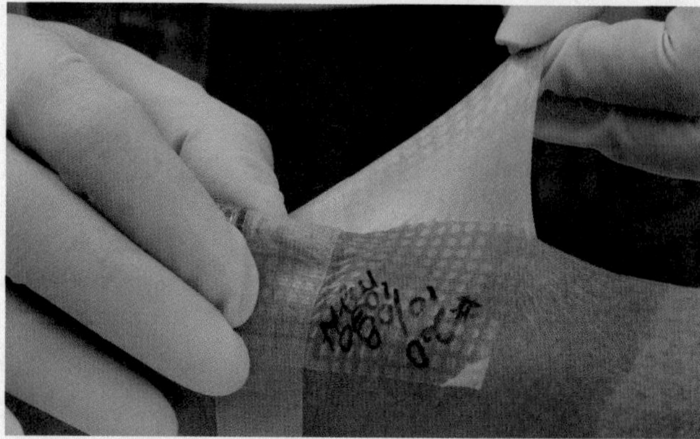

Step 4 Remove transparent dressing by pulling side laterally.

6. If IV is infusing properly, gently remove tape securing catheter. Stabilize catheter with one finger. Remove adhesive residue with adhesive remover, if necessary. *(Prevents catheter from dislodging.)*
7. Using circular motion, cleanse peripheral insertion site with antiseptic swab (see illustration), starting at insertion site and working outward, creating concentric circles. Allow antiseptic solution to dry completely. *(Allow antimicrobial solutions to air-dry completely to effectively reduce microbial counts* [INS, 2006]. *If antiseptic agents are used in combination, allow each to air-dry separately.)* *Option*: Apply skin protectant solution (Skin Prep or No Sting Barrier Film) to the area where the tape or dressing will be applied. Allow to dry.
8. Apply dressing.
   - **a.** Transparent dressing:
     - **(1)** Place transparent dressing over venipuncture site by smoothing dressing over IV site and catheter, up to the hub (refer to manufacturer's directions.) Do not cover the catheter hub or tubing junction with the dressing.

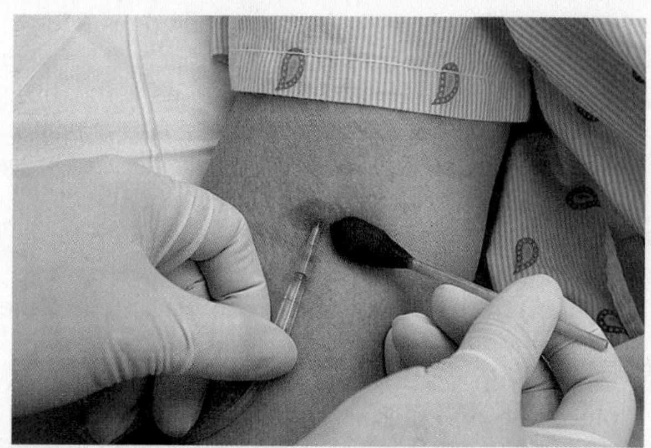

Step 7 Cleanse peripheral insertion site with antiseptic swab.

Continued

Skill 20-7 Maintaining an Intravenous Site—cont'd

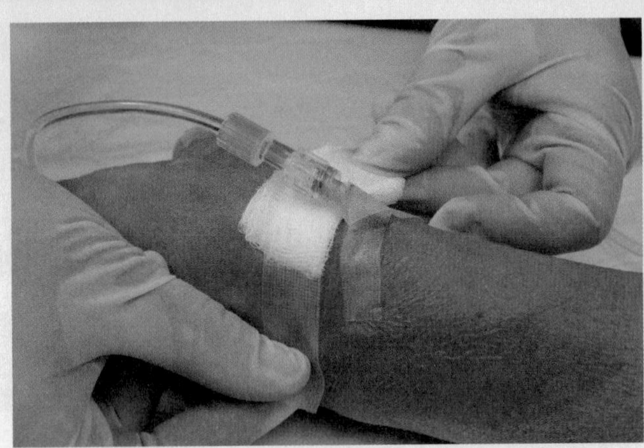
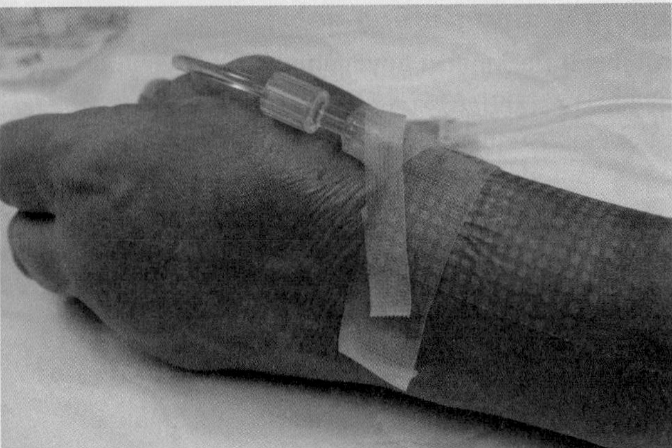

Step 8a(3) Apply chevron over tape.

(2) Take a 1-inch (2.5-cm) piece of tape and place it from end of hub of catheter to insertion site, over transparent dressing.

(3) Then apply a **chevron** (a piece of sterile tape that is ½ inch [1.5 cm] wide and about 4 inches [10 cm] long). Place the sterile tape carefully under hub of catheter with adhesive side up (see illustration), crisscross ends of tape over hub (see illustration) to make a chevron, and place only over tape, not over transparent dressing. *(Agencies that do not use chevrons cite the fact that the tape is nonsterile and wrapping it around the hub would promote possible infection).*

b. Gauze dressing:

(1) Place single 4-inch (10-cm) strip of sterile ½-inch (1.5 cm) nonallergenic tape under peripheral catheter hub with sticky side up. Crisscross tape over catheter hub to anchor it to skin. *(Chevron secures catheter to skin.)* Do not cover insertion site. If desired, place a second piece of sterile tape across catheter at hub.

(2) Place a 2 × 2 gauze over venipuncture site and catheter hub. Secure all edges with tape. Do not cover the connection between IV tubing and catheter hub with the dressing. *(Use occlusive gauze dressings to prevent airflow. Access to catheter hub is needed in an emergency and when changing tubing.)*

9. Fold a 2 × 2 gauze in half, and cover with tape 1 inch (2.5 cm) wide extending about an inch (2.5 cm) from each side of gauze. Place under the tubing and catheter hub junction. Curl a loop of tubing alongside the outside of the arm, and place a second piece of tape directly over the tubing and the 2 × 2, securing the tubing in two places. *(Securing the tubing at two places prevents catheter movement and dislodgment that increase the risk of phlebitis and infiltration. Placing tape on tape makes tubing removal easier and decreases the skin irritation.)* When using a transparent dressing, avoid placing tape directly over dressing. *(Tape application loosens transparent dressings.)*

10. Label the dressing with date and time of insertion, date and time of dressing change, gauze and length of catheter, and identification of nurse (see illustration in step 4). *(Allows easy recognition of type of device and time interval for site rotation.)* *Option*: Apply armboard, hand board, or commercial housing device if venipuncture site or dressing is affected by the motion of the elbow or wrist. *(Reduces the risk of phlebitis and infiltration from motion of the joint.)*

11. Discard used supplies, remove gloves, and perform hand hygiene.

12. Refer to standard steps 10 to 17.

Changing Infusion Tubing

1. Refer to standard steps 1 to 9.

2. Assemble equipment:

Continuous infusion:

- Microdrop or macrodrip infusion tubing as appropriate
- Filter and extensive tubing if necessary. *(Different types of tubing are used to administer medications or IV fluids. A solution given rapidly needs to be infused with macrodrip tubing, which delivers large drops (standard drop size is 10 to 15 gtt*/mL depending on the manufacturer) so that the prescribed rate can be maintained. In contrast, microdrip tubing provides a standard drop size of 60 gtt/mL. Microdrip tubing is used to allow precise regulation of IV fluids even at slow rates. In addition, patients sometimes require IV extension tubing to increase mobility, decrease manipulation*

*gtt, Drops.

and potential contamination at insertion site, or facilitate changes in position.)
- Tubing label

Intermittent saline or heparin lock:
- Injection cap or prn adapter
- Loop or short extension tubing (if necessary)
- Sterile 2 × 2 gauze pads
- 5-mL syringe filled with normal saline or heparin flush solution (check agency policy)
- Clean gloves
- Additional equipment as needed if application of new IV dressing is required (see Changing the Peripheral IV Dressing, steps 4 to 7 on p. 549)

3. Assessment:
   a. Determine when new infusion set is needed (e.g., according to agency policy, or after contamination or puncture of infusion tubing).
   b. Observe for occlusion in tubing such as kinking, drug or mineral precipitate, or blood. *(Infusion of incompatible medication potentially leads to precipitate formation. Retrograde blood flow from vein is possible that will adhere to tubing. Infusion of viscous blood components sometimes causes adherence to walls of tubing and decreases size of lumen.)*
   c. Determine patient's need for continued IV infusion.
4. Open new infusion set, and connect add-on pieces such as filters or extension tubing. *(Separation of infusion tubing increases the risk of air emboli, hemorrhage, and infection.)* Keep protective covering over spike and distal adapter. *(Protective covers reduce entrance of microorganisms.)* Secure all junctions with Luer-Loks, clasping devices, or threaded devices. Avoid the use of tape.
5. If catheter hub is not visible, remove IV dressing as directed in Changing the Peripheral IV Dressing, steps 3 and 4 on p. 549. Do not remove tape securing catheter to skin (if gauze dressing was used). *(Movement of catheter will sometimes cause it to dislodge.)* If transparent dressing has to be removed, place small piece of sterile tape across hub to temporarily anchor catheter during disconnection.
6. For existing continuous infusion:
   a. Close roller clamp on new tubing.
   b. Slow rate of infusion to keep vein open (KVO) on existing IV by regulating roller clamp on old tubing.
   c. Compress and fill drip chamber of old tubing.
7. Remove IV container from pole, invert container, and remove old tubing from solution. Carefully hold container while hanging or taping the drip chamber on IV pole 36 inches (90 cm) above IV site. *(Fluid in drip chamber will run slowly to keep catheter patent.)*
8. Place insertion spike of new tubing into old fluid container opening. Hang container on IV pole, compress and release drip chamber on new tubing, and fill drip chamber one third to one half full (see illustration).

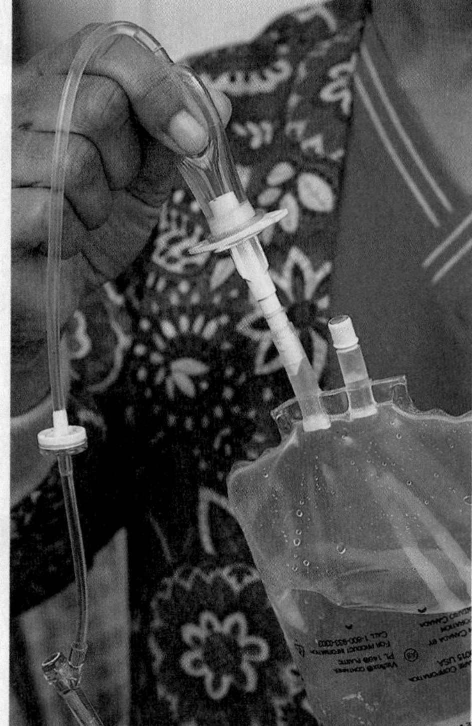
Step 8 Squeeze drip chamber to fill with fluid.

9. Slowly open roller clamp, remove protective cap from adapter (if necessary), and flush new tubing with solution. Stop infusion, and replace cap. *(Slow flush of solution into tubing reduces formation of air bubbles in tubing.)*
10. Turn roller clamp on old tubing to "off" position. *Option:* Place 2 × 2 gauze under catheter hub. *(Prevents tubing from accidentally contacting skin and collects blood that may leak from catheter hub.)*
11. Stabilize hub of catheter, and apply pressure over vein just above catheter tip (at least 1½ inches above insertion site). Gently disconnect old tubing from catheter hub, and quickly insert adapter of new tubing into catheter hub (see illustrations). *(Keeps loss of blood to a minimum as tubing is changed.)*
12. Open roller clamp on new tubing, allowing solution to run rapidly for 30 to 60 seconds, and then regulate IV drip according to physician's orders and monitor rate hourly (see illustration). *(Clears catheter of any blood in lumen, preventing occlusion.)*
13. Attach a piece of tape or a preprinted label with date and time of tubing change onto tubing below the drip chamber. *(Provides reference to determine next time for tubing change.)*
14. Remove and discard 2 × 2 gauze (if used) and old IV tubing. If necessary, apply new dressing. Dispose of gloves.

Continued

Skill 20-7 Maintaining an Intravenous Site—cont'd

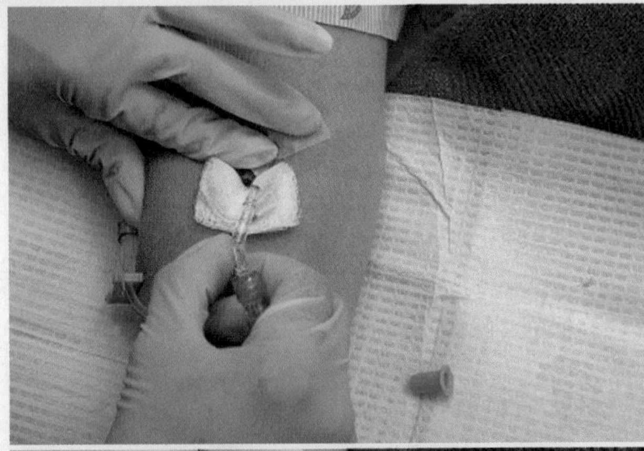

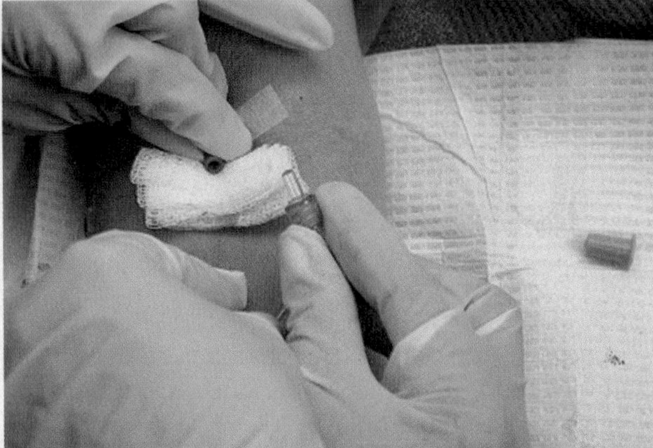

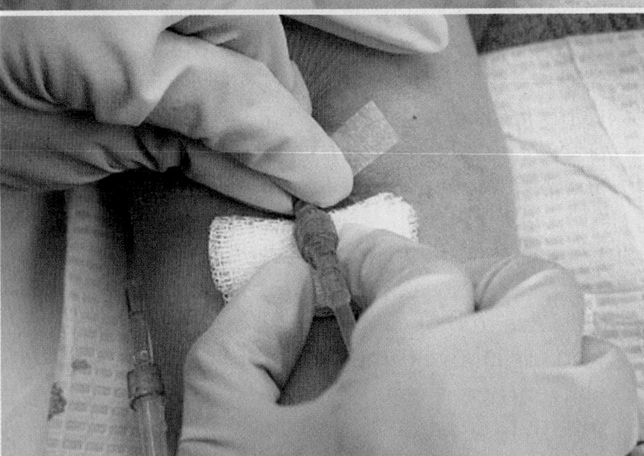

Step **11** Changing infusion tubing.

15. Form a loop of tubing, and secure it to patient's arm with a strip of tape. *(Prevents accidental pulling against site and catheter movement.)*
16. Refer to standard steps 10 to 17.

Changing Fluid Container

1. Refer to standard steps 1 to 9.
2. Assemble equipment:
   - Bottle or bag of IV solution as ordered by physician
   - Time tape
   - Pen

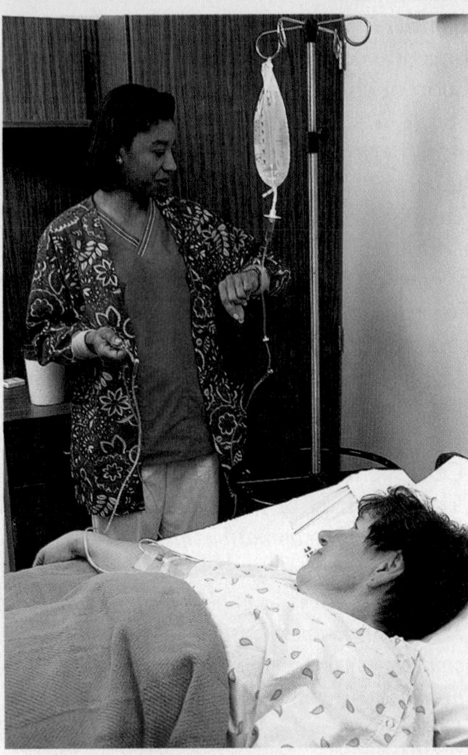

Step **12** Changing infusion tubing.

3. Assessment:
   a. Check physician's orders. *(Ensures that correct solution will be used and that the order is complete.)*
   b. If order is written for KVO, contact physician for clarification of the rate of infusion. Note date and time when solution was last changed. *(Orders for KVO do not provide complete information and have potential to result in fluid overload or deficit and electrolyte imbalance. A KVO order is required to contain a specific infusion rate; check agency policy.)*
   c. Verify patient's identification. *(Ensures right patient receives ordered IV fluid.)*
   d. Determine the compatibility of all IV fluids and additives by consulting appropriate literature or the pharmacy. *(Patency of the inside of catheter depends on prevention of chemical interactions. Precipitation is possible because of concentration of drugs in solution. When pH changes through contact between solutions or medications, formation of a precipitate is possible.)*
   e. Determine patient's understanding of need for continuing IV therapy.
   f. Assess patency of current IV access site. Check for blood return and/or free flow of infusion.
4. Prepare next solution at least 1 hour before needed. If prepared in pharmacy, be sure it has been delivered to the patient's location. Check

that the solution is correct and properly labeled. *(Ensures no disruption in fluid therapy to patient.)* Check solution expiration date. Observe for precipitate and discoloration.

5. Change solution when fluid remains only in neck of container or when new type of solution has been ordered. *(Prevents waste of solution.)*
6. Move roller clamp to stop flow rate, and remove old IV fluid container from IV pole.
7. Quickly remove spike from old container, keeping it sterile. Remove protective cover from new fluid container. Without touching tip of spike, insert it into new bag or bottle. *(Ensures sterility of solution.)*
8. Hang new bag or bottle of solution on IV pole.
9. Check for air in tubing. If bubbles form, it is possible to remove them by closing the roller clamp, stretching the tubing downward, and tapping the tubing with the fingers (the bubbles rise in the tubing to the drip chamber). For larger amounts of air, swab port with antiseptic swab, allow to dry, and connect a syringe to an injection port below the air and aspirate the air into the syringe. *(Infusion of air in tubing potentially results in air embolus, which is sometimes fatal.)* (Tell patient the "champagne-type of bubbles" inside the tubing are not a problem. They will be removed by the filter in the line.)
10. Make sure drip chamber is one third to one half full. If drip chamber is too full, gently pinch off tubing below the drip chamber, hang container, and release the tubing. *(If chamber is completely filled, you are not able to observe drip rate.)*
11. Regulate flow to prescribed rate.
12. Place time label on the side of container, and label with the time hung, the time of completion, and appropriate interval. If using plastic bags, mark only on the label and not on the container.
13. Refer to standard steps 10 to 17.

Discontinuing IV Medications

1. Refer to standard steps 1 to 9.
2. Assemble equipment:
   - Clean gloves
   - Sterile cap or cover for infusion tubing
   - 0.5-mL syringe filled with normal saline or heparin flush solution (check agency policy)
   - 10-mL syringe filled with normal saline or heparin flush solution (check agency policy)
   - Antiseptic swabs
   - Injection cap replacement (if needed)
3. Assessment:
   a. Observe fluid container for complete infusion of all medications.
   b. Review care plan for any blood samples required after medication infusion. *(Monitoring of serum concentration of some IV medications is required to prevent reaching toxic levels. Dosage adjustment or alterations of timing for next dose are sometimes required; check agency policy.)*
   c. Continue to monitor patient's response to medications. *(Enables evaluation of medication's effects.)*
4. Move roller clamp on infusion tubing to the "off" position.
5. Remove any clasping devices, and disconnect medication delivery tubing from injection port. *(If tubing spike, connector end, fluid pathway, or fluid container is contaminated, a new tubing set or fluid container is required.)*
6. Remove the needle or needleless adapter on the infusion tubing; discard appropriately in receptacle, and replace with a sterile cap or cover, as required. *(Infusion tubing is possible to reuse with next ordered medication.)*
7. Swab injection port or prn adapter on main IV tubing with antiseptic swab (see illustration). *(Ensures sterility of port.)*
8. For intermittent medication piggybacked into a continuous infusion, attach 5-mL saline-filled syringe to injection port, and flush the line gently. Regulate fluid flow of the continuous infusion as ordered. *(Saline flush prevents incompatible medications from coming into contact in the infusion tubing. There is no way to know how much pressure is exerted inside catheter lumen. A 5-mL syringe generates less pressure than a 3-mL syringe. Do not force irrigation if resistance is felt.)*
9. For intermittent medications through a saline or heparin lock, attach saline-filled 5- to 10-mL syringe to injection port and flush catheter gently, or attach syringe filled with heparin flush solution to injection port and flush gently, if necessary (check agency policy). Attach sterile injection port cover, if necessary. *(Flushing with 3 to 10 mL of saline after each medication is crucial. Volume of flush depends on lumen size, catheter length, and medication infused.)* **Approach flushing of any IV catheter carefully. If you meet resistance, first assess mechanical causes (e.g., closed clamps, kinked tubing, position of extremity). Never forcefully attempt to flush.** ***(Fibrin formation, drug precipi-***

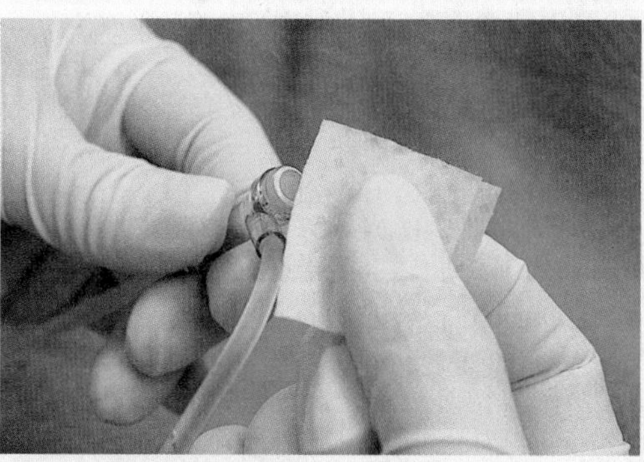

Step 7 Cleanse injection port.

Continued

Skill 20-7 Maintaining an Intravenous Site—cont'd

tates, and blood clots will sometimes occlude catheter lumen. Forceful flush against these occlusions has the potential to cause fracture of catheter and possible embolus formation.) Use size of syringe for flushing in accordance with manufacturer's guidelines for pounds per square inch (INS, 2006).

10. Prepare patient for obtaining blood samples after medication infusion, if necessary.
11. Refer to standard steps 10 to 17.

Discontinuing Peripheral IV Access

1. Refer to standard steps 1 to 9.
2. Assemble equipment:
   - Clean gloves
   - Sterile 2 × 2 or 4 × 4 gauze pad
   - Tape
   - Antiseptic swab
3. Assessment:
   a. Observe existing IV site for signs and symptoms of infection, infiltration, or phlebitis. *(Indications of need to discontinue IV).*
   b. Review physician's orders for discontinuation of IV therapy. *(Physician order is required to discontinue IV therapy. The specific wording will sometimes not include removal of catheter, but this is implied.)*
   c. Determine patient's understanding of the need for removal of peripheral IV catheter.
4. Explain procedure to patient. Explain that it is necessary to hold affected extremity still, and how long procedure will take. *(Keeps patient's anxiety and discomfort to a minimum.)*
5. Turn IV tubing roller clamp to "off" position. Remove tape securing tubing.
6. Remove IV site dressing and tape while stabilizing catheter. *(Movement of catheter will cause discomfort.)* (Never use scissors to remove the tape or dressing because it is possible to accidentally cut the catheter.)
7. With dry gauze or alcohol swab held over site, apply light pressure and withdraw the catheter, using a slow steady movement, keeping the hub parallel to the skin (see illustration). *(Changing the angle of the catheter inside the vein sometimes causes additional vein irritation, increasing the risk of postinfusion phlebitis.)*
8. Apply pressure to the site for 2 to 3 minutes, using a dry, sterile gauze pad. Secure the tape. *(Dry pad causes less irritation to the puncture site. Subcutaneous hematoma is a common complication. When needle is removed, vein wall contracts to stop bleeding. Contraction is enhanced by pressure to site for at least 2 to 3 minutes.)*

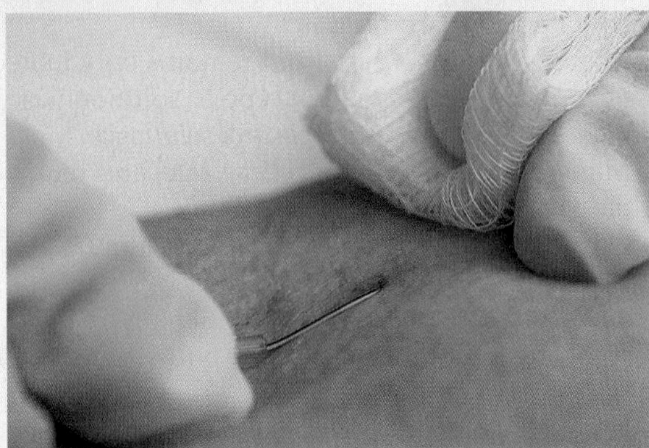

Step 7 Withdraw IV catheter.

9. Inspect the catheter for intactness, noting tip integrity and length. *(Tips of catheter sometimes break off, causing an embolus, an emergency situation. Notify physician if tip is broken.)*
10. Discard used supplies.
11. Remove and discard gloves, and perform hand hygiene.
12. Instruct patient to report any erythema, pain, drainage, or edema that occurs after catheter removal. *(Postinfusion phlebitis sometimes occurs within 48 to 96 hours after catheter removal.)*
13. Refer to standard steps 10 to 17.

Notes for Recording and Reporting

1. Record time peripheral dressing was changed, reason for dressing change, type of dressing material used, patency of system, and observation of venipuncture site.
2. Record changing tubing on patient's record, including the rate of infusion. A special IV flow sheet is sometimes used.
3. Record amount and type of fluid infused and amount and type of new fluid according to agency policy. A special flow sheet is sometimes used for parenteral fluids.
4. Record time of discontinuing medication and flushing infusion tubing and catheter, including amount and type of flush solution and condition of site.
5. Record time peripheral IV is discontinued. Include site assessment information and gauge and length of catheter removed.
6. Report to nurse in charge or oncoming nurse that the dressing was changed, any significant information about IV site or IV system, the time you discontinued the medication or IV, and the time you obtained any blood samples.

Dressings used to cover IV insertion sites help prevent the introduction of microorganisms. The two most common types of dressings for IV sites are gauze and transparent dressings. The advantages of transparent dressings are easy visualization of the site and their lower likelihood than gauze of becoming soiled or damp. Follow your agency's policy and recommendations for routine IV dressing changes (usually every 48 to 72 hours) (Potter & Perry, 2009). However, it is always necessary to change IV dressings if they become wet, soiled, or loose (INS, 2000).

There are several types of IV solution containers, including plastic and glass. You will change these containers on a routine basis according to agency policy, which in turn is dictated by the type of solution, the type of container, and whether or not the IV is a standard peripheral IV or an ambulatory infusion device (Potter & Perry, 2009).

Also follow agency policy regarding tubing changes. The INS (2000) recommends changing tubing every 72 hours for continuous infusions unless the facility is experiencing higher than a 5% IV-related infection and phlebitis rate, in which case the recommended interval is reduced to every 48 hours. For patients with intermittent infusions or infusions through an injection or access port, the INS recommends tubing changes every 24 hours.

It is best to use gowns made for patients with IVs that have snaps across the shoulders. With patients wearing regular gowns or their own clothes, never disconnect the tubing when assisting with the gown or clothing change. Instead, thread the IV solution container and tubing through the sleeve as you do with the patient's arm (Elkin et al., 2007). See Box 20-5 for nursing diagnoses for the patient receiving intravenous therapy.

Box 20-5 Nursing Diagnoses for the Patient Receiving Intravenous Therapy

Risk for infection:
- Related to invasive procedure

Impaired skin integrity:
- Related to invasive procedure

Risk for fluid volume, excess or deficit:
- Related to alterations in regulatory mechanisms of hydration
- Related to fluid and electrolyte imbalance

Risk for injury:
- Related to presence of IV catheter acting as a foreign body
- Related to adverse events
- Related to IV medications

Knowledge, deficient:
- Related to lack of exposure to information

Data from North American Nursing Diagnosis Association International (NANDA-I). (2009). *NANDA-I nursing diagnoses: Definitions and classification 2009-2011*. Oxford, United Kingdom: Author.

SKILLS FOR RESPIRATORY DISORDERS

OXYGEN THERAPY

Oxygen therapy is one method of preventing or relieving tissue hypoxia. Oxygen therapy must be ordered by a physician and closely monitored by the nurse to ensure proper administration (see Coordinated Care box on oxygen administration). Oxygen is treated as a drug; therefore, it is important to follow the six rights of drug administration when administering oxygen (see Chapter 23). Oxygen administration is expensive and poses the risk of serious side effects, such as oxygen toxicity or atelectasis (Potter & Perry, 2009).

The element oxygen is a colorless, odorless, and tasteless gas that will not burn or explode. However, if combined with other factors, such as an electrical spark or fire, oxygen will support combustion and ignite. Be sure to observe all safety precautions (Box 20-6).

Coordinated Care

Collaboration

OXYGEN ADMINISTRATION

- The skill of oxygen administration by nasal cannula or mask requires the critical thinking application unique to a nurse. You are responsible for correctly administering oxygen, including adjusting oxygen flow rate and assessing patient response to oxygen therapy.
- Correct placement and adjustment of oxygen devices is acceptable to delegate to assistive personnel. Instruct the care provider in possible unexpected outcomes associated with oxygen delivery and the need to report these to you if they occur.

Box 20-6 Safety Precautions during Oxygen Use

- Place "No Smoking" and/or "Oxygen in Use" signs in conspicuous locations.
- Instruct the patient, the family, and visitors that smoking is not permitted, because oxygen supports combustion (burning).
- Avoid the use of electrical appliances, such as razors, blankets, and heating pads.
- Secure portable oxygen delivery systems, such as cylinders, to prevent their falling or accidentally being tipped over.
- Avoid placing oxygen cylinders near sources of heat, such as lamps or radiators.
- Avoid clothing that is not fire resistant.
- Ensure that all electrical equipment is functioning appropriately and is well grounded. Avoid frayed, tangled, or cluttered cords, and do not overload circuits with too many appliances.
- Know the institution's fire procedure and location of fire extinguishers.
- Administer oxygen as ordered by a physician; the physician determines the method of administration and the flow rate of oxygen (O_2).
- Avoid use of petrolatum products such as petroleum jelly.

Oxygen therapy is frequently initiated by a respiratory therapist, who is a health care professional licensed to deliver treatment that will improve a patient's ventilation and oxygenation needs.

The signs and symptoms manifested by patients who have a possible need for supplemental oxygen will vary according to the degree of oxygen deficiency (Box 20-7, Skill 20-8, Figure 20-12, and Life Span Considerations for Older Adults, Patient Teaching, and Home Care Considerations boxes on oxygen therapy).

Box 20-7 Signs and Symptoms of Hypoxia

- Apprehension, anxiety, restlessness
- Decreased ability to concentrate
- Decreased level of consciousness
- Increased fatigue
- Vertigo
- Behavioral changes
- Increased pulse rate: as hypoxia advances, bradycardia results, which in turn results in decreased oxygen saturation by pulse oximetry
- Increased rate and depth of respiration: as hypoxia progresses, shallow, slow respirations develop
- Elevated blood pressure; if O_2 deficiency is not corrected, blood pressure will decrease
- Cardiac dysrhythmias
- Pallor
- Cyanosis
- Clubbing (with chronic hypoxia)
- Dyspnea

Transtracheal Oxygen Delivery

A newer method of oxygen delivery is the transtracheal catheter, which is inserted directly into the trachea between the second and third tracheal cartilages.

 **Life Span Considerations**

Older Adults

Oxygen Therapy

- Normal arterial oxygen levels sometimes decrease with age. It is possible that a 70-year-old will have a normal arterial Po_2 between 75 and 80.
- The drive to breathe in patients who have chronically increased CO_2 levels such as in chronic emphysema is based on their oxygen status. Oxygen flow rates greater than 2 L/min are to be given with great caution in these individuals.
- The older adult is often at increased risk for skin impairment. Frequent monitoring for erythema over the ears is necessary. Early interventions such as loosening the straps, repositioning the tubing, or adding padding over the ears will often prevent impairment.

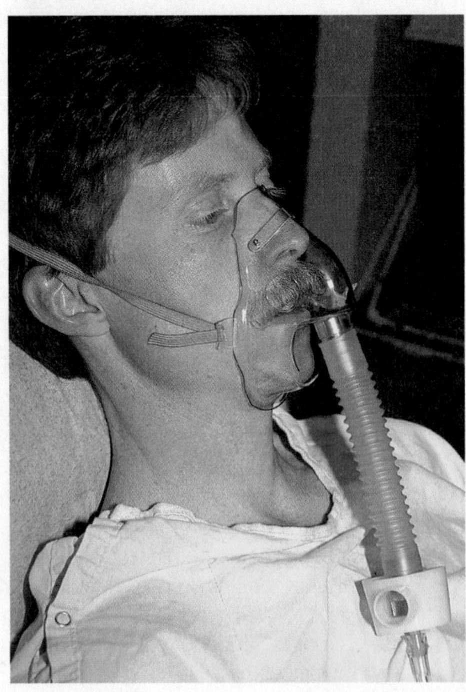

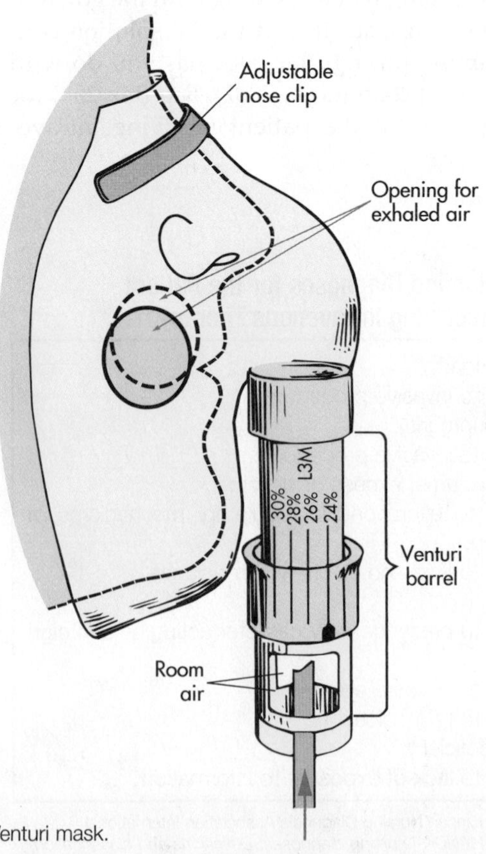

FIGURE 20-12 Venturi mask.

Skill 20-8 Oxygen Administration

Nursing Action *(Rationale)*

1. Refer to standard steps 1 to 9.
2. Assemble equipment:
   - Specific oxygen delivery system (e.g., mask, cannula, or tent, which is used primarily for pediatric patients)
   - Oxygen tubing (consider extension tubing)
   - Source of oxygen
   - Flowmeter
   - Humidifier bottle and sterile water
   - "Oxygen in Use" sign
   - Clean gloves
   - Stethoscope
3. Explain necessary precautions during oxygen therapy (see Box 20-6). *(Promotes safety.)*
4. Position patient in Fowler's or semi-Fowler's position. *(Allows for maximum lung expansion.)*
5. Assess patient's airway. *(Enables you to confirm patent airway and determine need for oxygen.)* Assess patient for signs and symptoms of hypoxia (results from hypoxemia, which is a deficiency of oxygen in the arterial blood) and respiratory distress (see Box 20-7). Take laboratory reports of arterial blood gas levels into account. Suction any secretions obstructing the airway, and reassess lung sounds with stethoscope (see Skill 20-11).
6. Fill humidifier container to designated level, and if needed, humidify for flow rates greater than 4 L/min; use sterile water or as prescribed. *(Provides moisture to prevent drying of the nasooropharyngeal mucosa.)*
7. Attach flowmeter to humidifier and insert in proper oxygen source; most institutions have a central source of oxygen with a specifically designed outlet. Verify that water is bubbling. *(Presence of bubbling indicates that oxygen is humidified before delivery to patient. It is necessary to properly secure flowmeter to oxygen source for adequate delivery of O_2.)*
8. Administer oxygen therapy:
   a. **Nasal cannula** (see illustration): A simple, two-pronged plastic device that is used to deliver low concentrations of oxygen. A nasal cannula allows patient to eat and talk normally and is appropriate for all age-groups. Observe caution to properly place prongs to prevent oxygen from coming in direct contact with nasal mucosa. Oxygen has a drying effect on mucosa and interferes with moistening and warming air inhaled through nasal passages, making breathing uncomfortable for patient. It is your responsibility to maintain method, flow rate, comfort, and safety of a patient receiving oxygen therapy.

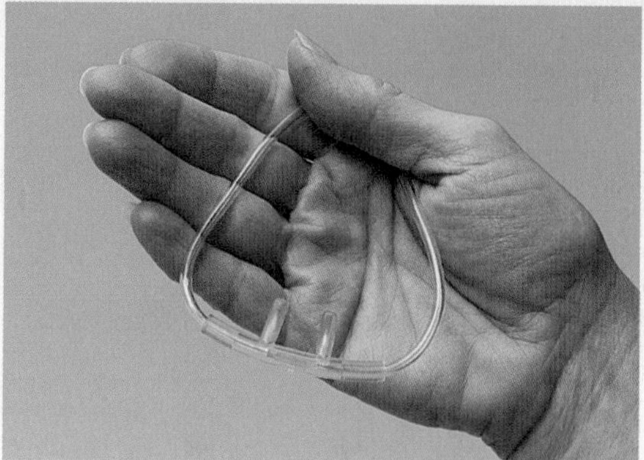

Step 8a Nasal cannula.

   (1) Attach nasal cannula to oxygen tubing (if it is not preattached), and then attach to flowmeter. *(It is necessary for oxygen delivery system to be continuous to ensure adequate supply of amounts of oxygen.)*
   (2) Place prongs in cup of water. Adjust flowmeter to 6 to 10 L/min to flush tubing and prongs with oxygen. *(Enables you to determine patency and removes any microscopic particles possibly in tubing.)* If water bubbles, tubing and prongs are patent. Wipe off water.
   (3) Adjust flow rate to prescribed amount. *(Ensures delivery of oxygen flow rate as directed by the physician.)*
   (4) Place a nasal prong into each nostril of the patient (see illustration). *(Directs flow of oxygen into patient's upper respiratory tract.)* Adjust liter flow per physician's order; usually 2 L/min is prescribed.
   (5) Adjust straps of cannula over the ears and tighten under the chin (see illustration). *(Proper fit is snug and comfortable to prevent displacement of prongs.)*
   (6) Place padding between strap and ears. Use lamb's wool, gauze, or cotton balls. *(Prevents skin irritation.)*
   (7) Provide slack of tubing, and secure to patient's garment. *(Reduces risk of prong(s) causing pressure on the nares, as well as of displacement as patient moves or is repositioned.)*
   (8) Maintain regular assessment. *(Ensures delivery of prescribed oxygen flow rate.)*
      (a) Assess cannula frequently for possible obstruction.

Continued

Skill 20-8 Oxygen Administration—cont'd

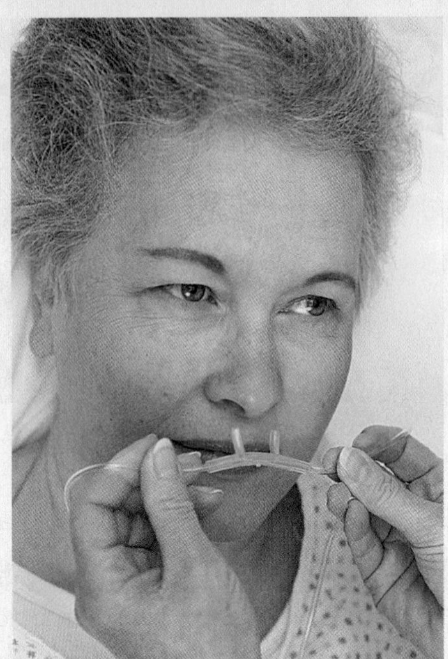
Step **8a(4)**

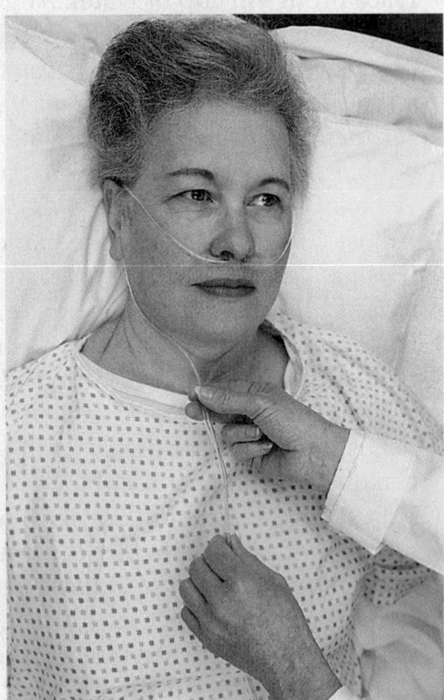
Step **8a(5)**

(b) Observe external nasal area, nares, and superior surface of both ears for skin impairment every 6 to 8 hours.

(c) Assess nares and prongs and cleanse with cotton-tipped applicator as needed.

(d) Apply water-soluble lubricant to nares. *(Prevents drying.)*

(e) Refer to physician's orders for any prescribed changes in flow rate.

(f) Maintain solution in humidifier container, if used, at appropriate level at all times. *(Prevents inhalation of dehumidified oxygen.)*

(g) Auscultate lung sounds. *(Verifies adequate oxygenation.)*

(h) Consult with physician regarding need for pulse oximetry if patient's oxygen level is unstable.

b. Face mask: Depending on patient's respiratory condition, physician will sometimes prescribe oxygen to be administered by oxygen mask (see illustration). The mask is designed to fit snugly over patient's nose and mouth. Different types of masks will be used according to patient's needs, such as the Venturi mask (see Figure 20-12), the partial-rebreathing mask (step 8b[5][a]), the nonrebreathing mask (step 8b), and the simple face mask.

(1) Adjust flow rate of oxygen per physician's order. Usually 6 to 10 L/min, which is measured in percentages, is prescribed. The respiratory therapist is usually responsible for maintaining proper flow. Observe for fine mist or bubbling in humidifier.

(2) Allow patient to hold mask, and place your hand over patient's hand. *(Placing mask over patient's face sometimes causes feeling of suffocation and apprehension. This action allows patient to become accustomed to mask and to have some control over placing it on face.)*

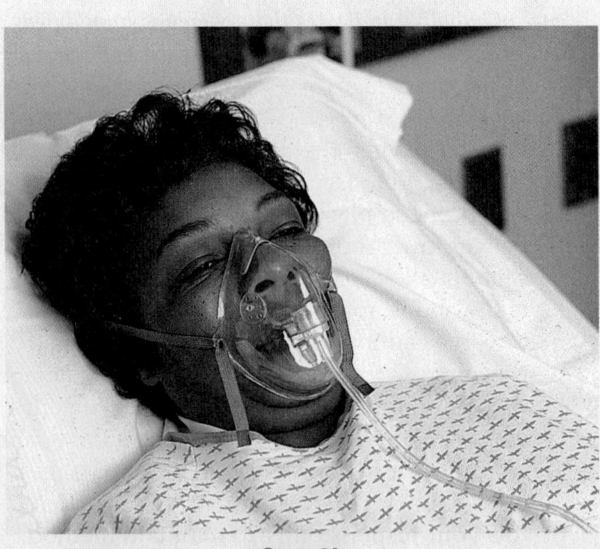
Step **8b**

(3) Place mask over bridge of nose, and then cover mouth. *(This method is less threatening to the patient.)*

(4) Adjust straps around patient's head and over ears. Place cotton ball or gauze over ears under elastic straps. *(Provides comfort and prevents skin impairment.)*

(5) Observe reservoir bag if one is attached to mask. *(Mask's expanding and collapsing with patient's breathing confirms appropriate fit is maintained.)*

(a) **Partial-rebreathing mask:** When functioning properly, the reservoir will fill on exhalation and almost collapse on inhalation (see illustration).

(b) **Nonrebreathing mask:** When functioning properly, the reservoir will fill on exhalation and will never totally collapse on inhalation.

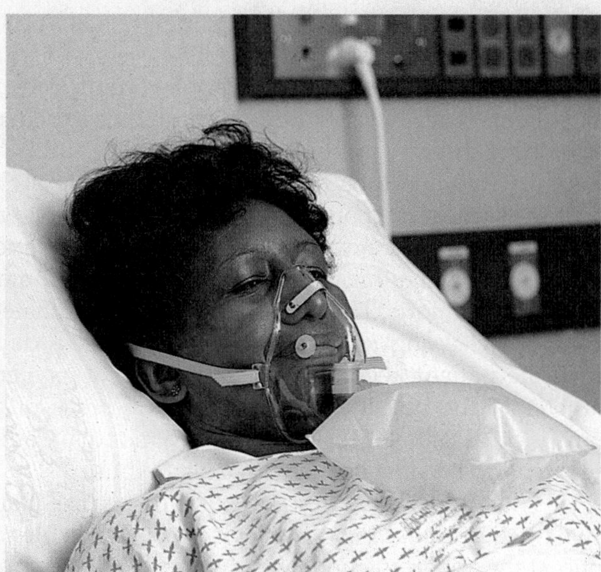

Step **8b(5)(a)**

(6) Maintain regular assessments. *(Ensures that specialized face masks are working properly.)*

(a) Remove mask and cleanse and dry skin every 1 to 2 hours. *(Removes condensation and other debris that may form.)*

(b) Refer to physician's orders for prescribed flow rate and any changes.

(c) Maintain solution in humidifier container, if used, at appropriate level at all times. Oxygen is not humidified with a flow rate of ½ to 3 L/min except with infants, and even with a flow rate of ¼ L/min, oxygen is always humidified. Oxygen is always humidified with a flow rate of 3 to 6 L/min. Above a flow rate of 6 L/min, a simple mask, Venturi mask, or nonrebreather mask is used and the oxygen is not humidified. Always use sterile water, never tap water, because sterile water decreases the growth of microorganisms.

9. Refer to standard steps 10 to 17.
10. Document: *(Verifies performance of procedure and ensures continuity of care.)*
    - Date
    - Time
    - Flow rate
    - Method of oxygen delivery
    - Respiratory assessment
    - Patient's response
    - Changes in physician's orders
    - Adverse reactions or side effects
    - Patient teaching (see Patient Teaching and Home Care Considerations boxes on oxygen therapy)

 Patient Teaching

Oxygen Therapy

- Teach how to apply the oxygen equipment, such as the cannula or mask.
- Discuss safety precautions for oxygen use (see Box 20-6).
- It is important to stress the dangers of changing the oxygen flow rate from the prescribed flow rate. Emphasize that it is possible for the patient to be short of breath because of reasons other than hypoxemia and to contact physician if increased shortness of breath occurs.
- Instruct on frequent ambulation or position changes to mobilize secretions.
- Encourage to practice deep breathing and coughing techniques to facilitate air exchange.
- Teach to maintain adequate fluid intake to help liquefy secretions. Recommend fluids that are caffeine and sugar free. Drinks high in sugar and caffeine sometimes cause dehydration. Avoid dairy products, which tend to thicken secretions.
- Good medication teaching addresses the rationale for prescribed medications, as well as side effects.
- Teach that performing oral hygiene at regular intervals will help rid the mouth of any bad taste from secretions coughed up or expectorated.

Home Care Considerations

Oxygen Therapy

- If oxygen is used at home, instruct the patient's family to post a "No Smoking" sign on the door of the house.
- When oxygen cylinders are used, it is necessary to secure them so that they will not fall over. Oxygen cylinders are stored upright, chained on appropriate holders.
- In home settings, oxygen tubing will sometimes be as long as 50 feet.
- Instruct patient's family on safety measures of oxygen therapy (see Box 20-6).
- Teach patient and family members how to use home equipment.
- Instruct patient and family members to observe level of oxygen in canister tanks and to use portable tanks when patient is not at home.
- Instruct patient and family members to fill plastic humidity bottle with distilled water every 24 hours. Make sure they know never to use tap water.
- Provide two complete sets of tubing so one set of equipment is available for use while the other is being cleaned or repaired.
- Assess home for availability of a three-pronged outlet for the compressor to prevent electric shock.
- Teach to maintain constant flow rate; change flow rate only with order of a physician.
- Assess home for appropriate storage of equipment.
- Assess family's willingness to assist patient with home delivery system.
- Teach patient and family deep breathing and coughing exercises.
- Teach patient and family nutritional and adequate hydration needs.

Transtracheal oxygen delivery was pioneered by Henry J. Heimlich.

Unlike a tracheostomy tube, a transtracheal catheter (Figure 20-13) does not interfere with drinking, eating, or talking. The nasal cannula delivers oxygen only during inhalation, but the transtracheal oxygen delivery system delivers oxygen throughout the respiratory cycle. No oxygen is lost to the atmosphere; therefore oxygen delivery is less expensive. Additional humidification is unnecessary because the nasopharynx, the area most in need of supplemental humidity, is bypassed. This allows the flow rate to be decreased for some patients. Those patients who require 2 L/min with a cannula will need only 1 L/min with a transtracheal catheter. The low flow rates enable patients to use portable oxygen delivery systems longer between refills. Transtracheal oxygen delivery is recommended for patients with heart failure or chronic obstructive pulmonary disease.

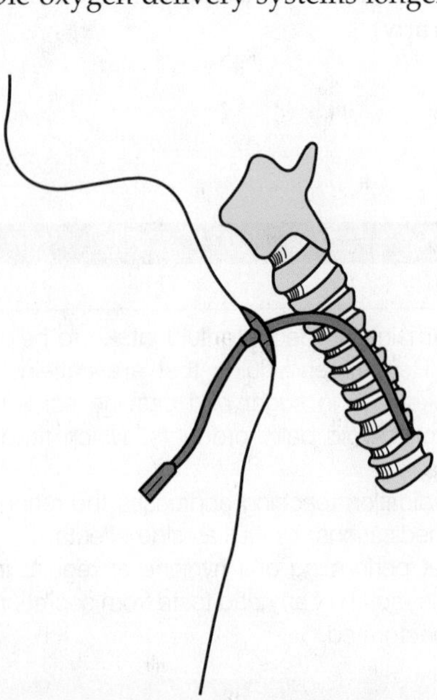

FIGURE 20-13 A transtracheal catheter is possible to insert into the trachea between the second and third tracheal cartilages.

A small oxygen tube (8 or 9 F) is inserted through the transtracheal tract opening, through which oxygen is administered. Remove the tube for cleaning, and administer oxygen through the nose in the meantime. Use clean technique. The transtracheal oxygen catheter will need cleaning as often as several times a day. Have the patient keep an extra transtracheal oxygen catheter at the bedside. Avoid continued reuse of a transtracheal catheter for longer than 3 months. Catheters tend to become brittle with extended use.

This method is especially suited for home use. It allows the individual to be active. It is even possible to conceal the apparatus under a shirt and tie. Make sure the patient knows to inspect the transtracheal tract opening regularly for erythema, edema, or excessive exudate. (Small amounts of clear exudate are expected.) The area is cleaned twice daily with a cotton-tipped applicator. Suggest using hydrogen peroxide to wash the neck and remove dried exudate. The transtracheal tract (like a tracheostomy) never truly heals as long as it is kept open for oxygen delivery. If tube replacement is delayed more than 30 minutes, the opening will sometimes seal over.

Care of the Tracheostomy

The term **tracheostomy** means "an artificial opening made by a surgical incision into the trachea." After the surgical procedure is performed, the physician inserts a tracheostomy tube into the opening and secures it in place by cotton tapes around the patient's neck. This provides the patient with a patent airway. Sterile gauze is placed around the opening, under the flange of the outer tube, for skin protection. Use wipes that are free of lint around the tracheostomy opening. Inhaled lint irritates respiratory passages and often causes undue coughing. The primary nursing responsibilities are to maintain a patent airway, keep the inner cannula clean, prevent impairment of surrounding tissue, and provide a means of communication for the patient (Skill 20-9). An endotracheal or a tracheostomy (or "trach") tube provides a direct route for introduction of pathogens into the lower airway, increasing the risk of infection (Figures 20-14 and 20-15). It is essential that the following preventive nursing interventions be consistently implemented:

1. Minimize infection risk:
   a. Assess the patient regularly for excess secretions and suction as often as necessary.

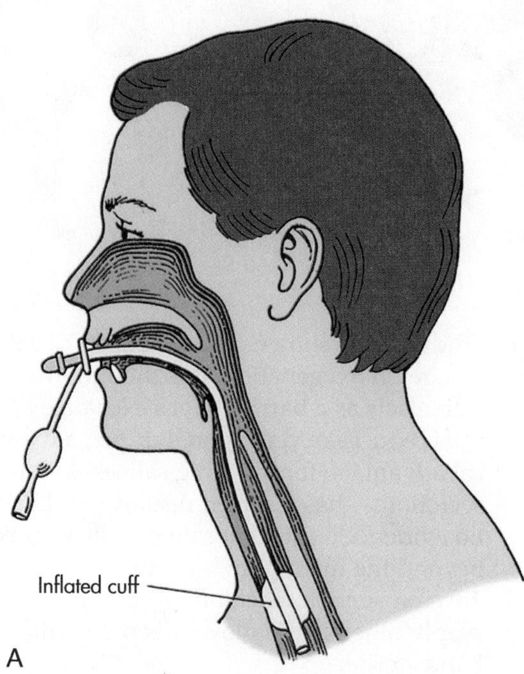

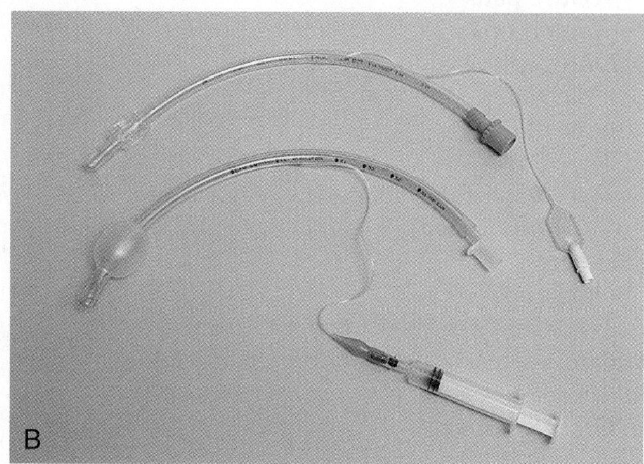

FIGURE 20-14 **A,** Endotracheal (ET) tube with inflated cuff. **B,** ET tubes with uninflated cuffs and syringe for inflation. Patient is unable to speak while tube is in place because air cannot flow through the vocal cords.

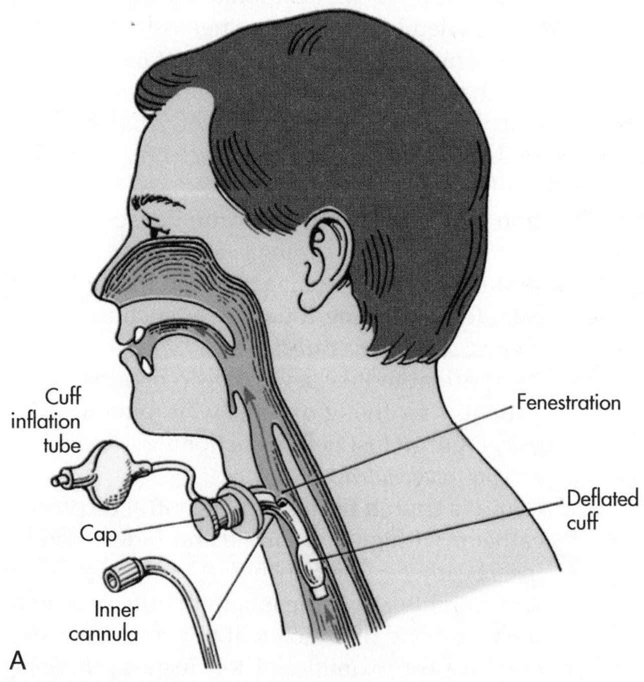

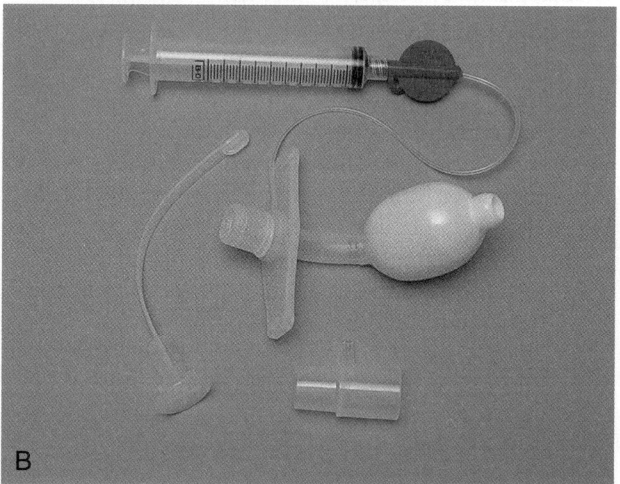

FIGURE 20-15 **A,** Trach tube (fenestrated) with inner cannula removed and cap in place to allow speech. **B,** Trach tube with obturator for insertion and syringe for inflation of cuff.

Skill 20-9 Tracheostomy Care and Suctioning

Nursing Action *(Rationale)*

1. Refer to standard steps 1 to 9.
2. Assemble equipment:
   - Paper and pencil
   - Sterile towel or prepackaged drape
   - Suction apparatus (wall mount or portable)
   - Sterile suction catheter kit
   - Sterile disposable tracheostomy "trach" kit, which contains:
     —Two basins
     —Pipe cleaners
     —Forceps
     —Gauze pads
     —Cotton tips
   - Hydrogen peroxide
   - Sterile water or normal saline
   - Sterile gloves
   - Clean gloves
   - Clean, water-repellent gown, goggles, and mask (if indicated)
   - Scissors
   - Stethoscope
3. Assess patient's tracheostomy for sanguineous exudate, edema, and respiratory obstruction. *(Allows you to identify potential need for further nursing interventions.)*
4. Position patient in semi-Fowler's position. *(Allows for optimum lung expansion.)*
5. Provide paper and pencil for patient. (Because patient cannot speak, this offers means of communication.)
6. Position self at head of bed facing patient. Always face patient while cleaning a tracheostomy. *(Enables close observation for respiratory difficulty and coughing, which create possibility of expelling cannula.)*
7. Auscultate lungs. *(Provides a baseline assessment.)*
8. Place towel or prepackaged drape under tracheostomy and across chest. *(Protects patient's gown and the bed linens.)*
9. Prepare equipment and supplies on overbed table (see illustration). *(Organizes procedure.)*
   a. Open suction catheter, leaving it in its wrapper (maintains sterility), and attach it to suction machine.
   b. Pour cleansing solution in one basin and rinsing solution in another basin. The first basin will hold hydrogen peroxide. *(Serves to cleanse mucus and secretions from inner cannula.)* The second basin will contain normal saline. *(Serves to rinse cannula.)* If basins are prepackaged with sterile gloves, use one-glove technique to remove basins and pour solution with ungloved hand.

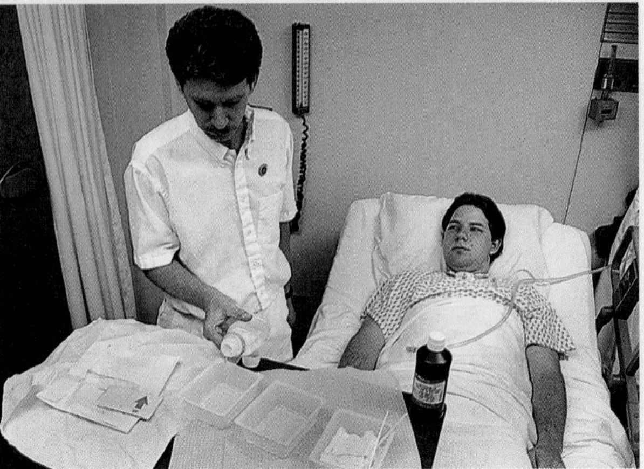

Step **9**

   c. Studies have shown adverse effects of saline lavage on oxygenation. It is thought that saline acts as a barrier to gas exchange and thus reduces oxygenation. Further, a theoretical advantage for instilling saline—to loosen secretions—has received no support. Little or no evidence exists that saline is distributed beyond the main stem bronchi.
   d. Turn on suction machine.
   e. Apply other sterile glove. Keep dominant hand sterile.
10. Unlock and remove inner cannula; place in hydrogen peroxide cleansing solution. Place fingers on tabs of outer cannula. *(Prevents movement that has potential to irritate surrounding tissue and cause pain and coughing.)* ***NEVER*** remove outer cannula. If it is expelled by patient, use hemostat to hold tracheostomy open and call for assistance. Always have a sterile packaged hemostat, as well as an extra sterile tracheostomy set, available at the bedside. *(Ensures that emergency equipment is close at hand.)*
11. Suction inner aspect of outer cannula (see illustration). *(Aids in maintaining patent airway.)*
   a. Withdraw sterile rinsing solution through catheter by placing thumb over suction control. *(Moistens catheter.)*
   b. Ask patient to take several deep breaths, or if patient is receiving oxygen, wait to remove oxygen until just before suctioning. *(Keeps patient oxygenated.)*
   c. Remove thumb from suction control or pinch catheter with gloved thumb and index finger; insert catheter 5 to 6 inches. (Depth of catheter will roughly equal the length of outer cannula, the distal end of which will protrude from the opening approximately 1 to 2 inches.) *(Keeping thumb off of suction vent or pinching the catheter*

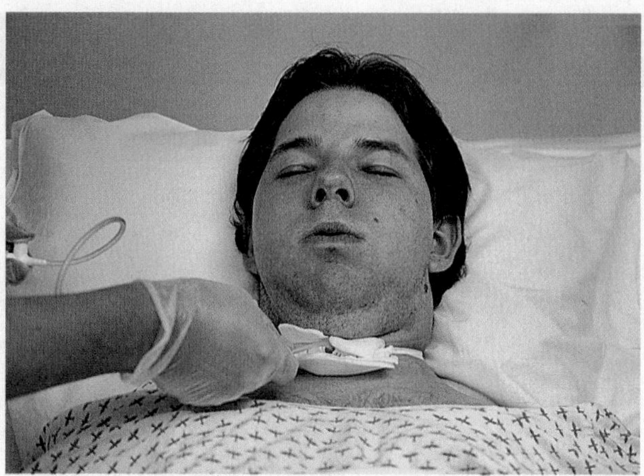

Step **11**

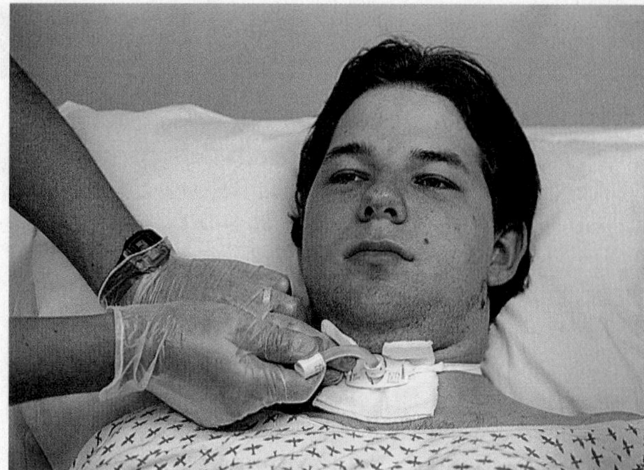

Step **13d**

prevents suctioning while inserting catheter, which has potential to damage the mucosa.)

d. Apply intermittent suction by placing thumb on and off suction control, and gently rotate catheter as it is withdrawn.

e. Suction for a maximum of 10 seconds at a time, never longer. *(Prolonged suctioning depletes oxygen supply.)* For a good idea of the patient's experience of not breathing, try holding your own breath until you are uncomfortable.

f. Rinse catheter with sterile solution and repeat steps c and d if needed.

g. Allow patient to rest between each suctioning effort. If patient was previously receiving oxygen, reapply it at the prescribed rate between each stint. *(Suctioning is often exhausting and frightening for patient. Resting helps regain depleted oxygen and renew strength.)*

h. Turn off suction and dispose of catheter appropriately.

12. Apply second sterile glove, if one-glove technique is used, or apply new pair of sterile gloves. *(Reduces spread of microorganisms.)*

13. Clean inner cannula. *(Removes secretions and hydrogen peroxide from inner cannula.)*

a. Use pipe cleaners and brush to clean inside and outside of inner cannula.

b. Place inner cannula in sterile normal saline solution. *(Rinses away the hydrogen peroxide.)*

c. Inspect inner and outer areas of inner cannula. Remove excess liquid (see step 13a).

d. Insert inner cannula and lock in place (see illustration). *(Secures inner cannula and reestablishes oxygen supply.)*

14. Clean skin around tracheostomy and tabs of outer cannula with hydrogen peroxide and cotton-tipped swabs. Use wipes that are free of lint around the tracheostomy opening. *(Inhaled lint [from cotton balls, etc.] irritates the respiratory passages and tends to cause undue coughing. Special tracheostomy dressings are available.)*

15. Thoroughly rinse cleansing solution from skin. *(Aseptically removes secretions from stoma site.)* Place dry, sterile dressing around tracheostomy face plate (see illustration). *(Prevents skin impairment from flange of tracheostomy tube rubbing against the peristomal skin.)*

16. Change cotton tapes. *(Always do this last to prevent cannula from being expelled.)* Only attach clean tape when necessary.

a. Untie one side of cotton tape from outer cannula and replace with clean one. It is advisable to obtain the assistance of another person who will stabilize the tracheostomy tube while you remove and replace one set of ties. *(Provides more room for threading the clean ties and prevents accidental expulsion of outer cannula.)*

b. Bring clean tape under back of neck. *(Securely holds tracheostomy tube in place to prevent movement of cannula that will potentially stimulate coughing and expel cannula.)*

c. Untie other side from outer cannula and replace with clean tape.

d. Tie ends of two clean cotton tapes together and position knot at side of neck. *(Avoid*

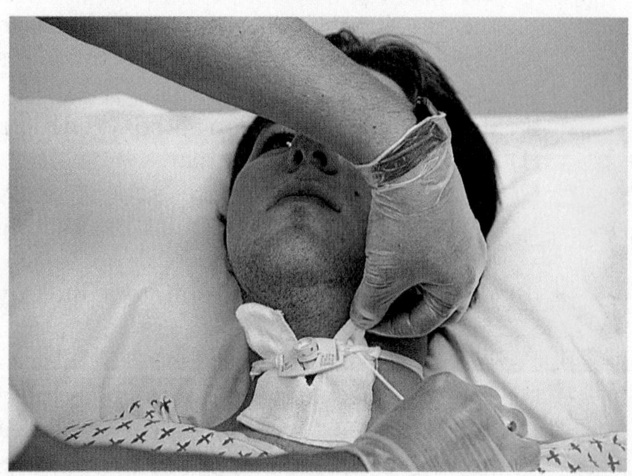

Step **15**

Continued

Skill 20-9 Tracheostomy Care and Suctioning—cont'd

placing knot at back of neck, which often causes pressure and discomfort to cervical vertebrae.)

17. Auscultate lung sounds. *(Enables you to determine any change from baseline assessment.)*
18. Provide mouth care. *(Promotes good oral hygiene. Patients with tracheostomies often have halitosis.)*
19. Refer to standard steps 10 to 17.
20. Place call light, paper, and pencil within easy reach. *(Enables patient to communicate needs.)*
21. Reassess patient's tracheostomy for signs of bleeding, edema, and respiratory obstruction. *(Patients with tracheostomy frequently have bloody secretions for 2 to 3 days after procedure or for 24 hours after each tracheostomy tube change.)*
22. Document: *(Verifies performance of procedure and ensures continuity of care.)*
    - Tracheostomy care performed
    - Patient's response
    - Respiratory assessment
    - Suction performed
    - Adverse reactions
    - Condition of tracheal stoma and peristomal skin
    - If oxygen is administered, note flow rate and method used
    - Patient teaching (see Home Care Considerations box on tracheostomy care)
23. Skill 20-10 describes how to care for a cuffed tracheostomy tube.

b. Provide constant airway humidification.
c. Change all respiratory therapy equipment every 8 hours.
d. Remove water that condenses in equipment tubing.
e. Provide frequent mouth care (apply moisturizing agents to dry, cracked lips).
f. Maintain nutritional levels.
   (1) Patients with endotracheal tubes are allowed nothing by mouth. It will be necessary to provide nourishment parenterally or enterally.
   (2) Patients with a tracheostomy are not limited in regards to drinking fluids and eating. Some sources suggest inflating the cuff on a tracheostomy tube to prevent aspiration during eating or drinking, but other sources suggest that this causes difficulty swallowing as a result of the cuff bulging into the esophagus (Regan & Dallachiesa, 2009). Some physicians will order the cuff to be inflated for 30 minutes after meals. Nursing assessment or physician orders will determine which technique is used.
g. Ensure adequate ventilation and oxygenation.
   (1) Assess lung sounds regularly.
   (2) Turn and reposition the patient every 2 hours for maximum ventilation and lung expansion.
   (3) Assess the effects of respiratory therapy frequently.
h. Provide safety and comfort.
   (1) Assess tube placement at regular intervals—tracheostomy tubes are secured around neck with tapes or specially designed ties.
   (2) Change the tapes or ties whenever soiled to lessen the chances of skin impairment.
   (3) Always keep a spare tracheostomy tube at the bedside.

2. Reduce **sensory deprivation** (the enforced absence of usual and accustomed sensory stimuli [the absence of normal stimuli]) to a minimum.
   a. Organize questions so that the patient is able to give simple yes or no responses by nodding the head or using hand signals.
   b. Assess whether the patient is able to use an erasable board (e.g., Magic Slate) or notepad to communicate.
   c. Always talk to the patient and explain all procedures. While preparing patient, explain: "Suctioning will help clear your secretions and make you more comfortable. Try to cough deeply. Take two or three deep breaths after I suction you and replace your oxygen."
   d. Reorient the patient frequently.
   e. Encourage family and friends to talk to the patient.
   f. Keep a call light (or tap bell) within patient's reach.

With today's knowledge and new materials, a single-cannula tracheostomy is used. This type of tracheostomy tube is referred to as the cuffed tracheostomy tube (see Figure 20-15). It is made of plastic and has an inflatable cuff around the middle of the distal portion of the tube. The physician will sometimes order a cuffed tracheostomy tube to be used initially until the healing process of the tracheal stoma is complete. The cuffed tube is commonly employed for temporary use, to hold the tube in place during special treatments (e.g., ventilation or intermittent positive-pressure breathing [IPPB]), and to prevent aspiration during such activities as eating or taking medications.

IPPB is a mechanical method for assisting pulmonary ventilation that employs a device that administers air or oxygen for the inflation of the lungs under positive pressure. Exhalation is usually passive.

Although nursing interventions for patients with endotracheal and tracheostomy tubes is similar, patients with tracheostomies have additional nursing care needs (see Home Care Considerations and Coordinated Care boxes on suctioning for tracheostomy care). To prevent depression of the respiratory center, it is advisable to give analgesics and sedatives with caution. The patient is suctioned as often as necessary, possibly every 5 minutes during the first few postoperative hours (when respirations are noisy and pulse and respiratory rates are increased, the patient needs to be suctioned). Patients who are conscious are usually able to indicate when they need to be suctioned. A patient who is able to expectorate secretions will require suctioning less frequently. The amount of mucus decreases gradually, and you will perform suctioning less frequently. However, the patient remains apprehensive and needs constant attendance and reassurance (Box 20-8).

 Home Care Considerations

Tracheostomy Care

- Some patients with an artificial airway who are at home will have permanent tracheostomy, as well as a T-piece or T-tube or tracheostomy collar.
- Patients need to be able to perform tracheostomy care and suctioning techniques.
- Assess patient's home environment for presence of respiratory irritants, cleanliness, and location in which to clean suctioning equipment and hang it up to drain.
- Confirm that humidifier is present—added moisture is important.

 Coordinated Care

Collaboration

SUCTIONING FOR TRACHEOSTOMY CARE

- The skill of suctioning, other than oropharyngeal suctioning (Yankauer), requires the critical thinking and knowledge application unique to a nurse or other licensed health care professional.
- Oropharyngeal suctioning is possible to delegate to assistive personnel (AP), including the patient and family when appropriate.
- In special situations the skill of performing a permanent tracheostomy tube suctioning is possible to delegate to AP. These situations include stable patients with permanent tracheostomy tubes after head and neck surgery and patients receiving mechanical ventilation at home.
- You are responsible for assessing the patient's airway patency and response to airway suctioning.

Box 20-8 Nursing Diagnoses to Promote Oxygenation

Ineffective airway clearance:
- Related to ineffective cough
- Related to excessive secretions

Ineffective breathing pattern:
- Related to respiratory muscle weakness
- Related to fatigue
- Related to abnormal breathing patterns

Disturbed thought processes:
- Related to inadequate oxygenation and carbon dioxide retention

Activity intolerance:
- Related to imbalance between oxygen supply and demand

Anxiety, fear, or hopelessness:
- Related to dyspnea and feelings of suffocation
- Related to fear of dying

Impaired verbal communication:
- Related to presence of tracheostomy
- Related to intubation

Data from North American Nursing Diagnosis Association International (NANDA-I). (2009). *NANDA-I nursing diagnoses: Definitions and classification 2009-2011.* Oxford, United Kingdom: Author.

Care of the Patient with a Tracheostomy Collar and T-Piece or T-Tube

Since a tracheostomy bypasses the upper airway that normally filters and humidifies air upon inspiration, patients with artificial airways must have constant humidification. A T-piece/tube and tracheostomy collar are examples of two devices that supply humidified oxygen to an artificial airway (Perry & Potter, 2009). Both help supply humidified oxygen or room air to the airway.

The T-piece or T-tube is a T-shaped device with a 0.6-inch (15-mm) connection with large-lumen tubing (Figure 20-16). The recommended flow rate is 10 L/min (Skill 20-10). Tracheostomy collars supply humidification to the lower respiratory tract. The collar is curved and has an adjustable strap that extends around the patient's neck (Figure 20-17). The tracheostomy collar

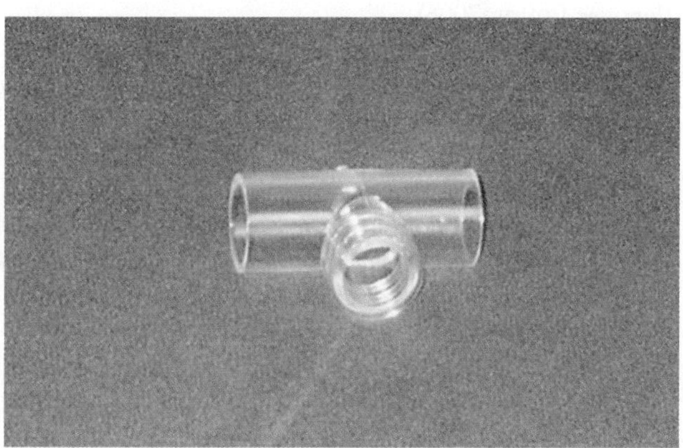

FIGURE 20-16 T-piece or T-tube.

Skill 20-10 Care of the Patient with a Cuffed Tracheostomy Tube

Nursing Action *(Rationale)*

1. Refer to standard steps 1 to 9.
2. Suction patient as in Skill 20-9, steps 1 to 11.
3. Connect syringe to pilot balloon valve (see illustration). *(Provides inflation and deflation of tube balloon.)*
4. Position stethoscope in sternal notch or above tracheostomy tube, and listen for minimal amount of air leak at end of inspiration (see illustration). *(Allows you to confirm proper cuff inflation.)*

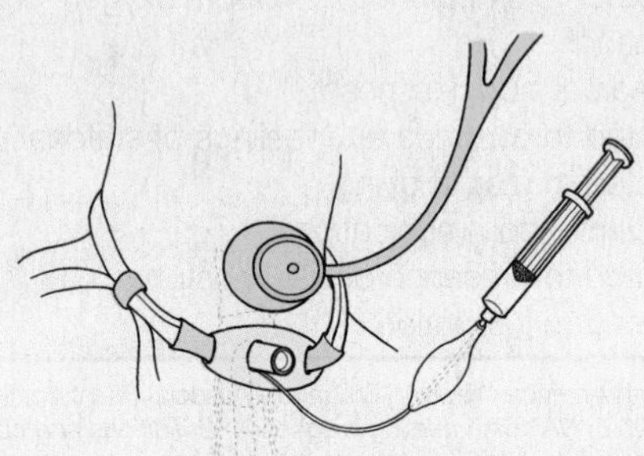

Steps **3 and 4**

5. Remove all air from cuff if no air leak is auscultated. *(Releases excessive air pressure.)*
6. While listening with stethoscope, slowly inflate cuff with 0.5 to 1 mL of air at a time. When no air leak is heard, stop injecting air and slowly withdraw up to 0.5 mL of air until air leak is auscultated with stethoscope.
7. If excessive air leak is heard, slowly add air as in step 6. *(Air leak will sometimes prevent lung expansion and increases risk of aspiration.)*
8. Remove stethoscope and cleanse diaphragm with alcohol swab. *(Reduces spread of microorganisms.)*
9. Do not leave syringe attached to pilot balloon valve; remove syringe and either discard in proper container or store per agency's policy. *(Causes valve to break or "stick open"; when valve is removed, air is lost from cuff.)*
10. Follow steps 17 to 22 in Skill 20-9.

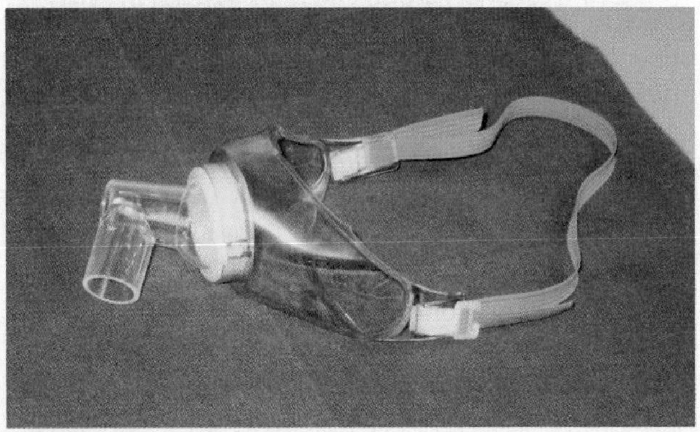

FIGURE 20-17 Tracheostomy collar.

provides oxygen with the flow meter set at 10 L/min (Perry & Potter, 2006).

When caring for the patient's tracheostomy collar or T-piece or T-tube, the following procedure is recommended:

1. Perform hand hygiene to reduce transmission of microorganisms.
2. Position the patient for comfort, usually in a semi-Fowler's position.
3. Inspect the rate of flow and the solution level for humidification often during the course of the patient's oxygen therapy to ensure adequate oxygenation.
4. Provide nose and mouth care to keep the mucosa lubricated, moist, clean, and fresh during the course of the patient's therapy.
5. Secure the collar or T-piece at the neck over the tracheostomy. Make certain all tubing connections are secure.
6. Adjust the oxygen flow rate according to the physician's order.
7. Adjust the temperature of the humidified oxygen.
8. Use large-lumen tubing from the oxygen source to the patient.
9. Condensation occurs within the tracheostomy collar or T-piece, so observe frequently.
10. The collar or T-piece and tubing should be removed frequently to be drained and cleaned to prevent aspiration of the moisture. Excessive water accumulates more often at higher humidity.
11. As moisture collects, suction the tracheostomy and provide tracheostomy care as often as necessary.
12. Make sure you are always able to see the mist of the humidified oxygen.

See Skill 20-11 for the procedure for clearing a patient's airway.

SKILLS FOR URINARY OR REPRODUCTIVE TRACT DISORDERS

URINARY ELIMINATION

Urinary elimination is a natural process that individuals take for granted until it is altered by some uncontrollable physiologic factor. Patients needing assistance with urinary elimination will often require physiologic

Skill 20-11 Clearing the Airway

Nursing Action *(Rationale)*

1. Refer to standard steps 1 to 9.
2. Assemble equipment:
   - Appropriate suction catheter
   - Sterile gloves
   - Clean gloves as indicated
   - Sterile equipment (suction kit)
   - Unsterile equipment (unsterile basin or cup)
   - Tap water, sterile water, or normal saline
   - Towel
   - Portable or wall suction apparatus
   - Connecting tubing
   - Face shield, if indicated
3. Assess need for suctioning. *(Physical signs will indicate need to perform this procedure.)*
   - Gurgling respirations
   - Restlessness
   - Vomitus in mouth
   - Drooling
4. Explain that coughing, sneezing, or gagging is expected. *(Encourages cooperation and reduces risks and associated anxiety to a minimum.)*
5. Position patient.
   a. If patient is alert and conscious, place in semi-Fowler's position (head to one side is the position of choice). *(Placing head to one side promotes drainage of secretions and facilitates insertion of the suction catheter.)*
   b. If patient is unconscious, place in side-lying position facing you.
      (1) Place towel lengthwise under patient's chin and over pillow. *(Protects bed linens from contamination.)*
6. Pour sterile normal saline solution into sterile container. *(For moistening and cleansing catheter.)*
7. Turn on suction machine, and select appropriate suction pressure. Never suction with any more vacuum pressure than needed to remove the secretions, and use the smallest catheter that will remove the secretions well. *(Elevated pressure setting or using a too-large catheter increases risk of trauma to oral and nasal mucosa.)* Connect suction catheter to tubing (see illustration).
   Common vacuum settings for wall suction units:
   - Infants: 50 to 95 mm Hg
   - Children: 95 to 110 mm Hg
   - Adults: 110 to 150 mm Hg

   Common catheter sizes:
   - Infant: 6 to 8 F
   - Children: 8 to 10 F
   - Adults: 12 to 16 F
8. Aspirate solution through catheter by placing thumb over open end of connector or over vent. *(Enables you to check patency of suction catheter and suction pressure and moistens catheter for ease of insertion.)*

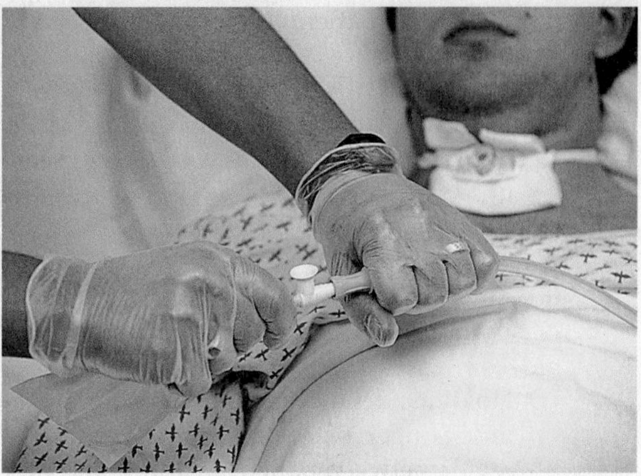

Step **7** Note the white vent.

9. Remove thumb from Y-connector opening, or pinch catheter with thumb and index finger; if using suction catheter with vent, remove thumb from vent opening. *(Prevents injury to mucous membrane while catheter is being inserted.)*
10. Insert catheter. (See specific suction guidelines.) *(Catheter provides continuous suction.)*
    a. **Oropharyngeal suctioning** (wearing clean gloves is acceptable)
       (1) Gently insert Yankauer or tonsillar tip suction catheter (see illustration) into one side of mouth. *(Gentleness prevents tissue trauma.)*
       (2) Glide Yankauer toward oropharynx without suction. *(Prevents tissue trauma.)*
       (3) Apply suction and move Yankauer tonsillar tip catheter around mouth until secretions are cleared.

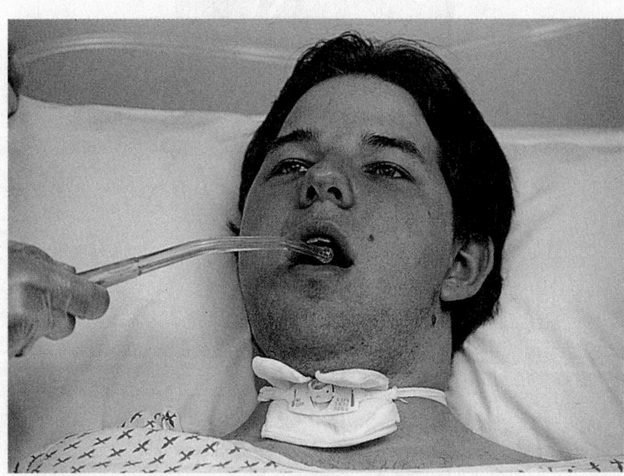

Step **10a(1)**

Continued

Skill 20-11 Clearing the Airway—cont'd

(4) Encourage patient to cough. *(Moves secretions from lower airway into mouth and upper airway.)*

(5) Rinse Yankauer with water in cup or basin until connecting tubing is cleared of secretions. Turn off suction. *(Rinses catheter and reduces probability of transmission of microorganisms.)*

(6) Repeat procedure as necessary.

b. **Nasopharyngeal suctioning** (wear sterile gloves):

(1) Holding suction catheter with thumb and index finger, place nasal catheter near region between patient's earlobe and tip of nose. Do not touch side of face, nose, or earlobe. *(Marks correct length of catheter for insertion. Distance from earlobe to tip of nose approximates depth of insertion.)*
Length of insertion:
- Adults: 16 cm
- Older children: 8 to 12 cm
- Infants and young children: 4 to 8 cm

(2) Lubricate catheter with water-soluble jelly. *(Water-soluble lubricant dissolves, thus preventing possible buildup hindering airway.)*

(3) Hold catheter to note its natural curvature, and gently insert catheter into one side of nasal passage (see illustration). *(Using the natural curvature of the catheter and gentleness facilitates easier and less traumatic insertion.)*

c. **Nasotracheal suctioning** (wear sterile gloves):

(1) Holding suction catheter with thumb and index finger, place nasotracheal catheter near region between earlobe to tip of nose and extend to trachea. Do not touch side of face, nose, or earlobe. *(Maintains sterility. Marks correct length of catheter for insertion.)*
Length of insertion:
- Adults: 20 to 24 cm
- Older children: 14 to 20 cm
- Young children and infants: 8 to 14 cm

(2) Lubricate catheter with a water-soluble jelly. *(Facilitates gliding catheter past nasal turbinates.)*

(3) Ask patient if either side of nose is obstructed; use unobstructed side. Hold catheter to note its natural curvature, and gently insert catheter into one side of nasal passage. *(Using the natural curvature of catheter and gentleness facilitates easier and less traumatic insertion.)*

(4) Stimulate coughing reflex, or ask patient to cough to guide catheter into trachea. If no cough reflex is present or if patient is not able to assist, insert catheter when patient inhales (see illustration of step 10b[3]). *(Helps prevent displacement of catheter into esophagus.)*

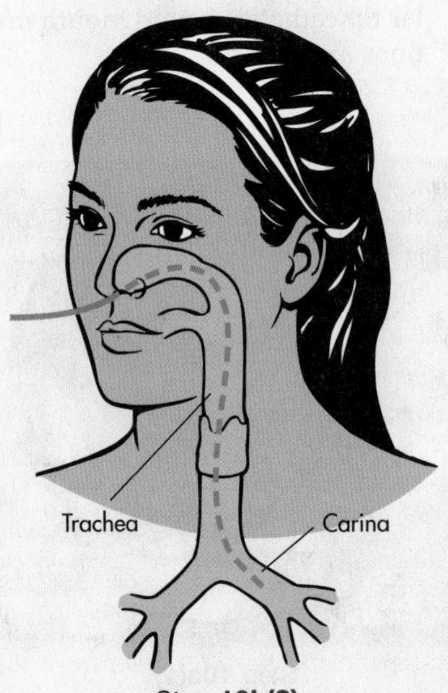

Step **10b(3)**

11. Apply intermittent suction by placing thumb over suction opening; withdraw catheter as you rotate it gently. *(Intermittent suction and gentle rotation of the catheter prevents injury to mucosa.)*
12. Observe patient closely, and limit suction to 10 to 15 seconds. (Suctioning longer than 10 to 15 seconds risks causing cardiopulmonary compromise.)
13. Repeat suctioning if needed.
14. Allow 1 to 2 minutes of rest between suctioning if it is necessary to repeat procedure. If oxygen is administered by nasal cannula, mask, or other means, reapply oxygen during rest period. *(Provides rest and comfort and allows patient to regain oxygen supply. Time needed for patient to rest between suctioning will vary from 1 to 2 minutes to 20 to 30 seconds, depending on patient's ability to tolerate procedure.)*
15. If patient is alert and is able to cooperate, request patient to breathe deeply and cough. *(Coughing moves secretions from lower airway into mouth and upper airway.)*
16. When suctioning is complete, suction between cheeks and gum line and under tongue; suction mouth last to prevent contaminating catheter. *(Ensures all secretions have been removed.)*
17. Place catheter in solution and apply suction. *(Flushes secretions from catheter and tubing to maintain patency in the event it is necessary to repeat procedure.)*

18. Discard catheter and used suction catheters: wrap catheter around gloved hand; pull glove off hand and over catheter. Remove face shield, if worn. Perform hand hygiene. *(Reduces the transmission of microorganisms and prevents direct contact with equipment and secretions.)*
19. Place sterile, unopened catheter at patient's bedside. *(Provides quick access to suction equipment if patient needs suctioning immediately.)*
20. Provide mouth care. *(Promotes patient comfort.)*
21. Assess patient's breathing patterns. Assess for decrease in anxiety, fatigue, vital signs, and level of consciousness and color. *(Identifies patient's response to suction procedure.)*
22. Refer to standard steps 10 to 17.
23. Document: *(Verifies performance of procedure and ensures continuity of care.)*
    - Date
    - Time
    - Method of suctioning
    - Amount, consistency, color, and odor of secretions
    - Respiratory assessment
    - Patient's response
    - Patient teaching

and psychological assistance from you. Physiologic support will at times involve an invasive procedure, such as the insertion of a urinary catheter into the bladder. Some patients need psychological assistance to help them adjust to a visible urine collection drainage bag. Therefore it is important for you to be competent in performing technical skills and sensitive to a patient's psychological needs (Coordinated Care box on urinary catheterization). The urinary tract is susceptible to infections, particularly when invaded, as is the case when a sterile catheter is inserted. Therefore it is necessary for you to be able to apply the principles of sterile asepsis.

Urine clears the body of waste materials and aids in the maintaining the balance of electrolytes. Conditions that interfere with urinary drainage have the capacity, therefore, to create a health crisis. It is important to reestablish urine flow as soon as possible to prevent the buildup of toxins in the bloodstream. Patients at risk for difficulty with urine elimination include those who have undergone surgical procedures of the bladder, the prostate, or the vagina; patients with primary urologic problems, such as urethral stricture; and those who are critically ill with multisystemic problems.

Coordinated Care

Delegation

URINARY CATHETERIZATION

- The skill of urinary catheterization is acceptable to delegate to assistive personnel (AP) in some settings (see agency policy). First-time catheterization or catheterization of patients in an acute care setting or patients with urethral trauma requires the critical thinking and knowledge application unique to a nurse, and delegation is inappropriate.
- The skill of removing a retention catheter is possible to delegate to AP; however, assessment and teaching require the critical thinking and knowledge application unique to a nurse. Instruct AP to measure first voiding and to report time and amount to you.
- The skill of obtaining catheterized specimens for residual urine is acceptable to delegate to AP in some settings (see agency policy). Initial patient assessment and coordination of repeated catheterization require the critical thinking and knowledge application unique to a nurse, and delegation is inappropriate.
- The skill of catheter irrigation requires the critical thinking and knowledge application unique to a nurse. Delegation to AP is inappropriate.
- The skill of caring for a newly established suprapubic catheter requires the critical thinking and knowledge application unique to a nurse. Delegation to AP is inappropriate.

Maintaining Adequate Urinary Drainage

Most catheters are made of soft plastic or rubber and are used for both treatment and diagnosis. Urinary catheters are used to maintain urine flow, to divert urine flow to facilitate healing postoperatively, to introduce medications by irrigation, and to dilate or prevent narrowing of some portions of the urinary tract. Catheters are used for both intermittent and continuous urinary drainage. It is possible to introduce urinary catheters into the bladder, the ureter, or the kidney. **Catheterization** of the bladder involves introducing a rubber or plastic tube (a **urinary catheter**) through the meatus and the urethra and into the urinary bladder. The type and size of urinary catheter used are determined according to the location and the cause of the urinary tract problem. Catheters are measured by the French (F or Fr) system. Urethral catheters range in size from 14 to 24 F for adult patients. Ureteral catheters are usually 4 to 6 F. The physician always inserts ureteral catheters. You will usually be responsible for the insertion of urethral catheters.

Types of Catheters

Different types of catheters are used for different purposes (Figure 20-18). The coudé catheter, which has a tapered tip, is selected for ease of insertion when enlargement of the prostate gland is suspected. The curved stylet is used to assist the physician in the insertion of a urethral catheter in a male patient. The Foley catheter is designed with a balloon near its tip that is possible to inflate after insertion, holding the catheter in the urinary bladder for continuous drain-

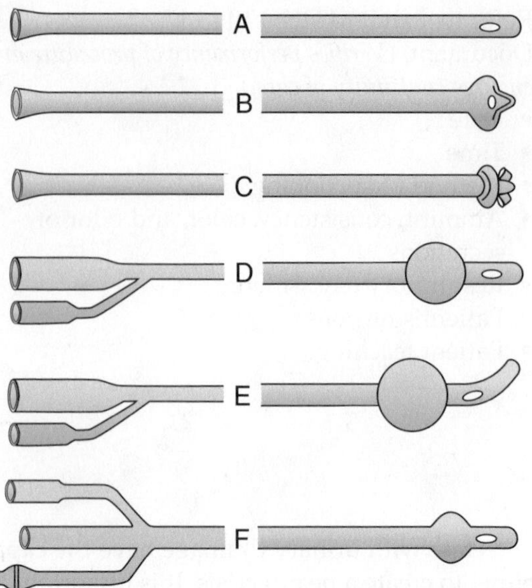

FIGURE 20-18 Different types of commonly used urinary catheters. **A,** Simple urethral catheter. **B,** Mushroom or de Pezzer (can be used for suprapubic catheterization). **C,** Winged-tip or Malecot. **D,** Indwelling with inflated balloon. **E,** Indwelling with coudé tip or Tiemann. **F,** Three-way indwelling (the third lumen is used for irrigation of the bladder).

age. Malecot and de Pezzer or mushroom catheters are used to drain urine from the renal pelvis of the kidney. The Robinson catheter has multiple openings in its tip to facilitate intermittent drainage. Ureteral catheters are long and slender to pass into the ureters. The whistle-tip catheter has a slanted, larger orifice at its tip to be used if there is blood in the urine. The cystostomy, the vesicostomy, or the suprapubic catheter is introduced through the abdominal wall above the symphysis pubis to create a temporary urinary diversion. This catheter diverts urine flow from the urethra as needed to treat injury to the bony pelvis, the urinary tract, or surrounding organs; strictures; or obstruction. The catheter is inserted via surgical incision or puncture of the abdominal and bladder walls with a trocar cannula. The catheter is connected to a sterile closed drainage system and secured to avoid accidental removal; the wound is covered with a sterile dressing. When the lower urinary tract has healed, the patient's ability to void is tested by clamping the catheter so that the patient will try to void naturally. When the measured residual urine is consistently less than 50 mL, the catheter is usually removed and a sterile dressing placed over the wound.

Condom Catheters

Medical supply companies manufacture and sell different types of condom-styled drainage systems sometimes referred to as a condom catheter (or a Texas catheter), with various features. For its effective and safe use, it is best to follow the manufacturer's instructions that accompany the device. A main drawback for using this device is that it sometimes becomes too constrictive. Maintain careful, close assessment. Explain the procedure even if the patient is comatose because it is possible that he will be able to hear.

This device is not a catheter but rather a drainage system connected to the external male genitalia (Figure 20-19). This noninvasive appliance is used for the incontinent male to keep skin irritation from urine to a minimum. The appliance is removed daily for cleansing and inspection of the skin. Never use tape to secure the device since this is likely to limit circulation to the penis, leading to necrosis of the surrounding skin and penis (Elkin et al., 2007). Use of the external catheter allows for a more normal lifestyle for the patient.

Nursing Interventions

Nursing interventions for the patient with a urinary drainage system include employing a number of principles to prevent and detect infection and trauma (Skills 20-12, 20-13, and 20-14; Figure 20-20).

1. Follow aseptic technique to avoid introduction of microorganisms from the environment. Never rest the collecting bag on the floor (Figure 20-21).
2. Record intake and output (I&O) (Figure 20-22). For precision monitoring, such as hourly urine output, add a urometer to the drainage system. If urine output falls to less than 50 mL/hr, first

Text continued on p. 579

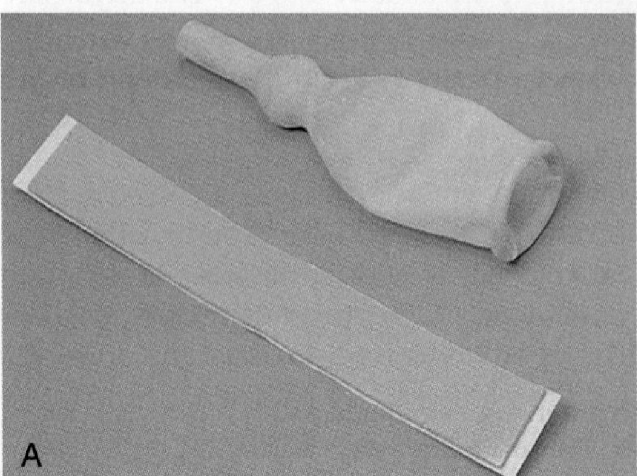

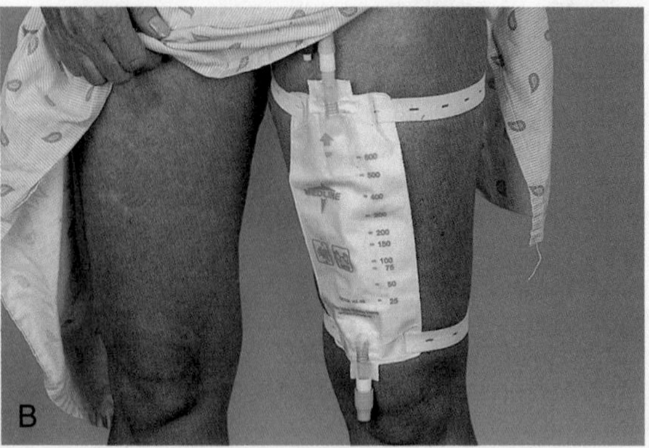

FIGURE 20-19 **A,** Condom catheter. **B,** Condom catheter attached to leg bag.

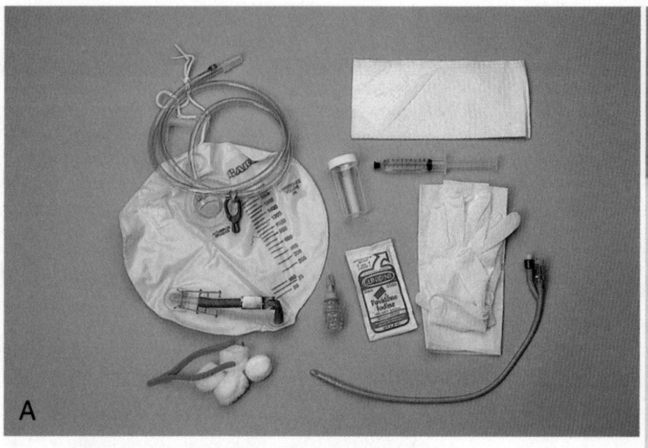

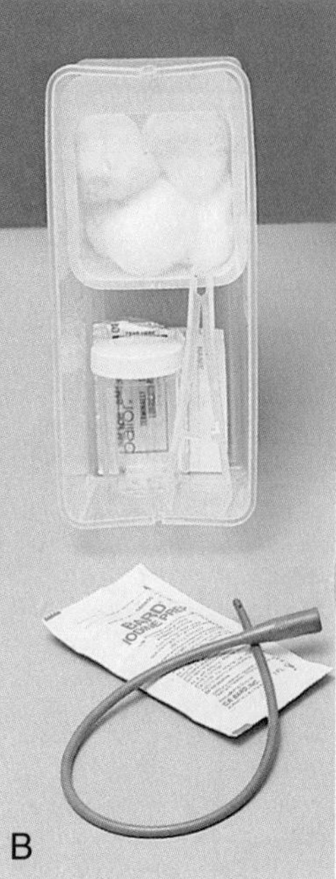

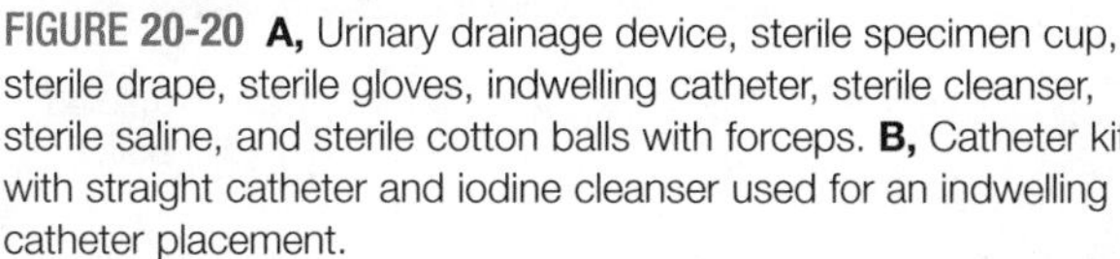
FIGURE 20-20 **A,** Urinary drainage device, sterile specimen cup, sterile drape, sterile gloves, indwelling catheter, sterile cleanser, sterile saline, and sterile cotton balls with forceps. **B,** Catheter kit with straight catheter and iodine cleanser used for an indwelling catheter placement.

Skill 20-12 Catheterization: Male and Female

Nursing Action *(Rationale)*

1. Refer to standard steps 1 to 9.
2. Assemble equipment:
   - Sterile Foley catheterization or straight catheterization tray:
     —Sterile gloves, if not in tray
     —Bed protector
     —Drape
     —Lubricant
     —Antiseptic cleansing unit
     —Cotton balls and pickup forceps
     —Prefilled syringe of sterile water
     —Catheter of correct size and type for procedure
     —Sterile drainage tubing and collection bag
     —Tape
     —Safety pins
     —Receptacle or basin (usually bottom of catheterization tray)
     —Specimen container (optional)
   - Light (flashlight or penlight)
   - Bath blanket
   - Disposable gloves, basin of warm water, soap, towel, and disposable washcloth
3. Assessment: *(Enables you to determine need for procedure and special interventions.)*
   a. When patient last voided.
   b. Level of awareness.
   c. Mobility and physical limitation of patient.
   d. Patient's sex and age.
   e. For distended bladder.
   f. For any pathologic conditions that are likely to impair passage of catheter (especially enlarged prostate gland in males).
   g. For allergies (to antiseptic [iodine], tape, rubber, and lubricant).
   h. Patient's knowledge of the purpose of catheterization.
4. Arrange for extra nursing personnel to assist if needed. *(Patients are not always able to assume positioning for procedure.)*
5. Position patient.
   a. Male: Supine position with thighs slightly abducted. *(Allows relaxation of muscles and easy access to urinary meatus.)*
   b. Female: Dorsal recumbent position with knees flexed, or soles of feet flat on bed, and knees about 2 feet apart (see illustration). *(Allows relaxation of muscles and easy access to urinary meatus.)*
6. Drape patient with bath blanket, covering upper body and shaping over both knees and legs, leaving genital area exposed. *(Prepares patient for procedure and provides for patient's privacy.)*
7. Place waterproof absorbent pad under patient's buttocks. *(Protects bed linens.)*
8. Arrange supplies and equipment on bedside table. Provide a good light. *(Easy access prevents possible contamination.)*
9. Don clean gloves, and wash perineal area with mild soap and warm water with disposable washcloth. *(Decreases microorganisms at the site.)*

Continued

Skill 20-12 Catheterization: Male and Female—cont'd

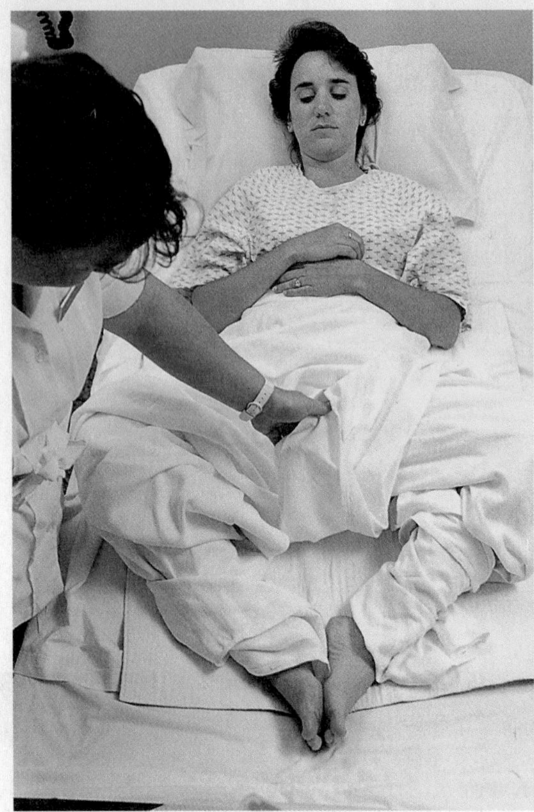
Step 5b

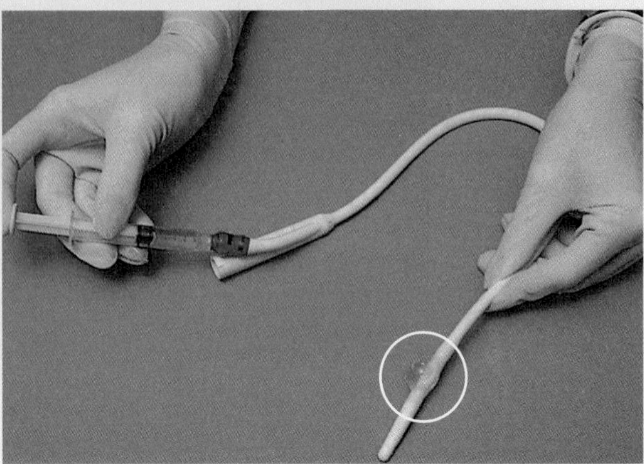

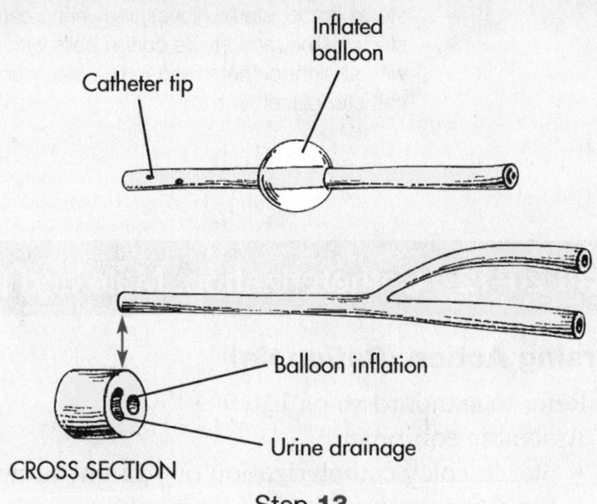

Step 13

10. Remove disposable gloves and place in proper receptacle. *(Reduces the spread of microorganisms.)*
11. Facing patient, stand on left side of bed if right-handed (on right side if left-handed). *(Successful catheter insertion requires you to assume comfortable position with all equipment close by.)*
12. Open packaging using sterile technique. Don sterile gloves (see illustration). *(Allows you to handle sterile supplies without contamination.)*
13. If indwelling catheter is used, test balloon by injecting normal saline or sterile water into balloon lumen until balloon is inflated; then aspirate saline or sterile water (see illustration). *(Assesses integrity of balloon. If balloon fails to inflate, obtain another sterile catheter.)*

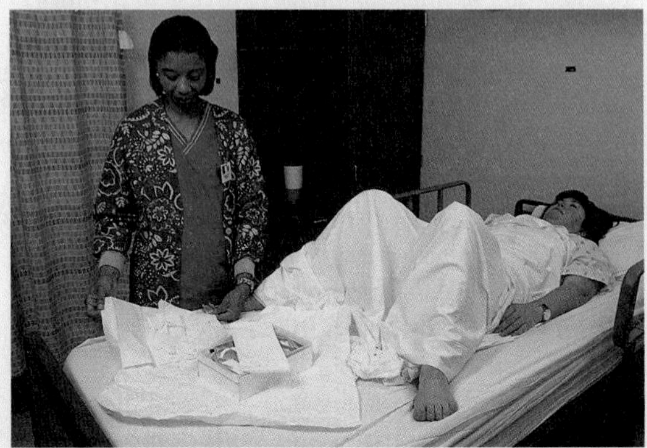
Step 12

14. Add antiseptic to cotton balls; open lubricant container. Lubricate catheter about 1½ to 2 inches (3.5 to 5 cm) for female; about 6 to 7 inches (15 to 18 cm) for male. *(Maintains principles of surgical asepsis and organizes work area. Lubricating catheter reduces the chance of friction causing trauma to the delicate mucous membranes of the urethra.)*
15. Wrap edges of sterile drape around gloved hands and request patient to raise hips; then slide drape under patient's buttocks. *(Protects hands from contamination while placing towel under edge of patient's buttocks.)*
16. Cleanse perineal area using forceps to hold cotton balls soaked in antiseptic solution. *(Cleansing reduces number of microorganisms at urethral meatus.)*
    a. **Male** (see illustration): If male is not circumcised, retract foreskin with nondominant hand. **Be certain to replace foreskin when procedure has been completed.** If erection occurs, discontinue procedure momentarily. This is normal but often embarrassing to

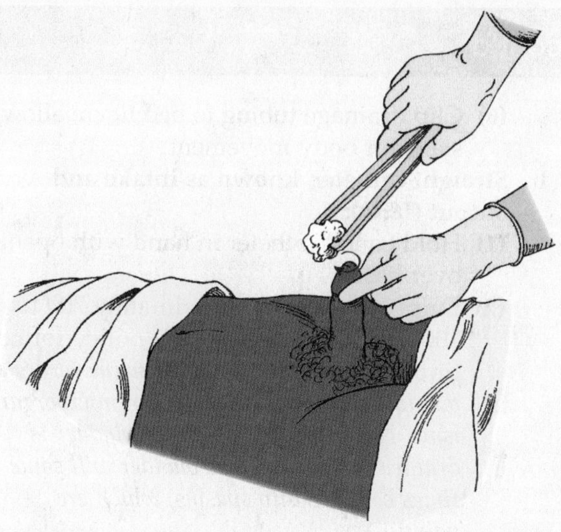

Step 16a

patient. React in a professional manner. *(Accidental release of foreskin or dropping of the penis during cleansing requires process to be repeated because area has been contaminated.)*

(1) Grasp penis at shaft below glans with one hand; continue to hold throughout insertion of catheter.

(2) With other hand, use forceps to hold cotton balls soaked in antiseptic solution.

(3) Cleanse meatus in circular motion. *(Decreases introduction of organisms into bladder.)*

(4) Repeat cleansing two more times using sterile cotton balls each time. *(Cleansing in this manner ensures optimal reduction of microorganisms from the area.)*

b. Female:

(1) Spread labia minora with thumb and index finger of nondominant hand to expose meatus; continue to hold throughout insertion of catheter.

(2) With other hand, use forceps to hold cotton balls soaked in antiseptic solution.

(3) Cleanse area from clitoris toward anus, using a different sterile cotton ball each time—first to the right of the meatus, then to the left of the meatus, then down the center over meatus (see illustration). *(Full visualization of the meatus is provided. Full separation of labia prevents contamination of meatus during cleansing. If closure of labia occurs, it is necessary to repeat the procedure.)*

17. Pick up catheter with free sterile-gloved hand near the tip; hold remaining part of catheter coiled in hands; place distal end in basin. *(Placing distal end of catheter in basin allows for urine collection. Coiling catheter in hand and holding near the tip allows easier manipulation during insertion.)*

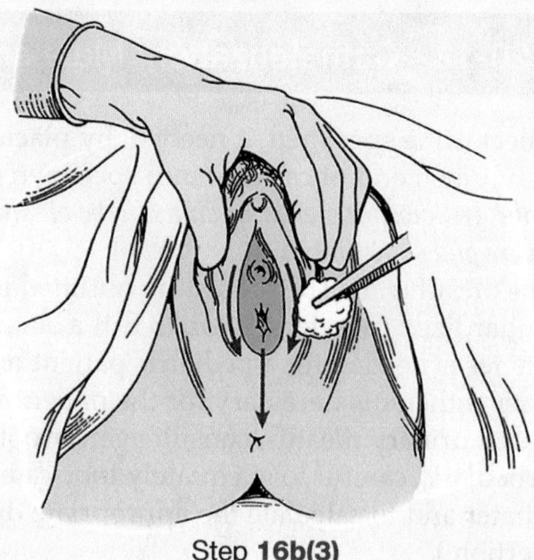

Step 16b(3)

18. Insert catheter gently, about 6 to 7 inches (15 to 18 cm) for male or 2 to 4 inches (5 to 10 cm) for female (see illustration). If, when inserting an indwelling catheter, urine flow is established, insert catheter 1½ inches (3.5 cm) farther; inflate balloon with 10 mL sterile water, watching patient's face for grimacing (a sign that balloon is inflating in urethra; if this occurs, deflate balloon and reposition catheter as above). Gently pull back on catheter until resistance is felt as balloon rests at orifice of urethra (see Figure 20-21, *A*). *(Asking patient to bear down gently as if to void causes relaxation of external sphincter, which aids in insertion of catheter. Advancement of catheter ensures bladder placement.)* If no urine returns in a few minutes, observe whether catheter has been inserted by mistake into vagina. If so, leave catheter in place as landmark indicating where not to insert, and insert another sterile catheter. *(Use of the same catheter will introduce a host of microorganisms into the bladder.)*

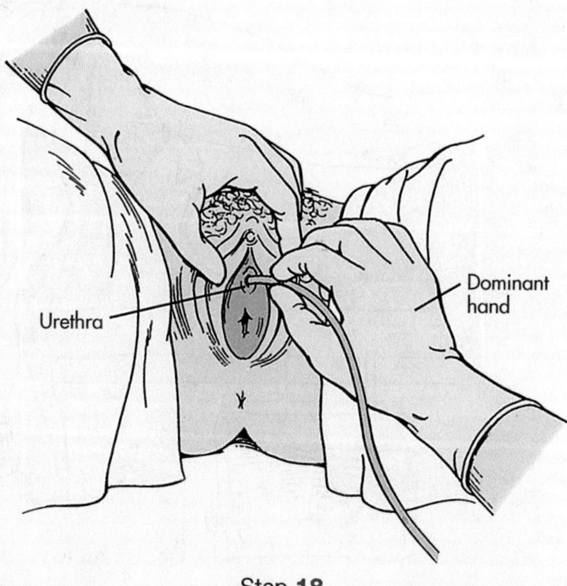

Step 18

Continued

Skill 20-12 Catheterization: Male and Female—cont'd

19. Collect urine specimen, if needed, by placing open lumen end of catheter into specimen container. *(Allows for sterile specimen to be obtained for culture and sensitivity.)*
20. Type of catheter. (The procedure outlined is for standardized catheters, 16 or 18 F. If a smaller catheter is needed for a pediatric patient or if a larger catheter is necessary for the patient with dilated urinary meatus, consult agency policy. Be particularly careful to adequately lubricate the catheter and to calculate the appropriate depth of insertion.)
    a. **Indwelling catheter:**
        (1) Inflate balloon with required amount of normal saline or sterile water (see Figure 20-21, *A*).
        (2) Pull gently to feel resistance.
        (3) Attach end of catheter to collecting tube of drainage system, holding drainage bag below bladder level. *(Most catheters are presealed to the collecting tube of the drainage system.)*
        (4) Attach collection bag to side of bed (see Figure 20-21, *B*).
        (5) Secure catheter to patient (see illustrations). *(Keeps tension and trauma to urethral opening to a minimum.)*
        —**Male:** Tape catheter to inner aspect of thigh or up over pubis or apply leg strap (depends on physician's order); allow slack for body movement.
        —**Female:** Tape catheter to inner thigh or apply leg strap; allow slack for body movement.
        (6) Clip drainage tubing to bed linen; allow slack for body movement.
    b. **Straight catheter, known as intake and output (I&O):**
        (1) Hold coiled catheter in hand with opening over basin.
        (2) Empty bladder (approximately 700 to 1000 mL). Refer to agency policy for continuing to drain. *(Retained urine serves as possible reservoir for growth of microorganisms. Note that if a distended bladder is drained too rapidly, the bladder will sometimes collapse into spasms, which are painful.)*
        (3) Withdraw catheter slowly. *(Keeps patient discomfort to a minimum.)*
21. Dry perineal area. (Maintains patient comfort.)
22. Refer to standard steps 10 to 17.
23. Label urine specimen with patient's name, date, physician's name, and other possibly pertinent information. Transport to laboratory. *(Verifies correct specimen for laboratory.)*
24. Assess flow of urine and drainage tubing setup. *(Determines whether urine is flowing adequately.)*
25. Document: *(Verifies performance of procedure and ensures continuity of care.)*
    - Type and size of catheter
    - Amount of solution to inflate balloon
    - Characteristics of urine
    - Amount of urine
    - Reason for catheterization
    - Specimen collected
    - Patient's response to procedure (any resistance met)

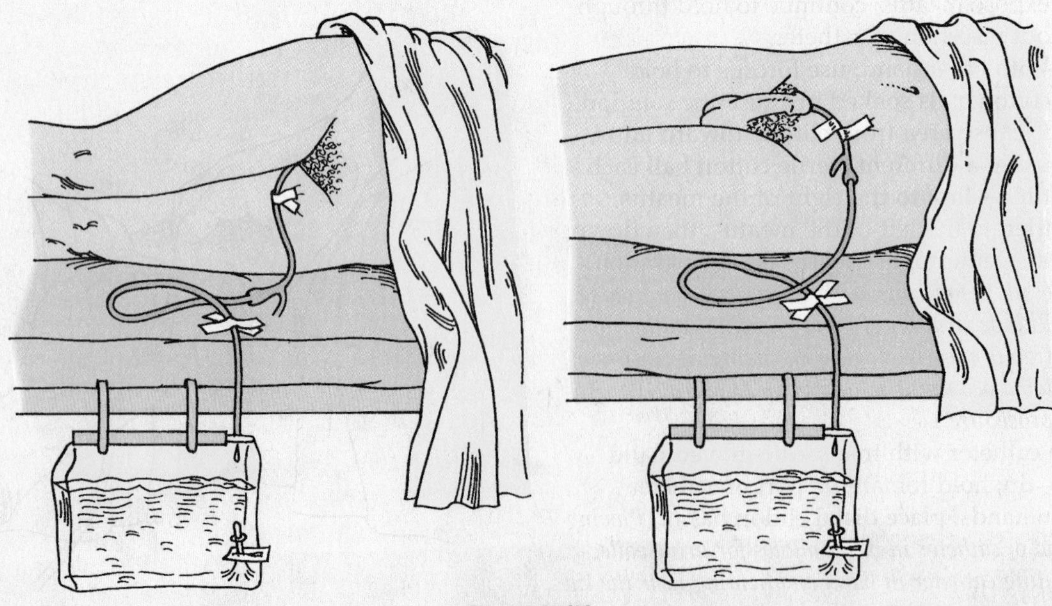

Step **20a(5)**

- Patient teaching (see Life Span Considerations for Older Adults box on catheterization)

26. Report any unusual findings immediately:
- No urine output
- Bladder discomfort despite catheter patency
- Leakage of urine from catheter
- Inability to insert catheter *(Necessary to assess further; if it is not possible to advance catheter, report immediately. Discomfort indicates possible infection. Leakage around catheter indicates possibility of improper catheter placement or inflation of balloon.)*

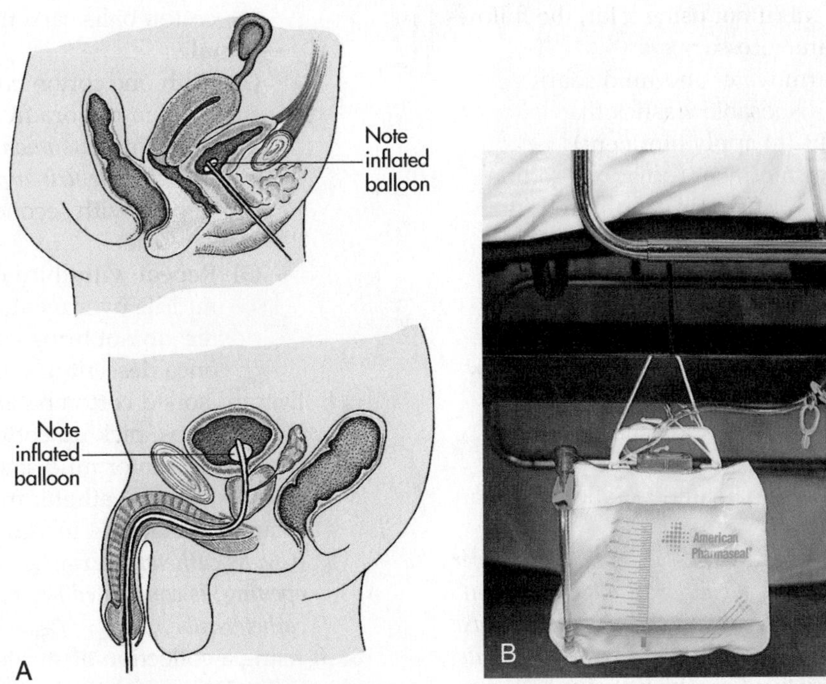

FIGURE 20-21 **A,** Balloon inflation in both male and female. **B,** It is essential to keep drainage system below the level of the bladder. Do not place bag on side rails or allow it to rest on the floor. Attach drainage bag to bed or IV pole while ambulating.

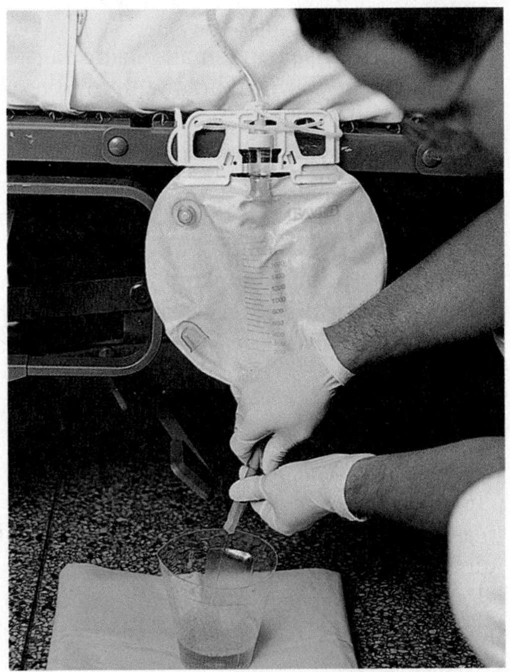

FIGURE 20-22 Empty and record urine output from Foley catheter into clean graduated container. Clean the drainage port before draining and before recapping.

Skill 20-13 Performing Routine Catheter Care

Nursing Action *(Rationale)*

1. Refer to standard steps 1 to 9.
2. Assemble equipment.
   - Disposable gloves
   - Bed protector
   - Bath blanket
   - Catheter care kit (if not using a kit, the following supplies are necessary):
     —Basin of warm water and mild soap
     —Towel and disposable washcloth
     —Sterile swabs (to apply ointment)
     —Antiinfective ointment (povidone-iodine [Betadine] or Neosporin), if ordered (not often used any more)
   - Small plastic bag for trash
3. Assess patient. *(Enables you to determine the patient's condition.)*
   a. How long catheter has been in place (follow agency policy).
   b. For any encrustations or discharge around urethral meatus.
   c. For complaints of pain and for allergies to antiseptic ointment.
   d. Patient's temperature. *(Assess temperature every 4 hours for 24 hours if odor or exudate is present.)*
   e. Patient's intake. *(Maintain adequate fluid intake, contingent on the patient's overall condition; this is essential to ensure free-flowing urine.)*
4. Position patient.
   —**Male:** supine position in bed.
   —**Female:** dorsal recumbent position in bed (see Skill 20-12, step 5b).
5. Place waterproof disposable pad under patient's buttocks and to the side from which catheter care will be given.
6. Drape patient with bath blanket, exposing only perineal area.
7. If using sterile catheter care kit:
   a. Open supplies using sterile technique and arrange on bedside table. *(Organizes procedure.)*
   b. Don sterile gloves. *(Prevents transmission of microorganisms.)*
   c. Place cotton balls in sterile basin near you and saturate with solution. *(Having supplies nearby prevents accidental contamination. Adhering to the principles of surgical asepsis reduces the possibility of introducing pathogens into the urinary tract.)*
   d. With one hand, expose urethral meatus:
      —**Male:** Retract foreskin, then hold penis erect; hold position.
      —**Female:** Gently retract labia minora away from urinary meatus and hold in position.
   e. Wash the area at the meatus and around catheter with cotton balls.
      —**Male:**
      (1) With one cotton ball, cleanse around meatus and catheter in a circular motion.
      (2) Repeat twice more, using different cotton balls each time.
      —**Female:**
      (1) With one cotton ball, swab to one side of labia minora from anterior to posterior. *(Prevents microorganisms from rectum entering the urinary system.)*
      (2) Repeat with second cotton ball on opposite side.
      (3) Repeat with third cotton ball down middle over meatus and around catheter; do not bring cotton ball back up once descent has begun.
   f. Discard soiled cotton balls in other basin in kit.
   g. With forceps, pick up cotton ball soaked in antiseptic solution or mild soap and water and cleanse around catheter from urethral opening to approximately 4 inches (10 cm) of catheter. *(Cleans catheter of exudate. The meatus [urethral opening] is considered less contaminated than the catheter tube.)*
8. If using a collection of sterile supplies:
   a. Open separate sterile packages, observing sterile technique.
   b. Don clean gloves. *(Prevents accidental contamination. Adhering to principles of surgical asepsis reduces the possibility of introducing pathogens into the urinary tract.)*
   c. Arrange refuse bag (small plastic bag).
   d. Cleanse the perineal area with mild soap and warm water. Pat dry.
      —**Male:** Retract foreskin; then hold the penis erect and hold in position.
      —**Female:** Gently retract labia away from urinary meatus and hold in position.
   e. Apply an appropriate amount of sterile ointment (if used) on sterile cotton-tipped applicator and gently apply around catheter at site of insertion.
   f. Release labia of female patient; replace foreskin of male patient. *(If foreskin is not replaced, serious consequences are possible.)*
9. Observe meatus, catheter, and surrounding tissue to assess normal or abnormal condition. Determine presence or absence of inflammation, edema, malodorous exudate, color of tissue, and burning sensation. *(Determines need for more aggressive therapy.)*

10. Dispose of equipment and linens, according to standard precautions and agency policy; remove gloves and dispose of in proper receptacle. Perform hand hygiene. *(Reduces spread of microorganisms.)*
11. Retape catheter to thigh. *(Prevents trauma and pain from tension and pulling.)*
12. Refer to standard steps 10 to 17.
13. Assess flow of urine through tubing. Assess the urine in the drainage tubing, not the accumulation in the collecting receptacle. *(One small clot has the potential to discolor the whole collection of urine. Assessing urine in the drainage tubing promotes accurate assessment of urine.)* If the drainage tubing becomes cloudy or stained, change the tubing to aid accurate observations of urine. Empty drainage receptacle at least every 8 hours or as necessary to prevent backup of urine into the tubing (and up into the bladder).
14. Document: *(Verifies performance of procedure and ensures continuity of care.)*
    - Time
    - Procedure
    - Assessment of urinary meatus
    - Character of urine
    - Patient response (if pertinent)
    - Patient teaching
15. Report any unusual findings immediately. *(Further therapy is sometimes required.)*

Skill 20-14 Catheter Irrigation: Open, Intermittent, Continuous, and Bladder Instillation

Nursing Action *(Rationale)*

1. Refer to standard steps 1 to 9.
2. Assemble equipment (exact equipment will depend on method used):
    - Irrigation setup
    - Sterile gloves
    - Sterile solution
    - Sterile calibrated container
    - Sterile Asepto syringe
    - Sterile basin
    - Antiseptic cleanser
    - Waterproof pad
    - Clean gloves
    - Sterile plug
    - Medication for instillation
3. Assessment: *(Enables you to determine patient's condition.)*
    a. Color of urine and presence of mucus or sediment.
    b. Patency of drainage tubing.
    c. Patient's intake and output record.
    d. Patient for presence of bladder spasms and discomfort.
    e. Patient's knowledge regarding purpose of the catheter irrigation.
4. Position patient:
    —**Male:** supine in bed
    —**Female:** dorsal recumbent position in bed
5. Drape patient with bath blanket, exposing perineal area; remove and dispose of gloves. *(Exposes catheter.)*
6. Place waterproof absorbent pad under patient's buttocks and to the side from which bladder irrigation will be done. *(Protects bed linens from soiling.)*
7. Arrange supplies and equipment at bedside on overbed table. *(Easy access prevents possible contamination.)*
8. Perform irrigation:
    a. **Open method** (not as popular as in the past):
        (1) Pour sterile irrigating solution (sterile normal saline is used as an irrigating solution unless otherwise specified) into sterile graduated container and recap solution bottle. Have irrigating solution at room temperature.
        (2) Don sterile gloves. *(Maintains the sterile field.)*
        (3) Place sterile basin between patient's legs, close to perineal area.
        (4) Disconnect catheter from drainage system and plug drainage tubing with sterile plug.
        (5) Draw 30 mL of sterile solution into syringe.
        (6) Cleanse catheter end with antiseptic swab.
        (7) Place tip of syringe into end of catheter and gently insert solution. *(Maintains sterility of equipment.)*
        (8) Withdraw syringe and allow solution to drain into basin by gravity.
        (9) If solution does not return, turn patient on side facing you. Refer to agency policy for further action if solution does not return.
        (10) Repeat injection of solution until amount ordered is injected and returned.
        (11) Remove plug from drainage tubing, and connect tubing to catheter. Do not touch

Continued

Skill 20-14 Catheter Irrigation: Open, Intermittent, Continuous, and Bladder Instillation—cont'd

ends of catheter and tubing because this will contaminate the system.

(12) Measure solution (to determine amount returned and amount of urine expelled). *(Using sterile supplies and adhering to sterile technique reduces the chance of urinary tract infection. A gentle approach reduces incidence of bladder spasms but clears catheter of obstruction. Drainage usually returns by gravity. Change in position sometimes moves tip of catheter in bladder, increasing the likelihood that instilled fluid will flow out.)*

b. **Closed intermittent method** (repeat steps 1 through 7 as described). *(Maintaining a closed system ensures against contamination resulting in a urinary tract infection.)*

(1) Pour sterile irrigating solution into graduated container. *(Sterile normal saline is used as an irrigating solution unless otherwise specified.)*

(2) Draw up sterile solution into syringe.

(3) Clamp catheter below injection port.

(4) Cleanse port with antiseptic.

(5) Insert needle of syringe into port.

(6) Inject solution into catheter slowly. *(Helps prevent bladder spasm; dislodges clots, sediment, or other material.)*

c. **Closed continuous method** (continuous bladder irrigation [CBI]): The physician has to order the solution, the strength, and the flow rate. If the physician specifies only solution, check with agency policy for protocol for strength and rate. The irrigation solution infuses continuously through one port while the second port drains urine and irrigation solution.

(1) Set up irrigating solution by attaching tubing to bag.

(2) Clamp off tubing so no solution flows through.

(3) Suspend bag on IV pole.

(4) Open clamp and allow solution to flow through tubing.

(5) Cleanse irrigating lumen on end of triple-lumen catheter (see Figure 20-23, *A*). *(The third catheter lumen or Y-connector provides means for irrigating solution to enter bladder. Necessary for system to remain sterile.)*

(6) Connect irrigating solution tubing to catheter lumen.

(7) Restore flow as ordered; calculate drip rate. *(Ensures continuous, even irrigation of catheter system. Prevents accumulation of solution in bladder, which will possibly cause bladder distention and injury.)*

(8) Deduct solution from urine in drainage bag when emptying. *(Allows you to compute true I&O.)*

d. **Bladder instillation:**

(1) Disconnect catheter from tubing—stabilize tubing to prevent touching the floor. NOTE: Using triple-lumen catheter makes it unnecessary to disconnect catheter from drainage tubing (see Figure 20-23, *B*).

(2) Cleanse end of catheter with antiseptic swab.

(3) Draw medication or solution into syringe. *(Prepares for instillation.)*

(4) Place tip of syringe into end of catheter and slowly inject medication or solution. *(Proceeding slowly prevents trauma to bladder mucosa.)*

(5) Clamp off end of catheter for necessary period. *(Allows medication or solution to be absorbed by bladder.)* Then reconnect catheter and tubing, making certain the system is tightly connected. *(Decreases risk of infection.)*

(6) Measure solution. *(Enables you to determine amount returned and amount of true urine for accurate recording of I&O.)*

9. Assess flow of urine through drainage tubing (see Figure 20-23, *B*). *(Data serve as baseline to judge patient response to therapy.)*
10. Refer to standard steps 10 to 17.
11. Document. Record urine output on I&O sheet.
    - Solution used as irrigant
    - Amount of solution used
    - Amount returned as drainage
    - Character of drainage
    - Patient teaching (see Patient Teaching boxes on catheter care and removing a urinary catheter)
12. Report any unusual findings immediately. *(More aggressive therapy is sometimes necessary.)*
    - Occlusion if present
    - Sudden bleeding
    - Infection
    - Increased pain
    - If irrigant does not return
    - Unrelieved bladder spasms

check the drainage system for proper placement and function.

3. Adequately hydrate the patient to flush the urinary tract.
4. Do not open the drainage system after it is in place except to irrigate the catheter, and then only with a specific order from the physician. It is important to maintain a closed system to prevent urinary infections (Figure 20-23).
5. Perform catheter care twice daily and as needed, using standard precautions (see Skill 20-13).
6. Assess the drainage system daily for leaks. Know agency policy on replacing the system.
7. Avoid placing the urinary drainage bag above the level of the catheter insertion, which will cause urine to reenter the drainage system and contaminate the urinary tract (see Figure 20-21).

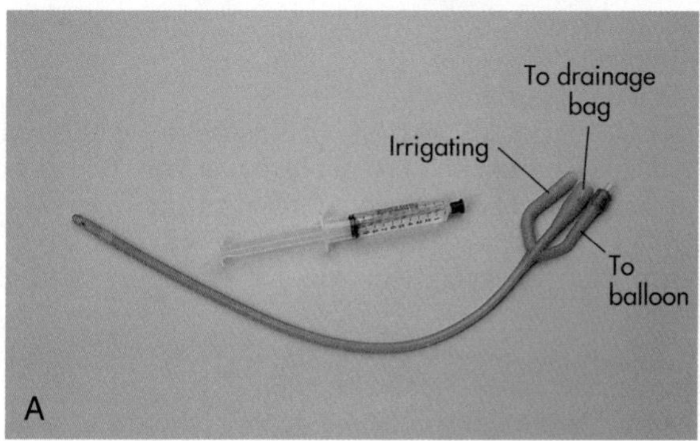

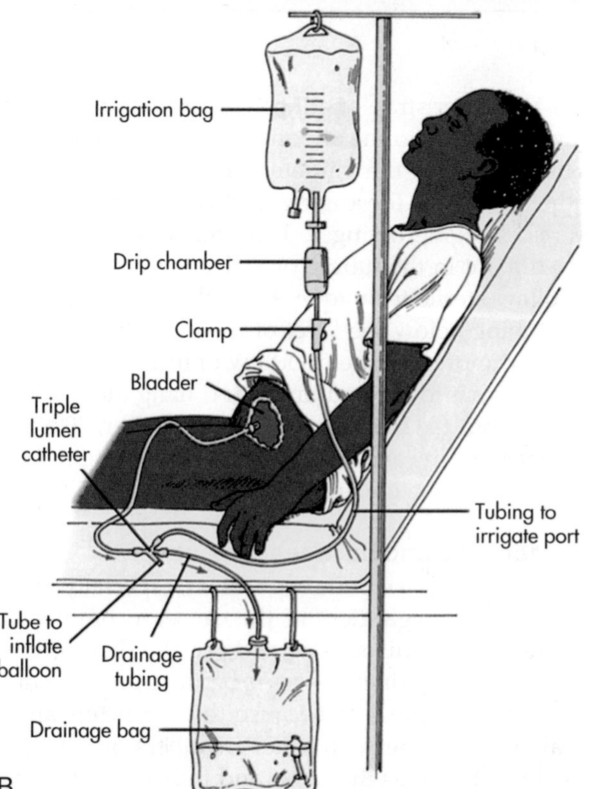

FIGURE 20-23 **A,** Triple-lumen catheter with sterile syringe to inflate catheter balloon. Note the port for inflating the balloon. **B,** Continuous sterile bladder irrigation setup.

8. Prevent tension on the system or backflow of urine while transferring the patient.
9. Ambulate the patient, if possible, to facilitate urine flow. If it is necessary to restrict the patient's activity, turn and reposition patient every 2 hours.
10. Avoid kinks or compression of the drainage tube that tend to cause pooling of urine within the urinary tract. Gently coil excess tubing, secure to the bottom bed linens with a clamp or pin to avoid dislodging the catheter, and release the tubing before transferring or repositioning the patient.
11. Gently inspect the entry site of the catheter for blood or exudate that indicates possible trauma or infection. Observe the color and composition of the urine to note any blood or sediment. During drainage of the collection bag, note the presence of any odor.
12. When ordered, collect specimens from the catheter by cleansing the drainage port with alcohol, then withdrawing the urine by using a sterile needle and a sterile 10-mL syringe using standard precautions. Send the urine specimen immediately to the laboratory (see Chapter 19).
13. Be sensitive to the patient's feelings regarding the catheter and the constant drainage system (see Life Span Considerations for Older Adults box on catheterization and Home Care Considerations box on urinary catheter care).

After the urinary catheter is removed, some patients have difficulty voiding until bladder tone and sensation return. If the patient complains of urinary retention, institute the following measures:

1. If necessary, try stimulating urination by running water, placing the patient's hands in water, or pouring water over the perineum. If the latter method is attempted, make sure to subtract the amount of water used when calculating the amount voided.
2. If the patient's condition permits, it is preferable for a female to sit on a bathroom stool or commode and for a male to stand to void.

The patient will in some cases experience some dribbling of urine after voiding as a result of dilation of the sphincter from the catheter. Record the time, the amount, and the color of the urine output.

Self-Catheterization

Self-catheterization is possibly the intervention of choice for the patient who experiences spinal cord injury or other neurologic disorders that interfere with urinary elimination. Intermittent self-catheterization promotes independent function for the patient. At home there is less risk of cross-contamination than in the hospital, so it is possible to modify the catheterization procedure as a clean technique, although it is necessary to instruct the patient using strict surgical asep-

Life Span Considerations

Older Adults

Catheterization

- A patient with a catheter is especially vulnerable to urinary tract infections (UTIs). The frail older adult patient who is physically compromised runs the additional risk of developing septicemia, a life-threatening infection that has spread to the blood. Do not routinely catheterize the patient who is incontinent.
- An adequate oral fluid intake of 2000 mL/day and assisting the older adult to toilet on a regular, timed basis will help bladder retraining and prevent the need for excessive catheterization.
- Attached equipment such as a catheter tends to make it less likely that the older adult will be fully ambulatory, thereby increasing the risks associated with decreased mobility. When catheters are required, make sure they are removed as soon as the patient's condition allows.
- Have patients who are at home or in long-term care use a leg bag during the day and switch to a large-volume bag at night so that sleep is not interrupted.
- Patients at home, and some who are in long-term care, are sometimes able to catheterize themselves on an intermittent basis using clean technique. Self-catheterization has been shown to be successful in maintaining continence and results in fewer infections than with the use of indwelling catheters.
- External catheters are recommended for patients with prostatic obstruction.
- Use of internal catheters is contraindicated in patients with prostatic obstruction.
- It is necessary to carefully evaluate patients with neuropathy before application of an external catheter and at more frequent intervals, at least twice daily.
- The skin on the penis will be very delicate on the older person and prone to tearing; extreme caution is needed with the adhesives.

Home Care Considerations

Urinary Catheter Care

- Assess patient and primary caregiver to determine ability and motivation:
  —To maintain accurate records of intake and output (I&O)
  —To participate in routine catheter care
  —To perform catheter irrigation when necessary
- Provide patient and primary caregiver with appropriate containers and I&O chart. I&O measurements require conversion chart for household measures to metric measures. Demonstrate proper method for measuring I&O.
- Provide opportunity for patient and primary caregiver to demonstrate understanding of procedure for measuring I&O (see Chapter 22).
- Instruct on appropriate catheter care (see Skill 20-13).
- Explain how to care for catheter and drainage systems.
- Teach signs and symptoms of urinary tract infection:
  —Urgency
  —Frequency
  —Hesitancy
  —Burning
  —Bladder spasms
- Disposable supplies are best. If it is necessary to reuse catheters, have patient and primary caregiver learn boiling techniques. (Boil rubber catheter 20 minutes and wrap in clean cloth.)
- Teach catheterization technique, if necessary (see Skill 20-12).
- Assess patient's environment for appropriate storage space for materials needed for procedure.
- Consider referral to home care agency to follow up and reinforce teaching concepts.

sis in the hospital because of the risk of infection there. Emphasize the need for the patient to be alert for signs of infection and to have periodic evaluations by the physician. Follow institutional guidelines for catheter insertion technique.

Routine Catheter Care

In order to prevent urinary tract infections, it is important that patients receive perineal hygiene. At least every 8 hours, patients need catheter care including perineal care (see Skill 20-13) and cleansing of the first 2 inches of the catheter, with care to remove any secretions or encrustations. When providing perineal care, also assess for inflammation at and around the urethral meatus. In addition, note any swelling or discharge from the area. Avoid use of powders and lotions in the perineal area of patients with catheters since it leads to the growth of microorganisms that will potentially enter the urinary tract and cause urinary tract infections (Potter & Perry, 2009). Patients who are catheterized and who are incontinent of stool will need cleaning after bowel movements.

If a catheter strap or adhesive tape was in use to secure the tubing to the abdomen or leg in order to prevent pulling of the catheter, replace it after giving catheter care. If the tubing and collection device requires changing owing to leakage, odor, or collection of sediment in the tubing or collection device, be sure to follow sterile technique. Keep the collection device and tubing below the level of the bladder at all times in order to prevent the backflow of urine. Loop tubing and secure it to the bed linen, and hang the collection device from the bed frame (Perry & Potter, 2009) (see Patient Teaching and Home Care Considerations boxes on urinary catheter care).

Incontinence and its Management

Incontinence is a common problem, especially among older adults. Regardless of the cause, incontinence is psychologically distressing and socially disruptive.

Urinary incontinence occurs because pressure in the bladder is too great or because the sphincters are too weak. Collaborate with other members of the health care team to assess the cause and the extent of incontinence and to assist in managing the problem. The physical therapist, for example, will be able to assess

Patient Teaching

Urinary Catheter Care

- As you position the patient, explain, "First I will position you as comfortably as I can. I want you to lie still so that you do not accidentally contaminate the sterile equipment. I will let you know before I actually begin to insert the catheter."
- As you prepare to cleanse the area explain to the patient, "You will feel cold and wet."
- As you are about to insert the catheter explain to the patient, "I want you to bear down gently as if you were passing urine. This may burn and you may feel pressure."
- Explain the need for the patient to drink fluids to flush the urinary system.
- Explain the need for meticulous catheter care and perineal care.
- Answer patient's questions about procedures.
- Instruct patient about proper transfer from bed, chair, or stretcher.
- Teach the principles of catheter care.
- Instruct the patient about Kegel exercises.
- Identify the side effects that are possible, and explain the need to report them immediately (e.g., blood in the urine).
- Caution patient not to lie on tubing.
- Explain the importance of holding the catheter drainage receptacle at arm's length while ambulatory.
- Teach patient that using powders or lotion on the perineum is contraindicated because of the risk of growth of microorganisms that will be able to ascend the urinary tract.
- External catheters sometimes contribute to urinary tract infections; therefore, teach the caregiver signs and symptoms of infection and again emphasize medical asepsis.
- Encourage using a leg bag during the day and a bedside drainage bag at night.
- Loose-fitting clothing is sometimes needed to promote adequate drainage.
- Long-term use of external catheters is inadvisable because skin impairment (breakdown) becomes a major problem.

the extent of musculoskeletal involvement and determine methods of treatment.

Incontinence sometimes involves a small leakage of urine when the person laughs, coughs, or lifts something heavy. It is helpful to teach the patient exercises to strengthen muscles around the external sphincters to manage this type of incontinence. Pelvic floor exercises (Kegel exercises) involve tightening of the ring of muscle around the vagina and the anus for several seconds. (See discussion in the next section.) Persistent urge, stress, or overflow incontinence will usually necessitate referral for urologic evaluation.

When paralyzed patients have overflow incontinence, Credé's method is helpful. This involves applying manual pressure over the lower abdomen to express urine from the bladder at regular intervals. Credé's method requires a measure of expertise to prevent injury to the bladder.

Incontinence characterized by urine or fecal flow at unpredictable times requires the use of disposable adult undergarments or underpads as the primary means of management. Some incontinence products are designed for small amounts of leakage. Alert patients need an incontinence product that is discreet and promotes self-care.

Urine and feces are highly irritating to the skin. Skin that is continuously exposed quickly becomes inflamed and irritated. Cleansing the skin thoroughly after each episode of incontinence with warm, soapy water and drying it thoroughly help prevent skin impairment (Box 20-9). Urostomy care is discussed elsewhere in this chapter.

Avoid all negative verbal and nonverbal expressions. Cleanse the perineum in a professional, caring, and matter-of-fact manner. Under no circumstances is it acceptable to reprimand or humiliate (scold) a patient for having an "accident."

Box 20-9 Nursing Diagnoses for the Patient with a Urinary Tract Disorder

Functional urinary incontinence:
- Related to sensory deficits
- Related to cognitive deficits
- Related to mobility deficits

Risk for impaired skin integrity:
- Related to presence of urine

Situational low self-esteem:
- Related to inability to control passage of urine

Stress urinary incontinence:
- Related to degenerative change in pelvis muscles and structural support associated with increased age

Urge urinary incontinence:
- Related to decreased bladder capacity due to abdominal surgeries or indwelling urinary catheters

Risk for infection:
- Related to inadequate personal hygiene
- Related to lack of knowledge of care of a urinary stoma

Data from North American Nursing Diagnosis Association International (NANDA-I). (2009). *NANDA-I nursing diagnoses: Definitions and classification 2009-2011.* Oxford, United Kingdom: Author.

Bladder Training

When urinary incontinence results from decreased perception of bladder fullness or impaired voluntary motor control, bladder training is often helpful. Bladder training is possible to modify according to different problems.

In preparation for the removal of a urethral catheter, the physician will sometimes order a clamp-unclamp routine to improve bladder tone. Bladder training often involves developing the use of the muscles of the perineum to improve voluntary control over voiding. The patient with stress incontinence will learn to exercise the muscles of the perineum to assist in stopping urine flow. Instruct the patient to perform Kegel, or pubococcygeal, exercises by tightening the muscles of the perineal floor. One way for the patient to develop awareness of the appropriate muscle group is by trying to stop the flow of urine during voiding. Once the patient has identified the correct muscles and the feeling of their contraction, direct him or her to tighten the muscles of the perineum, hold that tension for 10 seconds, and then relax for 10 seconds. The exercises are best done initially in groups of 10, building to groups of 20, four times a day. Because muscle control develops gradually, it will sometimes take 4 to 6 weeks to develop control of leakage.

Skill 20-15 Removing an Indwelling Catheter

Nursing Action *(Rationale)*

1. Refer to standard steps 1 to 9.
2. Assemble equipment:
   - 10-mL syringe without a needle or larger depending on volume of fluid used to inflate balloon (see illustration.)
3. Assessment:
   a. Note length of time catheter has been in place. *(The longer the catheter has been in place, the greater the risk for decreased bladder muscle tone and inflammation of the urethra.)*
   b. Assess the patient's knowledge of what to expect. *(Many patients anticipate discomfort or have fears about ability to void successfully after removal of the catheter.)*
4. Provide privacy. Position the patient supine and place a waterproof pad under the catheter. *(Protects the bed linens.)* Females will need to abduct their legs with the drape between their thighs (see step 5b of Skill 20-12). It is acceptable for drape to lie on male's thighs.
5. Insert hub of syringe into inflation valve (balloon port) and aspirate until tubing collapses. *(Indicates that entire contents of balloon have been removed.)*
6. Remove catheter steadily and smoothly (females have catheter in about 2 to 3 inches [5 to 7.5 cm] and males about 6 to 7 inches [15 to 18 cm]). *(Facilitates procedure that has no discomfort.) Catheter will usually slide out very easily. Do not use force. If any resistance is noted, repeat step 5 to remove remaining water. (Prevents trauma to the urethra.)*
7. Wrap catheter in waterproof pad. Unhook collection bag and drainage tubing from the bed. *(Prevents any leakage from the catheter onto the patient, you, or bed linens.)*
8. Measure urine, and empty drainage bag. *(Promotes accurate reporting and recording.)*
9. Record output. *(Communicates patient care.)*
10. Cleanse the perineum with soap and water, and dry area thoroughly. *(Promotes comfort and a feeling of cleanliness.)*
11. Explain to patient:
    a. It is important to have a fluid intake of 1.5 to 2 L/day unless contraindicated.
    b. Instruct patient of need to void within 8 hours and that each voiding will be into the "hat" and measured. Most facilities and physicians want the patient to void 3 times in substantial amounts to verify adequate emptying of the urinary bladder. *(Confirms the ability of the patient to empty the bladder adequately.)*
    c. Explain that many patients experience mild burning or discomfort with first voiding, which soon subsides.
    d. Inform the patient to report any signs of urinary tract infection: urgency, burning, frequency, excreting small amount and pain or discomfort, which are most likely to develop in 2 to 3 days.
12. Place the urine hat on the toilet seat (see Chapter 19). *(Facilitates accurate assessment of patient's output.)*
13. Refer to standard steps 12 to 17.
14. Document and report: *(Promotes continuity of patient care.)*
    - Time catheter was removed
    - Teaching related to increasing fluid intake and signs and symptoms of urinary tract infection
    - Time, amount, and characteristics of first voiding
    - Complete I&O record

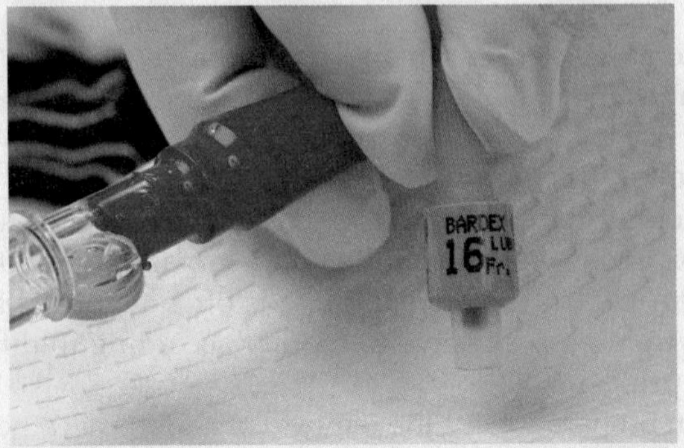

Step 2 Note size of balloon printed on catheter.

Habit training involves establishing a voiding schedule and provides cooperative patients with opportunity to achieve continence by voiding at regular intervals (every 1½ to 2 hours). Monitor the patient's voiding for a few days to identify patterns, or schedule voiding times to correlate with the patient's activities. Typical voiding times are upon rising, before each meal, and at bedtime. Assist the patient to void as scheduled. Periodically ask patients if they are wet or dry, check them for wetness, remind or assist them to the toilet as scheduled, and praise them for appropriate toileting. After a few days, evaluate the scheduled voiding pattern by identifying its effectiveness in keeping the patient continent. Then modify the schedule until continence is established. Fluid intake and medications will typically influence voiding patterns (e.g., a patient will often need to void 30 minutes after the ingestion of coffee or furosemide in response to the diuretic effect). Limiting fluids after the evening meal reduces the need for nighttime voiding and helps keep the patient dry.

REMOVAL OF AN INDWELLING CATHETER

It is always best to remove an indwelling catheter as soon as possible, because its presence increases the risk for urinary tract infection (Skill 20-15). Following surgery, you will usually remove the catheter after 8 to 24 hours, depending on the type of surgery. In some situations, the catheter will remain in place for days or even weeks. The longer a catheter has been in place, the greater the risk that the patient will have difficulty voiding after its removal. A patient who has had an overdistended bladder or who has altered sensory perception because of regional anesthesia, such as a spinal or epidural block, is also likely to have difficulty voiding following catheter removal. Expect most patients to void adequately no more than 8 hours after catheter removal.

Urinary tract infection, which is one of the most common types of **iatrogenic** (caused by treatment or diagnostic procedures) infections, often develops 2 or more days after catheter removal. With early discharge, patients need to be informed of the risk for infection, prevention measures, and signs and symptoms (urgency, frequency, burning, excreting in small amounts, and pain) that are necessary to report to the physician (see Patient Teaching box on removing a urinary catheter).

VAGINAL IRRIGATION

The douche/internal vaginal irrigation (pericare is the external douche) is not performed or ordered as commonly as in the past. Secretions from the vaginal membranes are there to protect the area from infection so it is desirable *not* to wash these protective agents away unless necessary as in preparation for surgery. The physician will order the solution to use, such as saline, sterile water, or medication solutions. Commercially prepared douches are also available for one-time use.

 Patient Teaching

Removing Urinary Catheter

Instruct the patient on the following when an indwelling catheter has been removed:

- Explain that it will take time for the urinary bladder to reestablish voluntary control of urine.
- Describe how to collect and measure urine output and the need for same.
- Explain the need to drink at least 2 L (eight 8-oz glasses/cups) per day of fluids (usually indicated to reduce risk of infection).
- Explain that it is common to feel some burning or discomfort in the meatal area when first voiding.
- Identify the side effects that are possible, and explain the need to report them immediately. (Sometimes patients void in small amounts frequently and complain of burning or pain; this indicates possible urinary retention or urinary infection.)
- Instruct regarding the use of over-the-counter medications that have potential to cause urinary retention, such as nasal decongestants and anticholingeric medications.

 Coordinated Care

Delegation

VAGINAL IRRIGATION

- The skill for administering a vaginal irrigation is acceptable to delegate to assistive personnel in some settings (check agency policy). Initial patient assessment requires the critical thinking unique to a nurse, and delegation is inappropriate.
- Female patients often develop vaginal infections necessitating topical application of antiinfective agents. Vaginal medications are available in foam, jelly, cream, and suppository forms (see Chapter 23). It is also possible to give medicated irrigations or douches; however, their excessive use sometimes leads to irritation of the vaginal mucosa (see Skill 20-16).

Advise the patient to seek guidance from the primary caregiver (Skill 20-16 and Coordinated Care box on vaginal irrigation).

SKILLS FOR GASTROINTESTINAL DISORDERS

INSERTING AND MAINTAINING NASOGASTRIC TUBES

A **nasogastric (NG) tube** is a flexible, hollow tube that is passed into the stomach via the nasopharynx. The NG tube serves either to remove gastric contents or to administer fluids or nutrients into the stomach. The primary purpose of the NG tube is for decompression or removal of flatus and fluids from the stomach. The NG tube helps prevent vomiting and distention caused by reduced peristalsis resulting from general anesthesia, manipulation of the viscera during surgery, or obstruction of the operative site by edema. When used for decompression, the NG tube is usually connected to an intermittent gastric suction device. You will

Skill 20-16 Performing a Vaginal Irrigation or Douche

Nursing Action *(Rationale)*

1. Refer to standard steps 1 to 9.
2. Assemble equipment:
   - Drape
   - Bedpan and tissues
   - Waterproof pad
   - Douche kit
   - Solution container, tubing, and nozzle
   - Wash basin, disposable washcloths, and towel
   - Clean disposable gloves
   - Ordered solution (1000 to 1500 mL at body temperature or commercially prepared solutions in smaller amounts)
   - Bath blanket
3. Assist patient to the dorsal recumbent position. *(Position allows for easy access to and good exposure of vaginal orifice.)*
4. Prepare patient:
   a. Drape patient's abdomen and lower extremities. *(Keeps patient's embarrassment to a minimum.)*
   b. Position patient on bedpan with waterproof pad underneath. *(Allows hips to be higher than shoulders so that solution will reach posterior fornix of vagina and distend the vaginal wall, ensuring solution reaches between the folds [rugae]. Bedpan collects solution and pad protects the bed linens.)*
   c. Be certain vaginal orifice is well illuminated by room light or gooseneck lamp. *(Ensures visualization of external genitalia for proper insertion.)*
5. Assessment: *(Findings provide baseline to monitor effect of therapy.)*
   a. Condition of external genitalia and vaginal canal (is possible to do just before insertion).
   b. For symptoms of pruritus, burning, or discomfort.
   c. For possible discharge and odor. *(A thick, white, patchy, curdlike discharge clinging to the vaginal walls is a sign of yeast infection, a common female disorder.)* Perineal care is sometimes necessary before administering the douche (see Chapter 18).
   d. For signs of inflammation, erythema, or edema.
6. Prepare equipment. *(Organizes procedure.)* Have solution at body temperature. *(Prevents burning the delicate mucosa of the vagina.)* Allow some solution to drain down the tubing out through the nozzle into bedpan. *(Removes air from tubing and moistens nozzle.)*
7. Gently retract labial folds and maintain position. Direct nozzle toward the sacrum, following the floor of the vagina. *(Allows correct position of nozzle.)*
8. Raise the container approximately 12 to 20 inches (30 to 50 cm) above level of vagina. Insert nozzle 3 to 4 inches (7 to 10 cm). Allow solution to flow while inserting and rotating nozzle. Instruct patient to tighten perineal muscles as if to suppress urination and then relax. Repeat four or five times during procedure. Administer all of the solution. *(Allowing solution to flow during insertion moistens the vaginal orifice, thus reducing friction. Rotating the nozzle allows irrigation of all areas in the vagina. Periodic contracting and relaxing of perineal muscles allows solution to flow between rugae.)*
9. Withdraw nozzle and assist patient to a comfortable position while she remains on the bedpan. *(The remaining solution will drain by gravity. The bedpan will collect solution.)*
10. Refer to standard steps 10 to 17.
11. Allow patient to remain on bedpan a short time (10 minutes), then don clean gloves; remove bedpan, assessing results; and dispose of remaining solution in proper manner (know agency policy). Cleanse patient or allow patient to cleanse herself with basin of warm water, towel, and washcloth. Assist patient to a comfortable position. Remove gloves, discard them in proper receptacle, and perform hand hygiene. *(Reduces spread of microorganisms and provides for patient comfort.)*
12. Document: *(Verifies performance of procedure and ensures continuity of care.)*
    - Time
    - Type, amount, and temperature of solution
    - Assessment of external genitalia and vagina *(Documented description provides baseline to determine change in patient's condition.)*
    - Patient's response
    - Patient teaching:
      —Value of and technique for regular perineal hygiene. A daily douche for cleansing purposes is not recommended because it depletes the vaginal vault of the normal secretions.
      —Cleansing the perineal area from pubis (anterior) to rectum (posterior) prevents transfer of microorganisms from rectal area to vaginal or bladder area.
      —When instructing the patient on the douche procedure at home, teach patient to recline in the bathtub while administering the douche.
      —Sitting on the toilet forces the douche solution uphill and will not distend the rugae of the vaginal vault.
13. Report unusual findings. *(Female patients often develop vaginal infections requiring topical application of antiinfective agents.)*

routinely measure contents of the suction container to monitor intake and output. The tubes most commonly used for decompression are the Levin and Salem sump tubes. The Levin tube has one lumen and several openings near the tip. The Salem sump tube is a double-lumen tube: one lumen provides an air vent, and the other is for removal of gastric contents (Figure 20-24).

The patient with an NG tube presents several nursing challenges. Box 20-10 lists selected nursing diagnoses for the patient who has been intubated. One of the greatest challenges is maintaining patient comfort. Some patients state that the discomfort from the tube exceeds the pain from the surgical incision. NG tubes continually irritate the nasal mucosa. To lessen this discomfort, secure the tube with a nose guard (a tube fixation device using a shaped adhesive patch) to the nose and then to the gown with a pin to prevent unnecessary movement (Skill 20-17 and Patient Teaching box on nasogastric tubes). Other comfort measures include removing excess secretions from around the nares (nostrils) and lubricating the nostrils and the tube with a water-soluble lubricant to prevent crusting of secretions.

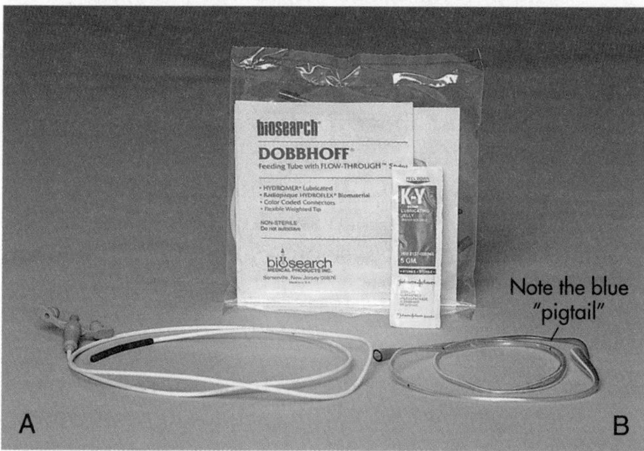

FIGURE 20-24 **A,** Small-bore feeding tube. **B,** Salem sump tube. Note the blue "pigtail."

Box 20-10 Nursing Diagnoses for the Patient with Intubation

Imbalanced nutrition, less than body requirements:
- Related to insufficient intake

Impaired swallowing:
- Related to neuromuscular impairment

Risk for aspiration:
- Related to choking
- Related to inability to swallow

Diarrhea:
- Related to altered intake associated with tube feedings

Constipation:
- Related to altered intake associated with tube feedings

Data from North American Nursing Diagnosis Association International (NANDA-I). (2009). *NANDA-I nursing diagnoses: Definitions and classification 2009-2011.* Oxford, United Kingdom: Author.

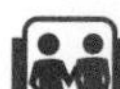 Patient Teaching

Nasogastric Tube

- Explain role of a nasogastric tube in supplementing nutrition.
- Explain how the decompression tube will prevent nausea, vomiting, and abdominal distention.
- Teach patient and family how to care for the nasogastric tube at home.
- Explain the need to maintain moist mucous membranes with special mouth care.
- Explain to patient how to relax and communicate during tube insertion. For example, "Now I will explain each step as we go along. The tube will cause a burning pain as it passes through your nose. I want you to raise one finger to tell me when it really hurts so that I can be gentle and at the same time get this done as quickly as possible."
- Explain that now you are about to insert the feeding tube. Let patient know how he or she can assist. For example, "I will insert the tube through your nose toward the back of your throat. Once the tip is in the back of your throat, I will ask you to begin to swallow. We may use water (ice chips) (if allowed) if you find it hard to swallow. I will tell you when to stop swallowing."
- Ensure adequate lubrication of tube to decrease discomfort, especially with older adults, some of whom will have decreased oral or nasopharyngeal secretions.

Skill 20-17 Inserting a Nasogastric Tube

Nursing Action *(Rationale)*

1. Refer to standard steps 1 to 9.
2. Assemble equipment:
   - Bath towel
   - 14 or 16 F nasogastric (NG) tube (smaller bore for child) or feeding type of tube (see Figure 20-24)
   - Water-soluble lubricating jelly
   - Stethoscope
   - Tongue blade
   - Flashlight
   - Asepto bulb or cone-tip syringe
   - Nose guard
   - Safety pin and rubber band
   - Clamp
   - Suction container
   - Suction machine
   - Glass of water with straw
   - Facial tissues
   - Normal saline
   - Tincture of benzoin (optional)
   - Unsterile gloves

Continued

Skill 20-17 Inserting a Nasogastric Tube—cont'd

3. Assess patient for condition of oral cavity. *(Enables you to determine need for special nursing measures and for oral hygiene after tube placement.)* Palpate patient's abdomen. *(This determination will later serve as comparison after tube is inserted.)*
4. Position patient in high Fowler's position with pillow behind head and shoulders. *(Promotes patient's ability to swallow during procedure.)*
5. Stand at right side of bed if right-handed and left side if left-handed. *(Best allows for easy manipulation of tubing.)*
6. Place bath towel over patient's chest; give tissues to patient. *(This prevents soiling of gown. Tube insertion through nasal passages sometimes causes eyes to tear up.)*
7. Instruct patient to relax and breathe normally while occluding one nostril. Repeat this action for other nostril. Select nostril with greater airflow. *(The tube passes more easily through nostril that is more patent.)* Many institutions have nasogastric tubes cooled in ice or saline, which stiffens them to facilitate passage.
8. Measure distance to insert tube. Measure total distance from tip of nose to earlobe and from there to xiphoid process of sternum (see illustration). Tube should extend from nostril to stomach; distance varies with each patient. *(This measurement provides distance from nose to stomach in 98% of patients.)*
9. Mark off length of tube to be inserted with piece of tape, or note distance from next tube marking. *(Helps ensure correct length of tubing will be inserted.)*
10. Curve 14 to 16 inches (10 to 15 cm) of end of tube tightly around index finger; release. *(Curving tube tip aids insertion.)*
11. Lubricate 3 to 4 inches (7.5 to 10 cm) of end of tube with water-soluble lubricating jelly. *(Minimizes friction against nasal mucosa.)*
12. Initially instruct patient to extend neck back against pillow; insert tube slowly through nostril with curved end pointing downward (see illustration). *(Facilitates initial passage of tube through nostril and maintains clear airway for open nostril.)*
13. Continue to pass tube along floor of nasal passage, aiming down toward ear. When resistance is felt, apply gentle downward pressure to advance tube (do not force past resistance). *(Reduces discomfort of tube rubbing against upper nasal turbinates. Resistance is caused by posterior nasopharynx. Downward pressure helps tube curl around corner of nasopharynx.)*
14. If resistance continues, withdraw tube, allow patient to rest, relubricate tube, and insert into other nostril. *(Forcing against resistance has potential to cause trauma to mucosa. Pause also helps relieve anxiety.)*
15. Continue insertion of tube until just past nasopharynx by gently rotating tube toward opposite nostril.
    a. Stop tube advancement, allow patient to relax, and provide tissues. *(Relieves anxiety; tearing is natural response to mucosal irritation.)*
    b. Explain that the next step requires swallowing. *(Tube is about to enter esophagus.)*
16. With tube just above oropharynx, instruct patient to flex head forward and dry swallow or suck in air through straw. Advance tube 1 to 2 inches (2.5 to 5 cm) with each swallow. While advancing the tube in an unconscious patient (or in a patient who cannot swallow), stroke the patient's neck. *(Encourages the swallowing reflex and facilitates passage down the esophagus.)* If patient has trouble swallowing and is allowed fluids, offer glass of water. Advance tube with each swallow of water. *(The flexed position closes off upper airway to trachea and opens esophagus. Swallowing closes epiglottis over trachea and helps move tube into esophagus. Swallowing water reduces gagging or choking.)*

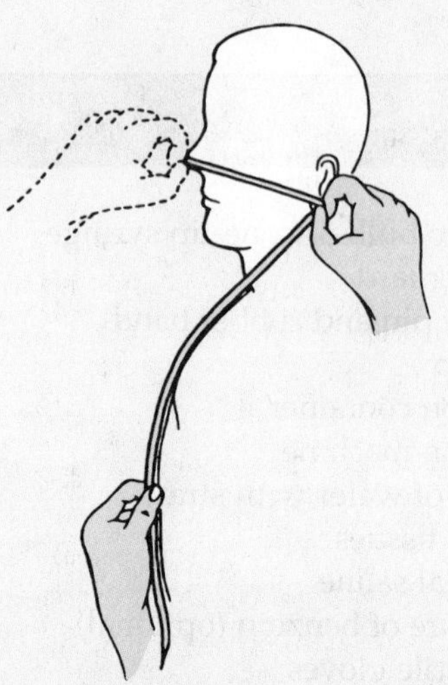
Step **8**

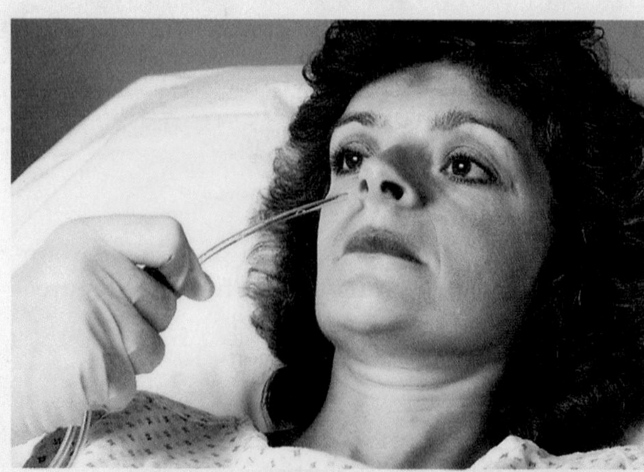
Step **12**

17. If patient begins to cough, gag, or choke, stop tube advancement. Instruct patient to breathe easily and take sips of water. *(Tubing sometimes accidentally enters larynx and initiates cough reflex. Gagging is eased by swallowing water.)*
18. If patient continues to cough, pull tube back slightly. *(It is possible for tube to enter the larynx and obstruct airway.)*
19. If patient continues to gag, assess back of pharynx using flashlight and tongue blade. *(It is possible for tubing to accidentally enter larynx and initiate cough reflex.)*
20. After patient relaxes, continue to advance tube desired distance. *(It is necessary for tip of tube to be in the stomach to provide proper decompression.)*
21. Ask patient to talk. *(Patient will be unable to talk if tube is passed through vocal cords.)*
22. Assess posterior pharynx for presence of coiled tube. *(The tube is pliable and there is potential for it to coil up in back of pharynx instead of advancing into esophagus.)*
23. Attach cone-tipped syringe to end of tube. Aspirate gently back on syringe to obtain gastric contents. *(Begins determination of whether tube is correctly in place in the stomach.)*
24. Measure pH of aspirate with color-coded pH paper with range of whole numbers from 1 to 11. Gastric aspirates have decidedly acidic pH values, preferably 4 or less (see Chapter 21, Skill 21-1). *(Determines whether tube is correctly in place in the stomach. Insufflation of air into tube followed by auscultation of sounds is no longer considered most effective in determining tube placement. Sounds transmitted by insufflation of air are sometimes transmitted from pleural space to upper abdomen, giving false impression of placement. Know agency policy for preferred method. X-ray study is the most reliable method for determining correct tube placement.)*
25. If tube is not in the stomach, advance another 1 to 2 inches (2.5 to 5 cm) and repeat steps 23 and 24. *(Assesses for tube placement.)*
26. After tube is properly inserted, clamp end or connect it to suction. *(Intermittent suction is most effective for decompression.)* You will often clamp tube for short periods such as during ambulation. *(Patients going to operating room often have tube clamped.)*
27. Secure tube to nose with a nose guard. Avoid putting pressure on nares (see illustration). *(Anchors the tube securely.)* Clean the skin over the nose with alcohol to remove any skin oils or soil and coat with Skin Prep before applying the nose guard.
28. Fasten end of tube to gown by looping rubber band around tube in slip knot. Pin rubber band to gown (see illustration). *(Reduces chance of putting pressure on nares by tube moving. Pinning provides slack for movement.)*

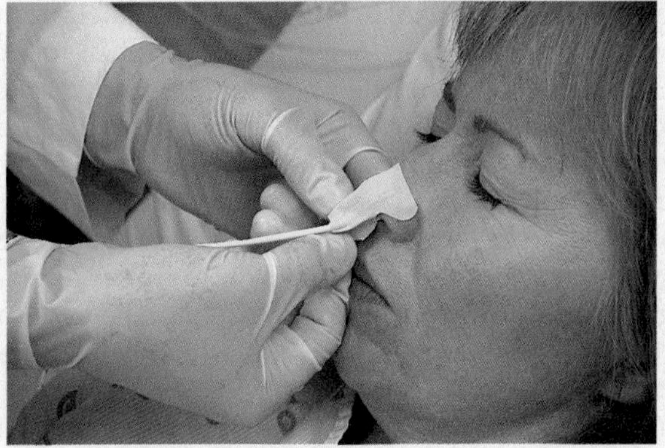

Step **27**

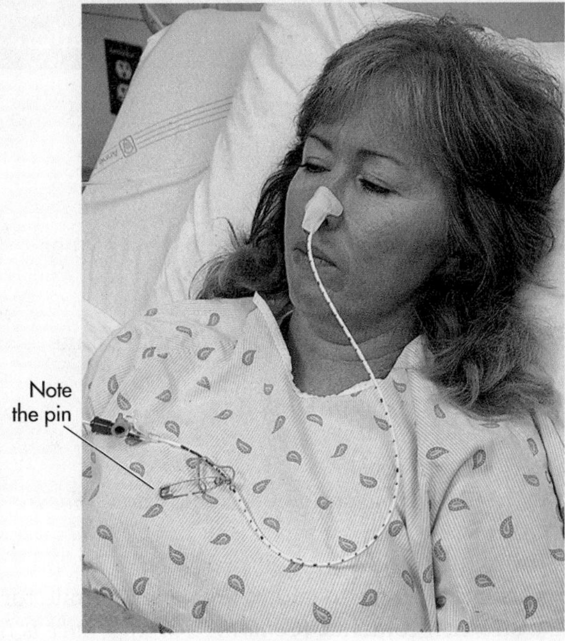

Note the pin

Step **28**

29. Unless physician orders otherwise, elevate head of bed 30 degrees. *(Helps prevent esophageal reflux and keeps to a minimum irritation caused by tube against posterior pharynx.)*
30. Refer to standard steps 10 to 17.
31. Document: *(Verifies performance of procedure and ensures continuity of care.)*
    - Time and type of tube inserted
    - Tolerance to procedure
    - Confirmation of placement
    - Character and amount of gastric contents
    - Whether tube is clamped or connected to suction
    - Patient teaching (see Patient Teaching box on nasogastric tubes)
32. Report abnormalities:
    - Inability to advance tube. *(Additional interventions or therapies are sometimes necessary, such as smaller-bore tube, chest x-ray study, or airway suctioning.)*

Patients are inclined to breathe through their mouth owing to the nasal occlusion from the tube, and the lips and tongue will often become dry and cracked. Provide mouth care at least every 2 hours to keep dehydration to a minimum. Rinsing the mouth with cool water usually provides some comfort; however, it is important to ensure that the patient does not swallow any water. Check the physician's orders to see if it is all right to allow the patient to chew gum to increase salivation or suck on small ice chips, which helps relieve throat dryness. An ice bag placed on the external throat is another method that often provides some relief of the discomfort.

Another nursing challenge is maintaining patency of the tube. Sometimes the tube becomes occluded with secretions or the internal tip of the tube will become occluded if the end of the tube is pressing against the gastric mucosa. Irrigate the nasogastric tube regularly with normal saline and an Asepto (bulb-tipped or piston-tipped) syringe (Skill 20-18). Turning the patient facilitates draining the stomach. If necessary, try either advancing the tubing further or withdrawing it somewhat in order to reposition it. However, only a physician is permitted to reposition the tube when certain surgical procedures have been performed. For

Skill 20-18 Nasogastric Tube Irrigation

Nursing Action *(Rationale)*

1. Refer to standard steps 1 to 9.
2. Assemble equipment:
   - Syringe
   - Irrigation set with either bulb- (Asepto) or piston-tipped syringe
   - Container for irrigant
   - Irrigation solution, usually normal saline
   - Clamp
   - Towel or waterproof pad
   - Stethoscope
   - Clean gloves
3. Place patient in semi-Fowler's position. *(Facilitates procedure.)*
4. Verify that tube is in right place:
   - Attach syringe to end of tube and aspirate for stomach contents. *(Confirms that tip of tube is in the stomach.)*
5. Assess abdomen. *(Provides baseline data for later comparison.)*
6. Pour normal saline into container; draw up 30 mL (or amount ordered) into bulb (Asepto) or piston syringe. *(Use of saline keeps loss of electrolytes from stomach fluid to a minimum.)*
7. Clamp connection tubing distal to connection site for drainage or suction apparatus. Disconnect tubing and lay end on a towel. *(Reduces backflow of secretions and soiling of patient's gown and bed linens.)*
8. Insert tip of irrigating syringe into end of nasogastric (NG) tube. Hold syringe with tip pointed toward the floor, and instill 30 mL or ordered amount of saline slowly and evenly. Do NOT force solution. Never use air vent or pigtail on tubing of Salem sump for irrigation. *(Position of syringe prevents introduction of air into vent tubing, which has potential to cause gastric distention. Solution introduced under pressure has potential to cause gastric trauma.)*
9. If resistance is met, assess tubing for kinks, change patient's position, and repeat attempt; if resistance continues, confer with registered nurse (RN) or physician. *(Ensures that tip of tubing is not lying against wall of stomach. Buildup of secretions will cause distention.)*
10. Withdraw fluid into syringe and measure; continue irrigating with ordered amount of saline until purpose of irrigation has been accomplished. *(Clears the tubing.)*
11. Reconnect NG tube to suction to prevent leakage of fluid from airway vent of Salem sump tubes; introduce 30 mL of air into airway lumen to clear air vent tubing. Secure airway lumen above level of stomach to prevent siphoning effect. *(Reestablishes drainage collection.)*
12. Note amount of saline instilled and withdrawn. Subtract amount instilled from amount withdrawn and record difference as output. *(Fluid remaining in stomach is measured as intake.)*
13. Refer to standard steps 10 to 17.
14. Document: *(Description of gastric contents provides baseline to determine any change.)*
    - Time
    - Type and amount of solution
    - Character and volume of aspirate
    - Patient teaching (see Patient Teaching box on nasogastric tubes)
    - Record balance of fluid instilled and aspirated on intake and output (I&O) sheet *(Balance reflects fluid gain or loss.)*
15. Report abnormalities. *(Findings indicate need to reposition tube or administer additional therapies.)*
    - Failure of tube to drain
    - Abdominal distention
    - Unusual characteristic of drainage (blood)

example, do not reposition an NG tube yourself for a patient who has had gastric or esophageal surgery.

States and agencies vary on policy for who is authorized to insert NG tubes (see Coordinated Care box on nasogastric tubes). Some states have endorsed the LPN/LVN Certification Course, which enables a licensed practical nurse or licensed vocational nurse (LPN/LVN) to insert NG tubes (see Skill 20-17) (know agency policy). Most agencies allow the LPN/LVN to irrigate the NG tube (see Skill 20-18), administer feedings (see Chapter 21, Skill 21-1), care for the NG tube (Skill 20-19), and remove the NG tube (Skill 20-20) (know agency policy).

 Coordinated Care

Collaboration

NASOGASTRIC TUBE

- The skill of inserting a nasogastric tube requires the critical thinking and knowledge application unique to a nurse. Assistive personnel (AP) is permitted to measure and record the drainage from the NG tube and provide oral and nasal hygiene. Also teach AP how to properly secure the NG tube.
- The skill of irrigating an NG tube requires the critical thinking and knowledge application unique to a nurse and is not appropriate to delegate to AP.
- The skill of removing an NG tube requires the critical thinking and knowledge application unique to a nurse and is not appropriate to delegate to AP.

BOWEL ELIMINATION

Elimination of bowel wastes **(defecation)** is a basic human need and is essential for normal body function. Normal bowel elimination depends on several factors: a balanced diet, including high-fiber foods; a daily fluid intake of 2000 to 3000 mL; and activity to promote muscle tone and peristalsis (rhythmic contractions of the intestine that propel gastric contents through the GI tract). Normal stool **(feces)** is described for documentation as moderate in amount, brown, and soft in consistency and is expelled every 1 to 3 days. However, each patient has an individual pattern of defecation.

Promotion of normal patterns of elimination includes establishing a routine time for defecation, heeding the urge to defecate, sitting on a commode, and having privacy during elimination. Many people have their own established ritual to promote elimination, such as drinking warm water with lemon juice or drinking black coffee with breakfast.

Bowel elimination is a private activity. Affording the patient privacy is your responsibility. Respect the patient's embarrassment, provide supportive nursing measures, and allow as much privacy as possible.

In many cultures, squatting is the usual position for females for defecation and urination. For males, squat-

Skill 20-19 Gastric and Intestinal Suctioning Care

Nursing Action *(Rationale)*

1. Refer to standard steps 1 to 9.
2. Assemble equipment:
   - Asepto syringe
   - Towel
   - Suction apparatus, if used
   - Clean gloves
   - Emesis basin
   - Stethoscope
3. Assess suction apparatus. *(Enables you to determine whether suctioning apparatus is functioning.)*
   a. **For suction machine** (Gomco):
      (1) Machine is plugged in securely.
      (2) Light is blinking on and off.
      (3) Tubing connections are secured.
      (4) Setting is correct.
   b. **For wall suction:**
      (1) Pressure gauge connections are tight.
      (2) Pressure indicated on gauge is as ordered or according to agency policy, 80 to 100 mm Hg. *(Pressure above 120 mm Hg leads to gastric bleeding.)*
      (3) Suction is set on intermittent or continuous as ordered.
4. Assess patient: *(Enables you to determine need for any special care.)*
   a. Oral and nasal cavities.
   b. Abdomen for bowel sounds and extent of distention. *(Provides baseline for further assessments and may indicate tube malfunction.)*
   c. Patient is on nothing-by-mouth (NPO) status.
   d. Lips and oral mucosa; keep moist. *(Prevents drying.)*
5. Ensure that tubing is not kinked and that patient is not lying on tubing. *(Verifies that the patient or tube itself is not causing obstruction.)*
6. Pin nasogastric (NG) tube to patient's gown with enough slack to allow movement (see illustration for step 28 of Skill 20-17). *(Prevents dislodging tube and patient discomfort.)*
7. Verify that drainage is moving through tubing to drainage collection bottle. *(Indicates that stomach or intestinal contents are being removed.)*
8. For Salem sump tube, see that vent is pointing upward. *(There is potential that vent pointing downward will promote drainage through vent via gravity.)* Listen at opening of blue air vent. *(Hissing sound indicates air vent is patent.)* If you

Continued

Skill 20-19 Gastric and Intestinal Suctioning Care—cont'd

hear no hissing sounds, instruct patient to cough or reposition patient in the right or left Sims' or the supine position. *(Helps move distal opening of tube [in the stomach] away from the mucosa wall and enable the suction to resume.)* It may be necessary to momentarily disconnect the NG tube from the suction tubing; be certain to reconnect immediately.

9. Measure amount of drainage in bottle, noting color; empty when becoming full and at end of each shift. *(Provides baseline for further assessments, prevents overflow, and provides for accurate measurement.)*
10. Refer to standard steps 10 to 17.
11. Document: *(Description of gastric contents provides baseline to determine any change.)*
    - Procedure
    - Time
    - Observations
    - Amount, color, and consistency of drainage
    - Abnormalities
    - Patient teaching (see Patient Teaching box on nasogastric tubes)
12. Report any abnormalities to physician. *(Findings will indicate any need to reposition tube or administer additional therapies.)*
    - Failure of tube to drain
    - Abdominal distention
    - Unusual characteristics of drainage (blood)

Skill 20-20 Nasogastric Tube Removal

Nursing Action *(Rationale)*

1. Refer to standard steps 1 to 9.
2. Assemble equipment:
    - Facial tissues
    - Towel or waterproof pad
    - Plastic bag
    - Clean gloves
    - Clamp (optional)
    - Mask and goggles if spillage is expected (optional)
3. Reassure that removal is less distressing than insertion. *(Reduces patient's anxiety and promotes cooperation.)*
4. Assess:
    - **a.** Patient's abdomen for bowel sounds. *(Provides baseline data of abdomen for future comparison.)*
    - **b.** Patient's nasal and oral cavity. *(Enables you to determine need for special interventions.)*
5. If tube is attached to suction, turn off suction and disconnect tubing, remove nose guard, and unfasten pin from gown. *(Decreases patient's discomfort.)*
6. Place towel or waterproof pad across patient's chest and give patient tissues. *(Protects bed linens. Patients often wish to wipe eyes and blow nose after tube removal.)*
7. Instruct patient to take deep breath and hold it; pinch tube with fingers or clamp. *(Prevents aspiration from any leakage.)* Quickly and smoothly remove tube while patient is holding breath. *(If patient begins to gag, continue to remove tubing, because it is the tubing that is causing the patient to gag. Airway will be temporarily obstructed during tube removal.)*
8. Place tubing in plastic bag or towel. *(Plastic bag or towel covers and conceals tube, which is not usually a pleasant sight.)*
9. Provide oral and nasal care; position patient for comfort. *(Promotes comfort.)*
10. Dispose of tube and equipment; measure drainage; note color and write down for documentation later. *(Provides accurate measure of fluid output. Reduces transfer of microorganisms.)*
11. Refer to standard steps 10 to 17.
12. Document: *(Verifies performance of procedure and ensures continuity of care.)*
    - Removal of nasogastric (NG) tube and condition of tube
    - Patient's tolerance of procedure
    - Presence of bowel sounds
    - Abdominal distention
13. Inspect condition of nares and oral cavity. Report abnormalities. *(Findings will indicate any need to administer additional therapies.)*
    - Erythema
    - Tenderness
    - Excoriation
    - Complaints of severe sore throat
    - Irritation during swallowing
    - Nasal fullness
    - Absence of bowel sounds
14. Palpate abdomen periodically, noting any distention, pain, or rigidity; auscultate abdomen for bowel sounds. *(Determines success of abdominal decompression and the return of peristalsis.)*

ting is the usual position during defecation and standing is the custom for urinating. For the patient confined to bed, it is impossible to assume the customary positions; instead, to the extent possible, facilitate the upright position. Some adults will resist using a bedpan or urinal because of the emphasis on privacy. Children will often find the equipment unfamiliar and threatening. See Chapter 18 for further discussion on assisting the patient with a bedpan or urinal.

Box 20-11 Nursing Diagnoses for Altered Bowel Elimination

Constipation:
- Related to dehydration
- Related to decreased activity
- Related to a postsurgical ileus
- Related to inadequate dietary fiber

Acute pain:
- Related to bowel distention

Deficient knowledge:
- Related to ostomy self-care
- Related to irrigation management

Disturbed body image:
- Related to presence of ostomy

Risk for impaired skin integrity:
- Related to irritation of peristomal skin

Anxiety:
- Related to bowel function
- Related to rejection by friends

Ineffective coping:
- Related to daily ostomy care requirements

Data from North American Nursing Diagnosis Association International (NANDA-I). (2009). *NANDA-I nursing diagnoses: Definitions and classification 2009-2011*. Oxford, United Kingdom: Author.

During the physical assessment for admission, assess the patient's abdomen to determine nursing diagnoses related to alterations in bowel elimination, including patterns and habits (Box 20-11).

Be alert to patient habits that are detrimental to normal bowel function. Long-term, routine use of laxatives and cathartics (substances that produce bowel movements) eventually causes the intestines to lose the ability to respond to the presence of stool, often resulting in chronic constipation. The routine use of mineral oil tends to cause reduced absorption of fat-soluble vitamins. Overcoming cathartic dependency is often difficult to accomplish and requires you to teach the patient (see Life Span Considerations for Older Adults box on altered bowel elimination).

CARE OF THE PATIENT WITH HEMORRHOIDS

Hemorrhoids are a source of discomfort that have the capacity to lead to an alteration in elimination. Hemorrhoids appear both internally and externally; as hard stool passes through the irritated rectum, the patient experiences pain. One of the main goals for patients with hemorrhoids is for the patient to have soft stools. Ways to accomplish this are to maintain a proper diet, obtain adequate fluid intake, and participate in regular exercise. If the hemorrhoids are swollen, localized heat often provides relief. A common form of heat application for hemorrhoids is a sitz bath. Use extreme caution when inserting rectal thermometers, suppositories, or rectal tubes for patients with hemorrhoids, and use a liberal amount of lubricant during insertion. Make sure you are able to directly visualize the anus before inserting any object into the anus and rectum.

Life Span Considerations

Older Adults

Altered Bowel Elimination

- Many older adult patients are especially prone to dysrhythmias and other problems related to vagal stimulation; monitor heart rate and rhythm closely.
- At least 28% of older adults are constipated as a result of insufficient dietary bulk, inadequate fluid intake, laxative abuse, diminished muscle tone and motor function, decreased defecation reflex, mental or physical illness, and presence of tumors or strictures.
- For an older adult, instituting a diet adequate in dietary fiber (6 to 10 g/day) adds bulk, weight, and form to stool and improves defecation.
- Consider development of a regular toileting routine that includes responding to the urge to defecate.
- Consider having patient or family member keep a week's diary of meals and fluid intake. Determine if dietary pattern contributes to constipation. Recommend a diet adequate in fiber.
- In long-term care, maintenance of activity is usually important in maintaining peristalsis.
- Evaluate the older adult's cognitive status and capacity to understand ostomy self-care instructions.
- Evaluate the older adult's motor and visual ability to prepare ostomy equipment. For patients who are unable to custom-cut the size of their skin barriers, consider having barriers precut by the ostomy equipment supplier or using a precut two-piece system.
- Avoid hot water and harsh soaps when washing the peristomal skin.
- Teach older adult patients about the change in the number of eliminations (from an incontinent ostomy) that will be normal on a daily basis.
- Financial concerns about the cost of ostomy supplies and reimbursement are often an important issue for patients on Medicare; aid is available.
- Some older adults become upset if they do not have a daily bowel movement. With some irrigation routines, irrigation is not done daily; therefore the patient will not have a daily bowel movement. Patient needs to understand and accept this.

FLATULENCE

Flatulence (presence of air or gas in the intestinal tract) typically arises when a person consumes gas-producing liquids and foods such as carbonated beverages, cabbage, or beans; swallows excessive amounts of air; or is constipated. In hospitalized patients, flatulence is often caused by decreased peristalsis, abdominal surgery, some narcotic medications, and decreased physical activity. Flatulence sometimes causes distention (swelling) of the stomach and abdomen and in some cases mild to moderate abdominal cramping and pain. One of the most effective measures to promote peristalsis and passage of flatus is walking. When the discomforts of flatulence are not relieved by eliminating the possible causes or by walking, use of a rectal tube is possible. The presence of the tube in the rectum stimulates peristalsis and the movement of flatus (Skill 20-21).

ADMINISTERING AN ENEMA

The primary reason for an enema is promotion of defecation. An enema serves to introduce a solution into the colon via the anus, through the rectum, and into the colon. Enemas are given for a number of reasons, such as cleansing the colon or breaking up a fecal mass. A cleansing enema helps to completely empty the colon of feces by instilling large volumes of solution, which stimulates peristalsis. Caution patients to limit the number of enemas they use since the defecation reflex becomes dependent on an enema with repeated use, thus causing constipation. Therefore, it is necessary to determine the cause of bowel irregularity or constipation in order to treat the cause rather than relying on enemas (Skill 20-22).

Enema administration is considered an "evil" practice in some cultures, and this has potential to introduce a conflict when the patient needs an enema. It is common for young children to be frightened by administration of an enema.

Fecal Incontinence and Impaction

The first step in care of the patient with fecal incontinence is to assess if fecal impaction is the cause and to remove the impaction. An impaction is a collection of feces in the rectum that forms a mass that becomes so large or hard that the patient is unable to pass it voluntarily. The patient will be experiencing discomfort and inability to defecate and having loose, watery stool that leaks around the mass.

Sometimes an oil retention enema used alone will suffice to treat a fecal impaction, and sometimes you will use one in conjunction with manual digital removal (Skill 20-23 and Coordinated Care box on impaction removal). This type of enema softens the feces and lubricates the rectum and colon in order to ease the passage of the feces (Elkin et al., 2007).

Skill 20-21 Inserting a Rectal Tube

Nursing Action *(Rationale)*

1. Refer to standard steps 1 to 11.
2. Assemble equipment:
   - Stethoscope
   - Protector pad (Chux)
   - Gloves
   - Water-soluble lubricant
   - Commercial kit with water-soluble lubricant, gloves, rectal tube, sponges, basin, and waterproof pad
3. Assess bowel sounds. *(Provides basis for determining effectiveness of therapy.)*
4. Have patient assume left Sims' (side-lying) position. Arrange gown and top linens to prevent soiling while still covering patient. *(Facilitates procedure and provides for patient privacy.)*
5. Place waterproof pad under buttocks. *(Protects bottom linen.)*
6. Don gloves. Lubricate tube well with water-soluble lubricant. *(Reduces spread of microorganisms and facilitates the insertion of tube.)*
7. Expose anus. Insert tube 4 to 6 inches (10 to 15 cm) in the same manner as for an enema (see Skill 20-22).
8. Insert drainage end into receptacle or use commercially prepared set. *(The receptacle will contain any expelled stool.)*
9. Instruct the patient to lie quietly to prevent dislodging tube; leave tube in place no more than 30 minutes. If flatulence persists, notify the physician.
10. Remove tube and assist patient to bedpan, bedside commode, or toilet as necessary; stimulation of peristalsis often results in bowel movement.
11. Provide for patient hygiene; assess bowel sounds, and assist patient to bed or chair.
12. Refer to standard steps 12 to 17.
13. Document: *(Verifies performance of procedure and ensures continuity of care.)*
    - Time of insertion
    - Results
    - Patient reaction
14. If flatulence, abdominal discomfort, or distention continues, reinsert tube as required or as ordered by physician. *(Continued use of rectal tubes has potential to cause irritation and eventual skin impairment of the anus and the rectal mucosa.)*

Skill 20-22 Administering an Enema

Nursing Action *(Rationale)*

1. Refer to standard steps 1 to 9.
2. Assemble equipment:
   - Prepared kit or enema set (see illustration)
   - Solution
   - Clean gloves
   - Toilet tissue
   - Water-soluble lubricant
   - Bath blanket
   - Bedpan, bedside commode, or access to toilet
   - Wash basin, washcloth, towel, soap
   - IV pole
3. Assessment: *(Determines need for enema.)*
   a. Last bowel movement.
   b. Presence or absence of bowel sounds.
   c. Ability to control rectal sphincter. *(It is necessary to place patients with no sphincter control on a bedpan because patient will not be able to retain enema solution.)*
   d. Presence or absence of hemorrhoids. *(Will possibly obscure the rectal opening and cause discomfort or bleeding.)*
   e. Abdominal pain. *(Possibly affects patient's ability to tolerate enema. Never give an enema to patients with possible appendicitis because rupture of the appendix is possible result.)*
   f. Patient's level of understanding and previous experience with enemas. *(Enables you to provide for appropriate teaching measures.)*

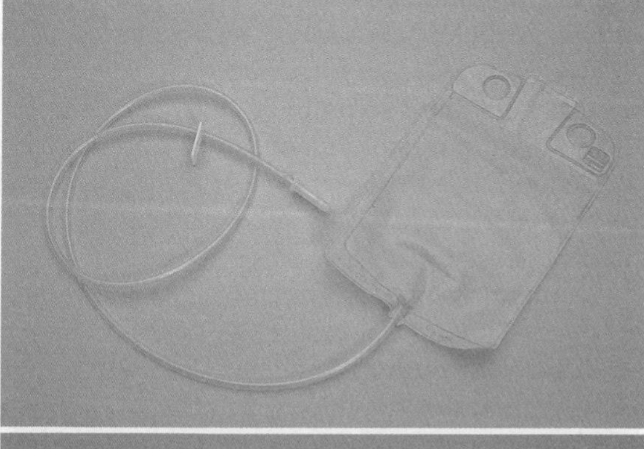

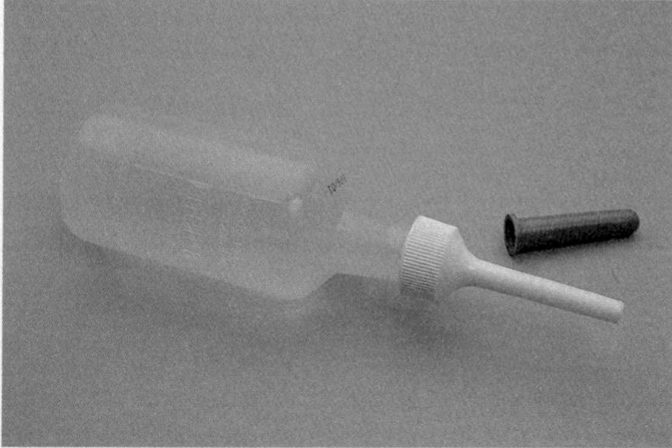

Step 2

4. Prepare solution. There are several types of enema solution. Cleansing enemas include tap water, normal saline, low-volume hypertonic solution, and soapsuds solution. (Considering the reports of soap damage to colonic mucosa [Schmelzer et al., 1993], it seems prudent to use alternatives such as saline, plain tap water, or a prepackaged enema.) *(Prepares equipment for procedure.)*
5. Arrange equipment at bedside. *(Organizes procedure.)*
6. Assist patient to the Sims' position. *(Allows enema solution to flow downward by gravity along natural curve of sigmoid colon and rectum, thus improving retention of enema.)* When giving an enema to a patient who is unable to contract the external sphincter, position the patient on the bedpan. Giving the enema with the patient sitting on the toilet is unsafe because it is possible for the inserted rectal tubing to abrade the rectal wall, and the enema solution is being forced uphill.
7. Place waterproof pad under patient. *(Protects bed linens.)*
8. Place bath blanket over patient and fanfold linen to foot of bed; adjust patient's gown to keep it from being soiled while it still provides privacy. *(Protects bed linens and patient's gown from soiling and provides warmth.)*
9. Clamp tubing; fill container with correctly warmed solution (usually 750 to 1000 mL at 105° F [41°C]) and any additives (see illustration for step 2, top); read disposable package instructions. *(Hot water has capacity to burn intestinal mucosa. Cold water has capacity to cause abdominal cramping and is difficult to retain.)* Administer a child's enema at 100° F to avoid burning rectal tissue. Release clamp, allowing solution to flow through tubing to remove any air from the tubing; reclamp.
   Suggested maximum volumes:
   —Infant: 150 to 250 mL
   —Toddler: 250 to 500 mL
   —School-age child: 500 mL
   —Adolescent: 500 to 700 mL
   —Adult: 750 to 1000 mL
   Or
   For commercially prepared enema (see illustration for step 2, bottom), the following steps replace steps 9 through 14. Rejoin the standard procedure at step 15.
   a. Remove cover from tip of enema (tip is prelubricated but add additional lubricant if needed); insert entire tip into anus. See step 10.
   b. Squeeze container until it is empty. Usually a small amount of solution will remain in con-

Continued

Skill 20-22 Administering an Enema—cont'd

tainer. Most containers hold about 250 mL. Continue to squeeze the container to prevent siphoning solution back into the container.

c. Encourage patient to retain solution at least 5 minutes. *(Retention of solution promotes peristalsis and enhances defecation.)*

10. Lubricate 4 inches (10 cm) at end of the tubing; spread patient's buttocks to expose anus; while rotating tube, gently insert it 3 to 4 inches (7 to 10 cm). Instruct patient to breathe out slowly through mouth. *(Breathing out promotes relaxation of external rectal sphincter. Presence of hemorrhoids obscures location of rectum. Probe gently with gloved finger to locate rectal opening as necessary.)*
11. Elevate container 12 to 18 inches (30 to 45 cm) above level of anus (see illustration). *(Allows solution to flow at adequate rate. Raising container too high causes rapid infusion and possibly painful distention of colon. Holding container too low leads to inadequate instillation of enema solution.)*

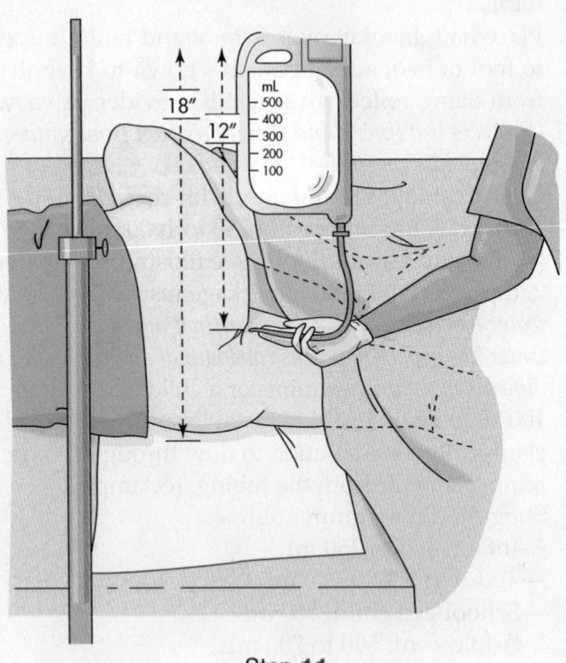

Step 11

12. Release clamp; allow more solution to flow slowly while holding clamp; usually solution will flow for 5 to 10 minutes. *(Allowing solution to instill slowly enables patient to retain all of solution and keeps discomfort to a minimum.)*
13. Lower container or clamp tubing if patient complains of cramping; encourage slow, deep breathing. Do not remove tubing tip. *(Temporary cessation of infusion reduces cramping to a minimum and promotes ability to retain all of the solution.)* If severe cramping, bleeding, or sudden severe abdominal pain occurs and is unrelieved by temporarily stopping or slowing flow of solution, stop enema and notify physician.
14. Clamp and remove tube when all of the solution has been administered. Encourage patient to retain solution at least 5 minutes. *(Retention of solution promotes peristalsis and enhances defecation.)*
15. When patient is no longer able to retain solution, assist to bedpan, bedside commode, or bathroom. *(Normal squatting position promotes defecation; longer retention promotes more effective stimulation of peristalsis and defecation.)*
16. Instruct patient to call you to inspect results before flushing stool. Observe characteristics of feces or solution. *(When enemas are ordered "until clear" in preparation for surgery, enemas are repeated until patient passes fluid that is clear and contains no fecal matter. Usually three consecutive enemas are adequate.)* If after three enemas the water is highly colored or contains solid fecal material, notify physician before continuing. *(Excessive loss of electrolytes is a dangerous possibility.)*
17. Refer to standard steps 10 to 17.
18. Provide for patient hygiene; assist patient to bed or chair. *(Patient will sometimes need assistance to cleanse anal area [wear gloves]. Fecal contents tend to irritate skin. Hygiene promotes patient comfort.)*
19. Document: *(Verifies performance of procedure and ensures continuity of care.)*
    - Type and volume of enema
    - Temperature of solution
    - Characteristics of results
    - How patient tolerates procedure

Coordinated Care

Collaboration

IMPACTION REMOVAL

The skill of removing an impaction requires critical thinking and knowledge unique to a nurse and is not appropriate to delegate. Instruct assistive personnel to inform you if the patient is able to pass a normal stool after the procedure is complete.

Management of fecal incontinence includes educating the patient about dietary measures, abdominal exercises, and physical activity.

OSTOMIES

A **colostomy** is the surgical creation of an artificial anus on the abdominal wall by incising (cutting) the colon and bringing it out through a stoma on the ab-

Skill 20-23 Digital Examination with Removal of Fecal Impaction

Nursing Action *(Rationale)*

1. Refer to standard steps 1 to 9.
2. Assemble equipment:
   - Bedpan
   - Water-soluble lubricant
   - Waterproof pad
   - Toilet tissue
   - Towel, washcloth, soap, and basin
   - Clean gloves
   - Bath blanket
3. Assessment: *(Determines need for procedure.)*
   a. Last bowel movement.
   b. Seepage of liquid stool (frequently a sign of fecal impaction).
   c. Inability to defecate even when the desire is there.
   d. Painful defecation.
   e. Bowel sounds and abdominal distention.
4. Assist patient to assume the Sims' position, and place waterproof pad under patient's buttocks. *(Protects the bed linens.)*
5. Place the bedpan on the bed close to the patient's buttocks.
6. Arrange patient's gown and top linens. *(Prevents soiling yet exposes only what is necessary.)* Drape patient with bath blanket. *(Provides warmth.)*
7. Don gloves; lubricate forefinger well with petroleum or water-soluble lubricant. *(Reduces irritation.)* Use the index finger of your dominant hand.
8. Insert finger gently; slowly but gently move finger into and around the fecal mass; as pieces of the mass are broken off, remove them to bedpan. At this time, instruct patient to take slow deep breaths. Breathe slowly with the patient. *(This procedure is often very uncomfortable for the patient. Excess rectal manipulation has potential to cause irritation to the mucosa, bleeding, and stimulation of the vagus nerve, which results in a reflex slowing of the heart rate.)*
9. Continue procedure until impaction is removed. *(Completes procedure.)*
10. Stop procedure for a few minutes if patient complains of severe discomfort. *(Gives patient opportunity to rest.)* Reassess the patient's heart rate and observe for signs of fatigue. Stop procedure if heart rate drops or rhythm changes or if bleeding occurs.
11. After removal is complete, wash and dry perineal area. Assist the patient to toilet or position on the bedpan if urge to defecate develops. Sometimes a small-volume cleansing enema will be in order. *(Promotes patient's sense of comfort and well-being.)*
12. Refer to standard steps 10 to 17.
13. Document: *(Verifies performance of procedure and ensures continuity of care.)*
    - Patient's tolerance to procedure
    - Amount and consistency of stool removed
    - Any adverse effects, such as blood on gloved finger or in stool
    - Patient teaching
14. Report abnormalities. *(More aggressive treatment will sometimes be necessary.)*

dominal surface. The colostomy diverts stool through the stoma. The stool may be liquid, semiformed, or formed, depending on the area of the colon incised. The procedure is performed for patients with cancer of the colon, intestinal obstructions, intestinal trauma, or inflammatory diseases of the colon. Some colostomies are permanent and some are temporary measures used until intestinal healing occurs.

An **ileostomy** is the surgical formation of an opening of the ileum onto the surface of the abdomen through which fecal matter is emptied. It is performed for patients with inflammatory bowel conditions and cancer of the large intestine. Although the stoma looks like that of a colostomy, it is somewhat smaller and is located lower on the abdomen. After surgery, the patient wears a pouch to collect the semiliquid fecal matter. Ileostomies are temporary or permanent, depending on the reason for performing the surgery.

A **urostomy** is the diversion of urine away from a diseased or defective bladder through a surgically created opening or stoma in the skin (see Chapter 50).

Colostomy Irrigation

Colostomy irrigation is less frequently performed than in the past. However, some patients desire regulation of a descending or sigmoid colostomy, and irrigation is sometimes necessary to achieve this. The patient needs to be prepared to devote 60 to 90 minutes per day in the bathroom for colostomy irrigation.

Special equipment is required, including a cone-tipped irrigation device (see step 7 of Skill 20-25) in order to prevent puncturing the intestinal mucosa with the enema equipment, as well as prevent the backflow of solution. Additional equipment includes an irrigation sleeve that is placed over the stoma with the end of the sleeve terminating in the commode. The effluent (stool that is discharged from a colostomy) and solution is contained by the sleeve as it passes into the commode. For adults, the irrigation solution ranges in

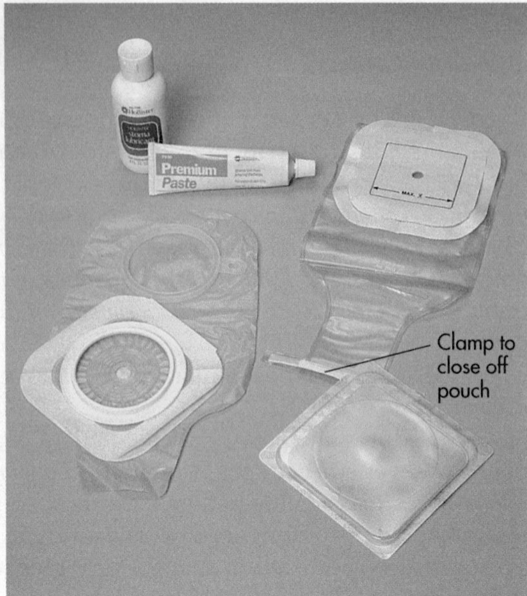

FIGURE 20-25 Ostomy pouches and skin barriers.

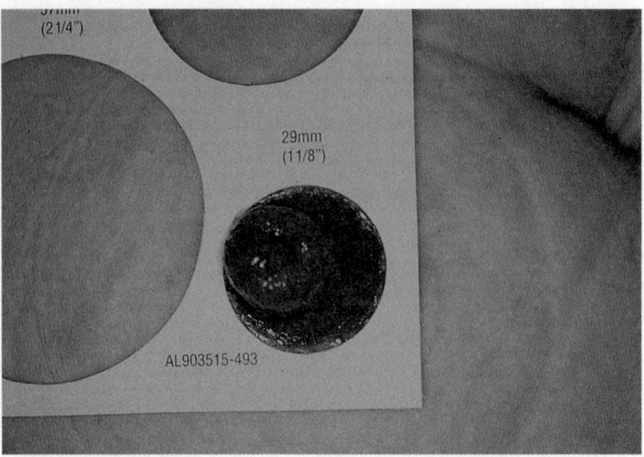

FIGURE 20-26 Measuring an ostomy using a measuring card.

amount from 500 to 700 mL of tap water, depending on the ordered amount, and takes approximately 5 to 10 minutes to instill. After removing the cone-tipped irrigator device, the patient remains on the commode with the sleeve in place for approximately 30 to 35 minutes until the effluent stops draining. Following irrigation, the stoma should be covered with either a pouching device or stoma cap (Hyland, 2004).

There are various types of pouching systems and skin barriers available to patients. There are one-piece and two-piece systems for patients to choose from. One-pouch systems have a skin barrier that is preattached to the pouch; two-piece systems have a pouch that is separate from the skin barrier. Some skin barriers are precut, whereas others are necessary to cut. The patient or the caregiver will cut the material to the proper size either by eye or using a "die cut" (Elkin et al., 2007). These customized devices, sized and ordered after allowing a 6- to 8-week period for healing, are not expensive to make and save the patient a great deal of effort in attempting to cut the barrier to the perfect size and shape each time. For proper fit, it is necessary to coordinate and purchase the skin barrier and the flange in the two-piece system from the same manufacturer. To be able to provide patients with optimum care, it is important for you to know the correct use of various products used for colostomy care (Figures 20-25 and 20-26, Skills 20-24 and 20-25, Patient Teaching boxes on ostomy care and on urostomy care, and Home Care Considerations and Coordinated Care boxes on ostomy care).

CONCLUSION

Always individualize nursing interventions to the patient's level of health, age, lifestyle, and needs. You will use many nursing skills to help the patient achieve a maximum level of functional health patterns.

Patient Teaching

Ostomy Care

- Include family members or significant other in teaching, because this tends to facilitate patient's readiness to learn.
- Use every pouch change as an opportunity to teach even if patient does not appear interested. Do not force patient to look at stoma—allow for a period of adjustment.
- Reinforce positive performance. "You did very well. Remember, it helps to hold the cone so that the solution runs easily. Next time you can show me how to insert it."
- You will often be able to judge patient's readiness to learn by willingness to look at stoma and asking questions, among other signals. If patient is apprehensive about touching or looking at stoma, have patient hold gauze pad over stoma and clean around stoma.
- Some patients acknowledge stoma with minimal emotional difficulty; some will never completely adjust to it. Individualize care according to patient's situation and circumstances.
- Teach to avoid constipation by eating a balanced diet or using a daily stool softener.
- If patient has limitations affecting dexterity, select pouching system that can be most easily managed.
- Give patient a teaching manual with clearly stated steps, or audiotaped instructions. With patient who has a learning disability, a "picture book" of the steps will sometimes be more appropriate.
- Give patient a list of equipment and the name, address, and phone number of a supplier in patient's community.
- Patients will in most cases be able to wear usual clothes, because peristalsis pushes stool out of stoma, and snug clothing will not interfere.
- Instruct patients not to leave pouches in extremely hot or cold locations, because temperature has potential to affect the barrier and adhesive materials.

 Patient Teaching

Urostomy Care

- Teach patient and caregivers to avoid touching the stoma with adhesive solvents to prevent irritating the stoma.
- Teach patient and caregivers to wick the urine with an absorbent, lint-free material to prevent a constant flow of urine while changing the appliance.
- Teach patient and caregivers to remove hair from the stomal area with scissors or an electric razor to prevent hair follicles from becoming irritated when the pouch is removed. Suggest that the procedure be performed in the morning before fluids are consumed and when urine flows more easily.
- Teach patient and caregivers that the properly applied appliance is able to remain in place 3 to 5 days.
- Teach patient and caregivers to empty appliance through the drain valve when it is one third to one half full to prevent the weight of the urine from loosening the seal around the stoma.
- Teach patient and caregivers to connect the appliance to a urine-collection container at night to prevent urine from stagnating in the appliance.
- Teach sanitary and dietary measures that will protect the peristomal skin and control odor.
- Offer positive reinforcement and written instructions, perhaps even videos.

See Patient Teaching box on ostomy care for further instructions.

 Coordinated Care

Collaboration

OSTOMY CARE

- The skill of pouching a stoma requires the critical thinking and knowledge application unique to a nurse. Some agencies permit delegation of the pouching of an established ostomy. In this case, instruct the care provider in the expected amount, color, and consistency of drainage from the ostomy. In addition, teach the care provider to report changes in the stoma and surrounding skin integrity.
- The skill of pouching an incontinent urinary diversion (see Chapter 50) requires the critical thinking and knowledge application unique to a nurse. In some agencies, a stoma nurse specialist is available to provide this care. Assistive personnel who provide personal care receive instructions to report any leakage of urine and/or breakdown of skin integrity to the nurse.
- The skill of irrigating a newly established colostomy requires the critical thinking and knowledge application unique to a nurse. However, in some settings assistive personnel are trained to perform irrigations on established ostomies. Review agency policy.

 Home Care Considerations

Ostomy Care

- Provide a referral to a home health agency or a visiting nurse before patient's hospital discharge.
- Pouches that wear well in the hospital will not necessarily wear well when the patient resumes a normal routine.
- A visiting nurse is often able to help achieve compliance with irrigation routine and assist in problem solving when necessary (colostomies are no longer routinely irrigated). A typical suggestion from the visiting nurse perspective is to hang the irrigation solution container from a hook on the wall or from a shower curtain rod instead of an intravenous pole.
- Urostomy, colostomy, and ileostomy products are usually available for purchase at local pharmacies.
- Encourage the patient to become involved with local ostomy organizations.
- Teach the patient and caregivers to routinely inspect the appearance of the stoma and the surrounding skin. The proper appearance of the stoma is moist, shiny, and dark pink to red, with minimal if any bleeding around it. Teach to report excessive bleeding, abnormal color, or swelling to you or the physician.
- Teach the patient and caregivers to avoid using alcohol around the stoma because alcohol dilates capillaries, causing bleeding.
- Teach the patient and caregivers not to use cold creams around the stoma because they tend to prevent pouches from adhering.
- Teach the patient and caregivers not to use peroxide on or around the stoma because it irritates tissue.
- Instruct the patient and caregivers to wash skin with mild soap and water. (Be certain to rinse thoroughly because soap is often irritating to the peristomal skin.) Pat or blot dry the skin thoroughly.
- Evaluate the patient's home toileting facilities. Evaluation includes the following:
  —The presence of adequate functioning and accessible toileting facilities
  —Number and location of toileting facilities
  —Number of other people living with the patient who have to share the toileting facilities
  —Identification of the pattern of use of the toileting facilities by the other people living with the patient (time of day and amount of time spent in bathroom)
- Evaluate the patient ostomy routine in relationship to usual lifestyle after discharge.
- Caution the patient that it is not possible to flush most ostomy pouches and barriers down the toilet; they clog the system. Dispose of used ostomy pouches according to local sanitation regulations.
- Make sure patient understands that it is not necessary to use sterile gauze to cleanse the stoma. Using a washcloth made of any soft material is fine.
- Review the patient's dietary pattern. Help patient and family members learn the types of foods to avoid so as to prevent problems with effluent (discharge or drainage of liquid, solid, or gas from the stoma) or odor.
- Teach patients that if water is not drinkable, they should not use it for irrigations (e.g., patients traveling to another country).

Skill 20-24 Performing Colostomy, Ileostomy, and Urostomy Care

Nursing Action *(Rationale)*

Ostomy Care

1. Refer to standard steps 1 to 9.
2. Assemble equipment (see Figure 20-25):
   - Pouch with attached wafer seal
   - Measuring guide
   - Barrier paste
   - Pouch clamp
   - Clean gloves
   - Basin with warm water
   - Disposable washcloth
   - Scissors
   - Skin sealant wipes (Skin Prep)
   - 1-inch-wide paper tape (optional)
   - Bedpan or trash bag
3. Assessment: *(Enables you to determine need for pouch change.)*
   a. Pouch leakage and length of time in place.
   b. Stoma for healing and color.
   c. Abdominal incision. *(Pouches require changing every 3 to 7 days to prevent skin impairment. Proper stoma appearance is moist and reddish pink. Ileostomy drainage is most damaging to the skin. Pouches also collect gas, which is necessary to expel, because it can disrupt skin care.)*
4. Arrange supplies and equipment at bedside or in bathroom (see Figure 20-25). *(Promotes smoothness of procedure.)*
5. Position patient supine and make comfortable. *(When patient is in the supine position, there are fewer skinfolds and wrinkles.)*
6. Unfasten and remove belt, if worn; carefully remove wafer seal from skin (adhesive solvent is sometimes needed). *(Reduces trauma; jerking irritates the skin and sometimes causes skin impairment.)* Not all patients wear a belt.
7. Place reusable pouch in bedpan or disposable pouch in plastic bag. *(Reduces the transmission of microorganisms.)*
8. Cleanse skin with warm water; pat dry. *(Not rubbing helps prevent skin impairment. Avoid use of soap because it leaves a residue on the skin that interferes with pouch adhesion to skin.)*
9. Measure stoma using measuring device (see Figure 20-26). *(Ensures proper fit.)*
10. Place toilet tissue over stoma; use gauze for ileostomy. *(Prevents expelled stool from causing skin impairment.)* Note color and viability of stoma. If using Skin Prep, apply to skin and allow to dry.
11. Apply protective skin barrier about 1⁄16 inch from stoma (e.g., Stomahesive, Hollihesive, Karaya paste). *(Creates wrinkle-free, secure seal; decreases chance of skin irritation from adhesive on skin.)*
12. Apply protective wafer with flange, cutting an opening in the center of wafer to 1⁄16 inch larger than stoma. *(Ensures proper fit.)*
13. Gently attach pouch to flange by compressing the two together. *(Ensures appropriate collection of feces and application of pouch reservoir.)*
14. Remove tissue or gauze from stoma and backing from protectant; center opening over stoma and press against skin for 1 to 2 minutes. *(Establishes contact between barrier adhesive and skin and ensures pouch adherence.)*
15. Fold over bottom edges of pouch once to fit clamp. Secure clamp. If bottom edge of pouch is folded over more than once, the plastic will be too thick for the clamp, thus springing the clamp and causing spillage of fecal matter. *(Creates secure seal to prevent leaking.)*
16. If patient uses belt, attach at this time. *(Supports pouch and enhances feelings of security.)*
17. Assist patient to comfortable position in bed or chair; remove equipment from bedside. *(Promotes comfort.)*
18. Empty, wash, and dry reusable pouch. *(Reduces odor and extends usefulness.)*
19. Refer to standard steps 10 to 17.
20. Document: *(Verifies performance of procedure and ensures continuity of care.)*
    - Procedure and observation
    - Type of pouch
    - Skin barrier
    - Amount and appearance of feces
    - Condition of stoma and peristomal skin
    - Patient's level of participation
    - Patient teaching (see Patient Teaching boxes on urostomy and ostomy care; and Home Care Considerations on ostomy care)

Urostomy Care

Follow steps 1 to 5 of ostomy care procedure. Then observe the following:

1. Empty urine into graduated pitcher; write down amount and characteristics of urine for later documentation. *(Ensures accurate recording.)*
2. Carefully remove wafer seal from skin (use adhesive solvent if necessary), and place pouch in plastic bag. *(Reduces trauma; jerking movements irritate the skin and tend to cause skin impairment.)*
3. Cleanse skin with warm water and pat dry. *(Not rubbing helps prevent skin impairment. Avoid using soap because it may irritate the skin.)*
4. Measure stoma using measuring device (see Figure 20-26); note color and viability of stoma. *(Ensures accurate fit. Careful assessment provides data for later comparison.)*

5. Place gauze over stoma. *(Prevents urine from contacting skin.)*
6. If using Skin Prep, apply to skin and allow to dry; apply protective stoma paste about 1⁄16 inch from the stoma. *(Ensures a tight/snug fit.)*
7. Apply protective wafer with flange, cutting an opening in the center of wafer 1⁄16 inch larger than stoma. *(Creates wrinkle-free seal; decreases chance of skin impairment occurring.)*
8. Refer to steps 13 through 20 of ostomy care procedure to complete urostomy care.

Skill 20-25 Performing a Colostomy Irrigation

Nursing Action *(Rationale)*

Note that colostomy irrigation is no longer done on a routine basis, but only to help patients with a descending or sigmoid colostomy to achieve some regularity of elimination.

1. Refer to standard steps 1 to 9.
2. Assemble equipment and supplies:
   - Irrigation set
   - Container
   - Tubing with clamp
   - Catheter with cone
   - Irrigation sleeve with or without belt
   - Clamp
   - Water-soluble lubricant
   - New pouch and wafer seal with flange
   - Clean gloves
   - Bedpan or toilet
   - Bed protector
   - Disposable washcloth and towel
   - Warm water and basin
3. Assessment: *(Enables you to determine need for procedure.)*
   a. Level of comfort (using a scale of 0 to 10) and need for pain management (see Chapter 16).
   b. Condition for appropriateness of irrigation as a management option. *(Only patients with a descending or sigmoid colostomy are appropriate candidates because stool is more formed and less liquid.)*
   c. Ability to manipulate irrigation equipment and to understand concepts of bowel management.
   d. Readiness to learn self-irrigation of colostomy.
4. Position patient:
   - Bathroom: Instruct patient to sit on toilet or on a chair in front of the toilet.
   - Bed: Have patient lie comfortably with head of bed slightly elevated. *(Do not overexpose patient because chilling might occur.)*
   - NOTE: As many of the following steps as possible should be performed by the patient with the nurse teaching and assisting as needed. Independence will come. Be alert to patient readiness.
5. Remove pouch, cleanse skin, and place irrigation sleeve over stoma; attach belt if patient uses one; place end of sleeve in toilet. *(Provides for patient cleanliness. Make sure irrigation sleeve is correctly attached. End of sleeve must be in toilet or bedpan to prevent spillage of feces.)*
6. Close clamp on irrigation tubing; fill irrigation container with 1000 mL tepid water (or as otherwise ordered). It is acceptable to hang container on a hook at patient's shoulder level. *(This position prevents too high a pressure and reduces possibility of bowel damage.)* Allow a small amount of water to flow through tubing. *(Solution that is too hot poses risk of burning bowel. If too cold, has potential to cause cramps. Allow some solution to fill tubing to express air, which is otherwise forced into the bowel, causing cramps.)*
7. Attach cone to tubing; lubricate cone; insert cone into stoma through top of sleeve (see illustration). Do not force cone into stoma. Use gentle pressure to hold tip in place in stoma. *(To prevent trauma to bowel, do not insert entire length of cone into stoma. Too little pressure will cause the irrigation solution to flow out alongside of cone and not into patient. Too much pressure has capacity to block flow of irrigation solution into patient.)*
8. While holding cone in place, allow solution to flow slowly into colon (500 to 1000 mL over 15 minutes). If patient complains of cramping, stop flow without removing cone until cramps

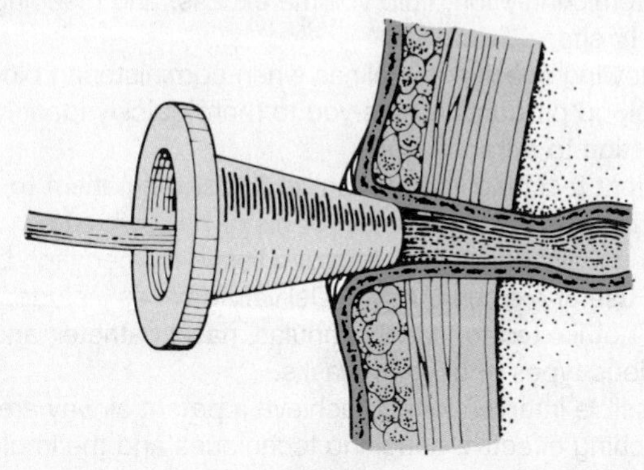

Step 7

Continued

Skill 20-25 Performing a Colostomy Irrigation—cont'd

subside. *(Too-rapid instillation of irrigation solution is likely to have adverse effect on patient.)*

9. After all solution is instilled, remove cone and close top of sleeve. *(Proper use of irrigation equipment will prevent spillage of feces.)*
10. Instruct patient to sit about 15 to 20 minutes while returns flow into toilet. *(It is acceptable to close the end of the irrigation sleeve with a clamp and allow the patient to be up and walk around the room, because exercise stimulates the bowel.)*
11. Drain sleeve; rinse and remove it. *(Some irrigation sleeves are reusable.)*
12. Observe patient and results of irrigation; flush toilet. *(Provides data for documentation.)*
13. Perform colostomy care (see Skill 20-24). *(Completes procedure and provides for patient comfort.)*
14. Refer to standard steps 10 to 17.
15. Document: *(Verifies performance of procedure and ensures continuity of care.)*
    - Solution used
    - Amount of solution
    - Results
    - Observations
    - Patient's tolerance

Get Ready for the NCLEX® Examination!

Key Points

- When applying heat or cold therapy, properly assess the patient's ability to sense varying temperatures, know factors that place the patient at risk for complications, and understand the physiologic effects of the applications in order to use the therapies safely.
- Irrigations of the eye are not usually to provide actual wound care, but rather to relieve local inflammation of the conjunctiva, apply antiseptic solution, or flush out exudate or caustic or irritating solutions.
- Using a small syringe and solution at body temperature, you will be able to cleanse a patient's external auditory canal of excess cerumen or exudate from a lesion or inflamed area.
- The nurse practice act of each state legally defines the nurse's qualification for and scope of practice in administering parenteral therapy and inserting nasogastric tubes.
- Knowledge of various complications of intravenous therapy and nursing interventions is required of any nurse administering these therapies.
- IV therapy poses the risk of several complications, including infiltration, phlebitis, infection at the IV site or systemic infection, fluid volume excess, and bleeding at the IV site.
- Following specific guidelines when administering blood or blood products allows you to more quickly identify a reaction to a transfusion.
- Patient teaching is important to assist the patient to learn to take responsibility for his or her own care.
- It is usually possible to improve tissue oxygenation by the use of oxygen therapy. Delivery devices include, but are not limited to, nasal cannulas, nasal catheter, and various types of oxygen masks.
- Possible interventions to achieve a patent airway are teaching effective coughing techniques and the implementation of suctioning.
- Even when an ostomy pouch is adhering well, it is best to change it at least every 5 to 7 days or according to pouch recommendations to allow for observation of the stoma and the peristomal skin.
- Emotional support of the patient (ostomate) is important for eventual acceptance of the change in body image.
- Consistency of the feces is directly affected by which portion of the colon is brought out to the stoma.
- Closed bladder drainage systems necessitate the use of aseptic technique during care.
- Intermittent urinary catheterization has a lower risk of infection than an indwelling urinary catheter owing to the relatively shorter time the catheter remains in the bladder.
- Strict asepsis is necessary when caring for a closed urinary drainage system.
- It is possible to use closed urinary drainage systems for instillation of sterile solutions or medications into the bladder.
- Patients with urostomies are at a high risk of skin impairment at the peristomal site due to nearly continuous urine drainage.
- When inserting a nasogastric tube, it is necessary to lubricate the tube well with a water-soluble lubricant to prevent trauma to the mucous membrane and to avoid lipid pneumonia.
- It is imperative for you to assess for proper nasogastric tube placement before an irrigation or tube feeding.
- Proper administration of an enema consists of the slow instillation of the correct volume of a warm solution.
- Irrigation of an ostomy follows the same principles as an enema administration, except that a special irrigating tube is needed and the patient is not able to control the passage of feces.
- Vagal stimulation and traumatization of the rectal mucosa are possible as a result of digital removal of stool.
- Skin impairment is possible after repeated exposure to liquid stool. This is especially true in patients who have a stoma.

Additional Learning Resources

Go to your Companion CD for an audio glossary, animations, video clips, and more.

evolve Be sure to visit the Evolve site at http://evolve.elsevier.com/Christensen/foundations/ for additional online resources.

Review Questions for the NCLEX® Examination

1. Which method will determine the correct distance to insert a nasogastric tube?
   1. Measure from center of forehead to top of nose to end of sternum.
   2. Measure from tip of nose to tip of earlobe to end of sternum.
   3. Measure from lips to tip of ear to just below the umbilicus.
   4. Measure from tip of ear to midway between end of sternum and umbilicus.

2. After inserting a nasogastric tube, it is possible to be certain it is in the proper place if:
   1. the patient no longer complains of pain or nausea.
   2. it is possible to inject 30 mL of normal saline with ease.
   3. bubbles occur when the tube is submerged into water.
   4. gastric contents are aspirated with cone-tipped syringe.

3. A patient diagnosed with throat cancer is 2 days postoperative and has a tracheostomy. Which part of the tracheostomy tube is removed for cleaning?
   1. Outer cannula
   2. Inner cannula
   3. Single-lumen tube
   4. Double-lumen tube

4. What safety precaution must be taken for a patient who has a tracheostomy tube?
   1. Keep a crash cart in the room.
   2. Be prepared to put him on a ventilator.
   3. Keep curved hemostat at the bedside.
   4. Be prepared to remove the tube.

5. If, when suctioning the patient, it becomes necessary to repeat the interventions, it is recommended that the nurse wait at least 3 minutes to allow for:
   1. overcoming fatigue.
   2. numbing of mucous membranes.
   3. replenishing oxygen.
   4. subsiding of pain.

6. Preoperatively the physician orders "enemas until clear." The maximum number of enemas the nurse can give without further orders is:
   1. two.
   2. three.
   3. five.
   4. unlimited.

7. The most serious problem that is possible to develop with the use of a condom catheter is:
   1. skin impairment resulting from accumulation of moisture.
   2. restriction of blood supply to the penis.
   3. patient will perhaps not be able to keep the catheter as clean as necessary.
   4. urine leakage resulting from an ill-fitting catheter.

8. What is the most suitable method for the nurse to use to prevent transmission of HIV or hepatitis B, C, and D during procedures associated with intravenous therapy?
   1. Wear gloves.
   2. Wear goggles.
   3. Use povidone-iodine for preparing the skin.
   4. Use sterile tape for dressings over venipuncture site.

9. Ear irrigation is a common procedure implemented to remove cerumen from the external ear canal. When irrigating the ear:
   1. proceed in a gentle manner.
   2. insert the entire tip of the syringe into the ear canal.
   3. use enough force to remove the wax or foreign body.
   4. position the patient on the unaffected side.

10. A patient is receiving oxygen at a rate of 1.5 L/min via nasal cannula. Which nursing intervention is indicated because the patient has a nasal cannula?
    1. Assess nares for skin impairment every 6 hours.
    2. Assess patency of the cannula every 2 hours.
    3. Inspect the oral cavity every 6 hours.
    4. Check oxygen flow and orders every 24 hours.

11. A more precise oxygen concentration is possible to achieve using a:
    1. nasal cannula.
    2. simple face mask.
    3. Venturi mask system.
    4. plastic face mask and inflated reservoir bag.

12. The unit manager orienting a new staff nurse evaluates which technique as appropriate for nasotracheal suctioning?
    1. Placing the patient in a supine position
    2. Preparing for a clean or unsterile technique
    3. Suctioning the oropharyngeal area first, then the nasotracheal area
    4. Applying intermittent suctioning for 10 seconds during catheter removal

13. What is a priority for the nurse when teaching a family about home oxygen therapy?
    1. Pathophysiology of the patient
    2. Use of the equipment
    3. Oximetry readings
    4. Length of time the oxygen is to be used

14. What is important in the site selection for a new intravenous line?
   1. Starting with the most proximal site
   2. Looking for hard, cordlike veins
   3. Using sites away from a dialysis graft
   4. Selecting the dominant arm

15. A patient has IV therapy for the administration of antibiotics and states that the IV site hurts and is swollen. Which data will tend to confirm phlebitis, as opposed to infiltration?
   1. Intensity of pain
   2. Warmth of skin surrounding IV site
   3. Amount of subcutaneous edema
   4. Skin discoloration resembling bruising

16. A patient complains of a headache and nausea and vomiting during a blood transfusion. Which action is it necessary for the nurse to take immediately?
   1. Check the vital signs.
   2. Stop the blood transfusion.
   3. Slow down the rate of blood flow.
   4. Notify the physician and the blood bank personnel.

17. Which is the least invasive alternative to urethral catheterization?
   1. Suprapubic catheterization
   2. Reinsertion of a Foley catheter
   3. Catheter irrigation
   4. Condom catheterization

18. What is appropriate for the nurse to incorporate into the teaching plan for a patient with an incontinent urinary diversion?
   1. The patient will need to order special clothing to fit around the stoma.
   2. A stomal pouch will need to be worn only at night.
   3. Special skin care is a priority.
   4. A reduction in physical activity will be planned.

19. The nursing instructor is supervising a student during the catheterization of a female patient. What is determined to be an appropriate part of the technique?
   1. Keeping both hands sterile throughout the procedure
   2. Reinserting the catheter if it was initially misinserted into the vagina
   3. Inflating the balloon to test it before catheter insertion
   4. Advancing the catheter 7 to 8 inches

20. A bladder retraining program for a patient in an extended care facility will properly include:
   1. providing negative reinforcement when the patient is incontinent.
   2. having the patient wear adult diapers as a preventive measure.
   3. putting the patient on a q2h toilet schedule during the day.
   4. promoting the intake of caffeine to stimulate voiding.

21. When irrigating a colostomy, the nurse will use a cone that fits properly to prevent:
   1. introducing air into the colon.
   2. leaking of the solution from the stoma.
   3. administering the solution too rapidly.
   4. introducing bacteria into the stoma.

22. The nurse recognizes which as true concerning ostomies?
   1. An ileostomy patient will have solid, formed stool.
   2. A double-barrel ostomy refers to one created for the ileum and one for the colon.
   3. Some patients will have control over when they can evacuate their colon.
   4. Family members or significant others will need to learn the care.

23. To secure a condom catheter to the penile shaft appropriately, it is important to apply the device so that the catheter is:
   1. tight and drained well.
   2. dependent and draining well.
   3. secured with adhesive tape applied in a circular pattern.
   4. snug and secure, but does not cause constriction to blood flow.

24. In order to maintain proper drainage of an indwelling catheter, it is important to:
   1. irrigate the catheter every 2 to 4 hours.
   2. ensure that the collection device is below bladder level.
   3. place the tubing under the patient's leg to prevent pulling on the bladder neck.
   4. demonstrate to the patient how to disconnect the device while ambulating.

25. Fecal impactions are best treated by:
   1. a clear liquid diet.
   2. cleansing enemas.
   3. limiting the patient fluid intake.
   4. oil-retention enemas.

26. For optimal results, in which position will the nurse place the patient when administering a cleansing enema?
   1. Supine
   2. Dorsal recumbent
   3. Left Sims'
   4. Prone

27. Which nursing intervention is the most important in preventing the introduction of microorganisms to the patient when initiating an IV?
   1. Hand hygiene
   2. Checking the identification of the patient
   3. Ensuring the six rights of medication administration
   4. Carefully checking the order for the correct IV solution

28. When assessing an IV site, indications that phlebitis has occurred include:

1. paleness and coolness.
2. bleeding from the site.
3. slowing of the flow of solution.
4. pain and erythema.

29. The ideal needle gauge for a rapid whole blood transfusion is:

1. 14- to 16-gauge.
2. 18- to 20-gauge.
3. 22- to 24-gauge.
4. 26- to 28-gauge.

30. It has been 15 minutes since a unit of blood infusion was initiated. Which is most indicative that the patient is experiencing a blood transfusion reaction?

1. The patient's blood pressure decreases.
2. The patient feels an urgent need to void.
3. The patient's skin is pale at the infusion site.
4. Localized edema is noticed at the infusion site.

31. The nurse is administering a routine enema to an adult patient. The patient complains of cramping and the urge to defecate. Which nursing intervention is the best to carry out?

1. Quickly finish instilling the rest of the solution.
2. Briefly stop the instillation.
3. Instruct the patient to hold his or her breath and bear down.
4. Immediately discontinue the instillation and withdraw the enema tubing from the rectum.

32. When providing indwelling catheter care, what areas are most important to be cleansed?

1. The perineal area
2. The area surrounding the urinary meatus
3. The labia majora and the labia minora
4. The perineal area and 2 inches of the catheter

33. Which patient will be at the greatest risk of complications from heat or cold therapy?

1. A diabetic patient with peripheral neuropathy
2. A cardiac patient with peripheral vascular disease
3. A patient who is unconscious following a motor vehicle accident
4. A patient who is hard of hearing and is unable to speak

34. The Infusion Nurses Society (INS) suggests changing IV tubing on peripheral lines in a facility with an IV-related infection rate of 3% every:

1. 24 hours.
2. 48 hours.
3. 72 hours.
4. 96 hours.

chapter

21 Basic Nutrition and Nutrition Therapy

evolve

http://evolve.elsevier.com/Christensen/foundationsadult

Kristen Kartchner Maughan

Objectives

1. Discuss the role of the nurse in promoting good nutrition.
2. Explain how to use diet planning guides in the assessment and planning of a diet.
3. List the six classes of essential nutrients, and identify those that provide energy.
4. List the functions and food sources of protein, carbohydrates, and fats.
5. List food sources and possible health benefits of dietary fiber.
6. Distinguish between saturated, unsaturated, and *trans* fats and cholesterol; identify current recommendations for dietary intake of fats and cholesterol.
7. Discuss key vitamins and minerals, their role in health, and their food sources.
8. Discuss changes in nutrient needs throughout the life cycle, and suggest ideas to ensure adequate nutrition during each stage of life.
9. Identify the effects of common medications on nutritional status.
10. Identify standard hospital diets and modifications for texture, consistency, and meal frequency.
11. List medical and surgical conditions that require a high-kilocalorie and high-protein diet, and suggest ways to increase kilocalories and protein in the diet.
12. Define obesity, and list components of an effective weight management program.
13. Describe the diet in the management of type 1 and type 2 diabetes mellitus.
14. Distinguish among anorexia nervosa, bulimia nervosa, and binge-eating disorder.
15. List conditions requiring a fat-modified diet, and identify limitations that accompany this diet on foods and certain food preparation methods.
16. Identify medical and surgical conditions necessitating modifications in sodium, potassium, protein, or fluid intake, and describe the dietary adjustments necessary in these conditions.
17. Define enteral nutrition and parenteral nutrition, and list medical and surgical conditions in which nutritional support is often indicated.

Key Terms

amino acids (ă-MĒ-nō ĂS-ĭdz, p. 611)
anabolism (ă-NĂB-ŏ-lĭzm, p. 612)
anorexia nervosa (ăn-ō-RĔK-sē-ă nŭr-VŌ-să, p. 635)
basal metabolic rate (BMR) (BĀ-săl mĕt-ă-BŎL-ĭk rāt, p. 631)
body mass index (BMI) (p. 632)
bulimia nervosa (bū-LĒ-mē-ă nŭr-VŌ-să, p. 636)
catabolism (kă-TĂB-ŏ-lĭsm, p. 612)
cholesterol (kŏ-LĔS-tŭr-ŏl, p. 610)
dietary fiber (p. 609)
dumping syndrome (p. 640)
enteral nutrition (ĔN-tŭr-ăl nū-TRĬ-shŭn, p. 646)
essential nutrients (p. 608)
glycogen (GLĪ-kŏ-jĕn, p. 609)
hydrogenation (hī-drŏ-jĕn-Ā-shŭn, p. 610)
kilocalorie (kcal) (kĭl-ō-KĂL-ō-rē, p. 608)
lipids (LĬ-pĭdz, p. 610)
lipoproteins (lī-pō-PRŌ-tēnz, p. 611)
medical nutrition therapy (p. 629)
nitrogen balance (p. 612)
nutrient (p. 608)
nutrient-dense foods (p. 621)
obesity (p. 632)
parenteral nutrition (pă-RĔN-tŭr-ăl nū-TRĬ-shŭn, p. 652)
pernicious anemia (pŭr-NĬSH-ŭs ă-NĒ-mē-ă, p. 616)
residue (p. 630)
satiety (să-TĪ-ĕ-tē, p. 610)
therapeutic diet (p. 629)
total parenteral nutrition (TPN) (p. 652)
tube feeding (p. 646)
vegan (VĒ-găn, p. 612)

Prevention—perhaps this word best describes why nutrition is becoming increasingly important in health care. Nutrition is the total of all processes involved in taking in and using food substances for proper growth, functioning, and maintenance of health. More and more evidence points to the fact that nutrition plays a role in many disease states, and that in many cases proper nutrition has the potential to help prevent or delay the onset of certain diseases. It has long been known that optimal nutrition ensures proper growth in children, teens, and pregnant women. But nutrition is important at every age, not only for growth but also quality of life. Nutrition is vital for the proper functioning of the cardiovascular, renal, pulmonary, nervous, digestive, and immune systems, among others. In short, nutrition plays a role directly or indirectly in all body processes. Never overlook its importance.

ROLE OF THE NURSE IN PROMOTING NUTRITION

Because you are most directly involved with the patient, the patient looks to you as a source of health information. Therefore you need to have a basic knowledge of nutrition. Although the dietitian is the nutrition expert, you will have opportunities to apply nutrition knowledge and promote good nutrition in a number of ways:

- Help the patient understand the importance of the diet, and encourage dietary compliance
- Serve meal trays to patients in a prompt and positive manner
- Assist some patients with eating
- Take and record patient weights
- Record patient intakes
- Observe clinical signs of poor nutrition and report them
- Serve as a communication link among the patient, dietitian, physician, and other members of the health care team
- Apply nutrition knowledge in your personal life. What better reason is there for understanding nutrition?

BASIC NUTRITION

DIET PLANNING GUIDES

MyPyramid

A number of sources in the United States have contributed guidelines that help people plan for optimal nutrition. The U.S. Department of Agriculture's (USDA) MyPyramid (Figure 21-1, p. 606) symbolizes a personalized approach to healthy eating and physical activity. MyPyramid emphasizes key concepts regarding activity and eating. The person climbing the stairs represents the concept of *activity* and serves as a reminder of the importance of daily physical activity. The narrowing of each food group from bottom to top conveys the idea of *moderation.* The wider base stands for foods with little or no solid fats or added sugars. Optimally, people select from these more often. The narrower top area represents foods containing more added sugars and solid fats. Those who are more active will typically be able to fit more of these foods into their diet. The six color bands representing the food groups of the pyramid symbolize *variety* and remind us that we need foods from all groups each day for good health. The different widths of the food group bands stand for *proportionality.* The widths suggest how much food a person should choose from each group. To personalize MyPyramid, enter your age, sex, and activity level on the MyPyramid page of the USDA's interactive website at www.mypyramid.gov. It is also possible to use Table 21-1 to find the amounts of foods, based on caloric needs, to consume from each group daily.

Dietary Guidelines for Americans

The U.S. Department of Health and Human Services (US DHHS) and the USDA (2005) have developed dietary guidelines specifically for the U.S. population.

Table 21-1 General Guidelines for Food Intake Patterns from MyPyramid: How Much Do You Need Each Day?

	SEDENTARY OLDER WOMEN AND CHILDREN	SEDENTARY OLDER MEN/ACTIVE ADULT WOMEN AND CHILDREN	SEDENTARY ADOLESCENT AND ADULT MEN/ACTIVE ADOLESCENT WOMEN AND OLDER MEN	ACTIVE ADOLESCENT AND ADULT MALES
Calorie level	1600	2000	2400	2800
Grains	5 oz	6 oz	8 oz	10 oz
Vegetables	2 cups	2½ cups	3 cups	3½ cups
Fruits	1½ cups	2 cups	2 cups	2½ cups
Milk	3 cups	3 cups	3 cups	3 cups
Meat and beans	5 oz	5½ oz	6½ oz	7 oz
Oils	5 tsp	6 tsp	7 tsp	8 tsp
Discretionary calories	132	267	362	426

Discretionary calorie allowance is the remaining amount of calories in a food intake pattern after accounting for the calories needed for all food groups—using forms of foods that are fat-free or low-fat and with no added sugars.

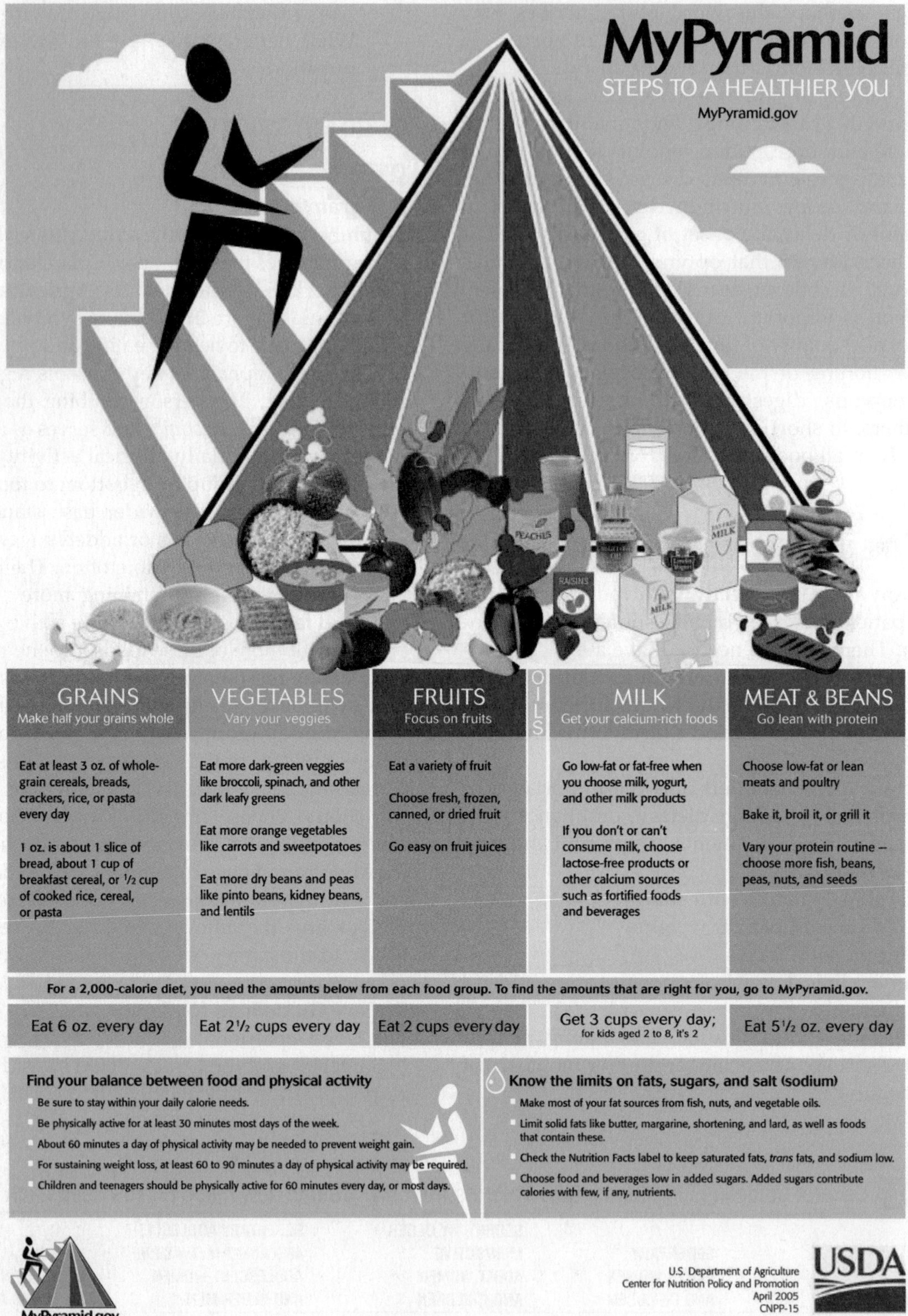

FIGURE 21-1 MyPyramid, a personalized guide to daily food choices and number of servings based on individual factors of age, sex, and activity levels.

These guidelines form the foundation of U.S. federal nutrition policy and directly affect federal nutrition programs such as food stamps, school breakfast and lunch programs, and the Special Supplemental Nutrition Program for Women, Infants, and Children (WIC). The government developed these guidelines to address the importance of adequate nutrition, as well as the prevention of overnutrition and chronic disease. They are intended for healthy children (ages 2 years and older) and adults of any age (Box 21-1).

Box 21-1 2005 Dietary Guidelines for Americans*

KEY RECOMMENDATIONS FOR THE GENERAL POPULATION

Adequate Nutrients within Calorie Needs

- Consume a variety of nutrient-dense foods and beverages within and among the basic food groups, while choosing foods that limit the intake of saturated and *trans* fatty acids, cholesterol, added sugars, salt, and alcohol.
- Meet recommended intakes within energy needs by adopting a balanced eating pattern, such as the U.S. Department of Agriculture (USDA) MyPyramid or the Dietary Approaches to Stop Hypertension (DASH) eating plan.

Weight Management

- To maintain body weight in a healthy range, balance calorie intake from foods and beverages with calories expended.
- To prevent gradual weight gain over time, make small decreases in food and beverage calorie intake and increase physical activity.

Physical Activity

- Engage in regular physical activity and reduce sedentary activities to promote health, psychological well-being, and a healthy body weight.
- To reduce the risk of chronic disease in adulthood, engage in at least 30 minutes of moderate physical activity, above usual activity, at work or at home on most days of the week.
- Most people will be able to obtain greater health benefits by engaging in physical activity of more vigorous intensity or longer duration.
- To help manage body weight and prevent gradual, unhealthy body weight gain in adulthood, engage in approximately 60 minutes of moderate to vigorous activity on most days of the week while not exceeding calorie intake requirements.
- To sustain weight loss in adulthood, participate in at least 60 to 90 minutes of daily moderate physical activity while not exceeding calorie intake requirements. Some people will need to consult with a health care provider before participating in this level of activity.
- Achieve physical fitness by including cardiovascular conditioning, stretching exercises for flexibility, and resistance exercises or calisthenics for muscle strength and endurance.

Food Groups to Encourage

- Consume a sufficient amount of fruits and vegetables while staying within calorie intake requirements. Two cups of fruit and 2½ cups of vegetables per day are the recommendation for a person with a 2000-calorie intake requirement, with higher or lower adjustments depending on the calorie level.
- Choose a variety of fruits and vegetables each day. In particular, select from all five vegetable subgroups (dark green, orange, legumes, starchy vegetables, and other vegetables) several times a week.
- Consume 3 or more ounce-equivalents/day of whole-grain products, with the rest of the recommended grains coming from enriched or whole-grain products. In general, at least half the grains should come from whole grains.
- Consume 3 cups/day of fat-free or low-fat milk or equivalent milk products.

Fats

- Consume less than 10% of calories from saturated fatty acids and less than 300 mg/day of cholesterol, and keep consumption of *trans* fatty acids as low as possible.
- Keep total fat intake between 20% and 35% of calories, with most fats coming from sources of polyunsaturated and monounsaturated fatty acids, such as fish, nuts, and vegetable oils.
- When selecting and preparing meat, poultry, dry beans, and milk or milk products, make choices that are lean, low fat, or fat free.
- Limit intake of fats and oils high in saturated and/or *trans* fatty acids, and choose products low in such fats and oils.

Carbohydrates

- Choose fiber-rich fruits, vegetables, and whole grains often.
- Choose and prepare foods and beverages with little added sugar or caloric sweeteners, such as amounts suggested by the USDA MyPyramid and the DASH eating plan.
- Reduce the incidence of dental caries by practicing good oral hygiene and decreasing consumption of sugar- and starch-containing foods and beverages.

Sodium and Potassium

- Consume less than 2300 mg/day of sodium (approximately 1 teaspoon of salt).
- Choose and prepare foods with little salt. At the same time, consume potassium-rich foods, such as fruits and vegetables.

Alcoholic Beverages

- If you choose to drink alcoholic beverages, do so sensibly and in moderation—defined as the consumption of no more than one drink per day for women and two drinks per day for men.
- Do not consume any alcoholic beverages if you are not able to restrict your alcohol intake, as well as if you fall into any of these categories: women of childbearing age who may become pregnant, pregnant and lactating women, children and adolescents, individuals taking medications that have potential to interact with alcohol, and those with specific medical conditions.
- Avoid consuming alcoholic beverages if you engage in activities that require attention, skill, or coordination, such as driving or operating machinery.

Food Safety

- To avoid microbial food-borne illness:
  —Clean hands, food contact surfaces, and fruits and vegetables. Do not wash or rinse meat and poultry.
  —Separate raw, cooked, and ready-to-eat foods while shopping and preparing or storing foods.
  —Cook foods to a safe temperature to kill microorganisms.
  —Chill (refrigerate) perishable food promptly, and defrost foods properly.
  —Avoid consuming raw (unpasteurized) milk or any products made from unpasteurized milk; raw or partially cooked eggs, or foods containing raw eggs; raw or undercooked meat and poultry; unpasteurized juices; and raw sprouts.

From U.S. Department of Health and Human Services and U.S. Department of Agriculture. (2005). *Dietary guidelines for Americans, 2005.* (6th ed.). Washington, DC: U.S. Government Printing Office, January 2005.

*The *Dietary Guidelines for Americans, 2005* contains additional recommendations for specific populations. The full document is available at www.health.gov/DietaryGuidelines/dga2005/document/default.htm.

Dietary Reference Intakes

Dietary reference intakes (DRIs) refer to a set of nutrient-based values that serve for both assessing and planning diets. The DRIs replace and expand on the recommended dietary allowances (RDAs), which have been used for more than 50 years in the United States. They are the basis for daily values used in the Nutrition Facts labels on foods. The purpose of DRIs is to help individuals optimize their health, prevent disease, and (where data are available) avoid consuming too much of a nutrient. Like the former RDAs, each DRI refers to the average daily nutrient intake of apparently healthy individuals over time. The amount of intake will often vary substantially from day to day without ill effect in most cases. Information listing DRIs for individuals is available from the USDA, available at www.nutrition.gov.

ESSENTIAL NUTRIENTS

Basic Functions

A **nutrient** is a chemical compound or element found in food that is necessary for good health. **Essential nutrients** are those that our bodies are not able to make in the amounts essential for good health, and that are therefore necessary to obtain through diet or other sources. There are six classes of essential nutrients: carbohydrates, fats, proteins, vitamins, minerals, and water. Each is necessary for life. Nutrients perform any or all of these basic functions: (1) provide energy, (2) build and repair tissue, and (3) regulate body processes.

Provide Energy

A **kilocalorie (kcal)** is a measurement of energy, much as a pound is a measurement of weight. When we say a certain food has so many kilocalories, we are actually saying it will provide energy. The more kilocalories in a food, the greater its energy-giving potential. Of the six essential nutrients, three provide energy—carbohydrate, fat, and protein. Alcohol, although not a nutrient, provides energy as well. Carbohydrate and protein provide approximately 4 kcal/g, whereas fat provides 9 kcal/g. Alcohol supplies 7 kcal/g. Authorities recommend obtaining about 45% to 65% of daily kilocalories from carbohydrate, 20% to 35% from fat, and 10% to 35% from protein. This distribution is called the **caloric distribution** of the diet. Vitamins, minerals, and water do not provide energy (kcal).

Build and Repair Tissue

Many nutrients are necessary for building and repairing tissue. Examples include protein, a vital constituent of muscle, blood, organs, epithelium, and other tissues; calcium and phosphorus, necessary nutrients in bone structure; iron, a major constituent of hemoglobin in the red blood cells; and fat, a component found in all cell walls.

Regulate Body Processes

Metabolism is the combination of all chemical processes that take place in living organisms. Nutrients play various roles in metabolism and thereby help regulate certain body processes. For example, the presence of carbohydrates is required for fat to be used correctly and completely. The B vitamins are necessary for the body to derive energy from foods. Water is an integral part of almost all chemical reactions in the body.

Carbohydrates

Carbohydrates are any of a certain group of organic compounds containing carbon, hydrogen, and oxygen, the most important of which are sugar, starch, cellulose, and gum. The main function of carbohydrates is to provide energy. Carbohydrates are also important in adequate amounts to spare protein from being used as an energy source. Carbohydrates are classified as either simple or complex (Table 21-2).

Simple Carbohydrates

Chemically, carbohydrates are made of molecular units called **saccharides,** or sugar units. The simple carbohydrates (often called **simple sugars**) include the

Table 21-2 Summary of Carbohydrate Classification

CHEMICAL CLASS	CLASS MEMBERS	DIETARY SOURCES
SIMPLE CARBOHYDRATE		
Monosaccharides	Glucose	Dextrose, corn syrup
	Fructose	Fruit, honey, high-fructose corn syrup
	Galactose	Milk (only found in lactose)
Disaccharides	Sucrose	Table sugar, sugarcane, beet sugar, powdered and brown sugar, fruit
	Lactose	Milk
	Maltose	Malted grain products
COMPLEX CARBOHYDRATE		
Polysaccharides	Starch	Grains and grain products (e.g., cereals, breads, crackers, pasta, rice, legumes, corn, potatoes, vegetables)
	Glycogen	No significant dietary source (storage form of carbohydrate in animal tissue)
	Dietary fiber	Whole grains, legumes, fruits, vegetables, nuts, seeds

monosaccharides and the disaccharides. Monosaccharides have only one sugar unit. Fructose, the sugar found naturally in fruits, is a monosaccharide. Disaccharides are made up of two sugar units bonded together. Table sugar (sucrose) and the sugar found naturally in milk (lactose) are examples of disaccharides (see Table 21-2).

Simple carbohydrates are part of a healthy diet; in the United States, however, it is refined sugar whose consumption is high. Table sugar and sweeteners such as honey and corn syrup are high in kilocalories, are virtually devoid of nutrients, and contribute to dental caries (cavities). The current recommendation is to reduce sugar consumption to less than 10% of total daily kilocalories. Simple sugars are found naturally in many nutritious foods such as milk and fruit. It is important not to exclude these from the diet. Rather, to limit sugar intake, encourage people to use moderation in their consumption of added sugars, sweets, and soft drinks.

Complex Carbohydrates

Complex carbohydrates are termed **polysaccharides** because they are made of long chains of glucose (sugar) units. They include starch, glycogen, and dietary fiber. Starch is found in many plant foods such as grains, legumes, and vegetables, particularly starchy vegetables such as corn and potatoes. Glycogen, a polysaccharide, is not generally consumed in the diet but is the body's storage form of carbohydrate. It is found mainly in the liver, and some is stored in the muscles.

Dietary fiber is a generic term for nondigestible chemical substances found in plants. It, like polysaccharides, is made of long chains of bonded glucose units; however, fiber is bonded in such a way that the body cannot digest it completely. Therefore most of the fiber we consume is eventually excreted in the feces. Foods containing dietary fiber include a combination of both water-soluble and water-insoluble fiber. Both types of fiber provide health benefits.

Insoluble fibers are found most abundantly in vegetables, wheat, and most whole grains. Insoluble fiber appears to be effective in softening stools, speeding transit of foods through the digestive tract, and reducing pressure in the colon. Thus it may help relieve constipation and reduce the risk of certain gastrointestinal (GI) disorders such as diverticulosis or hemorrhoids.

Water-soluble fibers are found in greater amounts in fruits, oats, barley, and legumes. Soluble fiber binds with the bile acids and cholesterol in the digestive tract, preventing their absorption and thereby helping to lower blood cholesterol, thus reducing the risk of atherosclerotic cardiovascular disease. It also helps delay gastric emptying and provides a feeling of fullness. Both types of fiber seem to aid in reducing the risk of type 2 diabetes, and in weight management and diabetic control. Often, it enhances weight reduction efforts to include fiber-rich foods in the diet in place of high-fat and high-kilocalorie foods. Fiber may delay glucose absorption and increase insulin sensitivity, thereby improving blood sugar control in people with diabetes.

It is best for complex carbohydrates, including sources rich in fiber, to make up the bulk of the diet. Encourage patients to choose at least five servings of fruits and vegetables and six servings of grains, cereals, pasta, or rice each day. By choosing foods closer to their whole state rather than in a refined or processed state, people are able to increase the fiber content of their diet. Current recommendations for fiber intake are between 21 and 38 g/day. There may be hazards to consuming too much fiber, and benefits from fiber supplementation are not well documented. Therefore it is recommended that most people get fiber from foods rather than supplements. It is also important that fluid intake be adequate as well as the increase in fiber. Information concerning the fiber content of selected foods can be found on Nutrition Facts labels. Table 21-3 shows how to estimate fiber intake.

Digestion and Metabolism of Carbohydrates

All carbohydrates except fiber are broken down in the digestive tract into monosaccharides (single-sugar units) before they are absorbed and eventually converted to glucose. Glucose circulates in the bloodstream and is used by the cells for energy. The brain derives almost all its energy from glucose.

Table 21-3 Do You Eat Enough Fiber in a Day?

FOOD GROUP	NUMBER OF DAILY SERVINGS* FROM EACH GROUP	MULTIPLY BY THE FIBER	
Dry beans, peas, lentils	____ servings	× 6 g =	____
Fruits, vegetables, whole grains, nuts	____ servings	× 2.5 g =	____
Refined grain products (white bread, white rice, regular pasta)	____ servings	× 1 g =	____
Other grain products (including breakfast cereal)	____ servings†	× ____ g† =	____
	Total daily grams of fiber (add up column)	= ____ g	

Adapted from American Institute of Cancer Research. (2001, rev. 2004). *The facts about fiber*. Available online at www.aicr.org/site/PageServer?pagename=pub_facts_fiber. Accessed September 9, 2009.
*For serving size description, see Table 21-1.
†Check the label for number of grams of fiber per serving.

If the body meets its energy needs, it will store carbohydrates as glycogen. Once glycogen stores are full, the body will convert further excesses of carbohydrate to fat and store them as adipose tissue (body fat).

Fats (Lipids)

Lipids are a group of organic substances of a fatty nature that are insoluble in water and necessary for good health. Fats and cholesterol are both lipids.

Fat is composed of fatty acids and occurs in various forms or consistencies ranging from oil to tallow. It performs a number of functions in the body. Fat provides the most concentrated source of energy of all the nutrients (9 kcal/g). The body is able to use for energy both the fat in foods and that stored as adipose tissue. **Adipose tissue** is the body's storage form of fat and helps insulate the body from temperature extremes. It serves as a cushion to protect organs and other tissues from being bumped or jarred. In addition, fat is a component in all cell membranes.

Dietary fat provides **satiety,** a feeling of fullness and satisfaction from food. It adds flavor and aroma to foods. Fat provides the body with essential fatty acids—linoleic acid and linolenic acid. It also carries the fat-soluble vitamins, A, D, E, and K. Most dietary fat consists of triglycerides. Triglycerides are composed of glycerol, a three-carbon chain with three fatty acids attached to it, hence the name **triglyceride.** Fatty acids are classified as either saturated or unsaturated. All fats and oils contain a combination of saturated and unsaturated fatty acids in various proportions.

Saturated Fatty Acids

A saturated fatty acid is one whose chemical bonds are completely filled, or saturated, with hydrogen. Saturated fats share similar characteristics. They are generally of animal origin and solid at room temperature. Fats that contribute the greatest amounts of saturated fat to the diet are listed in Table 21-4. Saturated fats tend to increase blood cholesterol levels, thus increasing the risk of atherosclerosis (the buildup of fatty deposits on the artery walls).

Unsaturated Fatty Acids

An unsaturated fatty acid has one or more places on its chemical chain where hydrogen is missing. These are called *points of unsaturation.* A fatty acid with only one point of unsaturation is called a **monounsaturated fatty acid.** Fatty acids with two or more points of unsaturation are termed **polyunsaturated.** Unsaturated fats are usually from plant sources and are liquid at room temperature. Sources of monounsaturated fats and polyunsaturated fats are listed in Table 21-4. Unsaturated fats, especially monounsaturated fats, are thought to have a blood cholesterol–lowering effect at moderate levels of intake and in combination with lowered saturated fat intake.

Table 21-4 Food Sources of Fatty Acids

FATTY ACID CLASS	FOODS CONTRIBUTING SIGNIFICANT AMOUNTS TO THE DIET
Saturated	Coconut, palm, and palm kernel oils (tropical oils) Fat in and on meats and poultry Egg yolk Butter, cream, milk fat Cocoa butter Olive oil, olives
Monounsaturated	Canola oil Peanuts and peanut oil Most other nuts Avocados
Polyunsaturated	Safflower oil Sunflower oil Cottonseed oil Soybean oil Corn oil Most fish oils
Trans	Partially hydrogenated plant and fish oils Stick margarines, shortening Commercial fats used for frying, baking

***Trans* fatty acids.** *Trans* fatty acids are unsaturated fatty acids that vary slightly in their chemical configuration from naturally occurring unsaturated fatty acids. Synthetic *trans* fatty acids are produced during **hydrogenation,** a process in which hydrogen is added to vegetable oil to make it more solid and stable, and less susceptible to becoming rancid. These are present in foods containing partially hydrogenated vegetable oils such as some deep-fried restaurant foods; packaged cookies, crackers, and other baked goods; some margarines; and shortening. Naturally occurring *trans* fatty acids are found in smaller amounts in dairy products and some meats. *Trans* fatty acids in the diet tend to increase blood cholesterol levels.

Current recommendations for healthy individuals older than 2 years are to obtain 20% to 35% of total calories from fat, with less than 10% of total calories from saturated fats and keeping *trans* fatty acid intake to a minimum. Because fat is an essential nutrient, a minimum intake of at least 15 g/day is recommended to prevent essential fatty acid deficiency. Suggestions for fat-controlled diets are discussed later in the chapter.

Cholesterol

Cholesterol is a lipid belonging to a class of chemical substances called **sterols.** Sterols are present in small quantities in many fruits, vegetables, nuts, seeds, cereals, vegetable oils, and other plant sources (see www.ific.org). Cholesterol performs specific functions in the body; however, it provides no energy (kilocalories). It is synthesized in the liver and is found in foods of animal origin. Plant foods and oils do not contain cholesterol. In fact, plant sterols will sometimes decrease cholesterol levels in the blood. The highest amounts of **dietary cholesterol** (the cholesterol found in foods) come from organ meats and egg yolks. It is also present in smaller but significant amounts in seafood, meats, poultry, and dairy products. Low-fat dairy products have less cholesterol than their higher-fat counterparts. The recommended intake of dietary cholesterol is an average of no more than 300 mg/day. Decreasing the intake of animal fats will achieve a parallel decrease in dietary cholesterol. Dietary cholesterol is thought to increase blood cholesterol levels, but not as greatly as saturated fats or *trans* fatty acids.

Digestion and Metabolism of Fat

For fat to be digested, it has to be emulsified, or pulled into suspension, with digestive juices. Bile, a secretion of the liver, is necessary to emulsify fat. Bile is stored in the gallbladder and dispensed into the duodenum when fat is present. Once emulsified, the body is able to break down and absorb fats. The body uses fat for various functions mentioned previously or for energy. It will store excess dietary fat as adipose tissue.

After absorption, lipids are packaged as lipoproteins. **Lipoproteins** are molecules made of lipid surrounded by protein. They facilitate the transport of lipids in the bloodstream. Types of lipoproteins include chylomicrons, high-density lipoproteins (HDLs), low-density lipoproteins (LDLs), and very-low-density lipoproteins (VLDLs). Of particular interest in cardiovascular disease are the LDLs and the HDLs. Both of these kinds of lipoproteins carry cholesterol in the bloodstream; however, it appears that the cholesterol found in the LDLs increases the risk of atherosclerosis by contributing to plaque buildup on the artery walls. In contrast, HDL cholesterol seems to have the opposite effect. It appears that HDLs transport cholesterol from the bloodstream to the liver to be degraded and excreted. LDLs are sometimes referred to as carrying the "bad" cholesterol, whereas HDLs carry the "good" cholesterol.

Goals for the American population stress maintaining or reducing total **serum cholesterol** (the cholesterol found in the bloodstream) to less than 200 mg/dL. Focus your teaching in particular on reducing LDL cholesterol levels and increasing or maintaining HDL levels. Table 21-5 classifies the blood cholesterol values used to determine health risk. The major food components that raise LDL cholesterol are saturated fats, *trans* fatty acids, and to a lesser extent, dietary cholesterol. Dietary factors that lower LDL cholesterol include polyunsaturated fatty acids, monounsaturated fatty acids, and to a lesser extent, soluble fiber and soy protein. In addition, sustained weight reduction will lower LDL levels in some individuals. Food components that sometimes lower HDL levels include *trans* fatty acids and, in some individuals, simple sugars. Factors that increase HDL cholesterol include monounsaturated fatty acids and regular physical activity.

Table 21-5 Classification of LDL, Total, and HDL Cholesterol (mg/dL)

LDL CHOLESTEROL	
<100	Optimal
100-129	Near or above optimal
130-159	Borderline high
160-189	High
≥190	Very high
TOTAL CHOLESTEROL	
<200	Desirable
200-239	Borderline high
≥240	High
HDL CHOLESTEROL	
<40 men; <50 women	Low

Source: National Cholesterol Education Program (NCEP). (2001, rev. 2004). ATP III Executive Summary; and Toth, P.P. (2005). The "good cholesterol": High-density lipoprotein. *Circulation*, 111:e89.
HDL, High-density lipoprotein; *LDL*, low-density lipoprotein.

Protein

The human body contains thousands of different proteins. Proteins make up the bulk of the body's lean tissues and organs. In contrast to either carbohydrate or fat, protein has numerous functions in the body. Carbohydrates, fat, and protein all contain carbon, hydrogen, and oxygen, but protein is unique in that it also contains nitrogen. Nitrogen is a necessary element in the formation of any type of protein. Proteins are necessary for tissue growth, repair, and wound healing. Collagen, a vital connective tissue, is made of protein. Some hormones, including thyroxine and insulin, are proteins. Enzymes are proteins produced by living cells that catalyze chemical reactions without being changed in the process. They are necessary for digestion and metabolism. The plasma proteins aid in fluid balance within the body. Albumin, a plasma protein, attracts water and has the capacity to pull fluid from one body compartment to another to attain balance. Hemoglobin in the red blood cells carries oxygen throughout the body. Immunoglobulins (antibodies) are also made of proteins, emphasizing the role protein plays in immune function. If necessary, the body will use protein for energy. It supplies 4 kcal/g; however, if the body uses protein as an energy source, it is no longer available for any other function.

Proteins are made of smaller units called **amino acids** (the building blocks of protein). Approximately 20 amino acids are used by the human body. A variety of ways of bonding them results in the formation of different proteins. The body uses all these amino acids, but only 9 of them are considered **essential amino acids;** that is, since the body does not make them in sufficient quantity to sustain health, it is necessary to obtain them from the diet. The body is able to manufacture adequate amounts of the other amino acids from those that are essential.

The recommendation is for 10% to 35% of total daily calories to come from protein. The DRI for protein in healthy adults is 0.8 g/kg of body weight/day.

Complete Proteins

Food proteins are classified as either complete or incomplete. A complete protein is one that contains all nine essential amino acids in sufficient quantity and ratio for the body's needs. Complete proteins are generally of animal origin and are found in foods such as meat, poultry and fish, milk, cheese, eggs, and soy.

Incomplete Proteins

Incomplete proteins are those that are lacking in one or more of the essential amino acids. Incomplete proteins are of plant origin. This includes the protein in grains, legumes, nuts, and seeds. When a person consumes a variety of incomplete proteins in the diet, the body is able to obtain the necessary balance of the essential amino acids.

Vegetarian Diets

There is no single vegetarian eating pattern. A vegetarian diet is made up of mainly plant foods; however, some vegetarian diets will include dairy products or eggs as well. The **vegan,** or strict vegetarian, diet completely excludes all animal products. Studies of vegetarians indicate that they may be at lower risk for various chronic diseases such as coronary artery disease, colon cancer, obesity, and type 2 diabetes. It is possible to meet protein needs with a vegetarian diet. The long-taught principle of eating specific plant proteins in combination (complementary proteins) is unnecessary as long as a wide variety of plant foods are included in the diet and caloric intake is adequate to meet energy needs. Strict vegetarians need to include a reliable source of vitamin B_{12} in the diet such as fortified breakfast cereal or a vitamin supplement. Vitamin B_{12} is found exclusively in animal foods.

Digestion and Metabolism of Protein

It is necessary to break down proteins to smaller amino acid units or individual amino acids before absorption.

Once absorbed, amino acids are disassembled and used for energy or reassembled into new proteins to be used for the body's various needs. Protein metabolism—how the protein is used by the body—is determined by what type of nitrogen balance the body is in. **Nitrogen balance** is the amount of nitrogen that is consumed compared with the amount of nitrogen excreted in a given time.

Nitrogen is obtained from eating foods and drinking beverages that contain protein or through intravenous (IV) feedings. Nitrogen is excreted in urine, feces, and sweat. Other losses of nitrogen occur with the sloughing off of dead skin and intestinal cells and in hair and fingernails.

If kilocalorie intake is adequate, the body uses the nitrogen in protein to perform the functions listed earlier. If, however, inadequate kilocalories are being consumed, the body is forced to use dietary protein for energy. When protein is used for energy, the nitrogen is wasted and not available to build or maintain tissues. Similarly, during times of increased kilocalorie and protein needs such as during illness or after surgery or trauma, the body will sometimes have to use its protein (lean tissue) stores for energy. When lean body tissue is broken down for energy, the nitrogen is excreted. If the body loses more nitrogen than it is consuming, it is in *negative nitrogen balance.* This is also typically defined as **catabolism** (the breaking-down or destructive phase of metabolism).

However, during periods of growth, such as during infancy, childhood, and adolescence, during pregnancy, or in recovery periods, the nitrogen (protein) consumed is used to build tissues and therefore is retained by the body. In this case, the amount of nitrogen consumed is greater than the amount excreted. This is called *positive nitrogen balance,* or **anabolism** (the building-up or constructive phase of metabolism). Zero nitrogen balance, or nitrogen equilibrium, occurs when the amount of nitrogen consumed is equal to the amount excreted. Healthy adults who maintain their weight might be at zero nitrogen balance. When protein is consumed in amounts greater than body needs, the amino acids will be chemically changed, converted to fat, and stored as adipose tissue. Therefore more dietary protein does not necessarily make more muscle.

Excess dietary protein is sometimes unhealthy. Those consuming high-protein diets tend to excrete more calcium, putting them at a potentially increased risk for osteoporosis. Too much dietary protein also tends to place an excessive burden on the kidneys, possibly leading to health problems.

Protein-Energy Malnutrition

When individuals suffer from a lack of energy or protein intake, protein-energy malnutrition (PEM) will sometimes result. PEM is fairly common in both children and adults in developing countries, and malnutrition is associated with over half the deaths of children less than 5 years of age worldwide. In developed countries, PEM is found most often in hospital settings, is usually associated with disease, and is more commonly seen in older adults. Two types of PEM exist—marasmus and kwashiorkor.

Marasmus occurs secondary to severe restrictions in both kilocalories and protein. It is a chronic condition characterized by wasting of body tissues. As the disease progresses, subcutaneous fat stores and then muscle stores are depleted, leaving the victim with a "skin and bones" appearance.

Kwashiorkor occurs as a result of severe protein restriction in the presence of other calories. It is seen most often in children in developing countries, with onset at the time the child is weaned from breastfeeding. Kwashiorkor is characterized by edema in the feet and legs, and often in the abdomen, the face, and the hands. Because of this edema, the child sometimes appears "fat" and the parents regard the child as well-fed. PEM is usually accompanied by multiple nutrient deficiencies and leads to stunted growth and impaired cognitive development in children, reduced mental and physical capacity, and lowered resistance to infections.

Vitamins and Minerals

Vitamins are organic compounds that are essential in small quantities for normal physiologic and metabolic functioning of the body. **Minerals** differ from vitamins in that they are inorganic and they are single elements rather than compounds. Both vitamins and minerals are needed in much smaller amounts than carbohydrates, proteins, and fats, yet they are just as essential. Neither vitamins nor minerals provide energy (calories) themselves, but they work in conjunction with other nutrients in the body to regulate many processes, including energy production.

Because vitamins and minerals are needed in such small amounts, these nutrients do pose a possibility for overconsumption. **Toxicity** is a condition that results from exposure to excess amounts of a substance that does not cause adverse effects in small amounts. Toxicity generally occurs from use of large supplemental doses of vitamins or minerals and not from consumption of food sources.

Americans tend to be very interested in vitamins and minerals. There have been claims of these nutrients helping reduce stress, preventing colds, increasing sexuality, increasing energy, improving physical performance, and reducing the risk for certain diseases. Many people believe that if some is good, more is better. The simple truth is that for most people, vitamins and minerals are best obtained from a balanced, varied diet. Except in certain cases, supplementation is not necessary. For those who like to use a supplement as "insurance" against an imperfect diet, a simple multivitamin and mineral supplement providing about 100% of the U.S. DRI should suffice. It is best to avoid large doses, or megadoses, of nutrients and the taking of numerous types of supplements, except for therapeutic purposes and while under a physician's care.

Because they are compounds, vitamins are susceptible to destruction by heat, light, and exposure to air. Sometimes they are lost when foods are cooked in water. It is not possible for minerals to be destroyed as vitamins are because they are single elements rather than compounds. However, they are sometimes lost in cooking water. Thus methods of preparation and storage have the potential to affect the final nutrient content of foods (Box 21-2).

Box 21-2 Methods of Preserving the Nutrient Content of Foods

- Expose food to as little water as possible: steam, microwave, stir-fry, or bake rather than boil.
- Expose food to as little air as possible: keep prepared vegetables, fruits, and juices covered and airtight; cut and manipulate food as little as possible; and keep lids on pans while cooking.
- Avoid very high temperatures, long cooking times, and keeping foods hot for an extended time, as in a buffet line.
- Keep and use the cooking water.
- Store fruits and vegetables cold.
- Keep milk in opaque containers.
- Use foods in whole form whenever possible.

Vitamins

Vitamins are classified by whether they are soluble in fat or soluble in water. Vitamins A, D, E, and K are fat soluble. They are usually carried in the fatty portions of food. The body is able to store fat-soluble vitamins. It is possible for an excess of these to reach toxic levels in the body.

The water-soluble vitamins include the B vitamins and vitamin C. The body is not readily able to store these vitamins since they are water soluble. Excesses are generally excreted in the urine. Daily intake of these vitamins is necessary because body reserves are minimal. Table 21-6 lists all the vitamins with their food sources, functions, and deficiency and toxicity symptoms.

Antioxidant vitamins. Certain vitamins are of particular interest in medical treatments and disease. The antioxidant vitamins, as they are sometimes called—vitamins E and C, and vitamin A in the previtamin form of beta-carotene—have a possible link to reduced risks of certain cancers and heart disease. Antioxidants function by delaying or preventing the destruction or breakdown of cell membranes in the presence of oxygen.

Most links between these nutrients and disease involve dietary intake, and blood levels that are the result of food choices rather than supplements. Thus a focus on diet, such as eating more fruits and vegetables, is the currently recommended strategy to prevent disease.

Vitamin C. Vitamin C supplementation has become a common practice because of claims that it helps prevent the common cold and prevents or cures cancer. Although it is true that adequate vitamin C is necessary for proper immune function, large supplemental doses of the vitamin have not been consistently and conclusively shown to be of greater value than what

Table 21-6 **Vitamins**

NAME	FOOD SOURCES	FUNCTION	CLINICAL EFFECTS OF INADEQUATE INTAKE: DEFICIENCY SIGNS AND SYMPTOMS	ADVERSE EFFECTS FROM HIGH DOSES: TOXICITY SIGNS AND SYMPTOMS
Vitamin A (beta-carotene is a previtamin; it is converted to vitamin A in the body)	Egg yolks, liver, milk Carrots, winter squash, sweet potatoes, spinach, collards, kale, broccoli, apricots, cantaloupe	Vision, epithelial tissue integrity, growth, reproduction, embryonic development, immune function	Night blindness, xerophthalmia, increased infections, follicular hyperkeratosis	Fatigue, headache, nausea, vomiting, blurred vision, liver abnormalities, bone and skin change
Vitamin D (calciferol)	Fortified milk, fortified margarine, egg yolks, liver, fish oils Sunlight on skin	Maintain blood calcium and phosphorus balance	Rickets (children): abnormal shape and structure of bones Osteomalacia (adults): weakening and softening of bones	Calcification of soft tissues
Vitamin E (α-tocopherol)	Vegetable oils, dark green leafy vegetables, wheat germ, nuts	Antioxidant; protection of cell membranes		Increased tendency to hemorrhage
Vitamin K	Green leafy vegetables, milk, dairy products, liver, meat, egg yolks, green tea (synthesis by intestinal bacteria)	Formation of blood clotting factors	Increased prothrombin time; in severe cases, hemorrhaging	None exhibited
Thiamine (vitamin B_1)	Unrefined whole grains, enriched and fortified grains and cereals, liver, pork, legumes, nuts	Carbohydrate metabolism	Beriberi: mental confusion, anorexia, muscle weakness and wasting, found in association with chronic alcoholism	None exhibited
Riboflavin (vitamin B_2)	Milk, meats, poultry, fish, enriched and fortified grains and cereals	General metabolism	Ariboflavinosis: sore throat, cheilosis (a disorder of the lips and mouth characterized by scales and fissures), glossitis, dermatitis	None exhibited
Niacin	Meat, poultry, enriched and fortified grains and cereals (high-protein foods that contain tryptophan)	General metabolism	Pellagra: dermatitis, constipation or diarrhea, dementia, depression	Nausea, vomiting, flushing, pruritus (itching) of the skin, abnormal liver function
Vitamin B_6 (pyridoxine)	Meat, poultry, fish, eggs, brown rice, wheat, oats, soybeans	Amino acid metabolism, general metabolism	Anemia, convulsions, dermatitis, depression, confusion	Peripheral neuropathy, irregular muscle coordination
Folic acid	Liver, green leafy vegetables, legumes, fruits, enriched grain products	Nucleic acid synthesis, amino acid metabolism	Macrocytic (large-cell) anemia, elevated homocysteine	Will sometimes mask vitamin B_{12} deficiency; interferes with the anticonvulsant drug phenytoin (Dilantin)
Vitamin B_{12} (cyanocobalamin)	Animal products (meat, fish, poultry, milk, dairy products, eggs)	New cell synthesis, maintenance of nerve cells	Pernicious anemia: macrocytic megaloblastic anemia	None exhibited
Biotin	Liver, egg yolks, soy flour, cereals, yeast (synthesis by intestinal bacteria)	General metabolism	Dermatitis, conjunctivitis, alopecia, depression (rare)	None exhibited

Table 21-6 Vitamins—cont'd

NAME	FOOD SOURCES	FUNCTION	CLINICAL EFFECTS OF INADEQUATE INTAKE: DEFICIENCY SIGNS AND SYMPTOMS	ADVERSE EFFECTS FROM HIGH DOSES: TOXICITY SIGNS AND SYMPTOMS
Choline	Richest sources are liver, kidney, wheat germ, brewer's yeast, and egg yolks	Maintenance of cell membranes, memory retention, muscle control, lipid metabolism	Liver damage	Hypotension, sweating, diarrhea, fishy body odor
Pantothenic acid	Widespread in foods; abundant in animal tissue, whole grains, and legumes	General metabolism	Listlessness and fatigue (rare)	Diarrhea and water retention
Vitamin C (ascorbic acid)	Citrus fruits and juices, strawberries, kiwi fruit, melons, broccoli, peppers, tomatoes, potatoes, fortified beverages	Antioxidant; wound healing, tissue growth and maintenance, proper immune function, absorption of iron	Scurvy: gingivitis, bleeding gums, easy bruising, increased infections, poor wound healing, rough skin, joint pain, muscle atrophy, fatigue	Abdominal cramps and diarrhea

can be obtained solely through diet. The adult DRI for vitamin C is 90 mg/day for men and 75 mg/day for women. An additional 35 mg/day is recommended for those who smoke cigarettes because smoking increases metabolic turnover of the vitamin. The upper limit is set at 2 g/day. Intakes above this level pose the risk of diarrhea and GI disturbances. It is easy to meet the DRI through wise dietary choices (Table 21-7).

Table 21-7 Vitamin C Content of Selected Foods*

FOOD	SERVING SIZE	VITAMIN C (mg)
Orange juice, fresh squeezed	1 cup	124
Cantaloupe	1 cup	59
Orange juice, from concentrate	1 cup	97
Strawberries, whole	1 cup	98
Grapefruit juice, from concentrate	1 cup	83
Kiwi	1 medium	71
Green pepper	1	96
Orange	1 medium	96
Broccoli, cooked	½ cup	74
Brussels sprouts, cooked	½ cup	71
Grapefruit, pink	½ medium	38
Watermelon	1 wedge	23
Tomato juice	1 cup	45
Cauliflower, cooked	1 cup	55
Potato, baked	1	20
Tomato	1	23
Spinach, cooked	½ cup	18

Data from U.S. Department of Agriculture. (n.d.). USDA national nutrient database for standard reference, release 22. Vitamin C. Available at www.ars.usda.gov/SP2UserFiles/Place/12354500/Data/SR22/nutrlist/sr22w401.pdf. Accessed December, 2009.

*The adult recommended daily allowance (RDA) for vitamin C is 90 mg/day for men and 75 mg/day for women.

Vitamin D. Vitamin D will be a nutrient of concern for some older adult patients in long-term care facilities. Vitamin D is obtained in two ways: from small amounts in liver, egg yolks, and some fish, and, most commonly, from dietary sources including fortified milk and milk products. The body also has the capacity to make vitamin D from exposure to sunlight. A patient in long-term care who is confined indoors and does not drink milk or consume milk products is likely to be at risk for inadequate vitamin D. Vitamin D is necessary for calcium metabolism.

Vitamin K. Vitamin K plays a role in blood clotting. Optimally, patients who are taking antiplatelet drugs or anticoagulants will consume consistent amounts of vitamin K from day to day. Large fluctuations in vitamin K intake have potential to alter the effects of the anticoagulant drug. Liver disease, and not just the diet, will affect vitamin K production.

Folate (folic acid). Adequate folic acid before and during pregnancy plays a possible role in reducing the risk of neural tube defects in the infant. Therefore the recommendation for women who are capable of becoming pregnant is to take 400 mcg/day of folate from fortified foods or a supplement in addition to the folate found naturally in a varied diet.

Vitamin B_{12}. Groups at risk for low intake of vitamin B_{12} include strict vegetarians, people over age 50, and individuals who have had stomach surgery. Because vitamin B_{12} is found primarily in foods of animal origin, those who follow a strict vegetarian diet (vegans) will not always receive adequate vitamin B_{12} from foods and are likely to benefit from a supplement. Approximately 10% to 30% of people older than 50 years of age will have difficulty absorbing vitamin B_{12} from foods because of low stomach acid secretion. Supplemental vitamin B_{12} is more readily absorbed in these individuals; therefore it is recommended that individuals older than age 50 receive the majority of their vitamin B_{12} from fortified foods or supplements containing B_{12}.

Vitamin B_{12} requires a special **intrinsic factor** produced in the lower portion of the stomach for absorption. When the intrinsic factor is missing, for example, after stomach excision or resection, **pernicious anemia** (a progressive macrocytic megaloblastic anemia, affecting mainly older people) develops. Pernicious anemia results because B_{12} is not absorbed. Treatment of pernicious anemia requires B_{12} injections for a lifetime.

Minerals

Minerals are classified as either major or trace minerals. Major minerals are those needed in amounts greater than 100 mg/day. They include calcium, phosphorus, magnesium, sulfur, sodium, potassium, and chloride. The trace minerals are needed in much smaller amounts. Trace minerals include iron, zinc, iodine, selenium, copper, manganese, fluoride, chromium, and molybdenum. Other trace minerals thought to be essential, but of which less is known, include arsenic, boron, nickel, and silicon. Table 21-8 lists the

Table 21-8 Minerals

NAME	FOOD SOURCES	FUNCTION	DEFICIENCY SIGNS AND SYMPTOMS	ADVERSE EFFECTS OR TOXICITY FROM HIGH DOSES
Calcium	Milk, cheese, milk products, green leafy vegetables, broccoli, legumes, fish with bones, fortified cereals	Formation and maintenance of bones and teeth, blood clotting, nerve conduction, muscle contraction	Osteoporosis (adults): weak, more porous bones Stunted growth in children	Constipation, increased risk in males for urinary stone formation, reduced absorption of iron and zinc
Phosphorus	Milk, meat, poultry, fish, grains, food additives, found in almost all foods	Essential component of bone, energy metabolism, acid-base balance	Rare, but sometimes occurs in patients using aluminum hydroxide antacids	Calcification of nonskeletal tissues
Magnesium	Nuts, legumes, whole grains, green leafy vegetables, fortified cereals	Bone mineralization, muscle contraction and relaxation, general metabolism, blood pressure regulation	Nausea, muscle weakness, confusion, tetany (rare, usually caused by other disease states)	Diarrhea
Sulfur	All foods containing protein	Essential constituent of proteins, metabolism	None exhibited except in severe protein deficiency	None exhibited
Sodium	Salt, processed foods, small amounts in whole unprocessed foods	Fluid and acid-base balance, nerve conduction, muscle contraction	Cramps, mental confusion, apathy, appetite loss (usually secondary to diarrhea or disease)	Hypertension in susceptible individuals, increased calcium excretion
Potassium	Sweet potatoes, fruits, vegetables, fresh meat, legumes, milk	Nerve conduction; muscle contraction, including the heart; fluid and acid-base balance	Severe: cardiac dysrhythmias, muscle weakness, glucose intolerance Moderate: increased blood pressure, risk of kidney stones, increased bone turnover	Cardiac arrest
Chloride	Salt, processed foods, water supply	Fluid and acid-base balance	Metabolic alkalosis	None exhibited
Iron	Clams, liver, oysters, meat, poultry, fish, legumes, whole and enriched grains, fortified cereals	Part of hemoglobin and myoglobin; necessary for oxygen transport and use in the body; part of some enzymes; energy metabolism	Microcytic, hypochromic anemia: fatigue, weakness, headache, apathy, pale skin, decreased immune function In children: reduced attention span, decreased ability to learn	Tissue damage, constipation, decreased zinc absorption Accidental poisoning in children: nausea, vomiting, diarrhea, rapid heartbeat, weak pulse, dizziness, shock, disorientation
Zinc	Red meat, liver, eggs, seafood, cereal, whole grains, legumes	Part of many enzymes involved in metabolism	Loss of appetite, growth retardation, skin changes, immune system dysfunction	Impaired immune response, impaired copper status, reduced HDL cholesterol

HDL, High-density lipoprotein.

Table 21-8 Minerals—cont'd

NAME	FOOD SOURCES	FUNCTION	DEFICIENCY SIGNS AND SYMPTOMS	ADVERSE EFFECTS OR TOXICITY FROM HIGH DOSES
Iodine	Iodized salt, seafood, plants grown in iodine-rich soil	Part of thyroxin, which helps regulate metabolism, growth, and development	Goiter: enlarged thyroid gland, weight gain, skin and hair changes Cretinism: mental and physical retardation of fetus	Enlarged thyroid gland
Selenium	Meat, poultry, fish, bread, grains, seeds	Antioxidant	Cardiomyopathy	Nail and hair changes, nausea, diarrhea, skin rash, garlic breath odor, fatigue
Copper	Organ meats, seafood, nuts, seeds, whole grains, cocoa	Necessary for utilization of iron	Anemia, vascular skeletal problems	Nausea, vomiting, liver damage
Fluoride	Water supply, plants grown in fluoride-rich soil	Increases tooth resistance to decay, stimulates new bone formation	Increased susceptibility to tooth decay	Fluorosis: mottled tooth enamel, altered bone health
Chromium	Whole grains, liver, nuts, cheese	Maintenance of normal glucose metabolism	Impaired glucose tolerance, diabetes-like symptoms	None exhibited
Manganese	Widely distributed in food; richest in whole grains, cereals, fruits, vegetables	General metabolism, formation of bone	Dermatitis, reduced bone mineralization, altered lipid and carbohydrate metabolism	Central nervous system pathology

minerals with a summary of their food sources, function, and deficiency and toxicity signs and symptoms.

Calcium. Calcium has a protective effect against both osteoporosis and hypertension. **Osteoporosis** is an abnormal reduction in bone density leading to bone pain, fractures, loss of stature, and deformities. In the United States alone, 1.5 million bone fractures are attributed to this bone disease annually. Women are affected more than men. Many hip fractures are the result of osteoporosis. Besides pain, hip fractures often result in dramatic lifestyle changes, disability, and loss of independence. An estimated 12% to 20% of people with hip fractures die from complications within 1 year of the fracture.

The causes of osteoporosis are multiple. Peak bone mass is determined not only by calcium intake but also by genetic influences, sex, hormone levels, physical activity, and dietary intake of vitamin D, fluoride, and other trace minerals. In the United States, high-sodium, high-protein, and low-potassium diets appear to contribute to osteoporosis by increasing the amount of calcium that is excreted in the urine. Growth and mineralization of bone occur from birth until early adulthood. Peak bone mass is achieved during the age span of 19 to 30 years. A higher peak bone mass reached in young adulthood lowers the risk of bone fractures at a later age. Therefore calcium intake in childhood, adolescence, and young adulthood is important. The time to start preventing osteoporosis is at a very young age. Calcium is also necessary in adulthood for bone maintenance and to prevent excessive bone loss. In women, menopause greatly accelerates the rate of bone loss.

The recommended intake of calcium is similar for both men and women, but it varies across age-groups. The requirement for older children and adolescents is set at 1300 mg/day. The suggested intake for adults is 1000 mg/day up to age 50 and 1200 mg/day for adults 51 years of age and older. No increases in calcium intake are recommended during pregnancy and lactation. Additional dietary calcium does not appear to have any influence on the changes seen in maternal bone mass during pregnancy and lactation, and women's calcium absorption increases during this period. The calcium recommendation for those with osteoporosis is 1500 mg/day.

The amount of calcium recommended for good health is often difficult to achieve from diet alone. Many foods, such as orange juice and breakfast cereals, are fortified with calcium. It is also possible to take calcium supplements, but they are best when they remain just that—supplemental—and are never allowed to replace calcium-rich foods in the diet. Foods provide not only calcium but also other nutrients that are beneficial in disease prevention (Table 21-9).

Calcium absorption and excretion may be affected by physiologic circumstances and dietary factors. Box 21-3 discusses factors that influence calcium absorption and excretion.

Sodium. Sodium is a mineral essential to health. In the body it functions as an **electrolyte** (a compound

Table 21-9 Calcium Content of Selected Foods

FOOD	SERVING SIZE	CALCIUM (mg)
Milk	1 cup	291-316
Yogurt	1 cup	274-415
Ice cream	1 cup	176
Cheddar cheese	1 oz	306
American cheese	1 oz	348
Processed cheese	1 oz	159-219
Cottage cheese	½ cup	77
Sardines	3 oz	371
Salmon with bones (canned)	1 oz	167
Tofu (processed with calcium)	3 oz	225
Collard greens (cooked)	1 cup	148-357
Broccoli (cooked)	1 cup	94-177

Box 21-3 Factors Affecting Calcium Absorption and Excretion

FACTORS THAT IMPROVE CALCIUM ABSORPTION FROM THE GASTROINTESTINAL TRACT
- Increased physiologic need (e.g., infancy, childhood, adolescence, pregnancy)
- Acidic conditions in the stomach (presence of food in the stomach increases stomach acid secretion)
- Small doses (less than 500 mg) of calcium are better absorbed than large doses

FACTORS THAT DECREASE CALCIUM ABSORPTION FROM THE GASTROINTESTINAL TRACT
- Calcium absorption decreases with age
- Calcium is poorly absorbed from foods rich in oxalic or phytic acids (spinach, sweet potatoes, rhubarb, beans, seeds, nuts, grains)

DIETARY FACTORS THAT INCREASE EXCRETION (LOSS) OF CALCIUM IN URINE
- High-sodium diets
- Low-potassium diets
- High-protein diets
- Caffeine

that, when dissolved in water or another solvent, dissociates into ions and is able to conduct an electrical current). Sodium is needed in very small amounts for good health and is found naturally in almost all foods. Therefore dietary sodium deficiency is virtually unheard of in the United States. Of greater concern is the possibility that excess sodium has the potential to be detrimental to health. Salt (sodium chloride) is the largest contributor of sodium to the diet. The major adverse effect of too much sodium is elevated blood pressure. Approximately 65 million, or 31% of American adults, suffer from hypertension. Diets low in salt have been shown to lower blood pressure. Sodium attracts water; because of this, a high-sodium diet has the potential to exacerbate edema (fluid retention). High-sodium diets are linked to increased urinary calcium excretion. Dietary reference intakes for sodium suggest an adequate intake (AI) of 1500 mg/day for younger adults, 1300 mg for adults, and 1200 mg for older adults. The upper limit of intake is set at 2300 mg/day. Most adults in the United States consume significantly greater amounts than this. Specifics concerning the sodium content of various foods and food groups is available from many nutritional information sources and on Nutrition Facts labels.

Potassium. Potassium, also an electrolyte, is needed for normal cellular function. A severe deficiency of potassium leads to hypokalemia (blood potassium level less than 3.5 mmol/L)—a life-threatening state. Individuals on potassium-wasting diuretics and chronic laxative users need to achieve adequate potassium intake through diet and/or supplementation.

The DRIs for potassium suggest an AI of 4700 mg/day for all adults. At present, most Americans consume much less than this. Studies indicate that a moderate potassium deficiency (in the absence of hypokalemia) will possibly lead to increased blood pressure, increased risk of kidney stones, and increased bone loss. Therefore adequate potassium intake is likely to help in controlling blood pressure and improving bone health.

Potassium is found naturally in many foods, especially fruits, vegetables, and milk. Potassium is easily lost during food processing. At the same time, processed foods almost always have added salt or other sources of sodium. Encouraging patients to eat more foods in their natural states and fewer processed foods will help in reducing sodium intake and increasing potassium intake. Consuming at least five servings/day of fruits and vegetables is perhaps the best way to increase potassium intake. Potassium supplementation is not recommended, except when prescribed by a physician, because toxicity sometimes leads to cardiac arrest. Specifics concerning the potassium content of various foods and food groups can be found in many nutritional information sources.

Iron. Iron is a part of hemoglobin, myoglobin, and a number of enzymes. Hemoglobin is part of the red blood cell and carries oxygen to the cells. Myoglobin is a similar compound in the muscle tissue.

Iron deficiency anemia manifests itself as a microcytic (small cell size) hypochromic (less cell color) anemia. Not all anemia is caused by a marginal intake or excess loss of iron, but iron deficiency anemia is a major health problem around the world. Symptoms include fatigue, weakness, headaches, apathy, and pale skin and mucous membranes. Immune function is also decreased sometimes. It is difficult to measure the effects of anemia, but work capacity and job performance tend to be greatly diminished. In children, iron deficiency has been associated with a short attention span, irritability, and a reduced ability to learn.

Children 6 months to 4 years, adolescents, menstruating women, and pregnant women are at greatest risk for iron deficiency anemia. Dietary requirements for adult women are higher than for men because of the monthly blood loss of menstruation. Iron DRIs are set at 15 mg/day for adolescent girls and 18 mg/day for premenopausal adult women. Postmenopausal women, adult men, and children have a DRI of 8 mg/day of iron. Pregnant women have an iron requirement set at 27 mg/day. To meet this requirement, encourage supplementation.

Food sources of iron include meat (especially organ meats), poultry, fish, whole grains, soy foods, and fortified and enriched grain products. Best sources listed in dietary guidelines are clams, fortified cereals, oysters, and soybeans. Dietary iron is found in two forms—heme and nonheme. Heme iron is well absorbed. Much of the iron in animal tissues (meats, poultry, and fish) is heme iron. Nonheme iron is not well absorbed from the GI tract. The iron in plant products is nonheme. Supplemental iron also seems to be poorly absorbed. Iron absorption from the GI tract may be enhanced or inhibited by certain dietary factors (Box 21-4).

Iron can be toxic and even fatal. Iron poisoning is seen each year in children who overdose on iron-containing vitamin and mineral supplements. Immediate medical attention is necessary if a child ingests large amounts of iron-containing supplements.

Chromium. Chromium is necessary for glucose metabolism and seems to work with insulin in regulating blood glucose. Adequate intake of chromium is thought to be particularly important for those suffering from type 2 diabetes mellitus. However, anyone receiving chromium supplementation for diabetes needs to be under medical supervision.

Box 21-4 Factors Affecting Iron Absorption

FACTORS THAT ENHANCE IRON ABSORPTION

- Meat, fish, and poultry, which have a factor, sometimes called the MFP factor, that enhances iron absorption
- Vitamin C (ascorbic acid), when eaten in the same meal with iron-containing foods

FACTORS THAT INHIBIT IRON ABSORPTION

- Bran and some fibers, which contain phytates that bind iron in the gastrointestinal (GI) tract so that it is not absorbed
- Polyphenols, which are compounds found in coffee, tea, and red wine
- Some medications, such as antacids
- Calcium in milk and supplement form
- Vegetable proteins, especially soy protein

It is possible to obtain adequate chromium through diet alone. Rich food sources include whole grains, cheese, liver, eggs, peas, apples, and nuts.

Water

Water is the nutrient most vital to life. Lack of this nutrient will bring detrimental effects more rapidly than any other. Water makes up approximately 60% of adult body weight and 80% of infant weight. Water performs many functions. It provides form and structure to body tissues. It acts as a solvent and is necessary for most of the body's chemical processes to occur. Water transports nutrients and other substances throughout the body by way of the blood, body secretions, and tissue fluids. It lubricates and protects moving parts of the body such as joints. It also lubricates food and aids in digestion. Water is necessary to regulate body temperature. If fluid needs are not met, dehydration will result. When more than 10% of body weight is lost through dehydration, it is a life-threatening situation. Signs of dehydration include poor skin turgor; flushed, dry skin; dry mouth; decreased urine output; irritability; and disorientation.

About 80% of our total water intake comes from drinking water and other beverages, and 20% comes from the water contained in foods. The need for water varies depending on factors such as body size, age, activity level, metabolic needs, and temperature, so it is not possible to give a specific recommendation; however, a suggested daily intake of 9 cups (women) to 13 cups (men) of fluids from drinking water and other beverages will be adequate for most adults. Pregnant and lactating women have increased water needs. Infants tend to be at a greater risk of dehydration because they have a higher percentage of water as body weight and are more susceptible to greater skin losses of water. In the young infant, breast milk and formula normally provide adequate fluid, but extra fluids will often be needed in warmer weather. Older adults have a decreased sensitivity to thirst and are at greater risk for dehydration. It is necessary to pay special attention to this population to make certain fluid needs are met.

LIFE CYCLE NUTRITION

PREGNANCY AND LACTATION

Nutrient needs during periods of intensive growth, such as pregnancy and infancy, are greater than at any other time during the life cycle.

Evidence has always pointed to the fact that optimal nutrition during pregnancy reduces the risk of complications, premature deliveries, and low birth weight. Even the mother's nutrition before conception plays a likely role in the final outcome of a pregnancy. Always encourage women of childbearing age to consume a healthy diet and use care in the con-

Table 21-10 Nutrient Needs during Pregnancy and Lactation

AMOUNT (DIETARY REFERENCE INTAKES)				
NONPREGNANT ADULT NEED	**PREGNANCY NEED**	**LACTATION NEED**	**REASONS FOR INCREASED NUTRIENT NEED IN PREGNANCY**	**FOOD SOURCES**
PROTEIN				
46-50 g	60 g	65 g	Rapid fetal tissue growth Amniotic fluid Placental growth and development Maternal tissue growth: uterus, breasts Increased maternal circulating blood volume: • Hemoglobin increase • Plasma protein increase Maternal storage reserves for labor, delivery, and lactation	Milk, cheese, eggs, meat, grains, legumes, nuts, soy products
CALORIES*				
2200	2500	2700	Increased basal metabolic rate, energy needs Protein sparing	See individual foods
MINERALS				
Calcium†				
1000 mg	1000 mg	1000 mg	Fetal skeleton formation Fetal tooth bud formation Increased maternal calcium metabolism Maternal blood pressure control	Milk; yogurt; cheese; fortified soy milk; dark green leafy vegetables
Iron				
18 mg	27 mg	9 mg	Increased maternal circulating blood volume, increased hemoglobin Fetal liver iron storage High iron cost of pregnancy	Liver, meats, eggs, whole or enriched grain, leafy vegetables, nuts, legumes, dried fruits, fortified cereals
IODINE				
150 mcg	220 mcg	290 mcg	Increased basal metabolic rate Increased thyroxine production	Iodized salt
MAGNESIUM				
310 mg	350 mg	310 mg	Coenzyme in energy and protein metabolism Enzyme activator Tissue growth, cell metabolism Muscle action	Nuts, soybeans, cocoa, seafood, whole grains, dried beans and peas
VITAMINS				
B_6 (Pyridoxine)				
1.3 mg	1.9 mg	2 mg	Coenzyme in protein metabolism Increased fetal growth requirement	Milk, wheat, corn, liver, meat
Folic Acid				
400 mcg	600 mcg	500 mcg	Increased red blood cells Prevention of macrocytic anemia Prevention of neural tube defects	Green leafy vegetables, oranges, artichokes, broccoli, asparagus, liver, fortified grain products
Vitamin C				
75 mg	85 mg	120 mg	Tissue formation and integrity Formation of connective tissue Enhanced iron absorption	Citrus fruits, strawberries, broccoli, tomatoes, raw green leafy vegetables
Vitamin A				
700 mcg	770 mcg	1300 mcg	Vitamin content in breast milk Embryonic development Breast milk production	Milk, egg yolks, organ meats, deep orange and green fruits and vegetables

*Provision of adequate nonprotein calories so that protein is available for tissue synthesis and maintenance rather than utilized for energy needs.
†Calcium absorption increases during pregnancy and lactation, so no additional dietary calcium is advised.

sumption of alcohol and caffeine. You have an opportunity to help educate the patient regarding a healthy diet during pregnancy (see Patient Teaching box on nutrition during pregnancy). Broaden the focus of maternal care to include preconceptional, as well as prenatal, nutrition care. Many women are unaware of their pregnancy during the first weeks after conception. Similarly, most women do not attend prenatal information classes until the later months of their pregnancy. Although any prenatal education is positive, the ideal is to provide information before conception or within the first few weeks of pregnancy. During these early weeks of pregnancy, adequate folic acid is thought to greatly reduce the risk of neural tube defects, such as spina bifida, in the infant. For this reason, advise women of childbearing age to consume 400 mcg/day of folate from fortified foods in addition to natural food sources.

During pregnancy, nutrient needs increase more than calorie needs. Therefore, encourage women to select **nutrient-dense foods** (foods that contain large amounts of nutrients relative to kilocalories). For a detailed discussion on nutrient needs in pregnancy and sample menus for pregnancy, see Tables 21-10 and 21-11.

Table 21-11 Sample Menus for Diet during Pregnancy

MENU 1	MENU 2
BREAKFAST	
1 cup high-fiber ready-to-eat cereal	2 eggs, scrambled in 1 tsp vegetable oil with ½ cup chopped onion, pepper, mushroom, tomato
1 slice wheat toast	1½ oz shredded cheese
1 tsp vegetable oil spread	1 bran muffin
1 banana	1 tbsp vegetable oil spread
1 cup 1% or skim milk	6 oz orange juice
SNACK	
1 apple	½ cup mixed nuts and dried fruit
2 Tbsp peanut butter	
LUNCH	
2 oz turkey on 2 slices wheat bread	1 cup black bean and vegetable soup
1 tsp mayonnaise	2 slices corn bread
1 cup spinach salad	1 tbsp vegetable oil spread
6 whole-grain crackers	2 tsp honey
1 cup skim or 1% milk	1 cup fresh strawberries
	1 cup skim or 1% milk
SNACK	
½ cantaloupe with ½ cup low-fat cottage cheese	3 cups popcorn
DINNER	
Pork-vegetable stir-fry:	4 oz grilled chicken breast
3 oz lean pork	1 baked potato
1½ cups fresh vegetables	2 tbsp sour cream and chives
2 tsp olive oil	1 cup steamed broccoli
Seasonings	½ cup pasta salad with vinegar and oil dressing
1 cup steamed brown rice	1 dinner roll
Water	1 tsp vegetable oil spread
	Water
SNACK	
2 oatmeal raisin cookies	1 cup low-fat yogurt topped with ⅓ cup granola
1 cup 1% or skim milk	
APPROXIMATE NUMBER OF SERVINGS PROVIDED PER MENU	
Grain group	8
Fruit group	3
Vegetable group	4
Milk group	3
Meat group	6 oz
Fats, oils, and sweets	5-6

Concerns in Pregnancy

Weight Gain

Weight gain in pregnancy is important. Recommended weight gains vary based on a woman's prepregnancy weight. Optimal weight gain for normal-weight women is 25 to 35 pounds. Underweight women will preferably gain between 28 and 40 pounds, in contrast to the 15 to 25 pounds recommended for overweight women. Encourage young adolescents and African-American women to strive for gains at the upper end of the recommended range. Advise short women to aim for the lower end of the range.

Under no circumstances is weight loss to be attempted in pregnancy. Mothers who do not gain adequate weight in pregnancy risk giving birth to a low-birth-weight (LBW) infant, one with a birth weight of less than 5.5 pounds (2500 g). These babies have a greater risk of complications during and after birth. Mortality rates are higher for LBW infants, except when the birth weight is primarily related to maternal or paternal size.

Patient Teaching

Nutrition during Pregnancy

- Explain the need for adequate but not excessive calories during pregnancy.
- Caution against weight loss during pregnancy.
- Teach the use of the MyPyramid website (www.mypyramid.gov) as a guide to a healthy diet.
- Discuss the importance of nutrient-dense foods to provide adequate nutrients for fetal development.
- Stress the importance of adequate fluid intake during pregnancy.
- Encourage consistency in taking any prenatal supplements prescribed by the patient's physician.
- Discourage the use of alcohol at any time during pregnancy.

Discomforts and Complications

Many women experience discomforts during pregnancy. Common among these is nausea and vomiting, often referred to as morning sickness. Women who were taking a multivitamin at the time of conception tend to be less likely to need medical attention for vomiting. Vitamin B_6 is safe and effective in the treatment of nausea and vomiting of pregnancy, and supplemental ginger has been shown to have beneficial effects. Advise women to discuss with their physician any supplementation during pregnancy. Mild nausea and vomiting as well as other discomforts often can be alleviated with the safe and simple dietary alterations listed in Box 21-5.

Occasionally, pregnancy will bring about medical conditions that pose potential dangers for both the mother and the fetus. Hypertensive disorders of pregnancy include chronic hypertension, preeclampsia-eclampsia (sometimes called *toxemia*), and gestational hypertension. These disorders are the second leading cause of maternal death in the United States and contribute significantly to stillbirths and neonatal complications. Those at increased risk are women older than 40 years of age; women of African-American ethnicity; those who are nulliparous or multiparous; patients with preexisting conditions (e.g., hypertension, renal disease, diabetes); and those with a family history. Obese women are three times more likely to develop preeclampsia than nonobese women. Be careful, if you work in outpatient, home care, and acute care settings, when monitoring a pregnant patient's blood pressure so that you help identify and treat any problems early on. Signs sometimes include not only high blood pressure, but edema and proteinuria as well. Proper nutrition is vital both before and throughout pregnancy and has some potential to help in blood pressure management. Ideally, those at high risk will choose a diet rich in fruits, vegetables, and milk products, adequate in protein, and moderate in sodium. Contrary to old practices, severe sodium restriction is contraindicated in the presence of preeclampsia.

With the incidence of diabetes on the rise in the United States, more women are expected to enter pregnancy with preexisting diabetes or to develop diabetes during their pregnancy. Preexisting diabetes during pregnancy is associated with increased risk of congenital abnormalities, miscarriage, and maternal and/or fetal death. Gestational diabetes appears in the latter half of pregnancy (after 24 weeks) and increases the risk of infant macrosomia, or gigantism (an abnormal condition characterized by excessive size and stature), leading to a difficult labor. Those with gestational diabetes have increased rates of cesarean delivery and often develop type 2 diabetes after pregnancy. Make sure all women undergo screening for gestational diabetes during pregnancy. For women with preexisting diabetes, achieving good blood glucose control both before and during pregnancy is important. Gestational diabetes is often controlled through nutrition therapy and moderate exercise, but for women who are unable to achieve glycemic control, insulin therapy will often be necessary. Diabetes is discussed in greater detail later in this chapter.

Anemia is another common nutritional problem in pregnancy. Both iron deficiency and folacin deficiency anemia are possible. Adequate diet—including meats, poultry, and fish; green leafy vegetables; and a variety of fruits and other vegetables—should be consumed, along with a prenatal supplement containing iron and folic acid.

Box 21-5 Nutritional Suggestions to Relieve Some Discomforts of Pregnancy

NAUSEA, VOMITING, GASTRIC DISTRESS

- To reduce nausea, eat soda crackers or other dry grain products before getting out of bed.
- Consume five or six small meals that include protein each day.
- Avoid letting your stomach become empty.
- Drink plenty of fluids during the day; however, drink liquids before or after meals to avoid feeling too full.
- Avoid high-fat or fried foods in excess.
- Limit foods with strong odors during times of nausea. Avoid odors that bother you.
- Allow time after eating before lying down or going to bed to prevent epigastric distress.

CONSTIPATION

- Drink plenty of fluids, especially water.
- Include fiber-rich foods at each meal.
- Include moderate daily exercise.

Practices to Avoid

Some dietary practices are best to avoid during pregnancy, especially alcohol consumption. Alcohol contributes to an increased risk of mental and physical retardation of the fetus. *Fetal alcohol syndrome* (FAS) is the name given to the cluster of signs and symptoms seen in many infants whose mothers consumed alcohol during her pregnancy. It includes not only physical and mental retardation but also characteristic facial and body deformities. There has been no determination of a safe level of alcohol consumption during pregnancy, and most nutrition experts favor total abstinence. The American Medical Association goes one step further in recommending that women of childbearing age abstain from drinking alcohol as soon as they plan to become pregnant.

High caffeine consumption is associated with delayed conception, increased risk of spontaneous abortion, and low birth weight. Advise pregnant women to avoid caffeine intake in excess of 300 mg/day (approximately three servings of coffee, or 300 mg from colas, teas, etc.). For more information on caffeine, see the section on nutrient-drug interactions later in this chapter.

Smoking, although not a dietary factor, is best to discourage. Low birth weight occurs more frequently in infants of mothers who smoke. Advise women to avoid taking drugs of any kind, including over-the-counter medications and herbal and botanical supplements, except under the advice of a physician. The risk of foodborne illness is higher for pregnant women and their fetuses. Encourage pregnant women to follow food safety guidelines from the US DHHS–USDA Dietary Guidelines (see Box 21-1) and limit fish intake to 12 ounces/week or less. Advise against eating shark, swordfish, king mackerel, or tilefish because of the possibility of mercury intake. Dieting for weight reduction is also contraindicated during pregnancy.

Lactation

During lactation, a woman does well to follow a diet similar to that followed during pregnancy. Kilocalorie needs and many nutrient needs are actually higher than during pregnancy (see Table 21-10). An increase of 500 kcal/day is recommended. Fluid needs are increased in lactation and are possible to obtain through the consumption of water, milk, juices, and other beverages. Advise moderation in any consumption of coffee, tea, and alcohol, because caffeine and alcohol can enter the breast milk.

During lactation, adequate nutrition is vital. A poor kilocalorie and nutrient intake will decrease the quantity of milk produced. Nutritional quality of a woman's milk remains fairly constant except in cases of severe nutrient deficiency. Therefore it is essential for the lactating mother to be properly nourished to ensure that lactation continues and milk supply is adequate. If a lactating mother complains that she is unable to produce "enough" milk for the infant, ask about her dietary and fluid intake.

INFANCY

The time from birth to 1 year of age is one of rapid growth and development. The average infant's birth weight triples by the first birthday. Obviously, nutrition is important for proper growth and development.

Breast milk or iron-fortified infant formula is generally recommended in the first year of life. Breast milk contains several antiinfective factors, which lead to a lower incidence of infections in breastfed infants. Encourage breastfeeding whenever possible; however, if a woman prefers to feed her infant formula, support her in that decision.

Consumption of regular cow's milk (whole, low-fat, or skim) is inappropriate during the first year of life. Unlike adults, infants need a high percentage of kilocalories from fat. Skim or low-fat milk provides inadequate fat, is more difficult to digest, and places undue physiologic stress on the kidneys. Whole milk from cows supplies low amounts of iron, essential fatty acids, and vitamin E, and excess amounts of sodium, potassium, and protein, relative to an infant's needs. During the first year, the only acceptable alternative to breast milk is iron-fortified infant formula. Whole milk is acceptable after the first year, but skim and low-fat milk are inappropriate until the child is 2 years of age. In the first 6 months, water, juice, and other solid foods are generally unnecessary for infants. Introducing solid foods too early increases the risk for food allergies and choking.

At approximately 4 to 6 months of age, depending on the infant's development, it is possible to introduce solid foods into the diet. Table 21-12 gives a summary of eating skills, hunger and fullness cues, and appropriate food textures for children 0 to 24 months of age. There are a few principles to follow when introducing solid foods. Choose and introduce single-ingredient foods one at a time at weekly intervals. This will allow sufficient time to detect any food-related allergies. Because foods high in iron are recommended as weaning foods, iron-fortified cereals and pureed meats are good first foods. If the family has a history of food allergies, it is generally best to withhold wheat cereal, wheat products, and egg whites until 1 year of age.

Most commercially prepared baby foods in the United States are nutritious, safe, and of high quality. However, it is important to read labels and use foods without added salt and sugar. Single-ingredient foods are better choices than the mixed, dinner-type baby foods because they have fewer fillers. If baby foods are prepared at home, it is important to take care to reduce the risk of foodborne illness by having a sanitary preparation area and proper storage conditions.

There is no nutritional indication to feed juice to infants younger than 6 months. Offering juice before solid foods are introduced into the diet poses a risk of having juice replace breast milk or infant formula in the diet. This tends to reduce the intake of protein, fat, vitamins, and minerals such as iron, calcium, and zinc. It is prudent to give juice only to infants who are able to drink from a cup. Prolonged exposure of the teeth to the sugars in juice is a major contributing factor to dental caries. Discourage the practice of allowing children to carry a bottle, cup, or box of juice around throughout the day, which leads to excessive exposure of the teeth to carbohydrate.

CHILDHOOD

At approximately 1 year of age, appetite generally tapers off, and the growth rate slows from that of infancy. Children still need adequate nutrition, although nutrient needs relative to weight are generally less

Table 21-12 Summary of Physical and Eating Skills, Hunger and Fullness Cues, and Appropriate Food Textures for Children Ages 0 to 24 Months

NEWBORN	HEAD UP	SUPPORTED SITTER	INDEPENDENT SITTER	CRAWLER	BEGINNING TO WALK	INDEPENDENT TODDLER
PHYSICAL SKILLS						
Needs head support	More skillful head control with support emerging	Sits with help or support On tummy, pushes up on arms with straight elbows	Sits independently Able to pick up and hold small object in hand Leans toward food or spoon	Learns to crawl Possibly pulls self to stand	Pulls self to stand Stands alone Takes early steps	Walks well alone Runs
EATING SKILLS						
Baby establishes a suck-swallow-breathe pattern during breast- or bottle feeding	Breastfeeds or bottle feeds Tongue moves forward and backward to suck	Possibly pushes food out of mouth with tongue, gradually decreasing this behavior with age Moves pureed food forward and backward in mouth with tongue to swallow Recognizes spoon and holds mouth open as spoon approaches	Learns to keep thick purees in mouth Pulls head downward and presses upper lip to draw food from spoon Tries to rake foods toward self into fist Able to transfer food from one hand to the other Able to drink from a cup held by feeder	Learns to move tongue from side to side to transfer food around mouth and push food to the side of the mouth to mash it Begins to use jaw and tongue to mash food Plays with spoon at mealtime, sometimes brings it to mouth, but does not use it for self-feeding yet Able to feed self finger foods Holds cup independently Holds small foods between thumb and first finger	Feeds self easily with fingers Able to drink from a straw Able to hold cup with two hands and take swallows More skillful at chewing Dips spoon in food rather than scooping Demands to spoon-feed self Bites through a variety of textures	Chews and swallows firmer foods skillfully Learns to use a fork for spearing Uses spoon with less spilling Able to hold cup in one hand and set it down skillfully

BABY'S HUNGER AND FULLNESS CUES						
Cries or fusses to show hunger Gazes at caregiver, opens mouth during feeding indicating desire to continue Spits out nipple or falls asleep when full Stops sucking when full	Cries or fusses to show hunger Smiles, gazes at caregiver, or coos during feeding to indicate desire to continue Spits out nipple or falls asleep when full Stops sucking when full	Moves head forward to reach spoon when hungry May swipe the food toward the mouth when hungry Turns head away from spoon when full May be distracted or notice surroundings more when full	Reaches for spoon or food when hungry Points to food when hungry Slows down in eating when full Clenches mouth shut or pushes food away when full	Reaches for food when hungry Points to food when hungry Shows excitement when food is presented when hungry Pushes food away when full Slows down in eating when full	Expresses desire for specific foods with words or sounds Shakes head to say "no more" when full	Combines phrases with gestures, such as "want that" and pointing Can lead caregiver to refrigerator and point to a desired food or drink Uses words such as "all done" and "get down" Plays with food or throws food when full
APPROPRIATE FOODS AND TEXTURES						
Breast milk or infant formula	Breast milk or infant formula	Breast milk or infant formula Infant cereals Thin pureed foods	Breast milk or infant formula Infant cereals Thin pureed baby foods Thicker pureed baby foods Soft mashed foods without lumps 100% juice	Breast milk or infant formula 100% juice Infant cereals Pureed foods Ground or soft mashed foods with tiny soft noticeable lumps Foods with soft texture Crunchy foods that dissolve (such as baby biscuits or crackers) Increase variety of flavors offered	Breast milk, infant formula, or whole milk 100% juice Coarsely chopped foods, including foods with noticeable pieces Foods with soft to moderate texture Toddler foods Bite-sized pieces of foods Bites through a variety of textures	Whole milk 100% juice Coarsely chopped foods Toddler foods Bite-sized pieces of foods Becomes efficient at eating foods of varying textures and taking controlled bites of soft solids, hard solids, or crunchy foods by 2 years

From Butte, N., et al. (2004). The start healthy feeding guidelines for infants and toddlers. *Journal of the American Dietetic Association, 104*(3), 442.

than in infancy. The www.mypyramid.gov website offers an appropriate guide for children's diets (see Figure 21-1). Obviously, the younger child will typically need smaller serving sizes than adults, and as the child grows, serving sizes will increase.

Childhood is a critical time for instilling good dietary habits. It is also a time for children to test their independence (Figure 21-2). Food is often a source of contention at mealtime, with the parents resorting to coaxing to get the child to eat or arguing with the child to gain compliance. Often the more pressure that is placed on the child at mealtime, the more negative the experience, and the more resistant to developing sound eating habits the child will become. In general, if children are offered nutritious foods in pleasant surroundings and in nonthreatening ways, they will most likely be adequately nourished. A good rule of thumb is for parents and caregivers to decide which foods to serve and at what time. The child gets to decide what and how much to eat (see Health Promotion box).

ADOLESCENCE

The adolescent years are years of both physical and emotional growth. In making food choices, teenagers are influenced greatly by peer pressure and social acceptance. Their diets are often filled with kilocalorie-rich and nutrient-poor snack foods. Fast foods make up a large portion of the diet, and although these foods do not lack nutrients, the fast-food diet often completely lacks fruits and vegetables and sometimes milk. Common dietary inadequacies in adolescence include iron and calcium (particularly in girls) and vitamins A and C and folic acid. Iron needs increase with the onset of menstruation in girls, and anemia is a common problem. Boys' nutritional intakes are generally better than are girls'. During adolescence, many teenagers experiment with alcohol and drugs, and these substances typically have detrimental effects on nutritional status.

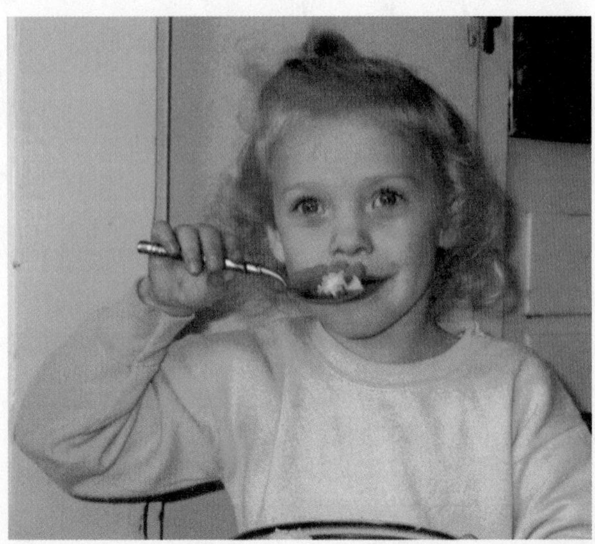

FIGURE 21-2 Self-feeding toddler.

Health Promotion

Ways to Encourage Good Dietary Habits in Children

- Encourage children to eat meals and snacks at regular times and usually at the table. By having set eating times, children will learn that they cannot eat continually all day.
- Try to make meals relaxed and enjoyable. Children need time to eat correctly, and mealtimes should be a positive experience.
- Offer a variety of foods from all six food groups, and give children a choice from what you offer them.
- Remember, physical growth and appetite come in spurts. Do not force children to eat more than they want to eat.
- Give small servings, or teach children how to serve themselves small servings. Then let them have seconds if still hungry.
- Offer new foods, but do not force children to eat foods they dislike. If the child will not eat a new food, quietly remove the food and offer it again at another time.
- Encourage children to help with food selection and preparation.
- Keep nutritious snacks available, such as fruit, cheese, crackers, raw vegetables, and bread. Most children need to snack.
- Limit sweets, and do not use sweets and foods as rewards or bribes.
- Encourage children to be physically active.
- As adults, set a good example by practicing sound dietary and exercise habits.

Obesity in the young is a common problem in U.S. society. As mentioned, these years are a time of growth, and although obesity is not ideal, restrictive diets sometimes cause harm by suppressing development and even leading to eating disorders. Focus attention on healthy eating habits and moderation of soft drinks and sugar- and fat-laden snack foods, and emphasize adequate physical activity. Limiting television viewing and computer usage is one way to help increase physical activity (at least 60 min/day) and thus increase the amount of energy expended. It is best to attempt weight-reduction diets only under the advice of a physician and with the guidance of a dietitian.

ADULTHOOD

During adulthood, nutrient needs change little in comparison with the necessary adjustments called for during the years of growth and development. Energy needs, however, decrease with age. At the same time, many adults decrease activity levels. The combined effects of decreased energy needs and reduced physical activity often result in weight gain. As adults advance in years, it is important for them to eat nutrient-dense foods and thereby receive adequate nutrition with fewer kilocalories. Place emphasis on maintaining an active lifestyle.

With age comes the increasing likelihood of age-related illness. Because many older Americans suffer

Life Span Considerations

Older Adults

Aging and Nutrition

- Aging often affects the eating process. Changes in dentition, decreased saliva production, and alterations in swallowing all have the potential to affect nutrient intake. It is sometimes necessary to adjust food consistency to facilitate food intake. Chopped, ground, pureed, and liquid diets tend to be less appealing to the older person; serve them in as palatable a manner as possible.
- The aroma and taste of foods is sometimes affected by normal changes of aging. In addition, many older adults are on special diets that restrict the use of salt, sugars, and fats. This leads to a possibly inadequate nutrient intake. The use of flavorings, seasonings, and spices to enhance flavor and aroma is often helpful.
- Older adults experience changes in digestive secretions, gastrointestinal mucosa, and enzyme production. This affects how food is digested, absorbed, and excreted. Water, dietary fiber, and adequate physical activity play an important role in preventing constipation in older adults.
- Aging often leads to loss of muscle mass, thereby reducing basal metabolic rate. Kilocalorie needs decrease approximately 5% for each decade between 55 and 75 and 7% for each decade after age 75.
- Older adults may have a greater need for certain nutrients, including protein, riboflavin, vitamin B_6, folic acid, vitamin B_{12}, vitamin D, and calcium. A multivitamin and mineral supplement supplying 100% of the recommended daily allowance (RDA) will often be beneficial for individuals with a low kilocalorie intake or during periods of poor intake. In addition, many older adults will not need as much vitamin A as younger adults. Advise patients not to consume large doses of any nutrient unless under a physician's supervision.
- Older adults often take numerous medications. Many medications tend to affect nutritional status. Be aware of drug-nutrient interactions and side effects that have potential to influence dietary intake.
- Because of illness, restricted mobility, or financial limitations, or some combination of these, older adults sometimes have difficulty obtaining and preparing nutritious food.
- Age-related social and mental changes such as forgetfulness, loneliness, and apathy are likely to affect the eating habits of older adults.
- Increased incidence of chronic medical conditions in older adults often necessitates the use of therapeutic diets. The most common conditions include diabetes mellitus, cardiovascular disease, renal insufficiency, osteoporosis, diverticulosis, anemia, and lactose intolerance. The older adult who has long-standing dietary preferences and habits will often find diet modification difficult. Always assess individual needs and situations before determining the most appropriate nutrition therapy.

from heart disease, arthritis, osteoporosis, diabetes, kidney disease, and other disorders, nutrient needs vary greatly from individual to individual (see Life Span Considerations for Older Adults box).

Nutritional Concerns of Adults in Long-Term Care Facilities

Malnutrition is a common problem among nursing home residents and profoundly influences physical health and quality of life. Poor nutritional status is related to a number of factors:

- Residents of long-term care facilities sometimes experience cognitive or physical impairment, disease processes, and emotional disturbances, all of which have possible effects on nutritional intake and status.
- Many, if not most, residents in the nursing home environment need some assistance or encouragement with eating and drinking. Staffing ratios at these facilities are not always adequate; consequently, residents do not always receive the attention they need when it comes to dietary intake. In addition, when staffing ratios are inadequate or health care providers are not well trained in feeding techniques, inappropriate force-feeding methods are sometimes used to ensure that patients consume their food.
- Many long-term care facility residents are on restricted diets. Excessive sodium or fat restrictions often reduce the palatability of food and thereby contribute to poor nutritional intake.
- Inadequate fluid intake and dehydration sometimes occur secondary to decreased thirst sensation, decreased independence, dysphagia (difficulty swallowing), and incontinence.
- **Pressure sores** occur in many nonambulatory residents, increasing kilocalorie, protein, and nutrient needs.

See the Coordinated Care box for managing the feeding of nursing home residents.

Coordinated Care

Collaboration

FEEDINGS IN LONG-TERM CARE FACILITIES

- Nursing assistants or dietary aides are most likely to be aware of the amount and types of food consumed by older adults.
- Data that are more specific than the typical good/fair/poor ratings or even percentage are important for good care planning.
- It is essential for assistants to report on the foods consumed in terms of both type and amount (e.g., the amount of meat and vegetables versus the amount of applesauce and dessert).
- Teach the nursing assistant how to properly feed the resident when you are unable to do so.

The enjoyment of food is often the last remaining pleasure of many long-term care facility residents. Make every effort to see that residents are offered familiar foods that taste good. Many long-term care facilities have adopted a liberalized older adult diet. This diet has mild salt, fat, and concentrated sweets restrictions, but avoids severe restrictions. Thus palatability is balanced with diet therapy.

It is important to take cultural and personal food preferences into account so that choice is offered in food selection. Liquid nutritional supplements often help to increase kilocalorie, protein, and nutrient intake; however, the use of these supplements will detract from the patient's quality of life if they are used as a substitute for regular food.

Offer fluids to residents at all meals and between meals to ensure adequate intake. It is important for both you and other staff members to watch for signs of dehydration such as nausea and vomiting, elevated temperature, decreased urination, dry mucous membranes, poor skin turgor, constipation, hypotension, swollen tongue, sunken eyes, and chronic infections.

Actively supervise dining areas, and help educate employees and family members of residents in safe and effective feeding techniques. Family involvement helps increase residents' dietary intake; encourage it whenever possible. Above all, make sure you and other employees understand the value of mealtime as a pleasant social experience, and advocate for adequate staffing ratios in long-term care facilities.

Nutrient-Drug Interactions

Medical conditions and disease states often necessitate drug therapy. Many older adults take a number of prescription medications daily. Added to these medications are over-the-counter drugs, which people purchase and use without a prescription. Many medications have the capacity to adversely affect a person's nutritional status.

Drugs have the potential to alter food intake by either increasing or decreasing appetite or the ability to eat. In many instances, they also affect the absorption, metabolism, and excretion of certain nutrients. Conversely, food intake and vitamin or mineral supplementation sometimes affects the absorption, distribution, metabolism, and action of some medications (Table 21-13).

Caffeine

Caffeine is a drug. It is a central nervous system stimulant and a diuretic. It has potential to cause nervousness, irritability, anxiety, insomnia, and heart dysrhythmias and palpitations. It also tends to affect blood pressure, circulation, and gastric acid secretion. In children, caffeine consumption sometimes goes unnoticed as a source of "hyperactive" behavior. Often older people are not able to tolerate caffeine as well as they were able to when they were younger. The effects of caffeine vary from individual to individual. One person will consume large amounts of caffeine with no apparent side effects, and another person will be highly sensitive to caffeine. Advise older people to use moderation in their intake of caffeine, as well as to be aware of its possible effects, which will resemble an anxiety attack in some people. In those who complain of these symptoms, assess caffeine consumption. Reducing caffeine intake often alleviates these negative effects and will possibly avert the use of yet another

Table 21-13 Common Medications and Their Effect on Nutrition

DRUG TYPE	POSSIBLE DIETARY SIGNIFICANCE
Antacids	Reduced phosphorus, vitamin A, and iron absorption.
Antibiotics	Nausea, vomiting, and diarrhea, leading to reduced absorption from vomiting and increased excretion of multiple nutrients from diarrhea. Long-term therapy may decrease vitamin K synthesis.
Anticoagulants (e.g., warfarin)	Vitamin K counteracts medication. Consistent intake of vitamin K is essential. Avoid high-dose supplements of vitamins A and E.
Aspirin	In long-term therapy: increased excretion of and decreased serum levels of ascorbic acid (vitamin C); possible GI bleeding leading to loss of iron; vitamin K depletion. Encourage diet rich in vitamin C.
Antihypertensives	Vitamin B_6 depletion. Vitamin B_6 (hydralazine) supplementation is encouraged for those with marginal diets.
Diuretics (e.g., furosemide, chlorothiazide, hydrochlorothiazide)	Increased electrolyte excretion leading to potassium, magnesium, and calcium depletion. Potassium-rich diet is encouraged. May require potassium supplements.
Diuretics (spironolactone)	Decreased potassium excretion—avoid supplements and salt substitutes.
Laxatives	Decreased absorption of calcium, potassium, fat-soluble vitamins (especially vitamin D). Encourage fiber- and fluid-rich diets. Encourage physical activity (may reduce the need for laxatives).

Table 21-14 Caffeine Content of Selected Beverages and Foods

BEVERAGE	SERVING SIZE	AVERAGE AMOUNT OF CAFFEINE (mg)
COFFEE		
Brewed, drip	8 oz	184
Starbucks Brewed (Grande)	16 oz	320
Starbucks Vanilla Latte (Grande)	16 oz	150
Brewed, percolated	8 oz	128
Instant	8 oz	96
Decaffeinated	8 oz	5
TEA		
Brewed 5 minutes	8 oz	80
Instant	8 oz	48
Iced tea	12 oz	70
Snapple, regular and diet	16 oz	42
SOFT DRINKS		
Coca-Cola, regular and diet	12 oz	45
Dr. Pepper, regular and diet	12 oz	40
Mountain Dew	12 oz	54
Pepsi, regular and diet	12 oz	37
Lemon-lime, orange, root beer	12 oz	0
ENERGY DRINKS		
Spike Shooter	8.4 oz	300
Monster Energy	16 oz	160
Red Bull	8.3 oz	80
SoBe Essential Energy	8 oz	48
HOT COCOA	8 oz	6
CHOCOLATE MILK	8 oz	5
MILK CHOCOLATE	1 oz	6
DARK CHOCOLATE, SEMISWEET	1 oz	20

Modified from Lecos, C. (1993). Caffeine jitters: some safety questions remain. *FDA Consumer* (Jan); American Dietetic Association. (1988). *Manual of clinical dietetics*. Chicago: The Association; and Center for Science in the Public Interest (2007).

drug, this time to relieve anxiety. The caffeine content of selected foods and beverages is shown in Table 21-14. General recommendations are to limit caffeine intake to less than 300 mg/day.

MEDICAL NUTRITION THERAPY AND THERAPEUTIC DIETS

Medical nutrition therapy is the use of specific nutrition techniques to treat an illness, injury, or condition. It involves modifying diets in such a way as to meet the requirements created by disease or injury. A diet used as a medical treatment is called a **therapeutic diet.** If a patient needs a special diet, the physician will prescribe the diet and write the diet order in the medical record. The therapeutic diet is planned and instruction is given by the dietitian. You will often serve and monitor the therapeutic diet. It is important to consider cultural and religious preferences when implementing a therapeutic diet (see Cultural Considerations box). Consult with the physician when conditions necessitate a possible change in diet order.

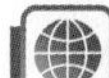 **Cultural Considerations**

Culture and Nutrition

A trauma patient was injured in an automobile accident and stayed at a small medical facility in the Midwestern United States. The patient was Muslim and for a time was fed intravenously. When oral feedings were again resumed, the patient requested a vegetarian diet. Being unfamiliar with the dietary customs of this religious group, the nutrition department prepared and sent a typical vegetarian diet excluding all animal foods. There was some concern over whether the patient would receive adequate calories and protein for recovery while on this diet. A visit with the patient revealed that he had asked for a vegetarian diet to avoid pork; however, he was amenable to consuming milk products, poultry, and fish. With this knowledge, it was easy to adjust his diet to provide adequate nutrition and respect his religious preferences as well.

There is much to consider when dealing with patients of varied cultural, social, or religious backgrounds:

- Food habits are among the oldest and most deeply rooted aspects of many cultures.
- Food plays an important role in quality of life. The loss of culturally related foods during hospitalization or long-term care has great potential to affect the patient both emotionally and physically.
- Never make assumptions. Be specific when asking questions regarding the patient's dietary preferences.
- The patient is likely to need help in marking the menu if he or she speaks another language or is unfamiliar with foods on the menu. Pictures of food are often helpful when there is a language barrier.
- Communication between the nursing staff and nutrition services is key. Inform nutrition services if poor intake is noted so that the diet can be individualized.
- Patients often have strong beliefs regarding certain foods or food combinations. Unless these beliefs are injurious to the patient, work to ensure that staff respects them.
- In long-term care facilities, it is important to make every effort to work with the patient or family to provide special foods for observance of holidays, festivals, and other occasions.
- Occasionally the family of a patient will be permitted (with the physician's approval) to bring in food for the patient if the facility is unable to provide that food. Take special care to ensure food safety.

CONSISTENCY, TEXTURE, AND FREQUENCY MODIFICATIONS

The term *therapeutic diet* often brings to mind nutrient-modified diets such as low-fat or low-sodium diets. But modifications in textures, consistencies, and meal frequency are also therapeutic in some cases. Most hospitals have standard diets based on consistency, specifically liquid, soft, and regular diets.

Liquid Diets

The two types of liquid diets are clear liquid and full liquid. The clear liquid diet is a nonirritating diet consisting of liquids that are easily digested and absorbed and leave little residue in the GI tract. **Residue** is food, fiber, and other substances that remain in the colon after digestion is completed. The clear liquid diet is typically used before diagnostic tests, particularly tests on the GI tract, or before surgery. It is commonly used postoperatively until the bowel resumes activity and is also used during some times of vomiting or diarrhea. The clear liquid diet is low in kilocalories, protein, and most nutrients. It is to be used temporarily, preferably for 3 days or less.

The full-liquid diet is used as a transition diet after a clear liquid diet. A full-liquid diet is more nutritionally complete than a clear liquid diet but is still lacking in some nutrients, such as iron, zinc, and fiber. This diet, too, is best used only temporarily (Box 21-6).

Liquid nutritional supplements are sometimes used for patients who are likely to require liquid diets for longer periods. These supplemental formulas contain a concentrated source of kilocalories, protein, and essential nutrients. They are generally lactose free (and sugar free for diabetics) and readily digested and absorbed. These supplements also lend themselves to use in addition to a regular or therapeutic diet to help increase kilocalorie and nutrient intake.

Soft and Low-Residue Diets

Soft diets often serve as an intermediate step when the patient is progressing from a liquid to a regular diet. Soft diets and low-residue diets will also be used for many people with conditions affecting the GI tract, such as diverticulitis, inflammatory bowel disease, gastritis, and esophageal varices, and during periods of indigestion or diarrhea.

A soft diet is generally low in fiber and in some facilities is called a *low-fiber diet*. It includes foods from all food groups, including meat, fish, poultry, eggs, milk, grains, fruits, and vegetables. Foods excluded are whole grains and high-fiber cereals; nuts; seeds; bran; fried foods; legumes, peas, corn, and gas-producing vegetables such as cabbage; raw fruits (except bananas); and raw vegetables. Usually, foods with strong spices will also be limited. This diet is nutritionally adequate, with the exception of fiber. The low-residue diet is similar to the soft diet but also includes restrictions on milk and milk products because they leave more residue in the colon. If milk is omitted, take care that the patient receives adequate calcium from other sources.

The mechanical soft diet is specifically for those with chewing or swallowing difficulties. This diet eliminates foods that are difficult to chew or swallow. Other foods are sometimes chopped, pureed, or liquefied. This diet is necessary to individualize based on the extent of the patient's chewing or swallowing difficulties.

Box 21-6 Foods Included in Liquid Diets

CLEAR LIQUIDS
- Bouillon
- Fat-free broth
- Grape, apple, cranberry juice
- Fruit drinks
- Popsicles
- Gelatin
- Tea, coffee
- Ginger ale, lemon-lime soda
- Supplemental formulas

FULL LIQUIDS
- All clear liquids
- Strained cereals
- Strained soups
- Fruit and vegetable juices
- Milk, milk shakes
- Ice cream, sherbet
- Custard
- Puddings
- Supplemental formulas

High-Fiber Diets

The high-fiber diet is a variation of the regular diet and is sometimes used therapeutically. It serves as a treatment for some GI disorders and sometimes has a preventive effect against some diseases. High-fiber diets are used in the treatment of constipation. With adequate fluids, fiber has the capacity to reduce constipation in the young, as well as the older adult, which helps reduce or eliminate the need for laxatives. A high-fiber diet is recommended for patients with diverticulosis, the presence of pouchlike herniations through the muscular walls of the colon. A high-fiber diet often helps lessen the severity of symptoms and inflammation (diverticulitis). If diverticulitis occurs, sometimes the patient will need to follow a low-residue diet for a short time until symptoms subside and then gradually return to eating a high-fiber diet.

For most people, doubling the intake of dietary fiber is a reasonable goal to achieve a high-fiber diet. Advise using foods with high fiber content in place of similar foods with little or no fiber, for example, whole-grain rather than refined products. Recommend using fresh-cooked or raw fruits and vegetables rather than canned or processed varieties. Advise patients who are just beginning a high-fiber diet to increase intake gradually so that the body has the chance to become accustomed to larger amounts of fiber. Adequate fluid intake is essential with a high-fiber diet.

Meal Frequency Modifications

Often, especially in GI-related disorders, treatment includes small, frequent meals rather than three larger meals. The patient will consume as many as six to eight small meals or snacks daily. Smaller meals place a lighter workload than large meals on the GI tract, the cardiovascular system, and the respiratory system.

Small, frequent meals are often indicated for GI disorders, such as hiatal hernia and epigastric distress, during periods of nausea or indigestion, for reflux esophagitis, and in pancreatitis. Some physicians will also prescribe them after myocardial infarction or when patients experience decreased appetite.

KILOCALORIE MODIFICATIONS

The body requires a specific amount of energy each day to carry out its tasks. Energy intake includes foods and beverages consumed daily. Energy output includes the amount necessary to maintain vital functions in the body at rest, determined by the basal metabolic rate (BMR). Other energy expenditures fuel physical activity and digestion of food. Perhaps a better way to understand energy balance is to imagine a balance scale with energy intake on one side and energy output on the other (Figure 21-3). When intake equals output, the body is in zero energy balance, or equilibrium. During zero energy balance, weight will remain constant. If energy intake exceeds energy output, the energy balance becomes positive. Positive energy balance results in weight gain. Conversely, if intake is less than output, the energy balance becomes negative, leading to weight loss.

High-Kilocalorie and High-Protein Diets

During times of physiologic stress, such as after surgery, bone fractures, sepsis, burns, or pressure ulcers, and in some forms of cancer, the body's energy and protein needs are increased. Medical trauma has potential to greatly increase the BMR, so that if energy needs are not met by diet, negative energy balance and negative nitrogen balance will result. The patient will lose protein stores and weight.

Many trauma and cancer patients suffer from **anorexia,** or lack of appetite, and sometimes also have difficulty with the eating process. This further complicates the problem of nutritional inadequacies. Dietary treatment does best to aim at restoring energy and nitrogen balance in the normal-weight patient or creating a positive energy and nitrogen balance in the underweight patient. High-kilocalorie and high-protein diets provide increased amounts of kilocalories and protein in a small volume. Suggestions to help increase intake of kilocalories and protein are listed in Box 21-7.

Of course, it is still necessary for the diet to provide a balance of foods from all the food groups. Keep in mind that the appearance of the food and how it is served are often the deciding factor in whether or not the patient eats it. Make sure those serving foods do so with a positive attitude and encouragement. Make meals as attractive as possible. Serve beverages, especially liquid nutritional supplements, in glasses, not cans. Serve foods at the correct temperature: serve meals promptly, and refrigerate snacks and supplements if necessary.

If a patient is not able to consume adequate kilocalories, caregivers will often consider nutritional support in the form of tube feedings or IV feedings. This is discussed later in the chapter.

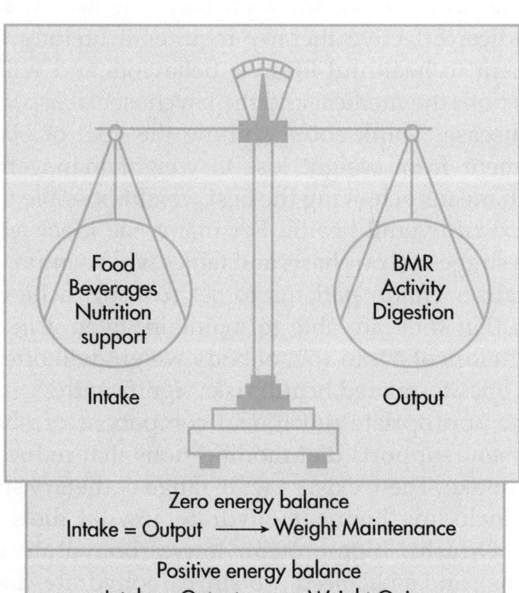

FIGURE 21-3 Energy balance.

Kilocalorie-Controlled and Low-Kilocalorie Diets

Kilocalorie-controlled and low-kilocalorie diets are useful in the treatment of obesity and in the prevention of excess weight gain.

Obesity

The prevalence of obesity has reached epidemic proportions in the United States and is a growing health concern in both developed and developing countries.

Box 21-7 Suggestions for Increasing Kilocalories and Protein

- Add powdered milk or protein powder to milk shakes, beverages, soups, puddings, and cooked cereals.
- Spread peanut butter on crackers, fruit, or celery.
- Add cheese to casseroles, soups, and sauces.
- Use extra meat, chicken, or fish in casseroles and soups.
- Add sugar to foods when reasonable (this adds only kilocalories).
- Use generous amounts of kilocalorie-dense foods such as butter, vegetable oils, mayonnaise, cream cheese, sour cream, and cream in recipes, as spreads, or as dips.
- Add nuts and dried fruits to cereals, breads, or desserts.
- Have snacks available at all times.
- Encourage the patient to eat high-kilocalorie foods first and eat the lower-kilocalorie foods if still hungry.

In the United States, nearly 35% of adults and over 16% of children and adolescents are obese. Obesity increases the risk for many diseases and health conditions including hypertension, coronary heart disease, stroke, type 2 diabetes, dyslipidemias, osteoarthritis, gallbladder disease, some cancers, and sleep apnea. In addition to physical health risks, those who are obese often suffer from social prejudice and psychological issues related to their disease. Obesity dramatically affects quality of life and reduces average life expectancy.

Measurement of obesity. Obesity is defined as an excess of adipose tissue or body fat above the level considered healthy. In the simplest terms, it is overfatness. Body mass index (BMI) has become the medical standard that defines overweight and obesity. BMI is determined by dividing weight (in kilograms) by height (in meters squared). Figure 21-4 lists and classifies the BMIs for various heights and weights. A BMI between 18.5 and 24.9 is associated with the lowest health risk. Those with BMIs between 25 and 29.9 are considered overweight, and those with BMIs of 30 or greater are considered obese. A BMI of less than 18.5 qualifies as underweight and is also associated with health risks.

When using BMI to evaluate health status, it is important to consider **body composition** (the percentage of weight that comes from body fat versus lean tissue). The location and amount of body fat in combination with BMI will sometimes be better predictors of health risk than BMI alone. Excess body fat in the upper body and the abdominal area in particular (central adiposity) increases the risk of cardiovascular disease and diabetes, whereas excess weight in the hips and the lower body poses a lesser risk. For example, a muscular individual will perhaps score in the overweight category on the BMI but have a healthy body fat percentage and thus be at a lower health risk than someone who has the same BMI with a high amount of body fat. The World Health Organization (WHO) (2000) defines obesity as a body fat percentage of 25% or higher in men and 35% or higher in women. Both **waist circumference** and **waist-to-hip ratio** are indices used to identify central adiposity. Waist circumference is measured at the midpoint between the lowest rib and the iliac crest (top of the hip). A waist circumference of 40 inches (102 cm) of more in men and 35 inches (88 cm) of more in women indicates abdominal obesity. Waist-to-hip ratio is calculated by dividing the waist measurement by the hip measurement. A waist-to-hip ratio of more than 0.90 in men and more than 0.85 in women is indicative of abdominal obesity.

Etiology of obesity. Simply put, obesity is caused by the chronic energy imbalance that results when more energy is consumed than expended. There is, however, nothing simple about obesity. It is a complex disease, and much remains to be learned regarding its etiology. Most experts agree that genetic, environmental, and behavioral factors contribute to obesity. The body has a powerful and multifaceted system that regulates energy intake and expenditure. Genetic, hormonal, and metabolic factors combine to control and regulate appetite and energy metabolism. Many obese individuals have a probable predisposition toward obesity that is precipitated by the environment in which they live and the choices they make based on that environment.

Sedentary lifestyles are common in the United States. Only half of adults achieve the recommended amount of physical activity each day, and 25% report no leisure-time physical activity at all. There are fewer jobs requiring physical activity, and many spend their entire workday seated behind a desk. Some schools have cut physical education classes and recess time so children are less physically active at school, and both children and adults often spend their free time in front of a television or computer. In addition, the design of many communities discourages physical activity. For example, it will be unsafe to walk or bike to work or school if there are no sidewalks or bike paths available. The typical American diet is also a factor in the etiology of obesity. Presented with an abundant food supply, it becomes easier to overeat. Food is readily available at any time of day and is possible to eat almost anywhere. High-fat, high-calorie prepackaged foods and sugar-laden soft drinks are readily accessible, and both restaurants and supermarkets serve up increasingly larger portions and package sizes. Rather than sit down to eat at the family or lunchroom table, more people are consuming meals and snacks on the run, in the car, or in front of the computer or television. One frequent consequence of this lifestyle is loss of the ability to recognize feelings of fullness and satisfaction from food, the state of satiety.

Treatment of obesity. Obesity should be treated as a complex, chronic, relapsing disease, and it is necessary to administer treatment with empathy and without prejudice. Effective therapy requires a lifelong commitment to healthful lifestyle behaviors and will address both the medical and the psychosocial aspects of the disease. Think about shifting the goal of obesity treatment from weight loss to weight management, which means achieving the best weight possible in the context of overall health. For many, the ideal weight goals suggested on charts and tables will be impossible to realize. Guide patients to set realistic, achievable goals that they are able to maintain. Even a modest weight loss of 5% to 15% of body weight will often reduce obesity-related health risks significantly.

The appropriate nutritional component of obesity treatment supports diet modifications that reduce energy intake. There exists a wide range of dietary strategies, including high-carbohydrate, low-fat diets (Pritikin, Ornish); high-protein, low-carbohydrate diets (Atkins); and a balanced protein, carbohydrate, and fat diet (Weight Watchers, The Zone, DASH). Each of these diets can lead to successful weight loss under certain conditions. The critical factor is to find the nutrition plan that is most acceptable to the individual and that

Body mass index (BMI) is usually measured with the Quetelet index as follows: weight divided by height squared (W/H^2 [kg/m^2]).
To use the table, find the appropriate height in the left-hand column. Move across to a given weight. The number at the top of the column is the BMI at that height and weight. Pounds have been rounded off.

Body Mass Index	19	20	21	22	23	24	25	26	27	28	29	30	31	32	33	34	35	36	37	38	39	40	41	42	43	44	45	46	47	48	49	50	51	52	53	54
Height (inches)	**Body Weight (pounds)**																																			
58	91	96	100	105	110	115	119	124	129	134	138	143	148	153	158	162	167	172	177	181	186	191	196	201	205	210	215	220	224	229	234	239	244	248	253	258
59	94	99	104	109	114	119	124	128	133	138	143	148	153	158	163	168	173	178	183	188	193	198	203	208	212	217	222	227	232	237	242	247	252	257	262	267
60	97	102	107	112	118	123	128	133	138	143	148	153	158	163	168	174	179	184	189	194	199	204	209	215	220	225	230	235	240	245	250	255	261	266	271	276
61	100	106	111	116	122	127	132	137	143	148	153	158	164	169	174	180	185	190	195	201	206	211	217	222	227	232	238	243	248	254	259	264	269	275	280	285
62	104	109	115	120	126	131	136	142	147	153	158	164	169	175	180	186	191	196	202	207	213	218	224	229	235	240	246	251	256	262	267	273	278	284	289	295
63	107	113	118	124	130	135	141	146	152	158	163	169	175	180	186	191	197	203	208	214	220	225	231	237	242	248	254	259	265	270	278	282	287	293	299	304
64	110	116	122	128	134	140	145	151	157	163	169	174	180	186	192	197	204	209	215	221	227	232	238	244	250	256	262	267	273	279	285	291	296	302	308	314
65	114	120	126	132	138	144	150	156	162	168	174	180	186	192	198	204	210	216	222	228	234	240	246	252	258	264	270	276	282	288	294	300	306	312	318	324
66	118	124	130	136	142	148	155	161	167	173	179	186	192	198	204	210	216	223	229	235	241	247	253	260	266	272	278	284	291	297	303	309	315	322	328	334
67	121	127	134	140	146	153	159	166	172	178	185	191	198	204	211	217	223	230	236	242	249	255	261	268	274	280	287	293	299	306	312	319	325	331	338	344
68	125	131	138	144	151	158	164	171	177	184	190	197	203	210	216	223	230	236	243	249	256	262	269	276	282	289	295	302	308	315	322	328	335	341	348	354
69	128	135	142	149	155	162	169	176	182	189	196	203	209	216	223	230	236	243	250	257	263	270	277	284	291	297	304	311	318	324	331	338	345	351	358	365
70	132	139	146	153	160	167	174	181	188	195	202	209	216	222	229	236	243	250	257	264	271	278	285	292	299	306	313	320	327	334	341	348	355	362	369	376
71	136	143	150	157	165	172	179	186	193	200	208	215	222	229	236	243	250	257	265	272	279	286	293	301	308	315	322	329	338	343	351	358	365	372	379	386
72	140	147	154	162	169	177	184	191	199	206	213	221	228	235	242	250	258	265	272	279	287	294	302	309	316	324	331	338	346	353	361	368	375	383	390	397
73	144	151	159	166	174	182	189	197	204	212	219	227	235	242	250	257	265	272	280	288	295	302	310	318	325	333	340	348	355	363	371	378	386	393	401	408
74	148	155	163	171	179	186	194	202	210	218	225	233	241	249	256	264	272	280	287	295	303	311	319	326	334	342	350	358	365	373	381	389	396	404	412	420
75	152	160	168	176	184	192	200	208	216	224	232	240	248	256	264	272	279	287	295	303	311	319	327	335	343	351	359	367	375	383	391	399	407	415	423	431
76	156	164	172	180	189	197	205	213	221	230	238	246	254	263	271	279	287	295	304	312	320	328	336	344	353	361	369	377	385	394	402	410	418	426	435	443

FIGURE 21-4 Body mass index.

he or she is best able to follow. Generally, good diets will provide no fewer than 1200 kcal/day. On diets of less than 1500 kcal/day, a multivitamin and mineral supplement is recommended. Caution patients against the use of very-low-calorie and semistarvation diets unless they are under the strict care of a physician.

It is advisable for diet therapy to address strategies for maintenance once weight loss is achieved, since regaining weight is a common problem in obesity treatment. Most individuals will have decreased caloric needs after achieving a lower body weight; therefore, caloric intake will most likely have to remain lower for a lifetime. Discuss this with patients as "lifestyle changes," not "a diet." The word *diet* has negative connotations.

Physical activity is an integral part of any weight loss effort and is critical for weight maintenance after initial loss. Recommend the inclusion of approximately 60 to 90 minutes of physical activity most days of the week for initial weight loss, and encourage 60 minutes per day for weight maintenance. This amount of physical activity will perhaps seem daunting to those who have been previously inactive, but encourage a gradual increase of physical activity until the goal of 60 to 90 minutes is achieved. It is possible to accumulate this physical activity in shorter increments throughout the day rather than in one 60- to 90-minute session. Recreational activities such as sports and gardening count toward the physical activity total. Aerobic (oxygen-using) exercises such as brisk walking, jogging, cycling, cross-country skiing, and cross-training appear to be most helpful in decreasing body fat. Resistance training (weight lifting, calisthenics) is also beneficial in maintaining lean body mass and bone density. BMR decreases when muscle mass is lost; therefore, resistance training tends to help prevent a reduction of BMR. As with the diet, encourage people to find a physical activity that they enjoy and will be able to stick with. Exercise need not be extreme; in fact, moderate intensity exercise is more sustainable with less risk of injury.

Effective psychological interventions in the treatment of obesity foster a more healthful attitude about eating and body image. This usually includes counseling about self-esteem, body image, body acceptance, and coping with societal pressures. Patients often need to practice mindfulness and body awareness, learning to sense feelings of fullness by responding to internal, rather than external cues. Through this process, many patients are able to reduce their focus on weight loss and food and establish a more constructive focus on life and good health. A support system of family, friends, or a support group is also beneficial.

Bariatric surgery for the treatment of obesity is becoming more common, and evidence to support the effectiveness of this approach is growing. Candidates for bariatric surgery are usually morbidly obese (BMI ≥40) or have a BMI of 35 or higher with comorbid conditions such as cardiovascular disease or type 2 diabetes. Patients achieve substantial weight loss after surgery, and long-term maintenance of weight loss is greater than with any other treatment. The majority of patients with preexisting diabetes, hyperlipidemia, hypertension, and/or sleep apnea experience improvement or complete resolution of these conditions. In addition, mortality rates of surgically treated obese patients appear to be lower than in those who receive treatment with traditional methods. For most patients, the benefits of bariatric surgery will outweigh the risks; however, as with any major surgery, risks do exist and include nutrition-related complications such as nutrient deficiencies, dumping syndrome, and diarrhea. Strict adherence to dietary protocol and supplement prescriptions usually helps prevent nutritional complications. The proper diet after bariatric surgery emphasizes nutritional balance and variety. Because of the small amount of food that it is possible to eat, the physician will usually prescribe a multivitamin and mineral supplement, along with other nutritional supplements as needed. The most common nutritional deficiencies include iron, folate, and vitamin B_{12}. Eating behavior guidelines after bariatric surgery include small portion sizes, eating slowly and chewing foods completely, consuming beverages and food at separate times, and avoiding foods that are poorly tolerated. As with other weight-management approaches, physical activity is a key component of therapy after bariatric surgery. These patients need to undergo a psychiatric evaluation before surgery.

Pharmacotherapy involves the use of prescription drugs or the many over-the-counter medications currently available for treatment. If patients use weight-loss drugs, it is important to make these drugs part of a comprehensive program including diet therapy and physical activity for those with a BMI of 30 or greater or patients with a BMI of 27 or greater with one or more concomitant risk factors. Over-the-counter medications will sometimes help suppress appetite; however, the effect is usually temporary.

EATING DISORDERS

The three most common eating disorders are anorexia nervosa, bulimia nervosa, and binge eating. These are complex psychiatric disorders related to a number of factors, including individual mental and emotional processes, family relationships, cultural values, and genetic predisposition. Eating disorders are serious, potentially life-threatening conditions affecting emotional and physical health. Approximately 90% of anorexia nervosa and bulimia nervosa cases occur in preadolescent to young adult women. However, increasing numbers of affected boys, older women, and men are emerging. Binge-eating disorder is seen in almost as many men as women. Because of the secretiveness and shame associated with eating disorders, many cases may go unreported. Early detection and treatment of eating disorders increase the likelihood of recovery. Table 21-15 lists diagnostic criteria used to identify eating disorders.

Table 21-15 Comparison of Eating Disorder Diagnoses

	ANOREXIA NERVOSA	BULIMIA NERVOSA	BINGE-EATING DISORDER
Body weight and other physical indicators	Body weight at or below 85% of normal for age, sex, and height Amenorrhea (in women)	Possibly underweight, normal weight, or overweight	Usually obese
Eating behaviors	1. Restricting type: self-imposed starvation or semistarvation 2. Binge-eating or purging type: regular episodes of binge eating (eating an amount of food the patient considers to be excessive)	Recurrent episodes of binge eating—the compulsive eating of an excessive amount of food while feeling a lack of control over eating Binge eating or purging occurs at least twice per week for a period of 3 months or more	Recurrent episodes of binge eating—the compulsive eating of an excessive amount of food while feeling a lack of control over eating Episodes occur at least twice per week for a period of 6 months and are associated with at least three of the following: 1. Eating until uncomfortably full 2. Eating when not physically hungry 3. Eating rapidly 4. Eating alone because of embarrassment 5. Feeling guilt, disgust, or depression after overeating
Compensatory behaviors (purging)	1. Restricting type: may use excessive exercise 2. Binge-eating or purging type: regular episodes of self-induced vomiting or misuse of laxatives, diuretics, or enemas	1. Purging type: regular episodes of self-induced vomiting or the misuse of laxatives, emetics, diuretics, or enemas 2. Nonpurging type: use of fasting or excessive exercise	None
Psychological indicators	Distorted body image—patient perceives herself or himself as fat Intense fear of becoming fat Denial of the problem and its seriousness	Feelings of self-worth disproportionately based on body weight, shape, and size Usually aware that there is a problem	Poor self-esteem, possible depression Aware that there is a problem

Eating disorders are relatively new in medical science, and their prevalence seems to be increasing. These disorders occur almost exclusively in developed nations. Many factors contribute to the development of eating disorders; however, it appears that our society, with its focus on thinness, has contributed to the rise in their occurrence.

Recognizing and treating eating disorders early offers some hope of lessening their effects. Table 21-16 lists some danger signs of these disorders. Above all, it is essential to place the greatest focus on prevention. As a society, we need to concentrate on good health rather than on thinness. Each individual needs to respect and value her or his uniqueness.

Anorexia Nervosa

Anorexia nervosa is an eating disorder characterized by self-imposed starvation. It typically develops in the early to middle stages of adolescence.

Certain characteristics and behaviors are common in individuals with this disorder, including an intense drive for thinness, an intense fear of gaining weight or becoming fat, and a distorted body image such that individuals view themselves as fat even when their weight is much less than average for their height. Some patients exhibit obsessive-compulsive behaviors toward food, attempting to maintain strict control over intake by counting calories meticulously, practicing unusual food behaviors and rituals, making excuses to avoid eating, and hiding food she or he claims to have eaten. Some will vicariously enjoy food by cooking it, serving it, or being around it without eating it. Periods of starvation, compulsive exercising, and purging after meals are among the most common behaviors. Common purging behaviors are self-induced vomiting and the misuse of diuretics, laxatives, emetics, and enemas.

Weight loss and maintenance of weight at or below 85% of goal weight are apparent physical symptoms. Other physical symptoms include cessation of menstruation in women, loss of sexual drive, cold intolerance, the growth of fine hair on the body and the face (lanugo), hypotension, and heart irregularities. Bone

Table 21-16 Signs and Symptoms of Eating Disorders

CATEGORY	SIGNS OR SYMPTOMS
Emotional	Change in attitude or performance Inability to concentrate Body image complaints or concerns: • Refers to self as fat, gross, ugly; overestimates body size; believes he or she is fat when of normal weight or thin • Unable to accept compliments • Constantly compares self to others; self-disparaging comments • Mood affected by thoughts about appearance; seeks outside reassurance about looks Appears sad, depressed, anxious; expresses feelings of worthlessness Obsessed with maintaining low weight to enhance performance in sports, dance, acting, modeling, and the like
Physical	Sudden weight loss, gain, or fluctuation in a short time Abdominal pain; feeling full or "bloated"; bouts of constipation or diarrhea Feeling fatigue or faint, weak, or dizzy Dry hair or skin, dehydration, poor circulation in hands and feet Cold intolerance Lanugo hair (fine hair on body and face) Edematous glands in the neck or beneath the jaw Erosion of tooth enamel, cavities, tooth pain, changes in tooth appearance Amenorrhea in women in childbearing age Insomnia
Behavioral	Caloric restriction and preoccupation with dieting Chaotic food intake; skips meals; exhibits peculiar eating rituals Extreme preoccupation with food; constantly talks about food Secretive eating; binge eating Carries own food; eats small amounts or nothing in front of others Wears baggy clothes: • To hide a very thin body • To hide weight gain • To hide a normal-sized body because of distorted body image Spends increasing amounts of time alone; withdraws from family and friends Displays compulsive or obsessive behaviors Spends frequent and increasing amount of time in the bathroom Abuses laxatives, diuretics, enemas, or diet pills Excessive amounts of exercise

Adapted from National Eating Disorders Association. (2006). *Eating disorder signs and symptoms specific to a school setting.* Available at www.nationaleatingdisorders.org. Accessed December, 2009.

density is compromised, which leads in some cases to compression of vertebrae and stress fractures. The GI tract is affected, causing delayed gastric emptying, slowed peristalsis, and severe constipation. The lining of the digestive tract often deteriorates so that on refeeding, the patient experiences malabsorption, flatulence, and diarrhea. This further compounds the negative perception of food. The brain activity is affected, leading to altered thinking patterns, disturbed sleep, and bad dreams. There is also evidence of structural brain abnormalities (tissue loss), some of which will perhaps be irreversible. Personality and emotional changes are often pronounced. Depression and apathy are possible.

A multidisciplinary approach to treatment is best and involves nutrition therapy and counseling along with psychological and family counseling. Nutritional goals include increasing and improving dietary intake to reverse nutrient deficiencies, achieving a healthy weight for height, and reestablishing normal eating patterns.

Bulimia Nervosa

Bulimia nervosa is an eating disorder characterized by periods of binge eating followed by purging or inappropriate compensatory behavior to prevent weight gain. A binge is the compulsive eating of an amount of food that is considered excessive in normal circumstances. A bulimic person is dominated by a sense of **lack of control** over the eating. Binge eating is followed by purging—self-induced vomiting and the misuse of diuretics, laxatives, emetics, and enemas—or by other compensatory behaviors such as severe caloric restriction, excessive exercising, or the use of diet pills.

Those with bulimia are usually within a normal weight range. Most are aware that their eating patterns are abnormal. They often experience fear of not being able to stop eating and experience depression, guilt, and remorse after a binge. In addition, bulimia tends to occur in combination with other psychiatric disorders such as depression, obsessive-compulsive disorder, substance abuse, and self-injurious behavior. Clinical symptoms of bulimia include possible tooth erosion, calloused knuckles, swollen parotid (salivary) glands, broken blood vessels in the eyes or face, stomach lacerations, and esophageal and sinus infections from excessive vomiting. Electrolyte imbalances are possible and lead to muscle weakness and cramps, abnormal heart rhythms, cardiac complications, and occasionally, sudden death. The use of syrup of ipecac to induce vomiting is extremely dangerous. Syrup of ipecac is cardiotoxic.

Proper treatment for bulimia, like that for anorexia nervosa, is multidisciplinary. Psychological counseling and therapy are necessary. Nutritional goals include improving dietary intake to correct nutritional deficiencies and electrolyte imbalances, and cessation of binge-purge behavior with reestablishment of normal eating. If the patient is overweight, it is best to delay weight loss until eating is normalized.

Binge-Eating Disorder

Binge-eating disorder is a recently recognized disorder sometimes referred to as compulsive overeating. Some believe that this is the most common eating disorder, affecting millions of Americans. Binge-eating disorder is characterized by frequent, recurrent episodes of binge eating; that is, eating a larger amount of food than normal during a short time (within a 2-hour period) and feeling a lack of control over eating during the binge episode. Unlike bulimia nervosa, binge-eating disorder is not associated with purging or inappropriate compensatory behavior.

People with binge-eating disorder are often obese; advise them to consider treatment that focuses on their binge-eating behavior before they attempt to lose weight. Treatment will typically include some combination of cognitive-behavioral therapy, interpersonal psychotherapy, antidepressants, and self-help groups.

CARBOHYDRATE-MODIFIED DIETS

Diabetes Mellitus

The most common type of carbohydrate-modified diet serves in the treatment of diabetes mellitus. Diabetes mellitus is a disease in which the body does not produce or properly use insulin. Insulin is a hormone that is needed to convert sugar, starches, and other food into the energy needed for daily life. The cause of diabetes is unknown, although both genetics and environmental factors such as obesity and lack of exercise appear to play a role.

There are two major types of diabetes. Type 1 diabetes, most often occurring in children and young adults, is a disease in which the body does not produce any insulin. People with type 1 diabetes are required to take daily insulin injections to stay alive. Type 1 diabetes accounts for 5% to 10% of diabetes cases. Type 2 diabetes mellitus is a metabolic disorder resulting from the body's inability to make enough or properly use insulin. It is the most common form of the disease. Type 2 diabetes accounts for 90% to 95% of the incidence of diabetes. Type 2 diabetes is nearing epidemic proportions because of an increased number of older Americans and a greater prevalence of obesity and sedentary lifestyles.

Nutrition Therapy for Diabetes Mellitus

The primary goals for medical nutrition therapy in the treatment of diabetes mellitus are as follows:

1. Improve metabolic outcomes by achieving and maintaining optimal blood glucose, blood lipid, and blood pressure levels.
2. Prevent or slow the rate of development of the chronic complications of diabetes (obesity, dyslipidemia, cardiovascular disease, hypertension, nephropathy, and retinopathy) by modifying nutrient intake and lifestyle.
3. Address individual nutritional needs, taking into consideration personal and cultural preferences and willingness to change.
4. Maintain the pleasure of eating by only limiting food choices when indicated by scientific evidence.

Achieving nutrition-related goals calls for a coordinated team effort including physician, nurse, diabetic educator, registered dietitian, patient, and patient's family. It is necessary to individualize nutrition therapy for diabetes for each patient. Discourage the use of standardized preprinted diet sheets. All patients with diabetes need the opportunity to develop a realistic and achievable eating plan with a professional diet counselor. Lifestyle, current eating and exercise patterns, caloric and nutrient needs, the presence of other diseases, and the use of insulin or oral antidiabetic medication are all necessary to take into consideration when developing an eating plan for the patient with diabetes.

Nutrition recommendations for a healthy lifestyle for the general public are also appropriate for people with diabetes. What differs for those with diabetes is the need to more closely monitor and control carbohydrate intake. If a patient is using insulin or oral diabetic medications, consistency is necessary to achieve a proper balance between the timing and carbohydrate content of meals and snacks and medications. Advise inclusion in the diet of foods containing carbohydrate from whole grains, fruits, vegetables, and low-fat milk. Base the amount of dietary carbohydrate on individual needs. In the past, the prevalent belief regarding diabetes concerned the supposed need to avoid sugars. This belief rested on the theory that since sugars are more rapidly digested and absorbed, they aggravate hyperglycemia. There is, however, little scientific evidence to support this theory. In the context of a healthy diet, it is fine to consume some sugars and sugar-containing foods. The *total amount* of carbohydrate in meals and snacks is more important than the source or type of carbohydrate. Encourage consumption of a variety of fiber-containing foods; however, there is no reason to recommend that those with diabetes consume a greater amount of fiber than you do for any person in the general population.

The primary dietary fat goal for people with diabetes is to limit saturated fat and dietary cholesterol to help control blood lipid levels. Recommendations are to limit saturated fat to less than 7% of calories and dietary cholesterol to less than 200 mg/day. In addition, recommend keeping the intake of *trans* fatty acids to a minimum. Recent evidence shows that the use of monounsaturated fats in place of some carbohydrates will often help lower blood triglyceride levels and improve glycemic control. Two or more servings of fish per week (excepting commercially fried filets) are recommended.

Type 1 diabetes. The diet in type 1 diabetes represents the goal of balancing carbohydrate intake with insulin administration. Determine an acceptable meal plan based on the individual's usual food intake. Then integrate insulin injections or the insulin pump dosage into the usual plan of eating and exercise patterns. Initially, consistent timing and content of meals and snacks is essential to determine insulin requirements. Individuals will then be able to monitor blood glucose levels and learn to make adjustments in insulin dosages based on blood glucose patterns. Because most patients with type 1 diabetes are still in childhood or adolescence at the time of diagnosis, it is necessary for the eating plan to provide adequate kilocalories for normal growth and development and be as flexible as possible.

Type 2 diabetes. The primary goals of nutrition therapy for type 2 diabetes are to provide a nutritionally adequate meal plan that achieves and maintains desirable weight, normal blood cholesterol concentration, and normal blood glucose levels. Because many people with type 2 diabetes are overweight and insulin resistant, it is helpful to encourage lifestyle changes that result in reduced energy intake and increased physical activity. Mild to moderate weight loss (5% to 7% of starting weight) has been shown to improve metabolic control, even if desirable weight is not achieved. Increased physical activity can aid in weight reduction and lead to improved blood glucose levels, decreased insulin resistance, and reduced cardiovascular risk factors.

Diabetic Diet Tools

Exchange lists are often used in diabetic meal planning. Because of the flexibility and variation allowed with exchange lists, they are often used in weight-reduction programs as well. Foods are divided into groups based on carbohydrate, protein, and fat content. Typically, the patient receives instructions to include a certain number of servings from each food group at a particular meal or snack. Helping patients to identify correct serving sizes and the nutrient components of food groups, enables them to better control their carbohydrate, fat, and kilocalorie intake throughout the day. Food groups and serving sizes for diabetic meal planning are found in Box 21-8.

Carbohydrate counting is a meal-planning approach that focuses on the total amount of carbohydrates eaten

Box 21-8 Food Groups and Serving Sizes* for Diabetic Meal Planning

CARBOHYDRATE-CONTAINING CHOICES
Each serving contains approximately 15 g carbohydrate

Grains
Representative servings: ½ cup cooked cereal, ½ cup rice or pasta, 1 oz bread product (1 slice), ¾ cup ready-to-eat cereal (about 1 oz)

Milk and Milk Products
Representative servings: 1 cup skim milk, 1% milk, or buttermilk, 6 oz plain, nonfat yogurt, 1 cup plain soymilk
(NOTE: Cheese included in meat substitutes)

Nonstarchy Vegetables
(contains only 5 g carbohydrate per serving)
Representative servings: ½ cup cooked vegetables or vegetable juice; 1 cup raw vegetables, 2 cups raw leafy greens

Fruit
Representative servings: 1 medium-sized piece fresh fruit, ½ cup canned fruit, ½ cup fruit juice, 1 cup cubed melon or berries, ½ banana

Starchy Vegetables
Representative servings: ½ cup starchy vegetables (potato, corn, peas, winter squash, dried beans and other legumes)

Discretionary Carbohydrates
Representative servings: ½ cup ice cream, 3-inch cookie, 4 oz soft drink, ½ cup pudding, 1/12 angel food cake

MEAT AND FAT CHOICES
Contain little if any carbohydrate per serving

Meat and Meat Substitutes
(NOTE: Beans included in starchy vegetables)
Lean: 1 oz lean meat or fish, 1 oz skinless poultry, ¼ cup cottage cheese
Medium-fat: 1 oz ground meat or poultry with skin, 1 egg, ½ cup tofu
High-fat: 1 oz sausage or hot dog, 1 oz natural cheeses, 2 tbsp peanut butter

Fats and Oils
Monounsaturated fat: 1 tsp oil (olive, canola, peanut, sesame), 4 to 6 nuts, 8 large olives, 2 tbsp avocado
Polyunsaturated fat: 1 tsp margarine, mayonnaise, or oil (corn, soybean, cottonseed, safflower), 1 tbsp salad dressing
Saturated fat: 1 tsp butter or shortening, 1 tbsp cream or cream cheese, 2 tbsp sour cream, half and half, gravy, coconut, 1 slice bacon

*Serving sizes adapted for carbohydrate content from www.MyPyramid.gov.

at meals and snacks. The primary premises of carbohydrate counting are that carbohydrate found in foods is the primary nutrient affecting blood glucose levels, and that careful attention to carbohydrate quantity and distribution offers improved metabolic control in diabetes. Patients are taught to identify carbohydrate-containing food groups: starch and bread, fruit, milk, and other carbohydrates. Patients are given a certain number of carbohydrate choices at each meal and snack. One carbohydrate choice is equal to 15 g of carbohydrate. In addition to carbohydrate choices, patients learn to eat established amounts of protein and fat each day for good health, but they are allowed to eat them anytime throughout the day. A sample menu using MyPyramid and carbohydrate counting is found in Table 21-17.

Other Nutritional Considerations

If a person taking insulin fails to consume adequate carbohydrate, a drop in blood glucose levels is possible, causing hypoglycemia (low blood glucose). Symptoms of hypoglycemia include headache, disorientation, weakness, perspiration, shallow breathing, nervousness, visual disturbances, and vertigo, and it sometimes leads to unconsciousness. Sometimes the person experiencing hypoglycemia gives the mistaken impression of being intoxicated. It is advisable to wear proper medical identification to prevent such a mistake. It is necessary to treat hypoglycemia with immediate administration of glucose or any carbohydrate that contains glucose. A good strategy for patients is to practice the 15-15 rule: take 15 g of carbohydrate, wait 15 minutes, and test blood glucose to see if the response to the carbohydrate is adequate. In the event unconsciousness has occurred, intravenous administration of glucose is essential.

Acute illness in persons with type 1 diabetes increases the risk of diabetic ketoacidosis. Insulin requirements continue and sometimes even rise during illness. It is important to continue insulin, carefully monitor blood glucose levels, drink adequate amounts of fluids,

Table 21-17 Sample Menu Using MyPyramid and Carbohydrate Counting*

FOOD ITEM	FOOD GROUP	NUMBER OF CARBOHYDRATE CHOICES	TOTAL CARBOHYDRATE CHOICES PER MEAL
BREAKFAST			
1 cup oatmeal w/ cinnamon	Grain	2	
2 tbsp raisins	Fruit	1	
½ cup skim milk	Milk	½	
1 cup tea			
			3½
LUNCH			
Sandwich (2 slices whole wheat bread, 2 oz tuna, 1 tbsp salad dressing)	Grain Lean meat Oils	2	
Potato salad (½ cup potatoes, 1 tbsp salad dressing)	Starchy vegetable Oil	1	
			3
SNACK			
1 fresh peach	Fruit	1	
6 oz sugar-free vanilla yogurt	Milk	1	
			2
DINNER			
3 oz grilled skinless chicken	Lean meat		
1 cup rice pilaf	Grain	2	
2 cups lettuce salad with fresh vegetables	Nonstarchy vegetable	⅓	
1 tbsp Italian dressing	Oil		
1 cup green beans	Nonstarchy vegetable	⅔	
½ cup strawberry ice cream	Discretionary carbohydrate	1	
			4
SNACK			
1 medium apple	Fruit	1	
1 oz whole-grain crackers	Grain	1	
1 oz cheddar cheese	Meat substitute		
			2

*This menu provides 1700 kcal and 220 g carbohydrate.

and ingest carbohydrates, especially if the blood glucose level falls below 100 mg/dL. Beverages such as juices and punch, Popsicles, flavored gelatin, crackers, puddings, and ice cream all contain carbohydrates and tend to be more palatable to the sick person.

For people with diabetes, the guidelines for alcohol use are the same as for the general population. If individuals choose to drink alcohol, teach them to limit intake to one drink per day for adult women and two drinks per day for adult men. Because alcohol increases the risk of hypoglycemia, consuming it with food is best.

Dumping Syndrome

Dumping syndrome is possible after surgery in which a portion or all of the stomach is removed (partial or total gastrectomy) or after bariatric surgery for weight reduction. After partial or total gastrectomy, the stomach contents sometimes empty too rapidly into the jejunum. The body reacts by sending water to the intestinal tract, thus reducing blood pressure. The load in the intestinal tract increases peristalsis, leading to diarrhea. Signs and symptoms occur shortly after meals and include cramping, weakness, diaphoresis, vertigo, nausea, and possibly vomiting.

Diet therapy involves giving small, frequent meals that are higher in protein and fat and lower in carbohydrates. Advise the patient to avoid concentrated sweets, and to take fluids 30 to 60 minutes before or after a meal. The dumping syndrome diet will in some cases be needed only temporarily until the body adjusts to the changes caused by surgery.

Lactose Intolerance

Lactose intolerance occurs as a result of a lack of the digestive enzyme **lactase.** Because of this lack, the GI tract is unable to break down lactose, the milk sugar. Symptoms occur after ingestion of milk products and include nausea, cramps, a bloated feeling, flatulence, and diarrhea.

Diet for lactose intolerance excludes milk and milk products, such as ice cream, puddings, cheese, and powdered milk. The person often needs to avoid foods with milk added, such as biscuit or muffin mixes, some soups, and other prepared foods.

Some individuals have a deficiency rather than a total absence of lactase. These individuals are often able to tolerate small amounts of milk products, especially yogurt and cheese. Lactase enzyme–containing preparations are available to take before consuming dairy products. Lactose-free milks and milk products are available in most grocery stores.

FAT-MODIFIED DIETS

Fat- and cholesterol-controlled diets help reduce the risk of atherosclerosis and certain cancers. Dietary fat intake is also modified in the treatment of some diseases.

Fat-Controlled Diets

A fat-controlled diet is desirable for the prevention and treatment of **atherosclerosis** (a disorder characterized by buildup of cholesterol and lipids on the artery walls), heart disease, and **hyperlipidemia** (elevated levels of blood lipids such as cholesterol and triglycerides). Diabetic diets also incorporate fat control. A fat-controlled diet limits total fat, saturated fat, and *trans* fatty acids (Table 21-18).

The American Heart Association (AHA) promotes dietary guidelines for the general population to enhance health and reduce the risk of cardiovascular disease. The National Cholesterol Education Program has developed the Therapeutic Lifestyle Changes (TLC) diet. The TLC diet is the first step in treatment of patients with elevated blood lipids and existing cardiovascular disease (Table 21-19).

Table 21-18 Some Characteristics of Cholesterol-Lowering Diets

NUTRIENT	AMERICAN HEART ASSOCIATION DIETARY GUIDELINES	NATIONAL CHOLESTEROL EDUCATION PROGRAM (NCEP) THERAPEUTIC LIFESTYLE CHANGES (TLC) DIET
Total fat	≤30% of total kcal	25%-35% of total kcal
Saturated fat (including *trans* fatty acids)	≤10% of total kcal	≤7% of total kcal
Polyunsaturated fat	Up to 10% of total kcal	Up to 10% of total kcal
Monounsaturated fat	Remaining total fat kcal	Up to 20% of total kcal
Cholesterol	≤300 mg/day	≤200 mg/day
Carbohydrate	5 or more fruits and vegetables and 6 or more grain servings per day	50%-60% of total kcal
Fiber	Choose whole grains and high-fiber fruits and vegetables	20-30 g/day
Total calories	Match intake of total energy to overall energy needs	Balance energy intake with expenditure to maintain desirable body weight/prevent weight gain
Sodium	<2400 mg/day	<2400 mg/day
Other	Two servings of fish per week	

Data from American Heart Association. (2000). Dietary guidelines. *Circulation, 102,* 2284; and National Heart, Lung, and Blood Institute. (2001). The Third Report of the NCEP Expert Panel on Detection, Evaluation, and Treatment of High Blood Cholesterol: Executive summary. *JAMA, 285*(19), 2490.

Table 21-19 Guidelines for Following the Therapeutic Lifestyle Changes (TLC) Diet

FOOD GROUPS	CHOOSE . . .	GO EASY ON . . .
Meat, poultry, and fish (<5 oz/day; 2 servings of fish/week) **Eggs** (<2 egg yolks/week) **Dry beans and nuts**	• Lean fresh meats, extra lean ground beef, and lean deli meats* • Poultry without the skin, ground turkey made from white meat • Fish and shellfish • Eggs (limit yolks to 2/week; substitute 2 egg whites for 1 egg in recipes) • Dry beans and peas, fat-free refried beans, tofu • Nuts* (in moderation)	• Meats with visible fat and marbling • Regular ground beef • Processed meats: sausage, bacon, frankfurters, cold cuts • Organ meats • Duck and goose • Deep-fried meats, poultry, or fish • Some shellfish is high in cholesterol—use moderate portions
Milk, yogurt, and cheese (2-3 servings/day)	• Fat-free (skim) or 1% milk, buttermilk, soy milk • Fat-free or reduced-fat cheeses* (3 g of fat or less per oz) • Low-fat or nonfat cottage cheese* • Low-fat or fat-free yogurt	• Whole or 2% milk, half-and-half • Whole-milk yogurt • Full-fat cheese with more than 3 g fat per oz
Fruits and vegetables (5 or more servings/day)	• Fresh, frozen, canned, or dried fruits and vegetables • Add more vegetables to meat dishes, casseroles, or soups • Keep fresh fruits and vegetables readily available for snacks • Use fruit as dessert	• Vegetables with high-calorie sauces • Fruits with added sugar • Deep-fried vegetables (including French fries) • Limit juices, instead choosing whole fruits and vegetables for more fiber
Breads, cereals, rice, pasta, and other grains (6 or more servings/day depending on energy needs)	• Breads, bread products, and cereals made from whole grains such as whole wheat, buckwheat, bulgur (cracked wheat), oats, rye, millet, quinoa, bran • Brown rice, wild rice • Whole-grain pastas • Popcorn	• White breads and products made with refined grains that are lower in fiber (check label) • Baked goods made with added fat and eggs, such as muffins, biscuits, croissants and butter rolls
Fats and oils (Limited total amount; replace saturated fats with unsaturated fats; read labels to identify saturated and *trans* fat content)	• Liquid vegetable oils (canola, corn, olive, peanut, safflower, sesame, soybean, and sunflower) • Margarines with liquid vegetable oils as first ingredient (soft tub, liquid, or vegetable oil spreads) • Light or nonfat mayonnaise and salad dressing • Reduced-fat sour cream, cream cheese, and whipped toppings	• Butter, lard, fatback, bacon drippings • Margarines with hydrogenated or partially hydrogenated oil as the first ingredient (read label for *trans* fat) • Solid shortening • Coconut milk; coconut, palm and palm-kernel oils • Full-fat sour cream, cream cheese, whipped cream
Sweets, snacks, condiments (To be used occasionally based on caloric needs)	• Low-fat ice cream, frozen yogurt, sorbet, sherbet, or low-fat puddings • Angel food cake; low-fat brownies • Fat-free or low-fat cookies such as animal crackers, vanilla wafers, gingersnaps, graham crackers • Whole-grain snack crackers*	• Regular ice cream; pudding made with whole or 2% milk • Doughnuts and pastries • Pie, regular cakes and cookies • Snack crackers with high-fat content

Adapted from National Heart, Lung, and Blood Institute. *Tip sheet: TLC daily food guide*. Available at www.nhlbisupport.com/chd1/S2Tipsheets/foodgroup.htm.
*Sometimes contain high levels of sodium.

Individuals who are reducing saturated and *trans* fatty acids in the diet are still able to choose low-fat foods from all the food groups. Encourage them to choose low-fat dairy products, lean meats, skinless poultry, and fish. Advise limiting eggs to four or fewer per week, and organ meats, such as liver, to one serving per week or less. Limits are also necessary on added fats, such as butter, stick margarine, mayonnaise, cream, and sour cream.

The inclusion of monounsaturated fats in the diet often helps lower blood cholesterol and triglyceride levels. Likewise, the cardiovascular benefits of **omega-3 fatty acids**—a particular type of unsaturated fat found in fatty fish, flaxseed oil, and soy products—have emerged. Therefore, encourage patients to substitute unsaturated fatty acids from fish, vegetables, legumes, and nuts in place of saturated and *trans* fatty acids. Many people are unfamiliar with these products or have avoided these foods in the past and will need to learn ways to include these foods in the diet, as well as new shopping and food preparation techniques. Teach patients to identify food sources of these fats such as fish, olive oil, canola oil, peanut oil, flaxseed oil, soy products, and nuts.

As medical professionals, we must not forget the qualities fat possesses and the pleasure it offers. Many Americans believe that to have a low-fat diet, it is necessary to completely eliminate all high-fat foods. This is not so. Choosing a low-fat and low-cholesterol diet does not mean "never eat cheese because it contains fat" or "never eat egg yolks because they contain cholesterol." It is the *total* amount of fat, saturated fat, and cholesterol that matters. Besides, foods such as cheese and egg yolks contribute important nutrients to the diet. Sometimes eliminating all high-fat foods compromises the diet's overall nutritional value. For example, consider an older woman who has been prescribed a low-fat, low-cholesterol diet. In an effort to reduce fat and cholesterol, she decides to eliminate dairy products from her diet. Although she is consuming less saturated fat and cholesterol, she is also receiving less protein, calcium, riboflavin, and vitamin B_{12}. Although she has reduced her risk for heart disease, she has increased her risk for osteoporosis.

Rather than totally eliminating high-fat foods, encourage moderation. Balance high-fat foods with other foods that contain less fat and cholesterol. For example, if patients desire ice cream after dinner, which is high in fat, they should choose a low-fat entrée such as broiled fish or chicken. Educate patients to read nutrition labels and nutrition information materials and to become familiar with the amounts of fat in various food items. They will then be able to monitor portion sizes and budget their fat intake to be less than or equal to their daily fat allowance. By adhering to balance, variety, and moderation, patients are still able to enjoy some of their favorite foods while following a healthy, fat-controlled diet.

Metabolic Syndrome

The metabolic syndrome is a constellation of metabolic risk factors, including abdominal obesity, dyslipidemia (elevated triglycerides and low HDL cholesterol), elevated blood pressure, and insulin resistance. This combination of risk factors appears to directly promote the development of atherosclerotic cardiovascular disease (ASCVD) and type 2 diabetes. The most important of these risk factors appears to be abdominal obesity (waist circumference of 40 inches or more in men and 35 inches or more in women) and insulin resistance (fasting blood sugar of 100 mg/dL or higher). The prevalence of metabolic syndrome has increased dramatically in recent years with an estimated 50 million cases in the United States. For those without established diabetes, metabolic syndrome doubles the risk of developing ASCVD; for those with diabetes, the risk is increased fivefold. Thus, the early diagnosis and treatment of metabolic syndrome promises to help reduce the incidence of ASCVD. Criteria used in the diagnosis of metabolic syndrome are listed in Table 21-20.

Lifestyle therapy is the first-line intervention in the treatment of metabolic syndrome. Major lifestyle interventions include cessation of cigarette smoking, weight loss in overweight or obese individuals, increased physical activity, and a fat-controlled diet (Box 21-9).

Table 21-20 Diagnostic Criteria for Metabolic Syndrome

MEASURE*	CATEGORICAL CUT POINTS
Elevated waist circumference	≥102 cm (≥40 inches) in men ≥88 cm (≥35 inches) in women
Elevated triglycerides	≥150 mg/dL (1.7 mmol/L) *Or* Drug treatment for elevated triglycerides
Reduced HDL cholesterol	<40 mg/dL (<1.3 mmol/L) in men <50 mg/dL (<1.3 mmol/L) in women *Or* Drug treatment for reduced HDL
Elevated blood pressure	≥130 mm Hg systolic blood pressure *Or* ≥85 mm Hg diastolic blood pressure *Or* Drug treatment for hypertension
Elevated fasting blood glucose	≥100 mg/dL *Or* Drug treatment for elevated glucose

From Grundy, S.M., et al. (2005). Diagnosis and management of the metabolic syndrome. *Circulation, 112*(17), e285.
HDL, High-density lipoprotein.
*NOTE: Any three of the five criteria constitutes a diagnosis of metabolic syndrome.

Box 21-9 Treatment of Lifestyle Risk Factors in Metabolic Syndrome

ABDOMINAL OBESITY

Goal: Reduce body weight by 7% to 10% during first year of therapy. Continue weight loss thereafter to extent possible with goal to ultimately achieve desirable weight (BMI <25).

PHYSICAL INACTIVITY

Goal: Regular moderate-intensity physical activity; at least 30 minutes of continuous or intermittent (preferably 60 minutes) 5 days/week, but preferably every day.

ATHEROGENIC DIET

Goal: Reduced intakes of saturated fat, *trans* fat, and cholesterol (use Therapeutic Lifestyle Changes [TLC] diet)

From Grundy, S.M., et al. (2005). Diagnosis and management of the metabolic syndrome. *Circulation, 112*(17), e285.

Depending upon the severity of risk factors, the need for more aggressive treatments is possible, including the use of therapeutic drugs.

Low-Fat Diets

Low-fat diets differ from fat-controlled diets in that all fats are limited, regardless of saturation. Any time fat malabsorption occurs, a need to limit dietary fat is possible. GI diseases that involve malabsorption of fat include cystic fibrosis, inflammatory bowel disease, pancreatitis, and short-bowel syndrome (secondary to bowel resection). Those with cystic fibrosis (CF) experience pancreatic insufficiency and thus, malabsorption of fat. However, the use of oral enzyme therapy before meals and snacks helps reduce malabsorption, allowing CF patients to consume a diet higher in fat. Gallbladder disease often calls for a low-fat diet. Some patients with gallbladder disease will be overweight or obese. Weight reduction is indicated for these individuals and has the potential to reduce symptoms of disease.

Low-fat diets sometimes restrict fat to as little as 25 g/day. With this severe fat restriction, no visible fats are allowed (e.g., butter, cream, oil). Only nonfat dairy products and lean meat, fish, and poultry (no more than 5 oz/day) are allowed. Emphasize adequate grains, cereals, fruits, and vegetables.

Some patients are unable to digest regular fats (long-chain triglycerides). Occasionally the use of a special type of fat called medium-chain triglycerides (MCTs) is necessary. This type of fat is absorbed readily and requires minimal digestion. MCTs are expensive and generally available only in special supplemental formulas.

PROTEIN-, ELECTROLYTE-, AND FLUID-MODIFIED DIETS

Protein-Restricted Diets

In disease states, increased protein intake is often considered to facilitate healing. However, in the presence of defects in protein metabolism or excretion, it is best to reduce or at least control protein intake. Two such conditions—chronic renal failure and cirrhosis of the liver—sometimes warrant protein restrictions.

In renal failure, the kidney is unable to excrete protein waste products. These waste products will sometimes build up in the bloodstream, leading to a condition known as azotemia. If a patient is experiencing renal failure, sometimes a modest protein restriction is beneficial in delaying the need for dialysis (a medical procedure for the removal of certain elements from the blood). Protein restriction in renal failure involves limiting the total amount of protein consumed and emphasizing the use of high-quality proteins. High-quality proteins are complete proteins found in eggs, meat, poultry, fish, and milk products. Incomplete proteins, those found in plant products such as dried beans and whole grains, contribute to azotemia and will be limited. Once a patient has been placed on renal dialysis, protein needs are greater than for the normal population; however, the dietary emphasis is still on complete proteins.

During cirrhosis (a chronic degenerative disease of the liver), scar tissue develops in the liver, hampering its effectiveness in removing ammonia (a waste product of protein metabolism), which builds up in the bloodstream. If not controlled, high ammonia levels have the potential to lead to hepatic coma, brain damage, and death. In the presence of cirrhosis, keep protein intake initially at or above the DRI to facilitate healing and tissue regeneration. However, if blood ammonia levels become elevated, the patient will need to follow a low-protein diet. Special nutritional support formulas with modified protein content have been developed for both renal failure and hepatic coma.

Sodium-Restricted Diets

Sodium restrictions are used to treat a number of medical conditions. Hypertension is often responsive to a lowered sodium intake. The Dietary Approaches to Stop Hypertension (DASH) diet (National Institutes of Health & National Heart, Lung, and Blood Institute, 2001) has been found to effectively lower blood pressure. It involves limiting sodium intake to either 2400 or 1500 mg/day. The DASH diet also emphasizes fruit and vegetable intakes of 8 to 12 servings per day and 2 to 4 servings of low- or nonfat milk products. Information on the DASH diet is available from the National Heart, Lung, and Blood Institute (www.nhlbi.nih.gov).

Sodium is also restricted when water retention or edema is present. In the presence of congestive heart failure, a decrease in sodium intake is necessary to alleviate pulmonary and peripheral edema. Directly after a myocardial infarction, sodium, fluid, kilocalorie, and fat restrictions are often implemented. These restrictions are to reduce the workload on the heart to a minimum. As recovery progresses, the diet will be liberalized as the individual's condition permits. If cirrhosis is accompanied by ascites, reduce sodium intake. In chronic renal failure, sodium restriction is necessary for blood pressure control and to reduce feelings of thirst.

Sodium-restricted diets vary in degree. The no-added-salt (NAS) diet is the least restrictive, allowing 2000 to 3000 mg/day of sodium. This diet allows the use of most foods with the exception of highly salted snack foods and prepared foods. Patients following this diet will have to read nutrition labels to assess the sodium content of food products and determine which will be appropriate for their diet. Advise the addition of little or no salt in cooking or at the table (Box 21-10). Permitted amounts on other sodium-restricted diets range from 2000 mg/day (2 g) to as little as 500 mg/day of sodium.

Box 21-10 What to Limit in Sodium-Restricted Diets

- Salt in cooking or at the table
- Salt-preserved foods, such as smoked or cured meats or pickled foods
- Regular canned soups, broths, and bouillon
- Spices and condiments that contain sodium, such as soy sauce, barbeque sauce, Worcestershire and steak sauces, meat tenderizers, monosodium glutamate (MSG), spice salts, and salad dressings
- Leavening agents such as baking soda and powder
- Canned vegetables (fresh and frozen are lower in sodium)
- Salty snack foods such as pretzels, popcorn, and chips
- Processed cheeses
- Commercial mixes such as pasta, stuffing, muffins, and potatoes

NOTE: Generally, the more processed or "instant" a food is, the more sodium it will contain.

In the presence of cystic fibrosis, the sweat glands produce excessive amounts of sodium and chloride. In this special condition, there is no restriction on sodium intake; indeed, encourage generous amounts of sodium and salt to compensate for the large losses of sodium through sweat.

Potassium-Modified Diets

An increased intake of potassium sometimes helps with blood pressure control. The American Heart Association and proponents of the DASH diet encourage a diet that emphasizes fruits, vegetables, and low-fat dairy products. This diet is rich in potassium, magnesium, and calcium and helps reduce blood pressure in many cases. People taking potassium-wasting diuretics need larger amounts of potassium or potassium supplements.

In end-stage renal disease and other kidney disease, it is sometimes necessary to restrict potassium intake to as little as 2000 mg/day. During renal failure, potassium is retained, leading to a buildup of potassium in the bloodstream. If dietary intake is not controlled, blood potassium levels will potentially increase to the point of causing dysrhythmias and sudden cardiac arrest.

Fluid-Modified Diets

Fluid in a number of forms is part of the diet. Of course, all beverages—milk, juice, coffee, and tea—add fluid to the diet. Other dietary fluid sources include gelatins, ice cream, sherbet, puddings, Popsicles, fruit ices, and soups.

During end-stage renal disease and other kidney disease with low urine output, fluid is restricted to 500 to 750 mL/day (approximately 2 to 3 cups) plus an amount equal to daily urine output. Fluid restrictions are also common for patients during congestive heart failure, directly after a myocardial infarction, or in hepatic coma or ascites.

In the hospital, fluid restrictions are often divided between the nursing and the dietary departments. For example, if a patient is on a 1000-mL fluid restriction, the dietary department will sometimes be allowed to provide the patient with 600 mL, and the nursing department will give 400 mL/day. The amount of fluid allowed for nursing depends on the patient's IV and medication needs.

While patients have fluid restrictions, they often experience excessive thirst. Some suggestions to help alleviate thirst include rinsing the mouth with cold mouthwash, putting lemon into cold water to make it more refreshing, freezing fluid so it takes longer to consume, eating cold fruits and raw vegetables, chewing gum, sucking on breath mints or hard candies (in moderation), brushing teeth often, and limiting sodium intake (see Patient Teaching box on fluid restrictions).

Increased fluid intake is a common dietary treatment for renal calculi (kidney stones) and urinary tract infection. Additional fluid helps dilute the urine and increase urinary output. Fluid needs are also higher during periods of diarrhea, vomiting, or malabsorption, such as in inflammatory bowel disease. To prevent dehydration, the patient needs to take care to replace fluids that are lost.

A burn victim loses a large volume of fluids from the wounds. Immediately after a severe burn, fluids, electrolytes, and protein are given intravenously rather than orally, because burn patients experience a temporary loss of bowel function. Once bowel activity resumes, adequate fluids are a necessary part of dietary treatment. Burn victims also require enormous amounts of protein, kilocalories, and certain vitamins and minerals.

Most conditions requiring diet therapy involve combinations of therapeutic diets. To summarize, Table 21-21 lists different medical conditions and their commonly prescribed diets.

Patient Teaching

Fluid Restrictions

The physician and dietitian will determine the exact fluid restriction. You have the opportunity to help teach and reinforce the fluid restriction in the following ways:

- Explain the rationale for the fluid restriction.
- Indicate whether the restriction is temporary.
- Identify the various sources of fluid intake (e.g., IV fluids, fluid with medications, fluid in foods such as soup, ice cream, or gelatin).
- Teach what "mL" represents, and compare to measures with which the patient is familiar. For example, "You are allowed 1000 mL of fluid per day. This is about the same as 1 quart or 4 cups."
- Show patients the volume of fluid they are allowed.
- Suggest ways to alleviate thirst without drinking fluids.
- Discuss the consequences of overconsumption of fluids.

Table 21-21 Summary of Diet Modifications

CONDITION	POSSIBLE DIET MODIFICATIONS
Acquired immunodeficiency syndrome (AIDS)	High kilocalorie and protein; increased fluid intake; mechanical soft diet; possible tube feeding or TPN
Atherosclerosis	Fat controlled; high fiber; when necessary, kilocalorie or sodium restricted
Burns	High kilocalorie and protein; increased fluid intake; vitamin/mineral therapy
Cancer	High kilocalorie and protein (in some forms); dietary adjustments made based on symptoms; possible tube feeding or TPN
Cirrhosis, hepatic coma	Protein restricted; possible sodium, fat, and fluid restriction; no alcohol; vitamin and mineral supplementation
Congestive heart failure	Sodium restricted; fluid restricted; small, frequent feedings; soft diet; possible kilocalorie restriction
Constipation	High fiber; increased fluid intake
Cystic fibrosis	High kilocalorie and protein; generous sodium; vitamin and mineral supplementation, enzyme replacement therapy
Diabetes mellitus	Carbohydrate controlled; fat controlled; high fiber
Diverticulitis	Soft, low residue
Diverticulosis	High fiber
Dumping syndrome	Carbohydrate restricted; no concentrated sweets; small, frequent feedings
Gallbladder disease	Low fat; when necessary, kilocalorie restricted
Gastritis	Low residue
Hepatitis	High kilocalorie and protein
Hiatal hernia	Small, frequent feedings; low fat; bland; when necessary, kilocalorie restricted
Hyperlipidemia	Fat controlled; when necessary, kilocalorie restricted; carbohydrate controlled
Hypertension	Sodium restricted; high potassium; kilocalorie controlled, limit alcohol
Hypoglycemia	No concentrated sweets; small, frequent feedings; higher protein
Inflammatory bowel disease	Low residue; low fat; high kilocalorie and protein; fluid and electrolyte replacement; vitamin and mineral supplementation; possible lactose restriction, possible bland diet; tube feeding or TPN
Lactose intolerance	Lactose restricted for lactose intolerance
Malabsorption	Low fat; high kilocalorie and protein; fluid and electrolyte replacement
Mouth	Mechanical soft diet; possible tube feeding
Broken jaw or oral surgery	Mechanical soft diet
Dental caries, periodontal disease, ill-fitting dentures, missing teeth	Mechanical soft diet
Dry mouth	Mechanical soft diet; increased fluid intake
Dysphagia (difficulty swallowing)	Individualize diet; possible tube feeding
Ulcers of mouth or gums	Mechanical soft diet; limit acidic and spicy foods
Heart attack	Low sodium; kilocalorie restricted; soft, frequent feedings; fat controlled; fluid restricted (temporary); moderate-temperature foods
Nausea	Soft; small, frequent feedings
Obesity	Kilocalorie restricted; fat controlled; high fiber
Pancreatitis	Low fat; small, frequent feedings; possible tube feedings or TPN
Reflux esophagitis	Small, frequent feedings; low fat
Renal calculi (kidney stones)	Increased fluid intake; possible calcium controlled
Renal failure	
Acute	Protein restricted; high kilocalorie; fluid, sodium, and potassium controlled
Chronic	Protein controlled; low sodium; potassium, fluid, and phosphorus restricted; vitamin and mineral supplement
Underweight	High kilocalorie and protein
Vomiting	Fluid and electrolyte replacement
Wound healing, pressure ulcers	High protein, adequate kilocalorie, adequate fluid, possible supplementation of vitamin C and zinc

Modified from Cataldo, C.B., et al. (1989). *Nutrition and diet therapy: principles and practice.* (2nd ed.). St. Paul, Minn: West.
TPN, Total parenteral nutrition.

NUTRITIONAL SUPPORT

Occasionally a patient is unable to consume an oral diet. For whatever reason, alternative feeding methods are available in the form of tube feedings or IV feedings.

TUBE FEEDINGS

A tube feeding is the administration of nutritionally balanced liquefied foods or formula through a tube inserted into the stomach, the duodenum, or the jejunum by way of a nasoenteric tube or a feeding ostomy. The feeding is sometimes referred to as enteral nutrition (administration of nutrients into the GI tract) support. Tube feedings are typically indicated when a patient is unable to chew or swallow, such as after oral surgery or facial trauma; when a patient has no appetite or refuses to eat; in times of great nutritional need, such as in the patient suffering burns or trauma; in the comatose patient; or during periods of moderate malabsorption or diarrhea.

Tube feedings will be used only when all or at least part of the GI tract is functioning. Tube feedings are most commonly administered by way of a nasogastric tube, that is, a tube that is passed through the nose and into the stomach (Figure 21-5). If regurgitation is common or gastric residual is high, a nasojejunal or nasoduodenal tube (a tube that is passed through the nose and into the jejunum or the duodenum) will sometimes be used to reduce the risk of aspiration.

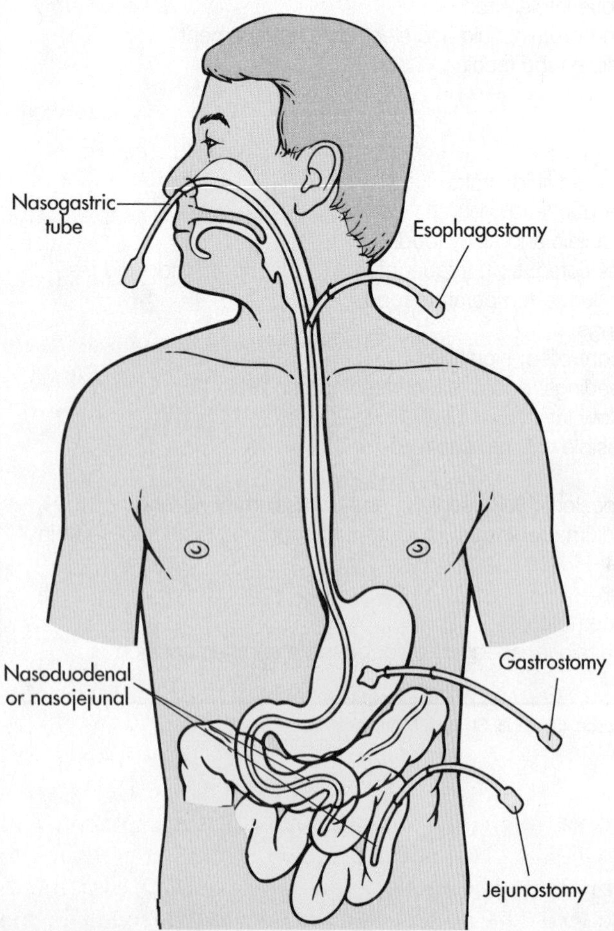

FIGURE 21-5 Tube feeding sites.

In cases in which long-term tube feedings are necessary, such as in a patient with a gastrectomy or intestinal resection or in a patient with an upper GI obstruction, feeding ostomies are sometimes employed. Feeding ostomies are surgical openings through which a feeding tube passes. It is possible to make ostomies into the esophagus (esophagostomy), the stomach (gastrostomy), or the jejunum (jejunostomy) (see Figure 21-5). Ostomy feeding need not be continuous but are possible to give intermittently, permitting more freedom of movement.

In the hospital, tube feedings on a continuous basis are possible, using a continuous drip pump that administers the formula slowly over 16 to 24 hours. Feedings are also possible to give intermittently. This involves giving a specific volume of formula over a short time, about 20 to 30 minutes. This will usually be done four to six times daily. Intermittent feeding is preferred by many long-term tube-fed patients. Bolus feedings (giving a 4- to 6-hour volume of formula in a matter of minutes) are also given sometimes, but most patients tolerate them poorly.

Tube feedings are considered to be aggressive nutrition therapy, and it is necessary to monitor them closely. Distention, diarrhea, and nausea usually indicate that the formula strength, volume, or rate is too great. Dumping syndrome is also possible with rapid and concentrated formula delivery. Complications arise at times, including diarrhea; contamination of formula; infection; aspiration; overhydration or dehydration; abnormalities of blood concentrations of electrolytes, glucose, and other nutrients; and development of liver abnormalities (Table 21-22). See the Home Care Considerations box for patients receiving enteral feeding.

Nasogastric Tube Feedings

Checking for placement of a feeding tube before administering medication or tube feeding is critical to

Home Care Considerations

Patients Receiving Enteral Feeding

- Teach the patient or primary caregiver (1) to assess the placement of the tube before administering formula; (2) the method of gastrointestinal (GI) fluid pH measurement and the expected range; (3) *not* to administer a feeding if there is any doubt concerning tube placement; and (4) to administer feedings at room temperature.
- Teach the patient to report any adverse signs and symptoms, such as diarrhea, abdominal cramps, nausea and vomiting, or respiratory distress.
- Teach the patient to care for the gastrostomy or jejunostomy tube site and about adverse signs and symptoms to report (such as drainage, redness, swelling, or tube displacement).

Table 21-22 Common Problems and Nursing Interventions Associated with Administering Tube Feedings

PROBLEM	NURSING INTERVENTION
Irritation of oral mucous membranes	Oral mucous membranes often become dry and irritated when the patient is unable to take nourishment by mouth and is receiving nourishment by gavage. Frequent oral hygiene helps prevent this problem; administer it at least four times a day.
Acute otitis media	Otitis media is possible when the nasogastric tube presses against the eustachian tube, which causes obstruction and edema. It is best prevented by turning the patient from side to side frequently, at least every 2 hours, and by using as small a nasogastric tube as possible.
Irritation of nasal and palate tissues	Tissue irritation occurs as a result of pressure on tissues by the nasogastric tube. Some procedures include that the tube be removed a few inches every day, coated with an antibiotic ointment, and then reinserted.
Diarrhea	Diarrhea is commonly caused by introducing nourishment too rapidly or using formula or nourishment that is too concentrated. The usual care is to decrease the strength of the nourishment and administer it more slowly. An antidiarrheal drug will sometimes be ordered.
Nausea	Nausea is commonly caused by introducing nourishment too rapidly. It is also possible that the formula of the nourishment is unsatisfactory. Usual care is to administer nourishment more slowly and possibly change the formula.
Abdominal distention	Abdominal distention commonly occurs when the stomach empties too slowly. Omit the nourishment if the amount aspirated from the stomach before feeding is 100 to 150 mL. In some instances, the physician orders the feedings to be stopped, at least temporarily.
Aspiration	Aspiration is best prevented by ensuring that the tube is in the stomach before introducing the nourishment and by keeping the head of the patient's bed elevated between 30 and 45 degrees. Suction of the mouth and throat are sometimes called for when regurgitation and vomiting are present.
Clogged tube	An occluded tube is prevented by keeping a constant flow rate when nourishment is given continuously and by flushing the tube well after single feedings. It is acceptable to gently irrigate the tube after obtaining a medical order. If irrigation does not relieve the obstruction, sometimes it is necessary to remove and replace the tube.
High electrolyte blood levels	High electrolyte blood levels are usually the result of the patient receiving insufficient fluids. Water is usually offered through the tube at a rate of 100 mL every 4 to 6 hours (exact amount will vary by physician's order).

safe patient care. A feeding tube is improperly positioned when it is accidentally placed in the lung, the esophagus, or even the stomach when proper placement is in the small bowel. It is all too easy to place tubes in the wrong position or allow them to migrate into the esophagus and the lung. Complications such as aspiration pneumonia, pneumothorax, and peritonitis have potential to develop if the tube placement is incorrect and feedings are subsequently administered.

The most dependable means of checking tube placement is through radiologic confirmation. Chest x-ray films are considered the standard of care, especially for confirming placement of small-diameter tubes. Unfortunately, not all institutions have policies mandating this method. X-ray studies are also not usually performed for large-diameter nasogastric (NG) and nasointestinal (NI) tubes because most clinicians feel the tubes are less likely to enter the lung undetected. The next best method for confirming feeding tube placement is through pH measurement. By testing the pH of fluid aspirated from a newly inserted feeding tube, it is possible to make reasonable assumptions about the tube's location. Traditionally, the auscultatory method has been used to determine NG tube placement. It was long thought possible to confirm proper tube placement by insufflating air with a syringe through a tube and then using a stethoscope to listen for a gurgling sound over the epigastric region. Today the reliability of this method appears highly questionable (air in a tube inadvertently placed in the lungs, the pharynx, or the esophagus will transmit sound similar to that entering the stomach). It is not a good method to use on its own to rule out inadvertent respiratory positioning of feeding tubes.

Many potential complications are possible with administration of tube feedings. The cost of managing the ensuing complications and infections is high. Complications are sometimes related to the tube itself, such as placement of the tube in the lung, frequent tube clogging, or the tube inadvertently being pulled out. Complications also occur when the administered tube feeding causes delayed gastric emptying, bloating, diarrhea, or aspiration pneumonia.

Skill 21-1 includes the administration of the tube feeding via bolus and continuous drip via gravity or infusion pump, and Skill 21-2 includes the administration of enteral feedings via gastrostomy or jejunostomy tube. It is important to check placement of NG and NI tubes before initiating feedings. Using good hand hygiene technique and clean equipment, and hanging formula only for the recommended time to prevent spoiling are critical to avoiding contamination of the system and subsequent infection in the patient.

Text continued on p. 652

Skill 21-1 Administering Nasogastric Tube Feedings

Nursing Action *(Rationale)*

1. Refer to medical record, care plan, or Kardex for special interventions. *(Provides a basis for care. Many nursing interventions require a physician's order. Verification is ensured when nurse reviews medical record. The physician's order will state formula, rate, route, and frequency of feeding.)*
2. Introduce self. *(Decreases patient anxiety.)*
3. Identify patient. *(Ensures procedure is performed with correct patient.)*
4. Explain the procedure and the reason it is to be done in terms the patient is able to understand, and allow time for the patient to ask questions. Advise patient of any unpleasantness that will possibly be experienced. *(Enlists patient's cooperation; decreases patient's anxiety and prepares patient.)*
5. Assess need for and provide patient teaching during procedure. *(Promotes patient's independence.)*
6. Assess patient. Assess abdomen for distention or tenderness. Auscultate for active bowel sounds before each feeding. *(Absence of bowel sounds indicates inability of the GI tract to digest or absorb nutrients and provides baseline information for later comparisons.)*
7. Wash hands and don clean gloves according to agency policy and guidelines from the CDC and OSHA. *(Reduces spread of microorganisms.)*
8. Assemble equipment and complete necessary charges. Know agency policy. Organize procedure. *(Some equipment is disposable and charged to the patient as used.)*
   - Disposable feeding bag and ready-to-hang system
   - 30-mL or larger Luer-Lok or catheter-tip syringe
   - Stethoscope and pH indicator strips
   - Infusion pump (required for intestinal feedings; be certain to use pump designed for tube feedings)
   - Prescribed enteral feedings
   - Gloves
   - Equipment to obtain blood glucose for fingerstick (some agencies allow only laboratory personnel to do fingersticks)
9. Prepare patient for intervention:
   a. Close door or pull privacy curtain. *(Provides privacy and promotes patient's comfort.)*
   b. Raise bed to a comfortable working height; lower side rail on side nearest you. *(Promotes proper body mechanics by keeping muscle strain in caregivers to a minimum and preventing injury or fatigue.)*
   c. Elevate head of bed to put patient in Fowler's position, at least 30 degrees, or reverse Trendelenburg position if spinal injury is present. *(Reduces risk of aspiration during feeding with head higher than stomach or lower than stomach in spinal injury patients.)*
10. Determine tube placements and gastric residual. Let patient know the purpose of the test: "I'm checking the fluid from your stomach to make sure that the tube is in the right place. I put a drop on this paper strip, and the value tells me the tube is where it belongs." Radiographic evidence of placement is the most accurate, but cost and radiation exposure prohibit frequent checks many times per day. *(Presence of gastric secretions indicates that the distal end of the tube is in the stomach. Residual volume indicates if gastric emptying is delayed. A possible indication of delayed gastric emptying is the presence of 150 mL or more remaining in patient's stomach.)*
    a. Aspirate gastric or intestinal contents with appropriate cone-tipped syringe inserted into end of tube (see illustrations). (If patient has a small-bore feeding tube, aspirate slowly to prevent collapse. Gastric secretions are usually green, brown, or tan to off-white (see illustration); intestinal fluid is medium to deep

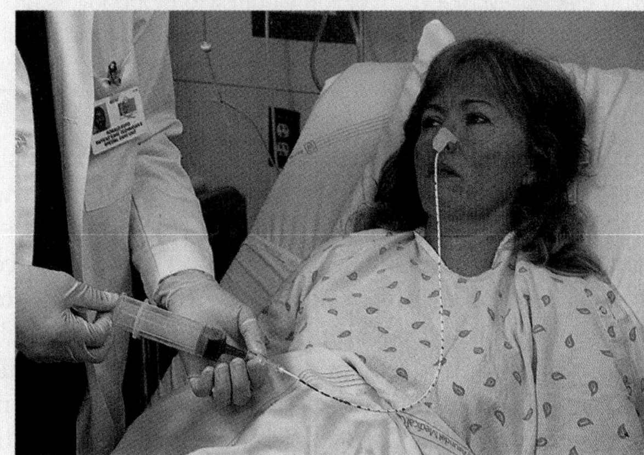

Step **10a,** A

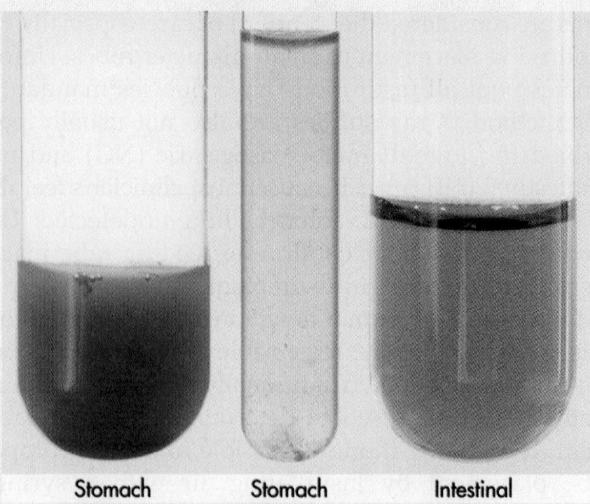

Step **10a,** B

golden brown or bile stained. Pleural fluid is pale, clear yellow, and watery.)

b. Place drop of GI contents on pH test paper for measurement (see illustration). *(Gastric contents will usually have a pH range of 0 to 4; tracheobronchial and pleural secretions will usually have a pH greater than 6, and intestinal contents will usually have a pH of 7 or greater. Visual inspection of fluid helps differentiate gastric from intestinal fluids.)*

c. If tube is inserted nasally, inspect oral cavity for tube kinking or curling in back of throat. *(Indicates that tube is no longer correctly positioned in the GI tract. Alert patients will gag, but unconscious patients or those without a gag reflex are not able to do so.)*

d. If unable to aspirate, suspect the tube is occluded or kinked, and attempt to flush it with 30 mL of tap water. *(Using a small syringe [3- to 6-mL] generates a large force and has the potential to rupture small feeding tubes. A small-bore feeding tube in the intestine will not necessarily have residual volume.)*

11. Readminister residual volume to patient by allowing it to flow from syringe into tubing. If volume of residual is large, administer slowly. *(Helps prevent fluid and electrolyte imbalance. Slow administration keeps nausea to a minimum.)* If residual amounts are greater than last infusion or 150 mL, hold feeding 1 hour and reassess residual. *(Some physicians will order to reduce feeding by the amount of aspirate. Refer to medical record and nursing care plan.)*

12. Prepare formula for administration:

a. If pouring directly from a can, check expiration date and wipe off top of can (see illustration).

b. If using premixed base, check date and time of mixing, as well as correct strength (full, half strength). Some physicians or agencies require formula to be at room temperature. *(Cold formula sometimes causes gastric clamping and discomfort because the liquid is not warmed by mouth or esophagus as food is when consumed orally.)*

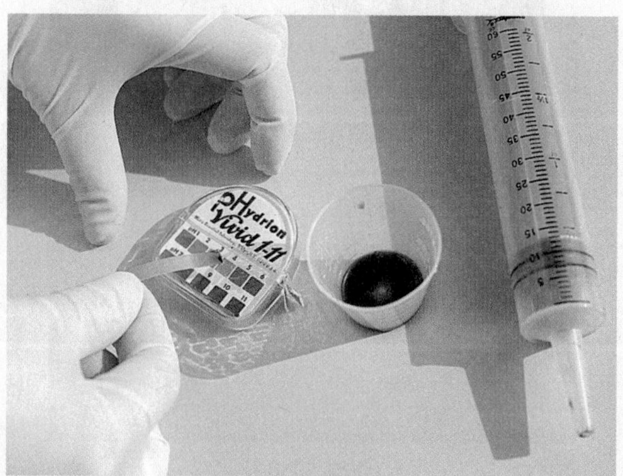

Step **10b**

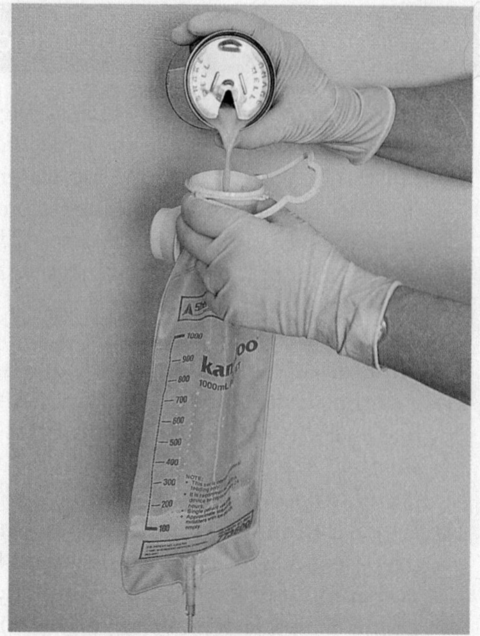

Step **12a**

13. Administer feeding.

a. **Bolus or intermittent feedings:**

(1) Administer the tube feeding with 60-mL bulb or plunger syringe.

(2) Remove cap or plug from end of feeding tube and pinch closed. *(Pinching the tubing prevents leakage and air from entering the patient's stomach.)*

(3) Attach syringe by removing bulb or plunger and inserting tip into end of tube. Elevate to no more than 18 inches (45 cm) above insertion site (see illustration).

(4) Fill syringe with formula, release tube, and allow syringe to empty gradually, refilling until prescribed or ordered amount has been administered. *(Slow delivery of tube feeding [50 to 100 mL/min] is better tol-*

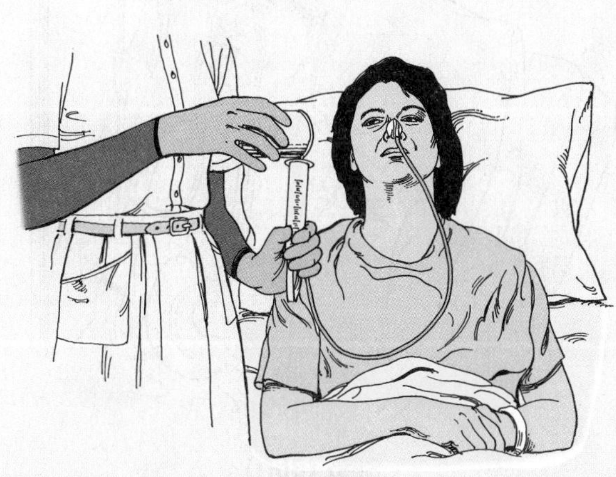

Step **13a(3)**

Continued

Skill 21-1 Administering Nasogastric Tube Feedings—cont'd

erated. Continuous draining from syringe helps prevent air entry and gas production.)

(5) Flush tube with 30 to 60 mL tap water (or ordered amount) when feeding is complete. *(Prevents tube clogging with thicker feeding.)*

(6) Recap or plug tube. *(Prevents leakage and prevents air from entering the stomach between feedings.)*

b. Continuous drip method:

(1) Administer the tube feeding with gavage bag (see illustration). *(Easily tolerated in the stomach. Allows periods for patient to be unattached to a feeding system.)*

(2) Prepare administration set: Clamp tubing, prepare gavage bag with prescribed type and amount of formula, unclamp and prime tubing to remove air, and then reclamp tubing. *(This method is designed to deliver prescribed hourly rate of feeding. With patients who receive continuous drip feedings, check residuals every 4 hours and verify tube placement.)*

(3) Label bag with tube feeding type, strength, and amount. Include date, time, and initials. *(Communicates essential information to all staff.)*

(4) Pinch end of feeding tube. Remove plug or cap, and securely attach gavage tubing to end of feeding tube.

(5) Set rate by adjusting roller clamp on tubing. Usually this type of tube feeding infuses for 30 to 60 minutes three to six times per day.

(6) Flush tube with 30 to 60 mL tap water (or ordered amount) when feeding complete. *(Prevents tube clogging.)*

(7) Recap or plug tube. *(Prevents leakage and prevents air from entering the stomach.)*

c. Feeding via infusion pump:

(1) Administer the tube feeding as a continuous drip via infusion pump (see illustration). *(Allows a smaller volume of feeding to be delivered continuously. There is less risk of aspiration or missed feedings.)*

(2) Prepare administration set, with type and amount of formula to last no more than 8 hours. Clamp tubing, spike bag, and unclamp and prime tubing. Reclamp tubing. *(Helps prevent spoilage. Prefilled vacuum packages are available from the manufacturer and are less likely to spoil.)*

(3) Label bag with tube feeding type, strength, and amount. Include date, time, and initials. *(Communicates essential information to all staff.)*

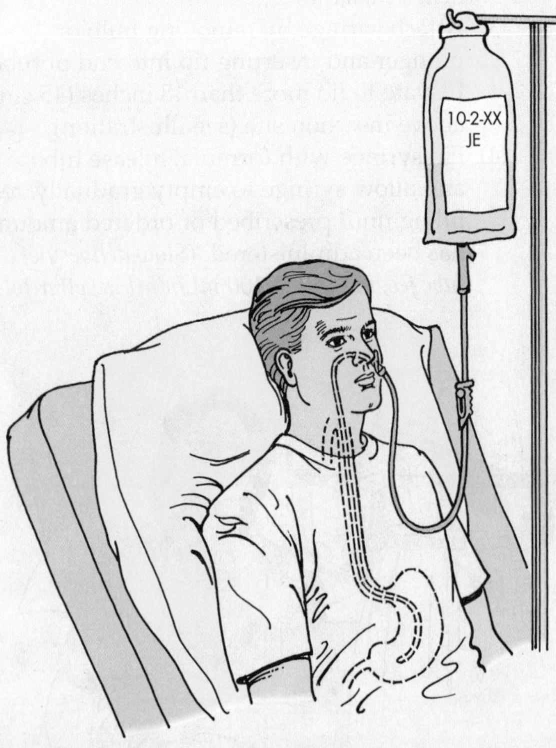

Step **13b(1)**

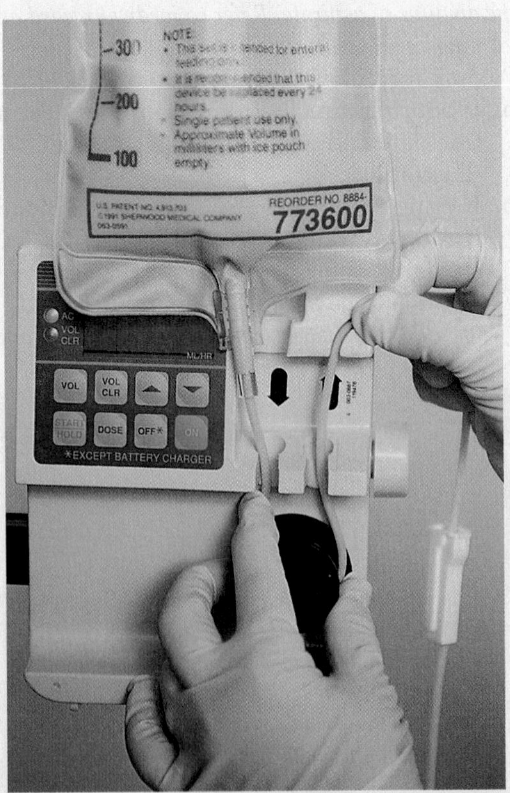

Step **13c(1)**

(4) Hang tube feeding set on IV pole with infusion pump. Connect tubing to pump and set rate.
(5) Pinch end of feeding tube. Remove plug or cap. Connect infusion tubing to patient feeding tube. *(Prevents air from entering the stomach.)*
(6) Open roller clamp on infusion tubing. Turn infusion pump on.
(7) Check residual volumes every 4 hours by aspirating with 60-mL syringe. *(Ensures that tube feeding is continuing to infuse through the GI system.)*

14. Fill a 60-mL syringe with ordered volume of water (usually 30 to 50 mL). Inject into feeding tube to flush after bolus or as ordered with continuous drip. *(Helps prevent tube becoming clogged. Water replacement is vital to help patient maintain adequate fluid and electrolyte balance.)*
15. Flush tube with water every 4 to 8 hours as described in step 13b(6), and clamp tubing if feedings are not infusing.
16. Rinse syringe or bag and tubing with warm water after all bolus and gavage feedings. Remove and discard gloves and wash hands. *(Rinsing removes formula left in equipment, reduces potential for bacterial growth, and allows for reuse of equipment. Most agencies require replacement with new equipment every 24 hours.)*
17. Ask if patient is comfortable while infusion is continuing. *(Complaints of cramping possibly indicate tube feeding is too cold or is infusing too fast.)* Report any diarrhea to the physician. *(It is possible that patient needs antidiarrheal agents [Kaopectate, Lomotil].)*
18. When infusion is complete, assist patient to a position of comfort and place needed items within easy reach. Be certain patient has a means to call for assistance and knows how to use it. *(Promotes safety.)*
19. Raise side rails, and lower bed to lowest position. *(Promotes safety.)* Some alert patients may have side rails down during the daylight hours. Some agencies do not allow for side rails—know agency policy.
20. Remove gloves, dispose of used supplies, and wash hands. *(Reduces spread of microorganisms.)*
21. Document:
    - Amount of feeding
    - Type of feeding
    - Status of feeding tubes
    - Patient's tolerance
    - Any adverse effects
    - Patient teaching
22. Monitor weight and laboratory values daily. *(Improving laboratory values and weight gain are indications of improved nutritional status. However, a sudden weight gain of more than 2 lb in 24 hours usually indicates fluid retention.)*
23. Observe and assess patient for shortness of breath, low oxygenation saturation, and presence of feeding from airway. See Table 21-22 for common problems associated with administering tube feedings and their nursing interventions.

Skill 21-2 Administering Enteral Feedings via Gastrostomy or Jejunostomy Tube

Nursing Action *(Rationale)*

Observe all guidelines for nasogastric tube feedings and follow steps 1 through 9 of Skill 21-1; then continue with the following steps.

1. Verify tube placement (see Skill 21-1, step 10).
    a. **Gastrostomy tube:** Aspirate gastric secretions; assess their appearance and check pH; return aspirated contents to stomach unless the volume exceeds 150 mL. *(Gastric fluid is usually cloudy and grassy green or tan to off-white; in contrast, intestinal fluid is usually deep golden yellow and clearer than gastric fluid.)*
    b. **Jejunostomy tube:** Aspirate intestinal secretions, observe their appearance, and check pH. *(Presence of intestinal fluid indicates that the end of the tube is in the small intestine [i.e., duodenum or jejunum]. Generally the intestinal residual is very small [10 mL or less]. If fluid tests acidic on pH test or looks like gastric fluid, or the residual volume is large [more than 10 mL], it is possible that displacement of the tube into the stomach has occurred.)*
2. Flush tube with 30 mL of tap water.
3. Initiate feedings.
    a. **Syringe feedings** (see Skill 21-1, step 13a): Usually gastrostomy and jejunostomy feedings are given continuously to ensure proper absorption. However, you will sometimes give initial feedings by bolus to assess patient's tolerance to formula.
        (1) Pinch proximal end of gastrostomy tube.
        (2) Remove plunger and attach barrel of syringe to end of tube, and then fill syringe with formula.
        (3) Allow syringe to empty gradually. Refill until prescribed amount has been delivered to patient. *(Too-rapid instillation has potential to cause complications.)*

Continued

Skill 21-2 Administering Enteral Feedings via Gastrostomy or Jejunostomy Tube—cont'd

b. Continuous drip method (see Skill 21-1, step 13b).
 (1) Fill feeding container with enough formula for 4 hours of feeding.
 (2) Hang container on IV pole, and clear tubing of air.
 (3) Thread tubing on pump according to manufacturer's directions.
 (4) Connect tubing to end of feeding tube.
 (5) Begin infusion at prescribed rate.

4. Assess skin around tube exit site. Make sure to cleanse the skin around the tube daily with warm water and mild soap. Dressings around the exit site are usually not recommended. *(Report any drainage, erythema, edema, or displacement of the tube to the physician.)*

5. Dispose of supplies. Wash hands. *(Prevents transmission of microorganisms.)*

6. Monitor fingerstick blood glucose every 6 hours until maximum administration rate is reached and maintained for 24 hours. *(Alerts you to patient's tolerance of glucose.)*

7. Monitor intake and output every 24 hours. *(Intake and output are indications of fluid balance or fluid volume excess.)*

8. Weigh patient daily until maximum administration rate is reached and maintained for 24 hours; then weigh patient three times per week. *(Weight gain is indicator of improved nutritional status; however, a sudden gain of more than 2 pounds in 24 hours usually indicates fluid retention.)*

9. Observe return of normal laboratory values. *(Improving laboratory values [albumin, transferrin, prealbumin] indicate an improved nutritional status.)*

10. Inspect site for signs of pressure. *(Enteral tubes sometimes cause uncomfortable pressure areas on patient's skin.)*

11. Document (see Skill 21-1, step 21).

12. Monitor weight and laboratory values (see Skill 21-1, step 22).

13. Observe for any adverse reactions (see Skill 21-1, step 23).

PARENTERAL NUTRITION SUPPORT

Parenteral nutrition, or **hyperalimentation,** is the term used to describe intravenous feedings. Parenteral nutrition is possible to administer through peripheral veins, such as those in the arms or the legs. When you administer parenteral nutrition by this route, it is called **peripheral parenteral nutrition (PPN).**

Total parenteral nutrition (TPN) refers to the administration of a hypertonic solution into a large central vein. In TPN, you will usually infuse the solution into the superior vena cava via a catheter threaded through either the subclavian or the internal jugular vein (Figure 21-6). TPN and PPN formulas are composed of glucose, amino acids, vitamins, minerals, and

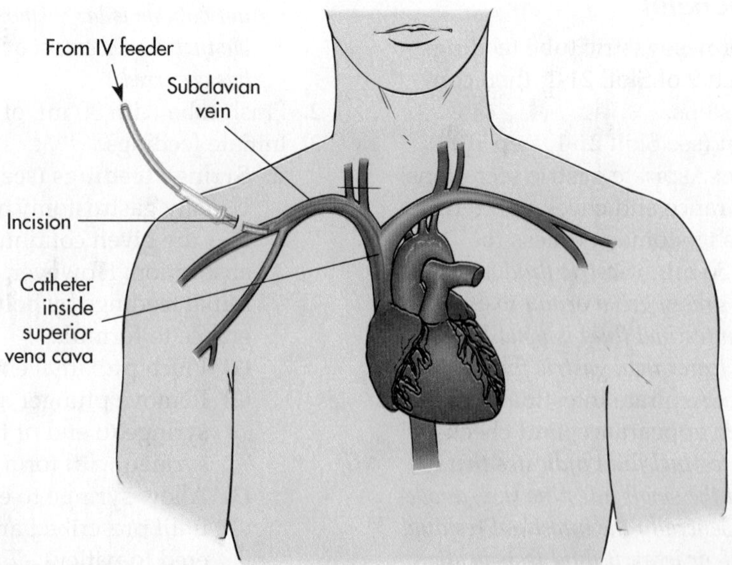

FIGURE 21-6 Central venous catheter placement during administration of parenteral nutrition.

electrolytes. Fat, in the form of triglycerides, is also given as a supplement to the main formula. It is administered separately through a Y-connector tube or into a peripheral vein.

Parenteral nutrition support is indicated for the patient with a nonfunctioning or dysfunctioning GI tract. When IV nutrition is necessary, use PPN as the first choice of administration if possible. PPN carries less risk of complications, necessitates less monitoring, and costs less than administration by the central venous route. Candidates for PPN are those needing 3000 kcal/day or less, those needing supplementation to oral diet, or those requiring short-term therapy (less than 3 weeks).

TPN is indicated for patients needing a highly concentrated formula, such as those who need more kilocalories than can be administered peripherally or those requiring fluid restriction—a concentrated formula delivers more kilocalories and nutrients in a smaller volume. Other candidates for TPN include those who have to be on IV feedings for more than 3 weeks and those with unsuitable or unavailable peripheral veins.

TPN necessitates constant medical care. Surgical placement of a catheter in one of the central veins is necessary to establish central venous access. This imposes significant risks on the patient, including sepsis (major infection), pneumothorax (air in the pleural cavity), hemothorax (blood in the pleural cavity), phlebitis (inflammation of the vein), or thrombosis (blood clots). It is necessary to keep the catheter site aseptic and feeding solutions sterile. Constant monitoring of the biochemical and clinical status of the patient is essential.

Some patients receiving TPN will experience fluid and electrolyte imbalances, hyperglycemia or hypoglycemia, metabolic disturbances, and bone disorders such as osteomalacia (softening of the bones). For this reason, you will have to monitor blood chemistries frequently. Check blood glucose several times each day. Administer regular insulin on a sliding scale to maintain blood glucose levels below 200 mg/dL.

FEEDING THE PATIENT

Some patients are not able to feed themselves. Weakness, paralysis, casts, and other physical limitations often make self-feeding impossible. You and your coworkers will feed these patients.

It is necessary to create a relaxed mood so the patient does not feel rushed. Many people pray before eating, so be sure to provide the time and privacy to do so if the patient wishes. This demonstrates caring and respect for the patient. Ask the patient about the order he or she wants you to offer foods and fluids. Use a spoon, because spoons are less likely than forks to cause injury. Fill the spoon only one third full so that the patient can easily chew and swallow the mouthful.

Patients who are not able to feed themselves will sometimes feel angry, humiliated, and embarrassed. Some of them will not like depending on others. Some are depressed and resentful, and others may refuse to eat. Allow these patients to try to feed themselves as much as possible. However, make sure they do not exceed activity limits ordered by the physician. Do provide them with all possible support and encouragement.

Visually impaired patients are often keenly aware of food aromas. Often they can identify some foods served; still, always tell the patient what foods and fluids are on the tray. When feeding a visually impaired patient, identify what you are offering each time. For patients who feed themselves, identify foods and fluids and indicate their location on the tray by referring to the numbers on a clock (Figure 21-7).

Meals provide social contact with others. Engage the patient in pleasant conversation while giving the patient enough time to chew and swallow food. Also, sit facing the patient. Sitting is more relaxing and shows the patient that you have time to feed the patient comfortably. Standing communicates nonverbally that you do not have time and that you are in a hurry. By facing the patient, you are also able to see how well the patient is eating and whether the patient has problems swallowing.

Observe the steps shown in Skill 21-3 when assisting patients with eating.

SERVING MEAL TRAYS

Weakness and illness will often affect a patient's ability to eat. Odors, unpleasant equipment, an uncomfortable position, the need for oral hygiene, the need to

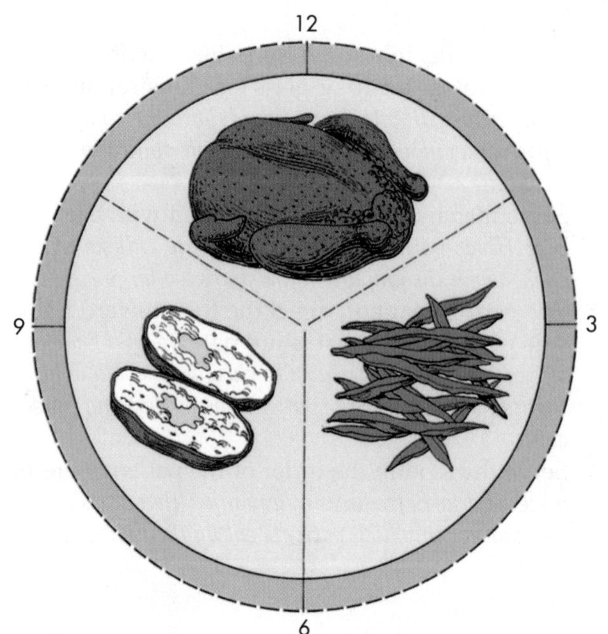

FIGURE 21-7 For the visually impaired patient: "The potatoes are at 9 o'clock."

Skill 21-3 Assisting Patients with Eating

Nursing Action *(Rationale)*

1. Complete or delay care that will interfere with eating. *(It is best for the patient to eat food at its appropriate serving temperature.)*
2. Provide a period of rest or quiet before meals. Offer the patient a bedpan or urinal before mealtime. *(A tired or excited patient is usually in no mood to eat.)*
3. Provide the patient with an opportunity for handwashing, and offer mouth care before eating. *(Refreshment before eating encourages appetite.)*
4. Remove any soiled articles or clutter from the room. *(An unattractive environment tends to decrease the desire to eat.)*
5. Make the patient comfortable for eating; use pain relief techniques if needed. *(It is easier for the patient to enjoy food if the patient is comfortable.)*
6. Raise the head of the bed to a sitting position if possible. *(The sitting or semisitting position usually makes swallowing easier and choking less likely than does the lying position.)*
7. Cover the patient's upper chest with a napkin or towel. *(Use of an absorbent substance keeps the bedclothes and linens from becoming soiled.)*
8. Sit beside the patient. Avoid appearing hurried. *(Tension interferes with chewing and digestion. Make the time spent relaxing; it also provides an opportunity to gather more data or do informal teaching.)*
9. Encourage patients to take part in their eating as much as possible and to the extent that their condition permits. *(Developing independence is a goal of nursing. Most adults feel childlike when they are fed by someone else.)*
10. Provide a flexible straw for patients who are unable to use a cup or glass (see illustration). *(A straw helps patients direct liquids into their mouth at a pace and amount that matches their ability to swallow.)*
11. Serve manageable amounts of food with each bite. *(Even patients who are sitting up will sometimes choke when the amounts of food are too large.)*
12. For a stroke patient, direct the food toward the side of the mouth that is not paralyzed. *(The stroke patient is better able to chew and swallow food that is placed where the patient has feeling and muscle control.)*
13. Serve the food in the order of the patient's preference. *(Perform feedings in a manner that simulates the manner in which patients eat by themselves when able.)*
14. Give the patient time to chew thoroughly and swallow the food. *(Chewing aids the first step in digestion by breaking up food and mixing it with saliva and enzymes in the mouth. Large pieces of food have potential to obstruct the airway if swallowed.)*
15. Modify utensils and the texture of food if the patient has to remain flat while eating. Use a child's training cup or a large syringe with a flexible rubber tube. Puree or grind foods if necessary. *(A flat position decreases the patient's ability to control food in the mouth and increases the risk of choking.)*
16. If you have begun to feed a patient, do not leave until he or she has finished eating. Do not interrupt a meal. *(Food and beverages change temperatures with delays, which makes them unappealing.)*
17. Talk with the patient about pleasant subjects. Eating is a social situation. *(Focusing on problems tends to interfere with the patient's appetite.)*
18. Follow the suggestions in Skill 21-4 for removing a tray.

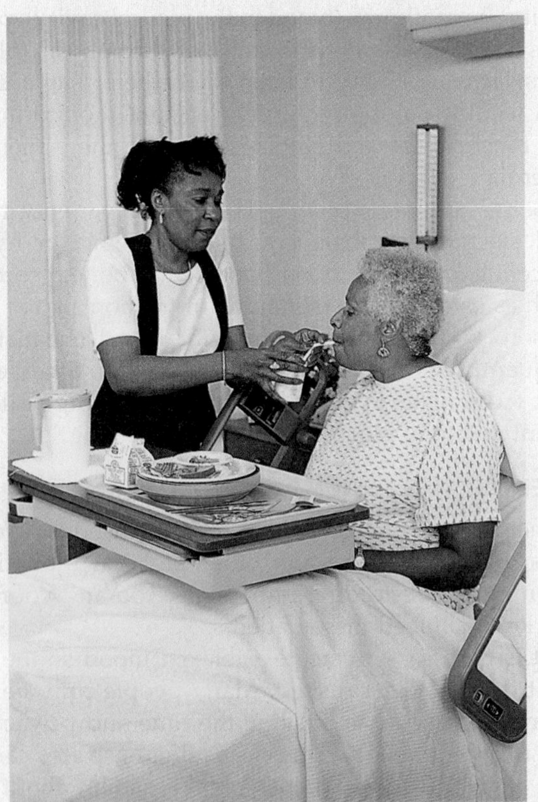

Step **10**

void, and the presence of pain are some factors that affect appetite. One way you and your colleagues are able to control these factors is by getting the patient ready for meals.

In hospitals, food is usually served in the patient's room. Some patients eat in dining rooms, the cafeteria, or lounges. Food is served in containers that keep hot and cold foods at the correct temperature. You will serve meal trays after preparing patients for meals. You will be able to serve trays promptly if patients are ready to eat. Serving trays help keep food at the right temperature.

Observe the steps shown in Skill 21-4 when serving and removing patients' trays.

Skill 21-4 Serving and Removing Trays

Nursing Action *(Rationale)*

1. Be available when trays arrive from the dietary department. *(Delay in serving food alters the serving temperature.)*
2. Clear the area where the patient will eat. *(Clutter is likely to cause the tray or the patient's belongings to fall or become misplaced.)*
3. Check the general appearance of the tray for spilled liquids, missing items, or ordered food that is missing. *(Make sure the tray is complete, orderly, and tidy so that eating can be enjoyed.)*
4. Compare the name on the tray with the name on the patient's identification bracelet. *(A tray served to the wrong patient is an error with potentially serious consequences.)*
5. Ensure that patients who are undergoing special tests have food withheld or provided according to test directions. *(Some tests necessitate that patients fast or eat specific types of foods, such as a fat-free meal.)*
6. Check to see that the patient is not being served foods to which he or she is allergic or that he or she is not able to tolerate. *(A patient's condition is sometimes made worse by eating foods that his or her system is not able to tolerate.)*
7. Place the tray so that it faces the patient, and remove the food covers (see Skill 21-3, step 10). *(Positioning the tray and removing the covers allows easy access for the patient.)*
8. Open milk cartons and cereal boxes, butter the toast, cut the meat, and otherwise assist as necessary. *(Some patients will have difficulty doing these simple tasks even if they are not disabled.)*
9. Serve trays that have been kept warm last to those patients who need help with eating. *(Having cold food waiting at bedside is unappetizing and often annoying for the patient.)*
10. Note the kinds and amounts of food that the patient is *not* eating. *(Consider ordering substitutes for uneaten food or whether there are other problems you are able to solve, such as loose dentures, that interfere with eating.)*
11. Observe whether or not the patient feels satisfied with the amount of food served. It is best to make serving sizes match appetite. *(Serving large portions to a patient with a minimal appetite tends to reduce food consumption.)*
12. Follow agency policies about serving food brought from home. Ensure that the food is covered, labeled, and refrigerated or stored properly. *(As long as the food is appropriate for the patient's diet, there usually is not a problem. Spoiled or misplaced food offends those who made special efforts to prepare it.)*
13. Be considerate, and visit with patients who are on a special diet and may be denied food they like because of a health problem. *(The patient needs the nurse's help, support, and understanding with unwanted changes in lifestyle.)*
14. Encourage patients to eat, but do not scold those who feel that they are not able to do so. *(Insisting that patients eat or implying that they are uncooperative is not a good nursing approach.)*
15. Remove trays as soon as possible, and restore the cleanliness of the eating area. *(Being left clean and comfortable after eating is pleasant for the patient.)*
16. Assist or offer the patient an opportunity to brush and floss teeth. *(Oral hygiene after eating helps prevent dental caries.)*
17. Record how the patient ate, and enter the amount of fluid consumed if appropriate. *(Helps you evaluate whether the nutritional and fluid needs of the patient are being met.)*
18. Always assess the patient's appetite during your first assessment of the day. Ask how much he or she ate for breakfast, and so on. *(Helps you make your nutritional assessment objectively.)*
19. Use fractions or percentages (such as ¼, ⅓, ½; or 35%, 50%, 100%), or follow agency policy. *(It is necessary to state nutritional assessment in objective terms.)*

Get Ready for the NCLEX® Examination!

Key Points

- Nurses play an important role in promoting good nutrition.
- Nutrients are necessary for the proper functioning of all life processes in the body.
- There are food planning guides to help plan and assess diets for nutritional adequacy.
- Essential nutrients include protein, carbohydrate, fat, vitamins, minerals, and water.
- Deficiencies or excesses of nutrients will often lead to disease or dysfunction of various body systems.
- For healthy Americans, it is possible for well-planned diets to provide adequate nutrition without supplementation.
- Nutrient needs change throughout the life cycle, and people need to adjust their diet to meet those needs.
- Medications have potential to affect nutritional status. Be aware of drug-nutrient interactions.
- Medical nutrition therapy involves using the diet as medical treatment for disease or injury.
- Diets will often be altered in consistency or frequency when GI function prohibits the use of a regular diet.
- Kilocalorie modifications are used when patients need to gain or lose weight. High-kilocalorie and high-protein diets will sometimes be necessary for weight maintenance in patients with increased metabolic needs.
- Obesity is a complex disorder; individualized treatment is necessary, but when done properly, any treatment involves a healthful diet with physical activity and addresses psychological issues.
- The eating disorders anorexia nervosa and bulimia nervosa call for multidisciplinary treatment efforts, including nutritional, family, and psychological therapy. Place an emphasis on the prevention of these disorders in youth by promoting good health and the value of individuality.
- Carbohydrate-controlled, fat-controlled, high-fiber diets are used in the treatment of diabetes mellitus.
- Fat-controlled diets emphasize reduction of total fat, saturated fat, and *trans* fatty acids. They are used in the treatment of heart disease, atherosclerosis, obesity, diabetes, and metabolic syndrome. Low-fat diets restrict all fats and are sometimes needed in the treatment of malabsorption syndromes and gallbladder disease.
- Sodium-restricted diets are used in the treatment of hypertension, congestive heart failure, and renal disease. They are also sometimes used when edema is present.
- Protein- and electrolyte-modified diets are used to treat renal disease and cirrhosis.
- Fluid restrictions are necessary when urine output is decreased, when edema is present, or during heart failure. Adequate fluid is necessary to prevent dehydration, particularly in older adults.
- Nutritional support (tube feedings or parenteral nutrition) is often necessary when oral intake is impossible or inadequate. GI function usually indicates which type of feeding is appropriate.
- When feeding a patient or resident, ask about the preferred order in which to offer foods and fluids.
- Serve meal trays after preparing patients for meals.

Additional Learning Resources

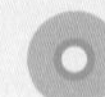

Go to your Companion CD for an audio glossary, animations, video clips, and more.

evolve Be sure to visit the Evolve site at http://evolve.elsevier.com/Christensen/foundations/ for additional online resources.

Review Questions for the NCLEX® Examination

1. A 35-year-old patient is healthy but wishes to lose weight because her BMI is 27. Which suggestions are most appropriate for her?
   1. This BMI is too low for good health; the patient will possibly need to supplement her diet to increase her weight.
   2. This is an acceptable BMI, and it is best to maintain weight at this level for continued good health.
   3. Appropriate weight loss is possible with a healthy, reduced-calorie diet and incorporating at least 30 minutes of physical activity into each day.
   4. This BMI is elevated to the point that adjunct treatments, such as surgery, will be of possible benefit.

2. A 10-year-old has an elevated BMI. Which suggestions are most appropriate to help him with his weight management?
   1. Encourage a low-calorie diet that allows for moderate weight loss of no more than 2 pounds per week.
   2. Encourage the avoidance of sweets and snack foods and limit eating to only three meals per day.
   3. Encourage using the www.mypyramid.gov website to help plan a healthy diet, and suggest limiting TV viewing time.
   4. Encourage family therapy to assess the reasons for excessive weight gain in such a young person.

3. A patient takes medication for hypertension and asks if there is anything possible to do with his diet to help reduce his blood pressure. The best response is:
   1. "A low-fat, low-cholesterol diet with only a limited amount of simple sugars will have the greatest effect on your blood pressure."
   2. "A salt-free diet will have the greatest effect on your blood pressure. Don't add salt in your cooking or at the table."
   3. "Adequate calcium and potassium intake, as well as lower sodium intake, offers some possibility of helping your blood pressure. Eat plenty of fruits, vegetables, and low-fat milk products."
   4. "Discontinue the use of processed foods, and buy only natural foods. That way, you will have less sodium in your diet."

4. A cancer patient is experiencing anorexia and weight loss. Which suggestions are most likely to help him increase intake and prevent weight loss?
   1. Encourage him to eat double portions at each meal.
   2. Suggest he snack often on high-kilocalorie foods.
   3. Encourage him to eat the lower-kilocalorie foods first.
   4. Suggest that he decrease his exercise.
5. A patient with type 2 diabetes obese and has an elevated blood cholesterol. Which goals for nutrition therapy are most appropriate for this patient?
   1. Encourage her to focus her efforts on achieving healthy blood glucose and lipid levels and to include regular exercise.
   2. Educate her on how to adjust her insulin injections to better integrate with her usual eating and exercise patterns.
   3. Train her on how to recognize and treat hypoglycemia.
   4. Encourage her to reduce sodium intake and increase potassium intake to help control blood pressure.
6. A patient with lactose intolerance still wants to include dairy products in her diet. Which suggestions offer the possibility of enabling her to do this?
   1. Consume vitamin C at the same time as dairy products to increase absorption.
   2. Take calcium supplements with each meal.
   3. Consume small portions of fermented dairy products such as cheese or yogurt.
   4. Use skim milk rather than whole milk products.
7. A patient with iron deficiency anemia started taking iron supplements but is also trying to increase iron absorption. What will enhance iron absorption?
   1. Drinking milk or taking calcium supplements at the same time as eating iron-rich foods
   2. Taking iron supplements with coffee, tea, or red wine
   3. Consuming vitamin C–rich foods at the same meal with iron-containing foods
   4. Taking iron supplements with a high-fiber bran cereal
8. A patient with arthritis has been using aspirin on a daily basis for the past 5 years. What effect does aspirin sometimes have on nutritional status?
   1. It will sometimes increase energy metabolism, thus increasing kilocalorie needs.
   2. It will sometimes cause loss of appetite and taste bud changes.
   3. It will sometimes lead to decreased excretion of potassium.
   4. It will sometimes increase excretion of vitamin C and possibly lead to loss of iron from the GI tract.
9. A newly married patient planning for pregnancy has heard that some experts recommend folic acid supplements for women of childbearing age. What is the reason for this recommendation?
   1. Folic acid may help prevent neural tube defects in the developing fetus.
   2. Folic acid provides extra kilocalories for the synthesis of new cells.
   3. It is impossible to receive adequate amounts of folic acid in the diet.
   4. Folic acid will help increase iron absorption in the GI tract.
10. A patient is trying to substitute unsaturated fats in place of saturated fats in his diet. He asks how to identify an unsaturated fat. What are properties of unsaturated fats that will help him?
    1. They are bonded together with chemical bonds that the body is not able to digest.
    2. They include tropical oils and hydrogenated fats and are solid at room temperature.
    3. They are from plant sources and are liquid at room temperature.
    4. They contain dietary cholesterol.
11. A nurse is caring for a patient who has just been diagnosed with type 2 diabetes mellitus. The patient is concerned about the dietary changes she will need to make for her condition and asks the nurse to tell her about the diet. Which actions are appropriate and within the scope of practice for a nurse?
    1. Review the patient's chart, and recommend a calorie and carbohydrate intake based on blood glucose and lipid values.
    2. Discuss the rationale for and the general principles of the diabetic diet with the patient, and then communicate the patient's concerns to the registered dietitian and physician.
    3. Locate the physician's diet order in the medical chart, and then obtain a preprinted diet sheet showing the exchange lists for meal planning and a menu pattern based on the prescribed calorie level.
    4. Decline to comment on the diet because the nurse is not a trained professional in the area of nutrition; refer all questions to a registered dietitian.
12. A 40-year-old patient was recently diagnosed with type 2 diabetes. He is in the hospital for tests and is receiving a diabetic diet. His wife expresses concern because she notices cookies on his lunch tray. Which response best describes current recommendations for the use of concentrated sweets in the diabetic diet?
    1. "Sugars and sweets are permitted in moderation in the diabetic diet. The important thing is that the total carbohydrate content of the meal is controlled and balanced with your husband's medication and nutrient needs."
    2. "I can understand your concern. Sugars are more rapidly absorbed and have the capacity to raise blood glucose levels more quickly than other carbohydrates. I will check with the kitchen and see if your husband received the wrong tray."
    3. "I'm sure that if the cookies were on the meal tray that they must be allowed in the diet. They are probably low in sugar. There is likely no need for concern."
    4. "Sugar is used to treat hypoglycemia—low blood sugar. Perhaps your husband had a low blood sugar reading before breakfast, and the dietitian sent up the cookies to give him some extra sugar on his lunch meal tray."

13. The physician has recommended that the patient increase the amount of fiber in her diet to help control her blood cholesterol levels. Which guidelines are most appropriate for increasing water-soluble fiber in the diet?
    1. Choose a daily fiber supplement that contains no artificial additives and preservatives; follow the instructions on the container, and be sure to drink plenty of water.
    2. Choose foods that are closer to their whole state rather than refined or processed, including more fruits, oats, and legumes to increase soluble fiber; and drink plenty of water.
    3. Choose more vegetables, vegetable juices, whole wheat, and whole wheat products to increase soluble fiber; and drink plenty of water.
    4. Choose more fruit juices to provide both fluid and fiber; and include iron-fortified breakfast cereals to enhance the absorption of fiber from the fruit juice.

14. A patient is controlling his blood cholesterol through diet. He is familiar with food sources of saturated fat and cholesterol, but is confused about *trans* fatty acids. Which group of foods contributes the most *trans* fatty acids?
    1. Butter, cream, fats in meats, and tropical oils such as palm and coconut oils
    2. Fish oils, nuts and seeds, and vegetable oils such as olive oil and canola oil
    3. Stick margarines, shortening, deep-fried restaurant foods, and commercially prepared baked goods
    4. Liquid margarines, vegetable oil spreads, and vegetable oils such as corn, soybean, and cottonseed

15. A patient with a family history of osteoporosis is taking calcium supplements and practicing good health habits to reduce her risk of developing osteoporosis. Which practice would negatively affect calcium balance?
    1. Taking small doses of calcium throughout the day rather than one large dose
    2. Choosing plenty of milk products, and avoiding excess caffeine intake
    3. Consuming a high-protein diet
    4. Consuming a diet that is moderate in sodium

16. A 14-year-old patient is a good student and has been actively involved in school activities and sports. Currently her weight is in an appropriate range for her age and height; however, her mother has been concerned that the patient is developing an eating disorder and describes some of her behaviors to the nurse. Which set of symptoms and signs will give cause to investigate the possibility of an eating disorder?
    1. Change of peer groups. Spending less time at home and participating in fewer family meals. Staying out past curfew with friends. Challenging the family rules.
    2. Increased interest in appearance—spending long periods in the morning getting ready for school. Feeling embarrassed about changes in her body. Consuming more fast foods and snack foods and eating less at mealtimes.
    3. Increased competitive drive to perform well in both athletics and school with increased amount of time spent in training for sports. Choosing to eliminate meat from her diet. Criticism of family meal choices.
    4. Increased interest in preparing foods for others and calorie counting. Exhibiting peculiar eating rituals at the table. Expressing disgust with body size. Gradual withdrawal from friends and social activities.

17. A 14-year-old trauma patient has just been started on nasogastric tube feedings. Shortly after administration of the formula begins, the patient complains of nausea and abdominal cramps. What should the nurse suspect?
    1. The formula rate, strength, or volume is possibly too great.
    2. The temperature of the formula is too high, and it is best to chill the formula before administration.
    3. Gastric emptying has been delayed, and it is necessary to stop the tube feeding.
    4. Perhaps the feeding tube is emptying into the lung rather than the stomach.

18. A patient in the early stages of pregnancy is experiencing some nausea and vomiting. Which suggestion would NOT be appropriate for the nurse to recommend?
    1. Limit foods with strong odors, and avoid food odors that bother you.
    2. Take a high-dose vitamin B_6 supplement three times a day.
    3. Try consuming five or six smaller meals each day, and include a source of protein in each meal.
    4. Try not to let your stomach get completely empty. Eat before you are overly hungry.

19. A patient has been breastfeeding her infant, who is now 4 months old. She has a family history of food allergies and asks the nurse for advice regarding the introduction of solid foods. Choose the best response in this situation.
    1. "When your baby can sit with help or support, it is all right for you to begin introducing solid foods. Be sure to introduce the foods one at a time and wait a few days before introducing another food to observe for any allergic reactions."
    2. "Keep feeding only breast milk to your baby for as long as possible. Then begin by introducing fruit juices in a bottle to supplement your breast milk."
    3. "When your baby learns to sit up without help or support, it is all right for you to start introducing solid foods. Begin with wheat cereals and egg products, and supplement meals with whole cow's milk from a cup."
    4. "As soon as your baby is able to crawl, it is all right for you to begin introducing solid foods. Be sure to avoid all foods for which you know your family has allergic reactions."

20. The public health nurse is conducting a screening for metabolic syndrome. Which patient has a cluster of risk factors that meets the diagnostic criteria for metabolic syndrome?

1. Mrs. J.P.: Blood pressure of 146/78 mm Hg; triglycerides of 85 mg/dL; HDL cholesterol of 46 mg/dL; fasting blood glucose of 64 mg/dL; waist circumference of 32 inches.
2. Mrs. L.B.: Waist circumference of 42 inches; fasting blood glucose of 102 mg/dL; blood pressure of 128/80 mm Hg; triglycerides of 148 mg/dL; HDL cholesterol of 46 mg/dL.
3. Mr. B.: Triglycerides of 78 mg/dL, on lipid-lowering medication; HDL cholesterol of 55 mg/dL; blood pressure of 110/66 mg/dL; waist circumference of 36 inches; fasting blood glucose of 90 mg/dL.
4. Mrs. M.: Waist circumference of 38 inches; fasting blood glucose of 96 mg/dL, on glucose-lowering medication; blood pressure of 136/72 mm Hg; triglycerides of 160 mg/dL; HDL cholesterol of 40 mg/dL.

21. Adequate nutrition is important in a patient's recovery and overall health. An older adult stroke patient who has lost the use of his dominant hand is having trouble eating without help. In this situation, which of the following actions will be the most helpful to encourage intake?

1. Tell the patient where each food is located on his plate by using the numbers on a clock as a reference.
2. Ask the patient which foods he desires assistance with. Encourage the patient to take part in his eating as much as possible.
3. Alter the consistency of the food by pureeing or grinding the foods for ease of chewing.
4. Stand close to the patient and face him while you feed him.

22. A middle-age patient is in the early stage of renal failure. His physician has recommended that he limit his protein intake to slow the progression of his renal disease. To keep his protein intake adequate, but not excessive, his dietitian has recommended that he choose high-quality protein sources to meet his needs. Which group of foods contains the most high-quality (or complete) proteins?

1. Legumes, whole wheat products, oats
2. Nuts and seeds, peanut butter, gelatin
3. Olive oil, canola oil, flaxseed oil
4. Eggs, meats, milk

23. A patient has just started a weight-reduction diet and is aware that increasing physical activity is important for weight loss. She asks the nurse how much and what type of exercises are best for her to incorporate into her weight-reduction efforts. Select the answer that best reflects current guidelines:

1. "For weight loss, it is recommended that you include 60 to 90 minutes of physical activity on most days of the week. It may sound like a lot, but you don't have to do it all at once. it is fine to include two or three shorter bouts of activity during the day if it's easier for you. A variety of activities, such as walking, gardening, and weight lifting, can count toward your total."
2. "Try to accumulate at least 30 minutes of moderate physical activity most days of the week. Aerobic activities will be the most important for burning calories. Exercises like walking, swimming, cycling, and jogging are aerobic."
3. "For weight loss, it is recommended that you engage in 30 to 60 minutes of vigorous aerobic activity on most days of the week. Vigorous activity will burn the most calories, so it is important to really push yourself in order to reach a point where you are burning fat calories during your workout. One long bout of exercise is probably better than multiple shorter bouts."
4. "When you diet, you often lose muscle mass. As muscle mass decreases, your basal metabolic rate (BMR) may also decrease. The best exercise would be about 30 minutes of daily weight lifting to help prevent muscle loss and keep your BMR from dropping."

24. An 80-year-old retired farmer is normally congenial and alert, but when the home health nurse visits he is irritable and appears disoriented. The nurse notices that his eyes appear sunken, he has poor skin turgor, and his mouth is dry. What is the most likely cause of these symptoms?

1. Heart attack
2. High blood pressure
3. Dehydration
4. Alcohol abuse

chapter

22 Fluids and Electrolytes

evolve

http://evolve.elsevier.com/Christensen/foundationsadult

Barbara Lauritsen Christensen

Objectives

1. List, describe, and compare the body fluid compartments.
2. Discuss active and passive transport processes and give two examples of each.
3. Discuss the role of specific electrolytes in maintaining homeostasis.
4. Describe the cause and effect of deficits and excesses of sodium, potassium, chloride, calcium, magnesium, phosphorus, and bicarbonate.
5. Differentiate between the roles of the buffers, the lungs, and the kidneys in maintaining acid-base balance.
6. Compare and contrast the four primary types of acid-base imbalances.
7. Discuss the role of the nursing process in maintaining fluid, electrolyte, and acid-base balances.
8. Discuss how the very young, the very old, and the obese patient are at risk for fluid volume deficit.

Key Terms

acid-base balance (p. 673)
active transport (p. 664)
adenosine triphosphate (ATP) (ă-DĔN-ŏ-sēn trī-FŎS-fāt, p. 663)
anions (ĂN-ī-ŏnz, p. 665)
bicarbonate (bī-KĂHR-bō-nāt, p. 673)
blood buffers (p. 674)
calcium (p. 669)
cations (KĂT-ī-ŏnz, p. 665)
chloride (p. 668)
diffusion (p. 663)
electrolytes (ĕ-LĔK-trō-lītz, p. 665)
extracellular (ĕks-tră-SĔL-yū-lăr, p. 661)
filtration (p. 664)
homeostasis (hō-mē-ō-STĀ-sĭs, p. 662)
hypertonic (hī-pŭr-TŎN-ĭk, p. 664)
hypotonic (hī-pō-TŎN-ĭk, p. 664)
interstitial (ĭn-tŭr-STĬSH-ăl, p. 661)
intracellular (ĭn-tră-SĔL-yū-lăr, p. 661)
intravascular (ĭn-tră-VĂS-cyū-lăr, p. 662)
ions (Ī-ŏnz, p. 665)
isotonic (ī-sō-TŎN-ĭk, p. 664)
magnesium (p. 672)
milliequivalent (mEq) (mĭl-ē-ĕ-KWĬV-ă-lĕnt, p. 665)
osmosis (ŏz-MŌ-sĭs, p. 664)
passive transport (p. 663)
phosphorus (FŎS-fŭ-rŭs, p. 671)
potassium (pŏ-TĂS-ē-ŭm, p. 666)
sodium (p. 665)

In this chapter you will find a discussion of body fluids and electrolytes, their normal values, the mechanisms that operate to keep them normal, and some of the more common types of fluid and electrolyte imbalances.

FLUIDS (WATER)

Water has many functions. It provides an extracellular transportation route to deliver nutrients to the cells and carry waste products from the cells. Once inside the cells, it provides a medium in which chemical reactions, or metabolism, is able to occur. Water also acts as a lubricant for tissues. Two other important functions of water are to aid in the maintenance of acid-base balance and to assist in heat regulation by evaporation.

Water is critically important to the body. Water constitutes the largest percentage of body weight. This percentage depends on several factors and varies with each individual. First, age affects the amount of water in the body. A newborn's body weight is comprised of 70% to 80% water. That percentage increases in a premature infant to as high as 90%. The infant begins to lose body fluid most rapidly in the first 6 months, and by 12 years the proportion approaches that of an adult. The percentage water makes up in the body declines from that highest percentage at birth to 50% to 60% in adults and 45% to 55% in the older adult.

Another important influence on the amount of water in the body is the amount of fat in the individual. There is a correlation between water content and fat content; fat contains relatively little water. A woman has proportionately more body fat than a man, which means the woman has less body fluid than the man. The more obese an individual, the smaller the percentage of body water. Both obese and older adults are at risk for complications of illness from dehydration or fluid shifts because they have less fluid reserve in their bodies (see Life Span Considerations for Older Adults

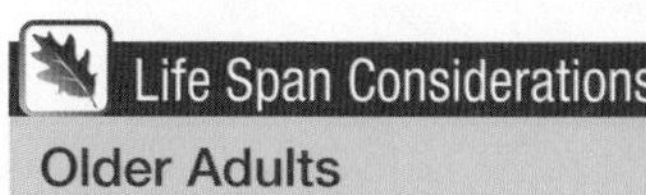

Older Adults

Dehydration

Older adults are at increased risk of dehydration because of the following factors:

- Fat replaces lean muscle as aging progresses, leading to a decrease in total body fluid.
- The aging kidney is less able to concentrate urine, so more fluid is lost.
- Decreases in mobility and diminished sense of thirst often result in decreased fluid intake.
- Incontinent older individuals sometimes restrict fluid intake to reduce the frequency of urination.
- To compensate for changes in taste, older adults often oversalt their food, resulting in electrolyte and fluid imbalances.
- Physiologic changes in the skin and mucous membranes make them less reliable indicators of dehydration.
- Dehydration will sometimes first manifest as mild disorientation.
- Signs and symptoms of dehydration include thirst, dry mucous membranes, increased heart rate, decreased blood pressure, poor skin turgor, and flat neck veins.
- Dehydration increases the risk of orthostatic hypotension.
- Decreased fluid intake increases the likelihood of constipation.
- Because the aging kidney is less efficient at excretion, giving intravenous (IV) infusions or supplements containing sodium or potassium increases the risk of electrolyte imbalance.
- Monitor the complete blood count carefully to detect changes in the hematocrit as it relates to hemoglobin. Decreased plasma volume elevates the hematocrit, whereas the hemoglobin level remains constant.

box). Infants are also at risk for dehydration. More than half of an infant's fluid is **extracellular** (outside the cells) (Figure 22-1). Extracellular fluid is lost from the body more rapidly than **intracellular** (inside the cells) fluid. Very young, very old, and obese patients are at a higher risk for developing a deficient fluid volume. A loss of 10% of body fluid is serious in an adult, and a 20% loss is fatal. In an infant those figures are even more significant. A loss of 5% is serious, 10% is very serious, and 15% is fatal.

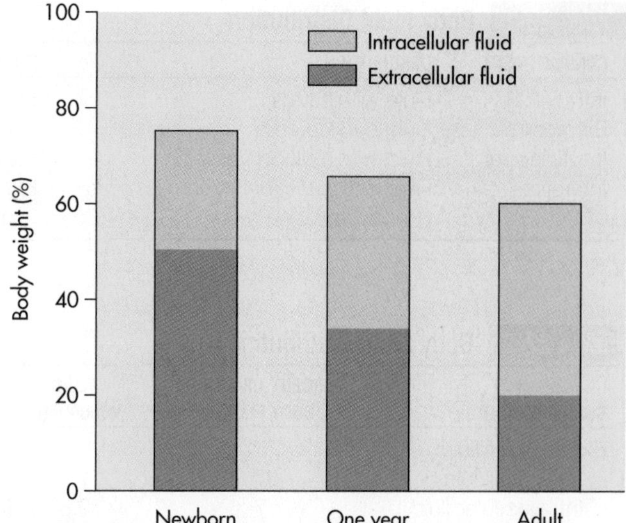

FIGURE 22-1 In the newborn, more than half of total body fluid is extracellular. As the child grows, proportions gradually reach adult levels.

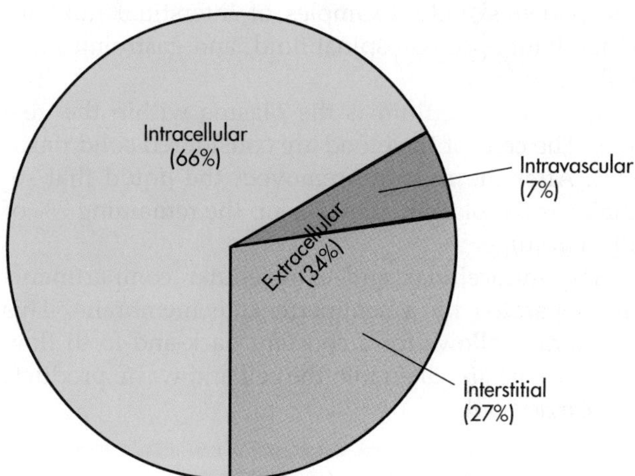

FIGURE 22-2 Volumes of body fluids in each fluid compartment.

FLUID COMPARTMENTS

The locations of fluids in the body are identified by categorizing them into compartments. However, *compartment* is an abstract term because rather than being contained in a compartment in a specific area, the fluids are in constant motion throughout the body to carry out their functions.

The body has two primary fluid compartments: intracellular and extracellular (Figure 22-2). Even though each is specific in its location and functions, there is constant interaction between the compartments.

The fluid compartments (Tables 22-1 and 22-2) are as follows:

1. Intracellular
2. Extracellular
   a. Interstitial
   b. Intravascular

The intracellular fluid compartment is the larger of the two compartments, comprising 66% of the body's fluid. It contains the fluid inside the billions of cells within the body.

The extracellular compartment contains any fluid outside the cells. This compartment is further divided into the interstitial and the intravascular fluid compartments.

Interstitial fluid is between the cells, or in the tissues. It accounts for approximately 27% of the fluid in

Table 22-1 Body Fluid Distribution

COMPARTMENT	DESCRIPTION	FLUID
Intracellular	Fluid within cells	Intracellular fluid (ICF)
Extracellular	Fluid outside cells	Extracellular fluid (ECF)
Intravascular	Fluid within blood vessels	Plasma
Interstitial	Fluid in tissues (between cells or in body spaces)	Examples: interstitial fluid, lymph, cerebrospinal fluid, intraocular fluid, gastrointestinal (GI) secretions, urine, perspiration, exudates

Table 22-2 Body Fluid Distribution

COMPARTMENT	PERCENT OF TOTAL BODY FLUID	FLUID VOLUME (L)
Extracellular fluid		
Interstitial fluid	27	11.2
Intravascular fluid (plasma)	7	2.8
Intracellular fluid	66	42

Table 22-3 Normal Fluid Intake and Output in an Adult Eating 2500 Calories per Day (Approximate Figures)

ROUTE	GAIN (mL)	ROUTE	AMOUNT OF LOSS (mL)
Water in food	1000	Skin	500
Water from oxidation	300	Lungs	350
Water as liquid	1200	Feces	150
		Kidney	1500
Total	2500	Total	2500

the patient's body. Examples of interstitial fluid include lymph, cerebrospinal fluid, and gastrointestinal (GI) secretions.

Intravascular fluid is the plasma within the vessels. The cells of the blood are considered solid particles. After the cells are removed, the liquid that remains is the plasma. It makes up the remaining 7% of fluid volume.

The intracellular and extracellular compartments are separated by a semipermeable membrane. This membrane allows for a constant back-and-forth flow as nutrients are taken into the cell and waste products are carried out.

INTAKE AND OUTPUT

As water moves through all parts of the body, it is constantly being lost. Fluid leaves the body through the kidneys, the lungs, the skin, and the GI tract. To maintain homeostasis, the normal daily loss must be met by the normal daily intake. **Homeostasis** is a relative constancy in the internal environment of the body, naturally maintained by adaptive responses that promote healthy survival. In order to maintain homeostasis, it is necessary that bodily fluids and electrolytes remain within the exact limits of normal (Lewis et al., 2007). Daily water intake and output (I&O) is approximately 2500 mL (Table 22-3).

Water loss is replenished in two ways—first, by ingestion of liquids and food, and second, by metabolism, both of food and in body tissues. Intake includes all fluids entering the body. Fluids are either liquids taken orally or those consumed in food, including foods that assume a liquid consistency at room temperature. Additional intake includes tube feedings and parenteral intake such as intravenous (IV) fluids, blood components, and total parenteral nutrition (TPN).

Liquid output includes all fluids leaving the body, including those lost through perspiration and expiration. Urine, diarrhea, vomitus, nasogastric suction, and chest tube drainage are examples of measurable output. Drainage from surgical wounds and drainage collected in surgical receptacles such as the Jackson-Pratt, Davol, or Hemovac systems are also considered liquid output. The determination of exact amounts of fluid loss and fluid replacement is not possible as part of nursing interventions, so you will use approximations. Because it is possible to measure fluid I&O, the importance of accurate record keeping cannot be overemphasized when determining a patient's fluid needs.

The kidneys play an extremely important role in fluid balance. If the kidneys are not functioning properly, the body has great difficulty with regulating fluid balance. The nephrons are the functioning units of the kidney. The nephrons filter blood at a rate of 125 mL/min, or about 180 L/day. This is called the **glomerular filtration rate** and leads to an output of 1 to 2 L (1000 to 2000 mL) of urine per day. The nephrons reabsorb the remaining 178 L or more of fluid.

If the body loses even 1% to 2% of its fluid, the kidneys conserve fluid by reabsorbing more water from the renal filtrate, which results in a more concentrated urine.

It is necessary for the kidneys to excrete a minimum of 30 mL/hr of urine (720 mL/24 hr) to eliminate waste products from the body. The kidneys react to fluid excesses by excreting a more dilute urine; this rids the body of excess fluid and conserves electrolytes.

A simple and accurate method of determining water balance is by weighing the patient under exact conditions, for example, same time of day, same amount of bed clothing, same type of gown, and same

Skill 22-1 Measuring Intake and Output (I&O)

Nursing Action *(Rationale)*

1. Identify patient. *(Ensures accuracy.)*
2. Explain procedure. *(Enlists patient's cooperation and promotes patient participation.)*
3. Instruct patient to inform staff of all oral intake. Provide a marked intake and output (I&O) container. *(Facilitates accurate I&O measurement.)*
4. Instruct patient not to empty any output collection receptacles and to notify you after elimination. *(Contributes to accurate I&O measurement.)*
5. Alert all staff and remind patient of need to measure I&O. *(Promotes accurate compliance.)*
6. Measure and record all fluids taken orally, gastric tube feedings, and all fluids administered parenterally. *(Helps ensure accurate measurement of intake.)*
7. Wash hands and don gloves. *(Prevents transmission of microorganisms.)*
8. Measure and record output in Foley drainage system, diarrhea stools, nasogastric suction, emesis, ileostomy, and output in surgical wound receptacles such as Davol, Jackson-Pratt, and Hemovac. Measure and record output from chest tube drainage in water-sealed container by marking with felt-tip pen. *(Ensures accurate measurement and proper disposal of output.)*
9. Remove gloves and wash hands. *(Prevents cross-contamination.)*
10. Compute and document I&O on patient's record. *(Ensures accurate documentation of total I&O.)*
11. Be vigilant to maintain accurate I&O when ordered.

attached equipment, such as electrodes. Empty all drainage bags before weighing the patient. **Because 1 L of fluid equals 2.2 pounds (1 kg), a weight change of 2.2 pounds will reflect a loss or gain of 1 L of body fluid** (Skill 22-1). To determine a patient's hydration or dehydration levels, performance of urine specific measurements is appropriate. A urine specific gravity of more than 1.030 indicates concentrated urine (seen in conditions of dehydration), whereas a measurement of less than 1.010 indicates dilute urine (seen in conditions of hydration) (Lewis et al., 2007).

MOVEMENT OF FLUID AND ELECTROLYTES

Substances entering the body begin their journey in the extracellular fluid. However, to carry out their functions, they have to cross the semipermeable membrane surrounding each body cell and enter the cell. The fat and protein molecules that make up the membrane are arranged so that some substances can enter the cells and others cannot. Several methods are used to move fluids, electrolytes and other solutes, or dissolved substances from one compartment to another.

A number of processes allow this mass movement of substances into and out of cells. These transport processes are classified under two general headings:

1. Passive transport processes
2. Active transport processes

As implied by their name, active transport processes necessitate the expenditure of energy by the cell, and passive transport processes do not. The energy required for active transport processes is obtained from an important chemical substance called adenosine triphosphate (ATP). ATP is produced in the mitochondria from nutrients and is capable of releasing energy that in turn enables the cell to work. For active transport processes to occur, the breakdown of ATP and the use of the related energy are required.

The details of active and passive transport of substances across cell membranes is much easier to understand if you keep in mind the following two key facts: (1) in passive transport (the movement of small molecules by diffusion across a cell membrane) processes, no cellular energy is required to move substances from a high concentration to a low concentration; and (2) in active transport processes, cellular energy is required to move substances from a low concentration to a high concentration.

PASSIVE TRANSPORT

The primary passive transport processes that move substances through the cell membranes include the following:

- Diffusion
- Osmosis
- Filtration

DIFFUSION

Water is able to move freely from one compartment to another by diffusion. Diffusion is the movement of particles in all directions through a solution or gas (Table 22-4). In diffusion, solutes move from an area of higher concentration to an area of lower concentration, which eventually results in an equal distribution of solutes within the two areas. Diffusion occurs, for example, when ink is dropped into a glass of water. The ink will disperse in all directions until it is evenly distributed throughout the fluid. When diffusion occurs in the body, the molecules have the same action as the ink spreading through the water. With each inhalation by the patient, oxygen enters the lungs and moves into

Table 22-4 Passive Transport Processes

PROCESS	DESCRIPTION	EXAMPLES
Diffusion	Movement of particles through a membrane from an area of high concentration to an area of low concentration—that is, down the concentration gradient	Movement of carbon dioxide out of all cells; movement of sodium ions into nerve cells as they conduct an impulse
Osmosis	Diffusion of water through a selectively permeable membrane in the presence of at least one impermeable solute	Diffusion of water molecules into and out of cells to correct imbalances in water concentration
Filtration	Movement of water and small solute particles, but not larger particles, through a filtration membrane; movement occurs from area of high pressure to area of low pressure	In the kidney, water and small solutes move from blood vessels but blood proteins and blood cells do not, thus beginning the formation of urine

From Thibodeau, G.A., & Patton, K.T. (2008). *Structure and function of the human body.* (13th ed.). St. Louis: Mosby.

the intravascular compartment and into the cells by diffusion. Gases, including oxygen, nitrogen, and carbon dioxide, leave the capillaries and diffuse into the cell membrane and become distributed throughout the body (Lewis et al., 2007).

OSMOSIS

Osmosis is the movement of water from an area of lower concentration to an area of higher concentration (see Table 22-4). Osmosis equalizes the concentration of ions or molecules on each side of the membrane (Lewis et al., 2007). The flow of water will continue until the number of ions or molecules on both sides of the membrane is equal. What happens when you boil a hot dog in water is an example of osmosis. The water passes through the hot dog skin, which is a semipermeable membrane, in an attempt to equalize the number of molecules on both sides of the membrane. Finally, when the hot dog is able to hold no more water, the skin, or semipermeable membrane, ruptures.

The red blood cells offer an example of the osmotic process in the body. If extracellular fluid is more concentrated than intracellular fluid, the fluid from inside the cell moves out to the extracellular fluid, causing the red blood cell to shrink. If the fluid among the compartments is in equilibrium, fluid will enter and leave the cell at the same rate and the cell size will not change. Another example is when extracellular fluid is less concentrated than the fluid in the red blood cells. Fluid moves into the cell, causing it to enlarge. The process will sometimes continue until the cell ruptures.

Solutions are classified in the body as hypertonic, isotonic, or hypotonic according to the electrolyte concentration. The concentration of the solution will cause the cells of the body to react the same way the red blood cell does. **Hypertonic** (a solution of higher osmotic pressure) solutions pull fluid from the cells; **isotonic** (a solution of same osmotic pressure) solutions expand the body's fluid volume without causing a fluid shift from one compartment to another; and **hypotonic** (a solution of lower osmotic pressure) solutions move into the cells, causing them to enlarge. Each of these actions occurs through the mechanism of osmosis.

FILTRATION

Filtration is the transfer of water and dissolved substances from an area of higher pressure to an area of lower pressure. An example of filtration occurs at the capillary level of the circulation. A force behind filtration is called **hydrostatic pressure,** which is the force of fluid pressing outward on a vessel wall (see Table 22-4). The pumping action of the heart is responsible for the amount of force, the hydrostatic pressure, that causes water and electrolytes to move from the capillaries to the interstitial fluid.

ACTIVE TRANSPORT

The fluid movements discussed to this point necessitate no energy expenditure by the body; they are examples of passive transport. **Active transport** requires energy; it is a force that moves molecules into cells without regard for their positive or negative charge and against concentration factors that will prevent entry into the cell via diffusion. Active transport moves fluid and electrolytes from an area of lower concentration to an area of higher concentration.

Substances actively transported through the cell membrane include sodium, potassium, calcium, iron, hydrogen, and amino acids. The movement of glucose into the cells occurs through the process of active transport. Insulin provides the transport for glucose to leave the intravascular compartment and move into the cells, where the glucose can then be used for energy.

ELECTROLYTES

As water moves through the compartments of the body, it contains substances that are sometimes called **minerals** or **salts** but which are technically known as **electrolytes.** Electrolytes are substances that when in solution, separate (or dissociate) into electrically charged particles. Electrolytes develop tiny electrical charges when they dissolve in water and break up into particles known as ions. Ions develop either a positive or negative electrical charge. Ions with a positive charge are called cations. Ions with a negative charge are called anions.

The following are examples of cations:
- Sodium (Na^+)
- Potassium (K^+)
- Calcium (Ca^{++})
- Magnesium (Mg^{++})

The following are examples of anions:
- Chloride (Cl^-)
- Bicarbonate (HCO_3^-)
- Sulfate (SO_4^-)
- Hydrogen phosphate (HPO_4^-)

A balance exists among the electrolytes. The principal electrolytes must be present in proper quantities for normal metabolism and function in the body. For this balance to occur, there must be a negatively charged anion for each positively charged cation.

A sample of plasma is taken to measure the electrolytes. The measurement is expressed in milliequivalents (mEq). Rather than electrolytes being measured by their weights, they are measured by their electrical activity. A milliequivalent (mEq) is a measure of the chemical activity or chemical combining power of an ion. The chemical activity of an electrolyte is compared with the chemical activity of hydrogen. One milliequivalent of any electrolyte has the same chemical combining power as 1 mEq of hydrogen. In each fluid compartment in the body, the cations and anions balance each other with their chemical combining power to maintain electrical neutrality, which again keeps the body in homeostasis.

Although the electrolytes move freely among the fluid compartments, each has a primary location. The location and the function of each electrolyte become important in understanding disease processes. The healthy body maintains homeostasis by correcting any excesses or deficiencies of the electrolytes.

Sodium

The normal blood level of sodium (Na^+), a cation and the most abundant electrolyte in the body, is 134 to 142 mEq/L. It is the major extracellular electrolyte, and because the plasma sample used to measure electrolyte levels comes from the extracellular fluid, the level is high. In contrast, the intracellular level of sodium is approximately 10 mEq. The major source of sodium comes from the diet. That is true of all the electrolytes. However, unlike the other electrolytes, sodium is a substance that it is frequently necessary to limit in the diet rather than encourage. The kidneys are the primary excretion route for sodium. It is important to know that many electrolytes, such as sodium, not only pass into and out of the body, but also move back and forth between a number of body fluids during each 24-hour period. Figure 22-3 shows the large volumes of sodium-containing internal secretions that are produced each day. During a 24-hour period, more than 8 L of fluid containing 1000 to 1300 mEq of sodium are poured into the digestive system. This sodium, along with most of that contained in the diet, is almost completely reabsorbed. Some major dietary sources of sodium are cheese, table salt, seafood, processed meat, canned vegetables, canned soups, ketchup, and snack foods, such as pretzels and potato chips. Precise regulation and control of sodium levels is required for survival.

The functions of sodium include regulation of the water balance. Sodium controls the extracellular fluid volume mainly through osmotic pressure, because water follows the sodium in the body (where sodium is, water will follow). It also increases cell membrane permeability. Sodium stimulates conduction of nerve impulses and helps maintain neuromuscular irritability. Sodium is important in controlling contractility of muscles, especially the heart.

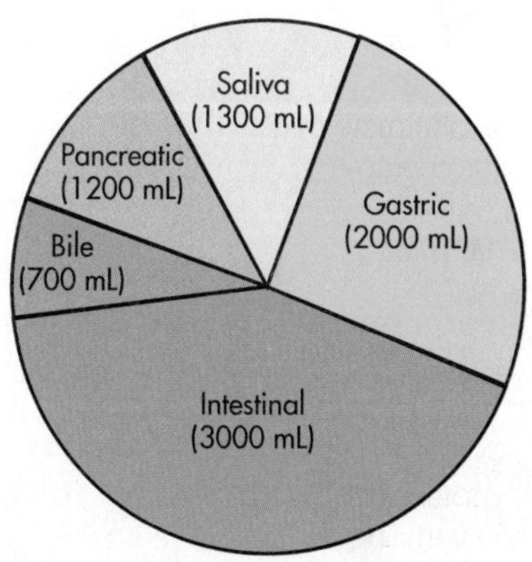

FIGURE 22-3 Sodium-containing internal secretions produced every day.

Hyponatremia

A less-than-normal concentration of sodium in the blood is called **hyponatremia.** This is possible when there is a sodium loss or a water excess (Box 22-1). Hyponatremia occurs when the sodium drops to less than 134 mEq/L in the extracellular fluid.

When a deficiency results from sodium loss, the body attempts to compensate by decreasing water excretion. Hyponatremia occurs because water is being retained in the body, which has a diluting effect on all of the blood components. The signs and symptoms of hyponatremia depend on the cause and also on how rapid and severe the sodium loss is. As sodium levels decrease in the extracellular fluid, water is pulled into the cells, causing them to become edematous, and as the fluid moves into the cells, potassium is shifted out; therefore the patient is likely to also have a potassium imbalance.

Hypernatremia

Hypernatremia is a greater-than-normal concentration of sodium. The sodium level exceeds 145 mEq/L. It is caused by an excess of sodium or a decrease in body water (Box 22-2). The body attempts to correct the imbalance by conserving water through renal reabsorption. Hypernatremia causes fluid to shift from the cells to the interstitial spaces, resulting in cellular dehydration and an interruption in cellular processes. Again, a potassium imbalance frequently occurs. In sodium retention, potassium is excreted.

Potassium

The normal blood serum level of **potassium** (K^+), the dominant intracellular cation, is 3.5 to 5 mEq/L. The level of potassium in the extracellular fluid is low because potassium is an intracellular electrolyte. The intracellular level of potassium (usually not measured) is much higher at 150 mEq/L. Of the body's potassium, 98% is in the cells and 2% is in the extracellular fluid.

A well-balanced diet usually provides adequate potassium. Approximately 65 mEq of potassium is required each day. Potassium is widely distributed in natural foods; fruits, such as oranges, bananas, apricots and cantaloupe; legumes; leafy vegetables; potatoes; mushrooms; tomatoes; carrots; and meat are sources of potassium (Box 22-3). The average daily intake of potassium is 60 to 100 mEq.

The routes of potassium excretion are the kidneys (80% to 90%) and in the feces and perspiration (10% to 20%). The kidneys control the excretion of potassium. Sodium and potassium seem to pair off against each other, and the kidneys prefer to conserve sodium, even when both electrolytes are depleted. In both normal and abnormal situations, sodium will be reabsorbed and potassium will be excreted. Because the major route of excretion of potassium is the kidneys, any

Box 22-1 Hyponatremia: Causes, Signs and Symptoms, and Nursing Interventions

CAUSES
- Inadequate sodium intake
- Loss of GI fluids
- Vomiting
- Diarrhea
- GI or biliary drainage via nasogastric tube or T-tube
- Fistulas
- Loss through skin
- Diaphoresis
- Large open lesions (burns)
- Shifting of body fluids
- Massive edema
- Ascites
- Burns
- Small bowel obstruction
- Lengthy hydrotherapy

SIGNS AND SYMPTOMS
- Headache*
- Irritability
- Muscle weakness, muscle twitching, tremors
- Fatigue*
- Apathy
- Postural hypotension*
- Nausea and vomiting
- Abdominal cramps
- Apprehension

Severe or Prolonged Deficit
- Shock
- Altered level of consciousness (lethargy, confusion)
- Seizures
- Coma
- Altered level of consciousness usually accompanies a serum sodium level less than 125 mEq/L and indicates that the patient's condition is deteriorating

NURSING INTERVENTIONS
- Monitor I&O of patients receiving diuretic medications
- Monitor and record vital signs, especially blood pressure and pulse
- Monitor neurologic status frequently; report any change in level of consciousness
- Weigh patient daily
- Monitor skin turgor at least every 8 hours
- Restrict fluid intake as ordered, because this is primary treatment for dilutional hyponatremia; post a sign about fluid restriction in the patient's room
- Observe for abnormal GI, renal, or skin losses
- Replace fluid loss with fluids containing sodium, not plain water

GI, Gastrointestinal; *I&O*, intake and output.
*Most common signs and symptoms.

Box 22-2 Hypernatremia: Causes, Signs and Symptoms, and Nursing Interventions

CAUSES
- More water than sodium is lost from the body
- Abnormally large intake of sodium
  - —Taking too many salt tablets
  - —Overuse of table salt
  - —IV saline infused too rapidly
  - —Prepared foods: frozen, canned, smoked
  - —Dairy products in large amounts
  - —Consumption of antacids containing sodium

SIGNS AND SYMPTOMS
- Dry, tenacious mucous membranes
- Low urinary output
- Firm, rubbery tissue turgor
- Restlessness, agitation, confusion, flushed skin

Severe or Prolonged Excess
- Manic excitement
- Tachycardia
- Death

NURSING INTERVENTIONS
- Monitor and record vital signs, especially blood pressure and pulse
- Provide a safe environment for confused or agitated patient
- Monitor I&O
- Weigh daily to check for body fluid loss
- Decrease sodium intake in diet
- Monitor water loss from fever, infection, increased respiratory rate
- Monitor serum sodium level

I&O, Intake and output; *IV*, intravenous.

Box 22-3 Foods Rich in Potassium

FRUITS (INCLUDING JUICES)
- Apricots
- Bananas
- Grapefruit
- Melon
- Cantaloupe
- Honeydew
- Dried fruits, figs, dates, raisins
- Oranges

PROTEIN FOODS
- Beef
- Chicken
- Liver
- Pork
- Veal
- Turkey
- Milk
- Nuts, peanut butter

VEGETABLES
- Asparagus
- Dried beans
- Broccoli
- Cabbage
- Carrots
- Celery
- Mushrooms
- Dried peas
- Potatoes (especially skins): white, sweet
- Spinach
- Squash
- Tomatoes

BEVERAGES
- Cocoa
- Cola drinks
- Instant tea and coffee

condition that causes a decrease in urine output also causes potassium retention. Serum potassium levels increase in kidney failure (Lewis et al., 2007). A rise in potassium necessitates continuous monitoring. An important consideration in homeostasis is that kidney function will determine the potassium level in the body. Too little or too much potassium affects the heart muscle and has potential to result in a life-threatening disturbance in cardiac rhythm (dysrhythmia).

The main function of potassium is regulation of water and electrolyte content within the cell. With sodium and calcium, it promotes transmission of nerve impulses and also skeletal muscle function. Potassium assists in the cellular metabolism of carbohydrates and proteins. Another function of potassium is to control the hydrogen ion concentration. When potassium moves out of the cell, sodium and hydrogen ions move in. The result is the regulation of acid-base balance.

Hypokalemia

A decrease in the body's potassium to a level less than 3.5 mEq/L is known as **hypokalemia.** Because the normal range for a serum potassium level is narrow (3.5 to 5 mEq/L), a slight decrease has profound consequences. The major cause of potassium loss is renal excretion (Box 22-4). The kidneys do not conserve potassium and excrete it even when the body needs the potassium. Intestinal fluids contain large amounts of potassium. In excessive GI losses from gastric suctioning or prolonged vomiting, potassium tends to become depleted. Severe diarrhea, fistulas, ileostomy, villous adenoma (tumor of the intestine that produces potassium-containing mucus), and excessive diaphoresis will also sometimes result in potassium loss. The use of diuretics, such as thiazides or furosemide (Lasix), promotes hypokalemia. Conditions that cause injury to the cells in turn cause the release of potas-

Box 22-4 Hypokalemia: Causes, Signs and Symptoms, and Nursing Interventions

CAUSES
- Decreased potassium intake
- Increased potassium loss
  - —Increased aldosterone activity
  - —GI losses (vomiting, diarrhea, GI suctioning)
  - —Ileostomy
  - —Potassium-losing diuretics
  - —Loss from cells, as in trauma, burns, fistulas
  - —Skin losses, diaphoresis
- Conditions causing very large urine output
- Potassium shift into cells
  - —Treatment of acidosis
  - —Metabolic alkalosis
  - —Villous adenoma (tumor of the intestine that produces potassium-containing mucus)

SIGNS AND SYMPTOMS
- Skeletal muscle weakness (especially in lower extremities), leg cramps*
- Paresthesias, hyporeflexia
- Decreased bowel sounds, cramps, and constipation, anorexia, nausea, vomiting*
- Diminished deep tendon reflexes, lethargy, confusion; paralysis involving the respiratory muscles; coma
- Orthostatic hypotension
- Cardiac dysrhythmias; weak, irregular pulse
- ECG changes
- Polyuria

Severe or Prolonged Deficit
- Flaccid paralysis
- Kidney damage
- Paralytic ileus
- Cardiac or respiratory arrest

NURSING INTERVENTIONS
- Carefully assess patients taking digitalis glycosides, especially if also taking a diuretic, for hypoglycemia, which has capacity to potentiate the action of the digitalis glycoside medication and cause toxicity
- Administer potassium chloride (KCl) supplement as prescribed by the physician (oral or IV)
- Whether through a peripheral or central catheter, it is necessary to administer IV potassium with care to prevent serious complications
- IV potassium is always diluted and delivered using an infusion controller
- Encourage increased intake of foods high in potassium
- Monitor bowel sounds
- Monitor serum potassium level
- Monitor I&O (about 40 mEq of potassium is lost in each liter of urine; diuresis has potential to put the patient at a risk for potassium loss)
- During treatment with potassium, it is necessary for the patient's urinary output to be at least 600 mL/day. If urinary output is less than 20 mL/hr for 2 consecutive hours, interrupt the infusion and immediately notify the physician. If renal function is impaired, there is a significant risk of hyperkalemia.†
- Monitor telemetry

ECG, Electrocardiogram; *GI*, gastrointestinal; *I&O*, intake and output; *IV*, intravenous.
*Most common signs and symptoms.
†From Burger, C. (2004). Hypokalemia—averting crisis with early recognition and intervention. *American Journal of Nursing, 104*(11), 61.

sium from the cells to the interstitial spaces and ultimately to the kidneys. If renal function is normal, the potassium will be excreted. Because the normal amounts of potassium are so small, fluctuations have the potential to develop into serious problems. Hypokalemia has the capacity to affect skeletal and cardiac function. The resulting muscle weakness causes life-threatening cardiac conduction abnormalities.

Hyperkalemia

An increase in the body's serum potassium level greater than 5 mEq/L is known as **hyperkalemia.** Because the normal range for a serum potassium level is narrow (3.5 to 5 mEq/L), a slight increase poses the risk of serious consequences. Potassium is gained through intake and lost by excretion. This condition is not as common as hypokalemia as long as renal function is normal. The major cause of potassium excess is renal disease, in which potassium is not excreted adequately (Box 22-5). When severe tissue damage occurs, potassium is released from the cells. Shock often accompanies this damage, resulting in reduced kidney output. The result is an elevated potassium level.

Excessive intake of foods high in potassium, especially with decreased urine output, may cause an increased serum potassium level. Other causes of hyperkalemia include (1) excessive use of salt substitutes (most of which use potassium as a substitute for sodium); (2) potassium supplements (oral or IV); (3) infusion of a large volume of blood nearing its expiration date (serum concentration increases the longer donated blood is stored); (4) drugs such as beta blockers, which inhibit potassium shifts into cells; (5) potassium-sparing diuretics such as spironolactone; (6) chemotherapy, which causes cell death or lysis with release of high levels of intracellular potassium into the blood; (7) angiotensin-converting enzyme inhibitors; (8) nonsteroidal antiinflammatory drugs; and (9) aminoglycosides.

Although hyperkalemia is less common than hypokalemia, it is often more dangerous because of cardiac arrest, which is caused by overstimulation of the cardiac muscle. A serum potassium level of 7 mEq/L or greater risks serious cardiac dysrhythmias.

Chloride

The normal blood level of **chloride** (Cl^-), an extracellular anion, is 96 to 105 mEq/L. It is the chief anion in

Box 22-5 Hyperkalemia: Causes, Signs and Symptoms, and Nursing Interventions

CAUSES

NOTE: Hyperkalemia may be the most dangerous of the electrolyte disorders.

- Potassium intake (parenteral or oral) in excess of kidney's ability to excrete
- Excessive use of salt substitutes
- Renal failure
- Adrenal insufficiency
- Potassium enters the bloodstream from injured cells with extensive trauma (shift of potassium out of the cells into extracellular fluid)
- Metabolic acidosis
- Infusion of large volume of blood nearing expiration date
- Beta blockers
- Potassium-sparing diuretics
- Tumor lysis syndrome after chemotherapy
- Angiotensin-converting enzyme inhibitors
- Nonsteroidal antiinflammatory drugs
- Aminoglycosides

SIGNS AND SYMPTOMS*

- Signs and symptoms are often nonspecific; serum potassium level and electrocardiogram (ECG) tracings are often the best clinical indicators
- Irritability
- Nausea, vomiting†
- Diarrhea, colic†
- Cardiac dysrhythmias†
- ECG changes
- Irregular pulse rate
- Hypotension
- Numbness, tingling
- Paresthesias
- Skeletal muscle weakness, especially of lower extremities

Severe or Prolonged Excess

- Flaccid paralysis
- Cardiac arrest† (serious dysrhythmias become especially dangerous when the serum potassium level reaches 7 mEq/L or more [normal serum potassium level ranges from 3.5 to 5 mEq/L])
- Anuria

NURSING INTERVENTIONS

- Decrease intake of foods high in potassium
- Administer Kayexalate (sodium polystyrene sulfonate) as prescribed by the physician (Kayexalate is possible to give orally, through a nasogastric tube, or as a retention enema); keep in mind when giving Kayexalate that serum sodium level will sometimes rise—watch for congestive heart failure
- Loop diuretics
- Decrease or stop medications associated with high potassium level
- Monitor underlying disorders leading to high potassium level
- Assess vital signs
- Monitor telemetry to detect dysrhythmias
- Monitor I&O (report an output of less than 30 mL/hr; an inability to excrete potassium in the urine will potentially lead to dangerously high potassium level)
- Hemodialysis in acute symptomatic hyperkalemia
- Monitor bowel sounds and number and character of bowel movements
- Monitor serum potassium level

*Prolonged potassium excess results in signs and symptoms similar to those of hypokalemia.
†Most common signs and symptoms.

interstitial and intravascular fluid. Even though chloride accounts for more than two thirds of the anions in the body, it is usually not considered alone. Chloride has the ability to diffuse quickly between the intracellular and extracellular compartments and combines easily with sodium to form sodium chloride or with potassium to form potassium chloride. It is more often linked with sodium.

The daily requirement of chloride is equal to that of sodium (3.65 to 10.85 g/day). Foods containing sodium also contain chloride. The main route of excretion is through the kidneys.

Chloride is necessary for the formation of hydrochloric acid in gastric juice. It is also a valuable electrolyte in regulating the osmotic pressure between the compartments and assisting in the regulation of acid-base balance.

Hypochloremia

Hypochloremia usually occurs when sodium is lost, because sodium and chloride are frequently paired. The most common causes of hypochloremia are vomiting and prolonged nasogastric or fistula drainage.

Hyperchloremia

Hyperchloremia rarely occurs but is possible when bicarbonate levels fall. The increase in chloride anions represents an attempt to compensate and maintain equal numbers with the cations in the body fluid. Because chloride imbalances rarely occur independently of other electrolytes, there are no specific signs and symptoms to identify a chloride imbalance.

Calcium

The normal blood level of calcium (Ca^{++}), a positively charged ion, is approximately 4.5 mEq/L. Of the 1200 g of calcium in the body, 99% is concentrated in the bones and the teeth, where it is physiologically inactive. The remaining 1% is found in the soft tissue and the extracellular fluid. Calcium is deposited in the bones and mobilized as needed to keep the blood level constant during any period of insufficient intake. Three considerations are important in the blood calcium level:

1. Deposition and resorption of bone
2. Absorption of calcium from the GI tract
3. Excretion of calcium in urine and feces

Vitamin D, calcitonin, and parathyroid hormone (parathormone) are necessary for the absorption and utilization of calcium.

The best food sources of calcium are milk and cheese. Other sources include beans, nuts, cauliflower, lettuce, and egg yolks. The average daily intake is 200 to 2500 mg. The dietary reference intakes (DRIs) vary from 360 mg for infants to 1200 mg for females 15 to 18 years of age. During pregnancy and lactation, 1300 mg is required. Prevention of osteoporosis focuses on adequate calcium intake (1000 mg/day in premenopausal women and postmenopausal women taking estrogen and 1500 mg/day in postmenopausal women who are not receiving supplemental estrogen). Calcium is removed from the body via the urine and feces.

Calcium is required for the formation and maintenance of strong bones and teeth. It is also necessary for normal blood clotting. Calcium has a depressing or sedative effect on neuromuscular irritability and thus promotes normal transmission of nerve impulses; it also helps regulate normal muscle contraction and relaxation. It helps hold body cells together by establishing the thickness and strength of cell membranes. One of its most important functions is to act as an enzyme activator for chemical reactions in the body.

Hypocalcemia

Hypocalcemia develops when the serum level is less than 4.5 mEq/L. Possible deficiencies arise from a variety of problems (Box 22-6):

- Infusion of excess amounts of citrated blood (citrates bind to the calcium)
- Excessive loss through diarrhea
- Inadequate dietary intake of calcium or vitamin D
- Surgical removal of parathyroid glands
- Decreased parathyroid function
- Pancreatic disease
- Small bowel disease

The signs and symptoms of hypocalcemia are neuromuscular irritation and increased excitability. As neuromuscular signs and symptoms increase, tetany is possible. Tetany is a condition characterized by excessive muscle cramps, laryngeal spasms, stridor, carpal spasms (Trousseau's sign), pedal spasms, and contraction of facial muscles (Chvostek's sign) (Figure 22-4).

Hypercalcemia

Hypercalcemia occurs when calcium levels exceed 5.8 mEq/L. It may occur when calcium stored in the bone enters the circulation, for example, in patients who are immobilized (Box 22-7). An increased intake of calcium or vitamin D also causes hypercalcemia.

Box 22-6 Hypocalcemia: Causes, Signs and Symptoms, and Nursing Interventions

CAUSES
- Excess binding of calcium ions
- Large amount of citrated blood
- Excess alcohol
- Alkalosis
- Dietary deficiency of calcium and vitamin D
- Chronic renal failure
- Pancreatic disease
- Disease of small bowel; malabsorption
- Severe diarrhea
- Anticonvulsants, such as phenobarbital and phenytoin (Dilantin)
- Diuretics (Lasix, Edecrin)
- Draining intestinal fistulas
- Deficiency of parathyroid hormone or vitamin D
- Increased magnesium
- Thyroid surgery (surgical removal of parathyroid glands, removal of parathyroid tumor)
- Injury or disease of parathyroid gland
- Severe burns
- Low serum albumin levels

SIGNS AND SYMPTOMS
- Anxiety, confusion, irritability
- Osteoporosis, pathologic fractures
- Tingling around nose, mouth, ears, fingers, toes*
- Twitching
- Muscle spasm of feet and hands*
- Tetany (note positive Trousseau's or Chvostek's sign [see Figure 22-4])
- Laryngeal spasms
- Nausea, vomiting*
- Hyperactive deep tendon reflexes
- Diarrhea*
- Cardiac dysrhythmias, cardiac arrest
- Calcium deposits in body tissues
- Diminished response to digitalis glycosides

NURSING INTERVENTIONS
- Monitor vital signs; monitor respiratory status, including rate, depth, and rhythm; be alert for stridor, dyspnea, or crowing (laryngeal spasms)
- Monitor pertinent laboratory values including calcium, albumin, and magnesium
- Encourage intake of a diet high in calcium-rich foods, vitamin D, and protein
- Administer calcium and vitamin D as prescribed by the physician
- Monitor treatment of underlying causes
- Acute hypocalcemia necessitates either IV calcium gluconate or calcium chloride
- For acute hypocalcemia, keep a tracheotomy tray and resuscitation bag at bedside in case of laryngeal spasms
- Monitor telemetry
- Monitor serum calcium, albumin, and magnesium levels
- Monitor I&O

I&O, Intake and output; *IV*, intravenous.
*Most common signs and symptoms.

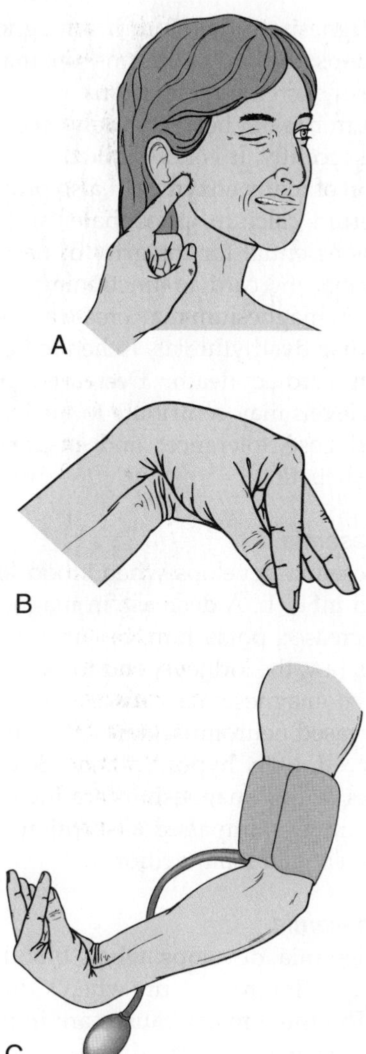

FIGURE 22-4 Tests for hypocalcemia. **A,** Chvostek's sign is a contraction of facial muscles in response to a light tap over the facial nerve in front of the ear. **B,** Trousseau's sign is a carpal spasm induced by **C,** inflating a blood pressure cuff above the systolic pressure for a few minutes.

Box 22-7 Hypercalcemia: Causes, Signs and Symptoms, and Nursing Interventions

CAUSES

- Loss from bone
- Immobilization
- Metastatic bone cancer
- Multiple myeloma
- Excess intake
- Dietary
- Antacids containing calcium
- Increased absorption
- Increased parathyroid hormone
- Increased vitamin D

SIGNS AND SYMPTOMS

- Anorexia, nausea, vomiting
- Behavioral changes, including confusion
- Thirst, polyuria*
- Renal calculi
- Decreased deep tendon reflexes
- Constipation
- Paralytic ileus
- Lethargy, coma
- Cardiac dysrhythmias, cardiac arrest
- Hypertension
- Decreased muscle tone*
- Decreased GI motility
- Bone pain

NURSING INTERVENTIONS

- Assist in the promotion of excretion of calcium in the urine
- Administer diuretics as ordered by the physician
- Encourage drinking 3000 to 4000 L of fluids per day
- Monitor I&O
- Be aware that in life-threatening hypercalcemia, measures to increase calcium secretion will sometimes include hemodialysis or peritoneal dialysis

GI, Gastrointestinal; *I&O,* intake and output.
*Most common signs and symptoms.

Neuromuscular activity is depressed, and renal calculi may develop because of the excretion of high levels of calcium by the kidneys.

Phosphorus

The normal blood level of phosphorus, chiefly present as hydrogen phosphate (HPO_4^-), an intracellular anion, is approximately 4 mEq/L. Phosphorus and calcium have an inverse relationship in the body: An increase in one causes a decrease in the other. As blood calcium levels increase, a decrease in phosphorus levels is necessary, and vice versa. The majority (70% to 80%) of phosphorus is found combined with calcium in an individual's bones and teeth, 10% is in an individual's muscle, and the remaining 10% is in the nerve tissue of the body.

Dietary intake of phosphorus is usually 800 to 1500 mg/day. The minimum daily requirement is 800 mg. Higher intake during pregnancy and lactation is needed. An adequate intake of vitamin D is necessary for the absorption of both calcium and phosphorus. Because a generous amount of phosphorus is present in many foods, a deficiency seldom occurs. Foods especially high in phosphorus include beef, pork, fish, poultry, milk products, and legumes. The kidneys are responsible for approximately 90% of the excretion of phosphorus. The remainder is excreted in the feces.

With calcium, phosphorus contributes to the support and maintenance of bones and teeth. It is important in many chemical reactions and acts as a buffer to regulate the body's acid-base balance. It promotes the effectiveness of many of the B vitamins, assists in normal nerve and muscle activity, and participates in carbohydrate metabolism.

Hypophosphatemia

Hypophosphatemia is possible as a result of a dietary insufficiency, impaired kidney function, or maldistribution of phosphate. Muscle weakness, especially affecting the respiratory muscles, sometimes occurs.

Hyperphosphatemia

Hyperphosphatemia most commonly occurs as a result of renal insufficiency. Another cause is increased intake of phosphate or vitamin D. Signs and symptoms of tetany, numbness and tingling around the mouth, and muscle spasms develop.

Magnesium

The normal blood level of **magnesium** (Mg^{++}), the second most abundant cation in the intracellular fluid, is 1.5 to 2.4 mEq/L. Although only small amounts of magnesium are in the blood, it is important in maintaining normal body function. The majority (60%) is found in the bone, 39% in the muscle and the soft tissue, and 1% in the extracellular fluid, most of which is in the cerebrospinal fluid.

Dietary intake is usually 200 to 400 mg daily. The minimum daily requirement is 250 mg for the average adult, 150 mg for an infant, and 400 mg for a female during pregnancy and lactation. Magnesium is another electrolyte commonly distributed in foods. Whole grains, fruits, vegetables, meat, fish, legumes, and dairy products are dietary sources.

The major route of magnesium excretion is the kidneys. There is a correlation between the amount of magnesium and the amount of potassium excreted. The kidneys do not conserve potassium, but they do conserve magnesium; therefore if a magnesium deficiency develops, the body will conserve magnesium at the expense of excreting potassium.

Magnesium has not been a widely recognized electrolyte until recently. It is now linked as a cofactor in the activation of many enzymes. It also promotes regulation of serum calcium, phosphate, and potassium levels and is essential for integrity of nervous tissue, skeletal muscle, and cardiac functioning.

Diets low in magnesium may create a risk for hypertension, cardiac dysrhythmias, ischemic heart disease, and sudden cardiac death. Decreased intracellular magnesium levels may contribute to the hypertension, abnormal glucose tolerance, and insulin resistance common in diabetics.

Hypomagnesemia

Hypomagnesemia develops when blood levels fall to less than 1.5 mEq/L. A decrease in magnesium often parallels decreased potassium, because if the magnesium level is low, the kidneys tend to excrete more potassium. Hypomagnesemia causes signs and symptoms of increased neuromuscular irritability similar to those observed with hypocalcemia (Box 22-8). The major causes of low magnesium are increased excretion by the kidneys, impaired absorption from the GI tract, and prolonged malnutrition.

Hypermagnesemia

Hypermagnesemia develops when blood levels exceed 2.5 mEq/L. It rarely occurs when kidney function is normal. The three major causes are impaired renal function, excess magnesium administration, and dia-

Box 22-8 Hypomagnesemia: Causes, Signs and Symptoms, and Nursing Interventions

CAUSES

- Decreased intake
  - —Prolonged malnutrition
  - —Starvation
- Impaired absorption from GI tract
  - —Alcoholism
  - —Hypercalcemia
  - —Diarrhea
  - —Draining intestinal fistulas
- Conditions causing large losses of urine
- Prolonged IV feedings without magnesium supplementation

SIGNS AND SYMPTOMS

- Anorexia
- Mental changes*
- Agitation, depression, confusion
- Dysphagia
- Hyperactive deep tendon reflexes
- Nausea and vomiting
- Paresthesias*
- Tetany
- Tremors
- Seizures
- Ataxia
- Cramps, spasticity, tetany
- Tachycardia
- Hypotension
- Cardiac dysrhythmias

NURSING INTERVENTIONS

- Monitor vital signs
- Assess neuromuscular status
- Assess dysphagia
- Increase intake of magnesium-rich foods
- Administer magnesium supplements as prescribed by the physician
- Monitor I&O
- Monitor telemetry
- Institute seizure precautions
- Monitor respiratory status

GI, Gastrointestinal; *I&O*, intake and output; *IV*, intravenous.
*Most common signs and symptoms.

Box 22-9 Hypermagnesemia: Causes, Signs and Symptoms, and Nursing Interventions

CAUSES
- Renal failure
- Diabetic ketoacidosis with severe water loss

SIGNS AND SYMPTOMS
- Hypotension*
- Vasodilation*
- Heat
- Thirst
- Nausea and vomiting
- Loss of deep tendon reflexes
- Respiratory depression

Prolonged or Severe Excess
- Coma
- Cardiac arrest

NURSING INTERVENTIONS
- Promote urine excretion
- Administer diuretics as prescribed by the physician
- Decrease intake of foods or medications high in magnesium
- Monitor I&O

I&O, Intake and output.
*Most common signs and symptoms.

betic ketoacidosis when there is severe water loss (Box 22-9). An excess of magnesium severely restricts nerve and muscle activity.

Bicarbonate

The normal level of bicarbonate (HCO_3^-), one of the main anions in the extracellular fluid, is 22 to 24 mEq/L. It is an alkaline electrolyte whose major function is the regulation of the acid-base balance, also called *acid-alkaline balance.* Bicarbonate acts as a buffer to neutralize acids in the body and maintain the 20:1 bicarbonate to carbonic acid ratio needed to keep the body in homeostasis. The kidneys selectively regulate the amount of bicarbonate retained or excreted.

ACID-BASE BALANCE

Acid-base balance means homeostasis of the hydrogen ion (H^+) concentration in the body fluids. The hydrogen ion concentration is determined by the ratio of carbonic acid (H_2CO_3) to bicarbonate (HCO_3^-) in the extracellular fluid. The ratio needed for homeostasis is 1 part carbonic acid to 20 parts bicarbonate. The symbol used to indicate hydrogen ion balance is pH. When pH is measured, it is actually the hydrogen ion concentration in the patient's body that is measured. A sample of extracellular fluid, specifically arterial blood, is used to determine the body's pH.

Arterial blood gases will reveal whether the blood is acid, neutral, or alkaline. The more hydrogen ions in a solution, the more acid the solution. The fewer hydrogen ions in a solution, the more alkaline the solution. The terms *base* and *alkaline* are interchangeable; a base is an alkaline substance. An inverse relationship exists between hydrogen ion concentration and the pH level: As the numbers of hydrogen ion increase, the acidity of the solution increases and the pH decreases. The opposite happens with alkalinity—the number of hydrogen ions decreases and the pH increases. A pH of less than 7.35 is acid. A pH of greater than 7.45 is alkaline. The normal pH of arterial blood is approximately 7.45, whereas the normal pH of venous blood and interstitial fluid is approximately 7.35. Between 7.35 and 7.45 is considered normal blood pH. A pH lower than 6.8 or higher than 7.8 is usually fatal (Figure 22-5).

Two general types of disturbances can cause a pH imbalance. One imbalance arises from an increase or a

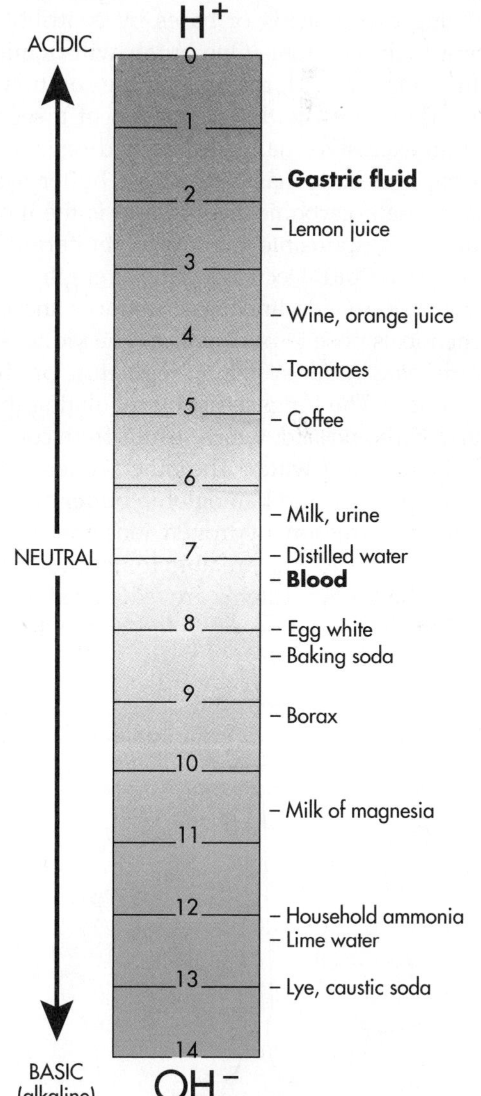

FIGURE 22-5 The pH scale. A pH of 7 is considered neutral. Values toward the top (less than 7) are acidic (the lower the number, the more acidic). Values toward the bottom (greater than 7) are basic (the higher the number, the more basic). Representative fluids and their approximate pHs are listed at the side of the figure.

decrease in the base substance—bicarbonate. The other imbalance results from adding or subtracting the acid substance—carbonic acid. The body's metabolism affects the base side of balance—so a bicarbonate imbalance causes metabolic acidosis or alkalosis. The body's respiratory system affects the acid side of the balance—so a carbonic acid imbalance causes respiratory acidosis or alkalosis. The four primary types of acid-base imbalance (discussed later in the chapter) are **respiratory acidosis, respiratory alkalosis, metabolic acidosis,** and **metabolic alkalosis.** Figure 22-6 shows the carbonic acid/bicarbonate ratio and pH.

The body has three systems that work to keep the pH in the narrow range of normal: the blood buffers, the respiratory system, and the kidneys. These systems are the body's three lines of defense that are constantly working to maintain a normal pH.

Try thinking of the **blood buffers** as chemical sponges. They circulate throughout the body in pairs, neutralizing excess acids or bases by contributing or accepting hydrogen ions. One buffer will dominate if the solution is too acid; the other if the solution is too alkaline. They work within a fraction of a second to prevent an excessive change in the hydrogen ion concentration. The body has four major buffer systems. The bicarbonate–carbonic acid system is the most important. It is responsible mainly for buffering blood and interstitial fluid. Decreasing the strength of potentially damaging acids and bases reduces the danger these chemicals pose to pH balance. The kidneys assist the bicarbonate buffer system in regulating production of bicarbonate. The lungs assist by regulating the production of carbonic acid, which results from combining carbon dioxide and water. The other systems are the phosphate, protein, and hemoglobin buffer systems.

For every 1 million hydrogen ions that enter the body, the buffer systems are able to neutralize all but five. Once the buffer systems are exhausted, the body calls on the second line of defense: the lungs. By speeding up or slowing down respirations, the lungs have the capacity to increase or decrease the amount of carbon dioxide in the blood. Removing carbon dioxide from the blood lowers the carbonic acid level; this is the mechanism by which the respiratory system regulates pH. Whereas it took seconds for the buffer systems to work, it takes minutes for the lungs to begin to adjust the pH. Even though the respiratory system is slower than the buffers, however, the lungs are able to eliminate large amounts of acid (in the form of carbon dioxide) from the body. Just enough carbon dioxide is retained in the blood to maintain a normal pH level. If the pH drops suddenly from the normal range of 7.35 to 7.45 to 7, the respiratory system is able to return the pH to about 7.2 to 7.3 within 1 minute. Chemoreceptors in the medulla of the brainstem provide the stimulus to increase respirations; however, as the hydrogen ion concentration approaches normal, the stimulus is lost. The buffers will accomplish the remaining adjustments needed to return the level to normal.

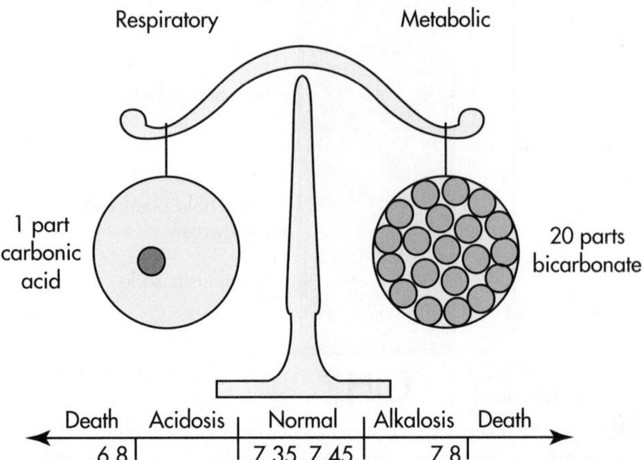

FIGURE 22-6 Carbonic acid to bicarbonate ratio and pH. The normal plasma range is 7.35 to 7.45. A normal pH is maintained by a ratio of 1 part carbonic acid to 20 parts bicarbonate.

The third line of defense is the kidneys. The action of the lungs in coping with an imbalance is simple: We breathe more slowly or more quickly. The kidneys have much more selective control. They are able to excrete varying amounts of acid or base into the urine. If the acidity of blood rises above normal, the kidneys will selectively eliminate more acids so the hydrogen ion concentration increases in the blood. If the blood becomes too alkaline, the kidneys will selectively eliminate more bases, especially bicarbonate. Normal urine is acidic because the body produces excess acids in the metabolic processes that occur continuously in the body. The kidneys are the slowest of the systems, but they are efficient enough to return the pH to exactly normal. Their response takes hours to days.

The three systems work closely together to maintain a normal hydrogen ion concentration. The buffers are immediate and continuous in contributing or accepting hydrogen ions. The respiratory system has the capacity to come into play within minutes, regulating the carbon dioxide level in the blood and thus controlling carbonic acid. The kidneys are the third line of defense, and although they work more slowly than the other two systems, they are able to eliminate either hydrogen ions or bicarbonate ions, which means they can either increase or decrease pH.

ACID-BASE IMBALANCE

Acid-base balance means homeostasis of the hydrogen ion concentration. A steady acid-base balance is normally maintained in the body (Lewis et al., 2007). An upset in acid-base balance results in either acidosis (when blood pH is less than 7.35), or alkalosis (when blood pH is greater than 7.45). The lungs and the kidneys are the two major organs responsible for regulation of the acid and base substances in the body. When imbalances occur, they represent an imbalance in the function of the lungs, the kidneys, or both. Many diseases create a potential for acid-base imbalances as well as fluid and electrolyte problems. Diseases that pose a risk for these imbalances include diabetes mellitus, chronic obstructive pulmonary disease (COPD), and end-stage renal disease, as well as severe vomiting and diarrhea (Lewis et al., 2007).

There are four primary types of acid-base imbalances: respiratory acidosis, respiratory alkalosis, metabolic acidosis, and metabolic alkalosis (Table 22-5).

RESPIRATORY ACIDOSIS

Any condition that impairs normal ventilation causes respiratory acidosis (Box 22-10). Retention of carbon dioxide occurs with a resultant increase of carbonic acid in the blood. As pH falls and the normal 20:1 bicarbonate to carbonic acid ratio is upset, the Pco_2 (partial carbon dioxide) level increases. Shallow respirations result because of the retained carbon dioxide. The patient will also experience a depression of central nervous system activity. Because the lungs are responsible for the respiratory parameters of the acid-base balance, the kidneys, which are responsible for the metabolic parameters, will attempt to compensate by retaining the base substance bicarbonate. During respiratory acidosis, it takes 24 hours for the kidneys to respond in a compensatory mechanism by retaining bicarbonate (Lewis et al., 2007).

Treatment for respiratory acidosis is aimed at improving ventilation. The primary goal is to support the patient's respirations. Intermittent positive-pressure breathing (IPPB) to promote exhalation of carbon dioxide, antibiotic administration for any respiratory infection, adequate hydration (2 to 3 L/day) to keep the mucous membranes moist and aid in removal of secretions, and use of bronchodilators to help reduce bronchial spasms will be possible elements of the treatment regimen. Therapy is also directed at correcting the primary condition responsible for the imbalance.

Table 22-5 Acid-Base Imbalances and Compensatory Mechanisms

ACID-BASE IMBALANCE	MODE OF COMPENSATION
Respiratory acidosis	Kidneys will retain increased amounts of HCO_3^- to increase pH
Respiratory alkalosis	Kidneys will excrete increased amounts of HCO_3^- to lower pH
Metabolic acidosis	Lungs "blow off" CO_2 to raise pH
Metabolic alkalosis	Lungs retain CO_2 to lower pH

From Pagana, K., & Pagana, T. (2006). *Mosby's diagnostic and laboratory test reference.* (6th ed.). St. Louis: Mosby.

RESPIRATORY ALKALOSIS

Respiratory alkalosis is caused by hyperventilation (Box 22-11). Respirations that increase in rate, depth, or both have the potential to result in the loss of excessive amounts of carbon dioxide with a resultant lowering of the carbonic acid level in the blood. The pH rises because of the decrease in carbonic acid, which is blown off with each exhalation.

Box 22-10 Respiratory Acidosis: Causes, Common Clinical Signs and Symptoms, and Laboratory Data

CAUSES
- Compromise in any of the three essential parts of breathing—ventilation, perfusion, or diffusion
- Chronic obstructive pulmonary disease
- Pneumonia
- Respiratory failure
- Atelectasis
- Barbiturate or sedative overdose
- Paralysis of respiratory muscles (Guillain-Barré syndrome, poliomyelitis, myasthenia gravis)
- Traumatic injuries to the thorax (flail chest)
- Obesity
- Airway obstruction
- Head injuries
- Stroke (CVA)
- Drowning
- Cystic fibrosis

COMMON CLINICAL SIGNS AND SYMPTOMS

Central Nervous System
- Lethargy
- Disorientation
- Occipital headache
- Decreased deep tendon reflexes
- Dizziness
- Decreasing level of consciousness
- Seizures
- Coma

Cardiopulmonary System
- Dyspnea
- Tachycardia
- Hypotension
- Cardiac dysrhythmias

Musculoskeletal System
- Tremors
- Weakness

LABORATORY DATA
- pH less than 7.35
- $Paco_2$ greater than 45 mm Hg (unless the patient has chronic obstructive pulmonary disease)
- Pao_2 normal or less than 80 mm Hg, depending on severity of acidosis
- O_2 saturation normal or less than 95%, depending on severity of acidosis
- HCO_3^- normal in early respiratory acidosis
- K^+ greater than 5 mEq/L

CVA, Cardiovascular accident.

Box 22-11 Respiratory Alkalosis: Causes, Common Clinical Signs and Symptoms, and Laboratory Data

CAUSES
- Hyperventilation (caused by hypoxia, pulmonary emboli, anxiety, fear, pain, exercise, fever)
- Anemia
- Hypermetabolic states
- Disorders of the central nervous system (head injuries, infections)
- Drugs (aspirin overdose)
- Asthma
- Pneumonia
- Inappropriate mechanical ventilator settings

COMMON CLINICAL SIGNS AND SYMPTOMS

Central Nervous System
- Anxious appearance
- Irritability
- Confusion
- Tingling of the extremities
- Fainting
- Dizziness
- Seizures

Cardiopulmonary System
- Tachypnea
- Cardiac dysrhythmias

Musculoskeletal System
- Tetany
- Muscle weakness

LABORATORY DATA
- pH 7.45 or greater
- $Paco_2$ less than 35 mm Hg
- Pao_2 normal
- O_2 saturation normal
- HCO_3^- 22 to 24 mEq/L (normal)
- K^+ less than 3.5 mEq/L

The common treatment for respiratory alkalosis is sedation and reassurance. If the cause is anxiety, it helps to make the patient aware of the abnormal breathing pattern. Instruct the patient to breathe slowly to retain and accumulate carbon dioxide in the body. Another effective treatment is for the patient to breathe into a paper bag, which will cause rebreathing of the exhaled carbon dioxide.

METABOLIC ACIDOSIS

Metabolic acidosis is possible as a result of either a gain of hydrogen ions or a loss of bicarbonate—in other words, retaining too many acids (H^+ ions) or losing too many bases (HCO_3^-) (Box 22-12). Examples of metabolic acidosis include diabetic ketoacidosis from ketone accumulation, lactic acid elevation (seen in shock), and acidosis from loss of too many bases (as in severe diarrhea or renal failure) (Lewis et al., 2007).

Without sufficient bases, the pH of the blood falls below the normal 7.35 to 7.45. With the loss of base substances, the bicarbonate level will also drop. The

Box 22-12 Metabolic Acidosis: Causes, Common Clinical Signs and Symptoms, and Laboratory Data

CAUSES
- Starvation
- Dehydration
- Diabetic ketoacidosis
- Lactic acidosis
- Renal failure
- Shock
- Severe diarrhea
- Drugs (methanol, ethanol, formic acid, paraldehyde, aspirin)
- Renal tubular acidosis
- Renal failure

COMMON CLINICAL SIGNS AND SYMPTOMS

Central Nervous System
- Lethargy
- Headache
- Decreasing level of consciousness
- Coma

Cardiopulmonary System
- Kussmaul's respirations (deep, rapid respirations)
- Dysrhythmias
- Warm, flushed skin

Gastrointestinal System
- Anorexia
- Nausea
- Vomiting
- Diarrhea
- Abdominal pain

Musculoskeletal System
- Weakness

LABORATORY DATA
- pH less than 7.35
- $Paco_2$ normal, or less than 35 mm Hg if lungs are compensating
- Pao_2 normal, or less than 35 mm Hg if lungs are compensating
- O_2 saturation normal
- HCO_3^- less than 22 mEq/L
- K^+ greater than 5 mEq/L

effect of metabolic acidosis is hyperventilation, occurring as the lungs attempt to compensate by blowing off carbon dioxide to lower the Pco_2 level. A patient with diabetic ketoacidosis will often develop Kussmaul's respirations (deep, rapid breathing), which serve to blow off carbon dioxide in an attempt to reverse the condition of metabolic acidosis (Lewis et al., 2007). Administration of sodium bicarbonate is the usual treatment for acidosis.

METABOLIC ALKALOSIS

Metabolic alkalosis results when a significant amount of acid is lost from the body or an increase in the bicarbonate level occurs (Box 22-13). The most common causes of metabolic alkalosis are vomiting gastric con-

Box 22-13 Metabolic Alkalosis: Causes, Common Clinical Signs and Symptoms, and Laboratory Data

CAUSES
- Excessive vomiting
- Prolonged gastric suctioning
- Electrolyte disturbance
- Cushing's disease
- Drugs (steroids, sodium bicarbonate, diuretics); overdose of baking soda, excessive use of antacids such as Mylanta
- Hyperaldosteronism

COMMON CLINICAL SIGNS AND SYMPTOMS

Central Nervous System
- Headache
- Irritability
- Lethargy
- Decreases in level of consciousness
- Seizures

Cardiopulmonary System
- Atrial tachycardia
- Slow, shallow respirations with periods of apnea
- Cardiac dysrhythmias (related to hypokalemia)

Gastrointestinal System
- Nausea
- Vomiting
- Anorexia

Musculoskeletal System
- Numbness and tingling of extremities
- Tremors
- Hypertonicity of muscles, muscle cramps
- Tetany

LABORATORY DATA
- pH greater than 7.45
- $Paco_2$ normal or greater than 45 mm Hg if lungs are compensating
- Pao_2 normal
- O_2 saturation normal
- HCO_3^- greater than 26 mEq/L
- K^+ less than 3.5 mEq/L

tent (normally high in acid) and gastric suction. Metabolic alkalosis is also possible in patients who ingest excess amounts of alkaline agents, such as bicarbonate-containing antacids (e.g., Alka-Seltzer, soda bicarbonate). Metabolic alkalosis depresses the central nervous system. The respiratory rate is decreased, thus decreasing the amount of carbon dioxide exhaled and raising the level of plasma CO_2 (Lewis et al., 2007). Again, as with the other acid-base imbalances, treatment is aimed at the cause.

NURSING PROCESS

The role of the licensed practical nurse/licensed vocational nurse (LPN/LVN) in the nursing process as stated is that the LPN/LVN will:
- Participate in planning care for patients based on patient needs
- Review patient's plan of care and recommend revisions as needed
- Review and follow defined prioritization for patient care
- Use clinical pathways, care maps, or care plans to guide and review patient care

Assessment

During assessment of fluid, electrolyte, and acid-base balances, you will identify patients at risk for imbalances, the presence of any alterations, and the extent to which body systems are involved. Assessment helps you anticipate the patient's needs for nursing interventions. Gathering assessment data also helps determine the effectiveness of therapies and any adverse reactions to them.

The assessment includes the nursing history; physical examination; measuring and recording of I&O; laboratory studies; and consideration of factors influencing fluid, electrolyte, and acid-base balances.

Nursing Diagnosis

In the areas of fluid, electrolyte, and acid-base balances, it is particularly important that you be skilled and use critical thinking to formulate nursing diagnoses. Use the following nursing diagnoses for fluid, electrolyte, and acid-base alterations:
- Risk for deficient fluid volume
- Imbalanced nutrition: less than body requirements
- Deficient fluid volume
- Risk for imbalanced fluid volume
- Excess fluid volume
- Impaired or risk for impaired skin integrity
- Impaired tissue integrity
- Impaired oral mucous membrane
- Ineffective tissue perfusion
- Decreased cardiac output
- Impaired gas exchange
- Ineffective breathing pattern

The assessment data that establish the risk for or the actual presence of a nursing diagnosis in these areas will often be subtle. Typically, patterns and trends will emerge only when you consciously look for them, because many body systems are involved. For example, relevant assessment data for the nursing diagnosis of deficient fluid volume will perhaps include the presence of insufficient oral intake, weight loss, dry skin and mucous membranes, inelastic skin turgor, decreased blood pressure, and increased heart rate. The serum sodium will possibly be elevated. The urine will potentially be dark, with an elevated specific gravity. In some cases, the volume of the urine will be decreasing over a period of days. The omission of any of these data will lead you to formulate an incomplete picture of the patient's condition and perhaps result in an incorrect diagnosis.

In addition to the accurate clustering of assessment data, it is essential that you precisely identify the related factor for the nursing diagnosis to plan appropriate nursing interventions. For example, for the nursing diagnosis of deficient fluid volume, the related factor is sometimes diarrhea, and sometimes vomiting or difficulty swallowing. This nursing diagnosis is not present if the patient is receiving nothing by mouth (NPO) as part of the treatment regimen. If the related factor is diarrhea, you will administer ordered antidiarrheal medication and provide oral fluids that contain electrolytes and glucose. You will teach the patient to use careful handwashing and to avoid dairy products. In contrast, if the related factor is vomiting, you will administer antiemetics, remove sights and odors that have the potential to induce nausea, and provide a small amount of fluids containing electrolytes. If the related factor is difficulty swallowing, you will attempt to ensure that the patient is maximally stimulated; position the patient in a high Fowler's position or on the side during times of intake; provide foods and fluids with a soft, pureed, or thickened consistency; provide 5-mL amounts with each mouthful; and investigate the need for enteral or total parenteral nutrition.

Expected Outcomes and Planning

The first step in the planning process is setting priorities. Many nursing diagnoses in the areas of fluid, electrolyte, and acid-base balance represent high-priority patient problems. The consequences are potentially serious, even life threatening (e.g., seizures, dysrhythmias, or coma).

During the planning process, you will formulate nursing interventions for use to prevent or treat fluid, electrolyte, and acid-base imbalances. It is important to collaborate with the patient and the family during this part of the assessment and planning processes. The family will be helpful in identifying the subtle changes in behavior associated with these imbalances, such as anxiety, confusion, or irritability. During the planning process, it is important to remember that the patient and the family need to know preventive measures, signs and symptoms to report, and measures that are possible to implement if an imbalance occurs. When medications, special diets, or oral or IV fluids are administered in the home, the patient and the family need careful teaching to be able to perform these interventions safely. Consider the patient's preferences and resources during each step of the planning process (e.g., if the patient needs to be encouraged to increase oral intake, determine the patient's favorite beverages and incorporate them into the plan of care). In the hospital, anticipate the needs of the patient and family for specific information and initiate teaching before discharge so they will be ready for these procedures. The home health nurse continues the teaching plan and evaluates the effectiveness of the home interventions.

You will also work closely with other members of the health care team, such as the physician, the dietitian, or the physical therapist. For example, when you collect new assessment data that suggest the patient is developing a fluid, electrolyte, or acid-base imbalance, you will consult with the physician to determine the need for dietary, pharmacologic, IV fluid, or other therapy. Your responsibilities also include ongoing monitoring of the patient's fluid, electrolyte, and acid-base status to determine the safety of implementing physician and nursing orders and any need for a change in the plan of care. For example, perhaps the physician will order an oral potassium supplement to be given to the patient three times each day. Before administering the first dose each day, verify that the serum potassium level is normal and that the urine output is adequate. Withhold the dose of potassium and consult the physician if the serum level is elevated or if the urine output has decreased.

After priority setting and collaboration with the patient, family, and health care team, you will develop a care plan with your colleagues that is individualized according to the patient's acute or chronic fluid, electrolyte, or acid-base status. The plan is based on one or more of the following goals:

Goal: The patient's fluid, electrolyte, and acid-base balances are restored and maintained.

Outcomes:

The patient's vital signs will return to baseline normal.

The patient will have normal skin turgor.

The patient will have moist oral mucous membranes.

The patient's weight will be stable at baseline normal.

The patient will have no edema.

The patient will have clear breath sounds.

The patient's serum and urine electrolyte and chemistry results and arterial blood gas values will be normal.

The patient's urine output will equal intake.

Implementation

Prevention of fluid, electrolyte, and acid-base imbalances is important. When imbalances occur, you will remove or treat the cause of the imbalance if possible. Other nursing interventions aim to correct the imbalances.

When a patient's fluid volume is depleted, it is possible to replace fluids and electrolytes orally, with IV administration of fluids and blood components, or through total parenteral nutrition if the fluid deficit is caused by malnutrition. For patients with fluid volume excess, implement measures to reduce fluids, such as fluid intake restrictions, reduced sodium intake, and use of diuretics. When the patient has an electrolyte imbalance, provide an appropriate diet and administer supplements when ordered. For patients with acid-base imbalances, initiate such measures as reducing anxiety, improving pulmonary function, controlling the loss of GI content, or ensuring the control of conditions such as diabetes mellitus or renal failure.

Evaluation

Evaluate the interventions by comparing the patient's responses to the expected outcomes of the established goals. Be prepared to revise the plan of care based on the evaluation. Evaluative measures typically include the following:

Goal: Patient's fluid and electrolyte balances are restored and maintained.

Evaluative measures:
Obtain daily weight and monitor.
Obtain patient's vital signs.
Measure all routes of intake and output.
Auscultate for adventitious lung sounds.
Assess oral mucous membranes for dryness or moistness.
Assess tissue turgor for tenting or edema.
Monitor serum electrolytes.

Get Ready for the NCLEX® Examination!

Key Points

- Water is the primary fluid in the body.
- The two fluid compartments are the intracellular and extracellular compartments. The extracellular compartment is composed in turn of the interstitial and intravascular areas.
- Fluid movement takes place by means of three passive transport systems—diffusion, osmosis, and filtration—and one active transport system—active transport by ATP energy.
- Electrolytes are chemical compounds that carry either a positive or negative charge. Positive ions are called cations; negative ions are called anions. To maintain homeostasis, it is necessary for the cations and the anions to balance each other in the body fluids.
- Sodium is the major extracellular cation in the body. Water follows sodium as it moves from one fluid compartment to another.
- Potassium is the major intracellular cation in the body. Imbalances in potassium, either high or low levels, have potential to cause life-threatening cardiac conditions.
- The four types of acid-base imbalance are respiratory acidosis, respiratory alkalosis, metabolic acidosis, and metabolic alkalosis.
- Arterial blood has a normal pH range of 7.35 to 7.45. A pH less than 7.35 is considered abnormally acidic; a pH greater than 7.45 is considered abnormally alkaline. A pH lower than 6.8 or higher than 7.8 is usually fatal.
- Any process that interferes with normal ventilation and causes a decrease or an increase in the excretion of volatile acids poses the risk of causing respiratory acidosis or respiratory alkalosis.
- Any process that interferes with normal production or excretion of nonvolatile hydrogen ions poses the risk of causing metabolic acidosis or metabolic alkalosis.
- Respiratory acidosis or alkalosis will result when the lungs fail to regulate the carbonic acid concentration in the blood. Metabolic acidosis or alkalosis will result when the kidneys fail to regulate the bicarbonate concentration in the blood.
- If the lungs are unable to reassert their function and correct respiratory acidosis, the kidneys will respond in an attempt to correct the imbalance. If the kidneys are unable to reassert their function and correct metabolic acidosis, the lungs will respond in an attempt to correct the imbalance.

Additional Learning Resources

Go to your Companion CD for an audio glossary, animations, video clips, and more.

evolve Be sure to visit the Evolve site at http://evolve.elsevier.com/Christensen/foundations/ for additional online resources.

Review Questions for the NCLEX® Examination

1. A 66-year-old patient has recently been experiencing excessive edema in his feet. The nurse discusses with the patient the dietary changes that are perhaps causing the water retention associated with the patient's edema. Which electrolyte has the greatest influence on water balance in the body?
   1. Sodium (Na^+)
   2. Potassium (K^+)
   3. Chloride (Cl^-)
   4. Calcium (Ca^{++})
2. Which regulatory system is the body's first line of defense in keeping the pH within normal limits?
   1. Buffers in the blood
   2. Respiratory system
   3. Renal system
   4. Blood pressure
3. The most accurate method to use in determining water balance in the body is to:
   1. weigh the patient daily at the same time each day.
   2. record an accurate 24-hour I&O.
   3. ask the patient to document on an I&O form left at the bedside.
   4. have the same nurse care for the patient each day.
4. A patient is concerned about giving her family adequate amounts of potassium in their diets. She asks the nurse to help plan a meal containing foods with the most potassium. Which diet contains foods with the most potassium?
   1. Baked chicken, green salad, and fresh fruit plate
   2. Macaroni and cheese, cornbread, and gelatin
   3. Tacos, chips and salsa, and ice cream
   4. Seafood plate, marinated vegetables, sponge cake

5. The major route of excretion of all electrolytes from the body is via the:
   1. skin.
   2. lungs.
   3. kidneys.
   4. feces.

6. Fluid movement in the cells equalizes the ions or the molecules on each side of the semipermeable membrane. The movement of water from an area of lower concentration to an area of higher concentration occurs through:
   1. diffusion.
   2. filtration.
   3. active transport.
   4. osmosis.

7. The largest fluid compartment in the body is the:
   1. intracellular.
   2. extracellular.
   3. interstitial.
   4. intravascular.

8. Diffusion, osmosis, and filtration are all examples of:
   1. active transport.
   2. passive transport.
   3. ATP energy.
   4. Krebs cycle.

9. The term used to indicate hydrogen ion concentration in the body is:
   1. mEq.
   2. ATP.
   3. pH.
   4. mL.

10. The most common cause of hypocalcemia involves a dysfunction of:
    1. antidiuretic hormone.
    2. growth hormone.
    3. parathyroid hormone.
    4. thyroid hormone.

11. A patient has a positive Chvostek's sign. The nurse will expect laboratory tests to reveal:
    1. total serum calcium of less than 8.9 mEq/L.
    2. total serum calcium of greater than 10.1 mEq/L.
    3. ionized calcium of greater than 5.1 mg/dL.
    4. total serum potassium of less than 3 mEq/L.

12. Potassium is responsible for:
    1. building muscle mass.
    2. building bone structure and strength.
    3. neuromuscular and cardiac function.
    4. maintaining normal blood glucose levels.

13. Neuromuscular signs and symptoms of hypokalemia include:
    1. confusion and irritability.
    2. diminished deep tendon reflexes.
    3. parkinsonian type of tremors.
    4. carpopedal spasms.

14. Medications to be given when treating hyperkalemia include:
    1. sodium succinate and mannitol.
    2. mannitol and regular insulin.
    3. sodium polystyrene sulfonate (Kayexalate).
    4. antacids.

15. Because 1 L of fluid equals 2.2 lb (1 kg), a weight change of 2 kg (4.4 lb) will reflect a loss or gain of ________ body fluid.

16. When the body senses hypoxemia or hypercapnia (greater than normal amounts of carbon dioxide in the blood), the chemoreceptors in the medulla of the brainstem respond by:
    1. slowing the respiratory rate.
    2. decreasing the heart rate.
    3. increasing the depth and rate of respirations.
    4. lowering the blood pressure.

17. Which statements concerning a patient with severe hyperkalemia are correct?
    1. Cardiac arrest is possible, especially when serum potassium levels reach 7 mEq/L.
    2. Administer Kayexalate as prescribed by the physician.
    3. Report a urinary output less than 30 mL/hr.
    4. Monitor vital signs every 12 hours.

18. In acute respiratory acidosis, the renal compensatory mechanisms begin to operate within:
    1. 4 to 6 hours.
    2. 24 hours.
    3. 2 to 3 days.
    4. 1 to 2 hours.

19. Daily water intake and output (I&O) is approximately how many mL?
    1. 1500
    2. 3500
    3. 6500
    4. 2500

20. It is necessary for the kidneys to secrete a minimum of how many mL/hr of urine to eliminate waste products from the body?
    1. 30 mL/hr
    2. 60 mL/hr
    3. 20 mL/hr
    4. 100 mL/hr

21. The normal pH of blood is approximately ________.

22. Ketoacid accumulation in diabetic ketoacidosis often results in which type of respirations?
    1. Cheyne-Stokes respirations
    2. Kussmaul's respirations
    3. Bradypnea
    4. Apnea

Mathematics Review and Medication Administration

chapter 23

evolve

Barbara Lauritsen Christensen

http://evolve.elsevier.com/Christensen/foundationsadult

Objectives

1. Confidently use basic mathematics skills to solve dosage problems accurately.
2. Set up and work problems using the following formula: (Desired dose/Available dose) × Amount.
3. Set up and work problems using the proportion method.
4. Use "key" equivalents of metric and apothecary measurement systems in dosage problems.
5. Convert measurement units within the metric system.
6. Convert between measurement units of the metric system and the apothecary system.
7. Determine the appropriateness of dosage orders for children by the use of Young's, Clark's, and Fried's rules and the body surface area nomogram.
8. Explain each phase of drug action.
9. Explain the importance of decreased hepatic and renal functioning.
10. Discuss drug dosage.
11. Discuss minimal dosage.
12. Discuss maximal dosage.
13. Discuss toxic dosage.
14. Discuss lethal dosage.
15. Discuss potentiation.
16. Explain the importance of an antagonist counteracting an agonist.
17. Describe factors to consider in choosing routes of administration of medication.
18. Discuss the nurse's role and responsibilities in medication administration.
19. List the "six rights" of medication administration.
20. Discuss the use of The Joint Commission's abbreviations to prevent medication errors.
21. Describe five factors that affect drug action in patients.
22. Discuss "safety tips from nurse experts."
23. Describe the importance of accurate transcription of medication orders.
24. Define the following terms and give the order of priority they indicate: stat, ASAP, now, and prn.
25. Explain what is meant by a controlled substance.
26. List three ways medication orders are given.
27. Discuss the three preferred choices for intramuscular injections.
28. Discuss the correct technique for locating intramuscular injection sites.

Key Terms

adverse drug reaction (p. 693)
agonist (ĂG-ŏ-nĭst, p. 693)
anaphylactic shock (ăn-ă-fĭ-LĂK-tĭk, p. 731)
antagonist (ăn-TĂG-ŏ-nĭst, p. 693)
body surface area (p. 691)
buccal (BŬK-ŭl, p. 712)
compatibility (p. 692)
cumulative (p. 692)
denominator (p. 682)
dimensional analysis (DA) (p. 688)
drip factor (p. 731)
drug interaction (p. 692)
enteral (ĔN-tŭr-ŭl, p. 702)
enteric-coated (ĕn-TĔR-ĭk, p. 702)
extremes (p. 687)
gauge (gāj, p. 716)
graduated (p. 704)
idiosyncratic (ĭd-ē-ō-sĭn-KRĂT-ĭk, p. 693)
intermittent venous access device (ĭn-tŭr-MĬT-ĕnt VĒ-nŭs, p. 728)
lumen (LŪ-mĕn, p. 716)
means (p. 687)
meniscus (mĕ-NĬS-kŭs, p. 704)
metabolite (mĕ-TĂB-ŏ-līt, p. 692)
milliequivalent (mĭll-ē-ĕ-KWĬV-ă-lĕnt, p. 689)
numerator (p. 682)
parenteral (pă-RĔN-tŭr-ŭl, p. 712)
patient-controlled analgesia (PCA) (p. 729)
percent (p. 686)
percutaneous (pŭr-kyū-TĀ-nē-ŭs, p. 707)
pharmacology (p. 692)
potentiation (pō-tĕn-shē-Ā-shŭn, p. 692)
proportion (p. 687)
pulverize (p. 704)
ratio (p. 687)
souffle cup (sū-FLĀ cŭp, p. 706)
sublingual (sŭb-LĬNG-gwŭl, p. 712)
therapeutic (p. 692)
tolerance (p. 693)
topical applications (p. 707)

One of your roles as a nurse is to accurately calculate drug dosages to provide safe medication administration to each patient. The basic mathematics section of this chapter provides you with a review of basic math, three measurement systems, two methods of solving dosage problems, and methods of determining the appropriateness of children's drug orders.

MATHEMATICS REVIEW AND PRINCIPLES

FRACTIONS

Are you afraid of fractions? Many students are. It helps to understand what fractions are. What is a fraction? A fraction is a "part" of a whole number. For example:

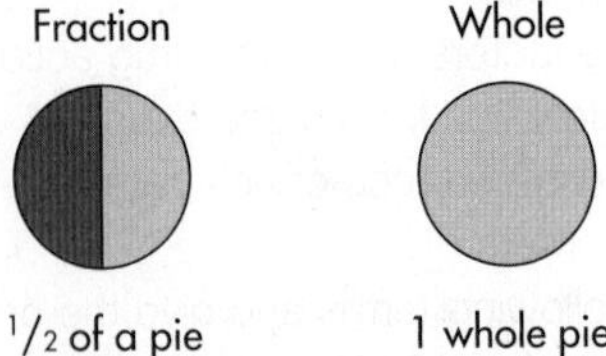

Numerator: the "top" number of a fraction
Denominator: the "bottom" number of a fraction

TYPES OF FRACTIONS

Proper fractions—the numerator is less than the denominator.

EXAMPLE: $\frac{1}{2}$ Numerator / Denominator

Improper fractions—the numerator is larger than the denominator.

EXAMPLE: $\frac{2}{1}$ Numerator / Denominator

Mixed fractions—consist of a whole number plus a fraction.

EXAMPLE: $1\frac{1}{2}$ 1 is the whole number, $\frac{1}{2}$ is the fraction

CHANGING AN IMPROPER FRACTION TO A WHOLE OR MIXED NUMBER

RULE 1: Divide the denominator (bottom number) into the numerator (top number).

EXAMPLE: 1. Change $\frac{10}{5}$ to a *whole* number.

$10 \div 5 = 2$ (a WHOLE number)

2. Change $\frac{40}{5}$ to a *whole* number.

$40 \div 5 = 8$ (a WHOLE number)

EXAMPLE: 3. Change $\frac{20}{7}$ (an improper fraction) to a *mixed* number.

$$20 \div 7 = 7\overline{)20} = 2\frac{6}{7} \text{ (a MIXED number)}$$

$$\begin{array}{r} 2 \\ 7\overline{)20} \\ \underline{14} \\ 6 \\ \hline 7 \end{array}$$

4. Change $\frac{54}{5}$ to a *mixed* number.

$$\begin{array}{r} 10 \\ 54 \div 5 = 5\overline{)54} \\ \underline{50} \\ \frac{4}{5} = 10\frac{4}{5} \text{ (a MIXED number)} \end{array}$$

CHANGING A MIXED NUMBER TO AN IMPROPER FRACTION

RULE 1: Multiply the denominator (bottom number) by the whole number.
RULE 2: Add the numerator to the product; this sum is now the new numerator.

EXAMPLE: a. Change $2\frac{6}{7}$ (a mixed number) to an improper fraction.

Multiply the denominator 7 by the whole number 2.

$7 \times 2 = 14$ (The answer from numbers multiplied is called the **product.**)

b. Add the original numerator to the product.

$6 + 14 = 20$ (The answer from numbers added is called the **sum.**)

c. Place the sum, 20, over the original denominator, 7, to obtain an improper fraction.

$$\frac{20}{7}$$

The mixed $2\frac{6}{7}$ number is now the improper fraction $\frac{20}{7}$.

REDUCING FRACTIONS TO THE LOWEST TERM

You will commonly reduce fractions to the lowest term in which they can be expressed, because it is easier to work with smaller numbers. For example, you will be able to reduce both $\frac{20}{80}$ and $\frac{25}{100}$ to $\frac{1}{4}$, which is more convenient to use in calculation.

RULE 1: Find a number that will evenly divide into the numerator *and* the denominator.

EXAMPLE: $\frac{2}{10}$

What number will divide into the numerator, 2?
2 will divide evenly into the numerator, 2, one time.
2 will divide into the denominator, 10, five times.

$\frac{2}{10} = \frac{1}{5}$ (Reduce all fractions to their lowest terms.)

EXAMPLE: $\frac{16}{60} = \frac{4}{15}$ (The number 4 divides evenly into both the numerator and the denominator.)

DETERMINING WHICH FRACTION IS LARGER

RULE 1: If the denominators are the *same*, the fraction with the *larger numerator* is the larger fraction.

PROBLEM: Which is larger, $\frac{4}{6}$ or $\frac{2}{6}$?

ANSWER: $\frac{4}{6}$ is larger

RULE 2: If the denominators are *different*, such as $\frac{2}{5}$ and $\frac{1}{3}$, first find a "common denominator." (Finding a common denominator means to find a number into which both denominators can be divided.) Common, or equivalent, numerators will also be found.

PROBLEM: Which is larger, $\frac{2}{5}$ or $\frac{1}{3}$?

Find a common denominator for $\frac{2}{5}$ and $\frac{1}{3}$.

HINT: Try multiplying the denominators to get a common denominator.

$\frac{2}{5} = \frac{?}{15} \quad \frac{1}{3} = \frac{?}{15}$

RULE 3: After you find the common denominator, find an equivalent numerator for each fraction.

$\frac{2}{5} = \frac{?}{15} \quad \frac{1}{3} = \frac{?}{15}$

Find an equivalent numerator by dividing the first denominator into the equivalent denominator; multiply the answer by the first numerator.

EXAMPLE: 1. $\frac{2}{5} = \frac{6}{15}$ $(15 \div 5 = 3; 3 \times 2 = 6)$

2. $\frac{1}{3} = \frac{5}{15}$ $(15 \div 3 = 5; 5 \times 1 = 5)$

RULE 4: Compare the two fractions; the one with the larger numerator is the larger fraction.

PROBLEM: Which is larger, $\frac{6}{15}$ or $\frac{5}{15}$?

ANSWER: $\frac{6}{15}$ is larger

EXAMPLE: Which is larger, $\frac{2}{3}$ or $\frac{6}{8}$?

$\frac{2}{3} = \frac{16}{24} \quad \frac{6}{8} = \frac{18}{24}$

ANSWER: $\frac{6}{8}$ is larger

ADDING FRACTIONS WITH THE SAME DENOMINATOR

RULE 1: Add the numerators, and place this sum of the numerators over the denominator and reduce the new fraction if possible.

EXAMPLE:

$$\begin{array}{r} \frac{1}{6} \\ +\frac{1}{6} \\ \hline \frac{2}{6} = \frac{1}{3} \end{array}$$

ADDING FRACTIONS WITH DIFFERENT DENOMINATORS

RULE 1: Find common denominators for all fractions in the problem.

EXAMPLE:

$$\begin{array}{r} \frac{1}{3} = \frac{?}{12} \\ +\frac{2}{4} = \frac{?}{12} \\ \hline \end{array}$$

(3 and 4 will divide into 12; 12 is the common denominator.)

RULE 2: Find the equivalent numerators.

EXAMPLE: 1.

$$\begin{array}{rl} \frac{1}{3} = \frac{4}{12} & (12 \div 3 = 4; 4 \times 1 = 4) \\ +\frac{2}{4} = \frac{6}{12} & (12 \div 4 = 3; 3 \times 2 = 6) \\ \hline \frac{10}{12} = \frac{5}{6} & \end{array}$$

2.

$$\begin{array}{r} \frac{6}{20} = \frac{6}{20} \\ +\frac{12}{20} = \frac{12}{20} \\ \hline \frac{18}{20} = \frac{9}{10} \end{array}$$

ADDING MIXED NUMBERS

RULE 1: Add the fractions of the mixed number. Then add the sum of the fractions to the whole numbers.

EXAMPLE: 1.

$$\begin{array}{r} 1\frac{2}{3} \\ +2\frac{1}{3} \\ \hline 3\frac{3}{3} = 4 \end{array}$$

2.

$$\begin{array}{r} 1\frac{3}{5} = 1\frac{6}{10} \\ +4\frac{5}{10} = 4\frac{5}{10} \\ \hline 5\frac{11}{10} = 5 + 1 \text{ whole} + \frac{1}{10}, \end{array}$$

$$\text{which} = 6\frac{1}{10}$$

SUBTRACTING FRACTIONS WITH THE SAME DENOMINATOR

RULE 1: Subtract the numerators, and place the answer over the denominator in the answer.

EXAMPLE: 1.

$$\begin{array}{r} \frac{3}{5} \\ -\frac{1}{5} \\ \hline \frac{2}{5} \end{array}$$

2.

$$\begin{array}{r} \frac{4}{7} \\ -\frac{2}{7} \\ \hline \frac{2}{7} \end{array}$$

SUBTRACTING FRACTIONS WITH DIFFERENT DENOMINATORS

RULE 1: First find a common denominator, and then subtract.

EXAMPLE: 1.

$$\begin{array}{r} \frac{3}{4} = \frac{9}{12} \\ -\frac{1}{3} = \frac{4}{12} \\ \hline \frac{5}{12} \end{array}$$

2.

$$\begin{array}{r} \frac{2}{3} = \frac{4}{6} \\ -\frac{1}{2} = \frac{3}{6} \\ \hline \frac{1}{6} \end{array}$$

SUBTRACTING MIXED NUMBERS

RULE 1: When the numerator of the top fraction is smaller than that of the bottom fraction, borrow one whole number from the whole number of the mixed fraction and express it as a fraction.

PROBLEM:

$$\begin{array}{r} 3\frac{9}{15} \\ -2\frac{10}{15} \\ \hline \end{array}$$

EXAMPLE: $3 = 2\frac{15}{15}$

RULE 2: Add the fraction of the original mixed number to the new fraction.

EXAMPLE: $3\frac{9}{15} = 2\frac{15}{15} + \frac{9}{15} = 2\frac{24}{15}$

RULE 3: Subtract fractions and whole numbers, if any.

$$\begin{array}{r} 2\frac{24}{15} \\ -2\frac{10}{15} \\ \hline \frac{14}{15} \end{array}$$

EXAMPLE: 1. $5\frac{6}{10} = 4\frac{10}{10} + \frac{6}{10} = 4\frac{16}{10}$

2. $-3\frac{8}{10} = 3\frac{8}{10}$

$$\begin{array}{r} 4\frac{16}{10} \\ -3\frac{8}{10} \\ \hline 1\frac{8}{10} \text{ or } 1\frac{4}{5} \end{array}$$

MULTIPLYING FRACTIONS

RULE 1: Multiply the numerators by each other; multiply the denominators by each other.

EXAMPLE: 1. $\frac{1}{2} \times \frac{3}{4} = \frac{1 \times 3}{2 \times 4} = \frac{3}{8}$

2. $\frac{4}{8} \times \frac{1}{3} = \frac{4 \times 1}{8 \times 3} = \frac{4}{24} = \frac{1}{6}$

MULTIPLYING FRACTIONS AND MIXED NUMBERS

RULE 1: Change the mixed number to an improper fraction. (See the section on changing mixed numbers to improper fractions.)

PROBLEM: Multiply $3\frac{1}{2}$ by $1\frac{2}{3}$

EXAMPLE: a. Change $3\frac{1}{2}$ and $1\frac{2}{3}$ to improper fractions.

$$3\frac{1}{2} = \frac{7}{2} \qquad 1\frac{2}{3} = \frac{5}{3}$$

b. Multiply.

$$\frac{7 \times 5}{2 \times 3} = \frac{35}{6} = 6\overline{)35} = 5\frac{5}{6}$$

$$\begin{array}{r} 5 \\ 6\overline{)35} \\ 30 \\ \hline 5 \\ \hline 6 \end{array}$$

PROBLEM: Multiply $1\frac{2}{3}$ by $2\frac{3}{4}$

EXAMPLE: $1\frac{2}{3} = \frac{5}{3} \quad 2\frac{3}{4} = \frac{11}{4}$

$$\frac{5}{3} \times \frac{11}{4} = \frac{55}{12} = 4\frac{7}{12}$$

DIVIDING FRACTIONS

RULE 1: Write the problem down *correctly.*
RULE 2: Invert the second fraction, and multiply; and then reduce to lowest terms.

PROBLEM: Divide $\frac{1}{2}$ by $\frac{3}{4}$

EXAMPLE: a. Write the problem down *correctly.*

$$\frac{1}{2} \div \frac{3}{4}$$

b. Invert the second fraction; change the division sign to a multiplication sign; multiply.

$$\frac{1}{2} \times \frac{4}{3} = \frac{4}{6}$$

c. Reduce to the lowest terms.

$$\frac{4}{6} = \frac{2}{3}$$

DIVIDING FRACTIONS AND WHOLE NUMBERS

RULE 1: Change the whole number to a fraction.
RULE 2: Divide, and then reduce to lowest terms.

PROBLEM: Divide 4 by $\frac{3}{5}$

EXAMPLE: a. Change 4 to a fraction. Make 4 the numerator and use 1 as the denominator.

$$\frac{4}{1}$$

b. Invert second fraction; multiply.

$$\frac{4 \times 5}{1 \times 3} = \frac{20}{3}$$

c. Reduce to lowest terms.

$$\frac{20}{3} = 6\frac{2}{3} \qquad 3\overline{)20} = 6,\ 20 - 18 = 2,\ \text{remainder } \frac{2}{3}$$

DECIMAL FRACTIONS

The decimal fraction is a type of fraction whose denominator is always some multiple (or division) of ten. The placement or position of the decimal point determines whether the denominator is 10, multiples of 10, or divisions of 10.

NAMES OF DECIMAL PLACES

.00001	One hundred thousandths
.0001	Ten thousandths
.001	Thousandths
.01	Hundredths
.1	Tenths
1.	Unit (whole numbers)
10	Tens
100	Hundreds
1000	Thousands
10,000	Ten thousands
100,000	One hundred thousands

RULE 1: A decimal point found to the left of a whole number means that the number is a *fraction* of a whole number.

EXAMPLE: 0.1 "Point one" is $\frac{1}{10}$ of the whole number 1.

HINT: Place a zero to the left of the decimal point to prevent mistaking .1 for 1.

Correct placement of decimal points in drug dosages is *critical.*

RULE 2: A decimal point found *after* (to the right of) a number means that it is a whole number.

EXAMPLE: 5. = 5

RULE 3: A number *without* a decimal point is understood to have an "invisible" decimal point following it.

EXAMPLE: 1 = 1.

ADDING DECIMALS

RULE 1: Align the decimal point of each decimal fraction in a column.
RULE 2: Add.

PROBLEM: Add 3.34 and 0.6

EXAMPLE:

```
  3.34   Align decimal point in column; add.
+ 0.6
  3.94
  ↑ Make sure that the decimal point is
    aligned properly in the answer.
```

SUBTRACTING DECIMALS

RULE 1: Align the decimal points of each decimal fraction in a column.
RULE 2: Subtract.

PROBLEM: Subtract 7.45 from 15.

EXAMPLE:

```
 15.00   Align decimal point in column; subtract.
− 7.45
  7.55
  ↑ Make sure that the decimal point is
    aligned properly in the answer.
```

ROUNDING A NUMBER

RULE 1: Round up a number that follows the decimal point if it is 5 or larger, so as to increase the number before it by one whole number.

EXAMPLE: 7.55 = 7.6 or 8
HINT: There are times when it is practical to round a volume of medication.

PROBLEM: How is it possible to give 7.55 minims easily?
ANSWER: Round 7.55 to 8; give 8 minims.
NOTE: Minims are very small units of measurement. Milliliters and cubic centimeters are not rounded in this manner because it would alter the drug dosage significantly. The use of minims is becoming obsolete.

MULTIPLYING DECIMALS

RULE 1: Multiply. You do not have to align decimal points in the problem.
RULE 2: Determine the location of the decimal point in the answer by adding up how many numbers are found to the right of the decimal points in the numbers multiplied.

EXAMPLE:

$$\begin{array}{r} 5.50 \\ \times\ 2.15 \\ \hline 2750 \\ 550 \\ 1100 \\ \hline 11.8250x \end{array}$$

(There are two numbers found after the decimal points on the top and two on the bottom.)

x = 11.8250 or 12 (rounded)

NOTE: A small "x" hereafter indicates the unexpressed decimal after a whole number or a decimal point that has been moved from one place to another.

DIVIDING DECIMALS

RULE 1: Change a decimal fraction in the divisor to a whole number by moving the decimal point *all* the way to the right.
PROBLEM: Divide 2.5 by 1.5.

EXAMPLE: a. (divisor) 1.5)2.5 (dividend)

b. 1.5x)2.5 (15)2.5)

RULE 2: Move the decimal point in the dividend the *same number of places moved in the divisor.*

EXAMPLE: 1.5x)2.5 The decimal point in the divisor is unexpressed after it is moved.

RULE 3: Place the decimal point in the answer directly over the decimal point in the dividend after moving the decimal point in the dividend.

EXAMPLE: 15)25.

RULE 4: If a decimal point is in the divisor, but not in the dividend (such as .5)15), move it the same number of places as the divisor. Remember there is an unexpressed decimal point at the right of all whole numbers.

EXAMPLE: .5x)15.x 5)150.

RULE 5: If the dividend contains a decimal fraction and the divisor does not, leave the divisor as it is.

EXAMPLE: 5)2.5 would remain unchanged.

CHANGING FRACTIONS TO DECIMALS

RULE 1: Divide the numerator (the top number) by the denominator (the bottom number).

PROBLEM: Change $\frac{3}{4}$ to a decimal fraction.

EXAMPLE: $\frac{3}{4} = 4\overline{)3.00}$ = .75

$$\begin{array}{r} .75 \\ 4)\overline{3.00} \\ 28 \\ \hline 20 \\ 20 \\ \hline \end{array}$$

CHANGING A DECIMAL FRACTION TO A COMMON FRACTION

Decimal fractions are based on 10s, multiples of 10, and divisions of 10. The position or place of the decimal point indicates the denominator.
RULE 1: To change a decimal fraction to a common fraction, give the decimal fraction a denominator according to the position of the decimal point in the decimal fraction.

PROBLEM: Change .1 to a common fraction.

EXAMPLE: a. 0.1 (The decimal point is in the "tens" place; 10 is the denominator.)

$\overline{10}$

b. Now that the denominator is 10, place the 1 over it to make a common fraction.

$\frac{1}{10}$

PERCENTS

The word percent and its symbol, %, mean "hundredths." A hundredth is a fraction of a whole number; therefore a number followed by % is a **fraction.** The denominator of the fraction is understood to be 100.

EXAMPLE: 25% is the same as $\frac{25}{100}$

Reduce $\frac{25}{100}$ to $\frac{1}{4}$

CHANGING A PERCENT TO A DECIMAL FRACTION

RULE 1: Remove %; move the decimal point two places to the left to indicate "hundredths."

PROBLEM: Change 25% to a decimal fraction.

EXAMPLE: 0.25

CHANGING A FRACTION TO A PERCENT

RULE 1: Change a fraction to a percent by dividing the numerator by the denominator.
RULE 2: Multiply the answer by 100.
RULE 3: Label the answer with the percent symbol.

EXAMPLE: $\frac{3}{4} = 4\overline{)3.00}$ = 0.75

```
     0.75
  4)3.00
    28
     20
     20
    100
  × 0.75
    500   (There are two decimal
   700     places in this problem, move
  75.00x   the decimal point in the
           answer two places to the left.)
```

75% Therefore $\frac{3}{4} = 75\%$

MULTIPLYING BY PERCENT

RULE 1: Change percent to a decimal (move decimal point two places to the left).
RULE 2: Multiply.

PROBLEM: Multiply 80 by 7.5%.

EXAMPLE: 7.5% is .075

```
     80
  × .075
    400
   560
   00      (Move decimal point three
  6.000x   places to the left = 6)
```

RATIOS

Ratio shows the relationship of one number or quantity to another number or quantity. Numbers of a ratio are separated by a colon. A ratio is also a fraction. The value of a ratio is not changed if both terms are multiplied or divided by the same number.

EXAMPLE: 2 : 4 is the same as 1 : 2 or 4 : 8

When you write numbers in ratio, you must express them all in the same units.

EXAMPLE: Express 1 liter, 2 ounces, and 30 milliliters (mL) all in the same way: 1000 mL : 60 mL : 30 mL.

You may write a fraction as a ratio.

EXAMPLE: $\frac{1}{25} = 1 : 25$ $\quad \frac{3}{4} = 3 : 4$

Ratio is an important concept that is used in the following methods of calculating dosages.

PROPORTIONS

Proportion shows that the relationship between two ratios has equal value.

EXAMPLE: 1 is to 2 as 4 is to 8 or 1 : 2 :: 4 : 8

Means are the inner terms of the proportion.
Extremes are the outer terms of the proportion.

EXAMPLE: 1 : 2 :: 4 : 8 (means: 2 and 4) $\quad$ 1 : 2 :: 4 : 8 (extremes: 1 and 8)

Set up the left side of the proportion as the "known" side using information that is known or given. The known information will be:

EXAMPLE: a. An equivalent such as 60 milligrams = 1 grain (60 mg : 1 gr)
or
b. A physician's medication or intravenous (IV) order, such as "give 1000 mL in 8 hr" (1000 mL : 8 hr)
or
c. A drug dosage on hand or available, such as information on a drug label that reads "50 mg/mL" (50 mg : 1 mL)

PROBLEM: The physician orders Demerol 25 mg q 3-4 hr as needed (prn) for pain. On hand is a vial labeled "50 mg/1 mL."

RULE 1: Set up the known side.

EXAMPLE: 50 mg : 1 (given on the label)

RULE 2: Set up the unknown side. Use x for what you are trying to find, such as "How many mL are needed to give 25 mg?"

	Known		Unknown
EXAMPLE:	50 mg : 1 mL	::	25 mg : x mL

RULE 3: Set up the units, such as mg and mL, in the *same position on each side* of the problem.

EXAMPLE: ___ mg : ___ mL :: ___ mg : ___ mL

RULE 4: Multiply the means.

RULE 5: Multiply the extremes.

PROBLEM: 50 mg : 1 mL :: 25 mg : x mL

EXAMPLE: a. Multiply the means.

$$50 \text{ mg} : 1 \text{ mL} :: 25 \text{ mg} : x \text{ mL} = 25$$

b. Multiply the extremes.

$$50 \text{ mg} : 1 \text{ mL} :: 25 \text{ mg} : x \text{ mL} = 50x$$

c. Express the proportion.

$$50x = 25$$

RULE 6: Solve for *x* (divide the number with the *x* into the number on the opposite side of the problem).

EXAMPLE: 50 mg : 1 mL :: 25 mg : x mL

$$50x = 25 \quad = \quad 50\overline{)25.0}^{\;.5}$$
$$x = 0.5$$

RULE 7: Label the answer with the unit of measurement that accompanies the *x* in the problem.

EXAMPLE: 50 mg : 1 mL :: 25 mg : x mL

$$50x = 25$$
$$x = 0.5 \text{ mL}$$

REVIEW OF PROPORTION METHOD

1. Set up problems in the *same order* on both sides.
2. Multiply the means; multiply the extremes.
3. The number multiplied with the *x* is always that number with the *x* to the right of it.

   EXAMPLE: 2 mg : 1 mL :: 5 mg : x mL
4. Divide the number with the *x* into the number on the other side of the problem.
5. Label the problem by looking to see what unit of measurement the *x* is with the proportion.

$$\frac{\text{Desired dosage}}{\text{Available dosage}} \times \text{Amount}$$

Many nurses use the following method of solving dosage problems.

RULE 1: Place the dose that the physician wants given over the dose that you have available (on hand).

PROBLEM: The physician orders 40 mg of furosemide (Lasix). You have an ampule (small glass container that usually contains a single dose of a solution) of furosemide labeled Lasix 20 mg/mL.

EXAMPLE:
$$\frac{(\text{Desired dosage})\ 40 \text{ mg}}{(\text{Available dose})\ 20 \text{ mg}} \times \frac{1 \text{ mL}}{1} = \frac{40}{20}$$
$$= 40 \div 20 = 2 \text{ mL}$$

PROBLEM: The physician orders 15 mg of diazepam (Valium). You have Valium tablets that contain 5 mg/tablet.

EXAMPLE:
$$\frac{(\text{Desired dosage})\ 15 \text{ mg}}{(\text{Available dose})\ 5 \text{ mg}} \times \frac{1 \text{ tab}}{x \text{ tab}} = \frac{15}{5x} = x$$
$$= 15 \div 5 = 3 \text{ tab}$$

DIMENSIONAL ANALYSIS*

The **dimensional analysis (DA)** method (also called *factor labeling* or the *label factor* method) calculates dosages using the following three factors:

1. Drug label factor: The form of the drug dose *(V)* with the equivalence in units *(H)*; for example, 1 capsule = 500 mg.
2. Conversion factor *(C)*: It will help to memorize the following common conversions (see the section on the Apothecary System with its abbreviations for a discussion of grains [gr]):

   1 g = 1000 mg   1 g = 15 gr
   1000 mg = 15 gr   1 gr = 60 mg
3. Drug order factor: The dosage desired *(D)*.

These three factors are set up in an equation that allows you to cancel the units, obtaining the correct units for delivery.

$$V = \frac{V\,(\text{vehicle})}{H\,(\text{on hand})} \times \frac{C\,(H)}{C\,(D)} \times \frac{D\,(\text{desired})}{1}$$

(drug label)   (conversion factor)   (drug order)

With dimensional analysis, the conversion factor is built into the equation and is included when the units of measurement of the drug order and drug container differ. If the two are of the same units of measurement, the conversion factor is eliminated from the equation.

EXAMPLE: Order calls for acetaminophen (Tylenol) gr xv, po, prn (15 grains, by mouth, as needed)

Available:

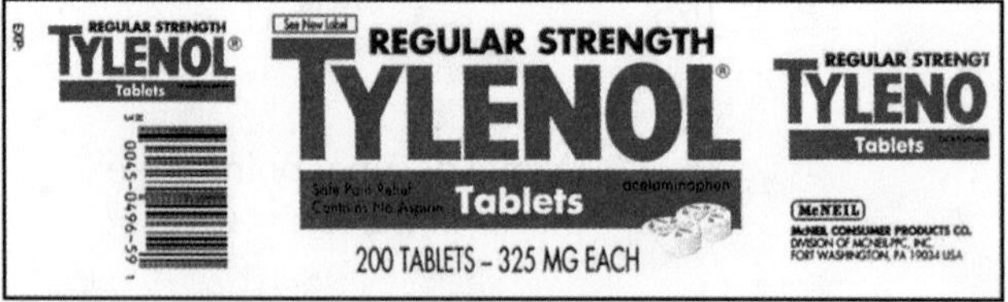

Factors: 325 mg = 1 tablet (from drug label)
15 gr/1 (from drug order)
Conversion factor: 1000 mg = 15 gr
How many tablet(s) should be given?

$$\text{Tab} = \frac{1 \text{ tab}}{325 \text{ mg}} \times \frac{1000 \text{ mg}}{15 \text{ gr}} \times \frac{15 \text{ gr}}{1} = \frac{1000}{325} = 3.07 \text{ tab or } 3 \text{ tab}$$

*From Kee, J.L., & Hayes, E.R. (2007). *Pharmacology: a nursing process approach.* (5th ed.). Philadelphia: Saunders.

Box 23-1 Nursing Responsibilities in Solving Dosage Problems

- Do not allow for any errors in calculating dosages.
- Check math work with another nurse.
- Work problems systematically and carefully on paper.
- Reduce distractions while working problems.
- Recheck calculations.
- Is the answer reasonable?

See Box 23-1 for the nurse's responsibilities in solving dosage problems accurately.

THE METRIC SYSTEM

The metric system is the preferred system of weights and measures. It is more accurate and easier to use in calculating dosage problems.

Similar to the U.S. monetary system, which is based on the dollar, the metric system is also based on the decimal system. The decimal system uses the divisions and multiples of a unit that is always in ratios of tens.

EXAMPLE: 1 dollar = 10 dimes
10 dimes = 20 nickels
20 nickels = 100 pennies

All these units are multiples or divisions of tens.

The metric system uses the following basic units of volume, weight, and length:

liter (L) volume (amount) of fluids
gram (g) weight of solids
meter (m) measure of length

Smaller units are designated by the following prefixes:

deci 0.1 of the unit; tens (liter, gram, meter)
centi 0.01 of the unit; hundredths
milli 0.001 of the unit; thousandths

Larger units are designated with the following prefixes:

deka 10 times the unit (liter, gram, meter)
hecto 100 times the unit
kilo 1000 times the unit

Units of Volume

1 liter (L)	= 1000 milliliters (mL)
0.001 liter (L)	= 1 milliliter (mL)
1 milliliter (mL)	= 1 cubic centimeter (cc)

Units of Weight

1 gram (g)	= 1000 milligrams (mg)
0.001 gram (g)	= 1 milligram (mg)
1 kilogram (kg)	= 1000 grams (g)
0.001 kilogram (kg)	= 1 gram (g)

In addition to the preceding units of measurement, you will often encounter the term **milliequivalent,** abbreviated mEq. Milliequivalent refers to the concentration of electrolytes in a certain volume of solution, expressed as milliequivalents per liter (mEq/L). Potassium chloride (KCl) is an electrolyte that is sometimes ordered as an IV additive to a liter (1000 mL) of fluid.

EXAMPLE: The doctor orders the following:
Add 40 mEq KCl to 1 L D_5W to run at 125 mL/hr.

APPROXIMATE EQUIVALENTS OF THE METRIC SYSTEM AND THE APOTHECARY SYSTEM

The apothecary system is a system of measurement that is still used by some physicians and hospitals. It is being replaced by the metric system. Because its use does continue today, you will occasionally need the following equivalents to convert dosages from one system to another. The conversions are only approximations, but they are acceptable equivalents with which to work. Convert from one system to another to work dosage problems in the same measurement units.

Volume

Metric		*Apothecary*
1 milliliter (mL)	=	15 or 16 minims (♍ XV/XVI) (minims are rarely used
4 or 5 milliliters (mL)	=	1 fluid dram (f ʒ i̇)
30 milliliters (mL)	=	1 fluid ounce (f ℥ i̇)
500 milliliters (mL)	=	1 pint (O i̇ or 1 pt)
1000 milliliters (mL) or 1 liter (L)	=	1 quart (1 Qt)

The following are symbols for the apothecary units:

Minim = ♍
Fluid dram = ʒ
Fluid ounce = ℥
Pint = O or pt
Quart = Qt

The symbols appear in front of the number (which is written in Roman numerals).

EXAMPLE: 16 minims is written ♍ XVI. You will almost never use minims in the current health care system. More commonly, you will use the metric system of the apothecary system.

EXAMPLE: Instead of 8 minims (♍ VIII), you will usually state 0.5 mL.

Weight

Metric		*Apothecary*
60 milligrams (mg)	=	1 gr (gr is the symbol for grain)
1000 milligrams (mg)	=	15 grains (gr XV)
4 grams (g or Gm)	=	1 dram (ʒ i̇)
30 grams (g)	=	1 ounce (℥ i̇)
0.45 kilogram (kg)	=	1 pound (lb)
1 kilogram (kg)	=	2.2 pounds (lb)

METRIC MEASUREMENTS OF LENGTH

The basic unit of length in the metric system is the meter. The meter is equal to 39.37 inches, about 3½ inches longer than 1 yard (36 inches). Some of the tasks that you will perform using the metric measurements of length will be the following:

- Measure area size for topical applications
- Measure results of intradermal skin tests (size of drug or allergen reaction on the skin)
- Measure wound size
- Measure pressure ulcers
- Measure height, length, and head circumference (common tasks in obstetrics and pediatrics)
- Measure abdominal girth (obstetrics and patients with ascites and heart failure)

0.001 meter	= 1 millimeter (mm)
0.01 meter	= 1 centimeter (cm)
0.1 meter	= 1 decimeter (dm)
10 meters	= 1 decameter (dam)
100 meters	= 1 hectometer (hm)
1000 meters	= 1 kilometer (km)

Most frequently used equivalents are the following:

1 meter (m)	= 1000 millimeters (mm)
0.001 meter (m)	= 1 millimeter (mm)
1 meter (m)	= 100 centimeters (cm)
1 centimeter (cm)	= 10 millimeters (mm)
1 millimeter (mm)	= 0.1 centimeter (cm)

BIG TO SMALL RULE

Whatever method is used to solve dosage problems, always convert the units of measurement in the problem to the same unit of measurement.

Some students find it difficult to convert dosages that contain decimal fractions. This section discusses a quick, easy method called the "big to small" rule. It is useful in converting dosages **within the same system** (the metric system).

Because there are 1000 mL in 1 L (and 1000 mg in 1 g), you will be able to convert milliliters to liters (and milligrams to grams) by this method. Likewise, convert liters to milliliters (and grams to milligrams) by this method.

CONVERTING LARGER UNITS OF MEASUREMENT TO SMALLER UNITS OF MEASUREMENT (GRAMS TO MILLIGRAMS; LITERS TO MILLILITERS)

RULE 1: Write down BIG ⟶ SMALL.

RULE 2: Place the large unit under the word *BIG* and the small unit under the word *SMALL*.

EXAMPLE: BIG ⟶ SMALL
2.5 g = ___ mg

RULE 3: Move the decimal point three places in the direction of the arrow; add zeros.

EXAMPLE: BIG ⟶ SMALL
2.500 = 2500 mg

CONVERTING SMALLER UNITS OF MEASUREMENT TO LARGER UNITS OF MEASUREMENT (MILLIGRAMS TO GRAMS; MILLILITERS TO LITERS)

RULE 1: Write down the big-to-small rule formula.

EXAMPLE: BIG ⟶ SMALL

RULE 2: Reverse the direction of the arrow.

EXAMPLE: BIG ⟵ SMALL

RULE 3: Place the large unit under the word *BIG* and the small unit under the word *SMALL*.

EXAMPLE: BIG ⟵ SMALL
x g = 2500 mg

RULE 4: Move the decimal point three places in the direction that the arrow points.

EXAMPLE: BIG ⟵ SMALL
2.5 g = 2.500

PEDIATRIC CONSIDERATIONS

Pediatric dosage refers to the determination of the correct amount, the correct frequency, and the total number of doses of a medication you are going to administer to a child or infant.

It is necessary to consider age, weight, body surface area, and the ability of the child to absorb, metabolize, and excrete medication when administering medication to a child.

It is the physician's responsibility to determine medication orders and dosage for a pediatric patient, but you need to be able to recognize appropriate and inappropriate drug dosages and orders.

It is essential for you to be knowledgeable about the four standard formulas for calculating children's dosages. These are Young's rule, Clark's rule, Fried's rule, and the body surface area method.

YOUNG'S RULE

Young's rule is a method to calculate the appropriate dose of a drug for a child 2 years of age or older.

YOUNG'S RULE is as follows:

$$\frac{\text{Age of child}}{\text{Age of child} + 12} \times \text{Average adult dose} = \text{Child's dose}$$

This rule applies to children up to the age of 12.

PROBLEM: The average adult dose of a particular medication is 50 mg. What is an appropriate dose of this medication for an 8-year-old child?

$$\frac{8\text{ yr}}{8+12} \times 50\text{ mg} = \frac{8}{20} \times \frac{50}{1} = \frac{400}{20} = 20\overline{)400} = 20\text{ mg}$$

(long division: 400 ÷ 20 = 20; 40, 0, 0)

ANSWER: 20 mg is an appropriate dose.

CLARK'S RULE

Clark's rule is a method of calculating the approximate pediatric dosage of a drug for a child.

CLARK'S RULE is as follows:

$$\frac{\text{Weight of child in pounds}}{150} \times \text{Average adult dose} = \text{Child's dose}$$

This rule uses the child's weight to determine dosage.

PROBLEM: The average adult dose of a particular medication is 25 mg. What is an appropriate dose of this medication for a child who weighs 40 pounds?

EXAMPLE:

$$\frac{40\text{ lb}}{150} \times 25\text{ mg} = \frac{40}{150} \times \frac{25}{1} = \frac{1000}{150} = 150\overline{)1000.00}$$

6.66
900
1000
900
1000

= 6.7 mg or 7 mg

ANSWER: 6.7 or 7 mg is an appropriate dose.

FRIED'S RULE

This rule is used for infants less than 2 years of age.

FRIED'S RULE is as follows:

$$\frac{\text{Age in months}}{150} \times \text{Average adult dose} = \text{Child's dose}$$

PROBLEM: The average adult dose of a particular medication is 25 mg. What is an appropriate dose of this medication for a child who is 22 months of age?

EXAMPLE:

$$\frac{22}{150} \times 25\text{ mg} = \frac{550}{150} = 150\overline{)550.00} = 3.7 \text{ or } 4\text{ mg}$$

3.66
450
1000
900
1000

ANSWER: 3.7 or 4 mg is an appropriate dose.

ESTIMATING BODY SURFACE AREA IN CHILDREN

Body surface area is defined as the total area exposed to the outside environment. For pediatric patients of average size, it is acceptable to estimate body surface area with the scale shown in Figure 23-1. Match weight to the corresponding surface area. For other pediatric patients, use the other scale. Lay a straight edge on the correct height and weight points for your patient, and observe the point where it intersects on the surface area scale at center.

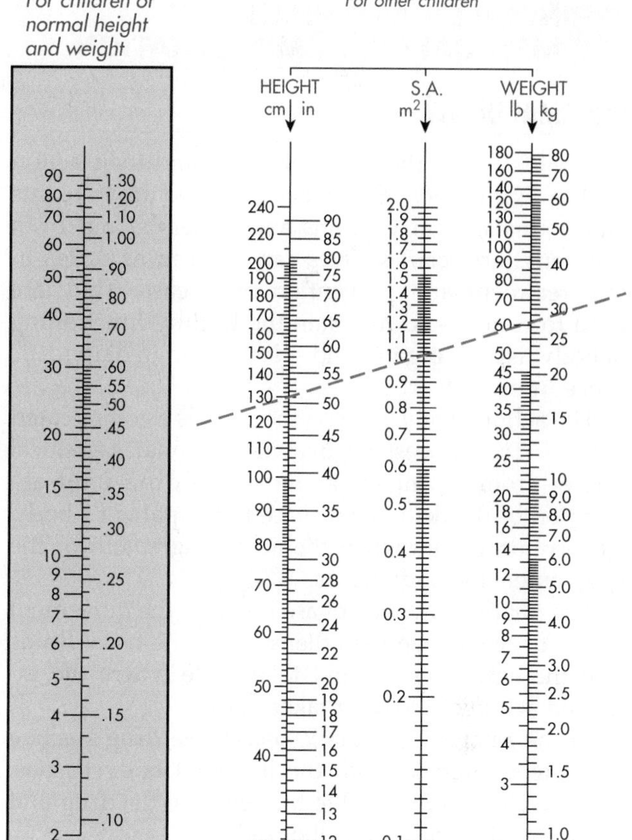

FIGURE 23-1 Estimating body surface area in children.

PROBLEM: Trey, an 8-year-old, weighs 60 pounds and is 51 inches tall. His body surface area (as determined by using the nomogram in Figure 23-1) is 1.0. If an adult dose is 50 mg, how many mg should Trey receive?

EXAMPLE: Use the formula:

$$\frac{SA(m2)}{1.73\text{ m}2} \times \text{Adult dose} = \text{Child's dose}$$

(Trey's surface area expressed in square meters = 1.0)

$$\frac{1.0}{1.73} \times 50\text{ mg} = \frac{1.0}{1.73} \times \frac{50}{1} = \frac{50}{1.73}$$

$$= 1.73\overline{)50.00.00} = 29\text{ mg}$$

28.9
356
1440
1384
1560
1557
3
173

ANSWER: 29 mg is appropriate for a child of Trey's height and weight.

Body surface area is used for determining pediatric dosages for burn patients in particular and also for determining radiation dosages.

PRINCIPLES AND PRACTICE OF MEDICATION ADMINISTRATION

PHARMACOLOGY

Pharmacology is the study of drugs and their action on the living body. Substances derived from plants and animals, from vitamins and minerals, and from synthetic (artificial) sources can be used as drugs in the treatment and prevention of disease. They are used to restore and maintain the healthy functioning of body tissues, organs, and systems and in diagnostic procedures.

The action of any drug on the body is a complicated process. This process begins with the pharmaceutical phase—from the manufacture of the drug until absorption of the drug takes place in the patient's body. Absorption occurs when the active ingredient of the drug enters the body fluids.

The pharmacokinetic phase involves the movement of the drug's active ingredients from the body fluids into the entire system and to the site where the intended action of the drug takes place.

In the pharmacodynamic phase, the drug's active ingredient interacts with the intended body tissues. The body's cells respond to the action of the drug and change as the drug is metabolized.

The liver is the main organ that inactivates and metabolizes drugs; the kidneys are the principal organs that eliminate the metabolites of drugs from the body. A metabolite is a substance produced by metabolic action, which results in the breakdown of the drug.

You need to understand the process of drug action and elimination from the body, because each patient will be affected differently by the medications prescribed. It is necessary to assess and consider each patient's hepatic (liver) and renal (kidney) functions, because decreased hepatic or renal function have potential to prolong the length of time a drug stays in the body.

Drugs that are not excreted in the urine, feces, sweat, tears, breast milk (in lactating mothers), and expired air will possibly build up in the body. A drug that builds up in the body is said to have a cumulative (increasing by incremental steps with an eventual total) effect, which sometimes leads to toxic (harmful) or even lethal (deadly) effects (Box 23-2).

Box 23-2 Terms Used with Dosages

Minimal dose: The smallest amount of a drug that produces a therapeutic effect
Maximal dose: The largest amount of a drug that it is possible to give safely
Toxic dose: The amount of a drug that produces signs and symptoms of poisoning
Lethal dose: The amount of a drug that will cause death

DRUG DOSAGE

Dosage is the amount of a drug prescribed for the patient by the physician in a given amount of time or at a given frequency—for example, "Give 100 mg Dilantin po tid." A **dose** of medicine refers to a single administration of a drug, given at one time. The dose ordered in the example is 100 mg. You will give a 100-mg dose (one capsule) of Dilantin by mouth (po; Latin, *per os*) three times a day, for a total daily dosage of 300 mg (given in divided doses). Make sure to familiarize yourself with therapeutic (beneficial) dosages of frequently used drugs to confidently and correctly administer doses of medication to each patient (see Box 23-2).

DRUG ACTIONS AND INTERACTIONS

There are two general types of drug action—local and systemic. Drugs that have a local action produce an effect only on the area where the drug is placed. Systemic drug action affects the entire body, because the drug enters the systemic circulation.

When one drug alters the action of another drug, it is called a drug interaction (a modification of the effect of a drug when administered with another drug). When two or more drugs are given together, the combined actions of the drugs will sometimes produce a totally different effect than the expected effect of either drug. These effects are sometimes beneficial and sometimes harmful. When one drug increases the action or the effect of another drug, it is called potentiation, or **synergism.** Drug combinations are often used with the express purpose of "boosting" the action of one or the other of the drugs administered.

Some drugs do not combine chemically or physically—or both—with other drugs. This is called drug **incompatibility.** For example, when two drugs are mixed and the solution changes color, becomes cloudy, or forms a precipitate (solid mass), incompatibility is suspected. Compatibility (the quality or state of existing together in harmony) charts allow quick reference to determine whether it is acceptable to give one drug along with another drug in the same syringe or intravenous infusion.

Drug interactions are more likely to occur with drugs that are especially potent (strong), such as digitalis. The cardiotonics (drugs that slow and strengthen the heart), antihypertensives (drugs that lower blood pressure), hypoglycemic agents (oral medications that lower blood glucose [sugar]), insulin (injectable medication that lowers blood glucose), and heparin (medication that decreases the clotting of blood) are all powerful agents that are important to be familiar with before you give them. In drug interactions, the effect will sometimes be an increase or a decrease in the action of either substance, and other times an adverse effect that is not normally associated with either drug.

The particular interaction is usually the result of incompatibility between the two drugs or of a change in the rate of absorption or the quantity absorbed in the body.

Drug interactions are a frequent cause of adverse effects, decreased patient compliance, and prolonged hospitalizations. Continual awareness of the possibility of interactions and observation for these complications are the responsibility of all health professionals. Watch for changes in level of consciousness such as slurred speech or ataxia (unsteady gait) and for changes in vital signs. Listen to what the patient says about the medication's effects. The licensed practical nurse or licensed vocational nurse (LPN/LVN) reports observations to the registered nurse (RN) and documents these observations objectively in the nursing notes. Physicians depend on the ongoing nursing assessment of each patient's response to drug therapy.

Knowledge of agonistic and antagonistic drug action is helpful to the nurse and the physician. A drug that produces a predictable response at the intended site of action is called an agonist. An antagonist is a drug that will block the action of another drug. Antagonistic drugs are used to counteract the effects of a previously given drug. For example, naloxone HCl (Narcan) works against the central nervous system–depressant effects of meperidine HCl (Demerol) and other central nervous system depressants by blocking the action of the depressant.

Because each patient responds differently to medications, always be alert to the possibility of idiosyncratic drug reactions. An idiosyncratic response to a drug is an individual's unique hypersensitivity to a particular drug. It is an unexpected response to a medication. Idiosyncratic reactions are thought to have a genetic basis. For example, an idiosyncratic reaction to a sedative that was given to produce calmness will perhaps unexpectedly cause the patient to become agitated and restless. For this reason, it is important to observe and assess patients for signs of overdose, toxicity, and unexpected drug reactions even though they are receiving the correct therapeutic dose.

Some patients will be hypersensitive or allergic to a drug. Assess the patient's drug history *before* giving a drug. Has the patient taken the drug before? Does the patient have any known allergies to medications? If so, withhold the drug and report this information to the charge nurse. *When in doubt, "Don't."*

A reduced response to a drug over time is called drug tolerance. The patient who has developed tolerance to a drug requires a larger dose of the drug to achieve the same effect that a smaller therapeutic dose once gave. Drug tolerance is either acquired from taking increasing dosages of the drug over time or results from genetic factors unique to the individual.

It is essential to observe each patient's reaction to drug therapy, particularly when the patient receives a drug for the first time. Assess the patient's mental and physical status before a new medication is started to establish a baseline reference. Report changes in mental or physical status to the RN. Causes of the change are likely to be an adverse drug reaction (a harmful, unintended reaction to a drug administered at a normal dosage), drug hypersensitivity, or drug intolerance.

Drug administration is a tremendous nursing responsibility. Never give any unfamiliar medication to a patient without first looking it up in a drug reference book. The *Physicians' Desk Reference (PDR)* is a book you will usually be able to find in the nurses' station. Use it to find therapeutic dosage, indications for use of the drug, **contraindications** (conditions in which the drug should not be used), side effects, available formulations and routes of administration, generic and trade names, a list of poison control centers, and information for managing overdoses. The *PDR* is published annually.

The following factors affect how patients respond to medication and are necessary to consider in patient assessment:

- **Age.** Very young and very old people generally react more acutely to drugs than others. Older adults tend to have a higher ratio of fat tissue to muscle tissue, and the higher fat percentage will typically affect the distribution and accumulation of fat-soluble drugs. Prolonged drug action is likely to occur in older adults, because renal and hepatic function is often decreased (Table 23-1). The very young do not have fully developed renal and hepatic functions; therefore, drugs are inefficiently metabolized and excreted.
- **Weight.** Overweight people often require higher drug dosages than those of average weight. Underweight individuals usually require lower drug dosages. Body surface area, height, and weight are important factors in determining drug dosages in children.
- **Physical health.** People in poor physical health do not tolerate average dosages as well as those in good health. Disease processes alter dosage requirements, particularly in patients with renal, hepatic, cardiovascular, and gastrointestinal (GI) dysfunctions.
- **Psychological status.** Stress, emotional conflict, anxiety, and fear have the capacity to alter the response to drug therapy. Also, if the patient has faith in the drug, the hospital, the physician, and you, he or she is more likely to adhere to the medication therapy. Your actions, attitudes, and skills affect the patient's response to drug therapy as well.
- **Environmental temperature.** Heat will sometimes increase the rate at which the body metabolizes a drug, as cold will decrease it.

Table 23-1 Influence of Aging on Drug Actions in Older Adults

AGE-RELATED PHYSIOLOGIC CHANGE	EFFECT ON DRUG ACTION AND PATIENT RESPONSE	NURSING INTERVENTIONS
GASTROINTESTINAL TRACT		
Oral Cavity		
Loss of elasticity in oral mucosa, which becomes dry and easily abraded	Difficulty in swallowing tablets or capsules; sensitivity to drugs that cause dryness of mouth, susceptibility to gum disease and dental caries	Have patient rinse oral cavity frequently with clear tepid water, floss daily, and brush teeth and gums gently. Recommend synthetic substitute saliva.
Esophagus		
Delayed esophageal clearance because of weakened contractions and failure of lower esophageal sphincter to relax	Difficulty in swallowing large tablets or capsules; tissue erosion caused by drugs such as aspirin and uncoated potassium chloride	Position patient upright. Administer full glass of liquid with drug. Crush tablets and mix with food (if gastric pH does not affect absorption).
Stomach		
Decrease in gastric acidity and peristalsis	Potentiation of irritating effects of highly acidic drugs (e.g., aspirin)	Have patient drink full glass of water and take medication with nonfat snack to reduce gastric distress.
Large Intestine		
Reduced colon muscle tone; loss of defecation reflex; decreased intestinal blood flow	Slowing of drug excretion; overuse and abuse of laxatives by patient; delayed drug absorption	Provide normal fluid intake. Instruct patient to eat bulk-forming foods and avoid use of constipating drugs.
SKIN AND VASCULAR SYSTEM		
Reduced subcutaneous skinfold thickness in extremities (less body fat); reduced elasticity in skin and vascular system; increased fragility of blood vessels	Patient prone to bleeding after injections	Avoid using veins in hand for intravenous (IV) injections. Apply pressure to injection sites after administration. Observe injection sites for bleeding.
Liver		
Reduced liver size; decline in hepatic blood flow	Longer biotransformation time; longer-than-normal duration of drug action; greater risk for drug sensitivity and toxicity	Monitor for signs and symptoms of liver impairment (jaundice, pruritus, dark urine). Monitor blood chemistry values for hepatic toxicity.
Kidneys		
Reduced glomerular filtration; decreased tubular function and renal blood flow	Risk of drug accumulation and toxicity	Prevent urinary retention (keep catheters flowing freely and observe frequency of urination). Monitor for signs and symptoms of renal impairment (reduced output and difficulty in urinating). Provide normal fluid intake. Monitor blood urea nitrogen (BUN) and serum creatinine levels.

- **Sex.** Women tend to have a higher percentage of body fat than men, whereas men have a higher percentage of body fluid. Because some drugs are fat soluble, women with high body fat percentage tend to accumulate fat-soluble drugs in their bodies. It is important to advise pregnant and lactating women that the substances taken during pregnancy have the capacity to pass through the placenta and adversely affect the fetus. It is also possible for drugs to pass to infants through breast milk.
- **Amount of food in the stomach.** Drugs taken on an empty stomach reach the bloodstream faster than those taken on a full stomach. Irritating drugs are given after or with meals so that they will not irritate the GI tract.
- **Dosage forms.** Dosage forms influence the onset, intensity, and duration of a drug. Drugs in intravenous and intramuscular formulations act more quickly than drugs taken orally.

It is important to continually assess and evaluate drug action in each patient. Use judgment before giving medications, because any drug has the potential to cause harm.

Make sure to be knowledgeable about the basics of drug action, how drug orders are written, how to interpret them, and how they are transcribed. Always follow the basic practices and principles of safe medication administration. High personal and professional standards protect the patient and prevent you from making medication errors.

MEDICATION ORDERS

You are ethically and legally responsible for ensuring that the patient receives the correct medication as ordered by the physician. Physicians write medication orders during patient admissions, during morning and evening rounds, after surgery, and any other time throughout the day or night as needed. As soon as possible after a physician writes an order, see that you read and interpret the order. Then transcribe the drug order to the Medex (a small card listing the name, dose, and schedule of administration of each patient's medication used in dispensing drugs to each patient) (or Kardex, depending on your facility's policy) or place the drug order in the computer, exactly the same way that the order appears on the order sheet. If the handwriting is illegible, ask another nurse to interpret or call the physician for clarification.

You will send the medication request for the patient's medications to the pharmacy. The pharmacist will prepare and send the medications to the patient's unit.

DRUG DISTRIBUTION SYSTEMS

There are various systems used for storing and distributing medications. Institutions such as hospitals and long-term care facilities have designated areas for stocking and dispensing medications. All storage areas which house medications always remain locked when unattended. The **unit-dose system** is based on a portable cart with drawers, containing a 24-hour supply of medications for each patient. Each medication is individually wrapped in a unit-dose, which is the ordered dose of medication the patient is to receive at each prescribed time. Typically, you will be able to transport the medication cart from room to room to administer the medication at designated times. The medication cart is always locked when not attended. In some institutions, there is a locked cabinet in each patient's room where their medications are stored (Elkin et al., 2007).

Computer-controlled dispensing systems are a combination of unit-dose and floor stock systems. Pyxis Corporation supplies the MedStation, which is a system containing various medications placed in individual compartments. You use the computerized screen to request a specific medication. You have a security code that allows you access only to those medications specifically prescribed for a patient. The system's computer records all medications removed from the MedStation as given, and facilitates automatic charges to the appropriate patient as well (Figure 23-2) (Elkin et al., 2007).

Whether a unit-dose or multidose system is used, it is your responsibility to properly store medications on the nursing unit. Follow the storage instructions for each drug; some require refrigeration, whereas others have to be kept in a dark or cool area. It is essential to safely and securely store opioids, barbiturates, and other controlled drugs that have a high potential for abuse in a locked box with its own unique key.

Frequently, the drug the nursing unit receives from the pharmacy will have a different name than that ordered by the physician. Each drug has several names; the two most common types are the trade name and the generic name. The trade name is the brand name given to it by the manufacturer for use especially by consumers and care providers. It is followed on the package by the symbol ®. The trade name is usually short and easy to spell and to pronounce, such as "Lasix." It is capitalized. The generic name, frequently used, is usually longer, is not capitalized, and is typically used by the manufacturer and researchers. The generic name for Lasix is furosemide.

Make certain that the drug you have received is the same drug that was ordered. Consult the pharmacist if there is a question about the identity of a drug. Once assured that the medication is the correct one, clearly and accurately transcribe the medication name, dosage, times, and stop date on the Medex or the computer. In many facilities, unit clerks transcribe drug orders. The RN or LPN/LVN who transcribes or verifies the order writes her or his signature and title and the time and date immediately after the last order on the order sheet. The nurse draws a line after the last order to indicate the end of that physician's particular order.

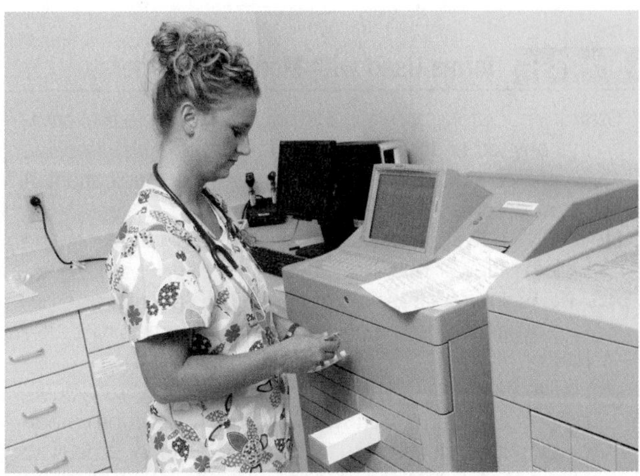

FIGURE 23-2 Nurse using computer-controlled dispensing system.

Medication orders properly include the following:
- Patient's name (on physician's order sheet)
- Patient's date of birth
- Date and time of the order (usually on the left side of the order sheet); written by the physician
- Name of drug
- Dosage of the drug, including dose size and frequency (e.g., give acetaminophen 650 mg q 4 hr prn [or, every four hours as needed])
- Route of administration, as prescribed by the physician
- Signature of the physician
- Any special instructions regarding any aspect of administering the drug (e.g., give acetaminophen 650 mg q 4 hr if temperature >101° F)

The RN will sign off on one-time-only orders, such as "stat," "now," or "ASAP," on the physician's order sheet as soon as possible after the medication has been given (Box 23-3). Doing so prevents another nurse from "double-dosing" the patient as a result of poor communication between nurses. If the order is written on the Medex or the medication administration record (MAR) (Figure 23-3, *A* and *B*), it is necessary to properly transcribe the order and discontinue the order immediately after giving the medication (see Medex examples in Figure 23-3).

CONTROLLED SUBSTANCES

Opioids, barbiturates, and other controlled drugs that have a high possibility for abuse or addiction are kept under a double lock. In cases when a computerized system has not been implemented, the "narcotic keys" are kept by designated nurses each shift. It is those nurses' responsibility to see that each controlled drug used that shift is logged in the narcotic log book. At the end of each shift, controlled drugs in the locker are carefully counted by a designated nurse of the outgoing shift and the nurse of the incoming shift. The number of drugs given, according to the log book, and the actual number of medications contained in the locker are required to be exactly the same. The staff are not dismissed until the narcotic count is done. If the count is incorrect, it is necessary to find the error or the missing drug before anyone is dismissed. It is essential not to allow the nurse to take the keys home by mistake.

Many agencies now use computerized systems for medication access and distribution. Computerized storage has eliminated the need to do the narcotic count at the end of each shift.

Always have a witness to any "wasting" (disposal) of a controlled medication. The witness and the person wasting the medication are required to sign the log book to indicate that the medication was wasted. Controlled substances are handled only by people with licenses, such as an RN, an LPN/LVN, or a student nurse under the supervision of the nurse educator (Box 23-4).

TYPES OF ORDERS

Standing Orders

Standing orders are those that are already written by a physician for a patient on a particular unit or area. You will carry them out without having to call the physician for confirmation, and whether or not the physician is present. A copy of the orders is kept on the unit. Know where the orders are located, be knowledgeable about handling orders, and use assessment and judgment skills in implementing these orders. It sometimes causes unnecessary stress or discomfort to a patient if you are unaware that the physician has left standing orders. If

Box 23-3 Terms Used with Medication Orders

Stat: Immediately; number one priority; give before executing any other type of order. To prevent mistakes, be careful to document that you gave the medication. A "stat" order is a one-time-only dose.

Now: Give now; number two priority; give before executing orders of lower priority. Cancel order after giving.

ASAP: As soon as possible; number three priority; give before executing orders of lower priority. Cancel order after giving.

prn: Give as necessary; the patient is permitted to request prn medication, or you will sometimes offer a prn medication; it is necessary for prn medication orders to specify a definite time interval between permitted repeat administrations.

Box 23-4 Guidelines for Safe Administration and Control of Opioids and Other Controlled Substances

- Store all opioids and other controlled substances in a locked, secure cabinet or container. (Computerized, locked cabinets are now available.)
- Designated nurses keep special keys (or a special computer entry code) for the cabinet that contains opioids and other controlled substances.
- During an institution's change of shift, the nurse going off duty counts all opioids and other controlled substances with the nurse coming on duty. Both nurses sign the opioid record to indicate that the count is correct.
- It is obligatory to report discrepancies in opioid counts immediately.
- A special inventory record is used each time an opioid or other controlled substance is dispensed.
- The record is used to document the patient's name, birth date, room number, date, time of drug administration, name of drug, dosage, and signature of nurse dispensing the drug.
- The form provides an accurate, ongoing count of opioids and other controlled substances used and remaining.
- If only one part of a premeasured dosage of a controlled substance is given, a second nurse witnesses disposal of the unused portion and documents such on the record form.

A

ADDRESSOGRAPH

GREAT PLAINS REGIONAL MEDICAL CENTER

MEDEX

ALLERGY: Morphine sulfate

DIAGNOSIS: HF

RD - RIGHT DELTOID
LD - LEFT DELTOID
RG - RIGHT GLUTEUS UPPER, OUTER QUADRANT
LG - LEFT GLUTEUS UPPER, OUTER QUADRANT
RLT - RIGHT LATERAL THIGH
LLT - LEFT LATERAL THIGH
VG - VENTROGLUTEAL

*SITE ABBREVIATIONS ARE TO BE CIRCLED.
*DRUGS REQUIRING NURSING INTERVENTION BEFORE ADMINISTRATION, ENTER ASSESSMENT FINDING, THE TIME & YOUR INITIALS IN THE APPROPRIATE DATE COLUMN.

MEDICATION ADMINISTRATION RECORD

DATE	MEDICATION/DOSE FREQUENCY	ROUTE	MEDICATION SCHEDULE	ID	DATE: 1-9-10			DATE: 1-10-10			DATE: 1-11-10		
					23 - 7	7 - 15	15 - 23	23 - 7	7 - 15	15 - 23	23 - 7	7 - 15	15 - 23
12-9-10	Isopto Carpine 4% Ṫ gtt	Rt eye	qid 09-13-17-21	JR		09 BC							
12-9	Isopto Carpine 4% Ṫ gtt	Left eye	Bedtime 2100	JR			021 BC						
12-9	Peri-Colase ṪṪ	PO	Every day 0900	JR		09 BC							
12-9	Calan 40 mg	PO	Bid 09-21	JR		09 BC							
12-9	Ceftin 250 mg	PO	tid 09-13-21	JR		09 BC							
12-9	Lanoxin 0.125 mg	PO	Daily 0900	JR		09 BC							
12-9	Capoten 25 mg	PO	Bid 09-21	JR		09 BC							
PRN MEDICATION													
12-9	Dulcolax Supp.	R	prn	JR			19 EK						
12-9	Restoril 15 mg Ṫ	PO	Bedtime prn sleep	JR			21 EK						
12-9	Bancap HC Ṫ	PO	q 4 hr prn	JR		13 EK							

INITIALS / FULL SIGNATURE /TITLE

BC Barbara Christensen RN MS

EK Elaine Kockrow RN MS

ID = PERSON TAKING OFF ORDERS / RN

ROOM: NAME:

FIGURE 23-3 **A,** Medication administration record.

Continued

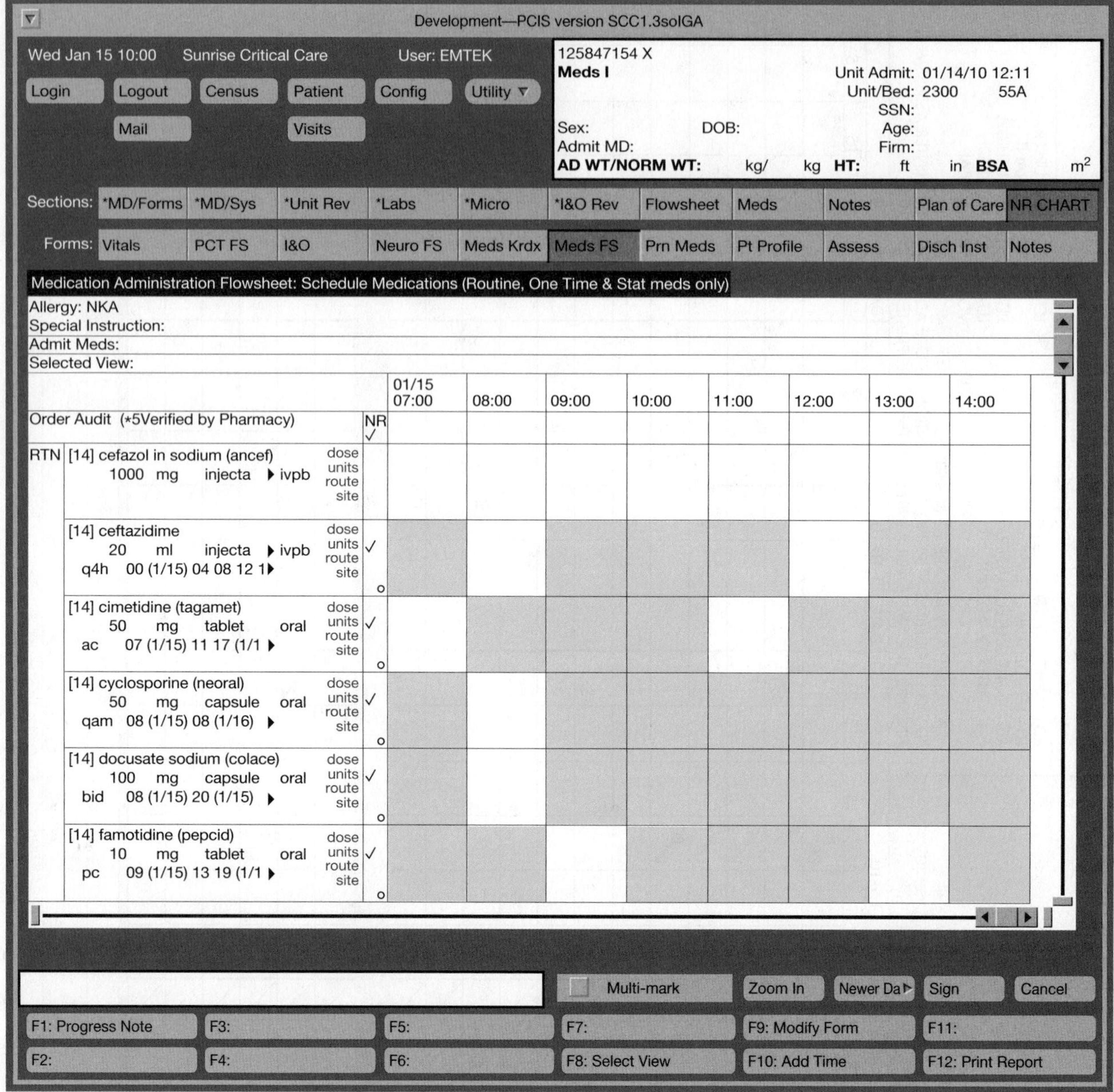

FIGURE 23-3, cont'd B, Computer list of ordered medications.

there is any question about a standing order, get verification or clarification from the physician who wrote them. Each physician leaves different standing orders; you are obliged to know the physicians' orders.

There are two types of standing orders:

1. **Standing order with expiration.** The order is written and kept in a folder at the nurses' station. The order will be either discontinued or reordered on or before the expiration date.
2. **Standing order without expiration.** The order is written and kept in a folder at the nurses' station, but no expiration date is given and the order remains valid until further notice from the physician.

Verbal Orders

The physician gives a verbal order in the presence of an LPN/LVN or an RN directly or over the telephone. Observe hospital policy for LPNs/LVNs taking verbal and telephone orders. Write verbal orders on the physician's order sheet exactly as the physician gave them. Have the physician sign the order as soon as possible. Be alert and careful when taking verbal orders. If the order is unclear or confusing, do not hesitate to ask the physician about the order. Always repeat the order to the physician to make sure that what was heard is what the physician actually said.

"SIX RIGHTS" OF MEDICATION ADMINISTRATION

Use each step of the nursing process in carrying out the responsibilities of medication administration. Medications are administered in a variety of ways. Regardless of the route by which a drug enters the body, the same practices and principles of medication administration apply.

Following the "six rights," performing the "three label checks," using standard precautions, and practicing good hand hygiene and aseptic technique ensure excellent drug administration practice.

Follow the "six rights" every time you give a drug (Box 23-5).

RIGHT MEDICATION

The Joint Commission (TJC) formally known as the Joint Commission on Accreditation of Healthcare Organizations (JCAHO) added medication reconciliation as a national safety goal for 2005. The protocol includes obtaining a complete list of the patient's current medications, and reviewing and documenting these medications with the patient and family involved. You will review the medications the patient is receiving in the hospital compared to those on the patient's list. Upon transfer to another service health care setting or dismissed home, you are again obliged to reconcile the list of medications the patient is on (Elkin et al., 2007).

Make sure the drug to be given is the correct drug, and perform "the three label checks": check the label on the drug's container three times—before, during, and after preparation. Take the medication to the patient's bedside in its original packaging, and open the packaging immediately before giving the dose (Box 23-6).

Never give a medication that another person has prepared, and *never* prepare or use a medication that is not labeled. In both cases it is impossible to know for sure what medication was prepared or what medication was in the unlabeled container.

Check the physician's order to verify the Medex or computer printout if there is a question about a medication. It is important to become familiar with generic and trade names of frequently used medications. Consult the *PDR* or the pharmacist if necessary.

Box 23-5 The "Six Rights" of Medication Administration

1. Right medication
2. Right dose
3. Right patient
4. Right time
5. Right route
6. Right documentation

Box 23-6 The Three Label Checks of Medication Administration

1. Check the label when taking the medication from its storage area.
2. Check the label before removing the medication from its container.
3. Check the label before discarding or replacing the medication container and before giving the medication to the patient.

RIGHT DOSE

Check the Medex or computer printout to verify the dosage of a drug. If there is a question, check the physician's order. Always check the label on the container for the dose per milliliter (dose/mL) or the dose per tablet, and consult with another nurse to check calculations or clarify a dosage (milliliters [mL] and cubic centimeters [cc] are sometimes used interchangeably).

The chance of an error occurring increases when a medication is prepared from a dose formulation other than what is ordered. Always compare the calculation of a dose with a second nurse who has calculated the dose independently. Calculations are even more important if there is an unusual calculation or when they involve a potentially toxic drug. Always use the correct measuring devices while preparing medications. Use a medicine cup marked in mL or a syringe to measure liquid preparations. Most pediatric medications are accompanied with a sealed dropper (Elkin et al., 2007).

It is also necessary to asses the appropriateness of the dose: Is the dose consistent with the age of the patient, the diagnosis of the patient, and the sex of the patient? Look at the number of tablets that constitute the dose or the number of milliliters that make up the dose. Does the number of tablets or the number of milliliters in the syringe look and sound reasonable? It is important to check the decimal place in the dosage ordered and your calculations: A decimal in the wrong place will potentially cause a serious drug error.

RIGHT TIME

You are responsible for putting the drug order into effect on the right schedule. Hospitals generally specify a standardized schedule. As explained by Elkin and colleagues (2007), "Medications to be given three times a day (tid) may be routinely scheduled for 0800, 1400, and 2000; or 0900, 1300, and 1900, depending on the agency policy. A drug may also be ordered every 8 hours (q 8 hr), which is also three times a day. The medication ordered q 8 hr needs to be given around the clock (ATC) to maintain adequate therapeutic levels and would, for example, be given at 0800, 1600, and 2400." Work any medication order into the standardized schedule as soon as possible. Table 23-2 lists commonly used abbreviations.

Table 23-2 Commonly Used Abbreviations

ABBREVIATION	MEANING	EXAMPLE
bid *(bis in die)*	Two times a day	0900-2100
tid *(ter in die)*	Three times a day	0900-1300-1700
qid *(quater in die)*	Four times a day	0800-1200-1600-2000
ac *(ante cibum)*	Before meals	Varies with hospital or unit
pc *(post cibum)*	After meals	Varies with hospital or unit

Make sure to administer all routinely ordered medications within 30 minutes of the scheduled time—no earlier than 30 minutes beforehand and no later than 30 minutes afterward. Some variance is allowed depending on the medications being administered. Some facilities are allowing administration 60 minutes before or 60 minutes after the scheduled time. Be certain to know the policy of the agency in which you are employed (Elkin et al., 2007). In particular, give antibiotics on time to maintain therapeutic blood levels.

Do not give medications to be administered as required (prn; Latin, *pro re nata*) before the time specified by the physician's order. Check the date that the drug order was written to be sure that the drug, the intravenous infusion, or the blood product is started and given on the right day and at the right time. Check the order sheet and the Medex or computer printout for dates and times to be sure that the medication has not been discontinued (d/c).

RIGHT ROUTE

The route chosen for administering a drug depends on the drug's properties and desired effect and the patient's physical and mental condition. It is necessary to place the route of administration on all prescribed medication orders. If the route of administration is not stated, clarify the specific route by contacting the prescriber immediately (Elkin et al., 2007). You will frequently be involved in judging the best route for a medicine. If an injection is prescribed, only parenteral liquids are acceptable to use. All parenteral medications are labeled "for injectable use only." Serious complications will result if a liquid intended for oral use is injected, possibly a sterile abscess or even fatal systematic effects (Elkin et al., 2007). When the medication preparation is parenteral (intramuscular [IM], subcutaneous [Sub-Q or subQ], intradermal [ID], or intravenous [IV]), be absolutely certain to inject the drug into the tissue specified.

RIGHT PATIENT

Make sure to give the medication to the right patient by systematically identifying the patient in every situation: check the patient's identification bracelet, including the name and date of birth, against the Medex or computer printout. Always take the MAR into the patient's room during medication administration. Having the MAR in hand lets you double-check medication and order before administering. Ask the patient to state his or her full name and date of birth. Sometimes you will also ask the patient to spell his or her name as you check the identification band. Identification of the patient is not to include the patient's room or bed number (TJC, 2005).

An unconscious patient is not able to provide self-identification, so the unconscious patient's safety depends on you. A family member or visitor will sometimes be at the bedside, but do not rely on others to identify the patient. Always check the identification band on conscious or unconscious patients, and never give medications to or perform procedures on a patient who does not have an identification band. After patient identification, always check for medication allergies. Nursing homes typically present a special challenge for a nurse who does not know the residents well. These residents usually do not wear identification bracelets and are sometimes confused or unable to respond to their name. Some nursing homes post the resident's name on the door for identification. Many nursing homes have a photo of each resident with the individual MAR.

After the six rights have been observed and the three label checks have been done, the nurse uses standard precautions (see Chapter 12).

RIGHT DOCUMENTATION

Make a notation of the drug's administration on the patient's chart or in the computer *immediately* after you give the drug. In cases of emergency and when you give medications used only occasionally, it is especially important not to overlook this step. Institutional policy will sometimes require that the chart notation of intramuscular medications also include the site of the injection and any complaints made by the patient at the time of administration. In the chart or computer notation, identify the drug given, the dosage, and the time you actually give it (not the time it is supposed to be given). In ambulatory care settings where immunizations are given, policy sometimes requires you to chart the lot number listed on the bottle. In your progress notes, include description of any response the patient has to the medications or their administration. Note any complaints or adverse effects in the chart, and report them to the head nurse and the physician. Never record on the chart any medications that you did not give or record them before you give them (see Box 23-8 and Safety Alert box).

It is clear that if all these principles are followed, it is essential to ***never*** give medication prepared by another nurse, even when you and your colleagues are very busy, when emergencies occur, or when you are interrupted. It is impossible to assume that all the "rights" are followed unless the person who prepares the medication is the one who gives the medication. Occasionally a physician will ask you or another nurse to prepare the medication for the physician to give. It is then acceptable for you to prepare the medication, but go along with the physician to see that the medication is given as ordered. Clearly document that the physician gave the medication.

Following institutional policy, using common sense, and remembering the high standards of care and ethical integrity that are essential for nurses to maintain will reduce the chance for medication error (Boxes 23-7 and 23-8). If an error is made, honesty in discussing the problem and prompt action to correct any damage

 Safety Alert!

The Joint Commission's "Do Not Use" List of Abbreviations

Each health care facility is obliged to develop and adhere to a "Do Not Use" list of abbreviations, acronyms, and symbols that must include those banned by The Joint Commission (TJC; formerly JCAHO) on April 1, 2004. These abbreviations are prohibited on all clinical documentation. Each health care facility is permitted to add its own entries to the list of banned abbreviations.

Starting in 2005, the TJC abbreviations were banned from inclusion in any documentation, including preprinted forms and computer software; however, patient safety always takes priority over adherence to these restrictions. For example, if an order containing a banned abbreviation is otherwise clear and complete and taking time to contact the prescriber will endanger your patient, carry out the order then confirm the term as soon as possible.

TJC's required minimum list of abbreviations not to use follows:

Abbreviation	***Potential Problem***	***Preferred Term***
U for unit	Mistaken as 0 (zero), 4, or cc	Write "unit"
IU for international unit	Mistaken as I.V. (intravenous) or 10	Write "international unit"
q.d. for once daily	Mistaken for each other	Write "daily" and "every other day"
q.o.d. for every other day	The period after the q or the o can be mistaken for "i" (q.i.d. means four times per day).	Write "every other day"
Trailing zero (9.0 mg)	Overlooked decimal point can lead to tenfold overdose	Never write a zero by itself after a decimal point (9 mg).
Lack of leading zero (.9 mg)	Overlooked decimal can lead to overdose	Always use zero before a decimal point (0.9 mg)
MS MSO_4 $MgSO_4$	Confused for one another Can be interpreted as morphine sulfate or magnesium sulfate	Write "morphine sulfate" or "magnesium sulfate"
H.S. (for half-strength or Latin abbreviation for bedtime)	Mistaken for either half-strength or hour of sleep (at bedtime) qH.S. mistaken for every hour All can result in a dosing error	Write "half-strength" or "at bedtime"

Data from The Institute for Safe Medication Practices. (n.d.). Retrieved from www.ismp.org; and The Joint Commission. *The official "Do Not Use" List.* (2005). Retrieved August 28, 2009 from www.jointcommission.org/PatientSafety/DoNotUseList.

Box 23-7 Safety Tips from Nurse Experts

The nurses at the Institute for Safe Medication Practices frequently learn about errors and potentially hazardous conditions via the USP-ISMP Medication Errors Reporting Program. They have translated these lessons into routine safeguards for clinical practice:

- **Enlist the patient's help to protect against errors.** Teach the patient about medications and the importance of proper identification before receiving medications or undergoing a procedure.
- **Make pharmacists part of the team.** Rely on them as ready sources of drug information, and send them important patient information so they can screen all medication orders for safety.
- **Take the medication administration record (MAR) to the bedside.** Prepare only one patient's medications at a time and leave drugs in their labeled packages. Compare each drug with the MAR one last time before you administer it, verify the patient's name and birth date on the MAR, and document drug administration at the bedside.
- **Keep calculations to a minimum.** If you are obliged to make calculations, however, have another nurse independently calculate the dose and the rate, and compare your answers. Even if you use a dosing table to determine infusion rate, have another nurse check your infusion pump settings.
- **Ask for an independent double-check of high-alert drugs before administration.** Double-checking all medications is impractical, but high-risk drugs and doses for high-risk patients warrant a second look by another nurse.
- **Do not sacrifice safety for timeliness.** Outside of emergencies, the need to quickly administer drugs does not outweigh the safety benefit of having a pharmacist review the order. Be realistic about pharmacy turnaround time for routine medications.
- **Always report errors.** Only through insightful information from people who have made errors will your facility be able to review system-based causes and devise remedies. Support colleagues who have made and reported errors.
- **Review the literature for error reports from other facilities.** Take error reports to staff meetings, discuss the likelihood of similar errors in your practice setting, identify possible system-based causes, and suggest ways to remedy them. To report an error, call the USP-ISMP Medication Errors Reporting Program at 1-800-23-ERROR.

From Institute for Safe Medication Practices. (2001). ISMP medication safety alert. *Nursing*, *31*(12), 43.

Box 23-8 Safety Tips for Medication Administration

- Follow the six rights of medication administration (see Box 23-5).
- Be sure to read labels at least three times (comparing medication administration record [MAR] with label): when removing drug from storage, before taking to patient's room, before giving drug (see Box 23-6).
- Use at least three patient identifiers (e.g., name band, patient pronouncing name, patient giving date of birth), whenever administering a medication.
- Do not allow any other activity to interrupt the administration of medication to a patient.
- Do not interpret illegible handwriting; clarify with prescriber.
- Question unusually large or small doses.
- Document all medications as soon as you give them.

Data from Elkin, M.K., et al. (2007). *Nursing interventions and clinical skills.* (4th ed.). St. Louis: Mosby.

Home Care Considerations

Drug Safety

Instruct the patient to do the following:

- Keep each drug in its original labeled container.
- Protect drugs from exposure to heat and light, as required.
- Check that labels are legible.
- Discard outdated medications.
- Always finish a prescribed drug unless otherwise instructed, and never save a drug for future illnesses.
- Dispose of drugs in a sink or toilet, and never place drugs in the trash within reach of children.
- Never give a family member or friend a drug prescribed for another person.
- Refrigerate drugs that require it.
- Read labels carefully, and follow all instructions.
- Notify physician or practitioner of any side effects.

are especially important in protecting the patient from harm (Clayton & Stock, 2008).

IMPORTANT CONSIDERATIONS OF MEDICATION ADMINISTRATION

While handling equipment during medication administration, always follow the principle of "sterile to sterile and clean to clean." It is essential to wash hands before and after caring for each patient. Keep work spaces and equipment clean and orderly, and work with your agency to establish practices that will keep staff members and patients safe. Do not take shortcuts, and never deviate from principles that are effective (or look on other staff members to do so). Apply the following rules:

1. If you did not pour it, do not give it.
2. If you gave it, chart it.
3. Do not chart for someone else or have someone else chart for you.
4. Do not transport or accept a container that is not labeled.
5. Do not put down an unlabeled syringe; keep it in your hand or label it before you put it down.
6. If given a verbal order, write it down or enter it into the computer, then repeat the order to the physician. The only time you are permitted to repeat a spoken order without first writing it is when reading it back is not feasible, such as during surgery or a code.
7. If you make an error, report it immediately to the charge nurse or supervisor, or if you are in charge, notify the physician. It is essential to analyze each error reported with an emphasis on how the system allowed the error to reach the patient, not on who made the error. Reporting errors helps identify and correct recurring problems.
8. Never leave a medication tray or cart unattended or unlocked.
9. Do not leave a medication with a patient or family member. Watch the patient take and swallow the medication.
10. Always return to assess the patient's response to the medication.
11. Chart as soon as possible after giving medication.
12. If a patient refuses medication, do not force it; chart "Refused medication because of [state reason patient refused medication]."
13. If you elect to omit a dose based on your nursing judgment, let another nurse help make the decision. If you do not give the medication, document "Dose omitted because [state reason dose omitted]." Be objective and exact in charting. Report your decision to the physician (see Home Care Considerations box).

ROUTES OF ADMINISTRATION

Drugs enter the body through three general routes—enteral, percutaneous, and parenteral. The drugs that enter the body by these routes come in various forms, or formulations.

ENTERAL ADMINISTRATION

Drugs that enter through the **enteral** (by the GI tract) routes are given in these forms:

1. **Powders.** Often mixed with a liquid (diluent) before administration
2. **Pills.** Round, solid drug form that has to break down into solution form (dissolution) in the stomach
3. **Tablets.** Round, spherical, or oddly shaped forms that dissolve in the stomach
   a. *Scored.* Indented to allow tablet to be broken in half
   b. **Enteric-coated.** Candylike coated shell encases tablet to keep tablet from being absorbed in

the stomach; absorption takes place in the intestine. **Enteric** pertains to the small intestine.

c. *Capsule.* Powders or pellets enclosed in a gelatin-like, elongated, spherical form; encapsulated because (1) substance is bad tasting or (2) substance is a spansule with time-release pellets to delay the action of the drug

d. *Lozenge* or *troche.* A sweet mucilage type of tablet that dissolves in the mouth to release medication

4. **Liquids and suspensions.** Solid particles and liquid are necessary to shake to disperse solid particles throughout the liquid portion before absorption by the body is possible
5. **Suppositories.** Drugs mixed with lubricated substance molded to insert into body cavities such as the rectum; have to melt at body temperature to be absorbed

These dosage forms are given by the enteral routes. The enteral routes are as follows:

- **po:** by mouth
- **Tubal:** by nasogastric, gastrostomy, or jejunostomy tube
- **Suppository:** by rectum or vagina
- **Enema:** by rectum

Preparation of Tablets, Pills, and Capsules

Medications in tablet, pill, and capsule form that enter the GI tract are absorbed more slowly into the bloodstream than those taken by any other route. The slow absorption rate makes the po (by mouth; oral) route relatively safe.

If an error is made, report it immediately to the RN. Make out an incident report to document the error. Do not hesitate to report an error, because prompt intervention will possibly prevent adverse effects to the patient.

Also be aware that some po medications are irritating to the patient's GI tract and that larger tablets will be difficult for some patients to swallow (Skill 23-1).

Preparation of Liquid Medications

Liquid medication is often the chosen formulation for children; for patients who are not able to swallow tablets, pills, or capsules; and for older adult patients. It is possible to give liquids po or via a nasogastric, gastrostomy, or jejunostomy tube.

Never give liquids to unconscious patients because of the possibility of their aspirating (inhaling) the medication into the respiratory tract.

Be aware that some liquid medications are not to be followed with water and that some medications, such

Skill 23-1 Administering Tablets, Pills, and Capsules

Nursing Action *(Rationale)*

1. Follow the six rights (see Box 23-5). *(Prevents medication errors.)*
2. Perform the three label checks (see Box 23-6). *(Prevents medication errors.)*
3. Follow standard precautions (see Chapter 12, Box 12-5). *(Prevents spread of microorganisms.)*
4. Perform hand hygiene. *(Prevents spread of microorganisms.)*
5. If using unit-dose package (see illustration), place unopened package in medicine cup. *(Prevents medication errors.)*

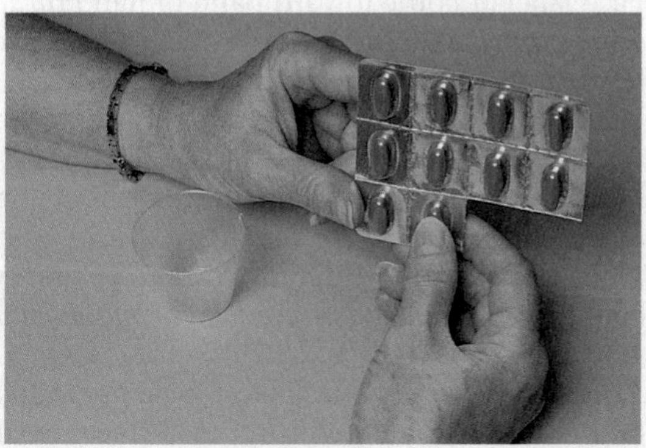

Step 5

6. If using a multidose bottle, pour tablet, without touching it, into cap of bottle. *(Prevents contamination.)*
7. Pour tablet from cap into medicine cup.
8. If using medicine tray (for several patients), set it up from left to right, front to back, with labels with patient's name and room number. *(Prevents errors.)*
9. If pouring from multidose bottle and patient is to receive several tablets, use separate cup for medications such as digitalis. If the patient's pulse is less than 60 bpm, withhold the medication and report this to the RN; the physician will then be notified. *(By placing digitalis in a separate cup marked with a red heart, it will be identified easily.)*
10. If a tablet has to be broken in half to administer half the dose, use a gloved hand or a cutting device. Score the tablet along the manufactured line in the center of the tablet. Destroy the remainder of the tablet, or save it in its original container, depending on your agency's protocol (Elkin et al., 2007).
11. To crush oral tablets if a patient has swallowing problems, use a mortar and pestle or pill-crushing device (Elkin et al., 2007). It is important not to crush drugs that are capsules, enteric-coated, long-acting, or slow-release. These drugs are

Continued

Skill 23-1 Administering Tablets, Pills, and Capsules—cont'd

made to prevent stomach irritation or destruction by gastric acids as well as control the rate of release of the drug. Do not crush medications if there is a notation on them such as "extended release," "sustained release," or "XL," "SR," or "CD" (Miller, 2000).

12. If you drop any pills, tablets, or capsules on the floor (happens more commonly with medications that come from multidose bottles), discard them. *(Prevents contaminated medications being administered to patient.)*
13. Take medication to the room.
14. Identify patient by checking identification bracelet and asking patient's name and birth date. Compare with MAR. *(Prevents medication errors.)*
15. Explain procedure to patient.
16. Document administration of medication on Medex or computer with time, date, and name.
17. Return to assess patient's response to medication. *(Enables you to determine effectiveness of medication and any occurrence of adverse reactions.)*
18. Document assessment in nursing notes.

as iron, will sometimes stain the teeth. Look for and follow any instructions on the label (Skill 23-2).

Tubal Medications

Nasogastric (NG) tubes are used to administer liquid medications to unconscious patients, dysphagic patients (patients who have difficulty swallowing), and those who are too ill to eat. It is also possible to use a gastrostomy tube (placed through the abdominal wall and into the stomach) or jejunostomy tube (placed through the abdominal wall and into the jejunum) in the same manner as the NG tube.

Many medicines come in liquid form. If they do not, you will sometimes **pulverize** (crush to a powder) solid tablets, using a mortar and pestle. Mix the crushed tablet with 30 mL of water, and give the mixture through the tube. It is also possible to open capsules, mix the contents with 30 mL of water, and administer this mixture (Skill 23-3). Not all tablets are safe to be crushed, and not all capsules are safe to be opened (e.g., medications that are time released). Doing so creates the risk of toxic effects (see Skill 23-1, Step 11). Check the correct clinical pharmacology reference or the *PDR* to verify safety of pulverizing tablets or opening capsules.

Suppositories

A suppository is a cone-, egg-, or spindle-shaped medication made for insertion into the rectum or the vagina. Suppositories dissolve at body temperature and are absorbed directly into the bloodstream. Suppositories are useful for babies, patients who cannot take oral preparations, and patients with nausea and vomiting (Skill 23-4).

Store suppositories in a cool place so that they do not melt. It is acceptable to place them in the refrigerator.

Skill 23-2 Administering Liquid Medications

Nursing Action *(Rationale)*

1. Follow the six rights (see Box 23-5). *(Prevents medication errors.)*
2. Perform the three label checks (see Box 23-6). *(Prevents medication errors.)*
3. Follow standard precautions (see Chapter 12, Box 12-5). *(Prevents spread of microorganisms.)*
4. Perform hand hygiene. *(Prevents spread of microorganisms.)*
5. Remove liquid preparation from patient's drug box or bin (or from medication cabinet).
6. Check dose/mL and total volume of medication in container.
7. Calculate dosage; if the dose ordered is different from the dose/mL stated on the label, calculate correct dose; if ordered medication is labeled according to a different measurement system, convert by using appropriate equivalent. Work problem on paper.
8. Check calculations with another nurse. *(Helps prevent errors.)*
9. Obtain **graduated** (has markings indicating marked amount) medicine cup (total volume of cup is 30 mL or 1 oz) or appropriate syringe. *(For accuracy.)*
10. Face label of bottle toward palm of hand *(to avoid soiling label)*; if label becomes soiled, return the bottle to the pharmacy. Do not give medication if label is unreadable. *(Maintains accuracy and prevents errors.)*
11. Place medicine cup on flat surface or hold at eye level while pouring. *(Maintains accuracy.)*
12. Place cap of bottle with inner rim up to prevent contaminating inside of cap *(and thus contaminate remaining contents of bottle).*
13. Read dosage amount at lowest level of **meniscus** (curve formed by liquid's upper surface; see illustration) (for accuracy).

14. Transport medication to patient's room.
15. Identify patient by checking identification bracelet and asking patient's name and birth date. Compare with MAR. *(Prevents medication errors.)*
16. Explain procedure to patient.
17. Document administration on Medex or computer with time, date, and name.
18. Return to assess patient's response to medication. *(Enables you to determine effectiveness of medication and any occurrence of adverse reactions.)*
19. Document assessment in nursing notes.

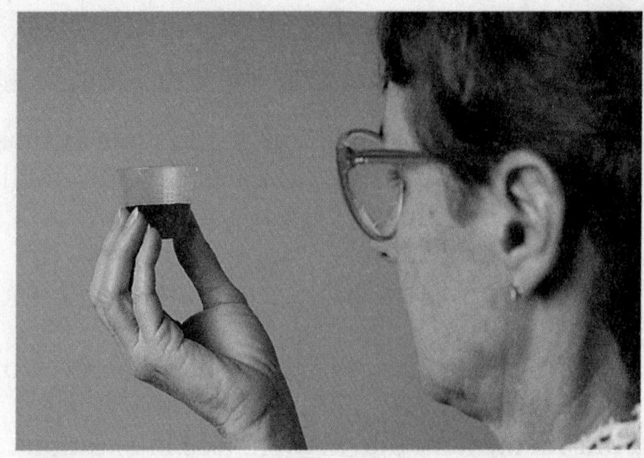
Step **13**

Skill 23-3 Administering Tubal Medications

Nursing Action *(Rationale)*

1. Follow the six rights (see Box 23-5). *(Prevents medication errors.)*
2. Perform the three label checks (see Box 23-6). *(Prevents medication errors.)*
3. Follow standard precautions (see Chapter 12, Box 12-5). *(Prevents spread of microorganisms.)*
4. Perform hand hygiene. *(Prevents spread of microorganisms.)*
5. Prepare medication using the same procedure as for liquid medications.
6. Gather equipment. *(Organizes procedure.)*
   - Disposable gloves
   - 10-mL syringe
   - Towel
   - Stethoscope
   - Bulb or Asepto syringe
   - Tap water
7. Take equipment and medication to patient's room.
8. Identify patient by checking identification bracelet and asking patient's name and birth date. *(Prevents medication errors.)*
9. Explain procedure; answer questions patient may have about the procedure. *(Establishes trust.)*
10. Place patient in high Fowler's position.
11. Put towel over patient's chest. *(Protects clothing and bed linens.)*
12. Don disposable, unsterile gloves. *(Reduces spread of microorganisms.)*
13. Check and recheck placement and patency of tube using at least two methods (see also Chapter 21, Skill 21-1, step 10). *(Ensures that tube is in the stomach and not in the respiratory tract.)*
    a. **Method A:** Attach piston or Asepto syringe to end of nasogastric (NG) tube (see illustration). Pull plunger back or release suction of bulb syringe to aspirate stomach contents. If stomach contents are seen, instill 10 to 20 mL of water before medication administration to clear tube; proceed with medication. Because of the difficulty in withdrawing fluid from small-bore feeding tubes, nurses often rely incorrectly on the auscultatory method to confirm NG feeding tube placement. In the meantime, keep a high index of suspicion for tube displacement in patients at risk and use meticulous assessment skills.

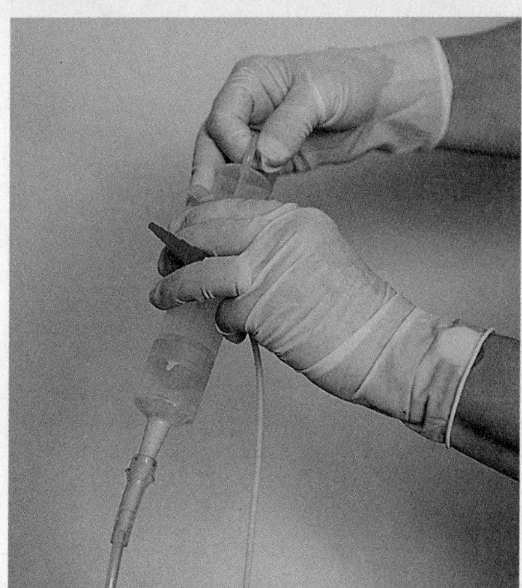
Step **13a**

    b. **Method B:** Place stethoscope over stomach. Push 10 mL of air through NG tube with syringe. *(The rush of air is heard in stomach with stethoscope if tube is in stomach. Proceed with medication.)*
    c. **Method C:** Many authorities now recommend the litmus test instead of the auscultatory (air-instillation) method. *(Sounds created by instillation of air may be transmitted from the pleural space to the upper abdomen, giving false impression of placement. Know agency policy for preferred method.)* Measure pH of aspirate with color-

Continued

Skill 23-3 Administering Tubal Medications—cont'd

coded pH paper with range of whole numbers from 1 to 11. Gastric aspirates have decidedly acidic pH values, preferably 4 or less.

14. Clamp tube with rubber-tipped hemostats or other clamping device. *(Prevents leakage of fluid from tube.)*
15. Attach syringe to end of tube (with plunger out of syringe).
16. Pour medication into syringe (see illustration).

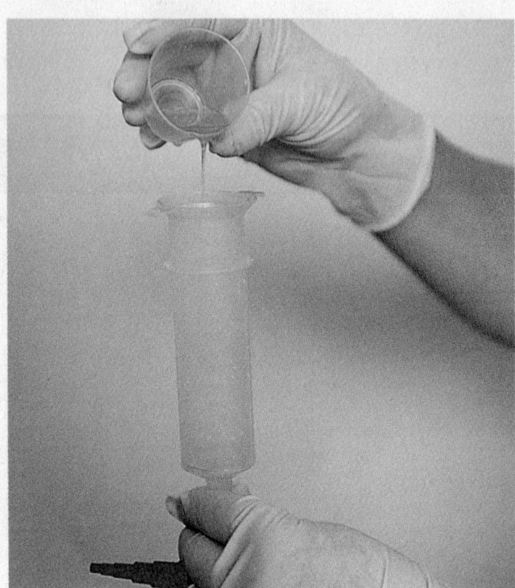

Step **16**

17. Unclamp tubing to allow medication to slowly flow by gravity.
18. Follow medication with 30 to 50 mL of water. *(Flushes the medication into stomach. Water is essential to enhance absorption of medication and is used to clean and maintain patency of NG tube.)*
19. Clamp tubing: secure tube after medication is given.
20. If NG tube is attached to suction, do not reconnect suction for 30 minutes. *(The medication will then have time to absorb because medication will not be aspirated through tube.)*
21. Remove towel from patient.
22. Remove gloves.
23. Leave patient in comfortable position.
24. Gather equipment; clean up patient and area.
25. Perform hand hygiene. *(Prevents spread of microorganisms.)*
26. Document administration of NG medication in Medex or computer with time, date, and name. Remember to document the amount of fluid used for medication administration as intake on intake and output (I&O) sheet. *(Ensures accurate I&O.)*
27. Return to assess patient's response to medication. *(Enables you to determine effectiveness of medication and any occurrence of adverse reactions.)*
28. Document assessment in nursing notes.

Skill 23-4 Administering Rectal Suppositories

Nursing Action *(Rationale)*

1. Follow the six rights (see Box 23-5). *(Prevents medication errors.)*
2. Perform the three label checks (see Box 23-6). *(Prevents medication errors.)*
3. Follow standard precautions (see Chapter 12, Box 12-5). *(Prevents spread of microorganisms.)*
4. Gather equipment. *(Organizes procedure.)*
   - Gloves or finger cot
   - Lubricant
   - Suppository
   - Souffle cup
5. Perform hand hygiene. *(Prevents spread of microorganisms.)*
6. Obtain suppository from refrigerator or from patient's medication bin.
7. Place unopened suppository into medicine cup or **souffle cup** (ungraduated disposable paper cup).
8. Take disposable, unsterile gloves or finger cot (single-digit plastic finger cover) to room.
9. Introduce yourself; explain procedure to patient. *(Enlists patient's cooperation and establishes trust.)*
10. Identify patient by checking identification bracelet and asking patient's name and birth date. *(Prevents medication errors.)*
11. Provide privacy.
12. Position patient in Sims' position (on left side with upper leg flexed at knee). *(Position exposes anus and helps patient to relax external anal sphincter. Left-side positioning lessens the likelihood of the suppository or feces being expelled.)*
13. Unwrap suppository.
14. Maintain privacy; expose buttocks.
15. Don gloves. *(Protects you from fecal material and reduces the spread of microorganisms.)*
16. Assess anus externally and gently palpate rectal vault as needed. *(Enables you to determine presence of active rectal bleeding as well as note whether rectum contains feces, which potentially cause problems with suppository placement.)* Do not palpate a patient's rectum following rectal surgery. If a patient has hemorrhoids, always use a generous amount of a lubricating gel and gently manipulate the tissues to visualize the anus for insertion

of the suppository. If a patient has active rectal bleeding or diarrhea, insertion of a rectal suppository is usually contraindicated (McKenry & McKenry, 2008).

17. Apply lubricant, such as KY jelly, to tapered end of suppository. *(Lubrication reduces friction as suppository enters rectal area.)*
18. Ask patient to take deep breath; insert beyond internal anal sphincter. Insert suppository as patient exhales to relax anal sphincter. *(Forcing suppository through constricted sphincter causes discomfort.)*
19. Ask patient to retain suppository as long as possible. *(This allows the medication to completely dissolve and absorb through mucous membranes of rectum into capillaries of systemic circulatory system.)* Hold the buttocks together to help patient retain suppository. *(Provides sufficient time for the effects of the suppository to reach the maximum effectiveness.)*
20. Discard gloves.
21. Help patient assume comfortable position.
22. Perform hand hygiene. *(Reduces spread of microorganisms.)*
23. Document administration of suppository in Medex or computer with time, date, and name.
24. Return to assess patient's response to medication. *(Enables you to determine effectiveness of medication and any occurrence of adverse reactions.)*
25. Document assessment in nursing notes.

PERCUTANEOUS ADMINISTRATION

Dosage forms used with the **percutaneous** route (through the skin or mucous membranes) include lotions, ointments, creams, and powders.

The percutaneous routes are as follows:

1. **Topical.** Applied to the skin
2. **Instillation.**
   a. Applied to the mucous membranes of the mouth
      (1) *Sublingual* (under the tongue)
      (2) *Buccal* (in the cheek)
   b. Applied to the mucous membranes of eye, ear, nose, and vagina
3. **Inhalation.** Aerosolized liquids, gases

The percutaneous routes are those routes by which medications are absorbed through the skin or the mucous membranes. Most percutaneous medications produce a local action, but some produce a systemic action.

The percutaneous routes include **topical applications** (applied to the skin), instillations, and inhalations. Absorption is rapid but of short duration.

Topical medications include ointments, creams, powders, lotions, and transdermal patches.

Ointments

An ointment is an oil-based semisolid medication; you will apply it to the skin or a mucous membrane. Nitroglycerin (NTG) is a commonly used ointment that produces an effect of longer duration than the sublingual form. Apply NTG ointment topically by using applicator paper; place the paper on the skin with the ointment side on the skin. Hold the applicator paper in place with paper tape. Do not touch the NTG side of the applicator paper or the NTG side of the disk.

Sites you will commonly use for NTG applications are chest, flank, and upper arm. Remove ointments with cottonseed oil and gauze.

Creams

Creams are semisolid, nongreasy emulsions that contain medication for external application. Gently rub creams into the area; they are easy to remove with water and gauze. Certain creams are prescription medications, and it is necessary to follow directions for application carefully to prevent overdosage.

Lotions

Lotions are generally aqueous preparations that are used as soothing agents to relieve pruritus or that protect the skin, cleanse the skin, or act as astringents. Lotions contain suspended particles that are necessary to bring into solution by shaking before application. Gently pat (do not rub) lotions onto the skin; remove them with soap and water (Skill 23-5).

Transdermal Patches (Topical Disk)

Adhesive-backed medicated patches applied to the skin provide sustained, continuous release of medication over several hours or days. Examples of transdermal patches are analgesic, NTG, nicotine, and estrogen. Choose a clear, dry area of the body that is free of hair. Do not attempt to apply the patch on skin that is oily, burned, or excoriated or has any impairment of skin integrity (Figure 23-4).

Eyedrops and Eye Ointments

Eyedrops and ointments are sterile. Take care to keep all ophthalmic (eye) preparations sterile by not touching the dropper or the tube of ointment to the eye. Check the container to ensure that the medication is

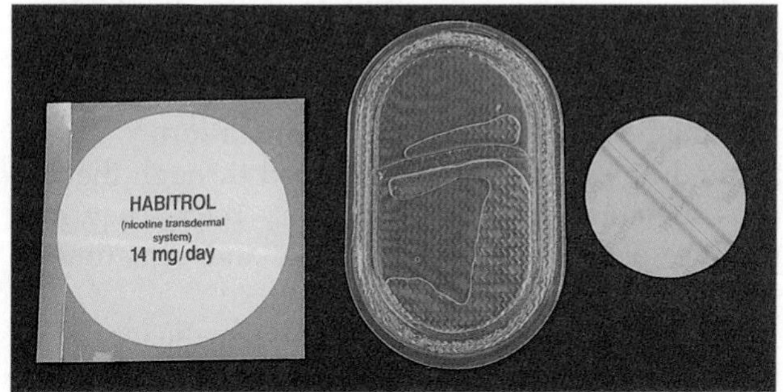

FIGURE 23-4 A variety of medications are available as transdermal patches.

Skill 23-5 Applying Topical Agents

Nursing Action *(Rationale)*

1. Follow the six rights (see Box 23-5). *(Prevents medication errors.)*
2. Perform the three label checks (see Box 23-6). *(Prevents medication errors.)*
3. Follow standard precautions (see Chapter 12, Box 12-5). *(Reduces spread of microorganisms.)*
4. Gather equipment. *(Organizes procedure.)*
   - Gloves
   - Medication
   - Washing materials
5. Perform hand hygiene. *(Reduces spread of microorganisms.)*
6. Transport medication to room.
7. Identify patient by checking identification bracelet and asking patient's name and birth date. *(Prevents medication errors.)*
8. Introduce yourself; explain procedure to patient. *(Establishes trust.)*
9. Provide privacy; place patient in comfortable position that allows exposure of selected site.
10. Don gloves. *(Reduces spread of microorganisms and prevents absorption of topical agent into your skin.)*
11. Read prescription instructions carefully. *(For accuracy.)*
12. Prepare medicinal agent (ointments, creams, and lotions sometimes have to be squeezed or removed with a tongue blade, depending on preparation used).
13. Wash affected area, removing debris, encrustations, and previous medications. *(Removal of debris enhances penetration of topical drug through skin. Cleansing removes microorganisms resident in remaining debris.)*
14. Apply paper applicator, disk (see Figure 23-4), lotion, ointment, or cream. Be certain to remove plastic from disk before applying to skin. *(Essential for absorption of medication.)*
15. Remove gloves.
16. Leave patient properly draped or clothed in comfortable position.
17. Answer patient's questions, and teach patient to perform self-applications if appropriate.
18. Clean work area.
19. Wash hands. *(Reduces spread of microorganisms.)*
20. Record administration in Medex or computer with time, date, and name.
21. Return to assess patient's response to medication. *(Enables you to determine effectiveness of medication and any occurrence of adverse reactions.)*
22. Document assessment in nursing notes.

marked "for ophthalmic use." Only use ophthalmic medications for one patient, and do not share them (Skill 23-6).

Eardrops

Containers of solutions to be used as eardrops will be labeled "otic." It is necessary to have them at room temperature when applying. Use an individual bottle for each patient (Skill 23-7).

Nose Drops

Nose drops are for individual use only (Skill 23-8).

Nasal Sprays

Because nasal sprays are absorbed quickly, less medication is used and wasted when you administer them in this manner. Nasal sprays are for individual use only (Skill 23-9).

Administering Medications by Inhalation

Some drugs are able to be absorbed through the mucous membranes of the respiratory tract. They may produce a relatively limited effect and sometimes a systemic effect.

Respiratory therapy departments use the inhalation route routinely, as do anesthesiologists and nurse anesthetists.

Your participation in inhalation therapy will in all likelihood be limited to helping patients use metered-dose inhalers (MDIs) that contain bronchodilators or corticosteroids. Read and follow directions for use of these inhalers, because methods of use may vary among manufacturers.

Drugs administered with handheld inhalers are dispersed through an aerosol spray, mist, or powder that penetrates lung airways. The alveolar-capillary network absorbs medications rapidly. The purpose of most MDIs is to produce local effects such as bronchodilation. However, some medications have the capacity to create systemic side effects.

Patients who receive drugs by inhalation frequently suffer from chronic respiratory disease such as chronic asthma, emphysema, or bronchitis. Drugs given by inhalation provide these patients with control of airway obstruction, and because these patients depend on medications for disease control, they need to learn about them and the ways to administer them safely.

An MDI delivers a measured dose of drug with each push of a canister. Approximately 5 to 10 pounds of pressure are necessary to activate the aerosol. However, hand strength diminishes with age and from chronic respiratory disease. A three-point or lateral hand position is effective in activating a canister. Some

Text continued on p. 712

Skill 23-6 Administering Eyedrops and Eye Ointments

Nursing Action *(Rationale)*

1. Follow the six rights (see Box 23-5). *(Prevents medication errors.)*
2. Perform the three label checks (see Box 23-6). *(Prevents medication errors.)*
3. Follow standard precautions (see Chapter 12, Box 12-5). *(Prevents spread of microorganisms.)*
4. Gather equipment. *(Organizes procedure.)*
   - Eyedrops
   - Gloves
   - Cotton ball or tissue
   - Sterile saline
5. Perform hand hygiene. *(Prevents spread of microorganisms.)*
6. Transport medication to room. Confirm medication is ophthalmic preparation.
7. Identify patient by checking identification bracelet and asking patient's name and birth date. *(Prevents medication errors.)*
8. Introduce yourself; explain procedure. *(Establishes trust.)*
9. Provide privacy; position back of patient's head on pillow; direct patient's face upward toward ceiling.
10. Determine which eye (or both) is to receive the medication.
11. Don gloves. *(Reduces spread of microorganisms.)*
12. Remove exudate; clean eye as needed using sterile solution of saline; use cotton balls to wipe away exudate; use one cotton ball per stroke, wiping from inner canthus outward. *(Cleansing eye from inner to outer canthus avoids introducing microorganisms into lacrimal ducts. Soaking allows easy removal of dried exudate that harbor microorganisms.)*
13. To apply drops, expose lower conjunctival sac by having patient look upward while gentle traction is applied to lower eyelid (see illustration).
14. Put prescribed number of drops into conjunctival sac, not onto eyeball. *(Therapeutic effect of drug is obtained only when drops enter sac.)*
15. Conjunctival sac normally holds one or two drops. *(Applying drops to conjuctival sac provides even distribution of medicine across eye.)*

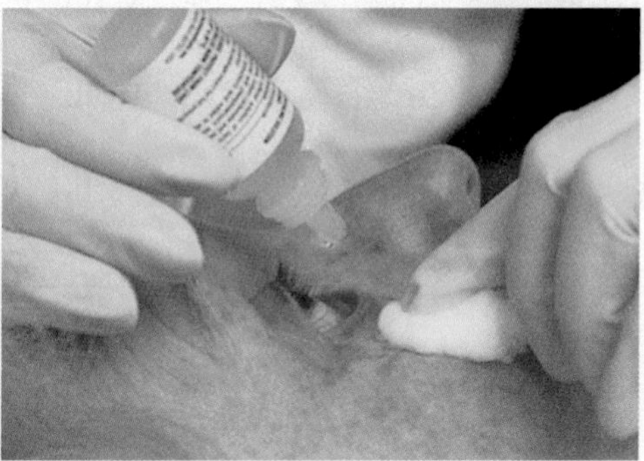

Step **13**

16. Using a cotton ball or tissue, apply gentle pressure above bone at inner corner of eyelid for 1 to 2 minutes (see illustration). *(Minimizes absorption into circulatory system.)*
17. Apply sterile dressing, if ordered.
18. To apply ointment, expose lower conjunctival sac by having patient look upward while gentle traction is applied to lower eyelid (see illustration).
19. Squeeze ointment into lower conjunctival sac.
20. Ask patient to close eye and move it around in circular motion. *(Spreads medication evenly.)*
21. Apply sterile dressing, if ordered.
22. After applying drops or ointment to an eye, leave patient in comfortable position; clean up the work area.
23. Remove gloves and wash hands. *(Reduces spread of microorganisms.)*
24. Answer patient's questions and, if appropriate, teach patient to perform self-care.
25. Record administration of medications in the Medex or computer with time, date, and name.
26. Return to assess patient's response to medication. *(Enables you to determine effectiveness of medication and any occurrence of adverse reactions.)*
27. Document assessment in nursing notes.

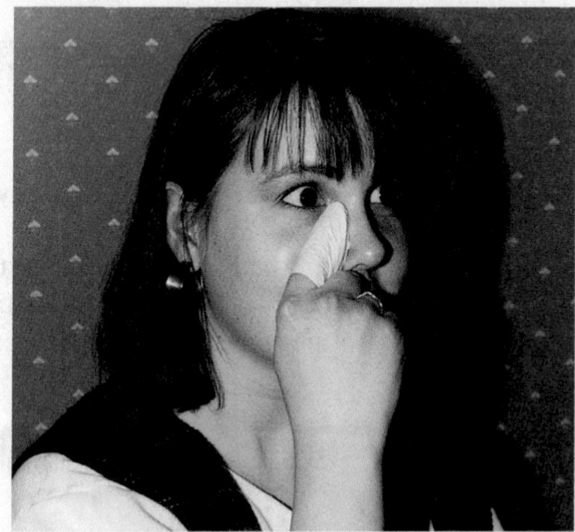

Step **16**

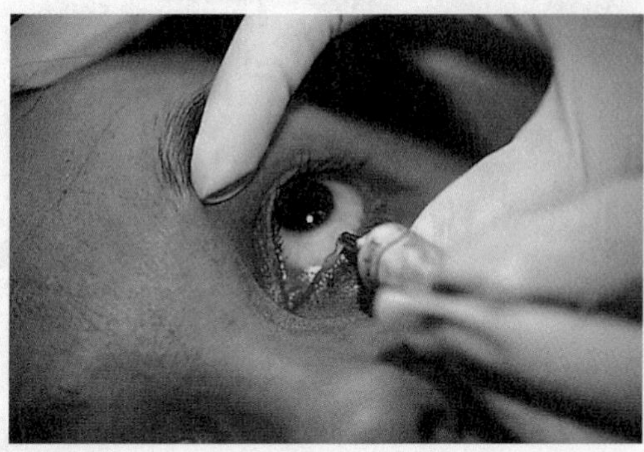

Step **18**

Skill 23-7 Administering Eardrops

Nursing Action *(Rationale)*

1. Follow the six rights (see Box 23-5). *(Prevents medication errors.)*
2. Perform the three label checks (see Box 23-6). *(Prevents medication errors.)*
3. Follow standard precautions (see Chapter 12, Box 12-5). *(Prevents spread of microorganisms.)*
4. Gather equipment. *(Organizes procedure.)*
   - Eardrops
   - Gloves
   - Cotton ball
5. Perform hand hygiene. *(Prevents spread of microorganisms.)*
6. Transport medication to room. Confirm medication is otic preparation.
7. Identify patient by checking identification bracelet and asking patient's name and birth date. *(Prevents medication errors.)*
8. Introduce yourself; explain procedure. *(Establishes trust.)*
9. Provide privacy; position patient with affected ear upward.
10. Determine which ear (or both) is to receive the medication.
11. Don gloves. *(Reduces spread of microorganisms.)*
12. Remove external exudate from ear; it is necessary to obtain an order before irrigating the ear. *(Drainage harbors microorganisms and sometimes impedes distribution of medication into the canal.)*
13. Draw medication into dropper.
14. Instill drops:
    a. **For adults and for children older than 3 years old:** Turn head and affected side up; pull earlobe upward and back to straighten external auditory canal; give drops without touching ear with dropper (see illustration). *(Straightening of ear canal provides direct access to deeper external structures.)*
    b. **For children younger than 3 years old:** Turn head with affected side up; pull earlobe downward and back; instill drops without touching ear with dropper (see illustration). *(Straightening of ear canal provides direct access to deeper external structures.)*
15. Tell patient to remain in same position for 5 to 10 minutes to allow medication to drain into ear by gravity. *(To promote distribution of drops in ear canal.)*
16. Place a cotton ball loosely into ear as needed. *(Prevents escape of medication when patient sits or stands.)*
17. Remove gloves.
18. Leave patient in comfortable position; clean work area.
19. Answer patient's questions and, if appropriate, teach patient self-care.
20. Perform hand hygiene. *(Reduces spread of microorganisms.)*
21. Record administration in Medex or computer with time, date, and name.
22. Return to assess patient's response to medication. *(Enables you to determine effectiveness of medication and any occurrence of adverse reactions.)*
22. Document assessment in nursing notes.

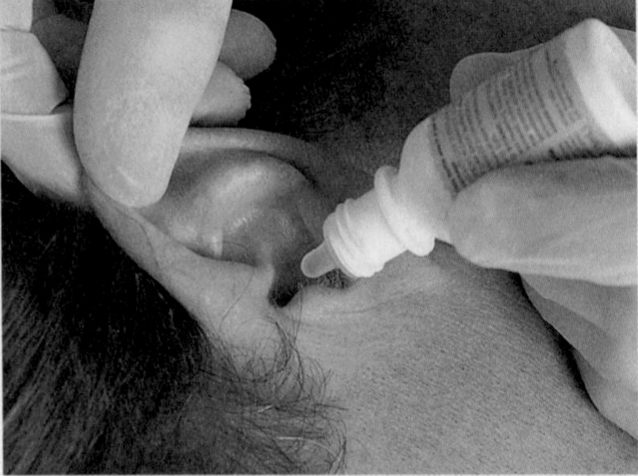

Step **14a**

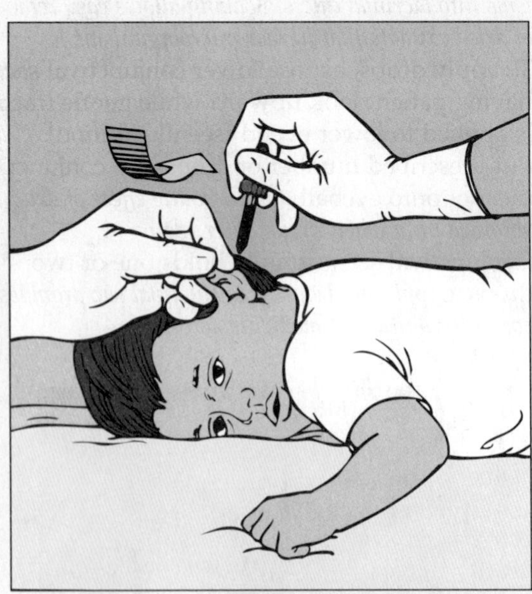

Step **14b**

Skill 23-8 Administering Nose Drops

Nursing Action *(Rationale)*

1. Follow the six rights (see Box 23-5). *(Prevents medication errors.)*
2. Perform the three label checks (see Box 23-6). *(Prevents medication errors.)*
3. Follow standard precautions (see Chapter 12, Box 12-5). *(Prevents spread of microorganisms.)*
4. Gather equipment. *(Organizes procedure.)*
   - Nose drops
   - Gloves
   - Tissues
5. Perform hand hygiene. *(Prevents spread of microorganisms.)*
6. Transport medication to room.
7. Identify patient by checking identification bracelet and asking patient's name and birth date. *(Prevents medication errors.)*
8. Introduce yourself; explain procedure. *(Establishes trust.)*
9. Provide privacy.
10. Don gloves. *(Reduces spread of microorganisms.)*
11. Ask adult or older child to clear nose of accumulations by blowing gently into tissue. *(Allows absorption of medication.)*
12. Determine which nostril (or both) is to receive the medication.
13. Position patient:
    a. **Adult:** Have patient lie down, hanging head backward over edge of bed (if condition permits) or with pillow under shoulders to hyperextend the neck if patient can tolerate it. *(Promotes absorption of medication.)*
    b. **Younger child:** Position child on bed with head backward and downward. *(Promotes absorption of medication.)*
    c. **Infant:** Hold infant with head backward and downward. *(Promotes absorption of medication.)*

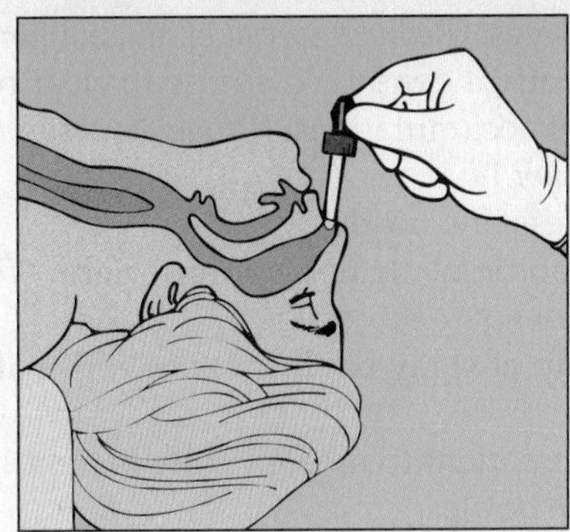

Step 14

14. After drawing medication into dropper, instill medication while holding dropper above nostril being treated (see illustration).
15. If ordered, repeat procedure to instill drops in other nostril.
16. Tell patient to hold position for a few minutes. *(Allows medication to remain in place.)*
17. Remove gloves.
18. Tell patient to refrain from blowing nose immediately after instillation. *(Prevents removal of medication.)*
19. Offer tissues for later use.
20. Leave patient in comfortable position; clean work area.
21. Answer patient's questions and, if appropriate, teach patient self-care.
22. Perform hand hygiene. *(Reduces spread of microorganisms.)*
23. Record administration in Medex or computer with time, date, and name.
24. Return to assess patient's response to medication. *(Enables you to determine effectiveness of medication and any occurrence of adverse reactions.)*
25. Document assessment in nursing notes.

Skill 23-9 Administering Nasal Sprays

Nursing Action *(Rationale)*

1. Follow the six rights (see Box 23-5). *(Prevents medication errors.)*
2. Perform the three label checks (see Box 23-6). *(Prevents medication errors.)*
3. Follow standard precautions (see Chapter 12, Box 12-5). *(Prevents spread of microorganisms.)*
4. Gather equipment. *(Organizes procedure.)*
   - Nasal spray
   - Gloves
   - Tissues
5. Perform hand hygiene. *(Prevents spread of microorganisms.)*
6. Transport medication to patient.
7. Determine which nostril (or both) is to receive the medication.
8. Identify patient by checking identification bracelet and asking patient's name and birth date. *(Prevents medication errors.)*
9. Introduce yourself; explain procedure. *(Establishes trust.)*
10. Provide privacy; position patient upright.

Continued

Skill 23-9 Administering Nasal Sprays—cont'd

11. Don gloves. *(Reduces spread of microorganisms.)*
12. Have patient gently blow nose to clear nasal passages of accumulations. *(Promotes absorption of medication.)*
13. Compress one nostril.
14. Shake bottle while holding it upright. *(To mix solution.)*
15. Insert tip of spray bottle into patient's patent nostril.
16. Instruct patient to inhale; while patient inhales, squeeze bottle.
17. If ordered, repeat procedure for other nostril.
18. Tell patient to refrain from blowing nose for a few minutes; offer tissues for later use. *(Promotes absorption of medication.)*
19. Answer patient's questions and, if appropriate, teach self-administration.
20. Remove gloves and wash hands. *(Reduces spread of microorganisms.)*
21. Record administration in Medex or computer with time, date, and name.
22. Return to assess patient's response to medication. *(Enables you to determine effectiveness of medication and any occurrence of adverse reactions.)*
23. Document assessment in nursing notes.

patients will require two hands or an adapted inhaler device.

Proper administration of an MDI calls for coordination during the breathing cycle. Some patients who have difficulty with this coordination will spray only the back of the throat and not receive a full dose. A device called a spacer **(AeroChamber)** fits onto the MDI and improves a patient's ability to deliver a proper dose of medication. Do not let patients inhale too quickly; do not let them hold the inhaler upside down or sideways; do not have them deliver more than one puff with each inspiration. Do have patients sit up straight, and do assess their ability to hold and manipulate the inhaler and depress the canister (Skill 23-10).

Sublingual Administration

Sublingual (the area beneath the tongue) administration of a drug (usually in tablet form) is achieved by placing the tablet beneath the tongue until the tablet dissolves. It is also acceptable to squeeze liquid out of a capsule if it is ordered by sublingual route. Tell the patient not to eat, drink, or smoke while the tablet is dissolving in the mouth. After dissolution, the active ingredient, such as NTG, is rapidly absorbed into the bloodstream. Drugs given by the sublingual route bypass the liver, which reduces the time it takes for the drug to produce its desired action. If NTG is self-administered by the patient sublingually, stress to the patient the importance of notifying personnel for documentation of time administered and effect of the drug.

Nitroglycerin is a common sublingual medication. It is usually ordered to be left at the bedside so the patient is able to take it ad lib (as desired). The patient is allowed to take the NTG tablets to the diagnostic imaging department or to any other diagnostic testing area in case a tablet is needed for anginal pain. Instruct the patient to notify the nurse of any usage of NTG and its effect. Teach the patient to wet the tablet with saliva before putting it under the tongue to speed absorption (*Ins and outs of giving drugs transmucosally*, 2003).

Follow the same procedure to prepare the administration of sublingual tablets as for solid oral medication, with the exceptions noted in Skill 23-11.

Buccal Administration

Buccal administration is achieved by placing a tablet between the cheek and the teeth, or between the cheek and the gums. It is left there until it dissolves. Absorption into the capillaries of the mucous membranes of the cheek gives rapid onset of the drug's active ingredient because of its direct entry into the systemic circulation.

Use the same procedure for buccal administration as for solid tablet administration or sublingual administration (Skill 23-12).

PARENTERAL ADMINISTRATION

The parenteral routes are those other than the digestive system route. They are usually thought of as the needle route. Dosage forms are liquids that are contained in the following:

- **Ampules.** Ampules are glass containers that are opened by snapping off the top part of the ampule. They are intended for unit-dose use.
- **Vials.** Vials are glass containers sealed with a metal cap with a rubber diaphragm in the middle of the cap. The rubber diaphragm permits a needle to enter the vial for either unit-dose or multidose use (depending on the contents of the vial).

Large volumes of fluids are contained in plastic or glass containers, such as intravenous (IV) fluid bags. IV fluid bags or bottles range in capacity from 50 to 1000 mL.

The parenteral routes are as follows:

- **IM:** intramuscular (within the muscle)
- **Sub-Q or subQ:** subcutaneous (under the dermis; fatty tissue)
- **ID:** intradermal (within the dermis)
- **IV:** intravenous (within the vein)

Skill 23-10 Administering Inhalants

Nursing Action *(Rationale)*

1. Follow the six rights (see Box 23-5). *(Prevents medication errors.)*
2. Perform the three label checks (see Box 23-6). *(Prevents medication errors.)*
3. Follow standard procedures (see Chapter 12, Box 12-5). *(Prevents spread of microorganisms.)*
4. Gather equipment. *(Organizes procedure.)*
   - Gloves
   - Inhaler
   - Canister
   - Spacer device
5. Perform hand hygiene. *(Prevents spread of microorganisms.)*
6. Transport medications to room.
7. Identify patient by checking identification bracelet and asking patient's name and birth date. *(Prevents medication errors.)*
8. Introduce yourself; explain procedure. *(Establishes trust.)*
9. Provide privacy.
10. Don gloves. *(Reduces spread of microorganisms.)*
11. Allow patient opportunity to manipulate inhaler, canister, and spacer device (e.g., AeroChamber). Explain and demonstrate how canister fits into inhaler. *(Patient needs to be familiar with how to assemble and use equipment.)*
12. Explain what metered dose is and warn patient about overuse of inhaler, including drug side effects. *(Patient needs to know the dangers of excessive inhalations because of risk of serious side effects. If drug is given in recommended doses, side effects are minimal.)*
13. Remove mouthpiece cover from inhaler. Shake inhaler well. *(Ensures mixing of medication in canister.)*
14. Position inhaler:
    a. **Without AeroChamber (spacer):** Have patient open lips and place inhaler ½ to 1 inch (1 to 2 cm) from mouth with opening toward back of pharynx. Lips will not touch inhaler (see illustration). *(Prevents rapid influx of inhaled medication and subsequent airway irritation. Positioning the mouthpiece 1 to 2 cm from the mouth is considered the best way to deliver the medication without a spacer.)*
    b. **With AeroChamber (spacer):** Have patient exhale fully, then grasp mouthpiece with teeth and lips while holding inhaler with thumb at the mouthpiece and fingers at the top (see illustration). *(Spacers are recommended because the device allows particles of the medication to "ride" the breath into the airways rather than hit the back of the pharynx.)*

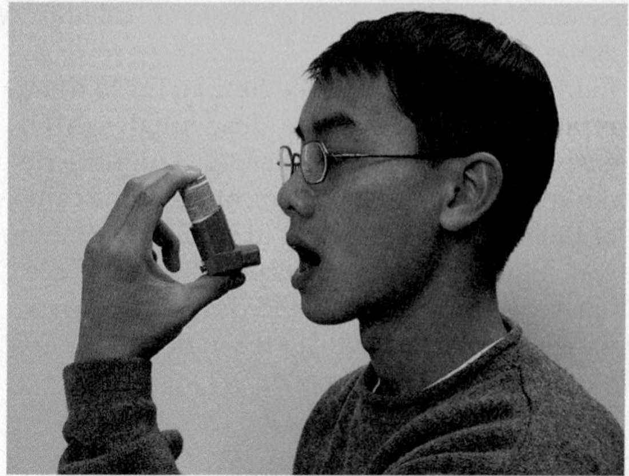

Step **14a**

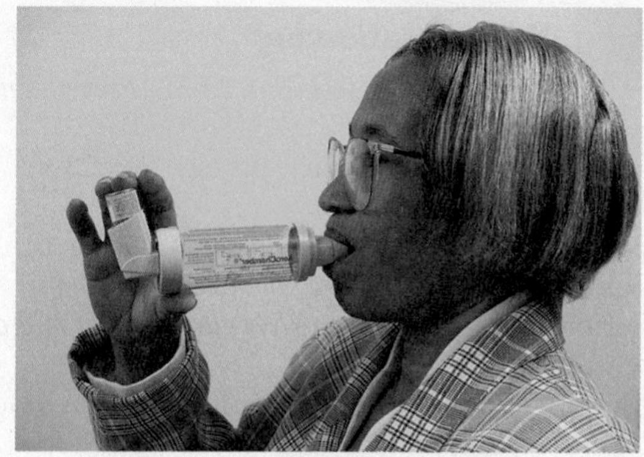

Step **14b**

15. Instruct patient to press down on inhaler to release medication while inhaling slowly and deeply through mouth.
16. Instruct patient to breathe in slowly for 2 to 3 seconds, and to hold breath for approximately 10 seconds. *(Holding breath allows tiny drops of aerosol spray to reach deeper branches of airway.)*
17. Instruct patient to exhale through pursed lips.
18. Instruct patient to wait 2 to 5 minutes between puffs. More than one puff is usually prescribed. *(First inhalation opens airways and reduces inflammation. Second or third inhalation penetrates more deeply into airways.)*
19. If more than one type of inhaled medication is prescribed, wait 5 to 10 minutes between inhalations or as ordered by physician. *(Drug administration is prescribed at intervals during day to promote bronchodilation and keep side effects to a minimum.)*
20. Explain that patient will sometimes feel gagging sensation in throat caused by droplets of medication on pharynx or tongue.
21. Instruct patient in removing medication canister and cleaning inhaler in warm water. *(To remove*

Continued

Skill 23-10 Administering Inhalants—cont'd

residue that can interfere with proper distribution of medication.)

22. **Evidenced-based practice for patient to determine when their metered-dose inhaler (MDI) is empty:** In the past, patients were taught to determine the remainder of medication in the canister of their MDI by floating it in water. This method was found to be very inaccurate owing to the variety of canister sizes and designs. Patients used different methods to try to determine if a canister was empty, and tended to use the medication canister much longer than its intended duration. Rubin and Durotoye (2005) recommended that, when MDIs do not have built-in dose counters, it is best to instruct the patient in how to count doses still available in the canister by calculating the number of puffs used per day to calculate the number of days to expect the inhaler to last.

Skill 23-11 Administering Sublingual Medications

Nursing Action *(Rationale)*

1. Follow the six rights (see Box 23-5). *(Prevents medication errors.)*
2. Perform the three label checks (see Box 23-6). *(Prevents medication errors.)*
3. Follow standard precautions (see Chapter 12, Box 12-5). *(Prevents spread of microorganisms.)*
4. Perform hand hygiene. *(Prevents spread of microorganisms.)*
5. Identify patient by checking identification bracelet and asking patient's name and birth date. *(Prevents medication errors.)*
6. Don gloves and place tablet under patient's tongue. *(Reduces spread of microorganisms and prevents absorption of medication into your skin.)*
7. Do not follow with water. *(Water reduces absorption of medication.)*
8. Instruct patient not to swallow tablet, but to let it dissolve. *(Swallowing reduces absorption of medication.)*
9. Teach patient how to place medication under tongue when self-administering. Instruct patient to let it dissolve.
10. Remove gloves and wash hands. *(Reduces spread of microorganisms.)*
11. Document sublingual administration in Medex or computer with time, date, and name.
12. Return to assess patient's response to medication. *(Enables you to determine effectiveness of medication and any occurrence of adverse reactions.)*
13. Document assessment in nursing notes.

Skill 23-12 Administering Buccal Medications

Nursing Action *(Rationale)*

1. Follow the six rights (see Box 23-5). *(Prevents medication errors.)*
2. Perform the three label checks (see Box 23-6). *(Prevents medication errors.)*
3. Follow standard precautions (see Chapter 12, Box 12-5). *(Prevents spread of microorganisms.)*
4. Perform hand hygiene. *(Prevents spread of microorganisms.)*
5. Identify patient by checking identification bracelet and asking patient's name and birth date. *(Prevents medication errors.)*
6. Don gloves to place medication between patient's cheek and gum. *(Prevents spread of microorganisms.)*
7. Do not follow with water. *(Reduces absorption of medication.)*
8. Instruct patient not to swallow tablet, but to let it dissolve.
9. Teach patient how to place medication between gum and cheek when self-administering.
10. Remove gloves and wash hands. *(Reduces spread of microorganisms.)*
11. Document buccal administration in Medex or computer with time, date, and name.
12. Return to assess patient's response to medication. *(Enables you to determine effectiveness of medication and any occurrence of adverse reactions.)*
13. Document assessment in nurse's notes.

Parenteral actually refers to all routes other than the GI, or enteral, routes. Parenteral routes are used for the following reasons:

- Some medications, such as insulin, are altered by the secretions of the GI tract.
- Some patients are not able to take medications by mouth, such as those who are intubated; are severely dysphagic (unable to eat); or have full-thickness burns, shock, nausea, or vomiting.
- The parenteral route gives a more rapid onset of action than the oral route.
- The duration of the effects of parenteral administration is shorter than that of oral administration.
- Smaller doses of parenteral drugs are possible to use because active drug ingredients are not changed or lost in the GI tract and liver.
- Intravenous administration of a drug is possible to regulate closely. Immediate entry into the bloodstream gives immediate onset of the drug's action.

Always wash hands thoroughly before selecting and handling syringes, needles, and other equipment. Use aseptic technique, because the skin is penetrated (which makes a portal of entry into the body for pathogenic organisms).

It is necessary to perform parenteral medication administration skillfully and accurately. Exact dosages are essential, as is selection of the proper site for the injection.

Equipment

Syringes

A syringe consists of a barrel, a plunger, and a tip (Figure 23-5). The outside barrel is calibrated in milliliters, insulin units, and in some agencies, heparin units.

Barrel sizes range from 1 to 50 mL. The outside of the barrel is not sterile, but the inside is. The tip of the barrel is either the plain or the Luer-Lok kind. The needle slips directly onto the plain barrel tip, whereas it is necessary to turn the Luer-Lok needle to the right as you place it onto the barrel.

The plunger inside of the barrel is also sterile; avoid touching the plunger anywhere except the tip. Use the plunger to draw up and inject medication from the syringe. The plunger has a rubber stopper on the end that is inside the barrel. Read the volume of a medication at the area of the rubber stopper nearest the needle.

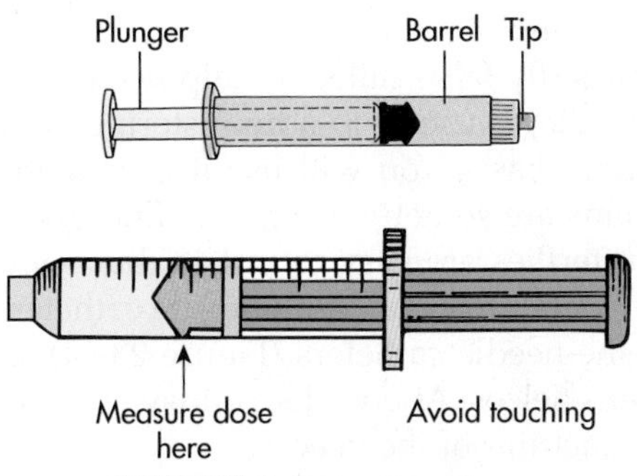

FIGURE 23-5 Parts of a syringe.

The most commonly used syringe sizes are 1 mL (tuberculin syringe), 3 mL, and 5 mL.

Tuberculin syringe. The tuberculin syringe (Figure 23-6) holds a total volume of 1 mL. It is used to give volumes of medication of 1 mL or less. It is used for giving small doses of epinephrine, intradermal skin tests, and subcutaneous medication.

The tuberculin syringe is measured in milliliters (mL). The long lines represent 0.1 (1⁄10) mL, the shorter lines represent 0.05 (5⁄100) mL, and the shortest lines represent 0.01 (1⁄100) mL.

Insulin syringe. Only use the insulin syringe for insulin, because it is calibrated in units (Figure 23-7). Most

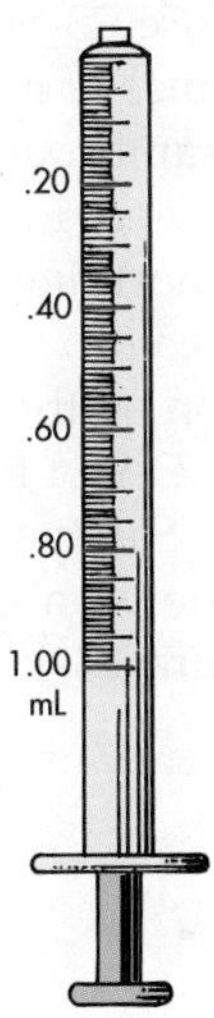

FIGURE 23-6 Tuberculin syringe calibration. Tuberculin syringe is marked in 0.01 (hundredths) for doses of less than 1 mL.

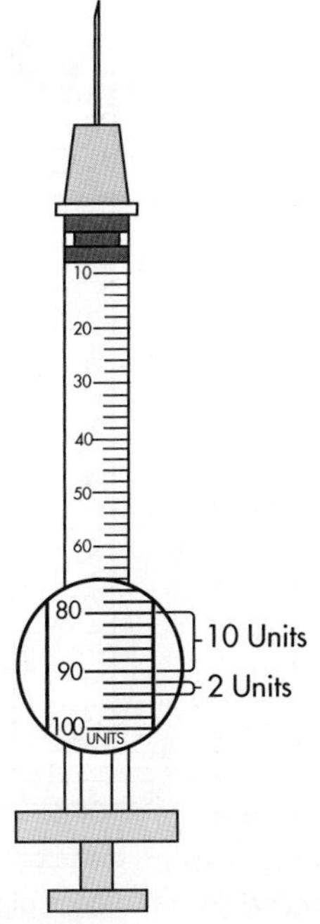

FIGURE 23-7 Calibration of U100 insulin syringe.

insulin is made in the concentration of U100. The U100 syringe holds 100 units of insulin per 1 mL. The U50 syringe holds 50 units of insulin per 0.5 mL. There is also a U30 syringe in 0.3-mL size. The unit scale on the barrel of the syringe usually differs with syringe size. The 1-mL syringe is usually marked in 2-unit increments. The 0.5-mL syringe is marked in 1-unit increments. The 0.3-mL syringe is marked in either 1- or 0.5-unit increments and is preferred for use in children and those who require small doses of insulin. Because the graduations on the 0.3-mL syringe are farther apart and easier for patients to read, this syringe is particularly useful for patients with vision problems. Always check all insulin dosages with another nurse before administering the medication to the patient. It is necessary for both of you to document that you checked the insulin dose.

3-mL syringe. The most frequently used syringe is the 3-mL syringe (Figure 23-8). The 3-mL syringe is chosen for giving volumes of medication of 1 to 3 mL. It is used for most intramuscular (IM) injections. The 3-mL syringe is calibrated in mL or cc, which are equivalent units. The short lines represent 0.1 mL; the longer lines represent 0.5 mL.

Base syringe selection on the volume of medication that are giving (Figure 23-9, *A* to *C*).

Safety-Glide syringes. Safety-Glide syringes to prevent needlesticks are now on the market (see Figure 23-9, *A* to *C* and Figure 23-10). Most hospitals and long-term care facilities use syringes with safety glides to protect personnel from needlestick injuries.

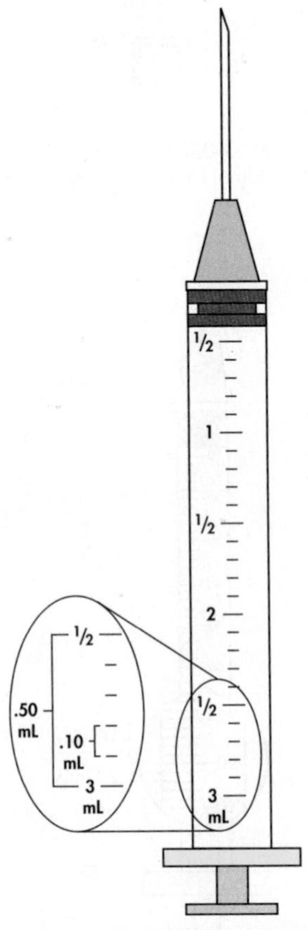

FIGURE 23-8 Reading the calibrations of a 3-mL syringe.

Disposable injection units. Disposable, single-dose, prefilled syringes are available for some medications. Check the dose you need, and expel any unneeded portion of the contents before injecting the patient.

The Tubex and Carpuject injection systems include reusable plastic or metal syringes that hold prefilled, disposable, sterile cartridge-needle units (Figure 23-11). Slip the cartridge into the mechanism, secure it (per package directions), and check for air bubbles. Advance the plunger to obtain the correct dosage and then to expel the medication, as in a regular syringe.

Needles

The parts of a needle are the hub, the shaft, and the beveled tip (Figure 23-12). The opening at the needle's beveled tip reveals the lumen (the inside of the hollow shaft). The diameter of the lumen determines the gauge (a standard or scale of measurement) of the needle (Figure 23-13). The smaller the gauge, the larger the diameter of the needle. Needle gauge selection is based on the viscosity (thickness) of the medication. The thicker the medication, the smaller the gauge (the larger the lumen) required. A 20- to 22-gauge needle is usually adequate for most nonviscous IM injections. A 16- to 18-gauge needle is appropriate for blood administration, emergency IV routes, and surgical cases. A 25- to 26-gauge needle is frequently used for infants and children and for intradermal injections, and 27- to 28-gauge needles are available for subcutaneous injections. Insulin-syringe needles are typically 29 and 30 gauge.

Needle length. You will select needle length based on the depth of the tissue into which you need to inject the medication. Intradermal (ID) injections require only ⅜- to ⅝-inch needle length, whereas an IM injection will often require 1- to 1½-inch needle length, depending on the amount of muscle tissue the patient has. Needle length for subcutaneous injections is usually ⅝ to ½ inch, based on depth of appropriate tissue (see Figure 23-13). Insulin-syringe needles are available in a standard ½-inch length and a 5⁄16-inch length. The shorter needle tends to be less intimidating, and many diabetic patients perceive them to be less painful than standard-length needles.

Intravenous needles. Two types of needles made especially for IV use are the butterfly and the over-the-needle catheter.

The butterfly (also called a scalp needle or a wing-tipped needle) is useful in administering IV fluids on a short-term basis. You will use it in pediatric cases, where veins are sometimes hard to find except in the scalp. Butterflies are easy to put in, but some health care providers prefer over-the-needle catheters.

Over-the-needle catheters (Figure 23-14) are called Angiocaths, Jelcos, Abbocaths, or Insytes, according to the manufacturer of the needle.

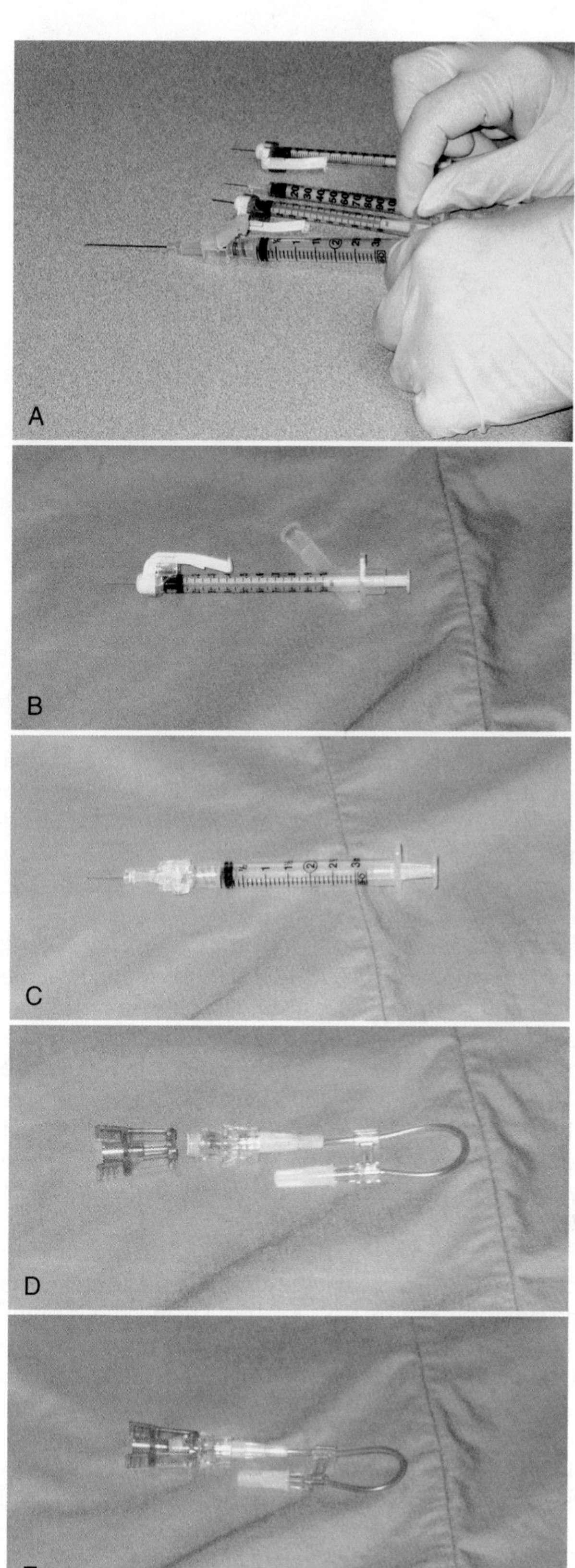

FIGURE 23-9 Types of syringes. **A** (top to bottom), Disposable Safety-Glide insulin syringe, tuberculin syringe, 3-mL intramuscular syringe. **B,** Safety-Glide tuberculin syringe. **C,** Safety-Glide 3-mL syringe (subcutaneous). **D,** Saline lock with needleless adapter. **E,** Saline lock showing the needleless adapter snapped into place.

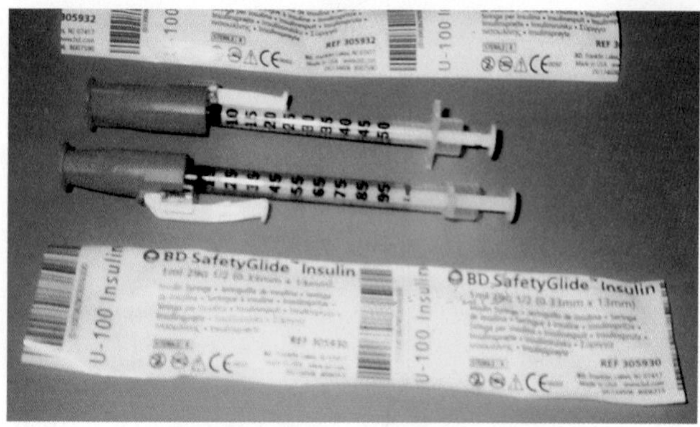

FIGURE 23-10 Safety-Glide syringe.

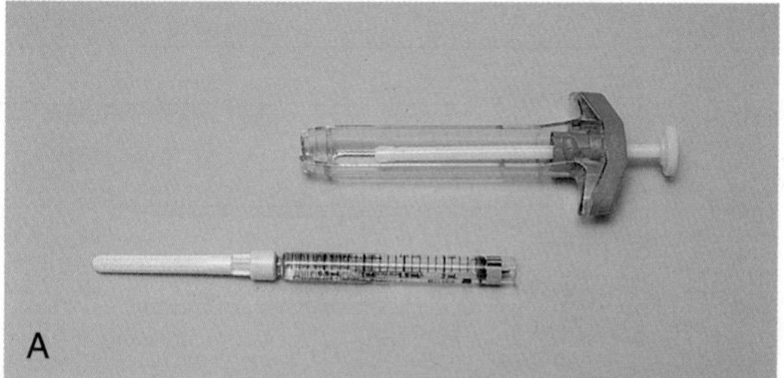

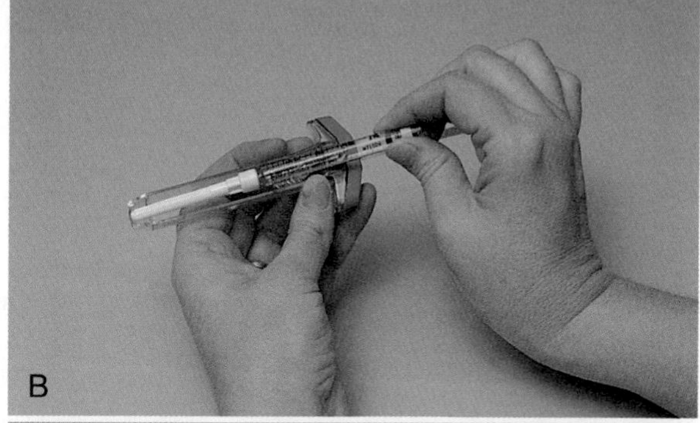

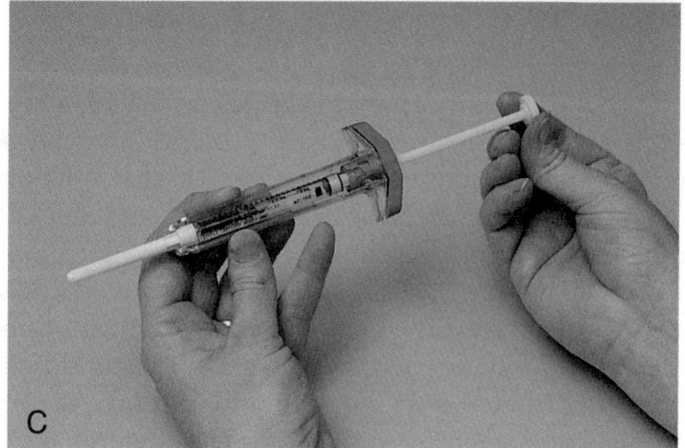

FIGURE 23-11 A, Carpuject syringe and prefilled sterile cartridge with needle. **B,** Assembling the Carpuject. **C,** Cartridge slides into syringe barrel, turns, and locks at needle end. Plunger then screws into cartridge end.

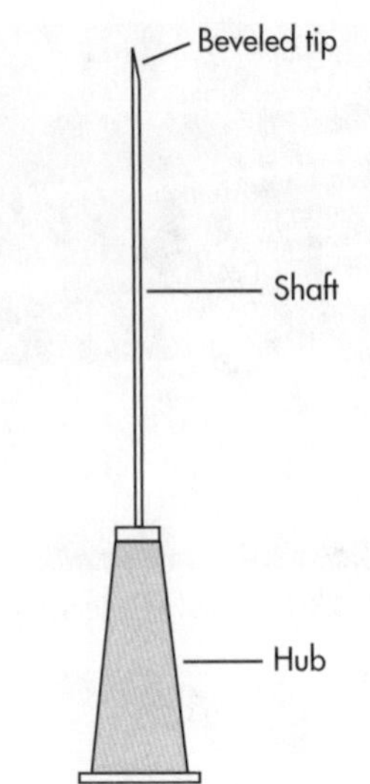

FIGURE 23-12 Parts of a needle.

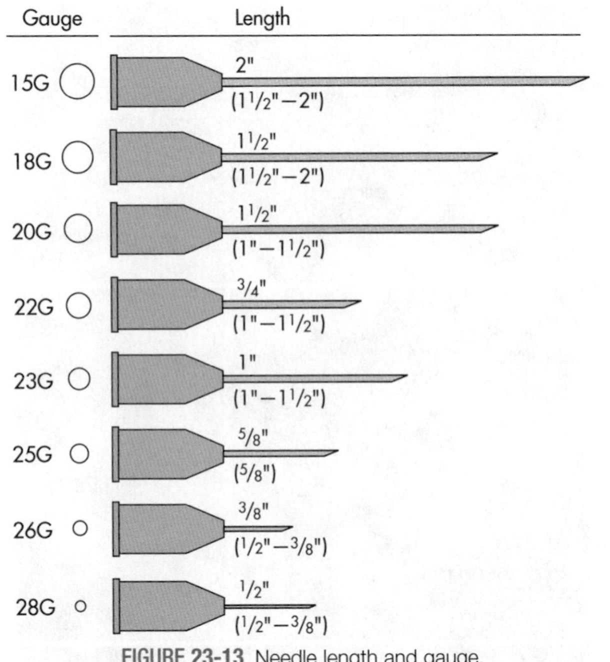

FIGURE 23-13 Needle length and gauge.

Over-the-needle catheters are preferred for emergency situations, surgery cases, blood and blood product transfusions, intensive care cases, transporting situations (e.g., helicopters, ambulances), thick IV infusions, and total parenteral nutrition.

Angiocaths are plastic catheters over a stainless steel needle stylet. A stylet is a sharp, bevel-tipped metal guide that is used to pierce the skin and vein. Once the catheter is in the vein, blood return is seen and the stylet is removed. The plastic catheter is left in the vein. The catheter is preferred for long-term IV use because it is more flexible and better withstands patient movement (see Figure 23-14, *B*).

It is not possible to use butterflies and Angiocaths for an indefinite length of time. Assess them every shift for patency (openness) and intactness or complications.

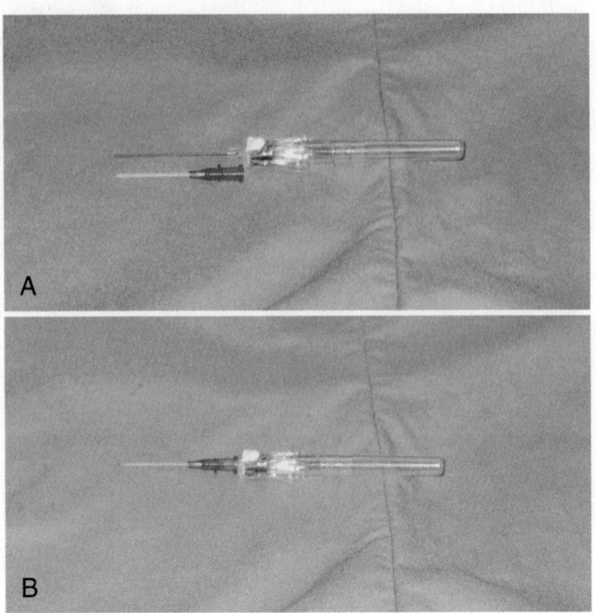

FIGURE 23-14 **A,** Over-the-needle catheter. **B,** Needle is removed with the plastic cannula, which remains in the vein.

Intracaths are similar to Angiocaths, except that they are much longer. Physicians insert Intracaths for long-term IV administration or for IV nutritional feedings (total parenteral nutrition). See Skill 23-13 for preparation of parenteral medications.

Needleless Devices

Approximately 600,000 to 1,000,000 accidental needlesticks and sharps injuries occur annually in health care settings. These injuries commonly occur when nurses forget and recap needles, mishandle IV lines and needles, or contact stray needles left at a patient's bedside. The risk of exposure of health care workers to bloodborne pathogens has led to the development of needleless devices, or special needle safety devices (OSHA, 2009).

Special syringes are designed with a sheath or guard that covers the needle after it is withdrawn from the skin (see Figure 23-9, *A* to *C*). The needle is immediately covered, eliminating the chance for a needlestick injury. The syringe and sheath are disposed of together in a receptacle. The Centers for Disease Control and Prevention (CDC) and Occupational Safety and Health Administration (OSHA) have recommended use of needleless devices to reduce the risk to health care workers from needlesticks and sharps injuries (OSHA, 2009).

IV catheters have been developed with blunt-edged cannulas, valves, or needle guards to reduce the occurrence of injuries during IV insertion or medication delivery (see Figure 23-14, *A* and *B*). In addition, there is now IV tubing with recessed and shielded needle connectors, further reducing needlesticks (see Figure 23-9, *D* and *E*).

Skill 23-13 Preparing Parenteral Medications

Nursing Action *(Rationale)*

1. Follow the six rights (see Box 23-5). *(Prevents medication errors.)*
2. Perform the three label checks (see Box 23-6). *(Prevents medication errors.)*
3. Follow standard precautions (see Chapter 12, Box 12-5). *(Prevents spread of microorganisms.)*
4. Perform hand hygiene before handling equipment and prepare medication in clean area. *(Prevents spread of microorganisms.)*
5. Maintain sterility of sterile parts of syringe and needle. Use aseptic technique throughout preparation. *(Prevents contamination.)*
6. Compare drug and dosage ordered with drug and dose on hand; check expiration date, dose/mL, and total volume of solution in vial or ampule. Look for contaminants or defects in vial or ampule.
7. Calculate drug dosage and check calculations with another nurse. *(Prevents drug errors.)*
8. Check compatibility chart or consult pharmacy if mixing two medications. *(It is essential that any medications mixed are compatible.)*
9. Don gloves. *(Prevents spread of microorganisms.)*
10. Prepare medication syringe:
    a. **Withdrawing medication from a vial:**
    (1) Remove metal cap from top of vial; wipe rubber diaphragm briskly with alcohol sponge. *(Not all drug manufacturers guarantee that seals of unused vials are sterile. Therefore it is necessary to swab seals before drawing up medication.)*
    (2) Pull plunger of syringe back to aspirate air into syringe equal to amount of drug to be withdrawn. *(It is necessary to inject air into the vial to prevent buildup of negative pressure in vial when aspirating medication.)*
    (3) Insert needle into inverted vial; inject air and withdraw volume of solution to be given. Keep needle under solution. *(Prevents aspiration of air into syringe.)*
    (4) Push plunger gently to disperse solution to tip of needle. Remove air bubbles by gently tapping syringe.
    b. **Withdrawing medication from an ampule:**
    (1) Tap the top of ampule to move solution from top of ampule to bottom of ampule (see illustration).
    (2) Cover neck of ampule with an alcohol sponge; break off top of ampule; deposit top of glass ampule in sharps container (see illustration). *(Prevents injury.)*

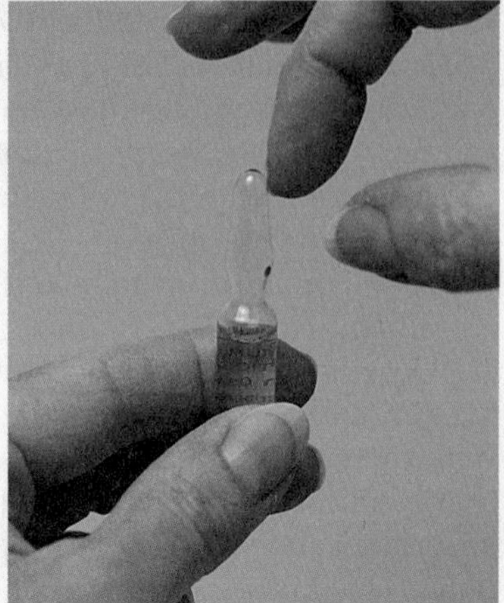

Step **10b(1)**

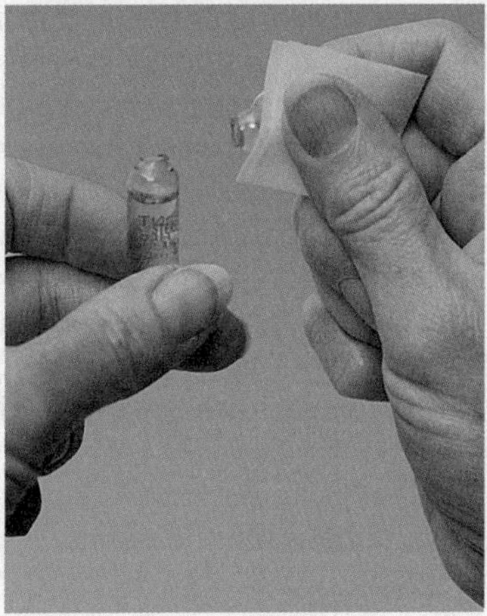

Step **10b(2)**

    (3) Use a filter needle to aspirate medication from ampule. *(Filter or aspiration needles catch particles of glass that may be in the solution from the broken ampule.)*
    (4) Insert filter needle into open neck of ampule; invert ampule to withdraw correct dose.
    (5) Replace filter needle with needle appropriate for purpose and viscosity of solution.
    (6) Push plunger gently until the plunger measures the correct dose.
    c. **Reconstituting a powdered dosage form:**
    (1) Follow instructions on manufacturer's box and drug insert. The instructions will specify the type and the amount of diluent to use (e.g., add 10 mL of bacteriostatic saline to prepare a ratio of 500 mg/mL).
    (2) Remove the protective cap from diluent and cleanse vial with alcohol pad; withdraw diluent using sterile technique.

Continued

Skill 23-13 Preparing Parenteral Medications—cont'd

(3) Withdraw needle from diluent vial.
(4) Inject diluent into vial of powdered drug; remove syringe and needle. Gently shake and tap vial. *(Dissolves powder into solution.)*
(5) Label solution with the following:
  (a) Date and time mixed
  (b) Name of person who mixed drug and diluent
  (c) Dose/mL obtained (concentration)
  (d) Amount and type of diluent used
(6) Withdraw correct dose (see illustration); change needle with a new needle of appropriate gauge and length for patient. *(It is necessary to exchange the needle with the needle for injection into patient's tissue. Needles become dull as they enter rubber stopper. Changing needles also prevents tracking of medication through patient's tissues, keeping pain caused to a minimum.)*

d. Placing two medications into one syringe (insulin example used):
(1) Check compatibility of two drugs with a compatibility chart or call pharmacy.
(2) Check and compare label of each drug ordered with label of each drug on hand.
(3) Compare each label with medication order.
(4) Roll long- and intermediate-acting insulin between the palms. *(Resuspends insulin.)* Do not shake any insulin. *(Causes air bubbles.)* (NOTE: Do *not* mix long-acting insulin glargine [Lantus] with regular insulin. *(Lantus is acidic and will affect action of regular insulin.)*
(5) Briskly wipe tops of both vials with separate alcohol swabs. *(Prevents contamination.)*
(6) Pull back plunger of syringe to amount equal to volume of longer-acting insulin to be given. *(Prevents buildup of negative pressure.)*
(7) Insert needle and inject air into vial of longer-acting insulin.
(8) Withdraw needle from vial without having removed insulin.
(9) Pull back plunger of syringe to amount equal to volume of shorter-acting (regular or rapid) insulin to be given.
(10) Insert needle through rubber stopper of second vial; inject air into vial.
(11) Invert vial; withdraw volume of shorter-acting (regular or rapid) insulin first. *(Prevents contamination of regular or rapid insulin by intermediate or long-acting insulin.)*
(12) Check dosage in syringe against medication order, as well as with another nurse. *(Prevents insulin error.)*
(13) Wipe rubber stopper of longer-acting insulin; insert needle of the syringe containing shorter- or rapid-acting insulin, and withdraw ordered dose of longer-acting insulin. Check dose in syringe against medication order with second nurse. *(Prevents insulin error.)*
(14) Remove needle or syringe from vial.
(15) Check labels of both vials against medication order. *(Ensures accuracy.)*
(16) Pull plunger back enough to allow space in barrel of syringe for insulin to be gently mixed. Mix by tilting syringe back and forth; remove air. Administer mixtures of insulin within 5 minutes of preparation. *(Regular insulin binds with [NPH] and the action of regular insulin is reduced.)*

11. Identify room, bed, patient's name, and patient birth date. *(Prevents medication errors.)*
12. Don gloves. *(Prevents spread of microorganisms.)*
13. Prepare injection site and inject according to prescribed route and method (see Skills 23-14 through 23-17).

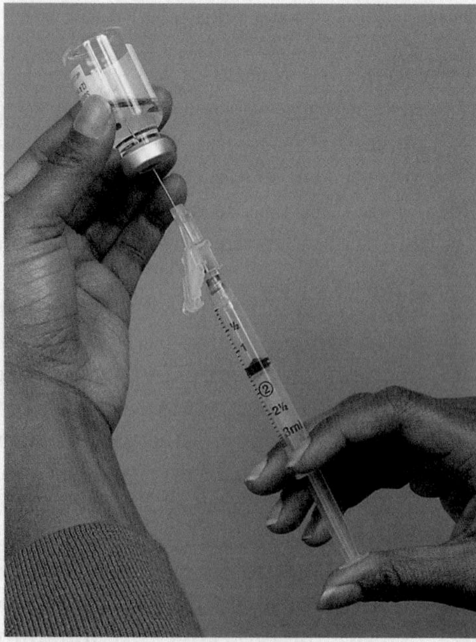

Step **10c(6)**

Intramuscular Injections

An IM injection involves inserting a needle into the muscle tissue to administer medication. Because muscle tissue has a large blood supply, absorption of an IM medication is faster than a subQ medication. The most commonly used sites are the ventrogluteal area, the vastus lateralis of the thigh, and the deltoid muscle of the arm.

When selecting an IM site, ensure that the site is free of pain, infection, necrosis, ecchymosis, and abrasions. Other important factors to consider are the location of underlying bones, nerves, and major blood vessels, as well as the amount of solution to be injected. The various sites have advantages as well as disadvantages (Elkin et al., 2007). Formerly, the dorsogluteal muscle site was frequently used; however, because the sciatic nerve and superior gluteal artery are near, this muscle is no longer recommended as an injection site. Permanent or partial paralysis of the involved leg is possible if a needle hits the sciatic nerve (Nicoll et al., 2002).

For adults and children older than 7 months, the ventrogluteal site is preferred for IM injections. The advantages of this site are that it (1) provides the greatest thickness of gluteal muscle, (2) does not have nerves and blood vessels penetrating it, (3) has the most consistent and thinnest layer of adipose tissue covering it, and (4) has very few documented injuries associated with its use (Rodger et al., 2000). You will develop skill in the proper location for giving an IM injection by palpating anatomical landmarks correctly and being knowledgeable of the location of underlying nerves and blood vessels (Boxes 23-9 and 23-10) (Elkin et al., 2007).

Intramuscular injections for analgesia are given much less often because of the frequent use of patient-controlled analgesia (PCA) and patient-controlled epidural (PCE). IM injections are painful and more prone to complications.

Site Selection

Ventrogluteal site. The gluteal sites are the ventrogluteal and the dorsogluteal. The **ventrogluteal site** (Figure 23-15) is located by using three landmarks—the greater trochanter, the anterior iliac spine, and the iliac crest (the hip bone).

With the palm of your hand on the lateral portion of the greater trochanter and your index (pointer) finger on the anterior superior iliac spine, extend your middle finger to the iliac crest. Inject medication into the V formed by your index and middle fingers. The best position for the patient is prone. Muscle relaxation is promoted by turning the patient's toes inward. It is also possible to use a side-lying position, with muscle relaxation promoted by flexing the upper leg. The dorsogluteal muscle is no longer recommended as an injection site owing to its proximity to the sciatic nerve (Nicoll et al., 2002).

Vastus lateralis muscle. The vastus lateralis muscle (Figure 23-16) is the preferred site for children younger than 3 years of age because it is free of nerves and blood vessels. It is also used in adults. The vastus is located on the anterior lateral thigh. Have the patient in a supine or sitting position. Place one hand above the patient's knee and one hand below the greater trochanter. Make the IM injection in the area between your two hands. Depending on development of this muscle, it is possible to inject up to 3 mL of medication. The ventrogluteal site is now also used for IM injections for children older than 7 months.

Rectus femoris muscle. The rectus femoris muscle (Figure 23-17) is located by the same manner as the vastus lateralis. The rectus femoris is medial to the

Box 23-9 Characteristics of Intramuscular Sites

VASTUS LATERALIS MUSCLE

- This large, developed muscle lacks major nerves and blood vessels and is the most fully developed muscle in the newborn.
- Preferred site for administration of biologic substances (e.g., immunizations) to infants younger than 12 months of age,* but also used in adults.
- Rapid drug absorption occurs.

VENTROGLUTEAL MUSCLE

- Involves the gluteus medius and the gluteus minimus.
- Situated deep and away from major nerves and blood vessels and is a safe site for all patients.
- Ventrogluteal site not associated with injuries such as fibrosis, nerve damage, abscess, tissue necrosis, muscle contraction, gangrene, and pain, as seen with other intramuscular (IM) sites.*
- Preferred injection site for infants, children, and adults.

DORSOGLUTEAL MUSCLE

- You run the risk of striking the underlying sciatic nerve, the greater trochanter, or major blood vessels.
- No longer recommended as an intramuscular site.*

DELTOID MUSCLE

- This site is easily accessible, but the muscle is not well developed in most patients.
- Use only for small volumes (0.5 to 1 mL) of medication, and for administration of routine immunizations in toddler, older children, and adults.*
- Give hepatitis B vaccine only in the deltoid.†
- Avoid using the deltoid muscle in infants or children with underdeveloped muscles.

*Nicoll, L.H., et al. (2002). Intramuscular injection: an integrative research review and guideline for evidence-based practice. *Appl Nurs Res, 16*(2), 149.
†Elkin, M.K., et al. (2007). *Nursing interventions and clinical skills.* (4th ed.). St. Louis: Mosby.

Box 23-10 Locating Sites for Intramuscular Injections

VENTROGLUTEAL SITE

1. Position patient on either side, with knee bent and upper leg slightly ahead of the bottom leg. It is also acceptable for the patient to remain supine or lie on abdomen. Instruct patient to relax muscles where you are placing injection.
2. Palpate the greater trochanter at the head of the femur and the anterior superior iliac spine. To locate the proper site, use your left hand when the patient lies on the left side and your right hand when the patient lies on the right side.
3. Using your right hand for the left hip and your left hand for the right hip, place the heel of your hand over the greater trochanter of the patient's hip. Point your thumb toward the patient's groin, point your index finger toward the anterior superior iliac spine, and extend your middle finger back along the iliac crest toward the buttock as far as possible (NOTE: A "V" is formed between the index and middle finger) (see Figure 23-15).
4. The injection site is the center of the triangle formed by the index and middle fingers.
5. Spread skin taut to give injection. Use your dominant hand to give injection (see Figure 23-15).

VASTUS LATERALIS SITE

1. Position patient lying supine or sitting with site well exposed. If patient is supine, have patient flex knee on side where medication will be given.
2. Use the greater trochanter and the knee as landmarks for injection site. Place one hand above the knee and one hand below the greater trochanter of the femur.
3. Locate the middle third of the muscle and the midline of the anterior thigh and the midline of the thigh's lateral (outer) side.
4. The injection site is located within a rectangle formed by these boundaries (see Figure 23-16).

DELTOID SITE

1. Position patient sitting or lying down, exposing the upper arm and shoulder. Remove any tight-fitting sleeves rather than rolling them up.
2. Ask patient to relax the arm at the side with the elbow flexed. Instruct patient to place the lower arm across the abdomen or the chest.
3. Palpate the lower edge of the acromion process, which forms the base of a triangle in line with the midpoint of the lateral aspect of the upper arm (see Figure 23-18).
4. Place four fingers across the deltoid muscle, with the top finger along the acromion process.
5. The injection site is in the center of the triangle, about 3 to 5 cm (1 to 2 inches) below the acromion process (see Figure 23-18).

From Elkin, M.K., et al. (2007). *Nursing interventions and clinical skills*. (4th ed.). St. Louis: Mosby.

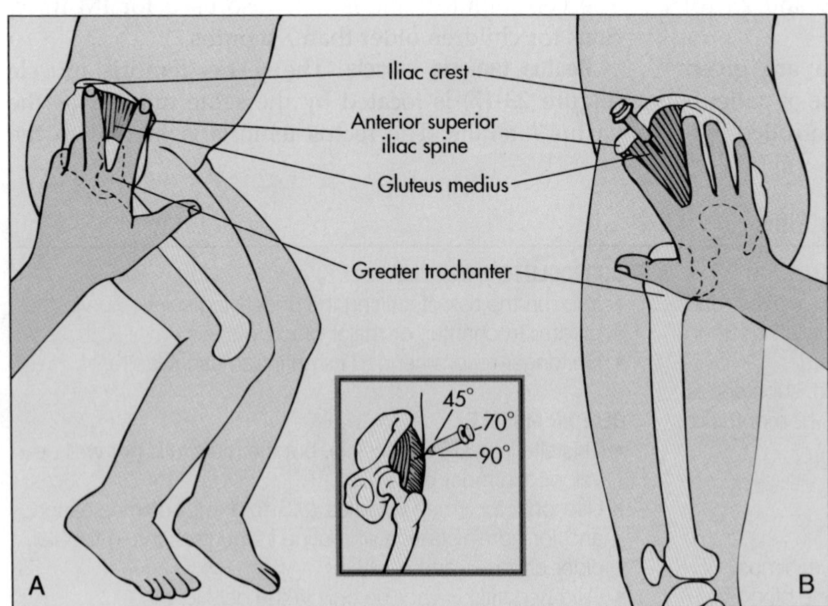

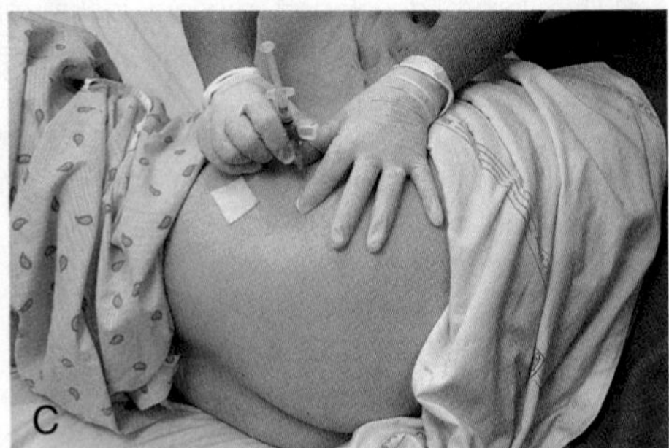

FIGURE 23-15 Ventrogluteal site. **A,** Child and infant. **B,** Adult. **C,** Locating IM injection for ventrogluteal site.

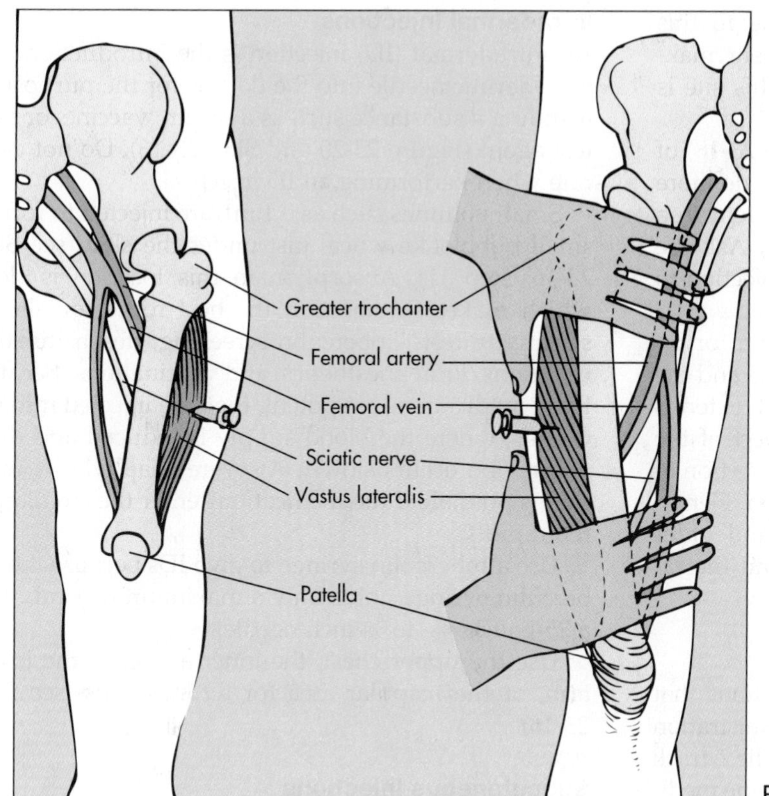

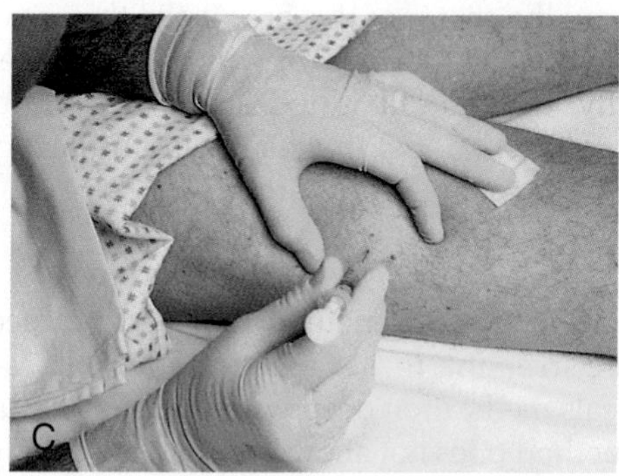

FIGURE 23-16 Vastus lateralis muscle. **A,** Child and infant. **B,** Adult. **C,** Giving IM injection in vastus lateralis site on adult.

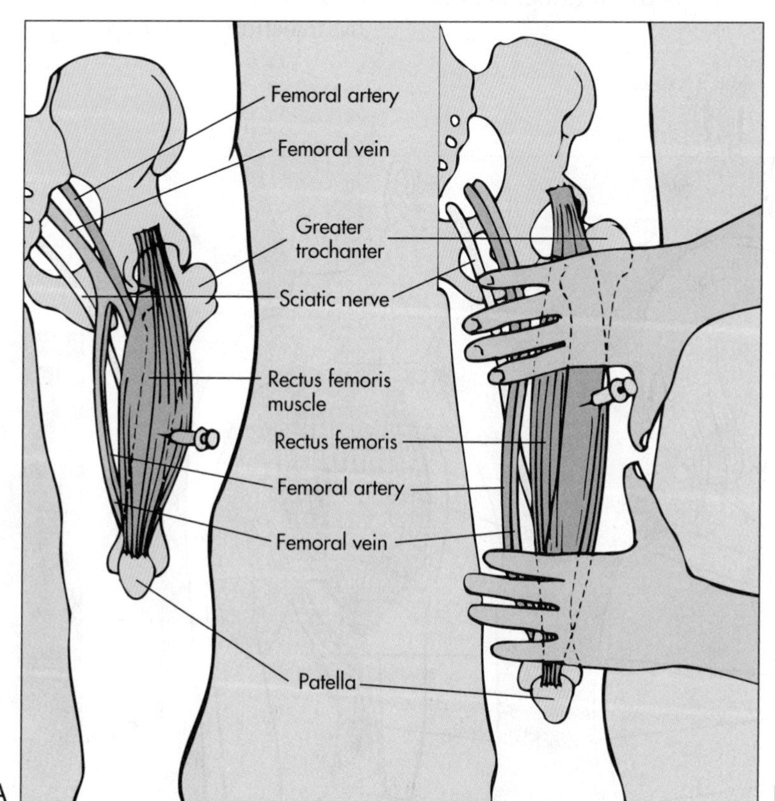

FIGURE 23-17 Rectus femoris muscle. **A,** Child and infant. **B,** Adult.

vastus lateralis. The sciatic nerve lies close to this muscle, and major blood vessels are also present, making the site potentially dangerous to use. This site is rarely used.

Deltoid muscle. The deltoid muscle (Figure 23-18) of the upper arm is a relatively small area. Inject no more than 1 mL into this muscle. Position the patient in a sitting, standing, prone, or supine position. Ask the patient to relax his or her arm during the injection to decrease discomfort.

The landmarks for locating the proper area for injection are the acromion process of the scapula and the axillary fold. Draw an imaginary line that extends from the axillary fold across the lateral aspect of the arm; the center of this area is the thicker midportion of the muscle, where you will give the injection. Generally, the deltoid is too small in children and older adults. Also, the brachial vein and artery and the radial nerve are in this area (Skill 23-14).

Z-Track Method

Use the Z-track method for injecting medications that are irritating to the tissues. Z-track IM administration seals medication deep within muscle tissue. The Z-track method does not allow staining or tracking of the medication into the tissue as the needle is withdrawn. The Z-track method of IM injection keeps tissue irritation to a minimum by sealing the drug within muscle tissues (Figure 23-19). Use this method when giving IM iron (Skill 23-15) or hydroxyzine (Vistaril). Select an IM site in larger, deeper muscles such as the ventrogluteal or dorsogluteal.

Intradermal Injections

An intradermal (ID) injection is the introduction of a hypodermic needle into the dermis for the purpose of instilling a substance such as a serum, vaccine, or skin test agent (Figure 23-20 and Skill 23-16). Do not aspirate when performing an ID injection.

Small volumes such as 0.1 mL are injected to form a small bubblelike wheal just under the skin (see Skill 23-16, step 11). Absorption in this location is slow, which makes ID injection the best route for allergy sensitivity tests, tuberculin screening, desensitization injections, local anesthetics, and vaccinations. Because these medications are potent, they are injected into the dermis, where the blood supply is reduced and drug absorption occurs slowly. A severe anaphylactic reaction is possible if the medications enter the circulation too rapidly.

Use a tuberculin syringe to give IDs because the tuberculin syringe holds only a maximum of 1 mL. Use a 25-gauge, ⅜- to ⅝-inch needle.

Use the upper chest, the inner aspect of the lower arm, or the scapular area for ID injections (see Skill 23-16).

Subcutaneous Injections

You will give insulin, heparin, Lovenox, Fragmin, Epogen, and Neupogen by the subQ route. Make these injections into the loose connective tissue between the dermis and the muscle layer. Because subcutaneous tissue is not as richly supplied with blood as the muscles, drug absorption is somewhat slower than with IM injections. The outer aspect of the upper arms, the

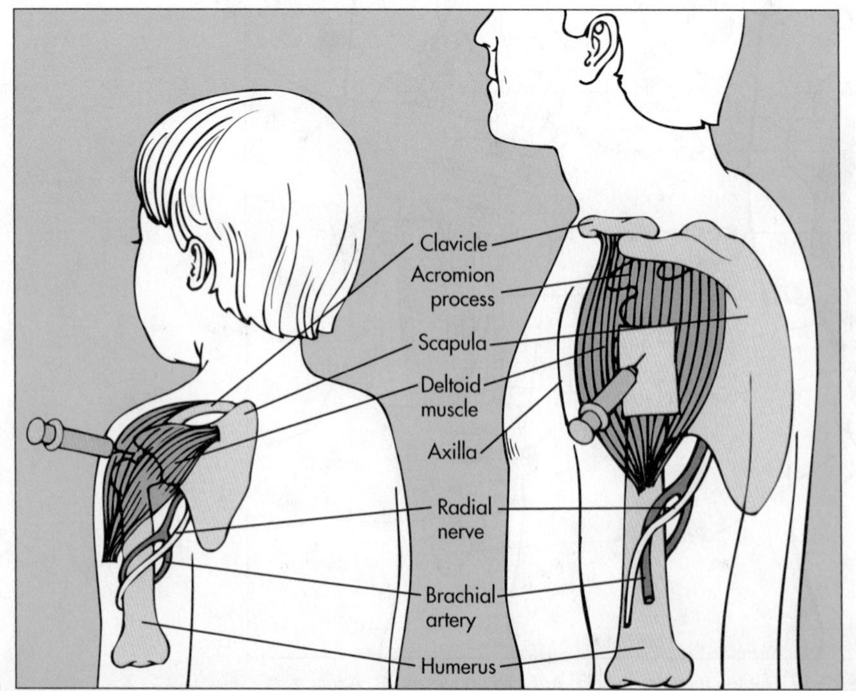

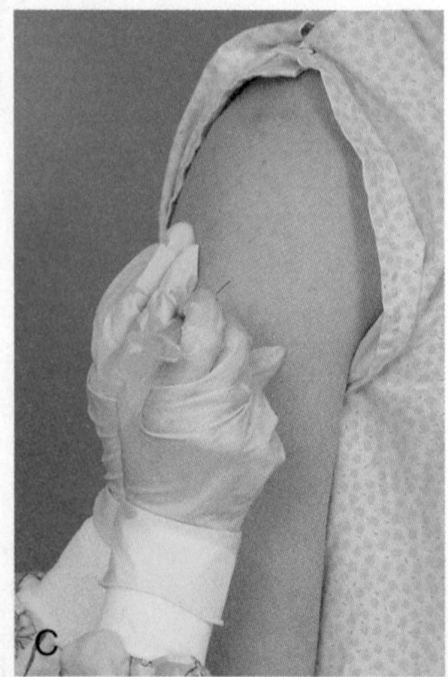

FIGURE 23-18 Deltoid muscle site. **A,** Child and infant. **B,** Adult. **C,** Giving IM injection in deltoid site.

Skill 23-14 Giving an Intramuscular Injection

Nursing Action *(Rationale)*

1. Follow the six rights (see Box 23-5). *(Prevents medication errors.)*
2. Perform the three label checks (see Box 23-6). *(Prevents medication errors.)*
3. Follow standard precautions (see Chapter 12, Box 12-5). *(Prevents spread of microorganisms.)*
4. Perform hand hygiene. *(Prevents spread of microorganisms.)*
5. Prepare medication according to standard procedure for injectables (see Skill 23-13).
6. Don gloves. *(Prevents spread of microorganisms.)*
7. Identify patient by checking identification bracelet and asking patient's name and birth date. *(Prevents medication errors.)* Explain the procedure.
8. Select and expose site (according to intramuscular [IM] site selection procedure); provide privacy.
9. Clean skin with alcohol swab (from center outward), spread skin tight with thumb and index finger; let dry. *(Mechanical and chemical action removes microorganisms.)*
10. Ask patient to take a deep breath and exhale slowly to relax muscle as needle is inserted. *(Lessens pain from injection.)*
11. Insert needle at a 90-degree angle quickly in a dartlike motion. *(Quickness reduces discomfort.)*
12. Maintain needle's position in muscle; gently aspirate (pull back plunger) to be certain needle is in muscle (and not in a vein or an artery). Aspirate 5 to 10 seconds. *(Aspirating for 5 to 10 seconds is adequate to ensure needle is not in a small blood vessel.)*
    a. If blood is seen, needle is in a vein or an artery. Withdraw needle and discard medication; prepare new medication (see Skill 23-13). Select another site for new attempt and begin again from step 8.
13. Slowly inject medication into muscle to lessen discomfort. *(A slow, steady injection rate of medication promotes comfort and minimizes tissue damage.)*
14. Withdraw needle quickly without bending or twisting it. *(Minimizes tissue injury.)*
15. Use pressure gauze (2 × 2) to stop any bleeding. Apply gentle pressure. *(Massaging site can cause tissue irritation.)*
16. Do not recap needle; discard directly into sharps container. *(Prevents needlesticks.)*
17. Remove gloves and wash hands. *(Prevents spread of microorganisms.)*
18. Record administration of medication in the Medex or computer with time, date, and name. Chart site used and amount and type of medication (e.g., meperidine [Demerol] 50 mg given IM left ventrogluteal). *(Remember, a quick, dartlike insertion followed by slow injection of the medication is much less painful to the patient.)*
19. Return to assess patient's response to medication. *(Enables you to determine effectiveness of medication and any occurrence of adverse reactions.)*
20. Document assessment in nursing notes.

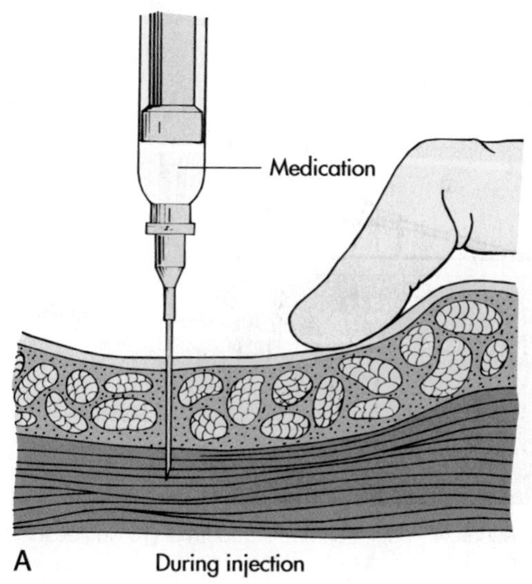

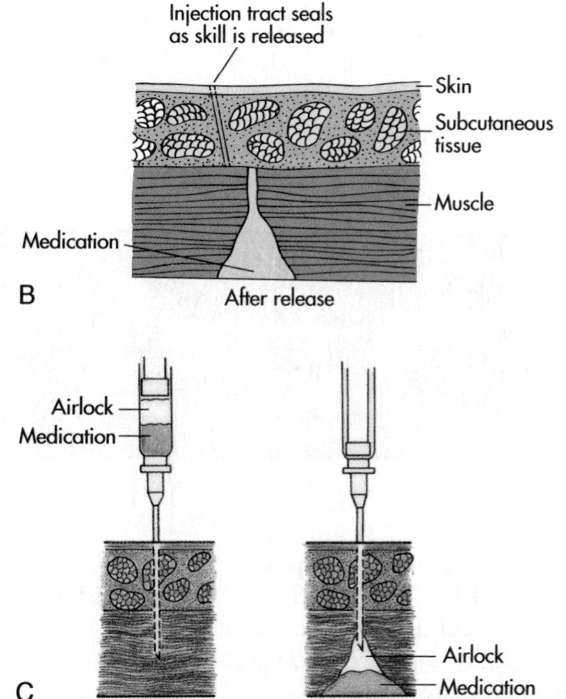

FIGURE 23-19 **A,** Z-track method. **B,** Using an airlock. **C,** Administering IM injection by airlock technique.

Skill 23-15 Giving a Z-Track Injection

Nursing Action *(Rationale)*

1. Follow the six rights (see Box 23-5). *(Prevents medication errors.)*
2. Perform the three label checks (see Box 23-6). *(Prevents medication errors.)*
3. Follow standard precautions (see Chapter 12, Box 12-5). *(Prevents spread of microorganisms.)*
4. Perform hand hygiene. *(Prevents spread of microorganisms.)*
5. Prepare medication according to standard procedure for injectables (see Skill 23-13).
6. Don gloves. *(Prevents spread of microorganisms.)*
7. Use one needle to withdraw dose from container. Use another needle (1½ to 2 inches) to inject medication so that no solution remains on the outside of needle shaft.
8. Draw up 0.2 mL of air to create an airlock.
9. Identify patient by checking identification bracelet and asking patient's name and birth date. *(Prevents medication errors.)*
10. Expose and locate dorsogluteal or ventrogluteal site according to intramuscular (IM) site selection procedure; provide privacy.
11. Clean site with an alcohol swab. *(Mechanical and chemical action removes microorganisms.)*
12. Ask the patient to take a deep breath and to slowly exhale. *(Relaxes the muscle.)* Pull skin tightly in a lateral direction (move skin at least 1 to 1½ inches laterally) to one side. Hold the skin taut with the nondominant hand. *(Z-track technique reduces discomfort and leakage of medication into tissue.)*
13. Insert needle at a 90-degree angle; aspirate. *(It is necessary to insert a needle at 90-degree angle for it to enter muscle.)*
    a. If blood is seen, needle is in a vein or artery. Withdraw needle and discard medication; prepare new medication (see Skill 23-13). Select another site for new attempt and begin again from step 13.
    b. If no blood is seen, inject medication and air slowly; wait 10 seconds to allow the medication to disperse slowly.
14. Withdraw needle quickly. Allow skin to return to its normal position, which leaves a zigzag path that seals the needle track wherever tissue planes slide across each other. *(The drug is not able to escape from the muscle tissue.)* (See Figure 23-19.)
15. Use a 2 × 2 gauze pad or bandage as needed.
16. Do not massage site. *(Massaging sometimes causes tissue irritation.)*
17. Do not recap needle; discard directly into sharps container. *(Prevents needlesticks.)*
18. Remove gloves and wash hands. *(Prevents spread of microorganisms.)*
19. Record administration of medication in the Medex or computer with time, date, and name. Chart site used, Z-track method used, and amount and type of medication given.
20. Return to assess patient's response to medication. *(Determines effectiveness of medication and occurrence of adverse reactions.)*
21. Document assessment in nursing notes.

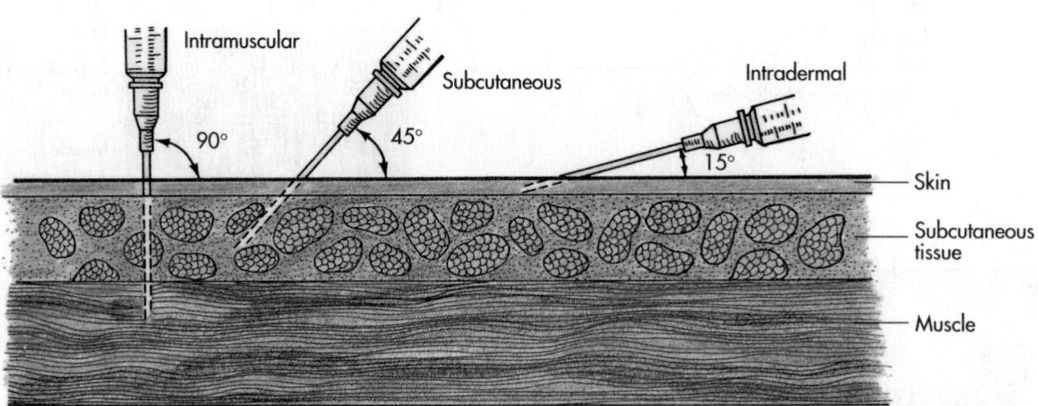

FIGURE 23-20 Angles of insertion for intramuscular (90 degrees), subcutaneous (45 degrees), and intradermal (15 degrees) injections.

abdomen, the thighs, and the scapula are sites used for subQ injections. Inject no more than 1 mL of solution into these sites, and always carefully chart the injection. Rotate sites of repeated injections to prevent tissue damage and discomfort.

Give subQ injections at a 45-degree angle if the patient is thin or at a 90-degree angle if the patient has ample subcutaneous tissue. Use your judgment in selecting sites for injection and in determining the angle of injection. Select needle length so that the medication

Skill 23-16 Giving an Intradermal Injection

Nursing Action *(Rationale)*

1. Follow the six rights (see Box 23-5). *(Prevents medication errors.)*
2. Perform the three label checks (see Box 23-6). *(Prevents medication errors.)*
3. Follow standard precautions (see Chapter 12, Box 12-5). *(Prevents spread of microorganisms.)*
4. Perform hand hygiene. *(Prevents spread of microorganisms.)*
5. Prepare medication according to standard procedure for injectables (see Skill 23-13).
6. Don gloves. *(Prevents spread of microorganisms.)*
7. Identify patient by checking identification bracelet and asking patient's name and birth date. *(Prevents medication errors.)*
8. Select arm and expose inner aspect of lower arm.
9. Clean site gently with alcohol swab from center outward; let dry. *(Mechanical and chemical action removes microorganisms.)*
10. Two injections are made if test is for sensitivity. *(One injection is a control using sterile water or bacteriostatic saline; the other is test substance.)* Insert a 25-gauge needle with bevel up directly under skin. Advance needle through epidermis to approximately ⅛ inch (3 mm) below the skin surface. You will be able to see the needle tip through the skin.
11. Make a small, bubblelike wheal with test solution. *(Creation of bleb shows placement of needle is correct.)* Insert needle at approximately a 15-degree angle (see illustration). Do not inject into subcutaneous tissue. Inject control of saline into another site for comparison with test substance after designated time interval.
12. Do not massage site. *(Massage will most likely disperse medication into underlying tissue layers and alter test results.)*
13. Draw a circle around skin test with a marker; label area with time, date, and name of test. Another method is to make a diagram in patient's chart to indicate location of site. *(Facilitates assessment of site and reading of test results.)*
14. Remove gloves and wash hands. *(Prevents spread of microorganisms.)*
15. If an indurated (hardened) erythematous area is observed, measure indurated area and record results in millimeters with metric ruler.
16. Compare control bleb with agent bleb; document results in chart.
17. Return to assess patient's response to medication. *(Enables you to determine effectiveness of medication and any occurrence of adverse reactions.)*
18. Document assessment in nursing notes.

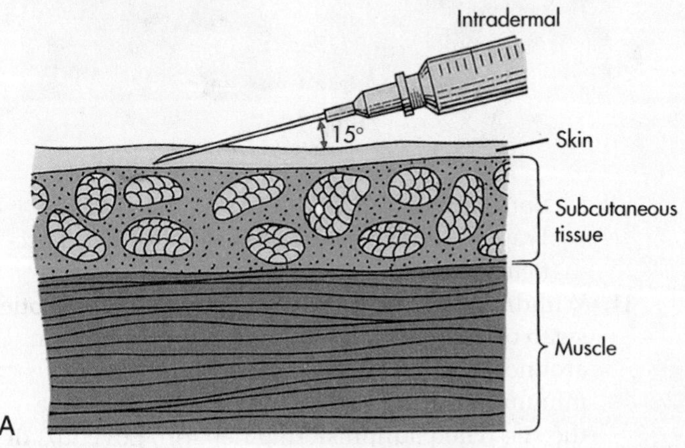

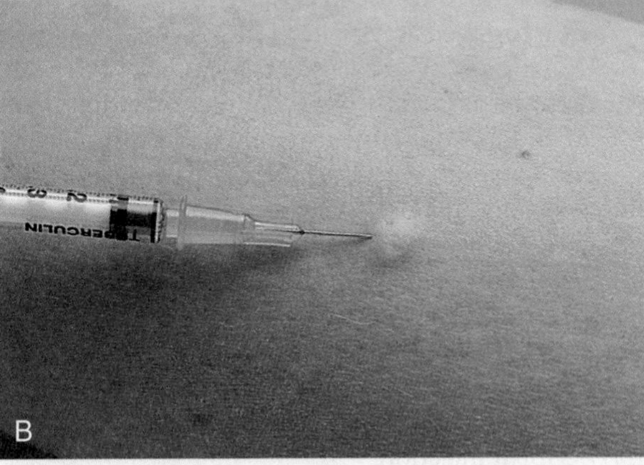

Step 11

will be injected into subcutaneous tissue and not muscle tissue. Usual needle length is ½ to ⅝ inch, and a 25-gauge needle is the one of choice (Figure 23-21 and Skill 23-17).

Intravenous Therapy

The IV route of administration has become a more frequently used one as nurses assume more responsibility in IV therapy. Advances in technology of IV equipment also enable nurses and physicians to deliver IV fluids and medications more safely.

The IV route serves to (1) provide fluid and electrolyte maintenance, restoration, and replacement; (2) administer medications and nutritional feedings; (3) administer blood and blood products; (4) administer chemotherapy to cancer patients; (5) administer patient-controlled analgesics; and (6) keep a vein open for quick access.

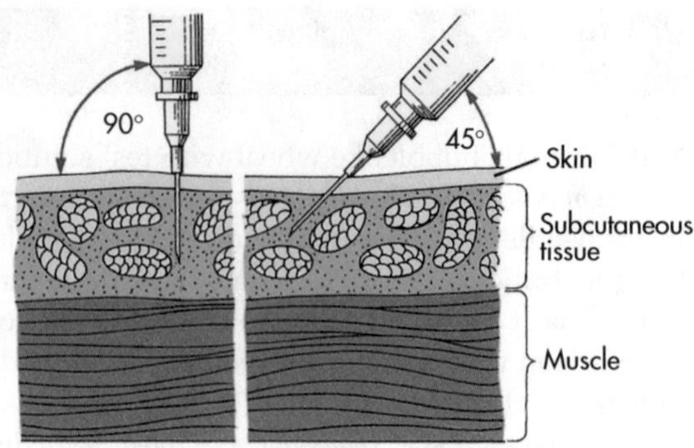

FIGURE 23-21 Subcutaneous injection. Angle and needle length depend on thickness of the skinfold.

Methods of Intravenous Administration

IV medications are possible to administer by several methods.

IV push. Give the medication directly into a vein or by means of a heparin or saline lock or injection port of an existing IV tubing set.

Intermittent venous access device. An intermittent venous access device (commonly called a heparin or saline lock) is an IV infusion device with male adapters covered by rubber diaphragms for the administration of intermittent infusions and as an access site for emergency drugs (see Figure 23-9, *D* and *E*). Intermittent venous access devices provide ready access for IV antibiotic therapy and other IV drug therapies without causing the unnecessary pain of a restick with every dose. They have revolutionized IV therapy. They also come into use in a wide variety of diagnostic tests. An

Skill 23-17 Giving a Subcutaneous Injection

Nursing Action *(Rationale)*

1. Follow the six rights (see Box 23-5). *(Prevents medication errors.)*
2. Perform the three label checks (see Box 23-6). *(Prevents medication errors.)*
3. Follow standard precautions (see Chapter 12, Box 12-5). *(Prevents spread of microorganisms.)*
4. Perform hand hygiene. *(Prevents spread of microorganisms.)*
5. Prepare medication according to standard procedure for injectables (see Skill 23-13).
6. Don gloves. *(Prevents spread of microorganisms.)*
7. Identify patient by checking identification bracelet and asking patient's name and birth date. *(Prevents medication errors.)*
8. Select and expose site (check which site was used previously and rotate site). The abdomen is the usual preferred site when administering heparin, Lovenox, or Fragmin.
9. Clean site with an alcohol swab from center outward in circular motion; let dry. *(Mechanical and chemical action removes microorganisms.)*
10. Perform injection:
    a. **Method A: Thin patient or child:** Spread skin of selected site taut and hold firmly; insert needle at 45-degree angle and aspirate. *(Angle ensures that medication reaches subcutaneous tissue rather than muscle.)* Inject medication slowly. Do not aspirate if giving heparin, Lovenox, or Fragmin (see illustration). *(Slow injection reduces pain and trauma.)*
    b. **Method B: Average size or obese patient:** Grasp and press together skin of selected site so that it forms roll between fingers. Insert needle at a 90-degree angle and aspirate. Do not aspirate if giving heparin, Lovenox, or Fragmin. Inject medication slowly. *(Slow injection reduces pain and trauma.)*

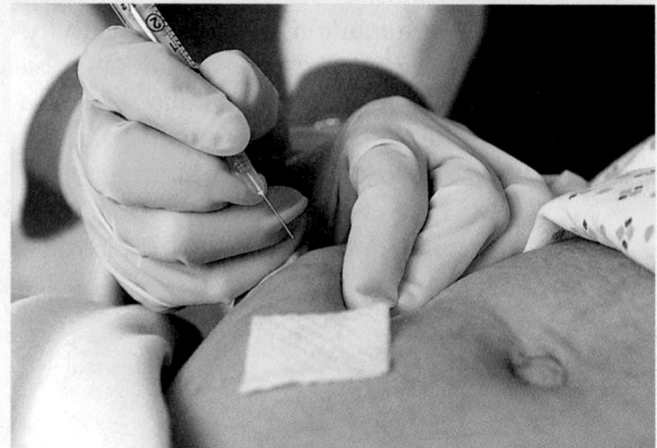
Step **10a**

11. Withdraw needle quickly, and apply an antiseptic swab or a 2 × 2 gauze sponge. Supporting skin around injection site keeps discomfort to a minimum during withdrawal. Do not massage the site when administering heparin, Lovenox, or Fragmin. *(Massage will increase local bleeding, and ecchymosis will occur.)*
12. Do not recap needle; discard directly into sharps container. *(Prevents needlesticks.)*
13. Remove gloves and wash hands. *(Prevents spread of microorganisms.)*
14. Chart site used and amount and type of medication.
15. Return to assess patient's response to medication. *(Enables you to determine effectiveness of medication and any occurrence of adverse reactions.)*
16. Document assessment in nursing notes.

RN or an LPN/LVN who is certified in IV therapy performs the procedure, depending on the nurse practice act for each state.

Intermittent venous access devices attach onto a needleless hub. Once attached, the intermittent venous access device is filled with the anticoagulant heparin or normal saline. This keeps the vein open and makes it possible to administer IV medication at intervals without requiring a continuous infusion of fluid to ensure patency.

The intermittent venous access device prevents the mixing of incompatible drugs or fluids. Practitioners continue to have unanswered questions regarding the best solution to maintain the patency of intermittent infusion devices (heparin versus saline flushes). It is now widely accepted that normal saline is as effective as heparin as a flush for intermittent infusion devices.

Intermittent infusion (or piggyback). IV piggybacks (IVPBs) are drug infusions that are given at intervals, such as qid (four times a day). It is possible to connect them either to heparin or saline locks or to the injection port of the IV tubing (see Figure 23-22, *C* and *D*). Once the medication has infused, you will remove the piggyback from the heparin or saline lock or IV tubing. This is a common way to administer antibiotics.

Continuous infusions. Medication is added to a bag of IV fluid and infuses over the same period as the IV fluid.

Electronic pumps and controllers. Pumps and controllers regulate the flow rate of infusions. Pumps deliver the fluid via pressure whereas controllers deliver the infusion with the aid of gravity. Controllers monitor the flow rate of fluid by a photoelectric eye (see Figure 23-22, *A* and *B*).

Patient-controlled analgesia. Patient-controlled analgesia (PCA) is a drug-delivery system that dispenses a preset IV dose of an opioid analgesic into a patient's vein when the patient pushes a switch on an electric cord (Figure 23-23). It is administered by a programmable pump that the patient controls. The RN programs the pump according to the physician's order, which specifies the amount of an opioid the patient receives per dose. The pump also controls the total amount of drug that it is possible to receive over a specific period. A lockout interval device automatically inactivates the system if a patient tries to increase the amount of an opioid within a preset time period.

You are responsible for programming the computerized pump and for loading the vial of morphine, Fentanyl, Dilaudid, or Buprenex into it. You are responsible to do the following:

- Instruct patients to press or release button when analgesia is needed. (Have patients demonstrate or verbalize understanding.) Reassure them that they will not receive too much medication.
- Maintain PCA therapy:
  —Monitor number of doses received by patient
  —Monitor respirations and blood pressure of patient for signs of oversedation

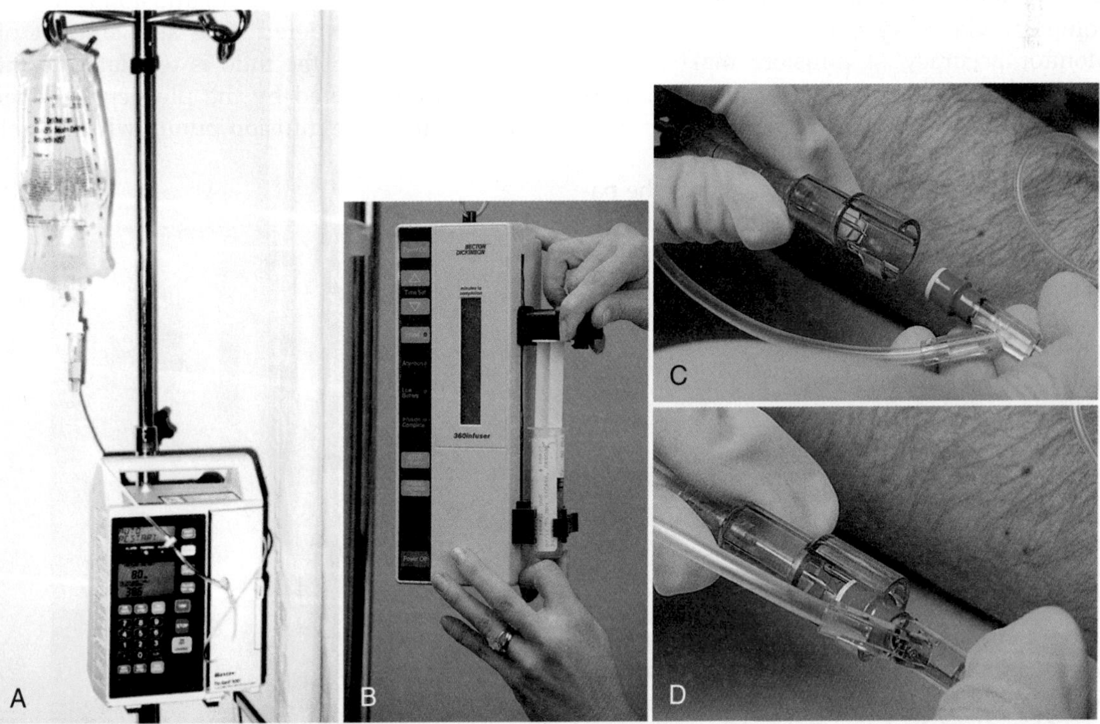

FIGURE 23-22 Intravenous therapy. **A,** IV fluid container attached to an electronic infusion pump. **B,** A flow rate controller device. These devices are attached to the IV system to mechanically control and maintain a precise rate of flow. If the pump or controller alarm sounds, the nurse will attend to the device. **C** and **D,** Injection port of IV tubing is used for drug infusion.

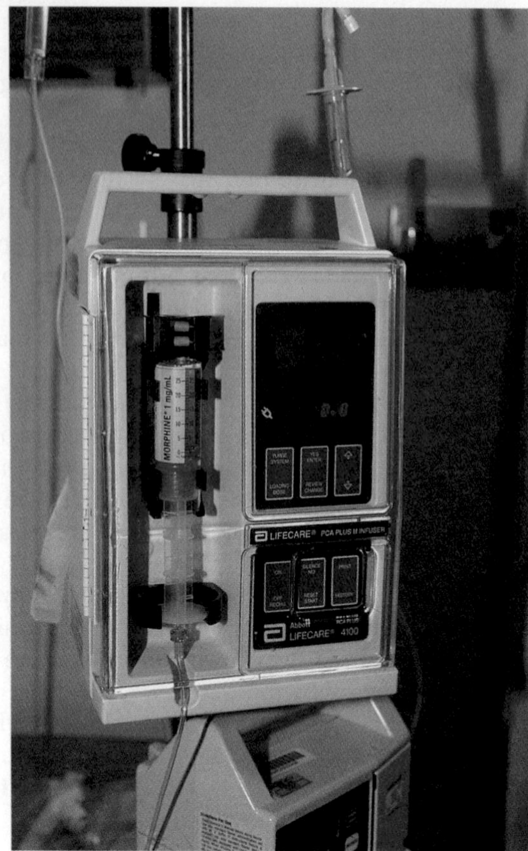

FIGURE 23-23 PCA infusion pump.

—Monitor patient for relief of pain (if possible, always use pain assessment scale)
—Document total volume infused and remaining volume in vial every shift
—Monitor accuracy of infusion; make certain that the opioid antagonist naloxone (Narcan) is readily available to use if physician orders

- Lock the machine.
- Do not let others administer doses unless the patient is not able to push the button and clearly communicates that a dose is needed and wanted.

Two RNs are needed to verify the PCA pump settings against the order. Check the patient's name, the drug, route, and concentration, dose volume limits; lockout interval and frequency; and 4-hour limit. Recheck settings every time the syringe, the parameters, or the caregiver changes.

Meperidine (Demerol) is not recommended for administration via PCA because it has neurotoxic potential (Pullen, 2003).

PCA medication infusion is considered by many to provide more pain relief with less medication. Also, the patient is more in control of medication administration, which often helps lessen anxiety and pain. The PCA is an effective and efficient method for administration of analgesic medications. Dose rates and limits are programmed according to physician's orders, and the patient self-administers the medication by pressing a button.

Special PCA order sheets are used by the physician to specify the following:

1. Type and strength of medication
   EXAMPLE: Morphine sulfate 1 mg/mL
2. Loading dose (an optional larger-than-usual dose to give initial pain relief)
   EXAMPLE: Range: 1 to 5 mL
   Usual: 1 to 2 mL
3. Maintenance dose (dose dispensed each time patient presses control button)
   EXAMPLE: Range: 0.1 to 5 mL
   Usual: 0.5 to 1 mL
4. Lockout interval (minimum time between doses)
   EXAMPLE: Range: 5 to 99 minutes
   Usual: 6 to 15 minutes
5. Four-hour limit (maximum volume delivered in 4 hours)
   EXAMPLE: Range: 5 to 30 mL in 5-mL increments
   Usual: 10 to 20 mL

Volumetric chambers. A volumetric chamber consists of IV tubing with a chamber that holds a prescribed amount of fluid; it is separate from the drip chamber. Medication such as oxytocin (Pitocin) or lidocaine is possible to add to the fluid in the chamber. Careful control over the delivery of the medication to the patient is possible when this method is used (Figure 23-24).

Nursing Responsibility

The physician orders the amount and type of IV fluid and length of time that the infusion is to run. You ensure that the ordered type and amount of fluid is started and that the fluid is regulated to infuse over the period ordered by the physician. Generally you will be using an infusion pump, which eliminates the

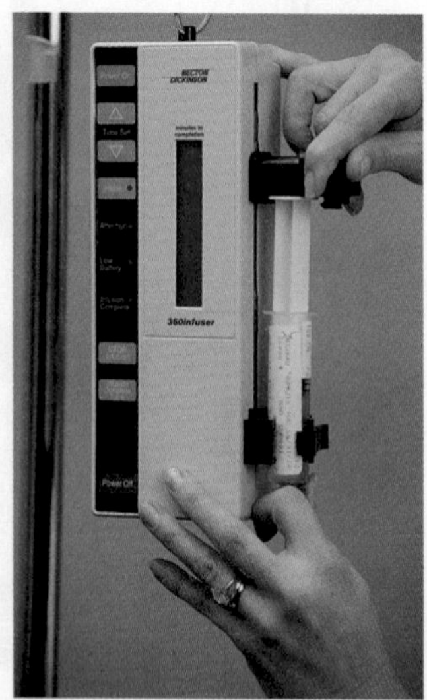

FIGURE 23-24 Volumetric chamber.

need to count drops. However, if you are not using an electronic infusion pump, you will regulate the IV infusion by knowing the number of drops per minute that it will take for the entire volume of fluid to infuse over the specified time ordered by the physician.

To find the number of drops per minute (the **drip rate**), you need to know which type of IV tubing will be used with the infusion. Look on the IV tubing box for the drip factor (an apparatus that is used to deliver measured amounts of IV solutions of specific flow rates based on the size of drops of the solution). The box will indicate whether the IV tubing is calibrated to deliver macrodrops or microdrops. To change mL to drops to calculate IV flow rates, you need to know the drip factor. Macrodrop sets deliver 10, 15, or 20 drops per 1 mL of fluid; microdrop, or minidrop, sets deliver 60 drops per 1 mL of fluid.

For example, a physician orders 1000 mL of D_5 ½ normal saline (NS) with 20 mEq KCl to be infused over an 8-hour period. How will you know how many drops have to drip from the drip chamber every minute for 8 hours to make the fluid run out in 8 hours? To find drops per minute, change milliliters to drops by multiplying milliliters by the drip factor (on tubing set).

EXAMPLE: 1000 mL (total volume to be infused)
× 15 (drip factor)
5000
1000
15,000 gtt (drops)

Thus 15,000 gtt will drip over 8 hours. Change hours to minutes.

EXAMPLE: $1 \text{ hr} : 60 \text{ min} :: 8 \text{ hr} : x \text{ min}$
$1x = 480$
$x = 480 \text{ min}$

To regulate the infusion, how many drops will have to drip over 1 minute?

EXAMPLE: $15{,}000 \text{ gtt} : 480 \text{ min} :: x \text{ gtt} : 1 \text{ min}$
$480x = 15{,}000$
$x = 15{,}000 \div 480$
$x = 31 \text{ gtt/min}$

The rate of fluid flow is regulated by adjusting the volume control clamp until 31 drops drip from the chamber in 1 minute. In 8 hours, the infusion should be completed as ordered.

EXAMPLE: The physician orders 1000 mL D_5 ¼ NS with 1 ampule of multiple vitamins to be infused over an 8-hour period. The drip factor on the box is 10 drops per 1 mL of fluid. Divide the amount to infuse (1000 ml) by the time (8 hours). This will give the mL/hr.

$$\begin{array}{r} 125 \text{ mL/hour} \\ 8 \text{ hours} \overline{)1000 \text{ mL}} \end{array}$$

To reduce the milliliters per hour to drops per minute, compute the following formula:

$$\frac{\text{Amount} \times \text{Drip factor}}{\text{Time}}$$

$$\frac{125 \text{ (mL) (amount)} \times 10 \text{ (drip factor)}}{60 \text{ sec (time)}}$$

$$\frac{1250}{60} \qquad \begin{array}{r} 20/21 \text{ drops/min} \\ 60 \text{ sec}\overline{)1250} \end{array}$$

ANSWER: 20/21 gtt/min

Most facilities use electronic infusion pumps, which record the volume of the fluid infused. An infusion pump is designed to deliver a measured amount of fluid over a period of time (e.g., mL/hr). The pump has a drop sensor, and an alarm that will sound if drops are not detected at the appropriate rate. There are also alarms to alert you to increased system pressure that can occur with an infiltration (IV seeping into the tissue instead of the vascular space; see Figure 23-22). An accurate intake of all intravenous therapy is recorded.

Monitoring intravenous therapy. Check the infusion and the IV needle site at least every hour, looking at the flow of fluid, which will sometimes be altered or stopped by air in the tubing, kinked tubing, or clotted blood in the tubing. It is necessary to keep the tubing patent (open) to keep the venous site open. If the fluid flow is obstructed or significantly slowed, the needle will become occluded with coagulated blood. You will have to select another IV site and perform another venipuncture. Never allow the tubing to get air in it as a result of an IV bag running dry. If bags are near completion, reporting to the RN or the LPN/LVN is necessary, depending on the state nurse practice act.

Observe the IV site every time you check the infusion, looking for erythema, wetness, and edema. Inflammation often means the onset of phlebitis (inflamed vein), and edema, coolness to touch, pallor, and pain indicates a possible infiltration (the process whereby a fluid passes into the tissues) of fluid into the tissue. Report these conditions to the head nurse. In addition, report the following:

- A patient with sudden onset of chills, fever, headache, nausea, and vomiting
- An anxious, dyspneic patient with a weak and rapid pulse

These factors sometimes indicate complications of IV therapy that require immediate medical intervention.

Allergic reactions are possible as a result of IV medication administration. Reactions range from a mild rash to anaphylactic shock (a severe, life-threatening hypersensitivity reaction). Signs and symptoms sometimes appear suddenly and sometimes appear as long as 30 to 60 minutes after an infusion of an IV medication. Report the following if it occurs:

- Respiratory distress from bronchospasms such as restlessness, dyspnea, wheezing, and cyanosis (bluish coloration of the skin)
- Skin reactions such as pruritus (itching) or urticaria (hives)
- Signs of circulatory collapse, such as rapidly falling blood pressure, weak and rapid (thready) pulse, or vertigo
- GI signs and symptoms such as nausea, vomiting, and diarrhea
- Change in mental status

Anaphylactic shock necessitates immediate intervention. Notify the RN immediately if you or any other staff members observe any allergic signs or symptoms.

 NURSING PROCESS

The role of the licensed practical nurse/licensed vocational nurse (LPN/LVN) in the nursing process as stated is that the LPN/LVN will:

- Participate in planning care for patients based on patient needs
- Review patient's plan of care and recommend revisions as needed
- Review and follow defined prioritization for patient care
- Use clinical pathways, care maps, or care plans to guide and review patient care

Assessment

You will assess many factors to determine the need for and potential response to drug therapy. These factors include the patient's medical history, diet, and allergy history. Also assess the patient's current physical and mental status. Coordination limitations will sometimes interfere with the patient's ability to prepare doses and take medications correctly. Also consider the patient's knowledge and understanding of drug therapy. It is important for you to know as much as possible about each drug given, including normal dosages, purpose, action, routes, side effects, and interaction with other drugs.

Nursing Diagnosis

Use assessment findings to determine actual or potential problems with drug therapy. Certain data reveal nursing diagnoses. These may include the following:

- Anxiety
- Health-seeking behaviors (specify)

Life Span Considerations

Older Adults

Medications and Aging

- All phases of pharmacokinetics are affected by aging. Give older people the lowest dosage of medication necessary to achieve the desired therapeutic benefits.
- Dry mouth often contributes to difficulty swallowing medications. Sipping water before attempting to swallow the medication or covering the medication with a moist food such as applesauce tends to facilitate swallowing.
- It is necessary to take more precautions when administering parenteral medication to older adults because of a decreased amount of muscle and subcutaneous tissue. Examine sites for suitability, and rotate them. Carefully select needles of the proper length based on the selected site and a tissue assessment of the individual.
- Because of decreased tolerance to intravenous (IV) medications, it is necessary to carefully assess the older adult for toxicity.
- Polypharmacy (use of excessive numbers of different medications) is a common problem for older adults. Each medication taken increases the risk of interactions or toxicity. Teach older adults to refrain from taking any medication unless it is approved by the primary physician.
- Teach the older person to keep accurate and current records of all prescription and over-the-counter medications, and to present this list each time the person seeks medical attention.
- Because of decreased renal, cardiac, and hepatic functioning, the older adult is at greater risk of becoming adversely and possibly fatally affected by medications. Also, hospitalized older adults often have one or more chronic illnesses for which they take multiple medications.
- Be aware of and observe for signs and symptoms of decreased drug excretion, cumulative effects of drugs, drug potentiation, and drug incompatibilities. Only by frequent observations and careful, thoughtful assessments of the older patient will you help prevent toxic, lethal, and even fatal effects.
- Some older adults do not hear, see, communicate, or move about as well as younger patients. Some will also be disoriented and perhaps even more so at night; therefore, when you medicate older patients, take more time to carefully assess their level of consciousness beforehand and afterward.
- Carefully observe the list of medications prescribed for each patient, and ascertain whether there have been any incompatibilities or incorrect dosages or whether any medications are possibly adversely affecting the patient.
- Any medication has the potential to cause adverse effects in the older adult, whether it is an antihistamine, an opioid, or any other. Observe carefully and immediately for drug interactions and side effects. Report and document all signs and symptoms you detect. You will often be the first to notice a change in a patient's condition.
- The prevention of drug-related problems is the combined responsibility of the nurse, the physician, the pharmacist, and others who care for the patient. Solid communication between the health care team, the patient, and the patient's family is necessary to safely and effectively medicate the older adult.

- Risk for injury
- Deficient knowledge (specify)
- Impaired physical mobility
- Noncompliance: drug regimen
- Disturbed sensory/perception (specify) (auditory, gustatory, kinesthetic, olfactory, tactile, visual)

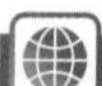

Cultural Considerations

Navajo Indian Medicine Men and Women

- Herbalists are those specialized practitioners who use herbs to treat patients and who may also diagnose illness and causes of ailments.
- Medicine men and medicine women have *jish,* or medicine bundles, containing symbolic and sacred items, including corn pollen, feathers, stones, arrowheads, and other instruments used for healing and blessing.
- Many of these sacred objects and plants are found on the sacred mountains that border the Navajo reservation and are gathered by medicine people.*
- There is a great effort on the part of the Indian Health Service and traditional Navajo healers to work together in a collaborative and cooperative way.
- It is not uncommon to observe a medicine man or medicine woman in the hospital speaking with a physician regarding the care of a patient. When medically indicated, sometimes patients also receive passes to participate in a healing ceremony held outside the hospital.
- There has been a continued and sustained mutual respect on the part of these two groups for the expertise of the other.*

Data from Giger, J., & Davidhizar, R. (2008). *Transcultural nursing assessment and intervention.* (4th ed.). St. Louis: Mosby; and Sanchez, T.R., Plawecki, J.A., & Plawecki, H.M. (1996). The delivery of culturally sensitive health care to Native Americans. *Journal of Holistic Nursing, 14:*295-307.
*Navajo Health Systems Agency. (1985).

Expected Outcomes and Planning

Focus the plan of care on the safe administration of drugs. Use the time during drug administration to teach patients about their medications. Collaborate with the patient's family and significant others about drug regimens after discharge.

The plan of care is likely to include the following goal and outcome:

Goal: Patient and family understand drug therapy.

Outcome: Patient and family describe information about the drug, dosage, schedule, purpose, and adverse effects.

Implementation

Identify factors that have the potential to improve or diminish a patient's health and well-being. Physical limitations, economic status, cultural beliefs, values, and habits tend to influence a patient's compliance with medication schedules (see Cultural Considerations box). You are responsible for knowing about medications and their potential adverse effects on the patient, especially if there are multiple prescriptions. The capabilities and limitations of the older adult are especially important considerations (see Life Span Considerations for Older Adults box).

Evaluation

Use evaluative measures to determine whether patient outcomes were met. Always be prepared to revise the care plan based on the evaluation.

Goal: Patient and family understand drug therapy.

Evaluative measure: Ask patient or family to describe purpose, dosage, and adverse effects of each prescribed medication.

Get Ready for the NCLEX® Examination!

Key Points

- Accurately calculate drug dosages to provide safe medication administration to each patient.
- A ratio shows the relationship of one number or quantity to another number or quantity.
- A proportion shows that the relationship between two ratios has equal value; extremes are the outer terms of the proportion, whereas means are the inner terms of the proportion.
- There is no room for error in calculating dosages; make sure to check math work with another nurse, reduce distractions while working problems, and recheck calculations.
- The metric system is the preferred system of weights and measures; it is more accurate and easier to use in calculating dosage problems.
- Whatever method you use to solve dosage problems, always convert the units of measurement in the problem so they are all the same.
- Age, weight, body surface area, and the ability of the body to absorb, metabolize, and excrete medication are necessary to consider when administering medication to a child.
- It is necessary to be knowledgeable about the four standard formulas for calculating children's dosages: Young's rule, Clark's rule, Fried's rule, and body surface area method.
- When preparing medications, check the medication container label against the medication administration record or computer printout three times.
- The "six rights" of medication administration ensure accurate preparation and administration of medication dosages.
- Only administer medications you prepare.

- Never administer medication without accurately identifying the patient by room number, bed, patient's name, and birth date.
- Chart medications immediately after administration.
- Never leave a prepared medication unattended.
- Failure to select injection sites by anatomical landmarks poses the risk of tissue, bone, or nerve damage.
- You are ethically and legally responsible for ensuring that the patient receives the correct medication ordered by the physician.
- Each medication order is required to include the patient's name and date of birth; order; date; medication name, dosage, route, and frequency of administration; and physician's signature.
- Always have a witness to the "wasting" (disposal) of a controlled substance or medication, and make sure both persons sign the log book to indicate that the medication was wasted.
- Medications enter the body through oral, sublingual, buccal, parenteral, percutaneous, inhalation, and topical (skin and mucous membranes) routes.
- Medications administered parenterally are absorbed more quickly than medications administered by other routes.
- The Z-track method for intramuscular injections (such as iron preparations) minimizes irritation and prevents discoloration of tissue by sealing the medication in muscle tissue.
- Intramuscular injections for analgesia are given less frequently these days because of the use of PCA and PCE pumps.
- You will give intradermal injections for skin testing (e.g., tuberculin screening and allergy tests).
- Because of decreased renal, cardiac, or hepatic functioning, the older adult is at greater risk of becoming adversely and possibly fatally affected by medications.

Additional Resources

Go to your Companion CD for an audio glossary, animations, video clips, and more.

evolve Be sure to visit the Evolve site at http://evolve.elsevier.com/Christensen/foundations/ for additional online resources.

Review Questions for the NCLEX® Examination

Work the following problems. Use the proportion method or desired dose/available dose formula, key equivalents, and the big to small rule.

1. The physician has ordered 0.5 g of ceftriaxone (Rocephin). The nurse has available a vial labeled 250 mg/mL. How many mL will the nurse give the patient?
   1. 2 mL
   2. 0.2 mL
   3. 0.05 mL
   4. 0.5 mL

2. Digoxin (Lanoxin) 0.125 mg is ordered. On hand is Lanoxin 0.5 mg/mL. How many mL will the nurse give?
   1. 3 mL
   2. 0.25 mL
   3. 2.5 mL
   4. 0.025 mL

3. The patient's mother is to give her child 6 mL of a liquid medication. Her only measuring tool in her new apartment is a teaspoon. How many teaspoons of the medication will she give?
   1. 1 tsp
   2. 2 tsp
   3. 3 tsp
   4. ½ tsp

4. The pediatrician has requested the pediatric patient's weight in kilograms. The scales say that the patient weighs 30 lb. How many kilograms will be reported to the physician?
   1. 20.6 kg
   2. 15 kg
   3. 13.6 kg
   4. 22 kg

For questions 5 through 7, use the proportion method. Multiply milliliters by the drip factor to convert milliliters to drops.

5. Ordered is 1 L of D_5 ½ NS to run over 8 hours. The drip factor stated on the IV tubing is 15 gtt/mL. How many milliliters will be infused every hour?
   1. 100 mL/hr
   2. 125 mL/hr
   3. 150 mL/hr
   4. 175 mL/hr

6. An IV of 1 L of D_5 ½ NS is to run at 150 mL/hr. How long will this IV run?
   1. 6 hours
   2. 6.6 hours
   3. 7.5 hours
   4. 8 hours

7. At 1500, an 8-hour bag of 1 L D_5 LR (lactated Ringer's), which was started at 0900, has 100 mL left in it. Does this infusion have to run slower or faster, or is it running at the correct rate?
   1. Has to infuse slower
   2. Has to infuse faster
   3. Is at the correct rate
   4. Has to be discontinued

8. Which intramuscular injection site is no longer recommended to be used because of the nearness of the sciatic nerve to the muscle and potential for permanent or partial paralysis of the involved leg?
   1. Ventrogluteal site
   2. Deltoid site
   3. Vastus lateralis site
   4. Dorsogluteal site

9. The physician ordered 125 mg of acetaminophen (Tylenol) for a 2-month-old infant who weighs 10 pounds. Is this appropriate (the average adult dose of Tylenol is 500 mg)?

1. It is appropriate.
2. It is a little too much.
3. It is an extreme overdose.
4. It is not enough.

10. The average dose of a medication is 0.4 mg (gr 1⁄150) for an adult. What is the dosage for a 12-year-old?

1. 2 mg
2. 0.002 mg
3. 0.02 mg
4. 0.2 mg

11. An adult dose of diazepam (Valium) is 5 mg. How many mL is appropriate for a child who weighs 27 kg?

1. 2 mg
2. 1.5 mg
3. 3 mg
4. 2.5 mg

12. A 71-year-old patient with hypertension, heart failure (HF), anxiety, and a productive cough is to receive his medications at 8 AM daily. Which medication will be given last?

1. Lasix tablet
2. Coreg tablet
3. Robitussin cough syrup
4. Paxil tablet

13. The LPN is asked by an RN to take an unlabeled container of solution to the operating room. The LPN's best response is to say:

1. "Of course, I'll take it right away!"
2. "What is in the container?"
3. "I will have the orderly take it."
4. "I am not permitted to transport an unlabeled container."

14. After a possible exposure to tuberculosis, a 25-year-old health worker receives a TB skin test. The skin test will be given by the following type of injection:

1. Intramuscular
2. Intradermal
3. Subcutaneous
4. Intravenous

15. The physician orders vitamin B_{12} IM for a 70-year-old with a history of pernicious anemia. The nurse is choosing from the following gauges of needles. Which one is most appropriate?

1. 22-gauge
2. 25-gauge
3. 18-gauge
4. 16-gauge

16. Insulin is to be given to a well-nourished 55-year-old man admitted for diabetes mellitus. His insulin is to be given via subcutaneous injection. What angle is acceptable for the injection?

1. 45 degrees
2. 90 degrees
3. 15 degrees only
4. 35 degrees only

17. The nurse is deciding on the angle used in delivering subcutaneous heparin. The decision will be based on the:

1. amount of solution in the syringe.
2. length and the gauge of the needle.
3. amount of subcutaneous tissue of the patient.
4. needle length and the amount of subcutaneous tissue available.

18. The patient complains of nausea after having a total abdominal hysterectomy. The nurse prepares an injection of promethazine (Phenergan) 25 mg for IM injection and selects a needle length of:

1. 1 to 1½ inches
2. 3⁄8 inch
3. 5⁄8 inch
4. ¼ inch

19. A 6-month-old is to be immunized for diphtheria, tetanus, and pertussis. His IM injection will be given in which muscle?

1. Deltoid
2. Ventrogluteal
3. Gluteus maximus
4. Vastus lateralis

20. Epinephrine contained in 0.3 mL is ordered for an 18-year-old who had an anaphylactic reaction to a bee sting. Which syringe is the best choice for delivering this volume of fluid?

1. 1-mL tuberculin syringe
2. 100 units per 1-mL syringe
3. 3-mL syringe
4. 5-mL syringe

21. A 96-year-old nursing home resident is to receive several medications at 2100. These medications are for emphysema, peripheral vascular disease, and heart failure. The nurse realizes that the dosages for an older adult are:

1. the same as for pediatric patients.
2. the same as average adult dosages.
3. higher than average adult dosages.
4. lower than average adult dosages.

22. When obtaining information about a specific drug, what book is published annually and contains information from drug manufacturers?

1. *Nurse's Drug Handbook*
2. *Drug Facts and Comparisons Guide*
3. *Physicians' Desk Reference (PDR)*
4. *Pharmacy Policy Manual*

23. What is the acceptable time range to administer an 8 AM medication?
   1. 0800 to 1000
   2. 0700 to 0900
   3. 0800 to 0830
   4. 0730 to 0830

24. What is true regarding nursing responsibilities with controlled substances?
   1. Medications that have a high degree of addiction or abuse are double-locked.
   2. It is the nurse's responsibility to count all controlled substances between shifts.
   3. If another nurse is not available when you are discarding an unused portion of a controlled substance, it is acceptable to tell the other nurse about it later or have the other nurse co-sign.
   4. Only statements 1 and 2 are true.
   5. Statements 1, 2, and 3 are true.

25. Documentation of medication administration is extremely important. What information will the nurse include in the documentation? *(Choose all that apply.)*
   1. Drug name, dose, and time of administration
   2. Patient's response to all prn medications
   3. Location of intramuscular injections
   4. All of the above

26. The first action to take when a medication error takes place is to:
   1. call the physician.
   2. call the supervisor.
   3. complete an incident report.
   4. check the patient.

27. If a medication is ordered orally, and the patient is NPO (nothing by mouth), which action does the nurse take?
   1. Give the medication by injection.
   2. Give the medication rectally.
   3. Omit the medication and note on chart.
   4. Consult the nurse in charge.

28. The physician orders 1 g of kanamycin sulfate po every 6 hours for a 60-year-old hospitalized patient. The patient's last dose of kanamycin was at 0600. The nurse in this situation is legally responsible for: *(Choose all that apply.)*
   1. administering 1 g of kanamycin by mouth to the patient at noon.
   2. knowing the expected action and average dose of kanamycin and the reason that the patient is receiving the drug.
   3. discontinuing the kanamycin if the patient complains of nausea.
   4. documenting the administration of kanamycin and evaluating the therapeutic effect.

29. When reading a medication label, the nurse should: *(Choose all that apply.)*
   1. check the expiration date.
   2. compare the medication order with the label.
   3. read the label when removing the medication from the container.
   4. request a second nurse to check dosage on label.

30. The physician writes the order for oxycodone (Roxicodone) one or two tablets orally q 3-4 hr prn for pain. How will the nurse interpret this order?
   1. Administer the Roxicodone every 3 to 4 hours around the clock.
   2. Administer the Roxicodone whenever the patient asks for it, because it is prn.
   3. Administer the Roxicodone only if the patient asks for it.
   4. Inform the patient that the medication is available to take every 3 to 4 hours as needed for pain.

31. Prescribed medications are prepared and administered during which phase of the nursing process?
   1. Assessment
   2. Planning
   3. Implementation
   4. Evaluation

32. A patient hospitalized with newly diagnosed hypertension is on enalapril (Vasotec) 5 mg po bid. His next dose is at 0900. When taking his vital signs, the nurse discovers the patient's blood pressure is 90/42. What should the nurse do?
   1. Hold the medication and inform the physician of a change in the patient's blood pressure.
   2. Give the medication on time (the blood pressure is within normal limits).
   3. Ask the patient how he is feeling; if he is not having adverse signs or symptoms of low blood pressure, give him the medication.
   4. Give half the dose ordered.

chapter 24

Emergency First Aid Nursing

Barbara Lauritsen Christensen and Cynthia Steury-Lattz

evolve

http://evolve.elsevier.com/Christensen/foundationsadult

Objectives

1. List the priorities of assessment to be performed when arriving at a situation where first aid is necessary.
2. Discuss moral, legal, and physical interventions involved in performing first aid.
3. List the reasons for performing cardiopulmonary resuscitation (CPR).
4. Discuss the legal implications of CPR.
5. List the steps in performing one-rescuer and two-rescuer CPR on an adult victim.
6. List the steps in performing CPR on an infant or child.
7. Name the steps in performing the abdominal thrusts on conscious and unconscious victims and pregnant victims.
8. Discuss management of airway obstruction in a child and an infant.
9. Discuss the signs and symptoms of shock.
10. List nursing interventions to treat shock.
11. Discuss three methods of controlling hemorrhage.
12. Discuss the five general types of open wounds: abrasions, incisions, lacerations, punctures, and avulsions.
13. Discuss treatment of wounds.
14. Discuss methods of treating four common types of poisonings.
15. List the characteristics of assessment of bone, joint, and muscle injuries.
16. Discuss emergency care for suspected injuries.
17. Define three types of burns.
18. Discuss the nursing interventions in the first aid treatment of burns.
19. Describe the nursing interventions of heat and cold emergencies.
20. Discuss features that should alert you to the possibility of a bioterrorism-related outbreak.
21. Discuss high-risk syndromes of bioterrorism.

Key Terms

ABCs (p. 740)
air embolism (ĔM-bŏ-lĭzm, p. 748)
biologic death (p. 739)
bioterrorism (p. 761)
brain death (p. 739)
cardiac arrest (p. 741)
cardiopulmonary resuscitation (CPR) (kăr-dē-ō-PŬL-mō-nă-rē rē-sŭs-ĭ-TĀ-shŭn, p. 738)
clinical death (p. 739)
contusions (kŏn-TŪ-zhŭnz, p. 750)
crepitus (KRĔP-ĭ-tŭs, p. 758)
cyanosis (sī-ă-NŌ-sĭs, p. 746)
ecchymoses (ĕk-ĭ-MŌ-sēz, p. 750)
emergency medical services (EMS) (p. 737)
endemic (ĕn-DĔM-ĭk, p. 761)
epidemic (ĕp-ĭ-DĔM-ĭk, p. 761)
epistaxis (ĕp-ĭ-STĂK-sĭs, p. 749)
epistaxis digitorum (ĕp-ĭ-STĂK-sĭs dĭj-ĭ-TŎR-ŭm, p. 749)
flail chest (p. 752)
Good Samaritan laws (p. 738)
hematemesis (hē-mă-TĔM-ĕ-sĭs, p. 750)
hematuria (hē-mă-TŪ-rē-ă, p. 750)
hemoptysis (hē-MŎP-tĭ-sĭs, p. 750)
hemothorax (hē-mō-THŌ-răks, p. 751)
melena (MĔL-ĕ-nă, p. 750)
oliguria (ŏl-ĭ-GŪ-rē-ă, p. 747)
pleural space (PLŪR-ăl spās, p. 751)
pneumothorax (nū-mō-THŌ-răks, p. 751)
shock (p. 746)
stridor (STRĪ-dŏr, p. 745)
tachycardia (tăk-ĕ-KĂR-dē-ă, p. 747)
terrorism (p. 761)
tetanus toxoid (TĔT-ă-nŭs TŎKS-ŏyd, p. 750)
triage (TRĒ-ăhzh, p. 738)

First aid is the immediate, **temporary** assistance given to a person who is injured or has become ill. First aid includes assessing the victim for life-threatening conditions, performing appropriate interventions to sustain life, and keeping the person in the best possible physical and mental condition until the assistance of emergency medical services (EMS) (a national network of services that provides coordinated aid and medical assistance from primary response to definitive care) is obtained. It is important to remember that first aid does not replace medical care but is used to preserve life until medical help is obtained. Because minutes are precious in preventing permanent disability and injury, be prepared to handle emergency conditions and administer first aid. In the case of multiple injuries, survey patients quickly for severity of injuries so you are able to treat life-threatening problems first. This process of classifying a group of patients according to the severity of injury and need of care is called triage. The triage process is based on the premise that it is important to treat patients who have a threat to life, vision, or limb before other patients. In disaster medicine, triage is a process in which a large group of patients is sorted so it is possible to concentrate care and resources on those who are likely to survive.

OBTAINING MEDICAL EMERGENCY AID

Your ability to recognize the need for medical assistance and knowledge of how to obtain medical emergency aid will sometimes mean the difference between life and death to an injured or ill person. It is important to know the right phone number to call, both in the community and in the institutional setting. In most communities the emergency medical number is 911; however, numbers for the fire department, the police department, or the local hospital will be the most correct number to call for assistance in some localities. Box 24-1 provides information to convey when calling in a medical emergency from the community.

It is essential that health care providers be prepared to provide cardiopulmonary resuscitation (CPR) (basic emergency procedure for life support) if needed until emergency medical assistance arrives. All health care providers need to maintain CPR certification. Most health care institutions provide training. CPR certification is also available from local fire departments and local chapters of the American Red Cross and the American Heart Association.

The guidelines for administering CPR undergo periodic review and are subject to change. This chapter discusses CPR based on the most current guidelines provided by the American Heart Association at the time of this text's publication.

Box 24-1 Information to Convey in a Medical Emergency

1. Name of the person making the call
2. Location of the emergency
3. What has happened (either by direct observation or by gathering data from others)
4. Report whether an immediate threat still exists such as a fire, flood, or physical threat by someone else such as use of a gun or knife
5. Number of people who need assistance
6. The victim's or victims' name(s) and age(s)
7. Obvious injuries and the victim's or victims' apparent condition
8. First aid measures that have already been administered
9. Presence of medical-alert bracelet or any known history
10. The physical characteristics of the rescue (stairs, elevators)

NOTE: Always hang up when instructed to do so by the emergency services operator.

MORAL AND LEGAL RESPONSIBILITIES OF THE NURSE

Good Samaritan laws (legal stipulation for protection of those who give first aid in an emergency situation) have been enacted in most states to protect health professionals from legal liability when providing emergency first aid. If you follow a reasonable and prudent course of action, the chances of legal problems are very small. The licensed practical nurse (LPN) or licensed vocational nurse (LVN) is obliged to obtain permission to treat any patient, even in an emergency situation. Before you administer first aid, obtain verbal permission from the victim; the victim also has the right to refuse first aid. The law assumes consent from an unconscious person. After you have initiated first aid, there is a moral and legal obligation to continue the aid until someone with comparable or better training is able to care for the victim; for example, an emergency medical technician (EMT) or a physician will perhaps arrive at the scene and take over the first aid care of the victim.

ASSESSMENT OF THE EMERGENCY SITUATION

Assessment of life-threatening problems is the first priority in an emergency situation. Sometimes you will need someone to help to care for victims of some injuries or illnesses, or to call EMS. If necessary, shout several times to get someone's attention, or call 911 or another emergency number. Not all areas use the 911 system. While seeking help, continue the primary survey by assessing for (1) an open airway, (2) breathing, and (3) circulation (pulse and severe bleeding). This is known as assessing for the ABCs (discussed later in the chapter). An immediate life-threatening situation of highest priority is arrested or abnormal breathing. To assess whether the victim is breathing properly, open the airway with a head-tilt/chin-lift maneuver unless you suspect neck injury. If you suspect cervical spine injury, use a jaw thrust without head tilt to open the airway. Use caution not to move the neck out of proper alignment. Never use hyperextension of the head and neck to establish an airway because of the potential for causing or exacerbating a cervical spine injury.

Determine whether the chest is rising, listen for breath sounds, and place your cheek near the victim's mouth to feel the passage of air from the victim's breathing. Assess rhythm, depth, and rate of respirations. The following are signs that the victim is having problems breathing: cyanosis, gasping, wheezing, stridor, and snoring.

An arrested or abnormal pulse is also a life-threatening situation. Assess the rate, rhythm, and strength of the carotid pulse for no longer than 10 seconds. It is important to observe for signs of external bleeding and internal bleeding, which potentially lead to shock. Monitor the person's skin color, temperature, pupil reaction, pulse, and respiration. Poisonings are also life threatening. Observe for burns or stains in and around the person's mouth or hands. Depressed respirations and circulatory collapse are other possible results of poisoning.

After the initial assessment for life-threatening problems, observe the victim for indications of skull injury and brain or spinal cord damage, which call for attention as soon as possible. Decreasing level of consciousness, abnormal pupil reaction, and lack of movement in the arms or the legs indicates possible injury to the head or spinal cord. Attend to fractures, dislocations, and superficial ecchymoses or wounds after treating the more serious conditions.

CARDIOPULMONARY RESUSCITATION (CPR)

ETHICAL IMPLICATIONS

Reasons that individuals choose not to become involved in performing CPR include (1) lack of motivation, (2) fear of doing harm, (3) lack of knowledge, and (4) fear of contracting communicable diseases. However, once you or anyone else starts CPR, do not discontinue it *except* for the following reasons:

- The victim recovers.
- The rescuer is exhausted and is not able to continue CPR.
- Trained medical personnel arrive on the scene and take over CPR.
- A licensed physician arrives on the scene, pronounces the victim dead, and orders CPR to be discontinued.

When you as an LPN/LVN are providing emergency care to a patient, stay with the patient until care is assumed by a registered nurse (RN), physician, or emergency medical personnel.

EVENTS NECESSITATING CPR

Many situations require resuscitation efforts (Box 24-2). CPR is indicated in any syndrome in which respiration or respiration and circulation are absent. There are two purposes of CPR:

1. To keep the lungs supplied with oxygen when breathing has stopped
2. To keep the blood circulating and carrying oxygen to the brain, the heart, and other parts of the body

Clinical death means that heartbeat and respiration have ceased. **Biologic death** results from permanent cellular damage caused by lack of oxygen. The brain is the first organ to suffer from this lack of oxygen. If initiated before 4 minutes of cardiopulmonary arrest have elapsed, in many cases CPR holds the promise of reversing clinical death. After 10 minutes without CPR, brain death is certain. Therefore it is extremely important that CPR is begun as quickly as possible. **Brain death** is an irreversible form of unconsciousness characterized by a complete loss of brain function

Box 24-2 Events Necessitating Cardiopulmonary Resuscitation

- **Cardiac arrest.** The most common cause of cardiac arrest is myocardial infarction (MI). In addition, shock from hemorrhage, trauma to the heart, respiratory arrest, and drugs have potential to precipitate a cardiac arrest.
- **Drowning.** Children are common victims of drowning and boating accidents. People using alcohol or other drugs near bodies of water are often victims of drowning. It is important to note that near-drowning victims sometimes recover completely after long periods of submersion. The low water temperature that produces hypothermia reduces the metabolic rate and decreases oxygen demands. Because of this, it is necessary to initiate cardiopulmonary resuscitation (CPR) even when 4 to 6 minutes are known to have elapsed.
- **Electrical shock.** People who come near sources of high-voltage electricity run the risk of accidental electrocution. Electrical shock will sometimes paralyze the breathing muscles and cause cardiac arrest by interfering with the normal rhythm of the heart. It is essential for the rescuer who is initiating CPR to be careful not to inadvertently come into contact with the electric current. The rescuer needs to ensure that the current is de-energized before beginning CPR.
- **Anaphylactic reaction.** Exposure to a known allergen (e.g., food, poisons, drugs) or an insect bite has the capacity to produce the severe allergic reaction known as anaphylaxis. This reaction often causes spasms or edema of the upper airway and will in some cases progress to cardiovascular collapse. CPR is necessary to initiate immediately, as with any other emergency situation.
- **Asphyxiation.** Asphyxiation or suffocation caused by inhaling a gas other than oxygen is possible as a result of fires, chemical spills, or gas leaks. In addition, children and adults will sometimes suffer respiratory arrest and ultimately cardiac arrest from choking on food or small objects that are placed in the mouth. Abdominal thrusts and CPR are performed in this instance.
- **Drug overdose.** Intentional or accidental abuse of alcohol and drugs pose a risk of respiratory and cardiac arrest. Besides treating this as a poisoning emergency, perform CPR as necessary.
- **Sudden infant death syndrome (SIDS).** SIDS is the unexpected and sudden death of an apparently normal and healthy infant that occurs during sleep and with no evidence of disease on physical examination or autopsy. Readiness to perform early CPR and home monitoring systems to detect prolonged apnea are aspects of prevention.

while the heart continues to beat. The legal definition of this condition varies from state to state. The usual clinical criteria for brain death include the absence of reflex activity, movements, and respiration. The pupils are dilated and fixed. Because hypothermia, anesthesia, poisoning, or drug intoxication have the capacity to cause a deep physiologic depression that resembles brain death, a diagnosis of brain death requires that the electrical activity of the brain be evaluated and shown to be absent on two electroencephalograms performed 12 to 24 hours apart. Cerebral blood flow studies are permitted in some states to evaluate whether brain death has occurred. Brain death is also called **irreversible coma.**

INITIAL ASSESSMENT AND RESPONSE

The initial assessment task when determining the need for CPR is to determine responsiveness. Do this by gently shaking the victim and shouting, "Are you OK?" This precaution will prevent you from injuring a person who is alert but sleeping. "OK" is a word that is understandable in any language.

Immediately call for help when beginning a rescue. It is imperative to access the EMS as quickly as possible. Shouting for help, directing another person to make a telephone call, or making the call oneself is recommended. It is vitally important to obtain an automatic external defibrillator (AED) if there is one available. Return to the victim, and immediately begin CPR and use the AED to treat defibrillation if it is required.

For the most successful treatment of cardiac arrest, it is best to start CPR as well as the use of an AED within the first 3 to 5 minutes. AEDs are available in numerous nonhospital settings such as airports, schools, and business locations for use by laypersons who witness an incidence of cardiac arrest (Figure 24-1). Basic life support education for health care providers as well as non–health care providers will include instruction in CPR as well as how to use an AED.

THE ABCs OF CPR

To remember the steps of one- or two-rescuer CPR, remember the ABCs, a mnemonic for assessing status of emergency patients:

Airway
Breathing
Circulation

Airway

Assess the victim's airway to confirm the absence of breathing and to establish a patent airway. If there is no evidence of head or neck trauma, use the head-tilt/chin-lift maneuver to open the airway. This method consists of placing one hand on the victim's forehead and applying firm backward pressure to tilt the head back. Place the fingers of the other hand under the jaw (avoiding the soft tissue under the chin) to lift the chin forward (Figure 24-2).

CAUTION: If a neck injury is suspected, establish the airway using the jaw thrust (or chin lift) without the head tilt. The jaw thrust is possible to accomplish by grasping the angle of the victim's lower jaw with your hands on both sides of the jaw and bringing the mandible forward, keeping the neck in straight alignment and not tilting the head back.

To determine breathlessness, do the following:

- Look for the rise and fall of the chest.
- Listen for sounds of breathing.
- Feel for the warmth of the victim's mouth against your cheek (see Figure 24-2).

Breathing

Mouth-to-mouth ventilation is the quickest method of supplying oxygen to the victim's lungs. The rescuer's exhaled air has enough oxygen to supply the victim's

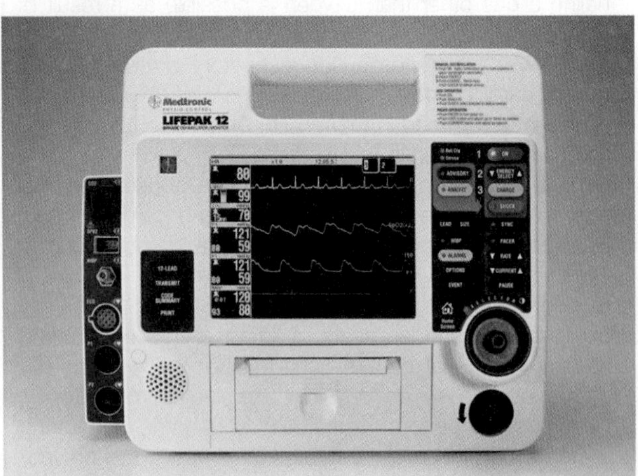

FIGURE 24-1 Automatic external defibrillator (AED) located at an airport.

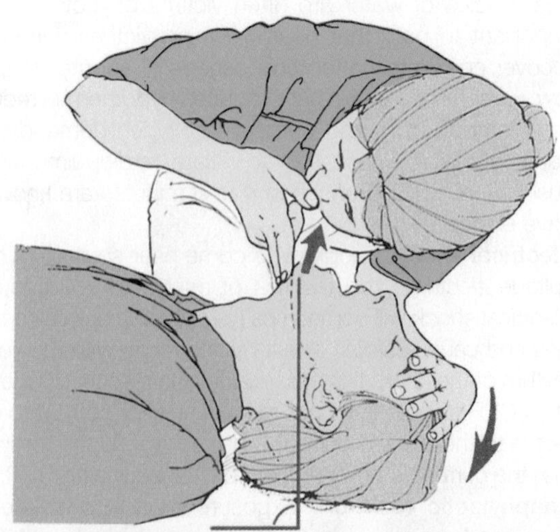
FIGURE 24-2 Head-tilt/chin-lift maneuver.

needs until life-support systems take over. It is necessary to maintain the head-tilt/chin-lift position and an airtight seal throughout rescue breathing.

To preserve the open airway, place yourself at the victim's shoulders. Use the thumb and the index finger of the hand you are using to maintain the head tilt to gently pinch the nostrils closed. Then take a deep breath, seal your lips around the outside of the victim's mouth (creating an airtight seal), and give two full breaths lasting 1 second each (Figure 24-3). This keeps gastric distention to a minimum and decreases the potential of the victim vomiting, which sometimes result from giving rapid breaths and excessive air volume. Allow the victim to exhale passively.

If the initial attempt to ventilate the victim is unsuccessful, reposition the head and again attempt to ventilate. Improper chin and head position is the most common reason for difficulty with ventilation. If the second attempt at ventilation is also unsuccessful, proceed with foreign body airway obstruction management procedures (see later discussion).

Circulation

Once you have performed the initial ventilations, it is important to assess for the presence of the pulse. Pulselessness (cardiac arrest) indicates the need for external cardiac compressions. Respiratory arrest is possible without cardiac arrest. Performing external cardiac compressions on a victim with a pulse has the potential to result in severe physical damage. If the victim has a pulse, initiate rescue breathing at a rate of one breath every 5 to 6 seconds, or 10 to 12 times per minute for the adult (see separate discussion of CPR for infants and children). Cardiac arrest will follow if respiratory arrest continues.

To determine pulselessness, the carotid pulse is the most reliable and accessible for the CPR rescuer. While the head tilt is maintained with one of your hands on the victim's forehead, locate the victim's thyroid cartilage (Adam's apple) with two or three fingers of your other hand. Then gently slide these fingers into the groove between the trachea and the muscles on the side of the neck until you feel the carotid pulse. Palpate the pulse gently on one side so as not to obliterate the artery. The absence of a pulse confirms the diagnosis of **cardiac arrest** (sudden cessation of functional circulation).

Performing external cardiac compressions will circulate blood to the heart, the lungs, the brain, and the rest of the body. If external cardiac compressions are performed properly, it is possible to maintain 20% to 50% of the normal output of the heart. This will bring enough oxygen to the body to sustain life. Proper hand position will enable as much blood to be circulated as possible. Position your hands as follows:

1. Compress the lower half of the victim's sternum in the center (middle) of the chest, between the nipples.
2. Place the heel of your hand on the sternum in the center (middle) of the chest between the nipples, and then place the heel of your second hand on top of the first so that your hands overlap and are parallel.
3. It is acceptable to extend or interlace your fingers, but in any case keep them off the chest (Figure 24-4).

Proper compression technique is important to deliver the appropriate amount of force to simulate the pumping action of the heart. Compression techniques are as follows:

1. Lock your elbows in place, with your arms straight and your shoulders positioned over your hands so that the thrusts of external cardiac compressions are in a downward motion. Some of the force of the compressions will be lost if there is a rolling or rocking motion.

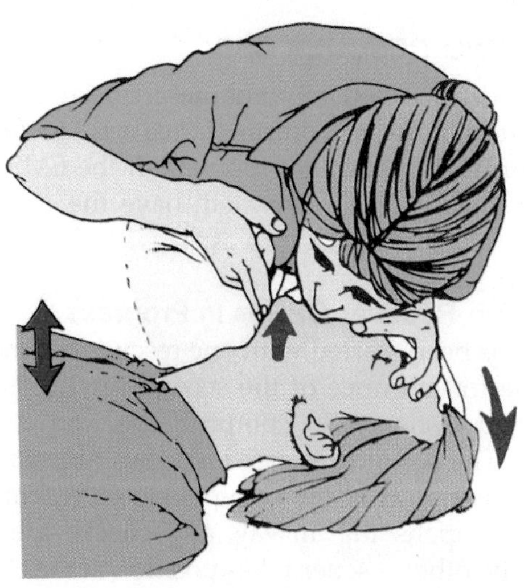

FIGURE 24-3 Mouth-to-mouth ventilation.

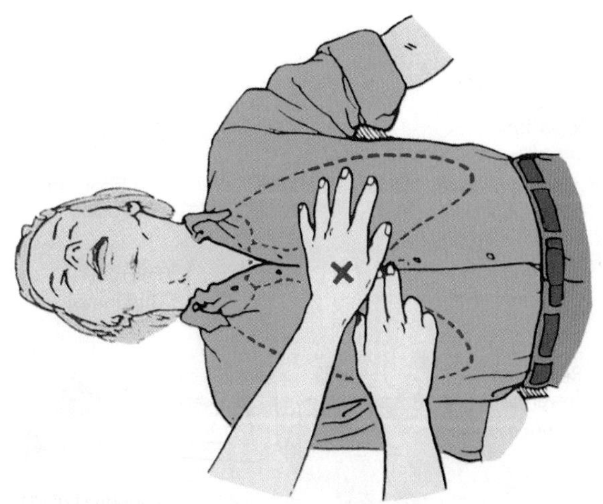

FIGURE 24-4 Position of hand for external cardiac compressions.

2. Lean forward and push, creating pressure to depress the sternum 1½ to 2 inches (3.5 to 5 cm) in the adult (see the section on pediatric CPR for the correlated information for children). This is difficult to estimate, but you will feel some give in the sternum. The motion is smooth, never rolling or jerking (Figure 24-5).
3. Release external chest compression pressure completely to allow the chest to return to position. This allows blood to flow into the heart. (Complete chest recoil allows venous return to the heart, is necessary for effective CPR, and is to be emphasized in training. Get some practice to ensure you know how to deliver good chest compressions. During a two-person rescue, trade off with another rescuer every few minutes to reduce the contribution of fatigue to inadequate chest compression depth and rate.) Keep the time you allow for compression approximately equal to the time for chest recoil or relaxation. Do not pause between compressions. The proper compression rate is approximately 100 compressions per minute.
4. Maintain your hand position at all times—do not lift your hands or move them in any way. Keep your hands in contact with the chest.
5. Complications of external chest compressions include lacerated liver, fractured ribs, and fractured sternum, as well as bruising or bleeding of the liver, the lung, and the spleen.

Do not let any concern for possible injuries from CPR interfere with prompt and energetic application.

The sequencing of breathing to external compressions in one-rescuer and two-rescuer CPR is discussed next.

STEPS FOR ADULT ONE-RESCUER CPR

Airway

1. Determine unresponsiveness.
2. Call for help. Activate the EMS system.
3. Position the victim (and yourself).
4. Open the airway.

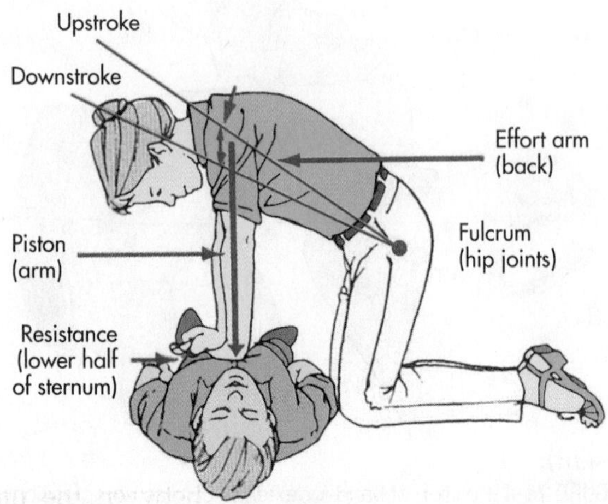

FIGURE 24-5 Positioning for proper compression techniques.

Breathing

1. Determine breathlessness. Look, listen, and feel.
2. If victim is not breathing, give two slow breaths. Allow for exhalation between breaths.
3. If unable to give two breaths, reposition the head and reattempt to ventilate.
4. If still unable, proceed with foreign body airway obstruction management procedures.

Circulation

1. Determine pulselessness.
2. If pulse is present, continue rescue breathing about 10 to 12 times per minute, or one breath every 5 to 6 seconds. Activate the EMS system.
3. If pulse is not present, perform 30 chest compressions at a rate of about 100 per minute. Count "1 and, 2 and, 3 and, 4 and, 5 and . . ." until you have done 30 compressions, and follow them with two slow breaths.
4. Continue with 30 compressions and two slow breaths for two more cycles (30:2, about 1 minute).
5. *Reassessment*. After two cycles, reevaluate the victim for the following:
   - Return of pulse (count for 5 seconds). If absent, pick back up with CPR, beginning with compressions.
   - Return of breathing (assess for 3 to 5 seconds). If present, monitor breathing and pulse closely. Keep the victim in a side-lying position. If breathing is not present, continue rescue breathing, with one breath every 5 seconds, or about 10 to 12 per minute.

If the victim has spontaneous return of breathing and heart function and if no trauma is present, place him or her in a side-lying "recovery position" to protect the airway. If not, continue CPR, checking for return of pulse and breathing every few minutes.

ADULT TWO-RESCUER CPR

Because of the need to combine artificial ventilation with external cardiac compressions, it is less fatiguing to perform CPR with two rescuers. If the EMS system has not already been activated, have the second rescuer do so before starting to assist with CPR.

When One-Rescuer CPR Is in Progress

If CPR has been started with one rescuer, the most logical time for entrance of the second rescuer is after a completed cycle of 30 compressions and two slow breaths. The second rescuer identifies himself or herself by saying, "I know two-person CPR," moves to the head, opens the airway, and checks the carotid pulse. The other rescuer takes position at the chest and finds the proper hand placement for chest compressions. This should take no longer than 5 seconds.

The compression:ventilation ratio for two-person CPR is 30 chest compressions for every two breaths. Pause for 1 second to allow for ventilation (inspiration). Exhalation occurs during chest compressions. The compression rate for two-person CPR is 100 per minute. The rescuer performing chest compressions is more likely to become fatigued. This rescuer will initiate the switching procedure.

When No CPR Is in Progress

If both rescuers arrive at the scene at the same time, and both acknowledge that they know two-person CPR, it is important to establish priorities. Have one rescuer activate the EMS system, while the other initiates one-rescuer CPR. If a third person is available to activate the EMS system, proceed with the two-rescuer method as follows. Have one rescuer go to the victim's head and do the following:

1. Determine unresponsiveness.
2. Position the victim.
3. Open the airway.
4. Assess for breathing.
5. If breathing is absent, say, "No breathing," and give two ventilations.
6. Assess for pulse.
7. If pulse is absent, say, "No pulse."

Have the second rescuer, at the same time, do the following:

1. Find the location for external cardiac compressions.
2. Assume proper hand position.
3. Begin external cardiac compressions after the "No pulse" statement is made by the first rescuer; the sequencing remains 30 compressions for every two breaths.

It is the responsibility of the ventilator (rescuer performing rescue breathing) to evaluate the effectiveness of chest compressions by assessing the carotid pulse during chest compressions (normally, a pulse will be felt on each compression) and monitoring for the spontaneous return of circulation and breathing.

Switching Places

Switching the positions of the ventilator and the compressor prevents fatigue of both rescuers and allows time for the ventilator to evaluate the effectiveness of CPR. The switch is initiated by the rescuer performing chest compressions at the end of the 30:2 sequence. After giving a breath, the ventilator moves to the chest and gets into position to give compressions. The compressor moves to the victim's head and checks the pulse for 5 seconds. If no pulse is felt, she or he gives a breath and gives the command "Resume CPR."

PEDIATRIC CPR—CHILD OR INFANT

The basic steps of CPR and foreign body airway obstruction management are the same whether the victim is an infant, a child, or an adult. For the purpose of basic life support (BLS), an infant is defined as anyone younger than 1 year of age. A child is defined as anyone between ages 1 and 8 years.

Airway

Determine unresponsiveness. Gently shake the child. With an infant, try gently tapping the infant's heels.

If there is no response, shout for help. If someone responds, send the person to activate the emergency medical system and get an AED (if available). The new guideline is to perform BLS for 2 minutes before activating the EMS system. If you are performing a one-person rescue for an unresponsive child or infant victim, provide 5 cycles of CPR before leaving the child or infant victim to activate the emergency response system. Most pediatric arrests are respiratory in nature.

Position the victim on a firm, flat surface for the best CPR effectiveness. If, however, you are able to obtain help more quickly by performing CPR while carrying the infant, it will sometimes be advantageous. However, this technique is not as effective.

Use the head-tilt/chin-lift or jaw thrust technique to open the airway of a child. However, take care not to hyperextend an infant's neck because this sometimes leads the shorter trachea to become occluded. Do not tilt the head in the case of a head injury; use the jaw thrust instead. Caution is necessary with suspected neck injuries in infants and children, as it is in adult cases.

Breathing

After the airway is open, look for movement of the chest, listen for breath sounds, and feel for exhaled airflow. If there is no breathing, inhale, pinch the child's nostrils closed, and seal the child's mouth.

Give two breaths (1 second per breath), with a pause between breaths. The volume of air in an infant's lungs is smaller than that in an adult's, so adjust your breaths to allow for appropriate rise and fall of the chest. A good rule of thumb is usually to use the amount of air for the infant that an adult is able to hold in the cheeks. The creation of gastric distention is common in infants and children during CPR as a result of overinflation of the lungs.

Circulation

Make an assessment of the pulse on the carotid artery of the child and the brachial artery of the infant. If there is a pulse, continue rescue breathing at a rate of one breath every 3 to 5 seconds. If there is no pulse, it is necessary to perform external cardiac compressions as well.

When performing external cardiac compressions in the infant, do the following (this technique is preferred for infants when two health care providers are present):

1. Visualize an imaginary line between the nipples.

2. Use a two-thumb, encircling-hands compression technique, performing compressions with the thumbs (Figure 24-6).
   a. Place both thumbs side by side or one on top of the other over the lower half of the infant's breastbone (sternum) about one fingerbreadth below the nipple line.
   b. Make sure your thumbs do not compress on or near the bottom of the sternum (xiphoid process).
   c. Encircle the infant's chest with the remaining fingers of both hands. Use both hands to compress the infant's sternum.
3. The breastbone is compressed to a depth of ½ to 1 inch at a rate of at least 100 times per minute. Count aloud very quickly: "one, two, three, four, five." Perform the compression-and-release action smoothly. It has been recommended to "think" the count rather than counting aloud—it is easy to lose count because the rate is so fast.
4. At the end of each compression, release pressure and allow the sternum to return to normal position without removing your hands from their placement. Keep your movements smooth, not jerky.
5. The sequence of compressions to ventilation is 30:2 (30 compressions to two breaths).
6. After 20 cycles of 30:2 (about 1 minute), recheck for signs of circulation. If no signs of circulation are present, continue 30:2 cycles, beginning with chest compressions.

When performing cardiac compressions in the child, do the following:

1. Palpate the lower margin of the child's ribcage with your middle and index fingers while maintaining the head tilt with the other hand.
2. Locate the xiphoid process (where the ribs and breastbone meet).
3. With the middle finger on this notch, place your index finger next to your middle finger.

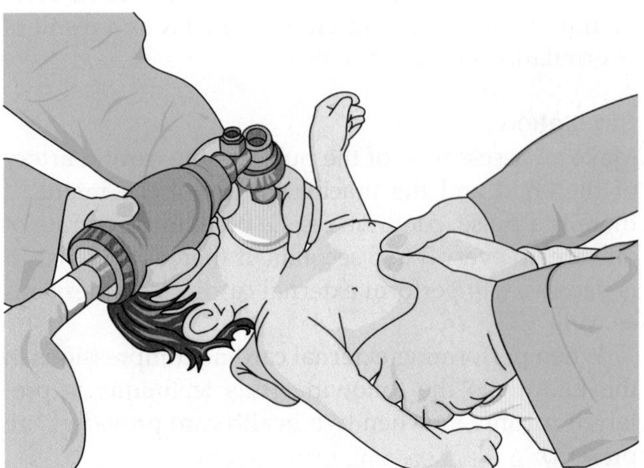

FIGURE 24-6 Position of fingers for proper compression techniques in infants.

4. Looking at the landmark, place the heel of your hand next to where your index finger was.
5. Compress the chest with the heel of one hand at a depth of 1 to 1½ inches 100 times per minute. Make sure your fingers do not touch the ribs.
6. Keep the compressions smooth, allowing the chest to return to the natural position after each compression.
7. The sequence is 30 compressions to 2 breaths.
8. If the child is older or large, use the adult method of CPR.

HANDS-ONLY CPR

The American Heart Association (AHA) issued a "call to action" statement on March 31, 2008. It recommends that bystanders who are not trained in conventional CPR use only their hands, without the rescue breathing, in the crucial moments after they witness an out-of-hospital sudden cardiac arrest. The AHA recommends that if there is a witness to a sudden collapse of an adult and the victim is unresponsive, it is best to call 911 and start chest compressions "hard and fast" in the middle of the chest. Many times people nearby do not help because they are not confident in what they are doing and fear that they will hurt the victim. If the bystander is not trained in CPR or is not confident in being able to perform rescue breathing, performing hands-only CPR is the best response. Optimally this will continue until emergency medical assistance arrives or an AED is made available.

If the bystander is trained in CPR and is confident in being able to provide rescue breaths with minimal interruptions to chest compressions, performing either CPR with a 30:2 ratio of chest compressions to breaths or hands-only CPR is acceptable. This should continue until an AED is made available or emergency medical providers arrive to help.

Newer studies have found that in people with out-of-hospital cardiac arrest, survival numbers were comparable between those who received chest compressions only and conventional CPR (Colihan, 2008).

FOREIGN BODY AIRWAY OBSTRUCTION MANAGEMENT

Food, particularly meat, is the most common cause of choking or airway obstruction in the adult. Factors that contribute to this include large or poorly chewed pieces of food, the ingestion of alcohol, and loose-fitting dentures. Foreign objects (e.g., marbles, beads, buttons, and food) are the most common cause of airway obstruction in children.

If the victim is able to cough forcibly, the air exchange is good, although there may be wheezing between coughs. **Do not interfere** with the victim at this point. However, do monitor the victim closely, because it is possible that he or she will regress to a state of poor air exchange.

The victim experiencing poor air exchange is likely to have a weak, ineffective cough; make a high-pitched, "crowing" noise while inhaling; have increased respiratory difficulty; and develop cyanosis. With complete airway obstruction, the victim is not able to speak, breathe, or cough, and will sometimes clutch the neck (Figure 24-7). This sign is the universal distress signal. To assess the inability to speak, ask the victim, "Are you choking?" Complete airway obstruction will prevent oxygen from entering the lungs and being circulated to the brain and vital organs. Unless prompt action is initiated, the victim will become unconscious and death will result.

The following maneuver is the most effective method of removing foreign body airway obstructions.

CONSCIOUS VICTIM

Abdominal thrusts given below the diaphragm, an emergency procedure for dislodging a bolus of food or other obstruction from the trachea to prevent asphyxiation, are recommended for relieving foreign body airway obstruction. These thrusts put pressure on the diaphragm, forcing air from the lungs to move and expel the foreign object. If the victim is in a sitting position, stand behind the victim and wrap your arms around the victim's waist. Then make a fist with one hand and place the thumb of your fist against the middle of the victim's abdomen slightly above the navel and well below the tip of the xiphoid process. Wrap your other hand over the fist to provide added force. Then press your fist into the victim's abdomen with a quick upward thrust (Figure 24-8). Repeat each thrust until the foreign body is expelled or the victim becomes unconscious. It is sometimes necessary to repeat the maneuver 6 to 10 times. If the victim is pregnant or obese, chest thrusts are acceptable instead of abdominal thrusts. Keep your hands in the same position as for chest compressions in CPR.

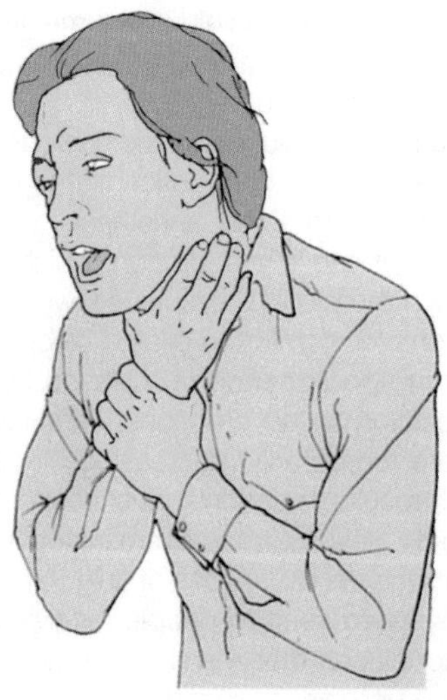

FIGURE 24-7 Victims typically clutch the neck when experiencing airway obstruction.

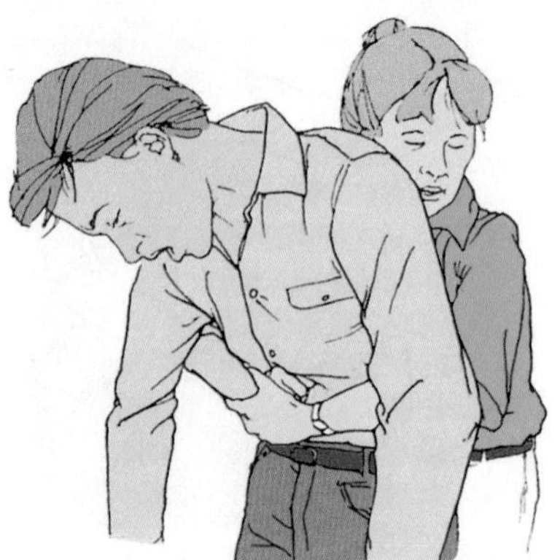

FIGURE 24-8 Abdominal thrusts.

UNCONSCIOUS VICTIM

If a victim becomes unconscious, lie him or her down in a face-up (supine) position. Because regurgitation is common in an unconscious victim, perform a finger sweep. To perform the finger sweep, open the victim's mouth by grasping both the tongue and the lower jaw between your thumb and fingers and lifting upward. This draws the tongue from the back of the throat and away from the foreign body. Insert the index finger of your available hand along the side of the cheek and deeply into the throat to the base of the tongue. Use a hooking motion to dislodge the object and bring it into the mouth, where you will be able to grasp and remove it. Take care not to push the foreign body farther down into the throat with this maneuver.

Then open the airway and attempt to ventilate (if you have successfully dislodged the foreign body, the victim will need artificial respirations and possibly external cardiac compressions). If ventilation is unsuccessful, perform five abdominal thrusts. To perform abdominal thrusts on an unconscious victim, kneel astride the victim's thighs and place the heel of one hand against the victim's abdomen, in the midline slightly above the navel but well below the tip of the xiphoid process. Keep the second hand on top of the first hand for additional force. Press into the abdomen with a quick, upward thrust. Open the victim's mouth again, and perform another finger sweep. Repeat all these steps until the foreign body is dislodged and spontaneous breathing is restored. If spontaneous breathing is not restored, initiate CPR.

INFANT

Of all deaths from foreign body aspiration, 65% are in the infant age-group. Aspirated materials include food, such as candies and nuts, and small objects. Infants and children experience acute respiratory distress with coughing, gagging, and **stridor** (harsh sound during respirations, high-pitched and resembling the blowing of wind, caused by obstruction of the air passage). The victim will often become unconscious.

Treat the child in a manner similar to the adult with performance of abdominal thrusts. However, there is a

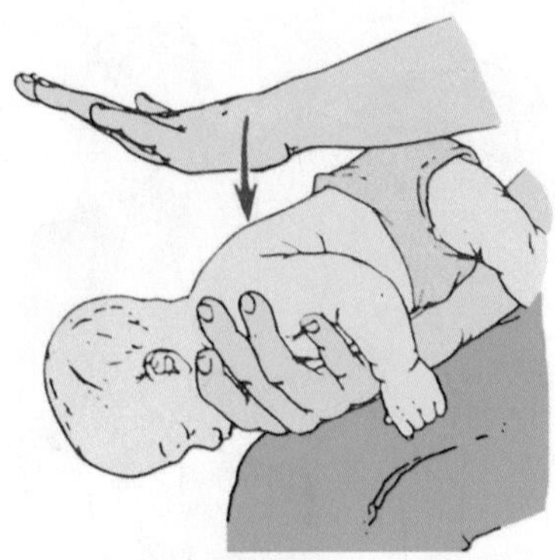

FIGURE 24-9 Clearing airway obstruction in an infant.

potential for injury in using this maneuver in the infant. Use a combination of back blows and chest thrusts with an infant, as follows:

1. Straddle the infant over your arm with the head lower than the trunk and the face down, and support the infant firmly at the jaw.
2. Rest the arm holding the infant on your thigh, and deliver five back blows between the infant's shoulders with the heel of the hand of your other arm (Figure 24-9).
3. Place your free hand on the infant's back so that the victim is sandwiched between the two hands, one supporting the neck, jaw, and chest while the other supports the back.
4. While continuing to support the head and neck, turn the infant and place the infant on your thigh, with the head lower than the trunk.
5. Perform five chest thrusts with your hands in the same position as when performing external cardiac compressions (see Figure 24-6).
6. Never use the blind finger-sweep technique, because it is possible to cause the foreign body to become lodged more deeply because of the shortened trachea of the infant. However, if you are able to see the object when the infant's mouth is open, remove it.

SHOCK

Shock is an abnormal condition of inadequate blood flow to the body's peripheral tissues (decreased tissue perfusion). The cardiovascular system fails to provide sufficient blood circulation (oxygen, nutrients, hormones, and electrolytes) to the body's tissues, and metabolic waste removal is decreased. Shock results in life-threatening cellular dysfunction, hypotension, and oliguria. To maintain circulatory homeostasis, the following mechanisms are necessary: a functioning heart to circulate blood and a sufficient volume of blood. The capability of the vascular system (accommodating blood flow to the capillaries and cells for perfusion and thus providing oxygen and glucose, as well as returning carbon dioxide to the right side of the heart) is also necessary to maintain adequate circulation. Inability of the body to compensate for failure of one or more of these mechanisms results in shock.

CLASSIFICATION OF SHOCK

Shock is classified according to its cause. The most common causes of shock are severe loss of blood, intense pain, extensive trauma, burns, poisons, emotional stress or intense emotions, extremes of heat and cold, electrical shock, allergic reactions, and a sudden or severe illness. Box 24-3 provides several examples of types of shock.

ASSESSMENT

The signs and symptoms of shock are sometimes disguised by other signs of injury; some will often appear only in the late stages of shock. Be aware of the following when assessing the victim for shock:

- *Level of consciousness.* The victim tends to experience changes in behavior, restlessness, anxiety, disorientation, syncope, and agitation. As the condition worsens, the victim becomes more lethargic. Coma and death are possible.
- *Skin changes.* The skin becomes cool, clammy, pale, and ashen. As shock progresses, cyanosis

Box 24-3 Types of Shock

- **Anaphylactic shock.** Anaphylaxis (an exaggerated hypersensitivity reaction to a previously encountered antigen) results from a sudden, severe, allergic reaction to a foreign substance. Shock occurs because of the sudden decrease in the amount of circulating blood caused by the sudden release of histamine, which creates capillary hyperpermeability, which in turn causes the release of plasma through the capillary walls.
- **Cardiogenic shock.** Results from poor heart function caused by various cardiovascular abnormalities. The heart is unable to maintain sufficient blood pressure to all body parts.
- **Hypovolemic shock** (also known as hemorrhagic shock). Caused by a decrease in fluid volume from bleeding, prolonged vomiting, or diarrhea, or by loss of fluid owing to surgery, trauma, or burns.
- **Neurogenic shock.** Caused by the nervous system's failure to maintain normal contraction of the blood vessels. Common causes are spinal anesthesia, quadriplegia, or medications that cause vasodilation, which create a condition in which the blood pressure is lower because there is not enough blood to fill the dilated blood vessels.
- **Psychogenic shock syncope.** Caused by the nervous system's reaction to an emotional stimulus. The blood vessels dilate temporarily, decreasing blood flow to the brain, which results in unconsciousness, or syncope.
- **Septic shock.** Results from severe infection. Toxins from the microorganisms cause loss of fluid through the blood vessel walls; often seen in people receiving chemotherapy or in conditions that result in immunocompromised functioning, such as acquired immunodeficiency syndrome (AIDS).

(slightly bluish, grayish, slatelike, or dark purple discoloration of the skin, especially of the lips and nailbeds, due to an excess of deoxygenated hemoglobin in the blood) develops, and the victim appears dehydrated.

- *Blood pressure.* Initially the blood pressure is often normal, but as shock progresses, there is a steady decrease in blood pressure and capillary refill time is delayed. In hypovolemic shock, hypotension is a late manifestation.
- *Pulse.* The pulse rate usually increases (tachycardia, abnormal rapidity of heart action, usually defined as a heart rate of more than 100 beats per minute in an adult) in all types of shock. The pulse also becomes weak and thready in character.
- *Respirations.* The respiratory rate increases. Respirations are also frequently shallow, rapid, labored, or irregular as a result of vasoconstriction in the lungs, which causes fluid to accumulate.
- *Urinary output.* With decreased circulation of fluid volume, the amount of urinary output is decreased (oliguria, diminished amount of urine formation, less than 500 mL in every 24 hours).
- *Neuromuscular changes.* Decreased oxygen to the tissues results in weakness or tremors of the arms and legs. Eyelids close, and the pupils dilate.
- *Gastrointestinal effects.* Because of loss of fluids and fluid shifts, the victim will complain of thirst. Nausea, vomiting, and dry mucous membranes are also possible.

NURSING INTERVENTIONS

It is essential to treat shock immediately. Priority interventions are to establish an airway, control bleeding, and reduce pain. Place the patient in a supine position with the legs elevated (Figure 24-10, *A*). This position will help improve venous flow to the right side of the heart as well as cardiac output. Oxygen therapy is often required to assist the patient in meeting oxygenation needs (Laskowski-Jones, 2006e).

When a patient is in shock, hypotension is possible. Most clinicians usually do not recommend the use of the Trendelenburg position, which risks interfering with pulmonary function as well as increasing intracranial pressure (Lewis et al., 2007). If you suspect head, neck, or spinal injuries, it is essential to keep the victim flat and not move him or her, unless it is absolutely necessary to prevent further injury (see Figure 24-10, *B*). If the victim is unconscious or is vomiting or bleeding around the nose and mouth, position him or her on the side to allow the airway to clear and to encourage drainage. Elevate the head and shoulders if the victim is having problems breathing (see Figure 24-10, *C*).

Maintain the shock victim's body temperature: Keep the victim warm and dry by placing blankets or other coverings under the victim to prevent heat loss from underneath. Cover the victim with any available

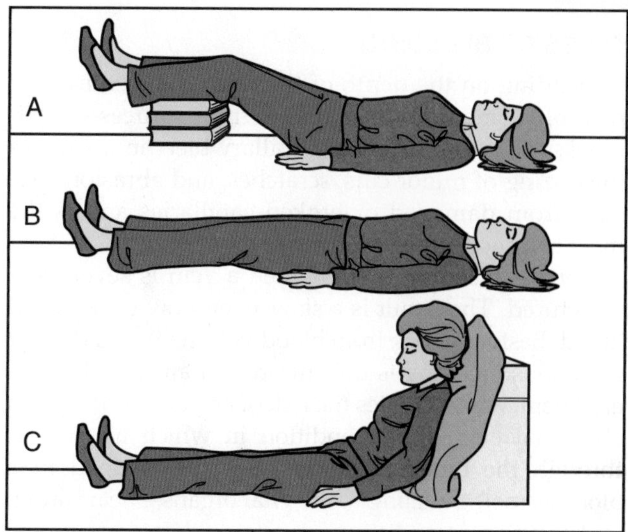

FIGURE 24-10 Body positions for shock. **A,** Supine position with patient's legs elevated 6 to 8 inches (15 to 20 cm). **B,** Position for patients with suspected head, neck, or spinal injuries. **C,** Position for patients with breathing problems.

material, such as a blanket or clothing; however, avoid overheating. Never give the victim anything to eat or drink because the presence of internal injuries is possible, immediate surgery is often needed, and many patients aspirate the fluid. A moistened cloth will relieve dry mouth or mucous membranes. In a clinical setting, make certain the patient has venous access, usually with two large-bore IV catheters (ideally 14- to 16-gauge) to facilitate rapid fluid and blood product administration, if needed.

Take measures to relieve pain in the shock victim. Nursing interventions include avoiding rough handling, and adjusting tight or uncomfortable clothing or bandages. It is important not to give analgesics or drugs unless directed by a physician. Do not allow others to attempt to give alcoholic substances to a victim. Because the victim is likely to be very frightened, it is essential to give emotional support and reassurance.

BLEEDING AND HEMORRHAGE

An average adult man has approximately 12 pints of blood circulating in his bloodstream. Blood is necessary to transport oxygen and nutrients to all parts of the body.

EFFECTS OF BLOOD LOSS

The loss of blood (hemorrhage) from internal or external bleeding causes a decrease in oxygen supply to the body tissues. Decreased blood volume also causes the blood pressure to fall; thus the heart is called on to pump faster to compensate for the decrease in blood volume and blood pressure. The body will attempt to clot the blood to halt bleeding. Clotting usually requires 6 to 7 minutes. If uncontrolled, bleeding can result in shock and death.

TYPES OF BLEEDING

Depending on the depth of the wound, bleeding will possibly come from one or all of three sources—capillaries, veins, and arteries. Capillary bleeding, such as the oozing of minor cuts, scratches, and abrasions, results from damaged or broken capillaries and is the most common type of external hemorrhage.

Venous bleeding occurs when a vein is severed or punctured. The result is a slow, even flow of dark red blood. Besides shock from blood volume loss, a danger of venous bleeding is the entrance of air into the severed vein, which creates the risk of an **air embolism** (an abnormal circulatory condition in which air travels through the bloodstream and becomes lodged in a blood vessel) traveling to the vital organs—heart, lung, and brain.

Arterial bleeding is the least common type of injury, because arteries are located deep in the body and are usually protected by bones, fat, and other structures. When an artery is severed or punctured, the bleeding is characterized by the heavy spurting of bright red blood in the rhythm of the heartbeat. The most common arteries that it is possible to affect in this way are the following:

- Femoral (in the upper thigh and groin)
- Radial (in the lateral aspect of the lower arm)
- Brachial (in the medial aspect of the upper arm)
- Carotid (on either side of the neck)

NURSING INTERVENTIONS

Direct Pressure

The most effective general treatment of bleeding is to apply direct pressure over the bleeding site. This is possible to accomplish by placing a dressing or the cleanest material possible over the wound and applying firm pressure with your gloved hand (Figure 24-11). Then apply a bandage, with the knot tied snugly over the wound to exert direct pressure. If bleeding continues after the bandage is applied, resume pressure with your gloved hand as well as the bandage. Bleeding will usually be controlled in 10 to 30 minutes. Do not allow anyone but a physician to remove the bandage supplying direct pressure, even if it becomes saturated with blood. Instead, place another layer of dressing on top and continue to exert firm pressure.

Raising the bleeding part of the body above the level of the heart will decrease blood flow and increase the body's ability to clot at this site. Use this technique *only* if there are no suspected or known fractures or conditions that are possible to exacerbate by this maneuver. It is acceptable to elevate a splinted fracture, however, if no other contraindications are present.

Indirect Pressure

If direct pressure and elevation do not control bleeding, it is possible to apply indirect pressure to any of the pressure points situated along main arteries (Figure 24-12). To apply indirect pressure, use the fingers or the heel of your hand to compress the artery against the underlying bone located between the heart and the wound. Do this only if there are no suspected fractures beneath the area where you have to apply pressure. The most common pressure points are over the carotid, subclavian, brachial, and femoral arteries.

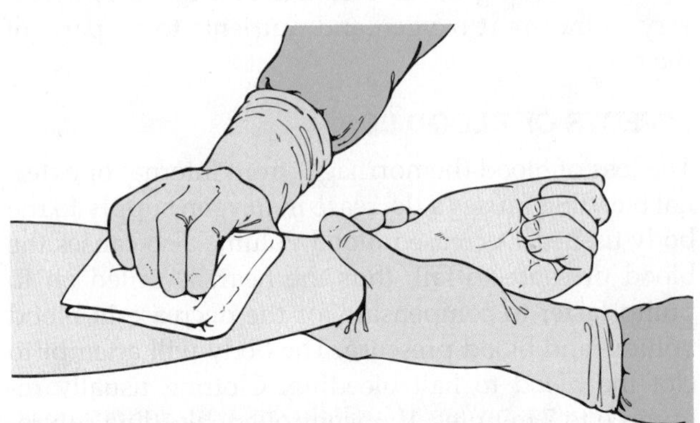

FIGURE 24-11 Applying pressure to a wound site.

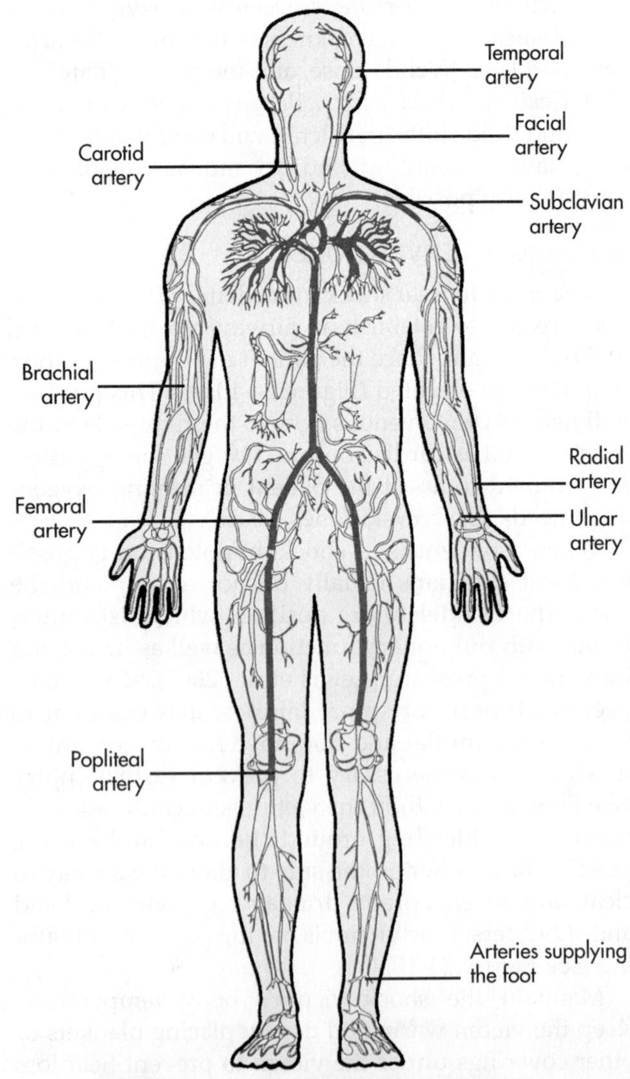

FIGURE 24-12 Pressure points for bleeding control.

Application of a Tourniquet

Bleeding is almost always possible to control by the three-step measure of **direct pressure, elevation,** and **indirect pressure.** Use a tourniquet *only* when these methods have failed and the victim's life is in danger. Extensive damage to the affected part is possible because of the cessation of arterial blood flow to the area. Consider using a tourniquet only if risking a limb is necessary to save a life (Laskowski-Jones, 2006e). A tourniquet also has the capacity to damage nerves and vessels directly below or under the tourniquet. An improperly, loosely applied tourniquet will not stop arterial flow but will hinder venous flow. Tourniquet use is often considered beyond the scope of first aid and those acting in good faith, such as a Good Samaritan, and is usually restricted to professionals such as physicians and paramedics. Skill 24-1 provides techniques to follow when applying a tourniquet.

EPISTAXIS

Epistaxis (nosebleed) is common but is seldom a serious emergency. However, profuse bleeding from the nose does have the potential to lead to shock. Epistaxis has several causes: trauma (especially a direct blow to the nose); epistaxis digitorum (self-inflicted local digital trauma from nasal picking); infections, including the common cold; snorting cocaine; overuse of nasal sprays; high blood pressure; strenuous activity; and low humidity in winter months. Epistaxis in an older adult may be caused by underlying conditions, such as hypertension. Always assess an older adult's blood pressure if epistaxis is present.

Nursing Interventions

Keep the person with epistaxis quiet in a sitting position, leaning forward. If the victim is unable to sit up, it is best that he or she remain supine with the head and shoulders raised (if this position is not contraindicated by other injuries).

Other interventions include the following:

- Keep the victim's head tilted slightly forward so that blood will not run down the back of the throat and cause choking or vomiting.
- With your thumb and forefinger, apply steady pressure to both nostrils for 10 to 15 minutes before releasing.

Skill 24-1 Applying a Tourniquet*

Nursing Action *(Rationale)*

1. Use a strong, wide, flat piece of material, if possible (e.g., towel, necktie, wide belt). *(Never use rope or wire, which has the potential to cut the skin.)*
2. Place pressure on the nearest pressure point. *(Controls bleeding while you are applying the tourniquet.)*
3. Apply a pad (piece of cloth, handkerchief, dressing) over the artery to be compressed. *(Prevents damage to the skin.)*
4. Place the tourniquet between the wound and the heart; allow some uninjured skin between the wound and the tourniquet. *(Prevents undue pressure on the injured site.)* Wrap the material around the limb twice, and tie a half-knot on the upper surface of the limb. *(Secures tourniquet in place.)*
5. Place a stick or rod (approximately 6 inches long) over the knot, and secure it in place. *(Enhances effect of tourniquet.)*
6. Twist the stick enough times to stop the bleeding. *(A tighter twist poses a risk for additional injury.)*
7. Secure the stick firmly with the free ends of the tourniquet. Do not cover the tourniquet (see illustration). *(Tourniquet must be clearly visible to medical personnel.)*
8. Write "T" or "TK" (meaning tourniquet) and the time it was applied, on the victim's forehead. Attach a note to the victim's clothing describing the time and location of the tourniquet application. *(Ensures further interventions. A tourniquet allowed to remain in place too long poses the risk of further injury.)*
9. Treat for shock and transport to the nearest medical facility. *(Ensures timely interventions.)*
10. Never loosen a tourniquet once it has been applied. Always seek medical attention once a tourniquet has been applied. *(Consistent treatment is necessary.)*

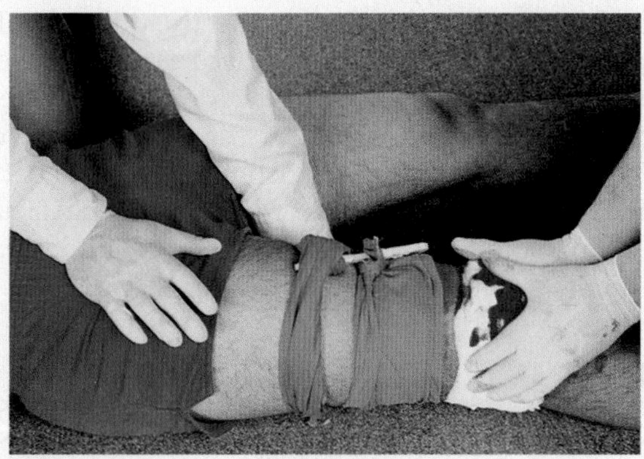

Step 7

*Note that tourniquet use is often considered beyond the scope of first aid and those acting in good faith, such as a Good Samaritan, and is usually restricted to professionals such as physicians and paramedics.

- Remind the victim to breathe through the mouth and to expectorate any accumulated blood.
- Apply ice compresses over the nose, which may help control bleeding.
- Look in the victim's mouth at the back of the throat to assess for bleeding from a posterior site.

If bleeding continues despite interventions, seek medical assistance, because it is possible that the victim is bleeding from a posterior site, possibly making fluid replacement necessary, as well as surgery.

INTERNAL BLEEDING

Internal bleeding is a potentially life-threatening situation. It is difficult to diagnose and often progresses rapidly. Common causes of internal bleeding include fractures, knife or bullet wounds, crush injuries, organ injuries, and medical conditions such as ruptured aneurysms.

Assessment

All the signs and symptoms of shock will often be present. Initially, some victims experience only vertigo (dizziness). The victim will sometimes also expectorate blood (hemoptysis) or vomit blood (hematemesis). Dark, tarry stool (melena) or blood in urine (hematuria) are sometimes present. Pain, tenderness, or a dislocation at the site of a suspected injury indicates possible internal bleeding, as does obvious bleeding from the mouth, the rectum, or any other body opening.

Nursing Interventions

Internal bleeding is a priority medical emergency; make every effort to obtain medical care immediately. Victims on anticoagulant therapy are likely to have significant blood loss from minor injury. Significant blood loss also occurs in some victims with a history of alcohol abuse, as well as those victims with blood dyscrasias.

Place the victim on a flat surface with legs slightly elevated if this is not contraindicated by other injuries. Establish an airway, and institute treatment for shock. Position a cold compress or ice on the area of the suspected injury. Never apply ice directly to the skin because it can "burn" the tissue. Place a towel or clean cloth between the ice and the skin. Maintain body temperature with blankets, and assess vital signs every 5 minutes. Do not give the victim anything to eat or drink. Administer oxygen as ordered by the physician. By giving support and reassurance you will decrease the victim's fear and anxiety.

WOUNDS AND TRAUMA

A **wound** is an injury to the internal or external soft tissues of the body. The basic rules for first aid treatment after the ABCs are as follows:

1. Stop bleeding.
2. Treat for shock.
3. Prevent infection.

CLOSED WOUNDS

Closed wounds involve the underlying tissues of the body; the top layer of skin is not broken. Examples of closed wounds are ecchymoses (discolorations of an area of the skin or mucous membrane caused by the extravasation of blood into the subcutaneous tissues; also called a **bruise**), contusions (injuries that do not break the skin, caused by a blow and characterized by edema, discoloration, and pain), strains, and sprains. They most commonly occur as a result of falls, automobile accidents, or contact sports.

The following signs and symptoms are most likely to occur with a closed wound: (1) **edema** usually appears within 24 to 48 hours; (2) **discoloration** is likely to occur as a result of the formation of a hematoma (swelling containing blood)—initially the discoloration is blackish blue and then turns to green or yellow within a few days; (3) **deformity** of the limbs is caused by fractures and dislocations; (4) **shock** often follows from the force of the trauma; (5) **pain** and **tenderness** at the site are possible; and (6) signs of **internal bleeding** will sometimes be present.

Nursing Interventions

If the wound is small, applying ice packs is one possibility, along with padding, an elastic bandage, or a 4-inch by 4-inch abdominal dressing used for pressure. If the wound is large, monitor the patient for shock; also apply cold compresses and a pressure bandage. Obtain medical assistance immediately.

OPEN WOUNDS

Open wounds are openings or breaks in the mucous membrane or skin. Regardless of the type, there is always danger of bleeding or infection. Infection is more common in wounds that do not bleed freely, because active bleeding tends to flush microorganisms from the wound. Following are five general types of open wounds—abrasions, incisions, lacerations, punctures, avulsions—and their nursing interventions.

A tetanus toxoid (an active immunizing agent prepared from detoxified tetanus toxin that produces an antigenic response in the body, conferring active immunity to tetanus infection) injection is necessary as a general treatment for all open wounds. It is necessary to readminister the tetanus vaccine every 10 years to maintain immunity. The attending physician will ultimately decide on administration in a given case, especially for those wounds that have occurred as a result of a soiled object or are themselves dirty.

Abrasions

Abrasions are caused by a rubbing or scraping of the outer layers of the skin. Bleeding is limited to oozing of blood; there is danger of infection from contamination with dirt and microorganisms. Examples of abrasions include rope and road burns, scratches, and scrapes of knees and elbows.

Nursing Interventions

Remove all dirt, if possible. Do not use strong antiseptics because they often irritate the skin. There is no one solution to use in cleaning wounds. The solution is not as important as the technique used. Clean the wound from the inside out. Normal saline is safe and effective and will remove debris with copious irrigation. Unless properly diluted, povidone-iodine will actually cause tissue necrosis because it is too harsh. Cover the abrasion with a sterile dressing.

Advise the victim as to the signs and symptoms of infection, such as edema, erythema, pain, and purulent exudate. Also instruct the victim to seek medical attention if these signs and symptoms occur.

Puncture Wounds

Puncture wounds are piercing wounds of the skin. They are typically made by knives, nails, wood, glass, or other objects that penetrate the skin. A puncture will often force dirt and microorganisms deep into the tissues. If the object remains firmly in the skin, do not remove it, rather leave it in place for a physician to remove. Removal has the potential to cause significant bleeding necessitating emergent surgical intervention.

Nursing Interventions

Thoroughly irrigate all puncture wounds to remove as much debris and microorganisms as possible. Patients often require a tetanus booster.

Incisions

Incisions are smoothly divided wounds made by sharp instruments. Infection is not as likely to occur, because blood flows freely from the wound. However, bleeding is sometimes extensive, and muscle, tendon, and nerve damage is possible. Common examples of incisional wounds include cuts from knives, broken glass, razors, or paper edges.

Nursing Interventions

Carefully clean the incision and cover it with a sterile dressing; use an antiseptic only at a physician's recommendation. Typically, you will use a butterfly bandage, Steri-Strips, or sutures to hold the edges of the wound together. Control bleeding by applying pressure. Seek medical attention if the incision is deep, bleeding is profuse, and function is limited.

Lacerations

Lacerations are wounds that are torn with jagged, irregular edges. Bleeding is often profuse, and tissue destruction and infection are possible. Auto accidents, blunt objects, and heavy machinery accidents are common causes of lacerations.

Nursing Interventions

Carefully clean the laceration. Control bleeding by applying pressure (see Figure 24-11). Use adhesive strips, Steri-Strips, or butterfly bandages to close the edges of the laceration. Cover the wound with a sterile dressing, and see that the victim goes to a physician for treatment.

Avulsions

An avulsion is a torn piece of tissue that results in a section being completely removed or left hanging by a flap. Avulsions are sometimes minor, with only a small amount of displaced skin, but sometimes they include large areas of tissue, with exposure of underlying bones, tendons, or muscles. Avulsions are often more difficult to heal than other types of wounds because wound edges are sometimes not well approximated when repaired.

Nursing Interventions

Control bleeding by direct pressure. After thorough cleansing, suturing will often be necessary to repair an avulsion wound. Closely monitor the wound site for healing without complications.

Chest Wounds

Chest wounds are extremely dangerous and necessitate immediate medical attention. In many chest wounds, air or blood escapes into the **pleural space** (the potential space between the visceral and parietal layers of the pleurae). Normally this space is a vacuum; therefore air **(pneumothorax)** or blood **(hemothorax)** entering this space has potential to cause an increase in pressure, which will often result in collapse of lung tissue.

Assessment

Assess the following factors:

- Sharp pain at the site of the injury
- Pain associated with breathing
- Difficult and labored breathing
- Failure of one or both sides of the chest to expand normally with inspiration
- Expectorating bright red or frothy blood (hemoptysis)
- Signs and symptoms of shock: rapid, weak, thready pulse; vertigo; and hypotension
- Cyanosis of the skin and mucous membranes
- A sucking or hissing sound as air flows in and out of the chest
- Distention of the neck and arm veins
- Anxiety
- Tracheal deviation

Nursing Interventions

For the first aid treatment of penetrating chest wounds, if the chest wall has been penetrated by a sharp object, do *not* remove the object; this will sometimes result in further bleeding and the entrance of air into the chest wound. Immobilize the object with dressings and tape. Employ the ABCs of treatment. Treat the victim; however, it will sometimes be necessary to elevate the victim's head slightly to facilitate breathing.

If there is a sucking chest wound (without the penetrating object in place), apply an airtight dressing. Any available material is acceptable to use—gauze, plastic wrap, clothing, or even your hand, if that is the only thing available. It is necessary for this dressing to be large enough so that it is not sucked into the hole in the victim's chest, and as airtight as possible. Monitor the victim for any signs and symptoms of developing pneumothorax. Any signs of increased respiratory distress indicate the possible development of a tension pneumothorax. In that case, leave one side of the dressing untaped. Withhold liquids, because aspiration is possible.

For the first aid treatment of crushing chest wounds, it is important to know that the most common injury to the chest is fractured ribs. Severe blunt trauma sometimes results in **flail chest** (two or more ribs fractured in two or more places, resulting in instability in part of the chest wall) with associated hemothorax, pneumothorax, and pulmonary contusion (Figure 24-13). Paradoxic motion develops as a result of the instability this brings about in part of the chest wall, with the lung underlying the injured area contracting on inspiration and bulging on expiration. If uncorrected, respiratory distress and hypoxia will result. Elevate the victim's head and shoulders to facilitate breathing if spinal injury is not suspected. Apply dressings carefully to any open wounds to avoid any pressure to the chest that has potential to impair breathing.

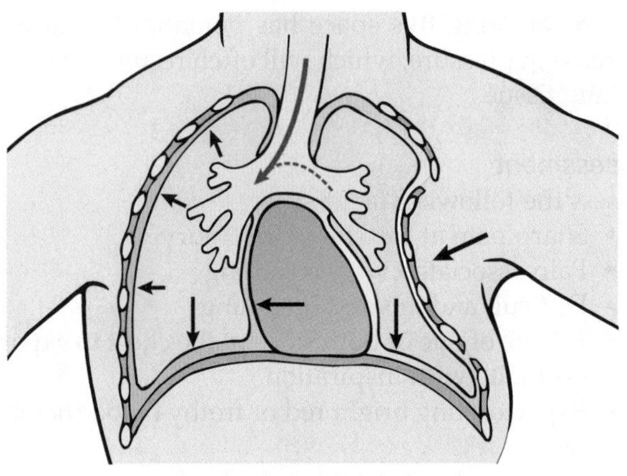

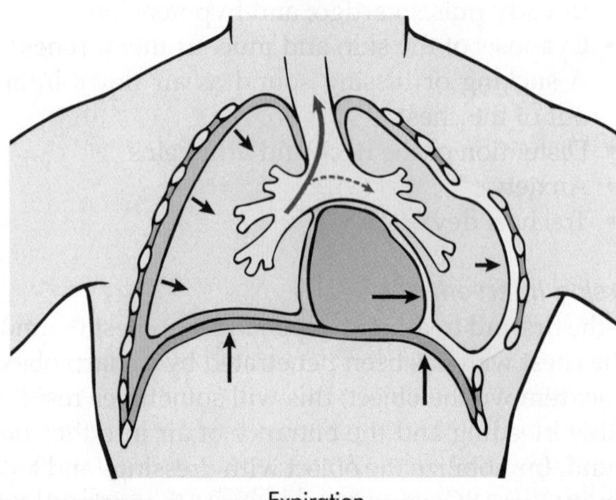

FIGURE 24-13 Flail chest.

DRESSINGS AND BANDAGES

General Principles of Bandaging

First control bleeding before applying the bandage. Open the dressing carefully, using sterile materials if possible. If sterile equipment is not available, use the cleanest material possible. See that the dressing covers the entire wound. Bandage wounds firmly but not too tightly; tight bandages tend to interfere with circulation to the tissue and have the potential to act as a tourniquet, causing tissue and nerve damage.

Loose ends sometimes catch on objects. Always bandage the part in the desired alignment; never bend a joint after it is bandaged. Leave the tips of the fingers and the toes exposed, if possible, to make it possible to check for circulation. Frequently assess for edema and circulation. Tie knots over the top of open wounds to help apply pressure and control bleeding unless this is contraindicated.

Application of Common Types of Bandages

Bandage Compress

The bandage compress is the most common type of dressing. It consists of several thicknesses of gauze, covered with tape or gauze.

Triangular Bandage

The triangular bandage is made of a piece of cloth that is folded diagonally and cut along the fold. You will use this most commonly as a sling to support injured bones. Skill 24-2 describes the application of an arm sling using a triangular bandage.

Gauze Roller Bandage

Use the gauze roller bandage to support an injured part, apply pressure to a dressing for control of bleeding, or secure a splint to immobilize a part (Figure 24-14). Apply gauze roller bandages uniformly to ob-

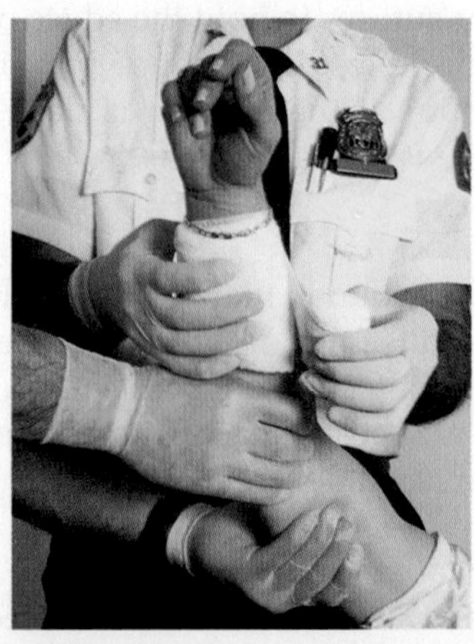

FIGURE 24-14 Use of a roller bandage.

Skill 24-2 Applying an Arm Sling Using a Triangular (Sling and Swathe) Bandage

Nursing Action *(Rationale)*

1. Place one end of the base of the open triangle over the uninjured shoulder. *(Prevents undue pressure on injured side.)*
2. Place the apex of the triangle behind the elbow of the injured arm. *(Facilitates usefulness of sling.)*
3. Bend the arm at the elbow with the hand elevated slightly (4 to 5 inches). *(Enables venous return from hand and forearm, and facilitates drainage from edema.)*
4. Bring the forearm across the chest and over the bandage (see illustration). *(Establishes position of arm in sling.)*
5. Take the lower end of the triangle, and bring it over the shoulder of the injured side. Tie the bandage on the neck at the uninjured side so that the knot is on the side of the neck. *(Prevents pressure on cervical spine.)*
6. Twist the remaining end of the bandage, and tuck it in at the elbow. *(Secures sling.)*
7. Remember to keep fingertips exposed. *(Secures sling and allows for easy assessment of circulation.)*

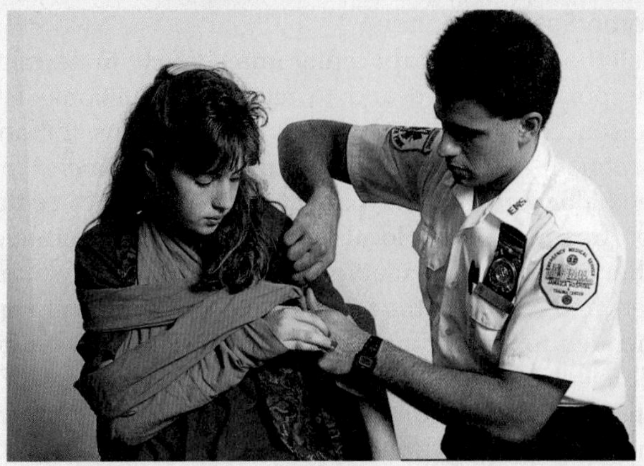

Step 4

tain even pressure. Cover the skin completely; it is safer to use a greater number of evenly spaced overlapping turns than fewer, tighter turns of the bandage. Start the gauze roller bandage at the point of dressing or at the part of the limb with the smallest circumference (e.g., the wrist or the ankle). Fasten the gauze roller bandage with either tape or a square knot. Use circular or spiral roller bandages to cover a cylindrical part. A figure-8 bandage is another option, especially useful if splints are necessary or when dressing an ankle (see Chapter 20).

POISONS

Each year thousands of people die from self-inflicted or accidental poisonings. Of these people, the majority are children. A **poison** is any substance (solid, liquid, or gas) that even in small amounts causes damage to the body or interferes with the function of its systems. Poison control centers throughout the United States are equipped to give information about poisons and methods of treatment on a 24-hour-a-day, 7-day-a-week basis. Most poisons act rapidly and thus necessitate immediate first aid.

Poison control centers need the following information:

- Weight of patient
- Age of patient
- Substance ingested, inhaled, or injected
- How much was taken
- When it was taken
- If patient takes other drugs and by which routes
- Status of patient at present

GENERAL ASSESSMENT OF POISONINGS

Acute signs and symptoms of poisonings are sometimes delayed for hours. The following are possible indications of poisonings: respiratory distress; pulmonary edema; bronchospasm; severe nausea, vomiting, or diarrhea; seizures, twitching, or paralysis; decreased level of consciousness or unconsciousness; restlessness, delirium, agitation, or panic; color changes; pale, flushed, or cyanotic skin; signs of burns or edema around the mouth or other areas of the body; pain, tenderness, or cramps on swallowing; characteristic odor on the breath; unusual urine color (red, green, bright yellow, black, bronze); slow, labored breathing or wheezing; abnormal constriction or dilation of pupils; abnormal eye movements, such as nystagmus (constant, involuntary, cyclic movement of the eyeball); skin irritation, erythema, or edema; and shock or cardiac arrest.

INGESTED POISONS

Poison ingestion by mouth is the most common type of poisoning, especially in children. Common substances include household cleaning products such as drain cleaners, oven cleaners, laundry detergents, floor or furniture polish, rat poison, cockroach sprays and baits, diaper pail deodorants, garden and garage supplies (e.g., insecticides, gasoline), drugs, medications, food, and plants, such as poinsettias. Older adults sometimes require special precautions (see Life Span Considerations for Older Adults box).

Immediate Response

Call the poison control center immediately to describe the poison ingested and to receive instructions. The poison control center will give instructions for any treatment to start in the home and/or recommend immediately bringing the patient to an emergency center for treatment. The local poison control center telephone number is available with other emergency numbers in the front of the telephone directory. It is recommended to place the poison control center number by all telephones in the home (Hockenberry et al., 2007). The American Academy of Pediatrics does not recommend keeping syrup of ipecac in the home to induce vomiting (American Academy of Pediatrics, 2003).

Treat for shock and administer CPR if needed. Make sure the substance's container and any vomitus is brought to the medical facility to help identify and treat the poison. Never give an antidote until you have consulted the poison control center.

INHALED POISONS

Poisons that are possible to inhale are often present without anyone knowing, and thus there is no advance warning of a problem. Once inhaled they are absorbed very rapidly, so prompt first aid measures are important. Common sources of inhaled poisons include carbon monoxide (from automobiles, fires, heating systems, propane engines, and paint remover), carbon dioxide (from sewers or industry), and refrigeration gases. Chlorine (used in cleaning and industry) and fumes from sprays and other liquid chemicals also have the potential to give off poisonous fumes, typically when cleaning chemicals are mixed together and create poisonous fumes.

Nursing Interventions

First assess the danger. Remove the victim from the area of exposure as soon as possible, but only if there is no danger to you or other rescuers. Loosen clothing from the victim's throat and chest. Maintain an airway, and ascertain whether it is necessary to start CPR. Keep the victim quiet and inactive while immediate transport to the nearest medical facility takes place.

 Life Span Considerations

Older Adults

Accidental Overdose

- Older adult patients are sometimes the victims of accidental overdose for the following reasons:
  - —Poor eyesight potentially leads to ingesting the wrong medication. Be sure all medications and other substances are clearly marked in large lettering.
  - —Confusion potentially leads to accidentally repeating a medication. Use of medication boxes in which medications are set up for a week at a time helps eliminate duplicate doses.
- Older patients are often receiving several medications. Be sure to get a good health history, including all medications, when providing emergency treatment.

ABSORBED POISONS

Poisons, caustic chemicals, and poisonous plants that come in contact with the skin are often rapidly absorbed, causing burning, skin irritation, allergic responses, or severe systemic reactions. Most signs and symptoms occur within 1 to 2 hours after absorption. Signs and symptoms include nausea, vomiting, diarrhea, flushed skin, dilated pupils, cardiovascular abnormalities, and central nervous system (CNS) and respiratory reactions. Poison ivy, poison oak, and poison sumac are the most common plants that have the capacity to elicit a poison response.

Nursing Interventions

The first action necessary is to quickly remove the source of the irritation and then to wash the contacted area with soap and water. Skin preparations that are effective in the treatment of contact poisonings include baking soda, Burow's solution, and oatmeal. Calamine lotion and hydrocortisone cream (5%) are effective to relieve pruritus.

INJECTED POISONS

Injections of drugs to which an individual is allergic and venomous stings from insects, reptiles, and animals will cause allergic reactions ranging from mild to severe. Emergency care involves keeping to a minimum any poison traveling to the heart.

Minor Reactions to Insect Bites

If the individual has been stung by a bee, remove the stinger with the **side** of a knife or credit card in a scraping motion. If you attempt to grasp the barbed stinger with tweezers, you will sometimes force venom further into the skin. Nursing interventions include washing the bite with soap and water and applying cold packs to relieve pain and slow the absorption of the poison. A paste of baking soda and water sometimes relieves pruritus at the site. Do not use a paste of meat tenderizer, because it will often irritate tissues if the skin is not intact.

Severe Reactions to Insect Bites

Within as little as 60 minutes or up to several hours afterward, a victim of a bite or sting will sometimes experience a severe allergic reaction. Urticaria, wheezing, edema of the lips and tongue, generalized pruritus, and respiratory arrest are the most common signs and symptoms of anaphylactic shock (severe allergic reaction).

Nursing Interventions

Have the victim lie down in a supine position with the legs elevated to promote venous return to the heart.

Immobilize the area of the bite. Remove rings and jewelry.

Then apply a wide (4- to 5-inch; 10- to 12.5-cm) constricting band proximal to the wound. Do not release the constricting band once applied because doing so will release a bolus of toxin into the patient. The properly applied band will stop only venous, not arterial, blood flow; therefore, make sure you are able to detect a pulse below the constriction. Keep the affected part in a dependent position, below the level of the heart. Have the victim transported to the hospital immediately, and if possible, identify the type of animal or insect that caused the bite. Keep the patient on nothing-by-mouth (NPO) status. People who know that they are allergic sometimes wear medical-alert tags and carry an epinephrine pen, an anaphylaxis kit, or antihistamines such as diphenhydramine (Benadryl) to take after a bite. Self-administration is possible. Only give this medication yourself if directed to do so by the physician.

Table 24-1 Blood Alcohol Concentration (BAC) and Related Effects

BAC* mg/dL (mg%)	PSYCHOPHYSIOLOGIC EFFECT
20 (0.02)	Light and moderate drinkers begin to feel some effects. Approximate BAC is reached after one drink.
40 (0.04)	Most people begin to feel relaxed.
60 (0.06)	Judgment is mildly impaired. People are less able to make rational decisions about their capabilities (e.g., driving skills).
80 (0.08)	Definite impairment of muscle coordination and driving skills occurs. Person is legally intoxicated in some states.
100 (0.10)	Clear deterioration of reaction time and control is observed. Person is legally intoxicated in most states.
120 (0.12)	Vomiting occurs unless this level is reached slowly.
150 (0.15)	Balance and movement are impaired. Equivalent of one half pint of whiskey is circulating in the bloodstream.
300 (0.30)	Many people lose consciousness.
400 (0.40)	Most people lose consciousness, and some die.
450 (0.45)	Breathing stops; person eventually dies.

From Lewis, S.L., et al. (2007). *Medical-surgical nursing: assessment and management of clinical problems.* (7th ed.). St. Louis: Mosby.
*Blood alcohol concentration (BAC) is generally recorded in milligrams of alcohol per deciliter (mg/dL) of blood or milligrams percent (mg%). Percentage is used for legal definitions of intoxication. BAC is dependent on how much alcohol is consumed, how fast it is consumed, and the person's weight and sex. Alcohol affects women differently than men. Expect women to have substantially more alcohol-caused impairment than men at equivalent levels of consumption.

DRUG AND ALCOHOL EMERGENCIES

Drugs (including alcohol) are chemical substances that have the potential to affect body functioning and are subject to abuse and overdose.

ALCOHOL

Alcohol is the most commonly abused drug in the world. It is a CNS depressant that has the capacity to cause many signs and symptoms, even death (Table 24-1).

Assessment

Signs and symptoms of **mild** intoxication include nausea, vomiting, diarrhea, lack of coordination, and poor muscle control. Flushing, erythema of the face and eyes, visual disturbances, and rapid mood swings are often present. Slurred or inappropriate speech, inappropriate behavior, and lethargy (sleepiness) are also typical.

Serious alcohol intoxication is usually caused by consuming a large quantity of alcohol over a short period. Signs and symptoms include drowsiness that progresses to coma; rapid, weak pulse; and depressed, labored breathing or respiratory arrest. Loss of control of urinary and bowel functions, and disorientation, restlessness, and hallucinations are possible, as are tremors that have the potential to progress to grand mal seizures, nausea, vomiting, expectorating blood from the respiratory tract, and diarrhea. Some people will also experience loss of memory, visual disturbances, lack of muscle coordination, and depressed reflexes.

DRUGS

Abuse of drugs is a major problem in the world today. Not only are illegal drugs abused, but so are prescription and over-the-counter medications. In assessing the drug abuser, observe for signs and symptoms of loss of reality orientation, hallucinations, and varying degrees of consciousness; coma and death are possible results. Slurred speech, extremes in mood swings, inappropriate behavior, and anxiety are also present in some cases. Sometimes the victim will have a fever and flushed skin and be experiencing diaphoresis (sweating). Lack of coordination and impaired judgment typically makes safety a real problem. Depending on the drug, the pulse and blood pressure will often increase or decrease, the pupils constrict or dilate, and the appetite increases or decreases. Obvious hypodermic needle marks on arms, legs, hands, feet, and neck are often present. Many victims complain of diarrhea or pain in the abdomen, legs, or joints, and also experience tremors or seizures.

Nursing Interventions

Because an accurate nursing history is important, obtain as much information as possible about the substance ingested, and keep the containers if possible. Handle any life-threatening situations first, ensuring an open airway is established and maintained. If the victim is unconscious, turn him or her to the side. Loosen clothing to assist ventilation. If the victim is having muscle twitching and is drowsy, do not attempt to arouse him or her, because this will sometimes precipitate a seizure. If a fever is present, attempt to reduce it by applying cool, wet compresses. Protect the victim from self-injury during a seizure or hallucination by removing harmful objects from the patient's vicinity. Do not attempt to restrain a victim during seizure activity.

Be calm, supportive, and nonjudgmental, especially if the patient is very agitated or excited. Never leave the intoxicated person alone. Frequently perform a careful assessment of mental status and vital signs. It is possible for a substance abuse victim to go into respiratory arrest very quickly. It is necessary to transport the victim promptly to a medical facility.

THERMAL AND COLD EMERGENCIES

HEAT INJURIES

Excessive heat affects the body in several ways. In a hot environment, heat builds up in the body. The body automatically attempts to get rid of the excessive heat by producing an increased amount of perspiration and slowing down muscular activity. If this mechanism fails for any external (environmental) or internal reason, heatstroke or heat exhaustion is the possible result. Heat exhaustion and heatstroke represent different reactions to excessive heat; for this reason signs, symptoms, and treatment are also different.

Heat Exhaustion

Heat exhaustion is the most common type of heat injury and is the result of prolonged perspiration and the loss of large quantities of salt and water. It occurs most often in hot, humid weather, when people do not adequately replace fluids (common in older adults who have a diminished thirst mechanism despite dehydration).

Nursing assessment of the victim of heat exhaustion includes observing for signs and symptoms such as headache, vertigo, nausea, weakness, and diaphoresis.

Mental disorientation and brief loss of consciousness sometimes occur. The victim has a normal body temperature with pale, cold, clammy skin. Some victims complain of abdominal cramps and loss of appetite. Breathing will typically be rapid and shallow, and the pulse weak and rapid. Blood pressure will sometimes drop but usually returns to normal when the person assumes a recumbent position.

Nursing Interventions

It is essential to cool the victim off as quickly as possible; move the victim to a cool area, but avoid chilling. Remove as much clothing as possible, and loosen constrictive clothing to allow the circulation of air to cool the body. Have the victim lie down with the feet 8 to 12 inches higher than the head. Use cold, wet compresses to cool the victim, as well as a fan or air conditioner if available.

If the victim is completely conscious and alert, give one half glass (120 mL) of water every 15 minutes for 1 hour. The use of salted water is controversial in the treatment of heat emergencies. Follow the advice of the physician when administering salted water. If the victim is drowsy or vomiting, do not give any fluids by mouth. In the clinical setting, IV fluids are given. Have the victim transported to a medical facility as soon as possible.

Heatstroke

Heatstroke is the more serious heat injury; death is possible if heatstroke goes untreated. The most common cause of heatstroke is vigorous physical activity in a hot, humid environment. The body becomes overheated, but the cooling mechanism of perspiration does not operate because of the hot, humid conditions. Deprived of this mechanism, the body stores excessive heat. Body temperature will sometimes rise to 106° F (41° C) or greater. Brain and CNS damage will possibly result.

Assessment

The signs and symptoms of heatstroke include rapidly rising body temperature; hot, dry, erythemic skin; and no visible perspiration. The pulse is rapid initially, then slows and weakens as the blood pressure falls. Breathing becomes deep and rapid. The victim complains of headache, dry mouth, nausea, and vomiting; some victims experience vertigo and decreased level of consciousness, and collapse. Muscle twitching and convulsions are possible.

Nursing Interventions

It is important to cool the victim as quickly as possible, moving him or her to a cool area. Establishing and maintaining an airway are priority nursing interventions. Undress the victim (retaining undergarments only). Cool the victim's bare skin as quickly as possible with cold water or ice compresses. It is acceptable to place cold packs around the neck, under the axillae, on the inguinal area, and around the ankles to cool the blood in the main arteries. Use a fan or air conditioner if available. Continue treatment until the victim's temperature falls below 100° F (37.7° C). Monitor the victim for chilling (control shivering because this will only increase temperature) as the body temperature falls, and check the temperature every 10 to 15 minutes to ensure that it does not rise again. Continue cooling efforts until the victim is able to obtain medical assistance.

EXPOSURE TO EXCESSIVE COLD

When the body is exposed to severe cold, body heat is lost, blood vessels constrict, and destruction of tissue sometimes results. Cold, moist air, fatigue, smoking, drugs, alcohol, dehydration, age, and some disease entities (such as diabetes mellitus) accelerate the potential for injury. People with darker skin are more prone to frostbite.

Hypothermia

Hypothermia is a body temperature lower than the normal level of 95° F (35° C). The brain, the heart, the lungs, and other vital organs are affected by this drop in temperature. Hypothermia occurs most frequently when the air is windy, cold, and moist or when precipitation is present. Many victims are exhausted, intoxicated, or using illicit drugs. Older adults or persons living in a poorly heated environment are subject to hypothermia. Older adults do not tolerate cold as well as younger adults. The older adult will often experience hypothermia at warmer temperatures than a younger adult.

Assessment

Initially, the victim is likely to shiver uncontrollably; shivering ceases when the body temperature is less than 90° F (32.2° C). Speech becomes slow, slurred, and incoherent, and the victim tends to demonstrate memory lapses, disorientation, stupor, decreased reflex response, and poor judgment. Safety is a problem, because the gait becomes uncoordinated, and muscle activity will sometimes decrease or even cease. The skin appears mottled and edematous, and the patient complains of generalized numbness. A weak, irregular pulse develops with hypotension and a depressed respiratory rate. The victim becomes lethargic, with decreasing levels of consciousness. The functioning of the liver, the kidneys, and the digestive system slows down. This often results in problems of coagulation, abdominal distention, and paralytic ileus, as well as acute renal failure (Beattie, 2006). Finally there is a loss of all reflexes, and the victim appears to be dead. Severe problems with electrolyte disturbances create the risk of serious dysrhythmias and cardiac arrest.

Nursing Interventions

Although a person in the final stages of hypothermia will sometimes appear to be dead because of the effects of the lowered metabolic rate, it is possible to revive many such victims. Always attempt to treat hypothermia by instituting first aid. Initiate CPR if necessary, even if the victim appears dead. Continue CPR until the body is warmed. Place the victim in a supine position with the head lower than the feet. Warm the victim *slowly;* rapid exposure to warmth tends to precipitate shock. Move the victim to a warm area, and remove all wet clothes and replace them with dry ones. Cover the victim with warm blankets. In treating a patient in the final stages of hypothermia, active internal rewarming in addition to passive external rewarming will effectively raise the core body temperature. One method is to administer warm humidified oxygen per mask or per ventilator; another method is to use heated IV fluids such as D_5 NS at 104° to 113° F (40° to 45° C). Patients with final stages of hypothermia sometimes develop atrial fibrillation and therefore will need continuous electrocardiographic (ECG) monitoring during treatment and immediately afterward (Beattie, 2006).

If the victim is completely conscious, it is acceptable to provide warm fluids to drink. *Never* give alcohol because of its vasodilatory effect on the peripheral vessels, which causes the central core temperature to drop further. It is essential to obtain medical help as soon as possible.

Frostbite

Frostbite is the most common and dangerous local cold injury involving freezing and damaging of body cells. Ice crystals actually form in the body fluid and underlying tissues. These crystals draw water from the cells, causing destruction of tissue integrity. Common areas affected by frostbite are the ears, nose, fingers, and toes. Hypothermia sometimes accompanies frostbite.

Assessment

Initially the frostbitten skin takes on a red flush, and the victim typically complains of numbness, tingling, or pain. Progressively the part becomes hard and loses all sensation. The color of the part changes to grayish white as circulation diminishes further. If thawing occurs, the color will often change to blue-purple or black, indicating severe damage to or death of tissues. Edema often develops, followed by blisters. If frostbite damage is severe, complete loss of function of the part is possible.

Nursing Interventions

If there is a possibility that the part will become refrozen after it has been thawed, it is better to leave it frozen until the victim arrives at a medical facility. Severe tissue damage is possible as a result of thawing and refreezing a frozen part. Treat the victim for shock and hypothermia, and establish and maintain an airway. Remove any constricting clothing to encourage circulation.

If there is no risk of the part being refrozen, warm it in the following manner: Immerse the frozen part in warm water (preferably a bathtub) at 104° to 110° F (40° to 43.3° C) for 20 to 45 minutes. Check the water temperature frequently, and do not allow it to cool. If a tub is not available, use a hot, moist towel. **Be very careful not to rub the part;** you create the risk of bruising and damaging the underlying tissue by friction. If water is not available, warm the part by placing it against a warm part of your body—the axilla, the abdomen, or between the legs. Never place the frozen part near an open flame or oven. Gentle warming is necessary to prevent burns and damage.

Once the part is warmed, encourage the victim to gently move the part. If the legs or feet are involved, however, do not allow the victim to walk. Wrap the thawed part in clean towels or bulky dressings, and elevate it. Keep the entire body warm, and offer warm fluids to drink. Once again, never give alcohol; and do not allow the victim to smoke because this will cause further vasoconstriction. Never place ice, snow, or cold sources on a frostbitten area. Have a physician evaluate all frostbite injuries, no matter how minor.

BONE, JOINT, AND MUSCLE INJURIES

The four major types of injuries that occur to bones, tendons, ligaments, and muscles are fractures, dislocations, sprains, and strains.

FRACTURES

A **fracture** is a break in the continuity of a bone. Fractured bones are seldom an immediate threat to life, although they do have the potential to cause serious complications. In administering first aid to an injured victim, establishing an airway and treating hemorrhage are priorities. Fractures sometimes cause considerable blood loss (750 to 3000 mL from a fractured pelvis and 500 to 3000 mL from a fractured femur).

There are several types of common fractures:

- **Open or compound fractures:** An open wound exists over the fracture site. Often the affected bone is visible as it protrudes through the skin.
- **Closed fracture:** The skin overlying the injury is intact.
- **Comminuted fracture:** The bone is shattered into two or more fragments or pieces.
- **Greenstick fracture:** An incomplete break, occurring most commonly in children because their bones are pliable.
- **Spiral fracture:** Fracture resulting from a twisting force.
- **Impacted fracture:** Fracture resulting from trauma that causes the bone ends to jam together.
- **Compressed fracture:** Fracture to the vertebrae as the result of pressure.
- **Depression fracture:** Results from blunt trauma to a flat bone, causing an indentation in the bone.

Assessment

The physician, using x-ray diagnostic procedures, will determine whether a bone is fractured. Fracture is suspected if there are pain and tenderness in the area of the fracture; pain also develops during movement, and the victim complains of an inability to move the affected part. A deformity of the limb may be obvious, with edema and discoloration (cyanosis, erythema) of the area. Fragments of bone will sometimes protrude through the skin. If the affected part is moved, a grating sound is heard. This is called **crepitus** and is caused by the broken bones scraping against each other. Sometimes the victim will report having heard or felt the bone snap.

Nursing Interventions

Do not move the victim unless he or she is in danger. The ABCs of first aid take priority. Next, control bleeding in open fractures by cutting away the clothing around the wound and covering the wound with a large, sterile pressure dressing. Do not attempt to reduce the fracture; you will possibly cause further damage to the bone and tissue. Treat the victim for shock.

Immobilize the fracture, but make no attempt to realign the bone. The rule is, "Splint the part where it lies." It is possible to change a fracture from a simple break to a comminuted or splintered one by moving it improperly. Use a lightweight but rigid splint. It has to be long enough to extend past the joints above and beyond the fracture, and be wider than the thickest part of the injury. Make sure the splint is padded on the inner surface to prevent contact with the skin. Support the fracture while gently sliding the splint under the limb. Use a roller bandage or similar material to secure the limb in place (Figure 24-15). Monitor circulation in the limb by assessing color, temperature, and pulses below the injury; complaints of numbness and tingling; and evidence of edema. Apply ice or cold packs to reduce edema (swelling).

DISLOCATIONS

Dislocations occur in joints. They usually result from a blow or fall. Common sites of dislocations are the jaw, the shoulder, the elbow, the wrist, the finger, the hip, and the ankle.

Assessment

The victim will usually complain of pain and edema in the area of the dislocation. Sometimes you will be able to observe a deformity of the part. Sometimes the part will be rigid, and the victim unable to move it.

Nursing Interventions

Never attempt to reduce a dislocation or push the joint back into place; this will further damage delicate ligaments, tendons, nerves (especially the olecranon elbow), and the bone. It is necessary to splint the joint in

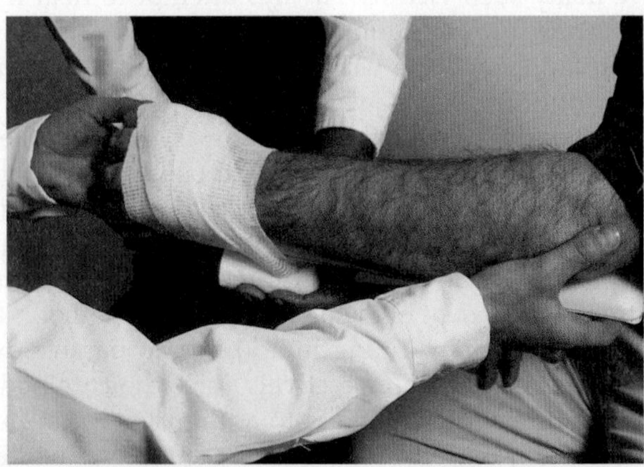

FIGURE 24-15 Immobilization of a fractured arm.

the same manner as a fracture. Make sure the splint is large enough to support the limb in the line of the deformity. Bind the limb to the body or support it in a sling. This is useful in dislocations of the shoulder and elbow. Apply ice or cold packs to reduce edema (swelling) to surrounding tissues.

STRAINS AND SPRAINS

Strains are injuries to muscle tissue that result from stretching and tearing from overexertion. Sprains are injuries to joints resulting from stretched or torn ligaments, typically caused by twisting the joint beyond the normal range of motion. The most commonly affected joints are the knee and the ankle. Permanent damage to the tissue and joint are possible if sprains are left untreated.

Assessment

Injuries to muscle or ligaments result in the following signs and symptoms:

- **Strains:** Spasms or muscle "knots," acute pain, stiffness, and weakness on movement; back pain radiating down the leg; discoloration
- **Sprains:** Pain or tenderness around a joint; immobility of the joint; rapid and marked edema; discoloration around the joint

Nursing Interventions

Treat any suspected musculoskeletal injury as a fracture until fracture is definitely ruled out. In the treatment of sprains and strains, remember the acronym **RICE**, which stands for *r*est, *i*ce, *c*ompression, and *e*levation:

R **Rest** the affected extremity.

I **Ice** is applied to the part but not directly to the skin until the edema and pain subside (24 to 72 hours is most common). Follow this with warm compresses to encourage healing by increasing the blood flow. Assess the victim's skin frequently for any evidence of burns.

C **Compression:** Use an Ace bandage or compression bandage to support the injured part.

E **Elevation:** Elevate the part above the level of the heart to promote venous flow and reduce edema.

SPINAL CORD INJURIES

Assessment

To assess for paralysis, ask the victim if he or she is able to move the hands and feet and if any pain or sensation is felt. Test for sensation by touching or pinching the victim's skin. Any abrasions and ecchymosis, especially on the shoulders, back, and abdomen, indicate possible injury to the victim's spinal cord.

Nursing Interventions

Take spinal cord precautions in all cases of head trauma and multiple traumas. There is a high correlation between neck and spinal cord injuries in patients with facial lacerations. Establish an airway, keeping the head in a neutral position (never hyperextending the neck). If the victim vomits, have several people, acting together as one unit, move the victim onto his or her side to allow drainage.

Administer CPR if necessary. Treat hemorrhage and shock. Always keep the head and neck in line with the body when moving the victim. Even a slight movement of the individual's head creates the potential of causing spinal damage. Do not attempt to move the victim without at least three assistants (Skill 24-3). Make sure the technicians are trained in emergency medical care (i.e., EMTs).

BURN INJURIES

Burns are a leading cause of accidental injuries, especially among children. Burns are caused by heat from fire or steam, electricity from faulty wiring, chemicals such as lye, strong cleaning products, acids, solar radiation, and radioactive materials. The initial management of the burn patient begins at the time of injury. The first priority is to stop the burning process.

Burns are often classified according to their depth or the extent of the body surface area burned. The principal complications of all burns are shock from loss of fluids and electrolytes, and trauma and infection due to the loss of the skin as a barrier. Calculate the extent of burns using the rule of nines (Figure 24-16).

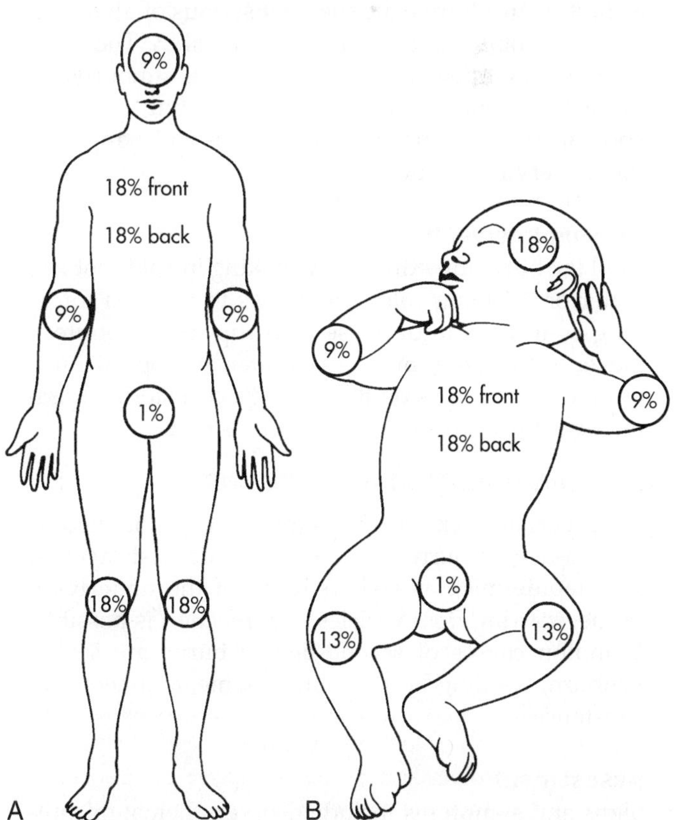

FIGURE 24-16 Rule of nines. **A,** Adult. **B,** Child.

Skill 24-3 Moving the Victim with a Suspected Spinal Cord Injury

Nursing Action *(Rationale)*

1. Carefully roll the victim, supporting the entire length of the body, just enough to slip a solid board underneath the victim. It is necessary for the board to extend beyond the victim's head and feet (see illustrations). *(Supports the entire spine.)*
2. While another person steadies the victim's head, place a towel or padding in the space underneath the victim's neck (never put the head on a pillow). *(Immobilizes the head and neck.)*
3. Place additional padding (rolled-up blankets, towels, sandbags) around the head and neck, keeping the neck in line with the body. Using a cervical collar is acceptable. *(Holds the head in place.)*
4. Secure the victim to the backboard with bandages, or improvise these. Tape the head in place. *(Immobilizes the entire body.)*
5. In the event of an emergency situation in which the victim is wearing a helmet, immobilize the victim with the helmet left in place. *(Prevents further injury.)*

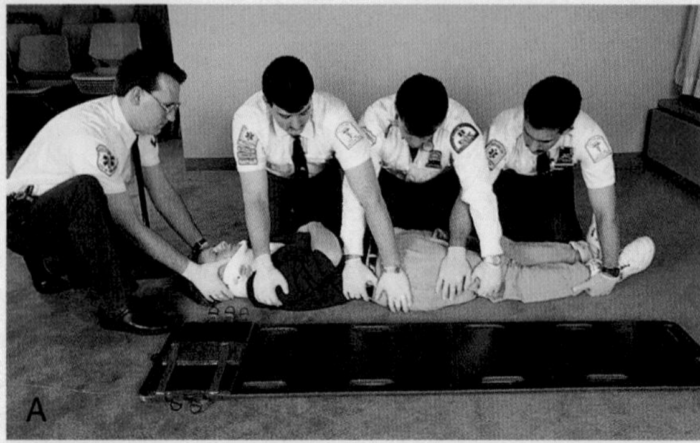

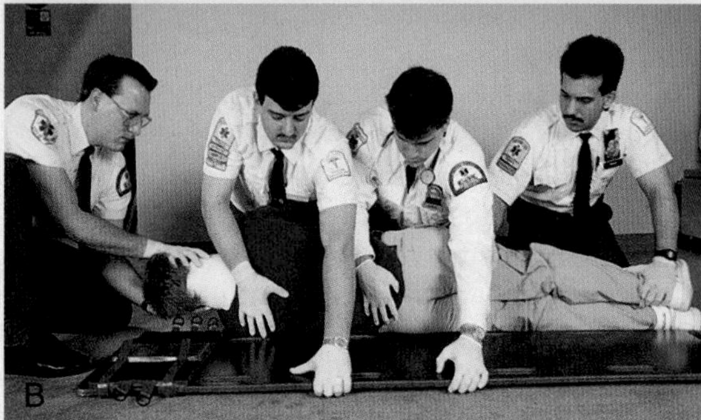

Step 1

SHALLOW PARTIAL-THICKNESS BURNS

Shallow partial-thickness burns (previously classified as first-degree burns) are the least serious of all burns, involving only the outer layer of the skin. The most common first-degree burns are simple sunburns or burns from contact with hot objects. Healing is usually spontaneous and uncomplicated. Signs and symptoms include erythema and pain.

Nursing Interventions

Cool the burn immediately by soaking in cold (not ice) water or applying cold compresses to the area for as long as it takes to decrease pain (up to 30 minutes). Never put grease, butter, saltwater, or topical burn ointments or sprays on the burn. Place a sterile dressing over the burn site to prevent infection.

DEEP PARTIAL-THICKNESS BURNS

Deep partial-thickness burns (previously classified as second-degree burns) fully involve the first layer of skin (epidermis), as well as some of the underlying tissue; scarring from vesicles and infection is possible. Common causes of second-degree burns are severe sunburn, scalding liquids, direct flame, and chemical substances.

Assessment

Signs and symptoms include deep erythema, or mottled skin with blister formation. Considerable edema often results, lasting several days. Fluid will typically weep through the skin surface (loss of plasma), and the patient will complain of intense pain.

FULL-THICKNESS BURNS

Full-thickness burns (previously classified as third-degree burns) involve destruction of the skin and underlying tissue, including fat, muscle, and bone. The area is usually charred, and healing is difficult. The skin will usually be thick and leathery, with black or dark brown, cherry red, or dry and milky white colors. Often the victim will not complain of pain, because nerve endings are sometimes severed by the burn. There is a hyperpermeability of capillaries, with plasma seeping into the interstitial spaces resulting in edema and vesiculation (blistering). The larger the burned area involved, the greater the shift of fluid from the intravascular area into the interstitial area. Fluid loss causes a fluid and electrolyte imbalance to occur. Hypovolemic shock and infection are common complications. Medical attention is urgent. Common causes of full-thickness burns are direct flame (ignited clothing), explosions, and gasoline or oil fires.

Nursing Interventions for Moderate to Severe Burns (Deep Partial-Thickness and Full-Thickness Burns)

It is crucial to establish an airway before edema occurs. Assess respiratory and cardiac function. Airway, breathing, and circulation are the priority concerns. Remove all of the victim's clothing, shoes, and jewelry, which may be constricting and even smoldering. It is possible to cause more severe burns by leaving clothing on. Administer CPR if necessary. Treat the victim for shock. Keep the victim warm, with the burned area elevated. Inspect for burns or soot around the mouth and nose, which have the potential to affect respiratory status. Immediately flush chemical burns with copious amounts of water.

If medical help will be arriving within 15 to 30 minutes, withhold oral fluids. If medical help is delayed, it is acceptable to give one half a glass of water mixed with one half a teaspoon of salt plus one half a teaspoon of baking soda to replace electrolytes. If vomiting occurs, do not give fluids.

Cool a partial-thickness burn immediately, using cool compresses; do not do this for other types of burns. Cool compresses will sometimes cause hypothermia in victims with more extensive burns. Remove clothing from the burned area. Always remove the victim's shoes; often heavy boots will be smoldering and will cause a more severe burn. Do not break vesicles (blisters), and avoid touching the burn with anything except sterile dressings. Do not apply antiseptics, ointments, sprays, or creams on the burn; this will potentially interfere with medical treatment and cause further complications. Apply loose, sterile dressings over the burn. Check the victim frequently to be sure that edema has not caused further constriction of the area near the burn.

TERRORISM AND BIOTERRORISM

TERRORISM

Terrorism, or the possibility of a terrorist attack, is a new environmental health threat. Terrorism is a violent or dangerous act used to intimidate or coerce a person or government in furtherance of a political or social agenda. Before 1990 and the Gulf War, the possibility of the United States coming under attack from terrorist groups using biological, chemical, or nuclear weapons seemed remote. After the terrorist attacks on The World Trade Center in New York City and the Pentagon on September 11, 2001, the Homeland Security Act of 2002 was implemented. Its purpose was to create a single agency to oversee the development of a comprehensive approach to any large domestic incident. Today, more than ever, we are concerned about an attack by an individual or small group on one of our cities, a large sporting event, or a unit of our military forces.

BIOTERRORISM

Bioterrorism, or the use of biological agents to create fear and threat, is the most likely form of terrorist attack to occur. It is essential for health care facilities to be prepared to treat mass casualties from such an attack. A facility's emergency management plan provides details on how to respond to a terrorist attack, for example, determining the agent used, determining the time and location of the attack and the affected population, obtaining and delivering supplies, and providing treatment. Nurses need to prepare themselves through education and training to respond to an attack by taking the necessary steps to initiate an agency's emergency management plan.

Bioterrorist Attacks

Although the occurrence of a bioterrorist attack has been limited to the anthrax deaths following September 11, 2001, the threat is considerable. Nurses need to be prepared to make accurate and timely assessments in any type of setting. If an attack occurs, it will most likely involve the use of biological agents such as anthrax, botulism, smallpox, or bubonic plague. A bioterrorist attack will likely resemble a natural outbreak initially, but it is necessary to recognize the possibility that the microorganisms used have been modified for increased virulence or have resistance to antibiotics or vaccines. Biological attacks are either overt (announced) or covert (unannounced). Overt attacks necessitate rapid assessment of the reality of their occurrence and their nature, followed by an appropriate response. Covert attacks become obvious only after victims present themselves requesting medical care, after the incubation period has passed and clinical signs begin to appear. In both cases it is essential for you to know and recognize **high-risk syndromes** (groups of signs and symptoms resulting from a common cause or appearing together, to present a clinical picture of a disease) (Box 24-4). Acutely ill patients representing the earliest cases after a covert attack will seek care in emergency departments. Patients who are at the onset of an illness and are less ill are likely to seek care in primary care settings or try to manage the signs and symptoms on their own.

It is possible to use basic **epidemiologic** (the distribution and determinants of health-related states and events in populations) principles to assess whether or not a patient's presentation of symptoms is typical of an endemic (the expected or normal incidence native to or occurring naturally to a specific area or environment) disease or is an unusual event that properly raises a red flag. Features that will alert you to the possibility of a bioterrorism-related outbreak include the following:

- A rapidly increasing incidence of a disease (e.g., within hours or days) in a normally healthy population
- An unusual increase in the number of people seeking care, especially with fever, respiratory, or gastrointestinal complaints
- An epidemic disease rapidly emerging at an uncharacteristic time or in an unusual pattern
- Lower attack rates among patients who had been indoors, in areas with filtered or closed ventilation, compared with people who had been outdoors

Box 24-4 High-Risk Syndromes

Anthrax (acute infectious disease caused by *Bacillus anthracis,* a spore-forming, gram-positive bacillus). Humans become infected through skin contact, ingestion, or inhalation. Person-to-person transmission of inhalational disease does not occur. Direct exposure to vesicle secretions of skin anthrax sometimes results in secondary cutaneous infection.

Clinical Features: Pulmonary: flulike symptoms; possible brief interim improvement; within 2 to 4 days, abrupt onset of respiratory failure and hemodynamic collapse. Gram-positive bacilli on blood culture tests. *Cutaneous:* local skin involvement, common on the head, the forearms, or the hands; localized itching followed by a papular lesion that turns vesicular and within 2 to 6 days becomes a depressed black eschar. *Gastrointestinal:* abdominal pain, nausea, vomiting, and fever after eating contaminated food (usually meat); bloody diarrhea, hematemesis; gram-positive bacilli on blood culture. Symptoms begin within 1 day to 8 weeks (average 5 days) depending on exposure route and amount of agent.

Botulism (caused by *Clostridium botulinum,* an anaerobic gram-positive bacillus that produces a potent neurotoxin). Foodborne botulism is the most common form. An airborne form of botulism is also possible.

Clinical Features: Foodborne botulism causes abdominal cramping, diarrhea, and other gastrointestinal symptoms. Both foodborne and inhalation botulism cause responsive patient with absence of fever; drooping eyelids, weakened jaw clench, and difficulty swallowing or speaking; blurred vision and double vision; symmetric paralysis of arms first, followed by respiratory muscles, and then legs; respiratory dysfunction from respiratory muscle paralysis. **No sensory deficits.** Neurologic symptoms of botulism begin 12 to 36 hours after ingestion and 24 to 72 hours after inhalation. The disease is not transmitted from person to person.

Plague (an acute bacterial disease caused by the gram-negative bacillus *Yersinia pestis*). A bioterrorism-related outbreak is generally expected to be airborne.

Clinical Features: Fever, cough, chest pain, hemoptysis, mucopurulent or watery sputum with gram-negative rods in a Gram stain test. X-ray film shows bronchopneumonia. Person-to-person transmission is possible via large aerosol droplets. Symptoms usually appear within 1 to 3 days.

Smallpox (an acute viral illness caused by the *variola virus*). Disease has the potential to cause severe morbidity in a nonimmune population, and it is transmissible via the airborne route. A single case of smallpox is a public health emergency.

Clinical Features: Symptoms are similar to other acute viral illnesses such as the flu. Skin lesions appear, quickly progressing from macules to papules to vesicles. Other symptoms include 2 to 4 days of fever and myalgia; rash is most prominent on face and extremities (including palms and soles); rash scabs over in 1 to 2 weeks. Smallpox is transmitted by large and small respiratory droplets. Person-to-person transmission is likely from airborne and droplet exposure, and by contact with skin lesions or secretions. Symptoms begin in 7 to 17 days (average 12 days).

Adapted from Potter P.A., & Perry A.G. (2007). *Basic nursing: essentials for practice.* (6th ed.). St. Louis: Mosby.

- Clusters of patients arriving from a single locale
- Large numbers of rapidly fatal cases
- Any patient with a disease that is relatively uncommon and has bioterrorism potential

You need to be able to recognize a biological casualty and to carry out your role and responsibilities quickly and efficiently. Timely communication is critical for alerting both the medical and the general communities at large to a bioterrorist attack. Health care agencies' emergency plans will outline the predetermined departments to contact in the event of an attack and who is responsible for reporting the suspected occurrence to the local public health authorities.

Infection prevention and control practices are critical in the event of a biological attack. All patients with suspected or confirmed bioterrorism-related illnesses are necessary to manage using standard precautions (see Chapter 12). For certain diseases, such as smallpox or pneumonic plague, airborne and contact isolation precautions will be needed. Although a number of infections associated with biological agents are not transmitted from patient to patient, in general it is best to limit the transport and movement of patients to movement that is essential for treatment and care. It is also obligatory for staff to ensure that they are using all safety precautions to protect themselves as well as those in the immediate surroundings.

TERRORISM BY NUCLEAR EXPOSURE

The threat of nuclear terrorism is real. One projected example is an attack on a domestic nuclear weapon facility. Another is the use of a so-called "dirty bomb," which is a radiation dispersal device that has nuclear waste coupled with a conventional bomb.

The source of radiation on the contaminated patient is carried on the body or clothing, or it has been ingested or absorbed through a skin opening. The effects on the patient are determined by the amount of radiation absorbed (absorbed radiation is measured by the gray [Gy], equal to 100 rads). When less than 0.75 Gy is absorbed, patients usually do not have any symptoms. Patients who absorb 8 Gy will usually die, and an absorption of 30 Gy is always fatal. The Occupational Safety and Health Administration (OSHA) (2005) requires that hospitals have an emergency plan for treating patients contaminated with radioactive substances. A decontamination unit is set up near the emergency department.

The patient who absorbs more than 0.75 Gy will possibly develop acute radiation syndrome; the severity of symptoms will vary, depending on the amount of radiation absorbed. The following symptoms are noted:

- **Hematopoietic:** Deficiency of white blood cells and platelets, which leads to bleeding, anemia, infections, impaired wound healing, and immunodeficiency
- **Gastrointestinal:** Loss of mucosal barrier and cells lining the intestine, which results in fluid and electrolyte loss, vomiting, hematemesis, diarrhea, melena, loss of normal flora, and sepsis
- **Cerebrovascular and central nervous system:** Cerebral edema, hyperpyrexia, hypotension, confusion, and disorientation
- **Skin:** Loss of epidermis and possibly the dermis

During the prodromal phase immediately following exposure, signs and symptoms in more than one of these areas appear. The latent phase follows in a day or two when all symptoms generally disappear for a few days to a few weeks. Then, in the illness phase, the signs and symptoms reappear and intensify. Following the peak in the illness phase, the patient will either begin to recover or will die. Death typically occurs from infection or other complications.

CHEMICAL TERRORISM

The following are several types of agents that may be used in chemical terrorism.

- **Pulmonary agents:** Include the gases chlorine (Cl), phosgene, ammonia, and hydrochloric acid. These agents cause shortness of breath, chest tightness, and wheezing and often lead to pulmonary edema. Symptoms sometimes take 2 to 24 hours to appear. Fluid in the lungs leads to hypovolemia and hypotension. Patient will possibly require mechanical ventilation and supportive care.
- **Incapacitating agents:** Include BZ (a glycolate anticholinergic compound) and agent 15 (an Iraqi version of BZ). These agents impair rather than kill or seriously injure victims. The effects include understimulation of organs, hyperthermia, hallucinations, altered perceptions, and erratic behavior.
- **Cyanide agents:** Hydrogen cyanide is one example; these agents form cyanide when metabolized and can be either ingested or inhaled. A patient in severe respiratory distress without cyanosis has probably been exposed to cyanide. Cyanide has a pungent odor similar to bitter almonds or peaches. When an individual is exposed to a high concentration, death will occur within 5 to 10 minutes.
- **Nerve agents:** Taubin (GA), Sarin (GB), Soman (GD), and V-agents (VX) are some of the most toxic nerve agents, and they cause death in a matter of minutes. Symptoms include increased saliva production, chest pressure, rhinorrhea, vomiting, muscle weakness, incontinence, and convulsions. Appearance of symptoms is possible up to 10 hours following exposure to a low concentration.
- **Vesicant agents:** Sulfur mustard (H), distilled mustard (HD), nitrogen mustard (HN 1, 3), mustargen (HN 2), lewisite (L), and phosgene oxime (OX) are in this group. Vesicants are more lethal than pulmonary agents and cyanide agents because they will sometimes remain in the environment for weeks, which results in a continuing source of exposure. Sulfur mustard smells like mustard or garlic, but another agent smells like geraniums, and yet another has a peppery smell. Vesicants affect the skin, the eyes, and the airway, and large doses damage the bone marrow. These agents have the capacity to cause vesicles that progress to severe tissue necrosis and sloughing. Symptoms of sulfur mustard exposure appear in 4 to 8 hours, but cellular damage occurs in 2 minutes with agents like lewisite and phosgene oxime.

❖ NURSING PROCESS

The role of the licensed practical nurse/licensed vocational nurse (LPN/LVN) in the nursing process as stated is that the LPN/LVN will:

- Participate in planning care for patients based on patient needs
- Review patient's plan of care and recommend revisions as needed
- Review and follow defined prioritization for patient care
- Use clinical pathways, care maps, or care plans to guide and review patient care

■ Assessment

Patients requiring first aid are possibly suffering from a variety of injuries, not just the immediately visible problem. It is necessary to perform a complete head-to-toe assessment on all patients to determine the extent of injury. Give primary consideration to the ABCs—airway, breathing, and circulation. Quick and accurate assessment of the situation is vital.

Suspect all patients who have sustained head trauma of having spinal injuries. Automobile accidents and falls are injuries that often result in spinal injuries. Even though no visible injury is noted, severe damage is possible in the absence of proper immobilization.

Also assess the emotional status of patients needing first aid. Even minor accidents will often cause emotional distress. This is true not only for the patient, but also for the patient's family and friends.

■ Nursing Diagnosis

A nursing diagnosis provides the basis for developing a plan of care for the patient. Emergency care patients will often have a variety of problems that it is necessary to address. You will then be able to plan care of the patient. Possible nursing diagnoses for first aid may include the following:

- Acute confusion
- Ineffective tissue perfusion (cerebral, cardiopulmonary, renal, gastrointestinal, peripheral)

- Anxiety
- Decreased cardiac output
- Hyperthermia
- Hypothermia
- Impaired skin integrity
- Impaired spontaneous ventilation
- Ineffective airway clearance
- Acute or chronic pain
- Post-trauma syndrome
- Risk for infection

Expected Outcomes and Planning

Focus the plan for patients needing first aid on life-threatening emergencies as a priority. Specific, measurable goals and outcomes are important to prevent further injury to the patient. Be prepared to provide care quickly and efficiently and be aware of complications as they become apparent.

The plan of care relates to the specific nursing diagnosis. Examples include the following:

Goal 1: Identify interventions to prevent the risk of infection.

Outcome: No signs or symptoms of infection are noted.

Goal 2: Patient remains free of complications such as brain damage.

Outcome: Core body temperature is within normal range.

Implementation

Depending on the patient's injuries, a variety of measures are possible to implement to meet the patient's needs (Nursing Care Plan 24-1). Priorities are always maintaining an open airway, ensuring that the patient is breathing or providing artificial respiration, and maintaining circulation. Ensuring cardiac functioning will sometimes involve giving cardiac compression. Severe bleeding, such as arterial spurting, is possible to control by direct pressure, indirect pressure, or a tourniquet as a last resort. Stabilization of the spine in suspected spinal injuries is possible to accomplish through the use of neck immobilizers and backboards.

Patients needing first aid care will also need emotional support. Family and friends are also likely to need your understanding and comforting. Keeping the patient and family informed of procedures and the arrival of emergency aid will help them keep their anxiety levels under control. See the Cultural Considerations and Home Care Considerations boxes for additional information regarding emergency nursing interventions.

Evaluation

Evaluation is an ongoing process. Injuries are not always visible on initial assessment. It is essential to constantly reevaluate the situation until the patient's condition is stable. You will update the plan of care

Nursing Care Plan 24-1 The Patient with a Laceration

Ms. Tan, 75 years of age, is living in a long-term care facility. She accidentally cut herself with a knife during dinner. On examination, the nurse finds a 2-cm laceration to the patient's left hand that is actively bleeding.

NURSING DIAGNOSIS *Impaired skin integrity, related to trauma*

Patient Goals and Expected Outcomes	Nursing Interventions	Evaluation
Bleeding wound will be controlled within 15 minutes Patient's wound will heal without complication within 7 to 10 days	Assess extent of wound, amount and type of bleeding, presence of dirt or contaminating substances. Cleanse wound using normal saline. Apply direct pressure to control bleeding. Dress wound with sterile dressings.	Superficial 2-cm laceration to the palm of the left hand, moderate amount of bleeding noted. No visible dirt or food particles in wound. Wound irrigated with normal saline; bleeding controlled after 5 minutes of direct pressure. Wound dressed with a sterile 4-inch by 4-inch gauze secured with tape.

NURSING DIAGNOSIS *Risk for infection, related to laceration*

Patient Goals and Expected Outcomes	Nursing Interventions	Evaluation
Wound will heal within 7 to 10 days without signs of infection	Cleanse wound every shift with normal saline. Keep covered with sterile dressings until wound heals.	Wound edges well approximated; no bleeding, redness, swelling, or drainage from site.

Critical Thinking Questions

1. Ms. Tan's wound was superficial. In contrast, what would be the nurse's actions if the wound appears to be deep or was spurting blood?
2. What safety measures are indicated to ensure Ms. Tan is not injured again?

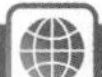

Cultural Considerations

Effect of Culture during Emergencies

- At a time of emergency, patients will often fall back on their language of origin. An interpreter will be able to help with language barriers.
- Emergency equipment is frightening to many people. Be sure patients understand what you are doing and the purpose of any equipment.
- Some cultures believe in the use of a local medicine person and are distrustful of Western medical practitioners. Try to work within a patient's beliefs rather than contradicting them outright. In an emergency, patients will look toward what they know best.

depending on the evaluation. Refer to the goals and outcomes when planning care, and perform procedures designed to meet those goals. Examples of goals and evaluative measures are as follows:

Goal 1: Bleeding from open wound is controlled.

Evaluative measure: No visible bleeding is noted after application of direct pressure.

Goal 2: Patient has no apparent spinal cord injury.

Evaluative measure: Patient is neurologically intact after immobilization of spine.

Home Care Considerations

Emergencies in the Home

- If ice is not available in the home, look for a bag of frozen vegetables. Peas work especially well.
- Have patients keep a list of medications, allergies, and special needs with their list of emergency numbers. This often saves time and provides valuable information for emergency medical personnel.
- Advise all patients to equip their homes with an emergency first aid kit kept in an easily accessible place. Properly supplied kits include adhesive bandages, antiseptic, gauze dressings, tape, tweezers, scissors and antibiotic ointment. It is also a good idea to include directions for what to do in an emergency.
- Prevention is the key to eliminating emergencies in the home. Advise patients to "accident-proof" their homes. Advise patients to keep cleaning products and poisons, as well as medications, out of the reach of children. Hand rails, nonskid surfaces, and adequate lighting help prevent falls. Advise older adults to avoid decorating with throw rugs and other objects that can cause them to trip. Keep electrical cords in good repair with no frayed cords.

Get Ready for the NCLEX® Examination!

Key Points

- First aid serves to preserve life until medical help arrives, not to replace medical care.
- Airway problems, circulatory problems, profuse bleeding, and poisonings are life-threatening situations that necessitate priority emergency care.
- Suspect shock in all situations involving traumatic injuries, diseases, and physical and emotional stress.
- Reactions to a poisonous bite will often take a few minutes to several hours to appear. Take first aid measures immediately.
- Always splint a fractured part in the position it is in, and never attempt to realign it.
- Take spinal cord precautions in all cases of head trauma and multiple traumas. Even a slight movement of the individual's head creates the potential for causing spinal damage.
- The dangers from burn injuries are shock, loss of fluids, and infection.
- In heat emergencies, it is important to cool the victim as soon as possible.
- Personnel trained in CPR and a rapid-response EMS system will often be able to resuscitate victims of cardiac arrest or apparent sudden death.
- All health care providers need to maintain current CPR certification.
- It is necessary for rescuers to perform CPR according to the standards designated by the American Heart Association or the American Red Cross.
- There is a moral obligation to continue CPR once it has been initiated unless the rescuer is exhausted and is not able to continue, trained medical personnel take over CPR, or a licensed physician pronounces the victim dead.
- Airway, breathing, and circulation (the ABCs) are the three steps to remember in one- or two-rescuer CPR.
- If external cardiac compressions are performed accurately, it is possible to supply enough oxygen to the heart, the lungs, the brain, and the rest of the body to sustain life.
- Two fingers are used during chest compressions in the infant.
- If a victim is choking but has good air exchange (is coughing forcibly), do not interfere.
- Performing abdominal thrusts is the most effective method of removing a foreign body obstructing the airway.
- Do not use the finger-sweep technique when managing foreign body airway obstruction in the infant.
- A relatively new potential environmental health threat is the possibility of a terrorist attack.
- Bioterrorism, or the use of biological agents to create fear and threat, is the most likely form of terrorist attack to occur.

Additional Learning Resources

Go to your Companion CD for an audio glossary, animations, video clips, and more.

evolve Be sure to visit the Evolve site at http://evolve.elsevier.com/Christensen/foundations/ for additional online resources.

Review Questions for the NCLEX® Examination

1. The priority assessment to make of a victim at the scene of a car accident is whether or not:
   1. the victim is actively bleeding.
   2. the victim has a patent airway.
   3. there is an apical pulse.
   4. there are signs of head trauma.

2. When caring for a victim who has a head injury and is developing shock, the nurse should:
   1. elevate the victim's head.
   2. lower the victim's feet.
   3. elevate the victim's upper body.
   4. leave the victim in a flat position.

3. The nurse finds an unconscious woman in a car that is on fire. She is breathing, her arm is fractured, and she has several lacerations that are bleeding profusely. What should the nurse do first?
   1. Splint the fractured arm.
   2. Get the woman out of the car.
   3. Give mouth-to-mouth resuscitation.
   4. Stop the bleeding.

4. A neighbor tells the nurse that her 12-year-old daughter has been burned with scalding water. The arm is red and starting to blister. In addition to advising her to see a doctor, what will the nurse tell the neighbor to apply to the burn?
   1. Hydrogen peroxide
   2. Petroleum jelly
   3. Cool compresses
   4. Saltwater compresses

5. A patient is found on the floor of her room. She fell while crawling over the side rails of her bed. She is unconscious and has a large laceration to the head that is bleeding profusely. The nurse's first priority is to:
   1. notify the physician.
   2. apply direct pressure to the laceration to the patient's head.
   3. check the patient's vital signs.
   4. ensure that the patient has an open airway.

6. A man is found walking next to his car after an automobile accident. He is breathing rapidly and has cool, clammy skin. The man is possibly suffering from:
   1. shock.
   2. head trauma.
   3. peripheral vascular injury.
   4. spinal injury.

7. The nurse is swimming at the lake and hears people calling for help. On arrival, the nurse finds that a 12-year-old boy was water-skiing when he lost control and was hit in the head with a ski. He is lying on the shore, unconscious. The nurse notices that the boy is cyanotic and has a laceration on his head that is bleeding. The first priority is to:
   1. control the bleeding.
   2. immobilize the neck and spine.
   3. move him to a warmer area.
   4. ensure there is an open airway.

8. The nurse comes across a one-car automobile accident. The driver of the car is walking around with a dazed look on his face. He states that he was wearing his seatbelt, but is unsure of what happened exactly. He has no visible injury. After checking his vital signs, the nurse finds BP 84/56, P 110, R 32. Another bystander says that an ambulance is on the way. The nurse's first priority will be to:
   1. complete a neurologic assessment.
   2. instruct him to get back in the car and rest.
   3. position him on his back on the ground with feet elevated.
   4. assess for any wounds.

9. The nurse is told in report that one of the patients has been very depressed lately. On checking the unit, the nurse finds the patient in the bathroom with one wrist bleeding profusely. The patient states that she broke a glass and used it to cut her wrist in a suicide attempt. After sending someone to call for help, the nurse should:
   1. attempt to find out what has been causing her depression.
   2. apply a tourniquet above the injury.
   3. use 4-inch by 4-inch gauze pads to apply direct pressure.
   4. thoroughly wash the wound.

10. A 44-year-old patient is brought to the emergency department with a gunshot wound to the chest. On examination, the nurse finds that he is conscious and complaining of pain. There is slight bleeding at the entrance wound, and there is no exit wound. Vital signs are BP 100/76, P 100, R 40. If the patient complains of having difficulty breathing, the nurse's first priority will be to:
    1. obtain pulse oximetry reading and start oxygen via nasal cannula.
    2. give morphine sulfate to control the pain.
    3. position him flat on his back with feet elevated.
    4. apply pressure to the entrance wound.

11. A neighbor tells the nurse that her 5-year-old son has ingested one of her liquid cleaning supplies. The child is in no distress at this time. The mother shows the nurse the bottle; the nurse is unfamiliar with the ingredients. The nurse's first priority would be to:
    1. give syrup of ipecac to induce vomiting.
    2. give milk to neutralize any acids.
    3. give water to dilute the poison.
    4. call the poison control center.

12. A new potential environmental health threat is the possibility of:
    1. bioterrorism.
    2. noise pollution.
    3. water pollution.
    4. air pollution.

13. When giving one- or two-person CPR to adults and children, the nurse should use the universal compression:ventilation ratio of _______ chest compressions for every _______ breaths.

14. The compression rate for one- or two-rescuer CPR for adults and children is approximately ________ compressions per minute.

15. In the case of multiple injuries, patients are quickly surveyed for severity of injuries so that life-threatening problems can be treated first. This process is called:
    1. secondary survey.
    2. high-resource intensity.
    3. triage.
    4. collaborative care.

16. Shock is best defined as:
    1. cardiovascular collapse.
    2. loss of sympathetic tone.
    3. inadequate tissue perfusion.
    4. blood pressure less than 90 mm Hg systolic.

chapter

25 Health Promotion and Pregnancy

evolve

http://evolve.elsevier.com/Christensen/foundationsadult

Elaine Oden Kockrow

Objectives

1. Explain the physiology of conception.
2. Discuss the anatomical and physiologic alterations that occur during pregnancy.
3. Identify the components of antepartal assessment.
4. Differentiate among the presumptive, possible, and positive signs of pregnancy.
5. Discuss the common discomforts of pregnancy.
6. List the danger signs that might occur during pregnancy.
7. Discuss cultural practices and beliefs that may affect ongoing health care during pregnancy.
8. Describe nutritional requirements during pregnancy.
9. Identify nursing diagnoses relevant to care of the prenatal patient.

Key Terms

amniocentesis (ăm-nē-ō-sĕn-TĒ-sĭs, p. 783)
antepartal (ăn-tē-PĂR-tăl, p. 785)
ballottement (bă-LŎT-mĕnt, p. 786)
blastocyst (BLĂS-tō-sĭst, p. 769)
chorionic villi (kō-rē-ŎN-ĭk VĬL-ī, p. 769)
ectoderm (ĔK-tō-dĕrm, p. 770)
ectopic pregnancy (ĕk-TŎP-ĭk PRĔG-năn-sē, p. 769)
endoderm (ĔN-dō-dĕrm, p. 770)
flagellation (flăj-ĕ-LĀ-shŭn, p. 768)
Goodell's sign (p. 786)
gravida (GRĂV-ĭ-dă, p. 788)
Hëgar's sign (p. 786)
implantation (p. 769)
intrapartal (p. 785)
lanugo (lă-NŪ-gō, p. 781)
mesoderm (MĔZ-ō-dĕrm, p. 770)
morula (MŎR-ū-lă, p. 769)
para (p. 788)
perinatal (p. 785)
postpartal (p. 785)
prenatal (p. 785)
teratogenic agents (tĕr-ă-tō-JĔN-ĭk Ā-gĕntz, p. 770)
trimesters (p. 785)
ultrasonography (ŭl-tră-sŏ-NŎG-ră-fē, p. 782)
villi (VĬL-ī, p. 769)
Wharton's jelly (p. 770)
zygote (ZĪ-gōt, p. 769)

Few experiences in life are as exciting and challenging as childbearing. Profound and dramatic changes occur in a relatively short time. Childbearing is a challenge to the new mother, to the newly developing or changing family unit, to society, and to the nurse who assists in the childbearing process. The maternity nurse is in a unique position of providing care to the unborn.

The goal of maternity care is a healthy pregnancy with a physically safe and emotionally satisfying outcome for both mother and infant. Consistent health supervision and surveillance are of utmost importance. Many pregnant women and their families are unfamiliar with the changes that accompany pregnancy. The knowledgeable maternity nurse can help a pregnant woman recognize the relationship between her physical status and her care plan. Sharing information encourages the pregnant woman to participate in her own care, depending on her interest, need to know, and readiness to learn.

PHYSIOLOGY OF PREGNANCY

Understanding the physiologic changes of pregnancy begins with understanding the normal anatomy and physiology of the male and female reproductive systems. It is particularly important to review the menstrual cycle and related hormonal activity. It is also important to recognize that specific cells (ova in the female and sperm in the male) carry genetic messages to their offspring. These cells are united to form a new individual with a unique genetic makeup, parts of which come from each parent.

FERTILIZATION

During sexual intercourse sperm carried in the male's ejaculatory semen enter the female's vagina. By **flagellation** (whiplike movement) the sperm travel through the mucus of the cervical canal (if the mucus is receptive), enter the uterine chamber, and move into the ampulla—the outer third of the fallopian tube. If the timing is right, an ovum has been produced and is also within the ampulla of the tube; in such cases fertilization may occur. Fertilization takes place when the sperm joins or fuses with the ovum; this is also called **conception.** The fusion of the sperm into the ovum requires approximately 24 hours. Once fertilization has occurred, the new cell is referred to as a zygote (cell formed by the union of two reproductive cells) or a fertilized ovum. This cell carries 46 chromosomes (44 autosomes and two sex chromosomes). At the moment of fertilization the sex of the zygote and all other genetic characteristics are determined and do not change.

IMPLANTATION

The zygote moves through the uterine tube by ciliary action and some irregular peristaltic activity. It takes 3 or 4 days to enter the uterine cavity. During this time the zygote is in a phase of rapid cell division called **mitosis.** Further changes result in formation of a structure called the morula (developmental stage of the fertilized ovum in which there is a solid mass of cells resembling a mulberry), which develops into the blastocyst (the embryonic form; a spherical mass of cells having a central fluid-filled cavity surrounded by two layers of cells). Stem cells are derived from the inner cell mass of the blastocyst (Box 25-1). After the blastocyst is free in the uterine cavity for 1 or 2 days, the exposed cell walls of the blastocyst (called the **trophoblast**) secrete enzymes that are able to break down protein and penetrate cell membranes. These enzymes allow the blastocyst to enter the endometrium and implant. The action of the enzymes normally stops short of the myometrium but may cause slight bleeding in some individuals. This is called **implantation bleeding.** Although this bleeding is rarely more than spotting, it may confuse some women, who think that they had a very light and short menstrual cycle when really they are pregnant.

The condition of the uterine lining is critical for implantation (embedding of the fertilized ovum in the uterine mucosa) of the zygote. During the secretory phase of the menstrual cycle the endometrium has an enriched vascular bed with enlarged blood vessels and an increased store of glycogen. This will support development of the embryo if implantation occurs. Implantation usually occurs in the fundus of the uterus on either the anterior or posterior surfaces. If uterine conditions are not suitable, implantation is unlikely to occur. If intrauterine vascular or hormonal conditions cannot sustain the implanted embryo, a spontaneous abortion occurs. Most spontaneous abortions occur during the first 8 weeks of pregnancy for these reasons. Ectopic pregnancy, in which implantation occurs outside of the uterine cavity, also poses serious problems. These conditions are discussed further in Chapter 28.

Box 25-1 Stem Cells

Stem cells are able to divide for indefinite periods and can differentiate into the many different types of cells that make up an organism. Embryonic stem cells are derived from the blastocyst before it implants in the uterine wall. A zygote is described as totipotent because it has the potential to produce all the cells and tissues that compose an embryo and to support its in utero development. The term *pluripotent* is used to describe stem cells that generate cells derived from the three embryonic germ layers: endoderm, mesoderm, and ectoderm. The embryonic stem cell is pluripotent.

Human stem cells were derived and maintained for the first time in 1988 by Thomson and colleagues, using blastocysts donated by couples undergoing in vitro fertilization. Potential uses of human embryonic stem cells include transplant therapy, in which tissues damaged by disease or injury are replaced or restored, as for example, in diabetes, Parkinson's disease, heart disease, and multiple sclerosis. Stem cell research raises ethical concerns related to the source of human embryonic stem cells (embryos left over from in vitro fertilization and aborted fetuses).

On May 9, 2009, President Obama lifted an 8-year ban on embryonic stem cell research, calling it "an important step in advancing the cause of science in America."

Data from National Institutes of Health. (2001). *Stem cells: Scientific progress and future research directions*. Department of Health and Human Services, June, 2001. Available online at http://stemcells.nih.gov/info. Accessed September, 2009; Hockenberry, M.J., et al. (2007). *Wong's maternal-child nursing care.* (8th ed.). St. Louis: Mosby; and Lite, J. (2009). Obama ends embryonic stem cell research ban. Available online at www.scientificamerican.com/blog/60-second-science/post.cfm?id=obama-ends-embryonic-stem-cell-rese-2009-03-09. Accessed September 24, 2009.

During the first few weeks after implantation, primary villi (short vascular processes or protrusions growing on certain membranous surfaces) appear. These villi use maternal blood vessels as a source of nourishment and oxygen for the developing embryo. The villi nourish the embryo from the time of implantation (about 2 weeks after conception) until the seventh or eighth week. Also during these first few weeks the first stages of the chorionic villi (tiny vascular protrusions on the chorionic surface that project into the maternal blood sinuses of the uterus and help form the placenta) occur. Chorionic villi secrete human chorionic gonadotropin (HCG), a hormone that stimulates the continued production of progesterone and estrogen by the corpus luteum. This is why ovulation and menstruation cease during pregnancy. Primary villi also synthesize protein and glucose for approximately 12 weeks, until the fetus is adequately developed to meet its own needs. The chorionic villi become the fetal portion of the placenta.

EMBRYONIC AND FETAL DEVELOPMENT

Until the time of implantation (the germinal phase), the cell mass is referred to as the zygote. During this period the fertilized ovum develops from the two original cells into a many-celled organism. The zygote develops two separate and distinct cavities: the amniotic cavity and the yolk sac. The amniotic cavity has walls lined with the ectoderm (outer layer of embryonic tissue giving rise to skin, nails, and hair) and is filled with amniotic fluid. The yolk sac is lined with the endoderm (the innermost of the cell layers, which develop into the lining of cavities and passages of the body and the covering of most internal organs). The yolk sac supplies nourishment until implantation. A third layer of primary cells, the mesoderm (embryonic middle layer of germ cells giving rise to all types of muscles, connective tissue, bone marrow, blood, lymphoid tissue, and all epithelial tissue), is located between the two cavities. The embryo develops at the point at which these three layers meet, called the **trilaminar embryonic disk.**

The embryonic stage begins with implantation and encompasses approximately the first 8 weeks of pregnancy. During the embryonic stage, the three primary cell layers differentiate into tissue and layers, which form the placenta, embryonic membranes, and the embryo itself. Cell growth is rapid. A simple heart begins beating, and rudimentary (basic, initial, or primary) forms of all the major organs and systems develop. By the end of this stage, the embryo has acquired a human appearance. Starting with the ninth week the embryo is referred to as the **fetus,** and the fetal stage begins. (See Chapter 31 and Figure 31-1 for fetal circulation.)

Many structures develop simultaneously in the embryo; therefore when an infant is born with one birth defect or abnormality, the physician checks for others that are likely to be present. During the early weeks of pregnancy, often before a woman even knows that she is pregnant, teratogenic agents (any drug, virus, or irradiation that can cause malformation of the fetus) can cause serious harm. For example, rubella, or German measles, is a known **teratogen** (a nongenetic factor that causes malformations and disease syndromes in utero). Although rubella is usually a mild childhood disease, at this stage of pregnancy the virus can affect all of the germ layers and cause serious anomalies such as cardiac defects, deafness, and cognitive impairment.

The prenatal calendar (Table 25-1) describes fetal development and maternal changes throughout pregnancy.

EMBRYONIC AND FETAL PHYSIOLOGY

Placenta

The **placenta** (Greek, "flat plate") is a disklike organ made up of about 20 sections called **cotyledons.** It is a unique structure, present only during pregnancy. From a few beginning cells, this organ develops rapidly. At full term the placenta looks like a large red disk with a diameter of 8 inches (20 cm) and a thickness of 1 inch (2.5 cm). It normally weighs between 1 pound and 1 pound, 5 ounces (450 and 600 g). The bulk of the placenta is fetal in origin. The side attached to the uterine wall ("Dirty Duncan") appears dark red and has a rough surface; the cotyledons are apparent as distinct lobes with clefts or divisions between each lobe. The Duncan presentation is associated with blood expulsion with the placenta. The fetal side is smooth and shiny ("Shiny Schultze"). It consists of the membranes of the amniotic sac that encases the fetus. A small gush of blood precedes the placenta when the Schultze side is presenting. On delivery, assess the placenta and determine the presenting side, then examine the placenta for intactness. Document your findings.

As mentioned, the placenta functions as an endocrine gland secreting HCG and the steroidal hormones estrogen and progesterone, which maintain the pregnancy. In addition, the placenta is the site of the exchange of nutrients, oxygen, and waste products between the fetus and the maternal circulation. The placenta allows transfer of oxygen and nutrients through such processes as diffusion and active transport, and it also blocks the transfer of certain substances. This is called the placental barrier. Some viruses are able to cross the placental barrier, but most bacteria are too large to cross. Some drugs do not cross the placenta, but most do and can cause serious harm to the growing embryo or fetus. After delivery the placenta is of no further use and is expelled.

Fetal Membranes

The amniotic sac is composed of two layers, both originating in the zygote. The outer layer, the **chorion,** attaches to the fetal portion of the placenta. The inner layer, the **amnion,** blends with the fetal umbilical cord. These membranes appear fragile, but in fact they are strong enough to contain the fetus and amniotic fluid even at full term.

Umbilical Cord

The umbilical cord joins the embryo to the placenta. It originates in the fetal portion of the placenta and is normally attached near the center. The cord is typically 20 to 22 inches (50 to 55 cm) long and less than 1 inch (2.5 cm) in diameter at the time of delivery. Umbilical cords can vary widely in appearance. The major part of the cord is a pale white, gelatinous-mucoid substance called Wharton's jelly (a gelatinous tissue that remains when the embryonic body stalk blends with the yolk sac within the umbilical cord). This substance prevents compression of the blood vessels. Normally two arteries and one vein are apparent and may give the cord a ropelike appearance. The vein carries oxygenated blood to the fetus; the arteries carry deoxygenated blood back to the placenta. The cord has no pain receptors, so cutting at the time of delivery does not cause pain.

Amniotic Fluid

Amniotic fluid acts as a cushion against mechanical injury, helps regulate fetal temperature, and allows the developing embryo or fetus room for growth. The amount of fluid changes from about 30 mL (1 oz) at

Text continued on p. 781

Table 25-1 Fetal Development and Maternal Events during Pregnancy and Drug Substances to Avoid

WEEK 1	WEEK 2	WEEK 3	WEEK 4	WEEK 5	WEEK 6	WEEK 7	WEEK 8
BABY'S DEVELOPMENT							
The ovum becomes fertilized, divides, and burrows into the uterus.	The embryonic disk (ectoderm, endoderm, mesoderm) is formed. These three primitive germ layers will generate every organ and tissue in the baby's body.	The first body segments appear, which will eventually form the primitive spine, the brain, and the spinal cord.	Heart, blood circulation, and digestive tract take shape. The embryo is now 0.2 inch long; the head is a third of its total length.	The heart starts to pump blood; limb buds appear. Major divisions of the brain can now be discerned.	Eyes begin to take shape; external ears develop from skinfolds.	Development proceeds rapidly. The face is now complete with eyes, nose, lips, and tongue—even primitive milk teeth. Tiny bones and muscles appear beneath the thin skin.	The embryo is now a little more than 1 inch long.
MATERNAL EVENTS							
Ovaries increase production of the pregnancy-maintaining hormone, progesterone.	The first period is missed.	Placenta grows to cover one fifteenth of the uterine interior. Breasts may begin to feel tender. There is no weight gain.			Exchange of fetal and maternal metabolites across the placenta begins, yet the two circulations are completely separate.	No noticeable weight gain occurs.	The placenta now covers about one third of the uterine lining.
COMMON MATERNAL DISCOMFORTS							
		Morning sickness occurs because increased hormonal activity slows down the digestive system, apparently to enhance the absorption of nutrients for the baby.	Fatigue is thought to be caused by a change in ovarian hormone production (progesterone and relaxin), the purpose of which is to relax pelvic ligaments, stimulate breast growth, and soften the cervix.		Urinary frequency is caused by the uterus compressing the bladder against the pelvic bones, thus reducing its capacity, and also by hormonal changes that affect the water balance in the body.		

Continued

Table 25-1 Fetal Development and Maternal Events during Pregnancy and Drug Substances to Avoid—cont'd

WEEK 1	WEEK 2	WEEK 3	WEEK 4	WEEK 5	WEEK 6	WEEK 7	WEEK 8
REMEDIES							
		Eat a few dry crackers before rising. Eat frequent, small, low-fat meals during the day to help. Drink liquids.	Exercise regularly and get plenty of sleep with frequent naps during the day.		Decrease pressure on the bladder at night by sleeping on the side. Also, drink no fluids after 6 PM.		
DRUG SUBSTANCES TO AVOID							
		Antiemetics: cyclizine (Marezine), meclizine (Antivert, Bonine), trimethobenzamide (Tigan). (Avoid throughout pregnancy.)	Stimulants: amphetamines, excessive caffeine. (Avoid throughout pregnancy.)				
ACCEPTABLE ALTERNATIVES							
None: Avoid all drugs not prescribed by a physician for a specific condition. Avoid x-rays.							

WEEK 9	WEEK 10	WEEK 11	WEEK 12	WEEK 13	WEEK 14	WEEK 15	WEEK 16
BABY'S DEVELOPMENT							
Genitalia are now well defined; the baby's sex is determined. Eyelids finish forming and seal shut. The embryo has become a fetus. 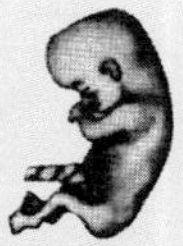	The fetus assumes a more human shape as the lower body rapidly develops. Blood and bone cells form. The first movements begin. 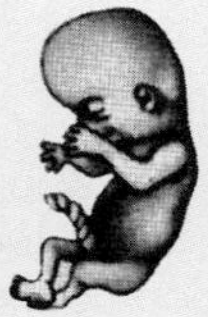	Organs begin to function. The pancreas produces insulin; the kidneys produce urine. 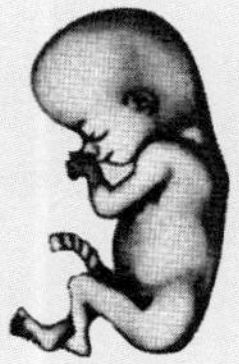	The lungs have taken shape; primitive breathing motions begin. The swallowing reflex has been mastered as the fetus sucks its thumb while floating weightlessly in the amniotic fluid. 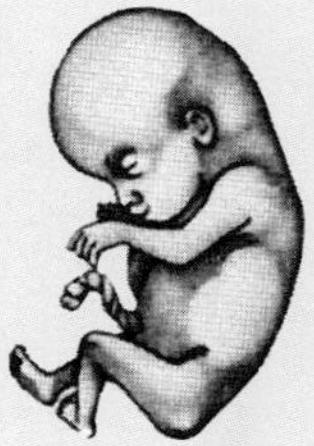	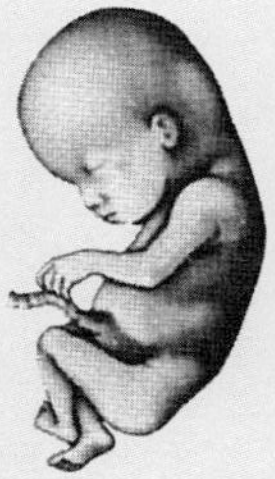	The musculoskeletal system has matured. The nervous system begins to exercise some control over the body; blood vessels rapidly develop. 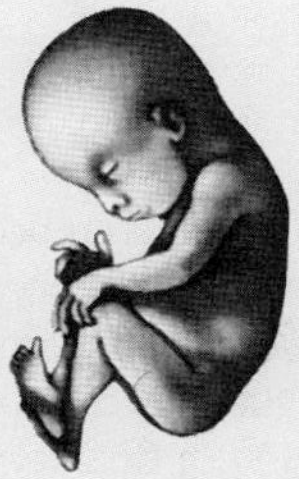	With hands ready to grasp, the fetus, now weighing about 7 ounces, kicks restlessly against the amniotic sac. 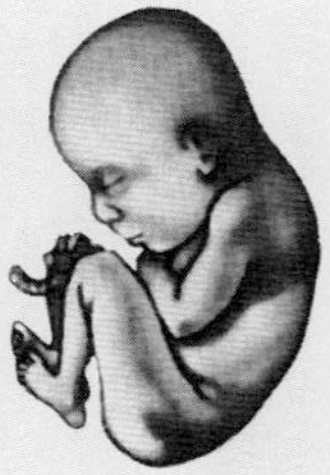	All organs and structures have been formed, and a period of simple growth begins. 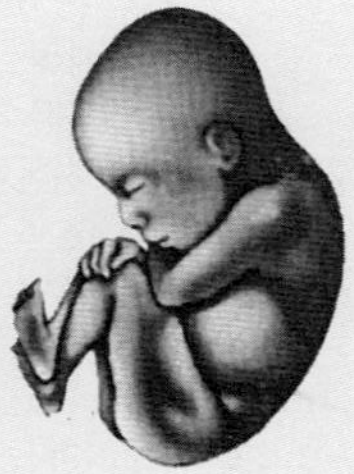
MATERNAL EVENTS							
Maternal blood volume has increased 30% to 40%.	Some women describe the sensation of these first movements as if something were blowing bubbles through a straw in their stomachs.	There is a 2- to 3-pound weight gain and a possible increase in perspiration.	The placenta has reached complete functional maturity, acting as the baby's lungs, kidneys, liver, and digestive and immune systems.		There is a 3- to 4-pound weight gain, and her belly begins to show.		The fetal heartbeat can now be heard with an amplified stethoscope. Placenta begins producing the estrogen hormone.

Continued

Table 25-1 Fetal Development and Maternal Events during Pregnancy and Drug Substances to Avoid—cont'd

WEEK 9	WEEK 10	WEEK 11	WEEK 12	WEEK 13	WEEK 14	WEEK 15	WEEK 16
COMMON MATERNAL DISCOMFORTS							
	Sleeplessness may result from the discomfort or anxieties of pregnancy.				Vaginal secretions are the result of an increased supply of blood and glucose to the vaginal mucosa. Severe pruritus, irritation, and malodor suggest infection. If infection is suspected, consult a professional.		Headaches may occur while her body adjusts to changes in blood volume and vascular tone. Emotional tension may also be a factor.
REMEDIES							
	Take warm shower before sleeping. Support body parts with pillows.				Cleanse daily with warm water, keeping the area dry to prevent chafing. Apply yogurt for vulvar pruritus.		Change body positions slowly. Resting with a damp cloth on the forehead may help. Drink milk or eat a small snack to obtain some relief.
DRUG SUBSTANCES TO AVOID							
	Tranquilizers, narcotics, antihistamines, alcohol, barbiturates. (Avoid throughout pregnancy.)				Vaginal antiinfectives: metronidazole (Flagyl). (Avoid throughout pregnancy.)		Analgesics: salicylates (aspirin), phenacetin-caffeine, propoxyphene (Darvon), indomethacin (Indocin). Tranquilizers. (Avoid throughout pregnancy.)

	WEEK 17	WEEK 18	WEEK 19	WEEK 20	WEEK 21	WEEK 22	WEEK 23	WEEK 24
ACCEPTABLE ALTERNATIVES	None: Avoid all drugs not prescribed by a physician for a specific condition. Avoid x-rays.					Sufaniliamide (AVC Cream), nystatin (Mycostatin) vaginal tablets, miconazole (Monistat) vaginal cream.		Tylenol brand acetaminophen.
BABY'S DEVELOPMENT		An oily coating protects the fetus. Fine hair covers the body and keeps the oil on the skin.	Eyebrows, eyelashes, and head hair develop.	The fetus is now following a regular schedule of sleeping, turning, sucking, and kicking and has settled on a favorite position in the uterus.		The skeleton is developing rapidly as the bone-forming cells increase their activity.	Eyelids begin to open and close.	The fetus now weighs about 27 ounces.

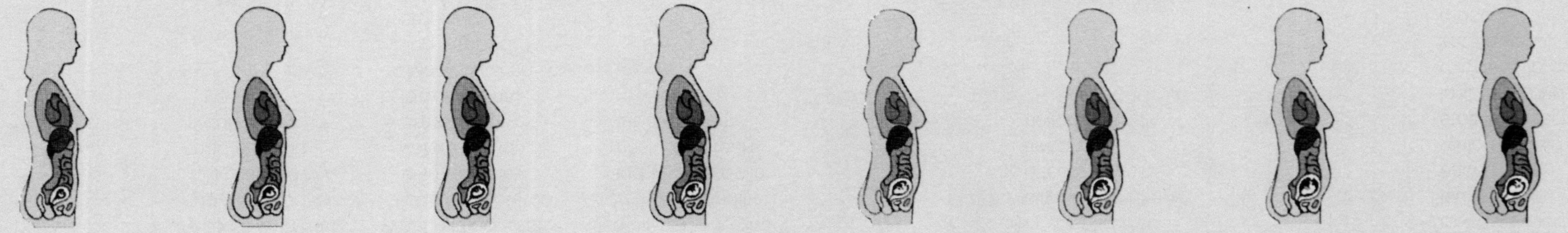

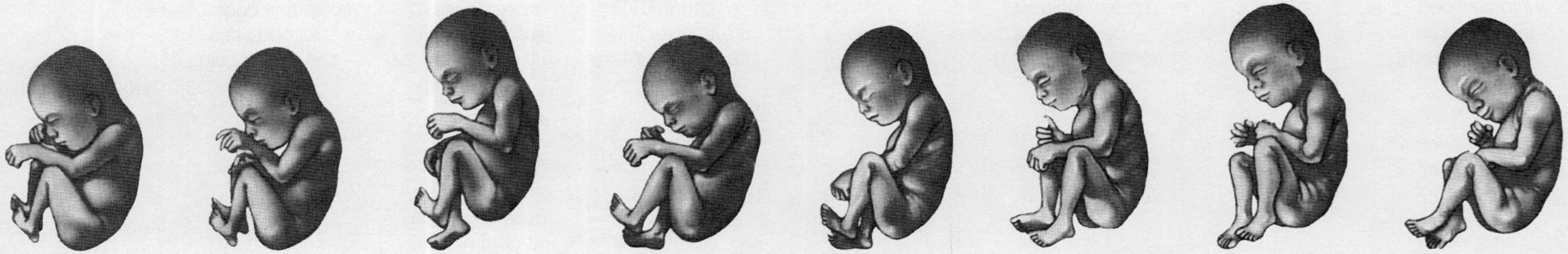

Continued

Table 25-1 Fetal Development and Maternal Events during Pregnancy and Drug Substances to Avoid—cont'd

WEEK 17	WEEK 18	WEEK 19	WEEK 20	WEEK 21	WEEK 22	WEEK 23	WEEK 24
MATERNAL EVENTS							
	There is a 3- to 4-pound weight gain.	Breasts begin secreting colostrum in preparation for nursing.	Placenta reaches its largest size relative to fetus, covering half the uterine lining. The amniotic sac contains 400 mL of fluid.		There is a 3- to 4- pound weight gain.		The placenta becomes thicker rather than wider. Mother can now sense when baby is awake.
COMMON MATERNAL DISCOMFORTS							
	Faintness or dizziness occurs when standing suddenly, caused by reduced blood flow to the brain as the body adjusts to new circulatory patterns. Shortness of breath may occur.	Varicose veins are often the result of rising blood pressure in the lower extremities. This is caused by the enlarged uterus cutting off blood flow back from the legs to the heart.	Allergies, such as hay fever, are a common problem.		Skin changes such as darkened nipples, stretch marks, splotches on cheeks and forehead, acne, and redness on palms and soles are due to increased hormone levels in the blood.		Epistaxis sometimes occurs because of increased blood volume and nasal congestion.
REMEDIES							
	Try to sit with feet up when possible; rise slowly and support yourself.	When sitting, rest legs on footstool with feet elevated; avoid pressure on lower thighs. (Many women find support stockings helpful.)	Use air conditioning (with a clean filter) and wear a pollen mask to screen out allergens.		Be patient. (Virtually all of these effects subside soon after childbirth.)		Apply a little petroleum jelly in each nostril, which should stop the bleeding. Use a humidifier. Do not irritate nasal mucosa.
DRUG SUBSTANCES TO AVOID							
	Tranquilizers, alcohol. (Avoid throughout pregnancy.)		Most antihistamines: hydroxyzine (Atarax), trimeprazine (Temaril). (Avoid throughout pregnancy.)		Tetracycline (for acne). (Avoid throughout pregnancy.)		

	WEEK 25	WEEK 26	WEEK 27	WEEK 28	WEEK 29	WEEK 30	WEEK 31	WEEK 32
ACCEPTABLE ALTERNATIVES		Smelling salts, aromatic spirits of ammonia.		Chlorpheniramine for congestion; nasal spray for stuffy nose, occasionally; calamine lotion for rashes.		If nipples or abdomen itch, a lanolin-based cream or baby oil can provide relief. A mild soap can remove the excessive facial oil produced by acne.		Pseudoephedrine or nasal spray may be used occasionally for stuffy nose, if necessary.
	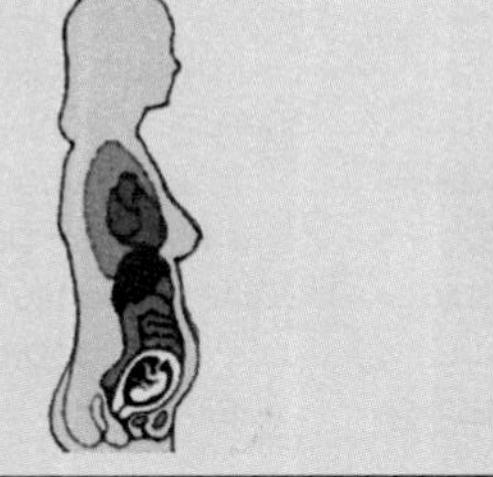	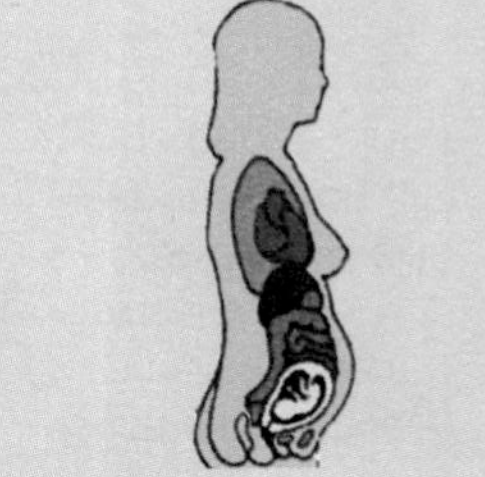	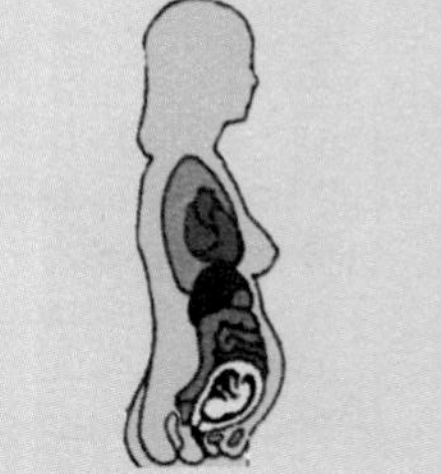	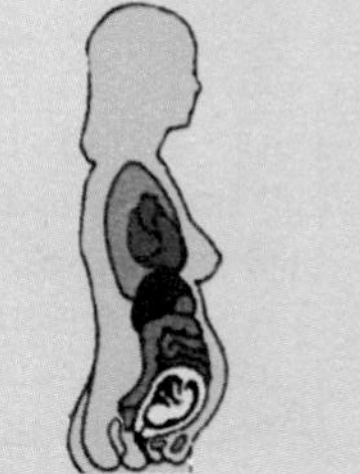	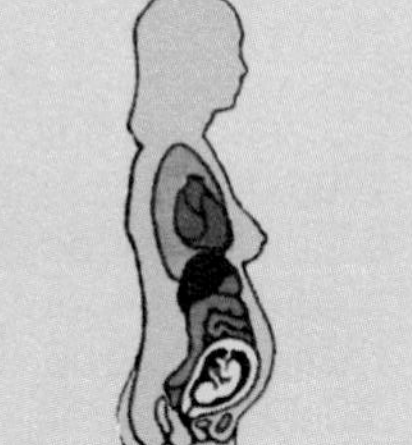	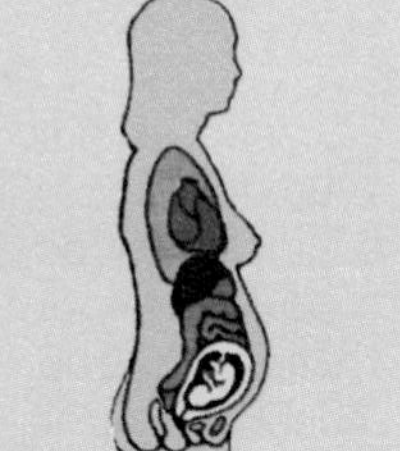	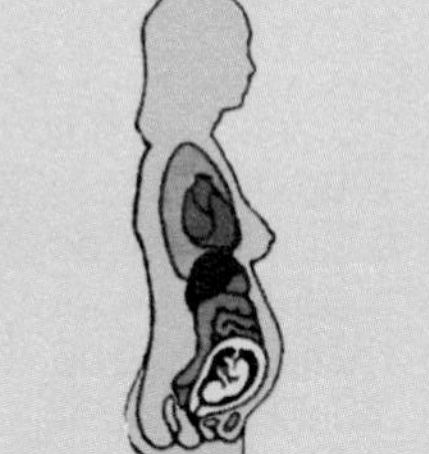	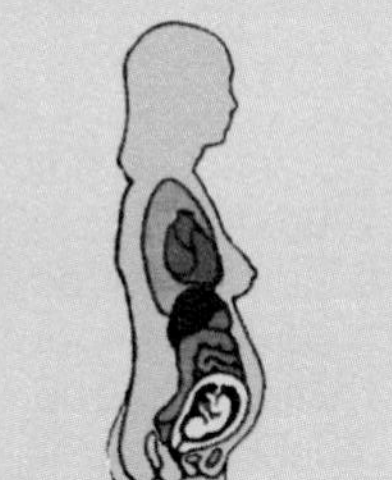
BABY'S DEVELOPMENT		To a certain extent, the fetus can now breathe, swallow, and regulate its body temperature, but it still depends greatly on maternal support.	A substance called surfactant forms in the lungs, preparing them to function independently after birth.	Fetus is two thirds grown.	Fat deposits are building up beneath the skin to insulate the fetus against the abrupt change in temperature at birth.	The digestive tract and the lungs are now nearly fully matured, and the skin becomes less red and wrinkled.	The fetus has grown to about 14 inches.	
	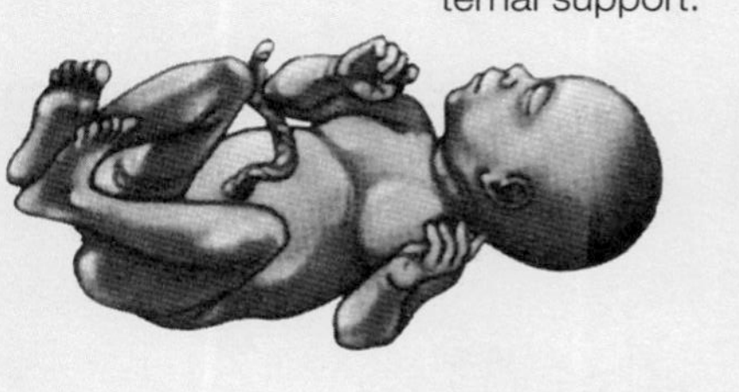		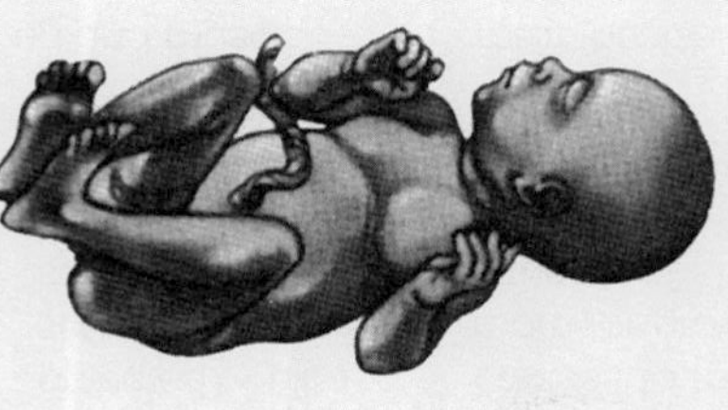			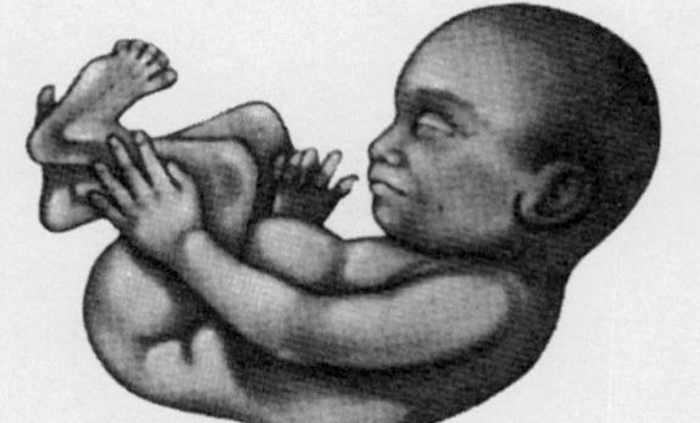		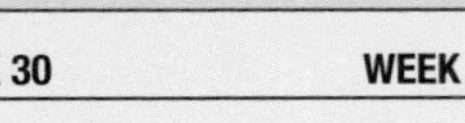 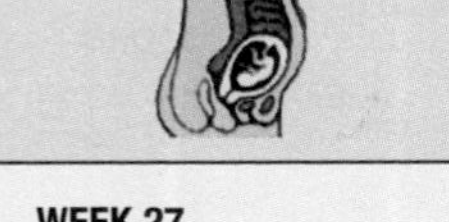

Continued

Table 25-1 Fetal Development and Maternal Events during Pregnancy and Drug Substances to Avoid—cont'd

WEEK 25	WEEK 26	WEEK 27	WEEK 28	WEEK 29	WEEK 30	WEEK 31	WEEK 32
MATERNAL EVENTS							
	There is a 3- to 4-pound weight gain.	Respiratory movements can be detected by ultrasound. Mother sometimes feels baby's breathing as "hiccups."	The volume of amniotic fluid decreases to make room for growing fetus.		There is a 3- to 5-pound weight gain.		
COMMON MATERNAL DISCOMFORTS							
		Leg and muscle cramps may be caused by fatigue, pressure exerted on the nerves by the uterus, or too little calcium or too much phosphorus in the diet.	Pyrosis (heartburn) often occurs because the stomach emptying time is delayed, causing a burning sensation in the throat.		Edema of ankles occurs. The pressure of the uterus on the large veins returning blood to the heart may induce water retention.	Constipation is another result of the decelerated digestive process. As food moves slowly through the intestines, more water is extracted, leaving the stool drier and harder.	Mother may have trouble sleeping because of baby's activity. Hemorrhoids may also develop.
REMEDIES							
		Exercise regularly, especially walking. Elevate legs and flex toes when resting. Increase milk consumption.	Drink milk between small, frequent meals. (This problem will disappear soon after the baby's birth.)		Elevate legs, once or twice a day for an hour or so, level with the hips. Sleep on the left side.	Eat foods containing roughage, such as raw fruits, vegetables, and cereals with bran. Drink liquids and exercise frequently.	Soak in a warm bath or sit on soft pillows to soothe the symptoms.
DRUG SUBSTANCES TO AVOID							
		Salicylates (aspirin), tranquilizers. (Avoid throughout pregnancy.)	Antacids: calcium carbonate, magnesium trisilicate (Gaviscon), sodium bicarbonate (baking soda), cimetidine (Tagamet). (Avoid throughout pregnancy.)		Most diuretics ("water pills"). (Avoid throughout pregnancy.)	Laxatives: mineral oil, castor oil. (Avoid throughout pregnancy.)	

ACCEPTABLE ALTERNATIVES

Calcium supplements with little or no phosphorus.

Maalox, Mylanta (also for "gas").

For constipation: Metamucil, Senokot, teaspoon of milk of magnesia at bedtime.

For hemorrhoids: dibucaine (Nupercainal) suppositories or cream, hydrocortisone (Anusol), benzocaine (Medicone).

WEEK 33 — **TO TERM**

BABY'S DEVELOPMENT

Virtually the entire uterus is now occupied by the fetus, and its activity is restricted.

Maternal antibodies against measles, mumps, rubella, whooping cough, and scarlet fever are transferred to the baby, providing protection for about 6 months until the infant's own immune system can take over.

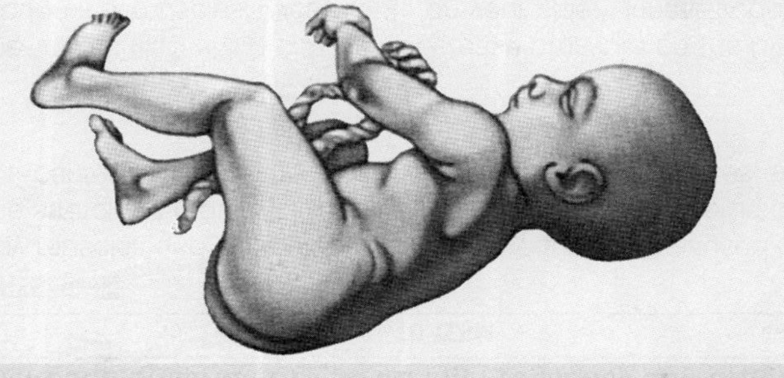

MATERNAL EVENTS

The placenta is nearly four times as thick as it was 20 weeks before and weighs about 20 ounces.

Preparing for birth, the fetus descends deeper into the mother's pelvis. There is a 3- to 5-pound weight gain.

In 9 months, the miracle is complete; a single, microscopic fertilized cell has transformed into a 6 trillion–celled human being.

Continued

Table 25-1 Fetal Development and Maternal Events during Pregnancy and Drug Substances to Avoid—cont'd

WEEK 33	TO TERM	
COMMON MATERNAL DISCOMFORTS		
Backaches are often caused by muscles and ligaments relaxing in preparation for the stretching required in delivery and by the added off-center weight of the enlarged uterus.	Urinary frequency is caused (for the second time in pregnancy) by the uterus compressing the bladder against the pelvic bones, thus reducing its capacity.	Uterine contractions become perceptible as the cervix and lower uterine segment prepare for labor.
REMEDIES		
Do back exercises, such as the "pelvic tilt," which can help strengthen back and abdominal muscles. Wear low-heeled shoes or flats; avoid heavy lifting.	Decrease pressure on the bladder at night by sleeping on your side. Urinate frequently.	
DRUG SUBSTANCES TO AVOID		
Analgesics: salicylates (aspirin), propoxyphene (Darvon), phenacetin-caffeine, indomethacin (Indocin), codeine. (Avoid throughout pregnancy.)		
ACCEPTABLE ALTERNATIVES		
	Tylenol brand acetaminophen (occasional use).	

10 weeks to as much as 1 L at delivery. This slightly alkaline fluid is changing continuously. Amniotic fluid contains albumin, urea, uric acid, creatinine, bilirubin, **lecithin** (phospholipids for fat metabolism), **sphingomyelin** (a compound of lipids and sphingosine, found in high concentrations in the brain and other tissues of the nervous system), fructose, fat, leukocytes, proteins, epithelial cells, enzymes, and strands of lanugo (downy, fine hair characteristic of the fetus between 20 weeks of gestation and birth; most noticeable over the shoulders, forehead, and cheeks but found on nearly all parts of the body except for the palms and the soles). Amniocentesis (discussed later) can be done in the later stages of pregnancy to help determine the development, maturity, health, and sex of the fetus.

FETAL WELL-BEING

A variety of technologic and assessment tools can be used to evaluate fetal well-being. These tools are used to evaluate maternal and fetal health problems, fetal congenital anomalies, and fetal growth and maturity (Table 25-2).

Assessing Fetal Heart Tones

The fetal heart shows activity by the seventh week of gestation. Practitioners can auscultate fetal heart tones between 10 and 12 weeks by using Doppler mode (Figure 25-1). To hear the fetal heart tones, place the instrument in the midline, just above the symphysis pubis, and apply firm pressure. Offer the woman and her family the opportunity to listen to the fetal

Table 25-2 Assessment Tools to Evaluate Fetal Well-Being

DIAGNOSTIC TEST OR ASSESSMENT TOOL	DESCRIPTION AND PURPOSE
Ultrasonography (US)	High-frequency sound waves visualize fetus to help determine gestational age, monitor fetal growth, see number of fetuses and location of placenta, estimate volume of amniotic fluid, note presence of anomalies.
Maternal serum alpha-fetoprotein (AFP) screening	Blood test to identify birth defects and anomalies such as Down syndrome (low levels) or neural tube defect (high levels).
Chorionic villus sampling (CVS)	Aspiration of small amount of tissue from the placenta to detect genetic disorders.
Amniocentesis	Aspiration of small amount of amniotic fluid to reveal sex and chromosomal abnormalities, health status, and maturity of fetus. Performed at 16th week of pregnancy to detect abnormalities; performed later in pregnancy to determine fetal lung maturity.
Nonstress test (NST)	Fetal movement and fetal heart rate recorded by external fetal monitors to evaluate the response of the fetal heart rate to fetal movement. Performed when risk is present for placental insufficiency, after the 27th to 30th week of pregnancy by stimulation of uterine contractions.
Contraction stress test (CST)	The response of fetal heart rate to decreased oxygen supply during uterine contractions measured via external fetal monitoring. Performed after 32nd week of pregnancy by stimulation of uterine contractions.
Magnetic resonance imaging (MRI)	Noninvasive tool provides images of soft tissue. Vascular structures within the body may be seen without the use of iodinated contrast medium, without biologic risk. Interference from skeletal, fatty, or gas-filled structures is not a problem as it is in ultrasonography.
Biophysical profile (BPP)	Fetal status assessment by evaluation of NST, fetal breathing movements, fetal muscle tone, fetal movements, and amniotic fluid volume (see Table 25-3).
Nipple-stimulated contraction test (NST)	Measurement of uterine contractions caused by oxytocin released by the posterior pituitary gland during nipple stimulation. Be careful to avoid hyperstimulation. Contractions longer than 80 seconds or more frequent than four in a 10-minute period are considered hypertonic. Methods of nipple stimulation include application of warm, moist compresses to the breast tissue and tactile stimulation. Nipple massage for 10 minutes or twice for 5 minutes, repeated as necessary, may also be used. Once sufficient contractions to perform the test have occurred, halt the stimulation.
Daily fetal movement count (DFMC) (kick count)	Measurement of fetal movement as an indicator of fetal health. Advantages of the test include that it is simple, low cost, noninvasive, and fast. Instruct woman to count fetal movements for 1 hour two or three times daily. No exact number of movements has been identified as a "failing test." However, fewer than three fetal movements in a 1-hour period or the absence of fetal movements for 12 hours is an indication for further evaluation (see Patient Teaching box on guidelines for counting fetal movements). Daily fetal movement count can be done to evaluate the fetus in high-risk pregnancies for complications related to reduced oxygenation.

Data from Lowdermilk, D.L., & Perry, S.E. (2007). *Maternity and women's health care.* (9th ed.). St. Louis: Mosby; Druzin, M., Gabbe, S., & Reed, K. (2002). Antepartum fetal evaluation. In S. Gabbe, J. Niebyl, & J. Simpson (Eds.), *Obstetrics: Normal and problem pregnancies.* (4th ed.). Churchill Livingstone: New York; and Armour, K. (2004). Antepartum maternal-fetal assessment: Using surveillance to improve maternal and fetal outcomes. *AWHONN Lifelines, 8*(3):232-240.

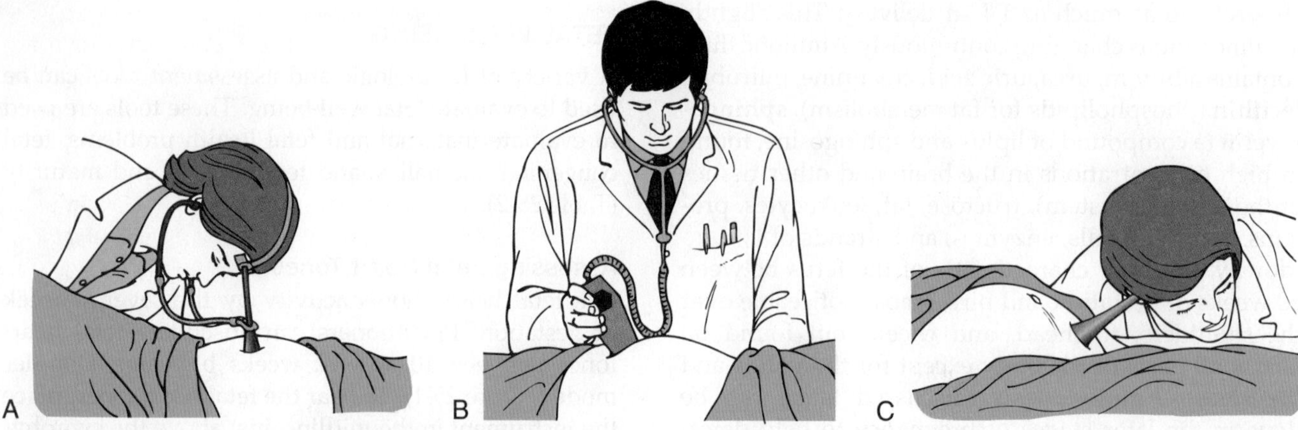

FIGURE 25-1 Detecting fetal heartbeat. **A,** Fetoscope (18 to 20 weeks). **B,** Doppler ultrasound stethoscope (12 weeks). **C,** Pinard's stethoscope. NOTE: Hands should not touch stethoscope while the nurse is listening.

heart tones. Assess the fetus's health status at each visit for the remainder of the pregnancy.

Assessing Fundal Height

During the second trimester the uterus becomes an abdominal organ. The fundal height, or measurement of the height of the uterus above the symphysis pubis, is one indicator of fetal growth. The measurement also provides a gross estimate of the duration of pregnancy. During the second and third trimesters (weeks 18 to 30) the height of the fundus in centimeters is approximately the same as the number of weeks of gestation, if the woman's bladder is empty at the time of measurement. In addition, measurement of fundal height may aid in identification of high-risk factors. A stable or decreased fundal height may indicate intrauterine growth restriction; an excessive increase could indicate multifetal gestation or hydramnios.

A paper tape measure or a pelvimeter may be used to measure fundal height. To increase the reliability of the measurement, the same person should examine the pregnant woman at each of her prenatal visits. Often this is not possible, so establish a protocol that specifies the measurement technique, including the woman's position on the examining table, the measuring device, and the method of measurement used (Figure 25-2).

Ultrasonography

During **ultrasonography,** high-frequency sound waves are used to visualize the fetus. Because soft tissue is visualized, this noninvasive tool can be used to determine gestational age, monitor fetal growth, determine the number of fetuses and the location of the placenta, estimate the volume of amniotic fluid, and detect anomalies. It can also be used in conjunction with invasive tests such as amniocentesis. A growing number of nurses perform ultrasound scans and biophysical profiles (BPPs; a system of estimating current fetal status by analyzing five variables via ultrasonography and nonstress testing). However, most nurses are involved mainly in counseling and educating women about the procedure (see Patient Teaching box on ultrasound examination).

Maternal Serum Alpha-Fetoprotein Screening

Maternal serum alpha-fetoprotein screening is used to identify certain birth defects and chromosomal anomalies. Serum testing should be done between 16 and 18 weeks of gestation. Elevated levels are suggestive of

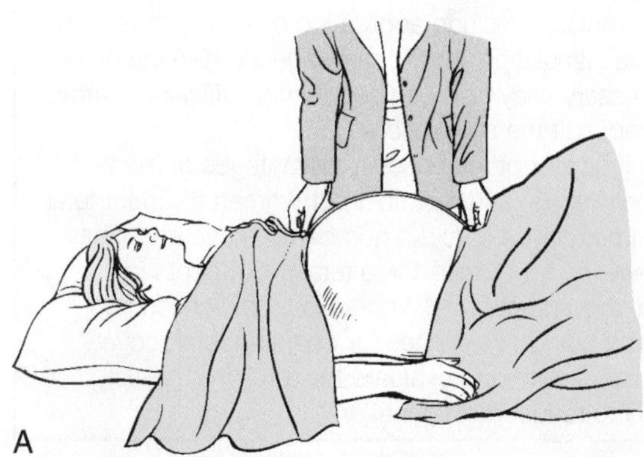

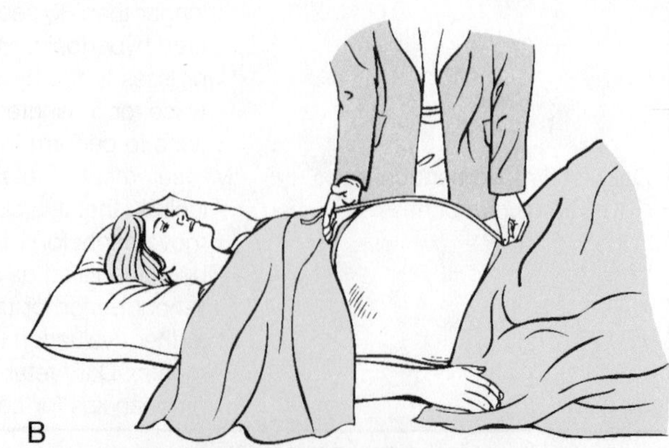

FIGURE 25-2 Measurement of fundal height from symphysis that, **A,** includes the upper curve of the fundus and, **B,** does not include the upper curve of the fundus. Note position of hands and measuring tape.

Patient Teaching

Preparing for Ultrasound Examination

Inform the woman that she will need to have a full bladder for an abdominal ultrasound because this allows better imaging of the fetus. Position her comfortably, with pillows under her head and knees while the test is conducted. Apply ultrasonic gel to the abdomen and pass the scanner over it while images are reproduced. The woman and her partner can watch if they wish. The woman should not feel any discomfort.

For a transvaginal ultrasound, tell the woman that she may either be in a lithotomy position or have her pelvis elevated. These positions are optimal for imaging the pelvic structures. Introduce a transducer with a protective sheath covering into the vagina. If the woman wants to insert it herself, allow her to do so. The angle of the probe or the tilt of the table may be altered during the examination, but the procedure should not be painful.

neural tube defects, whereas low levels may suggest a fetus with Down syndrome (trisomy 21).

Chorionic Villus Sampling

Chorionic villus sampling is a relatively new test to detect genetic disorders of the fetus. It is usually performed at 8 to 12 weeks of gestation and requires aspiration of a small amount of tissue from the chorion of the placenta.

Amniocentesis

Amniocentesis involves removing a small amount of amniotic fluid by passing a needle through the abdominal wall (Figure 25-3). This procedure is usually conducted in conjunction with abdominal ultrasound, which enables the physician to visualize the location of the fetus, the placenta, and a pocket of amniotic fluid. Laboratory examination of the amniotic fluid can reveal valuable information regarding genetic factors such as sex and chromosomal abnormalities, health status, and maturity of the fetus.

Early amniocentesis is performed at approximately the 16th week of pregnancy and is used to detect biochemical or chromosomal abnormalities. Testing at this time allows the mother to consider termination of the pregnancy before the legal point of viability (22 weeks) is reached. The fetus's ability to survive outside the uterus is known as *viability*. Because of advances in technology and maternal and neonatal care, the gestational age at which the fetus is viable has decreased from 28 weeks to as early as 20 weeks (Lowdermilk & Perry, 2007). Later in pregnancy amniocentesis is primarily used to determine fetal lung maturity. It is sometimes performed to detect intrauterine infection or fetal distress.

Nonstress Test

The nonstress test (NST) is done to evaluate how the fetal heart rate responds to periods of fetal movement. It is indicated when there is a risk for placental insufficiency such as pregnancy-induced hypertension, diabetes, postmaturity, maternal smoking, or inadequate maternal nutrition. With a baseline fetal heart rate of 120 to 160 bpm, the fetal heart rate normally accelerates at least 15 bpm for at least 15 seconds with fetal movement. Testing is done using external fetal monitors (see Chapter 26), with the tocotransducer recording fetal movement and the ultrasound transducer recording the fetal heart rate. A reactive result indicates a healthy

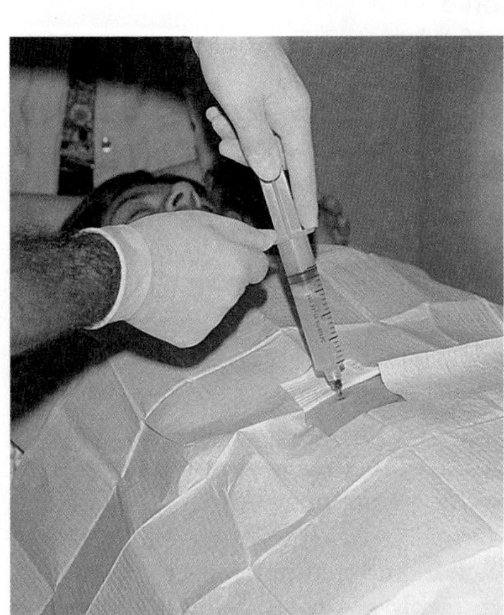

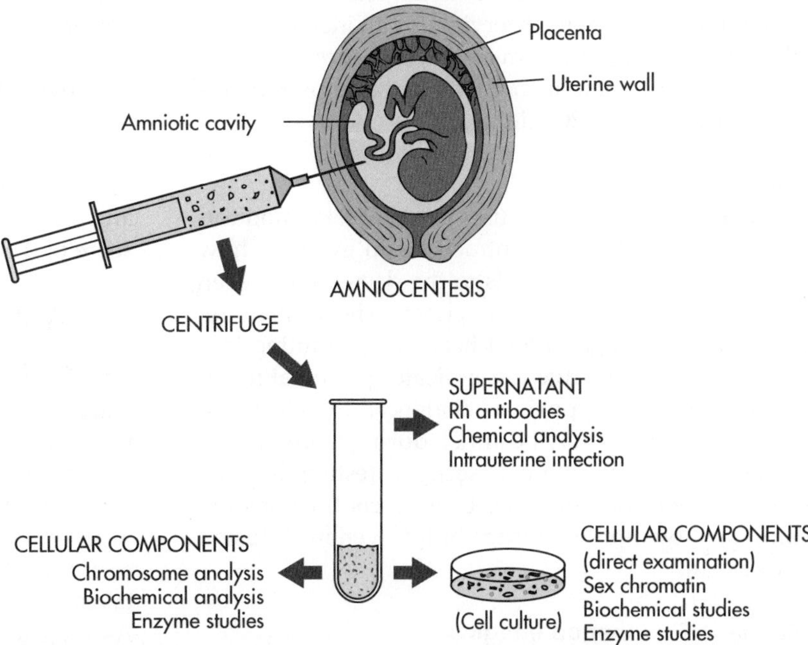

FIGURE 25-3 Transabdominal amniocentesis.

Table 25-3 Interpretation of Biophysical Profile Score Variables

FETAL VARIABLE	NORMAL BEHAVIOR (SCORE = 2)	ABNORMAL BEHAVIOR (SCORE = 0)
Fetal breathing movements (FBM)	Intermittent multiple episodes of more than 30-second duration, within 30-minute BPS time frame. Hiccups count. With continuous FBM for 30 minutes, exclude fetal acidosis.	Continuous breathing without cessation. Completely absent breathing or no sustained episodes.
Body or limb movements	At least four discrete body movements in 30 minutes. Continuous active movement episodes count as a single movement. Includes fine motor movements, rolling movements, and so on, but not REM or mouthing movements.	Three or fewer body or limb movements in a 30-minute observation period.
Fetal tone and posture	Demonstration of active extension with rapid return to flexion of fetal limbs and brisk repositioning or trunk rotation. Opening and closing of hand, mouth, kicking, and so on.	Low-velocity movement only. Incomplete flexion, flaccid extremity positions, abnormal fetal posture. Must score 0 when FM completely absent.
Cardiotocogram (CTG)	Normal mean variation (computerized FHR interpretation), accelerations associated with maternal palpation of FM (accelerations graded for gestation), 20-minute CTG.	Fetal movement and accelerations not coupled. Insufficient accelerations, absent accelerations, or decelerative trace. Mean variation <20 on numerical analysis of CTG.
Amniotic fluid evaluation	At least one pocket >3 cm with no umbilical cord.	No cord-free pocket >2 cm or elements of subjectively reduced amniotic fluid volume deficit.

From Harman, C.R. (2008). Assessment of fetal health. In R.K. Creasy, R. Resnik, & J.D. Iams (Eds.), *Maternal-fetal medicine: principles and practice.* (6th ed.). Philadelphia: Saunders.
BPS, Biophysical profile score; *FHR,* fetal heart rate; *FM,* fetal movement; *REM,* rapid eye movement.

fetus. A nonreactive NST may indicate a compromised fetus and requires further evaluation with another NST, a BPP, or a contraction stress test. Testing is done after the 27th week.

Nursing responsibilities include explaining the procedure to the patient, assuring the patient that no discomfort is associated with the NST, encouraging the patient to verbalize her fears, having the patient eat before the test to elevate serum glucose levels, having the patient empty her bladder and then assume a Sims' position, applying the external fetal monitors to the patient's abdomen, observing for an increase in fetal heart rate with fetal movement, and stimulating fetal activity by external methods if the fetus remains quiet for more than 20 minutes.

Contraction Stress Test

The contraction stress test uses external fetal monitoring and stimulation of contractions to evaluate how the fetal heart rate responds to the decreased oxygen supply during uterine contractions. The desired response is no change in fetal heart rate, resulting in a negative test. A positive test indicates placental insufficiency and fetal hypoxia as evidenced by late decelerations. The fetus may be at risk during labor and require delivery by cesarean section. Testing is done after 32 weeks of gestation. Uterine contractions are stimulated by nipple massage or intravenous infusion of oxytocin.

Magnetic Resonance Imaging

Magnetic resonance imaging (MRI) is a noninvasive tool that can be used for obstetric and gynecologic diagnosis. As with computed tomography (CT), MRI provides excellent pictures of soft tissue. Unlike CT, ionizing radiation is not used; thus vascular structures within the body can be evaluated without injecting an iodinated contrast medium, thereby eliminating any known biologic risk. As with sonography, MRI is noninvasive and can provide images in multiple planes, but interference from skeletal, fatty, or gas-filled structures is not a problem. Also, imaging of deep pelvic structures does not depend on a full bladder. Although this procedure has many advantages, its total safety has not been accurately determined.

Biophysical Profile

The BPP assesses fetal status by evaluating several factors (Table 25-3). These include the NST, fetal breathing movements, fetal muscle tone, fetal movements, and amniotic fluid volume. Each category is given a score of 0 or 2; a total score of 8 or more is reassuring.

MATERNAL PHYSIOLOGY

HORMONAL CHANGES

Estrogen and progesterone levels remain elevated for the first 8 to 10 weeks of pregnancy as a result of HCG, which supports the corpus luteum, a structure that grows on the surface of the ovary within the ruptured ovarian follicle after ovulation. During pregnancy, it secretes progesterone. After this time the placenta takes over production and maintains necessary levels. As long as these levels are high, follicle-stimulating hormone, luteinizing hormone, and ovulation are suppressed, as is menstruation.

UTERUS

The uterus enlarges during pregnancy as a result of hormonal stimulus, increased vascularity, hyperplasia (new muscle fiber and tissue), and hypertrophy (enlargement of existing fiber and tissue). The nonpregnant uterus is pear shaped and weighs approximately 2 ounces (50 g). By the third trimester (the last 3 months of a 9-month pregnancy), it is egg shaped and has increased in weight to 2.2 pounds (1000 g). At term it can hold a fetus, a placenta, and amniotic fluid totaling more than 8½ pounds (4000 g).

The consistency of the tissue changes also. Changes in the cervix and fundus, along with an altered position in the pelvis, are early signs of pregnancy. The uterus, which in a nonpregnant state is a pelvic organ, rises to the base of the ribcage. The superior aspect of the uterus (the fundus) is located at the level of the xiphoid process by the end of the third trimester.

BREASTS

Changes in the breasts during pregnancy include hypertrophy of the mammary glandular tissue and increased vascularization, pigmentation, size, and prominence of nipples and areolae. These breast changes are all caused by hormonal stimulation.

MATERNITY CYCLE

The maternity cycle, which is discussed in this and successive chapters, is divided into three distinct periods. The first portion of the cycle is called the antepartal period (from Latin root *ante,* "before," and *parere,* "to bring to bear") or prenatal period (from Latin root *pre,* "before," and *natal,* "birth"). The antepartal period begins with conception and ends with the onset of labor.

The next portion of the cycle is referred to as the intrapartal period (from Latin *intra,* "within," and *parere,* "to bring to bear"). This period begins with the onset of labor and ends with delivery of the placenta. The same period is sometimes called the perinatal portion (from Latin *peri,* "around," and *natal,* "birth").

The final stage of the cycle is the postpartal period (from Latin *post,* "after" and *parere,* "to bring to bear"). This period starts after the delivery of the placenta and lasts for approximately 6 weeks or until the reproductive organs return to the prepregnancy state.

Pregnancy spans 9 months, approximately 40 weeks. Pregnancy is also divided into 3-month periods, or trimesters. The first trimester covers weeks 1 through 13; the second, weeks 14 through 26; and the third, weeks 27 through term gestation (38 to 40 weeks).

ANTEPARTAL ASSESSMENT

GENERAL PHYSICAL ASSESSMENT

Prenatal care and assessment should begin when pregnancy is planned or as soon as the first menstrual period is missed. Ideally the woman has been receiving regular medical attention and is already known by the health care provider. Unfortunately, because of cost or frequent changes of residence, many people do not receive regular, routine health care. Many women also seek the attention of a specialist, an obstetrician, a nurse practitioner, or a midwife during pregnancy. This requires establishing a new relationship with a primary care practitioner and total review of the health history.

On the first visit, obtain **demographic** (the statistical and quantitative study of characteristics of the human population) data such as age, occupation, and marital status, along with insurance information. The basic information helps the primary care practitioner identify potential areas of concern. For example, an adolescent who is 15, single, unemployed, and a high school dropout with no insurance presents a different set of concerns from a 25-year-old, married, college graduate with comprehensive insurance.

Obtain a basic family and personal medical history. To anticipate any problems, the primary care practitioner must be aware of any genetic diseases in either the mother's or the father's family. A family history that includes genetic diseases may worry the pregnant woman until she is assured that her baby is normal. If serious genetic problems are known, many couples seek genetic counseling before they consider having children.

GENETIC COUNSELING

Rapid expansion in the identification, understanding, and diagnosis of genetic disease has only led to effective medical or surgical therapies for a small number of patients. For most genetic conditions, therapeutic or preventive measures are nonexistent or disappointingly limited. Consequently, the most useful means of reducing the incidence of these disorders is by preventing their transmission. As more becomes known about genetic disorders, more accurate predictions can be made about the probability of a couple passing a disorder to their offspring. At present the best way to reduce the number of children born with genetic defects is for health professionals to provide families with genetic information and services.

Assessment begins with a personal medical history and a review of systems. Obtain information about chronic diseases such as cardiac problems, hypertension, diabetes mellitus, and infectious diseases (e.g., rubella, acquired immunodeficiency syndrome, or other sexually transmitted infections). Document any history of accidents or previous surgeries. Significant findings in these areas may indicate the potential for problems and the need for early medical and nursing intervention. High-risk pregnancies are discussed in Chapter 28.

Assess lifestyle patterns, including recreational activities; nutrition and eating habits; use of prescription medications, street drugs, alcohol, or tobacco; and work exposure to hazardous conditions. Early detection and correction of problem situations can reduce hazards to the woman and prevent detrimental effects on the fetus.

A basic physical examination is completed (Box 25-2). All these tests increase the data available and enable the primary care practitioner to plan comprehensive care.

OBSTETRIC ASSESSMENT

In addition to the general health history and physical examination, obtain information about the woman's gynecologic, menstrual, and obstetric history. This includes the use of contraceptives and the regularity of the menstrual period, including frequency, duration, amount of flow, presence of pain, and any other significant comments. Review any history of gynecologic surgery, vaginal discharge, or herpes infection. The physician may ask questions regarding exposure to diethylstilbestrol (DES), since daughters of women who took DES during pregnancy have an increased risk of spontaneous abortion caused by incompetent cervix.

Discuss the number of pregnancies the patient has had and their outcomes. This includes the course of the pregnancy with special attention to any complications, the type of delivery (vaginal or cesarean), any complications during delivery, the use of forceps or other medical assistance, the type of anesthetic used, the condition of the newborn, and any complications of the postpartal period.

GYNECOLOGIC EXAMINATION

The gynecologic examination is also performed at this time. The nurse is often called on to prepare the necessary equipment and assist in this examination. Also provide explanations and emotional support to the patient (Box 25-3).

Box 25-2 Basic Prenatal Physical Examination

- Measurement of vital signs, height, and weight
- Assessment of heart, lungs, and reflexes
- General physical inspection of skin and mobility
- Basic bloodwork (hemoglobin; hematocrit; serology tests for detection of syphilis, human immunodeficiency virus, and hepatitis virus; blood typing; Rh factor; rubella titer)
- Routine urinalysis for glucose, protein, ketones
- Pregnancy tests if pregnancy has not already been confirmed

Box 25-3 Gynecologic Examination

- Palpation and auscultation of the abdomen
- Visualization of the cervix and vagina
- Evaluation of the bony pelvis
- Palpation of the uterus externally or bimanually
- Examination of the vulva, the perineum, the anus, and the rectum
- Sometimes a Papanicolaou's (Pap) smear (done at the beginning of the examination)

DETERMINATION OF PREGNANCY

Many times a woman comes to a physician's office because she suspects she is pregnant. After the entire history and physical examination have been done, the physician can determine with varying degrees of certainty whether she is or not.

PRESUMPTIVE SIGNS

The presumptive signs are indicators that a woman may be pregnant, but these signs may also indicate other conditions not related to pregnancy:

- **Amenorrhea:** Absence of menstruation.
- **Nausea and vomiting**
- **Frequent urination**
- **Breast changes:** Swelling, tingling, and tenderness of the breasts are common during pregnancy, along with changes in pigmentation of the areolae. The sebaceous material secreted from the ducts of the glands to the skin of each areola lubricates and protects the breasts from infection and trauma during breastfeeding.
- **Change in the shape of the abdomen**
- **Quickening:** The subjective sensation of fetal movement first occurs at about 16 to 18 weeks of gestation.
- **Skin changes:** Pigment changes, such as darkening of some areas of the body such as the areolae, may occur.
- **Chadwick's sign:** During the pelvic examination the physician may note that the vagina, the cervix, and sometimes the vulva have a violet or purplish discoloration.

PROBABLE SIGNS

The probable signs indicate a high likelihood that the woman is pregnant. These signs are not, however, 100% reliable indicators:

- **Changes in the reproductive organs:** Enlargement of the uterus indicates a high probability of pregnancy, particularly if accompanied by changes in the consistency of the isthmus of the uterus (the segment between the fundus and the cervix). A softening of this segment is called **Hëgar's sign** (Figure 25-4). This change and a softening or increased pliability of the cervix called **Goodell's sign** are most commonly seen in pregnancy. **Ballottement,** which may be used at approximately 16 to 18 weeks of gestation, is a technique that involves palpating the uterus in such a way that the examiner feels the rebound of the floating fetus (Figure 25-5).
- **Positive pregnancy tests:** Using either blood or urine to measure the level of HCG, many of these tests are available over the counter in drugstores. However, the reliability of these products depends on the technique used in collecting the urine specimen and performing the test. Tests

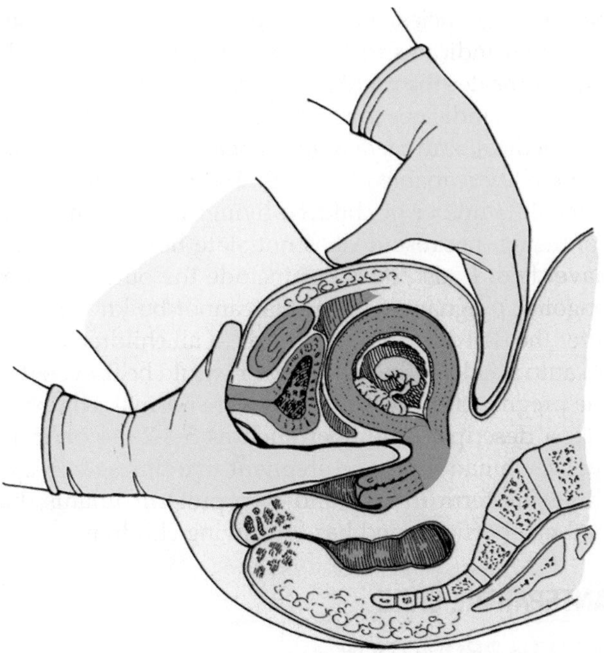

FIGURE 25-4 Hëgar's sign. Bimanual examination for assessing compressibility and softening of isthmus (lower uterine segment) while the cervix is still firm.

administered by the primary care practitioner are generally between 95% and 99% accurate. The greatest advantages of pregnancy tests are that they can be administered early in pregnancy and are reasonably inexpensive. If the test results are positive and other indicators such as uterine changes are abnormal, the primary care practitioner may suspect complications such as an ectopic (outside the uterus) pregnancy or hydatidiform mole (abnormal growth of a fertilized ovum in which a large vascular mass, but no fetus, develops). Hydatidiform mole frequently results in a highly reactive pregnancy test, and the test may continue to indicate positive results even after surgical removal.

Box 25-4 Positive Signs of Pregnancy

- **Visualization:** The fetal skeleton seen on x-ray examination is a positive sign of pregnancy, but use of radiation is generally limited during pregnancy because of possible danger to the fetus. Ultrasonic tracing of the fetus is also a positive indication of pregnancy.
- **Fetal movement:** Fetal movement may be detected by a trained observer (the primary care practitioner).
- **Auscultation of fetal heart tone:** Fetal heart activity can be detected by ultrasound at 6 weeks; tones heard by Doppler at 10 to 17 weeks and by stethoscope at 17 to 19 weeks.

POSITIVE SIGNS

Positive signs are those that occur only with pregnancy and are not present at any other time (Box 25-4).

DETERMINATION OF THE ESTIMATED DATE OF BIRTH

Normal human pregnancy, counting from the first day of the last menstrual period, is about 280 days, 40 weeks, 10 lunar months (28 days each), or slightly more than 9 calendar months.

The estimated date of birth (EDB), or estimated date of delivery (EDD)—often known as the "due date"—involves calculations based on the woman's menstrual cycle. The most common method is called **Nägele's rule:** Start with the first day of the woman's last menstrual period and count back 3 months, then add 7 days. For example, if the first day of the last menstrual period was June 14, counting back 3 months to March 14 and then adding 7 days would yield an EDB of March 21. Studies reveal that only a small percentage of infants are actually born on the date predicted; most deliveries, however, do occur within 10 days before or after the EDB.

If the woman does not keep a menstrual record, calculation of the EDB may be more difficult. The primary care practitioner must then rely on observations

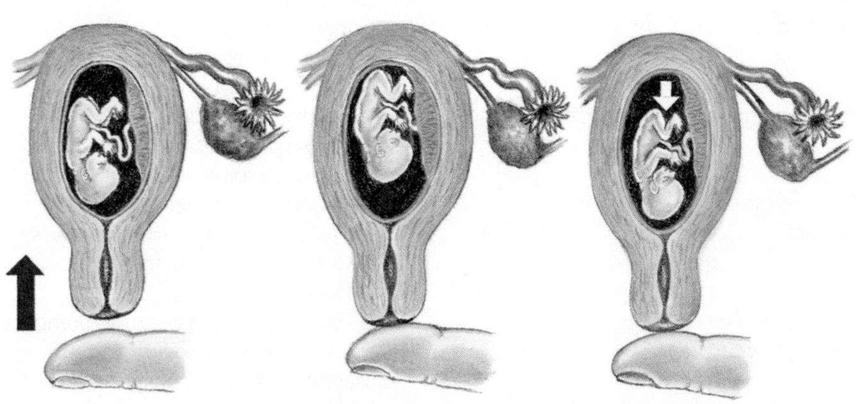

FIGURE 25-5 Internal ballottement (18 weeks).

such as quickening, estimation of fetal size by palpation, or ultrasonic tests, all of which can be unreliable. If it is essential for the primary care practitioner to know the level of fetal maturity, he or she can perform specialized tests later in the pregnancy.

OBSTETRIC TERMINOLOGY

Specific terms are used in obstetrics to describe the number of times a woman has been pregnant and has given birth. Gravida (from the Latin root *gravidus*, "heavy") indicates a pregnant woman. Latin numerical prefixes are added to this term to indicate number of pregnancies, such as **primigravida** (one), **nulligravida** (none), and **multigravida** (multiple). Similarly, prefixes are added to the Latin root para ("to bring forth") to indicate the number of births, such as **primipara** (one), **nullipara** (none), and **multipara** (multiple). Many facilities use a shorthand method of keeping track of a patient's obstetric history; for example, "1/0" indicates one pregnancy with no viable births.

A more detailed five-part description is sometimes used (Box 25-5). The first digit represents the total number of pregnancies, including the present one; the second digit indicates the number of term deliveries; the third indicates the number of premature deliveries; and the fourth indicates the number of abortions. **Abortion** is a medical term meaning loss of a fetus before the age of viability (capable of living). The fifth number indicates the number of children living. This is sometimes confusing, because it does not state how a child may have died. It also does not include the outcome of an ongoing pregnancy, since this cannot be known until after the delivery. In other words, if all children died in an auto accident, the last number would be 0, even if all the pregnancies and deliveries were normal. For example, a descriptive number such as 5-3-2-0-4 indicates that a woman has been pregnant five times, delivered three full-term infants and two preterm infants, has had no abortions, and has four living children.

Box 25-5 Defining Parity

FIVE-DIGIT SYSTEM: GTPAL
G: Gravidity
T: Term births
P: Preterm births
A: Abortions
L: Living children

FOUR-DIGIT SYSTEM: TPAL
T: Term births
P: Preterm births
A: Abortions
L: Living children

ANTEPARTAL CARE

HEALTH PROMOTION

Most pregnant women want to learn more about pregnancy, childbirth, and motherhood (provided they have no serious problems in the area of role relationship, coping, or self-perception). Pregnancy is one time in life when most women see the importance of regular medical supervision and are willing to make changes in their habits. They think of their baby first and do everything that is best for the infant.

A checklist for antepartal needs throughout pregnancy is a valuable teaching tool. It provides the team of care providers with a communication tool to prevent gaps and to identify areas of repeated concerns for patients. Sharing the checklist with patients reassures them that other pregnant women and their families face the same issues. Reading the checklist also reminds patients of information they might otherwise forget (Box 25-6).

Box 25-6 A Trimester Checklist

- Schedule and events of visits
- Counseling for self-care
- Adaptations and discomforts
  —Dyspnea
  —Insomnia
  —Psychosocial responses and family dynamics
  —Gingivitis
  —Urinary frequency
  —Perineal discomfort and pressure
  —Braxton Hicks contractions
  —Leg cramps
  —Ankle edema
- Safety (balance)
- Exercise and rest
- Relaxation
- Nutrition
- Sexuality
- Personal hygiene
- Danger signs, general
- Danger signs, preterm labor
- Fetal growth and development
- Preparation for baby
  —Feeding method
  —Nipple preparation
- Preparation for labor
  —Recognition: false versus true
  —Prenatal classes
  —Control of discomfort
  —Hospital tour
  —Provision for other family members
- Preparation for homecoming
- Diagnostic tests (specify)
- Other

Once pregnancy is determined, prenatal care is instituted. Nursing interventions follow the nursing process: assessment, analysis, formulation of nursing diagnoses, planning, implementation, and evaluation.

Pregnancy is an excellent time to establish good general health practices. Until they become pregnant, many women do not have regular physical examinations or Papanicolaou's (Pap) smears or do not do home screening tests such as breast self-examination (BSE). The high motivation level makes this a good time to teach patients about health maintenance practices.

Early in pregnancy the woman often begins to seek information and make choices regarding how and where she wishes to give birth. Provide information regarding the options available in a particular community (see Chapter 26).

Routine care during pregnancy begins with the initial examination and history, as previously described. Appointments are recommended once a month through the seventh month, once every 2 weeks for the next month, and then once every week until delivery. If any problems occur or the primary care practitioner suspects anything unusual, such as a multiple pregnancy, the schedule of visits may be altered. Dental care should continue during pregnancy. Any major dental work, such as oral surgery or extractions, is usually delayed until after delivery.

Smoking during pregnancy can be dangerous to the developing fetus. Oxygen deprivation can lead to decreased intrauterine growth and low birth weight. Drinking alcoholic beverages during pregnancy is also contraindicated, particularly during the first trimester. Fetal alcohol syndrome is discussed in Chapter 28.

Women should avoid taking any medication or drugs during pregnancy, including over-the-counter drugs (Box 25-7). As mentioned, most drugs are able to cross the placenta and are transmitted to the fetus. Only medications prescribed by the primary care practitioner should be taken. Street drugs such as marijuana and cocaine are dangerous to both mother and fetus and must be avoided. Complementary and alternative therapies may also be used during pregnancy, but as with medications the mother should be extremely cautious about herbal remedies (Box 25-8).

Embryonic and fetal development is vulnerable to environmental teratogens. Many potentially dangerous chemicals are present in the home, yard, and workplace, including cleaning agents, paints, sprays, herbicides, and pesticides. The soil and water supply may be unsafe. Therefore the woman should (1) read all labels for ingredients and proper use of product; (2) ensure adequate ventilation with clean air; (3) dispose of wastes appropriately; (4) wear gloves when handling chemicals; and (5) change job assignments or workplace as necessary.

Today many women continue to work throughout pregnancy. It is important that the work environment be checked for chemicals and other hazards. The Occupational Safety and Health Administration has numerous guidelines for hazards in the workplace. Address working conditions such as lifting and standing or sitting for long periods. Encourage the woman to take frequent rest periods.

DANGER SIGNS DURING PREGNANCY

Although pregnancy involves many changes and normal discomforts, certain conditions signal the need for

Box 25-7 Food and Drug Administration Drug Categories

The rational use of any medication requires a risk-versus-benefit assessment. Among the many risk factors that complicate assessment, pregnancy is one of the most perplexing. The U.S. Food and Drug Administration has established five categories to indicate the potential of a systemically absorbed drug for causing birth defects. The key differences among the categories are the degree (reliability) of evidence and the risk:benefit ratio. Pregnancy category X is particularly notable; it is assigned to a drug if there are any data that indicate the drug is a teratogen and the risk:benefit ratio does not support use of the drug. Category X drugs are contraindicated during pregnancy.

PREGNANCY CATEGORY AND DEFINITION

A: Adequate studies in pregnant women have not demonstrated a risk to the fetus in the first trimester of pregnancy, and there is no evidence of risk in later trimesters.

B: Animal studies have not demonstrated a risk to the fetus, but there are no adequate studies in pregnant women; or animal studies have shown an adverse effect, but adequate studies in pregnant women have not demonstrated a risk to the fetus during the first trimester of pregnancy, and there is no evidence of risk in later trimesters.

C: Animal studies have shown an adverse effect on the fetus, but there are no adequate studies in humans; the benefits from the use of the drug in pregnant women may be acceptable despite its potential risks; or there are no animal reproduction studies and no adequate studies in humans.

D: There is evidence of human fetal risk, but the potential benefits from the use of the drug in pregnant women may be acceptable despite its potential risks.

X: Studies in animals or humans demonstrate fetal abnormalities, or adverse reaction reports indicate evidence of fetal risk. The risk of use in a pregnant woman clearly outweighs any possible benefit.

NR: Not rated

Regardless of the designated pregnancy category or presumed safety, no drug should be administered during pregnancy unless it is clearly needed and potential benefits outweigh potential risks.

Modified from Skidmore-Roth, L. (2010). *Mosby's 2010 nursing drug reference.* (23rd ed.). St. Louis: Mosby.

Box 25-8 Complementary and Alternative Therapies Used in Pregnancy

MORNING SICKNESS AND HYPEREMESIS
- Acupuncture
- Acupressure
- Shiatzu
- Herbal remedies: Some herbs can cause miscarriage, preterm labor, or fetal or maternal injury. Pregnant women should discuss use in pregnancy with the health care provider and with an expert in the use of the herb.
  —Lemon balm
  —Peppermint
  —Spearmint
  —Ginger root
  —Raspberry leaf
  —Fennel
  —Chamomile
  —Hops
  —Meadowsweet
  —Wild yam root

RELAXATION AND MUSCLE-ACHE RELIEF
- Yoga
- Biofeedback
- Reflexology
- Therapeutic touch
- Massage

From Lowdermilk, D.L., & Perry, S.E. (2007). *Maternal and women's health care.* (9th ed.). St. Louis: Mosby.

immediate medical attention (Box 25-9). Teach the pregnant woman these danger signs and how to monitor fetal movements (see Patient Teaching box for guidelines for counting fetal movements). Stress the importance of contacting the primary care practitioner promptly if any of these signs is present.

NUTRITIONAL AND METABOLIC HEALTH PATTERN

See Chapter 21 for information about basic nutrition and nutritional therapy for the life cycle, stages of pregnancy, and lactation.

Box 25-9 Danger Signs and Symptoms During Pregnancy

- Visual disturbances: diplopia (double vision), blurring, or spots
- Headaches, severe, sudden, or continuous
- Edema: swelling of the face, presacral area, or fingers
- Rapid weight gain, in excess of normal gain for gestation
- Pain: severe abdominal or epigastric pain
- Signs of infection: fever, chills, diarrhea, changes in vaginal drainage, pain or burning with urination
- Vaginal bleeding (no matter how slight)
- Vaginal drainage (aside from normal mucus)
- Persistent vomiting
- Muscular irritability or convulsions
- Absence or decrease in fetal movement once felt

 **Patient Teaching**

Guidelines for Counting Fetal Movements (Kick Counts)

- The patient should choose a time of day when she can sit or lie quietly.
- Teach the patient the different counting strategies:
  —Starting at 9 AM, count the baby's movements until 10 movements are counted. If 10 movements have not been counted in 12 hours, notify the primary health care provider immediately.
  —Count four movements, three times a day after meals. Most people count four movements in 1 hour. If four movements are not felt, count for 1 more hour. If, at the end of 2 hours, the patient has not felt four movements, she should notify the primary health care provider immediately.

Modified from Hockenberry, M.J., et al. (2007). *Wong's maternal-child nursing care.* (8th ed.). St. Louis: Mosby.

Pica

Pica is craving and eating substances that are not normally considered edible. The reason for this condition is unknown, but it is more common in certain cultural groups and regions of the country. It may be seen in children and occasionally during pregnancy. Substances ingested include clay or laundry starch. Although not toxic, they may interfere with iron absorption, resulting in anemia. Large amounts of clay may also result in fecal impaction.

Common Discomforts

Many pregnant women experience some discomforts of the gastrointestinal tract during pregnancy. Some women have excessive salivation (ptyalism), presumably in response to the high levels of estrogen during pregnancy. Although it may be uncomfortable and awkward at times, ptyalism causes no serious problems and disappears late in pregnancy or after delivery. Using astringent mouthwash, chewing gum, or sucking on hard candy may provide relief.

Nausea is common in the early stages of pregnancy. It typically occurs when the woman awakens in the morning; hence the name "morning sickness." It can, however, occur at any time of the day. Nausea is thought to be caused by increased HCG levels and changes in carbohydrate metabolism. Mild nausea can usually be controlled by slowly eating a few soda crackers or dry toast before rising from bed. Other suggestions are eating smaller, more frequent meals and avoiding spicy or greasy food. Morning sickness rarely lasts beyond the fourth month. If it lasts longer, if it is more severe, and particularly if it involves vomiting, the primary care practitioner should be contacted. The most severe form is called **hyperemesis gravidarum.** Its cause is not clear, but if left untreated, it can lead to dehydration, fluid and electrolyte imbalance, acid-base imbalance, altered kidney and cardiac function, and even fetal death. Hospitalization with close medical supervision, including feeding, may be required (see Chapter 28).

Pyrosis (heartburn) from gastric reflux into the esophagus can be caused by the increasing size of the fetus in the abdominal cavity, which displaces the stomach. Increased progesterone level, which leads to relaxation of the cardiac sphincter, and decreased gastric mobility, which delays the stomach's emptying time, can also contribute to the problem. Smaller, more frequent meals; decreased fat intake; low-sodium antacids; and avoidance of lying down after meals often give relief (see Chapter 21).

Skin Changes

Changes in pigmentation often occur during pregnancy as a result of increased amounts of melanocyte-stimulating hormone. The changes occur primarily in areas that already have greater pigmentation, such as the areolae; nipples; vulva; perianal area; and linea alba (midline of the abdomen from pubis to umbilicus), which darkens and is called the **linea nigra.**

Chloasma, the mask of pregnancy, is an irregular darkening of the cheeks, forehead, and nose. These changes are often more obvious in women with darker hair and skin and may be worsened by sun exposure. This generally disappears or fades significantly soon after delivery.

Striae gravidarum, or stretch marks, are reddish, wavy streaks that can appear on the thighs, the abdomen, and the breasts. They are more common with distention but may occur even in relatively thin women. They usually fade after delivery. Because integumentary system changes vary greatly among women of different racial backgrounds, note the color of a woman's skin along with any changes that may be attributed to pregnancy when performing physical assessment.

Spider nevi (a branched growth of dilated capillaries on the skin) and **palmar erythema** (reddened palms) are sometimes seen. These conditions are caused by increased blood flow resulting from high estrogen levels. Both usually disappear when the pregnancy ends.

Hair and nail growth are frequently accelerated during pregnancy, with **hirsutism** (excessive body hair in a masculine distribution pattern as a result of heredity, hormonal dysfunction, or medication) commonly reported. Oily skin and acne may occur in some women, whereas others report a clearing of their skin. This is usually temporary unless other physiologic problems are active.

Occasionally, decreased emptying of the gallbladder may result in subclinical jaundice, which causes generalized pruritus (itching). This and other concerns are noted in Table 25-4.

Changes in the Cardiovascular System

Maternal adjustments to pregnancy involve extensive changes in the cardiovascular system, both anatomical and physiologic. Changes can result in episodes of orthostatic hypotension. An increase of platelets and fibrinogen increases the woman's risk for blood clots. Cardiovascular adaptations protect the woman's normal physiologic functioning, meet the metabolic demands of pregnancy, and provide for fetal development and growth (Table 25-5).

Changes in the Respiratory System

Structural and ventilatory adaptations during pregnancy provide for maternal and fetal needs. Maternal oxygen requirements increase in response to the accelerated metabolic rate and the need to add to the tissue mass in the uterus and breasts. In addition, the fetus requires oxygen and a way to eliminate carbon dioxide. Elevation of estrogen causes the ligaments of the ribcage to relax, permitting increased chest expansion (Table 25-6).

Changes in the Musculoskeletal System

The gradually changing body and increasing weight of the pregnant woman cause noticeable alterations in her posture (Figure 25-6) and the way she walks late in pregnancy. The great abdominal distention that gives the pelvis a forward tilt, decreased abdominal muscle tone, and increased weight bearing create a realignment of the spinal curvature. The woman's center of gravity shifts forward. An increase in the normal lumbosacral curve (lordosis) develops, and a compensatory curvature in the cervicodorsal region (exaggerated anterior flexion of the head) develops to help her maintain her balance. Aching, numbness, and weakness of the upper extremities may result. Large breasts and a stoop-shouldered stance further accentuate the lumbar and dorsal curves. Walking is more difficult, and the pregnant woman's waddling gait (called "the proud walk of pregnancy" by Shakespeare) is well known. The ligamentous and muscular structures of the middle and lower spine may be severely stressed. These and related changes often cause musculoskeletal discomfort, especially in older women or those with a back disorder or a faulty sense of balance. With large or multiple gestation pregnancies, overdistention may cause the abdominal wall muscles to separate **(diastasis recti abdominis**). Management of this condition is typically conservative, but severe cases may require surgical repair (Lowdermilk & Perry, 2007).

Slight relaxation and increased mobility of the pelvic joints are normal during pregnancy. They are a result of the exaggerated elasticity and softening of the connective tissue caused by increased circulating steroid sex hormones, especially estrogen. Relaxin, an ovarian hormone, assists in the relaxation and softening. These adaptations permit enlargement of pelvic dimensions to facilitate labor and birth. The degree of relaxation varies, but considerable separation of the symphysis pubis and the instability of the sacroiliac joints may cause pain and difficulty in walking. Obesity and multifetal pregnancy tend to increase the pelvic instability.

Table 25-4 Discomforts and Concerns Related to Maternal Adaptations during the Third Trimester

DISCOMFORT	PHYSIOLOGY	TEACHING FOR SELF-CARE
Shortness of breath and dyspnea in 60% of pregnant women	Expansion of diaphragm limited by enlarging uterus; diaphragm elevated approximately 1½ inches (4 cm); some relief after lightening (when the fetus settles lower in the true pelvis, leaving more space in the upper abdomen)	Good posture; sleep with extra pillow; avoid overloading stomach; stop smoking; refer to physician if symptoms worsen to rule out anemia, emphysema, and asthma
Insomnia (later weeks of pregnancy)	Fetal movements, muscular cramping, urinary frequency, shortness of breath, or other discomforts	Reassurance; conscious relaxation; back massage or effleurage (deep or gentle stroking); support of body parts with pillows; warm milk or shower before retiring
Psychosocial responses: mood swings, mixed feelings, increased anxiety	Hormonal and metabolic adaptations; feelings about impending labor, delivery, and parenthood	Reassurance and support from significant other and nurse; improved communication with partner, family, and others
Return of urinary frequency and urgency	Vascular engorgement and altered bladder function caused by hormones; bladder capacity reduced by enlarging uterus and fetal presenting part; lightening	Kegel exercises (see Patient Teaching box on Kegel exercises [p. 794]); limit fluid intake before bedtime; reassurance; wear perineal pad; refer to physician for pain or burning sensation
Perineal discomfort and pressure	Pressure from enlarging uterus, especially when standing or walking; multifetal gestation	Rest, conscious relaxation, and good posture; maternity girdle; refer to physician for assessment and treatment if pain is present; rule out labor
Braxton Hicks contractions	Intensification of uterine contractions in preparation for work of labor	Reassurance; rest; change of position; practice breathing techniques when contractions are bothersome; effleurage; rule out labor
Leg cramps (gastrocnemius spasm), especially when reclining	Compression of nerves supplying lower extremities because of enlarging uterus; reduced level of diffusible serum calcium or elevation of serum phosphorus; aggravating factors: fatigue, poor peripheral circulation, pointing toes when stretching legs or when walking, drinking more than 1 quart (1 L) of milk per day; cause unclear	Rule out blood clot by checking for Homans' sign; use massage and heat over affected muscle; stretch affected muscle until spasm relaxes; physician-prescribed oral supplementation with calcium carbonate or calcium lactate tablets; aluminum hydroxide gel, 1 oz, with each meal removes phosphorus by absorbing it
Ankle edema (nonpitting) to lower extremities	Edema aggravated by prolonged standing, sitting, poor posture, lack of exercise, constrictive clothing (e.g., garters), or hot weather	Ample fluid intake for "natural" diuretic effect; put on support stockings before rising; rest periodically with legs and hips elevated; exercise moderately; refer to physician if generalized edema develops (diuretics are contraindicated)

Table 25-5 Cardiovascular Changes in Pregnancy

PARAMETER	CHANGE
Heart rate	Increases 10 to 15 bpm
Blood pressure	Remains at prepregnancy levels in first trimester (systolic) Slight decrease in second trimester (systolic and diastolic) Returns to prepregnancy levels in third trimester (diastolic)
Blood volume	Increases by 1500 mL or 40% to 50% above prepregnancy level
Red blood cell mass	Increases 17%
Hemoglobin	Decreases
Hematocrit	Decreases
White blood cell count	Increases in second and third trimesters
Cardiac output	Increases 30% to 50%

Adapted from Lowdermilk, D.L., & Perry, S.E. (2007). *Maternal and women's health care.* (9th ed.). St. Louis: Mosby.

Table 25-6 Respiratory Changes in Pregnancy

PARAMETER	CHANGE
Respiratory rate	Unchanged or slightly increased
Tidal volume	Increased 30% to 40%
Vital capacity	Unchanged
Inspiratory capacity	Increased
Expiratory volume	Decreased
Total lung capacity	Unchanged to slightly decreased
Oxygen consumption	Increased 15% to 20%

Adapted from Lowdermilk, D.L., & Perry, S.E. (2007). *Maternal and women's health care.* (9th ed.). St. Louis: Mosby.

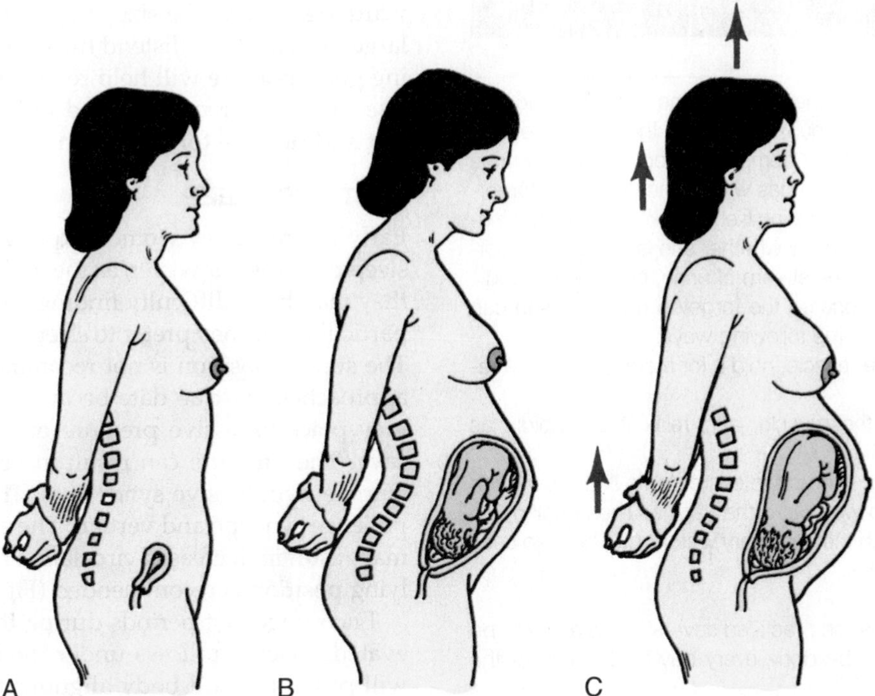

FIGURE 25-6 Postural changes during pregnancy. **A,** Nonpregnant. **B,** Incorrect posture during pregnancy. **C,** Correct posture during pregnancy.

Hygiene Practices

Bathing or showering during pregnancy should continue as part of routine hygiene. Increased perspiration is common, and good personal hygiene is important to prevent body odor. Tub bathing may become difficult in the later months of pregnancy because of changes in mobility and balance. Some primary care practitioners restrict tub baths in the last month because the cervix may have begun to dilate.

Most primary care practitioners recommend that women avoid hot tubs, sauna baths, and spas during pregnancy because maternal hyperthermia during the first trimester may result in central nervous system defects of the fetus. Because early in the first trimester a woman may not be aware she is pregnant, those not taking measures to prevent pregnancy should probably also avoid hyperthermic baths.

Douching is not recommended, even though the woman may have increased vaginal discharge. If vaginal drainage causes pruritus or other symptoms, this should be reported to the primary care practitioner.

Pregnant women do not have to buy special clothing, but should choose garments that are comfortable and do not restrict movement. It is important to avoid circulation-restricting clothing such as garters. Larger bras may be necessary as breasts enlarge; a too-snug bra may interfere with breathing.

ELIMINATION

Gastrointestinal System

Slowing of intestinal peristalsis can result in abdominal distention, flatulence, and constipation. Constipation can also be related to the iron supplements the woman is taking.

Hemorrhoids can result from straining as a result of constipation. They can also be caused by the enlarged uterus putting pressure on the pelvic blood vessels, slowing venous return from the lower extremities. Women with a history of cholelithiasis may experience problems with this as a result of an increased cholesterol level, which is common during pregnancy. Adequate fluid intake, dietary roughage, and exercise may help reduce problems related to constipation.

Urinary System

Frequency of urination is a common complaint of pregnancy. During pregnancy the mother must excrete not only her own waste products but also those of the fetus. Urinary output increases, and the specific gravity of urine decreases. Early in pregnancy the enlarging uterus irritates the bladder by putting pressure on it. This continues until the uterus rises into the abdominal cavity. Later in pregnancy, when the presenting part descends into the pelvis, the pressure and symptoms return. Teach the patient Kegel exercises to help tone the muscles of the perineum and prevent stress incontinence (see Patient Teaching box on Kegel exercises).

The ureter and kidneys may become dilated, particularly on the right side, as a result of placental progesterone and pressure from the enlarging uterus. Restricted circulation in the pelvis as the uterus enlarges increases the risk of bladder trauma and urinary tract infection.

ACTIVITY AND EXERCISE

Patients should continue normal activity throughout an uncomplicated pregnancy. If a woman regularly participates in a fitness program or sport, she probably

Patient Teaching

Kegel Exercises

- The muscles that stop the flow of urine are the pubococcygeal muscles. These muscles support the pelvic floor, the bladder, and the urethra. Attempts to stop the flow of urine or forestall the expulsion of gas will aid the woman in targeting the involved muscles. Doing Kegel exercises during urination helps the woman know whether she is doing them correctly. If she can stop the stream of urine, her tone is good.
- After a woman has located the targeted muscles, she can do Kegel exercises in the following ways:
  —**Slow:** Tighten the muscle, hold it for a count of 3, and relax it.
  —**Quick:** Tighten the muscle, and relax it as rapidly as possible.
  —**Push out, pull in:** Pull up the entire pelvic floor as though trying to suck up water into the vagina. Then bear down as if trying to push the imaginary water out. This also uses abdominal muscles.

PRACTICE

- Kegel exercises must be practiced several times a day to be effective. They must be done every day for the rest of the woman's life.
- These exercises can be done 10 times in a row at least three times or more per day. Although some people recommend doing this as many as 100 times in a row, this only fatigues the pelvic floor muscles.
- A good time to practice is during trips to the bathroom, but additional practice at other times is even more beneficial.

can continue with most activities. This should be discussed with the primary care practitioner if she has any doubts. High-risk activities or those that require a great deal of balance and coordination are discouraged. Common sense is the best guide.

Fatigue is a common complaint during pregnancy. The woman must pace herself and not overdo tiring activities.

Changes in balance and posture occur as the fetus increases in size. To compensate for the shifting center of gravity, the lumbodorsal curve increases (lordosis). This may result in low backaches. Hormonal influence on pelvic bones, resulting in joint relaxation, can lead to a waddling gait. Footwear with low heels and the use of good body mechanics will help reduce discomfort.

Leg cramps are common, perhaps related to pressure on the pelvic blood vessels and nerves or altered calcium and phosphorus balance. Dorsiflexion of the foot may help reduce these cramps. Dependent edema and varicose veins can also result from increasing intraabdominal pressure. Many women wear support hose to reduce edema; resting with legs elevated is also helpful.

Round ligament pain or tenderness in the lower abdomen is a result of stretching of the ligaments by the enlarging uterus. There is no way to prevent this, but using good body mechanics reduces the discomfort.

Dyspnea (shortness of breath) may be experienced as the uterus enlarges and pushes the diaphragm upward, decreasing the size of the chest cavity. Avoiding large meals, which distend the stomach, and maintaining good posture will help relieve this problem. Exercises are often recommended to help reduce discomfort and prepare for childbirth (Box 25-10).

REST AND SLEEP

Early in pregnancy women experience few changes in sleep patterns. However, as the abdomen grows larger, they may have difficulty finding a position of comfort, particularly if they prefer to sleep in the prone position. The supine position is not recommended as a woman approaches her due date because the enlarged uterus may place excessive pressure on the aorta and vena cava. The pressure can result in vena cava syndrome (supine hypotensive syndrome). The woman may experience syncope and vertigo. The supine position also may result in decreased circulation for the fetus. A side-lying position is recommended (Figure 25-7).

Encourage rest periods during the day with feet elevated. Placing pillows under the legs and abdomen will promote good body alignment and rest. Naps at intervals during the day can be helpful, but these are not always possible with busy lifestyles.

SEXUALITY AND REPRODUCTIVE SYSTEM

Breast Changes

Breast changes begin early in pregnancy. Many women complain of tingling and a feeling of fullness. Increased sensitivity is also common. Generally the breasts grow in preparation for lactation. Nipples and areolae darken. Colostrum may be secreted by the nipples in late pregnancy.

Sexual Activity

Sexual desire and activity may change during pregnancy. Unless the pregnancy has complications or the bag of waters has ruptured, there is no physiologic reason to limit sexual activity during pregnancy. Many factors have a strong influence on the frequency and type of sexual activity, including cultural, religious,

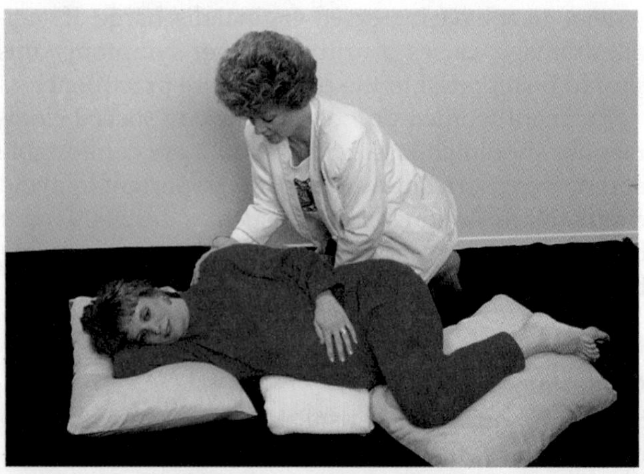

FIGURE 25-7 During the third trimester, pillows supporting the abdomen and back provide a comfortable position for rest.

Box 25-10 Exercise Tips for Pregnant Women

- Consult your health care provider when you know or suspect you are pregnant. Discuss your medical and obstetric history, your current regimen, and the exercises you would like to continue throughout pregnancy.
- Seek help in determining an exercise routine that is well within your limit of tolerance, especially if you have not been exercising regularly.
- Consider decreasing weight-bearing exercises (jogging, running), and concentrate on non–weight-bearing activities such as swimming, cycling, or stretching. If you are a runner, you may wish to walk instead, starting in your seventh month.
- Reduce exercise sharply 4 weeks before your due date. Strenuous exercise during the last few weeks of pregnancy increases the risk of low birth weight, stillbirth, and infant death.
- Avoid risky activities such as surfing, mountain climbing, sky diving, and racquetball. Activities requiring precise balance and coordination may be dangerous.
- Exercise regularly at least three times a week, as long as you are healthy, to improve muscle tone and increase or maintain your stamina. Sporadic exercises may put undue strain on your muscles.
- Limit activity to shorter intervals. Exercise for 10 to 15 minutes, rest for 2 to 3 minutes, then exercise for another 10 to 15 minutes.
- Decrease your exercise level as your pregnancy progresses. The normal alterations of advancing pregnancy, such as decreased cardiac reserve and increased respiratory effort, may produce physiologic stress if you exercise strenuously for a long time.
- Take your pulse every 10 to 15 minutes while you are exercising. If it is more than 140 bpm, slow down until it returns to a maximum of 90 bpm.
- Avoid becoming overheated for extended periods. It is best not to exercise for more than 35 minutes, especially in hot, humid weather. As your body temperature rises, the heat is transmitted to your fetus. Prolonged or repeated fetal temperature elevation may result in birth defects, especially during the first 3 months.
- Warm-up and stretching exercises prepare your joints for more strenuous exercise and lessen the likelihood of strain or injury to your joints.
- A cool-down period of mild activity after exercising will help bring your respiratory, heart, and metabolic rates back to normal and avoid pooling of blood in the exercise muscles.
- Rest for 10 minutes after exercising, lying on your left side. As the uterus grows, it puts pressure on a major vein carrying blood to your heart on the right side of your abdomen. Lying on your left side takes the pressure off and promotes return circulation from your extremities and muscles to your heart, increasing blood flow to your placenta and fetus.
- Drink two or three 8-oz glasses of water after you exercise to replace the body fluids you lost through perspiration. While exercising, drink water whenever you feel the need.
- Increase your caloric intake to replace the calories burned during exercise. Choose such high-protein foods as fish, cheese, eggs, or meat.
- Take your time. This is not the time to be competitive or train for activities requiring long endurance.
- Wear a supportive bra. Your increased breast weight may cause changes in posture and put pressure on the ulnar nerve.
- Wear supportive shoes. As your uterus grows, your center of gravity shifts and you compensate by arching your back. These natural changes may make you feel off balance and more likely to fall.
- Stop exercising immediately if you experience shortness of breath, dizziness, numbness, tingling, abdominal pain, or vaginal bleeding, and consult your health care provider.

and psychological influences. It is important for the partners to communicate their fears, concerns, and needs to each other. Many women experience a decrease in desire as a result of hormonal changes and discomfort. Change in body shape and body image may also cause concern. Discussion of various coital positions and sexual activity that does not include intercourse is appropriate. The primary care practitioner may promote this discussion by introducing the topic during routine prenatal care.

Increased vaginal secretions are common during pregnancy. **Leukorrhea,** an increase in vaginal mucus, results from hormonal changes. If the discharge changes in color or odor, the physician should be informed at once.

Vaginal Bleeding

Vaginal bleeding at any time during pregnancy should be reported to the physician at once. Sexual activity should cease until the cause of the bleeding is determined and should be resumed only when the physician determines that no danger exists.

COPING AND STRESS TOLERANCE

Pregnancy is a developmental landmark. Physiologically it marks the onset of adulthood, no matter what the woman's age. As with other significant developmental changes, anxiety is normal. All the physical and hormonal changes of pregnancy place additional stress on the woman. Fears are plentiful. Will the labor and delivery be painful? Will the baby be normal? Will she be able to provide proper care? Will there be enough money? Mood swings and ambivalence (conflicting emotions) are common as the woman works through her fears and comes to grips with the reality of pregnancy and how it will affect her life.

Women use problem-solving skills and methods of coping that worked in the past in an attempt to adjust to this new situation. Provide support as this problem solving occurs and help the woman work through her unique situation. Explain the normal physiologic changes and discomforts. Listening and allowing the woman adequate time to verbalize her fears can also help reduce anxieties.

ROLES, RELATIONSHIPS, AND ADAPTATION

The expectant woman has generally held several roles in her life, such as child, student, employee, and wife. Pregnancy introduces a totally new role, that of mother. The woman often looks to her own life for role models and tends to seek guidance from family and friends. Culture has much to do with how she defines her role (Box 25-11).

Dynamics also change between the woman and the baby's father, particularly with the first pregnancy. The mother is no longer just a wife or girlfriend; she is also a mother. While she is coping with the role change to mother, he is coping with the role change to father (Box 25-12).

SELF-PERCEPTION AND SELF-CONCEPT

The rapid changes in body shape and size can lead to changes in self-image. Many women feel unattractive when they are pregnant. They may also feel a loss of control related to the changes taking place. They are no longer free to do as they please because all their actions may affect the growing fetus.

Box 25-11 Maternal Adaptation

Adaptation to the maternal role involves a complex social and cognitive learning process. Pregnancy functions as a rite of passage and indicates that physiologic maturity has been reached. Reva Rubin began studying maternal role adaptation in the 1960s. She described the developing tasks of pregnancy as accepting the pregnancy, identifying the role of mother, reordering the relationships between her mother and herself and between herself and her partner, establishing a relationship with the unborn child, and preparing for the birth experience.

Women who are prepared to accept a pregnancy seek medical validation early. When pregnancy is confirmed, a woman's emotional responses may range from delight to shock, disbelief, and despair. A general state of well-being predominates, but emotional lability is common. These rapid mood changes include increased irritability, explosions of tears and anger, and feelings of great joy and cheerfulness. Such changes are often attributed to hormonal changes.

Rubin describes changes in pregnancy as follows. The subjective experience of time and space changes during pregnancy; early in pregnancy, nothing seems to be happening, and the woman spends much time sleeping. With quickening (feelings of fetal movement) in the second trimester, there is a reduction of time and space, both geographic and social, as the woman turns her attention inward to her pregnancy. She examines or fosters relationships with her mother and other women who have been or are pregnant. With the third trimester, there is a slower pace and a sense that time is running out as the women's activities are curtailed. A mother's reaction to her daughter's pregnancy signifies her acceptance of the grandchild and of her daughter. If the mother is supportive, the daughter has an opportunity to discuss pregnancy and labor and her feelings of joy or ambivalence with a knowledgeable and accepting woman.

The partner's emotional support is an important factor in successfully accomplishing the developmental tasks of pregnancy. Pregnant women express two major needs concerning their partner: feeling loved and valued, and having the child accepted. The addition of a child changes forever the nature of the bond between partners. The partner can be a stabilizing influence, a good listener to expressions of doubts and fears, and a source of physical and emotional reassurance. The partner can also feel jealous of the unborn baby. Lesbian and unpartnered women have received little attention in the literature. Some suggest that a woman partner may be better able to understand and nurture her partner. An unpartnered woman may seek out her mother or other women friends to meet her dependence needs.

Data from Mercer, R. (1995). *Becoming a mother.* New York: Springer. In Hockenberry, M.J., et al. (2007). *Wong's maternal-child nursing care.* (8th ed.). St. Louis: Mosby.

Box 25-12 Paternal Adaptation

A man's emotional response to becoming a father, his concerns, and his informational needs change during the course of pregnancy. There are three styles of involvement and one style of relative noninvolvement that men can experience during pregnancy (May, 1980, 1982). Men may be relatively uninvolved in pregnancy as observers, avoiding direct involvement in activities such as parent education classes and decisions about breastfeeding. Others are more involved and expressive, displaying a strong emotional response to pregnancy and a desire to be a full partner in the project. Some expectant fathers experience the *couvade syndrome* and have pregnancy-like symptoms such as nausea, other gastrointestinal complaints, and fatigue (couvade is a custom in some non-Western cultures whereby a husband goes through mock pregnancy and labor). Some fathers adopt the instrumental style, performing tasks in their role as manager of the pregnancy. They feel responsible for the outcome of pregnancy and are protective and supportive of their partners.

The father's beliefs and feelings about the ideal mother and father and his cultural expectation of appropriate behavior during pregnancy affect his response to his partner's need for him. One man may engage in nurturing behavior; another may feel lonely and alienated as the woman becomes physically and emotionally engrossed in the unborn child. The man may seek comfort and understanding outside the home, or become interested in a new hobby or involved with his work. Some men view pregnancy as a proof of their masculinity and their dominant role. To others, pregnancy has no meaning in terms of responsibility to either mother or child. For most men, however, pregnancy is a time of preparation for the parental role, of fantasy or great pleasure, and of intense learning.

Data from Hockenberry, M.J., et al. (2007). *Wong's maternal-child nursing care.* (8th ed.). St. Louis: Mosby.

COGNITIVE AND PERCEPTUAL CHANGES

Although sensory changes are uncommon with pregnancy, blurring or diplopia (double vision) may indicate problems with gestational hypertension (formerly termed pregnancy-induced hypertension; see Chapter 28).

PREPARATION FOR CHILDBIRTH

Prenatal education is important. Most primary care practitioners give explanations during routine visits, but the time available is too brief to meet all of the average woman's needs. The nurse plays an important role in prenatal education. Many low-cost pamphlets are available and should be provided whenever possible. Libraries and bookstores also have many good books on prenatal care. Special classes are offered by hospitals, public health agencies, private organizations, and the Red Cross to help the childbearing family understand and prepare for the demands of pregnancy, labor, the newborn, and parenthood.

CHILDBIRTH PREPARATION CLASSES

Communities often have a variety of courses that complement one another and meet the differing needs of specific segments of the population (Figure 25-8). Some classes are general, whereas others are targeted toward specific groups such as adolescents, those having cesarean or vaginal birth after cesarean delivery, siblings, or grandparents (Box 25-13).

Common methods of prepared childbirth include Dick-Read, which focuses on progressive relaxation techniques and avoidance of analgesics; Bradley, which stresses control of environmental factors, such as lighting, temperature, and noise, to provide a calm, supportive environment for childbirth; Leboyer, which uses a warm water bath to reduce the trauma of birth; and Lamaze, which uses breathing, distraction, and focusing techniques to mentally control pain. It requires disciplined training throughout the pregnancy. The Patient Teaching box on safety during pregnancy provides activity and environmental guidelines.

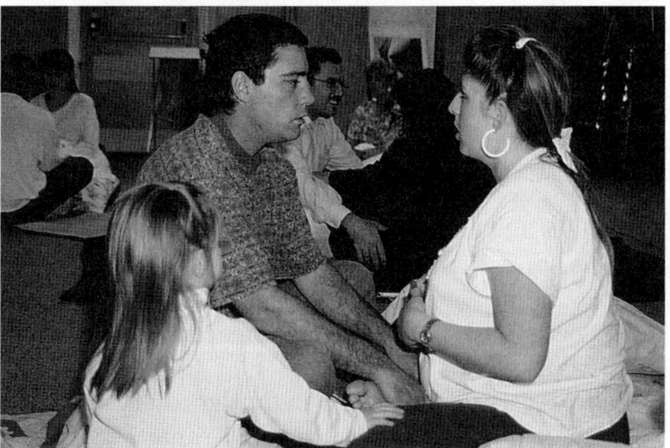

FIGURE 25-8 Entire family participating in a childbirth preparation course.

Box 25-13 Areas Typically Discussed in Childbirth Preparation Classes

- A review of reproductive anatomy and physiology
- Physical and emotional changes commonly observed during pregnancy
- Fetal growth and development
- Nutrition
- Routine aspects of prenatal hygiene and exercise
- Danger signs during pregnancy
- The birth process, both vaginal and cesarean
- Analgesia and anesthesia during labor and delivery
- Care of the newborn infant
- Breastfeeding
- Sibling preparation
- Changing family dynamics
- Postpartal exercises

Patient Teaching

Safety during Pregnancy

Changes in the body due to pregnancy include relaxation of joints, alteration of the center of gravity, faintness, and discomfort. Problems with coordination and balance are common. Therefore the woman should follow these guidelines:

- Use good body mechanics.
- Use safety features on tools or vehicles (safety seatbelts, shoulder harness, headrests, goggles, helmets) as specified.
- Avoid activities requiring coordination, balance, and concentration.
- Take rest periods; reschedule daily activities to meet rest and relaxation needs.

CULTURAL VARIATIONS IN PRENATAL CARE

It is imperative that the practitioner determine and explore cultural practices and beliefs with the patient (see Cultural Considerations box) (see Chapter 8 for further discussion of the cultural aspects of nursing).

❖ NURSING PROCESS *for Normal Pregnancy*

The role of the licensed practical nurse/licensed vocational nurse (LPN/LVN) in the nursing process as stated is that the LPN/LVN will:

- Participate in planning care for patients based on patient needs
- Review patient's plan of care and recommend revisions as needed
- Review and follow defined prioritization for patient care
- Use clinical pathways, care maps, or care plans to guide and review patient care

Cultural Considerations

Pregnancy

- Many cultural and religious factors affect the pregnant woman. It is important not to generalize when giving care. Not all members of a cultural group behave in exactly the same way. Discuss beliefs with each individual to determine her unique cultural practices. If the practices do not cause harm, include them in planning care.
- Because of cultural and other factors, such as lack of money, lack of transportation, and poor communication on the part of health care providers, many women do not participate in the prenatal care system. Do not misinterpret their behavior as uncaring, lazy, or ignorant.
- A concern for modesty is also a deterrent for prenatal care for many people. Exposing one's body parts, especially to a male practitioner, is a major violation of modesty. Thus many women prefer a midwife over the male practitioner. Too often health care providers assume women lose this modesty during pregnancy and labor. Most women value and appreciate efforts to maintain modesty.
- Virtually all cultures emphasize the importance of a socially harmonious and agreeable environment. Absence of stressful relationships is important for a successful outcome for mother and baby.
- Foster harmony with other persons. Visits from extended family members may be required to demonstrate continued pleasant and noncontroversial relationships. If discord exists in any relationship, the nurse and other staff must deal with it in culturally prescribed ways.
- In some belief systems, taboos are related to magical thinking. Some Hispanics believe that, during pregnancy, witnessing an eclipse of the moon may cause a cleft palate in the infant; exposure to an earthquake may result in preterm delivery or miscarriage (the lay term for a spontaneous abortion); and a breech presentation may occur if the earthquake was exceptionally strong. Some blacks believe a pregnant woman must not ridicule someone with an affliction or her child may be born with the same handicap. There is a widely held folk belief that raising one's arm above one's head or tying knots may cause the umbilical cord to wrap around the baby's neck and become knotted.
- Some cultures of the Southwest may wear amulets (charm, talisman, fetish, lucky piece), spirit medals, and beads to ward off evil spirits.
- Pregnant Filipino women are cautioned that any activity is dangerous, and others willingly take over their work. Inactivity constitutes a protection for mother and child. The mother is encouraged to simply produce the succeeding generation. This behavior should not be misinterpreted as laziness or noncompliance.

Assessment

Assessment begins when the woman visits the physician's office or clinic during the early part of her pregnancy. The first visit includes obtaining demographic data, taking a health history, and performing a general physical assessment, as well as an obstetric assessment. The general assessment includes lifestyle patterns, body system examination, and laboratory screening of blood and urine. Also explore the woman's perceptions of her condition, cultural and ethnic influences, experiences with other caregivers, lifestyle, and patterns of coping. A symptom diary, in which the woman records emotions, behaviors, physical symptoms, diet, and exercise and rest patterns, is a useful diagnostic tool. The obstetric assessment includes a gynecologic and obstetric history and a gynecologic examination with Pap smear, if needed.

Nursing Diagnosis

Nursing assessment helps identify the needs of the pregnant patient. Care can be then based on these needs. Possible nursing diagnoses for a normal pregnancy include the following:

- Disturbed body image
- Imbalanced nutrition: less than body requirements
- Risk for injury
- Activity intolerance
- Stress urinary incontinence
- Constipation
- Sleep deprivation
- Fatigue
- Deficient knowledge (specify)
- Interrupted family processes
- Fear
- Risk for impaired parenting

Expected Outcomes and Planning

The care plan should focus on the pregnant patient's needs and the nurse's ability to address those needs effectively (Nursing Care Plan 25-1). Each patient has different needs, and care must be individualized accordingly.

The care plan focuses on goals and outcomes specific to the nursing diagnosis. Examples include the following:

Goal 1: Patient will use self-care behaviors to maintain optimal levels of wellness for herself and the fetus.

Outcome: Patient keeps all prenatal appointments, does not smoke or drink alcoholic beverages, and does not use other drugs unless prescribed by her physician.

Goal 2: Patient will become knowledgeable about needs and concerns experienced during each trimester.

Outcome: Patient keeps a symptom diary and discusses it on each visit to the primary caregiver. Patient attends prenatal classes regularly.

Nursing Care Plan 25-1 The Patient with a Normal Pregnancy

Ms. Pullman is a 23-year-old gravida 1, para 0 at 30 weeks of gestation. She has gained 12 pounds since the beginning of her pregnancy. She has a full-time job at an insurance company and plays tennis twice a week. She is a vegetarian but does eat some fish. She takes prenatal vitamins daily. She complains of some constipation, although her bowel habits were normal before her pregnancy.

NURSING DIAGNOSIS *Imbalanced nutrition: less than body requirements, related to dietary habits*

Patient Goals and Expected Outcomes	Nursing Interventions	Evaluation
Patient will meet nutritional needs	Assess weight at regular intervals. Review the MyPyramid food guide.	Patient meets her nutritional needs as evidenced by recommended weight gain.
Patient will know about additional nutritional needs during pregnancy and how to fulfill them	Provide information related to nutritional needs during pregnancy. Have patient keep dietary diary.	Patient displays knowledge of additional nutritional needs by eating a well-balanced diet as evidenced by dietary diary and appropriate weight gain.
	Encourage patient to drink 6 to 8 glasses of water daily to aid in bowel regularity.	Patient reports water intake of 6 to 8 glasses daily.

NURSING DIAGNOSIS *Risk for impaired parenting or attachment, related to developmental stressors of pregnancy and to lack of knowledge and skill*

Patient Goals and Expected Outcomes	Nursing Interventions	Evaluation
Patient will follow a lifestyle that is conducive to a positive pregnancy outcome	Discuss measures that promote a healthy pregnancy outcome, including nutrition, physical activity, rest, stress reduction, and lifestyle changes. Encourage patient to ask questions and express concerns.	The patient makes necessary lifestyle changes to promote a positive pregnancy outcome. Patient uses effective coping strategies regarding stressors of pregnancy.
Patient will express ability to cope with the changes and stressors of pregnancy	Provide encouragement for effective coping strategies used. Encourage patient to keep a symptom diary and bring it with her to each prenatal visit. Inform parents of community resources to assist and support them as needed. Help parents develop realistic expectations of newborn behaviors and demands. Assess parents' plans to incorporate the newborn into the family circle. Offer opportunity for demonstration of baby skills, with return demonstration.	Patient keeps symptom diary and brings it to each prenatal visit; feels free to discuss concerns. Parents complete infant bathing, diapering, cord care, and feeding appropriately in return demonstration.

Critical Thinking Questions

1. How should the nurse respond to Ms. Pullman if she expresses concern about her dietary practices and their effect on her baby? What suggestions can the nurse give her to ensure that her diet is adequate to support the pregnancy?
2. Ms. Pullman states that she is concerned about having to reduce her activity schedule, particularly tennis, which she enjoys. She is worried she will begin to resent her baby because of the need to alter her activities. How should the nurse respond to her concerns? What suggestions should the nurse give her?

Implementation

Nursing interventions during the prenatal period may include the following:

- Identify factors that may interfere with health maintenance.
- Provide information to the patient to promote health maintenance.
- Assess and counsel on nutritional habits and weight gain.
- Stress safety issues regarding risk of injury as the pregnancy progresses.

Health Promotion

Prenatal Health Maintenance Measures

Health maintenance is an important aspect of prenatal care. Patient participation in the care ensures prompt reporting of problematic responses to pregnancy. Patient responsibility for health maintenance is strengthened by a readiness to learn and by the nurse's understanding of maternal adaptations to the growth of the unborn child.

The expectant mother needs information about many topics. Be observant, listen, and know the typical concerns of expectant parents to anticipate what questions will be asked and prompt mothers and their partners to discuss what is on their minds. Provide printed literature to supplement the individualized teaching; women often avidly read books and pamphlets related to their own experience. Read the literature before distributing it, and point out areas that may not correspond to local health care practices. Patients who receive conflicting advice or instruction may grow frustrated with members of the health care team and the care provided.

Topics to discuss with pregnant women may include the following.

EMPLOYMENT

- Employment of pregnant women usually has no adverse effects on pregnancy outcomes. Job discrimination that is based solely on pregnancy is illegal. However, some job environments pose potential risk to the fetus (e.g., dry-cleaning plants, chemical laboratories, and parking garages).
- Discourage activities that require a good sense of balance, especially during the last half of pregnancy.
- Commonly, excessive fatigue is the deciding factor in the termination of employment.
- Women in sedentary jobs need to walk around at intervals and should neither sit nor stand in one position for long periods. This will counter sluggish leg circulation, which can cause varices and thrombophlebitis. Women should also avoid crossing their legs at the knees because this also fosters such conditions. Standing for long periods increases the risk of preterm labor.
- The pregnant woman's chair should provide adequate back support. Use of a footstool can prevent pressure on veins, relieve strain on varicosities, and reduce swelling of feet.

CLOTHING

- Comfortable, loose clothing is best. Washable fabrics (e.g., absorbent cottons) are often preferred. Maternity clothes may be purchased new or found in good condition at thrift shops or garage sales. Tight bras and belts, stretch pants, garters, tight-top kneesocks, panty girdles, and other constrictive clothing should be avoided because tight clothing over the perineum encourages vaginitis and miliaria (heat rash), and impaired circulation in the legs can cause varices.
- Maternity bras are constructed to accommodate the increased breast weight, chest circumference, and size of breast tail tissue (under the arm). These bras have drop-flaps over the nipples to facilitate breastfeeding. A good bra can help prevent neckache and backache.
- Elastic hose are comfortable and promote greater venous emptying in women with large varicose veins. Ideally the woman should put on support stockings before getting out of bed in the morning.
- Comfortable shoes that provide firm support and promote good posture and balance are advisable. Tall high heels and platform shoes are not recommended because of the woman's changed center of gravity, which can cause her to lose balance. In addition, the woman's pelvis tilts forward in the third trimester, increasing her lumbar curve. The resulting leg aches and cramps will be aggravated by shoes that do not provide good support.

TRAVEL

- Travel is not contraindicated for low-risk pregnant women, but those with high-risk pregnancies are advised to avoid long-distance travel after fetal viability has been reached, to avoid the economic and psychological consequences of delivering a preterm infant far from home.
- Travel to areas where medical care is poor, water is untreated, and malaria is prevalent should be avoided if possible.
- Women who contemplate foreign travel should be aware that many health insurance carriers do not cover birth in a foreign setting or even hospitalization for preterm labor.
- Pregnant women who travel long distances should schedule periods of activity and rest. While sitting, she can practice deep breathing, foot circling, and alternately contracting and relaxing different muscle groups. She should avoid becoming fatigued.
- Although travel in itself is not a cause of adverse outcomes such as miscarriage or preterm labor, certain precautions are recommended while traveling in a car. The woman should always use automobile restraints, generally a combination lap belt and shoulder harness. The lap belt is worn low across the hip bones and as snug as is comfortable. The shoulder belt is worn above the pregnant uterus and below the neck to avoid chafing. The pregnant woman should sit upright and use the headrest to avoid a whiplash injury.
- Maternal death as a result of injury is the most common cause of fetal death. The next most common cause is placental separation. This occurs because body contours change in reaction to the force of a collision. The uterus as a muscular organ can adapt its shape to that of the body, but the placenta lacks the resiliency to change. At the impact of collision, placental separation can occur.
- Airline travel in large commercial jets usually poses little risk to the pregnant woman, but policies vary from airline to airline. The pregnant woman is advised to inquire about restrictions or recommendations from her carrier. Magnetometers (metal detectors) used at airport security checkpoints are not harmful to the fetus. Cabins of commercial airlines are maintained at 8% humidity, which may result in some water loss; hydration (with water) should be maintained under these conditions. Sitting in a cramped seat of an airliner for prolonged periods may increase the risk of superficial and deep thrombophlebitis. A pregnant woman is encouraged to take a 15-minute walk around the aircraft cabin during each hour of travel to minimize this risk.

- Teach the importance of pacing activities.
- Review the importance of adequate fluid intake.
- Review patterns of elimination and any changes that have occurred.
- Teach ways to position body for sleep promotion and rest.
- Provide information on prenatal classes.
- Explain discomforts and danger signs.
- Encourage verbalization of fears and concerns.
- Incorporate patient's cultural values into the care plan.

See Health Promotion box for self-care prenatal health maintenance measures.

Evaluation

Continually evaluate the success of the interventions. As the pregnancy progresses, the focus and interventions will change. Refers to the goals and outcomes to determine whether the care plan was successful and the outcomes were met. Be assured that care has been effective when the woman reports improvements in the quality of her life, skill in self-care, and a positive self-concept and body image.

Get Ready for the NCLEX® Examination!

Key Points

- Pregnancy is a normal process that involves many complex physiologic changes in the mother.
- Over a period of 280 days, two initial cells join and develop into a unique, viable human being.
- Unique structures such as the placenta, membranes, the umbilical cord, and amniotic fluid protect and support the developing fetus. These structures are discarded when the pregnancy is completed and they are no longer necessary.
- All aspects of the mother's lifestyle can potentially affect her developing fetus.
- Many drugs and viruses can cross the placenta and present serious hazards to the developing embryo, particularly during the first trimester of pregnancy.
- Sophisticated diagnostic tests are often performed to identify genetic or developmental problems during pregnancy. Early identification of problems may influence a woman's decisions regarding a pregnancy.
- Although pregnancy is a normal process, regular and ongoing health care is important throughout pregnancy.
- At present the best means of reducing the number of children born with genetic defects is for health professionals to provide families with genetic information and services.
- Many signs and symptoms of pregnancy are similar to those manifested by other medical conditions. The positive signs of pregnancy are visualization of the fetus, fetal motion detected by a trained observer, and auscultation of fetal heart sounds.
- Every pregnant woman should be aware of the danger signs during pregnancy and contact her physician if any of them are present.
- The rational use of any medication requires a risk-versus-benefit assessment. Among the many risk factors that complicate assessment, pregnancy is one of the most perplexing.
- Nutritional needs change during pregnancy. To support normal growth and development of the fetus, the woman requires increased calories, minerals, and vitamins.
- Many discomforts may occur during pregnancy. Be aware of measures that can reduce these discomforts without harming the mother or the fetus.
- Pregnancy is a time of role adjustment for both prospective parents. All family members are affected by the addition of a new member.
- Adequate preparation enables the woman to become a knowledgeable participant in the entire childbearing process. Be aware of classes available in the community and the materials covered in these classes.
- The nurse and the patient are influenced by cultural and personal values and beliefs during the patient's pregnancy. Careful assessment is imperative.

Additional Learning Resources

Go to your Companion CD-ROM for an audio glossary, animations, video clips, and more.

evolve Be sure to visit the Evolve site at http://evolve.elsevier.com/Christensen/foundations/ for additional online resources.

Review Questions for the NCLEX® Examination

1. A 25-year-old woman comes to the clinic and says she thinks she is pregnant. Her last period was July 20. Based on this fact, what would be the expected date of birth (EDB)?
   1. April 13
   2. April 27
   3. May 20
   4. March 27

2. The patient reports experiencing nausea, vomiting, and breast tenderness along with missing her period. These symptoms are considered to be what type of signs of pregnancy?
   1. Probable
   2. Positive
   3. Presumptive
   4. Possible

3. A pregnant patient at her third office visit asks the nurse, "What can I do when my leg goes into a cramp?" The patient demonstrates understanding of the nurse's instruction regarding relief of leg cramps if she:
   1. wiggles and points her toes during the cramp.
   2. applies cold compresses to the affected leg.
   3. extends her leg and dorsiflexes her foot during the cramp.
   4. avoids weight bearing on the affected leg during the cramp.

4. The patient asks the nurse how she will know when she first feels the baby move. The best explanation is that the movement:
   1. will feel like cramps.
   2. is rhythmic and called Goodell's sign.
   3. is flutterlike and is called quickening.
   4. is like a thud and is called Hëgar's sign.

5. While giving a health history to the nurse, the patient reports that she usually has a glass of wine with dinner. What is the safe level of alcohol intake for her during her pregnancy?
   1. No alcohol
   2. Wine only—one or two glasses daily with meals
   3. Up to 4 ounces daily
   4. Beer or wine only after the first trimester

6. The nurse explains to the patient that she should contact her health care provider if she experiences any of the danger signs of pregnancy. Which symptom is a danger sign during pregnancy?
   1. Urinary frequency
   2. Severe headaches
   3. Backache
   4. Heartburn

7. During the third trimester, patients often complain of various discomforts. Which discomfort would not be expected at this time?
   1. Dyspnea
   2. Insomnia
   3. Ankle edema
   4. Dysuria

8. A test that may be done in late pregnancy to determine fetal well-being is the nonstress test. This test is based on which phenomenon?
   1. Fetal heart rate increases in connection with fetal movement.
   2. Braxton Hicks contractions cause an increase in fetal heart rate.
   3. Fetal heart rate slows in response to contractions.
   4. Fetal movement causes an increase in maternal heart rate.

9. Constipation is a frequent complaint as a pregnancy progresses. Which measure would be best to recommend to relieve constipation?
   1. Drink 6 to 8 glasses of water daily.
   2. Take an over-the-counter laxative.
   3. Take an iron supplement only every other day.
   4. Take mineral oil at bedtime.

10. At one of her prenatal visits, the patient is scheduled for a sonogram. Sonography cannot be used to assess:
    1. number of fetuses.
    2. gestational age of fetus.
    3. Down syndrome.
    4. congenital anomalies.

11. Which symptom would be considered a first-trimester warning sign and should be reported immediately to the health care provider?
    1. Nausea with occasional vomiting
    2. Fatigue
    3. Urinary frequency
    4. Vaginal bleeding

12. A pregnant woman at 10 weeks of gestation jogs three or four times per week. She is concerned about the effect of exercise on the fetus. The nurse should inform her that:
    1. "You do not need to modify your exercising anytime during your pregnancy."
    2. "Stop exercising because it will harm the fetus."
    3. "You may find that you need to modify your exercising to walking later in your pregnancy, around the seventh month."
    4. "Jogging is too hard on your body; switch to walking now."

13. A woman at 23 weeks of gestation calls to tell the nurse she thinks she is leaking fluid from her vagina. The nurse should tell her:
    1. "As long as the baby is still moving around, there is nothing to worry about."
    2. "Come to the office right away."
    3. "Call me back in 2 hours, and tell me if there is any change in the leakage."
    4. "We can wait until your next appointment to check you."

14. A woman admitted in labor has an obstetric history indicating that she has had three children, all of whom are living. One was born at 39 weeks of gestation, another at 34 of weeks of gestation, and another at 35 weeks of gestation. What are her gravidity and parity using the five-digit GTPAL system?
    1. 4-1-1-1-3
    2. 4-1-2-0-3
    3. 3-0-3-0-3
    4. 3-1-2-0-3

15. The nurse teaches a pregnant woman about the presumptive, probable, and positive signs of pregnancy. The woman demonstrates understanding of the nurse's instructions if she states that a positive sign of pregnancy is:
    1. a positive pregnancy test.
    2. fetal movement palpated by the primary caregiver.
    3. Braxton Hicks contractions.
    4. nausea and vomiting.

Fill in the Blank

Fill in the blank using the correct medical vocabulary.

16. ____________ Woman who is pregnant

17. ____________ Woman who is pregnant for the first time

18. ____________ Woman who has had two or more pregnancies

19. ____________ Capacity to live outside the uterus

20. An expectant father confides in the nurse that his pregnant wife (10 weeks of gestation) is driving him crazy. "One minute she seems happy and the next minute she seems unhappy, and the next she is crying over nothing at all. Is there something wrong with her?" The nurse's best response would be:

1. "This is normal behavior and should begin to subside by the second trimester."
2. "She may be having difficulty relating to the pregnancy. I will refer her to a counselor I know."
3. "This is called emotional lability and is related to hormone changes and anxiety during pregnancy. The mood swings will subside as she adjusts to being pregnant."
4. "You seem impatient with her. Perhaps this is precipitating her behavior."

21. When planning a diet with a pregnant woman, the nurse's first action would be to:

1. review the woman's dietary intake.
2. teach the woman about the MyPyramid food guide.
3. caution the woman to avoid large doses of vitamins, especially those that are fat soluble.
4. instruct the woman to limit the intake of fatty foods.

22. A pregnant woman at 32 weeks of gestation complains of feeling dizzy and lightheaded while her fundal height is being measured. Her skin is pale and moist. The nurse's initial response would be to:

1. assess the woman's blood pressure and pulse.
2. have the woman breathe into a paper bag.
3. raise the woman's legs.
4. turn the woman on her side.

23. When obtaining a reproductive health history from a female patient, the nurse should:

1. limit the time spent on exploration of intimate topics.
2. explain the purpose of questions asked and how they will be used.
3. avoid asking questions that may embarrass the patient.
4. use only acceptable medical terminology when referring to body parts and functions.

24. After admitting a new patient to the maternity unit, the nurse writes a care plan. This process of determining outcomes and interventions is which stage of the nursing process?

1. Assessment
2. Planning
3. Implementation
4. Evaluation

chapter

26 Labor and Delivery

evolve

http://evolve.elsevier.com/Christensen/foundationsadult

Elaine Oden Kockrow

Objectives

1. Discuss birth planning.
2. Discuss birth setting choices.
3. Explain the five factors that affect the labor process.
4. Discuss the signs and symptoms of impending labor.
5. Distinguish between true and false labor.
6. Discuss fetopelvic disproportion.
7. Describe the "powers" involved in labor and delivery.
8. Identify the mechanisms of labor.
9. Identify the stages of labor.
10. Describe the assessment for labor and delivery.
11. Explain breathing techniques beneficial for the patient in labor.
12. Identify nursing diagnoses relevant to the woman in labor.
13. Outline medical interventions related to labor and delivery.
14. Discuss nursing interventions related to labor and delivery.

Key Terms

amniotomy (ăm-nē-ŎT-ō-mē, p. 837)
attitude (p. 809)
Braxton Hicks contractions (p. 806)
descent (p. 816)
effacement (ĕ-FĀS-mĕnt, p. 806)
engagement (ĕn-GĀJ-mĕnt, p. 816)
episiotomy (ĕ-pĭs-ē-ŎT-ō-mē, p. 819)
expulsion (p. 816)
extension (p. 816)
external rotation (p. 816)
fetal lie (p. 809)
fetal position (p. 809)
fetal presentation (p. 809)
fetopelvic disproportion (fē-tō-PĔL-vĭk, p. 838)
flexion (FLĔK-shŭn, p. 809)
hypoxia (hī-PŎK-sē-ă, p. 826)
internal rotation (p. 816)
lightening (p. 805)
meconium (mĕ-KŌ-nē-ŭm, p. 826)
oligohydramnios (ŏl-ĭ-gō-hī-DRĂM-nē-ŏs, p. 809)
oxytocin (ŏks-ē-TŌ-sĭn, p. 819)
restitution (p. 816)
surfactant (sŭr-FĂK-tănt, p. 827)
uterine inertia (YŪ-tĕr-ĭn ĭn-ĔR-shă, p. 837)

BIRTH PLANNING

Teaching provided to a family expecting the birth of a child should include an in-depth discussion of the options available during the labor, delivery, and postpartum periods. The family should assess priorities and begin to set goals. The tool that women can use to communicate choices for the child's birth is known as a birth plan. The first trimester is the optimal time to initiate the dialogue regarding the available options. Customize teaching for the facility selected for the birth. As the pregnancy progresses, encourage the expectant family to review the plan and modify it as desired. The birth plan is subject to change; stress that the plan will be implemented only if the health care needs of the mother and baby are not compromised. Events in the later part of the pregnancy or during labor may require changes in the plan to ensure safe, effective care of the mother and baby (Lowdermilk & Perry, 2007).

BIRTH SETTING CHOICES

Selecting the environment in which to give birth is an important decision for the expectant family. Three primary options are available: (1) hospital, (2) birthing center, or (3) home. Review individual care needs—including availability and preference of the selected health care provider, qualities of the birth site, health condition of the mother and the child, and regulations imposed by the health coverage provider—to make the best decision about the birthing location (Lowdermilk & Perry, 2007).

Hospitals

It is estimated that an overwhelming 99% of all deliveries in the United States occur in a hospital setting (Martin et al., 2005). Hospitals offer varying services for expectant families. Options may include labor and delivery in a traditional labor unit with transfer to a postpartum unit after delivery. The newborn care unit may be combined with the postpartum unit or be free standing. The combination unit is referred to as a mother-baby unit. Some facilities offer single-room services in which the woman labors, delivers, and receives postpartum care in one area. This arrangement is known as a labor, delivery, recovery, postpartum (LDRP) unit. Freestanding birthing facilities normally provide care using the LDRP format (Lowdermilk & Perry, 2007).

Birthing Centers

Some hospitals have birthing centers that emphasize family-focused care and try to incorporate the family and significant others into the care plan. The LDRP format is traditionally used in birthing centers. The popularity of these centers is growing. A freestanding birthing center offers childbirth outside of a hospital, but typically nearby to allow for easy access in the event of complications. Care in a birthing center is cost effective and is provided by nurse-midwives and physicians. Eligibility for childbirth in a freestanding center is limited to those women considered to be low risk for development of complications (Lowdermilk & Perry, 2007).

Home

Women interested in a more relaxed, family-centered, and relatively low-cost delivery experience may consider a home birth. The risk of infection also is lower in a home birth. Home delivery is only an option for a woman in good health with a reasonable expectation of a positive outcome for both mother and baby. A home delivery must be carefully considered by all parties and must be approved by the attending physician and nurse-midwife (Lowdermilk & Perry, 2007).

NORMAL LABOR

ONSET

In most pregnancies the fetus reaches maturity and the uterus begins the process of labor at exactly the right time. Although this process has been occurring throughout human history, researchers are still trying to discover the exact cause for the onset, or beginning, of labor. The theories fall into two main categories: those based on mechanical changes and those based on hormonal changes.

One mechanical theory involves uterine stretching. It is based on the principle that once a hollow-body organ reaches a certain state of distention, it will spontaneously contract and empty. For example, a full bladder will empty by incontinence and a distended stomach will empty by vomiting. It is hypothesized that when the uterus stretches to a certain size it will empty spontaneously. However, the wide variation of uterine size between different pregnancies in the same woman makes this a weak theory. For example, a woman may have one pregnancy in which she delivers a 6-pound baby at term. In her next pregnancy she may again reach term but deliver twins each weighing 6 pounds.

Several hormonal theories for the onset of labor are based on either an increase or a decrease in hormones. In some of the theories, the source of the hormones is the mother; in other theories it is the fetus. Some of the more common (but still unproven) theories relating to hormones are (1) oxytocin stimulation, (2) progesterone withdrawal, (3) estrogen stimulation, and (4) fetal cortisol.

SIGNS OF IMPENDING LABOR

Although we do not know what causes labor, we can recognize when labor is about to begin by watching for certain signs. As early as 2 weeks before the onset of labor the woman may notice that the fetus seems to have settled, or "dropped," into the pelvis. This is called **lightening** and is seen most often in nulliparas. Once lightening has occurred, the woman often notices that urinary frequency returns. She may be able to breathe more normally because the abdominal cavity has more space. Multiparas may not experience this change until they are in active labor.

Occasionally a woman may have a seepage or sudden outflow of fluid from the vagina. This may be urine, or it may be amniotic fluid, indicating a rupture of the amniotic sac. A simple test with Nitrazine paper can distinguish between these (Box 26-1). Without washing the area, the paper is moistened with the discharge. If the paper reacts (turns blue), the discharge is

Box 26-1 Nitrazine Test for Rupture of Membranes

- Explain the procedure to the woman or the couple.
- Perform the procedure.
  —Wash hands.
  —Use Nitrazine test paper, a dye-impregnated test paper for determining pH (differentiates amniotic fluid, which is slightly alkaline, from urine and purulent material [pus], which are acidic).
  —Wearing a sterile glove lubricated with water, place piece of test paper on cervical opening.
  OR
  —Use a sterile, cotton-tipped applicator to dip deep into vagina to pick up fluid; touch applicator to test paper. (Procedure may be done during speculum examination.)
- Read results:
  —Membranes probably intact: identifies vaginal and most body fluids that are acidic:
  Yellow pH 5.0
  Olive-yellow pH 5.5
  Olive-green pH 6.0
  —Membranes probably ruptured: identifies amniotic fluid that is alkaline:
  Blue-green pH 6.5
  Blue-gray pH 7.0
  Deep blue pH 7.5
  —False test results are possible because of presence of bloody show, insufficient amniotic fluid, or semen.
- Provide pericare as needed.
- Remove gloves and wash hands.
- Document results (positive or negative).

probably amniotic fluid. If the test is nonreactive, the membranes are probably intact. The amniotic sac generally ruptures after labor has begun. If it ruptures before labor starts, medical attention is essential. If labor does not occur within a few hours of the rupture of the membranes, the physician usually attempts to start labor by administering medication. Delivery should occur 18 to 24 hours after membranes rupture. Prolonged rupture of membranes puts the woman and her fetus at risk for infection.

The amount of vaginal drainage typically increases as term approaches, and blood-tinged mucus called **bloody show** may be observed. This is the mucus that occluded the opening of the cervix during pregnancy (mucous plug). Vaginal examination may reveal that the cervix has begun to change consistency. The cervix begins to soften, and in true labor it also begins to thin (efface) and open (dilate).

Backache and contractions of the uterus, called **Braxton Hicks contractions** (irregular tightening of the pregnant uterus that begins in the first trimester and increases in frequency, duration, and intensity as pregnancy progresses), are common as the pregnancy approaches term. The severity of these contractions varies from mild to moderate. They remain irregular and do not dilate the cervix.

Some women notice a slight loss of weight (1 to 3 pounds) a few days before labor, and others report a last-minute burst of energy.

True labor is marked by the onset of regular, rhythmic contractions that cause progressive cervical dilation and **effacement** (thinning and shortening or obliteration of the cervix that occurs during late pregnancy, labor, or both).

FALSE LABOR VERSUS TRUE LABOR

Because many women fear that they will go to the hospital at the wrong time, explain how true labor differs from false labor (Table 26-1). Stress that, when there is any doubt, they should obtain medical attention. At times even experienced professionals find it difficult to differentiate the early stages of true labor from false labor.

LABOR AND DELIVERY

STANDARD PRECAUTIONS DURING CHILDBIRTH

Birth is a time when nurses and other health care providers are exposed to a great deal of maternal and newborn blood and body fluids. Observing standard precautions helps prevent transmission of infection through contact with body fluids. The standard precautions applicable to childbirth include the following:

- Wash hands before donning gloves and after performing procedures and removing gloves.
- Wear gloves (clean or sterile, as appropriate) when performing procedures that require contact with the woman's genitalia and body fluids, including bloody show (e.g., during vaginal examination, amniotomy, hygienic care of the perineum, insertion of an internal scalp electrode and intrauterine pressure monitor, and catheterization).
- When assisting with a birth, wear a cover gown and a mask with a shield or protective eyewear. Cap and shoe covers are worn for cesarean birth but are optional for vaginal birth in a birthing room. The primary health care provider who is attending the birth should wear a sterile gown with a waterproof front and sleeves.
- Drape the woman with sterile towels and sheets as appropriate. Explain to the woman what can and cannot be touched.
- Help the woman's partner put on appropriate coverings for the type of birth, such as cap, mask, gown, and shoe covers. Show the partner where to stand and what can and cannot be touched.
- Wear gloves and gown when handling the newborn immediately after birth.
- Use an appropriate method to suction the newborn's airway, such as a bulb syringe, mechanical wall suction, or DeLee oral suction device that

Table 26-1 Comparison of True and False Labor

TRUE LABOR	FALSE LABOR
Contractions follow a regular pattern.	Contractions rarely follow a pattern.
Contractions come closer together, are stronger, and tend to last longer.	Contractions vary in length and intensity.
Contractions get stronger with ambulation.	Contractions frequently stop with ambulation or position change.
Contractions seem to start in the lower back and then travel to the lower abdomen.	Contractions may be felt in the back, but are most often noticed in the fundus.
[illegible]ntractions are usually not stopped by controlled breathing, [illegible]ation, or other relaxation interventions.	Contractions eventually stop with relaxation interventions.
[illegible] softens, effaces, and dilates.	The cervix may soften, but there is little or no change in effacement or dilation.
[illegible]s continues descent into the pelvis.	There is no significant change in the fetal position.

prevents the newborn's mucus from getting into the user's mouth or airway.

PROCESS OF LABOR AND DELIVERY

To understand the complex process of labor and delivery, examine each of the factors involved. These factors are frequently called the five Ps:

- **Passageway:** The pelvis and soft tissues
- **Passengers:** The fetus and placenta
- **Powers:** Contractions
- **Position of mother:** Standing, walking, side lying, squatting, on hands and knees
- **Psyche:** Psychological response

Passageway

Pelvis

The superior portion of the pelvis (iliac segment of the innominate bones) supports the uterus and fetus during the late months of pregnancy. These bones aid in directing the fetus into the inferior (lower) portion of the pelvis, which is called the **true pelvis.** The two sections are divided by an imaginary line called the **linea terminalis,** or pelvic inlet.

The size and shape of the true pelvis are more important than those of the false pelvis because the fetal head must be able to pass through this section of the pelvis for vaginal delivery to occur. Four different types of pelves are recognized, each with a unique shape and characteristics (Table 26-2).

The true pelvis is further divided into three segments: the inlet; the cavity, or midpelvis; and the outlet (Figure 26-1). The primary care practitioner can use several methods for evaluating the size of the true pelvis:

- **Palpation:** Externally, the primary care practitioner can use a pelvimeter to determine the distance between the ischial tuberosities. This helps estimate the distance between the ischial spines, which can otherwise be obtained only by pelvic x-ray examination. Internally, the primary care practitioner can palpate additional bony prominences to determine pelvic adequacy.

Table 26-2 Comparison of Pelvic Types

CHARACTERISTIC	GYNECOID	ANDROID	ANTHROPOID	PLATYPELLOID
Percent of women	50%	23%	24%	3%
Brim	Slightly ovoid or transversely rounded Round	Heart shaped, angulated Heart	Oval, wider anteroposteriorly Oval	Flattened anteroposteriorly, wide transversely Flat
Depth	Moderate	Deep	Deep	Shallow
Side walls	Straight	Convergent	Straight	Straight
Ischial spines	Blunt, somewhat widely separated	Prominent, narrow interspinous diameter	Prominent, often with narrow interspinous diameter	Blunted, widely separated
Sacrum	Deep, curved	Slightly curved, terminal portion often beaked	Slightly curved	Slightly curved
Subpubic arch	Wide	Narrow	Narrow	Wide
Usual mode of delivery	Vaginal • Spontaneous • Occiput anterior position	Cesarean Vaginal • Difficult, with forceps	Vaginal • With forceps or spontaneous • Occiput posterior or occiput anterior position	Vaginal • Spontaneous

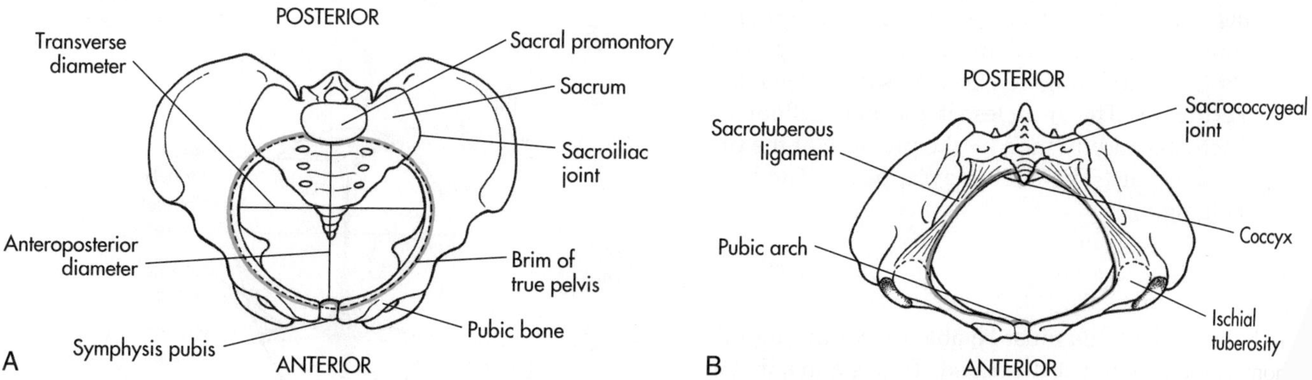

FIGURE 26-1 Female pelvis. **A,** Pelvic brim (inlet, linea terminalis, or iliopectineal line) from above. **B,** Pelvic outlet from below.

- **Pelvimetry:** With x-ray films from different views, the primary care practitioner can accurately measure the bony prominences. However, this measurement is for women who are not pregnant but have an injury or known developmental problem, such as rickets. Pelvimetry is not routinely done during pregnancy because the radiation may harm the fetus.
- **Ultrasonography:** Sound waves above the range of human hearing can also be used to estimate pelvic adequacy. Because ultrasound does not involve the use of radiation, it is generally regarded as safe for the fetus. In more than 20 years of obstetric use, no detrimental effects have been observed. Ultrasound can visualize soft tissue and helps gather information regarding fetal growth, multiple pregnancy, placental location, and abnormal presentation that may complicate delivery.

It is important to understand that adequacy of the pelvis is relative. For each delivery the primary care practitioner must determine whether the pelvis is adequate to allow passage of the fetus. Although certain measurements are considered "normal," the size and position of the fetus make each situation unique.

Soft Tissues

During labor the uterus, the cervix, the vagina, and the muscles of the perineum change in consistency and shape to allow passage of the fetus in the following ways:

- **Uterine tissues:** During labor the walls of the upper section of the uterus have a thickened musculature that provides the force during contractions. The muscle walls of the lower section become thinner and act as a passive tube. Located between the two sections is a band of tissue, the physiologic retraction ring.
- **Cervical tissues:** As contractions of the muscular upper segment apply downward pressure, the uterine contents (fetal presenting part) efface and dilate the cervix.
- **Vagina:** In response to hormonal changes during pregnancy, the vagina undergoes many changes. Increased blood supply (vascularity), increased thickness of the mucosa, loosening of the connective tissue, and enlargement (hypertrophy) of smooth muscle cells all make the vagina capable of stretching (dilating) to allow passage of the fetus.
- **Perineum:** The muscles of the pelvic floor are stretched and thinned by the pressure of the presenting part. The anus may appear dilated and bulging.

ngers

ne fetus must be able to exit through the geway just described. This is a major chal- ause at term the fetus often weighs 7 pounds and is 20 to 21 inches long.

Fetal skull. The fetal skull is usually the largest part of the body, so delivery of the head is of greatest concern. The shoulders and the pelvis, which are more mobile, generally do not cause problems.

The bones of the fetal skull are not rigidly joined (fused). This allows the bony plates to move and overlap as they progress through the maternal pelvis. This reshaping of the skull bones in response to pressure against the maternal pelvis is called **molding.**

The major bones of the skull are the two frontal bones, the two parietal bones, the two temporal bones, and the occiput. They are joined by membranous spaces called **sutures.** Where sutures meet, there are larger membranous areas called **fontanelles** (Figure 26-2). The anterior fontanelle (bregma) is formed by four bones and thus tends to be larger and diamond shaped. The posterior fontanelle is formed by three bones and is smaller and triangular. By palpating the sutures and the fontanelles through the cervix, the primary care practitioner can determine the presentation of the fetus during labor. The largest transverse diameter of the skull is the biparietal measurement. If this is

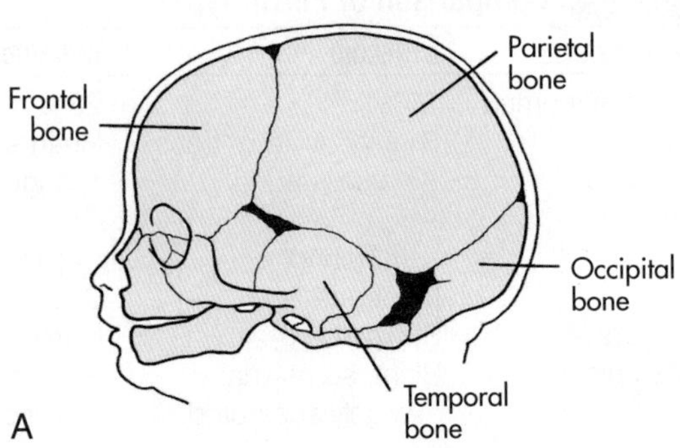

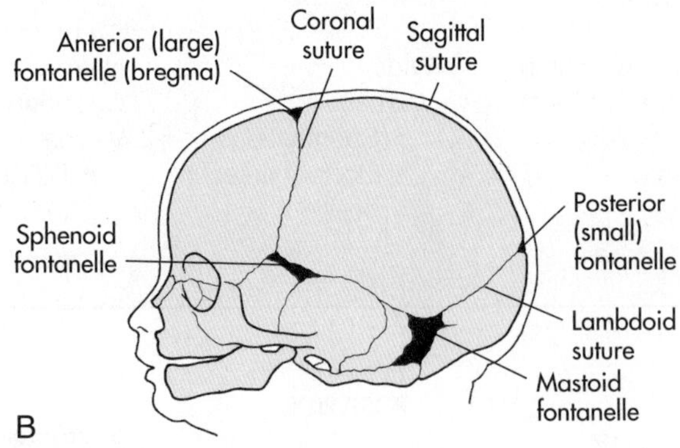

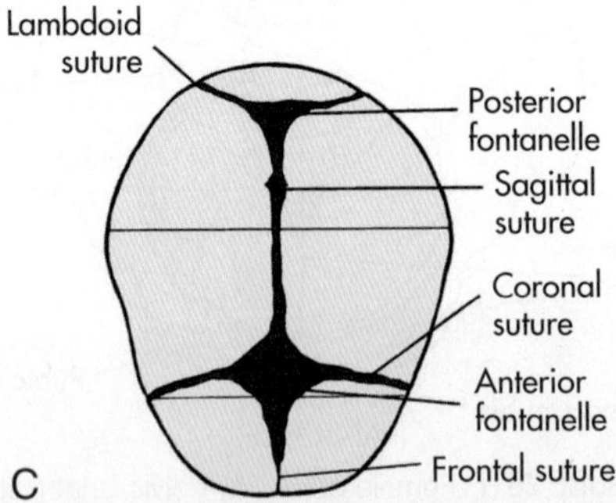

FIGURE 26-2 Fetal head at term. **A,** Bones. **B,** Fontanelles. **C,** Sutures.

too large, the skull may not be able to enter the mother's pelvis.

Fetal attitude. The relationship of fetal body parts to one another is called attitude. At term, the ideal attitude for the fetal body is flexion. The back is bowed outward, the chin is touching the sternum, the arms are crossed on the chest, and the thighs are flexed on the abdomen. This is called the fetal position (the relationship of the occiput, sacrum, chin, or scapula of the fetus to the front, back, or sides of the mother's pelvis). This attitude takes up minimal space and allows the best angle of approach to the pelvis. If the fetus does not have enough room because of too little or no amniotic fluid (oligohydramnios; often indicative of fetal urinary tract defect), multiple pregnancies, or anatomical variations in the mother, the attitude may be altered, leading to complications of labor or delivery.

Fetal lie. Fetal lie is the relationship of the cephalocaudal (head-to-buttocks) axis of the fetus to the cephalocaudal axis of the mother. If the spine of the fetus is parallel to the spine of the mother, the lie is called **longitudinal.** The presentation could be cephalic (head down) or breech (buttocks down). The lie is longitudinal in 99% of deliveries. If the spine of the fetus is perpendicular to that of the mother, it is called **transverse lie.** Only 1% of deliveries involve a transverse lie. This is most common in women who have had many pregnancies (resulting in weakened abdominal walls), maternal pelvic contracture, or placenta previa (see Chapter 28). While the fetus is small, it changes lie frequently. By term the fetal lie seldom changes because space is limited.

Fetal presentation. Fetal presentation (that part of the fetus [head, face, breech, or shoulders] that first enters the pelvis and lies over the inlet) describes the part that will be in contact with the cervix. This is determined by both attitude and lie. In about 96% of deliveries the presentation is cephalic. In cephalic presentation some part of the fetal head is in contact with the cervix. Cephalic presentation is divided into four types: vertex (region between the fontanelles), brow, face, and mentum (chin).

In about 3% of deliveries the presentation is breech. Either the buttocks or legs are in contact with the cervix. Three types of breech presentation are possible: complete breech, in which the buttocks present and the thighs are well flexed on the abdomen; frank breech, in which the buttocks present and the thighs are extended across the abdomen and chest; and footling breech, in which there is no flexion and one foot or two feet present. Breech presentations are more difficult to deliver vaginally. To decrease risks to the fetus, the majority of breech births are delivered surgically (see Cesarean Delivery, p. 838).

In about 1% of deliveries some other body part presents. These occur when the fetus has been in a transverse lie. The shoulder, hand, elbow, and iliac crest are possible presenting parts. These cases also require a cesarean birth.

Fetal position. Position is the relationship of the presenting fetal part to a quadrant of the maternal pelvis. Fetal position can be determined by abdominal inspection and palpation (Leopold's maneuvers, Figure 26-3), vaginal or rectal examination, auscultation of fetal heart tones, or ultrasound or x-ray examination. Once the position is determined, it is expressed in abbreviated form. For example, the most common position for delivery is left occiput anterior (LOA), in which the occiput of the fetus points toward the left anterior segment of the maternal pelvis. The right occiput anterior (ROA) position is the next most common position. Many combinations are possible (Figures 26-4 and 26-5).

A longitudinal lie, well-flexed attitude, and vertex presentation are the ideal. This position best enables the fetal skull bones to mold as they progress through the maternal pelvis. The fetal skull also provides a smooth, round surface, which is most effective in effacing and dilating the cervix. The smooth, regular shape also fills the cervix and prevents the umbilical cord from prolapsing, or coming before the fetus. Cord prolapse is dangerous because pressure on the vessels in the cord can restrict blood flow to the fetus.

If a part other than the vertex presents, labor is generally longer, more tiring to the mother, and more likely to require surgical intervention.

Prompt recognition of a prolapsed umbilical cord is important because fetal hypoxia resulting from prolonged cord compression (occlusion of blood flow to and from the fetus for more than 5 minutes) usually

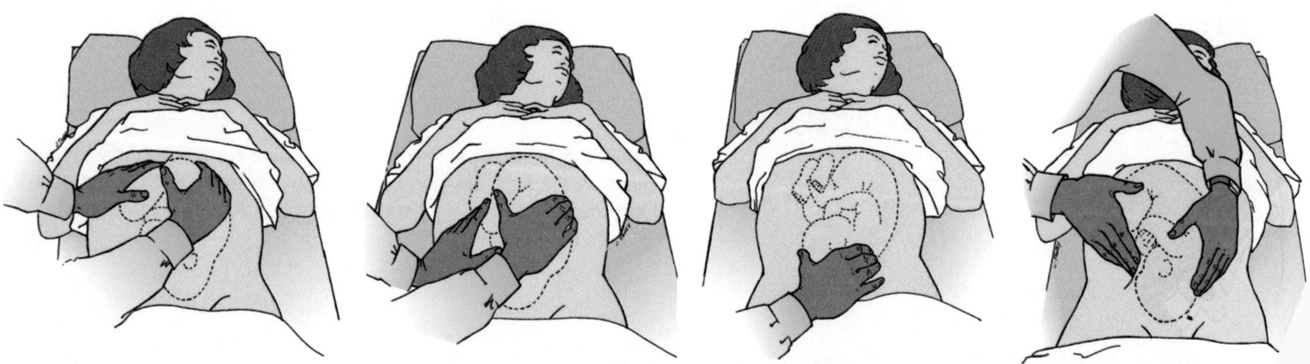

FIGURE 26-3 Leopold's maneuvers.

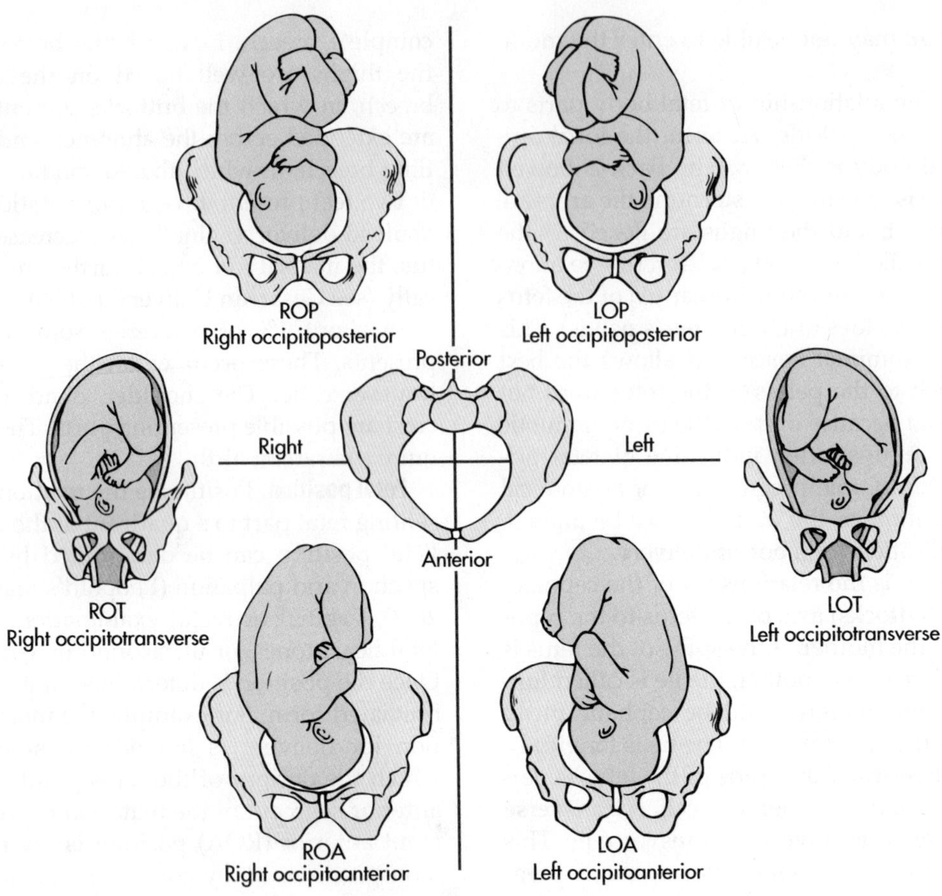

FIGURE 26-4 Cephalic positions. Examples of fetal vertex (occiput) presentation in relation to front, back, and side of maternal pelvis.

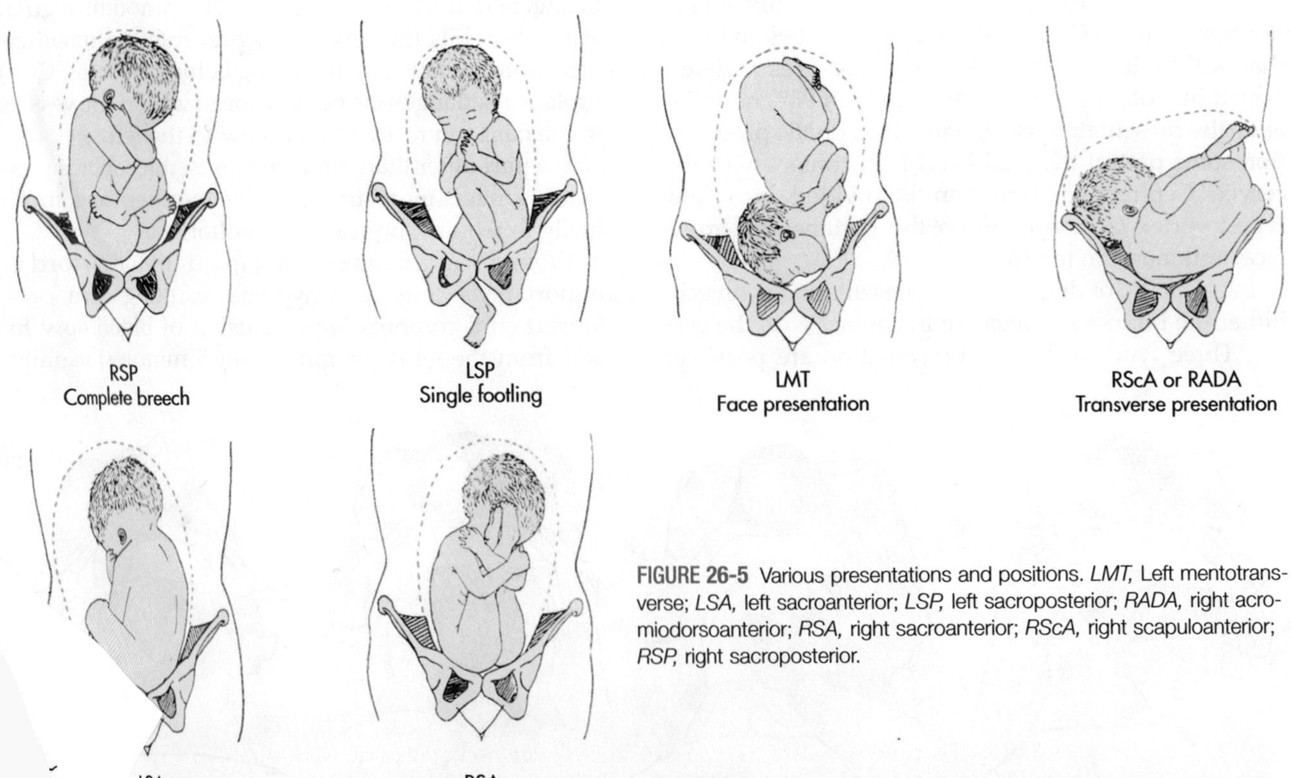

FIGURE 26-5 Various presentations and positions. *LMT,* Left mentotransverse; *LSA,* left sacroanterior; *LSP,* left sacroposterior; *RADA,* right acromiodorsoanterior; *RSA,* right sacroanterior; *RScA,* right scapuloanterior; *RSP,* right sacroposterior.

results in central nervous system damage or death of the fetus. The examiner can relieve pressure on the cord by putting a sterile gloved hand into the vagina and holding the presenting part off of the umbilical cord (Figure 26-6, *A* and *B*). The woman is assisted into a position such as a modified Sims' (Figure 26-6, *C*), Trendelenburg's, or knee-chest (Figure 26-6, *D*) position, so that gravity keeps the pressure of the presenting part off of the cord. If the cervix is fully dilated, forceps- or vacuum-assisted delivery can be performed for the fetus in a cephalic presentation; otherwise a cesarean birth is likely. Nonreassuring fetal status, inadequate uterine relaxation, and bleeding can also occur as a result of a prolapsed umbilical cord.

Placenta

The placenta is also referred to as a passenger. After the fetus is delivered by strong uterine contractions, the placental attachment site is significantly smaller. This reduced size causes the placenta to separate from its attachment. Normally the first few strong contractions 5 to 7 minutes after the birth of the baby shear the placenta from its base. A placenta will not easily be freed from a flaccid (relaxed) uterus because the placental attachment site is not reduced in size.

Placental separation is indicated by the following signs (Figure 26-7):

- A firmly contracting fundus
- A change in the uterus from discoid (disklike) to globular ovoid (egg shape) as the placenta moves to the lower segment
- A sudden gush of dark blood from the introitus (the entrance into the vagina)
- Apparent lengthening of the umbilical cord as the placenta gets closer to the introitus
- A vaginal fullness (the placenta) noted on vaginal or rectal examination or fetal membranes seen at the introitus

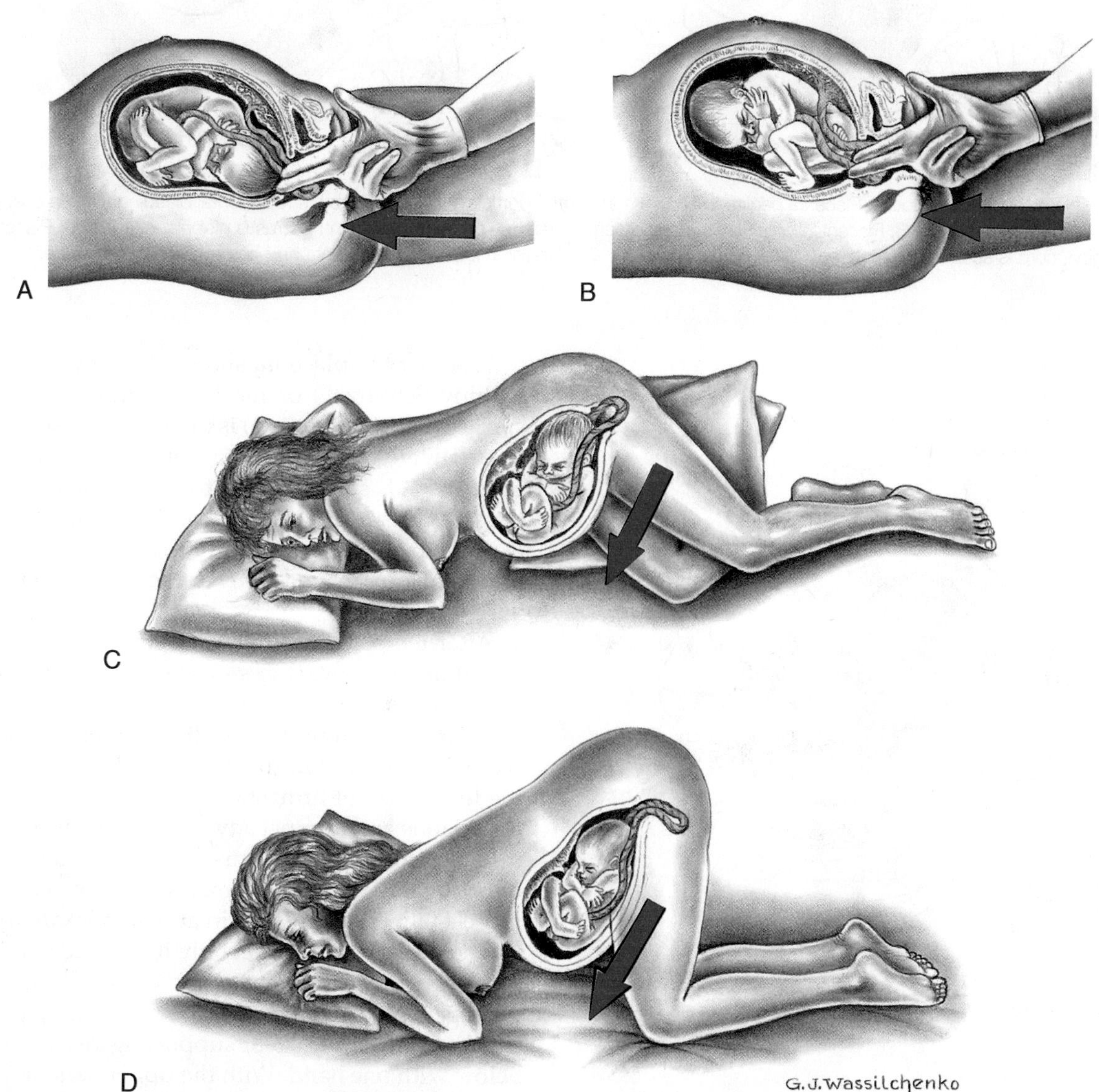

FIGURE 26-6 *Arrows* indicate direction of pressure against presenting part to relieve compression of prolapsed umbilical cord. Pressure exerted by examiner's fingers in, **A,** vertex presentation and, **B,** breech presentation. **C,** Gravity relieves pressure when woman is in modified Sims' position with hips elevated as high as possible without pillows. **D,** Knee-chest position.

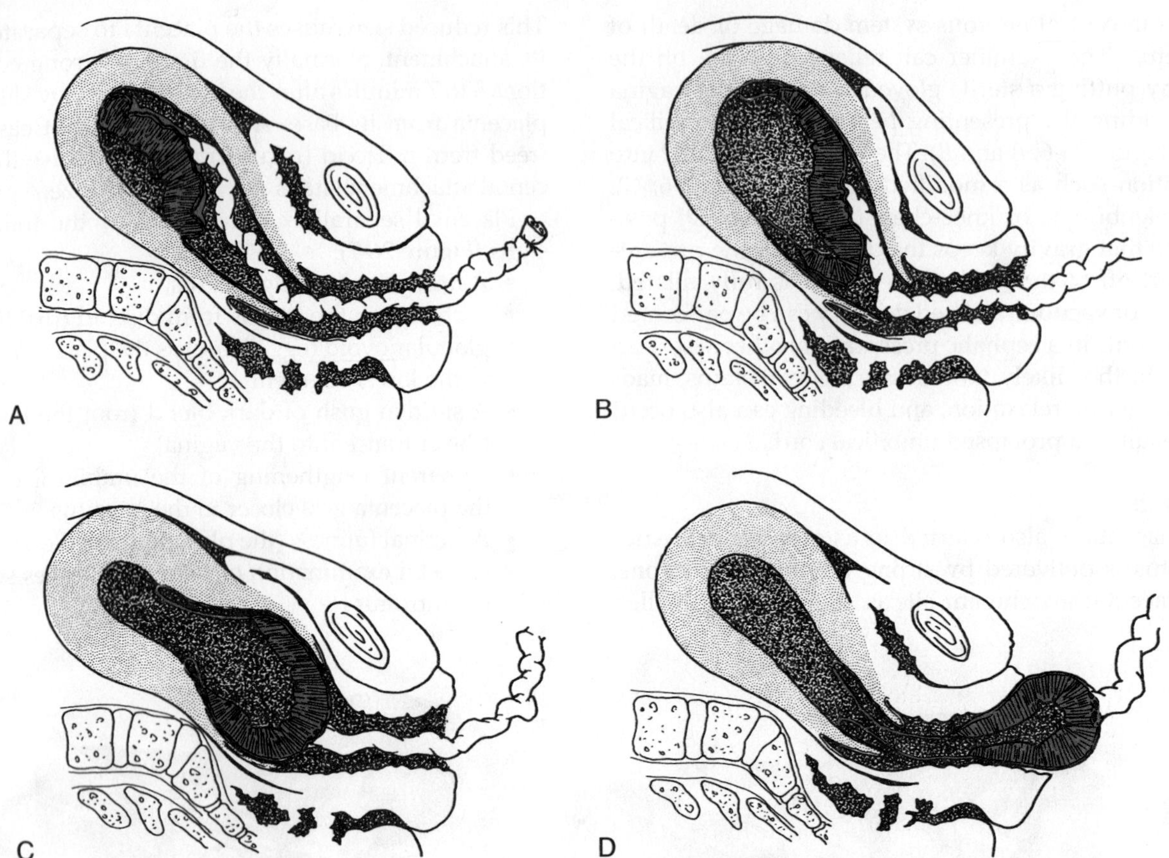

FIGURE 26-7 Third stage of labor. **A,** Placenta begins to separate in central portion accompanied by retroplacental bleeding. Uterus changes from discoid to globular shape. **B,** Placenta completes separation and enters lower uterine segment. Uterus is globular shaped. **C,** Placenta enters vagina, cord is seen to lengthen, and bleeding may increase. **D,** Expulsion (delivery) of placenta and completion of third stage.

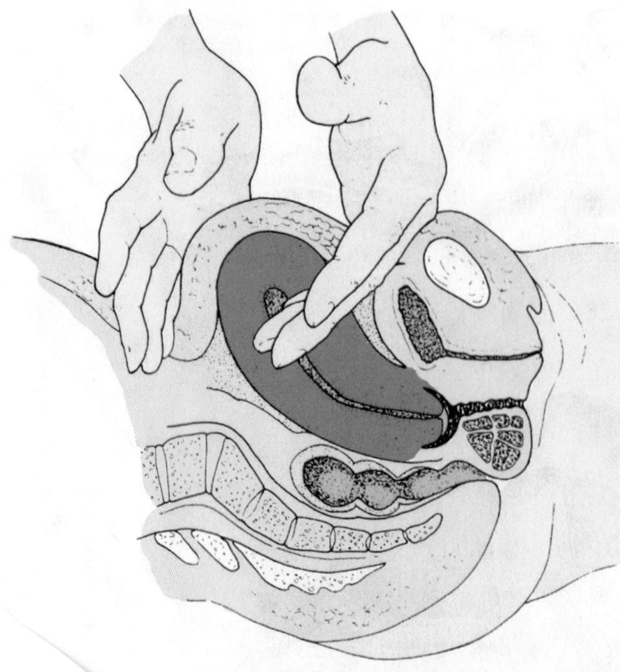

[FIGURE] 26-8 Palpating fundus of uterus during first hour after delivery.

Whether the placenta shows its shiny fetal surface ("Shiny Schultze") or its dark, roughened maternal surface ("Dirty Duncan") is of no clinical significance. The delivery of the placenta completes the third stage of labor. This stage lasts 15 to 30 minutes or longer if the health care practitioner waits for the mother to express the placenta herself. When the delivery of the placenta is managed actively, it can take less than 5 minutes.

After the placenta (with its membranes) emerges, it is examined for intactness to be certain that no portion of it remains in the uterine cavity. The goal of this stage of labor is the prompt separation and expulsion of the placenta, achieved in the easiest and safest manner. If the fundus is not firm, stimulate the uterine muscle to regain tone and to expel any clots before measuring the distance from the umbilicus. Palpate the uterus gently only until it is firm; overstimulation causes uterine muscle fatigue and results in atonia (relaxation).

The uterus can contract only if it is free of intrauterine clots. Take care to avoid inversion of the uterus during expulsion of clots. To expel clots, place the hands as in Figure 26-8, supporting the uterus from below with one hand. With the upper hand apply firm pressure downward toward the vagina while observing the perineum for the number and size of expelled clots. While performing these assessments, teach the patient the rationale for the assessment and how to maintain uterine tone by self-palpation.

Powers

Involuntary and voluntary contractions combine to expel the fetus and the placenta from the uterus. Involuntary uterine contractions, called primary powers, signal the beginning of labor. Once the cervix has dilated, the woman's voluntary bearing-down efforts, called secondary powers, augment the force of the involuntary contractions.

Primary Powers

The involuntary contractions originate at certain pacemaker points in the thickened muscle layers of the upper uterine segment. From the pacemaker points, contractions move downward over the uterus in waves, separated by short rest periods.

The primary powers are responsible for the effacement and dilation of the cervix and descent of the fetus. Effacement is the shortening and thinning of the cervix during the first stage of labor. The cervix, normally 2 to 3 cm long and about 1 cm thick, is obliterated or "taken up" by shortening of the uterine muscle bundles in advancing labor. Only a thin edge of the cervix can be palpated when effacement is complete. In a first pregnancy, effacement generally occurs at term before significant dilation occurs. In subsequent pregnancies, effacement and dilation of the cervix tend to progress together. Degree of effacement is expressed in percentages from 0% to 100% (e.g., a cervix 50% effaced) (Figure 26-9).

Dilation of the cervix is the enlargement of the cervical opening and the cervical canal that occurs once labor has begun. The diameter of the cervix increases from less than 1 cm to full dilation (approximately 10 cm) to allow birth of a term fetus. When the cervix is fully dilated (and completely retracted), it can no longer be palpated. Full cervical dilation marks the end of the first stage of labor.

Dilation of the cervix occurs by the drawing upward of the musculofibrous components of the cervix as a result of strong uterine contractions. Pressure from the amniotic fluid while the membranes are intact, and the force applied by the presenting part, also promote cervical dilation. Scarring of the cervix as a result of prior infection or surgery may slow cervical dilation.

In the first and second stages of labor, increased intrauterine pressure caused by contractions places pressure on the descending fetus and the cervix. When the

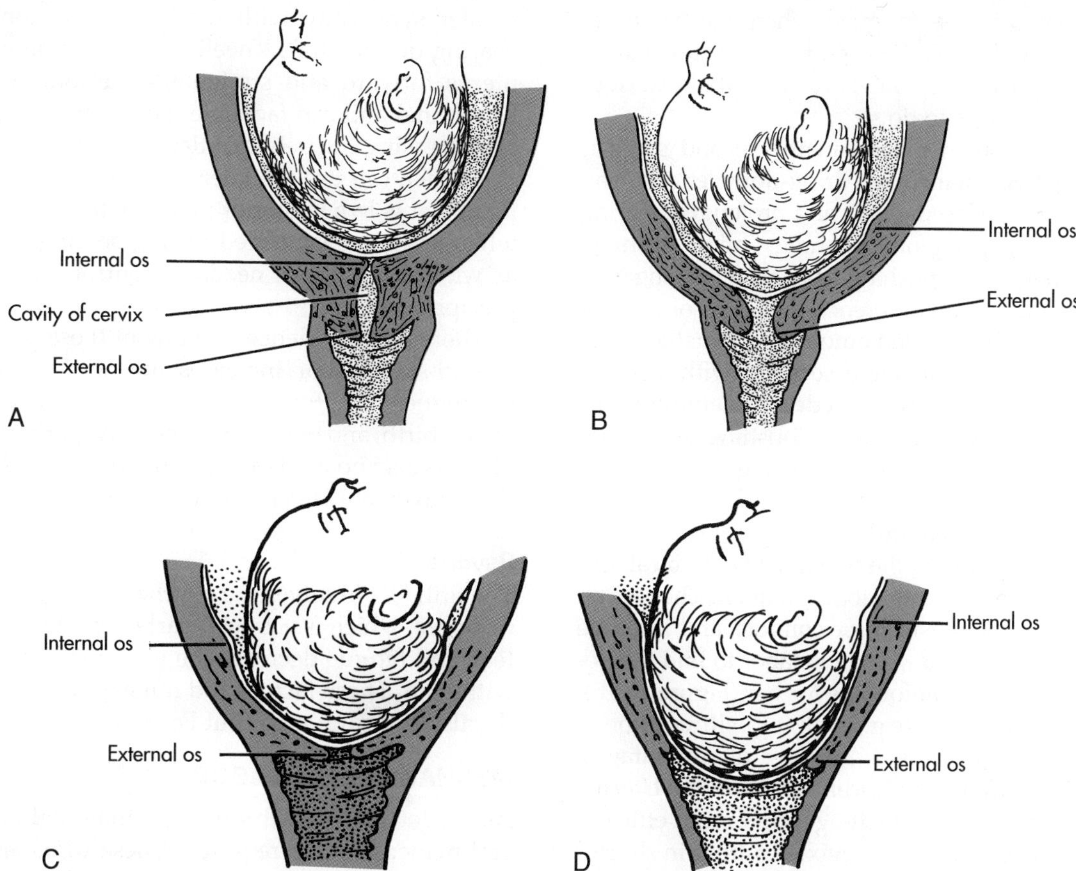

FIGURE 26-9 Cervical effacement and dilation. Note how cervix is drawn up around presenting part at the internal opening. Membranes are intact, and head is not well applied to cervix. **A,** Before labor. **B,** Early effacement. **C,** Complete effacement (100%). Head is well applied to cerv **D,** Complete dilation (10 cm). Some overlapping of cranial bones. Membranes still intact.

presenting part of the fetus reaches the perineal floor, mechanical stretching of the cervix occurs. Stretch receptors in the posterior vagina cause release of exogenous oxytocin that triggers the maternal urge to bear down, or Ferguson's reflex.

Uterine contractions are involuntary and usually independent from external forces. For example, laboring women who are paraplegic have normal uterine contractions. Uterine contractions may temporarily become less frequent and intense when the woman receives narcotic analgesic medication or epidural analgesia early in labor. The relationship between prolonged labor and epidural analgesia is still under investigation.

Secondary Powers

As soon as the presenting part reaches the pelvic floor, the contractions change in character and become expulsive. The woman experiences an involuntary urge to push. She uses secondary powers (bearing-down efforts) as she contracts her diaphragm and abdominal muscles, and pushes. These bearing-down efforts result in increased intraabdominal pressure that compresses the uterus on all sides and increases the expulsive forces.

The secondary powers have no effect on cervical dilation, but they are important in expelling the infant from the uterus and vagina after the cervix is fully dilated. Pushing in the second stage is more effective, and the woman is less fatigued when she begins to push only after she has the urge to do so rather than beginning to push when she is fully dilated but does not yet have the urge to do so.

The way a woman pushes in the second stage is much debated. Spontaneous bearing-down efforts, Valsalva's maneuver (closed glottis and prolonged bearing down), pushing, open glottis pushing, "mini" pushing, and forced methods of pushing have been investigated. Although no significant differences in length of second-stage labor have been found among these methods, fetal hypoxia and acidosis are associated with directed pushing. Continued study is needed to determine the effectiveness and safety of various pushing techniques in relation to maternal and fetal outcome.

Position of the Woman in Labor

Maternal position affects the woman's anatomical and physiologic adaptations to labor. Frequent changes in position relieve fatigue, increase comfort, and improve circulation. Encourage a woman in labor to find the positions that are most comfortable for her (Figure 26-10).

An upright position (e.g., walking, sitting, kneel- or squatting) offers a number of advantages. ...y can promote the descent of the fetus. Uterine ...ons are generally stronger and more efficient ...nd dilating the cervix, resulting in shorter ...ght position is also beneficial for the ...diac output, which normally increases during labor as uterine contractions return blood to the vascular bed. Increased cardiac output improves blood flow to the uteroplacental unit and the maternal kidneys. An upright position also helps reduce pressure on the descending aorta and ascending vena cava and prevents their compression. Compression of these vessels would compromise cardiac output and lead to supine hypotension and decreased placental perfusion. If the woman wishes to lie down, a lateral position is suggested.

The "all fours" position (on hands and knees) may be used to relieve backache if the fetus is in an occipitoposterior position. It also may assist in anterior rotation of the fetus.

The woman's preference may determine positioning for second-stage labor, but the decision is also affected by the condition of the woman or fetus, the environment, and the health care provider's confidence in assisting in a birth in a specific position. For physician-attended births in the United States, the lithotomy position is predominant. Alternative positions and position changes are most commonly practiced by nurse-midwives.

A woman in a semirecumbent position needs adequate body support to push effectively because her weight is on her sacrum, moving the coccyx forward and causing a reduction in the pelvic outlet. In a sitting or squatting position, abdominal muscles work in greater synchrony with uterine contractions during bearing-down effort. Kneeling or squatting moves the uterus forward and straightens the long axis of the birth canal and can facilitate the second stage of labor by increasing the pelvic outlet.

Women can use the lateral position to help rotate a fetus that is in a posterior position. It can also be used when less force is needed during bearing down, such as when the woman needs to control the speed of a precipitous birth.

There is no evidence that any of these positions for second-stage labor increases the need for operative techniques (e.g., forceps- or vacuum-assisted birth, cesarean birth, and episiotomy) or cause perineal trauma. There is also no evidence that use of any of these positions adversely affects the newborn.

Psyche

The fifth "P" involves the psyche, or the psychological response, which is a crucial part of childbirth. Anxiety, fear, and fatigue decrease the woman's ability to cope with pain. These factors and nursing interventions are discussed throughout Unit Four.

MECHANISMS OF LABOR

As the fetus moves through the maternal pelvis, several maneuvers are required. These turns and adjustments are called the **mechanisms of labor.** The mechanisms of labor in the vertex position are as follows.

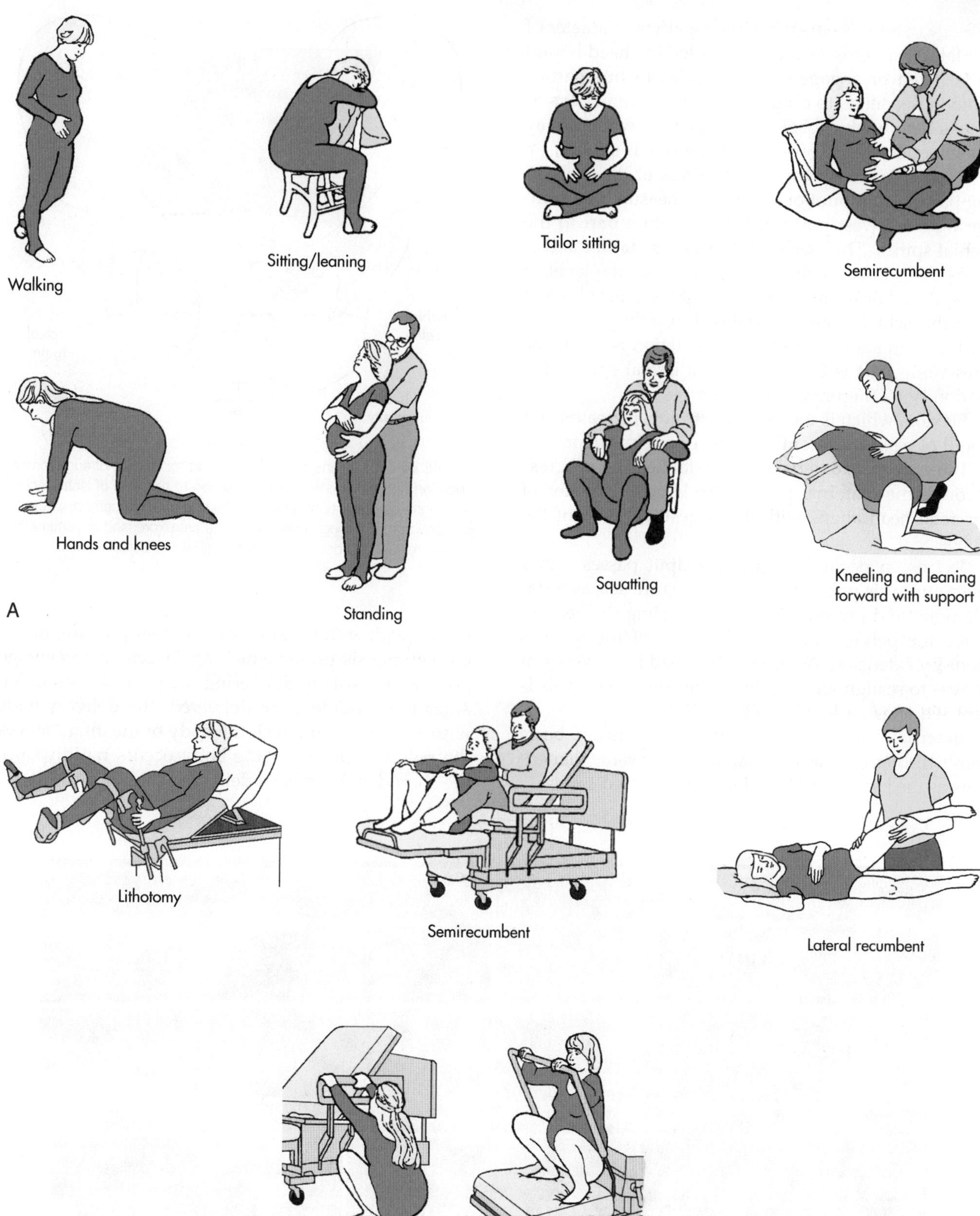

FIGURE 26-10 **A,** Positions for labor. **B,** Positions for birth.

Engagement occurs when the biparietal diameter of the fetal head crosses the pelvic inlet; the head is said to be fixed or engaged in the pelvis. In nulliparous women this tends to occur early, often several days or weeks before labor begins. Multiparous women may not experience engagement until labor has started.

Descent is the downward progress of the presenting part. The amount of progress is measured by comparing the lowest point of the presenting part to the ischial spines. This is referred to as the **station** and is measured in centimeters above or below the level of the spines. For example, if the presenting part is even with the ischial spines, the station is 0; if the presenting part is 2 cm above the spines, the station is −2; if the presenting part is 2 cm below the ischial spines, the station is +2 (Figure 26-11).

Flexion, which is the normal attitude, increases as a result of resistance from the cervix or pelvic floor.

Internal rotation enables the fetal head to progress through the maternal pelvis. The largest diameter of the fetal head aligns with the largest diameter of the pelvis.

Extension occurs when the occiput passes under the symphysis pubis. This bony structure acts as a stable point and provides leverage, enabling the head to leave the pelvis. The actual delivery of the head is done by extension. As soon as the head is delivered, it moves to realign with the body and shoulders. This is referred to as restitution (Figure 26-12).

External rotation occurs as the shoulders and body move through the birth canal, using the same maneuvers as the head. The shoulders are delivered similarly to the head, with the anterior shoulder pressing under the symphysis pubis, which again acts as a leverage point and assists in delivering the posterior shoulder. After the shoulders are delivered, the delivery ends with expulsion, in which the body of the infant leaves the pelvis. Delivery of the body occurs rapidly once the shoulders have been delivered (Figure 26-13).

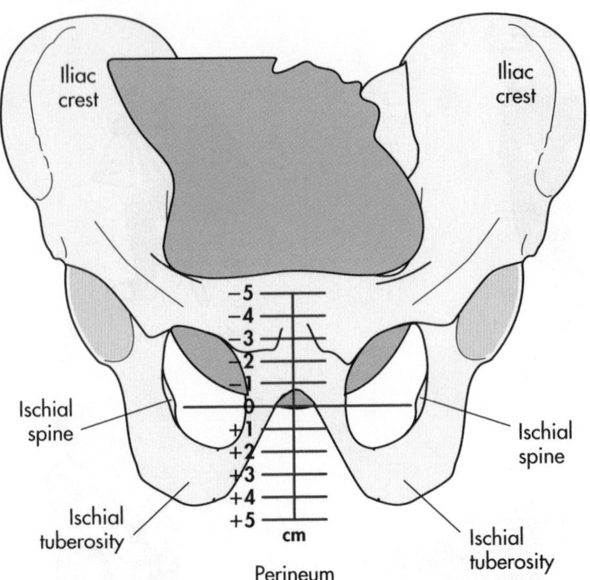

FIGURE 26-11 Stations of presenting part, or degree of engagement. Location of the presenting part in relation to the level of ischial spines is designated station and indicates degree of advancement of the presenting part through pelvis. Stations are expressed in centimeters above (minus) and below (plus) the level of the ischial spines.

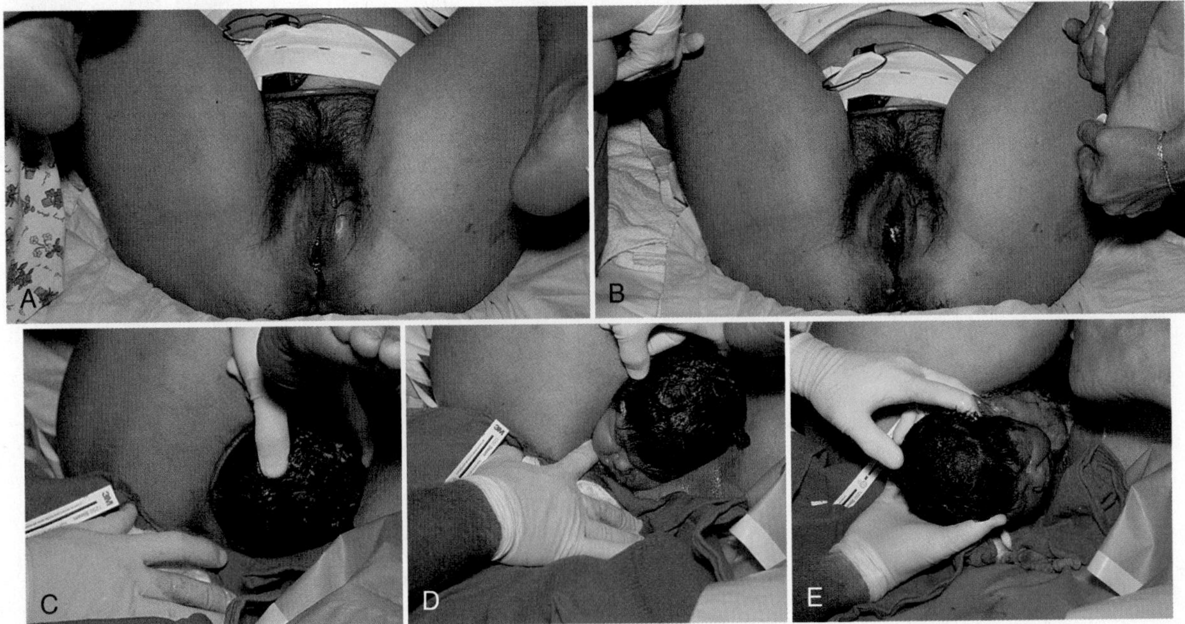

FIGURE 26-12 Normal vaginal birth. **A,** Anteroposterior slit. Vertex visible during contraction. **B,** Oval opening. Vertex presenting. **C,** Crowning. **D,** Nurse-midwife using the Ritgen maneuver as head is born by extension. **E,** After nurse-midwife checks for nuchal cord, she supports head during external rotation and restitution.

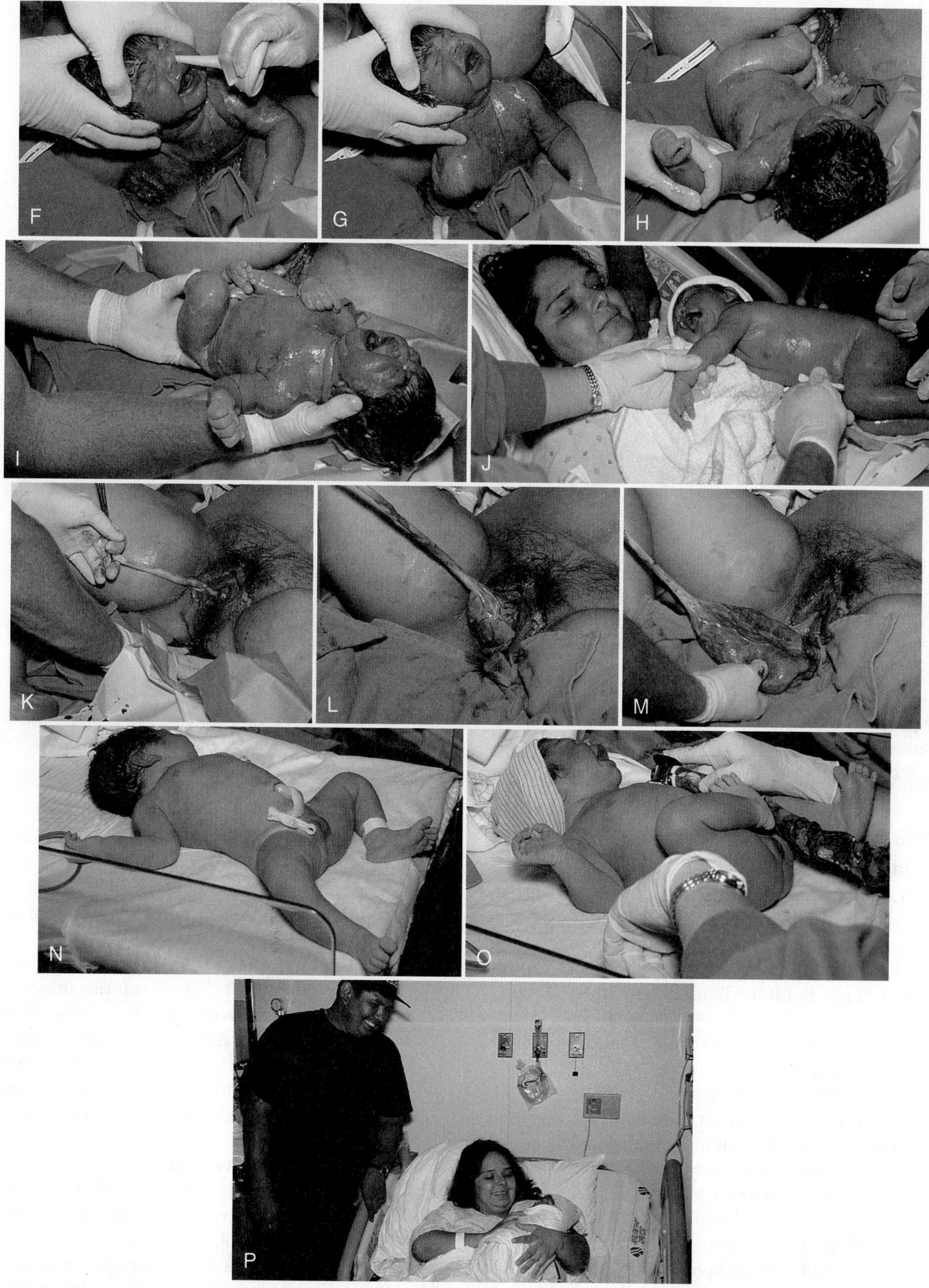

FIGURE 26-12, cont'd **F,** Note the use of bulb syringe to suction mucus. **G,** Birth of posterior shoulder. **H,** Birth of newborn by slow expulsion. **I** and **J,** Second stage complete. Note that newborn is not completely pink yet. **K,** Note increased bleeding as placenta separates. **L,** Expulsion of placenta. **M,** Expulsion is complete, marking the end of the third stage. **N,** Newborn awaiting assessment. Note that color is almost completely pink. **O,** Newborn assessment under radiant warmer. **P,** Parents admiring their newborn.

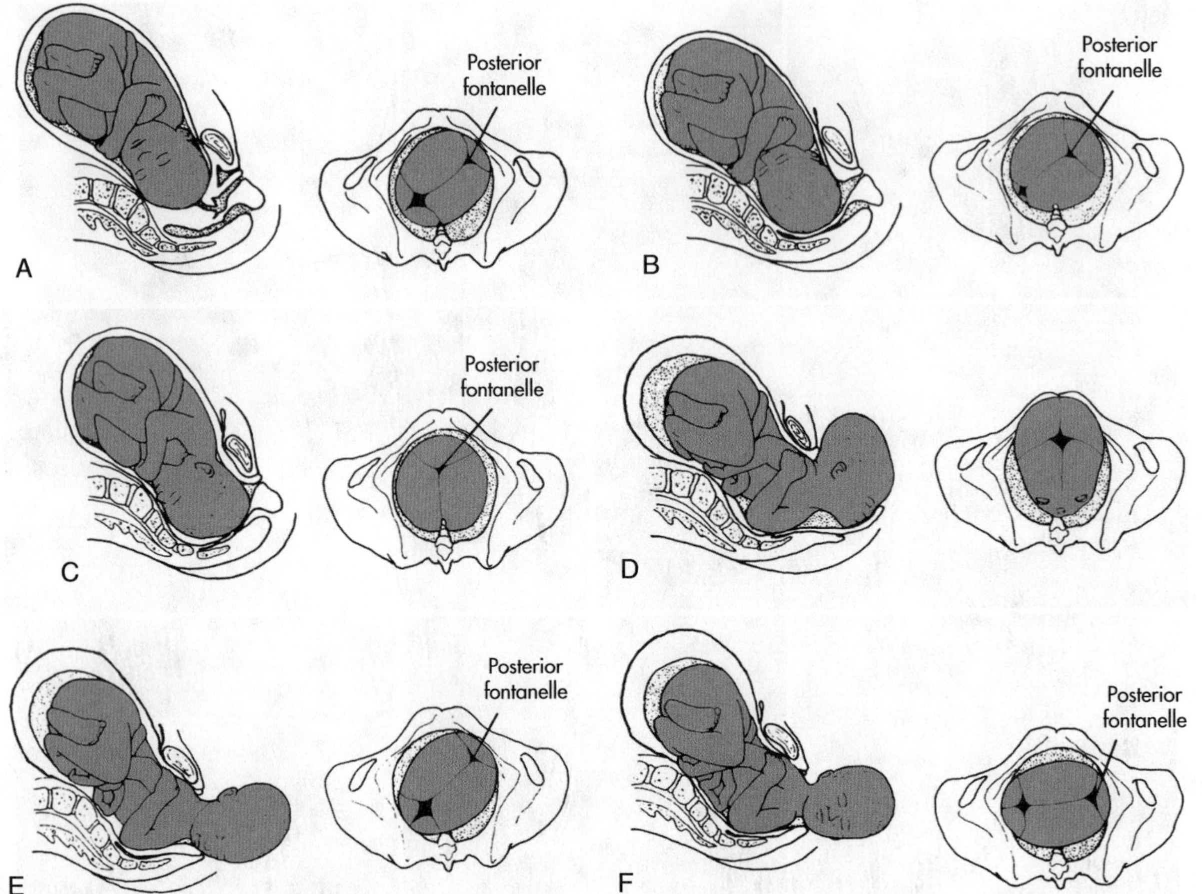

FIGURE 26-13 Mechanism of labor in left occipitoanterior (LOA) presentation. **A,** Engagement and descent. **B,** Flexion. **C,** Internal rotation to OA. **D,** Extension. **E,** Restitution. **F,** External rotation.

STAGES OF LABOR AND DELIVERY

First Stage: Dilation

The first stage begins with the onset of regular contractions and ends with complete dilation of the cervix. This is generally the longest stage of labor, averaging 10 to 12 hours in nulliparas and 6 to 8 hours in multiparas. This stage is often divided into the following three phases:

1. **Early latent phase,** 0 to 3 cm dilation; contractions occurring 5 to 8 minutes apart and lasting 20 to 35 seconds. The woman generally is alert, frequently is talkative, and tends to be receptive to coaching on breathing techniques. The nurse or a significant other may be the coach, reviewing techniques learned in prenatal classes. Pain tends to be mild and easily controlled. Backache is common. Many women, particularly multiparas, prefer to remain home during this stage. If the bag of waters has not ruptured, many women walk during this stage. The nulliparous woman may be anxious about her ability to cope with childbirth.
2. **Middle or active phase,** 4 to 7 cm dilation; contractions occurring at 3- to 5-minute intervals and lasting 40 to 60 seconds. The woman becomes less talkative and focuses on breathing techniques learned during prenatal classes. If she has not already learned breathing techniques, teach them to her during labor. The intensity of the pain increases but still may be manageable without medication.
3. **Transitional phase,** 7 to 10 cm dilation; contractions occurring at 2- to 3-minute intervals and lasting up to 80 seconds. The woman is deeply focused and may not wish to communicate with the nurse or significant other. If the woman has not requested pain medication earlier, she may desire it at this time. Nausea is common.

Second Stage: Delivery of the Fetus

The second stage of labor begins with complete dilation at 10 cm and ends with the birth of the baby. This stage lasts an average of 30 minutes to 2 hours in nulliparas and 20 minutes to 90 minutes in multiparas. Contractions continue to last 80 to 90 seconds or slightly less. (If any woman in labor states "The baby is coming!" anticipate an immediate birth.)

Once the cervix is completely dilated, the woman usually feels the urge to push and is anxious to do so. Pushing is hard work, and the woman requires ongoing encouragement from the coach and nurse. Resting between contractions, if possible, is important to conserve energy.

During this stage the primary care practitioner may provide anesthesia and perform an episiotomy. The episiotomy is a surgical incision of the perineum at the end of the second stage of labor to allow easier delivery and to avoid laceration of the perineum (Figure 26-14). The most common type of episiotomy is a midline, or median, incision that separates the tissues of the perineum at an anatomical junction. If the perineum is too small, the primary care practitioner may perform a mediolateral incision in which muscle must be cut. This is generally more uncomfortable and is done only when necessary.

Immediately after delivery the baby's airway is established (see Response of the Newborn to Birth, p. 826) and the umbilical cord is clamped with two clamps and then severed between the clamps. If everything is normal, show the baby to the parents. Then either give the infant to the mother to hold or position him or her in a warming unit that allows for close observation and care. If any problems occur with the infant, administer care immediately. This emergency care may need to be performed in the delivery area. Remain calm and supportive to the parents. Be aware that the parents may be alarmed and require support and explanations to allay their fears for the newborn.

Third Stage: Delivery of the Placenta

The third stage begins with the delivery of the infant and ends with the delivery of the placenta. The average for both primiparas and multiparas is 5 to 20 minutes.

Generally, the mother is less interested in the third stage; she is focused on the newborn. Many women wish to inspect and possibly breastfeed the infant. When the placenta detaches from the uterine wall, blood suddenly pours out of the vagina. The cord protruding from the vagina lengthens, and the uterus becomes more rounded and firm. The woman may again experience contractions. The size and consistency of the placenta usually permit delivery with one or two pushes. Some women are curious to see the placenta; if so, show it to them. During this time the primary care practitioner repairs the episiotomy if one was performed. Total blood loss is normally 200 to 300 mL; it is considered excessive if more than 500 mL of blood is lost during delivery. It is common for an oxytocic medication, such as oxytocin (Pitocin) or methylergonovine maleate (Methergine), to be administered during this stage (Table 26-3). An **oxytocic** (oxytocin is a hormone produced by the pituitary gland) is a drug that stimulates uterine contractions, thus accelerating childbirth and preventing postdelivery hemorrhage. These medications cause the uterus to contract firmly, compressing blood vessels inside the uterus and keeping blood loss to a minimum.

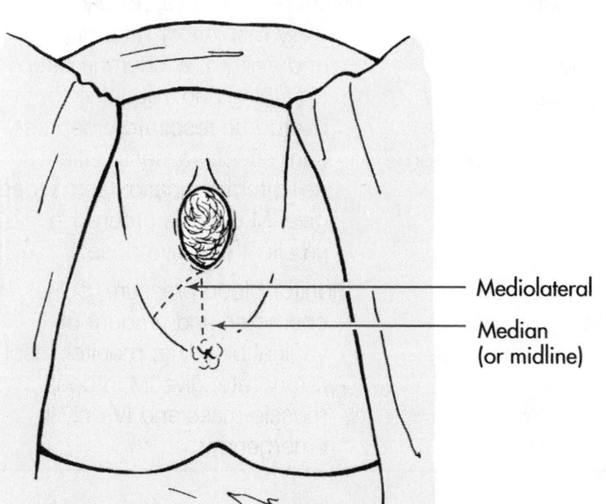

FIGURE 26-14 Types of episiotomies.

Fourth Stage: Stabilization

The time immediately after delivery is critical as the mother's body attempts to recover from the efforts of labor. Usually the mother is monitored closely for 2 to 4 hours after delivery in the birthing room or in a recovery room. Some women, particularly those who had a long or difficult labor and delivery, are exhausted and wish only to rest. Others seem euphoric and wish to talk about the experience or spend time with the baby and their significant other.

Monitor physiologic changes closely during the fourth stage. Assess vital signs, uterine tone, vaginal drainage, and the perineal tissue. During the first hour perform assessments every 15 minutes. If observations are within normal limits, assessments are done every 30 minutes for the next hour. If all observations remain normal, the woman is transferred to a patient room for the remainder of her hospitalization (unless she is in a birthing center, where she may remain until discharge).

MONITORING FETAL STATUS

The process of labor is stressful to the fetus, and it is important to monitor the fetus continuously during this time. Fetal heart rate (FHR) is a good indicator of the fetus's condition. The normal FHR range is 120 to 160 bpm. An increase or decrease of 30 bpm may indicate fetal distress and should be reported immediately (Box 26-2).

Auscultate the FHR, using a fetoscope or a Doppler instrument, every 15 to 30 minutes during the first stage of labor and every 5 minutes during the second stage. Also assess the FHR immediately after rupture of the membranes, particularly if the head is not engaged (i.e., not firmly settled into the pelvis).

Electronic Fetal Monitoring (EFM)

Frequently, continuous electronic monitors, either internal or external, are applied. Monitors can detect subtle changes of condition before they can be recognized by auscultation. The external, or indirect, mode

Table 26-3 Medications for Normal Labor and Delivery

Generic (Brand)	Action	Side Effects	Nursing Implications
Butorphanol (Stadol) (not commonly used)	Synthetic, centrally acting analgesic, providing relief of moderate to severe pain during labor	Drowsiness, sedation, headache, vertigo, dizziness, weakness, confusion, insomnia, nervousness, respiratory depression, change in blood pressure, palpitations, bradycardia, nausea, clammy skin, tingling, flushing and warmth, diaphoresis, skin rash, pruritus, increased urinary output Neonatal: respiratory depression, disorganized infant behavior, tendency to cry a lot	Monitor for respiratory depression; do not give if respiratory rate is <15 breaths/min; monitor vital signs; observe neonate for respiratory depression; observe safety precautions due to sedation and dizziness.
Misoprostol (synthetic prostaglandin E; Cytotec)	Used most widely to prevent nonsteroidal antiinflammatory drug–induced gastric ulcer in patients at high risk	Headache, nausea, dyspepsia, vomiting, constipation, flatulence	Some physicians use it to induce labor, especially in the event of fetal demise, at a dose of 200 mcg administered vaginally in the posterior fornix. It is easier on the mother because labor and delivery can be over in as little as 45 minutes. To induce labor when there is not fetal demise, administer 25 mcg vaginally into the posterior fornix. The tablets come in 100 mcg; are quartered, resembling a fine white powder; and then are inserted vaginally.
Magnesium sulfate	Decreases acetylcholine in motor nerve terminals, which is responsible for seizure prevention in preeclampsia and eclampsia	Diarrhea; side effects are related to magnesium levels: with >3 mg/dL, depressed central nervous system, blocked neuromuscular transmission leading to anticonvulsant effects; with >5 mg/dL, depressed deep tendon reflexes; with >12.5 mg/dL, respiratory paralysis	Obtain vital signs every 15 minutes after IV dose; do not exceed 150 mg/min; monitor cardiac function; time contractions and monitor fetal heart rate; monitor intake and output (should remain ≥30 mL/hr).
Meperidine (Demerol)	Synthetic morphine-like compound, producing comparable analgesic effects and providing relief of moderate to severe pain	Pruritus, dizziness, sedation, weakness, euphoria, respiratory depression, hypotension, palpitations, bradycardia or tachycardia, dry mouth, nausea, constipation, oliguria, urinary retention Neonatal: respiratory depression	Being used less and less frequently. Monitor vital signs closely, especially respiratory rate, depth, and rhythm; encourage deep breathing and coughing to overcome respiratory depressant effects; assess patient's need for medication as needed; give IM or IV as ordered in smallest effective dose.
Methylergonovine maleate (Methergine)	Stimulates uterine contraction, decreases bleeding	Headache, dizziness, nausea, vomiting, chest pain, palpitations, hypertension, tinnitus, sweating, rash	Monitor blood pressure, pulse, character, and amount of vaginal bleeding; monitor respiratory rate; give IM in deep muscle mass and IV only in emergency.

IM, Intramuscularly, intramuscular; *IV*, intravenously, intravenous.

Table 26-3 Medications for Normal Labor and Delivery—cont'd

Generic (Brand)	Action	Side Effects	Nursing Implications
Oxytocin (Pitocin, Syntocinon)	Acts directly on myofibrils, producing uterine contractions; stimulates milk ejection by breasts	Anaphylaxis, postpartum hemorrhage, cardiac arrhythmias, nausea, vomiting, premature ventricular contractions, hypertension, convulsions Fetal: bradycardia, arrhythmias, jaundice, hypoxia, intracranial hemorrhage	Monitor intake and output ratio, contractions, fetal heart rate, blood pressure, pulse, and respirations.
Prostaglandin E (dinoprostone [Prepidil, Cervidil])	Stimulates uterine contractions like those seen in normal labor	Uterine contractile abnormalities, nausea, vomiting, diarrhea, back pain, warm feeling in vagina, fever Fetal: heart rate abnormalities, bradycardia	Use caution to prevent contact with skin; wash thoroughly after administration; bring to room temperature before administering; do not force warming process; have patient remain supine for 15-30 minutes after insertion.
Ritodrine hydrochloride (Yutopar)	Uterine beta$_2$-adrenergic receptor–stimulating effect, which reduces uterine contractions	Erythema, rash, dyspnea, hyperglycemia, headache, restlessness, anxiety, chills, tremor, nausea, vomiting, diarrhea, constipation, altered maternal and fetal heart rates	Being used less and less frequently. Monitor maternal and fetal heart tones during infusion; watch intensity and length of uterine contractions; monitor fluid intake to prevent overload; monitor blood glucose level in diabetic patients.
Fentanyl citrate (Sublimaze) (epidural)	Binds with opiate receptors in the central nervous system, altering both perception of and emotional response to pain through an unknown mechanism	Sedation, euphoria, vertigo, headache, confusion, anxiety, depression, seizures, blood pressure deviations, nausea, vomiting, respiratory depression	Used occasionally. Monitor circulatory and respiratory status and urinary function. Monitor arterial oxygen saturation.
Carboprost tromethamine (Hemabate)	Produces strong, prompt contractions of uterine smooth muscle; used in postpartum hemorrhage due to uterine atony not managed by conventional methods	Headache, anxiety, weakness, arrhythmias, eye pain, nausea, vomiting, uterine rupture, backache, leg cramps, wheezing, fever, chills	Used only by trained personnel in a hospital setting. May be injected into the uterus.
Promethazine hydrochloride (Phenergan)	Prevents but does not reverse histamine-mediated responses; at high dose exhibits local anesthetic effects; used as adjunct to analgesics	Sedation, blood pressure deviations, blurred vision, nausea, vomiting, urine retention, seizures	Used most of the time for postoperative cesarean delivery. Inject deep into large muscle mass. Often used as an adjunct to analgesics. May be mixed with meperidine in the same syringe.
Nalbuphine hydrochloride (Nubain)	Binds with opiate receptors in the central nervous system, altering perception of and emotional response to pain through an unknown mechanism	Headache, sedation, vertigo, syncope, restlessness, crying, confusion, blood pressure variations, bradycardia, blurred vision, nausea and vomiting, urinary urgency, respiratory depression, asthma Neonatal: disorganized infant behavior, fussiness, refusal to nurse	Usually administer one or two doses and then begin an epidural. Monitor circulatory and respiratory status and bladder and bowel function; withhold dose and notify physician if respirations become shallow or fall below 12 breaths/min. Stool softeners may be ordered.

Continued

Table 26-3 Medications for Normal Labor and Delivery—cont'd

Generic (Brand)	Action	Side Effects	Nursing Implications
Hydroxyzine (Vistaril)	Antianxiety antepartum and postpartum adjunctive therapy	Drowsiness, dry mouth, marked discomfort at IM injection site	Being used less frequently. Aspirate IM injection carefully to prevent inadvertent IV injection. Inject deeply into a large muscle mass. Observe for sedation.
Naloxone hydrochloride (Narcan)	Thought to displace previously administered narcotic-opioid analgesics from their receptors (competitive antagonism); indicated for use in known or suspected narcotic-induced respiratory depression in neonates (asphyxia neonatorum)	Tremors, seizures, blood pressure variations, nausea, vomiting Can cause seizure when used with street drugs (of which the health care worker is sometimes unaware)	Not used as often as once was. Respiratory rate increases within 1-2 minutes. Monitor respiratory depth and rate. Be prepared to provide oxygen, ventilation, and other resuscitation measures. Administer IV into umbilical vein. May be repeated every 2-3 minutes.

Box 26-2 Changes in Fetal Heart Rate

NORMAL BASELINE RATE
- 120 to 160 bpm

TACHYCARDIA
- Moderate increase to 160 to 180 bpm
- Marked increase greater than 180 bpm; significant if variability is absent and late or variable decelerations (a decrease in the speed or velocity of an object or reaction) are present

Nursing Interventions*
- Interventions depend on the cause.
- Reduce maternal fever with antipyretics as ordered and cooling measures.
- Oxygen at 8 to 10 L/min per face mask may be of some value.
- Carry out health care provider's orders to alleviate cause.

BRADYCARDIA
- Moderate decrease to 100 to 120 bpm
- Marked decrease to fewer than 100 bpm; significant if variability is decreased or absent or if late or variable decelerations are present

Nursing Interventions*
- Interventions depend on the cause.
- Intervention is not warranted in fetus with heart block diagnosed by electrocardiogram.
- Oxygen at 8 to 10 L/min per face mask may be of some value.
- Carry out health care provider's orders to alleviate cause.
- Scalp stimulation may be performed to determine whether the fetus is able to compensate physiologically for stress (fetal heart rate [FHR] will accelerate).

VARIABILITY
- Measures the normal fluctuation of the FHR from the baseline
- Absent or minimal variability possibly indicative of fetal distress
- Variability classified as long-term variability (LTV) or short-term variability (STV)

DECELERATIONS
- Periodic decrease in the FHR in response to contractions; classified as early, late, or variable (see Figure 26-18)
- Early decelerations: caused by pressure on fetal skull; tend to be uniform; onset, shape, and recovery correspond to contractions
- Late decelerations: caused by decreased oxygen and blood flow to fetus through the placenta; usually noted at or after the peak of the contraction; may indicate fetal distress, particularly if associated with changes in baseline FHR and absence of variability
- Variable decelerations: caused by compression on the umbilical cord; occur randomly and onset may be sudden; FHR decreases below normal range

Nursing Interventions*
- Notify the primary caregiver immediately and initiate appropriate treatment when patient has a prolonged deceleration.

*See Box 26-3 for care of the woman being monitored electronically for fetal status during labor.

uses external transducers on the maternal abdominal wall to assess FHR and uterine activity (Figure 26-15). An ultrasound transducer uses high-frequency sound waves to reflect movement of the fetal heart ventricles. A tocotransducer monitors uterine activity and records frequency and duration of contractions. A strip chart prints out both FHR (upper part of the strip) and uterine activity (lower part of the strip) (Figure 26-16, *A*). External monitoring can be used in both the antepartal and the intrapartal periods. It does not require rupture of membranes or cervical dilation; however, the tocotransducer cannot assess the intensity of contractions. Maternal position can affect the accuracy of the recordings.

Internal monitoring uses a spiral electrode applied to the presenting part to monitor the FHR (Figure 26-17). An intrauterine catheter is used to monitor frequency, duration, intensity, and resting tone of uterine contractions. This catheter is compressed during contractions, placing pressure on a strain gauge or pressure transducer. FHR and uterine pressure are reflected on a strip chart (Figure 26-16, *B*). Internal monitoring can be used only during the intrapartal period because membranes must be ruptured and the cervix dilated 2 to 3 cm. Display of FHR and uterine activity is accurate regardless of maternal position. Box 26-3 lists guidelines for care of the woman being monitored electronically for fetal status during labor.

FHR is monitored in relation to the contractions. A decrease in FHR occurs in response to the contractions and is called a **deceleration.** Decelerations can be early, late, or variable (Figure 26-18) (see Box 26-2).

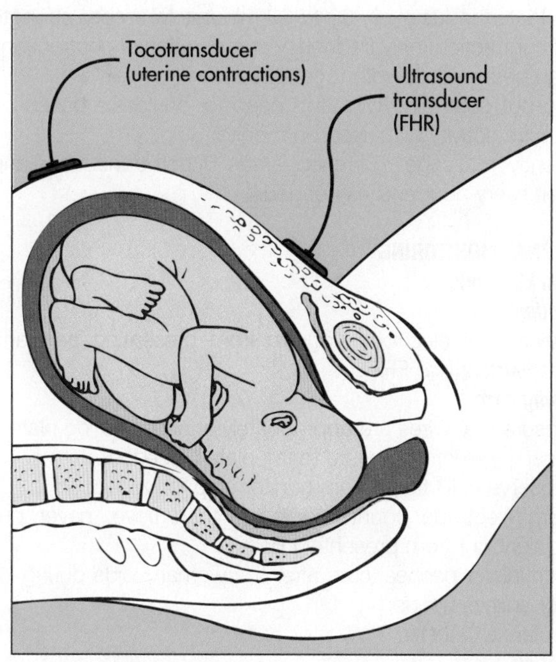

FIGURE 26-15 Diagram of external noninvasive fetal monitoring with tocotransducer and ultrasound transducer, with ultrasound transducer placed below umbilicus and tocotransducer placed on uterine fundus position. *FHR,* Fetal heart rate.

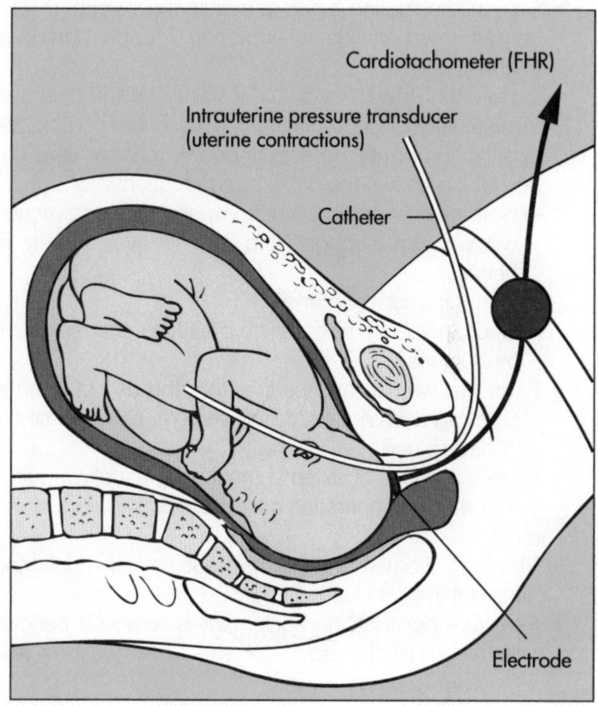

FIGURE 26-17 Diagram of internal invasive fetal monitoring with intrauterine catheter and spiral electrode in place (membranes ruptured and cervix dilated). *FHR,* Fetal heart rate.

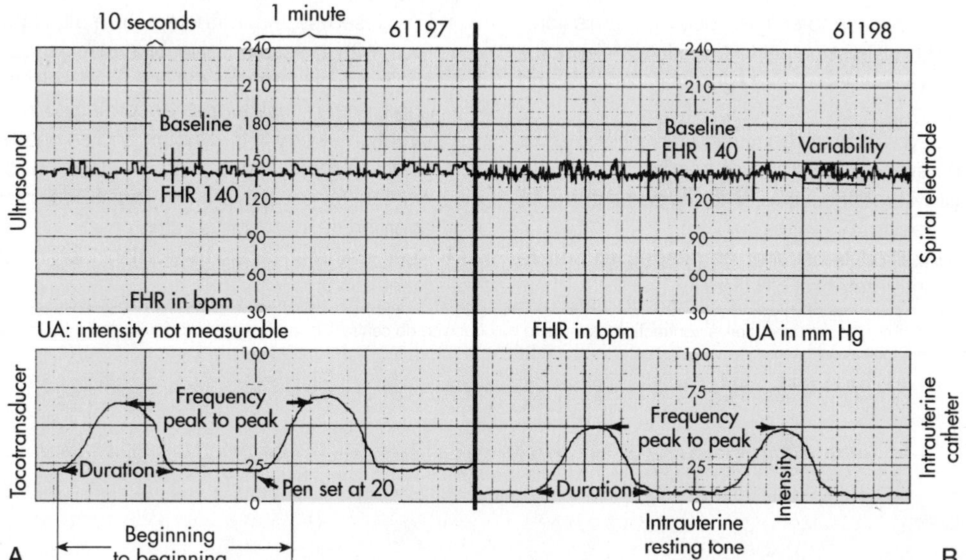

FIGURE 26-16 Display of fetal heart rate *(FHR)* and uterine activity *(UA)* on chart paper. **A,** External mode with ultrasound transducer and tocotransducer as signal sources. **B,** Internal mode with spiral electrode and intrauterine catheter as signal sources.

Box 26-3 Care of the Woman Using Electronic Fetal Monitoring

The following guidelines relate to patient teaching and the functioning of the monitor.

- Explain that fetal status can be continuously assessed by electronic fetal monitoring (EFM), even during contractions.
- Explain that the lower tracing on the monitor strip paper shows uterine activity; the upper tracing shows the fetal heart rate (FHR).
- Reassure woman and partner that prepared childbirth techniques can be implemented without difficulty.
- Explain that during external monitoring effleurage can be performed on sides of abdomen or upper portion of thighs.
- Explain that breathing patterns based on the time and the intensity of contractions can be enhanced by the observation of uterine activity on the monitor strip paper, which shows the onset of contractions.
  —Note peak of contraction; knowing that a contraction will not get stronger and is half over usually is helpful.
  —Note diminishing intensity.
  —Coordinate with appropriate breathing and relaxation techniques.
- Reassure woman and partner that the use of internal monitoring does not restrict movement, although she is confined to bed.*
- Explain that use of external monitoring usually requires the woman's cooperation during positioning and movement.
- Reassure woman and partner that use of monitoring does not imply fetal jeopardy.
- Reassure her that the equipment is removed periodically to permit the applicator site to be washed and other care to be given.

EXTERNAL MONITORING

Ultrasound Transducer

Function

Monitors FHR with high-frequency sound waves.

Nursing care

- Tap transducer before use to ensure sound transmission.
- Apply ultrasound transmission gel to transducer, clean abdomen and transducer, and reapply gel every 2 hours and as needed.
- Massage reddened skin areas gently and reposition belt or adhesive device every 2 hours and as needed.
- Auscultate FHR with stethoscope or fetoscope if in doubt as to validity or tracing.
- Position and reposition transducer as needed to ensure receipt of clean, interpretable FHR data.

Tocotransducer

Function

Monitors uterine activity via a pressure-sensing device placed on the maternal abdomen.

Nursing care

- Position and reposition every 2 hours and as needed on the fundus, where there is the least maternal tissue.
- Keep abdominal strap snug but comfortable for the laboring woman.
- Adjust pen-set between contractions to print between 10 and 20 mm Hg on the monitor strip paper.
- Palpate fundus every 30 to 60 minutes to assess strength of contraction; only frequency and duration of contractions can be assessed with tocotransducer.
- Do not determine woman's need for analgesia based on uterine activity displayed on monitor strip.
- Gently massage reddened areas under transducer and belt every hour and as needed.

INTERNAL MONITORING

Spiral Electrode

Function

Obtains fetal electrocardiogram from presenting part and converts it into FHR.

Nursing care

- Ensure that wires are appropriately attached to leg plate.
- Reapply electrode paste to leg plate if needed.
- Observe FHR tracing on monitor strip for variability.
- Turn electrode counterclockwise to remove; never pull straight out from presenting part.
- Administer perineal care after the woman voids during labor and as needed.

Intrauterine Catheter

Function

Catheter (solid or fluid filled) that monitors intraamniotic pressure internally.

Nursing care

- Flush open system catheter with sterile water before insertion and as needed.
- Ensure that the length line on catheter is visible at introitus.
- For closed-system catheters, turn off stopcock to woman, then with pressure valve of strain gauge released, flush strain gauge, remove syringe, and set stylus to 0 line of chart paper; test further according to manufacturer's instructions every 3 to 4 hours and as needed.
- Check proper functioning by tapping catheter, asking woman to cough, or applying fundal pressure; observe appropriate inflection on strip chart.
- Keep catheter taped to woman's leg to prevent dislodgment.

*Portable telemetry monitors allow the FHR and uterine contraction patterns to be observed on centrally located electronic display stations. These portable units permit ambulation during electronic monitoring.

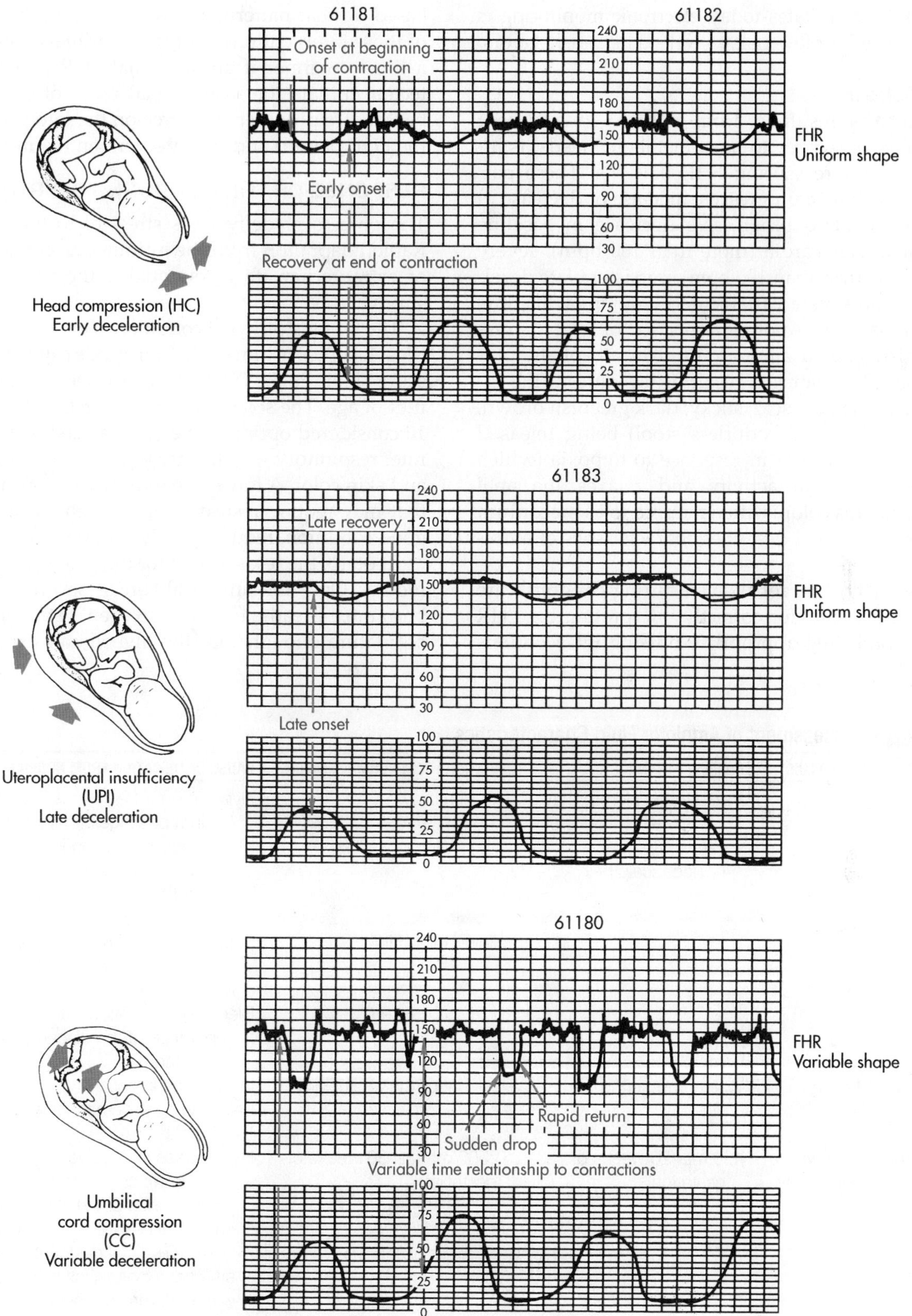

FIGURE 26-18 Summary of periodic changes. *FHR,* Fetal heart rate.

In the United States today, electronic monitoring is routinely used for low-risk, as well as high-risk, labors.

Fetal Distress

Fetal distress resulting from **hypoxia** (insufficient availability of oxygen to meet metabolic needs) is indicated by nonreassuring FHR patterns. These patterns can include a progressive increase or decrease in the baseline FHR, progressive decrease in baseline variability, tachycardia (more than 160 bpm), severe bradycardia (less than 100 bpm), persistent late decelerations, and severe variable decelerations with slow return to baseline. Another indication of fetal distress is greenish-stained amniotic fluid in a cephalic presentation. The color is a result of **meconium** (the infant's first stool, a viscid, sticky; dark greenish brown, almost black; sterile, odorless stool) being released from the fetal rectum in response to hypoxia (which increases intestinal activity and relaxes the anal sphincter). This color is often referred to as **meconium staining.** Table 26-4 describes characteristics of amniotic fluid.

Nurses who care for women during childbirth are legally responsible for correctly interpreting the FHR pattern, indicating appropriate nursing interventions based on that pattern, and documenting the outcome of those interventions. Notify the primary caregiver in a timely manner if an abnormal FHR pattern is detected. Initiate the institutional chain of command if health care providers disagree on the interpretation of the FHR pattern and the intervention required.

RESPONSE OF THE NEWBORN TO BIRTH

The process of delivery is stressful to the newborn. Rapid adaptation from the intrauterine climate to that of extrauterine life is essential if the newborn is to survive.

The infant's physical condition is evaluated at birth. Most facilities use an evaluation guide called the **Apgar score** (Table 26-5). This scoring is done at 1 and 5 minutes of age. The score can range from 0 to 10, with 8 to 10 considered optimal. The criteria used include heart rate, respiratory effort, muscle tone, reflex irritability, and skin color. A low score indicates serious problems that may require resuscitation. A high score indicates good condition, requiring only routine care.

In utero, the fetus's need for oxygen was met by the mother. Once the umbilical cord is severed, the newborn must breathe to obtain oxygen. Fetal lungs must be mature enough that the alveoli can expand ade-

Table 26-4 Assessment of Amniotic Fluid Characteristics

CHARACTERISTIC OF FLUID	NORMAL FINDING	DEVIATION FROM NORMAL FINDING	CAUSE OF DEVIATION FROM NORMAL
Color	Pale, straw colored; may contain white flecks of vernix caseosa, lanugo, scalp hair	Greenish brown	Hypoxic episode in fetus results in meconium passage into fluid May be normal finding in breech presentation, related to pressure exerted on fetal abdominal wall during descent
		Yellow-stained fluid	Fetal hypoxia ≥36 hours before rupture of membranes; fetal hemolytic disease; intrauterine infection
		Port-wine colored	Bleeding associated with premature separation of the placenta (abruptio placentae)
Viscosity and odor	Watery; no strong odor	Thick, cloudy, foul smelling	Intrauterine infection Large amount of meconium making fluid thick
Amount (normally varies with gestational age)	400 mL (20 weeks of gestation)	>2000 mL (32-36 weeks of gestation)	Hydramnios (excessive amount of amniotic fluid): associated with congenital anomalies of the fetus when fetus cannot drink or fluid is trapped in the body (e.g., fetal gastrointestinal obstruction or atresias); increased risk with maternal pregestational or gestational diabetes mellitus
	1000 mL (36-38 weeks of gestation)	<500 mL (32-36 weeks of gestation)	Oligohydramnios (a condition in which the volume of amniotic fluid is <300 mL in the third trimester): associated with incomplete or absent kidney; obstruction of urethra; fetus cannot secrete or excrete urine

Adapted from Lowdermilk, D.L., & Perry, S.E. (2007). *Maternity and women's health care.* (9th ed.). St. Louis: Mosby.

Table 26-5 Apgar Scoring Chart

SIGN	0	1	2
Heart rate	Absent	Slow—<100 bpm	>100 bpm
Respiratory effort	Absent	Slow—irregular	Good crying
Muscle tone	Flaccid, limp	Some flexion of extremities	Active motion
Reflex irritability	No response	Grimace	Vigorous cry, cough, or sneeze
Color*	Pale blue	Body pink, extremities blue	Completely pink

*Skin color or its absence may not be a reliable guide in nonwhites, although melanin (the pigment that gives color to the skin) is less apparent at birth than later.

quately. The infant produces a substance called **surfactant,** which decreases surface tension within the alveoli and permits inflation. At the time of delivery a combination of chemical, thermal, tactile, and mechanical changes initiates the first breath.

The airway must be cleared of fluids that are in the lungs. Some fluids are forced from the lungs as the thorax passes through the pelvis during delivery. Use a bulb syringe to remove excess fluid from the mouth and nasopharynx (Box 26-4). Positioning of the infant is also important (Figure 26-19).

Warmth is necessary to prevent a rapid drop in body temperature. The environment in utero is approximately 99° F (37.2° C); the external environment in the delivery room is usually about 70° F (21.1° C). To prevent hypothermia, immediately dry the infant to help reduce heat loss from evaporation. Then place the baby in contact with the mother's skin, especially if she wishes to breastfeed, or transfer the baby to a radiant warming unit.

Box 26-4 Suctioning with a Bulb Syringe

- Suction the mouth first to prevent the infant from inhaling pharyngeal secretions by gasping as the nares are touched.
- Compress the bulb (see figure) and insert it into one side of the mouth. Avoid the center of the infant's mouth because this could stimulate the gag reflex.
- Suction the nasal passages one nostril at a time.
- When the infant's cry does not sound as though it is through mucus or a bubble, stop suctioning. The bulb syringe should always be kept in the infant's crib.
- Give the parents demonstrations on how to use the bulb syringe and ask them to perform a return demonstration.

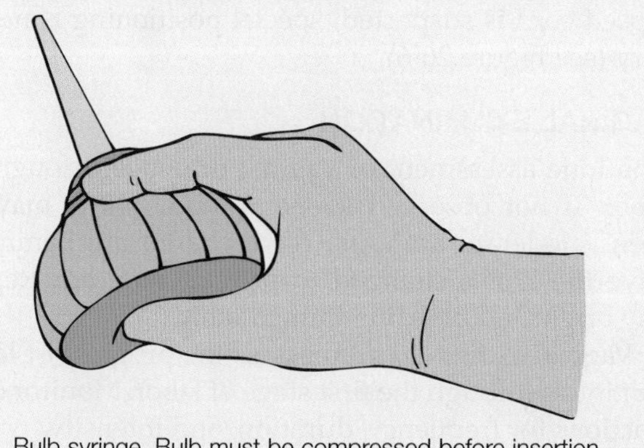

Bulb syringe. Bulb must be compressed before insertion.

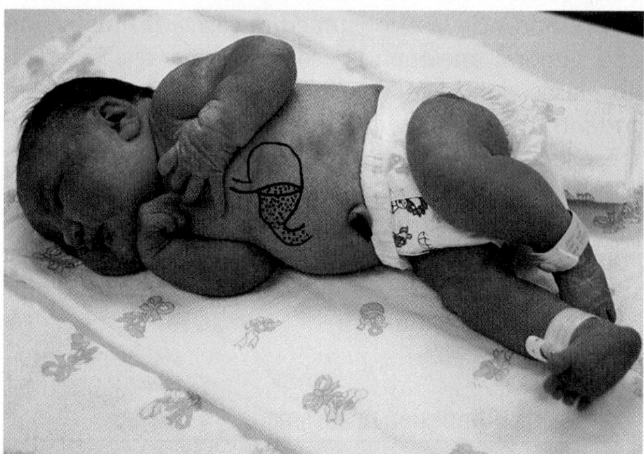

FIGURE 26-19 Infant is turned to right side and supported in this position to facilitate drainage from mouth and to promote emptying of stomach contents into the small intestine.

If there are no complications, the infant remains in the mother's view until her care is completed. Place identification bracelets on both mother and baby before they leave the delivery room. A bracelet is also worn by the baby's father or other person designated by the mother at many institutions. These are used to verify infant identification and match it with that of the mother until discharge. Footprinting the infant is another method of identification; this may be done in the delivery area or in the nursery.

NURSING ASSESSMENT AND INTERVENTIONS

HEALTH PERCEPTION AND HEALTH MANAGEMENT

Find out how well prepared for childbirth the woman is. The woman who has attended classes and practiced breathing techniques requires a different level of explanation and support than one who has had no preparation. If a hospital delivery is planned, admission is generally prearranged and much of the paperwork completed ahead of time to minimize delays. If home delivery is anticipated, the primary care practitioner will give directions for the family.

When hospitalization is anticipated, it is a good idea for the prospective parents to prepare a suitcase with necessary items well in advance of the date of delivery. Making a trial run to the hospital also can reduce fears of not getting to the hospital on time. If children are at home, parents should make plans for their care. Advise the parents-to-be to anticipate as many problems as possible and make several alternate plans. On admission, begin the assessment (Box 26-5).

NUTRITIONAL AND METABOLIC PATTERN

Gastrointestinal motility and absorption decrease during labor and delivery. Food eaten before labor may remain in the digestive tract and lead to complaints of nausea and vomiting. Once active labor begins, solid foods are generally withheld. Find out when food was last consumed in case administration of a general anesthetic becomes necessary. In addition, assess fluid intake. Increased physical exertion and mouth breathing are common during labor. When these factors are combined with restricted oral intake, a fluid deficit may result. Some primary care practitioners allow small amounts of ice chips or clear beverages during labor. Orders for intravenous fluids, such as a 5% dextrose solution, to prevent fluid imbalance are common.

Box 26-5 Admission Assessment

- **Review the prenatal record,** including general medical history, obstetric history, and the history of the current pregnancy. This record should include information about allergies and any current health problems, such as respiratory tract or other types of infection.
- **Interview the patient** for signs and symptoms of the onset of labor, such as the nature and frequency of contractions, level of discomfort, and the presence of vaginal discharge such as bloody show or loss of amniotic fluid. If these data indicate that the woman is in labor, obtain information regarding the type of preparation for childbirth, support person present, special cultural practices or expectations, type of anesthesia planned, method of infant feeding desired, and name of pediatrician.
- **Perform the physical examination,** including a complete set of vital signs and fetal heart tones. These data will function as a baseline for further assessment. Auscultate heart and lung sounds. Inspect the face, the hands, the legs, and the sacrum for signs of edema. Palpate the abdomen to determine the fetal lie and presentation. Assess the status of the membranes. If there is any question regarding ruptured membranes, perform a Nitrazine test (see Box 26-1) before the vaginal examination, since solutions used may make the test results unreliable. Time contractions to determine frequency, regularity, duration, and intensity. A vaginal examination is performed to determine the progress of labor, including position, dilation, effacement, and station.
- **Perform diagnostic tests,** including a urinalysis to check for glucose, protein, or ketones, which may indicate potential complications. If blood analyses were not performed during pregnancy, they should be done at this time. Information about hemoglobin and hematocrit levels, blood type and Rh factor, and antibody titer and screening for sexually transmitted infections help in assessment of actual or potential problems.

ELIMINATION

Depending on the amount of fluid intake, urinary output may be normal or decreased. Voiding every 2 hours is desirable. **A full bladder can interfere with the progress of labor.** When membranes are intact, use of the toilet is permitted. Once membranes are ruptured, the bedpan is preferred. If the presenting part is compressing the urethra, catheterization may be ordered.

Assess bowel elimination. Some women experience diarrhea with the onset of labor. Careful hygiene technique is important to reduce the possibility of contamination. Enemas were once routinely administered to empty the colon and maximize space in the pelvic cavity; today they are given only when specifically ordered. Large-volume enemas are sometimes used to stimulate or strengthen labor. **Enemas should not be given if there is vaginal bleeding or premature labor, if the presenting part is not engaged, or if the presentation is not vertex.** If membranes are ruptured, the enema should be expelled into a bedpan.

The urge to defecate during labor may indicate the start of the second stage. Before the woman attempts to have a bowel movement, inspect the perineum and assess dilation for progress of labor.

ACTIVITY AND EXERCISE

Encourage ambulation as long as the membranes have not ruptured. Ambulation may also be permitted if the membranes have ruptured and the presenting part is fully engaged. Walking provides distraction and tends to strengthen the effectiveness of labor. If ambulation becomes too uncomfortable, or if the mother has been given analgesics, she usually is advised to rest. Positioning becomes important; encourage the woman to assume the position most comfortable for her. Some women prefer sitting or semiseated positions. Low back pain is common. A side-lying position is frequently more comfortable than supine. Changing position may help reduce discomfort. If the patient is allowed to be up, a warm shower provides much relief for low back pain during labor. Side-lying positions reduce pressure on the vena cava. The left side is recommended if the FHR shows late deceleration or if the woman experiences hypotension (Figure 26-20). If prolapsed cord is suspected, special positioning is necessary (see Figure 26-6).

VAGINAL EXAMINATION

Continue assessment of vaginal drainage throughout labor. If not observed sooner, bloody show may be seen. Moderate amounts of discharge are common; have the linens changed to provide comfort. Report any bright-red bleeding immediately.

Vaginal examination to assess the progress of labor continues through the first stage of labor. Monitor contractions for frequency, duration, and intensity.

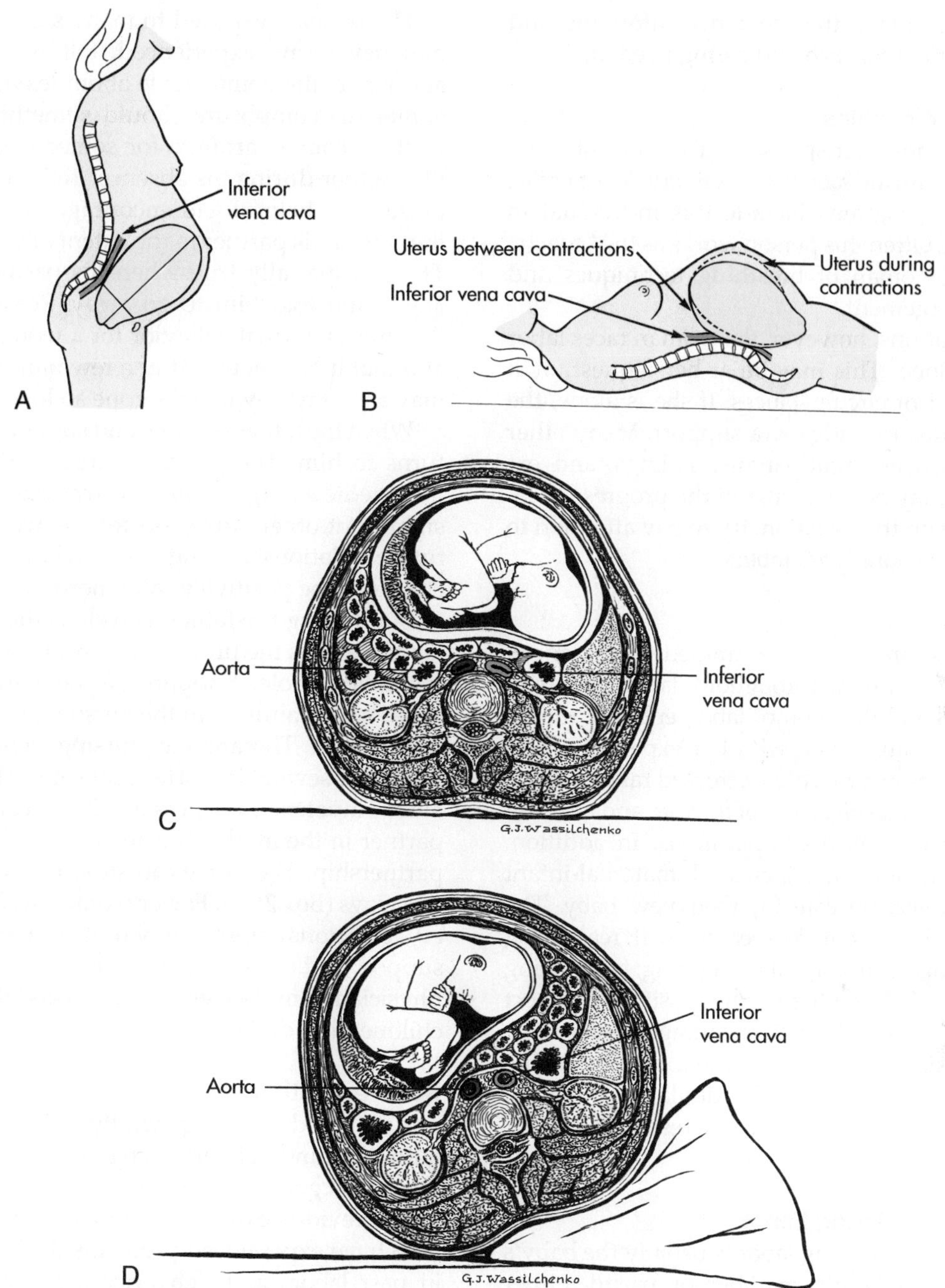

FIGURE 26-20 Supine hypotension. Note relationship of gravid uterus to ascending vena cava in standing posture **(A)** and in supine posture **(B)**. **C,** Compression of aorta and inferior vena cava with woman in supine position. **D,** Relieved by use of a wedge pillow placed under woman's right side.

PSYCHOSOCIAL ASSESSMENT

Coping and Stress Tolerance

During labor and delivery many women, particularly primigravidas, express fears. They may have unrealistic expectations and believe that they should be able to control their labor. Controlled breathing techniques help, but the involuntary nature of labor troubles many women. Encouragement and support in breathing exercises, along with explanations regarding the progress of labor, are helpful. Fatigue and pain lower the woman's ability to cope. It is important to understand the cultural and religious background of each woman, since these factors may strongly influence her behavior.

Pay attention to the support person's reaction. Often the woman's significant other also experiences fears and anxieties. The father in particular may exhibit concerns about the process of labor and the pain the mother is experiencing. At times fathers express guilt about their role, either in not being able to help enough or in being responsible for the pregnancy. Tell the father that he is an important participant, not an unwanted guest, in the process of childbirth. Encourage him to help make the woman comfortable and provide the companionship and caring needed.

Roles and Relationships

Many women want their spouse or a significant other to be with them during labor and delivery. Most childbirth education programs include this individual in the preparation. Often this person works as the "coach" to remind the woman of breathing techniques and provide encouragement.

In some situations, however, the woman faces labor and delivery alone. This may be at her request, or it may be a matter of circumstances. If she is alone, the nursing staff must provide extra support. Many other individuals, such as grandparents, siblings, and extended family, may be interested in the progress of labor. Depending on the situation, try to pay attention to the needs of these family members.

Doulas

The continuous presence of a trained, experienced woman, called a **doula,** throughout labor can help reduce the pain and duration of labor, enhance the laboring woman's satisfaction with her experience, and improve outcomes in terms of a decreased rate of operative delivery (cesarean birth, use of forceps, and vacuum extraction) and childbirth complications. In addition, women often demonstrate increased maternal-infant bonding and ability to care for their new baby. The doula supports the woman by speaking soft, reassuring words; by touching, stroking, and hugging; by walking with her; and by helping her change position. Support of the woman's partner through encouragement, praise, and role modeling is also an essential activity of the doula. The nurse works with the doula in providing supportive care but retains the overall responsibility for patient care.

Father or Partner during Labor

The support partner during labor is usually the baby's father, although a family member or friend, either male or female, may perform this role. (This discussion refers to the partner as the father.) No matter whom the support partner is, include that person in the circle of communication while caring for the woman in labor. He often is able to provide comfort measures and touch that the laboring woman needs. When the woman becomes focused on her pain, sometimes the father can persuade her to try nonpharmacologic variations of comfort measures. He usually is able to interpret her needs and desires to staff members. He may be focused and involved with the woman, or he may be more passive because of cultural norms or fear. Assess his level of comfort in asking questions and in being present and involved during the second-stage labor and birth. This helps determine what level of support to provide to the couple.

The father is exposed to many sights and smells he may never have experienced. Tell him what to expect and make him comfortable about leaving the room to gather his composure should something shock him. First, of course, arrange for someone else to support the mother during his absence. Tell the father that his presence is helpful and encourage his involvement in the care of his partner to the extent of his comfort level. This is especially true when his partner has become angry and told him to go away. Reassure the father that this is normal behavior for a woman in transition and that if he reenters after a few minutes, the woman may ask him why he was gone so long.

When the father is active and supportive, the mother turns to him. The primary care practitioner remains the medical-surgical expert without taking on the significant-other surrogate role as well. The couple's future relationship and their relationship with the child may be positively influenced.

Supporting the father as well as the mother during labor elevates the nurse's role from custodial care to a therapeutic role. Support of the father reflects the nurse's commitment to the person, the family, and the community. Therapeutic nursing actions convey to the father several important concepts: (1) he is of value and competent as a person, (2) he can learn to be a partner in the mother's care, and (3) childbearing is a partnership. The nurse can support the father in various ways (Box 26-6). Fewer women suffered postdelivery emotional upsets when their partners received support and assistance from parent education classes, physicians, midwives, and nurses throughout the childbearing cycle.

Self-Perception

The prepared mother generally feels more able to deal with labor and delivery than the unprepared one. Multigravidas generally have more confidence, since they have previous experience on which to draw. Women who have experienced problems during pregnancy or in past labors and deliveries may need reassurance that they can be successful. Even an unprepared woman can participate in simple breathing exercises with coaching from the nurse.

Women with a History of Sexual Abuse

Memories of sexual abuse can be triggered during labor by undergoing intrusive procedures such as vaginal examination; losing control; being confined to bed and "restrained" by monitors, intravenous lines, and epidurals; being watched by students; and experiencing intense sensations in the uterus and genital area, especially while pushing the baby out. Women who are survivors of abuse may fight the labor process by reacting in panic or anger toward care providers, may take control of everyone and everything related to their childbirth, may surrender by being submissive

Box 26-6 Supporting the Father

- Regardless of the degree of involvement desired, orient the father to the maternity unit, including the woman's labor room, the cafeteria, the waiting room, the nursery, and names and functions of personnel present.
- Respect his or their decisions as to his degree of involvement, whether the decision is active participation in the delivery room or just being kept informed. When appropriate, provide information on which he or they can base decisions; offer choice as opposed to coercion. This is their experience and their baby.
- Let him know when his presence has been helpful, and continue to reinforce this throughout labor.
- Offer to teach him comfort measures to the degree he wants to know them. Reassure him that he is not assuming the responsibility for observation and management of his partner's labor but supporting her as she progresses.
- Communicate with him frequently regarding her progress, procedures to be performed, what to expect from procedures, and what is expected of him.
- Prepare him for changes in her behavior and physical appearance.
- Remind him to eat; offer snacks and fluids if possible.
- Relieve him as necessary; offer blankets and a pillow if he is to sleep in a chair by the bedside. Acknowledge the stress of the situation on each partner and identify normal responses. The nonjudgmental attitudes of staff members help the father and the mother accept their own and the other person's behavior.
- Try to modify or eliminate unsettling stimuli (e.g., extra noise, extra light, chatter).

and dependent, or may retreat by mentally dissociating themselves from the sensations of labor and birth.

Help these women associate the sensations they are experiencing with the process of childbirth and not their past abuse. Maintain the woman's sense of control by explaining all procedures and why they are needed, validating her needs and paying close attention to her requests, proceeding at the woman's pace by waiting for her permission to touch her, accepting her reactions to labor, and protecting her privacy by limiting the exposure of her body and the number of people involved in her care. It is recommended that all laboring women be cared for in this manner, since they may choose not to reveal a history of sexual abuse.

Cognitive and Perceptual Issues

Pain is a major concern during labor and delivery. Breathing exercises help reduce discomfort, but as the intensity of labor increases, most women require some form of analgesia or anesthesia. The physician prescribes these medications with caution, since they pass through the placenta and affect the fetus. Timing is critical to prevent diminished or depressed respiratory effort at the time of birth. Carefully assess the condition of mother and fetus before and after medication administration.

The most commonly used analgesics are meperidine hydrochloride (Demerol) and butorphanol tartrate (Stadol), which may be given intramuscularly or intravenously. Antianxiety medications such as hydroxyzine (Vistaril) and diazepam (Valium) may be administered to reduce apprehension and anxiety. These medications also potentiate the effects of narcotics. Occasionally, sedative-hypnotics such as pentobarbital (Nembutal) and secobarbital (Seconal) are given in early labor to promote relaxation and rest.

The form of anesthesia used depends on the patient's wishes and the primary care practitioner's assessment of maternal and fetal need. Anesthetics are classified as general, regional, and local. Most vaginal deliveries today include a form of regional anesthetic (Figure 26-21). Regional anesthetics include paracervical, epidural, spinal, and pudendal blocks (Table 26-6; Figures 26-22 and 26-23).

GENERAL ANESTHESIA

General anesthesia is systemic pain control that involves loss of consciousness. It is rarely used for vaginal births, but still has a place in cesarean deliveries. Some women either refuse or are not good candidates for epidural or subarachnoid block, but require surgery. Occasionally a planned epidural or subarachnoid block proves inadequate for surgical anesthesia, or it may be necessary to perform a cesarean birth so quickly that no time is available to establish either type of regional block. General anesthesia may be required for emergency procedures at any stage of pregnancy, such as to repair injury from an accident or domestic violence.

Technique

Before induction of anesthesia, the woman breathes oxygen for 3 to 5 minutes or four deep breaths to increase her oxygen stores and those of her fetus for the short period of apnea during anesthesia induction. A wedge is placed under the woman's right side (or the operating table is tilted toward her left side) to displace the uterus from the aorta and inferior vena cava, promoting placental blood flow.

Adverse Effects of General Anesthesia

Major adverse effects are possible with the use of general anesthesia. **Maternal aspiration of gastric contents** can occur. Regurgitation with aspiration of acidic gastric contents is a potentially fatal complication. Aspiration of food particles may result in airway obstruction. Aspiration of acidic secretions causes chemical injury to the airways (aspiration pneumonitis). Infection often occurs after the initial lung injury. For purposes of general anesthesia, anesthesia providers assume a pregnant woman has a full stomach.

Respiratory depression may occur in either the mother or infant but is more likely in the baby if delivery is delayed after starting anesthesia.

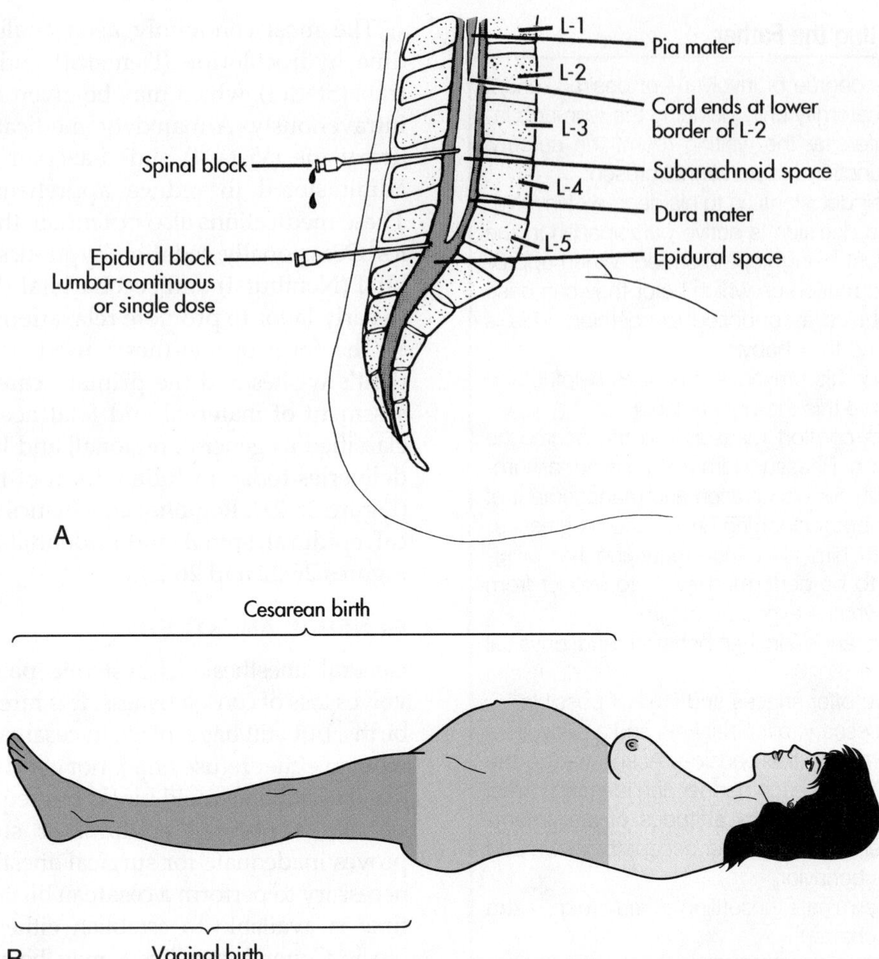

FIGURE 26-21 **A,** Regional anesthesia in obstetrics. **B,** Level of anesthesia necessary for cesarean delivery and vaginal delivery.

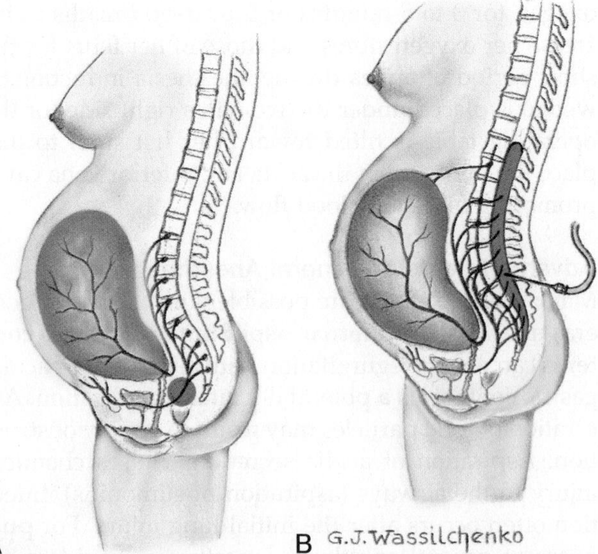

FIGURE 26-22 Pain pathways and sites of pharmacologic nerve blocks. **A,** Pudendal block: suitable during second and third stages of labor and for repair of episiotomy or lacerations. **B,** Epidural block: suitable for all stages of labor and for repair of episiotomy or lacerations.

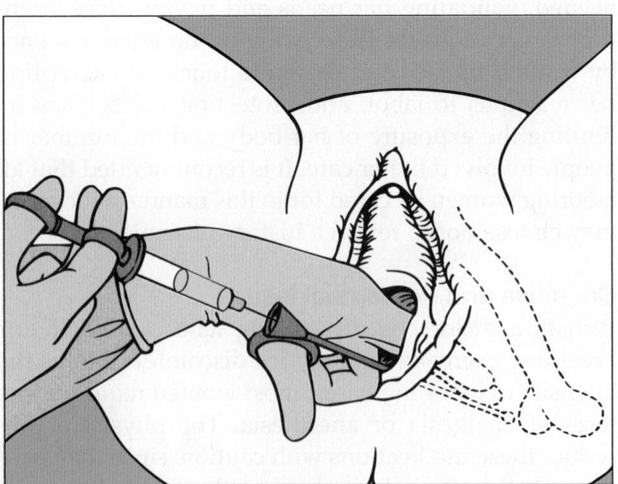

FIGURE 26-23 Pudendal block. Use of needle guide (Iowa trumpet) and Luer-Lok syringe to inject medication.

Table 26-6 Anesthesia for Labor and Delivery

TYPE OF ANESTHESIA	USUAL DOSAGE	ADMINISTRATION	AREA ANESTHETIZED OR EFFECTS	POSSIBLE SIDE EFFECTS		NURSING INTERVENTIONS AFTER ADMINISTRATION
				MOTHER	FETUS	
REGIONAL						
Paracervical block	5-10 mL of 1% solution of a "caine" drug	Injection, either side of cervix at 4 cm dilation	Cervix and uterus	Can slow labor	30% incidence of temporary slowing of fetal heart rate	Closely monitor fetal heart tones and maternal vital signs and contractions.
Pudendal block (see Figures 26-22 and 26-23)	5-10 mL of 1% solution of a "caine" drug	Injection into area of pudendal nerves for birth	Perineum	None unless allergic to drug	None	Provide reassurance and explanation; monitor fetal heart tones and maternal vital signs closely.
Caudal and lumbar epidural (see Figure 26-22)	5-15 mL of 1%, 1.5%, or 2% solution of a "caine" drug	Caudal canal Epidural space at 4 cm dilation	Pelvic region	Hypotension; cannot "push" for delivery; may slow labor if started too early	Slowing of fetal heart and fetal heart deceleration	Monitor fetal heart tones and maternal vital signs closely; use excellent aseptic techniques.
Saddle block (low spinal)	1-1.5 mL of solution; concentration dependent on "caine" drug used	Injection under dura of spinal cord for birth	Pelvic region	Postspinal headache, hypotension	None	Intravenous injection and oxygen are usually used.
GENERAL INHALATION						
Nitrous oxide		Inhaled through mask	Complete body	Could aspirate if vomits	Respiratory depression; hypoxia	Be alert and prepared for vomiting (with aspiration of food) and excessive uterine bleeding owing to uterine relaxation.
OTHER SIMILAR AGENT						
Thiopental sodium (Pentothal)	4 mg/kg	Intravenous	Complete body	Vomiting with aspiration, respiratory depression, arrhythmias	None	Monitor respiratory status closely.
INHALANT ANALGESIA						
Methoxyflurane (Penthrane)	0.3%-0.5% in first stage or at time of delivery	Volatile inhalant	Relieves pain	Hypotension; shallow, slow respirations	Hypoxia and central nervous system depression	Inform woman of what she will experience; allow her to administer as needed; do not hold mask for her. Check vital signs frequently.

Uterine relaxation can occur with some inhalational anesthetics. This characteristic is desirable for treating some complications, such as replacing an inverted uterus. However, postpartum hemorrhage may occur if the uterus relaxes after birth.

Methods to Minimize Adverse Effects

Measures to reduce the risk of maternal aspiration (or of lung injury, if aspiration occurs) include the following:

- Restrict intake to clear fluids or maintain nothing-by-mouth status if surgery is expected, such as with a scheduled cesarean birth.
- Administer drugs to raise the gastric pH and make secretions less acidic, such as sodium citrate and citric acid (Bicitra), ranitidine (Zantac), cimetidine (Tagamet), or famotidine (Pepcid).
- Administer drugs to reduce secretions, such as glycopyrrolate (Robinul).
- Use cricoid pressure (Sellick's maneuver) or block the esophagus by pressing the rigid trachea against it.

Avert neonatal respiratory depression by (1) reducing the time from induction of anesthesia until the umbilical cord is clamped and (2) keeping use of sedating drugs and anesthetics to a minimum until the cord is clamped.

To reduce the time from induction of anesthesia to cord clamping, prepare and drape the woman and alert the physicians before anesthesia is begun. Before cord clamping, the anesthesia is so light that the woman may move on the operating table as the incision is made, but she rarely remembers the experience or does not recall it as painful. The anesthesia level is deepened after the cord is clamped.

Values and Beliefs

Cultural beliefs and practices have implications for labor and delivery, as they do in all aspects of life. Respect the values and beliefs of women in labor. Seek information about specific cultural practices, values, and beliefs and incorporate these in the care plan (see Cultural Considerations box).

Non–English-Speaking Woman in Labor

A woman's level of anxiety in labor rises when she does not understand what is happening to her or what is being said. English-speaking women may feel some stress from a misunderstanding, but the effect on a non–English-speaking woman is more dramatic because she may feel a complete loss of control over her situation if no health care providers speak her language. She can panic and withdraw or become physically abusive when someone tries to do something she perceives might harm her or her baby.

Sometimes a support person is able to serve as a translator, though ideally a bilingual nurse will care for the woman. Alternatively, contact an employee or volunteer translator for assistance. If no one in the hospital is able to translate, call a translation service to translate over the telephone. For some women, a female translator may be more acceptable. If no translator is available, the labor and birth unit staff can prepare a set of cards with graphic depictions that illustrate common situations. Even when the nurse has limited ability to communicate verbally with the woman, in most instances efforts to communicate are meaningful and appreciated by the woman.

Cultural Considerations

Traditional Birth Practices of Various Cultural Groups

- Southeast Asia (China, Japan, Korea): Father usually not present; stoic response to pain; side-lying position preferred; may eat during labor; cesarean birth not desired; postpartum, ambulation is limited, and shower and bathing prohibited
- Laos: Squat for birth; prefer female attendants; father may or may not be present
- India: Father not present; natural childbirth methods used; female relatives present as caregivers
- Iran: Father not present; female caregivers and support people present at birth
- Hispanic: Stoic about pain until second stage; father and female relatives present; loud behavior in labor
- Native Americans: Birth may be attended by whole family; herbs may be used to promote uterine activity; prefer female attendant; birth may occur in the squatting position; herbs used to stop postpartum bleeding; bury placenta for good luck
- African American: May arrive at hospital in advanced labor; emotional support often provided by other women, especially the woman's mother; postpartum vaginal bleeding may be seen as sickness; tub baths and shampooing of hair prohibited; varied emotional responses: some cry out, some display stoic behavior to avoid calling attention to self

Data from D'Avanzo, C., & Geissler, E. (2003). *Pocket guide to cultural health assessment.* (3rd ed.). St. Louis: Mosby.

Precipitous Labor and Emergency Birth

Precipitous labor is defined as labor that lasts less than 3 hours from the onset of contractions to the time of birth. Precipitous labor may result from hypertonic uterine contractions that are tetanic-like in intensity. Maternal and fetal complications can result. Maternal complications include uterine rupture, lacerations of the birth canal, amniotic fluid embolism, and postpartum hemorrhage. Fetal complications include hypoxia resulting from decreased periods of uterine relaxation between contractions and intracranial hemorrhage related to rapid birth.

Women who experience precipitous labor often describe feelings of disbelief, alarm, panic, and finally relief when they arrive at the hospital. They express frustration when nurses do not believe that they are ready to push. Some women have difficulty remembering the details of their labor and birth and require others, including caregivers, to help them fill in the gaps in their memory. If the baby is responsive, a good intervention is to place the baby at the mother's breast. This will stimulate the uterus to contract.

❖ NURSING PROCESS *for Normal Labor*

The role of the licensed practical nurse/licensed vocational nurse (LPN/LVN) in the nursing process as stated is that the LPN/LVN will:

- Participate in planning care for patients based on patient needs
- Review patient's care plan and recommend revisions as needed
- Review and follow defined prioritization for patient care
- Use clinical pathways, care maps, or care plans to guide and review patient care

■ Assessment

Assessment begins with admission of the patient to the labor and delivery unit. Take a nursing history, including current labor, birth plan, current pregnancy and complications, previous pregnancies and complications, general medical history, and support system. Assess uterine contractions for frequency, duration, intensity, and resting tone. Assess FHR for baseline and decelerations. Assess cervical changes, condition of the membranes, and vaginal discharge. Also assess the patient's general physical status, including degree of pain or discomfort, and her psychosocial reaction to labor. The assessments, except for the history, are ongoing, with findings changing as the labor progresses.

■ Nursing Diagnosis

Nursing assessment helps identify the needs of the laboring patient. Care can then be based on these needs (Nursing Care Plan 26-1). Possible nursing diagnoses for a laboring patient include but are not limited to the following:

- Acute pain
- Fatigue
- Risk for infection
- Ineffective tissue perfusion (maternal)
- Risk for deficient fluid volume
- Impaired urinary elimination
- Risk for injury
- Deficient knowledge
- Anxiety
- Fear
- Social isolation
- Ineffective coping

■ Expected Outcomes and Planning

The care plan focuses on the needs of the laboring patient and the nurse's ability to meet those needs effectively. Each patient has differing needs, and care must be individualized accordingly. The care plan focuses on goals and outcomes specific to the nursing diagnosis. Examples include the following:

Goal 1: Patient will use techniques learned in prenatal childbirth classes to cope with pain during labor.

Outcome: Patient demonstrates ability to relax between contractions and effectively perform breathing techniques during contractions.

Goal 2: Patient's level of anxiety will remain mild to moderate as labor progresses.

Outcome: Patient participates in anxiety-reducing activities and dozes between contractions.

■ Implementation

Nursing interventions during labor include the following:

- Provide emotional support to both the patient and her coach or significant other.
- Maintain a supportive environment.
- Give physical care to provide comfort to the patient.
- Explain all procedures performed.
- Identify any factors that may indicate interference with labor.
- Provide encouragement throughout the labor process.
- Encourage verbalization of fears and concerns.
- Continually monitor the progress of the labor to ensure the safety and well-being of the mother and fetus.

■ Evaluation

Continually evaluate the effectiveness of the interventions. As the labor progresses, the focus and interventions will change. Refer to the goals and outcomes to determine whether the care plan was effective and the outcomes met. Examples include the following:

Goal 1: Patient will use techniques learned in prenatal childbirth classes to cope with pain during labor.

Evaluative measure: Observe the patient correctly performing breathing techniques during contractions.

Goal 2: Patient's level of anxiety will remain mild to moderate as labor progresses.

Evaluative measure: Ask patient to demonstrate relaxation techniques used to reduce anxiety (Box 26-7).

MEDICAL INTERVENTIONS

Although labor and delivery are essentially normal processes, sometimes complications arise. At times the physician needs to intervene to protect the mother or fetus.

Nursing Care Plan 26-1 The Patient with Spontaneous Rupture of Membranes

Ms. Grither is a 27-year-old gravida 2, para 1 at 39½ weeks of gestation who appears on the labor and delivery unit with spontaneous rupture of membranes and regular contractions every 3 minutes. She has had a normal pregnancy without complications and has an insignificant medical history. Her first pregnancy ended with a vaginal delivery of a 7-lb, 8-oz boy after a 10-hour labor.

NURSING DIAGNOSIS *Acute pain, related to the process of labor and birth*

Patient Goals and Expected Outcomes	Nursing Interventions	Evaluation
Patient will use techniques learned in prenatal classes to cope with pain of labor and birth Patient will have reduced pain with use of relief measures	Provide comfort measures to reduce anxiety, enhance relaxation, and increase the effectiveness of pain relief measures (see Table 26-3): • Back massage with sacral counterpressure • Cold, moist cloth to forehead • Frequent change of position • Hygienic care: sponge bath, perineal care Use alternative measures for pain relief: • Effleurage • Relaxation, guided imagery, focal points • Breathing Administer analgesics safely. Encourage use of techniques and provide positive reinforcement.	Patient performs breathing techniques during contractions. Patient uses techniques and expresses their effectiveness. Patient expresses pain reduction with use of analgesics and other pain relief measures.

NURSING DIAGNOSIS *Anxiety, related to the childbirth experience*

Patient Goals and Expected Outcomes	Nursing Interventions	Evaluation
Patient's level of anxiety will be maintained at a mild to moderate level Patient will participate in anxiety-reducing activities	Encourage use of childbirth relaxation techniques (see Box 26-7). Review birth plan with patient and coach. Use comfort measures to facilitate relaxation (see Box 26-7). Use calm, confident, caring approach. Encourage expression of feelings. Inform patient and coach of progress and procedures. Maintain privacy. Administer medications as necessary.	Patient's anxiety is reduced through breathing techniques and guided imagery with assistance of coach. Patient dozes between contractions.

Critical Thinking Questions

1. Ms. Grither's labor is progressing normally with continuous monitoring. Suddenly the fetal heart rate drops to 90 bpm with late decelerations with each contraction. What should the nurse do now? Explain the reason for these actions.
2. Ms. Grither and her coach have been working well together to manage her labor, using a focal point, breathing techniques, and guided imagery. Suddenly she becomes irritable and tells her coach, "Don't touch me!" Her coach is bewildered by this change in behavior. How should the nurse explain Ms. Grither's behavior to her coach? How can the nurse help the coach continue to be effective during this time?

INDUCTION

As discussed, the exact cause of labor is unknown. Induction is an attempt to start labor at a chosen time, rather than waiting for it to begin spontaneously. This intervention may be necessary when membranes have been ruptured for longer than a few hours, in cases of severe pregnancy-induced hypertension, or in a post-term pregnancy. Occasionally an elective induction is performed when the woman has a history of precipitous labor (lasting less than 3 hours). This is done to prevent an emergency out-of-hospital delivery.

The primary care practitioner assesses each woman carefully to determine that she is a good candidate for induction and that no harm will come to either mother or fetus. The medically approved methods of inducing labor include amniotomy, prostaglandin gel application, and oxytocin stimulation.

Box 26-7 Nurse's Role in Relaxation and Breathing Techniques

FIRST STAGE

Goal: Promote Relaxation of Abdominal Muscles

- Provide support during contractions: coach breathing, give back rubs, provide cool cloths.
- Provide distracting activities: guided imagery, focal point, effleurage (rhythmic stroking of abdomen by woman), progressive muscle relaxation, breathing techniques, music.
- Provide support and reminders for previously learned breathing techniques. If no specific method has been learned, encourage the following pattern:
  —Early, or latent, phase: slow, deep chest or abdominal breathing, six to nine breaths/min; inhale through nose and out through pursed lips.
  —Middle, or active, phase: Slow acceleration, then deceleration of breaths through contraction; breaths shallow; approximately 16 to 20 breaths/min.
  —Transitional phase: four to six pants followed by a blow for duration of contraction.
- Remind patient to use breathing techniques only during contractions and normal breathing patterns between contractions.
- Remind patient to take deep, cleansing breath before and after contraction to increase oxygen intake.
- Remind patient to avoid rapid breathing, which leads to hyperventilation, because this can result in decreased oxygenation to fetus, as well as symptoms for the mother.

SECOND STAGE

Goal: Increase Abdominal Pressure and Assist in Expelling Fetus

- Assist patient with natural bearing-down effort (BDE) or urge to push.
- Help patient into a position that will facilitate BDE during contractions: upright (squatting on bed), semirecumbent with shoulders curved and knees bent, lateral (raise and support upper leg during BDE).
- Assist patient with breathing during BDE:
  —Two deep, cleansing breaths at contraction onset; take a breath, hold a few seconds, then push while exhaling in short (7-second) periods.
  —Two deep, cleansing breaths at contraction end.
- Help patient into a position of comfort between contractions.
- Provide encouragement for effort and encourage relaxation techniques between contractions.
- Remind patient to pant during contraction if BDE is to be avoided.

Amniotomy

If the amniotic membranes have not ruptured, the primary care practitioner may use a sterile hook-shaped instrument to open the sac and allow the fluid to drain; this procedure is called an **amniotomy** (or artificial rupture of the fetal membrane). Measure FHR immediately before and after this procedure. Assess the amount and color of amniotic fluid. If all criteria for induction are met, labor typically starts within 6 to 8 hours.

Prostaglandin Gel Application

After assessment of the mother and fetus, the primary care practitioner applies prostaglandin E (PGE) gel intracervically using a plastic catheter (see Table 26-3). Contractions normally begin within an hour of instillation of the gel. Carefully monitor vital signs, FHR, and contractions. It is common for an amniotomy to be performed in conjunction with the gel application. An internal fetal monitor is also routinely applied when PGE gel is used. In most facilities the LPN/LVN does not apply this gel but does monitor and assess labor progress.

Oxytocin Stimulation

Use of oxytocin is indicated to induce labor or to stimulate a labor that is not making adequate progress because of **uterine inertia** (absence or weakness of uterine contractions). A dilute form of the medication is administered intravenously. Pitocin is most commonly used, although Syntocinon, a synthetic form of oxytocin, is occasionally used (see Table 26-3). These medications are powerful and are started by the primary care practitioner or a specially trained nurse, if hospital policies permit. After induction, monitor the progress of labor. Because the contractions that result from oxytocin can be very strong, monitor the FHR and contractions carefully and document care. Stop the infusion and contact the primary care practitioner if there are signs or symptoms of complications, such as changes in FHR; bradycardia; tachycardia; arrhythmias; or excessive frequency, duration, or pressure of contractions.

FORCEPS DELIVERY

Forceps are a spoonlike device that fits around the fetal head to aid in expulsion. As with induction, certain criteria must be met before the primary care practitioner uses forceps. The nurse assisting in the delivery is responsible for providing the type of forceps requested by the primary care practitioner. Closely monitor the FHR before and during the forceps maneuvers. Also explain to the mother that these actions will help the baby.

VACUUM EXTRACTION

An alternative to forceps delivery is vacuum extraction, which involves attaching a vacuum cup to the fetal head and applying negative pressure. Criteria for this procedure include vertex presentation, ruptured membranes, complete dilation of the cervix, and lack of cephalopelvic disproportion. During this procedure assess the FHR frequently and encourage the mother to remain active in the birth process by pushing with contractions. The most common neonatal findings after this procedure are caput succedaneum, edema of the scalp, and circular bruising of the scalp. Reassure the parents that these conditions are temporary.

CESAREAN DELIVERY

Cesarean birth is delivery through an abdominal and uterine incision. This type of delivery may be anticipated or be performed in cases of emergency. The number of cesarean deliveries has increased greatly during the past 30 years. Despite concerns in the medical community and the media about this trend, more than 25% of all deliveries continue to take place by the cesarean route.

Indications for cesarean birth can be maternal or fetal. The major maternal indications for cesarean delivery are (1) **fetopelvic disproportion** (also called cephalopelvic; the head of the fetus is larger than the pelvic outlet), so that the fetus is unable to pass through the maternal pelvis; (2) previous cesarean delivery; (3) breech presentation; (4) medical conditions that would endanger the mother's health, such as cardiac complications; (5) abnormal conditions of the placenta, such as placenta previa; (6) infections of the vaginal canal; and (7) pelvic abnormalities. The major fetal indicators are (1) fetal oxygen deprivation (hypoxia); (2) prolapse of the umbilical cord; (3) breech presentation; (4) malpresentations, such as transverse; and (5) congenital anomalies. These conditions are discussed in greater depth in Chapter 28.

Current medical practice is rethinking at least one of these criteria. The old rule was "once a cesarean, always a cesarean." Today many women who have previously delivered by cesarean are candidates for vaginal birth after cesarean (VBAC). Depending on the woman's medical history, the nature of this pregnancy, and the reason for the earlier cesarean, the primary care practitioner may permit a trial labor. In these cases the woman must be carefully monitored, and the facility must be prepared to perform an emergency cesarean if complications arise (Box 26-8).

To perform a cesarean delivery, the primary care practitioner makes incisions in both the abdominal and the uterine walls. Depending on the technique used, several different incisions may be employed.

Nursing diagnoses and interventions for the patient delivering by cesarean include but are not limited to the following:

Nursing Diagnoses	Nursing Interventions
Risk for infection, related to a surgical procedure	Monitor and document vital signs and FHR. Maintain good aseptic technique during vaginal examinations, catheterization, and preoperative skin preparation. Monitor blood loss and white blood cell count. Administer antibiotics as ordered. Monitor and encourage fluid intake.
Situational self-esteem, related to change in birth plan	Discuss changes in birth plan, including the reason for the changes. Encourage patient to verbalize feelings about cesarean birth. Provide positive reassurance. Involve patient in decision making. Accept patient's own pace in working through grief or crisis situations.

Box 26-8 Vaginal Birth After Cesarean Birth

Approximately 60% to 80% of women with one low transverse uterine incision from a previous cesarean birth have successful vaginal births. Women who had their previous cesarean for a nonrecurring reason, such as breech presentation, are more likely to have a successful vaginal birth after cesarean birth (VBAC) than women who had their previous cesarean for dystocia. Women who have had a vaginal birth before or since the prior cesarean birth are more likely to have successful VBAC.

Candidates for VBAC include the following:

- A woman who has one or two previous low transverse uterine incisions but no other uterine scars (e.g., removal of fibroid tumors) or a previous uterine rupture
- A pelvis that is clinically adequate for the estimated fetal size

Management of women who plan VBAC includes the following considerations:

- External cephalic version may be as successful for women having a previous cesarean as for women with an unscarred uterus.
- Epidural analgesia and anesthesia may be used.
- Induction and augmentation of labor with oxytocin may be done. Use of prostaglandin gel appears to be safe. Misoprostol (Cytotec) is currently contraindicated.
- Most authorities recommend electronic fetal monitoring.
- Immediate availability of a physician during active labor if an emergency cesarean is needed.
- Availability of anesthesia and personnel to perform an emergency cesarean.

Adapted from McKinney, E.S., et al. (2005). *Maternal-child nursing.* (2nd ed.). St. Louis: Mosby.

Get Ready for the NCLEX® Examination!

Key Points

- Although various theories have been proposed, the process that starts labor has not been determined.
- True labor and false labor can be confusing to the patient and health care personnel; even knowledgeable individuals can be mistaken.
- The birth process can occur in a variety of settings. The most important concern is protecting the welfare of both the mother and the newborn.
- Vaginal delivery involves a complex interrelationship of the passageway, the passengers, and the powers.
- The first stage of labor is usually the longest. Both mother and fetus face significant risks during this time and must be carefully and continually assessed.
- Fetal monitoring, using internal or external sensors, enhances the nurse's ability to monitor labor and recognize signs of fetal distress.
- Many women are trained in specific breathing techniques designed to reduce pain and facilitate control of the birthing process. Be prepared to assist with these.
- The fourth stage of labor, the time of stabilization, requires careful nursing assessment of the mother. Assess vital signs and perform fundal checks to detect excessive blood loss.
- Episiotomies may be performed and lacerations may occur even during "normal" childbirth. Their appropriate and prompt repair is essential.
- The Apgar scoring system is used 1 and 5 minutes after birth to assess the newborn's condition.
- Modification of functional health patterns occurs during labor and delivery. Assess all areas to detect problems quickly and report them promptly.
- In some cases the primary care practitioner may have to intervene in the process of labor and delivery and use forceps or surgical means to deliver a healthy newborn.
- Facilitate mother-infant attachment by meeting the new mother's physical, support, and teaching needs.
- If any laboring woman states "The baby is coming!" anticipate an immediate birth.

Additional Learning Resources

Go to your companion CD for an audio glossary, animations, video clips, and more.

evolve Be sure to visit the Evolve site at http://evolve.elsevier.com/Christensen/foundations/ for additional online resources.

Review Questions for the NCLEX® Examination

1. A 23-year-old primigravida arrives on the labor unit in early labor. Which assessment finding would indicate that labor has begun?
   1. Decreased vaginal secretions
   2. Weight gain of 1 to 3 pounds
   3. Bloody show
   4. Increased fetal movement

2. To determine fetal lie, presentation, and position, the caregiver uses which assessment technique?
   1. Abdominal ultrasonography
   2. Fetal heart tone auscultation
   3. Palpation of contractions
   4. Leopold's maneuvers

3. During the initial assessment, the nurse determines that the fetal position is ROA. Where is the fetal presenting part in relation to the maternal pelvis?
   1. The occiput is facing the right side and the front of the maternal pelvis.
   2. The mentum is facing the right side and the front of the maternal pelvis.
   3. The occiput is facing the left side and the back of the maternal pelvis.
   4. The sacrum is facing the right side and the front of the maternal pelvis.

4. A woman is having regular contractions. To assess the frequency of her labor contractions, time:
   1. the interval between the peaks of the contractions.
   2. the beginning of one contraction to the beginning of the next.
   3. the end of one contraction to the beginning of the next.
   4. how many contractions she has in a 15-minute period.

5. A woman asks the nurse when she will have an internal fetal monitor applied. The best answer is:
   1. "Because you have had a low-risk pregnancy, you are not considered a candidate for internal monitoring."
   2. "Your health care provider decides when to apply the internal monitor."
   3. "Your cervix must be 2 to 3 cm dilated and your membranes ruptured before an internal monitor can be applied."
   4. "We can apply the internal monitor at any time after your membranes rupture."

6. A woman tells the nurse she thinks her membranes have ruptured. What action by the nurse will best validate rupture of membranes?
   1. Feel the drawsheet for wetness.
   2. Perform a Nitrazine test.
   3. Insert a Foley catheter into her bladder.
   4. Have her cough.

7. A woman has progressed through her labor without difficulty. However, the fetal heart rate has been decreasing with each contraction for the past 15 minutes. The rate decreases from 150 to 125 bpm after the peak of the contraction and returns to 150 bpm 15 seconds after the contraction is finished. The nurse concludes that the patient is having:
   1. variable decelerations.
   2. early decelerations.
   3. late decelerations.
   4. combination decelerations.

8. When the woman enters the transition phase to active labor, which behaviors would the nurse expect to see?
   1. A desire for personal contact and touch
   2. Sleepiness and quietness, with a desire for touch
   3. Responsiveness to teaching
   4. Irritability, resistance to touch, withdrawal

9. As the woman's labor progresses, which assessment finding would indicate that the second stage of labor has begun?
   1. Passage of a mucous plug
   2. Bearing-down reflex
   3. Dilation of the cervix to 7 cm
   4. Change in shape of the uterus

10. Which fetal heart rate finding would be a concern during the woman's labor?
    1. Accelerations
    2. Early decelerations
    3. Average FHR of 126 bpm
    4. Late decelerations

11. Which maternal cardiovascular finding is expected during labor?
    1. Increased cardiac output
    2. Increased pulse rate
    3. Decreased white blood cell count
    4. Decreased blood pressure

12. The nurse notes accelerations with fetal movement. These:
    1. are reassuring.
    2. are caused by umbilical cord compression.
    3. warrant close observation.
    4. are caused by uteroplacental insufficiency.

13. The patient delivers an 8-pound, 1-ounce boy. Ten minutes later there is a sudden gush of blood from her vagina. At the same time the woman's uterus becomes globular in shape and the umbilical cord lengthens. What do these findings probably indicate?
    1. Separation of the placenta
    2. Uterine hemorrhage
    3. Cervical or vaginal laceration
    4. Uterine involution

14. A woman pregnant for the first time is dilated 3 cm, with contractions every 5 minutes. She is groaning and perspiring excessively and states that she did not attend childbirth classes. The most important nursing action is to:
    1. notify the woman's health care provider.
    2. administer the prescribed narcotic analgesic.
    3. ensure that her labor will be overseen.
    4. give simple breathing and relaxation instructions.

15. When planning care for a woman whose membranes have ruptured, the nurse recognizes that the woman's risk for which of the following has increased?
    1. Intrauterine infection
    2. Hemorrhage
    3. Precipitous labor
    4. Supine hypotension

True Labor or False Labor

Identify each of the following as true labor (TL) or false labor (FL).

16. _____ Contractions rarely follow a pattern.

17. _____ Contractions frequently stop with ambulation or position change.

18. _____ Contractions seem to start in the lower back and then travel to the lower abdomen.

19. _____ The cervix softens, effaces, and dilates.

20. _____ There is no significant change in fetal position.

chapter

27

Care of the Mother and Newborn

evolve

Elaine Oden Kockrow

http://evolve.elsevier.com/Christensen/foundationsadult

Objectives

1. Describe postpartum assessment of the mother.
2. Identify the physiologic changes that occur in the post-partum period.
3. Discuss the nursing responsibilities during the postpartum period.
4. Explain the importance of teaching personal and infant care.
5. Discuss the psychosocial adaptations that occur after birth.
6. Discuss interventions to prevent infant abductions.
7. Describe the assessment of the normal newborn.
8. Identify the physical characteristics of the normal newborn.
9. Identify normal reflexes observed in the newborn.
10. Explain common variations that may be observed in the newborn.
11. Describe the behavioral characteristics of the newborn.
12. Discuss nursing interventions for the circumcised newborn.
13. Explain parent-child attachment (bonding).
14. Discuss nutritional needs and feeding of the newborn.
15. Discuss quieting techniques for the fussy newborn.
16. Discuss discharge teaching and postpartum home care.

Key Terms

acrocyanosis (ăk-rō-sī-ă-NŌ-sĭs, p. 867)
autolysis (aw-TŎL-ĭ-sĭs, p. 842)
circumcision (p. 875)
colostrum (kŏ-LŎS-trŭm, p. 874)
cryptorchidism (krĭp-TŎR-kĭ-dĭz-ĕm, p. 869)
diaphoresis (dī-ă-fŏ-RĒ-sĭs, p. 844)
diuresis (dī-ŭr-RĒ-sĭs, p. 844)
engorgement (ĕn-GŎRJ-mĕnt, p. 857)
fontanelles (FŎN-tă-nĕlz, p. 867)
gynecomastia (jĭn-ĕ-kō-MĂS-tē-ă, p. 869)
harlequin sign (HĂR-lĕ-kwĭn, p. 867)
Homans' sign (p. 857)
involution (p. 842)
lactation (p. 844)
lanugo (p. 867)
latch-on (p. 858)
lochia (LŌ-kē-ă, p. 842)
meconium (p. 876)
parent-child attachment (bonding) (p. 877)
polydactyly (pŏl-ē-DĂK-tĕ-lē, p. 869)
prolactin (p. 844)
pseudomenstruation (sū-dō-mĕn-strū-Ā-shŭn, p. 869)
puerperium (pū-ĕr-PĔR-ē-ŭm, p. 841)
syndactyly (sĭn-DĂK-tĕ-lē, p. 869)
vernix caseosa (VĔR-nĭks kăs-ē-Ō-să, p. 867)

The postpartum period, also called the **puerperium,** lasts from the time the woman delivers the placenta until the reproductive organs return to approximately the nonpregnant size and position. The puerperium lasts about 3 to 6 weeks and consists of two stages. The immediate postpartum period, lasting up to 6 hours after delivery, is sometimes called the **fourth stage of labor,** or the recovery stage. The new mother requires special care and attention after the difficulties of delivery. This is a time for close observation and assessment to ensure that no problems occur. The later postpartum stage follows the stage of recovery and lasts until about 6 weeks after delivery.

During the postpartum period the mother's body makes rapid physiologic adaptations. The anatomical and physiologic changes that took place over 9 months reverse within just 6 weeks. Many psychological changes also occur as the woman and her family adjust to the new family member or members.

ANATOMIC AND PHYSIOLOGIC CHANGES OF THE MOTHER

REPRODUCTIVE ORGANS

Uterus

After the birth of the baby and delivery of the placenta, the uterus contracts in response to **oxytocin** (a hormone produced by the posterior pituitary gland that stimulates uterine contractions and release of milk in the mammary glands [let-down reflex]). This contraction compresses blood vessels at the site where the placenta separated from the uterine wall. This site, an area 3 to 4 inches (8 to 10 cm) in diameter, has open venous sinuses. If the uterus does not contract adequately, the woman may lose too much blood. The placental site heals through exfoliation, in which necrotic tissue is sloughed from the uterine lining, leaving a fresh layer of endometrial tissue free from scars. This process is necessary for successive pregnancies to occur.

Immediately after delivery the uterine fundus is about midway between the umbilicus and symphysis pubis or slightly higher. It weighs approximately 2 pounds (907 g). Within 12 hours it rises to the level of the umbilicus at midline. After 24 to 48 hours it begins a gradual descent, and within a week it will be barely palpable at the level of the symphysis pubis and weigh 1 pound (453 g). Within 6 weeks the uterus will again be a pelvic organ approximately the nonpregnant size of 2 ounces (57 g). This decrease in size is called **involution** (Figure 27-1).

After contracting, the muscle fiber does not return to its original length but remains slightly shortened. This unique attribute of uterine muscle aids in preventing postdelivery hemorrhage and results in involution.

Involution is carried out by a process called autolysis. **Autolysis** (the self-dissolution or self-digestion that occurs in tissues or cells by enzymes in the cells themselves) is a result of sudden withdrawal of estrogen and progesterone, which releases proteolytic enzymes into the endometrium. These enzymes cause the cells to lose protein materials and thereby shrink. The number of muscle cells remains the same, but the size of each cell changes dramatically.

The fluid waste discharged after delivery is called **lochia** and consists of blood, tissue, and mucus. As the uterine lining is shed, the necrotic tissue, blood, and mucus leave the body through the vagina. Lochia has a fleshy odor similar to that of menstrual discharge. For the first day or two after delivery, the lochia is made up mostly of blood, resulting in a bright red drainage called **lochia rubra.** As the placental site heals, the discharge becomes pink to brown and is called **lochia serosa.** After the seventh day the drainage is slightly yellow to white and is called **lochia alba.** This continues for another 10 days to 2 weeks. If

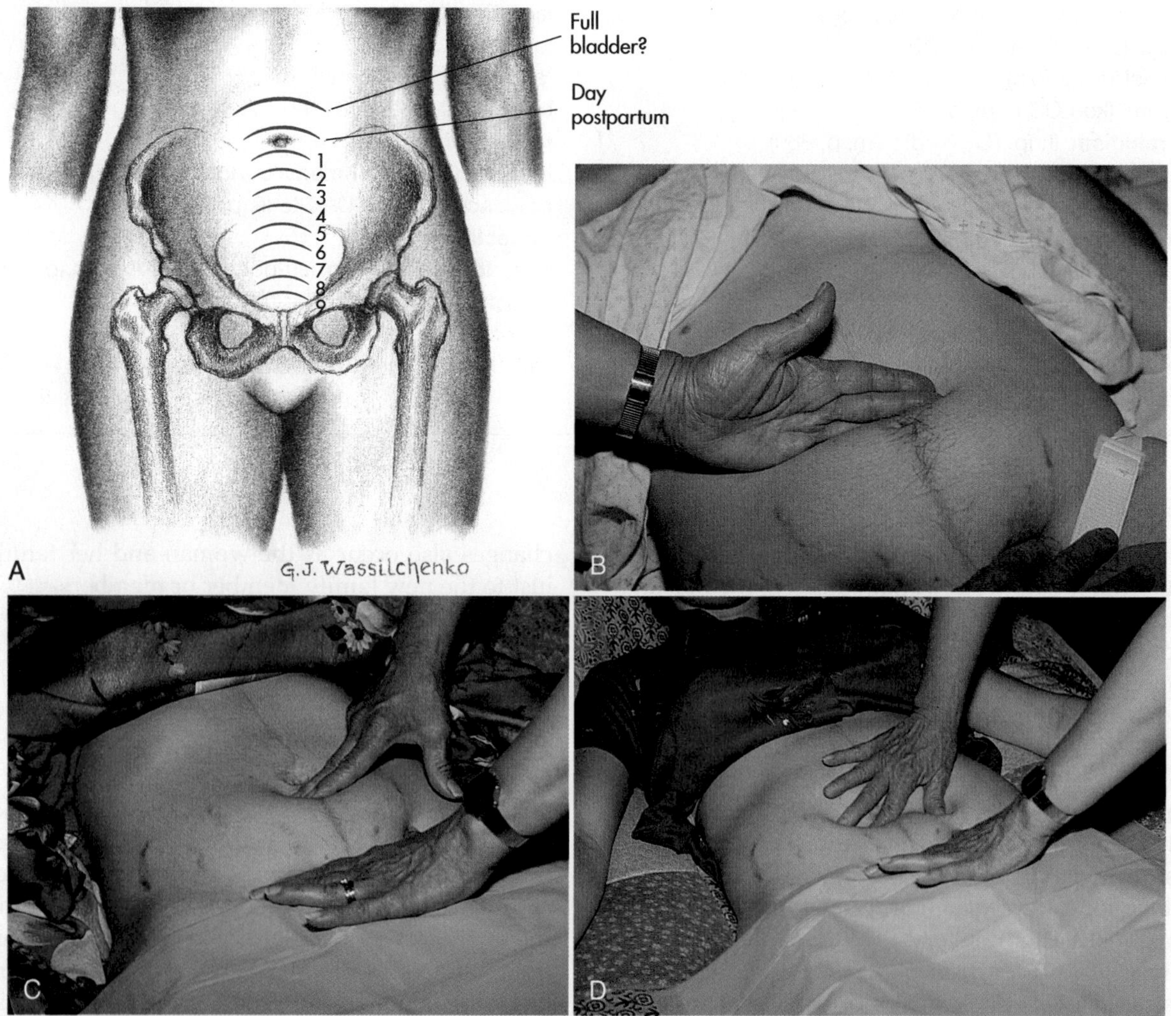

FIGURE 27-1 Assessment of involution of uterus after delivery. **A,** Normal progress, days 1 through 9. **B,** Size and position of uterus 2 hours after delivery. **C,** Two days after delivery. **D,** Four days after delivery.

fragments of the placenta remain in the uterus, the uterus will not be able to contract and seal blood vessels adequately. This can result in excessive blood loss and may require surgical intervention (Table 27-1). See Box 27-1 for signs and symptoms of hypovolemic shock and nursing interventions.

Cervix, Vagina, and Perineum

The cervix appears edematous, with bruising. The external cervical os has a ragged, slitlike appearance instead of being round as seen in the nulliparous woman. The vagina is thin and dry, with an absence of rugae. Vaginal mucus production returns with the return of estrogen production. Rugae reappear in 4 weeks.

The perineum may have some edema and bruising also. The episiotomy (if present) should be free of erythema, with the edges well approximated and without discharge. It should heal in 2 to 3 weeks. Lacerations of the perineum are classified from first to fourth degree, depending on depth of involvement. The repaired laceration should also have well-approximated edges and no drainage. Healing time depends on laceration depth. Return of these areas to the nonpregnant state should be complete in 6 to 8 weeks.

Lacerations of the Genital Tract

Lacerations of the cervix, the vagina, and the perineum are also causes of postpartum hemorrhage. Hemorrhage related to lacerations should be suspected if bleeding continues despite a firm, contracted uterine fundus. This bleeding can be a slow trickle, an oozing, or frank hemorrhage.

Factors that can lead to obstetric lacerations of the lower genital tract include operative birth, precipitous birth, congenital abnormalities of the maternal soft parts (vulva perineum), and a contracted pelvis. Other causes include size, abnormal presentation, and position of the fetus; relative size of the presenting part to the size of the birth canal; scarring from prior vaginal infections, injury, or surgery; and vulvar, perineal, and vaginal varicosities. Extreme vascularity in the labia and periclitoral area often results in profuse bleeding if laceration occurs. Pelvic hematomas (i.e., a collection of blood in the connective tissue) may be vulvar, vaginal, or retroperitoneal in origin. Vulvar hematomas are the most common. They usually are visible and painful. Vaginal hematomas are typically associated with a forceps-assisted birth, episiotomy, or primigravidity. Retroperitoneal hematomas are the least common but are life threatening. They are caused by laceration of one of the vessels attached to the hypogastric artery, usually because of the rupture of a cesarean scar during labor.

Most acute injuries and lacerations of the perineum, the vagina, the uterus, and their support tissues occur

Table 27-1 Lochia and Nonlochia Bleeding

LOCHIA	NONLOCHIA BLEEDING
Lochia usually trickles from the vaginal opening. The steady flow is greater as the uterus contracts.	If the blood discharge spurts from the vagina, there may be cervical or vaginal tears in addition to the normal lochia.
A gush of lochia may result as the uterus is massaged. If it is dark in color, it has been pooled in the relaxed vagina, and the amount soon lessens to a trickle of bright red lochia (in the early puerperium).	If the amount of bleeding continues to be excessive and bright red, a tear may be the source.

Box 27-1 Hypovolemic Shock

SIGNS AND SYMPTOMS

- Woman has persistent significant bleeding (perineal pad soaked within 15 minutes); this may not be accompanied by a change in vital signs or maternal color or behavior.
- Woman states she feels weak, lightheaded, "funny," "sick to my stomach," or "sees stars."
- Woman begins to act anxious or exhibits air hunger.
- Woman's skin turns ashen or grayish.
- Skin feels cool and clammy.
- Pulse rate increases.
- Blood pressure declines.

INTERVENTIONS

- Notify primary health care provider.
- If uterus is atonic, massage gently and expel clots to cause uterus to contract; compress uterus manually, as needed, by using two hands. Add oxytocic agent to intravenous (IV) drip, as ordered.
- Give oxygen by face mask or nasal prongs at 8 to 10 L/min.
- Tilt the woman to her side or elevate the right hip; elevate her legs to at least a 30-degree angle.
- Provide additional or maintain existing IV infusion of lactated Ringer's solution or normal saline solution to restore circulatory volume.
- Administer blood or blood products, as ordered.
- Monitor vital signs.
- Insert an indwelling urinary catheter to monitor perfusion of kidneys.
- Administer emergency drugs, as ordered.
- Prepare for possible surgery or other emergency treatments or procedures.
- Chart incident, medical and nursing interventions instituted, and results of treatments.

during childbirth. Some injuries to the supporting tissues, whether they were acute or nonacute and whether they were repaired or not, may lead to gynecologic problems later in life (e.g., pelvic relaxation, uterine prolapse, cystocele, and rectocele). Immediate repair promotes healing, limits residual damage, and decreases the possibility of infection.

The tendency to sustain lacerations varies with each woman; in some women the soft tissue may be less distensible. Heredity may be a factor in this. For example, the tissue of light-skinned women, especially those with reddish hair, is not as readily distensible as that of darker-skinned women, and healing may be less efficient.

Perineal lacerations. Perineal lacerations are the most common of all injuries in the lower genital tract. They usually occur when the fetal head is being born. The extent of the laceration is defined in terms of its depth:

- **First degree:** Laceration extends through the skin and structures superficial to muscles.
- **Second degree:** Laceration extends through muscles of perineal body.
- **Third degree:** Laceration continues through the sphincter muscle.
- **Fourth degree:** Laceration also involves the anterior rectal wall.

Perineal injury is often accompanied by small lacerations on the medial surfaces of the labia minora below the pubic rami and to the sides of the urethra and the clitoris. Lacerations in this vascular area often result in profuse bleeding; such lacerations must be repaired with absorbable suture.

Pay special attention to third- and fourth-degree lacerations so that the woman retains fecal continence. Take measures to promote soft stools for a few days to increase the woman's comfort and to foster healing. Antimicrobial therapy may be used in some cases.

Vaginal and urethral lacerations. Vaginal lacerations often occur in conjunction with perineal lacerations. Vaginal lacerations tend to extend up the lateral walls (sulci) and, if deep enough, involve the levator ani muscle. Additional injury may occur high in the vaginal vault near the level of the ischial spines. Vaginal vault lacerations may be circular and may result from forceps rotation, especially when there is cephalopelvic disproportion, rapid fetal descent, or precipitous birth. Lacerations can also occur around the urethra (periurethral) and in the area of the clitoris.

Cervical injuries. Cervical injuries occur when the cervix retracts over the advancing fetal head. These cervical lacerations occur at the lateral angles of the external os; most are shallow, and bleeding is minimal. Larger lacerations may extend to the vaginal vault or beyond the vault into the lower uterine segment; serious bleeding may occur. Extensive lacerations may follow hasty attempts to enlarge the cervical opening artificially or to deliver the fetus before full cervical dilation is achieved. Injuries to the cervix can have adverse effects on future pregnancies and childbirths.

Nursing interventions for episiotomy, lacerations, and hemorrhoids are listed in Box 27-2.

Breasts

Breast changes begin early in pregnancy. Increased amounts of estrogen stimulate enlargement of breast size by increasing adipose tissue and fluid retention. Estrogen also stimulates the growth of the milk ducts to prepare for **lactation** (function of secreting milk or period during which milk is secreted). Milk production is necessary if a woman plans to breastfeed her infant. This is a basic yet complex process.

The first secretion produced by the breast is colostrum. This precursor to milk is thin, watery, and slightly yellow. It is rich in protein, calories, antibodies, and lymphocytes. Women, particularly multigravidas, may produce colostrum as early as the second trimester of pregnancy. Its production continues for about 2 days after delivery, when true milk production begins.

Lactation is a combination of hormonal, neurologic, and psychological responses. After delivery, estrogen and progesterone levels diminish rapidly. As they drop, the level of prolactin increases. **Prolactin,** a hormone secreted by the anterior pituitary gland, is responsible for stimulating milk production in the mammary alveolar cells. Stimulation of the nipples, particularly by the infant's sucking, causes the release of oxytocin from the posterior pituitary gland. Oxytocin stimulates contraction of the mammary ducts, and milk is ejected from the breast. This cycle is called the **let-down reflex.**

OTHER BODY SYSTEMS

Cardiovascular

Blood volume is reduced to nonpregnant levels by 2 to 4 weeks after delivery. **Diuresis** (the increased formation and secretion of urine) and **diaphoresis** (the secretion of sweat, especially when profuse) account for most of the fluid loss. Blood loss during delivery accounts for an additional 300 to 500 mL (600 to 800 mL with cesarean delivery). Cardiac output also declines rapidly. The patient is at risk for thrombus formation as a result of elevation of platelets in the early postpartum period.

Urinary

As a result of trauma, increased bladder capacity, and the effects of conduction anesthesia, after childbirth women have a decreased urge to void. In addition, pelvic soreness caused by forceps used during labor, vaginal lacerations, or the episiotomy reduces or alters the voiding reflex. Decreased voiding combined with postpartal diuresis may result in bladder distention. Immediately after giving birth, the woman may bleed excessively if the bladder becomes distended because

Box 27-2 Interventions for Episiotomy, Lacerations, and Hemorrhoids

CLEANSING
- Wash hands before and after cleaning perineum and changing pads.
- Explain procedure.
- Wash perineum with mild soap and warm water at least once daily.
- Cleanse from symphysis pubis to anal area.
- Apply peripad from front to back, protecting inner surface of pad from contamination.
- Wrap soiled pad and place in covered waste container.
- Change pad with each void or defecation or at least four times per day.
- Assess amount and character of lochia with each pad change.

ICE PACK
- Apply a covered ice pack to perineum from front to back:
  —During first 2 hours to decrease edema formation and increase comfort
  —After the first 2 hours following the birth to provide anesthetic effect

SQUEEZE BOTTLE
- Demonstrate for and assist woman; explain rationale.
- Fill bottle with tap water warmed to approximately 100.4° F (38° C) (comfortably warm on the wrist).
- Instruct woman to position nozzle between her legs so that squirts of water reach perineum as she sits on toilet.
- Explain that it will take whole bottle of water to cleanse perineum.
- Remind her to blot dry with toilet paper or clean wipes.
- Remind her to avoid contamination from anal area.
- Apply clean pad.

SITZ BATH

Built-in Type
- Prepare bath by thoroughly scrubbing with cleaning agent and rinsing. Pad with towel before filling.
- Explain procedure.
- Fill one half to one third with water of correct temperature (100.4° to 105° F [38° to 40.6° C]). Some women prefer cool sitz baths; add ice to lower the temperature to a comfortable level.
- Encourage woman to use at least twice a day for 20 minutes.
- Place call bell within easy reach.
- Teach woman to enter bath by tightening gluteal muscles and keeping them tightened and then relaxing them after she is in the bath.
- Place dry towels within reach.
- Ensure privacy.
- Check on woman in 15 minutes; assess pulse as needed.

Disposable Type
- Clamp tubing and fill bag with warm water.
- Raise toilet seat, place bath in bowl with overflow opening directed toward back of toilet.
- Place container above toilet bowl.
- Attach tube into groove at front of bath.
- Loosen tube clamp to regulate rate of flow; fill bath to half full; continue as above for built-in sitz bath.

DRY HEAT
- Inspect lamp for defects.
- Cover lamp with towels.
- Position lamp 50 cm from perineum; use three times a day for 20-minute periods.
- Provide draping over woman.
- If same lamp is being used by several women, clean it carefully between uses.
- Teach woman regarding use of 40-watt bulb at home.

TOPICAL APPLICATIONS
- Apply anesthetic cream or spray; use sparingly three or four times a day.
- Offer witch hazel pads (Tucks) after voiding or defecating; woman pats perineum dry from front to back, then applies witch hazel pads. Explain rationale.

it pushes the uterus up and to the side and prevents the uterus from firmly contracting. Later in the puerperium, overdistention can make the bladder more susceptible to infection and delay the return of normal voiding. With adequate emptying of the bladder, bladder tone is usually restored 5 to 7 days after childbirth, with daily urinary output of up to 3 L common.

Neurologic

Neurologic changes during the puerperium result from a reversal of maternal adaptations to pregnancy or from trauma during labor and childbirth. Pregnancy-induced neurologic discomforts abate after birth. Through diuresis, edema is eliminated, relieving carpal tunnel syndrome by easing compression of the medial nerve. The periodic numbness and tingling of fingers that affect 5% of pregnant women usually disappear after birth, unless lifting and carrying the baby aggravate the condition.

Headache requires careful assessment. Postpartum headaches may be caused by various conditions, including gestational hypertension, stress, and leakage of cerebrospinal fluid into the extradural space during placement of the needle for epidural or spinal anesthesia. Depending on the cause and effectiveness of the treatment, the headaches can last from 1 to 3 days to several weeks.

Gastrointestinal

Appetite generally returns to normal immediately after delivery. However, gastric motility may continue to decline, leading to constipation. Normal bowel elimination should resume within 2 or 3 days after delivery. Decreased abdominal tone and tenderness from the episiotomy or hemorrhoids may make the patient reluctant to strain for a bowel movement.

Endocrine

Placental hormone levels rapidly fall after delivery and are soon undetectable or at their nonpregnant values. Estrogen and progesterone levels drop markedly after expulsion of the placenta, reaching their lowest levels 1 week into the postpartum period. Decreased estrogen levels are associated with breast engorgement and with the diuresis of excess extracellular fluid that has accumulated during pregnancy. The estrogen levels in nonlactating women begin to rise by 2 weeks after birth and are higher by postpartum day 17 than in women who breastfeed. The anterior pituitary secretes prolactin, but only in response to nipple stimulation. Other endocrine glands (thyroid, adrenal, and pancreas) return to prepregnant size and function.

Musculoskeletal

Abdominal muscle tone returns and joint stabilization occurs over a 6- to 8-week period after delivery. The return of muscle tone depends on previous tone, proper exercise, and the amount of adipose tissue. Some pelvic joints may never fully return to their prepregnant position. Patients may feel discomfort in the joints immediately after delivery because of secretion of the hormone relaxin. However, even when all other joints return to their normal pregnant state, those of the parous woman's feet do not. The new mother may notice a permanent increase in shoe size.

Integumentary

Chloasma of pregnancy usually disappears at the end of pregnancy. Hyperpigmentation of the areola (the area encircling the nipple) and linea nigra (a dark line on the abdomen of a pregnant woman, usually extending from the symphysis pubis midline to the umbilicus) may not disappear completely after childbirth. Some women have permanent darker pigmentation of those areas. Striae gravidarum (stretch marks) on the breasts, the abdomen, and the thighs may fade but usually do not disappear.

Vascular abnormalities such as spider angiomas (nevi), palmar erythema, and epulis generally regress as estrogen rapidly declines after the end of pregnancy. For some women, spider nevi persist indefinitely.

The abundance of fine hair seen during pregnancy usually disappears after giving birth; however, any coarse or bristly hair that appears during pregnancy usually remains. Fingernails return to their prepregnancy consistency and strength.

Profuse diaphoresis in the immediate postpartum period is the most noticeable change in the integumentary system. This is common, especially at night during the first week postpartum.

Immune

No significant changes in the maternal immune system occur during the postpartum period. Determine whether the mother needs a rubella vaccination or Rh_o(D) immune globulin (RhoGAM) for prevention of Rh isoimmunization.

TRANSFER FROM THE RECOVERY AREA

After the initial recovery period of 1 to 2 hours, the woman may be transferred to a postpartum room in the same or another nursing unit. In labor, delivery, recovery, postpartum (LDRP) room settings, the nurse who provided care during the recovery period usually continues caring for the woman. In the labor, delivery, recovery (LDR) room or a traditional setting, the woman is transferred to a separate unit where the postpartum nursing staff provides her care. Women who have received general or regional anesthesia must be cleared for transfer from the recovery area by a member of the anesthesia care team. In some settings the baby remains with the mother wherever she goes. In other facilities the baby is taken to the nursery for several hours of observation during the mother's initial recovery period.

In preparing the transfer report, the recovery nurse uses information from the admission record, the birth record, and the recovery record. Information that is communicated to the postpartum nurse includes health care provider; gravidity and parity; age; anesthetic used; medications given; duration of labor and time of rupture of membranes; oxytocin induction or augmentation; type of birth and repair; blood type and Rh status; state of rubella immunity; syphilis and hepatitis serology test results; intravenous (IV) infusion of any fluids; physiologic status since birth; description of fundus, lochia, bladder, and perineum; infant's sex and weight; time of birth; pediatrician; chosen method of feeding; any abnormalities noted; and assessment of initial parent-infant interaction.

Most of this information is also documented for the nursing staff in the newborn nursery. In addition, provide specific information on the infant's Apgar scores, weight, voiding, and feeding since birth. Also record nursing interventions that have been completed (e.g., prophylaxis, vitamin K injection).

NURSING ASSESSMENT OF AND INTERVENTIONS FOR THE MOTHER

HEALTH MANAGEMENT AND HEALTH PERCEPTION

Women with uncomplicated deliveries remain in the hospital a short time after giving birth. It may be only hours, or it may be 1 or 2 days after delivery. Even women who delivered by cesarean are rarely kept more than 5 to 7 days. This may be a result of financial concerns, type of insurance coverage, or personal preference. Early discharge is usually a patient's choice. Some choose to go home as early as 36 hours after delivery. Because early discharge is increasingly common, it is important to assess the woman's ability to meet her own needs and those of her infant. Parent-newborn relationship assessments are vital.

Discuss the home situation. If any aspect of the home situation appears unsafe or questionable, make an appointment with a social worker before discharge. Also review self-care concerns, including postpartum danger signs (Box 27-3) and the importance of medical follow-up. Review infant and self-care activities and family planning information.

Parent-Newborn Relationships

The mother's reaction to the sight of her newborn may range from excited laughing, talking, and even crying to apparent apathy. A polite smile and nod may acknowledge the comments of nurses and primary care practitioners. Occasionally the mother appears angry or indifferent, turns away from the baby, concentrates on her own pain, or makes hostile comments. These varying reactions can arise from pleasure, exhaustion, or deep disappointment. Whatever the reaction and cause may be, the mother needs continuing acceptance and support from all the staff. A written form accompanying the baby's chart should record the parents' reaction at birth. How did the parents look? What did they say? What did they do? (Box 27-4.)

Childbearing practices and rituals of other cultures may be different from standard practices associated with bonding in the Anglo-American culture. For example, Chinese families traditionally use extended family members to care for the newborn so the mother can rest and recover, especially after a cesarean birth. In some cultures, women do not initiate breastfeeding until their breast milk comes in. In other cultures, families do not name their babies until after the confinement month. The amount of eye contact also varies among cultures.

Become knowledgeable about the childbearing beliefs and practices of diverse cultural and ethnic groups. Because individual cultural variations exist within groups, clarify with the patient and family members or friends what cultural norms the patient follows. Incorrect judgments may be made about mother-infant bonding if you do not practice culturally sensitive care.

Some warning signs of possible difficulties in parent-child relationships, apparent immediately after delivery, are listed in Box 27-5.

Maternal Self-Image

An important assessment concerns the woman's self-concept, body image, and sexuality. How a new mother feels about herself and her body during the puerpe-

Box 27-4 Assessing Attachment Behaviors

- When the infant is brought to the parents, do they reach out for the infant and call the infant by name? (Recognize that in some cultures parents may not name the infant in the early newborn period.)
- Do the parents speak about the infant in terms of identification: Whom the infant looks like, what appears special about their infant compared with other infants?
- When parents are holding the infant, what kind of body contact is there: Do parents feel at ease changing the infant's position? Do they use fingertips or whole hands? Are there parts of the body they avoid touching or parts of the body they investigate and scrutinize?
- When the infant is awake, what kinds of stimulation do the parents provide: Do they talk to the infant, to each other, or to no one? How do they look at the infant: direct visual contact, avoidance of eye contact, or looking at other people or objects?
- How comfortable do the parents appear in terms of caring for the infant? Do they express any concern regarding their ability or disgust for certain activities, such as changing diapers?
- What type of affection do they demonstrate to the newborn, such as smiling, stroking, kissing, or rocking?
- If the infant is fussy, what kinds of comforting techniques do the parents use, such as rocking, swaddling, talking, or stroking?

Box 27-3 Postpartum Maternal Danger Signs

- Fever with or without chills
- Malodorous vaginal discharge
- Excessive amount of vaginal discharge
- Bright red vaginal bleeding after it has changed to pink or rust
- Edema; erythematous or painful area on the legs
- Pain or burning sensation with urination or an inability to void
- Breast changes such as localized pain, heat, edema, or malodorous drainage
- Pain in the perineal or pelvic area

Box 27-5 Postpartum Danger Signs for Parent-Newborn Relationships

- Passive reaction, either verbal or nonverbal (Parents do not touch, hold, or examine baby or talk in affectionate terms or tones about baby.)
- Hostile reaction, either verbal or nonverbal (Parents make inappropriate verbalization, glances, or disparaging remarks about child's physical characteristics.)
- Disappointment over sex of baby
- Lack of eye contact
- Nonsupportive interaction between parents (If interaction seems questionable, talk to nurse and physician involved with delivery for further information.)

Box 27-6 Resumption of Sexual Intercourse

- A woman can safely resume sexual intercourse by the second to fourth week after birth when bleeding has stopped and the episiotomy has healed. For the first 6 weeks to 6 months postpartum, the vagina does not lubricate well.
- The physiologic reactions to sexual stimulation for the first 3 months after birth will be slower and less intense. The strength of the orgasm is reduced.
- A water-soluble gel, cocoa butter, or a contraceptive cream or jelly might be used for lubrication. If some vaginal tenderness is present, the partner can insert one or more clean, lubricated fingers into the vagina and rotate them within the vagina to help relax it and to identify possible areas of discomfort. A position in which the woman has control of the depth of the insertion of the penis also is useful. The side-by-side or female-on-top position may be more comfortable.
- The presence of the baby influences postbirth lovemaking. Parents hear every sound made by the baby; conversely they may be concerned that the baby hears every sound they make. In either case, any phase of the sexual response cycle may be interrupted by hearing the baby cry or move, leaving both partners frustrated and unsatisfied. In addition, the amount of psychological energy expended in child care activities may lead to fatigue.
- Some women report feeling sexual stimulation and orgasms when breastfeeding their babies. Breastfeeding mothers often are interested in returning to sexual activity before nonnursing mothers.
- Instruct the woman to correctly perform Kegel exercises to strengthen the pubococcygeal muscle. This muscle is associated with bowel and bladder function and with vaginal feeling during intercourse.

rium may affect her behavior, adaptation to parenting, and sexuality.

Feelings related to sexual adjustment after childbirth often cause concern for new parents. Women who have recently given birth may be reluctant to resume sexual intercourse for fear of pain or damage to healing perineal tissue. Because many new parents are anxious for information but reluctant to bring up the subject, postpartum nurses should matter-of-factly include the topic of postpartum sexuality during their routine physical assessment. While examining the episiotomy site, for example, the nurse can say, "I know you are sore right now, but it probably won't be long until you [you and your partner] are ready to make love again. Have you thought about what that might be like? Would you like to ask me questions?" (Box 27-6). This approach assures the woman and her partner that resuming sexual activity is a legitimate concern for new parents and indicates the nurse's willingness to answer questions.

Promoting Parenting Skills

Parents are responsive to praise of their newborn. Many require reassurance that the baby's blue appearance after delivery is normal until respirations are well established. Review the reason for the molding of the baby's head. Repeat information about the hospital's routine for future parent-child contacts. Encourage siblings to get acquainted with the new family member (Figure 27-2). The hospital staff, by their interest and their concern, can do much to make this experience satisfying for parents, family, and significant others.

One of the main concepts to stress is that parenthood is a learned role. As such, parenthood takes time to master, improves with experience, and evolves gradually and continually as the needs of the parent and child change. Parents first become acquainted with their new baby as the nurse performs a physical examination and describes any normal variations. Nurses act as role models by providing loving, attentive care (Boxes 27-7 and 27-8). As one nurse described it:

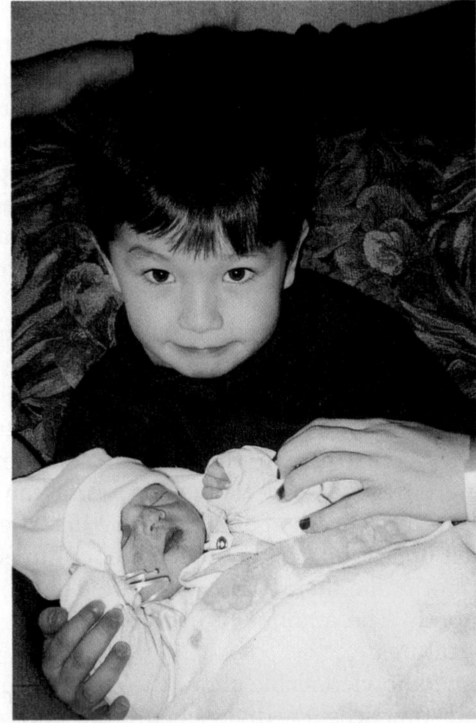

FIGURE 27-2 Sibling involvement.

> I found the mother crying and distraught as she wrapped and unwrapped her baby. She said, "I don't seem to be doing anything right." I took the baby from her and talked to him, "What are you doing to your mother? You have her all upset!" The baby alerted to my voice and looked at me. Then I said to the mother, "Now you talk to him." She said, "You're a big, lovely boy; don't cry so much." The baby hearing her voice, promptly turned his head to look at her. I said, "You see, he knows his mother's voice and prefers it to mine." The mother was surprised and seemed very pleased and excited. We then reviewed how to wrap a baby snugly.

Box 27-7 Postpartum Maternal Teaching Summary

FUNDUS (HEIGHT, MASSAGE)
- Fundus height will go down one fingerbreadth a day.
- It will be back into pelvis in 10 days.
- It feels firm, like a softball.
- Report bogginess to primary care practitioner immediately.
- May have cramping with nursing.

LOCHIA (AMOUNT, CHANGES, WARNING SIGNS)
- First 3 days, lochia will be dark red, like menstrual flow; 2 or 3 days after this, it will be pinkish brown.
- Moderate flow: four to eight lightly saturated pads a day.
- Flow continues for 3 to 4 weeks.
- The last couple of weeks, it will be a yellowish color with a musty, stale odor.
- Report any foul-smelling or bright red discharge or large clots.
- If overactive, flow may increase. Rest; if flow does not subside, notify primary care practitioner.

PERINEUM (EPISIOTOMY CARE, CLEANSING, HEALING, DOUCHING, TAMPONS)
- Take sitz baths two or three times daily with vaginal delivery.
- Cleanse from front to back.
- Use perineal spray water bottle after voiding.
- Change pad frequently—after each voiding and when soiled.
- Do not douche or use tampons until after first office visit when primary care practitioner says it is okay.
- Continue using witch hazel (Tucks pads) for discomfort and to aid in healing.
- Episiotomy will heal in approximately 3 weeks (when the lochia has stopped).

BREASTS
- **Breastfeeding** (nipple care, engorgement, feeding techniques, breast pump)
  —Air dry; use proper technique to break infant's suction to the nipple; use Massé Breast cream if ordered; wear a good supportive bra.
  —Can become pregnant while nursing; use a contraceptive.
  —For engorgement, apply heat, warm shower; may pump to enable baby to latch on.
  —Feeding techniques: demonstrate proper use; advise where to purchase materials; demonstrate manual expression; expressed milk may be frozen in plastic bottles or bags for up to 2 weeks.
  —May take a mild analgesic 1 hour before nursing.
- **Dry breasts** (engorgement, fluid intake)
  —Wear supportive, well-fitting bra.
  —Avoid breast stimulation (warm showers).
  —Apply ice bags for 20 minutes four times a day.
  —It takes about 5 days to suppress lactation.
  —Do not drink excessive amounts of fluids (normal: six to eight 8-ounce glasses).

NUTRITION (NURSING, DIETING)
- Continue prenatal vitamins until gone.
- Nursing: need 500 kcal more than prepregnant diet; need increased protein, 400 mg calcium each day, 8 to 10 glasses of fluid each day; avoid onions, cabbage, chocolate, spices, and foods that may distress infant; no dieting during breastfeeding.

SEXUALITY (SEXUAL ACTIVITY) (See Box 27-6)
- Forty-five percent of nonnursing mothers resume menses by sixth week.
- Breastfeeding does not protect against pregnancy.
- Avoid sexual activity until after first postbirth office visit and approval by primary care practitioner.
- If episiotomy is not healed and sexual activity is resumed, there is increased discomfort and chance of infection.

EXERCISE (WHEN, HOW MUCH)
- Increased lochia or pain means you need to reevaluate activity.
- Do not resume strenuous exercises until primary care practitioner approves.
- Gradually increase activity.

EMOTIONS (BONDING, "BABY BLUES")
- Parent-child attachment (bonding): schedule time to enjoy baby; use eye contact, cuddling, and caressing; enjoy infant feedings.
- Postpartum blues:
  —May be tearful or anorexic and have difficulty sleeping.
  —Hormonal factors and fatigue are often responsible.
  —Notify primary care practitioner if prolonged, increased, or unmanageable.

CESAREAN BIRTH (INCISION, ACTIVITY)
- Notify primary care practitioner of any redness, drainage, separation of incision, temperature greater than 100.4° F (38° C).
- Do not lift anything heavier than baby, gradually increase activity.
- Take pain medications as ordered and needed.

REPORT TO PRIMARY CAREGIVER
- Temperature greater than 100.4° F (38° C).
- Chills.
- Change in lochia: foul odor, return to bright red, excessive amount.
- Calf pain, tenderness, or swelling.
- Evidence of mastitis: breast tenderness, cracking, redness, or a feeling of discomfort or uneasiness.
- Urinary urgency, burning, or frequency.
- Severe or incapacitating depression.

SAFETY (CAR SEAT SAFETY FILM, CAR SEAT DEMONSTRATION)
- Review infant safety from baby discharge sheet.
- Review car seat safety film if available.
- Volunteers have car seats to rent.
- Demonstrate proper use of car seat.

NOTE: Many facilities give a booklet to each new mother titled *The New Mom's Handbook.* Written material enhances verbal instruction.

Box 27-8 Newborn Teaching Summary

SECURITY

- Know the caregiver. Check references.
- Ask others who are trusted to babysit.
- Do not leave baby alone on flat surface because the baby could roll over and off the surface.
- Do not lay baby on abdomen; place on the side or back to prevent sudden infant death syndrome (SIDS).
- Car seat safety and law:
  - —Use until age 4 years or 40 pounds.
  - —Infant in car seat should be secured in back seat facing the rear of the car.
  - —This is the law in most states; if you are stopped, you could be fined.

BATH DEMONSTRATION AND NORMAL SKIN CONDITIONS

- Skin should be soft, pinkish, and dry.
- Clean perineum from front to back to prevent urinary tract infections.
- Use hypoallergenic soap. Most babies need bathing only every other day.
- Keep diaper area as clean as possible. (Use no powder.)
- Keep head clean, rinsing well after each shampoo to prevent cradle cap.

UMBILICAL CORD CARE

- Use alcohol on cord stump daily. (Be careful to prevent alcohol from dripping down to perineal area.)
- Keep area dry; fold diaper down with plastic side on outside to prevent moisture retention.
- Sponge bathe for 7 to 10 days until umbilical cord comes off. (Do not soak in bath water.)
- Report any redness, drainage, or foul odor coming from umbilical area.

CIRCUMCISION CARE

- If a Gomco or Mogan clamp was used, apply petroleum jelly–covered gauze to penis after every diaper change. Keep area clean to prevent infection; cleanse penis carefully with warm water at least every 4 hours.
- If a Plastibell is used, the plastic rim remains in place for about a week while healing takes place, after which the Plastibell will fall off. Petroleum gauze is not necessary.
- Do not allow pressure on circumcised area. Loose diapering is necessary.
- Do not be alarmed when a yellowish crust forms; this is part of the normal healing process. Do not attempt to remove this crust; it will last only 2 or 3 days. Fanfold the diaper so that it does not press on the area.

EYE CARE

- Wash with water from inner to outer corner with a different area of the washcloth for each eye.
- Note that a special treatment was administered to baby's eyes on delivery. This may cause some swelling and redness. Do not be alarmed; this is normal.

DIAPER AREA CARE

- Change diaper as soon as possible.
  - —Wash from front to back, especially on girls, to prevent urinary tract infection.
- Cleanse with warm water and mild soap; dry well
- If rash persists, call the physician.
- Use no powder. If possible, have diaper area open to the air.

FEEDING METHOD

Breast

- Position: Entire body of infant should face the breast.
  - —Feed baby before he or she gets frantic and very hungry.
  - —Lightly brush the infant's lips with the nipple to start the rooting reflex.
  - —Alternate breasts with each feeding.
  - —Direct the nipple into infant's mouth with as much of the areola tissue in the baby's mouth and over the tongue as possible.
  - —Gently hold breast away from baby's nostrils; babies are nose breathers.
  - —To break suction, place finger under nipple; do not pull breast away from baby.
  - —Mothers who have cesarean births need to support infant so that he or she does not rest on the abdomen for long periods.
- Burping baby:
  - —Burp between breasts, over the shoulder, sitting up supported by your hands, or lying across your lap.
- Length of time to nurse:
  - —Feed for 10 to 15 minutes from each breast.
  - —It is important to empty both breasts because an empty breast signals the woman's body to produce more milk.
- Supplement: You may pump your breast while away from baby; keep breast milk cold during transport.
  - —Breast milk can be safely stored in a refrigerator for 24 to 48 hours.
  - —If breast milk will not be used within 48 hours, it should be frozen immediately after being expressed. Breast milk may be frozen for 2 weeks.
  - —To thaw, gently shake container under warm tap water or place breast milk in a container of warm water. Thawed breast milk should be used immediately. It should not be refrozen. Do not use a microwave to thaw or heat breast milk.
  - —After the milk supply is established, an occasional bottle will not affect lactation or breastfeeding.
- Stooling pattern: Stools of breastfed babies are loose. Some infants have a stool with each feeding.

Bottle

- Positions:
  - —Never prop the bottle.
  - —Hold the bottle so that fluid fills the nipple and none of the air in the bottle is allowed to enter the nipple.
  - —Avoid overfeeding; be alert to infant cues that enough formula has been taken (e.g., falls asleep, turns head to side, or ceases to suck).
- Burping baby:
  - —Burp baby every 0.5 to 1 oz of milk.
  - —Position baby over the shoulder, sitting up supported by your hands, or lying across your lap.
- Preparing bottles:
  - —Purchase formula in ready-to-use powder or in liquid concentrate to be mixed with water.

Box 27-8 Newborn Teaching Summary—cont'd

—Prepare formulas with scrupulous cleanliness unless home conditions or the water supply is unsafe (such as from a private well); then water should be boiled for 15 minutes.
—Many helpful pamphlets on formula preparations are available.
—Give formula at room temperature; test formula temperature on inner wrist or back of hand.
—Opened container of ready-to-feed or concentrated formula should be discarded after 24 hours; date the opened container.
—After feeding, position baby on right side to discourage regurgitation.

CLOTHING
- Dress infant for the season.
- Dress infant in soft, comfortable clothing.
- Dress infant as you are dressed.

VAGINAL AND BREAST SECRETIONS
- As the maternal hormones clear the infant's bloodstream, the infant may have a mucuslike, bloody vaginal discharge.
- Both girl and boy babies may have a swelling of the breast tissue, and sometimes a thin discharge may be seen; this will subside as the mother's hormones are eliminated from infant's body.

BULB SYRINGE
- Squeeze out air to establish suction by compressing the bulb and holding it in.
- Gently insert tip of syringe into the side of infant's mouth and release; then suction the nares.
- Clean well after each use.

INFANT CARDIOPULMONARY RESUSCITATION
- Be sure to see film before dismissal if available.
- Teaching:
  —Give fingertip compressions (5 to 1).
  —Give puffs for breaths (1 to 5).
  —Cover baby's nose with cheek as you cover mouth.
  —Avoid stretching back too far in the head-tilt/chin-lift.

PHENYLKETONURIA, BIOTINIDASE, AND THYROID TESTING
- These tests should be performed on all newborns.
- Undetected abnormalities could lead to brain damage or death. With early detection and proper treatment, these are preventable.

AFTER DISCHARGE
- Keep, read, and refer to pamphlets if you have any questions.
- Use medication prescribed only by a physician. (Do not use nose drops because aspiration may result in lung complications.)

WHEN TO CALL PHYSICIAN
- If baby develops sudden fever, rash, excessive vomiting, diarrhea, distended abdomen, or bleeding from circumcision, call the physician.
- Normal body temperature ranges from 97.6° to 99° F (36.4° to 37.2° C) when taken via the axillary route. This method is recommended until age 6 years.

NUTRITIONAL AND METABOLIC ISSUES

Recovery Stage

After the time and exertion involved in labor and delivery, the mother is often hungry. Most physicians allow a meal after delivery if the woman is alert and not nauseated. Fluids are important during the recovery phase to replace the fluids and blood lost during delivery; offer a variety of fluids such as water and juices. If the physician orders IV fluids, administer them promptly. When a general anesthetic has been used, such as during a cesarean delivery, verify the **presence of bowel sounds** before giving solid food.

If the woman has been using mouth-breathing techniques during labor, she may have dry mucous membranes, cracked lips, and noticeable breath odor. Good oral hygiene relieves these symptoms and reduces discomfort. A complete sponge bath enhances well-being and comfort by removing perspiration and other waste products from the skin.

Later Postpartum Stage

Diet remains an important concern postpartum. Many women are concerned about the weight gained during pregnancy and wish to lose the excess as soon as possible. It is important that dieting not deprive the woman of necessary nutrition. If the woman has not gained excessive weight during pregnancy, she usually returns to her prepregnant weight in 6 to 8 weeks without dieting. Most physicians do not recommend any weight-loss diets until after this time. Women who are not breastfeeding should continue to eat well-balanced diets that follow MyPyramid suggestions (see Figure 21-1). Women who are breastfeeding generally continue the diet recommended during pregnancy, since the body requires extra calories, vitamins, and minerals for lactation. The breastfeeding mother should maintain the increased caloric intake of 300 to 500 kcal/day as part of a well-balanced diet and should maintain a daily fluid intake of 2 to 3 L.

HYGIENE

During the postpartum stage, excessive perspiration and a slight odor from drainage are common. Encourage regular bathing (showers are preferred) to minimize odors and promote comfort. Most women are permitted to be up ad lib and prefer to shower and shampoo by themselves. They may experience vertigo as a result of vascular shifts related to the heat of the shower. If this occurs while standing in the shower, the woman may experience syncope and injure herself. The first time the newly delivered woman takes a shower, provide for safety by instructing her on use of the emergency call signal and the length of shower time recommended, and provide a chair in the shower room. Also check the patient frequently during her first shower to verify she is safe. Tub baths are not recommended until after the postpartum examination at 6 weeks so that no water that has been contaminated with body wastes enters the vaginal canal or uterus until healing is completed.

The physician sometimes orders sitz baths to reduce discomfort and promote healing of the perineum. Vasodilation from the warm water helps reduce edema and speed tissue repair. Instruct the patient about water temperature and length of time. As with a shower, vascular changes may occur; check on the patient regularly to promote safety. It is important that proper cleaning of equipment take place between patients if community facilities are used (Figure 27-3). Some facilities use a personal, portable sitz bath that the patient can take home at discharge.

If the woman has delivered by cesarean, she has an abdominal incision with sutures or staples. Assess this incision in the same manner as any other surgical incision. It should remain approximated with no erythema, little exudate, and no malodor (foul odor). The incision may be left open to the air or a surgical dressing applied, depending on the physician's orders. Some physicians apply Steri-Strips rather than a dressing over the incision. If no dressing is used to protect the wound, care should be taken so clothing does not irritate the incision. Usually the patient may shower with a plastic cover over the incision.

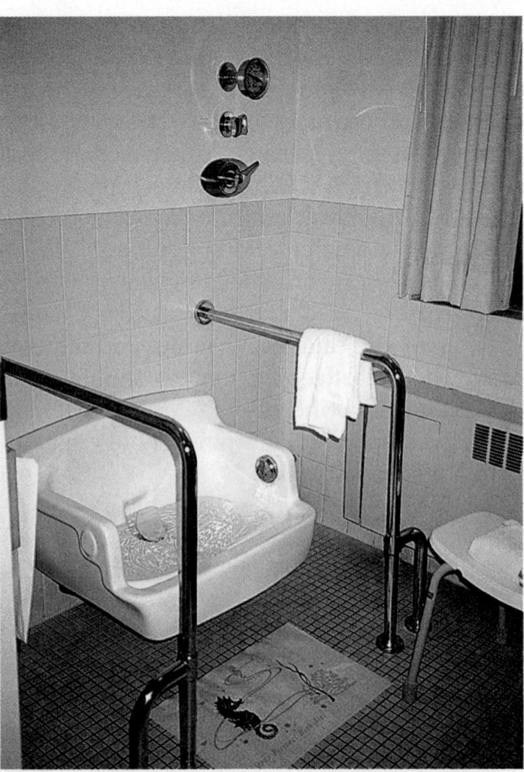
FIGURE 27-3 Sitz bath for perineal care.

ELIMINATION

Recovery Stage

Diuresis and diaphoresis are common immediately after delivery. If the woman received IV fluids, urinary output may be increased. Support the bladder above the symphysis pubis and palpate it to check for fullness. Encourage voiding, since a full bladder may interfere with complete contraction of the uterus, potentially causing hemorrhage.

Many times the tissue edema from the delivery makes voiding difficult. The initial voiding should occur within 4 to 6 hours after delivery. Some agencies have a policy to assess voidings three times in measurable amounts of 300 mL or more after delivery to determine urinary elimination. Try measures to stimulate voiding. If these are unsuccessful, catheterization may be required. An indwelling catheter is routinely inserted before cesarean delivery and may remain in place for 1 or 2 days after delivery.

Later Postpartum Stage

Because most women are fatigued and the perineum is still painful, you must encourage the woman to void at regular intervals of 2 to 4 hours. If the woman is voiding frequently and in small amounts (less than 100 mL), suspect retention with overflow. Also question the patient about any symptoms of urgency, frequency, or dysuria. If any of these is noted, report it promptly. Incomplete emptying of the bladder prevents the uterus from contracting normally; it also predisposes the patient to urinary tract infections.

Review proper cleansing technique after delivery. Instruct the woman to gently cleanse and pat dry from the anterior to posterior of the perineum. This method of cleansing prevents microorganisms from the rectal area being transported to the cleaner urinary or vaginal areas. After each urination or bowel movement she should do proper cleansing using a plastic squeeze bottle with a pointed tip filled with warm (100° F [37.7° C]) water. Cleansing with toilet tissue is discouraged until the episiotomy or laceration is healed.

Ideally, bowel elimination should occur before discharge from the hospital. Fear of discomfort because of an edematous, painful episiotomy or hemorrhoids may result in the woman's resisting the urge to defecate. Bowel peristalsis may continue to be slowed. When this fact is combined with decreased activity and loss of abdominal tone, constipation may result. To prevent this, many physicians order bulk enhancers or stool softeners. Occasionally, suppositories are administered to promote bowel evacuation. Inspect the perineum to detect problems and assure the patient that no harm will come from normal elimination. Stress the importance of adequate bulk in the diet and adequate fluid intake. Sitz baths can also soothe the perineum and promote bowel elimination.

Cesarean birth patients, particularly those who received general anesthesia, are likely to develop problems with bowel function. The combination of general anesthesia and lost abdominal tone increases the risk of ileus, so pay close attention to bowel function and report any abnormal observations promptly. To promote bowel function, assist with and encourage the patient to ambulate periodically throughout the day.

Perineal pads, worn to absorb vaginal drainage, should be changed after each urination or defecation. Teach the woman the importance of correct application and changing of the pad. Pads should be applied and removed from anterior to posterior and secured so as not to move about. If they are not correctly worn, contaminated areas could touch cleaner areas of the perineum and increase the risk of infection. Stress correct and scrupulous handwashing to prevent cross-contamination.

MAINTENANCE OF SAFETY

ACTIVITY AND EXERCISE

Recovery Stage

Monitor vital signs every 15 minutes for 2 hours during the recovery stage (Table 27-2). Ensure the mother is settled comfortably in bed. A patient who has just given birth may need to remain in bed for a time to allow her body systems to adjust to fluid volume changes. Decide the appropriate time for the first ambulation, considering baseline blood pressure, amount of blood lost, type and amount of analgesic or anesthetic medications administered during labor and birth, level of pain evident in the woman's movements, and patient's desire to ambulate. The rapid decrease in intraabdominal pressure after birth results in a dilation of the blood vessels supplying the intestines (known as splanchnic engorgement), causing blood to pool in the viscera. This contributes to orthostatic hypotension; when a woman who has recently given birth stands up, she may faint or feel lightheaded.

Keep aromatic ammonia ampules on hand; these can be easily broken to revive the patient who is ambulating for the first time. Caution the patient to use her call bell to summon help before she attempts to get out of bed. Assess her color, pulse, and level of consciousness (LOC) in response to conversation and then assist her in ambulating to the bathroom. Once the woman has reached the bathroom, remain outside the door and inquire as to her well-being every minute or so. If there is no answer, enter the bathroom to assess the woman's condition. Have a wheelchair available in the room or just outside in the case the woman feels too weak to walk back to bed. Encourage her to rest after the ambulation, so that she can regain her strength.

Table 27-2 Vital Signs and Blood Pressure After Delivery

NORMAL FINDINGS	DEVIATIONS FROM NORMAL FINDINGS AND PROBABLE CAUSES
TEMPERATURE	
During first 24 hours, temperature may rise to 100.4° F (38° C) as a result of dehydrating effects of labor. After 24 hours the woman should be afebrile.	A diagnosis of puerperal sepsis is suggested if a rise in maternal temperature to 100.4° F (38° C) is noted after the first 24 hours after delivery and recurs or persists for 2 days. Other possibilities are mastitis, endometritis, urinary tract infections, and other systemic infections.
PULSE	
Bradycardia is common for the first 6 to 8 days after delivery. It is caused by increased cardiac output and stroke volume. The pulse returns to nonpregnant levels by 3 months after delivery. A pulse rate between 50 and 70 bpm is considered normal.	A rapid pulse rate or one that is increasing may indicate hypovolemia as a result of hemorrhage.
RESPIRATIONS	
Respirations should fall to within the woman's normal predelivery range.	Hypoventilation may follow an unusually high subarachnoid (spinal) block.
BLOOD PRESSURE	
Blood pressure is altered slightly if at all. Orthostatic hypotension, as indicated by feelings of vertigo or syncope immediately after standing up, can develop in the first 48 hours as a result of the splanchnic engorgement (the excessive filling or pooling of blood within the visceral vasculature after removal of pressure from the abdomen) that may occur after delivery.	Low or falling blood pressure may reflect hypovolemia secondary to hemorrhage. However, it is a late sign, and other symptoms of hemorrhage usually alert the staff. An increased reading may result from excessive use of vasopressor or oxytocic medications. Because gestational hypertension can persist into or begin in the postpartum period, routinely evaluate blood pressure. If a woman complains of headache, rule out hypertension as a cause before administering analgesics. If the blood pressure is elevated, confine the woman to bed and notify the physician.

The patient who has received conduction anesthesia (epidural block) is kept in bed until she is able to fully move, feels sensation in her legs, and has blood pressure and pulse within normal limits. Assess her ability to communicate, her LOC, and her vital signs for stability (within normal limits) before allowing her to get out of bed. Check that the patient is wearing slippers before she ambulates to prevent slipping or sliding.

The patient who has received analgesics needs to be observed closely until she is fully recovered from the medication (i.e., vital signs are stable within her normal range and she is fully awake).

The woman's temperature may be slightly elevated if she is dehydrated. A temperature higher than 100.4° F (38° C) is significant and should be reported. Many women feel chilled after giving birth and appreciate an extra blanket or one that has been warmed. Sometimes offering a beverage such as hot tea or warm milk provides comfort. Tell the patient this chilling is a normal reaction to the stress of labor.

Slight bradycardia, 50 to 70 bpm, is sometimes observed and is not considered abnormal if the other vital signs are within normal limits. Tachycardia may also occur in response to increased blood loss or physical exertion.

Blood pressure may be slightly elevated from exertion, from excitement, and possibly from the oxytocic medications. If the blood pressure is consistently elevated, or if the patient also complains of headache or visual disturbances, complications related to gestational hypertension could be occurring. These often persist even after delivery. Notify the physician immediately. Decrease in blood pressure could be caused by altered intraabdominal pressure or hemorrhage. Watch changes closely and report them.

Most mothers are not very active during this stage. They wish to rest, hold the baby, or visit with their significant others.

Later Postpartum Stage

Vital signs normally stabilize within the first 2 hours after delivery; report immediately any abnormality persisting longer than this. If vital signs have not stabilized within this time, continue to monitor them and report significant changes.

A temperature of 100.4° F (38° C) or higher on 2 successive days during the first 10 days after delivery (not including the first 24 hours) is considered indicative of puerperal infection. Closely monitor any signs and symptoms of infection during the postpartum stage. Use good aseptic technique when caring for the postpartum patient. Review the signs and symptoms of infection with the new mother before discharge, and stress the importance of contacting the physician promptly if any of these occur (see Box 27-3).

Also assess pulse and blood pressure. Bradycardia may persist up to 10 days after delivery. Elevated blood pressure readings or a continued decrease in blood pressure may be significant and should be reported promptly.

Most women try to get as much rest as possible while in the hospital. This is important, but activity is also needed to prevent complications such as thrombophlebitis of the lower extremities. Encourage new mothers to get out of bed and move about in the room. If the baby is kept in a nursery away from the mother's room, this is a good target for ambulation. If the perineum is uncomfortable, teach the woman to stand using the muscles of the legs while squeezing the buttocks together. This technique also helps when she attempts to sit. If she appears unsteady, accompany her when she ambulates. Ambulation is important for women who delivered by cesarean birth; think of them as surgical patients and encourage ambulation as soon as possible. Remember that inactivity predisposes patients to development of thrombophlebitis.

The flow of lochia may increase suddenly when the patient gets out of bed; secretions that pooled in the vagina drain out of the body when she stands. Once the lochia has changed to **serosa** or **alba,** excessive exercise or activity may result in the lochia's changing back to **rubra.** This is a sign to slow down and increase activity gradually.

The physician will indicate when to begin postpartum exercises suitable for the new mother, whether she delivered vaginally or by cesarean. The woman should begin gradually and avoid vigorous exercise until after the 6 weeks' examination, when the physician releases her to do so. Teach her isometric exercises that help toning without causing undue exertion.

REST AND SLEEP

Rest and sleep are important through the postpartum period. After the difficulties most women encounter at the end of pregnancy, it is a pleasure to sleep in any position desired. Many women report that the night after delivery, they get the best sleep they have experienced in weeks.

Hospital noises interrupt the sleep of many new mothers; keep environmental noise to a minimum to promote rest and sleep. Do not disturb the patient's sleep unless it is necessary to protect her well-being.

If she is breastfeeding, the new mother may choose to feed the infant at intervals through the night. This interrupted sleep pattern may persist for weeks until the infant is capable of sleeping for 5 or 6 hours without a feeding. Instruct the patient on the importance of naps and rest periods during the day to compensate for lost sleep. If sleep deprivation is prolonged, it may interfere with milk production and the let-down reflex.

REPRODUCTIVE ISSUES

Recovery Stage

Check the fundus and lochia every 15 minutes for the first 1 or 2 hours after delivery. The fundus should remain contracted, firm, and midline. This is critical, since severe bleeding may result if the uterus does not tightly constrict the placental site. As discussed earlier, a full bladder can displace the uterus and prevent its contraction. Encourage the patient to empty her bladder before checking the fundus. Palpate the uterus by placing one hand over the lower segment of the uterus near the pubic bone. Use the side of the other hand to feel the location and consistency of the uterus (see Figures 26-8 and 27-1).

If the fundus is not firm, it will be difficult to locate. An atonic uterus, one that has lost muscle tone, feels soft or boggy. Gently massage the fundus to increase contractility. Frequently small clots are expressed during this maneuver, and the uterus regains good contracted tone. If this does not result in contraction, the physician may order oxytocic medication—commonly oxytocin (Pitocin) or methylergonovine maleate (Methergine). These are usually administered intravenously to obtain prompt response. Methylergonovine may also be administered intramuscularly or orally. Monitor vital signs closely if these medications are given, since they may cause elevated blood pressure, bradycardia, nausea, headache, vertigo, and other side effects (Table 27-3).

Table 27-3 Medications for the Mother and Newborn

Generic (Brand)	Action	Side Effects	Nursing Implications
Codeine (with acetaminophen) (Tylenol #3) Oxycodone terephthalate (with acetaminophen) (Percocet)	Pain reliever, narcotic	Drowsiness, sedation, nausea, vomiting, constipation, respiratory depression, urinary retention, allergic reactions, rash, urticaria	Avoid concomitant use of alcohol or other central nervous system–depressant drugs; tell patient to avoid driving or other hazardous tasks while taking these medications; warn patient that extended use may result in dependency; avoid overdosing mother on acetaminophen.
Ibuprofen (Advil, Motrin, Nuprin)	Nonsteroidal antiinflammatory with antipyretic and analgesic properties	Heartburn, nausea, pruritus, lightheadedness, gastrointestinal bleeding	Give 1 hour before or 2 hours after meals; with gastrointestinal intolerance, give with meals; instruct patient to avoid taking aspirin or acetaminophen concurrently; teach patient to avoid alcohol intake and to report gastrointestinal distress or bleeding.
Methylergonovine maleate (Methergine)	Oxytocic agent, stimulates uterine contraction, used to control postpartum bleeding	Headache, dizziness, nausea, chest pain, tachycardia, hypertension	Contraindicated in patients sensitive to ergot derivatives.
Oxytocin (Pitocin)	Oxytocic agent, stimulates uterine contractions	*Mother:* nausea, vomiting, uterine spasm or rupture, water intoxication, seizures, cardiac arrhythmias, hypotension *Fetus:* cardiac arrhythmias, central nervous system or brain damage	Carefully monitor intake and output; fetal heart tones; and length, duration, and force of uterine contractions.
Simethicone (Mylicon)	Antiflatulent	None	Instruct patient to chew tablet thoroughly before swallowing; give after meals.
Rh_o(D) immune globulin (RhoGAM)	Gamma globulin solution containing immunoglobulins (IgG); provides passive immunity by suppressing antibody response and formation of anti-Rh(D) in Rh-negative individual exposed to Rh-positive blood	Injection site irritation; slight fever and lethargy	Check lot number, administer IM only to mother, using deltoid muscle within 72 hours of pregnancy termination.

IgG, Immunoglobulin G; *IM*, intramuscularly.
NOTE: Hepatitis B vaccine is no longer given at birth while still in the hospital but in the physician's office, as determined by the health care provider.

Continued

Table 27-3 Medications for the Mother and Newborn—cont'd

Generic (Brand)	Action	Side Effects	Nursing Implications
Rubella vaccine	Live virus vaccine	Rash, joint pain, pain at site Does not harm breastfeeding mothers	Administer IM in deltoid muscle during postpartum period; warn patient to avoid pregnancy for at least 3 months. Obtain informed consent.
Vitamin, prenatal (Materna)	Vitamin supplement	Nausea, vomiting	Tell patient it is important that pregnant women take prenatal vitamins and not regular vitamin supplements and that prenatal vitamins contain extra folic acid, which is needed for normal fetal development.
Witch hazel (Tucks pads, cream)	Astringent	Local irritation	Instruct mother that it is for external use only; use for relief of perineal discomfort.
Dibucaine ointment (Nupercainal)	Topical anesthetic	Allergic reactions, burning, stinging	Instruct mother that it is for external use only (application to severely denuded tissue may result in systemic absorption).
Vitamin K (AquaMEPHYTON)	Antidote for inadequate absorption and synthesis of vitamin K in neonate	With a large dose: hyperbilirubinemia, hemolytic anemia, kernicterus	Administer 0.5 to 1 mg IM in the middle third of the infant's vastus lateralis muscle of thigh after delivery. Stabilize leg firmly.
Purified lanolin cream	Retains the skin's natural moisture and protects the mother's nipple from further abrasions	None; does not need to be washed off for the next feeding	Applied to the mother's nipple. Mothers with a history of wool allergy should not use lanolin before a skin test can be done.
Erythromycin ophthalmic ointment or drops (Ilotycin)	Ophthalmic antibiotic agent	Irritation of eye that lasts 24-48 hours Vision may be blurred temporarily	Apply to conjunctival sacs of baby. Wear gloves. Cleanse eye first, if necessary. Spread the ointment from the inner canthus to the outer canthus on lower lid. Do not touch the tube to the eye. After 1 minute, wipe off excess ointment. Observe eyes for irritation.
Benzocaine (Dermaplast spray or ointment)	Local anesthetic that inhibits conduction of nerve impulses from sensory nerves, temporarily reducing perception of local discomfort	Urticaria, edema, contact dermatitis	Cleanse area with clear, warm water after each trip to the toilet. Hold spray 6-12 inches from affected area and spray liberally. Use up to four times a day.

IM, Intramuscularly.

While palpating the uterus, observe the amount of lochia. If the uterus is contracting well, small to moderate amounts of drainage are observed. If tone is poor, the amount of lochia is increased. Learn what is considered scant, light, moderate, and heavy amounts. This is usually determined by number of absorbent pads saturated in a period, such as pads per hour (Figure 27-4). The time factor is important when assessing lochia. One pad saturated in 30 minutes is more serious than one pad saturated in 4 hours. Pay particular attention to the patient who has a small but steady trickle of lochia; the blood loss may be significantly greater than in those who seem to bleed larger amounts (see Table 27-1). Also be sure to check under the but-

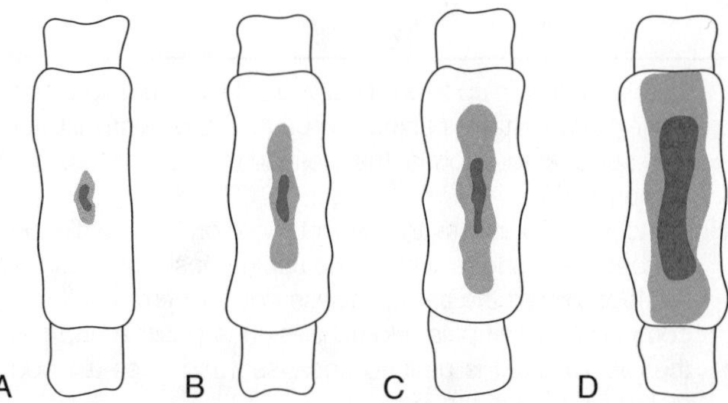

FIGURE 27-4 Suggested guidelines for assessing lochia volume. The pad may also be weighed and compared with the weight of a clean, dry pad (1 g of weight equals 1 mL). **A,** Scant, less than 1 inch (2.5 cm). **B,** Light, less than 4 inches (10 cm). **C,** Moderate, less than 6 inches (15 cm). **D,** Heavy, saturated pad within 1 hour.

tocks of the patient who remains in the supine position; many times gravity causes drainage to miss the pad and pool under the patient.

Later Postpartum Stage

Perform daily assessments of the breasts, the fundus, lochia, the perineum, the rectum, and the vascular condition of the legs. These are often called the postpartum checks.

As in the recovery stage, assess the location and consistency of the uterine fundus for the normal signs of involution. It is normally located at the level of the umbilicus on the day of delivery. The first day postpartum it may be one fingerbreadth above or at the level of the umbilicus; after that it normally descends at the rate of one fingerbreadth per day (see Figure 27-1, *A*). When assessing the fundus of a woman who delivered by cesarean, carefully palpate the sides of the incision to determine uterine tone and position.

As during the early recovery stage, the fundus should remain firmly contracted. Manage any atony as described. If massage does not result in adequate contraction, notify the physician. Lochia may begin to change within the first 2 days from the rubra to the serosa form. Assess the amount of drainage. Frequently less lochia is observed after cesarean deliveries because the uterine cavity is suctioned as part of the surgical procedure. The odor of the lochia should remain fleshy. If there is a fetid odor, infection may be present; report this promptly.

Inspect the perineum and the rectum by having the woman assume a lateral position with the upper leg drawn toward the chest. The perineum should be approximated. If an episiotomy was performed, the tissue may appear edematous. Erythema is common. Ecchymosis is also common, particularly after a difficult delivery. Many physicians order some form of topical anesthetic, such as witch hazel (Tucks pads) or dibucaine (Nupercainal) ointment, to soothe the perineum (see Table 27-3). This should be applied to the perineum by means of a clean, lint-free tissue, not the fingers.

If localized edema, discoloration, and intense pain are observed in the perineal area, a hematoma may be present. This hematoma is caused by excessive bleeding into the tissue. A hematoma is most common after deliveries in which forceps were used. Hematomas may be obvious or may be concealed in the vaginal canal. If the woman complains of persistent perineal pain or fullness in the vagina, notify the physician. This problem requires medical attention and perhaps surgical intervention.

Although the rectum and legs are not part of the reproductive system, these areas are typically included in postpartum assessments. Hemorrhoids (varicosities of the rectum) usually disappear quickly after delivery if there is no longstanding history of this problem. Use topical anesthetics to relieve pain if ordered by the physician. Sitz baths also provide relief and should be offered if the physician has ordered them. Suppositories may be ordered for hemorrhoid treatment.

Examine the patient's legs by stretching and straightening each leg, then dorsiflexing the foot. Pain in the calf is a positive **Homans' sign,** which indicates inflammation of the blood vessels of the leg and possible thrombophlebitis. Notify the physician promptly.

The postpartum assessment can be organized as a head-to-toe assessment using the eight letters BUBBLE-HE (Box 27-9).

Lactation and Breastfeeding

Advise all new mothers to wear a bra, even if the breasts are not overly large. The bra should be comfortable and fitted to provide support. Encourage breastfeeding mothers to use bras large enough to accommodate the growth that occurs with lactation. Nonnursing mothers need a bra that provides adequate compression to inhibit lactation without being uncomfortable.

With the bra removed, inspect and palpate the breasts. Observe for erythema, heat, edema, and engorgement.

Engorgement is an uncomfortable fullness of the breasts that occurs when the milk supply initially comes in. It is a result of venous and lymphatic stasis that occurs during lactation. Filling of the breast with milk usually begins in the axillary region, so palpate both the body and the tail of the breast. Engorgement is usually observed about the third day postpartum and resolves in about 48 hours. Because most patients are home by the time engorgement occurs, teach the new mother the symptoms of engorgement and methods of obtaining relief. If the patient is breastfeeding, interventions such as manual expression of milk and application of warm, moist heat are most useful. If the patient is not breastfeeding, compression of the breasts with a firm bra, wrapped ice packs, and analgesics are most often recommended.

Inspect the nipples for inflammation, fissures, or tenderness. The nipples generally do not cause prob-

Box 27-9 Postpartum Assessment: BUBBLE-HE

Breast: To assess the breast, have the patient lie down and remove her bra. Palpate both breasts for engorgement or nodules. Inspect nipples for pressure, soreness, cracks, or fissures.

Uterus: The top of the uterus, the fundus, should remain very firm. If it becomes soft, the uterine muscles probably are not contracting properly or the uterus has retained placental fragments. Both conditions predispose the patient to hemorrhage. Gently massage the uterus to help the muscles contract and expel placental fragments.

Bladder: The new mother may urinate frequently the first few days after giving birth. Be alert for signs and symptoms of infection. Also note any dysuria or urinary retention.

Bowel: Because of early discharge from the hospital, many women leave without having had a bowel movement. Assess for bowel sounds, encourage activity with rest periods, and encourage adequate fluid intake.

Lochia: Lochia has a definite fleshy scent, but if it has a fetid odor, it may indicate infection. Assess carefully.

Episiotomy: Most new mothers have an episiotomy and in some cases, a laceration. (NOTE: There is a move away from doing an episiotomy on the side—either left or right—and possibly even away from doing episiotomies at all, but midline is the site of choice. For a lateral episiotomy, use the following procedures.) Position the patient on her affected side. Instruct her to flex her top leg at the knee and draw it up toward her waist. Use a flashlight and wear gloves. Stand behind the patient and gently lift her top buttock to expose the perineum. Also assess for hemorrhoids.

Homans' sign: To assess the patient, position the legs flat on the bed while she reclines in the supine position. Dorsiflex her foot toward the ankle. Assess both extremities. If she complains of calf pain, Homans' sign is positive and further assessment is needed because it indicates a blood clot in a vessel in the leg.

Emotional status: Consider the three phases most new mothers pass through:

1. The first is "taking in"—the time immediately following birth. She sleeps, depends on others for nurturing and food, and relives the events surrounding the birth.
2. Over the next few days she will be "taking hold." She is preoccupied with the present and concerned about her health and her baby's condition. She cares for herself and wants to learn to care for her newborn.
3. The next phase, "letting go," comes later in the postpartum period. She reestablishes relationships with other people.

Monitor the patient's emotional status, noting how she interacts with her family, her level of independence, sleep and rest patterns, mood swings, irritability, or crying.

Modified from Ferguson, H. (1987). Planning letter-perfect postpartum care, *Nursing, 17*(5), 50.

lems for nonlactating mothers; however, if the patient is breastfeeding, the nipples should be kept soft and supple. Most physicians recommend avoiding soap or other chemicals because they dry the skin and may be ingested by the infant. Plain water and air-drying may prevent problems. Some physicians recommend allowing the nipples to dry after feeding without removing the milk residue. If additional moisturizer is needed, small amounts of unscented lanolin or a nipple cream may be used to soften and soothe dry, tender nipples. Modifications in the positioning of the baby may be needed if tender or cracked nipples continue to be a problem.

In addition to assessing the breasts, help the breastfeeding mother succeed in establishing lactation. To establish the lactation response, the breast must be adequately stimulated so prolactin can be released by the anterior pituitary. Once the milk supply is established, prolactin production decreases, and it is primarily oxytocin, released as the baby suckles, that maintains the supply of milk.

The mother may feel a tingling or prickling sensation, known as the **let-down reflex,** when feeding time approaches. If the mother nurses the baby at regular, frequent intervals and empties the breasts, the supply of milk increases in response to the baby's demands. If the breast is not adequately stimulated, the lactation response may not be established. This can happen when the baby has a weak suck or is not put to breast often enough. If the breast is not emptied adequately, the pressure of the milk in the alveoli can also suppress milk production. Incorrect placement at breast may also lead to problems. If the baby's mouth grasps only the nipple and does not apply pressure on the lactiferous glands (mammary glands or Montgomery's glands, consisting of 20 to 24 glands in the areolae of the nipples), milk will not be released and the needed stimulation will not occur. This also may lead to nipple trauma and soreness.

Become knowledgeable about correct breastfeeding techniques so you can instruct the breastfeeding mother. These include correct position and placement of the nipple and areola in the baby's mouth, stimulation of the infant to enable correct latch-on (attachment of the infant to the breast for feeding), frequency and length of nursing, and care of the breasts. Also assist the mother's efforts by providing support and encouragement. Lactation consultants, teaching videos, and support groups such as La Leche League are excellent resources that supplement and reinforce teaching by the nurse (Figures 27-5 and 27-6).

Manual pumping of the breasts may be necessary in some cases. The mother whose infant is unable to suckle at breast at birth may pump to establish lactation and provide milk that can be fed to her baby by alternate means. The mother who must spend an ex-

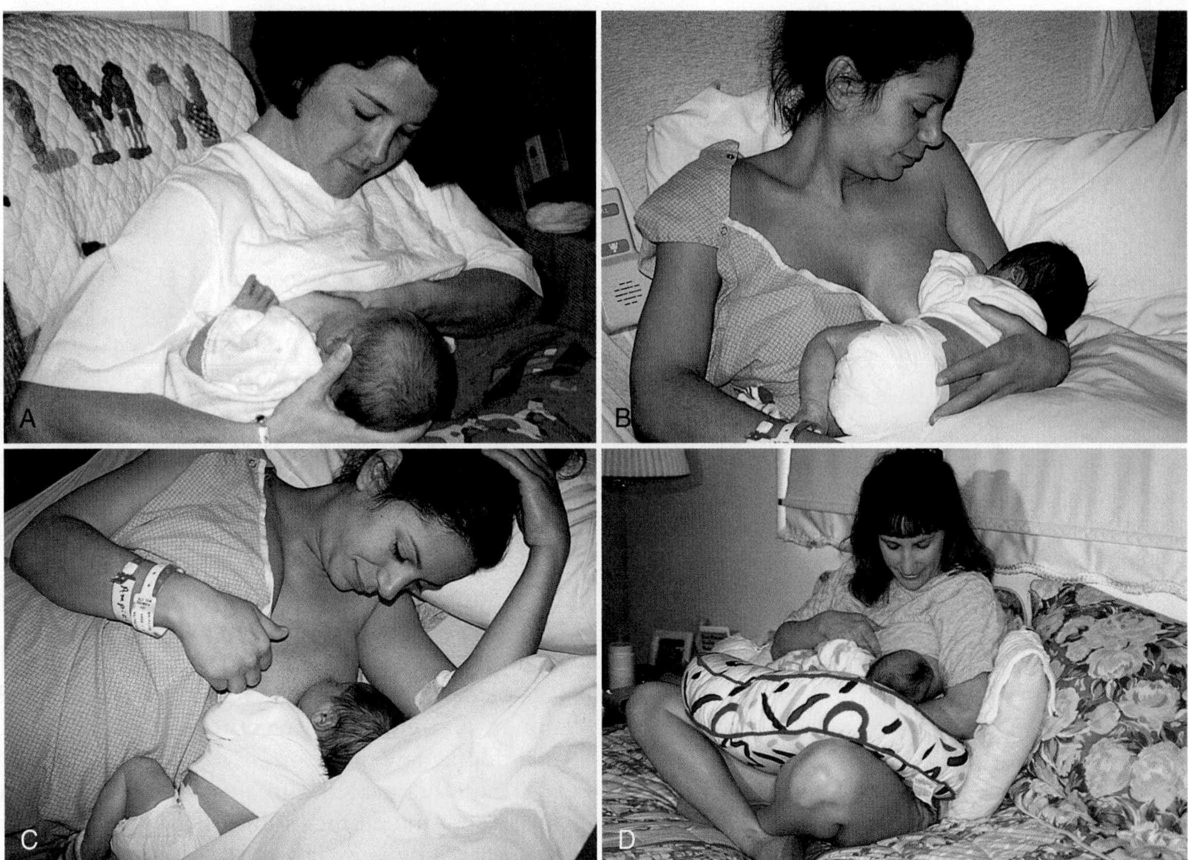

FIGURE 27-5 Positioning the baby for breastfeeding. **A,** Football hold. **B,** Cradling. **C,** Lying down. **D,** Across the lap.

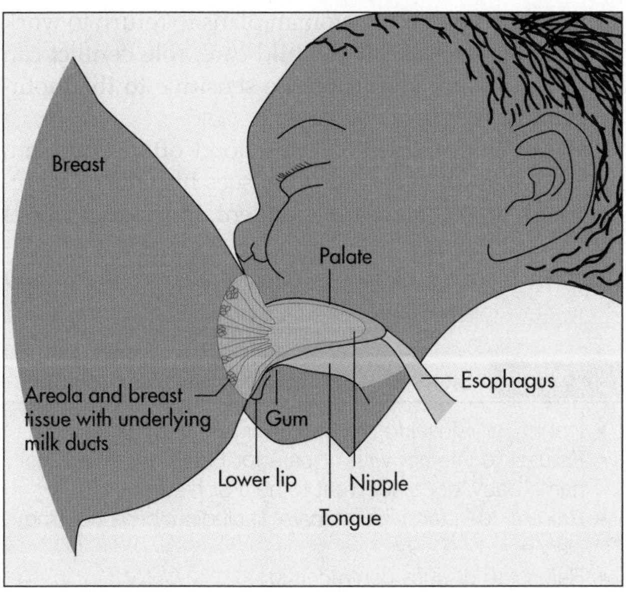

FIGURE 27-6 Correct attachment (latch-on) of infant at breast.

Box 27-10 Advantages of Breastfeeding

- **Antiinfective properties:** Immunoglobulins, lymphocytes, and other immune components that are present in breast milk protect the infant against infection. The bifidus factor in breast milk encourages growth of normal bacterial flora in the infant's gastrointestinal tract.
- **Nutrition:** Breast milk is specifically made for the human infant. Its protein, carbohydrate, and fat ratio is thought to be ideal for growth and development. It is well digested and readily absorbed.
- **Growth and development:** Breastfeeding promotes better tooth and jaw alignment. It may be less likely to produce obesity in the child, and it may favor optimum bonding between mother and infant.
- **Allergy:** Breastfeeding may reduce the incidence of allergies in infants at high risk for allergic conditions.
- **Maternal benefits:** Hormones produced in breastfeeding help contract and shrink the uterus. Breastfeeding requires no formula preparation or bottle sterilization and is more economical than formula feeding.

tended time away from her infant, such as while at work, may pump to maintain lactation and provide breast milk for her baby during her absence.

Breastfeeding has many benefits for the mother (Box 27-10). The release of oxytocin during breastfeeding stimulates contraction of the uterus, so it undergoes more rapid involution. There is a lower incidence of breast cancer in women who have nursed for at least 3 months. Also, many women who breastfeed report a special closeness to their infants, since they are providing important nourishment. Human milk provides many factors that are uniquely suited to the infant and enhance growth and development. Human milk has antibacterial and antiviral properties, immunoglobulins, and antiallergy factors that protect the infant against many infections and diseases. Mother's milk also contains growth factors, digestive enzymes, and proteins that foster the maturation process begun in utero.

Nursing diagnoses and interventions for the breastfeeding patient include but are not limited to the following:

Nursing Diagnoses	Nursing Interventions
Imbalanced nutrition: less than body requirements, related to nutritional demands during lactation	Review dietary choices. Instruct patient to continue diet recommended during pregnancy. Arrange consultation with a dietitian. Inform patient of Women, Infants, and Children (WIC) supplemental food program.
Anxiety, related to initiating feedings due to inexperience	Evaluate patient's readiness to initiate feedings. Initiate feedings as soon as possible. Position mother and infant for comfort. Initiate correct latch-on and position correctly. Support and encourage mother in breastfeeding attempts.

Bottle feeding is another choice for the new mother. If she chooses not to breastfeed, lactation must be suppressed. This can be accomplished by mechanical means, starting before milk production begins. The woman wears a supportive bra within 4 to 6 hours after delivery. Ice to the breasts also decreases the discomfort that may result from engorgement. She should avoid any form of breast stimulation, such as pumping the breasts, and avoid applying heat to the breasts, such as turning her back to the hot water when showering. Do not restrict maternal fluid intake.

PSYCHOSOCIAL ASSESSMENT

COPING AND STRESS TOLERANCE

Many new mothers feel overwhelmed by the responsibility of motherhood. They feel intimidated by the nurses' capability and skill with the newborn. They often feel inept and may not wish to ask questions that might be viewed as unintelligent. Establishing rapport, listening, and anticipating fears and anxieties are important nursing measures. False reassurances are not helpful; thorough teaching and encouragement are far more beneficial.

Often women experience a period of depression after delivery that is triggered by rapid hormonal shifts. This so-called postpartum depression, or "blues," may be mild or severe. It often appears between 2 and 7 days postpartum. Prepare the woman for the possibility of this and plan a course of action if it occurs.

SIGNS OF POTENTIAL PROBLEMS

No assessment of psychosocial needs is complete without assessing for signs of potential problems. Not all potential psychosocial problems are easily identified. However, some signs may indicate a need for further evaluation by a caregiver skilled in that area (Box 27-11). The presence of one or more of these signs does not prove that a problem exists, but may indicate a need for further assessment (see Chapter 28).

ROLES AND RELATIONSHIPS

The addition of a new family member has a major effect on roles and relationships. These changes are most obvious when the first child is born, but adjustments take place whenever another child joins a family. Time, money, and emotional resources must be divided to include the new member.

The mother faces the greatest number of changes. In our society the mother still fills the role of the child's primary caregiver. The responsibility of this role, 24 hours a day, 7 days a week, is overwhelming to many women. Today, because many women are independent wage earners, the loss of freedom is a difficult adjustment. Even if the woman plans to return to work and arranges for excellent child care, role conflict can lead to guilt and confusion. Be sensitive to the mother's concerns.

The responsibilities of fatherhood often become a reality when the father actually sees his child. The realization that a totally dependent individual needs him is frightening to many men. The financial concerns of feeding, clothing, and sheltering his family

Box 27-11 Signs of Potential Psychosocial Problems

- Inability or refusal to discuss labor and birth experience
- Refusal to interact with or care for baby (e.g., does not name baby, does not want to hold or feed baby)
- Refusal to attend infant care (including breastfeeding) classes
- Refusal to discuss contraception
- References to self as ugly and useless
- Excessive preoccupation with self (body image)
- Marked depression
- Lack of support system
- Partner or other family members reacting negatively to baby
- Expression of disappointment over baby's sex
- View of baby as messy or unattractive
- Baby reminding mother of family member or friend she does not like

take on new significance. A two-income family may have only the father's wages, at least temporarily. Even if the mother returns to work, there are new expenses for child care. The wife is now also a mother, and many times the child's needs take priority over the husband's needs or wishes. Freedom and spontaneity give way to a life circumscribed by feeding schedules, diaper bags, and babysitters.

Because many men have little knowledge or experience in caring for infants, simple things such as feeding, changing diapers, or even carrying a baby may be intimidating. Help alleviate these fears by including the father in teaching whenever possible and by allowing him to verbalize his fears and concerns. Fathers go through a predictable three-stage process during the first 3 weeks of their transition to parenthood (Table 27-4).

Additional role adjustments relate to friends and the extended family. Friendships and socialization may take lower priority. Siblings assume a new position in the family order. Parents now become grandparents, and in-laws share grandchildren. These are all dynamic situations, and each family makes a variety of accommodations in incorporating their new roles.

SELF-PERCEPTION

It is common for the new mother to wish to discuss her perception of the labor and delivery. Allow time for her to verbalize and work through her experiences. Reality may differ greatly from her expectations, and she needs explanations to clarify things in her mind. The new mother may spend considerable time with friends or in telephone conversation relating her experiences through labor and delivery.

The new mother may be passive for the first day or two. This is called the taking-in stage (see Box 27-9). During this time the mother needs supportive care. Her primary focus may be on herself and on personal needs such as sleep, food, and attention. She may defer to the nurses and let others care for the baby. This is followed by the taking-hold stage, when the woman is ready to assume greater authority and responsibility for herself and her baby.

Mood swings are common early in the postpartum period, related to recent stresses, fatigue, and rapid hormonal changes. Explain this to the new mother so that she does not become unduly concerned.

It is common for new mothers, particularly primiparas, to expect that they will regain their prepregnancy figure quickly after delivery. Many bring clothes that they hoped to wear home, only to be sadly disappointed. Be supportive and explain that it takes time for the body to regain the prepregnancy tone and shape.

Table 27-4 Transition to Fatherhood: A Three-Stage Process

STAGE	CHARACTERISTICS
Stage 1: Expectations	Father has preconceptions about what life will be like after baby comes home.
Stage 2: Reality	Father realizes that expectations are not always based on fact. Common feelings experienced are sadness, ambivalence, jealousy, and frustration. Father has overwhelming desire to be more involved. Some fathers are pleasantly surprised at ease and fun of parenting.
Stage 3: Transition to mastery	Father makes conscious decision to take control and become more actively involved with infant.

COGNITIVE AND PERCEPTUAL ISSUES

Control of discomfort during the postpartum period is necessary for the woman to resume a normal activity level and get adequate rest. The most common discomforts experienced are perineal pain from the episiotomy and **afterbirth pains.** Afterbirth pains are cramping sensations resulting from the contraction of the uterus. They are more common and may be more severe in multiparas.

Most physicians prescribe analgesics for these discomforts. Acetaminophen is commonly used, with or without codeine. Codeine is generally effective but is a controlled substance and also has side effects, such as constipation and vertigo, that may be undesirable in the postpartum patient (see Table 27-3). Salicylates, such as aspirin, are usually avoided because they may interfere with clotting mechanisms. Recently ibuprofen (Motrin) has been popular. Ibuprofen is an analgesic, an antiinflammatory, and a prostaglandin inhibitor. It is often effective in reducing the severity of the cramping without altering the contraction of the uterine muscle. **Caution:** Ibuprofen is to be used with caution in people with kidney or heart disease or those taking diuretics.

Another major challenge of the postpartum period involves learning how to care for herself and the newborn. This can be overwhelming for the first-time mother. The nurse has limited time to teach all the necessary information. Most hospitals have teaching lists and printed handouts or booklets that cover all the key areas (see Box 27-7). To prevent the woman from becoming overwhelmed, pace teaching throughout the hospital stay, rather than leaving it until discharge. Also document newborn teaching (see Box 27-8).

❖ NURSING PROCESS *for the Postpartum Mother*

The role of the licensed practical nurse/licensed vocational nurse (LPN/LVN) in the nursing process as stated is that the LPN/LVN will:

- Participate in planning care for patients based on patient needs

- Review patient's care plan and recommend revisions as needed
- Review and follow defined prioritization for patient care
- Use clinical pathways, care maps, or care plans to guide and review patient care

Assessment

Assessment begins with admission of the patient to the postpartum unit from the labor and delivery unit. Review the prenatal history for obstetric history, prenatal care, and health status during the pregnancy. Also review the events of labor, delivery, and recovery, including the onset of labor, the mother's physical and emotional status during labor, progress of labor, status of fetus, birth, and status of neonate. A physical and psychosocial assessment should follow. Areas assessed should include reproductive system, cardiovascular status, nutrition, elimination, activity and rest, maternal self-concept, knowledge level, parenting role, attachment, home environment, and support system. Physical and psychosocial assessments are ongoing during the postpartum stay.

Nursing Diagnosis

Nursing assessment helps identify the needs of the postpartum patient. Care can then be based on these needs. Possible nursing diagnoses for the postpartum patient include the following:

- Risk for deficient fluid volume
- Risk for infection
- Impaired urinary elimination
- Constipation
- Imbalanced nutrition: less than body requirements
- Imbalanced nutrition: more than body requirements
- Acute pain
- Impaired tissue integrity
- Disturbed sleep pattern
- Deficient knowledge
- Anxiety
- Risk for impaired parenting
- Interrupted family processes
- Impaired parenting
- Situational low self-esteem

Expected Outcomes and Planning

The care plan focuses on the needs of the postpartum patient and the nurse's ability to meet those needs effectively (Nursing Care Plan 27-1). Each patient has differing needs; care must be individualized accordingly.

The care plan focuses on goals and outcomes specific to the nursing diagnosis. Examples include the following:

Goal 1: Patient will experience relief of pain at episiotomy site.

Outcome: Patient uses appropriate pain relief measures, such as a sitz bath, topical anesthetic spray, and medication as required.

Goal 2: Patient will provide appropriate, safe care to infant.

Outcome: Patient demonstrates competence in bathing, feeding, diapering, and comforting infant.

Implementation

Nursing interventions during the postpartum period include the following:

- Assess progress of involution by monitoring vital signs, breasts, fundus, lochia, episiotomy.
- Administer oxytocics, analgesics, and stool softeners as ordered.
- Use aseptic techniques, good handwashing, and standard precautions when caring for patient and baby.
- Teach or demonstrate the following (see Boxes 27-7 and 27-8):
  - —Breast care measures
  - —Signs and symptoms of infection and prevention measures
  - —Nutritional and dietary requirements for healing and lactation
  - —Postpartum exercises
  - —Infant care techniques
- Provide comfort and pain relief measures.
- Encourage patient and family to express feelings.
- Make referrals to community agencies as appropriate.

Implementation of nursing care involves putting into practice specific activities that should result in the expected outcomes planned for each individual patient.

Evaluation

Continually evaluate the success of the interventions. As the postpartum period progresses, the goals and interventions may change. Refer to the goals and outcomes to determine whether the plan was successful and the outcomes met. Examples include the following:

Goal 1: Patient will experience relief of pain at episiotomy site.

Evaluative measures: Patient uses sitz bath twice a day, applies topical anesthetic spray with each peripad change, and requests analgesics for episiotomy pain.

Goal 2: Patient will provide appropriate, safe care to infant.

Evaluative measures: Patient demonstrates appropriate infant bathing techniques, use of infant car seat, and feeding techniques.

VALUES AND BELIEFS

Cultural beliefs and practices are important determinants of parenting behaviors. They influence the inter-

Nursing Care Plan 27-1 The Mother with a Newborn

Baby Caleb is a 39-week-gestation male neonate, 7 pounds, 3 ounces, and 21 inches long (Figure 27-7), born today to Philip and Anne Pearson. Caleb was born by vaginal delivery after a 7-hour labor. Ms. Pearson had epidural anesthesia. Her pregnancy and medical history were unremarkable. Caleb is the Pearsons' first child, and Ms. Pearson has begun breastfeeding. Caleb will be circumcised tomorrow. He has been nursing every 3 hours for approximately 20 minutes with a strong suck. At the initial assessment of Caleb 1 hour after birth, findings were all within normal limits. He was given 0.5 mL vitamin K (AquaMEPHYTON) in the left anterolateral thigh, and erythromycin (Ilotycin) was placed in both eyes. His temperature on admission to the nursery was 97.5° F (36.4° C) axillary. After an hour under the radiant warmer, his temperature was 98.6° F (37° C) axillary and he was given his initial bath. Caleb is currently rooming with his mother, who is asking numerous questions about his care.

INFANT NURSING DIAGNOSIS *Risk for imbalanced body temperature, hypothermia, related to exposure to cool environment*

Patient Goals and Expected Outcomes	Nursing Interventions	Evaluation
Stable infant temperature will be established and maintained	Dry infant immediately after birth. Wrap infant in warm blanket. Place under radiant warmer on admission to nursery. Place cap on infant's head. Keep infant away from drafts, exterior walls, and windows. Keep infant off cold surfaces. Monitor temperature every 30 minutes until normal, then every 4 hours. Delay bath until temperature is above 97.7° F (36.5° C) axillary.	Infant's temperature remains greater than 97.7° F (36.5° C) axillary. Infant is placed under radiant warmer on admission to nursery. Infant is properly dressed Infant shows no signs of cold stress.

MATERNAL NURSING DIAGNOSIS *Deficient knowledge, maternal, related to being a first-time parent*

Patient Goals and Expected Outcomes	Nursing Interventions	Evaluation
Mother will verbalize understanding of infant care Mother will demonstrate infant bath and diaper change Mother will verbalize correct safety practices Mother will use correct breastfeeding techniques	Demonstrate and encourage return demonstration of infant bath, including umbilical cord care, circumcision care, and dressing. Demonstrate diaper change and cleaning of genital area. Teach correct positioning of infant. Teach techniques for breastfeeding. Teach methods to maintain infant's temperature.	Mother correctly bathes and diapers infant. Mother practices safe technique when handling infant. Mother successfully breastfeeds infant using correct techniques.

Critical Thinking Questions

1. Even though Caleb is nursing well at each feeding, Ms. Pearson is anxious about her ability to successfully breastfeed. She asks how she will know whether Caleb is getting enough breast milk and whether she should supplement with formula, juice, or cereal. How should the nurse answer her?
2. A Gomco circumcision is performed on Caleb. After the procedure is completed, Caleb is returned to his mother's room. What should the nurse tell Ms. Pearson in response to her questions regarding diaper changes and care of the circumcision? How should the nurse describe the expected appearance of the circumcised penis?

actions with the infant and the parent's or family's caregiving style. For example, Asian mothers may remain at home with the baby for at least 30 days after birth and are not supposed to engage in household chores, including care of the infant. Many times the grandmother takes over the baby's care immediately, even before discharge from the hospital. Similarly, Jordanian mothers might have a 40-day lying-in after birth during which their mothers or sisters care for the baby. Hispanics may practice a 40-day period after birth during which the mother is expected to recuperate and get acquainted with her infant. Traditionally this involves many restrictions concerning food (spicy or cold foods, fish, pork, and citrus are avoided; tortillas and chicken soup are encouraged); exercise; and activities, including sexual intercourse. Abdominal binding is a traditional practice, and many grown women avoid tub bathing and washing their hair. Traditional Hispanic husbands do not expect to see their wives or infants until both have been cleaned and dressed after birth.

People in all cultures desire and value children. In Asian families, children are valued as a source of family strength and stability, are perceived as wealth, and

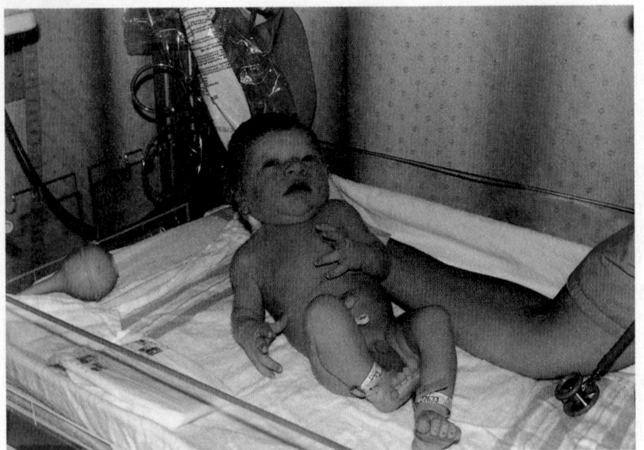

FIGURE 27-7 Newborn in a radiant warmer.

are objects of parental love and affection. In the Yup'ik culture of the Alaskan Eskimos, where sharing has traditionally been necessary for survival, children are looked on as security. There is no concept of illegitimacy; every child is welcomed and loved. Adoption is common and is usually within the extended family.

Differing cultural values can influence parents' interactions with health care professionals; for example, Asians are taught to be humble and obedient. They are brought up not to question authority figures (such as a nurse), to avoid confrontation, and to respect the yin-yang balance in nature. Because of these learned values, an Asian mother might not confront the nurse about the length of time it takes to receive the medication requested for her episiotomy pain. A mother may nod and say "Yes" in response to the nurse's directions for using an iced sitz bath but then not use the bath. The "Yes," in this case, is a courtesy, meaning "I'm listening," rather than an indication of agreement. The mother does not use the iced sitz bath because of her traditional avoidance of bathing and cold in the puerperium.

Because all members of a cultural group do not necessarily adhere to traditional practices, validate which cultural practices are important to individual parents. Knowledge of cultural beliefs can help with accurate assessments and diagnoses of observed parenting behaviors. For example, nurses may become concerned when they observe cultural practices that appear to reflect poor maternal-infant bonding. Algerian mothers may not unwrap and explore their infants as part of the acquaintance process because in Algeria, babies are wrapped tightly in swaddling clothes to protect them physically and psychologically. A Vietnamese woman may care for her infant but refuse to cuddle or further interact with her child. This apparent lack of interest in the newborn is this cultural group's attempt to ward off "evil spirits" and actually reflects an intense love and concern for the child. Asian mothers might be criticized for almost immediately relinquishing care of infants to grandmothers and not even attempting to hold their babies when they are brought to the room. However, extended family members show their support for a new mother's rest and recuperation by assisting with the care of the baby. Contrary to the guidance given to mothers in the United States about "nipple confusion," a mix of breastfeeding and bottle feeding is standard practice for Japanese mothers. This is out of concern for the mother's rest during the first 2 to 3 months and does not interfere with lactation; breastfeeding is widespread among Japanese women.

In helping new families adjust to parenthood, follow principles that facilitate nursing practice within transcultural situations (see Cultural Considerations box).

PREVENTING INFANT ABDUCTION

An unfortunate but essential nursing role is protecting the infant from abduction (kidnapping). Precautions include teaching parents how to recognize the picture identification badge worn by birth facility personnel.

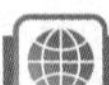

Cultural Considerations

Postpartum Period

- Many cultures emphasize certain postpartum rituals for mother and baby. In some cultures, including Chinese, Mexican, Korean, and Southeast Asian, these may include bathing, activity, and dietary restrictions designed to restore the hot-cold (yin-yang) balance of the body:
  - —The mothers may observe a long period of seclusion and rest with avoidance of physical activity. Household responsibilities and infant care are provided by other female family members. Period of seclusion may last from 2 weeks to 40 days.
  - —They avoid cold and maintain increased body warmth; avoid bathing, hair washing, exercise, and exposure to wind for 7 to 30 days after childbirth; and add extra heat (cover with blankets).
  - —The women avoid cold and raw foods and water. They eat only warm foods and drink hot beverages to replace blood loss and to restore the balance of hot and cold in the bodies. Traditional foods of culture are encouraged.
  - —These women may wear abdominal binders. They may prefer not to give their babies colostrum.
- In other cultures, breastfeeding practices are not established until after milk comes in because of belief that colostrum is "bad" for the baby.
- Low-income mothers may need to contend with stressors that distract them from developing a relationship with their babies. Inability to pay for infant supplies or child care, chaotic home situations, and worry over eligibility for social and health care services deplete these women's mental and physical energy.
- Arabic women eat special meals designed to restore their energy.
  - —They are expected to stay at home for 40 days after delivery to avoid illness resulting from exposure to the outside air.
- Haitian women may request to take the placenta home to bury or burn.

Provide parents with written and oral information, including a picture of staff identification badges. Caution parents to never give their infant to anyone who does not have proper identification.

Staff members who are working temporarily on the unit are assigned special identification badges that are carefully monitored so that they cannot be removed from the premises without alerting the staff. In some agencies, an electronic sensor is attached to each infant by a bracelet or tag. The sensor activates an alarm if it goes near an exit or if it is cut or removed from the infant. With some systems, all exits lock automatically if an alarm is activated.

Entrances to the maternity unit should be in areas where staff can watch people entering and leaving. Unit doors may be locked at all times. Entrance requires knocking, pressing a call signal, or using a card key or a code on the lock. Visitors to maternity units may be required to check in with security guards or other staff members and wear special visitor identification tags. Remote exits are locked and often equipped with video cameras and alarms. Staff must respond quickly whenever a door alarm sounds.

Newborns are usually abducted by women who are familiar with the birth facility and its routines. They are of childbearing age, are often overweight, and may live near the birth facility. They usually visit several times to learn the routines so that they can impersonate birth facility staff to gain access to a newborn. They often know the layout of the facility and the locations of exits well. The woman may have had a previous pregnancy loss or is unable to get pregnant. She may want an infant to solidify her relationship with her husband or boyfriend. Although the woman plans the kidnapping scheme, she waits for an appropriate opportunity to take any infant (Box 27-12).

DISCHARGE: BEFORE 24 HOURS AND AFTER 48 HOURS

Early postpartum discharge, shortened hospital stays, and *1-day maternity stays* are all terms for the length of hospital stays of mothers and their babies after a low-risk birth. The trend of shortened hospital stays is based largely on efforts to reduce health care costs, coupled with consumer demands to have less medical intervention and more family-focused experiences.

Laws Relating to Discharge

Health care providers have expressed concern with shortened stays because some medical problems do not show up in the first 24 hours after birth. New mothers do not have sufficient time to learn how to care for their newborns and identify problems such as jaundice and dehydration related to breastfeeding difficulties.

The concern for the potential increase in adverse maternal-infant outcomes from hospital early discharge practices led the American College of Obstetricians and Gynecologists, the American Academy of Pediatrics, and other professional health care organizations to promote the enactment of federal and state maternity length-of-stay bills to ensure adequate care for both the mother and the newborn. The Newborns' and Mothers' Health Protection Act of 1996 provides minimum federal standards for health plan coverage for mothers and their newborns. The act requires all health plans to allow the new mother and the newborn to remain in the hospital for a minimum of 48 hours

Box 27-12 Precautions to Prevent Infant Abductions

- All personnel must wear appropriate identification that is easily visible at all times. No one without appropriate identification should handle or transport infants.
- Enlist parents' help in preventing kidnapping. Teach them to allow only hospital staff with proper identification to take their infants from them.
- Teach parents and staff to transport infants only in their cribs and never by carrying them. Question anyone walking in the hallway carrying an infant.
- Investigate anyone with a newborn near an exit or in an unusual part of the facility.
- Be suspicious of anyone who does not seem to be visiting a specific mother or who asks detailed questions about nursery or discharge routine.
- Be suspicious of unknown people carrying large bags or packages that could contain an infant.
- Respond immediately when an alarm sounds signaling that a remote exit has been opened or an infant has been taken to an unauthorized area.
- Never leave infants unattended at any time. Teach parents that infants must be observed at all times. If no family members are present, the mother can take her infant into the bathroom with her or send the infant back to the nursery if she wishes to nap.
- Take infants to mothers one at a time. Never leave an infant in the hallway unsupervised.
- When infants are left in mothers' rooms, place the cribs away from the doorways.
- If entrances to the maternity unit or nurseries are equipped with locks that open to codes or card keys, protect them from others.
- When a parent or a family member comes to the nursery to take an infant, always match the infant and adult identification bracelet numbers. Never give an infant to anyone without the correct identification bracelet or other proper identification.
- Alert hospital security immediately of any suspicious activity.
- Suggest that parents not place announcements in the paper or signs in their yard that might alert an abductor that a new baby is in the home.

after a normal vaginal birth and 96 hours after a cesarean birth unless the attending provider, in consultation with the mother, decides on early discharge.

MATERNAL FOLLOW-UP CARE

After delivery the woman is instructed to make a follow-up appointment with her health care provider in 6 weeks. Some birthing units require this appointment be made before discharge. If the nurse schedules the appointment, the patient needs prompt notification of the date and time of the appointment. Women experiencing complications may be seen sooner.

WELL-BABY FOLLOW-UP CARE

Healthy infants are seen by the physician at 2 weeks of age. Babies who are discharged before 48 hours of age are traditionally seen by the health care provider within 3 to 5 days after discharge. The purpose of this appointment is to review nutritional status, elimination, and the presence of jaundice. The schedule of appointments for a well baby is every 2 to 3 months until age 18 months. Milestone visits are planned for ages 2 and 3 and then every 2 years. These visits focus on preventive care such as health education, nutritional assessments, review of growth and development, and routine immunizations (see Chapter 29).

ANATOMY AND PHYSIOLOGY OF THE NORMAL NEWBORN

ASSESSMENT IMMEDIATELY AFTER DELIVERY

In addition to Apgar scoring (see Chapter 26), which is done immediately after delivery, perform other assessments to establish the newborn's gestational age. Gestational age is the actual number of weeks since conception. It is important because many problems observed in newborns are age related. Because many women are unsure of the exact date of conception, calendar-based gestational age is unreliable. Physical and neurologic assessments based on established criteria are more reliable. Evaluate physical characteristics within the first few hours of life. Neurologic assessment is done 24 hours later, after the nervous system has had the opportunity to stabilize from the trauma of delivery.

CHARACTERISTICS

Body Size and Shape

The newborn's head is disproportionately large for his or her body. The abdomen is prominent, with a smaller chest and narrow hips. The body is usually held in a moderately flexed position. There is a wide variation of size in normal newborns. The average newborn weighs 7 pounds, 8 ounces (3400 g) and is approximately 20 inches (50 cm) long. Charts are available for plotting height and weight. The head circumference averages 13 to 14 inches (33 to 35.5 cm) and is generally about 1 inch (2.5 cm) larger than the chest circumference, which averages 12 to 13 inches (30.5 to 33 cm).

Vital Signs

Respiratory rate averages 30 to 60 breaths/min with brief periods of apnea. Breathing is diaphragmatic and should be effortless, without evidence of respiratory distress. Rate and rhythm vary with activity. Pulse rate averages 120 to 160 bpm with higher and lower variations depending on activity.

The heartbeat should have a regular rate and rhythm. Auscultate the apical beat between the fourth and fifth intercostal spaces. This is best done when the infant is asleep. Murmurs are common in the newborn. The physician determines whether they are significant. The blood pressure averages 60 to 80/40 to 50 mm Hg and should be approximately the same in all four extremities. A drop in systolic blood pressure (about 15 mm Hg) in the first hour after birth is common. Crying and moving usually cause increases in systolic blood pressure. The axillary temperature of the newborn should be between 97.6° and 98.6° F (36.4° and 37° C), with stabilization of temperature occurring within 8 to 10 hours after birth.

Skin

The infant's skin can exhibit a wide range of rashes and color changes (Box 27-13). Most are not significant and disappear within a few days. However, parents may be concerned until the changes are explained.

Box 27-13 Common Skin Observations in the Newborn

- **Milia** are small white spots usually seen on the nose and chin. They are a result of occluded sebaceous glands and disappear spontaneously within a few weeks.
- **Newborn rash,** or erythema toxicum neonatorum, is an elevated, hivelike rash that may result in small white vesicles. It is not contagious and, like milia, disappears without treatment.
- **Telangiectatic nevi,** "stork bites," are flat, pink or red marks often seen on the eyelids, nose, or nape of the neck. These are dilated capillaries that become more vivid when the infant cries. They are not significant to the health of the infant and disappear at 1 to 2 years of age.
- **Mongolian spots** are areas of increased pigmentation. The lumbar dorsal area is the most common location. The area may appear bluish black. These are most often seen in darker-skinned people.
- **Nevus flammeus,** port-wine stain, is a reddish purple discoloration often seen on the face. This is a capillary angioma below the epidermis. Unfortunately, these will not disappear spontaneously. Medical techniques have been developed that reduce or remove port-wine birthmarks.
- **Strawberry birthmarks,** nevus vasculosus, are capillary hemangiomas. These may continue to increase in size for several months. They normally then begin to shrink spontaneously and usually disappear early in childhood.

Color

The white newborn is usually pink to slightly reddish in appearance. The black newborn may appear pinkish or yellowish brown. Newborns of Spanish descent may have an olive tint or a slight yellow cast to the skin. Newborns of Asian descent may be a rosy or yellowish tan. The color of Native American newborns depends on the tribe and can vary from a light pink to a dark, reddish brown. By the second or third day, the skin turns to its more natural tone and is drier and flakier. The ruddiness results from normally elevated red blood cell concentration.

The hands and feet may appear slightly blue; this is called acrocyanosis and is caused by poor peripheral circulation. Acrocyanosis can last for 7 to 10 days. It is most commonly observed when the infant becomes cold. Mottling, a lacy pattern with dilated vessels on pale skin, is also common. Another normal variation is called the harlequin sign; half of the newborn's body appears deep red and the other half appears pale as a result of vasomotor disturbance, with some vessels constricting while others dilate. When the infant is placed on one side, the dependent half is noticeably pinker than the superior half. This may last for up to 20 minutes. Although disturbing to view, it is not harmful.

Jaundice, a yellow discoloration caused by deposits of bile pigments and also known as **icterus neonatorum,** is first detected over bony prominences on the face and the mucous membranes. This is abnormal during the first 24 hours of life. After 24 hours it is not necessarily abnormal. The newborn's hemoglobin and hematocrit levels frequently are elevated; hemoglobin may range from 14 to 24 g/dL and hematocrit from 44% to 64%. After 24 hours, the newborn may develop physiologic jaundice (jaundice occurring 48 hours or later after birth, gradually disappearing by the seventh to tenth day, and caused by the normal reduction in the number of red blood cells), since the excessive levels of hemoglobins are no longer required for oxygen transport. Further assessment of jaundice is required. The physician may order laboratory and diagnostic tests to determine the nature of the problem and begin treatment to prevent complications. Causes of jaundice are discussed further in Chapter 28.

Appearance

At birth the skin is covered with a yellowish white, cream cheese–like substance called vernix caseosa. This substance protects the infant's skin from the amniotic fluid. When the vernix caseosa is removed, the skin may appear dry and may crack, flake, and peel. Another common finding is lanugo (downy, fine hair characteristic of the fetus, between 20 weeks of gestation and birth); lanugo is most noticeable over the shoulders, forehead, and cheeks, but it is found on nearly all parts of the body except the palms, soles, and scalp.

Good turgor and tissue elasticity are normally observed. Desquamation of the skin of the term infant does not occur until a few days after birth. Its presence at birth is an indication of postmaturity.

Head

The fontanelles (broad area or soft spot consisting of a strong band of connective tissue contiguous with [touching] cranial bones and located at the junction of the bones) should be palpable. The **anterior fontanelle** is normally large and diamond shaped and closes at approximately 18 months of age. The **posterior fontanelle** is smaller and triangular and normally closes at 2 months of age. The sagittal suture may be felt by running the fingers between the two fontanelles (see Chapter 26, Figure 26-2).

The newborn's head may manifest many variations. Most of these are a result of the birth process and disappear without treatment shortly after the delivery:

- **Molding** is overlapping of the bones of the skull. The head may appear elongated and misshapen; this is a result of compression during delivery and normally disappears within a day or two.
- **Caput succedaneum** is commonly seen with molding. It is the result of edema in the soft tissue of the scalp. The tissue feels spongy and may be felt over suture lines. This also disappears without treatment (Figure 27-8, *A*).
- **Cephalhematoma** is caused by bleeding within the periosteum of a cranial bone. It is confined to a particular bone and does not cross suture lines. This is usually a result of difficult labor. Cephalhematomas generally appear 1 or 2 days after birth. These normally absorb without treatment. Large hematomas may lead to anemia and jaundice, which require medical intervention (Figure 27-8, *B*).

Face

The newborn's chin is receding and the nose relatively flat. Fat pads make the cheeks appear full and round. Movements of the face should be symmetric. The mouth should open freely, and the oral cavity should be intact with a closed palate. Small white nodules called **Epstein's pearls** may be observed on the hard palate. These are a result of epithelial cells and disappear spontaneously within a few weeks. Rarely, an infant is born with teeth; this should be watched closely because they may become loose and be aspirated. The oral cavity should be clean and free from lesions. A fungal infection may be acquired during passage through the birth canal if the mother is infected with *Candida albicans.* This results in thrush, a white, patchy coating of the mucous membranes that cannot be wiped off. Treatment with antifungal medications such as nystatin or gentian violet is required.

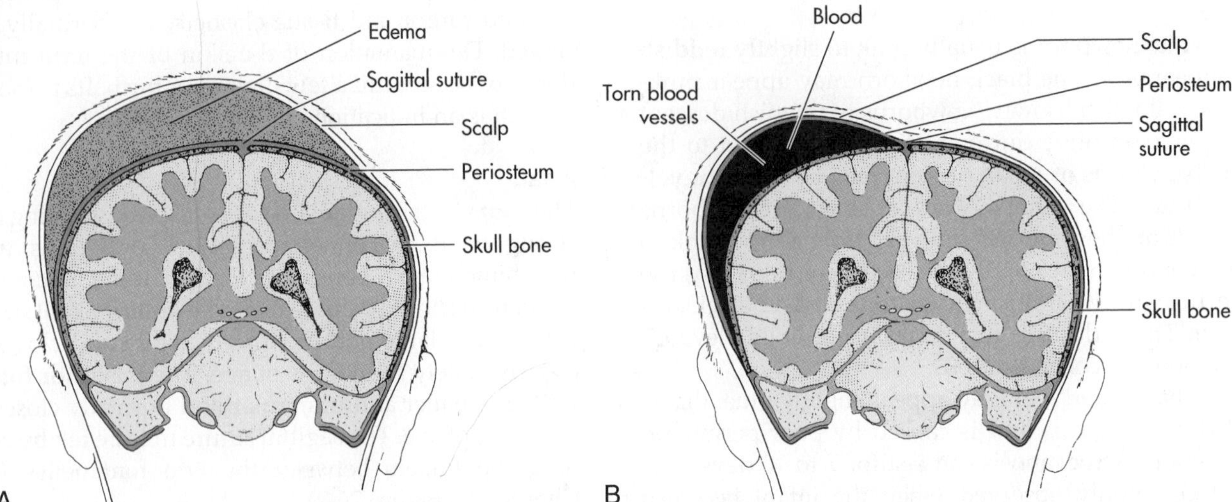

FIGURE 27-8 Differences between caput succedaneum and cephalhematoma. **A,** Caput succedaneum: edema of scalp noted at birth; crosses suture line. **B,** Cephalhematoma: bleeding between periosteum and skull bone appearing within first 2 days; does not cross suture lines.

Eyes

The eyelids may appear edematous because of prophylactic antibiotic medication that was applied to the eyes after birth to prevent **ophthalmia neonatorum** (infection in the neonate's eyes, usually resulting from gonorrheal or other infection contracted when the fetus passes through the birth canal [vagina]). The eyes appear wide set. **Strabismus** (crossed eyes) and **nystagmus** (abnormal motion of the eyes) are commonly seen as a result of the newborn's immature nervous system. Most white infants have slate-gray to blue irises at birth; in darker-skinned infants the irises may appear darker. The newborn does not produce tears because the lacrimal structures have not fully matured. Vision has been found to be more acute than previously believed. Newborns are nearsighted and can see objects best at 8 to 10 inches; most prefer simple patterns in black and white and human faces. Make certain the parents know this because eye contact with the baby is an important part of bonding.

Ears

The ears are normally positioned with the upper insertion of the pinna located even with the outer canthus of the eye. Low-set ears may indicate a chromosomal disorder. Newborns are most attentive to high-pitched sounds and the mother's voice. The fetus becomes familiar with the mother's voice in utero.

Umbilical Cord

The umbilical cord is whitish blue-gray with three vessels (one vein and two arteries) and contains a gelatinous tissue called Wharton's jelly. Inspect the cord for the number of vessels because a two-vessel cord may indicate congenital anomalies. In Figure 27-9, note the cord stump in *A* and the cord stump in *B* (triple dye gives it the purplish color).

Providing Cord Care

Check the cord for bleeding or oozing during the early hours after birth. The cord clamp must be securely fas-

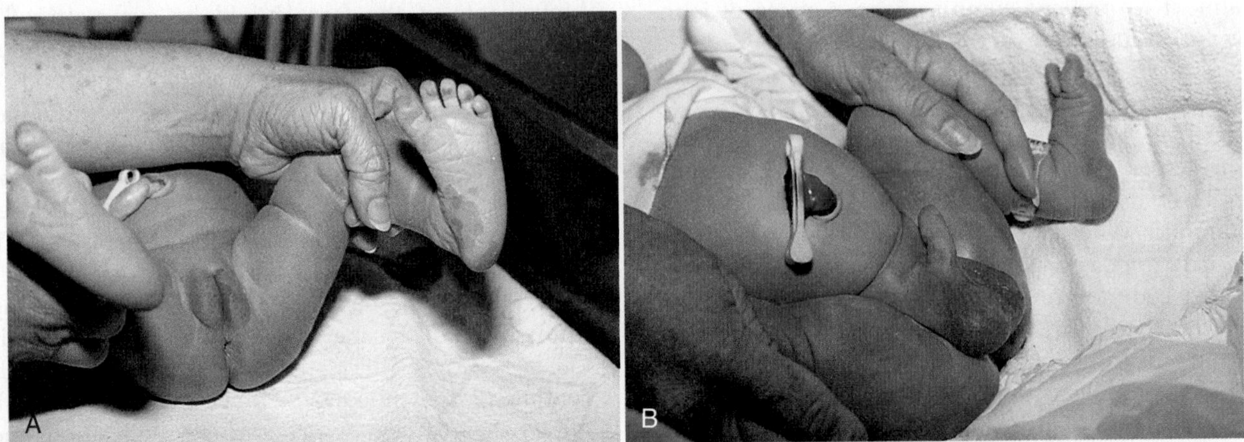

FIGURE 27-9 External genitalia. **A,** Genitalia in female term infant. Note mucoid vaginal discharge. **B,** Genitalia in male infant. Uncircumcised penis. Rugae cover scrotum, indicating term gestation. Cord has been swabbed with ethylene blue to prevent infection.

tened with no skin caught in it. Purulent drainage or redness or edema at the base indicates infection. The cord becomes brownish black within 2 or 3 days and falls off in about 10 to 14 days.

Care of the cord varies in different agencies. It may be treated with a bactericidal substance such as triple-dye solution (see Figure 27-9, *B*), antibiotic ointment, or alcohol three times a day, or allowed to dry naturally. None of the treatments commonly used is better at keeping the cord clean and dry than the others. When soiled, the cord should be cleaned with water. This natural treatment of cords may shorten the time to cord separation and does not lead to increased infections. The diaper is folded below the cord to keep the cord dry and free from contamination by urine.

Remove the cord clamp about 24 hours after birth if the end of the cord is dry (Figure 27-10). Although the base of the cord is still moist, it will not bleed if the end is dry and crisp.

Reflexes

Normal newborns exhibit a wide variety of reflexes (Table 27-5). Some are protective reflexes, such as the rooting, sucking, gag, swallow, blink, burp, hiccup, and sneeze reflex. Other reflexes, such as the Babinski, Moro, tonic neck, and stepping, are related to the immature nervous system. Many are present for a limited time and then disappear.

Genitalia

The genitalia in female newborns may be edematous (see Figure 27-9, *A*). Discharge of blood-tinged mucus from the vagina, called **pseudomenstruation,** may occur in response to maternal hormones. Either sex may have enlarged breasts. This is called **gynecomastia** and is also a result of maternal hormones. The labia majora cover the minora in term infants (see Figure 27-9, *A*). The scrotum in the male may be enlarged and edematous, indicating a hydrocele. The testicles are normally descended in term infants (see Figure 27-9, *B*); in preterm infants they may not be descended **(cryptorchidism).** Inspect the penis for position of the urethral meatus. Abnormal placement may result in problems with voiding. Circumcision (the surgical removal of the foreskin) is not normally done if there is any malplacement, since the foreskin may be used as part of the surgical correction.

Spine

The spine should be straight without curves. The normal cervical and lumbar curves develop once the infant begins to stand. Also examine the spine for dimples, tufts of hair, and masses that may indicate abnormalities of spinal column development.

Extremities

The arms and hands are generally flexed against the body. Both arms should move evenly. Trauma during delivery may result in fracture of the clavicle or in brachial palsy. Both hands should be free from webbing (**syndactyly;** malformation of digits, commonly seen as webbing or fusion of two or more digits to form one structure) or extra digits **(polydactyly).** A single crease in the palm of the hand, a simian line, may indicate chromosomal disorders such as **Down syndrome** (mongolism or trisomy 21, caused by an extra chromosome 21 in the G group) (see Chapter 31). Nails often extend beyond the fingertips. Legs should be equal in length. If one leg appears longer or if the gluteal or popliteal folds are **asymmetric** (unequal in size or shape), congenital hip dysplasia may be suspected. The hips should move freely.

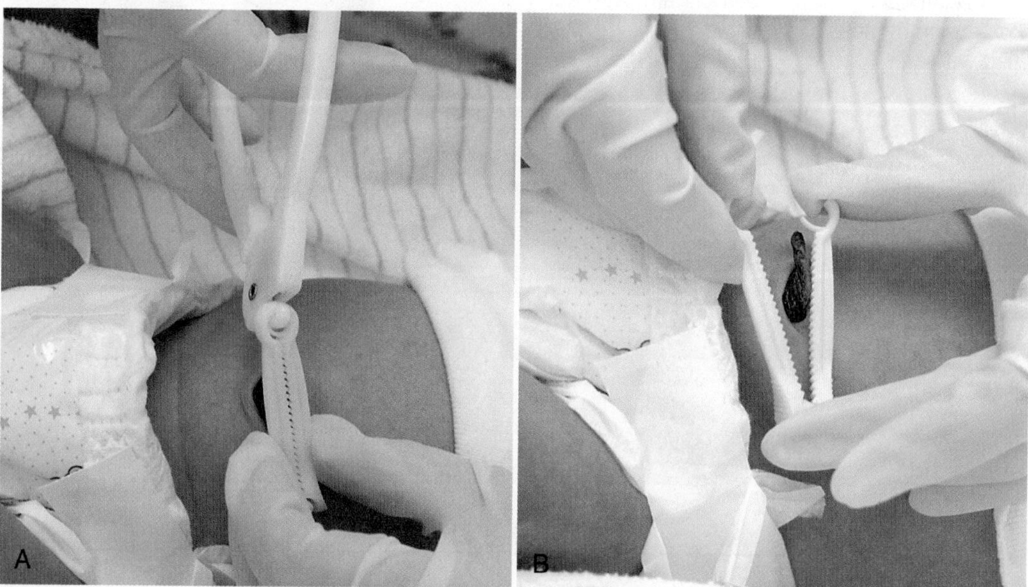

FIGURE 27-10 The cord clamp is removed when the end of the cord is dry and crisp. The clamp is cut **(A)** and separated **(B).** NOTE: No triple dye was used; the diaper is folded down away from the cord area.

Table 27-5 **Assessment of Reflexes in the Normal Newborn**

EXPECTED BEHAVIORAL RESPONSE	COMMENTS	
MORO (STARTLE) REFLEX Sudden jarring or change in equilibrium causes extension and abduction of extremities and fanning of fingers, with index finger and thumb forming a C shape, followed by flexion and adduction of extremities; legs may weakly flex; infant may cry.	Elicit reflex by holding the infant above the examining table in a supine position with one hand beneath the sacrum and the other supporting the upper back and head; then allow the infant's head to suddenly fall about 30 degrees. Disappears after 3 to 4 months; usually strongest during first 2 months.	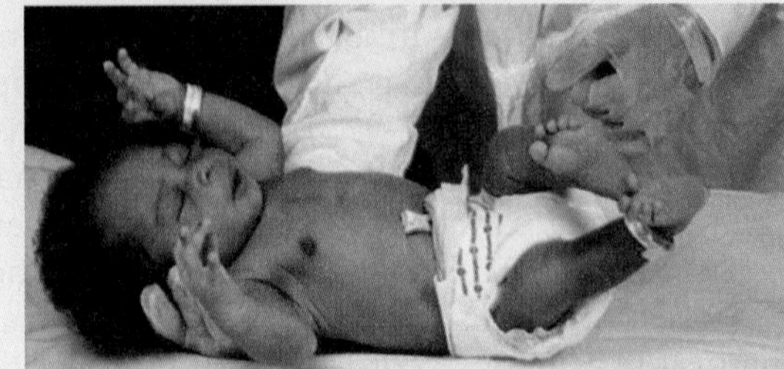 Moro reflex.
TONIC NECK REFLEX When infant's head is quickly turned to one side, arm and leg will extend on that side, and opposite arm and leg will flex; posture resembles a fencing position.	Disappears by 3 to 4 months of age, to be replaced by symmetric positioning of both sides of body.	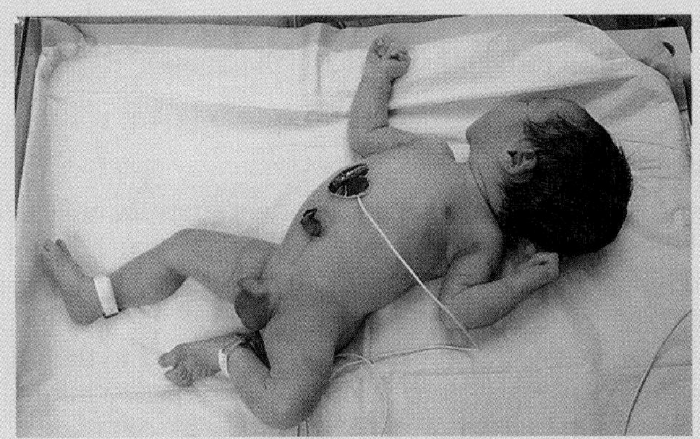 Tonic neck reflex.
CRAWLING When placed on abdomen, infant will make crawling movements with the arms and legs.	Disappears at about 6 weeks of age.	
DANCE OR STEPPING REFLEX If infant is held so that sole of foot touches a hard surface, there will be a reciprocal flexion and extension of the leg, simulating walking.	Disappears after 3 to 4 weeks, to be replaced by deliberate movement.	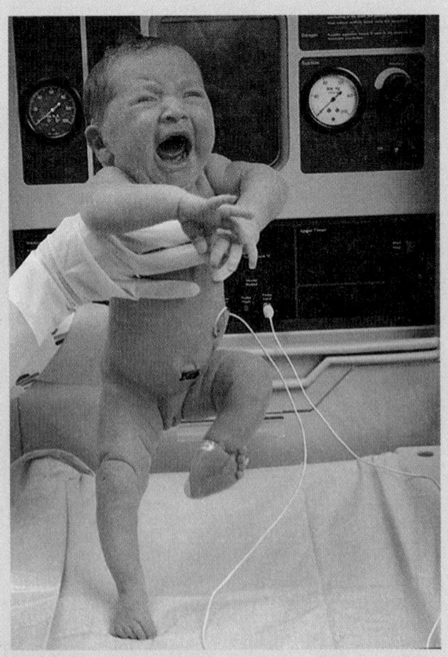 Step reflex.

Table 27-5 Assessment of Reflexes in the Normal Newborn—cont'd

EXPECTED BEHAVIORAL RESPONSE	COMMENTS	
BABINSKI REFLEX When the sole of the foot is stroked along side of sole beginning at heel and then moving across ball of foot to big toe, toes will fan out with dorsiflexion of big toe.	Disappears by 1 year. Absence laterally indicates central nervous system damage.	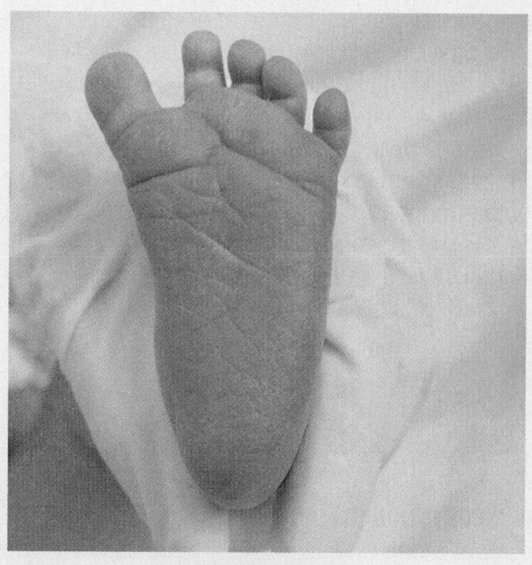 Babinski reflex.
GRASP REFLEX **Palmar.** Place finger in the palm of the hand. Infant's fingers curl around examiner's fingers.		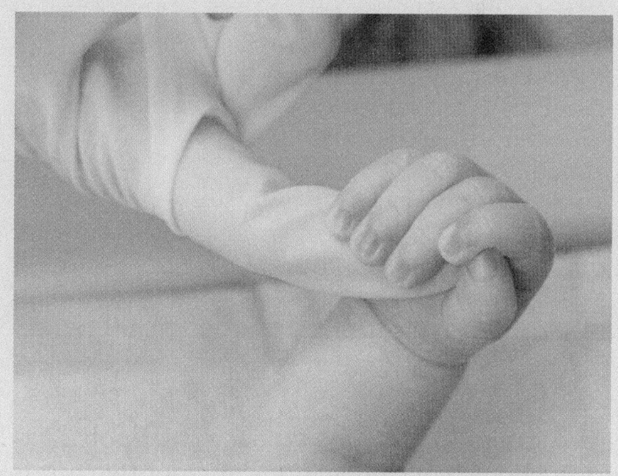 Palmar grasp reflex.
Plantar. Place fingers at the base of the toes. Toes curl downward.		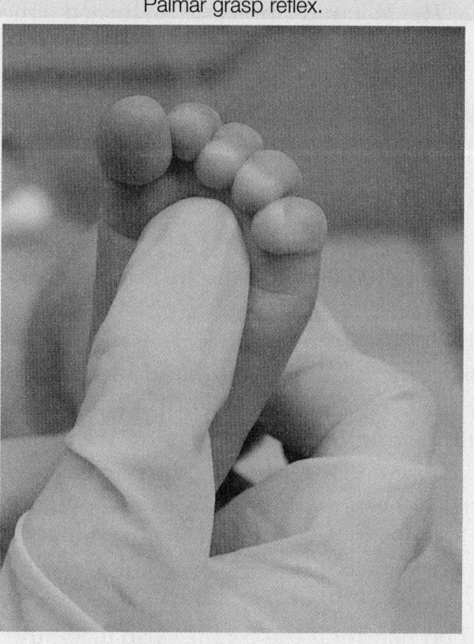 Plantar grasp reflex.

Continued

Table 27-5 Assessment of Reflexes in the Normal Newborn—cont'd

EXPECTED BEHAVIORAL RESPONSE	COMMENTS	
PULL TO SIT (TRACTION) REFLEX		
Pull infant up by the wrist from supine position with head in midline. Head lags until infant is in upright position, then head is held in the same place with chest and shoulder momentarily before falling forward; infant will attempt to right head.		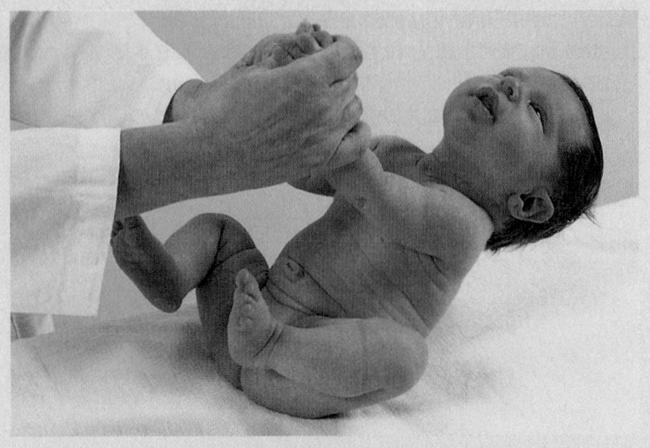 Pull to sit.
TRUNK INCURVATION (GALANT REFLEX)		
Place infant prone on flat surface; run finger down back about 1½ to 2 inches lateral to the spine, first on one side and then on the other. In response, infant flexes the trunk and swings his or her pelvis toward the stimulated side.	The response disappears by the fourth week. Absence of response suggests general depression of nervous system.	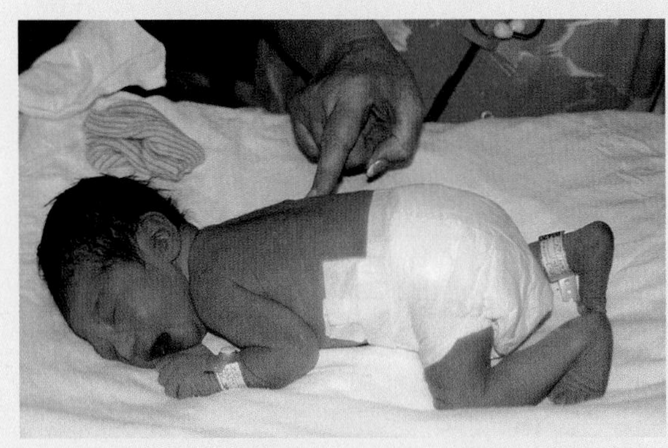 Galant reflex.

Also assess the feet for syndactyly or polydactyly. Creases should cover at least the anterior two thirds of the sole. The feet may appear to be turned abnormally, often the result of the newborn's position in utero.

NURSING ASSESSMENT AND INTERVENTIONS FOR THE NEWBORN

HEALTH MANAGEMENT AND HEALTH PERCEPTION

Before giving the newborn to the mother, check identification bracelets to prevent the possibility of giving the baby to the wrong mother.

Instruct the mother about hand hygiene when caring for the baby to prevent the spread of microorganisms; this is important when going from performing personal hygiene to caring for the infant.

Instruct the new mother in safety practices to reduce the likelihood of injury to the infant. Demonstrate positions that provide head support while carrying and burping (Figure 27-11). The large head requires care when handling the infant. Also teach the mother to never leave the baby unattended in an unsafe location, such as on a table or a bed. The environment should be kept free of hazards, such as pins or other sharp objects. Demonstrate bathing techniques and temperature taking. Teach the mother to position the infant on his or her side after feeding to reduce the possibility of aspiration if the baby regurgitates. A rolled-up bathing or baby blanket may be placed along the back of the baby to aid in maintaining the side-lying position. Advise the mother not to place the baby in the prone position after eating because of the danger of vomiting and aspiration. Bottles should never be propped for feeding, since this may lead to choking or aspiration. The use of infant car seats is now mandatory in most states.

NUTRITIONAL AND METABOLIC ISSUES

State laws require that certain diagnostic tests be performed on the newborn. Know the laws of your state. These tests are done to detect conditions that result in serious complications, such as neurologic disorders and cognitive impairment. With early detection and proper treatment, many complications can be eliminated or reduced. Most of the diseases tested for involve inborn errors of metabolism in which the newborn is unable to metabolize various nutrients. Some

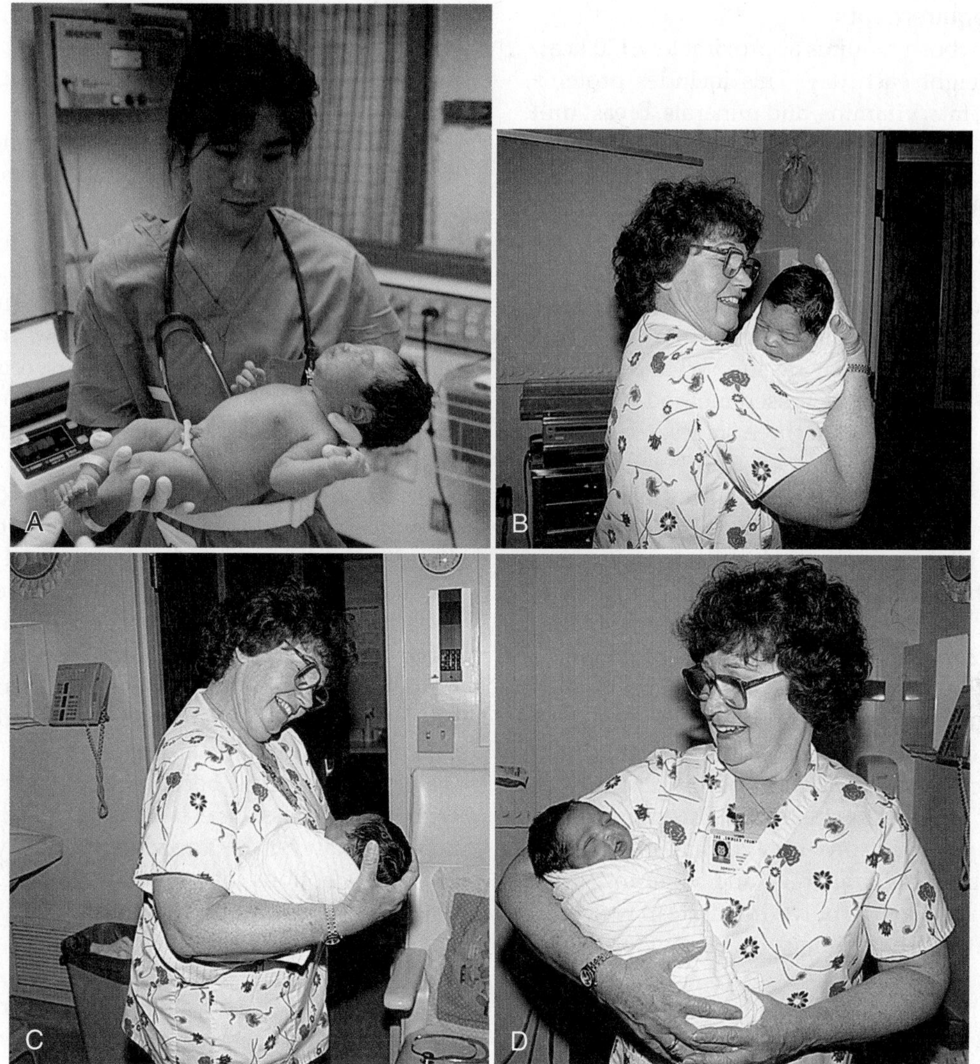

FIGURE 27-11 Holding baby securely with support for head. **A,** Holding newborn while moving from one place to another. **B,** Holding newborn upright in burping position. **C,** Football hold. **D,** Cradle hold.

of the more common tests are done to detect phenylketonuria, maple sugar urine disease, galactosemia, and hypothyroidism. These tests involve either blood or urine samples. For most test results to be meaningful, the newborn must have consumed an adequate amount of either human milk or cow's milk formula. Because of early discharge of mothers and newborns, this may not occur before the newborn goes home. If the tests are performed before the neonate is discharged from the hospital, completion of the necessary bloodwork should be verified and noted on the chart before the newborn is allowed to leave. If the tests are done later, usually at 2 to 5 days of age, the newborn returns to the hospital or physician's office. Be certain that the parents understand the importance of the tests and when the newborn is to be tested (Table 27-6).

Newborns have low prothrombin levels at birth and are at risk for hemorrhage. Because they are not able to synthesize vitamin K in the colon until they have adequate intestinal flora, a vitamin K injection (AquaMEPHYTON) is routinely administered. Injections are best administered in the vastus lateralis muscle because it is more developed than the newborn's other muscles.

Table 27-6 Standard Laboratory Values in a Full-Term Infant*

PARAMETER	VALUE
Hematocrit	14-24 g/dL
Glucose	40-60 mg/dL
Bilirubin, direct	0-1 mg/dL
Hemoglobin	14-24 g/dL

*Heelstick capillary blood.

Monitor weight daily. A newborn normally loses up to 10% of his or her body weight in the first week of life, from a combination of factors. More weight is lost through the passing of meconium and urine than is taken in by the newborn. This is particularly true in breastfed babies. Most newborns regain their birth weight within the second week.

Nutritional Requirements

The normal newborn requires approximately 120 kcal/kg of body weight each day. This includes proteins, carbohydrates, fats, vitamins, and minerals. Breast milk and prepared formulas are balanced to meet the newborn's needs. Because newborns cannot concentrate urine efficiently, fluid intake needs are high; 140 to 160 mL/kg/day is necessary (1 kg = 2.2 pounds).

With the improved formulas available today, the infant's fluid and nutritional needs can be met by either breastfeeding or bottle feeding. The mother can choose the method she prefers. Provide support and teaching appropriate to the mother's chosen method.

Breast milk is produced in three stages. **Colostrum,** the first substance produced, is thin, watery, and slightly yellow. It is rich in protein and calories in addition to antibodies and lymphocytes. It also contains high levels of immunoglobulins, which transfer some immunity to the newborn. The mother begins producing colostrum in the last trimester of pregnancy and continues for 2 to 4 days after delivery; she then produces transitional milk for about 1 week. This may appear thinner and more watery but is high in fats, lactose, and water-soluble vitamins and contains more calories than colostrum. Mature milk is generally established by 2 weeks after delivery. This may appear very thin and watery. It provides 20 kcal/oz and contains lactose, proteins, minerals, and vitamins. If the mother is eating properly, only vitamin D may need to be supplemented. The primary care provider should be consulted.

Because human milk is uniquely designed to meet the needs of the human infant, it is used as the standard for all infant feedings. Infants who are not breastfed should be given commercial formulas. Low-income families usually are eligible for services through the WIC program, which provides iron-fortified infant formula.

Bovine milk (cow's milk) is the basis of most formulas. Infants with an allergic reaction to cow's milk formula may experience diarrhea, rash, colic, vomiting, and, in extreme cases, failure to thrive. Soy milk formula is acceptable for some of these infants, but others are allergic to soy protein. If hypersensitivity to cow's milk protein is suspected, a hydrolyzed casein formula may be effective; however, these special formulas are expensive.

Formulas are produced by modifying cow's milk to make it more similar to human milk. It appears thicker and richer but also contains 20 kcal/oz. Formulas are available in ready-to-feed, powdered, and concentrated forms. Instruct the mother in proper preparation and storage to prevent nutritional or digestive problems in her infant.

In bottle-fed infants, the first feeding is normally 15 to 30 mL of sterile water. This must be given with caution to verify that the infant is able to swallow normally and has no anomalies of the digestive tract. If the infant takes the water without difficulty, begin bottle feeding. Breastfed newborns can be put to breast to nurse immediately after birth, without a sterile water feeding.

It is normal for infants to regurgitate mucus after the first few feedings. Food intake is necessary to prevent hypoglycemia, which is stressful to the newborn. Some facilities have a policy requiring a blood glucose determination test. Excessive maternal glucose results in fetal hyperglycemia and fetal hyperinsulinism. After birth, the neonate's high levels of insulin will deplete the glucose stores, and hypoglycemia will result. If the infant's blood glucose level is 40 mg/dL or less, sterile glucose water is given in the first hours after birth.

The frequency of feeding depends on the type of feeding. Breastfed babies tend to do best on an "on demand" schedule, generally nursing at 1- to 3-hour intervals. Bottle-fed babies tend to eat less frequently, usually every 2 to 4 hours, because formula is digested more slowly. Each baby establishes a pattern over time. It is important not to overfeed, particularly with bottle-fed babies, because this can lead to regurgitation. Breastfed infants are not normally given glucose water supplements because doing so may interfere with the process of establishing lactation, since the neonate may not be adequately hungry when put to breast. Exceptions may be made in cases in which the newborn's blood glucose is low.

Both bottle-fed and breastfed babies need to be burped at intervals. While sucking, the baby normally swallows air; if this air is not cleared from the stomach, the infant may feel satisfied and stop eating. When the air clears the stomach, the infant may again appear hungry.

Before starting, the mother should choose a feeding position that is comfortable and that facilitates the flow of milk into the stomach. Many different positions are suitable for breastfeeding or bottle feeding (see Figure 27-5).

Hypothermia

Maintenance of body temperature is a major concern when caring for newborns. Prolonged exposure to a cold environment can result in increased oxygen consumption and depleted glycogen reserves. Newborns have a relatively large surface area and a limited amount of protective adipose tissue. They lose heat through radiation, evaporation, conduction, and convection. Be aware of this and take precautions to reduce the losses (Table 27-7).

Monitor temperature with a skin sensor or thermometer. Verify that the anus is patent. The rectal method of temperature assessment is used less often because of the chance of rectal irritation or perforation. Most facilities use the axillary route because it is considered safe. The normal axillary temperature is 97.6° to 98.6° F (36.4° to 37° C). Mercury thermometers are

Table 27-7 **Precautions to Minimize Heat Loss in Infants**

TYPES OF HEAT LOSS	NURSING INTERVENTIONS TO PREVENT HEAT LOSS
Radiation: Loss that occurs when heat transfers from the body to cooler surfaces and objects not in contact with the body	Keep body well wrapped to prevent radiant loss. Work quickly to avoid excessive time with skin exposed. Use radiant warmer to minimize loss. Locate crib away from outside wall.
Evaporation: Loss when water is converted into a vapor	Dry infant thoroughly after delivery and promptly when bathing.
Conduction: Loss of heat to a cooler surface by direct skin contact	Pad surfaces under infant, including tables and scales. Warm other equipment, such as stethoscopes, before use.
Convection: Loss of heat to cooler air currents	Reduce drafts from open doors, windows, or air conditioning; wrap newborn to protect from cold.

rarely used in health care settings today, although they may still be used in the home.

Hygiene

Inspection and bathing of the neonate take place after the body temperature has stabilized. The frequency and type of baths depend on facility policies. Bathing serves a number of purposes: complete cleansing, observation of the infant's condition, comfort, and parent-child socialization.

Gather all bathing articles and the infant's change of clothing before bathing. The room temperature should be 75° F (24° C), and the bathing area should be free of drafts to prevent heat loss. The bath water should be approximately 100° F (38° C). Heat loss in the infant is greater than heat loss in the adult because of the relatively large ratio of the skin surface to body mass in the newborn. To conserve the infant's energy, control heat loss by bathing the infant quickly, padding cold surfaces, exposing only a portion of the body at a time, and thoroughly drying the infant. Until the initial bath is completed, wear gloves when handling the newborn.

Centers for Disease Control and Prevention regulations related to standard precautions against human immunodeficiency virus and other bloodborne pathogens have increased the use of soap solutions for bathing newborn infants. Use a nonmedicated mild soap for the initial bath. Shampoo the hair and use a brush or a comb to remove dried blood and vernix caseosa. Use cotton balls, not gauze, to cleanse the nostrils and ears. Careful drying may decrease the risk of infection. The order of the bath is essentially the same as for an adult, beginning with the eyes, the face, and the head and ending with the anal region. Reassess the temperature 30 minutes after completion of the bath.

After the initial bath, washing with warm water is sufficient for the first week. However, the perineal area should be carefully washed with nonmedicated mild soap and warm water and carefully dried with each diaper change.

The infant's fragile skin can be injured by vigorous cleansing. Do not vigorously remove vernix caseosa (the white material that looks like cold cream) because it is attached to the upper, protective layer of the skin. Vernix caseosa may be left on for 48 hours; if it persists beyond that time, wash if off gently. Some nurses advocate massaging the vernix caseosa gently into the skin. To date, no studies have confirmed the benefits or disadvantages of this technique.

Questions have arisen about some routine practices: use of soap, oils, powder, lotion, and sponging. According to Wong and colleagues (2006):

> One of the most important considerations in skin cleansing is preservation of the skin's pH, which is about 5 soon after birth. The slightly acidic skin surface has bacteriostatic effects. Consequently, only warm water with a mild soap should be used for the bath. Alkaline soaps such as Ivory, oils, powder, and lotions are not used because they alter the pH, thus providing a better environment for bacterial growth. Talcum has the added risk of aspiration if applied too close to the infant's face.

Discuss the choice of cloth or disposable diapers with parents. Cloth diapers today are different from those used years ago with plastic or rubber pants. Using disposable diapers exclusively is the most expensive and most popular method. Over 1 or 2 years, the cost can be considerable, particularly if more than one child is wearing diapers. However, some disposable diapers may help prevent diaper dermatitis.

Pay special attention to care of the umbilical area. At delivery the cord is moist. Over the next few days a drying process called **mummification** (producing a dry, hard mass) begins. Avoid getting the cord wet during bathing. Most facilities have a routine to promote drying by use of alcohol or other substances (triple dye) that inhibit microbial growth. Odor or exudate from the cord is abnormal and should be reported promptly. Delay tub bathing until the fully dried cord drops off at about 10 days of age.

Give the mother a demonstration of temperature taking and bathing the newborn. If possible, encourage her to bathe the infant while you observe. This will help her gain confidence and provides an opportunity to answer questions about care. It is also a good time to demonstrate safe methods of holding and positioning the infant.

Circumcision refers to the surgical removal of the foreskin. Many parents elect to have the procedure performed on their newborn infants. In a policy statement published in 1999 and reaffirmed in 2005, the

American Academy of Pediatrics (AAP) acknowledges the health benefits of circumcision but does not believe these are a reason for all male infants to have the procedure. The AAP further states that analgesia should be used if a circumcision is performed; a consent form for both is required.

If circumcision is performed, keep the area clean and assess it for bleeding every hour for the first 12 hours postoperatively. Apply gentle pressure to the bleeding area with a folded gauze pad. Sterile petroleum gauze is usually applied to the penis after a Gomco or Mogan circumcision and is left in place for 24 hours; it is replaced if it becomes dislodged prematurely. If a Plastibell circumcision is performed, the petroleum gauze is not needed because the plastic bell that covers the glans will not stick to the diaper.

Wash the penis gently at diaper changes to remove urine and feces, and reapply fresh sterile petroleum gauze. Do not attempt to remove the dried yellow exudate that forms in 24 hours and persists for 2 to 3 days; this is part of the normal healing process. Cloth diapers may be recommended during the healing period (about 1 week). Avoid positioning the infant on the abdomen for the first few hours after the procedure. Loose diapering is necessary. If bleeding is not controlled, continue application of intermittent pressure, notify the physician, and prepare for blood vessel ligation. If the infant has undergone this procedure without anesthesia, he should be comforted until he is quieted and then returned to his crib. These infants usually are fussy for about 2 to 3 hours and may refuse a feeding.

It is important to teach the parents appropriate home care before discharge of the newborn. Teaching should include measures to promote hygiene, thus reducing the risks of infection. Educate the parents to report immediately any unusual signs and symptoms such as edema; purulent, malodorous discharge; elevated temperature; and delayed healing.

ELIMINATION

The newborn should void within 24 hours of delivery. If this does not occur, notify the physician. The average newborn voids small amounts of poorly concentrated urine; it is normally clear and odorless. Occasionally a small pink or brownish discharge may be observed as a result of uric acid crystals that were formed in the bladder in utero. As fluid intake increases and kidney function improves, urination becomes more frequent and assumes the normal color.

Bowel elimination should occur within 24 hours of birth. The newborn's initial stools are odorless, black-green, and sticky. This is called **meconium** and is made up of vernix, strands of lanugo, mucus, and other substances from the amniotic fluid. Occasionally the first stool is encased in mucus and called a **meconium plug.** If no stool is observed, notify the physician so that an examination can be performed to determine the problem. Once the infant begins to take nourishment, the stool changes. Transitional stools, which occur on about the second day, tend to be greenish and loose. These are seen until about the fourth day, when the milk stool is seen. Breastfed babies tend to pass stool frequently, sometimes with every feeding. The stool is pale yellow and sweet smelling. Small curds may be observed. Babies who are bottle fed tend to have fewer stools, usually two or three per day after the first 2 weeks. These are bright yellow and pasty in consistency; the odor may be slightly stronger than that of breastfed babies. This type of stool continues until solid food is introduced. Very watery stools, green stools (after the transition), or stools expelled with force may indicate gastrointestinal irritation or infection and should be reported promptly. Newborns can lose a great deal of fluid rapidly and become dehydrated (see Box 27-14 for stooling patterns of newborns). (It should be noted that newborns normally give the impression of straining with a stool because their muscles are underdeveloped. This can cause parents undue concern if they are not advised about it. The straining subsides as growth and maturity continue.)

The skin of the perineum and buttocks can become irritated if waste products are left in contact for too long. Teach the parents to wash the skin, wiping from anterior to posterior, after each voiding or stool, and to change diapers promptly. Recommend minimal use of creams, which can irritate the skin. Disposable or cloth diapers may be chosen.

Box 27-14 Change in Stooling of Newborns

MECONIUM

- Infant's first stool is composed of amniotic fluid and its constituents, intestinal secretions, shed mucosal cells, and possibly blood (ingested maternal blood or minor bleeding of alimentary tract vessels).
- Passage of meconium should occur within the first 24 to 48 hours, although it may be delayed up to 7 days in very low–birth-weight infants.

TRANSITIONAL STOOLS

- Transitional stools usually appear by the third day after initiation of feeding.
- They are greenish brown to yellowish brown, thin, and less sticky than meconium; they may contain some milk curds.

MILK STOOL

- Milk stools usually appear by the fourth day.
- In *breastfed* infants, stools are yellow to golden, are pasty in consistency, and have an odor similar to that of sour milk.
- In *formula-fed* infants, stools are pale yellow to light brown, are firmer in consistency, and have a more offensive odor.

REST AND SLEEP

Most newborns spend 16 to 20 hours per day sleeping. They may be observed to startle and make sucking motions during sleep. Breathing may be regular and even or irregular, depending on the sleep state. The time awake is spent crying, eating, or in quiet alertness. Each infant establishes a unique pattern, which may be erratic but stabilizes over time as the nervous and digestive systems mature. Most infants do not exceed 5 continuous hours of sleep for some months, which can be disruptive to the mother's sleep.

ACTIVITY AND EXERCISE

Maintenance of a clear airway is critical. Many infants require suctioning to remove mucus from the nose and mouth. Newborns are obligate (necessary or required) nose breathers; they must be able to breathe through their nose while suckling. Therefore the nasal passageway must be kept open and free from mucus. A small bulb syringe is commonly used. Compress it before insertion and then gently release it to suction secretions. Explain to parents the use of the bulb syringe before the first feeding. For the first few days a bulb syringe should always be kept with the newborn, particularly during feeding.

Crying is the newborn's only means of communication. The cry can indicate hunger, pain, the need for attention, or fussiness. The newborn's cry should be strong, vigorous, and of medium pitch. As mother and infant become more adept at interpreting each other's behavior, some mothers state that they are able to distinguish the reason for crying. The following report indicates that mother and baby are communicating effectively:

> I can tell when she's hungry. Crying starts in a plaintive [sorrowful, sad] way and then becomes more and more demanding. When she is hurt she lets out a startled yell as though she couldn't believe it was happening to her. Sometimes when she is put down to sleep, she starts a kind of talking cry, jerky and demanding: it gets louder, and if nothing happens, fades away in little spurts. The fussy cry is the hardest to take—nothing seems to work; like a complaining that goes on and on.

A high-pitched cry may indicate neurologic problems and should be observed further and evaluated by a physician. See Patient Teaching box for infant quieting techniques.

PARENT-CHILD ATTACHMENT

The human infant is born defenseless and could not survive without a caregiver. The parents are responsible for the infant's physical and psychological development.

Parenting is not instinctive; a new parent must bond with the baby first. **Parent-child attachment (bonding)** is defined as the initial phase in a relationship characterized by strong attraction and a desire to interact (Figure 27-12). Without bonding, parents would find it difficult to maintain the energy required to meet the newborn's needs. The nurse cannot make bonding occur but can facilitate its development.

 Patient Teaching

Infant Quieting Techniques

- Many newborns feel insecure in the center of a large crib. They prefer a small, warm, soft space that reminds them of intrauterine life. Try a smaller bed, such as a bassinet, portable crib, buggy, or cradle, or use a rolled-up blanket to turn a corner of the big crib into a smaller place.
- Carry your baby in a frontpack or backpack.
- Swaddle your newborn snugly in a receiving blanket. Swaddling keeps your newborn's arms and legs close to his or her body, similar to the intrauterine position. It makes the newborn feel more secure.
- Prewarm the crib sheets with a hot water bottle or heating pad that you remove before putting your baby to bed. Some babies startle when placed on a cold sheet.
- Some newborns need extra sucking to soothe themselves to sleep. Breastfeeding mothers may prefer to let their infant suckle at the breast as a soothing technique. Other mothers choose to use a pacifier. Stroke the pacifier against the roof of the baby's mouth to encourage him or her to suck it during the first 2 weeks. Around age 3 months, infants can find and suck their thumbs as a way of self-consoling.
- A rhythmic, monotonous noise simulating the intrauterine sounds of your heartbeat and blood flow may help your infant settle down. Some parents have found it helpful to put a fussy baby in a portable crib beside the dishwasher or washing machine.
- Movement often helps quiet a baby. Take your baby for a ride in the car or an outing in a stroller or carriage. Rock your baby in a rocking chair or cradle.
- Place your baby on his or her stomach across your lap; pat and rub his or her back while gently bouncing your legs or swaying them from left to right.
- Babies enjoy skin-to-skin contact. A combination of this and warm water often helps soothe a fussy baby. Fill your tub with warm water. Get in and let the baby lie on your chest so that the baby is immersed in the water up to his or her neck. Cuddle the baby.
- Let your baby see your face. Talk to your baby in a soothing voice.
- Your baby may simply be bored. Bring him or her into the room where you and the rest of your family are. Change your baby's position; many babies like to be upright, such as being held up on your shoulder.

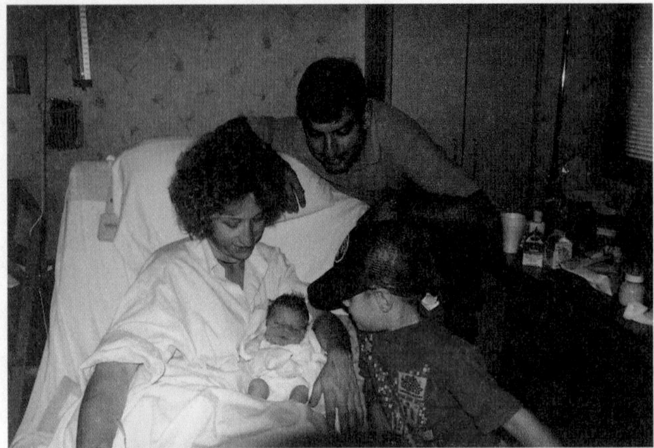

FIGURE 27-12 Parents and sibling interacting with a newborn.

Early contact with the infant is important to establish bonding. A new mother normally wishes to touch and explore her baby. Holding the infant close and looking eye to eye (the en face position) helps bonding occur (Figure 27-13). It is normal for a new mother to talk in high-pitched tones to the baby. Encourage early and frequent interaction between the newborn and the parents (Figure 27-14). Attachment increases when the infant begins to respond.

The newborn has amazing capabilities. The infant is a socially responsive human being who can probably learn better on the first day of life than ever again. Immediately after birth, the baby stares intently at the parents' faces and sees them. In fact, the newborn prefers looking at the mother's face, especially the eyes, than at other objects. The newborn also can recognize an approaching object as a threat and turns away to avoid it. He or she reaches for an object and usually come close to touching it. The newborn imitates another person's facial expressions such as sticking out the tongue, opening the mouth, and pursing the lips. Newborn babies are active stimulus seekers where repetition and the level of stimulation are important.

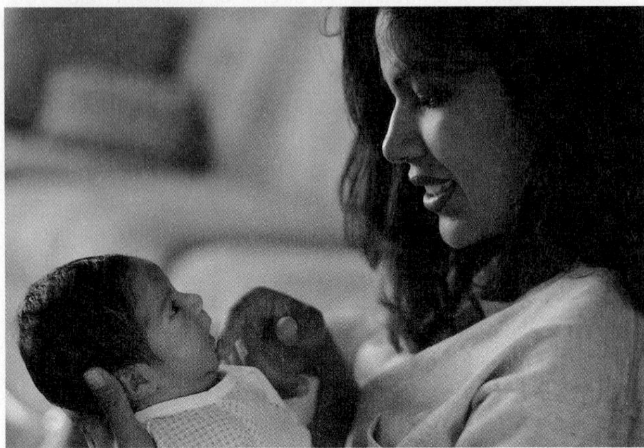

FIGURE 27-13 The infant is quiet and alert during the initial sensitive period. The newborn gazes at the mother and responds to her voice and touch.

The baby is capable of shutting out stimuli and may even turn his or her head at the sound of the mother's voice.

Indeed, babies are not passive and unresponsive creatures to be hurried off to the hospital nursery after birth. The affectionate bond between parents and child begins at the moment of birth (see Figures 27-13 and 27-14). As long as the newborn is responding normally, immediate skin-to-skin contact with the parents is important in bonding. The newborn has difficulty opening the eyes under bright spotlights but will look around if the lights are dimmed. (If necessary, dim the main lights in the delivery area and keep a light focused over the perineum for episiotomy repair or other procedures.) Shielding the infant's face with a hands or a blanket also provides enough protection from the light to encourage the baby to open the eyes. Objects are in clearest range for the newborn at about 8 to 10 inches. Newborns prefer faces over other patterns. Refraining from using prophylactic eyedrops and weighing and measuring the baby for 30 minutes

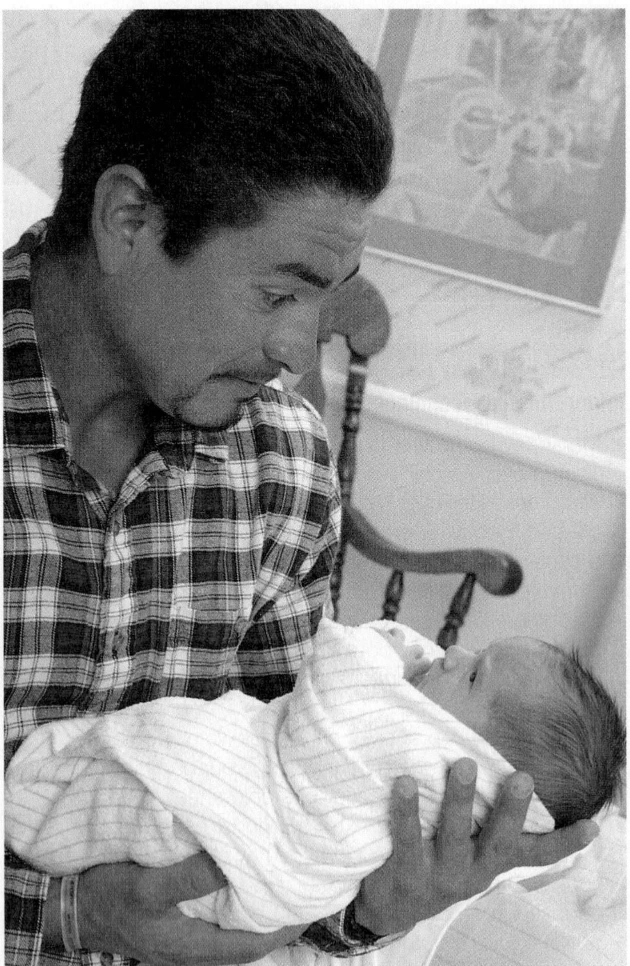

FIGURE 27-14 Fathers' behavior at initial contact with their infants often corresponds to maternal behaviors. The intense fascination that fathers exhibit is called engrossment. Note eye-to-eye contact between father and infant.

to 1 hour after birth allows the parents time alone with their baby so that the attachment process can proceed without interruption. The mother may wish to breastfeed in the first hour after birth; the nurse or the father can assist her.

Periods of quiet alertness are best for interaction. Explain the different levels of alertness to the parents so they can recognize them. Time care so that the mother is available to enjoy quiet moments with her newborn.

Nursing diagnoses for the newborn infant may include the following:

- Risk for ineffective airway clearance
- Risk for ineffective thermoregulation
- Risk for injury
- Risk for infection
- Health-seeking behaviors (desire for information about infant care)
- Ineffective breathing pattern
- Acute pain

Get Ready for the NCLEX® Examination!

Key Points

- During the 6 weeks after delivery, the reproductive organs return to approximately the prepregnant size and location.
- The new mother should avoid dieting and excessive activity during the early postpartum period.
- Postpartum fatigue and depression are common as a result of hormonal and physiologic changes.
- Complications can occur during the postpartum period. It is essential to assess each woman carefully.
- Before discharge, provide instruction concerning the danger signs of the postpartum period and verify that the woman knows when and how to contact her physician.
- Hormonal changes enable the woman to produce enough milk to meet the nutritional needs of the growing infant. Nutritional needs of the lactating woman are similar to those during pregnancy.
- Motherhood is a learned skill. The new mother requires extensive teaching and encouragement about parenting skills.
- Early discharge requires that the nurse provide essential teaching in a brief period. Be careful to document teaching.
- Supplement teaching with written materials so the new mother has something to refer to when at home.
- Conduct assessment of the newborn in a head-to-toe format. Thoroughly review each body system.
- Newborns exhibit a wide range of normal variation. Verify any questionable observations with another nurse or physician.
- Hypothermia and infection are two major areas of concern when providing care to the newborn.
- Circumcision is an elective surgical procedure.
- The newborn has social as well as physical needs.
- Injuries to the cervix can have adverse effects on future pregnancies. Repair should be immediate.
- In preparing the transfer report, the recovery nurse uses information from the admission record, the birth record, and the recovery record.
- In helping new families adjust to parenthood, provide culturally sensitive care following principles that facilitate nursing practice within transcultural situations.
- Infant abduction from hospitals in the United States has been in the increase. Parents and nurses must work together to ensure the safety of newborns in the hospital environment.
- Provide demonstration and teaching to educate the mother about the newborn's hygiene needs.
- Whether or not this is the couple's first baby, parents appreciate anticipatory guidance in the care of their child.
- Parent-child attachment (bonding) is the process by which parent and child come to love and accept each other.

Additional Learning Resources

Go to your Companion CD for an audio glossary, animations, video clips, and more.

evolve Be sure to visit the Evolve site at http://evolve.elsevier.com/Christensen/foundations/ for additional online resources.

Review Questions for the NCLEX® Examination

1. A woman has delivered her first baby, a boy, vaginally after 6 hours of labor. She had an uneventful pregnancy and is in good general health. She is transferred from the recovery room to the postpartum unit. Routine care of the postpartum patient includes all the following except:
   1. maintaining intake and output until the patient is voiding in sufficient quantities.
   2. massaging the fundus firmly every 15 minutes.
   3. assessing the emotional status of the new mother.
   4. checking breasts for engorgement and cracking of nipples.

2. The nurse is performing a routine postpartum assessment. Before measuring the height of the patient's fundus, the nurse should:
   1. massage the uterus.
   2. apply pressure to the fundus to check for clots.
   3. elevate the head of the bed.
   4. ask the patient to empty her bladder.

3. The nurse finds bright red bleeding on a patient's peripad. The stain is about 6 inches long. What is the correct description of the character and amount of lochia?
   1. Lochia rubra, moderate
   2. Lochia serosa, heavy
   3. Lochia rubra, heavy
   4. Lochia serosa, light

4. The nurse is teaching breast care for the lactating woman. It should include all the following except:
   1. exposing the nipples to air for 20 to 30 minutes daily.
   2. wearing a supportive bra 24 hours a day for the first few weeks.
   3. washing breasts and nipples with soap and water before each feeding.
   4. avoiding use of plastic liners in bra.

5. A woman asks the nurse how she will know her baby is getting enough milk. The nurse's response is based on her knowledge that a good determinant is the baby:
   1. awakens every 4 to 6 hours to eat.
   2. stops nursing when full.
   3. has 6 to 10 wet diapers per day.
   4. will cry when hungry.

6. In evaluating maternal adjustment, which behavior would lead the nurse to believe that the patient is still in the taking-in phase? She:
   1. states she is "starving" and can't wait to eat.
   2. spends the majority of her time talking about her delivery experience.
   3. takes a shower and washes her hair.
   4. asks to learn how to give her baby a bath.

7. A baby boy is 1 hour old when admitted to the newborn nursery. He weighs 7 pounds, 3 ounces; is 21 inches long; has irregular respirations of 42 breaths/min with adequate chest movement, a heart rate of 145 bpm, and a temperature of 35.6° C, axillary; and is acrocyanotic. What would be an appropriate goal for this baby within the next 2 hours, based on these findings?
   1. Color will remain unchanged.
   2. Respirations will slow.
   3. Temperature will stabilize at 36.5° to 37° C.
   4. Heart rate will decrease to 100 bpm.

8. When teaching parents how to bathe their baby, which point should the nurse stress?
   1. Do not immerse the baby in water until after the umbilical cord has fallen off.
   2. Use only mild medicated or scented soap.
   3. Apply baby powder after the bath to keep the skin dry.
   4. Apply baby oil after the bath to keep the skin soft and smooth.

9. The nurse teaches parents about care of the umbilical cord. What is not a part of this care?
   1. Cleaning the cord with an alcohol swab
   2. Keeping the diaper folded below the cord
   3. Applying triple dye to the cord
   4. Keeping the cord moist to promote healing

10. A baby has a Gomco circumcision. What instruction would the nurse give his parents for care of the circumcised penis?
    1. Soak the penis in warm water daily.
    2. Cover the glans with a petroleum gauze dressing.
    3. Clean the glans with alcohol to promote healing.
    4. Remove any yellowish exudate that forms within 24 hours.

11. On examining a woman who gave birth 5 hours previously, the nurse finds that the woman has saturated a perineal pad within 15 minutes. The nurse's first action is to:
    1. increase the drip rate of an IV infusion of Ringer's lactate solution.
    2. assess the patient's vital signs.
    3. call the patient's primary health care provider.
    4. palpate the woman's fundus.

12. A woman gave birth 48 hours ago to a healthy baby girl. She has decided to bottle feed. During the assessment, the nurse notices that both breasts are swollen, warm, and tender on palpation. The patient should be advised that this is best treated by:
    1. running warm water over her breasts during a shower.
    2. applying ice to the breasts for comfort.
    3. expressing small amounts of milk from the breasts to relieve pressure.
    4. wearing a loose-fitting bra to prevent nipple irritation.

13. A first-time mother is to be discharged from the hospital tomorrow with her baby girl. Which behavior indicates a need for further intervention by the nurse before she can be discharged? The woman:
    1. leaves the baby on her bed while she takes a shower.
    2. continues to hold and cuddle her baby after she has fed her.
    3. reads a magazine while her baby sleeps.
    4. changes her baby's diaper, then shows the nurse the contents of the diaper.

14. The nurse observes several interactions between a postpartum woman and her new son. Which behavior, if exhibited by this woman, would the nurse identify as maladaptive regarding parent-infant attachment?
    1. Talks and coos to her son
    2. Seldom makes eye contact with her son
    3. Cuddles her son close to her
    4. Tells visitors how well her son is feeding

15. The nurse can help a father in his transition to parenthood by:
    1. pointing out that the infant turned to his voice.
    2. encouraging him to go home to get some sleep.
    3. taping the baby's diaper a different way.
    4. suggesting that he let the baby sleep in the bassinet.

16. When performing a postpartum assessment, the nurse should:
    1. assist the patient into a lateral position with upper leg flexed forward to facilitate examination of her perineum.
    2. assist the patient into a supine position with her arms above her head and her legs extended for the examination of her abdomen.
    3. instruct the patient to avoid urinating just before the examination since a full bladder will facilitate funda position.
    4. wash hands and put on sterile gloves before beginning.

17. The nurse helps the breastfeeing woman change her newborn's diaper after the baby's first bowel movement. The mother expresses concern since there is a large amount of sticky, dark green—almost black—stool. She asks the nurse if something is wrong. The nurse's best response is to:

1. tell the woman not to worry since all breastfed babies have this type of stool.
2. explain that this type of stool is called meconium and is expected for the first few bowel movements of all newborns.
3. ask the woman what she ate at her last meal before giving birth.
4. suggest that the mother ask her pediatrician to explain newborns' stool patterns.

18. ________ refers to the process whereby an infant's behavior and characteristics call forth a corresponding set of maternal behaviors and characteristics.

19. ________ refers to the face-to-face position in which a parent's and infant's faces are approximately 20 cm apart and on the same plane or level.

20. ________ is a term applied to a parent's absorption, preoccupation, and interest in his or her infant; the term typically is used to describe the father's intense involvement with his newborn.

21. ________ is the phase of maternal postpartum adjustment characterized by a woman's need to review her labor and birth experiences with the nurse who cared for her while she was in labor. Other behaviors exhibited include reliance on others to help her meet needs, excitement, and talkativeness.

chapter

28 Care of the High-Risk Mother, Newborn, and Family with Special Needs

evolve

http://evolve.elsevier.com/Christensen/foundationsadult

Elaine Oden Kockrow

Objectives

1. List conditions that increase maternal and fetal risk.
2. Compare and contrast abruptio placentae and placenta previa, noting signs and symptoms, complications, and nursing and medical management.
3. Identify diagnostic tests used to determine high-risk situations.
4. Describe the HELLP syndrome.
5. Discuss gestational hypertension.
6. Identify the management priorities of eclamptic seizures.
7. Identify preexisting maternal health conditions that influence pregnancy.
8. List the infectious diseases most likely to cause serious complications.
9. Discuss the care of the pregnant adolescent.
10. Discuss the problems created by alcohol and drug abuse.
11. Identify concerns related to preterm infants.
12. Explain the hemolytic diseases of the newborn.
13. Discuss nursing diagnoses related to high-risk conditions of the mother and the newborn.
14. Identify nursing interventions for the pregnant woman with a cardiac disorder.
15. Explain the care of a pregnant woman with a pulmonary disorder.

Key Terms

anasarca (ăn-ă-SĂR-kă, p. 896)
atony (ĂT-ō-nē, p. 894)
brown fat (p. 916)
cerclage (sĕr-KLĂHZH, p. 890)
direct Coombs' test (p. 919)
dizygotic (dī-zī-GŎT-ĭk, p. 886)
eclampsia (ĕ-KLĂMP-sē-ă, p. 896)
erythroblastosis fetalis (ĕ-rĭth-rō-blăs-TŌ-sĭs fĕ-TĂL-ĭs, p. 918)
gestational diabetes mellitus (GDM) (jĕs-TĀ-shŭn-ăl dī-ă-BĒ-tēz MĔL-ĭ-tŭs, p. 905)
gestational hypertension (GH) (jĕs-TĀ-shŭn-ăl hī-pĕr-TĔN-shŭn, p. 895)
glycosylated hemoglobin (glī-KŌ-sĭ-lāt-ĕd HĒ-mō-glō-bĭn, p. 906)
high-risk pregnancy (p. 882)
hydramnios (hī-DRĂM-nē-ŏs, p. 894)
hyperbilirubinemia (hī-pĕr-bĭl-ĭ-rū-bĭ-NĒ-mē-ă, p. 918)
incompetent cervix (p. 889)
indirect Coombs' test (p. 919)
kernicterus (kĕr-NĬK-tĕr-ŭs, p. 918)
kick count (p. 899)
monozygotic (mŏn-ō-zī-GŎT-ĭk, p. 886)
morbidity (p. 883)
mortality (p. 883)
phototherapy (p. 920)
placental barrier (plă-SĔN-tăl, p. 918)
preeclampsia (prē-ĕ-KLĂMP-sē-ă, p. 896)
severe preeclampsia (p. 896)
TORCH (p. 902)

Approximately 500,000 of the 4 million births that occur in the United States each year are categorized as high risk because of maternal or fetal complications. Prevention of morbidity and mortality among mothers and infants depends on identification of the risk, along with appropriate and timely intervention during the perinatal period.

With the changing demographics in the United States, more women and families are at risk for complications because of factors that are not physiologic. For example, an increasing number of homeless, single, or uninsured pregnant women have no access to prenatal care during any stage of pregnancy. Behaviors and lifestyles that pose a risk to the health of the mother and fetus also contribute to the problem (Box 28-1).

Although most pregnancies proceed normally, complications and high-risk situations can occur at any stage of the childbearing process. The nurse must be aware of these so that appropriate, timely actions can be taken (see Cultural Considerations box on high-risk pregnancies). Two lives are involved, and the care provided must protect the welfare of both.

COMPLICATIONS OF PREGNANCY

All members of the obstetric team and other medical personnel collaborate closely to care for the high-risk patient. A **high-risk pregnancy** is one in which the life or health of the mother or the infant is jeopardized by a disorder that is associated with or exists at the same

Box 28-1 Classification of High-Risk Factors of Pregnancy

BIOPHYSICAL

- **Genetic considerations:** Genetic factors may interfere with normal fetal or neonatal development, result in congenital anomalies, or create difficulties for the mother.
- **Nutritional status:** Adequate nutrition, without which fetal growth and development cannot proceed normally, is one of the most important determinants of pregnancy outcome.
- **Medical and obstetric disorders:** Complications of current and past pregnancies, obstetric-related illnesses, and pregnancy losses put the patient at risk.

PSYCHOSOCIAL

- **Smoking:** A strong, consistent, causal relationship has been established between maternal smoking and reduced birth weight.
- **Caffeine:** Birth defects in humans have not been related to caffeine consumption. High intake (three or more cups of coffee per day) has been related to a slight decrease in birth weight.
- **Alcohol:** Alcohol exerts adverse effects on the fetus, resulting in fetal alcohol syndrome, fetal alcohol effects, learning disabilities, and hyperactivity.
- **Drugs:** The developing fetus may be adversely affected by drugs through several mechanisms. They can cause metabolic disturbances, produce chemical effects, or depress or alter central nervous system function. This category includes medications prescribed by a health care provider or bought over the counter, as well as commonly abused drugs such as heroin, cocaine, and marijuana.
- **Psychological status:** Childbearing triggers profound and complex physiologic, psychological, and social changes, with evidence to suggest a relationship between emotional distress and birth complications. This risk factor includes conditions such as specific intrapsychic disturbances and addictive lifestyles.

SOCIODEMOGRAPHIC

- **Low income:** Poverty underlies many other risk factors and leads to inadequate financial resources for food and prenatal care, poor general health, increased risk of medical complications of pregnancy, and greater prevalence of adverse environmental influences.
- **Lack of prenatal care:** Failure to diagnose and treat complications early is a major risk factor arising from financial barriers or lack of access to care; cultural beliefs that do not support this need; and fear of the health care system and its providers.
- **Age:** Women at both ends of the childbearing age spectrum have a higher incidence of poor outcomes; however, age may not be a risk factor in all cases.
  —*Adolescents:* More complications are seen in young mothers (less than 15 years old), who have a 60% higher mortality rate than those over age 20, and in pregnancies occurring less than 3 years after menarche. Complications include anemia, gestational hypertension (GH), prolonged labor, and contracted pelvis and cephalopelvic disproportion. Long-term social implications of early motherhood are lower educational status, lower income, increased dependence on government support programs, higher divorce rates, and higher parity.
  —*Mature mothers:* The risks to mothers over 35 years old are not from age alone but from other considerations such as number and spacing of previous pregnancies, genetic disposition of the parents, medical history, lifestyle, nutrition, and prenatal care. Medical conditions more likely to be experienced by mature women include hypertension and GH, diabetes, extended labor, cesarean birth, placenta previa, abruptio placentae, and death. Her fetus is at greater risk for low birth weight.
- **Parity:** The number of previous pregnancies is a risk factor that is associated with age and includes all first pregnancies, especially a first pregnancy at either end of the childbearing age spectrum. The incidence of GH and dystocia is higher with a first birth.
- **Marital status:** The increased mortality and morbidity rates for unmarried women, including a greater risk for GH, are often related to inadequate prenatal care and a younger childbearing age.
- **Residence:** The availability and quality of prenatal care varies widely with geographic residence. Women in metropolitan areas have more prenatal visits than those in rural areas, who have fewer opportunities for specialized care and consequently a higher incidence of maternal mortality.
- **Ethnicity:** Although ethnicity itself is not a major risk factor, race is an indicator of other sociodemographic risk factors. Nonwhite women are more than three times as likely as white women to die of pregnancy-related causes. Black babies have the highest rates of prematurity and low birth weight, with an infant mortality rate more than double that for whites.

ENVIRONMENTAL

- Various environmental substances can affect fertility and fetal development, the chance of a live birth, and the child's subsequent mental and physical development. Environmental influences include infections; radiation; chemicals such as pesticides, therapeutic drugs, illicit drugs, industrial pollutants, and cigarette smoke; stress; and diet.
- Paternal exposure to mutagenic agents in the workplace has been associated with an increased risk of spontaneous abortion.

time as the pregnancy. For the mother the high-risk status extends (based on medical judgment) through the puerperium, that is, 6 weeks after delivery. Postdelivery maternal complications are usually resolved within a month, but perinatal **morbidity** (state of being diseased) may continue for months or years.

A better understanding of human reproduction has greatly reduced morbidity and **mortality** (quality or state of being subject to death). Knowledge of the fetus and neonatal disorders has increased dramatically in the past 15 to 25 years. As a result, infant mortality rates have improved, dropping from 26 per 1000 live

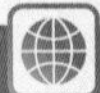

Cultural Considerations

High-Risk Pregnancies

- Providers must consider culturally based differences that could affect the treatment of diverse groups of women, and women must share practices and beliefs that could affect their nursing care or their willingness to comply. Health care providers are obligated to respect their patients' various sources of information and beliefs about sickness and health.
- Some women value privacy to such an extent that they are reluctant to disrobe and avoid physical examination unless absolutely necessary.
- Some women rely on their husbands to make major decisions, including those affecting the woman's health.
- Religious beliefs may dictate a care plan (e.g., with birth control measures or blood transfusions).
- Folk medicine, homeopathy, prayer, or a combination of these may be preferred to traditional Western medicine. Even the perceived effectiveness of medications may be affected by route of administration or color of pills.

births in 1960 to a historic low of 6.8 deaths per 1000 live births in 2001. However, less significant improvements have occurred in perinatal morbidity and mortality rates when only high-risk pregnancies are considered. Furthermore, the U.S. mortality rate remains higher than that of many other industrialized countries. Infant mortality rates vary widely by racial and ethnic groups and geographically, with the highest rate among infants born to black mothers in the largest U.S. cities (Centers for Disease Control and Prevention, 2002). Understanding the high-risk patient allows individualized therapeutic nursing interventions. Nurses can be instrumental in educating the public about the importance of obtaining early and regular care during pregnancy. See Box 28-2 for factors that place the postpartum woman and neonate at high risk.

HYPEREMESIS GRAVIDARUM

Etiology

When a woman vomits so much during pregnancy that it causes electrolyte, metabolic, and nutritional imbalances, the condition is termed **hyperemesis gravidarum.** Although mild morning sickness is common, hyperemesis gravidarum (also called **pernicious vomiting**) is a serious complication.

Hyperemesis is associated with weight loss, dehydration, acidosis from starvation, elevated blood and urine ketones, alkalosis from loss of hydrochloric acid in gastric juices and fluid, and hypokalemia. Short-term hepatic dysfunction with elevated liver enzymes may occur. Thiamine deficiency can cause encephalopathy.

The exact cause of this condition is not known. Hormones, particularly human chorionic gonadotropin (HCG), might be to blame. Hyperemesis is more common with conditions involving high levels of HCG, such as hydatidiform mole. Psychogenic factors may also play a role. Hyperemesis gravidarum is one of the most common nutrition-related discomforts of pregnancy. It is more common among unmarried white women during first pregnancies and in multifetal pregnancies. More recently the organism that causes peptic ulcer disease, *Helicobacter pylori,* has been associated with hyperemesis.

Clinical Manifestations

The mother with hyperemesis gravidarum experiences vomiting and retching far worse than the usual morning sickness. Women may border on starvation

Box 28-2 Factors that Place the Postpartum Patient and the Newborn at Risk

MOTHER

- Hemorrhage
- Traumatic labor or birth
- Infection
- Psychosocial factors
- Abnormal vital signs
- Previous medical conditions (e.g., diabetes, cardiovascular disease)

INFANT (FACTORS FOR ADMISSION TO NEONATAL INTENSIVE CARE UNIT)

High-Risk Category

- Continuing or developing signs of respiratory distress syndrome
- Asphyxiation (Apgar score, 6 at 5 minutes); resuscitation required at birth
- Preterm infants; dysmature infants
- Cyanosis or suspected cardiovascular disease; persistent cyanosis
- Major congenital malformations requiring surgery; chromosomal anomalies
- Convulsions, sepsis, hemorrhagic diathesis (constitutional predisposition to certain disease conditions), or shock
- Meconium aspiration syndrome
- Central nervous system depression for longer than 24 hours
- Hypoglycemia
- Hypocalcemia
- Hyperbilirubinemia

Moderate-Risk Category

- Dysmaturity (premature weight between 2000 and 2500 g)
- Apgar score of less than 5 at 1 minute
- Feeding problems
- Multifetal birth
- Transient tachypnea
- Hypomagnesemia or hypermagnesemia
- Hypoparathyroidism
- Jitteriness or hyperactivity
- Cardiac anomalies not requiring immediate catheterization
- Heart murmur
- Anemia
- Central nervous system depression for less than 24 hours

and become severely dehydrated. Many serious complications that endanger both the mother and fetus can result. Acid-base imbalance related to the loss of excessive amounts of hydrochloric acid or intestinal juices may result in alkalosis or acidosis. Potassium may become depleted, leading to cardiac arrhythmias. Vitamin deficiencies can lead to jaundice and hemorrhage.

Assessment

Assess, record, and report the frequency, amount, and character of emesis. Carefully measure fluid intake and output (I&O). Assess skin turgor and mucous membranes. Psychosocial assessment includes asking the woman about anxiety, fears, and concerns related to her own health and the effects on her pregnancy. Assess family members' anxiety and their role in supporting the woman.

Assessment of the fetal status is also important. Monitor fetal heart rate (FHR) regularly and immediately report any significant changes (see Chapter 26).

Medical Management

Medical treatment is directed at meeting nutritional needs, thereby maintaining acid-base and electrolyte balance. Monitor intravenous (IV) feeding closely. Solid intake is restricted until vomiting stops and the woman feels capable of trying solid food. Slowly introduce bland solids, such as toast and crackers, and assess the woman's ability to tolerate these foods. In severe cases total parenteral nutrition may be necessary.

Observe the patient for any signs of complications such as metabolic acidosis, jaundice, premature labor, or hemorrhage. Alert the physician if these occur.

Nursing Interventions and Patient Teaching

The patient is hospitalized and given parenteral fluids. Oral hygiene is essential, because the mouth may be irritated by the vomitus. Weigh the woman daily during acute illness and test her urine for ketones. Weight loss and ketones in the urine suggest that fat stores and protein are being metabolized to meet energy needs. A consultation with a dietitian is recommended (see Chapter 21 for further diet modification suggestions). Take steps to reduce the mother's emotional distress; commonly she fears for herself and her fetus. Provide emotional support and explanations. Include the family in the care plan whenever possible. Their participation may help alleviate some of the emotional stress associated with hospitalization.

After several days of treatment in the hospital, most women return home, taking nourishment by mouth. A few women continue to experience intractable nausea and vomiting throughout pregnancy. Rarely, it may be necessary to maintain a woman on enteral, parenteral, or total parenteral nutrition to provide adequate nutrition for the mother and fetus.

Nursing diagnoses and interventions for the patient with hyperemesis gravidarum include but are not limited to the following:

Nursing Diagnoses	Nursing Interventions
Imbalanced nutrition: less than body requirements, related to nausea and persistent vomiting secondary to pregnancy	Monitor food intake; caloric record may be desirable. Offer dry crackers and bland food as tolerated. Provide a pleasant atmosphere at meals. Administer antiemetics as ordered. Measure and record I&O. Weigh daily at same time. Encourage oral fluids, slowly increasing amount as tolerated. Maintain a calm, compassionate, and sympathetic manner. Encourage patient to discuss concerns. Encourage family participation.
Fear, related to possibility of harm to fetus or self	Convey acceptance of patient's perception of fear. Help patient identify personal strengths and previous coping mechanisms. Help patient identify sources of support. Provide opportunities to verbalize fears. Provide continuity of care. Refer to social worker as indicated.

Patient teaching includes (1) arranging for dietary consultation; (2) educating patient regarding condition, including signs of improvement or deterioration, and treatment measures; (3) teaching patient how to assist with her own treatment (e.g., eating small, frequent meals with high carbohydrate content); and (4) providing referrals for follow-up treatment, such as psychological counseling, or for social worker support.

Prognosis

In most instances hyperemesis gravidarum responds to therapy, and the prognosis is good. If untreated, hyperemesis gravidarum can result in maternal and fetal death.

MULTIFETAL PREGNANCY

Etiology

Pregnancy involving twins occurs in approximately 1 of 85 births in the United States. Triplets occur in approximately 1 in 8100 births. Pregnancies involving more than three fetuses are even rarer. Women carrying three or more embryos often took fertility drugs.

Twins are classified as monozygotic or dizygotic. Monozygotic twins begin with one fertilized ovum; the embryonic disk divides, causing identical twins. Because the genetic message is identical, the twins are of the same sex and carry an identical genetic code. They sometimes share a placenta, but each has a separate umbilical cord. Dizygotic twins are the result of two separate ova being fertilized at the same time. These twins almost always have separate placentas. The sexes can be different, and the genetic makeup varies; they are no more closely related than siblings born at different times (Figure 28-1). Dizygotic twinning may be hereditary in some families, presumably because the woman inherited a tendency to release more than one ovum per cycle.

Pathophysiology

Maternal and fetal risks increase during multiple pregnancy. Spontaneous abortions, maternal anemia, GH, hydramnios, and bleeding from placenta previa or abruptio placentae are more common in women with twins. The fetuses are more likely to have congenital anomalies, problems with entangled cords, and growth problems. An incomplete separation of the embryonic disk can result in conjoined (Siamese) twins.

Labor may be complicated by the loss of uterine tone that results from overstretching of the musculature, abnormal presentations, and preterm labor. Many twin pregnancies and almost all with more than two fetuses require a cesarean delivery.

Because of overdistention of the uterus, twins usually deliver before term and may have extended hospital stays. Twins may be double joy, but they are also double the responsibility and expense of one baby. The parents need a great deal of support both before and after the twins arrive. It is possible to breastfeed twins. However, the woman who plans to do this needs help with her other responsibilities because breastfeeding consumes a lot of time and energy.

Clinical Manifestations

Multiple pregnancy is suspected when uterine enlargement exceeds the norm. Abdominal palpation using Leopold's maneuvers, auscultation of two distinct heart tones, and ultrasonography reveal the presence of multiple fetuses.

HYDATIDIFORM MOLE (MOLAR PREGNANCY)

Hydatidiform mole (molar pregnancy) is a gestational trophoblastic disease. Hydatidiform moles come in two distinct types: complete (or classic) mole and partial mole.

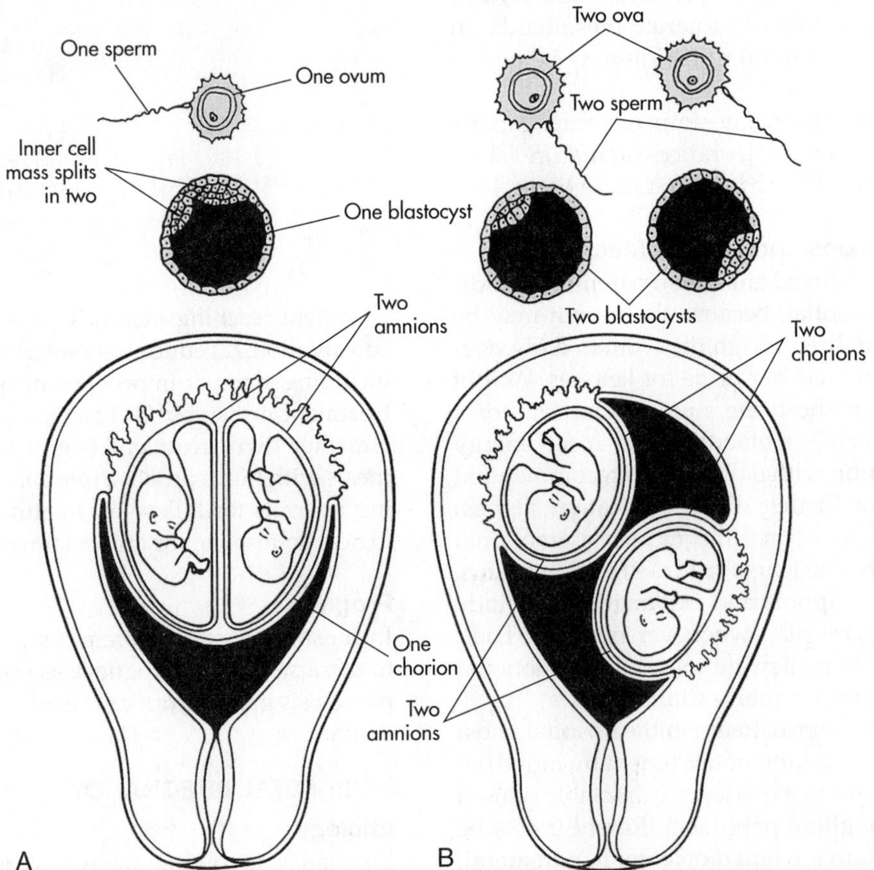

FIGURE 28-1 Multiple pregnancies. **A,** Identical twins develop from one ovum and one sperm. **B,** Fraternal twins develop from two ova and two sperm.

Etiology

Hydatidiform mole formation occurs in 1 of every 1500 to 2000 pregnancies in the United States and Europe, but a higher incidence has been reported in Asian countries. The etiology is unknown, although an ovular defect or nutritional deficiency (such as carotene or protein) may occur. Women are at higher risk for hydatidiform mole formation if they have undergone ovulation stimulation with clomiphene (Clomid), are in their early teens, or are older than 40 years of age. The risk of a second mole is 1% to 2%.

Pathophysiology

The complete mole results from fertilization of an egg whose nucleus has been lost or inactivated. The nucleus of a sperm (23X) duplicates itself (resulting in the diploid number 46XX) because the ovum has no genetic material or the material is inactive. The mole resembles a bunch of white grapes. The fluid-filled vesicles grow rapidly, causing the uterus to be larger than expected for the duration of the pregnancy. Usually the complete mole contains no fetus, placenta, amniotic membranes, or fluid. With no placenta to receive maternal blood, hemorrhage into the uterine cavity and vaginal bleeding occur. About 20% of cases of complete mole progress toward choriocarcinoma.

Clinical Manifestations

The signs and symptoms of a complete hydatidiform mole in the early stage cannot be distinguished from those of normal pregnancy. Later, vaginal bleeding occurs in almost 95% of cases. The vaginal discharge may be dark brown (resembling prune juice) or bright red and either scant or profuse. It may continue for a few days or off and on for weeks. Early in pregnancy the uterus in approximately half of affected women is significantly larger than expected based on the date of the last menstrual period. The percentage of women with an excessively enlarged uterus increases as the pregnancy advances. Approximately 25% of affected women have a uterus smaller than would be expected from menstrual dates.

Anemia from blood loss, excessive nausea and vomiting (hyperemesis gravidarum), and abdominal cramps caused by uterine distention are relatively common findings. Preeclampsia occurs in about 15% of cases, usually between 9 and 12 weeks of gestation, but any symptoms of GH before 20 weeks of gestation may suggest hydatidiform mole. Hyperthyroidism and pulmonary embolization of trophoblastic elements occur infrequently but are serious complications of hydatidiform mole. Partial moles cause few of these symptoms and may be mistaken for an incomplete or missed abortion.

Passages of vesicles (grapelike clusters) may occur around 16 weeks of gestation. There is no fetal movement, FHR, or palpable fetal parts. Some women have signs and symptoms of hyperthyroidism.

Diagnostic Measures

Diagnosis can be made by ultrasonography, amniography, and measurement of HCG level in the blood. In most cases the mole is discovered when abortion is threatened or in progress.

Medical Management

Although most moles abort spontaneously, suction curettage offers a safe, rapid, and effective method of evacuating a hydatidiform mole if necessary. Induction of labor with oxytocic agents or prostaglandins is not recommended because of the increased risk of embolization of trophoblastic tissue. Rh_o(D) immune globulin is administered to women who are Rh negative to prevent isoimmunization. Women who have experienced a molar pregnancy must avoid becoming pregnant for a year. Even with removal of the products of conception, cells may remain behind and develop into a malignancy. The patient requires frequent evaluation of serum HCG levels because elevations are associated with the development of cancer (Lowdermilk & Perry, 2007).

Nursing Interventions and Patient Teaching

Provide the woman and her family with information about the disease process, the necessity for a long course of follow-up, and the possible consequences of the disease. Help the woman understand and cope with pregnancy loss and recognize that the pregnancy was abnormal. Encourage the woman and her family to express their feelings, and provide information about support groups or counseling resources if needed. Explain the need to postpone a subsequent pregnancy for 6 months to 1 year, and provide contraception counseling to emphasize the importance of consistent, reliable use of the method chosen.

ECTOPIC PREGNANCY

Etiology

In ectopic pregnancy implantation occurs somewhere other than within the uterus, most commonly the fallopian tube. The incidence of ectopic pregnancy has increased dramatically throughout the world in the past 20 years. Ectopic pregnancy rates are higher in nonwhite and older women, particularly those over age 35 years. The rapid increase in incidence is attributed to the growing number of women of childbearing age who have fallopian tubes scarred by pelvic infection, inflammation, or surgery. Pelvic infection or inflammation (pelvic inflammatory disease) is often caused by a sexually transmitted infection (STI). Pelvic infection may also occur after induced abortion or childbirth.

About 95% of all ectopic pregnancies occur in the fallopian tube (Figure 28-2). Other sites include the abdominal cavity (Figure 28-3), an ovary, ligaments, and the cervix. Tubal pregnancy occurs when for some reason the progress of the fertilized ovum through the

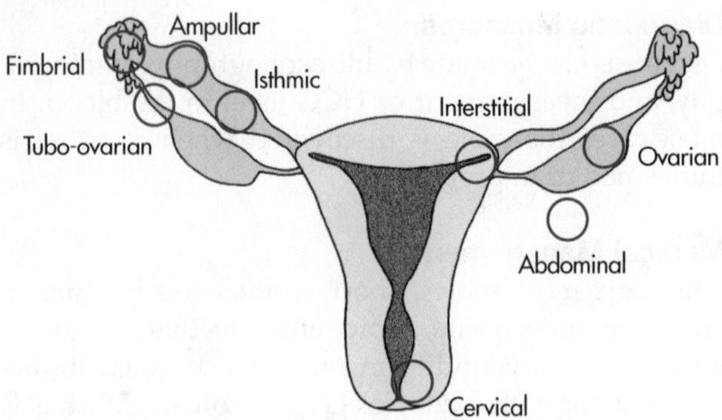

FIGURE 28-2 Sites of implantation of ectopic pregnancies in order of frequency of occurrence: ampulla, isthmus, interstitium, fimbria, tubo-ovarian ligament, ovary, abdominal cavity, and cervix (external os).

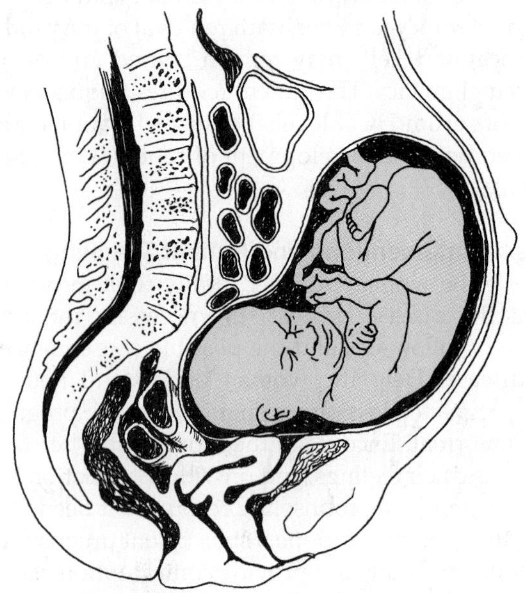

FIGURE 28-3 Ectopic pregnancy, abdominal.

fallopian tube is slowed or obstructed. Women who require assisted reproductive techniques to conceive have a greater risk of ectopic pregnancy. This is probably due to the underlying cause of infertility. Additional risk factors include use of an intrauterine device for contraception, anatomical or functional defects in the fallopian tubes, cigarette smoking, and vaginal douching.

Pathophysiology

When the fertilized ovum implants and begins to develop in the fallopian tube, it soon grows too large to be contained. This results in rupture of the tube and bleeding into the abdominal cavity. Approximately 1 out of every 100 reported pregnancies is ectopic. At least three fourths of ectopic pregnancies become symptomatic and are diagnosed during the first trimester. Ectopic pregnancy is a significant cause of maternal morbidity and mortality even in developed countries.

Clinical Manifestations

The patient may have slight vaginal bleeding and hypovolemic shock. Signs of peritoneal irritation include sharp, localized, one-sided pain or pain referred to the shoulder. The abdomen may become rigid and tender. Early diagnosis can be made by ultrasound and laboratory testing.

Medical Management and Nursing Interventions

The woman with an ectopic pregnancy almost always requires rapid surgical treatment (**salpingectomy,** removal of the tube; or **salpingostomy,** repair of the tube) and blood replacement therapy. Medical therapy, in the form of a single or multiple doses of methotrexate, has been effective in treating unruptured ectopic pregnancy. Methotrexate is a folic acid antagonist that has been used for years to treat actively proliferating trophoblastic disease. It destroys the rapidly dividing cells. Medical management may allow preservation of the tube, thus improving the chance of future fertility. Pregnancies can still occur when only one tube is present, although the likelihood of fertility decreases. In addition, the same conditions that caused the ectopic pregnancy in the tube that was removed may exist in the other tube.

The woman and her family often need support to resolve emotions that may include anger, grief, guilt, and self-blame. The woman also may be anxious about her ability to become pregnant. Be aware that these women may feel an acute sense of loss similar to that of women suffering miscarriage. Clarify the physician's explanation and use therapeutic communication techniques that help the woman deal with her anxiety and grief.

Prognosis

The prognosis varies. Maternal death from ectopic pregnancy occurs in about 1 in 800 cases in North America. The rates of maternal morbidity and secondary surgery are high, however, principally because of inaccurate or delayed diagnosis. The physician must rule out uterine abortion, ruptured corpus luteum cyst, appendicitis, salpingitis, ovarian cysts, torsion of the ovary, and urinary tract infection. The perinatal mortality rate in ectopic pregnancy is virtually 100%. Ectopic pregnancy recurs in approximately 10% of women, but more than 50% of women who have had an ectopic pregnancy achieve at least one normal pregnancy thereafter. The diagnosis and management of this condition are rapidly changing as technology improves.

SPONTANEOUS ABORTION

Etiology

Abortion is the termination of pregnancy before the age of viability—or 20 weeks of gestation in the United States. There are two types of abortion: (1) spontaneous abortion results from natural causes, and (2) therapeutic abortion (including elective abortion) is the interruption of the pregnancy for medical or personal reasons. Spontaneous abortion is generally referred to by the lay public as a miscarriage. Most spontaneous abortions occur during the first trimester of pregnancy. It is estimated that as many as 10% to 15% of all pregnancies end in first-trimester spontaneous abortion. Many of these go unrecognized, with the woman merely thinking that her menstrual period was delayed.

More than half of all spontaneous abortions are caused by abnormal embryonic development, chromosomal defects, and inheritable disorders. Most other spontaneous abortions result from maternal causes such as advancing maternal age and parity, chronic infections, chronic debilitating diseases, poor nutrition, and recreational drug use. The reasons for the remainder are open to speculation.

Pathophysiology

The pathophysiology depends on the specific cause.

Clinical Manifestations

The main presenting symptom is bleeding, which may or may not be accompanied by cramps or backache. Spontaneous abortions are classified as follows:

- **Threatened:** Unexplained bleeding and cramping occur. The fetus may or may not be alive. Membranes remain intact, and the cervical os remains closed.
- **Inevitable:** Bleeding increases and the cervical os begins to dilate. Membranes may rupture.
- **Complete:** All products of conception are expelled from the uterus.
- **Incomplete:** Some, but not all, of the products of conception are expelled.
- **Missed:** The fetus dies and growth ceases, but the fetus remains in utero. Amenorrhea continues, but no uterine growth is measurable. In fact, the uterus may decrease in size.
- **Septic:** Malodorous bleeding, elevated temperature, and cramping may be present; cervical os is opened; and abdominal tenderness is typical.
- **Habitual:** This is often referred to as recurrent spontaneous abortion, when the woman has spontaneously aborted in three or more consecutive pregnancies; emotional trauma is increased, especially with subsequent pregnancies.

Medical Management

When a spontaneous abortion occurs, administer IV fluids and replace blood loss with transfusions, as ordered. A dilation and curettage (D&C) or dilation and evacuation (suction) (D&E) may be indicated to remove retained placental tissue (Box 28-3). If significant blood loss occurred, iron supplementation may be ordered.

Box 28-3 Types of Spontaneous Abortion and Therapeutic Management

- **Threatened:** Decreased activity, sedation, and avoidance of stress and orgasm are recommended. Further treatment depends on patient's course.
- **Inevitable, incomplete:** Prompt termination of pregnancy is accomplished, usually by dilation and evacuation (D&E).
- **Complete:** No further intervention may be needed if uterine contractions are adequate to prevent hemorrhage and if there is no infection.
- **Missed:** If spontaneous evacuation of the uterus does not occur, pregnancy is terminated by method appropriate to duration of pregnancy. Blood clotting factors are monitored until uterus is empty. Disseminated intravascular coagulation (DIC) and incoagulability of blood with uncontrolled hemorrhage may develop in cases of fetal death after 12th week if products of conception are retained for longer than 5 weeks (see discussion of DIC).
- **Septic:** Pregnancy is immediately terminated by method appropriate to duration of pregnancy. Cervical culture and sensitivity studies are done, and broad-spectrum antibiotic therapy (e.g., ampicillin) is started. Treatment for septic shock is initiated if necessary. If there are signs of uterine infection, such as an elevated temperature, vaginal discharge with a foul odor, or abdominal pain, evacuation of the uterus is delayed until antibiotic therapy is initiated.

Patient Teaching

Patient teaching should include the need for rest (see Patient Teaching box on spontaneous abortion).

INCOMPETENT CERVIX

A cause of late abortion is incompetent cervix, which traditionally was defined as passive and painless dilation of the cervix during the second trimester. This

Patient Teaching

Spontaneous Abortion

- Refer patient to appropriate support groups, clergy, or professional counseling.
- Advise patient to report any heavy, profuse, or bright red bleeding to physician.
- Reassure patient that a scant, dark discharge may persist for 1 to 2 weeks.
- Instruct patient not to use tampons or douches until bleeding has stopped.
- Instruct patient to avoid sexual intercourse until bleeding has stopped.
- Acknowledge that patient has experienced a loss and that time is required for recovery. She may experience mood swings and depression.
- Instruct patient to take antibiotics as prescribed.
- Advise patient to postpone attempts at pregnancy for at least 2 months to allow her body to recover.

definition assumes an "all or nothing" role for the cervix; it is either competent or incompetent. Newer thinking contends that cervical competence is variable and is determined in part by cervical length. Other related factors include composition of the cervical tissue and the individual circumstances associated with the pregnancy, such as maternal stress and lifestyle.

Etiology

Etiologic factors include a history of cervical lacerations during childbirth, excessive cervical dilation for curettage or biopsy, or the patient's mother's ingestion of diethylstilbestrol during pregnancy with the patient. Other instances may result from a congenitally short cervix or cervical or uterine anomalies. Reduced cervical competence is a clinical diagnosis, based on a history of short labors and recurring loss of the pregnancy at progressively earlier gestational ages. Ultrasound is used to diagnose this condition objectively. A short cervix (less than 20 mm long) is indicative of reduced cervical competence. Often, but not always, the short cervix is accompanied by effacement of the internal cervical os.

Medical Management

Women with a history of painless cervical dilation and effacement in a previous pregnancy or with a previous second-trimester loss in which short cervix and effacement were documented by ultrasound are candidates for prophylactic cerclage, a technique that uses suture material to constrict the internal os of the cervix (Figure 28-4). Prophylactic cerclage is placed at 10 to 14 weeks of gestation, after which the woman is told to refrain from intercourse, prolonged (more than 90 minutes) standing, and heavy lifting. She is monitored over the course of her pregnancy with ultrasound scans to assess for cervical shortening and effacement. The cerclage is electively removed (usually an office or clinic procedure) when the woman reaches 37 weeks of gestation, or it may be left in place and a cesarean birth performed. Approximately 80% to 90% of pregnancies treated with cerclage result in live, viable births. If removed, the cerclage must be replaced with each successive pregnancy.

A woman whose reduced cervical competence is diagnosed during the current pregnancy may undergo emergency cerclage placement. Risks of the procedure include premature rupture of membranes, preterm labor, and **chorioamnionitis** (an inflammatory reaction in fetal membranes to bacteria or viruses in amniotic fluid). Because of these risks, and because bed rest and **tocolytic therapy** (drugs used to relax the uterus) can be used to prolong the pregnancy, cerclage is rarely performed after 26 weeks of gestation.

After a cervical cerclage is performed, monitor the woman for contractions, signs of rupture of membranes, and infection. Make referrals as appropriate for assistance once she is discharged to her home. Make certain she understands the rationale for the treatment and needed follow-up care. Because the diagnosis of reduced cervical competence is usually not made until the woman has lost one or two pregnancies, she may feel guilty or to blame for this impending loss. Therefore assess the patient for previous reactions to stress and appropriateness of coping responses. She needs the support of her health care providers and her family. If management is unsuccessful and the fetus is born before viability, provide appropriate grief support. If the fetus is born prematurely, appropriate anticipatory guidance and support are necessary.

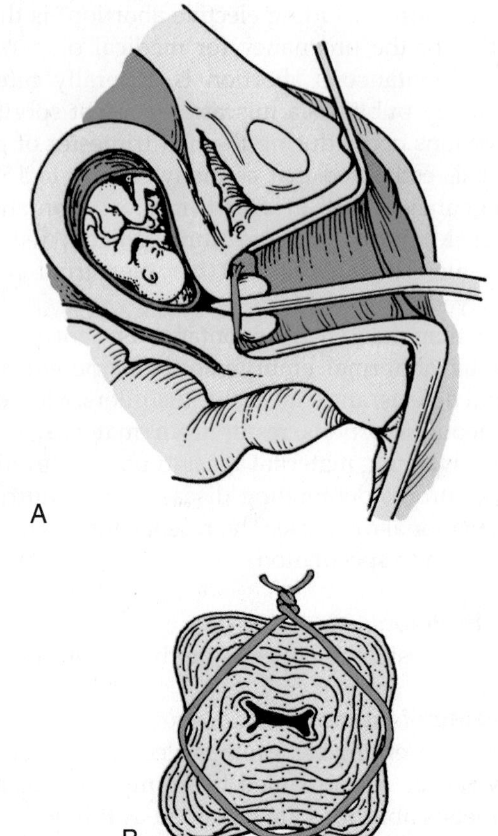

FIGURE 28-4 **A,** Cerclage correction of recurrent premature dilation of cervix. **B,** Cross-section of closed internal os.

Prognosis

Prognosis for the patient with an incompetent cervix is good.

BLEEDING DISORDERS

Vaginal bleeding during pregnancy is an indication that problems exist; instruct the patient to contact her physician if any bleeding occurs. Depending on the stage of pregnancy, several different conditions may cause the bleeding.

PLACENTA PREVIA

Etiology

Placenta previa occurs when the placenta implants in the lower uterine segment. Placenta previa is described by the degree to which the placenta covers the internal cervical os: complete with total coverage; partial with incomplete coverage; and marginal, which indicates that only an edge of the placenta approaches the internal os (Figure 28-5). The term **low implantation** is used when the placenta is situated in the lower uterine segment away from the internal os. In the second trimester approximately 45% of all placentas are implanted in the lower uterine segment. As the lower uterine segment lengthens (stretches), the placenta seems to move upward.

Placenta previa occurs in 1 in 200 pregnancies. The cause is unknown. The most important risk factor is previous cesarean birth, possibly related to endometrial scarring. The risk increases with the number of previous cesarean births; in women with four or more, the risk of previa is nearly 10%. Other risk factors include multiple gestation (because of the larger placental area), closely spaced pregnancies, and advanced maternal age (older than 35 years).

Pathophysiology

In the last trimester of pregnancy, uterine size increases and the cervix begins to dilate and efface. As the placenta separates from the uterus at the internal os of the cervix, sinuses at the site begin to bleed. The amount of bleeding depends on the amount of separation that occurs.

Clinical Manifestations

The main presenting symptom of placenta previa is painless, bright red, vaginal bleeding occurring after 20 weeks of gestation. The bright red bleeding may be intermittent, may occur in gushes, or more rarely may be continuous. It may start while the patient is resting or in the midst of any activity. Severe hemorrhage almost never occurs unless vaginal or rectal examination initiates violent bleeding before or during early labor.

The detachment of placenta previa is painless. If the first bleeding coincides with the onset of labor, the patient may experience discomfort because of uterine contractions.

Abdominal examination usually reveals a soft (relaxed), nontender uterus of normal tone.

Obstetric ultrasound is the diagnostic method of choice. The vaginal examination, known as the **double setup procedure,** is a serious undertaking. A sterile vaginal examination is performed in an operating room, with personnel and equipment ready to effect an immediate vaginal or cesarean birth. Because manipulation of the lower uterine segment or cervix may result in profound hemorrhage, preparation for immediate delivery is necessary.

Medical Management

Because of the relative safety of cesarean birth today, this is usually the treatment of choice for placenta previa. Some obstetricians may decided to "wait and see" and eventually deliver the baby vaginally.

The patient diagnosed with placenta previa remains in the hospital under close supervision. Blood, typed and crossmatched, is usually available for emergency use. Delivery is delayed, if possible, until after the 36th week.

If the patient is at home, the care plan includes bed rest, the presence of a responsible adult at all times, and ready transportation to the hospital. Teach the patient and the family the importance of (1) assessing vaginal discharge or bleeding after each urination or bowel movement, or more often as needed; (2) counting fetal movements daily; (3) assessing uterine activity daily; and (4) forgoing sexual intercourse to prevent disruption of the placenta. The woman or the family should report any change at once.

Blood loss may cease with delivery of the infant. However, the interlacing muscle bundles contracting around open vessels so characteristic of the upper part

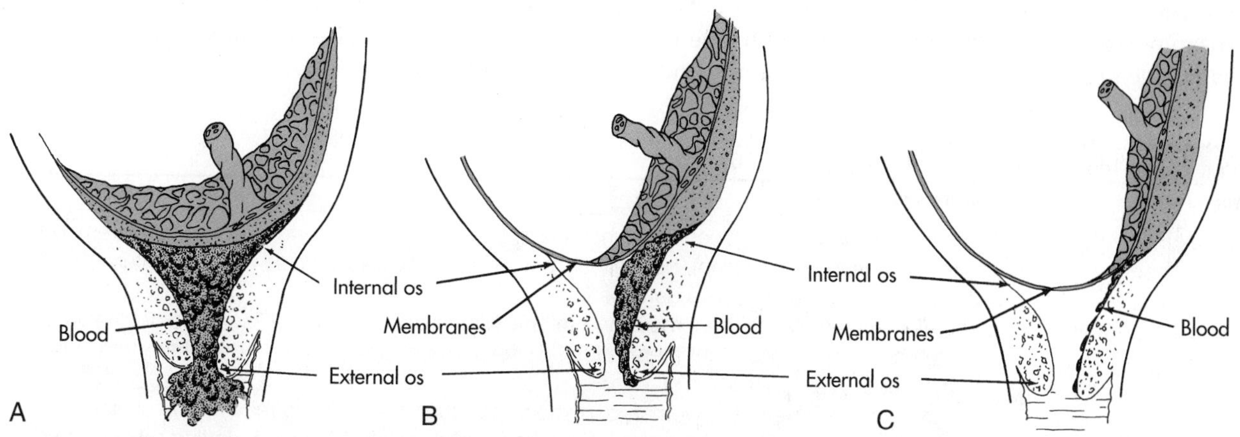

FIGURE 28-5 Types of placenta previa after onset of labor. **A,** Complete, or total. **B,** Incomplete, or partial. **C,** Marginal, or low lying.

of the uterus are absent in the lower part of the uterus. Therefore postpartum hemorrhage may occur even if the fundus is contracted firmly. Hemorrhage and the possible results of anemia increase the risk of infection—both placentitis and puerperal (postpartum) infection. If bleeding cannot be controlled, a hysterectomy may be necessary. During emergency preparations, constantly provide reassurance to reduce the woman's anxiety and that of her family.

Prognosis

Maternal mortality rate in placenta previa dropped almost 50%, to about 0.6%, during the past two decades in most areas in North America because of conservative therapy. The perinatal mortality rate (resulting primarily from preterm birth) still approaches 20% in most hospitals.

ABRUPTIO PLACENTAE

Etiology

Abruptio placentae is premature separation of the normally implanted placenta from the uterine wall. This generally occurs late in pregnancy, frequently during labor. Abruptio placentae occurs in about 1% of all pregnancies. The cause is unknown. Predisposing factors include trauma, chronic hypertension, and GH. Abruptio placentae is three times more likely to occur in women with gravidity of more than five. Women who use cocaine during pregnancy have a significant incidence of premature separation of the placenta. Blunt external abdominal trauma, usually the result of motor vehicle accidents or maternal battering, is an increasingly significant cause of placental abruption.

Pathophysiology

When the placenta separates from the uterine wall, bleeding from uterine sinuses occurs, as in placenta previa. The most common classification of placental abruption is according to type and severity (Table 28-1).

Clinical Manifestations

The major symptoms of abruptio placentae are sudden, severe pain accompanied by uterine rigidity. The uterus may also increase in size as a result of the hemorrhage. The first sign during labor may be strong and constant contractions (tetany). Symptoms vary with the degree of separation.

Assessment

When any vaginal bleeding occurs during pregnancy, assess the following:

- **Duration, amount, color, and characteristics of the bleeding:** This includes assessing (1) the time since the onset of bleeding; (2) what, if any, activity preceded the bleeding episode; (3) the number of pads saturated per hour; and (4) the color of the bleeding (bright red, dark red, or brown). If a clot or tissue is passed, save it for examination by the physician.
- **Vital signs:** Depending on the origin and severity of the bleeding, signs of shock may be present. In addition to pulse and blood pressure, observe for pallor; diaphoresis; cool, clammy skin; and dyspnea. These physical signs will seem out of proportion to the amount of bleeding if the hemorrhage is concealed, as in central abruptio placentae.
- **Pain:** Note the location, nature, and duration of pain and whether bleeding is painless. This will help the physician determine the cause of the bleeding.
- **FHR:** Depending on the stage of pregnancy, measure FHR with a fetoscope or Doppler amplifier. If pregnancy is in the early stages, fetal heart sounds may not be heard. In labor when there is uteroplacental insufficiency, the fetus, in its struggle to obtain more oxygen, may be restless and active. The FHR either greatly accelerates or slows.
- **Emotional response:** In addition to a physical assessment, address the emotional response of the expectant mother and her partner. They will most likely be anxious, fearful, confused, and overwhelmed by the activity. They may have little knowledge of medical management and may not realize that the fetus must be delivered as quickly as possible and that a surgical procedure is necessary. Moreover, they may fear for the life of the woman and the fetus. Also the baby may be dead when the mother is admitted, adding shock and grief to their anxiety.

Table 28-1 Classification of Placental Abruption

TYPE	SEVERITY
Grade I (mild—1)	The woman has vaginal bleeding perhaps with uterine tenderness and mild tetany (extremely prolonged uterine contraction), but neither mother nor baby is in distress. Approximately 10% to 20% of placental surface is detached.
Grade II (moderate—2)	The woman has uterine tenderness and tetany, with or without external evidence of bleeding. The mother is not in shock, but there is fetal distress. Approximately 20%-50% of the total surface is detached.
Grade III (severe—3)	Uterine atony is severe, the woman is in shock (although the bleeding may not be obvious), and the fetus is dead. Often the woman has coagulopathy (defect in blood-clotting mechanisms). More than 50% of the placental surface area is detached.

Diagnostic Tests

The most common laboratory tests include measurement of hemoglobin and hematocrit levels to determine the amount of blood lost. Blood typing and crossmatching are ordered in case blood replacement is necessary. Hormone studies may be ordered to determine fetal death. Ultrasound scans may be done to determine placental location and fetal life. Vaginal and rectal examinations are avoided because they may increase the bleeding.

Medical Management

Abruptio placentae in its more severe form is an obstetric emergency. The treatment often, but not always, includes delivery by cesarean birth and blood replacement.

A modified side-lying position with a wedge placed under the patient's right hip facilitates uterine-placental perfusion. Carefully monitor blood and fluid replacement therapy. Insert a retention catheter to monitor urinary output. The fetus is monitored and delivered when indicated. If signs of fetal compromise such as hypoxia are present or if the expectant mother exhibits signs of excessive bleeding, either obvious or concealed, the fetus is delivered immediately. Intensive monitoring of both the woman and the fetus is essential because rapid deterioration of either can occur.

A woman undergoing immediate cesarean delivery may feel powerless as the health care team hurriedly prepares her for surgery. If possible, explain anticipated procedures to the woman and her family to reduce their fear and anxiety.

Nursing Interventions

Nursing measures are structured to support and promote optimal physical and psychological functioning.

Oxygen should be available. If blood loss is significant, oxygen-carrying capability is decreased; oxygen may be ordered to prevent maternal or fetal hypoxia.

IV or blood replacement therapy may be required, so be prepared for this. Possible loss of the pregnancy is a crisis. Be supportive of the patient's and family's emotional needs. Remain with the woman as much as possible, listen to her concerns, give clear explanations about medical treatment, and prepare her for the possible loss.

Nursing diagnoses and interventions for the patient with abruptio placentae include but are not limited to the following:

Nursing Diagnoses	Nursing Interventions
Decreased cardiac output, related to excessive bleeding secondary to abruptio placentae	Monitor and record vital signs every 15 minutes until stable, then every hour as indicated. Measure and record I&O. Weigh daily. Assess skin turgor and mucous membranes. Help patient ambulate. Monitor blood replacement therapy.
Anticipatory grieving, related to possible loss of pregnancy	Allow time for patient to verbalize concerns about loss. Assist with grieving processes. Encourage contact with support system. Encourage session with spiritual advisor if patient so desires. Foster active participation of significant other.

Prognosis

Premature separation of the placenta is a serious disorder and accounts for about 15% of all perinatal deaths. Maternal mortality rate approaches 1% in abruptio placentae; this condition remains a leading cause of maternal death. The mother's prognosis depends on the extent of placental detachment, overall blood loss, degree of disseminated intravascular coagulation (DIC), and time between the placental separation and delivery.

Approximately one third of infants of women with premature separation of the placenta die. More than 50% die as a result of preterm delivery, and many others die as a result of intrauterine hypoxia.

DISSEMINATED INTRAVASCULAR COAGULATION

Etiology

Disseminated intravascular coagulation (DIC) is a potentially life-threatening disorder that results from alterations in the normal clotting mechanism. DIC is always a secondary diagnosis. It may be seen with abruptio placentae, incomplete abortion, hypertensive disease, or infectious process. It may occur with a post-term delivery. Coagulation defects do not usually occur unless fetal death occurs after the first trimester.

Pathophysiology

In DIC the body's attempts to prevent excessive blood loss put stress on the coagulation processes. The body produces excessive amounts of thrombin, stimulating the conversion of fibrinogen to fibrin. Elevated fibrin levels result in multiple small clots forming in small blood vessels, which may lead to obstruction of vessels, ischemia, and damage to vital organs. This clot formation also traps platelets and can result in generalized hemorrhage.

Clinical Manifestations

The onset of symptoms is sudden. The patient may complain of chest pain or dyspnea and become extremely restless and cyanotic, occasionally expectorating frothy, blood-tinged mucus. Profound circulatory shock from hemorrhage may occur rapidly. Fetal and maternal death may result.

Assessment

All women with complications that may result in DIC should be observed closely for signs of bleeding such as epistaxis (nosebleeds); bleeding gums; or petechiae, particularly around the blood pressure cuff on the patient's arm. Excessive bleeding may occur from a site of slight trauma, such as venipuncture sites, intramuscular or subcutaneous injection sites, nicks from shaving of perineum or abdomen, and injury from insertion of urinary catheter. Continue to monitor the maternal and fetal conditions by assessment of vital signs, FHR, and I&O and by general careful assessment.

Diagnostic Tests

Blood testing includes determination of hemoglobin and hematocrit. Clotting factor studies, such as fibrinogen levels, platelet counts, prothrombin time (PT), and partial thromboplastin time (PTT), are typically ordered for the patient. Laboratory tests may reveal various degrees of anemia and decreased fibrinogen and platelet counts. Prolonged PT and PTT are also typical.

Medical Management

Emergency care for DIC includes IV administration of fibrinogen, blood, and other substances that will help restore normal clotting mechanisms. Paradoxically, DIC therapy may include heparin by continuous infusion pump (although its use is controversial) and oxygen therapy by a tight-fitting mask at 10 to 12 L/min. If the fetus is not yet born, delivery should occur as soon as possible. Carefully monitor urinary output (it must be maintained at more than 30 mL/hr) because renal failure is one consequence of DIC.

If the woman is still pregnant, position her in a side-lying tilt to maximize blood flow to the uterus.

Nursing Interventions

Nursing interventions are directed at supporting medical treatment. Report signs and symptoms promptly and completely. Use caution when providing care to minimize the risk of additional trauma to tissue, which may lead to further bleeding. Recognize and support the emotional needs of the patient and the family.

Prognosis

Prognosis depends on the degree and extent of the underlying disorder, as well as the response of the woman to prompt and proper treatment.

POSTPARTUM HEMORRHAGE

Etiology

Postpartum hemorrhage (PPH) occurs in two stages. Early PPH is blood loss greater than 500 mL after vaginal childbirth or 100 mL after cesarean birth. However, this amount of blood loss is not unusual during childbirth. Estimating blood loss is difficult, especially when bleeding is brisk or hemorrhage is concealed. It is one of the leading causes of maternal morbidity and mortality in the first 24 hours after delivery; late PPH occurs after the first 24 hours. At least 5% of women suffer PPH.

The most common causes of early hemorrhage are (1) uterine **atony** (lack of normal tone or strength), often related to excessive distention of the uterus from multiple pregnancy, **hydramnios** (excessive amount of amniotic fluid), or a large infant (atony is also more common in grand multiparas or when labor is prolonged or traumatic); (2) retained placenta or fragments of the placenta; and (3) lacerations of the perineum. The most common cause of late PPH is retained placental fragments.

Pathophysiology

The major action that prevents hemorrhage is contraction of the uterus, which seals off the uterine sinuses. Hemorrhage results when loss of tone or tissue remaining in the cavity prevents adequate uterine contraction.

Assessment

Nursing assessment of uterine contraction and lochia is part of routine postpartum assessment. If the uterus is boggy (soft, uncontracted) or the flow of lochia is heavy, suspect hemorrhage. Vital signs may also change if blood loss is substantial. Report any alteration promptly.

PPH can progress rapidly to shock; therefore assess the patient carefully and thoroughly. Review the history for factors that predispose to PPH.

For the first 24 hours after childbirth the uterus should feel like a firmly contracted ball roughly the size of a large grapefruit. It should be easily located at about the level of the umbilicus. Lochia should be dark red and moderate in amount. Saturation of more than one peripad per hour is considered a large amount, and saturation of more than one peripad in 15 minutes is excessive. Realize that, although bleeding may be profuse and dramatic, a constant trickle or dribble is just as dangerous.

Assess the bleeding color, amount, and, if possible, source. Note the time of the last pad change. If the pad is loose, blood may pool under the patient, so assessment must include checking under the patient.

Vital signs may not be reliable indicators of shock in the immediate postpartum period because of physiologic adaptations of this stage. Data should include assessment for bladder distention, since a full bladder lifts and displaces the uterus and prevents effective contraction of the uterine muscles. Help the mother urinate or catheterize her as necessary.

Medical Management

The medical treatment for retained placental fragments is D&E to surgically remove the tissue. For perineal lacerations, lacerations are identified and repaired. The medical management for uterine atony is performing fundal massage, keeping the bladder empty, and administering oxytocics. Failure to control bleeding may necessitate a hysterectomy. Blood transfusions are administered if hemorrhage is severe.

Nursing Interventions

Nursing interventions are directed at reducing blood loss. Initial care includes fundal massage; normally this increases the uterine tone and decreases bleeding. If the uterus remains atonic, the physician typically prescribes an oxytocic. Monitor vital signs carefully when oxytocin is administered. If bleeding continues, placental fragments may have been retained. If a dilation and evacuation (D&E) is required, prepare the patient for surgery. Explain the necessity of surgery to reduce anxiety.

Other surgical preparations include obtaining signed consent forms; verifying that laboratory data are on the chart, the patient has had nothing by mouth, and identification and allergy bands are in place; completing skin preparations as ordered; having the patient empty her bladder or inserting an indwelling catheter; removing jewelry, contact lenses, and dentures; obtaining vital signs; administering preoperative medication as scheduled; monitoring safety with side rails up; and documenting all preoperative care.

Administer oxytocin or other drugs to stimulate uterine contraction. Labor and birth units have standing orders or protocols for the nurse to implement interventions, such as starting IV infusions and administering medications.

Trauma

If the fundus is firm but bleeding is excessive, the cause may be laceration of the cervix or birth canal. Inspect the perineum for a laceration in that area. Lacerations of the cervix or vagina are not visible, but bleeding when the uterus is contracted suggests a laceration. This sign warrants examination of the vaginal walls and the cervix by the health care provider (see Chapter 27 and Box 27-2).

If the mother complains of deep, severe pelvic or rectal pain or if vital signs or skin changes suggest hemorrhage but excessive bleeding is not obvious, the cause may be concealed bleeding and the formation of a hematoma. Examine the vulva for a bulging mass or skin discoloration. A hematoma in the vagina or in the retroperitoneal area will not be obvious. Notify the health care provider.

Keep the woman on bed rest to increase venous return and maintain cardiac output. The Trendelenburg position may interfere with cardiac function and is not advised. Continue assessments; call for assistance; and save all pads, linen savers, and linen so that blood loss can be estimated accurately. Assistance is necessary so that one nurse can continue to massage the uncontracted uterus and perform and record assessments while the other notifies the health care provider of the mother's condition.

The unusual activity of the hospital staff may make the mother and her family anxious. Keeping the family informed is one of the most effective ways of reducing anxiety.

Nursing diagnoses and interventions for the patient with PPH include but are not limited to the following:

Nursing Diagnoses	Nursing Interventions
Deficient knowledge, related to signs of hemorrhage	Select teaching strategies appropriate to patient's need and willingness to learn. Demonstrate postpartum checks of fundus and lochia. Observe patient performing self-check. Review importance of contacting the physician if signs are abnormal or questionable.
Deficient fluid volume, related to hypovolemia secondary to excessive blood loss	Perform fundal massage until firm. Monitor vital signs and I&O closely. Assess blood loss by pad saturation. Monitor fluid replacement therapy. Monitor for signs and symptoms of infection. Teach patient fundal massage. Encourage fluids by mouth unless contraindicated.

Patient Teaching

Because today's patients leave the hospital in a relatively short time, teach them how to perform the postpartum checks of the fundus and lochia. Late PPH, which typically occurs without warning 7 to 14 days after delivery, can be dangerous for the unsuspecting mother. Alert her to call the physician if bleeding is excessive or persists longer than expected.

Prognosis

Although all possible medical, surgical, and nursing interventions are attempted, there still may be maternal mortality.

GESTATIONAL HYPERTENSION

Etiology

Gestational hypertension (GH), formerly referred to as pregnancy-induced hypertension, is a disease encountered during pregnancy or early in the puerperium, characterized by increasing hypertension, albuminuria, and generalized edema. GH includes (1) preeclampsia, which may be mild or severe; and (2) eclampsia, the most severe form of GH, which places both the mother and the fetus at risk.

The cause of GH is unknown. Many theories have been proposed, but to date none has been proven. This condition was formerly called **toxemia** because it was thought that a toxin caused the symptoms. This condition is seen most often in primigravidas, particularly those younger than 20 or older than 35 years of age. It is also more common in women from lower socioeconomic groups or patients with poor nutritional status. A woman with a multiple pregnancy, diabetes mellitus, or family history of GH is also at increased risk. GH is a disease process unique to pregnancy. The only known cure is termination of the pregnancy.

Pathophysiology

Complex hormonal and vascular changes occur with GH; these lead to increased blood pressure, decreased placental perfusion, decreased renal perfusion, altered glomerular filtration rate, and fluid and electrolyte imbalance.

Clinical Manifestations

The classic signs of GH, in order of appearance, are (1) edema, (2) hypertension, and (3) proteinuria. These signs generally appear after the 20th week of pregnancy. GH is a progressive disease. Depending on the severity of the symptoms, GH is classified as preeclampsia (which is further subdivided into mild or severe forms) and eclampsia.

Mild Preeclampsia

Early preeclampsia has few clinical symptoms. Change in the blood pressure readings—an increase of 30 mm Hg systolic and 15 mm Hg diastolic, or a reading of 140/90 mm Hg in a woman whose blood pressure has been normal—indicates a problem. This is why it is important to establish baseline readings early in pregnancy. Generalized edema may be evident in the face, the hands, and the ankles. Weight may increase as much as 3 pounds (1.4 kg) per month in the second trimester and 1 pound (0.5 kg) per week in the third trimester. Urine testing frequently shows 1+ to 2+ albumin readings. The urinary output is at least 500 mL/24 hr.

Severe Preeclampsia

The symptoms of severe preeclampsia may appear suddenly. Blood pressure readings increase; readings of 160/110 mm Hg or higher on two separate occasions 6 hours apart with the pregnant woman on bed rest are common. Edema becomes increasingly obvious and may be observed in the face, the hands, the sacral area, the abdomen, and throughout the lower extremities. Weight increases dramatically. The woman may gain as much as 2 pounds (0.9 kg) in a matter of a few days or a week. Urine testing for albumin shows 3+ to 4+ readings. The urinary output is less than 500 mL/24 hr.

Eclampsia

Eclampsia is the most severe form of GH. The most dramatic characteristic is seizures, with tonic (pertaining to or characterized by muscular tension) and clonic (spasmodic alteration of muscular contractions) phases. This is generally followed by a coma that lasts from minutes to hours. Other signs are elevated blood pressure, albuminuria, and oliguria. If untreated, this sequence of seizure-coma may repeat, and death may follow.

Assessment

Assess blood pressure routinely throughout pregnancy, labor, delivery, and the postpartum period. GH can occur any time after the 20th week and persist until 2 days after delivery. Record weight at each prenatal visit and compare it with norms. Excessive or rapid weight gain, particularly when accompanied by edema, should be reported promptly. Assess for edema at each visit (Figure 28-6). Edema is typically described using a scale of 1+ to 4+:

1+ Minimal edema on pedal and pretibial area
2+ Obvious edema of lower extremities
3+ Edema of face, hands, sacrum, and abdomen
4+ Massive, generalized edema (anasarca)

Test urine for albumin using dipstick reagents at each visit and on admission for labor. (If the bag of waters is ruptured, these dipstick readings may be inaccurate.) Certain symptoms, such as continuous headache, drowsiness, or mental confusion, indicate poor cerebral perfusion and may be precursors of convulsions. Visual disturbances, such as blurred or double vision or spots before the eyes, indicate arterial spasms and edema in the retina. Some symptoms such as epigastric pain or "upset stomach" are particularly ominous because they indicate distention of the hepatic capsule and often warn that a convulsion is imminent. Decreased urinary output indicates poor perfusion of the kidneys and may precede acute renal failure.

If the patient is hospitalized for GH, monitor deep tendon reflexes (Table 28-2, Figure 28-7) and urinary output; also electronically monitor FHR.

Diagnostic Tests

Typical tests include hematocrit, blood urea nitrogen, complete blood cell count, clotting studies, liver en-

Table 28-2 Assessing Deep Tendon Reflexes

DEGREE	GRADING
Hyperactive response (brisk with intermittent or transient clonus)	4+
More than normal (brisk), slightly hyperactive	3+
Normal, active, expected response	2+
Sluggish or diminished	1+
No response	0

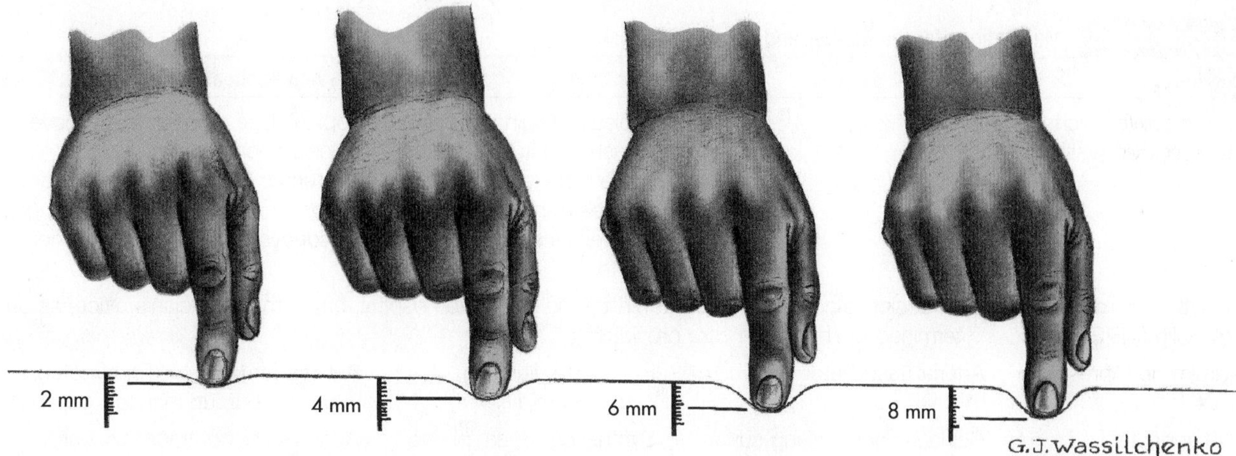

FIGURE 28-6 Scale for pitting edema depth.

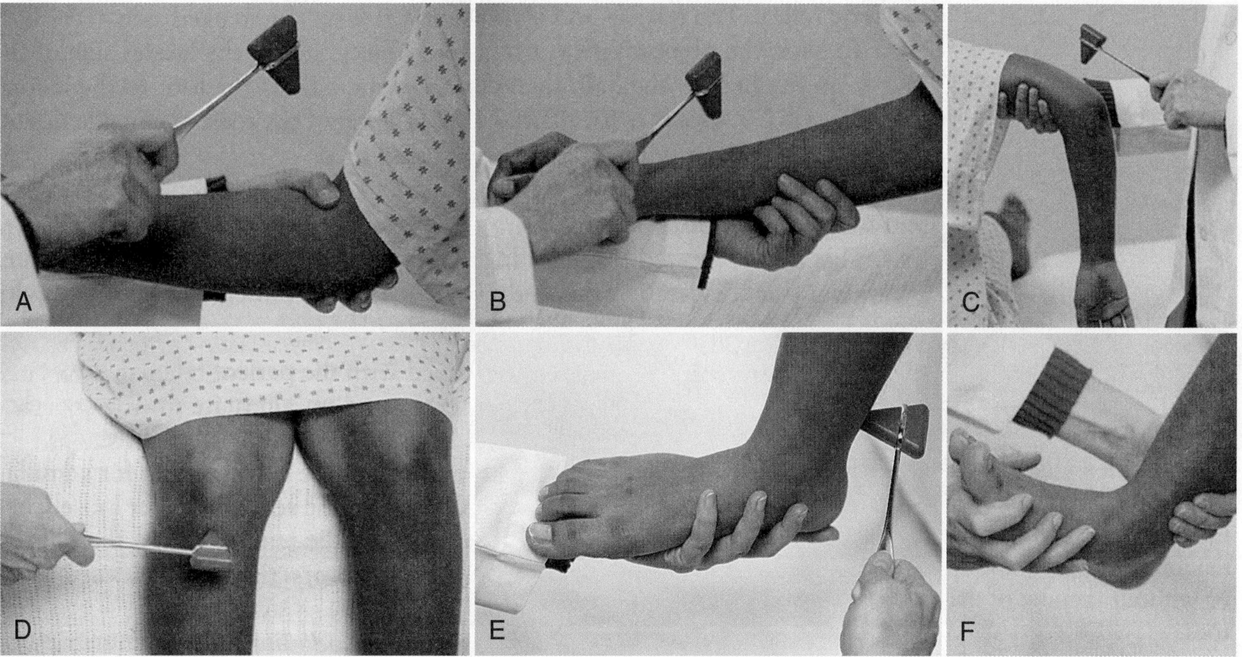

FIGURE 28-7 Location of tendons for evaluation of deep tendon reflexes. **A,** Biceps. **B,** Brachioradial. **C,** Triceps. **D,** Patellar. **E,** Achilles. **F,** Evaluation of ankle clonus.

zymes, type and screen, possible crossmatch, and urine tests for specific gravity and protein. Often a 24-hour urine collection is obtained to measure creatinine and protein clearance. Electrolyte panels are commonly drawn. If symptoms indicate severe preeclampsia or eclampsia, liver function and platelet count evaluations are also done. If the physician decides on early induction of labor, tests for fetal maturity and well-being, including estriol levels, amniocentesis, ultrasonography, and stress tests, may be done.

Medical Management

The woman may or may not need to be hospitalized depending on the severity of symptoms. Mild preeclampsia may be managed at home, but more severe symptoms require hospitalization. Bed rest is typically ordered, preferably in the left lateral recumbent position, which reduces pressure on the inferior vena cava and promotes venous return. A well-balanced diet with adequate protein is important. Moderate sodium intake is allowed, but high-sodium foods should be avoided. Meals are allowed as long as the woman is alert and has no signs of impending convulsions. IV therapy may be initiated to keep a line open for emergency medications. IV electrolytes may also be administered. In cases of severe preeclampsia or eclampsia, medications may be prescribed. Magnesium sulfate may be prescribed parenterally to prevent seizures in preeclampsia. Sedatives and antihypertensives may also be ordered (Table 28-3).

Table 28-3 Medications for the Mother and Newborn at Risk

Generic (Brand)	Action	Side Effects	Nursing Implications
Valacyclovir (converts to acyclovir) (Valtrex)	Antiviral	Topical: Stinging, burning, rash, pruritus Systemic: Headache, seizures, renal toxicity, phlebitis at intravenous site	Topical: Use glove to apply, cover lesion completely. Systemic: Ensure adequate hydration to prevent crystallization in kidneys; give IV dose for 1 hour.
Hepatitis B immune globulin (HBIG)	The vaccine is no longer given at birth while still in the hospital, but in the physician's office, as determined by the health care provider.		
Hydralazine (Apresoline)	Arterial vasodilator	Headache, flushing, tachycardia	Assess for tachycardia, hypotension, urinary output; maintain bed rest.
Lung surfactant Colfosceril palmitate (Exosurf [synthetic]) Beractant (Survanta [natural lung surfactant])	Replaces natural lung surfactant that maintains lung inflation and prevents lung collapse; used to treat and prevent respiratory distress syndrome in premature neonates	Synthetic: Apnea, pulmonary hemorrhage, pulmonary air leak Natural: Transient bradycardia, oxygen desaturation, hypotension, apnea	Administer endotracheally only; suction before administration (drug may reflux into endotracheal tube during administration); slow or stop administration until tube is clear.
Magnesium sulfate ($MgSO_4$)	See Chapter 26		
Oxytocin (Pitocin)	See Chapter 26		
Rh_o(D) immune globulin (RhoGAM)	See Chapter 27		
Ritodrine (Yutopar)	See Chapter 26		
Rubella vaccine	See Chapter 27		
Naloxone hydrochloride (Narcan)	Reverses central nervous system and respiratory depression caused by narcotics (opiates) Competes with narcotics at receptor sites	If given to an infant of a mother addicted to drugs, causes withdrawal and may cause seizures	Prepare the syringe before birth by drawing up more than is needed. After birth, remove excess from the syringe and give the amount according to the estimate of the infant's weight. Inject rapidly. Monitor for response and be prepared to give repeated doses if necessary. Use resuscitation measures as necessary.
Terbutaline (Brethine)*	Stimulates beta-adrenergic receptors of the sympathetic nervous system Results primarily in bronchodilation and inhibition of uterine muscle activity Increases pulse rate and widens pulse pressure	Maternal and fetal tachycardia, palpitations, cardiac arrhythmias, chest pain, wide pulse pressure, dyspnea, tremors, weakness, dizziness, headache, hyperglycemia, nausea, vomiting, skin flushing and diaphoresis	Explain common side effects, which are usually well tolerated. Assess fetal heart rate (FHR), usually with continuous fetal monitoring. Assess maternal pulse, respirations and blood pressure by the same schedule as for FHR. Maintain adequate hydration. Encourage patient to urinate every 2 hours. Report any significant or unacceptable side effects. Repeat continuing or recurrent uterine activity. Teach signs and symptoms of recurrent preterm labor and follow-up medical care after discharge.

*Not approved by the U.S. Food and Drug Administration (FDA) for inhibiting uterine activity, although it is widely used for this purpose; research has been mixed regarding the drug effects of terbutaline for this purpose, but its lower risk for adverse side effects, combined with some efficacy, has maintained its use.

Table 28-3 Medications for the Mother and Newborn at Risk—cont'd

Generic (Brand)	Action	Side Effects	Nursing Implications
Nifedipine (Procardia)	Relaxes smooth muscles (tocolytic) Inhibits uterine contractions in preterm labor Not approved by the FDA for inhibiting uterine activity, although it is widely used for this purpose		See nursing implications for terbutaline.
Penicillin	Used for group B streptococcus Administered after culture and sensitivity is completed	Interferes with contraception usage	Assess for allergies; hypersensitivity reaction may be delayed. Assess respiratory system for abnormalities such as rate, status, character, any tightness in chest.

Nursing Interventions

The goal of nursing interventions is to be alert for signs and symptoms of preeclampsia, such as complaints of headache, edema, and blurred vision.

In mild cases monitor routine I&O; in severe cases it may be necessary to insert an indwelling catheter and record hourly urinary output. Monitor fetal condition carefully. In mild cases routine auscultation of FHR is adequate; in severe cases fetal monitors give more accurate information. Monitor I&O levels carefully to avoid fluid overload from IV infusions and magnesium sulfate toxicity.

Some practitioners request a **kick count,** a daily count of fetal movements felt in 1 hour while the mother is resting. Fetal activity of less than three kicks per hour is considered serious and must be reported. Fetal activity decreases if hypoxia develops.

Record daily weight and I&O to determine the amount of fluids eliminated from the body. Monitor blood pressure every 4 hours or more frequently if condition indicates. Encouraging compliance with treatment can help prevent the patient from convulsing. Because stress may exacerbate this condition, keep the environment quiet and nonstressful. Maintaining a stress-free environment is difficult, however, since enforced bed rest may last for several weeks. Enforced bed rest or hospitalization can be highly disruptive for the patient and her family; there are financial implications, and the woman's condition can seriously affect family dynamics. Explain the necessity of treatment and the care and the treatment that will be given (Box 28-4).

Emotional and psychological support is essential in helping the woman and her family cope. Their perception of the disease process, the reasons for it, and the care received will affect their compliance with and participation in therapy. The family needs to use coping mechanisms and support systems to help them through this crisis. Also remember that, although this woman has a high-risk condition, she is first of all having a baby. A care plan designed for the woman with preeclampsia must be integrated with the nursing care all women need during labor and birth.

Box 28-4 Eclamptic Seizure Precautions and Interventions

- Keep the environment quiet and nonstimulating, with subdued lighting.
- For seizure precautions, use padded side rails and have suction and oxygen administration equipment and airway ready to use.
- Keep the call button within easy reach.
- Emergency medication tray is immediately accessible.
  - —Hydralazine (antihypertensive vasodilator) and magnesium sulfate in or adjacent to woman's room
  - —Calcium gluconate immediately available in a well-labeled syringe at the bedside as an antidote to magnesium sulfate toxicity
- Emergency birth pack is accessible.
- Reduce noise when the door must be opened or closed.
- Keep noise to a minimum, including blocking incoming telephone calls or visitors.
- Group nursing assessments and care to allow the woman periods of undisturbed rest.
- Move carefully and calmly around the room and avoiding bumping into the bed or startling the woman.
- Collaborate with the woman and her family to restrict visitors.

Protecting the Woman and Fetus during a Convulsion

The nurse's primary responsibilities to protect the woman and the fetus during a convulsion include the following:

- Remain with the woman and press the emergency bell for assistance.
- If she is not on her side already, attempt to turn the woman onto her side when the tonic phase begins. A side-lying position permits greater circulation through the placenta, and it may help prevent aspiration.

- Note the time and sequence of the convulsion.
- Insert an airway after the convulsion, and suction the woman's mouth and nose to clear secretions and prevent aspiration. Provide oxygen by mask at 8 to 10 L/min to increase oxygenation of the placenta and all maternal body organs.
- Observe fetal monitor patterns for nonreassuring signs, such as bradycardia, tachycardia, or decreased variability. These usually resolve within a few minutes as maternal oxygenation is restored.
- Notify, or have another nurse notify, the physician that a convulsion has occurred. Administer medications and prepare for additional medical interventions as directed by the physician.

Providing Information and Support for the Family

Explain to the family what has happened without minimizing the seriousness of the situation. A convulsion is frightening for anyone who witnesses it, and the family is often reassured when the nurse explains that the convulsion lasts only a few minutes and that the woman will probably not be conscious for some time afterward. Acknowledge that the convulsion indicates worsening of the condition and that the physician will need to determine future management; this may include delivery of the infant as soon as possible. Vaginal birth is preferred if the maternal and fetal conditions permit because of abnormalities in the coagulation and other body systems.

Nursing diagnoses and interventions for the patient with GH include but are not limited to the following:

Nursing Diagnoses	Nursing Interventions
Deficient diversional activity, related to environmental lack of stimulation	Find out about hobbies or interests that the woman can perform while resting. Involve patient in conversation while performing care. Encourage family to visit and bring books or other recreational items. Provide change of scenery if possible. Encourage relaxation techniques. Encourage listening to music. Gentle exercise (range of motion, stretching, Kegels, pelvic tilt) is important in maintaining muscle tone, blood flow, regularity of bowel function, and a sense of well-being.

Nursing Diagnoses	Nursing Interventions
Risk for injury, related to elevated blood pressure and central nervous system irritability	Determine prepregnant baseline vital sign values. Monitor blood pressure every 4 hours (or more frequently as necessary) in supine and lateral recumbent positions. Assess for headache and visual disturbances. Weigh patient daily. Monitor I&O. Assess deep tendon reflexes for clonus. Monitor urine for protein. Observe for pitting edema of upper extremities, periorbital area, and face. Monitor laboratory values. Maintain bed rest as needed.

Patient Teaching

Teach all pregnant women the danger signs of complications in pregnancy and the importance of regular medical supervision. Many of the symptoms of GH, particularly the mild, early symptoms, are only detected by maintaining regular physician contact. If GH is diagnosed, explain the consequences of failure to comply.

Encourage high-quality protein, vitamin, and mineral intake. Salt restriction below the normal dietary levels (4 to 6 g/24 hr) is usually not recommended.

Be certain that the patient understands that bed rest is vital because it slows metabolism and relieves dependent edema.

Prognosis

Immediate and continuous care by the obstetric team is mandatory to prevent maternal and fetal morbidity and mortality.

HELLP SYNDROME

The **HELLP syndrome** (*H*, hemolysis; *EL*, elevated liver enzymes; *LP*, low platelet count) represents an extension of the pathology of severe preeclampsia and eclampsia. The initial symptoms of the HELLP syndrome usually appear early in the third trimester, though they may appear in the early postpartum period.

For a woman to be diagnosed as having the HELLP syndrome, her platelet count must be less than 100,000/mm^3, her liver enzyme levels (aspartate aminotransferase and alanine aminotransferase) must be elevated, and some evidence for intravascular hemolysis must be present. The hemolysis accounts for the large drop in hematocrit, out of proportion to blood loss, that occurs in most new mothers with HELLP syndrome during the postpartum period. A unique form of coagulopathy (not DIC) occurs with the HELLP syndrome.

Recognition of the clinical and laboratory findings of the HELLP syndrome is essential to initiate early, aggressive therapy and prevent maternal and fetal mortality.

The prominent symptom of the HELLP syndrome is pain in the right upper quadrant, the lower chest, or the epigastric area. The woman may have tenderness due to liver distention. Additional signs and symptoms include nausea, vomiting, and severe edema. Avoid traumatizing the liver by abdominal palpation, and use care in transporting the woman. A sudden increase in intraabdominal pressure, including a seizure, could lead to rupture of a subcapsular hematoma, resulting in internal bleeding and hypovolemic shock (see Chapter 27 and Box 27-1).

Women with HELLP syndrome should be managed in a setting with full intensive care facilities available. Their treatment is the same as for preeclampsia or eclampsia. After delivery, most women begin recovering within 72 hours.

Intrapartum nursing care of the woman with severe preeclampsia or HELLP syndrome involves continuous monitoring of maternal and fetal status as labor progresses. Continue the assessment and prevention of tissue hypoxia and hemorrhage, both of which can lead to permanent compromise of vital organs, throughout the intrapartum and postpartum period.

An unfavorable (uneffaced and undilated) cervix and the aggressive nature of this disorder support the need for cesarean birth. Prolonged induction of labor could increase maternal morbidity. Fresh-frozen plasma may be needed if bleeding occurs and persists. The major laboratory manifestations of the disease, however, may not appear until the early postpartum period (48 to 72 hours). Delayed transfusion of packed red blood cells (RBCs) and platelets often is necessary because of the continued hemolysis. Attempt to lower the blood pressure if the diastolic pressure is consistently greater than 110 mm Hg. However, blood pressure may be normal or slightly elevated; thus it is not an adequate indicator of the severity of the disease. Hypoglycemia may be present in the woman with HELLP syndrome and, when the blood glucose is less than 40 mg/dL, is associated with a high maternal mortality rate.

COMPLICATIONS RELATED TO INFECTION

Both mother and fetus must be considered in the assessment of maternal infection. In some diseases, such as tuberculosis, the fetus almost always is spared, even though the mother may be dying. With other infections, such as rubella, the fetus may be critically compromised, while the mother is only slightly ill.

Pregnancy is generally regarded as an immunosuppressed condition. It is still an immunologic mystery that a fetus is not rejected during pregnancy. Altered immune responses during pregnancy may decrease maternal ability to fight infection. In addition, genital tract changes may affect susceptibility. As pregnancy advances, vaginal walls engorge, the cervix enlarges, and vaginal pH decreases, contributing to susceptibility.

Some consequences of maternal infection, such as infertility and sterility, last a lifetime. Psychosocial problems as a result of maternal infections may include altered interpersonal relationships and lowered self-esteem. Other conditions, such as a congenitally acquired infection, often affect a child's length and quality of life.

Education and counseling are important in the prevention of maternal infections. Adolescent mothers are at risk because of earlier onset of intercourse and increased likelihood of multiple partners. The recent trend of exchanging sex for drugs is contributing to a rise in infection rates, especially among urban, poor, and minority women.

The prevention of disease and reduction of maternal and neonatal complications continue to be enormous challenges. Many microorganisms can increase maternal and fetal risk. There is an increase in mortality and morbidity rates when infection is present; thus it is important to prevent infection or at least recognize and treat it promptly.

MASTITIS

Mastitis, an infection of the lactating breast, occurs most often during the second and third weeks after childbirth, although it may develop at any time. It usually affects only one breast.

Mastitis is often caused by *Staphylococcus aureus.* The bacteria are typically carried on the hands of the mother or agency staff or in the newborn's mouth. The organism may enter through an injured area of the nipple, such as a crack or blister, although there may be no sign of injury. Nipple soreness may result in insufficient emptying of the breast.

Engorgement and stasis of milk frequently precede mastitis, often when a feeding is skipped, when the infant begins sleeping through the night, or when breastfeeding is suddenly stopped. Constriction of the breasts from a tight bra may interfere with emptying all of the ducts and may lead to infection. The mother who is fatigued or stressed or who has other health problems that compromise her immune system is at increased risk for mastitis.

Initial symptoms may be flulike with fatigue and aching muscles. Symptoms progress to include fever of 101.1° F (38.3° C) or higher, chills, malaise, and headache. Mastitis is characterized by a localized area of redness and inflammation.

Antibiotic therapy, antiinfective agents (antimicrobial agents), and continued emptying of the breast by breastfeeding or breast pump constitute the first line of treatment. With early antibiotic treatment, mastitis usually resolves in 24 to 48 hours. Approximately 5% of women develop a breast abscess, which is treated with surgical drainage and antibiotics.

Supportive measures include application of heat or ice packs, breast support, and analgesics. The mother should continue to breastfeed from both breasts. If the affected breast is too sore, she can use a breast pump. Regular emptying of the breast helps prevent abscess formation. If an abscess forms and ruptures into the breast ducts, breastfeeding on that side should be discontinued and a breast pump used to empty the breast temporarily. Milk obtained should be discarded.

Nursing Interventions and Patient Teaching

Mastitis rarely occurs before discharge from the birth facility, so provide information for prevention. Measures to prevent mastitis include correctly positioning the infant and avoiding nipple trauma and milk stasis. The mother should breastfeed every 2 to 3 hours. She should avoid formula supplements and nipple shields, and she should change nursing pads when they are wet. She should also avoid continuous pressure on the breasts from tight bras or infant carriers.

Once mastitis occurs, nursing measures are aimed at increasing comfort and helping the mother maintain lactation. Moist heat promotes comfort and increases circulation. A shower or hot packs should be used before feeding or pumping the breasts. Cold packs can be used between feedings to reduce edema. The woman should complete the entire course of antibiotic therapy to prevent recurrence or a breast abscess.

The woman should completely empty the breast at each feeding to prevent stasis of milk, which can result in an abscess. If she is too sore to breastfeed on the affected side or if she is taking medications that are contraindicated during lactation, instruct her to express the milk or use a pump to empty the breasts. Breastfeeding or pumping every 1½ to 2 hours makes the mother more comfortable and prevents stasis. Starting the feeding on the unaffected side causes the milk-ejection reflex to occur in the painful breast and makes the process more efficient. Massage over the affected area before and during the feeding helps ensure complete emptying. The mother should stay in bed during the acute phase of her illness. Her fluid intake should be 3000 mL/day. Analgesics may be required to relieve discomfort.

The mother with mastitis is likely to be discouraged and may decide to stop breastfeeding because of the discomfort involved. Weaning during an episode of mastitis may increase engorgement and stasis, leading to abscess formation or recurrent infection. Therefore encourage the mother to continue breastfeeding.

TORCH INFECTIONS AND HUMAN IMMUNODEFICIENCY VIRUS

TORCH infections—or *T*oxoplasmosis, *O*ther infections such as hepatitis, *R*ubella virus, *C*ytomegalovirus, and *H*erpes simplex viruses—are a group of organisms capable of crossing the placenta and adversely affecting the development of the fetus (Box 28-5).

Transmission of human immunodeficiency virus (HIV), a retrovirus, occurs primarily through the exchange of body fluids. Severe depression of the cellular immune system characterizes acquired immunodeficiency syndrome (AIDS) (Box 28-6). Although the populations at high risk have been well documented, assess all women for the possibility of HIV exposure. HIV infection in women is commonly reported at a later stage in the disease, and they usually enter the hospital for initiation of treatment when the illness is more severe. The delay may be due in part to the fact that the symptoms are different from those in men. Chronic vaginitis and candidiasis are common presenting problems.

It is difficult to determine obstetric risk in people with HIV infection because so many other factors are often present. Many HIV-positive women also suffer from drug and alcohol addiction, poor nutrition, limited access to prenatal care, or concurrent STIs. HIV-positive women are probably at risk for preterm labor and birth, premature rupture of membranes, intrauterine growth restriction (IUGR), perinatal mortality, and postpartum endometritis (see Chapter 56).

Etiology

Numerous infectious diseases may cause complications during pregnancy. Some are airborne or ingested, but most are spread by direct contact, usually through sexual transmission. Others are contracted by use of contaminated needles or blood transfusions.

Nursing Interventions

The presence of infection is not always evident. Because of the increased incidence of serious infectious diseases, the Centers for Disease Control and Prevention recommend that standard precautions be taken for all patients. These precautions are most important when dealing with blood and body fluids. Those caring for mothers and newborns are frequently exposed to blood and body fluids and must be particularly alert. Wear gloves, masks, gowns, and glasses during procedures that involve splashing of body fluids, such as amniotomy. Use gloves when cleaning or assessing the breasts or perineal area. Also use gloves when performing the initial newborn bath or changing diapers. Thorough handwashing, as always, is essential. Suction or resuscitate the infant using mechanical barriers or equipment such as mouth shields, suction devices,

Box 28-5 TORCH Infections

T—TOXOPLASMOSIS

- Toxoplasmosis is caused by a protozoan, *Toxoplasma gondii,* which can be contracted by eating raw, contaminated meats or having contact with the feces of infected cats.
- Toxoplasmosis is one of the common accompanying opportunistic infections of acquired immunodeficiency syndrome (AIDS). The mother may be free of symptoms or may develop myalgia, enlarged posterior cervical lymph nodes, malaise, and rash that disappear in a matter of days. Acute infection in pregnancy produces flulike symptoms and lymphadenopathy.
- Diagnosis is confirmed by blood studies, and women in at-risk groups should have toxoplasmosis titer evaluated.
- The effects on the fetus can be profound: spontaneous abortion, stillbirth, neonatal death, blindness, retardation, and a wide range of congenital anomalies.
- Teach all pregnant women to avoid undercooked meats.
- If cats are present in the environment, the woman should wear gloves whenever chance of contact with feces exists.

O—OTHER

- The primary infection included in this category is hepatitis. Hepatitis A is a virus spread by droplets or hands and is associated with poor handwashing after defecation.
- Pregnancy effects include spontaneous abortion and flulike signs and symptoms: fever, malaise, and nausea. If the fetus is exposed in the first trimester and is untreated, possible effects include fetal anomalies, preterm birth, fetal or neonatal hepatitis, and intrauterine death. Gamma globulin vaccination is given to mothers and newborns for prophylaxis.
- Hepatitis B is a virus transmitted in a manner similar to that of human immunodeficiency virus (HIV). Routes of transmission include contaminated needles, syringes, or blood products; sexual intercourse; and body fluid exchange.
- During pregnancy, common signs and symptoms include fever, rash, anorexia, malaise, myalgias, and jaundice if the liver is acutely affected. Fetal and newborn effects are the same as those listed for hepatitis A. Vaccination during pregnancy is not thought to pose a risk to the fetus. All mothers and neonates are encouraged to receive hepatitis B vaccine.
- The "other" group includes other miscellaneous infections that may affect the mother or fetus (or both).
  —Urinary tract and vaginal infections can cause fever, chills, dysuria, pain, malaise, and changes in vaginal drainage. Report any of these symptoms promptly to the physician. Culture and sensitivity tests usually reveal the specific organism. The physician bases treatment on the causative organism and the severity of the problem. Treatment must be done cautiously because of the possibility of teratogenic effects from the antibiotics.
  —Sexually transmitted infections are also a serious concern. Syphilis can also cross the placental barrier and infect the fetus. Chlamydia may cause pneumonia or eye infections in the newborn. Gonorrhea can cause pelvic inflammatory disease in the mother and eye infections in the newborn.

R—RUBELLA, GERMAN MEASLES, OR 3-DAY MEASLES

- Rubella is a viral infection transmitted by droplets. Fever, rash, and mild lymphedema usually are seen in the affected mother. If contracted during the first trimester, rubella can cause a wide range of congenital defects, including congenital heart disease, mental retardation, deafness, and cataracts.
- Diagnosis is made by serologic tests for rubella titer.
- Immunization should ideally be given before a woman reaches childbearing age. If a pregnant woman does not have immunity, caution her to avoid risk of exposure to the disease.
- Because this immunization involves administration of an attenuated (diluted to reduce virulence of pathogenic microorganism) virus, it is given after delivery, frequently just before discharge. This is one time the physician can be certain that the woman is not pregnant.
- Further caution the woman to avoid becoming pregnant for 2 to 3 months after vaccination, because the attenuated virus used for immunization may still be present.

C—CYTOMEGALOVIRUS

- Cytomegalovirus (CMV) is a virus and belongs to the herpesvirus group.
- CMV is a common infection that can be spread by close contact, breastfeeding, sexual relations, and kissing.
- More than half of all adults have antibodies to the virus.
- This virus is capable of crossing the placental barrier and causing serious damage to the fetus, including cognitive impairment, hearing problems, and congenital anomalies. It is unusual in that the mother may be totally asymptomatic and it does not always cause fetal complications.
- Pregnant health care providers should observe standard precautions to avoid exposure to droplets of infected secretions such as saliva, urine, and respiratory discharges.

H—HERPES GENITALIS

- Herpes genitalis is also called herpesvirus type 2. It causes painful lesions on the external genitalia and can also involve the cervix.
- Intrauterine infection of the fetus can occur if the membranes rupture or vaginal delivery takes place when active lesions are present. If the virus is not treated, the neonatal mortality rate is extremely high.
- Diagnosis is made on the basis of maternal symptoms and a culture of the lesions.
- Women with active herpes infection should deliver by cesarean birth.
- The pregnancy effects of primary genital herpes infection include spontaneous abortion, preterm labor, and intrauterine growth restriction.
- Health care providers with herpes simplex virus (HSV) infections should take precautions. Anyone with oral HSV lesions should wear a mask if in close contact with newborns, and anyone with skin lesions should not give direct care until lesions are dried and crusted. Scrupulous handwashing is essential.

Box 28-6 Acquired Immunodeficiency Syndrome

- Acquired immunodeficiency syndrome (AIDS) is a major health concern. It has had a significant effect on all areas of health care, including maternal nursing.
- The causative organism is the human immunodeficiency virus (HIV), which enters the body through blood, blood products, or sexual contact. It is capable of crossing the placental barrier and infecting the fetus in utero, causing congenital defects such as microcephaly (abnormal smallness of the head) and facial deformities.
- Because of the long incubation period, infants born to HIV-seropositive mothers may show no indication at birth but develop signs of the infection later. These include failure to thrive, recurrent infection, interstitial pneumonia, and neurologic abnormalities.
- Studies place the risk of perinatal transmission at 20% to 50%. Most children diagnosed with AIDS die within the first few years of life.
- All pregnant women diagnosed with HIV benefit from antiretroviral therapy. The majority of mother-to-fetus transmissions occur in the final weeks of pregnancy.
- There is rapid HIV testing for women who come in for delivery without having had prenatal care. Results are rapidly available and allow for safer management of mother and baby.
- Vaginal birth is strongly discouraged and cesarean delivery is advisable. Cesarean births have been shown to reduce contact with maternal virus.

and ventilators. Take care when handling needles and syringes; dispose of these in special containers without breaking or recapping.

During the birthing process every effort should be made to decrease the neonate's exposure to infected maternal blood and secretions. If feasible, the membranes should be left intact until the birth. Women who give birth within 4 hours after membrane rupture are less likely to transmit the virus to their neonates than women who experience a longer interval between rupture and birth. Avoid fetal scalp electrodes and scalp pH sampling because these procedures may result in inoculation of the virus into the fetus. Likewise, avoid the use of forceps and a vacuum extractor when possible. Episiotomy and cesarean birth do not seem to greatly influence the infection rate.

The cleansed neonate can be with the HIV-infected mother after birth, but breastfeeding is discouraged because of possible HIV transmission in breast milk. (The World Health Organization has not discouraged breastfeeding in nonindustrialized nations because of the decreased availability of infant formula and hygiene risks in the preparation of formula but may be changing its recommendation.) After discharge, the woman and her infant are referred to physicians who are experienced in the treatment of AIDS and associated conditions.

Psychological support is important to the patient with an infectious disease. Because many of these diseases are life threatening to the mother, the fetus, or the newborn, fear and anxiety are common. If the infection results in fetal mortality or defects, the mother may express guilt. The nurse must also cope with his or her own feelings about these serious infectious diseases. Caring for mothers and newborns with AIDS and other such diseases can create judgmental feelings in the nurse that he or she must resolve.

Patient Teaching

Education on prevention of infection should start long before pregnancy. Infections acquired by a woman before she becomes pregnant can seriously affect the outcome of pregnancy. Immunization for rubella before childbearing years is essential; stress to all new mothers the importance of having children routinely immunized. Review hygiene practices such as careful handwashing and proper storage and preparation of meats. Discuss safer sex practices, including use of condoms, with individuals at risk, and stress the importance of regular medical care and treatment.

Counseling the pregnant woman with a vaginal infection should also include measures to deal with the discomfort (Box 28-7).

Prognosis

The success of the prevention measures depends on the conscientious effort of the health care worker in carrying out all recommended procedures carefully and the patient's willingness to comply with preventive measures or prescribed therapy.

PULMONARY TUBERCULOSIS

Pulmonary tuberculosis results from infection by *Mycobacterium tuberculosis.* It is transmitted by aerosolized droplets of liquid containing the bacterium that are inhaled by a noninfected individual and taken into the lung. Initially most people are asymptomatic. Screen women obtaining prenatal care for tuberculosis by administering an intradermal injection of mycobacterial protein (purified protein derivative). If the reaction is positive, protect the woman's abdomen with a lead shield while a radiograph is taken of her chest. The di-

Box 28-7 Comfort Measures for the Pregnant Woman with a Vaginal Infection

- Pour warm water over the urethra and vulva.
- Take warm sitz baths for 15 minutes three to five times daily.
- Avoid strong deodorant soaps, creams, and ointments.
- Dry the genital area with a blow-dryer. (To prevent burning, beware of high temperatures.)
- Wear 100% cotton underwear.
- Do not wear tight-fitting jeans.
- Do not wear panties or pantyhose with nylon inserts.
- Obtain early and regular Papanicolaou's (Pap) smears.
- Avoid any sexual contact during outbreaks.

agnosis is confirmed by isolating and identifying the bacterium in the sputum.

Symptomatic people have general malaise, fatigue, loss of appetite, weight loss, and fever. These symptoms occur in the late afternoon and evening and are accompanied by night sweats. As the disease progresses, patients develop a chronic cough and produce mucopurulent sputum.

Tuberculosis is associated with poverty, malnutrition, and HIV infection. Worldwide it is responsible for more deaths than any other communicable disease. Moreover, the incidence is increasing in inner-city areas and among homeless people. It is also prevalent among immigrants from Southeast Asia and Central and South America.

Although perinatal infection is rare, it may be acquired as the fetus swallows infected amniotic fluid or is exposed through the umbilical vein. The diagnosis is made by finding the bacilli in a gastric aspirate of the neonate or in placental tissue. Signs of congenital tuberculosis include failure to thrive; lethargy; respiratory distress; fever; and enlargement of the spleen, the liver, and lymph nodes. If the mother remains untreated, the newborn is at high risk for acquiring tuberculosis by inhaling infectious respiratory droplets from the mother.

Medical Management

Multidrug therapy is used to protect the woman and her fetus. Management of the infant involves preventing the disease or treating early infection. Federal guidelines recommend not allowing the infant to be exposed to the mother after birth until cleared by the health department requirements. This may also influence the discharge of mother and infant. Prevention focuses on teaching family members how the disease is transmitted so that they can protect the infant from airborne organisms. The infant should be skin tested at birth and may be started on preventive therapy. Repeat skin testing at 3 to 4 months. Therapy is usually continued for at least 9 months. The infant's tuberculosis medication may stop if the mother and family members are well treated and show no additional disease. If the skin test result converts to positive, a full course of drug therapy should be given.

COMPLICATIONS RELATED TO EXISTING MEDICAL CONDITIONS

DIABETES MELLITUS

Etiology

Before the discovery of insulin in 1920, diabetic women rarely gave birth to a healthy baby. Many diabetic women of childbearing age were infertile or sterile, and the majority of those who became pregnant were unable to carry to term. The perinatal mortality rate was approximately 65%, with stillbirth being the largest cause of fetal death.

Diabetes mellitus is an endocrine disorder that affects metabolism and the utilization of glucose. This disease is not curable and is often difficult to control. In pregnancy, hormonal changes and stresses placed on all the maternal body systems result in even more complex medical and nursing management. Diabetes is a risk factor in approximately 1% to 2% of pregnancies.

Pathophysiology

In diabetes mellitus the pancreas does not produce adequate amounts of insulin to metabolize glucose normally. Because glucose does not enter the cells without adequate insulin, blood glucose levels remain high. The cells release stored fat and protein for energy, leading to ketosis and a negative nitrogen balance.

Diabetes is classified into various forms. Type 1 (formerly called insulin-dependent diabetes mellitus) requires regular administration of insulin for control. Type 2 (formerly called non–insulin-dependent diabetes mellitus) is most often controlled by diet or oral hypoglycemics. **Pregestational diabetes mellitus** is the label sometimes given to type 1 or type 2 diabetes that existed before pregnancy.

Gestational diabetes mellitus (GDM) is the inability to produce enough insulin to maintain normal glucose levels during pregnancy. Increased dietary glucose needs, along with insulin resistance from placental hormones, cortisol, and insulinase, result in hyperglycemia and GDM. The patient with GDM is usually diagnosed in the middle of the pregnancy and may have sustained hyperglycemia in the early months of the pregnancy. Thus she may be at greater risk for fetal complications than a woman with preexisting diabetes.

Improved control of this disease process has reduced the risk to both mother and fetus; however, the incidence of complications is still significant. Maternal complications include infections (urinary tract and vaginal), difficult labor related to increased fetal size (which frequently results in cesarean birth), vascular complications (including retinopathy), azotemia, ketoacidosis, hypertensive disorders such as preeclampsia, and cesarean birth. Fetal complications include stillbirth, spontaneous abortion, hydramnios (excessive amniotic fluid), large placenta, alteration in size for gestational age (macrosomia), congenital anomalies, neonatal hypoglycemia, neonatal hyperbilirubinemia, respiratory distress syndrome, and fetal or neonatal death.

Clinical Manifestations

Alteration in blood glucose levels is the major manifestation of the disease. Blood glucose levels greater than 120 mg/dL significantly increase the risk of complications. When blood glucose levels are elevated, the classic symptoms of diabetes—polyuria, polydipsia, and polyphagia—may be observed (Box 28-8).

Box 28-8 Signs and Symptoms of Maternal Hypoglycemia and Hyperglycemia

HYPOGLYCEMIA
- Shakiness (tremors)
- Sweating
- Pallor; cold, clammy skin
- Disorientation, irritability
- Headache
- Hunger
- Blurred vision

HYPERGLYCEMIA
- Fatigue
- Flushed, hot skin
- Dry mouth, excessive thirst
- Frequent urination
- Rapid, deep respirations; odor of acetone on breath
- Drowsiness, headache
- Depressed reflexes

Assessment

Perform urine testing at all prenatal visits. If testing indicates the presence of glucose, additional testing is required. For the known diabetic, assess diet, activity, and medication compliance. Assess the vascular system regularly for possible complications, and watch the patient closely for signs of infection. Also assess the condition of the fetus by serial ultrasonography and other medical measures.

Diagnostic Tests

A 1-hour diabetes screening test or glucose tolerance tests may be ordered. If the woman is known to have diabetes mellitus, carefully monitor blood glucose levels throughout the pregnancy. **Glycosylated hemoglobin** (a combination of hemoglobin and blood glucose, making up about 4% to 8% of the total hemoglobin; i.e., the hemoglobin chains have glucose attached to them) tests are used to monitor glucose control up to 3 months prior to the test. Fingerstick blood testing is also useful.

Diagnostic techniques for fetal surveillance often are performed during pregnancy complicated by diabetes mellitus. Tests to evaluate fetal well-being include nonstress test, contraction stress test, alpha-fetoprotein, biophysical profile (see Table 25-3), and serum estriols (the major estrogen secreted by the placenta, measured to determine placental functioning). Try to determine the estimated date of birth. A baseline ultrasound scan is done to assess the fetus's gestational age. Follow-up ultrasound examinations are performed as often as every 4 to 6 weeks to monitor fetal growth and development and to assess for congenital abnormalities. Biochemical analysis of amniotic fluid is performed to ascertain fetal lung maturity, typically in the third trimester. Amniocentesis earlier in gestation may be used to diagnose congenital anomalies.

Nursing Interventions

Nursing care is directed at maintaining the patient in a euglycemic (normal blood glucose) status. The patient's insulin requirements change significantly throughout pregnancy, labor, and delivery. Assess the patient carefully at each visit, complete all blood glucose level evaluations as ordered, and report any abnormalities to the physician promptly. Because of possible teratogenic effects, oral hypoglycemics are usually discontinued. Insulin may be required by both type 2 and GDM patients to control blood glucose levels.

Nursing diagnoses and interventions for the patient with GDM include but are not limited to the following:

Nursing Diagnoses	Nursing Interventions
Risk for injury, related to improper insulin administration	Assess patient's understanding of insulin needs. Explain purpose of insulin, effect on body, and possible side effects. Review symptoms of hypoglycemia and peak action of insulin. Stress importance of following regimen, including diet, exercise, and insulin administration. Demonstrate correct technique for self-monitoring blood glucose. Explain how to adjust insulin dosage. Demonstrate correct withdrawal and administration of insulin, including site rotation.
Risk for ineffective health maintenance, related to deficient knowledge of the effects of pregnancy on diabetes control	Review pathophysiology of the disease. Assist the patient in formulating questions for the physician. Clarify misconceptions. Teach home monitoring of blood glucose levels. Review effects of diabetes on the pregnant patient. Explain in simple terms the advantages to the fetus of maintaining a normal maternal blood glucose level. Advantages include an optimal pattern of growth, the increased likelihood that the baby will be born near term, and fewer complications associated with prematurity.

Nursing Diagnoses	Nursing Interventions
	Teach danger signs of diabetes and whom to notify (provide written as well as oral instructions). Stress importance of weekly prenatal visits during second half of pregnancy. Refer patient to community diabetic support groups.

Patient Teaching

The need for teaching differs with the classification of the disease and the patient's willingness to learn. A woman who has been diagnosed before pregnancy needs reinforcement of diet, medication, and health practices. Also explain the effects pregnancy has on diabetes throughout the course of pregnancy, labor, delivery, and the postpartum period. For the gestational diabetic, stress the necessity of good control of the disease, including all the teaching normally given to a new diabetic.

Be an active listener and allow time for the woman and her family to express concerns and feelings. Convey acceptance of expressed feelings whether they are negative or positive. Sharing emotions will help the woman cope with her anxiety and frustration and thus promote her active participation in her care.

Prognosis

Blood glucose control is essential in pregnancy. Insulin will not cross the placental barrier (placental tissue limits passage of certain substances); consequently, control of the mother's diabetes is vital to the health of the fetus. Most women benefit from praise when diabetic control is well maintained. They feel competent and trusted by the health care team and motivated to continue.

CARDIAC DISEASE

Pregnancy increases the demands on the cardiovascular system. This is not a problem for the normal, healthy heart, which is able to adapt to the increased demands. However, women who have preexisting cardiac disease face increased risk when cardiac function is challenged by pregnancy. About 1% of pregnancies are complicated by heart disease. The degree of disability is often more important than the type of cardiovascular disease in the treatment and prognosis during pregnancy.

Etiology

The most common cardiac problems of maternity patients result from rheumatic heart disease, congenital heart defects, or mitral valve prolapse. Occasionally a condition called peripartum **cardiomyopathy** (disease of the myocardium, especially due to primary diseases of the heart muscle) is observed in pregnant patients who have no history of cardiac problems. This may be seen in the last month of pregnancy or during the postpartum period. The symptoms are similar to those of congestive heart failure.

With successful treatment of congenital cardiac anomalies or mitral stenosis resulting from rheumatic heart disease, many girls are now reaching childbearing age and bearing children. Rheumatic heart disease, a complication of streptococcal infection, is not common in the United States but may be found in recent immigrants. Hypertensive heart disease, often a secondary effect of obesity, can be expected to affect more childbearing women because of the growing incidence in the general population. Cardiomyopathy is a disorder of the muscle structure of the heart that may have any of several causes. Congestive heart failure may be secondary to underlying heart disease or a result of treatment for other conditions.

Pathophysiology

During pregnancy increased blood volume, heart rate, and cardiac output are normal. In the woman with existing cardiac problems, the muscle, the valves, or the vessels are overly stressed by these changes. Symptoms of the underlying pathologic condition are exacerbated, resulting in cardiac decompensation, congestive failure, and other medical problems.

Clinical Manifestations

The symptoms depend on the underlying pathologic condition. Edema, cyanosis, tachycardia, palpitations, arrhythmias, chest pain, dyspnea, and fatigue may occur. Physical exertion may increase the severity of the symptoms. Clinical findings are those of heart failure (left ventricular failure). The patient has decreased cardiac output and pulmonary congestion, with fluid collecting in the lungs. Pulmonary edema and pleural effusion also occur, and pulmonary crackles, hemoptysis, and cough may be present.

Assessment

At each prenatal visit measure the patient's vital signs and evaluate her ability to participate in activities. Unusual fatigue with activity may reveal problems. Monitor for edema, weight gain, murmurs, cough, dyspnea, or abnormal lung sounds. Compare these data with normal changes during pregnancy. The patient with preexisting heart disease should also be followed by her cardiologist during her pregnancy.

The pregnant woman with cardiac disease requires detailed assessment to determine the potential for optimal maternal health and a viable fetus throughout the peripartum period. If she chooses to continue the pregnancy, assess the high-risk pregnant woman's condition as often as weekly.

Diagnostic Tests

Chest x-ray evaluation, electrocardiograms, echocardiograms, and auscultation are used to determine the type and severity of the cardiac problem. Blood gas analysis may be performed if severe decompensation is observed. A woman's sudden inability to perform activities that she previously was comfortable doing may indicate cardiovascular decompensation.

Nursing Interventions

Nursing care is directed at helping the woman maintain normal physical and psychosocial function. During pregnancy teach the importance of diet, medications, paced activity, and adequate rest. This includes education about the specific disease and its management. Iron intake must be adequate to prevent anemia, which will further stress the heart. Sodium may be restricted to control the fluid volume and decrease cardiac stress. Stool softeners may be prescribed to decrease use of the Valsalva maneuver (holding the breath while bearing down) when defecating. The activity level is dictated by the severity of the cardiac problem. Be aware of the medical recommendations and help the woman incorporate these into her daily life. Patients with more severe cardiac problems require the greatest adjustments. Be highly sensitive to personal and family needs.

If cardiopulmonary arrest occurs during pregnancy, cardiopulmonary resuscitation may be performed within certain guidelines (Box 28-9).

During labor, the semi-Fowler's or side-lying position with the head elevated enhances respiratory effort and improves circulation. During every contraction 300 to 500 mL of blood shifts from the uterus and placenta into the central circulation. This extra fluid causes a sharp rise in cardiac workload; therefore careful management of IV administration is essential to prevent fluid overload. The efforts of labor may require oxygen administration to increase the blood oxygen saturation, which is monitored by pulse oximetry. Administer medications such as cardiotonics, diuretics, prophylactic antibiotics, sedatives, and analgesics as directed by the physician. Reduce discomfort to a minimum. Also try to eliminate unnecessary activity by the patient during labor. Resting between contractions and using shorter, open-glottis pushing are recommended to conserve energy. Closely monitor fetal condition for any signs of distress, using a fetal monitor for continuous assessment. Calmly explain everything to decrease anxiety.

A vaginal delivery is recommended for a woman with heart disease unless there are specific indications for a cesarean birth. Vacuum extraction or outlet forceps are often used to minimize the mother's use of the Valsalva maneuver when pushing during the second stage.

Box 28-9 Cardiopulmonary Resuscitation for the Pregnant Woman

AIRWAY

- Determine unresponsiveness.
- Activate emergency medical system and get the automated external defibrillator (AED) if available.
- Position woman on flat, firm surface with uterus displaced laterally with a wedge (e.g., a rolled towel placed under her hip) or manually, or place her in a lateral position.
- Open airway with head-tilt/chin-lift maneuver.

BREATHING

- Determine breathlessness (look, listen, feel).
- If the woman is not breathing, give two slow breaths.

CIRCULATION

- Determine pulselessness by feeling carotid pulse.
- If there is no pulse, begin chest compressions at rate of 100 per minute. Chest compressions may be performed slightly higher on the sternum if the uterus is enlarged enough to displace the diaphragm into a higher position.
- After four cycles of 15 compressions and two breaths, check her pulse. If pulse is not present, continue cardiopulmonary resuscitation.

DEFIBRILLATION

- Use an AED according to standard protocol to analyze heart rhythm and deliver shock if indicated.

RELIEF OF FOREIGN-BODY AIRWAY OBSTRUCTION

- If the pregnant woman is unable to speak or cough, perform chest thrusts. Stand behind the woman and place your arms under her armpits to encircle her chest. Press backward with quick thrusts until the foreign body is expelled.
- If the woman becomes unresponsive, follow the steps for victims who become unresponsive, but use chest thrusts instead of abdominal thrusts.

Modified from Stapleton, E., et al. (2001). *Fundamentals of BLS for healthcare providers*. Dallas: American Heart Association.

Postpartum care varies according to the severity of the cardiac problem. Explore methods of incorporating care of the infant into the mother's activities. Because extravascular fluid returns to the bloodstream after delivery, the mother is at risk for developing cardiac decompression during the 48 hours after the birth.

To promote normal parent-child attachment, establish contact as early as possible. Discuss breastfeeding with the physician, since the physical effort may be excessive for the mother and the transfer of medications in the breast milk may be harmful to the infant. As in all other areas of nursing, continue to assess the patient's status and give explanations for all care.

Amnioinfusion

Amnioinfusion, an infusion of fluids directly into the amniotic sac, may be performed during pregnancy to treat patients experiencing **oligohydramnios,** a deficit in the level of amniotic fluid. During labor, amnioinfusion may be performed with saline or lactated Ringer's solution to manage women with cord compression resulting in variable decelerations. Amniotic fluid provides buoyancy to the fetus, preventing cord compression and promoting musculoskeletal development.

Prognosis

In cardiac complications the maternal mortality rate has been estimated in the range of 30% to 60%; the infant mortality rate is approximately 10%. The prognosis is good if cardiomegaly is not persistent after 6 months. The prognosis for women whose hearts remain enlarged is not as favorable. Future pregnancies usually result in some cardiac failure (50% to 88%). The mortality rate may be as high as 60%. Oral contraceptives are contraindicated because of the risk of thromboembolism.

COMPLICATIONS RELATED TO AGE

ADOLESCENTS

Adolescent patients present the nurse with a unique challenge. A significant number are sexually active and in need of contraceptive counseling; many become pregnant. The pregnant adolescent, her family, and her partner require sensitive, competent nursing interventions. The young woman may choose to terminate the pregnancy or carry it to term. She may place the infant up for adoption or elect to keep the baby. The nurse plays a vital role in helping the patient make informed decisions and in supporting her, both physically and emotionally, in carrying out her chosen option. The nurse should never recommend a choice.

Growth and Development

The period of adolescence is divided into three stages: early, middle, and late. The higher the developmental level, the greater the readiness to accept responsibility for self and others.

Adolescent development is characterized by physical, cognitive, and behavioral development approximating chronologic age. Adolescents are egocentric, concrete thinkers and have feelings of invincibility, which leads to risky behaviors, such as smoking, drug and alcohol abuse, and unprotected sex with multiple partners.

Before the child can become a mature adult, he or she must accomplish the developmental tasks of adolescence, including acceptance of body image, acceptance of sexual identity, development of a personal value system, preparation for making a living, independence from parents, development of decision-making skills, and development of an adult identity. These tasks vary from culture to culture and with individual adolescents and their goals.

Pregnancy interrupts work on identity formation and developmental tasks. Attempting to accomplish developmental tasks of pregnancy and of normal adolescence simultaneously may be overwhelming. The psychological burden may lead to depression and to postponement in attaining an adult identity. The pregnant adolescent faces further developmental tasks of parenthood. These tasks are as important to the new adolescent parents as they organize ways to behave in their environment as they are for the adult (see life span discussion in Chapter 9).

Although the number of adolescent pregnancies in the United States has not increased in the past 5 to 10 years, pregnancies have significantly increased among very young adolescents (ages 10 to 14). This trend is attributed to many sociologic factors, including breakdown of the traditional family and changes in social mores resulting in earlier sexual activity. Teenagers account for an increasingly large percentage of births and abortions. Physiologic immaturity, incomplete education, and unresolved developmental tasks are complicating factors.

Several physiologic concerns are associated with the young pregnant adolescent. These include an increased risk for GH, cephalopelvic disproportion resulting in cesarean birth, abruptio placentae, low birth weight, IUGR, anemia, infection, preterm delivery, and perinatal death. Pregnant teenagers also commonly fear or deny the pregnancy and go without medical attention until late in pregnancy. Lack of prenatal care increases the risk to the pregnant teenager and her infant.

Sociocultural concerns are seen in both educational and economic arenas. The pregnancy frequently ends the adolescent's formal education, which leads to reduced job opportunities because of lack of training. This results in an increased poverty risk with potentially prolonged dependence on public assistance.

Assessment

Assessment of all health patterns for each adolescent is essential. When prenatal care is initiated early and consistently, and confounding variables (e.g., socioeconomic factors) are controlled, very young pregnant adolescents are at no greater risk (nor are their infants) for an adverse outcome than older pregnant women. The nurse's role in reducing the risks and consequences of adolescent pregnancy is twofold: to encourage early and continued prenatal care, and to refer the adolescent, if necessary, for appropriate social support services, which can help reverse the effects of a negative socioeconomic environment.

Nursing Interventions

When caring for the pregnant adolescent, be aware of the patient's unique nature and incorporate both physical and psychological interventions into the care plan. An understanding of adolescent growth and development is necessary to successfully relate to and care for this patient.

Nursing diagnoses and interventions for the pregnant adolescent patient include but are not limited to the following:

Nursing Diagnoses	Nursing Interventions
Deficient knowledge, related to choices regarding pregnancy, childbirth experiences, and parenthood	Examine own views regarding sexuality to be able to maintain nonjudgmental approach. Listen and give honest answers. Create a safe and stable environment that engenders trust. Evaluate which stage of development the adolescent is experiencing. Teach the adolescent about pregnancy choices, childbirth, and parenthood. Encourage questions and verbalization of fears and concerns. Compliment teens on the questions asked and efforts made to learn about issues. Encourage support personnel to attend and participate in prenatal care. Refer to childbirth and parenthood class and community support and information groups.
Imbalanced nutrition: less than body requirements, related to inadequate diet	Perform 24-hour diet recall to establish dietary habits. Assess height and weight and compare to norms for age. Assess for frequent dieting, eating disorders, smoking, alcohol use, and substance abuse. Assess fat content of diet. Assess fluid intake for caffeine levels. Explain fetal need for weight gain. Refer to dietitian for nutrition counseling. Provide sample menus, including increased vitamins, minerals, and calories. Refer to the Women, Infants, and Children (WIC) program for dietary supplements.

Labor and Birth

The very young adolescent may be frightened of needles, pelvic examinations, noises from other women in labor or from equipment, and birth rooms. Provide single, private rooms when possible. Ensure the patient has the support of a knowledgeable coach, whether husband, friend, parent, or nurse. Many teenagers come to labor lacking preparation; they are frightened and often alone. If they are admitted early in the first stage, teach about relaxation with contractions, ambulation, side-lying positions, and comfort measures. The adolescent is more concerned with how the baby will get out than with fetal well-being.

Pregnant young adolescents are often still growing, so there is an increased chance of cephalopelvic disproportion and cesarean birth. This provides an additional fear for the laboring adolescent. Be prepared to provide the necessary support and encouragement required. Always provide anticipatory guidance and explain procedures. Many adolescents keep their infants and are responsive to staff members' sharing their delight. For these young parents, efforts to promote parent-child attachment are particularly important.

Postpartum Care

Physically, the adolescent mother requires the same care as any woman who has given birth. Provide explicit directions for self-care and infant care. Most adolescents view the care of the infant as their primary area of concern. Continue to assess the new mother's parenting abilities during the postpartum period. In addition, continue to support the patient by involving grandparents or other family members, making home visits, and referring to group sessions for discussion of infant care and parenting problems. Outreach programs concerned with self-care, parent-child interactions, child injuries, and failure to thrive, as well as those that provide prompt and effective intervention, prevent more serious problems.

Postpartum contraception is a high priority for almost every young adolescent. The risk of repeat pregnancy in adolescence is high, and all the accompanying risks of adolescent pregnancy increase with each subsequent pregnancy. Almost universally, postpartum adolescents say that they will never have sex again and therefore need no birth control. Nonetheless adolescents need to leave the hospital with barrier methods (foam and condoms) and the knowledge of how and when to use them. Very young adolescents may be shy or embarrassed about touching their genitalia to use barrier methods. In addition, they are not likely to anticipate intercourse. For these reasons, some health care providers send adolescents home on a regimen of oral contraceptives. This practice is controversial because of the increased risk of thromboembolic disease in the immediate postpartum period (first 4 weeks). Thus the decision must be based on the individual adolescent and her life situation. Medroxyprogesterone (Depo-Provera) and levonorgestrel (Norplant) are currently strongly encouraged as contraceptives for adolescents. Cultural values and practices also should be taken into account.

Adolescent males need to be considered and included in any interventions in sexuality education, family planning, and parent education.

The adolescent mother needs support if she is considering adoption for her child. Avoid using phrases that give negative connotations to the adoption process. Phrases such as "put up for adoption" and "give up for adoption" imply the biologic parents are uncaring. Neither should the terms "real parents" or "natural parents" be used exclusively for genetic parents. The adoptive parents are the "real parents" because they care for the child. Neutral language, such as "arranging for an adoption," "biologic parent" or "birth mother," and "adoptive parent," is preferred. Give the mother the option of either remaining on the postpartum floor or transferring to another unit. Assure her that she will have as much access to the baby as she desires.

Grief results from actual or perceived loss. The adolescent may experience grief from thoughts about adoption, the birth of a preterm infant who may be in intensive care, or the infant's death. Help the patient move through the grieving process. The adolescent who gives birth to a preterm infant or one who is small for gestational age may find it difficult to reconcile this tiny, scrawny infant with her fantasized "Gerber baby." She may be afraid of caring for the child introduced to her in the intensive care unit. The confidence in her abilities gained during the prenatal period may be replaced by feelings of being overwhelmed and incompetent. Intensive teaching and continual support programs are essential to keep the young mother and her vulnerable infant from becoming estranged.

Many young mothers pattern their parenting on what they themselves experienced. Therefore it is vital to determine the kind of support that those close to young mothers are able or prepared to give and the kinds of community aid that can supplement this support. The adolescent may have conflict with dependence versus independence issues as she performs her mothering role within the framework of her family of origin. The adolescent's family also may need help adapting to their new roles.

Adolescent Father

The adolescent father also faces immediate developmental crises: completing the developmental tasks of adolescence and making a transition to parenthood and, sometimes, to marriage. These transitions can be stressful. Begin interacting with the adolescent father by asking his pregnant partner to bring him to the clinic with her so that he may participate in the birth. With the pregnant teen's agreement, the father also may be contacted directly.

To include the young father in all aspects of the care, assess four areas: (1) the couple's relationship; (2) levels of stress, concern, and coping; (3) educational and vocational goals; and (4) level of health care knowledge. Like all fathers, adolescent fathers need support to discuss their emotional responses to the pregnancy. The nurse's nonjudgmental attitude is essential for open communication. Recognize the father's feelings of guilt, powerlessness, or bravado and their negative consequences for both parents and child. Counseling must be reality oriented. Discuss topics such as finances, child care, parenting skills, and the father's role in the birth experience. Teenage fathers also need knowledge of reproductive physiology and birth control options.

The adolescent mother's partner and family affect how she deals with her pregnancy, labor, birth, and subsequent parenthood. The adolescent father may continue to be involved with the young mother. In many instances he plays an important role in the decisions she faces in pregnancy, including whether to continue the pregnancy, have an abortion, keep the child, or arrange for adoption.

Support the young father by helping him develop realistic perceptions of his role as "father of a child." Encourage his use of coping mechanisms that are not detrimental to his, his partner's, or his child's well-being. Enlist support systems, parents, and professional agencies on his behalf. Encourage mutual responsibility for birth control.

Patient Teaching

Education of the pregnant adolescent is essential. To work effectively with adolescents, be sensitive, nonjudgmental, and knowledgeable about the stages of adolescence. Because no two adolescents are alike, use a wide range of skills to reach each individual (Figure 28-8; Patient Teaching box on adolescent parents). Pa-

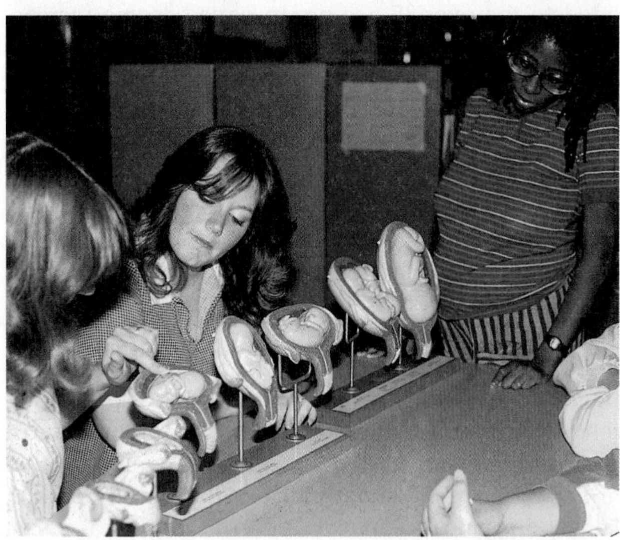

FIGURE 28-8 Pregnant adolescents review fetal development.

Patient Teaching

Adolescent Parents

- Nutrition is a major area of concern for the teenager. The young teen is often still growing herself, and her nutritional intake must meet her own needs and those of the fetus. Fad diets and food idiosyncrasies are common in teenagers; take this into account when teaching nutrition. Body image disturbance is a problem even for a mature woman. The teenager, particularly one who has not yet accepted the fact of pregnancy, may limit food intake to avoid gaining weight. This can be exceedingly dangerous to both mother and infant.
- Preparation for labor and delivery is also essential. Many adolescents have little knowledge of human anatomy and have fears and misconceptions about the process of childbirth. They may have heard stories from friends that increase their anxiety. Be factual without being harsh when describing the birth process.
- Many adolescents plan to raise their infants; therefore instruction should include child care, growth, and development. Refer the women to community agencies that will provide ongoing support.
- Do not ignore the adolescent father. Consider the effect of pregnancy on him, particularly if he remains meaningfully involved with the teenage mother. Counseling is important for both, since the physical, financial, and emotional consequences of the pregnancy will affect both of them for the rest of their lives.

tient teaching may need to be directed toward the adolescent mother, who is often the primary caregiver. Efforts should be made to keep the adolescent in school. Many high schools have programs to assist adolescent parents in their educational endeavors.

OLDER PREGNANT WOMAN

At the other end of the reproductive cycle are women who have their first child after they are 35 years of age. These women have a somewhat increased risk of maternal and fetal complications. Issues and concerns related to the over-35 age-group have become increasingly prominent in the past decade. Some women have always borne children at a later age either by choice or because of lack or failure of contraception during the perimenopausal years. Today this group also includes women who have postponed pregnancy because of careers or other reasons, and women with infertility problems who become pregnant through technologic advances that have expanded alternatives for couples desiring children.

Many women become aware of the so-called biologic clock as menopause approaches and wish to have a child while they are still able to do so. The potential for infertility increases with age. Although most women who wait until later in life are well educated and have consciously decided to become pregnant, conception and pregnancy are not always easy. The incidence of ectopic pregnancy, placenta previa, and various medical conditions such as diabetes or hypertension increases with age. If the woman does become pregnant, each year after age 35 increases the risk of conceiving a child with Down syndrome or other chromosomal anomalies (Arias et al., 2003). Amniocentesis and chorionic villus sampling are commonly done to detect genetic problems. Detection of genetic disorders can raise ethical dilemmas regarding aborting or raising a disabled child.

However, older women who are without medical problems have much lower risks for problems than previously thought. Those who do have some complications can often have a successful pregnancy with good medical and nursing care.

As women maintain better overall health and fitness, increased age appears to be less of an impediment to a normal pregnancy. Most first-time mothers older than 35 years have waited and chosen this specific time for pregnancy; this choice is influenced by their awareness of the increasing possibility of infertility or of genetic defects in the infants of older women. Such women seek information about pregnancy from books and friends. They actively try to prevent fetal disorders and are careful in searching for the best possible maternity care. They identify sources of stress in their lives. They are concerned about having enough energy and stamina to meet the demands of parenting and their new roles and relationships.

Psychosocial adjustment to parenthood at this time of life depends greatly on the individual and her situation. Changes in income, lifestyle, and work routines can present challenges that are stressful, even if the pregnancy is desired.

Peer support may be less available for the mature primigravida. Many friends have teenage children and do not relate to the concerns of a new mother. Younger mothers have some of the same concerns, but they often do not share the perspective of older mothers. Family support may also be lacking. The woman's parents are usually in their sixties or seventies and may not be able to assist with child care to the extent that younger grandparents can.

Mature gravidas also worry about complications that may affect the fetus or their own health. They are aware that they may not have another opportunity for pregnancy because of their age. They may be concerned about their ability to balance their career with increased family responsibilities.

Studies have identified certain factors that can influence parental responses in this older group (Tough et al., 2002). Fatigue and the need for more rest seem to be the major concerns of older parents with newborns. Many of these mothers are less resilient than younger women and need to stay in the hospital longer, rather than be forced to an early discharge as some third-party payers request.

Emphasize measures to assist the mother in regaining strength and muscle tone (e.g., prenatal and postnatal exercises). Some older mothers may find that the care of the newborn infant exhausts their physical capabilities. Many women might benefit from referral to supportive resources in the community.

ADOPTION

Some women carry the pregnancy to term and then give up the newborn to the care of another family for adoption. The decision to place the infant for adoption is a painful one that can produce long-lasting feelings of ambivalence and sorrow. On the one hand, the birth mother may be satisfied that the infant is going into a stable home where a child is wanted and will receive excellent care. On the other hand, the social pressures and personal feelings against giving up one's child are often intense.

The relationship between the birth mother and the adoptive parents varies greatly. The adoptive parents may be unknown to the birth mother, or she may have chosen them. Some adoptive mothers participate in the birth. The birth mother may never see the infant again or may keep in contact and participate in the child's life.

Nurses are sometimes unsure of how to communicate with the woman who is giving up her infant. First, the nursing staff who come into contact with the woman must be informed of her decision to place the infant for adoption. Information prevents inadvertent comments that could cause distress. Second, remember that adoption is an act of love, not one of abandonment, as the woman gives the newborn to a family who is better able to provide financial and emotional support.

Also be prepared to respect any special wishes that the mother may have about the birth. For instance, most birth mothers want to know all about the infant. They may want to see and hold the newborn and give it a name. Many take photographs or save the crib card. Such actions provide memories of the infant and help the mother through the grieving process that may accompany adoption of the child.

Try to establish rapport and a trusting relationship with the mother. It is helpful to acknowledge the situation at the initial contact with the woman: "Hello, my name is Claire, and I'll be your nurse today. I understand the adoptive family is coming this morning. What can I do to help you get ready?" This communication is more helpful than ignoring the event that is of primary concern to the mother. It also provides an opening for her to express feelings such as attachment to the infant, ambivalence about her decision, and profound sadness.

Nurses also teach adoptive families how to care for the newborn and what to expect in growth and development. Teaching requires adequate time and a private place. This family benefits from all the teaching provided to other new parents. They may be anxious, and demonstrations as well as return demonstrations are appropriate.

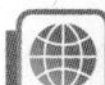 Cultural Considerations

Contraception

- Birth control as a government mandate for mainland China has been lifted. Previously, most Chinese women had an intrauterine device inserted after the birth of their first child. Some Chinese women do not want hormonal methods of contraception because they fear putting these medications in their bodies, but many now choose birth control because of the benefits of having only one child.
- Saudi Arabian and Hispanic women will likely choose the rhythm method because of religious beliefs.
- (East) Indian men are encouraged to have voluntary sterilization by vasectomy.
- Muslim couples may practice contraception by mutual consent as long as its use is not harmful to the woman. Acceptable contraceptive methods include foam and condoms, the diaphragm, and natural family planning.
- Hmong women highly value and desire large families, which limits birth control practices.
- Arabic women value large families, and sons are especially prized.

CONTRACEPTION

Contraception refers to actions taken to avoid becoming pregnant. Women and men actively engage in family planning and determine when to attempt to conceive a child or avoid pregnancy. A wide variety of birth control products are available. Selection of one involves a review of personal preferences and consideration of the woman's medical history and age. When caring for a woman and her partner seeking contraceptive devices, provide information about the use, effectiveness in preventing pregnancy, cost, potential protection from STIs, and pros and cons of the method selected (Lowdermilk & Perry, 2007). A visit with her primary care provider or health care professional is advised. Also take into account cultural values and practices (see Cultural Considerations box on contraception).

POSTPARTUM THROMBOPHLEBITIS

Development of a blood clot in the interior of a blood vessel resulting from inflammation or obstruction of a vessel is known as a **thrombosis.** The postpartum period may be affected by three types of thrombosis:

- **Superficial venous thrombosis:** Venous inflammation just below the skin's surface
- **Deep vein thrombosis:** A blood clot in a vein deep within the body, usually in the lower extremities
- **Pulmonary embolism:** Occlusion of the pulmonary artery by a blood clot traveling from elsewhere in the body

Incidence and Etiology

Thromboembolic disease is seen in less than 1% of postpartum women. Early ambulation after childbirth helps reduce the incidence. Risk factors of thromboembolic disease are increasing age, obesity, surgery, multiparity, and immobility.

Clinical Manifestations

Pain and tenderness in the lower extremities, along with warmth, redness, and hardening over the involved vessel, are common manifestations of superficial venous thrombosis.

During pregnancy, calf tenderness or leg pain and swelling may indicate deep vein thrombosis. The positive Homans' sign is not considered a definitive test, since it may be associated with other conditions. Be alert for the respiratory changes of dyspnea and tachycardia, which may signal pulmonary embolism.

Diagnosis is not based solely on the physical examination. Doppler ultrasound provides a noninvasive means to confirm the presence of thromboembolic disease. Invasive procedures such as venography are avoided out of concern for the well-being of the fetus (Lowdermilk & Perry, 2007).

Medical Management

A conservative approach is used to manage superficial venous thrombosis. Pharmacologic management includes the use of nonsteroidal antiinflammatory medications. Administer pain medications as needed, and limit activity. The goal is to rest the affected extremity in an elevated position. Heat applications and elastic stockings are also recommended.

The acute phase of treatment for deep venous thrombosis includes intravenous anticoagulant therapy, activity restriction, leg elevation, and pain management. Once the symptoms have eased, elastic stockings are applied and the woman is able to ambulate. Begin administering oral anticoagulant medications during this phase. Oral therapy can be anticipated for 3 months.

Management of a pulmonary embolism involves IV heparin therapy. After the acute phase of the illness, the patient takes subcutaneous heparin or oral anticoagulant therapies for 6 months. The use of aspirin is contraindicated in patients taking anticoagulant medications because of the increased risk for bleeding (Lowdermilk & Perry, 2007).

Nursing Interventions

To assess the woman with a thrombosis, observe and gently palpate the affected area, palpate peripheral pulses, measure the circumference of the leg for comparison, observe for signs of bleeding, and determine the presence of crackles or respiratory distress.

Evaluate the effectiveness of anticoagulant therapy in part by laboratory values. The PT or PTT is drawn and reviewed throughout the therapy. Report to the physician any laboratory values falling outside the recommended therapeutic range.

The patient's ability to provide self-care is limited during the acute phase of the illness; therefore she will need assistance to perform self-care activities. While she is on bed rest, advise the woman to avoid positions that sharply flex the legs, since it will cause pooling of the blood. In addition, instruct her to change positions frequently (Lowdermilk & Perry, 2007).

Nursing care of a woman experiencing a thrombosis involves patient and family education and ongoing assessment. Teach the patient about the diagnosis and treatment plans. Activity limitations may be difficult, so educate the patient about the risks associated with noncompliance. Massage of the thrombus is contraindicated because it may cause the clot to break free and travel to vital body organs.

Discharge teaching should also include information about the prescribed medication regimen and follow-up appointments with the laboratory and the physician. Medication education includes scheduling, dosages, potential side effects, and problems to report. Laboratory monitoring is needed throughout the therapy. The risk for injury is increased as a result of the anticoagulant therapy, so advise her to use a soft toothbrush and electric razor. Warfarin is associated with birth defects, so have a frank discussion about the need for contraception (Lowdermilk & Perry, 2007).

COMPLICATIONS RELATED TO THE NEWBORN

NEWBORNS AT RISK

Many maternal conditions can place the newborn in increased danger of illness or death. Identify any maternal risk factors as soon as possible to decrease the risk to the fetus or the newborn. Once these risks are identified, all medical and nursing measures possible should be undertaken to minimize the consequences to both the mother and the newborn.

When risk factors are identified early, care providers can prepare to meet the needs of the newborn at risk. New equipment, such as fetal monitors and more sensitive diagnostic tests, has made it easier to recognize problems during labor and delivery. Despite all progress, however, many infants still are born in need of special attention.

Assess the newborn at the time of delivery. The Apgar score gives important information about the newborn's status at 1 and 5 minutes after delivery (see Chapter 26). This is followed by a more detailed assessment of size related to gestational age. Distinguish between infants who are preterm and those who are small for gestational age. Although both groups are at risk, the problems they present are different.

GESTATIONAL AGE

Gestational age is a significant factor in neonatal mortality and morbidity (Figures 28-9 and 28-10). Both

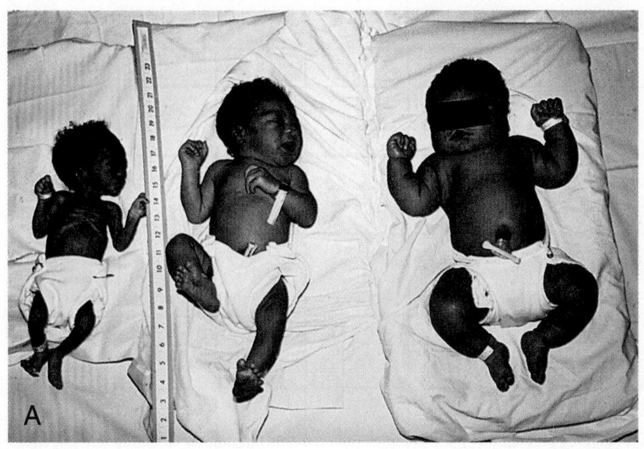

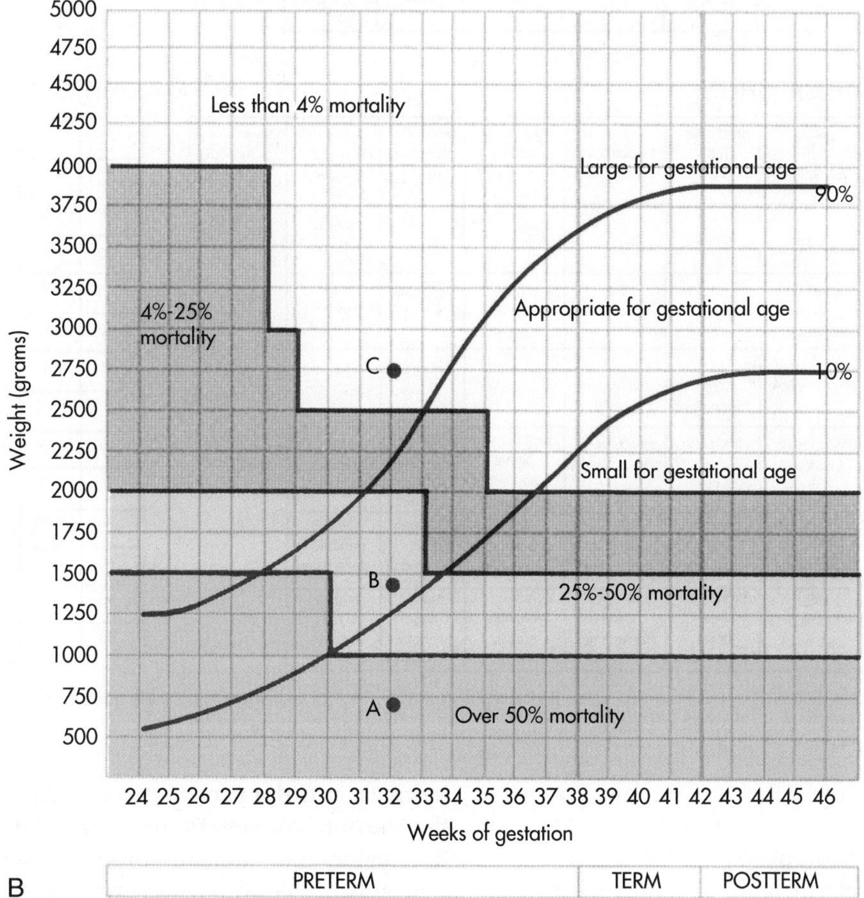

FIGURE 28-9 **A,** Three babies of the same gestational age, with weights of 600, 1400, and 2750 g, respectively, from left to right. Their weights are plotted in **B** at points *A, B,* and *C.* **B,** Intrauterine growth status for gestational age and according to appropriateness of growth.

preterm and postterm infants are at risk. Gestational age is classified as follows:

- **Preterm:** 0 to 37 complete weeks of pregnancy
- **Term:** 38 to 41 complete weeks of pregnancy
- **Postterm:** 42 or more weeks of pregnancy

Physical assessment procedures to determine gestational age are based on the method devised by Lilly and Victor Dubowitz, South African physicians. Their method is based on 21 strictly defined physical and neurologic signs and provides the correct gestational age ±2 weeks in 95% of infants. Most birthing facilities have this scale or ones similar for determining gestational age. Ideally the tests are performed between 2 and 8 hours of age. For the first hour the infant is recovering from the stress of birth, and this is reflected in muscle movements; for example, the arm recoil is slower in a fatigued infant. After 48 hours some responses change significantly. The plantar creases on the soles of the feet appear to increase in number and become visible as the skin loses fluid and dries. Figure 28-9 shows newborn maturity rating and classification.

NEUROMUSCULAR MATURITY

	−1	0	1	2	3	4	5
Posture							
Square Window (wrist)	> 90°	90°	60°	45°	30°	0°	
Arm Recoil		180°	140° - 180°	110° - 140°	90° - 110°	< 90°	
Popliteal Angle	180°	160°	140°	120°	100°	90°	< 90°
Scarf Sign							
Heel to Ear							

PHYSICAL MATURITY

Skin	sticky friable transparent	gelatinous red, translucent	smooth pink, visible veins	superficial peeling or rash, few veins	cracking pale areas rare veins	parchment deep cracking no vessels	leathery cracked wrinkled
Lanugo	none	sparse	abundant	thinning	bald areas	mostly bald	
Plantar Surface	heel-toe 40-50 mm: -1 <40 mm: -2	>50 mm no crease	faint red marks	anterior transverse crease only	creases ant. 2/3	creases over entire sole	
Breast	imperceptible	barely perceptible	flat areola no bud	stippled areola 1-2 mm bud	raised areola 3-4 mm bud	full areola 5-10 mm bud	
Eye/Ear	lids fused loosely: -1 tightly: -2	lids open pinna flat stays folded	sl. curved pinna; soft; slow recoil	well-curved pinna; soft but ready recoil	formed & firm instant recoil	thick cartilage ear stiff	
Genitals (male)	scrotum flat, smooth	scrotum empty faint rugae	testes in upper canal rare rugae	testes descending few rugae	testes down good rugae	testes pendulous deep rugae	
Genitals (female)	clitoris prominent labia flat	prominent clitoris small labia minora	prominent clitoris enlarging minora	majora & minora equally prominent	majora large minora small	majora cover clitoris & minora	

MATURITY RATING

score	weeks
-10	20
-5	22
0	24
5	26
10	28
15	30
20	32
25	34
30	36
35	38
40	40
45	42
50	44

FIGURE 28-10 Estimation of gestational age. New Ballard scale for newborn maturity rating. Expanded scale includes extremely premature infants and has been refined to improve accuracy in more mature infants.

PRETERM INFANT

Etiology and Pathophysiology

The exact causes of preterm labor are unknown. In some cases it is related to maternal or placental problems, but in other cases the cause cannot be determined. The end result is delivery of an infant at 37 weeks or less of gestation.

The preterm infant is developmentally immature. The lungs do not produce enough surfactant to allow adequate oxygenation. Circulation may not have adapted from fetal to neonatal as it usually does in a term infant, leading to oxygenation problems.

Problems with heat conservation stem from lack of subcutaneous fat, a large surface area relative to body weight, and poor reserves of glucose and **brown fat** (a source of heat unique to neonates that is capable of greater thermogenic [heat-producing] activity than ordinary fat; deposits are found around the adrenals, the kidneys, and the neck; between scapulae; and behind the sternum for several weeks after birth). The digestive system is formed, but problems with absorption of nutrients are common. The renal system is immature and ineffective. Fluid and acid-base imbalance is frequently observed. The infant is also neurologically immature; the gag, suck, and swallow reflexes may be weak or absent, and other normal reflexes may be absent or atypical.

The preterm infant is at risk because of immaturity of organ systems and lack of reserves. The morbidity and mortality rate for preterm infants is three to four times higher than that of older infants of comparable weight. The potential problems and care needs of the preterm infant of 2000 g differ from those of the term, postterm, or postmature infant of equal weight.

Preterm infants are at a distinct disadvantage when they face the transition from intrauterine to extrauterine life. The degree of disadvantage depends primarily on their level of maturity. Physiologic disorders and anomalous malformations affect their response to treatment as well. In general, the closer they are to the normal term infant in gestational age and birth weight, the easier will be their adjustment to the external environment.

Clinical Manifestations

The preterm newborn's posture is froglike or flaccid. The color is usually ruddy, and cyanosis may be present immediately following birth and for the first few hours of life. The head appears large in proportion to the body, and the bones of the skull are pliable with large, flat fontanelles. The skin is thin and translucent with obvious blood vessels and little subcutaneous fat. A layer of fine hair (lanugo) may coat large areas of the body. Cartilage in the ears is pliable, and the ears can be easily folded. The genitalia in boys are small, and frequently the testes are undescended. In girls the labia majora are small and less prominent than the labia minora. The cry is weak, and reflexes are immature or absent.

Assessment

Assess all systems of the preterm newborn carefully and continually; changes occur rapidly and require continuous monitoring. Preterm infants are typically placed in an intensive care nursery and receive care from nurses specially trained to meet their needs.

The preterm infant's greatest potential problem is respiratory distress syndrome, resulting from an immature respiratory system (see Chapter 31). The first symptom of respiratory distress is usually grunting on expiration, followed by nasal flaring, circumoral cyanosis, substernal retractions, and tachypnea. It is treated with oxygen therapy and artificial surfactant. Providing periods of rest and maintaining body temperature are important components of treatment.

An accurate assessment of gestational age is a good indicator of the problems a preterm newborn is likely to experience. Follow a systematic approach in assessment. The preterm infant's response to extrauterine life is different from that of the term infant. Knowing the physiologic basis of these differences helps assess these infants, understand their responses, and determine which potential problems are most likely to occur.

Diagnostic Tests

A wide range of diagnostic tests may be performed, based on the newborn's specific needs.

Nursing Interventions

The specifics of care of the preterm newborn are beyond the scope of this text. The major goals include maintaining and stabilizing preterm newborns until they mature adequately. Respiratory regulation, thermoregulation, fluid and electrolyte regulation, sensory stimulation, and promotion of bonding with the parents are all major areas of concern for the nurse.

Nursing diagnoses and interventions for the preterm infant include but are not limited to the following:

Nursing Diagnoses	Nursing Interventions
Risk for ineffective thermoregulation, related to immature temperature regulation center, large body surface in relation to body weight, and minimal brown fat stores	Use skin probe to measure skin temperature and take steps to maintain it at 97° to 98° F (36.1° to 36.7° C). Monitor heart rate and rhythm. Keep infant well covered and wrapped in blankets. Pad cold surfaces. Use radiant warmer if infant is uncovered for extended periods. Keep skin dry. Avoid drafts. Keep crib, warmer, or Isolette away from windows and cold external walls. Monitor for signs and symptoms of cold stress: decreased temperature, lethargy, and pallor (cold stress increases oxygen requirements). Avoid taking rectal temperature. Obtain axillary temperatures and compare with registered skin probe temperature every 30 minutes for 2 hours and until stable.
Risk for anxiety (parental), related to preterm birth, separation, and breastfeeding	Encourage parents to stay with baby in the neonatal intensive care unit. Encourage parents to actively participate in all aspects of care, if possible. Encourage parents to hold baby and examine baby en face. Encourage mother to breastfeed. Explain the use of all equipment being used. Discuss baby's behavioral cues and physical characteristics. Encourage parents to express their feelings about the pregnancy, the labor, and the birth.

Continued

Nursing Diagnoses	Nursing Interventions
Risk for anxiety (parental), related to preterm birth, separation, and breastfeeding—cont'd	Discuss parents' feeding decisions. Facilitate milk expression and storage by providing equipment or referral for lactation consultation.

POSTTERM INFANT

The postterm infant may show signs of placental insufficiency because the aging placenta was not fully functioning. Fetal malnutrition may occur as a result of deteriorating metabolic exchanges in the aging placenta. The infant may also be at increased risk for perinatal mortality resulting from intrauterine hypoxia during labor and birth. This infant is at risk for asphyxia, respiratory distress, and hypoglycemia.

GESTATIONAL SIZE

Newborns are also classified according to their weight at any given gestational age. An infant may be:

- **Small for gestational age (SGA):** Weight is less than the 10th percentile for age.
- **Appropriate for gestational age (AGA):** Weight is between the 10th and 90th percentiles.
- **Large for gestational age (LGA):** Weight is greater than the 90th percentile.
- **Low birth weight:** Weight is 2500 g or less at birth.

An SGA infant may be preterm, term, or postterm; an AGA infant may be preterm, term, or postterm; and an LGA infant may be preterm, term, or postterm.

The SGA infant may be small because of problems in the first trimester, such as infections or chromosomal abnormalities, or a later reduction in the fetal oxygen supply and fetal nutrition as a result of smoking, maternal hypertension, or malnutrition. Problems seen with SGA infants include asphyxia, meconium aspiration syndrome, hypoglycemia, and hypothermia. LGA infants often have hypoglycemia, respiratory distress, birth injuries, and asphyxia.

INFANT OF A DIABETIC MOTHER

The infant of a diabetic mother, whether preterm, term, or postterm, is at risk. This infant frequently exhibits macrosomia (excessive size and stature), hypoglycemia, perinatal asphyxia, hypocalcemia, respiratory difficulties, and hyperbilirubinemia. The infant of the gestational diabetic may also have congenital anomalies as a result of the uncontrolled maternal blood glucose levels in early pregnancy.

HEMOLYTIC DISEASES

Etiology

Hemolysis may result from basic incompatibility of blood groups, such as ABO or Rh incompatibility, or from a transfer of antibodies through the placenta.

Pathophysiology

Understanding Rh incompatibility requires an understanding of basic genetics. Rh incompatibility occurs only when the mother is Rh negative and the fetus is Rh positive. For this to occur, the father of the fetus must be Rh positive (Figure 28-11).

The term **Rh negative** indicates that the woman does not possess a specific blood antigen. If the woman is sensitized (i.e., exposed to the antigen), she produces antibodies. Exposure can occur through blood transfusion of incompatible blood or during pregnancy, when some fetal blood cells enter the maternal circulation. This transfer of antigen may occur in cases of abortion or abruption or at the time of delivery. Once the mother develops Rh antibodies, they remain in her blood, as do other antibodies.

When the woman becomes pregnant, maternal antibodies may cross the placental barrier (the boundary provided by placental tissue between the fetal and maternal circulations; small substances, excluding blood cells, may cross this barrier). If the fetal RBCs contain the Rh antigen, the maternal Rh antibodies cause hemolysis (destruction) of the fetal RBCs. The higher the level of maternal antibodies, the greater the destruction of fetal RBCs. This destruction of fetal RBCs results in pathologic jaundice, which occurs within the first 24 hours after birth.

Because sensitization most often occurs at delivery, the firstborn fetus generally has no signs of hemolysis; successive fetuses are most likely to be affected. Today serious problems related to Rh incompatibility, such as erythroblastosis fetalis (a type of hemolytic anemia that occurs in newborns as a result of maternal-fetal blood group incompatibility, especially involving the Rh factor and ABO blood groups), are usually prevented by administration of a special gamma globulin, Rh_o(D) immune globulin (RhoGAM).

ABO incompatibility is also an antigen-antibody process. Type O blood naturally contains anti-A and anti-B antibodies. These antibodies cross the placenta and cause hemolysis if the fetus has blood types A or B. Incompatibility is also possible if the mother is A and the infant B or if the mother is B and the infant A. No sensitization is required, and it may affect the first and all successive pregnancies.

Clinical Manifestations

The mother shows no clinical symptoms. Hemolysis may occur in utero, and detection must be made by diagnostic tests on amniotic fluid, suspected by changes in fetal condition, or maternal diagnostic tests. Jaundice present at birth or in the first 24 hours of life is considered an indicator of a pathologic condition. Kernicterus (an abnormal toxic accumulation of bilirubin in central nervous system tissues caused by hyperbilirubinemia [an excess of bilirubin in the blood of the newborn]) may result in neurologic damage or death. Anemia caused by RBC destruction is also possible.

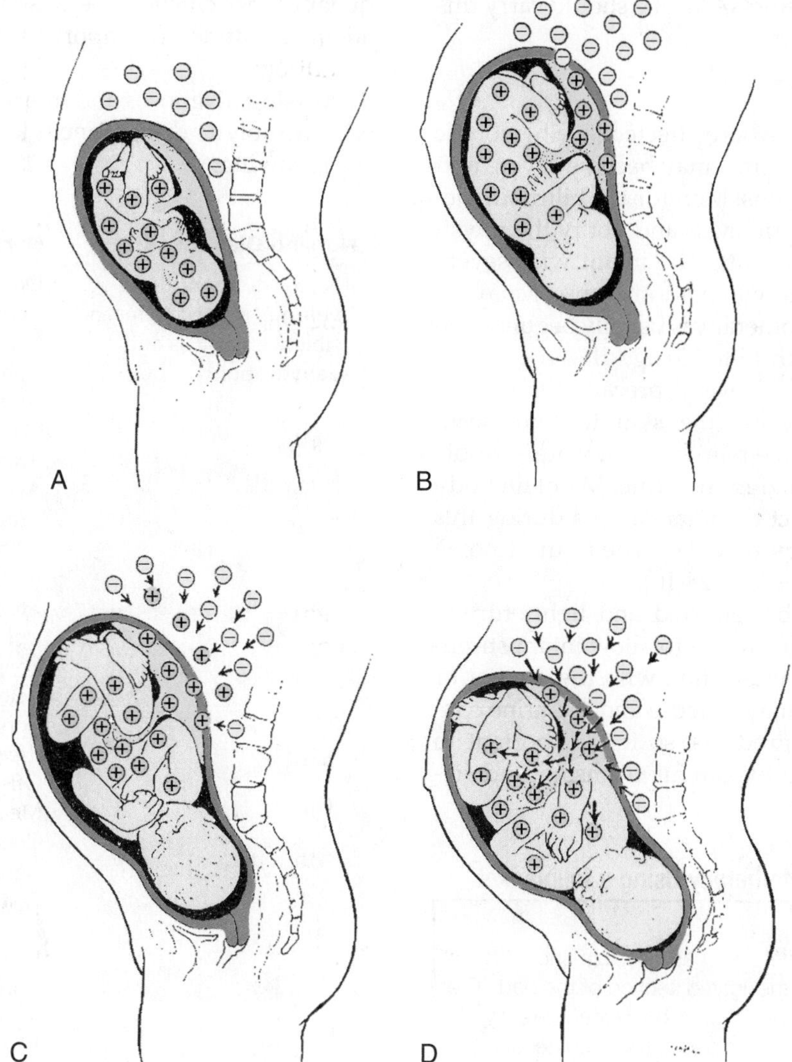

FIGURE 28-11 Mechanisms of erythroblastosis fetalis, which is caused by Rh incompatibility. **A,** Rh-positive fetus is carried by Rh-negative mother. **B,** Rh protein crosses placental barrier and invades mother's bloodstream. **C,** Mother's system manufactures antibodies to destroy foreign Rh protein. **D,** Antibodies cross back over placenta and destroy fetus's blood cells, which are intimately associated with Rh protein.

Assessment

Determine the maternal blood type and Rh factor during pregnancy. If the mother is Rh negative, find out the father's blood type. If he is also Rh negative, no Rh-based problem will occur. If the father is Rh positive, problems are possible. Also assess the woman's history for any events that may have caused sensitization, such as previous pregnancy, birth, abortion, or amniocentesis and transfusion with Rh-positive blood, which causes immediate sensitization. Even premature separation of the placenta and trauma may cause sensitization.

Diagnostic Tests

Blood typing reveals situations that require follow-up. An **indirect Coombs' test** of maternal blood measures the number of maternal antibodies. Antibody titer tests determine the level of maternal antibodies. If the titer exceeds 1:16, amniocentesis may be performed to obtain fluid for further testing. Optical density studies, which measure bilirubin level, can be done on this fluid to assess fetal condition. (If the fetus is determined to be in grave danger, intrauterine transfusion may be necessary.) After delivery, a **direct Coombs' test** is done on infant blood to determine the presence of antibody-coated RBCs. Bilirubin levels of infant blood indicate the extent of RBC destruction.

Nursing Interventions

Maternal

If the results of an Rh-negative mother's indirect Coombs' test are negative, the mother is given an intramuscular injection of RhoGAM. This is currently recommended at 28 weeks of pregnancy and again within 72 hours of delivery. RhoGAM provides passive antibodies and prevents development of naturally occurring maternal antibodies. RhoGAM should also be given to an Rh-negative mother in cases of abortion, ectopic pregnancy, and amniocentesis. Give the mother an identification card with vital information, including date of last injection of RhoGAM. She should carry this card with her at all times.

Newborn

Carefully observe the newborn affected by a hemolytic process; jaundice and anemia may become severe and lead to other complications. Monitor the bilirubin, hemoglobin, and hematocrit levels and notify the physician of any abnormal results. The infant with severe jaundice may be treated with phototherapy or may require transfusion. Phototherapy is usually begun when the bilirubin levels reach 12 to 15 mg/dL.

Phototherapy requires several precautions. **Phototherapy** involves exposing the skin to fluorescent lights, which converts the bilirubin to a water-soluble form that can be excreted in the urine. Maintain body temperature and protect the infant's eyes during this treatment. Phototherapy may be carried out at home by the use of biliblanket (Box 28-10).

Eyepatches should be removed and lights turned off during feedings and bathing to allow infant stimulation and face-to-face interaction with the mother or other caregiver. Stools may be loose and the urine contains excessive waste products, so it is important to maintain skin integrity by careful cleansing and frequent diaper changes. Because fluid loss is increased, adequate fluids are important to maintain necessary hydration.

Nursing diagnoses and interventions for the patient with hemolytic disease include but are not limited to the following:

Nursing Diagnoses	Nursing Interventions
Risk for deficient fluid volume, related to insensible weight loss and dehydration	Do not clothe infant; diapering is questionable. Maintain thermoneutral phototherapy environment. Maintain axillary temperature at 97.7° F (36.5° C). Assess axillary temperature at least every 2 hours and as needed. Avoid exposure of skin temperature probe to phototherapy lights. Weigh infant daily unclothed at the same time on the same scale before feeding. Offer pacifier as needed. Measure accurate I&O. Check urine specific gravity every shift. Test strength of bililight according to hospital's and manufacturer's policy. Note neurologic signs of kernicterus and report immediately.
Risk for impaired parenting, related to disruption of parent-infant interaction secondary to phototherapy	Explain need to provide adequate fluid intake, including water between feedings. Discuss signs and symptoms to report to physician, such as recurrence of jaundice or persistent diarrhea. Emphasize importance of having laboratory tests done as ordered. Emphasize importance of follow-up care. Encourage parent participation in infant care activities such as feeding, bathing, and cuddling. Review care of infant with hyperbilirubinemia as necessary with parents. Permit siblings to visit according to hospital policy.

Box 28-10 Home Phototherapy Using a Biliblanket

Information for parents:
- As much of the infant's skin as possible should be in direct contact with the lighted section of the pad. The infant's back or chest should be placed directly on the pad, with the tip of the pad at the shoulder and the cable at the feet.
- Follow the equipment supplier's instructions regarding safety and use of the phototherapy unit.
- Phototherapy can be discontinued for brief periods without harming your baby.
- Temperature instability may occur when starting and stopping phototherapy and when collecting laboratory specimens.
- Effects of phototherapy may include changes in frequency and color of the infant's stools and rash due to an increase in the number of loose stools.

Notify your child's health care provider if:
- A notable change is seen in activity level.
- The infant's temperature is not maintained at 97° or 100° F (33.3° to 37.7° C).
- The infant is feeding poorly.
- The infant is not voiding six times per day or does not void within a 6-hour period.
- Infant vomits two or more feedings.

Notify your home care agency if:
- Phototherapy is discontinued.
- An equipment malfunction occurs.

From University of California San Francisco Home Health Care. (2001). *Guidelines for home therapy*. San Francisco: University of California. In D.L. Lowdermilk & S.E. Perry (Eds.). (2007). *Maternity and women's health care.* (9th ed.). St. Louis: Mosby.

Nursing Diagnoses	Nursing Interventions
	When parents visit, turn off lights and remove eyeshields for the time period ordered by physician. Reinforce explanation of phototherapy, reasons for particular interventions, and care plan.

Patient Teaching

Rh-negative women should be aware of the process involved in Rh sensitization. Answer all questions that the woman or her partner may have. Phototherapy is likely to be disturbing to the parents and can interfere with parent-child attachment. Explain the reasons for treatment and provide opportunities for maternal-infant interaction. Today many newborns are sent home receiving this form of therapy. Many insurance companies recognize the therapeutic value of phototherapy at home and include phototherapy in their policies. Teach the parents correct use of the equipment and the special care required by the infant.

SUBSTANCE ABUSE

The use of legal substances, such as alcohol and tobacco, or illicit drugs, such as cocaine and marijuana, increases the risk for medical complications in the mother and poor birth outcomes in the infant. Approximately 1 in 10 infants is exposed to one or more mood-altering drugs during pregnancy. Although tobacco, alcohol, and marijuana are the most commonly abused drugs, the use of cocaine and heroin has had a major effect on health care for pregnant women and their offspring.

When the pregnant woman takes a substance, the fetus experiences the same systemic effects as the expectant mother but often more severely. For instance, cocaine raises the blood pressure of the woman and the fetus and puts both at risk for intracranial bleeding. A drug that causes intoxication in the woman causes it for prolonged periods in the fetus. The fetus cannot metabolize drugs efficiently and experiences the effects long after they have disappeared in the woman. Maternal, fetal, and neonatal effects of commonly abused substances are summarized in Table 28-4.

Nursing Interventions

Nursing care for the infant is directed at preventing further injury, particularly during the withdrawal phase. Infants of known drug and alcohol users are generally placed in a neonatal intensive care unit. Physical care includes careful temperature regulation and monitoring of vital signs. Observe the newborn to detect increasing instability. Provide small feedings, and observe the infant for diarrhea, regurgitation, and vomiting. Positioning on the right side helps prevent aspiration. IV therapy may be required. Administer medications as ordered to prevent the most serious withdrawal symptoms. Reduce stimuli that may aggravate seizures. These infants are often inconsolable, which makes caring for them difficult and stressful.

Include the newborn's parents in care whenever possible. Depending on the severity of the problems encountered, the infant may remain in the hospital, be discharged to the parent, or be placed in the custody of social services. It is a major challenge to establish a therapeutic relationship with the chemically dependent parent. Consult with social welfare or other departments that are best able to protect the newborn and also help the parent obtain the treatment needed to overcome an addiction.

COMPLICATIONS RELATED TO POSTPARTUM MENTAL HEALTH DISORDERS

Mental health disorders have implications for the mother, the newborn, and the entire family. Such conditions can interfere with attachment to the newborn and family integration, and some may threaten the safety and well-being of the mother, the newborn, and other children. Because birth is usually thought to be a happy event, a new mother's emotional distress may confuse family and friends and leave them unable to act. At a time when she most needs the caring attention of loved ones, they may either criticize or withdraw because of their own anxiety.

MOOD DISORDERS

Mood disorders are the predominant mental health disorder in the postpartum period, typically occurring within 4 weeks of childbirth. The majority of women with mood disorders experience a mild depression, or "baby blues," after the birth of a child. Others can have more serious depression that can eventually incapacitate them to the point of being unable to care for themselves or their babies. Postpartum depression (PPD) leads to moderate to severe disturbances in the interaction of mothers and infants, which are predictive of poorer infant learning outcomes. In rare cases, a disturbed mother may kill her infant, herself, or other family members. Nurses are strategically positioned to offer anticipatory guidance, to assess the mental health of new mothers, to offer therapeutic interventions, and to provide referrals when necessary. Failure to do so may have tragic consequences.

Many women feel guilty about being depressed at a time when they believe they should be happy. They may be reluctant to discuss their symptoms or their negative feelings toward the child. A prominent feature of PPD is rejection of the infant, often caused by abnormal jealousy. The mother may be obsessed by

Table 28-4 Maternal and Fetal or Neonatal Effects of Commonly Abused Substances

SUBSTANCE	MATERNAL EFFECTS	FETAL OR NEONATAL EFFECTS
Caffeine (coffee, tea, cola, chocolate, cold remedies, analgesics)	Stimulation of CNS and cardiac function, vasoconstriction, mild diuresis; half-life triples during pregnancy	Crosses placental barrier and stimulates fetus; teratogenic effects are undocumented
Tobacco	Decreased placental perfusion, anemia, PROM, preterm labor, spontaneous abortion	Prematurity, LBW, fetal demise, developmental delays, increased incidence of SIDS, pneumonia
Alcohol (beer, wine, mixed drinks, after-dinner drinks)	Spontaneous abortion	Fetal demise, IUGR, FAS (facial and cranial anomalies, developmental delay, mental retardation, short attention span), fetal alcohol effects (milder form of FAS)
Cocaine ("crack")	Hyperarousal state, generalized vasoconstriction, hypertension, increased incidence of spontaneous abortion, abruptio placentae, preterm labor, cardiovascular complications (stroke, heart attack), seizures, increased STIs	Tachycardia; stillbirth; prematurity; LBW; tremors; IUGR; irritability; decreased ability to interact with environmental stimuli; poor feeding reflexes; nausea, vomiting, diarrhea; decreased intellectual development; distended, flabby, creased abdomen (prune-belly syndrome) caused by absence of abdominal muscles
Narcotics (heroin, methadone, morphine)	Spontaneous abortion, PROM, preterm labor, increased incidence of STIs, HIV exposure, hepatitis, malnutrition	IUGR, perinatal asphyxia, intellectual impairment, neonatal abstinence syndrome, neonatal infections, fetal or neonatal death (SIDS, child abuse, and neglect)
Sedatives (barbiturates, tranquilizers)	Lethargy, drowsiness, CNS depression	Neonatal abstinence syndrome, seizures, delayed lung maturity, possible teratogenic effect
Amphetamines ("speed," "crystal," or "ice" when processed in crystals to smoke)	Malnutrition, tachycardia, withdrawal symptoms (lethargy, depression)	Increased risk for IUGR, prematurity, cardiac anomalies, cleft palate, abruptio placentae, hypoglycemia, sweating, poor visual tracing, "glassy-eyed" look, lethargy, feeding problems
Marijuana ("pot" or "grass")	Often used with other drugs (alcohol, cocaine, tobacco), increased incidence of anemia and inadequate weight gain	Unclear, more study needed; believed related to prematurity, IUGR, tremors, sensitivity to light

From McKinney, E.S., et al. (2005). *Maternal-child nursing.* (2nd ed.). St. Louis: Elsevier.
CNS, Central nervous system; *FAS,* fetal alcohol syndrome; *HIV,* human immunodeficiency virus; *IUGR,* intrauterine growth restriction; *LBW,* low birth weight; *PROM,* premature rupture of membranes; *SIDS,* sudden infant death syndrome; *STIs,* sexually transmitted infections.

the notion that the offspring will take her place in her partner's affections. Attitudes toward the infant may include disinterest, annoyance with care demands, and blaming because of her lack of maternal feeling. The woman may appear awkward in her responses to the baby. Obsessive thoughts about harming the child frighten her. Often she does not share these thoughts because of embarrassment, but when she does, other family members become frightened as well.

Medical Management

The natural course is one of gradual improvement over the 6 months after birth. Supportive treatment alone is not effective for major PPD; pharmacologic intervention is needed in most instances. Treatment options include antidepressants, anxiolytic agents (a sedative or minor tranquilizer), and electroconvulsive therapy. Psychotherapy focuses on the mother's fears and concerns regarding her new responsibilities and roles, as well as monitoring for suicidal or homicidal thoughts. For some women, hospitalization is necessary.

NURSING PROCESS *for the Mother and Newborn at Risk*

The role of the licensed practical nurse/licensed vocational nurse (LPN/LVN) in the nursing process as stated is that the LPN/LVN will:

- Participate in planning care for patients based on patient needs
- Review patient's care plan and recommend revisions as needed
- Review and follow defined prioritization for patient care
- Use clinical pathways, care maps, or care plans to guide and review patient care

Assessment

Nursing process for the patient at risk begins with assessment, which focuses on the history of the pregnancy and the patient's symptoms. Assessment includes both physical and psychological arenas. Specific assessment items depend on the patient's disorder. Assessment should also include past medical history, obstetric history, and social history.

Nursing Diagnosis

Nursing assessment helps identify the needs of the high-risk patient. Care can then be based on these needs. Nursing diagnoses depend on the high-risk condition and symptoms observed (see nursing diagnoses throughout the chapter).

Expected Outcomes and Planning

The care plan focuses on the needs of the high-risk patient and the nurse's ability to meet those needs effectively. Each patient has different needs, and care is individualized accordingly. The care plan focuses on goals and outcomes specific to the nursing diagnosis. Examples include the following:

Goal 1: The patient with hyperemesis gravidarum will maintain caloric intake adequate to provide for fetal health and growth.

Outcome: Patient eats and retains 1800 kcal/day and drinks 2000 mL of fluid per day.

Goal 2: The preterm neonate will maintain skin temperature of 97.5° to 98.6° F (36.4° to 37° C) axillary while in an open crib.

Outcome: Neonate's temperature is 97.8° to 98.6° F (36.6° to 37° C) axillary on three successive occasions 4 hours apart.

Implementation

Nursing interventions for the high-risk patient are determined by the nursing diagnosis and goals for the specific condition being treated.

Evaluation

Continually evaluate the success of the interventions. As the high-risk patient's situation changes, so may the goals and interventions. Refer to the goals and outcomes to determine whether the plan was successful and the outcomes met. For example:

Goal 1: The patient with hyperemesis gravidarum will maintain caloric intake adequate to provide for fetal health and growth.

Evaluative measures: Patient ate six small meals totaling 1500 kcal with one emesis of 200 mL. Fluid intake of water and tea was 1200 mL.

Goal 2: The preterm neonate will maintain skin temperature of 97.5° to 98.6° F (36.4° to 37° C) axillary while in an open crib.

Evaluative measure: Neonate's temperature was 98.6° F (37° C) axillary at 0600, 98.2° F (36.8° C) axillary at 1000, and 98.9° F (37.2° C) axillary at 1400.

Get Ready for the NCLEX® Examination!

Key Points

- Complications can occur during any stage of the childbearing process.
- Continually assess pregnant women and newborns for any signs of complications.
- Educate all pregnant women about danger signs that indicate complications, stressing the importance of prompt medical attention.
- Hemorrhage is a danger sign both during pregnancy and after delivery.
- Bleeding disorders of pregnancy are medical emergencies that demand expert teamwork from health care professionals.
- Premature separation, or placental abruption, is characterized by painful vaginal bleeding. A concealed bleed is possible depending on the location of the separation. Concealed bleeding is associated with abdominal rigidity.
- Placenta previa results from an abnormal location of implantation of the placenta, completely or partially covering the cervical os. This is associated with third trimester and painless vaginal bleeding.
- The type of spontaneous abortion determines the management.
- The cause of GH is unknown, and there are no known reliable tests for predicting women at risk for preeclampsia.
- Magnesium sulfate, the anticonvulsant agent of choice for preventing eclampsia, requires careful monitoring of reflexes, respirations, and urinary output; its antidote, calcium gluconate, should be at the bedside.
- A wide range of infectious diseases present a threat to the mother and the newborn.
- The Rh-negative mother may require special interventions to prevent sensitization, which may have an effect on future pregnancies.
- Preexisting health conditions, such as cardiac problems or diabetes mellitus, increase the risks of childbearing.
- Routine screening for GDM is performed for most women during the second trimester. Women with increased risk factors or those who are suspected of having diabetes-related issues may be tested earlier in gestation.
- The mother's age is significant in childbearing. Both the very young and the older mother are at increased risk.
- Adolescents can develop trusting relationships with helping professionals whom they respect.
- Drug and alcohol use have a serious impact on the developing fetus.
- Infant mortality rates have shown improvement, dropping from 26 per 1000 live births in 1960 to 6.8 per 1000 live births in 2001.
- Approximately 80% to 90% of pregnancies treated with cerclage result in live, viable births.

- The woman who is addicted to narcotics may have infections that compound the risk to the infant, including hepatitis; septicemia; and STIs, including AIDS.
- Newborns born to drug- or alcohol-abusing mothers may manifest a variety of anatomical and neurologic defects.
- Infants born preterm or postterm and SGA or LGA are at greater risk for complications.
- Preterm infants are physiologically immature and at risk for respiratory distress syndrome, hypoglycemia, hyperbilirubinemia, and thermoregulation problems.

Additional Learning Resources

Go to your Companion CD for an audio glossary, animations, video clips, and more.

evolve Be sure to visit the Evolve site at http://evolve.elsevier.com/Christensen/foundations/ for additional online resources.

Review Questions for the NCLEX® Examination

1. A patient is admitted to the hospital with a diagnosis of hyperemesis gravidarum. What is the cause of this condition?
1. Neurologic disorder
2. Inadequate nutrition
3. Unknown cause
4. Hyperglycemia

2. A patient is admitted to the hospital with a 3-day history of right abdominal pain. Her admitting diagnosis is suspected ectopic pregnancy. The nurse knows an ectopic pregnancy occurs:
1. outside the uterus.
2. in the fallopian tube.
3. early in ovulation.
4. during cervical implantation.

3. A patient has been diagnosed with placenta previa. Which symptom is considered the classic diagnostic criterion for placenta previa?
1. Irregular fetal heartbeat
2. Uterine irritability
3. Elevation of temperature
4. Painless vaginal bleeding

4. A patient is in labor and suddenly complains of sharp fundal pain. She begins to have vaginal bleeding as well. What is the most likely cause of her symptoms?
1. Preterm labor
2. Abruptio placentae
3. Pelvic inflammatory disease
4. Placenta previa

5. A patient is diagnosed with an inevitable abortion. Which assessment finding distinguishes an inevitable abortion from a threatened abortion?
1. Uterine cramping
2. Vaginal bleeding
3. Cervical dilation
4. History of previous abortions

6. A patient is suspected of having gestational hypertension. Which assessment step should the nurse take?
1. Assess her deep tendon reflexes.
2. Determine when she last ate.
3. Perform a Nitrazine test.
4. Do a vaginal examination to check for cervical dilation.

7. What is the most common cause of postpartum hemorrhage?
1. Cervical lacerations
2. Uterine atony
3. Cesarean birth
4. Disseminated intravascular coagulation

8. A baby boy was born at 38 weeks of gestation to a mother with type 1 diabetes. Into which category would this infant most likely fall?
1. Premature
2. Average for gestational age
3. Intrauterine growth restriction
4. Large for gestational age

9. A baby girl was born at 34 weeks of gestation. At 3 hours old she is diagnosed with respiratory distress. What is an early symptom of respiratory distress?
1. Nasal flaring
2. Expiratory grunting
3. Cyanosis
4. Substernal retractions

10. A patient is Rh negative and delivers an infant with Rh-positive blood. The nurse gives her RhoGAM to:
1. stimulate formation of maternal blood antigens.
2. stimulate production of maternal blood antibodies.
3. prevent production of maternal blood antibodies.
4. prevent production of fetal blood antigens.

11. After giving birth to a healthy baby boy, a primiparous woman, age 16, is admitted to the postpartum unit. An appropriate nursing diagnosis for her at this time is *risk for impaired parenting,* related to deficient knowledge of newborn care. In planning for the woman's discharge, the nurse should include what in the care plan?
1. Tell the woman how to feed and bathe her baby.
2. Give the woman written information on bathing her baby.
3. Advise the woman that all mothers instinctively know how to care for their babies.
4. Provide time for the woman to bathe her baby after she views a baby bath demonstration.

12. A newborn is jaundiced and receiving phototherapy. An appropriate nursing intervention when caring for an infant with hyperbilirubinemia who is receiving phototherapy would be to:
1. apply an oil-based lotion to the newborn's skin to prevent drying and cracking.
2. limit the newborn's intake of milk to prevent nausea, vomiting, and diarrhea.
3. place eyeshields over the newborn's eyes.
4. change the newborn's position every 3 to 4 hours.

13. A 26-year-old pregnant woman, gravida 2, para 1, is 28 weeks pregnant when she experiences bright red, painless vaginal bleeding. On her arrival at the hospital, what would be an expected diagnostic procedure?
    1. Amniocentesis for fetal lung maturity
    2. Ultrasound for placental location
    3. Contraction stress test
    4. Internal fetal monitoring

14. In planning care of a 30-year-old woman with pregestational diabetes, the nurse recognizes that the most important factor affecting pregnancy outcome is the:
    1. mother's age.
    2. number of years since diabetes was diagnosed.
    3. amount of insulin required prenatally.
    4. degree of blood glucose control during pregnancy.

15. When caring for a pregnant woman with cardiac problems, the nurse should be alert for signs and symptoms of cardiac decompensation, which include:
    1. regular heart rate, hypertension.
    2. increased urinary output, tachycardia, dry cough.
    3. shortness of breath, bradycardia, hypertension.
    4. dyspnea, crackles, irregular weak pulse.

16. Human immunodeficiency virus (HIV) may be perinatally transmitted:
    1. only in the third trimester from maternal circulation.
    2. only through the ingestion of infected amniotic fluid.
    3. through the ingestion of breast milk from an infected mother.
    4. through improper handling of a meconium-filled diaper.

17. _______________ would be the immediate focus for the care of a pregnant woman at 38 weeks of gestation with marginal placenta previa who has just given birth to a healthy newborn boy.

18. _______________ is the gestation of twins, triplets, quadruplets, or more than four infants.

19. _______________ is the birth of the fetus through a transabdominal incision of the uterus.

20. _______________ has a major effect on the health and well-being of the postpartum woman, her newborn, and the entire family. It is characterized by intense pervasive sadness and mood swings.

chapter 29

Health Promotion for the Infant, Child, and Adolescent

evolve

http://evolve.elsevier.com/Christensen/foundationsadult

Barbara Lauritsen Christensen

Objectives

1. Identify the 10 leading health indicators cited in *Healthy People 2010.*
2. List three benefits of regular physical activity in children.
3. State the American Academy of Pediatrics' recommendations for immunization administration in healthy infants and children.
4. State three strategies to promote dental health.
5. State the causes and prevention of accidental poisonings.
6. Describe four strategies to prevent aspiration of a foreign body.
7. Discuss the proper use of infant safety seats in motor vehicles.
8. Identify six health benefits associated with exercise, activity, and sports.
9. List 10 safety precautions important in educating parents to prevent environmental injuries to children.

Key Terms

anticipatory guidance (p. 926)
botulism (p. 936)
nursing bottle caries (p. 935)

The focus of health promotion is to assist individuals to realize their full potential. It takes active participation by patients and family to develop and maintain a lifestyle that optimizes wellness. Traditionally, the primary care of children has fostered health promotion through health supervision and health maintenance visits, immunizations, screenings and surveillance, and anticipatory guidance (psychological preparation, based on developmental stage, of a person for an event expected to be stressful, as in preparing a child for surgery by explaining what will happen and what it will feel like; also used to prepare parents for normal growth and development of their children). Health promotion activities are essential in identifying risks and encouraging healthy behaviors in children and their families.

One of the major roles in nursing is promoting wellness and disease prevention. Pediatric nursing provides many unique opportunities to participate in this role. The pediatric population offers several challenges not found in the adult population. As a pediatric nurse, you will have to use a multidisciplinary approach to meet the demands related to the promotion of wellness and disease prevention concerning the pediatric population.

This chapter identifies health promotion and disease prevention factors unique to the pediatric population. The primary focus of this chapter is on the indicators identified in *Healthy People 2010* (U.S. Department of Health & Human Services, 2000), as well as dental health, poisoning, aspiration, and burn injuries related to children.

HEALTHY PEOPLE 2010

Healthy People 2010: Understanding and Improving Health was published by the U.S. Department of Health & Human Services (HHS) in 2000.* This document identifies 10 "leading health indicators" that reflect current areas of major concern in the United States:

1. Physical activity
2. Overweight and obesity
3. Tobacco use
4. Substance abuse
5. Responsible sexual behavior
6. Mental health
7. Injury and violence
8. Environmental quality
9. Immunizations
10. Access to health care

Eight of the indicators include specific target goals related to children and adolescents (Table 29-1). Environmental quality and access to health care do not have specific target goals that address the pediatric

*Note: All statistics in this chapter are from *Healthy People 2010,* unless otherwise cited.

Table 29-1 **Leading Health Indicators Adapted from *Healthy People 2010***

LEADING HEALTH INDICATOR	*HEALTHY PEOPLE 2010* TARGET GOAL
Physical activity	Increase the percentage of adolescents who participate in regular, vigorous exercise to 85%
Overweight and obesity	Reduce the percentage of children who are overweight or obese to 5%
Tobacco use	Reduce the percentage of adolescents who smoke cigarettes to 16%
Substance abuse	Increase the percentage of children who refrain from alcohol and drug use to 89%
Responsible sexual activity	Increase the percentage of adolescents who abstain from sexual activity or use condoms to 95%
Mental health	Reduce the percentage of adolescents who attempt suicide to 2% and reduce the relapse rate for adolescents with eating disorders
Injury and violence	Reduce the death rate of children related to motor vehicle accidents and homicides
Environmental quality	Reduce exposure to ozone to 0% and reduce exposure to environmental tobacco smoke to 45%
Immunizations	Increase the percentage of children who receive immunizations to 80%
Access to health care	Increase the percentage of coverage to 100%

Data from U.S. Department of Health and Human Services. (2000). *Healthy people 2010: Understanding and improving health, objectives for improving health, tracking* Healthy People 2010. Washington, DC: U.S. Government Printing Office.

population; however, goals for the population in general are included (see Health Promotion box).

PHYSICAL ACTIVITY

Physical activity is essential for the healthy growth and development of children and adolescents; however, not all children receive the needed amount of physical activity (Figure 29-1). According to *Healthy People 2010*, only 65% of adolescents were engaging in the recommended amount of physical activity. Regular physical activity lowers death rates in adults and reduces the risk for developing heart disease, high blood pressure, diabetes mellitus, and colon cancer. In children, regular physical activity increases bone and muscle strength and helps decrease body fat. Psychological benefits of regular physical activity include improvement in self-esteem and reduction in stress and depression.

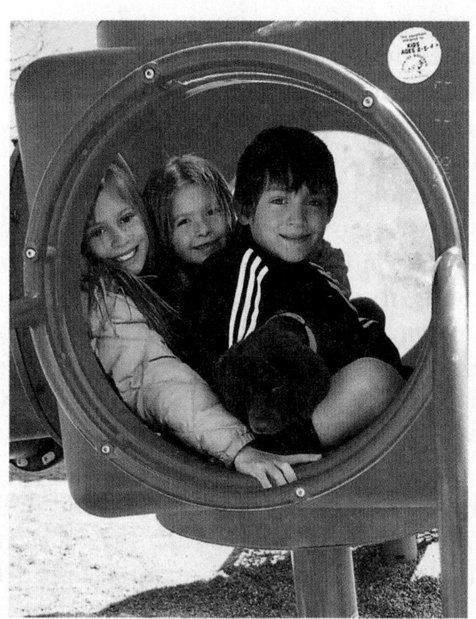

FIGURE 29-1 Children engaging in physical activity.

You have the opportunity to promote physical activity in the pediatric population by educating parents, teachers, school administrators, and daycare providers. Physical activity in children is often reflective of the adults within their environment. Another way you help is by being a good role model for both children and other adults by participating in regular physical activity.

OVERWEIGHT AND OBESITY

Children with a body mass index (BMI) between the 85th and 95th percentiles are considered overweight, and obesity is defined as a BMI greater than the 95th percentile. Children in the 99th percentile are considered to be extremely obese (Paoletti, 2007).

The number of overweight children in the United States is increasing and seems to be approaching epidemic status. In economically developed countries, the most common disease seen in childhood and adolescence is now obesity (Paoletti, 2007). In the 1990–2000 National Health and Nutrition Examination Survey, data indicated that 15% of children and teens between 6 and 19 years were overweight. The prevalence of childhood obesity in the United States is estimated to be about 17%. Twice as many children and almost three times as many adolescents are now considered to be above ideal weight compared with their counterparts in 1980 (Paoletti, 2007).

The goal of *Healthy People 2010* is to reduce this number to 5%. Physical risks associated with excess weight include high blood pressure, high cholesterol, type 2 diabetes mellitus, fatty liver disease, heart disease, stroke, gallbladder disease, arthritis, sleep apnea, and problems breathing. Psychological risks associated with excess weight include discrimination, social stigmatization, lowered self-esteem, social isolation, and feelings of depression and rejection.

Many factors contribute to the excess weight carried by children today. Some of the most common are lack

Health Promotion

Encouraging Healthy Behaviors in the Infant, the Toddler and Child, and the Adolescent

INFANT

- Encourage parental bonding.
- Monitor growth and development through well-baby clinic appointments.
- Encourage breastfeeding, if appropriate.
- Use prescribed baby formula to provide necessary nutrients and vitamins.
- Introduce baby foods as recommended: Begin with rice cereal and introduce one new food per week to monitor for allergic reactions.
- Monitor transitioning stools as the gastrointestinal system matures.
- Provide age-appropriate play to encourage physical and mental development.
- Transport in child carrier facing the rear of the car (birth to 20 pounds).
- Maintain immunization schedule as recommended.

TODDLER AND CHILD

- Encourage a healthy diet to include high-nutrient foods such as fruits, vegetables, whole grains, and low-fat dairy and protein products (both child and adolescent).
- Continue to provide health care including immunizations and dental care.
- Encourage developmentally appropriate play.
- Remember that autonomy and initiative are paramount and offer toddler and child choice of nutritionally dense foods.
- Teach parents and child appropriate methods for good hygiene include handwashing, covering mouth when coughing or sneezing, etc.
- Mandate use of seatbelts while riding in vehicle.
  —Toddler 20 to 40 pounds, front-facing safety seat secured in rear seat.
  —Child more than 40 pounds to be secured in booster seat with lap and shoulder belt.
- Wear protective helmets when riding tricycles and bicycles.
- Maintain immunization schedule as recommended.

ADOLESCENTS

- Instruct parents to monitor adolescent for use of drugs and/or alcohol by noting changes in behavior.
- Wear protective helmets when riding bikes, motorcycles, or skateboarding.
- Provide nutritionally dense foods and snacks to support this period of growth.
- Allow privacy in telephone use and interactions with friends.
- Allow the child to establish an identity even if it is different from that of the parents.
- Insist on mandatory use of seatbelts when in vehicle.
- Maintain immunization schedule as recommended.
- Encourage dental care.
- Encourage safe sun practices
  —Teach that long-term effects of sun exposure, such as tanning, include premature aging of the skin, increased risk of skin cancer, and, in susceptible individuals, phototoxic reactions.
  —Teach that the long-term effects of tanning machines are similar to those of the sun; dermatologists do not recommend suntanning by this means.
  —Provide education on the use of sunscreens, including hypoallergenic products, with a sun protective factor (SPF) of at least 15 and a nonalcohol base without lanolin or fragrance is important.

of physical activity, increased fast food consumption, working mothers, and poverty. Although not all of these factors are possible to eliminate, many of them are amenable to significant improvement.

Exercise

Decreased physical activity is clearly related to increased body mass and an increased risk of obesity. Our society has changed to include a more sedentary lifestyle. Children in the United States spend an average of 6 hours and 32 minutes per day with various media, including television, computers, video games, and electronic games (American Academy of Pediatrics [AAP], 2001). In U.S. households, 32% of 2- to 7-year-olds and 65% of 8- to 18-year-olds have a television in their bedroom. Think of the effect on children's physical activity, and thus on their BMI, if they reduced by half the amount of time spent per day with various media!

Nutrition

Families today are often pressed for time. The convenience of fast food combined with the increase in families with two working parents has contributed to poor eating habits for many children. Children's diets contain an estimated 11% to 15% of calories from saturated fat instead of the American Heart Association's recommendation of a maximum of 7%. Children tend to consume high-calorie, poorer-quality diets that do not meet federal dietary recommendations for healthy growth and development. Childhood obesity results from a diet high in calories from saturated fat and lack of exercise (Paoletti, 2007).

In contrast, the *Dietary Guidelines for Americans* (2005), written jointly by the U.S. Department of Health and Human Services and the U.S. Department of Agriculture, recommends that children ages 2 and older consume a diet that has an assortment of foods that includes fruits, vegetables, grains (especially whole grains), fish, lean meats, poultry, and beans. Fat restriction is not appropriate for toddlers; 30% of their calories will optimally come from fat. Whole milk or 2% milk is recommended for toddlers (American Academy of Pediatrics, 2001). It is acceptable for the child and the adolescent to consume low-fat or fat-free milk products.

Promoting Lifestyle Changes

Your most important role in relation to overweight and obese children comes in the area of education. Education of children and parents concerning dietary choices is essential. The *Dietary Guidelines for Americans* recommends that children get at least 60 minutes of physical activity per day. It is important to teach about the optimal types and amounts of physical activity. Many parents do not realize the magnitude of this problem; however, simply by acquiring an awareness of the need, many parents are motivated to make significant lifestyle changes for their children.

TOBACCO USE

Cigarette smoking continues to be the single most preventable cause of death and disease in the United States. A significant number of children and teenagers still begin or continue to smoke today. According to the Centers for Disease Control and Prevention (2005), in 2004, 21.8% of senior high school students in the United States smoked cigarettes. Nationwide, 22% of young people initiate smoking by 13 years of age (Logan & Carlini-Marlatt, 2004). Many states have implemented laws restricting the sale of tobacco products to minors. Cigarettes are considered to be a gateway drug, and teenagers who smoke are 11.4 times more likely to use illicit drugs.

Other forms of tobacco exposure that also arouse concern include smokeless tobacco, cigar smoking, and environmental tobacco smoke, commonly referred to as secondhand smoke. Adolescents rarely understand the risks involved in smokeless tobacco. These risks include lip, gum, throat, and stomach cancers. Cigar smoking became more popular in the 1990s, especially among women. Environmental tobacco smoke results in increased risk for heart and lung disease, particularly asthma and bronchitis in children. Parents often point out that they do not smoke in front of their child; however, the damaging smoke is often trapped in clothing, drapes, and household furnishings.

The American Cancer Society (ACS), as well as many other organizations, offers excellent programs and resource materials aimed at educating children and adolescents concerning the dangers involved in tobacco use. These programs are available at no cost to schools, civic organizations, and health care professionals. Some teens volunteer with these programs to discourage tobacco use. Knowledge of available resources and the ability to promote their use is part of every pediatric nurse's toolbox and professional responsibility.

SUBSTANCE ABUSE

In 1999, approximately 79% of adolescents between ages 12 and 17 reported that they had not used illicit drugs or alcohol in the past month. *Healthy People 2010* established a target goal of 89% of adolescents who will refrain from illicit drug or alcohol use. Adolescents are the group at greatest risk of regular drug abuse; approximately 1% to 2% of teens use hard drugs regularly (U.S. Department of Health and Human Services, 2008). Substance abuse is associated with many social problems found in the United States. These problems include domestic violence, sexually transmitted infections (STIs), teen pregnancy, school failure, motor vehicle accidents (MVAs), increased health care costs, decreased worker productivity, and increased homelessness. Adolescents are currently experimenting with marijuana, cocaine, crack, heroin, acid (LSD), inhalants, methamphetamines, ecstasy, other street drugs, and misuse of prescription drugs. Recently, abuse of prescription and synthetic drugs has become a concern for professionals who work with children and adolescents. In addition, health professionals are concerned about the use of alcohol and volatile substances that are inhaled to achieve altered sensorium (such as gasoline, spray paint, antifreeze, and organic solvents). The good news reported in *Healthy People 2010* is that substance abuse among adolescents remains below the all-time high reported in 1979. However, there has been an increase in children ages 12 and 13 who are experimenting with drugs. This is of particular concern because the younger a person is when drug use (abuse) becomes habitual, the stronger the addiction, and the more difficult the task of breaking it.

Encourage parents to talk with their children about the risks of substance abuse, and to plan appropriate child care and supervision. Children who are left unattended are more likely to experiment with drugs. After-school programs are available in many areas. Also help educate parents regarding the signs of drug use in their children that will potentially crop up.

TELEVISION, VIDEO GAMES, AND THE INTERNET

Parents and child development specialists are concerned about the influence that television has on child development and behavior (Hockenberry & Wilson, 2007). Although television is capable of producing positive learning outcomes, the values and attitudes represented on television are often not realistic, and at times they clash with the values that the child has been taught. Television seldom represents the actual daily experiences that a child faces. Sixty-one percent of television shows depict acts of violence, the use of violence to solve problems, carrying weapons as a normal behavior, and criminals going unpunished (AAP, 2001). If children are to benefit from watching television, parents have to carefully monitor the child's selection of programs, view programs with their children, and have a discussion concerning the program content after the program is finished (AAP, 2001; Hamilton, 2000).

There is sufficient evidence that exposure to violence on television is not conducive to the well-being of children (Cantor, 2000; Grossman, 2000). Research is showing more aggressive behavior as well as increased fearfulness and decreased sensitivity on the part of some children who watch violent television programs (AAP, 2001; Grossman, 2000). It has also been noted that children who view violent television are less likely to prevent or stop a fight. They also have nightmares, obsessive thoughts, and sleep disturbances (Cantor, 2000).

There are both critics and supporters concerning the effect of video games on children and adolescents. Critics argue that video games have detrimental effects that include preventing children from completion of their homework, producing tension and violence, and causing sleeplessness. Critics also suggest video games have potentially negative physical and psychological results. Adverse physical effects possibly include triggering of epileptic seizures. It is interesting to note, however, that there is some possibility that video games have a positive influence on the child with dyslexia (American Psychological Association, 2005). Supporters feel video games improve eye-hand coordination, inductive reasoning skills, and perception. They also suggest that video games are a positive substitute for the passivity involved in watching television (Hockenberry & Wilson, 2007).

In the United States, 71% of families who have children ages 8 to 17 have computers. Computers and the Internet provide valuable educational as well as recreational information, but just as in television programming, there are many dangers. Children are sometimes exposed to dangerous or illegal material and negative contact with others through e-mail or in chat rooms. Sharing personal data or meeting with strangers puts the child and the family at both financial and physical risk (McColgan-Giardino et al., 2005). Parents and children need to be educated about the potential risks involved in accessing the Internet, and the child always needs adult supervision (Hockenberry & Wilson, 2007).

Parents and teachers can provide safeguards by limiting the amount of time that children are allowed to watch television, play video games, or be online. Advise them to monitor content and to increase access to educational alternatives (Hockenberry & Wilson, 2007).

RESPONSIBLE SEXUAL BEHAVIOR

Healthy People 2010 reported good news related to responsible sexual behavior among young people. In the prior 6 years, there was an increase in all youth who were abstaining from sexual activity, as well as an increase in the use of condoms among those youth who were sexually active. The major risks associated with irresponsible sexual behavior include unintended pregnancy, STIs, and human immunodeficiency virus and acquired immunodeficiency syndrome (HIV/AIDS). Approximately one half of all new HIV cases in the United States occur among people younger than 25 years of age.

Although abstinence is the only protection that is 100% effective, proper use of condoms helps prevent unintended pregnancies and transmission of STIs. This topic has always been a controversial issue with parents, school officials, and health care professionals. It does not matter who provides the education: The bottom line is the necessity of teaching adolescents about responsible sexual behavior, because it is, often enough, a matter of life and death.

MENTAL HEALTH

Healthy People 2010 cites two target areas related to adolescents and mental health: a decrease in the number of adolescents who attempt suicide and a reduction in the relapse rate for adolescents with eating disorders. The teenage years are among the most difficult times of a person's life. Teenagers want to fit in. They need to belong. They want to look and act like others their age. Parents often forget how difficult this time is for the adolescent.

Mental health issues are often considered less important than physical illnesses. It is all too common for nurses who feel confident to help with physical symptoms to feel powerless when confronting matters concerning mental health.

If you become a pediatric nurse today, you will be obliged to treat your patients holistically. This means addressing both physical and mental health. Nurses often underestimate the effect they are able to have on their patients' mental health. Keep these mental health issues in mind in your practice of pediatric nursing: depression, suicide, eating disorders, and substance abuse. If you do not think that you possess the skills necessary to provide mental health care in any given situation, make referral to the appropriate health care professionals.

INJURY AND VIOLENCE

Injuries have historically been a problem in the pediatric population. Common injuries found in children and adolescents involve MVAs, accidental poisonings, suffocation, drowning, falls, aspiration of foreign bodies, and burns. Accidental firearm injuries have occurred for decades in the pediatric population. Sad to say, premeditated, intentional shootings are also occurring more frequently among today's adolescents.

The target goals related to injury and violence involving children and adolescents include a reduction in pediatric deaths caused by MVAs and homicides. You will contribute to these goals by encouraging proper use of child safety restraints and seatbelts. Advise parents of the following guidelines:

- Use infant car seats designed according to federal safety guidelines:
  - —Birth to 20 pounds: rear-facing safety seats secured in the rear seat
  - —Toddlers 20 to 40 pounds: front-facing safety seats secured in the rear seat (Figure 29-2)

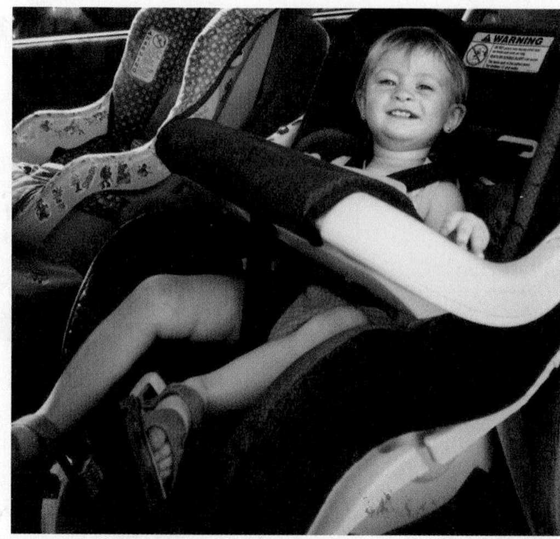

FIGURE 29-2 Toddler in front-facing safety seat, secured in rear seat.

—Children more than 40 pounds secured in booster seats with lap and shoulder belts. The properly fitted shoulder belt lies across the chest and the lap belt sits below the hip bones to prevent internal injuries in the event of a vehicular accident.

- Teach the child pedestrian safety: "Stop, Look, Listen" at crosswalks; use sidewalks; wear light-colored clothing at night.
- Supervise children when playing outdoors—no playing at the curb or behind parked cars.
- Insist that the child wear an approved helmet when riding tricycles, bicycles, scooters, mopeds, and skateboards (Figure 29-3). Protective wrist, elbow, and knee pads are necessary during play involving skateboards and while roller-skating or in-line skating.
- Reinforce the danger of using drugs or alcohol when driving, and insist that no child ride in a car with a person who has been drinking alcohol or using drugs.
- Emphasize rules for safe driving with the adolescent driver.

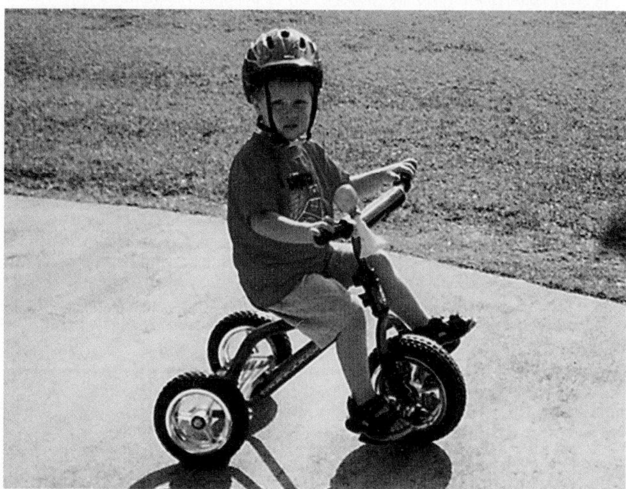

FIGURE 29-3 Proper use of a safety helmet begins at an early age.

Your role as pediatric nurse in the reduction of pediatric deaths by homicide includes assessment for potential violent behaviors and mental health disorders. Encourage parents to monitor their children's activities. Parents need to be aware of where their children are going, and with whom. As mentioned, advise parents to monitor computer and Internet access. Encourage teachers, parents, and students to report strange behavior or threats made by other students.

There are other significant injury prevention concepts that call for your awareness and concern. Poisoning, aspiration, and burn injuries in children are addressed later in this chapter.

ENVIRONMENTAL QUALITY

Environmental quality concerns specific to children and adolescents include exposure to environmental tobacco smoke (ETS), ozone (outdoor) standards, and (for infants and young children) exposure to lead-based paint. Make sure parents are aware of potential exposure to lead-based paint in older housing and possibly furniture, such as cribs. They need additional education with regard to proper testing for lead level in children, who are in some circumstances at risk for lead poisoning.

See the earlier section on tobacco for a discussion of exposure to ETS and the potential problems related to it. Your responsibilities regarding ozone standards include being aware of any danger in your area and of possible measures to take for prevention or avoidance, and sharing this information with others.

IMMUNIZATION

Immunizations are an excellent way to prevent the occurrence and spread of certain infectious diseases. Currently 73% of all children in the United States have received a full schedule of recommended immunizations. *Healthy People's* target related to immunizations is the goal of immunizing 80% of all children in the United States. Immunization standards offer a challenge for the pediatric nurse because these standards often change. With modern advances in medical research, new immunizations are developed. The most recent recommended childhood immunization schedule for the United States, valid as of 2008, was approved by the Advisory Committee on Immunization Practices (ACIP), the American Academy of Pediatrics (AAP), and the American Academy of Family Physicians (AAFP) (Figures 29-4, 29-5, and 29-6). Children who follow the recommended immunization schedule are protected against 10 vaccine-preventable childhood diseases by age 2.

Gardasil and Cervarix are 3-dose vaccines to prevent infection from human papillomavirus (HPV), the main

Text continued on p. 935

Recommended Immunization Schedule for Persons Aged 0 Through 6 Years—United States • 2009

For those who fall behind or start late, see the catch-up schedule

Vaccine ▼ Age ►	Birth	1 month	2 months	4 months	6 months	12 months	15 months	18 months	19–23 months	2–3 years	4–6 years
Hepatitis B[1]	HepB	HepB		*see footnote 1*		HepB					
Rotavirus[2]			RV	RV	*RV*[2]						
Diphtheria, Tetanus, Pertussis[3]			DTaP	DTaP	DTaP	*see footnote 3*	DTaP				DTaP
Haemophilus influenzae type b[4]			Hib	Hib	*Hib*[4]	Hib					
Pneumococcal[5]			PCV	PCV	PCV	PCV				PPSV	
Inactivated Poliovirus			IPV	IPV		IPV					IPV
Influenza[6]								Influenza (Yearly)			
Measles, Mumps, Rubella[7]						MMR			*see footnote 7*		MMR
Varicella[8]						Varicella			*see footnote 8*		Varicella
Hepatitis A[9]								HepA (2 doses)		HepA Series	
Meningococcal[10]										MCV	

Range of recommended ages

Certain high-risk groups

This schedule indicates the recommended ages for routine administration of currently licensed vaccines, as of December 1, 2008, for children aged 0 through 6 years. Any dose not administered at the recommended age should be administered at a subsequent visit, when indicated and feasible. Licensed combination vaccines may be used whenever any component of the combination is indicated and other components are not contraindicated and if approved by the Food and Drug Administration for that dose of the series. Providers should consult the relevant Advisory Committee on Immunization Practices statement for detailed recommendations, including high-risk conditions: http://www.cdc.gov/vaccines/pubs/acip-list.htm. Clinically significant adverse events that follow immunization should be reported to the Vaccine Adverse Event Reporting System (VAERS). Guidance about how to obtain and complete a VAERS form is available at http://www.vaers.hhs.gov or by telephone, 800-822-7967.

1. Hepatitis B vaccine (HepB). ***(Minimum age: birth)***

At birth:

- Administer monovalent HepB to all newborns before hospital discharge.
- If mother is hepatitis B surface antigen (HBsAg)-positive, administer HepB and 0.5 mL of hepatitis B immune globulin (HBIG) within 12 hours of birth.
- If mother's HBsAg status is unknown, administer HepB within 12 hours of birth. Determine mother's HBsAg status as soon as possible and, if HBsAg-positive, administer HBIG (no later than age 1 week).

After the birth dose:

- The HepB series should be completed with either monovalent HepB or a combination vaccine containing HepB. The second dose should be administered at age 1 or 2 months. The final dose should be administered no earlier than age 24 weeks.
- Infants born to HBsAg-positive mothers should be tested for HBsAg and antibody to HBsAg (anti-HBs) after completion of at least 3 doses of the HepB series, at age 9 through 18 months (generally at the next well-child visit).

4-month dose:

- Administration of 4 doses of HepB to infants is permissible when combination vaccines containing HepB are administered after the birth dose.

2. Rotavirus vaccine (RV). ***(Minimum age: 6 weeks)***

- Administer the first dose at age 6 through 14 weeks (maximum age: 14 weeks 6 days). Vaccination should not be initiated for infants aged 15 weeks or older (i.e., 15 weeks 0 days or older).
- Administer the final dose in the series by age 8 months 0 days.
- If Rotarix® is administered at ages 2 and 4 months, a dose at 6 months is not indicated.

3. Diphtheria and tetanus toxoids and acellular pertussis vaccine (DTaP). ***(Minimum age: 6 weeks)***

- The fourth dose may be administered as early as age 12 months, provided at least 6 months have elapsed since the third dose.
- Administer the final dose in the series at age 4 through 6 years.

4. *Haemophilus influenzae* type b conjugate vaccine (Hib). ***(Minimum age: 6 weeks)***

- If PRP-OMP (PedvaxHIB® or Comvax® [HepB-Hib]) is administered at ages 2 and 4 months, a dose at age 6 months is not indicated.
- TriHiBit® (DTaP/Hib) should not be used for doses at ages 2, 4, or 6 months but can be used as the final dose in children aged 12 months or older.

5. Pneumococcal vaccine. ***(Minimum age: 6 weeks for pneumococcal conjugate vaccine [PCV]; 2 years for pneumococcal polysaccharide vaccine [PPSV])***

- PCV is recommended for all children aged younger than 5 years. Administer 1 dose of PCV to all healthy children aged 24 through 59 months who are not completely vaccinated for their age.
- Administer PPSV to children aged 2 years or older with certain underlying medical conditions (see *MMWR* 2000;49[No. RR-9]), including a cochlear implant.

6. Influenza vaccine. ***(Minimum age: 6 months for trivalent inactivated influenza vaccine [TIV]; 2 years for live, attenuated influenza vaccine [LAIV])***

- Administer annually to children aged 6 months through 18 years.
- For healthy nonpregnant persons (i.e., those who do not have underlying medical conditions that predispose them to influenza complications) aged 2 through 49 years, either LAIV or TIV may be used.
- Children receiving TIV should receive 0.25 mL if aged 6 through 35 months or 0.5 mL if aged 3 years or older.
- Administer 2 doses (separated by at least 4 weeks) to children aged younger than 9 years who are receiving influenza vaccine for the first time or who were vaccinated for the first time during the previous influenza season but only received 1 dose.

7. Measles, mumps, and rubella vaccine (MMR). ***(Minimum age: 12 months)***

- Administer the second dose at age 4 through 6 years. However, the second dose may be administered before age 4, provided at least 28 days have elapsed since the first dose.

8. Varicella vaccine. ***(Minimum age: 12 months)***

- Administer the second dose at age 4 through 6 years. However, the second dose may be administered before age 4, provided at least 3 months have elapsed since the first dose.
- For children aged 12 months through 12 years the minimum interval between doses is 3 months. However, if the second dose was administered at least 28 days after the first dose, it can be accepted as valid.

9. Hepatitis A vaccine (HepA). ***(Minimum age: 12 months)***

- Administer to all children aged 1 year (i.e., aged 12 through 23 months). Administer 2 doses at least 6 months apart.
- Children not fully vaccinated by age 2 years can be vaccinated at subsequent visits.
- HepA also is recommended for children older than 1 year who live in areas where vaccination programs target older children or who are at increased risk of infection. See *MMWR* 2006;55(No. RR-7).

10. Meningococcal vaccine. ***(Minimum age: 2 years for meningococcal conjugate vaccine [MCV] and for meningococcal polysaccharide vaccine [MPSV])***

- Administer MCV to children aged 2 through 10 years with terminal complement component deficiency, anatomic or functional asplenia, and certain other high-risk groups. See *MMWR* 2005;54(No. RR-7).
- Persons who received MPSV 3 or more years previously and who remain at increased risk for meningococcal disease should be revaccinated with MCV.

The Recommended Immunization Schedules for Persons Aged 0 Through 18 Years are approved by the Advisory Committee on Immunization Practices (www.cdc.gov/vaccines/recs/acip), the American Academy of Pediatrics (http://www.aap.org), and the American Academy of Family Physicians (http://www.aafp.org).

DEPARTMENT OF HEALTH AND HUMAN SERVICES • CENTERS FOR DISEASE CONTROL AND PREVENTION

FIGURE 29-4 Recommended schedule for childhood (ages 0 to 6) immunization in the United States.

Recommended Immunization Schedule for Persons Aged 7 Through 18 Years—United States • 2009

For those who fall behind or start late, see the schedule below and the catch-up schedule

Vaccine ▼ Age ▶	7–10 years	11–12 years	13–18 years
Tetanus, Diphtheria, Pertussis[1]	*see footnote 1*	Tdap	Tdap
Human Papillomavirus[2]	*see footnote 2*	HPV (3 doses)	HPV Series
Meningococcal[3]	MCV	MCV	MCV
Influenza[4]		Influenza (Yearly)	
Pneumococcal[5]		PPSV	
Hepatitis A[6]		HepA Series	
Hepatitis B[7]		HepB Series	
Inactivated Poliovirus[8]		IPV Series	
Measles, Mumps, Rubella[9]		MMR Series	
Varicella[10]		Varicella Series	

Range of recommended ages

Catch-up immunization

Certain high-risk groups

This schedule indicates the recommended ages for routine administration of currently licensed vaccines, as of December 1, 2008, for children aged 7 through 18 years. Any dose not administered at the recommended age should be administered at a subsequent visit, when indicated and feasible. Licensed combination vaccines may be used whenever any component of the combination is indicated and other components are not contraindicated and if approved by the Food and Drug Administration for that dose of the series. Providers should consult the relevant Advisory Committee on Immunization Practices statement for detailed recommendations, including high-risk conditions: http://www.cdc.gov/vaccines/pubs/acip-list.htm. Clinically significant adverse events that follow immunization should be reported to the Vaccine Adverse Event Reporting System (VAERS). Guidance about how to obtain and complete a VAERS form is available at http://www.vaers.hhs.gov or by telephone, 800-822-7967.

1. Tetanus and diphtheria toxoids and acellular pertussis vaccine (Tdap). ***(Minimum age: 10 years for BOOSTRIX® and 11 years for ADACEL®)***
- Administer at age 11 or 12 years for those who have completed the recommended childhood DTP/DTaP vaccination series and have not received a tetanus and diphtheria toxoid (Td) booster dose.
- Persons aged 13 through 18 years who have not received Tdap should receive a dose.
- A 5-year interval from the last Td dose is encouraged when Tdap is used as a booster dose; however, a shorter interval may be used if pertussis immunity is needed.

2. Human papillomavirus vaccine (HPV). ***(Minimum age: 9 years)***
- Administer the first dose to females at age 11 or 12 years.
- Administer the second dose 2 months after the first dose and the third dose 6 months after the first dose (at least 24 weeks after the first dose).
- Administer the series to females at age 13 through 18 years if not previously vaccinated.

3. Meningococcal conjugate vaccine (MCV).
- Administer at age 11 or 12 years, or at age 13 through 18 years if not previously vaccinated.
- Administer to previously unvaccinated college freshmen living in a dormitory.
- MCV is recommended for children aged 2 through 10 years with terminal complement component deficiency, anatomic or functional asplenia, and certain other groups at high risk. See *MMWR* 2005;54(No. RR-7).
- Persons who received MPSV 5 or more years previously and remain at increased risk for meningococcal disease should be revaccinated with MCV.

4. Influenza vaccine.
- Administer annually to children aged 6 months through 18 years.
- For healthy nonpregnant persons (i.e., those who do not have underlying medical conditions that predispose them to influenza complications) aged 2 through 49 years, either LAIV or TIV may be used.
- Administer 2 doses (separated by at least 4 weeks) to children aged younger than 9 years who are receiving influenza vaccine for the first time or who were vaccinated for the first time during the previous influenza season but only received 1 dose.

5. Pneumococcal polysaccharide vaccine (PPSV).
- Administer to children with certain underlying medical conditions (see *MMWR* 1997;46[No. RR-8]), including a cochlear implant. A single revaccination should be administered to children with functional or anatomic asplenia or other immunocompromising condition after 5 years.

6. Hepatitis A vaccine (HepA).
- Administer 2 doses at least 6 months apart.
- HepA is recommended for children older than 1 year who live in areas where vaccination programs target older children or who are at increased risk of infection. See *MMWR* 2006;55(No. RR-7).

7. Hepatitis B vaccine (HepB).
- Administer the 3-dose series to those not previously vaccinated.
- A 2-dose series (separated by at least 4 months) of adult formulation Recombivax HB® is licensed for children aged 11 through 15 years.

8. Inactivated poliovirus vaccine (IPV).
- For children who received an all-IPV or all-oral poliovirus (OPV) series, a fourth dose is not necessary if the third dose was administered at age 4 years or older.
- If both OPV and IPV were administered as part of a series, a total of 4 doses should be administered, regardless of the child's current age.

9. Measles, mumps, and rubella vaccine (MMR).
- If not previously vaccinated, administer 2 doses or the second dose for those who have received only 1 dose, with at least 28 days between doses.

10. Varicella vaccine.
- For persons aged 7 through 18 years without evidence of immunity (see *MMWR* 2007;56[No. RR-4]), administer 2 doses if not previously vaccinated or the second dose if they have received only 1 dose.
- For persons aged 7 through 12 years, the minimum interval between doses is 3 months. However, if the second dose was administered at least 28 days after the first dose, it can be accepted as valid.
- For persons aged 13 years and older, the minimum interval between doses is 28 days.

The Recommended Immunization Schedules for Persons Aged 0 Through 18 Years are approved by the Advisory Committee on Immunization Practices (www.cdc.gov/vaccines/recs/acip), the American Academy of Pediatrics (http://www.aap.org), and the American Academy of Family Physicians (http://www.aafp.org).

DEPARTMENT OF HEALTH AND HUMAN SERVICES • CENTERS FOR DISEASE CONTROL AND PREVENTION

FIGURE 29-5 Recommended schedule for adolescent (ages 7 to 18) immunization in the United States.

Catch-up Immunization Schedule for Persons Aged 4 Months Through 18 Years Who Start Late or Who Are More Than 1 Month Behind—United States • 2009

The table below provides catch-up schedules and minimum intervals between doses for children whose vaccinations have been delayed. A vaccine series does not need to be restarted, regardless of the time that has elapsed between doses. Use the section appropriate for the child's age.

Vaccine	Minimum Age for Dose 1	Minimum Interval Between Doses			
		Dose 1 to Dose 2	Dose 2 to Dose 3	Dose 3 to Dose 4	Dose 4 to Dose 5
CATCH-UP SCHEDULE FOR PERSONS AGED 4 MONTHS THROUGH 6 YEARS					
Hepatitis B[1]	Birth	4 weeks	8 weeks (and at least 16 weeks after first dose)		
Rotavirus[2]	6 wks	4 weeks	4 weeks[2]		
Diphtheria, Tetanus, Pertussis[3]	6 wks	4 weeks	4 weeks	6 months	6 months[3]
Haemophilus influenzae type b[4]	6 wks	**4 weeks** if first dose administered at younger than age 12 months **8 weeks (as final dose)** if first dose administered at age 12-14 months **No further doses needed** if first dose administered at age 15 months or older	**4 weeks[4]** if current age is younger than 12 months **8 weeks (as final dose)[4]** if current age is 12 months or older and second dose administered at younger than age 15 months **No further doses needed** if previous dose administered at age 15 months or older	**8 weeks (as final dose)** This dose only necessary for children aged 12 months through 59 months who received 3 doses before age 12 months	
Pneumococcal[5]	6 wks	**4 weeks** if first dose administered at younger than age 12 months **8 weeks** (as final dose for healthy children) if first dose administered at age 12 months or older or current age 24 through 59 months **No further doses needed** for healthy children if first dose administered at age 24 months or older	**4 weeks** if current age is younger than 12 months **8 weeks** (as final dose for healthy children) if current age is 12 months or older **No further doses needed** for healthy children if previous dose administered at age 24 months or older	**8 weeks (as final dose)** This dose only necessary for children aged 12 months through 59 months who received 3 doses before age 12 months or for high-risk children who received 3 doses at any age	
Inactivated Poliovirus[6]	6 wks	4 weeks	4 weeks	4 weeks[6]	
Measles, Mumps, Rubella[7]	12 mos	4 weeks			
Varicella[8]	12 mos	3 months			
Hepatitis A[9]	12 mos	6 months			
CATCH-UP SCHEDULE FOR PERSONS AGED 7 THROUGH 18 YEARS					
Tetanus, Diphtheria/ Tetanus, Diphtheria, Pertussis[10]	7 yrs[10]	4 weeks	**4 weeks** if first dose administered at younger than age 12 months **6 months** if first dose administered at age 12 months or older	**6 months** if first dose administered at younger than age 12 months	
Human Papillomavirus[11]	9 yrs	Routine dosing intervals are recommended[11]			
Hepatitis A[9]	12 mos	6 months			
Hepatitis B[1]	Birth	4 weeks	8 weeks (and at least 16 weeks after first dose)		
Inactivated Poliovirus[6]	6 wks	4 weeks	4 weeks	4 weeks[6]	
Measles, Mumps, Rubella[7]	12 mos	4 weeks			
Varicella[8]	12 mos	**3 months** if the person is younger than age 13 years **4 weeks** if the person is aged 13 years or older			

1. Hepatitis B vaccine (HepB).
- Administer the 3-dose series to those not previously vaccinated.
- A 2-dose series (separated by at least 4 months) of adult formulation Recombivax HB® is licensed for children aged 11 through 15 years.

2. Rotavirus vaccine (RV).
- The maximum age for the first dose is 14 weeks 6 days. Vaccination should not be initiated for infants aged 15 weeks or older (i.e., 15 weeks 0 days or older).
- Administer the final dose in the series by age 8 months 0 days.
- If Rotarix® was administered for the first and second doses, a third dose is not indicated.

3. Diphtheria and tetanus toxoids and acellular pertussis vaccine (DTaP).
- The fifth dose is not necessary if the fourth dose was administered at age 4 years or older.

4. *Haemophilus influenzae* type b conjugate vaccine (Hib).
- Hib vaccine is not generally recommended for persons aged 5 years or older. No efficacy data are available on which to base a recommendation concerning use of Hib vaccine for older children and adults. However, studies suggest good immunogenicity in persons who have sickle cell disease, leukemia, or HIV infection, or who have had a splenectomy; administering 1 dose of Hib vaccine to these persons is not contraindicated.
- If the first 2 doses were PRP-OMP (PedvaxHIB® or Comvax®), and administered at age 11 months or younger, the third (and final) dose should be administered at age 12 through 15 months and at least 8 weeks after the second dose.
- If the first dose was administered at age 7 through 11 months, administer 2 doses separated by 4 weeks and a final dose at age 12 through 15 months.

5. Pneumococcal vaccine.
- Administer 1 dose of pneumococcal conjugate vaccine (PCV) to all healthy children aged 24 through 59 months who have not received at least 1 dose of PCV on or after age 12 months.
- For children aged 24 through 59 months with underlying medical conditions, administer 1 dose of PCV if 3 doses were received previously or administer 2 doses of PCV at least 8 weeks apart if fewer than 3 doses were received previously.
- Administer pneumococcal polysaccharide vaccine (PPSV) to children aged 2 years or older with certain underlying medical conditions (see *MMWR* 2000;49[No. RR-9]), including a cochlear implant, at least 8 weeks after the last dose of PCV.

6. Inactivated poliovirus vaccine (IPV).
- For children who received an all-IPV or all-oral poliovirus (OPV) series, a fourth dose is not necessary if the third dose was administered at age 4 years or older.
- If both OPV and IPV were administered as part of a series, a total of 4 doses should be administered, regardless of the child's current age.

7. Measles, mumps, and rubella vaccine (MMR).
- Administer the second dose at age 4 through 6 years. However, the second dose may be administered before age 4, provided at least 28 days have elapsed since the first dose.
- If not previously vaccinated, administer 2 doses with at least 28 days between doses.

8. Varicella vaccine.
- Administer the second dose at age 4 through 6 years. However, the second dose may be administered before age 4, provided at least 3 months have elapsed since the first dose.
- For persons aged 12 months through 12 years, the minimum interval between doses is 3 months. However, if the second dose was administered at least 28 days after the first dose, it can be accepted as valid.
- For persons aged 13 years and older, the minimum interval between doses is 28 days.

9. Hepatitis A vaccine (HepA).
- HepA is recommended for children older than 1 year who live in areas where vaccination programs target older children or who are at increased risk of infection. See *MMWR* 2006;55(No. RR-7).

10. Tetanus and diphtheria toxoids vaccine (Td) and tetanus and diphtheria toxoids and acellular pertussis vaccine (Tdap).
- Doses of DTaP are counted as part of the Td/Tdap series
- Tdap should be substituted for a single dose of Td in the catch-up series or as a booster for children aged 10 through 18 years; use Td for other doses.

11. Human papillomavirus vaccine (HPV).
- Administer the series to females at age 13 through 18 years if not previously vaccinated.
- Use recommended routine dosing intervals for series catch-up (i.e., the second and third doses should be administered at 2 and 6 months after the first dose). However, the minimum interval between the first and second doses is 4 weeks. The minimum interval between the second and third doses is 12 weeks, and the third dose should be given at least 24 weeks after the first dose.

Information about reporting reactions after immunization is available online at http://www.vaers.hhs.gov or by telephone, 800-822-7967. Suspected cases of vaccine-preventable diseases should be reported to the state or local health department. Additional information, including precautions and contraindications for immunization, is available from the National Center for Immunization and Respiratory Diseases at http://www.cdc.gov/vaccines or telephone, 800-CDC-INFO (800-232-4636).

DEPARTMENT OF HEALTH AND HUMAN SERVICES • CENTERS FOR DISEASE CONTROL AND PREVENTION

FIGURE 29-6 Catch-up schedule for immunization (ages 4 months to 18 years) in the United States.

cause of genital warts and cervical cancer (U.S. Food and Drug Administration, 2009). Gardasil offers coverage against HPV types 6, 11, 16, and 18; Cervarix is effective against HPV types 16 and 18. The National Institute of Allergy and Infectious Diseases (NIAID) (2009) recommends that girls and young women up to age 26 be vaccinated before becoming sexually active. These vaccines are not effective after exposure to HPV.

Barriers to proper immunization include lack of insurance and funding, lack of transportation, lack of education about the importance of immunizations, and personal and cultural beliefs. Vaccination assistance programs provide vaccinations to children whose parents are unable to pay (Hockenberry & Wilson, 2007). Make sure you know the current recommended immunization schedule and are able to answer parents' concerns regarding immunizations.

ACCESS TO HEALTH CARE

Many Americans do not have any type of health care insurance. Approximately 11 million children in the United States are uninsured. Many individuals who do have some type of coverage are underinsured. This raises a sometimes impassable obstacle for people seeking health care services. Other common barriers associated with access to health care, in addition to the financial one, include lack of primary care providers, cultural and spiritual differences, language barriers, discrimination, and concerns about confidentiality. All health care providers have a responsibility to improve health care access to all people.

DENTAL HEALTH

A multidisciplinary approach to all aspects of pediatric health promotion is fundamental to safeguarding the physical and emotional health of all children. Dental health promotion, an aspect of proper health care, is best to begin with the eruption of the primary teeth, usually at about 6 months of age; advise parents to begin it no later than when the child has reached 2½ years of age, the average age when deciduous dentition is complete. Although the incidence of dental caries has decreased considerably since the introduction of fluorides and increased dental health education and promotion, nursing bottle caries continues to be a significant concern for infants and toddlers. **Nursing bottle caries** is tooth decay that is the result of prolonged nursing after the infant has been put to bed, when the milk, juice, or other fluid is allowed to bathe the teeth, thus providing sugar to oral bacteria for growth. During sleep, decreased salivary flow prevents clearance of the liquid from the mouth, and the liquid pools on the teeth (Figure 29-7). You are in a unique position to prevent these and other problems by promoting good dental health through counseling and education.

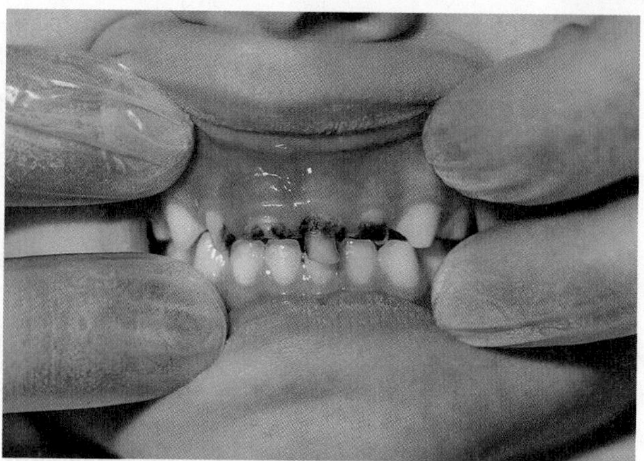

FIGURE 29-7 Nursing bottle caries.

STRATEGIES TO PROMOTE DENTAL HEALTH

Make early institution of good dental hygiene and practices to prevent dental caries a part of the anticipatory guidance for all children and their parents. Help children and parents by teaching them to employ the following strategies:

- Begin cleansing the oral cavity in infancy by wiping the teeth and gums with a damp washcloth (Figure 29-8). A toothbrush will usually be too harsh for an infant's tender gums. As an infant

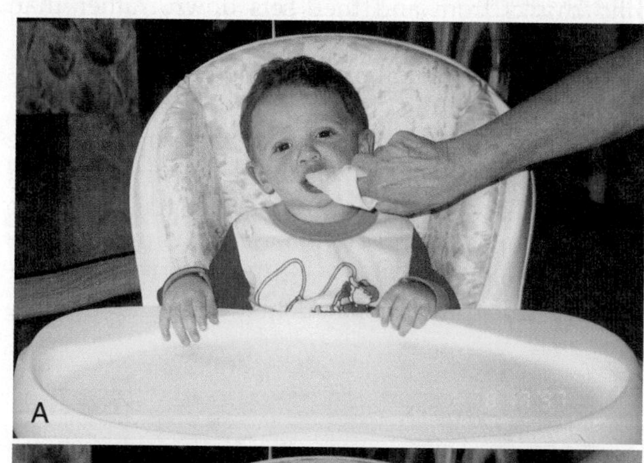

A

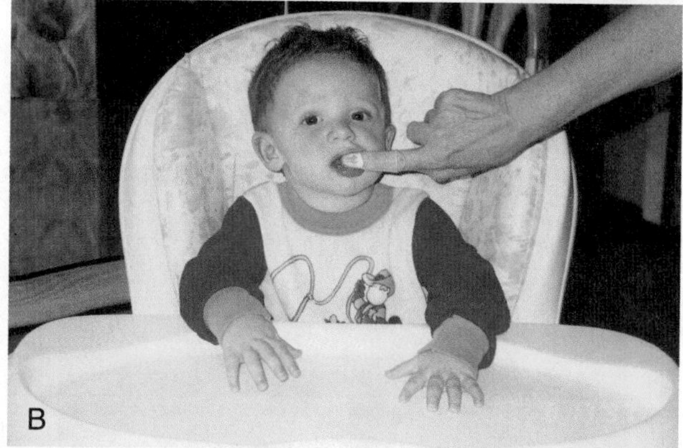

B

FIGURE 29-8 For the infant, wipe the oral cavity and teeth with a damp washcloth. **A,** Cleansing with a damp washcloth. **B,** Cleansing with a fingercot toothbrush.

gets more teeth, use a small soft-bristled toothbrush with plain water to cleanse the teeth and gums. Avoid using toothpaste during this age, especially if fluoridated, because swallowing by the infant will lead to ingestion of excessive amounts of fluoride.
- Initiate fluoride supplementation at 6 months of age if the water in the infant's residential area is not fluoridated. Fluoride supplementation is no longer recommended for infants under 6 months of age.
- Encourage proper nutrition during infancy and childhood to promote good dental health. Avoid, or use sparingly, food with concentrated sugars. In addition, advise against using honey during the first year of life because some cases of infant botulism (an often fatal form of food poisoning caused by an endotoxin produced by the bacillus *Clostridium botulinum*) have been associated with it. Other foods that are associated with an increased incidence of dental caries include molasses, corn syrup, and dried fruits such as raisins.

Specific interventions are possible to prevent nursing bottle caries. Give the last bottle *before* bedtime, with proper cleansing of the teeth and gums *before* putting the child down to sleep. Use water in the bedtime bottle instead of juice or milk. Do not use sugar- or honey-coated pacifiers. Offer juice in cups, which the child drinks from and then sets down, rather than bottles.

After infancy, dental hygiene and health care needs continue through the various stages of development.
- For preschool children, when the eruption of the deciduous teeth is complete, continued good dental hygiene is important. Parental assistance and supervision is required with brushing; also teach parents to perform flossing (Figure 29-9). See that professional dental care and fluoride supplementation continues. Encourage proper nutrition (see Chapter 21).
- Eruption of permanent teeth begins during the school-age years. Good dental hygiene and professional dental supervision are especially important during this period. Screening for malocclusion problems that result from abnormal eruption of permanent teeth is also important. Teach or reinforce correct brushing and flossing techniques. Have children brush teeth after meals and snacks and at bedtime. Encourage the child to decrease the ingestion of high-sugar foods.
- Although the rate of caries formation slows during the adolescent years, continuing good dental practices is still important. Adolescence is often a time when orthodontic appliances are applied to correct malocclusions. Adolescents are typically concerned with body image and often need to be reminded of the temporary nature of these devices and their proper use and care.

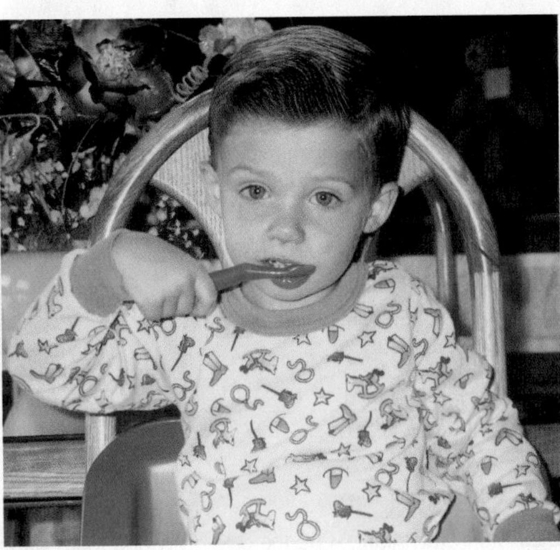

FIGURE 29-9 Young children can participate in toothbrushing, but parents need to brush all the child's teeth thoroughly.

INJURY PREVENTION

Injuries in children are associated with age, developmental level, and the physical and cognitive skills of the child. The inexperience of infants with the environment and their immature motor skills leave them vulnerable to falls and suffocation. Toddlers and preschoolers are at increased risk of injuries from water-related accidents, poisoning, and burns as they acquire new skills. School-age children become more competitive in their activities, and will sometimes suffer injuries from bicycle accidents, MVAs, and skating accidents. In their struggle to gain independence and freedom, adolescents become more vulnerable to injuries and death from MVAs and accidents involving firearms, alcohol, and illegal drugs. **Anticipatory guidance** education has been the most widely used approach to educate parents in accident prevention. Use every opportunity to educate parents in injury prevention (see the Safety Alert).

POISONING

The ingestion of harmful or poisonous substances is a common cause of morbidity and mortality in children younger than age 5. Children in the 1- to 2-year age-group are at increased risk because of their natural curiosity to explore their environment once they become mobile. The Poison Prevention Packaging Act of 1970, which requires childproof packaging of medications, has greatly reduced the incidence of poisoning; however, continued strategies and educational efforts are needed to reduce the morbidity and mortality of this preventable cause. Children are vulnerable to becoming poisoned from a variety of causes, including pharmaceuticals (especially acetaminophen, cough and cold preparations, iron, vitamins, and oral contraceptives) and nonpharmaceuticals (cleaning products,

Safety Alert!

Infant, Toddler and Child, and Adolescent

INFANT

- Keep your hands on the infant at all times when crib rail is down.
- Use an infant car safety seat restraint that has been federally approved.
- Always place an infant weighting less than 9 kg (20 pounds) or who is younger than 1 year of age in a rear-facing child safety seat in the back seat of the automobile. Never place an infant in the front seat of a vehicle.*
- Leave no gaps between crib side and mattress.
- Place infants on their backs to sleep. There is an increased risk of sudden infant death syndrome (SIDS) in infants placed in side-lying or prone position.
- Check all toys for small parts to reduce risk of choking or wounds.
- Support head, and shield head from injury.
- Do not prop bottle.
- Place infant in upright position when feeding solid foods
- Use clean bowl and spoon to feed, and do not feed directly from jar; this prevents contamination of food
- *Never* leave infant unattended in or near water.
- *Never*, under any circumstances leave infant unsupervised in bathtub.
- Apply a sunscreen when infant is exposed to sunlight (year-round).

TODDLER AND CHILD

- Use a toddler car safety seat restraint that has been federally approved; it is acceptable to switch the safety seat restraint to forward facing once the child weighs more than 20 pounds and is older than 1 year.*
- Use car booster seats, also known as belt-positioning devices, for child less than 4 feet 9 inches tall and weighing more than 40 pounds, typically between 4 and 8 years.
- *Never* leave toddler unattended in vehicle or shopping cart.
- Protect from falls, burns, and collisions with objects that result from running and climbing.
- Use washable toys without small parts or sharp edges.
- Supervise closely when near any source of water.
- *Never* leave unsupervised in a bathtub.
- Cover electrical outlets with protective plastic caps.
- Do not allow toddler or child to play on curb or behind a parked car.
- Supervise tricycle and bicycle riding; have child wear helmet.
- Teach child to obey pedestrian safety rules.
- Never leave infant or toddler unattended in high chair.
- Supervise at playgrounds; select safe play areas.
- Apply a sunscreen when toddler or child is exposed to sunlight (year-round).
- Stress danger of open flames.
- Always check bath water temperature; adjust water temperature to 120° F (48.9° C) or cooler (infants, toddlers, children).
- Place all potentially toxic agents out of reach or in a locked cabinet.
- Discard all unused refrigerators, ovens, and other appliances; if storing an old appliance, remove door.
- Keep venetian blind cords out of toddler or child's reach.
- Teach child to never go with strangers.
- Teach child to tell parents if anyone makes child feel uncomfortable in any way.

ADOLESCENT

- Adolescents feel indestructible and tend to be more prone to deliberate (suicide) or nondeliberate accidents such as in the use of guns, drugs, or motor vehicles.
- Emphasize and encourage safe pedestrian behavior.
  —At night, walk with a friend.
  —Do not walk in secluded area; take well-traveled walkways.
- Provide competent driver education; encourage judicious use of vehicle; discourage drag racing, "playing chicken"; maintain vehicle in proper condition (brakes, tires, etc.).
- Teach and promote safety and maintenance of two-wheeled vehicles.
- Promote use of seatbelts.
- Promote and encourage wearing of safety apparel such as helmet, long trousers.
- Reinforce the dangers of using drugs, including alcohol, when operating a motor vehicle.
- Teach nonswimmer to swim.
- Teach basic rules of water safety; stress the need to make sure water is of sufficient depth for diving.
- Reinforce proper behavior in areas involving contact with burn hazards (gasoline, electrical wires, fires).
- Advise regarding excessive exposure to natural or artificial sunlight (ultraviolet burn), encourage use of sunscreen.
- Discourage use of all tobacco products.
- Educate in hazards of drug use, including alcohol.
- Promote acquisition of proper instruction in sports and use of sports equipment.
- Instruct in safe use of and respect for firearms and other devices with potential danger (e.g., power tools, fireworks).

*Data from Hockenberry, M.J., & Wilson, D. (2007). *Wong's nursing care of infants and children.* (8th ed.). St. Louis: Mosby.

lead, plants, insecticides and pesticides, mouthwashes, and cosmetics).

Prevention

All parents need to be educated to prevent accidental poisoning. Despite parents' best efforts, children are still at risk, especially when visiting the homes of relatives or friends. Parents must know the number of the poison control center (PCC) in their area. Advise parents to place the PCC telephone number close to each telephone in the home and program it into their cell phones. The PCC hotline number is usually found in the front of the telephone directory (Hockenberry & Wilson, 2007). The U.S. Poison Control Center no longer recommends syrup of ipecac for routine treatment of poisoning. Help parents institute prevention strategies by instructing them to do the following:

- Never refer to medicines as candy; medicines are drugs. Store them with childproof caps, and keep them out of reach or in a locked cabinet.

- Place cleaning supplies and other toxic substances, including batteries, up high and out of reach of curious youngsters or in a locked cabinet.
- Do not keep large quantities of toxic agents (e.g., pesticides, cleaning fluids, drugs) in the home.
- Inspect your home for possible sources of lead contamination, including lead-based paint on windowsills, stair rails, door moldings, and peeling wall paint.
- Keep toxic plants out of reach of small hands.
- Remember that many grandparents will be taking medications, and they, too, need to keep them in a locked cabinet or up high and out of the reach of children. Keep purses out of the child's reach.
- Educate older children and adolescents about the dangers of drugs and alcohol.

A nursing diagnosis and interventions for the patient with poisoning include but are not limited to the following:

Nursing Diagnosis	Nursing Interventions
Risk for poisoning, related to lack of knowledge of safeguarding child's environment from harmful, poisonous substances	Counsel parents to store medicines with childproof caps. Teach parents to store harmful substances out of child's reach and in a locked cabinet. Educate parents to contact health care facility and poison control center immediately if suspected ingestion of harmful substance is noted.

ASPIRATION OF A FOREIGN BODY

In children younger than 1 year of age, the leading cause of fatal injury is asphyxiation by aspiration of foreign materials into the respiratory tract. Although all children younger than age 3 are at risk, the older infant 6 months to 1 year of age is at greatest risk because of the normal hand-to-mouth activities common in this age-group. The severity of respiratory tract obstruction depends on the location and the type of material aspirated. Foods that pose the greatest danger are usually round, such as hot dogs, round candy, nuts, grapes, popcorn, peanuts, cookies or biscuits, other meats, carrots, apples, peanut butter, and beans. Common objects that are easily aspirated include buttons on clothing or toys, beads, coins, balloons, pins, and barrettes. Toys with small or loosely attached parts and pacifier nipples that become detached from the shield are also dangerous. More recently, the caps of medication syringes have also been implicated when caretakers forget to remove them before administering medication to a child.

Families need to be cognizant of choking hazards for small children. You are in an excellent position to counsel families in prevention strategies. Box 29-1 summarizes areas to discuss with parents during routine health supervision visits.

BURN INJURIES

Burns are the third leading cause of accidental death in children 1 to 4 years of age, the second in children ages 5 to 9, and third in ages 10 to 14 years old. Up to 75% of all burn injuries occur in the home, with children younger than age 2 experiencing more scald burns and children older than 5 being more frequently involved in flame burns. Burns are the result of thermal damage to skin and tissues. Severity is related to the temperature and length of time the skin is exposed to the heat source. Burns occur as a result of flames, chemicals, hot objects, radiation, or electricity.

Prevention

As infants and children acquire new motor skills, they are more vulnerable to accidental burn and other injuries. You have a unique opportunity to educate parents to avoid risks and provide a safe environment for their children. Teach the following safety precautions:

- Keep the hot water heater set at no more than 120° F (49° C).
- Turn all pot handles on the stove toward the back of the stove.
- Keep hot objects, such as cigarettes, coffee pots, and hot liquids or foods, out of the reach of small hands.
- Remove hanging tablecloths and electrical cords, especially around children who crawl or walk.
- Teach older children safe cooking and emphasize that it is never acceptable to wear loose clothing near the stove or other heat source (e.g., fireplace, wood-burning stove).
- Use guardrails or guards around fireplaces, space heaters, and other heating sources.
- Use and maintain smoke detectors in the home.

Box 29-1 Foreign Body Aspiration Prevention Strategies

- Keep small objects and toys away from infants and young children who are developmentally unable to obey restrictions; small objects also have the potential to be introduced into the nose or the ear by the child, causing obstruction.
- Inform parents of the dangers of round foods to children too young to chew these foods properly—they are acceptable to introduce when the child is older.
- When administering medications by syringe, stress to parents the need to remove the cap first.
- Encourage parents to choose one-piece pacifiers that do not come apart and cause aspiration. Have the parents check the pacifier frequently by pulling on the nipple. If it becomes separated from the shield, it is to be discarded.

- Keep electrical wires hidden and out of the reach of children.
- Use plastic caps to cover electrical outlets.
- Keep small, hot appliances such as curling irons and steam irons out of the reach of children.
- Keep a fire extinguisher in the home and know how to operate it.
- Use a cool mist rather than a hot mist vaporizer.
- Use a hat and sunscreen on children when outdoors, especially during peak sun hours.
- Teach older children the potential of burn hazards such as gasoline, matches, barbecue grills, candles, and fireworks (including Roman candles, etc.).
- Have parents map out an escape route in the home and practice fire drills with family members.
- Keep the telephone numbers of the fire and rescue squads near the telephone (911 in most areas). Teach small children "nine-one-one" (911), because how to dial nine-eleven will not necessarily be a concept they are able to grasp.

Get Ready for the NCLEX® Examination!

Key Points

- Anticipatory guidance is education of parents to prepare them for normal growth and development of their children. It is also psychological preparation of a person for an event expected to be stressful, as in preparation of a child for surgery by explaining what will happen and what it will feel like.
- *Healthy People 2010* identified 10 leading health indicators for health promotion and disease prevention.
- Initiate fluoride supplementation at 6 months of age if the water in the infant's residential area is not fluoridated.
- The development of immunizations against communicable diseases has significantly reduced the morbidity and mortality associated with many diseases.
- Injuries in children are associated with age, developmental level, and the physical and cognitive skills of the child.
- Use infant safety seats designed according to federal safety guidelines: birth to 20 pounds—rear-facing safety seats secured in the rear seat; toddlers 20 to 40 pounds—front-facing safety seats secured in the rear seat; children over 40 pounds—secured in booster seats with lap and shoulder belts per federal safety protocol.

Additional Resources

Go to your Companion CD for an audio glossary, animations, video clips, and more.

evolve Be sure to visit the Evolve site at http://evolve.elsevier.com/Christensen/foundations/ for additional online resources.

Review Questions for the NCLEX® Examination

1. When counseling the parents of a 6-month-old about dental health, the nurse will include which statement(s)? *(Select all that apply.)*
   1. "Begin cleansing the oral cavity by wiping teeth and gums with a damp washcloth."
   2. "Avoid toothpaste at this age, especially if it is fluoridated."
   3. "Initiate fluoride supplementation at 6 months of age if infant's home water supply is not fluoridated."
   4. "It is acceptable to prop a bottle with juice or milk for the infant."
2. Many children and adolescents in the United States are overweight or obese. One important factor for the pediatric nurse to consider is:
   1. because more mothers work outside the home, children and adolescents eat only fast foods.
   2. obese children always become obese adults.
   3. being overweight or obese sometimes results in major physical and psychological health problems.
   4. it is best for families to have more meals at home.
3. Responsible sexual behavior among young people includes:
   1. having sexual activity only with someone you know.
   2. abstaining from sexual activity or properly using condoms.
   3. having sexual activity only once a month.
   4. requiring sexual partners to be tested for HIV.
4. A 15-year-old male patient states that he does not smoke; however, he does use chewing tobacco. It is the nurse's responsibility to inform him that he:
   1. is at great risk for lung cancer.
   2. is at great risk for lip, gum, and throat cancer.
   3. will be at great risk for becoming a smoker later in life.
   4. absolutely has to stop using all tobacco products immediately.
5. The U.S. Poison Control Center (PCC) no longer recommends ______________ for home treatment of poisoning.
6. For infants less than 20 pounds, the car safety seat should face the ______________ of the car.
7. It is acceptable for children weighing more than ______________ pounds to ride in a booster seat facing the front of the car.

8. The parents of a 10-month-old are concerned about motor vehicle safety. In counseling them, the nurse is aware that:
   1. children weighing more than 35 pounds need to be secured with a lap and shoulder belt.
   2. infants from birth to 20 pounds need to be in a rear-facing safety seat.
   3. when using a lap and shoulder belt, have the lap belt rest above the hip bones.
   4. when using a lap and shoulder belt, have the shoulder belt fit across the upper abdomen.

9. The parents of a 6-year-old girl want to enroll her in a soccer league. Which statement will the nurse include in advice regarding sports participation for the early school-age child?
   1. "A preparticipation sports physical is not necessary at this age."
   2. "Your daughter should be encouraged to join ballet or tennis and not a team sport."
   3. "Sports participation for this age-group should focus on enjoyment rather than competition."
   4. "Your daughter should not participate in team sports until she is 9 years old."

10. Proper counseling of the parent of a 1-year-old regarding safety includes which instruction(s)? *(Select all that apply.)*
    1. Fence pools with a self-locking gate.
    2. Keep drapery cords out of children's reach.
    3. Place infant on back to sleep.
    4. Do not tie pacifiers on a string around the infant's neck.

11. Human papillomavirus (HPV) vaccine is now recommended for girls between what ages? *(Select all that apply.)*
    1. 13 to 26 years, if vaccine not received previously
    2. 5 to 8 years
    3. 11 to 12 years
    4. 18 months to 4 years

12. HPV is a leading cause of:
    1. sterility in women.
    2. menorrhagia.
    3. pneumonia.
    4. cervical cancer.

chapter 30

Basic Pediatric Nursing Care

Barbara Lauritsen Christensen

evolve

http://evolve.elsevier.com/Christensen/foundationsadult

Objectives

1. Identify events that had a significant effect on the health care of children in the United States in the twentieth century.
2. Discuss the works of Dr. Abraham Jacobi and Lillian Wald.
3. Describe the purposes and outcomes from 1909 to the 1980s of the various White House conferences on children.
4. Discuss the personal characteristics and professional skills of a pediatric nurse.
5. Identify key elements of family-centered care.
6. Describe areas in which the pediatric nurse uses principles of growth and development.
7. Discuss how to use the head-to-toe method for the physical assessment of a child.
8. Describe metabolism in the child and its relationship with nutrition.
9. List general strategies to consider using when talking with children.
10. Outline several approaches for making the hospitalization of children a positive experience for them and their families.
11. Discuss pain management in infants and children.
12. Explain the needs of parents during their child's hospitalization.
13. Discuss common pediatric procedures.
14. Discuss administration of pediatric medications.
15. Identify each category of age and behavior as it pertains to accidents and hazards, and accident prevention in the pediatric population.

Key Terms

anterior fontanelle (fŏn-tă-NĔL, p. 965)
anticipatory guidance (p. 947)
birth defects (congenital anomalies) (kŏn-JĔN-ĭ-tăl ă-NŎM-ă-lēz, p. 943)
body surface area (BSA) (p. 973)
children with special needs (p. 944)
cognitive impairment (p. 946)
en face position (ăhn FĂS, p. 952)
family-centered care (p. 944)
morbidity (mŏr-BĬD-ĭ-tē, p. 977)
mortality (mŏr-TĂL-ĭ-tē, p. 941)
primary (deciduous) teeth (dĕ-SĬD-ū-ŭs, p. 952)
vastus lateralis muscle (VĂS-tŭs lăt-ŭr-Ă-lĭs, p. 975)
weaning (p. 955)

HISTORY OF CHILD CARE—THEN AND NOW

For centuries, children were considered miniature adults. In medieval art, you will see the bodies of children painted with adultlike proportions and musculature rather than with physical characteristics of infants and children. Childhood was considered an unimportant stage of life.

In colonial America, children had to assume adult responsibilities as soon as they were able. The value of children was related directly to the work they could perform. Infant and childhood mortality (the condition of being subject to death) rates were high. Epidemic diseases were common, and there was no control over or treatment for smallpox, diphtheria, measles, dysentery, mumps, chickenpox, yellow fever, cholera, or whooping cough. Farm accidents and burns from open fireplaces and gunpowder also contributed to high mortality rates.

With industrialization in America, the population shifted in numbers from rural to urban settings, where people lived in overcrowded and unsanitary conditions. Some unsanitary conditions were caused by lack of knowledge about how disease occurs. For instance, milk was not refrigerated and contained hundreds of millions of bacteria, which contributed to the development of diarrhea and tuberculosis.

Children continued to be looked on as little adults as they worked in factories 12 to 14 hours a day. They had no legal rights, and there were no work laws. Family life was sacrificed, and the real issue was survival.

Children's health care needs were not considered to be different from those of adults until 1860. At that time Dr. Abraham Jacobi, a New York physician referred to as the "father of pediatrics," first lectured to medical students on special diseases and health problems of children. With several other physicians, Dr. Jacobi pioneered the scientific and clinical investigation of childhood diseases. One outstanding achievement during Dr. Jacobi's era was the establishment of "milk stations," where infants were weighed and mothers were taught how to prepare milk before giving it to their babies. Mothers also had access to nurses who taught them the benefits of fresh air, clean water, adequate clothing, and satisfying the recreational needs of children. This crusade for pure milk resulted in improved sanitation, the pasteurization of milk, and increased interest in infant care. Despite a remarkable decline in infant mortality rate, and health care efforts notwithstanding, 20% of children still died before their second birthday, and 50% died before age 21.

During the late 1800s, increasing concern developed for the social welfare of children, especially those who were homeless or employed as factory laborers. Children in orphanages and foundling homes were subjected to cruel and inhumane treatment by caregivers. Reformer Lillian Wald (1867–1940) founded the Henry Street Settlement in New York City, which provided nursing service, social work, and an organized program of social, cultural, and educational activities. She is regarded as the founder of public health or community nursing. Thus her work had far-reaching effects on child health and nursing.

As medical and scientific advances revealed more causes of disease, emphasis came to be placed on isolation and asepsis. In the early 1900s, children with contagious disease were isolated from adult patients. Parents were prohibited from visiting because of the possibility of transmitting disease to and from home. It was not until the 1940s and the famous works of Spitz (1945) and Robertson and Robertson (1990) on institutionalized children that health care professionals began to recognize how isolation and maternal deprivation affected children. The growing interest in the psychological health of children resulted in changes for hospitalized children, such as rooming in, prehospitalization, parent education, and hospital schooling.

Influenced by social reformers such as Lillian Wald, national leaders began to take action to improve children's living conditions. In 1909, President Theodore Roosevelt called the first White House Conference on Children. It focused on such issues as child labor, dependent children, and infant care. In 1912, the U.S. Children's Bureau was established as a direct result of that conference. Its charge was to investigate all aspects of child care, including infant mortality, child labor laws, conditions of social agencies, and the country's birthrate.

The second White House Conference on Children convened in 1919, after the end of World War I. It addressed the socioeconomic situation of mothers and children. The first federally supported health programs for mothers and children were established. The depression of 1929 paralyzed the United States and resulted in devastating social and economic conditions, which had their greatest impact on children. A White House Conference on Children was called in 1930 to study the economic effects of the depression on the health and well-being of children. Thereafter a conference was held at the beginning of each decade until the 1980s. These conferences have been responsible over the years for many changes in child health and welfare, including funding for essential programs, legislation, and a shift from treating diseases to preventive health care. Attendees were professionals who worked with children, representatives of federal and state agencies and volunteer organizations, and members of various citizens' groups. Although the group did not have legislative powers, together its members raised the consciousness of public officials and private citizens regarding the status of children and families.

The United States did not recover from the Great Depression for many years. In the interim, the Children's Bureau was able to propose legislation that affected children. The most remarkable pieces of legislation were those authorized by the Social Security Act of 1937, which was signed by President Franklin D. Roosevelt. The health care needs of children were incorporated into the provisions of Title V, Maternal and Child Health Services, which among other accomplishments recognized for the first time the needs of disabled children. Another important milestone was the Women, Infants, and Children (WIC) program, which opened its first distribution site in 1974. WIC offers assistance with food and nutrition counseling for low-income pregnant, breastfeeding, and non-breastfeeding postpartum women and infants and children under the age of 5 years (Hockenberry & Wilson, 2007).

Today the Office of Child Development, established in 1967, oversees children's programs. It houses the Children's Bureau and the Bureau of Child Development Services, which operates such programs as Head Start. The Secretary of Health and Human Services is the cabinet officer responsible for all their activities. In December 1987, Congress and President Ronald Reagan created the National Commission on Children to serve as a forum on behalf of the children of the nation. In May 1991, after 2½ years of intensive investigation and deliberation, the 34-member commission concluded that the United States is failing many of its children. For example, the proportion of children who are not adequately immunized for preventable childhood diseases has increased dramatically since the early 1980s. Lack of immunization resulted in 26,500 cases of measles and 60 deaths from measles in 1990. The commission's final report listed numerous recommendations for addressing pressing children's issues, such as the need to ensure income security, improve health, increase educational achievement, prepare adolescents for adulthood, strengthen and support families, and protect vulnerable children and their families.

Child health and child care shows an increase in access to and a more equitable distribution of services in the 1960s. In the late 1970s and the 1980s, the emphasis moved to cost containment. Cost containment and access to care continue to be major issues for those addressing health care reform in the twenty-first century.

Indeed, children are the focus of many of our century's reform initiatives, and solutions are sure to emphasize collaboration between various disciplines. For example, violence, once considered solely a criminal justice problem, is now acknowledged as a preventable public health problem. The most effective solutions for this and other multifaceted problems will require the expertise of health care professionals, as well as law enforcement and criminal justice officials, social workers, economists, and educators.

PEDIATRIC NURSING

The nursing of infants and children is consistent with the revised definition of nursing proposed by the Social Policy Task Force of the American Nurses Association (ANA) in 2003. The definition states that "nursing is the prevention of illness, the alleviation of suffering, and the protection, promotion, and restoration of health in the care of individuals, families, groups, communities, and populations" (ANA, 2003). This definition incorporates the four essential features of nursing practice:

1. Attention to the full range of human experiences and responses to health and illness without restriction to a problem-focused orientation
2. Integration of objective data with knowledge gained from an understanding of the patient or group's subjective experience
3. Application of scientific knowledge to the processes of diagnosis and treatment
4. Provision of a caring relationship that facilitates health and healing (ANA, 2003)

The purpose of pediatric nursing is to promote the highest possible state of health in each child by (1) preventing disease or injury; (2) assisting children, including those with a permanent disability or health problem, to achieve and maintain an optimum level of health and development; and (3) treating or rehabilitating children who have deviations from an optimal state of health.

CHARACTERISTICS OF A PEDIATRIC NURSE

Pediatric nursing is different from other clinical specialties in nursing. First is the requirement that you as a nurse enjoy working with children of all ages. A great deal of time is spent with an individual child. Second, when a child has a health problem, the child, the family, and the disease become a nursing concern; none can be separated from the other two. Pediatric nursing is family-centered nursing in its truest sense. It is very important for the family to be totally involved and have a feeling of control over the decision making concerning their child's health care. It is crucial that you establish a therapeutic rapport with the child as well as the parent while establishing professional boundaries to more effectively meet their needs (Hockenberry & Wilson, 2007).

Your keen observation skills are a must, especially when caring for infants and toddlers or children who are critically ill or cannot communicate in the traditional language-based sense. You will have to be the one to interpret signals of pain, thirst, and other discomforts. By watching children play or perform certain tasks, you will be able to assess their developmental ages. In addition, not all **birth defects (congenital anomalies)** (any abnormality present at birth, particularly a structural one, that is possible to inherit genetically, acquire during gestation, or acquire during the parturition [process of giving birth]) are diagnosed in the newborn period; sometimes you will have the opportunity to identify a problem as a result of your nursing assessment. When children are very ill, minor changes in their physical status sometimes result in a variety of complications, and therefore it is important that you note any changes as early as possible. These examples typify the role observation plays in clinical practice.

Often you will be involved in supporting a child through a difficult procedure or serious illness. Such an endeavor not only includes preparation for the event, it requires establishing a level of trust, which permits children to express their fear, apprehension, and anxiety. To establish a trusting relationship, convey respect to children, talk with them at a level they are able to understand, and most importantly, be honest.

Teaching is ongoing in pediatrics. The forms it takes range from explaining the effects of a medication to an 8-year-old to helping parents learn how to give a subcutaneous injection to their child. There also are innumerable opportunities to help children and parents adapt to a chronic illness or disorder, which requires a nurse's knowledge of community resources or volunteer agencies available for equipment or support.

You also need to be aware of the indirect teaching that occurs through example. A pediatric nurse serves as a role model for children by demonstrating appropriate health promotion and prevention behaviors, such as maintaining good nutrition, a healthy lifestyle, and personal hygiene, or for parents by exhibiting age-appropriate responses to children.

Another role you will fill is that of child and family advocate, whether the situation involves ethical decision making or has more to do with the quality of care given. Sometimes this will take the form of coordinating the activities of a health team and collaborating with members of different disciplines to provide a child with the expert care that is required.

Being able to communicate effectively with a child is essential. However, to enjoy and continue working in pediatrics, what you will need most is the ability to recognize and appreciate the uniqueness that each child or adolescent brings to a nurse-patient relationship. It is that special quality—uniqueness—that anyone who provides care for children is called on to understand, respect, and cherish.

CHILDREN WITH SPECIAL NEEDS

Medical advances over the past two decades have resulted in significant changes in the pediatric population. Fragile or premature infants and children with severe injuries or disabilities are now being saved, children who never would have survived in the past. This progress has not been won without cost: Many of these children are left with chronic or disabling conditions, some with very severe and involved complications. The definition of **children with special needs** includes infants and children with congenital abnormalities, malignancies, gastrointestinal (GI) diseases, and central nervous system (CNS) anomalies. Many of these children depend on technology.

Children with special needs make up approximately 35% of the youngsters hospitalized today. However, many forms of technology previously found only in hospital settings have been adapted for home use. With appropriate services and support, even children with very severe disabilities are living at home with their families and attending school with their peers.

FAMILY-CENTERED CARE

The term **family-centered care,** although present in the nursing literature for many years, has recently undergone redefinition and clarification (Box 30-1). Family-centered care is a philosophy of care that recognizes the family as the constant in the child's life and holds that systems and personnel are called on to support, respect, encourage, and enhance the strengths and competence of the family. Nurses and others in the community support families in their natural caregiving and decision-making roles by building on the family's and individual members' unique strengths.

Three key components of family-centered care are respect, collaboration, and support. Families receive support for their caregiving and decision making when health care professionals build on families' unique strengths and acknowledge their expertise in caring for their child—both within and outside the hospital setting.

Two basic concepts in family-centered care are enabling and empowerment. Professionals **enable** families by creating opportunities for all family members to make use of their abilities and competencies and to acquire new ones that are necessary to meet the needs of the child and the family. **Empowerment** describes the interaction of professionals with families to bring about or cement families' sense of control over their lives. Empowerment frees families to foster their own strengths, abilities, and actions and thus enables them to make positive changes in their lives.

The **parent-professional partnership** is a powerful mechanism for enabling and empowering families.

Box 30-1 Key Elements of Family-Centered Care

- Recognizing that the family is the constant in a child's life; whereas the service systems and personnel within those systems fluctuate
- Facilitating parent-professional collaboration at all levels of health care:
  —Care of an individual child
  —Program development, implementation, and evaluation
  —Policy formation
- Honoring the racial, ethnic, cultural, and socioeconomic diversity of families
- Recognizing family strengths and individuality and respecting different methods of coping
- Sharing with parents, on a continuing basis and in a supportive manner, complete and unbiased information
- Encouraging and facilitating family-to-family support and networking
- Understanding and incorporating the developmental needs of infants, children, and adolescents and their families into health care systems
- Implementing comprehensive policies and programs that provide emotional and financial support to meet the needs of families
- Designing accessible health care systems that are flexible, culturally competent, and responsive to family-identified needs

From Shelton, T.L., & Stepanek, J.S. (1994). *Family-centered care for children needing specialized health and developmental services.* Bethesda, MD: Association for the Care of Children's Health.

Parents serve as respected equals with professionals and have the right to decide what is important for themselves and their family. The professional supports and strengthens the family's ability to nurture and promote family development. Professionals also need to work together as a team to benefit the children and their families.

In a parent-professional partnership, all persons contribute their knowledge, skills, and resources toward the well-being of the patient. The family needs to feel free to contribute according to its strengths and needs. As a pediatric nurse, you will be in a position to assist every family to identify its strengths and use those strengths in a therapeutic manner (Hockenberry & Wilson, 2007).

Children are vulnerable to the major stressors inherent in being hospitalized, such as separation from family and familiar environment, loss of control, bodily trauma, and pain. Many factors influence the child's response to the illness and hospitalization. These factors include the child's developmental age, past experiences with illness or hospitalization, family support system, and coping skills, as well as the gravity of the diagnosis (Hockenberry & Wilson, 2007).

To better understand family-centered care, it helps to compare the typical handling of a particular situation in the past with today's family-centered approach to care. In the past, parents were usually denied access to their child's medical records or hospital chart. With a family-centered care approach, parents have the same access to information about their child as all other members of the child's health care team. Other changes, such as hospitals welcoming parents 24 hours a day, reflect increased acknowledgment of the importance of family.

A family-centered approach to care is an important concept in the nursing care of all children. However, it is crucial for optimum care of children with special needs, who will likely experience repeated contact with the health care system throughout their lives.

PARTNERSHIPS WITH PARENTS

Related to family-centered care is the concept of partnerships with parents. Parental involvement in children's care has evolved since the days when they relinquished their role to institutions; today parents play the role of planners, in addition to recipients, of services.

The best way to promote this role is to establish a partnership between parents and nurses, other caregivers, and service providers. In a true partnership, parents are respected as equals and enjoy their rightful role in deciding what is important for themselves and their family. Your role as a nurse is to support and strengthen the family's ability to nurture and promote its members' development.

Mutual respect is the foundation for effective partnerships with parents. Parents know their child better than anyone else and are able to provide you with important information that you will not be able to obtain in any other way. Parents of children with special needs also often become experts on their child's condition. The tradition of the authoritarian nurse has been replaced by a system where nurses are consultants to the parents, sharing their unique knowledge and decision-making responsibility (Box 30-2).

FUTURE CHALLENGES FOR THE PEDIATRIC NURSE

The present shift in focus from treatment of disease to promotion of health is likely to further expand nurses' roles in ambulatory care, with prevention and health teaching receiving a major emphasis. The need for home care and community health services will make it imperative for nurses to become more independent and acquire skills well beyond those needed in traditional care settings.

Technologic advances will open up new areas of technical skills for pediatric nurses to master and use in patient care. Likewise the demand for computer know-how in work settings will favor nurses with a technology-related expertise.

Changing demographics will also affect you as a pediatric nurse; the adult population is growing faster than the pediatric population. Accompanying this trend is a decrease in the numbers of younger children and an increase in those of older children, as well as a decrease in the white population with an increase in minority groups. Such changes will affect the delivery of health care, with problems of adolescents and minority groups taking on greater significance. You will need to keep abreast of developments in adolescent medicine and continually adapt your care to the cultural environment in which you practice.

Box 30-2 Implementing Family-Centered Care

Although professionals readily accept the concept of family-centered care, they have been slow to implement practices that embody "the family as the patient." This lag has occurred in part because family-centered care requires a shift in orientation regarding the provision of services. The philosophy behind family-centered care requires stretching beyond clinical practices that have become traditional because of their convenience to the institution and personnel.

- Common examples of **system-based care** are exclusionary policies such as not allowing family members to stay with their children during a procedure and restricting visiting hours, as well as the number and the age of visitors.
- Family-centered care means putting families at the center of the caregiving process, with their input serving as the major determinant of the interventions provided. For example, exclusionary policies are replaced with **family-based care,** such as parental and child **choice** regarding separation during procedures, open visiting hours, and no limitations on the age or the number of visitors, except per family request. In fact, the question arises: Aren't we misusing the word *visitor* altogether? Family members certainly are not visitors to their child; nurses and other staff are.
- Even **child-based care** is not synonymous with family-based care. For example, often the hospital dietary service will provide selections for children but fail to provide inexpensive meals for parents or consider family cultural and religious traditions. Primary nurses will at times focus on the child's needs but place little emphasis on the family's concerns.

In your practice, what policies can be considered system-, child-, or family-based care? How can those that are not family based be changed? What reasons do staff give for preferring system-based care?

- Compare your agency's policies with its mission statement and purpose. Fortunately, models of family-centered care do exist and have documented benefits:
  —Families experience greater feelings of confidence and competence and less stress in caring for their children.
  —The dependence of families on professional caregivers decreases.
  —Costs of care decrease.
  —Professionals experience greater job satisfaction.
  —Both parents and providers are empowered to develop new skills and expertise.

NURSING IMPLICATIONS OF GROWTH AND DEVELOPMENT

It is important for you to know the basic principles of normal growth and development to understand what infants and children are like, what can be expected from them, what their needs are, and why they behave as they do. Although each child is unique, groups of children of the same age are more alike than they are different. For example, a number of general statements can be made about the babies in a newborn nursery and yet there are significant differences among them. In knowing their similarities, you will be better able to perform assessments, develop interventions, identify problems, and promote normal development (see Health Promotion box).

Growth and development are complex processes that occur in stages as the body grows and the mind and the personality unfold. The newborn moves through infancy, toddlerhood, preschool age, school age, and adolescence, and each stage consists of predictable, orderly events that are accomplished sequentially. When you know the normal milestones a 6-year-old typically accomplishes, for example, it is easier to identify a delay in the 6-year-old who has not mastered the expected developmental milestones. It is important to realize that there are differences in the rate or the timing with which a child accomplishes a particular task. One infant will sit up at 5 months of age, perhaps, and another at 7 months. However, most infants do so at 6 months of age. As you will probably expect, illness or a lack of stimulation interferes with normal development. Other variables that affect development include a baby's genetic makeup and a host of environmental factors, such as ethnic background, religion, family size, socioeconomic bracket, and education.

A student in pediatric nursing does well to ask why growth and development are important aspects of studying children. One of the nurse's primary responsibilities is to identify an infant or child who is demonstrating cognitive impairment (the preferred term for mental retardation). The earlier intervention takes place, the greater the likelihood of achieving improvement or remediation. You will also have a chance as a pediatric nurse to play a significant role in other types of interventions. For example, you will caution expectant mothers on the hazards of consuming alcohol or smoking while pregnant, refer children with suspected delays to early interventionists, teach parents therapeutic activities and exercises to use with their children, and become knowledgeable about resources in the community that serve children and their families.

Knowledge of child development will allow you to use a developmental rather than a chronologic approach to pediatric nursing care. A developmental approach emphasizes the child's abilities and strengths rather than disabilities and weaknesses. It considers children's individuality and personalities and builds on what they *are able* to do rather than concentrating on what they *are not able* to do.

Understanding normal growth and development will enable you to select age-appropriate toys for the infant or young toddler and devise activities that appeal to the school-age child or adolescent. Children learn through every opportunity that is made available to them. One need only observe a 2-year-old playing with a large four-sided box to appreciate a child's curiosity and creativity. The things you will see that

Health Promotion

Characteristics of the Infant, the Toddler and Child, and the Adolescent: Encouraging Healthy Behaviors at Each Stage

INFANT

- Doubles weight by 6 months; triples weight by 1 year
- Vision at birth is 20/300; by 12 months is 20/100
- Play requires stimulation activities involving motor skills, language, and social skills
- Likes toys that bang, shake, or can be pulled; enjoys playing "peek-a-boo"
- Likes verbal praise and encouragement

Guidance

- Encourage parents not to use baby talk but to pronounce words correctly.
- Sleep is usually established by the spacing of feedings. Encourage parents to give care during awake times either before or after feedings.

TODDLER AND CHILD

- Weight gain from 1 to 3 years is about 5 pounds per year. Usually four times birth weight by 3 years of age
- Period of intense activity and exploration
- Will take one or two naps a day and sleep up to 9 to 12 hours a night
- Bowel and bladder control usually achieved by 3 years of age
- Practices parallel play
- Cognition regarding thinking and reasoning based on magical or egocentric processes
- Experiences physiologic anorexia, which allows the child to either binge or be picky depending on individual growth spurts and plateaus

ADOLESCENT

- Needs to be more independent, and will vacillate between independent and dependent roles, which may be reflected in mood swings
- Will exhibit logical thought and reasoning; often questions values of parents
- Prefers being with peers to establish identity

Guidance

- Recommend milk as drink of choice because of increased needs for calcium.

Table 30-1 Children's Concepts of Illness

INFANTS	PRESCHOOLERS	SCHOOL-AGE CHILDREN	ADOLESCENTS
Perceive illness as generalized discomfort and pain	Conceive of illness as a punishment for bad thoughts or behavior; believe that adults have the power to magically cure the illness if they want to	Sometimes perceive illness as a result of bad or indiscreet behavior; sometimes have an accurate awareness of the location of body parts and a beginning understanding of body processes and functions	Focus on discrete symptoms rather than overall effect of illness; often intellectually question and deal with information about illness; will at times use denial of illness or overcompensate in areas not affected

child think to do with that box will stun and amaze you, or for that matter, any adult.

Age and developmental level influence the ways in which children perceive and make sense of experiences such as illness or disability, and therefore make an impact on their ability to cope. With this knowledge, you will be better prepared to develop appropriate nursing care plans. There are some generalizations that are possible to make regarding children's concept of illness at different stages of development (Table 30-1). Keep in mind that children, particularly very young ones, sometimes change very rapidly in both the physical and developmental senses. Therefore make sure to continually reassess and modify nursing care plans to reflect these changes.

For a pediatric nurse, knowledge of growth and development also is the basis for anticipatory guidance with parents. **Anticipatory guidance** (psychological preparation of a patient for an event expected to be stressful, as you do when preparing a child for surgery by explaining what will happen and what it will feel like; also used to prepare parents for normal growth and development of their children) means to teach parents (and children when they are old enough to understand) what is likely to occur in the coming weeks and months so that it is possible to lay the groundwork now to protect and promote the child's well-being at that time. For example, parents will learn that their 9- or 10-month-old will begin to crawl from one place to another. It is normal, it is expected, and it needs to be allowed. However, parents will have to remove any harmful objects from the child's reach.

Once a child becomes mobile, it is important to "childproof" the environment, making it a safe one for the curious crawler. Play is the work of childhood. It is best done in a safe environment, using toys that are safe. You will play an important role in assisting parents to understand the physical and behavioral changes that occur rapidly in the developing infant or toddler. These principles also are useful in working with school-age children, who will be exposed to many new experiences once they start school, or preadolescents, who need to be ready to manage the hormonal and growth changes they will experience. The parents of the adolescent are usually as confused and perplexed as the youngster is about changes and behavior at this stage of development. Nurses, again, play an important role in supporting and guiding both parent and adolescent through this trying time of life.

PHYSICAL ASSESSMENT OF THE PEDIATRIC PATIENT

The child's rate of growth, level of understanding, and means of communicating differ from their equivalents in the adult. Each stage of childhood is unique, with its own set of characteristics. The challenges that children present to a nurse are constant, exciting, and satisfying. You will find it necessary to use different skills with children of different age-groups.

As in the adult, the sequence of assessing a child follows a head-to-toe direction. Sometimes you will need to alter the sequence to accommodate the child's developmental needs, but document your findings in the traditional way nonetheless.

To prepare a child for a physical assessment, use developmental and chronologic age as the main criteria for the choice of method to assess each body system (Boxes 30-3 and 30-4).

GROWTH MEASUREMENTS

Measurement of physical growth is a key element in evaluation of the health status of children. The growth parameters include weight, height, and head circumference and sometimes skinfold thickness and arm circumference. You will plot the child's measurements by percentiles on growth charts and compare them with those of the general pediatric population to determine deviations from the norm.

The most commonly used growth charts in the United States are from the National Center for Health Statistics (NCHS). The growth charts have been revised to include body mass index for age (BMI-for-age) charts, 3rd and 97th smoothed percentiles for all charts, and the 85th percentile for the weight-for-stature and BMI-for-age charts.

Children whose growth you will probably investigate further include the following:

- Children whose height and weight percentiles are widely disparate (e.g., height in the 10th percentile and weight in the 90th percentile, especially with above-average skinfold thickness).
- Children who fail to show the expected growth rates in height and weight, especially during the rapid growth periods of infancy and adolescence.

Box 30-3 Guidelines for Performing Pediatric Physical Assessment

- Perform examination in appropriate, nonthreatening area:
  - —Have room well lit and decorated with neutral colors
  - —Have room temperature comfortably warm
  - —Place all strange and potentially frightening equipment out of sight
  - —Have some toys, dolls, stuffed animals, and games available for child
  - —If possible, have rooms decorated and equipped for children of different ages
  - —Provide privacy, especially for school-age children and adolescents
- Provide time for play and becoming acquainted.
- Look for behaviors that signal child's readiness to cooperate:
  - —Talking to nurse
  - —Making eye contact
  - —Accepting offered equipment
  - —Allowing physical touching
  - —Choosing to sit on examining table rather than parent's lap
- If you observe no signs of readiness, use the following techniques:
  - —Talk to patient; gradually focus on a favorite object, such as doll
  - —Make complimentary remarks about child, such as appearance, dress, or a favorite object
  - —Tell a funny story or play a simple magic trick
  - —Have a nonthreatening "friend" available, such as a hand puppet, to "talk" to child for the nurse
- If child refuses to cooperate, use the following techniques:
  - —Assess reason for uncooperative behavior; consider that a child who is unduly afraid has perhaps had a previous experience that was traumatic
  - —Try to involve child and parent in process
  - —Avoid prolonged explanations about examining procedure
  - —Use a firm, direct approach regarding expected behavior
  - —Perform examination as quickly as possible
  - —Have attendant gently restrain child
  - —Minimize any disruptions or stimulations: limit number of people in room; use isolated room; use quiet, calm, confident voice
- Begin examination in a nonthreatening manner for young children or children who are fearful:
  - —Use approaches such as "Simon says" to encourage child to make a face, squeeze a hand, stand on one foot, and so on
- Use "paper-doll" technique:
  1. Lay child supine on an examining table or floor that is covered with a large sheet of paper
  2. Trace around child's body
  3. Use body outline to demonstrate what will be examined, such as drawing a heart and listening with the stethoscope before performing the activity on child.
- Involve child in examination process:
  - —Provide choices, such as sitting on the bed or the chair
  - —Allow child to handle or hold equipment
  - —Encourage child to use equipment on a doll, family member, or examiner
  - —Explain each step of the procedure in simple language
  - —Examine child in a comfortable and secure position: sitting in parent's lap; sitting upright if in respiratory distress
  - —Proceed to examine the body in an organized sequence (usually head to toe) with the following exceptions: Examine painful areas last; in emergency situation, examine vital functions (airway, breathing, and circulation) and injured area first
  - —Reassure child throughout examination, especially about bodily concerns that arise during puberty
  - —Discuss findings with family at end of examination
  - —Praise child for cooperation during examination; give reward such as small toy, stickers, or sucker

Box 30-4 Assessing Body Systems by Age

Using developmental and chronologic age as the main criteria for the choice of method to assess each body system accomplishes several goals:

- Minimizes stress and anxiety associated with assessment of various body parts
- Fosters a trusting nurse-child-parent relationship
- Allows for maximum preparation of the child
- Preserves the essential security of the parent-child relationship, especially with young children
- Maximizes the accuracy and reliability of assessment findings

- Children who show a sudden increase, except during puberty, or a decrease in a previously steady growth pattern.

Because growth is a continuous but uneven process, the most reliable evaluation lies in comparison of growth measurements of each child over a prolonged time (Table 30-2).

Table 30-2 Expected Growth Rates at Various Ages

AGE	EXPECTED GROWTH RATE PER YEAR (cm)	(in)
1 to 6 months	18-22	7.2-8.8
6 to 12 months	14-18	5.6-7.2
Second year	11	4.4
Third year	8	3.2
Fourth year	7	2.8
Fifth to tenth years	5-6	2-2.4

You will measure head circumference in children up to 36 months. The area you measure is usually above the eyebrows and pinna of the ears and around the occipital prominence at the back of the skull (Figure 30-1).

Length refers to measurements taken when children are supine. Until children are 2 years old, you will measure recumbent length. Have someone assist by holding the child's head in midline while you extend the child's legs to take a measurement.

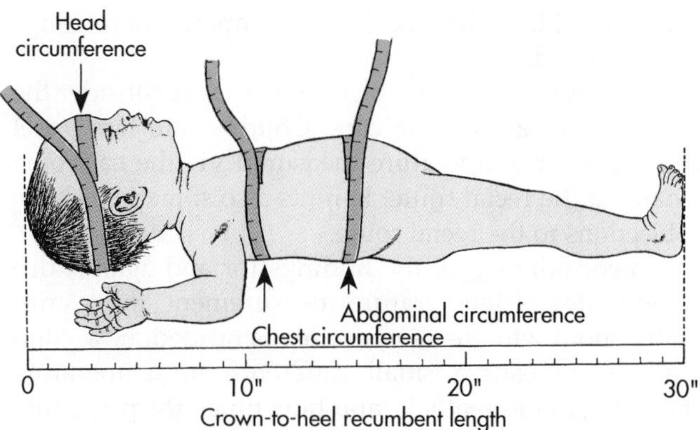

FIGURE 30-1 Measurement of head, chest, and abdominal circumference and crown-to-heel measurement (recumbent length).

Height refers to a measurement when a child stands upright.

Weight

A child's weight will reflect fluid loss and inadequate calories, especially in the infant and the toddler. Use the same scale and weigh the child at the same time every day. Perform weight measurements in a warm room. What children wear and what is attached to them will affect weight. For example, the weight of a naked infant (birth to 36 months) with a nasogastric (NG) tube, electrodes, and intravenous (IV) armboard differs significantly from that of the infant without these attachments. If equipment has been added or removed, document this on the graphic sheet. Usually you will weigh older children with underpants or a light gown (Figure 30-2). In any case, respect the privacy of all children.

Skinfold Thickness

Determine skinfold thickness at one site, taking at least two measurements for the greatest reliability (Box 30-5).

Box 30-5 Measuring Triceps Skinfold Thickness

- With child's right arm flexed 90 degrees at elbow, mark midpoint between acromion and olecranon on posterior aspect of arm.
- With arm hanging freely, grasp a fold of skin between thumb and forefinger 1 cm above midpoint.
- Gently pull fold away from underlying muscle and continue to hold through the remaining steps until measurement is completed.
  —Place caliper jaws over skinfold at midpoint mark; if a plastic catheter (e.g., Ross Adipometer) is used, apply pressure with thumb to align lines on caliper; follow directions for using other calipers.
  —Estimate reading to nearest millimeter, 2 or 3 seconds after applying pressure.
  —Take measurements until you obtain two readings that agree within 1 mm.

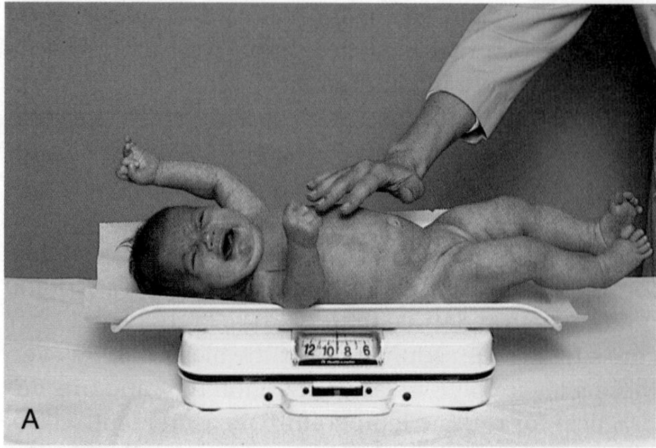

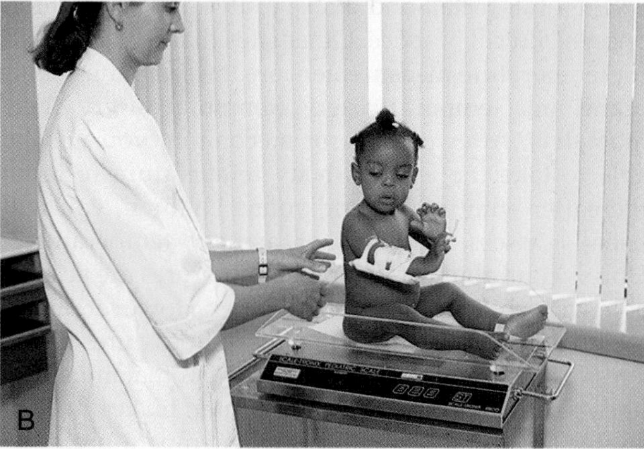

FIGURE 30-2 A, Infant on scale. **B,** Toddler on scale.

Arm circumference measures muscle mass. Follow the same procedure as for skinfold thickness except measurement is made with a tape.

VITAL SIGNS

Key elements in evaluating physical status are vital signs—temperature, pulse, respiration, and blood pressure. (For best results in taking vital signs of an infant, count respirations first, before the infant is disturbed; take pulse second, and temperature last.)

Body temperature, which also reflects metabolism, is fairly stable from infancy through adulthood. Following the unstable regulatory ability in the neonatal period, heat production steadily declines as the infant grows into childhood. In an air-conditioned delivery room, the newborn's temperature will sometimes drop to 97° F (36.1° C) or lower, which accounts for the use of radiant warmers for newborns after delivery. Newborns also tend to have difficulty dissipating heat in an overheated environment, which increases the risk of hyperthermia.

Despite the ability to regulate their temperatures, infants and toddlers are prone to wide variations, especially after crying for extended periods or after active play. Temperature elevations also occur rapidly in young children when infections are present.

Beginning at approximately 12 years of age, girls display a temperature that remains relatively stable, whereas the temperature in boys continues to fall for a few years longer. Females maintain a temperature slightly above that of males throughout life (for normal temperature in children see Table 30-3).

The primary purpose of measuring body temperature is to detect abnormally high or low values. In febrile patients, the chief concern is the temperature of the brain, because very high temperatures have the capacity to cause neural damage. Thus the best sites for measuring temperature are those closest to the brain, which reflect central, or core, body heat. Other core sites are the esophagus and the bladder. However, these sites involve invasive thermometry and are impractical for routine temperature measurement.

The oral, rectal, and axillary sites are all common ones in clinical practice. Other sites that are now used for temperature measurement are the tympanic membrane and temporal artery (temporal artery thermometry). After passage of meconium, you will be able to take the infant's body temperature rectally; thereafter with infants and young children, you will usually assess tympanic or axillary temperatures. Unless contraindicated, oral temperatures are acceptable with children 6 years and older. However, many facilities are now using tympanic temperatures for all ages. The ear's proximity to the hypothalamus, the body's temperature-regulating center, makes it a desirable area for reflecting true core temperature.

In comparisons with rectal, oral, or axillary temperature assessments in children, tympanic membrane measurements are fairly insensitive in detecting fevers and should be used with caution for children younger than 3 years of age.

In addition, the size of the probe has the potential to influence the reading. Many ear probes are too large to be correctly placed in the canal. An infrared ear thermometer, the Ototemp Pedi-Q, features a small (2.5 mm) probe that fits in the infant's ear and gives a reliable tympanic membrane temperature.

Technique is also a very important factor. For the sensor to detect heat from the drum, not from the cooler canals, you will have to straighten the ear canal, as when using an otoscope. With the ear pulled back and down and the probe tip pointing at the midpoint between the eyebrow and the sideburn on the opposite side of the face, higher temperature readings are obtained.

Finally, in deciding which route to use, consider the principle of atraumatic care. Children are less upset having their temperature measured via the ear route than via the rectal route. Parents also sometimes have objections to the rectal route.

In considering all the findings for and against different sites of temperature measurement, think critically about why the temperature is needed, how clinically significant a small difference in temperature between routes really is, and how much the procedure upsets the child and the caregiver. Remember, we are not even sure what normal body temperature is. The gold standard of 98.6° F (37° C) in adults has been questioned since it varies among individuals.

Heart Rate or Pulse

Great variations also exist in the heart rates of children. Although the apical beat of a newborn sometimes reaches 152 per minute, the heart rate gradually slows to 72 to 75 beats per minute by adolescence (Table 30-4). The presence of infection increases the heart rate, as does physical activity. During sleep, a child's pulse is at its slowest rate.

Take note of the rhythm and any irregularities in rate. Count the pulse rate for 1 full minute. Whereas you will take an apical pulse on infants and young children, with children 5 years of age and older you will often take a radial pulse. An apical pulse measurement, heard at the apex of the heart (located at the fifth intercostal space on the left side), is more reliable if you take it while the patient is asleep. To assess for murmurs of the heart, listen at the second intercostal space.

Respiration

Count respirations in the same manner as you do in the adult. Newborns are obligate nasal breathers, which means they breathe only through their noses; they will not breathe through the mouth until they reach 3 or 4 weeks of age. The infant's respirations are primarily diaphragmatic; use the abdominal movements you observe for your count. In children younger than 7 years of age, respiratory movements are abdominal or dia-

Table 30-3 Normal Temperature in Children

	TEMPERATURE	
AGE	(° F)	(° C)
3 months	99.4	37.5
6 months	99.5	37.5
1 year	99.7	37.7
3 years	99.0	37.2
5 years	98.6	37.0
7 years	98.3	36.8
9 years	98.1	36.7
11 years	98.0	36.7
13 years	97.8	36.6

Table 30-4 Vital Signs (Averages)

AGE	HEART RATE PER MINUTE	RESPIRATIONS PER MINUTE	BLOOD PRESSURE
Newborn	120	35	70/50
1-11 months	120	30	90/60
2 years	110	25	96/68
4 years	100	23	100/70
6 years	100	21	105/70
10 years	90	20	108/70
12 years	88	20	110/70
16 years	70	20	120/70

phragmatic. In older children, respirations are chiefly thoracic. The respiratory rate also slows as a child progresses from infancy to adolescence.

A newborn's respiratory rate is extremely erratic, so for accuracy it is necessary to count it for 1 full minute to take account of any irregularities. Assess the rate, the depth, and the quality of respirations. The rate in the newborn will sometimes be as rapid as 40 to 50 breaths per minute, gradually slowing to 25 to 32 per minute by 36 hours of age (see Table 30-4 for normal respiratory rate in children).

Blood Pressure

You will measure blood pressure in children 3 years of age and older (Box 30-6). Blood pressure is low in a newborn. Gradually it rises, so that by the end of adolescence it is about 120/78 mm Hg (see Table 30-4). Any child with symptoms of hypertension, or those in intensive care, at high risk, and in emergency departments, need to have their blood pressure measured.

To ensure accuracy when doing a blood pressure reading, it is important to use the correct cuff size. Make sure the cuff covers two thirds of the length of the upper arm or leg (Box 30-7).

See sites for measuring children's blood pressure in Figure 30-3.

The technique for measuring blood pressure in children is the same as that for an adult. Because children are easily upset by unfamiliar procedures, it is best to explain each step. For preschool and early school-age children, explain how the cuff will feel, such as "tight feeling," "arm hug," or "I want to feel your muscle." Use an explanation such as, "I want to see how strong your muscle is."

Box 30-6 Calculating Normal Blood Pressure

Use the following quick formula to calculate normal systolic blood pressure:

- 1 to 7 years: Age in years + 90
- 8 to 18 years: (2 × age in years) + 83

Use the following quick formula to calculate normal diastolic blood pressure:

- 1 to 5 years: 56
- 6 to 8 years: Age in years + 52

Box 30-7 Correct Blood Pressure Cuff Size

- In choosing cuffs, use an appropriately sized one
- Cuff of proper size will cover two thirds of the length of the upper arm or leg
- If a cuff of the correct size is not available, use an oversized cuff rather than an undersized one, or use another site that more appropriately fits the cuff size
- Do not choose a cuff based on the name of the cuff (e.g., an "infant" cuff will be too small for some infants)

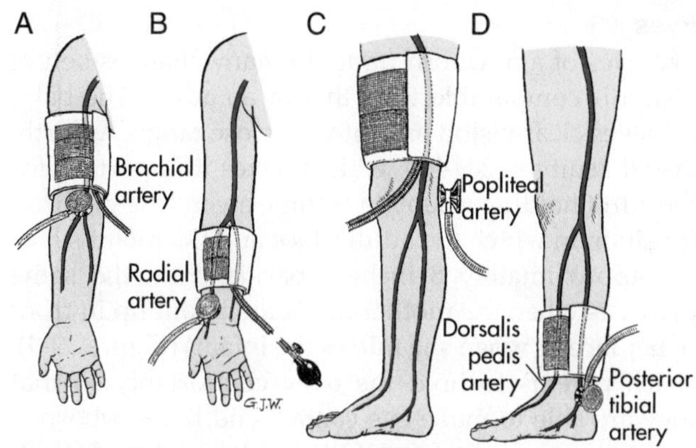

FIGURE 30-3 Sites for measuring blood pressure. **A,** Upper arm. **B,** Lower arm or forearm. **C,** Thigh. **D,** Calf or ankle.

Because results are best when the child is quiet and relaxed during the procedure, measure blood pressure before performing any anxiety-producing procedures. Infants and small children are often quieter if you take the reading while they are sitting on the parent's lap. Never place the blood pressure cuff on any limb with an intravenous site.

HEAD-TO-TOE ASSESSMENT

Skin

Genetic factors influence assessment of skin color, as do physiologic factors. Edema decreases intensity of skin color, sometimes producing false pallor. Pallor is a sign of potential anemia, chronic disease, edema, or shock. Compare pallor or cyanosis (bluish tone) against the color change normally produced by blanching, using the nonpigmented nail: press down on the free edge of the nail and observe return blood flow. Apply pressure to the lips or gums of dark-skinned individuals to observe color change. A yellow tint sometimes indicates jaundice.

Erythema will usually be the result of increased temperature, local inflammation, or infection. Normal skin texture in the young child is smooth, soft, and slightly dry to the touch.

Accessory Structures

Scalp hair is usually lustrous, silky, and elastic. Genetic factors influence the appearance of hair. Tufts of hair anywhere along the spine, especially the sacrum, are significant because they sometimes mark the site of spina bifida occulta.

Normal nails are pink, convex, smooth, and hard but flexible, not brittle. Dark-skinned individuals sometimes have more deeply pigmented nailbeds. Variation in color, such as blueness, suggests cyanosis.

Each individual has a distinct set of handprints and footprints. The palm normally shows three flexion creases. If grossly abnormal lines or folds are observed, sometimes a specialist will investigate further. It is important to note that the skin and accessory structures change with the aging process of an individual.

Eyes

The eyes of a newborn undergo many changes before vision is comparable with that of an adult. The baby achieves clear vision only at very close range. At birth, visual acuity is 20/400, which makes it important for the adult holding a baby to assume an **en face position** (position in which the adult's face and the infant's face are approximately 8 inches apart and on the same plane, as when the mother holds the infant up in front of her face or when she nurses the infant) (Figure 30-4). Teach parents to hold the baby comfortably so that they are able to make eye contact and the newborn is able to gaze on the face of the holder. Although tears are absent immediately after birth, by the second week of life tear glands begin to function. Newborns develop the ability to follow bright, colorful objects by the second or third week of life.

Although visual acuity is 20/200 by the fourth or fifth month, depth perception does not develop before the ninth or tenth month. One-year-olds, who enjoy playing with large objects (blocks, toys, and boxes), often bump into obstacles because their vision is only 20/100. Vision improves to 20/30 to 20/22 by age 2 to 3 years. When a child starts school, **accommodation** (changes in ciliary muscle and the lens in bringing light rays from various distances to focus on the retina) and **refraction** (the production by the normal eye of the proper image of the object on the retina) also are present. It takes almost 6 years of continual development for the parts of the eyes to function as they do in an adult.

Ears

Inspect the ear for general hygiene. If the ear canal appears free of **cerumen** (a waxy substance produced by the ceruminous gland in the outer portion of the canal), ask about ear-cleaning methods. It is best to question the parent and child about ear cleaning by remarking on how clean the ears are and asking how they remove wax. This approach will more likely yield an honest answer. Advise parents and children to clean the ears with a washcloth and, if they use a swab, to gently wipe only the outer portion of the external canal. Also advise that they will be able to soften any cerumen that is hard by instilling 2 or 3 drops of mineral oil into the ear for a few days and then rinsing the external canal with an ear syringe.

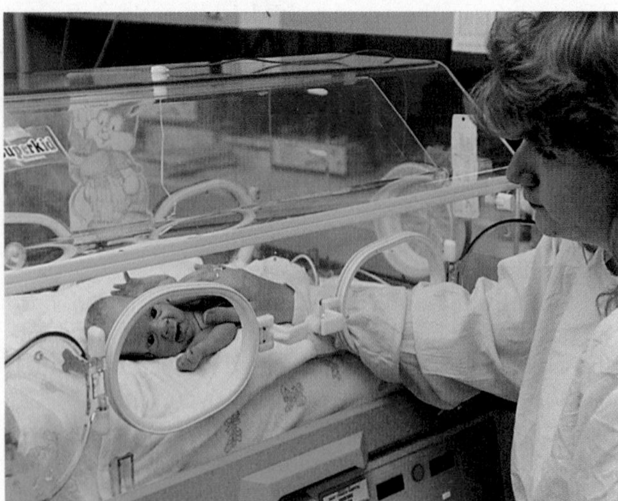

FIGURE 30-4 Sometimes a mother has to overcome a physical barrier to achieve the en face position.

Nose, Mouth, and Throat

The nose normally lies from the center point between the eyes to the notch of the upper lip. Normally there is no discharge from the nose. It is important to inspect the lining of the mouth. Ask the child to open the mouth wide, to move the tongue in different directions, and to say "Ahh," which depresses the tongue for full view of the mouth.

Infants and toddlers, however, usually resist and will not open their mouth. If the child resists, pinch the nostrils closed; this forces the child to open the mouth to breathe. Place the tongue blade along the side of the tongue, not the center, where the gag reflex is elicited. You will frequently see protrusion of the tongue in children with cognitive impairment.

It is also important to check the number of teeth. The **primary (deciduous) teeth** (baby teeth; the set of 20 teeth that normally appear during infancy) begin to descend between the sixth and ninth months of life. The central incisors are the first teeth to appear. By a child's third birthday, all 20 primary teeth are present. The exact mechanisms responsible for the eruption of teeth are not fully understood. The eruption of teeth is distressing to most babies, whose gums become erythematous and edematous. The fussiness demonstrated sometimes results in a refusal to eat. A cold teething ring and numbing (locally anesthetizing) agents provide some relief to painful gums. Good dental hygiene begins as soon as the primary teeth erupt. See Figure 30-5 for the sequence of eruption of primary teeth.

Permanent teeth begin to appear at about 6 years, and most are present by 12 years.

Lungs

Guidelines for effective auscultation of lung sounds in children are seen in Box 30-8 and Figure 30-6.

Chest

During infancy, the chest is almost circular. As the child grows, the chest size normally increases in a transverse direction. Asymmetry in the chest indicates the possibility of serious underlying problems such as cardiac enlargement (bulging on left side of ribcage) or pulmonary dysfunction. Most often asymmetry in the adolescent is a sign of **scoliosis** (lateral curvature of the spine). In an older child, a barrel-shaped chest

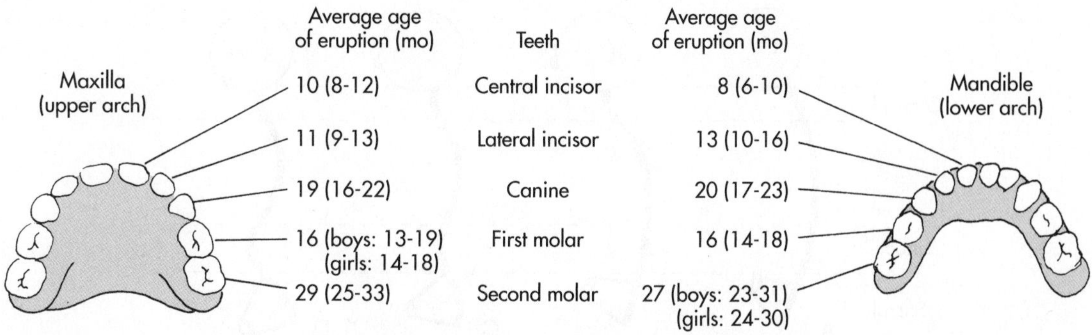

FIGURE 30-5 Sequence of eruption of primary teeth.

Box 30-8 Guidelines for Effective Auscultation of Lungs

- Make sure child is relaxed and not crying, talking, or laughing. Record if child is crying.
- Check that room is comfortable and quiet.
- Warm the stethoscope before placing it against skin.
- Apply firm pressure on chestpiece but not enough to prevent vibrations and transmission of sound.
- Avoid placing stethoscope over hair or clothing, moving it against skin, breathing on tubing, or sliding fingers over chestpiece, all of which often cause sounds that falsely resemble pathologic findings.
- Use a symmetric and orderly approach to compare sounds.
- Ask child to "blow out" the light on an otoscope or pocket flashlight; discreetly turn off the light on the last try so that the child feels successful (see Figure 30-6).
- Place a cotton ball in child's palm; ask child to blow the ball into the air and have parent catch it.
- Place a small tissue on the top of a pencil and ask child to blow the tissue off.
- Have child blow a pinwheel, a party horn, or bubbles.

sometimes indicates chronic obstructive pulmonary disease such as cystic fibrosis or asthma.

Back

The back of a newborn is C-shaped. As growth occurs, the typical S-shaped curve is seen in the older child and the adult. Marked curvature in posture is abnormal. Scoliosis is an important childhood problem, especially in females (Figure 30-7).

Abdomen

Examination of the abdomen involves the following:

- **Inspection** done while the child is erect and supine. Normally in infants and young children, the abdomen is cylindric. In the supine position, it is flat.
- **Auscultation**—unlike listening to heart or the lung sounds with a stethoscope gently on the skin, to hear bowel sounds it is necessary to press the diaphragm of the stethoscope firmly against the abdominal surface.

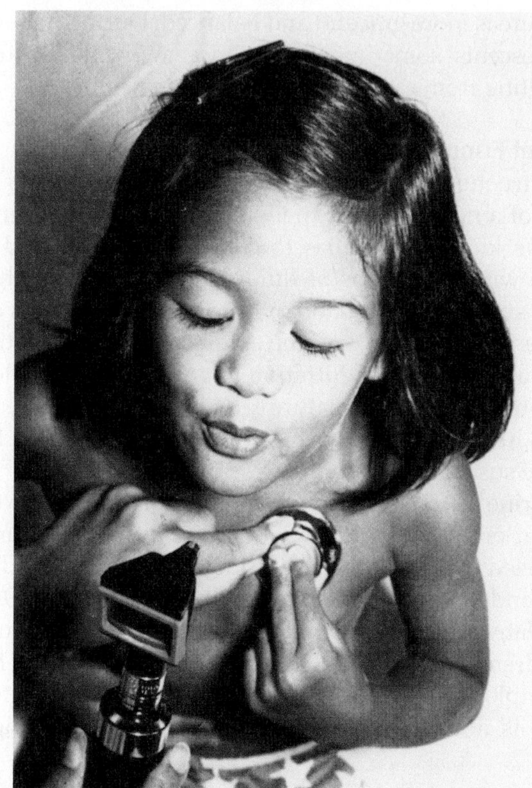

FIGURE 30-6 Auscultating lungs while child "blows out" otoscope light.

The most important sound to listen for is peristalsis, which you will possibly hear every 10 to 30 seconds, depending on when the child last ate. Normal peristalsis sounds like metallic clicks and gurgles. Loud grumbling noises usually denote hunger. Always report absence of bowel sounds or hyperperistalsis, because either usually denotes an abdominal disorder.

Extremities

Examine the extremities at birth for symmetry, range of motion, and signs of malformation. Count fingers and toes to be certain of normal numbers. As a toddler begins to walk, the legs are usually bowlegged until lower body and leg muscles develop. It is also important to observe the infant and the toddler for arch development and correct gait. By school age, the walking

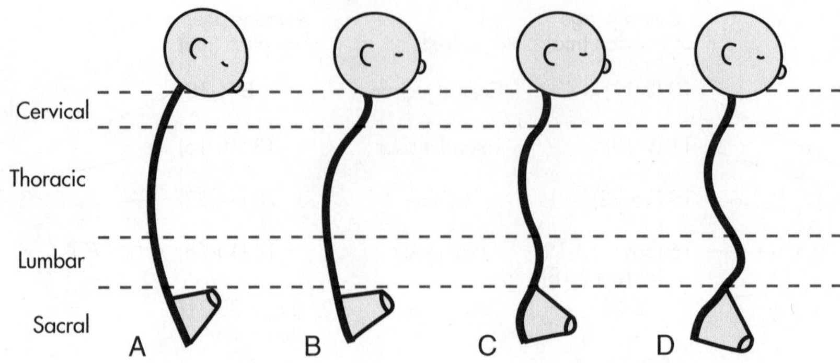

FIGURE 30-7 Development of spinal curvatures. **A,** Newborn. **B,** Cervical secondary curvature. **C,** Lumbar secondary curvature. **D,** Lordosis.

posture is more graceful and balanced. During puberty, adolescents sometimes experience awkward posture resulting from rapid growth of extremities.

Renal Function

All structural components are present in the renal system of a newborn, but there is a functional deficiency in the kidneys' abilities to concentrate urine and to cope with conditions of fluid and electrolyte fluctuation, such as dehydration or fluid overload. Infants are more prone to fluid volume excess and to dehydration because glomerular filtration and absorption are low as a result of the immature kidney function. The kidneys in children are not protected by padding and become susceptible to injury.

Urine output varies and depends on the size of the infant or child. Table 30-5 identifies average volumes excreted at given ages. The urine is colorless and odorless and has a specific gravity of approximately 1.020.

Many tests done in adults are not done in young children because of the immature kidney function. For example, urea clearance is impaired in young children, so it is not measured in infants or toddlers younger than 2.

Anus

It is important to check a child's anal sphincter. Note history of bowel movements for diarrhea, constipation, or rectal bleeding, which will aid in establishing what is normal. Inspect the skin around the anal area for lesions, the most common of which are caused by diaper rash. If the child complains of perianal itching, test for pinworms.

Table 30-5 Kidney Function and Urine Output

AGE	VOLUME OF URINE OUTPUT
Preterm newborn	1-3 mL/kg/hr
Full-term newborn	3-4 mL/kg/hr
6 months	12 mL/hr
1 year	22 mL/hr
5 years	28 mL/hr
12 years	33-35 mL/hr

Genitalia

Genitalia examination is usually uneventful for infants or toddlers but can be anxiety producing for older preschoolers, school-age children, and adolescents.

The genital examination is an excellent time for eliciting questions concerning body functions or sexual activity. It provides an opportunity to increase or reinforce the child's knowledge of reproductive anatomy and explain its function.

During the male genital examination, assess the external appearance of the glans and the shaft of the penis, the prepuce, the urethral meatus, and the scrotum. Edema, skin lesions, inflammation, or other irregularities are possible signs of underlying disorders, especially sexually transmitted infections (STIs). You will usually limit your examination of the female genitalia to inspection and palpation of external structures.

FACTORS INFLUENCING GROWTH AND DEVELOPMENT

NUTRITION

Looking at the child holistically prompts you to add your awareness of his or her nutritional heritage to your assessment of current family nutrition. Nutrition is probably the single most important influence on growth. During infancy and childhood, the demand for calories is great because of rapid increase in height and weight. Growth is uneven during infancy and adolescence. A child's appetite fluctuates in response to growth spurts. The average child (e.g., 6- to 10-year-old child) expends 55% of energy metabolized for maintenance of body functions, 25% for physical activity, 8% in fecal loss, and 12% for growth. Good nutrition begins before conception and is closely related to good health throughout life.

Infants begin life outside the womb nursing at the breast or ingesting formula or breast milk by bottle or tube. Human milk is the most desirable complete diet for the infant for the first 6 months of life. Until 12 months of age, it is best for infants to receive only breast milk or formula. Advise against giving whole cow's milk until the child passes the 12-month mark, because it can cause occult GI bleeding and iron deficiency anemia in young infants. Skim or low-fat milk is not recommended because the essential fatty acids are inadequate and the solute concentration of protein and electrolytes, such as sodium, is too high.

Most infants are given solid foods at 4 to 6 months of age when they begin to need more iron in the diet and their teeth begin to erupt. Iron-fortified cereal is the first solid food most parents give to a baby. Rice cereal is easily digested and has low allergenic potential, so it is a common choice. However, oatmeal and barley are high-protein cereals and make good options as well. After several months of breast milk or formula, the addition of solid foods to an infant's diet is a significant developmental step.

Although the order of introduction of foods other than cereal is arbitrary, the usual sequence is strained fruits, fruit juices, strained vegetables, and strained meats. As more teeth erupt, suggest offering finger food such as zwieback. This helps infants develop a hand-to-mouth cycle, which is basic to feeding themselves.

It is important for each new food to be introduced at weekly intervals so that it is possible to recognize any food allergies (an allergic response sometimes takes several days to appear). Development of a rash, wheezing, or diarrhea is a common sign indicating the presence of an allergy to a food.

By 9 months, several teeth have erupted, and it is possible to offer junior foods, which are of much coarser texture. These fruits, vegetables, and meats taste different, and their different texture encourages the infant to chew. Good choices of finger foods to give at this time include pieces of fruit (excluding grapes, which could choke the infant) and cooked vegetables.

The cost of baby foods is significant; therefore as the infant acquires more teeth and does not experience difficulty eating solids, encourage parents to prepare these foods at home. Canned foods other than those prepared for infants often contain excessive sodium or sugar. If sweetening is needed, refined sugar is acceptable to use, but advise against using honey and corn syrup because of the risk of infant botulism. Encourage cooking fresh or frozen foods and using a blender or food processor. By 12 to 15 months, toddlers are usually eating table food prepared for the family. Although using a spoon is messy, typical toddlers become angry and frustrated when they are "ready" to feed themselves and parents continue to feed them.

Weaning (gradually eliminating breastfeeding or bottle feeding and instituting cup and table feedings) is a major accomplishment of toddlerhood. The earlier method of feeding has provided the child with a great deal of pleasure and satisfaction, and giving it up is sometimes difficult for child and parent alike. Solid foods also are pleasing to the taste buds, but when toddlers feed themselves with a spoon, turning it upside down as they navigate the utensil toward their mouth, they lose much of the food. The same occurs with a cup. A plastic cup with a spout decreases the amount of milk or juice that is spilled. Most 9- or 10-month-old infants who are able to sit in their high chairs begin to demonstrate a readiness to wean. They become much more active and squirm when they are held for feedings. In addition, they observe siblings and adults drinking from cups or glasses and desire to do the same. Gradually, parents will replace bottle feedings or breastfeedings with the cup. Usually the bedtime feeding is the last one parents discontinue. Never allow a child to take a bottle of milk or any sweetened liquids to bed, because this is a major cause of dental caries in deciduous teeth. If the child requires a bottle at bedtime, have the parent give water.

Ideally, concentrated sugars and high-carbohydrate snacks are absent from the young child's diet. The form of sugar in foods is important. Cariogenic foods are those that are sticky and hard and remain in the mouth longer (e.g., lollipops). Help parents plan meals and snacks including foods less damaging to teeth.

As children move through toddler and preschool stages, they often develop fads with strong preferences. Teach the school-age child and parent the value of a diet balanced to promote growth. Adolescent problems include dietary imbalance and excesses. Excess intake of calories, sugar, fat, cholesterol, and sodium are common. Inadequate intake of certain vitamins is evident among girls and teens of low socioeconomic status. In combination with other factors, these dietary patterns tend to result in increased risk of chronic disease such as heart disease, osteoporosis, and some types of cancer later in life. At least once during the teen years, provide total cholesterol screening for adolescents whose parents have a serum cholesterol level greater than 240 mg/day; also provide it when an adolescent passes the 19th birthday.

Each year, approximately 41 per 1000 adolescents become pregnant (Centers for Disease Control and Prevention [CDC], 2009). The pregnant teen exhibits food preferences, eating behaviors, and lifestyle habits similar to nonpregnant peers. Frequent snacking on foods high in fat and sugar and low in essential nutrients (calcium, iron, zinc, folate, and vitamins B_6, A, and C) cause special concerns during pregnancy. Nurses play a central role in meeting the needs of pregnant teenagers. You are frequently the one the young girl will turn to for help and guidance in her dilemma and the one she relies on for support and reassurance. Focus your nutritional assessment on the dietary adequacy of iron, calcium, and multivitamins with folic acid.

METABOLISM

Metabolic needs vary among individuals. The rate of metabolism is highest in the newborn infant because the ratio of total body surface area to body weight is much greater in the infant than it is in the adult. This proportion decreases as the child grows and matures. The basal metabolic rate (BMR) is a measure of metabolism when the body is at rest, and it changes dramatically as the body increases in size. If you consider that newborns double their birth weight by 5 to 6 months and triple it by about 1 year of age, you will better appreciate the rapid rate at which metabolism occurs in very young children.

The body uses energy provided by foods. Whereas the energy requirements for an infant are highest during the first 6 months of life, they are fairly constant from 4 to 10 years and vary in adolescence, depending on the teen's physical development (Table 30-6).

Because metabolism is so high in infants and children, their ability to recover from surgery or a fractured bone is swift compared with that of an adult. With the accelerated rate of all bodily functions, healing occurs quickly, provided all necessary nutritional components are in place. For example, a fractured femur at birth is united in 3 weeks, but an 8-year-old with the same type of fracture requires 8 weeks for union, and a 20-year-old takes 20 weeks to heal.

SLEEP AND REST

Children spend less total time sleeping as they mature. The newborn sleeps much of the time not occupied with feeding and other aspects of care. Most babies are sleeping through the night by the latter part of their first year and take one or two naps a day. Most 12- to 18-month-olds usually nap once a day. The 3-year-old child has usually given up all daytime naps.

The best way to prevent sleep problems with the infant and child is to establish bedtime rituals that do not foster problematic patterns. One of the most constructive ways is to place the infant awake in his or her own crib or bed. Advise using the bed for sleeping only—not as a playpen.

Table 30-6 Daily Caloric Needs of Infants, Children, and Adolescents

AGE-GROUP	CALORIC NEEDS (kcal/kg)
INFANTS	
Birth to 6 months	108
6-12 months	98
CHILDREN	
1-3 years	102
4-6 years	90
7-10 years	70
ADOLESCENTS	
Males	
11-14 years	55
15-18 years	45
Females	
11-14 years	47
15-18 years	40

Modified from Food and Nutrition Board. (1989). *Recommended daily allowances.* (10th ed.). Washington, DC: National Academy Press.

SPEECH AND COMMUNICATION

Crying at birth is the earliest evidence of speech, wordless though it is. Infants use this method of communicating when they are hungry, in pain, or need to be changed. Crying is gradually followed by other sounds, such as cooing, laughing, or babbling. By 9 months, infants practice the noises they are able to make and painstakingly repeat them. Infants enjoy the sounds of their own voice. While they begin to express themselves, they also begin to imitate the vocal sounds of an adult. It is possible to have an actual conversation with the infant. Although no formal words are exchanged, it is a pleasant experience. The adult speaks, the infant responds, the adult answers, and so on. While each takes a turn at contributing to this verbal exchange, the "conversation" usually ends with laughter. As the infant begins to enjoy experimenting with these sounds, it is important to encourage these vocalizations; it is positive reinforcement for oral communication.

A 1-year-old has a three- or four-word vocabulary. It usually includes **mama** and **dada.** In toddlerhood, more words are understood than expressed. Children usually know 25 to 50 words by 18 months, but by 2 years they often know more than 250 words. Speech develops rapidly at this stage, as children practice and learn new words and their meanings. Soon they are able to say a two- or three-word sentence. Preschoolers have a fairly extensive vocabulary to convey their wants, needs, and desires.

Speech ability is determined by the child's stage of development, the amount of stimulation or encouragement received from adults, the child's health status, and many other factors. In addition, the development of language does not occur in isolation. It is related to the physiologic, neurologic, and psychosocial progress that is occurring simultaneously. Children learn the complex symbol system of language with astonishing speed.

Make sure you know what typifies speech at certain stages of childhood. That knowledge helps you identify any problems. For example, the lack of babbling or the inability of a 9-month-old to imitate sounds is a possible indication of deafness or hearing impairment. All babies make verbal sounds until 6 or 7 months of age, but then the child who is unable to hear will decrease these verbalizations in favor of gesturing or some expression of body language (or nonverbal communication).

You will use verbal communication in a variety of ways in your practice. Talking softly to infants while cuddling them is an important part of establishing trust in a relationship with babies. Although the toddler is leery of strangers, if you talk with a parent first, the 2-year-old senses the trusting attitude of the adult and begins to participate in the conversation. As a result of improving verbal skills, preschoolers and school-age children understand more and share their concerns more easily. Teaching 8- and 10-year-olds is particularly satisfying because they are eager to learn. On the other hand, adolescents who have refined their verbal abilities communicate a significant amount of information nonverbally through body language, gestures, or facial expressions. General strategies to consider when talking with children include the following:

- Use a calm, unhurried, and confident voice.
- Speak clearly, be specific, and use as few words as possible. As a general guide, use sentences whose sum of words is equal to the child's age in years plus one.
- State directions and suggestions in a positive way; for example, say, "You need to stay very still," rather than, "Don't move."
- Because children see things only in relation to themselves and from their viewpoint, focus communication on them.
- After greeting the child, continue to talk to both the child and the parent while pursuing activities that do not involve the child directly.
- Use play as a strategy for getting to know the child. For example, if the child has a doll or a stuffed animal, begin by speaking to the toy. Then initiate conversation with the child by asking simple questions about the toy.
- Listen to and observe the child at play. Often children will express important information, such as complicated or difficult feelings, through this familiar medium.
- Look for opportunities to offer the child choices, but offer them only when they really exist. (It is confusing to children to have a choice offered when there actually is none.) For example, when it is necessary for a child to change into a gown, a statement such as, "I need your dress off so I can listen to your chest. Shall I help you take it off?" gives the child an explanation, a choice, and some control.
- Be honest with children. However, be careful about creating overly scary impressions. Instead of saying, "This will hurt" before a procedure, it is better to prepare the child with a statement such as, "Children tell me different things about how this feels. Some say it feels like a chicken pecking or a cat scratching. Afterward, will you tell me what it felt like for you?"
- Use direct and concrete communication with young children because they are unable to work with abstractions or to separate fact from fantasy. For example, they attach literal meanings to such common phrases as "a frog in the throat" or "hold your horses."
- Avoid using a phrase that is open to a young child's misinterpretation. For example, the statement, "Let's see how warm your body is," is preferred to, "Let's take your temperature," because young children may wonder what you are going to do with their temperature once you have it and if you are planning to give it back. Words such as "shot" are frightening if a child envisions a shot from a gun. Instead substitute, "putting some medicine under the skin."
- Children between 5 and 8 years want concrete explanations and reasons for everything, because they rely more on what they know than what they see when faced with new problems. Continue to use relatively simple explanations, remembering that their expanding vocabulary will facilitate communication.

One of the most important points to remember is to speak with a child according to the child's stage of development (see Communication box). How you talk with a 2-year-old differs greatly from the conversation you will have with a 12-year-old. To be successful in establishing relationships with children and to be effective in teaching or sharing information, be sure to communicate with them at the appropriate level.

Nonverbal Communication

Young children become very adept at understanding nonverbal communication. They sense anxiety or fear by the rise in pitch of the parent's voice. Nodding of the head, using direct eye contact, tapping finger or foot, avoiding eye contact, and using sign language are nonverbal symbols. Sometimes you will need to use nonverbal behaviors yourself to receive confirmation from the children in return. Children are very sensitive to nonverbal cues.

HOSPITALIZATION OF A CHILD

Hospitalization is an anxiety-producing experience for children and their families, primarily because of a basic fear of not knowing what will occur. It creates an interruption in the child's normal development. Every member of the family is affected by the hospitalization because of the disruption it brings about in routines. Hospitalization is often the first crisis children face. How a child deals with this crisis will be influenced by developmental age, previous illness experience, separation coping skills, seriousness of the illness, and support of parents and staff. It is sometimes possible to make such an experience less traumatic by **anticipatory guidance,** explanations, and preparation to help relieve fear and anxiety. However, infants and toddlers are not able to understand. Therefore separation is especially painful for them. Preparation for a scheduled admission is possible; however, emergencies arise, and unplanned hospitalizations occur. In those instances, always give explanations whenever possible and as soon as feasible to avoid aggravating an already traumatic situation.

Communication

Developmental Considerations: Communicating Effectively with Young Children

INFANTS

- Consider your body language, such as gestures and posture, as well as pitch, intonation, and intensity of your voice.
- Nonverbal approaches work especially well for infants, with cuddling, patting, or some other form of gentle physical contact often quieting them.
- Maintain a calm voice and avoid sudden, loud noises. The actual words spoken are not as important as the way they are spoken.
- Because infants often begin fearing strangers at ages as young as 6 months, holding out the hands and asking the older infant to "come over" is seldom successful. If handling is necessary, the best approach is to pick up the infant firmly without using gestures.
- Infants are usually more at ease when upright and in visual contact with and proximity to their parents.

PRESCHOOL AND YOUNG SCHOOL-AGE CHILDREN

- Avoid quick approaches with preschool and young school-age children. Let them make the first move whenever possible.
- Broad smiles and other facial contortions sometimes have a threatening appearance.
- Avoid extended eye contact until after the child is comfortable.
- Position yourself at the child's eye level. You will appear less threatening to the child, and you will play down the child's smallness.
- Children are often more responsive when remaining close to the parent, such as sitting on the parent's lap.
- New or intimidating situations, such as hospitalization, are potentially stressful and make it even more difficult for children to grasp the new words they will encounter in this environment, as well as even simple words that express unfamiliar ideas. Avoid using expressions with dual meanings, such as "put to sleep."
- Substitute words that have potentially threatening interpretations with words that are less emotionally charged, such as replacing "stick" with "gently slide," or "hurt" with "feel uncomfortable."

OLDER SCHOOL-AGE CHILDREN

- Give children an opportunity to express their thoughts, concerns, and feelings. Listen and respond to underlying messages rather than just verbal content. Be attentive, try not to interrupt, and avoid making comments that convey disapproval or surprise.
- Avoid prying, asking embarrassing questions, and lecturing when giving advice.

ADOLESCENTS

- Be prepared to deal with a wide range of emotions and behaviors with adolescents. Give concrete explanations that focus on the teenager's concerns, even though the adolescent's capacity to think in abstract terms increases with age.
- It is not necessary to be fluent in teen jargon, but ask for clarification when necessary.
- To enhance communication, exchange information without using questions that back the teenager into a corner. Initially confine discussions to less threatening topics to allow time for trust to develop.
- Ask broad, open-ended questions before specific questions, such as "How's school?" before asking, "What is the best (or worst) thing about school?"

Modified from Clutter, L., et al. (1987). Communicating effectively with young children. *Child Nurse*, 5(4), 1.

Adequate preparation makes the transition from the security of a home to the unfamiliar atmosphere of a hospital less difficult. When it is best to begin preparation and how much information is right to give will vary. The age of the child will have a significant influence. A physician provides a family with details about a treatment plan, the length of stay, and expected results or outcomes. Parents are then able to reinforce the information by providing explanations to the child, using simple, age-appropriate terms. Usually there is time and opportunity before the actual admission for the child to talk about what is going to occur.

PREADMISSION PROGRAMS

Many hospitals have orientation programs for children who are to be admitted. In some hospitals, nurses conduct preadmission programs; other hospitals use **child life specialists** (health care professionals with extensive knowledge of child growth and development and the special emotional needs of children who are hospitalized).

The programs are based on the child's level of understanding and stage of development, with the purpose of familiarizing the child with hospital surroundings. These programs help to dismiss the child's fantasies and correct misconceptions. The programs include tours and audiovisual aids, such as movies, videos, and puppet shows. The child is given simple explanations of equipment used during surgery and hospitalization.

It is helpful for children to handle some of the items they will see while hospitalized, such as masks and gowns, stethoscopes, anesthesia masks, and syringes (without the needles attached). Make sure there is time for questions. Encourage children to talk about what they have seen or heard. By doing so, you will be able to identify problem areas or areas of concern. Some hospitals distribute coloring books or storybooks that focus on the information covered in the orientation program. This material reinforces information and also helps parents answer their children's questions. Many programs send the parents away with a brochure that describes hospital routines and lists items the hospital permits children to bring with them to the hospital. Keep written information simple, clear, and at an understandable level.

Timing of the orientation is important. There has to be enough advance time for the child to be able to assimilate the information after the program, but not so much time that the child will forget the information. Generally, the younger the child, the shorter the period between when the child is told about pending hospitalization and the actual admission date. Usually, a toddler is told only days before. However, school-age children have a better understanding of time and the future; it is therefore possible to tell them that they are going to the hospital "in 2 weeks." Tell adolescents as far in advance as possible to allow them time to inform peers and solicit their support.

It is necessary to allow children to prepare for this new experience in their own way. This preparation involves telling friends and selecting pictures of family members, toys, or clothes they wish to take, if they are permitted. Packing a bag with these items reinforces the event's reality.

Parents also benefit from such orientation programs. They receive information that is helpful in answering a child's questions at home. Printed materials provide parents a reference guide for reviewing what the child has been told.

Emergency Admission

An emergency admission, in contrast to a well-planned and well-prepared-for admission, thrusts the child into an unknown environment with strange equipment, frightening sounds, and many unfamiliar adults all around. The incident that results in the hospitalization usually is sudden, serious, and possibly painful. The speed with which a health team responds to the emergency is critical, and there is little time for explanations. Whenever possible, explain to the child and family what is happening. This can prevent an escalating crisis situation. When the child is stable and awake, assess the child's perception of what happened, correct any misconceptions, and provide information not given initially.

ADMISSION

Large hospitals often assign children to a nursing unit according to their age-group. For example, a 2-year-old will be on the toddler unit and a teenager on the adolescent unit. Smaller community hospitals attempt to group children of similar ages in rooms large enough to accommodate two to four children.

Confidentiality is of great importance when interviewing the hospitalized pediatric patient. It is particularly important with adolescents when they have concerns related to issues such as substance use or sexual behaviors.

Adolescents are more likely to participate in health care services when caring, respectful professionals are the ones providing them. Characteristics of good providers include compassion, warmth, understanding, an ability to communicate with the adolescent, a willingness to be straightforward and honest, and competency.

Pediatric units are usually bright, colorful, and cheery areas with cartoon figures on the walls (or ceilings of treatment rooms), many pictures, and large photographs of sports figures and popular singers. Often the unit or room will be decorated to reflect the age-group admitted there. For example, an infant and toddler unit will usually have many age-appropriate toys, high chairs, playpens, and strollers. In a typical adolescent area, you will find a lounge with a television, video games, VCR or DVD player, a CD player, and computers with age-appropriate software and Internet access. To decrease anxiety, most hospitals try to make the pediatric environment different from adult units and include many items that are found in the child's normal home or school environment.

First impressions are important and have the potential to color the child's entire hospital stay. Make sure, therefore, to greet children warmly and welcome them by name when they arrive on the unit. After they get to see their room and meet their roommate(s), give them a tour of the unit. Two important locations to point out are the area in which snacks or liquid refreshments are available and the playroom (or activity room when speaking to adolescents) where they will spend time when allowed out of bed. The play area is a safe, secure place for children. It contains an assortment of toys, games, and crafts for diversional activities. Newly admitted children also need explanations about when meals are served, how to operate their beds, and how to communicate with nurses by using a call bell or intercommunication system.

Sometimes anxiety levels about a hospital admission are high. Perhaps heart surgery is to occur or a brain tumor is suspected. In those instances, sometimes you will elect to postpone a tour or an in-depth orientation. The development of a therapeutic relationship with the family will very possibly seem more important, because it has the potential to affect the entire course of a hospitalization. Inform parents that a tour and further orientation are available and that the timing of such events is the parent's choice.

After the child is admitted, obtain a nursing history. An identification bracelet, usually worn on the wrist, is important to verify identity when medications are given or procedures are done. Often you will place these bands on the ankles of infants and toddlers because they are curious of items on their wrists. When you apply the band, allow enough space for one finger to fit between the band and the skin. Make sure the band is not constrictive, and check the skin underneath for its integrity.

Assess vital signs, including blood pressure. Measure and record the height (or length for infants) and weight. These are important baseline data. You will use height and weight in calculating a child's body surface area, especially when treating a child with burns or in calculating fluid and electrolyte requirements. Most medical centers use body weight in kilograms to compute drug dosages. An important nursing responsibility is identifying the scale used to weigh a child, if more than one is available, so that all staff will use the same scale for subsequent weighings.

A laboratory technician will draw routine blood samples on all newly admitted infants and children. Some hospitals make efforts to reduce the number of "sticks" a child receives by coordinating various physician requests whenever possible. You will also collect a urine specimen. The laboratory values provide a physician with baseline information and are sometimes diagnostic. The physician will order additional x-ray examinations or procedures as appropriate to the child's specific health problem.

HOSPITAL POLICIES

Changes in hospitals' policies over recent years reflect their changed attitude toward parents: Most hospitals no longer consider parents "visitors" and welcome their presence at all times throughout the child's hospitalization. Many hospitals have developed a system of family-centered care. This philosophy of care validates the integral role of the family in a child's life and acknowledges the family as an essential part of the child's care and illness experience. In this kind of system, the family becomes a partner in the care of the child.

Hospitalization is especially traumatic to very young children, and the presence of supportive parents increases their feelings of security. The typical fear and apprehension children experience when they are isolated from their parents and family is known as *separation anxiety* and causes major stress for the hospitalized child, especially between ages 15 to 30 months. That is why having parents and other family members present during hospitalization is so therapeutic for this age-group (Hockenberry & Wilson, 2007). Some hospitals have facilities that allow one parent to live in or room in, which means a parent is able to stay 24 hours a day. Make parents aware that beds, meals, and shower facilities are available for their use.

Parents who are involved in care have a sense of contributing to the child's recovery, which is an important consideration. Having a parent present increases the teaching opportunities you will have. It also enables you to assess a family's strengths, needs, and potential problem areas. However, parents need time to relax and to get away from the child's bedside periodically. Rooming-in is sometimes an exhausting experience. Parents need breaks and relief to remain effective in supporting the child. Hospitals with a family-centered philosophy set aside a room or other specified area on the nursing unit for parents where they have the chance to socialize, support each other, and share their thoughts. Note that the presence of parents does not mean that nurses give up their responsibilities in caring for these children.

Certain hospitals allow children to wear their own clothes; this is especially important for a hospitalized adolescent. However, if a child is scheduled for surgery or needs an IV line, hospital gowns are required because of the possibility of clothing loss or damage.

DEVELOPMENTAL SUPPORT FOR THE CHILD

Hospitalization not only interrupts children's normal routines, it also threatens their normal developmental process. It is not unusual for children to regress when hospitalized. For instance, some young school-age children will resume the practice of thumb-sucking. Often regression persists for several months after a child is discharged.

There are several ways for you to alleviate or even eliminate some of the traumatic effects of hospitalization on a child's normal development. A child's developmental level influences his or her understanding and response to hospitalization. Strategies for supporting children are likely to be more effective when they take developmental concerns and needs into account (Table 30-7).

Take particular care to meet the psychosocial needs of children with special needs who are hospitalized. Because of the nature of their conditions, there is an even greater likelihood that these children will experience invasive and traumatic procedures during frequent and lengthy hospital stays. These factors result in a group of children more vulnerable to the emotional and developmental consequences of hospitalization.

PAIN MANAGEMENT

Health care professionals, including nurses, tend to underestimate pain in children. Some people falsely believe that infants or young children are not able to feel pain. Another explanation for this tendency is a misconception of what playing or reading or any other activity means about a child's comfort level. We now know to assume that anything will be painful to infants and children if it is painful to adults. We also know that children, like adults, will engage in activities for distraction, as a method of coping with pain. These behaviors do not signal the absence of pain.

Pain has taken on recognition as the fifth vital sign, and it is necessary to document it during each shift assessment (Gilbert & Green, 2000). A critical component in managing pain is its assessment. However, pain assessment, especially for children who have limited cognitive and language skills, continues to be a challenge for health care providers. Often it will be difficult for you to ascertain when a child is in pain and how intense the pain is. Infants are not able to tell you that they are in pain or the pain's location. You have to rely on physiologic variables and behavioral variables, such as vocalization, facial expressions, and body movements, and keep in mind that whatever is painful for an adult will likely be painful for a person of any age. There have been some improvements over the last few years in methods to measure pain

Table 30-7 Age-Related Concerns and Needs of Children Who Are Hospitalized

CONCERNS	POSSIBLE RESPONSES	POSITIVE PARENT AND NURSE RESPONSES
INFANCY		
The infant needs to have parents close by; parents are seen as powerful. Parents' presence and reactions provide best support in handling fear, pain, and separation.	Inappropriate bonding; development of distrust; anxiety due to separation and new environment; delayed skills development	Maintain proximity to child (rooming-in); make frequent contact with child; stroke, cuddle, and rock child; talk and sing; read; communicate love for child.
TODDLER		
Separation from parents is a major issue. Loss of control is viewed in terms of physical restriction, loss of routine and rituals, and dependency. The toddler fears bodily injury and pain.	Regression: Lack of cooperation; not eating; no interaction with others; protest (e.g., verbal cries for parent; verbal attack on others; kicking, biting, hitting, pinching; possibly tries to escape to find parent; clings to parent); despair (e.g., passive, depressed, disinterested in environment; uncommunicative; loss of newly learned skills); negativism, temper tantrums; resistance	Praise for appropriate behavior (e.g., putting on slippers without help); restate reasons for hospitalization; rooming-in; continue with usual home routine (e.g., read a bedtime story); communicate love for child.
PRESCHOOL		
The presence of parents continues to be of primary importance. Hospitalization is perceived as rejection or punishment. Fears of mutilation are possible. Treatment is sometimes seen as hostile or punishment. Child is concerned with bodily penetration by surgery or injections.	Anger toward primary caretaker (parent); acting out (e.g., throwing toys, inappropriate verbalizations); refusal to listen to or look at or speak to parent; refusal to participate in hygiene and play activities; protest (less direct and aggressive than toddler, sometimes will displace feelings on others); despair and detachment; physical and verbal aggression; dependency; withdrawal; feelings of fear, anxiety, guilt, shame, physiologic responses; immature behavior	Accept and provide outlets for child's anger; communicate love for child; maintain behavior limits (appropriate discipline); restate reasons for hospitalization; use play conversation to continue hospital experience explanation. Reassure child that hospitalization is not a punishment.
SCHOOL AGE		
The school-age child is primarily concerned with lack of body control and mastery. Feelings of inadequacy are possible. The child may become demanding and rebellious to maintain semblance of control. Knowledge about illness is effective in handling anxiety.	Regression: Inability to complete some tasks; anger related to confinement, inability to be mobile, lack of contact with friends; refusal to ambulate; loneliness; boredom; isolation; withdrawal; depression; displaced anger; hostility; frustration; excessive sleeping or TV watching; information seeking	Establish consistent visiting pattern; implement plan for continued education and teacher visit; set limits for self-care tasks that are attainable; praise for appropriate behavior (e.g., completing homework); arrange peer visit.
ADOLESCENCE		
Hospitalization is sometimes viewed as a threat to independence. Conflicts over control issues become a focal concern. Separation from family and peers will interfere at times with developmental task mastery and lead to feelings of abandonment that substantiate a sense of worthlessness. There is concern about status in peer group after hospitalization.	Rejection; uncooperativeness; withdrawal; self-assertion; self-control; cooperativeness; fear; anxiety; overconfidence; will sometimes capitalize on gains from pain; depression; loneliness; withdrawal; boredom	Support the adolescent's need for independence, confidentiality, and decision making. Encourage opportunities to meet normal developmental tasks within the hospital (e.g., schoolwork, visits with peers).

Data from Association for the Care of Children's Health. (1980). *Guidelines for adolescent units*. Washington, D.C.: Association for the Care of Children's Health; Magrab, P. (1985). Psychosocial development of chronically ill children. In N. Hobbs & J.M. Perrin (Eds.), *Issues in the care of children with chronic illness*. San Francisco: Jossey-Bass; Pass, M., & Pass, C. (1987). Anticipatory guidance for parents of hospitalized children. *J Pediatr Nurs, 2*(4), 250; Hockenberry, M.J., et al. (2007). *Wong's nursing care of infants and children.* (8th ed.). St. Louis: Mosby.

(Hockenberry & Wilson, 2007). Pain assessment tools such as the Wong-Baker FACES Pain Rating Scale (Figure 30-8) will help you assess pain in children. Remember that some children will be reluctant to let you know they are experiencing pain for fear of getting pain medication by injection. Advocate for IV analgesic administration, particularly when IV lines are already in place, and promote oral analgesic administration as soon as possible.

Reasons other than inaccurate pain assessment also lead to undertreatment of pain in children. Fear of respiratory depression or addiction sometimes means that a child does not receive an adequate amount of analgesic, does not receive it often enough, or is not considered a candidate for certain opioids. Although respiratory depression is a possible side effect with opioids in children older than 3 months of age (and possibly younger), opioids cause no greater respiratory depression than in adults. As for addiction, there is no indication that children are at any increased risk of physiologic or psychological dependence from the use of opioids for pain management.

In addition to learning to accurately assess pain in children and advocating for and administering adequate analgesics, encourage parental presence and use sensitive care practices to lessen children's pain. Try integrating soothing talk or musical tapes into care practices. Infants often derive benefit from pacifiers, swaddling, rocking, or simply being held. Take care, whenever possible, to let the child's needs determine the timing of care routines, procedures, and tests. Also take appropriate action to reduce noise and other disturbing sensations to create a soothing and calming environment for the child in pain.

SURGERY

Undergoing a surgical procedure tends to be an especially stressful event for children and their families. Children facing surgery without information and preparation often develop misconceptions about the surgical event or any of the series of events leading up to or after surgery. Fantasies built on misconceptions typically lead to fears, which in turn often lead to negative reactions and long-term consequences, such as behavioral problems or an inability to trust others. Preparing a child for surgery entails providing information to parents and child about what will happen and what the child will experience. Addressing the events surrounding surgery that are most difficult for children is a good place to begin. Six stress points are common for children undergoing surgery: (1) admission, (2) blood tests, (3) the afternoon of the day before surgery, (4) injection

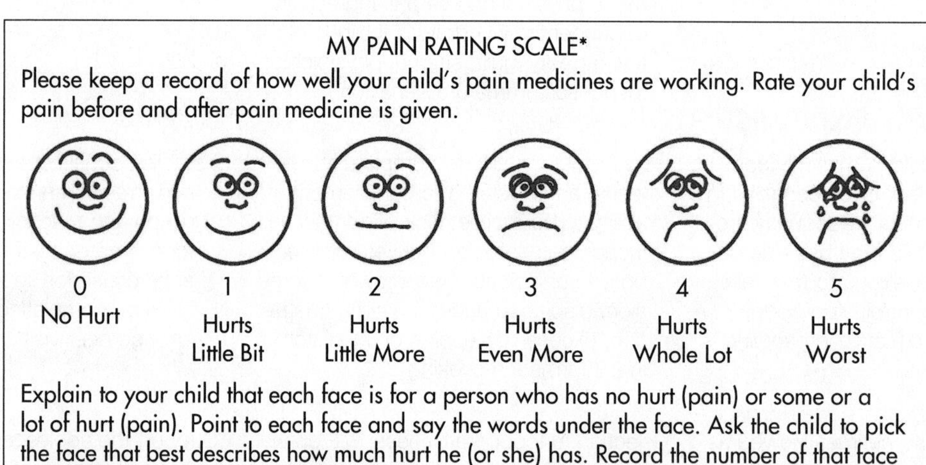

MY PAIN RATING SCALE*

Please keep a record of how well your child's pain medicines are working. Rate your child's pain before and after pain medicine is given.

Explain to your child that each face is for a person who has no hurt (pain) or some or a lot of hurt (pain). Point to each face and say the words under the face. Ask the child to pick the face that best describes how much hurt he (or she) has. Record the number of that face in the Pain Rating column. If your child's pain is above 2, or if you have other concerns with pain, let your nurse or physician know.

Date and time	Pain rating	Medicine I took	Side effects, such as drowsiness or upset stomach

FIGURE 30-8 Wong-Baker FACES Pain Rating Scale. Explain to the patient that each face is for a person who feels happy because he has no pain (hurt) or sad because he has some or a lot of pain. Face 0 is very happy because he does not hurt at all. Face 1 hurts just a little bit. Face 2 hurts a little more. Face 3 hurts even more. Face 4 hurts a whole lot. Face 5 hurts as much as you can imagine, although you do not have to be crying to feel this bad. Ask the patient to choose the face that best describes now how he or she is feeling. Recommended for people age 3 years or older.

of preoperative medication, (5) the moments before and during transport to the operating room, and (6) return from the postanesthesia care unit (PACU). Think through each stress point from the child's perspective, and develop an individualized preparation plan. Explain the hospital system to the parents and inform them of the operation's progress.

Age influences the types of fears and concerns regarding surgery a child is likely to experience. Table 30-8 lists common age-related fears and effective interventions. Using children's ages as a guide increases the likelihood that children will be adequately prepared for surgery and all the surrounding events.

PARENT PARTICIPATION

It is essential to establish an effective working relationship with parents as soon as possible. Parents are the most significant individuals to a child. Also, they know their child better than anyone else and often play an important role in assessing the child's responses. Therefore, take care to project a positive attitude toward parents: give them a warm greeting, smile, and establish eye contact. Gain the trust of the parents by (1) reviewing and interpreting information from the physician as needed, (2) asking the parents whether they have any questions, (3) conveying concern for the parents' well-being, (4) listening and being available, and (5) respecting them as experts on their child and soliciting their input. These activities are time consuming, and yet for a nurse who works with families, they are some of the most satisfying.

In obtaining a nursing history, it is important to select a quiet place on the unit to listen to parents' responses and to provide them with opportunities to ask questions. Even if the physician sees the reason for hospitalization as minor, in some cases a parent will perceive it as very serious. Parents experience fear and anxiety because of the seriousness of the illness, the procedures involved, or the pain the child will experience. Their apprehension then is transmitted to the child. Therefore it is important to convey interest and concern and try to decrease their anxieties.

Parents experience a series of reactions when a child is hospitalized. They too are in an unfamiliar environment, meeting different groups of people who ask many questions and give them much information. Perhaps the tests or procedures mentioned are unknown to them. It is possible for them to become frustrated because they do not understand much of what is being told to them. Parents often do not know hospital rules and regulations and what is expected of them. They lose control in this setting and feel powerless. To this point, they alone have cared for their son or daughter. Now a nurse assumes control over the child's care. If an accident is the cause for hospitalization, parents will sometimes be blaming themselves and feeling guilty.

On admission, parents need specific information on routines, hospital policies that affect them, any limitations that exist, and what is expected of them. When parents receive information that they can apply immediately, their anxiety levels decrease and they feel more comfortable. When you succeed in meeting the emotional needs of a parent, that parent is better able to support the child (Box 30-9).

Later, make sure to explain to the parents any diagnostic tests, medications, or procedures that the physician plans. Keep in mind that anxiety and the sheer volume of information they have to absorb will sometimes result in parents becoming confused or forgetting

Table 30-8 Age-Related Fears Associated with Surgery

AGE	PRIMARY CONCERNS	INTERVENTION
Younger than 5 years	What will happen when I wake up? Where will I be? Who will be with me?	Show recovery room, if possible. Tell when parents will visit after surgery. Encourage parents to be with child as soon as possible.
School age	Anesthesia	Show mask.
• Younger	That I might wake up during surgery	Explain "gas" or "medicine" and how it works.
• Older	How doctor knows when, or if doctor knows how, to awaken me	Stress concept of "special sleep." Explain that it is a special person's job to control the sleep.
	Same as above plus the following: Operation itself Mutilation Possible death	Same as above Provide knowledge about procedure.
Adolescents	Same as above plus the following: Special anxiety for change in body image Loss of control while under anesthesia (in terms of behavior and for body integrity) Peer reaction to scars Effect on sexuality Effect on adolescent mode of dress	Same as above Reassure that only what is supposed to be done will be performed. Introduce to peer with similar surgery.

Box 30-9 Factors Affecting Parents' Reactions to Their Child's Illness

- Seriousness of the threat to the child
- Previous experience with illness or hospitalization
- Medical procedures involved in diagnosis and treatment
- Available support systems
- Personal ego strengths
- Previous coping abilities
- Additional stresses on the family system
- Cultural and religious beliefs
- Communication patterns among family members

what they have heard. Any change in plans has the potential to generate anxiety and result in a parent being unable to process the information. Make sure, therefore, to thoroughly explain the tests and treatments. Offer information several times to the parents, if necessary, so you are certain they fully comprehend it.

As the parents' comfort increases, they become more involved in meeting their child's physical needs. Mothers tend to spend more time with their hospitalized children and participate early in providing care. Fathers are often more reluctant, so encourage them to become involved. When parents participate, they are contributing to the child's recovery. Another strategy is to ask for parents' assistance in establishing goals or revising a care plan.

The equipment that surrounds a child is often overwhelming, with the strange-sounding alarms or with electrodes placed on different parts of the child's body (Figure 30-9). When you explain the function of a monitor or some other device, it often becomes less threatening. However, it is important to use terms the parent can understand.

Initially, perhaps, a parent will watch you suction the child, perform chest physical therapy, or change a dressing. If you use these opportunities to describe what you are doing and why, parents become more interested. Eventually you will sometimes hear, "Do you think I can suction Billy today?" The information that has been exchanged between you and a parent, the demonstrations that have occurred, and the teaching that you have done have motivated this parent to perform a procedure he or she has not done before. Parents often become skillful in performing a variety of technical skills if you teach them in a patient, nonthreatening manner and encourage questions. Some activities in which parents become involved include gastrostomy tube feedings, tracheostomy suctioning, and subcutaneous injections.

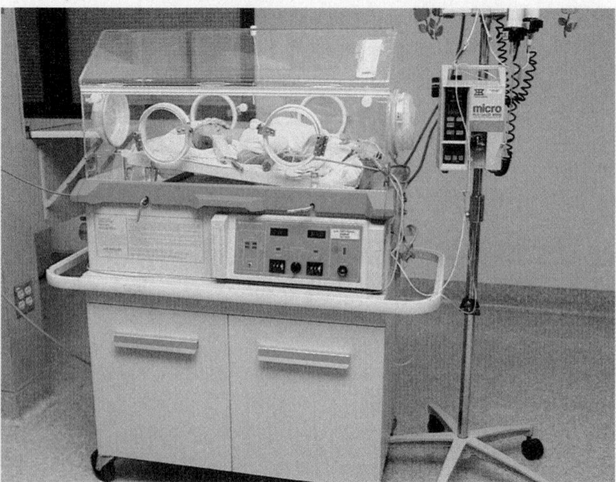

FIGURE 30-9 It is easy for a parent to feel overwhelmed by the equipment that surrounds an infant.

Make sure parents are confident in their ability to perform given tasks in their child's care, and encourage them to participate only in as many activities as they feel comfortable performing. Generally, the extent of parental involvement also is a good measure of your effectiveness as a teacher.

The last phase of adaptation for parents of a child who is hospitalized relates to discharge. Do not postpone teaching until the time of discharge. Teaching begins at admission and is an ongoing process throughout the hospitalization. The child will often have some activity restrictions, but after you have instructed them and ascertained their competence, parents will usually be able to provide any nursing interventions that are required at home.

COMMON PEDIATRIC PROCEDURES

Some of the following procedures are for general care of children, procedures healthy children experience in the home. Others take place primarily in health care settings. Many events that are common in health care settings will sometimes be frightening for children. Depending on the child's age, prepare children and their parents for all procedures, even those that you consider insignificant. Preparing children for procedures increases their cooperation, helps them cope, and promotes a sense of self-esteem and mastery.

A sensation-based approach is the most effective method of preparation. Provide information about what the child is likely to feel, see, smell, hear, or taste, along with emotions commonly experienced. For example, children scheduled for x-ray examinations or computed tomography (CT) scans will perhaps feel frightened, anxious, guilty ("Am I being punished for being bad?"), powerless, or curious. The sights they see probably include a "big machine" or "camera" over them and a lead shield or apron on themselves, the x-ray technician, and a parent if present. They will hear noises of the machine "buzzing" and the sliding of x-ray plates. The room and the table will most likely feel cold, and the lead shield heavy.

Timing is important in preparing the child. It is usually best to prepare young children close to the time of the procedure. It is possible to prepare older children further in advance. Preparation just before less complicated procedures, such as injections, fingersticks, or taking vital signs, is acceptable for children of all ages.

BATHING

Bathing the child provides you with the opportunity to do a complete skin assessment. When giving a bath, protect the infant from drafts and chilling. Usually you will bathe the child before a feeding to avoid stimulating regurgitation or vomiting by doing so afterward. Check the water temperature. If the umbilical cord is still attached, give a sponge bath. Clean the cord and the area around it with alcohol, which helps drying.

Use only water to clean areas around the eyes. Use a mild soap on the rest of the body, and bathe it starting with the face and moving on down the trunk. Expose, wash, rinse, and dry one section of the body thoroughly before bathing another anatomical part. A baby's creases need special attention. Babies have very short necks, and if you do not clean and dry them thoroughly, skin impairment is possible.

If you give a sponge bath at the bedside, place the infant across the width of the bed facing you. This practice allows greater control of any movement by the baby and decreases the likelihood of the baby rolling out of the crib. Never use cotton-tipped applicators to clean the ear canal, because injuries are possible with any sudden movement. A washcloth is adequate. Give special care to the genitalia. In females, separate the labia and wash them in the anterior-to-posterior direction. Wash the penis and the scrotum of a circumcised male. In an uncircumcised male, external washing and rinsing on a daily basis are all that is necessary. It is best not to attempt to retract the foreskin because it is almost always attached to the glans. Forcing the foreskin back risks harm to the penis, causing pain, bleeding, and possibly adhesions. No ointments or powders are usually advisable.

Infants enjoy being placed in basins or bathtub seats for baths. After washing the baby's face, lather the trunk and extremities. Using dry hands, which enables you to pick up the infant more securely, place the infant in the basin. The head needs the support of one hand; use your other hand to rinse the infant. Allow the baby to play and splash the water, which encourages development. After being removed from the basin, wrap the infant in a towel and dry it thoroughly.

Hold the infant "football style" when washing the infant's head. In this position, the infant's hip rests on your hip. Your hand supports the baby's head, and the baby's back rests on your forearm. This position allows the infant to look at your face while the hair is washed. After the hair is lathered well, rinse the head over the basin at the bedside. Sometimes parents ask about the baby's soft spot (**anterior fontanelle**; a space, roughly diamond shaped, covered by tough membranes between the bones of an infant's cranium; the posterior fontanelle is triangular). Assure them that the area will not be injured by shampooing.

Most toddlers love to be placed in a tub for their baths. Provide toys for the child to use in splashing, water play, and bathing. For most young children, it is enough to allow them to enjoy themselves in a tub for 15 to 30 minutes. It is important to remember that water is fascinating to a toddler because it has no shape or form. Safety is an issue: **Never** leave a child in a tub without supervision.

The school-age child will sometimes be reluctant to bathe, and many are not accustomed to a daily bath. With your encouragement, children who are feeling fairly well will usually participate in their daily care. Use your judgment of the child's physical and mental condition and advice from the child's parents to determine how much supervision a particular child requires.

Most adolescents gradually become accustomed to bathing or showering as part of their daily routine. The need for an underarm deodorant usually becomes evident during puberty. Privacy when bathing and dressing is of paramount importance during the teenage years.

FEEDINGS

Breastfeeding

Health care providers give preference for breast milk for providing nutrition for the full-term infant (Hockenberry & Wilson, 2007), and often a mother will wish to continue breastfeeding her baby who is ill or hospitalized. Assist the mother by providing a quiet environment and a comfortable chair for her to sit in when nursing her baby. Some mothers are unable to be present for every feeding, or the baby is unable to take milk directly from the breast. Encourage the mother in this case to use a breast pump, and provide a private place for this activity. It is possible to freeze bottles of breast milk and give them later by bottle or tube feeding.

Bottle Feeding

The correct position for feeding an infant is one that is comfortable for both adult and infant. Have the caregiver hold the infant securely. Place a table or stand within arm's reach so it is possible to set the bottle aside while **burping** (inducing belching or eructation) the baby. If a burp is not elicited by one position, try another.

Hold the bottle so formula fills the nipple entirely to decrease the amount of air the baby will swallow in the course of the feeding. Infants are not able to voluntarily push the bottle away when finished, so feed them only as much as they actively consume to prevent overfeeding. During the feeding, remove the bottle and burp the infant periodically. Newborns need burping more often than older babies. With experience, you will learn to recognize the infant's cues, such as squirming, that signal the infant's need to burp.

Burping and Finishing a Feeding

There are three common methods of burping an infant. One way is to place the infant in a sitting position on your lap. With one hand over the infant's chin and chest supporting the body as the infant leans forward, use the other to gently pat or rub the infant's back from the waist to the shoulders. It is also possible to place the infant flat across your lap, facedown, using one hand to rub or pat the back and the other hand to secure the body. The third position is with the baby upright against your body, looking backward over your shoulder. Your one arm holds the baby, and the other hand is free to rub the infant's back from the waist to the shoulders. Once the baby has released any trapped air, resume the feeding if the baby hasn't yet finished. Repeat this process until the infant has consumed the desired amount, ending with burping.

After feeding, position the infant on the right side. This permits the feeding to flow toward the lower end of the stomach and allows any swallowed air to rise above the fluid and through the esophagus. Place infants only on their back to sleep; this measure helps prevent sudden infant death syndrome (SIDS). The Academy of Pediatrics (2005) has recommended the use of a pacifier at naptime and bedtime as a protective mechanism against the incidence of SIDS during the first year of life. The reduction of SIDS with the use of a pacifier outweighs the pacifier's possible negative effects of developing dental problems or inhibiting breastfeeding (Hockenberry & Wilson, 2007).

Solids

When the infant starts solid food, assist the parent to learn the proper feeding position. Have them feed the infant in an infant seat. Always secure the safety strap. In an infant seat, the baby is able to focus the eyes on the adult, while both hands of an adult are free to introduce solids to the infant. Once an infant achieves control, it is acceptable for caregivers to hold the baby in their arms. Older infants (8 or 9 months old) will be able to eat in a high chair with a safety strap in place. It will sometimes be necessary to provide additional support. Try rolling up baby blankets and placing them on either side of the infant's trunk.

> It is important to wait to start solid foods until your baby is ready. Children do better with feeding if they have some control over the process, which is usually somewhere around 6 months of age. *The semireclining baby will have very little control over the spoon-feeding process.* The sitting baby can look at the spoon, feel the food with his fingers, get his fingers to his mouth. . . . He can open his mouth and lean forward if he wants to eat; he can close his mouth and turn his head away if he is not interested. It is easy for a parent to pick up and understand feeding cues from a sitting up baby who is eating solid food. It is much harder if you are starting out with one who is really too little, lying back in his infant seat.
>
> Once a toddler has begun walking, placement in a high chair is a confinement that might be vigorously resisted. In climbing out of a high chair, a toddler may fall and sustain a significant injury, despite the fact that a safety strap was used. There are two points to remember when dealing with a toddler. First, the toddler's appetite decreases at this age (physiologic anorexia), which is normal. Second, resistance to the high chair may be intense, and an injury can occur. It may be advantageous to try an alternative. Although they take in less solid food, toddlers continue to drink liquids freely.
>
> Not all walking babies vigorously resist high chairs. There are individual children who do, but this does not include all older babies. Eventually all babies/toddlers will resist a high chair, but base the timing on when to quit using the high chair on each individual baby. There are alternatives such as a booster seat, or pushing the high chair up to the table, or stools with backs/arm rests. Make sure the toddler's feet are supported—not dangling. Make sure he is at a height where he does not have to reach "up" to get his food and make sure he is close enough to the table to be somewhat confined so his attention is on eating. Ideally the family eats at the same time as the toddler; therefore, there is less risk for injury because parents can prevent the child from climbing all over his chair. (Sometimes ideal doesn't always occur.)
>
> It is usually not a good idea to put food on a chair and let the child "stroll by" and eat! First of all, the parent better know a good carpet and upholstery cleaner—the child is going to have food all over the house. Also—more seriously—children, even babies, need limits. They should learn that you eat at the table, you eat at regular times, and you eat with the family (ideally), you learn behavior standards at the table (manners)—toddlers learn these gradually.
>
> Parents should have three regular meals and planned snacks each day so the child eats about every 2 to 3 hours.
>
> Also, children should sit down to eat. Choking is more likely if children eat on the run.
>
> —*Kristen Maughan, RD; educator and mother of four*

Gavage

Some infants and children need gavage feedings. This involves passing a feeding tube through the nose or mouth, down the esophagus, and into the stomach. Although in many health care settings nurses are required to have additional training before performing this function, you will usually assist with the tube placement and are permitted to perform the actual tube feedings.

To measure the tube before placing it, a qualified staff member will use one of the following procedures: (1) measure from the nose to the distal area of the earlobe and then to the end of the xiphoid process or (2) measure from the nose to the earlobe and then to a point midway between the xiphoid process and the umbilicus.

Some restraint of infant activity is likely to be necessary when passing the tube. Pulling up the bottom of the shirt over both arms is often all that is needed to restrain the newborn. Some infants will perhaps need to be wrapped in a mummy type of safety reminder device before proceeding. (See the description of the mummy safety reminder device in a later section.) In the unlikely event that a premature infant requires restraint, a small towel folded across the chest and secured beneath the shoulders is usually sufficient; take care not to compromise breathing.

Because infants are nose breathers, the mouth is the preferred route for tube insertion. The tube will often be passed through the nose for older infants and children. Ask children who are able to understand, to swallow while the tube is being inserted. A tube that will be indwelling is almost always inserted through the nose; to prevent irritation, use alternate nostrils for reinsertion. Once inserted, tape the tube in place. If inserted through a nostril, tape the tube to the cheek, not to the forehead, to prevent possible structural and cosmetic damage to the nostril.

Before feedings, check tube placement by both (1) aspirating for stomach contents and (2) injecting a small amount of air (0.5 to 1 mL in premature or very small infants to 5 mL in larger children) through the syringe into the tube while simultaneously listening with a stethoscope over the stomach area for sounds of gurgling or growling. If there is any doubt about tube placement, do not proceed with feeding, and consult the practitioner. Sometimes radiographic data are necessary to confirm proper tube placement (see Chapters 20 and 21).

Whenever possible, hold the infant during the feeding. If this is impossible, position the infant or child on his or her back or toward the right side with the head and chest elevated. Give infants a pacifier during feedings to encourage sucking and help them associate sucking with satisfying hunger. Warm the formula to room temperature and, after a gentle push with the plunger, allow it to flow into the stomach by gravity. To prevent nausea and regurgitation, use rates of no more than 5 mL every 5 to 10 minutes in premature and very small infants and 10 mL per minute in older infants and children. At the completion of the feeding, flush the tube with sterile water (using from 1 or 2 mL for small tubes to 5 mL or more for large ones). Clamp or cap indwelling tubes after feeding. If the tube is to be removed, pinch it firmly to prevent escape of fluid and withdraw it quickly. Keep the child positioned on the right side for at least 1 hour to keep the possibility of regurgitation and aspiration to a minimum. Burp the infant if his or her condition permits. Record the type and the amount of feeding given and the child's response.

Gastrostomy

A gastrostomy tube (G tube) is often used in children when passing a gastric tube is contraindicated or in children who require tube feeding over an extended period. The physician places the tube during surgery when the child is under general anesthesia, or percutaneously using an endoscope with the child under local anesthesia. The practitioner inserts the tube through the abdominal wall into the stomach and secures it with a purse-string suture, as well as anchoring the stomach to the peritoneum at the operative site. Feeding is carried out in the same manner and rate as in gavage feeding. After feedings, place the child on the right side or in Fowler's position. The tube will be left open and suspended or clamped between feedings, depending on the child's condition.

Total Parenteral Nutrition

When feeding by way of the GI tract is impossible, inadequate, or hazardous, total parenteral nutrition (TPN; also called IV alimentation or hyperalimentation) is an option. A highly concentrated solution of protein, glucose, and other nutrients intravenously through conventional tubing with a special filter attached to remove particulate matter and microorganisms. Wide-diameter vessels, such as the subclavian vein, are the usual sites of infusion. In most health care settings, the nurse is required to have additional training before assisting with TPN. Nursing responsibilities include control of sepsis, monitoring of the infusion rate, and continuous observations. **Never** confuse this method of feeding with the use of "kangaroo" feedings in which you will use a mechanical pump to regulate the volume and rate of continuous gastric feedings per gastrostomy tube.

SAFETY REMINDER DEVICES

For safety reasons, children will sometimes need to be restrained after surgery or during a procedure or examination. Safety reminder devices (SRDs) are used only as a last resort. The safety reminder device is used to ensure that safe care is given to the patient. The following clinical situations allow for the use of safety reminder devices:

- Maintaining oxygen therapy without interruption
- Protection from harm if child has an indwelling catheter, IV tubes, pacemaker wire, or sutures
- Patients who are confused, agitated, or unable to comprehend instructions (Hockenberry & Wilson, 2007)

Make absolutely sure to apply the SRD correctly, and closely monitor circulation and skin integrity. Remove the SRD every 2 hours to permit exercise of the body area. If you need to restrain the extremities, release them one at a time so that the child cannot pull out an IV or NG tube. Attach the ties of all SRDs to bed frames only, not to side rails.

Elbow Safety Reminder Devices

Elbow SRDs prevent flexion or bending of elbows. They allow an infant or toddler to move the upper extremities but prevent them from touching the head and neck area; thus, for example, they protect the newly repaired cleft lip or palate or scalp vein infusion site. Slip clean tongue blades into the parallel pockets of a wraparound SRD. Pull the shirt or pajama sleeve down to the wrist, and place the elbow in the center of this SRD. Wrap the SRD around the arm and tie it securely. Cuff the sleeve over the bottom of the SRD to protect the skin. Check both the axilla and the wrist periodically for skin impairment.

Mummy Safety Reminder Device

A mummy SRD is used when it is necessary to immobilize head, neck, trunk, and upper and lower extremities. A jugular venipuncture or the insertion of an NG tube will sometimes call for this type of SRD. Place a square baby blanket on a crib, and fold over one corner. Place the infant on its back on the blanket so the shoulders are at the level of the fold and arms are at the sides. Wrap one corner of the blanket over the right arm, and tuck it under the infant's left side. Place the opposite corner over the left arm, and place it securely under the right side of the body (Figure 30-10). A commercially prepared mummy SRD is also available.

A modified version will sometimes be needed so it is possible to expose the chest. While you place one corner of the blanket around the right arm and tuck it under the baby's body, encircle the left arm with the opposite corner and secure it, too. Bring the corner beneath the feet up to the abdomen and pin it, thereby leaving the chest exposed.

Clove-Hitch Safety Reminder Device

This type of four-point SRD is for use on all extremities of a child. It is possible to use rolls of Kerlix, roller bandage, or strips of muslin. Pad the wrists and ankles with gauze squares or other soft material. A clove hitch is not a square knot. Make a figure-8 with the material, slip it over the padded wrist or ankle, and tighten it gently (see Chapter 14). Check each SRD frequently to be sure that circulation is not affected and pressure is not excessive. Use a slip knot to tie the ends of this SRD to the bed frame.

Jacket Safety Reminder Device

You will sometimes use a jacket SRD to keep an extremely active older infant or toddler safely in bed or in a high chair. It resembles a vest and has ties in the back. Pull the child's arms through the jacket, and tie the jacket in the back. Attach the long ties to a bed frame or under the seat of a high chair. Although children are able to move all body parts, it is not possible for them to climb out of beds or high chairs.

URINE COLLECTION

Collecting a urine specimen when the child is not toilet trained is sometimes a major problem in pediatrics. It is often a routine part of the admission procedure and provides important information. In addition, kidney infections are common, so it is necessary to collect and examine urine often.

Qualified personnel will sometimes perform suprapubic bladder aspiration on newborns and infants (Figure 30-11). Contamination is a minimal concern using this method. Place an infant in a froglike position for the procedure, similar to the position described later for femoral venipunctures. A physician prepares the skin above the bladder and inserts a 20- or 21-gauge needle into the bladder and removes several milliliters of urine. Gently prevent the legs from excessive movement, which has the potential to cause injury at the insertion site, by holding the infant's legs in a froglike position. Usually the best time for the procedure is 30 to 60 minutes after voiding.

You will also sometimes use plastic urine collection bags. It is important to apply them correctly. Applying skin preparation to the area increases the adhesiveness of these bags (Figure 30-12). In girls, give special attention to the narrow area between the vagina and the

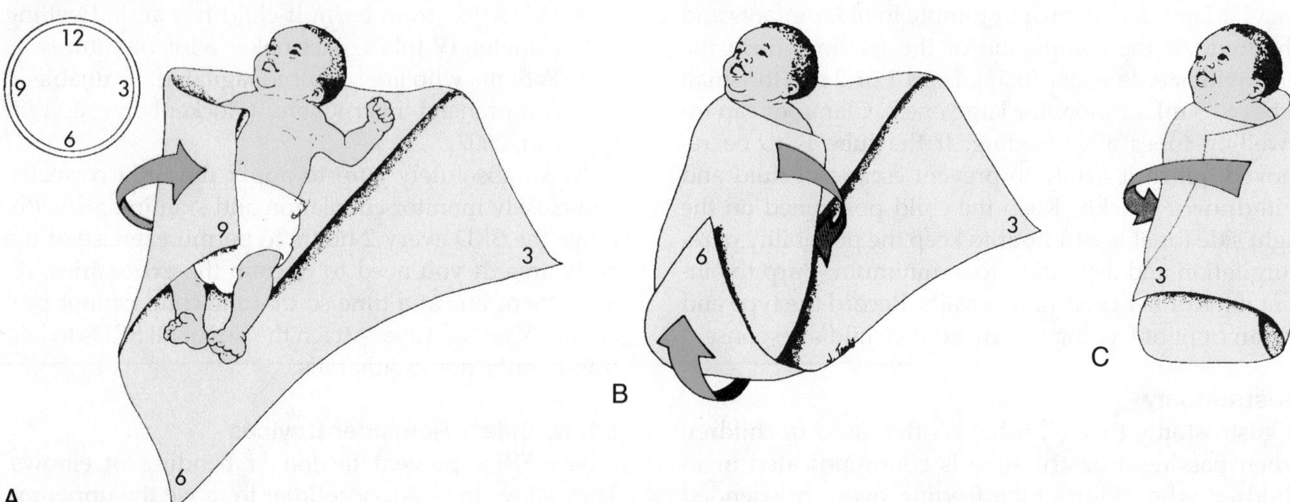

FIGURE 30-10 Mummy restraint. **A,** Fold material over the right arm, and then tuck the corner under the left side. **B,** Fold the bottom up and the opposite corner over the infant's left arm. **C,** Tuck it under the right side to secure it.

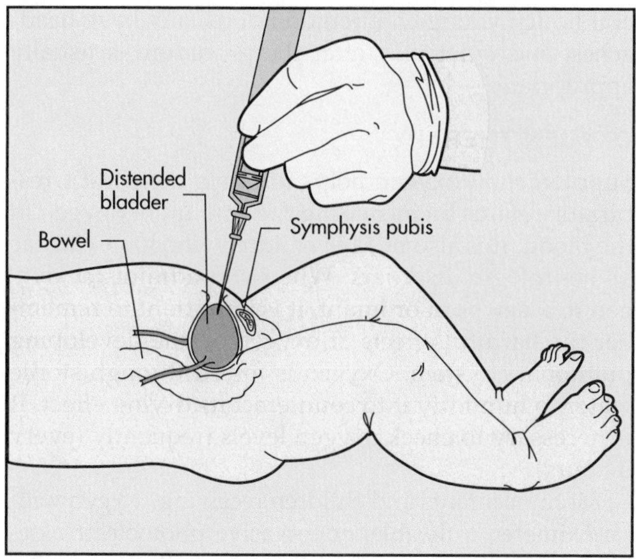

FIGURE 30-11 Suprapubic bladder aspiration.

rectum. If the adhesive backing is not attached securely to this area, you will cover the anus. As a result, it is possible for stool to contaminate the specimen.

When the bag is in place, cut a slit into the disposable diaper before it is placed on the child. By doing so, you will be able to pull the urine bag through to the outside so you can monitor it. As soon as the child voids, remove the bag, so there is less chance of losing the urine specimen.

Catheterizations are done occasionally. Because of the high possibility of contamination, especially in regard to introducing organisms into the urinary system, practitioners use this procedure as little as possible.

If urethral catheterization is necessary, it is recommended to apply a 2% lidocaine lubricant with applicator to the meatus. Advise the child that the lubricant is there to reduce any discomfort associated with inserting the catheter (Gerard et al., 2003).

VENIPUNCTURES TO OBTAIN BLOOD SPECIMENS

In infants and young children, the physician will sometimes use a jugular or femoral vein to obtain a blood specimen. It is your responsibility to prepare, position, and restrain the child. Holding the head or lower extremities absolutely immobile is critical.

When a jugular vein is used, you will place the child in a mummy SRD beforehand. Place the child's body on the examining table so that the shoulders are at the edge of the table. Turning the infant's head 45 degrees provides the best angle for successful entry (Figure 30-13). For a femoral venipuncture, place the infant on the back with both legs in a froglike position (Figure 30-14).

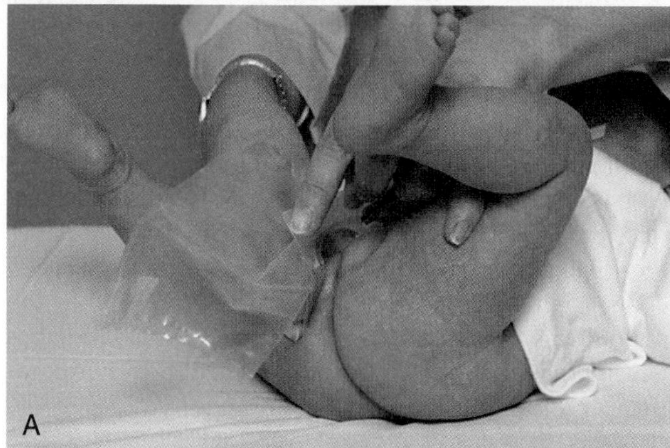

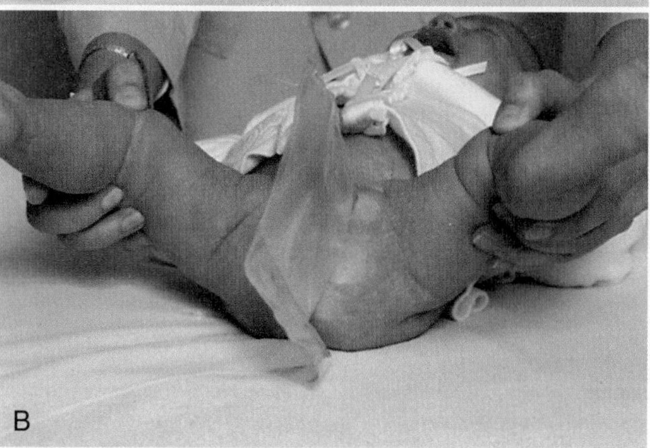

FIGURE 30-12 Application of a urine collection bag. **A,** On female infant, apply adhesive portion to exposed and dried perineum first. **B,** Bag adheres firmly around perineal area to prevent urine leakage.

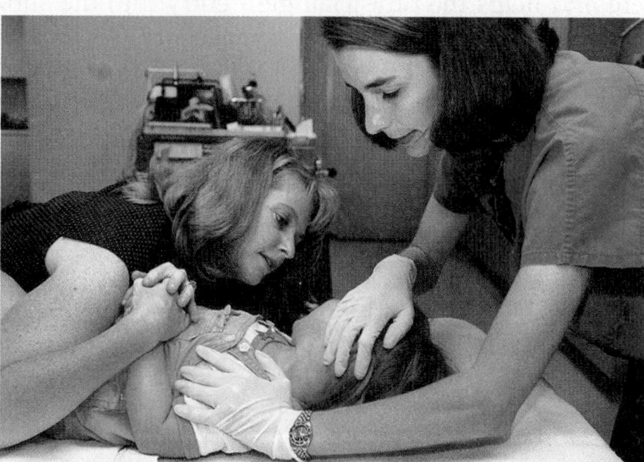

FIGURE 30-13 Correct position for jugular venipuncture procedure.

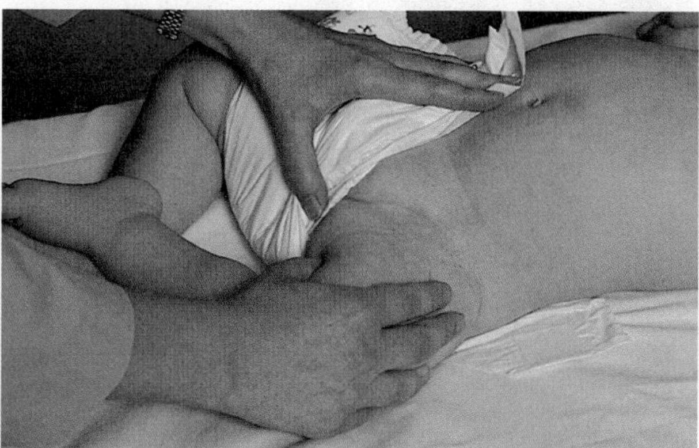

FIGURE 30-14 Position for femoral venipuncture procedure.

It is necessary to apply gentle pressure to both knees to restrict movement. Once the needle has been removed from the vein, apply pressure to the site to prevent the formation of a hematoma.

Sometimes the chosen site for venipuncture will be one of the veins of the extremities, especially the arm and the hand. Older children, with appropriate explanation, preparation, and support, will usually require only minimal if any restraint. One way of restraining younger children is to have the technician on one side of the child's bed and you on the other. Lean across the child's upper body to prevent movement, and immobilize the venipuncture site with an arm.

LUMBAR PUNCTURE

Lumbar punctures are often frightening for both children and parents. Explain the procedure to the parents and the child (if old enough to understand), and answer any questions they have. It is usually permitted to apply EMLA (eutectic mixture of local anesthetics), a local anesthetic cream, to the lumbar area. However, it is necessary to apply the EMLA cream at least 1 hour before the procedure.

This procedure requires positioning the child at the edge of the examining table or bed, on the side, facing you. Often you will place an infant in a sitting position. Gently flex the neck and the legs, as demonstrated in Figure 30-15. This angle increases the spinal curvature and helps the physician gain entry into the subarachnoid space of the lumbar spinal canal. It is important to observe the child for any signs of difficulty. You may have to wrap a toddler's legs in a blanket to decrease activity. Hold the child gently and securely in that position until the physician completes the spinal tap. Label the spinal fluid specimen immediately, and send it to the laboratory for analysis (Hockenberry & Wilson, 2007).

Normal spinal fluid pressure ranges from 60 to 180 mm Hg, the lower end of the range being typical in infants. Help adolescents avoid headache after a lumber puncture by advising them to lie flat for several hours; young children do not usually have headaches, and quiet play after the procedure is usually appropriate.

OXYGEN THERAPY

Supplemental oxygen helps improve the child's respiratory status by increasing the amount of oxygen in the blood. It is also used in children who have cardiac or neurologic disorders. When you administer oxygen to a newborn or infant, it is important to remember the harmful effects of oxygen on the developing pulmonary system. Oxygen is forced through sterile water to humidify it to counteract its drying effect. It is necessary to check oxygen levels frequently (every 2 hours).

Monitor infants and children receiving oxygen with an oximeter, a flexible, noninvasive photoelectric device with adhesive backing that you will place on the foot or the hand of an infant or the finger of an adolescent. The monitoring screen gives an instant reading of the oxygen saturation of blood. Correlation is high between this measurement and the arterial oxygenation. Table 30-9 presents advantages and disadvantages of various oxygen delivery systems.

Hood and Incubator

Oxygen often is delivered to small infants through a plastic hood that fits over the baby's head (Figure 30-16). It is an efficient method of providing oxygen at well-controlled levels. More important, the body is accessible for starting an IV line or performing a procedure.

A less efficient method of delivering oxygen to an infant is to use a closed incubator. However, incubators have imperfectly fitted lids, uncovered vents, and portholes that must be opened to perform an activity on the infant, all of which contribute to fluctuations in oxygen levels. Maintaining a constant temperature within the incubator is a problem, as well. As an infant's metabolism increases in an effort to maintain body temperature, larger amounts of oxygen are required.

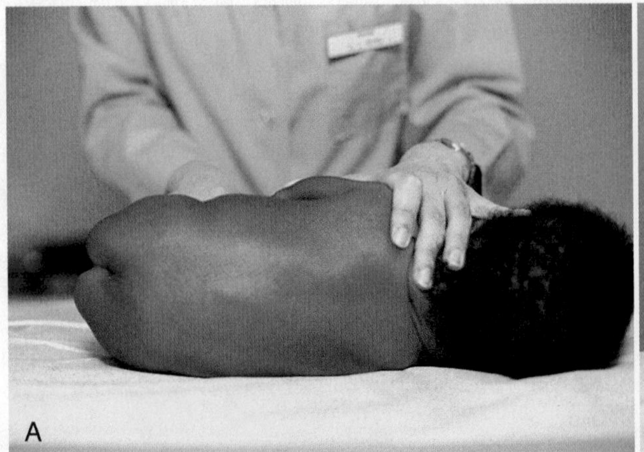

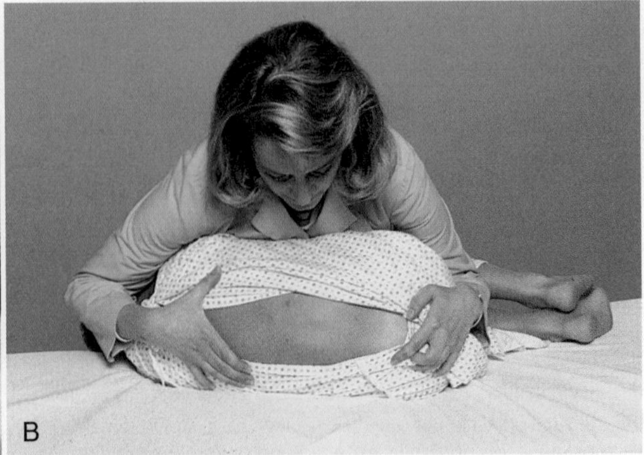

FIGURE 30-15 **A,** Modified side-lying position for lumbar puncture. **B,** Older child in side-lying position.

Table 30-9 Advantages and Disadvantages of Various Oxygen-Delivery Systems

SYSTEM	ADVANTAGES	DISADVANTAGES
Oxygen masks	Various sizes available Ability to provide a predictable concentration of oxygen (with Venturi mask) whether child breathes through nose or mouth	Skin irritation Fear of suffocation Accumulation of moisture on face Possibility of aspiration of vomitus Difficulty in controlling O_2 concentrations
Nasal cannula	Provision of constant oxygen flow even while child eats and talks Possibility of more complete observation of child because nose and mouth remain unobstructed	Discomfort for the child Possibility of causing abdominal distention and discomfort or vomiting Difficulty of controlling O_2 concentrations if child breathes through mouth Inability to provide mist if desired
Oxygen tent	Achievement of lower O_2 concentrations Child receives increased inspired O_2 concentration even while eating	Necessity for right fit around bed to prevent leakage of O_2 Cool and wet tent environment Poor access to patient—inspired O_2 levels will fall whenever tent is entered
Oxygen hood, face tent	Achievement of high O_2 concentrations Free access to patient's chest for assessment	High-humidity environment Need to remove patient for feeding and care

Modified from Hazinski, M.F. (Ed.). (1992). *Nursing care of the critically ill child.* (2nd ed.). St. Louis: Mosby.

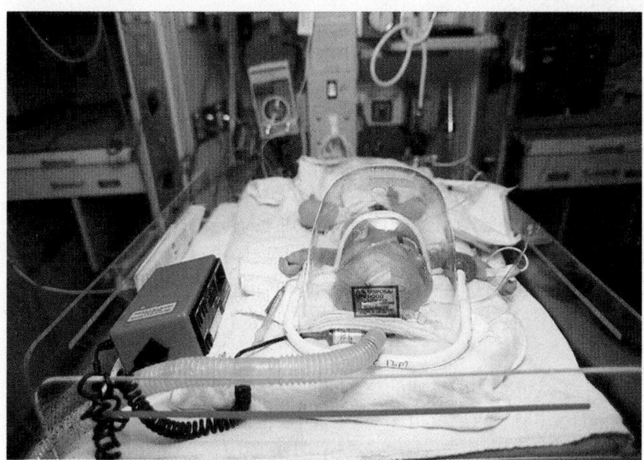

FIGURE 30-16 Oxygen is administered to an infant by means of a plastic hood (Oxy-Hood).

Mist Tents

The purpose of using a mist tent is to improve a child's respiratory status by liquefying pulmonary secretions. You will easily be able to observe the child through the plastic canopy. All of the device's working parts are outside of the tent, which is a distinct advantage when a toddler needs this form of therapy. Compressed air or oxygen runs through sterile water to form the therapeutic mist. A disadvantage is that you have to open the canopy for treatments and procedures, which lowers the concentration of the mist.

Take care to organize all activities and thus to limit the number of times the tent is opened, to make it possible to maintain desired concentrations and give the child longer rest periods. Tuck the tent under the mattress of a crib to maintain humidity levels. If the tent is functioning efficiently, dampness within it is significant, and frequent (every 3 to 4 hours) linen and clothing changes will often be necessary.

Nasal Cannula

Delivering oxygen to newborns and all ages of children is possible by means of a nasal cannula. It is a mode of delivery commonly used with infants suffering from bronchopulmonary dysplasia (abnormal development of the bronchi and the lungs). Maintaining the cannula's placement is often problematic in the infant, whose random head and hand movements disturb its position. Placing clear plastic tape around the oxygen tubing and over the nose and cheek helps prevent this. Adjusting the device at the back of an infant's head allows you to fit the tubing to the child, and hooking it over the pinnae helps stabilize it. In older children, keep the nasal cannula in place by using the adjustable elastic straps on the child's head.

SUCTIONING

Maintaining a patent airway sometimes necessitates suctioning. It is more common for air passages in children to become occluded because of the small size of their respiratory tract structures. Signs that a child possibly needs suctioning include pallor; restlessness or anxiety; increased pulse, respiration, and temperature; dyspnea; bubbling (copious amounts of thin secretions); rattling (thick, tenacious secretions); drooling; mouth breathing; nasal flaring; grunting; gasping; retractions; cyanosis; and erythema (flushed face). Infants often have an anxious look in their eyes or fidget constantly. An older child will perhaps constantly seek attention with no explanation, toss and turn in bed, or finger the edge of a blanket.

Use suctioning when secretions are audible in the airway or when signs of airway obstruction or oxygen deficit are present. It is possible to use various devices to suction children, such as a bulb syringe or a straight suction catheter of the proper size for the child. In nonemergency situations, demonstrate how the suction machine operates by suctioning some water from a cup. Reassure the small child that the machine is only suctioning excess fluid from the mouth or nose, not body contents. Recommended pressures for airway suctioning using wall suction range from 50 to 95 mm Hg for infants to 95 to 110 mm Hg for children.

The use of artificial airways has become a routine life-sustaining measure in the pediatric and neonatal population. Depth, timing, and frequency are important considerations when suctioning a tracheostomy or endotracheal tube:

- **Depth:** Approximately ¼ to ½ inch beyond the tip of the artificial airway; determine placement by placing an appropriately sized suction catheter into an artificial airway of the same size, insert the catheter to the appropriate depth, mark with tape, and keep at the bedside as a reference.
- **Timing:** Limit suctioning to not more than 5 seconds.
- **Frequency:** Allow 30 seconds between suctioning attempts (two or three attempts at most).

INTAKE AND OUTPUT

Many health disorders necessitate accurate monitoring of the amount of solids and liquids taken in and the amount excreted. For example, measuring and recording intake and output (I&O) is extremely important in infants with diarrhea, toddlers with burns, or adolescents with renal disorders. Infants who are hospitalized because they fail to thrive or to grow as expected are placed on "calorie counts," which call for the careful recording of all food ingested and liquids given. This intake is recorded at the bedside, and a nutritionist calculates the calories the child actually consumes. It is helpful in determining whether the cause is organic or the result of an inadequate intake. These causes are ruled out before a maternal-infant problem is considered.

All fluids given to a child are documented on a record kept at the bedside. Adolescents are usually able to assume this responsibility after an explanation.

A number of fluids are acceptable for encouraging fluid intake in the hospital and at home. They include diluted fruit juices, liquid or solid gelatin, sweetened tea, flavored ice pops, and sports electrolyte replacement drinks (e.g., Gatorade) and infant solution (e.g., Pedialyte).

Persuading a reluctant child to drink fluids is often quite a nursing challenge. Offer fluids in small amounts at frequent intervals to prevent dehydration. Do not force them, and do not awaken the child from rest for this purpose.

When you teach parents about fluid management, it is always wise to determine whether they understand the concept of clear liquids. It is important to emphasize that milk is not a liquid, because it forms curds when it comes in contact with the stomach lining. Caution parents about including broths, because most are high in sodium.

Encourage parents to relax any pressure on a child to eat during an acute illness. They need to understand that liquids provide necessary fluid and calories.

Infants and children who are unable or not permitted to take fluids by mouth face obligatory parenteral fluid therapy. Before an IV infusion is started, prepare the child and the family for this stressful procedure.

An understanding of the child's feeding habits will often help you increase consumption after you are able to step up the diet from fluids to solids. Once the child feels better, appetite begins to improve. It is best to take advantage of any hungry period by serving high-quality foods and snacks. With the permission of the physician, encourage parents to help by bringing in food items from home. This is especially important if the family's cultural eating habits differ from what hospital food services provide. The importance of recording all intake is key to preventing complications.

You will also measure all urine voided before discarding it. You will sometimes have to remind older children to save all urine. Measuring urine output in the infant or toddler who is not toilet trained is sometimes a challenge. Most hospitals require routine weighing of diapers (before and after voiding) of all children who are not toilet trained. Subtract the weight of a dry disposable diaper from the weight of the wet diaper. The difference in the weight in grams equals the milliliters voided: 1 g equals 1 mL of urine.

MEDICATION ADMINISTRATION

A critical responsibility of a pediatric nurse is the administration of pediatric medications. Make sure you know how to compute the dose correctly and administer it properly. For safety, have a second nurse check all computed dosages. Don't forget the "six rights" of medication administration discussed in Chapter 23: Give the *right* medication and the *right* amount of the right medication to the *right* child at the *right* time and by the *right* route with the *right* documentation. Also remember to assess and document the child's response to the drug. Factors related to growth and maturation alter the child's capacity to metabolize and excrete drugs (see the Safety Alert).

Immaturity or defects in all or part of the process of absorption, distribution, or excretion have the potential to alter the effect of a drug. Newborn and young children are more susceptible than adults to the toxic effects of certain medications because of their immature organ system's limited ability to detoxify or eliminate drugs. The side effects and toxic signs and symptoms are difficult to evaluate in a preverbal child.

Unit-doses are not used in pediatrics because children are of various ages and weights. Methods of calculating dosages for children consider age, body weight,

Safety Alert!

Administering Medication to the Infant, the Toddler and Child, and the Adolescent

INFANT

- It is the physician's responsibility to prescribe drugs in the correct dosage to achieve the desired effect without endangering the health of the child.
- You need to have an understanding of the safe dosage of medications you administer to children, as well as the expected action, possible side effects, and signs of toxicity.
- Calculate dosage for all medications by use of body surface area (BSA) in kilograms of weight. Any small differences in dosage have the potential to result in toxemia.
- It is essential for safety to have a second nurse check all computed dosages.
- When an ordered dose is outside the usual range or if there is some question regarding the preparation or the route of administration, always check with the prescribing practitioner before proceeding with the administration. You are legally liable for any drug administered.
- The vastus lateralis muscle is an acceptable injection site because it is the most developed and not located close to any major circulatory or nerve structures.
- The ventrogluteal muscle is situated away from major nerves and blood vessels. You will be able to identify it easily by a prominent bony landmark. Research of injection sites in children does not reveal any complications associated with the ventrogluteal site, and it is the preferred site for injections in children of all ages, including newborns (Cook, 2006).
- Administer oral medications with a disposable plastic syringe (remove needle), releasing them slowly into buccal pouch; it is also acceptable to place medication in an empty nipple and allow the infant to suck.

TODDLER AND CHILD

- Usually 1 mL is the maximum volume that is acceptable to administer parenterally (intramuscular [IM] or subcutaneous [subQ]) in a single site to small children.
- The ventrogluteal site is relatively free of major nerves and blood vessels, is a relatively large muscle, and is a safe injection site for young children.
- Allow toddler or child choices of drink to consume with oral medications.
- If possible, allow child to choose chewable or liquid medication if available.
- Never mix oral medications with essential foods, liquids, or honey (owing to risk of botulism); use nonessential foods like applesauce or pudding.
- Use childproof tops on all medications for safety.
- Provide for sufficient help in restraining young child before giving IM or subQ injections; children are often unable to cooperate, and their behavior is usually unpredictable.
- Apply EMLA (eutectic mixture of local anesthetics, a topical anesthetic) over IM site if time permits (at least 60 minutes, and preferably 2 to 2½ hours before giving injection). Applying LMX cream (lidocaine) is possible if time interval has to be shorter.

ADOLESCENT

- The adolescent is capable of logical thought and reasoning and requires an explanation of hospital routine and purpose of treatments and medications.
- Older children and adolescents usually pose few problems in selecting a suitable site for IM injections.
- When administering medications to an adolescent, follow the same protocol as for an adult.
- The ventrogluteal site is the preferred site for IM injections for the adolescent.

and **body surface area (BSA)** (total area exposed to the outside environment).

Calculating the proportional amount of BSA to body weight is the most reliable method for determining children's dosages. Use the height and weight of the child to estimate the BSA. This information is then applied to a formula to obtain dosage, such as the following:

$$\frac{\text{BSA of child}}{\text{BSA of adult}} \times \text{Adult dose} = \text{Estimated child's dose}$$

Also see Chapter 23 for a detailed explanation of pediatric considerations in medication administration.

Oral Medications

When administering liquids, take care to prevent aspiration. With the infant held in a semireclining position, place the medicine in the mouth using a spoon, plastic cup, plastic dropper, or plastic syringe (without the needle). Place the dropper or syringe along the side of the infant's tongue and administer the liquid slowly, waiting for the infant to swallow between deposits. Another option is to use an empty nipple to deposit liquid medication. Remove the nipple as soon as the infant consumes all of the medication. Young children who refuse to cooperate or who resist despite explanation will need mild physical coercion at times. If this is necessary, carry it out quickly, kindly, and carefully. Remember the possibility that a crying child will aspirate medication when lying on his or her back.

To encourage the child's acceptance of oral medications:

- Give the child an ice pop or small ice cube to suck to numb the tongue before giving the drug.
- Mix the drug with a small amount (about 1 tsp) of a sweet-tasting substance such as honey (except in infants because of the risk of botulism), flavored syrups, jam, fruit purées, or ice cream; avoid using essential food items, because the child may later refuse to eat them.
- Give a "chaser" of water, juice, a soft drink, or an ice pop or frozen juice bar after the drug.

- If nausea is a problem, give a carbonated beverage poured over finely crushed ice before or immediately after the medication.
- When medication has an unpleasant taste, have the child pinch the nose and drink the medicine through a straw. Much of what we taste is associated with smell.

Many pediatric medications are given by drops or dropper. A misunderstanding of these terms on parents' part creates a risk of overdose. In addition, many droppers that come with medications are marked in tenths of cubic centimeters. If parents use a syringe instead, which is marked in cubic centimeters, they run the risk of administering 4 cc instead of 0.4 cc. Parents also do not realize that cubic centimeters (cc) and milliliters (mL) are considered the same. If the prescription is written in cubic centimeters, parents often won't know what to do when droppers are in milliliters. Provide education to parents on correct methods for measuring and giving medication. Demonstrate the technique.

Table 30-10 Needle and Site Recommendations for Selected Injections

NEEDLE	SITE
INTRADERMAL (ID)	
3/8-1/2 inch	Primary: ventral forearm
25 to 27 gauge	
Short bevel	
SUBCUTANEOUS (SubQ)	
3/4-5/8 inch	Primary: upper arm; lower abdomen; anterior thigh
23 to 26 gauge	
Medium bevel	
INTRAMUSCULAR (IM)	
5/8-1 inch	Primary: 0-2 years—vastus lateralis, ventrogluteal
20 to 25 gauge	2-12 years—vastus lateralis; ventrogluteal
Medium bevel	

Modified from Elliott, M. (1991). Administering intradermal, subcutaneous, and intramuscular injections. In D. Smith (Ed.), *Comprehensive child and family nursing skills*. St. Louis: Mosby.

Intradermal, Subcutaneous, and Intramuscular Medications

Injections are a source of pain and fear for children, so drugs are usually given by injection only when other routes cannot be used. Table 30-10 lists recommendations for injection sites and needles. The primary site for IM injections are the vastus lateralis muscle (Figure 30-17) and the ventrogluteal muscle (Figure 30-18). The deltoid muscle is possible to use in children who are 18 months or older as a site for intramuscular injections and also in infants who are receiving their hepatitis B vaccine (Hockenberry & Wilson, 2007) (Figure 30-19). If time permits, apply EMLA, a local anesthetic cream, to the injection site at least 1 hour before the injection. Wear gloves to prevent anesthesia to your fingers.

Injections administered with care seldom produce trauma to the child. Repeated use of a single site has been associated with fibrosis of the muscle and subsequent muscle contracture. Most children are unpredictable, and few cooperate totally when receiving an

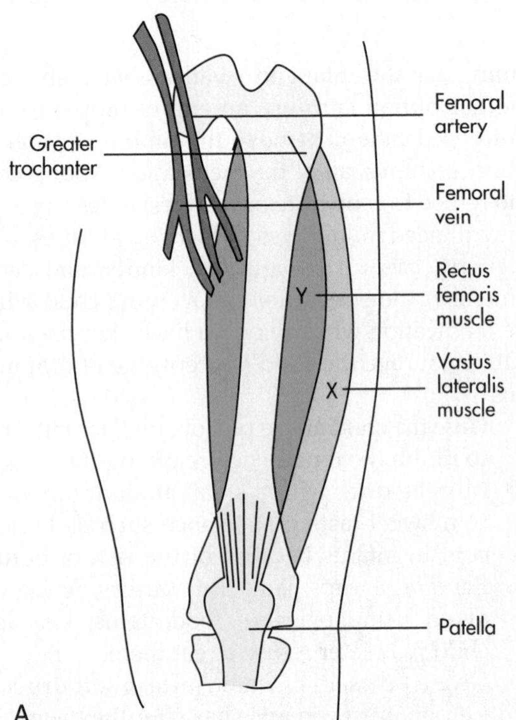

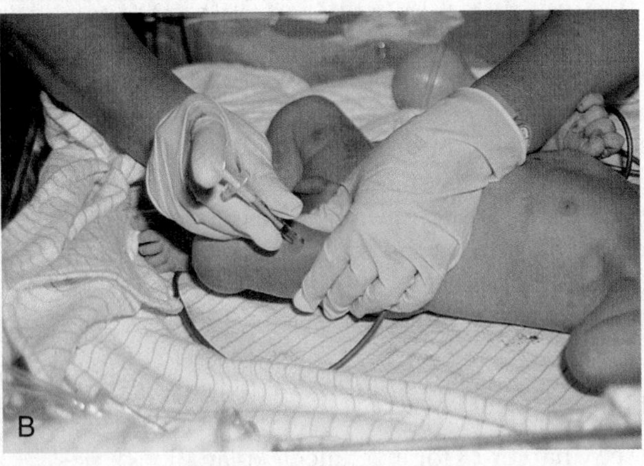

FIGURE 30-17 Intramuscular injection sites. **A,** The middle third of the vastus lateralis muscle is the primary site for intramuscular injections in the thigh. **B,** Infant's leg is stabilized for intramuscular injection. The needle penetrates the midlateral thigh on a front-to-back course.

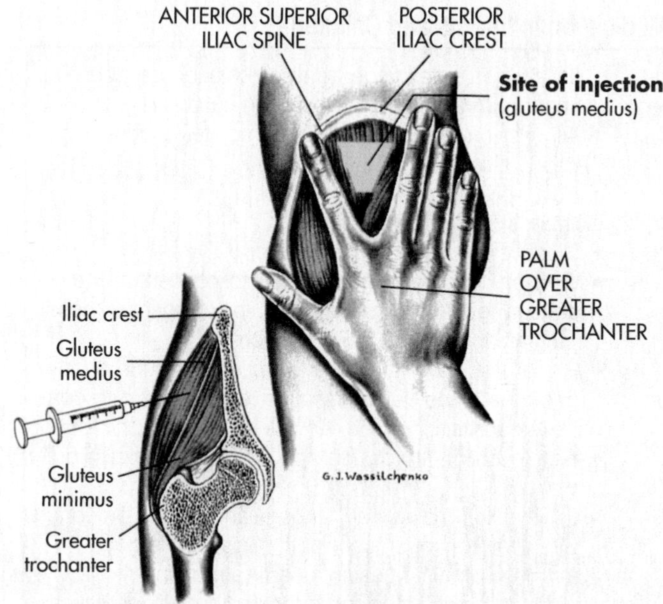

FIGURE 30-18 Ventrogluteal site for intramuscular injection.

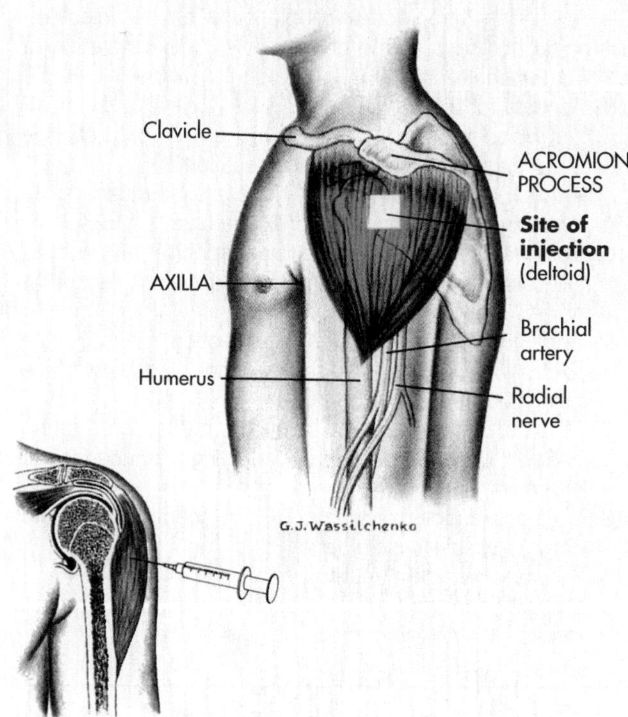

FIGURE 30-19 Deltoid site for intramuscular injection.

injection. It is advisable to have someone available to help gently restrain the child.

To estimate the needle length for IM injections, first grasp the **vastus lateralis muscle** (the largest of the four muscles of the quadriceps femoris, situated on the lateral side of the thigh) (Figure 30-17, *A*) or the deltoid muscle (Figure 30-19), and choose a needle length that is approximately half the distance between your thumb and your index finger. With the ventrogluteal site, grasp only subcutaneous tissue, so choose a needle length that is slightly more than half the distance (Figure 30-18). Needle length should allow for a small portion of the needle to be exposed at the skin surface as a precaution if the needle breaks off from the hub.

Factors to consider when selecting a site for IM injection on an infant or child include the following (Box 30-10):

- The amount and character of the medication to be injected
- The amount and the general condition of the muscle mass
- The frequency or number of injections to be given during the course of treatment
- The type of medication being given
- Factors that will possibly impede access to or cause contamination of the site
- The ability of the child to assume the required position safely

Intravenous Medications

The IV route of administering a medication is often selected for the following reasons:

- Medication is almost immediately distributed to tissues, and prompt physiologic action occurs.
- With consecutive doses, it is possible to achieve predictable drug levels and maintain therapeutic effects.
- After initial insertion, IV administration is more comfortable for the child than other types of parenteral injections.
- The IV sites in children differ from those of adults. A superficial scalp vein is commonly used in infants younger than 9 months of age because these veins have no valves, so it is possible to insert a needle in either direction. In addition, the child is able to move the head from side to side without dislodging the needle. Any accessible vein is acceptable to use in older children. The use of peripheral lines in a child's lower extremities will impede ambulation.
- You will sometimes convert an infusion line to a saline lock when a child does not require additional IV fluids but still needs additional medications, such as antibiotics or pain medication. With a saline lock, a child is able to move about except for those brief periods when drugs are infused. Irrigate the tube regularly to keep the line open as per agency policy.

OCULAR, OTIC, AND NASAL ADMINISTRATION

There are few differences in administering eye, ear, and nose medication to children or adults. Gaining children's cooperation is necessary for these procedures, as employing restraining techniques will also be at times.

Instilling eyedrops in infants is sometimes difficult because they often clench their lids together. One ap-

Box 30-10 Guidelines for Intramuscular Administration of Medication in Infants and Children

1. Use all usual safety precautions in administering medication (e.g., check child's identification). Apply EMLA cream (eutectic mixture of local anesthetics, a topical anesthetic) over site if time permits.
2. Prepare medication.
   - Select needle and syringe appropriate to the following:
     —Amount of fluid to be administered (syringe size)
     —Viscosity of fluid to be administered (needle gauge)
     —Amount of tissue to be penetrated (needle length)
   - Maximum volume to be administered in a single site is 1 mL for older infants and small children.
3. Determine the site of injection, and make certain muscle is large enough to accommodate volume and type of medication.
   - Older children: select site as with adult patient; allow child some choice of site, if feasible.
   - Vastus lateralis muscle and ventrogluteal muscle are acceptable sites for infants and small or debilitated children.
   - Dorsogluteal muscle is insufficiently developed to be a safe site for infants and small children. **The dorsogluteal muscle is not used for infants or children of any age.**
4. Administer medication.
   - Provide for sufficient help in restraining child; children are often uncooperative, and their behavior is usually unpredictable.
   - Explain briefly what is to be done and, if appropriate, what child can do to help.
   - Expose injection area for unobstructed view of landmarks.
   - Select a site where skin is free of irritation and danger of infection; palpate for and avoid sensitive or hardened areas. With multiple injections, rotate sites.
   - Place child in a lying or sitting position; child is not allowed to stand for the following reasons:
     —Landmarks are more difficult to assess
     —Restraint is more difficult
     —It is possible that child will faint and fall
   - Use a new, sharp needle with smallest diameter that permits free flow of the medication.
   - Grasp muscle firmly between thumb and fingers to isolate and stabilize muscle for deposition of drug in its deepest part; in obese children, spread skin with thumb and index finger to displace subcutaneous tissue, and grasp muscle deeply on each side.
   - Allow skin preparation to dry completely before penetrating skin.
   - Have medication at room temperature.
5. Decrease perception of pain:
   - Distract child with conversation.
   - Give child something on which to concentrate (e.g., squeezing a hand or bed rail, pinching own nose, humming, counting, yelling "Ouch").
   - Place a cold compress or wrapped ice cube on site about a minute before injection, or apply cold to contralateral site.
   - Say to child, "If you feel this, tell me to take it out, please."
   - Have child hold a small bandage and place it on puncture site after intramuscular (IM) injection is given.
6. Insert needle quickly, using a dartlike motion.
7. Avoid tracking any medication through superficial tissues:
   - If withdrawing medication from an ampule, use a needle equipped with a filter that removes glass particles; then use a new, nonfilter needle for injection.
   - Use the Z-track or air-bubble technique as indicated.
   - Do not depress the plunger at all during insertion of the needle.
8. Aspirate for blood.
   - If blood is found, remove syringe from site, change needle, and reinsert into new location.
   - If no blood is found, inject into a relaxed muscle.
9. Inject medication slowly (over 20 seconds).
10. Remove needle quickly; hold gauze sponge firmly against skin near needle when removing it to avoid pulling on tissue.
11. Apply firm pressure to site after injection; massage site to hasten absorption unless contraindicated, as with irritating drugs.
12. Place a small bandage on puncture site; with young children, decorate bandage by drawing a smiling face or other symbol of acceptance.
13. Hold and cuddle young child and encourage parents to comfort child; praise older child.
14. Allow expression of feelings.
15. Discard syringe and uncapped needle in puncture-resistant container located near site of use.
16. Record time of injection, drug, dose, and injection site.

proach is to place drops in the nasal corner where the lids meet. When the child opens the lids, medication flows into the conjunctiva. For younger children, playing a game tends to be helpful. If both eye ointment and eyedrops are ordered, give drops first, wait 3 minutes, and then apply the ointment to allow each drug to work. When possible, administer eye ointments before bedtime or naptime, because the child's vision will be blurred for a while.

Instill eardrops with the child restrained. For children 3 years of age and younger, straighten the external auditory canal by pulling the pinna downward and back. For children older than 3 years of age, pull the pinna upward and back. After instillation, have the child remain lying on the opposite side for a few minutes. Gentle massage of the area in front of the ear usually facilitates entry of the drops. Sometimes you will place sterile cotton loosely in the ear to prevent infected material from being forced into the mastoid area.

For nasal administration, position the child with the head hyperextended to prevent the strangling sensations caused by medication trickling into the pharynx rather than up into the nasal passages.

Table 30-11 Guidelines for Administration of Enemas to Children

AGE	AMOUNT	INSERTION DISTANCE
Infant	120-240 mL	1 inch
2-4 years	240-360 mL	2 inches
4-10 years	360-480 mL	3 inches
11 years	480-720 mL	4 inches

RECTAL ADMINISTRATION

The rectal route is less reliable but sometimes is used when the oral route is difficult or contraindicated. Lubricate the suppository with water-soluble jelly or warm water, and insert it quickly and gently into the rectum beyond the rectal sphincters. Then hold the buttocks together firmly to relieve pressure on the anal sphincter until the urge to expel the suppository has passed (5 to 10 minutes).

Enema

The procedure for an enema for a child does not differ essentially from that for an adult (Table 30-11). Use an isotonic solution in children. Do not use plain water because, being hypertonic, it has the potential to cause rapid fluid shift and overload.

Proper insertion of the catheter tip, especially in infants, is essential to prevent rectal damage and perforation. If insertion of the enema tip causes discomfort, remove the tip and notify the physician.

SAFETY

Protecting a child from harm is a major issue in pediatrics. Anticipatory guidance for parents of infants and toddlers and health teaching for school-age children and adolescents are two methods of preventing accidents. However, hazards and dangers are everywhere—in the home, at the playground, at school, and in the hospital.

Injuries cause more deaths and disabilities in children than all causes of disease combined. The risk-taking activities of adolescents also contribute to the **morbidity** (an illness or an abnormal condition or quality) and mortality of adolescence. Table 30-12 identifies common developmental characteristics, potential haz-

Table 30-12 Preventing Accidents

BEHAVIOR OR AGE-RELATED FACTOR	ACCIDENT OR HAZARD	PREVENTION
NEWBORN		
Sleeping	Suffocation	Do not tuck blankets in.
Poor head control		Do not use pillows.
Somewhat capable of moving body around		Do not use plastic bags in crib.
		Avoid soft, moldable mattresses.
		Place healthy infants in supine or side-lying positions for sleep.
	Accidents	Use an approved car seat and follow manufacturer's instructions.
		Check crib slats—have them no more than 2⅜ inches apart.
	Burns	Test bath water temperature.
		Never smoke or drink hot liquids while holding baby.
	Falls	Never leave baby alone or unattended on bed, sofa, or counter.
		Always have one hand on baby.
		Carry newborn with two hands.
	Lead poisoning	Eliminate or reduce the child's exposure to any surfaces or substances containing lead.*
1-6 MONTHS		
Head control improving	Suffocation	Keep crib free of plastic bags.
		Do not use pillows.
Placing objects in mouth	Foreign body aspiration	Inspect all toys; remove button eyes or detach small wheels.
	Injury from toys: loose parts or sharp edges	Do not offer foods that pose risk of choking, such as grapes, nuts, potato chips, and raisins.
		Remove open safety pins, needles, and nails from baby's reach.
Moving body from one place to another	Falls	Do not leave baby unattended on bed, sofa, or counter.
Beginning to pull self to sitting position	Burns	Test bath water; hold infant securely.
		Keep hot liquids in cups away from child's grasp.

*Continued attention to this precaution is necessary throughout childhood.

Continued

Table 30-12 Preventing Accidents—cont'd

BEHAVIOR OR AGE-RELATED FACTOR	ACCIDENT OR HAZARD	PREVENTION
7-12 MONTHS		
Sitting up	Falls, drownings	Never leave infant unattended in high chair, on bed, or in tub.
Crawling	Accidents	Use gates at bottom and top of stairs.
		Place guards around fireplaces; never leave infant alone near space heater.
	Suffocation	Do not leave plastic bags or balloons in crib or playpen or within infant's reach.
Feeding self	Aspiration, ingestion	Do not offer foods on which child is likely to choke, such as popcorn; small, hard candies; gum; or hot dogs.
		Lock up all medications and poisonous household substances.
		Purchase medicines and household cleaners in childproof containers.
		Keep number of local poison control center by telephone.
		Childproof the entire house, including placing poisonous houseplants out of reach.
1-2 YEARS		
Holding on or walking	Falls, lacerations, abrasions	Keep furniture with sharp edges and glass tabletops out of child's way or protect with special corner protectors.
		Keep sharp kitchen utensils and garden equipment out of reach or locked up.
Exploring environment	Electrical injuries	Always know where the toddler is playing.
		Supervise all outdoor play activities.
Running		Do not allow child to run with objects in mouth.
		Begin teaching safety outdoors, including dangers of traffic, climbing, and walking in front of swings at playgrounds.
	Motor vehicle accidents	Always use an approved car seat and follow manufacturer's instructions.
		Keep toddler in fenced area.
		Install childproof locks on car doors.
		Teach child to cross street holding an adult's hand.
		Keep car doors locked in garage or driveway.
		Do not allow play in driver's seat without adult present.
	Ingestion, inhalation	Keep insecticides, medications, and all harmful cleaners locked up.
	Suffocation	Supervise play with balloons.
		Do not allow plastic bags in play.
		Remove doors of refrigerators or chain shut before discarding.
	Drowning	Keep bath water level low in tub.
		Never leave child alone in tub or wading pool; empty wading pool after use.
		Supervise child closely at beach.
		Never allow child near water without an adult.
		Fence around swimming pool.
		Enroll toddler in swimming class.
	Burns	Remove matches and lighters from reach.
		Teach fire safety.
		Keep handles of pots toward center of stove when cooking.
		Keep child away from stove while preparing meals.
		Keep child away from charcoal fires.
3-5 YEARS		
Climbing	Falls, lacerations, and abrasions	Check yard, playground, and daycare center for potential hazards.
Running		Begin teaching: safety in using playground equipment; dangers of pushing and shoving playmates; and avoiding strangers.
Exploring environment outside the home		Supervise child using scissors, tricycles, and Big Wheels.
Improving motor skills		Discourage approaching animals without an adult present.
		Teach child his or her own name, address, and telephone number.

Table 30-12 Preventing Accidents—cont'd

BEHAVIOR OR AGE-RELATED FACTOR	ACCIDENT OR HAZARD	PREVENTION
3-5 YEARS—cont'd		
	Drowning	Supervise action-related activities, such as swimming. Never leave child alone in bathtub or wading pool. Never allow child near water without an adult.
	Motor vehicle and pedestrian accidents	Use car seat or safety belts in car according to department of transportation (DOT) standards. Review acceptable behavior in a moving car. Review crossing street at corner, watching lights and flow of traffic.
	Assault, abuse	Teach child to keep parent informed of whereabouts. Confine play to yard; do not allow to play in street.
	Burns	Practice fire drills in the home. Implement other practices similar to those for 1- to 2-year-olds.
	Firearms	Never keep loaded guns or rifles in house or garage. Keep service guns locked. Instruct child never to touch gun or bullets.
6-11 YEARS		
Motor skills continuing to improve Enjoying large muscle activities Becoming increasingly independent Engaging in competitive sports, unsupervised activities	Motor vehicle and pedestrian accidents, injuries, fractures	Review traffic safety. Use safety belts. Teach skateboard safety—control speed; refrain from jumping; use helmet, knee, and elbow pads. Teach bicycle safety—rules of the road, use of reflectors, proper signaling, use of helmets. Review safety regarding use of lawn mowers, farm equipment, and tools. Teach child not to hide in or play near cars.
	Assault, abuse	Caution child about playing in vacant buildings, quarries, or sand pits. Teach proper use of protective gear in competitive sports. Teach child not to throw objects at people or moving vehicles. Teach child how to call fire department, police, and emergency medical assistance.
	Drownings	Review swimming and boating safety. Do not allow ice skating on pond unless its safety has been determined. Never allow the child to swim or skate alone.
	Inhalation, ingestions	Evaluate health education programs at school. Emphasize the hazards of glue sniffing and drug or alcohol use. Encourage family discussions about substance abuse.
12-18 YEARS		
Rapid growth spurt Demonstrating risk-taking behaviors Demonstrating increased independence Engaging in extracurricular activities Reacting to peer group influence Driving a car	Motor vehicle, motorcycle, and bicycle injuries and fractures	Evaluate the high school's safety and health education programs. Review bicycle and motorcycle safety, including use of helmets. Enroll child in driver education classes. Establish limits regarding care, use, and consequences of drinking alcohol and driving.
	Sporting injuries	Encourage group participation in outdoor activities, such as running or jogging. Supervise competitive sports activities. Encourage enrolling in first aid classes. Maintain a physical conditioning program.
	Drownings	Review water safety in seasonal activities. Discourage risk-taking behaviors at pool or beach. Discuss dangers of swimming and skating alone.
	Firearms	Keep guns empty and locked up. Teach proper care of firearms. Supervise target practice in isolated areas.

ards, and preventive measures that help decrease the incidence of accidents and injuries.

Parents and children need to talk and listen to each other to prevent many accidents. Maintaining open communication between and among all members of a family is one method of prevention. The adult who is a role model, who thinks about safety, and who identifies potential dangers in the environment or a particular activity has immense power to influence a child.

Get Ready for the NCLEX® Examination!

Key Points

- It is important to know basic principles of normal growth and development to understand what infants and children are like, what it is possible to expect from them, what their needs are, and why they behave as they do.
- Knowledge of physical assessment using the systematic (head-to-toe) method is important for accurate documentation.
- Metabolism is highest in the newborn.
- Nutrition is probably the single most important influence on growth and is closely related to good health throughout life.
- By understanding that hospitalization is an anxiety-producing experience for the child and the family, you will be better able to address the needs of both.
- The medical and psychosocial needs of the child were considered unimportant before the twentieth century.
- The goal of the pediatric nurse is to promote the highest state of health in each child.
- Family-centered care is a philosophy of care that recognizes the family as the constant in the child's life and holds that systems and personnel are called on to support, respect, encourage, and enhance the strengths and competence of the family.
- By understanding parents' responses to hospitalization of a child, you will be better able to address the parents' needs.
- Children in different age categories show varying concerns and needs while hospitalized.
- One way to decrease the traumatic effects of a child's hospitalization is to have the child and his or her parents attend a preadmission orientation program.
- Rooming-in facilities allow a parent to become as involved as desired and provide the child with the security of an adult who is known, trusted, and loved.
- Preparing children for pediatric procedures increases their cooperation, helps them cope, and promotes a sense of self-esteem and mastery.
- Always provide explanations to children at an age-appropriate level so the child is able to understand them. Age and developmental level influence the ways in which children perceive and make sense of experiences such as illness or disability, and therefore make an impact on their ability to cope.
- The administration of pediatric medications is a serious responsibility.
- The preparation of medication for a child requires precise computation of dosage.
- Accidents are a leading cause of death in children and adolescents, and it is necessary to identify potential hazards and avoid them.

Additional Learning Resources

Go to your Companion CD for an audio glossary, animations, video clips, and more.

evolve Be sure to visit the Evolve site at http://evolve.elsevier.com/Christensen/foundations/ for additional online resources.

Review Questions for the NCLEX® Examination

1. Nursing students learn in class that the man known as the father of pediatrics is:
   1. Hippocrates.
   2. Abraham Jacobi.
   3. James Mott.
   4. R.E. Behrman.

2. The nurse who founded the Henry Street Settlement in New York City was:
   1. Florence Nightingale.
   2. Mari MacPhee.
   3. Lillian Wald.
   4. Linn Rogers.

3. The purpose of pediatric nursing is best stated as:
   1. treating psychological conditions in children.
   2. providing social welfare of children.
   3. promoting the highest possible state of health in children.
   4. emphasizing isolation and asepsis.

4. The first White House Conference on Children focused on issues of child labor, dependent children, and infant care. As a result, what was established in 1987 on behalf of children?
   1. U.S. Children's Bureau
   2. Office of Child Development
   3. National Commission on Children
   4. Women, Infants, and Children program

5. Hospitalization is an anxiety-producing experience for children and families. A 4-year-old child is to be hospitalized for the first time. His parents are apprehensive about the unknown. The nurse will best address their concerns by:
   1. providing information only as needed.
   2. providing an orientation to all children before hospitalization.
   3. providing a tour of the entire hospital.
   4. beginning to provide anticipatory guidance explanations and preparation on first contact.

6. The single most important influence on growth in the child is thought to be:
   1. high metabolism.
   2. nutrition.
   3. ethnic background.
   4. genetics.
7. The most effective method to prepare a child for a pediatric procedure is the:
   1. problem-solving approach.
   2. sensation-based approach.
   3. symbol-based approach.
   4. autonomy-based approach.
8. A 16-month-old child was admitted to the pediatric floor following surgery to repair a cleft palate. An elbow SRD was being used for what purpose?
   1. To monitor excessive pressure to sutures
   2. To provide movement in bed
   3. To prevent injury to operative area
   4. To allow jugular vein puncture with nasogastric tube insertion
9. It is essential to know that in pediatric medication administration:
   1. children and adults are susceptible to toxic effects of medication at the same rate.
   2. there are unit-doses for children.
   3. BSA is the most reliable method of calculating children's medication.
   4. the route of choice is the rectal route.
10. A family-centered approach to care is important when caring for any children but is crucial for optimum care for:
    1. school-age children.
    2. children having minor surgery.
    3. children with special needs.
    4. children receiving routine immunizations.
11. A 7-year-old is about to have a fingerstick. The best statement by the nurse to prepare her for the event is:
    1. "It will hurt but you are a big girl, so you can just grin and bear it."
    2. "It will hurt a lot, and you can cry if you want to."
    3. "Some children tell me it feels like a chicken pecking or a cat scratching."
    4. "Close your eyes, don't look, and it will be over in a minute."
12. An 18-month-old is hospitalized for surgery in the morning. The most helpful intervention to relieve the child's stress associated with hospitalization is:
    1. maintaining a normal routine.
    2. providing opportunities for play.
    3. encouraging parental presence and rooming in.
    4. encouraging self-care activities.
13. The parent of a 6-month-old states that the child's grandmother has expressed concern that the child may be "slow," because she is not crawling. The nurse's role is to:
    1. assure the parent that grandmothers are often overly concerned when it comes to grandchildren.
    2. ask the mother at what age her other children began crawling.
    3. refer the mother for additional evaluation, because most children do crawl by 6 months of age.
    4. assure the mother that children develop at their own rate, but most children do not crawl at age 6 months.
14. An accurate apical heart rate measurement is possible to assess at the _______________ intercostal space.
15. A new patient is 4 years old. On entering the patient's room for the first time, the nurse will:
    1. speak only to the parents, because the child will be very scared.
    2. explain all procedures in great detail, because the child will want to know what is going on.
    3. be careful not to use words that might be misinterpreted by the child, such as "take your temperature."
    4. tell the parents they must leave the room until the physical assessment is complete.
16. A 5-month-old has had abdominal surgery. With regard to pain management, the nurse will consider that:
    1. the infant will perhaps be comforted by sucking on a pacifier, being swaddled, or being rocked.
    2. analgesics are best given only if the child will not stop crying.
    3. at 5 months of age the infant has immature pain receptors, and therefore will not require analgesics.
    4. the child will have less pain if left alone in the bed for all activities.
17. What is true regarding the toddler's nutrition?
    1. The toddler needs to eat twice as much as a 6-month-old infant.
    2. Toddlers can be given solid foods at 4 to 6 months of age.
    3. The toddler is too busy to eat, so give finger foods like hot dogs, grapes, and nuts.
    4. The toddler has no risk of food allergies.
18. The most accurate method to measure urine output in an infant is to:
    1. weigh the diaper before and after the infant voids.
    2. weigh the infant after each wet diaper.
    3. have the parents try to catch the urine in a plastic cup.
    4. insert a Foley catheter for all infants who are not potty trained.

19. What is true of intramuscular injections in children younger than 2 years old? *(Select all that apply.)*
   1. Not possible to give because of poor muscular development
   2. Possible to give in the vastus lateralis muscle
   3. Possible to give in the ventrogluteal muscle
   4. Possible to give in the deltoid muscle

20. The most common asymmetry with lateral curvature of the spine in the adolescent is known as ______.

21. To examine a 6-month-old child's ear with an otoscope, the nurse pulls the ear:
   1. up and back.
   2. down and forward.
   3. up and forward.
   4. down and back.

chapter 31

Care of the Child with a Physical Disorder

evolve

Barbara Lauritsen Christensen

http://evolve.elsevier.com/Christensen/foundationsadult

Objectives

1. Describe etiology and pathophysiology, types of defects, clinical manifestations, diagnostic tests, and medical management of congenital heart defects.
2. Describe etiology and pathophysiology, clinical manifestations, diagnostic tests, medical management, nursing interventions, and patient teaching for children with iron deficiency anemia, sickle cell anemia, and aplastic anemia.
3. Discuss etiology and pathophysiology, clinical manifestations, diagnostic tests, medical management, nursing interventions, patient teaching, and prognosis for children with the coagulation disorders of hemophilia and idiopathic thrombocytopenia purpura.
4. Describe etiology and pathophysiology, clinical manifestations, diagnostic tests, medical management, nursing interventions, patient teaching, and prognosis for children with leukemia.
5. Demonstrate an understanding of etiology and pathophysiology, clinical manifestations, diagnostic tests, medical management, nursing interventions, patient teaching, and prognosis for children with acquired immunodeficiency syndrome (AIDS).
6. Discuss etiology and pathophysiology, clinical manifestations, diagnostic tests, medical management, nursing interventions, patient teaching, and prognosis for children with juvenile rheumatoid arthritis.
7. Discuss etiology and pathophysiology, clinical manifestations, diagnostic tests, medical management, nursing interventions, patient teaching, and prognosis for children with disorders of the respiratory system, including respiratory distress syndrome, bronchopulmonary dysplasia, pneumonia, sudden infant death syndrome, upper respiratory tract infections, tonsillitis, croup, bronchitis, respiratory syncytial virus, pulmonary tuberculosis, cystic fibrosis, and bronchial asthma.
8. Describe etiology and pathophysiology, clinical manifestations, diagnostic tests, medical management, nursing interventions, patient teaching, and prognosis for children with disorders of the gastrointestinal system, including cleft lip and cleft palate, dehydration, diarrhea, gastroenteritis, constipation, gastroesophageal reflux, hypertrophic pyloric stenosis, intussusception, and Hirschsprung's disease.
9. Discuss the parent teaching necessary to prevent urinary tract infection in infants and children.
10. Discuss etiology and pathophysiology, clinical manifestations, diagnostic tests, medical management, nursing interventions, patient teaching, and prognosis for children with disorders of the genitourinary system, including nephrotic syndrome, acute glomerulonephritis, and Wilms' tumor.
11. Describe etiology and pathophysiology, clinical manifestations, diagnostic tests, medical management, nursing interventions, patient teaching, and prognosis for children with disorders of the endocrine system, including hypothyroidism, hyperthyroidism, and diabetes mellitus.
12. Discuss etiology and pathophysiology, clinical manifestations, diagnostic tests, medical management, nursing interventions, patient teaching, and prognosis for children with disorders of the musculoskeletal system, including hip dysplasia, Legg-Calvé-Perthes disease, osteomyelitis, talipes, Duchenne's muscular dystrophy, and septic arthritis.
13. Discuss etiology and pathophysiology, clinical manifestations, diagnostic tests, medical management, nursing interventions, patient teaching, and prognosis for children with disorders of the nervous system, including meningitis, encephalitis, hydrocephalus, cerebral palsy, seizures, spina bifida, neonatal abstinence syndrome, and neuroblastoma.
14. Describe etiology and pathophysiology, clinical manifestations, diagnostic tests, medical management, nursing interventions, patient teaching, and prognosis for children with lead poisoning.
15. Discuss etiology and pathophysiology, clinical manifestations, diagnostic tests, medical management, nursing interventions, patient teaching, and prognosis for children with disorders of the integumentary system, including contact dermatitis, diaper dermatitis, eczema, seborrheic dermatitis, acne vulgaris, herpes simplex virus type I, tinea infections, candidiasis, and parasitic infections.
16. Discuss etiology and pathophysiology, clinical manifestations, diagnostic tests, medical management, nursing interventions, patient teaching, and prognosis for children with disorders of the sensory system, including otitis media, refractive errors (myopia, hyperopia), strabismus, periorbital cellulitis, and allergic rhinitis.

Key Terms

acquired heart disorders (p. 984)
alpha-fetoprotein (AFP) (fē-tō-PRŌ-tēn, p. 1047)
amblyopia (ăm-blē-Ō-pē-ă, p. 1063)
chelation therapy (kē-LĀ-shŭn, p. 1049)
congenital heart disease (CHD) (p. 984)
"currant jelly" stools (p. 1023)
glomerulonephritis (glō-mĕr-ū-lō-nĕ-FRĪ-tĭs, p. 1028)
Gowers' sign (p. 1039)
Legg-Calvé-Perthes disease (lĕg–kăl-vă–PĔR-tēz, p. 1036)
lichenification (lī-kĕn-ĭ-fĭ-KĀ-shŭn, p. 1052)
neural tube (NŪ-răl, p. 1047)
Nissen fundoplication (NĬS-ĕn fŭn-dō-plĭ-KĀ-shŭn, p. 1021)
nuchal rigidity (NŪ-kăl, p. 1041)
pica (PĪ-kă, p. 1049)
pneumothorax (nū-mō-THŌ-răks, p. 1004)
priapism (prī-ă-PĬZ-ĕm, p. 993)
prodromal (prō-DRŌ-măl, p. 1058)
sickled cell (SĬK'ld sĕl, p. 993)
subluxation (sŭb-lŭk-SĀ-shŭn, p. 1034)

Many of the health problems that affect children differ from those of adults, and management of these problems is likely to be quite different as well. Nurses need to be aware of the unique way they provide care to children and their families. In providing nursing interventions to children, it is important to include parents as much as possible, delegating to them any interventions that are appropriate. It is also necessary to provide them with resources within their community so they are able to provide for the continued health of their child after discharge.

This chapter proposes to provide the reader with a thorough understanding of the unique physical problems affecting children. Although it is dedicated to the understanding of the most prevalent health issues affecting children, it is beyond the scope of this chapter to address all disorders that may affect children. Refer as needed to other chapters within this comprehensive text that address specific disorders, many of which have pediatric implications.

DISORDERS OF CARDIOVASCULAR FUNCTION

Many cardiovascular disorders in children are the result of **congenital heart disease (CHD)** (an abnormality or anomaly of the heart present at birth). Consequences of many of these defects include heart failure, predisposition to infection, hypoxia, and alterations in growth. Another group of cardiovascular disorders, **acquired heart disorders,** comprises abnormalities occurring after birth that compromise the heart's function.

Any type of cardiovascular disorder tends to be frightening to the child and parents. It is important to educate and prepare them regarding the disorder and its management.

CONGENITAL HEART DISEASE

It is estimated that 5% to 10% of term newborns have a congenital heart disease. The rate is even higher in infants born prematurely.

Etiology and Pathophysiology

The etiology of most congenital heart defects is unknown (Hockenberry & Wilson, 2007). There are several probable environmental and genetic risk factors for the various types of defects. Environmental factors include intrauterine rubella exposure, maternal alcoholism, diabetes mellitus, advanced maternal age, and maternal drug ingestion (e.g., lithium, thalidomide, or phenytoin [Dilantin]). Genetic risk factors include a sibling or parent with a congenital heart disease, chromosomal anomalies (trisomy G [21, Down syndrome], trisomy D [13-15, Patau syndrome], and monosomy X [Turner syndrome]), and the presence of other noncardiac congenital anomalies.

Principles of Fetal and Postnatal Circulation

During fetal development, the placenta is the source of oxygen and nutrients. Oxygenated blood is brought to the fetus by the umbilical vein and enters the fetal heart via the inferior vena cava. The fetal lungs, which are collapsed and full of fluid, pose a strong resistance to the right side of the heart, increasing the pressures in the right atrium and the right ventricle. Because of the increased pressure in the right side of the heart, blood entering the heart from the inferior vena cava is directed across the right atrium through the foramen ovale to the left atrium. This blood is then ejected from the left ventricle into the aorta. Thus the blood richest in oxygen is pumped through the aorta to the coronary arteries, the brain, and the upper extremities. Venous blood returning from this region returns to the right atrium through the superior vena cava and is directed downward through the tricuspid valve into the right ventricle. From there it is pumped into the pulmonary artery, where the majority of the blood is shunted to the descending aorta through the ductus arteriosus and perfuses the lower body (Figure 31-1). Only a small amount enters the fetal lungs owing to high pulmonary resistance (Figure 31-2, *A*).

At delivery, with the first breath, the newborn's lungs expand and the fluid within them is absorbed

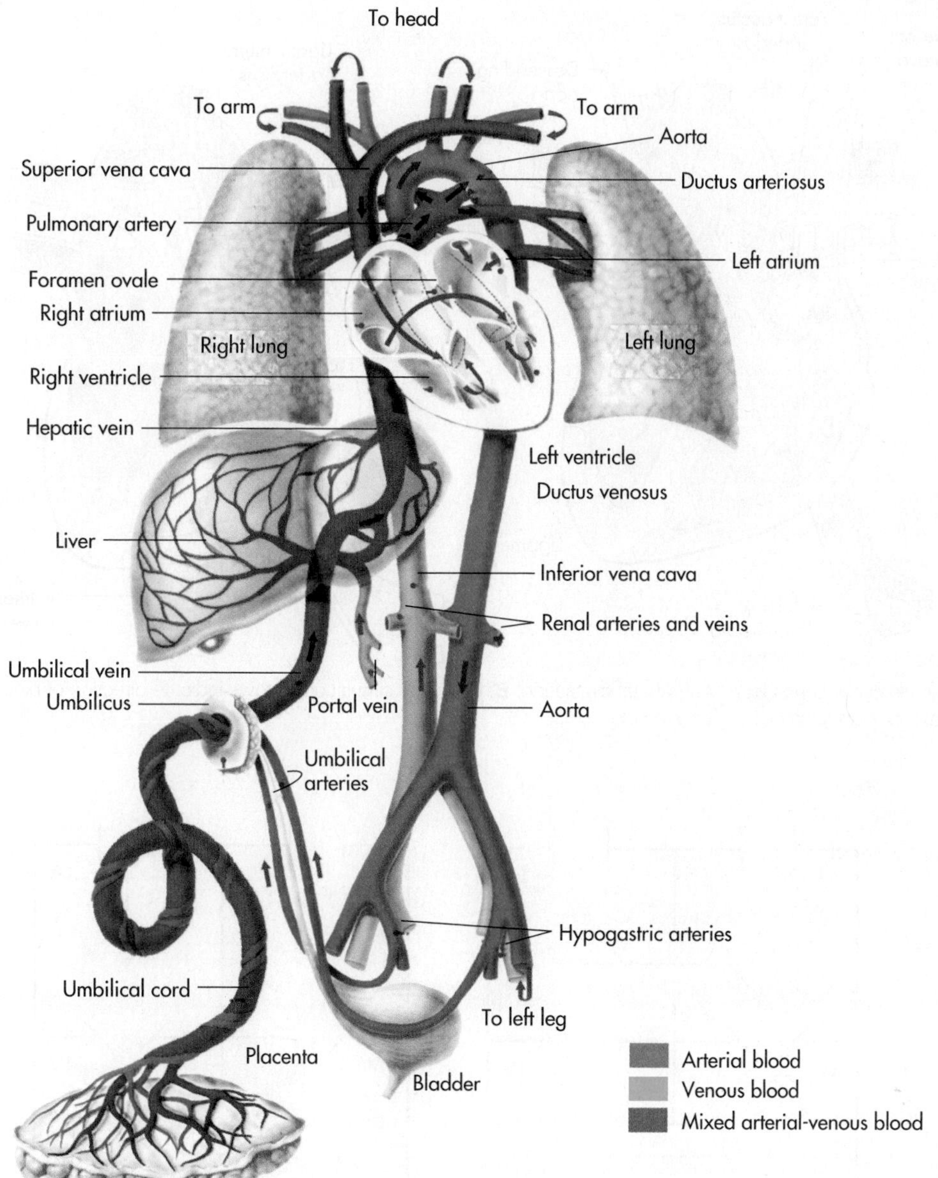

FIGURE 31-1 Fetal circulation.

into the pulmonary circulation. As a result, pulmonary and right heart pressures fall and, with the removal of the placenta, systemic pressures rise. The foramen ovale closes as the pressure in the left atrium exceeds the pressure in the right atrium. The ductus arteriosus closes with the increased oxygen content of the newborn's blood (Figure 31-2, *B*).

Types of Defects

In the past, health care providers proceeded on the basis of a classification into two basic categories of CHD: disorders related to symptoms of color (cyanotic or acyanotic) and disorders related to the direction of blood flow (left-to-right shunt or right-to-left shunt). These categories have sometimes been difficult for the pediatric nurse to understand because it was not possible to classify all disorders by these criteria.

Recently, a new classification system of CHD has emerged. The most current CHD categories are related to four physiologic characteristics: increased pulmonary blood flow, decreased pulmonary blood flow, obstruction to systemic blood flow, and mixed blood flow.

Figure 31-3 illustrates hemodynamics related to these categories. The figure does not illustrate the mixed blood flow, which includes a number of possible combinations of the mixing of oxygenated and unoxygenated blood in the heart or great vessels.

This chapter discusses several of the major CHDs, clinical manifestations, and medical management. See also the nursing care plan and critical thinking activities related to the child with CHD.

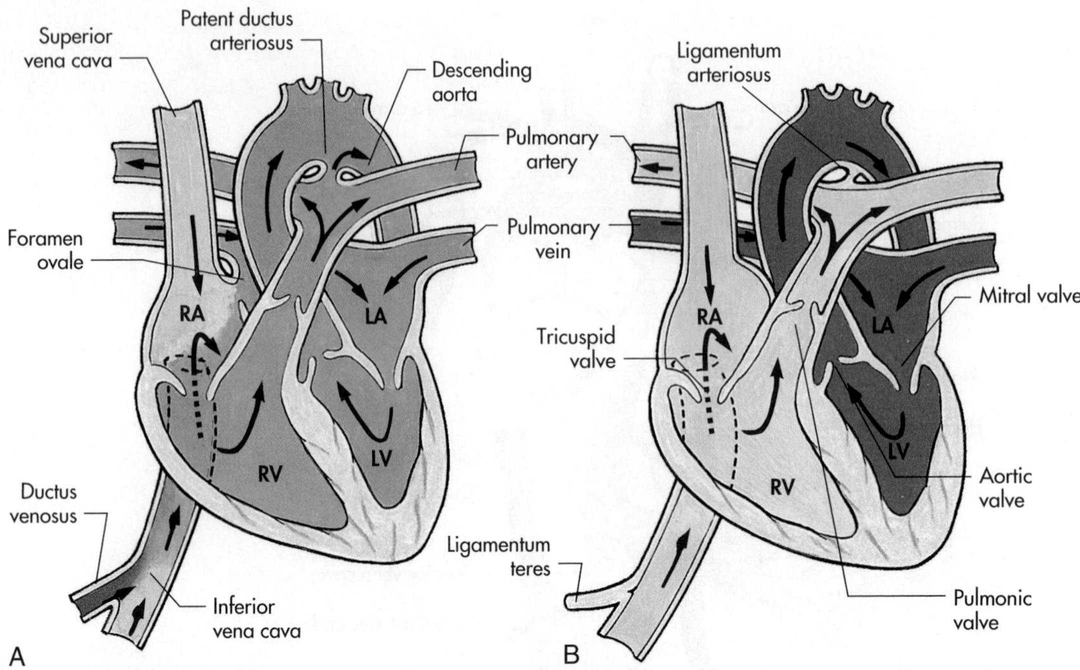

FIGURE 31-2 Changes in circulation at birth. **A,** Prenatal circulation. **B,** Postnatal circulation. Arrows indicate direction of blood flow. *RA,* Right atrium; *LA,* left atrium; *RV,* right ventricle; *LV,* left ventricle.

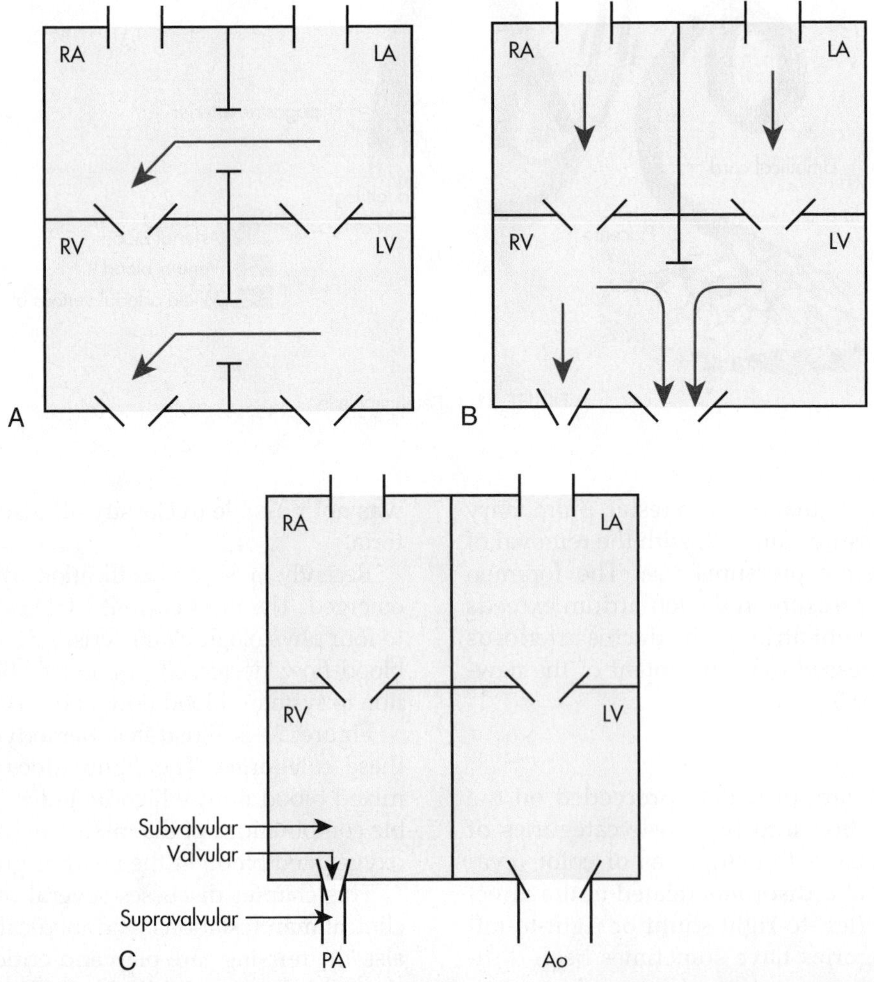

FIGURE 31-3 Hemodynamics in congenital heart disease. **A,** Increased pulmonary blood flow. **B,** Decreased pulmonary blood flow. **C,** Obstruction to systemic blood flow.

Clinical Manifestations

The child with suspected cardiac dysfunction will possibly exhibit cyanosis, pallor, cardiomegaly, pericardial rubs, murmurs, additional heart sounds (S_3 or S_4), discrepancies between apical and radial pulses, tachypnea, dyspnea, grunting, digital clubbing, hepatomegaly, splenomegaly, discrepancies between upper and lower extremity blood pressures, crackles, and wheezing. (See the discussion of specific clinical manifestations of common congenital heart defects later in this chapter.)

Diagnostic Tests

Many invasive and noninvasive tests are available to diagnose cardiovascular disorders. Which studies the physician orders will vary according to the nature of the suspected disorder. The more frequently conducted tests include urine culture, arterial blood gases (ABGs), electrocardiogram, echocardiogram, fluoroscopy, angiography, cardiac catheterization, and cardiac magnetic resonance imaging (MRI).

DEFECTS WITH INCREASED PULMONARY BLOOD FLOW

Defects with increased pulmonary blood flow are the most common CHD. In this type of defect, there is a communication of some type between the right and the left sides of the heart. Because of the increased pressure of the left side of the heart, some of the blood is pushed back to the right side of the heart. The increased blood on the right side of the heart is then moved to the lungs. The size of the defect and the amount of increase in blood volume determine to what degree the child develops symptoms of heart failure.

The most common defects with increased pulmonary blood flow are patent ductus arteriosus (PDA), atrial septal defect (ASD), and ventricular septal defect (VSD). The next sections present the clinical manifestations and medical management of each (Nursing Care Plan 31-1).

Patent Ductus Arteriosus

The ductus arteriosus is a fetal artery that connects the pulmonary artery to the aorta (see Figure 31-1). Failure of the ductus arteriosus to close within the first weeks of life allows blood to shunt from the high-pressure aorta (oxygenated blood) to the low-pressure pulmonary artery (unoxygenated blood) (Figure 31-4).

Clinical Manifestations

Children with small PDAs are sometimes asymptomatic. Children with larger defects will often exhibit signs and symptoms of heart failure. Other possible

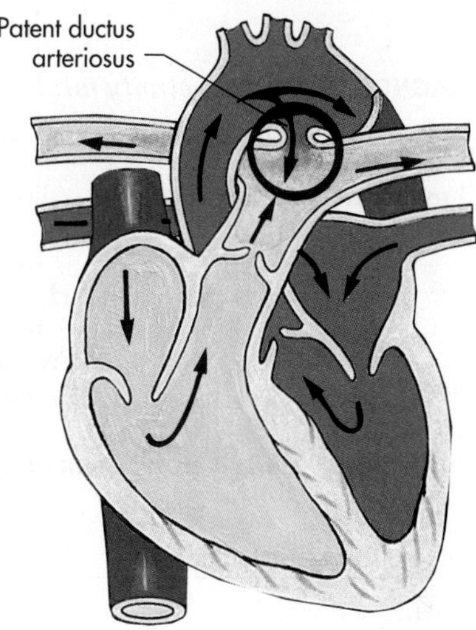

FIGURE 31-4 Patent ductus arteriosus.

Nursing Care Plan 31-1 The Child with Congenital Heart Disease

Dora is a 9-month-old female infant with a ventricular septal defect. She has a loud, harsh systolic murmur. She weighs 15 lb (her birth weight was 7 lb). The family has been told the septal defect will require open heart surgery when she is 18 to 24 months of age.

NURSING DIAGNOSIS *Decreased cardiac output, related to structural defect*

Patient Goals and Expected Outcomes	Nursing Interventions	Evaluation
Patient will exhibit improved cardiac output; heartbeat will be strong, regular, and within normal limits for age	Administer digoxin (Lanoxin) as ordered, using established precautions to prevent toxicity; check dosage with another nurse for safety. Count apical pulse for 1 full minute before giving drug. Withhold medication and notify practitioner if pulse rate is less than 90 to 110 bpm (infants) or 75 to 85 bpm (older children), depending on previous pulse readings. Monitor serum potassium levels (decrease in levels enhances digoxin toxicity).	Patient's heartbeat is strong and regular.

Continued

Nursing Care Plan 31-1 The Child with Congenital Heart Disease—cont'd

NURSING DIAGNOSIS ***Risk for infection, related to debilitated physical status***

Patient Goals and Expected Outcomes	Nursing Interventions	Evaluation
Patient will exhibit no evidence of infection	Use meticulous hand hygiene. Avoid contact with infected people. Monitor for signs of infection, including elevated temperature and elevated white blood cell (WBC) count, which indicate possible infection. Provide frequent rest periods. Provide adequate nutrition; assess nutritional status, including daily weight. Be alert for signs of complications: • Heart failure • Digitalis toxicity • Increased respiratory effort • Hypoxemia • Cerebral thrombosis • Cardiovascular collapse	No evidence of infection is noted; temperature and WBC count remain within normal limits.

NURSING DIAGNOSIS ***Risk for activity intolerance, related to imbalance between oxygen supply and demand***

Patient Goals and Expected Outcomes	Nursing Interventions	Evaluation
Patient will maintain adequate energy levels	Allow for frequent rest periods. Encourage quiet games and activities for age. Help child select activities appropriate to age, condition, and capabilities. Avoid extremes of environmental temperatures.	Patient is receiving adequate rest periods and is maintaining adequate energy levels.

NURSING DIAGNOSIS ***Delayed growth and development, related to inadequate oxygen and nutrients to tissues; social isolation***

Patient Goals and Expected Outcomes	Nursing Interventions	Evaluation
Patient will achieve normal growth and development	Provide a diet high in nutrition. Provide pleasant environment for eating. Encourage small, frequent feedings. Provide snacks several times a day. Provide frequent rest periods between feedings and activities. Encourage activities appropriate to the child's age and developmental level. Monitor for signs of heart failure and decreased cardiac output during activities. Arrange for continued family involvement during the child's hospitalization.	Patient is achieving normal growth and developmental milestones.

NURSING DIAGNOSIS ***Risk for injury, related to cardiac condition and therapies***

Patient Goals and Expected Outcomes	Nursing Interventions	Evaluation
Parents will recognize early signs of complications and institute appropriate action	Teach family to recognize signs of complications: • Heart failure • Digoxin toxicity • Vomiting (earliest sign) • Bradycardia • Dysrhythmias	Parents demonstrate knowledge of recognizing signs of complications of child's heart defect and demonstrate appropriate interventions during hypercyanotic spells.

Nursing Care Plan 31-1 The Child with Congenital Heart Disease—cont'd

Patient Goals and Expected Outcomes	Nursing Interventions	Evaluation
	• Increased respiratory effort—tachycardia, retention, grunting, cough, cyanosis • Hypoxemia—cyanosis, restlessness, tachycardia • Cerebral thrombosis—compensatory polycythemia (in cyanotic heart disease) is particularly hazardous when child is dehydrated • Cardiovascular collapse—pallor, cyanosis Teach family to intervene during hypercyanotic spells: • Place child in knee-chest position with head and chest elevated • Remain calm • Call practitioner	

NURSING DIAGNOSIS *Deficient knowledge, related to the disorder and methods of treatment*

Patient Goals and Expected Outcomes	Nursing Interventions	Evaluation
Family will demonstrate an understanding of the disorder and its treatments	Assess the family's understanding of the diagnosis. Reinforce the physician's explanation of the child's disorder and its treatments. Provide written instructions regarding medication schedules and treatment protocols. Encourage the family to verbalize questions, fears, and concerns. Allow the family to participate in the child's care when appropriate. Provide emotional support to the child and the family.	Family demonstrates understanding of child's cardiac condition as evidenced by verbal responses and therapeutic interventions.

Critical Thinking Questions

1. You enter Dora's room and notice her mother sitting at her bedside crying. She states, "I don't know how I will deal with her having heart surgery." What would be an appropriate initial response to Ms. Barnason?
2. Ms. Barnason states that Dora has a very poor appetite. What might be two helpful suggestions to educate the mother?
3. Ms. Barnason mentions that she is concerned Dora will get an infection and become acutely ill. What are two therapeutic nursing interventions for patient teaching?

clinical manifestations include a typical machinelike murmur audible at the upper left sternal border, widened pulse pressure, and bounding pulses.

Medical Management

Administration of indomethacin (a prostaglandin inhibitor) has been effective in closing the ductus arteriosus in full-term and premature newborns. Surgical correction involves ligating the ductus arteriosus through a thoracotomy incision (surgical opening into the thoracic cavity).

Currently, practitioners are using a new surgical technique in some cases. In this procedure, the surgeon makes three small incisions on the left side of the chest, and then uses a thoracoscope and instruments to place a clip on the ductus arteriosus.

Atrial Septal Defect

An ASD is an abnormal opening in the atrial septum, which enables blood to flow from the higher-pressure left atrium (oxygenated blood) to the lower-pressure right atrium (unoxygenated blood) (Figure 31-5).

Clinical Manifestations

Although some children will be asymptomatic, others typically have manifestations of heart failure. A characteristic harsh systolic murmur is possible to auscultate over the third intercostal space.

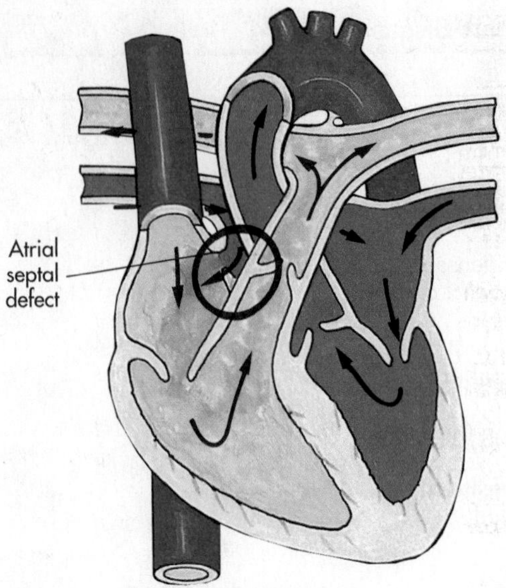

FIGURE 31-5 Atrial septal defect.

Medical Management

Surgical correction consists of open heart surgery with cardiopulmonary bypass. The surgeon repairs small defects with purse-string sutures, and moderate to large defects with a Dacron patch.

Ventricular Septal Defect

A VSD is an abnormal opening in the interventricular septum, resulting in the flow of blood from the higher-pressure left ventricle (oxygenated blood) to the lower-pressure right ventricle (unoxygenated blood). The possible scope of the defect ranges from a pinhole-sized opening to absence of the entire septum (single ventricle) (Figure 31-6).

Clinical Manifestations

Initially children are sometimes asymptomatic, but signs of heart failure eventually manifest. Other clinical manifestations include a loud, harsh systolic murmur and a palpable thrill.

Medical Management

Approximately 50% of VSDs close spontaneously; the remainder necessitate open heart surgery. A palliative procedure, known as a pulmonary artery banding, is possible to perform in symptomatic infants. This procedure involves impeding the flow of blood from the right ventricle to the pulmonary circulation, thus reducing pulmonary congestion. Complete surgical repair involves open heart surgery with the use of cardiopulmonary bypass. The surgeon usually repairs the defect with a Dacron patch; smaller defects sometimes necessitate only observation, and sometimes surgical closure with sutures.

DEFECTS WITH DECREASED PULMONARY BLOOD FLOW

Defects with decreased pulmonary blood flow result when there is some type of obstruction to the lungs or if there is no connection between the right side of the heart and the lungs. Examples of defects with decreased pulmonary blood flow include pulmonary stenosis, pulmonary atresia, and tetralogy of Fallot. The amount of obstruction or lack of connection determines the symptoms. The most common CHD resulting in decreased pulmonary blood flow is tetralogy of Fallot.

Tetralogy of Fallot

Tetralogy of Fallot (TOF) involves a combination of four defects: (1) pulmonary stenosis, (2) ventricular septal defect (VSD), (3) right ventricular hypertrophy, and (4) overriding aorta (Figure 31-7).

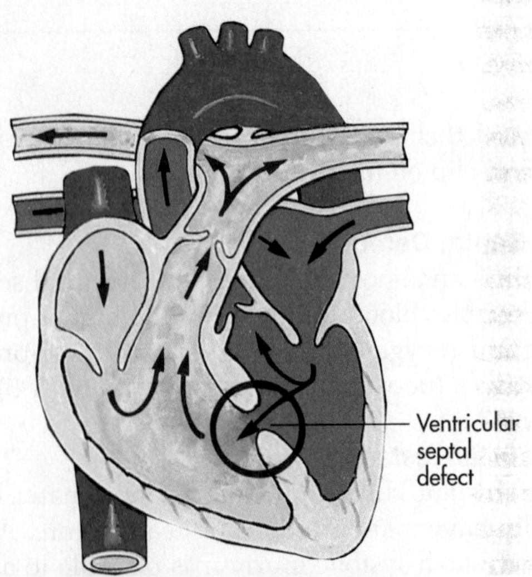

FIGURE 31-6 Ventricular septal defect.

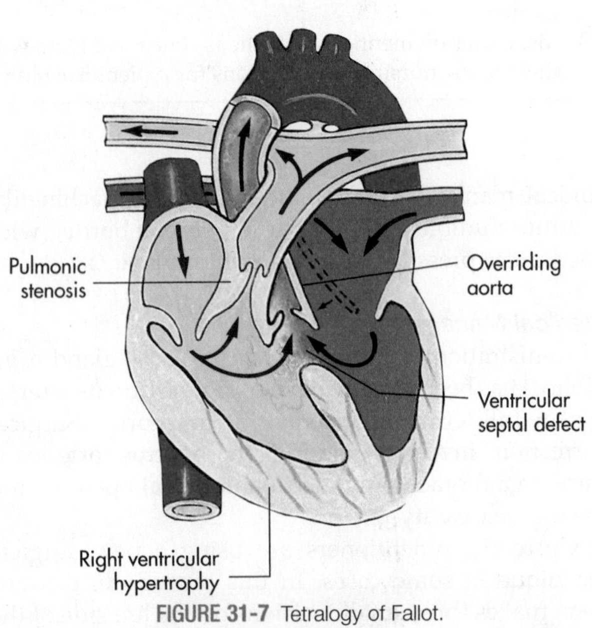

FIGURE 31-7 Tetralogy of Fallot.

Clinical Manifestations

Infants tend to be profoundly cyanotic at birth and often experience acute episodes of severe cyanosis and hypoxia (blue spells). Children with TOF will sometimes exhibit a systolic ejection murmur, clubbing of the nailbeds, dyspnea, squatting, poor growth, mental slowness, syncope (fainting), and stroke.

Medical Management

Usually the physician will perform a palliative procedure in infants with profound cyanosis and hypoxia. This temporary procedure, most commonly a Blalock-Taussig shunt, creates an artificial connection between the pulmonary artery and the aorta and thus redirects blood flow back to the lungs to allow for oxygenation. Complete surgical correction involves closure of the VSD, a pulmonic valvotomy, and repair of the overriding aorta.

MIXED DEFECTS

Mixed defects include those that do not fit into one of the other categories. These defects often include the mixing of oxygenated and unoxygenated blood in the heart or the great vessels. Symptoms are specific to the type of defects present. Examples of mixed defects include transposition of the great vessels, truncus arteriosus, and hypoplastic left heart syndrome.

Transposition of the Great Vessels

In transposition of the great vessels (TGV), the pulmonary artery arises from the left ventricle and the aorta arises from the right ventricle. Therefore venous blood returning to the right side of the heart exits through the aorta without being oxygenated, and oxygenated blood returning from the pulmonary system is returned via the pulmonary artery to the lungs (Figure 31-8). Some infants are born with associated defects that allow for communication between the two circulations.

Clinical Manifestations

Infants born with minimal communication between the two circulations have profound cyanosis. Those who are born with an associated defect such as PDA, ASD, or VSD sometimes have less cyanosis and experience manifestations of heart failure. Cardiomegaly is usually apparent on x-ray study.

Medical Management

Initially, the physician performs palliative procedures to provide mixing, either by enlarging an already present ASD or creating one by pulling a balloon catheter through the atrial septum. Complete correction of TGV entails open heart surgery and involves switching the great vessels to their proper positions.

DEFECTS WITH OBSTRUCTION TO SYSTEMIC BLOOD FLOW

Defects with obstruction to systemic blood flow result in the blood being unable to reach the body from the heart. Children with this type of defect show symptoms of lack of oxygenation and decreased peripheral blood flow due to the obstruction, as well as symptoms of heart failure, because the blood backs up into the lungs. Defects resulting in obstruction to systemic blood flow include aortic stenosis, pulmonary stenosis, and coarctation of the aorta.

Coarctation of the Aorta

Coarctation of the aorta (COA) is a narrowing of the lumen of the aorta (usually at the site of the ductus arteriosus), resulting in increased pressure proximal to the defect (head and upper extremities) and decreased pressure distal to the defect (body and lower extremities) (Figure 31-9).

FIGURE 31-8 Transposition of the great vessels.

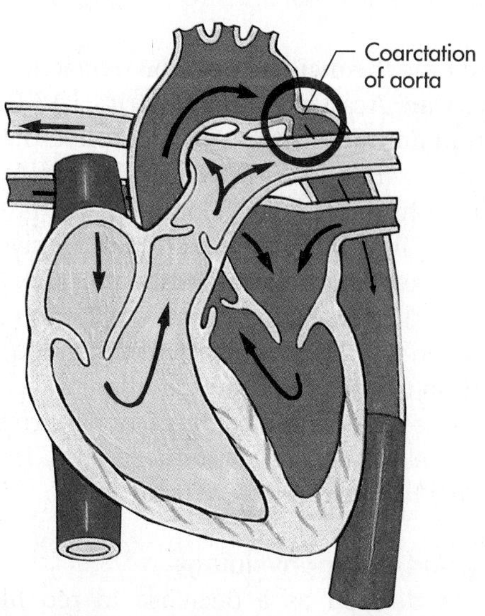

FIGURE 31-9 Coarctation of the aorta.

Clinical Manifestations

The blood pressure in the arms will be 20 mm Hg higher than that in the legs (reversal of normal pattern). Other manifestations include bounding pulses in the lower extremities, signs of heart failure, leg cramping on exertion in older children, and epistaxis.

Medical Management

Surgical correction involves removal of the narrowed portion of the aorta with an end-to-end anastomosis (a connection between two vessels) or graft replacement if the narrowing is extensive.

ACQUIRED HEART DISEASE

Acquired heart disease refers to those disorders whose onset comes after birth. They result from a variety of reasons, including autoimmune processes, infection, familial tendencies, and environmental factors. One disease that has experienced a resurgence in recent years and has caused concern to health professionals is rheumatic fever.

DISORDERS OF HEMATOLOGIC FUNCTION

Childhood blood disorders encompass wide ranges of etiology, severity, treatment, and prognosis; however, the majority of hematological disorders occurring in infants and children stem from chronic systemic illness, nutritional deficits, and inherited blood disorders.

ANEMIAS

IRON DEFICIENCY ANEMIA

Iron deficiency anemia is the most prevalent blood disorder in infancy and early childhood, with peak incidence occurring between 6 and 24 months in lower-income children. However, the prevalence has decreased, probably in part because of families' participation in the Women, Infants, and Children (WIC) program, which provides iron-fortified formula for the first year of life.

To decrease the incidence of iron deficiency anemia, the American Academy of Pediatrics (AAP) recommends human milk as the most complete diet for the infant's first 6 months of life (AAP, 2005c). A good alternative to human milk is commercial iron-fortified formula. An iron supplement should be given to infants who are being breastfed only after 6 months because of the decrease that occurs in the iron content of most women's milk. It is also recommended to delay the addition of cow's milk to the infant's diet because of pasteurized whole milk's deficiency in iron and the increased risk of occult gastrointestinal (GI) bleeding (AAP, 2004; Hockenberry & Wilson, 2007).

Etiology and Pathophysiology

Anemia is defined as a decrease in red blood cell (RBC) volume, a decrease in hemoglobin, or both. Anemia reduces the oxygen-carrying capacity of the blood and sometimes results in tissue hypoxia. Anemia is possible to classify as either **hypoproliferative** (defective erythrocyte production) or **hemolytic** (premature destruction of erythrocytes).

Iron deficiency anemia becomes apparent at about 6 months of age in the full-term infant and about 3 months of age in the premature infant, when the maternal stores of iron become depleted and the infant becomes dependent on dietary sources of iron. Infants develop iron deficiency anemia because (1) milk is a poor source of iron and these infants drink milk to the exclusion of solid foods and (2) infants who drink cow's milk have a 50% chance of increased fecal loss of blood. Most infants with iron deficiency anemia are underweight; however, many will be overweight (chubby) because of excessive milk consumption (Kliegman et al., 2007; Kwiatkowski et al., 1999). These infants are pale with poor muscle tone and have an increased risk for infection (Hockenberry & Wilson, 2007).

Premature infants are especially at risk because of their lower fetal iron supply. Adolescents are also at risk for iron deficiency anemia because of their rapid growth rate combined with poor eating habits. The most common cause of this disorder in this age-group is an inadequate intake of dietary iron, which is essential for hemoglobin synthesis. All races and ethnic groups are vulnerable to developing iron deficiency anemia (Kahn et al., 2002; White, 2005). Other causes include acute or chronic blood loss and malabsorption of dietary iron secondary to chronic diarrhea or malabsorption syndromes.

Clinical Manifestations

The clinical signs and symptoms of mild to moderate anemia (hemoglobin: 6 to 10 g/dL) are often vague and nonspecific and include irritability, weakness, decreased play activity, and fatigue. When hemoglobin falls below 5 g/dL, the child will have anorexia, skin pallor, pale mucous membranes, glossitis, concave or "spoon" fingernails, inability to concentrate, tachycardia, and systolic murmurs. Children with chronic, long-term anemia are often subject to growth retardation and developmental delays.

Diagnostic Tests

The diagnostic evaluation begins with an accurate history, including the child's diet, appetite, activity, weight and rate of growth, and any recent blood loss. Initial laboratory tests include a complete blood count (CBC), reticulocyte count, serum ferritin (a major iron-storage protein), serum iron concentration (SIC), and total iron-binding capacity (TIBC).

Medical Management

Therapeutic management involves iron replacement therapy, nutritional counseling, and treatment of any underlying conditions (hemorrhage or malabsorption). The health care provider usually prescribes oral iron supplementation of Fer-In-Sol (ferrous sulfate) until the hemoglobin level returns to normal. Advise giving citrus fruits or juices with iron supplements, because ascorbic acid enhances iron absorption. The child will receive parenteral iron only if the child has problems with the absorption of oral iron, and packed red blood cells only if the child is severely anemic (Hockenberry & Wilson, 2007). Permanent dietary changes are essential to prevent recurrence. Encourage breastfeeding, iron-fortified formulas, and iron-rich solid foods.

Nursing Interventions

Dietary counseling is of primary importance, and your assistance to the family in choosing iron-rich foods is valuable. Advise giving oral preparations of iron three times daily between meals with citrus fruits or juices to enhance iron absorption. Also inform parents that their child will have dark, tarry green stools while on oral iron therapy. To avoid staining of the teeth with liquid preparations of iron, teach the family to administer the medication with a syringe placed toward the back of the mouth for infants; older children are able to take the preparation through straws.

Patient Teaching

A primary nursing objective is to educate the family in how to prevent nutritional anemia. Discuss with parents the importance of using iron-fortified formula and the introduction of solid foods at the appropriate age. The best solid food source of iron is commercial infant cereals.

A difficulty encountered in discouraging the parents from feeding milk to the exclusion of other foods is dispelling the popular myth that milk is a perfect food. Many parents believe that milk is best for the infant and equate the weight gain with a healthy child and good mothering. They may not be concerned about providing other foods as long as the child continues to take milk. Also stress that overweight is not synonymous with good health.

Diet education of teenagers is especially difficult because teenage girls are particularly prone to follow weight-reduction diets. Emphasizing the effects of anemia on appearance (pallor) and energy level (difficulty maintaining popular activities) is sometimes useful.

Prognosis

Generally the prognosis for the child with iron deficiency anemia is good. However, if the iron deficiency is severe and prolonged, some children will have mild cognitive dysfunction as well as delayed growth and development and impaired immune function (Bogen et al., 2000; Harris, 2004).

SICKLE CELL ANEMIA (SCA)

Sickle cell anemia is one of a group of diseases collectively termed hemoglobinopathies, in which normal adult hemoglobin (hemoglobin A [HbA]) is partly or completely replaced by abnormal sickle hemoglobin (HbS). Sickle cell anemia is a genetic disorder characterized by an abnormal form of hemoglobin within the erythrocyte. In the United States, the disease is most common in the black population, with an incidence of 1 in 400 to 1 in 500 live births. Sickle cell anemia is classified as either sickle cell trait or active sickle cell disease. Sickle cell trait rarely results in clinical manifestations; however, children with sickle cell trait are carriers of sickle cell anemia. The rest of this discussion will focus on active sickle cell disease, which is the most severe and potentially fatal form of the disorder.

Etiology and Pathophysiology

When oxygen is released into the tissues, the abnormal hemoglobin becomes more viscous and crystallizes, causing the erythrocyte to change from its characteristic round shape to an elongated, crescent shape (sickled cell). As sickled cells clump, circulation slows, resulting in obstructions with severe tissue hypoxia and necrosis. Sickling is an intermittent phenomenon; the usual precipitating factors are infection, fever, hypoxemia, dehydration, high altitudes, cold, or emotional stress.

Clinical Manifestations

Children with sickle cell disease tend to first experience pallor, irritability, fatigue, and jaundice. Growth impairment becomes apparent as the child's height and weight fall below average. Cardiomegaly and heart failure develop in response to hypoxia and decreased cardiac output. In the older child, the joints and surrounding tissue often become edematous and painful. Strokes are possible if sickling causes cerebral occlusion, resulting in sensory deficits, paralysis, or death. Persistent penile erection (priapism) sometimes occurs in response to occluded penile veins. Severe sickling leads to recurrent sickle cell crisis, an acutely painful period that occurs intermittently throughout the life of a child with sickle cell anemia (Figure 31-10). It is possible to classify crises as one of three types: vasoocclusive, sequestration, or aplastic (Box 31-1).

Diagnostic Tests

Newborn screening for sickle cell anemia is mandatory in most of the United States so that it is possible to identify affected infants before symptoms occur. Institutions frequently use the sickle-turbidity test (Sickledex) for screening purposes. It is possible to perform on blood from a fingerstick and yields accurate results in 3 minutes. If the test is positive, the next step is to perform hemoglobin electrophoresis to determine sickle cell trait or sickle cell disease.

Medical Management

The treatment is primarily palliative and is outlined in Box 31-1.

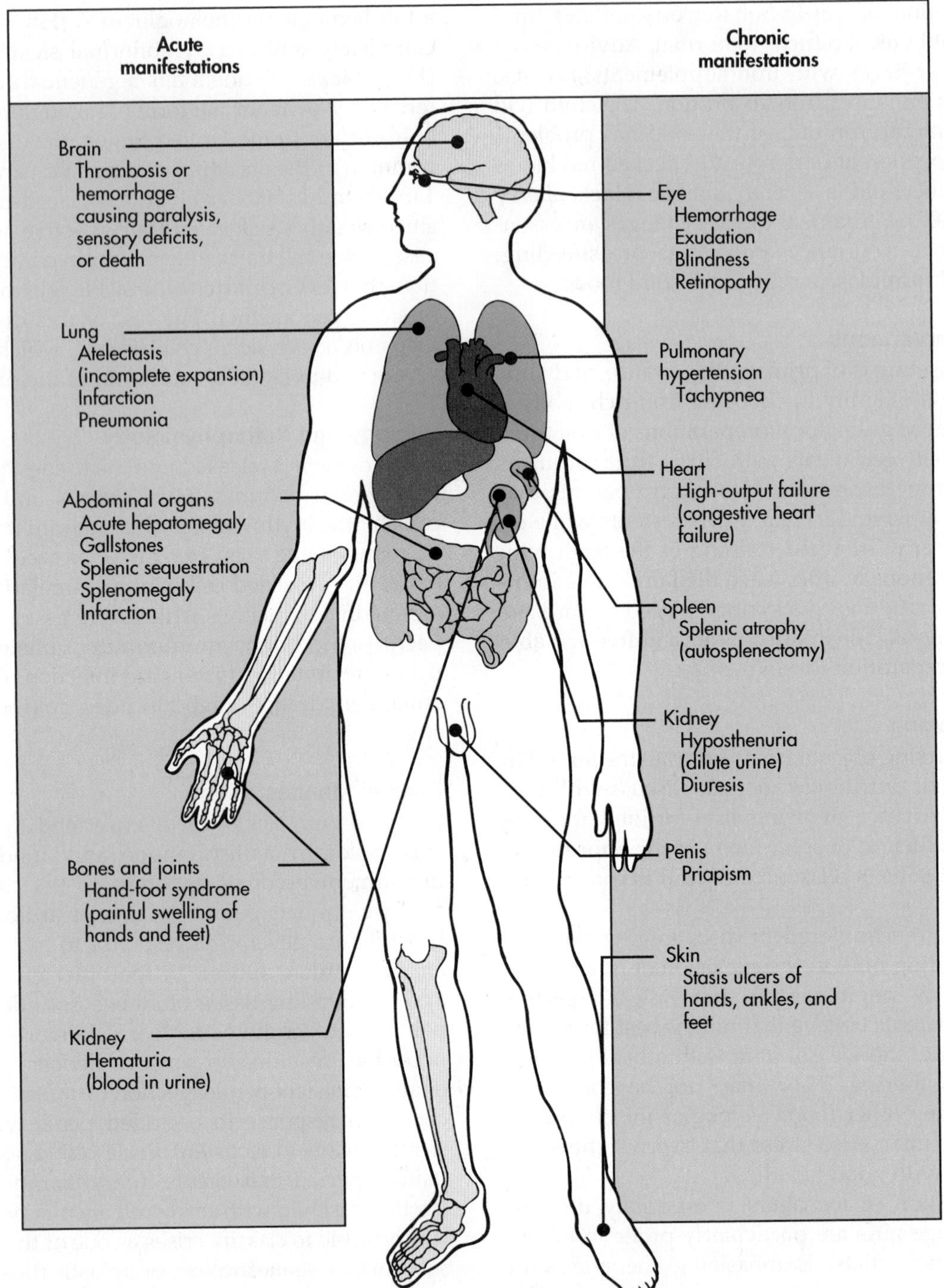

FIGURE 31-10 Clinical manifestations of sickle cell disease.

Nursing Interventions and Patient Teaching

Nursing interventions for the child in sickle cell crisis include maintaining adequate hydration to prevent further sickling, administering analgesics as ordered, providing adequate oxygenation, and applying comfort measures such as warm baths and local heat.

Teach families of children with sickle cell anemia to avoid situations that lead to hypoxia and sickling: infection, dehydration, emotional stress, and strenuous physical activity. Recommend the use of a medical-alert bracelet.

Prognosis

Most persons with sickle cell anemia live to be in their 50s. Children under the age of 5 are at the highest risk of death, which in most cases is the result of severe infections. As the child becomes an adolescent, crises are less frequent and less severe; however, death in early adulthood is not uncommon. Sickle cell anemia is a se-

Box 31-1 Types and Medical Management of Sickle Cell Crises

- **Vasoocclusive crisis:** Obstruction of the small blood vessels of the hands and feet, resulting in edema, impaired range of motion, and pain
  —Medical management: palliative (analgesics, hydration, oxygen)
- **Sequestration crisis:** Blood pools in the spleen and the liver, resulting in hepatosplenomegaly; sometimes progresses to cardiovascular collapse and death
  —Medical management: analgesics, volume expanders, transfusions; recurrent episodes treated by splenectomy
- **Aplastic crisis:** Caused by premature destruction of erythrocytes, resulting in profound anemia
  —Medical management: transfusion of packed red blood cells

rious, chronic illness often with a grave outcome (Buchanan, 2004; Dover & Platt, 2009; Gribbons, 1995).

APLASTIC ANEMIA

Aplastic anemia is due to the failure of the cell-generating capacity of the bone marrow. All formed elements of the blood are defective, underdeveloped, or absent, resulting in severe anemia, leukopenia, and thrombocytopenia (pancytopenia). It arises in some instances as a result of neoplastic disease of the bone marrow or, more commonly, from destruction of the bone marrow by exposure to toxic chemicals, ionizing radiation, or certain antibiotics or other medications. A failure of cell-producing capacity by aspirated bone marrow is diagnostic for aplastic anemia. In aplastic anemia, red blood cells, white blood cells, and platelets are deficient, and the red bone marrow becomes yellow, fatty marrow.

Treatment aims at restoring the function of the marrow by the use of (1) immunosuppressive treatment to manage the immunologic problem causing the failure of the formed elements in the marrow and (2) bone marrow transplantation to replace the defective marrow. The treatment of choice for severe aplastic anemia is bone marrow transplantation, if a suitable donor is available (Hockenberry & Wilson, 2007). Bone marrow transplantation is associated with a 69% 15-year survival rate (Hockenberry & Wilson, 2007).

COAGULATION DISORDERS

Coagulation disorders in children characteristically involve abnormal bleeding into the skin or from internal organs, secondary to clotting factor defects, platelet dysfunction, or vascular compromise.

HEMOPHILIA

Etiology and Pathophysiology

Hemophilia is a serious, lifelong bleeding disorder inherited as an X-linked recessive disorder. Hemophilia is transmitted by female carriers and affects male offspring in 1 in 10,000 male births. Classic hemophilia (type A) is caused by a deficiency in factor VIII, which is a necessary component of blood coagulation.

Clinical Manifestations

It is usually possible to make a diagnosis after infancy. In toddlerhood, when children typically become more active, hemophilic boys tend to have more episodes of oral bleeding and bruising. By age 4, 90% of these children have demonstrated persistent bleeding from minor lesions. The most frequent types of internal bleeding occur within the joints (hemarthrosis) and the muscles. Pain intensifies as the bleeding continues to fill the joint cavity, limiting movement to the point where the child refuses to use the affected joint. Recurrent episodes of hemarthrosis lead to bone deformities with resulting contractures and crippling. Intracranial hemorrhage, either spontaneous or secondary to head trauma, is life threatening and accounts for more hemophilic deaths than any other bleeding. Hematomas in the spinal cord have the capacity to cause paralysis.

Diagnostic Tests

Laboratory findings include a normal prothrombin time (PT) and International Normalized Ratio (INR), a normal bleeding time and platelet count, and a prolonged partial thromboplastin time (PTT). For specific determination of factor deficiencies, assay procedures normally performed in specialized laboratories are necessary. Factors VIII and IX are deficient or absent.

Medical Management

For minor external bleeding, pressure and cold packs are sometimes all that is necessary. The physician will sometimes also prescribe nonopioid or opioid analgesics. Therapeutic management of hemophilia involves replacing the deficient clotting factor. The two factor VIII concentrates now available for use in some cases are (1) high purified factor VIII concentrate (monoclonal) and (2) recombinant factor VIII concentrate. It is imperative for the patient to receive immediate replacement therapy with these factor concentrates to prevent the chronic joint problems from joint bleeding (Hockenberry & Wilson, 2007). The National Hemophilia Foundation advises the use of these products only, and no longer recommends using cryoprecipitate to treat factor VIII deficiency.

Nursing Interventions

It is very important to recognize early signs and symptoms of internal bleeding and aggressively treat them with factor concentrate replacement therapy. Listen to the child's symptoms for information to pass along to the examiner regarding the location of the bleed (Hockenberry & Wilson, 2007).

Nursing interventions focus on teaching the child and the family to avoid injury and control bleeding.

Advise using age-appropriate toys without rough or sharp edges, and removal of throw rugs and placement of barriers to stairs. Make sure playtime is supervised to minimize hazards and injuries. Encourage physical activity, such as swimming, softball, bicycling, hiking, bowling, golf, and running, to promote muscle development and psychological well-being. Advise against contact sports, such as football, hockey, or soccer, because of their potential for injury. Early dental visits with a dentist knowledgeable about hemophilia help keep the risk of one potential bleeding source to a minimum. Have children with hemophilia wear medical-alert bracelets. Also inform the family about the National Hemophilia Foundation, which is a good resource for financial, medical, and psychological assistance.

Patient Teaching

Teach parents to protect the child without being overprotective. When external bleeding occurs, instruct parents to apply pressure and cold. Teaching includes the RICE method of treatment: **r**est, **i**ce, **c**ompression, and **e**levation (Hockenberry & Wilson, 2007). Also instruct and encourage the child and family in safely administering factor products at home. Instruct parents to seek emergency medical care if the child has signs of increased intracranial pressure, which sometimes indicates an intracranial bleed—severe headache, slurred speech, vomiting, disorientation, and loss of consciousness.

Prognosis

With the two factor VIII concentrates now available and the ability to perform home infusion therapy, treatment of hemophilia has improved greatly and has greatly reduced associated morbidity (Montgomery et al., 2003). Children with hemophilia have a normal life expectancy but are greatly inconvenienced by their tendency to bleed (Hockenberry & Wilson, 2007). Unfortunately, those who were treated before use of the present purification techniques (before 1985) are at risk for human immunodeficiency virus (HIV) exposure. Half of those patients younger than 21 years of age will possibly have seroconverted to HIV positive, and a large number have developed AIDS. Persons with hemophilia who were diagnosed in the 1990s and have been treated with recombinant factor products have no risk of developing HIV infections (Hockenberry & Wilson, 2007).

Scientists are working to develop gene therapy as a possible treatment option in this century (Hockenberry & Wilson, 2007). This therapy involves introducing a working copy of the factor VIII gene into a patient who has a flawed copy of the gene.

IDIOPATHIC THROMBOCYTOPENIA PURPURA

Etiology and Pathophysiology

Idiopathic (cause unknown) thrombocytopenia purpura (ITP) is characterized by a marked decrease in the amount of circulating platelets with resultant bleeding beneath the skin. ITP is the most common thrombocytopenia of childhood, occurring most frequently in the 2- to 10-year age-group. It occurs in either acute or chronic form. As its name implies, the cause of ITP is unknown; however, it is believed to be an autoimmune response to disease-related antigens. The acute form of ITP usually follows a viral infection (such as a respiratory infection, rubella, rubeola, mumps, or chickenpox; or after infection with parvovirus B19) and is self-limiting; the chronic form has periods of remission.

Clinical Manifestations

Other than bleeding, the child appears well. The platelet count drops to below 20,000/mm^3, so there is impairment in clotting. Platelet counts less than 10,000/mm^3 will be potentially life threatening. Ecchymoses and a pinpoint petechial rash are usually the first signs of ITP, and the areas most commonly involved are over bony prominences. Other manifestations include bleeding gums, bleeding lips, and epistaxis (nosebleeds). The most serious complication of ITP is intracranial hemorrhage (bleeding into the subdural, the subarachnoid, or the intracerebellar space), and characteristic signs are hematuria (blood in urine), hemarthrosis, melena (black, tarry stools), hematemesis (blood in emesis), and menorrhagia (abnormally heavy menstrual periods).

Diagnostic Tests

Criteria indicating the possibility of this diagnosis are clinical manifestations. The platelet count is reduced to less than 20,000/mm^3. Microscopic examination reveals not only a decreased number of platelets but also platelets that are large. Bleeding time and clot reaction time are prolonged, and the tourniquet test for capillary fragility, in which a blood pressure cuff is inflated to 100 mm Hg and left in place for 5 minutes, will be positive (that is, with more than 15 petechiae present).

Medical Management

ITP is a self-limiting illness in the majority of cases, and about three fourths of children recover without complications within 3 months. In most cases, health care providers allow ITP to run its course with supportive management. Some will use a short course of corticosteroids to suppress the immune attack on platelets, thereby reducing the severity of the disease. Transfusions of packed RBCs are sometimes necessary in treating severe, life-threatening hemorrhage. Use of intravenous (IV) gamma globulin (IVGG) and anti-D antibody therapy has had some success in treating chronic cases of ITP. Anti-D antibody therapy is a relatively new treatment that is much less expensive than IVGG. Symptomatic children with recurrent or chronic ITP that fails to respond to treatment for a year or longer usually undergo splenectomy, which eliminates the site of antiplatelet antibody production. Splenectomy removes the risk of hemorrhage, as well as the need for parents to closely monitor their child's activities. Before considering splenectomy, health care providers generally recommend waiting until the child is more than 5 years of age because of the increased risk of bacterial infection. In general, physicians will order pneumococcal and meningococcal vaccines before splenectomy. The child also receives penicillin prophylaxis after splenectomy. The length of prophylactic therapy is controversial, but the usual recommendation is for a minimum of 3 years.

Nursing Interventions and Patient Teaching

Nursing interventions are largely supportive. Preventing bruising and controlling bleeding are of primary importance in managing ITP. Offer education and emotional support; in fact, the majority of these children will receive no treatment other than supportive therapy.

Teach families to protect the child while the platelet count is less than 100,000/mm^3 and to restrict activity and avoid injury. It is best for children with ITP not to participate in any contact sports, bike riding, skateboarding, in-line skating, gymnastics, climbing, or running. In addition, counsel the family never to use salicylate drugs (e.g., aspirin) for pain because salicylates inhibit platelet function. Teach them always to use salicylate substitutes such as acetaminophen (Tylenol) instead. Also instruct parents to notify their physician immediately if the child experiences acute head trauma and especially if the child exhibits symptoms of intracranial hemorrhage: headaches, visual disturbances, lethargy, vomiting, or disorientation.

Prognosis

For most children, the course is self-limited with complete recovery within 6 months. Occasionally, some children will develop a chronic form of ITP. A splenectomy is helpful in the chronic form of ITP to modify the disease and eliminate symptoms (Hockenberry & Wilson, 2007).

NEOPLASTIC DISORDERS

Neoplastic disorders are the leading cause of death from disease in children past infancy. Although therapeutic advances in drug treatment (chemotherapy), radiation therapy, and surgical techniques have increased the potential for a normal life span, the diagnosis of cancer remains a catastrophic, emotionally devastating occurrence for the child and family.

LEUKEMIA

Leukemia is the name given to a group of malignant diseases of the bone marrow and the lymphatic system. Leukemia is the most common malignancy of childhood, is more common in males than in females, and has a peak incidence occurring in children between 2 and 6 years of age. It is one of the forms of cancer that has demonstrated dramatic improvement in survival rates. Current long-term disease-free survival for children with acute lymphoid leukemia approaches 80%, whereas acute nonlymphoid leukemia has a 40% survival (Hockenberry & Wilson, 2007).

Etiology and Pathophysiology

The most common leukemia seen in children is acute lymphoid leukemia (ALL) followed by acute nonlymphoid (myelogenous) leukemia (ANLL or AML). Although its etiology is unknown, its pathologic characteristic is the uncontrollable proliferation of blast cells (immature white blood cells [WBCs]), which accumulate in the marrow and cause crowding and depression of other healthy cells (mature WBCs, RBCs, and platelets).

It is important to note that there is an overproduction of WBCs in leukemia; however, in the acute form of the disease, the WBCs are low. The bone marrow and peripheral blood smear disclose numerous elevated immature WBCs or blasts. The normal blood cells and vascular tissue are not directly destroyed by the leukemic cells, however, the leukemic cells infiltrate and crowd the normal cells thus depriving them of essential nutrients necessary for metabolism. Three problems and their associated effects develop as a result: (1) the decrease in RBCs causes anemia, (2) neutropenia leads to infection, and (3) the decrease in platelets causes bleeding (Hockenberry & Wilson, 2007). As nonfunctional blast cells infiltrate the lymph nodes, the liver, the kidney, and the spleen, they cause these organs to enlarge, producing the clinical manifestations seen in acute leukemia.

Clinical Manifestations

Anemia with pallor and fatigue is often severe and often provides the first sign. Other signs are leukopenia with fever and infection and thrombocytopenia with bleeding and petechiae. Blast cells also invade bones at times, causing bone pain, limping, and joint pain with edema. The infiltration of leukemic cells in the bone marrow results in a weakening of the bone and a tendency toward pathologic fractures (Hockenberry & Wilson, 2007). Hepatosplenomegaly and enlarged lymph nodes are often present at diagnosis. An important site of involvement is the central nervous system (CNS) secondary to leukemic infiltration, which sometimes causes increased intracranial pressure.

Diagnostic Tests

The physician will consider the diagnosis of leukemia after review of the patient's history and clinical manifestations (Hockenberry & Wilson, 2007). A CBC typically indicates pancytopenia (decreased RBCs, WBCs, and platelets). Examination of bone marrow aspirate and peripheral blood smear is diagnostic when it essentially shows immature blastic leukocyte cells. Performing a lumbar puncture is an option to determine if infiltration of the CNS has occurred.

Medical Management

The physician will institute a highly individualized treatment protocol immediately following diagnosis. Because many of the drugs used to bring about a remission have the capacity to cause a serious depletion of blood elements, the period immediately following remission tends to leave the child vulnerable to serious infection and hemorrhage. Supportive therapy is critical until the bone marrow recovers.

Almost immediately after confirmation of the diagnosis, induction therapy will begin and last for 4 to 6 weeks. The principal drugs that serve for induction in ALL are corticosteroids (especially prednisone), vincristine, and L-asparaginase, with or without doxorubicin. Drug therapy for ALL includes doxorubicin or daunorubicin (or daunomycin) and cytosine arabinoside.

To prevent the development of leukemia within the central nervous system (CNS leukemia), prophylactic treatment has become a standard protocol. Because the blood-brain barrier prohibits most systemic drugs from penetrating the CNS, the intrathecal route is the route of choice for CNS prophylaxis; that is, the physician injects the drugs directly into the cerebrospinal fluid via lumbar puncture. The drug of choice is methotrexate, given both intrathecally and intravenously, but other chemotherapeutic agents, such as triple intrathecal agent (consisting of methotrexate, cytarabine, and hydrocortisone), are also an option. Once remission has occurred, the physician will begin maintenance therapy in an effort to maintain remission and further reduce leukemic cells. The protocol includes daily doses of 6-mercaptopurine (6-MP), weekly doses of methotrexate, and monthly doses of prednisone and vincristine for 2 to 3 years.

Nursing Interventions

An important nursing intervention in dealing with children with any type of childhood cancer is to be available for family, especially in the early phases of diagnosis and treatment.

Nursing diagnoses and interventions for the child with cancer include but are not limited to the following:

Nursing Diagnoses	Nursing Interventions
Risk for infection, related to impaired immune system	Provide private room; use reverse isolation if necessary. Restrict all visitors and health care providers with active infection. Use strict hand hygiene technique. Monitor temperature. Use aseptic technique for all skin punctures. Administer granulocyte colony-stimulating factor (GCSF) subcutaneously, as prescribed, to reduce the incidence and duration of infection in children receiving chemotherapy treatment for cancer. In some research centers, special germ-free environments are available during complete myelosuppression from intensive chemotherapy or for bone marrow transplants. Screen all visitors and staff for signs of infection.
Risk for impaired skin integrity, related to treatment-induced changes	Use sheepskin, waffle pads, or flotation devices to prevent pressure areas. Clean mouth with soft-sponge toothbrush or cotton applicator to prevent mucosal bleeding. Give frequent mouth rinses.
Risk for imbalanced nutrition: less than body requirements, related to: • nausea • vomiting • anorexia	Encourage frequent, small meals of any food tolerated; plan to improve quality of food selections when appetite increases. Take advantage of hungry period; serve small snacks. Fortify foods with nutritious supplements, such as powdered milk or commercial supplements. Allow child to be involved in food preparation and selection when appropriate.
Anxiety, related to unknown outcome	Instruct patient and family about treatments. Promote atmosphere of open communication. Encourage patient and family to ventilate feelings. Recognize developmental fears associated with illness and procedures and disturbance in self-esteem.

Patient Teaching

When you work with families of children with cancer, you have a significant supportive role in helping them understand the therapies, preventing or managing expected side effects or toxicities, observing for late effects of treatment, and helping the child and family live as normal a life as possible and cope with the emotional aspects of the disease. Education is a constant feature of the nursing role, especially in terms of new treatments, clinical trials, and home care. You will help monitor all children closely following completion of treatment to evaluate for possible recurrence or to note any long-term complications as a result of the treatment (Hockenberry & Wilson, 2007).

Prognosis

Children diagnosed between 2 and 9 years of age have consistently demonstrated a better outlook than those diagnosed before 2 or after 10 years of age, and females appear to have a more favorable prognosis than males. About 95% of children with ALL achieve initial remission through a number of chemotherapeutic agents and irradiation (Shusterman & Meadows, 2000).

HODGKIN'S LYMPHOMA

Hodgkin's lymphoma is a malignant lymphoma distinguished by painless, progressive enlargement of lymphoid tissue. Five out of every 1 million children, most of whom are adolescents, develop Hodgkin's lymphoma (Hockenberry & Wilson, 2007). Although the exact etiology is still unknown, it is believed to occur in one specific site with spread to nearby lymph nodes through lymphatic routes. Performance of lymph node biopsy serves to determine the presence of Reed-Sternberg cells, the main diagnostic feature of Hodgkin's lymphoma. A bone marrow biopsy is useful in staging (Hockenberry & Wilson, 2007).

The incidence of Hodgkin's lymphoma is higher in males than females and rarely occurs in children under 5 years of age, with the incidence peaking between 15 and 19 years of age. Treatment depends on the staging process and follows the same protocols as for adult patients (Hockenberry & Wilson, 2007).

Prognosis

More than 90% of those diagnosed with early-stage Hodgkin's lymphoma and up to 75% of those with advanced disease will expect long-term survival, but some will possibly have a recurrence of their original malignancy or develop a second malignancy. The most common second malignancies are osteosarcoma, breast cancer, thyroid carcinoma, or leukemia. A patient who has a relapse has a 20% to 40% chance of achieving a complete remission. A bone marrow transplant may provide a cure (Lanzkowsky, 2000).

DISORDERS OF IMMUNE FUNCTION

Immunodeficiency disorders are the result of impaired immune function with alteration of the immune (self-defense) response. Immunodeficiency disorders are classified as primary or secondary. Primary immunodeficiency disorders result from genetic or congenital abnormalities and include X-linked agammaglobulinemia (defect in B cell development), DiGeorge syndrome (congenital absence of thymus and parathyroids), and severe combined immune deficiency (absence of both B and T lymphocytes and phagocytic cells). Secondary immunodeficiency disorders, the most common form of immunodeficiency, are acquired disorders associated with certain drug therapies such as corticosteroids, cancer chemotherapy, and antibiotics; radiation therapy; splenectomy; and viral infections. The common indicator in all immunodeficiency disorders is the development of unusual or recurrent, severe infections.

HUMAN IMMUNODEFICIENCY VIRUS AND ACQUIRED IMMUNODEFICIENCY SYNDROME

Etiology and Pathophysiology

Acquired immunodeficiency syndrome AIDS is a chronic and usually fatal disease caused by an acquired dysfunction of the immune system. AIDS is caused by HIV, which has been found in blood and in varying amounts in body fluids (semen, vaginal secretions, breast milk, tears, saliva, and urine). Disease in the majority of children (91%) with AIDS in the United States is due to perinatal infection by an HIV-infected mother while in utero, during parturition, or through breastfeeding. Less common, children have also become infected through the use of blood or blood product transfusions before 1985 and during sexual contact in child abuse. Adolescents often participate in high-risk behaviors, such as IV drug use and unsafe sex, which increases their risk of HIV infections (Hockenberry & Wilson, 2007).

The HIV virus has an attraction for the cells that have the CD_4^+ molecules on their surface such as the T-helper lymphocytes. These cells are targeted because they have more CD_4^+ receptors on their surfaces than any other cells. Immune dysfunction occurs owing to the destruction of T-helper cells by the HIV virus. A normal CD_4^+ lymphocyte count is 600 to 1200 per microliter (μL) of blood. The immune system remains healthy with CD_4^+ counts greater than 500 cells/μL. Severe immune problems occur when the CD_4^+ count falls below 200/μL, creating a high risk of opportunistic diseases and death from AIDS (Hockenberry & Wilson, 2007).

Three factors have resulted in a two thirds decrease in perinatal transmission of the HIV virus: (1) zidovudine therapy, (2) elective cesarean delivery, and (3) no breastfeeding for HIV-infected mothers and their newborns (Merchant et al., 2005; Kliegman et al., 2007). U.S. Public Health Service guidelines mandate pregnant women infected with HIV to obtain zidovudine treatment to reduce prenatal HIV transmission (Centers for Disease Control and Prevention [CDC], 1994; Hockenberry & Wilson, 2007).

Clinical Manifestations

Symptoms of HIV infection in children range from no symptoms to severe, life-threatening illnesses. Signs and symptoms commonly associated with AIDS include failure to thrive; progressive neurologic disease; developmental disabilities; deficits in motor skills, communication, and behavioral functioning; and frequent viral and bacterial infections (cytomegalovirus, herpes simplex virus, otitis media, sinusitis, enterocolitis, recurrent pneumonia, and septicemia).

The greatest threat to an HIV-infected infant younger than 1 year of age is *Pneumocystis jiroveci* (formerly *carinii*) pneumonia, which is sometimes life threatening. Unique findings in the pediatric AIDS population include lymphocytic interstitial pneumonia (LIP), oral and diaper-area candidiasis, and chronic ear infections. One of the most common causes of CNS mass lesions in HIV-infected children is malignant CNS lymphoma. In contrast to adult HIV infection, children rarely contract Kaposi's sarcoma. In adolescents, both males and females follow more adult-oriented symptomatology, with females exhibiting gynecologic manifestations similar to those seen in adult females. However, if you are caring for an HIV-infected adolescent, remember that he or she is still a child and still developing cognitively, physically, and emotionally.

Diagnostic Tests

In the child older than 18 months of age, the health care provider will make the diagnosis of HIV infection by using the same serologic enzyme-linked immunosorbent assay (ELISA) and Western blot testing for the presence of serum HIV antibodies as in adults. The individual's blood is tested with ELISA or enzyme immunoassay (EIA), antibody tests that detect the presence of HIV antibodies. If the EIA is positive for HIV, then the same blood is tested a second time. If the second EIA is positive, a more specific confirming test such as the Western blot is done. Blood that is reactive or positive in all three steps is reported to be HIV positive. But the diagnosis of the child younger than 18 months of age is complicated by the fact that in the seropositive mother, maternal HIV antibodies cross the placenta to the fetus. Most exposed infants up to 18 months of age will test positive for HIV antibodies, but it is unclear whose antibodies are being detected during this time.

However, for infants younger than 18 months a polymerase chain reaction (PCR) test, which actually tests for HIV, not for the antibody, is available to definitively diagnose HIV infection early in this age-group. The benefits of this type of testing include early identification and treatment of the HIV-infected infant, as well as decreased anxiety and waiting time for parents with HIV-exposed infants who are HIV negative.

Medical Management

Current treatment of the HIV-positive patient is aimed at slowing the growth of HIV, keeping the viral load low, preventing opportunistic infections and cancer, optimizing or restoring normal growth and development, improving quality of life, and increasing chances for survival (Hockenberry & Wilson, 2007).

Combined antiretroviral drugs help to prevent reproduction of new virus particles. Antiretroviral therapy does not cure the HIV-infected patient but assists in preventing further destruction of the immune system. These antiretroviral drugs are listed and organized by category in Box 31-2. The physician will order combinations of at least two but often three antiretroviral drugs or more to make it more difficult for the virus to develop resistance to the drugs. There are many drugs

Box 31-2 Antiretroviral Drugs

NUCLEOSIDE REVERSE TRANSCRIPTASE INHIBITORS
- Zidovudine
- Didanosine
- Stavudine
- Zalcitabine
- Lamivudine
- Abacavir

NONNUCLEOSIDE REVERSE TRANSCRIPTASE INHIBITORS
- Nevirapine
- Delavirdine
- Efavirenz

NUCLEOTIDE REVERSE TRANSCRIPTASE INHIBITOR
- Adefovir

PROTEASE INHIBITORS
- Indinavir
- Saquinavir
- Ritonavir
- Nelfinavir
- Amprenavir
- Fosamprenavir
- Lopinavir-ritonair

ADJUNCTIVE ANTIRETROVIRAL
- Hydroxyurea

Data from Hockenberry, M.J., & Wilson, D. (2007). *Wong's nursing care of infants and children.* (8th ed.). St. Louis: Mosby.

in development for treatment of the HIV-positive patient (Hockenberry & Wilson, 2007). Therapy is lifelong, making adherence difficult. Laboratory markers (CD_4^+ lymphocyte count, viral load) assist in monitoring both disease progression and response to therapy.

Immunization against common childhood diseases is recommended for all children exposed to and infected with HIV (Kliegman et al., 2007). Production of antibodies to vaccines is less than effective in some cases, and in others it decreases with time; therefore, prophylaxis after exposure to several diseases such as varicella, measles, mumps, and rubella is advisable if there is no evidence of severe immunocompromise (CDC, 1999; Kliegman et al., 2007). Another recommendation is for children to receive pneumococcal and influenza vaccines (Hockenberry & Wilson, 2007).

Nursing Interventions

The nursing interventions are basically the same for the adult and pediatric populations. However, it is necessary to monitor the HIV-infected child closely for signs of abnormal growth and development, which are common in this group. Complications of HIV-related infections often cause severe failure to thrive and numerous nutritional deficiencies. It is often difficult, because of recurrent illness with anorexia, nausea, and diarrhea, to maintain adequate nutrition. If the child has weight loss and slowing of growth and development, the health care provider will initiate intensive nutritional interventions (Hockenberry & Wilson, 2007). If there is family involvement, direct nursing interventions at supporting the family. Whenever possible, make arrangements for the intervention of social services and home health and nutritional services, such as Women, Infants, and Children (WIC).

Nursing diagnoses and interventions for the child with HIV include but are not limited to the following:

Nursing Diagnoses	Nursing Interventions
Risk for infection, related to: • impaired body defenses • presence of infective organisms	Restrict contact with people who have infections, including family, other children, friends, and members of staff. Observe thorough hand hygiene. Place child in room with noninfectious children; restrict visitors with active illnesses. Advise visitors (and hospital personnel) to practice thorough hand hygiene. Promote body's remaining natural defenses (e.g., good nutrition).
Impaired social interaction, related to: • physical limitations • hospitalizations • social stigma toward AIDS	Administer medication as prescribed. Assist child in identifying personal strengths. Educate school personnel and classmates about AIDS. Encourage child to participate in activities with other children.
Anticipatory grieving, related to having a child with a potentially fatal illness	Identify stage of grieving process family is experiencing. Provide opportunities for family to express emotions. Help parents deal with their feelings, allowing them more emotional reserve to meet the needs of their children. Encourage parents to share their moments of sorrow with their children. Facilitate family's assistance with child's care.

Patient Teaching

The adolescent population is increasingly contracting HIV infection. Changing moral standards, increased sexual freedom, increased IV drug use, and misinformation about the disease in this age-group render adolescents at high risk for exposure to the disease. As a patient advocate, you will become involved in educating these youngsters directly by counseling them on matters such as avoiding casual sex and using a condom during intercourse. Also consider helping promote educational messages in the media (Figure 31-11) (e.g., radio and MTV) and in places that youths frequent.

Prognosis

Perinatally infected infants generally have more rapid disease progression than children infected at an older age or adults. It has been reported that the risk of dying is higher for children who are diagnosed with AIDS early in life and in those who develop *P. jiroveci* (formerly *carinii*) pneumonia (PCP). The mean survival time from birth to death is about 9.4 years. Early recognition and improved medical treatments have changed the course of HIV infection in children from a rapidly fatal to a chronic but still terminal disease of childhood. The ultimate prognosis for perinatal HIV infection depends strongly on counseling pregnant women about HIV infection, voluntary testing, and the methods currently in practice for the prevention of perinatal transmission.

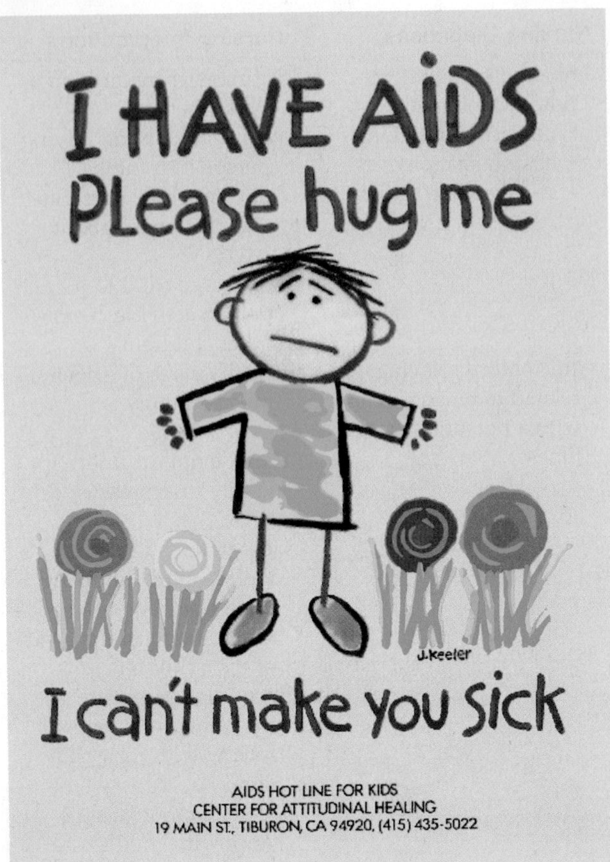

FIGURE 31-11 Using one medium to promote educational messages about AIDS.

JUVENILE RHEUMATOID ARTHRITIS (JUVENILE IDIOPATHIC ARTHRITIS)

Etiology and Pathophysiology

Juvenile idiopathic arthritis (JIA)—formerly known as *juvenile rheumatoid arthritis (JRA)*—is chronic arthritis that occurs during childhood (Hockenberry & Wilson, 2007). Because you will see both terms in research literature and in practice, the chapter discusses them jointly. JRA-JIA affects the joints and the tissues and manifests in 1 of every 1000 children. The disorder is idiopathic (cause unknown). Females are affected twice as often as males, with the highest incidence of the disease occurring between 1 and 3 years and 8 and 10 years (Hockenberry & Wilson, 2007).

In JRA-JIA there is chronic inflammation of the synovium with joint effusion. This inflammatory process leads to erosion, destruction, and fibrosis of the articular cartilage. We do not know the exact etiology of the inflammatory process, but the supposition is that the tissue injury arises from a previous infectious process.

Clinical Manifestations

JRA-JIA affects a single joint in some cases, and numerous joints in others. The joint(s) involved are stiff, edematous with loss of motion, and warm to the touch but not usually erythematous (Hockenberry & Wilson, 2007). The signs and symptoms that appear in acute systemic onset include daily afternoon and late-night temperature spikes, macular rash on the trunk and the extremities, and joint involvement. Other systemic conditions include pericarditis, pleuritis, lymphadenopathy, hepatosplenomegaly, iridocyclitis, and anemia. Systemic involvement occurs in only 10% of all patients. A significant number of JRA-JIA patients tend to "burn out," meaning the disease process becomes inactive (Hockenberry & Wilson, 2007).

Diagnostic Tests

JRA-JIA is a clinical diagnosis; there are no specific tests for diagnosing JRA-JIA. The latex fixation test, which identifies rheumatoid arthritis in the adult, is negative in 90% of juvenile cases. Depending on the degree of inflammation, the erythrocyte sedimentation rate (ESR) is sometimes elevated. In some types of JRA-JIA, antinuclear antibodies (ANAs) will be present. Radiographic findings in early-onset JRA-JIA sometimes show the widening of joint spaces and, later, fusion and articular destruction.

Medical Management

The goals of management include the prevention of joint contractures, preservation of joint function, and relief of signs and symptoms. There is no specific cure for JRA-JIA. Nonsteroidal antiinflammatory drugs (NSAIDs) are the first line of drug treatment. These include tolmetin (Tolectin), naproxen (Naprosyn), indomethacin (Indocin), ibuprofen (Motrin), diclofenac (Voltaren), and nabumetone (Relafen). Aspirin was once the drug of choice for treatment of JRA-JIA, but use is currently rare in children. The physician will usually add slower-acting antirheumatic drugs (SAARDs) to the drug therapy when one or two of the NSAIDs no longer effectively control signs and symptoms. The SAARDs include methotrexate (Rheumatrex), sulfasalazine (Azulfidine), and hydroxychloroquine (Plaquenil). Use of corticosteroids and biologic agents such as etanercept to treat JRA-JIA is an option these days when the child has significant physical disability and other medications have proven ineffective (Hockenberry & Wilson, 2007). Symptomatic treatment includes the application of moist heat to facilitate movement and physical therapy. Surgical intervention is sometimes necessary for some children unresponsive to therapy.

Nursing Interventions

Discuss potential problems in the school environment such as stairs and strenuous activities and facilitate planning with the school nurse to arrange for medication administration and rest periods. JRA-JIA strongly affects the normal activities of daily living (ADLs) of children afflicted with the disorder. Support and help the family in expressing their fears and concerns, and guide them in a daily program of rest, exercise, medication administration, and pain management. Encourage the child to perform ADLs (bathing, dressing, grooming) with little or no help from the family to enhance self-esteem. Also suggest support groups for the child and the parents that provide the necessary education and resources to effectively cope with a chronic, debilitating illness. Referrals to the Arthritis Foundation and the American Juvenile Arthritis Foundation can provide this assistance.

Nursing diagnoses and interventions for the child with JRA-JIA include but are not limited to the following:

Nursing Diagnoses	Nursing Interventions
Chronic pain, related to joint inflammation	Provide as much relief as possible with antiinflammatory medication and other therapies to help child tolerate the pain and cope as effectively as possible (although desirable, complete pain relief is probably unattainable). Apply moist heat to relieve pain and stiffness (the most efficient and practical method is tub baths).
Impaired physical mobility, related to: • joint discomfort • stiffness	Promote ADLs to provide satisfactory exercise and increase mobility. Encourage lying in the prone position to straighten hips and knees. Instruct patient and family in the purpose and correct use of any splints and appliances. Instruct in use of raised toilet seat for independent toileting.

Patient Teaching

Nursing interventions consist of educating the child and the family in the disease process and management. Teach parents to perform gentle range-of-motion (ROM) exercises to promote joint mobility, administer medications, apply heat to relieve pain (warm baths are often very effective), and encourage normal play activity to promote exercise and increase joint mobility.

Prognosis

The course of JRA-JIA is highly variable. Some 30% to 40% of patients have active disease 10 years after diagnosis, have substantial disability as adults, and require long-term drug therapy.

DISORDERS OF RESPIRATORY FUNCTION

Acute respiratory infections are extremely common in infants and children. The possibilities range from minor to life-threatening illnesses. Most respiratory illnesses involve viral pathogens. Bacterial infections most commonly involve group A β-hemolytic streptococci (GABHS), *Staphylococcus aureus,* and *Haemophilus influenzae.*

RESPIRATORY DISTRESS SYNDROME

Etiology and Pathophysiology

Respiratory distress syndrome (RDS), idiopathic respiratory distress syndrome (IRDS), and **hyaline membrane disease (HMD)** are terms that refer to the severe lung disorder that is the major cause of morbidity and mortality in the neonatal period. RDS is caused by a deficiency of surfactant and occurs almost exclusively in the preterm, low-birth-weight infant. RDS occurs more often in males and in infants delivered by cesarean section. Other predisposing factors include infants of diabetic mothers, asphyxia, maternal hemorrhage, and shock. Surfactant reduces the surface tension of fluids that line the alveoli, thereby permitting expansion of the lungs and alveolar inflation. Without sufficient production of surfactant, the infant is unable to keep the lungs inflated and the alveoli collapse at the end of expiration, resulting in hypoxia, atelectasis, and respiratory acidosis.

Clinical Manifestations

Respiratory signs and symptoms become apparent immediately after birth. Signs and symptoms include nasal flaring; expiratory grunting; intercostal, subcostal, or substernal retractions; dusky color; tachypnea (up to 80 to 120 breaths/min) initially, dyspnea; and low body temperature. Manifestations as the disease progresses include apnea, flaccidity, absent spontaneous movement, unresponsiveness, and mottling. In severe cases, infants will sometimes die within hours of the onset of signs and symptoms; those who survive gradually show improvement by the fourth day.

Diagnostic Tests

Criteria for the diagnosis of RDS consist of the clinical presentation and the radiographic examination. Blood gas analysis indicates the degree of respiratory and metabolic acidosis.

Medical Management

The treatment of RDS is entirely supportive and aims to correct imbalances. Supportive measures include maintaining a neutral thermal environment, providing adequate oxygenation either by increasing ambient (pertaining to the surrounding area) oxygen concentration or by ventilatory assistance, and correction of respiratory and metabolic acidosis. To prevent hypoxia and the toxic effects of high concentrations of oxygen, it is necessary to continually evaluate oxygen therapy by measuring arterial oxygen. The physician will order nutritional support through parenteral therapy during the early acute stage to prevent aspiration. Nipple and gavage feeding are contraindicated in any situation that creates a marked increase in respiratory rate because of the greater hazards of aspiration.

The administration of exogenous (originating outside the body) pulmonary surfactant to infants at high risk of developing or who have developed RDS has greatly reduced the morbidity and mortality associated with the disorder. Administration of exogenous surfactant occurs via an endotracheal (ET) tube directly into the infant's trachea and lungs shortly after birth. Additional doses are sometimes given. In some cases, administration of corticosteroids, such as betamethasone, to the mother before delivery helps increase the production of surfactant in the preterm infant.

Nursing Interventions and Patient Teaching

The primary nursing consideration in caring for the infant with RDS is observing and assessing the infant's response to therapy. Continuous monitoring and assessment are essential so that you are able to adjust oxygen concentrations and ventilator settings in response to the infant's blood gas measurements and pulse oximetry readings. Perform frequent respiratory assessments, observe the infant's behavior, and observe for signs of respiratory complications and sepsis. You will perform suctioning as needed, based on assessment of the neonate (auscultation, increased infant irritability, excessive moisture in the endotracheal tube). You will never carry out suctioning on a routine basis. Frequent vigorous suctioning creates the risk of bronchospasm, airway damage, infection, **pneumothorax** (a collection of air or gas in the pleural space causing the lung to collapse), hypoxia, and increased intracranial pressure that potentially leads to intraventricular hemorrhage in the neonate. Help the infant maintain an open airway by positioning the infant on the side with the head supported in alignment. Assess the infant's skin frequently, and protect the skin from impairment by frequent repositioning and the use of water mattresses or pillows and sheepskin. Use a water-soluble ointment to reduce irritation to the nares or around the mouth, and perform frequent oral hygiene with water to help relieve dryness caused by oxygen therapy.

Parents will need emotional support; encourage them to discuss their anxieties and concerns so that you have the opportunity to clarify information. Also encourage parents to touch, hold, and talk to the infant and participate in the care whenever possible to promote bonding.

Prognosis

RDS is a self-limiting disease. Infants with RDS who survive the first 96 hours have a reasonable chance of recovery. Surfactant replacement therapy tends to improve the survival rate and reduce the severity of RDS.

Prevention

Preventing premature delivery due to elective early delivery and cesarean birth is the most effective method of avoiding RDS. Adequate surfactant formation is reasonably possible to determine by amniocentesis, which allows assessment of the maturity of the fetal lungs (Hockenberry & Wilson, 2007).

BRONCHOPULMONARY DYSPLASIA

Etiology and Pathophysiology

Bronchopulmonary dysplasia (BPD) is a chronic pulmonary disorder that develops in premature infants. BPD arises in association with meconium aspiration, RDS, high concentrations of oxygen, positive pressure ventilation, and endotracheal intubation. Chronic lung changes include thickening and necrosis of alveolar walls with impairment of oxygen diffusion from the alveoli to the capillaries. Edema and inflammation of the capillary bed have the potential to cause some alveoli to collapse, some to hyperinflate, and others to rupture. Diffuse infiltrates, hyperinflation, and chronic pulmonary insufficiency characterize the disorder.

Clinical Manifestations

The clinical signs and symptoms of BPD vary widely. Most infants show evidence of respiratory distress (wheezing, retracting, nasal flaring, irritability, abundant secretions, and cyanosis when stressed). These children are vulnerable to upper respiratory infections and frequently require hospitalization because of poor respiratory status.

Diagnostic Tests

No specific signs or symptoms or laboratory data confirm a diagnosis of BPD. Radiographic examination and ABG determinations are often helpful in contributing to the diagnosis. Pulmonary function tests typically help determine the degree of lung dysfunction.

Medical Management

Medical management involves taking precautions to prevent RDS and reduce ventilation and oxygen requirements. When ventilation and oxygen are necessary, meticulous management is necessary in using the lowest concentration of oxygen and ventilatory pressures to maintain adequate gas exchange to avoid further damage of lung tissue. During weaning, use of bronchodilators is possible to decrease airway resistance and increase lung compliance. Management includes nutritional support, initially provided by total parenteral nutrition (TPN) and later by nasogastric, gavage, or breastfeeding or bottle feeding.

Nursing Interventions and Patient Teaching

Plan rest periods to decrease respiratory effort and conserve energy. When it is time to begin oral feedings, provide small, frequent feedings to prevent overdistention of the stomach, which has the capacity to interfere with respiratory effort. You are instrumental in supporting parents; encourage them to participate in their infant's care.

Also counsel parents about ways to reduce the risk of respiratory infections, and instruct them to notify their physician at the first sign of a respiratory infection in their child. Teach parents cardiopulmonary resuscitation and how to manage any other possibly anticipated emergency.

Prognosis

There is a high mortality rate in the first year. Infants who survive are at risk for chronic lung disease. The use of exogenous surfactant in neonates with RDS has greatly reduced the incidence of BPD and its morbidity in at-risk infants.

PNEUMONIA

Etiology and Pathophysiology

Pneumonia is an acute inflammation of the pulmonary parenchyma (tissue), small airways, and alveoli. Classification of pneumonia is by the causative agent: bacterial, viral, mycoplasmal, or foreign body aspiration. Pneumonia is common throughout childhood, occurs more frequently in infants and young children, and is usually associated with an upper respiratory infection. Pneumonias are most common in the winter months from November through March. Viral pneumonias are more common than bacterial pneumonias, with respiratory syncytial virus (RSV) accounting for the largest percentage of infections in infants and young children. Bacterial pneumonias most common in infants and children are caused by streptococcal, staphylococcal, pneumococcal, or *H. influenzae* organisms.

Clinical Manifestations

The clinical manifestations of viral and bacterial pneumonias are given in Box 31-3.

Diagnostic Tests

Radiographic examination establishes the location and the extent of infection. Peripheral blood tests sometimes reveal an elevated WBC count, with bacterial infection showing a greater elevation in WBC count than viral infection. Identification of the causative organism includes culture and Gram stain of respiratory secretions and the blood, and diagnostic thoracentesis if fluid is suspected in the pleural cavity. The laboratory identifies RSV by examining nasal or nasopharyngeal secretions for RSV antigen detection. If no bacterial microorganism is identified, the pneumonia is considered to be viral.

Box 31-3 Clinical Manifestations of Pneumonia in Children

- Cough
- Wheeze or crackles
- Respiratory distress
- Chest pain
- Anorexia
- Irritability
- Malaise
- Lethargy
- Headache
- Fever
- Myalgia
- Abdominal pain
- Nasal discharge

Medical Management

The goal of therapy in the management of pneumonia is to improve oxygenation and prevent dehydration. Treatment includes antibiotic therapy, oxygen therapy, chest physiotherapy, suctioning, fluid administration, and bronchodilators. Many physicians will order antipyretics to control fever.

To prevent RSV infection in premature neonates, there is a new protocol whereby high-risk infants are given monthly infusions of RSV immune globulin, which provides them with antibodies to RSV. The infant receives these infusions in an outpatient setting during RSV season, which runs from November through April.

The U.S. Food and Drug Administration (FDA) has approved a genetically engineered RSV monoclonal antibiotic called palivizumab for monthly intramuscular administration for high-risk children. Health care providers favor palivizumab over intravenous RSV immune globulin because it has few complications and does not interfere with the measles-mumps-rubella or varicella vaccinations (AAP, 2003d).

Nursing Interventions and Patient Teaching

Observation of respiratory status, including skin color and respiratory effort, and monitoring of cardiovascular status are two important nursing measures. You will follow infection control measures according to hospital protocol. Supportive nursing management includes providing for adequate rest periods to conserve energy, maintaining hydration by monitoring prescribed IV fluids, administration of oxygen and antibiotics as prescribed, and gentle suctioning with a bulb syringe when necessary. Use caution when giving oral fluids, if allowed, to help prevent aspiration and to decrease the possibility of aggravating a fatiguing cough.

Encourage parents to participate in their child's care, guiding them in the proper methods to feed and hold their child while in the mist tent to prevent dislodgement of IV catheters.

Prognosis

Prognosis for pneumococcal and streptococcal pneumonias is generally good, with rapid resolution when detection and treatment occur early. Staphylococcal pneumonias typically run a longer course, but early detection and treatment are usually effective.

SUDDEN INFANT DEATH SYNDROME

The sudden, unexpected, and unexplained death of a healthy infant evokes a variety of familial responses ranging from hysteria and denial to stoicism (being impassive, indifferent to joy or pain). Nurses assume an important role in assisting the family through the death and grieving process.

Etiology and Pathophysiology

Sudden infant death syndrome (SIDS) is the sudden, unexpected death of a healthy, normal infant younger than 1 year of age in which a postmortem examination, investigation of the death scene, and review of the case history fail to establish a cause of death. In the United States, mortality from SIDS has declined more than 40% since 1992. The incidence was 0.7 death per 1000 live births in 2002. SIDS still claimed the lives of 2295 infants in 2002, with peak incidence occurring between 2 and 4 months of age (AAP, 2003; Hockenberry & Wilson, 2007). Health care providers attribute the dramatic decrease to the Back to Sleep campaign. SIDS always occurs during sleep and is the third leading cause of death among infants aged 1 to 12 months.

SIDS occurs more often in males and in siblings of SIDS victims (Hockenberry & Wilson, 2007). Incidence is increased in winter months, with peak incidence occurring in January. Native Americans and blacks are most often affected, and there is an increased occurrence in lower socioeconomic classes. SIDS is often associated with premature birth and low birth weight, low Apgar scores (evaluation of an infant's physical condition, usually performed 1 minute and 5 minutes after birth), multiple births, and CNS and respiratory dysfunctions. There is also an association between SIDS and maternal smoking, drug addiction, and maternal age of less than 20 years. Breastfed infants have a lower incidence of SIDS. The cause of SIDS remains unknown, although there are numerous theories. Abnormalities include prolonged sleep apnea, depressed ventilatory response to increased carbon dioxide or decreased oxygen, increased frequency of short apneic episodes, and excessive periodic breathing. Other studies show a relationship between sleep position and SIDS (Malloy, 2002). Sleeping in a prone position possibly predisposes the infant to oropharyngeal obstruction or affects ventilatory arousal. Soft, polystyrene-filled mattresses or pillows have the potential to cause suffocation in the infant sleeping in a prone position. (See the Safety Alert box on preventing SIDS.)

Clinical Manifestations

Death occurs during sleep, and there is no audible outcry or sign of distress.

Diagnostic Tests

Confirmation of the diagnosis occurs at postmortem examination, which reveals pulmonary edema and intrathoracic hemorrhages.

Medical Management

Therapeutic management aims toward assisting the family that has just lost an infant to SIDS.

Nursing Interventions

The death of an infant from SIDS propels the family into a crisis situation. The initial response is one of extreme shock and disbelief. As parents try to cope, they often experience feelings of guilt and blame. Typically, it is the mother who finds her infant dead in the crib. The appearance of the dead infant indicates that some activity has taken place before death. The infant is most often positioned with the blankets over the head

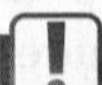 Safety Alert!

Preventing Sudden Infant Death Syndrome (SIDS)

- Maternal smoking, both prenatally and postnatally, is a possible cause of SIDS that some have proposed, as well as poor prenatal care and low maternal age.
- Co-sleeping, or bed sharing, has been reported to have a possible association with SIDS, especially in cases of maternal smoking (Kemp, 2000). Unlike cribs, whose design has to meet safety standards for infants, adult beds or sofas do not meet such specifications and potentially create a risk for accidental entrapment and suffocation.
- Overheating is a potential cause of SIDS that some have proposed; therefore, dress infants in light clothing and keep the room temperature at a comfortable range for a lightly dressed adult; avoid overbundling the infant (Mesich, 2005).
- The most compelling data come from studies that link sleep habits with an increased risk of SIDS. Sleeping in the prone position perhaps causes oropharyngeal obstruction or affects the thermal balance or arousal state. Potential mechanisms for cause of death that some have suggested are rebreathing of carbon dioxide by the prone infant and impaired arousal from active and quiet sleep when sleeping prone (Malloy, 2002).
- The AAP Task Force on Sudden Infant Death Syndrome (2005) recommended the use of a pacifier when infants are put down to sleep; for breastfed infants, delay pacifier use until infant is 1 month of age to allow for establishment of breastfeeding.
- The AAP (2000) recommends placing healthy infants to sleep in the supine (on the back) position. The AAP no longer recommends the side-lying and prone positions.
- Do not use soft bedding such as pillows or quilts under the infant for bedding.
- Remove bedding items such as stuffed animals or towels from the crib while the infant is asleep to prevent possible asphyxia.

and huddled in a corner of the crib. The infant's hands are sometimes clutching the sheets or blanket.

Frothy, blood-tinged secretions are noted in the mouth and the nostrils. The infant's appearance and the shock of an unexpected death lead many parents to believe that their infant has suffocated, and they become filled with self-blame. Be aware of these circumstances so that you will be able to assist and support the family effectively in this time of crisis. The first people to respond to a SIDS event are the police and ambulance personnel, who generally have knowledge of SIDS. When talking with the parent, their task is to be nonjudgmental, ask few questions, and provide support to the family. On the family's arrival in the emergency department, you will most likely be the first person to interact with them. Stay with the parent, listening to and supporting the family. Emergency department personnel ask only factual information about the event. If there was a resuscitation attempt at home, the child will sometimes have bruises and broken ribs, which will possibly arouse a false suspicion of physical abuse. The physician examines the infant and pronounces death. At this time, hospital personnel will discuss autopsy to establish the cause of death; otherwise it is not possible to lay to rest the circumstances surrounding the death. If you are working in the emergency department, you become instrumental in assisting families with grief and mourning. You will clean the infant, wrap the child in a sheet or blanket, and tidy the room where the family will be able to spend time with their dead infant. In coming to terms with the death, ensure that the parents' last moments with their infant are quiet, peaceful, and as meaningful as possible. Offer to stay with the family, or allow them private time if they wish. Pack the baby's belongings and give them to the family on their departure.

Patient Teaching

Arrange for a visiting nurse to visit the family as soon as possible after the death to decrease feelings of isolation, help them in understanding the SIDS phenomenon, and assist with siblings' feelings. A referral to the Sudden Infant Death Syndrome Alliance is always helpful.

UPPER RESPIRATORY TRACT INFECTIONS

ACUTE PHARYNGITIS (SORE THROAT)

Etiology and Pathophysiology

Acute pharyngitis is an inflammation of the pharynx. Approximately 80% of acute pharyngitis cases are viral in origin, whereas 20% are bacterial (GABHS). Acute pharyngitis occurs frequently between 4 and 12 years of age, when children are increasingly exposed to infections outside the home. The infecting organism in children less than 3 years of age with pharyngitis is usually *Haemophilus influenzae*. It is necessary to watch these children for neurologic signs and symptoms indicating possible meningitis; however, with the use of Hib vaccine, infections involving this organism are beginning to decline. Acute cases of pharyngitis are more common in later winter and early spring.

Clinical Manifestations

Viral pharyngitis causes low-grade fever, malaise, anorexia, pharyngeal erythema, and throat soreness. Many children also complain of headache, cough, hoarseness, rhinitis, and conjunctivitis. Streptococcal pharyngitis causes high fever, throat soreness, white exudates on the posterior pharynx and tonsillar region, vomiting, and abdominal pain.

Diagnostic Tests

Although 80% to 90% of all cases of acute pharyngitis are of viral origin, a throat culture is performed to rule out GABHS.

Medical Management

Viral pharyngitis is treated symptomatically with lozenges, gargles, and acetaminophen. It is necessary to treat streptococcal pharyngitis with a 10-day course of antimicrobial therapy to prevent complications (acute rheumatic fever and acute glomerulonephritis). Penicillin is the drug of choice for streptococcal pharyngitis. Other medications that also serve to treat streptococcal pharyngitis include erythromycin, azithromycin, clarithromycin, cephalosporins, and amoxicillin.

Nursing Interventions and Patient Teaching

Help relieve throat discomfort in both viral and bacterial infections with saline gargles, lozenges, warm compresses to the neck, and acetaminophen. Encourage cool liquids (nonacid) until the throat feels better; then introduce soft, bland foods. Emphasize follow-up care of streptococcal pharyngitis to ensure eradication of the causative organism.

Instruct the family in antimicrobial therapy, emphasizing the need to completely finish the medication even though the child feels better. When a child has a positive throat culture for streptococcal infection, remind the child to discard his or her toothbrush and replace it with a new one after taking antibiotics for 24 hours.

Prognosis

The prognosis of acute pharyngitis is usually excellent. Inadequately treated streptococcal infections sometimes trigger a response in the heart (rheumatic fever) or kidneys (acute glomerulonephritis).

TONSILLITIS

Etiology and Pathophysiology

The tonsils are masses of lymphoid tissue located in the pharyngeal cavity believed to protect the respiratory and alimentary tracts from invasion by pathogenic microorganisms. They probably also play a role in antibody formation. Tonsillitis usually occurs as a result of pharyngitis and has either viral or bacterial (streptococcal) causes.

Clinical Manifestations

The signs and symptoms of viral and bacterial tonsillitis are similar and include sore throat, headache, edematous and tender cervical lymph glands, fever, hoarseness, and cough. Additionally, in streptococcal tonsillitis, many children exhibit vomiting, complain of muscle aches, and have difficulty swallowing or breathing.

Diagnostic Tests

A CBC will sometimes indicate a significantly elevated WBC count. You will perform a throat culture to detect streptococcal tonsillitis.

Medical Management

The treatment for bacterial and nonbacterial tonsillitis includes the comfort measures described in acute pharyngitis. Additionally, treatment for bacterial tonsillitis comprises a 10-day course of penicillin (or erythromycin) to prevent complications. Tonsillectomy is not a recommended measure to treat chronic tonsillitis, and the American Academy of Otolaryngology—Head and Neck Surgery (2000) states that an indication for tonsillectomy or adenotonsillectomy is "three or more infections of the tonsils or adenoids per year despite adequate medical therapy." Surgery is possible to decrease the occurrence of hearing loss or deafness secondary to otitis media, but the positive potential effects are often not sufficient to justify the risk of surgery. In clinical practice, the majority of health care providers consider each patient on an individual basis and do not use a specific set of eligibility criteria for performing a tonsillectomy or adenotonsillectomy (Paradise et al., 2002).

Nursing Interventions

The nursing interventions for children with tonsillitis are the same as those described for acute pharyngitis. Before any indicated surgery, prepare the child psychologically. as Also assess the child for signs of infection and loose teeth and check the child's laboratory data, including the bleeding and clotting studies. Postoperatively, keep the child in a semiprone position to facilitate drainage; also monitor the child frequently for excessive bleeding, which will cause frequent swallowing even while asleep; give analgesics as prescribed; and, after recovery from analgesia, provide fluids (with the exception of acidic, grape, red, or chocolate drinks so you will be able to distinguish fresh or old blood in emesis from ingested liquid). A soft diet follows. Some health care providers advise against the use of straws because sucking sometimes precipitates bleeding; however, not all practitioners agree. Postoperative hemorrhage is unusual but possible. Therefore, observe the throat directly for evidence of bleeding, using a good source of light and, if necessary, carefully inserting a tongue depressor. Signs of hemorrhage include increased pulse (greater than 120 bpm), pallor, frequent clearing of the throat or swallowing by a younger child, and vomiting of bright red blood. Restlessness, an indication of hemorrhage, is sometimes difficult to differentiate from general discomfort after surgery. Decreasing blood pressure is a late sign of shock.

Patient Teaching

Appropriate discharge instructions include the following:

- Avoid foods that are irritating or highly seasoned.
- Avoid the use of gargles or vigorous toothbrushing.
- Discourage the child from coughing or clearing the throat.
- Use mild analgesics or an ice collar for pain.
- Do not use aspirin.
- Alert parents that hemorrhaging is possible 5 to 10 days after surgery as a result of tissue sloughing from the healing process. Any signs of bleeding necessitate immediate notification of the physician.

Prognosis

The prognosis is generally excellent. Improperly treated streptococcal infections potentially result in rheumatic fever or acute glomerulonephritis.

CROUP

Croup is an acute viral disease of childhood, marked by a resonant barking cough, suffocative and difficult breathing, and laryngeal spasm.

Laryngotracheobronchitis and Acute Epiglottitis

Etiology and Pathophysiology

Laryngotracheobronchitis (LTB) is the most common form of croup affecting children 3 months to 3 years of age and is usually viral in origin. LTB usually follows an upper respiratory infection that descends to the lower respiratory tract and has a gradual, progressive onset.

Acute epiglottitis is a severe, potentially life-threatening bacterial infection of the epiglottis in older children and is usually caused by *H. influenzae* type B. However, with the use of Hib vaccine, episodes of epiglottitis caused by *H. influenzae* have been decreasing. The inflamed epiglottis becomes cherry-red and edematous, which has the potential to lead to total airway obstruction.

Clinical Manifestations

The child with LTB initially demonstrates hoarseness; inspiratory stridor; tachypnea; nasal flaring; suprasternal, substernal, and intercostal retractions; and characteristic barking cough. Body temperature is usually normal or mildly elevated. Nursing assessment will include checking for the four Ds: drooling, dyspnea, dysphonia, and dysphagia (McKinney et al., 2005).

The child with epiglottitis is acutely ill with high fever, muffled voice, drooling, progressive respiratory distress, anxiety, and fear.

Diagnostic Tests

Diagnostic criteria for LTB consist of a history of a preceding upper respiratory infection, CBC with differential, the clinical signs and symptoms, and physical examination.

Clinical signs and symptoms serve to establish a tentative diagnosis of acute epiglottitis, considered a medical emergency. It is necessary to take the child to the operating or ambulatory surgery room, where emergency equipment is available for immediate intubation or tracheostomy in the event of further obstruction during examination of the pharynx. The physician will sometimes obtain lateral neck radiographs in the operating room to observe for soft tissue edema and area of obstruction. Skilled personnel with the equipment necessary to perform immediate intubation or tracheostomy never leave the child's side. The trend away from early intubation of children with LTB emphasizes the importance of nursing observation and the ability to recognize impending respiratory failure so that implementation of intubation is possible without delay. The child is put under anesthesia for visual examination of the pharynx and invasive procedures such as blood collection and insertion of IV lines. The laboratory will perform culture and sensitivity testing on tracheal secretions collected at the time of intubation.

Medical Management

Management of both LTB and epiglottitis focuses on maintaining an open airway. The child with LTB receives high cool-mist humidity with low-concentration oxygen (30%) by mist tent. Administration of epinephrine by aerosol helps to decrease airway edema by vasoconstriction and improve oxygenation by bronchodilation. The effects of epinephrine are short lived, and the child will most likely need repeated doses if and when the airway edema returns a few hours after administration. Therefore it is necessary to monitor children receiving epinephrine very closely. During the acute phase, the child receives nothing by mouth (NPO; from Latin, *nil per os*) because the typically rapid respirations predispose to aspiration. IV administration of fluids serves to accomplish adequate hydration. The use of sedatives is contraindicated because they mask restlessness, which is a clinical indication of hypoxia and a deteriorating condition.

Immediate treatment of the child with acute epiglottitis includes an artificial airway. Respiratory care includes humidification, gentle oral suctioning, and constant observation of respiratory status. Sometimes the physician will order oxygen for moderate respiratory distress, and aerosolized epinephrine to decrease airway edema by local vasoconstriction. You will begin IV antibiotics and fluids as ordered. Epiglottal edema usually decreases after 24 hours of antibiotic therapy. By the third day, the epiglottis is nearly normal in size, and it is safe to extubate the child at this time.

Nursing Interventions and Patient Teaching

LTB or acute epiglottitis tends to be a frightening experience for the child and the family. Never attempt to examine the mouth or throat in LTB since this will result in epiglottal spasm and stopped breathing. Respond quickly in a calm manner, supporting and reassuring parents that everything possible is being done for their child. Continually assesses the child for signs of response to therapy or increasing obstruction. Your observations will often provide the basis for any treatment changes. Maintain the child in Fowler's position, and monitor respirations for rate, depth, retractions, and nasal flaring. Also monitor the child's cardiac status, because restlessness and tachycardia are signs of increasing hypoxia. Check vital signs frequently. Keep intubation and tracheostomy sets at bedside for possible respiratory failure. Carefully plan nursing interventions to provide for frequent rest periods to conserve energy.

Keep parents informed of their child's progress, and encourage them to participate in care.

Prognosis

In most children, LTB is relatively mild. Gradual improvement to recovery occurs in 3 to 7 days. The most serious complication, and the one responsible for most deaths from croup, is laryngeal obstruction.

Without prompt diagnosis and treatment, the rapid course of epiglottitis has the potential to cause death within a few hours.

LOWER RESPIRATORY TRACT INFECTIONS

BRONCHITIS (TRACHEOBRONCHITIS)

Etiology and Pathophysiology

Bronchitis (tracheobronchitis) is an inflammation of the large airways, the trachea, and the bronchi. It usually follows an upper respiratory infection and is almost always viral in origin. The most common cause is rhinovirus, although parainfluenza, adenovirus, and RSV are other known causes. *Mycoplasma pneumoniae* is a common cause of bronchitis in children more than 6 years of age. Bronchitis occurs mainly in the winter months, primarily in children younger than 4 years of age (although it has potential to affect any age-group).

Clinical Manifestations

The onset is gradual with signs and symptoms of an upper respiratory tract infection (cough, coryza, little or no fever). After 2 to 3 days, the nonproductive, hacking cough becomes productive and worsens at night.

Diagnostic Tests

It is necessary to perform a radiographic examination of the chest for the child with severe signs and symptoms. For the majority of children, chest radiographs are normal.

Medical Management

Treatment is basically palliative. If the cough interferes with resting or eating, cough drops, lollipops, and pediatric cough preparations are usually effective. Cough suppressants are contraindicated in bronchitis unless the condition significantly affects sleep. Sometimes the health care provider will prescribe acetaminophen for fever. Antibiotics are not necessary in viral bronchitis. If the cough lasts beyond 10 days, there is a strong suspicion of a secondary bacterial infection.

Patient Teaching

Suggest the use of a cool-mist humidifier to relieve the child's cough and help liquefy secretions. Encourage fluids to decrease viscosity of secretions and prevent dehydration.

Prognosis

Acute bronchitis is self-limiting.

RESPIRATORY SYNCYTIAL VIRUS AND BRONCHIOLITIS

Etiology and Pathophysiology

Bronchiolitis is an acute viral inflammation of the smaller airway passages, the bronchioles, which become inflamed, causing edema. The accumulation of mucus and exudate has potential to partially or completely obstruct the lumen. Respiratory syncytial virus (RSV) is the organism responsible for the vast majority of cases. Bronchiolitis occurs in children younger than 2 years of age, with a peak incidence at 6 months of age. Bronchiolitis usually begins in the fall and has the highest incidence in the winter. Respiratory secretions from contamination of hand, nose, or other mucous membranes are the usual mode of transmission. RSV is able to survive for hours in paper tissues, countertops, or on gloves (Chavez-Bueno et al., 2005).

Clinical Manifestations

Upper respiratory infection signs and symptoms predominate during the first few days, followed by worsening signs and symptoms of respiratory distress. The infant exhibits retractions, tachypnea, nasal flaring, paroxysmal nonproductive coughing, and wheezing. Some infants will have low-grade or very high fever; be irritable, fussy, and anxious; and have difficulty eating. Respiratory distress becomes progressively more severe during the first 72 hours. Severe disease is followed by a rise in arterial carbon dioxide tension ($Paco_2$) (hypercapnia), leading to respiratory acidosis and hypoxemia.

Diagnostic Tests

The health care provider bases the diagnosis on the age of the child and the clinical signs and symptoms. Radiographic examination of the chest shows areas of atelectasis and hyperinflation. Tests providing positive identification of RSV are either enzyme-linked immunosorbent assay (ELISA) or rapid immunofluorescent antibody (IFA) from direct aspiration of nasal secretions or nasopharyngeal washings.

Medical Management

High humidity via mist tent serves to loosen secretions. If hypoxemia is present, the health care provider will order oxygen therapy with mist therapy. IV fluids are necessary if the infant is unable to tolerate oral feedings. Use of bronchodilators is sometimes an aspect of management in severe cases of bronchiolitis.

Medical therapy for bronchiolitis is controversial. Bronchodilators, corticosteroids, cough suppressants, and antibiotics are not effective in uncomplicated disease, and health care providers do not recommend them for routine use. The only drug the FDA has approved for treatment of the hospitalized child is ribavirin, an antiviral agent; however, ribavirin aerosol treatment is highly controversial because of its high cost, the potential toxic effects on exposed health care providers, and conflicting data on the results (Chavez-Bueno et al., 2005; Kliegman et al., 2007).

Nursing Interventions and Patient Teaching

Follow respiratory isolation precautions. Practice and encourage thorough hand hygiene to prevent cross-contamination, along with the use of contact precautions (gloves, gowns, masks, and goggles). Another infection control measure includes making patient assignments so that nurses assigned to children with RSV do not take care of other, high-risk patients. Acute nursing interventions focus on promoting adequate oxygenation, frequent monitoring of respiratory status, and maintaining hydration. As with any respiratory condition, parents will need reassurance and support during this stressful period.

Prognosis

The disease lasts 3 to 10 days, and the prognosis is generally good.

PULMONARY TUBERCULOSIS

Etiology and Pathophysiology

Pulmonary tuberculosis (TB) is a chronic bacterial lung infection caused by the bacillus *Mycobacterium tuberculosis*. TB remains a leading cause of death in many underdeveloped countries. It continues to be a public health problem in the United States primarily because of immigration of foreign-born people, the AIDS epidemic, and multiresistant strains of TB. More than one third of newly diagnosed cases of tuberculosis in children 14 years and younger in the United States are foreign born (AAP, 2003d). The most important risk factor in the progression of TB infection into active disease is an inadequate immune response caused by age or an impaired immune system, such as with young infants, the elderly, or those infected with HIV. Immunocompromised children and children less than 3 years of age are at greatest risk for TB, with the risk again increasing during the postpubertal adolescent years. The primary source of TB infection in children is exposure to an infected adult, usually a family member, babysitter, or frequent visitor.

Clinical Manifestations

Most children do not exhibit any clinical signs and symptoms when first infected. Signs and symptoms are extremely variable and develop so gradually that they often go unnoticed until the disease has significantly progressed.

Diagnostic Tests

Although not diagnostic, the tuberculin skin test (TST), formerly the Mantoux test, is the most important screening measure in identifying infected children at risk for disease. To confirm the diagnosis, positive bacteriologic sputum cultures for *M. tuberculosis* are essential. Infants and young children do not cough and expectorate sputum. Instead, mucus from the respiratory tract is usually swallowed. Therefore the best way to obtain sputum samples from infants and children is by gastric aspiration. Chest radiographs are also important in determining the presence and the extent of active lesions. The medical management and nursing interventions are basically the same as in the adult with active TB.

Patient Teaching

Because the success of therapy depends on compliance with the drug regimen, it is necessary to instruct parents regarding the importance of giving medications as often and for as long as ordered. The optimum duration of therapy is unknown, but the usual course of treatment is no less than 12 months for an initial treatment or 18 to 24 months for more serious forms of the disease.

Prognosis

The prognosis for most children is good, and it is even possible for a child to recover from TB infection without anyone ever diagnosing the disease. Children under the age of 2 years and adolescents and children infected with HIV have a more serious form of the disease. The very young child has a greater tendency to have widespread distribution of the tubercle bacillus affecting the lung, the bones, the kidney, or the brain. Tuberculosis meningitis potentially results in death. Antibiotic therapy has decreased the mortality rate (Hockenberry & Wilson, 2007).

CYSTIC FIBROSIS

Etiology and Pathophysiology

The child with cystic fibrosis (CF) has inherited the defective gene from both parents, and the odds of a child whose parents are both carriers developing CF are 1 in 4 (Hockenberry & Wilson, 2007). This is a disorder of the exocrine (mucus-producing) glands, with the characteristic presence of excessive thick mucus that obstructs the lungs and the gastrointestinal (GI) system. CF is a multiorgan disease, but death is usually caused by pulmonary failure. It is the most common fatal genetic disorder, occurring in about 1 out of every 3500 births in whites, 1 in 17,000 births in blacks, and 1 in 90,000 births in Asians (Hockenberry & Wilson, 2007).

CF affects both sexes equally and is most common in white populations. The abnormally thick mucus that collects in the lung airways and organ ducts causes obstruction. Bronchiolar obstruction predisposes the lung to infection, bronchiectasis, and cystic dilations. Complications include bronchial and bronchiolar obstruction, pulmonary hypertension, and cor pulmonale. Obstruction of the pancreatic ducts leads to dilation and fibrosis and a decrease in pancreatic enzymes (lipase, amylase, and trypsin), which results in malabsorption. The earliest manifestation of CF is meconium ileus in the newborn, in which the small intestine is occluded with tenacious puttylike, mucilaginous meconium. Obstruction in the hepatic system leads to biliary cirrhosis, portal hypertension, and splenomegaly. Elevated sodium chloride concentrations in the sweat and the saliva occur as a result of the abnormal reabsorption of chloride by epithelial cells.

Clinical Manifestations

Pancreatic insufficiency and malabsorption result in steatorrhea (bulky, foul-smelling, fatty stools), growth failure, protruding abdomen, and thin, wasted extremities. Rectal prolapse is a common GI manifestation of CF. Appetite is often increased early in the illness in response to poor absorption. Malabsorption also has the potential to lead to a vitamin K deficiency, resulting in bleeding disorders, esophageal varices, and ecchymoses. Diminished subcutaneous fat results in sallow, transparent skin. Pulmonary complications constitute the most serious threat to life in children with CF. Many children demonstrate respiratory symptoms before 1 year of age; others will sometimes not develop symptoms for weeks, months, or years. Pulmonary involvement is evident in chronic cough, wheezing, sputum production, and dyspnea resulting in hypoxia, clubbing of the fingers and toes, and cyanosis. Hyperinflation of the lungs will sometimes produce a barrel chest.

Diagnostic Tests

Diagnostic criteria for CF consist of a family history of the disorder, absence of pancreatic enzymes, chronic pulmonary involvement, and a positive sweat test. A sweat test greater than 60 mEq/L of chloride is diagnostic for CF. Normal sweat chloride is less than 40 mEq/L. A chest x-ray film will demonstrate patchy atelectasis and evidence of obstructive emphysema. Pulmonary function tests (PFT) will measure ventilation and diffusion of gas across the alveolar capillary membrane and provide evidence of pulmonary problems (Hockenberry & Wilson, 2007).

Medical Management

The goals of therapy include good nutrition, prevention and control of respiratory infections, and providing as normal a lifestyle as possible for the child. Pulmonary therapy is the single most important aspect of treatment. Chest physiotherapy (CPT) and high-frequency chest wall oscillations have improved both the health of the child and compliance by the caregiver (Hockenberry & Wilson, 2007). Encourage breathing exercises to improve aeration. Inhalation therapy with bronchodilators before CPT facilitates secretion removal. The use of expectorants, mucolytic agents, and antibiotics helps to relieve obstruction and resolve infections. Another medication delivered via aerosol is a recombinant human deoxyribonuclease called DNase, known generically as donase alfa (Pulmozyme). This drug reduces the viscosity of mucus and is well tolerated (Hockenberry & Wilson, 2007). The drug causes improvement in pulmonary function tests and perceptions of well-being, as well as reduction in the viscosity of sputum. Performance of chest physiotherapy is usually necessary twice daily (on rising and in the evening) and sometimes more frequently, especially during pulmonary infection. The **Flutter mucus clearance device** serves to increase expectoration of sputum and clear the airway in 5 to 15 minutes. It is a small, handheld plastic pipe with a stainless-steel ball on the inside that promotes removal of mucus and is possible for the child to use without assistance (Hockenberry & Wilson, 2007). Digestive and nutritional therapy includes pancreatic enzyme replacement, administration of fat-soluble vitamins (A, D, E, and K), and a diet high in calories, protein, and salt.

Nursing Interventions

Nursing interventions for the child with CF are highly complex and will be a challenge for you. Management focuses on improving pulmonary function and facilitating lung clearance, preventing or managing respiratory infections, promoting normal growth and development, optimizing nutritional status, educating about the illness and its management, planning for home care and community support, referring for counseling when needed, providing long-term support and follow-up, and encouraging medication compliance.

Improving pulmonary function involves CPT, breathing exercises, and inhalation treatment. CPT performed two or more times daily helps loosen secretions in the lung with high-frequency chest wall oscillations, and postural drainage facilitates the removal of these thick secretions. To encourage breathing exercises, suggest blowing bubbles or pinwheels to help prevent tracheobronchial obstruction. You or the respiratory therapist will sometimes carry out nebulizer treatments. Assess the child's tolerance to therapy and monitor its effectiveness. Institute infection control measures to prevent cross-contamination, and teach the family to protect the child from exposure to people with respiratory infections. Strongly recommend yearly influenza immunizations. Early in the course of the illness, some children will exhibit excessive appetite; as the disease progresses, the appetite decreases and the child will usually experience anorexia. Before meals and snacks, administer a mix of pancreatic enzymes, needed to digest proteins, fats, and carbohydrates, together with a carbohydrate.

Children with CF will have frequent hospitalizations, which are likely to interfere with normal development and impair socialization; address these issues with psychological support and appropriate activities. One of the most critical aspects in providing care to the CF child and family is assisting them with positive coping strategies and providing emotional support. Support groups are often a source of great comfort and assistance to newly diagnosed children and their families. The Cystic Fibrosis Foundation provides education and services to families and professionals.

Patient Teaching

Instruct the family in improving the nutritional status of their child to ensure adequate growth and development. You and your colleagues are responsible for coordinating counseling, referrals to community support, and home care services, as well as for educating the child and the family in the disease process and its management. All of the recommended childhood vaccinations as well as the influenza vaccine are appropriate for children with CF, along with a yearly influenza booster (Hockenberry & Wilson, 2007).

Prognosis

Cystic fibrosis is a chronic, incurable disease. According to the Cystic Fibrosis Foundation Patient Registry 2006 Annual Report, treatment of the disease has improved substantially over the past 25 years. The median survival rate in 2006 was 36.9 years compared to 25 years in 1985. Forty-five percent of the CF population are 18 years or older. The outlook for the patient with CF is more positive with new therapies, such as gene therapy, as well as improved pulmonary therapy, aerosolized antibiotic therapy and more nutritional education. With advances in treatments, parents and adolescents are challenged to set goals that include college, careers, and social relationships (Hockenberry & Wilson, 2007).

BRONCHIAL ASTHMA

Etiology and Pathophysiology

Asthma is a chronic inflammatory disorder of the airways in which many cells (mast cells, eosinophils, and T lymphocytes) play a role. Bronchial asthma is a reversible obstructive respiratory disorder. Asthma accounts for the greatest number of school absences and visits to the emergency department by children. It is the most common chronic disease in children and the third leading cause of hospital admissions in children under 15 years of age (Hockenberry & Wilson, 2007).

Bronchial asthma has a familial tendency and frequently occurs in association with allergic rhinitis and atopic dermatitis. A common cause of bronchial asthma is an allergic hypersensitivity to environmental factors. Although allergens play an important role in asthma, 20% to 40% of children with asthma have no evidence of allergic disease. The common factors associated with bronchial asthma include bronchospasm, mucosal edema, and increased mucosal secretions (Figure 31-12). Bronchospasm of the bronchial smooth muscle causes bronchial edema with a decrease in the diameter of the bronchi and bronchioles; edematous mucous membranes produce thick, tenacious secretions, which causes a further narrowing of the air passages. Mucous plugs that occlude the smaller air passages cause obstruction and air trapping distal to the obstruction, resulting in hypoxemia and increased respiratory effort.

The National Heart, Lung, and Blood Institute (1995) classifies asthma based on symptoms, which indicate the severity of the disease. The classifications are (1) mild intermittent, (2) mild persistent, (3) moderate persistent, and (4) severe persistent (Hockenberry & Wilson, 2007). These categories aid in the medical and environmental treatment of asthma.

Pulmonary function tests are useful in children after age 5 or 6 years. These tests help evaluate the presence and the degree of lung disease and responses to therapy. Health care providers often order skin testing for allergens on children with asthma to help identify and treat specific allergens.

Clinical Manifestations

Initially, many children complain of tightness in the chest, and it is possible to detect an audible expiratory wheeze. As the attack progresses, other signs and symptoms join these: shortness of breath, inspiratory and expiratory wheezing, tachypnea, dyspnea, coarse breath sounds, prolonged expiration, restlessness, anxiety, deep dark red color to lips, cyanosis, paroxysmal cough progressing from dry and hacking to productive, fatigue, and diaphoresis.

Diagnostic Tests

The health care provider will make the diagnosis primarily on the basis of clinical signs and symptoms,

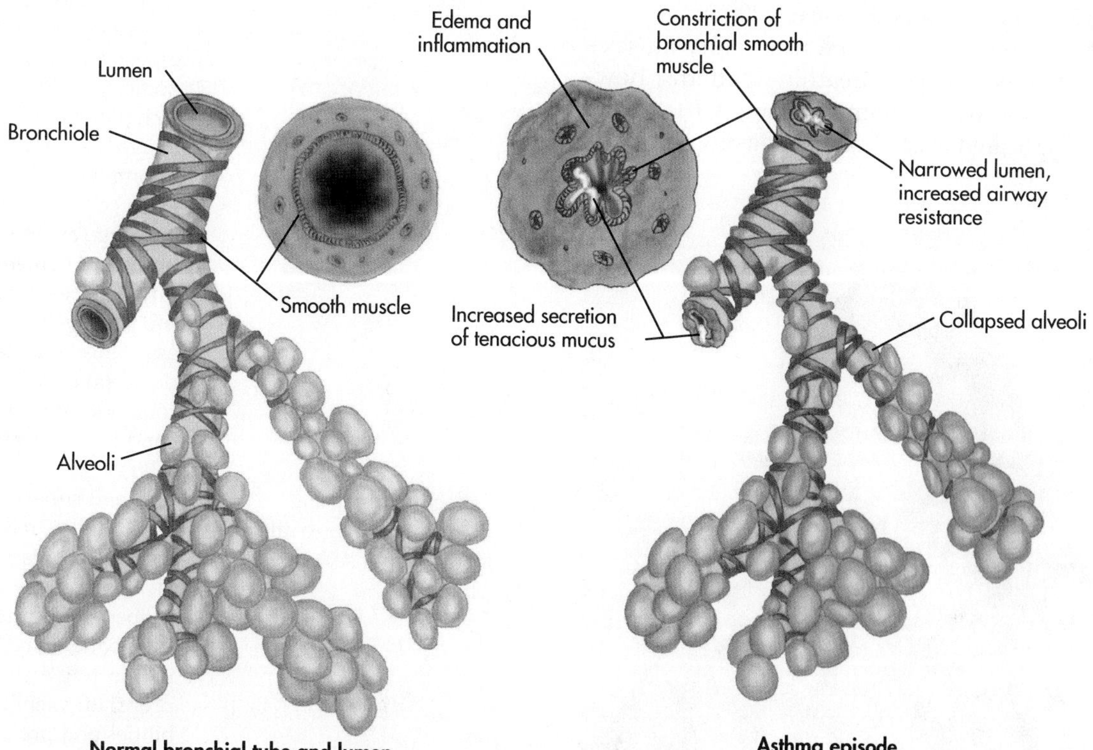

FIGURE 31-12 Comparison of a normal bronchial tube and a bronchial tube during an asthma episode. In bronchial asthma, the bronchiole is obstructed by muscle spasm, edema of the mucosa, inflammation, and thick secretions.

history, physical examination, pulmonary function tests, and serum laboratory tests such as ABGs and CBC. Radiographic examination of the chest is standard to rule out other pathology. Generally, chronic cough in the absence of infection or diffuse wheezing during the expiratory phase of respiration is sufficient to establish a diagnosis.

Medical Management

Medications that serve to treat asthma fall into two classes: long-term control medications (preventive medications) and quick-relief medications (rescue medications). Metered-dose inhalers (MDIs) often figure in the treatment of asthma. The health care provider will typically use nebulized medications for infants and young children who are not able to use a metered-dose inhaler. In the young school-age child, using a spacer helps ensure that the child receives the full dose prescribed. The spacer provides a reservoir for the medication to allow the child time to inhale the full dose (Figure 31-13).

Medications for treatment of asthma include inhaled corticosteroids, cromolyn sodium, and nedrocromil sodium. Long-acting β-adrenergic agonists, methylxanthines, and leukotriene modifiers are among the long-term control medications that are effective. Quick-relief medications include short-acting β_2-agonists, anticholinergics, as well as systemic corticosteroids. Bronchodilators, which relax the smooth muscle in the bronchial tree and dilate the respiratory airways, serve for both quick relief and long-term control. These bronchodilators include β_2-agonists, methylxanthines, and anticholinergics (Hockenberry & Wilson, 2007).

CPT is used to help strengthen respiratory muscles and develop more efficient breathing patterns; however, clinicians do not recommend using CPT during acute, uncomplicated exacerbations of asthma.

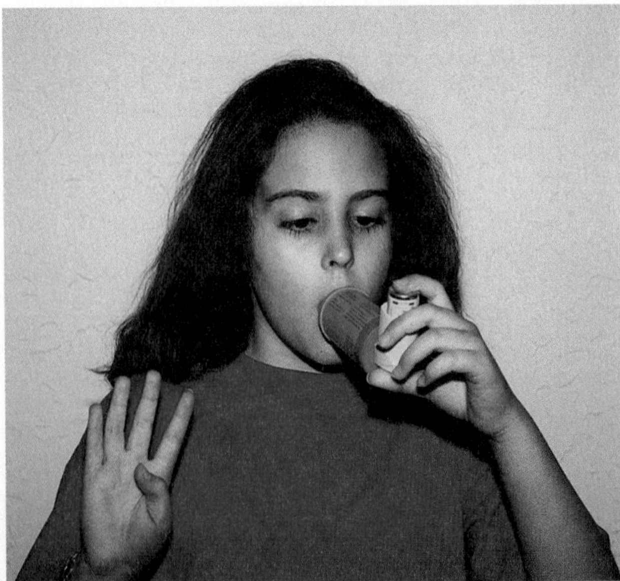

FIGURE 31-13 Child using a metered-dose inhaler with spacer.

Nursing Interventions

Nursing interventions include frequent monitoring of vital signs. Maintain adequate hydration to replace insensible loss through diaphoresis and hyperventilation. To facilitate optimal ventilation, keep the child in high Fowler's position, provide for rest periods, and teach breathing exercises. It is extremely important to provide a calm atmosphere and reassurance for the anxious child and family. Parents and children need to understand the illness and how to avert or prevent attacks at home. It is possible to identify allergens through skin testing and then institute measures to eliminate or avoid them.

Nursing diagnoses and interventions for the child with bronchial asthma include but are not limited to the following:

Nursing Diagnoses	Nursing Interventions
Risk for suffocation, related to interaction between individual and allergen(s)	Teach patient and family correct use of bronchodilators, corticosteroids. Teach patient and family how to avoid conditions or circumstances that precipitate asthmatic attack. Teach family meal planning to eliminate allergenic foods. Encourage removal of furry pets. Instruct family in modification of environment, "allergy-proofing" home, especially no smoking in home. Teach patient and family to avoid extremes of environmental temperature. Encourage avoidance of undue excitement or physical exertion. Help parents in obtaining assistance in installing device(s) to control environment (humidifier, air conditioner, electronic air filter).
Ineffective breathing pattern, related to allergenic response in bronchial tree	Teach and supervise breathing exercises and controlled breathing. Teach correct use of prescribed medications. Assist patient and family in selecting activities appropriate to child's capabilities and preferences. Encourage regular exercise.

Nursing Diagnoses	Nursing Interventions
	Encourage good posture. Encourage physical exercise involving stop-and-start activity that does not overtax the respiratory mechanism. Discourage physical inactivity.

Patient Teaching

Parents need to understand the nature of the disease and, when the allergens are determined, know how to avoid or relieve asthmatic attacks. Teach parents and the older child how to use the medications prescribed to relieve bronchospasms (see Figure 31-13). Teach early signs and symptoms of an impending attack so control is possible before symptoms become distressful. Older children who use a nebulizer or an aerosol device to deliver adrenergic drugs need instruction on how to use a metered-dose inhaler. Teach the parents to avoid exposing the child to excessive cold, wind, or other extremes of weather and to smoke, sprays, or other irritants. Self-care is a hallmark of effective asthma management, and self-management programs are important in helping the child and the family cope with the disease.

Prognosis

The outlook for children with asthma varies widely. Many children lose their signs and symptoms at puberty, but no known factor predicts which children will "outgrow" their asthma. Although death from asthma is rare, the death rate has been rising steadily during the last decade despite improvements in treatment.

It is necessary to assess children with asthma carefully and treat them aggressively. Asthma is increasing in prevalence, morbidity, and mortality in the United States, with the black population in particular demonstrating an increase. The increased incidence of asthma is possibly the result of underdiagnosis, undertreatment, unavailability of proper medical care, and a worsening of air pollution (Hockenberry & Wilson, 2007).

DISORDERS OF GASTROINTESTINAL FUNCTION

The primary function of the GI tract is the absorption and metabolism of nutrients necessary to support and promote optimal growth and development. Because the GI tract is responsible for processing nutrients for all parts of the body, an alteration in GI function has potential to affect other body systems. Failure to diagnose or treat a GI problem is likely to affect the overall health of the child. Conversely, any disease process has potential to result in manifestations of GI disturbance, even if it does not directly affect the GI tract.

CLEFT LIP AND CLEFT PALATE

Clefts of the lip and the palate are facial malformations that occur during embryologic development. A combination of cleft lip and palate is more common than an isolated occurrence of either. The incidence of cleft lip or cleft palate (or both) is 1 in 1000 live births.

Etiology and Pathophysiology

Cleft of the lip is due to a failure of the medial nasal and maxillary processes to join; it is caused by abnormal development of the external nose, the nasal cartilages, the nasal septum, and the medial nasal and maxillary processes. Both unilateral or bilateral clefts occur (Hockenberry & Wilson, 2007) (Figure 31-14). Cleft of the palate is caused by a failure of the palatal shelves to fuse. Cleft palates sometimes involve only the soft palate and sometimes extend into the hard palate.

The etiology of cleft lip and palate is consistent with a multifactorial inheritance. There is a linkage between several factors and the development of clefts in humans, such as the following: (1) folic acid deficiency in the maternal diet, (2) maternal intake of alcohol, and (3) smoking during pregnancy. Research demonstrates smoking early in pregnancy increases the risk of orofacial clefts, especially a one and one half- to twofold increase in the incidence of isolated clefts. The risk of orofacial clefts increases with the number of cigarettes smoked (Hockenberry & Wilson, 2007). Mistakenly, some folklore has attempted to link the cause of cleft lip and palate to prenatal influences (see Cultural Considerations box).

Clinical Manifestations

Feeding from the breast or the bottle will in some cases not be difficult in infants with less severe cleft lip and intact palate. More extensive cleft lips and clefts of the palate usually involve feeding difficulties; infants tend to have an ineffective suck, and saliva and feedings will sometimes leak into the nasal cavity, causing gagging and choking and leading to aspiration as the infant breathes.

There is in some cases also a delay in speech and, after it does develop, it is sometimes hypernasal with poor articulation. Children with cleft palate also tend to be predisposed to recurrent otitis media or persis-

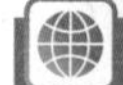 Cultural Considerations

Cleft Lip

Beliefs in folklore and superstitions have always surrounded pregnancy and birth. Some groups believe that prenatal influences affect the outcome of an unborn child, specifically with regard to birth defects. Some groups believe that if a pregnant woman encounters a rabbit or hare during her gestation, her child will be born with a "harelip" (cleft lip).

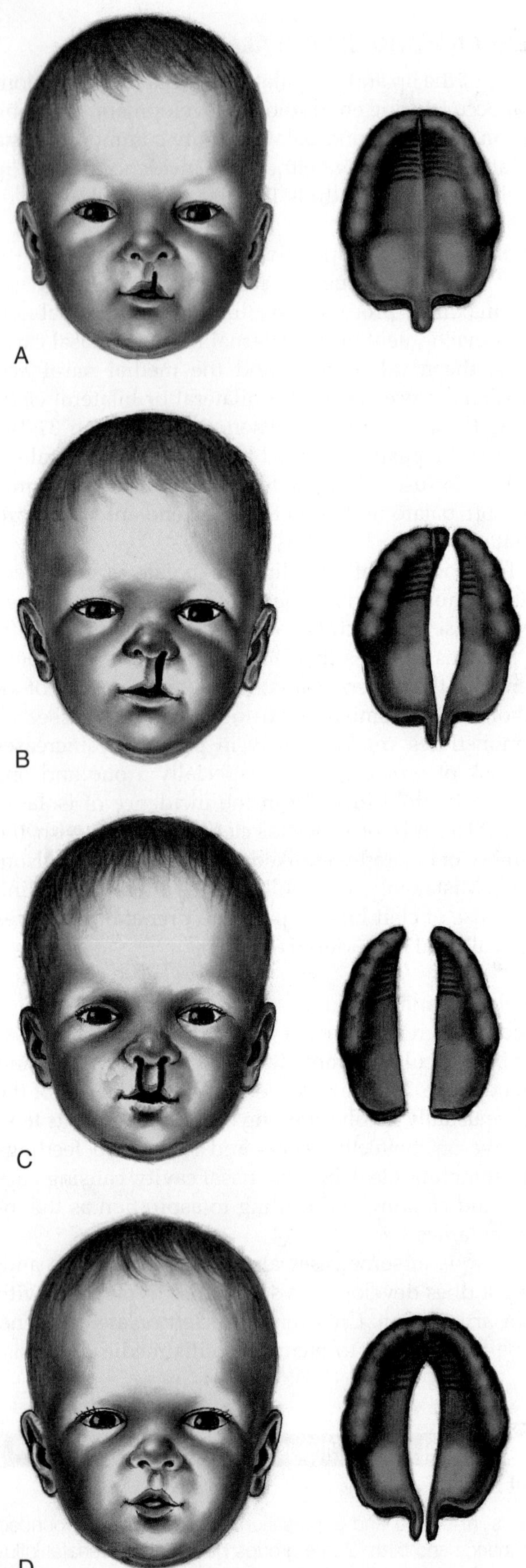

FIGURE 31-14 Variations in clefts of lip and palate at birth. **A,** Notch in vermilion border. **B,** Unilateral cleft lip and palate. **C,** Bilateral cleft lip and palate. **D,** Cleft palate.

tent otitis media with effusion as a result of eustachian tube dysfunction. It is common for the older child with cleft lip and palate to experience psychological difficulties because of the cosmetic appearance of the defect and problems with impaired speech and faulty dentition.

Diagnostic Tests

Cleft lip and most cases of cleft palate are apparent at birth, and the facial appearance of the infant is of immediate concern to the parents.

Medical Management

The surgeon will usually close the cleft lip, whether in isolation or in association with cleft palate, at 1 to 2 months of age, when the infant has shown satisfactory weight gain and is free of any oral, respiratory, or systemic infections. The surgical technique used is Z-plasty. This method involves the use of a staggered suture line to minimize notching of the lip from retracted scar tissue. The surgeon applies a Logan bow (a thin, arched metal bar that is taped to the cheeks) immediately after the surgery to prevent tension on the suture line when the child cries, and will order safety reminder devices (SRDs) to restrain the infant's arms to prevent the baby from rubbing the incision.

Repairs of clefts of the palate usually take place before 1 year of age. Surgical repair during this period allows for palatal changes associated with normal growth. For the most positive outcome after surgical repair, interventions involve a multidisciplinary health care team that includes the pediatric plastic surgeon, the orthodontist, the otolaryngologist, the speech and language pathologist, the audiologist, nurses, and social workers. The child will require long-term treatment and often will have lasting problems with speech and facial appearance (Hockenberry & Wilson, 2007).

Nursing Interventions

Nursing interventions for the child with cleft lip and palate are initially focused on ensuring adequate nutritional support for the infant and assisting the parents in dealing with the diagnosis. Before surgical correction of cleft lip and palate, feeding is often a considerable problem. The primary goals for nursing are to ensure an adequate intake of food and to prevent aspiration. The best method for feeding is to support the infant's head in an upright position and to use care and patience during each feeding. Because infants with cleft lip and palate cannot generate the suction required to feed through a normal nipple or breast, you will help the parents to use special feeding devices. There are a variety of special "cleft-palate" nipples that have had some success. However, large, soft nipples with large holes or long, soft lamb's nipples appear to offer the best means for nipple feeding (Figure 31-15). Breastfeeding is possible in some cases if the mother uses a breast shield with a special cleft-lip

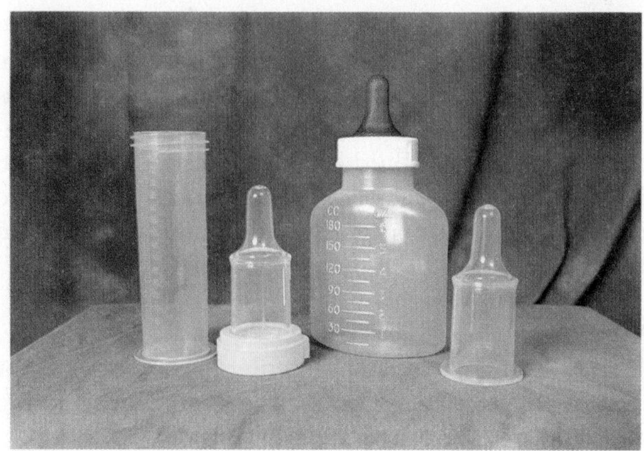

FIGURE 31-15 Some devices used to feed an infant with a cleft lip and palate.

nipple. A feeding technique that significantly increases the weight of a child with cleft lip and/or palate before surgery is called the ESSR feeding technique (Hockenberry & Wilson, 2007). ESSR stands for the following:

Enlarge the nipple
Stimulate the suck reflex
Swallow fluid appropriately
Rest when infant signals with facial expression.

During feedings, these infants require frequent burping because they tend to swallow large amounts of air.

Another important goal is to assist the parents in dealing with the diagnosis of cleft lip and palate and to promote bonding between the parents and the infant. To accomplish this goal, try emphasizing positive aspects of the infant's appearance and behavior. Another option is to show the parents photographs of children who have had cleft lip and palate repairs to illustrate the positive results of surgical intervention.

Postoperative nursing interventions include protecting the integrity of the suture line, promoting optimal nutrition, and continuing support of the child and parents. Position infants only on their sides or back; positioning on the abdomen allows them to rub the face on the sheets. Place SRDs on the child's elbows to prevent touching or rubbing of the suture line. Periodically remove the SRDs to enable movement of the arms, to provide an opportunity to observe the skin underneath for signs of impairment or pressure, and to cuddle the infant.

Immediately following surgery, you will usually keep the infant with cleft lip NPO until the effects of the anesthesia have disappeared. Then introduce the infant gradually to liquids, beginning with clear liquids (water and dextrose water) and gradually progressing to formula. A soft rubber-tipped feeder is generally preferred; slip the rubber tip of the feeder into the side of the infant's mouth carefully, avoiding contact with the suture line. Breastfeeding is usually contraindicated. Support the mother if she wishes to pump her breasts to promote the continued production of milk until the infant is able to feed directly from the breast. After feedings, gently cleanse the suture line with a saline-soaked cotton-tipped swab. Then place the infant in an infant seat or on the right side to promote digestion and prevent aspiration of regurgitated formula. In addition, careful aspiration of the oral and nasopharyngeal cavities is sometimes necessary to remove collections of mucus, blood, and saliva and to prevent aspiration. Administer analgesics as ordered.

Postoperative care after surgical repair of cleft palate is similar to that of cleft lip repair. Allow the child with cleft palate repair to lie on the abdomen because this will facilitate drainage of mucus and serosanguineous exudate from the oral cavity. Administer analgesics as ordered. You will usually provide liquid nourishments by cup. Use of straws, pacifiers, and eating utensils is not advisable because they may injure the suture line. Gradually advance the child from a liquid diet to a blenderized diet, and instruct parents to continue this diet after discharge until the surgeon instructs them otherwise.

Patient Teaching

Assist the family if possible by providing them with information on agencies that provide services, information, and support to families with a child who has cleft lip and palate. These agencies include the Cleft Palate Foundation and the March of Dimes–Birth Defects Foundation. Throughout the child's development, an important goal is the development of a healthy personality and self-esteem.

Prognosis

Most children with cleft lip or palate continue to have problems with speech impairments and middle ear infections postoperatively. Teach parents how to assist the child in developing normal speech patterns, be vigilant in seeking early treatment when symptoms of an upper respiratory tract infection develop, and obtain assistance if they note any hearing impairment (Hockenberry & Wilson, 2007).

DEHYDRATION

When the body loses more fluid than it absorbs, as in the presence of diarrhea, or when it absorbs less water than it excretes, as in the presence of vomiting, dehydration occurs. Basically, dehydration occurs whenever the total fluid intake is less than the total fluid output. The most accurate method to assess a child's degree of dehydration is by noting changes in the body weight. Mild, moderate, and severe dehydration correspond to fluid deficits of 5%, 10%, and 15%, respectively.

Etiology and Pathophysiology

Dehydration is the result of a number of possible disease processes that cause abnormal losses through the skin, respiratory, renal, and (most commonly) GI systems.

Clinical Manifestations

The physical signs of dehydration are primarily the result of a deficit in fluid volume. Because accurate recorded weight before the episode of dehydration is not always available for comparison, it is easier to diagnose the degree of dehydration based on its clinical manifestations (Table 31-1).

Diagnostic Tests

The health care provider will make the diagnosis of dehydration on the basis of observed clinical manifestations (see Table 31-1). Laboratory tests to support diagnosis and determine severity include serum sodium, serum glucose, serum bicarbonate, and blood urea nitrogen (BUN). In general, weighing the child daily also provides useful information about the degree and severity of dehydration.

Medical Management

Refer to the discussion on medical management of diarrhea (following section).

Nursing Interventions and Patient Teaching

Careful nursing assessment and intervention are important in the clinical detection and management of dehydration. It is an essential nursing function to assess for any clinical manifestations of dehydration. Begin this assessment with a general survey of the child and continue with specific observations.

Observation includes the measurement of intake and output (I&O). This measurement comprises oral and parenteral intake and losses from sweat, wound drainage, urine, stools, vomiting, nasogastric (NG) drainage, and fistulas. For children who are not toilet trained, weigh wet diapers to assess the amount of output. By subtracting the weight (in grams) of a dry diaper from the weight of the wet diaper, you will be able to calculate the actual fluid content of the diaper. The volume of fluid in milliliters is equal to the weight of the fluid measured in grams. Other observations that assist in the assessment of dehydration include vital signs, body weight, skin color, temperature and turgor, capillary refill, presence or absence of edema, moisture and color of mucous membranes, sensation of thirst, and in infants, assessment of the fontanelles.

Table 31-1 Clinical Manifestations of Dehydration

ASSESSMENT	SIGNS AND SYMPTOMS
Skin	Cold, dry, gray, loss of turgor
Mucous membranes	Dry
Eyes	Sunken
Fontanelle	Sunken
Behavior	Lethargic
Pulse	Rapid, weak
Blood pressure	Low
Respirations	Rapid

Teach the parents that infants and young children have a greater need for water than adults and are more vulnerable to alterations in fluid and electrolyte balance. Compared with older children and adults, infants have a greater fluid intake and output relative to size. Water and electrolyte disturbances occur more frequently and more rapidly, and infants and children adjust less promptly to these alterations.

Prognosis

Shock is common in severe depletion of extracellular fluid. With effective medical management and nursing interventions, the prognosis is favorable.

DIARRHEA AND GASTROENTERITIS

Diarrhea is one of the most common disorders affecting children; it has the capacity to quickly render the child vulnerable to fluid deficits and electrolyte imbalances. Diarrhea is a disturbance in intestinal motility, characterized by an increase in frequency, fluid content, and volume of stools. The diarrhea is sometimes acute and sometimes chronic, and either infectious or noninfectious. Diarrhea caused by an inflammatory process, such as infection, is called **gastroenteritis.**

Etiology and Pathophysiology

Although diarrhea results from a variety of causes, the most common is bacterial or viral invasion of the intestinal mucosa. The most prevalent bacterial pathogens are *Salmonella, Shigella, Campylobacter jejuni, Yersinia enterocolitica, Rotavirus, Giardia lamblia,* and *Clostridium difficile.* Many factors can predispose a child to diarrhea. Infants have a greater susceptibility to diarrhea, and the results are more serious because infants have a small extracellular fluid reserve. When this reserve is suddenly and quickly depleted, dehydration rapidly ensues. Children who are malnourished, debilitated, or immunocompromised are more prone to diarrhea. Poor hygiene, contaminated food or water, warm weather, and crowded and substandard living conditions also predispose children to diarrhea. Other common causes of diarrhea are the ingestion of large quantities of fruit juices such as apple juice, food sensitivities, antibiotics, and formula intolerance.

When a pathogen invades the intestinal mucosa, the resulting enterotoxins stimulate an inflammatory reaction. As a result, water and electrolytes are secreted and there is invasion and destruction of the epithelial cells of the GI mucosa. Serious disturbances, such as renal failure, dehydration, metabolic acidosis, shock, and circulatory collapse, will possibly follow.

Clinical Manifestations

There are other clinical manifestations of diarrhea in addition to the increased number of stools and the increased fluid content of stools (Box 31-4). Assess for these, as well as for any signs of dehydration, which is a common complication of diarrhea (see Table 31-1).

Box 31-4 Clinical Manifestations of Diarrhea

- Cool, pale skin
- Lethargy
- Sunken eyes
- Sunken fontanelles
- Poor skin turgor
- Rapid pulse and respirations
- Low blood pressure
- Normal or elevated temperature
- Irritability progressing to lethargy
- Weight loss
- Vomiting
- Malodorous stools

Diagnostic Tests

Obtain a careful history including information regarding recent travel, exposure to infected agents, personal contact, allergies, food or formula sensitivities, living conditions, and contact with contaminated water or food. Laboratory evaluation typically includes a stool culture and examination of the stool for ova and parasites, WBC count, and *Clostridium difficile* toxin.

Medical Management

The goals of management are to restore the fluid and electrolyte balance and to treat the underlying cause. The AAP no longer recommends withholding food or fluids for 24 hours following the onset of diarrhea or administering the traditional BRAT diet (bananas, rice, applesauce, and toast or tea). It is acceptable to offer an oral rehydration solution, such as Pedialyte or Rehydralyte, in small amounts for the first 4 to 6 hours following the onset of diarrhea. Have the infant who is breastfeeding continue doing so as a supplement to the oral rehydration solution. Administer an oral maintenance solution (Pedialyte or Infalyte) for the remaining first 24 hours. An older child is permitted to take clear liquids. When the number and fluid content of stools have decreased, gradually advance the infant to full-strength formula. In older children, offer solid foods when rehydration is complete. Initially, offer foods that are nonirritating to the bowel. These may include bananas, rice, applesauce, cereal, vegetable juice, crackers, pretzels, and toast (modified BRAT diet). Gradually resume a regular diet.

In cases of severe diarrhea, hospitalization and IV therapy are required. IV administration of a saline solution containing 5% dextrose serves for rehydration. This solution provides the child with fluid, sodium, and calories. Once kidney function has been verified, it is acceptable to add potassium to the IV solution to correct any potassium depletion. It is necessary to continue IV rehydration until the diarrhea improves. Once rehydration has begun and the severe effects of the diarrhea and dehydration have improved, the focus of management shifts to employing measures to detect and treat the underlying cause. This includes antimicrobial therapy where indicated.

Nursing Interventions and Patient Teaching

Nursing interventions for the infant or child with diarrhea focus on assessment, including the careful recording of I&O; promotion of rehydration; correction of electrolyte imbalances; provision of age-appropriate nutrition; prevention of the spread of the diarrhea; prevention of complications; and support of the child and family.

Nursing diagnoses and interventions for the child with diarrhea and gastroenteritis include but are not limited to the following:

Nursing Diagnoses	Nursing Interventions
Deficient fluid volume, related to excessive GI losses in stool	Offer oral fluids as indicated and as tolerated. Monitor IV fluids as prescribed. Maintain strict record of I&O (urine and stool); monitor urine specific gravity. Weigh child daily. Assess vital signs, skin turgor, mucous membranes, and mental status every 4 hours or as indicated.
Impaired skin integrity, related to irritation caused by frequent, loose stools	Change diaper frequently. Cleanse buttocks gently with bland, nonalkaline soap and water or immerse child in a bath for gentle cleansing. Apply protective ointment (type of ointment often varies according to individual child, and sometimes a trial period is necessary). Expose slightly erythematous intact skin to air whenever possible; apply protective ointment to very irritated or excoriated skin. Observe buttocks and perineum for infection, such as *Candida*.
Anxiety, related to: • separation from parents • unfamiliar environment • distressing procedures	Provide mouth care and pacifier for infants who are on nothing-by-mouth (NPO) status. Encourage family visitation and appropriate participation in care. Touch, hold, and talk to child as much as possible. Provide sensory stimulation and diversion appropriate for child's developmental level.

Instruct parents to avoid the use of antidiarrheals such as diphenoxylate (Lomotil) or kaolin and pectin (Kaopectate). Also caution them to wash their hands thoroughly after changing diapers to prevent the spread of infection. It is necessary to properly dispose of or thoroughly clean soiled diapers, bed linens, and clothes.

Prognosis

Parents manage mild or moderate diarrhea at home by simple methods. Severe diarrhea necessitates hospitalization with IV fluid therapy. With treatment, prognosis is usually excellent.

CONSTIPATION

Constipation is best defined as the passage of hardened stools, and it often occurs in association with failure to completely evacuate the colon with defecation. It is possible for constipation to manifest as a primary disorder or in association with a wide variety of GI tract or systemic disorders.

Etiology and Pathophysiology

Constipation is possible in children of any age. In the newborn period, the infant normally passes a first meconium stool within 24 to 36 hours. Failure to do this indicates possible intestinal atresia (congenital closure of a body part usually open, in this case any part of the intestine) or stenosis (constriction or narrowing of a passage or orifice), Hirschsprung's disease, meconium ileus (ileus of the newborn caused by obstruction of the bowel with meconium), or a meconium plug. In formula-fed infants, constipation will possibly result from a high fat or protein content or inadequate fluid in the formula. In children, constipation sometimes occurs in connection with environmental factors such as medications (e.g., iron supplements, anticonvulsant therapy, low-fiber diet, or antacids) or results from a learned repression of the urge to defecate. In children who have constipation, passage of hardened stools is painful. As a result, the child may repress the urge to defecate. Continuous repression results in dilation of the rectum, reduced sensation of the need to defecate, and decreased muscle tone in the lower rectum. This cycle results in chronic, incomplete evacuation of the colon, and the child becomes severely constipated. Episodes of diarrhea or **encopresis** (leakage around the firm stool in the rectum) often lead to accidents or soiling.

Clinical Manifestations

In infancy, constipation sometimes occurs in association with hard stools or evidence of fresh blood in the stools. Children with functional constipation sometimes experience cramping abdominal pain, anal fissures, pain on defecation, loss of appetite, and irritability.

Diagnostic Tests

Diagnosis of constipation depends on a careful history. Ask parents to describe the infant's or child's bowel patterns. The physician will perform a physical examination of the anus and rectum.

Medical Management

In the newborn, simple measures often effectively alleviate the problem. Modifying the formula with addition of more fluid or carbohydrates sometimes corrects the situation. For older infants, beyond 5 to 6 months, adding foods with bulk (fruits and vegetables) and increasing fluid intake sometimes corrects the problem. If the constipation is due to a tightened anal sphincter or anal stenosis, the physician will sometimes instruct parents to manually dilate the sphincter two or three times daily until sufficient dilation is attained. The management of simple constipation in children focuses on emptying the rectum completely of stool with the use of mild laxatives or enemas and instituting dietary modifications, such as increased fluid intake and addition of high-fiber foods, to prevent further constipation. The treatment of chronic constipation in children aims at complete evacuation of the rectum and toileting retraining therapy. It is usually possible to achieve complete evacuation of the rectum by using enemas, manual disimpaction, and stool softeners. After complete evacuation is attained, the care provider will institute bowel retraining therapy to sustain evacuation. This generally consists of behavioral modification, using positive reinforcement for toilet sitting and defecation, and emotional support.

Nursing Interventions and Patient Teaching

Nursing interventions begin with a careful history of bowel patterns, including stool characteristics (color, consistency, frequency, and associated pain), diet, and concomitant medications. If dietary modifications are to be instituted, it will be necessary to educate the parents regarding these and ensure their understanding. Sometimes parents also need instruction about normal stool patterns and what constitutes constipation. It will in some cases be important to discuss with parents their expectations and attitudes regarding toileting, and sometimes both parents and the child need emotional reassurance.

Instruct parents to avoid the use of raw or unpasteurized honey and corn syrup (Karo syrup) as a home remedy for constipation in young infants. Use of these products may be associated with the development of infant botulism.

Prognosis

Simple measures ordinarily correct constipation, but successful resolution depends on the age of the child and the underlying cause. In the more complex situations, counseling and bowel retraining are often necessary.

GASTROESOPHAGEAL REFLUX

Gastroesophageal reflux (GER) is possible to define as effortless regurgitation of the gastric contents into the esophagus. We term the passage of the gastric esophageal contents into the oropharynx *regurgitation,* whereas *vomiting* is the expulsion of refluxed gastric contents from the mouth. The health care provider diagnoses gastroesophageal reflux disease (GERD) when gastric contents reflux into the esophagus or oropharynx and produce symptoms (Hockenberry & Wilson, 2007). GER usually begins within 1 week of birth, and regurgitation occurs immediately after a feeding or when the infant is laid down after a feeding.

Etiology and Pathophysiology

GER is primarily due to an incompetent lower esophageal (or cardiac) sphincter. As a result, gastric contents are allowed to regurgitate into the esophagus.

Clinical Manifestations

Vomiting or spitting up is the primary manifestation in the first week of life. Aspiration of the gastric contents has potential to lead to respiratory signs such as apnea, choking or gagging after feedings, and aspiration pneumonia. In young children a chronic cough, wheezing, and recurrent pneumonia are common. Growth and weight gain are a problem with a majority of children. Continuous irritation of the esophageal lining with gastric acid will possibly lead to esophageal ulceration and bleeding. This usually manifests as anemia, hematemesis, or blood in the stools.

Diagnostic Tests

A carefully obtained history and growth measurements sometimes suffice to make the diagnosis in mild cases. In more severe or complex cases, diagnosis is possible by observation of reflux during barium esophagography, monitoring esophageal pH with an esophageal probe, upper endoscopy, or esophageal scintigraphy (detects radioactive substances in the esophagus after a feeding of the compound and assesses gastric emptying). Other possible tests include Hemoccult, chest radiography, and bronchoscopy.

Medical Management

Treatment of GER involves small, frequent feedings that have been thickened with infant cereal. If the infant is breastfeeding, have the mother manually express milk and mix it with cereal for feedings.

The prone position improves gastric emptying and decreases GER; however, the American Academy of Pediatrics (2000) recommends nonprone positioning during sleep. Prone positioning can only be used while the infant is awake, especially following feedings. Careful supervision of the infant is imperative (Hockenberry & Wilson, 2007).

Pharmacologic therapy is a possible adjunct therapy to treat infants and children with persistent symptoms of GER. H_2-histamine receptor antagonists, such as cimetidine (Tagamet), ranitidine (Zantac), or famotidine (Pepcid), are effective in reducing the amount of acid present in gastric content and will sometimes prevent esophagitis. It is also possible to give metoclopramide (Reglan) before meals and at bedtime to accelerate gastric emptying. Surgical management of GER is sometimes indicated in severe cases. A **Nissen fundoplication,** which involves wrapping the fundus of the stomach around the distal esophagus to prevent reflux of the stomach contents into the esophagus, is the most commonly performed surgical procedure. The most recent surgical advance is the introduction of the laparoscopic Nissen fundoplication.

Nursing Interventions and Patient Teaching

The goals of nursing include assisting in the recognition of signs of possible GER; providing care for the child undergoing a surgical procedure, if applicable; and providing emotional reassurance that GER is a disorder and not the result of faulty feeding practices.

An important aspect of teaching is educating parents about formula or breast milk thickened with cereal and proper positioning after feedings.

Prognosis

The majority of infants affected have mild GER and achieve normal function by 6 to 7 weeks of age. Generally 90% improve by about 1 year of age; they require only medical therapy. If GER is severe and remains unsuccessfully treated, multiple complications such as esophageal strictures and recurrent respiratory distress with aspiration pneumonia are possible.

HYPERTROPHIC PYLORIC STENOSIS

Hypertrophic pyloric stenosis (HPS) is an obstructive disorder in which the gastric outlet is mechanically obstructed by a congenitally hypertrophied pyloric muscle. It is also the most common reason for an abdominal operation during the first 6 months of life. HPS is present in approximately 1 in 250 live births. Males are three to four times more likely to be affected than females (Milla, 2004).

Etiology and Pathophysiology

We do not know the cause of HPS. There is an increased incidence in siblings and offspring of affected people. The circular muscle that surrounds the valve between the stomach and the duodenum becomes diffusely enlarged as the result of hypertrophy and hyperplasia (Figure 31-16). As a result, the passage becomes more narrow and it is difficult for the stomach to empty. At approximately 4 to 6 weeks of age, infants with HPS begin to vomit almost immediately after feedings. As the condition progresses, the vomiting grows more forceful and becomes projectile, the hallmark sign of HPS.

Clinical Manifestations

Initially, the signs begin as regurgitation that progresses to projectile vomiting 30 to 60 minutes after feeding. Lethargy, weight loss, poor skin turgor, sunken fontanelles, and loss of subcutaneous tissue often become apparent as dehydration ensues (Box 31-5).

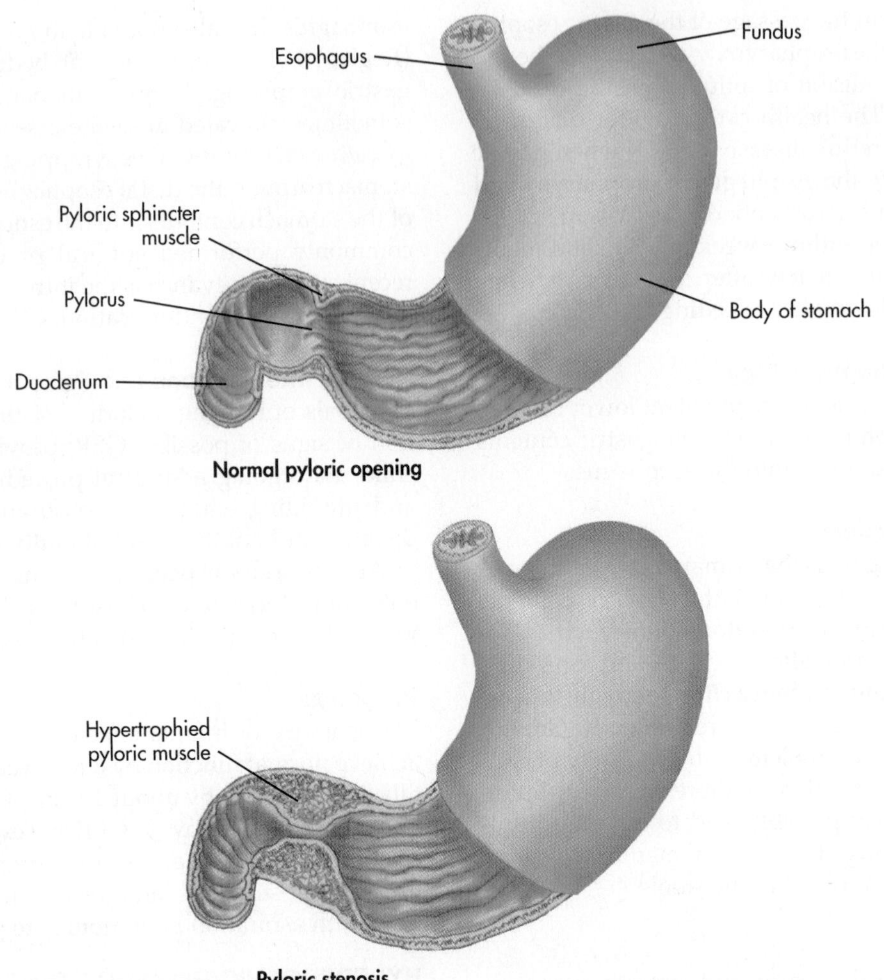

FIGURE 31-16 Comparison of normal pyloric opening with evidence of pyloric stenosis.

Box 31-5 Clinical Manifestations of Hypertrophic Pyloric Stenosis

- Projectile vomiting: will sometimes be ejected 3 to 4 feet from the child when in a side-lying position, 1 foot or more when in a back-lying position
  —Usually occurs shortly after feeding (may not occur for several hours)
  —May follow each feeding or appear intermittently
  —Nonbilious (no bile) vomitus; may be blood tinged
- Infant hungry, avid nurser; eagerly accepts a second feeding after vomiting episode
- No evidence of pain or discomfort except that of chronic hunger
- Weight loss
- Signs of dehydration
- Distended upper abdomen
- Readily palpable olive-shaped mass in the epigastrium just to the right of the umbilicus
- Visible gastric peristaltic waves that move from left to right across the epigastrium

Diagnostic Tests

Examination of the abdomen is likely to assist in the diagnosis and reveal key signs of HPS. Visible peristaltic waves that move from left to right across the epigastric region are sometimes evident, and palpation sometimes reveals an olive-shaped mass in this area to the right of the midline. If it is not possible to establish the diagnosis after history and physical examination, usually an ultrasonic examination is indicated. Ultrasonography will demonstrate an elongated sausage-shaped mass with an elongated pyloric channel. If ultrasound fails to demonstrate a hypertrophied pylorus, the physician will order upper GI radiography to rule out other causes of vomiting.

Medical Management

Surgical relief of the pyloric obstruction as soon as establishment of the diagnosis is the standard treatment for HPS. The surgical correction of HPS is accomplished by performing a **Fredet-Ramstedt procedure.** This operation (a pyloromyotomy) involves surgically splitting the pylorus muscle down to, but not including, the submucosa, allowing for a larger lumen. This procedure has a high success rate when the infant receives careful preoperative preparation to correct fluid and electrolyte imbalances.

Nursing Interventions and Patient Teaching

Nursing interventions of the infant with HPS primarily involve assisting with the establishment of a diagnosis, providing adequate nutrition, managing preoperative and postoperative care, and supporting the family. A carefully obtained history with assessment for signs and symptoms of HPS is essential for the prompt diagnosis. Correction of any metabolic disturbances and dehydration before surgery is essential. Generally this is possible through IV administration of fluid and electrolytes. It is necessary to keep the infant NPO to eliminate vomiting. Careful assessment of I&O is necessary to monitor fluid replacement and rehydration. Postoperative nursing interventions are focused on preventing complications by monitoring I&O, observation of physical signs, and instituting oral feedings. Usually you will begin feedings of glucose water 4 to 6 hours postoperatively, and then, if feedings are retained for 24 hours, start full feedings. Encourage parents to express their concerns and visit their infant frequently, participating in the care when appropriate. Barring complications, infants are usually discharged within 1 to 2 days after surgery.

Most parents need support and reassurance that the condition is caused by a structural problem and is no way a reflection of their parenting skills and capacities.

Prognosis

Most infants recover completely and rapidly following pyloromyotomy. Postoperative complications include persistent pyloric obstruction and wound dehiscence. Approximately 15% of infants with HPS also have gastroesophageal reflux.

INTUSSUSCEPTION

Intussusception is the most common cause of intestinal obstruction in children between 3 months and 6 years of age. It is twice as common in male children. Generally, health care providers are unable to determine the cause of intussusception.

Etiology and Pathophysiology

Intussusception is the result of the telescoping of one portion of the intestine into another (Figure 31-17). The site most commonly affected is the ileocecal valve, at the juncture of the distal ileum and the proximal colon. As the ileum telescopes into the colon, the passage of intestinal contents distal to the defect becomes obstructed. Subsequently, as the mucosa of the intestinal walls rub against each other, blood and mucus from the mucosa leak into the intestinal lumen and form "currant jelly" stools (feces that is mixed with blood and mucus from the intestinal mucosa), a hallmark sign of intussusception. Serious complications include peritonitis, intestinal ischemia, infarction, perforation, and shock. If the condition does not receive treatment, death of the child within 2 to 5 days is possible.

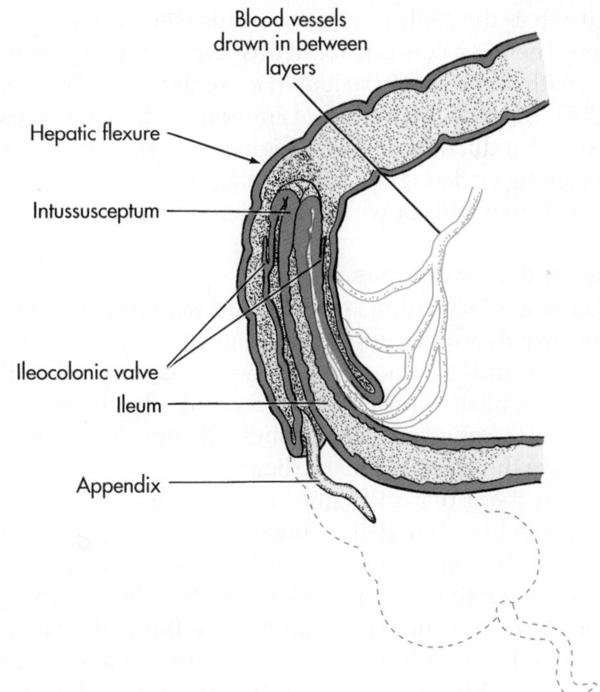

FIGURE 31-17 Ileocolic intussusception.

Clinical Manifestations

In most cases there is a sudden onset of severe abdominal pain in a previously well child. The child will assume a fetal position in an effort to guard the abdomen. Vomiting and lethargy usually occur. Within 12 hours of the onset of abdominal pain, the child usually passes the characteristic "currant jelly" stool.

Diagnostic Tests

The history and physical signs are usually diagnostic. The physician orders an abdominal radiograph called a flat plate of the abdomen initially to note the presence of any intraperitoneal air (free air under the diaphragm), which indicates a bowel obstruction. Free air under the diaphragm is a contraindication to administering a barium enema. A digital rectal examination will reveal blood and mucus. A barium enema or water-soluble contrast medium that demonstrates an obstruction to the flow through the intestine will give a definitive diagnosis of an intussusception (Hockenberry & Wilson, 2007).

Medical Management

It is often possible to relieve intussusception with hydrostatic reduction, using barium at the time of diagnostic evaluation. The force exerted by the flowing barium from the enema sometimes successfully forces the telescoped portion of the bowel into its correct position. A large number of radiologists are using a water-soluble contrast medium with air pressure instead of barium as the contrast agent to reduce the intussusception. There is a concern about possible barium peritonitis with the use of barium (Hockenberry & Wilson, 2007). Surgical treatment of intussusception involves manual reduction of the invagination (the process of becoming enclosed in a sheath) and, if necessary, resection of nonviable bowel with end-to-end anastomosis.

Nursing Interventions

Nursing interventions for the child with intussusception involve obtaining a thorough history from the parents and observing for physical signs that will help establish a prompt and accurate diagnosis. As soon as the physician establishes a diagnosis, begin to prepare the parents for the diagnostic barium enema. Inform them that in many cases this procedure will be corrective, but if it is unsuccessful, surgery will possibly be required. After the hydrostatic reduction, observe for the passage of barium and the return of normal bowel movements. Observe the child for at least 24 hours following the procedure to assess for the possibility of recurrence. If surgery is indicated, you will keep the child NPO with an NG tube set to intermittent low suction, and begin an IV infusion to supply adequate hydration and electrolytes. Postoperative care of the child involves obtaining vital signs, monitoring the operative site, and assessing for the return of bowel sounds. When peristaltic function has returned, it is appropriate to gradually introduce oral feedings.

Prognosis

Many patients with intussusception will obtain successful treatment with hydrostatic reduction. Surgery is required for patients in whom the water-soluble contrast medium enema with air pressure was unsuccessful. If untreated, 90% of patients will worsen or die of complications such as perforation, peritonitis, and sepsis. With early diagnosis and treatment, serious complications and death are rare.

HIRSCHSPRUNG'S DISEASE

Hirschsprung's disease, also known as **megacolon** (congenital aganglionic megacolon), is a functional intestinal obstruction caused by the absence of parasympathetic ganglion cells in a portion of the colon. The incidence is 1 in 5000 live births, with a predominance in males. It is more common in children with trisomy 21 (a congenital condition characterized by varying degrees of cognitive impairment and multiple defects [Down syndrome]), and a small number of cases follow a familial pattern (Wyllie & Hyams, 2006).

Etiology and Pathophysiology

In Hirschsprung's disease there is an absence of innervation to a segment of the bowel. In most cases, the lower portion of the sigmoid colon just above the anus is affected. As a result, there are no peristaltic waves in the affected portion of the colon to propel the fecal contents, causing an intestinal obstruction and distention of the bowel proximal to the defect (Figure 31-18).

Clinical Manifestations

Clinical manifestations often vary according to age. Early observation of the neonate will typically reveal a failure to pass meconium within 48 hours and signs of partial or complete intestinal obstruction, such as abdominal distention, vomiting, and poor feeding. Infants sometimes have a history of constipation or intermittent constipation and diarrhea. Dehydration, failure to thrive, abdominal distention, and fever are other possible manifestations. In the older child, there is an association between Hirschsprung's disease and chronic constipation; abdominal distention; ribbon-like, foul-smelling stools; poor weight gain; malnourishment; anemia; palpable fecal mass; and visible peristalsis.

Diagnostic Tests

A carefully obtained history, associated clinical manifestations, and a barium enema assist in making a diagnosis of Hirschsprung's disease.

Medical Management

Immediate treatment involves surgical removal of the affected portion of the bowel. The surgeon will proceed in two stages. The first-stage surgery involves placement of a temporary colostomy in the portion of normal, innervated colon just proximal to the defect. This will allow for a period of rest during which the normal bowel will regain its tone. The second-stage

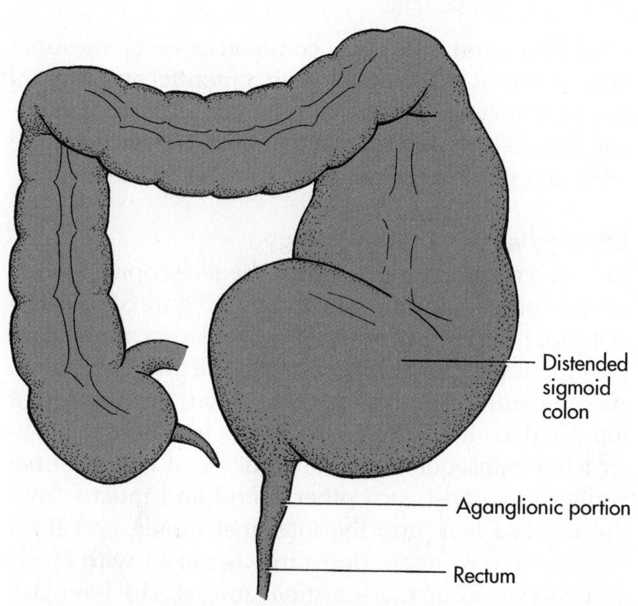

FIGURE 31-18 The affected bowel in Hirschsprung's disease.

surgery involves excising the affected segment and pulling the normal, innervated segment down through the anus, anastomosing it to the anal canal. The surgeon will usually perform this procedure, known as the **Soave endorectal pull-through,** when the child reaches a weight of 20 pounds.

Nursing Interventions and Patient Teaching

Focus your nursing interventions for the infant or child with Hirschsprung's disease on assisting the parents to adjust to the diagnosis, promoting parent-infant bonding, preparing the parents for surgery, and educating them regarding colostomy care. Preoperatively, direct nursing interventions toward restoring the child's nutritional status by providing a low-fiber, high-protein, high-calorie diet or, in severe cases, TPN. Sometimes you will have to evacuate the bowel with daily enemas and stool softeners. Administer oral antibiotics, if prescribed, to decrease intestinal flora. Measure abdominal girth daily. It is important to prepare the parents and child, when developmentally appropriate, for the colostomy. Stress that this is a temporary procedure unless a large portion of the bowel is involved, necessitating a permanent ileostomy. Postoperative care includes assessing vital signs and bowel sounds, observing for the passage of flatus and stools, and monitoring the operative site. The surgeon will generally place an NG tube set to low intermittent suction during the surgery and will order its removal as soon as peristalsis has returned, usually within 24 hours, and it is possible to introduce a regular diet for age.

Before discharge, parents need instruction regarding colostomy care; refer them as needed to a visiting nurse for assistance in caring for the colostomy.

Prognosis

After stabilizing the condition of the patient with Hirschsprung's disease with fluid and electrolyte replacement, the surgeon creates a temporary colostomy, followed by one or more complete corrective surgeries. It is usually possible to close the colostomy following the final surgery, after which most children are able to attain satisfactory defecatory function (Hockenberry & Wilson, 2007).

HERNIAS

A **hernia** is the protrusion of organs or portions of an organ through a structural defect or weakened muscle wall. A complication of herniation arises when the circulation to the protruding organ is impaired (known as a strangulated hernia) or when the pressure of protruding organs impairs the function of other organs. Incarceration of a hernia occurs when the hernia is not possible to reduce manually. Figure 31-19 and Table 31-2 illustrate and describe hernias affecting the diaphragm and the abdominal wall.

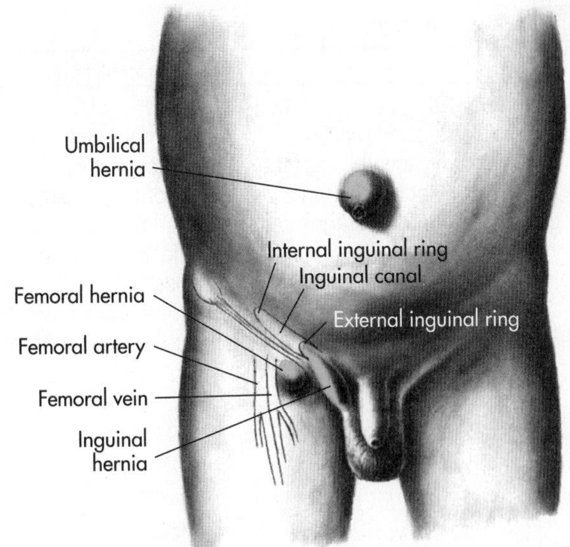

FIGURE 31-19 Location of hernias.

DISORDERS OF GENITOURINARY FUNCTION

Disorders of the genitourinary (GU) tract are common in children and arise from a variety of etiologic factors. The GU system is responsible for maintaining fluid and electrolyte balance within the body. Disorders of the GU system alter the delicate balance of fluid and electrolytes within the body and sometimes become life threatening.

URINARY TRACT INFECTION

Urinary tract infections (UTIs) affect the upper urinary tract (kidneys and ureters), the lower urinary tract (bladder and urethra), or both. They are more prevalent in females, uncircumcised males, and sexually active adolescents. UTIs are primarily caused by bacteria, most frequently gram-negative organisms. A shorter urethra in females (2 cm [0.8 in] in young girls and 4 cm [1.6 in] in mature women) provides a short access route to the bladder for organisms that are common to the perineal and perianal regions. Another factor that sometimes leads to UTIs is urinary stasis. Normally, the urine is sterile, but the warm climate within the bladder provides an excellent growth medium for bacteria. Teaching parents correct perineal cleansing is imperative. In infant boys, it is necessary to retract and cleanse the foreskin with each diaper change. When older male children begin bathing themselves, it is necessary for parents to monitor this cleaning. For females, cleansing the perineal area from front to back will prevent UTIs from *Escherichia coli*. Some children also have a congenital anomaly such as urethral stenosis or vesicoureteral reflux (backward flow of urine from the bladder to the ureters) that will potentially lead to urinary stasis and cause a UTI. Signs and symptoms of UTIs are often subtle, and it is possible that parents will not realize anything is wrong with the child. Especially initially,

Table 31-2 Hernias

TYPE	CLINICAL MANIFESTATIONS AND DIAGNOSTIC TESTS	INTERVENTIONS
DIAPHRAGMATIC		
Protrusion of a portion of the abdominal organs through the foramen of Bochdalek (and opening in the diaphragm)	Respiratory distress within hours of delivery; cyanosis, tachypnea, retractions, dyspnea, respiratory acidosis, and absent breath sounds on the affected side (presence of bowel sounds is possible) Abdominal pain, vomiting Diagnosis made by radiography	*Medical* Immediate surgical repair of the diaphragm with replacement of the herniation; placement of chest tubes *Nursing* *Preoperative:* Support respiratory function; provide comfort; place in semi-Fowler's position; perform suctioning, give oxygen, and monitor IV fluids *Postoperative:* Maintain routine postoperative care and monitoring, place in semi-Fowler's position; check physiotherapy and positive pressure ventilation; monitor oxygenation; provide comfort; support parents
HIATAL		
Intermittent protrusion of the stomach through the esophageal opening in the diaphragm	Vomiting, dysphasia, dyspnea, gastroesophageal reflux, respiratory distress, bleeding Diagnosis made by history and radiography	*Medical* Surgical repair of the esophageal opening *Nursing* Routine preoperative and postoperative care, as above
INGUINAL		
Loop of intestine prolapses through the inguinal ring above the scrotal sac because of muscle weakness; either unilateral or bilateral is possible	Hydrocele or undescended testes sometimes also present. Inguinal hernias are usually asymptomatic and are found only in the course of routine examination. However, it is possible for a hernia to become strangulated or incarcerated (i.e., a portion of the intestine becomes tightly caught in the hernia sac, restricting blood supply).	*Medical* Hernia is usually possible to reduce by gently manipulating the strapped intestine; when surgery is done (herniorrhaphy), overnight hospital stay is not necessary. *Nursing* Apply ice to the scrotum to reduce edema; comfort and quiet the child with an incarcerated (trapped) inguinal hernia so the surgeon is able to reduce the incarceration; do not use diapers postoperatively even if the child is not toilet trained; instruct parents not to give tub baths until healing is complete.
UMBILICAL		
Protrusion of the intestine through a weakness in the abdominal wall around the umbilicus	Inspection and palpation of abdomen High incidence in black infants Spontaneous closure at 1-2 years of age	*Medical* Spontaneous closure by 2 years of age in small defects (less than 2 cm); surgical closure if condition persists after age 2-5 or for defects larger than 2 cm *Nursing* Discourage use of home remedies (i.e., coins, belly bands, abdominal taping); reassure parents

the manifestations are likely to be subtle or not even present. In infants, fever, weight loss, failure to thrive, feeding difficulties, vomiting, and diarrhea are common. In children, urinary frequency, pain during urination, foul-smelling urine, incontinence in a toilet-trained child, abdominal or flank pain, hematuria, and vomiting are common signs and symptoms.

NEPHROTIC SYNDROME (NEPHROSIS)

Nephrotic syndrome is a clinical state characterized by proteinuria, edema, hyperlipidemia, and hypoproteinemia. Nephrotic syndrome is possible in three forms: (1) idiopathic or primary; (2) secondary (occurring as a result of glomerular damage caused by a known etiology); or (3) congenitally acquired. In children, the idiopathic form is seen most commonly.

Etiology and Pathophysiology

For most children (90%), the cause of the syndrome is unknown. Some health care providers have implicated autoimmune processes and a hypersensitivity to an antigen-antibody reaction as possible causes. The underlying pathologic abnormality is proteinuria resulting from glomerular damage that renders the glomerulus permeable to protein (proteinuria). Loss of protein in the urine causes a decrease in the level of protein in the blood (hypoproteinemia), which causes a decrease in colloidal osmotic pressure in the capillaries. This results in hyperpermeability of the capillaries and causes fluid to leak into the interstitial spaces (edema). With loss of fluid into the interstitial spaces, there is a decrease in blood volume (hypovolemia) (Hockenberry & Wilson, 2007). In compensation, the kidneys retain sodium and water, leading to yet a greater potential for edema. The mechanism by which the level of lipids in the blood increases is poorly understood.

Clinical Manifestations

The development of manifestations is subtle. Initially, children often develop periorbital edema, which is primarily noticed on waking from sleep. Abdominal distention is sometimes apparent as fluid accumulates in the abdominal cavity (ascites). As the syndrome progresses, the edema becomes generalized and severe (anasarca) (Figure 31-20). Vomiting, anorexia, diarrhea, and irritability are common. Increased body weight, decreased urine output, and marked edema are hallmark signs. Other signs include white nails, lusterless hair, and soft ear cartilage.

Diagnostic Tests

The diagnosis of nephrotic syndrome results from history and clinical manifestations, such as weight gain, generalized edema, proteinuria, hypoalbuminemia, and hypercholesterolemia (Hockenberry & Wilson, 2007). Analysis of the urine reveals marked proteinuria with a high specific gravity. The urine is frequently dark and frothy. RBCs, hyaline casts, and fat bodies will possibly also be present. Serum protein levels are reduced, and serum lipid levels are elevated. Performance of a renal biopsy is possible to determine the extent of glomerular damage and evaluate the response to therapy.

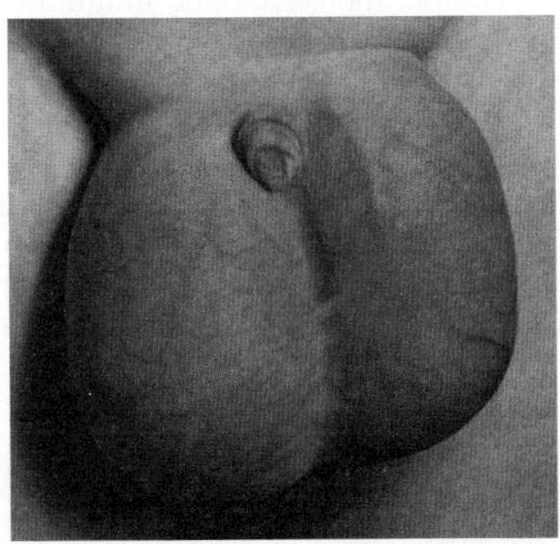

FIGURE 31-20 Child with nephrotic syndrome.

Medical Management

The principal goal of management of nephrotic syndrome is to reduce the edema. Steroid therapy is the primary means to accomplish this. The physician will order adrenocortical steroids (prednisone) to reduce the proteinuria and subsequently the edema. This response usually occurs within 7 to 21 days of initiation of the therapy; administration of the steroids slowly tapers over a period of several weeks and discontinues when the child is asymptomatic. Usually you will encourage bed rest in the acute phase of the illness, with progression to ambulation as the edema subsides. You will generally also place the child on a low-sodium diet during the period of severe edema. The child with nephrotic syndrome will not receive diuretics because they will decrease the circulating blood volume, which is already a concern for these children. Treatment for relapses consists of a repeated course of high-dose steroid therapy.

Nursing Interventions and Patient Teaching

Nursing interventions focus on clinical observation of the child in the acute phase and monitoring the effects of therapeutic interventions. Careful monitoring of I&O, body weight, and abdominal girth is essential in assessing the status of fluid retention or excretion. Provide meticulous skin care to prevent impairment of edematous skin and secondary infections. Frequent monitoring of vital signs is necessary to detect early signs of complications such as infection or shock. Because the child with nephrotic syndrome has a poor appetite, eating is likely to be a challenge. It is essential that the child have a good protein intake to offset the loss of protein through the urine. Offer preferred foods frequently in small amounts and serve them in an attractive manner. Dietary restrictions include a low-salt diet and fluid restriction. Because increased susceptibility to infection is a common side effect of steroid therapy, it is necessary to keep the child free of exposure to communicable diseases and sources of infection. As the edema decreases, it is appropriate to increase the child's activity. Provide continuous support of the family during the acute phase of the illness and while the child recovers.

Instruct parents in testing urine for albumin, administration of medications, diet restrictions (if any), and the common effects of steroid therapy. Also instruct parents regarding avoiding contact with infected playmates, but it is permissible for the child to attend school. Teach parents how to assess for signs of relapse, and tell them to seek immediate medical attention if this occurs.

Prognosis

The prognosis for ultimate recovery in most cases is good. A satisfactory response is more likely when detection of any relapses and institution of therapy occur promptly. Remissions are prolonged when instructions are carried out faithfully. It is estimated that approximately 80% of affected children will have a favorable prognosis.

ACUTE GLOMERULONEPHRITIS

Glomerulonephritis is an inflammation of the glomeruli of the kidney. Most commonly, it occurs as a postinfection phenomenon and is associated with pneumococcal, streptococcal, and viral infections. **Acute poststreptococcal glomerulonephritis** (APSGN) is the most common of the postinfection forms. APSGN primarily affects early school-age children, with a peak age of onset of 6 to 7 years, and has a 2:1 predominance in males (Hahn et al., 2005).

Etiology and Pathophysiology

APSGN follows a streptococcal infection of the throat or skin. Immune complexes that develop as a result of infection with certain strains of group A β-hemolytic streptococci become fixed to the basement membrane of glomeruli. Most streptococcal infections do not cause APSGN. A latent period of 10 to 21 days occurs between the streptococcal infection and the onset of clinical manifestations. The glomeruli become edematous and infiltrated with WBCs. As a result, the glomerular filtration rate decreases, causing an accumulation of sodium and water in the blood, which leads to circulatory congestion and edema. Inflammation and damage to the glomeruli result in increased permeability, allowing protein molecules to escape into the urine (proteinuria).

Clinical Manifestations

Manifestations of APSGN usually appear 10 to 14 days after the streptococcal infection. Initial characteristics are a sudden onset of hematuria, proteinuria, and oliguria. The child's urine sometimes appears cloudy, smoky brown, or what parents describe as tea or cola colored. Edema, abdominal pain, pallor, low-grade fever, anorexia, vomiting, and headache are sometimes present. Hypertension and heart failure are possible results of hypervolemia. Fluid retention does not completely explain the hypertension associated with acute glomerulonephritis. Overproduction of renin also sometimes occurs.

Diagnostic Tests

Urinalysis reveals proteinuria, hematuria, and elevated specific gravity. Half of patients have impaired glomerular filtration with resultant azotemia, which reveals an elevated BUN and creatinine levels (Hockenberry & Wilson, 2007), and urine culture is negative. Cultures of the throat or skin are positive for the streptococcal organism. The **antistreptolysin O titer** (antibodies formed against streptococcus) is elevated, indicating that there has been a recent infection with streptococcus.

Medical Management

The acute phase of glomerulonephritis generally lasts 1 to 2 weeks. During this time, the practitioner usually recommends bed rest, although many children will set their own limits based on their tolerance to activity. A diet of restricted fluid, sodium, potassium, and phosphate is initially required. Regular measurement of vital signs, body weight, and I&O is necessary to monitor the progression of the disease and detect any complications. It is necessary to anticipate acute hypertension and identify it early. The use of antihypertensive medications and diuretics serves to control hypertension. Antibiotic therapy is indicated only for children who have a persistent streptococcal infection.

Nursing Interventions and Patient Teaching

Nursing interventions focus on promoting rest and adequate nutrition, preventing and detecting complications, and supporting the child and family. During the acute phase of the illness, some health care providers will place the child on bed rest. Provide activities that require minimal energy expenditure and will keep the child's interest. Make sure meals reflect the child's preferences while adhering to any dietary restrictions the physician has ordered. Measurement of vital signs, body weight, and I&O will provide information about the disease's progression and detect the presence of complications.

Educate the parents about the disease and its therapy, and allow them to express their feelings and concerns.

Prognosis

Most children with APSGN recover completely, with few or no complications. Specific immunity is conferred, so that subsequent recurrences are uncommon.

WILMS' TUMOR (NEPHROBLASTOMA)

Wilms' tumor (or nephroblastoma) is the most common renal and intraabdominal malignant tumor of childhood, accounting for 20% of solid tumors in children. The peak age of incidence of these tumors is 2 to 3 years with 80% of patients diagnosed before 5 years of age (Hockenberry & Wilson, 2007).

Etiology and Pathophysiology

Wilms' tumor most commonly affects the left kidney. Both kidneys are affected in 10% of the cases. Wilms' tumor has both hereditary and nonhereditary origins.

The most common sites for metastasis are the lungs, the lymph nodes, the liver, the brain, and the bone.

Clinical Manifestations

Most Wilms' tumors manifest as enlarging, asymptomatic, and firm abdominal masses. Other manifestations of the tumor include abdominal pain, hematuria, fever, hypertension, weight loss, and fatigue. If there has been metastasis of the Wilms' tumor, dyspnea, cough, and chest pain will possibly be present.

Diagnostic Tests

Parents detect many tumors when they feel an enlarged abdominal mass while bathing, dressing, or carrying the child. In addition to a thorough history and physical examination, diagnostic studies include radiographic studies, abdominal ultrasound, abdominal and chest computed tomography, MRI, and hematological and chemistry studies. The physician will base the definitive (final) diagnosis on surgical biopsy. Because the tumor is encapsulated, it is important not to palpate the child's abdomen more than is necessary for diagnosis. This will keep to a minimum the possibility of rupture of the capsule and spillage of the malignant cells into the abdominal cavity.

Medical Management

Treatment of Wilms' tumor involves surgical resection as soon as possible after diagnosis, usually within 24 to 48 hours of admission. During surgery, the surgeon performs an exploration of the abdomen to determine the extent of the disease and whether there has been metastasis of the tumor. If one kidney is affected, the surgeon removes the tumor, the kidney, and the adrenal gland, employing meticulous care during resection to avoid rupture of the capsule and spread of cancer cells throughout the abdomen. The other kidney is examined for evidence of disease. If both kidneys are involved, the surgeon removes part of the kidney on the less affected side, and the entire kidney on the opposite side. Most children receive radiotherapy following surgery. Chemotherapy is indicated for all children. The usual course of treatment ranges from 6 to 15 months.

Nursing Interventions and Patient Teaching

Preoperative nursing interventions involve preparing the child and family for surgery. This is a challenging responsibility for you because most surgeries will take place within 24 hours of diagnosis. Postoperative nursing interventions are similar to those provided to the child undergoing abdominal surgery. Direct special attention toward monitoring bowel sounds and assessing renal function. Be sensitive to the parents' feelings about their child's diagnosis; it is common for parents to feel that they should have identified the mass earlier.

The overall objective in discharge planning is to return the child to a normal preoperative lifestyle. Emphasize the usual needs for discipline and moderate protection from infection. Help plan treatment schedules to allow uninterrupted school attendance. Because the child is left with one kidney, recommend certain precautions, such as avoiding contact sports, to prevent injuring the remaining organ. Prompt detection and treatment of any genitourinary signs or symptoms is mandatory.

Prognosis

Reinforce to parents that prognosis is excellent and survival rates have improved with the development of new treatment protocols. Children with localized tumor (stages I and II) have a 90% chance of cure with appropriate therapy.

STRUCTURAL DEFECTS OF THE GENITOURINARY TRACT

Structural defects of the GU tract have serious implications for the psychological well-being of the child. Prompt correction is necessary to avoid a negative psychological impact on the child, as well as to prevent physical complications. The major structural defects and their medical management are presented in Table 31-3 and Figure 31-21.

Nursing Interventions and Patient Teaching

Focus nursing interventions for the child with a defect of the GU tract on assisting with diagnosis and preparing the child and family for procedures and corrective surgeries. Provide the child and the parents with emotional support and opportunities to express their concerns, questions, and fears.

Prognosis

Satisfactory surgical repair is successful for the more common disorders and will take place or begin as early as possible.

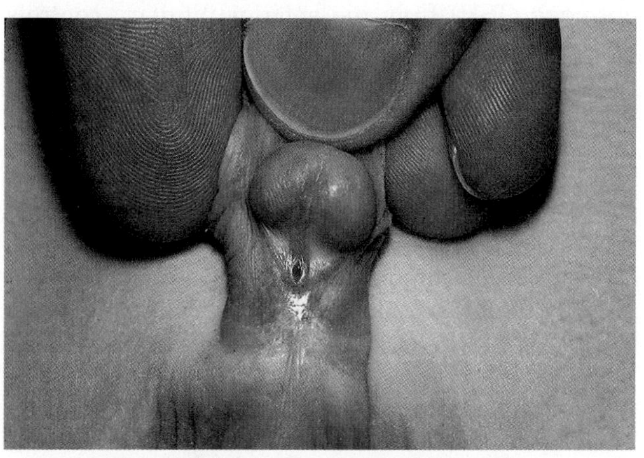

FIGURE 31-21 Hypospadias.

Table 31-3 **Defects of the External Genitourinary Tract**

DEFECT	MEDICAL MANAGEMENT
HYPOSPADIAS	
Urethral opening located along the ventral (anterior) surface of the penile shaft (see Figure 31-21)	Surgical correction involves extending the urethra to a normal position. After repair, the child is expected to have normal reproductive and urinary function.
EPISPADIAS	
Urethral opening located along the dorsal (posterior) surface of the penile shaft	Surgical correction involves penile and urethral lengthening and possibly bladder neck reconstruction.
PHIMOSIS	
Narrowing or stenosis of the opening of the foreskin	Mild cases are treated with manual retraction. Severe cases are treated with circumcision.
HYDROCELE	
Fluid in scrotal sac	Surgical correction indicated if spontaneous resolution has not occurred in 1 year.
CRYPTORCHIDISM	
Failure of one or both of the testes to descend into the scrotum	Medical management involves administration of human chorionic gonadotropin. Surgical correction: orchiopexy, which is surgical fixation of a testes. Treatment is aimed at preventing testicular damage and malignancies.
INGUINAL HERNIA	
Protrusion of the abdominal organs through the inguinal canal and into the scrotal sac (see Figure 31-19)	Surgical correction involves closure of the inguinal canal.

DISORDERS OF ENDOCRINE FUNCTION

The endocrine system is responsible for the production and secretion of the major chemical regulators of the body, namely the hormones. Disorders are caused primarily by an undersecretion or oversecretion of these hormones. Endocrine system dysfunctions affect all aspects of body function, including appearance, growth, and physical and psychological well-being.

HYPOTHYROIDISM

Hypothyroidism results from a deficient production of thyroid hormone (TH) by the thyroid gland. The main function of the thyroid gland is to regulate metabolism by the production of thyroxine (T_4), triiodothyronine (T_3), and calcitonin. Thyroid-stimulating hormone (TSH) from the anterior pituitary controls the secretion of these hormones.

Etiology and Pathophysiology

Both primary and acquired hypothyroidism are possible. Primary causes include (1) congenital defects or (2) defective synthesis resulting from an autoimmune process. Acquired causes of hypothyroidism include (1) insufficient stimulation of the gland by the pituitary or the hypothalamus or (2) systemic resistance to TH.

Clinical Manifestations

The clinical manifestations of hypothyroidism are described in Box 31-6.

Box 31-6 **Clinical Manifestations of Hypothyroidism**

CONGENITAL	ACQUIRED
• Prolonged jaundice	• Growth delay
• Lethargy	• Dry skin
• Poor appetite	• Puffy eyes
• Poor sucking reflex	• Constipation
• Dyspnea	• Lethargy
• Hypothermia	• Mental slowness
• Cool, mottled skin	

Diagnostic Tests

It is also possible to detect hypothyroidism when there is a decrease in serum levels of TH (T_4 and T_3) and an increase in serum TSH levels (if the defect is in the thyroid) or a decrease in serum TSH levels (if the defect is in the pituitary). A screening test for hypothyroidism is mandatory at birth.

Medical Management

The treatment of choice for congenital and acquired hypothyroidism is oral thyroid hormone replacement therapy. Prompt treatment is especially critical in the infant with congenital hypothyroidism to avoid permanent **cognitive** (the process of knowing) impairment.

Nursing Interventions and Patient Teaching

In addition to assisting in detection of the condition and implementation of TH replacement therapy, nursing interventions focus on assisting the child and family in compliance with the medical regimen and periodic monitoring of its effects. As soon as the child grows and matures, it is appropriate to place responsibility for the disorder and its treatment with the child.

Following diagnosis and implementation of thyroid hormone therapy, stress the importance of compliance and periodic monitoring of the response to therapy to the parents and to the child, when old enough.

Prognosis

If congenital hypothyroidism is present, it is necessary to start treatment shortly after birth for normal physical and intellectual growth to occur. The most significant factor adversely affecting eventual intelligence appears to be inadequate treatment, which in some cases will be related to noncompliance.

HYPERTHYROIDISM

Hyperthyroidism is generally rare in young children, primarily affecting young adolescents. The most common form of childhood hyperthyroidism is Graves' disease.

Etiology and Pathophysiology

Although we do not know the exact causal mechanism, the most accepted theory is an autoimmune process resulting in the production of immunoglobulins that have thyroid-stimulating properties.

Clinical Manifestations

The clinical manifestations of hyperthyroidism are described in Box 31-7.

Diagnostic Tests

In addition to clinical manifestations, the health care provider will make the diagnosis of hyperthyroidism based on increased serum levels of T_4, T_3, and radioactive iodine uptake (RAIU).

Box 31-7 Clinical Manifestations of Hyperthyroidism

- Nervousness
- Irritability
- Hyperactivity
- Tremors
- Excessive appetite
- Weight loss
- Exophthalmos (protruding eyeballs)
- Palpable thyroid gland
- Advanced bone age
- Tachycardia
- Tachypnea
- Hypertension
- Warm skin
- Accelerated growth
- Heat intolerance
- Thyroid storm: rapid onset—severe hyperthermia, vomiting, diarrhea, severe tachycardia; may advance to delirium, coma, death

Medical Management

The management of hyperthyroidism aims to decrease the rate of TH secretion. To accomplish this, the child receives antithyroid medications, including propylthiouracil (PTU) and methimazole (Tapazole), subtotal thyroidectomy, or radioactive iodine administration (iodine-131[^{131}I]).

Nursing Interventions and Patient Teaching

Focus nursing interventions for the child with hyperthyroidism on intervening with the physical manifestations of the disease. Sudden episodes of crying or elation exemplify the emotional lability typical of many affected children. Promote rest, and provide a quiet, nonstimulating environment in the initial phase of treatment. Alleviate heat intolerance by dressing the child in lightweight clothing, altering the room temperature, and offering lightweight blankets for sleeping comfort. Dietary modifications include increased calories and daily vitamin supplementation. If surgery is recommended, provide the child and family with explanations about the nature of the surgery, where the incision will be located, and what to expect postoperatively. Postoperative care includes strict observation of bleeding and complications. Keep the neck slightly flexed and supported to prevent strain on the suture line.

On discharge, make a referral to a public health, school, or home health nurse to facilitate continuity of care and increase compliance with the medical regimen.

Prognosis

Generally, after drug treatment, you will note some improvement within the first 2 weeks. In many children, a complete remission of the disorder will follow an initial treatment course of 1 to 2 years. Those who relapse sometimes benefit from a second course of medication therapy, but some of them will also be candidates for surgical intervention.

DIABETES MELLITUS

Diabetes mellitus (DM) is a syndrome characterized by a deficiency of insulin resulting in alterations in protein, carbohydrate, and fat metabolism. Type 1 diabetes mellitus is the most frequently seen endocrine disorder in children.

The terms the health care profession now uses for diabetes mellitus are *type 1* and *type 2*, with Arabic symbols to prevent confusion (e.g., it is possible to misread *type II* as *type 11* [eleven]) (American Diabetes Association, 2001). The previous classifications were insulin-dependent diabetes mellitus (IDDM), or type 1, and non–insulin-dependent diabetes mellitus (NIDDM), or type 2. These classifications were confusing because treatment is variable and sometimes the disease name ended up contradicting the actual treatment (some people with NIDDM will require insulin); and the terms do not reveal the underlying problem (Hockenberry & Wilson, 2007). Therefore, the profession now uses *type 1* and *type 2* to classify the type of diabetes the patient has (Hockenberry & Wilson, 2007).

Type 1 Diabetes

Type 1 diabetes usually begins in children or young adults but is possible to occur in adults. In type 1 diabetes, there is destruction of the pancreatic beta cells that produce insulin, which generally results in total insulin deficiency. In type 1 diabetes, a person with a genetic predisposition that is exposed to a precipitating event—such as a viral infection—will experience autoimmune destruction of the beta cells.

Type 2 Diabetes

In the past, type 2 diabetes was most common in persons who were older than 35 years, had a family history of diabetes, were overweight, and had a sedentary lifestyle. Type 2 diabetes results from insulin resistance and the body's improper use of insulin with relative insulin deficiency, not absolute insulin deficiency. In type 2 diabetes, some people have mostly insulin resistance with some insulin deficiency, and others have mostly deficiency in insulin secretion with some insulin resistance (Hockenberry & Wilson, 2007).

Changes in food consumption and activity levels have increased the rate of type 2 diabetes mellitus in children and adolescents in the United States. The number of children with elevated cholesterol or type 2 diabetes has at least tripled in the past 5 years. In the past 30 years, the percentage of children who are overweight has quadrupled, to 16% (Brosnan et al., 2001). The result is a rise in cholesterol levels, hypertension, and type 2 diabetes (in part from exercising too little and changes in food consumption).

Etiology and Pathophysiology

If there is a deficiency of insulin, glucose cannot enter the cell and the level of glucose in the bloodstream increases, known as *hyperglycemia*. The metabolism of carbohydrates, fats, and proteins requires insulin to allow these substances to enter the cell—with the exception of nerve cells and vascular tissue. A glucose level greater than 180 mg/dL exceeds the renal threshold, and glucose spills into the urine (glycosuria). This causes an osmotic diversion of water and thus excessive passage of urine (polyuria), which is a cardinal sign of diabetes. The polyuria results in loss of essential electrolytes (Hockenberry & Wilson, 2007).

Without glucose entering the cells, the body breaks down protein to convert to glucose in the liver (glucogenesis); this glucose increase contributes to the hyperglycemia. The body depletes fat and protein stores to meet its energy needs because in the face of insulin deficiency, it is not possible to use carbohydrates. The body's hunger mechanism is stimulated, which causes an increased food intake (polyphagia). The increase of food intake, in turn, further increases the hyperglycemia (Hockenberry & Wilson, 2007).

Ketoacidosis

When glucose is unavailable owing to the absence of insulin, the need arises for another source of energy. The breakdown of fats for energy produces fatty acids and glycerol in the fat cells and the liver, which are converted to ketone bodies. These ketone bodies are an alternative source of fuel; however, the rate of their use in the cells is limited. The body eliminates excess ketone bodies in the urine (ketonuria) or the lungs (acetone breath). The excessive ketone bodies in the blood (ketonemia) create strong acids that decrease the serum pH, thus resulting in ketoacidosis. Hyperventilation, which is characteristic of metabolic acidosis, results from the respiratory system's attempt to remove the excess carbon dioxide by increasing the depth and rate of respirations (Kussmaul's respirations) (Hockenberry & Wilson, 2007).

Diabetic ketoacidosis (DKA) is a grave condition. The child will be admitted to an intensive care unit, and the staff will immediately institute insulin therapy and correction of fluid and electrolyte imbalance (see Chapter 22). If treatment does not begin immediately, progressive deterioration with dehydration, electrolyte imbalance, ketoacidosis, coma, and death will result (Hockenberry & Wilson, 2007).

Diagnostic Tests

Diagnosis is made on the basis of test results, including an 8-hour fasting glucose level of greater than 126 mg/dL and a random blood glucose level of greater than 200 mg/dL, accompanied by classic signs of diabetes, such as (1) glycosuria, polyuria, weight loss despite good appetite and (2) manifestations of metabolic acidosis with or without stupor or coma. The level of glycosylated hemoglobin (hemoglobin A_{1c}) is another important parameter. Nondiabetic hemoglobin A_{1c} levels are between 4% and 6.5%. A hemoglobin A_{1c} value of 6.5% to 7.5% is acceptable for diabetes control for the child. Diagnostic criteria for ketoacidosis are hyperglycemia (blood glucose level greater than 330 mg/dL), ketonemia (strongly positive), ABGs revealing metabolic acidosis (pH less than 7.30; ketones are strong acids that lower serum pH), glycosuria, and ketonuria (Hockenberry & Wilson, 2007).

Medical Management

Medical management of DM in the child calls for a multidisciplinary approach that includes the family, the child (if appropriate), and a team of professionals including a pediatric endocrinologist, diabetic nurse educator, dietitian, and exercise physiologist. The child will require replacement of the insulin he or she is unable to produce (Hockenberry & Wilson, 2007). There are four types of therapeutic insulin: rapid, short, intermediate, and long acting. All insulins are prepared in 100 units/mL strength. The dosage of insulin for each child varies according to levels of glucose in the blood. To measure the serum glucose, put a drop of the child's blood on a test strip and read the color change by comparing it with a color chart or by inserting the strip into a glucose monitor. For glucose monitoring, puncture the side of the finger pad where there are fewer nerve endings and more blood vessels. Use the thumb or the ring finger because blood flows more freely to these areas (Hockenberry & Wilson, 2007).

The appropriate daily insulin dosage depends on food intake and activity and exercise levels. Management for most children involves a twice-daily insulin protocol combining rapid-acting (lispro) or short-acting (regular) and intermediate-acting (neutral protamine Hagedorn [NPH] or Lente) insulins. The child receives the injections of insulin before breakfast and before dinner. It is necessary to adjust the insulin dosage during growth spurts, increased exercise, illnesses, infections, and surgery.

The insulin pump, whose designers sought to more closely mimic the release of the insulin hormone from the islet cells of the pancreas, is also available for children with DM. The insulin pump delivers predetermined amounts of regular or lispro insulin continuously (Olohan & Zappitelli, 2003). It is necessary to measure blood glucose levels at least four times per day, and intensive education and supervision are necessary for maximum effectiveness and control of the infusion pump (Hockenberry & Wilson, 2007).

The device includes a syringe with a supply of insulin, a plunger, and a pump that pushes the plunger to deliver the correct dosage of insulin. The insulin moves from the syringe into a needle that rests within the subcutaneous tissue on the abdomen or thigh (Hockenberry & Wilson, 2007). It is necessary to change the needle aseptically every 48 hours. Although the insulin pump has advantages over daily insulin injections, one major disadvantage is impossibility of removing it for more than 2 hours under any circumstance.

Since the management of DM in children also centers on nutrition, make sure a nutritionist is available to discuss nutritional needs and restrictions with the child and family. Children with DM have essentially the same nutritional requirements as children who do not have DM, except for the need to remove concentrated sugars from the diet (Hockenberry & Wilson, 2007). Generally, management involves teaching children and their families to follow the American Diabetes Association (ADA) food plan. Based on an exchange system, this balanced diet incorporates the U.S. Department of Agriculture's MyPyramid recommendations. MyPyramid's purpose is to illustrate foods that should be included in a healthful diet and in what proportion (see Figure 21-1). Nutritional education includes instruction in eating meals and snacks when the peak insulin action is occurring. It is important to consider the total number of calories and the proportions of basic nutrients every day (Hockenberry & Wilson, 2007).

Encourage exercise because it has the capacity to lower blood glucose levels. Once again, it is always necessary to adjust food intake and insulin requirements to the child's activity level.

Nursing Interventions and Patient Teaching

Focus your nursing interventions for the child with DM on educating the child and the family about the disease and its treatment and possible complications, along with providing support and reassurance. Because the treatment of DM relies on principles of self-management, it is essential that the child and the family understand the disease and its treatment. Encourage the parents and the child to express their questions, fears, and concerns about the disease and its management. Support the child and the family in their adjustment to the disease, and provide them with concrete suggestions about managing the disease that will have a positive effect on their attitudes about DM and its management.

It is important that the child and family receive instruction about meal planning from a nutritionist, and for you to reinforce these instructions. The child and family need to be educated about the action of insulin, including the onset, peak, and duration of action, as well as manifestations of hyperglycemia and hypoglycemia. Make sure they are also aware of how to recognize manifestations of diabetic ketoacidosis. Instruct both the child and the family in the proper techniques of insulin injections. Teach them to develop a rotation pattern so that they do not give injections repeatedly in the same sites. Also teach the parents and the child the principles and techniques of home glucose monitoring (see Health Promotion box).

Prognosis

DM is a chronic metabolic disease, but compliance with treatment improves quality of life. Long-term complications involve the small, as well as larger, blood vessels. The most common microvascular complications affect the kidney (nephropathy) and the retina of the eye (retinopathy). Pathologic vascular consequences are possible as soon as 2½ to 3 years after diagnosis if there is poor control. If diabetes is well-controlled, it is possible to postpone vascular changes for 20 years or longer (Hockenberry & Wilson, 2007).

DISORDERS OF MUSCULOSKELETAL FUNCTION

Musculoskeletal problems in childhood are common and are a result of genetics, rapid growth, or the child's natural tendency toward active mobility. Many mus-

Health Promotion

Child with Diabetes Mellitus

- Self–blood glucose monitoring (SBGM) has improved diabetes management and is used successfully by children from the onset of their diabetes. By testing their own blood, children and parents are able to adjust their insulin regimen to maintain the glucose level in the normal range of 80 to 120 mg/dL. Diabetes management depends to a great extent on SBGM.
- Essentially, the nutritional needs of children with diabetes are no different from those of unaffected children. Children with diabetes require no special foods or supplements. They need sufficient calories to balance daily expenditure for energy and to satisfy the requirement for growth and development. They also need consistent intake and timing of food, especially carbohydrates.
- There is no one diet for diabetes. General guidelines exist, such as to eat less fat and saturated fat and to eat more whole grains, fruits, and vegetables. Sugars and sweets, or simple sugars, do not raise blood glucose any more quickly than starches, or "complex carbohydrates." Provide healthy nutrition advice—eat sugars and sweets in moderation. It is important to base diabetes meal plans on individual needs and develop them with expert assistance from a registered dietitian.
- Encourage exercise, and never restrict it unless other health conditions indicate the need to do so, because it lowers blood glucose levels. It is part of diabetes management, and planning it around the child's interest and capabilities is important. However, in most instances, children's activities are not rigidly scheduled. Compensate for the inevitable decreases in the blood glucose level by providing extra snacks before (and, if prolonged, during) the activity. Besides providing a feeling of well-being, regular exercise aids in the body's use of food and often decreases insulin requirements.
- Even a child with well-controlled diabetes typically experiences occasional mild symptoms of hypoglycemia, but if the child and caretakers recognize the signs and symptoms early and relieve them promptly by appropriate therapy, it is not usually necessary to interrupt the child's activity for more than a few minutes.
- Families need to understand the treatment method and the insulin prescribed, including the effective duration, onset, and peak action. They also need to know the characteristics of the various types of insulins, and the proper mixing and dilution of insulins. Insulin, after is has been opened, is necessary to discard in 1 month (even if refrigerated). Unopened insulin is good until the expiration date on the bottle.
- Never store insulin at very cold (less than 36° F [2.2° C]) or very hot (more than 86° F [30° C]) temperatures. Extreme temperatures destroy insulin.
- The site selected for insulin injection will sometimes depend on whether the child or parent administers the insulin. The upper arms, the thighs, the hips, and the abdomen are usual injection sites for insulin. The child is able to reach the thighs, the abdomen, and part of the hip and arm easily, but will sometimes require help to inject other sites. For example, have a parent pinch a loose fold of skin on the arm while the child injects the insulin.
- Some children are candidates for continuous subcutaneous insulin infusion with a portable insulin pump. The practitioner will teach the child and the parents to operate the device, including the mechanics of the pump, battery changes, and alarm systems. They learn how to load the syringe, insert the catheter, adjust the insulin flow for routine needs and for illnesses, and connect and disconnect the catheter. If you work where insulin pumps are part of the therapeutic regimen, make sure to become familiar with the operation of the specific device your facility uses and the protocol of the regimen.
- Self-management techniques the child and the family need to master are the testing of blood, administration of insulin, and adjustment of insulin and diet with alterations in day-to-day activities and unusual occurrences.

culoskeletal conditions are temporary, and ultimately, normal function returns.

DEVELOPMENTAL DYSPLASIA OF THE HIP

Etiology and Pathophysiology

Developmental dysplasia of the hip (DDH) is a developmental abnormality of the femoral head, the acetabulum, or both. DDH is associated with such conditions as first pregnancy, spina bifida, and breech presentation. The defining characteristic of subluxation of the hip is incorrect position, or partial dislocation, of the femoral head in the acetabulum. **Subluxation** is the degree of DDH most common in infants. Dislocation occurs when the femoral head has no contact with the acetabulum.

Clinical Manifestations

In the infant, there is shortening of the femur on the affected side; thigh and gluteal folds are uneven (or increased on the affected side) when the infant is placed in the prone position, and there is limited abduction of the hip on the affected side (Figure 31-22). The older, weight-bearing infant will sometimes have the affected leg shorter than the other, a waddling gait, or limping.

Diagnostic Tests

Early diagnosis of DDH in the newborn tends to make treatment more successful and less complicated. Nursing assessment of the previously listed manifestations alerts the physician to the possibility of DDH. In addition, sonography or radiographic examination is sometimes helpful in establishing the diagnosis.

Medical Management

Once diagnosed, treatment begins immediately. Any delay in treatment is likely to result in a worsening deformity and poorer prognosis. Treatment will depend on the severity of the dysplasia and the age of the infant. Treatment for infants younger than 6 months of

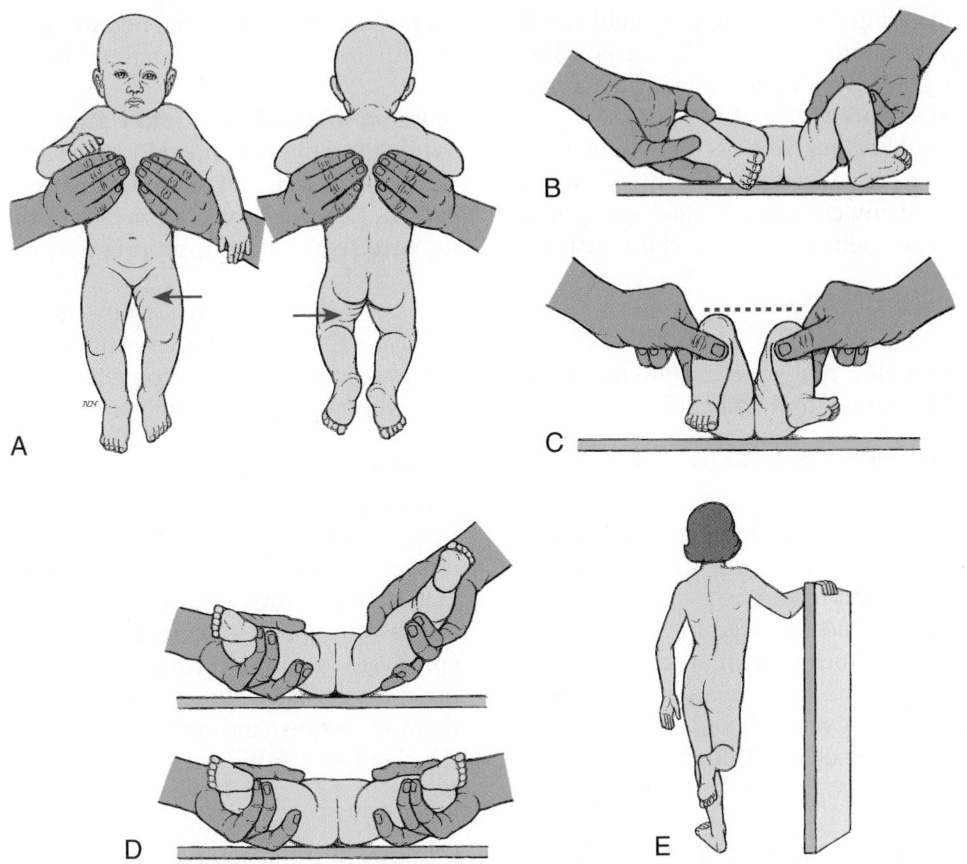

FIGURE 31-22 Signs of congenital dislocation of the hip. **A,** Asymmetry of gluteal and thigh folds. **B,** Limited hip abduction, as seen in flexion. **C,** Apparent shortening of femur, as indicated by level of knees in flexion. **D,** Ortolani's click (if infant is under 4 weeks of age). **E,** Positive Trendelenburg's sign or gait (if child is weight bearing).

age consists of positioning the head of the femur within the acetabulum and maintaining the hip in abduction for 4 to 6 months with the use of a Pavlik harness (Figure 31-23). Once this therapy achieves abduction, a hip spica cast will serve to maintain positioning for several months until the hip is stable. Infants diagnosed between ages 6 and 18 months will require skin traction reduction and casting until the hip is stable. Surgical open reduction will be necessary in some cases if soft tissue obstructs the head of the femur from entering the acetabulum. Immobilization in a hip spica cast follows open reduction. The management of children diagnosed after 18 months is more extensive because adaptive changes have taken place. Open surgical reduction, osteotomy, and arthroplasty are sometimes necessary.

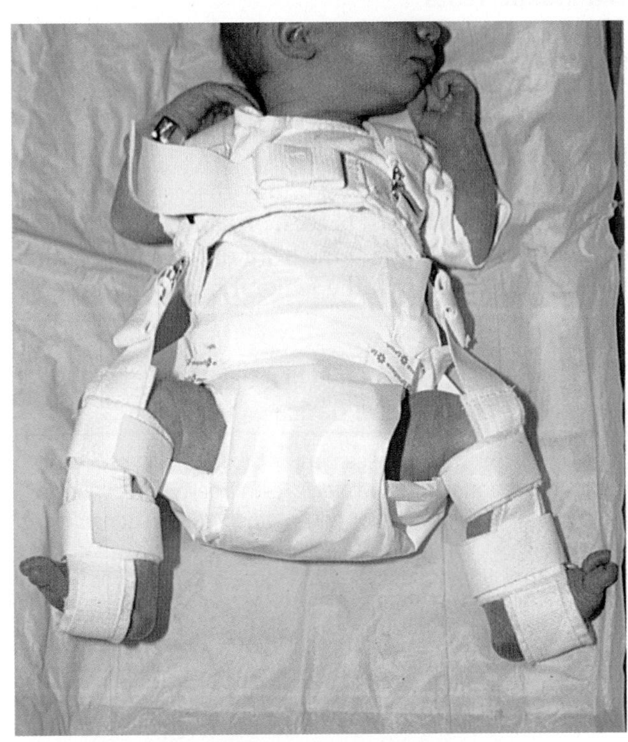

FIGURE 31-23 Child in Pavlik harness.

Nursing Interventions and Patient Teaching

Nurses play an important role in identifying signs of DDH and other congenital defects in newborns, and the earlier identification and treatment of the defect occur, the better the chance for a favorable outcome. The primary goals in caring for a child in a corrective device or cast are to maintain the position of the hip joint, prevent complications, and provide the stimulation necessary for the developing infant or child. As early as possible, involve parents in caring for their baby to build confidence in their ability to provide care at home. Box 31-8 provides general guidelines for the nursing interventions for a child in a corrective device or cast.

Parents and all other caregivers need to understand that children in corrective devices need involvement in all the activities of any child in the same age-group. Do not allow confinement to exclude children from family activities.

Prognosis

With early treatment, the prognosis is more favorable to the restoration of normal body function.

LEGG-CALVÉ-PERTHES DISEASE (COXA PLANA)

Etiology and Pathophysiology

Legg-Calvé-Perthes disease (coxa plana) is a disorder caused by decreased blood supply to the femoral head, which results in epiphyseal necrosis and degeneration of the femoral head followed by regeneration or calcification. It occurs four times more often in boys and affects children from 3 to 12 years of age (Kliegman et al., 2007). The cause of the disorder is unknown, and the disease process itself is self-limited.

Clinical Manifestations

Signs and symptoms are usually insidious. The child will usually complain of pain, exhibit a limp on the affected side, and have limited ROM. The condition is aggravated by activity and improves with rest.

Diagnostic Tests

The presence of the aforementioned signs raises the suspicion of Legg-Calvé-Perthes disease. Radiographic examination confirms the diagnosis.

Medical Management

Treatment of Legg-Calvé-Perthes disease consists of bed rest, traction, casts, braces, or harnesses. The goal of therapy is to maintain the head of the femur within the acetabulum so that the femoral head will preserve its normal shape as it regenerates. If this effort is successful, full ROM can be maintained.

Box 31-8 Care of the Child in a Cast or Corrective Device

- Do neurovascular assessment of the five Ps (impairments to be reported immediately): *p*ain, *p*allor or cyanosis, *p*aresthesia (numbing or tingling, decrease in sensation), *p*ulselessness, *p*uffiness.
- Monitor skin frequently for erythema or tenderness.
- Wash and dry skin at least daily.
- Smooth or pad sharp cast or brace edges with gauze or adhesive tape.
- Teach cast or brace maintenance and cleaning.
- Assess circular dressings for excessive tightness.
- Stimulate circulation with gentle massage over pressure areas.

Nursing Interventions and Patient Teaching

While the child is in traction or in casts, braces, or harnesses, skin care and neurovascular assessment are essential. Refer to Box 31-8 for care of the child in a cast or corrective device. Appropriate education of the family and child includes purpose, function, application, and care of the corrective device. It is essential that the child and the parents understand how important it is to achieving the desired outcome to use the corrective device correctly (Hockenberry & Wilson, 2007).

Prognosis

With patient compliance, the prognosis is excellent. Legg-Calvé-Perthes disease is self-limiting, and early, efficient treatment and the age of onset are important factors in a positive outcome. Younger children have the best prognosis for complete recovery because their epiphyses are more cartilaginous, whereas if the diagnosis occurs later, more damage has occurred before therapy begins and the outcome is less favorable (Hockenberry & Wilson, 2007).

SCOLIOSIS

Etiology and Pathophysiology

The most common skeletal deformity of adolescence is scoliosis. The condition is a lateral curvature of the spine that causes changes in the spine, the chest, and the hips. Severe curvature has the potential to affect cardiopulmonary and neurologic function and result in a negative self-image. Scoliosis is possible at any age but is more common in adolescent females.

Clinical Manifestations

The child with idiopathic scoliosis will have unequal hip height and shoulder height, scapular and rib prominence, and a posterior rib hump that is visible when the child bends forward at the waist (Figure 31-24).

Diagnostic Tests

Early identification and treatment of scoliosis are vitally important for a good prognosis. Routine screening of children from 10 to 15 years of age involves posterior observation of the undressed child (bending forward at the waist with arms and head hanging downward) for curvature, asymmetry, and rib hump. Radiographs confirm the diagnosis.

Medical Management

Curvatures of less than 20 degrees necessitate no treatment. Treatment for moderate curvatures consists of bracing, which will potentially slow the progression of scoliosis until the spine is mature. Two types of braces are used to treat scoliosis: the Boston brace and the thoracolumbosacral orthotic (TLSO) brace (Figure 31-25).

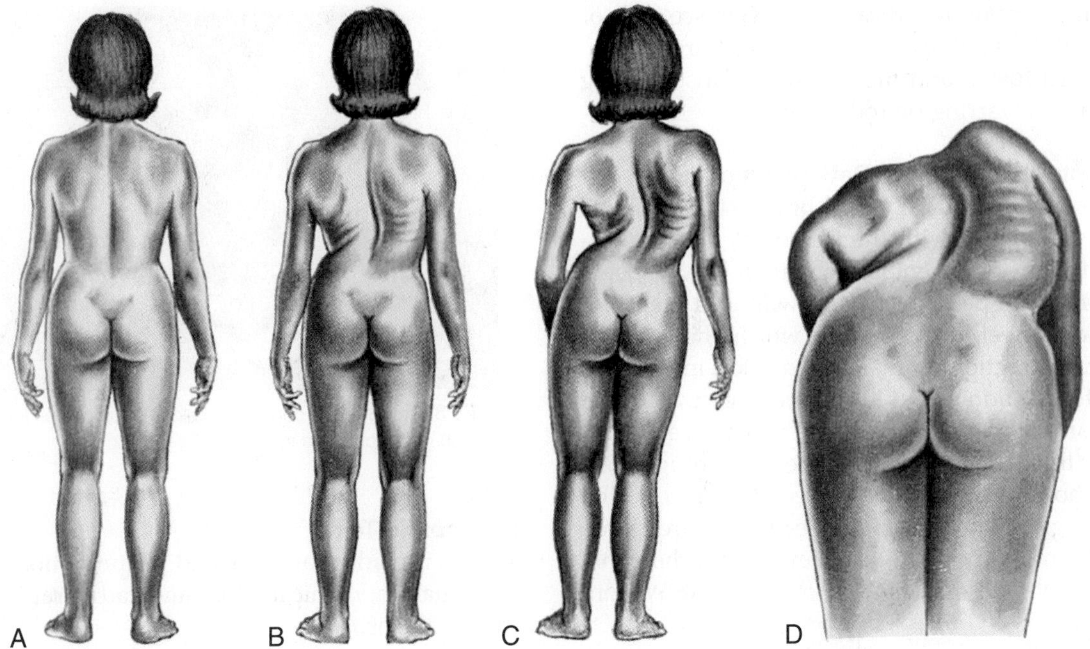

FIGURE 31-24 Scoliosis in children. Normal spinal alignment and abnormal spinal curvatures associated with scoliosis. **A,** Normal. **B,** Mild. **C,** Severe. **D,** Rotation and curvature.

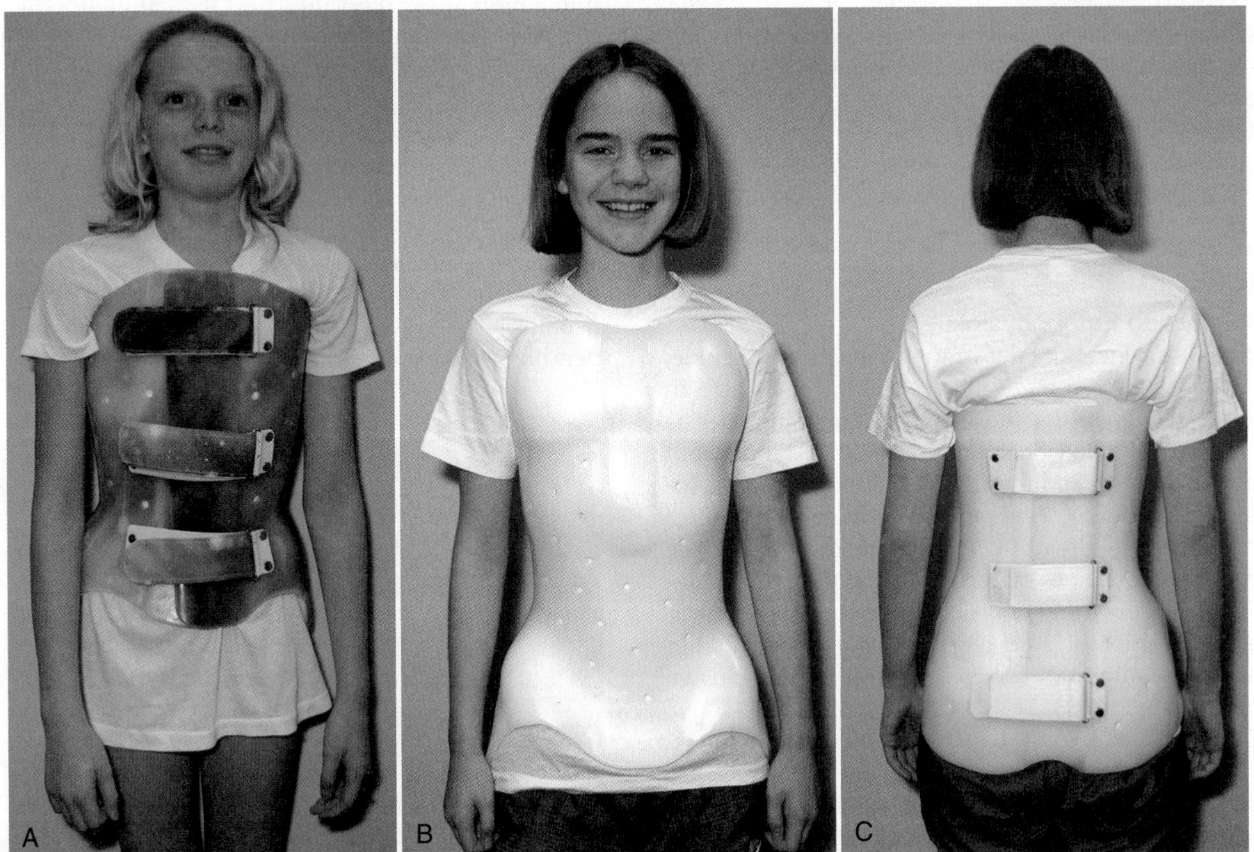

FIGURE 31-25 **A,** Standard thoracolumbosacral orthotic (TLSO) brace for idiopathic scoliosis. Note the color and design incorporated into the brace to make it more acceptable to children and adolescents. **B,** Variation of a standard TLSO brace that fastens in the back **(C)** to provide needed support for the spine curvature.

Surgical intervention is indicated in severe scoliosis or scoliosis that does not respond to bracing. Surgery consists of spinal fusion and the insertion of a stabilizing rod such as the Harrington rod or L-rod.

Nursing Interventions and Patient Teaching

The adolescent who has to wear a brace will often have difficulty complying with the treatment plan. Developmentally, the adolescent is trying to fit in with peers by conforming to peer norms and will need plenty of reassurance to feel attractive and worthwhile during treatment. Instruction on maintaining skin integrity is essential for the adolescent in a brace or cast. Box 31-8 outlines care for the child in a corrective device or cast. Make sure the parents and child receive thorough education in how the appliance corrects the defect, the therapy program, the anticipated results, the freedoms and constraints imposed by the device, and their role in achieving the desired goal (Hockenberry & Wilson, 2007).

Prognosis

Scoliosis if often treated throughout a long period of the child's growth, and prognosis depends on the severity of the condition and compliance with treatment (Hockenberry & Wilson, 2007).

OSTEOMYELITIS

Osteomyelitis is an infection within the bone. In children, the metaphysis of the femur, the tibia, and the humerus are the areas most commonly affected. Although osteomyelitis is possible at any age, the peak incidence in children occurs between ages 3 and 15 years, and boys are affected twice as often as girls (Frank et al., 2005).

TALIPES (CLUBFOOT)

Etiology and Pathophysiology

Talipes is a congenital deformity of the foot and ankle, of which there are many types. The incidence is 1 in every 1000 live births and is twice as high in males as in females. We do not know the cause of talipes, but theories point to an inherited or environmental disorder. The incidence of talipes is also higher in families where there is already a child with the defect. The more flexible talipes deformities are thought to develop from environmental conditions, such as intrauterine positioning and restricted movement within the uterus, although the evidence is not conclusive (Gilmore et al., 2003).

Clinical Manifestations

Talipes varies in severity. Clubfoot sometimes involves one foot (more common) and sometimes both feet. The most common type of clubfoot, **talipes equinovarus,** is when the foot is pointed downward and inward (Figure 31-26).

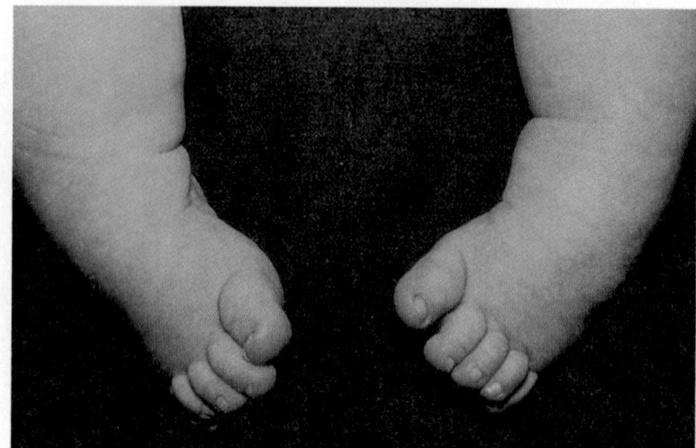

FIGURE 31-26 Bilateral congenital talipes equinovarus (congenital clubfoot) in 2-month-old infant.

Diagnostic Tests

Talipes is evident at birth, and the practitioner will use examination, manipulation, and radiographs to make the diagnosis.

Medical Management

Treatment of talipes consists of manipulation and the application of a series of short leg casts (Figure 31-27). The earlier the treatment begins, the more favorable the outcome. Serial casting begins shortly after birth. The health care provider gently manipulates the foot into a more normal position and then applies a cast to maintain the correction. The practitioner changes the cast weekly to allow for further manipulation and to accommodate the rapidly growing infant. The manipulation and the application of casts continues until marked overcorrection is reached. After completion of the casting series and correction of the deformity, the foot (or feet) will require a combination of passive stretching exercises and corrective splints or shoes to prevent the deformity from recurring. The child will usually have to wear a brace or corrective shoes depending on the surgeon's preference.

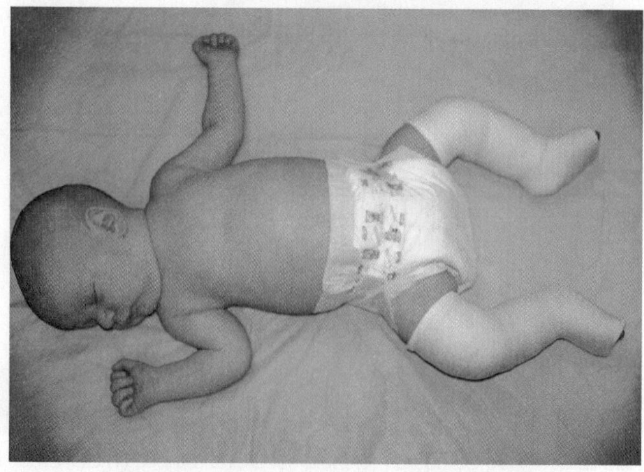

FIGURE 31-27 Feet casted for correction of bilateral congenital talipes equinovarus.

Nursing Interventions and Patient Teaching

After the diagnosis of talipes, parents will need support and education. Very often, parents will need time to adjust to the distressing fact that their child has a deformity. Take every opportunity to educate parents while encouraging them to express their feelings and concerns. Nursing care of the infant with casts is the same for any child in a cast (see Box 31-8). Often neonates receive the cast before discharge from the hospital. Keeping casts clean and dry is relatively easy with a small infant. Have the parents inspect cast edges carefully for rough edges, which will irritate newborn skin. Observe the toes frequently for coldness, pain, blueness, or edema, which, if present, is necessary to report to the physician immediately. Casts are cumbersome and heavy. Assist the parents to find comfortable positions for feeding, playing, and cuddling. Sponge baths are necessary until the infant no longer needs casting. Casts also tend to hinder the infant's ability to kick, move the legs, or roll over. During this time of limited activity, suggest that parents provide audio, visual, and tactile stimulation to encourage normal development. Treatment and follow-up care usually take place on an outpatient basis.

Nursing responsibilities include the teaching of passive stretching exercises with a return demonstration by the parent, if this is part of the treatment plan. Teach parents about cast care and how to handle the infant. Have them perform stretching exercises several times a day; many parents find it easier to remember to do the exercises if they do them together with another regular activity such as diaper changing or after feedings.

Prognosis

Some feet respond to treatment rapidly; some respond only to prolonged, vigorous, and sustained efforts; and the improvement in others remains disappointing even with maximum effort on the part of all concerned. Serial casting achieves the most reliable correction of talipes equinovarus.

DUCHENNE'S MUSCULAR DYSTROPHY

Etiology and Pathophysiology

Duchenne's muscular dystrophy (DMD) is a sex-linked inherited disorder whose defining characteristic is gradually progressive skeletal muscle wasting and weakness. DMD is the most severe and most common form of all dystrophies. The onset of signs and symptoms occurs between ages 2 and 4.

Clinical Manifestations

Initial signs and symptoms, which are mild and progress gradually, are easy to overlook. Parents tend to be the first to notice that the child is clumsy, frequently falls, has a waddling gait, and experiences difficulty running, climbing, and riding a bicycle. The muscles of the pelvic girdle are frequently involved, and the child shows evidence of this weakness by rising from the floor in a classic manner. The child lies on the side and flexes the knees (or gets on all fours), then extends the knees and uses the hands to "walk up" the thighs (Gowers' sign). As the disorder progresses, there is severe muscle wasting, resulting in contractures and deformities. By 12 years of age, ambulation is no longer possible. Respiratory tract infection usually occurs in the final stages when the diaphragm and the accessory muscles used in respiration become affected.

Diagnostic Tests

The health care provider considers the possibility of DMD based on the clinical signs and symptoms and the family history. Electromyogram (EMG), elevated serum creatine phosphokinase (CPK), elevated aspartate aminotransferase (AST), and muscle biopsy that reveals fibrous and fatty tissue confirm the diagnosis.

Medical Management

There is no effective treatment to arrest DMD. Therefore the goals are to maintain ambulation and independence for as long as possible. Physical therapy serves to optimize ROM and delay muscle atrophy; the use of braces sometimes helps to provide additional support; and surgical intervention to release contractures is another element of management.

Nursing Interventions and Patient Teaching

The most important nursing consideration in the care of a child with DMD is to assist the child and the family in developing positive coping strategies to deal with the progressively debilitating aspects of the illness and reduce anticipatory grieving. The goal is to maintain independence for as long as possible. Because of the progressive nature of the illness, you will need to assess the child's capabilities frequently. The care of a child with DMD, or any child with a chronic, debilitating terminal illness, is extremely demanding and stressful for the family. You are in a position to help the family lessen their anxiety and fears through teaching and active listening. A referral to the Muscular Dystrophy Association of America opens the door to a number of supplementary services to patients and their families.

Help the family plan an exercise program to encourage muscle strength and delay the onset of some of the physical disabilities. Counsel the family about good nutrition to prevent obesity, which will sometimes cause the child to become prematurely wheelchair bound.

Prognosis

Children rarely live past age 20, with death resulting from respiratory or cardiac complications.

SEPTIC ARTHRITIS (SEPTIC JOINT, SUPPURATIVE ARTHRITIS)

Etiology and Pathophysiology

Septic arthritis (septic joint, suppurative arthritis) is an infection of a joint, which possibly arises from bacteria in the blood or as a direct extension of an existing infection such as osteomyelitis. Bites (human, cat, dog, rat, or tick) are a frequent cause of septic arthritis. The infection causes joint irritation and damage to the synovial membrane; synovial fluid increases and causes distention within the joint. As the infection progresses, pus accumulates and breaks down the articulating cartilage (which does not have the capacity to regenerate) and leads to permanent damage. In infancy, the incidence of septic arthritis occurs equally among boys and girls; in the adolescent age-group, it occurs predominantly in males. The joints most commonly affected are hip, knee, shoulder, wrist, and ankle. In the neonatal group, the causative organisms include group B streptococci and gram-negative enterics (pertaining to the intestine); in the 6 months to 5 years age-group, *H. influenzae* (incidence has decreased in recent years owing to the *H. influenzae* vaccine); over 5 years of age, *S. aureus;* and in adolescents, *Neisseria gonorrhoeae.*

Clinical Manifestations

The affected joint is erythematous, edematous, warm, and exquisitely painful. There is usually limited ROM. The child maintains the extremities in a flexed position. If the lower extremities are involved, the child will often limp or refuse to walk. Except in infants, fever is usually present. Septic arthritis occurs very rapidly and is considered a medical emergency.

Diagnostic Tests

Radiographic examination will possibly reveal joint edema. The health care provider will aspirate the joint, and send purulent matter for Gram stain examination and culture. Performance of a blood culture is necessary. A peripheral blood smear will show leukocytosis and elevated ESR in children; infants do not always demonstrate this finding.

Medical Management

Joint aspiration and surgical irrigation are essential to managing the condition. Surgical drainage and irrigation ensure that the joint will be decompressed, safeguarding the vasculature, and will clear the joint of destructive purulent matter, eradicate the infection, and prevent secondary bloodborne spread of infection. The practitioner will initiate broad-spectrum IV antibiotic therapy and switch it to more specific antibiotics once the laboratory has identified the organism. IV therapy will continue for 10 to 14 days; once there is a good IV response, it is possible to change over to oral antibiotics. Oral therapy will continue to complete a 4-week course.

Nursing Interventions

The nursing interventions are the same as that for the child with osteomyelitis.

Prognosis

If the hip joint is involved, where it is possible for avascular necrosis to develop and cause deformity, long-term disability will possibly result.

FRACTURES

Although it is possible to fracture any bone, the most common fracture sites in children include the long bones of the extremities, the clavicles, the wrists, the fingers, and the skull. Fractures vary from complete (bone and periosteum separate completely) to incomplete or greenstick (the bone splits but does not completely break). Spiral fractures affect the length rather than the width of the bone and are frequently the result of child abuse.

Nursing Interventions

It is essential for health care providers to diligently remain alert for signs of the physical abuse of a child. Physical abuse has the potential to result in fractures and dislocations.

Assessing the child with a possible traumatic injury involves assessment of the injury and soft tissue damage. The first priority is to calm and reassure the child and the parents so that the assessment is possible. Once the child has calmed down, assess for pain and point of tenderness, color, sensation, motion, and pulses distal to the injury. If the injury necessitates casting, you will have specific nursing measures to institute. It is also necessary to address pain; alleviate it with the use of comfort measures and analgesics ordered by the physician. If the injury requires correction by traction, nursing interventions include maintaining skin integrity and monitoring skeletal traction sites for infection. Also observe for complications of immobility, especially circulatory compromise and muscle spasms. Encourage deep-breathing exercises; blowing bubbles or balloons (under supervision) offer a way to make this activity fun for the child.

DISORDERS OF NEUROLOGIC FUNCTION

Disorders that affect neurologic function fall into three major categories: (1) increased intracranial pressure, (2) hypoxia, and (3) seizure activity. The residual effects of neurologic disorders often have profound effects on the child's function and future performance. It is essential to identify neurologic impairments at an early stage so that it is possible to properly diagnose them and institute interventions.

MENINGITIS

Meningitis is a significant cause of illness in the pediatric age-group. Meningitis is an infection of the meninges. Most cases affect children younger than 5 years of age. Its importance lies primarily in the frequency with which it occurs in infancy and childhood and the unnecessarily high death rates and residual damage caused by undiagnosed and untreated or inadequately treated cases.

Etiology and Pathophysiology

Although a number of bacterial, viral, and fungal organisms have the capacity to cause meningitis, bacterial meningitis is the most common. The advent of antimicrobial therapy has had a marked effect on the course and prognosis of bacterial meningitis, although the use of vaccine against *H. influenzae* type B (Hib vaccine), beginning in 1990, led to the most dramatic decrease in bacterial meningitis of the *H. influenzae* type. However, bacterial meningitis caused by other organisms remains a serious illness in children. Organisms generally spread to the meninges following an upper respiratory infection, by lymphatic drainage, or by direct deposit through a lumbar puncture or skull fracture. Following invasion of the meninges by an organism, it enters the cerebrospinal fluid (CSF) and travels throughout the subarachnoid space, spreading the infection. As the meninges become infected, an inflammatory process ensues, causing a thick exudate and WBC accumulation. With continued inflammation, CSF flow becomes occluded and the brain becomes hyperemic (increased blood to a part) and edematous.

Clinical Manifestations

The manifestations of meningitis sometimes occur insidiously and sometimes suddenly, beginning with fever, vomiting, headache, irritability, photophobia, and nuchal rigidity (pain and stiffness in the neck when flexed) or opisthotonos (arched back); the manifestations progress in some cases to decreased level of consciousness and seizures. Infants typically exhibit a bulging fontanelle and a characteristic high-pitched cry. Classic signs of meningeal irritation include a positive **Kernig's sign** (resistance to knee extension in the supine position with the hips and knees flexed against the torso) and a positive **Brudzinski's sign** (flexion of the knees and hips when the neck is flexed rapidly onto the chest). Meningococcal meningitis, the most readily transmissible type of meningitis, sometimes also produces petechiae and rapidly progresses to death without prompt initiation of proper treatment.

Diagnostic Tests

The physician makes the diagnosis of meningitis through a carefully obtained history and physical and by analysis of CSF obtained by a lumbar puncture. The practitioner will obtain a CSF sample for culture and sensitivity. Findings that indicate a bacterial infection include presence of a bacterial organism, elevated WBC count, elevated protein level, and decreased glucose level. The physician will obtain a CT scan of the head if there is evidence of increased intracranial pressure, signs of which include papilledema, neurologic deficits, and bulging fontanelle. Increased intracranial pressure contraindicates the performance of a lumbar puncture owing to the possibility of causing herniation of the brainstem (Hockenberry & Wilson, 2007).

Medical Management

The management of bacterial meningitis involves immediate IV administration of appropriate antibiotic therapy. Therapy usually continues for at least 10 days or until the CSF culture is negative. Usually, the child will be in the intensive care unit and in isolation until appropriate antibiotic therapy has been under way for at least 24 hours.

The physician will order antibiotic agents, fluids, and antiseizure medications via an intravenous infusion (Hockenberry & Wilson, 2007). The choice of antibiotic is based on the known sensitivity. Appropriate hydration, antipyretics, and comfort measures are an important aspect of management. Closely observe the child for complications of meningitis, including seizures, disseminated intravascular coagulation syndrome, and shock. Institute safety measures, because the child will possibly develop seizures. After discharge, the health care provider will follow the child closely to assess for any sequelae of the disease, such as hearing impairments and cognitive, perceptual, language, and behavioral problems.

Nursing Interventions and Patient Teaching

Initial nursing interventions focus on rapid identification of the child with meningitis and prompt institution of appropriate antibiotic therapy. If meningitis is suspected, the priority nursing intervention is to administer antibiotics as soon as possible after they have been ordered (Hockenberry & Wilson, 2007). An hour before the performance of a lumbar puncture, apply EMLA (eutectic mixture of local anesthetics), a topical anesthetic cream, to the skin overlying L3 to L5 vertebrae. It reduces pain for children undergoing this procedure. Take all necessary isolation precautions to prevent the spread of the disease to yourself and others.

Promote rest for the child in the initial phase of the disease, and keep environmental stimuli (especially noise and bright lights) to a minimum. The child is likely to be most comfortable without a pillow and with the head of the bed elevated. Observe vital signs, level of consciousness, I&O, and neurologic signs at frequent intervals. Support families throughout the course of the disease; they are usually unprepared for the sudden acuteness of the disease and will perhaps feel guilty for not recognizing it earlier.

Prevention

The spread of bacterial meningitis is possible to avoid in the exposed siblings by prescribing prophylactic rifampin. Primary prevention strategies consist of vaccine administration.

There are several meningitis immunizations now available including *H. influenza* type b and pneumococcal conjugate for children beginning at 2 months of age. Vaccine for types A, C, Y, and W-135 meningococci is available. Meningococcal polysaccharide vaccination is available for children 2 years and older (Pichichero, 2005). The FDA licensed the new quadrivalent meningococcal conjugate vaccine (Menactra) in January 2005 for children and adults from 11 to 55 years (Pichichero, 2005). The mortality rate associated with bacterial meningitis is high, but early immunization promises to spare families from experiencing the tragic death of a child from this cause. You will play a significant role in educating families regarding preventive measures such as early *H. influenzae* type b vaccinations.

Prognosis

Although antimicrobial therapy will often have a significant effect on the course of meningitis, it remains a potentially life-threatening disease. The age of the child, the type of causative organism, the severity of the infection, the duration of the illness before the onset of therapy, and the sensitivity of the organism to antimicrobial drugs are important factors in the prognosis. Residual deficits are possible, including communicating hydrocephalus and possible hearing loss, blindness, seizures, learning disorders, and attention deficit disorder.

ENCEPHALITIS

Encephalitis is defined as an inflammation of the CNS, namely, the brain tissue and the spinal cord. The course of the disease closely resembles that of meningitis, and the care for each is similar.

Etiology and Pathophysiology

A variety of organisms have the capacity to cause encephalitis, such as bacteria, spirochetes, fungi, protozoa, and viruses. Most cases of encephalitis occur as a result of direct invasion of the CNS by a virus or from postinfectious involvement after a viral illness, such as measles, mumps, or varicella.

Clinical Manifestations

The manifestations of encephalitis sometimes begin gradually and sometimes suddenly and possibly include malaise, fever, headache, dizziness, nuchal rigidity, nausea, vomiting, ataxia, tremors, seizures, and coma, and in some cases proceed to death.

Diagnostic Tests

The physician bases the diagnosis of encephalitis on clinical manifestations associated with the disease and, if possible, identification of the virus. Laboratory detection of the virus is possible through serologic tests or CSF cultures.

Medical Management

The practitioner will promptly hospitalize the child suspected of having encephalitis for strict observation and supportive care. Treatment is primarily supportive. Management focuses on controlling fever, ensuring adequate hydration and nutrition, monitoring vital signs, and observing for complications.

Nursing Interventions and Patient Teaching

Nursing interventions for the child with encephalitis are the same as those for the child with meningitis. The major focus of care is on administering medication, controlling fever, monitoring neurologic status and vital signs, and providing emotional support to the child and the family.

Follow-up care with periodic reevaluation and rehabilitation are important for survivors with residual effects of the disease. Encourage the parents to keep appointments for follow-up examinations.

Prognosis

The prognosis depends on the child's age, the type of organism, and any residual neurologic damage. Children younger than 2 years of age sometimes exhibit increased neurologic disability, including learning disabilities and seizure disorders.

HYDROCEPHALUS

Hydrocephalus is a condition whose defining characteristic is an excess of fluid within the cranial vault, the subarachnoid space, or both. It is caused by an imbalance between the production and the absorption of CSF within the ventricular system. Development of hydrocephalus is possible during infancy (as a congenital lesion) and through adulthood.

Etiology and Pathophysiology

Hydrocephalus is caused by increased production of CSF, by obstruction within the ventricular system (noncommunicating hydrocephalus; no passage of fluid between the ventricles), or by defective reabsorption of the CSF (communicating hydrocephalus; passage of CSF between the ventricles). Overproduction of CSF arises most commonly owing to a tumor in the choroid plexus. Obstruction within the ventricular system is most frequently due to atresia (the absence of a normal body opening, duct, or canal), most commonly along the aqueduct of Sylvius (Figure 31-28). Other causes of obstruction include a hemorrhage, a growing tumor, or an infection. Defects in the body's reabsorptive process are sometimes caused by an extensive hemorrhage within the subarachnoid space, which obscures the absorptive surface of the membrane.

As CSF accumulates within the cranium, the brain is compressed against the skull and the ventricular system becomes dilated, increasing intracranial pressure (see Figure 31-28). If hydrocephalus occurs before

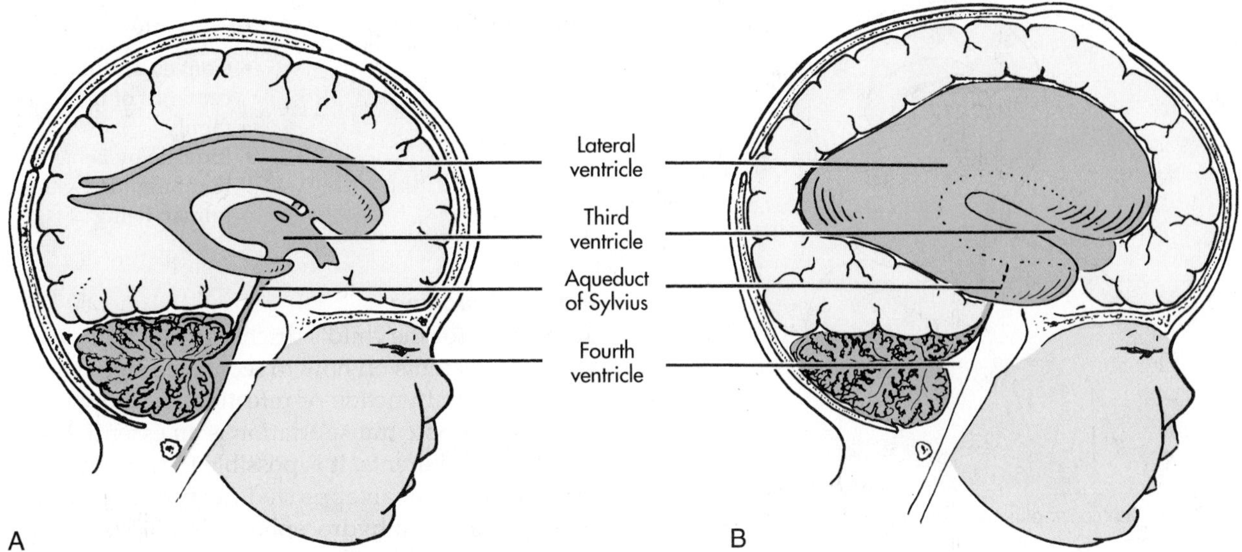

FIGURE 31-28 Hydrocephalus: an occlusion in flow of cerebrospinal fluid. **A,** Patent cerebrospinal fluid circulation. **B,** Enlarged lateral and third ventricles caused by obstruction of cerebral spinal fluid circulation—at the aqueduct of Sylvius.

the fusion of the cranial sutures, the skull becomes markedly enlarged (Figure 31-29).

Clinical Manifestations

In early infancy, manifestations of hydrocephalus include widening and bulging of the fontanelles, separation of the cranial sutures, dilation of scalp veins, thin and shiny scalp, and rapidly increasing head circumference. As CSF accumulation continues, frontal bossing (prominence of the forehead) becomes apparent. Other manifestations are depressed eyes with setting sun sign (sclera is seen above the iris), slow pupil response to light, irritability, high-pitched cry, difficulty in being consoled, lethargy, altered level of consciousness, and difficulty in sucking and feeding. In children, manifestations will possibly include headache on awakening, hyperactive reflexes, strabismus, unsteady gait, irritability, papilledema (edema of the optic disk), lethargy, disorientation, and progression to stupor.

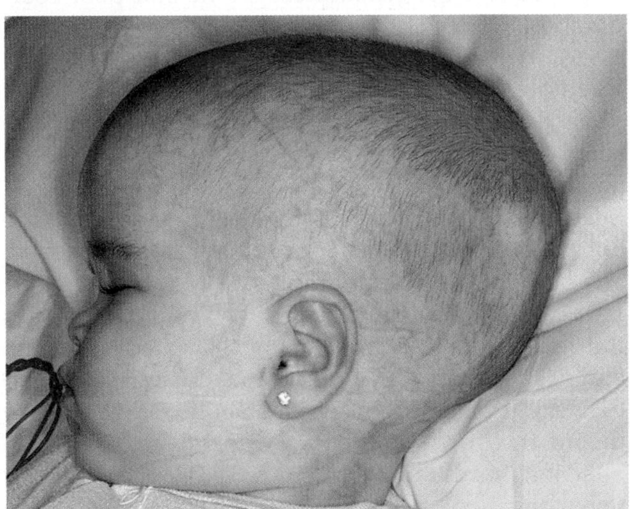

FIGURE 31-29 Child with enlarged head caused by hydrocephalus.

Diagnostic Tests

In infants, measurement of the head circumference is the most important diagnostic technique. It is important to measure the head circumference routinely in all infants. Any measurement that crosses one or more grid lines within a 2- to 4-week period is suggestive of hydrocephalus. Other diagnostic assessments include observation of neurologic signs that indicate the possibility of increased intracranial pressure, computed tomography (CT) scan, and MRI.

Medical Management

Treatment of hydrocephalus involves therapy to relieve ventricular pressure, treatment to correct the cause of the ventriculomegaly, treatment of complications, and assistance with the problems resulting from the effect of hydrocephalus on psychomotor development (Hockenberry & Wilson, 2007). If a tumor is the cause of hydrocephalus, the surgeon will remove it. If the cause of the hydrocephalus is obstruction, the treatment involves surgical shunting of excess CSF from the ventricles to the peritoneum with a ventriculoperitoneal shunt (VP shunt) (Figure 31-30). Revisions in the VP shunt are needed when the shunt malfunctions, becomes infected, or becomes too short as the child grows.

Nursing Interventions

Nursing interventions for the child with hydrocephalus involve assisting with prompt diagnosis, observing for complications of the disease and shunt placement, and providing support and education to the family. Nutrition is likely to become an issue if intracranial pressure increases. Avoid handling the child before,

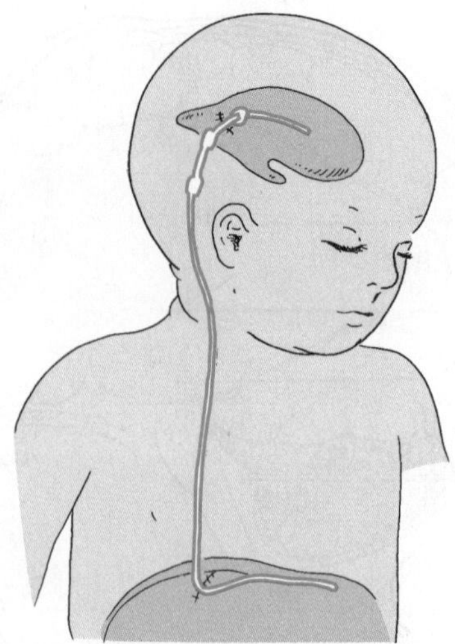

FIGURE 31-30 Ventricular peritoneal shunt. Catheter is threaded subcutaneously from small incisions at the sites of ventricular and peritoneal insertions.

during, and after feedings because it will sometimes lead to vomiting. Small, frequent feedings are usually better tolerated, and it is best to place infants on their sides after feedings to avoid aspiration. Postoperatively, observe the child for signs of increasing intracranial pressure, assess vital signs, and closely monitor I&O. Usually you will place the child on the nonoperative side to avoid putting pressure on the shunt site. Perform meticulous skin care, especially to the scalp, both preoperatively and postoperatively. Place a sheepskin under the child's head, and change the child's position every 2 hours. Support the family during the hospitalization and prepare them for discharge.

Nursing diagnoses and interventions for the child with hydrocephalus include but are not limited to the following:

Nursing Diagnoses	Nursing Interventions
Risk for infection, related to presence of mechanical drainage system	Perform hand hygiene before contact with patient. Limit visitors to reduce the number of organisms in patient's environment, and restrict visitation by individuals with any type of infection. Encourage adequate diet to maintain optimal nutritional status. Maintain asepsis for dressing changes and wound care.
Interrupted family processes, related to situational crisis (child with a physical defect)	Facilitate family's acceptance of infant: • Allow expression of feelings • Convey attitude of acceptance of infant and family • Indicate by behavior that infant is a valuable human being

Patient Teaching

To prepare for the child's discharge and home care, instruct the parents on how to recognize signs that indicate shunt malfunction or infection and how to pump if necessary. Safe transportation is an essential issue to discuss with parents. It is possible to restrain small infants reclining in an approved car bed. It is important to emphasize that hydrocephalus is a lifelong problem and that the child will require evaluation on a regular basis. The overall aim is to establish realistic goals and an appropriate educational program that will assist the child to achieve optimal potential.

Prognosis

The prognosis of children with treated hydrocephalus depends largely on the rate at which hydrocephalus develops, the duration of raised intracranial pressure, the frequency of complications, and the cause of hydrocephalus. With prompt diagnosis and proper shunt functioning, the survival rate for children with hydrocephalus is 80%.

CEREBRAL PALSY

Cerebral palsy (CP) is the most common permanent physical disability of childhood, affecting 1.2 to 3 in every 1000 live births (Ashwal et al., 2004). CP is a general term for a group of nonprogressive disorders of motoneuron impairment that result in motor dysfunction. In addition, the affected child will also sometimes exhibit intellectual, visual, language, and neurologic impairments. The primary manifestations of CP involve abnormal muscle tone and poor coordination.

Etiology and Pathophysiology

Many antenatal, perinatal, and postnatal factors share some of the responsibility in the etiology of CP. Antenatal factors include maternal nutritional deficiencies, infections, maternal drug ingestion, maternal metabolic disturbances, maternal hemorrhage, toxemia, and blood incompatibilities. Perinatal factors include cerebral trauma and anoxia during birth. Anoxia plays the most significant role in the pathology of brain damage. Anesthesia or analgesia during labor and delivery, prematurity, and metabolic or electrolyte disturbances are also factors. Postnatal factors include infection, head trauma, cerebrovascular accident, and poisoning.

Clinical Manifestations

The clinical manifestations of CP range from moderate to severe and are described in Box 31-9.

Diagnostic Tests

The diagnosis of CP is based on history and physical examination. A careful antenatal and birth history is necessary to obtain from the mother and documented. A thorough neurologic examination is an essential component of the physical examination process and often aids in establishing a diagnosis of CP. Additional tests will possibly include CT scan, cranial sonogram, electroencephalogram (EEG), and a serum metabolic screening.

Medical Management

There is no specific treatment for CP. Children with CP benefit from the integrated efforts of occupational, physical, and speech and hearing therapists. Care for the child is provided in the home and at an early-intervention center where children benefit from specialized services and parents have the opportunity to support each other. Some orthopedic abnormalities, such as functional scoliosis and tendon lengthening, sometimes necessitate corrective surgery, casting, or bracing in order to accomplish the following (Hockenberry & Wilson, 2007):

1. Development of ambulatory strength
2. Promotion of self-care
3. Functional independence
4. Integration of motor function
5. Improvement of appearance
6. Lessening of associated defects to the extent possible
7. Assistance in providing educational experiences according to the child's needs
8. Encouragement of socialization with unaffected and affected children

Botulinum toxin (Botox) has become an important drug in the treatment of spasticity for CP. Botox is injected into the muscle, where it acts to inhibit the release of acetylcholine into a specific muscle group, thereby preventing muscle movement. When administered early in the course of the disease, it is often possible to prevent contractures, particularly in lower extremities, and prevent surgical procedures with possible adverse effects. The goal is to allow stretching of the muscle as it relaxes and permit ambulation with an ankle-foot orthosis (AFO). The major reported adverse effect of Botox injection is pain at the injection site.

Intrathecal baclofen therapy is best suited for children with severe spasticity that interferes with activities of daily living and ambulation. A neurosurgeon performs the implantation procedure in the operating room, optimally in a multidisciplinary setting in which rehabilitation specialists are readily available and consistently involved in the patient's ongoing care (Hockenberry & Wilson, 2007).

Box 31-9 Clinical Manifestations of Cerebral Palsy

- Delayed gross motor development
- Involuntary movements
- Hypertonic muscles
- Poor sucking
- Feeding difficulties
- Persistence of primitive reflexes
- Exaggerated deep tendon reflexes
- Arching of back
- Vision and hearing impairments
- Extension and scissoring of lower extremities
- Developmental disabilities

Nursing Interventions

Nursing interventions for the child with CP focus on early recognition and prompt institution of interventions aimed at providing optimum development. Facilitate eating with the use of adaptive eating utensils. Encourage self-feeding and a high-calorie diet. It is important to encourage mobilization. Devices such as braces, wheeled scooters, and walkers are available to assist with mobility. Encourage use of protective headgear when a child is first learning to walk. It is important to praise children when goals are attained and encourage them to be as independent as possible within their limitations.

Nursing diagnoses and interventions for the child with CP include but are not limited to the following:

Nursing Diagnoses	Nursing Interventions
Impaired physical mobility, related to neuromuscular impairment	Encourage sitting, crawling, and walking at appropriate ages. Carry out therapies that strengthen and improve control. Assist child in using appropriate leg motions when learning to walk. Provide incentives to locomote. Ensure that the child is rested before attempting locomotion activities. Incorporate play that encourages desired behavior. Employ aids that facilitate locomotion such as parallel bars, crutches.

Continued

Nursing Diagnoses	Nursing Interventions
Self-care deficit, bathing/hygiene, feeding, toileting, related to physical disability	Encourage child to assist with care as age and capabilities permit. Select toys and activities that allow maximum participation by child and that improve motor function and sensory input. Assist with jaw control during feeding. Adapt utensils, foods, and clothing to facilitate self-help (e.g., large-bowled spoon with padded handle; finger foods and foods that adhere to, rather than slip from, utensil; and clothing that opens in front with self-adhering closings rather than buttons). Assist parents in toilet training child.

Patient Teaching

Teach parents proper handling of their children and how to assist them with ADLs. Teach the family to perform stretching and passive ROM exercises and to select play activities that provide for maximum stimulation and participation. Also educate parents about the disorder and the resources available to them so that they are able to ensure optimal development for their child.

Prognosis

CP is a chronic neurologic disability. There is no cure, but promotion of an optimal developmental course is vital so that the child is able to realize full potential within the limits of the brain dysfunction.

SEIZURE DISORDERS

Etiology and Pathophysiology

The term *seizure* refers to a sudden, excessive, disorderly discharge of abnormal electrical impulses by the brain's neurons, causing a temporary alteration in CNS function. Most seizures are idiopathic (no identifiable cause). Some seizures are acquired and result from such conditions as tumors, trauma, hypoxia, infections, poisons, fever, and metabolic disturbances. Children are most prone to seizures during the period between birth and 2 years. Approximately 5% of children will experience at least one seizure before adolescence. Epilepsy or recurrent seizures affect 1% to 2% of all children (Hockenberry & Wilson, 2007). The current classification system divides seizures into two major categories: partial and generalized. All children with seizure activity will have an EEG, which is the most useful tool for evaluating seizure disorders.

Medical Management

The treatment of seizure disorders primarily involves drug therapy. Anticonvulsants that are most valuable in controlling partial or generalized seizures include carbamazepine (Tegretol), phenytoin (Dilantin), fosphenytoin (Cerebyx), and valproic acid (Depakote or Depakene). The drugs of choice for absence seizures are ethosuximide (Zarontin) and valproic acid. Reducing polypharmacy helps provide a better quality of life, therefore experts currently recommend single-drug therapy. Several new drugs that give increased seizure control in many children include gabapentin (Neurontin), lamotrigine (Lamictal), and felbamate (Felbatol). The use of felbamate is controversial because of the side effects of aplastic anemia and hepatic failure. The initial treatment of status epilepticus focuses on supporting and maintaining vital functions, including securing a patent airway, administering oxygen, establishing venous access, providing hydration, and administering lorazepam (Ativan), diazepam (Valium), or phenobarbital, as ordered. After the continuous seizure is stopped, the child will possible receive a loading dose of phenytoin to ensure sustained control of seizures.

Anticonvulsant therapy continues for a prolonged period. The physician will modify the dosage as the child grows. In children with a normal EEG who have been seizure free for at least 2 years, it is possible to discontinue anticonvulsant medications without increasing the risk of seizure recurrence. Discontinuing the medication gradually over 1 to 2 weeks is best. Abrupt withdrawal of anticonvulsants has the potential to result in an increase in the number and severity of seizures and sometimes even precipitates an episode of status epilepticus.

Nursing Interventions

Nursing interventions for the child with a seizure disorder involve assisting with the diagnosis, providing acute care during a seizure, providing for long-term management of the seizure disorder, and supporting and assisting the child and the family. To assist with the diagnosis of a seizure disorder, it is essential to observe the child during a seizure and carefully document events, including any precipitating factors, if known or suspected; behavior before the seizure; time seizure began and ended; clinical manifestations of the seizure; and postseizure behavior and signs and symptoms. It is important to recognize precipitating factors and prevent or reduce to a minimum the child's exposure to them. It is important to protect the child from injury during a seizure. Measures to prevent injuries during a seizure include padding the bed side rails and keeping the side rails upright, easing the child to the floor from a sitting or standing position, moving furniture out of the way, loosening restrictive clothing, and turning the child's head to the side to prevent aspiration of secretions. It is important not to force an object (e.g., tongue blade, airway) between the child's teeth during a seizure because doing so sometimes causes oral trauma. Staying with the child during and after a seizure and providing reassurance, emotional support, and explanations will help keep the child's anxiety to a minimum. A significant nursing goal is to promote a positive self-image in the child through encouragement and identification of the child's strengths and assets. Providing emotional support to the family is also essential. Encourage parents to express their fears and concerns and assist them to understand their child's condition. The family needs education regarding the nature of the disorder and possible precipitating factors, seizure precaution measures, dosage and side effects of medications, and the importance of maintaining as normal a lifestyle as possible.

Patient Teaching

It is important to impress on the family the need to continue the medication regularly, without interruption, for as long as required. Help the parents plan the administration of the medication at convenient times to keep disruption of family routine to a minimum. Most neurologists prefer patients to take anticonvulsant medications in tablet or capsule form for more equal and accurate distribution of the medication. During periods of growth, medication dosage will need adjustment.

Prognosis

It is possible to control or greatly reduce the incidence of seizures in the majority of children, and new studies hold the promise of progress in future treatment. Seizures will not shorten the life of the child, and the child is able to attend school, marry, and elect to have children.

SPINA BIFIDA (MYELOMENINGOCELE)

Spina bifida is a term that describes a variety of congenital defects of **neural tube** (tube formed from the fusion of the neural folds from which the brain and spinal cord arise) closure. When the neural tube fails to close during embryonic development, a defect arises that will involve anything from a small area of the neural tube to its entire length. In spina bifida occulta, the infant will likely have a tuft of hair, cleft, or small, fatty mass over the defect. Myelomeningocele is one form of spina bifida whereby portions of the spinal cord, the meninges, spinal fluid, and nerves protrude through the neural tube defect.

Etiology and Pathophysiology

The etiology of neural tube defects is generally unknown. Poor nutrition and advanced maternal age have been implicated as contributing factors. Evidence supports the theory that neural tube defects arise out of the interaction of a genetic predisposition with an essential nutrient deficiency (folic acid) and that multivitamins containing folic acid taken during the first 6 weeks of pregnancy will prevent (by more than 50%) their occurrence (AAP, 1999).

Clinical Manifestations

Because the spinal cord most commonly ends at the defect, all motor and sensory function beyond the defect is absent. Most myelomeningoceles involve the lumbar and lumbosacral areas. Depending on the level of the defect, the infant will usually have flaccid paralysis and sensory deficits of the lower extremities, bowel and bladder incontinence, clubfoot defects, and a subluxated hip (a partial or incomplete dislocation of the hip). Hydrocephalus is present in 80% of affected infants.

Diagnostic Tests

It is sometimes possible to detect a neural tube defect prenatally. Uterine ultrasound and elevated maternal **alpha-fetoprotein (AFP)** (antigen present in the human fetus that helps in evaluating fetal development) level sometimes indicate the presence of a myelomeningocele. After birth, the health care provider makes the diagnosis on the basis of clinical manifestations. In some cases, the practitioners will order a CT scan to assess for the presence of hydrocephalus.

Medical Management

Treatment for the infant with myelomeningocele involves surgery to replace the neural contents within the sac to eliminate the possibility of infection. Sometimes it is necessary to insert a VP shunt to provide relief from hydrocephalus. Corrective surgeries are sometimes necessary to manage hip and lower extremity deformities. Additional measures include continuous neurologic assessments and assisting the family to deal with the diagnosis and surgery.

Nursing Interventions and Patient Teaching

Nursing interventions for the child with myelomeningocele focus on preventing infection and complications, providing postoperative care, and supporting and educating the family. Box 31-10 describes nursing interventions for the child with myelomeningocele.

Box 31-10 Nursing Interventions for the Child with Myelomeningocele

PREOPERATIVE

- Position child on abdomen.
- Cover sac with sterile, saline-soaked gauze.
- Protect sac from contact with feces and urine.

POSTOPERATIVE

- Position child on abdomen for 10 to 14 days (until incision is healed).
- Monitor vital signs.
- Observe for signs of bleeding and infection.

Parents will need explanations regarding their child's condition and the surgery it necessitates. Encourage family members to express their fears and concerns, and advise them of resources within their community that provide support and services for families of children with spinal defects.

Because the parents will continue at home the care that began in the hospital, they will need instruction on positioning, feeding, bowel training, bladder catheterization, and physical exercises.

Prognosis

The early prognosis for the child with myelomeningocele depends on the neurologic deficits present at birth, including motor ability, bladder and bowel innervation, and the presence of associated cerebral anomalies. Improved surgical techniques do not alter the major physical disability and deformity, nor the chronic urinary tract and pulmonary infections and constipation that affect the quality of life for these children.

NEONATAL ABSTINENCE SYNDROME

Because opioids readily cross the placental membrane, women who use drugs while they are pregnant cause a passive addiction in their unborn children. Opioids commonly abused by women during pregnancy include cocaine, "crack," heroin, and methadone. Shortly after birth, the infant exhibits signs and symptoms of drug withdrawal, including irritability, disturbed sleeping and feeding patterns, tremors, seizures, hyperreflexia (increased reflex reaction), clonus (abnormal neuromuscular activity characterized by rapidly alternating involuntary contraction and relaxation of skeletal muscles), high-pitched cry, hypertonic muscles, tachypnea, frantic sucking of hands, vomiting, diarrhea, and inability to maintain body temperature. Signs and symptoms of opioid withdrawal sometimes persist for 3 to 4 months. Usually the health care provider will order infants suspected of having opioid abstinence syndrome to have their urine analyzed for metabolites of the drug. It is essential to obtain a urine sample from the infant immediately after birth because the by-products of the drugs are quickly cleared from the body.

Infants who are experiencing neonatal abstinence syndrome are most comfortable in a nonstimulating environment that is free from bright lights and loud noises. They often prefer to be tightly swaddled in a blanket, with a pacifier to satisfy their vigorous sucking needs. It is essential to monitor the infant's I&O and vital signs. Organize nursing interventions in a manner that reduces the amount of disturbance to the infant.

On discharge, infants will need referral to an early intervention program because they are at risk for neurologic problems; parent-infant bonding difficulties; and developmental, behavioral, and learning disabilities. Mothers will need referral for parental education and drug treatment programs to enable an optimal outcome for both the child and family.

NEUROBLASTOMA

Neuroblastoma is a malignant tumor composed principally of cells resembling neuroblasts that give rise to cells of the sympathetic nervous system. After brain tumors, neuroblastomas are the most common solid tumors in childhood, with an incidence of approximately 1 per 10,000 children per year. More than 50% of the cases occur in children younger than 2 years, and 75% are encountered during the first 4 years of life. Neuroblastoma is a malignant tumor that has a high rate of dissemination, with 70% of patients having metastasis at the time of presentation (Weinstein et al., 2003).

Etiology and Pathophysiology

These tumors originate from embryonic neural crest cells that normally give rise to the adrenal medulla and the sympathetic ganglia. Consequently, the majority of tumors develop in the adrenal gland or the retroperitoneal sympathetic chain. Other sites include the head, neck, chest, and pelvis. The most common sites for metastatic disease include the liver, skin, lymph nodes, bone, and bone marrow.

Clinical Manifestations

The clinical manifestations of neuroblastoma depend on the location of the tumor. The most common location is the abdomen, and manifestations will possibly include a palpable, firm, irregular mass that crosses the midline; anorexia; bowel and bladder alterations related to compression by the tumor; and spinal cord compression. If the tumor is located in the upper chest, manifestations include dyspnea, difficulty swallowing, and neck and facial edema. Many of the manifestations at the time of diagnosis are the result of metastatic disease. Manifestations of metastasis are hepatomegaly, splenomegaly, anemia, bone and joint pain, skin nodules (especially in infants), periorbital edema, weight loss, pallor, and weakness.

Diagnostic Tests

Initial diagnostic studies focus on locating the primary tumor site and areas of metastasis. In addition to a complete history and physical, other studies include skeletal survey, bone scan, CT scan, abdominal ultrasound, MRI, bone marrow aspiration and biopsy, and urine collection for catecholamine (biologically active amines, epinephrine, and norepinephrine) metabolites (adrenal tumors will stimulate the production of catecholamines). A biopsy of the tumor provides a definitive (final) diagnosis and staging information.

Medical Management

The management of neuroblastoma involves a combination of surgery, radiation therapy, and chemotherapy. If the tumor is localized, the surgeon will remove the tumor, and radiation therapy will follow. If there is widely disseminated disease, the surgeon will remove as much of the tumor as possible, and the child receives follow-up chemotherapy and radiation therapy.

Nursing Interventions and Patient Teaching

Initial nursing interventions focus on preparing the child for diagnostic and operative procedures. Postoperative care is similar to that for any child undergoing abdominal surgery, including observation for any postoperative complications. Psychological support of the family is essential and involves helping them to prepare for the diagnostic and operative procedures and postoperative complications. Parents will need an opportunity to express their fears and concerns. Because of the high incidence of metastasis at diagnosis, parents will sometimes feel guilty that they did not seek medical attention sooner.

Parents will need to be educated about any chemotherapy or radiation therapy that is needed.

Prognosis

Because the tumor is so frequently invasive, the prognosis for neuroblastoma is poor. Generally, the younger the child at diagnosis (especially younger than 1 year of age), the better the survival rates. Also, neuroblastoma is one of the few tumors that may spontaneously regress, possibly as a result of maturity of the embryonic cell or the development of an active immune system.

LEAD POISONING

Lead poisoning is one of the most common, preventable, serious health care problems affecting children in the United States today. The Centers for Disease Control and Prevention (CDC) defines **lead poisoning** as a blood lead level of greater than 10 mg/dL. Lead levels too low to produce symptoms nonetheless can insidiously cause neurologic deficits. Lead levels as low as 10 micrograms per deciliter (mcg/dL) may cause significant health concerns in children, including long-term cognitive and behavioral problems.

Etiology and Pathophysiology

Environmental lead that is either ingested or inhaled continues to be the most important contributing factor in lead poisoning. The primary sources of lead exposure are lead-based paint or caulking chips, lead-contaminated soil and dust, and drinking water that has traveled through lead or lead-soldered pipes. Since 1978, the use of lead in household paint has been illegal in the United States; however, older homes that have deteriorating lead-based paint still pose a problem (Hockenberry & Wilson, 2007).

Ingested lead is slowly excreted from the body through the GI and GU tracts. Any lead that is retained is stored in the bone, where it remains inactive. When the level of lead exceeds the amount that bone can absorb, lead travels through the circulatory system and causes anemia. Children who have iron deficiencies absorb lead more readily than those who do not (Hockenberry & Wilson, 2007). Lead poisoning can cause serious, irreversible damage to the CNS, and the developing brain of younger children is particularly susceptible (Hockenberry & Wilson, 2007).

Clinical Manifestations

Manifestations of lead poisoning include anemia, anorexia, abdominal pain, lethargy, aggression, impulsiveness, irritability, learning difficulties, delinquency, decreased attention span, decreased curiosity, hearing deficits, growth and developmental failure, and pica (craving to eat nonfood substances). Neurocognitive effects are possible results from lead poisoning and lead to long-term complications such as lowered intelligent quotient (IQ) scores, developmental delays, speech and language problems, reading deficits, lower academic achievements, visual-spatial problems, and visual-motor problems (Hockenberry & Wilson, 2007).

Diagnostic Tests

Direct measurement of blood levels remains the primary diagnostic technique in the assessment of lead poisoning. In addition, a complete history and physical examination and an environmental assessment provide valuable information that will identify exposed children and environments at highest risk. Supplemental diagnostic studies include an x-ray examination of the abdomen, which will sometimes show recently ingested paint chips in the intestinal tract; long bone x-ray studies, which sometimes reveal lead lines (areas of increased density) near the epiphyseal lines; and urine studies to detect proteinuria, ketonuria, and glycosuria, which are possible results of lead-induced kidney damage.

Medical Management

The management of lead poisoning varies according to the child's blood level of lead. The primary objective of treatment is to remove lead from the body and prevent further exposure to lead. Pharmacologic treatment, such as chelation therapy (in toxicology, to use a compound to grasp a toxic substance and make it nonactive and thus nontoxic) is a key intervention for children who have excessive lead levels. The precise course of therapy and the chelating agent depend on the preference of the practitioner and the severity of the child's condition. There is also an emphasis on improving nutritional deficiencies and preventing infection.

Nursing Interventions and Patient Teaching

The challenges of lead poisoning provide a unique opportunity to pediatric nurses. With a shift toward primary prevention, you will have the opportunity to be instrumental in the quest to end childhood lead poisoning. The main goal of prevention strategies is to identify and deal with lead sources for the population of children at risk and the communities in which they live. The CDC (2005) recommends that state and local health departments assess local data on lead risks and develop lead screening recommendations for health care providers in their jurisdiction. To do this, a thorough environmental and health questionnaire should be completed at each routine health visit to assess a child's potential risk for lead exposure. Because lead is everywhere in the environment, essentially all children are at risk for lead poisoning. Therefore the CDC (2005) recommends screening all children between ages 6 months and 6 years for lead poisoning, except in communities where large numbers of screened children indicate that there is not an excessive lead burden (lead levels less than 10 mcg/dL). Parents also require support and understanding. Provide them with resources and referrals to help them access resources to help them with this problem.

Parent guidelines for reducing lead in the child's environment are described in Box 31-11.

Prognosis

Although most of the pathophysiologic effects of lead are reversible, the most serious consequences of both high- and low-level lead exposure are the effects on the CNS. In children with lead encephalopathy, permanent brain damage results in cognitive impairment, behavior changes, possible paralysis, and seizures. However, low-dose exposure also has the potential to cause permanent neurologic deficits. The neurologic deficits common with lead exposure include impulsivity, short attention span, distractibility, learning disabilities, and failure in school. Treatment for children with moderate levels of lead poisoning sometimes results in cognitive improvement (Hockenberry & Wilson, 2007).

DISORDERS OF INTEGUMENTARY FUNCTION

Skin function is affected by genetic factors, cleanliness, hydration, and nutrition. Dermatologic disorders in children are the reason for a significant proportion of children's visits to physician's offices and clinics. Many of these disorders are painful for the child, as well as distressing for the family.

NONINFECTIOUS DISORDERS OF THE SKIN

CONTACT DERMATITIS

Etiology and Pathophysiology

Contact dermatitis is an inflammatory, delayed immune response of the skin resulting from contact with environmental antigens to which a person is hypersensitive. Contact dermatitis has the highest incidence in infants and toddlers, and frequently there is a family history of allergy. The most commonly affected areas include face, neck, hands, feet, and legs. The allergens that are most commonly responsible in children include soaps, detergents, bubble baths, shoe components, metals, chemicals, cosmetics, and plants such as poison ivy, oak, and sumac.

Clinical Manifestations

The contact area becomes erythematous, edematous, and pruritic. Papules (solid, red, raised areas less than 0.5 cm in diameter) and vesicles (circumscribed raised areas filled with serous fluid and less than 0.5 cm in diameter) form and can weep and ooze if scratching breaks open the area.

Box 31-11 Parent Guidelines for Reducing Blood Lead Levels

- Make sure child does not have access to peeling paint or chewable surfaces painted with lead-based paint, especially window sills and wells.
- If house was built before 1960 and has hard-surfaced floors, wet mop them at least once a week with a high-phosphate solution (e.g., trisodium phosphate [available in hardware stores]). Wipe other hard surfaces (such as window sills and baseboards) with a similar solution. Do not vacuum hard-surfaced floors or window sills or wells, because this spreads dust. Use vacuum cleaners with agitators to remove dust from rugs rather than vacuum cleaners with suction only.
- Wash child's hands and face before eating.
- Wash toys and pacifiers frequently.
- If soil around home is likely to be contaminated with lead (e.g., if home was built before 1960 or is near a major highway), plant grass or other ground cover; plant bushes around outside of house so that child is not able to play there.
- During remodeling of older homes, be sure to follow correct procedures. Be certain children and pregnant women are not in the home, day or night, until work is completed. After deleading, thoroughly clean house using wet mopping before inhabitants return.
- In areas where lead content of water exceeds the drinking water standard, run water for at least 2 minutes from cold-water tap for drinking, cooking, and making formula; use first-flush water for purposes other than consumption.
- Do not store food in open cans, particularly if cans are imported.
- Do not use pottery or ceramic ware that was inadequately fired or is meant for decorative use for food storage or service.
- Avoid folk remedies that contain lead.
- Make sure that home exposure is not occurring from parental occupations or hobbies. Have household members employed in occupations such as lead smelting shower and change into clean clothing before leaving work.
- Make sure child eats regular meals, because more lead is absorbed on an empty stomach.
- Make sure child's diet contains plenty of iron, calcium, protein, and zinc.

Modified from Centers for Disease Control and Prevention. (1991). *Preventing lead poisoning in young children*. Atlanta: CDC.

Diagnostic Tests

The health care provider makes the diagnosis by observing the pattern and the location of the rash and by taking an accurate history to identify the causative agent. Skin testing is also helpful at times in the identification of suspected plants, foods, or animals.

Medical Management

Because the hypersensitive reaction is usually self-limiting, in most cases the practitioner directs treatment toward identifying and eliminating the cause and relieving signs and symptoms. Cool, wet dressings dipped in Burow's solution (solution of aluminum acetate, used as a drying agent for weeping skin lesions) or Aveeno baths help soothe the affected area. Advise parents not to use Caladryl lotion because the diphenhydramine (Benadryl) component is absorbed and has potential to result in toxicity. Recommend calamine lotion for children. These are all available without prescription. It is acceptable to apply topical, over-the-counter steroid creams to mild contact dermatitis. In more severe cases, the provider will often prescribe systemic corticosteroids. Oral antihistamines such as diphenhydramine (Benadryl) are helpful in controlling pruritus.

Nursing Interventions and Patient Teaching

Advise the family to keep the child's fingernails clipped short to prevent scratching from causing a secondary bacterial infection. Loose, lightweight clothing during the healing phase is also comforting and decreases irritation.

Teach parents to keep an accurate history of possible causative agents. Once it is clear what the primary irritant is, teach them to avoid it. If the skin does come in contact with the causative agent, teach parents to wash the affected area with a mild soap and water and dry it thoroughly. It is best to avoid talcum powder, overheating, and hot baths. Teach the parents to apply topical medications only as directed by a physician.

Prognosis

The reaction is usually self-limiting and normally resolves within 2 weeks.

DIAPER DERMATITIS

Etiology and Pathophysiology

Diaper dermatitis is one of the most common skin disorders in infancy and the cause of great concern for many parents. Diaper dermatitis is a form of contact dermatitis and usually caused by an external irritant. The most common irritating agents include prolonged exposure to urine or feces; inadequate cleaning of the diaper area; soaps, detergents, or fabric softeners used to wash diapers; excessive use of powders or ointments; and the use of plastic pants. Fair-complexioned infants tend to have more sensitive skin and are more vulnerable to diaper rash than darker-complexioned infants. The peak age of occurrence is 9 to 12 months of age, and the incidence is higher in bottle-fed than in breastfed infants.

Clinical Manifestations

The rash appears as erythematous papular lesions (similar in appearance to a scald) on the buttocks, the labia or the scrotum, the inner thighs, and the mons pubis—areas that come into direct contact with the diaper. Skinfolds are frequently spared. In many cases, a excoriated perianal area will be due to frequent diarrhea. The inflammation does not take on a specific configuration; rather, a variety of patterns are possible. The moist, warm, dark environment created by the diaper also tends to promote the growth of secondary bacterial or fungal infections. The infant with diaper dermatitis is usually uncomfortable and is likely to be fussy, irritable, and restless.

Diagnostic Tests

Clinical observation of the characteristics and the location of the rash and an assessment of possible irritants lead to the diagnosis of diaper dermatitis. Bacterial or fungal cultures will sometimes be necessary to investigate persistent secondary infections.

Medical Management

Keeping the diaper area *clean and dry* is of primary importance. Measures to promote healing and prevent diaper dermatitis from recurring include changing diapers as soon as they become soiled, thoroughly cleansing the diaper area with a mild soap and water and gently drying at each diaper change, exposing the affected area to the air several times a day, and avoiding occlusive plastic pants. For more severe cases, a topical glucocorticoid will sometimes be required.

Nursing Interventions and Patient Teaching

The prophylactic use of protective ointments such as Desitin, A&D ointment, or zinc oxide is often helpful. Keep diaper area clean. An excessive amount of powder is contraindicated because in the presence of moisture, the powder will cake, hold the moisture, and excoriate the skin (Box 31-12).

Teach parents the basics of diaper and skin care as outlined previously. To prevent the infant's inhalation of powder dust, instruct parents to put a small amount in their hand and apply it to the baby's diaper area (see Box 31-12).

Prognosis

Quick recognition with prompt therapy leads to a good prognosis.

ATOPIC DERMATITIS (ECZEMA)

Etiology and Pathophysiology

Atopic dermatitis is a pruritic, allergic response common in infancy and childhood. *Atopy* refers to an allergy for which there is a genetic or inherited predis-

Box 31-12 Parent Guidelines for Controlling Diaper Rash

- Keep skin dry.
  - —Use superabsorbent disposable diapers to reduce skin wetness. If using cloth diapers, use only overwraps that allow air to circulate; avoid using rubber pants.
  - —Change diapers as soon as soiled, especially with stool, whenever possible, and preferably once during the night.
  - —Expose healthy or only slightly irritated skin to air, not heat, to dry completely.
- Apply ointment, such as zinc oxide or petrolatum, to protect skin, especially if skin is very erythematous or has moist, open areas.
  - —When soiled, wipe off top layer of ointment and reapply.
  - —To completely remove ointment, especially zinc oxide, use mineral oil; do not wash vigorously.
- Avoid overwashing the skin, especially with perfumed soaps or commercial wipes that are potentially irritating. It is acceptable to use a moisturizer or nonsoap cleanser, such as cold cream or Cetaphil, to wipe urine from skin. Gently wipe stool from skin using water and mild soap, such as Dove.

position. A familial history of asthma, allergic rhinitis, or dry skin is often present. The disease also occurs in association with hypersensitivity to histamine. We do not know the exact cause, but food allergies and abnormal skin function are implicated by association. Infantile atopic dermatitis is possible between 2 and 5 months of age and sometimes continues to be problematic to age 2 or 3 years, when many children seem to "outgrow" the illness. Childhood atopic dermatitis usually occurs at age 2 or 3 years and will persist to 5 years of age in some cases. Adolescent atopic dermatitis is usually seen at 12 years of age and in some cases lasts indefinitely.

Clinical Manifestations

In infantile eczema, the primary lesions consist of erythema, vesicles, and papules, which typically ooze and form crusts. They appear most often on cheeks, scalp, trunk, and extensor surfaces of the extremities. In childhood eczema, the lesions appear as erythematous, scaly patches on trunk, elbows, knees, ankles, hands, and feet and behind the ears. The skin becomes thick and leatherlike **(lichenification).** In adolescent eczema, the lesions are the same as in childhood but the distribution involves mainly hands, feet, neck, and face. At any age, the unaffected skin is usually very dry, and the pruritus possibly extremely intense. The child will often be uncomfortable and restless. Infants unable to scratch will often rub their faces on linens or clothing in an effort to relieve the itch. Scratching or rubbing has the potential to also lead to secondary infections, and children with atopic dermatitis often have an increased susceptibility to bacterial *(Staphylococcus aureus),* viral (herpes simplex), and fungal skin infections. The signs and symptoms are better in humid climates and worse in fall and winter, when homes are heated and environmental humidity is lower.

Diagnostic Tests

The health care provider bases the diagnosis on clinical observation of the type and distribution of the lesions, a positive family history of allergy, and severity of pruritus. In general, skin testing is important in more severe cases to help determine specific allergens.

Medical Management

The therapeutic management includes hydration of the skin, controlling pruritus, decreasing inflammation, and preventing secondary infections. Skin hydration is possible to accomplish in a variety of ways. Tepid baths followed by the administration of an unscented cream or lotion help trap moisture in the skin. The application of occlusive creams or ointments helps relieve dry skin. To decrease inflammation, the practitioner will order thin applications of topical steroid creams or lotions. The strength and the type of topical steroid vary according to the degree of inflammation and the age of the child. Oral antihistamines such as diphenhydramine (Benadryl) or hydroxyzine (Atarax) are useful in controlling pruritus. Appropriate systemic antibiotics are necessary for secondary bacterial infections.

Nursing Interventions

Your role in caring for the child with atopic dermatitis involves measures to control pruritus, promote skin integrity, and provide support to the child and family. Compresses with Burow's solution (aluminum acetate) soothe itching and moisten skin. Discourage hot baths or showers because of their drying effect on the skin. Suggest adding cornstarch to tepid bath water to provide some relief from itching, as well as hydrate skin. Teach the child and the family to use only a mild, unscented soap such as Ivory (99% pure) or Neutrogena, if they use any soap at all. To prevent new lesions or secondary infection, it is essential to keep scratching to a minimum. For the infant, covering the hands with mittens or socks helps reduce scratching. For the older child, gloves allow for more dexterity. At times, it will perhaps be necessary to use safety reminder devices to discourage scratching; however, it is important that the infant or child be free from these restrictions periodically.

Patient Teaching

Overheating will usually intensify itching; therefore parents need to understand that dressing their child in lightweight, loose clothing made from cotton or cotton blends is preferable. Have them wash and double-rinse clothing, linens, and blankets to ensure removal of all soap residue. It is important for parents to understand that they have to apply lubricants frequently, especially after bathing while the skin is still damp to seal in moisture. Teach parents to keep fingernails and toenails clipped short and clean to keep the risk of infection to a minimum. At any age, keeping hands busy with play activities provides the distraction needed to discourage scratching. The appearance, discomfort, and irritability displayed by children with atopic dermatitis is often very upsetting for family members. Encourage parents to verbalize their feelings and provide reassurance. Teaching stress-reduction techniques is often helpful to both the child and the parents because stress tends to aggravate the severity of the condition.

Prognosis

Atopic dermatitis is possible to control but not cure. The majority of affected children (90%) outgrow atopic dermatitis by adolescence (Boguniewicz, 2005). Some may continue to have atopic dermatitis into adulthood.

SEBORRHEIC DERMATITIS

Etiology and Pathophysiology

Seborrheic dermatitis, or cradle cap, is a chronic inflammatory reaction of the skin common in infancy. Although we do not know the cause of the illness, its relation to sebaceous gland activity is suspect. Often there is no family history of allergy.

Clinical Manifestations

Seborrheic dermatitis most commonly affects the scalp and appears as thick, white or yellowish, crusty or scaly patches. Mild pruritus sometimes accompanies the disorder. Other commonly affected areas include the eyebrows or eyelids (blepharitis), the postauricular (behind the ear) area, the external ear (otitis externa), the nasolabial (nose and lip) folds, and the inguinal region (seborrheic diaper dermatitis).

Diagnostic Tests

Diagnosis rests on clinical observation of the characteristics and location of crusty patches.

Medical Management

Management of seborrheic dermatitis consists of treating the signs and symptoms and simple preventive measures. It is possible to remove crusty, scaly patches by applying mineral oil to soften the affected areas (except the eyelids) and help loosen crusts, followed by shampooing with a mild, tear-free shampoo and thoroughly rinsing. Then use a soft baby brush or a soft toothbrush to brush the hair and remove flakes from the hair. A fine-tooth comb also works well. Preventive measures include daily shampooing with an antiseborrheic shampoo. Topical corticosteroids are rarely needed.

Nursing Interventions and Patient Teaching

Soak crusts with warm water and cotton (or clean washcloth) compresses until loosened. Then cleanse the eye area with clean cotton (or a clean washcloth) and warm water, starting at the inner canthus and continuing to the outer canthus. For each stroke, use a clean piece of cotton (or clean area on the washcloth) (Table 31-4).

Often parents need reassurance that shampooing their infant's hair will not cause harm to the fontanelles. A demonstration on how to shampoo the hair will sometimes be necessary. If cradle cap is extensive, inform parents that several treatments will possibly be necessary to loosen and remove all crusts. If the eyelids are involved, teach the parents how to safely clean these areas.

Prognosis

The appearance of lesions is possible shortly after birth and until old age, with periods of remissions and exacerbations.

ACNE VULGARIS

Acne is an inflammatory process of the skin common in adolescence. It is slightly more common in males. Peak incidence occurs between 16 and 17 years of age in females and 17 and 18 years in males, although it is possible to note lesions as early as age 9 or 10 years (Hockenberry & Wilson, 2007). Acne is a disease that involves the pilosebaceous follicles (the hair follicles and sebaceous gland complex) of the face, the neck, the shoulders, the back, and the upper chest.

Medical Management

Treatment success depends on commitment from the adolescent. Before prescribing treatment, it is best to determine the adolescent's level of comfort and readiness to begin treatment.

Tretinoin (Retin-A) is the only drug that effectively interrupts the abnormal follicular keratinization that produces microcomedones, the invisible precursors of the visible comedones. Tretinoin alone is usually sufficient for management of comedonal acne. Do not apply the medication for at least 20 to 30 minutes after washing to decrease the burning sensation. It is important o emphasize the need to avoid sun and use sunscreen daily, because sun exposure has potential to result in severe sunburn. Advise adolescents to apply the medication at night and to use a sunscreen with a sun protection factor (SPF) of at least 15 in the daytime.

Topical benzoyl peroxide is an antibacterial agent that inhibits the growth of *Propionibacterium acnes* organisms. It is effective against both inflammatory and noninflammatory acne and is an effective first-line agent. This medication is available as a cream, lotion, gel, or wash.

When inflammatory lesions accompany the comedones, the health care provider will sometimes prescribe a topical antibacterial agent. These agents serve to prevent new lesions as well as to treat preexisting acne. Clindamycin, erythromycin, metronidazole, azelaic acid, and the combination of either benzoyl perox-

Table 31-4 Nursing Diagnoses and Nursing Interventions for the Child with a Disorder of Integumentary Function

NURSING DIAGNOSES	NURSING INTERVENTIONS
Impaired skin integrity, related to irritation	Assess for signs of scratching. Advise parents to keep the child's fingernails short or to cover hands with mittens or socks. Keep affected areas clean and dry. Apply medications as directed.
Chronic pain, related to pruritus	Encourage rest. Encourage well-balanced diet. Protect skinfolds and surfaces that rub together. Keep clothing and linens clean and dry. Remove adhesives and occlusive dressings carefully. Maintain careful hand hygiene. Wear gloves when indicated. Assess degree of discomfort. Administer antihistamine and glucocorticoid medications as directed to reduce pruritus and inflammation. Recommend loose, lightweight clothing to promote comfort. Apply cool compresses to soothe skin. Reduce external stimuli that aggravate discomfort, such as clothing or bed linens. Teach child to recognize agents or circumstances that produce reaction.
Risk for infection, related to scratching and skin impairment	Assess for signs of infection. Change diapers as soon as soiled. Administer appropriate antibiotics as directed. Implement standard precautions (see Chapter 12). Maintain careful hand hygiene. Teach and reinforce positive habits of hygienic care.
Disturbed body image, related to perceptions of appearance	Encourage child to express feelings about personal appearance and perceived reactions of others. Hold child (remember that there is no substitute for the stimulation and comfort of human contact). Touch and caress unaffected area. Teach self-care where appropriate. Involve child in planning treatment schedules. Support and encourage child in efforts to deal with multiple problems that sometimes occur in association with disorder, including discomfort, rejection, discouragement, and feelings of self-revulsion. Encourage child to maintain usual activities.
Interrupted family processes, related to having a child with a severe skin condition (e.g., eczema, psoriasis)	Teach family skills needed to carry out therapeutic program. Provide written instructions. Inform family of expected and unexpected results of therapy and a course of action to follow. Help devise special techniques to carry out therapy. Be aware of overprotectiveness and restrictiveness, which tend to stifle child's emotional growth. Allow and encourage family members, particularly the one who cares for the child most of the time, to express negative feelings, such as anger, frustration, and perhaps guilt. Stress that negative feelings are normal, acceptable, and expected, but that an outlet for them is necessary if family members are to remain healthy. Encourage family in efforts to carry out plan of care. Provide assistance when appropriate. Refer to agencies and services that assist with social, financial, and medical problems.

ide and erythromycin (Benzamycin) or benzoyl peroxide and glycolic acid are options for topical antibacterial therapy. The combination of 5% benzoyl peroxide and 3% erythromycin is especially beneficial. Tretinoin improves the penetration of other topical agents, and combination therapy with tretinoin and an antibacterial is helpful.

The practitioner will sometimes turn to systemic antibiotic therapy when moderate to severe acne does not respond to topical treatments. Oral antibiotics are considered safe to use to treat acne. These antibiotics include tetracycline, erythromycin, minocycline, doxycycline, clindamycin, and trimethoprim-sulfamethoxazole.

Females with mild to moderate acne sometimes respond well to topical treatment and the addition of an oral contraceptive pill (OCP). OCPs reduce the endogenous androgen production, which results in decreased acne.

Isotretinoin, 13-*cis* retinoic acid (Accutane), is a very potent and effective oral agent that is reserved for severe cystic acne that has not responded to other treatments. Isotretinoin is the only agent available that affects factors involved in the development of acne. However, it is essential for a dermatologist to manage any course of treatment with isotretinoin. Adolescents with multiple, active, deep dermal or subcutaneous cystic and nodular acne lesions receive treatment for 20 weeks. Multiple side effects are possible, including dry skin and mucous membranes, nasal irritation, dry eyes, decreased night vision, photosensitivity, arthralgia, headaches, mood changes, aggressive or violent behaviors, depression, and suicidal ideation. It is necessary to monitor adolescents on this drug for depression, depressive symptoms, and suicidal ideation. It is important to give this drug *only* at the recommended dosage for no longer than the recommended duration. The most significant side effects of this drug are the teratogenic (any substance that can cause developmental abnormalities in the fetus) effects. Isotretinoin is *absolutely contraindicated* in pregnant women. Sexually active young women are required to be using an effective contraceptive method during treatment and for 1 month after treatment. Also monitor patients receiving isotretinoin for elevated cholesterol and triglyceride levels. Significant elevation sometimes necessitates discontinuation of the medication (Hockenberry & Wilson, 2007).

Nursing Interventions and Patient Teaching

Inform the adolescent that benzoyl peroxide and retinoic acid are incompatible together, and thus the prescriber will direct the adolescent to use them on alternate days or to use one in the morning and the other at night. Also inform the adolescent of the side effects of topical medications, especially the erythematous skin that will sometimes result from compliance with the regimen prescribed by the dermatologist. Assess the psychosocial effect of acne on the adolescent's self-image. Depression, anxiety, and low self-esteem sometimes occur during the adolescent's developmental task of developing identity. The adolescent with acne will need a great deal of emotional support in dealing with feelings of self-consciousness and frustration, especially during periods of exacerbations. For adolescents who insist on wearing makeup, advise that water-based preparations are preferred. Emphasize meticulous skin care, including removal of cosmetics at night. Involving the adolescent in developing the plan of care is sometimes the key to ensuring successful compliance with the measures prescribed for resolution.

Although the disease is self-limited and not life threatening, its significance to the adolescent is great, and it is a mistake to underestimate the effect it sometimes has on young people. See Table 31-4 for nursing diagnoses with nursing interventions for a child with a disorder of integumentary function.

Prognosis

Acne will resolve spontaneously over a variable period, depending on the individual.

PSORIASIS

Psoriasis is a chronic, proliferative skin disorder characterized by thick, scaly patches and inflammation. Psoriasis is not usually seen in children younger than 6 years of age. The disorder has characteristic remissions and exacerbations. People are otherwise healthy. Humidifiers sometimes help in winter.

TRAUMATIC INJURIES

Animal, insect, and human bites in children account for a considerable number of visits to clinics and physicians' offices. Most bites from dogs or cats are from pets belonging to the family or neighbors. Dog bites involve lacerations or tissue avulsion injuries, whereas cats inflict more puncturelike wounds. Boys are bitten more often by dogs; girls are bitten more often by cats. Animal bites most often occur on the child's face, scalp, and upper extremities because children tend to keep their heads close to the animal during play. Human bites occur in young children during rough or aggressive play or when they become frustrated; bites are also possible as the result of child abuse. The most common traumatic injuries in children and their manifestations, management, and nursing interventions are outlined in Table 31-5.

INFECTIOUS DISORDERS OF THE SKIN

BACTERIAL INFECTIONS

Impetigo, folliculitis, and cellulitis are common bacterial infections in childhood. The assessment of systemic signs and symptoms, areas involved, and appearance of lesions are helpful in establishing the type of infection. Table 31-6 on p. 1057 reviews the etiology, the clinical manifestations, the management, and the nursing interventions for these infections.

Prognosis for bacterial infections of the skin is good but becomes guarded in the more complex and puzzling cases.

HERPES SIMPLEX VIRUS TYPE 1

Herpes simplex virus type 1 (HSV-1) is a common infection. HSV-1 is transmitted by direct contact of infected body fluids with nonintact skin or mucous

Table 31-5 Traumatic Injuries

CLINICAL MANIFESTATION	MANAGEMENT	PREVENTION
ANIMAL BITES (DOGS, CATS)		
Lacerations, punctures, tissue avulsion	Wound care	Supervise children during play with pets. Educate children in appropriate ways to handle pets. Teach understanding of animal behavior and respect for animals. Never leave infants alone with pet.
HUMAN BITES		
Lacerations	Wound care	Supervise young children at play.
INSECT BITES (FLEAS, MOSQUITOES, FLIES, GNATS)		
Hypersensitive reactions; papular urticaria; firm papules	Cool compresses, topical antihistamines, Caladryl lotion	Use insect repellents (should not contain greater than 10% *N,N*-Diethyl-meta-toluamide [DEET]). Remove source by treating furniture, mattresses, carpets, and pets.
INSECT STINGS (HORNETS, WASPS, BEES)		
Nonhypersensitive: local erythema, edema, tenderness, pruritus	Carefully scrape off stinger, if present; cleanse with soap and water; use cool compresses, antipruritic agents	Avoid insect breeding or nesting areas. Wear clothes that cover the extremities and feet.
Hypersensitive: systemic reactions and anaphylaxis	Intramuscular epinephrine and immediate medical attention; epinephrine kits available for home and school to prevent anaphylactic shock and death	
SUNBURN		
Mild: erythema, tenderness, mild edema Severe: severe erythema, pain, edema, vesicular formation	Cool compresses, moisturizers Immediate medical attention	Use topical sunscreens containing para-aminobenzoic acid (PABA) and sun protection factor (SPF) 15 to 45. Limit time spent in sun during period of maximum exposure (11 AM to 3 PM); at higher elevations, limit time on fresh snow and water, especially when sun is directly overhead.

membranes. The children most susceptible to HSV are immunosuppressed children (those receiving steroid therapy or chemotherapy, with leukemia, or who are HIV positive), children with burns, and infants with diaper rash or eczema.

Prognosis for viral infections of the skin is usually good; however, the infection will sometimes be fatal in children with depressed immunity. Healing will occur without scarring unless secondary infection develops.

TINEA CAPITIS, TINEA CORPORIS, TINEA CRURIS, AND TINEA PEDIS (RINGWORM)

Tinea infections are common fungal infections of the skin in children. Classification of the infections follows the area of the body that is involved. Tinea capitis is a common infection of the scalp among school-age children. Tinea corporis occurs on the trunk and on the extremities in young children; tinea cruris ("jock itch") affects the inguinal area of pubescent males; and tinea pedis ("athlete's foot") occurs between the patient's toes.

Prognosis for fungal infections of the skin, with treatment, is good.

CANDIDIASIS (THRUSH)

Etiology and Pathophysiology

The fungus *Candida albicans* causes candidiasis, or thrush. The infection is a common disorder in infants younger than 6 months of age and is transmitted by contaminated hands, nipples, and pacifiers. In some neonates, candidal infection results from passage through the infected vagina. The candidal lesion begins as a pustule on an inflammatory base. As inflammatory cells accumulate, whitish yellow or whitish gray curd-like patches appear over the infected area. The incidence of candidiasis is higher in immunocompromised children, infants of diabetic mothers, and children with oronasal malformations (cleft lip or palate).

Clinical Manifestations

The white patches of *Candida* frequently appear on moist tissues, because the organism is not able to

Table 31-6 Bacterial Infections of the Skin

ETIOLOGY	CLINICAL MANIFESTATIONS	MANAGEMENT
IMPETIGO		
Staphylococcus aureus, group A streptococcus, or both	Erythematous papules progress to vesicles with exudative and honey-colored crusting stages; involves face, buttocks, and extremities; pruritus is common	Mupirocin topical or systemic treatment with penicillin, erythromycin, or cloxacillin *Nursing interventions:* Teach family measures to control spread of infection; instruct in careful hand hygiene.
FOLLICULITIS		
S. aureus	Pustule with surrounding erythema of the hair follicle of the scalp or extremities; possible progression to a furuncle (a boil from the primary folliculitis), with extension into the surrounding dermis Systemic effects: malaise, if severe	Topical antibiotics and local, warm, moist compresses; more severe cases sometimes necessitate incision and drainage, followed by antibiotic therapy *Nursing interventions:* Teach family measures to control spread of infection; hygiene measures, such as careful hand hygiene.
CELLULITIS		
S. aureus, group A streptococcus, *Haemophilus influenzae* type b	Possible anywhere on the body; area is erythematous, edematous, warm, and painful; adjacent tender lymph node enlargement; sometimes will progress to abscess formation Systemic effects: fever, malaise	Antibiotic therapy, rest, and warm, moist compresses. Neonates with herpes simplex virus type 1 are hospitalized; children younger than 3 years of age with facial cellulitis are usually hospitalized. *Nursing interventions:* Gently cleanse area with saline; observe for complications; administer antibiotics and analgesics as prescribed; institute wound drainage precautions if drainage develops; teach family measures to control spread of infection, such as careful hand hygiene.

grow on dry skin. Common areas affected include the tongue, the buccal cavity, the GI tract, and the vagina. Often, parents mistake thrush for a formula coating on the tongue. Generally, the condition is asymptomatic and easily treated. However, severe cases sometimes result in pain and refusal to eat or drink, causing risk of dehydration.

Diagnostic Tests

Diagnosis rests on careful history and clinical observation of the plaques. To distinguish thrush from formula, rinse the area with water or gently wipe the area with a wet washcloth. If the white coating remains, thrush is present. Scraping lesions is contraindicated because they bleed easily.

Medical Management

Nystatin suspension is the most common antifungal agent health care providers use to treat oral *Candida* infections. Administer nystatin suspension after feedings and apply it directly onto the lesions and to each side of the mouth before the child swallows. Other drugs useful in the treatment of thrush include amphotericin B, clotrimazole, fluconazole, and miconazole. Treating infections early will often prevent more serious complications such as candidal infections of the upper airway and the GI tract. When a child has oral candidiasis, it is important to also inspect the diaper area for signs of infection. The provider will prescribe nystatin cream for diaper candidiasis.

Nursing Interventions and Patient Teaching

Instruct parents to complete the full 7-day course of nystatin suspension even though candidal lesions will in many cases no longer be present. Prevention of reinfection includes teaching parents to sterilize bottles, nipples, pacifiers, and teethers. Emphasize hand hygiene. Instruct parents to report any oral discomfort that results in poor fluid intake. Review signs of dehydration with the family. If the mother is breastfeeding, advise her to wash her nipples with soap and water before and after feedings. Some practitioners will also recommend the application of nystatin cream.

Prognosis

Prognosis for candidiasis (thrush) is good with prescribed therapy.

PARASITIC INFECTIONS

Scabies and Pediculosis

Scabies is an infectious parasitic disorder caused by a mite. Scabies is most common in school-age children. The scabies mite burrows under the skin, leaving behind debris, feces, and eggs. The condition causes a

Box 31-13 Medical Management and Nursing Interventions for Parasitic Infections

- Lindane (Kwell) 1% lotion, cream, or shampoo
- Simultaneous treatment of family members
- Atarax or Benadryl for pruritus
- Hot-water cleansing of contaminated clothing and linens
- Teach parents to do the following:
  - —Carefully inspect the head (at the nape of the neck) of a child who scratches the head more than usual for bite marks, erythema, and nits
  - —Read directions carefully before beginning therapy
  - —Be aware of psychological effects, which can be highly stressful to children

NOTE: Have examiners wear gloves when assessing for head lice.

linear, papular rash and intense pruritus. Transmission occurs by direct contact with an infected person, bed linen, or clothing.

Pediculosis capitis (head lice) is a scalp infection that causes intense pruritus. It is common among preschool and school-age children. The adult louse attaches to the skin and feeds by sucking blood. On the hair shaft, the mature female louse lays her eggs (nits), which hatch in 7 to 10 days. The louse does not jump or fly and is not carried or transmitted by pets. Infestations usually occur as a result of sharing contaminated combs, brushes, hats, or clothing that comes in contact with the head. Box 31-13 outlines medical management and nursing interventions for scabies and pediculosis.

Patient teaching is as follows:

- Remove dead lice and remaining nits with a fine-tooth comb. Tweezers will be necessary to remove the nits if the comb is ineffective.
- Machine wash all washable clothing, towels, and bed linens in hot water and dry in a hot dryer for at least 20 minutes. Dry-clean nonwashable items.
- Thoroughly vacuum carpets, car seats, pillows, stuffed animals, rugs, mattresses, and upholstered furniture.
- Seal nonwashable items in plastic bags for 14 days if unable to dry-clean or vacuum.
- Soak combs, brushes, and hair accessories in lice-killing products for 1 hour or in boiling water for 10 minutes.

Prognosis is good with treatment.

COMMUNICABLE DISEASES AND IMMUNIZATIONS

The development and use of vaccines has significantly reduced the incidence of many communicable diseases and the serious complications associated with them (see Figures 29-4, 29-5, and 29-6). However, health professionals will occasionally encounter children with a preventable communicable disease. You will usually be the first person to observe signs of illness, such as a rash, that is perhaps related to a communicable disease. Make sure you are able to identify potentially infectious cases so that it is possible to institute measures to prevent exposure and transmission to others. In assessing the child with suspicious signs and symptoms, determine whether the child has had any recent exposure to a known case and whether the child is experiencing any **prodromal** (early sign of a developing condition or disease) symptoms. The immunization status of the child and determining whether the child has a history of the illness will often help rule out certain communicable diseases. The goals of nursing interventions for the child with a communicable disease are to prevent transmission of disease to others, prevent complications, and promote supportive management. Table 31-7 describes the common communicable diseases seen in childhood and their medical management, specific nursing interventions, and possible complications. With accurate diagnosis, prompt treatment, and prevention of complications, prognosis is usually good.

DISORDERS OF SENSORY ORGAN FUNCTION

Sensory impairment in young children poses the risk of serious adverse outcomes in growth and development. Prevention, early detection, and management are essential for favorable outcomes.

HEARING

OTITIS MEDIA

Etiology and Pathophysiology

Otitis media (OM), an infection of the middle ear, is a common infection in children from 6 months to 2 years of age and often follows an upper respiratory infection. A significant cause of OM is the accumulation of bacteria in the nasopharynx. In young children, the eustachian tube, which connects the nasopharynx and the middle ear, is shorter, more horizontal, and wider, allowing nasopharyngeal flora to pass and become trapped in the middle ear. Feeding practices have also been implicated in the incidence of OM. It is possible that bottle-fed babies have a higher incidence of OM than breastfed babies because of the more supine position assumed during bottle feeding. Always evaluate toddlers and young children for foreign bodies (pieces of toys, beads, pebbles, vegetables, and so on) in the ear canal, which have potential to lead to hearing loss and local infection.

Clinical Manifestations

The infant or young child with acute otitis media (AOM) is likely to experience otalgia (earache), fever, rhinitis, fussiness, irritability, and decreased appetite. Pulling, tugging, or rubbing the affected ear or rolling the head from side to side indicates possible AOM. Older children will usually complain of ear pain. Oc-

Table 31-7 Childhood Communicable Diseases

DISEASE	CLINICAL MANIFESTATIONS	MEDICAL MANAGEMENT	NURSING INTERVENTIONS
RUBEOLA (MEASLES)			
Etiology: Paramyxovirus *Transmission:* Direct contact from respiratory tract secretions, blood, or urine of infected person *Incubation:* 7-12 days *Communicable period:* 4 days before to 5 days after rash appears	*Prodrome:* Fever, malaise, cough, coryza, conjunctivitis; Koplik's spots (pinpoint red spots with central white speck in buccal cavity opposite lower molars) 3-4 days before rash *Acute phase:* Rash appears as irregular macular erythema; begins on face and behind ears and spreads to feet; rash lasts up to 7 days; child will possibly exhibit vomiting, diarrhea, anorexia, lymphadenopathy *Complications:* Otitis media, pneumonia, laryngotracheitis, encephalitis	*Supportive management:* Acetaminophen, fluids, and bed rest until fever subsides; dim lights or sunglasses if photophobic	Institute seizure precautions (high fever is possible [104° F (40° C)]). Cleanse eyes to remove crusting and decrease rubbing. Use a cool-mist humidifier for cough. Offer small, frequent meals of bland foods. Keep skin clean and dry; use tepid baths. Restrict to quiet activities until child feels better, usually by day 6 of rash. Use isolation to protect nonimmunized children or the immunocompromised from exposure. Teach and encourage good hand hygiene technique. Notify physician of ear pain, chest pain, difficulty breathing, headaches.
RUBELLA (GERMAN MEASLES)			
Etiology: Rubivirus *Transmission:* Direct contact with nasopharyngeal secretions of infected person; indirect contact with contaminated articles (fomites); transplacental transmission *Incubation:* 14-21 days *Communicable period:* 7 days before to 5 days after rash appears	*Prodrome:* Young children—possible lymphadenopathy; adolescents and adults—low-grade fever, headache, sore throat, anorexia, clear nasal discharge, cough, lymphadenopathy 1-5 days *Acute phase:* Pinkish red maculopapular rash beginning on face; spreads to trunk, then extremities—3 days *Complications:* Usually none; rare—arthritis, encephalitis; birth defects as virus crosses placenta (teratogenic)	*Supportive management:* Acetaminophen for fever or discomfort	Provide respiratory isolation to protect nonimmunized children, pregnant women. Teach and encourage good hand hygiene technique. Institute comfort measures as needed. Isolate child from pregnant women. Reassure parents of benign nature of illness in affected child.
VARICELLA (CHICKENPOX)			
Etiology: Varicella zoster virus (herpesvirus) *Transmission:* Direct contact with respiratory tract secretions; indirect contact with contaminated articles; airborne droplets *Incubation:* 10-21 days (usually 13-17 days) *Communicable period:* 1 day before eruption until all lesions crusted (1 week after onset)	*Prodrome:* Low-grade fever, malaise, anorexia—24 hours *Acute phase:* Pruritic rash 3-5 days, begins as macule, progresses to papule and then vesicle on erythematous base; vesicles rupture, causing oozing and crusting; all three stages present in various intensities; rash appears on trunk, face, proximal extremities, mucous membranes	*Supportive management:* Acetaminophen for fever; systemic or topical antipruritics or systemic antihistamines; skin kept clean and dry; antiviral treatment—acyclovir (Zovirax); varicella zoster immune globulin within 3 days of exposure in high-risk children (those who are immunocompromised or have leukemia; newborns)	Keep nails short and smooth; give daily baths without soap; use lightweight, loose clothing; administer antipruritics or antihistamines as ordered; teach child to apply pressure on itch rather than scratching; use mittens on young children. Use strict isolation in hospital.

Continued

Table 31-7 Childhood Communicable Diseases—cont'd

DISEASE	CLINICAL MANIFESTATIONS	MEDICAL MANAGEMENT	NURSING INTERVENTIONS
VARICELLA (CHICKENPOX)—cont'd			
	Complications: Children—secondary bacterial skin infections possible; adults—pneumonia, encephalitis, laryngeal edema, hemorrhagic varicella, thrombocytopenia		If child is at home, instruct parents to isolate ill child from siblings and high-risk children and adults until lesions dry. Teach and encourage good hand hygiene technique. Administer acetaminophen as ordered. Encourage fluids.
ROSEOLA INFANTUM (EXANTHEMA SUBITUM)			
Etiology: Human herpesvirus, type 6 *Transmission:* Unknown; occurs in children age 6-24 months *Incubation:* Unknown *Communicable period:* Unknown	Sudden-onset, persistent high fever, lasts up to 4 days; child appears well otherwise; fever rapidly falls to normal followed by rose-pink macular or maculopapular rash on trunk and spreads to rest of body; rash lasts 1-2 days and is nonpruritic *Complications:* Febrile seizures	*Supportive management:* Acetaminophen for fever; seizure precautions for the child prone to febrile seizures; encourage fluids	Teach parents how to lower fever safely. Reassure parents as to benign nature of illness. If child is prone to seizures, discuss appropriate precautions.
ERYTHEMA INFECTIOSUM (FIFTH DISEASE)			
Etiology: Human parvovirus B19 *Transmission:* Respiratory tract secretions and blood *Incubation:* 4-14 days but up to 20 days *Communicable period:* Unknown—most likely before signs and symptoms develop; communicability unlikely once rash develops	*Prodrome:* In children with aplastic crisis—fever, malaise, myalgia; rash usually absent *Acute phase:* Rash appears in three stages: first stage—red rash on face, "slapped cheek" appearance (fades in 1-4 days), circumoral pallor; second stage—maculopapular, lacelike rash on upper extremities spreading to trunk and thighs; lasts 1 or more weeks; third stage—possible for rash to recur periodically for weeks in response to heat, sunlight, cold *Complications:* Arthralgia, arthritis infrequently in children but common in adults; encephalitis, myocarditis (rare); maternal infection—low risk for fetal hydrops	*Supportive management:* Acetaminophen for fever; analgesics or antiinflammatories	For hospitalized child, use respiratory isolation and precautions for 7 days after onset: no isolation is necessary at home. Teach and encourage good hand hygiene technique. Institute comfort measures as necessary.

casionally there will be purulent discharge in the ear canal, which is indicative of a ruptured tympanic membrane. When this occurs, there is a sudden cessation of ear pain.

Diagnostic Tests

Visualization of the tympanic membrane by otoscopic examination, along with clinical signs and symptoms, usually confirms the diagnosis. If drainage is in the ear canal, it is possible to culture the material.

Medical Management

The management of AOM includes administration of antibiotics for 10 days and acetaminophen for fever and discomfort. On completion of antibiotic therapy, the practitioner examines the child to determine the

Table 31-7 Childhood Communicable Diseases—cont'd

DISEASE	CLINICAL MANIFESTATIONS	MEDICAL MANAGEMENT	NURSING INTERVENTIONS
SCARLET FEVER *Etiology:* Group A β-hemolytic streptococcus *Transmission:* Direct contact with respiratory tract secretions of infected person *Incubation:* 2-5 days (average 3 days) *Communicable period:* During incubation and acute illness phase	*Prodrome:* Sudden-onset high fever, vomiting, headache, chills, malaise *Acute phase:* Tonsillitis, pharyngitis, white strawberry tongue (tongue has white coating and papillae become red and edematous) by day 1 or 2; by day 4, white coating sloughs leaving red strawberry tongue; sandpaper-like red rash appears about 12 hours after prodrome and is intense in skinfolds; cheeks are flushed and circumoral pallor present; desquamation begins by end of first week and continues for 3 weeks or longer *Complications:* Otitis media, pneumonia, sinusitis, glomerulonephritis, carditis, peritonsillar abscess	*Antimicrobial treatment:* Full course of penicillin or erythromycin for those allergic to penicillin *Supportive management:* Bed rest, analgesics, fluids	Institute respiratory isolation precautions until completion of first 24 hours of antimicrobial treatment. Teach and encourage good hand hygiene technique. Offer soft diet if child is able to chew; encourage fluids. Restrict to quiet activities until child feels better. Offer lozenges, gargles, cool-mist humidifier for throat. Maintain good oral hygiene. Advise parents to consult practitioner if fever persists after beginning therapy. Discuss procedures for preventing spread of infection.
MUMPS (PAROTITIS) *Etiology:* Paramyxovirus *Transmission:* Direct contact with respiratory tract secretions of infected person *Incubation:* 16-18 days *Communicable period:* 1-2 days and up to 7 days before parotid edema to 5-9 days after onset of signs and symptoms	*Prodrome:* Fever, malaise, headache *Acute phase:* Unilateral or bilateral edema and tenderness of parotid glands by day 3; chewing aggravates "earlike" pain *Complications:* Meningoencephalitis, epididymo-orchitis, arthritis, sensorineural deafness, myocarditis, sterility in males is rare	*Supportive management:* Acetaminophen for fever, analgesics for pain; intravenous (IV) fluids sometimes necessary for the child who refuses to eat or drink	Institute respiratory isolation and precautions for 9 days after onset of edema or until edema has subsided. Teach and encourage good hand hygiene technique. Offer soft, bland diet; encourage fluids. Use warm or cool compresses for edema. Dress child in tightly fitting underpants or scrotal support for orchitis.
DIPHTHERIA *Etiology: Corynebacterium diphtheriae* *Transmission:* Direct contact with nose, eye, throat discharges or skin lesions of infected person; rarely: fomite transmission or foodborne outbreaks *Incubation:* 2-5 days	Clinical manifestations vary according to diphtheritic membrane affected: • Nasal: Nasal discharge—serosanguineous and mucopurulent, possible progression to epistaxis • White membrane on nasal septum	Antimicrobial treatment—penicillin or erythromycin; antitoxin, usually IV, preceded by skin testing for horse serum sensitivity; possible tracheostomy for respiratory obstruction	Institute strict respiratory isolation and precautions. Maintain bed rest. Offer liquid or soft diet. Perform gentle suctioning, as necessary.

Continued

effectiveness of treatment and observe for complications. An accumulation of fluid that remains in the middle ear space is often an indication for surgical insertion of tympanostomy tubes to drain the fluid and relieve the pressure. In chronic OM, some health care providers will opt for tympanostomy tubes to prevent hearing loss. Tympanostomy tubes remain in the ear an average of 6 months before being spontaneously rejected.

Nursing Interventions and Patient Teaching

Children usually begin to feel better after 48 to 72 hours of antibiotic therapy. The application of heat or cold (whichever provides the greatest comfort) over the af-

Table 31-7 Childhood Communicable Diseases—cont'd

DISEASE	CLINICAL MANIFESTATIONS	MEDICAL MANAGEMENT	NURSING INTERVENTIONS
DIPHTHERIA—cont'd *Communicable period:* Untreated person—2 weeks to several months	• Tonsillar or pharyngeal: pharyngitis; malaise; anorexia; fever (low grade) • Membrane over tonsils, pharynx; lymphadenitis; laryngeal: cough, fever, hoarseness *Complications:* Airway obstruction, thrombocytopenia, myocarditis, vocal cord paralysis		Observe for signs of respiratory distress or obstruction: dyspnea, apprehensiveness, cyanosis; report such findings to physician. Keep tracheostomy set at bedside. Regulate humidity for optimum liquefaction of secretions.
PERTUSSIS (WHOOPING COUGH) *Etiology: Bordetella pertussis* *Transmission:* Direct contact or droplet spread of respiratory tract secretions of infected person *Incubation:* 7-20 days *Communicable period:* From prodromal stage through fourth week	*Prodrome:* Upper respiratory tract infection signs and symptoms 1-2 weeks; cough, sneezing, little or no fever, headache, anorexia *Acute phase:* Paroxysmal stage—dry, hacking cough followed by prolonged inspiration ("whoop" sound) most often at night; paroxysms usually followed by vomiting of thick, stringy mucus; lasts 4-6 weeks; convalescent stage—decrease in coughing and whooping and lasts 1-2 weeks *Complications:* Pneumonia, hypoxia, atelectasis, otitis media, seizures, dehydration, weight loss, prolapsed rectum, hernia, hemorrhage (epistaxis, subconjunctival, cerebral edema, and central nervous system [CNS] disturbances)	*Antimicrobial treatment:* Erythromycin or trimethoprim-sulfamethoxazole (Bactrim, Septra) for 7-10 days *Antiseizure treatment:* For those experiencing seizures; phenytoin; supportive management—hospitalization required for infants or children with underlying pulmonary or cardiac disease, dehydration, or severe signs and symptoms; gentle suctioning to prevent choking, high humidified oxygen therapy; IV fluids; intubation set at bedside for emergency	Institute respiratory isolation and precautions. Enforce strict hand hygiene. Maintain bed rest if child is febrile; offer quiet activities. Offer liquids—small amounts frequently; if child vomits, refeed. Monitor cardiac and respiratory status. Observe for signs of airway obstruction—dyspnea, restlessness, cyanosis—and report such findings to the health care provider. Provide high humidity and gentle, frequent suctioning to prevent choking. Reassure parents during paroxysms. Teach parents in the use of a cool-mist humidifier to avoid triggers of paroxysms (dust, smoke, chilling, sudden change in temperature, excitement). Teach parents how to recognize signs of respiratory distress, and arrange for a public health nurse to visit after discharge from hospital.

fected ear with the child lying on the affected side often also helps alleviate pain. This position also facilitates drainage of the exudate if the eardrum has ruptured or after a myringotomy. If the ear is draining, it is possible to clean the external canal with sterile cotton swabs or pledgets soaked in hydrogen peroxide. If ear wicks or lightly rolled sterile gauze packs are placed in the ear after surgical treatment, be sure they are loose enough to allow accumulated drainage to flow out of the ear; otherwise it is possible to transfer the infection to the mastoid process. Keep the wicks dry during shampoos or baths.

Emphasize how important it is to take the medication for the fully prescribed course to ensure eradication of the infection. Educate parents in the prevention of otitis media by teaching them to hold their infants in an upright position when feeding. If the child has tympanostomy tubes, teach parents postoperative care.

They need to protect the ear during bathing, shampooing, and swimming because it is possible to introduce bacteria from the water into the ear.

Prognosis

With appropriate therapy, most children improve within 48 to 72 hours. The most common complication of OM is mild to moderate hearing loss as a result of chronic or recurrent effusion. The episodic (temporary) hearing loss that sometimes occurs during occasional bouts of OM is usually reversible; however, conductive hearing loss associated with chronic OM will in some cases be permanent and has potential to interfere with language and cognitive development.

VISION

REFRACTIVE ERRORS (MYOPIA AND HYPEROPIA)

Refractive errors occur when light rays entering the lens are bent and fall in front of or behind the retina, preventing the image from falling on a single point on the retina as it normally does. Two of the most common refractive errors in childhood are myopia (nearsightedness) and hyperopia (farsightedness), which results in loss of visual acuity. Screening tests that measure visual acuity assist in identifying refractive errors. Treatment consists of corrective lenses and periodic reevaluation. You play a vital role in ensuring vision screening, especially in the preschool years, to prevent school problems later on.

STRABISMUS

In strabismus, a lack of coordination in the extraocular musculature results in a cross-eyed appearance. Strabismus is caused by muscle imbalance, results from paralysis, or in some cases is congenitally acquired. The condition affects sometimes one and sometimes both eyes and results in the brain receiving two images (instead of one). Common clinical manifestations include squinting, closing one eye, tilting the head (to block out one image), and difficulty focusing or picking up objects. Medical management varies according to the cause of the strabismus. There is no treatment that will perfectly align the eyes. The goal is to realign them as close to normal as possible. The injection of botulinum toxin (Botox) into the extraocular muscle will temporarily relax muscles (Thompsen, 2008). Occlusion therapy (patching the stronger eye) is sometimes successful in the older child (11 to 15 years) (Mohan et al., 2004). It is difficult to keep an occlusive patch on a toddler's eye for prolonged periods. The newer treatment is patching the stronger eye for a few hours a day or performing surgical intervention earlier. Nursing intervention includes adequate explanation of the treatment plan, care of corrective lenses, instruction in eye exercises, and reinforcement of occlusive patches if they become loose.

Left untreated, the child is at risk for **amblyopia** (lazy eye; reduction or dimness of vision, especially in which there is no apparent pathologic condition of the eye), in which there is a loss in visual acuity. This complication is possible to prevent if the underlying problem is corrected before the child is 6 years of age.

PERIORBITAL CELLULITIS

Etiology and pathophysiology

Periorbital cellulitis is a serious inflammation of the eyelid and periorbital area. The condition is usually unilateral and has the potential to affect the eye and the CNS. Conjunctivitis, impetigo, insect bites, and trauma are all possible causes of periorbital cellulitis. Common causative organisms include *H. influenzae, S. aureus,* and group A β-hemolytic streptococci.

Clinical Manifestations

Children with periorbital cellulitis usually experience pain, tenderness, fever, erythema (of distinctive magenta color), and edema of the eyelids and periorbital area. Headache and purulent nasal discharge are also sometimes present.

Diagnostic Tests

Cultures of the eye, the nose, and the blood help identify the causative agent. Ultrasound and CT scan of the orbit are sometimes useful to rule out abscess.

Medical Management

Because of the emergent nature of the illness, the physician will admit the child for aggressive IV antibiotic administration. It is common to use analgesics and antipyretics for pain and fever. Warm compresses also help to relieve discomfort.

Nursing Interventions and Patient Teaching

As the edema decreases, the skin around the eye becomes dry and begins to peel. Preserving skin integrity involves the application of a thin layer of petrolatum to the area.

Reassure parents that eye discoloration sometimes persists for several days and that most children recover completely without complication.

Prognosis

The edema usually subsides within 36 hours of antibiotic therapy. With appropriate treatment, the prognosis is usually excellent.

NASAL CAVITY

ALLERGIC RHINITIS

Etiology and Pathophysiology

Allergic rhinitis occurs in about 20% to 40% of the pediatric population, most commonly in children older than age 5 (Kliegman et al., 2007). Allergic rhinitis is either seasonal or perennial, and there is a familial predisposition to allergy in affected children. Exposure to an inhaled allergen sets off the allergic response.

Clinical Manifestations

The signs and symptoms common in the pediatric population include congestion, sniffling, mouth breathing, itchy nose, and postnasal drip. Often there is a line across the nose from nasal rubbing (allergic salute). The medical management and nursing interventions for the child with allergic rhinitis are the same as those for the adult.

Get Ready for the NCLEX® Examination!

Key Points

- The most common skin disorders of infancy and childhood include diaper dermatitis, atopic dermatitis, and seborrheic dermatitis.
- Treatment initiated immediately on diagnosis often results in a better prognosis for many of the musculoskeletal disorders seen in infancy.
- Cleft lip and palate, the most common facial malformation, usually involves nutritional, dental, and speech alterations and calls for a multidisciplinary approach to treatment.
- Congenital heart defects are classified as either acyanotic or cyanotic.
- Nursing interventions in the care of a child with heart failure are to assist in improving cardiac function, decreasing cardiac demands, reducing respiratory distress, maintaining nutritional status, promoting fluid loss, and providing family support.
- The most common form of neoplasm in childhood is acute lymphoblastic leukemia.
- Nursing interventions for the child with hemophilia involve preventing bleeding by decreasing the risk of injury, recognizing and managing bleeding with factor replacement, preventing the crippling effects of joint degeneration, and preparing and supporting the child and the family for home care.
- Give oral preparations of iron to the child with iron deficiency anemia between meals with citrus fruits or juices to enhance absorption.
- Croup is a term describing a group of signs and symptoms of varied origin. Characteristic manifestations are obstruction or edema in the region of the larynx, producing inspiratory stridor, hoarseness, and a cough described as "barking."
- Most children do not exhibit any clinical signs or symptoms when first infected with *M. tuberculosis;* therefore routine skin screening is an important measure in diagnosis.
- Characteristic signs of hypertrophic pyloric stenosis are characteristic projectile vomiting, malnutrition, dehydration, and a palpable mass in the epigastrium, and pyloromyotomy typically relieves it.
- Diabetes mellitus is a syndrome whose primary characteristic is a deficiency of insulin, resulting in alterations in protein, carbohydrate, and fat metabolism.
- Early recognition of hearing, vision, and speech deficits in infants and children is possible to accomplish through periodic screening and assessment.
- Although a number of bacterial, viral, and fungal organisms cause meningitis, bacterial meningitis is the most common.
- Lead in the environment that is either ingested or inhaled continues to be the most important contributing factor in lead poisoning.
- Acquired immunodeficiency syndromes are associated with certain drug therapies, radiation, splenectomy, and viral infections.

Additional Resources

Go to your Companion CD for an audio glossary, animations, video clips, and more.

evolve Be sure to visit the Evolve site at http://evolve.elsevier.com/Christensen/foundations/ for additional online resources.

Review Questions for the NCLEX® Examination

1. What are the general features of nephrotic syndrome?
   1. Gross hematuria, albuminuria, temperature of 101° F (38.3° C) to 103° F (39.4° C)
   2. Elevated blood pressure, weight loss, hematuria
   3. Albuminuria, edema, puffiness of face
   4. Edema, albuminuria, hypertension

2. Which factor predisposes the urinary tract to infection?
   1. A short urethra in young females
   2. Frequent emptying of the bladder
   3. An increased fluid intake
   4. Ingestion of highly acidic juices

3. Which statement best describes acute glomerulonephritis?
   1. It is a syndrome in which there is impaired reabsorption of bicarbonate or excretion of hydrogen ions.
   2. It occurs after an antecedent streptococcal infection.
   3. It is a disorder manifested by gross bacteria.
   4. It is a disorder associated with a defect in the ability to concentrate urine.

4. Which statement regarding Wilms' tumor is true?
   1. The tumor manifests as a firm, nontender, intra-abdominal mass.
   2. The tumor is sometimes difficult to distinguish from the spleen.
   3. The tumor usually crosses the midline.
   4. If the surgeon successfully removes the tumor without a tear in its capsule, no chemotherapy is needed.

5. What is an important nursing intervention when caring for a child who is experiencing a seizure?

1. Describe and record the seizure activity observed.
2. Restrain the child when seizures occur to prevent bodily harm.
3. Place a tongue blade between the teeth if they become clenched.
4. Suction the child during a seizure to prevent aspiration.

6. What clinical manifestations are suggestive of hydrocephalus in a neonate?

1. Bulging fontanelle, dilated scalp veins
2. Depressed fontanelle, decreased blood pressure
3. Constant low-pitched cry, restlessness
4. Closed fontanelle, high-pitched cry

7. A newborn was admitted to the nursery with a complete bilateral cleft lip and palate. The physician explained the plan of therapy and its expected good results; however, the mother refuses to see or hold her baby. What is the most therapeutic initial approach to the mother?

1. Restate what the physician has told her about plastic surgery.
2. Encourage her to express her feelings.
3. Emphasize the normalcy of her baby and the baby's need for mothering.
4. Keep the baby and mother apart until the lip has been repaired.

8. How is Hirschsprung's disease best described?

1. Absence of parasympathetic ganglion cells in a segment of the colon
2. Passage of excessive amounts of meconium in the neonate
3. Results in excessive peristaltic movements within the gastrointestinal tract
4. Results in frequent evacuation of solids, liquids, and gas

9. Telescoping of one segment of bowel within another is called:

1. atresia.
2. stenosis.
3. herniation.
4. intussusception.

10. Which condition is often associated with severe infantile diarrhea?

1. Metabolic acidosis
2. Metabolic alkalosis
3. Respiratory acidosis
4. Respiratory alkalosis

11. A 3-year-old in the emergency evaluation unit has a spiral fracture of the femur. It is important to recognize that:

1. spiral fractures are often signs of child abuse.
2. spiral fractures are common in 3-year-olds.
3. the bone will heal quickly without intervention.
4. the child will have one leg that is much shorter than the other.

12. A 6-month-old is suspected to have cystic fibrosis. The diagnostic test most commonly used for cystic fibrosis is:

1. bronchoscopy, with pulmonary washings.
2. chest x-ray study.
3. upper GI series.
4. sweat test.

13. A 16-year-old is being treated for acne. The nurse knows that:

1. acne is not life threatening and will not affect the adolescent in any way.
2. acne, although not life threatening, is likely to have a psychological effect on the adolescent.
3. all teenagers have acne; therefore it is not of any significance.
4. acne is the major cause of psychological problems in adolescents.

14. A 5-year-old patient is admitted to the pediatric unit in sickle cell crisis. Which nursing intervention(s) will be included? *(Select all that apply.)*

1. Strenuous exercise of the extremities to increase oxygen to the area
2. Administration of IV fluids to improve circulation and hydration
3. Administration of analgesics as ordered
4. Administration of oxygen as ordered

15. Pharmacologic management of nephrotic syndrome usually involves which classification of medications?

1. Antibiotics
2. Diuretics
3. Antihypertensives
4. Corticosteroids

16. When interviewing parents of an infant with hypertrophic pyloric stenosis, the nurse will expect the parents to report the symptom of:

1. diarrhea.
2. projectile vomiting.
3. poor appetite.
4. constipation.

17. An 8-year-old is admitted to the health center with cystic fibrosis. She has a history of chronic pulmonary and sinus problems. The nurse knows that cystic fibrosis is a hereditary disorder where there is a generalized dysfunction of the exocrine glands. It especially involves the:

1. thyroid gland.
2. sebaceous glands.
3. mucous glands.
4. salivary gland.

18. Which assessment for a patient who is 2½ years old with Wilms' tumor will the nurse not perform?

1. Auscultate lung sounds
2. Palpate the abdomen
3. Check skin turgor
4. Palpate femoral and dorsalis pedis pulses

19. Which disorder is not contagious?

1. Impetigo
2. *Staphylococcus aureus* infection
3. Infantile eczema (atopic dermatitis)
4. Pediculosis

20. Which disorder presents the greatest risk to the child with hemophilia?

1. Hematuria
2. Hemarthrosis
3. Intracranial bleeding
4. Anemia

21. The highest incidence of iron deficiency anemia occurs in which age-group?

1. Early infancy
2. 6 and 24 months
3. The preschooler
4. The school-age child

22. In discussing an 11-month-old's diet, which statement by her mother indicates a possible cause for iron deficiency anemia?

1. "Formula is so expensive. We switched to regular milk early on."
2. "She almost never drinks water."
3. "She doesn't really like peaches or pears, so we stick to bananas for fruit."
4. "I give her a piece of bread now and then. She likes to chew on it."

23. A priority of postoperative nursing care for a 9-month-old infant who has a cleft palate repair is:

1. referral to a parent support group.
2. adequate nutrition.
3. keeping an intravenous line open.
4. continuous sedation.

24. Which statement made by a 7-year-old patient with type 1 diabetes mellitus indicates a need for more teaching?

1. "My pancreas is sick and needs insulin until it gets better."
2. "I will need to take my insulin every day."
3. "I need to keep a piece of candy in my pocket in case I start to feel shaky."
4. "My mom has to give me insulin shots twice a day."

chapter

32

Care of the Child with a Mental or Cognitive Disorder

Barbara Lauritsen Christensen

evolve

http://evolve.elsevier.com/Christensen/foundationsadult

Objectives

1. State five physical and behavioral indicators that normally will arouse suspicion of child abuse.
2. Identify six possible causes of cognitive impairment.
3. Describe the clinical manifestations of Down syndrome.
4. Discuss the appropriate nursing interventions for caring for a child with autism.
5. Demonstrate an understanding of the medical management and nursing interventions for the child with a learning disability.
6. Describe four nursing interventions for the child with attention-deficit/hyperactivity disorder.
7. Identify six clinical manifestations of depression in children.
8. Discuss three nursing interventions for the child who is suicidal.

Key Terms

attention-deficit/hyperactivity disorder (ADHD) (p. 1075)
autism (p. 1070)
child maltreatment (p. 1071)
cognitive impairment (p. 1067)
Down syndrome (p. 1068)
failure to thrive (p. 1073)
intelligence quotient (IQ) (p. 1067)
psychogenic (p. 1079)
savants (p. 1071)
school avoidance (p. 1074)
somatization disorders (p. 1077)

Emotional and cognitive disorders in children present many challenging diagnostic and management dilemmas for nursing. This chapter attempts to provide the reader with an understanding of the unique issues surrounding children with emotional and cognitive disorders. In it you will find a presentation of the psychological, biologic, and social etiologies as well as effective and practical management strategies.

Although a multitude of emotional and cognitive disorders affect children, it is beyond the scope of this chapter to address them all. Please also consult other chapters within these comprehensive texts where related topics have pediatric implications.

DISORDERS OF COGNITIVE FUNCTION

A child's mental health is an integral part of the total well-being of the child. A variety of factors influence the personality and the developmental capabilities of a child, including genetic composition, environment, social support, and culture. It is appropriate to assess children for emotional as well as physical problems during all visits with a health care provider. Children who have been diagnosed with a cognitive impairment (as well as their families) require prompt intervention by specialists in the field of mental health. You will be instrumental in providing appropriate referrals and offering support to the child and the family (see Health Promotion box).

COGNITIVE IMPAIRMENT

Cognitive impairment (whose former designation was mental retardation) is the most common developmental disability. It refers to significantly subaverage general intellectual functioning existing concurrently with deficits in adaptive behavior and manifested during the developmental period. Cognitive impairment falls into four general categories, each corresponding to a range of the **intelligence quotient (IQ)** (an index of relative intelligence determined through the subject's answers to arbitrarily chosen questions) spectrum: (1) **mild** (educable cognitive impaired), IQ of 50 or 55 to approximately 70; (2) **moderate** (trainable cognitive impaired), IQ of 35 or 40 to 50 or 55; (3) **severe,** IQ of 20 or 25 to 35 or 40; and (4) **profound,** IQ below 25.

Etiology and Pathophysiology

The causes of cognitive impairment are varied and include biochemical, infectious, genetic, endocrine, and idiopathic factors. Specific causes include chromosomal abnormalities such as Down syndrome, perinatal infections (e.g., cytomegalovirus, rubella, syphilis, toxoplasmosis), perinatal anoxia, maternal drug or alcohol

Health Promotion

Encouraging Healthy Behaviors for the Child with a Mental or Cognitive Disorder

CHILD ABUSE

- Organize neighborhood programs that support efforts to protect children.
- Provide educational programs for children to recognize unsafe conditions.
- Teach children to say no, and ask for help from parents and/or school officials.
- Prepare children to deal with bribes or threats.
- Eliminate secrets between parents and child.
- Teach child about inappropriate touching and how to control who touches them and how.

DOWN SYNDROME

- Provide parents with information on normal developmental milestones.
- Encourage stimulating play.
- Provide nutritionally dense foods.
- Encourage physical activity and exercise.
- Praise child for accomplishments.
- Provide consistency in matters relating to discipline.
- Screen children with Down syndrome for atlantoaxial instability with a neurologic examination and radiography after their second birthday, before they engage in physically energetic exercise or sports or rehabilitative procedures.*

ATTENTION-DEFICIT/HYPERACTIVITY DISORDER (ADHD)

- Provide a routine for daily activities.
- Maintain a nonstressful environment, but set limits and provide rewards.
- Allow child time to explain events or interactions to reduce stress.
- Encourage parents to continue therapeutic regimen and monitor for medication side effects.

DEPRESSION

- Provide a trusting family relationship.
- Review treatment plan with parents as needed, because treatment is slow and lengthy.
- Provide positive reinforcement when child participates in group activities to discourage social isolation.
- Identify support groups within the community.

SUICIDE

- Alert parents to signs that include depression, social isolation, social withdrawal, preoccupation with death, and changes in eating and sleeping habits.
- Stay in contact with school, peers, and relatives for support at this time.

*From Kliegman, R.M., Behrman, R.E., Jenson, H.B., et al. (Eds.) (2007). Nelson textbook of pediatrics, (18th ed.). Philadelphia: Saunders.

abuse, metabolic disorders such as phenylketonuria, lead poisoning, hypothyroidism, and prematurity.

Clinical Manifestations

Manifestations vary according to the child's age and degree of impairment. Children typically fail to achieve developmental milestones at appropriate ages. Generally, they tend to manifest delays in motor, social, cognitive, or language skills, or some combination.

Diagnostic Tests

It is important to begin assessment of the child suspected of having cognitive impairment as soon as the parents or the health care provider realizes the child is not developing normally. Diagnostic studies include neurologic examination, computed tomography (CT) scan, serum metabolic screening, developmental screening tests (e.g., Denver II), standardized intellectual tests (e.g., Stanford-Binet Intelligence Scale; Wechsler Intelligence Scale for Children, Revised), and chromosomal analysis and genetic screening.

Nursing Interventions

Nursing interventions for a child with a cognitive impairment focus on promoting optimal development and providing the family with support, education, and referrals. The family needs support at the time of initial diagnosis and encouragement to verbalize their fears and concerns. Encourage parents to enroll the child in an early intervention program that will facilitate the child's self-care abilities and assist the family with future needs. When teaching, break up each task into small, specific steps, because the child will not always be able to understand the task as a whole. Encourage parents to keep their focus on the normal needs of all children—including love, social interaction, and play—regardless of cognitive ability (see Safety Alert box).

Patient and Family Teaching

It is essential to provide parents with information on normal developmental milestones, stimulation techniques, safety, normal speech development, sexual development, and the role of positive self-esteem in motivating children to accomplish goals within their limitations.

Prognosis

Cognitive impairment is a chronic condition. In recent years, major changes have occurred in the philosophy of care toward people with cognitive impairment. Children with cognitive impairment are no longer automatically admitted into institutional settings but often remain at home.

DOWN SYNDROME

Varying degrees of cognitive impairment and multiple defects characterize **Down syndrome,** a congenital chromosomal abnormality. It is the most common chromosomal abnormality, affecting 1 in 600 to 800 live births (Kliegman et al., 2007).

Safety Alert!

The Child with a Mental or Cognitive Disorder

CHILD ABUSE

- Provide protective measures in the hospital in connection with alleged predators.
- Establish a routine for nursing interventions.
- Explain all procedures and treatments.
- Praise child for accomplishments.
- Avoid asking probing questions.
- Provide consistency in nursing staff assignments.

DOWN SYNDROME

- Provide radiologic evaluation for **atlantoaxial instability** in children participating in sports that potentially involve stress on the head and neck, such as gymnastics, diving, butterfly stroke in swimming, high jump, and soccer. Do not allow children with Down syndrome who also have a diagnosis of atlantoaxial instability to be involved in activities that put stress on the head and neck. Surgical intervention will be required in some cases.* Symptoms of the disorder include neck pain, weakness, and torticollis. Affected children are at risk for spinal cord compression, which places the child at risk of losing established motor skills and bladder or bowel control.
- Report immediately any child with the following signs of spinal cord compression:
  —Persistent neck pain
  —Loss of established motor skills and bladder or bowel control
  —Changes in sensation
- Monitor airway clearance.
- Measures to decrease respiratory infections include clearing the nose with a bulb type of syringe, rinsing the mouth with water after feedings, increasing fluid intake, and using a cool-mist vaporizer to keep the mucous membranes moist and the secretions liquefied. Other helpful measures include changing the child's position frequently, performing postural drainage with percussion if necessary, practicing good hand hygiene, and properly disposing of soiled articles such as tissues.
- Monitor for adequate nutritional and fluid intake. The protruding tongue also interferes with feeding, especially of solid foods. Parents need to know that the tongue thrust is not an indication of refusal to feed, but a physiologic response. Advise parents to use a small but long straight-handled spoon to push the food toward the back and side of the mouth. If the child thrusts the food out, the parent feeds it in again. Decreased muscle tone affects gastric motility, predisposing the child to constipation. Dietary measures such as increased fiber and fluid intake promote evacuation. It is important to supervise dietary intake. It will sometimes be necessary to scrutinize the child's eating habits to prevent obesity.

ATTENTION-DEFICIT/HYPERACTIVITY DISORDER (ADHD)

- Keep in mind that the child with ADHD is often easily distracted by extraneous stimuli and may have difficulty following directions.
- The child also may have difficulty sequencing, storing, or retrieving data.
- Use pictures, demonstrations, or written lists for teaching and learning.

DEPRESSION

- Assess for diminished affect, fatigue with reduced motor activity, solitary play or disinterest in play, tearfulness or crying, dependency and clinging behavior, aggressive and disruptive behavior.
- Identification of the depressed child with suicidal tendencies and making appropriate referrals are important nursing functions.

SUICIDE

- Hospitalization is sometimes necessary for self-protection.
- Provide constant monitoring to prevent self-injury.

*Data from Hockenberry, M., & Wilson, D. (2007). *Wong's nursing care of infants and children.* (8th ed.). St. Louis: Mosby.

Etiology and Pathophysiology

The majority of cases of Down syndrome (95%) are attributable to an extra chromosome on the twenty-first pair, hence the term **trisomy 21.** The risk of having a child with Down syndrome increases with maternal age, especially as women pass 35 years of age, with peak incidence (1 in 110) occurring in offspring of women older than 40 years (Hockenberry & Wilson, 2007).

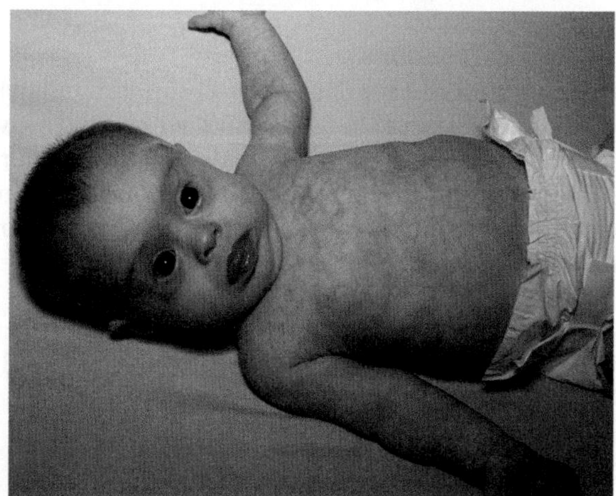

FIGURE 32-1 Down syndrome in infant. Note small, square head; upward slant to the eyes; flat nasal bridge; protruding tongue; mottled skin; and hypotonia.

Clinical Manifestations

Children with Down syndrome have a characteristic facial appearance (Figure 32-1). Most frequently, manifestations in the infant include a small, rounded skull with a flat occiput; upward-slanting eyes with epicanthal folds; broad, flat nose; protruding tongue; short, thick neck; hypotonic extremities; mottled skin; low-set ears; and a simian crease on the palmar side of the hand. All children with Down syndrome have some degree of intellectual impairment, ranging from low normal intelligence to severe cognitive impairment. Individual abilities vary greatly, but in general, children with Down syndrome typically display the following (Kliegman et al., 2007):

- Strengths in visual processing over auditory
- Weaknesses in grammar and language
- Delays in motor development

Children with Down syndrome are prone to upper respiratory infections and frequent otitis media, and many children have congenital heart defects, which are the chief cause of death, particularly during the first year of life. Other associated health problems include increased incidence of leukemia, dysfunction of the immune system, and thyroid dysfunction, especially congenital hypothyroidism.

Diagnostic Tests

As an adjunct to the characteristic manifestations indicating the diagnosis of Down syndrome, performance of a chromosomal analysis helps to confirm the chromosomal abnormality.

Medical Management

In addition to routine medical care, corrective surgery will be indicated in some cases for congenital heart defects. It is standard to conduct auditory and vision screening to assess for any sensory impairments. Treatment of otitis media is necessary to prevent auditory loss, which has potential to influence cognitive function. Most experts also recommend thyroid function tests. If growth is delayed, it is important to carefully monitor and document nutrition, height, and weight. In an attempt to increase height, health care providers give growth hormones in some cases. Plastic surgery to ameliorate the abnormal physical characteristics is another possibility (Hockenberry & Wilson, 2007).

Nursing Interventions

Care for the child with Down syndrome is similar to that discussed earlier for the child with a cognitive impairment. Primary nursing goals include supporting the family at the time of diagnosis and referring the child and family to agencies that provide support and services.

Patient and Family Teaching

The family will need education regarding their child's condition.

Prognosis

The life expectancy for people with Down syndrome has improved in recent years but remains lower than that for the general population. More than 80% of those afflicted survive to age 55 years and beyond (Hockenberry & Wilson, 2007). Down syndrome is associated with earlier aging. As the prognosis continues to improve for these individuals, it will be important to provide for their long-term health care, and social and leisure needs.

AUTISM

Autism is a complex developmental disorder of brain function that occurs in the presence of a broad range of intellectual and behavioral deficits, including impairment in social interaction, communication skills, and behavior (Thorne, 2007). Autism spectrum disorder (autism) varies in the severity of the disabilities that are possible and is manifested during early childhood, primarily during the period between 24 and 48 months of age (Hockenberry & Wilson, 2007). There is a high incidence of autism with estimates ranging from 1 in 500 to 1 in 150 persons (Pfeuffer, 2008). Autism occurs about four times more in males than females (although females are more severely affected) and is not related to socioeconomic level, race, or parenting style.

Etiology and Pathophysiology

The etiology of autism is unknown. However, considerable evidence supports multiple biologic causes (Muhle et al., 2004). Individuals with autism will possibly have abnormal electroencephalograms, epileptic seizures, delayed development of hand dominance, persistence of primitive reflexes, metabolic abnormalities (elevated blood serotonin), and hypoplasia of the cerebellar vermis (part of the brain involved in regulating motion and some aspects of memory). Brain overgrowth manifesting as a sudden increase in head size between 1 and 2 months and 6 to 14 months of age is an occasional phenomenon in children with autism.

There is strong evidence for a genetic basis. Conclusions of the Autism Genome Project, which studied autism genes, suggest that the presence of tiny, rare variations in genes increases the risk of autism spectrum disorder (Thorne, 2007). There is a 10% to 20% risk of recurrence of autism in families with one affected child.

Contrary to previous reports, autism does not appear to be caused by thimerosal-containing vaccines nor the measles-mumps-rubella (MMR) vaccine. Thimerosal is a mercury-based preservative used in most children's vaccines until the 1990s. Routinely given vaccines no longer use thimerosal as a preservative, or contain only trace amounts, with the exception of the influenza vaccine. Many have studied the relationship between childhood vaccinations with thimerosal preservative and the occurrence of autistic spectrum disorder without finding evidence of a relationship (Parker et al., 2004).

Recent reports have retrospectively tied autism to perinatal events such as a high incidence of uterine bleeding during pregnancy, as well as to lower maternal use of contraceptives and a higher incidence of neonatal hyperbilirubinemia. Researchers, however, urge caution in interpreting these findings (Muhle et al., 2004).

Clinical Manifestations and Diagnostic Tests

Children with autism demonstrate several peculiar and often seemingly bizarre characteristics, primarily in social interactions, communication, and behavior. One hallmark characteristic is the inability to maintain eye contact with another person. Parents of autistic children have noted difficulties their infants had at a very early age with eye contact and avoidance of body contact. Children with autism also display limited functional play and sometimes interact with toys in an unusual manner.

Autistic children often perform bizarre, repetitive, rapid motor activities such as flexing and extending the hand or fingers or performing distorted body movements (Hockenberry & Wilson, 2007). Some autistic children have significant gastrointestinal symptoms; constipation is a common one. Studies of these children at play suggest that deficits in social development are a primary feature of the illness. Autistic children lack socialization skills, which will sometimes be manifested by their inability to share enjoyment, achievements, or areas of interest with other persons (Hockenberry & Wilson, 2007).

Not all children with autism have the same manifestations. Some have mild forms necessitating minimal supervision, and some have severe forms in which self-abusive behavior is common. The majority (50% to 70%) of children with autism have some degree of cognitive disability, with scores typically in the moderate to severe range. More females than males tend to have very low intelligence scores. Despite their relatively moderate to severe disability, some children with autism excel in particular areas, such as art, music, memory, mathematics, or perceptual skills, such as puzzle building; they are known as **savants.**

Speech and language delays are also common in autistic children. The Practice Parameter Report of the American Academy of Neurology (Filipek et al., 2002) recommends immediate evaluation of any child who does not display such language skills as babbling or gesturing by 12 months, a single-word utterance by 16 months, and two-word phrases by 24 months. A sudden deterioration in expressive speech is also a red-flag event for further evaluation.

The report emphasizes early recognition, referral, diagnosis, and intensive early intervention to improve outcomes for children with autism. Unfortunately, it sometimes takes as long as 2 to 3 years after symptoms are first recognized for practitioners to reach a diagnosis.

Nursing Interventions

Therapeutic intervention for the child with autism is a specialized area involving professionals with advanced training. Although there is no cure for autism, there are numerous therapies to attempt. The most promising results have come through highly structured and intensive behavior modification programs. In general the objective in treatment is to promote positive reinforcement, increase social awareness of others, teach verbal communication skills, and decrease unacceptable behavior. Providing a structured routine for the child to follow is key in managing autism.

When these children are in the hospital, the parents are essential to planning care and ideally will stay with the child as much as possible. Recognize that not all children with autism are the same and that each one will require individual assessment and treatment. Decreasing stimulation by using a private room, avoiding extraneous auditory and visual distractions, and encouraging the parents to bring in possessions the child is attached to usually helps lessen the disruptiveness of hospitalization. Because physical contact often upsets these children, minimum holding and eye contact will sometimes be necessary to prevent behavioral outbursts. Take care when performing procedures on, administering medicine to, or feeding these children, because they are either fussy eaters who at times willfully starve themselves or gag to avoid eating, or are indiscriminate gorgers, swallowing any available edible or inedible items, such as a thermometer. Eating habits of autistic children tend to be particularly problematic for families and often involve food refusal, mouthing objects, eating nonedibles, and smelling and throwing food.

Children with autism need to be introduced slowly to new situations. Keep visits with staff caregivers short whenever possible. Because these children have difficulty organizing their behavior and redirecting their energy, they need to be told directly what to do. Keep communication at the child's developmental level, brief, and concrete.

Prognosis

Autism is usually a severely disabling condition. However, some children improve with acquisition of language skills and communication with others. Some ultimately achieve independence, but most require lifelong adult supervision. Aggravation of psychiatric symptoms occurs in about half of the children during adolescence, with girls having a tendency for continued deterioration.

Early diagnosis and treatment of autism is critical, and there tends to be a more positive outcome if the child has communication speech development by 6 years and an IQ greater than 50 (Hockenberry & Wilson, 2007).

CHILD MALTREATMENT

The maltreatment of children is a complicated and prevalent problem in today's society. The problem of maltreatment is not confined to one specific race, religion, or socioeconomic level. Although certain groups have higher reported rates of abuse, this problem occurs in every level of society. **Child mal-**

treatment is a broad term used to describe physical and emotional neglect and physical, emotional, and sexual abuse of children. In recent years the number of reported cases of child maltreatment has increased dramatically. In 2006, Child Protective Service (CPS) agencies in the United States confirmed documentation of just under 1 million cases of children suffering from maltreatment. In 2002, estimates indicated that 1400 children died as a result of child abuse and neglect (U.S. Department of Health and Human Services [US DHHS], 2006). Unfortunately, many cases of child maltreatment are insidious and go undetected and unreported.

CHILD NEGLECT

It is possible to divide **neglect** into two broad categories: physical neglect and emotional. **Physical neglect** is the failure of a parent or caretaker to supply a child with adequate food, clothing, shelter, education, or health care despite being financially able to do so or offered financial or other means to do so. **Emotional neglect,** in contrast, is the failure by a parent or caretaker to meet a child's needs for emotional nurturance, affection, and attention.

CHILD ABUSE

It is possible to divide child abuse into three broad categories: physical, emotional, and sexual. **Physical abuse** is the intentional infliction of physical injury upon a child, usually by the child's caregiver. **Emotional abuse** is the intentional attempt by a parent or caretaker to impair or destroy the mental or emotional state of a child. **Sexual abuse** is defined as commission of a sexual offense by a person responsible for the child's care, such as a parent, relative, acquaintance of the family, or babysitter, against a child who is dependent or developmentally immature, for the purpose of the perpetrator's own sexual stimulation or gratification.

Recent statistics reveal that 872,000 children in the United States suffered from abuse or neglect in 2004. The statistics also note that 62% suffered neglect, 17% physical abuse, 10% sexual abuse, 7% emotional abuse, and 2% medical neglect (Anbarghalami, 2007).

Etiology

Many factors contribute to the etiology of child maltreatment, including parental, child, and situational factors. Parental factors include the parent's own culture (see Cultural Considerations box), socialization history and history of having been an abused child, the parent's age and developmental level, attitudes toward the child and child rearing, knowledge of normal child behavior and development, and the parent's psychological state. Characteristics of the child sometimes place the child at risk for maltreatment. Many factors—including temperament, age, exceptional physical needs, disabilities, and health or behavior problems—have the potential to increase the potential for maltreatment by a parent or caretaker. Situational factors include sources of stress and support within the family's environment. Other factors sometimes present include marital problems, financial difficulties, drug and/or alcohol abuse, lack of social support or the inability of the parent or caretaker to ask for support, poor social network, and poor relationships with extended families. These factors have the power to increase the potential for an abusive reaction by adding stress to an environment in which a parent or caretaker is already lacking resources.

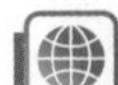
Cultural Considerations

Child Abuse

Uninformed health professionals run the risk of mistaking many cultural practices for evidence of child abuse. It is important to understand these practices and inform the family that they are possibly harmful and place them in jeopardy with child protective services. Examples of such practices include coining (repeatedly rubbing the edge of a coin on a child's skin, producing welts, to rid the body of a disease; primarily practiced by the Vietnamese) and moxibustion (a Southeast Asian practice of burning small areas of the skin to treat temper tantrums and enuresis).

Clinical Manifestations

Children who have been abused or neglected often manifest certain physical and/or behavioral indicators that suggest maltreatment. Table 32-1 summarizes these manifestations.

Nursing Interventions

The most important role for any health care provider, especially nurses, is the identification of a child who is being maltreated. Often you will be the first person to see the child and the parent. A thorough history and physical examination are the most effective diagnostic tools in recognizing a child who has been abused or neglected. Take your cue to investigate further from the presence of a behavioral or physical indicator of maltreatment, because these indicators rarely appear as single factors. Carefully document any manifestations of abuse in the medical record, along with the caretakers' explanation for these findings. When documenting, use direct quotes. It is important not to draw conclusions and to report only objective findings (Anbarghalami, 2007). Pay special attention to injuries that are unexplained or inconsistent with the parent or caretaker's explanation of how the injury was incurred.

If you suspect abuse, it is important to question the child and the parent separately. It is rare for a child to betray a parent and admit the abuse. Even the most battered of children remain loyal to the **perpetrators** (those guilty of committing the act). The use of drawings, play, diagrams, and anatomically correct dolls sometimes help a child to express what has happened.

Table 32-1 Clinical Manifestations of Possible Child Maltreatment

BEHAVIORAL INDICATORS	PHYSICAL INDICATORS
PHYSICAL NEGLECT	
Begging or stealing food Extended stays at school Fatigue or listlessness at school Delinquency Alcohol and/or drug abuse	**Failure to thrive**—the abnormal retardation of growth and development of the infant resulting from conditions that interfere with normal metabolism, appetite, and activity Lag in growth and development Consistent hunger Poor personal hygiene Inappropriate dress for season Unattended medical needs Abandonment
PHYSICAL ABUSE	
Frequent injuries explained as accidents Conflicting stories about the "accident" or injury from the parents or others Wary of contacts with parents or other adults Apprehension when other children cry Fear of parents or going home Wears concealing clothing to hide injuries Low self-esteem Suicide attempts	Ecchymosis, welts, and bite marks Ecchymosis reflecting the shape of object used to inflict injury (electrical cord, belt buckle, iron, radiator, or a hand) Evidence of human bites Lacerations or abrasions Burns that are symmetric and have no "splash marks" Cigar or cigarette burns on soles, palms, back, or buttocks Fractures: • To skull, nose or face • Multiple or spiral • Various stages of healing • Discovered in the course of examination, not reported by caretaker
SEXUAL ABUSE	
Provider will sometimes note nonspecific symptoms such as sleep disturbances or abdominal pain Promiscuous behavior Unwillingness to change for gym Withdrawal, fantasy, or infantile behavior Age-inappropriate sexual knowledge Poor peer relationships Delinquency Prostitution Forcing sexual acts on other children Fear of being touched Suicide attempts Low self-esteem Excessive or public masturbation Declining school performance	Difficulty in walking or sitting Torn, stained, or bloody underclothing Pain or pruritus in genital area Ecchymosis or bleeding in external genitalia, vaginal, or anal areas Ecchymosis to the hard or soft palate Sexually transmitted diseases in preteens Adolescent pregnancy Enuresis or encopresis Vaginal or penile discharge Foreign bodies in vagina or rectum Presence of semen Recurrent urinary tract infections
EMOTIONAL NEGLECT AND ABUSE	
Stranger anxiety Emotional withdrawal Inappropriate fearfulness Delinquency Lag in emotional and intellectual development Language difficulties Suicide attempts	Failure to thrive Feeding difficulties Enuresis or encopresis Sleep disturbances

All states have regulations for the mandatory reporting of child maltreatment when a health professional has reason to suspect that child abuse or neglect has occurred or is occurring. It is not necessary for the professional to be certain or prove that a child has been maltreated; it is enough for the reporter to distrust or doubt the caretaker's explanation of what has been observed in the child. Many states have a toll-free number where reports are taken by a state central registry and then referred to the social services office in the locality where the child resides. All health care providers are obliged to be alert to, assess, and report any abusive situations to proper authorities.

If the child requires hospitalization as a result of the abuse, it is important to maintain a nonjudgmental attitude toward the parents or caretakers. Establishing a rapport with the family will promote a trusting and open relationship between you and the parents. The hospitalization provides a unique opportunity to demonstrate positive caretaking activities and offer education through role modeling. It is important to provide consistency in the caregivers assigned to the child. Explain all procedures and treatment to the child to prevent the child from misinterpreting invasive or painful events. If the child is to return to the parents' care, integrate their participation into the daily routine. In this situation, it is essential for you to document interactions between the child and the parents in an objective and factual manner.

Preventing child maltreatment is an area in which you will be able to play an active role. During the prenatal period, you have the opportunity to identify families at risk for abuse and refer them for intervention. During the child's health care visits, be ready to identify families at risk when you observe behaviors that indicate a lack of understanding of the child's care requirements or when assessing the support systems available to the family in stress. Encourage parents to search for and make use of resources that will provide supportive services. Reinforcement of positive caretaking behaviors is an effective way of affirming positive parenting practices.

SCHOOL AVOIDANCE (SCHOOL PHOBIA, SCHOOL REFUSAL)

School avoidance occurs when a physically healthy child repeatedly stays home from school or is sent home from school for physical symptoms of an emotional origin. School avoidance is the most common cause of vague physical symptoms in school-age children. It affects approximately 5% of elementary schoolchildren and 2% of middle school students. It is possible that the incidence of school avoidance is decreasing as more mothers are in the workplace. This trend requires young children to master the conflict of separation at an earlier age.

Etiology and Pathophysiology

For some children, school avoidance is related to anxiety. Often they are worried about academic progress, peer conflicts, or marital discord in the home. Separation anxiety is also common among these children even after the normal age of mastery of this issue (3 to 4 years). These children tend to have an overprotective parent. Other children will perhaps not be anxious at all but receive secondary gains from their avoidance at school. These children will stretch out an illness until they get extremely behind in their studies. Parents of these children are sometimes too lenient, at other times place little value on education, and at still other times are unconcerned about the ramifications of missing school.

Clinical Manifestations

Children who are of the anxious type tend to have physiologic symptoms of anxiety, including headache, recurrent abdominal pain, vomiting, diarrhea, insomnia, pallor, palpitations, and hyperventilation. The child who receives secondary gains typically exaggerates or fabricates symptoms such as sore throat, leg pain, coughing tics, chest pain, and fatigue. Upon physical examination and laboratory testing, no organic cause is found. The child usually sounds very sick but appears to be well. Symptoms usually appear in the morning and decrease once the child is told he or she is not going to school.

Diagnostic Tests

Diagnostic tests are usually not indicated. Specific complaints will determine which laboratory tests, if any, may be indicated.

Medical Management and Nursing Interventions

Once the practitioner establishes the diagnosis, your primary role is to assist in convincing parents that their child is healthy, explain the diagnosis of school avoidance to them, and assist in returning the child to regular school attendance. Parents need to be educated that school avoidance occurs in "normal" children and that it is stress related and not a psychiatric disorder. Once parents are convinced that their child is healthy, it is necessary that the child immediately return to school. Tell parents to be firm in the morning if the child is refusing to go to school. It is important to bring any somatic complaints to the attention of the primary care provider, and if the condition is minor or without an organic cause, to then send the child to school. Reassure the child that nothing is physically wrong with him or her and that he or she is in good health. Explain to the child that attendance at school is nonnegotiable. Provide support and reassurance to the child who is anxious about peer or academic issues.

LEARNING DISABILITIES

It is estimated that learning disabilities (LDs) affect approximately 10% of all school-age children. LDs impair a child's ability to understand, assimilate, recall, or produce information. There are usually significant discrepancies on tests of academic achievement in mathematics, reading, writing, or some combination. The factors that underlie learning problems typically exist before school entry but often do not become apparent until academic demands are placed on the child.

Etiology and Pathophysiology

The etiology of learning disabilities is multifactorial, and often it is not possible to identify a specific cause. In some cases there is a positive family history. Learning problems are sometimes the result of various physiologic and/or environmental factors such as intrauterine exposure to drugs or infection; birth trauma; lead poisoning; seizures; attention deficit disorders; head trauma; seizures; malnutrition; and exposure to toxic substances, such as alcohol and lead. In many children, a coexisting psychiatric disorder underlies the learning disability. Hearing or vision impairments sometimes lead to learning problems, and it is important to include the necessary screening procedures in the diagnostic assessment before forming the diagnosis. Genetic syndromes such as fragile X syndrome or Prader-Willi syndrome sometimes occur in association with LDs.

Clinical Manifestations

Children with LDs typically manifest problems with speech, behavior, and/or motor coordination; failure to master basic, grade-appropriate academic skills in one or more subject areas; and a progressive decline in school performance. Other possible manifestations include delayed acquisition of language milestones, deficient social skills, avoidance behavior when confronted with challenging tasks, low frustration tolerance, disorganization, and somnolence.

Diagnostic Tests

A thorough history and physical examination sometimes provide specific indications to obtain a lead level, electroencephalogram (EEG), chromosomal studies, and hearing and vision screenings. General intelligence and achievement testing and neuropsychological testing offer assistance in identifying cognitive strengths and weaknesses and in developing a comprehensive educational plan.

Medical Management and Nursing Interventions

Management is primarily through appropriate educational referrals. Parents need to be educated about the special education process. Federal law requires that all schools provide a comprehensive evaluation on written request from the parents to the school principal. Therapeutic manipulation of the educational setting will perhaps include special arrangement within a regular classroom, alternative classroom placement, tutoring, and remediation assistance. Reevaluation for special education is required at least every 3 years. It is likely to be needed more frequently in certain situations of age, severity of disability, and academic progression. An important referral source for parents of a child with a learning disability is the National Center for Learning Disabilities (NCLD).*

Prognosis

With early identification, appropriate referrals, and proper educational interventions, the negative consequences of school failure are possible to avoid, and the child with an LD is usually able to function optimally within his or her limitations.

ATTENTION-DEFICIT/HYPERACTIVITY DISORDER

Attention-deficit/hyperactivity disorder (ADHD) is a group of behaviors—hyperactivity, inattentiveness, and impulsivity—that appear early in a child's life, persist throughout childhood and adolescence, and sometimes extend into adulthood. It is the most prevalent behavioral disorder of pediatrics, affecting 4% to 12% of school-age children. Males are affected more frequently (4:1).

Etiology and Pathophysiology

It is generally accepted that the etiology of ADHD is multifactorial. The incidence of ADHD in first-degree relatives is 25%. Studies of animals have led to theories of altered neurotransmitter profiles in children with ADHD. Certain environmental factors—including low socioeconomic status and parental psychopathology—also play a possible role in the development of ADHD. ADHD occurs much more frequently in families in which there is substance abuse, antisocial behaviors, cognitive disabilities, and depression (Hockenberry & Wilson, 2007).

Clinical Manifestations

Children with ADHD sometimes exhibit decreased attention span, impulsivity, failure to follow instructions, hyperactivity, poor self-regulation, noncompliance, aggression, fidgeting, immaturity during play, failure to follow rules of play games, lack of turn-taking during play, and easy distraction by extraneous stimuli. Associated problems include poor school performance; learning disabilities; antisocial behaviors such as lying, cheating, stealing; excessive anxiety; sleep disturbances; poor peer relationships; limited fine motor skills; and additional psychiatric diagnoses.

Diagnostic Tests

The report of characteristic behaviors made by multiple observers, over an extended period of time, and in various settings provides the proper basis for a diagnosis of ADHD. To accurately diagnose ADHD, it is necessary to conduct a thorough evaluation involving the pediatrician, the psychologist, the pediatric nurse, the classroom teacher, reading and math specialists, and special education teachers, as well as the child's parents (Hockenberry & Wilson, 2007). Many rating scales are available to assess ADHD.

Medical Management

Behavioral counseling, educational intervention, and pharmacotherapy are all essential components in the treatment of ADHD. Interventions aim at achieving

---

*National Center for Learning Disabilities, 381 Park Avenue South, Suite 1420, New York, NY 10016, (888) 575-7373, www.ncld.org.

optimal academic, emotional, social, and vocational outcomes and preserving good self-esteem.

Medications, especially central nervous stimulants, have proven to be highly effective in improving the behaviors of children with ADHD. Positive results include increased attention span, normalization of activity level, and reduced impulsiveness. Three of the most widely used medications are psychostimulants: methylphenidate (Ritalin), dextroamphetamine sulfate (Dexedrine), and pemoline (Cylert). These medications increase levels of dopamine and norepinephrine, which stimulate the inhibitory system of the central nervous system. Some 80% of children significantly improve while on one of these medications (American Academy of Pediatrics [AAP], 2001). Common side effects include insomnia, decrease in appetite, abdominal pain, dazed or withdrawn behavior, worsening of behaviors as medication wears off, and the development of tics. Tricyclic antidepressants, the atypical antidepressant bupropion (Wellbutrin), and alpha-2 agonists (clonidine [Catapres]) are second-line medications. Atomoxetine (Strattera), a presynaptic norepinephrine transport inhibitor, recently became available for use in children. Possible side effects will usually be dose related, and it is necessary to adjust dosages on an individual basis. Regularly scheduled evaluations of the child are essential with all of these medications.

Nursing Interventions

A critical role for the nurse is parent counseling. It is most important to allay any inappropriate feelings of guilt or responsibility the parents might have. Educate the parents on discipline. Teach them how to set limits that are appropriate and provide rewards. Encourage parents to establish a strict daily routine. Counsel the parents regarding the dangers of controversial therapies (e.g., megavitamin and herbal therapies). Stress the importance of accident prevention and safety. Explain to them the need for increased supervision while fostering additional responsibilities and independence. Assist in the development of the educational plan where appropriate. If the child is on medication, explain the reasons and minimal risks of such therapy with the child's teacher and school officials as needed. Parents also need to be informed of the importance of routine follow-up of children on medication. Make sure to check children for medication side effects every 6 months, and to assess the ongoing need for medication therapy every year or more often.

Prognosis

ADHD is relatively stable through early adolescence for most children. Symptoms sometimes persist into adulthood. Early identification of children with ADHD—and referral for appropriate medical, academic, and behavioral therapy—has demonstrated effective results (AAP, 2001).

OTHER DISORDERS

ANOREXIA NERVOSA AND BULIMIA NERVOSA

Anorexia and bulimia are eating disorders with significant underlying psychological and emotional issues. Although these are disorders that primarily affect adolescents, younger children are sometimes affected. For a thorough discussion of anorexia and bulimia, please refer to Chapter 21.

SUBSTANCE ABUSE

Substance abuse is primarily a problem of adolescence; however, it sometimes occurs in school-age children as well. In the child, substance abuse usually points to significant problems in the child, the family, or both, and warrants professional counseling. In the adolescent, the incentives are usually experimental and recreational. Drug, alcohol, and tobacco use by the adolescent tends to be symbolic of maturity or serve purposes of peer group acceptance, stress reduction, or rebellion (see Chapter 29).

DEPRESSION

Depression is generally defined as a mood disturbance with overall feelings of sadness, despair, worthlessness, or hopelessness. According to a survey by the Centers for Disease Control and Prevention (CDC, 2004), 36% of girls and 22% of boys in ninth through twelfth grades reported feeling "sad or hopeless almost every day for greater than or equal to 2 weeks in a row" in the previous 12 months. Almost 20% of these students reported seriously considering suicide during the past 12 months. Around 9% of U.S. high school students reported actually having attempted suicide during the previous 12 months, with girls (12%) being more likely than boys (5%) to have attempted suicide (CDC, 2004).

Etiology and Pathophysiology

The causes of major depression have not been established; however, possible risk factors are genetic or environmental. Many studies have shown a three to six times greater rate of depression in a child of a parent suffering from a major affective disorder. Cognitive theories attribute the development of depression to feelings of hopelessness and helplessness secondary to an actual or perceived loss. Psychosocial theories point to factors including disturbance in family dynamics or in the parent-child relationship, a family move, the death of a loved one, divorce, or abuse or maltreatment.

Clinical Manifestations

Depressive symptoms vary with age and developmental level of the child. In infancy, separation from the primary caretaker will possibly lead to protest (crying, panic) followed by apathy, blank staring, and sad facial expressions. School-age children often demonstrate sad facial expressions, irritability, crying easily, accident proneness, social withdrawal, and eating and sleeping disturbances. Some are also likely to manifest with anxiety symptoms, physical aggression, and academic underachievement. Adolescents typically show signs of impulsiveness, somatization disorders (characterized by recurrent, multiple physical complaints and symptoms for which there is no organic cause), eating disorders, drug or alcohol use, antisocial behavior, withdrawal, fatigue, and suicidal ideation.

Diagnostic Tests

Structured questionnaires or interviews (e.g., Children's Depression Inventory, Children's Depression Scale, Depression Self-Rating Scale) have demonstrated usefulness in diagnosing depression in children and adolescents. No definitive biologic tests are specific for depression.

Medical Management

Antidepressant medication along with psychological therapies is the mainstay of treatment of major depression. Tricyclic antidepressants or serotonin reuptake inhibitors (SRIs) such as fluoxetine (Prozac), trazodone (Desyrel), sertraline (Zoloft), bupropion (Wellbutrin), venlafaxine (Effexor), and paroxetine (Paxil) are helpful in alleviating symptoms. Parents need to be aware of suicidal tendencies during the first and second weeks of therapy. In 2004, the U.S. Food and Drug Administration (FDA) ordered pharmaceutical companies to add a "black box" warning on all antidepressants to alert health care providers of an increased risk of suicidal thoughts or ideation in pediatric patients. Since the decision, the AAP has been working to provide advice to its members who prescribe antidepressants. The AAP supports the FDA's decision but is asking them to reconsider and modify several points to protect patient safety and reduce concerns about potential liability. The AAP is concerned about several aspects of the FDA's recommended clinical monitoring program for all patients on these antidepressant medications. The follow-up monitoring program outlined by the FDA is perhaps too restrictive and threatens to diminish the number of primary care pediatricians willing to continue prescribing antidepressants. Recent estimates suggest 1 in 10 children suffer from mental illness severe enough to cause some level of impairment. Pediatricians prescribe approximately 15% of antidepressants used by children and adolescents (AAP, 2001).

Psychological therapies include play therapy; art therapy; and various talk therapies, including family therapy.

Nursing Interventions

Once the mental health professional and the primary health care provider establish the treatment plan, your role is to establish a trusting relationship with the child. In addition, provide support to the child's family, using open and honest communication.

Patient and Family Teaching

Review the treatment plan with the family and help them realize that recovery will in many cases be a slow, lengthy process.

Prognosis

For the child and family motivated to develop better supports and relationship skills, the prognosis will often be good. However, recurrence of depressive episodes is possible. (Also see Chapter 35 for further information on depression.)

Nursing diagnoses and interventions for the patient with depression include but are not limited to the following:

Nursing Diagnoses	Nursing Interventions
Social isolation, related to feelings of hopelessness	Encourage a therapeutic, trusting relationship. Provide supportive reassurance as needed. Provide positive reinforcement when child participates in group activities or interacts with others.
Deficient knowledge, child and/or family, related to lack of information about depression and its treatment	Assess child and family's understanding of depression and its treatment. Instruct child, family, and significant others about depression and its treatment. Identify support groups within their community.

SUICIDE

Suicide is defined as the deliberate act of self-injury with the intent that the injury result in death. Suicide is the third leading cause of death among 10- to 19-year-olds in the United States. Few prepubertal children actually kill themselves, although many of them are knowledgeable about suicide. Although females lead males in suicide attempts, males more often complete the act of suicide. Females tend to use more passive methods such as medication ingestion or carbon monoxide poisoning, whereas males traditionally use more violent methods such as hanging, firearms, or wrist slashing. Taking an overdose of drugs or other toxic substances is the most common method of suicide attempts (Hockenberry & Wilson, 2007).

Etiology and Pathophysiology

Suicide is not caused by a single factor; rather, suicide is the culmination of multiple factors. These include depression, which is a common preceding factor, loss of a loved one or relationship, and social isolation. The single most important individual factor is the presence of an active psychiatric disorder (e.g., depression, bipolar disorder, psychosis, substance abuse, or conduct disorder).

Comorbidity of an affective disorder and substance abuse also increase the risk of suicide. In addition, not having attained a sense of identity, a major task of adolescence, leads to self-doubt and low self-esteem.

Clinical Manifestations

Many completed suicides are the final result of previous attempts. Warning signs of suicide include depression, preoccupation with death, perceived or actual social isolation, withdrawal, poor school performance, drug and/or alcohol abuse, appetite and sleep disorders, and loneliness. Symptoms are usually present for at least 1 month before the suicide or attempt.

Diagnostic Tests

Diagnostic tests for depression (see earlier section on depression) are useful when early recognition of depressive symptoms is part of a comprehensive effort to prevent suicidal ideation and attempts.

Medical Management

It is best to share responsibility for a suicidal patient among as many people as possible. It indicates that others care. Individual, family, and group therapy seems to be most helpful for adolescents. Although ordinary practitioners are able to manage an acute depressive reaction without difficulty, it is important for the child or adolescent who has made a serious attempt or has a specific plan for suicide to receive immediate attention and competent psychiatric care.

Nursing Interventions

Mental health assessments of children and adolescents are a necessary part of every health visit. Children and adolescents will often be surprisingly open in communicating their feelings with a trusted nurse in a confidential setting. If you have any concerns, be direct by asking about thoughts of death or suicide, when the thoughts occurred, how long these thoughts lasted, and whether the patient has a plan. Any threat of suicide is necessary to take very seriously, particularly if the child has a plan, along with immediate evaluation by a mental health professional. Also help the child develop positive coping strategies in stressful situations (e.g., deep-breathing exercises, meditation, school or peer counseling) (Nursing Care Plan 32-1).

Nursing Care Plan 32-1 The Child Who Attempts Suicide

Samantha is a 12-year-old female who arrives at the hospital after taking 12 of her grandmother's antidysrhythmia pills in an attempt to end her life. She has been despondent since her mother died from breast cancer 6 months ago. Her school performance has been declining, and she has become increasingly isolated. She is admitted to the pediatric intensive care unit and then transferred to the adolescent psychiatric unit.

NURSING DIAGNOSIS *Risk for injury, related to poisoning and cardiac dysfunction*

Patient Goals and Expected Outcomes	Nursing Interventions	Evaluation
Patient will exhibit improved cardiac function	Maintain open airway and air exchange. Maintain cardiac function. Monitor patient for effects of the medications. Treat any dysrhythmias.	Telemetry reveals normal sinus rhythm; no dysrhythmias noted.

NURSING DIAGNOSIS *Ineffective coping, related to depression*

Patient Goals and Expected Outcomes	Nursing Interventions	Evaluation
Patient will develop and use healthy coping skills	Develop a therapeutic relationship. Encourage patient to verbalize feelings and concerns. Maintain a safe environment: • Remove potentially harmful objects. • Provide direct observation monitoring as needed. • Use physical restraints as needed to prevent self-injurious behaviors. Report any changes in affect or behavior. Reassure child and family of the plan to protect child from suicidal attempts.	Patient is beginning to verbalize great sadness and emptiness over mother's death.

Nursing Care Plan 32-1 The Child Who Attempts Suicide—cont'd

NURSING DIAGNOSIS *Situational low self-esteem, related to feelings of worthlessness*

Patient Goals and Expected Outcomes	Nursing Interventions	Evaluation
Patient will express feelings of positive self-worth	Encourage expression of feelings. Approach interactions with patient in a nonjudgmental manner. Provide positive feedback for all successes and reassurance after failures. Reinforce child and family's strengths.	Patient is making a list of her positive strengths.

NURSING DIAGNOSIS *Deficient knowledge, child and/or family, related to no previous experience with suicide*

Patient Goals and Expected Outcomes	Nursing Interventions	Evaluation
Patient and family will verbalize understanding of signs of potential risk of suicide	Assess current level of understanding. Make appropriate referrals as needed to psychiatrist or psychologist; social worker; peer support group; hot lines. Provide information about early warning signs of ineffective coping that potentially lead to suicidal attempt or gesture: insomnia, change in weight, excessive fatigue, isolating behaviors, thoughts of death, giving away belongings, disinterest in future, decreased social network. Encourage importance of follow-up and provide appointments and phone numbers.	Patient verbalizes willingness to attend follow-up counseling sessions.

Critical Thinking Questions

1. Upon entering Samantha's room the nurse notices that she is crying. She states, "I can't live without my mother; I want to be with her." What is an appropriate initial response?
2. Samantha's father is concerned about taking her home after discharge. What are two therapeutic nursing interventions for patient and family teaching?
3. Samantha begins to express interest in others and unit activities. What nursing interventions would be appropriate to encourage her?

Prognosis

Prognoses vary. The greatest risk lies in those children who verbalize suicidal thoughts and those who attempt suicide. It is possible for appropriate mental health care to help these children to alleviate depression and develop a more positive self-image.

PSYCHOGENIC ABDOMINAL PAIN (RECURRENT ABDOMINAL PAIN)

Recurrent abdominal pain (RAP) is usually multifactorial, organic, dysfunctional, or psychogenic in origin. Psychogenic RAP is most common in school-age and adolescent children and is a diagnosis that warrants consideration in children with episodes of recurrent abdominal pain occurring monthly for at least 3 consecutive months once other causes have been ruled out.

Etiology and Pathophysiology

Psychogenic RAP is often related to emotional factors in the child and/or family members such as poor self-esteem, anxiety, depression, school phobia, maternal depression, marital problems and divorce, or other health problems in family members. Consider organic causes—such as infections of the urinary tract, the gastrointestinal (GI) tract, and the reproductive tract—until proven otherwise.

Clinical Manifestations

The child is usually afebrile and will sometimes have occasional vomiting and constipation. The abdominal pain is usually nonspecific, or the child will complain of episodic periumbilical or epigastric pain that is unrelated to eating, defecation, or exercise.

Diagnostic Tests

For the child with recurrent abdominal pain, it is necessary to rule out organic causes. Obtain a complete blood count, sedimentation rate, urinalysis and culture, serum albumin and amylase, stool for occult blood, and culture for bacteria and parasites. In the adolescent female, also consider a pregnancy test.

Medical Management

Once the practitioner has ruled out organic causes, it is necessary to identify and address stressors in the child's life. Consultation with a mental health professional is often helpful. Children with psychogenic RAP sometimes need to be seen as often as once every 2 weeks to a month for pain evaluation and reassurance.

Nursing Interventions

Once the family has been advised that there is no organic cause for the abdominal pain, encourage parents to maintain a normal schedule for their child with regard to school, play, and exercise. Overprotective parents will need a great deal of emotional support in helping them deemphasize their child's complaints. Also give the family instructions to call if the child's symptoms worsen.

Prognosis

Once the stressors have been addressed, the prognosis is very good.

Get Ready for the NCLEX® Examination!

Key Points

- Cognitive impairment (whose former designation was mental retardation) is significantly below average general intellectual functioning existing concurrently with deficits in adoptive behavior and manifested during the developmental period.
- The majority of cases of Down syndrome are attributable to an extra chromosome on the twenty-first pair, hence the term trisomy 21.
- Autism is a complex developmental disorder of brain function that occurs in the presence of a broad range and severity of intellectual and behavioral deficits.
- Child maltreatment is a broad term that describes physical and emotional neglect and physical, emotional, and sexual abuse of children.
- All states have regulations for the mandatory reporting of child maltreatment when a health professional has reason to suspect that child abuse or neglect has occurred or is occurring.
- Learning problems are sometimes the result of various physiologic and/or environmental factors such as intrauterine exposure to drugs or infection, birth trauma, lead poisoning, seizures, attention-deficit disorders, head trauma, malnutrition, and exposure to toxic substances such as alcohol or lead.
- Medications, especially central nervous system stimulants such as methylphenidate (Ritalin), are highly effective in improving the behaviors of children with ADHD. Positive results include increased attention span, normalization of activity level, and reduced impulsiveness.
- Suicide is the third leading cause of death among 10- to 19-year-olds in the United States.
- Psychogenic recurrent abdominal pain (RAP) is often related to emotional factors in the child and/or family member such as poor self-esteem, anxiety, depression, school phobia, maternal depression, marital problems and divorce, or other health problems in family members.

Additional Resources

Go to your Companion CD for an audio glossary, animations, video clips, and more.

evolve Be sure to visit the Evolve site at http://evolve.elsevier.com/Christensen/foundations/ for additional online resources.

Review Questions for the NCLEX® Examination

1. The nurse is discussing possible causes of a 4-year-old child's cognitive impairment with his mother. Which should be included?
   1. Metabolic disorders, perinatal anoxia, hyperthyroidism
   2. Perinatal infection, metabolic disorders, and postmaturity
   3. Lead poisoning, prematurity, perinatal anoxia
   4. Iron overload, toxoplasmosis, maternal drug use

2. A 2-month-old infant is diagnosed with Down syndrome. Which clinical manifestation supports this diagnosis?
   1. Pointed nose
   2. Small, rounded skull with flat occiput; simian crease
   3. Small tongue
   4. Downward-slanting eyes

3. A 3-year-old girl has been sexually abused by her uncle. During her evaluation at the emergency department, which is an appropriate nursing intervention?
   1. Avoid touching the child without a parent's permission.
   2. Question the child only when the parent is present.
   3. Ask the child direct questions about the incident to gather factual information.
   4. Document any manifestations of abuse carefully in the medical record.

4. The current term used to describe subaverage intellectual function is:
   1. mental retardation.
   2. attention deficit.
   3. cognitive impairment.
   4. enuresis.

5. What are the three (3) broad categories of child abuse? *(Select all that apply.)*
   1. Physical
   2. Emotional
   3. Socioeconomic
   4. Sexual

6. When a child is beginning antidepressant medications, it is important for parents to be alert for signs of ______________ ______________ for the first 2 weeks of treatment.

7. The parents of a 12-year-old are concerned about the child's recent diagnosis of school avoidance. When supporting them, the nurse will:
   1. emphasize that the child is sick and needs to stay home from school.
   2. discuss the importance of the child returning to school.
   3. ignore any somatic complaints the child may have.
   4. instruct them that this is a psychiatric disorder.

8. A 14-year-old has tested positive for human immunodeficiency virus (HIV). If the patient expresses a wish to kill herself, the nurse's initial response or action will be to:
   1. tell her that they are very close to discovering a cure for HIV.
   2. encourage her to talk to her pastor.
   3. arrange a visit with another adolescent who is HIV positive.
   4. immediately report the threat to a mental health professional.

9. A 7-year-old has a diagnosis of recurrent abdominal pain (RAP). An important nursing intervention is to:
   1. encourage the parents to maintain a normal schedule for their child with regard to school, play, and exercise.
   2. support the parents in deemphasizing their child's complaints.
   3. educate the parents to contact the health care provider if symptoms worsen.
   4. all of the above.

10. A 3-year-old has received a diagnosis of a cognitive impairment. Which intervention is most important when dealing with the patient and her family?
    1. Encourage the family to enroll the child in an early intervention program.
    2. Discourage play with "normal" children to prevent feelings of inadequacy.
    3. Instruct the family not to discuss their feelings in front of the child.
    4. Educate the family that they should treat the child in a special manner because she is "slow."

11. If the mother of a child with Down syndrome expresses concerns about the child's physical health, the nurse should tell her that:
    1. children with Down syndrome are prone to upper respiratory infections.
    2. congenital heart defects are uncommon in children with Down syndrome.
    3. her child will need to be institutionalized before the age of 18.
    4. most children with Down syndrome develop leukemia.

12. The pediatric nurse understands the following about child abuse:
    1. Physical abuse rarely occurs to children who are strong willed or disabled.
    2. Sexual abuse is the only abuse that harms the child in the long term.
    3. Emotional abuse is as potentially harmful as physical and sexual abuse.
    4. Emotional abuse rarely has long-term effects on children.

13. Parents of children with ADHD should be taught that:
    1. discipline will not work for these children.
    2. accident prevention and safety is important for these children.
    3. medication is the answer for children with ADHD.
    4. ADHD will usually disappear before the child becomes an adolescent.

14. The health care provider has diagnosed a 14-year-old patient with depression. It is necessary for the nurse and the parents to recognize that:
    1. the patient will need to be placed in an inpatient mental health facility.
    2. the patient will have to stay on antidepressive medications for life.
    3. the recovery process for this patient is likely to be a slow, lengthy process.
    4. depression is nothing to worry about in a patient of this age.

15. What are the possible clinical manifestations seen in a child with autism? *(Select all that apply.)*
    1. The inability of the child to maintain eye contact with another person and avoidance of body contact
    2. Speech and language delays
    3. Deficits in social development
    4. High intelligence scores

16. The conclusion from numerous studies involving thousands of children receiving childhood vaccinations with thimerosal-containing vaccines and the development of autistic spectrum disorders are that:
    1. a high incidence existed.
    2. no relationship existed.

17. What percentage of U.S. high school students reported actually having attempted suicide during the previous 12 months?
    1. 2%
    2. 9%
    3. 12%
    4. 20%

chapter 33

Health Promotion and Care of the Older Adult

evolve

http://evolve.elsevier.com/Christensen/foundationsadult

Barbara Lauritsen Christensen and Martha E. Elkin

Objectives

1. Discuss health and wellness in the aging population of the United States in relation to the aims of *Healthy People 2010* (U.S. Department of Health and Human Services, 2000).
2. Identify some of the common myths concerning the older adult.
3. Describe biologic and psychosocial theories of aging.
4. Describe changes associated with aging for each of the body systems.
5. List methods of assessment used for each body system.
6. Identify nursing diagnoses appropriate to common health concerns of the older adult.
7. Describe appropriate nursing interventions for common health concerns of the older adult.
8. Compare how older adults differ from younger individuals in their response to illness, medications, and hospitalization.
9. Discuss how finances and housing are major concerns for the older adult.
10. Discuss changes that occur with aging in intelligence, learning, and memory.
11. Discuss common psychosocial events that occur with the older adult.
12. Identify ways to preserve dignity and to increase self-esteem of the older adult.

Key Terms

ageism (Ā-jĭzm, p. 1086)
akinesia (ă-kĭ-NĒ-zhă, p. 1112)
aphasia (ă-FĀ-zhă, p. 1112)
ataxia (ă-TĂK-sē-ă, p. 1111)
chronologic age (p. 1082)
claudication (klăw-dĭ-KĀ-shŭn, p. 1097)
dementia (dĕ-MĔN-shă, p. 1109)
dysarthria (dĭs-ĂHR-thrē-ă, p. 1112)
dysphagia (dĭs-FĀ-jă, p. 1092)
hemiplegia (hĕm-ĭ-PLĒ-jă, p. 1112)
kyphosis (kĭ-FŌ-sĭs, p. 1097)
nocturia (nŏk-TŪ-rē-ă, p. 1094)
orthostatic hypotension (ŏr-thō-STĂT-ĭk hī-pō-TĔN-shŭn, p. 1096)
presbycusis (prĕz-bē-KYŪ-sĭs, p. 1106)
presbyopia (prĕz-bē-Ō-pē-ă, p. 1105)
pruritus (prū-RĪ-tŭs, p. 1089)
senile (p. 1109)
shearing forces (p. 1089)

HEALTH AND WELLNESS IN THE AGING ADULT

OLDER ADULTHOOD DEFINED

Older adulthood begins at about age 65 and continues until death, a possible span of 40 years or more. Older adulthood is possible to divide into the **young-old** (ages 55 to 74) and the **old-old** (75 years old and older). The term **frail elderly** refers to those older than 75 years of age with health concerns. **Centenarians** are those older than 100 years of age.

Although older adulthood is tied to chronologic age, it is important to note that chronologic age (the age of an individual expressed as the time that has elapsed since birth) is an inadequate indicator of old age. Some individuals are "old" in their 50s, and others in their 90s are physically and mentally active, involved contributors to society. Generally, people do not see themselves or others as being old if they are active and healthy (Figure 33-1).

DEMOGRAPHICS

In the United States in 2007, there were 35.1 million persons 65 years of age and older, more than 12% of the population (U.S. Census Bureau, 2007) (Figure 33-2). In the past two decades, the older adult population (ages 65 and older) has grown twice as quickly as the rest of the population, and this increase is expected to continue in this century. Projections are that by the year 2030, more than 21% of the population will be older than 65 (Ebersole et al., 2008). Approximately 60% of these will be women and 40% men. The major-

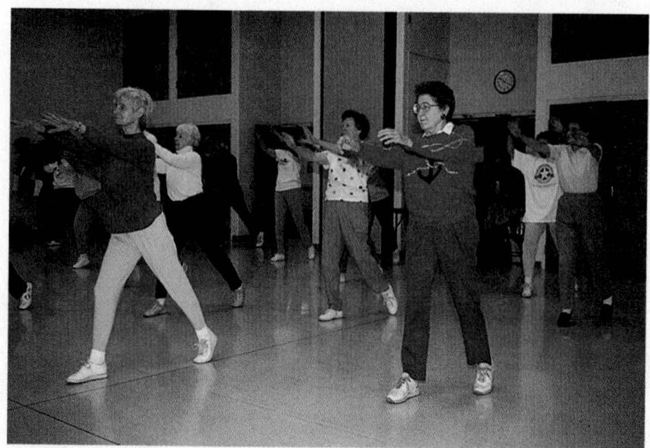

FIGURE 33-1 Exercise and activity contribute to a healthier lifestyle for older adults.

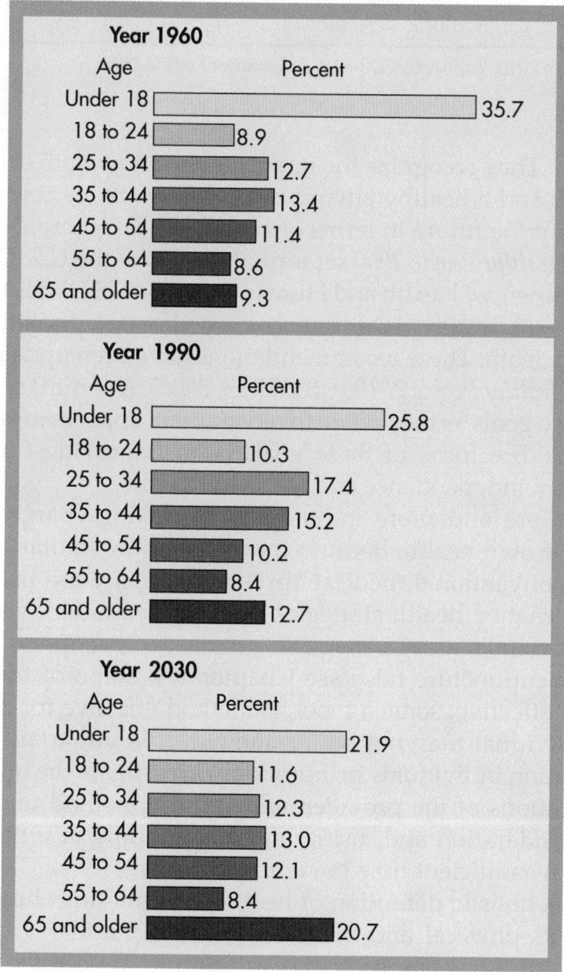

FIGURE 33-2 Age distribution of total U.S. population.

ity are white (90.5%). Blacks and other races make up 9.5% of older adults. In 2002, statistics projected a life expectancy in the United States of 79.7 years for females and 74.1 years for males; breaking down those overall statistics, life expectancy for black females was 75.6 years, and 68.8 years for black males (Ebersole et al., 2008). Japan has a life expectancy of 81.5 years and Sweden of 80.1 years, making them the two countries with the longest life expectancies (United Nations Population Division, 2002). Japan has an infant mortality rate of 3.3 deaths per 1000 live births, Sweden has 3.4 deaths per 1000 live births, and the United States has 6.8 deaths per 1000 live births. These statistics influence the longer life expectancy figures (Ebersole et al., 2008).

The health care delivery system relevant to the older population is becoming more complex for several reasons:

- Scientific advances often combine to delay life-threatening conditions of the past.
- Life expectancy has substantially increased.
- We place more focus today on ethical and legal issues related to life, disease, research, and dying.

Older adults are a diverse group in terms of age, life experiences, the aging process, health habits, attitudes, and response to illnesses. There is a definite need for nurses to acquire knowledge and skills for delivering age-appropriate care. This includes knowledge of normal aging versus what is abnormal aging; strong assessment skills not only with well older adults but also those with delirium, dementia, and depression; understanding of rehabilitation as it applies to promotion of functional ability in older adults; and the necessary sensitivity and patience to treat older adults with dignity and respect.

WELLNESS, HEALTH PROMOTION, AND DISEASE PREVENTION

The compelling holistic movement of our times is changing our understanding of health to comprise a broader definition of wellness than the mere absence of disease. Wellness is based on a belief that each person has an optimal level of function, and that even in chronic illness and dying some level of well-being is attainable. Wellness involves achieving a balance between an individual's emotional, spiritual, social, cultural, and physical state. Box 33-1 lists the traits of a

Box 33-1 Traits of a Healthy Person

Self-responsibility: Is attuned to body messages and knowledgeable about health status. Identifies health needs, defines a plan, and takes health-related action.

Nutritional awareness: Learns about foods that promote health and makes appropriate food selections.

Physical fitness: Identifies and practices a program of activity that works, including aerobics, balance, muscle flexibility, and muscle strength.

Stress management: Identifies sources of stress and identifies ways of coping, adaptation, and relaxation.

Environmental sensitivity: Designs personal space to include a healthy physical and social environment with opportunities for time with friends, supportive network, giving and receiving affection, and reinforcing wellness behaviors.

Data from U.S. Department of Health and Human Services (US DHHS). (2008). *Healthy People 2010.* Washington, DC: U.S. Government Printing Office.

Table 33-1 Suggested Screening for Preventive Health for People 50 Years Old and Older

EXAMINATION OR TEST	GROUP	FREQUENCY
Complete physical, including cholesterol	Men and women	Every 1-3 years to age 75, then annually
Blood pressure	Men and women	Every office visit
Pelvic examination, Papanicolaou (Pap) test, and breast examination	Women	Annually
Mammogram	Women	Every 1-2 years
Breast self-examination	Women	Monthly
Prostate examination	Men	Every 2 years
Testicular self-examination	Men	Monthly
Rectal examination	Men and women	Every 1-2 years
Stool for occult blood	Men and women	Annually
Eye examination	Men and women	Every 2 years
Glaucoma test	Men and women	Annually
Dental examination and cleaning	Men and women	Annually for those with own teeth; every 2 years for denture wearers
Hearing test	Men and women	Every 2-5 years

Data from U.S. Department of Health and Human Services (US DHHS). (2008). *Healthy People 2010.* Washington, DC: U.S. Government Printing Office.

healthy person. It is your role as a nurse to assist individuals to adapt to whatever situation exists so as to achieve this balance (Ebersole et al., 2008).

Health promotion focuses on a positive approach to health and emphasizes a person's strengths, resources, and abilities. Primary prevention stresses exercise for the prevention of cardiovascular disease, falls, and depression. Older people who quit smoking have the power to reduce their risk of heart disease, as well as improve lung function and circulation. A well-balanced diet without excess sugar, fat, or alcohol is another important aspect of primary prevention.

Secondary prevention in older adults focuses on early detection and treatment of disease. This includes screening for heart disease and hypertension, cancer, infectious disease, polypharmacy (misuse of multiple medications), nutrition, oral health, osteoporosis, falls, and social isolation (Table 33-1).

HEALTHY AGING

For the first time ever, it is very likely that most people in the United States will live into and beyond their 90s in good health—active up to and immediately before their death. The age of 65 is no longer considered particularly old. This reality changes the circumstances of life planning, social services, employment, and social policy as well as the focus of health care (Porter-O'Grady, 2001). Keeping this population healthy, active, and moving will require a high standard of assessment and health promotion.

The largest cohort in the United States, the baby boomers, is getting ready to age en masse. More than 1.5 million of them will live to 100 years of age. This group is extremely diverse and better educated, more mobile, and more aware of what is required to achieve and maintain good health than any previous generation. They recognize the importance of nutrition, exercise, and a healthy environment. Many are concerned about the future in terms of available health care.

Healthy People 2000 set forth the goals of the U.S. Department of Health and Human Services (US DHHS) to prevent health risks, unnecessary disease, disability, and death. These recommendations have been updated in *Healthy People 2010* (US DHHS, 2008). A summary of these goals as they relate to older adults appears in Box 33-2. The focus of these goals is on improving functional independence and the quality of life.

More and more individuals are taking charge of their own health. Because they are finding limitations in conventional medical approaches, many are using alternative health strategies such as meditation, visualization, massage, magnets, aromas, and acupressure or acupuncture (also see Chapter 17). Some of these are effective; some are not. A method effective for one individual may not be for another. It is important to caution individuals to thoroughly investigate the qualifications of the provider, research the method under consideration and, using only one therapy at a time, allow sufficient time to identify reactions.

A holistic definition of health does not limit health to its physical and mental aspects, but rather views health as a state of being, an attitude. It seems only natural to encourage older people to make decisions that affect their own lives, but health care providers frequently fail to do so. Given sufficient information, most individuals will make appropriate decisions.

Knowing the value others assign to us and having them treat us with respect builds self-esteem (Figure 33-3). It is inappropriate to address an older individual as "Gramps" or "Grandma" unless the person is your grandparent. It is important to call older adults by name or what they choose to be called; this indicates respect. It is also inappropriate to use the person's first

Box 33-2 ***Healthy People 2010***

GOALS

Goal 1: Increase quality and years of healthy life: To help individuals of all ages increase life expectancy and improve their quality of life

Goal 2: Eliminate health disparities: To eliminate health disparities among different segments of the population

GOALS, OBJECTIVES, AND FOCUS AREAS

Experts will be monitoring the nation's progress in achieving the two overarching goals of *Healthy People 2010* according to 467 objectives in 28 focus areas. Many objectives focus on interventions that aim to reduce or eliminate illness, disability, and premature death among individuals and communities. Others focus on broader issues, such as improving access to quality health care, strengthening public health services, and improving the availability and dissemination of health-related information. Each objective has a target for specific improvements to be achieved by the year 2010.

EXAMPLES OF FOCUS AREAS RELATING TO OLDER ADULTS

Heart Disease and Stroke

Goal: Improve cardiovascular health and quality of life through the prevention, detection, and treatment of risk factors: early identification and treatment of heart attacks and strokes; and prevention of recurrent cardiovascular events

Focus areas include coronary heart disease (CHD), stroke, blood pressure, and cholesterol.

12-1: Reduce coronary heart disease deaths. Target: 166 deaths per 100,000 population.
—Baseline: 208 coronary heart disease deaths per 100,000 population occurred in 1998.

12-7: Reduce stroke deaths. Target: 48 deaths per 100,000 population.
—Baseline: 60 deaths from stroke per 100,000 population occurred in 1998.

12-8 (Developmental): Increase the proportion of adults who are aware of the early warning symptoms and signs of a stroke.

2-9: Reduce the proportion of adults with osteoporosis. Target: 8%.
—Baseline: 10% of adults ages 50 years and older had osteoporosis as measured by low total femur bone mineral density (BMD) in 1988 to 1994. It is noted that there is a disparity between females and males, with females having a higher incidence.

5-10: Reduce the rate of lower extremity amputations in people with diabetes. Target: 1.8 lower extremity amputations per 1000 people with diabetes per year.
—Baseline: 4.1 lower extremity amputations per 1000 people with diabetes occurred in 1997.

15-27: Reduce deaths from falls. Target: 3 deaths per 100,000 population.
—Baseline: 4.7 deaths per 100,000 population were caused by falls in 1998.

15-28: Reduce hip fractures among older adults ages 65 and older.

Disparities

For example, it is noted that in 1998 the highest rate of coronary heart disease deaths was in black males at a rate of 257 per 100,000.

Target and Baseline

Objective	***Reduction in Hip Fractures***	***1998 Baseline (Rate per 100,000)***	***2010 Target (Rate per 100,000)***
15-28a	Females ages 65 years and older	1055.8	416
15-28b	Males ages 65 years and older	592.7	474

Data from National Hospital Discharge Survey (NHDS), CDC, NCHS. www.healthypeople.gov; U.S. Department of Health and Human Services. (2000). *Healthy People 2010: National health promotion and disease prevention objectives.* Washington, DC: U.S. Government Printing Office.

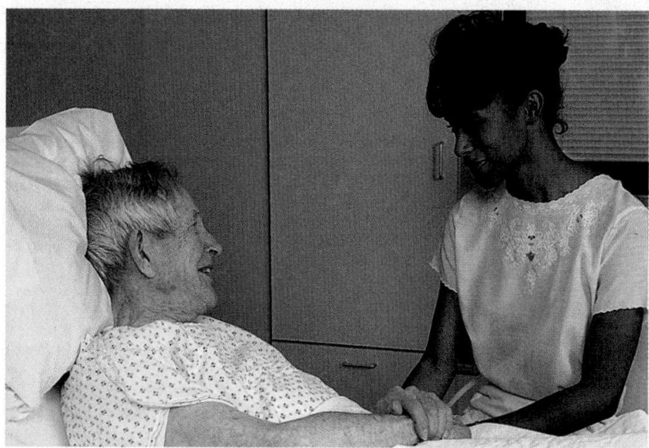

FIGURE 33-3 Self-esteem is vital for successful aging.

name unless the person so specifies. Forcing changes that exceed the individual's ability to cope will sometimes result in mental deterioration, physical illness, and even death. Your role as a nurse includes affirmation, enhancement, and support of each person's movement through the aging process, and encouraging health and wellness.

MYTHS AND REALITIES

The myths and stereotypes of aging and older adults are numerous (Box 33-3). Most myths are generalizations that focus on the negative aspects of aging. In many cases, research has proved such myths to be inaccurate.

THEORIES OF AGING

Our current knowledge about aging and the aging process is very limited. In an attempt to explain aging and a person's response to aging, experts have proposed a number of theories. Some of the biologic and psychosocial theories of aging are listed in Box 33-4. Biologic theories attempt to explain why the body ages; psychosocial theories try to give reasons for the responses and interactions older adults have with society during late adulthood (also see Chapter 9).

Box 33-3 Common Myths Associated with Aging

Myth: All people become senile when they become old.
Reality: Decline is not inevitable. Creativity and intelligence do not appear to change. Memory and learning ability sometimes show slight decline, because they are functions of the nervous system, which does experience some age-related changes. Serious decline in mental capabilities is generally a result of disease process—not age.
Myth: Older adults are isolated and alone.
Reality: The majority of older adults have at least weekly contact with family. Many live within a half-hour's drive of at least one family member. Although it is assumed that the family is the main support and source of social activity, many older people have also developed a network of friends who provide support and relationships.
Myth: Most older adults are in nursing homes or care facilities.
Reality: About 90% of older adults own and live in their own homes.
Myth: Older adults are poor.
Reality: Although the poverty rate for people older than 65 (12%) is higher than that of the rest of the population (10.5%), it is interesting to note that the median net worth of older households was more than $60,000, compared with the U.S. average for other households of $32,000. The net worth for 16% of older households was less than $5,000 and for 7% was more than $250,000.
Myth: Older adults are ill and disabled.
Reality: Most older people have at least one chronic condition, but these conditions generally do not limit their ability to manage their household and activities of daily living. In a study of noninstitutionalized older adults, approximately 7 of 10 individuals reported their health as "good" or "excellent" as compared with that of others their own age.

Box 33-4 Common Theories of Aging

BIOLOGIC

Programmed Aging
Cells in the body can reproduce only 40 to 60 times. Aging takes place when more and more cells no longer have the capacity to regenerate themselves.

Genetic Factors
People inherit a genetic program that determines their specific life expectancy.

Immunologic
The immune system becomes less effective and/or less able to distinguish between foreign and host cells, and aging is a result of the consequentially diminished protection from infection or disease, as well as the immune system destroying body cells that it misreads as defective or foreign.

Free Radical
In the course of the metabolic activity of the body that produces energy, extra electrons are released that build up in the body and combine chemically, damaging cells and interfering with normal body function, resulting in aging.

Wear and Tear
Cells of the body wear out from internal and external stress, including chemical damage, trauma, or dysfunction of body systems, and buildup of waste products.

PSYCHOSOCIAL

Erikson's Developmental Stages
In the last stage of life, the task is acceptance of life and one's own lifestyle, which potentially results in ego integrity. Inability to achieve a level of acceptance results in anger and despair.

Disengagement Theory
Aging is a process in which older adults and society gradually withdraw from each other to the mutual satisfaction of both.

Exchange Theory
Aging is reduced interaction between older adults and society as a result of the decreasing value that the interaction has for both.

Activity Theory
Older adults develop a positive concept of self as a result of maintaining ongoing social interactions. Well-being in later life is enhanced by substituting new roles in relation to family, recreation, and volunteer services for previous occupational roles.

Continuity Theory
Personality remains the same, and behavior becomes more predictable as people age.

AGEISM

Ageism is a term that describes a profound prejudice in American society against older adults. It reflects a deep-seated uneasiness on the part of younger people—a personal revulsion and distaste for growing old, disease, and disability, and fear of powerlessness, uselessness, and death. It is possible to see ageism as a process of systematic stereotyping of and discrimination against people because they are old, just as racism and sexism accomplish with skin color and sex. To combat this, a sense of hope, pride, confidence, security, and integrity have great power to enhance the quality of life for older adults. People of all ages are stakeholders in developing strategies and solutions to this end. We need to work together to eliminate the negative attitudes and discriminatory practices that harm us all.

LEGISLATION AFFECTING OLDER ADULTS

The first major legislation that attempted to provide financial security for older adults was the Social Security Act of 1935. At the time this law was passed, few people lived long enough to collect significant benefits. Over time, increasing numbers of politically active older adults sought and achieved major new legislation designed to benefit themselves (Table 33-2).

Table 33-2 Legislation that Has Helped Older Adults

YEAR	LEGISLATION
1935	Social Security Act
1965	Medicare and Medicaid established Administration on Aging established
1967	Age Discrimination Act passed
1972	Supplemental Security Income Program instituted Social Security indexed to reflect inflation, COLA Nutrition Act passed, which allows for provision of nutrition programs for older adults
1973	Council on Aging established
1978	Mandatory retirement age changed to age 70
1986	Mandatory retirement age eliminated for most employees
1987	Omnibus Budget Reconciliation Act (OBRA)
1988	Catastrophic health insurance established as part of Medicare
1990	Self-Determination Act: Responsibilities of care providers. Advance directives for health care provide legal clarification of an individual's wishes for limiting treatment in the event of acute illness and in dying
2004	Prescription drug plans instituted

In 2000, amendments to the Older Americans Act (OAA) included a 5-year reauthorization of the objectives aimed at preserving the rights and dignity of our nation's older citizens. The amendments retain the provisions for low-income minorities and add emphasis on older individuals residing in rural areas. The addition of the National Family Caregiver Support Program provided a means of addressing the nation's growing needs of caregivers. An additional new program was added to support caregivers of American Indian elders (Administration on Aging [AoA], 2000).

PSYCHOSOCIAL CONCERNS OF THE OLDER ADULT

STRESSES OF CAREGIVING

Older people receiving care may resent being burdens, feel anger and frustration in relinquishing roles, or become demanding in an attempt to regain control. Caregivers often experience role overload, finding themselves pulled in many directions. There simply may not be enough time to meet all demands. Caregivers are at high risk for stress-related problems including depression, anxiety, and increased vulnerability to physical health problems. It is important to assess the caregiver's coping style, how it affects caregiving, and the quality of the caregiver's support system. Conflict is possible between family members who live near an older person and those who live at a distance because of different perspectives. It is often helpful to remind distant family members not to let apparent differences between what they see and what the local caregiver has said discredit the caregiver. They also need to know that local caregivers often have to compromise with the older person and accept imperfect solutions to problems.

LOSS, GRIEF, AND DEPRESSION

Significant psychosocial changes experienced by older adults typically include personal, social, and economic losses. There are role changes and retirement, and the loss of significant others—parents, siblings, children, spouses, and friends. Physical changes often result in loss of independence and space. For some older adults, losses occur suddenly, concurrently, or within a short period. How well a person copes with grief related to loss and how long it takes for grief to be resolved depends on many factors. For some individuals, avoiding isolation and self-pity, helping others, joining groups, adopting a pet, setting goals, maintaining independence, and retaining a sense of humor are successful coping strategies for grief or isolation (also see Chapter 10).

For others, the stress and grief related to real and perceived losses lead to either short- or long-term depression. Fatigue, sadness, insomnia, anorexia, helplessness, crying, agitation, and hypochondria are frequent symptoms of depression in older adults. These symptoms are commonly misunderstood as changes that normally occur with aging. It is unfortunate that few older adults receive treatment for depression, although depression is more common in this age-group than any other. Older people who receive psychotherapy for depression show improvement.

Nursing diagnoses and interventions for older adults with loss, grief, or depression include but are not limited to the following:

Nursing Diagnoses	Nursing Interventions
Dysfunctional grieving, related to losses (specify)	Encourage verbalization of feelings regarding losses. Acknowledge reality of grief. Plan care to promote consistency and reduce stress. Encourage participation in activities to provide distraction. Refer to spiritual counselor or other sources of support. Spend time with isolated individual.
Powerlessness, related to personal, social, and economic losses	Allow older person to make choices whenever possible. Encourage person to do as much for self as possible. Adapt environment to support independence. Explain reasons for changes in plan of care.

END-OF-LIFE CARE

The nurse working with older adults is responsible for helping the entire health care team meet the physical, spiritual, and psychosocial needs of dying patients or residents. Caring for the families is an important part of this care. Knowledge about a person's culture and religious beliefs helps the team provide compassionate care.

Because dying people are often cared for in the nursing facility, it is necessary to understand the 1991 Patient Self-Determination Act (PSDA) as it relates to advance directives, living wills, durable powers of attorney, and do not resuscitate (DNR) orders. The health care team works closely with the patient or resident and the family to ensure that the patient's wishes are respected (see Chapter 10, Box 10-8).

THE AGING BODY

Physiologic changes affect a person's biologic, psychological, social, and environmental status. Physiologic changes in the aging process result in decreased immune response, a decrease in compensatory reserve, and loss of the body's ability to efficiently repair damaged tissue (Ebersole et al., 2008).

Numerous physiologic changes occur in all body systems during the natural aging process. Strong evidence cites disuse caused by inactivity as the most important contributor to declining physical mobility and function (Sullivan, 1987). Positive lifestyle modifications including physical activity and proper nutrition help to optimize physical abilities and promote healthier aging. The degree and rate at which changes occur vary among individuals, systems, and organs, as does a person's ability to compensate.

In this chapter, common nursing diagnoses and nursing interventions relating to each system are identified for selected age-related changes. In all cases, additional nursing diagnoses and nursing interventions will perhaps be appropriate to meet the individual needs of the older adult. See specific chapters for the discussion of nursing interventions that are appropriate regardless of age.

INTEGUMENTARY SYSTEM

Age-Related Changes

Aging skin is dry and thin and loses tone and elasticity, and with less fat under the skin, wrinkles become apparent. Hair grays and thins, and the distribution patterns often change, resulting in baldness. Nails grow slowly, and often become thicker and more brittle, develop ridges, and turn yellow. Touch sensation often changes because of thinner skin, response to medication, or disease. Aging skin is more susceptible to infection, ecchymosis, and tears, and wounds tend to heal more slowly (Danter, 2003). Age spots called **lentigo** are tan or brown macules brought on by sun exposure and are more common in middle-age or older people (Table 33-3).

Assessment

- Observe skin for signs of excessive dryness, or openings in the skin (tears or lesions). Note presence, location, and amount of exudate.
- Examine for lesions that have changed size, color, or shape. It is necessary for a dermatologist to examine lesions that are irregularly shaped, raised, crusty or pitted, or that bleed easily.
- Observe hair for excessive loss, dryness, or oiliness.
- Observe the nails for color, length, shape, symmetry, and cleanliness. Nursing interventions are indicated

Table 33-3 Integumentary Changes with Aging

PHYSIOLOGIC CHANGE	RESULTS
Decreased vascularity of dermis and decreased amount of melanin	Increased pallor in white skin
Decreased sebaceous gland function	Increased skin dryness
Decreased sweat gland function	Decreased perspiration
Decreased subcutaneous fat	Increased wrinkling
Decreased thickness of epidermis	Increased susceptibility to trauma
Increased localized pigmentation	Increased incidence of brown spots (senile lentigo)
Increased capillary fragility	Increased purple patches (senile purpura)
Decreased density of hair growth	Decreased amount and thickness of hair on head and body
Decreased melanin production in the hair bulb	Graying hair
Decreased hormone production	Decreased vaginal secretions and breast tissue mass as well as decreased speed of erection and the ability to maintain an erection Increased brittleness of nails
Decreased peripheral circulation	Increased thickening and yellowing of nails
Decreased rate of nail growth	Increased longitudinal ridges on nails
Increased androgen-to-estrogen ratio	Increased facial hair in women

to manage uncleanliness, excessive length, sharp edges, brittleness, increased thickening, and color changes.

Common Concerns and Nursing Interventions

Pruritus

Older people sometimes complain of dryness and itching (pruritus) of the skin, especially in cold dry weather, because of reduced glandular secretions and moisture. Soap tends to be drying, even special soap. It is necessary for older adults to use soap sparingly and rinse the residue completely away. Antibacterial soap is very drying and usually is not a good option.

In skilled nursing facilities, unless a resident has special skin problems, showers and shampoos take place twice a week. On other days, a partial bath includes face, hands, axillary region, and perineal area.

In general, less frequent bathing is recommended for sedentary older adults because the normal body oils and perspiration are less. It is best to use water- or light oil-based rather than alcohol-based substances. Applying water-based lotions to dry areas and after bathing will usually improve most individuals' comfort and help prevent the feeling of oil residue that some people find uncomfortable.

Moles

Most moles are benign; however, sun-related skin changes, including precancerous actinic keratoses, basal cell or squamous cell carcinoma, or malignant melanoma sometimes develop on sun-exposed areas. Have a dermatologist examine any suspicious lesion(s).

Nail Abnormalities

Bilateral clubbing indicates possible pulmonary or cardiac disease. Yellowing indicates possible fungal infection. Splintering indicates possible malnutrition, and pitting sometimes signals peripheral vascular disease, psoriasis, diabetes mellitus, or syphilis.

Pressure Ulcers

Pressure ulcers are a significant risk for older adults and patients with chronic disease. The National Pressure Ulcer Advisory Panel (NPUAP) estimates that more than 1 million Americans have pressure ulcers. Thin skin and lack of subcutaneous fat predispose older adults to pressure ulcer development when fragile skin is compressed between bony prominences of the body and other objects. The fragile skin also bruises and tears easily. Institute measures that will prevent pressure, friction, shearing forces (forces tending to produce injury by a shearing strain) that potentially produce injury to small blood vessels by sliding on a rough surface (Figure 33-4), and moisture (most commonly associated with incontinence). The best way to prevent pressure points is by repositioning at least every 2 hours. Many types of pads and aids are available. It is important to use aids that will reduce pressure to a minimum without restricting circulation or creating pressure on surrounding areas.

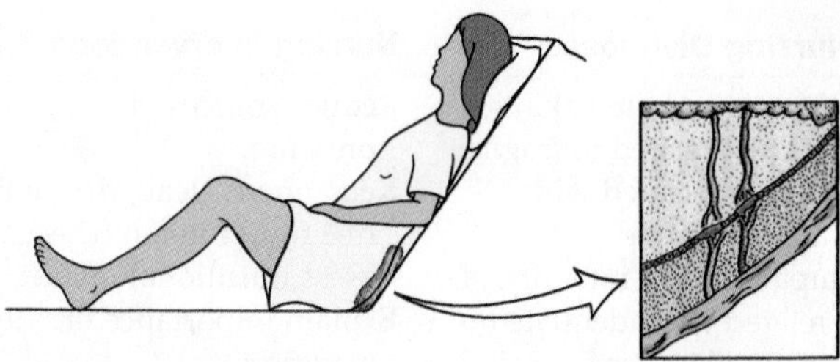

FIGURE 33-4 Shearing forces resulting from pressure against the skin impairs circulation to underlying tissues.

The most common situation resulting in friction occurs when fragile skin rubs against the bed sheets. In addition to the normal safety precautions taken to prevent injury to any patient, gentle handling during turning and transfer is required. It will probably be necessary in some cases to use additional assistance or equipment to adequately lift and move a resident rather than risk friction burns and tearing of the skin while repositioning in bed. Keep any use of tape on the skin of older adults to a minimum because it is easy to tear fragile skin in the process of removing tape. Urine, drainage, or fecal material left in contact with the skin even for a short period will potentially cause it to become impaired. This tends to accelerate the formation of pressure ulcers when it occurs at a pressure point such as the coccyx or hip. Remove urine, drainage, or fecal material, and wash the skin, rinse it with clear water, and pat it dry.

Prevention and healing of any pressure ulcer depend on good nutritional status. A well-balanced diet with attention to protein, vitamins, and minerals plays an important role in maintaining skin integrity in the older adult.

Nursing diagnoses and interventions for a resident with pressure ulcers include but are not limited to the following:

Nursing Diagnoses	Nursing Interventions
Risk for impaired skin integrity, related to fragile skin associated with aging	Perform daily skin inspection. Reduce frequency of bathing. Use mild, nondetergent soaps, and rinse thoroughly. Use emollients and lotions to maintain skin moisture. Turn and reposition frequently. Move and transfer carefully.

Continued

Nursing Diagnoses	Nursing Interventions
Risk for impaired skin integrity, related to fragile skin associated with aging—cont'd	Reduce sources of pressure. Keep linens clean, dry, and free from foreign objects.
Impaired skin integrity, related to inadequate nutritional intake	Assess nutritional intake. Explain importance of nutrition. Provide adequate protein, vitamins, minerals, and fluids.
Risk for infection, related to impaired skin integrity	Assess wounds daily including size, location, and depth. Obtain wound cultures if appropriate. Follow strict aseptic technique when performing wound care per physician's orders. Use photographs to document healing or changes in pressure ulcers.

GASTROINTESTINAL SYSTEM

Good nutrition is essential to health, function, and quality of life; unfavorable outcomes result from either undernutrition or overnutrition.

Nutritional problems account for one third to one half of all health problems in older adults, and many independently living older adults demonstrate nutritional deficiencies. Nutrition involves many complicated issues. Assessment and intervention relevant to nutrition issues has potential to assist the older adult to attain higher self-esteem, improved physical well-being, and a better quality of life (Maas et al., 2001).

Age-Related Changes

Older people experience a decreased secretion of saliva and a diminished gag response, which increases the chances of choking and aspiration. The physiologic changes in the stomach in the older adult include decreases in gastric motility, production of bicarbonate and gastric mucus, and production of intrinsic factor, which cause the body to become unable to utilize ingested vitamin B_{12} and lead to pernicious anemia (Ebersole et al., 2008).

Enzymes in the intestinal tract are also altered. The abdominal wall becomes less firm, and abdominal muscles weaken. Decreased tone of the intestine occurs, and decreased peristalsis is common leading to increased constipation (Table 33-4). The normal changes of aging are often intensified by medications commonly prescribed for other conditions, lack of fluids or dietary roughage or fiber, and lack of exercise. Liver function often decreases, making drug metabolism less efficient.

Table 33-4 Gastrointestinal Changes with Aging

PHYSIOLOGIC CHANGE	RESULTS
Increased dental caries and tooth loss	Decreased ability to chew normally Decreased nutritional status
Decreased gag reflex	Increased incidence of choking and aspiration
Decreased muscle tone at sphincters	Increased incidence of pyrosis (heartburn); esophageal reflux
Decreased gastric secretions	Decreased digestion
Decreased peristalsis	Increased constipation and bowel impaction

Assessment

- Assess oral cavity for presence of lesions; dental caries; loose, broken, or missing teeth; dentures that do not fit well; edematous gums; and halitosis.
- Assess ability to chew and swallow. Assess for complaints of heartburn and nausea.
- Assess dietary intake, especially of high-fiber foods, fat, and sodium. Note amount and type of food and fluid intake. Assess appetite.
- Assess weight. Compare with norms, and monitor for significant changes.
- Assess frequency, amount, odor, and consistency of bowel elimination. Assess abdomen for tenderness, distention, and active or diminished bowel sounds. Ask about complaints of intestinal cramping.
- Assess individual's ability to control defecation.
- Assess bowel elimination routines and use of laxatives.
- Annual fecal occult blood test is recommended for adults more than 50 years of age to detect colorectal cancer, the second leading cause of cancer deaths in the United States (Seidel et al., 2007)

Common Concerns and Nursing Interventions

Obesity

Defined as weighing at least 20% more than ideal body weight, obesity is common in older adults. It is prudent for older adults to consume less food than they did in their earlier, more physically active years. Adults 75 to 90 years of age need approximately 30 calories per kilogram of body weight (14 calories/pound), compared with 40 calories per kilogram (18 calories/pound) for people 20 to 37 years of age. This normally represents a diet of 1800 to 2400 calories daily, depending on sex and ideal weight. With the reduction in calories, older adults need to consume quality foods such as grains, vegetables, and fruits, which contain vitamins, minerals, roughage, and fiber to meet their daily needs without large amounts of sugars and fats. They also need foods that provide protein and are good sources of calcium.

Some foods will often not be tolerated as a result of changes in the digestive tract or difficulty chewing or swallowing. It is important to respect individual food preferences. A well-balanced diet is generally accepted as adequate without vitamin supplements. It is possible that vitamins A, C, E, and niacin help deter the aging process, counteract the effects of free radicals, and extend life.

Weight Loss

A very gradual weight loss over the later years is a normal response to loss of body mass. This typically occurs in association with changes in body composition of fat, muscle, and fluid. Decreased nutrient intake in aging as a result of decreased appetite, decrease in metabolic rate, and energy output also results in weight loss. A rapid weight loss indicates a possible illness and is necessary to be reported to the physician.

Fluids and Dehydration

Fluids are necessary for the body to function and remove waste products of metabolism. It is important for an older person to have a minimum of 1500 mL of fluids daily. Some older adults have a difficulty with hand grasp that affects pouring liquids as well as drinking from a cup. Older adults sometimes also decrease fluid intake in order to control incontinence (or due to illness such as congestive heart failure [CHF]), or because disabilities make it difficult to get to the bathroom and manage toileting.

When fluid deficit is caused by the older adult trying to control incontinence, the most appropriate interventions are to make fluids readily available and toilet facilities more easily accessible. Arranging the room so that access to the bathroom is unobstructed often helps. Sometimes it is necessary to assist the older adult to the bathroom on a schedule: usually every 2 hours during waking hours and every 4 hours at night. Keep a commode or urinal where the person can easily use it. Older adults who have a fluid deficit because of difficulty picking up a cup or bending the neck often find that one of the specially adapted cups with a double handle (Figure 33-5) or a cutout for the nose is a good solution. Some older adults who are disoriented will likely need to be prompted to drink, and those with severe impairments often need to be assisted to drink fluids on a scheduled basis.

Oral Hygiene

Inadequate oral hygiene, untreated periodontal disease, and the fact that today's older population matured before the introduction of many modern methods of dental prophylaxis are factors in the dental health of today's older population. In the future, with good oral hygiene practices throughout life, many people will maintain their natural teeth for life. Many people assume that it is normal to lose teeth during old age, but this is a misconception: It is *not* part of the normal aging process.

Missing teeth make chewing difficult and tiring. Loose-fitting dentures also tend to make chewing difficult and often allow food under the denture, resulting in lesions; both of these problems will decrease a person's desire to eat. Oral hygiene is essential to eliminate debris that has the potential to interfere with taste or cause lesions. Recommended mouth care for older

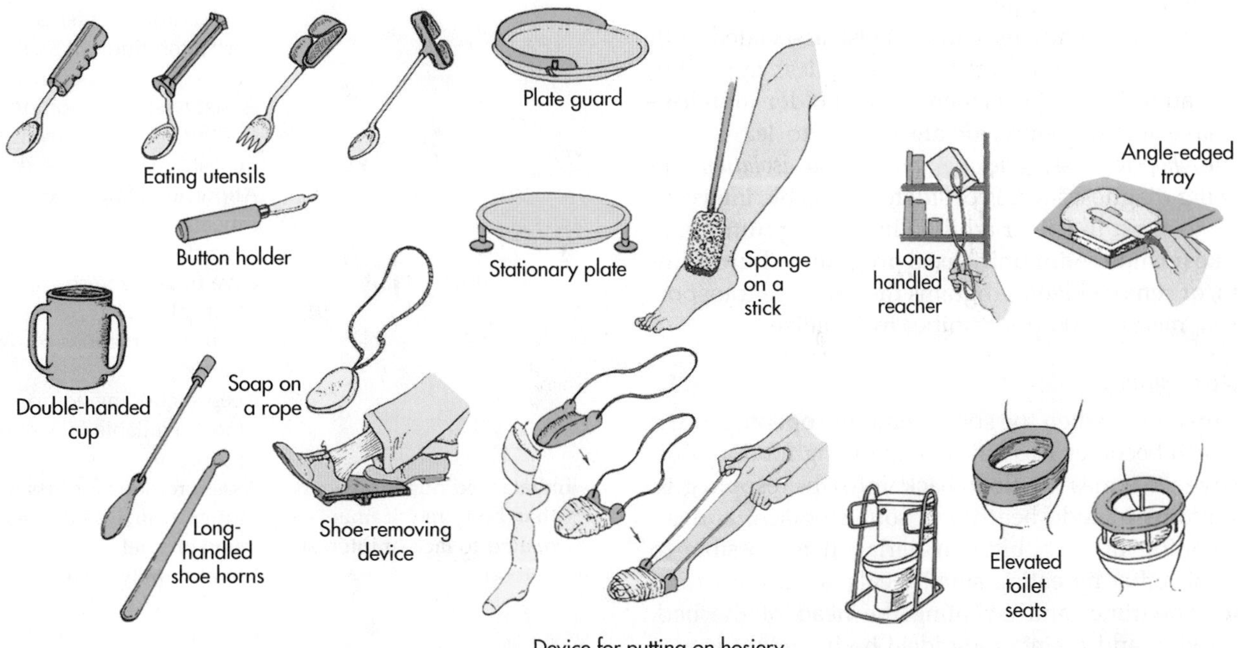

FIGURE 33-5 Assistive devices for older adults.

adults consists of a thorough cleansing of the entire mouth with a soft-bristled toothbrush or foam-stick applicator in the early morning and at bedtime. Mouth care is also important when an older adult has dentures. In addition to cleaning the dentures, brush the gums and the tongue, and rinse the mouth. If dentures are damaged, loose, or exert pressure on the oral mucous membranes, refer the person for dental services.

Loss of Appetite

Older adults frequently experience a loss of appetite. Changes in taste as a result of decreased saliva production and decreased number of taste buds sometimes make food unappealing. Decreased gastric motility occurs because of loss of smooth muscle in the stomach, which causes delay in empting time, distention, and early satiety. Anorexia and weight loss are often the result of these physiologic changes (Price & Wilson, 2002).

Interventions that are usually appropriate because of less taste or interest in food might include preparing the food using color and garnishes, using attractive dishes and table settings with good lighting and bright colors, and providing foods that have more seasoning if there are no restrictions. Preparing homemade frozen dinners from extra portions of a favorite meal is an easy and effective way to provide an interesting meal.

For individuals who have **impaired mobility** or **activity intolerance** that interferes with their ability to prepare food, community-based programs such as Meals-on-Wheels and home-delivered meals from a senior nutrition site are an option. Also, a wide variety of fresh, canned, and frozen foods in small or single servings are available in stores. Older adults need to check the sodium content in canned foods to avoid consuming excessive amounts.

For most individuals, eating is also associated with a social setting, and food tends to be less appealing when an individual eats alone. When older individuals have lost a spouse, or are unable to leave their home, *hopelessness, grieving,* and *social isolation* are nursing diagnoses to be considered. Possible interventions to assist the older adult in improving nutritional intake include community meal programs, church dinners, or senior citizen programs that provide transportation, meals, and opportunities to socialize.

Gastric Reflux

Reflux occurs when the sphincter at the opening to the stomach becomes less efficient, allowing food and digestive enzymes to flow back into the esophagus. Symptoms include heartburn, sour stomach, and regurgitation of sour, bitter material. It is possible to control reflux by eating small meals, avoiding eating before bedtime, and elevating the head of the bed. Achieving and maintaining ideal body weight is also helpful.

Food Intolerance

Lactose, primarily found in milk, is a common source of food intolerance. Dairy products are an important source of calcium, which is needed to prevent osteoporosis. Lactose-intolerant individuals need to replace milk with cheese and yogurt, which is processed and easier to digest.

Dysphagia

Difficulty swallowing (**dysphagia**) arises from many possible causes including a stroke or other neurologic dysfunction, local trauma, and obstruction with a tumor. Focus assessment on whether the dysphagia is with liquids, solids, or both, as well as the time frame for the progression of the symptoms. It is often more difficult for the older adult to swallow fluids or foods that contain firm foods in liquid such as soup, than it is to swallow semisolid or solid food.

Interventions for individuals who have difficulty swallowing include avoiding liquids, positioning, and verbal coaching. It is possible to add thickeners to liquids, which improves ability to control swallowing. The upright position, leaning slightly forward with the chin down, enlists the assistance of gravity to improve swallowing. Reducing distractions in the room and cueing the person to swallow are other ways to facilitate success.

Nursing diagnoses and interventions for the older adult with gastrointestinal system changes include but are not limited to the following:

Nursing Diagnoses	Nursing Interventions
Impaired swallowing, related to neurologic or vascular conditions	Refer to speech therapist for evaluation. Assess individual's unique needs and problems. Verify condition of teeth and/or fit of dentures. Assist to sitting position with chin flexed toward chest. Allow adequate time for meals. Feed slowly. Give frequent verbal cues to swallow. Reduce distractions during meals. Keep suctioning equipment available in case of problems.
Imbalanced nutrition: less than body requirements, related to lack of interest in food	Assess reasons for loss of interest, such as depression or grief. Monitor daily intake. Weigh weekly. Determine individual food preferences.

Nursing Diagnoses	Nursing Interventions
	Provide oral hygiene before meals. Serve meals in attractive manner; assist as needed. Supplement meals with nutritious snacks if permitted. Consult with dietitian. Provide for social interaction during meals.

Failure to Thrive

Failure to thrive in older adults is characterized by refusal to eat, loss of weight and lean body mass, and subsequent malnutrition. This is a complex situation associated with mental disorders such as dementia and depression as well as social and economic factors.

Specialized Nutritional Support

A patient or resident's inability to ingest, digest, or absorb nutrients is in some cases an indication for enteral tube feedings. It is possible to place feeding tubes into the stomach or the small intestine. Insertion through the nose (nasogastric or nasointestinal) or directly through the abdominal wall into the stomach (gastrostomy, percutaneous endoscopic gastrostomy [PEG]) are options, as is placement via radiology-assisted gastrostomy (RAG) or directly into the jejunum (jejunostomy).

Enteral formulas include standard (whole proteins and complex carbohydrates), modified protein (peptides) and elemental (amino acids) formulas. The practitioner will often order short-term enteral feeding following surgery, traumatic injury, or burns. Transition to an oral diet occurs as soon as is feasible.

Long-term use of feeding tubes contributes to increased health risks and discomfort (Kennedy, 2003). According to a recent study of nursing home residents with advanced cognitive impairment and the eating and swallowing problems that often accompany it, 33.8% had feeding tubes. This is a high percentage for a situation that is often possible to manage appropriately with hand-feeding (Figure 33-6).

Gastrointestinal Cancer

Medical investigation is indicated in the presence of the following "red flags" according to the American Cancer Society (Meiner & Lueckenotte, 2006):

- *Mouth:* A sore that does not heal, any lump, persistent red or white patch, difficulty or pain with chewing or swallowing
- *Stomach:* Persistent indigestion or heartburn, abdominal pain, or persistent nausea and/or vomiting
- *Elimination:* Any change in bowel habits, and presence of any blood in stool (black stools)

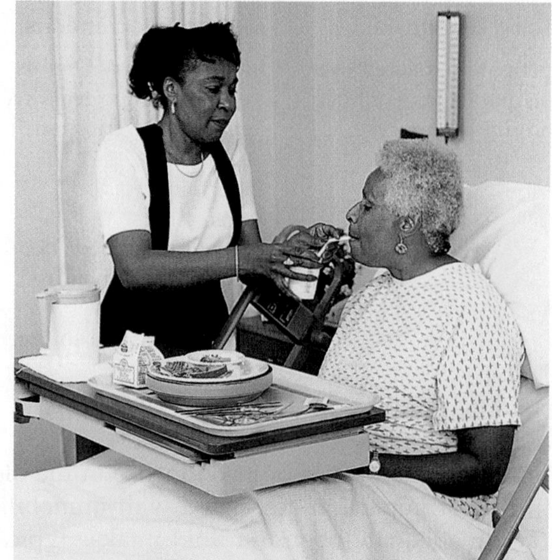

FIGURE 33-6 Hand-feeding will often avert the need for feeding tubes.

Constipation

Constipation has been broadly defined as an abnormally infrequent or difficult passage of hard, dry feces. Failure to relieve constipation creates the risk of a fecal impaction. It is possible for constipation to be acute or chronic. Attention to bowel function is known to be of increased concern to older adults. Problems often develop when there is a deviation from what is perceived as normal elimination, even when there are relatively minor physiologic changes. Assessment relating to constipation includes dietary intake of fiber and fluids, medications (antacids, iron preparations, anticholinergics, overuse of laxatives), mechanical obstruction (fecal impaction, volvulus, adhesions, strangulated hernia, cancer), activity and exercise patterns, and limitations such as inability to reach the toilet or a lack of privacy. Depression is a contributing factor in some instances.

Nursing interventions are to ensure adequate fluids, exercise, and a diet that contains fiber. If it is necessary to increase dietary fiber and the older adult is unable to eat enough vegetables and fruits, a good source of fiber is bran. Depending on the normal diet of the older adult, up to 10 g of bran per day is possible to include in the diet. This is achievable if the daily meals include two slices of whole-grain bread, two bran muffins or biscuits, and two spoonfuls of bran added to or sprinkled over other foods.

A nursing diagnosis and interventions for the older adult with constipation include but are not limited to the following:

Nursing Diagnosis	Nursing Interventions
Constipation, related to inadequate intake of fiber and fluids	Assess frequency and consistency of bowel movements.

Continued

Nursing Diagnosis	Nursing Interventions
Constipation, related to inadequate intake of fiber and fluids—cont'd	Increase dietary fiber by encouraging cereals such as bran and fruits such as prunes. Determine fluid preferences. Keep fluids at bedside, and offer them at frequent intervals. Administer stool softeners as ordered.

Fecal Incontinence

The most common cause of incontinence in the older adult is fecal impaction associated with immobilization and inadequate fiber and fluid intake. Typically there is a soft stool that oozes around the impaction, giving the appearance of diarrhea. Underlying diseases such as cancer, inflammatory bowel disease, colitis, and neurologic disease all have the potential to cause fecal incontinence. A digital rectal examination is sometimes required to determine the nature of the problem (Seidel et al., 2007).

Gastrointestinal Bleeding

Older people have less protective mucus secretion, and therefore they are more susceptible to gastrointestinal (GI) bleeding. Assess for blood in the stools in the presence of dizziness, pallor, tachycardia, or hypotension. Rectal bleeding is a sign of possible hemorrhoids, rectal fissures, or cancer. In older adults, consider a guaiac-positive stool an indication of pathologic disturbance until proven otherwise. The presence of some factors will yield a false guaiac-positive stool, including laxatives, iron supplements, cimetidine (Tagamet), anticoagulant, aspirin and nonsteroidal antiinflammatory drugs (NSAIDs); foods such as red meat also tend to yield a false positive.

GENITOURINARY SYSTEM

Age-Related Changes

Overall kidney function decreases with age (Table 33-5). Even with a decrease of 50%, the body has adequate reserve to support normal body functions unless kidney disease is present. Bladder capacity also decreases approximately 50%, so that it will in some people hold only 150 mL.

Incontinence occurs because bladder capacity decreases, urine residual increases, and bladder contractions increase. Sometimes a decrease of bladder tone also causes urine to remain in the bladder on emptying, causing a person to experience the sensation of a full bladder (frequency) within a brief period. Urinary tract infections sometimes trigger incontinence.

Affecting more than 17% of women and 11% of men older than age 65, urinary incontinence (UI) is embarrassing and debilitating. It is not a normal part of aging, although many believe that it is and do not seek treatment.

Table 33-5 Urinary Changes with Aging

PHYSIOLOGIC CHANGE	RESULTS
Decreased number of functional nephrons	Decreased filtration rate
Decreased blood supply	Decreased removal of body wastes Increased concentration of urine
Decreased muscle tone	Increased volume of residual urine, stress incontinence, nocturia
Decreased tissue elasticity	Decreased bladder capacity
Increased size of prostate	Increased risk of infection Decreased stream of urine Increased hesitancy, frequency, nocturia

Changes specific to women are related to perineal changes as estrogen levels decline. Intercourse possibly becomes painful as the vaginal opening constricts and the vagina shortens, loses tone, and dries. Abnormal postmenstrual bleeding sometimes indicates endometrial cancer, and is always necessary to investigate.

Changes specific to men involve enlargement of the prostate gland, which occludes the urethra and the flow of urine, and the scrotum becomes more pendulous. Although a man's libido does not normally decrease, erections may develop more slowly and orgasms become less intense.

Assessment

- Assess frequency, amount, odor, color, and consistency of urine.
- Assess individual's ability to control urination.
- Assess satisfaction with sexuality and affectionate relationships.

Common Concerns and Nursing Interventions

Nocturia

At least 50% of older men and 70% of older women have to get up two or more times during the night to empty their bladders, a condition known as **nocturia** (excessive urination at night). The most significant age-related change is the decrease in bladder capacity. Although nocturia does not jeopardize an individual's physical health, it is inconvenient, interferes with sleep, and tends to contribute to fatigue. In such situations, nursing interventions focus on limiting fluids in the evening, taking diuretic medications in the morning, and keeping to a minimum the hazards for falls when an individual has to get up to urinate. A history of nocturia or an increase in the number of episodes requires medical evaluation, because it sometimes indicates infection and the need for medical treatment.

Incontinence

Another related problem for many older individuals is incontinence. Some older adults will not leave their home for fear they will have an accident in public. There are several types of incontinence including stress, urge, overflow, and functional incontinence. These types may occur in combination, causing a mixed incontinence that is quite common in older adults.

Stress urinary incontinence is involuntary loss of a small amount of urine with increased abdominal pressure, such as coughing or sneezing; it is common in older women who have had multiple vaginal births or loss of muscle tone.

Urge urinary incontinence is associated with cystitis, urethritis, tumors, stones, and central nervous system (CNS) disorders such as stroke, dementia, and Parkinson's disease. Urge incontinence is characterized by involuntary urine loss after a sudden urge to void.

Overflow incontinence occurs when a chronically full bladder increases bladder pressure to a higher level than urethral resistance is able to counter, resulting in a loss of a small volume of urine. It is accompanied by a weak urine stream, difficulty starting to pass urine, interrupted voiding, or feeling of incomplete emptying. This is possible as a result of an atonic bladder from diabetic neuropathy, a side effect of anticholinergic medication, spinal cord injury, or mechanical obstruction (e.g., prostatic hypertrophy or a large cystocele).

Functional urinary incontinence occurs as a result of inability or unwillingness to toilet resulting from physical limitations, depression, or confinement to bed or use of restraints with dependence on a caregiver for assistance to the toilet.

Nursing interventions begin with an understanding that an older adult is *not* trying to get attention by requesting to go to the bathroom frequently and is not incontinent by choice. Never reprimand or humiliate an older adult for having to urinate or having accidents.

Careful evaluation of incontinence often helps identify *treatable* factors contributing to the incontinence. Treatment options include pharmacology, surgery, using urethral inserts, or transvaginal or transrectal electrical nerve stimulation. Pharmacologic treatment possibilities include newer, longer-acting versions of oxybutynin (Ditropan) and tolterodine (Detrol), which have fewer side effects. Behavioral therapies, such as pelvic floor–muscle training and bladder retraining, alone or in combination with medication, have the potential to improve UI without adverse effects. Bladder retraining encourages a gradual increase in the time between voidings by designating timed intervals between voidings, rather than responding to each urge to urinate. Pelvic floor–muscle training, also known as Kegel exercises, has been effective in some cases of stress incontinence among women who performed them daily. It is possible to use biofeedback techniques to teach the exercises to participants by providing observable information about the location and contraction of muscles of the pelvic floor (Engberg et al., 2003). It is appropriate to make certain that an older adult has frequent and easy access to a bathroom or a urinal or commode. When other treatments are unsuccessful, many ambulatory older adults feel comfortable going out in public if fitted with external collection devices, panty liners, or absorbent briefs. Never refer to an absorbent brief as a diaper when using it for an older adult.

A nursing diagnosis and interventions for the older adult with urinary system changes include but are not limited to the following:

Nursing Diagnosis	Nursing Interventions
Functional urinary incontinence	Collect baseline bladder diaries to establish the frequency of urinary accidents and what precipitates them. Assess caregiver's willingness to participate in a behavioral program to treat incontinence. Teach caregiver to implement a prompted voiding program, increasing awareness of the need to toilet and prompting to use the toilet at appropriate intervals. Assess daily fluid intake. If less than 6 to 8 glasses of fluid per day, instruct to increase fluid intake providing the bulk of the fluids during the day. Restrict caffeine intake, allowing no caffeine in the evening.

CARDIOVASCULAR SYSTEM

Age-Related Changes

In general, cardiovascular changes with aging involve loss of structural elasticity (Table 33-6). Because the chambers are less elastic, it takes longer for the heart to contract and/or the chambers to fill. The heart valves become thicker and more rigid. There is a decrease in pacemaker cells, and the electrical conduction is slowed or altered and can lead to dysrhythmias. With aging, the resting heart rate tends to decrease, and the heart loses some of its capacity to increase the rate in response to exercise. Arteriosclerosis develops as the blood vessels become less elastic and are lined with deposits, which results in increased blood pressure.

Table 33-6 Cardiovascular Changes with Aging

PHYSIOLOGIC CHANGE	RESULTS
Decreased cardiac output	Increased incidence of heart failure Decreased peripheral circulation
Decreased elasticity of heart muscle and blood vessels	Decreased venous return Increased dependent edema Increased incidence of orthostatic hypotension Increased varicosities and hemorrhoids
Increased atherosclerosis	Increased blood pressure Increased myocardial infarction

Hypertension in the older adult is defined as a pressure greater than 140/90 mm Hg (Seidel et al., 2007).

The leading cause of death in the United States is heart disease. There are two classifications for risk factors: nonmodifiable and modifiable. Age, sex, and family history are risk factors that it is not possible to modify. Smoking, high blood pressure, a high-fat diet, obesity, physical inactivity, and stress are amenable to change.

Disparities

Although stroke death rates have been decreasing, the decline among blacks has not been substantial. Stroke deaths are highest in black females born before 1950 and in males born after 1950. When adjusted for age, stroke deaths are almost 80% higher in blacks than in whites in all age-groups up to age 84 years and higher in males than in females throughout all adult age-groups. Strokes occur two and one-half times more often among blacks than among whites. Blacks also suffer more disability as a result of a stroke and are 200% more likely to die (McCance & Huether, 2010).

Assessment

- Assess for difficulty breathing (dyspnea or orthopnea) aggravated by exertion. Assess cough onset and duration.
- Assess for signs of pallor, rubor, or cyanosis.
- Assess for chest pain including onset, duration, relationship to activity, character (aching, burning, crushing), location, radiating, and severity using a scale of 0 to 10.
- Assess apical and peripheral pulses. Compare both extremities when assessing characteristics of peripheral pulses.
- Assess capillary refill time.
- Assess for presence of vertigo, syncope, and fatigue.
- Assess blood pressure in lying, sitting, and standing positions. Note any significant change between positions **(orthostatic hypotension)**.
- Assess for edema. Note location and severity.

Common Concerns and Nursing Interventions

Hypertension

Hypertension (HTN) contributes to coronary artery disease and stroke. It also contributes to the development of CHF, renal failure, and peripheral vascular disease. Pharmacologic treatment for hypertension in people older than age 60 has decreased the incidence of coronary events significantly.

Coronary Artery Disease

An elevated serum cholesterol is a major risk factor for coronary artery disease (CAD). A total cholesterol level of 150 mg/dL is where risk for cardiac disease increases. Decreasing saturated fat content in the diet is the first step in reducing cholesterol levels. Recommend getting no more than 10% of calories from saturated fat, and consuming no more than 300 mg of cholesterol per day (Seidel et al., 2007). The American Heart Association recommends 30 minutes of moderate intensive exercise four to five times a week. Advise older adults to begin an exercise program with a 10- to 15-minute warm-up to achieve 75% of their maximal heart rate safely. Walking is the best aerobic exercise for older adults. They are able to set their own pace and choose the location. Encourage older adults with CAD to participate in cardiac rehabilitation programs to restore their physical and mental health to the highest level of function. This often involves several phases beginning in the hospital and continued in an outpatient setting (see Patient Teaching box). A maintenance phase of counseling, exercise, and socialization is possible to continue indefinitely.

Dysrhythmias

Changes in the structure of and the blood supply to the heart and the pacemaker system sometimes make the heart more susceptible to irregular heart rhythms (dysrhythmias). Dysrhythmias will cause the heart to be less effective in supplying blood to the body and have the potential to lead to heart failure. Although the physician will treat the dysrhythmias and heart failure, nursing interventions are also necessary, such as observing the response to treatment by checking vital signs frequently; noting the rate, regularity, and strength of the pulse; accurately monitoring fluid intake and output (I&O); and observing and reporting an older person's response to medications. Other nursing interventions include keeping stress on the heart to a minimum by monitoring the response to activity and providing appropriate rest periods before and after activity.

Peripheral Vascular Disease

Vascular changes affect the arteries or veins of the older adult. Spasms or atherosclerosis allow insufficient amounts of oxygenated blood to circulate to tissues in the legs and feet. Some older adults have inadequate circulation to the muscles, resulting in cold feet,

Patient Teaching

Coronary Artery Disease

- Explain the disease, the healing process, and signs and symptoms of angina pectoris and myocardial infarction (MI).
- Explain the purpose, the dosage, the side effects, and special considerations of all prescribed medications.
- Instruct regarding these modifiable cardiac risk factors and actions that reduce the risks:
  —*Smoking:* Reduce or eliminate smoking; join a cessation program; and discuss the use of therapeutic aids with health care provider.
  —*Hypertension (HTN):* Take blood pressure measurements on a regular basis and maintain diet, activity, and medication treatment plan.
  —*Diabetes mellitus (DM):* Take glucose measurements on a regular basis and maintain diet, activity, and medication treatment plan.
  —*Obesity:* Maintain ideal weight for body build, size, and sex; join a weight-loss program; set realistic goals; and remain active.
  —*Inactivity:* Participate in progressive activity plan (e.g., walking); join a cardiac rehabilitation program; pace activities with rest periods; avoid heavy lifting; and resume sexual activity within 4 to 8 weeks.
  —*Poor diet:* Follow reduced cholesterol and reduced saturated fat diet; limit caffeine and alcohol intake; read labels; bake, broil, steam foods; and eat recommended amounts of fruits, vegetables, and grains.
  —*Stress:* Identify stressful situations and avoid them or modify reactions; walk to relieve anger; develop and use relaxation techniques as needed; and join a stress management group.

Modified from Meiner, S.E., & Lueckenotte, A. (2006). *Gerontologic nursing.* (3rd ed.). St. Louis: Mosby.

numbness, and intermittent **claudication** (cramping pain in the calves). Inadequate supply of arterial blood to the lower extremities results in a condition called peripheral vascular disease (PVD). Another common condition is varicose veins, involving failure of the valves to close adequately because of distention and weakening of the venous walls.

Nursing interventions include techniques to promote circulation, including walking to stimulate venous return, avoiding standing in one place for long periods, and not crossing the legs or knotting stockings to hold them up. For varicose veins, compression stockings offer a way to give veins needed support.

When inadequate circulation results in skin ulcerations and altered sensation (numbness), nursing interventions include compression stockings, pneumatic compression pumps, Unna boots, maintaining the cleanliness of the feet and legs; adequate shoes that will give protection, but not bind or rub; and teaching the older adult to be aware of situations that may cause injury, because sensation for hot and cold is decreased.

A nursing diagnosis and interventions for the older adult with peripheral vascular disease include but are not limited to the following:

Nursing Diagnosis	Nursing Interventions
Ineffective tissue perfusion, peripheral, related to circulatory changes with aging	Assess peripheral tissue for color, temperature sensation, movement, and the presence of pain. Assess rate, rhythm, and volume of peripheral pulses. Assess for the presence of edema. Apply antiembolism garments as ordered. Teach patient to avoid constrictive clothing. Establish a walking program to slowly and steadily increase walking distance without pain. Administer vasodilating or cardiotonic medications as ordered. Handle body tissues gently. Avoid temperature extremes. Discourage smoking.

RESPIRATORY SYSTEM

Age-Related Changes

The tissues of the lungs and bronchi become less elastic and more rigid with age. The ribs become less mobile, and osteoporosis and calcification of the cartilage lead to rigidity and stiffness of the thoracic cage. The oxygen-carrying capacity (hemoglobin) is often diminished in older adults. Muscles associated with respiration sometimes weaken, so that lung expansion and vital capacity are decreased. Older adults also tend to have a decrease in the number and effectiveness of cilia in the tracheobronchial tree, which results in increased difficulty in clearing secretions and increased risk of respiratory infections. This together with less elastic alveoli decreases vital capacity, which leads to shortness of breath with activity (Meiner & Lueckenotte, 2006).

In the presence of **kyphosis,** an abnormal curve in the upper spine sometimes called "dowager's hump," the chest wall is less able to expand because of changes in the skeletal system (Table 33-7). Overall, the older person's air exchange is reduced, and secretions as well as residual air remain in the lungs.

In addition there are *lifestyle factors* that affect lung function. Exercise has a positive effect on the respira-

Table 33-7 Respiratory Changes with Aging

PHYSIOLOGIC CHANGE	RESULTS
Decreased body fluids	Decreased ability to humidify air
Decreased number of cilia	Decreased ability to trap debris
Decreased tissue elasticity	Decreased gas exchange Increased pooling of secretions in lower lobes
Decreased number of capillaries	Decreased gas exchange
Increased calcification of cartilage	Increased rigidity of ribcage Decreased lung capacity
Possible development of kyphosis, an abnormal curve in the upper spine called "dowager's hump"	The chest wall is less able to expand because of changes in the skeletal system

tory and cardiovascular systems, and in turn, immobility has a negative effect. We have long known about the lung damage that smoking causes. Recently we have learned about the damaging effects of prolonged exposure to secondhand smoke in the lungs of nonsmokers. Obesity results in markedly reduced pulmonary function and increases breathlessness. Diminished cough and arousal reflexes increase the likelihood of aspiration during sleep. The increased sleep time of older adults increases the risk of both aspiration and oxygen desaturation due to diminished ventilatory drive and a loss of upper airway tone that predisposes to apnea or hypopnea.

Assessment

- Assess depth, rhythm, and rate of respiration at rest and with activity.
- Inspect the chest for shape and symmetry, body position, and use of accessory muscles for respiration.
- Assess breath sounds for adventitious sounds including crackles and wheezing (inspiratory or expiratory).
- Assess the amount of activity the individual is able to tolerate. Note activities that result in increased respiratory effort. Have patient or resident evaluate breathlessness on a scale of 0 to 10.
- Assess for the presence of cough. Note whether productive or nonproductive. Assess amount, frequency, and color of sputum production.

Common Concerns and Nursing Interventions

Chronic Obstructive Pulmonary Disease (COPD)

A common respiratory condition of older adults, COPD is not a single disease but commonly a combination of chronic bronchitis, chronic asthma, and emphysema in varying degrees that results in progressive changes that are seen as individuals become older. A smoking history increases the risk of debilitating COPD. Assessment reveals diminished breath sounds, crackles, and wheezes as well as a "barrel chest" characterized by an increased anteroposterior diameter. By 90 years of age, nearly everyone has some degree of COPD.

Nursing interventions for older adults with mild to moderate COPD include pulmonary hygiene, breathing retraining, chest physiotherapy, medications, smoking cessation, and exercise programs. Pulmonary hygiene includes hydrating to liquefy secretions and removing secretions by teaching deep diaphragmatic breathing and a variety of coughing techniques to improve airway clearance. Techniques such as pursed-lip breathing help empty the lungs of used air, which in turn promotes inhalation of adequate oxygen. Chest physiotherapy (CPT) includes chest percussion, postural drainage, and vibration and rib shaking. Postural drainage consists of positioning the patient in a head-down position to facilitate drainage of pulmonary secretions. Options for medication administration include giving them by mouth, metered-dose inhaler (MDI), or nebulizer (oxygen therapy is considered a medication). The patient and the family need to learn correct oxygen liter flow, when it is to be used, and care and use of the equipment.

It is important to teach patients how to adapt their lifestyles and activities of daily living (ADLs). Regular exercise of 30 minutes of moderate intensity 3 to 5 days a week reduces cardiovascular disease risks, improves musculoskeletal function, helps promote weight loss, and helps prevent bone loss in older adults. In the presence of COPD, it is necessary to start a program in very small increments, such as walking for 3 to 5 minutes daily. Appropriate exercise intensity maintains heart rate of at least 55% of the maximum rate for a patient's age, that is, a rate of 88 for a 60-year-old and 80 for a 75-year-old. Classes and exercise times usually allow for socialization with others, emotional support, and the opportunity to get out of the home.

Additional interventions include avoiding smoking and air pollution, preventing infections by avoiding crowds and people with upper respiratory infections, and using flu vaccines. Older patients with COPD often find it difficult, if not impossible, to stop smoking. Success partly depends on the support of family and friends. Programs are available through the American Lung Association and the American Cancer Society and many community hospitals.

Because respiratory function affects many other systems and the functional ability of the individual, other nursing diagnoses and interventions are likely to be appropriate for a patient with COPD.

Pneumonia

Age-related changes and decreased resistance to respiratory infections cause more older individuals to contract and die from pneumonia than younger people. Even with modern antibiotics and sophisticated medical treatment, pneumonia has the potential to be life threatening for the older adult. This is especially true if an older adult is hospitalized and has other chronic illnesses.

Older individuals do not always exhibit the usual signs and symptoms of pneumonia, such as high fever, cough, pain, and headache. In contrast, they often show signs and symptoms only of lethargy, disorientation, anorexia, and low or mild fever. Older adults showing such signs and symptoms need to consult a physician for diagnosis and treatment.

Interventions focus on liquefying secretions through adequate intake of fluids and prescribed medications, assisting removal of secretions by teaching proper coughing technique to improve airway clearance, and turning and deep breathing to improve gas exchange and prevent stasis of secretions (see Home Care Considerations box).

Nursing diagnoses and interventions for the older adult with respiratory changes include but are not limited to the following:

Nursing Diagnoses	Nursing Interventions
Ineffective airway clearance, related to excessive tenacious secretions	Assess respiratory patterns, effort, and lung sounds. Observe for signs of cyanosis. Teach effective breathing and coughing. Promote adequate hydration. Suction secretions if necessary. Administer supplemental oxygen and nebulizer treatments as ordered. Encourage use of spirometry as ordered.
Ineffective breathing pattern, related to inactivity	Assess respiratory patterns, effort, and lung sounds. Observe for signs of cyanosis. Position patient to maximize chest expansion. Maintain calm, restful environment. Administer sedatives or analgesics with caution.
Impaired gas exchange, related to elevated CO_2 (carbon dioxide)	Monitor oximetry readings for oxygen saturation. Administer oxygen per protocol.

Lung Cancer

Lung cancer is the leading cause of cancer deaths; it is rare in people less than 40 years of age and increases in incidence between ages 60 and 70. Risk factors for developing lung cancer include use of tobacco or marijuana; recurring inflammation; exposure to asbestos, talcum powder, or minerals or, less frequently, to radon; heredity; vitamin A deficiency; and air pollution. The leading cell types of lung cancer includes small-cell lung carcinoma (SCLC), which sometimes metastasizes to the central nervous system, the bones, and the liver. Often there are no signs or symptoms, or the signs are ignored or attributed to smoking or a preexisting lung disease. Common early signs and symptoms include cough, chest pain, and hemoptysis. The physician bases a diagnosis on the clinical history and chest x-ray studies or computed tomography (CT) scan of the chest. Lung cancer staging provides the basis for treatment. Stage I is treatable with surgery. Treatment modalities for other stages include surgery, radiotherapy, and adjuvant chemotherapy. Stage IV treatment is palliative and includes radiotherapy, chemotherapy, and laser therapy. Nursing interventions include relief of pain, emotional support, counseling, and discussion of options and alternatives.

Home Care Considerations

Respiratory Disorders

- Encourage homebound older adults with respiratory disease to drink 8 to 10 glasses of water a day, if not contraindicated.
- Encourage homebound older adults with respiratory disease to exercise within their capacity to promote thoracic muscle conditioning.
- Monitor homebound older adults for smoking and exposure to secondhand smoke. Encourage family members to not smoke in the presence of the older adult.
- Encourage homebound older adults to use pursed-lip breathing to control breathlessness and improve oxygenation.
- Monitor pulse oximetry to assess oxygenation.
- Encourage frequent small meals to reduce breathlessness associated with eating.
- If an older adult is using home oxygen, assess the home environment for potential safety hazards, including the possibility of the older adult tripping over oxygen tubing.
- Assess the older adult for confusion, occipital headaches, and forgetfulness. These symptoms may be indicative of carbon dioxide retention. Teach family caregivers these signs as well.

Modified from Meiner, S.E., & Lueckenotte, A. (2006). *Gerontologic nursing.* (3rd ed.). St. Louis: Mosby.

MUSCULOSKELETAL SYSTEM

Age-Related Changes

Some of the most obvious changes associated with aging occur in the musculoskeletal system. There is a gradual reduction in the number and the size of active muscle fibers, and there is decreased muscle tone, mass, and strength. The joints become less elastic and flexible with the loss and calcification of cartilage. There is an alteration in the equilibrium between bone deposition and resorption. For menopausal women, decreased estrogen increases bone resorption and decreases calcium deposition, resulting in bone loss and decreased bone density. The loss of bone density particularly affects the long bones and the vertebrae. In the spine, narrowing of the intervertebral spaces results in a loss of 1½ to 3 inches of height. The lumbar curve of the lower back changes, which results in a shift in the center of gravity. The gait changes as well, based on structural and postural changes. Changes in weight-bearing bones predispose to fractures (Seidel et al., 2007) (Table 33-8).

Assessment

- Assess joints, including both active and passive range of motion of each joint.
- Assess for stiffness and limitation of movement, edema or erythema, pain, and crepitus with particular motions. Assess functional abilities: (1) personal care (eating, bathing, dressing, grooming, elimination); (2) other activities (housework, driving, climbing stairs, caring for pets).
- Assess standing and gait, including balance, posture, base of support, size of steps, and ability to turn. Assess for limping, numbness or tingling, deformity or change in skeletal contour.
- Assess for muscle weakness, paralysis, tremors, spasms, clumsiness, muscle wasting, and muscle aches.
- Assess pain using a scale of 0 to 10, location, type, onset (sudden or gradual), aggravating or alleviating factors, and position of comfort.
- Assess history of falls, traumatic injury, surgeries on joint or bone, and back problems.

Common Concerns and Nursing Interventions

Arthritis

Two forms of arthritis sometimes occur in the older adult. Rheumatoid arthritis, a systemic inflammatory disease thought to be of immune factor origin, has the potential to affect people of any age but is most common in women after the age of 60. Osteoarthritis, or degenerative joint disease, is a noninflammatory disorder in which the cartilage in the joints deteriorates and new bone forms on the surface. This is the most common type of arthritis in older adults. Experts estimate that more than 90% of the population 40 years of age or older are affected, although a person will sometimes not experience signs or symptoms for many years (Ebersole et al., 2008). Affected joints most commonly include the distal and proximal interphalangeals, the knees, the hips, and the spine.

Because the chronic nature of osteoarthritis affects an individual's functional ability and lifestyle, interventions for older individuals with arthritis involve joint protection and energy conservation through a balance between rest and exercise. Simple measures such as a warm bath or shower in the morning often reduce early morning stiffness. Recommend range-of-motion and other forms of mild exercise to maintain muscle strength and joint motion. Heat or cold therapy and gentle massage usually help to control pain and muscle spasms. The health care provider will often prescribe NSAIDs and nonopioid analgesics. Injections of steroids into the joints two or three times yearly help with chronic pain.

In more advanced situations, use of assistive devices is common, such as splints, walkers, adapted utensils, and clothes with Velcro fasteners. With increasing disability and severe pain, many people consider surgical options. Joint arthroplasty, a surgical replacement of the involved joint, is successful in joints including shoulders, elbows, fingers, hips, and knees. Other surgical options include joint fusion, which increases function and decreases pain while eliminating some joint movement.

Table 33-8 Musculoskeletal Changes with Aging

PHYSIOLOGIC CHANGE	RESULTS
Decreased bone calcium	Osteoporosis Increased curvature of the spine (kyphosis)
Decreased fluid in intervertebral disks	Decreased height
Decreased blood supply to muscles	Decreased muscle strength
Decreased joint mobility	Decreased mobility and flexibility
Decreased muscle mass	Decreased strength Increased risk of falls

Hip Fractures

Because of age-related changes in the musculoskeletal system, falls pose an increased risk of fracture; in fact, about 5% of falls result in fracture (van Haastregt et al., 2000). The most frequently occurring fractures among older adults are hip, vertebral, and clavicular fractures. Fractures fall into two categories, open or closed, and vary according to location and type. The history of the patient with a fracture usually includes trauma followed by immediate local pain. Tenderness, edema, muscle spasm, deformity, bleeding, and loss of function are other manifestations common with fractures. Of these, hip fractures are the most disabling type for older adults. A significant percentage of patients with hip fracture die within 1 year following injury.

Clinicians use the locations of hip fractures to classify them. Intracapsular or subcapital fractures occur within the hip capsule. Extracapsular fractures occur below the capsule and include intertrochanteric and subtrochanteric (Figure 33-7).

After the injury that results in the fractured hip, the affected extremity is usually externally rotated and shortened. Tenderness and severe pain at the fracture site are often present. It is necessary to immobilize the joint, often with traction. Surgical repair is the preferred treatment when the patient's condition has stabilized. Surgery depends on the location and type of fracture and often includes open reduction and inter-

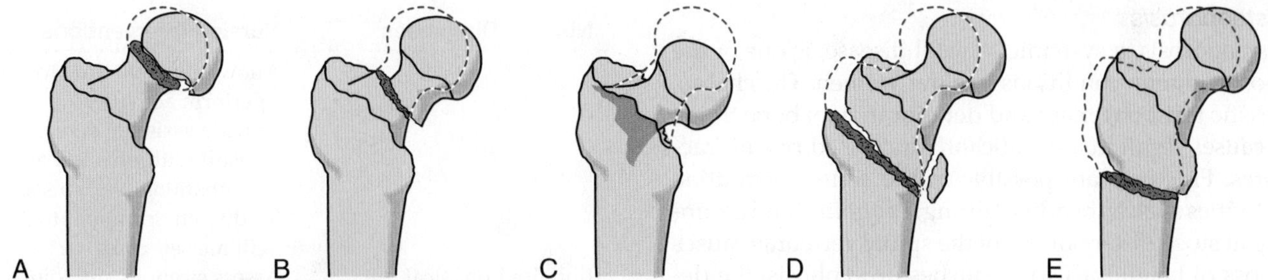

FIGURE 33-7 Types of fractures of the hip. **A,** Subcapital fracture. **B,** Transcervical fracture. **C,** Impacted fracture of the base of the neck. **D,** Intertrochanteric fracture. **E,** Subtrochanteric fracture.

nal fixation (ORIF) with pins, plates, and screws for extracapsular fractures (Figure 33-8, *A*) or prosthetic replacement of the femoral head for intracapsular fractures (bipolar or hemiarthroplasty) (Figure 33-8, *B*).

Nursing interventions postoperatively requires monitoring vital signs and I&O. Use turning, deep breathing, coughing, and an incentive spirometer to prevent respiratory complications. Monitor the operative site for signs of infection and bleeding. Assess movement, circulation, and sensation of the extremity to monitor for impaired circulation. Assess mental status. Postoperative delirium is possible from the anesthesia, the analgesic medications, pain, immobility, and loss of familiar surroundings. It is important to use opioid analgesics cautiously. Practitioners often use lower doses to prevent changes in mental status, respiratory depression, and oversedation.

Keeping the affected extremity in alignment helps keep pain to a minimum. Use pillows between the knees or an abduction splint to accomplish this. Patients who have hemiarthroplasty are at risk for dislocation, which is most likely to occur when the joint is adducted and internally rotated. Avoid movements such as crossing the legs and feet while seated, and adducting the legs when lying on the unoperated side. Instruct patients to use a raised toilet seat and a shower chair, and avoid activities that have potential to cause dislocation of the hip for 6 weeks or more until muscles surrounding the joint are healed and the joint has stabilized.

Comprehensive multidisciplinary rehabilitation focuses on the goal of returning the patient to the previous level of function. Specific areas of treatment include gait and transfer training, muscle strengthening through active assistive exercises, and teaching the use of assistive devices such as walkers and canes. It is important to prevent depression during the recovery time due to limited independence. Consistently point out the patient's strengths, give positive feedback, and reinforce progress.

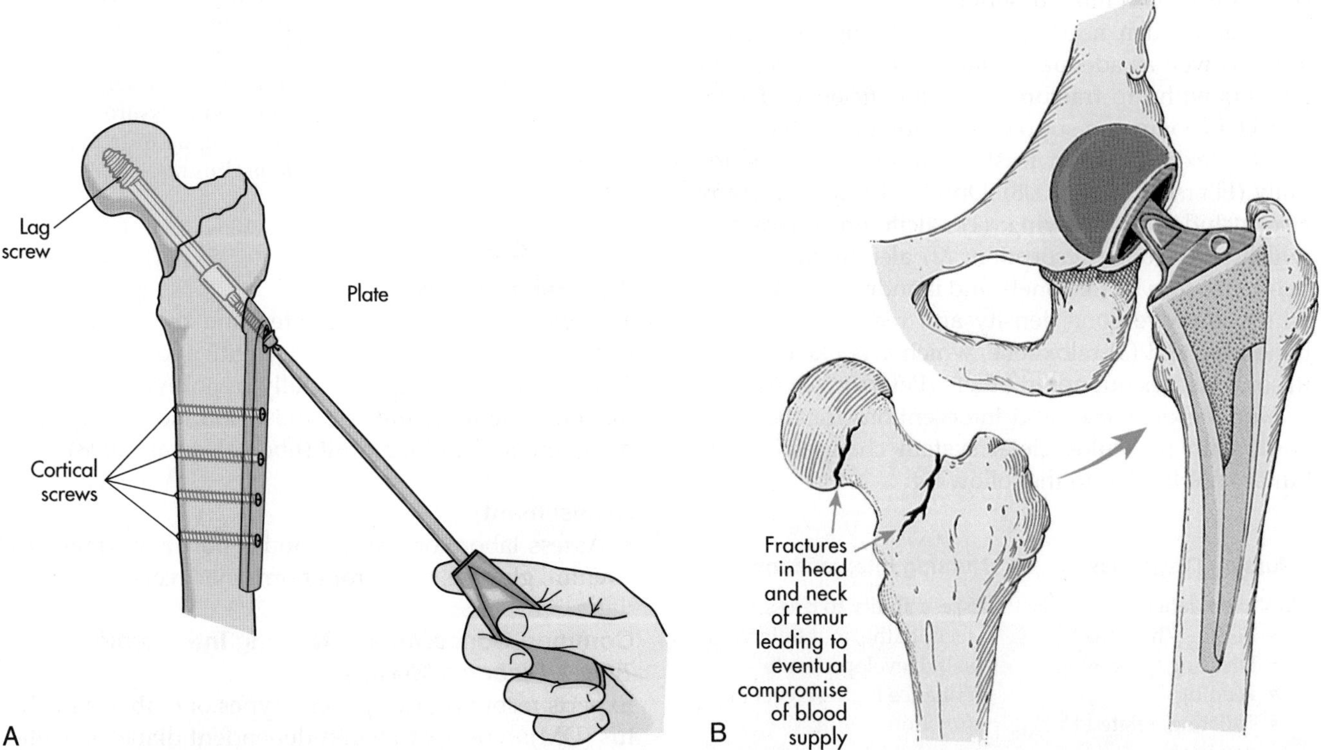

FIGURE 33-8 **A,** Open reduction and internal fixation (ORIF) with nails, screws, or rods. **B,** Bipolar or hemiarthroplasty.

Osteoporosis

Osteoporosis, a systemic skeletal disease, is one of the most common conditions in older women. The characteristic low bone mass and deterioration of bone tissue it causes result in a significantly increased risk of fractures. Fractures are possible in the course of routine activities such as bending, lifting, coughing, and straining at stool. Osteoporosis of the spinal vertebrae causes a loss of height of 1 to 2½ inches or kyphosis, the development of a C shape to the cervical vertebrae, which causes a stoop that is at times quite severe. The visible hump on the back is also called the dowager's hump. Although we tend to consider osteoporosis a disease of old age, it actually begins in younger women. Prevention begins with children and adolescents. A diet high in calcium and vitamin D as well as regular weight-bearing exercise lays the foundation for later life. Bone density testing helps identify older women at risk for fractures and points the way to instituting measures to prevent fractures. Advise all women to avoid smoking and excess alcohol and limit caffeine consumption. Additional information for osteoporosis education is available through the National Osteoporosis Foundation at www.nof.org.

Osteoporosis prevention for some women will include reducing estrogen deficiency related to perimenopause with hormone replacement therapy (HRT), but its use is controversial. Although HRT has a positive effect on calcium absorption, it possibly contributes to an increased incidence of endometrial cancer, an increased risk for breast cancer, and an increase in cardiovascular disease and stroke; therefore, practitioners generally do not prescribe estrogen for osteoporosis except in limited periods.

Older women need 1,000 to 1,500 mg of calcium daily as well as adequate vitamin D. Sixty percent of patients with hip fractures have a deficiency of vitamin D. Recommend supplementation unless the older adult is exposed to at least 15 minutes of sunshine daily (Ebersole et al., 2008). Options for drug therapy also include the following: (1) calcitonin (Miacalcin), which slows bone resorption; (2) alendronate (Fosamax), risedronate (Actonel), and ibandronate (Boniva), which improve bone density and reduce the rate of bone loss; and (3) raloxifene, which acts like estrogen in some tissues but not in others (Peterson, 2001).

Nursing diagnoses and interventions for the older adult with musculoskeletal system changes include but are not limited to the following:

Nursing Diagnoses	Nursing Interventions
Self-care deficit • Bathing/hygiene • Dressing/grooming • Feeding • Toileting, related to weakness	Assess ability to dress, feed, bathe, and toilet self. Develop plan to enhance highest level of function. Allow adequate time to perform activities. Provide assistive devices. Consult with physical and occupational therapists. Modify environment to facilitate self-care.
Impaired physical mobility	Assess strength and joint mobility. Teach maintenance of good body alignment.
Impaired bed mobility	Have patient change position. Consult with physical therapist.
Impaired walking	Provide assistive devices such as canes and walkers.
Risk for falls, related to age-related changes	Assess balance, gait, strength, medications that cause vertigo or drowsiness, sensory problems, and impaired mobility. Maintain a regular weight-bearing exercise routine that is enjoyable. Provide good lighting and assistive devices (walkers or canes) to assist balance. Eliminate environmental hazards, clutter, uneven walking surfaces, and scatter rugs. Encourage moving slowly from lying to standing to keep orthostatic hypotension (a sudden drop in blood pressure when standing up quickly) to a minimum.

ENDOCRINE SYSTEM

Age-Related Changes

The levels of hormones secreted and the response of body tissue to hormones change with age (Table 33-9). Thyroid disturbances, especially hypothyroidism and diabetes mellitus, are the most common endocrine disorders in the older adult (Ebersole et al., 2008).

Assessment

- Assess laboratory results and report abnormal calcium, glucose, or thyroid hormone levels.

Common Concerns and Nursing Interventions

Type 2 Diabetes Mellitus

Experts recognize two general types of diabetes mellitus (DM): type 1, or insulin-dependent diabetes mellitus (IDDM), in which the body fails to produce insulin;

Table 33-9 Endocrine Changes with Aging

PHYSIOLOGIC CHANGE	RESULTS
Decreased pituitary excretions of adrenocorticotropic hormone (ACTH) and steroids	Decreased muscle mass
Decreased production of thyroid-stimulating hormone	Decreased basal metabolic rate
Decreased production of parathyroid hormone (seen with osteoporosis)	Increased blood calcium levels
Decreased production and use of insulin	Increased blood glucose levels
Decreased release of testosterone, estrogen, and progesterone	Menopause in women and multiple system changes

and type 2, which we characterize as the body's inability to produce and utilize insulin appropriately. Of adults with diabetes, 85% to 90% have type 2 DM, which often begins in middle age. Patients do not always exhibit the usual signs or symptoms of thirst, increased appetite, and large amounts of urine, as seen in type 1 DM. In older adults, repeated infections, slow healing, and blurred vision, as well as weight gain or loss, tend to be more common signs or symptoms.

The goal for interventions in type 2 DM is to provide education and support to achieve and maintain a stable metabolic state through diet management, weight control, and exercise. Diabetic education includes topics such as medication, the disease process, monitoring blood glucose, signs and symptoms of hyperglycemia and hypoglycemia, sick-day management, foot care, eye care, and various other complications. To facilitate teaching, actively involve older adults and significant others in learning. Resources for patient educational handouts are available from the American Diabetes Association (ADA), and other sources.

When you are working with the older adult, assist in adapting the diet, with as little change as possible, to encourage compliance. Encourage obtaining a reasonable weight. Advise the person to balance intake with recommended amounts of protein, carbohydrates, fats, vitamins, and minerals. Encourage limiting refined sugar and choosing a high-fiber diet.

Older adults with DM are at a higher risk for foot problems because of changes in peripheral nerves and blood vessels. Inadequate blood flow to the feet and nerve damage contribute to the development of ulcers and infections. Hyperglycemia also plays a role because blood glucose levels of 200 mg/100 mL or greater are associated with an altered immune system leukocyte response. About 50% to 70% of all amputations of the feet are performed on individuals with DM (Meiner & Lueckenotte, 2006). **Peripheral neuropathy** is the presence of abnormal sensation, numbness, and burning sensations in the extremities. This condition increases with age, particularly in people who have diabetes mellitus. Decreased awareness of pain, temperature changes, and diminished circulation result in risk for injury. Undetected injuries become easily infected and, if untreated, in some cases necessitate eventual amputation. Activities that promote good circulation include avoidance of smoking, avoiding constricting footwear, and keeping legs uncrossed.

To prevent foot ulcers, recommend daily cleansing of the feet with nondrying agents and daily inspection of the feet for blisters, cuts, or infections using a mirror. It is best to cut nails straight across to prevent skin injury. Recommend regular visits to a physician or podiatrist. Counsel individuals with neuropathy of the feet, hyperglycemia, or a history of foot infections to seek care at the first sign of a foot injury or infection.

Hypothyroidism

Twenty percent of persons older than 65 years of age have thyroid problems, the most frequent of which is hypothyroidism (Ebersole et al., 2008). Decreased thyroid function often appears in a subclinical form, and the health care provider becomes aware of it through the results of routine serum testing. Almost all cases are inconspicuous and progress slowly toward thyroid failure. Signs frequently linked to hypothyroidism in older adults include unexplained elevation in triglycerides or plasma cholesterol, nonspecific cognitive impairment, slow metabolism, chest pain or atrial fibrillation, constipation, macrocytic anemia, vague arthritic complaints, cold intolerance, and depression with underlying apathy and withdrawal. The goal for interventions is stabilization of thyroid levels with medication (levothyroxine). The practitioner monitors the response to therapy through thyroid-stimulating hormone (TSH) levels. Nursing interventions center on patient and family education related to disease signs and symptoms as well as medication therapy. It is essential to carefully manage medication therapy. With treatment, patients generally experience increased energy and weight loss.

REPRODUCTIVE SYSTEM

Age-Related Changes

The major changes in the reproductive system related to aging are diminished levels of male and female hormones: estrogen and progesterone in women and androgen and testosterone in men. The process of aging diminishes sexual function but does not put a halt to it. Lack of the circulating hormone testosterone in men and estrogen, progesterone, and androgen in women results in changes in four aspects of the sexual system: arousal, orgasm, postorgasm, and extragenital changes. Although it takes longer for a man to be sexually aroused and achieve erection and ejaculation, men maintain the ability for sexual function into their 80s and 90s. For women, menopause is marked by a decrease in hormones, the inability to procreate, and tissue atrophy of ovaries, fallopian tubes, cervix, and vulva. There is a decrease in the amount of vaginal secretions, and the pH becomes more alkaline. Although age-related changes occur, they do not diminish the older woman's capacity to achieve orgasm and enjoy sexual relations (Table 33-10).

One of the greatest obstacles in assessing the sexuality of older adults is the failure on the part of many nurses to initiate the discussion (Meiner & Lueckenotte, 2006). To begin the assessment, consider making a general statement about the continuing sexual needs of older adults. Following this, open-ended questions regarding residents' sexuality are likely to be useful. For example:

"Tell me how you express your sexuality."

"What concerns do you have about fulfilling your continuing sexual needs?"

"In what ways has your sexual relationship with your partner changed as you have aged?"

The PLISSIT model has been used to assess and manage adults' sexuality. The model includes obtaining *p*ermission from the residents to initiate sexual discussion, providing the *l*imited *i*nformation they need to function sexually, giving *s*pecific *s*uggestions for individuals to proceed with sexual relations, and providing *i*ntensive *t*herapy regarding the issues of sexuality. The goal of assessment is to gather information that allows residents to express sexuality safely and to feel uninhibited by normal or pathologic problems.

Table 33-10 Reproductive Changes with Aging

PHYSIOLOGIC CHANGE	RESULTS
FEMALE	
Decreased estrogen levels	Vagina shortens, narrows, and loses some of its elasticity
	Decreased vaginal secretions
	Decreased pubic hair
	Increased vaginal tissue fragility and irritation
	Decreased size of uterus and vagina
	Increased pain with intercourse (dyspareunia)
	Decreased breast tissue mass
Increased vaginal alkalinity	Increased risk of infection
MALE	
Decreased testosterone	Decreased amount of facial and pubic hair
Decreased circulation	Decreased rate of ejaculation
	Decreased force of ejaculation
	Decreased speed gaining erection

It is common for nurses and nursing students to feel uncomfortable with assessing the sexual desires and functions of older patients. Regardless, a sexual assessment is a necessary part of the routine nursing assessment. Skill and comfort comes with practice.

Assessment

- Assess history of past experiences or difficulties as well as sexually transmitted diseases (STDs) and human immunodeficiency virus (HIV).
- Assess for signs of vaginal or penile ulceration, edema, or discharge.
- Assess for presence of lumps, dimpling, or drainage from the breast.
- Assess for information on alternative sexual orientations: lesbian, gay, bisexual, or transgender.

Common Concerns and Nursing Interventions

Sexual Function

The misconceptions that older adults are impotent and asexual or that they are perverse if they are sexually active are probably the most common reasons for sexual dysfunction in older adults. If individuals continue to be sexually active on a regular basis, they retain the capability to respond sexually. If an older adult indicates that sexual intercourse is difficult or uncomfortable because of vaginal dryness, suggest using estrogen creams or water-soluble lubricants to relieve the discomfort.

Research and information from a variety of sources indicate that aging individuals have the potential to be sexual, continue to have interest in sex, and are indeed sexual beings. For many older adults, the lack of a sexual partner is the main factor for decreased sexual activity.

Sexuality also encompasses sexual identity as a man or woman, intimacy (emotional closeness to others), and touch. Regardless of age, it is important to feel good about oneself as a male or female and to have close relationships with other people. Sexual intimacy is more than intercourse: it includes caressing, stroking and kissing, and being an emotional companion to the partner. Although sexual pleasure is not absolutely essential for a fulfilled later life, it has the power to add substantially to a higher quality of life (Maas et al., 2001).

To dispel misinformation, you will need to examine your own feelings about sexuality and aging and become informed about age-related changes in sexual function. It is also possible to support the sexuality of older adults by encouraging and helping them to look their best, complimenting them when they look nice, respecting and allowing them to have their privacy, allowing their expressions of affection for one another, and using touch to communicate acceptance. A pat on the arm or a hug is a potential way to communicate concern and caring to almost anyone.

A nursing diagnosis and interventions for the older adult with sexual dysfunction include but are not limited to the following:

Nursing Diagnosis	Nursing Interventions
Ineffective sexuality pattern, related to lack of privacy	Allow verbalization of concerns regarding sexual needs. Provide privacy for interaction between alert, consenting individuals. Assist individual to maintain good physical hygiene and meet cosmetic needs. Provide distraction and alternative activities for disoriented individual who masturbates; if unsuccessful, provide privacy.

SENSORY PERCEPTION

Age-Related Changes

The senses provide a link with the environment by receiving and interpreting various stimuli including but not limited to vision, hearing, taste, and smell (Table 33-11). Visual and hearing impairments interfere with communication, social interactions, and mobility, leading to social isolation. In the past, we recognized five senses: sight, hearing, taste, smell, and touch. Today, we acknowledge additional senses and categorize all senses into two major groups: general and special. General senses include touch, pressure, pain, temperature, vibration, and proprioception. Special senses are produced by highly localized organs and sensory cells including sight, hearing, taste, smell, and balance. Sensation, or perception, is the conscious awareness and interpretation of sensory stimuli by sensory receptors.

Table 33-11 Sensory Changes with Aging

PHYSIOLOGIC CHANGE	RESULTS
VISION	
Decreased number of eyelashes	Increased risk of eye injury
Decreased tear production	Increased risk of eye irritation
Increased discoloration of lens	Decreased color perception
Decreased tissue elasticity	Increased blurring
Decreased muscle tone	Decreased diameter of pupil Increased refractive errors Decreased night vision Increased sensitivity to glare
HEARING	
Decreased tissue elasticity	Decreased ability to distinguish high-frequency sounds
Decreased joint mobility	Decreased ability to distinguish high-frequency sounds Decreased hearing ability
Decreased number of hair cells in inner ear	Increased problems with balance
TASTE AND SMELL	
Decreased number of papillae on tongue	Decreased ability to taste
Decreased number of nasal sensory receptors	Decreased ability to detect smells

Vision

About one fifth of people older than age 70 have visual impairments that limit activity and increase the risk of falls. The four main causes of visual impairment are cataracts, glaucoma, macular degeneration, and diabetic retinopathy (Ebersole et al., 2008). Undiagnosed visual disorders are increasing among older adults, especially in ethnic and cultural minorities. In the next three decades, the number of blind and visually impaired older adults is expected to double, but with appropriate eye care, 40% of blindness and visual impairment is amenable to treatment or is preventable (Ebersole et al., 2008).

Age-related changes in vision include **presbyopia** (farsightedness resulting from a loss of elasticity of the lens of the eye), or narrowing of the peripheral field of vision, decreased ability to focus on near objects, and a decrease in visual acuity as the pupil becomes smaller and less responsive to light. There is some clouding of the eye's lens. Yellowing of the lens and changes in color perception cause older adults to have difficulty differentiating shades of the same color and colors such as green, blue, and violet. Depth perception is distorted, and vision in dim light becomes difficult. General vision screening for individuals who wear glasses or contact lenses involves observation of reading print from a newspaper. Note the distance from the eyes the person holds the newspaper, and verify the person's ability to see print clearly (Figure 33-9). Limited vision indicates the need for a more detailed eye examination. Although age-related changes decrease visual capability, blindness is not a normal result of aging.

Glaucoma

Glaucoma, the second leading cause of blindness in the United States, is caused by an occlusion in the drainage of the fluid in the anterior chamber of the eye, which produces an increase in intraocular pressure. Pressure transfers to the optic nerve, where damage or blindness is a possible result. Primary open-angle glaucoma, the most common type, makes up 90% of all cases of primary glaucoma. This type of glaucoma has the capacity to reduce vision so gradually and painlessly that a per-

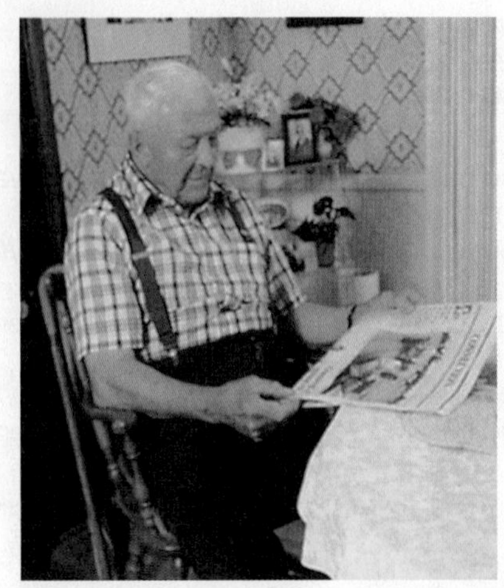

FIGURE 33-9 Vision screening using a newspaper.

son is unaware of a problem until the optic nerve is badly damaged. Visual loss begins with deteriorating peripheral vision. If the practitioner diagnoses the problem early, primary open-angle glaucoma is possible to control, thus preventing serious visual impairment (Ebersole et al., 2008).

In contrast, acute angle-closure glaucoma occurs suddenly as a result of complete occlusion in the path of the aqueous humor. Signs and symptoms of acute angle-closure glaucoma include severe eye pain, erythema, clouded or blurred vision, nausea and vomiting, rainbow halo surrounding lights, pupil dilation, and a steamy appearance of the cornea. Severe problems develop in acute angle-closure glaucoma when intraocular pressure rises above 50 mm Hg (normal range is 10 to 22 mm Hg). In the absence of emergency medical attention, severe vision loss will occur; blindness will result in 2 days. An iridectomy is a helpful option to reduce the intraocular pressure (Ebersole et al., 2008).

Medical follow-up and eye medication will be required for the rest of the person's life. Eyedrops are necessary to continue even in the absence of symptoms. After administration of eyedrops, pressure on the lacrimal duct for 1 minute prevents rapid systemic absorption. Use a medical-alert bracelet or card to identify glaucoma and the prescribed eyedrop solution.

Cataracts

Cataracts are the most common disorder found in the aging eye. They occur in 65% of people ages 50 to 59 and in 100% of people older than 80. A cataract is a clouding of the normally clear and transparent lens of the eye. Degenerative changes to the lens protein and fatty deposits (lipofuscion) in the lens are causative factors in the development of cataract (Ebersole et al., 2008). The lens focuses light on the retina to produce a sharp image. When a cataract forms, the lens sometimes become so opaque that the transmission of light to the retina becomes impossible. The size and the location of a cataract determine the amount of interference with sight. Symptoms reported include dimmed, blurred, or misty vision, the need for brighter light to read, and sensitivity to glare and light.

Interventions include surgery when vision loss interferes with normal ADLs, especially reading and driving. Several types of surgery exist, but the most recent technique involves the use of ultrasound to break the lens into small fragments, which allows removal from a tiny incision. A substitute lens is used to restore vision, which is a permanent, plastic intraocular lens. Cataract surgery is highly successful.

Hearing and Balance

It is possible to consider the organs of hearing and balance in three parts: the external ear, the middle ear, and the inner ear. The inner ear is involved in both hearing and balance. Hearing loss is not a normal part of aging and is necessary to further evaluate.

A third of older Americans have impaired hearing (Crews & Campbell, 2004). With age the eardrum loses elasticity, the ossicles of the middle ear become more rigid, and there is atrophy of auditory nerve and end-organs in the inner ear. Because of exposure to a variety of loud noises throughout life and age-related changes, older individuals often have hearing losses of different tones, causing some sounds to be distorted and others to be absent. Older adults often deny their hearing loss and need encouragement and support to explore various methods to improve hearing.

Cerumen impaction is a reversible, often overlooked cause of conductive hearing loss. Assess for itching and a feeling of ear fullness. Removal of the impaction sometimes restores hearing acuity and relieves symptoms associated with impaction. Removal includes instillation of a softening agent such as mineral oil or Debrox (nonprescription otic solution) twice daily for several days until wax softens. The health care provider then irrigates the ear using a syringe or Waterpik device on its low setting, finishing by draining excessive fluid from the ear.

Hearing impairment falls into three categories: conductive, sensorineural, or mixed. Conductive hearing loss results from interruption of the transmission of sound through the external auditory canal and middle ear and is usually related to cerumen impaction, otitis media, and fixation of the auditory ossicles.

Sensorineural hearing loss results when the inner ear, the auditory nerve, the brainstem, or the cortical auditory pathways do not function properly so that sound waves are not interpreted correctly. Mixed hearing loss is a conductive hearing loss superimposed on a sensorineural hearing loss.

Presbycusis is a sensorineural healing loss and the most common form of loss in older adults. Typically the loss is bilateral, resulting in difficulty hearing high-pitched tones and conversational speech. The sounds usually lost first are *f, s, th, ch,* and *sh.* As hearing loss progresses, the sounds of *b, t, p, k,* and *s* also become difficult to distinguish. The cause is unclear. Indications include behaviors such as increasing the volume on the television or the radio, tilting the head toward the person speaking, cupping a hand around one ear, trouble following conversation when more than one person is speaking, watching the speaker's lips, speaking loudly, and not responding when spoken to. Diagnosis involves audiometric evaluation. Treatment options include surgical placement with a cochlear implant, hearing devices, and auditory rehabilitation to facilitate communication.

Nursing interventions to improve communication when there is hearing loss include providing good visual contact to allow lip reading. Avoid situations in which there is glare or shadows on the person's field of vision. Reduce or eliminate background noise. Speak at a normal rate and volume. Do not overarticulate or shout. Use short sentences, and pause at the end of each sentence. Use facial expressions or gestures to give clues. Ask how you can help the listener, and be patient—stay positive and relaxed.

Touch

Touch involves tactile information involving pressure, vibration, and temperature. Age-related changes affecting the sense of touch and position include a decrease in the number of receptor cells throughout the skin and joints. Older adults have increasing difficulty sensing temperature and maintaining balance, which places them at risk for burns and falls. The most common disorders to affect tactile ability include stroke, peripheral vascular disease (PVD), and diabetic neuropathy. All these conditions involve decreased blood flow to various parts of the body. Direct nursing interventions toward preventing accidental trauma and injury in the affected limbs.

Smell and Taste

Olfactory receptors decline in number, which tends to reduce or alter a person's ability to smell. There is also a decrease in the number of taste buds, which often influences appetite and causes the person to use more seasoning.

Assessment

- Assess eyes for dryness, tearing, or signs of irritation.
- Assess ability of individual to see both close-up and at a distance. Ask about problems with or recent changes in vision.
- Assess hearing; note use of hearing aids and effectiveness.
- Assess for reported changes in taste or smell.

Common Concerns and Nursing Interventions

Decreased Vision

With increasing age comes decreasing visual capability. A number of interventions are possible to compensate for age-related changes in vision; make sure the patient's eyeglasses are clean and are available, increase the amount of light in the environment, reduce glare by using shades on windows and lights, and use night-lights to avoid abrupt light-to-dark changes. The use of low-vision aids such as large print, strongly contrasting colors (black on a white background), and magnifying glasses will help compensate for the decrease in visual acuity.

Decreased Hearing

The decreased ability to hear is frequently a frustration to both the older adults who are affected and the individuals who are trying to talk to them. Hearing aids sometimes help in situations in which amplification has the potential to improve hearing, but hearing aids do not compensate for nerve damage or effectively screen out other distracting noises. To communicate with an individual with a hearing loss, face the individual and speak at a normal or slightly slower pace without exaggerating or shouting, lower the tone of voice (because hearing loss is frequently in the higher tones), and eliminate background noise whenever possible. Another effective communication technique is using nonverbal communication such as gestures, smiles, nodding the head with the verbal message, and written communication. Even if the older person is frustrated when communication is difficult, carefully avoid expressing annoyance or impatience to the patient who has a hearing loss (Figure 33-10).

A nursing diagnosis and interventions for the older adult with altered senses include but are not limited to the following:

Nursing Diagnosis	Nursing Interventions
Disturbed sensory perception (specify)	Assess for sensory changes. Alert all caregivers to sensory problems of individual. Determine most effective methods of communicating with individual with sensory impairment. Modify environment to remove hazards and reduce risks. Verify that assistive devices such as hearing aids or glasses are clean and functional.

NERVOUS SYSTEM

Age-Related Changes

Structural and functional changes of the nervous system are intertwined and depend on a number of variables, including an individual's genetic makeup and the specific brain regions affected. Changes associated

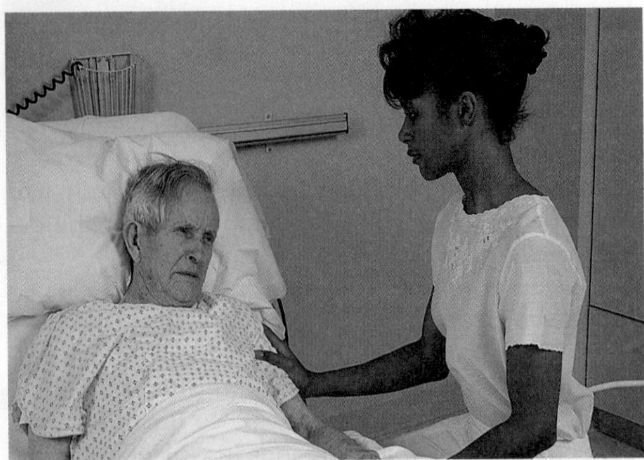

FIGURE 33-10 The nurse listens to the frustrated older adult with patience and compassion.

with aging include a decline in the number of brain cells and peripheral nerve cells and fibers, and synaptic changes that affect transmission and the sensitivity of target cells to neurotransmitters. Physiologically, nerve impulse transmission in the nervous system slows, resulting in a longer reaction time for older adults. Until recently, it was widely accepted that neuron death was an inevitable result of normal aging. Age-related declines in neuron numbers are not a significant part of normal aging. Unless pathologic degeneration occurs, changes in neuron size and weight bring few if any negative behavioral effects. Autonomic nervous system changes include decreased efficiency in maintaining normal body temperature and in the pulse returning to normal after exercise or stress (Table 33-12).

Functional ability in older people does not consistently decline. Changes in sensorimotor and motor function, memory, cognition, sleep patterns, and proprioception occur at varying rates. Personality—which we use here to mean stable, distinctive patterns of behavior, thought, and emotion—generally remains more consistent during normal aging (Meiner & Lueckenotte, 2006).

Memory

Common memory concerns for older adults include forgetting names, misplacing items, and poor recall of recent events or conversations. Short-term memory will perhaps decline with age, but long-term recall is usually maintained. Strategies for adapting, such as making lists or posting reminders, are useful to manage short-term memory loss.

Table 33-12 Neurologic Changes with Aging

PHYSIOLOGIC CHANGE	RESULTS
Decreased number of brain cells	Decreased reflexes
Decreased number of nerve fibers	Decreased coordination
Decreased number of neuroreceptors	Decreased perception of stimuli Decreased motor responses

Cognition

Cognitive function refers to the process by which information is acquired, stored, shared, and used. It has several components, including state of consciousness, general appearance and behavior, orientation, memory, language, intelligence, perception, insight and problem-solving ability, judgment, attention span, and mood and affect. Intellectual tasks such as thinking, remembering, perceiving, communicating, and calculating are all examples of cognitive function (Maas et al., 2001). Many people think that cognitive abilities decline in old age. Only some older people experience some deficits, and the decline occurs at different times in their lives. Generalizations about cognitive decline in older adults are inappropriate (Maas et al., 2001).

Although many older adults have perhaps had little formal education, they are often self-taught and also know many things from experience. Research indicates that most older people retain their intelligence and are capable of learning throughout their lives, although this will sometimes require more time because of age-related changes in the senses and nervous system.

Sleep

Sleep disturbances in the older adult sometimes occur as a result of changes in the reticular formation (RF). The RF is a small, thick cluster of neurons in the brainstem and extending into the cerebral cortex. Changes in the RF in the older adult have the potential to result in loss of deep sleep (stages 3 and 4). It takes longer for older adults to get the adequate amount of rest owing to the decrease in their "deep sleep" (Ebersole et al., 2008).

Proprioception

Proprioception, which we understand as the ability to maintain an upright position without falling, depends on the ability to use balance, posture, and movement. This requires much sensory input, motor output, and central integration of balance and locomotion. Aging results in slower reflexes, diminished strength of muscles for posture, and increased postural sway. Conditions such as damage to the structures of the inner ear may affect peripheral and central control of mobility and thus affect balance. The ability to achieve proprioception declines with age.

Personality

Personality remains stable during normal aging. Consider any signs of impaired emotional control, diminished initiative, or withdrawal as indicators of other problems or an initial sign of brain dysfunction.

Assessment

- Assess alertness level and level of consciousness including eye opening, verbal responses, and ability to follow simple commands.
- Assess appropriateness of behavior and responses.
- Assess mental status. Mental status examination tools vary depending on the setting. The Mental Status Questionnaire (MSQ) and Mini-Mental State Examination (MMSE) are examples. These assess orientation, immediate and recent memory, attention, calculation, and language and motor skills.
- Assess for the presence of pain. Note severity, location, quality, duration, and precipitating events.
- Assess sleep patterns. Note onset, duration, and quality of sleep as well as daytime napping.
- Assess laboratory results for electrolyte imbalance, anemia, liver function, thyroid function, drug levels, and vitamin B_{12}.
- Assess CT scan or magnetic resonance imaging (MRI) results if there is reason to suspect tumor, subdural hematoma, or stroke.

Common Concerns and Nursing Interventions

Insomnia

It is not unusual for older adults to state that they are not able to sleep. Studies of sleep patterns in various age-groups show that the sleep pattern changes with age (Fielo, 2001). With aging, there are fewer periods of deep sleep and frequent periods of wakefulness, giving the impression of sleeplessness even though the total sleep time is the same or only slightly reduced from that of young adulthood.

Many older people resort to hypnotics in an attempt to treat their insomnia. If the practitioner prescribes hypnotics, it is advisable not to use them longer than 10 days. Hypnotics often interfere with a person's normal sleep patterns, and they feel unrested and lethargic the following day (Ebersole et al., 2008).

Nursing interventions to help an older person sleep begin with encouraging a bedtime ritual. For most people this will typically include brushing the teeth, reading a book or the paper, using a favorite pillow, or listening to the radio. Exercise and activity during the day increase the likelihood of falling asleep easily at night. Research has also shown that the time it takes to fall asleep is related to the length of time from the last sleep period; therefore older adults sometimes find that they can fall asleep at night if they nap in the morning rather in the afternoon.

Delirium

Much of the emotional trauma of older adulthood arises from the misconception that most older adults become senile (the state of physical and mental deterioration associated with aging). The majority of causes of mental changes are reversible, and the state they induce is more accurately called **delirium.** It has a relatively rapid onset (hours to days) with a fluctuating and typically brief course (Meiner & Lueckenotte, 2006).

Delirium is not a disease of the nervous system; it is a syndrome resulting from a variety of causes. Multiple factors cause delirium. Environmental causes include social isolation, unfamiliar surroundings, sensory overload, immobilization, and sleep deprivation. Physiologic causes include metabolic, endocrine, and cardiovascular (inadequate oxygen to the brain) causes; cerebrovascular and nutritional causes; and infections, cerebral and extracranial neoplasms, and trauma. Toxic causes include medications, substance intoxication, and substance withdrawal. When an older adult has sudden mental changes, it is important to look for a cause. Once the practitioner identifies the cause and gives the delirium a specific diagnosis, it is possible to begin treatment. Research is focusing on identifying risk factors and prevention strategies (Meiner & Lueckenotte, 2006). See Table 33-13 for a comparison of characteristics associated with delirium, dementia, and depression.

Nursing interventions to prevent delirium include education of nursing staff to the signs and symptoms of delirium; orientation and communication; mobilization; environmental modifications; education of caregivers; pain control; management of elimination patterns; medication management; and discharge planning.

Reality Orientation

Reality orientation is a useful intervention for delirium. Guidelines for reality orientation include the following:

- Call patients or residents by their correct names or as they wish to be called.
- Make eye contact.
- Converse about familiar subjects.
- Provide familiar objects in the older adult's environment.
- Explain events and procedures in concise, simple language.
- Be honest.
- Set a routine and be consistent.
- Engage the older adult in familiar and simple activities that have a purpose, such as washing the face or brushing the teeth.

Dementia and Alzheimer's Disease

Experts define dementia as a progressive impairment of intellectual (cognitive) function that interferes with normal social and occupational activities. It is characterized by loss of memory and at least one other disturbance of intellectual function (e.g., orientation, attention, calculation, language, motor skills). Dementia affects short-term, intermediate, and long-term memory. The individual has difficulty with abstract thinking, and will, for instance, sometimes be unable to define the differences in objects or words. Aphasia (inability to understand words), agnosia (inability to

Table 33-13 Comparison of Characteristics Associated with Delirium, Dementia, and Depression

	DELIRIUM	DEMENTIA	DEPRESSION
Onset	Sudden	Insidious, relentless, or sporadic	Sudden; related to specific events
Duration	Hours to days	Persistent	Episodic or persistent
Time of day	Worse at night and when drug levels peak; sleep-wake cycle reversed	Stable or no change	Insomnia; sleeps during the day; early morning awakening
Cognitive impairment	Memory, attentiveness, consciousness, calculations	Abstract thinking, judgment, memory, thought patterns, calculations, agnosia; permanent and progressive	Complaints of memory loss, forgetfulness, and inability to concentrate
Activity	Increased or decreased; sometimes fluctuates; sometimes includes tremors and spastic movements	Unchanged from usual behavior	Lack of motivation or lethargic; restless or agitated
Speech and language	Slurred or rapid; manic rambling; incoherent	Disordered, rambling, or incoherent; struggles to find words	Slow, sluggish speech; slow processing and response to verbal stimuli
Mood and affect	Rapid mood swings; fearful and suspicious	Depressed, apathetic, uninterested	Extreme sadness, anxiety, and irritability
Delusions or hallucinations	Visual, auditory, tactile; hallucinations and delusions	Delusions but no hallucinations	Delusions about worthlessness; paranoid ideation
Associated factors and triggers	Physical condition, drug toxicity, head injury, change in environment, sensory deficits	Chronic alcoholism, vitamin B_{12} deficiency, Huntington's chorea, vascular disease, human immunodeficiency virus (HIV) infection, Alzheimer's disease	Loss of friends, family, health, and lifestyle
Reversibility	Potential	No; progressive	Potential

From Seidel, H.M., Ball, J.W., Dains, J.E., et al. (2007). *Mosby's guide to physical examination.* (6th ed.). St. Louis: Mosby.

recognize familiar objects), apraxia (problems manipulating things), and agraphia (difficulty writing and drawing) are all symptoms of dementia. Personality changes sometimes also become apparent (Meiner & Lueckenotte, 2006).

Alzheimer's disease is the most common cause of dementia. Dementia of the Alzheimer's type, whose cause we do not understand, is a progressive disorder in which the brain atrophies. Research has focused on genetic, viral, environmental, immunologic, and other causes. It usually arises in individuals older than 60 years of age; there is loss of cortical neurons, the ventricles are enlarged, and senile plaques and neurofibrillary tangles appear in the cortex of the brain. Experts divide the progression of Alzheimer's disease into three stages. In the early stage, there is a gradual onset of memory loss and difficulty focusing attention. The middle stage involves difficulty with language, object recognition, and judgment. In the terminal (final) stage there is some urinary and fecal incontinence, inability to ambulate or provide self-care, and inability to communicate. There is little or no response to surroundings or recognition of family members. In late stages, the individual becomes mute and bedridden. The average duration of the illness is 8 years, but it can last as long as 20 years or more.

Multi-infarct Dementia (MID)

MID is the second most common cause of dementia, accounting for 10% to 20% of cases (Elkin et al., 2007). This condition is related to vascular disorders within the brain that possibly result from stroke and severe hypertension; characteristics of the condition are periods of remission (absence of symptoms), preservation of personality, and mood swings. Risk factors for developing MID include arteriosclerosis, blood dyscrasias, cardiac decompensation, hypertension, atrial fibrillation, cardiac valve replacements, systemic emboli arising from other causes, DM, peripheral vascular disease, obesity, smoking, and vasospasms in the brain called transient ischemic attacks (TIAs). The usual progression of MID follows a stair-step decline rather than the slow steady decline of Alzheimer's disease. Symptoms depend on the location of the infarct. Abrupt-onset symptoms include confusion and problems with recent memory; wandering; getting lost in familiar places; moving with rapid shuffling steps; loss of bladder or bowel control; inappropriate display of emotions; and difficulty following instructions. Some intellectual impairment is common.

Transient Ischemic Attacks

The changes in the vascular system in older adults include thickening of the vessel walls and the presence to some degree of atherosclerosis and arteriosclerosis. Specific medical diagnoses related to arterial conditions common in the older adult are TIA and stroke.

TIAs are small spasms or occlusions in the cerebral vessels of the brain. Signs and symptoms of TIA vary, depending on the vessel's location in the brain. The most common signs and symptoms are changes in vision, headache, disorientation, ataxia (impaired ability to coordinate movement), and drop attacks (falling without losing consciousness). Symptoms sometimes last for as little as 20 minutes. Prompt treatment has the potential to prevent a stroke.

To prevent injury to the patient, you must provide a safe environment by removing hazards; use safety devices and mobility aids to prevent falls and assist balance; and use memory aids such as written instructions, schedules, and lists to assist the older adult in coping with disorientation. It is imperative for the patient with a TIA to have a neurologic examination and screening to determine if there are atherosclerotic plaque–like formations in the carotid arteries or other pathologic changes in the cerebral vasculature. The occurrence of strokes can be reduced greatly by identifying high-risk or stroke-prone older adults and providing the appropriate prophylactic interventions (Ebersole et al., 2008).

Other Dementia-Related Diseases

Dementia resulting from other diseases includes Huntington's disease, Creutzfeld-Jakob disease, and HIV (Table 33-14).

In managing dementia-related diseases, the goals are to maintain maximum self-care abilities and prevent injury. It is often necessary to break down ADLs such as dressing into small steps and explain what is happening at each step in very specific and simple terms. The individual will perhaps need coaching as to what to do when eating, and often it is better to give finger foods or only one item at a time. Keep the environment calm, and eliminate distracting stimuli. Care of an older adult with dementia or Alzheimer's disease requires patience. Routine is very important, and it is necessary to introduce changes very slowly. It is important to remember that the individual no longer thinks logically or understands the surroundings.

When understanding and communication become impaired, nonverbal communication becomes more important. Use a calm, pleasant tone of voice and gestures that correspond to the verbal message, maintain contact through touch, and use listening skills. Music has a positive influence including improved capacity to communicate, reminisce, and recall memories. Social reminiscence is a type of therapeutic interaction that uses active listening and observable feedback in a way that increases respect and empathy and decreases anxiety (Puentes, 2000). Avoid large groups and complex activities, because they are likely to cause the individual to become agitated or have a catastrophic reaction (become angry and display aggressive behavior).

Pain assessment is very difficult in the presence of cognitive impairment. Chronic pain has the capacity to cause depression, social isolation, and feelings of powerlessness. Of the pain assessment tools studied, the McGill pain scale is most effective for this population (using words such as *mild, distressing,* or *horrible*), and pointing to the affected person's own body is best to identify the pain's location (Kaasalainen, 2007).

Wandering is a behavior frequently associated with dementia. In some situations, it will be an attempt to find the bathroom or familiar surroundings; for some individuals, it will be their way of coping with anxiety. For individuals unable to locate the bathroom or their own rooms, easily read signs with universally accepted symbols and familiar objects are a means to help them find the way. Safety measures to prevent falls are essential.

Restraints and Safety Reminder Devices (SRDs)

Research is showing that the hazards of restraint use are greater than the perceived benefits (Ebersole et al., 2008). Experts have linked restraint use to limiting mobility, loss of muscle strength, incontinence, pressure ulcers, nerve injury, and infections. Accordingly, most health care facilities are moving toward becoming restraint-free environments. Since passage of the Nursing Home Reform Law of the Omnibus Budget Reconciliation Act (OBRA) in 1987, restraint use in nursing homes has declined dramatically. In order to receive Medicare licensure, all long-term care facilities are required to comply with statements from the Fed-

Table 33-14 Other Dementia-Related Diseases

DISEASE	CHARACTERISTICS
Huntington's disease	Age range at diagnosis is 5-70; not necessarily a disease of old age. Characterized by uncontrollable writhing movements and mental deterioration that terminate in severe dementia. Begins with disturbances of gait and slurred speech. Life expectancy after diagnosis is 16 years.
Creutzfeld-Jakob disease	Rare and rapidly progressive; associated with viral etiology, although isolation of a specific virus has not occurred. Average onset 50-60 years of age. Terminal within 6-12 months. No known treatment.
HIV-associated dementia	Characterized by forgetfulness, slowness, poor concentration, and difficulties in problem solving. Rapidly progressive.

eral Register (1991) that relate to physical and chemical restraints and abuse (Ebersole et al., 2008) (Box 33-5). The focus is now on assessing and identifying people at risk and implementing alternative strategies to prevent injury. Companionship, supervision, eliminating bothersome treatments, maintaining an appropriate environment, and social and physical activities are often successful alternatives to promote safety without restraint. Studies have shown that the risk of falling is highest soon after mechanical restraints are used (Capezuti, 2004).

Practitioners use several types of medication to help control symptoms such as agitation, anxiety, screaming, violence, and depression. Neuroleptics or antipsychotics are effective for some behavior problems. Benzodiazepines usually help reduce anxiety, and antidepressants help treat some behavior problems and sleep disturbances. Drugs at best delay progression of the disease and have potentially severe side effects. Researchers have as yet not determined long-term effects.

Parkinson's Disease

Parkinson's disease is the second most common disorder affecting the nervous system in the older adult. It is a progressive, degenerative disease whose defining characteristics are muscle rigidity, tremors, and **akinesia** (an abnormal state of motor and psychic hypoactivity). The individual has a masklike appearance, drooling, and shuffling gait and often experiences emotional instability. In most cases, stress and frustration increase signs and symptoms.

Medication therapy with levodopa, amantadine HCl (Symmetrel), and anticholinergics such as benztropine mesylate (Cogentin) and trihexyphenidyl HCl (Artane) sometimes help to slow the process of the disease or will in some cases temporarily improve a patient's condition, but side effects from the drugs also have potential to cause disorientation, blurred vision, delirium, and drowsiness.

Box 33-5 Statements on Use of Restraints and Abuse

- The resident has the right to be free from any physical or chemical restraints imposed for purposes of discipline or convenience, and not required to treat the resident's medical symptoms. The resident has the right to be free from verbal, sexual, physical, and mental abuse; corporal punishment; and involuntary seclusion.
- The facility is required to develop and implement written policies and procedures that prohibit mistreatment, neglect and abuse of residents.
- The facility is required to ensure that the resident environment remains as free of accidental hazards as possible, and that each resident receives adequate supervision and assistance devices to prevent accidents.

From *Federal Register* (V56187), Sept. 26, 1991, 48825.

Nursing interventions for an older adult with Parkinson's disease include observing the response to medication therapy and maintaining mobility through exercise and activity. Range-of-motion exercises and massage help to relieve muscle spasms and maintain joint mobility. Interventions for a safe environment such as removing throw rugs and furniture from walkways, providing hand rails and objects that are too stable to tip over easily, and good lighting are important because the lack of balance and other characteristics of the disease typically contribute to falls and injuries. Canes and walkers as well as adaptive aids for ADLs sometimes prolong the independence of an individual with Parkinson's disease.

Intellectual function is not impaired, but the tremors and involuntary movements cause difficulty in communication and much frustration for both the individual and others with whom he or she is trying to communicate. Giving the individual time to respond, encouraging efforts to communicate, and showing acceptance of the individual through actions and nonverbal communication sometimes help to alleviate some of the feelings of frustration.

Stroke

Stroke (brain attack) is the third leading cause of death in the United States and increases in likelihood after 55 years of age. Possible symptoms of a stroke include **hemiplegia** (paralysis of one side of the body), **dysarthria** (difficult, poorly articulated speech, resulting from interference in the control over the muscles of speech), **dysphagia** (difficulty in swallowing), sensory changes such as **hemianopia** (defective vision or blindness in half of the visual field), **aphasia** (an abnormal neurologic condition in which language function is defective or absent because of an injury to certain areas of the cerebral cortex), and intellectual and emotional changes. Research indicates that select patients with acute ischemic stroke will benefit from thrombolytics such as tissue plasminogen activator (t-PA, alteplase [Activase]). The results of one landmark study revealed that selected patients who are treated within 3 hours of the onset of symptoms are at least 30% more likely than patients who do not receive timely treatment to recover with little or no disability after 3 months (Sauer, 2002).

Nursing interventions immediately after the stroke involve support of life functions Although some of the initial neurologic involvement will possibly disappear in 3 to 6 months, most individuals will have some residual dysfunction. Interventions focus on rehabilitation to accomplish ADLs and to be as independent as possible. Older adults will sometimes need to learn to use the nondominant hand because of hemiplegia (Figure 33-11) and will often require adaptive and assistive devices for ADLs, such as special utensils, reaching devices, and pull-on or easily secured cloth-

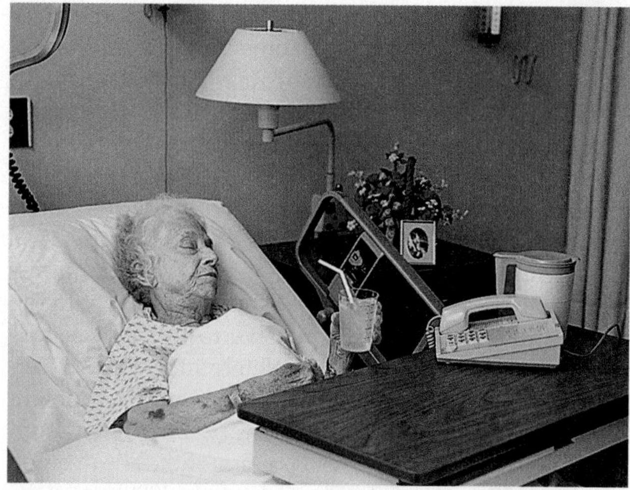

FIGURE 33-11 Hemiplegia of dominant right side necessitates learning to use nondominant hand for activities of daily living (ADLs).

ing. Wheelchairs and canes are sometimes necessary for weakness, loss of balance, and loss of leg control. Encourage or assist the patient to do the exercises and activities the therapist prescribes that will be most beneficial for progress. Communication techniques for older adults with aphasia include listening carefully, turning down or decreasing competing stimuli such as the radio or the television, using pictures and appropriate gestures, speaking slowly, using short direct statements, and not interrupting. With all interventions, make sure not to rush the older adult, and give encouragement and praise for effort as well as success in performing tasks. In many settings, physical therapy and occupational therapy provide a valuable role in assessment and treatment of changes related to neurologic problems.

Nursing diagnoses and interventions for the older adult with neurologic problems include but are not limited to the following:

Nursing Diagnoses	Nursing Interventions
Impaired verbal communication, related to memory loss and difficulty focusing attention	Assess communication patterns. Provide calm environment with minimal distraction. Use gestures to match simple verbal messages. Use touch to increase attention. Use familiar music to enhance recall.
Caregiver role strain, related to difficulty coping with cognitive losses and progressive deterioration of self-care abilities	Assess family support network and available resources. Establish opportunities for respite or time-out from caregiver role. Access community support groups. Provide stress management strategies. Assess for signs of depression.
Wandering, related to search for security	Provide continuity of care with same caregivers. Play familiar music. Massage to reduce generalized tension. Visit places of importance such as home and work sites. Use electronic ankle bracelet (activates an alarm if person nears exits). Provide personal attention with conversation and good eye contact. Provide outdoor walking daily with a buddy who converses during the walk.
Unilateral neglect, related to neurologic involvement	Position bed so people approach and provide care from the unaffected side. Ensure that affected body parts are safely positioned. Provide range-of-motion exercises to affected side. Adapt the environment to focus on the unaffected side (placement of personal items, television, or reading materials). Keep side rails up on affected side.

SAFETY AND SECURITY ISSUES FOR OLDER ADULTS

FINANCES

When asked what concerns them the most in their later years, older adults usually answer "health" and "finances." The two are frequently related. For older people, health care will often become a major expense and has the power to devastate their financial security. Because of chronic health problems in addition to acute episodes, older adults spend a greater percentage of their income on health care than younger individuals do. Most older adults are financially assisted by Medicare, Medicaid, or both. Older adults who are able to afford to pay the premiums for Medicare supplemental insurance have a coinsurance, which will pay the 20% of expenses that Medicare does not cover. A prescription drug plan is also available in which it is possible to take the premium out of the patient's Social Security check at a cost as low as $14.00 per month. Many have a fixed income from Social Security, retirement pensions, and only limited savings to pay for the rising costs of housing, food, and health care.

For individuals in lower socioeconomic groups, pensions are not always available, and low salaries and seasonal work prevent saving enough to provide basic needs later in life. Some women who never work outside the home depend entirely on their spouses financially and become impoverished when their husbands die.

Financial problems are all too possible when people have not planned carefully for retirement. Many people assume that adequate pensions will be available if they have to retire or if their spouses die and that Social Security pensions are available to everyone. Unfortunately, this is not true. Retirement planning, including financial planning, needs to begin early in life for both men and women. Because people live longer, sometimes retirement will last as long as 40 years. A number of agencies and senior programs in the community are available to help older adults who have limited resources. Such programs can include homemaking assistance, legal services, low-cost housing or housing improvement, heating assistance, multiservice senior programs, recreation programs, and information and referral services.

HOUSING

Housing represents a certain degree of self-concept and status. It is difficult for many of us to comprehend the insecurity that older adults feel when moving from one site to another in their later years. In addition to the stress of relocation and the initial anxiety of adapting to a new setting, older adults typically move to more restrictive environments, often against their wishes. Housing is often the largest expenditure in people's budgets; therefore it is a concern to many older adults.

When relocation is essential, it is best to match the environment as carefully as possible to the previous experience, and to make the new setting as unrestrictive as is feasible. One individual will be able to manage nicely in a small "mother-in-law" apartment. Another will be happy with a small cottage on the property of a child or a friend. Some few are able to remain in apartments where rent controls allow them to beat inflation costs. Many like mobile home living in small parks with central recreational and service areas that fit their needs and income. Some develop a "round-robin" tactic in which they live with each child for several months each year and never wear out their welcome before they move on to the next. Some remain in their own longtime residence (because of property tax advantages) or in homes they own outright. Some have a grandchild, other relative, or college student live on their premises, free of charge, who is able to provide them with some minimal assistance, company, and security. There are various arrangements for maintaining independent living, as long as people use some energy to creatively develop the plan (Ebersole et al., 2008).

Some older adults choose assisted living in a long-term care residence. These persons do not require 24/7 skilled nursing care, but they do require more assistance than they would receive in an independent living environment. It is more expensive to live in assisted-living facilities than in a completely independent setting; however, it is less costly than a skilled nursing home. Costs of assisted living vary, but range from $1200 per month to over $5000 per month. The average cost is $2627 per month (Ebersole et al., 2008).

FALLS

Falls are the leading cause of accidental death in individuals older than the age of 65. Approximately one third of people 70 years or older report falls in a single year. Generally, falls are caused by a combination of an environmental factor (e.g., a wet floor, stairs) and a physiologic problem (e.g., impaired vision or cognition, gait problems) (see Safety Alert box). Falls are possible as a result of disease processes and age-related changes. Decreased circulation to the brain; diminished coordination, space, and position perception; decreased

Safety Alert!

General Fall Prevention Guidelines

GENERAL CARE

- Wear low-heeled shoes with small wedge platforms.
- Wear leather or rubber-soled shoes.
- Leave night-lights on at night.
- Keep items within reach to prevent overreaching.
- Check the tips of canes and walkers for evenness.
- Paint the last step a different color, indoors and outdoors.
- Dangle the legs between positional changes, and rise slowly.
- Avoid the use of alcohol.
- Avoid rushing.
- Avoid risky behavior, such as standing on ladders unaided.

STEPS AND FLOOR SURFACES

- Be careful to avoid slippery floors and frayed carpets.
- Watch for the last step when descending the stairs.
- Count the number of steps as a cue while ascending and descending the stairs.
- Install and use sturdy banisters on both sides of staircases.
- Tack down throw rugs or remove them entirely.
- Remove obstacles in the path of traffic.
- On landings, use carpeting that has color contrast.

BATHROOM

- Install grab rails in the tub and shower and near the toilet.
- Avoid throw rugs; install carpeting.
- Apply oils to skin after showering or bathing.
- Avoid using bar soaps; use liquid soap from a dispenser mounted in the shower.

From Meiner, S.E., & Lueckenotte, A. (2006). *Gerontologic nursing.* (3rd ed.). St. Louis: Mosby.

ability to balance; decreased muscle strength; changes in gait; and slowed nervous system response are some of the major factors. Others include limited activity, side effects of medications, disorientation, and environmental hazards such as poor lighting and objects obstructing the pathway. In hospital or long-term care settings, insufficient staffing and lack of toileting programs increase the risk of falls (Ebersole et al., 2008).

Prevention *begins* with exercise that increases strength, balance, endurance, and body awareness. Exercise has to be weight bearing to maintain strength of muscles and bones and pleasurable in order to be continued in the long term.

To reduce the risk of falls to a minimum, it is essential to maintain an environment that is free of hazards. Some adaptations to prevent falls include providing assistive devices such as walkers and canes to aid balance, raised toilet seats, hand rails on stairs, grab bars in the bathroom, nonskid shoes, and removal of small scatter rugs. Teach older adults to sit on the side of the bed when they arise and to stand for a minute or so before walking as a technique to cope with orthostatic hypotension (sudden low blood pressure occurring when an individual assumes the standing posture) that sometimes arises owing to poor vascular perfusion or medications.

POLYPHARMACY

Although medications are often a powerful tool for improving the health of older adults, it tends to be a delicate balancing act to keep adverse effects and drug interactions to a minimum. The average older adult uses nearly five prescription medications and two nonprescription medications (Randall, 2006). Among commonly used medications are laxatives, analgesics, cardiovascular medications, vitamins and supplements, and psychoactive medications (Table 33-15).

Inappropriate use of multiple drugs has the potential to create a situation in which the risks outweigh the benefits. Older clients at risk are those who (1) take five or more prescription medications, (2) sometimes borrow medications, (3) use over-the-counter medications including vitamins, dietary supplements, or herbal preparations, (4) request refills without seeing the health care provider, (5) take medications whose prescriptions come from more than one health care provider, and (6) have prescriptions filled at more than one pharmacy. It is essential for assessment to include a review of all medications including over-the-counter medications. Ask the patient when each was prescribed, its purpose, and how it affects him or her. Encourage getting all medications at one pharmacy so the pharmacist is able to check for dangerous interactions (Brager, 2004).

Age-related changes in body function also contribute to some adverse reactions (Figure 33-12). Research indicates that the body's ability to absorb, transport, and eliminate medications is decreased with age because of impaired circulation, changes in vessel walls, and a decrease in the number and efficiency of the glomeruli in the kidneys (Williams, 2002). Metabolism of medications is also decreased as a result of decreased blood flow in the liver, fewer functioning liver cells, and a decrease in the liver enzymes that function to break down and transform medications. As a result of all the changes, many medications remain in the body longer than in a younger person. It is sometimes necessary to reduce dosages to prevent toxicity because the normal adult dosage is for a 150-pound, 20-year-old individual. Many older adults also have conditions such as HF or kidney disease that further impair the body's ability to metabolize and excrete medications.

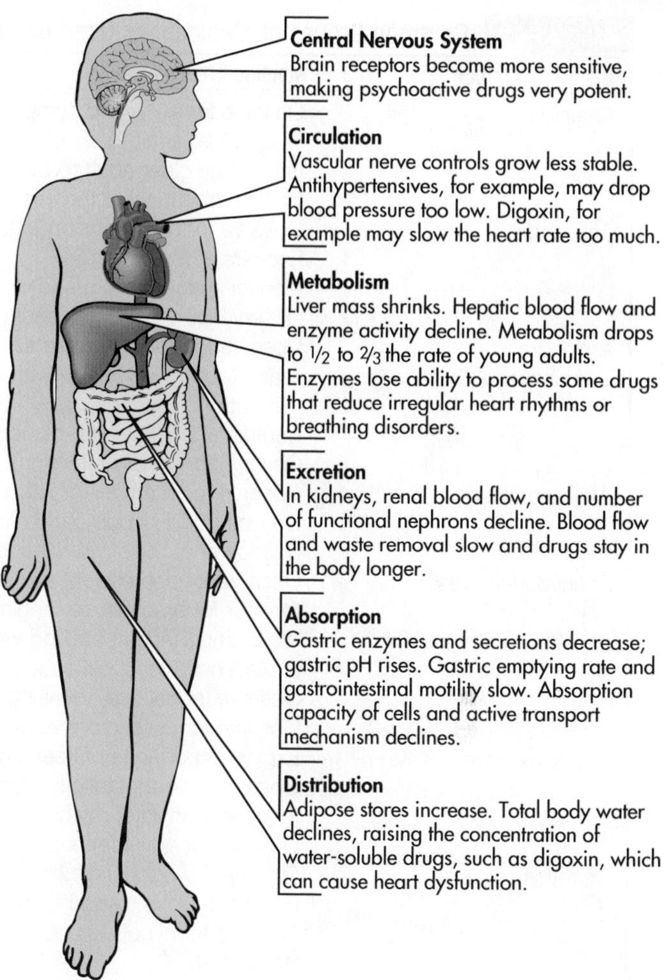

FIGURE 33-12 Changes in the aging body alter medication effects.

Probably 40% or more of adults use alternative pharmacotherapy, such as herbal remedies, and many of them believe that "natural" preparations are safe under all circumstances. Some of the alternative substances older adults commonly use include ginseng, *Ginkgo biloba*, garlic, and St. John's wort. Certain combinations, such as with anticoagulant agents or digoxin, have potential to alter their effectiveness or produce serious side effects. Encourage older adults to avoid taking any herb, supplement, or other over-the-counter products without contacting the health care

Table 33-15 Common Groups of Medications Used by the Older Adult

MEDICATION GROUP	NURSING INTERVENTIONS
Antacids	Observe for signs and symptoms of diarrhea, constipation. Teach older adult to check sodium and sugar content on the label. Encourage older adult to take antacid 1 hour after meals and not with other medications. Caution about use if there is a history of cardiac or renal conditions.
Antibiotics	Observe for disorientation, changes in hearing. Encourage fluid intake. Monitor weight, intake and output (I&O), specific gravity of urine. Observe for secondary yeast or fungal infections of mouth, vagina.
Antidepressants, antipsychotics	Observe for tremor, spasms. Teach techniques to use with vertigo when changing positions, and methods to counteract dry mouth. Caution about use with glaucoma, prostate, or cardiac conditions. Observe for urinary retention.
Antihistamines	Observe for changes in blood pressure. Observe for anticholinergic effects—restlessness, delirium. Caution about use with glaucoma, prostate, or cardiac conditions.
Antihypertensives	Observe for depression, anxiety, disorientation. Monitor for bradycardia, angina, hypotension.
Antiinflammatory agents	Teach importance of taking with food. Explain need for avoidance if there is a history of peptic ulcer. Observe for nausea, vomiting, gastrointestinal (GI) bleeding. Observe for psychological disturbances and masking of infections.
Cardiovascular agents	Explain importance of keeping appointments for laboratory examinations. Observe for orthostatic hypotension. Monitor heart rate, rhythm, and blood pressure. Observe for adverse reactions—disorientation, depression, vertigo, lethargy.
Diuretics	Observe for orthostatic hypotension, delirium, changes in mental function. Explain reasons for taking in the morning. Observe for hypokalemia. Weigh daily. Record I&O.
Opioids	Observe for hypotension. Observe for adverse or idiosyncratic reactions—hallucinations, agitation, disorientation. Monitor respiratory function.
Oral anticoagulants	Monitor prothrombin time (PT) and International Normalized Ratio (INR). Observe for bleeding. Explain importance of keeping appointments for laboratory examinations. Explain the need to avoid aspirin-containing products. Institute safety measures to prevent injury.
Oral hypoglycemic agents	Observe for signs of hypoglycemia—weakness, headache, malaise. Monitor blood glucose levels.
Tranquilizers and sedatives	Observe for signs of oversedation—lethargy, disorientation, agitation. Explain the need to avoid other depressants and alcohol. Observe for adverse and idiosyncratic reactions—delirium, orthostatic hypotension, cardiac dysrhythmia.

provider or a pharmacist who will review the complete drug profile (Brager, 2004).

Nursing interventions begin with assessing the older person's ability to take medications properly. Most older adults are interested in learning about the medications they are taking and appreciate techniques that will help them take the correct dose at the correct time, such as a chart or pill box with compartments labeled with the time and where the pills can be placed for each time they are to be taken. Also be alert to the possibility of medication interactions and signs and symptoms of toxicities, which are easy to misinterpret as "signs of old age." Disorientation, fatigue, anorexia, falls, and vertigo are frequently indications of a medication reaction, and it is necessary to report them to the physician for evaluation. Nursing actions and patient teaching for homebound older adults promote safe medication practices in the home environment (see Health Promotion box).

ELDER ABUSE AND NEGLECT

Abuse and neglect of the older adult refers to violence toward individuals older than the age of 65. Increasing concern has led the American Medical Association (AMA) to issue guidelines for the identification and treatment of abuse in five classifications: (1) physical

 Health Promotion

Medication Practices for Homebound Older Adults

- During each home visit, assess both the prescription and the nonprescription medications being taken by the homebound older adult.
- Document and notify the primary health care provider of the homebound older adult's medication regimen and of multiple physician sources for medications.
- Teach the possible complications and interactions of all over-the-counter medications to homebound older adults and their caregivers.
- Collaborate with social workers to identify community resources for financial assistance with pharmaceutical needs.
- Use laboratory parameters to monitor overuse and underuse of medications, as well as interactive states of medications.
- Monitor urinary output status of older adults because changes in renal excretion sometimes necessitate a decrease or increase in drug dosage.
- Teach the homebound older adult to set up a daily or weekly schedule of medications using a method or tool that fosters safe, independent administration.
- Reduce the chance of medication error by labeling or color coding medication bottles.
- Keep an accurate record of the homebound older adult's weight, because many medication dosages are calculated by body weight.
- Teach drug safety in the home environment by instructing older adults to do the following:
  —Keep drugs in original, labeled container.
  —Dispose of outdated medications in a sink or toilet only; never dispose of them in the trash within reach of children.
  —Never "share" drugs with friends or family members.
  —Always finish a prescribed medication; do not save it for a future illness.
  —Read labels carefully and follow all instructions.
- Instruct older adults who have difficulty opening childproof containers to request their health care providers ask for non-childproof containers when writing prescriptions.

Modified from Meiner, S.E., & Lueckenotte, A. (2006). *Gerontologic nursing.* (3rd ed.). St. Louis: Mosby.

or sexual abuse, (2) psychological abuse, (3) misuse of assets, (4) medical abuse (withholding necessary treatment or aids for ADLs), and (5) neglect. There are many reasons abuse and neglect are becoming more common. Some of these include frustration and exhaustion of a caregiver; alcoholism; turbulent lifestyles; and lack of financial, emotional, family, and community resources. The National Center on Elder Abuse identifies the two most important indicators of abuse as (1) an elder's frequent unexplained crying, and (2) an elder's unexplained fear of or suspicion of a particular person(s) in the home. Older adults are often afraid to admit that they are being abused or neglected. Most states now have mandatory laws requiring the reporting of older adult mistreatment. You are required to be aware of the reporting policies within your area of practice (Box 33-6).

Box 33-6 Types of Older Adult Abuse*

Physical abuse: The use of physical force that has potential to result in bodily injury, physical pain, or impairment.

Sexual abuse: Nonconsensual sexual contact of any kind with an older adult, including those persons unable to give consent.

Emotional or psychological abuse: The infliction of anguish, pain, or distress through verbal or nonverbal acts, including intimidation or enforced social isolation.

Neglect: The refusal or failure to fulfill any part of a person's previously agreed obligation or duties to an older adult dependent on the person for care or assistance.

Abandonment: The desertion of an older adult by an individual who had assumed the responsibility of providing care or assistance.

Medical abuse: Subjecting a person to unwanted medical treatments or procedures; medical neglect occurs when a medically necessary and desired treatment is withheld.

Financial or material abuse or exploitation: The illegal or improper use of older adult's funds, property, or assets.

Ebersole, P., Touhy, T., Hess, P., et al. (2008). *Toward healthy aging: Human needs and nursing response.* (7th ed.). St. Louis: Mosby.

*Older adult abuse implies that the recipient of the abuse is in a situation or condition in which there are limitations of some sort on the person's ability to protect herself or himself. Otherwise, it is more accurate to describe the actions as domestic violence, sexual assault, or fraud.

CONTINUUM OF OLDER ADULT CARE

With the steady growth in the number of older adults, you and your nursing colleagues are likely to spend most of your careers working with older adults. Adults older than age 50 consume nearly 45% of hospital services (Stanton & Rutherford, 2006). More than 80% of those older than age 65 have a chronic illness or functional disability, and those over the age of 75 often have three or four chronic illnesses including arthritis, hypertension, and heart disease as the most prevalent (Hazzard et al., 2003).

HOSPITALIZATION, SURGERY, AND REHABILITATION

Hospitals are dangerous places for older people, who are vulnerable to adverse drug reactions, falls, and infection. To deal with illness leading to hospitalization and surgical intervention, you need to have knowledge of the influence of aging as it relates to anesthesia and immobility. Although responses are individual, older adults have less reserve to cope physically and emotionally with the effects of hospitalization and surgery. They require longer postoperative recovery and convalescent periods. However, during these periods it is very important to keep to a minimum the normal effects of immobility on body systems, which tend to include stasis of secretions, orthostatic hypotension, and digestive and perceptual disorders. This is not to say that it is better for people in their 80s and 90s not to undergo surgery, but it is critical that their rehabilitation begin as soon after surgery as their condition stabilizes.

Especially important are measures to prevent complications of immobility and techniques to support coping skills and independence. Turning, deep breathing, coughing, or other techniques for ventilation, and removal of respiratory secretions are important with older adults because of the age-related changes in the respiratory tract that increase the risk of atelectasis and pneumonia. Depending on the type of surgery, it is best to ambulate older individuals within 8 to 24 hours to decrease the risks of stasis in the circulation, the kidneys and the bladder, and the respiratory tract. Getting up, even to stand or take a few steps, usually helps to stimulate peristalsis, peripheral vascular circulation, and muscle activity; expand the lungs; and improve mental outlook (Figure 33-13).

Encourage older individuals to perform self-care activities at their own level of tolerance and with rest periods. It is also important to remember that the hospitalization and the surgical intervention have potential to increase signs and symptoms of other chronic conditions, such as arthritis, which will sometimes be cause for complaints of discomfort or difficulty in ADLs.

DISCHARGE PLANNING

Older adults need to have the necessary knowledge, skill, and resources to meet self-care needs at home before discharge from a health care facility. Therefore, discharge teaching and planning are of utmost importance. Planning begins with assessment of the biophysical, psychosocial, educational, self-care, and environmental needs. Strategies depend on physical and emotional readiness to learn, educational level, and family and community resources available. Written and/or visual guidelines reinforce verbal instructions and should be provided. Learning is enhanced when the older adult is actively engaged in the learning process (see Patient Teaching box on discharge planning). Preserving as much of the older adult's autonomy as possible is a prime consideration. First consider the individual's physical strength and remaining functional abilities, not just the current disabilities, before making any modification to the home environment.

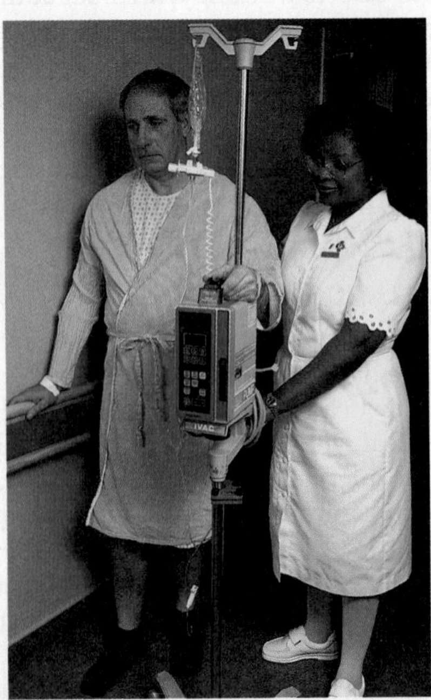

FIGURE 33-13 Ambulation decreases the risks of stasis in the circulation, the kidneys and bladder, and the respiratory tract.

HOME CARE

Many older adults are in need of services to maintain their independence in the community. Economic and technologic factors have combined to cause sicker patients to go home from the hospital sooner (Potter & Perry, 2005).

To be eligible for the Medicare home health benefit, it is necessary that an individual be homebound; have a condition that requires skilled, intermittent care; and have a referring physician who approves the plan of treatment in writing. The home health nurse assesses the physical, functional, emotional, socioeconomic, and environmental well-being of patients and works in collaboration with other members of the home health team including physical therapy, occupational therapy, speech therapy, social worker, and home health aide (HHA) or personal care attendant (PCA). Nurses initiate the plan of care and provide care requiring judgment and skill including health and self-care teaching; this teaching includes medications, medication administration, wound and decubitus care, urinary catheter care, ostomy care, postsurgical care, and care of the terminal patient. Some home health nurses provide intravenous therapy, enteral and parenteral nutrition, and chemotherapy. Once the registered nurse (RN) establishes the plan of care, licensed practical or vocational nurses (LPNs/LVNs) are per-

Patient Teaching

Discharge Planning for the Older Adult

- Teach when the older adult is alert and rested. Allow for several shorter sessions, watching for signs of fatigue.
- Involve the individual in discussion or activity.
- Focus on the person's strengths.
- Use approaches that adapt for the presence of pain and impaired range of joint motion, impaired reception of stimuli such as slower reaction time, muscular weakness, reduced pain and temperature perception, reduced depth perception and color discrimination, or reduced visual acuity.
- Consider need for adaptive devices, such as a syringe magnifier.
- As needed, enlist the help of the patient's significant other, and/or provide assistive personnel.

mitted to provide skilled nursing and HHAs to provide personal care such as ADLs, hygiene, vital signs, and other tasks ordinarily done by the patient or family. Families often hire PCAs for cases in which only a sitter is required, as opposed to personal or skilled care. They usually prepare meals, assist patients to the bathroom, assist with dressing and ambulation, and perform light housekeeping.

ASSISTED LIVING

Assisted living is one of the fastest growing industries in the United States. Placed between home health and the long-term care facility in the continuum of long-term care settings, assisted living offers meals, assistance with bathing and dressing, social and recreational programs, laundry and housekeeping services, transportation, emergency call system, health checks, and medication administration. Many services are purchased individually as needed by the resident.

Other options for living arrangements include retirement villages, senior housing apartments, single-family homes, group living, and sharing a home.

LONG-TERM CARE FACILITIES

Emphasis on reducing costs in the hospital setting through earlier discharge has led to the shift of more acutely ill residents to nursing facilities, traditionally referred to as nursing homes or long-term care facilities. Some of these facilities do not have enough professional nursing staff to provide the complex care these residents require.

Resident Characteristics

People living in nursing facilities are called residents. The facility is their temporary or permanent home, and some residents require nursing care until death. There are approximately 1.6 million individuals currently living in nursing homes in the United States. Estimates project a sharp increase in this number as the older population, particularly those over 85 years of age, grows exponentially over the next 30 years. Nursing facility residents tend to be women (95%), 75 years old and older (82%), white, and widowed (Ebersole et al., 2008).

Nursing home residents usually require 24-hour care, which is not possible to provide in the home environment because of the increased scope of needs and the family's inability to provide the necessary care (Ebersole et al., 2008). The facility usually provides medical, nursing, dietary, recreational, rehabilitative, social, and spiritual care. All care provided in nursing facilities must maintain or improve each resident's quality of life. Most residents require help in ADLs and have difficulty controlling both bowel and bladder.

Care Costs

The average cost of a nursing home was $74,000 per year in 2007 (American Elder Care Research Organization, 2009). Some Americans purchase long-term care insurance; however, individuals or state and federal Medicaid programs pay the majority of nursing home costs. Medicare will cover the cost of only the first 20 days of skilled and rehabilitative care. A significant co-pay from Medicare supplemental insurance is needed for the cost of care for the next 80 days if the need for care continues. Medicaid provides coverage for all levels of care, if the resident qualifies, but there is grave concern for the continuing ability of state and federal governments to support costs through the Medicaid programs (Ebersole et al., 2008).

Quality of Care

Nursing homes are highly regulated, but nursing homes' general lack of adequate funding has made it difficult to maintain the standards that have been legislated. The Omnibus Budget Reconciliation Act (OBRA) of 1987 and subsequent revisions aimed to improve the quality of care and certainly have had a positive outcome. OBRA requirements include comprehensive resident assessments, increased training requirements for certified nursing assistants (CNAs), elimination of the use of medical and physical restraints for discipline or convenience, greater number of nursing staff, availability of social workers, standards for nursing home administrators, and quality assurance activities (Ebersole et al., 2008).

There has also been legislation to protect the rights of residents of nursing homes, and it is mandatory to inform the residents of these rights. Staff is required to promote and protect these rights, which are posted in the long-term care facility so the residents are readily able to see them (Box 33-7). The Long-Term Ombudsman Program is a national effort to support the rights of the residents as well as the facilities. Each long-term care facility is obliged to post the name as well as the contact information of the ombudsman assigned to each facility (Ebersole et al., 2008).

Residents' rights include the following: the right to autonomy and active participation and decision making in their care and life, including the right to self-administer medications; the right to informed consent for the use of side rails and chemical and physical restraints; and the right to withdrawal or withholding of life-sustaining treatments.

Interdisciplinary functional assessment of residents is the cornerstone of clinical practice in long-term care. The minimum data set (MDS) is a tool intended to develop a complete picture of each resident. It includes a comprehensive assessment of background information, cognition, communication, hearing, vision, physical function, mood, behavior, activity, bowel and bladder continence, disease diagnoses, nutrition and dental status, skin condition, medication use, and special treatments and procedures. This information is used to develop an individualized, comprehensive plan of care for each resident.

Box 33-7 Bill of Rights for Long-Term Care Residents

- The right to voice grievances and have them remedied.
- The right to information about health conditions and treatments and to participate in one's own care to the extent possible.
- The right to choose one's own health care providers and to speak privately with one's health care providers.
- The right to consent to or refuse all aspects of care and treatments.
- The right to manage one's own finances if capable, or choose one's own financial advisor.
- The right to be transferred or discharged only for appropriate reasons.
- The right to be free from all forms of abuse.
- The right to be free from all forms of restraint to the extent compatible with safety.
- The right to privacy and confidentiality concerning one's person, personal information, and medical information.
- The right to be treated with dignity, consideration, and respect in keeping with one's individuality.
- The right to immediate visitation and access at any time for family, health care providers, and legal advisors; the right to reasonable visitation and access for others

NOTE: This list of rights is a sampling of federal and several states' lists of rights of residents or participants in long-term care. Check the rules of your own state for specific rights in law for that state.

Ebersole, P., Touhy, T., Hess, P., et al. (2008). *Toward healthy aging: human needs and nursing response.* (7th ed.). St. Louis: Mosby.

Get Ready for the NCLEX® Examination!

Key Points

- Although the efficiency of body systems declines with age, the body has reserves and compensatory mechanisms that normally, in the absence of disease, allow an individual to function well in late adulthood.
- Regardless of age, individuals have the same basic needs for physiologic function, safety, security, belonging, and self-esteem.
- Although older adults experience age-related changes, the rate and response to such changes are individual and necessitate individualized care.
- Individuals retain their intelligence, ability to learn, and memory throughout their lives as long as they remain free of disease that affects brain tissue or thought processes.
- The majority of older adults who consider themselves healthy nonetheless have one or more chronic conditions that will sometimes have acute episodic recurrences or will affect the treatment for other, nonrelated medical-surgical events.
- With advancing age, more coordinated and active interventions are required to support the physiologic and psychological equilibrium of the individual.
- Regardless of normal age-related changes or disease processes, supportive and restorative interventions are appropriate to maintain or improve the quality of life for an older adult.
- To assist the older adult to attain wellness potential, it is essential to recognize the importance of self-esteem, which enhances the individual's ability to cope as situations change.

Additional Learning Resources

Go to your Companion CD for an audio glossary, animations, video clips, and more.

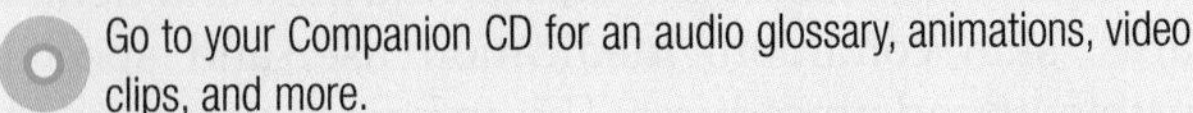

Be sure to visit the Evolve site at http://evolve.elsevier.com/Christensen/foundations/ for additional online resources.

Review Questions for the NCLEX® Examination

1. Which statement best describes demographic changes in relation to the aging population in the United States?
   1. The older adult population is growing twice as fast as the rest of the population.
   2. The most frequent cause of death for people older than 65 is heart disease.
   3. The term *frail elderly* refers to those more than 100 years of age.
   4. Of the population older than age 65, approximately 60% are men and 40% are women.

2. Which statement is a reality rather than a myth concerning older adults?
   1. Most people become senile when they become old.
   2. A majority of older adults in this society are lonely and isolated with less than monthly contact with family and friends.
   3. Approximately 70% of the older adult population reside in nursing homes.
   4. Most older people have at least one chronic condition and rate their health as "good."

3. According to the "disengagement theory," people who are aging:
   1. inherit a genetic program that determines their specific life expectancy.
   2. gradually withdraw from society.
   3. have the inability to achieve a level of acceptance, which results in anger and despair.
   4. experience a change of personality and behaviors related to illness and loneliness.

4. Which is the least likely result of normal aging?
   1. The integumentary system loses elasticity, the epidermis thins, and there is less subcutaneous fat.
   2. There is loss of muscle tone, which increases incidence of choking and aspiration.
   3. There is a gradual loss of weight due to loss of muscle tissue and fluid.
   4. There is increased resistance to infection due to improved immune response.

5. Which relates directly to assessment of adequate circulation to the brain?
   1. Assessment for vertigo or syncope
   2. Assessment for edema
   3. Assessment of apical and peripheral pulses
   4. Assessment of blood pressure

6. Which change is suggestive of osteoporosis?
   1. Decreased muscle strength and joint mobility
   2. Increased curvature of the spine and decreased height
   3. Loss of balance and unsteady gait
   4. Nocturia and sleep pattern disturbances

7. The term *dementia* refers to:
   1. a sudden change in mental status resulting from hypoxia, electrolyte imbalances, or some other treatable condition.
   2. a state of physical and mental deterioration associated with normal aging.
   3. loss of awareness of person, place, and time.
   4. a progressive loss of intellectual function most commonly related to Alzheimer's disease.

8. When administering medications to older adults, it is important for the nurse to keep in mind that:
   1. absorption, transport, and elimination of medications tends to decrease with age because of altered liver and kidney function and decreased circulation.
   2. doses will sometimes need to be increased to achieve desired effects.
   3. older people use a high percentage of over-the-counter (OTC) medications, which enhance the excretion of other drugs.
   4. brain receptors become less sensitive to drugs.

9. The most common response of the older adult to psychosocial changes such as loss of independence, spouse, and friends is:
   1. sleep disturbances.
   2. loss of appetite.
   3. depression.
   4. anger.

10. Farsightedness resulting from a loss of elasticity of the lens of the eye is called:
    1. aphasia.
    2. ataxia.
    3. presbyopia.
    4. pruritus.

11. Older adults often have an atypical response to illness or infection. What is an *atypical* response in previously active and alert older adults that is best to report?
    1. Disorientation, weakness, or incontinence
    2. Fever, loss of appetite, pain
    3. Cough, shortness of breath, and fever
    4. Falls, fainting spells, difficulty swallowing

12. A patient with three school-age children cares for her older adult mother who has Alzheimer's disease. Her mother's condition has become progressively worse to the point that she can no longer safely stay at home alone. A nursing diagnosis of *caregiver role strain* is made. Which nursing intervention is most appropriate?
    1. Provide a calm environment with minimal distraction.
    2. Access community support to provide opportunity for the caregiver to do errands and spend time with her children.
    3. Assess communication patterns.
    4. Encourage the use of gestures and touch to enhance communication.

13. Which would least likely be an appropriate nursing diagnosis for an older adult male with neurologic problems?
    1. Wandering
    2. Impaired verbal communication
    3. Impaired urinary elimination
    4. Risk for disturbed sensory perception

14. The primary reason for decreased sexual activity in many older adults is:
    1. painful sexual intercourse due to vaginal dryness or pain.
    2. loss of interest as a normal part of the aging process.
    3. treatment of other conditions with medications that induce impotence.
    4. lack of a sexual partner.

15. Aging often causes a decreased production of intrinsic factor from the stomach thus interfering with the body's ability to utilize vitamin B_{12}. What disease will develop from this deficiency?
    1. Iron deficiency anemia
    2. Aplastic anemia
    3. Pernicious anemia
    4. Sickle sell anemia

16. The normal range for intraocular pressure is:
    1. 50 to 60 mm Hg.
    2. 10 to 22 mm Hg.
    3. 22 to 32 mm Hg.
    4. 5 to 18 mm Hg.

17. Sleep disturbances may also be a normal part of aging resulting from changes in:
    1. center of Broca's area.
    2. cerebellar functioning.
    3. functioning of thalamus and globus pallidus.
    4. the reticular formation (RF) in the brainstem, and extending into the cerebral cortex.

chapter 34

Basic Concepts of Mental Health

evolve

http://evolve.elsevier.com/Christensen/foundationsadult

Anne W. Ryan

Objectives

1. Describe the mental health continuum.
2. Identify defining characteristics of people who are mentally healthy and those who are mentally ill.
3. Describe the parts of personality.
4. Describe the factors that influence an individual's response to change.
5. Identify factors that contribute to the development of emotional problems or mental illness.
6. Identify barriers to health adaptation.
7. Identify sources of stress.
8. Identify stages of illness behavior.
9. Identify major components of a nursing assessment that focuses on mental health status.
10. Identify basic nursing interventions for those experiencing illness or crisis.

Key Terms

adaptation (p. 1128)
anxiety (p. 1127)
behavior (p. 1122)
coping responses (p. 1128)
crisis (p. 1130)
defense mechanisms (p. 1128)
deinstitutionalization (p. 1124)
humoral theory (HŪ-mōr-ăl, p. 1123)
illness (p. 1129)
Linda Richards (p. 1124)
Martha Mitchell (p. 1124)
mental health (p. 1122)
mental health continuum (p. 1125)
mental illness (p. 1122)
mind-body link (p. 1128)
Omnibus Budget Reconciliation Act (OBRA) (p. 1124)
personality (p. 1126)
placebo effect (plă-SĒ-bō, p. 1129)
self (p. 1126)
self-concept (p. 1126)
stress (p. 1127)
stressor (p. 1127)

As a licensed practical nurse/licensed vocational nurse (LPN/LVN), you are likely to use mental health nursing principles in a variety of health care settings. Basic mental health concepts are useful in understanding a patient's behavioral responses to disease and dysfunction. It is possible to define **behavior** as the manner in which a person performs any or all of the activities of daily life. Individuals respond differently to changes in daily activities, such as the change created by illness and hospitalization. All individuals have unique personalities and resources that affect their behavior in dealing with changing situations and the changing environment. An individual's mental health will sometimes vary depending on the situation and the available support systems.

Let us define **mental health** as one's ability to cope with and adjust to the recurrent stresses of everyday living. Thus mentally healthy individuals are individuals who are able to enjoy life's activities, adapt successfully to changes, set realistic goals, solve problems, have satisfying working relationships, and maintain interpersonal relationships with family and friends (Figure 34-1).

Factors affecting mental health include inherited characteristics, childhood nurturing, and life's circumstances. The influence these factors have on the individual's response to daily stressors in life is sometimes positive and sometimes negative. Possible positive influences include inherent adequate coping ability, mother-child bonding at birth, success in school, good physical health, and financial security. Possible negative influences include cognitive impairment, schizophrenia, extreme sibling rivalry, parental rejection, deprivation of maternal love, poor physical health, poverty, and broken relationships.

Evidence of **mental illness** often consists of a pattern of behaviors that is conspicuous, threatening, and disruptive of relationships or that deviates significantly from behavior that is considered socially and culturally acceptable. Mental illness or disorder is a manifestation of dysfunction (behavioral, psychological, and biologic).

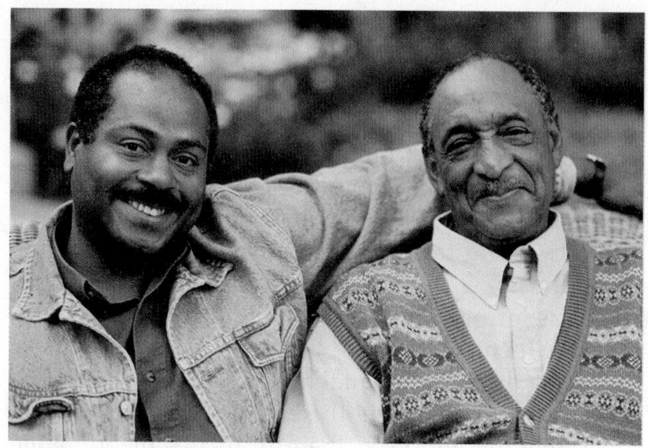

FIGURE 34-1 Maintaining interpersonal relationships with family members provides a positive influence that affects mental health.

Changes in society and in the economy have altered the status and situation of many individuals. It is estimated that one of every eight people in the United States is in need of mental health services. It is also estimated that one of every three people will develop a mental health problem at some point in life. In part, these statistics probably reflect our changing societal environment. You will find yourself in perhaps daily contact with battered spouses, abused children, homeless people, single parents, or substance abusers. Regardless of the practice setting, you will frequently find patients in need of emotional support.

Nurses are in a position to be a source of help to the patient. You will usually provide nursing interventions in a situation involving interpersonal exchange. Patients will express their feelings in a variety of ways. You have the responsibility of assessing and intervening while maintaining a caring relationship of trust with the patient. The emphasis of the mental health aspect of nursing is to assist the patient and family to achieve satisfying and productive ways of dealing with both the positive and the negative aspects of daily living and to cope with situations that call for a change in lifestyle.

This chapter does not pretend to be a comprehensive course in psychiatric nursing. The focus is on developing an awareness and understanding that regardless of the setting or the situation, the need for emotional wellbeing is a common thread in all patients.

HISTORICAL OVERVIEW

The history of mental health care dates to primitive times. During early history, people thought that a physically or mentally ill person was possessed by evil spirits. For mental illness, the shamans or medicine men focused on removing evil spirits by magical treatments such as spells, potions, noises, or sacrifices and physical treatments such as vomiting, bleeding, massage, and trephining (cutting holes in the skull to release evil spirits). If these tribal rites were unsuccessful, the tribe abandoned the individual to die by starvation or attack by wild animals.

Historical records show that there was an interest in mental health and illness and its treatment in the Greco-Roman era. The Greeks introduced the idea that it is possible to explain mental illness by observation of behavior. Hippocrates viewed mental illness as an imbalance of humors based on the fundamental elements of the world: air, fire, water, and earth. Each basic element corresponded to a particular fluid in the body: blood, yellow bile, black bile, and phlegm. This view of illness is called the **humoral theory** (pertaining to body fluids or substances contained in them). Roman physicians were interested in making their patients comfortable by providing physical care such as warm baths, massage, and music.

During the Dark Ages, or medieval times, about AD 500 to AD 1400, society lost track of this concept of mental illness. In the Dark Ages, the church became powerful and kept much knowledge locked away in the monasteries. Early Christians believed mental illness was punishment for sins committed, possession by the devil, or an effect of witchcraft. Exorcisms, physical punishment and imprisonment, or banishment became the treatment for mental illness. Toward the end of the Dark Ages, Arabic influences in Europe reawakened awareness of emotions and disease and medical treatment for mental illness. The first English institution for the mentally ill was Bethlehem Royal Hospital, founded in the sixteenth century under Henry VI. Our English word for a place of confusion and disorder, **bedlam,** originated from its nickname (Figure 34-2). We still use the term today. To raise money to run the institution, it was the custom to

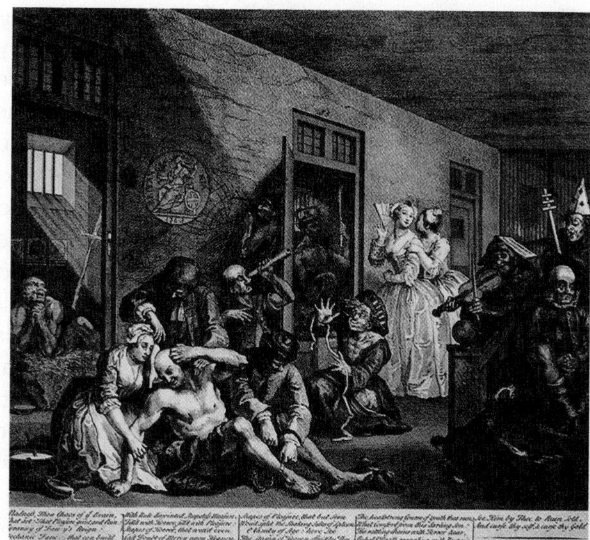

FIGURE 34-2 Bethlehem Royal Hospital, London, otherwise known as "Bedlam."

shackle or cage the residents and collect money from people who were curious to see these so-called subhuman creatures. This practice continued for several hundred years.

During the Renaissance and the Reformation (fifteenth and sixteenth centuries), little changed in the treatment of mental illness. The Reformation brought the closing of many Catholic institutions, which put the poor, the sick, and the insane back into the streets again.

The seventeenth and eighteenth centuries saw further growth of the sciences, literature, philosophy, and the arts, but conditions for the mentally ill were worse than ever. Bleeding, starving, beating, purging, and confinement were the treatments of the day. During the latter half of the eighteenth century, psychiatry became a separate branch of medicine.

Dr. Philippe Pinel, director of two Paris hospitals, changed the concept of care for the mentally ill. Pinel advocated humane care and maintenance of case history and conversation records. He classified illnesses by behaviors. In England about the same time, William Tukes, a Quaker, built an asylum similar to a Quaker household. His philosophy of care was to encourage acceptable behavior by providing a nurturing atmosphere. This concept of care became very popular.

In the United States, Dr. Benjamin Rush, a signer of the Declaration of Independence, established the Pennsylvania Hospital (1731) in Philadelphia for treatment of the mentally ill. Harsh treatment of the mentally ill still prevailed in the United States, as it did in Europe. Some newer therapies and devices (e.g., the tranquilizing chair) were used to encourage the rational mind to come forth. Dr. Rush used the newer, more humane therapies in his practice. He became known as the father of American psychiatry. The first public psychiatric hospital in the United States, Eastern Psychiatric Hospital, opened in 1773 in Williamsburg, Virginia.

The nineteenth century saw the flourishing of institutions and asylums. Overcrowding and bureaucracy brought the decline of care these institutions were able to provide. Dorothea Dix, a retired schoolteacher, was appalled by the care of the mentally ill and set out to do something about it. She surveyed jails, almshouses, and asylums throughout the United States, Canada, and Scotland and presented her findings to anyone who would listen—presidents, legislatures, civic groups, and concerned citizens. Her efforts brought millions of dollars toward the development of mental hospitals throughout the United States. In 1882, McLean Hospital in Waverly, Massachusetts, provided the first psychiatric training school for nurses. **Linda Richards,** who practiced in the 1880s, has been credited as the first psychiatric nurse.

The twentieth century ushered in the reform of mental health care, as a growing population became interested in social issues. Clifford Beers, a college student who had attempted suicide, spent 3 years as a patient in a mental hospital. Upon his release he wrote *A Mind That Found Itself,* which described the beatings, isolation, and confinement he experienced and witnessed while he was institutionalized. As a result of Beers' work, the Committee for Mental Hygiene formed in 1909. This committee focused on prevention of mental illness and removal of the stigma of mental illness. Around this same time, Dr. Sigmund Freud, a neurophysiologist now known as the father of psychiatry, was introducing his elaborate theories and treatment for mental illnesses.

During the 1930s, mental health practitioners developed electroconvulsive therapy (ECT) and insulin shock therapy and used them to treat schizophrenia. The field also saw the use of frontal lobotomy—a surgical procedure that severs the frontal lobes from the thalamus—to eliminate violent behaviors. By 1939, about half of all nursing schools offered psychiatric courses in their curriculum.

In the 1940s, the passage of the National Health Act and the establishment of the National Institute of Mental Health (NIMH) were among the most important developments in psychiatric medicine in the United States. The institute established research funding for the cause, the prevention, and the treatment of mental illnesses.

The 1950s brought about the introduction of psychotherapeutic drugs. This allowed the psychiatric patient to be treated in regular hospital settings. These drugs also allowed the individual to control his or her behavior and thus spend more time in the community, which was a primary goal of mental health care. At this time the government started the movement of **deinstitutionalization,** or release of institutional psychiatric patients to live and receive treatment in the community setting. During the 1960s and 1970s, legislatures brought about further changes in mental health treatment at the community level. A goal of community treatment is to return the individual to the home environment as soon as possible and to provide a support system within the community to facilitate treatment and bring about functioning as near to normal as possible.

President Jimmy Carter established the President's Commission on Mental Health in 1978. This commission assessed mental health care needs of the nation and made recommendations of action for the government to take. **Martha Mitchell,** a nurse educator and clinical specialist in psychiatric–mental health nursing, was among those appointed to this commission. This was the first time nursing had representation in a commission of this type. From this commission's recommendations, the most comprehensive mental health care bill in U.S. history, the Mental Health Care Systems Act, was passed in 1980.

President Ronald Reagan and his conservative administration passed the **Omnibus Budget Reconciliation Act (OBRA)** of 1981, drastically reducing funding for the mental health system and putting what moneys remained into block grants for use and disbursement at the community level. Rapid, if not indiscriminate, deinstitutionalization was one consequence of the severe fiscal cuts. Many mentally ill patients from state institutions were simply put out into the streets, where they were not able to find work and their families could not take care of them.

Now in the twenty-first century, health care providers put mental health concepts and principles into practice in a variety of settings, including public health and home health care facilities, outpatient settings, and acute care hospitals. Psychiatric and mental health care centers are not the only settings in which you will find the practice of mental health care. There are patients in need of emotional support in any and every health care setting. The community-based mental health movement and the holistic health movement have brought awareness to the public that all individuals, sick or well, have emotional needs to be met.

BASIC CONCEPTS RELATED TO MENTAL HEALTH

Nursing is a person-oriented profession. Every interaction that you have with a patient affords an opportunity for assessment of the patient's emotional state. It lies within your power and responsibility to create an environment that allows the patient to have as positive an experience as possible. Most people have an innate ability to heal themselves that is influenced by mental attitude. You can help the patient use this inner healing capacity through nursing interventions.

MENTAL HEALTH CONTINUUM

Consider mental health and mental illness as occupying opposite ends of a **mental health continuum** (Figure 34-3). On the illness side of the continuum, each of us is rarely in touch with reality. When on the healthy side on the continuum, we demonstrate a high level of wellness. This form of wellness includes an assertive communication style, acceptance of strengths and weaknesses, and available energy to deal with life's situations. The midpoint on the continuum represents normal mental health. Although a person occupying this point will probably display some lack of insight, this midpoint level is characterized by adequate coping skills, problem-solving ability, and satisfactory responses or adjustments to life changes with some growth or possibly some mild regression. Although many of us function in a relatively healthy manner, periods of crisis or biochemical imbalance have potential to decrease our functional capacity, moving us toward the illness end of the continuum (Box 34-1).

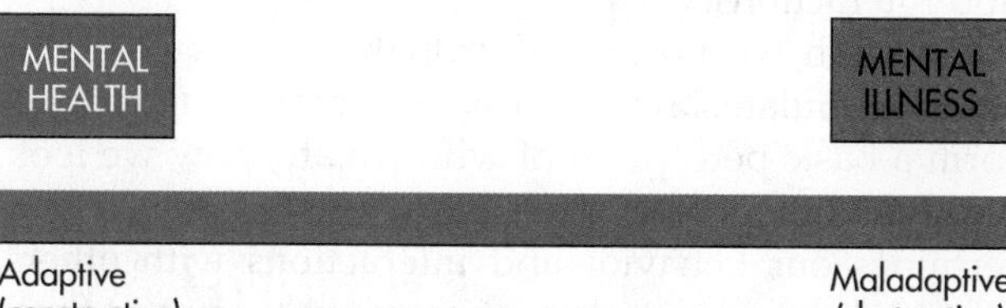

FIGURE 34-3 Mental health continuum.

To determine placement on the continuum, it is necessary to assess several components of mental health. These components include a positive self-concept, awareness of responsibility for one's own behavior and its consequences, maintenance of satisfying interpersonal relationships, adaptability to change, effective communication, awareness and acceptance of emotions and their expression, effective problem solving, and recognition and use of supportive systems (Figure 34-4).

The point at which we deem a person to be mentally ill is determined by the behavior the person exhibits, as well as the context in which the behavior occurs. Mental illness results from an inability to cope with a situation that we find overwhelming. The maladaptive behavior is often part of a response to acute anxiety (see Box 34-1).

Box 34-1 Characteristics Identified in Mental Illness

- Poor self-concept
- Feelings of inadequacy
- Dependent behavior due to feelings of inadequacy
- Pessimism that is constant
- Poor judgment
- Inability to cope
- Irresponsibility
- Inability to accept responsibility for actions
- Avoidance of problems (does not attempt to handle them)
- Inability to recognize own talents
- Inability to recognize limitations
- Inability to perceive reality
- Maladaptive behavior
- Demands or seeks immediate gratification
- Inability to establish a meaningful relationship

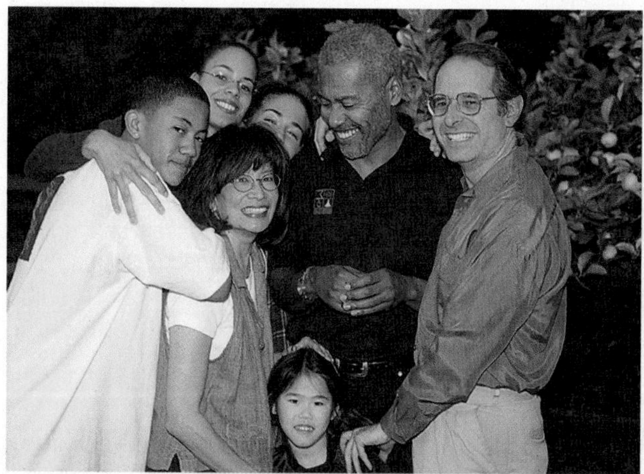

FIGURE 34-4 Recognition and use of a support system of family and friends is one of the mental health components that determines placement on the mental health continuum.

PERSONALITY AND SELF-CONCEPT

Personality refers to the relatively consistent set of attitudes and behaviors particular to an individual. Your personality consists of your unique patterns of mental, emotional, and behavioral traits, woven together. Thoughts, feelings, values, and beliefs evolve into a consistent set of traits that characterize you. Personality development comes under the influence of genetics and interactions with the environment. From infancy and throughout life, you have interactions that affect your personal security, values, personal identity, and relationships with others. Consider viewing personality as the total of our internal and external patterns of adjustment to life. There are many theories about growth process and the development of personality. All are attempts to explain why people behave the way they do as well as how each of us evolves emotionally and physically.

Erik Erikson provided a framework for understanding personality development in terms of task mastery (see Chapter 9). Erikson is one of the most widely read and influential theorists of development and his concepts of identity and identity crisis have had major professional influence throughout the social sciences. According to Erikson's framework, if a person does not master a given task, then it is possible to predict a certain set of behaviors.

Sigmund Freud described personality development as having three parts: id, ego, and superego (Box 34-2). The id functions on a primitive level and aims primarily at experiencing pleasure and avoiding pain. The ego functions to integrate and mediate between the self and the rest of the environment. It is the ego that experiences anxiety. The superego is the moralistic censoring force. It develops from the ego in response to reward or punishment from others. When all three substructures function in harmony, the individual experiences emotional stability; we consider that person to have a healthy self-concept. A mature, well-adjusted personality is under the leadership of the ego.

Box 34-2 Parts of the Personality

ID
- The basic innate drive for survival and pleasure
- Demands constant gratification
- Comprises the individual's entire personality at birth
- Is not changed by experience because it is not in contact with the external world
- Its goals are to reduce tension, to increase pleasure, and to keep discomfort to a minimum

EGO
- The reality factor
- Helps the individual perceive conditions accurately
- Decides how to act and when to act
- Is that portion of the psyche that is in contact with external reality—stands, so to speak, for reason and good sense, whereas the id stands for untamed passion

SUPEREGO
- The parental or societal value system
- Strives for perfection and morality
- Develops from the ego
- Serves as a judge or censor over thoughts and activities of the ego. Freud describes three functions of the superego: conscience, self-observation, and the formation of ideals

Freud delineated levels of awareness: conscious, preconscious, and unconscious. At the conscious level, experiences are within our awareness; we are aware of and able to control thoughts. *Preconsciousness* refers to thoughts, feelings, drives, and ideas that are outside our awareness but that we easily recall to consciousness. The preconscious state helps to screen certain thoughts and repress unpleasant thoughts and desires. The unconscious level holds memories, feelings, and thoughts that are not available to the conscious mind. This is the most significant level because of the effect it has on behavior.

Self is a complex concept comprising four distinct parts that influence behavior. The four areas of self are personal identity, body image, role, and self-esteem. Personal identity is the organizing principle of the self; it is the "I." A person with a strong identity knows who he or she is and is not. Body image comprises the picture of and the feelings toward your body. Body image includes feelings about the way you look, the way your body functions, sex, size, and whether your body image helps you realize personal gains. Manifestations of body image include stance, posture, clothing, and jewelry.

Role performance is the expected behavior of an individual in a social position. Roles are ascribed or assumed. An ascribed role—for example, being female or male—involves no personal choice. An assumed role (e.g., occupation) is selected by the individual. In a lifetime, each of us fills many overlapping roles, and we need to combine these roles to achieve an integrated pattern of functioning. Self-esteem is the assessment we make about personal worth. Self-esteem comprises the thoughts and feelings each of us holds about ourselves.

Self-concept is more than the total of the four parts of self. It is the frame of reference we use for all we know and experience. Self-concept includes all perceptions and values each of us holds and our behaviors and interactions.

Through the process of growth and development, we accumulate and process information that helps form a basic perception of who we are, how we look, and how others react to us. How we see ourselves determines our behavior and interactions with others. Disturbances in self-concept commonly arise in those of us with mental illness or emotional problems.

STRESS

Each of us is continually exposed to a variety of situations that produce stress. Our mental health fluctuates along with our ability to adapt and deal with life situations or events. Any event that requires change leads to stress. It is possible for the event to be either pleasant or unpleasant. **Stress** is the nonspecific response of the body to any demand made on it. Our response to a stressful situation or event is often a result of learned or conditioned behavior.

By contrast, a **stressor** is a situation, activity, or event that produces stress. Stressors are physical, social, economic, chemical, spiritual, or developmental, or some combination of all of these. The meaning we give to the stress determines whether we feel distress. Stress is highly subjective, uniquely perceived by the person experiencing it. Stress in itself is neither good nor bad; however, its has both positive and negative effects. Stress that facilitates individual growth and development and promotes change and adaptation brings positive results. Some stressors have potential to be overwhelming, yielding the negative results characteristic of ineffective coping.

Mental health nursing concerns itself with behavior, particularly a person's response to stressors. Health factors affect this response. The stress of being ill greatly influences a person's emotional well-being and coping ability. How we perceive stress determines whether the stress produces anxiety in us. It is important to remember that a person's response to a stressful situation or event is often a result of learned or conditioned behavior, and thus is, at least in theory, amenable to change. You have the opportunity to be a resource in helping a patient develop adaptive patterns of behavior.

ANXIETY

Anxiety is possible to define as a vague feeling of apprehension that results from a perceived threat to the self. Anxiety is said to be a universal emotion and is a response to a stressful event. It is a state of apprehension, a vague feeling whose source is often unknown. Anxiety is an internal process we experience when there is a real or perceived threat to our physical body or self-concept. Anxiety is a major component of all mental health disturbances. In mild forms, anxiety readies the body for action and reaction to danger. Mild levels of anxiety enable the body to meet stressful demands by promoting problem solving and constructive action. Higher levels of anxiety immobilize our coping skills and result in emotional chaos. In severe forms, anxiety interferes with daily activities.

Anxiety is usually described in terms of levels, and each level is associated with certain behaviors (Box 34-3). Signs of higher levels of anxiety include vocal changes; rapid speech; increased pulse, respirations, and blood pressure; tremors; restlessness; increased perspiration; nausea; decreased appetite; diarrhea; frequent urination; and occasionally vomiting.

Box 34-3 Levels of Anxiety

An individual's response in a given situation depends on the level of anxiety.

MILD
- Slight increase in vital signs and an awareness of danger
- Able to think and make connections; heightened awareness
- Is ready for action
- Motivation is increased

MODERATE
- Feels tension
- Perception has decreased
- Remains alert, but only to specific information
- Perhaps prone to arguing, teasing, or complaining
- Physical signs and symptoms often appear: headache, diarrhea, nausea, vomiting, low back pain, and increased vital signs

SEVERE
- Experiences a feeling of impending danger
- Perceptual field narrows significantly and becomes distorted
- Communication possibly distorted and difficult to understand
- Feels fatigued
- Changes in vital signs potentially evident on assessment

PANIC
- Feeling of extreme terror
- Possibly becomes immobilized
- Reality is distorted
- Personality will potentially disintegrate further
- Has potential to cause harm to self and others

Anxiety arises within each of us as the result of inner conflict, and subsequent behavior stems from the anxiety. Maladaptive behavior is often a defense against anxiety. We learn a variety of ways to respond to anxiety as we move through the various stages of growth and development. Behavior exhibited in response to stress and anxiety is the result of a combination of factors. The degree of anxiety we experience is influenced by the following:

- How we view the stressor
- The number of stressors we are handling at one time
- Previous experience with similar situations
- The magnitude of change the event represents for us

Events that have the potential to precipitate feelings of anxiety include the following:

- *Threats to physical integrity:* Decreased ability to perform activities of daily living; impending physiologic disability: surgery, diagnosis of a life-threatening disorder, pain, infection, trauma

- *Threats to self-esteem and insults to the identity:* Loss of significant relationships, loss of spouse, difficulty at work, loss of job, change in jobs, relocation to a new home

We relieve anxiety through various coping and mental mechanisms. These mechanisms are partly conscious and partly unconscious; they serve to protect us from situations perceived as dangerous. Anxiety is an inevitable part of life. Part of the emotional growth process is to learn to deal with stress and anxiety in an adaptive or corrective manner.

MOTIVATION

Motivation is the gathering of personal resources or inner drive to complete a task or reach a goal. We generate this inner drive by projecting the reward or the punishment we imagine we will receive when we have performed, or failed to perform, a task. Motivation is an important aspect in treating emotional problems. The motivation to participate in care helps the patient through the stages of recovery quickly.

FRUSTRATION

Frustration refers to anything that interferes with goal-directed activity. This concept is important in understanding the individual's response to frustration. Some people are more flexible and adaptable than others. When adaptive behavior fails, anxiety increases.

CONFLICT

Conflict is a struggle, usually a mental one, either conscious or unconscious. Conflict results from the simultaneous presence of opposing or incompatible thoughts, ideas, goals, or emotional forces, such as impulses, denials, or drives. Some conflicts we resolve easily, whereas others are more complicated and lead to serious levels of anxiety. An example of conflict is when a person is ill and needs to see a physician but does not for fear of getting bad news.

ADAPTATION AND COPING

Adaptation refers to our ability to adjust to changing life situations by using various strategies. Any kind of change in routines or patterns of living causes varying degrees of stress. Illness, family problems, lack of money, and inadequate transportation are all possible to view as stressful to any one of us. An inability to meet basic needs or role expectations has the power to precipitate emotional upheaval. Feelings and emotions are part of our behavior. An individual who develops ways to deal with stress and resolve it has adapted. Adaptation is possible to view as positive or negative. Both growth and regression are possible results of a stress experience.

Coping responses are the responses we use to reduce anxiety brought on by stress. Common coping responses include overeating, drinking, smoking, withdrawal, seeking out someone to talk with, yelling, exercising or other physical activity, fighting, pacing, or listening to music. Often we use coping responses both consciously and unconsciously to adjust to stress without changing our actual goal.

Use of defense mechanisms is another way of coping with anxiety. Defense mechanisms are unconscious, intrapsychic reactions that offer protection to the self from a stressful situation. **Defense mechanisms** are behavioral patterns that protect us against a real or perceived threat; we use them to block conscious awareness of threatening feelings. This type of behavior develops when we experience an unconscious conflict or a threat to our self-concept. All of us use defense mechanisms for self-protection (Table 34-1).

If we use defense mechanisms inappropriately or overuse them to cope, in mental health terms the behavior is maladaptive.

HOW ILLNESS AFFECTS MENTAL HEALTH

There is a misconception that mental health principles are applicable only in a mental health care facility or center. In reality you will address, along with every one of your colleagues, the mental health needs of each patient in your care. The stress of being ill greatly influences an individual's mental state and level of functioning.

Ordinarily, individuals feel in control of their lives. Illness reduces that control and sometimes creates instability, causing anxiety. When hospitalized, we leave behind the familiarity of home and work for the unfamiliar hospital setting. Upon entering the hospital setting, we exchange our clothes for hospital wear, submit our bodily fluids for testing and our body parts for imaging, endure the same questions again and again, sometimes enjoy only limited visitation with family and friends, and have to adapt ourselves to being one entry on someone else's scheduled daily duties—the nurse's.

Most people do not expect to become ill or have lifestyle alterations resulting from illness or accidents. Serious injury and illness have the capacity to dramatically alter our self-concept, body image, lifestyle, and role performance in family life, recreation, and work. Regardless of whether the situation is temporary or permanent, our mental and emotional states undergo a disturbance. As a nurse, you will only be able to provide effective nursing interventions if you take the patient's emotional state into consideration.

Meeting the psychosocial needs of the individual is a task for the health care team as a whole. Patients and their families remember the nurses who care for them. A memory of the nurse who showed a little extra consideration for the individual stays with them, as does that of the nurse who was short tempered or judgmental. One of the steps to meeting these needs is effective patient education. It helps to build trust and encourages the patient to have faith in the care you give. This promotes positive thinking, which affects the **mind-**

Table 34-1 Commonly Used Defense Mechanisms

MODE	DESCRIPTION
Compensation	An individual makes up for a "deficiency" in one area by excelling in or emphasizing another area. EXAMPLE: A boy who is small in stature places his emphasis on academics rather than attempting sports.
Conversion	Emotional conflicts are turned into a physical symptom, which provides the individual with some sort of benefit (secondary gain). EXAMPLE: The individual who witnesses a murder then experiences sudden blindness with no organic cause.
Denial	Reality is denied; it does not exist. EXAMPLE: The patient who has suffered a severe myocardial infarction is told that he will have to severely restrict his physical activity. The evening nurse finds him on the floor of his room, doing sit-ups and push-ups.
Displacement	Emotions are expressed toward someone or something other than the actual source of the emotion. Unconsciously, the individual does not feel safe expressing the feelings directly. EXAMPLE: The person has an argument with his employer and comes home and yells at his family.
Dissociation	Separation and detachment of emotional significance and affect from an idea or situation. EXAMPLE: The person who has been traumatically victimized retells her situation, while smiling and joking about it.
Identification	Individual incorporates a characteristic (thought or behavior) of another individual or group. The individual does not give up personal identity. EXAMPLE: A teenager who dresses like a favorite rock singer.
Introjection	A quality or attribute of another is internalized and becomes part of the individual. EXAMPLE: The child who follows her parents' instructions when the parents are not present (e.g., carefully crossing the street).
Projection	Attributing to other characteristics that the person does not want to admit possessing. Blaming personal shortcomings on someone else. EXAMPLE: A student who does poorly on an examination and states, "That test was unfair. The teacher did not present the material correctly."
Rationalization	A process of constructing plausible reasons to explain and justify one's behavior. The person denies actual thoughts and justifies actions by giving untrue, but seemingly more acceptable, reasons for the behavior. EXAMPLE: The young boy who was instructed to make up his bed and clean his room before leaving for school chooses to play instead. In the afternoon, when he and his mother arrive home and she becomes angry at noticing his disregard of her instructions, he states, "But Mom, Dad was in a hurry this morning and told me that if I wanted a ride to school, I'd better get in the car."
Reaction formation	The conscious behavior is completely opposite to the unconscious process. EXAMPLE: A person who is excessively polite to an individual who is disliked.
Regression	Behavior, thoughts, or feelings used at an earlier stage of development are exhibited. EXAMPLE: An 8-year-old who reverts to bed-wetting and thumb-sucking while hospitalized.
Repression	The unconscious process of barring from conscious thought of painful, disagreeable thoughts, experiences, and or impulses. Energy is expended so that the individual has less available energy. EXAMPLE: A patient who was incontinent after surgery represses the embarrassment and totally suppresses the event.
Sublimation	The discharge of sexual or aggressive energy and impulses in a socially acceptable way. EXAMPLE: The teenager who engages in many competitive sports.
Suppression	An intentional (conscious) exclusion of painful thoughts, experiences, or impulses. (Some do not consider this a defense mechanism.) EXAMPLE: A student who fails to keep an appointment for academic counseling.

body link of healing within. This placebo effect (positive response to treatment) on the body bolsters the immune system and has proven therapeutic power to augment your nursing interventions. Strong support is another factor that helps the patient stay in a positive frame of mind. Patient support groups, family connections, and community involvement are important to maintain during an illness. See Box 34-4 for psychiatric nursing diagnoses that you will often use to address the patient's psychosocial needs (see also Life Span Considerations for Older Adults box).

ILLNESS BEHAVIORS

Illness is a state of homeostatic imbalance. When we are ill or sick, we do not feel good. This is the body's way of saying, "Pay attention to my needs." The experience of being ill involves stages that are subjective and very personal. The illness experience starts with our awareness of symptoms that are not healthy. We then have to adjust and take on the sick role. The sick role allows us to be excused from everyday responsibilities and social responsibility in order to rest and heal. If an appropriate attempt at this stage does not cure the ailment, we go on to seek professional medical or other health care. The sick person receiving professional care assumes a dependent role—with the expectation of getting well. Keeping the patient informed and emotionally supported is a focus of professional care. Recovery and rehabilitation is the last stage of an illness event. You assist your patient by setting attainable short-term goals to enable the patient to be aware of his or her recovery and rehabilitation.

Box 34-4 NANDA-I Nursing Diagnoses for Psychiatric–Mental Health Nursing

Impaired adjustment
Anxiety
Disturbed body image
Impaired verbal communication
Ineffective coping
Decisional conflict
Ineffective denial
Interrupted family processes
Fear
Grieving
Hopelessness
Disturbed personal identity
Ineffective role performance
Risk for situational low self-esteem
Ineffective sexual patterns
Ineffective sleep pattern
Impaired social interaction
Risk for spiritual distress

Data from North American Nursing Diagnosis Association International (NANDA-I). (2009). *NANDA-I nursing diagnoses: definitions and classification 2009-2011.* Oxford, United Kingdom: Author.

Life Span Considerations

Older Adults

Aging and Mental Health

- Older people experiencing significant sensory changes in hearing or vision sometimes display behavioral changes that are easy to mistake for disorientation.
- Social isolation in the older adult is frequently a result of physical or financial limitations.
- The behavioral characteristics and personality of older people are often an exaggeration of their behavior at a younger age.
- Many losses—including loss of loved ones, home, job, and independence—occur with aging. These losses result in varying amounts of grief. The number of losses and the rapidity with which they occur have the potential to affect the coping ability of the older person and result in anxiety, fear, or depression.
- Relocation from home to hospital or even from room to room has potential to cause stress in the older person, which manifests as behavioral change.
- Hopelessness and helplessness are common in the older adult. These feelings sometimes lead older people to lose the will to live and even commit suicide.
- Reminiscence and life review are effective techniques to help the older adult cope with changing life circumstances.
- Alcoholism, often hidden or denied, is common among the older population. It is possible to use alcohol as an attempted means of coping with grief, depression, loneliness, or boredom. If unrecognized, it poses the risk of exacerbating medical conditions and leading to serious drug reactions.

Box 34-5 Behaviors Common with Illness

DENIAL

A refusal to admit being ill. Short-term denial is often useful in mobilizing internal resources, but long-term denial usually results in maladaptive behavior patterns.

ANXIETY

Feelings of apprehension and uncertainty about the illness. Fear has the capacity to produce sympathetic nervous response (fight-or-flight response). Assessing vital signs often helps assess level of anxiety.

SHOCK

An overwhelming emotion that paralyzes the individual's ability to process information. No decision making by the individual is possible. The individual is unable to sort through information received.

ANGER

A response to feeling mistreated, injured, or insulted. Anger behaviors are directed either inward or outward toward others, or both. Sometimes anger is an irrational response to minor events of the day and/or interrupts the person's social functioning.

WITHDRAWAL

Removes self from interaction with others and the environment. Withdrawal is often a sign of depression. Family members sometimes withdraw from an ill person or an ill person will sometimes isolate herself or himself from the family.

Crisis is a time of change or a turning point in life when we find it necessary to modify patterns of living to prevent our own disorganization or that of our family. Some of us have difficulty coping with an illness or crisis, and display denial, hostility, anger, vulgarity, noncompliance, aggression, manipulation, apathy, or depression.

The sick role often produces secondary gains as well as personal attention—for example, when a mother becomes very ill every time her daughter plans a trip out of town, or when a person obtains renewal of disability benefits because the injury flares up when reevaluation time comes around. It is possible for the sick role to become a way of life. Secondary gains are sometimes a ploy we use to manipulate and cope with various emotional conflicts. It is important for you to recognize this in order to plan appropriate interventions to meet emotional and psychological needs of the patient who feeds on the sick role in a destructive manner (Box 34-5).

Behavior is learned, and people bring their learned behavior patterns into the health care setting. All behavior has meaning. Humans behave to meet needs and to communicate. The behavior we exhibit is based on our experiences. Cultural and ethnic background affect the patient's and family's behavior during illness. For example, many men received the message as boys to "shake it off" when hurt. As adults, these men are less likely to seek medical treatment in the early stages of disease. A family will probably give home remedies that generations of their forebears have been used to treat colds and flu. American Indians view illness as a result of upsetting dead ancestors; rites and rituals are required to appease the ancestors. The United States is a land teeming with cultural diversity, obliging you to consider cultural influences on your patients' behavior (see Chapter 8). Your responsibility as a nurse is to note and to respond therapeutically to all behavior. By understanding the relationship of stressors, anxiety, and culture to behavior, you will be able to facilitate healthy adaptation.

CRISIS INTERVENTION

A serious illness, the breakup of a relationship, a car accident, or the death of a loved one all pose a risk of triggering a crisis response in an individual or family. An **identity** crisis is a condition of instability that arises from an emotional or situational upheaval and results in extreme or decisive change. A crisis represents potential opportunity as well as danger. From that period of vulnerability, we often develop personal growth and strength. Nurses deal with people in crisis nearly every day.

Phases of crisis are similar to stages in grief and dying (see Chapter 10). Initially there is a phase of confusion, disbelief, and high anxiety. This leads into a denial phase, with grasping onto the conviction that everything will be all right. Once the reality of the situation becomes evident, anger and remorse are generally expressed. Sadness and crying is a phase of grief seen during a crisis. It acknowledges and expresses the loss of what was and never will be again. The final phase of reconciliation is reached when it is accepted that life will continue but will be different than it was, and adaptation occurs.

Help the individual or family in your care get through a crisis by providing accurate information that aids in realistic perception of the situation (see Patient Teaching box).

Encouraging ventilation of feelings and providing empathic gestures such as silent physical closeness, holding a hand, or giving a hug when appropriate (do not attempt this with an angry, hostile patient) validates that individual's feelings of anger, denial, remorse, and grief as normal responses to crisis.

Identifying family supports and adequate coping mechanisms will help you recognize family communication patterns. Dysfunctional relationships will sometimes indicate a need to include other psychosocial professionals in the care of the individual and/or family in crisis. Active listening, restating the facts, and using other therapeutic communication techniques during family conferences are ways to help address the problem constructively. Offer as much flexibility in visiting hours as possible to reduce the frustration of separation in the individual and the family.

With or without crisis intervention, a crisis often tends to resolve itself over a 4- to 6-week period. The development of coping mechanisms and the redefinition of goals and roles in life often result from a crisis. The short-term active support you provide that focuses on problem solving helps facilitate a positive resolution to the crisis (Box 34-6).

Patient Teaching

Improving Mental Health

Teach patient to do the following:

- Recognize constructive aspects of mild or moderate anxiety in learning, growth, and movement toward self-actualization.
- Recognize personal characteristics that indicate presence of anxiety.
- Describe present state of anxiety.
- Analyze current expectations, goals, beliefs, and values in with the context of perceptions of what is actually happening.
- Recognize the healing power of positive thinking.
- Recognize sayings that support negative thinking, and change those sayings to reflect a positive feeling.
- Develop assertive communication skills.
- Develop problem-solving and decision-making skills.
- Use progressive muscle relaxation.
- Increase repertoire of strategies to reduce anxiety, including the following: talking or being with someone; simple, concrete tasks; walking; noncompetitive sports; professional assistance; listening to soothing music; meditating prayer; deep-breathing exercises; and relaxation exercises.

Box 34-6 Crisis Intervention

GOALS

1. Decrease emotional stress and protect the victim.
2. Assist the victim(s) to organize and mobilize resources.
3. Return to precrisis status or a higher functional level.

STEPS

1. Assess the situation and individual(s) involved in the crisis.
2. Determine possible interventions with input from a spiritual care provider, other family, significant others, or close friends, as well as health care providers.
3. Implement the intervention plan.
4. The crisis resolves and/or an anticipatory plan emerges from the solution to the problem.

APPLICATION OF THE NURSING PROCESS

In every setting, you will use the nursing process to meet the many needs of the patient. As an LPN/LVN, participate in the nursing process by observing pa-

Box 34-7 Assessment of Emotional Status

- **General appearance:** Describe dress, makeup, and hygiene.
- **General behavior:** Describe general activity level, posture, gait, and response to examination.
- **Speech pattern:** Describe rate, tone, loudness, and quantity content of speech (descriptions include: response to questions too detailed; extreme distractibility; unable to complete an answer; uses rhyming).
- **Content of thought:** Describe thinking: reality oriented, delusional, evidence of hallucinations, or evidence of ideas of reference or other non–reality-based thinking?
- **Mood and affect:** Describe overall feeling state and affect.
- **Sensorial function:** Describe orientation, memory, attention, ability to think abstractly.
- **Insight and judgment:** Does the individual understand the present situation? What is the individual willing to do about it?
- **Potential for danger:** Assess the individual's potential for violence or self-harm, degree of impulse control, previous history of violence or aggression toward others.

tient behavior and assisting in establishing the nursing diagnoses. Together with the registered nurse (RN), work on outlining appropriate nursing interventions for the individual. The LPN/LVN and RN implement the plan using therapeutic communication techniques and continue to observe and report behavior. Analysis of these observations makes it possible to make the appropriate adjustments in the plans of care.

Box 34-7 outlines basic nursing assessments of emotional status. Other possible assessments include observation for risk for violence, level of anxiety, use of defense mechanisms, and use of coping methods if the illness is severe or long lasting.

Get Ready for the NCLEX® Examination!

Key Points

- The historical view of mental health care shows the fear and ignorance of mental illness that have directly influenced the attitude toward mental illness that prevails today.
- Individuals have unique personalities. According to Freudian theory, the personality consists of the id, the ego, and the superego.
- All behavior has meaning. An individual's behavior is the best that person is capable of, given the present environment.
- Corrective emotional experiences assist the individual to change. Direct the therapeutic relationship to facilitate this.
- Personality refers to the relatively consistent set of attitudes and behaviors particular to an individual. Cultural and ethnic background influence personality development.
- Self is an important part of personality; self consists of identity, body image, role, and esteem.
- Anxiety is a universal response to a real or imagined threat to self.
- Defense mechanisms are automatic behaviors used to protect the personality in times of stress.
- Coping mechanisms are usually adaptive methods used to deal with feelings or stressors.
- Stress is the nonspecific response of the body to demands. Stressors are any factors causing stress. High stress or chronic stress have the potential to hamper the immune response to illness.
- It is possible to view mental health and illness as existing in a continuum.
- Physical illness affects the mental health of an individual. Behavior incorporating the sick role and dependency until recovery occurs allows the individual to cope with body image changes and keep the self intact.
- The use of therapeutic communication is a dynamic method of interaction with patients for problem solving and growth.
- Promoting the placebo effect—which is the patient's mind-body link of healing from within—augments nursing interventions.
- Observe and evaluate behavior to determine a patient's progress and the effectiveness of the care plan.

Additional Learning Resources

Go to your Companion CD for an audio glossary, animations, video clips, and more.

evolve Be sure to visit the Evolve site at http://evolve.elsevier.com/Christensen/foundations/ for additional online resources.

Review Questions for the NCLEX® Examination

1. In the eighteenth century, the English Quaker who advocated humane care and built an asylum to reflect a household was:
   1. Florence Nightingale.
   2. William Tukes.
   3. Sigmund Freud.
   4. Benjamin Rush.

2. The nurse who is credited for being the first psychiatric nurse in the United States is:
   1. Florence Nightingale.
   2. Dorothea Dix.
   3. Linda Richards.
   4. Clara Barton.

3. In the twentieth century, changes in the delivery of mental health care resulting from the development of electroconvulsive therapy and psychotherapeutic drugs brought about the phenomenon of:
    1. behavioral therapy.
    2. personality disorganization.
    3. deinstitutionalization.
    4. brain surgery.
4. Personality refers to:
    1. the level of mental health one attains in life.
    2. the relatively consistent set of attitudes and behaviors particular to an individual.
    3. the result of a positive self-concept and acceptable behavior.
    4. the ability to manage stress.
5. Stress is:
    1. a vague feeling of depression.
    2. an assumed role to protect the ego.
    3. a main reason for all mental illnesses.
    4. a response to any demand made upon the individual.
6. Anxiety is possible to define as:
    1. a vague feeling of apprehension.
    2. an assumed role to release the id.
    3. the main source of personality.
    4. emotional stability.
7. An assembly-line manager in a local auto parts factory was told that he would be laid off if his line did not meet the hourly quota. He promptly went to his workers and threatened to fire anyone who was found taking even 1 minute extra on their break. This is an example of:
    1. denial.
    2. regression.
    3. displacement.
    4. identification.
8. Punishment and abandonment were how people treated the mentally ill in the Dark Ages. These practices continued until the seventeenth and eighteenth centuries. Dr. Philippe Pinel of France advocated which practice of care that is still used today?
    1. Electroshock therapy for melancholy
    2. Humane care with record keeping of behaviors
    3. Psychoanalysis
    4. Home care in the community
9. Martha Mitchell, RN, worked with President Carter to develop the Mental Health Care Systems Act, which the U.S. Congress passed in 1980. This act established block grants for mental health care. What occurred as a result of this act?
    1. Deinstitutionalization
    2. Approved surgical treatment for schizophrenia
    3. Prohibition of electroshock therapy
    4. Increased construction of state facilities for residential mental health care
10. A 52-year-old suffered cardiac arrest from a myocardial infarction. During his acute care stay in the hospital, the patient flirts with all his female nurses. When he is asked to stop, he withdraws and later complains of chest heaviness. What is a possible explanation for the patient's behavior?
    1. Boredom from restricted activity
    2. Lack of motivation to recover
    3. Frustration from illness
    4. Threatened self-concept
11. A 14-year-old is having a difficult adolescence. Over the summer, she grew 3 inches and developed large breasts. One day, after boys teased her and imitated her figure, she went to the school nurse crying. What is the first step for the nurse to take?
    1. Call her parents.
    2. Have her tell in detail what happened.
    3. Ask who her friends are.
    4. Take her temperature and pulse.
12. The nurse is instructing a wife to give insulin injections to her husband. The wife is unable to sit still, frequently asks to repeat parts of the instruction for understanding, and sighs often with rapid respirations. What degree of anxiety is the wife experiencing?
    1. Mild
    2. Moderate
    3. Severe
    4. Panic
13. A CEO was admitted to the orthopedic ward with pelvic fracture, wrist fracture, and multiple contusions and abrasions from an auto accident. She yells for the nurse every 5 minutes, refuses to use her call light, and breaks out in tears when she does not get her way. This coping behavior is termed:
    1. regression.
    2. compensation.
    3. denial.
    4. displacement.
14. A college student is brought to the emergency department by her roommate. The roommate states that when the patient returned from her date she was crying and said she was raped. The patient recounts the evening's events, cracking jokes about her date's trouble keeping an erection and asking if the nurse knows where she can get a replacement for her favorite outfit, which has been torn. This defense mechanism is:
    1. displacement.
    2. compensation.
    3. denial.
    4. dissociation.

15. A teenager wrecks the family car by rear-ending a truck turning left. The teenager says, "It wasn't my fault. I came over the rise and that truck was just sitting there. It was his fault for turning left." What defense mechanism is the teenager using to deal with his situation?
    1. Compensation
    2. Conversion reaction
    3. Projection
    4. Rationalization

16. A 24-year-old is recovering from pelvic and leg fractures suffered in an auto accident. He has to be immobilized for 2 weeks and yells at the nurse, "Why does it have to take so long to heal?" What is the best approach in regard to managing stress to benefit the immune system to heal?
    1. Avoid all stress.
    2. Use the overhead trapeze bar for exercise for at least 1 hour.
    3. Confide in friends and family about frustrations.
    4. Use inanimate objects to vent anger.

17. After a few days of hospitalization, a patient is participating in plans to be transferred to a rehabilitation facility to continue therapies to enhance his activities of daily living (ADLs). Which statement indicates the patient is beginning to adjust to his new situation and future?
    1. "I know that once I can walk without assistance, I can go back to my own home."
    2. "My late wife would not want me to be by myself if I can't take care of myself."
    3. "I'm going to show everybody that I can make it on my own; just you wait!"
    4. "I don't know why everybody is making a big deal; I was by myself before I got sick."

18. A key tool the nurse uses when establishing a relationship with a patient with a psychiatric disorder is:
    1. self-disclosure.
    2. value judgments.
    3. self-reflection.
    4. countertransference.

19. A crisis occurs when a person:
    1. has no support system.
    2. suffers a stressor and responds with ineffective coping efforts.
    3. is exposed to a precipitating stressor.
    4. perceives a stressor to be threatening.

20. The highest priority in crisis intervention is:
    1. managing anxiety.
    2. identifying situational supports.
    3. patient safety.
    4. teaching specific coping skills the patient lacks.

21. Defense mechanisms are:
    1. irreversible.
    2. entirely pathological.
    3. means of managing conflict.
    4. predominantly conscious.

22. Assessment of an older adult patient will be enhanced if the nurse:
    1. identifies and accommodates physical needs first.
    2. pledges complete confidentiality on all topics to the patient.
    3. interprets information without consideration of the patient's spiritual or cultural background.
    4. adheres firmly to the sequence of questions on the standardized assessment tool.

chapter 35

Care of the Patient with a Psychiatric Disorder

Anne W. Ryan

evolve http://evolve.elsevier.com/Christensen/foundationsadult

Objectives

1. List the five axes of *DSM-IV-TR* used to examine and treat mental illnesses.
2. Identify and describe the major mental disorders.
3. List five warning signs of suicide.
4. Identify basic interventions for patients experiencing various mental health problems.
5. Describe the general care and treatment methods for patients experiencing mental health problems.
6. Name two alternative medicines used for mental disorders.

Key Terms

anxiety (p. 1145)
compulsions (p. 1146)
cyclothymic disorder (sī-klō-THĪ-mĭk, p. 1143)
delirium (p. 1140)
delusion (p. 1140)
dementia (dē-MĔN-shē-ă, p. 1140)
depression (p. 1142)
hallucination (hă-lū-sĭ-NĀ-shŭn, p. 1140)
hypomanic episode (hī-pō-MĂN-ĭk, p. 1143)
illusions (p. 1146)
mania (p. 1143)
multiaxial system (mŭl-tē-ĂK-sē-ăl, p. 1135)
neurosis (nū-RŌ-sĭs, p. 1135)
obsessions (p. 1146)
paraphilias (păr-ă-FĬL-ē-ă, p. 1147)
phobia (FŌ-bē-ă, p. 1146)
psychosis (sī-KŌ-sĭs, p. 1135)
schizophrenia (skĭt-sō-FRĒ-nē-ă, p. 1140)
serotonin syndrome (sĕr-ō-TŌ-nĭn, p. 1153)
somatization (sō-măt-ĭ-ZĀ-shŭn, p. 1148)
sundowning syndrome (p. 1140)

You are well advised to have a basic understanding of the classifications of human responses and treatment methods for mental illness. Many patients on a medical unit have, in addition to a physiologic disorder, a history of psychiatric problems. An even more common situation is the patient who is ill and is experiencing emotional disturbance from the effects of the illness. It is important to be able to interact therapeutically with both the physical and the emotional aspects of patient care.

Our ability to handle a stressful event depends on our psychological structure. **Neurosis** is a term describing ineffective coping with stress that causes mild interpersonal disorganization. People with a neurosis have insight that they have a psychiatric problem. A person with a neurosis remains oriented to reality but will perhaps have some degree of distortion of reality manifested by a strong emotional response to the trigger event. Various complaints of nervousness or emotional upset, compulsions, obsessiveness, and phobias are common with a neurosis. A neurotic person will often exhibit poor self-esteem and have social relationships that suffer some from the complaints noted. Treatment for patients with a neurosis is usually in outpatient facilities, if they seek treatment at all.

By contrast, a person suffering with **psychosis** is out of touch with reality and has severe personality deterioration, impaired perception and judgment, hallucinations, and delusions. A psychotic person does not recognize the fact of having a psychiatric illness. Treatment for psychosis often necessitates hospitalization with follow-up regularly through an outpatient facility. Some people seek voluntary admission for treatment. Involuntary admission (commonly called probating) is also possible; a judge, a clinical psychologist, or a physician has to carry out an involuntary admission if the individual is thought to be a danger to self or others.

The *Diagnostic and Statistical Manual of Psychiatric Disorders, IV-TR,* published by the American Psychiatric Association (APA, 2000), describes a **multiaxial system** that classifies mental disorders and outlines various disorders and descriptive references. Most hospitals and health care professionals in the United States today use the *DSM-IV-TR,* as it is commonly called, to facilitate medical diagnosis and to provide a guide to clinical practice.

This tool examines mental health illness according to five categories called axes (hence the term *multiaxial*):

Axis I: Identifying all major psychiatric disorders except developmentally delayed and personality disorders, such as depression, schizophrenia, anxiety, and substance-related disorders.

Axis II: Personality and developmental disorders, as well as prominent maladaptive personality features and defense mechanisms.

Axis III: General medical conditions that are potentially relevant to the understanding or management of the person's mental disorder.

Axis IV: Psychosocial and environmental disorders that have potential to affect the diagnosis, treatment, and prognosis of mental disorders.

Axis V: Global assessment of functioning that rates the overall psychological functioning of the person on a scale of 0 to 100.

The psychiatrist or physician makes a diagnosis based on stated criteria for each psychiatric disorder. Prescriptions for nursing interventions, as well as appropriate medications, are possible for conditions under axes I, II, or III. Axis IV serves to assess present stressors that are sometimes (and sometimes not) symptoms identified as necessitating additional nursing interventions. All five axes, when used together, facilitate a holistic assessment useful for comprehensive care. This classification system is an excellent resource and a valuable tool for psychiatric nurses and physicians.

Mental disorders discussed in this chapter include the following:

- Organic mental disorders (e.g., delirium and dementia)
- Thought process disorders (e.g., schizophrenia)
- Mood disorders
- Anxiety disorders
- Personality disorders
- Psychophysiologic disorders
- Eating disorders

You will find a basic description of each of the major disorders and a summary of treatment, prognosis, and related nursing diagnoses in Table 35-1.

ORGANIC MENTAL DISORDERS

Organic disorders differ from other mental health disorders. An identifiable brain disease or dysfunction is the basis for the behavior. These disorders affect cognitive or intellectual abilities. The effect ranges from mild lapses in memory to severe behavioral changes. A predominant characteristic of the type of disorder is disorientation.

Text continued on p. 1140

Table 35-1 The Patient with a Psychiatric Disorder

ORGANIC PSYCHIATRIC DISORDERS		
CHARACTERISTICS	**TREATMENT AND PROGNOSIS**	**ASSOCIATED NURSING DIAGNOSES**
Dementia		
Slow and progressive worsening of symptoms: impaired memory and judgment, personality changes, decreased cognitive function, impaired orientation	Treatment depends on the cause. Prognosis is poor; essential feature of this condition is the slow deteriorating rate of mental function.	Disturbed thought processes Fear Risk for injury Anxiety Bathing/hygiene self-care deficit Caregiver role strain
Delirium		
Acute, rapid onset of symptoms: disorientation, incoherent thought content, impaired cognitive function, symptoms worsen at night, illusions, hallucinations	Treatment depends on the cause. Prognosis is guarded.	Risk for injury Risk for other-directed violence Disturbed thought processes Bathing/hygiene self-care deficit

Nursing Interventions

Reality orientation techniques: Place large clock and calendar in view; keep curtains opened and lights on during the day; and use calm supportive approach.

Decrease sensory stimuli: Do not expose to crowds; give instructions one step at a time, and keep in simple terms.

Provide for safety: Place bed in lowest position; side rails useful to aid patient in turning. Be sure hallway rails, chair and bed alarms, and call light are within reach; place personal articles within reach; and ensure sufficient night lighting.

Adequate nutrition: Reduce dining distractions such as television; encourage snacks if unable to eat a sufficient amount at one time; monitor weight monthly; and have family bring in patient's favorite foods.

Self-care support: Assist as needed with activities of daily living (ADLs) and toileting; encourage mobility and other activities that use large muscle groups such as "Simon says" or armchair aerobics; try to keep the daily routine the same times of each day; and if possible have same group of staff assist with ADLs.

Table 35-1 The Patient with a Psychiatric Disorder—cont'd

THOUGHT PROCESS DISORDERS (SCHIZOPHRENIA)		
CHARACTERISTICS	**TREATMENT AND PROGNOSIS**	**ASSOCIATED NURSING DIAGNOSES**
Inappropriate emotional responses, bizarre behaviors, impaired communications, delusions, illusions, hallucinations, inability to relate to others, self-care deficit, symptoms present at least 6 months, with positive behaviors for 1 month or more	Treatment is milieu therapy (environment), psychotherapy, antipsychotic drug therapy, and long-term social support. Prognosis is variable and depends on the extent of the symptoms and responses to treatments. Patient with paranoid type is often reluctant to seek treatment.	Disturbed thought processes Disturbed sensory perception Anxiety Bathing/hygiene self-care deficit Dressing/grooming self-care deficit Impaired social interaction Ineffective role performance Interrupted family processes Disturbed sleep pattern Ineffective coping Disturbed personal identity

Nursing Interventions

Establish therapeutic relationship: Be available and listen actively; use clear, simple statements in communications; ensure that your body language is in tune with the message; and avoid hand gesturing when talking to prevent distraction from the message.

Reality orientation techniques: Use verbal reminding; place large clock and calendar in view; reduce stimuli to help patient focus on reality; and establish and reinforce a daily routine.

Reduce anxiety: Avoid having patient make choices; problem solve with patient on ways to reduce anxiety; encourage socialization by invitation not assignment; decrease sensory stimuli; and accept and support patient's feelings (empathy reduces anxiety).

Manage positive behaviors: Ask patient directly about his or her hallucinations; watch for cues that indicate the patient is hallucinating; focus on reality; do not argue with the patient or enter into the patient's hallucination; if the patient is having delusions, be open and honest in interactions to reduce suspicion; respond calmly and matter-of-factly to suspicions; have the patient describe who "they" are but do not argue the logic; and if the delusion is very strong, try to help the patient find a distraction from the delusion so as not to dwell upon it. Remember that hallucinations and delusions have the potential to provoke aggressive behavior. Watch for signs of growing agitation. Provide safety.

Manage negative behaviors: Encourage self-care, assist only as indicated; help patient recognize own feelings of the event that just occurred; and encourage social participation, but do not force it onto the patient.

Medication management: Be alert for early recognition of serious side effects; administer medications in liquid form if you suspect hoarding of pills; encourage the patient to take medications routinely to adjust to ideas of taking them for rest of life; and provide good nutrition.

AFFECTIVE (MOOD) DISORDERS		
CHARACTERISTICS	**TREATMENT AND PROGNOSIS**	**ASSOCIATED NURSING DIAGNOSES**
Major Depression		
Prolonged, intense unhappiness Symptoms include apathy, pessimism, multiple physical complaints, guilt feelings, anxiety, isolation, suicidal thoughts, appetite disturbance, fatigue, sleep disturbance, constipation, limited attention span, short-term memory disturbance	Treatment possibilities include antidepressant drug therapy, individual family or group psychotherapy, and electroconvulsive therapy (ECT) when drug therapy is ineffective or drugs are contraindicated. An estimated 50% of individuals have at least one additional episode of depression.	Risk for self-directed violence Hopelessness Ineffective coping Bathing/hygiene self-care deficit Dressing/grooming self-care deficit Impaired verbal communication Disturbed sleep pattern Powerlessness Risk for imbalanced nutrition Spiritual distress
Bipolar Affective Disorder		
Mood swings with manic episodes, alternating with or without episodes of depression. Symptoms of mania: grand or self-confident mood, overresponsiveness to stimuli, insomnia without fatigue, impaired judgment, irritability, psychomotor overactivity	Treatment possibilities include psychotherapy; antimanic drugs (lithium); and family and individual support, with education regarding drug use. Prognosis depends on response to medication and treatment.	Risk for injury Activity intolerance Risk for self-directed or other-directed violence Disturbed thought processes Impaired social interaction Risk for imbalanced nutrition: less than body requirements

Continued

Table 35-1 The Patient with a Psychiatric Disorder—cont'd

AFFECTIVE (MOOD) DISORDERS—cont'd

Nursing Interventions

Establish therapeutic relationship: Use a kind but firm manner in addressing the individual; be honest and consistent; and show compassion, composure, and patience. Remember that depressed individuals are slower in physical responses. Manic individuals are not able to stay focused.

Communications: *For depression:* Encourage expression of negative feeling; point out any specific improvement; reinforce assertive behavior; recognize and point out manifestations of self-destructive thoughts or behavior to the individual; and discuss and practice alternative ways to respond to stress. *For mania:* Keep directions specific and simple; use a calm approach; present reality without arguing; be consistent and keep to the rules; attempt to provide a focus in the conversation; interrupt to slow the individual down in conversation; and phrase questions that require a brief answer.

Planned activity: Avoid competitive activities that require the individual to continually pay attention in order to participate (e.g., volleyball). Bowling and a trip to a museum are better choices for group activities. When providing activities for the patient, do so in patient's room to reduce distractions. Small-group activities help build self-esteem. Allow for rest periods.

Nutritional risk: Select well-balanced meals and snacks, and include high-fiber foods in the diet to reduce constipation. Handheld foods (e.g., individual sandwiches, fresh vegetables and fruits, crackers) are good for the manic patient. Avoid junk food—snacks that are high in concentrated sugar and fats. Monitor for dehydration. Weigh weekly. DO NOT REMOVE SALT from the diet while a patient is on lithium. (Reduced salt intake is possible contributor to lithium toxicity.)

Drug therapy: Monitor lithium levels. Normal loading range is 1-1.5 mEq/L; and 0.6-1.2 mEq/L is common range for maintenance. Note presence or absence of adverse effects of lithium in charting. Note changes in individual's behavior and thoughts individual expresses. Document all behaviors possible to consider a suicide threat or action. Remind patient that antidepressant medications take about 2 to 4 weeks to show any effects.

ANXIETY DISORDERS

CHARACTERISTICS	TREATMENT AND PROGNOSIS	ASSOCIATED NURSING DIAGNOSES
Generalized Anxiety		
Characterized by a steady, pervasive level of anxiety; possible at any age but commonly occurs around ages 20-30; lasts 6 months or longer Symptoms: apprehension, irritability, insomnia, poor concentration, fear of unknown, preoccupied or neglectful self-care, autonomic hyperactivity; conversation dominated by physical complaints	Treatment possibilities include relaxation techniques, exercise, visual imagery, massage, biofeedback imagery, and antianxiety drug therapy. Prognosis is variable; condition sometimes lasts 6 months or longer.	Ineffective coping Anxiety Imbalanced nutrition: more (or less) than body requirements Fear
Panic Disorders		
Severe anxiety, intense fear; exhibits physical manifestations suddenly without apparent reason; onset frequently in late 20s; types of posttraumatic stress disorder are acute (occurs within 6 months of event), chronic (lasts more than 6 months), and delayed (starts 6 months or more after event)	Use treatments for generalized anxiety disorders. Attacks last minutes to hours and possibly recur several times a week. Debriefing techniques (as used by the military) are often helpful.	Anxiety Fear Ineffective coping Rape-trauma syndrome Interrupted family processes
Phobias		
Characterized by persistent and irrational fear of a specific object, situation, or activity; leads to lifestyle of self-protective avoidance; social phobias are more common in women	With desensitization, patient learns to relax while reentering phobia situation in imagination and then in real life. Anxiety and fear are kept to minimum. Prognosis is variable and depends on response to treatment.	Anxiety Ineffective coping Fear Interrupted family processes

Table 35-1 The Patient with a Psychiatric Disorder—cont'd

ANXIETY DISORDERS—cont'd

CHARACTERISTICS	TREATMENT AND PROGNOSIS	ASSOCIATED NURSING DIAGNOSES
Obsessive-Compulsive Disorders (OCDs)		
Anxiety condition characterized by inability to stop persistent, irrational, and uncontrollable acts (compulsions) or thoughts (obsessions) contrary to person's standards or judgment; usually appears after adolescence, resulting from fear, guilt, and anticipation of punishment; person is usually orderly, meticulous, dependable, and scrupulous, although with tendency to be rigid and stubborn; mild forms are common; equally distributed between men and women; increases with stress	Treatment often consists of psychotherapy, to uncover the basic fears and to help the person distinguish objective dangers from imagined dangers. Drug therapy using clomipramine (Anafranil) has been of great value. Prognosis is more severe than with other anxiety disorders; complete recovery is rare. However, complete disability usual only in a minority of cases.	Ineffective coping Anxiety Fear Altered thought processes Sleep pattern disturbance Posttrauma response Rape-trauma syndrome Social isolation

Nursing Interventions

Decrease environmental stimuli to reduce agitation. It is sometimes a good idea to restrict visitors to decrease stimuli, but allow the individual that control. Instruct about staff routine.

Encourage the individual to share thoughts and feelings. Be supportive and provide assistance. Encourage the individual to use more realistic thoughts, such as "Whatever happens, I can deal with it," or "I've been through this procedure before and I handled it."

Teach the individual relaxation techniques such as:

1. Abdominal or deep breathing.
2. Imagery: Comfortable position, use deep breathing, focus on a pleasant image and all the details of it.
3. For painful procedures, have the individual imagine how a favorite hero or role model would tolerate the procedure.
4. Brisk walks, back rubs, hot showers or baths, or a heating pad also help people relax.

Encourage self-care and simple decision making. Avoid reinforcing concerns over physical complaints, but do not ignore them without further assessment.

Include in therapeutic communications explanations of all procedures and treatments, and keep family informed about the hospital regulations (e.g., visiting hours) and the goals of the care provided (e.g., the need to reduce stimuli). Be punctual with treatments and medications. This builds trust. Anticipate needs.

PERSONALITY DISORDERS

CHARACTERISTICS	TREATMENT AND PROGNOSIS	ASSOCIATED NURSING DIAGNOSES
Possible to exhibit a range of behaviors, depending on the type of disorder present; common characteristics include poor impulse control (drinking, overeating, substance abuse, assaultive behavior), self-destructive acts such as self-mutilation, manipulation of others or dependency on others, inappropriate behavior for situation, disregard for rules; usually accompanied by denial of maladaptive behaviors	Treatment possibilities include psychotherapeutic drug therapy, support groups, and family counseling. Prognosis is guarded; antisocial personality disorder is the more socially malignant of the disorders and appears to have the most severe consequences.	Impaired social interaction Ineffective coping Interrupted family processes Risk for self-directed or other-directed violence Impaired parenting Relocation stress syndrome

Nursing Interventions

Maintain a therapeutic environment. Be firm and consistent. Set limits on behaviors. Establish consequences for violating limits. Provide positive feedback for appropriate behavior; encourage ventilation of feelings. Encourage decision making and patient participation. Discuss incidents with individual. Approach in a calm, confident manner. Know where patient is at all times. Be alert for manipulating behaviors.

DELIRIUM

Delirium is a rapid change in consciousness that occurs over a short time. Occurrence is possible at any age. Delirium is associated with reduced awareness and attention to surroundings, disorganized thinking, sensory misinterpretation, and irrelevant speech. Sleep patterns are often disturbed. Possible causes of delirium include physical illnesses such as fever, heart failure, pneumonia, azotemia, or malnutrition. Drug intoxication and anesthesia are also possible causes. Treatment for delirium is to determine the cause and correct it. If the cause is homeostatic imbalances such as hypoxemia, electrolyte imbalance, or malnutrition, focus treatment on the problem causing the imbalance. If the cause is chemical agents, withdraw the chemicals or drugs or reduce the dosage. A person with nocturnal delirium, or sundowning syndrome, displays increased disorientation and agitation only during the evening and nighttime.

DEMENTIA

Dementia is a term describing an altered mental state secondary to cerebral disease. Dementia is usually a slow and progressive loss of intellectual function that is often irreversible. Symptoms are often severe enough to interfere with activities of daily living (ADLs). Alzheimer's disease, diagnosed most often in older adults, is the most common type of dementia in the United States; vascular dementia is the second most common type. Using reality orientation techniques and providing a safe environment are two key aspects of nursing interventions (see Table 35-1).

THOUGHT PROCESS DISORDERS

SCHIZOPHRENIA

Characteristic of thought process disorders is bizarre, non–reality-based thinking. Schizophrenia is any one of a large group of psychotic disorders whose defining characteristics are gross distortion of reality; disturbance of language and communication; withdrawal from social interaction; and the disorganization and fragmentation of thought, perception, and emotional reaction. Schizophrenia is one of the most profoundly disabling mental illnesses you will ever encounter. Schizophrenia typically occurs in young adulthood. It strikes both sexes equally, and approximately 1% of the population will experience schizophrenia in their lifetimes. Schizophrenia is a chronic disorder with residual disability in functioning. The family typically experiences emotional and financial devastation. Schizophrenia is prone to aggravation from stresses in life. Schizophrenia is not the same as multiple personality disorder, which is rare.

Studies have indicated a biologic basis for the disease, dispelling the early theory of poor mother-child relationship as the cause, and researchers have noted brain tissue changes. The ventricles of the brain are larger, with the left ventricle larger than the right, and the cerebral cortex is smaller than normal. This is thought to account for the disorganized thinking, hallucinations, and delusions. The neurotransmitter dopamine is present in excess amounts in the brain with schizophrenia. Pupils differ in size, and blinking rate is sometimes faster or slower than normal. Clumsiness and difficulty in distinguishing the right and left sides of the body sometimes occur and are attributable to the enlarged ventricles of the brain.

Behaviors that schizophrenic individuals display fall into different categories: positive, or excessive, and negative, or absent. Prognosis for those individuals exhibiting positive behavior patterns is good, and there are fewer structural changes in the brain and better response to drug therapy. Positive behavior patterns include delusions, hallucinations, and disordered thinking.

Positive Behavior Patterns

A delusion is a false, fixed belief that is not possible to correct by feedback and that others in the same cultural context do not accept as true. The individual starts with a false premise, believing it to be true. The individual fits this false premise logically into his or her interpretation of reality. Because of the strong logic supporting the false premise, it is difficult for the individual to accept what is really true. There are several different types of delusions (Table 35-2).

A hallucination is a sensory experience without a stimulus trigger. Auditory hallucinations are the type people experience most often. Visual, olfactory, and tactile hallucinations are also possible in the schizophrenic individual.

Disordered thinking occurs when the individual is not able to interpret information being received in the brain. Loose association-making in speech sometimes makes this evident. Conversation does not flow logically. Also, **concreteness** is sometimes a sign of disordered thinking. For example, when someone is taking a picture and the schizophrenic individual hears, "Watch the birdie!" the individual will look up into the tree for the bird instead of smiling for the camera.

Negative Behavior Patterns

Negative, or absent, behavior patterns are also sometimes present together with positive behavior patterns. Negative behavior includes apathy (avolition), social withdrawal, alogia, blunted emotional responses, and anhedonia. **Apathy** is a lack of energy or interest, an acceptance of just sitting and doing nothing. An unkempt appearance is often a reflection of apathy. **Social withdrawal** occurs in an attempt to reduce stimuli to the brain. Some individuals are frightened or overwhelmed by the experience of trying to communicate with others and find it easier to withdraw from the contact. **Alogia** is defined as reduced content of speech.

Table 35-2 Types of Delusions

TYPES OF DELUSION	DEFINITION	EXAMPLE
Grandeur	Belief of being someone with great powers to control any situation	"I am God."
Ideas of reference	Belief that an event has special personal meaning	"The lady on TV is telling me to buy the soap."
Persecution	Belief that someone is out to harm him or her	"They put a transmitter in my tooth to monitor my every word."
Somatic delusions	False belief pertaining to bodily function or image	"I have leprosy."
Thought broadcasting	Belief that others know his or her ideas without action on his or her part to convey the thoughts	"You all know the thoughts I have been having today."
Thought insertion	Belief that ideas are put in his or her mind	"Janie put these thoughts in my head for her own pleasure."
Thought withdrawal	Belief that thoughts are being removed from his or her mind	"You have been stealing my thoughts."

Alogia sometimes occurs as part of the overload of information that occurs in conversation; the schizophrenic individual needs time to sort out the message received. Affect is the outward display or expression of emotion that is felt. **Flat affect** and **anhedonia** are terms describing the lack of expressed feelings. Flat affect is the lack of nonverbal expression of emotions, such as by means of facial expression or tone of voice. Anhedonia is the inability to experience happiness or joy. Sometimes the schizophrenic individual exhibits bizarre posturing or behaviors such as laughing when receiving news about a death in the family. Be aware that adverse effects of drugs also have the potential to produce negative or absent behaviors. It is important to assess the situation surrounding the behavior.

Subtypes of Schizophrenia

Schizophrenia is a cluster of behaviors. There are five subtypes of this category of illness:

1. *Disorganized:* Flat or inappropriate affect, incoherence; prognosis is poor.
2. *Paranoid:* Delusions, auditory hallucinations; prognosis is good with treatment.
3. *Catatonic:* Stupor, negativism, rigidity, excitement, posturing; prognosis is fair.
4. *Undifferentiated:* Delusions, hallucinations, incoherence, gross disorganization (does not fit criteria of other types); prognosis is fair.
5. *Residual:* Demonstrates typical signs and symptoms associated with schizophrenia without displaying evidence of gross disorganization, incoherence, delusions, and hallucinations; prognosis is poor.

Stages of Schizophrenia

The course of schizophrenia involves four stages and features acute episodes of psychosis alternating with periods of relatively normal function. The **prodromal phase** often begins in adolescence and begins with lack of energy or motivation and withdrawal. Other symptoms common in this stage are as follows: affect becomes blunted; beliefs and ideas become odd; the person sometimes develops an excessive interest in philosophy or religion; self-care and personal hygiene fall by the wayside; emotional lability is present; speech is difficult to follow; and the person often complains about multiple physical problems. Magical thinking, or believing that one's thoughts control events, is also a symptom.

Quiet, passive behavior is typical of the **prepsychotic phase.** The individual prefers to be alone. Hallucination and delusions sometimes occur in this stage. Odd, suspicious, or eccentric behavior patterns are present. Family members report that they feel the individual has changed into a stranger.

During the **acute phase,** signs and symptoms sometimes vary widely, but disturbances in thought, perception, emotion, and behavior are very apparent. Often, the individual loses contact with reality and is unable to function in the most basic ways.

The **residual phase** features a group of symptoms similar to that in the prodromal phase. The residual phase follows the acute phase. Following the residual phase is a remission period wherein the individual is able to experience some relief of symptoms and to manage some basic activities in life. Prognosis for recovery is fair to poor because of the complex aspects of this disorder.

Treatment for schizophrenia involves a number of psychotherapies to allow the individual self-expression, antipsychotic drug therapy to control symptoms, and a therapeutic relationship maintained over the years to provide continuity for the individual who suffers a lifelong illness.

MAJOR MOOD DISORDERS

Mood disorders, also known as affective disorders, are any of a group of psychotic disorders whose defining characteristics are severe and inappropriate emotional responses, prolonged and persistent disturbances of mood and related thought distortions, and other symptoms associated with either depressed or manic states. **Mood,** as defined by the *DSM-IV-TR*

(APA, 2000), is a prolonged emotion that affects a person's psyche. Extremes in mood range from depression to mania. Hereditary factors account for 60% to 80% of mood disorders. There is an insufficiency of the neurotransmitters norepinephrine and serotonin in depressed individuals and excess norepinephrine in manic individuals. Neurotransmitter insufficiency or excess is sometimes the result of heredity and sometimes of environmental factors such as prolonged stress or brain trauma. Most people experience both of these emotional states in their life; however, the individual with a mood disorder suffers for months or years without relief from these extreme moods.

DEPRESSION

Depression is a mood disturbance characterized by exaggerated feelings of sadness, despair, lowered self-esteem, loss of interest in former activities, and pessimistic thoughts. Depression is more than a state of mind; it is an illness that affects about 1 in every 20 people every year. Depression is found in all races, ethnic groups, age-groups, and socioeconomic levels. Women are affected twice as often as men.

Depression is so severe at times that an affected person will contemplate, or actually succeed at, committing suicide. Suicide is the eighth leading cause of death in the United States. It is possible to view many deaths supposedly due to accidental overdoses, automobile accidents, and refusal of medical care as hidden suicides even though they are not reported as such. Suicide attempts also do not make it into the statistics. Although the highest rate of suicide is among the older population, teen suicide is on the rise in this country. Teaching effective coping skills to our children is essential if we are to protect our greatest natural resource.

Because our culture basically does not accept suicide, there is great controversy over the terminally ill individual's right to commit suicide. Some people believe that ending one's life is a rational decision given certain circumstances, such as terminal illness; these people will defend the right to commit suicide. There is growing support for right-to-die legislation, which removes the criminal connotations from suicide and gives mature people the right to end their lives when they see fit. It is important to evaluate terminally ill individuals and treat them for depression, as well as for their physical disturbances, to ease their suffering and enhance their quality of life. Most people who commit suicide in the hospital setting have received the diagnosis of an incurable or painful illness.

To help prevent suicide, you need to recognize its warning signs and learn the kinds of actions that can often avert it (Box 35-1). Consider verbal statements such as "I wish I were dead," or "You won't see me coming back here again," or asking about specific methods of suicide as warning signals. Actions such as giving away possessions, drawing up a will, refusing medications, or neglecting hygiene are also possible warning signals. Many people experience anxiety due to moral conflict within themselves. Often the suicidal individual manages to leave that anxiety behind by making the decision to commit suicide.

Unipolar depression, or major depressive disorder, is defined as repeating, severe depressive episodes lasting more than 2 years. Estimates are that up to 15% of those with a diagnosis of major depressive disorder die from suicide. **Dysthymic disorder** is daily moderate depression that lasts more than 2 years. This disorder often ends up as a lifestyle in which the individual is able to function but not enjoy life.

Box 35-1 Suicide Warnings and Precautions

WARNING SIGNS OF SUICIDE

- Withdrawing from family or friends
- Talking about death, the hereafter, or suicide
- Giving away prized possessions
- Drug or alcohol abuse
- Personality changes, such as unusual anger, boredom, or apathy
- Signs of depression: unusual neglect of appearance; difficulty concentrating on work or school; complaints of physical problems that have no organic cause; disturbed sleeping or eating patterns; loss of self-esteem; feelings of helplessness, hopelessness, extreme anxiety, or panic.
- Previously failed attempts with verbalized regrets of failure.

SUICIDE PRECAUTIONS IN THE HOSPITAL ENVIRONMENT

- Remove articles that are possible to use for suicide: belts, straps, shoelaces, sheets, breakable items for sharp edges, razor blades, curtain cord, bed coils, and personal care items.
- Remove any furniture that is possible to use for self-injury as well as doors to closets. Make sure windows are shatterproof.
- Designate a room close to the front desk of the unit or a room with a closed TV monitor.
- Check the patient every 15 minutes around the clock.
- Instruct visitors not to leave gifts in the room until the staff examines them for anything that is possible to use for self-injury.
- Make sure the patient swallows all medications administered. Use liquid forms when available. Use injectables if patient refuses oral forms as ordered.
- Attend the patient during meals and keep track of eating utensils and dinnerware. Make sure used trays are not sitting where the patient has the opportunity to walk by and remove tableware.
- Make frequent therapeutic verbal contact.

BIPOLAR DISORDERS

Bipolar disorders, or manic-depressive disorders, feature sudden shifts between emotional extremes from depression to mania. Mania is a mood disorder whose signal characteristic is persistent, abnormal overactivity and a euphoric state. We often refer to the early phase of a manic episode as a hypomanic episode when symptoms are not severe. Often the manic person is engaging, outgoing, and charming, as well as achieving and successful, has excessive energy and optimism, and possibly a very productive member of the community. Unfortunately, a manic episode has potential to accelerate.

As it intensifies, the episode of mania changes from cheerfulness into excessive feelings of euphoria, talking rapidly, flight of ideas, unrealistic beliefs of abilities, no sleep, poor judgment, denial that anything will possibly go wrong, increased sex drive, and obnoxious or provocative behavior such as robbing a store without the fear of being caught. If untreated, delirium will possibly ensue, and death from exhaustion or accident is possible.

Cyclothymic disorder is a pattern that also involves repeated mood swings of hypomania and depression, although they are less intense. There are no periods of normal function with this condition. It is thought to be a muted version of bipolar disorder. Many individuals with cyclothymic disorder progress to bipolar disorder.

Other affective disorders are seasonal affective disorder (SAD) and postpartum depression. Both of these disorders are connected with hormonal imbalances and respond well to treatment. Practitioners treat SAD, also known as winter depression, with phototherapy. Postpartum depression often clears within days, but it is best to further investigate the problem if symptoms continue longer than 2 weeks.

MEDICAL TREATMENT

Medical treatment for mood disorders includes antidepressants and lithium, electroconvulsive therapy (ECT), and psychotherapy. Antidepressants, such as fluoxetine (Prozac), trazodone (Desyrel), amitriptyline (Elavil), and venlafaxine (Effexor), take 2 to 4 weeks to show lifting of the depression. Some antidepressants such as amitriptyline are best to take at bedtime because of a transient adverse effect of sedation; and this sometimes also helps normalize the sleeping pattern. Selective serotonin reuptake inhibitors (SSRIs), such as fluoxetine (Prozac) and paroxetine (Paxil), do not appear to cause as many of the anticholinergic and sedating side effects that sometimes cause patients to stop taking their medications. Some antidepressants, such as fluoxetine, are best to take in the morning to prevent the adverse effect of insomnia. *(See the later section on antidepressant medications for further discussion.)*

Practitioners use lithium to treat bipolar disorder. Lithium has a narrow therapeutic range, and close monitoring of the drug is necessary for safety.

Other drugs in the pharmacologic toolbox to treat mental illness symptoms include duloxetine (Cymbalta), bupropion (Wellbutrin), and mirtazapine (Remeron). Bupropion is also a first-line medication for smoking cessation.

Electroconvulsive therapy is an option to consider when drug therapy is ineffective or is contraindicated (Box 35-2) (Nursing Care Plan 35-1).

Box 35-2 Electroconvulsive Therapy (ECT)

ECT is administered on either an inpatient or outpatient basis.

PATIENT PREPARATION

1. Purpose of ECT: relief from depression. Patient signs consent for treatment forms.
2. Common side effects include headache, confusion upon awakening, short-term amnesia. Take Tylenol for persistent headache.
3. Patient needs to be on nothing-by-mouth (NPO) status for at least 8 hours before treatment.
4. Wear loose-fitting clothes with access to the arm for intravenous (IV) insertion.
5. Make sure patient arranges for someone to accompany him or her to and from the treatment. No treatment will take place if patient is unaccompanied.
6. Avoid driving or operating machinery for at least 1 day after treatment.
7. Avoid making any major decisions—about job, finances, relationships, and so forth—until the course of treatment is completed.
8. Take any prescribed medications on time.

TREATMENT

1. Take baseline vital signs.
2. Apply cardiac, blood pressure, and oximetry monitors to the patient.
3. Establish an IV line for administration of sedation and neuromuscular blockade.
4. Apply electroencephalogram (EEG) monitor to the patient.
5. After administration of IV drugs, the practitioner will establish an airway and deliver electrical shock for a few seconds.
6. A controlled seizure lasts 30 to 60 seconds. Neuromuscular blockade eliminates most body flexion, thereby reducing risk of spinal injury, bone fracture, or muscle tears.
7. The patient usually sleeps for about 1 hour after treatment.

POST-ECT CARE

1. Monitor vital signs and level of consciousness.
2. It is acceptable to discharge the patient with a responsible adult when alert and walking. Confusion is sometimes present, and some patients do not remember coming to and leaving the hospital for treatment.

Nursing Care Plan 35-1 The Patient with Depression

Mr. White is a 69-year-old widower whose wife died 9 months ago from cancer. He entered the open psychiatric unit with the diagnosis of major depression. Mr. White has an unmarried daughter who lives out of state and is a partner in a law firm. Mr. White has severe hypertension and early-stage chronic obstructive pulmonary disease (COPD). On admission, Mr. White states, "I just can't go on all alone like this . . . I have so little energy and I can't sleep like I used to." Mr. White has lost 32 pounds in the past 6 months; he weighs 145 pounds and is 5 feet 11 inches tall. Mr. White rarely leaves his home, although friends ask him out frequently. He is tearful at times, sighs often, and has poor eye contact during the admission interview. When asked, he admits to thoughts of killing himself. He states that he attempted to do so with an overdose of his hypertension medication, but he wanted to see his daughter one last time before he goes so he came to the emergency department.

NURSING DIAGNOSIS *Ineffective coping*

Patient Goals and Expected Outcomes	Nursing Interventions	Evaluation
Engage in reality-based interactions Express feelings directly and express anger or hostility outward in a safe manner	Establish a relationship; keep staff assignment as consistent as possible. Use a firm, kind manner; tell patient that you can see that he is sad but that he still needs to complete his personal hygiene and activities of daily living. If the patient is ruminating, convey that you will talk about reality or his feelings, but limit the attention you give to repeated expressions of rumination.	Evaluation is ongoing. Weekly care meetings of staff to discuss the patient's progress. Rely on good daily documentation that reflects the patient's progress or lack of progress. Patient is beginning to verbalize to staff his feelings of loss and grief due to his wife's death. Patient is expressing need to interact more with his daughter.

NURSING DIAGNOSIS *Impaired social interaction*

Patient Goals and Expected Outcomes	Nursing Interventions	Evaluation
Communicate with others Participate in activities	Initially, interact with the patient on a one-on-one basis. Progress to facilitating social interactions between patient and other patients, from small groups to larger groups. Encourage the patient to pursue personal interests, hobbies, and recreational activities. Encourage the patient to identify supportive people outside the unit and to develop these relationships.	Evaluation is ongoing. Patient is beginning to interact with other patients singularly as well as in small groups. Patient is beginning to become active in personal interests, such as attending a movie and reading a book.

NURSING DIAGNOSIS *Risk for self-directed violence*

Patient Goals and Expected Outcomes	Nursing Interventions	Evaluation
Avoid harming himself Identify alternative ways of dealing with stress and emotional problems	Determine appropriate level of suicide precautions, and institute the precautions immediately. Convey that you care about the patient and that you believe he is a worthwhile individual. Do not joke about death, belittle his wishes or feelings, or make insensitive remarks such as, "Everybody wants to live." Do not make moral judgments about suicide attempts or reinforce his feelings of guilt or sin. Refer to his spiritual resource person if indicated. Examine and remain aware of your own feelings about suicide. Talk with other staff members to deal with your feelings.	Evaluation is ongoing. Patient states that he does not intend to harm himself. Patient is verbalizing more acceptable ways of dealing with his depression with other staff members.

Nursing Care Plan 35-1 The Patient with Depression—cont'd

Patient Goals and Expected Outcomes	Nursing Interventions	Evaluation
	Involve the patient as much as possible in planning his treatment. Plan with the patient how he will recognize and deal with feelings and situations that have precipitated suicidal feelings in the past.	

NURSING DIAGNOSIS ***Imbalanced nutrition: less than body requirements***

Patient Goals and Expected Outcomes	Nursing Interventions	Evaluation
Maintain a regular, adequate eating pattern Maintain normal body weight	Monitor eating. Keep intake and output records. Encourage fluids (e.g., water, juices). Find out what foods the patient likes and dislikes. Try six small feedings per day. Discourage use of nonnutritional substances like artificial sweeteners, coffee creamers, diet soda, tea, or coffee.	Evaluation is ongoing. Patient is eating 50% to 60% of each meal. Patient is beginning to demonstrate interest in sitting down and eating with a group.

NURSING DIAGNOSIS ***Disturbed sleep pattern***

Patient Goals and Expected Outcomes	Nursing Interventions	Evaluation
Sleep 5 to 6 hours per night before discharge Verbalize ability to use relaxation techniques when awake at night	Plan physical activity while awake. Encourage planned naps only. Teach progressive relaxation exercises. Help patient establish a consistent sleep time.	Evaluation is ongoing. Patient is sleeping about 6 hours per night. Patient is going to sleep at a scheduled time each night.

Critical Thinking Questions

1. Mr. White is admitted to the psychiatric unit and placed on suicidal precautions. Mr. White sits stoically staring out the window and does not respond to the nurse's greeting. What safety interventions should the team incorporate into Mr. White's care to prevent his self-destruction?
2. Mr. White sleeps poorly, approximately 2 to 3 hours a night. What therapeutic interventions should be used to correct his sleep pattern disturbance?
3. Mr. White has had a weight loss of 32 pounds. What are some options for the staff to help Mr. White meet adequate nutritional requirements?

ANXIETY DISORDERS

Anxiety is a normal response to stress or threat. Anxiety is a state or feeling of apprehension, uneasiness, agitation, uncertainty, and fear resulting from the anticipation of some threat or danger. Experts describe many types of anxiety. **Signal anxiety** is a learned response to an event such as test taking. **Free-floating anxiety** is associated with feelings of dread that are not possible to identify. **Anxiety trait** is a learned aspect of personality. An individual with anxiety trait has anxious reactions to relatively nonstressful events. These individuals respond more quickly and more strongly to stress and are slower to level off than normal. (See discussion of normal anxiety response in Chapter 34.)

Generalized anxiety disorders (GADs) are characterized by a high degree of anxiety and/or avoidance behavior. An individual with GAD tends to worry or fret over many things and finds it difficult to concentrate on the task at hand.

Panic can be defined as an attack of acute, intense, and overwhelming anxiety accompanied by a degree of personality disorganization, such as being unable to solve problems or think clearly. In a panic attack, symptoms occur abruptly and peak within 10 minutes. Symptoms include at least four of the following: heart palpitations or accelerated heart rate; sweating, trembling or shaking; feelings of dyspnea or choking; chest pain; nausea or abdominal distress; feeling dizzy or faint; fear of losing control or going crazy; fear of dying; paresthesias (a sensation experienced as numbness, tingling, or "pins and needles"); and chills or hot flashes. Panic disorders are more common in women than in men.

Agoraphobia is considered to be a type of panic disorder. Agoraphobia is high anxiety brought on by situations in which a panic attack is possible. People with agoraphobia avoid people, places, or events that have potential to trigger an attack. Fear of not receiving any help or embarrassment when an attack occurs in a public place are characteristics of agoraphobia.

Treatment for panic disorders focuses on educating the individual on the nature of the disorder, assisting the individual to develop better coping mechanisms with anxiety, and blocking attacks pharmaceutically. Emotional support and reassurance are important nursing measures for individuals suffering with panic disorder.

PHOBIAS

A phobia is different from normal fear. A **phobia** is irrational fear in which the individual tends to dwell on the object of the phobia. The individual sometimes recognizes the irrational fear of the phobia but is still unable to control paralyzing anxiety. Characteristics of phobias vary with the culture. In some cultures, fear of hexes, magical spirits, snakes, and unseen forces have the power to trigger phobic fear reactions. Remember to consider the cultural background when assessing the individual's phobic response.

OBSESSIVE-COMPULSIVE DISORDER

Obsessive-compulsive disorder has two features. **Obsessions** are thoughts that are recurrent, intrusive, and senseless. These thoughts are anxiety producing and distressful in that they are uncontrollable. **Compulsions** are behaviors that are performed in response to an obsessive thought. The repetitive, ritualistic behaviors such as checking the locks 10 times before going to bed typically reduce the anxiety and tension produced by the obsession. The patient will sometimes recognize the behavior as absurd but is still compelled to perform the ritual to relieve tension. The patient tends to find it hard to express emotions and is often introspective. Stopping the repetitive act results in extreme anxiety. Depression is a feature that often occurs in association with this disorder. Isolation and undoing are mechanisms that often serve to ward off anxiety. Interpersonal relationships and occupations suffer because of the time-consuming behaviors.

Experts believe that activity addictions such as compulsive gambling, sexual promiscuity, excessive Internet use, or overeating arise from obsessive-compulsive behavior disorders. See Chapter 36 for more information concerning addiction.

POSTTRAUMATIC STRESS DISORDER

Posttraumatic stress disorder (PTSD), formerly called shell shock, describes a response to an intense traumatic experience that is beyond the usual range of human experiences. These experiences—such as war, rape, a major auto accident, observing someone tortured or being tortured, or witnessing a violent death—tend to evoke feelings of terror and helplessness. One example is witnessing the attack on New York City's World Trade Center on September 11, 2001. Those people who were able to escape the Trade Center towers before the collapse and emergency personnel who responded to the attack were the most likely to suffer from PTSD. The experience is often repeatedly relived in dreams or flashbacks. Flashbacks often arise in response to a trigger, a stimulus that resembles the experience or perhaps the anniversary of the event. Flashbacks sometimes include **illusions** (false interpretation of extreme sensory stimulus, usually visual or auditory, such as a mirage in the desert or voices on the wind) and hallucinations. Avoidance behavior associated with this disorder sometimes includes emotional detachment, guilt about being a survivor, amnesia of the event, insomnia, irritability, difficulty concentrating, and wariness. Physical response to severe anxiety occurs with each relived episode. Depression and substance abuse often occur in association with PTSD. Soldiers returning from war frequently suffer from PTSD.

There are three types of PTSD. In the acute type, symptoms occur within 6 months of the event and last about 6 months. The chronic type features symptoms that last 6 months or longer. The delayed type involves symptoms that start 6 months or more after the event.

Treatment for PTSD includes antidepressant or antiseizure medications; cognitive therapy, which focuses on breaking negative thought patterns; or behavioral therapy, which aims to break off a conditioned response that has become automatic. Debriefing people right after the event is one strategy practitioners recommend to prevent PTSD from occurring.

PERSONALITY DISORDERS

Personality disorders are inflexible, maladaptive patterns of behavior or thinking that accompany significant impairment of functioning. The disorder usually surfaces during adolescence or earlier and continues through adulthood. The associated behaviors are generally more troublesome to others than to the individual (Box 35-3).

Personality disorders are characterized by the following:

- Lack of insight, concrete thinking, poor attention, inability to understand the consequences of behavior or learn from them
- Distorted self-perception, either hatred or idealization of self
- Impaired relationships, projecting own feelings onto others, poor impulse control, inability to maintain healthy interpersonal relationships
- Inflexible behavioral response patterns that do not allow the individual to handle change easily

The *DSM-IV-TR* (APA, 2000) has classified 10 distinct personality disorders. These disorders are possible to cluster into groups of similar behavior: eccentric, erratic, and fearful (see Box 35-3).

Box 35-3 Personality Disorders

Abusive personality: An individual who uses violent or abusive behavior to cope with anxiety
Dependent personality: An individual who is overcooperative from a deep fear of abandonment; unable to carry out a task alone; unable to take responsibility for his or her own activities of daily living (ADLs); usually seeks overprotective, dominating, or abusive relationships
Paranoid personality: Characterized by suspicion, secretiveness, distortion of reality, and oversensitivity; thinks that others are "out to get" him or her
Borderline personality: Has not established self-identity; fears being alone; experiences mood swings over a short period; relationships with others reveal rapid shifts from adoring to cruel and punishing; impulsive
Antisocial personality: Has a history of difficulties with personal relationships; does not profit from experience or punishment; has no loyalties to any person, group, or code of ethics; has a tendency to rationalize behavior; relies on deceit and manipulation to get his or her way

From Morrison-Valfre, M. (2008). *Foundations of mental health nursing.* (4th ed.). St. Louis: Mosby.

SEXUAL DISORDERS

Sex is ranked as a basic need in Maslow's hierarchy of human needs. Human sexuality in our society is the sum of physical and psychological attributes that express one's gender identity and sexual behavior. Sexual disorders are of either physical or psychological origin, but often both physical and psychological factors play a part in the perceived disorder.

Defining normal sexual behavior is difficult against the inescapable backdrop of cultural influences, religious institutions, and societal laws that affect an individual's beliefs regarding acceptable and unacceptable sexual behavior. It is possible to view sexual behavior on a continuum from adaptive sexual behavior to maladaptive sexual behavior. Adaptive sexual behaviors occur in private between two consenting adults, and are satisfying and not forced upon each other. Maladaptive sexual behaviors are harmful to self or others and are possibly performed publicly and sometimes without the consent of all those involved.

Sexual orientation is one's preference or choice for a sex partner. **Heterosexual** is the term describing individuals who express their sexuality with members of the opposite sex. **Homosexual** (also gay or lesbian) is the term describing individuals who express their sexuality with members of the same sex. Historically speaking, heterosexual relationships have been the norm, but some cultures have also accepted homosexual relationships. For example, ancient Greek men regarded women as useful only for having babies and cleaning homes, and other men as desirable sex partners.

The *DSM-IV-TR* (APA, 2000) lists sexual and gender identity disorders in three main clusters: (1) sexual dysfunctions, (2) paraphilias, and (3) gender identity disorders. This list does not address sexual dysfunction caused by medical problems, such as impotence secondary to diabetic neuropathy.

Sexual dysfunction is a disturbance during sexual response. **Dyspareunia** (painful intercourse), hypoactive sexual desire, and premature ejaculation are examples of sexual dysfunction that have a possible psychological as well as a physical component. Some medications cause sexual dysfunction by altering sexual desire or the ability to perform. Medications are now available to treat men with erectile dysfunction (ED), if the dysfunction is due to physical causes.

Paraphilias are a group of sexually gratifying activities that are not common to the general public and are illegal in some countries, including the United States. The suffix *-philia* means "attraction to." Adding a descriptive prefix, such as *pedo-*, rounds out the descriptions of what the sexual attraction is to. **Pedophilia** means fondling and/or pursuing other sexual activities with a prepubescent child by an adult.

Other paraphilic disorders include **exhibitionism** (flashing), exposing one's genitals to an unsuspecting person(s) to achieve sexual arousal; **voyeurism,** obtaining sexual gratification by observing others during intercourse or viewing another's genitals; **frotteurism,** sexual arousal achieved by rubbing against or touching a nonconsenting individual; and **fetishism,** using an object, usually an article of clothing, to attain sexual arousal. Masturbation usually accompanies or follows fetishism. **Transvestic fetishism** involves wearing clothing of the opposite sex (cross-dressing) to obtain sexual gratification.

Other paraphilic disorders are sexual sadism and masochism. *Sadism* refers to achieving sexual arousal from inflicting pain or humiliation on another. Possible manifestations of sexual sadism vary from mild behavior such as spanking to more violent behavior such as stabbing or strangulation. *Sexual masochism* refers to sexual arousal by receiving mental or physical abuse. A diagnosis of sexual masochism is appropriate if punishment is necessary to achieve sexual gratification.

Gender identity is one of the first parts of personality development. With gender identity disorder, there is a conflict of biologic sex identity and gender perception. Many individuals truly believe that they were born with the wrong body. **Transsexualism** is a persistent desire to be the opposite sex and desire to have the body of the opposite sex. Transvestic fetishism is associated with this disorder. For a biologic sex change to take place, psychological counseling, hormone treatments, and major surgical procedures will possibly occur over the course of several years. The surgical procedure is not reversible, which is one of the reasons for the lengthy counseling.

Therapeutic interventions depend on the type of paraphilic disorder. Treatment for most individuals takes place on an outpatient basis. Some psychosexual problems are complex and require the skill of specially educated physicians, nurses, or sex therapists.

Many medical-surgical nurses encounter individuals who also have a sexual disorder. You need to be aware of your own attitudes and values about sexual behaviors. Your nonverbal messages of disapproval have the capacity to hinder development of a therapeutic relationship and affect the quality of nursing judgment.

PSYCHOPHYSIOLOGIC (SOMATOFORM) DISORDERS

Physical signs of emotional distress are sometimes very real. Just as eating too much at the Thanksgiving table will sometimes cause a person to be nauseated, so will receiving a very distressing piece of news. The term **psychosomatic illness** refers to a physical disorder arising as a result of a psychological trigger. This term developed a negative connotation as it acquired the implication that "it's all in your head." The more recent term **psychophysical illness** addresses the stress-related problems that have the potential to result in physical signs and symptoms. Psychophysiologic disorders are thought to have an emotional basis, manifested as a physical illness.

The body responds to continual or repeated stress by overactivating its stress response mechanism; this tends to result in many physical signs and symptoms such as diarrhea, heart palpitations, backaches, and headaches. The gastrointestinal tract appears to suffer the most from chronic stress.

Physical disorders thought to have psychological underpinnings include ulcerative colitis, irritable bowel syndrome, hypertension, cardiac disease, asthma, arthritis, some skin disorders, irregular menstruation, and migraine headache.

Somatization, or somatoform disorder, is a disorder whose typical characteristics are recurrent, multiple, physical complaints and symptoms for which there is no organic cause. It is a process whereby an individual's feelings, needs, and conflicts are manifested physiologically. Somatoform disorder diagnosis follows the ruling out of any possible physical causes of dysfunctions, any drug or other toxic substance reaction, or mental health problems that are possibly related to the symptoms. We also call somatization **Briquet's syndrome.**

EATING DISORDERS

Certain individuals develop nutritional problems that have a psychological component and are known as eating disorders. Two common eating disorders are anorexia nervosa and bulimia nervosa.

ANOREXIA NERVOSA

Anorexia nervosa is a severe form of self-starvation that potentially leads to death. It occurs predominantly in adolescent girls of above-average intelligence. They have an intense fear of obesity, bizarre attitudes toward food, and a disturbed self-image. Nursing interventions include the following: developing a trusting relationship, promoting better nutrition by having stress-free mealtimes, offering frequent small meals, setting limits to decrease manipulation and procrastination behavior, encouraging the person to express feelings, and offering unconditional acceptance of both negative and positive feelings the person expresses. It is important that the focus be not on food but on the underlying feelings. The etiology of the disease has nothing to do with food and everything to do with self-control and willpower.

BULIMIA NERVOSA

Bulimia nervosa, commonly known as bingeing, is closely related to anorexia nervosa. Characteristics of bulimia are episodes of overeating followed by purging through induced vomiting, laxatives, diuretics, fasting, or vigorous exercise. Bulimia occurs primarily in white females of high-school age, usually middle to upper class and well educated. Signs and symptoms of bulimia nervosa include feelings of low self-esteem, lack of control, and guilt. Anxiety and depression are also components of this disorder. Physical signs are hoarseness, esophagitis, dental erosion (primarily of front teeth), palate lacerations, and complaints of weakness or fatigue. Laboratory tests show electrolyte imbalance. Nursing interventions include building a trusting relationship, helping the person explore triggers for bingeing and better coping behaviors, and involving family members to recognize how their interactions support bingeing. The binge and purge cycle of behavior is difficult to break.

Behavior management, individual psychotherapy, family therapy, and psychopharmacology are all treatment modalities useful for eating disorders. Fluoxetine (Prozac) and sertraline (Zoloft) are helpful for treating patients with eating disorders. See Chapter 21 for more information about eating disorders.

OVERVIEW OF TREATMENT METHODS

COMMUNICATION AND THE THERAPEUTIC RELATIONSHIP

Therapeutic communication plays an important part of the therapeutic techniques practitioners use in treatment of psychiatric disorders. Psychiatric nursing is a science and an art. Each individual has unique value and potential for growth. As a nurse, you will apply your own self-concept in the context of a therapeutic relationship; to accomplish this, it is necessary to have self-knowledge.

The key component to psychiatric–mental health treatment is the development of a helping-trust relationship. The relationship maximizes the patient's strengths, maintains self-esteem, and assists the patient to develop and use coping skills. The helping-trust relationship is a therapeutic professional relationship; it is not social in nature. In a therapeutic relationship, you assist the patient in learning new ways of responding to people and situations.

Therapeutic communication is a dynamic process in which both participants (the nurse and the patient) share meaning and interact in the interests of problem solving and growth. To be therapeutic, it is necessary that communication assist with the corrective experiences that help the patient in meeting predetermined goals. Therapeutic techniques for communication are included in Chapter 3. These techniques are possible to use in every nursing situation. The therapeutic dialogues in the Communication box demonstrate therapeutic nurse-patient interactions.

There are different types of relationships. Most are social; that is, the participants are equally involved in exchanging information and meeting individual needs. In a therapeutic relationship, both participants agree on goals and work toward them. You assist the individual to learn new ways of interacting to function more effectively. You attempt to establish a rapport with the patient and gain trust to facilitate positive interactions that will lead to corrective behavior. In day-to-day interactions with a patient, you will find that the individual is more responsive and amenable to instruction if you have obtained the person's trust and the person sees you as a competent professional.

Psychotherapy

Treatment for psychiatric problems often consists of using one or more of the following psychological techniques. **Behavior therapy** serves to relieve anxiety through the conditioning and retraining of behavioral

Communication

Starting the Conversation

Possibilities for starting a conversation with a patient include several approaches:

- What circumstances brought you to the hospital?
- Tell me a little about what has been going on with you.
- Mrs. Jacobi, I am Linda, and I'll be your nurse today.
- Tell me how you are feeling.

THERAPEUTIC DIALOGUE 1

Mrs. Jacobi underwent a hysterectomy 1 week ago for several fibroid tumors. She is 32 years of age and has a 3-year-old child. She has been married 5 years. The nurse who admitted her after surgery enters the room and finds her crying.

Nurse: *(Walks over to Mrs. Jacobi and touches her arm and stands there quietly.)*

Patient: *(Continues to cry but looks up at the nurse and starts to quiet.)*

Nurse: You look upset; would you like to talk? *(Pulls up a chair and sits at eye level.)*

Patient: My whole life is ruined.

Nurse: Your life is ruined?

Patient: I wanted other children; we were going to have a large family.

Nurse: Tell me what a large family means to you.

Patients experiencing loss often need to cry. Crying begins to release emotion; the patient needs you to accept it. Your close physical presence and touch communicate acceptance. Acknowledgment of feelings encourages further expression, and then it is possible to explore the patient's sense of loss.

THERAPEUTIC DIALOGUE 2

Mr. Harowitz, 65 years of age, has been diagnosed with cancer of the lung. The day nurse is making initial patient rounds and enters the room. The nurse notices that Mr. Harowitz looks uncomfortable.

Nurse: *(Walks over to the bed.)* Good morning, Mr. Harowitz. You look uncomfortable.

Patient: I'm tired; I stayed awake all night.

Nurse: You had difficulty sleeping?

Patient: I have a lot on my mind. I couldn't sleep.

Nurse: *(Sits down next to the patient and pats his hand.)* Tell me what has been worrying you.

Encourage patients to talk (ventilate). Be observant for nonverbal communication and for underlying meanings in the stated words. Talking brings emotions to the surface where it is possible to identify and deal with them.

It is not possible to emphasize enough that both you and the patient bring your physiologic, psychological, developmental, and spiritual components into the therapeutic relationship. Other elements you bring into the relationship are previous life experiences, needs, aspirations, and frustrations. You have an opportunity to help the patient explore a life event and the meaning that it has for the individual.

THERAPEUTIC DIALOGUE 3

Mrs. Kim, who has been pacing the halls, is now staring out the window. She is toying with a ring on her finger. You notice that Mrs. Kim is vigorously tapping one foot on the floor.

Nurse: *(Walks over to patient and sits beside her.)* Mrs. Kim, I have noticed that you seem a little restless. Is something troubling you?

Patient: No, not really. Well, maybe I am a little upset.

Nurse: Is there something in particular that is upsetting you?

Patient: I don't know. I'm just anxious.

Nurse: Tell me how you feel.

Patient: I feel jittery and nervous.

Nurse: Is there something specific that is worrying you right now?

Patient: My husband is going to lose his job in another month, and here I am in the hospital. I just don't know how we'll pay the bills. It scares me.

Nurse: Have you and your husband discussed this situation?

Patient: *(Continues to share her feelings with the nurse.)*

Anxiety is an unpleasant feeling of tension and apprehension. A person experiencing anxiety will sometimes be unaware of the exact source of the tension. An array of physical and psychological symptoms usually accompany anxiety. Resolution of the anxiety begins with awareness of the anxiety's source. A person seeks ways to resolve the tension (problem solving) in order to be rid of the tension.

responses by repetition. It is often possible to resolve phobias with this technique. **Cognitive therapy** focuses on breaking negative thought patterns and developing positive feelings about memories or thoughts. **Group therapy** is often a useful modality in a hospital setting or day treatment programs. A group of patients with similar problems gain insight through discussion and role playing. **Play therapy** often helps children express themselves by using toys such as puppets as their "spokesperson" of feelings.

Hypnosis helps a person recover deeply repressed emotions and speed recovery. It also serves to help change habits such as smoking.

Psychoanalysis was developed by Sigmund Freud. It is a long-term and intense form of therapy that allows the individual to bring unconscious thoughts to the surface. **Free association** (speaking thoughts without censorship) and dream interpretation are among the tools in psychoanalysis.

Adjunctive therapies include occupational therapy, recreational therapy, music therapy, magnetic therapy, art therapy, and hydrotherapy. These types of therapy allow expression of feelings, help increase self-esteem, and promote positive interaction and reality orientation. Such forms of adjunctive therapy are possible to use in a group setting or individually.

Limits of Confidentiality

Confidentiality is sometimes a dilemma when therapeutic effectiveness of care depends on the patient's willingness to talk about feelings and thoughts. It is important that the patient knows that each member of the health care team will share any information he or she receives with the others. No one member of the team keeps any secrets from the others. This practice also curtails patients' manipulating the staff, or pitting one staff member or patient against another.

Just as you as a nurse have a duty to report child abuse, you also have a duty to warn. Sometimes a patient will express intent to kill someone when he or she is released, and it is obligatory that you notify the appropriate authorities. Families of victims have filed (and won) suits against health care workers for not warning the victim.

ELECTROCONVULSIVE THERAPY

In the late 1930s, two Italian physicians, Ugo Cerletti and Lucio Bino, introduced this technique to treat psychiatric disorders. Through the years, electroconvulsive therapy (ECT) has been refined. Muscle relaxants and anesthesia are now part of the therapy; these reduce the incidence of fracture, contusion, and sprains from the induced seizure.

Electroconvulsive therapy is a treatment for depression, mania, or schizoaffective disorders that do not respond to other treatment modalities. The course of ECT usually requires about 10 treatments over several weeks. Only a very small amount of electrical current is required to trigger a tonic-clonic (grand mal) seizure; thus there is no risk of electrocution. Temporary memory loss after treatment is expected and lasts from a few hours up to a few days. Confusion right after a treatment usually dissipates in a few hours.

ECT is usually an outpatient treatment. There is a potential danger with the treatment, and it involves a great deal of care. When administered properly, for the right illness, ECT can help as much as or more than any other treatment.

Before an individual receives ECT, it is necessary to perform several tests. A thorough physical examination—which includes a blood chemistry survey, complete blood count, and urinalysis—serves to detect any unsuspected conditions.

The practitioner completes a thorough mental examination. An electroencephalogram (EEG) rules out any existing electrical abnormalities. Chest and lumbosacral spine radiography serve to rule out any skeletal abnormalities. An electrocardiogram (ECG) is also necessary to perform because the treatment can put a strain on the heart.

In preparing the patient for ECT, treat the individual as a surgical candidate. In collecting data, make sure all tests have been completed and the physician has received the reports. Obtain vital signs, height, and weight. If the individual has a knowledge deficit about the procedure, it is necessary to answer all of the patient's questions before it is possible to sign a consent form. Describing the steps of the day, the room where the treatment is given, and where recovery takes place helps reduce anxiety.

Make sure the patient is on nothing-by-mouth (NPO) status for at least 8 hours before the treatment. Just before the treatment, instruct the patient to void. Make sure the patient has removed all watches, jewelry, glasses or contacts, dentures, and hairpins. If the individual is an outpatient, it is acceptable to wear loose clothing such as a sweat suit or a hospital gown.

Administer pre-ECT medications, usually including a sedative. Establish an IV line for the anesthesiologist to use during the treatment.

Post-ECT care is similar to that of any postsurgical patient in the recovery room. Once the patient is fully awake, give a light meal or snack with acetaminophen. Giving a warm bath or assisting with mobility after the patient regains consciousness is sometimes also be part of the care. Sometimes the patient will be confused afterward and need supervision and reassurance. Make sure family members understand the need for constant attendance on the individual because of the temporary confusion. Do not allow the individual to drive until the confusion is gone.

Continual reassurance, support, and attentiveness before and after each treatment help the individual deal with anxiety about ECT (see Box 35-2).

PSYCHOPHARMACOLOGY

Psychotropic (psychoactive) medications in conjunction with other therapies serve to help modify an individual's behavior. Medication helps to control symptoms. Monitoring for signs of effectiveness and evidence of side effects is a very important nursing responsibility. It is clearly part of your role as the nurse administering these medications to understand their use (Table 35-3).

Antidepressants

There are many antidepressant medications. In the newest class are the SSRIs, which include fluoxetine (Prozac), sertraline (Zoloft), venlafaxine (Effexor), citalopram (Celexa), and paroxetine (Paxil). As mentioned, both clinicians and patients tend to prefer these drugs over the other classes because they have fewer side effects. Other classes of antidepressants are tricyclics; monoamine oxidase inhibitors (MAOIs); and triazolopyradines, a group that is similar to tricyclics and includes trazodone (Desyrel). Bupropion (Wellbutrin) is of the aminoketone class.

These medications work in different ways in the brain to alleviate signs and symptoms of depression, such as decreased appetite or sleep pattern disturbances, prolonged sadness, and lack of concentration.

Table 35-3 Medications for Psychiatric–Mental Health Disorders

Generic (Trade)	Side Effects and Precautions	Nursing Implications
ANTIMANICS		
Lithium carbonate (Eskalith, Lithobid) Divalproex sodium (Depakote) Carbamazepine (Tegretol)	Indigestion, rashes, drowsiness, ataxia, aplastic anemia, agranulocytosis, kidney damage from long-term lithium use Lithium toxicity—serum levels >1.5 mcg/L Symptoms: Nausea, vomiting, abdominal cramps, polyuria, polydipsia, ataxia, tremor, slurred speech, disorientation, and seizures	Teach patient signs and symptoms of toxicity and to maintain high fluid intake and stable salt use. Blood tests to assess drug level will be periodically necessary. Risk for injury if drowsy or ataxic. Avoid alcohol use. Take with food if causing indigestion.
ANTIPSYCHOTICS		
Chlorpromazine (Thorazine) Thioridazine HCl (Mellaril-5) Trifluoperazine HCl (Stelazine) Fluphenazine HCl (Prolixin, Permitil) Perphenazine (Trilafon) Thiothixene (Navane) Haloperidol (Haldol)	Anticholinergic effects: Dry mouth, blurred vision, constipation, urinary retention, postural hypotension Extrapyramidal side effects (EPS): Akathisia (severe restlessness—cannot stand still, foot tapping) Parkinsonian effects: Rigidity, resting tremor, shuffling gait Dystonias: Bizarre movements of the face and neck, torticollis, oculogyric crisis Other side effects: Lowered seizure threshold, tardive dyskinesia (involuntary movements of lips, tongue, jaw after medications are stopped or decreased) Rare: Neuroleptic malignant syndrome (hyperthermia, muscle rigidity, labile blood pressure (BP), confusion, cardiovascular collapse)	Suggest sugarless candy or gum for dry mouth. Teach patient that it is important to take the medication on time and to avoid stopping the medication abruptly. Have patient wear sunscreen. Establish baseline vital signs and blood counts. Explain need to rise slowly from sitting to standing. Watch for developing ataxia, clumsiness, nervousness when dose increased. Watch for EPS, and use anticholinergic medications as ordered prn (Cogentin, Benadryl). Watch for neuroleptic malignant syndrome.
ATYPICAL ANTIPSYCHOTICS Used in treating resistant forms of schizophrenia; usually more expensive but also less occurrence of adverse effects		
Clozapine (Clozaril)	Low risk of EPS and tardive dyskinesia; 1%-2% incidence of agranulocytosis; weekly serum monitoring necessary	Suggest sugarless candy or gum for dry mouth. Explain need to rise slowly from sitting to standing.
Olanzapine (Zyprexa)	Significant improvement of negative behaviors; most common effects are dry mouth, dyspepsia, drowsiness, postural hypotension; no association with agranulocytosis	
Risperidone (Risperdal)	Low rate of extrapyramidal effects, and no association with agranulocytosis	

Continued

Table 35-3 Medications for Psychiatric–Mental Health Disorders—cont'd

Generic (Trade)	Side Effects and Precautions	Nursing Implications
ANTIANXIETY AGENTS Alprazolam (Xanax) Buspirone (Buspar) Chlordiazepoxide HCl (Librium) Clorazepate dipotassium (Tranxene) Lorazepam (Ativan) Oxazepam (Serax)	Drowsiness, ataxia, muscle weakness, occasionally disinhibition, "morning hangover," transient hypotension, potentially habit forming, aggravates depression or psychosis	Watch for increased side effects in older adults. Teach patient not to operate machines or drive if side effect of drowsiness is occurring. Avoid alcohol use. Do not stop medications abruptly. Explain need to rise slowly from sitting to standing.
ANTIDEPRESSANTS **Tricyclics** Amitriptyline (Elavil) Amoxapine (Asendin) Desipramine HCl (Norpramin) Imipramine HCl (Tofranil) Nortriptyline HCl (Aventyl, Pamelor)	Anticholinergic effects (see antipsychotics) Other precautions: Do not use in patients with severe liver disease or after myocardial infarction; administer with caution for people with cardiac disease Sudden stoppage sometimes causes sleep disturbance	Monitor BP for hypotension. Suggest sugarless candy or gum for dry mouth. Explain that appetite sometimes increases. Caution against strenuous exercise or high temperature because of reduced diaphoresis.
Monoamine Oxidase Inhibitors (MAOIs) Phenelzine sulfate (Nardil) Tranylcypromine sulfate (Parnate)	Orthostatic hypotension, headache, abnormal heart rate and rhythm, blurred vision, dry mouth, fatigue, nausea, vomiting, constipation, urinary hesitancy and retention Other precautions: Hypertensive crisis is possible result from eating foods containing tyramine (red wine, beer, aged cheese, chocolate, licorice, yogurt, caffeine-rich foods, liver, and broad beans)	Monitor BP; explain need to rise slowly from sitting to standing. Teach patient that tyramine-rich foods pose risk of life-threatening effects and are necessary to restrict. Consult physician before taking over-the-counter cough or cold medicines. Know drug interactions; consult resource when physician prescribes additional medications. Monitor intake and output.
Selective Serotonin Reuptake Inhibitors (SSRIs) Fluoxetine (Prozac) Fluvoxamine (Luvox) Paroxetine HCl (Paxil) Sertraline (Zoloft)	Anticholinergic effects (see antipsychotics), appetite loss, transient fatigue, weight loss, diarrhea or constipation, diaphoresis, anxiety, tremors, insomnia, tachycardia, sexual dysfunction	Because of insomnia, take medication in the morning and early afternoon. Avoid alcohol use. Call physician before taking other medications. Use cautiously in patients with renal or hepatic impairment. Monitor for symptoms of serotonin syndrome.
Other Antidepressants Venlafaxine (Effexor) Maprotiline (Ludiomil) Nefazodone (Serzone) Bupropion (Wellbutrin) Trazodone (Desyrel) Mirtazapine (Remeron)	See SSRI side effects	Same as above; take bupropion in three divided doses to minimize seizure risk. Trazodone acceptable to take with food to decrease vertigo. Do not take mirtazapine within 14 days of MAOI use; has potential to cause hypertension, seizures, and death. Assess complete blood count (CBC) and liver function periodically.

None of them take effect immediately; it will generally take 2 to 4 weeks to note any improvement. People often describe the change that drug therapy accomplishes in depression as a fog lifting. Antidepressant therapy is necessary to maintain for several months to a year to prevent symptom recurrence.

Serotonin Syndrome

Serotonin syndrome is a potentially life-threatening condition that occurs usually as a result of an interaction between an SSRI and another serotonergic agent. Occurrence is also possible in older adult patients taking only an SSRI. Symptoms include altered mental status, autonomic dysfunction, and neuromuscular abnormalities.

Confusion, delirium, agitation, and mutism are some of the altered mental states that practitioners sometimes fail to recognize as side effects in chronically ill older adults living in long-term care facilities, where the rate of depression is sometimes as high as 30% to 50%. Autonomic dysfunction can include blood pressure fluctuation, tachycardia, hyperthermia, marked pupil dilation (mydriasis), shivering, and diaphoresis. Possible neuromuscular symptoms include some that are similar to those that antipsychotic medications also produce (see the later, more detailed discussion of extrapyramidal symptoms): akathisia (a jittery feeling inside that causes restlessness), ataxia (incoordination), dystonia, dyskinesia, hyperreflexia, tremors, and seizures. Older adult patients are more likely to display neuromuscular side effects, raising their risk of injury from falls. This syndrome worsens Parkinson's disease. Laboratory work indicating serotonin syndrome shows elevated creatine phosphokinase (CPK) from muscle disintegration, elevated white blood cells (WBCs) and transaminases, and decreased serum bicarbonate level.

Treatment for serotonin syndrome is to slowly decrease the dosage of the drug. Sudden discontinuation has potential to cause dizziness, nausea, vomiting, muscle pain, headaches, fatigue, anxiety, crying spells, and irritability. Instruct the patient about calling for assistance to ambulate until side effects have subsided. In the home setting especially, it is a good idea for the home health nurse to encourage the patient to take an active role in managing medications by reporting even minor side effects or concerns. Also review any over-the-counter (OTC) medication the patient takes. Emphasize the importance of telling you and the prescribing health care provider when the patient uses an OTC medication.

Be familiar with each drug, possible drug interactions, and serious side effects when assessing the patient for efficacy of antidepressants.

Antimanics

Lithium carbonate is the chief drug health care providers use to stabilize the mood and behavior of a patient with mania. A therapeutic blood level is required and sometimes takes 7 to 10 days to achieve. During the interim, the practitioner will frequently use antipsychotic medications to control behavior. Toxicity is a problem that comes up with lithium. Poor fluid intake and salt restriction in the diet increase the risk of toxicity. Be aware of the signs of toxicity: nausea, vomiting, diarrhea, drowsiness, muscle weakness, and ataxia. If the patient does not stop taking the drug, toxicity will potentially lead to seizures and death. Patient education is an important factor in lithium administration. The therapeutic level of lithium is fairly narrow—0.4 to 1.3 mEq/L—and it is necessary to individually evaluate and carefully monitor all patients.

Antipsychotics

Antipsychotic medications or major tranquilizers serve for acute and chronic management of (1) schizophrenia, (2) organic mental disorders with psychosis, and (3) the manic phase of bipolar mood disorder. These drugs provide symptomatic control but are not a cure. Responses to these drugs are highly individualized. It is best, as usual, to use the lowest effective dose.

A number of dose-related side effects occur in association with antipsychotics. Postural hypotension and sedation are common when first starting the drugs. Consider implementing safety measures to prevent falls. Photosensitivity is another side effect. Make sure patients wear sunscreen, hats, clothing, and glasses to prevent sunburn. Autonomic reactions include urinary retention, dry mouth, constipation, edema, and weight gain. Increasing fluid intake not only relieves dry mouth but also actually triggers the body to release excess fluid from the tissues.

Various abnormal neuromuscular symptoms occur in association with these drugs. Pseudoparkinsonism (e.g., tremor with rigid posture); **akathisia,** or an inability to sit still, with continuous hand, mouth, or body movements (e.g., foot tapping); **dystonias,** or aberrant posturing (e.g., hand spasms); and **dyskinesia,** or involuntary movements (e.g., lip smacking or tongue protruding) are among the extrapyramidal symptoms. **Tardive dyskinesia** is an extrapyramidal reaction that occurs when reducing the medication dosage, and it sometimes has a permanent effect. It is necessary to take immediate action to combat extrapyramidal effects. Stoppage or reduction of the dose of the drug, administering parenteral diphenhydramine (Benadryl), and follow-up use of antiparkinsonian drugs such as trihexyphenidyl (Artane) or benztropine (Cogentin) are among the options to consider.

Antianxiety Agents

Antianxiety drugs (anxiolytics) or minor tranquilizers often help individuals experiencing moderate to severe anxiety. Practitioners use benzodiazepine sedatives such as lorazepam (Ativan) to relieve the tension without sacrificing motivation. Abuse of drugs in this category is common.

Ongoing maintenance for people with a severe persistent (chronic) mental illness will often be very challenging for the individual and the family. Rehospitalization, when it occurs, reminds them that a cure for the disorder has not taken place and that close monitoring is still necessary, even when the individual is relatively free of symptoms. The special needs of the long-term mentally ill individual are essential to address by community mental health care and support, partial hospital programs, and assisted living environments.

ALTERNATIVE THERAPIES

Use of natural or herbal medications has gained tremendous popularity (see Chapter 17). However, there has been relatively little integration of their use into the current system based on prescription and OTC drugs. The control and manufacture of these medications does not fall under the laws of the U.S. Food and Drug Administration (FDA); as a result, the quality and the potency vary from manufacturer to manufacturer. Claims and clinical study results are not always consistent. Still, millions of people use herbal medicine based only on advertising claims. Include inquiries about the use of herbs when obtaining a drug history from the patient.

St. John's wort (*Hypericum* spp.) is one of the most common weeds in the world, and studies have shown its possible effectiveness to treat mild depression with few side effects when the patient takes therapeutic doses. St. John's wort will potentially interact with MAOIs and has the capacity to trigger hypertension if taken with allergy medication containing monoamines or phenylalanine, or amino acid supplements containing tyrosine.

Kava *(Piper methysticum)* is an herb some people take to treat anxiety and insomnia because of its sedative effects. Scaly rash on the backs of hands and the forearms and on the soles of feet is a common side effect. Alcohol potentiates the sedative effect and, if taken with benzodiazepines, it produces toxicity and induces coma. Other side effects are neuromuscular abnormalities similar to the side effects of antipsychotics. Another herb useful in treating anxiety is gotu kola, an herb that practitioners of ayurvedic medicine use. The effectiveness of gotu kola is comparable to diazepam in reducing anxiety.

Ginkgo and ginseng are also popular herbs that some believe improve memory and boost energy. Ginkgo provides moderate memory and cognitive improvement in treatment of early Alzheimer's disease by promoting cerebral blood flow, but it sometimes potentiates the action of anticoagulant drugs such as aspirin and warfarin (Coumadin), which poses the risk of fatal hemorrhage. Ginkgo has the capacity to affect insulin secretion, and ginseng sometimes lowers blood glucose in diabetics.

Foods and beverages now often contain herbs. Even oatmeal boxes tout the healing properties of lowering cholesterol. Instruct the patient to read labels and avoid drug interactions with herbal additives. Encourage the patient to seek information about herbs from the pharmacist or physician before using any.

Aromatherapy has gained a foothold in the American way of life; however, its effects are limited. Its use is generally to enhance or potentiate another remedy. Use takes the forms of scented oils for massage, volatile oils to sniff or inhale, and scented candles or incense. Users believe that certain odors trigger chemical activity in the brain to relieve imbalance in the body.

Citrus essences, peppermint, cedarwood, rosemary, sandalwood, chamomile, and lavender are a few essential oils that many believe help relieve stress and anxiety. It is possible to use such oils in a variety of ways—for example, in chamomile tea, a sandalwood candle, or a hot bath with lavender oil. Aromatherapy focuses on the atmosphere of the moment and uses the body's senses to try to achieve balance within. It has a definite place in holistic care.

APPLICATION OF THE NURSING PROCESS

In the psychiatric setting, as every setting, you will use the nursing process to meet the many needs of the patient, including assessment, nursing diagnoses formulation, planning, intervention, and evaluation. As a licensed practical nurse/licensed vocational nurse (LPN/LVN), you will participate in the nursing process as a member of the mental health care team that includes nurses, therapists, and physicians. Your observation of patient behavior and therapeutic communications with the patient assist the registered nurse (RN) in collecting data to form nursing diagnoses. Your contributions in developing nursing diagnoses with the RN ensure appropriate interventions for the patient. You and the RN work together to implement the plan of care for a therapeutic nurse-patient relationship.

Focus health promotion interventions on preventing relapse and managing symptoms by practicing a healthy lifestyle. Simple, concrete, clear patient teaching will be most successful. Patients need to realize that it is possible to manage their behaviors by recognizing when these behaviors are becoming problematic, and talking with their health care provider and/or therapist.

Evaluation of the patient will be ongoing. At intervals or when the patient's response dictates, you and your colleagues will update the care plan. Examination of the documentation and personal observations are considerations when evaluating the plan of care.

It is essential to clearly document all phases of the nursing process. Most of the documentation methods you will use are ongoing and will include the assessment criteria the health care team uses. Keep your notes accurate and descriptive. Avoid terms such as "appears depressed." Instead, use terms such as "no eye contact noted during conversation." Documentation of the patient's actual conversation is very valuable.

Working with patients who have a mental disorder is always a challenge. Honesty with a caring attitude goes a long way in helping the person deal effectively with his or her problem.

Get Ready for the NCLEX® Examination!

Key Points

- *DSM-IV-TR* is a multiaxial system that serves in the diagnosis of psychiatric disorders. It comprises the physical, the psychiatric, and the social factors affecting the individual.
- You will use the nursing process in the psychiatric context; it includes assessment, nursing diagnoses formulation, planning, intervention, and evaluation. The care plan documents this process.
- To help prevent suicide, it is necessary to recognize its warning signs and learn the kinds of actions that are possible to avert it.
- Therapeutic communication is a dynamic method of interacting with patients for problem solving and growth.
- In psychiatry, medications serve to assist individuals with feelings and behaviors.
- You and the health care team will observe and evaluate behavior to determine a patient's progress and the effectiveness of the care plan.

Additional Learning Resources

Go to your Companion CD for an audio glossary, animations, video clips, and more.

evolve Be sure to visit the Evolve site at http://evolve.elsevier.com/Christensen/foundations/ for additional online resources.

Review Questions for the NCLEX® Examination

1. An 82-year-old was admitted to the long-term care facility with moderate to severe heart failure and is unable to take care of himself at home. After dinner, the patient becomes agitated and confused. There are no significant changes in vital signs, and he has received the same medications he had been taking at home. What cause of acute confusion should the nurse consider?
   1. Alzheimer's disease
   2. Sundowning syndrome
   3. Electrolyte imbalance
   4. Acute renal failure
2. A patient with Alzheimer's disease continually wanders. Which snack will best meet the patient's nutritional needs?
   1. Candy bars and ice cream sundaes
   2. Eggnog milk shakes and oatmeal-raisin cookies
   3. Celery sticks and rice cakes
   4. Root beer and potato chips
3. The psychiatrist makes a diagnosis using a multiaxial system guide called:
   1. the *Physicians' Desk Reference.*
   2. the *Diagnostic and Statistical Manual, IV-TR.*
   3. the hospital formulary.
   4. Freud's *The Ego and the Id.*
4. A delusional patient becomes agitated while watching television and states, "If I don't buy Crest toothpaste right now, I will have cavities." The nurse's best response is:
   1. "The advertisement on the TV is saying its product will reduce tooth decay if you use their product regularly."
   2. "Get your coat and let's go to the store now."
   3. "You can't believe everything you hear or see on TV."
   4. "Turn off the TV! That lady is projecting thoughts into your head! She works for the CIA!"
5. Negative, or absent, behavior patterns in the schizophrenic patient include:
   1. delusions.
   2. hallucinations.
   3. disordered thinking.
   4. apathy.
6. Besides feelings of sadness or despair, which is also a sign or symptom of depression?
   1. Extreme fatigue
   2. Restlessness
   3. Flight of ideas
   4. Hallucinations
7. The therapy of choice for bipolar, or manic-depressive, disorder is:
   1. chlorpromazine (Thorazine).
   2. lithium salts.
   3. electroconvulsive therapy.
   4. fluoxetine (Prozac).
8. A patient admitted to the emergency department is complaining of an anxiety attack. The nurse must be aware that signs of anxiety include:
   1. hypotension and bradycardia.
   2. lethargy and thready pulse.
   3. hyperventilation and tachycardia.
   4. hallucinations and apathy.

9. A 47-year-old is in the hospital for severe depression. She is unkempt and has lost 15 pounds in the past 2 months. Her family states that she always keeps a knife in her purse. The nurse will consider which intervention for this patient?

1. Suicide precautions to prevent self-injury
2. Occupational therapy to build self-esteem
3. Art psychotherapy to help her express feelings
4. Large-portioned meals to improve nutritional status

10. Antipsychotic medications have a number of side effects that discourage compliance by the patient. Which effect has potential to lead to serious permanent problems?

1. Photosensitivity
2. Postural hypotension
3. Chronic constipation
4. Tardive dyskinesia

11. A patient says the anchorwoman on the television news talks to him and told him that there was a car bombing in Israel today. What is the nurse's best response?

1. "No, she was talking to me, not you."
2. "She is reporting the world news to everyone in the room. It only appears she is looking at you but she is looking in a TV camera that sends a picture to the TV."
3. "If you look in the back of the TV console, you will see there is no person inside."
4. "You are delusional. That is only a projected image of a person reading the news to a camera far away."

12. An 87-year-old patient lives with her daughter's family and has been having gastroenteritis for 2 days. Her daughter became very concerned when the patient wanted to go home and see her mother and father in the country. The patient had never been confused before today and became more confused by the end of the day. Her daughter took her to the emergency department where the emergency department physician admitted her with a diagnosis of dehydration. This confusion is possible to diagnose as:

1. delirium.
2. delusions.
3. dementia.
4. hallucinations.

13. A 24-year-old was admitted for medication adjustment for her bipolar disorder. The patient has not slept for 2 days and is unable to sit for more than a few minutes at a time. She has lost 11 pounds in the past week. Which factor will facilitate the best nutrition for the patient while she is in her manic phase?

1. Have her take her meals in her room to reduce distracting stimuli.
2. Have the kitchen double her meal portions since she only eats half of the food served.
3. Allow the patient to snack on candy bars between meals to gain back her lost weight.
4. Keep sandwiches, granola bars, fruit, and noncaffeinated beverages available at the desk.

14. A patient who was sexually abused as a child recently married but finds sexual intercourse painful. She confides in her friend who is a nurse. What is the appropriate response from her friend?

1. "You should see your gynecologist right away in case you have torn tissues."
2. "It is normal to have pain at first, but you will adjust to your husband over time."
3. "You should seek counseling and make sure to get a good physical examination."
4. "Did you report this abuse to the police?"

15. A patient is a broker on Wall Street who smokes half a pack of cigarettes a day. He avoids caffeine because he has trouble sleeping. He also often complains of an aching lower back. His physician was not able to find anything wrong physically. What is a possible cause of his back pain?

1. Congenital anomaly
2. Psychophysiologic origins
3. Possible renal calculi forming
4. Dependent personality disorder

16. A 17-year-old is worried about her weight. When she is out with friends, she eats junk food until she vomits and then exercises the next day for 4 hours. If she does not have a daily bowel movement, she takes a laxative. Her dentist has noticed her front teeth have signs of erosion. Her family has noticed her hair falling out, and now they have decided to take her to the family physician. The physician diagnoses her with:

1. anorexia nervosa.
2. laxative addiction.
3. bulimia nervosa.
4. gastroenteritis.

17. A 37-year-old is not responding to drug therapy for depression. The physician has recommended ECT treatments for 1 week as an outpatient. The nurse will stress which point in his pretreatment teaching?

1. Have someone take you to and from the clinic.
2. Eat a good breakfast because you will sleep through lunch.
3. Scrub your forearms before coming to the clinic.
4. Take a laxative the night before so you won't have an accident during the treatment.

18. A 78-year-old is living in a long-term care facility. She had a stroke while living at home and fell, fracturing her hip. She became depressed and has been receiving several medications for depression and chronic pain syndrome. The nurse finds the patient staring at her food tray and wringing her hands. When the nurse asks what is wrong, the patient replies, "I just feel too nervous inside to eat. I don't know why I should be nervous. Maybe I need a nerve pill." What is a possible cause of the patient's nervousness?

1. Unconscious fear from the stroke
2. Residual effects from the stroke
3. Having suicidal ideation
4. Developing serotonin syndrome

19. A 27-year-old has schizophrenia and lives in a group home. The group home has a monthly recreational outing. Which activity is most appropriate?

1. Volleyball game with another group home
2. Bowling with family members
3. Fishing at the local dam's spillway
4. Trip to the library

20. A 17-year-old tells his mother he is writing a paper for class on all the rock stars who have killed themselves. In the past few months, he has let his hair grow long, bathes only once a week, and stays in his room when he is at home. He is tired and irritable. His mother asks a friend who is a nurse if this is normal teenage behavior. What is the best response?

1. "Yes, all teens go through a grunge stage."
2. "Yes, he is just tired from the rapid growth spurt during adolescence."
3. "No, and if he doesn't snap out of it, you might want to take him to a physician."
4. "No, he should see a physician or counselor right away."

21. A 70-year-old is in the hospital for pneumonia and has been taking sertraline (Zoloft) for 1 year for depression. On the third day of her hospitalization, the patient has a pulse rate of 100, demonstrates trembling in her hands, has an oral temperature of 103° F, and is diaphoretic. What is the nursing assessment?

1. High anxiety, related to hospitalization
2. Increased cranial pressure
3. Impaired airway
4. Serotonin syndrome

22. What is the appropriate nursing action in question 21?

1. Notify the physician immediately, and also report it to the nursing supervisor.
2. Give the patient her ordered prn medication for fever.
3. Record the patient's vital signs.
4. Call the patient's "responsible party" listed on the admission sheet.

23. To effectively communicate with a patient demonstrating manic, elevated mood behaviors, the nurse will:

1. provide detailed explanations to patient.
2. joke and use puns with patient.
3. be brief and concrete with patient.
4. offer prn medications to patient.

24. A priority nursing intervention when working with a patient with any personality disorder is:

1. encouraging group activity participation.
2. reassuring the patient that he or she is a "good person."
3. setting limits with the patient.
4. supporting the patient's decisions consistently.

25. Which risk factor for eating disorders comes up most often in the history of an adolescent with an eating disorder?

1. Dieting
2. Excessive exercise
3. Purging
4. Preoccupation with food

26. Nursing interventions helpful in lowering a patient's level of anxiety from severe to moderate include:

1. providing seclusion for the patient.
2. listening for similarities the patient expresses.
3. changing subjects until the patient calms.
4. allowing the patient to distort reality.

27. When providing care for a depressed patient, the highest nursing priority is:

1. anorexia and weight loss.
2. lowered self-esteem.
3. inability to care effectively.
4. suicidal ideation.

28. An 84-year-old admitted for a cerebral vascular accident (CVA) has been told that he can no longer live alone. The nurse enters the patient's room to find him attempting to get out of bed, with the top sheet knotted around his neck. What is the immediate nursing assessment for this patient?

1. Danger to self
2. Noncompliance
3. Depression
4. Impairment of self-esteem

29. After the nurse removes the sheet from the patient's neck and returns him to bed, what is the most appropriate nursing intervention?

1. Leave the room to report the patient's behavior.
2. Sit beside the patient's bed and ask if he would like to talk.
3. Tell the patient that he will not be able to stay in this room, but will be moved to a psychiatric unit.
4. Tell the patient that he should cheer up; he's still alive.

chapter

36 Care of the Patient with an Addictive Personality

evolve

http://evolve.elsevier.com/Christensen/foundationsadult

Anne W. Ryan

Objectives

1. Name two traits that characterize an addictive personality.
2. Describe the three stages of dependence.
3. Describe one legal effort that has decreased the incidence of substance abuse.
4. Describe three disorders associated with alcoholism.
5. Explain the two phases of recovery: detoxification and rehabilitation.
6. Identify six types of drugs of abuse.
7. Describe possible steps to help the chemically impaired nurse.

Key Terms

abuse (p. 1158)
addiction (p. 1158)
addictive personality (p. 1159)
Alcoholics Anonymous (AA) (p. 1164)
alcoholism (p. 1158)
amotivational cannabis syndrome (ā-mō-tĭ-VĀ-shŭn-ăl KĂN-ă-bĭs, p. 1170)
bruxism (BRŬK-sĭz-ĕm, p. 1169)
cannabis (KĂN-ă-bĭs, p. 1170)
club drugs (p. 1166)
delirium tremens (DTs) (p. 1161)
depressants (p. 1166)
detoxification (dĕ-tŏk-sĭ-fĭ-KĀ-shŭn, p. 1163)
gateway drug (p. 1160)
group therapy (p. 1164)
hallucinogens (hă-LŪ-sĭ-nō-jĕn, p. 1168)
Healthcare Integrity and Protection Data Bank (HIPDB) (p. 1173)
huffing (p. 1171)
inhalants (p. 1170)
peer assistance programs (p. 1173)
psychoactive drugs (sī-kō-ĂK-tĭv, p. 1159)
raves (p. 1166)
street drugs (p. 1166)
tolerance (p. 1159)

The treatment of patients with addictive behaviors is an important concern for nurses. In today's society, problems associated with the **abuse** or misuse of alcohol, tobacco, caffeine, nicotine, and other drugs consume a major proportion of health care dollars. Many patients who enter with other diagnoses into acute care hospitals, doctors' offices, and psychiatric hospitals sometimes also suffer from some type of addictive behavior. You are thus likely to encounter problems of substance abuse and addiction in patients suffering from other medical conditions. Patients often deny or hide their substance abuse problem. In your concern about the patient's medical condition, perhaps you will not consider substance abuse until withdrawal symptoms become apparent. Patients suffering with chronic pain have a high risk of developing tolerance and addiction to opioids. Patients suffering from anxiety and depression sometimes self-medicate with alcohol or marijuana. It is important to investigate what the patient does to relieve stress or pain when collecting data about the patient. These data often help identify addictive behavior patterns that can impede the patient's recovery from acute illness.

ADDICTION

The definition of **addiction** contains four elements: (1) excessive use or abuse, (2) display of psychological disturbance, (3) decline of social and economic function, and (4) uncontrollable consumption, indicating dependence. **Alcoholism** refers to addiction to alcohol. It is possible to suffer from more than one addiction at the same time. An example is the alcoholic person who is also a smoker and a compulsive gambler.

Of adults ages 18 years and older, 44% report having consumed 12 or more alcoholic drinks in the past year. About 10% of these current drinkers meet diagnostic criteria for alcohol addiction, and an additional 7% meet diagnostic criteria for alcohol abuse (Touhy & Jett, 2009). Age at the onset of drinking strongly predicts the development of alcohol dependence in the life span. Of those who start drinking at the age of 14 or younger, 44% will develop alcoholism. As our society ages, alcohol and drug abuse are increasing in the older population. The older adult sometimes turns to alcohol, prescription and nonprescription drugs, caffeine, and nicotine to help cope with physiologic and sociologic changes with aging. Aging causes changes in absorption, distribution, metabolism, and excretion of drugs, thus increasing the risk of misuse and abuse.

Alcohol is involved in 38% of all deaths caused by motor vehicle accidents and fatal intentional injuries such as suicides and homicides. About 100,000 deaths each year are related to alcohol consumption (Touhy & Jett, 2009).

The use of alcohol and drugs predates recorded history. Cultures from many parts of the world have used alcohol and drugs as medicine, in celebrations, and as a part of worship services. In the history of the United States, legal positions on the use of alcohol have varied. The temperance movement in the 1800s stressed moderation in the use of alcohol. Prohibition, which forbade the production and sale of alcohol beverages, was passed in 1919 and later repealed in 1933. There has been a decrease in alcohol use over the years that experts attribute to education of the public and laws set forth to limit availability to minors.

Although there has been a long-term drop in overall alcohol use, many people still use illicit drugs. In 1998 there were 13.6 million users (6.2%) in the United States. Some 60% of these illicit drug users admitted to abuse only of marijuana. Estimates are that there are 4.4 million chronic drug users nationally (National Institute on Drug Abuse [NIDA], n.d.). The goal of the Comprehensive Drug Abuse and Controlled Substance Act of 1970 (commonly referred to as the Controlled Substance Act) was to provide legal control over drugs that previous federal drug-related laws did not cover. The Bureau of Drug Abuse Control moved from the U.S. Food and Drug Administration (FDA) to the Justice Department, and later merged into the Drug Enforcement Agency (DEA); this last is today the leading agency responsible for enforcing the 1970 act. All prescribing physicians and dispensing pharmacies register with the DEA. Smuggling and other illegal activities provide the public with illicit drugs.

Certain common traits have been identified in addicted people. These traits have often been grouped under the term **addictive personality** (a person who exhibits a pattern of compulsive and habitual use of a substance or practice to cope with psychic pain from conflict and anxiety). These personality traits include low stress tolerance, dependency, negative self-image, feelings of insecurity, and depression. It is not clear whether these traits are present before the development of dependence or are a result of it.

STAGES OF DEPENDENCE

Psychoactive drugs, including alcohol, make the user feel good. Social use of drugs creates a relaxed atmosphere, encouraging people to share themselves more openly. Movies, television commercials, and other media have suggested that we "need a drink" after a hard day at the office. Unfortunately, every psychoactive drug, including caffeine and nicotine, has the potential to be abused or addicting. In the 1970s, alcoholism and drug addiction acquired recognition as diseases. Experts published diagnostic criteria and established treatment centers for addiction in the United States—a psychoactive drug–oriented society. When does substance abuse become a disease and a problem? The indicator appears to be the loss of control. The disease of dependence is a chronic, incurable, progressive one with three characteristic stages of dependence: early, middle, and late (Table 36-1).

EARLY STAGES

As a person uses an increasing amount of an addicting substance and uses it more frequently to achieve the same effect, **tolerance** develops. The user experiences the untoward effects of insomnia, anxiety, cramps, heart palpitations, changes in sexual libido, and accidental injury. Some users will decrease or stop to prove that they have control of their substance use. Family and friends will probably comment about their concern

Table 36-1 Stages of Dependence

EARLY STAGE	MIDDLE STAGE	LATE STAGE
Increased drug tolerance Strong denial Defends drug use to family concerns More socializing with users Increased tardiness or call-offs from work/school Possible legal problems Good prognosis for recovery, even without a treatment program	Moderate impairment Withdrawal signs with abstinence Uses to feel "normal" Established pattern of use Further alienation from family Drug-related behavior such as lying, stealing, mood swing Physical health declines Weight loss noticeable Blackouts Financial/legal problems Job loss or frequent job changes Few recover without treatment	Severe impairment in all areas of function Continuous use but cannot achieve "normal" feeling Medical problems worsen; organ involvement Malnutrition worsens Poor problem solving and judgment Manipulative, denies problems Unemployed Often homeless Must receive treatment for improvement

of the user's overinvolvement with drugs. The user will perhaps make light of the concern, or become hostile and defensive. Sometimes the user will avoid family and socialize only with other users. The user is prone to legal problems such as charges of driving while intoxicated. The user will sometimes miss work or show up late for work after a weekend off. A pattern of absenteeism emerges. If a student is a user, truancy and falling grades with an "I don't care" attitude are common. Mood swings, decreased self-esteem, shame, guilt, remorse, resentment, and irritability are typical, with a tendency for these feelings to focus on drug use. Financial difficulties arise in connection with greater expenditures for drug use. The prognosis with treatment is good in this early stage, and recovery without treatment is possible.

MIDDLE STAGE

In this stage, the dependent user is moderately impaired. With difficulty, the user makes efforts to decrease or stop, followed by heavier use. Abstinence brings on signs and symptoms of withdrawal. The user now uses just to feel "normal." The user has a pattern of using in regard to time, place, and situation. The user weakens family relationships and friendships by his or her drug-related behavior such as arguing, lying, stealing, incest, physical abuse, and child neglect. Physical health declines. Common problems that arise during this stage include weight changes; anorexia; malnutrition; gastrointestinal problems such as nausea, diarrhea, and gastritis; suicide attempts; blackouts of short-term memory; sexual problems; sexually transmitted infection; accidental injury; infections; and overdose. Job loss is common because of absenteeism, drug use on the job, and uncooperative attitudes. Employers sometimes ask the user to seek treatment. Social isolation increases, and the user continues to have legal and crime-related problems. Some dependent users stay in this stage a long time. If the user is a multidrug user, progression into the late stage is faster. Very few people in this stage recover without treatment.

LATE STAGE

In this stage, the dependent user displays severe impairment in all areas of function. Drug use is nearly continual in an attempt to avoid emotional and physical pain, but the user is not able to achieve a feeling of normalcy. Medical problems worsen. Along with malnutrition, liver disease, pancreatitis, toxic psychosis, kidney failure, sexual impotence, and stroke are possible. The user neglects personal hygiene. An intravenous user is at great risk to contract human immunodeficiency virus (HIV) or hepatitis B or C or to develop septicemia, abscesses, or infective endocarditis. The user will in some cases be suicidal or homicidal. The user is manipulative, is in denial of his or her problems, and has poor problem-solving ability and judgment. The user in this stage is usually unemployed, only associates with dealers or other users, and will perhaps be homeless. People in this stage will not improve without treatment.

ALCOHOL ABUSE AND ALCOHOLISM

Alcoholism is a national health problem surpassed only by heart disease and cancer. No one theory explains the cause of alcoholism. Several factors probably contribute to the development of alcoholism. Some believe that people are more likely to develop alcoholism because of some biologic reason, such as an inner urge controlled by the nervous system or a dysfunction of the endocrine system. Alcoholism is, in part, genetically determined. The incidence of alcoholism in members of alcoholic families is high: the sons of alcoholic men have a 30% to 50% risk of developing alcoholism over their lifetime (American Society of Addiction Medicine [ASAM], n.d.). Also, deficiencies in some hepatic enzymes necessary to metabolize alcohol contribute to the development of alcoholism in some people. Many Asians, American Indians, and Eskimos have deficiencies in these enzymes; alcoholism is higher in these ethnic groups than in the general public. Jews, Mormons, and Moslems have very low rates of alcoholism, whereas the French and the Irish have high rates.

Other theories rest on the belief that some part of the personality leads to the development of alcoholism. Some people still believe that alcoholism develops as a result of either a moral fault or a sin of the alcoholic. This theory provided the basis for much of the early treatment of alcoholics. Health care providers trained to provide treatment regimens based on this moral theory have difficulty assimilating newer biologic theories into their care.

Wide cultural differences concerning drug and alcohol use have been found in U.S. society. Most teenagers have their first drink between the ages of 12 and 15. Alcohol sometimes serves as an informal passage into adulthood. Drinking beer or other alcoholic beverages is the way we celebrate certain holidays (e.g., St. Patrick's Day). Experts consider drinking to be the leading health problem in the African-American community. Hispanics and many other ethnic groups celebrate life while drinking alcohol. Alcohol often falls into the category of a **gateway drug**; many multidrug users begin by abusing alcohol and later abuse other substances.

ETIOLOGY AND PATHOPHYSIOLOGY

Alcohol is a central nervous system (CNS) depressant. The so-called stimulating effect occurs because the first areas alcohol affects are the higher centers of the brain, including the frontal cortex, which govern self-control. Judgment is blocked, but memory of pleasure is retained. As a person continues to ingest alcohol, it affects the nucleus accumbens in the limbic system (the most primitive part of the brain; it regulates hunger, thirst, and sexual desire). Repeated alcohol consumption affects the basal ganglia of the brain, where it unbalances compulsion controls, leading to obsessive-compulsive behavior. Unconsciousness from rapid, large-quantity consumption is possible, during which respiration is sometimes affected. Death from acute alcohol poisoning is possible.

The active ingredient of alcoholic beverages is ethyl alcohol or ethanol. There are similar amounts of alcohol in 12 ounces of beer, 4 ounces of wine, and 1½ ounces of hard liquor. Alcohol does not require digestion, and the body absorbs it readily in the stomach and the intestine. An empty stomach increases the rate of absorption. After ingestion, the body loses small amounts through breathing and in the urine, but 90% is metabolized by the liver.

Alcohol has a diuretic effect. The urine of a heavy drinker sometimes contains increased amounts of electrolytes, especially potassium, magnesium, and zinc. Prolonged use of alcohol has a toxic effect on the intestinal mucosa that results in decreased absorption of thiamine (vitamin B_1), folic acid, and vitamin B_{12}.

Alcohol does not undergo conversion to glycogen; it does provide the body with calories but no minerals or vitamins. One ounce of alcohol provides 200 kcal but no other nutritional value. Blood alcohol levels depend on the amount of alcohol ingested and the size of the individual. Most states designate blood alcohol serum (BAS) levels of 80 mg/dL (0.08%) as the legal limit for driving a motor vehicle. Increasing blood alcohol levels have increasingly serious side effects (Table 36-2).

DISORDERS ASSOCIATED WITH ALCOHOLISM

Fetal Alcohol Syndrome

Fetal alcohol syndrome (FAS) is a congenital anomaly resulting from daily maternal ingestion of alcohol equivalent to 3 ounces of absolute alcohol per day. This syndrome is common in newborns whose mothers drank heavily during pregnancy. Birth defects related to alcohol use include mental retardation, growth disorders, wide-set eyes, malformed body parts, and spontaneous abortion or stillbirths. As few as two drinks per day have the potential to cause adverse effects in an infant.

Table 36-2 Blood Alcohol Levels and Related Side Effects

BLOOD ALCOHOL SERUM (BAS) LEVEL	SIDE EFFECTS
50-75 mg/dL (0.05%-0.075%)	Pleasant, relaxed state, mild sedation, loosening of inhibitions
100-200 mg/dL (0.10%-0.20%)	Overt signs of intoxication: loosening of the tongue, clumsiness, beginning emotional changes (legal limit in most states)
200-400 mg/dL (0.20%-0.40%)	Severe intoxication: difficulty speaking, stumbling, blurred vision, emotional lability
400-500 mg/dL (0.40%-0.50%)	Stupor, coma
>500 mg/dL (>0.50%)	Respiratory failure, usually fatal

Alcohol Withdrawal Syndrome

Alcohol withdrawal syndrome occurs in a person who has developed physiologic dependence and quits drinking for whatever reason. Alcoholics at risk for having alcohol withdrawal syndrome include older people, people who have previously suffered delirium tremens, malnourished people, and people suffering with another acute illness. The range of possible signs and symptoms varies from mild tremor and flulike signs and symptoms to severe agitation and hallucinations. Signs and symptoms associated with the cessation of alcohol consumption include diaphoresis, tachycardia, hypertension, tremors, nausea and/or vomiting, anorexia, restlessness, disorientation, hallucinations, and seizures.

The tremors from alcohol cessation are seen 6 to 48 hours after the last drink and sometimes last for 3 to 5 days. Usually tremors occur in the hands but are also possible in the tongue, the chin, the trunk, and the feet. Seizures are possible 12 to 24 hours after cessation. Usually these are tonic-clonic (grand mal) seizures and often are not preceded by an aura.

Delirium Tremens

Delirium tremens (DTs) is a complication of alcohol withdrawal. This acute psychotic reaction is a result of excessive alcohol consumption over a long period. The risk of death from this complication is as high as 15%, even with treatment. Signs of DTs are tremors, activity increased sometimes to the point of extreme agitation, disorientation, fear with an appearance of panic, hallucinations, and elevated temperature. DTs most often occur 1 to 4 days after cessation of alcohol and usually last from 2 days to a week.

Korsakoff's Psychosis and Wernicke's Encephalopathy

Korsakoff's psychosis and Wernicke's encephalopathy are two brain disorders that sometimes occur in chronic alcoholics. Characteristics of Korsakoff's psychosis are short-term memory loss, disorientation, muttering delirium, insomnia, hallucinations, polyneuritis, and painful extremities with footdrop affecting the gait. Wernicke's encephalopathy occurs in association with thiamine deficiency, causing brain damage in the temporal lobes of the brain. It features memory loss, aphasia, involuntary eye movement and double vision, lack of muscle coordination, and disorientation with confabulation (i.e., the patient fills in memory gaps with inappropriate words).

Because alcohol affects all tissues in the body, chronic alcohol ingestion has potential to cause dam-

Table 36-3 Disorders Associated with Alcoholism

SYSTEM	DISORDERS
Gastrointestinal (GI)	Gastritis; pancreatitis; cancer of mouth, esophagus, and stomach; esophageal varices; GI bleeding; malabsorption of nutrition; ascites
Hepatic	Hepatitis, cirrhosis, fatty liver, liver failure, hepatic encephalopathy
Cardiovascular and blood disorders	Hypertension, enlarged heart, high cholesterol, heart failure, portal hypertension, low blood sugar, anemia, poor clotting ability, increased susceptibility to infection
Respiratory	Decreased cough reflex, aspiration pneumonia
Uroreproductive	Prostatitis, impotence, urinary flow problems
Musculoskeletal	Myopathies, bone fractures from falls, joint damage from injury
Neurologic	Neuritis, organic brain diseases such as Wernicke's encephalopathy and Korsakoff's psychosis, nerve palsies, gait changes, short-term memory loss

age to all parts of the body. Table 36-3 presents other disorders arising from chronic alcohol use.

NURSING MANAGEMENT

ASSESSMENT

It is important to collect both subjective and objective data about the patient suffering from substance abuse or dependence. Collection of **subjective data** includes the person's normal using or drinking pattern, as well as the date and time of the last drink or use of a drug. The specific substance and the quantity the person used are important. Other complaints such as nausea, indigestion, sleep disturbance, or pain sometimes indicate the simultaneous occurrence of another disease process, not only side effects of substance abuse. Assessment of normal dietary patterns, the presence of any disease requiring treatment with prescribed medications, and regular use of any over-the-counter drugs help to complete the picture of the patient's present state of wellness. Obtain this information in as much detail as possible. Do not forget to ask about drug allergies or unusual responses to anesthesia, sedatives, or preoperative medications. Maintaining a concerned, nonjudgmental attitude when asking for details helps to reassure the patient, as does the promise of confidentiality about this very private part of his or her life.

Assess for any history of tremors, hallucinations, delusions, seizures, or DTs. Note any past periods of abstinence. Inquire about any problems with occupation, family, or legal matters. Assess for any family history of substance dependency. Remember that denial is very strong in the person with untreated substance abuse or dependence, and patient information will often not be accurate. It is helpful to validate information with families or significant others if possible. Another helpful questionnaire that is often useful in affirming alcohol abuse is the CAGE questionnaire, whose title arises from an acronym formed from among the tool's four questions (Box 36-1).

Collection of **objective data** includes height, weight, vital signs, and physical assessment. Note the presence of tremor or skin conditions, especially on the forearms. Needle tracks and small scabs on forearms, backs of hands, and insteps indicate intravenous use. Acne-like facial rash is possibly related to MDMA (ecstasy) use.

Frequent sniffing, stuffy nose, or harsh nonproductive cough is possibly related to drug use. Assess general behavior and cognitive abilities for impairment. The presence of tachycardia, hypertension, petechiae, and neuropathies is significant. The presence of ascites or a urine or blood sample positive for drugs or alcohol will alert you to the need for further investigation of the history.

DIAGNOSTIC TESTS

Blood and urine tests help screen for toxins. Some foods will at times cause a false-positive reading in a urine screen. If a person ate a poppy seed roll and later gave urine for a drug screen, it is possible that it will yield a positive result for heroin. Abnormalities in routine blood tests are sometimes directly related to alcoholism. Elevated liver enzymes, hypoglycemia, and abnormal blood protein levels occur with alcoholism. Magnesium levels will be decreased in some cases. It is not uncommon to find anemia and other evidence of poor nutrition in the addicted patient. Some practitioners will also order testing for hepatitis and HIV.

NURSING DIAGNOSES

Nursing diagnoses and interventions for the patient with an addiction cover emotional needs as well as physical needs (Table 36-4).

Box 36-1 CAGE Questions

Two or more affirmations to these questions indicate probable alcoholism:

1. Have you ever felt you ought to **c**ut down on your drinking?
2. Have people **a**nnoyed you by criticizing your drinking?
3. Have you ever felt bad or **g**uilty about your drinking?
4. Have you ever had a drink first thing in the morning to steady your nerves or for your hangover (i.e., **e**ye-opener)?

From Fortinash, K., & Holoday-Worret, P. (2008). *Psychiatric mental health nursing*. (4th ed.). St. Louis: Mosby.

Table 36-4 **Some Possible Nursing Diagnoses for Addiction**

PHYSICAL NEEDS	EMOTIONAL NEEDS	EDUCATIONAL NEEDS
Ineffective airway clearance	Ineffective coping	Deficient knowledge
Risk for aspiration	Ineffective denial	Disturbed personal identity
Activity intolerance	Anticipatory grieving	Noncompliance
Risk for falls	Family processes: alcoholism, dysfunctional	Disturbed sensory perception
Risk for imbalanced fluid volume	Hopelessness	Ineffective community or ineffective family therapeutic regimen management
Ineffective health maintenance	Risk for loneliness	Disturbed thought processes
Risk for infection	Impaired memory	
Risk for injury	Risk for powerlessness	
Nausea	Chronic low self-esteem	
Imbalanced nutrition: less than body requirements	Social isolation	
Self-care deficit: bathing/hygiene, dressing/grooming	Spiritual distress	
Sexual dysfunction	Risk for suicide	
Disturbed sleep pattern	Risk for violence	

Nursing Diagnoses–Definitions and Classifications 2009-2011 ©2009, 2007, 2005, 2003, 2001, 1998, 1996, 1994. NANDA International. Used by arrangement with Wiley-Blackwell Publishing, a company of John Wiley & Sons, Inc.

NURSING INTERVENTIONS

Care for the addicted patient starts with **detoxification,** the removal of the poisonous effects of a substance. A controlled setting where it is possible to closely observe and treat the patient for any complications is important during this acute phase of recovery.

Safety of the patient is a primary concern. If the patient is intoxicated, maintain a patent airway. Consider the side-lying position and oral suctioning if you think it will be possible to aspirate oral secretions or vomiting. If swallowing is intact, elevate the head of the bed at least 30 degrees to encourage better air exchange. Administration of intravenous (IV) fluids is possible to correct the patient's fluids and electrolyte balance. Monitor the IV site often, especially if the patient is restless. Institute your facility's seizure precautions, such as padded side rails, floor pads, and moving patient to a room close to the nurse's station.

The practitioner will usually treat tremors, nervousness, and restlessness with drugs such as chlordiazepoxide (Librium) or naltrexone (ReVia). Give scheduled doses on time. Reduce environmental stimuli. Allow the patient to ambulate or do whatever will help ease nervousness, but encourage the patient to refrain from overexertion. Attend the patient while ambulating if he or she is unsteady from coordination disturbance or lack of conditioning. As weakness subsides, include a regular exercise regimen in the care plan (Nursing Care Plan 36-1).

Cardiorespiratory distress is a possible result of stimulant abuse. The health care provider will sometimes prescribe beta-adrenergic agents such as propranolol (Inderal) and calcium blockers such as nifedepine (Procardia) and oxygen. Continuous cardiac monitoring and frequent checks on vital signs with respiratory assessment will help you detect any adverse changes early, before they have the chance to become life threatening.

Keep explanations simple, and speak in a calm voice. Plan for patient verbalization. Use therapeutic conversation techniques to assist the patient to understand himself or herself (self-realization). Reinforce teaching about the disease concept of addiction. Confront denial in a nonjudgmental manner. Encourage the family to participate in planning for sobriety. Counselors will sometimes initiate individual therapy to assist the patient into the rehabilitation phase of recovery.

If the patient is extremely restless, the physician will sometimes order magnesium sulfate to raise the seizure threshold or another anticonvulsant medication such as phenytoin (Dilantin). High doses of chlordiazepoxide have potential to cause urinary retention. Intake and output measurements will be appropriate in some cases.

Disorientation is possible, especially at night. Nightlights in the room and frequent nurse visits tend to help. If the patient is not able to sleep at night, have him or her sit up and have a snack; then give a back rub and encourage the patient to rest. Notify your supervisor if the patient appears fearful or panicky and unable to reacquire orientation to reality. Check vital signs (including temperature) before notifying the physician. Physical restraints have potential to escalate aggressive behavior but are sometimes necessary if the patient poses a risk for harm to self or others.

Often the patient is malnourished and is suffering from loss of appetite. Good food is good medicine. If the patient is not able to eat very much, find out favorite foods and provide them with snacks between meals. Administration of multivitamins and thiamine as ordered help the patient improve his or her nutritional state.

Nursing Care Plan 36-1 The Patient Who Abuses Alcohol

Jonathan, 56 years of age, has worked as an executive in a corporation. His employer confronted him about his increasing tendency to call in sick, last-minute rescheduling of meetings, and excessive alcohol use during luncheon meetings. Later, after the confrontation, the police cited him for driving while intoxicated for the third time and put him in jail. Sentencing included the requirement to complete a treatment program for alcoholism.

NURSING DIAGNOSIS ***Ineffective denial, related to inability to admit being an alcoholic***

Patient Goals and Expected Outcomes	Nursing Interventions	Rationale
Participate in program Identify negative effects of drinking on others Abstain from alcohol use Express acceptance of alcoholism as a disease Express acceptance of responsibility for own behavior Maintain abstinence after discharge	Confront the patient's denial by relating incidents and problems to its use. Reinforce teaching about the disease of alcoholism. Encourage the patient to identify behaviors that have caused problems in his or her life. Do not allow the patient to rationalize or blame others.	It is necessary to address the problem of alcoholism first. Providing knowledge about the disease and having the patient identify the relationship between alcohol and his or her problems will help the patient overcome denial. Blaming others is an excuse to continue drinking behavior.

NURSING DIAGNOSIS ***Ineffective coping, related to abnormal use of alcohol***

Patient Goals and Expected Outcomes	Nursing Interventions	Rationale
Express feelings directly and express anger or hostility outward in a safe manner Practice nonchemical alternatives to dealing with stress or difficult situations Verbalize increased self-esteem	Encourage the patient to explore alternative ways of dealing with a stressful situation. Involve the patient in a group to provide confrontation, positive feedback, and sharing of feelings. Avoid discussion of unanswerable questions, such as why he or she drinks.	Patient perhaps has minimal experience of dealing with stress without alcohol. Groups of peers are honest and supportive. Asking why when there is no answer is dwelling on the negative and in the past. Focus on positive and the future, where change has the power to make a difference.

Critical Thinking Questions

1. During Jonathan's assessment, the nurse notes that he has tremors, is agitated, and verbalizes visual hallucinations. What therapeutic interventions are appropriate to perform to prevent injury to the patient?
2. As Jonathan's physical condition improves, he discloses his hopelessness and lack of desire to continue living. What is an appropriate response by the nurse?
3. During group therapy, Jonathan states, "Now that I am physically better, I know I will be able to stop drinking. I don't need any help. There really isn't anything wrong with me." What is the appropriate staff intervention at this time?

REHABILITATION

After detoxification, the acute phase of recovery, it is time to start rehabilitation. The object of treatment is to assist the patient to abstain from substance abuse. Because there is no cure, abstinence is the practical equivalent to the control of the disease. Administration of disulfiram (Antabuse) is sometimes a way to encourage abstinence. It causes facial flushing, nausea, tachycardia, dyspnea, dizziness, and confusion when the patient consumes alcohol. The purpose is to reduce alcohol consumption by aversion. Treatment programs often include family in part of the treatment plan. These programs are sometimes inpatient programs, and sometimes outpatient or day-treatment programs.

Group Therapy

Group therapy is an often-used treatment modality. **Group therapy** provides a caring, emotionally supportive atmosphere where the patient is able to see the relationship of substance abuse and negative consequences in his or her life. The group tends to point out negative defense mechanisms such as denial or displacement and offer possible solutions to its members. Encourage families to attend support groups to help the patient and family to grow together, not apart. Group therapy sometimes continues after completion of an inpatient program. Group therapy is an important part of all recovery programs.

Alcoholics Anonymous

Alcoholics Anonymous (AA) is an international nonprofit organization that began in 1935 that consists of abstinent alcoholics helping other alcoholics to become and stay sober through group support, shared experiences, and faith in a power greater than themselves. There are regular meetings in most communities. You will often find listings of local AA chapters in the telephone book. The foundation of AA is a 12-step program that assists the dependent person in admitting powerlessness over alcohol (Box 36-2). Other groups have followed up on the success of AA, usually using similar models for rehabilitation; these groups include Overeaters Anonymous, Al-Anon, and Narcotics Anonymous.

Treatment Centers

Residential treatment centers provide the opportunity for detoxification. There is no direct medical intervention; instead, trained nurses provide close physical monitoring with the assistance of counselors and recovered peers. After detoxification, the patient enters a drug- and alcohol-free residence. A primary goal of this type of treatment is the rebuilding of social skills that do not involve drug use as the primary method of interaction. The length of the stay in a treatment center ranges from 1 to 6 months; most centers operate on an ability-to-pay basis, with some governmental funding.

Pain Management

Pain management sometimes involves the use of addicting substances, which sometimes complicates pain management for an addicted person. The medical community has greatly improved the regimen options for effective pain management using combinations of nonopioid, opioid, and antianxiety agents along with nonchemical interventions. Nursing interventions require not only careful assessment of pain but also observation for developing patterns of drug-seeking behavior that indicate the patient's tolerance or addiction to the drug. Encouraging the patient to practice and use nonchemical interventions to ease pain will reduce the risk of chemical dependency for relief (Box 36-3).

Box 36-2 Twelve Steps of Alcoholics Anonymous

1. We admitted we were powerless over alcohol—that our lives had become unmanageable.
2. Came to believe that a Power greater than ourselves could restore us to sanity.
3. Made a decision to turn our will and our lives over to the care of God *as we understood Him.*
4. Made a searching and fearless moral inventory of ourselves.
5. Admitted to God, to ourselves, and to another human being the exact nature of our wrongs.
6. Were entirely ready to have God remove all these defects of character.
7. Humbly asked Him to remove our shortcomings.
8. Made a list of all persons we had harmed, and became willing to make amends to them all.
9. Made direct amends to such people wherever possible, except when to do so would injure them or others.
10. Continued to take personal inventory and when we were wrong promptly admitted it.
11. Sought through prayer and meditation to improve our conscious contact with God *as we understood Him,* praying only for knowledge of His will for us and the power to carry that out.
12. Having had a spiritual awakening as a result of these steps, we tried to carry this message to alcoholics, and to practice these principles in all our affairs.

From Alcoholics Anonymous. (2001). *Alcoholics anonymous.* (4th ed.). New York: Alcoholics World Services, Inc.

Box 36-3 Addiction Issues to Consider

The medical community is overcoming its fear of addiction and starting to provide adequate pain management for acute and chronic pain conditions.

- Postoperative care using opioids in patient-controlled administration devices has shown that both opioid need and the severity of pain decrease. The patient is often using nonopioid medications for pain control by the third postoperative day. No development of tolerance or addiction occurs. However, the patient sometimes suffers undue fears of addiction when told that opioids will be used to control postoperative pain. Explanation of the pain management regimen usually helps allay the patient's fears of addiction. Encouraging the patient to use the self-medication before activities will help the patient heal more quickly.
- Chronic pain management involves more than just a pill to relieve pain. It is very important to use imagery, physical therapy, and other methods to help the patient relieve pain without chemical intervention. Side effects of high doses of NSAIDs* are not tolerated by some patients; in such cases, it is possible to use narcotics to control pain. Although opioid addiction is always a possibility, the physician will sometimes consider opioids to be cheaper and more effective than treating the serious side effects of high-dose NSAID therapy. If the patient is dying, addiction to opioid agents is not an issue, but close monitoring is necessary to avoid acute overdose.
- Acute pain management for addicts presents a challenge to the health care team. Accidents and surgery are usually the cause of the acute pain. Circumstances around an injury will sometimes trigger withdrawal symptoms within 24 hours of admission to an acute care facility. Most often, the physician orders medications to relieve pain and suppress withdrawal symptoms. Cross-tolerance and multisubstance abuse require you to carefully consider minor changes in the patient's condition. In the plan of care, discuss referral for rehabilitation, and the initial steps of rehabilitation will in some cases be part of the patient's acute phase of recovery.

*Nonsteroidal antiinflammatory drugs. This classification includes aspirin, ibuprofen, naproxen, and other drugs.

DRUG ABUSE

Although you will see alcohol abuse more frequently in patients fighting addiction or who you are helping to treat for another health problem, drug abuse is also rearing its ugly head in the health care setting. Many people think only of illegal drugs when drug abuse is mentioned. However, abuse of prescription and over-the-counter drugs is common. Older adults sometimes trade or share prescription drugs. Rationalizations such as, "If it worked for me, it will for my friend," and, "If one pill works, two pills will work better," often serve to deny or justify misuse or abuse of many prescription and over-the-counter drugs.

When a person takes drugs for other than medical reasons or in a higher-than-recommended dosage, we call this drug misuse or abuse. **Club drugs** refer to those drugs people frequently take for euphoric effect at parties, concerts, dance clubs, or all-night **raves** or "trances." Club drugs are often street drugs. **Street drugs** are substances that users buy from illegal drug dealers. Either they come from illegal manufacturers without strict controls, are illegally obtained prescription drugs, or are not approved for use in the United States. Chronic abuse has the potential to lead to psychological and/or physical dependence. Many commonly abused drugs act on the limbic system of the brain and potentially cause permanent damage to that area (Figure 36-1; Box 36-4). Commonly abused drugs this chapter discusses are depressants, opioids, stimulants, hallucinogens, cannabis, and inhalants (Box 36-5).

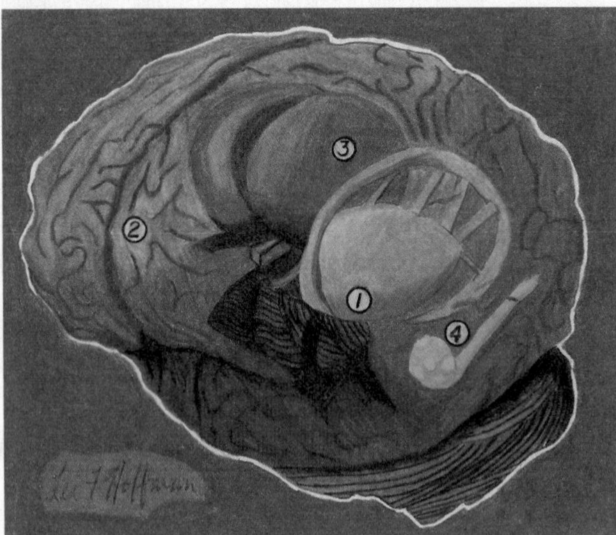

1-Nucleus Accumbens
- Most primitive brain center
- Location for drives for hunger, thirst, lust, and pleasure

2-Frontal Cortex
- Stores memory
- Makes judgments
- Controls impulses
- Encodes memory of pleasure experiences

3-Basal Ganglia
- Controls movement and repetitive tasks
- Obsessive/compulsive behaviors

4-Amygdala
- Triggers body response to stress

FIGURE 36-1 Limbic system. The limbic system is considered to be the emotional center of the brain. An emotional response to an incoming stimulus is produced and then stored in memory.

DEPRESSANTS

CNS **depressants** include alcohol, sedative-hypnotic medications, and opioid analgesics. The sedative-hypnotic medications most often abused include barbiturates and benzodiazepines (minor tranquilizers). People usually take them orally in tablet or capsule form. Box 36-6 lists the effects of depressants.

Barbiturates entered into medical use in the beginning of the twentieth century; they are useful in the clinical context for their sedative, hypnotic, anesthetic, and anticonvulsant effects. Problematic side effects include respiratory depression, rapid tolerance, and dependency, with untoward effects (e.g., seizures or status epilepticus) accompanying sudden withdrawal. In the 1960s, benzodiazepines became popular as a safer alternative to barbiturates. Flurazepam (Dalmane) and

Box 36-4 The Limbic System of the Brain

These structures, which some refer to as the limbic lobe, are involved in feeding, defense, reproduction, emotional responses, and the consolidation and retention of memory. The limbic lobe is not a separate structure; rather, it comprises border areas of the frontal, the parietal, and the temporal lobes with inner brain structures around the ventricles. Structures included are basal ganglia, amygdala, hippocampus, thalamus, hypothalamus, nucleus accumbens, cerebral cortex, olfactory cortex, and connecting nerve tracts.

Box 36-5 Commonly Abused Drugs and Their Street Names*

Amphetamines: Speed, truck driver, copilot, black beauties, crank, go
Barbiturates: Reds, blues, yellow jackets, rainbows, bluies
Benzodiazepines: Downers, chill pill, vitamin V
Chloral hydrate: Mickey Finn, mickey
Cocaine: Snow, crack, blow, coke, nose candy, toot, white dust, toot sweet
GHB: Soap, easy lay, Georgia homeboy, liquid ecstasy
Heroin: H, smack, scag, junk, caca
Ketamine: Special K, vitamin K
Lysergic acid diethylamide: LSD, acid, windowpane, gelcap, microdots, blotter, purple haze
Marijuana: Pot, reefer, grass, dope, weed, green, cannabis, Jamaican, Acapulco gold
Methamphetamine: Speed, crystal, ice
MDMA: Ecstasy, E, XTC, hug, love bug, beans, Adam
Nitrous oxide: Nitrous, whippets
PCP: Angel dust, rocket fuel, wack, ozone
Psilocybin: Shroom, magic mushroom
Rohypnol: Roofies, rough, rope, roach

GHB, Gamma-hydroxybutyrate; *MDMA*, 3,4-methylenedioxymethamphetamine; *PCP*, phencyclidine.
*Street names are usually regional and often change as slang language changes.

Box 36-6 Signs and Symptoms of Central Nervous System Depressants

- Decreased respirations
- Passiveness, listlessness
- Heaviness in extremities
- Pinpoint pupils (opioid effect)
- Reduced hunger or thirst
- Reduced sexual drive
- Memory loss
- Slurred speech
- Nausea and vomiting
- Ataxic gait (staggering)
- "Nod state"

chlordiazepoxide (Librium) were the first in this group, and diazepam (Valium) quickly followed them.

Valium soon became the most frequently prescribed antianxiety agent. The effects of addiction and overdose with benzodiazepines were not apparent at first, but by 1981, Valium dropped to the sixth most prescribed drug in the United States. In the 1990s, alprazolam (Xanax) was the most frequently prescribed benzodiazepine for treatment of acute anxiety (ASAM, 2009).

Another benzodiazepine that gained notoriety in the 1990s was flunitrazepam (Rohypnol). Perpetrators of sexual assault have frequently misused this drug, and people thus sometimes refer to it as a "date-rape drug." It is easy to mix it stealthily into an alcoholic drink, and then the victim consumes it unknowingly. Its effects include muscle relaxation and amnesia. Alcohol increases these effects; the two together are sometimes a lethal combination. Rohypnol is not legal for use in the United States.

Some people in the United States have abused GHB (gamma-hydroxybutyrate) for its euphoric, sedative, and bodybuilding (anabolic) effects. Its abuse as a synthetic steroid is common at fitness centers and gyms. As with Rohypnol, GHB has been associated with club drug use and sexual assault. Both Rohypnol and GHB are odorless, tasteless, and colorless. They are easy to mix with drinks and quickly cause unconsciousness. These drugs also rapidly cause relaxation of voluntary muscles and also potentially cause the victim to have long-term amnesia for events occurring while under the effect of the drug.

OPIOID ANALGESICS

Opioid analgesics are those drugs made from the opium poppy. Hippocrates sang the praises of the poppy's magical pain-relieving properties. During the sixteenth century, laudanum, an opium compound, was the most popular medication in Europe. Today heroin is the most widely abused opioid (opiate). There are an estimated 400,000 to 600,000 heroin addicts in the United States (Ries et al., 2009). Heroin is a schedule I drug that has no medical use. People take heroin by snorting, smoking, or injecting it into a vein. Morphine and its synthetic derivatives are schedule II drugs. They are possible to take orally or inject. Opioids replace natural endorphins in the CNS, which makes these drugs highly addictive. Besides being excellent pain suppressants, opioids act as cough suppressants, slow peristalsis in the gut, and mildly contract the bladder. Tolerance develops rapidly, but abstinence reverses tolerance. Cross-tolerance with other opioids is possible. Three general types of opioid abusers are (1) street abusers who get opioids illegally, (2) abusers of opioids from medical sources (prescription opioids), and (3) methadone abusers. Nurses often deal with people in the second group, who are predominantly middle-class older adults, health care professionals, women, and those with chronic pain syndrome.

Symptoms of acute opioid overdose include severe respiratory depression, pinpoint pupils, and stupor or coma. Aspiration is possible. Treatment involves supporting ventilation and administering naloxone (Narcan) as prescribed. The health care provider will sometimes prescribe clonidine (Catapres) to help reduce withdrawal symptoms. It is important to continue monitoring for recurrent toxic symptoms when naloxone is discontinued.

Morphine and heroin addicts who consume huge amounts typically begin with predictable withdrawal signs and symptoms approximately 6 hours after the last dose. Withdrawal symptoms include flulike signs and symptoms and body aches, watery eyes and runny nose, dilated pupils, vomiting, cramps and diarrhea, diaphoresis, tachycardia, hypertension, and chills and fever. The term "cold turkey" comes from the gooseflesh that is common during withdrawal. Intensity of signs and symptoms usually peaks in 2 to 3 days. Signs and symptoms subside within 5 to 10 days.

Methadone (Dolophine) is a synthetic opioid that helps suppress withdrawal symptoms in the morphine or heroin addict. Once the patient's condition stabilizes, the methadone dosage decreases daily until the addict is methadone free. Levo-alpha-acetylmethadol or LAAM (Orlaam) is a long-acting compound of methadone; it has been associated with better outcomes than has methadone. Methadone itself is sometimes a drug of abuse for former heroin addicts. Success of any cessation program depends on the motivation of the user.

STIMULANTS

CNS stimulants include a wide variety of substances. The category ranges from caffeine (the most widely consumed substance in the world) to cocaine and amphetamines. Box 36-7 lists the effects of stimulants.

Caffeine

Caffeine is present in foods and over-the-counter medications such as cold and sinus medications and appe-

Box 36-7 Signs and Symptoms of Central Nervous System Stimulants

- Mental alertness
- Insomnia
- Increased concentration
- Delirium and hallucinations
- Drug-induced psychosis
- Euphoria
- Elation
- Anxiety and paranoia
- Hostility and anger
- Anorexia
- Dilated pupils
- Bruxism (grinding of teeth)
- Tachycardia
- Peripheral vasoconstriction
- Hypertension
- Bronchodilation
- Hyperreflexia
- Twitching and tremors
- Nausea
- Diarrhea

tite suppressants. It is chemically related to theophylline, which is useful in the treatment of chronic obstructive pulmonary disease (COPD). Stimulant effects of caffeine are usually mild and typically last 5 to 7 hours after consumption. Habitual use of five to seven cups of caffeinated beverages per day has the capacity to cause withdrawal symptoms of headache, fatigue, and irritability. Coffee, tea, chocolate, and soft drinks are commonly consumed foods that contain moderate to large concentrations of caffeine. Caffeine will potentially aggravate anxiety disorders and schizophrenia as well as heart conditions.

Nicotine

Nicotine is a drug present in tobacco. Tobacco use is a legally sanctioned form of substance abuse. The number of Americans who smoke is declining, but the number of women smokers and underage smokers is rising. The effects of nicotine include increased alertness and concentration, appetite suppression, and vasoconstriction. Heavy or persistent smokers quickly develop tolerance and dependence. Smokers sometimes switch to smokeless, oral forms of tobacco (snuff or chew) to reduce hazards from smoke. If heavy users stop suddenly, withdrawal symptoms occur that include craving, irritability, restlessness, impatience, hostility, anxiety, confusion, difficulty in concentration, disturbed sleep, increased appetite, and decreased heart rate. Treatment for nicotine dependence includes use of agents that deliver decreasing doses of nicotine. These agents include nicotine gum, transdermal patches, or nasal spray; agents that block the reinforcing effect of smoking; an antidepressant, bupropion (Zyban); and combinations thereof. Behavioral therapy is also often beneficial in remaining smoke free. As many as 70% of people who quit smoking relapse within 1 year.

Cocaine

Cocaine is a white powder that is used as a topical, local, and regional anesthetic and as a vasoconstrictor for some types of surgery of the eye, the ear, the nose, and the throat. Crack cocaine is an inexpensive form of cocaine mixed with baking soda. Freebasing is a method of extracting cocaine. Drug abusers often smoke crack cocaine and freebase cocaine. To take powder cocaine, they make it into lines and snort it. Cocaine is possible to take intravenously. The rush is within 30 seconds but the effect is very short lived. The crash following the rush brings on intense craving, agitation, and moderate to severe depression. Crack cocaine addiction occurs rapidly. The cravings have the potential to persist months into abstinence, making treatment difficult. The use of powder and crack cocaine became epidemic in the 1980s and 1990s.

Cocaine is a strong CNS stimulant. Chronic abuse erodes the nasal septum and often causes sinusitis and rhinitis. Smoking freebase cocaine poses the risk of bodily injury from burns, and the caustic chemicals that people use to make it sometimes cause hemoptysis and pneumonitis. Overdose potentially produces cardiorespiratory distress and seizures. It is best to hospitalize the user to stabilize heart abnormalities and protect from suicide if profound depression occurs. Health care providers have used dopaminergic drugs such as amantadine (Symmetrel) and bromocriptine (Parlodel), which serve in the treatment of Parkinson's disease, to reduce the craving. If psychotic symptoms do not resolve in 3 days, it is appropriate to start conventional treatment. Neonates of addicted mothers ("crack babies") need close monitoring for complications. Swaddling or wrapping the baby snugly is often comforting; keep stimuli such as bright lights, loud noises, and excessive handling to a minimum.

Amphetamines

Amphetamines and their analogs (e.g., methylphenidate [Ritalin]) gained popularity as club drugs in the 1990s. Amphetamine is a powder that is possible to snort, smoke, or inject. People often mix it with other drugs such as heroin or marijuana. Methamphetamine is a potent, addictive amphetamine that causes powerful release of the neurotransmitter dopamine. Over time, dopamine depletion in the brain has the capacity to cause parkinsonian-like symptoms. Brain cell damage is sometimes permanent. CNS stimulation is so strong that hallucinations and paranoia are possible. Weight loss and malnutrition from the anorexia effect are sometimes severe. Overstimulation of the heart will sometimes raise blood pressure, which potentially causes damage to blood vessels, leading to heart attack or stroke. Brain damage at the cellular level and sudden death have occurred with amphetamine use. Treatment for withdrawal corresponds to the severity of the symptoms. Chronic abusers typically exhibit flat affect, forgetfulness, and difficulty in concentration due to irreversible brain damage after completing detoxification.

HALLUCINOGENS

Hallucinogens, which are either natural or synthetic, affect several areas of the brain. These drugs alter perception and thinking, and some of their effects sometimes last 6 to 12 hours. Deaths have occurred due to altered perceptions that have potential to trigger the fight-or-flight response, which then leads to possible cardiac arrest or dangerously altered thinking, such as having the ability to fly from the roof into the clouds.

Drugs in this group are phencyclidine (PCP); lysergic acid diethylamide (LSD); 3,4-methylenedioxymethamphetamine (MDMA), known as Ecstasy, and its parent drug, methylenedioxyamphetamine (MDA); ketamine; mescaline; and psilocybin.

PCP

PCP came onto the street scene in the 1960s and quickly gained a reputation of causing bad drug reactions. Experts consider it addictive with regular use. In low to moderate doses, symptoms of generalized numbness and poor coordination occur. Flushing and sweating occur with a rise in blood pressure and pulse. Some users report feelings of increased strength and power. Overdoses of PCP sometimes become apparent through symptoms of schizophrenia-like psychosis with extreme violence or attempted suicide. Seizures and coma are possible. At high doses, a drop in respirations, pulse, and blood pressure accompanies loss of balance, blurred vision, nausea, and vomiting. PCP is a powder that easily dissolves in water or alcohol; users often sprinkle it in other drugs such as marijuana. Some people take it without knowing, unaware that PCP is mixed into another street drug.

LSD

LSD also came onto the street scene in the 1960s. It is one of the most potent of the hallucinogens. Because its effects potentially last more than 12 hours, an LSD experience is referred to as a "trip." Dilation of pupils, sweating, loss of appetite, dry mouth, sleeplessness, and tremors occur. Crossover of sensory perception such as "hearing colors" and "seeing sounds" occurs. Altered perceptions such as melting walls and fear of insanity and death sometimes trigger panic attacks. Flashback of symptoms is possible, suddenly within a few days or more than a year after LSD use. These flashbacks usually occur in chronic users. Risks of LSD use include flashbacks, bad "trips," lingering mental disorders such as severe depression and schizophrenia, and general impairment of mental function. LSD does not produce compulsive drug-seeking behavior, and experts consider it nonaddictive.

MDMA (Ecstasy)

MDMA, also known as Ecstasy, has been a very popular club drug since the 1980s, with a reported increase in use from 40.1% in 1999 to 51.4% in 2000 (ASAM, 2009). It is considered a hallucinogenic stimulant that is neurotoxic, causing release of the neurotransmitter serotonin until it is depleted in the brain cells (Figure 36-2). Because serotonin is involved with regulating mood, aggression, sex drive, sleep, and pain perception, there are many risks of lingering problems. Normal growth and development are altered in adolescents.

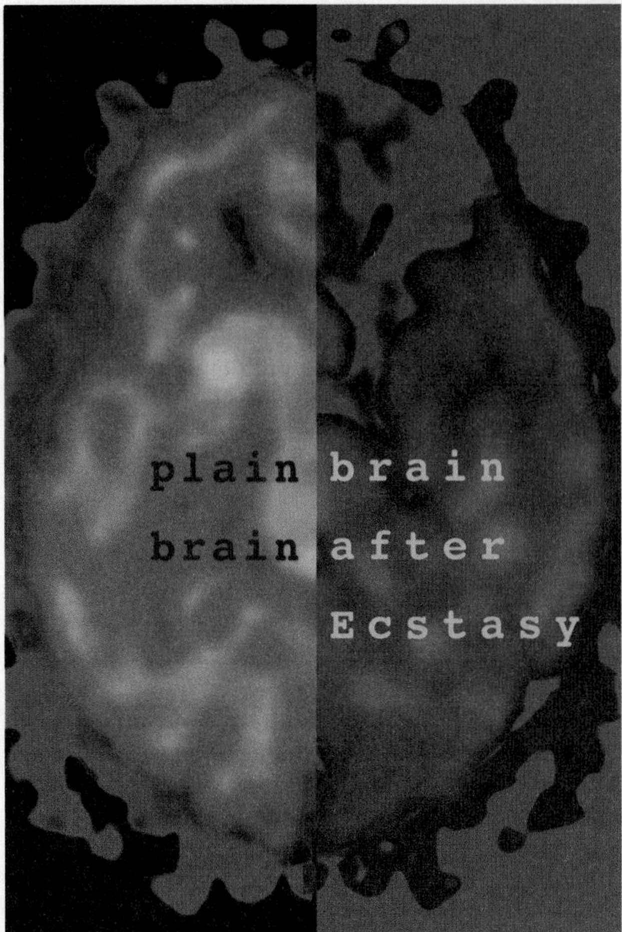

FIGURE 36-2 These brain scans show the sharp difference in human brain function for an individual who has never used drugs and one who has used the club drug Ecstasy (MDMA) many times, but has not used any drugs for at least 3 weeks before having the scan. The left, bright-reddish half shows active serotonin sites in the brain. The dark sections in the right half are serotonin sites that are not present even after 3 weeks without any drugs. In addition to these changes in serotonin sites, Ecstasy injures serotonin neurons. Although these have the capacity to regrow, they do not grow back normally and sometimes not in the right location.

MDMA produces physical symptoms of muscle tension, **bruxism** (grinding of the teeth), nausea, blurred vision, chilling or sweating, and faintness. In high doses, it has the potential to trigger malignant hyperthermia, which leads to kidney and heart failure. MDMA gives the user a feeling of euphoria, like being in love. Many people use baby pacifiers to ease the teeth-grinding effect. Heat exhaustion occurs due to physical exertion (movement eases muscle tension) and excess fluid loss. Drug effects potentially last 6 hours or longer. Users report drug craving as well as lasting psychological difficulties such as confusion, sleep disturbance, poor concentration, and anxiety.

MDMA's parent drug, MDA, has properties similar to those of MDMA and is related to the amphetamine group. Lingering parkinsonian-like tremor has been reported with regular use of this drug.

Ketamine

Ketamine is an anesthetic drug the FDA has approved for human and veterinary use. Most ketamine that people sell legally in the United States is intended for veterinary use. Ketamine users either snort or inject it. It produces a dreamlike state with hallucinations. At higher doses, amnesia, impaired motor function, and delirium are possible. Some people use it as a date-rape drug. Fatal respiratory problems have occurred. Emergency departments in the country's larger cities have reported increased use among youth during the past 5 years (ASAM, 2009).

Mescaline and Psilocybin

Mescaline and psilocybin are naturally occurring hallucinogens. Mescaline is derived from peyote cactus. When dried, the round cactus looks like a button. Descendants of the Apache American Indian tribe won the legal right to continue peyote use in their religious ceremonies. Psilocybin comes from a mushroom. Both produce the same types of hallucinations and side effects of LSD but are not as long lasting as LSD. The general lack of availability has made the abuse potentials of these drugs low.

CANNABIS

People have used **cannabis** or marijuana for thousands of years. Its first descriptions are in Chinese writings of 2700 BC. No other drug has evoked so much controversy over the appropriateness of legalizing and using it for medical purposes. Marijuana remains a schedule I drug because of its high abuse and addiction potential in the absence of proven medical use. Evaluation for therapeutic use as an analgesic, antiemetic for chemotherapy, tranquilizer, glaucoma medication, and antispasmodic for multiple sclerosis victims shows only fair results. Some county governments in Western states are challenging the federal law by allowing county law to regulate medical use.

Marijuana and hemp are common names for the herb *Cannabis sativa*. Hashish is the concentrated resin from the plant. THC (delta-9-tetrahydrocannabinol) is the main active ingredient present in marijuana. Users usually smoke marijuana in a cigarette (or "joint" or "nail") or in a pipe (or "bong"). It is possible to eat marijuana in foods such as brownies for a longer-lasting effect. Physical effects are short lived, but THC does potentially accumulate in the body because of its fat solubility. THC will sometimes remain in the body up to a month or longer after last use, allowing the person to test positive for this illegal drug for a long time.

Effects of marijuana include distorted perception; difficulty in problem solving, memory, and learning; euphoria; uncontrolled laughter; dreamy or sleepy affect, an effect that has earned the nickname being "stoned"; anxiety and panic attacks; dry mouth and dry eyes; increased sexual interest; loss of coordination; and increased heart rate.

Chronic abusers sometimes have some long-lasting effects. Some physical effects include stuffy nose, bronchitis and asthma, lung cancer, abnormal sleeping and eating patterns, decreased testosterone and sperm count, and decreased immune function. Accidents occur because of altered perception and judgment. Some observers report craving and drug-seeking behavior. Psychological effects include panic reactions, hallucinations, and delusions from acute toxicity; organic brain syndrome; and amotivational cannabis syndrome.

Characteristics of **amotivational cannabis syndrome** are decreased goal-directed activities, abrupt mood swings, abnormal irritability and hostility, apathy, and decline of personal grooming. Depression, paranoia, and suicidal thoughts or attempts are possible. Abstinence reverses this syndrome.

Research on marijuana use among people 18 years of age and younger has shown a trend of lower achievement than in nonusers, more acceptance of deviant and delinquent behavior, poorer relationships with parents, and greater rebelliousness. Some 50% of twelfth-graders have tried marijuana. Many continue to use marijuana into adulthood. It remains the most commonly used illicit drug in the United States.

Like alcohol, experts consider marijuana a gateway drug. Many drug abusers have reported starting with marijuana. Each year, more people enter treatment centers for their primary addiction to marijuana. Some people report withdrawal symptoms, suggesting that physical dependence as well as psychological dependence is possible.

INHALANTS

Inhalants are volatile chemicals that have the capacity to alter thinking and feeling when people inhale them. This group includes solvents, glues, aerosols, refrigerants, and anesthetic gases. Use of inhalants during religious rites and healing ceremonies dates back to ancient Egypt. Today, inhalants are favorite drugs of abuse among young people between the ages of 14 and 17. Inhalants serve, in some cases, as gateway drugs to more dangerous drug abuse.

In the 1960s, the number of reports of abuse using model airplane glue, lighter fluid, and cleaning fluids grew rapidly. The federal government banned the use of carbon tetrachloride after reports attributed a number of deaths to it and benzene. Use of inhalants has tapered off. Rates of use are higher among minorities such as Mexican Americans and American Indians. Men are more likely to abuse than women. Users in a group setting sometimes put solvents onto a cloth or into a paper or plastic bag and pass it around; they sometimes call this **huffing.** Effects are short lived and include a euphoric or intoxicated feeling, auditory hallucinations, feeling weightless or floating on air, ataxia, slurred speech, wheezing, cough, photophobia, irregular heartbeat, anorexia, and nausea. High doses pose the risk of respiratory arrest and irreversible damage to the brain, kidneys, or other organs. Most fatalities have occurred with butane, adhesive solvents, and cleaning fluid solvents containing toluene and other halogenated hydrocarbons.

Some people used anesthetic gases, chloroform, and ether as anesthetics and parlor entertainment until less flammable gases gained notoriety. Nitrous oxide (laughing gas), which dentists use today, is available as a street drug and in balloons at outdoor festival activities. After inhalation, its effects last only a few minutes. "Whippets" are nitrous oxide cartridges for commercial use. Amyl nitrate and butyl nitrate ("poppers"), whose proper use is to treat heart disease, are cloth-covered ampules that a user has to break and inhale.

Most inhalants do not show up in a routine drug screen, but chronic users sometimes develop organic brain disorders, general myalgia and neuritis, mood disorders, and cognitive impairment. Liver and kidney failure are possible results of chronic exposure to inhalants (Table 36-5).

Table 36-5 Acute Intoxication and Withdrawal of Psychoactive Substances

SIGNS AND SYMPTOMS	TREATMENT	WITHDRAWAL SYMPTOMS
ALCOHOL		
Behavior dependent upon blood serum levels: slurred speech; ataxia; blurred vision; decreased level of consciousness; possible nausea, vomiting, and diarrhea; loss of consciousness and respiratory depression with high levels	Maintain ventilation. Side-lying position if unconscious. Monitor vital signs every 30-60 minutes until stable. Check emesis and stool for occult blood. Offer fluids and small bland foods when swallowing ability is intact. Allow up as tolerated, but avoid overexertion. Give thiamine as ordered; possible to give IM or IV initially, then daily orally. Give sedative as ordered for tremor and restlessness; watch for urine retention with high dosage of chlordiazepoxide (Librium); physician sometimes orders naltrexone (ReVia). Seizure medications such as phenytoin (Dilantin) or magnesium sulfate possible to give if indicated. Provide teaching of health risks. Encourage to seek a recovery program such as AA.	Mild to severe tremors of the hands, jaw, torso Restlessness, pacing Illogical thinking Demanding, drug craving Manipulating Diaphoresis Chain smoking Visual and auditory hallucinations Confusion If unable to reorient, appears panicked, and temperature is elevated, suspect DTs
CNS DEPRESSANTS		
Relaxation to sleepiness to coma, depressed vital signs, pinpoint pupils, respiratory depression Includes barbiturates, benzodiazepines, narcotics	Lavage if recent ingestion. Maintain ventilation. Side-lying position if unconscious. Monitor vital signs every 15-30 minutes until stable. Administer drugs as ordered for cardiac dysrhythmias. Barbiturates necessary to wean down in decreasing dosages to reduce risk of status epilepticus. Methadone or LAAM possible to start for maintenance therapy. Clonidine possible to give for opioid withdrawal as well as naltrexone (ReVia). Provide teaching concerning health risks. Encourage to seek a recovery program.	Opioids: restlessness, yawning, lacrimation, diaphoresis, rhinorrhea, anorexia, abdominal cramping, body ache, tremors, gooseflesh, insomnia, drug craving, possible seizures with barbiturates, symptoms like DTs

AA, Alcoholics Anonymous; *DTs*, delirium tremens; *IM*, intramuscular (route); *IV*, intravenous (route); *LAAM*, levo-alpha-acetylmethadol.

Continued

Table 36-5 Acute Intoxication and Withdrawal of Psychoactive Substances—cont'd

SIGNS AND SYMPTOMS	TREATMENT	WITHDRAWAL SYMPTOMS
CNS STIMULANTS		
Elevated vital signs, cardiac dysrhythmias, flushing or pallor, agitation, paranoia, fever, convulsions, cardiac arrest Includes cocaine, amphetamines, MDMA effects	Monitor vital signs. Provide a quiet environment. Reorient to reality. Encourage fluids and nutrition. Give cardiac drugs as ordered; beta blockers (Inderal) and calcium channel blockers (Procardia) possible to administer for dysrhythmias. Amantadine (Symmetrel) and other antiparkinsonian drugs possible to give to reduce cocaine craving. Provide teaching concerning health risks. Encourage to seek a recovery program.	Mild withdrawal: apathy, somnolence, fatigue, irritability, depression Severe withdrawal: drug craving, "crashing," depression, paranoia, suicidal ideation, tachycardia, heart failure, malnutrition
HALLUCINOGENS		
Strong psychological effects; emotional lability (laughing or crying); acute panic attacks; acute psychosis from a "bad trip"; "flashback" episodes Includes LSD, PCP, ketamine, MDMA	Provide a quiet supportive environment. Remind patient that experience from drug will subside when the drug is out of the body. Monitor vital signs routinely. Physician sometimes orders an antianxiety drug for severe anxiety or agitation. Encourage fluids. Provide teaching concerning the health risks and possible permanent damage.	No evidence of withdrawal symptoms
CANNABIS		
Mild anxiety to panic attacks, emotional lability, appetite stimulant, dilated pupils, dry mouth, dry eyes, drowsiness	Provide supportive environment. Give antianxiety medication as ordered for agitation. Provide teaching concerning health risks and amotivational cannabis syndrome.	Mild withdrawal symptoms: drug craving, irritability, anorexia, insomnia
INHALANTS		
Usually short-acting effects, euphoria, intoxication	Usually chronic use impairs cardiopulmonary function as well as hepatic and renal failure. Provide teaching concerning health risks (e.g., plastic bags lead to possible suffocation death).	No withdrawal symptoms; drug craving by chronic users noted

CNS, Central nervous system; *LSD,* lysergic acid diethylamide; *MDMA,* 3,4-methylenedioxymethamphetamine; *PCP,* phencyclidine.

CHEMICALLY IMPAIRED NURSES

In 1982, the American Nurses Association (ANA) adopted a policy that recommends offering treatment to chemically impaired nurses before taking disciplinary action. Today, according to the National Council of State Boards of Nursing (2000), 37 states have programs that offer chemically impaired nurses the option to receive treatment and rehabilitation in order to keep their license.

Nurses are as vulnerable as the general public to substance abuse and addiction. Denial by the abuser as well as colleagues is very strong. Many of the same indicators of substance abuse that are evident in our patients crop up in addicted nurses. Family history, a chronic medical condition requiring opioid analgesics, physical signs and symptoms of use, memory loss, mood swings, and changes in work performance and work relationships sometimes point to substance abuse.

Some abusers request to work night shift or assignments that facilitate access to drugs. Behaviors indicating possible use on the job include frequent trips to the bathroom, with behavioral changes noted afterward, and sudden absence from the unit. Impaired nurses become illogical and careless in charting and/or performing duties. Discrepancies in narcotics counts, patients who feel less pain relief when that nurse is on duty, and unusual variation in the quantity of medications dispensed to the patients on the unit are indications of drug diversion by the impaired nurse.

Box 36-8 Warning Signs of Nurse Impairment

The Texas Peer Assistance Program for Nurses lists the following behavior patterns as warning signs that a nurse is possibly impaired by chemical dependence or a mental health disorder.

ALCOHOLISM
- Irritability, mood swings
- Elaborate excuses for behavior; unkempt appearance
- Blackouts (periods of temporary amnesia)
- Impaired motor coordination, slurred speech, flushed face, bloodshot eyes
- Numerous injuries, burns, bruises, and so on, with vague explanations for same
- Smell of alcohol on breath, or excessive use of mouthwash, mints, and so forth
- Increased isolation from others

DRUG ADDICTION
- Rapid changes in mood and/or performance
- Frequent absence from unit; frequent use of restroom
- Possibly works a lot of overtime; usually arriving early and staying late
- Increased somatic complaints necessitating prescriptions of pain medications
- Consistently signs out more or larger amounts of controlled drugs than anyone else; excessive wasting of drugs
- Often volunteers to medicate other nurses' patients; sometimes wears long sleeves all the time
- Increased isolation from others
- Patient reports that pain medication is not effective or that did not receive medication
- Excessive discrepancies in signing and documentation procedures of controlled substances

MENTAL HEALTH DISORDER
- Depressed, lethargic, unable to focus or concentrate, apathetic
- Makes many mistakes at work
- Erratic behavior or mood swings
- Inappropriate or bizarre behavior or speech
- Will sometimes also exhibit some of the same or similar characteristics as chemically dependent nurses

From Texas Peer Assistance Program for Nurses–Texas Nurses Association. Retrieved October, 2009 from www.texasnurses.org.

As addiction progresses, the impaired nurse will sometimes sign out medications and report spillage. Some will steal drugs from the patient's bedside after supply count for the shift is done. Some nurses have stolen entire deliveries with the sign-out sheets and then claimed that it was an accounting error (Box 36-8).

Impaired nurses put their patients at risk for injury, medication error, and slower recovery. It is important for nursing colleagues to report suspicious behavior. It is the duty of every nurse to uphold the standards of the profession. Most state boards of nursing will accept anonymous tips. Although it is easy to ignore or cover up the problem, reporting suspicious behavior anonymously or to the supervisor will begin the healing process for that impaired nurse. Report observations objectively, and keep a diary in case it becomes necessary to recall an event. When action is necessary, the supervisor or the state board of nursing contacts the peer assistance program. Sometimes mental illness will, upon investigation, turn out to be responsible for the behavioral manifestations rather than drug abuse. Either way, those in authority will approach the nurse and ask him or her to seek treatment.

Peer assistance programs (called *diversion programs* in some states) are usually under the jurisdiction of the state board of nursing. These programs administer contract agreements requiring that the nurse undergo treatment and monitoring for a period of several years in order to keep his or her license in good standing. Many have requirements of continued attendance to Alcoholics Anonymous or Narcotics Anonymous, with random drug screening as part of the monitoring during return to work. Some job modification will be necessary in some cases to reduce stress and decrease opportunity for relapse. These programs maintain confidentiality as much as possible, but it is necessary to notify employers of a nurse in the program. It is not permitted in most states to subpoena any records the program keeps.

In 1999 the U.S. Department of Health and Human Services established a national data bank, **Healthcare Integrity and Protection Data Bank (HIPDB).** It requires federal and state government agencies (including nursing boards and health agencies) to report all final adverse actions taken against a health care provider, supplier, or practitioner since August 1996. This provides incentive for the nurse to enter treatment and avoid any final action that is mandatory to report to the HIPDB.

Finally, if the nurse is suffering from addiction or another health problem that affects performance on the job, it is crucial that he or she be truthful and seek help. The nurse's action today will be a benefit to his or her own personal life and career, to the welfare of patients, and to the overall functioning of the health care setting.

Get Ready for the NCLEX® Examination!

Key Points

- Many patients who enter acute care facilities with other diagnoses also have problems of drug and alcohol abuse.
- *Substance abuse* and *drug dependency* are terms we often use interchangeably when referring to addiction.
- Alcoholism is a chronic, incurable, progressive disease.
- Common traits of an addictive personality include low stress tolerance, dependency, negative self-image, depression, and feelings of insecurity.
- The three distinct stages of dependence disease are early, middle, and late.
- Moral theories on alcoholism are falling from favor because of biologic findings. Changes in brain activity, hepatic enzyme deficiencies, and genetic links prove the existence of a disease process.
- Alcohol and drug use weaves its way into our multicultural society through family traditions, peer pressure, and mass media advertising.
- Chronic alcohol abuse is toxic to multiple organs; disorders develop due to chronic alcohol abuse.
- Denial and delusions are coping mechanisms common among untreated substance abusers.
- Maintaining a professional, nonjudgmental attitude when communicating about use sometimes allows the user to be honest about use.
- The goal of detoxification is to keep the patient free from complications while ridding the body of the substance.
- Safety is of primary concern during detoxification.
- Malnourishment occurs often in chronic alcohol and drug abusers.
- People abuse over-the-counter drugs and prescription drugs as well as illegal drugs.
- Street drugs pose a risk of severe side effects and sometimes permanent damage because there are no controls in the manufacturing of these drugs.
- Peer assistance programs are available for helping impaired nurses into recovery without taking away the privilege to practice nursing.

Additional Learning Resources

Go to your Companion CD for an audio glossary, animations, video clips, and more.

evolve Be sure to visit the Evolve site at http://evolve.elsevier.com/Christensen/foundations/ for additional online resources.

Review Questions for the NCLEX® Examination

1. An early age at the onset of drinking alcohol strongly predicts a high risk of developing:
   1. Alzheimer's disease.
   2. alcohol or substance abuse.
   3. resistance to chemical dependency.
   4. immunity to alcohol.

2. In all deaths due to motor vehicles and fatal intentional injuries, alcohol is involved in what percentage of them?
   1. 7%
   2. 10%
   3. 17%
   4. 38%

3. A patient is on his second postoperative day after surgical removal of renal calculi. He is agitated and asking to have the physician send him home. He states he cannot get any rest at the hospital and is only able to rest at home. Slight tremors in his hands are noted. The nurse checks the admission database and "no" was written in the section regarding alcohol and drug use. Which coping mechanism that users often practice is relevant and making it difficult to obtain accurate information concerning the use of alcohol or drugs?
   1. Denial
   2. Regression
   3. Guilt
   4. Hostility

4. A patient was found unconscious in his apartment with four empty bottles of whiskey and brought to the hospital by his family. Upon admission, he moans out loud and is having dry heaves and diarrhea. What is the best way to maintain his airway?
   1. Elevate the head of the bed to ease breathing, and place an emesis basin on the patient's lap.
   2. Place the patient in the side-lying position until the swallowing reflex is intact.
   3. Adjust the bed to the reverse Trendelenburg position until the patient regains consciousness.
   4. Tape an oral suction catheter in place to avoid aspiration.

5. A patient has entered an alcohol treatment center. He has tremors in his hands and chin and he appears anxious. He has trouble sitting down while going through the admission process. Which nursing intervention is possible to help relieve the patient's nervousness during detoxification?
   1. Restrict the patient to his room to reduce environmental stimuli.
   2. Allow the patient to attend an exercise class daily.
   3. Allow the patient up ad lib on the unit.
   4. Medicate the patient with antiseizure drugs.

6. The area of the brain that most psychoactive substances affect and potentially cause permanent damage to is the:
   1. brainstem.
   2. limbic system.
   3. cerebellum.
   4. callosum.

7. A patient's nervousness has escalated, and this evening he keeps looking over his shoulder. He shouts out, "There's a fire!" Upon entering his room, the nurse finds the patient huddled in a corner, diaphoretic and with a fearful expression. The nurse reassures him that there is no fire and assesses him, finding the following: BP 160/95, P 132, R 30, T 100. A sign that indicates delirium tremens is:
   1. fever.
   2. abdominal cramping.
   3. sedation.
   4. double vision.

8. A patient's family was killed in an auto accident last year. Her doctor prescribed diazepam (Valium) 10 mg three or four times daily po as needed, which she has taken daily for the past year. The physician has decided to discontinue her medication. What teaching point should the nurse stress about stopping a benzodiazepine?
   1. Call the office if you develop abdominal cramps or diarrhea.
   2. Take an over-the-counter drug for insomnia.
   3. Taper off the use of diazepam over the next week.
   4. Avoid caffeinated drinks in the evening.

9. A 25-year-old patient entered the hospital with diagnoses of septicemia and infective endocarditis. He admits to using IV heroin regularly. The nurse should observe for withdrawal symptoms, including:
   1. red rash similar to that of chickenpox.
   2. head cold and flulike signs and symptoms.
   3. intractable singultus.
   4. severe joint pain and back pain.

10. The benzodiazepine drug that is illegal in the United States and nicknamed the "date-rape" drug is:
   1. diazepam (Valium).
   2. flunitrazepam (Rohypnol).
   3. PCP.
   4. LSD.

11. Experts consider MDMA, also known as Ecstasy, neurotoxic because:
   1. serotonin is depleted in the brain, damaging neurons.
   2. dehydration causes neurologic damage.
   3. heart damage occurs from malignant hyperthermia.
   4. inner ear damage leads to deafness.

12. Amotivational cannabis syndrome—which is characterized by apathy, abnormal irritability, and decrease in personal hygiene—is a result of chronic use of:
   1. lysergic acid diethylamide (LSD).
   2. cocaine.
   3. marijuana.
   4. heroin.

13. Federal and state government agencies are required by law to report all final adverse actions taken against a health care provider, supplier, or practitioner to a national database called:
   1. National Health and Welfare Records Department.
   2. Healthcare Management Organization of the United States.
   3. Federal Drug Enforcement Agency.
   4. Healthcare Integrity and Protection Data Bank.

14. A patient is scheduled for abdominal surgery. He tells the nurse that his uncle became addicted to narcotics after his surgery; fearing that he too could become addicted, he does not want to receive any narcotics. What is the nurse's most appropriate response?
   1. "Don't worry. You can refuse to take them."
   2. "Usually narcotics are given in the first few days after surgery; then you will be given a milder pain reliever for your pain. You will not be given narcotics long enough to become addicted."
   3. "Your fear of addiction is unfounded, but I will tell your physician about your concern."
   4. "I've never heard of anyone getting hooked on narcotics after surgery."

15. The nurse is ready to give the end-of-shift report to the nurse in charge of the unit for the next shift. When the oncoming nurse arrives 15 minutes late, she does not make eye contact, she smells of mints, her hands are trembling, her uniform is disheveled, and her shoes are untied. She asks no questions regarding any patients, and leaves the room when the report is completed. What should the first nurse do?
   1. Go home because the shift is completed.
   2. Call the supervisor and report observations.
   3. Stay on the unit until she is sure the oncoming nurse has no questions regarding the patients.
   4. Call the state board of nursing and report the oncoming nurse's behavior.

16. A patient has begun a substance abuse outpatient treatment program and is allowed to return to work, with supervision. Which statement by the patient indicates that she is recovering from her substance abuse problem?
   1. "I wish I knew who turned me in to administration; I would like to give that nosy witch a piece of my mind!"
   2. "Just because I had a glass of wine with a meal before I came to work once or twice, I'm going to be watched like a hawk. What a pain!"
   3. "I realize that I'm going to have to regain the trust of my co-workers and administrators, but I can do that, one day at a time."
   4. "If other people took their jobs as seriously as I take mine, they wouldn't have time to rat on other people."

17. By which symptom is it possible to identify a long-term cocaine user?

1. Clear, constricted pupils
2. Red irritated nostrils
3. Conjunctival redness
4. Muscle aches

18. A person addicted to heroin is likely to exhibit which symptoms of withdrawal?

1. Nausea and vomiting, diarrhea, and diaphoresis
2. Tremors, insomnia, and seizures
3. Incoordination and unsteady gait
4. Increased heart rate and flushing

19. A patient has begun attending Alcoholics Anonymous (AA) meetings. Which statement reflects the purpose of their organization?

1. "They claim they will help me stay sober."
2. "I'll dry out in AA, and then I can have a social drink once in a while."
3. "AA is only for people who have reached the bottom."
4. "If I lose my job, AA will help me find another."

20. Symptoms of alcohol withdrawal include:

1. euphoria, hyperactivity, and insomnia.
2. depression, suicidal ideation, and hypersomnia.
3. diaphoresis, nausea and vomiting, and tremors.
4. unsteady gait, nystagmus, and severe disorientation to time and place.

chapter 37

Home Health Nursing

evolve

Barbara Lauritsen Christensen

http://evolve.elsevier.com/Christensen/foundationsadult

Objectives

1. Describe how home health care differs from community and public health care services.
2. List at least three types of home health agencies.
3. Summarize governmental financing possibilities for home health nursing.
4. Discuss new developments that are occurring in home health care, including remote electronic monitoring.
5. Relate seven steps to breaking through cultural barriers to communication.
6. List at least four services that are possible to provide by home health care.
7. Describe two major ways home care differs from hospital care.
8. Define skilled nursing services.
9. Describe the role of the LPN/LVN in the delivery of skilled nursing care.
10. Relate the nursing process to home health care practice.
11. List two sources of reimbursement for home care services.

Key Terms

accreditation (ă-crĕd-ĭ-TĀ-shŭn, p. 1180)
certification (sŭr-tĭ-fĭ-KĀ-shŭn, p. 1180)
diagnosis-related groups (DRGs) (p. 1179)
home health care (p. 1177)
Medicaid (p. 1187)
Medicare (p. 1187)

Home health care services enable individuals of all ages to remain in the comfort and security of their homes while receiving health care. Family support, familiar surroundings, and participation in the care process contribute to feelings of worth and dignity. Possible services include skilled nursing, physical therapy, psychiatric therapy, pain education and management, speech language therapy, occupational therapy, social services, intravenous therapy, nutritional support, respiratory therapy, acquisition of medical supplies and equipment, and home health aide, homemaker, pet-care assistance, and companion care.

Patients most often receive referrals for home health services upon discharge from the hospital; however, it is also possible for the patient, the family, or the health care provider to request home health care at other times.

To qualify for coverage by Medicare, a health maintenance organization (HMO), or various types of insurance, it is necessary for the patient to be "homebound," meaning unable to leave the home or requiring a great deal of effort to travel for appointments to see the health care provider. The patient also has to be in need of intermittent skilled nursing care.

Patients older than 65 years account for half of all home health patients. Patients of all ages with various diagnoses account for the other half. Hospitals are most likely to discharge those patients to home health care with a stroke, chronic obstructive pulmonary disease, fractured hips needing surgical interventions, and joint replacement procedures. Home health care includes services ranging from wound care to ostomy assistance, setting up oral medications, prefilling insulin syringes or administering injections of vitamin B_{12}, assisting patients postoperatively after undergoing total hip and total knee replacements, and monitoring patients with heart failure, diabetes, and hypertension (Lewis et al., 2007). The frequency and length of home health visits vary depending on the services needed. The visits occur sometimes as often as twice daily and as seldom as monthly.

Physicians have become more involved in home care. Advancing technology has allowed more care to be delivered in the home. Home health care is needed because Americans are living longer and thus have more disease conditions that require care. Also, hospital stays are, on the average, much shorter than in the past, so many patients still require nursing interventions on discharge from the hospital. Home health care is also essential because an increasing number of women work outside the home. Women who traditionally provided health care for their families are no longer available to provide this service. There is an increased mobility in our society and an increase in single-parent families with female heads of households. These factors have eroded the traditional support system of the family.

Recently there has been a shift to community-based care. This has led to an increased number of acutely ill home-care patients, changing demands on health care providers, and greater populations of the unserved and the underserved.

The best approach to patient care is one of teamwork and blending of disciplines. The licensed practical nurse/licensed vocational nurse (LPN/LVN) is a valuable member of this very important health care team. Registered nurses (RNs) are now primarily involved in the administration and management of agencies and the supervision of nursing interventions. Although home care has traditionally been a part of public and community health services, its focus is now much narrower.

HOME HEALTH CARE DEFINED

Home health care preserves individual independence and integrity and keeps families together. The following are definitions of home health care as viewed from four different perspectives:

- *Official:* A component of comprehensive health care in which individuals and their families receive services in their place of residence for the purpose of promoting, maintaining, or restoring health, or of minimizing the effects of illness and disability.
- *Patient:* Skilled and compassionate care provided on a one-to-one basis in the comforting and familiar surroundings of the home. Providers base care on individual needs and personalized schedules and do so over a given period to enable adjustment, change, and learning to take place effectively.
- *Family:* A means to keep the family together as a functioning, integrated unit. The goals are learning to adapt to change, preventing dysfunctional patterns from setting in, and attaining family wellness within the scope of an individual member's illness or disability. It provides needed emotional support and linkage with the larger community support systems.
- *Provider:* Challenges all disciplines involved to provide excellent care in often less-than-excellent conditions and surroundings. Independence, creativity, communication, and excellent clinical skills are integral aspects of daily practice. It is an opportunity for nurses to demonstrate the best of their profession and themselves in cooperation with the health care team to patients and families with physical and psychological needs.

HISTORICAL OVERVIEW

The former definition of home care was simply providing physical care to the sick in their homes, but the scope and the complexity of the concept and practice have grown. Roots of the concept go back to the New Testament of the Bible, which describes visiting the sick as a form of charity. Sixth-century monks practiced home care as an important aspect of their work in the community. One of the earliest organized systems for home care was developed in 1617 by St. Vincent de Paul, who organized the Sisterhood of the Dames de Charité to meet social welfare and visiting nursing needs. In the 1700s, families were the primary caregivers. The poor were hospitalized, whereas those with financial means were cared for in their homes by visiting physicians.

The first home care program in the United States came into being in 1796 as the Boston Dispensary. In 1859, William Rathbone of Liverpool, England, established the Metropolitan Nursing Association, the first organized district nursing service, because of the outstanding home care his dying wife received. He believed that many people with long-term illnesses had a better chance to receive the kind of care they desired in their own homes than in a hospital—a belief central to home care today.

Nurses provided care to all ages of people with both acute and chronic care needs in the first visiting nurse service in the United States, formed in Philadelphia in 1886. Lillian Wald and Mary Brewster developed a visiting nurse service for the poor in New York City in 1893 at the Nurses' Settlement House on Henry Street. The late 1800s and early 1900s saw the formalization of visiting nurse associations, and public health departments became widespread.

The Metropolitan Life Insurance Company had a major effect on the growth and nature of home services when, in 1909, it began offering nursing services to its millions of industrial policyholders. This initiated third-party payment for services. Payment until then had been primarily a matter of charity or the responsibility of the patient.

The Social Security Act of 1935 first provided governmental rather than local charitable funding for selected services such as maternal health, treatment for communicable diseases, and the training of public health professionals. The Act subsidized assistance for the poor and aged. Amendments to the Act in 1950 further defined services and opened the door to direct payment for providers.

A revolution, however, occurred in 1965 with the enactment of Title XVIII (known as Medicare) and Title XIX (known as Medicaid) amendments to the Social Security Act. Medicare provided direct federal monies for the health care of all citizens 65 and older (or disabled), regardless of socioeconomic status. The companion Medicaid bill covered the care needs of the poor and indigent of all ages. When Medicare became effective in 1966, it revolutionized home care by (1) changing it to a medical rather than nursing model of practice, (2) defining and limiting the services it reimbursed, and (3) changing the payment source and even changing the reason for providing home care (see Life Span Considerations for Older Adults box).

The next major influence on home care came in 1983. Congress enacted the prospective payment system (PPS) as a part of the Tax Equity and Fiscal Responsibility Act for hospitals receiving Medicare reimbursement. This system, based on major diagnostic categories and diagnosis-related groups (DRGs), pays a set rate (according to diagnosis) for the hospitalized patient's care rather than the "cost," or charges an institution traditionally bills according to its own schedule of fees. The net effect of the change was a major shift of patients out of hospitals and into their homes, extended-care facilities, or skilled nursing facilities. Discharge for such patients occurred earlier in their convalescence, and thus the patient required more nursing care. This created a challenge to home care in terms of volume of patients seen, of the need to provide more skilled nursing care over more intensive periods, and the evolution of highly technical procedures in the home. Existing agencies expanded, and new ones developed to meet the demand.

In an effort to control home health expenditures, Congress imposed new limits on home health payments through a provision of the Balanced Budget Act of 1997 (BBA) called the Interim Payment System (IPS). Until BBA, there were no limits on payment for covered home health services provided to qualifying patients as long as visit costs were within "reasonable" cost limits. To reduce the growth in home health, the IPS imposed lower per-visit limits and imposed a new agency-specific, aggregate per-beneficiary limit based on agencies' federal fiscal year spending in 1994.

The effects of IPS were more far reaching than either Congress or the Health Care Financing Administration (HCFA) intended, producing a 20% reduction in beneficiaries served and reduction in overall expenditures by 40%. The effect on individual agencies that were unable to maintain costs within per-visit and per-beneficiary limits was devastating. Of the 10,500 Medicare-certified home health agencies in existence in 1997, more than 2500 closed by September 1999 (St. Pierre & Dombi, 2000). On October 1, 2000, the HCFA implemented a new payment system for home health agencies to increase payment to patients (Gent et al., 2001).

BBA also provided the authority for development of a PPS for home health. Thus Medicare pays providers of home health services at fixed predetermined rates for services and supplies to cover an episode of care during a specific period. The goal of PPS is to produce new incentives for the home health provider to be more efficient in the delivery of home health services and still remain financially solvent (St. Pierre & Dombi, 2000). The PPS has not led to a decline in quality of care or negative outcomes in patient care (Centers for Medicare & Medicaid Services [CMS], n.d.). Congress and the administration expect the incentives for efficiency to continue to produce savings under IPS.

Home care visits and Medicare expenditures for home care quadrupled between 1980 and 1991. This was directly attributed to shorter hospitalizations, more seriously ill patients being discharged to home, and increased acceptance of the delivery of higher technology care in the home. Home health care grew five times faster than the average of other health care industries between 1990 and 1997 and accounted for more than 6% of health service jobs. The annual growth rate for home health care had been 16.4% in the years 1988 to 1993 and was the fastest growing segment of health care.

Life Span Considerations

Older Adults

Home Care Services

- The growing number of older adults has resulted in increased need for home health care services.
- Early-discharge policies have resulted in very ill older adults leaving the hospital. This increases the importance of patient teaching, early discharge planning, and appropriate referral to home health agencies by hospital staff nurses.
- Many older adults do not require total care but do require a limited amount of assistance. Home care reduces disruption of lifestyle and is more cost effective than institutional placement.
- Transfer to a hospital or nursing home even on a temporary basis increases the stress level of older people. Stress is decreased if they receive care in a familiar environment.
- It is crucial for caregivers to learn the importance of preserving the older adult's autonomy, and to make any modifications to the home environment with consideration of the older adult's physical strengths and remaining functional abilities, not just the patient's disabilities.
- A number of service agencies exist that are in a position to assist older adults in their communities. These include Meals-on-Wheels, home health aides, homemakers, and home-based physical therapy services. As a nurse, make sure you are familiar with home health services in your area, and help older people make arrangements for the appropriate services.

TYPES OF HOME CARE AGENCIES

In the broadest terms, delivery of home care services is possible by any individual, service group, organization, or agency with the desire to provide services to the older adult, disabled, or ill of any age. It is possible for the type and qualifications of personnel used, the quality of services delivered, and standards of care to vary widely, and these often depend on funding sources. The agency typically has to comply with federal, state, and local laws and regulations via the following:

- **Licensure by the state.** This gives legal permission to operate within that state only. Regulations vary widely. Not all states have such laws.

- **Certification by the state certifying body that the federal government designates.** The federal government set the rules governing certification (a process in which the government evaluates and recognizes an individual, institution, or educational program as meeting certain predetermined standards). Only certified agencies are permitted to receive Medicare payment. Many states piggyback Medicaid reimbursement to certification, as do some insurers.
- **Certificate of need: Some states grant this according to rules and formulas that state regulators devise.** Cost of starting and running the agency, availability of personnel, and need for their services are generally considered in this process.
- **Accreditation by an outside agency that evaluates and judges how well the agency meets certain standards that the accrediting organization sets.** An agency will sometimes obtain this accreditation (a process whereby a professional association or nongovernmental agency grants recognition to a school or institution for demonstrated ability in a special area of practice or training) from the National League for Nursing Community Health Accreditation Program, The Joint Commission, or the National Homecaring Council. Other groups sometimes grant accreditation to special programs or specialized agencies. Some of these national accrediting agencies are seeking "deemed status" from federal regulators, which will allow their accreditation to also serve as the required certification. This will eliminate the need for separate surveys for some agencies.

Before Medicare, the provision of home health care was primarily the task of visiting nurse associations, nursing divisions of state or local health departments, and hospitals. Now agencies are classified according to (1) *tax status,* for profit or not for profit; (2) *location,* freestanding or institution based; and (3) *governance,* private or public. Table 37-1 summarizes and describes the six generally accepted types of home health agencies. The structure of some of these agencies is subject to change and variation. For example, some visiting nurse associations have reorganized and placed their home health agencies into private, nonprofit structures to ensure reimbursement that will cover the cost of providing services.

Growth in number of agencies has mirrored the growth of home care. Although the late 1980s saw a decrease in agencies, the numbers rebounded, largely because of increases in hospital-based agencies and specialized agencies providing highly technical types of care. Such high-technology care will possibly include intravenous services, ventilator-dependent care services, and management of human immunodeficiency virus (HIV) patients in the home.

CHANGES IN HOME HEALTH CARE

Changes are occurring in home health care. The Joint Commission (TJC) is looking for agencies to establish ethics committees to handle ethical issues that arise in the home. Medicare is reimbursing psychiatric nurse clinicians for home visits. Psychiatric patients are required to be under the care of a psychiatrist and have a psychiatric diagnosis. The psychiatric nurse clinician provides therapy and education, as well as counsels family members.

Patients with acquired immunodeficiency syndrome (AIDS) represent a growing home health care population, with nearly 42,000 AIDS cases reported in 2005 (Centers for Disease Control and Prevention [CDC], 2007).

Social workers are taking a more active role in home health care. Social workers provide assistance with a patient's emotional, financial, and household problems, thus allowing the nurse more time to perform nursing interventions.

More home health agencies are employing nurse pain specialists to assess and manage pain control in the home. They are able to provide education to patients and staff and provide greater benefits in relief of pain as well as reduce the cost of ineffective pain management.

Most agencies are obtaining a separate Medicare certification to provide hospice care. Medicare-certified hospices receive per diem payments rather than a fee for visit. This method of payment is more economical for insurers and taxpayers.

Pet-care programs are emerging to reduce stress for home health patients who are too ill to care for their pets. A "durable power of attorney for pet care" allows a patient to make arrangements for pet care if he or she becomes hospitalized or dies. Some home health agencies provide special pet services, such as transporting pets to veterinarian appointments.

Electronic home visits have evolved. A computerized system now has the capacity to call a patient on the telephone at home and ask recorded questions such as, "What is your blood pressure?" The patient is able to respond by using the phone's keypad. In this way the nurse is able to efficiently review the patient's progress without making a home visit. Over the past several years, advances in technology and forward-thinking home health agencies have helped spur a jump in the adoption of telemonitoring for home health patients. A growing body of research indicates the extreme promise telemonitoring holds (Wright, 2003). Patients have a 70% reduced rehospitalization and emergency department use rate when their health care providers manage care not only with the help of telemonitoring such as standard vital sign measurement (e.g., temperature, heart rate, blood pressure, oxygen saturation, weight) but also though the various peripheral technologies available (such as blood glucose measurement, spirom-

Table 37-1 Home Health Agencies

STATUS	GOVERNANCE	SOURCE OF SUPPORT	SERVICES OFFERED	NATURE OF STAFF	TIME OF SERVICE	EXAMPLE
VOLUNTARY Public; nonprofit; freestanding	Community-based board of directors	Tax-deductible contributions; grants; fees from all sources	Community health; public health; home health	RN; LPN/LVN; aide; homemaker; social worker; therapists	Generally ½-8 hr	Visiting nurse association
OFFICIAL Public; nonprofit; freestanding	State, county, city, or other local unit of government and volunteer board representatives of the area	State, local, or county revenues; grants; fees from limited sources; charitable contributions	Community health; public health; home health	RN; LPN/LVN; aide; homemaker; social worker; therapists	Generally ½-4 hr	State health departments; county health departments; city health departments
COMBINATION Public; nonprofit; freestanding	Jointly operated by the two types of agencies above under a combined board of directors	State, local, or county revenues; grants; fees from limited sources; charitable contributions	Community health; public health; home health	RN; LPN/LVN; aide; homemaker; social worker; therapists	Generally ½-4 hr	County-based visiting nurse association
HOSPITAL Private; nonprofit or for profit; institution based; hospital	Hospital board of directors	Fees from all sources	Home health; community health (limited)	RN; LPN/LVN; aide; social worker; therapists	Generally ½-4 hr	XYZ hospital home health agency
PROPRIETARY Private; for profit; freestanding	Governed and owned by individual, corporation, or other organization; many paid boards of directors appointed by owner	Fees from most sources; some do and some do not participate in Medicare-Medicaid	Some offer limited home health; private duty; homemaker	RN; LPN/LVN; aide	1-24 hr	Home health care of XYZ
PRIVATE NOT FOR PROFIT Private; nonprofit; freestanding	Governed and owned by individual, corporation, or other organizational structure; board appointed by owner	Fees from most sources; some do and some do not participate in Medicare-Medicaid	Some offer limited home health services; private duty; homemaker	RN; LPN/LVN; aide	½-24 hr	ABC home health agency
OTHER Private; for profit or nonprofit; institution based	Based within formalized institution; governed by that board or designated board	Fees from all sources	Home health services; limited homemaker	RN; LPN/LVN; aide; therapists; may have homemaker; social worker	½-8 hr	ABC nursing home—home health agency; ABC rehabilitation facility home care

LPN/LVN, Licensed practical nurse or licensed vocational nurse; *RN*, registered nurse.

etry, electrocardiogram (ECG), prothrombin time or International Normalized Ratio (INR), digital cameras, and videophones). Any patient meeting Medicare certification standards is a candidate to benefit from daily vital sign monitoring via telemonitoring from the home to the home health agency (Bolch, 2004).

One of the most rapidly growing segments in home health is home infusion therapy; an increasing number of home health agencies are offering home infusion services in an effort to compete for patient referrals. Health care facilities are eager to have home health agencies provide this service, since home intravenous (IV) therapy fits right in with their cost-cutting strategies. A 30-day IV antibiotic regimen of one common cephalosporin, for example, costs about $5000 when the patient receives it in the hospital but just $1600 when the patient is at home.

Antibiotics, hydration, and total parenteral nutrition (TPN) are three of the most common forms of home IV therapy, and the practitioner often orders them for patients at home without any prior hospital admission. Other less frequently used therapies include IV analgesic medications, chemotherapy, and dobutamine (Dobutrex); dobutamine, whose administration once occurred only in the intensive care unit (ICU), now serves as palliative therapy for home care patients with severe refractory CHF and for those awaiting heart transplants.

SERVICE COMPONENTS

Most home health agencies follow the basic Medicare model of services they offer. State licensing boards and professional organizations dictate functions and scopes of practice. Primary services include the following:

- Skilled nursing
- Physical therapy
- Speech-language therapy
- Occupational therapy
- Medical social services
- Homemaker–home health aide

Other therapy services (e.g., respiratory) or professional services (e.g., nutritional counseling, pharmacy, podiatry, dentistry, and psychiatric or mental health) are sometimes among an agency's offerings. Provision of support services (e.g., homemaker, companion, and respite) is common but not directly reimbursable by Medicare. The service mix depends on patient diagnosis, patient and family needs, and availability of resources. The agency commonly provides medical supplies, including durable medical equipment (DME). Home medical equipment ranging from the traditional hospital bed to highly sophisticated items such as respirators and apnea monitors are possible to buy or lease from companies specializing in equipment provision (see Health Promotion box).

Medicare and Medicaid home care services are based on the medical model of treatment and depend on the physician for entry into the formalized system. Medicare requires a plan of treatment signed by the physician, outlining all disciplines, treatment, frequency, and duration. These orders are necessary to recertify every 60 days. Third-party payers sometimes do and sometimes do not have similar requirements. This chapter will explain only the primary services.

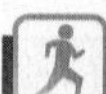 **Health Promotion**

Home Care

- The most common diagnoses for home care patients are diabetes mellitus, hypertension, heart failure, osteoarthritis, stroke, acute and chronic wounds, chronic obstructive pulmonary disease, heart disease, cancer, and psychiatric disorders.
- Commonly performed treatments in the home include administration of infusion therapy (i.e., antibiotic administration), patient-controlled analgesia for pain management, enteral feedings, parenteral nutrition, chemotherapy, hydration therapy, and psychiatric counseling and education.
- The nurse and a rehabilitation team member will at times also provide medical equipment in the home to facilitate medical treatment and safety, such as electrical beds, wheelchairs, commodes, walkers, and other assistive devices.

SKILLED NURSING

Currently licensed RNs provide and direct skilled nursing services. Some agencies require that nurses have a bachelor's degree in nursing, whereas others hire graduates of all types of RN programs and teach them agency policies and specific procedures. Not all nurses have the ability to be effective home health nurses. The LPN/LVN is permitted to provide basic nursing services under the supervision of the RN.

Service Goals

Skilled nursing services revolve around four major goals:

1. *Restorative:* The return to a previous level of functioning as appropriate and realistic
2. *Improvement:* Achieving better health and a higher level of functioning than at admission
3. *Maintenance:* Preserving functional capacities and independence by maintaining current level of health
4. *Promotion:* Teaching healthy lifestyles that keep the effect of illness or disability to a minimum and prevent the recurrence of illness

Provider Attributes

Nurses practicing in the home setting are caregivers, teachers, counselors, case managers, and advocates. To be a home health nurse, you need to be technically proficient and self-motivated, have expert organizational skills, be innovative, be an independent decision maker, and respond to problems promptly. Common sense, flexibility, compassion, empathy, patience, honesty, and dependability are essential. Assessment and teaching skills are crucial in caring for patients in their homes as well as in structured facilities. In home health nursing, you will not always have supplies readily available; to be successful, you will learn to improvise based on what materials are available. You will generally provide services in the patient's home; hence you will need to feel comfortable with the unknown, as well as accept differences in ethnic cultures and value systems. Nurses who depend on the security of the institutional setting, immediate medical direction, and frequent peer support find the independence of home care practice difficult.

If you are a home health nurse, it is necessary that you keep in mind the dominant role the patient and the family play. Unlike the hospital situation, home health nursing requires that nurses and other providers adapt to the patient, family, and home environment. You will be a visitor in the patient's home. The patient's and family's cultural values and beliefs are very important for you to acknowledge and respect. You will often encounter the use of home remedies and complementary and alternative therapies and have the responsibility to carefully guide the patient and family in their safe and effective use (Lewis et al., 2007).

Strong communication skills are essential for teaching, counseling, interviewing, and listening. A high energy level, cheerfulness, and a positive attitude are valuable attributes, because you will often be called on to work with patients and families who are under stress. Respect for the patient's dignity, privacy, and need of autonomy is an integral part of providing effective nursing services. Commitment to professional standards of practice, ongoing continuing education, and skills updates are important.

ROLE OF THE LPN/LVN

RNs have been the primary providers of skilled service by both tradition and regulation. However, skilled service has become a growing field of practice for the LPN/LVN as agencies cope with increased staffing needs, nursing shortages, and recognition of the many contributions the LPN/LVN makes to home care.

An RN has to supervise LPNs/LVNs. Although LPNs/LVNs are not empowered to make detailed patient assessments or clinical judgments, their observations, reporting, documentation, teaching, and technical care capabilities are important to home care. Chapter 38 also discusses the LPN/LVN's role as a member of the home health care team.

Provider Attributes

Personal and professional attributes described for RNs also apply to the LPN/LVN. Independent practice is not allowed, but self-direction, motivation, creativity, clinical proficiency, flexibility, compassion, empathy, and patience are all essential attributes. Good communication skills—both written and spoken—are necessary. The ability to work alone, follow directions, recognize important changes in condition, and assist in patient teaching is needed. Evaluation of care interventions and recommendations for alteration of the plan of care constitute a part of the role. It is important to understand and practice the concept of teamwork.

Functions

Depending on the agency, agency policies, and state practice acts, the LPN/LVN will sometimes provide the following services in the home as directed and supervised by the RN:

- Catheter care and teaching
- Ostomy care and teaching
- Wound care and sterile dressing changes
- Obtaining specimens for cultures
- Injection administration
- Prefilling insulin syringes
- Fingersticks for blood glucose readings
- Monitoring physical status (such as lung sounds, bowel sounds, pulses, edema, and weight)
- Teaching, monitoring, or setting up medications, including IV medications
- Nutrition; assessment of nutrition and hydration status; teaching about prescribed diet; administration of nasogastric, gastrostomy, and jejunostomy tube feedings, and teaching families about tube feedings
- Specimen collection
- Therapeutic diet teaching or reinforcement
- Respiratory care, management of oxygen therapy, mechanical ventilation, and physiotherapy
- Tracheostomy care, including suctioning

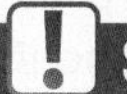 Safety Alert!

Home Oxygen Use

MASK OR CANNULA
- Ensure that the straps are not too tight
- Remove straps two or three times/day to wash, dry, and stimulate skin
- Pad any pressure points
- Observe tops of ears for skin impairment from pressure points

ORAL AND NASAL MUCOUS MEMBRANES
- Assess oral and nasal mucous membranes two or three times/day
- Use water-based gel on lips and nasal mucosa
- Provide frequent oral hygiene
- Provide humidification via humidifier or nebulizing device

DECREASING RISK FOR INFECTION
- Remove mask or collar and cleanse with water two or three times/day
- Cleanse skin carefully at this time and observe for cuts, scratches, and ecchymosis
- Change disposable equipment frequently
- Remove secretions that are expectorated

DECREASING RISK OF FIRE INJURIES
- Post "No Smoking" warning signs in home where they are clearly visible
- Do not allow open flames, wool blankets, or mineral oils in the area where oxygen is in use
- Do not allow smoking in the home

- Enemas for special conditions
- Insertion of urinary catheter, irrigation, and observation for infections
- Bowel and bladder training
- Pain management
- Emotional support
- Preventive health measures
- Patient and family teaching (Figure 37-1)
- Vital signs

Assistance with highly technical procedures—such as IV therapies, home dialysis, and respirator management—is occurring in home health care.

Home health care offers a new and challenging area of practice for the LPN/LVN who enjoys practicing nursing in a less restrictive environment. LPNs/LVNs employed in home health agencies cite satisfaction in terms of flexibility, pay, and one-on-one relationships with patients. The need for this level of nursing practice will continue to grow. Commitment to quality of care is a common thread through skilled nursing services; hence the LPN/LVN has the responsibility to also pursue frequent inservice updates and continuing education to ensure current practice.

PHYSICAL THERAPY

A qualified and licensed physical therapist is required to provide services. A physical therapy assistant under the supervision of the licensed therapist is permitted to deliver limited services. The goals of treatment have to be restorative for Medicare reimbursement but will in some cases be for maintenance or prevention for other payer sources. The therapist completes a detailed assessment of the patient and then determines treatment, education, and assistive devices needed for rehabilitation. These are included as a part of the physician-approved plan of treatment. Treatments range from muscle strengthening to transcutaneous nerve stimulation and ultrasound treatments. Patients who have orthopedic conditions, such as repair of a fractured hip, a total hip or total knee replacement, and those with neuromuscular diseases such as stroke, multiple sclerosis, or amyotrophic lateral sclerosis receive referral to a physical therapist (Lewis et al., 2007). The therapist actively teaches the patient and the family the rehabilitation plan to promote self-care and independence. Communication with the physician and the RN promotes continuity of care.

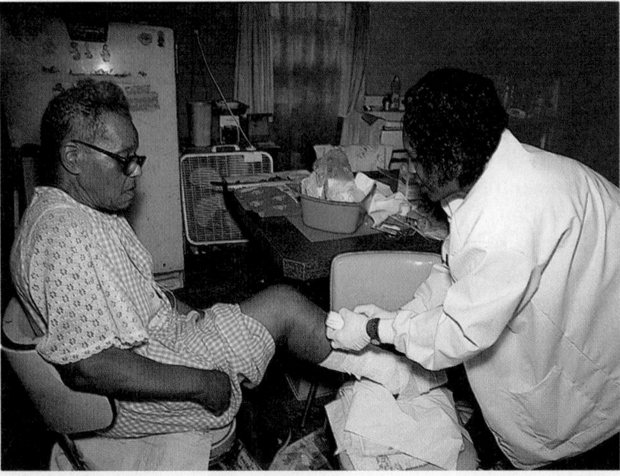

FIGURE 37-1 Educating the patient in the home setting.

SPEECH-LANGUAGE THERAPY

To be reimbursed by Medicare, a master's-prepared clinician who has been certified by the American Speech and Hearing Association is required to provide speech services. Other insurers sometimes accept a practitioner prepared at the bachelor's level. Therapy goals include reducing to a minimum communication disorders and their physical, emotional, and social impact. Independent functioning and maximum rehabilitation of speech and language abilities are primary treatment goals. Often the provision of services occurs after stroke or surgery. Possible therapies range from language relearning to working with eating or swallowing disorders or teaching lipreading to those with hearing disorders. Pathologists work closely with the patient and family for rehabilitation or adjustment to a new disability.

OCCUPATIONAL THERAPY

Occupational therapy services deal with life's practical tasks. Therapists have bachelor's level preparation and have the opportunity to earn the occupational therapist, registered (OTR) designation if they meet the registration requirements of the National Occupational Therapy Association. The certified occupational therapy assistant is permitted to provide some services under the supervision of the OTR. Based on a complete evaluation of functional level, the therapist will choose and teach therapeutic activities designed to restore functional levels. Services include the following:

1. Techniques to increase independence
2. Analysis of activities as they relate to patients' skin, their environment, their families, and their routines
3. Expanding the disease management approach into a lifestyle management approach
4. Design, fabrication, and fitting of orthotic or self-help devices
5. Assessment for vocational training

Occupational therapists assist patients to improve in their performance of activities of daily living (ADLs), as well as their sensory-motor, cognitive, and neuromuscular functioning (Lewis et al., 2007). Patient-centered education is an integral part of attaining independence in self-care.

MEDICAL SOCIAL SERVICES

Social workers prepared at the master's level provide medical social services. Workers with bachelor's degrees are permitted to provide services under the supervision of a social worker with a master's degree

(MSW). Their focus is on the emotional and social aspects of illness. The patient, the family, or other support systems undergo evaluation for social, emotional, and environmental factors. The care plan includes education, counseling, payment source identification, and referrals. Coping with stress and crisis intervention are also part of social worker services. Social services in home health are generally short term.

HOMEMAKER–HOME HEALTH AIDE

Medicare refers to the homemaker–home health aide (HM-HHA) as a home health aide (HHA). These workers are an integral part of the home health care team. They provide the basic support services that sometimes enable an elderly individual, disabled adult, or dependent child to remain at home. Medicare requires that a primary skilled or therapy service (speech or physical) be provided before HHA services are arranged. Medicaid and some insurers have less stringent requirements. Many insurers do not reimburse this care. Family members and individuals are often willing to pay privately to prevent institutionalization.

Most aide services fall into one of three categories: (1) *personal care,* or assistance with bathing, oral hygiene, eating, dressing, and toileting (see Coordinated Care box); (2) *physical assistance* with transfers, medications, and ambulation; or (3) *household chores,* or cooking, light housekeeping, shopping, and laundry. Medicare will not cover visits made solely for the third reason.

Although training of aides has long been required by Medicare, rules governing type, length, and content of preparation have been nonexistent; hence skills and standards were not uniform. Part of the Omnibus Budget Reconciliation Act of 1987 involved the formulation of new standards for training and competency evaluation that are now in effect.

Medicare and Medicaid require on-site supervision of the aide every 2 weeks, principally by an RN. Supervision by a licensed physical therapist is acceptable if skilled nursing is not involved. Private payers, however, often do not have such requirements. Aide services are sometimes provided in blocks of time ranging from 1 to 2 hours for Medicare to 8 to 24 hours for private or other payment sources.

 Coordinated Care

Delegation

PATIENT BATHING

Skills of bathing are often acceptable to delegate to assistive personnel (AP); however, skin and range-of-motion (ROM) assessment require the critical thinking and knowledge application unique to the nurse. As a nurse, do the following:

- Instruct the care provider what type of bath (complete, partial assist, tub, shower) is appropriate to the patient's diagnosis, needs, and ability.
- Remind the care provider to notify you of any skin integrity problems so you will make sure to inspect areas of impairment or potential impairment.
- Remind the care provider to use an organized approach and reassuring tone of voice so the patient feels safe and comfortable during bathing.
- Instruct the care provider to encourage the patient to report any concerns or discomfort during the bath.
- Instruct the care provider to encourage as much independence in the patient's self-care skills as appropriate and to provide positive feedback.

THE TYPICAL HOME HEALTH PROCESS

REFERRAL

The entry point to the home health care system is by referral. This comes from the patient, the family, a social service agency, the hospital, the physician, or another agency. Agencies have a variety of methods of intake for referrals, ranging from a formalized hospital discharge planning process with a central agency intake coordinator to a direct call from the patient's physician to the agency staff.

ADMISSION

An RN makes the initial evaluation and admission visit within 24 to 48 hours of the referral. Sometimes an RN will complete this in a formal role as admission nurse, and at other times a staff nurse who will serve as the primary nurse on the case will do so. The physician will often give general orders before this visit, but agencies sometimes make an evaluation visit without orders if agency policy permits. The evaluation and admission process generally includes at least the following:

1. Complete patient evaluation, including physical and psychosocial factors
2. Environmental assessment relating specifically to safety and ability to provide services effectively in the home
3. Identification of primary functional impairments
4. Identification of the impact of the disease or disability on the patient and the family
5. Assessment of the support system of the family or the significant other
6. Determination of knowledge and adherence to treatments and medications
7. Determination of desire for care and services
8. Involvement of the patient and the family in the development of the plan of care and goals
9. Notification to the patient of rights as a patient, along with information on costs, payment sources, and billing practices
10. Explanation of the patient's right to self-determination, including information and implementation policies for advanced directives
11. Provision of initial nursing interventions (it is necessary for the nurse to obtain an initial set of orders from the health care provider and pro-

ceed with providing the specific interventions ordered)

The admission process typically takes a minimum of 1 hour. It will take longer if the patient is disoriented or in need of nursing interventions. Some hospital-based agencies will initiate an abbreviated evaluation visit while the patient is still in the hospital.

CARE PLAN

If the agency is to admit the patient, it is necessary to contact the physician for specific orders before delivery of care. Agency staff drafts a treatment plan cooperatively with the physician. This plan describes the current physical status of the patient, medications, treatments, the disciplines needed to provide care, the frequency and the duration of services, the goals and outcomes, and the time frame for implementation. The physician is required to sign the plan of treatment, which serves as the traditional physician orders. The treatment plan is possible to alter at any time (based on patient needs) through additional written, signed orders, and it is obligatory to review and renew it on a regular schedule for Medicare and Medicaid patients. It is possible to write separate care plans that are discipline specific, such as nursing and physical therapy. A separate, detailed home health aide care plan is always required.

VISITS

Visits for interventions by the disciplines made in the orders serve to meet the patient-centered goals and make progress toward identified outcomes. Skilled nursing visits typically take 30 to 45 minutes but duration potentially increases to several hours for complex procedures. Therapy visits range from 30 minutes to 1 hour. With increasing federal pressure to decrease home care and hospice costs, and with the current Medicare PPS, clinical efficiency is critically necessary within the industry. The current method of developing individual care plans, that is, having a home care nurse visit a patient for a predetermined number of visits per week during each episode of care, is no longer tenable. Telemonitored patients are "seen" daily, thereby allowing agencies to plan home visits not for regular patient assessment (such as vital signs), but to provide hands-on intervention or face-to-face teaching when necessary. The purpose of telemonitoring is not to replace nurses, but to generate data that professional caregivers need to make critically important clinical decisions, allowing them to use their time and talents more effectively and efficiently (Bolch, 2004). Aide visits average 1 to 2 hours but sometimes will be longer, depending on needs and payment source. Revisions to the plan of care and referrals to other agencies occur during this period. Patients receive visits as infrequently as once a month for diabetic monitoring to several times a day over a short period to provide complex care. Some patients receive only skilled nursing services, and others receive visits by all disciplines. Greater and more frequent use of LPNs/LVNs is occurring when clinically appropriate. Patients will sometimes remain on the caseload for a week or years, but 60 to 90 days is common depending on the PPS payments authorized.

DOCUMENTATION

Throughout the care process, concise and complete documentation is essential. This documentation is sometimes handwritten and sometimes dictated or entered into a computer. A number of agencies use the problem-oriented record system—many in combination with the nursing diagnosis system.

Many agencies are beginning to use various problem classification schemes linked with nursing diagnoses (Box 37-1), specific interventions, and defined patient outcomes. Documentation that follows the nursing process model provides an accurate picture of the type and the quality of care. It reflects the effectiveness of the plan of care and progress toward goals and outcomes, or it reflects the nature of and the reasons for lack of progress or deterioration and includes alternative interventions. It is also necessary to document communications with the home care team and referral sources.

Other factors also influence documentation. Staff need to recognize the record as a legal document subject to close scrutiny at any time. Professional standards, accountability, and quality of care are closely

Box 37-1 Selected Nursing Diagnoses for Home Health Care

Risk for infection, related to:
- Inadequate primary or secondary defenses
- Inadequate acquired immunity
- Malnutrition

Deficient knowledge related to:
- Lack of experience
- Cognition limitation

Imbalanced nutrition, less than body requirements, related to:
- Inability to ingest or digest food
- Inability to absorb nutrients
- Economic deprivation

Bathing/hygiene self-care deficit, related to:
- Pain
- Musculoskeletal impairment
- Decreased endurance
- Neurologic impairment

Impaired skin integrity, related to:
- Physical immobility
- Radiation
- Impaired circulation (pressure)
- Inadequate nutrition

Pain, related to:
- Chronic illness (e.g., rheumatoid arthritis)
- Terminal cancer

linked to legal implications, as well as to internal evaluation purposes. Reimbursement sources have a major influence on documentation requirements by setting forth specific forms and formats that are necessary to follow. Medicare requires extensive paperwork. Private insurer requirements are generally less cumbersome.

DISCHARGE PLANNING

Discharge planning for home care, as in hospitals, begins with admission. When patient goals or other specific criteria are met, the discharge occurs. Agencies encourage patient and family participation in discharge planning. The agency consults the physician regarding the discharge, and he or she issues the final order. Many agencies follow up on a postdischarge basis to track patient progress and elicit patient satisfaction information. The purpose of discharge planning is to promote continuity of care in the patient's home.

QUALITY ASSURANCE, ASSESSMENT, AND IMPROVEMENT

Quality assessment programs provide documentation for outside organizations and for internal measures for improvements and refinements of policies and procedures. Assessing quality involves evaluating all aspects of the agency operation. Three major elements are included:

1. *Structural criteria:* The agency's overall organization, philosophy, policies, procedures, bylaws, personnel practices, supervision, orientation, contracts, and physical facilities
2. *Process criteria:* Evaluation of care delivery. Authorities scrutinize the activities of the health professionals and paraprofessionals and support in the management of patient care, documentation, and patient care conferences.
3. *Outcome criteria:* Measurement of change in patient behavior, the results of patient care in terms of changes, health indicators, and satisfaction. Care standards and expected outcomes are an integral part of this area.

Those responsible for quality assessment develop specific criteria and measures in each area and evaluate them for compliance and effectiveness. Evaluation is possible to accomplish in some areas by management, and in others by a multidisciplinary committee or by groups of outside professionals and consumers.

In the past, measures of quality of the agency, the care delivered, and the staff were subjective, with little standardization and agreement. Quality assessment plans now reflect standards, objectives, and measurable outcomes and include plans for remediation or improvement as an integral part of the process. There is a move by a national accreditation body (TJC) and many businesses to redefine quality assessment activities in terms of quality improvement. Terms such as **total quality management, continuous quality improvement,** and **quality improvement** (for home care) relate to an agency-wide commitment to excellence that covers clinical and nonclinical functions. The following major principles are involved:

- Quality of patient care and desired outcomes are possible to improve by assessing and improving governance, management, and clinical and support processes that affect patient outcomes.
- Processes are carried out by individuals (managers, clinicians, support) and jointly by these groups.
- It is necessary to coordinate and integrate processes.
- Employees of an organization are motivated and competent to carry out processes and it is appropriate to give them opportunities to continuously improve through continuing education and also cardiopulmonary resuscitation (CPR) certification.

Continued movement toward this philosophy of home care management is likely in these first years of the twenty-first century. It will have a direct effect on all staff and provide a different emphasis on how many agencies will operate.

REIMBURSEMENT SOURCES

Reimbursement for home health services comes from a variety of sources, and covered services and disciplines vary. Medicare and Medicaid are major sources of income for the majority of agencies, but reliance on these sources for reimbursement has decreased in recent years.

MEDICARE

Medicare is a federal program that requires agencies to be certified as meeting the federal conditions of participation, which set forth specific requirements for organization, staffing, training, types of services covered, and agency evaluation. Regulations further mandate eligibility requirements. Beneficiaries of services are required to be 65 or older, disabled, or have end-stage renal disease. In addition, they have to be (1) under the care of a licensed physician, (2) homebound, and (3) in need of skilled nursing or therapy services on an intermittent basis. Types of services covered and length of coverage are further delineated in guidelines developed by the Health Care Financing Administration (HCFA). Ten regional fiscal intermediaries, who act on behalf of the HCFA, receive claims for payment, process reimbursement, and determine coverage.

MEDICAID

The **Medicaid** program pays for home care services to indigent and low-income people of all ages. The state administers it, but both state and federal funding subsidizes it. Many states require Medicare certification for participation in the Medicaid program. Services covered vary from state to state, but most include the basic services covered by Medicare plus expansion of aide and personal care services. This program has received permission, through a waiver process, to pay for around-the-clock services to children who require high-technology care and equipment. Children who have lived in an institution are able to go home and be a part of the family unit (Figure 37-2).

THIRD PARTY

Third-party insurers pay for limited home care services. Coverage, requirements, and payment rates vary. Reimbursement is often tied to posthospitalization recoveries. A few progressive companies are paying for nursing and aide services for new mothers who return home within 24 hours of delivery.

There is wide practice of case management by or on behalf of insurance companies and worker compensation plans. A case manager (commonly a nurse or social worker) will determine and arrange for a mix of home care, therapy services, counseling, supplies, and equipment for a patient. The availability of these combined, paid-for services often allows earlier discharges and provides a planned approach to rehabilitation.

A similar approach to case management for the older adult is commonly the goal of Area Agencies on Aging, social service departments, community or public health agencies, independent case managers, or contracts with groups or companies providing such services. Costs are sometimes fully paid, depending on how the service is provided.

PRIVATE PAY

Individuals sometimes also pay directly for home health services. Possible charges range from the standard full charge to scaled-down rates based on the ability of the patient to pay.

OTHER SOURCES

Health maintenance organizations (HMOs) and preferred provider organizations (PPOs) have negotiated contracts with home health agencies to provide services to their patients. Both organizations are prepaid health plans operated independently or through employer groups. Again, requirements and coverage differ.

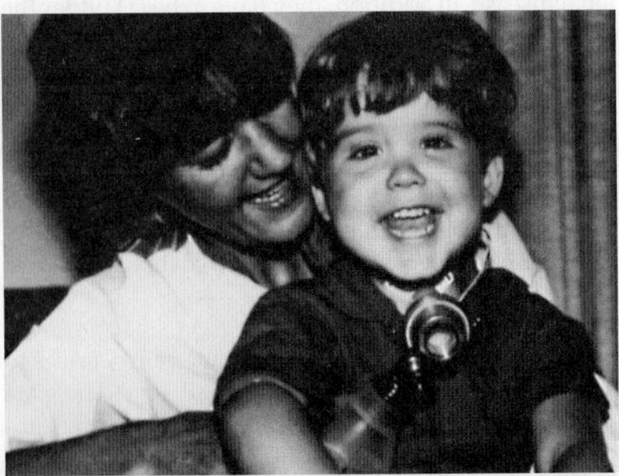

FIGURE 37-2 Child with Ondine's disease, chronic obstructive pulmonary disease, and collapsible airway syndrome. With the services of home health care, he has been able to recover at home.

CULTURAL CONSIDERATIONS

Nurses encounter great diversity in a variety of cultural interactions. It is very important to consider this factor when providing nursing interventions in the hospital, the nursing home, or the community. Culture is present in the lives of patients, families, and health care providers and is especially apparent in the home environment. Frustration occurs when values conflict, thus increasing the complexity involved in nursing interventions. As a nurse, you need to anticipate potential cultural problems and identify your own and other's values. Cultural health practices are acceptable to incorporate with traditional medical care in the home environment, provided it does not conflict with the prescribed treatment.

Apply all of the strategies you use to communicate with patients in general to patients from different cultures. In addition, there are several other steps to take to ensure clear and effective communication with patients from other cultures (see Cultural Considerations box; also see Chapters 3 and 8).

❖ NURSING PROCESS

The role of the licensed practical nurse/licensed vocational nurse (LPN/LVN) in the nursing process as stated is that the LPN/LVN will:

- Participate in planning care for patients based on patient needs
- Review patient's plan of care and recommend revisions as needed
- Review and follow defined prioritization for patient care
- Use clinical pathways, care maps, or care plans to guide and review patient care

Home health nursing uses the basic nursing process to assess the needs, establish a patient-centered plan of care, implement nursing actions, evaluate the effectiveness of actions, and plan for modification or resolution of identified problems. Possible interventions range from wound care to intravenous chemotherapy. Teaching will sometimes involve diabetes mellitus instruction or perhaps the management of complex support equipment in the home. Teaching is always patient centered, with the primary goals being self-care and independent functioning within the confines of the illness or disability (Figure 37-3). In the counseling role, you will sometimes provide emotional support to the dying patient and the family or provide skilled psychiatric interventions (if properly qualified). Case management possibly includes only supervision of the home health aide or will involve the coordination of complex care plans with services,

Cultural Considerations

Breaking through Cultural Barriers to Communication

Step 1: Assess your attitudes about people from other cultures.
- Review your personal beliefs and past experiences.
- Set aside any attitudes, values, and biases that are judgmental.

Step 2: Assess communications variables from a cultural perspective.
- Learn as much as possible about the patient's cultural customs and beliefs.
- Encourage the patient to reveal cultural interpretation of health, illness, and health care.
- Be sensitive to the uniqueness of the patient.
- Identify sources of discrepancy between the patient's and your own conceptions of health and illness.
- Communicate at the patient's level of functioning.
- Assess cultural factors that have the potential to affect your relationship with the patient, and respond appropriately.

Step 3: Modify communication to meet cultural needs.
- Be attentive to signs of fear, anxiety, and confusion in the patient. Be alert for feedback that the patient is not understanding.
- Respond in a reassuring manner in keeping with the patient's cultural orientation.
- Be alert to words the patient seems to understand, and use them frequently.
- Keep messages simple, and repeat them frequently.
- Avoid using medical terms and abbreviations that the patient perhaps does not understand.
- Be aware that in some cultural groups discussion with others concerning the patient will possibly cause offense and impede nursing practices.
- Use an appropriate language dictionary. A Spanish-English equivalency chart will help in some cases.

Step 4: Respect the patient and his or her communicated needs.
- Use a kind and attentive approach to convey respect.
- Learn how people signal that they are listening in the patient's culture; then use appropriate active listening techniques.
- Adopt an attitude of flexibility, respect, and interest to help bridge barriers imposed by culture.
- Be considerate of reluctance to talk when the subject involves sexual matters; be aware that in some cultures, people do not discuss sexual matters freely with members of the opposite sex.

Step 5: Communicate in a nonthreatening manner.
- Use a caring tone of voice and facial expression to help alleviate the patient's fears.
- Speak slowly and distinctly, but not loudly.
- Conduct the interview in an unhurried manner.
- Follow acceptable social and cultural amenities.
- Ask general questions during the information-gathering stage.
- Be patient when the respondent gives information that seems unrelated to the patient's health problem.
- Develop a trusting relationship by listening carefully, allowing time, and giving the patient your full attention.
- Use gestures and pictures to help the patient understand.
- Repeat the message in different ways if necessary.

Step 6: Use interpreters to improve communication.
- Ask the interpreter to translate the message, not just the individual words.
- Obtain feedback to confirm understanding.
- Use an interpreter who is culturally sensitive.

Modified from Giger, J.N., & Davidhizar, R.E. (2007). *Transcultural nursing: Assessment and intervention.* (5th ed.). St. Louis: Mosby.

supplies, and equipment provided by many different disciplines.

Assessment

Begin assessment by considering the patient and the family members and the patient's attitude toward the family. Also assess functions of the patient and the family. These include the ability of the family to provide emotional support for the patient, the ability to cope with the current health problem or situation, ways that goals are set, and progress everyone makes toward the achievement of goals. It is necessary to work within the structure of the family when providing care.

Nursing Diagnosis

The nursing diagnosis often focuses on the family's ability to cope with the illness of the family member. During times of acute illness, the family will in some cases become extremely distressed and will possibly focus solely on the patient, neglecting the needs of other members. While caring for a patient, sometimes you will learn of such difficulties and have the

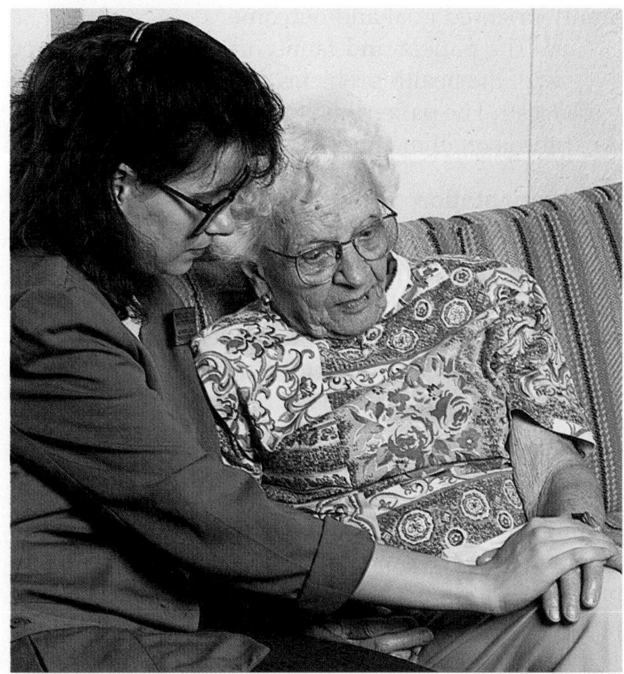

FIGURE 37-3 In the home, the nurse encourages the patient to use imagery to relax and relieve pain.

opportunity to help or refer the family to other resources. It is important to maintain a family nursing perspective. Possible nursing diagnoses related to the home health patient and family include the following:

- Interrupted family processes
- Impaired parenting
- Anxiety
- Caregiver role strain
- Constipation
- Impaired physical mobility
- Imbalanced nutrition: less than body requirements
- Acute confusion
- Ineffective airway clearance
- Risk for impaired skin integrity
- Compromised family coping
- Disabled family coping
- Fatigue
- Ineffective coping
- Ineffective management of therapeutic regimen
- Deficient knowledge
- Acute/Chronic pain
- Impaired home maintenance
- Risk for infection
- Social isolation
- Risk for caregiver role strain
- Risk for injury

Expected Outcomes and Planning

When planning nursing interventions for the patient, work with the patient and the family in setting goals. It is important for the patient and the family to understand and agree on the goals as you set them together. Also consider ways that the older adult affects family structure. The following is an example of a family-oriented goal and outcome:

Goal: The patient and family understand and cope with the health problems of its member.

Outcome: The patient and family are able to meet the needs of all members.

Implementation

After goal setting has taken place, assist the patient and family to learn health promotion practices. Providing accurate health information about the diagnosis and the prognosis helps the patient and the family members to understand the patient's experience and the best ways to be effective caregivers.

Evaluation

Be prepared to revise a plan of care depending on the findings of the evaluation. The nurse determines whether expected outcomes have been met. An example of a goal and evaluative measure related to the family follows:

Goal: The family understands and copes with the health problems of its members.

Evaluative measure: The family members are able to perform care measures correctly.

CONCLUSION

Current trends support the growth of home care as an economic, humane, preferred health delivery system for many types of care. Advances in medical knowledge, coupled with high-technology health care, have increased the number of individuals surviving birth traumas, prematurity, infectious diseases, acute illnesses, accidents, and other maladies that were formerly fatal.

Medical management and control rather than cure are the standard of care for many illnesses. This has increased the number of potentially debilitating chronic illnesses. Dependency and disability are more prevalent in all age-groups. Home care provides the assessment and evaluation of chronic illnesses necessary to prevent acute episodes. Aides and homemakers have the capacity to provide necessary support in ADLs to enable the patient to remain in the home.

The birth rate has declined, resulting in an aging population. In the 1900s, only 2% of the U.S. population was 65 or older. That figure was 12.3% (36 million people) in 2004 and is projected to reach 20% by 2030. Nearly 20% of this group fall into the categories of the poor or the near-poor. Some 80% of this group is estimated to have at least one chronic disability. The older-than-85 age-group is the fastest growing group today. About 40% of those 85 and older need help with physical activities (Federal Interagency Forum on Aging-Related Statistics, 2004). Assistance in daily living is essential to this group. Skilled nursing and therapy offer rehabilitation and prevention of deterioration, as well as methods to cope with physical changes.

Federal and private insurers are trying to cap the rapidly rising cost of health care by shortening hospital stays and controlling admissions. Home care agencies are filling the gap for patients who are released early but who still require complex care or rehabilitation. In many cases, home care services offer the means to prevent hospitalization by providing enteral, parenteral, intravenous, and blood transfusion services.

The movement toward deinstitutionalization of technology-dependent children and adults is now becoming feasible as Medicaid and third-party payers change reimbursement criteria. Home care support makes "family life" a reality for people who once thought of hospital personnel as parents.

Home health providers support an emphasis on healthy living and illness prevention as part of the plan of care. This one-on-one education teaches specific techniques to prevent recurrences of illness or deterioration of condition. Individuals want to be at home as long as possible. Care provided by home health agencies and support from social service agencies and others are now making this possible throughout the life span.

Get Ready for the NCLEX® Examination!

Key Points

- Home health care allows individuals to maintain personal control and to participate in the direction of their own care.
- Families are an important part of the success of home care services as health care workers provide care, supervision, assistance, and support in attaining the care plan goals.
- Home health care is not a new concept; however, legislative, regulatory, and current health care trends have changed the way it is provided.
- A number of different professional and paraprofessional disciplines provide home care services based on a coordinated plan of care approved by a physician. Teamwork is an essential component of the concept.
- Home health agencies are organized groups that employ or contract with professionals and paraprofessionals to provide services. Different types of agencies will usually be subject to varying federal, state, and local laws and regulations.
- Skilled nursing care is the most frequently provided service. RNs and LPNs/LVNs under the supervision of RNs provide direct care of different levels of complexity.
- Providers of care in the home need to possess special qualities to effectively practice in this nontraditional environment.
- Home health care agencies strive to provide the highest quality of services economically. Success is evaluated through quality assurance plans.
- Home health services are reimbursed by federal, state, local, group, and private sources.
- Congress imposed new limits on home health payments through a provision of the Balanced Budget Act of 1997 (BBA) called the Interim Payment System (IPS).
- Quality assessment of safe and effective care in the home is of great significance.
- Although some aspects of nursing interventions in the home are the same as those practiced in other health care settings, home health care nurses pay particular attention to interaction and cooperation among family members, the patient, and other members of the health care team.
- The acuity levels of patients requiring care in their homes continues to rise, and the technologic aspects of care, including use of mechanical equipment and invasive procedures such as intravenous therapies, are increasing in home care. These factors, when combined with shorter hospital stays, require extensive discharge planning to prepare patients and family for home health care.

Additional Learning Resources

Go to your Companion CD for an audio glossary, animations, video clips, and more.

evolve Be sure to visit the Evolve site at http://evolve.elsevier.com/Christensen/foundations/ for additional online resources.

Review Questions for the NCLEX® Examination

1. A 79-year-old patient recently fractured her hip and had a hemiarthroplasty (bipolar) hip repair. Her daughter works during the day but provides care in the evening. The most appropriate service agency to provide for this patient's daily care is a/an:
   1. private duty agency.
   2. home health care agency.
   3. nursing home facility.
   4. outpatient rehabilitation agency.

2. A student nurse asks her nurse educator why there is an increased demand for home health care. The most accurate response by the educator is that:
   1. more family members want to care for their ill members at home.
   2. there is a shortage of nurses who want to work in acute hospital care settings.
   3. there is an increase in the number of older patients with chronic illnesses.
   4. there is increased technology in hospitals, which provokes anxiety in many patients.

3. The nurse is assigned to home health care for an 83-year-old patient with a stroke who has right-sided hemiplegia, difficulty swallowing, and speech impairment. He is receiving care in his home from his wife and retired daughter. It is necessary for the nurse involved in administering care in their home to provide a:
   1. strict regimen and care plan.
   2. holistic, nonjudgmental philosophy.
   3. teaching plan for all family members.
   4. means of transporting the patient to his physician.

4. Nurses are aware that evolving future health care trends point to:
   1. decreased reimbursement for home health care services.
   2. keeping patients in the hospital longer because of the severity of their illnesses.
   3. increased high-technology procedures in the home setting.
   4. slowed growth in number of agencies involved in home care.

5. A 68-year-old patient is recovering from an abdominoperineal resection with a permanent colostomy. Her physician has ordered home health care nursing upon her discharge. A primary goal for home health care nursing for this patient will be to:
   1. return the patient to previous lifestyle.
   2. avoid dependency on medication therapy.
   3. establish self-care and independence.
   4. maintain a friendly relationship with family members.

6. It is necessary for a nursing supervisor for home health care to always be concerned with patient care and:

1. location of the home.
2. quality assurance.
3. method of payment.
4. number of children in the home.

7. When the home health care nurse makes arrangements for the patient to receive home care, data are collected from the:

1. home care agency.
2. patient and family members.
3. insurance company.
4. community volunteer agencies.

8. Which services does a home health agency generally provide? *(Select all that apply.)*

1. Skilled nursing
2. Nutritional support
3. Home health aide
4. Recreational therapy

9. A major influence on home health care began in 1983. This system, based on major diagnostic categories and diagnosis-related groups, paid a set rate for the hospitalized patient's care rather than the "cost," or charges traditionally billed by institutions. Such patients were discharged earlier in their convalescence and thus required more home nursing care. This system is called:

1. prospective payment system (PPS).
2. Medicaid.
3. Medicare.
4. Older American Act.

10. In 1997, Congress imposed new limits on home health payments through a provision of the:

1. Social Security Administration.
2. National Institutes of Health (NIH).
3. Balanced Budget Act (BBA).
4. Human and Health Services (HHS).

11. The effects of the 1997 congressional provision affected home health by:

1. increasing the number of patients served by home health.
2. decreasing the number of patients served by home health.

12. In 2000, the Health Care Financing Administration (HCFA) instituted:

1. a new payment system for home health agencies.
2. Medicare-certified agencies.
3. The Joint Commission.
4. rules governing certification of home health agencies.

13. Two major nursing considerations crucial for patients in their homes as well as in structured facilities are:

1. need for security and immediate medical direction.
2. assessment and teaching.
3. frequent peer support and independence.
4. need for administrators' and managers' availability and casual documentation.

14. The environment for home health care nursing is controlled by the:

1. physician.
2. home health nurse.
3. physical therapist.
4. patient and the family.

15. Over the past several years, technology advances have helped increase the adoption of ________ to monitor the patient's vital signs, oxygen saturation, and weight in the home for the home health agency.

16. To qualify for coverage for home health services by Medicare, an HMO, or other insurance, it is necessary to meet which criteria? *(Select all that apply.)*

1. The patient needs wound care.
2. The patient has to be homebound.
3. The patient has to need intermittent skilled nursing care.
4. The patient needs to receive a vitamin B_{12} injection every month.

chapter 38

Long-Term Care

evolve

Elaine Oden Kockrow and Patricia A. O'Neill

http://evolve.elsevier.com/Christensen/foundationsadult

Objectives

1. Describe settings of long-term care services.
2. Identify patients of long-term care services.
3. Discuss federal and state regulations related to long-term care.
4. Identify the sources of reimbursement for long-term care services.
5. Define chronic and acute health services.
6. Describe goals of long-term care health services.
7. Describe long-term care nursing services.
8. Describe services available from each type of agency: home health agency, hospice agency, adult daycare, assisted living facility, continuing care community, and long-term care facility.

Key Terms

activities of daily living (ADLs) (p. 1195)
adult daycare (p. 1196)
assisted living (p. 1197)
continuing care retirement community (CCRC) (p. 1198)
functional assessment (p. 1202)
hospice (HŎS-pĭs, p. 1196)
instrumental activities of daily living (IADLs) (p. 1197)
long-term care (p. 1193)
Medicaid (p. 1201)
Medicare (p. 1201)
minimum data set (MDS) (p. 1202)
Omnibus Budget Reconciliation Act (OBRA) (p. 1201)
palliative care (p. 1196)
quality of life (p. 1193)
resident assessment instrument (RAI) (p. 1202)
residential care (p. 1197)
restorative nursing care (p. 1200)
skilled nursing facilities (p. 1198)
subacute unit (p. 1198)

Long-term care is defined by the American Nurses Association (ANA) as the provision of physical, psychological, spiritual, social, and economic services to help people attain, maintain, and regain their optimum level of functioning. It encompasses a range of services, including health maintenance and care, to people who have lost their ability to function independently because of a chronic illness or condition. The need for long-term care services arises after the acute stage of an illness has resolved, and when the patient continues to need services to support and maintain physical and psychological status and functional abilities. Patients in need of long-term care are primarily older adults who are frail or disabled, but they are sometimes also young and middle-age adults, or even children with chronic illnesses, developmental disabilities, or traumatic injuries.

There are various settings for and a broad spectrum of long-term care services. What the setting is and for what services depends on the individual and unique needs of each patient. Caregivers need to use a patient-centered approach to achieve and maintain an individualized plan of care and to assist the patient in preserving a meaningful quality of life. It is possible to define quality of life as a measure of the optimum energy or force that endows a person with the power to cope successfully with the full range of challenges he or she encounters in the real world. Quality of life is important in maintaining self-esteem and a sense of well-being, as well as experiencing the pleasures of life (Figure 38-1). Furthermore, the *Healthy People 2010* initiative specifically addresses quality of life as one of its two broad goals: "to increase the quality and years of healthy life" (U.S. Department of Health and Human Services [US DHHS], 2000).

Culture is a system of values, beliefs, and practices that guide a person's behavior. Cultural influences play a large role in shaping patients' beliefs about health and illness, therefore greatly influencing health behaviors. Religion is one of the universal components of culture (see Cultural Considerations box on religion among older adult populations). Ethnicity is a person's identification with a certain ethnic group based on shared traditions, national origin, physical characteristics, and other markers such as language, religion, food, and dress. The composition of the older adult population is changing—racial and ethnic diversity is increasing (see Cultural Considerations box on diversity in the long-term care setting). For example, 4% of older adults in the United States are Hispanic; this number is expected

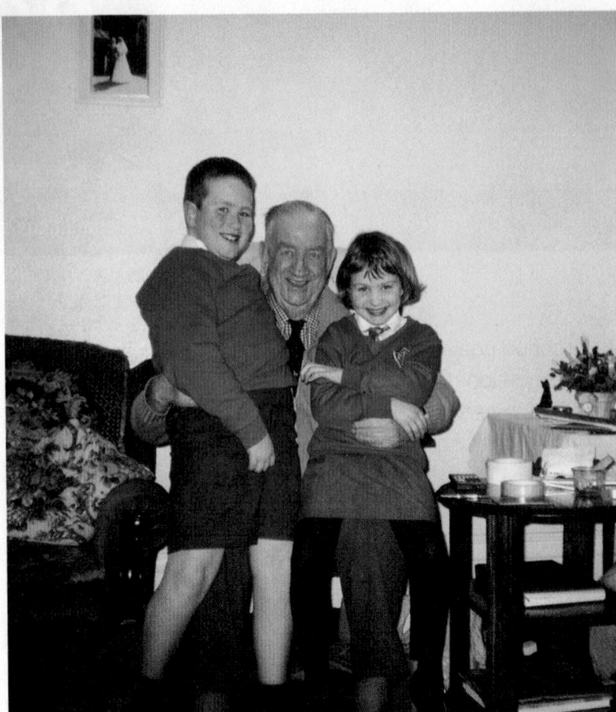

FIGURE 38-1 Family is important in helping to maintain quality of life for the older adult.

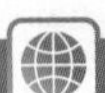

Cultural Considerations

Religion among Older Adult Populations

- In the long-term care facility, one goal of the interdisciplinary team is to provide opportunities for the resident to participate in worship services that support his or her religious beliefs. Worship services to meet spiritual needs are important; also encourage visitation and support from clergy of any denomination.
- Nursing, social services, and the dietary department provide support through an interdisciplinary team approach. The team discusses the care of the resident and the appropriateness of attendance at worship services.
- Dietary services take into consideration any food preferences or foods to avoid, based on the resident's culture and religion.
- The long-term care facility consistently provides opportunities to practice one's religious faith.

to increase to 16% by 2050 (US DHHS and Administration on Aging, 2003). Knowledge of cultural and ethnic groups is important to your ability to provide comprehensive nursing interventions (see O'Neill [2002] for a comprehensive discussion about culture and aging).

Historically, providers of long-term care have managed these services based on a medical model that includes expert nursing services and medical management. Patient safety in any setting has and always will be a priority. As the patient population changes, health care in the long-term care industry will evolve to meet the needs of older adults with functional impairments related to normal changes of aging, in addition to any health disorders they experience.

Cultural Considerations

Diversity in Long-Term Care Facilities

Although residents of long-term care facilities are predominantly white women, residents are becoming older and ethnically more diverse.

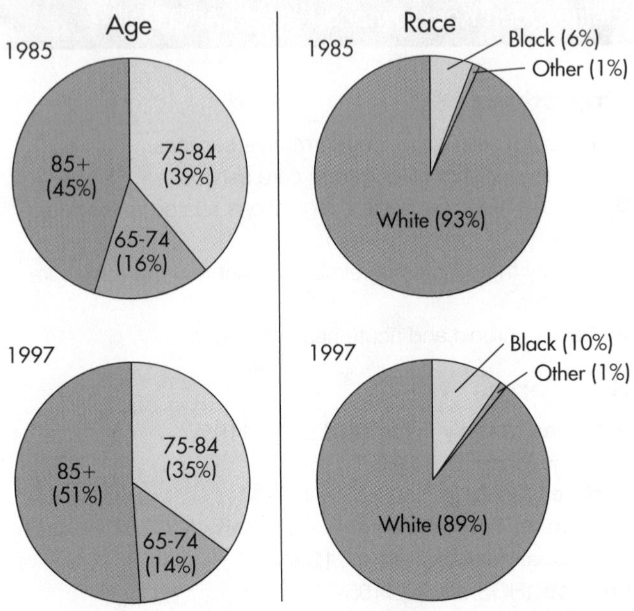

Data from Sahyoun, N.R., et al. (2001). *The changing profile of nursing home residents 1985-1997.* (No. 4). Hyattsville, MD: National Center for Health Statistics.

SETTINGS FOR LONG-TERM CARE

For the past several years, the long-term care system has been undergoing transformation, and numerous alternatives to long-term care facilities have emerged (Medicare.gov, 2007). Part of this transformation has been driven by consumer demand, a trend that experts expect will continue as the baby boomer generation ages and older adults demand greater attention on health care issues pertinent to their needs. The future of long-term care will continue to evolve over the coming years. At present, numerous settings provide long-term care, but they all fall under one of three basic categories, from least restrictive to most restrictive (Figure 38-2):

1. The home
2. Residential care settings
3. Institutional settings

THE HOME

Most older adults live in a home setting, with only a small percentage of those age 65 and older residing in an institutional setting. Of these, the majority (67%) live in a family setting, consisting of spouse, children, siblings, or other relatives. The remaining older adults who live in a home setting live either alone (30.6%) or with nonrelatives (2.7%) (Centers for Disease Control and Prevention [CDC], National Center for Health Statistics, 2004).

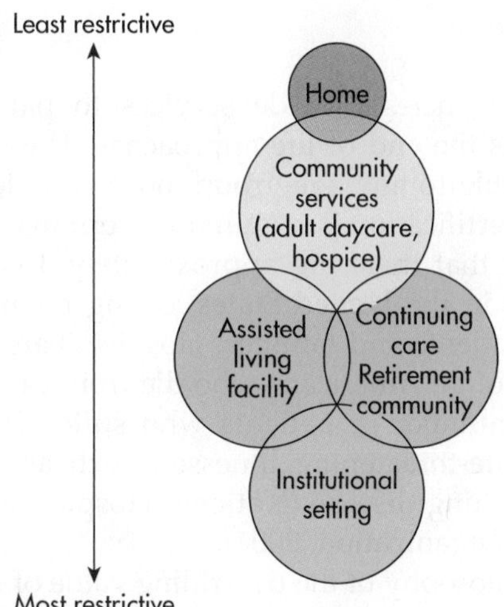

FIGURE 38-2 Available settings that provide long-term care services.

Care of the older adult at home sometimes involves a great deal of participation from loved ones. Much of the responsibility for care often falls on women. Older women will in some cases be caring for a spouse, children, grandchildren, and even great-grandchildren in a multigenerational household (Figure 38-3). Without the support of the family unit, there would undoubtedly be even more admissions to long-term care facilities, perhaps triple the current number. It is not possible to ignore the cost savings to society: It costs approximately half as much to care for an older adult at home as it would cost in a long-term care facility, unless the older adult has a great degree of physical impairment. Many of those caring for older adults at home rely on valuable community services to assist them (Box 38-1).

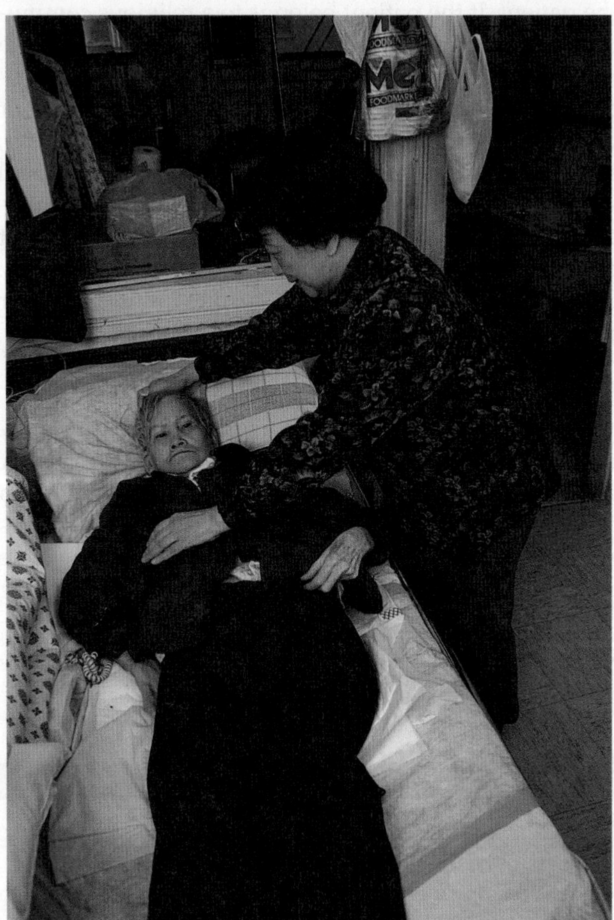

FIGURE 38-3 Caring for aging parents is one of the tasks of middle adulthood. Women who care for aging parents often find it difficult to balance their own needs and the needs of others.

One of these services, the home health agency, strives to fulfill the needs of the homebound patient in his or her home as long as possible (see Chapter 37). The growth of the over-65 population and the increase of the cost of institutional long-term care have stimulated interest in home health care. Although the typical home health patient is female, older than age 85, with circulatory or cardiac disorders (CDC, 2004), some home care patients require only minimal assistance, such as help with **activities of daily living (ADLs)**, those routines of hygiene, dressing and grooming, toileting, eating, and ambulating each person carries out independently throughout life; others are perhaps receiving complex medical therapies such as mechanical ventilation and renal dialysis.

Services that home health agencies provide focus on rehabilitation with physical therapy, occupational therapy, speech therapy, respiratory therapy, access to social services, nutritional support by a registered dietitian, the rental or purchase of durable medical equipment, and nursing services. Home health agencies offer nursing services from professionals including homemakers, shoppers, respite care workers, personal care attendants, certified nursing assistants (CNAs), home health aides (HHAs), licensed practical nurses and licensed vocational nurses (LPNs/LVNs), and registered nurses (RNs) to provide the more complex care and education.

Box 38-1 Services to Support Home Care Providers for Older Adults

- *Respite care:* Scheduled stays for the older adult needing care at a long-term care facility (e.g., 1 week every 4 months) to give caregiver and older adult with needs "time off."
- *Daycare:* A setting providing structured activities during the day, similar to daycare for children.
- *Home health care:* Including homemakers, shoppers, respite care workers, personal care attendants, home health aides, and nursing care staff.
- *Nutrition programs:* Congregate meals (at senior center) or home delivery of one hot meal per day (Meals-on-Wheels) for a nominal fee.
- *Senior centers:* Government-funded centers that provide recreational activities, lunch, health screening, classes, and transportation to and from the site if needed.
- *Transportation services:* Dial-a-Ride service to grocery shopping or medical appointments.

Adapted from O'Neill, P.A. (2002). *Caring for the older adult: a health promotion perspective*. Philadelphia: Saunders.

In recent years, Medicare has developed two programs that promise to allow older adults with health care needs to continue living at home while receiving services. These programs are called Program of All-Inclusive Care for the Elderly (PACE) and Social Managed Care Plan (Medicare.gov, 2007). The latter serves only four areas of the country at present and requires deductibles and co-pays, and most branches exclude patients with end-stage renal disease. PACE, on the other hand, has sites in 14 states and requires only that the patient be 55 years of age or older, live in a "service area," be screened by a group of health professionals, and sign and agree to enrollment terms. PACE offers and manages all of the "medical, social, and rehabilitative services their enrollees need to preserve or restore their independence, to remain in their homes and communities, and to maintain their quality of life" (Medicare.gov, 2007).

Role of the Licensed Practical Nurse/Licensed Vocational Nurse and the Registered Nurse

Often the role of the LPN/LVN in the home health care setting will involve private duty or shift work. His or her responsibilities will sometimes include home visits to gather data to evaluate care provided by the homemakers, personal care attendants, CNAs, and HHAs. The LPN/LVN also provides a valuable human resource as staffing coordinator, intake coordinator, or medical chart auditor or reviewer. The staffing coordinator receives information from the intake coordinator describing the requested home care for the patient. The staffing coordinator, based on established protocols, schedules the appropriate care provider to meet the needs of the patient and verifies financial coverage for the care. A medical chart auditor or reviewer uses knowledge of health care to fulfill the quality assurance documentation guidelines (see Coordinated Care box).

In home health care, the RN provides intermittent visits for holistic care, supervisory home visits, comprehensive assessments, referrals, nursing interventions, health care education, health maintenance, and home management. Within the home health care agency, the RN also functions as a manager and administrator.

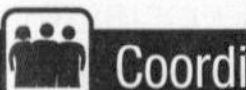

Coordinated Care

Delegation

THE LICENSED PRACTICAL OR LICENSED VOCATIONAL NURSE AS STAFF COORDINATOR

An important example of the LPN/LVN delegating care is when the LPN/LVN performs the role of staffing coordinator. As with any delegation, it is critical that the LPN/LVN consider the scope of practice and the individual abilities of the caregiver when scheduling and assigning care. In some states, LPNs/LVNs are not authorized to delegate; only RNs have the power to delegate, by regulation.

HOSPICE

Hospice agencies provide services to patients and families as the end of life approaches. These services are available to any age-group, not just older adults. Medical certification is required for terminal care. It is estimated that there are approximately 3200 hospice programs in the United States, caring for more than 885,000 patients and families. Hospices care for more than half of all Americans who die from cancer and a growing number of patients who suffer from other chronic, life-threatening illnesses, such as end-stage heart and lung disease (National Hospice and Palliative Care Organization, 2004).

The philosophy of the overriding value of maintaining comfort as death approaches is central to hospice care. **Palliative care** extends the principles of hospice care to a broader population that has the possibility to benefit from comfort care earlier in their illness or disease process. This agency provides nursing interventions to meet basic needs, ADLs, pain and symptom management, and spiritual and psychosocial support for the patient, the family, and significant others. Care providers include CNAs, HHAs, LPNs/LVNs, and RNs for case management. Volunteers provide respite relief for caregivers and socialization and companionship for the patient. If the patient belongs to a religious community, parish nurses sometimes serve as an adjunct to hospice care to assist the patient and family with psychosocial concerns and bereavement issues. Hospice or terminal care is possible to provide in the home setting; in an inpatient hospice unit located in an institutional setting, such as a long-term care facility; or in a standalone "hospice house." Patients enter into an inpatient hospice unit generally for one of the following reasons: pain or symptom management, respite for the family, or terminal care (see Home Care Considerations box).

ADULT DAYCARE

Adult daycare services are community-based programs designed to meet the needs of functionally or cognitively impaired adults through supervised health care and social and recreational activities (Alzheimer's Association, n.d.). These structured, comprehensive programs provide a variety of services, including physical care, mental stimulation, socialization, assistance with health maintenance, and health referrals, during any part of the day, but for less than 24 hours a

Home Care Considerations

Hospice Care

Providers of hospice care usually do so in the patient's home. Typically, a family member serves as the primary caregiver, with hospice staff on call 24 hours a day and making regular visits.

National Hospice and Palliative Care Organization. (2004). *What is hospice and palliative care?* Available at www.nhpco.org/i4a/pages/index.cfm?pageid=4648. Accessed December, 2009.

day (Box 38-2). These centers generally operate during regular business hours, with the patient returning home to family or caregivers at night, although some offer services during evening and weekend hours.

Adult daycare centers are designed to serve adults who require supervision, social opportunities, or assistance, owing to a physical or cognitive impairment. The typical adult attending daycare is disabled and averages 75 years of age. Many require assistance with one to three ADLs (Lucas et al., 2002).

Adult mental health centers and senior centers are additional places where families are able to turn for adult daycare services. These centers are sometimes located in churches or public-use areas within the community. Their staff includes a director, an activities coordinator, and a personal care attendant. The director of an adult daycare center is sometimes a social worker, and more preferably, an RN. It is appropriate for the activities coordinator to have specialized training and education in activities to promote maintenance of functional abilities and independence in the environment (Figure 38-4). The personal care attendant assists with ADLs. The CNA or personal care attendant has to meet state requirements of training in assistance with ADLs and basic observation skills.

In summary, numerous services are available for the older adult who wishes to live at home. The time often comes, however, when the older adult is no longer able to remain in the home environment despite the support of family and community services.

Box 38-2 Typical Services Offered by Adult Daycare Centers

- Transportation
- Social services
- Meals
- Nursing interventions
- Personal care
- Counseling
- Therapeutic activities
- Rehabilitation therapies

From National Adult Day Services Association, Inc. (2008). *Adult day services: overview and facts.* Available at www.nadsa.org/adsfacts/default.asp. Accessed December, 2009.

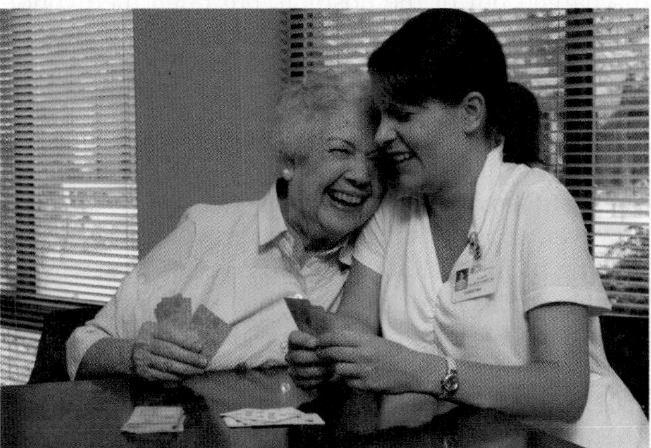

FIGURE 38-4 Social interaction and acceptance are important aspects of care for the older adult.

RESIDENTIAL CARE SETTINGS

Residential care settings serve primarily an older adult population, offering a wide variety of services. Among the most popular types of residential care facilities are assisted living facilities, congregate care facilities, and retirement communities (Caregivers USA, 2004). In the following section, we will examine two of the more popular types of settings that have flourished in the past decade: assisted living and continuing care retirement communities.

Assisted Living

Assisted living is a type of residential care setting in which the adult patient rents a small one-bedroom or studio-type apartment and has the option of receiving several personal care services such as bathing, dressing, and taking medications. Assisted living services are possible to provide in freestanding residences, near or integrated with skilled nursing homes or hospitals, as components of continuing care retirement communities, or at independent housing complexes. Virtually unheard of before 1990, assisted living facilities number more than 11,000 in the United States with more than half a million residents nationwide. The typical resident of an assisted living setting is an 80-year-old woman who is mobile but needs assistance with two ADLs (National Center for Assisted Living, 2006a).

Personal care services included in assisted living environments include housekeeping and laundry. The patient receives encouragement to partake in communal dining and various social activities. Some facilities offer transportation for organized recreational activity or personal business (Figure 38-5). Nursing care varies from minimal care for patients with impairments in ADLs or instrumental activities of daily living (IADLs), to more complex daily tasks such as shopping and using the telephone, as well as assistance with medications to more complex care such as tube feeding and oxygen therapy. Some facilities even con-

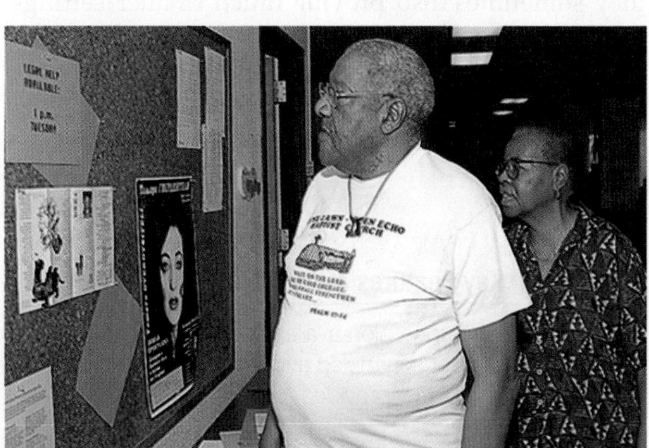

FIGURE 38-5 Bulletin board at a senior center showing times when legal help is available.

tract for outside hospice care. You will find key features of assisted living in Box 38-3.

Staffing requirements for caregivers in assisted living facilities vary from state to state. Many states have age and skill requirements for caregivers (e.g., first aid, cardiopulmonary resuscitation [CPR]) and sometimes require special credentialing such as CNA or HHA. Administrators are sometimes RNs or LPNs, and sometimes not, and many states require continuing education (National Center for Assisted Living, 2009). (A detailed listing of requirements, state by state, is available at www.ncal.org/about/2006_reg_review.pdf.) As of January 1, 2009, the state of Virginia will require all persons who administer medications in a Department of Social Service licensed assisted living facility to be a registered Medication Aide (registered with the Virginia Board of Nursing).

Continuing Care Retirement Communities

A **continuing care retirement community (CCRC)** offers a complete range of housing and health care accommodations, from independent living to 24-hour skilled nursing care. Usually, an older adult will enter a CCRC when he or she is in relatively good health and capable of living independently or with little assistance. In most cases, signing a contract to enter a CCRC is a lifetime commitment. The CCRC offers the resident this complete range of housing and care for the rest of his or her life, enabling the older adult the opportunity to experience a gradual transition from independent living to continuous skilled nursing care (if needed) while remaining at the same location. For an older couple, it is comforting to know that they will be able to stay together, even though one of them will possibly come to require long-term care.

There are more than 2000 CCRCs in the United States, serving approximately 625,000 older adults. The typical resident is a woman and 83 years of age, although most adults enter the CCRC at age 78. CCRCs offer apartments, townhomes, or detached dwellings, or a combination of these; they sometimes accommodate several hundred residents, although they sometimes also provide much smaller settings. Facilities range from luxurious settings with tennis courts, swimming pools, and hotel-style dining rooms to more modest facilities with similar but less plush amenities. Many CCRCs have long waiting lists for admission.

Box 38-3 Key Features of Assisted Living

- Services and supervision available 24 hours a day
- Services to meet scheduled and unscheduled needs
- Care and services provided or arranged to promote independence
- Emphasis on resident's dignity, autonomy, and choice
- Emphasis on privacy and a homelike environment

Nursing interventions a resident in a CCRC takes advantage of depend on the functional abilities of the older adult. With more independent residents, a personal care attendant, CNA, or HHA will perhaps provide assistance with ADLs or IADLs. Nursing interventions are possible to provide for residents requiring skilled nursing interventions by LPNs/LVNs or RNs. Some CCRCs contract with outside agencies to provide needed services, such as hospice care. Some CCRCs contract with nursing registries to provide personnel for long-term care in a resident's apartment. The reward of nursing in this setting is, again, the opportunity to care for a patient over a longer time frame.

INSTITUTIONAL SETTINGS

Subacute Unit

The **subacute unit** is a type of institutional setting that has become extremely popular since the late 1980s, when the advantage became clear of providing a less expensive alternative to acute care when patients have high-acuity medical and nursing intervention needs. The subacute unit is possible to view as a bridge between acute care and long-term care. Most subacute units are located in freestanding **skilled nursing facilities;** others are former hospital units that have been reclassified to provide subacute care. Subacute units have a stronger rehabilitative focus and shorter length of stay than a long-term care facility. The level of care that subacute units provide is at nearly the same acuity as in the hospital. In fact, the typical older adult in a subacute unit today corresponds to the typical medical-surgical patient of the 1980s.

Why is this happening? It is a combination of our increased life span and changes in hospital reimbursement. Modern medicine is saving lives that, before technologic advances, we were unable to save. This has led to a ripple effect: Those people who did not have a chance to survive before technologic advances are now occupying beds in the intensive care unit (ICU). People who used to occupy the ICU beds are now on the medical-surgical floor. Those who used to occupy beds on the medical-surgical floor are now discharged out of the hospital, but often their conditions are too complicated for home care; hence the evolution of the subacute unit.

In the acute care setting, strict rules about length of stay and limitations in cost reimbursement limit the amount of time it is possible to hospitalize an adult. These strict reimbursement rules for acute care do not, however, apply to subacute care provided in a skilled nursing facility setting. Therefore cost savings are an important reason for the growth of subacute care: The average cost saving per day is estimated to be 40% to 60% when compared with the hospital setting (O'Neill, 2002).

You will find older adults with numerous disorders in a subacute facility. Patients are able to receive numerous therapies, including intravenous medication administration via peripheral or central venous catheters, complex dressing changes, and even mechanical ventilation. The four most common patient care needs in subacute care are physical rehabilitation, stroke rehabilitation, wound care, and recovery from hip fracture. The nurse employed in a subacute unit needs to have a variety of assessment, rehabilitative, medical-surgical, and leadership skills. The assessment and technical skills of a medical-surgical nurse are required, along with the knowledge about reimbursement and interdisciplinary team skills of a long-term care nurse.

Long-Term Care Facility

The long-term care facility is the dominant setting for long-term care services. Commonly known as a nursing home or extended-care facility, this institutional setting provides services to adults, primarily older adults (older than 65). Long-term care facilities provide 24-hour care to individuals who do not require expensive inpatient hospital services but who do not have options for care at home or by other community agencies or services. Because the long-term care facility becomes a home for the older adult, either on a long-term or short-term basis, the older adult is referred to as a resident rather than patient. The average age of a long-term care resident is 81 years, and more than half of long-term care facility residents are age 85 or older (US DHHS, 2003).

Most residents of long-term care facilities have more than one health disorder when they are admitted, and more than half have three or more medical diagnoses. These are the most common disorders on admission:

- Cardiovascular disease, including hypertension and cerebrovascular accident
- Mental and cognitive disorders, including depression, anxiety, and dementia
- Endocrine disorders, including type 2 diabetes mellitus and hypothyroidism

It is a common misconception that the majority of older adults live in long-term care facilities; overall, only 4.5% of all adults older than age 65 reside in such a setting. With increasing age, however, the percentages increase dramatically: from 1.1% for those ages 65 to 74, to 4.7% for those ages 75 to 84, to 18.2% for those older than age 85 (Administration on Aging, 2004).

Although cardiovascular disorders are the most common diagnoses on admission, they are not necessarily the main reasons why an older adult enters into long-term care. Cognitive impairment, incontinence, inability to perform ADLs, and being single or widowed are also important factors determining placement into a long-term care facility. Patients with cognitive disorders, such as Alzheimer's disease, are difficult to manage at home or in other less restrictive care environments, owing to the patient's short-term memory loss, confusion, disorientation, restlessness, wandering, and hallucinations. A major safety event, such as forgetting to turn off the stove, is often the precipitating event in long-term care facility placement. As patients with Alzheimer's disease advance in age, they also experience a decline in their ability to participate in their ADLs, and eventually become totally dependent on others for care. In the final stages of the disorder, they become immobile.

Two categories of residents generally are found in a long-term care facility. The first category is the short-term resident, sometimes called the short-stay resident. Typically, this type of resident has been transferred from an acute care facility to which he or she had been admitted for an acute illness or the worsening of a chronic illness. The resident is admitted principally for rehabilitation and is expected to be discharged within 6 months. There are many similarities between this type of resident and the resident of a subacute unit. The second category is the traditional type of resident who lives in the facility on a long-term basis. Such a resident usually stays in the facility until he or she dies or is transferred to an acute care facility. This resident possibly has numerous nursing intervention needs and is perhaps cognitively impaired. Most residents in the typical long-term care facility are of the traditional category, although the trend is toward admitting more short-term residents. As a result, the overall nursing interventions of long-term care residents have become increasingly complex.

The long-term care facility industry is large and will continue to grow as the population ages, although it is changing. There are fewer, but larger, long-term care facilities today. The greatest population growth is occurring in the older adult group, the oldest-old or frail elderly, those older than age 85. The philosophy in a long-term care facility is to maintain and restore health and functional abilities to the resident's highest level and to provide a homelike atmosphere, promoting dignity, independence, restoration, maintenance, and assistance in ADLs, and skilled nursing interventions (Box 38-4).

The Long-Term Interdisciplinary Care Team

The long-term care facility is an interdisciplinary setting. In this setting, health care professionals work together as an interdisciplinary team to meet the needs of the older adult. Members of the team will possibly include the resident, nursing personnel (gerontologic clinical nurse specialists, RNs, LPNs/LVNs, CNAs), a physician, social worker, pharmacist, dietitian, activities director, and rehabilitation specialists (from the areas of physical therapy, occupational therapy, and speech therapy), as well as a podiatrist, psychiatrist, audiologist, and dentist. As mentioned, the long-term care industry is now challenged to provide a homelike environment and an individualized approach to residents with more complex care needs than this setting

Box 38-4 Selection of a Nursing Home

SIX ASPECTS OF QUALITY TO CONSIDER

An important step in the process of selecting a nursing home is to visit the nursing home. While looking around the nursing home, consider whether you observe these aspects of quality:

- *Home:* The nursing home does not feel like a hospital. It is a home, a place where people live. Staff encourages residents to personalize their rooms. Privacy is respected.
- *Care:* In addition to assistance with basic activities of daily living such as bathing, dressing, eating, oral hygiene, and toileting, staff assists residents with social and recreational activities. Residents are out of bed and dressed according to their preferences. Visitors are able to see the staff actively assisting and interacting socially with residents.
- *Family involvement:* Staff welcomes families when they visit the facility. Staff encourages family involvement, whether families wish to provide information, ask questions, participate in care planning, or assist with social activities or physical care.
- *Environment:* Residents, their clothing, their belongings, and their surroundings are clean. Staff are clean and well-groomed. There are no pervasive odors in the facility. Ample nonglare lighting, minimal noise, plants, comfortable furniture, and pets contribute to a homelike environment.
- *Communication:* Good communication among residents, families, and staff is necessary for quality care. Good communication is respectful and considerate.
- *Staff:* Members of the nursing home staff are attentive to resident requests and actively involved with assisting the residents. They focus on the person, not on the task. The assistance that they provide to residents includes assistance with social or recreational activities, as well as the performance of nursing duties.

Data from Potter, P.A., & Perry, A.G. (2007). *Basic nursing: essentials for practice.* (6th ed). St. Louis: Mosby; Rantz, M., Popejoy, L., & Zwygart-Stauffacher, M. (2001). *The new nursing homes: a 20-minute way to find great long-term care.* Minneapolis: Fairview Press.

used to accommodate. The interdisciplinary care planning meetings (often called ICPs) are mandated by OBRA to occur on a regular basis. The team meets regularly to review a resident's care plan, with each team member offering his or her unique perspective.

The goal is to have a plan of care that accurately reflects the resident's needs and goals and, as much as possible, retains life as it was at home. The care plan sometimes has many components and properly includes input from the direct care providers and CNAs, as well as nurses. In some states it is a requirement that the resident's family members or significant others also receive an invitation to attend these interdisciplinary team meetings. If nursing assistants are not part of the official meeting, it will be up to the LPN/LVN to communicate closely with them. It is important that LPNs/LVNs make sure their viewpoints are represented because they are usually the ones who work most closely with the older adults, performing the majority of physical care in the long-term care setting. Involving all categories is crucial to successfully implementing the interventions developed at the meeting.

Managing the long-term care facility is an administrator, and there is also a director of nursing (DON). The facility has nursing services, social services, dietary services, activities or recreation, rehabilitation or physical therapy, building maintenance, and housekeeping departments. These facilities and the provision of care are highly regulated by state and federal agencies to ensure quality services to a potentially vulnerable population, the frail older adult.

Nursing services is the largest department, as it is in most health care facilities. The structure of the department includes an RN as the DON. Depending on the size of the facility or the number of beds, the facility will sometimes have an assistant director of nursing (ADON), a staffing coordinator, and RNs as managers of nursing units and shift charge nurses. In many facilities, LPNs/LVNs function in these management roles, as well as provide direct nursing care. LPNs/LVNs are sometimes facility supervisors, medical record technicians, staff development assistants, and admission coordinators because of their nursing assessment and data collection abilities. Within the nursing department, CNAs provide the largest percentage of nursing care. The CNA receives educational preparation to encourage the patient's independence within the environment, offer restorative nursing interventions, and assist with ADLs. This group of nursing care providers also learns basic observation, reporting, and recording skills to support nursing care.

A unique member of the caregiving team in the long-term care facility setting, in some states, is the certified medication aide or certified medication technician (CMA/CMT). This caregiver is first required to be a CNA and then has the option to complete an educational course in administering medications. In the long-term care facility, medication administration is permitted by the RN, the LPN/LVN, or the CMA/CMT. In regard to medication administration, the difference between long-term care and acute care is the vast number of patients the medication administration person will sometimes administer medications to. In some states, this ratio is as high as one medication administration person to 60 residents; in long-term care there is a 2-hour window for legal administration of medications (1 hour before the scheduled time to 1 hour after), although it is important to check the individual facility's policy. Restorative nursing assistants are CNAs who have completed an educational program that focuses on **restorative nursing care**, or basic concepts of physical therapy for maintenance of functional mobility and physical activity.

Legal, Ethical, and Financial Issues

Legal and ethical issues among long-term care agencies are similar but have subtle differences depending on the provider setting. The majority of providers are subject to regulation by federal and state guidelines or use them as minimum standards for health care services, reimbursement, or quality indicators. The **Omnibus Budget Reconciliation Act (OBRA)** of 1987, also known as the nursing home reform legislation, was a landmark law affecting long-term care facilities. OBRA defines requirements for the quality of care given to residents and covers many aspects of institutional life, including nutrition, staffing, qualifications required of personnel, and many others. Some specific OBRA regulations can be found in Table 38-1.

Some of the positive outcomes of OBRA include empowerment of residents, focus on residents' rights, reduction or elimination of physical restraint use, and improved staffing, although many nurses believe that staffing continues to require greater improvement in many facilities. The enactment of OBRA led to the requirement for long-term care facilities to use greater numbers of licensed nursing staff; this led to greater opportunities for employment for the LPN/LVN. Other aspects of the OBRA law helped expand the role of the LPN/LVN to include areas such as intravenous therapy and team leading.

The Health Care Financing Administration (HCFA) administers and monitors the OBRA guidelines through institutional surveys. Surveyors are required by law to visit the long-term care facility unannounced (on an annual basis and as needed) to assess the quality of life for the residents by assessing each department and its services, the physical layout of the facility, and records. The HCFA makes available the information it obtains about quality of long-term care facilities to beneficiaries, providers, researchers, and state surveyors.

Long-term care facilities typically have not received funding to support the increasing costs of care. The long-term care facility is able to receive **Medicare** (a federally funded national health insurance program in the United States for people older than age 65) funding by adhering to the HCFA guidelines for reimbursement. **Medicaid** (a federally funded, state-operated program of medical assistance to people with low incomes), financial assistance provided to anyone who qualifies, is a large source of revenue for the long-term care facility. Only recently has insurance reimbursement for long-term care become available, so people primarily use private pay, with the result that older adults have to spend all their assets in a short time. The resident will sometimes then qualify for Medicaid to cover the continued costs of living in a long-term care facility.

Long-term care facilities, like all other health care providers, come under the regulation of the Occupational Safety and Health Administration (OSHA). The inclusion of long-term care facilities in the OSHA guidelines significantly increases the cost of care in this setting but ensures a safe environment for the personnel, which is mandatory today.

Resident rights are a universal priority in all long-term care settings (Box 38-5). Residents and staff of each agency receive communications about setting-specific interpretations as a part of orientation for the personnel and orientation to the services for the recipient of health care services. Advance directives are imperative and valuable in the long-term care facility. Do not resuscitate (DNR) orders from the physician are always the result of discussion with the resident, family, and significant others and documentation by the physician is required. These directions help promote dignity in the last stages of life.

Power of attorney, guardianship, and responsible party designation are all varying degrees of decision-making mechanisms for the resident. The legal system is the route to establish power of attorney and

Table 38-1 Applications of the Omnibus Budget Reconciliation Act of 1987

CATEGORY	REQUIREMENTS
Resident rights	The resident is fully informed in advance and participates in decisions about care and services or changes in care and services
Physical restraints	No restraints are applied for discipline or convenience
Resident assessment	Comprehensive resident assessment is performed and serves as the foundation of planning and delivery of care
Licensed nursing services	There is 24-hour licensed nursing service
Registered nurses	Registered nurse coverage 8 consecutive hours per day, 7 days per week
Nursing assistants	Nursing assistants are trained and competency tested

From O'Neill, P.A. (2002). *Caring for the older adult: a health promotion perspective.* Philadelphia: Saunders.

Box 38-5 Other Ethical Issues Related to Long-Term Care

- Adherence to a Patient's Bill of Rights
- Advance directives
- Do not resuscitate (DNR) orders
- Power of attorney
- Guardianship
- Responsible party designation

guardianship, and documentation (legal papers) in the resident's chart is necessary. A responsible party is a person the patient designates, not necessarily with legal formality, to take care of financial and business affairs.

Functional Assessment and Documentation

Several different types of nursing are present, then, in this setting: team nursing, functional nursing, total resident care, or a combination of these. The goal remains the same, that is, to provide nursing interventions to a special population over a long period, based on individual assessment and fulfillment of the resident's wishes and needs at this time in his or her life.

The interdisciplinary **functional assessment** of the resident is the cornerstone of clinical practice in this setting. OBRA prescribed the method of resident assessment and care plan development in an instrument known as the **resident assessment instrument (RAI).** The LPN/LVN is permitted to complete this assessment tool under the direction of the RN, but it has be signed by the RN. The RAI consists of three parts: the **minimum data set (MDS),** the resident assessment protocols (RAPs), and the utilization guidelines. The MDS provides a system for assessment of each resident's functional, medical, mental, and psychosocial status on admission to a facility and at regular intervals thereafter. It is an assessment instrument consisting of more than 400 items that usually help identify a resident's problems, strengths, needs, and preferences so that it is possible to maintain or enhance a resident's function.

After the nurse completes the MDS on a resident, responses to specific items trigger further assessment using the RAPs. RAPs are assessment guides that address common clinical problems, such as delirium, falls, and urinary incontinence. RAPs have accompanying utilization guidelines, the third component. These contain a wealth of clinical information to assist in assessment and care planning. The functional status of the resident is the ability to perform normal, expected, or required activities. In reference to the older adult, it is the capacity to perform self-care activities (ADLs), as well as the more complex personal, household, and social activities (IADLs) required for independent living. The MDS incorporates many of the same assessment factors as a functional assessment tool and requires input from nursing and social services within a specified time frame. The comprehensive assessment provided by the RAI is intended to lead to improved care planning and provision of care for long-term care facility residents.

In this setting, documentation of the resident's condition is different from that in the acute care setting. A summary, including vital signs and weights, is required only monthly. The exception to this charting is a condition change, acute illness, or incident reporting, which is necessary to document at or soon after the time of occurrence.

❖ NURSING PROCESS

The role of the licensed practical nurse/licensed vocational nurse (LPN/LVN) in the nursing process as stated is that the LPN/LVN will:

- Participate in planning care for patients based on patient needs
- Review patient's plan of care and recommend revisions as needed
- Review and follow defined prioritization for patient care
- Use clinical pathways, care maps, or care plans to guide and review patient care

The nursing process is used in long-term care on admission to the facility and is a continuing, ongoing process.

Assessment

The assessment of a long-term care resident occurs on admission and is an ongoing process for collecting data and information to meet a resident's needs. Communication with the resident, significant other, or family member is essential for complete data collection. The nursing assessment includes a health history, medication history (including herbal products and nutritional supplements) and current medication usage, a functional assessment related to ADLs, personal preferences (e.g., routines, likes and dislikes, hobbies), a physical assessment to document baseline information, and a mental status assessment. The MDS, as well as nursing admission forms, documents a great deal of this information. In long-term care, the interdisciplinary team reviews the resident's plan of care every 90 days for resolution of problems or revision of goals and interventions.

Nursing Diagnosis

You and the team will identify nursing diagnoses from the assessment. Prioritize risk nursing diagnoses for

Safety Alert!

Herbal Products and Nutritional Supplements

When eliciting a medication history and current medication usage patterns, it is crucial to ask about the use of herbs and nutritional supplements. These products, which are marketed as "safe" and "natural," are unregulated by the U.S. Food and Drug Administration (FDA) and potentially have actions and side effects similar to medications. They also have the potential to interact with medications the health care provider prescribes for the resident and in some cases affect medical conditions (either beneficially or detrimentally). Take a complete history of vitamin and mineral usage (and look at the label on the bottle if available); some multivitamin and multimineral products actually contain multiple herbs as well. The resident will sometimes be unaware that he or she is consuming herbal products.

the long-term care resident according to that individual's needs. Possible selections are available in the following list of nursing diagnoses (which is not all-inclusive):

- Risk for aspiration, related to impaired swallowing, ill-fitting dentures, musculoskeletal weakness, and medical conditions such as stroke
- Ineffective airway clearance, related to chronic respiratory conditions and musculoskeletal weakness
- Impaired gas exchange, related to chronic respiratory conditions
- Decreased cardiac output, related to cardiovascular disease
- Imbalanced nutrition: less than body requirements, related to decreased appetite and cognitive impairment
- Risk for deficient fluid volume, related to altered thirst mechanism
- Functional urinary incontinence, related to decreased bladder capacity
- Disturbed thought processes, related to cognitive impairment
- Chronic confusion, related to cognitive impairment
- Bathing/hygiene self-care deficit, related to musculoskeletal weakness
- Risk for injury, related to forgetfulness, impaired balance
- Impaired physical mobility, related to abnormal gait
- Risk for impaired skin integrity, related to malnutrition
- Chronic low self-esteem, related to physical impairment
- Dysfunctional grieving, related to multiple losses
- Anxiety, related to financial difficulties
- Social isolation, related to homebound status

Expected Outcomes and Planning

It is necessary for the planning process to be patient centered and individualized to meet the needs of the patient. Priorities begin with consideration of meeting basic physiologic needs (airway, breathing, and circulation) and go on to consider the patient's multiple conditions or needs. Emotional and psychosocial needs of the patient are also necessary to consider and include in the plan of care.

Properly formulated, the expected outcomes reflect the input of the patient, significant others, and the interdisciplinary team. Expected outcomes have to be measurable, be specific to the nursing diagnosis, and include a time element. Examples are as follows:

Expected outcome 1: Patient will have respirations of 16 to 20 breaths per minute during the next 90 days.

Expected outcome 2: Patient will have pulse rate between 60 and 100 beats per minute during the next 90 days.

Expected outcome 3: Patient will verbalize two positive attributes about his or her appearance within 2 days.

Implementation

Nursing interventions basic to long-term care include making rounds and monitoring for resident safety **every** 2 hours. The interpretation of this includes seeing the resident, changing his or her position, assessing for incontinence, providing skin care, and offering fluids. For example, the LPN/LVN or RN has the responsibility of assessing and intervening to support progress toward the first patient-centered expected outcome in the previous section with the following interventions. Assess the resident for the following:

- Respiratory rate, noisy respirations, signs of suprasternal or intercostal retractions, or nasal flaring
- Color of skin, lips, mucous membranes, and nailbeds; cyanosis
- Adventitious lung sounds: Describe character and phase of the respiratory cycle (inspiration or expiration) when they occur
- Oxygen administration: Note the method of oxygen delivery (nasal cannula versus mask); verify flow rate with physician order; post a "No Smoking" sign on room door; secure the tank for safety; assess tubing or mask for proper fit on resident's face; assess skin for impairment; maintain tubing off the floor
- Offer a sip of water cautiously to assess resident's ability to swallow fluids
- Assess for cough, sputum characteristics, and ability to expectorate
- Elevate the head of the bed to 30 degrees or greater
- Offer periods of rest between activities
- Alternate foods and fluid when assessing with meals

Evaluation

Although the RN is officially responsible for the evaluation and modification of the plan of care for the patient, the LPN/LVN's contribution is crucial. The data gathered, along with observation of changes in the patient, will make the difference in whether the plan of care is successful.

It is necessary to aim nursing evaluation directly at the patient outcomes. The outcomes identified earlier in the chapter are straightforward and objective, and they require nursing assessment and data gathering to evaluate progress. Evaluation of other outcomes will possibly require additional investigation, such as consulting various sources of information (including reading the progress notes, discussing the plan with the resident, speaking with family and significant others, listening to nursing report, and investigating laboratory data). In addition, the nursing evaluation also has to take into consideration individual interventions employed: which ones were effective and which ones were less useful. This written evaluation will be helpful for all nurses implementing the care plan.

The evaluation of care is based on questions such as the following: Was the expected outcome reached for and with the resident? Is the outcome what the resident wishes to accomplish? Are significant others and family members supportive of the outcomes developed by the interdisciplinary team with the resident? After consideration and analysis of the evaluative measures, using the nurse's knowledge base, the team makes a decision to continue the current regimen or to implement a change in the nursing interventions to better achieve the patient-centered expected outcome and offer a better quality of life the resident desires. For example:

Expected outcome 1: Patient will have respirations of 16 to 20 breaths per minute.

Evaluative measure: Is the resident experiencing shortness of breath during activity or rest? Is there a color change of lips during activity? What is the resident's respiratory rate before, during, and after activity?

The nursing services in long-term care center on functional assessment. It is also important to provide nursing interventions based on the following prioritized list of nursing needs: airway, breathing, circulation, nutrition, fluids, elimination, sexuality, safety and security, belonging, self-esteem, and self-actualization.

Get Ready for the NCLEX® Examination!

Key Points

- The need for long-term care services arises after the acute stage of an illness has resolved, when the patient continues to need services to maintain his or her current and changing physical and psychosocial status and functional abilities.
- Settings that provide long-term care include the home, residential care settings, and institutional settings.
- Services that assist those caring for older adults in the home include adult daycare, hospice, home health agencies, and other community agencies and services.
- Residential care settings offer a wide variety of services to the older adult; two of the more popular types are assisted living facilities and continuing care retirement communities.
- Institutional facilities include subacute units and long-term care facilities.
- The majority of long-term health care providers are under regulation by federal and state guidelines or use them as minimum standards for health care services, reimbursement, and quality indicators.
- Ethical issues related to long-term care services include adherence to a Patient's Bill of Rights, advance directives, DNR orders, power of attorney, guardianship, and responsible party designation.
- In the long-term care facility, the resident's plan of care is reviewed every 90 days for resolution of problems or revision of expected outcomes and interventions by the team.

Additional Learning Resources

Go to your Companion CD for an audio glossary, animations, video clips, and more.

evolve Be sure to visit the Evolve site at http://evolve.elsevier.com/Christensen/foundations/ for additional online resources.

Review Questions for the NCLEX® Examination

1. What defines long-term care?
   1. Nursing home care for 6 months
   2. Care provided after the acute stage of an illness has resolved
   3. Care provided in an institutional setting
   4. Care provided to someone older than age 65

2. Which patient will probably best benefit from long-term care services?
   1. A 98-year-old widow who lives at home independently, can perform ADLs and IADLs, but needs a ride to church every Sunday
   2. A 65-year-old widower who is recovering from a stroke and is unable to move his left side
   3. A 75-year-old woman who lives with her husband and has arthritis and osteoporosis with complaints of mild to moderate stiffness every morning
   4. A 70-year-old man who lives alone and has a history of coronary artery disease and hypertension

3. Which patient is an inappropriate candidate for hospice care?
   1. A 65-year-old woman who has metastatic lung cancer and receives home health services
   2. A 77-year-old man who has end-stage prostate cancer and lives in a long-term care facility
   3. A 44-year-old woman who has AIDS and lives in a continuing care retirement community
   4. A 70-year-old woman who had total knee replacement surgery 1 week ago

4. A 78-year-old patient is receiving hospice care for his end-stage cardiac disease. Which statement by his wife will the nurse report to the RN?
   1. "What are the side effects of my husband's pain medication?"
   2. "Are there support groups to help with the grieving process?"
   3. "My husband finally slept for more than two hours last night."
   4. "How will I know when it is time to call 9-1-1?"

5. What institutional setting is a bridge between acute care and long-term care?
   1. Subacute care
   2. Nursing home care
   3. Residential care
   4. Adult daycare

6. Which scenario best illustrates the effect OBRA has had on the professional practice of LPNs/LVNs in the long-term care setting? The LPN:
   1. is responsible for administering intravenous therapy.
   2. provides direct bedside resident care.
   3. performs dressing changes.
   4. functions as medication nurse.

7. Which correctly states one of the two broad goals of *Healthy People 2010?*
   1. Increase quality and years of healthy life.
   2. Stop Americans from smoking.
   3. Decrease the number of Americans admitted to long-term care facilities.
   4. Reduce deaths from falls and fall-related injuries.

8. Which is the best example of an interdisciplinary team?
   1. Director of nurses, charge nurse, staff nurse, CNA, resident
   2. Resident, nurses, physician, social worker, pharmacist, dietitian, activities director, rehabilitation specialists, podiatrist, psychiatrist, audiologist, dentist
   3. Attending physician, resident physician, intern, medical student
   4. Gerontologic clinical nurse specialist, physician, pharmacist, social worker, clergy, resident

9. Select the statement that best describes palliative care.
   1. Palliative care is usually provided in acute care facilities.
   2. Palliative care is typically recommended for individuals with less than 6 months' life expectancy.
   3. Palliative care is usually affiliated with a church and provided by parish nurses.
   4. Palliative care extends the principles of hospice care to a broader population that has the possibility to benefit from comfort care earlier in their disease process.

10. Most older adults in the United States live in a(n):
    1. long-term care facility.
    2. adult daycare facility.
    3. home setting.
    4. assisted living setting.

11. PACE and the Social Managed Care Plan are:
    1. exercise programs that attempt to help older adults meet the goals of *Healthy People 2010*.
    2. Medicare programs that allow older adults to continue living at home while receiving medical services.
    3. insurance fraud schemes that target older adults.
    4. classes offered by senior centers.

chapter

39 Rehabilitation Nursing

evolve

http://evolve.elsevier.com/Christensen/foundationsadult

Sharon K. Duffy

Objectives

1. Define the philosophy of rehabilitation nursing.
2. Describe the interdisciplinary rehabilitation team concept and the function of each team member.
3. Discuss characteristics of the nurse in the specialized practice of rehabilitation.
4. Discuss two major disabling conditions.
5. Provide nursing diagnoses, goals, interventions, and evaluation and outcome criteria for two major disabling conditions.
6. Discuss the importance of returning home and preparing for community reentry.
7. Recognize the importance and significance of family-centered care in rehabilitation.
8. Recognize the uniqueness of pediatric and gerontologic rehabilitation nursing.
9. Recognize polytrauma as a new and difficult challenge facing rehabilitation.
10. Recognize how important it is for the nurse on the rehabilitation team to be knowledgeable about posttraumatic stress disorder (PTSD) and assess for its presence.

Key Terms

chronic illness (p. 1207)
Commission on Accreditation of Rehabilitation Facilities (CARF) (p. 1211)
comprehensive rehabilitation plan (p. 1211)
disability (p. 1207)
family-centered care (p. 1212)
functional limitation (p. 1207)
gerontologic rehabilitation nursing (p. 1213)
handicap (p. 1207)
impairment (p. 1206)
interdisciplinary rehabilitation team (p. 1209)
multidisciplinary rehabilitation team (p. 1209)
pediatric rehabilitation nursing (p. 1212)
posttraumatic stress disorder (PTSD) (p. 1213)
spinal cord injury (SCI) (p. 1214)
transdisciplinary rehabilitation team (p. 1210)
traumatic brain injury (TBI) (p. 1217)

Rehabilitation nursing is really what holistic nursing is all about. In rehabilitation nursing, we assess and address every aspect of the individual's needs and care. Nursing has undergone many changes, but the one thing that has remained constant is the need for the implementation of comprehensive, compassionate, conscientious, and up-to-date theories of practice. This is exactly what rehabilitation nursing is. We practice the concepts of rehabilitation nursing throughout the continuum of care and across the life span of the patient.

Rehabilitation is possible to define in a variety of ways. For our purposes, it is the process of restoring the individual to the fullest physical, mental, social, vocational, and economic capacity of which he or she is capable. It involves relearning former skills—relearning the activities of daily living (ADLs)—and learning the new skills necessary to adapt and live fully within the context of an altered lifestyle. Rehabilitation means adjusting to a new set of needs by involving and applying previous knowledge and skills in combination with a variety of new ideas, knowledge, and skills.

Rehabilitation has to begin from the very onset of a traumatic event or diagnosis of a chronic illness. According to Ruth Stryker (1977), rehabilitation is a creative process that begins immediately with preventive care and continues throughout the course of the illness and through the restorative phase of care, and involves adaptation of the whole being to a new life.

NEED FOR REHABILITATION

Rehabilitation is required and valuable in a variety of circumstances. What precipitates the need for rehabilitation is impairment, disability, handicap, functional limitation, or chronic illness, or some combination of these. The World Health Organization (1980) defines these terms as follows:

- **Impairment:** Any loss or abnormality of psychological, physical, or anatomical structure or function.

- **Disability:** Any restriction or lack (resulting from an impairment) of an ability to perform an activity in the manner or within the range considered normal for a human being.
- **Handicap:** A disadvantage for a given individual resulting from an impairment or disability that limits or prevents the fulfillment of a role that is normal for that particular individual. The handicap one individual with a given disability faces may not be a concern or handicap for another individual with the same disability.
- **Functional limitation:** Any loss of ability to perform tasks and obligations of usual roles and normal daily life. See discussion later in the chapter regarding functional assessment.
- **Chronic illness:** An irreversible presence, accumulation, or latency of disease states or impairments that involve the total human environment for supportive care, function, and prevention of further disability.

It is important to recognize the difference and uniqueness of each of these terms. Recognize that the individual has a disability, with the focus being on the individual rather than on the disability. Thus rehabilitation nurses work with people who have disabilities, rather than the disabled.

CHRONIC ILLNESS AND DISABILITY

Although managing chronic illness and disability is one of the biggest health care problems facing developed countries, the U.S. health care system is not yet positioned to provide optimal care for the more than 125 million individuals who need it. The emphasis on acute care persists in spite of the fact that people with chronic illnesses constitute the largest group of health consumers. Projections indicate that by 2050, one in five Americans will have a chronic illness or disability, and associated medical costs will exceed $1 trillion (Merck Institute on Aging and Health, 2002). The U.S. Department of Health and Human Services (US DHHS) has addressed the need for a systematic approach to managing chronic illness and improving the quality of life for people with disabilities in a set of objectives outlining health goals titled *Healthy People 2010* (US DHHS, 2000). *Healthy People 2010* sets forth two overarching objectives: to eliminate disparities in health care delivery and to improve the length and quality of life. To accomplish these goals, the US DHHS has identified 28 focus areas encompassing 247 objectives. Of the 28 focus areas, 11 relate specifically to chronic illness and disability (Box 39-1). A concerned public, as well as committed and knowledgeable professionals, will be required to accomplish these goals.

It is necessary to educate health care providers to recognize the special needs of the person with a chronic illness or disability and to organize, plan, and provide care to meet these needs. To appreciate the need for a specific, unique approach to planning and providing care for individuals with chronic illnesses and disabling conditions, providers first need to understand the concepts of chronicity and disability.

Box 39-1 *Healthy People 2010* Focus Areas Related to Chronic Illness and Disability

- Access to quality health services
- Arthritis, osteoporosis, and chronic back conditions
- Cancer
- Chronic kidney disease
- Diabetes
- Disability and secondary conditions
- Heart disease and stroke
- Human immunodeficiency virus (HIV)
- Mental health and mental disorders
- Respiratory diseases
- Vision and hearing

CHRONICITY

Unlike acute illnesses, which are usually abrupt in onset and self-limiting (the illness is either resolved or death ensues), chronic illnesses have the potential to be either abrupt or insidious in onset and by definition persist for an extended and indefinite period. Theorists have developed many definitions of chronic illness. However, all definitions include one or more of the characteristics first outlined by the Commission on Chronic Illness (1957). These characteristics include any impairment or deviation from normal that has the following features:

- Is permanent
- Leaves a residual disability
- Is caused by a nonreversible pathologic condition
- Requires special training of the patient for rehabilitation
- Requires a long period of supervision, observation, or care

To define or understand any health-related condition, we have to understand where it comes into the overall experience of being human. It is important to recognize that the illness experience is just one aspect of being human. In fact, developing a chronic illness is the "norm" in an aging population. Emmanual (1982) referred to life as "the accumulation of chronic illness [to] which we eventually succumb" (Lubkin & Larsen, 2006).

DISABILITY

The Americans with Disabilities Act (ADA) became law in 1990. This landmark legislation provides protection against discrimination for people with disabilities. Universally accepted, the ADA defines an individual as disabled if he or she has a physical or mental impairment that substantially limits one or more major life activities, has a record of such an impairment, or is regarded as having such an impairment.

As is the case with chronic illness, it is important to recognize that having a disability is just one of many variants of the normal human experience. One way to look at it is to assert that all individuals are only temporarily able bodied, and that at some point in life we will all experience some form of disability. It is essential to develop this level of awareness to avoid labeling groups of people in ways that risk disenfranchising them.

People with disabilities, like people with chronic illnesses, are first and foremost people. They are not their illness or their disability. They are more than the sum of their parts, and identifying them as such is obligatory. The basis for planning care that promotes health and positively affects the quality of life is a holistic, person-first approach that honors the shared experience of being human along with the uniqueness of the individual and recognizes strengths as well as impairments.

Furthermore, providers are called on to offer interventions that address the need of people with chronic illnesses or disabilities to develop personally within the context of that illness or disability.

CROSS-CULTURAL REHABILITATION

In the new millennium, the world is in a state of transformation. Many countries are experiencing considerable demographic shifts along with an increasingly wide range of ethnic identification, religion, material reality, beliefs, and behaviors—all leading to rich diversity and cultural complexity. At the same time, health professionals are becoming much more aware of the need to become culturally competent in order to be most effective in their interaction with patients. Unfortunately, rehabilitation professionals, organizations, and systems have yet to adequately address the issue of cultural competence.

We are called on to engage in genuine collaboration with our patients and colleagues, including those trained in other disciplines and community-level workers, in order to obtain the best possible functional outcome for the patient. Disability exists in all societies, yet the definition and significance of disability and its significance in an individual culture depends upon that culture's values. Attitudes also vary toward individuals with a disability, concepts of rehabilitation, the sociocultural, biologic, and economic implications of disability, and policy affecting individuals with a disability. (See Chapter 8 for a detailed discussion of Culture and Ethnic Considerations.)

CULTURAL COMPETENCE

Cultural competence acknowledges and incorporates—at all levels—the importance of culture, the assessment of cross-cultural relations, vigilance toward the dynamics that result from cultural differences, the expansion of cultural knowledge, and the adaptation of services to meet culturally unique needs (Cross et al., 1989).

The following describes a culturally competent practitioner:

- Has the capacity for cultural self-assessment
- Values diversity, with an awareness, acceptance, and even celebration of differences in life view, health systems, communication styles, and other life-sustaining elements
- Is conscious of the dynamics of difference
- Institutionalizes cultural knowledge
- Adapts to diversity

In summary, what characterizes cultural competence is acceptance and respect for difference, continuing self-assessment regarding culture, vigilance toward the dynamics of difference, ongoing expansion of cultural knowledge and resources, and adaptability of services.

People develop *cultural proficiency* when they hold culture in high regard. The culturally proficient professional recognizes the need to conduct research, disseminate the results, and develop new approaches that promise to increase culturally competent practice. Rehabilitation professionals have an ethical responsibility to strive for cultural competence and cultural proficiency.

ISSUES IN REHABILITATION

In rehabilitation, several forces drive the rendering of care. The issues involved include but are not limited to the following:

- **Quality of life versus quantity of life:** Rehabilitation focuses on continually improving the quality of the person's life, not merely maintaining life itself.
- **Care versus cure:** Because of the suddenness and catastrophic effect of many conditions necessitating rehabilitation, it is necessary to consider the care of the individual versus the cure of the condition. Many conditions are irreversible; therefore, the focus of care is on adapting and accepting an altered life rather than resolving an illness.
- **High cost of interdisciplinary care versus long-term care:** Rehabilitation is expensive, mainly because the care is delivered by a team of highly trained professionals. In some cases, we view successful rehabilitation as a person's return to productive employment. Studies of resource allocation have shown that for every dollar we spend on rehabilitation, we save an average of three dollars if the individual is able to live independently and return to the workforce, eliminating the expense of a caregiver or residential long-term care. Remember, however, that in some cases a disability means that two people become unemployed—

the individual with the disability and the caregiver. Rehabilitation in this scenario is successful, and the savings still considerable, if the individual with the disability becomes independent enough to not require a caregiver even though he or she remains unable to return to work.

Rehabilitation is that process of outcome-focused patient care delivered by an interdisciplinary team of highly trained professionals with the goal of improving the total well-being of people with disabilities. The underlying philosophy of rehabilitation is to focus on abilities rather than disabilities, to continually make the most of the abilities that remain intact. The individual, the family, and the support system are the focus of all rehabilitation efforts. Quality rehabilitation will result in people who are continually striving to reach their highest potential of living independently in today's complex world.

GOALS OF REHABILITATION

Rehabilitation is, as mentioned, a goal-oriented (outcome-oriented) process. These goals are personal, and in each case we individualize them to meet the holistic needs of each person we serve. To determine goals, we engage in a collaborative goal-setting process that includes the members of the rehabilitation team, with the individual and the family at the center of the process.

It is appropriate to include the following criteria in all rehabilitation goals:

- The goals maximize the quality of life of the individual.
- The goals address the individual's specific needs.
- The goals assist the individual with adjusting to an altered lifestyle.
- The goals are directed toward promoting wellness and keeping complications to a minimum.
- All goals assist the individual in attaining the highest degree of function and self-sufficiency possible.
- The goals assist the individual with home and community reentry.

Make sure all rehabilitation efforts are outcome focused and comprehensive and constitute an educational process.

CORNERSTONES OF REHABILITATION

Rehabilitation is like a road, the road to recovery following a traumatic, life-changing event. The following building blocks or stepping stones pave the way as we travel along it:

- **Focus on the individual:** Center all efforts at rehabilitation around the individual's goals and objectives. When the individual sets or holds goals that are less than realistic, the team works with the individual in reshaping expectations.
- **Community reentry:** We consider rehabilitation successful if the individual is able to reenter the community through participation in social, vocational, and recreational activities.
- **Independence:** The goals of rehabilitation focus on promoting and maintaining physical and emotional independence.
- **Functional ability:** We measure progress in rehabilitation in terms of functional outcomes.
- **Team approach:** We achieve rehabilitation goals through the work of the rehabilitation team members, including the individual and the family.
- **Quality of life:** Goals focus on improving the quality of life rather than increasing the quantity of life.
- **Prevention and wellness:** Because many problems calling for rehabilitation are long term, our goals focus on preventing complications and maximizing function.
- **Change process:** All individuals and families who experience a disabling condition or chronic illness experience the change process. The rehabilitation team is responsible for directing the change in as positive a manner as possible.
- **Adaptation:** Although individuals with disabilities do not always accept their disability, learning to adapt to the circumstances created by the limits of their abilities is a positive method of coping.
- **Patient and family education:** Knowledge and skills are essential components of the rehabilitation program. Individuals with substantial disability have potential to gain a degree of independence through patient education, which enables them to direct their own care.

REHABILITATION TEAM

Because no one discipline offers the knowledge and expertise necessary to provide all the components of the rehabilitation program, the rehabilitation team is composed of people from multiple disciplines. The team coordinates the comprehensive rehabilitation program for each patient in an individualized manner (Table 39-1, Figure 39-1).

MODELS OF TEAM FUNCTIONING

Here we will briefly discuss three primary models of rehabilitation team functioning. One model, primarily of service in the past, is the **multidisciplinary rehabilitation team.** Characteristic of this model are discipline-specific goals, clear boundaries between disciplines, and outcomes that are the sum of each discipline's efforts. Effective communication is the key to success for this type of team.

The type of team most commonly used today in rehabilitation hospitals is the **interdisciplinary rehabilitation team.** This type of team collaborates to identify individuals' goals and features a combination of ex-

Table 39-1 Rehabilitation Team

MEMBER	ROLE	GOAL
Patient	Key member	Participates in goal setting; takes control of own life
Physiatrist	Rehabilitation physician	Team leader; coordinator of program
Rehabilitation RN	Coordinator, educator	Provides support; promotes independence
Rehabilitation LPN/LVN	Care provider; advocate	Assists in treatment plan and implementation
Physical therapist	Designs exercise program	Provides therapy; assesses needs; provides training
Occupational therapist	Assesses independent living needs	Recommends equipment modifications; adapts equipment
Speech pathologist	Designs rehabilitation communication program	Assists in regaining communication skills; educator
Therapeutic recreation therapist	Recreation planner	Activates leisure time; promotes interest in activities
Clinical psychologist	Emotional evaluator	Assists patient in developing realistic positive attitudes
Chaplain	Consultant	Provides support and guidance
Vocational rehabilitation counselor	Vocational planner	Helps obtain training and employment

LPN/LVN, Licensed practical nurse or licensed vocational nurse; *RN*, registered nurse.

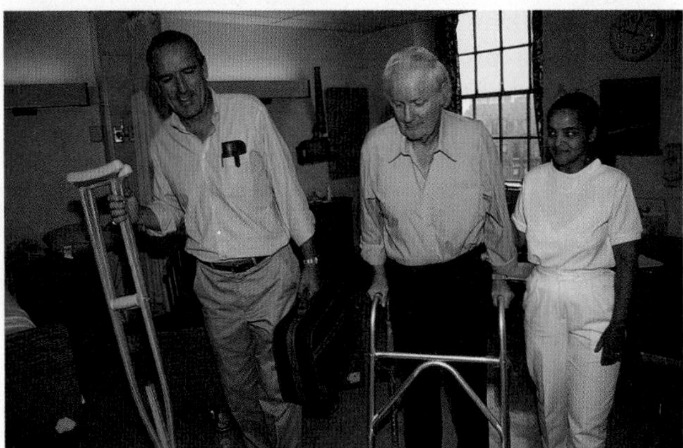

FIGURE 39-1 The nurse and the physical therapist, members of the rehabilitation team, helping a patient with ambulation.

panded problem solving beyond the boundaries of the individual disciplines together with discipline-specific work toward goal attainment.

A third type of team is the **transdisciplinary rehabilitation team.** What characterizes this model is the blurring of boundaries between disciplines, as well as cross-training and flexibility to reduce to a minimum any duplication of effort toward individual goal attainment.

Major strengths of the team method of care delivery are that it is well established, promotes good communication and collaboration among disciplines, addresses comprehensive aspects of care, energizes staff, and views the patient holistically.

Although these rehabilitation models provide a structure for delivery of rehabilitation services, it is still necessary to integrate services and ensure that they are comprehensive and appropriate. Rehabilitation nurses—diverse in expertise, roles, and work settings—play a critical role in models for rehabilitation.

REHABILITATION NURSE

Just what is your role on this team as a rehabilitation nurse? The nurse is in a unique position. You are the only member of the team who is with the patient on a 24-hour basis. As a rehabilitation nurse, you need to have a broad knowledge base of the pathophysiology of a wide range of medical-surgical conditions and a body of highly specialized knowledge and skills regarding rehabilitation.

However, rehabilitation nursing is an attitude in addition to a set of specialized knowledge and skills. If you practice in the area of rehabilitation, your work is predicated on the belief that individuals with functional disabilities have an intrinsic worth that transcends their disabilities. Estimates are that 50% of rehabilitation nursing is know-how; the other 50% is simple open-minded encouragement. William Barclay put it this way:

> One of the highest of human duties is the duty of encouragement. . . . It is easy to laugh at men's ideals; it is easy to pour cold water on their enthusiasm; it is easy to discourage others. The world is full of discouragers. . . . We have a duty to encourage one another. Many a time a word of praise or thanks has kept a man on his feet. Blessed is the man who speaks such a word.

Rehabilitation nurses are obliged to be those who offer encouragement on a regular basis. Your role as a rehabilitation nurse is to put the individual in charge of his or her own care rather than taking charge yourself.

The Association of Rehabilitation Nurses (n.d.) gives the following definition:

> Rehabilitation nursing is the diagnosis and treatment of human responses of individuals and groups to actual or potential health problems relative to altered functional ability and lifestyle. The goal of rehabilitation nursing is to assist the individual who has a disability and/or chronic illness in restoring, maintaining, and promoting his or her maximal health. This includes preventing chronic illness and disability.

You will need specialized training to become an effective team member. In reality, any successful rehabilitation will call on you to integrate the efforts of all team members into the total program. It is the rehabilitation nurse who reinforces teaching and training completed by the other disciplines on a 24-hour-a-day, 7-day-a-week basis. One hour of physical therapy is possible to undo, or to reinforce, 23 hours a day. Solid rehabilitation nursing is essential for a successful rehabilitation outcome.

You will have to wear many hats. Rehabilitation nursing roles include those of educator, caregiver, counselor, care coordinator, case manager, patient advocate, consultant, researcher, administrator or manager, and expert witness.

You will find rehabilitation nursing being practiced in a variety of settings across the continuum of care: primary care clinics, home health agencies, outpatient services, hospitals and rehabilitation facilities, skilled nursing facilities, subacute or transitional care facilities, residential facilities, daycare agencies, insurance companies, and private companies. The rehabilitation nurse is a vital member of the interdisciplinary rehabilitation team.

Your focus will be on enabling the individual to move from a totally dependent state to a level of independence. In the optimum scenario, each patient receives individual treatment from specific nurses and therapists so that bonds of trust and friendship have the opportunity to develop through the difficult rehabilitation process. Extensive family and patient education, modern adaptive equipment, numerous community integration activities, specialized programs, and professional, effective team therapies all combine to help the patients learn to make the most of their lives.

It is possible to use basic rehabilitation whether the patient is suffering from arthritis, multiple sclerosis, mental illness, brain attack or stroke, spinal cord injury (SCI), burn, or traumatic brain injury (TBI). Your responsibility is to apply appropriate concepts and techniques throughout the continuum of care. All basic nursing measures are essential, such as position changes and maintaining body alignment. This prevents skeletal and muscular deformities (contractures) and pressure ulcers.

Rehabilitation nursing is a challenge that requires knowledge, teamwork, coordination, planning, and patience. To care for people with disabilities, it is important for rehabilitation professionals to learn and stay abreast of current knowledge and techniques.

The phenomenon of change as it relates to the human experience is a central concept in nursing. This is especially true for rehabilitation nurses, who regularly interact with people experiencing great change. The focus of this chapter is the individual patient, the central member of the rehabilitation team. Understanding and promoting the change process is therefore an integral part of your role as a rehabilitation nurse.

All rehabilitation nurses are expected to engage in professional role activities appropriate to their education, position, and practice setting.

COMPREHENSIVE REHABILITATION PLAN

The more comprehensive the rehabilitation program, the better the chances for higher functional outcomes of the people served. According to the **Commission on Accreditation of Rehabilitation Facilities (CARF)** (a nonprofit, private, international standard-setting and accreditation body whose mission is to promote and advocate the delivery of quality rehabilitation), it is necessary to initiate an overall individualized **comprehensive rehabilitation plan** of care within 24 hours of admission and have it ready for review and revision by the team within 3 days of admission. The results of the interdisciplinary admission assessment provide the basis for developing the plan. Underlying it are individual goals incorporating the unique strengths, needs, abilities, and preferences of the person it serves. This plan will reflect the environment where the person will go upon discharge. It is necessary that goals are measurable, are described in functional or behavioral terms, have associated time frames for achievement, and list the responsible team member(s).

All clinicians treating the patient will use this comprehensive plan of care. Evaluation conferences and family conferences take place on a regular basis. The active participation of the people served is an integral part of planning and implementing the discharge process.

PATIENT EDUCATION

Patient education is crucial for the rehabilitation process to be comprehensive. Patient education is an ongoing and integral process by which patients and families build knowledge, skills, and confidence to regain physical and psychosocial functioning following an illness or injury. The following five-step approach is an option to guide this process:

1. Assess the patient's and the family's needs, abilities, and concerns.
2. Plan interventions based on these needs, abilities, and concerns.
3. Implement the educational plan.
4. Document the educational process.
5. Evaluate and revise the educational plan.

Guidelines for patient teaching are available from the following:

- Americans with Disabilities Act
- The Joint Commission
- CARF
- American Nurses Association and Association of Rehabilitation Nurses Nursing Standards of Practice
- Individual facility or unit standards
- Patient Care Partnership (Patient's Bill of Rights)
- State nurse practice acts
- National Health Planning and Resource Development Act

SCOPE OF INDIVIDUALS REQUIRING REHABILITATION

Rehabilitation is a bridge for the patient, spanning the gap between uselessness and usefulness, between hopelessness and hopefulness, between despair and happiness. The scope of conditions requiring rehabilitation is broad and spans the life continuum. Living longer in the United States presents an interesting paradox between retiring and enjoying the so-called golden years and a strong probability of acquiring one or more chronic, disabling conditions. Chronic illness and physiologic changes of aging increase the likelihood of physical limitations and disability disproportionately for older people compared with younger adults. However, families continue to care for most older people with disabling conditions; relatively few live in nursing homes. On the other hand, as many as 5 million older people who are hospitalized annually are candidates to benefit from rehabilitation services. Whether in the acute stage of an illness or injury or in the community, rehabilitation services for the older person are built around maintaining functional abilities, ensuring safety, promoting effective coping, preventing complications, and modifying the environment for maximum independence.

A disability has a number of potential effects on both the patient and the family, including behavioral and emotional changes and changes in roles, body image, self-concept, and family dynamics.

FAMILY AND FAMILY-CENTERED CARE

Family and **family-centered care** is a philosophy that recognizes the pivotal role of the family in the lives of children with disabilities or other chronic conditions. It is a philosophy that strives to support families in their natural caregiving roles by building on the parents' unique strengths as individuals. This perspective promotes normal patterns of living at home and in the community and views families and professionals as equals in a partnership committed to excellence at all levels of health care. The ability and willingness of nurses and health care providers to share knowledge and control of health resources with families, empowering them to act as advocates for themselves and their children, is an integral part of family-centered care.

The key elements of family-centered care include the following:

- Incorporating into policy and practice the recognition that the family is the constant in a child's life, whereas the service systems and support personnel within those systems fluctuate
- Facilitating family-professional collaboration at all levels of hospital, home, and community care
- Exchanging complete and unbiased information between families and professionals in a supportive manner at all times
- Encouraging and facilitating family-to-family support and networking
- Appreciating families as families and children as children; recognizing that they possess a wide range of strengths, concerns, emotions, and aspirations beyond their need for specialized health and developmental services and support

In summary, family-centered care is an evolving concept. Collaboration between family and professional is essential for providing appropriate and optimal care.

Family-centered care is not a blueprint but a process that will differ based on variations in situations, families, cultures, health care settings, and providers. Family-centered care requires learning new ways of relating to and working with families, in rehabilitation and throughout the continuum of care.

PEDIATRIC REHABILITATION NURSING

Pediatric rehabilitation nursing is a specialty practice area that also continues to grow within the field of rehabilitation. The field of pediatric rehabilitation has experienced marked development over the past century. Chronic disabling conditions have increased as a result of improved survival rates for illnesses and injuries that once were fatal.

Over the past 20 years, the field has evolved from a mere combination of pediatrics and rehabilitation into a true specialty committed to the care of children with disabilities or other chronic conditions and their families. Nurses in this field, in a collaborative relationship with the interdisciplinary team, provide a continuum of care so those children can become contributing members of society and function at their maximum potential. Infants, children, and adolescents with a variety of disabling conditions receive specialized care from hospital to home, from clinic to school. Physical, emotional, social, cultural, educational, developmental, and spiritual dimensions are all the subject of consideration in a holistic approach to care. The goal is to cherish and foster the unique qualities of each child.

The primary difference between rehabilitation of children and rehabilitation of adults is the developmental potential of the child. It is possible for the child or adolescent to receive an injury resulting in disability at any age, with very different consequences for his or her future depending on the age and developmental level at which the trauma occurred. Children who are born with genetic disorders, who are premature, or whose fetal development is affected by maternal disease, injury, or substance abuse require services focused on habilitation rather then rehabilitation. Whereas rehabilitation refers to the relearning of skills or behaviors lost as a result of disease or injury, habilitation refers to the process of acquiring skills and behaviors by an individual whose development has been affected by disease or other disabling conditions since birth or very early childhood.

In summary, in your roles as leader, advocate, and educator, you will have the power as a pediatric rehabilitation nurse to have a very positive influence on the lives of children with disabilities and chronic conditions, as well as on their families. By facilitating transition from hospital to home and community and offering counseling and support to families, you will provide assistance in meeting identified needs. By designing an individualized plan of care that incorporates the values and beliefs supported in rehabilitation, you have the opportunity to affect the quality of the child's life for the better and facilitate the child's interactions with family and friends within the greater community.

GERONTOLOGIC REHABILITATION NURSING

Gerontologic rehabilitation nursing is a specialty practice that focuses on the unique requirements of older adult rehabilitation patients. Because the needs of the older adult differ from those of the rest of the population, the knowledge and skill needed to provide quality patient care warrants special attention. The gerontologic rehabilitation nurse (GRN) is knowledgeable about both techniques of caring for the aged and rehabilitation concepts and principles. This unique type of nursing combines knowledge of both the aging process and rehabilitation practice in the specialized task of caring for the aging adult with a disability or long-term health problem.

Your main goal in gerontologic rehabilitation nursing is to assist older adult patients in achieving their personal optimal level of health and well-being by providing holistic care in a therapeutic environment. This aim is similar to that of the general rehabilitation nurse but with a special focus on the geriatric population, considering their special needs, roles, and social relationships, and the potential physical limitations that are possible as a result of the aging process.

GRNs strive not only to provide rehabilitative care but also to teach prevention. Thus GRNs have an opportunity to function within primary, secondary, and tertiary levels of care, with the universal goal of helping older adult patients to achieve optimum wellness and self-care.

POLYTRAUMA AND REHABILITATION NURSING

Soldiers wounded in conflicts, including those going on in Iraq and Afghanistan, pose new challenges to today's health care system. These soldiers are experiencing multiple traumas with variable patterns, known as polytrauma–blast related injury (PT/BRI), resulting from explosions. Nursing rehabilitative care in the military and Veterans Administration is thus responding to these challenges.

Blast injuries are categorized as primary, secondary, tertiary, or quaternary (miscellaneous) (Wrightman & Gladish, 2001). Air-filled cavities in the body (ears, lungs, and gastrointestinal tract) and organs enveloped by fluid-filled cavities (brain and spinal cord) are most susceptible to compression damage from high explosive blasts. These injuries fall into the primary injury category (Elsayed & Gorbunov, 2006). Airborne debris, bomb fragments, and shrapnel embedded in any body part comprise the secondary injury category. Any injury the soldier sustains from being thrown as the result of an explosive shock wave or dynamic overpressure is a tertiary injury. Examples include broken bones and traumatic head and spinal cord injuries. Inhalation and exposure to toxic chemicals, traumatic amputations of limbs, and burns are examples of quaternary injuries (Nelson, 2008).

In an effort to deal more effectively with PT/BRI, medical treatment of these soldiers is focusing on postacute care with the goal of reducing disabilities associated with these injuries (Scott et al., 2005). The rehabilitation teams for soldiers who have experienced PT/BRI gear their care toward discovering and treating additional injuries that were not detected during the postacute phase, as well as treating those originally identified injuries (Warden, 2006). The earlier the identification of injuries occurs, the more successful treatment outcomes and the lower costs incurred during treatment (Arlinger, 2003).

It is important to understand, identify, and treat PT/BRIs in order to avoid focusing care solely on the more visible injuries. Successful treatment of this newly identified group of injuries allows soldiers suffering from a variety of conditions, ranging from concussions causing cognitive and vestibular deficits to posttraumatic stress disorder, to receive necessary treatment (Gordon et al., 1998; Scott et al., 2005).

POSTTRAUMATIC STRESS DISORDER

Posttraumatic stress disorder (PTSD) is defined as a psychological reaction to the experience of trauma outside the normal range of human experience (American Psychological Association [APA], 2000). Studies indicate that 8% to 12% of the population has experienced the anxiety disorder of PTSD during some time in their lives (Stein et al., 2003).

The American Psychological Association first identified PTSD in 1980 (APA, 1980). Before 1980, the field described soldiers who experienced the symptoms now known as PTSD as suffering from "shell shock" or "war neurosis" (Glass, 1969), and many believed these soldiers were making up the symptoms in order to avoid being involved in further combat (Clark, 1997). Following the Vietnam War, PTSD received acceptance as a psychiatric diagnosis, and other forms of trauma, such as rape and natural disasters, were also identified as causes (APA, 1980).

Events such as the September 11, 2001, terrorist attacks in the United States, Operation Iraqi Freedom, and Hurricane Katrina have again brought attention to PTSD of survivors. However, doubt regarding the disorder still occurs among some family members and health care providers. PTSD remains difficult to diagnose because of its varying clinical features and the reluctance on the part of many sufferers to report symptoms for fear of being looked at as "psychotic" or "crazy" (Clark, 1997).

There is no definitive treatment modality identified for PTSD, but psychotherapy and pharmacotherapy are the most common forms of treatment of PTSD (Stein et al., 2003). Currently, studies show that a combination of cognitive and behavioral therapy is most effective in treating the disorder (Bisson & Andrew, 2005; Bradley et al., 2005).

As the nurse on the rehabilitation team, it is important that you be knowledgeable of the difference between PTSD symptoms and symptoms of grief and prolonged grief. These disorders differ not only in symptoms, but in treatment (Pivar, 2006; Rumpler, 2008). You will play a critical supportive role during rehabilitation. The therapeutic goal is patient empowerment, and you help the patient regain control over the symptoms of PTSD (Clark, 1997; Ferguson et al., 2004). You will play an integral role on the rehabilitation team through early assessment of PTSD symptoms and your use of therapeutic communication to assist patients in achieving the goal of treatment (Sheldon et al., 2006). Therapeutic communication techniques include listening, reframing, normalizing responses, and working to develop trust in the nurse-patient relationship (Bostrom & Schwecke, 2007; Clark, 1997). You also need to be aware of your own reactions, emotions, and communication skills when caring for trauma victims. Nurses who are feeling overwhelmed sometimes need to consult with a mental health care provider.

DISABLING DISORDERS

Following are two of the major conditions for which dedicated rehabilitation efforts are necessary.

SPINAL CORD INJURIES

SCIs occur mainly as a result of traumatic accidents, and the individuals paralyzed are primarily young males. Because of improved emergency and medical care, they now are more likely to survive the injury. Because of their youth, they have vocational potential. Injury level and the extent of damage to the spinal cord will largely determine functional disabilities. Functional limitations occur in nearly every aspect of an individual's life following an SCI.

The effect of SCI on the individual remains one of the most compelling challenges in the field of rehabilitation. People with SCI often require considerable motivation and reeducation to regain a satisfying quality of life and to ensure community reintegration. Crucial to rehabilitation is the communal effort of an interdisciplinary team whose members work together to meet the specific needs of both the individual and the family.

A **spinal cord injury (SCI)** is any injury in which the spinal cord undergoes compression by fracture or displaced vertebrae, bleeding, or edema. Each injury has its unique characteristics, but in general, the higher the injury point, the greater the loss of function. The body parts and the functions located above the injury point will continue to function as they should. Injury to the spinal cord is irreversible in that the cord is unable to repair itself. Spinal function will sometimes be present below the level of the lesion. In general, however, the effects of an injured spinal cord include paralysis, loss of normal bowel and bladder function, and loss of sensation. Terminology associated with SCI includes but is not limited to the following:

- **Complete injury:** No motor or sensory function below the level of injury
- **Incomplete injury:** Some or all motor or sensory function below the level of injury
- **Quadriplegia:** Damage to the cervical spine or the neck that involves weakness or paralysis in all four extremities
- **Paraplegia:** Damage below the cervical area that involves weakness or paralysis in the trunk and lower extremities
- **Paresis:** A slight paralysis, incomplete loss of muscular power, or weakness of a limb

It is possible to divide SCIs into the following categories:

- **Cervical cord injury:** Level of injury is at cervical spine C2 to C7 and involves paralysis of all extremities and trunk, respiratory failure, bladder and bowel disturbance, bradycardia, perspiration, elevated temperature, and headache.
- **Thoracic cord injury:** Level of injury is at thoracic spine T1 to T12 and involves paralysis of lower extremities. Initially muscles are flaccid (weak, soft, flabby, lacking normal muscle tone) and later become spastic (having spasms or other uncontrolled contractions of the skeletal muscles). Paralysis of bladder, bowel, and sphincters; pain in chest or back; abdominal distention; and loss of sexual function are other potential symptoms.
- **Lumbar cord injury:** Level of injury is at lumbar spine L1 to L2 with paralysis of lower extremities, bladder, and rectum and loss of sexual function (Figure 39-2).

Common medical complications experienced by patients with SCI include but are not limited to postural hypotension, autonomic dysreflexia, heterotopic ossification, and deep-vein thrombosis. Nursing diagnoses for a patient with SCI include but are not limited to those in Nursing Care Plan 39-1.

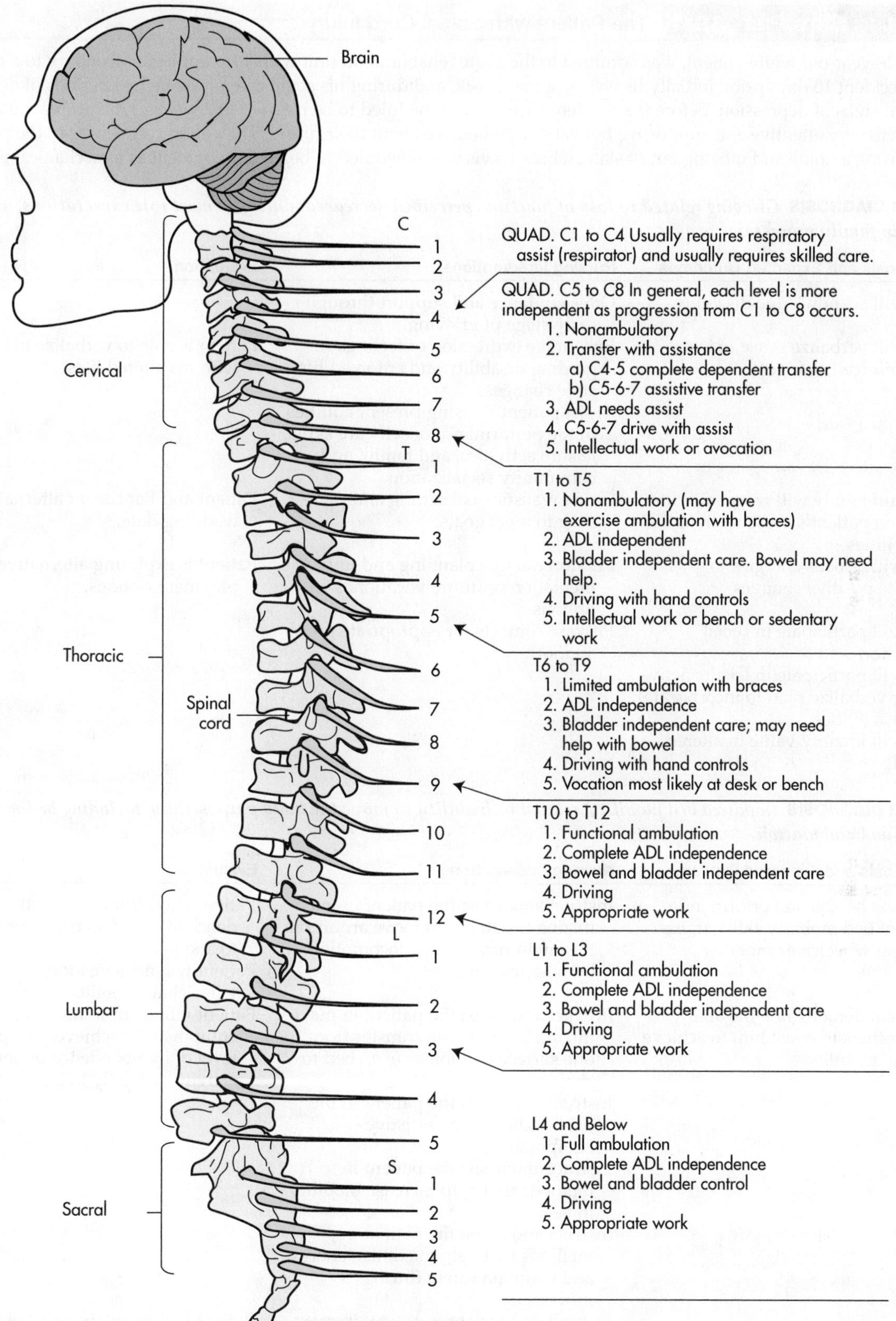

FIGURE 39-2 The level of injury on the spinal cord and the severity of the injury often help predict what a patient will be able to do. These are general guidelines, however; it is necessary to treat each patient individually.

Nursing Care Plan 39-1 The Patient with Spinal Cord Injury

Travis, a 26-year-old white patient, was admitted to the acute rehabilitation unit with T1 paraplegia secondary to a motor vehicle accident 10 days prior. Initially he was in spinal shock, and during his acute care phase he had periods of despondency and signs of depression. Before the accident, Travis was scheduled to be married in 2 weeks. His future wife and his family were very attentive and supportive but very apprehensive about their future. The young couple was in the process of purchasing a home and moving out of state, where Travis was scheduled to begin employment as a mechanical engineer.

NURSING DIAGNOSIS ***Grieving related to loss of function, perceived decreased ability to meet role expectations, and changes in family processes***

Patient Goals and Expected Outcomes	Nursing Interventions	Evaluation
Patient will acknowledge disability	Offer guidance and support through early stage of grieving.	
Patient will verbalize sense of loss from enforced changes	Encourage expression of feelings regarding disability and enforced lifestyle changes. Assist patient in using present abilities in the performance of self-care skills, leisure activities, and family and community socialization.	Patient is able to verbalize his distress with his altered lifestyle.
Patient and family will reorganize life based on patient's present strengths and abilities	Guide realistic goal setting and planning to meet goals.	Patient and fiancée set alternate wedding date.
Patient will refocus energies to promote positive changes	Reinforce active planning and implementation of future vocational options.	Patient is exploring alternative employment options.
Patient will participate in social interaction	Provide contacts for appropriate group support.	
Patient will participate in leisure activities or verbalize plan to incorporate leisure activities		
Patient will identify value in altered lifestyle		

NURSING DIAGNOSIS ***Impaired bed mobility, related to inability to move the body purposefully, including bed mobility, transfer, and ambulation***

Patient Goals and Expected Outcomes	Nursing Interventions	Evaluation
Patient will be able to perform independent bed mobility skills, transfers, and wheelchair mobility	Instruct and assist the patient in maximizing his ability to move around in the environment (e.g., locomotion by wheelchair).	Patient will achieve optimal independence in transfers from one surface to another. Patient will achieve independence in wheelchair mobility.
Patient will demonstrate the ability to direct others to assist him to achieve optimal mobility	Instruct and assist the patient in maximizing his ability to transfer from one surface to another (e.g., bed to chair). Instruct and assist the patient in the use of adaptive or assistive equipment. Instruct and assist the patient in methods that help increase mobility in bed. Instruct and assist the patient in methods that help maximize energy and maintain safety during movement.	Patient will learn to use adaptive equipment to achieve his optimal level of independence in performing activities of daily living.
	Instruct and assist the patient in maintaining optimal body alignment to promote skin integrity and prevent contracture.	Patient will maintain intact skin integrity. Patient will be free of contractures.

Nursing Care Plan 39-1 The Patient with Spinal Cord Injury—cont'd

Critical Thinking Questions

1. Describe the stimuli or precipitating factors associated with bowel functioning or management that have potential to cause autonomic dysreflexia and the appropriate interventions if it does occur.
2. A patient is a C5 quadriplegic. How is it possible to lessen the patient's potential for developing orthostatic hypotension?
3. While explaining orthostatic hypotension to a new nursing assistant, what commonly occurring signs and symptoms should the nurse describe, and what instructions should be given to the nursing assistant?

Postural Hypotension

Some spinal cord–injured individuals will at times have a marked drop in blood pressure while sitting in a wheelchair. It is common for many quadriplegic patients to have a blood pressure of 90/60 mm Hg (or lower) when sitting as a result of the pooling of the blood in the lower extremities and in the abdominal area. Returning the patient to the horizontal position will usually stop dizziness. To lessen hypotension, raise the head of the bed 15 to 20 minutes before placing the patient in the wheelchair. Use of elastic stockings (thromboembolic disease [TED] hose) and abdominal binders is also an option.

Autonomic Dysreflexia

Patients with spinal cord lesions above T5 sometimes experience sudden and extreme elevations in blood pressure caused by a reflex action of the autonomic nervous system. It is the result of some stimulation of the body below the level of the injury, usually a distended bladder from a blocked catheter. Any stimulation has potential to produce the syndrome, including constipation, diarrhea, sexual activity, pressure ulcers, position changes (from lying to sitting), and even wrinkles in clothing or bed sheets. In addition to high blood pressure, possible symptoms include diaphoresis, shivering or goose bumps, flushing of the skin, and a severe, pounding headache.

Treatment for autonomic dysreflexia is to find the source of irritation and remove it. Once the irritation is gone, the blood pressure will return to normal within a few minutes. Raise the patient into a sitting position immediately. This helps reduce the elevated blood pressure before damage occurs.

Heterotopic Ossification

Heterotopic ossification is the abnormal formation of bone cells in joints. It commonly arises in people with SCIs and occurs below the level of the lesion. The formation of extra bone in these joints usually results in limited range of motion. The most commonly affected joints are the hip and sometimes the knee. It occurs most frequently 1 to 4 months following injury and rarely occurs after 1 year. Symptoms include localized edema around the area; after several days, you will be able to feel a firm mass in underlying tissue. After several weeks, there is loss of range of motion. Treatment options involve aggressive range of motion, medications, and occasionally surgery.

Deep-Vein Thrombosis

Patients with spinal injuries have the potential to develop deep-vein thrombosis (DVT) in the lower extremities. DVT is a clotting of blood within vessels of the legs caused by slowing of the circulation or an alteration of the blood vessel walls. Clinical signs include localized swelling, redness, and heat in the involved area. If these signs are present, aggressive movement to that leg is unwise because it has potential to detach the blood clot, which in turn has potential to lodge in the lung (embolus). Anticoagulants (blood thinners) prevent DVT. Passive and active range-of-motion (ROM) exercises are other possible preventive measures.

TRAUMATIC BRAIN INJURIES

Every year an estimated 2 million Americans suffer from **traumatic brain injury (TBI)** ranging in nature from mild concussion to the more devastating kind that renders injured people comatose for the remainder of their lives. Although some people are fortunate enough to return to their previous functioning level shortly after receiving their injury, statistics related to TBI are rather depressing. Many of the 75,000 to 100,000 people who die each year from TBI are children and young adults. Of those individuals who do survive, 500,000 receive injuries severe enough to require hospitalization, and 90,000 of these injuries result in severe and permanent disability. Most brain-related disabilities, including physical, cognitive, and psychosocial difficulties, call for at least 5 to 10 years of difficult and painful rehabilitation; many require lifelong treatment and attention. When these statistics expand to include families of individuals with brain injuries, the number of people whose lives are forever altered by TBI rises to staggering proportions.

The primary goal of the rehabilitation professional treating the survivor of brain injury is to restore the person to the highest possible level of independent functioning.

Head injuries fall into two classifications, either penetrating or closed head injuries. In penetrating injuries, an object lacerates the scalp, fractures the skull, and injures the soft tissue in its path, thus destroying nerve cells. In a closed head injury, some application of force causes the brain to collide with an inner surface of the skull. There is often violent twisting action, which causes the upper section of the brain to rotate while the lower end remains securely anchored in a stationary position. This results in widespread damage called shearing (when the brain mass is rotated in the cranial vault). Brain injuries are also possible as a result of other traumas (e.g., electrocution, drug overdose).

Brain injuries are classified as **mild, moderate, severe,** or **catastrophic.** Brief or no loss of consciousness characterizes mild brain injury. This type constitutes the majority of head injuries. Neurologic examinations are often normal. Postconcussive syndrome sometimes persists for months, years, or indefinitely. Signs and symptoms include fatigue, headache, vertigo, lethargy, irritability, personality changes, cognitive deficits, decreased information processing speed, and memory, understanding, learning, and perceptual difficulties. These symptoms lead to feelings of incompetence, guilt, and frustration. Family members also become impatient and frustrated at times.

In the moderate brain injury, there is a characteristic period of unconsciousness ranging from 1 to 24 hours. There are usually cognitive impairments, which include planning, sequencing, judgment, reasoning, and computation skills. Generally there are some psychosocial problems, which include self-centeredness, denial, mood swings, agitation, depression, lethargy, sexual dysfunction, emotional lability, low frustration tolerance, poor judgment, or behavioral outbursts.

Patients with severe brain injuries experience unconsciousness or posttrauma amnesia in excess of 8 days. Cognitive, psychosocial, and behavioral disabilities result.

Catastrophic brain injury features a defining characteristic of a coma lasting several months or longer. These individuals sometimes appear to be awake. However, they generally never regain significant, meaningful communication with their environment.

In rehabilitative assessment of the patient with TBI, expect to see inconsistent performance, anger, and frustration; and ineffective behavior will be changeable (unless it is neurogenic in origin). Cognitive barriers to rehabilitative recovery include problems in thinking and reasoning (impaired memory), impaired concentration and attention, and impaired informational processing speed. Psychosocially there appears to be a lack of initiative. However, this is a normal consequence of a head injury. Egocentric (self-centered) behavior is 100% normal in a brain-injured individual, as is depres-

Nursing Care Plan 39-2 The Patient with Traumatic Brain Injury

Jeff is a 33-year-old single white male employed as a chemist for a large pharmaceutical company. He lives alone in a second-floor apartment. After not reporting to work for 2 days, he was found unconscious on the floor of his bathroom. He was taken to the hospital, where he remained in deep coma for 5 days as a result of electrocution that caused anoxic encephalopathy. After 4 weeks, Jeff was transferred to an acute rehabilitation unit.

NURSING DIAGNOSIS *Decreased intracranial adaptive capacity, related to neurologic deficits as demonstrated by the following:*

- *Disturbance in orientation*
- *Disturbance in memory*
- *Disturbance in attention/concentration*
- *Disturbance in judgment*
- *Disturbance in reasoning/problem solving*

Patient Goals and Expected Outcomes	Nursing Interventions	Evaluation
Patient will provide accurate responses to orientation testing	Provide reality orientation and testing.	Patient is able to consistently respond accurately when reality testing is done.
Patient will have increased attention span	Implement memory training program. Implement visual and auditory cues. Control environmental stimuli when working with patient.	Patient is able to follow a three-step command consistently. Patient is able to recall names and activities completed during the previous 3 days. Patient is able to complete a task once it is begun.
Patient will demonstrate appropriate behavior based on reality	Provide appropriate level of interactions with a gradual increase in socially appropriate interactions.	Patient is able to demonstrate good judgment in abstract problem-solving situations given to him.
Patient will demonstrate improved accuracy in problem solving	Cue patient on the focus of task before starting and reorient as required. Implement sensory stimulation program.	Patient is able to use information to reach appropriate conclusions.

Nursing Care Plan 39-2 The Patient with Traumatic Brain Injury—cont'd

NURSING DIAGNOSIS ***Risk for injury, related to neurologic deficit resulting in the following:***
- *Impaired judgment*
- *Impaired mobility*
- *Impaired coordination*
- *History of injuries*
- *Decreased sensation*
- *Omission of safety measures (e.g., locking of wheelchair, positioning feet)*

Patient Goals and Expected Outcomes	Nursing Interventions	Evaluation
Patient will demonstrate an awareness of potential safety hazards Patient will demonstrate safety in activities of daily living (ADLs) and mobility activities Patient will demonstrate knowledge and use of safety devices Patient will obtain assistance for activities appropriately to ensure safety Patient will remain injury free	Initiate appropriate safety precautions to protect patient from injury. Establish behavior modification program for isolated safety activities. Use verbal cueing to prevent injury in all activities. Reinforce use of appropriate measures to compensate for the patient's physical or cognitive deficits. Explain side effects of medications that have potential to affect the patient's safety. Anticipate the patient's needs (e.g., toileting, eating, and drinking) to keep impulsive movement to a minimum. Use calm, controlled, and consistent manner. Use short-term, goal-directed techniques. Assume nothing: review, review, review.	Periodically evaluate and document patient's progress toward prevention of injury. Consult with other health care professionals on methods to prevent patient from sustaining injury.

Critical Thinking Questions

1. Deficits with socialization, motivation, and sexual behaviors seen after brain injury are due to damage to which portion of the brain? Discuss appropriate nursing interventions for a patient with this type of injury.
2. A patient recovering from a traumatic brain injury has problems telling the difference between objects that have a similar shape. What is this type of deficit, and what nursing interventions are appropriate for a patient with this deficit?
3. What interventions are most appropriate to begin establishing communication with a patient who is just emerging from coma following a brain injury?

sion. Generally, the more the memory improves, the more the patient becomes depressed. Abstinence from alcohol is a primary injunction for any patient with a brain injury. Alcohol increases the chance of impulse and seizure activity.

Continuous and honest involvement of the family, as both a victim of the injury and an equal participant in the rehabilitation process, is critical to the successful rehabilitation of the patient with TBI. It is critical for rehabilitation professionals to be available and honest in reporting to families. Equal communication with all family members is important, as is encouraging the family to become involved in counseling and education. Encourage the family to be aware of each others' needs and interest. Assist them to become involved in a support group and to inform themselves of available community resources.

Regardless of personality types, any disability, particularly a TBI, is a crisis that threatens many aspects of the patient's and family's life: job income, pleasures, family, community ties, health, and life itself. The fears are very real.

Nursing diagnoses for a patient with TBI include but are not limited to those in Nursing Care Plan 39-2.

CONCLUSION

If you become a rehabilitation nurse, count on a career with a few key mandates and rewards: take your responsibility seriously as a professional who has the power to significantly affect the future of those with disabilities. Facilitate the change from resistance to openness, turning inertia into action. Keep your focus on the assets and the successes of people who have disabilities.

Ralph Waldo Emerson (1803–1882) summed it up succinctly when he wrote, "It is one of the most beautiful compensations of this life that no man can sincerely try to help another without helping himself."

Get Ready for the NCLEX® Examination!

Key Points

- Rehabilitation is the process of maximizing an individual's capabilities or resources to foster optimal independent functioning.
- The patient is the most important team member and is crucial to involve in planning the programs and learning in detail about the disabilities, the ways of accomplishing the goals, and the options available.
- Rehabilitation nursing aims toward preventing complications of disease or trauma and maintaining or restoring function.
- Basic rehabilitation is possible regardless of cause of disability. The rehabilitation team will individualize care by developing goal-directed, comprehensive care plans for each patient.
- A disability has a number of potential effects on both the patient and the family, including behavioral and emotional changes and changes in roles, body image, self-concept, and family dynamics.
- Use holistic nursing interventions to assist the patient in attaining an optimal level of functioning and well-being.
- A comprehensive rehabilitation plan is multifaceted and properly involves a functional assessment, an evaluation conference, and a family conference.
- Keep the focus of all rehabilitation on the patient's abilities, not on his or her disabilities.

Additional Learning Resources

Go to your Companion CD for an audio glossary, animations, video clips, and more.

evolve Be sure to visit the Evolve site at http://evolve.elsevier.com/Christensen/foundations/ for additional online resources.

Review Questions for the NCLEX® Examination

1. Rehabilitation of the older adult focuses on which aspect(s)? *(Select all that apply.)*
   1. Maintaining functional abilities
   2. Ensuring safety
   3. Promoting effective coping
   4. Preventing complications
   5. Maximizing independence
2. The goal of rehabilitation for older adult patients is to:
   1. return to work.
   2. teach safe mobility.
   3. improve quality of life.
   4. reduce cellular destruction.
3. A 19-year-old patient is seen in the emergency department after a diving accident. She is noted as having a spinal cord injury at the cervical level (C3). Which nursing diagnosis is likely?
   1. Ineffective breathing patterns, related to neurogenic injury
   2. Deficient fluid volume, related to osmotic diuresis
   3. Acute pain, related to disease process
   4. Deficient knowledge, related to disease process
4. An 11-year-old boy had a head injury from being struck in the skull by a baseball bat. He awoke in a hospital 3 weeks later. His head injury would be classified as a:
   1. mild brain injury.
   2. moderate brain injury.
   3. severe brain injury.
   4. catastrophic brain injury.
5. A patient has been in the intensive care unit for several days following a head injury. His condition is stable, but today he has shown no signs of improvement. Over the past shift, the patient's father has seemed increasingly upset over apparently minor concerns. Toward the end of the shift, he yells at the nurse when the intravenous (IV) alarm goes off. The most appropriate response is:
   1. "You sound upset."
   2. "I am going to get my supervisor for you."
   3. "You need a break."
   4. "Maybe you had better speak to the physician."
6. The pediatric rehabilitation nurse:
   1. advocates for the child and family.
   2. does not burden parents with decision making.
   3. realizes that children with disabilities will never be productive members of society.
   4. does not take cultural values of parents into consideration.
7. According to the World Health Organization (WHO), the disadvantage for a person that results from an impairment or a disability and limits that person's fulfillment of his or her normal roles is defined as a(n):
   1. disability.
   2. impairment.
   3. handicap.
   4. inconvenience.
8. According to the definition of rehabilitation nursing established by the Association of Rehabilitation Nurses, the major goal of rehabilitation nursing is to assist the individual in:
   1. achieving optimal physical functioning.
   2. obtaining therapy services.
   3. restoring and maintaining optimal health.
   4. identifying funding sources.
9. Rehabilitation nursing practice requires:
   1. specialized knowledge and skills.
   2. organized approaches to care.
   3. skills in all therapies that are provided.
   4. rigid mastery of tasks.
10. The first step to becoming culturally competent is to:
    1. know your own culture.
    2. learn about other cultures.
    3. practice what you know about other cultures.
    4. continue to learn about other cultures.

11. Which is a barrier to cultural competence?

1. Respect for the beliefs of others
2. Knowing all members of a cultural group are not necessarily alike
3. Believing that one's own culture is better than others
4. Not treating one group better than another based on culture or race

12. As part of the rehabilitation treatment team, the nurse is often the first professional to detect the presence of PTSD symptoms because:

1. nurses are more intuitive than other members of the team.
2. nurses are in the unique position of having extended time to talk with patients and hear their concerns, feelings, and needs.
3. nurses are the only members of the team knowledgeable about PTSD.
4. the rehabilitation team has no need to address this issue.

13. The classification levels of injuries that occur as a result of exposure to a blast are:

1. primary, secondary, and tertiary.
2. quaternary.
3. miscellaneous injuries.
4. All of the above.

14. Communication with families of patients with polytraumatic injuries properly includes:

1. clear, accurate, and comprehensive information of their loved ones' injuries.
2. supportive, empathetic, and sensitive manner to giving them the information.
3. reassurance there will be someone available to assist them in dealing with their own stress and anxiety.
4. All of the above.

chapter

40 Hospice Care

evolve

http://evolve.elsevier.com/Christensen/foundationsadult

Barbara Lauritsen Christensen

Objectives

1. Discuss the philosophy of hospice care.
2. Differentiate between palliative care and curative care.
3. Discuss four criteria for admission to hospice care.
4. Name the members of the interdisciplinary team and explain their roles.
5. List three common symptoms related to a terminal illness.
6. Develop a care plan with patient goals related to these symptoms.
7. Discuss the usefulness of pain assessments and when it is best to complete them.
8. Discuss the role of hospice in families' bereavement period.
9. Discuss two ethical issues in hospice care.

Key Terms

adjuvant (ĂJ-ŭ-vănt, p. 1228)
bereavement (bĭ-RĒV-mĕnt, p. 1226)
cachexia (kă-KĔK-sē-ă, p. 1231)
curative treatment (p. 1223)
holistic (hō-LĬ-stĭk, p. 1224)
hospice (HŎS-pĭs, p. 1222)
interdisciplinary team (p. 1224)
pain assessment (p. 1228)
palliative care (PĂL-ē-ă-tĭv, p. 1223)
primary caregiver (p. 1224)
psychosocial (p. 1226)
respite care (RĔS-pĭt, p. 1226)
terminal illness (p. 1222)
titrate (TĪ-trāt, p. 1229)

Hospice is a philosophy of care about providing support to patients with a **terminal illness** (a disease in an advanced stage with no known cure and poor prognosis) and their families. The philosophy of hospice is to promote comfort and use compassion, interest, and genuine concern to allow the patient to live a better lifestyle during the dying process (Lewis et al., 2007). With hospice support, the patient and the family recognize that dying is a natural part of life. Care and support are managed by an interdisciplinary team, and the goals are to maximize the quality of life and keep the patient as comfortable as possible in the home setting that he or she chooses (Box 40-1).

HISTORICAL OVERVIEW

Hospice is from the Latin word *hospitium,* meaning hospitality and lodging. The concept originated in Europe, where hospices were resting places for travelers. Monks and nuns believed that service to one's neighbor was a sign of love and dedication to God. Typical medieval hospices run by monks and nuns were a combination guesthouse and infirmary. They were places of refuge for the poor, the sick, and travelers on religious journeys. They provided food, shelter, and care to ill guests until they were strong enough to continue their journey or they died. As centuries passed and hospices developed into hospitals, the emphasis on physical care increased, with the spiritual care becoming less important.

The idea of hospice was renewed in the 1960s in London, when Dame Cicely Saunders, a nurse and physician, realized that the terminally ill needed a different kind of care. She had a patient who was dying of a terminal illness, and she found that quality of life was not the main emphasis of his care. She then devoted her life to improving pain management and symptom control for people who were dying. She believed it is important that each patient know his or her own contribution to life and that his or her life had meaning. She began her work at St. Joseph's Hospice, operated by the Irish Sisters of Charity. In 1968, St. Christopher's Hospice of London was opened, and this hospice continues to serve as a national and international education, training, and research center for professionals involved in the hospice approach to terminal care.

The philosophy of hospice migrated to the United States in the early 1970s, with the first hospice program opening in Connecticut in 1971. Since then physicians, nurses, clergy, social workers, and many nonprofessional volunteers have worked together to develop more than 3300 hospice programs serving nearly 950,000 patients throughout the United States (Lorenz, et al., 2004).

Box 40-1 A Hospice Nurse's Perspective

Frequently I am asked if it isn't depressing to work with the terminally ill and death every day. Frankly, I can't think of doing anything else. Death is as much a part of life as birth, and through hospice, I am challenged to find very individualized and innovative ways to give back the control dying patients have lost while being treated for various kinds of terminal illnesses.

As a hospice nurse, I am guided by a dedicated interdisciplinary team to achieve symptom control so quality of life can again be realized. Many hopes and dreams can become reality once a patient is comfortable. Frequently comfort enables our patients to take one more family trip, attend a great family reunion, go to a special wedding, graduation, or anniversary. What could be more rewarding than playing a part in that, and seeing the joy it brings? Together we rejoice in the celebration of life—see families reunited—see peace made with God—review each triumph and weep over each disappointment and loss. Families are enabled to say all the things they couldn't find words for before: the thank you's; the I'm sorry's; the forgive me's; the I love you's; and finally the good-byes.

Of course there is sadness, but there is also reconciliation, peace and beauty, for this is a part of life and these are the important things in life. Daily, I feel so personally grateful for every person I have known and loved and lost, for I know that I have learned far more about living from them than I could ever teach them about dying. Through it all, I've become closer to God, more compassionate, more open to people, and more sensitive to the needs of others. Hospice nursing has given me direction and hope.

Kathleen Carsten, CRNH
Hospice Nurse

Hospices vary in structure and organization. Some hospices are based in a hospital, and some in a home health agency or community-based organization. Hospice care usually occurs in the patient's home. Occasionally, the hospice patient goes into the hospital and receives hospice services for control of acute pain or respite care for the family or care provider. The patient will sometimes receive hospice care intermittently and sometimes on a continuous basis (Lewis et al., 2007). There are also freestanding hospices. If the hospice is a freestanding facility, the atmosphere is more like that of a friendly dormitory than that of a hospital. The patients usually wear their own clothes, move about the hospice as they choose, and socialize with each other and with the staff. The kitchen is always open for individually prepared food, as well as for conversation.

Skilled staff that include physicians, nurses, hospice aides, social workers, spiritual leaders, bereavement coordinators, and volunteers often make home visits, where the patient most often resides. The staff give comfort, as well as medications and therapy. The staff also educate the patient and the caregiver in disease processes, medication administration, and how to provide daily care. Expert help and support is available to the patient and the caregiver 24 hours a day either by phone or by home visits.

Life Span Considerations

Older Adults

Hospice Care

- Many older adult patients at home or in nursing homes will likely meet the criteria and benefit from hospice care.
- The Hospice Medicare Benefit covers all expenses for palliative care related to the terminal illness, including professional staff visits, medication, equipment, and respite and acute care.
- Hospice often provides the dying older adult with a higher level of control and dignity than other types of health care.
- The primary caregiver is often an older adult spouse.
- The Hospice Medicare Benefit provides for bereavement follow-up care for at least 1 year following the death.

The Medicare Hospice Benefit came into effect in 1983, and today hospice services are reimbursable through Medicare, Medicaid, and most private insurance companies. Medicare certification or state licensure ensures quality hospice services (see Life Span Considerations for Older Adults box).

PALLIATIVE VERSUS CURATIVE CARE

Palliative care, as defined by the World Health Organization (WHO), is the active, complete care of a patient whose disease has not responded to curative therapy. Palliative care emphasizes the control of pain, relief of symptoms, and provision of psychological, social, and spiritual assistance (WHO, n.d.). It is possible to begin palliative care earlier in the dying process, whereas hospice is usually available only in the last 6 months of life. As such, palliative care provides the framework for future hospice assistance (Lewis et al., 2007).

When a patient with a life-threatening illness has exhausted all treatment and the disease has not been arrested or cured, it is necessary for the patient to decide whether continued active therapy is feasible or beneficial. By this time, the patient will perhaps already have experienced many debilitating physical and emotional symptoms as a result of the treatments or the progression of the disease.

This situation leads the patient and family to decide whether to continue with curative or to transition to palliative measures. **Curative treatment** is aggressive care in which the goal and intent is curing the disease and prolonging life at all cost. Palliative care is not curative in nature but aims to relieve pain and distress and to control symptoms of the disease. Hospice care emphasizes quality and not quantity of life.

It is important to give the patient and caregiver honest and accurate information so that they are able to make appropriate decisions. Hospice care is appropriate when active, curative treatment is no longer effective and supportive measures are necessary to assist the terminally ill patient through the dying process. It offers the patient a supported and safe passage from life to death in a way that preserves dignity and important relationships. Hospice is appropriate mainly for those individuals who believe that how they live is more important than how long they live. Death and dying become realities affecting family roles, lifestyle patterns, and future goals of the patient and family.

Palliative care is not giving up hope; it is full of hope of a good, fulfilling life.

CRITERIA FOR ADMISSION

The patient is required to meet certain criteria to be admitted into hospice:

- The attending physician has to certify that the patient's illness is terminal and the patient has a prognosis of 6 months or less to live. The attending physician is required to be a doctor of medicine or osteopathy and be the patient's designated physician.
- For the patient to qualify for Medicare or Medicaid assistance, two physicians are required to verify that the patient is dying and has less than 6 months to live. The hospice patient who continues to live beyond the estimated time period will still qualify for Medicare providing hospice criteria are still met (Lewis et al., 2007).
- It is mandatory that the patient desires the services. The patient has to be willing to forgo any further curative treatment and be willing to seek only palliative care.
- The patient and caregiver are required to understand and agree that hospice staff will plan the care according to comfort and that they will not necessarily perform life-support measures.
- The patient and caregiver are required to understand the prognosis and be willing to participate in the planning of the care.

Most hospices in the United States request that the patient have a **primary caregiver** (one who assumes ongoing responsibility for health maintenance and therapy for the illness). The caregiver is sometimes an immediate family member and sometimes a significant other, a friend, or a hired caregiver. Caregivers become vital when patients are no longer able to care for themselves safely. If the patient resides in a freestanding hospice residence, a long-term care facility, or a residential home, the nursing staff is designated as the primary caregiver.

Once the criteria are met and the patient is admitted to hospice, the staff performs complete physical, psychosocial, and spiritual assessments, and those involved discuss the care openly. The patient and caregiver receive a complete explanation of the hospice program and the philosophy of hospice, along with the interdisciplinary team concept.

GOALS OF HOSPICE

To provide effective hospice care, you will need an understanding of the philosophy and its relationship with the patient's responses and points of view. The basic goals of hospice address the following:

- Controlling or alleviating the patient's symptoms
- Allowing the patient and caregiver to be involved in the decisions regarding the plan of care
- Encouraging the patient and caregiver to live life to the fullest
- Providing continuous support to maintain patient and family confidence
- Educating and supporting the primary caregiver in the home setting that the patient chooses

INTERDISCIPLINARY TEAM

This approach of hospice, defined as **holistic** (pertaining to the total patient care that considers the physical, emotional, social, economic, and spiritual needs of the person) care, is to use an interdisciplinary team to manage the problems. The **interdisciplinary team** (multiprofessional health team working together in caring for the terminally ill patient) develops and supervises the plan of care in conjunction with all those involved with the care. The core interdisciplinary team members are the medical director, the nurse coordinator, the social worker, and the spiritual coordinator. To provide support to the dying patient and the caregiver, the interdisciplinary team considers all aspects of the family unit. They include the family in all decisions and care planning, because families also experience the stresses of the terminal illness and death of the patient (Figure 40-1). These stresses also extend into the bereavement period after the patient dies.

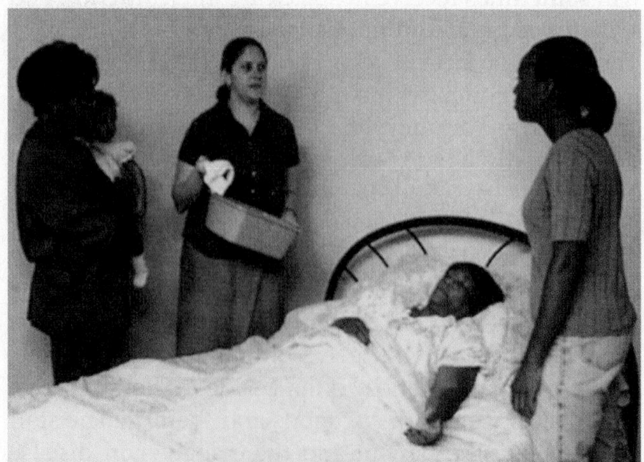

FIGURE 40-1 Family members are an important part of hospice, a philosophy of palliative and supportive care for the dying.

The hospice patient is assigned a primary team that consists of the patient's own attending physician, the primary hospice nurse, the social worker, a primary hospice aide, a primary volunteer, and a spiritual leader. This group of professionals, along with the interdisciplinary team, develops and is responsible for carrying out the plan of care. Regular and frequent team meetings are held to discuss the patient's physical, mental, and spiritual conditions, with revisions being made to the plan of care as needed. Discussions as to the effectiveness of the plan of care also take place. The team meeting is the place to bring together all members' observations and thoughts respectfully, and the team strives to function as a cohesive unit to use all expertise and resources in the interest of providing quality patient care (Tables 40-1 and 40-2).

MEDICAL DIRECTOR

The medical director is a doctor of medicine or osteopathy, and assumes overall responsibility for the medical component of the hospice patient's care program. The medical director does not take the place of the patient's attending physician but acts as a consultant for the attending physician. The medical director, with consultation from the interdisciplinary team, medically certifies the patient's eligibility for hospice care. The medical director is a mediator between the interdisciplinary team and the attending physician. He or she oversees the plan of care, ensuring that the care being provided and ordered is palliative in nature.

NURSE COORDINATOR AND HOSPICE NURSES

The nurse coordinator is a registered nurse who coordinates the implementation of the plan of care for each patient. The nurse coordinator will often do the initial assessment, admit the patient to the hospice program, and develop the plan of care along with the interdisciplinary team. The nurse coordinator also ensures that the plan of care is being followed, coordinates assignments of the hospice nurses and aides, facilitates meetings, and determines methods of payment.

Hospice nurses coordinate services of the hospice team, which includes hospice physicians, pharmacists, dietitians, physical therapists, social workers, clergy, certified nursing assistants, and hospice volunteers. Hospice nurses have to possess compassion, excellent

Table 40-1 Core Interdisciplinary Hospice Team

TEAM MEMBER	BACKGROUND	FUNCTION OR RESPONSIBILITY
Medical director	Licensed physician	Is a mediator between the hospice team and attending physician Provides consultation relative to the medical aspect of care
Nurse coordinator	Licensed registered nurse	Manages the patient care Explains the service, admits the patients, assigns the primary team
Social worker	Bachelor's degree in social work	Evaluates the psychosocial needs Is a resource for potential community services Assists with counseling in grief issues
Spiritual coordinator	Seminary degree	Liaison between the patient and spiritual community Coordinates spiritual support

Table 40-2 Primary Hospice Team

TEAM MEMBER	BACKGROUND	FUNCTION OR RESPONSIBILITY
Volunteer coordinator	Experience in volunteer work	Recruits and trains the volunteers Coordinates assignments of volunteers
Bereavement coordinator	Professional with grief experience	Assesses and supports the bereaved survivor Facilitates support groups
Hospice pharmacist	Licensed registered pharmacist	Provides drug consultation
Primary physician	Licensed physician	Responsible for the medical aspect of symptom control for patient
Primary nurse	Licensed registered nurse	Is a liaison between patient and caregiver, physician, and interdisciplinary team Evaluates patient's response to treatment Educates the patient and family in disease process and care Assesses symptom management Provides emotional support to patient and caregiver
Primary spiritual leader	As required by religious group	Supports patient and caregiver to cope with fears and uncertainty of spiritual issues
Hospice volunteer	Completion of volunteer training	Provides companionship for patient and caregiver Available for short periods of respite care
Hospice aide	Certified as a home health aide	Administers personal care and assistance with bathing

teaching skills, and the ability to adapt therapeutically to the hospice patients' many needs. It is also necessary for a hospice nurse to be especially adept in pain and symptom control (Lewis et al., 2007).

SOCIAL WORKER

The social worker is required to have at least a bachelor's degree, and in many agencies a master's degree, in social work. The social worker evaluates and assesses the **psychosocial** (a combination of psychological and social factors) needs of the patient. The social worker assists with accessing community resources and filing insurance papers, and also supports the patient and caregiver with emotional and grief issues. The social worker will also assist with counseling in some cases when communication difficulties are present. The social worker will provide these services under the direction of the physician and in accordance with the plan of care.

SPIRITUAL COORDINATOR

The spiritual coordinator is required to have a seminary degree, but affiliation with any church is acceptable. The spiritual coordinator is the liaison between the spiritual community and the interdisciplinary team. The spiritual coordinator assists with the spiritual assessment of the patient and, in keeping with patients' and families' beliefs, develops the plan of care regarding spiritual matters. If the patient desires spiritual assistance and does not have a spiritual home, the spiritual coordinator will assist in finding the spiritual support desired. The spiritual coordinator is vital in assisting the patient and caregiver to cope with fears and uncertainty. Possible support includes dealing with unfinished business and regrets and providing opportunities for reconciliation, prayer, and spiritual healing. Funeral planning and performing funeral services are also included in this role. Continued support for the family throughout the bereavement period is fulfilled by the spiritual coordinator. The spiritual coordinator is one resource to assist with cultural differences (see Cultural Considerations box).

The following sections describe additional members of the team that are needed to provide adequate care for the patient.

VOLUNTEER COORDINATOR

It is necessary for the volunteer coordinator to have experience in volunteer work. The volunteer coordinator assesses the needs of the patient and caregiver for volunteer services. When families are responsible for the total care of the patient in the home, caregiver "burnout" becomes a concern. This is when the services of volunteers become vital. They provide companionship, caregiver relief through **respite care** (a period of relief from responsibilities of caring for a patient), and emotional support. Appropriate services for the volunteer to provide are what we think of as typical of a good neighbor, perhaps reading to the patient, or sitting with the patient while the caregiver leaves the home for short periods, grocery shopping, or yard work. The volunteer coordinator ensures that the volunteer is adequately trained and prepared for working with the dying patient. Responsibilities also include assigning the proper volunteer to the appropriate patient. Each year, 400,000 hospice volunteers donate more than 5 million hours of time to hospice patients (Hospice Foundation of America, n.d.).

> **Cultural Considerations**
>
> **Death and Dying**
>
> - The United States is becoming more and more multicultural, and hospice care is challenged to meet the needs of people from other cultures.
> - Compassionate and empathic care bridges cultures, but it is necessary to learn as much as possible about the culture so it is possible to provide assistance. People all have different reactions and traditions regarding death and dying, but all experience grief.
> - Do not make a change regarding the plan of care without first discussing it with the whole family.
> - Often when working with Hispanic people you are working with a large, extended, extremely interdependent family. They tend to show great respect to elders, and many will defer decisions to the men in the family. Hispanics will sometimes want all the family members to view the body before it is removed from the home setting. Often that may mean a wait of several hours before the mortuary is able to remove the body.

BEREAVEMENT COORDINATOR

The **bereavement** (a common depressed reaction to the death of someone close) coordinator is a professional who has experience in dealing with grief issues. The bereavement coordinator assesses the patient and the caregiver at admission to the hospice program and identifies risk factors that have potential to be of concern following the death of the patient. The bereavement coordinator follows the plan of care for the bereaved caregiver for at least a year following the death. The bereavement coordinator facilitates support groups and assigns bereavement volunteers to visit the caregiver.

The bereavement coordinator will sometimes also provide counseling but has the option to refer the family to other counseling if the issues are too great. The goals of bereavement counseling for loved ones during the patient's illness and following the death are to (1) provide support and (2) assist survivors in the transition to a life without the deceased person. It is appropriate to incorporate grief support into the plan of care.

HOSPICE PHARMACIST

The hospice pharmacist is required to be a licensed pharmacist and available for consultation on the drugs the hospice patient may be taking. The pharmacist evaluates for drug-drug or drug-food interactions, appropriate drug doses, and correct administration times and routes. The pharmacist typically gives information and advice about common drugs used, administration time, and doses (Table 40-3).

DIETITIAN CONSULTANT

Licensed medical nutritional therapists (LMNTs) are available for hospice consultations and for diet counseling. The hospice nurse performs the nutritional assessment at admission. If the nurse notes nutritional problems, a referral to the LMNT is possible for assistance with diet counseling and meal planning. The LMNT also assists with educating the caregiver regarding nutritional issues in end-stage diseases.

HOSPICE AIDE

The hospice aide is a certified nurse assistant who works under the supervision of the hospice nurse. The hospice aide follows the plan of care that the interdisciplinary team develops and assists the patient with bathing and personal care, including hair, nail, oral, and skin care. The hospice aide will sometimes also assist the patient or the caregiver with light homemaker services. The patient and the hospice aide often develop a close relationship, and the patient will in some cases share feelings with the aide more easily than with any other member of the team.

OTHER SERVICES

Other services, if needed, are available from the physical therapist, the speech-language pathologist, and the occupational therapist. These services are not available for rehabilitative purposes, but to assist with improving the quality of life and care for the patient and the caregiver. The physical therapist is available to assist with teaching the caregiver transferring skills, exercises that are sometimes useful to relieve muscle cramps, wheelchair fittings, and other skills that serve in caring for the dying patient. The speech-language pathologist is available if difficulties arise with communication or swallowing. The occupational therapist is also available for positioning for comfort, providing adaptive equipment for the patient, or other assistance for comfort and for activities of daily living (ADLs).

PALLIATIVE CARE

The goal and emphasis of hospice is symptom management and palliative care. The team of caregivers routinely assesses, reassesses, and documents the severity, the treatment, and the control of symptoms of the illness.

PAIN

Of all the symptoms a dying patient experiences, pain is the most dreaded and feared; therefore pain is a priority for symptom management. It disrupts the quality, the activities, and the enjoyment of life. To the healthy person, pain is usually temporary and tolerable, but to the terminally ill patient it can be excruciating, constant, and terrifying. Pain takes many forms, such as physical, psychosocial, and spiritual, and becomes a major factor that it is right and proper to address and alleviate. Experts believe that it is possible to

Table 40-3 Medications for Hospice Care

Generic (Trade)	Indications	Side Effects	Nursing Interventions
Morphine sulfate—immediate-release (Roxanol)	Indicated for acute and severe pain	Constipation, nausea and vomiting, sedation	Assess pain control using pain assessment; instruct on administration routinely
Morphine sulfate—controlled-release (MS Contin)	Indicated for moderate and severe pain	Constipation, nausea and vomiting, sedation	Assess pain control and medication effectiveness
Fentanyl transdermal system (Duragesic patch)	Opioid for moderate and severe pain	Confusion, hypoventilation, nausea and vomiting, constipation	Instruct family to clean skin with water only and dry before application
Droperidol (Inapsine)	Antiemetic	Hypotension and tachycardia, drowsiness, dizziness	Ensure caregiver is giving the antiemetic appropriately and routinely
Prochlorperazine (Compazine)	Antiemetic	Extrapyramidal symptoms, dry mouth, depression	Assess control of nausea and ensure caregiver is giving the antiemetic appropriately and routinely
Senna (Senokot)	Constipation	Nausea and vomiting, diarrhea, abdominal cramping	Encourage fluids, assess gastrointestinal status, and give laxative routinely if patient is taking pain medication
Lorazepam (Ativan)	Antianxiety	Dizziness, drowsiness, orthostatic hypotension, tachycardia	Administer routinely; instruct in safety issues regarding rising slowly and not driving

Box 40-2 Pain Assessment Questionnaire

1. Throughout our lives, most of us have had pain from time to time such as minor headaches, sprains, and toothaches. Have you had pain other than everyday kinds of pain today?
2. Where is the pain? (The use of a body chart often helps the patient to identify the location.)
3. Using the scale of 0 to 10, with 0 being no pain and 10 being the worst pain imaginable, rate the pain at its worst in the past 24 hours.
4. Using the same scale of 0 to 10, rate the pain at its lowest point in the past 24 hours.
5. Using the same scale of 0 to 10, rate the pain on the average.
6. Describe your pain. (The words the patient uses to describe the pain help you to understand the type of pain for treatment purposes.)
7. What treatments or medications are you using to control the pain?
8. Using the scale of 0 to 10, with 0 being no relief and 10 being complete relief, rate the amount of relief received from the treatment.
9. What causes or increases the pain?
10. Does the pain interfere with any of the following:
    - General activity
    - Mood
    - Walking ability
    - Normal work
    - Relations with other people
    - Sleep
    - Appetite
    - Enjoyment of life

manage pain effectively 95% to 97% of the time. It is all too easy for the caregiver caring for people experiencing pain to become frustrated and feel helpless as he or she tries to control the discomfort, leading to further feelings of guilt and inadequacy.

Initially the physician will sometimes order diagnostic tests to determine the exact cause of the pain. It will possibly be related to tumor invasion, compression of organs or nerves, erosion of tissue, or other pathologic factors. Removing the cause will be impossible in some cases; therefore controlling the symptoms becomes central to the successful management of pain for the terminally ill. Assessments are vital to determining the plan of managing pain, and the patient is the primary source to go to for information. The patient's self-report of intensity, quality, and management of pain provides the most significant data. Make sure that **pain assessment** (evaluation of the factors that alleviate or exacerbate a patient's pain) includes the severity and the history of the pain and what brings relief to the patient. Begin pain assessment with the patient's self-report and have the patient rate the pain on a scale of 0 to 10, with 0 being having no pain at all and 10 being the worst imaginable pain. Any pain the patient rates at 5 or higher on the pain scale has a great effect on the quality of life.

Clinicians use many different pain assessments, such as the familiar OLD CARTS, which stands for *O* = onset, *L* = location, *D* = duration, *C* = character of pain, *A* = aggravating factors, *R* = relieving factors, *T* = treatments, *S* = severity. Use this type of assessment with the patient on every visit and every new complaint or increase in pain. Make sure that assessment of pain, considered the fifth vital sign, is ongoing; note any change in the intensity or type of pain that will necessitate changes to the plan of care (Box 40-2).

The answers to the questions in Box 40-2 serve to determine the appropriate mode of therapy that will be effective in managing the patient's pain. The goal of therapy is to prescribe a sufficient dose of effective drug to alleviate pain and at the same time allow the patient to remain alert enough to participate in activities of daily living (Box 40-3).

Box 40-3 Pain Control

- It is never right for a patient to suffer pain, often intolerable pain, because of the lack of adequate pain control. Try asking the question, "What is pain?" The answer is simple; pain is anything the patient says it is, whether real or perceived.
- Pain is treated with drugs (morphine) or a combination of drugs to provide maximum relief while at the same time avoiding maximum side effects.
- Proper pain relief is provided on a regular round-the-clock basis.
- The need for palliative care worldwide is enormous and will continue to increase. Symptom management and adequate pain control have to be the prime objective for you as a hospice nurse, at the same time you always strive to maintain the patient's dignity and capacity to contribute as a full human being.*

*Gordon, A. (2001). End of life issues. *Caring,* 20(21):6.

Three main types of pain are necessary to address. **Somatic pain** arises from the musculoskeletal system and is described as aching, stabbing, or throbbing. There are appropriate roles for nonsteroidal antiinflammatory drugs (NSAIDs), nonopioid drugs, and opioid drugs in treating somatic pain.

Pain that originates from the internal organs is called **visceral pain.** The words people commonly use to describe this are cramping, pressure, dull, or squeezing pain. Physicians typically prescribe anticholinergic medications alone or as an **adjuvant** (additional drug or treatment that is added to assist in the action of the primary pain treatment) to nonopioids or opioids.

Neuropathic pain arises from the nerves and the nervous system. Tingling, burning, or shooting pains are often due to neuropathic causes. The physician will sometimes order anticonvulsants to give as an adjuvant to assist with pain control.

Lifestyle considerations are important in determining the route and the type of medication to give for control of pain. Oral medications are preferable because they help the patient and the caregiver manage the scheduling and administration more easily. After determining the severity of pain and the type of medication to be used, it is important to **titrate** (slowly increase the amount of drug to find the therapeutic dose) the dosage of the medication. Mild to moderate pain is sometimes possible to manage with NSAIDs; as the pain increases in severity with progression of the patient's condition, the physician will often switch the analgesic over to an opioid drug with or without adjuvant drugs. Nonsteroidal drugs are possible to give along with the opioid to enhance the medication's effectiveness. Oral administration of analgesics is not always feasible because of nausea and vomiting, obstruction, or inability to swallow, and other routes enter into consideration, such as sublingual, subcutaneous, parenteral, rectal, or topical. Morphine derivatives are often the drugs of choice in caring for the hospice patient because it is possible to deliver them by all routes and the dose can be titrated to control the pain. Administer analgesic routinely, with a prn drug available for breakthrough pain so good control is possible to maintain.

Using long-acting medications such as MS Contin, Oxycontin, or Duragesic patches often provides better pain control and is more convenient for the patient and the caregiver. As the pain increases, it is important to monitor the amount and frequency of prn medications so the appropriate increase in the routine medications is possible.

As the patient's condition deteriorates and pain increases, the expert knowledge and skill of the hospice personnel in titrating and managing the pain is invaluable.

Ineffective pain management is usually associated with undermedication resulting from common myths and fears. The myths and fears are addiction, tolerance, and respiratory depression. With careful and expert monitoring by the hospice team, along with reassurance and support, these fears are possible to relieve.

Never rule out other effective methods in managing pain. Radiation therapy, nerve blocks, and psychological or physical methods are all options to try in appropriate circumstances. Hot or cold packs at the site of discomfort, repositioning the patient, music therapy, relaxation techniques, acupuncture, or even transcutaneous electric nerve stimulation (TENS) are sometimes good alternatives. If it works for the patient, do not overlook it.

Nursing Interventions and Patient Teaching

Your role as a nurse is to focus on the effectiveness of the plan, to ensure that the care plan achieves good control of the symptoms (Nursing Care Plan 40-1). It is necessary to constantly assess and reassess the pain and the symptoms to ensure that their management is adequate. Educate the patient and the caregiver in the appropriate administration, scheduling, and effects of the medication to help them become aware of increasing signs and symptoms of pain. Make sure the patient and the caregiver understand that it is possible to control pain and that using large doses of opioids is common and necessary to achieve that control. It is good to educate the patient and the caregiver that "the dose that works is the dose that works." Assist the caregiver in setting a schedule for administering the medications and then monitor the patient's response to and compliance with the established plan.

Patient education regarding other techniques of pain and symptom management are also a nursing responsibility. Possibilities include music therapy, relaxation methods, and other alternative methods. It is important to give encouragement and positive reinforcement to the patient and the family in their effort at following the plan.

NAUSEA AND VOMITING

Nausea and vomiting tend to be very upsetting to both the patient and the caregiver. Many patients consider nausea to be worse than vomiting because at times it is only noticeable to the patient and therefore flies under the radar of caregivers and health professionals. It is important to assess for the cause of nausea and vomiting, and remove it if at all possible. Nausea is a possible result of chemotherapy side effects, obstruction, tumor, uncontrolled pain, constipation, and even food smells. At times the treatment of the nausea is as simple as bringing in food already prepared so that the cooking smells do not bother the patient. Sometimes the drugs used for pain control cause nausea; giving antiemetics with the opioid analgesic is useful. Nausea is a common side effect with the initiation of opioid treatment. This side effect usually subsides after a time, and the best response is to use an antiemetic rather than discontinue the opioid. Anxiety has also been known to cause nausea, which then leads to vomiting. Patients who vomit are typically anxious about why they are vomiting, which often worsens the symptoms.

Nursing Interventions and Patient Teaching

Educate the patient and the caregiver regarding the cause or the prevention of nausea and vomiting. Encourage the patient to take the ordered antiemetics routinely, 30 minutes before meals and at bedtime. Try using antiemetic drugs such as prochlorperazine (Compazine) and promethazine (Phenergan) suppositories if possible until the nausea is controlled, and then use oral drugs prophylactically to prevent the nausea from returning. Metoclopramide (Reglan) is

Nursing Care Plan 40-1 The Hospice Patient with Metastatic Prostate Cancer

Mr. Bartucci is a 74-year-old with prostate cancer with bone metastasis. He complains of severe pain in his right leg and in his ribs, which he rates as a 7 to 8 on a scale of 0 to 10. Mr. Bartucci also has shortness of breath. He is on a regimen of MS Contin 20 mg every 12 hours with Roxanol 20 mg every 4 hours.

NURSING DIAGNOSIS ***Pain related to the cancer that has metastasized to the bone, manifested by complaints of pain***

Patient Goals and Expected Outcomes	Nursing Interventions	Evaluation
Pain will be controlled at 2 or less on a scale of 0 to 10	Assess pain control and pain level using the pain assessment scale of 0 to 10 every visit. Assess patient and caregiver understanding of medication administration. Assess for compliance with medication schedule. Assess for side effects of the medications, and educate accordingly. Notify the interdisciplinary team of any uncontrolled pain. Educate patient and caregiver of other pain control methods such as transcutaneous electric nerve stimulation (TENS), repositioning methods, and heat and cold treatments. Have the patient and caregiver keep a pain diary.	Patient relates pain is at 7 or 8 on the pain scale of 0 to 10.

NURSING DIAGNOSIS ***Ineffective breathing pattern, related to disease process***

Patient Goals and Expected Outcomes	Nursing Interventions	Evaluation
Patient will not complain of shortness of breath	Assess respiratory status and effort every visit. Patient to rate ineffective respiratory effort using the scale of 0 to 10 every visit. Assess need for oxygen use by performing an oximetry level as ordered prn. Administer oxygen per nasal cannula prn. Notify the interdisciplinary team of any complaints of respiratory distress. Educate patient and caregiver on methods that will ease respiratory distress (e.g., relaxation techniques, diaphragmatic breathing, medication usage, positioning). Provide emotional support to patient and caregiver at each visit.	Patient rates respiratory distress at 6 on a scale of 0 to 10. Oxygen administered at 3 L/min by nasal cannula.

Critical Thinking Questions

1. Mr. Bartucci's wife complains to the hospice nurse that her husband has not had a bowel movement in 3 days. What will be included in an appropriate nursing intervention that would provide relief for Mr. Bartucci?
2. The nurse notes that Mr. Bartucci is restless and notes dyspnea. She performs an oximetry check on Mr. Bartucci and notes an 83% oxygen saturation. List three nursing interventions to improve his respiratory distress.

effective in controlling mild to moderate nausea and vomiting. Because it increases gastric motility, its use is contraindicated in patients with suspected bowel obstruction. Benzodiazepines are not for use as single-agent antiemetics, but they are often extremely effective when used in conjunction with other antiemetics or for treating nausea and vomiting associated with anxiety. Drugs in this class, such as lorazepam (Ativan) or alprazolam (Xanax), reduce anxiety, although they tend to be sedating.

Eating slowly and in a pleasant atmosphere, with relaxation and rest periods after eating, is a good way to control the nausea. If vomiting occurs, discourage eating for a short time until peristalsis stabilizes. When the nausea and vomiting have subsided, have the patient begin drinking liquids to avoid dehydration or start eating soft, bland foods. Serve small, light, bland meals, avoiding sweet, greasy, spicy, or strong-smelling foods. If anxiety and fear are causing nausea and vomiting, verbalizing the fears is often helpful. Under no circumstances is it ever acceptable to force the patient to eat food or drink fluids if he or she has no desire to eat, because this also has potential to compromise dignity and be detrimental to the patient's well-being.

CONSTIPATION

One of the most common problems of the terminally ill patient is constipation. Constipation has many possible causes, and assessment as to the cause is fundamental to treating it adequately. Sometimes this problem causes more anxiety and discomfort than pain itself. Because constipation has the capacity to cause other symptoms, such as abdominal pain, nausea, or vomiting, prevention of the problem is important. Factors that contribute to constipation are poor dietary intake, poor fluid intake, hypercalcemia, hyponatremia, tumor compression of the bowel, use of opioids for pain control, and decrease in physical activity. Follow the initiation of opioids with the initiation of a stool softener and a stimulant as well. Some opioids are more likely to cause constipation than others; in such cases, a different opioid will perhaps be helpful. Changing the rate of administration sometimes also provides some relief. Transdermal fentanyl has proven to be associated with significantly less constipation than sustained-release oral morphine (the drugs were equally effective in treating pain) (Haughney, 2004). As with other drugs, if inability to swallow or nausea and vomiting are also a problem, consider other routes, such as suppositories or enemas. A rectal examination will sometimes be necessary to check for an impaction along with manual removal of stool. The Fleet enema helps soften and dissolve a hard impaction whose removal is otherwise a painful procedure.

Nursing Interventions and Patient Teaching

Supporting and educating the patient and the caregiver are your primary concerns. Make sure to cover the following points with the patient and the caregiver:

- A decrease in oral intake will also decrease the amount of stool expelled.
- Even though a patient does not have oral intake, bowel movements will still be possible in some cases.
- Opioids pose a risk of constipation, so it is necessary to give laxatives.
- Comfort is the all-important factor. If the patient has not had a bowel movement, assessment of discomfort, bowel sounds, and firmness of abdomen are necessary to do before any active treatment.

ANOREXIA AND MALNUTRITION

Anorexia and malnutrition are major anxiety-producing symptoms of terminal illness. Poor appetite potentially arises from nausea, vomiting, constipation, dysphagia, stomatitis, tumor invasion, general deterioration of the body, depression, or infections. These complications lead to difficulty in eating, which in turn causes loss of appetite. Odors of food cooking, inability to tolerate sweet foods, or a bitter taste in the mouth also contribute to the problem. This makes food less enjoyable, so the patient does not eat.

Disease processes change the body's metabolism and appetite, which sometimes lead to **cachexia** (malnutrition marked by weakness and emaciation), usually associated with a serious disease such as cancer and resulting in muscle weakness and weight loss. If poor oral intake of either food or fluids is affecting the quality of life, it is necessary to make adjustments to the plan of care.

Nursing Interventions and Patient Teaching

Complete nutritional assessments routinely and apply the findings to the hospice plan of care as appropriate. The nurse, as always, assesses and treats causes such as nausea and vomiting. If anorexia is related to stomatitis or infections, good oral hygiene is important. A technique to alleviate discomfort of the mouth is to use swabs or Toothettes soaked in flavored mouthwash. Small frequent drinks, crushed ice, or artificial saliva are often useful to relieve a dry mouth. If the odor of food causes anorexia, make sure the patient is not in the kitchen during meal preparation, or have family, friends, or volunteers bring in meals. Make the meals as attractive as possible, using foods the patient chooses. High-protein supplements are helpful when eating is difficult. Avoid weighing the patient because sometimes the patient will be depressed and discouraged by attention to weight loss. Often the caregiver needs additional support when a patient is not eating, because caregivers often think a reduced diet will hasten death and in contrast, if they manage to get the patient to eat, the food will prolong life. You will often have to reassure the patient and the caregiver that anorexia is part of the end-of-dying process and that forcing the patient to eat has some potential to be harmful. If the anorexia's cause is untreatable, such as tumor invasion, the patient and the caregiver are likely to need additional emotional support. Rarely do artificial hydration, total parental nutrition, and tube feedings come into consideration. These will perhaps slow the overall cachexic effect, but the long-term result and quality of life will not change.

DYSPNEA OR AIR HUNGER

Dyspnea is a symptom that arises from a variety of possible conditions, such as heart failure, dysrhythmias, infection, ascites, or tumor growth. Breathing effectively will be difficult for many patients, especially during the very end stages of the illness. Air hunger is sometimes caused by tumor pressure, fluid and electrolyte imbalance, or anemia. Anxiety resulting from fear or panic will potentially accompany this problem. Some respiratory distress will be relieved by oxygen, morphine, or bronchodilators. Oxygen will perhaps not actually relieve the dyspnea, but it often eases the anxiety of both the patient and the caregiver. Oral or nebulized morphine helps relax the patient's respiratory effort, thus allowing a greater respiratory efficiency. Bronchodilators sometimes ease respiratory obstructions and ease the respiratory distress. Often, 24 to 48 hours before death, the patient will exhibit the "death rattle," which is the result of an accumulation of mucus and fluids in the posterior area of the pharynx. The sound that air makes as it passes through the mucus is coarse and loud and very upsetting to the caregiver. Medications that are sometimes helpful in the prevention of excess secretions are the anticholinergic drugs such as transdermal scopolamine.

Nursing Interventions and Patient Teaching

Your main focus is in relieving the anxiety and supporting the patient and caregiver. Education on positioning, use of a fan to circulate air, use of morphine to decrease the work of respiration, use of tranquilizers to ease anxiety, and maintaining good oral hygiene will aid the patient. Keep suctioning at a minimum because it actually increases mucus production and is very uncomfortable to the patient. Only use suctioning if the patient is choking and unable to recover.

PSYCHOSOCIAL AND SPIRITUAL ISSUES

Spiritual unrest and issues are often interrelated with psychosocial problems and have the potential to surface especially when symptoms are uncontrolled. It is always necessary to respect any religious or spiritual concerns and meet the patient's wishes if at all possible. Spiritual assessments are meant to gather information regarding the patient's feelings and needs. Some patients will question their faiths and beliefs, and some will look to find support that they have never had, when confronted with a terminal illness. Many symptoms such as depression, the need to suffer, bitterness, anger, hallucinations, or dreams of fire are in some cases indicative of unmet spiritual needs.

Nursing Interventions and Patient Teaching

Refer spiritual issues to the spiritual coordinator, and do not use them as an opening for you to share your own feelings and beliefs unless specifically asked. It depends on the hospice organization whether the nurse or the spiritual coordinator does the spiritual assessment. It is essential for the assessor to be nonjudgmental and accepting of the patient's and the caregiver's spiritual beliefs. The social worker will possibly also assist with the relationship between the patient and the caregiver and provide counseling to resolve conflict. The social worker does not "fix" the conflicts but assists in finding solutions and problem solving. The development of trust is critical between the patient and the interdisciplinary team and is invaluable when dealing with these issues.

OTHER COMMON SIGNS AND SYMPTOMS

Weight loss and dehydration will sometimes lead to a decrease of soft tissue, especially on the bony areas of knees, hips, elbows, and buttocks, leading to skin impairment.

Increased weakness is also notable in the last stages of a terminal illness. With increased weakness, activity intolerance increases, and the patient spends most of the time reclining. This leads to risk for skin impairment and the formation of pressure ulcers. Along with weakness come safety issues of being unstable and falling. Patients often exhibit signs of depression and will perhaps make comments regarding suicide. Comments regarding suicide do not always come from the actual desire to kill oneself but are, in some cases, rather a statement of a desire for independence. Sleeplessness and insomnia sometimes occur as a result of an accumulation of signs and symptoms, and exhaustion has the potential to cause an exacerbation of all other signs and symptoms.

Nursing Interventions and Patient Teaching

It is important at this time to teach the patient and the caregiver the basics of good skin care. Cleanliness promoted by bathing is often refreshing, as well as therapeutic in promoting comfort and the feeling of self-worth. Inspect the skin frequently, and keep it as dry and clean as possible. Stress the need to avoid harsh soaps, strong detergents, and irritations from buttons,

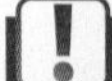 **Safety Alert!**

Prevention of Skin Impairment

Safety risks for hospice patients are many, owing to the debilitating nature of the terminal illness and other comorbidities many patients have. There is potential for skin impairment due to poor nutrition, decreased circulation, and decreased mobility. Frequent education to the family and the patient are required to promote integrity of the skin. Have the caregiver observe the patient's skin and report any erythema or impairment. Instruct the caregiver to reposition for comfort, use alternating air or eggcrate mattresses, and to perform good hygiene to prevent skin impairment.

snaps, or food crumbs. An eggcrate mattress, sheepskin, or air-flotation mattress, as well as heel and elbow protectors, help cushion the bony areas. The hospice aide will often be very helpful to the patient in assisting with personal care, hygiene, and bathing. If pressure ulcers occur, cleaning with normal saline, drying well, and applying a skin protector are helpful measures. An awareness of safety is essential in preventing falls and injuries, and providing information regarding home safety is important. Listening and providing emotional support is an important nursing intervention for depression and suicidal thoughts. The social worker is influential in these situations.

PATIENT AND CAREGIVER TEACHING

The hospice interdisciplinary team realizes that a terminal illness is potentially the most difficult time in a person's life. The team will take as honest and straightforward an approach as possible in all matters affecting the patient and caregiver. It is thought that the fear of the unknown is always greater than the fear of the known. Because of this, education is an important part of the care the team provides to the patient. Educating the caregiver in symptom management, hands-on care of the patient, caring for body functions, and teaching regarding the signs and symptoms of approaching death are important to help relieve fears (Table 40-4).

BEREAVEMENT PERIOD

Hospice care does not conclude once the patient dies but usually continues for at least 1 year with bereavement support. The family, especially the primary caregiver, continues to need support during the bereavement period after the patient dies. Even though the family feels they have prepared for the death, facing the future without the person who died is difficult. Many believe that four full seasons must pass before the bereaved are able to begin to think of the deceased without feeling intense emotional pain. The death of a loved one is a devastating agony that takes a long time to heal and subside. Depending on the size of the program, special bereavement teams with counselors will possibly be available for the caregiver and family. Some teams facilitate a bereavement support group that meets on a regular basis, providing these families the opportunities to communicate and share their feelings. Volunteers and pastors keep in touch by visits, phone calls, cards, and remembering the bereaved person on holidays and anniversaries.

The hospice staff also goes through a grieving period for each patient who dies. It is a good idea to encourage the team members to attend funeral services, attend memorials, or visit the caregivers as appropriate following the death to help ease their grief. Each hospice provides support to its staff with support meetings and time to vent their feelings and to heal.

Table 40-4 Signs and Symptoms of Approaching Death

SIGNS AND SYMPTOMS	NURSING INTERVENTIONS
The arms and legs of the body sometimes become cool to the touch and the underside of the body sometimes becomes darker.	Keep warm blankets on the patient to prevent feeling of coldness.
The patient sometimes spends more and more time sleeping during the day and at times will be difficult to arouse.	Assist caregiver in planning time to be with the patient when the patient is most alert.
The patient sometimes becomes increasingly confused about time, place, and identity of close and familiar people.	Reorient the patient as appropriate to the time of day and who is present. Do not upset the patient.
Incontinence of urine and bowel movements often happens when death is imminent. Sometimes there is a significant decrease in urine output.	Educate the caregiver in keeping the patient clean and dry. Provide pads or adult diapers as needed.
Oral secretions sometimes become more profuse and collect in the back of the throat. This produces the sound often referred to as the "death rattle."	Provide a cool-mist humidifier to increase the humidity in the room when oral secretions build up. Elevating the head of the bed with pillows or obtaining a hospital bed will make breathing easier.
Clarity of hearing and vision decrease slightly.	Keep lights on in the room when vision decreases and never assume that the patient is not able to hear you.
Restlessness, pulling at the bed linen, and having visions of people or things that do not exist sometimes occur.	Talk calmly and assuredly with the confused person so as not to startle or frighten the person further.
The patient will have a decreased need for food and drink.	Educate the caregiver that the patient will not starve to death or die of dehydration. Much reassurance is needed in this area.
Breathing patterns will change to an irregular pace; there are sometimes 10- to 30-second periods of no breathing, or apnea.	Elevating the head of the bed often relieves the person who has irregular breathing patterns. Oxygen sometimes is and sometimes is not beneficial.
Changes in vital signs occur, with decreased blood pressure and elevated pulse.	Educate the family that these changes are normal and expected and are not uncomfortable for the patient.

ETHICAL ISSUES IN HOSPICE CARE

Ethical issues that sometimes arise when dealing with hospice patients include withholding or withdrawing nutritional support, the right to refuse treatment, and do not resuscitate (DNR) orders. Families find it difficult to discontinue nourishment, even when death is clearly approaching. If the patient is unconscious, decisions regarding these issues sometimes fall on one family member, which has potential to create guilt feelings if other family members disagree. There are no simple answers to any of these concerns. It is helpful when the patient makes his or her wishes known in advance, such as in a living will or an advance directive, or assigns a durable power of attorney.

An advance directive is a document prepared while an individual is alive and competent. It provides guidance to the family and the health care team in the event the person is no longer capable of making decisions. The directive states the individual's preferences concerning life-support measures and organ donations and sometimes gives authority to another person to make decisions for the patient who is now perhaps in a coma.

It is imperative to be aware of your organization's ethics policies and procedures so that you and your colleagues are able to appropriately and correctly address any questions and concerns. No discrimination is ever tolerable for patients in hospice, regardless of sex, race, age, religion, and diagnosis. It is never acceptable for hospices to exclude or refuse high-cost patients; their mandate is to serve everyone regardless of ability to pay. Services are to be available 7 days a week, 24 hours a day.

A hospice patient has lost so much throughout the illness: health, job, independence, self-esteem, family, and financial security. Hospice attempts to assist the patient in maintaining dignity and control. Hospice places the emphasis on living and not dying. It is important for the hospice team to be sensitive to the patient's and the caregiver's needs and maintain honesty at all times. Make sure to include the patient and the caregiver in all aspects of care and decision making. Provide opportunities for expressing concerns and fears, because this will make the process less fearful and threatening. Allowing the patient and the caregiver to live fully, comfortably, and in dignity until death occurs naturally is the main goal of hospice care.

THE FUTURE OF HOSPICE

Trends indicate that as more patients and families are educated about its many benefits, hospice is growing as an attractive alternative to facing death in a clinical setting. Nevertheless, only a fraction of those who have the option of hospice care choose to participate in it. Physicians, patients, and family members are often unwilling to begin hospice care for several reasons. The patient or family sometimes believe that availing themselves of the services of hospice denotes giving up hope, and some physicians are hesitant to prescribe hospice care if they perceive the patient's worsening condition a personal failure on their part (Lewis et al., 2007). It is necessary for physicians and nurses caring for patients with terminal illnesses in clinical facilities to open the dialogue with families about the option of hospice and its possible benefits to patients and their caregivers. Until clinicians, patients, and families become more comfortable talking about the process of death and dying, hospice will remain too marginalized to fulfill its promise as an excellent option for accessing supportive services during an extremely difficult time ("The state of hospice in America," 2004).

Get Ready for the NCLEX® Examination!

Key Points

- Hospice is a philosophy of care about providing support to patients with a terminal illness and their families.
- *Hospice* is from the Latin word *hospitium*, meaning hospitality and lodging.
- Hospice care is appropriate when active treatment is no longer effective and supportive measures are necessary to assist the terminally ill patient through the dying process.
- The Hospice Medicare Benefit covers all expenses for palliative care related to the terminal illness, including professional staff visits, medication, equipment, and respite and acute care.
- Hospice care emphasizes quality, not quantity, of life.
- Palliative care is appropriate when a cure is not possible but care is still necessary.
- The goal of palliative care is to control pain and other symptoms for the prevention of distress.
- Palliative care is the active, complete care of a patient whose disease has not responded to curative therapy.
- Admission to a hospice program is the decision of a patient and family, because not all people need or desire hospice care.
- An important criterion for the patient to be admitted into hospice is certification that the patient has a prognosis of 6 months or less to live from the attending physician and a second physician.
- Hospice care consists of a blending of professionals and nonprofessionals to meet the total needs of the patient and family.
- An interdisciplinary team delivers hospice care, because no individual or individual profession is able to meet all the needs of terminally ill patients and families all the time.

- Hospice care takes all aspects of the lives of patients and their families into consideration. Stresses and concerns have the potential to arise in many ways when families are faced with a terminal illness.
- A hospice care program considers the patient and family together as the unit of care, because families experience much stress and pain during the terminal illness of one of their members.
- Family participation in caregiving is an important part of palliative care.
- Hospice care is available 24 hours a day, 7 days a week, because it is possible that needs will arise at any time.
- Hospice care is respectful of all patient and family belief systems, seeking resources to meet the physical, psychosocial, and spiritual needs of the family unit.
- Hospice care for the family continues into the bereavement period. Needs of the family continue after the patient dies.

Additional Learning Resources

Go to your Companion CD for an audio glossary, animations, video clips, and more.

evolve Be sure to visit the Evolve site at http://evolve.elsevier.com/Christensen/foundations/ for additional online resources.

Review Questions for the NCLEX® Examination

1. The doctor is explaining to a 74-year-old patient that his prostate cancer is progressing and that curative treatment is no longer an option. The doctor has recommended hospice to the patient and his wife with this explanation:
   1. "We can provide support and control your symptoms and discomfort so you have good quality days."
   2. "With hospice we would continue with aggressive curative care."
   3. "There is no hope left for you and you should just go home and wait to die."
   4. "We can no longer guarantee controlled symptoms or a dignified life, but we can still provide sympathy."

2. The patient's wife calls the hospice nurse and reports that her husband is complaining of pain in his leg and is not able to get comfortable. The hospice nurse will:
   1. tell the wife that pain will increase because of the progression of the disease and there is nothing to be done.
   2. ask the wife what the patient is rating his pain and if he had taken any prn medication for breakthrough pain.
   3. tell the wife that her husband must be a complainer.
   4. tell the wife to wait until morning and call the doctor.

3. When the nurse makes a home visit the patient is experiencing shortness of breath and has increased anxiety. The hospice nurse will:
   1. assess the respiratory status, check the oximetry, call the doctor for possible orders for oxygen, and increase morphine to assist in decreasing the respiratory distress.
   2. tell the patient that he is out of shape and needs to exercise.
   3. have the wife tell him that she is disappointed in him for complaining.
   4. sit and hold his hand.

4. The patient is experiencing a decreased appetite and is worried about his weight loss. The hospice nurse will:
   1. tell the wife to cook all of his favorite foods and maybe he will eat.
   2. tell the patient that he should really force himself to eat.
   3. tell the patient that decreased appetite is normal and it is okay for him to eat only what he feels like eating.
   4. bring the patient a pizza to stimulate his appetite.

5. The patient's wife is exhausted and expresses a need to get away for a short time. The volunteer coordinator has assessed the need for a volunteer and will:
   1. tell the wife a volunteer will not help the situation at all.
   2. tell the wife that it is best for her to just stay with her husband because he might die while she is away.
   3. assign a volunteer to sit with the patient for a couple of hours two or three times a week so that the wife is able to either take a nap or to leave for a short time to do errands.
   4. assign a volunteer to do errands so that the patient's wife does not have to leave.

6. As a part of the hospice program, the patient has a core interdisciplinary team that manages his care. This team is made up of a(an):
   1. accountant, pharmacist, priest, and nurse.
   2. physical therapist, occupational therapist, speech-language pathologist, and home health aide.
   3. nurse coordinator, medical director, social worker, and spiritual coordinator.
   4. volunteer, pastor, home health aide, and social worker.

7. The patient's wife tells the hospice aide that she is having problems meeting their financial obligations. The hospice aide will:
   1. tell no one because this is confidential information.
   2. ask her for permission to report this to the interdisciplinary team and have the social worker make a visit to see if it is possible to provide assistance.
   3. report this to the patient's church to see if there is some financial assistance available.
   4. tell the next-door neighbor.

8. The patient has an advance directive, but the nurse is not sure that she is able to follow his wishes. The nurse should:
   1. ignore the advance directive.
   2. call the patient's lawyer.
   3. discuss it with the interdisciplinary team and the organization's ethics committee.
   4. follow the directive even though the nurse is uncomfortable with the directions.

9. The patient is complaining of constipation. He has had very little food intake the past 4 days. The nurse should:

1. tell his wife to stop all food and water.
2. assess for bowel sounds, abdominal distention, and possible impaction.
3. tell him that due to his decreased intake, he will have very little stool.
4. tell him to bear down to assist in elimination of his stool.

10. The patient is complaining of pain at a 5 on a pain scale of 0 to 10. The nurse should:

1. assume that since the pain is a 5, no further treatment is necessary or no changes are appropriate.
2. ask the patient what he wants his pain goal to be; if it is below 5, then you will have to notify the physician.
3. explain that the patient needs to try to tolerate a pain rating 5 or less.
4. automatically give the patient an additional analgesic.

11. The ___________ is the mediator between the hospice team and the attending physician.

12. ___________ is considered the fifth vital sign and is important to assess with every hospice visit.

13. The patient is in the terminal stage of life. His wife, the caregiver, asks the nurse if it is still appropriate to turn the patient every 2 hours even though it causes the patient discomfort and stimulates restlessness. The nurse should:

1. reply, "You should always reposition the patient every 2 hours no matter what."
2. reply, "Yes, you do not want the patient to develop pressure ulcers."
3. educate the wife that her husband is actively dying and she does not have to position the patient unless he appears uncomfortable and a change of position would make him feel better.
4. None of the above.

14. The patient has never attended church and on admission requested no spiritual support. Now he is within days of death and voiced some spiritual concerns to the nurse. The nurse should:

1. share personal spiritual beliefs with him.
2. tell him that it is too late and no church would accept him.
3. report to the interdisciplinary team and have the spiritual coordinator make a home visit.
4. report information to the social worker.

15. The patient died peacefully and with dignity, but his wife is still having problems dealing with the death. The hospice program has:

1. continued bereavement support for her for the next year.
2. dismissed the wife from all hospice services.
3. told her to be grateful he died a peaceful death and get on with her life.
4. had the hospice aide continue with her visits to the home.

16. For the patient to qualify for assistance from Medicare or Medicaid for hospice care, which criteria are necessary? *(Select all that apply.)*

1. Physicians state the patient has less than 6 months to live.
2. The patient is receiving chemotherapy or radiation.
3. Two physicians verify the patient is dying.
4. The patient has less than 1 year to live.

17. The bereavement coordinator on the hospice team follows a plan of care for the bereaved caregiver for what length of time following the death of the patient?

1. 3 to 4 months
2. 9 to 10 months
3. At least 1 year
4. 3 years

18. What is included in the definition of palliative care according to the World Health Organization? *(Select all that apply.)*

1. Focusing on controlling pain and other symptoms as well as reducing psychological, social, and spiritual distress for the patient and the family
2. The active total care of patients whose disease is not responsive to curative treatment
3. The framework for hospice care
4. The active total care of patients by providing treatments to assist in improving patient prognosis

Introduction to Anatomy and Physiology

chapter 41

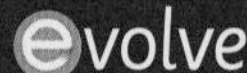

Barbara Lauritsen Christensen and M. Christine Neff

http://evolve.elsevier.com/Christensen/foundationsadult

Objectives

1. Define the difference between anatomy and physiology.
2. Define the term *anatomical position.*
3. List and define the principal directional terms and sections (planes) used in describing the body and the relationship of body parts to one another.
4. Use each word in a given list of anatomical terms in a sentence.
5. List the nine abdominopelvic regions and the abdominopelvic quadrants.
6. List and discuss in order of increasing complexity the levels of organization of the body.
7. Differentiate among tissues, organs, and systems.
8. Identify and define three major components of the cell.
9. Discuss the stages of mitosis and explain the importance of cellular reproduction.
10. Differentiate between active and passive transport processes that move substances through cell membranes, and give two examples of each.
11. Describe the four types of body tissues.
12. Discuss the two types of epithelial membranes.
13. List the 11 major organ systems of the body and briefly describe the major functions of each.

Key Terms

active transport (p. 1244)
anatomy (p. 1237)
cell (p. 1240)
cytoplasm (CĪ-tō-plăzm, p. 1242)
diffusion (dĭ-FŪ-zhŭn, p. 1245)
dorsal (p. 1237)
filtration (p. 1245)
homeostasis (hō-mē-ō-STĀ-sĭs, p. 1241)
membrane (p. 1248)
mitosis (mī-TŌ-sĭs, p. 1243)
nucleus (p. 1242)
organ (pp. 1241, 1248)
osmosis (ŏz-MŌ-sĭs, p. 1245)
passive transport (p. 1245)
phagocytosis (făg-ō-sī-TŌ-sĭs, p. 1244)
physiology (fĭz-ē-ŎL-ō-jē, p. 1237)
pinocytosis (pī-nō-sī-TŌ-sĭs, p. 1244)
system (p. 1241)
tissue (p. 1241)
ventral (p. 1237)

Caring for a person with a disease process requires an understanding of the normal functioning of the human body, so the nurse must know basic human anatomy and physiology. **Anatomy** is the study, classification, and description of structures and organs of the body. **Physiology** explains the processes and functions of the various structures and how they interrelate. The normal, healthy human body is like a finely tuned machine, with each part performing a special function to accomplish a goal. As with the machine, when the body malfunctions, the repairer must understand how it works. Without the necessary repairs to return the body to homeostasis, illness, disease, or death may result.

ANATOMICAL TERMINOLOGY

Study of the human body first requires one to master certain terms that aid in locating specific structures. To understand the following terms, consider the body in a normal anatomical position, that is, standing erect with the face and palms facing forward (Figure 41-1):

Anterior (or **ventral**): To face forward; the front of the body. The chest is located anterior to the spine (Figure 41-2).
Posterior (or **dorsal**): Toward the back. The kidneys are posterior to the peritoneum.
Cranial: Toward the head. The brain is located in the cranial portion of the body.
Caudal: Toward the "tail"; the distal portion of the spine. A caudal anesthetic may be given.
Superior: Toward the head or above. The neck is superior to the shoulders.
Inferior: Lower, toward the feet, or below another. The foot is inferior to the ankle.
Medial: Toward the midline. The sternum (breastbone) is located in the medial portion of the chest.

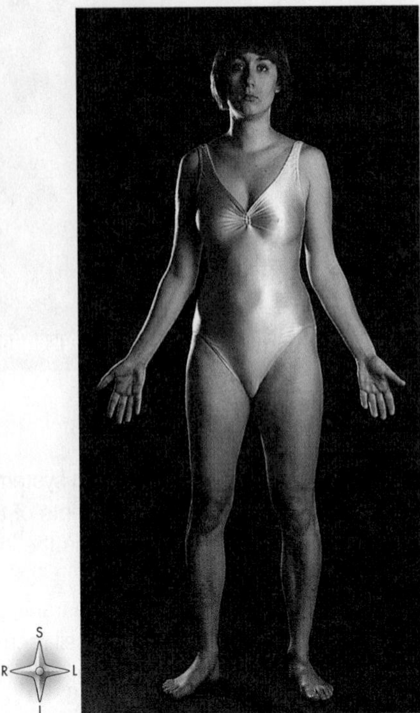

FIGURE 41-1 Anatomical position. The body is in an erect or standing posture with the arms at the sides and palms forward. The head and feet also point forward. The right and left sides of the body are mirror images of each other.

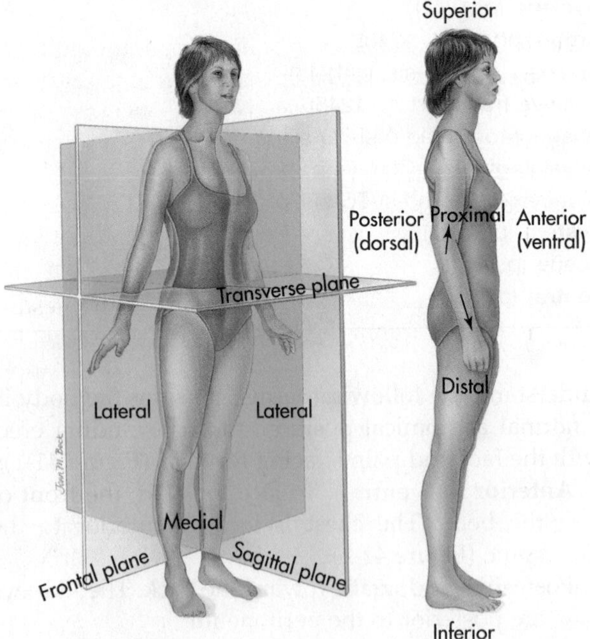

FIGURE 41-2 Directions and planes of the body.

Lateral: Toward the side. The outer area of the leg, the area located on the side, is called lateral.

Proximal: Nearest the origin of the structure; nearest the trunk. The elbow is proximal to the forearm.

Distal: Farthest from the origin of the structure; farthest from the trunk. The fingers are distal to the hand.

Superficial: Nearer the surface. The skin of the arm is superficial to the muscles below it.

Deep: Farther away from the body surface. The bone of the upper arm is deep to the muscles that surround and cover it.

BODY PLANES

To make it easier to study individual organs or the body as a whole, divide the body into three imaginary planes: the sagittal, the coronal (frontal), and the transverse (see Figure 41-2):

1. The **sagittal** plane runs lengthwise from the front to the back. A sagittal cut gives a right and a left portion of the body. A midsagittal cut gives two equal halves.
2. The **coronal** (frontal) plane divides the body into a ventral (front) section and a dorsal (back) section.
3. The **transverse** plane cuts the body horizontal to the sagittal and frontal planes, dividing the body into caudal and cranial portions.

BODY CAVITIES

From the outside, the body appears to be a solid structure, but it is not. It is made up of open spaces, or cavities, that contain compact, well-ordered arrangements of internal organs. The body has two major cavities that are, in turn, subdivided and contain compact, well-ordered arrangements of internal organs. The two major cavities are the ventral and the dorsal body cavities (Figure 41-3 and Table 41-1).

Ventral Cavity

The ventral cavity consists of the **thoracic** (or chest) cavity and the **abdominopelvic cavity** (see Figure 41-3), which are separated by the diaphragm (a muscle directly beneath the lungs).

The thoracic cavity contains the heart and the lungs. Its midportion is a subdivision of the thoracic cavity, the mediastinum, which contains the trachea, the heart, and the blood vessels. Its other subdivisions are the right and left pleural cavities, which contain the lungs.

The abdominal cavity contains the stomach, the liver, the gallbladder, the spleen, the pancreas, the small intestine, and parts of the large intestine. A subdivision called the **pelvic cavity** contains the lower portion of the large intestine (lower sigmoid colon, rectum), the urinary bladder, and the internal structures of the reproductive system. The abdominal and pelvic cavities are not separated by any structure and therefore are referred to as the abdominopelvic cavity (see Table 41-1).

Dorsal Cavity

The dorsal cavity is composed of the cranial and spinal body cavities. The cranial body cavity houses the brain, whereas the spinal cavity contains the spinal cord. The dorsal body cavity is smaller than the ventral cavity (see Table 41-1).

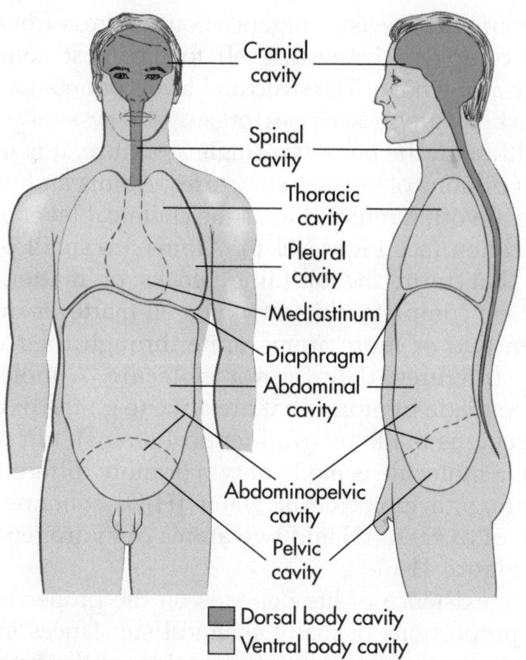

FIGURE 41-3 Location and subdivisions of the dorsal and ventral body cavities as viewed from the front (anterior) and the side (lateral).

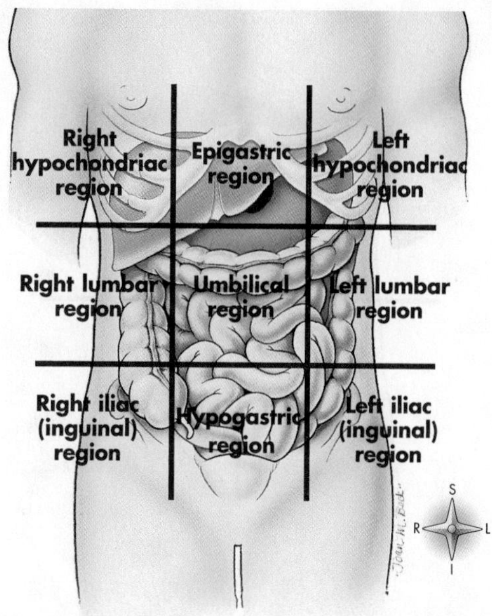

FIGURE 41-4 The nine regions of the abdominopelvic cavity. The most superficial organs are shown. Can you identify the deeper structures in each region?

Table 41-1 Body Cavities

BODY CAVITY	ORGAN(S)
VENTRAL BODY CAVITY	
Thoracic Cavity	
Mediastinum	Trachea, heart, blood vessels
Pleural cavities	Lungs
Abdominopelvic Cavity	
Abdominal cavity	Liver, gallbladder, stomach, spleen, pancreas, small intestine, parts of large intestine
Pelvic cavity	Lower (sigmoid) colon, rectum, urinary bladder, reproductive organs
DORSAL BODY CAVITY	
Cranial cavity	Brain
Spinal cavity	Spinal cord

ABDOMINAL REGIONS

For convenience in locating abdominal organs, anatomists divide the abdomen into nine imaginary regions. The nine regions (Figure 41-4), identified from right to left and from top to bottom, are the following:

1. Right hypochondriac region
2. Epigastric region
3. Left hypochondriac region
4. Right lumbar region
5. Umbilical region
6. Left lumbar region
7. Right iliac (inguinal) region
8. Hypogastric region
9. Left iliac (inguinal) region

The most superficial organs located in each of the nine abdominal regions are shown in Figure 41-4. The visible organs in each region are as follows: (1) right hypochondriac region, the right lobe of the liver and the gallbladder; (2) epigastric region, parts of the right and left lobes of the liver and a large portion of the stomach; (3) left hypochondriac region, a small portion of the stomach and large intestine; (4) right lumbar region, parts of the large and small intestine; (5) umbilical region, a portion of the transverse colon and loops of the small intestine; (6) left lumbar region, additional loops of the small intestine and a part of the colon; (7) right iliac region, the cecum and parts of the small intestine; (8) hypogastric region, loops of the small intestine, the urinary bladder, and the appendix; and (9) left iliac region, portions of the colon and the small intestine.

ABDOMINOPELVIC QUADRANTS

Health professionals frequently divide the abdomen into four quadrants to describe the site of abdominopelvic pain or locate an internal pathologic condition such as a tumor or abscess (Figure 41-5). Horizontal and vertical lines passing through the umbilicus (navel) divide the abdomen into **right** and **left upper quadrants** and **right** and **left lower quadrants.**

STRUCTURAL LEVELS OF ORGANIZATION

Before studying the structure and function of the human body and its many parts, think about how those parts are organized and how they might fit together into a functioning whole. Figure 41-6 illustrates the different levels of organization that influence body structure and

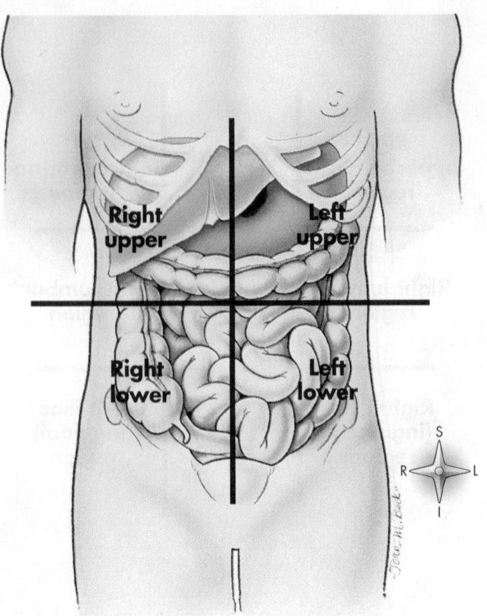

FIGURE 41-5 Horizontal and vertical line passing through the umbilicus (navel) divides the abdomen into right and left upper quadrants and right and left lower quadrants.

function. The levels of organization progress from the least complex (chemical level) to the most complex (body as a whole). The structural levels of organization in the body are cells, tissues, organs, and systems.

Although the body is a single structure, it is made up of billions of smaller structures. Atoms and molecules are often referred to as the chemical level of organization (see Figure 41-6). **Atoms** are small particles that form the building blocks of matter, the smallest complete units of which all matter is made. When two or more atoms unite through their electron structures, they form a **molecule.** A molecule can be made of atoms that are alike (e.g., the oxygen molecule is made of two identical atoms), but more often a molecule is made of two or more different atoms (e.g., a molecule of water [H_2O] contains one atom of oxygen [O] and two atoms of hydrogen [H]) (see Figure 41-6).

The existence of life depends on the proper levels and proportions of many chemical substances in the cytoplasm of cells. **Cells** are considered the smallest living units of structure and function in our body. Al-

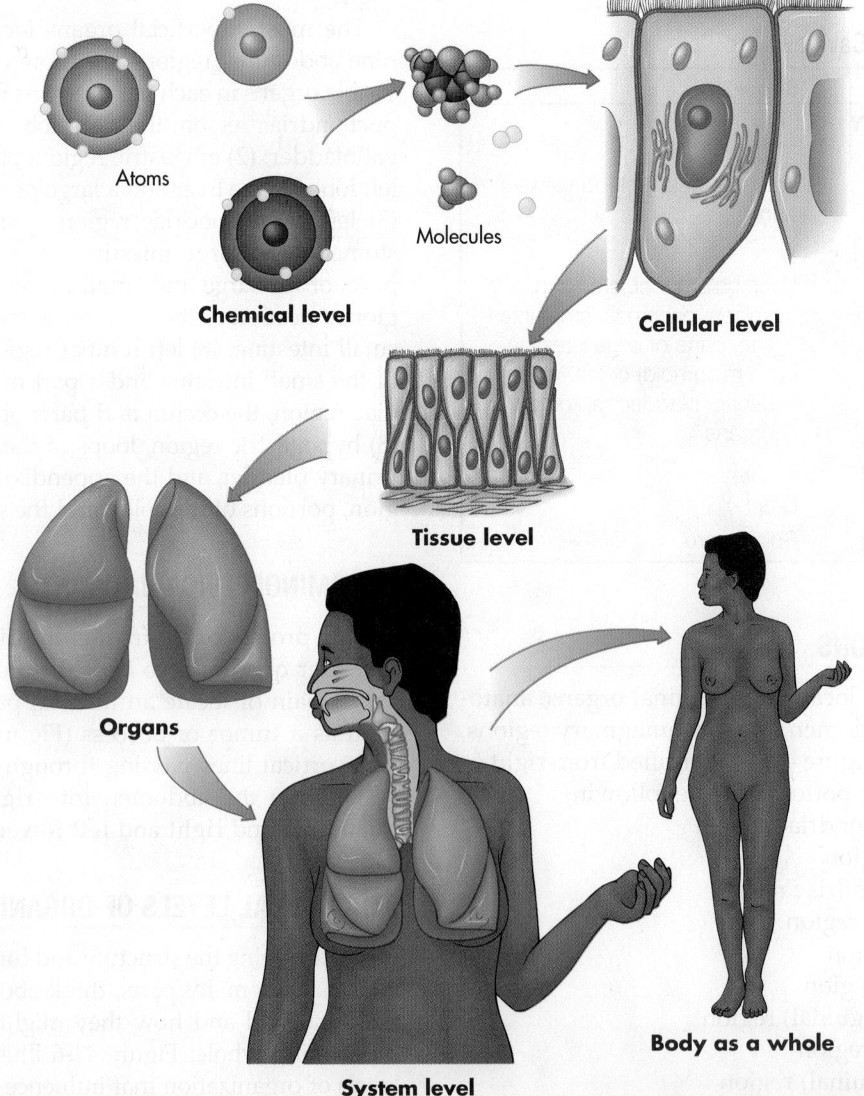

FIGURE 41-6 Structural levels of organization in the body.

though considered the simplest units of living matter, cells are far from simple; they are extremely complex.

Tissues are even more complex than cells. By definition a **tissue** is an organization of many similar cells that act together to perform a common function. Cells are held together and surrounded by varying amounts and types of gluelike, nonliving intercellular substances.

Organs are more complex than tissues. An **organ** is a group of several different kinds of tissues arranged to perform a special function. The lungs shown in Figure 41-6 are an example of organization at the organ level.

Systems are the most complex units that make up the body. A **system** is an organization of varying numbers and kinds of organs arranged to perform complex functions for the body. The organs of the respiratory system shown in Figure 41-6 permit air to enter the body and travel to the lungs, where oxygen and carbon dioxide are exchanged. Organs of the respiratory system include the nose, the windpipe (or trachea), and the complex series of bronchial tubes that permit passage of air into the lungs.

CELLS

Almost 350 years ago Robert Hooke discovered the first cell while examining plant fragments under the microscope. The structures reminded him of tiny, individual miniature prison cells, so he coined the term *cell* (the fundamental unit of all living tissue) (Figure 41-7). Many living things are so simple that they consist of just one cell. The human body, however, is so complex that it has trillions of these tiny powerhouses of life.

All cells are microscopic but differ widely in size and shape. Despite their differences, all cells exhibit five unique characteristics of life: growth, metabolism, responsiveness, reproduction, and homeostasis. **Homeostasis** is when the body's internal environment is relatively constant; this state is naturally maintained by adaptive responses that promote healthy survival.

Structural Parts of Cells

The three main parts of a cell are the plasma membrane, the cytoplasm, and the nucleus (see Figure 41-7).

Plasma Membrane

The plasma membrane encloses the cytoplasm and forms the outer boundary of the cell. It is an incredibly delicate structure—only about 7 nm (nanometers), or 3/10,000,000 inch, thick! Yet it has a precise, orderly structure.

Even though it seems fragile, the plasma membrane is strong enough to keep the cell whole and intact. It also performs other life-preserving functions for the cell, serving as a gateway between the fluid inside the cell and the fluid around it. The plasma membrane is **selectively permeable.** This means the membrane permits certain substances to enter and leave while not allowing other substances to cross. This membrane separates the cell contents from the dilute saltwater solution called interstitial fluid, or simply tissue fluid, which bathes every cell in the body. The plasma membrane also has distinct surface proteins that identify a cell as coming from one particular individual. This fact is the basis of **tissue typing,** a procedure performed before an organ from one person is transplanted into another. Carbohydrate chains attached to the surface of cells often help identify cell types.

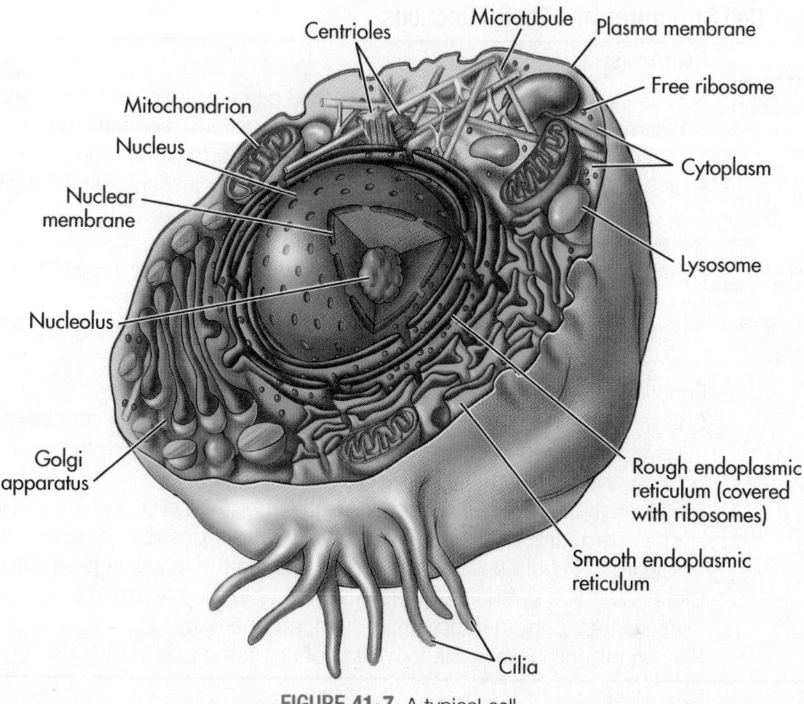

FIGURE 41-7 A typical cell.

Cytoplasm

Cytoplasm is the internal living material of cells. Cytoplasm (protoplasm) is a sticky, fluidlike substance that lies between the plasma membrane and the nucleus of the cell. Numerous organelles (tiny functioning structures) are located within the cytoplasm. Cells contain cytoplasm, or "living matter," a substance that exists only in cells. Cytoplasm is composed largely of a gel-like substance that contains water, food, minerals, enzymes, and other specialized materials. The term *cyto-* is a combining form from the Greek and denotes a relationship to a cell. These organelles were not discovered until the development of the powerful electron microscope.

Cytoplasm is composed of 70% water with traces of proteins, lipids, carbohydrates, minerals, and salts. (Table 41-2 lists major cell structures and their functions.)

Nucleus

The **nucleus** is the largest organelle within the cell. It is responsible for cell reproduction and control of the other organelles. The nucleus is surrounded by the nuclear membrane. It contains nucleoplasm, a refined form of cytoplasm. The nucleus contains two specialized structures: the nucleolus and the chromatin granules. The nucleolus is critical in the formation of protein. The chromatin granules are composed of protein and deoxyribonucleic acid (DNA). DNA contains the genetic code, or blueprint, of the body.

Endoplasmic Reticulum

Throughout the cytoplasm lies a system of membranes, or canals, called the endoplasmic reticulum (ER). ER functions as a miniature circulating system for the cell by carrying substances from one part of the cell to another. There are two types of ER: (1) smooth, which is found in cells that deal with fatty substances; and (2) rough, which is found in cells that manufacture proteins.

Ribosomes

Ribosomes are tiny structures floating free in the cytoplasm or attached to the rough ER. They are called **protein factories** because they produce enzymes and other proteins.

Mitochondria

The mitochondria are the powerhouses of the cells. They are bean shaped with a folded interior membrane. They take food and convert it to a complex energy form, adenosine triphosphate (ATP), for use by the cell. ATP is described as the "energy currency" of the cells because it supplies the energy for all activities.

Lysosomes

Lysosomes are small saclike structures containing enzymes that digest food compounds and microbes that have invaded the cell.

Golgi Apparatus

The Golgi apparatus is usually located near the nucleus. It is the "packaging plant" of the cell. It packages certain carbohydrate and protein compounds into globules. Then it moves outward through the cell membrane, where it breaks open and releases its contents.

Centrioles

The centrioles are paired, rod-shaped organelles. During cell division (mitosis) they aid in the formation of the spindle, a structure necessary for cell reproduction.

Table 41-2 Some Major Cell Structures and Their Functions

CELL STRUCTURE	FUNCTION(S)
Plasma membrane	Serves as the cell's boundary; protein and carbohydrate molecules on outer surface of plasma membrane perform various functions (e.g., serve as markers that identify cells of each individual or as receptor molecules for certain hormones)
Endoplasmic reticulum (ER)	Ribosomes attach to rough ER to synthesize proteins; smooth ER synthesizes lipids and certain carbohydrates
Ribosomes	Synthesize proteins; the cell's "protein factories"
Mitochondria	Synthesize adenosine triphosphate (ATP); the cell's "powerhouses"
Lysosomes	Serve as cell's "digestive system"
Golgi apparatus	Synthesizes carbohydrate, combines it with protein, and packages the product as globules of glycoprotein
Centrioles	Function in cell reproduction
Cilia	Short, hairlike extensions on the free surfaces of some cells capable of movement; often have specialized functions such as propelling mucus upward over cells that line the respiratory tract
Flagella	Single projections of cell surfaces, much larger than cilia; an example in humans is the "tail" of a sperm cell; propulsive movement makes it possible for sperm to "swim" or move toward the ovum once they are deposited in the female reproductive tract
Nucleus	Dictates protein synthesis, thereby playing an essential role in other cell activities, namely, active transport, metabolism, growth, and heredity
Nucleoli	Play an essential role in the formation of ribosomes

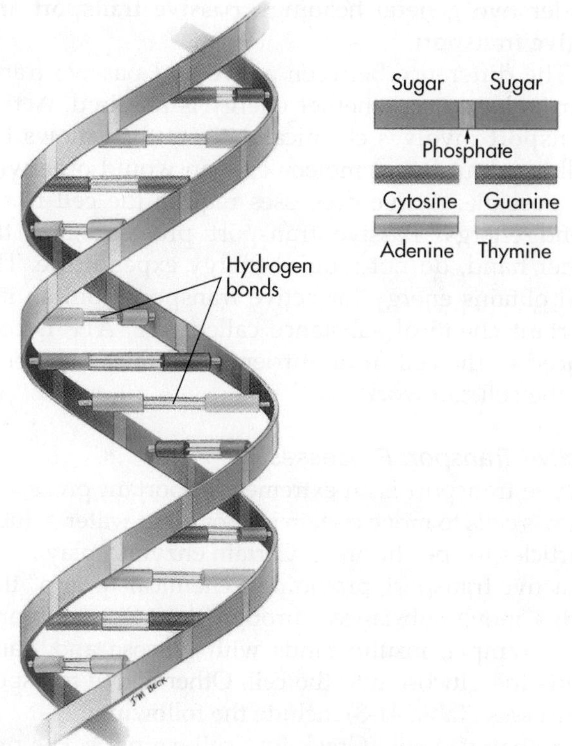

FIGURE 41-8 Deoxyribonucleic acid (DNA) molecule. Note that each side of the DNA molecule consists of alternating sugar and phosphate groups. Each sugar group is united to the sugar group opposite it by a pair of nitrogenous bases (adenine-thymine or cytosine-guanine). The sequence of these pairs constitutes a genetic code that determines the structure and function of a cell.

Protein Synthesis

Protein is a vital component of every cell in the body. Protein production relies on nucleic acids in the cell's cytoplasm and nucleus. Two important nucleic acids are (1) DNA (Figure 41-8), which is located in the nucleus; and (2) ribonucleic acid (RNA), which is located in the cytoplasm. The DNA encodes the message for protein synthesis and sends it to the RNA, which transports it to the ribosomes, where the protein is produced. Hence DNA is called the **chemical blueprint**, and RNA is called the **chemical messenger.**

Cell Division

All cells in the body, except sex cells, reproduce by **mitosis.** This is a type of somatic (pertaining to nonreproductive cells) cell division in which the original cell divides to form two daughters. Each daughter cell has the same characteristics (including both the nucleus and cytoplasm) as the original cell. Each daughter cell contains the same number of chromosomes as the parent cell. Each chromosome in the daughter cells contains the complete genetic information of the original chromosome because of duplication of the DNA molecule during interphase (Figure 41-9).

The chromosomes (spindle-shaped rods) in the cell's nucleus carry the genes that are responsible for the organism's traits, including such hereditary factors as hair and eye color. These chromosomes are composed of DNA. Each body cell in humans contains

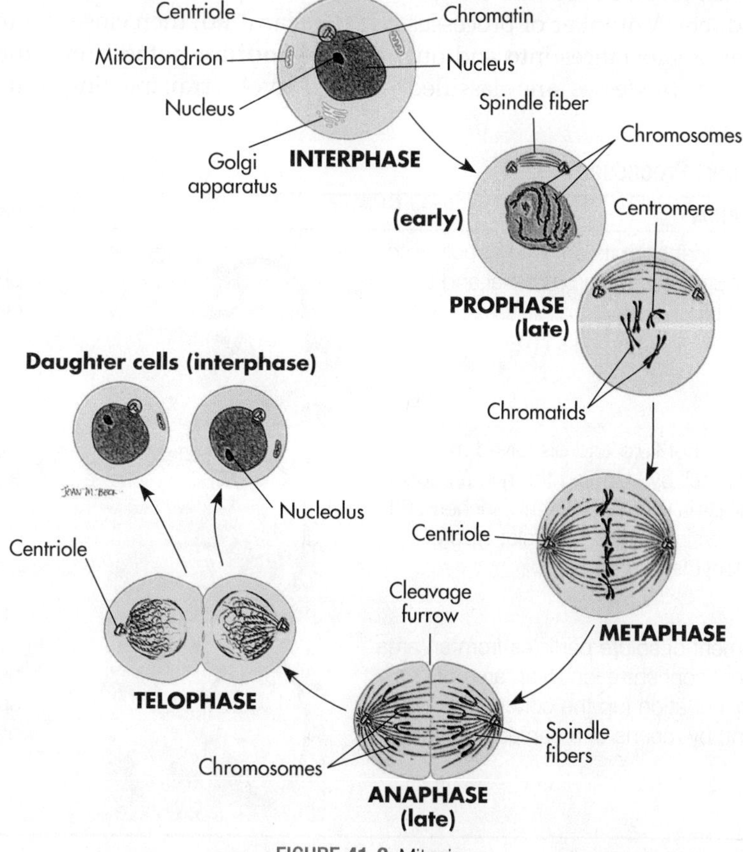

FIGURE 41-9 Mitosis.

46 chromosomes, which exist in pairs. At the time of fertilization, one member of each pair is received from the father and one is received from the mother. These paired chromosomes, except for the pair that determines sex, are alike in size and appearance and carry genes for the same traits.

During mitosis the cell goes through four phases: prophase, metaphase, anaphase, and telophase.

Prophase

In the nucleus the chromosomes form two strands called **chromatids.** In the cytoplasm the centrioles form a network of spindle fibers.

Metaphase

The nuclear membrane and nucleolus disappear, and the chromosomes are aligned across the center of the cell. The centrioles are at the opposite ends of the cell, and spindle fibers are attached to each chromatid.

Anaphase

The chromosomes are pulled to the opposite ends of the cell, and cell division begins.

Telophase

During this final phase of cell division, the two nuclei appear and the chromosomes disperse. At the end of the phase, two new daughter cells appear.

Movement of Materials Across Cell Membranes

For a cell to survive, it must receive food and oxygen and secrete its waste products. A number of processes allow for mass movement of substances into and out of the cells. These transport processes are classified under two general headings: **passive transport** and **active transport.**

The difference between active and passive transport is based on whether energy is required. **Active transport** involves chemical activity that allows the cell to admit larger molecules than would otherwise be possible. Active processes require the cell to expend energy. Passive transport processes, on the other hand, do not require energy expenditure. The cell obtains energy for active transport from an important chemical substance called ATP. ATP is produced in the cell from nutrients and releases energy so the cell can work.

Active Transport Processes

Active transport is an extremely important process. It allows cells to move certain ions or other water-soluble particles to specific areas. Certain enzymes play a role in active transport, providing a chemical "pump" that helps move substances through the cell membrane. For example, insulin binds with glucose and transports the glucose into the cell. Other active transport processes (Table 41-3) include the following:

- **Phagocytosis** (Greek for "cell-eating"): The process that permits a cell to engulf (or surround) any foreign material and to digest it. The white blood cells in the human body often perform this function.
- **Pinocytosis:** The process by which extracellular fluid is taken into the cell. The cell membrane develops a saclike indentation filled with extracellular fluid, then closes around it and digests it.
- **Sodium-potassium pump:** The process of actively transporting sodium ions (Na^+) out of

Table 41-3 Active Transport Processes

PROCESS	DESCRIPTION		EXAMPLES
Phagocytosis	Process that permits a cell to engulf or to surround any foreign material and to digest it		Trapping of bacterial cells by phagocytic white blood cells
Pinocytosis	Movement of fluid and dissolved molecules into a cell by trapping them in a section of plasma membrane that pinches off to form an intracellular vesicle; type of endocytosis		Trapping of large protein molecules by some body cell
Calcium pump	Movement of solute particles from an area of low concentration to an area of high concentration (up the concentration gradient) by means of a carrier molecule	ATP	In muscle cells, pumping of nearly all calcium ions to special compartments or out of the cell

Modified from Thibodeau, G.A., & Patton, K.T. (2007). *Anatomy and physiology* (6th ed.). St. Louis: Mosby.

ATP, Adenosine triphosphate. The energy required for active transport processes is obtained from ATP. ATP is in all active transport processes.

cells and potassium ions (K^+) into cells. The sodium-potassium pump maintains a lower sodium concentration in intracellular fluid than in the surrounding extracellular fluid. At the same time, this pump maintains a higher potassium concentration in the intracellular fluid than in the surrounding extracellular fluid. This active transport pump operates in the plasma membrane of all human cells and is essential for healthy cell survival.

- **Calcium pump:** Active calcium carriers in the membranes of muscle cells (for example) that allow the cell to force nearly all of the intracellular calcium ions (Ca^{++}) into special compartments or out of the cell entirely. This is important because a muscle cell cannot operate properly unless the intracellular Ca^{++} concentration is kept low during rest.

Active transport processes require cellular energy to move substances from a low concentration to a high concentration. In contrast, **passive transport** processes—the movement of small molecules across the membrane of a cell by diffusion—do not require cellular energy and move substances from a high concentration to a lower concentration.

Passive Transport Processes

The primary passive transport processes (Table 41-4) include the following:

- **Diffusion:** A process in which solid particles in a fluid move from an area of higher concentration to an area of lower concentration, resulting in an even distribution of the particles in the fluid (Figure 41-10).

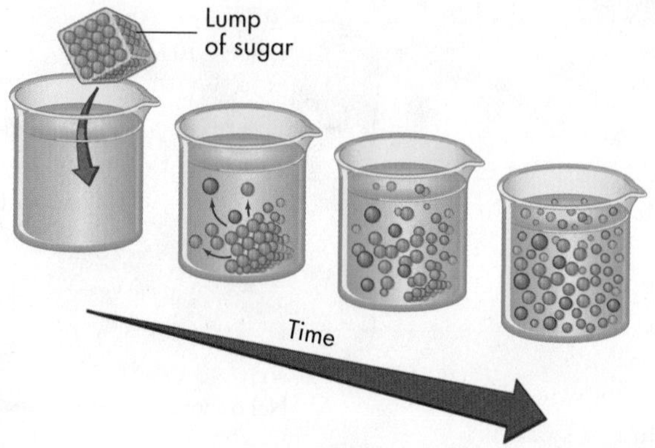

FIGURE 41-10 Diffusion. The molecules of a lump of sugar are very densely packed when they enter the water. As sugar molecules collide frequently in the area of high concentration, they gradually spread away from each other toward the area of lower concentration. Eventually the sugar molecules are evenly distributed.

- **Osmosis:** The passage of water across a selectively permeable membrane, with the water molecules going from the less concentrated solution to the more concentrated solution (Figure 41-11).
- **Filtration:** The movement of water and particles through a membrane by force from either pressure or gravity. This membrane contains spaces that allow liquid to pass but are too small to be permeated by solid particles. Movement is from areas of greater pressure to areas of lesser pressure.

TISSUES

Tissues are groups of similar cells that work together to perform a specific function. The body and its organs are composed of the following four main types of tissues (Table 41-5).

Table 41-4 Passive Transport Processes

PROCESS	DESCRIPTION	EXAMPLES
Simple diffusion	Movement of particles through phospholipid bilayer or through channels from an area of high concentration to an area of low concentration—that is, down the concentration gradient	Movement of carbon dioxide out of all cells; movement of sodium ions into nerve cells as they conduct an impulse
Filtration	Movement of water and particles through a membrane by force from either pressure or gravity; membrane contains spaces that allow liquid to pass but are too small to be permeated by solid material; movement from areas of greater pressure to areas of lesser pressure	During procedure called peritoneal dialysis, small solutes diffuse from blood vessels but blood proteins do not (thus removing only small solutes from the blood)
Osmosis	Passage of water across a selectively permeable membrane; water molecules move from a less concentrated solution to a more concentrated solution	Diffusion of water molecules into and out of cells to correct imbalances in water concentration

Modified from Thibodeau, G.A., & Patton, K.T. (2007). *Anatomy and physiology* (6th ed.). St. Louis: Mosby.

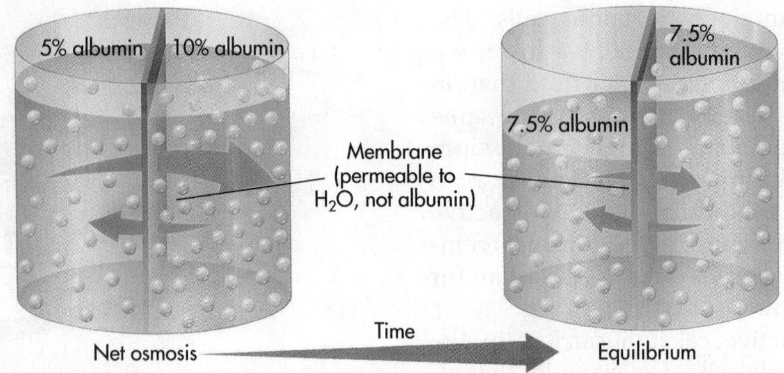

FIGURE 41-11 Osmosis. Osmosis is the diffusion of water through a selectively permeable membrane. The membrane shown in this diagram is permeable to water but not to albumin. Because there are relatively more water molecules in 5% albumin than in 10% albumin, more water molecules osmose from the more dilute into the more concentrated solution (as indicated by the *large arrow* in the diagram on the left) than osmose in the opposite direction. The overall direction of osmosis, in other words, is toward the more concentrated solution. Movement across the membrane continues until the concentrations of the solutions equalize.

Table 41-5 Tissues

TISSUE	LOCATION	FUNCTION
EPITHELIAL		
Simple squamous	Alveoli of lungs	Absorption by diffusion of respiratory gases between alveolar air and blood
	Lining of blood and lymphatic vessels	Absorption by diffusion, filtration, and osmosis
Stratified squamous	Surface of lining of mouth and esophagus	Protection
	Surface of skin (epidermis)	Protection
Simple columnar	Surface layer of lining of stomach, intestines, and parts of respiratory tract	Protection; secretion; absorption
Stratified transitional	Urinary bladder	Protection
CONNECTIVE*		
Areolar	Between other tissues and organs	Connection
Adipose (fat)	Under skin	Protection
	Padding at various points	Insulation; support; reserve food
Dense fibrous	Tendons; ligaments	Flexible but strong connection
Bone	Skeleton	Support; protection
Cartilage	Part of nasal septum; covering articular surfaces of bones; larynx; rings in trachea and bronchi	Firm but flexible support
	Disks between vertebrae	
	External ear	
Blood	Blood vessels	Transportation
Hematopoietic	Liquid matrix with dense arrangement of blood cell–producing cells located in red bone marrow	Blood cell formation
MUSCLE		
Skeletal (striated voluntary); see Figure 41-12, *A*	Muscles that attach to bones	Maintenance of posture, movement of bones
	Eyeball muscles	Eye movements
	Upper third of esophagus	First part of swallowing
Cardiac (striated involuntary); see Figure 41-12, *B*	Wall of heart	Contraction of heart
Smooth (nonstriated involuntary or visceral); see Figure 41-12, *C*	In walls of tubular viscera of digestive, respiratory, and genitourinary tracts	Movement of substances along respective tracts
	In walls of blood vessels and large lymphatic vessels	Changing diameter of blood vessels
	In ducts of glands	Movement of substances along ducts
	Intrinsic eye muscles (iris and ciliary body)	Changing diameter of pupils and shape of lens
	Arrector of muscles of hairs	Erection of hairs (gooseflesh)
NERVOUS	Brain; spinal cord; nerves	Irritability; conduction

*Connective tissues are the most widely distributed of all tissues.

1. Epithelial tissue
2. Connective tissue
3. Muscle tissue
4. Nervous tissue

Epithelial Tissue

Epithelial cells are packed closely together and contain no blood vessels. Epithelial tissue covers the outside of the body and some of the internal structures. The four types of epithelial tissue are (1) simple squamous, (2) stratified squamous, (3) simple columnar, and (4) stratified transitional (see Table 41-5).

Epithelial tissue serves several important functions in the body, including the following:

- **Protection:** Covering the body and many of its organs, it serves as a protective barrier against invasion.
- **Absorption:** Certain specialized epithelial cells can absorb material in the body (e.g., the lining of the small intestine can absorb digested nutrients).
- **Secretion:** Mucus is secreted in areas such as the respiratory and digestive tracts.

Connective Tissue

As the name suggests, connective tissue "connects," or joins, tissues or structures of the body, and it also supports and protects them. Connective tissue is the most abundant and widely distributed tissue in the body. It exists in varying forms: thin and delicate, tough and cordlike, or liquid (blood). Mast cells, plasma cells, and white blood cells are found in connective tissue; red blood cells are not unless blood vessels have been injured. Unlike the closely packed epithelial tissue, the connective tissue cells are spaced out and surrounded by intercellular fluid, which is composed of protein complexes and tissue fluid.

Some of the most important forms of connective tissue are **areolar** connective tissue, **adipose** (fat) tissue, **fibrous** connective tissue, **bone, cartilage, blood,** and **hematopoietic** tissue (see Table 41-5).

Muscle Tissue

Muscle tissue is composed of cells that contract in response to a message from the brain or the spinal cord. The three types of muscle cells are (1) **skeletal** (striated, voluntary), (2) **cardiac** (striated, involuntary), and (3) **visceral** (smooth, involuntary) (Figure 41-12).

Skeletal muscle cells are striated (have a striped appearance) and attach to bones to produce voluntary movement. Skeletal muscle is also known as **voluntary muscle** because a person has voluntary control over skeletal muscle contractions (see Figure 41-12, *A*).

Cardiac muscle cells are striated with fibers that branch to form many networks, or webs. These networks are found only in the walls of the heart, and the regular contractions of cardiac muscle produce the heartbeat. Generally, cardiac muscle cells are involuntary, that is, a person cannot contract them at will (see Figure 41-2, *B*).

Smooth (visceral) muscle cells are nonstriated and appear in the viscera, or internal organs, such as the walls of blood vessels, the stomach, the intestines, and the uterus. Contractions of smooth muscle propel food and fluid through the digestive tract and help regulate the diameter of blood vessels. Contraction of smooth muscle in the tubes of the respiratory system, such as the bronchioles in the lungs, can impair breathing and result in asthma attacks and labored respiration. Generally, smooth muscles are involuntary, but some control can be exerted through the use of biofeedback techniques (see Figure 41-12, *C*).

Nervous Tissue

Nervous tissue allows rapid communication between the brain or spinal cord body structures and control of body functions. Nervous tissue is composed of two

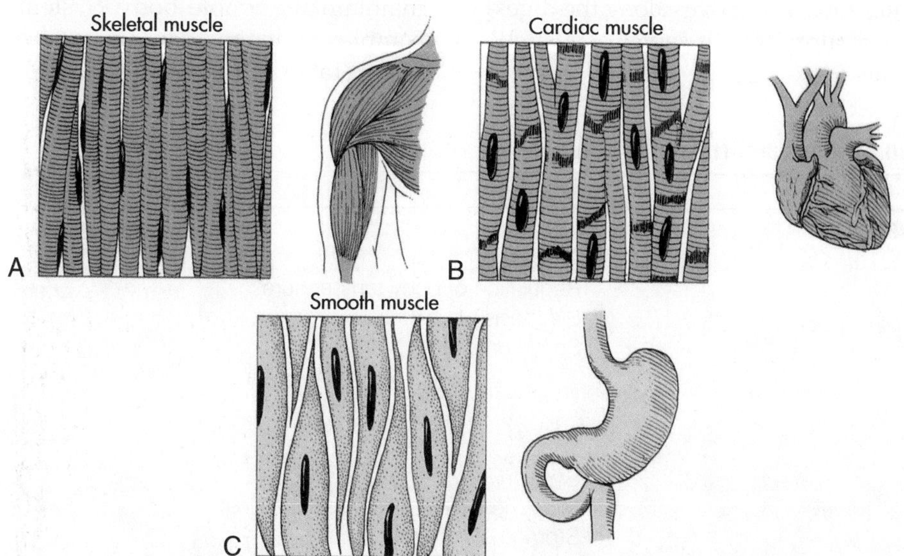

FIGURE 41-12 Types of muscles. **A,** Skeletal muscle. **B,** Cardiac muscle. **C,** Smooth muscle.

types of cells: neurons and glial cells. The neurons are the nerve cells and transmit impulses or messages. They are the system's functional or conducting units. The glial cells are connecting and supporting cells; they support and nourish the neurons.

Neurons have three parts: (1) dendrites, which carry impulses toward the cell body; (2) cell body; and (3) axons, which carry impulses away from the cell body (see Chapter 54, Figure 54-1).

MEMBRANES

Membranes are thin sheets of tissue that serve many functions in the body. They cover body surfaces, line and lubricate hollow organs, and protect and anchor organs and bones. The two major types of membranes are epithelial and connective tissue membranes.

Epithelial Membranes

Epithelial membranes are usually composed of a thin layer of epithelial cells with an underlying layer of connective tissue for strength. Epithelial membranes are divided into two subgroups: mucous membranes and serous membranes.

Mucous Membranes

Mucous membranes secrete **mucus** (a thick, slippery material), which keeps the membranes moist and soft and protects against bacterial invasion. Mucous membranes line the body surfaces that open to the outside environment. Examples include the nose; the mouth; and urinary, respiratory, gastrointestinal, and reproductive tracts. The type of epithelium in the mucous membrane varies, depending on its location and function. The esophagus, for example, contains a tough, abrasion-resistant, stratified squamous epithelium. A thin layer of simple columnar epithelium covers the walls of the lower segments of the digestive tract.

In addition to protection, the mucus produced by mucous membranes also serves other purposes. For example, it lubricates food as it moves along the digestive tract. In the respiratory tract it serves as a sticky trap for contaminants.

Serous Membranes

Serous membranes secrete a thin, watery fluid that prevents friction when organs rub against one another. These membranes line the body surfaces that do not open to the outside environment. Examples include the lungs (pleura), the intestines (peritoneum), and the heart (pericardium). Like epithelial membranes, serous membranes are composed of two distinct layers of tissue: (1) the epithelial sheet, a thin layer of simple squamous epithelium; and (2) the connective tissue layer, a very thin sheet that holds and supports the epithelial cells.

The serous membrane that lines body cavities and covers the surfaces of organs in those cavities is really a single, continuous sheet covering two different surfaces. The **parietal** membrane lines the wall of the cavity like wallpaper; the **visceral** membrane covers the surface of the viscera (organs within the cavity).

Connective Tissue Membranes (Synovial Membranes)

Connective tissue (or synovial) membranes are smooth and slick and secrete **synovial fluid** (a thick, colorless lubricating fluid). Synovial membranes line the joint spaces and prevent friction between the ends of the bones, thus allowing free movement of the joints. Synovial membranes also line small, cushionlike sacs called **bursae,** which are found between some moving body parts. Unlike serous and mucous membranes, connective tissue membranes do not contain epithelial components.

ORGANS AND SYSTEMS

When several kinds of tissues are united to perform a more complex function than any tissue alone, they are called **organs.** Examples are the heart, stomach, and kidneys. These organs working together for the same general purpose make up organ systems, which maintain the whole body. Systems perform a more complex function than any one organ can perform alone (Table 41-6).

Table 41-6 Organ Systems and Their Functions

STRUCTURE	FUNCTION
INTEGUMENTARY SYSTEM	
Skin	Protection
Hair	Regulation of body temperature
Nails	Synthesis of chemicals
Sense receptors	Sense organ
Sweat glands	
Oil glands	
SKELETAL SYSTEM	
Bones	Support
Joints	Movement (with joints and muscles)
	Storage of minerals
	Blood cell formation

Table 41-6 Organ Systems and Their Functions—cont'd

STRUCTURE	FUNCTION
MUSCULAR SYSTEM	
Voluntary or striated muscles Involuntary or smooth muscles	Movement Maintenance of body posture Production of heat
NERVOUS SYSTEM	
Brain Spinal cord Nerves Sense organs	Contains body's control center Responsible for all the coordination of body's activities Communication Integration Control Recognition of sensory stimuli System functions by production of nerve impulses caused by stimuli of various types Control is fast acting and of short duration
ENDOCRINE SYSTEM	
Pituitary gland Pineal gland Hypothalamus Thyroid gland Parathyroid glands Thymus gland Adrenal glands Pancreas Ovaries (female) Testes (male)	Secretion of special substances (hormones) directly into the blood Same as nervous system—communication, integration, control Control is slow and of long duration Examples of hormone regulation: growth, metabolism, reproduction, and fluid and electrolyte balance
CARDIOVASCULAR (CIRCULATORY) SYSTEM	
Heart Blood vessels	Transportation for nutrition, water, oxygen, and wastes Regulation of body temperature Immunity (body defense)
LYMPHATIC SYSTEM	
Lymph nodes Lymphatic vessels Thymus Spleen Tonsils	Protection Maintains body's internal fluid environment by producing, filtering and conveying lymph Production of various blood cellsTransportation
RESPIRATORY SYSTEM	
Nose Pharynx Larynx Trachea Bronchi Lungs	Exchange of waste gas (carbon dioxide) for oxygen in the lungs Area of gas exchange in the lungs called alveoli Filtration of irritants from inspired air Regulation of acid-base balance
DIGESTIVE SYSTEM	
Primary Organs	
Mouth Pharynx Esophagus Stomach Small intestine (duodenum, jejunum, ileum) Large intestine (ascending, transverse, descending, sigmoid) Rectum Anal canal	Mechanical and chemical breakdown (digestion) of food Absorption of nutrients Undigested waste product that is eliminated is called **feces**

Continued

Table 41-6 Organ Systems and Their Functions—cont'd

STRUCTURE	FUNCTION
DIGESTIVE SYSTEM—cont'd	
Accessory Organs	
Teeth	
Salivary glands	
Tongue	
Liver	
Gallbladder	
Pancreas	
Appendix	Appendix is a structural but not a functional part of digestive system
URINARY SYSTEM	
Kidneys	Clearing or cleaning blood of waste products; waste product excreted from body is called **urine**
Ureters	Electrolyte balance
Urinary bladder	Water balance
Urethra	Acid-base balance
	Urethra has urinary and reproductive functions (in male)
REPRODUCTIVE SYSTEM	
Male	
Gonads (testes)	Survival of species
Genital ducts (epididymis, vas deferens, ejaculatory duct, urethra)	Production of sex cells (male are sperm; female are ova)
	Transfer and fertilization of sex cells
Accessory glands (prostate, seminal vesicles, Cowper's glands)	Development and birth of offspring
	Nourishment of offspring
Supporting structures (penis, scrotum)	Production of sex hormones
Female	
Gonads (ovaries)	
Accessory organs (uterus, fallopian tubes [oviducts], vagina)	
External genitalia (vulva)	
Mons pubis	
Labia majora	
Labia minora	
Clitoris	
Accessory glands	
Skene's glands	
Bartholin's glands	
Mammary glands (breasts)	

Get Ready for the NCLEX® Examination!

Key Points

- Anatomy is the study, classification, and description of structures and organs of the body. Physiology explains the function of the various structures and how they interrelate.
- The normal anatomical position of the body is standing erect with the face and the palms of the hands forward.
- For the purposes of study, the body is divided into three imaginary planes: sagittal, coronal (frontal), and transverse.
- The body is divided into two large groups of cavities: the dorsal and the ventral. The dorsal cavity contains the cranial and spinal cavities. The ventral cavity contains the thoracic, abdominal, and pelvic cavities.
- For the purposes of study, the abdominal region is divided into nine regions: right hypochondriac region, epigastric region, left hypochondriac region, right lumbar region, umbilical region, left lumbar region, right inguinal region, hypogastric region, and left inguinal region.
- The cell's major structures are the cytoplasm, nucleus, ER, ribosomes, mitochondria, lysosomes, Golgi apparatus, and centrioles.
- Organization is a fundamental characteristic of body structure.
- Cells are considered to be the smallest living units of structure and function in the body. Although long recognized as the simplest units of living matter, cells are extremely complex.
- Tissues are groups of similar cells that work together to perform a specific function.
- Organs are structures made up of two or more kinds of tissues organized so they can perform a more complex function than they could alone.

- Systems are groups of organs arranged so they can perform a more complex function than they could alone.
- To receive nutrition and oxygen and to rid itself of wastes, the cell performs passive transport (diffusion, osmosis, filtration) and active transport (phagocytosis and pinocytosis).
- The body is composed of four main types of tissues: epithelial, connective, muscle, and nervous tissues.
- The major systems of the body are integumentary, skeletal, muscular, nervous, endocrine, cardiovascular (circulatory), lymphatic, respiratory, digestive, urinary, and reproductive.

Additional Learning Resources

Go to your Companion CD for an audio glossary, animations, video clips, and more.

evolve Be sure to visit the Evolve site at http://evolve.elsevier.com/Christensen/adult/ for additional online resources.

Review Questions for the NCLEX-PN® Examination

1. The anatomical term that refers to the distal portion of the spine is:
   1. medial.
   2. caudal.
   3. proximal.
   4. dorsal.

2. The trachea, the heart, the blood vessels, and the lungs are located in which body cavity?
   1. Dorsal
   2. Abdominopelvic
   3. Ventral
   4. Pelvic

3. A relative constant state in the body's internal environment naturally maintained by adaptive responses that promote healthy survival is called:
   1. homeostasis.
   2. mitosis.
   3. lysosomes.
   4. protein synthesis.

4. A process in which solid particles in a fluid move from an area of greater concentration to an area of lesser concentration, resulting in an even distribution of the particles in the fluid, is called:
   1. phagocytosis.
   2. pinocytosis.
   3. osmosis.
   4. diffusion.

5. The movement of materials across the membrane of a cell by means of chemical activity requiring the expenditure of energy by the cell is called:
   1. passive passport.
   2. active transport.
   3. telophase.
   4. transcription.

6. What type of tissue is composed of cells that contract in response to a message from the brain or spinal cord?
   1. Epithelial
   2. Connective
   3. Membrane
   4. Muscle

7. The thin sheets of tissue that secrete mucus and line the body surfaces that open to the outside environment are:
   1. mucous membranes.
   2. serous membranes.
   3. striated, involuntary.
   4. visceral, involuntary.

8. An active transport process that permits a cell to engulf or surround foreign material and digest it is called:
   1. mitosis.
   2. pinocytosis.
   3. phagocytosis.
   4. filtration.

9. A type of cell division of somatic cells in which each daughter cell contains the same number of chromosomes as the parent cell is called:
   1. flagella.
   2. mitosis.
   3. ER synthesis.
   4. mitochondria.

10. A group of several different kinds of tissues arranged so they can perform a special function together is called:
    1. cells.
    2. organ.
    3. tissue.
    4. system.

11. Groups of similar cells that work together to perform a specific function are called:
    1. cells.
    2. organ.
    3. tissue.
    4. system.

12. The hypogastric region of the abdominopelvic cavity is:
    1. inferior to the umbilical region.
    2. lateral to the left iliac region.
    3. medial to the right iliac region.
    4. both 1 and 3.

13. The two major cavities of the body are the:
    1. thoracic and abdominal.
    2. abdominal and pelvic.
    3. dorsal and ventral.
    4. anterior and posterior.

14. The structure that divides the thoracic cavity from the abdominal cavity is the:
    1. mediastinum.
    2. diaphragm.
    3. lungs.
    4. stomach.

Matching

Match the directional terms in Column B with its *opposite* term in Column A.

Column A	***Column B***
15. _____ Superior	**a.** posterior
16. _____ Distal	**b.** superficial
17. _____ Anterior	**c.** medial
18. _____ Lateral	**d.** proximal
19. _____ Deep	**e.** inferior

Match the function in Column B with the correct system in Column A.

Column A

20. _____ Integumentary
21. _____ Skeletal
22. _____ Muscular
23. _____ Nervous
24. _____ Endocrine
25. _____ Cardiovascular
26. _____ Lymphatic
27. _____ Respiratory
28. _____ Digestive
29. _____ Urinary
30. _____ Reproductive

Column B

a. Provides movement, body posture, and heat
b. Uses hormones to regulate body functions
c. Transports fatty nutrients from the digestive system to the blood
d. Makes physical and chemical change in nutrients and absorbs nutrients
e. Cleans the blood of metabolic wastes and regulates electrolyte balance
f. Protects underlying structures, provides for sensory reception, and regulates body temperature
g. Transports substances from one part of the body to another
h. Ensures the survival of the species rather than the individual
i. Uses electrochemical signals to integrate and control body functions
j. Exchanges oxygen and carbon dioxide and regulates acid-base balance
k. Provides a rigid framework for the body and stores minerals

chapter 42

Care of the Surgical Patient

Elaine Oden Kockrow and Barbara Lauritsen Christensen

evolve http://evolve.elsevier.com/Christensen/foundationsadult

Objectives

1. Identify the purposes of surgery.
2. Distinguish among elective, urgent, and emergency surgery.
3. Explain the concept of perioperative nursing.
4. Discuss the factors that influence an individual's ability to tolerate surgery.
5. Discuss considerations for the older adult surgical patient.
6. Describe the preoperative checklist.
7. Explain the importance of informed consent for surgery.
8. Explain the procedure for turning, deep breathing, coughing, and leg exercises for postoperative patients.
9. Differentiate among general, regional, and local anesthesia.
10. Explain conscious sedation.
11. Describe the role of the circulating nurse and the scrub nurse during surgery.
12. Discuss the initial nursing assessment and management immediately after transfer from the postanesthesia care unit.
13. Identify the rationale for nursing interventions designed to prevent postoperative complications.
14. List the assessment data for the surgical patient.
15. Identify the information needed for the postoperative patient in preparation for discharge.
16. Discuss the nursing process as it pertains to the surgical patient.

Key Terms

ablation (ăb-LĀ-shŭn, p. 1254)
anesthesia (ăn-ĕs-THĒ-zē-ă, p. 1273)
atelectasis (ă-tĕ-LĔK-tā-sĭs, p. 1285)
cachexia (kă-KĔK-sē-ă, p. 1284)
catabolism (kă-TĂB-ō-lĭsm, p. 1288)
conscious sedation (sĕ-DĀ-shŭn, p. 1276)
dehiscence (dē-HĬS-ĕns, p. 1284)
drainage (p. 1281)
embolus (ĔM-bō-lŭs, p. 1269)
evisceration (ĕ-vĭs-ĕr-Ā-shŭn, p. 1284)
extubate (ĕks-TŪ-bāt, p. 1281)
exudate (ĔKS-ū-dāt, p. 1281)
incentive spirometry (ĭn-SĔN-tĭv spī-RŎM-ĕ-trē, p. 1264)
incisions (ĭn-SĬZH-ŭn, p. 1271)
infarct (ĬN-făhrkt, p. 1269)
informed consent (p. 1260)
intraoperative (ĭn-tră-ŎP-ĕr-ă-tĭv, p. 1254)
palliative (PĂL-ē-ă-tĭv, p. 1254)
paralytic ileus (păr-ă-LĬT-ĭk ĬL-ē-ŭs, p. 1288)
perioperative (pĕr-ē-ŎP-ĕr-ă-tĭv, p. 1254)
postoperative (pōst-ŎP-ĕr-ă-tĭv, p. 1254)
preoperative (prē-ŎP-ĕr-ă-tĭv, p. 1254)
prosthesis (prŏs-THĒ-sĭs, p. 1277)
singultus (SĬNG-gŭl-tŭs, p. 1288)
surgery (p. 1253)
surgical asepsis (ā-SĔP-sĭs, p. 1280)
thrombus (THRŎM-bŭs, p. 1268)

Surgery is defined as that branch of medicine concerned with diseases and trauma requiring operative procedures. Surgery became a medical specialty in the mid-nineteenth century. It enabled physicians to treat conditions that were difficult or impossible to manage only with medicine. However, early surgeons had little knowledge of the principles of asepsis, and anesthetic techniques were primitive and unsafe. Indeed, a surgeon's success was based on speed. In the 1840s the discovery of anesthesia allowed surgeons to operate on a patient who was pain free. Nurses working in the first operating rooms (ORs) cleaned the rooms and equipment, performed technical tasks such as obtaining supplies, and occasionally accompanied the patient to the surgical ward to deliver nursing care.

With the advent of antiseptic and later aseptic practices, surgery became a treatment of choice for many conditions. Safer anesthetic gases allowed surgeons to conduct longer operative procedures. All surgery was conducted in hospital settings. Although modern-day suites have moved surgery from the Dark Ages, patients still often view the surgical process as mysterious and frightening.

Surgery is classified as elective, urgent, or emergency. Elective surgery is not necessary to preserve life and may be performed at a time the patient chooses. Urgent surgery is required to keep additional health problems from occurring. Emergency surgery is performed immediately to save the individual's life or preserve the function of a body part. Surgical procedures may also be labeled as either major or minor, although all surgeries have an element of risk.

Surgery is performed for various purposes, including diagnostic, **ablation** (amputation or excision of any body part or removal of a growth or harmful substance), **palliative** (therapy to relieve or reduce uncomfortable symptoms without cure), reconstructive, transplant, constructive, and cosmetic (Table 42-1). See Table 42-2 for frequently used surgical terminology.

Traditionally, surgical procedures were performed in hospitals. With the discovery of new technologies and today's emphasis on decreasing health care costs, the surgical suite may now be in a variety of settings. Although facilities use different terms for surgical settings and processes, some common variations exist (Box 42-1).

PERIOPERATIVE NURSING

Perioperative nursing refers to the nurse's role during the **preoperative** (before surgery), **intraoperative** (during surgery), and **postoperative** (after surgery) phases of a surgical experience. Perioperative nursing stresses the importance of providing continuity of care for the surgical patient using the nursing process. In many hospitals, perioperative nurses assess a patient's health status preoperatively, identify specific patient needs, teach and counsel, attend to the patient's needs in the OR, and then follow the patient's recovery. However, in other institutions, different nurses care for the patient during each phase. Nurses also may delegate certain aspects of perioperative nursing to appropriate personnel (Box 42-2). The nurse's major responsibility is safe, consistent, and effective nursing interventions during each phase of surgery.

Table 42-1 Classification for Surgical Procedures

TYPE	DESCRIPTION AND EXAMPLES
ADMISSION STATUS	
Ambulatory (outpatient)	Patient who enters setting, has surgical procedure, and is discharged on the same day (e.g., breast biopsy, cataract extraction, hemorrhoidectomy, scar revision)
Same-day admit	Patient who enters hospital and undergoes surgery on the same day and remains for convalescence (e.g., carotid endarterectomy, cholecystectomy, mastectomy, vaginal hysterectomy)
Inpatient	Patient who is admitted to hospital, undergoes surgery, and remains in hospital for convalescence (e.g., amputation, heart transplant, laryngectomy, resection of aortic aneurysm)
SERIOUSNESS	
Major	Involves extensive reconstruction or alteration in body parts; poses great risks to well-being (e.g., coronary artery bypass, colon resection, gastric resection)
Minor	Involves minimal alteration in body parts; often designed to correct deformities; involves minimal risks compared with those of major procedures (e.g., cataract extraction, skin graft, tooth extraction)
URGENCY	
Elective	Performed on basis of patient's choice (e.g., bunionectomy, plastic surgery)
Urgent	Necessary for patient's health (e.g., excision of cancerous tumor, removal of gallbladder for stones, vascular repair for obstructed artery [e.g., coronary artery bypass])
Emergency	Must be done immediately to save life or preserve function of body part (e.g., removal of perforated appendix, repair of traumatic amputation, control of internal hemorrhaging)
PURPOSE	
Diagnostic	Surgical exploration that allows physician to confirm diagnosis; may involve removal of tissue for further diagnostic testing (e.g., exploratory laparotomy [incision into peritoneal cavity to inspect abdominal organs], breast mass biopsy)
Ablation	Excision or removal of diseased body part (e.g., amputation, removal of appendix, cholecystectomy)
Palliative	Surgery for relief or reduction of intensity of disease symptoms; will not produce cure (e.g., colostomy, debridement of necrotic tissue)
Reconstructive	Restoration of function or appearance to traumatized or malfunctioning tissue (e.g., internal fixation of fractures, scar revision, breast reconstruction)
Transplant	Replacement of malfunctioning organs (e.g., cornea, heart, joints, kidney)
Constructive	Restoration of function lost or reduced as result of congenital anomalies (e.g., repair of cleft palate, closure of atrial-septal defect in heart)
Cosmetic	Alteration of personal appearance (e.g., rhinoplasty to reshape nose)

Table 42-2 Surgical Terminology

TERM	INTERPRETATION WITH EXAMPLE
Anastomosis	Surgical joining of two ducts or blood vessels to allow flow from one to another; to bypass an area (e.g., *Billroth I,* joins stomach and duodenum)
-ectomy	Surgical removal of (e.g., *cholecystectomy,* removal of the gallbladder)
Lysis	Destruction or dissolution of (e.g., *lysis of adhesions,* removal of adhesions)
-orrhaphy	Surgical repair of (e.g., *herniorrhaphy,* repair of a hernia)
-oscopy	Direct visualization by a scope (e.g., *cystoscopy,* direct visualization of the urinary tract by means of a cystoscope)
-ostomy	Opening made to allow the passage of drainage (e.g., *ileostomy,* formation of an opening of the ileum onto the surface of the abdomen for passage of feces)
-otomy	Opening into (e.g., *thoracotomy,* surgical opening into the thoracic cavity)
-pexy	Fixation of (e.g., *cecopexy,* fixation or suspension of the cecum to correct its excessive mobility)
-plasty	Plastic surgery (e.g., *mammoplasty,* reshaping of the breasts to reduce, lift, reconstruct)

Box 42-1 Common Surgical Settings

- **Inpatient:** Patient hospitalized for surgery
- **One-day (same-day surgery):** Patient admitted the day surgery is scheduled and dismissed the same day
- **Outpatient:** Patient, not hospitalized, admitted either to a short-stay unit or directly to the surgical suite (sometimes referred to ambulatory surgery)
- **Short-stay surgical center ("surgicenter"):** Independently owned agency; surgery performed when overnight hospitalization is not required (also called ambulatory surgical center or one-day surgery center)
- **Short-stay unit:** Department or floor where a patient's stay does not exceed 24 hours (sometimes referred to as outpatient/observation unit)
- **Mobile surgery units:** Units that move from place to place; go to the patient instead of the patient traveling to the unit

INFLUENCING FACTORS

Regardless of the surgical procedure, the process is stressful for the patient. Observing a patient's mannerisms and listening to questions help identify the patient's feelings and concerns. By helping patients express their concerns, the nurse can offer support, reassurance, and information—the best way to address fear of the unknown.

Numerous factors affect the individual's ability to tolerate surgery.

Age

The young and the old do not tolerate major surgical treatment as well as those in other age-groups. Their altered metabolic needs may not respond to physiologic changes quickly. Specific concerns center on the body's response to temperature changes, cardiovascular shifts, respiratory needs, and renal function. To assist patients in returning to their optimal level of health, nursing assessments and appropriate interventions should be ongoing (see Life Span Considerations box).

Box 42-2 Delegation Considerations in Perioperative Nursing

- The skills of assessment that are part of preparing the patient for surgery require the critical thinking and knowledge application unique to a nurse. For these skills, delegation is inappropriate. Assistive personnel (AP) may obtain vital signs and weight and height measurements. Instruct AP on proper precautions for these delegated procedures as needed.
- The skills of preoperative teaching require the critical thinking and knowledge application unique to a nurse. For this skill, delegation is inappropriate. AP can reinforce and assist patients in performing postoperative exercises.
  - —Review with AP any precautions for a particular patient (e.g., turning method).
  - —Be certain staff knows when to inform the nurse if the patient is unable to perform the exercises correctly.
- Coordinating the patient's preparation for surgery requires the critical thinking and knowledge application unique to a nurse. However, AP may administer an enema or douche; obtain vital signs; apply antiembolic stockings; and assist patient in removing clothing, jewelry, and prostheses.
  - —Instruct AP in proper precautions when preparing a patient for surgery.
  - —Instruct AP in proper observations and precautions if the patient has an IV catheter in place.
- The skills of sterile gowning and gloving can be delegated to a surgical technologist or the nurse who has acquired the proper skills.
- The skill of initiating and managing postoperative care of the patient requires the critical thinking and knowledge application unique to a nurse. AP may obtain vital signs, apply nasal cannula or oxygen mask, and provide basic comfort and hygiene measures.

Physical Condition

Healthy patients have smoother and faster recovery periods than patients who have coexisting health problems. Assess each body system to identify actual and potential problems, then select measures to prevent postsurgical complications (Box 42-3).

Life Span Considerations

Older Adults

Undergoing Surgery

- Older adults undergoing surgery have higher morbidity and mortality rates than younger people.
- Surgery places a greater stress on older people than on younger people. Carefully evaluate the older patient's physiologic status and coexisting conditions before surgery. Medical management is often preferred unless a condition is life threatening. However, age is no longer a factor for determining the benefit an individual can achieve from a surgical procedure. Consequently, nurses are caring for many more surgical patients of advanced age and are required to know the age-related factors that affect a surgical procedure.
- Older patients tend to recover more slowly from surgery compared with younger patients. Recovery is affected by the level of mental functioning, individual coping ability, and the availability of support systems.
- Risks of aspiration, atelectasis, pneumonia, thrombus formation, infection, and altered tissue perfusion are increased in the older adult.
- Disorientation or toxic reactions can occur in the older adult after the administration of anesthetics, sedatives, or analgesics. These reactions are often present for days after administration of the medication.
- Preoperative and postoperative teaching may require extra time. Provide teaching at the older adult's level of understanding. Repeat and reinforce directions.
- When communicating with older adult patients, be aware of any auditory, visual, or cognitive impairment that may be present.

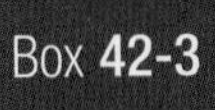

Box 42-3 ABCDE Mnemonic Device to Ascertain Serious Illness or Trauma in the Preoperative Patient

A Allergy to medications, chemicals, and other environmental products such as latex. All allergies are reported to anesthesia and surgical personnel before the beginning of surgery. Place an allergy band on the patient's arm immediately.

B Bleeding tendencies or the use of medications that deter clotting, such as aspirin or products containing aspirin, heparin, or warfarin sodium. Herbal medications may also increase bleeding times or mask potential blood-related problems.

C Cortisone or steroid use.

D Diabetes mellitus, a condition that not only requires strict control of blood glucose levels but is also known to delay wound healing.

E Emboli. Previous embolic events (such as lower leg blood clots) may recur because of prolonged immobility.

Patients whose immune systems are suppressed are at a much higher risk for development of postoperative infection and are less capable of fighting that infection.

Nutritional Factors

The body uses carbohydrates, proteins, and fats to supply energy-producing glucose to its cells. Carbohydrates and fats are the primary energy producers, and protein is essential to build and repair body tissue. During stressful conditions, the body's need for energy and repair increases. Nutritional needs are affected by a patient's age and physical requirements; patients who maintain a sound, nutritional diet tend to recover more quickly.

A complete diet history identifies the patient's usual eating habits, nutritional patterns, and food preferences. Dietary practices are influenced by a patient's ethnic, cultural, religious, and socioeconomic background. With this information, offer the patient appropriate foods that are high in energy-producing nutrients. Surgery may decrease a patient's appetite and alter metabolic functions, so observe the patient for signs of malnutrition. If malnutrition is promptly identified, tube feedings, intravenous (IV) therapy, or parenteral hyperalimentation can be initiated (see Chapter 21).

PSYCHOSOCIAL NEEDS

As patients and families plan for surgery, they frequently express concern and fears about possible outcomes (Box 42-4). Preoperative fear has been linked to postoperative behavior. The preoperative anxiety level influences the amount of anesthesia required, the amount of postoperative pain medication needed, and the speed of recovery from surgery. Determine each patient's perceptions, emotions, behavior, and support systems that may help or hinder their progress through the surgical period. Patiently and actively listening to the patient, the family, and significant others invites confidence and helps reduce anxiety levels (Figure 42-1).

While the patient attempts to understand the approaching surgery, family members and support people are also trying to cope. Families may have additional burdens, such as financial obligations, living changes, and added personal responsibilities. In addition to nursing and medical personnel, ministerial staff, social workers, or patient advocates can provide support for patients and families during this stressful time (see Patient Teaching box).

SOCIOECONOMIC AND CULTURAL NEEDS

The United States is a nation of diverse individuals from different social, economic, religious, ethnic, and cultural origins. Even geographic location affects the way a patient responds to surgery. Therefore it is im-

Box 42-4 Common Fears Associated with Surgery

- **Fear of loss of control** is associated primarily with anesthesia. The patient becomes almost totally dependent on the health care team during the surgical experience—even for basic needs such as breathing and life support—while under the influence of anesthesia.
- **Fear of the unknown** may result from uncertainty about the surgical outcome or a lack of knowledge regarding the surgical experience.
- **Fear of anesthesia** may include fears of unpleasant induction of or emergence from anesthesia. The patient may fear waking up during the operation and feeling pain while under anesthesia. This fear is often related to loss of control and fear of the unknown.
- **Fear of pain or inadequate postoperative analgesia** is common. Reassure the patient and significant others that the pain will be controlled.
- **Fear of death** is a legitimate fear. Even with the great strides in surgery and anesthesia, no anesthetic or operation is perfectly safe for all patients.
- **Fear of separation from the usual support group** may arise because the patient is separated from spouse, family, or significant others, as well as other support groups, and is cared for by strangers during this highly stressful period.
- **Fear of disruption of life patterns** relates to surgery and recovery interfering in varying degrees with activities of daily living, social activities, work, and professional activities.
- **Fear of change in body image and mutilation** is not unusual. Surgery disrupts body integrity and threatens body image.
- **Fear of detection of cancer** produces a high anxiety level.

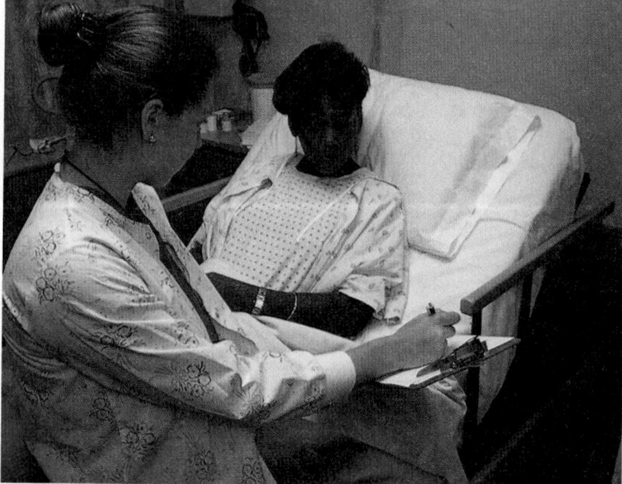

FIGURE 42-1 Often knowledge deficits occur when the patient is undergoing her first surgical experience.

portant to allow patients and families to express themselves openly.

Patients from different cultures (see Chapter 8) may react to the preoperative experience in different ways. A multicultural perspective helps nurses approach patients with respect and individually tailor care that promotes recovery (see Cultural Considerations box).

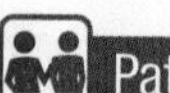

Patient Teaching

Preoperative Care

Examples of helpful information for preoperative patients and families are the following:

- Preoperative tests, reason, preparation
- Preoperative routines, sequence of events
- Special equipment needed
- Transfer to operating room (time, checking procedures)
- Medications
- Recovery room or postanesthesia care unit
  - —Place where the patient will awaken
  - —Frequent monitoring of vital signs
  - —Return to room when vital signs are stable
- Probable postoperative therapies
  - —Need for increased mobility as soon as possible
  - —Need to keep respiratory passages clear
- Anticipated treatments (e.g., intravenous line, dressing changes, incentive spirometry)
- Pain medication routines (timing sequence, "as needed" [prn] status), other modalities of management such as patient-controlled analgesia and patient-controlled epidural

MEDICATIONS

Review of the patient's current medication regimen is essential. Polypharmacy (concurrent use of multiple medications) occurs in all age-groups but is more common with older adults. Studies have shown that patients age 65 and older use an average of two to six prescribed medications and one to three over-the-counter medications. The use of multiple medications can lead to adverse drug reactions and interactions with other medications in the perioperative setting.

During the surgical experience, health care providers use medications in a number of pharmacologic categories, including anesthesia agents, antimicrobials, anticoagulants, hemostatic agents, oxytocics, steroids, diagnostic imaging dyes, diuretics, central nervous system agents, and emergency protocol medications. A seriously ill patient may receive as many as 20 medications in a perioperative setting at one time. Large numbers of medications increase the chance of interactions.

Patients also frequently use herbal remedies as alternative or complementary medicines. Ask patients about their use of herbal remedies, either as dietary supplements or as medicines. Unless specifically asked, some patients may not consider their natural remedies as medicines. Even though herbs are natural products, they act like medications and may interact with or potentiate other medications or interfere with surgical procedures (Table 42-3).

Some medications may be stopped when a patient goes to surgery. However, it is important to know the purposes and actions of drugs, since they may be critical for patients with diseases such as diabetes. The anesthesiologist, in collaboration with the patient's

Cultural Considerations

The Surgical Patient

- Use of the patient's language helps put an anxious patient at ease. Use an interpreter when possible; learn some key phrases in foreign languages; and use references such as medical dictionaries, which usually have key phrases listed in an appendix.
- Because some Southeast Asians and Native Americans may avoid eye contact and consider it disrespectful, consider limiting eye contact when dealing with such patients.
- Chinese-Americans may not ask for pain medication and may need teaching to help explain how comfort and relief from pain promote healing and a quicker recovery.
- Native Americans are often stoic when ill. Complaints of pain to the nurse may be in general terms such as, "I am uncomfortable." Undertreatment of pain is common. The patient may lack basic trust.
- Among Arab-Americans, verbal consent often has more meaning than written consent because it is based on trust. Fully explain the need for written consent. The patient is expressive regarding pain; pain may cause intense fear. Prepare the patient for painful procedures, and develop a care plan to prevent pain.
- Blacks may be open to expression of pain but may avoid medication because of fear of addiction. For a terminal diagnosis, news is best expressed in a family care conference or by speaking with the patient's religious representative.
- For Vietnamese-American patients, having an interpreter (often a hired one) is important, depending on the sensitivity of the subject under discussion, because of modesty. A female family member is expected to be at the bedside to provide care and comfort. Men are the decision makers and support the family; therefore speaking with the male head of the family may be necessary.
- Russian-American patients often prefer an amiable nurse who has a friendly smile. Use open, inviting, nonverbal postures. A Russian-American patient is more willing to follow instruction if the nurse providing it is sincere, competent, and trustworthy. Russian-American families usually have a principal patriarch.

Table 42-3 Preoperative Considerations for Commonly Ingested Herbs

HERB	COMMON USES	PREOPERATIVE CONSIDERATIONS
Echinacea	Treat cold symptoms	Possible negative impact on the liver Subsequent interference with hepatic metabolism of certain anesthesia medications
Ephedra sinica	Decongestant Weight loss	Increased risk of cardiac dysrhythmias May reduce effectiveness of medications used to treat hypotension
Feverfew	Migraine prevention	Has anticoagulation factors; potential for increased bleeding Preoperative assessment should include clotting studies Discontinue before surgery
Garlic	Improved immunity High blood pressure and cholesterol	Potential for increased bleeding
Ginger	Motion sickness Cough Menstrual cramps Intestinal gas	Risk of prolonged clotting times Preoperative assessment should include clotting studies Discontinue before surgery
Ginkgo biloba	Brain function and alertness Tension Erectile dysfunction	Potential for increased bleeding
Ginseng	Overall well-being Diabetes	May increase anesthetic agent requirements Potential for hypoglycemia in patients taking insulin or oral diabetes agents
Guarana	Mental alertness Fatigue	May reduce the efficacy of warfarin May potentiate sympathetic nervous system stimulants, leading to cardiac complications May decrease cerebral blood flow
Kava	Sleep aid Anxiety, tension	May potentiate muscle relaxants May increase effects of certain antiemetics Potential for serious liver damage and subsequent decreased hepatic metabolism of certain anesthetic agents
Licorice	Asthma, eczema, rheumatoid arthritis Expectorant Gastritis	May cause hypertension Potential for hypokalemia and associated cardiac dysrhythmias
St. John's wort	Antidepressant Antiviral properties Antiinflammatory action	Should not be used with other psychoactive drugs, monoamine oxidase inhibitors, or serotonin reuptake inhibitors Discontinue before surgery because of possible drug interactions
Valerian root	Sedative or tranquilizer effect Sleep aid	Should not be used with sedatives or anxiolytics May increase effects of central nervous system depressants

physician and surgeon, determines whether these medications should be taken the day of surgery and postoperatively.

Remember to assess for allergies to drugs that may be given during any phase of the surgery. If patients say they are allergic to a drug, ask them exactly what happened when they took it. Also ask about nondrug allergies, including allergies to foods, chemicals, pollen, antiseptics used to prepare the skin for surgery, and latex rubber products. Patients with a history of allergic responsiveness are more likely to have hypersensitivity reactions to anesthesia agents. Many facilities require such patients to wear an allergy identification band during surgery. Flag the front of the patient's chart to alert all health care providers to the allergy status.

EDUCATION AND EXPERIENCE

As individuals age, life experiences influence problem-solving abilities and coping methods. Tailoring information to a patient's educational level enables understanding to replace fear. Encourage patients to repeat or summarize what has been presented. This process double checks what patients heard and how they interpreted it.

PREOPERATIVE PHASE

Before surgery, patients require a thorough health assessment. Acute or chronic diseases hinder the body's ability to repair itself or adjust to surgical treatment. Disorders of the systems identified in Table 42-4 pre-

Table 42-4 Surgical Effects on Body Systems

DISEASE OR DISORDER	SURGICAL EFFECTS
CARDIOVASCULAR (Chapter 48)	
Recent myocardial infarction, dysrhythmias, and heart failure Hypertension	Hypotension and cardiac dysrhythmias are the most common cardiovascular complications of the surgical patient. Early recognition and management before these complications become serious enough to diminish cardiac output depend on frequent assessment of the patient's vital signs.
ENDOCRINE (Chapter 51)	
Liver disease	Liver disease alters metabolism and elimination of drugs administered during surgery and impairs wound healing because of alterations in protein metabolism.
Diabetes mellitus	Diabetes increases susceptibility to infection and may impair wound healing from altered glucose metabolism and associated circulatory impairment. Fluctuating blood levels may cause central nervous system malfunction during anesthesia.
GASTROINTESTINAL (Chapter 45)	
Hiatal hernia Ulcers	Preoperative and postoperative medication may be necessary to control gastric acidity.
Esophageal varices	Risk of hemorrhage may increase due to intubation.
IMMUNE (Chapter 55)	
Acquired immunodeficiency syndrome Allergies Immunodeficiency	Disease slows the body's ability to fight infection. Immunologic disorders increase risk of infection and delay wound healing after surgery. Hypothermia during surgery decreases immune function.
MUSCULOSKELETAL (Chapter 44)	Osteoporosis and increased risk for fractures in the older adult places patient at increased risk for injury.
NEUROLOGIC (Chapter 54)	
Seizures	Check the therapeutic levels of patient's medications.
Myasthenia gravis	Muscle relaxants may need to be excluded due to decreased ability to reverse their effects.
Cerebrovascular accident	Impaired verbal communication, defective perception of the body, paralysis, and visual disturbances place patient at high risk for injury.
Peripheral vascular disease	Patient has a decreased threshold for peripheral pain.
RESPIRATORY (Chapter 49)	
Tumors	Lung motility is decreased and gas exchange slowed.
Chronic obstructive pulmonary disease Emphysema Asthma	Anesthetic agents reduce respiratory function, increasing risk for severe hypoventilation.
URINARY (Chapter 50)	
Renal failure	Impaired kidney function decreases excretion of anesthesia and alters acid-base balance.
Tumors	Prostate enlargement may increase risk of urinary tract infection.

sent high-risk conditions for surgery. Each system is further affected by the patient's age, health, nutritional status, and mental state. Assessment questions regarding the patient's use of chemicals, alcohol, and recreational substances help the health team select medications. Postoperative care is also adjusted, when possible, to prevent potential complications. For example, a patient who smokes cigarettes may have impaired alveoli and reduced lung capacity. Mucus and anesthesia by-products may be trapped in the lung, causing atelectasis and pneumonia. After surgery, breathing exercises and treatments for the smoker aid in lung expansion and decrease the risk of respiratory complications.

Additional preoperative questions identify allergies, past surgeries, and infection and disease history. Ask the patient to name prescription drugs currently taken, over-the-counter drugs, and home remedies. Also record the patient's vital signs, height, and weight before surgery to have a baseline for postoperative comparison.

PREOPERATIVE TEACHING

Patient teaching before surgery helps decrease the patient's stress associated with fear of the unknown. Preoperative information helps reduce (1) anxiety, (2) the amount of anesthesia needed, (3) postsurgical pain, and (4) corticosteroid production. Decreasing postsurgical complications through preoperative teaching speeds wound healing.

In providing preoperative teaching, include the patient and family and remember that basic terminology and information are easier to understand than complex explanations. Stop frequently to verify the patient's understanding of information, ask questions, and encourage responses. Avoid questions that can be answered "yes" or "no." For example, "Do you have any questions?" is not as good as "What questions do you have?" If printed materials or videotapes are routinely used in preoperative teaching sessions, document what the patient read, heard, or saw. Older adults may have difficulty reading small print or hearing taped messages. If the patient does not understand English, an interpreter can explain information presented. Also emphasize that a nurse will be with the patient throughout the entire surgical experience.

For surgical procedures that have potential long-term effects, support groups can offer support preoperatively. Cancer organizations, amputation support groups, and enterostomal therapist associations are examples of large national organizations that offer peer support for surgical and nonsurgical patients.

Ideally, preoperative teaching is provided 1 or 2 days before surgery, when anxiety is not as high. In some instances, the patient may not be admitted to the hospital until early on the day of surgery. Most institutions have an established teaching program, often with a systematic preoperative teaching plan and checklist. Begin by clarifying the sequence of preoperative and postoperative events. Generally, instruct the patient about the surgical procedure, informed consent, the method of skin preparation, and the gastrointestinal (GI) cleanser to be used. Clarify what the physician has explained. Review the time of the surgery and information about the recovery area (e.g., previously assigned units, intensive care, specialty units, or outpatient area). If a transfer is planned, it is helpful to take the patient and family on a tour of the new unit. Reinforce that vital signs, dressings, and tubes are assessed every 15 to 30 minutes until the patient is awake and stable.

PREOPERATIVE PREPARATION

Preparation for surgery depends on the patient's age and physical and nutritional status, the type of surgery, and the surgeon's preference. For surgery in a short-stay or ambulatory setting, the workup normally occurs a few days in advance. If the patient is admitted to the hospital, testing may be conducted to assess for potential problems. Preparation frequently includes both in-hospital testing and evaluation of test results that were completed in the physician's office.

Laboratory Tests and Diagnostic Imaging

Testing before surgery depends on the institution's policies, the physician's directives, and the patient's condition. Follow standing orders in completing this overall process. Laboratory tests commonly reviewed before surgery include a urinalysis; a complete blood count; and a blood chemistry profile to assess endocrine, hepatic, renal, and cardiovascular functions. Serum electrolytes are evaluated if extensive surgery is planned or the patient has associated problems. One essential electrolyte examined is potassium; if not enough potassium is available, dysrhythmias can occur during anesthesia and the patient's recovery may be delayed by general muscle weakness. A chest x-ray evaluation and electrocardiogram are used to identify disease processes or existing respiratory or cardiac damage. Additional tests are conducted to assess the organ involved in surgery. Blood chemistry profile (lactate dehydrogenase, γ-glutamyltransferase, alkaline phosphatase, total bilirubin) and urine bilirubin levels are used to assess hepatic function.

Informed Consent

The Patient's Bill of Rights affirms that patients must give **informed consent** (permission to perform a specific test or procedure) before the beginning of any procedure. In signing the consent form, the patient must be competent and agrees to have the procedure that is stated on the form. Information must be clear, the risks explained, expected benefits identified, and consequences or alternatives for the presenting problem stated. Witnesses are required to meet the state's legal requirements. A witness only verifies that this is the person who signed the consent and that it was a voluntary consent. The witness (often a nurse) does not verify that the patient understands the procedure. Ideally, the surgeon discusses the surgical procedure with the patient in advance. In some institutions, the surgical consent is completed in the physician's office or in the admissions department before the patient is admitted to the unit. Informed consent should not be obtained if the patient is disoriented, unconscious, mentally incompetent, or, in some agencies, under the influence of sedatives. Know agency policy (see Chapter 2, Figure 2-1).

If the patient does not see or hear well, allow additional time to explain the surgery. For patients who do not understand English or are deaf, an interpreter may be necessary. Never coerce a patient into signing a consent that he or she does not understand or that contains information different from that originally given. If necessary, contact the physician and indicate that the patient does not understand the procedure.

In an emergency, the patient may not be able to give consent for surgery. Every effort is made to locate family members to assume this responsibility. Occasionally telephone permission may be obtained. Hospitals have standard guidelines for obtaining verbal consent. If the patient's life is in danger and family members cannot be located, the surgeon may legally perform surgery. If family members object to surgery that the physician believes is essential, a court order may be obtained for the procedure. This practice is used only in extreme circumstances, however (e.g., when a child's life is in danger). Know agency policy.

Gastrointestinal Preparation

At midnight before surgery, the patient is usually placed on nothing by mouth (NPO) status; this ensures the GI tract is empty when the patient is anesthetized, thereby decreasing the chance of vomiting or aspirating emesis after surgery. An NPO sign is posted over the patient's bed, and all fluids are removed from the room. Reinforce with both the patient and the family the importance of not ingesting foods or fluids. If the patient fails to comply with the NPO order, notify the physician. An order for NPO after midnight should apply to solid foods for patients scheduled for surgery in the morning. An early light breakfast is allowed for afternoon procedures. Clear liquid may be taken up to 3 hours before surgery.

Patients can have oral care while NPO, but caution them not to swallow fluids used. A wet cloth on the lips helps relieve dryness. If patients need to be hydrated or require special IV medications, the physician may order parenteral fluids or medication. Depending on the surgery, many patients resume foods and fluids the same day after surgery.

Because anesthesia relaxes the bowel, a bowel cleanser may be ordered to evacuate fecal material and lessen postoperative GI problems (nausea and vomiting). A cleansing enema or a general laxative is frequently used. A GI lavage solution, GoLYTELY (an isosmotic solution), rapidly evacuates the bowel. GoLYTELY is contraindicated, however, in patients with GI obstruction, gastric retention, bowel perforation, toxic colitis, or megacolon. If a bowel preparation is used, chart the type of preparation used, the patient's tolerance to the procedure, and results. Before bowel surgery, medication (neomycin, sulfonamides, erythromycin) may be given over a period of days to detoxify and sterilize the GI tract. This lessens the chance of fecal contamination during surgery.

Skin Preparation

Before surgery the patient may have hair removed at the surgical site. The operative site must be shaved carefully to remove the hair without injuring the skin (Skill 42-1). However, surgeons generally order hair removal only if it might interfere with exposure, closure, or dressing of the surgical site. Shaving the hair before surgery creates microscopic cuts that increase the risk of surgical site infection. The Centers for Disease Control and Prevention strongly recommends not removing hair at all unless it would interfere with the surgery (Nichols, 2001).

There is debate about the best method to remove hair. A lower rate of infection occurs with either no shave or use of electric clippers than with any other method. Use of a depilatory agent (a substance or procedure that removes hair) also has a low wound infection rate. In some cases, the patient showers after hair removal, unless contraindicated, using an antiseptic soap such as Hibiclens. If the surgical procedure involves the head, neck, or upper chest area, the patient also shampoos the hair.

If shaving is used, it should be performed close to the actual time of the surgical procedure to decrease the time for growth of bacteria and lower the potential for infection. Some surgical departments prepare the patient either in a surgical holding room or in the OR itself. Each agency or facility should have policies and protocols regarding the timing, the method, and the people responsible for the preoperative skin preparation of surgical patients.

Hospital policies differ regarding the description of skin areas to be prepped, or the surgeon may give specific orders. Review agency policy and the patient chart to determine the area to be shaved (Figure 42-2). Before the skin preparation, carefully assess the surgical site for skin impairment (e.g., infection, irritation, bruises, or lesions). Assess the patient for allergies. Record anything unusual and report it to the surgeon.

Once the patient is in the OR, scrub the skin thoroughly with a detergent solution and then apply an antiseptic solution to kill more adherent and deeper-residing bacteria. The surgeon may place a transparent sterile drape directly over the skin before making an incision.

Skill 42-1 Performing a Surgical Skin Preparation

Nursing Action *(Rationale)*

1. Refer to medical record, care plan, or Kardex for special interventions. *(Provides basis for care.)*
2. Obtain equipment. *(Organizes procedure.)*
   a. Appropriate light
   b. Operating room prep kit
      - Basin
      - Razor
      - Sponge with soap
      - Waterproof pad
      - Cotton-tipped applicators
   c. Clean gloves
3. Introduce self. *(Decreases patient's anxiety.)*
4. Identify patient. *(Identifies correct patient for procedure.)*
5. Explain procedure to patient. *(Seeks cooperation and decreases anxiety.)*
6. Wash hands and, if appropriate, don clean gloves. Know agency policy and guidelines from the Centers for Disease Control and Prevention (CDC) and the Occupational Safety and Health Administration (OSHA). *(Reduces spread of microorganisms.)*
7. Prepare patient for intervention:
   a. Close door to room or pull curtain. *(Provides privacy.)*
   b. Drape for procedure if necessary and position patient. *(Promotes proper body mechanics.)*
8. Raise bed to comfortable working level. *(Promotes proper body mechanics.)*
9. Place towel or waterproof pad under area to be shaved. *(Protects bed and linen from soiling.)*
10. Fill basin with warm water. *(Allows nurse to lather soap and rinse skin.)*
11. Place bath blanket over patient. *(Exposes only area to be shaved.)*
12. Adjust lighting. *(Allows thorough assessment of skin and helps decrease chance of skin impairment.)*
13. Lather skin with antiseptic soap and warm water. *(Cleanses skin, softens hair, and reduces friction from razor.)*

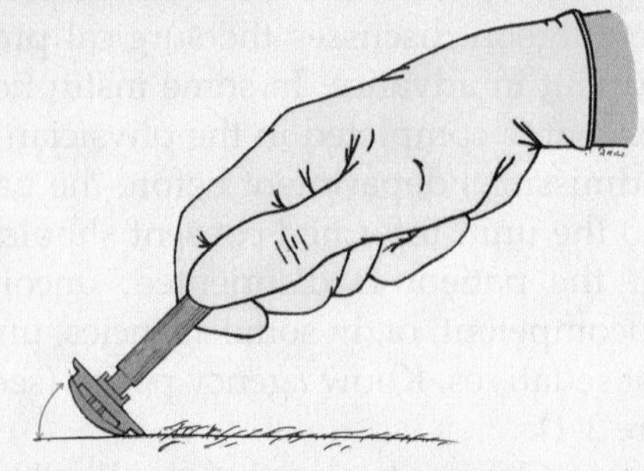

Step 14

14. Hold razor at a 30- to 45-degree angle to skin. *(Minimizes chances of cutting or nicking skin.)*
    a. Shave small areas while holding skin taut.
    b. Use short, smooth strokes. *(Prevents pulling skin.)*
    c. Shave hair in same direction it grows (see illustration). *(Removes hair close to skin surface.)*
15. Rinse razor frequently. *(Removes accumulation of hair from razor and prevents contamination from dirty water.)*
16. If entire area is shaved, cleanse it with a washcloth and clean, warm water. Dry skin. *(Removes excess shaved hair, body oils, and soil on skin. Reduces number of microorganisms. Promotes patient comfort.)*
17. Reassess skin for cuts, nicks, or hair. *(Prevents growth of microorganisms and possible infections from skin impairment.)*
18. Return patient to appropriate position. *(Provides patient comfort and safety.)*
19. Clean and dispose of equipment. *(Reduces spread of microorganisms.)*
20. Remove and dispose of soiled gloves and wash hands. *(Reduces spread of microorganisms.)*
21. Document. *(Verifies procedure.)*

Special concerns for patients undergoing a surgical skin preparation are as follows:

- Small children may be easily frightened by this procedure, and it may need to be done in the OR.
- Older adults need a detailed explanation to relieve their anxiety.
- Older adults have less subcutaneous tissue, less skin elasticity, and more delicate skin tissue. Take extreme care when shaving the older adult.
- Older adults are usually more susceptible to infections.

Latex Allergy Considerations

Focused assessment of risk factors helps identify patients with the nursing diagnosis of risk for latex allergy response. Assessing the patient's experience helps identify those at risk for a systemic reaction; for example, patients may relate stories of complicated anesthesia events, hives from blowing up a balloon, or severe swelling of the labia with a urinary catheterization.

With the advent of Universal Precautions (now called *Standard Precautions*) in the late 1980s, the use of latex gloves dramatically increased, and latex allergies became much more common. Basically, every health care

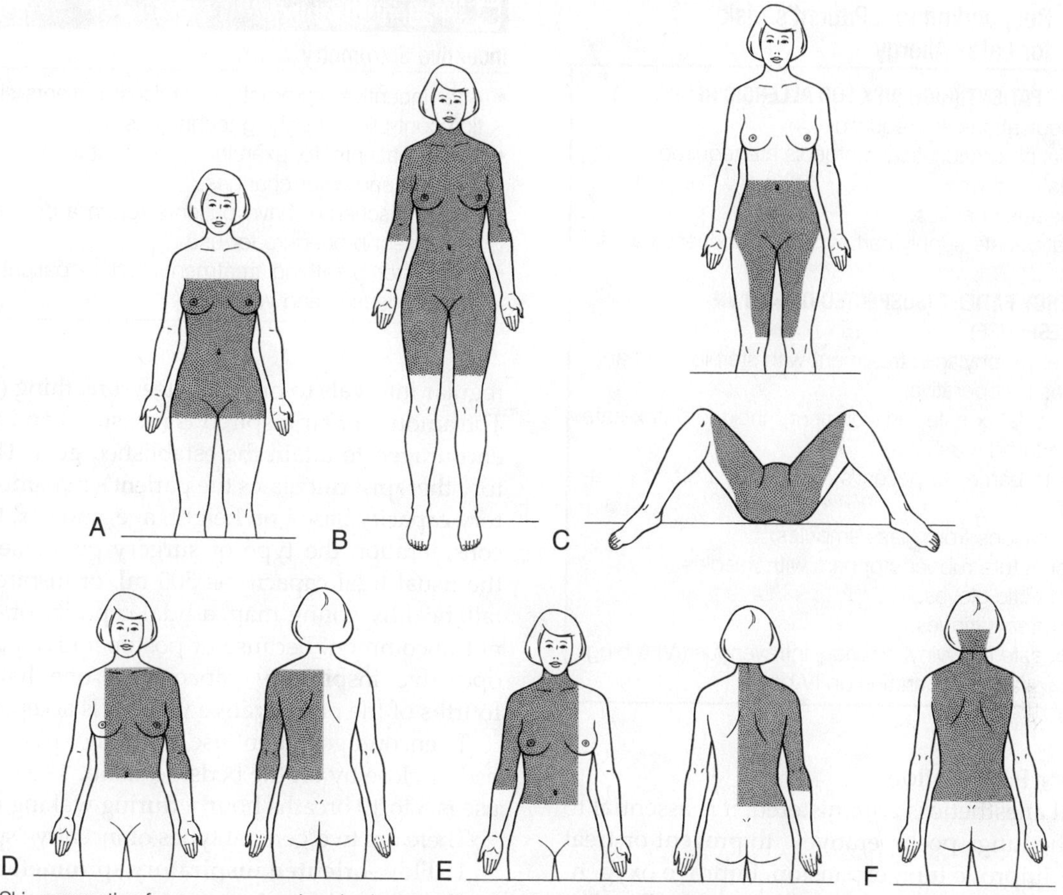

FIGURE 42-2 Skin preparation for surgery on various body areas. The shading indicates the area that could be shaved. **A,** Abdominal surgery. **B,** Open heart surgery. **C,** Perineal surgery. **D,** Chest or thoracic surgery. **E,** Breast surgery. **F,** Cervical spine surgery.

worker wears gloves. Most gloves are powdered to make them easier to put on. The powder absorbs protein allergens from the latex and deposits them on skin and into surgical wounds; it also aerosolizes the protein allergens. Aerosolized latex allergens are carried in ventilation systems, requiring further preventive measures.

Latex allergy is classified in three categories: irritant reaction and types IV and I allergic reactions. The irritant reaction, which is most commonly seen, is actually a nonallergic reaction. The type IV allergic reaction to latex is a cell-mediated response to the chemical irritants found in latex products. The true latex allergy is the type I allergic reaction, and it occurs shortly after exposure to the proteins in latex rubber. The type I reaction is an immunoglobulin E–mediated systemic reaction that occurs when latex proteins are touched, inhaled, or ingested.

Factors influencing the risk for latex allergy response are the person's susceptibility and the route, duration, and frequency of latex exposure. Risk factors include the following:

- History of anaphylactic reaction of unknown etiology during a medical or surgical procedure
- Multiple surgical procedures (especially from infancy)
- Food allergies (specifically kiwi, bananas, avocados, chestnuts)
- A job with daily exposure to latex (health care, food handlers, tire manufacturers)
- History of reactions to latex (balloons, condoms, gloves)
- Allergy to poinsettia plants
- History of allergies and asthma

To provide a latex-safe environment for susceptible patients, all surgical patients should be screened for the risk for latex allergy response before admission. Identification of patients at risk is the first step in preventing a reaction.

When a patient with a suspected or known latex allergy is scheduled for surgery, all latex use is avoided and the patient is admitted directly to the OR as the first case of the day, if possible. Many facilities have converted isolation rooms into latex-safe environments for patients with latex allergy. Ensure that everyone on the health care team is aware that a patient is, or may be, latex allergic. Place a medical alert or allergy band around the patient's wrist, and clearly flag the patient's status on the chart. Remove all natural rubber latex products from the area. Use latex-free measures to prepare the patient's medication. Have a crash cart standing by stocked with latex-free equipment, supplies, and drugs for treating anaphylaxis. As ordered, give preoperative prophylactic treatment with glucocorticoid steroids and antihistamines. Box 42-5 lists interventions for the perioperative care of patients with risk for latex allergy response.

Box 42-5 Responding to a Patient's Risk for Latex Allergy

LATEX-ALERT PATIENT (HIGH RISK FOR ALLERGIC RESPONSE)
- No premedications are required.
- No special pharmaceutical protocols are required.
- Use nonlatex gloves.
- Use latex-safe supplies.
- Keep a latex-safe supply cart available in patient's area.

LATEX-ALLERGY PATIENT (SUSPECTED OR KNOWN ALLERGIC RESPONSE)
- Administer prophylactic treatment with steroids and antihistamines preoperatively.
- Prepare a latex-safe environment, include latex-safe supply cart and crash cart.
- Apply cloth barrier to patient's arm under a blood pressure cuff.
- Use medications from glass ampules.
- Do not puncture rubber stoppers with needles.
- Wear synthetic gloves.
- Use latex-free syringes.
- Use latex-safe (polyvinyl chloride) intravenous (IV) tubing.
- Do not use latex preparation on IV bags.

Respiratory Preparation

If a general anesthetic is administered, it is essential to ventilate the lungs postoperatively to prevent or treat atelectasis, improve lung expansion, improve oxygenation, and prevent postoperative pneumonia. Because the lungs do not expand fully during surgery, mucus and gases remain in the lungs until expelled. Pulmonary exercises can assist in expanding the lungs and removing these by-products. Preoperative introduction to the use of the incentive spirometer is of great value to the patient.

In spirometry, referred to as **incentive spirometry,** the patient uses a device (spirometer) at the bedside at regular intervals to promote deep breathing (Skill 42-2). The amount of air inspired is measured and the patient encouraged to attain the established goal. The respiratory therapist calculates the patient's maximum inspiratory capacity based on height, age, and sex, taking into consideration the type of surgery performed. At rest, the usual tidal capacity is 500 mL of inspired air. In a tall, healthy young man, a tidal capacity of 4300 mL is not uncommon. Because of postoperative pain, a postoperative inspiratory capacity of one half to three fourths of the preoperative volume is acceptable.

To encourage patient use, place the spirometer in the bed or close by on the bedside stand. The usual rate of use is 8 to 10 breaths hourly during waking hours.

There are two general types of incentive spirometers:

1. **Flow-oriented inspiratory spirometer:** This type of incentive spirometer is inexpensive and measures inspiration. It contains one or more clear plastic cylinder chambers that contain freely movable, colored, lightweight plastic balls. Instruct the patient to place the mouthpiece in the mouth and inhale slowly and deeply; this raises the balls in the cylinders. Encourage the patient to keep the colored balls floating as long as possible. The degree of elevation is marked on the

Patient Teaching

Incentive Spirometry
- After incentive spirometry exercises, patients should practice controlled coughing techniques.
- Teach patients to examine their sputum for consistency, amount, and color changes.
- Before discharge, have patients return a demonstration of the correct procedure for use.
- Administer breathing treatments before patients' meals to prevent nausea and vomiting.

Skill 42-2 Incentive Spirometry or Positive Expiratory Pressure Therapy and "Huff" Coughing

Nursing Action *(Rationale)*

1. Refer to physician's orders, care plan, or Kardex. *(Health care facilities frequently require a medical order for incentive spirometry.)*
2. Assess patient's respiratory status and lung sounds. Indications for spirometry are (a) asymmetric chest wall movement, (b) increased respiratory rate, (c) increased production of sputum, and (d) diminished lung expansion postoperatively. *(Alerts health care personnel to those patients at risk for respiratory complications during illness or after surgery.)*
3. Explain procedure, and instruct patient in the correct use of the spirometer. Frequently the respiratory therapist will do this. However, it may be the nurse's responsibility to follow up and promote proper technique. *(Understanding improves compliance with use.)*
4. Obtain supplies and equipment. *(Organizes procedure.)*
   a. Incentive spirometer or positive expiratory pressure (PEP) therapy device
   b. Emesis basin
   c. Tissues
   d. Bedside trash bag
   e. Clean gloves (if soiling is likely)
5. Wash hands and don gloves (if soiling is likely). Know agency policy and guidelines from the Centers for Disease Control and Prevention and the Occupational Safety and Health Administration. *(Reduces spread of microorganisms.)*

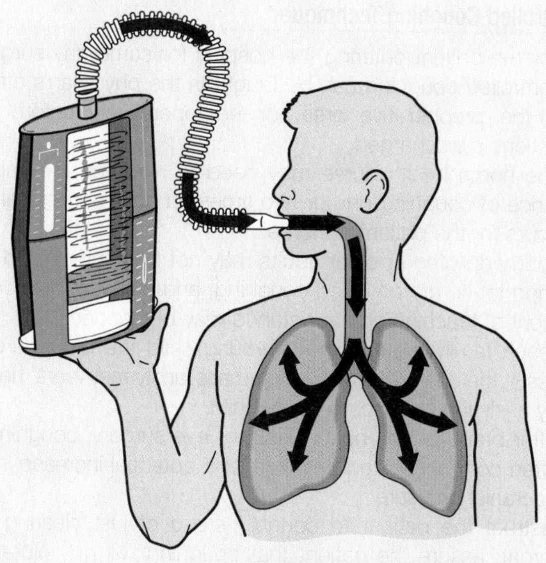
Step 9a

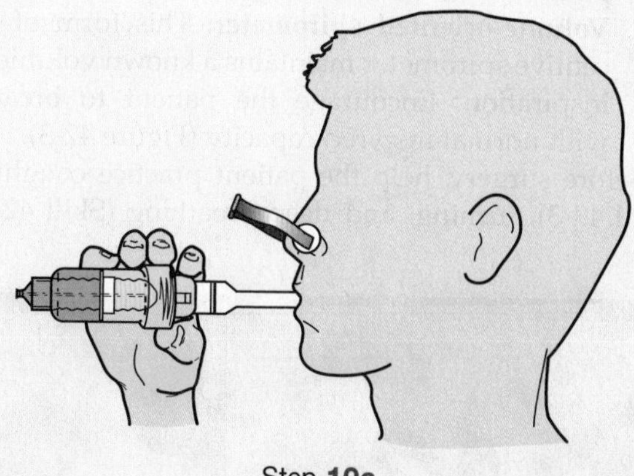
Step 10c

6. Place prescribed incentive spirometer at the bedside. *(Prepares equipment for procedure.)*
7. Place patient in semi-Fowler's or full Fowler's position. *(Promotes optimal lung expansion.)*
8. Place tissues, emesis basin, and bedside trash bag within easy reach. *(Enables sanitary disposal of respiratory secretions expectorated during procedure.)*
9. Incentive spirometry
   a. Instruct patient to completely cover mouthpiece with lips (use a noseclip if patient is unable to breathe through the mouthpiece) and to (a) inhale slowly until maximum inspiration is reached, (b) hold breath 2 or 3 seconds, and (c) slowly exhale (see illustration). *(Promotes maximum inspiration.)*
   b. Instruct patient to relax and breathe normally for a short time. *(Prevents patient from hyperventilating and prevents fatigue.)*
   c. Instruct and encourage patient to gradually increase depth of inspiration. *(Promotes maximum lung expansion.)*
   d. Offer oral hygiene after spirometry is completed. *(Patients often find this refreshing.)*
   e. Store spirometer in an appropriate place, such as the bedside table, until next scheduled time. *(Provides a convenient place for repeated use.)*
10. PEP therapy and "huff" coughing
    a. Wash hands. *(Reduces transmission of microorganisms.)*
    b. Set PEP device for setting ordered. *(The higher the setting, the more effort required.)*
    c. Instruct patient to assume semi-Fowler's or high Fowler's position, and place noseclip on patient's nose (see illustration). *(Promotes optimum lung expansion and expectoration of mucus.)*
    d. Instruct patient to place lips around mouthpiece and (1) take a full breath and exhale two or three times longer than inhalation and (b) repeat this pattern for 10 to 20 breaths. *(Ensures that all breathing is done through the mouth and that the device is used properly.)*
    e. Remove device from mouth, and have patient take a slow, deep breath and hold for 3 seconds. *(Promotes lung expansion before coughing.)*
    f. Instruct patient to exhale in quick, short, forced "huffs." *("Huff" coughing, or forced expiratory technique, promotes bronchial hygiene by increasing expectoration of secretions.)*
11. Position patient as desired or as ordered. *(Helps maintain patient comfort and promotes maximum chest expansion.)*
12. Place call light within easy reach. *(Maintains patient safety.)*
13. Remove and dispose of soiled gloves and wash hands. *(Reduces spread of microorganisms.)*
14. Assess respiratory status and evaluate patient's response to spirometry. *(Provides a basis for repeated use.)*
15. Document in nurse's notes patient's respiratory status before and after incentive spirometry, type of spirometry, and any adverse effects from the procedure. *(Verifies patient care. Some agencies require such documentation for third-party reimbursements.)*
16. Carry out patient teaching (see Patient Teaching box, Incentive Spirometry).

cylinders so that this, plus the length of time the patient maintains elevation, can be recorded.

2. **Volume-oriented spirometer:** This form of incentive spirometer maintains a known volume of inspiration. Encourage the patient to breathe with normal inspired capacity (Figure 42-3).

Before surgery, help the patient practice coughing (Skill 42-3), turning, and deep breathing (Skill 42-4).

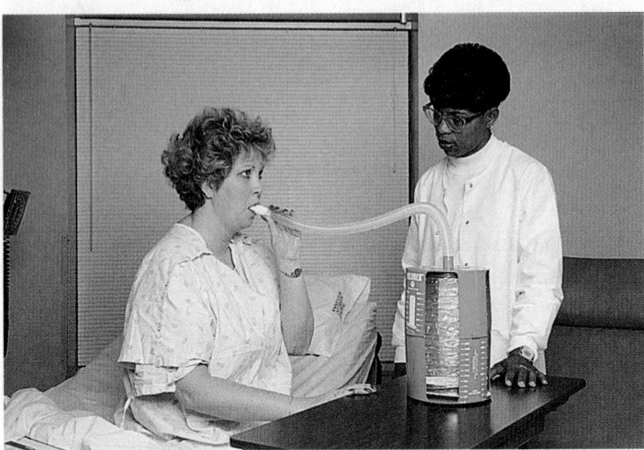

FIGURE 42-3 Volume-oriented spirometer.

Patient Teaching

Controlled Coughing Technique

- For the patient entering the hospital for same-day surgery, controlled coughing can be taught in the physician's office, in the preoperative area, or postoperatively before the patient is discharged.
- The home health nurse may need to reinforce the importance of coughing one or two times an hour during waking hours for the patient at home.
- Young children or older adults may not fully understand the importance of controlled coughing, and continual reinforcement of teaching and assistance may be needed.
- Teach family members of a young child the procedure to assist the child. This also helps meet family members' needs by assisting in the care of the child.
- After brain, spinal, head, neck, or eye surgery, coughing is often contraindicated because of a potential increase in intracranial pressure.
- Instruct the patient to cough instead of just clearing the throat; assure the patient that coughing will not injure the incision.
- Teach the patient to examine the sputum for odor, consistency, amount, and color changes.

Skill 42-3 Teaching Controlled Coughing

Nursing Action *(Rationale)*

1. Refer to medical record, care plan, or Kardex for special interventions. *(Provides basis for care.)*
2. Obtain equipment. *(Organizes procedure.)*
   a. Pillow or bath blanket
   b. Gloves
   c. Emesis basin
   d. Facial tissues
   e. Chair or bed
3. Introduce self. *(Decreases patient's anxiety.)*
4. Identify patient. *(Ensures correct patient for procedure.)*
5. Explain procedure. *(Seeks cooperation.)*
6. Wash hands and don clean gloves according to agency policy and guidelines from the Centers for Disease Control and Prevention and the Occupational Safety and Health Administration. *(Reduces spread of microorganisms.)*
7. Assist patient to upright position. Place pillow between bed or chair and patient. *(Facilitates deep breathing and optimum chest expansion.)*
8. Demonstrate coughing exercise for patient (see illustration). *(Allows patient to observe nurse and to ask questions.)*
   a. Take several deep breaths. *(Deep breaths expand lungs fully so that air moves behind mucus and facilitates effect of coughing.)*

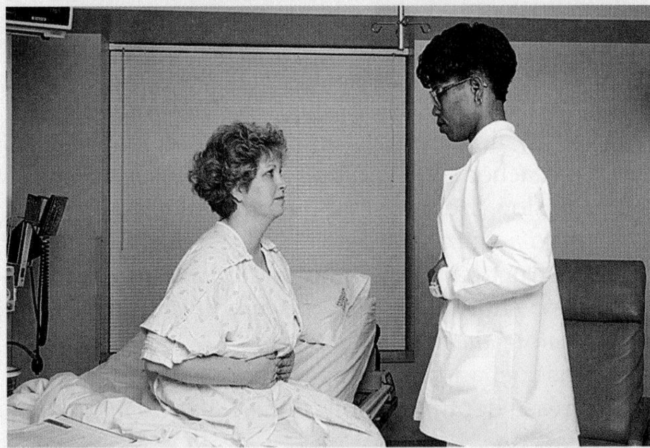

Step 8

   b. Inhale through nose.
   c. Exhale through mouth with pursed lips.
   d. Inhale deeply again and hold breath for count of three.
   e. Cough two or three consecutive times without inhaling between coughs. *(Consecutive coughs remove mucus more effectively and completely than one forceful cough.)*
9. Caution patient against just clearing the throat instead of coughing. *(Clearing the throat does not remove mucus from deep in airways.)*

10. Abdominal or thoracic incision can be splinted before coughing with hands, pillow, towel, or rolled bath blanket (see illustration). *(Surgical incision cuts through muscles, tissues, and nerve endings. Deep breathing and coughing place additional stress on suture line and cause discomfort. Splinting incision provides firm support and reduces incisional pulling.)*

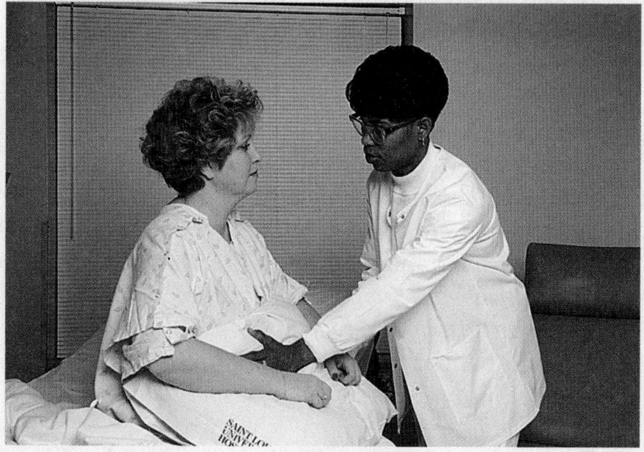

Step **10**

11. Encourage patient to practice coughing while splinting incisional area once or twice an hour during waking hours. Assist patient as indicated. *(Helps effectively expectorate mucus with minimal discomfort.)*
12. Remind patient to use tissues and emesis basin for any mucus expectorated. *(Reduces spread of microorganisms.)*
13. Teach patient to examine sputum for consistency, amount, and color change. *(Changes could indicate respiratory complications such as pneumonia.)*
14. Provide wash cloth and warm water for washing hands and face, provide for oral hygiene, and return patient to comfortable position. *(Provides for patient comfort.)*
15. Remove and dispose of soiled gloves and wash hands. *(Reduces spread of microorganisms.)*
16. Document exercises performed and patient's ability to perform them independently. *(Verifies care given and patient teaching.)*
17. Carry out patient teaching (see Patient Teaching box, Controlled Coughing Technique).

Skill 42-4 Teaching Postoperative Breathing Techniques, Leg Exercises, and Turning

Nursing Action *(Rationale)*

1. Refer to medical record, care plan, or Kardex for special interventions. *(Provides basis for care.)*
2. Obtain equipment. *(Helps organize procedure.)*
   a. Support pillow, towel, or folded bath blanket
   b. Gloves
   c. Emesis basin
   d. Facial tissues
3. Introduce self. *(Decreases patient's anxiety.)*
4. Identify patient. *(Verifies correct patient for procedure.)*
5. Explain procedure to patient. *(Improves cooperation and decreases anxiety.)*
6. Wash hands and don clean gloves. Know agency policy and guidelines from the Centers for Disease Control and Prevention and the Occupational Safety and Health Administration. *(Reduces spread of microorganisms.)*
7. Prepare patient for intervention.
   a. Close door to room or pull curtain. *(Provides privacy.)*
   b. Drape for procedure if necessary.
8. Raise bed to comfortable working level. *(Promotes proper body mechanics.)*
9. Premedicate with pain medication, if indicated. *(Elicits patient compliance.)*

Postoperative Breathing Techniques

10. Place pillow between patient and bed or chair. *(Allows for fuller chest expansion. [Bed or chair itself is too firm to provide expansion.])*
11. Sit or stand facing patient. *(Allows patient to observe nurse.)*
12. Demonstrate taking slow, deep breaths. Avoid moving shoulders and chest while inhaling. Inhale through nose. *(Prevents panting and hyperventilation. Moistens, filters, and warms inhaled air.)*
13. Hold breath for a count of three, and slowly exhale through pursed lips. *(Allows for gradual expulsion of air.)*
14. Repeat exercise three to five times. Have patient practice exercise. *(Allows patient to observe appropriate technique. Allows nurse to assess patient's technique and correct errors.)*

Continued

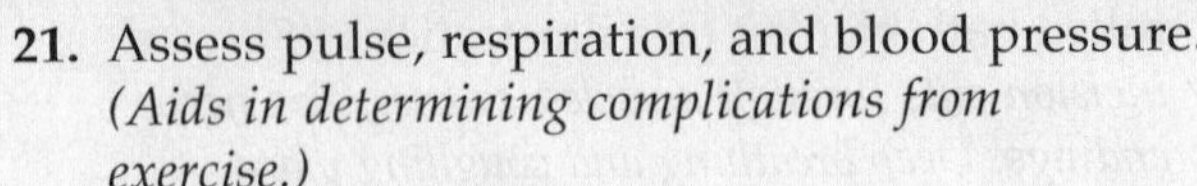

Skill 42-4 Teaching Postoperative Breathing Techniques, Leg Exercises, and Turning—cont'd

15. Instruct patient to take 10 slow, deep breaths every 2 hours until ambulatory. *(Helps prevent postoperative complications.)*
16. If there is an abdominal or chest incision, instruct patient to splint incisional area using pillow or bath blanket, if desired, during breathing exercises. *(Provides support and additional security for patient.)*

Leg Exercises

17. Lifting one leg at a time and supporting joints, gently flex and extend leg 5 to 10 times (see illustration). *(Stimulates circulation and helps prevent thrombi formation.)*
18. Repeat exercise with opposite extremity. Lifting leg while supporting joints, gently flex leg 5 to 10 times. *(Stimulates circulation and helps prevent thrombi formation.)*
19. Alternately point toes toward the chin and toward the foot of the bed four or five times. *(Uses additional muscle flexion and contraction to stimulate circulation.)*
20. Make circle with ankles of both feet four or five times to the left and four or five times to the right (see illustration). *(Further stimulates circulation through muscle contraction and flexion.)*
21. Assess pulse, respiration, and blood pressure. *(Aids in determining complications from exercise.)*

Turning Exercises

22. Instruct patient to assume supine position to right side of bed. Have side rails on both sides of bed in up position. *(Positioning begins on right side of bed so that turning to left side will not cause patient to roll toward bed's edge. Side rails in the raised position promote patient safety.)*
23. Instruct patient to place left hand over incisional area to splint it. *(Supports and minimizes pulling on suture line during turning.)*
24. Instruct patient to keep left leg straight and flex right knee up and over left leg. *(Straight leg stabilizes patient's position. Flexed right leg shifts weight for easier turning.)*
25. Instruct patient to turn every 2 hours while awake. *(Reduces risk of vascular and pulmonary complications.)*
26. Remove and dispose of soiled gloves and wash hands. *(Reduces spread of microorganisms.)*
27. Document. *(Records patient education and verifies procedure.)*

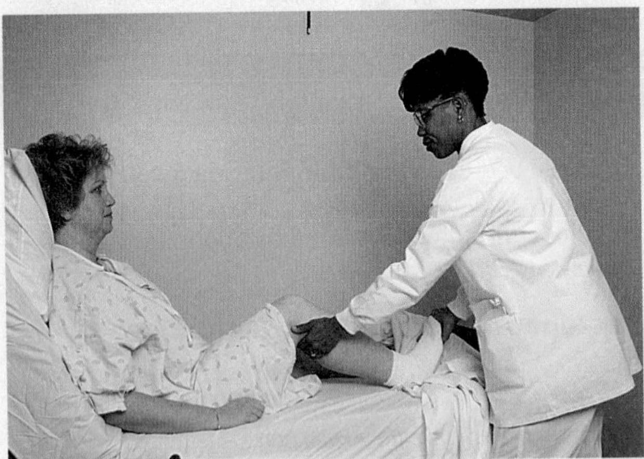

Step **17**

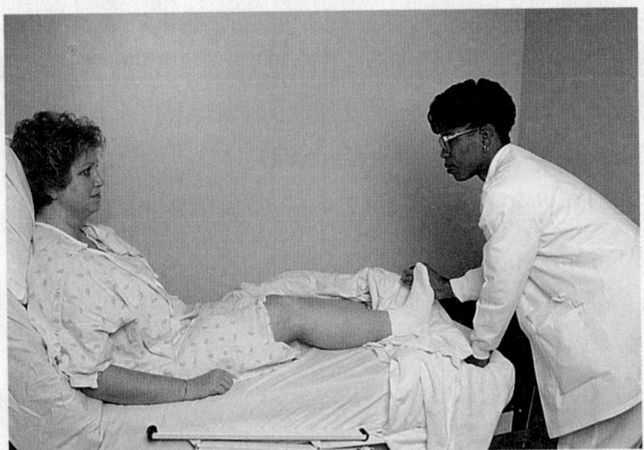

Step **20**

Because coughing increases intracranial pressure, it is usually contraindicated in cranial and spinal-related surgeries. Coughing is also contraindicated for patients having cataract surgery (Box 42-6). Some physicians believe coughing may actually cause alveolar collapse and order only incentive spirometry. Patients frequently ambulate within a few hours of surgery to return cardiovascular and respiratory functions to normal more quickly.

Cardiovascular Considerations

Accompanying the need to turn, cough, and deep breathe is the need to practice leg exercises (see Skill 42-4). Because blood stasis occurs when the patient lies flat, encourage him or her to do leg exercises to assist venous blood flow. With the venous blood slowing, a **thrombus** (an accumulation of platelets, fibrin, clotting factors, and cellular elements of the blood attached to the anterior wall of a vessel, sometimes oc-

Box 42-6 Surgeries for Which Coughing Is Contraindicated or Modified

- **Intracranial:** Coughing increases intracranial pressure (ICP), leading to cerebrospinal fluid leak.
- **Eye:** Coughing increases ICP, which then increases intraocular pressure, causing pressure on suture line.
- **Ear:** Mouth must be kept open if coughing occurs to prevent pressure backup through eustachian tube to middle ear, causing pressure on suture line.
- **Nose:** Mouth must be kept open if coughing occurs to prevent dislodgment of a clot with subsequent bleeding.
- **Throat:** Vigorous coughing may dislodge a clot with subsequent bleeding.
- **Spinal:** Coughing increases spinal canal pressure.

cluding the lumen) may form. If a thrombus is dislodged, it can travel as an **embolus** to the lungs, the heart, or the brain, where the vessel can be occluded. Without an adequate blood supply, an **infarct** (localized area of necrosis) can occur. Antiembolism stockings (thromboembolic deterrent stockings), a Jobst pump, or sequential compression devices (SCDs) with intermittent external pneumonic compression system may be ordered to provide support and to prevent venous thrombus in the lower extremities (Skill 42-5).

Consider the following points when applying antiembolism stockings.

Patient Teaching

Use of Thromboembolic Deterrent Stockings and Sequential Compression Devices

- Teach patient to correctly apply antiembolism stockings.
- Teach patient appropriate care of the stockings. (Wash in warm water and mild soap, do not wring dry, and lay over flat surface to dry.)
- Instruct patient not to massage legs because of the risk of dislodging a thrombus.
- Teach patient the signs of possible complications. (If stockings or devices are too restrictive, edema and pain could result.)

- Postoperative patients with abdominal or thoracic incisions will not be able to bend and pull on their own stockings.
- Stockings may be difficult to fit and maintain in obese or very thin patients.
- Stockings may be difficult to apply for elderly patients; the nurse or family members will need to assist.

Vital Signs

Vital signs mirror the body's response to anesthesia and surgery. Instruct the patient before surgery that it is normal for blood pressure, temperature, pulse, and respiration to be monitored until stable. The schedule

Skill 42-5 Applying Thromboembolic Deterrent Stockings and Sequential Compression Devices

Nursing Action *(Rationale)*

1. Refer to medical record, care plan, or Kardex for special interventions. *(Provides basis for care.)*
2. Obtain equipment. *(Organizes procedure.)*
   a. Thromboembolic deterrent stockings (TEDs) or sequential compression devices (SCDs)
   b. Clean gloves (when appropriate)
   c. Tape measure
3. Introduce self. *(Decreases patient's anxiety.)*
4. Identify patient. *(Identifies correct patient for procedure.)*
5. Explain procedure. *(Seeks cooperation and decreases anxiety.)*
6. Wash hands and, if appropriate, don clean gloves. Know agency policy and guidelines from the Centers for Disease Control and Prevention and the Occupational Safety and Health Administration. *(Reduces spread of microorganisms.)*
7. Prepare patient.
   a. Close door to room, pull curtain, and drape for procedure, if necessary. *(Provides privacy.)*
8. Raise bed to comfortable working level. *(Promotes proper body mechanics.)*
9. Examine legs and assess risk for conditions. *(Helps nurse determine presence of pigmentation around ankles, pitting edema, or peripheral cyanosis, which may indicate inadequate circulation.)*
10. Assess patient for calf pain or positive Homans' sign. *(May indicate presence of thrombophlebitis.)*
11. Measure legs for stockings according to agency policy, and order stockings. *(Promotes the correct size to accomplish purpose of stockings.)*

Thromboembolic Deterrent Stockings

12. Assist patient to supine position to apply stockings before patient rises. Patient should be recumbent for at least 30 minutes before application. *(Prevents veins from becoming distended or edema from occurring.)*
13. Turn stockings inside out as far as heel. Place thumbs inside foot part, and slip stocking on until heel is correctly aligned (Figure 42-4, *A* and *B*). *(Positions stocking for appropriate application.)*

Continued

Skill 42-5 Applying Thromboembolic Deterrent Stockings and Sequential Compression Devices—cont'd

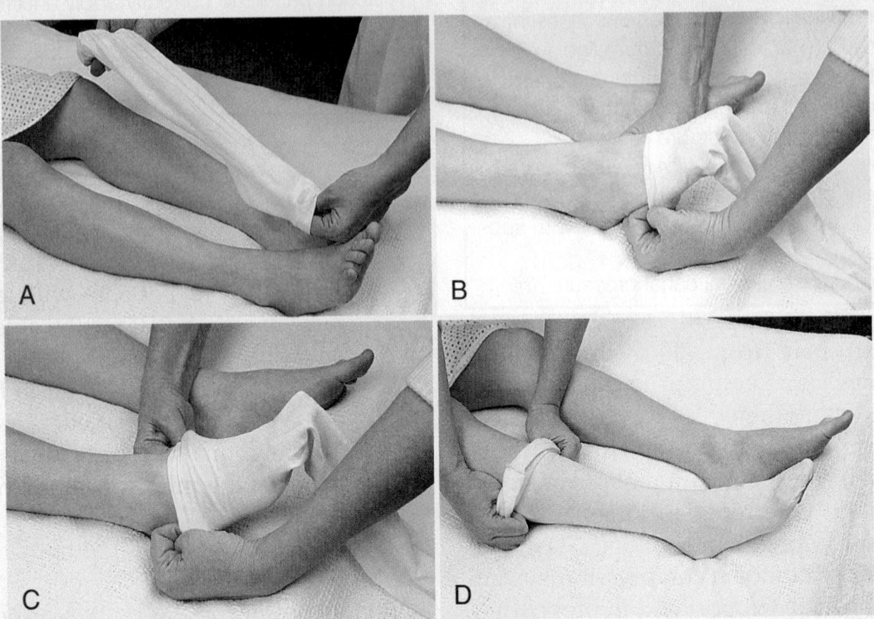

FIGURE 42-4 Applying antiembolism stockings. **A,** Turn the elastic stocking inside out by placing one hand into the sock, holding the toes of the sock with the other hand, and pulling. **B,** Place the patient's toes into the foot of the elastic stocking, making sure that the sock is smooth. **C,** Slide remaining portion of the sock over the patient's foot, making sure that the toes are covered. Sock will now be right-side out. **D,** Slide the sock up over the patient's calf until the sock is completely extended. Be sure that the sock is smooth with no ridges.

14. Gather fabric and ease it over ankle and up the leg (Figure 42-4, C). *(Prevents bunching of stocking, which can cause local pooling of blood.)*
15. Pull leg portion of stocking over foot and up as far as it will go, making certain that gusset lies over femoral artery. Adjust stocking to fit evenly and smoothly with no wrinkles (Figure 42-4, D). *(Allows appropriate fit and application, which are vital for maintaining even pressure. Prevents irritation and impediments to circulation.)*
16. Repeat steps 12 to 15 for opposite extremity. *(Ensures appropriate application.)*

Sequential Compression Devices (Figure 42-5)

17. Place sleeve under patient's leg, with fuller portion at top of thigh. *(Ensures correct fit.)*
18. Apply sleeve with opening at front of knee and closed portion behind knee. *(Ensures appropriate placement and desired effect.)*
19. When the SCD is in place, make sure there are no wrinkles or creases in stockings. Fold Velcro strips over to secure stockings. *(Allows proper functioning of stockings and prevents irritation.)*
20. Attach tubing to SCD after both sleeves are applied. Align arrows for correct connection and appropriate effect. Plug in unit. *(Allows air to inflate stockings in sequential order.)*

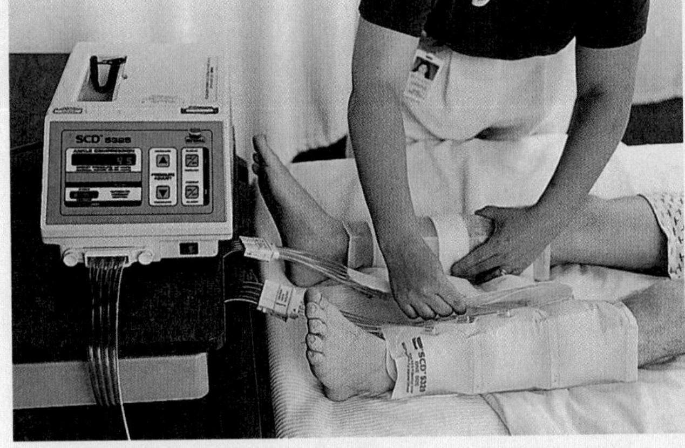

FIGURE 42-5 Application of sequential compression devices.

21. Assess patient periodically. *(Determines presence of edema or cyanosis.)*
22. Assess stocking at regular intervals. *(Ensures that top has not rolled down or loosened and that no wrinkles are present.)*
23. Remove and dispose of soiled gloves and wash hands. *(Reduces spread of microorganisms.)*
24. Document. *(Verifies patient care.)*
25. Carry out patient teaching (see Patient Teaching box, Use of Thromboembolic Deterrent Stockings and Sequential Compression Devices, p. 1269).

for monitoring vital signs depends on the hospital's protocol and the patient's stability. Preoperative vital signs serve as the baseline for deciding when stability has returned or problems arise. Postoperative vital signs are discussed later in this chapter.

Genitourinary Considerations

After general anesthesia, the urinary bladder's tone is decreased. Therefore you should know the patient's normal bladder habits and identify when the bladder is full and distended. Inform the patient preoperatively that the lower part of the abdomen will be palpated at intervals to check for bladder fullness (Figure 42-6). Once patients are awake and tolerating fluids, encourage an adequate intake. Occasionally a urinary catheter is inserted to monitor urinary output. This procedure is normally reserved for patients undergoing urinary surgery or those who may have difficulty voiding. The catheter is usually removed 1 or 2 days postoperatively to reduce the chance of bladder infection. Once it is removed, encourage the patient to drink 8 ounces of fluids per hour while awake unless contraindicated. Also, monitor intake and output (I&O) values until the patient's normal voiding pattern returns. Urinary retention and urinary tract infections are common postoperative complications.

Surgical Wounds

With today's technologies, **incisions** (cuts produced surgically by a sharp instrument to create an opening into an organ or body space) are closed in a variety of ways: sutures, staples, Steri-Strips, or transparent strips. Knowing the type of closure enables you to explain its appearance to the patient. Some surgeries require the removal of exudate, often with a drain. Explain the purpose of the drain and the need for close monitoring. Although not all incisions require dressings, assess the wound's appearance. Wound care, dressing changes, and drainage systems are described in more detail in Chapters 12, 13, and 20.

Pain

Patients fear pain more than any other postsurgical complication. Emphasize to the patient that pain relief is an important part of care. Various methods are used to reduce discomfort. If the patient is considering nonpharmacologic analgesia (e.g., imagery, biofeedback, relaxation techniques), review these techniques and allow practice time. The majority of patients choose traditional analgesia. Postoperative pain is what the patient says it is, so it is important to reassure patients that addiction to analgesics rarely occurs in the time frame needed for comfort. For the patient who is apprehensive about intermittent injections, patient-controlled analgesia (PCA) and opioids injected into the epidural space (patient-controlled epidural) are safe and effective for postoperative pain management. When the patient is allowed oral intake, oral analgesics coupled with nontraditional methods are often effective (see Chapter 16).

Tubes

Depending on the surgery, patient teaching includes information about nasogastric (NG) tubes, wound evacuation units, and IV and oxygen therapy. Allowing patients to view the equipment and apparatus and understand their purposes lessens the fear associated with each. (See Chapters 13 and 20 for more detailed discussion of the tubes and drains used in the postoperative patient.)

Preoperative Medication

Preoperative medication reduces the patient's anxiety, decreases the amount of anesthetic needed, and reduces respiratory tract secretions. Provide the patient with information on what to expect from preoperative medications. Barbiturates and tranquilizers (phenobarbital and diazepam [Valium]) are sometimes given for sedation to reduce the amount of the anesthetic required. Opioid analgesics (meperidine and morphine) may be administered by intermittent injection or PCA if the patient has pain before surgery; this also reduces the amount of anesthetic required. An introduction to PCA preoperatively helps patients understand the concept and how the equipment works. Anticholinergics such as atropine reduce spasms of smooth muscles and decrease gastric, bronchial, and salivary secretions (Table 42-5).

The patient frequently becomes drowsy, notices a dry mouth, and experiences vertigo after receiving the

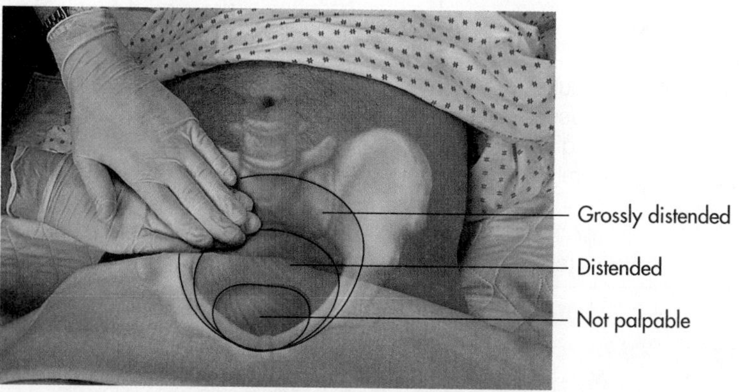

FIGURE 42-6 Assess the bladder by palpating the lower abdomen for distention.

Table 42-5 Medications for the Perioperative Period

Generic (Trade)	Dose and Route	Action	Nursing Implications
BENZODIAZEPINES			
Midazolam (Versed, Valium, Ativan)	Dose depends on the amount of adequate sedation necessary for surgery	Decreases anxiety and produces sedation Induces amnesia	Monitor for respiratory depression, hypotension, drowsiness, and lack of coordination.
Diazepam	5-20 mg po		
Lorazepam	44 mcg/kg to 2 mg IV		
OPIOID ANALGESICS			
Morphine (Morphine) Fentanyl citrate (Sublimaze)	5-15 mg IM, IV 50 mcg/mL IM or slow IV	Decreases anxiety Allows decreased anesthetics	Monitor for respiratory depression, nausea, vomiting, orthostatic hypotension, and pruritus.
H_2 RECEPTOR ANTAGONISTS			
Famotidine (Pepcid) Ranitidine (Zantac)	20 mg IV 50 mg IV	Reduces gastric acid volume and concentration	Monitor for confusion and dizziness in older adults.
ANTIEMETICS			
Metoclopramide (Reglan) Droperidol (Inapsine) Ondansetron HCl (5-HT_3 receptor antagonist) (Zofran)	10 mg IV or IM 2.5-10 mg 4 mg IV	Enhances gastric emptying Tranquilizer Prevents postoperative nausea and vomiting	Monitor for sedation and extrapyramidal reaction (involuntary movement, muscle tone changes, and abnormal posture). Instruct patient to report any difficulty breathing.
ANTICHOLINERGICS			
Atropine sulfate (Atropine sulfate) Glycopyrrolate (Robinul)	0.4-0.6 mg IM or IV 0.1-0.3 mg IM or IV	Reduces oral and respiratory secretions to decrease risk of aspiration Decreases vomiting and laryngospasm	Monitor for confusion, restlessness, and tachycardia. Prepare patient to expect dry mouth.
ANTIBIOTICS			
Cefazolin sodium (Ancef)	1-2 g q6h Maximum 12 g/day	Bactericidal Wound infection Minimizes risk of wound infection	If large doses are given, therapy is prolonged or patient is at high risk, monitor for signs and symptoms of superinfection, including abdominal pain, moderate to severe diarrhea, severe anal or genital pruritus, and severe mouth soreness. Determine patient's history of allergies. If dosing continues, space drug evenly around the clock. Advise patient to complete therapy.
Cefotaxime sodium (Claforan)	1 g IM or IV 30-90 min preoperative	Bactericidal	
Ceftriaxone (Rocephin)	1 g IM or IV 0.5-2 hr preoperative	Bactericidal as perioperative prophylaxis	
ADRENOCORTICAL STEROID			
Methylprednisolone (Depo-Medrol, Solu-Medrol)	Adults: 10-250 mg (succinate) IV q 4-6 hr Oral 2-60 mg in 4 divided doses IM 10-80 mg (acetate)	Decreases inflammation	Determine whether patient has hypersensitivity to drug. Determine whether patient has diabetes mellitus, and anticipate an increase in antidiabetic drug regimen because of raised blood glucose level.

Table 42-5 Medications for the Perioperative Period—cont'd

Generic (Trade)	Dose and Route	Action	Nursing Implications
NONSTEROIDAL ANTIINFLAMMATORY DRUG (NSAID)			
Ketorolac (Toradol)	50 mg/mL IM; 30 mg/mL IV push over at least 15 sec	Reduces intensity of pain Reduces inflammation	Assess the duration, location, onset, and type of pain the patient is having. Evaluate patient for therapeutic response.
ANTICOAGULANTS			
Enoxaparin sodium (Lovenox)	30 mg/0.3 mL to 150 mg/mL subQ in prefilled syringes	Produces anticoagulation Prevents new clot formation or secondary embolic complications	Do not give IM, but give subQ. Tell the patient not to take aspirin or similar over-the-counter drugs.
Heparin sodium (Heparin)	10 units/mL to 15,000 units/ 500 mL subQ Heparin sodium flush syringes: 10 units/ mL, 100 units/mL; vials (most use saline for the flush) 10 units/mL ≤100 units/mL; vials 10-100 units/mL		Cross-check heparin dose with another nurse before administering. Use constant rate IV infusion pump. Monitor the patient's partial thromboplastin time diligently. Assess patient's gums for erythema and gingival bleeding; skin for bruises or petechiae; and urine for hematuria.
Warfarin sodium (Coumadin)	5 mg vials IM; 1-10 mg po tablets or IV		Observe patient for evidence of hemorrhage such as abdominal or back pain, decreased blood pressure, increased pulse rate, and severe headache. Urge patient to not ingest alcohol or make drastic dietary changes. If administration continues, urge patient to notify the physician if he or she experiences black stools; bleeding; brown, dark, or red urine; coffee-ground vomitus; or red-speckled mucus from a cough.

preoperative medication. Ask the patient to void beforehand. If preoperative medication is given on the nursing unit, the patient must remain in bed. Institute safety measures, such as putting the bed in low position and raising side rails, and monitor the patient every 15 to 30 minutes until the patient leaves for surgery. Reassure the patient and provide a quiet environment on the nursing unit while waiting for transport to the surgical suite. In many institutions, the preoperative medication is given by the anesthesiologist or anesthesia provider in the preoperative holding area.

Surgery cancels all medications ordered before surgery, except for medications for long-term conditions, such as phenytoin (Dilantin) for seizure control (Table 42-6). The surgeon reorders medication necessary after surgery.

Anesthesia

Anesthesia means the absence of feelings (pain) (*an,* meaning "without," plus *esthesia,* meaning "awareness of feeling"). Anesthesia is divided into three categories: general, regional, and local.

General Anesthesia

Modern anesthetics are much easier to reverse and allow the patient to recover with fewer unwanted effects than in the past. **General anesthesia** results in an immobile, quiet patient who does not recall the surgical procedure. The patient's amnesia acts as protection from the unpleasant events. General anesthesia is used for major surgery requiring extensive tissue manipulation.

An anesthesiologist gives general anesthetics by IV and inhalation routes through the four stages of anesthesia. In **Stage I** the patient is awake and the administra-

Table 42-6 Medications with Special Implications for the Surgical Patient

DRUG CLASS	EFFECTS DURING SURGERY
Antibiotics	Antibiotics potentiate action of anesthetic agents. If taken within 2 weeks before surgery, aminoglycosides (gentamicin, tobramycin, neomycin) may cause mild respiratory depression from depressed neuromuscular transmission.
Antidysrhythmics	Antidysrhythmics can reduce cardiac contractility and impair cardiac conduction during anesthesia.
Anticoagulants	Anticoagulants alter normal clotting factors and thus increase risk of hemorrhaging. They should be discontinued at least 48 hours before surgery. Aspirin is a commonly used medication that can alter clotting mechanisms.
Anticonvulsants	Long-term use of certain anticonvulsants (e.g., phenytoin [Dilantin], phenobarbital) can alter metabolism of anesthetic agents.
Antihypertensives	Antihypertensives interact with anesthetic agents to cause bradycardia, hypotension, and impaired circulation. They inhibit synthesis and storage of norepinephrine in sympathetic nerve endings.
Corticosteroids	With prolonged use, corticosteroids cause adrenal atrophy, which reduces the body's ability to withstand stress. Before and during surgery, dosage may be temporarily increased.
Insulin	Diabetic patient's need for insulin after surgery is reduced because nutritional intake is decreased. Stress response and intravenous administration of glucose solutions can increase dosage requirements after surgery.
Diuretics	Diuretics potentiate electrolyte imbalances (particularly potassium) after surgery.
Nonsteroidal antiinflammatory drugs (NSAIDs)	NSAIDs inhibit platelet aggregation and may prolong bleeding, increasing susceptibility to postoperative bleeding.
Herbal therapies (ginger, ginkgo, ginseng)	These herbal therapies can affect platelet activity and increase susceptibility to postoperative bleeding. Ginseng may increase hypoglycemia with insulin therapy. (See Chapter 17, Complementary and Alternative Therapies.)

Adapted from Potter, P.A., & Perry, A.G. (2007). *Basic nursing: essentials for practice* (6th ed.). St. Louis: Mosby.

tion of anesthetic agents begins. The stage is completed when the patient loses consciousness. **Stage II** begins with the loss of consciousness and ends with the onset of regular breathing and loss of eyelid reflexes. This is referred to as the excitement or delirium phase because it is often accompanied by involuntary motor activity. The patient must not receive any auditory or physical stimulation during this period because it can stimulate a release of catecholamines, which can raise heart rate and blood pressure. **Stage III** begins with the onset of regular breathing and ends if respirations cease This stage is known as the operative or surgical phase. **Stage IV** begins with the cessation of respirations and must be avoided, or it will necessitate the initiation of cardiopulmonary resuscitation and may lead to death. These stages were defined in the past when ether was used and may be less clear with newer anesthetic agents.

A more useful designation of stages includes the three phases of induction, maintenance, and emergence. The **induction phase** includes the administration of agents and endotracheal intubation. The **maintenance phase** includes positioning the patient, preparing the skin for incision, and performing the surgery. Appropriate levels of anesthesia are maintained during this phase. During the **emergence phase,** anesthetics are decreased and the patient begins to awaken. Because of the short half-life of today's medications, emergence often occurs in the OR.

Anesthesia is often induced intravenously, although an inhalation agent may be used. The patient is unconscious 10 to 20 seconds after the dose. Barbiturates provide sedation, amnesia, and hypnosis but must be used with other agents to relieve pain and relax muscles. To prevent aspiration and other respiratory complications, the anesthesiologist puts an endotracheal tube into the patient's airway. Endotracheal intubation is usually performed after administration of short-acting or, occasionally, long-acting muscle relaxants (Figure 42-7).

An anesthesia provider or OR nurse may assist with cricoid pressure during induction of general anesthesia and endotracheal cuff inflation during intubation. Cricoid pressure reduces the risk of aspirating stomach contents by compressing the esophagus to prevent passive regurgitation. (This technique cannot, however, stop active vomiting.) The maneuver is begun while the patient is awake. Patient reassurance is important during this period of mild discomfort. Once initiated, pressure must be held constant until the cuff has been inflated or aspiration can happen rapidly.

When induction is completed, anesthesia may be maintained through a combination of inhalation and IV medications. The patient also receives a continuous supply of oxygen and adjunct medications such as opioid analgesics and muscle relaxants. A combination of smaller amounts of several medications can mean a significant reduction in the dose compared with using a single medication.

The duration of anesthesia depends on the length of surgery. Surgical risks influence the duration of surgery. The greatest risks from general anesthesia are the side effects of anesthetic agents, including cardiovascular depression or irritability, respiratory depression, and liver and kidney damage.

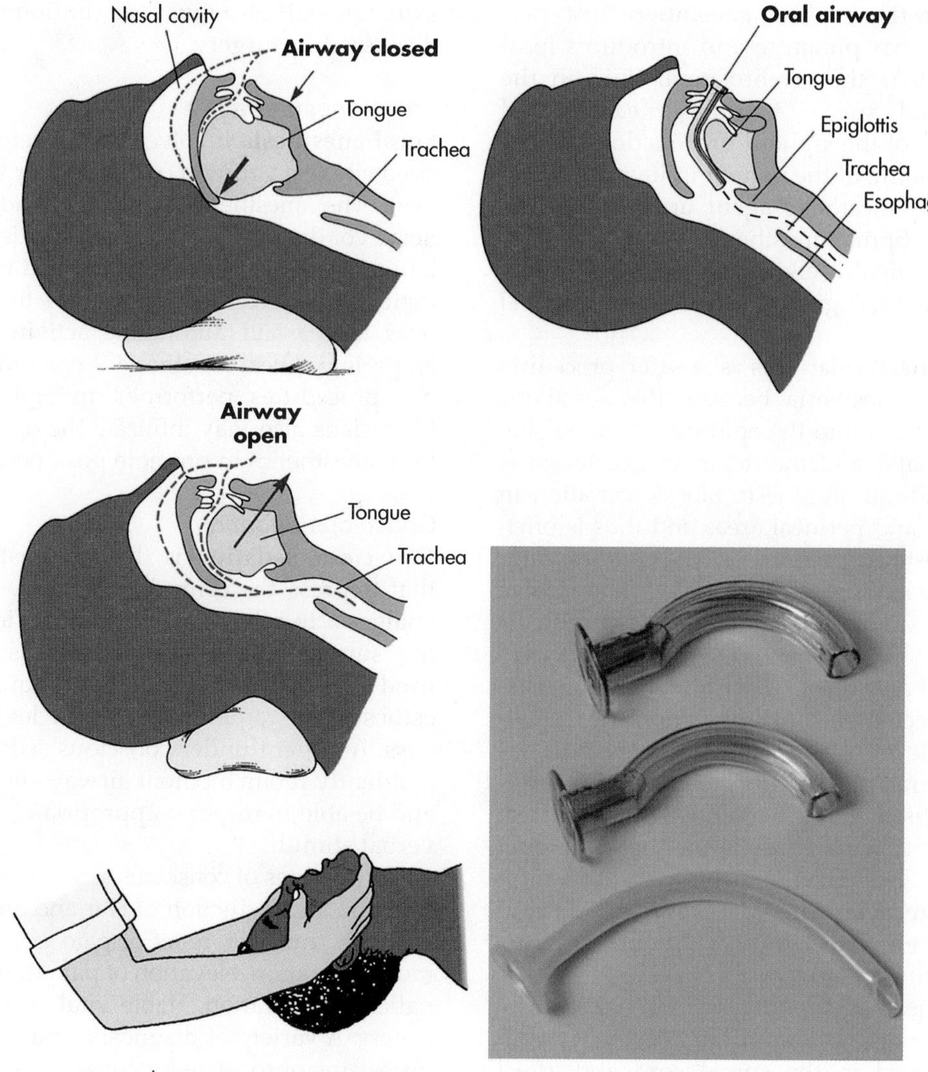

FIGURE 42-7 Possible airways used during surgery.

Emergence from anesthesia occurs when the procedure is completed and reversal agents are given. The oropharynx is suctioned to decrease the risk of aspiration and laryngeal spasm after extubation. Extubation is often accomplished before transfer to the postanesthesia care unit (PACU).

Regional Anesthesia

Induction of **regional anesthesia** results in loss of sensation in an area of the body. The portion of sensory pathways that is anesthetized depends on the method of induction. The patient does not lose consciousness with regional anesthesia, but is usually sedated. The anesthesiologist gives regional anesthetics by infiltration and local application. Figure 42-8 demonstrates common locations for the induction of medication to achieve the regional block.

Infiltration of anesthetic agents may involve one of the following induction methods:

- **Nerve block:** Local anesthetic is injected into a nerve (e.g., brachial plexus in the arms), blocking the nerve supply to the operative site.

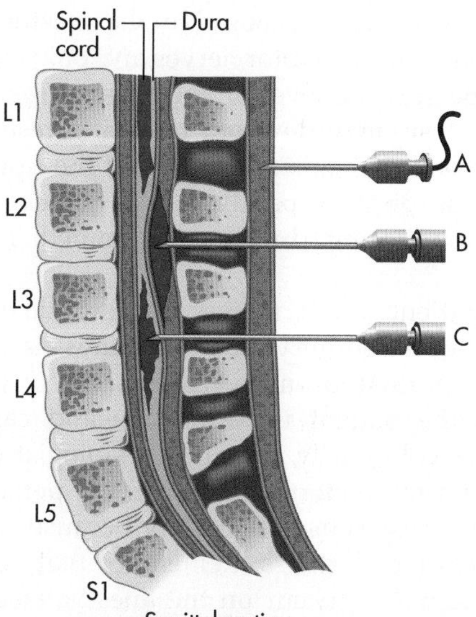

FIGURE 42-8 Spinal column—side view with spinal and epidural anesthesia needle placement. *A,* Epidural catheter. *B,* Single injection epidural. *C,* Spinal anesthesia. (Interspaces most commonly used are L4-L5, L3-L4, and L2-L3.)

- **Spinal anesthesia:** The anesthesiologist performs a lumbar puncture and introduces local anesthetic into the cerebrospinal fluid in the subarachnoid space. Anesthesia can extend from the tip of the xiphoid process down to the feet. Positioning of the patient influences movement of the anesthetic agent up or down the spinal cord. Spinal anesthesia is often used for lower abdominal, pelvic, and lower extremity procedures; urologic procedures; or surgical obstetrics.
- **Epidural anesthesia:** This is a safer procedure than spinal anesthesia because the anesthetic agent is injected into the epidural space outside the dura mater and the depth of anesthesia is lighter. Epidural anesthesia blocks sensation in the vaginal and perineal areas and thus is often used for obstetric procedures. The epidural catheter may be left in so that the patient can receive medication via continuous epidural infusion after surgery.
- **IV regional anesthesia (Bier block):** Local anesthetic is injected via an IV line into an extremity below the level of a tourniquet after blood has been withdrawn. The drug is allowed to infiltrate only tissues in the intended surgical area. The extremity is pain free while the tourniquet is in place. Advantages include a short onset and short recovery time. However, the tourniquet may be inflated for only 2 hours or tissue damage will occur.

Infiltrative anesthesia involves risks, particularly with spinal anesthesia, because the anesthetic agent may move upward in the spinal cord and affect breathing. This migration of anesthetic depends on the drug type and amount and patient position. The patient's blood pressure may suddenly drop due to extensive vasodilation caused by the anesthetic block to sympathetic vasomotor nerves and pain and motor nerve fibers. If the level of anesthesia rises, respiratory paralysis may develop, requiring resuscitation by the anesthesiologist. Elevation of the upper body prevents respiratory paralysis. The patient requires careful monitoring during and immediately after surgery.

The patient under regional anesthesia is awake throughout the surgery unless the physician orders a tranquilizer that promotes sleep and/or amnesia. Because the patient is responsive and capable of breathing voluntarily, the anesthesiologist does not need to use an endotracheal tube. OR personnel often gain a false sense of security because of the patient's relative alertness. Remember that burns and other trauma can occur on the anesthetized part of the body without the patient being aware of the injury. It is therefore necessary to frequently observe the position of extremities and the condition of the skin. OR staff also must use caution regarding topics discussed in surgery.

Local Anesthesia

Local anesthesia involves loss of sensation at the desired site (e.g., growth on the skin or the cornea of the eye). The anesthetic agent (e.g., lidocaine) inhibits nerve conduction until the drug diffuses into the circulation. It may be injected or applied topically. The patient loses sensation of pain and touch, and control over motor and autonomic activities (e.g., bladder emptying). Local anesthesia is commonly used for minor procedures performed in ambulatory surgery. Physicians also may infiltrate the operative area with local anesthetics to promote postoperative pain relief.

Conscious Sedation

Conscious sedation is the administration of drugs that depress the central nervous system or provide analgesia to relieve anxiety or provide amnesia during surgical diagnostic procedures. It is routinely used for procedures that do not require complete anesthesia but rather a depressed level of consciousness. A patient under conscious sedation must independently retain a patent airway and airway reflexes and be able to respond appropriately to physical and verbal stimuli.

Advantages of conscious sedation include adequate sedation and reduction of fear and anxiety with minimal risk, amnesia, relief of pain and noxious stimuli, mood alteration, elevation of pain threshold, enhanced patient cooperation, stable vital signs, and rapid recovery. A variety of diagnostic and therapeutic procedures are appropriate for conscious sedation; these include burn dressing changes, cosmetic surgery, and pulmonary biopsy and bronchoscopy.

Nurses assisting with the administration of conscious sedation must be knowledgeable about anatomy, physiology, cardiac dysrhythmias, procedural complications, and pharmacologic principles related to the administration of individual conscious sedation agents. Nurses must also be able to assess, diagnose, and intervene in the event of untoward reactions and demonstrate skill in airway management and oxygen delivery. Resuscitation equipment must be readily available.

Positioning the Patient for Surgery

During general anesthesia the nursing personnel and surgeon often wait to position the patient until he or she is completely relaxed. The choice of position is usually determined by the surgical approach (Figure 42-9). Ideally the patient's position provides good access to the operative site and sustains adequate circulatory and respiratory function. It should not impair neuromuscular structures. The patient's comfort and safety must be considered. The team must

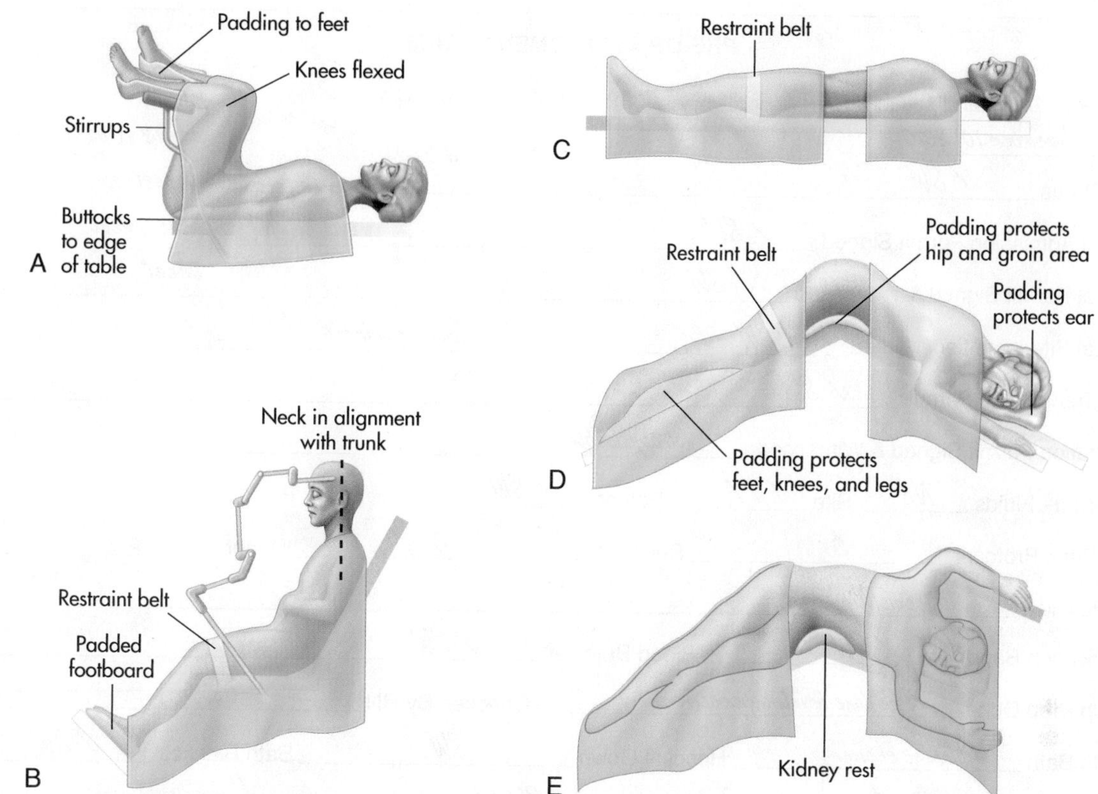

FIGURE 42-9 Common perioperative positions and the padding provided to relieve pressure in each position. **A,** Lithotomy position, used for vaginal and perineal procedures. **B,** Sitting position, used for neurologic procedures. **C,** Supine position (the most common position). Potential pressure points are the occiput, scapula, olecranon, thoracic vertebrae, sacrum, coccyx, and calcaneus. **D,** Jackknife position, used for gluteal and anorectal surgeries. **E,** Lateral kidney position, used for procedures requiring a retroperitoneal approach.

take into account age, weight, height, nutritional status, physical limitations, and preexisting conditions and document them for staff who care for the patient postoperatively. Sometimes nurses in postoperative divisions fail to appreciate the discomfort a patient may feel after surgery (e.g., discomfort of the left arm or side of a patient whose right kidney was removed).

An alert person maintains normal range of joint motion by pain and pressure receptors. If a joint is extended too far, pain reminds the person that muscle joint strain is too great. In a patient who is anesthetized, however, normal defense mechanisms cannot guard against joint damage, muscle stretch, and strain. The muscles are so relaxed that it is relatively easy to place the patient in a position he or she could not assume while awake. The patient often remains in a given position for several hours. Although it may be necessary to place a patient in an unusual position, attempt to maintain correct alignment and protect the patient from pressure, abrasion, and other injuries (e.g., corneal abrasion). Attachments to the OR table allow protection and padding of extremities and bony prominences. Positioning should not interfere with normal movement of the diaphragm or circulation to body parts. If restraints are necessary, pad the area to be restrained to prevent skin trauma (see Chapter 14).

Preoperative Checklist

Complete the preoperative checklist before the patient leaves the nursing unit (Figure 42-10). Signing the preoperative checklist means that you assume responsibility for all areas of care included on the list. If the preoperative medication is to be given on the nursing unit, complete the preoperative checklist before administering the medication. Any **prosthesis** (an artificial replacement for a missing part of the body), contact lenses, dentures, jewelry, and other valuables are removed and either given to family members or placed in a secure area. Some hospitals allow dentures to be worn while in surgery and removed later. If the patient wears rings, they should be secured with tape and noted in the chart. The patient should void before the preoperative medication is administered, or 1 hour before surgery is scheduled. Although most patients become drowsy after administration of a preoperative medication, a few either become hyperactive or demonstrate no side effects. Remind the patient to remain in bed, and raise the side rails. Place the call light within reach and point it out to the patient.

PRE-OP ASSESSMENT FORM

(Please check carefully and initial)

Date *November 10, 2010*

Extra copies on back of post-op assessment sheet

1. DNR Status *✓SW*
2. Medical Admission Permit Signed *✓SW*
3. Surgical Permit Signed & Witnessed *✓SW*
4. Surgical Site Identified/Marked *✓SW* *Left lower quadrant*
5. Blood Transfusion Permit *✓SW*
6. Sterilization Permit Signed & Witnessed *not applicable*
7. IV Started - Fluids *NS* Site *L.7.A* Patent *✓SW*
8. Bone Bank Protocol *ø* Recipient *ø* Donor *ø*
9. Allergies, list: *penicillin*
10. Identification Band *✓SW* Blood Bracelet *✓SW*
11. Pre-Op Prep Done *to be done in intraoperative* Checked By RN ———
12. Pre-Op Bath *Hibiclens shower* Hospital Gown *✓SW* Bath Blanket *✓SW*
13. Remove: Dentures *ø* Glasses/Contacts *✓SW* Jewelry/Nail Polish/Hairpins/Makeup *✓SW*
14. TED stockings when ordered *✓SW* Side Rails Up *✓SW* Patient Labels *✓SW*
15. Pre-Op Vital Signs Time: *1000* T *98⁶* P *80* R *20* BP *120/80* Pain Intensity 0-10 *ø SW*
16. Pre-Op Medications *to be administered in intraoperative*
17. Insert Foley Catheter *✓SW*
18. Physical Disability, such as Amputations, Glass Eye, etc. *ø*
19. Systemic Diseases *type 2 diabetes mellitus* *SW*
20. History and Physical *✓SW*

See Guidelines for pre-op testing policy number 600 - P 118. Testing completed per policy.

21. Lab Reports: *CBC, Basic metabolic profile*

ECG *on chart* *SW* Chest X-Ray *on chart* *SW*

NURSING STAFF IDENTIFICATION

SW Susan Welker RN

22. Infectious Process Present ___ Yes *X* No
Type of Infection ———
23. Additional Comments *pre- & post-op nursing interventions explained*
24. Chart Signed Off *✓SW RN*

Great Plains Regional Medical Center
601 West Leota Street - P.O. Box 1167
North Platte, Nebraska 69103-1167

LABEL

FIGURE 42-10 Preoperative assessment form.

Eliminating Wrong Site and Wrong Procedure Surgery

In 2006, The Joint Commission (TJC) established Universal Protocol guidelines to prevent surgeons from performing surgery on the wrong site or performing the wrong procedure (TJC, 2009a). If an invasive surgical procedure is planned, this protocol must be implemented regardless of location (ambulatory surgery centers, hospital, or health care provider's office). The protocol consists of three main principles:

1. Obtain a preoperative verification that guarantees all relevant documents and studies are available and that they meet the patient's expectations.
2. Mark the operative site with indelible ink, including marking left or right, multiple structures (e.g., toes), and levels of the spine.
3. Just before the start of the procedure, all members of the surgical and procedure team have a time-out to verify they have the correct patient, procedure, site, and any implants.

A legally designated representative or an active patient must be included in all the protocol steps. If the representative or patient refuses to allow marking of the operative site, this must be noted on the procedure checklist (Ridge, 2008).

Transport to the Operating Room

Personnel in the OR notify the nursing unit when it is time for surgery. The transporter checks the patient's identification bracelet against the patient's medical record to be sure the correct person is going to surgery. For transportation on a gurney, the nurses and transporter help the patient safely transfer from bed to gurney. The ambulatory surgery patient may walk to the OR, allowing more control over the event. The trip to surgery should be as smooth as possible so that the sedated patient does not experience nausea or dizziness.

Allow the family to visit before the patient is transported to the OR, then direct the family to the appropriate waiting area. If family members plan on leaving the facility during the procedure, ensure there is a way to contact them and give them phone numbers of the nurse's station and patient's room.

Preparing for the Postoperative Patient

If the patient was hospitalized before surgery and will return to the same nursing unit, prepare the bed and room for the patient's return. Arrange furniture so that the gurney can easily be brought to the bedside. Place the bed in the high position with the bed rails down on the receiving side and up on the other side. A postoperative bedside unit should include the following:

- Sphygmomanometer, stethoscope, and thermometer
- Emesis basin
- Clean gown
- Wash cloth, towel, and facial tissues
- IV pole and pump
- Suction equipment
- Oxygen equipment
- Extra pillows for positioning
- Bed pads to protect bed linen from drainage
- PCA pump

INTRAOPERATIVE PHASE

Intraoperative (within the surgical suite) care centers on care and protection of the patient. When the patient enters the OR (Figure 42-11), identify the patient both verbally and by the identification band and medical records. Nursing interventions include warm, personal contact with the patient to humanize the OR's often cold, aseptic, and highly technical environment. During surgery and particularly anesthesia, patients cannot protect themselves from many sources of possible harm. Essential elements for monitoring and promoting patient safety are being aware of the potential for harm, recognizing body areas most susceptible to injury, strictly adhering to principles of positioning and asepsis, and monitoring sites for impairment or early signs of injury. Do not leave small or potentially dangerous objects such as needles and syringes near the patient. Use side rails and safety straps, even for the fully conscious patient; safety reminder devices may be necessary to protect the delirious, semicomatose, or disoriented patient from injury.

HOLDING AREA

In many hospitals the patient enters a surgical care unit called a **preanesthesia care unit** (or holding area) outside the OR, where the nurse completes the preoperative preparations. Nurses in this unit are usually part of the OR staff and wear surgical scrub suits.

The nurse or anesthesiologist inserts an IV catheter into the patient's vein to establish a route for fluid re-

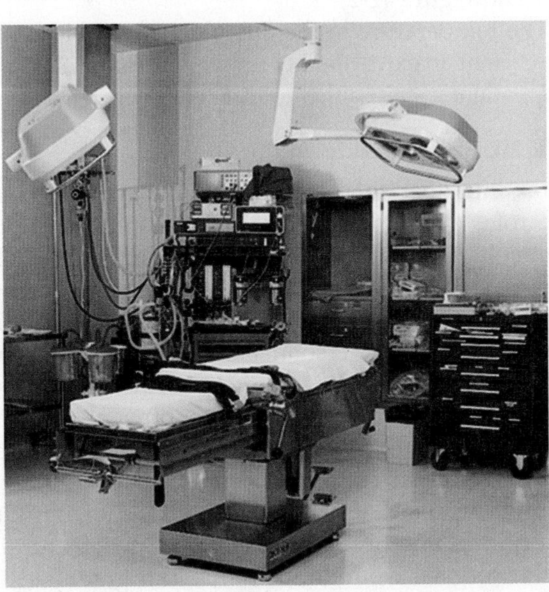

FIGURE 42-11 Traditional operating room.

Box 42-7 Responsibilities of the Circulating Nurse and the Scrub Nurse

RESPONSIBILITIES OF THE CIRCULATING NURSE

- Prepares operating room with necessary equipment and supplies and ensures that equipment is functional
- Arranges sterile and unsterile supplies; opens sterile supplies for scrub nurse
- Sends for patient at proper time
- Visits with patient preoperatively; explains role, identifies patient, verifies operative permit, and answers any questions
- Performs patient assessment
- Confirms patient assessment
- Checks medical record for completeness
- Assists in safe transfer of patient to operating room table
- Positions patient on operating room table in accordance with type of procedure and surgeon's preference
- Places conductive pad on patient if electrocautery is to be used
- Counts sponges, needles, and instruments with scrub nurse before surgery
- Assists scrub nurse and surgeons by tying gowns
- May prepare patient's skin
- Assists scrub nurse in arranging tables to create sterile field
- Maintains continuous astute observations during surgery to anticipate needs of patient, scrub nurse, surgeons, and anesthesiologist
- Provides supplies to scrub nurse as needed
- Observes sterile field closely for any breaks in aseptic technique, and reports accordingly
- Cares for surgical specimens according to institutional policy
- Documents operative record and nurse's notes
- Counts sponges, needles, and instruments when closure of wound begins
- Transfers patient to gurney for transport to recovery area
- Accompanies patient to the recovery room and provides a report

RESPONSIBILITIES OF THE SCRUB NURSE

- Performs surgical hand scrub
- Dons sterile gown and gloves aseptically
- Arranges sterile supplies and instruments in manner prescribed for procedure
- Checks instruments for proper functioning
- Counts sponges, needles, and instruments with circulating nurse
- Gowns and gloves surgeons as they enter operating room
- Assists with surgical draping of patient
- Maintains neat and orderly sterile field
- Corrects breaks in aseptic technique
- Observes progress of surgical procedure
- Hands surgeon instruments, sponges, and necessary supplies during procedure
- Identifies and handles surgical specimens correctly
- Maintains count of sponges, needles, and instruments so none will be misplaced or lost in wound

placement and IV medications. Use a large-bore IV catheter for optimal infusion of all fluids and possible blood products. Administer preoperative medications.

If hair around the surgical site needs to be removed, this is done in a private area near the OR immediately before surgery. Consult the physician's order sheet and the agency policy and procedure manual (see Skill 42-1 and Figure 42-2).

The temperature in the OR is usually cool, so offer the patient an extra blanket for warmth and relaxation. The patient's stay in the holding area is brief.

THE NURSE'S ROLE

In the intraoperative phase, the nurse assumes one of two roles during the surgical procedure: scrub nurse or circulating nurse (Box 42-7). Everyone (nurses, physicians, anesthesia providers) in the OR must prevent contamination of sterile items and aid in maintaining aseptic conditions. Personnel practice **surgical asepsis** (using sterile technique to protect against infection before, during, or after surgery) to prevent microbial contamination of the operative site. The goal of surgical asepsis is to prevent or minimize postoperative wound infections. The patient is at risk for introduction of infecting organisms through catheters, drains, or the surgical wound. Standards and guidelines for surgical scrubs and skin preparation should be strictly followed. The operation's success and ease greatly depend on group dynamics as professionals work to achieve common goals (Figure 42-12).

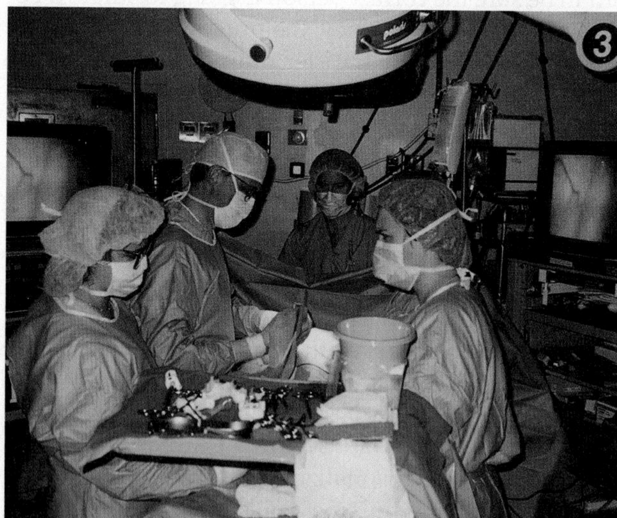

FIGURE 42-12 Safe, effective intraoperative care requires a team effort.

POSTOPERATIVE PHASE

IMMEDIATE POSTOPERATIVE PHASE

During the postoperative phase the OR nurse assists in transferring the patient to the PACU (Figure 42-13), the recovery room, or the intensive care area. Review with

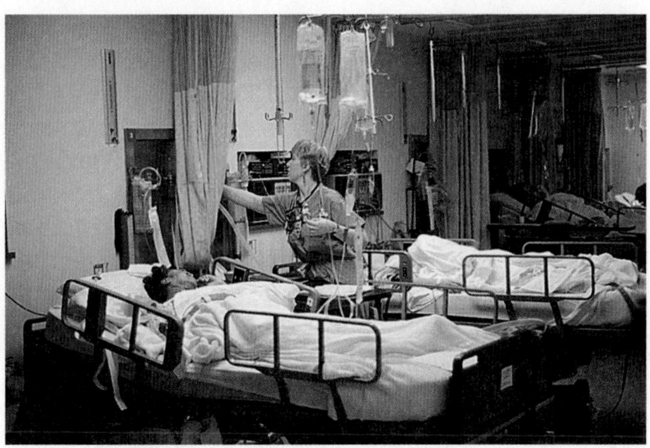

FIGURE 42-13 Nurse in a postanesthesia care unit.

the staff information about the patient's status, including IV fluids, medications, and blood products administered; the surgical dressing; any complication in the OR; and unusual risks for hemorrhage or cardiac irregularities. The OR nurse is an important resource in planning the patient's postoperative care.

Immediate postoperative observation and interventions follow the ABCS of airway, breathing, consciousness, circulation, and systems (Table 42-7). Assess vital signs every 15 minutes during the recovery period, and monitor respiratory and GI functions. Evaluate the wound for any **drainage** (the removal of fluids from a body cavity, wound, or other source of discharge by one or more methods) or **exudate** (substances [e.g., perspiration, pus, serum] that slowly seep from cells or blood vessels through small pores or breaks in cell membranes). Once the patient has a patent airway and stable vital signs, is conscious, and responds to stimuli, the anesthesia provider or surgeon approves transfer to the nursing unit. As the patient regains consciousness, relief of pain is often the first need expressed. Frequently, medication is given in the recovery area. Staff on the nursing unit review documentation from the surgical suite and recovery room to assess how well the patient tolerated the surgical process.

Carefully monitor body temperature. Hypothermia, a core temperature of less than 98.6° F (37° C), occurs in 60% to 80% of all postoperative patients. Contributing factors include body exposure in a cold OR, the effects of cold solutions, and a consequence of some anesthetics. The heat loss that occurs in the OR can continue in the PACU if the patient is not warmed sufficiently. Warm blankets are used, especially around the feet; adding warmth around the head is helpful. A newer method is convective warming therapy, in which a disposable cover inflated with warm air from a heating unit is placed over the patient; warm air passes out through the underside, so the warm air is constantly

Table 42-7 Interventions Associated with the ABCS of Immediate Recovery

ASSESSMENT MODE	INTERVENTION
A: Airway	Maintain patency: keep head tilted up and back; may position on side with the face down and the neck slightly extended. Note presence or absence of gag or swallowing reflex; stay at bedside until gag reflex returns. Suction until awake and alert. Provide oxygen if necessary.
B: Breathing	Evaluate depth, rate, sounds, rhythm, and chest movement. Assess color of mucous membranes. Place hand above patient's nose to detect respirations if shallow. Initiate coughing and deep breathing exercises as soon as patient is able to respond. Chart time oxygen is discontinued. Monitor oxygen saturation levels (SaO_2) by pulse oximetry checks.
C: Consciousness	**Extubate** patient (remove endotracheal tube from airway). Patient responds to commands. Patient verbalizes responses. Patient reacts to stimuli.
C: Circulation	Monitor temperature, pulse, respirations, and blood pressure every 10 to 15 minutes; take axillary, tympanic, or rectal temperature if warranted. Assess rate, rhythm, and quality of pulse. Evaluate color and warmth of skin and color of nailbeds. Check peripheral pulses as indicated. Assess incision and dressing (monitor wound drainage output). Monitor intravenous lines: solution, rate, site. Cardiac monitors are usually in place for patients who had general anesthesia.
S: System review	Assess neurologic functions, muscle strength, and response. Monitor drains, tubes, and color and amount of output. Check for pressure, type, and condition of dressings. Evaluate pain response; may need to give analgesic and monitor patient response. Observe for allergic reactions. Assess urinary output if Foley catheter is in place.

moving. In the PACU, monitor the patient's temperature and vital signs every 15 minutes until vital signs are stable, or more frequently if they are unstable. The frequency and duration of monitoring are dictated by facility PACU policy. Patients are monitored until they are discharged from the PACU, usually at least 1 hour. Before discharge, their minimum temperature must be greater than 96.8° F (36° C). Warming requires the maintenance of temperature without overwarming and excessive vasodilation, which can cause fluid shifts and a decrease in blood pressure.

The PACU nurse must be aware that malignant hyperthermia can occur in the PACU and repeatedly assess the patient for signs of this condition. Malignant hyperthermia is a genetic disorder characterized by uncontrolled skeletal muscle contractions leading to potentially fatal hyperthermia. It occurs in patients predisposed to the disorder when they receive a combination of certain anesthetic agents. Unless the triggering event is stopped and the body is cooled, death results.

LATER POSTOPERATIVE PHASE

Immediate Assessments

When the patient returns to the nursing unit, a thorough postsurgical assessment follows. Review vital signs, the IV and incisional sites, any tubes, and postoperative orders. A review of each body system identifies when body functions return and provides a guideline for further assessments. Unless otherwise indicated, monitor vital signs and make general assessments using the "times-four" factor—every 15 minutes times 4 (for 4 hours); every 30 minutes times 4; every hour times 4; then every 4 hours, or until assessments are within expected ranges. The times-four gauge is the maximal time that should elapse between assessments. Table 42-8 details body temperature responses to surgery. A postoperative flow sheet (Figure 42-14) is frequently used to document the patient's progress. Significant observations are critical for the patient after surgery.

Although the patient may respond, the level of functioning is impaired. Keep the side rails up and the call light within reach. Until the patient is fully conscious, do not place a pillow under the head. Either position the patient on the side, depending on the type of surgery, or raise the head of the bed to a 45-degree angle. Positioning the head higher than the chest reduces the chance of the patient aspirating vomitus. Because nausea and vomiting are normal in the first 12 to 24 hours, keep an emesis basin at the bedside. If the patient vomits, measure the amount and carefully describe it in the documentation. Report any red or coffee-ground emesis immediately. Frequently the patient remains on NPO status for the first few hours after surgery. Introduce fluids gradually. The physician usually orders ice chips followed by clear or full liquids.

Postoperative complications can occur suddenly; therefore note any change. Because the patient is often

Table 42-8 Temperature Assessment and Intervention

CAUSE	ASSESSMENT AND INTERVENTION
HYPOTHERMIA	
Within First 12 Hours	
Response to surgery, anesthesia, and body exposure	Monitor temperature readings. Assess for warmth. Provide warm blankets. Do not expose for long periods. Assess orientation.
HYPERTHERMIA	
24-48 Hours	
Dehydration Decreased lung activity Inflammatory response to surgery	Monitor temperature readings. Monitor intravenous rate. Encourage fluids. Assess intake and output (I&O). Have patient turn, cough, and breathe deeply. Provide incentive spirometer. Assess lung sounds. Observe incision.
After Day 2	
Infection: respiratory, wound, urinary, or circulatory	Monitor temperature readings. Assess lung sounds and expectoration of sputum. Evaluate incision and drainage. Monitor I&O. Encourage fluids of 6-8 oz/hr unless contraindicated. Note urine color, odor, amount, and consistency, and patient's complaints of burning on micturition. Perform leg exercises every 2 hours, and ambulate every 4 hours.

POST-OP ASSESSMENT FORM

SURGEON: Dr. J. Bernard	REPORT FROM: S Welker RN		ALLERGIES: NKA
Date: 1-27-10	Anesthesia Note: General	PROCEDURE: Reverse colostomy-sigmoid colostomy resection (seg mem)	
ARRIVAL ON FLOOR 1440	BLOCK LEVEL:	CBI CREDIT ———	

PRE-OP MEDS	INTRA OP MEDS	POST OP MEDS	CBI INTAKE ———	IV FLUIDS & CREDITS
Versed 2 mg	Fentanyl 250 mcg	Versed 1 mg	OUTPUT Foley 650 mL	NS - 125 mL
pepcid 20 mg	Flagyl 750 mg	Morphine 1 mg		700 mL
	Zofran 4 g	q 10 min/6 mg/	DRAINS Jackson Pratt Ø	EBL ———
			PACKS NA	IV INTAKE 3300 mL

Time	BP-P-R		TEMP	PAIN INTENSITY 0-10	SAO_2	NURSING OBSERVATIONS
1440	144/83	84-12	96^{6}	Ø	95%	1440 Returned from pacunit to Room 356 B per gurney—awake—alert—
1500	166/82	86-16	96^{8}	5	94%	oriented x 4. Color pink—skin warm and dry. Normal saline infusing in left
1515	152/82	86-16			96%	wrist @ 125 mL/hr with MS. PCA present. Site without edema or erythema.-
1530	145/78	84-18	96^{9}	4	96%	Pedal pulses 4 bilaterally. Capillary refill < 2 seconds.
1545	140/79	86-16	96^{3}	4	96%	Lung sounds clear. O2 4L per nasal Cannula. Incentive spirometer to 1500 mL.—
1600	139/73	86-18	96^{4}	4	97%	Abd. dressings dry & intact c̄ SM am't of serosanguineous exudate. Area
1630	144/80	87-18	96^{8}	4	95%	marked. Bowel sounds absent. 44 Jackson Pratt draining serosanguineous —
1730	149/78	87-18	97^{2}	4	90%	exudate. Foley catheter draining light, yellow urine. TED hose on bilaterally –
1830	129/71	86	97^{5}	4	99%	flowtrons in place.
						1600 active ROM to lower extremities.
						1730 Walked 100 feet c̄ assistance. C/o dizziness & nausea —
						returned to bed.
						1800 IV NS changed to D5 ½ NS @ 125 mL/hr. Site s̄
						erythema or edema. Luann Richardson SPN —
						1900 Above assessment remains unchanged.
						Luann Richardson SPN.

NURSING STAFF SIGNATURE AND INITIALS

LR Luann Richardson SPN

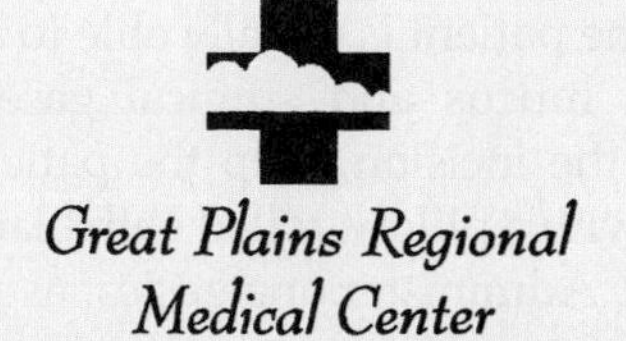

Great Plains Regional Medical Center

601 West Leota Street - P.O. Box 1167
North Platte, Nebraska 69103-1167

N-12 (Rev. 7/03) | topel | LABEL

FIGURE 42-14 Postoperative assessment form.

Box 42-8 Possible Causes of Postoperative Shock

- Movement of patient from operating table to gurney
- Patient (gurney) being jarred during transport
- Reactions to drugs and anesthesia
- Loss of blood and other body fluids
- Cardiac dysrhythmias
- Cardiac failure
- Inadequate ventilation
- Pain

cold, provide additional blankets for comfort, without leading to sweating. Vital signs, coupled with the patient's behavior, are first-line observations. A pulse that increases and becomes thready—coupled with a declining blood pressure, cool and clammy skin, reduced urinary output, and restlessness—may signal hypovolemic shock. Hypovolemic shock in the postoperative period is frequently caused by internal hemorrhage, a life-threatening emergency (Box 42-8). A drop in blood pressure slightly below a patient's preoperative baseline reading is common after surgery. However, a significant drop in blood pressure, accompanied by an increased heart rate, may indicate hemorrhage, circulatory failure, or fluid shifts. Do not diagnose impending hypovolemic shock on the basis of one low blood pressure reading. If you are concerned about a dropping blood pressure, measure pressure every 5 minutes for 15 minutes to determine the variability. Decreased blood pressure can also mean that the anesthetic is wearing off or that the patient is experiencing severe pain.

In addition to hypotension, manifestations of shock include tachycardia; restlessness and apprehension; and cold, moist, pale, or cyanotic skin. When a patient appears to be going into shock, take the following steps: (1) administer oxygen or increase its rate of delivery, (2) raise the patient's legs above the level of the heart, (3) increase the rate of IV fluids (unless contraindicated because of fluid excretion problems), (4) notify the anesthesia provider and the surgeon, (5) provide medications as ordered, and (6) continue to assess the patient and response to interventions.

Incision

Monitor the incisional dressing, since bleeding or excessive drainage may also signal postoperative hemorrhage. Normally dressings are not changed but are reinforced during the first 24 hours. To accurately measure the amount of drainage, circle the drainage markings on the dressing and write the time and date. **Dehiscence** (the separation of a surgical incision or rupture of a wound closure) may occur 3 days to more than 2 weeks postoperatively. Wound separation in the first 3 days is usually related to technical factors, such as the sutures. Separation from 3 to 14 days postoperatively is usually associated with postoperative complications such as distention, vomiting, excessive coughing, dehydration, or infection. Wound separation after

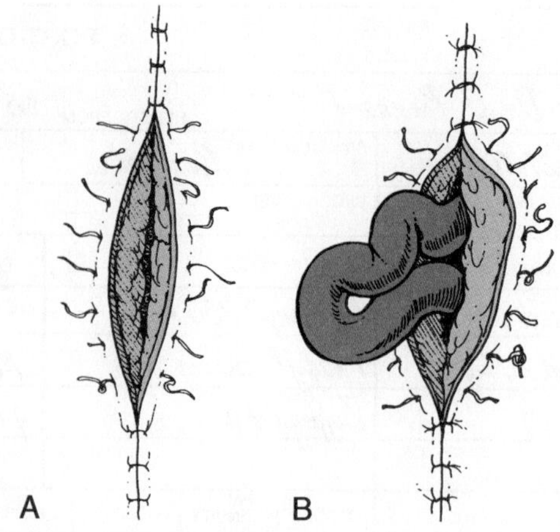

FIGURE 42-15 **A,** Wound dehiscence. **B,** Evisceration.

2 weeks is usually associated with metabolic factors, such as **cachexia** (ill health, malnutrition, and wasting as a result of chronic disease), hypoproteinemia, increased age, malignancy, radiation therapy, and obesity. Wound **evisceration** (protrusion of an internal organ through a wound or surgical incision, especially in the abdominal wall) may also occur. Both wound dehiscence and evisceration require prompt attention (Figure 42-15). If the patient feels a sudden "give," sutures may have broken. Contact the physician immediately. Cover the wound with a sterile towel moistened with sterile physiological saline (warm). Tension on the abdomen may be decreased by placing the patient in Fowler's position with the knees slightly flexed. Reassure the patient regarding the situation, and tell him or her that surgery will be required. Prepare the patient for surgery. Sterile technique procedures—including dressing change and care of the surgical incision with phases of wound healing—are discussed in Chapters 12 and 13.

Ventilation

Immediate postoperative hypoventilation can result from drugs (anesthetics, narcotics, tranquilizers, sedatives), incisional pain, obesity, chronic lung disease, or pressure on the diaphragm. Inadequate ventilation leads to hypoxemia. Monitor arterial oxygenation saturation (Sao_2), either by arterial blood gas measurements or by pulse oximetry.

Because lung ventilation is vital, help the patient turn, cough, and breathe deeply every 1 to 2 hours until the chest is clear. Having practiced this combination preoperatively, the patient is usually able to adequately remove trapped mucus and surgical gases. To ease the pressure on the incision, help the patient support the surgical site with a pillow, rolled bath blanket, or the heel of the hand. Administer analgesics, as prescribed, to control pain before coughing and deep breathing exercises. Early mobility and frequent position changes facilitate secretion clearance and improve the ventilation and perfusion in the lungs. Respiratory infections are frequently caused by shallow breathing and poor coughing. Listen for wheezing or crowing sounds from patients who have undergone head or neck surgery; this response occurs when edema places pressure over the trachea, resulting in respiratory insufficiency.

If the patient feels chest pain or has a fever, productive cough, or dyspnea, **atelectasis** (an abnormal condition characterized by the collapse of lung tissue) or pneumonia may be developing. Sudden chest pain along with dyspnea, tachycardia, cyanosis, diaphoresis, and hypotension is a sign of a pulmonary embolism. Raise the head of the bed to decrease dyspnea, and immediately report signs and symptoms. Frequently oxygen therapy is instituted to assist with breathing.

Whenever air exchange is reduced, postoperative recovery slows. Medication, suctioning, and oxygen therapy may be needed to assist the patient in respiratory distress. Mechanical devices, such as incentive spirometers, are used to stimulate deep breathing (see Skill 42-2). Frequently the incentive spirometer is used when the patient can deep breathe independently; the instrument visually measures the amount of air inhaled. Volume-oriented spirometers assist patients in deep breathing. Patients are encouraged to take 10 deep breaths every hour while awake.

If respiratory complications develop, the physician may order respiratory therapy to provide intermittent positive pressure breathing (IPPB) treatments to deliver a mixture of air and oxygen; medication can be added to enhance respirations. Chest percussion and postural drainage—a form of chest physiotherapy that combines positioning and percussion movements to lung areas to help dislodge and move secretions—are also used. Do not leave patients unattended during postural drainage, since they may experience respiratory distress.

Box 42-9 Postoperative Comfort Measures for Pain

DECREASE EXTERNAL STIMULI
- Darken room; close drapes.
- Keep TV and radio off or low.
- Monitor hall traffic and noise.
- Assess staff interruptions.
- Check room for noise—dripping water, buzzing lights, constant intercom messages.

REDUCE INTERRUPTIONS
- Plan care to allow rest.
- Post "Do Not Disturb" sign.
- Unplug telephone.
- Restrict visitors.
- Pull curtains around bed.

ELIMINATE ODORS
- Discuss offending odors and assess elimination.
- Remove from room all dressings that are soiled with exudate.
- Post "No Smoking" sign.
- Alert housekeeping to omit room-cleaning products.
- Install air-circulating unit.
- Alert dietary department to reduce foods with odors.

NURSING INTERVENTIONS
- Ask patient about normal relaxation patterns and practices.
- Have patient practice deep-breathing and relaxation techniques.
- Plan rest periods.
- Provide back rub.
- Engage patient in conversation; ask about concerns and fears.
- Encourage diversional activities.
- Reposition and support with pillows, bed rolls.
- Check tube placement.
- Offer warm fluids if indicated.
- Reduce room clutter.
- Provide restful environment.

Pain

Internal organs do not have many nerve endings, but a skin incision produces painful responses. Because pain is normal postoperatively, offer patients prescribed analgesics. Ask patients every 3 to 4 hours if they need something for pain because some patients will not ask for an analgesic. Acute pain begins to subside within 24 to 48 hours, and pain medication is adjusted as necessary. In the early stages of recovery, comfort interventions help ease pain. Anxiety may affect pain perception. After the acute phase, comfort measures may be the only interventions required (Box 42-9).

A patient's level of pain can be difficult to evaluate. Ask the patient to rate the pain on a scale of 0 to 10. There are standard pain indexes (restlessness, moaning, grimacing, diaphoresis), but some patients may not outwardly exhibit signs. Objective pain factors are signs that the body is responding to "pain"; these include vital sign changes (blood pressure lowers in the immediate postoperative period and elevates in response to pain after about 12 hours, and pulse increases), restlessness, diaphoresis, and pallor. The patient's description of discomfort represents subjective pain factors. The way the pain affects the patient emotionally is termed **suffering.** Pain behaviors are influenced by the patient's culture and past experiences. Behaviors include moaning, grimacing, and favoring a body area.

The effectiveness of analgesic measures differs with each person; if relief is not obtained, changing the medication or administration schedule may provide effective pain control. Each patient interprets pain differently and has a personal pain tolerance level. Remember that only the patient bearing the pain is an expert about that pain. McCaffery and Pasero (1999) states, "Pain is whatever the experiencing person says it is, existing whenever he says it does."

The success of pain management depends on the surgery, the patient's emotional state, and postopera-

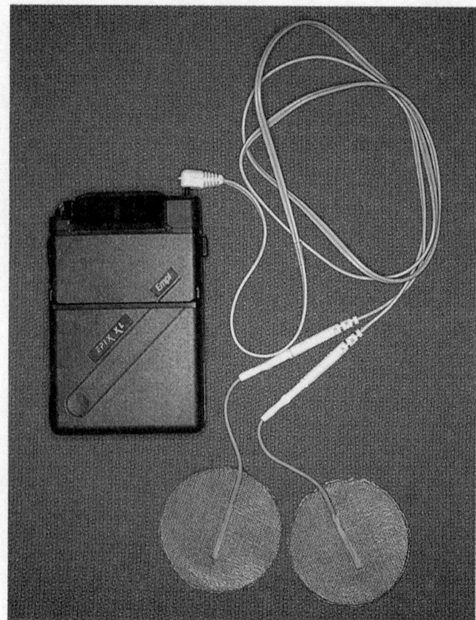

FIGURE 42-16 Transcutaneous electric nerve stimulation (TENS) unit.

tive complications. Patients experiencing chronic pain may have more difficulty obtaining relief than individuals with acute episodes. Commonly used analgesic measures are nurse-administered narcotics, patient-controlled IV medications (see Chapter 16), and pain control via a transcutaneous electric nerve stimulation (TENS) unit (Figure 42-16). Attached to the skin, the TENS unit applies electric impulses to the nerve endings and blocks transmission of pain signals to the brain. The PCA system is a pump that is programmed to dispense only a given amount of medication. The patient can self-administer an analgesic by pressing a control button. Monitor the PCA system every 3 to 4 hours.

Urinary Function

Anesthesia retards urinary function. Assess the bladder area every 2 hours for distention and changes in renal function. It routinely takes 6 to 8 hours for voiding to occur after surgery. If patients do not void within 8 hours, catheterization may be necessary, but it should be used as a last measure. Have the patient listen to running water, place the hands in warm water, or walk to the bathroom, if able, to facilitate voiding. Helping male patients stand often encourages voiding. Serum blood urea nitrogen may be measured daily until patient has recovered. Usually I&O are measured while a Foley catheter is in place, while the patient is receiving IV therapy, and immediately after a Foley catheter has been removed. Continue urine measurement until the patient is voiding without difficulty.

Fluid deficit may result from inadequate replacement of body fluids lost during surgery or from continued fluid losses. Fluid excess may occur from large amounts of IV fluids when kidney function is inadequate (evidenced by oliguria). A urinary output of 30 mL per hour is considered acceptable postoperatively. Unless the patient has had urinary tract surgery, urine should be clear and yellow and have an ammonia odor.

Venous Stasis

Venous stasis (a disorder in which the normal flow of fluid through a vessel of the body is slowed or halted) is the underlying cause of thrombus formation. Performing leg exercises every 2 hours and using intermittent pneumatic compression devices and compression stockings aid the circulatory system and help prevent deep-vein thrombosis. Assessment of the feet and legs includes palpating for pedal pulse and noting the skin's color and temperature. If edema, aching or cramping, sensitivity, or pain occurs in the calf (Homans' sign) or leg, the patient will complain of calf pain on dorsiflexion of the foot, and a thrombus should be suspected. Have the patient remain in bed until the physician can perform an evaluation. Teach the patient not to cross legs when in bed, and encourage sitting up as another means of preventing venous stasis. Do not use a knee gatch.

Surgical patients are at the greatest risk of developing life-threatening deep-vein thrombosis and pulmonary embolism. Not only does surgery injure blood vessels, but anesthesia and inactivity also cause venous stasis. Surgery, however, is not the only risk factor. Others include pregnancy, myocardial infarction, heart failure, stroke (brain attack), cancer, sepsis, and immobility. The most effective method of preventing deep-vein thrombosis is with low-dose subcutaneous heparin therapy. Heparin is an anticoagulant but is contraindicated in trauma and general surgery patients. Antiembolism stockings and ambulation are also useful preventive measures.

The external intermittent pneumatic compression system (SCD) (see Skill 42-5) is used on patients who are at risk of developing deep-vein thrombosis and pulmonary embolism. This device includes an air pressure pump and cuffs, one for each calf or foot. Continuous inflation and deflation of the cuffs decreases pooling of venous blood in the legs and improves venous return to the heart. The pressure cuffs automatically inflate to 40 mm Hg or the prescribed setting and deflate in cycles, with inflation lasting about 12 seconds and deflation lasting about 48 seconds. This system is contraindicated for any patient with acute thrombophlebitis or deep-vein thrombosis.

When ambulating the patient, disconnect the pump tubing, although sometimes the cuffs are kept in place on the calves. Do not disconnect the device for more than 30 minutes. If the patient has diagnostic examinations that require leaving the nursing unit for longer than 30 minutes, the compression pump, the cuffs or sleeves, and the instructions on operation should travel with the patient.

The treatment continues for 72 hours postoperatively or until the patient is ambulating well. Remove the cuffs once a day to assess skin integrity and provide skin care. Document the use of the intermittent external pneumatic compression system and any reaction such as numbness or tingling (see Figure 42-5).

Activity

Early ambulation is a significant factor in hastening postoperative recovery and preventing postoperative complications. The exercise of getting in and out of bed and walking during the early postoperative period has numerous benefits (Box 42-10). Ambulation is usually contraindicated for patients with severe infection or thrombophlebitis.

Assessment

Before helping the patient ambulate for the first few times after major surgery, assess the following:

1. Level of alertness: Ask the patient simple questions or to follow simple commands.
2. Cardiovascular status (orthostatic hypotension)
   a. Assess pulse and respiratory rate and depth while patient is supine, then after sitting.
   b. Observe skin color for pallor while patient is sitting.
   c. Note complaints of vertigo while patient is sitting.
3. Motor status
   a. Assess muscle strength of patient's legs.
   b. Assess sitting ability.
      (1) Help patient to sitting position on side of bed.
      (2) Ask patient to maintain an erect position while being gently pushed sideways.

It is also important to know of any preoperative limitations to ambulation. The patient with arthritis or arteriosclerosis may take longer to move and to adjust to standing and walking. The patient who used a walker preoperatively needs assistance for a longer time before using the walker again. Family members are important in assisting patients with any physical limitation and in providing emotional support during postoperative recovery.

Nursing Interventions

Nursing interventions are as follows:

1. Encourage muscle-strengthening exercises before ambulation:
   a. Have patient bend knees, lower knees, press back of knees hard against bed.
   b. Have patient alternately contract and relax calf and thigh muscles 10 times using the following cycle: contract, relax, rest.
2. Have patient sit on side of bed (legs dangling) to become accustomed to upright position before ambulating the first time. Be certain that pulse has stabilized (returned to baseline) before patient attempts ambulation.
3. Clamp NG tube while patient ambulates, and then reconnect.
4. Keep urinary tube connected to drainage bag; carry bag or pin bag to inside of robe. Keep drainage receptacle below level of bladder to prevent reflux of urine.
5. Attach IV bag to a movable pole.
6. Use two people to assist in ambulating an unsteady patient receiving IV fluids (Figure 42-17).
7. Encourage patient to walk farther at each ambulation.

Box 42-10 Effects of Early Postoperative Ambulation

- Increased rate and depth of breathing
  —Prevention of atelectasis and hypostatic pneumonia
  —Increased mental alertness from increased oxygenation to brain
- Increased circulation
  —Nutrients required for healing are more available to wound
  —Prevention of thrombophlebitis
- Increased micturition (urinary elimination)
  —Increased kidney function
  —Prevention of urinary retention
- Increased metabolism
  —Prevention of loss of muscle tone
  —Restoration of nitrogen balance
- Increased peristalsis
  —Promotion of expulsion of flatus
  —Prevention of abdominal distention and gas pain
  —Prevention of constipation
  —Prevention of paralytic ileus

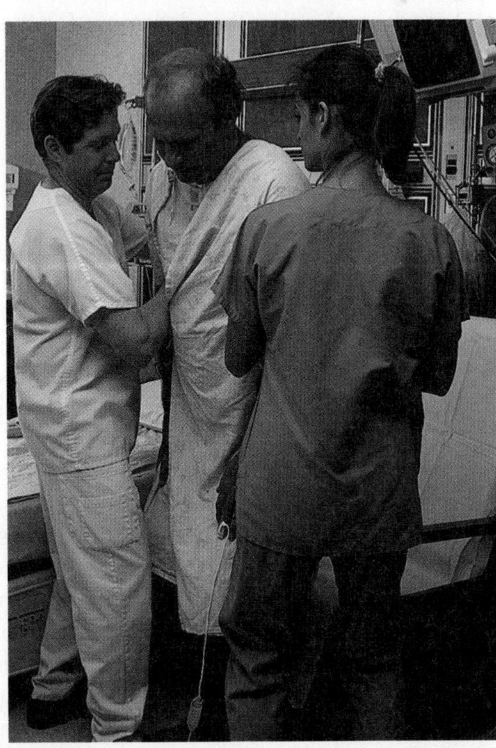

FIGURE 42-17 Progression in levels of postoperative activity promotes tissue perfusion.

The word ***ambulate*** means to move from place to place—to walk. Sitting in a chair is not ambulation. After ambulating, the patient may sit in a chair, but should be advised to stand and walk at intervals and to elevate the legs while sitting to prevent venous pooling in the extremities. The patient should avoid sitting in a chair for long periods. Also see Chapter 15.

GASTROINTESTINAL STATUS

Abdominal distention frequently occurs after surgery. Because anesthesia and surgical manipulation slow peristalsis, it may take 3 or 4 days for bowel activity to return. Ask the patient if he or she is nauseated or hungry (a more accurate assessment of gastrointestinal activity than the presence of bowel sounds). Listening for bowel sounds in the lower abdomen can help gauge the return of function. Normal peristalsis is indicated by hearing 5 to 30 gurgles per minute. Listen for bowel sounds in all four quadrants for 1 minute. A **paralytic ileus** (a decrease in or absence of intestinal peristalsis that may occur after abdominal surgery, peritoneal trauma, severe metabolic disease, and other conditions) may also develop. If inactivity continues, the physician usually orders an NG or nasointestinal tube to be placed to help remove the gas formed in the stomach and small intestine. When listening for bowel sounds in patients who have an NG or nasointestinal tube, turn off the suction machine but *never* leave the room without turning the machine back on.

Verify abdominal distention by measuring the patient's abdominal girth. To ensure the measurement is accurate, mark on the skin the placement for the tape measure, which is at the level of the umbilicus. Assess and chart the expelling of flatus, bowel sounds, and abdominal girth. Occasionally analgesics (meperidine) and other medications may slow peristalsis; charting the patient's GI habits helps identify etiologic factors.

Encouraging movement (turning every 2 hours, early ambulation) assists in restoring GI activity. A rectal tube may be inserted, or the physician may order an "up and down" flush (Harris flush) to relieve pain from intestinal gas. A Harris flush is a mild colonic irrigation using 100 to 200 mL of enema solution. After instillation, the enema container is lowered and the solution siphoned back into the container. This process may be repeated. For the patient who has difficulty with flatus, limiting iced beverages and offering warm liquids may help resolve the discomfort. The patient may have fluids and food withheld until flatus is expelled. As the patient returns to previous eating habits, bowel function slowly resumes its preoperative state. Constipation is also a frequent problem after surgery. The same aids for abdominal distention assist in alleviating constipation. If the patient does not pass feces within 2 or 3 days after resuming solid foods, a suppository or tap water enema may be ordered. Again, encourage ambulation to promote peristalsis.

Singultus (hiccup) is an involuntary contraction of the diaphragm followed by rapid closure of the glottis. Singultus results from irritation of the phrenic nerve. The condition is seen most often in men. Sedatives may be necessary in extreme cases. Because abdominal distention may be the cause, assess the patient's abdomen for proper GI function. Abdominal distention usually is caused by gas in the intestinal tract, but may be related to internal bleeding. Evaluate the patient for signs of shock: vital signs, skin condition, and level of consciousness.

FLUIDS AND ELECTROLYTES

Fluid is lost during surgery through blood loss and increased insensible fluid loss through the lungs and skin. For at least the first 24 to 48 hours after surgery, the body retains fluids as part of the stress response to trauma and the effect of anesthesia.

Sodium and potassium depletion can occur after surgery as a result of the loss of blood or body fluids during surgery or the loss of GI secretion because of vomiting and NG tubes. Potassium is also lost during **catabolism** (tissue breakdown), especially after severe trauma or crush injuries. Loss of gastric secretions can result in chloride loss, producing metabolic alkalosis. Electrolytes are often added to the IV solution in the form of potassium chloride (KCl). However, potassium may irritate the vein when administered by an IV route. Advise the patient that a stinging sensation may occur.

Closely monitor fluid tolerance and electrolyte values during the postoperative period. When the patient returns from the recovery room, therapy will be in progress. Until the patient is past the nausea and vomiting period and can tolerate oral fluids, maintain parenteral therapy. Observe the IV line for patency and ordered fluid rate, and monitor the IV site for erythema, edema, heat, and pain. The IV solution may become infiltrated because of movement or inadvertent dislodgment of the needle when the patient ambulates; therefore it is necessary to assess the site every 1 to 2 hours or when the patient complains of discomfort. The assessment for rate of infusion is extremely important for older patients, who may quickly experience fluid overload and pulmonary edema.

Muscles and nerves require ongoing nourishment to function adequately, and parenteral fluids contain the necessary glucose and electrolytes. Depending on the type of surgery and the patient's nutritional needs, IV therapy lasts from a few hours to a few days. As long as the patient is receiving parenteral fluids, record the patient's I&O. If the patient's overall nutritional state is in question, weigh the patient daily. Also see Chapter 22.

As oral fluids are introduced, encourage patients to drink small amounts frequently (6 to 8 ounces per hour). Review the diet history to note fluids normally enjoyed. Unless otherwise ordered, patients usually begin by ingesting clear liquids (7-Up, water, tea, broth, gelatin) and progress as the GI system returns to normal functioning. If the patient has difficulty drinking the amount of fluid recommended, offer fluids more frequently and without a straw. (A straw, although convenient, reduces the amount of fluids ingested.) Unless the patient has other problems (e.g., decreased renal excretion because of renal failure or advanced age), encourage the patient to drink 2000 to 2400 mL in 24 hours. Because iced and carbonated beverages cause GI disturbances in some individuals, patients should avoid these fluids until active peristalsis is noted. If nausea and vomiting persist, an antiemetic such as promethazine (Phenergan), benzquinamide (Emete-Con), or prochlorperazine (Compazine) is usually ordered to be administered intravenously or rectally.

NURSING PROCESS *for the Surgical Patient*

The role of the licensed practical nurse/licensed vocational nurse (LPN/LVN) in the nursing process is that the LPN/LVN will:

- Participate in planning care for patients based on patient needs.
- Review patients' care plans and recommend revisions as needed.
- Review and follow defined prioritization for patient care.
- Use clinical pathways, care maps, or care plans to guide and review patient care.

Assessment

General assessment of the preoperative patient includes obtaining a nursing history. This consists of any prior surgery, allergies, current medications, use of other drugs or alcohol, and smoking status. Also assess the patient's physical condition, at-risk data, emotional status of the patient and family members, and preoperative diagnostic data. It is important for the patient and family to understand the surgical procedure and the expected outcomes. In the intraoperative stage, complete any procedures such as skin preparation or catheterization. During surgery and recovery, continually assess the patient's condition. Also provide postoperative care to prevent and detect complications and return the patient to wellness.

Nursing Diagnosis

Nursing diagnoses establish direction for the care that is provided during one or all surgical phases (Boxes 42-11 and 42-12). Nursing diagnoses may focus on preoperative, intraoperative, and postoperative risks. Preventive care is essential for effective management of the surgical patient.

Box 42-11 Preoperative Nursing Diagnoses

- **Airway clearance, ineffective,** related to:
  - —Diminished cough
  - —Increased pulmonary congestion
- **Anxiety (specify level),** related to:
  - —Knowledge deficit of impending surgery
  - —Threat of loss of body part
- **Coping, compromised family,** related to:
  - —Temporary role change of patient
  - —Impending severity of surgery
- **Fear,** related to:
  - —Impending surgery
  - —Anticipation of postoperative pain
- **Knowledge, deficient regarding implications of surgery,** related to:
  - —Lack of experience with surgery
  - —Information misinterpretation
- **Nutrition, imbalanced: less than body requirements,** related to:
  - —Preoperative malnourishment
- **Nutrition, imbalanced: more than body requirements,** related to:
  - —Excess intake of food
- **Powerlessness,** related to:
  - —Emergency nature of surgery
- **Skin integrity, risk for impaired,** related to:
  - —Preoperative radiation
  - —Immobilization during surgery
- **Sleep deprivation,** related to:
  - —Fear of surgery
  - —Preoperative hospital routines

Expected Outcomes and Planning

The care plan begins before surgery and follows through the postoperative period to provide the best nursing interventions possible. It is important to include the patient in health care planning. A patient informed about the surgical experience is less likely to be fearful and is better able to prepare for expected outcomes.

Goals and expected outcomes for the surgical patient may include the following:

Goal: Patient achieves physical comfort.
Outcome: Patient verbalizes relief of pain.

Implementation

Nursing interventions before surgery physically and psychologically prepare the patient for the surgical procedure. Act as an advocate for the patient during and after surgery to ensure that the patient's dignity and rights are protected at all times (see Nursing Care Plan 42-1).

Evaluation

Evaluate the effectiveness of the care plan and revise the plan as needed. An example of a goal and an evaluative measure is the following:

Goal: Patient achieves physical comfort.
Evaluative measure: Observe patient for nonverbal signs of discomfort, such as guarding the painful area and grimacing.

Box 42-12 Postoperative Nursing Diagnoses

- **Airway clearance, ineffective,** related to:
  - —Diminished cough
  - —Retained secretions
  - —Prolonged sedation
- **Body temperature, hypothermia,** related to:
  - —Lowered metabolism
- **Breathing pattern, ineffective,** related to:
  - —Incisional pain
  - —Analgesia effects on ventilation
- **Communication, impaired verbal,** related to:
  - —Endotracheal tube placement
  - —Airway tube placement
- **Coping, ineffective,** related to:
  - —Constraints imposed by surgery
  - —Postoperative therapies
- **Fluid volume, risk for deficient,** related to:
  - —Wound drainage
  - —Inadequate fluid intake
- **Grieving, anticipatory,** related to:
  - —Patient's critical condition
- **Infection, risk for,** related to:
  - —Surgical wound incision
  - —Presence of Foley catheter and wound drainage tubes
- **Mobility, impaired bed,** related to:
  - —Pain
  - —Postoperative activity restrictions
  - —Casts or dressings
  - —Surgical incision
  - —Nasogastric (NG) tube placement
- **Oral mucous membrane, impaired,** related to:
  - —Irritation of NG or endotracheal tube
  - —NPO status
- **Self-care deficit, bathing/hygiene, dressing/grooming, feeding, toileting,** related to:
  - —Postoperative activity restrictions
  - —Pain
- **Skin integrity, risk for impaired,** related to:
  - —Wound exudate
  - —Impaired mobility
  - —Decrease in nutritional intake

Nursing Care Plan 42-1 The Postoperative Patient

Mr. Sanders is a 40-year-old obese patient weighing 280 lb, who was admitted with bowel obstruction and a scheduled right hemicolectomy. Mr. Sanders has hypertension and a history of poor wound healing.

NURSING DIAGNOSIS *Ineffective airway clearance, related to incisional pain*

Patient Goals and Expected Outcomes	Nursing Interventions	Evaluation and Rationale
Patient will cough deeply in 24 hours	Medicate with analgesia to control pain.	Providing pain relief enables patient to cough and breathe deeply without discomfort.
Patient's lung sounds will clear after coughing	Raise head of bed to full Fowler's position during exercises.	In Fowler's position the diaphragm falls, which permits lung expansion.
	Splint incision with rolled bath blanket.	Splinting incision provides abdominal support during coughing.
	Have patient turn, cough, and deep breathe every hour while awake.	Turning, coughing, and deep breathing aid in mobilizing secretions.
	Use incentive spirometer hourly.	Adequate lung expansion can prevent atelectasis.
	Take vital signs q4h and note evidence of dyspnea or restlessness.	
	Monitor intravenous fluids.	
	Offer sips of fluid every hour if permissible.	Increased fluid intake helps prevent thickening of mucus.

NURSING DIAGNOSIS *Ineffective breathing pattern, related to poor body mechanics*

Patient Goals and Expected Outcomes	Nursing Interventions	Evaluation and Rationale
Patient will effectively use incentive spirometer	Encourage deep breathing q1-2h while awake.	Adequate lung expansion helps prevent atelectasis.
Patient's respirations will be even and unlabored	Reposition q2h; support joints and incision.	Turning promotes lung expansion.
	Continue oxygen at 2 L per cannula; cleanse nares q4h; post "No Smoking" sign.	Additional oxygen ensures adequate tissue oxygenation. "No Smoking" sign promotes safety.
	Encourage use of incentive spirometer.	Adequate lung expansion helps prevent atelectasis.

Nursing Care Plan 42-1 The Postoperative Patient—cont'd

Patient Goals and Expected Outcomes	Nursing Interventions	Evaluation and Rationale
	Record respirations q4h, noting depth, rate, and quality.	Regular assessments helps detect early signs and symptoms of respiratory complications.
	Assess skin and nailbed q4h; report slow blanching color and condition.	A change in color of skin and nailbeds signals poor oxygenation.
	Darken room; decrease stimuli, monitor pain, and offer analgesic prn.	Comfort measures promote rest and relaxation and decrease pain level.

NURSING DIAGNOSIS ***Risk for infection, related to open surgical incision and draining wound***

Patient Goals and Expected Outcomes	Nursing Interventions	Evaluation and Rationale
Patient's wound will not be erythematous or produce purulent exudate	Use good handwashing technique.	Handwashing helps prevent transmission of microorganisms.
Patient's vital signs will remain within normal range	Monitor wound q4h, noting amount and color of drainage; assess skin for warmth, color, and sensation.	Regular assessments reveals early signs and symptoms of wound infection.
	Mark drainage on dressing q4h; reinforce prn.	Containing wound drainage within dressing provides comfort to the patient and enables the nurse to correctly determine the type of drainage.
	Use surgical asepsis when changing dressing.	Surgical asepsis prevents the transmission of microorganisms.
	Monitor vital signs q4h.	Regular assessments of vital signs reveal early signs and symptoms of wound infection.
	Monitor white blood cell (WBC) level as ordered.	Elevation of WBCs indicates an infectious process and its severity.

Critical Thinking Questions

1. On the second postoperative day, Mr. Sanders is taking shallow breaths and having difficulty complying with coughing and deep breathing. His temperature is 101.8° F (38.8° C), and he has adventitious breath sounds bilaterally in the bases. List several nursing interventions to assist Mr. Sanders.
2. In his third postoperative day Mr. Sanders has an erythematous incision with moderate amounts of purulent exudate from the Penrose drain site. List the correct nursing interventions.
3. What signs and symptoms would the nurse note when assessing Mr. Sanders for dehydration secondary to elevated temperature and decreased fluid intake?

DISCHARGE: PROVIDING GENERAL INFORMATION

Preparation for the patient's discharge is an ongoing process throughout the surgical experience, beginning during the preoperative period. The informed patient is therefore prepared as events unfold and gradually assumes greater responsibility for self-care during the postoperative period. As discharge approaches, be certain the patient has vital information (Box 42-13). If the physician has not provided information about diet or activity prescriptions or restrictions, either obtain this information or encourage the patient to do so. Attention to complete discharge instruction may prevent needless distress for the patient. Written instructions are important for reinforcing verbal information. Specifically document in the record the discharge instructions provided to the patient and family (Figure 42-18). Document information related to patient's mental status (ability to understand importance of teaching for patient and family members). For the patient, the postoperative phase of care continues into the recuperative period. Assessment and evaluation of the patient after discharge may involve a follow-up call or a visit from a home health nurse.

AMBULATORY SURGERY DISCHARGE

The patient leaving an ambulatory surgery setting must be able to provide a degree of self-care and must be mobile and alert. Postoperative pain and nausea and

Box 42-13 Vital Information for the Discharged Patient

- Care of wound site and any dressings
- Action and possible side effects of any medications; when and how to take them
- Activities allowed and prohibited; when various physical activities can be resumed safely (e.g., driving a car, return to work, sexual intercourse, leisure activities)
- Dietary restrictions or modifications
- Symptoms to be reported (e.g., development of incisional tenderness or increased drainage, discomfort in other parts of the body)
- Where and when to return for follow-up care

vomiting must be controlled. Overall, the patient must be stable and near the same level of functioning as before surgery. On discharge, give the patient and family both specific and general instructions—verbally and reinforced with written directions. The patient may not drive and must be accompanied by a responsible adult at the time of discharge. Telephone the patient for a follow-up evaluation and to address any specific questions and concerns.

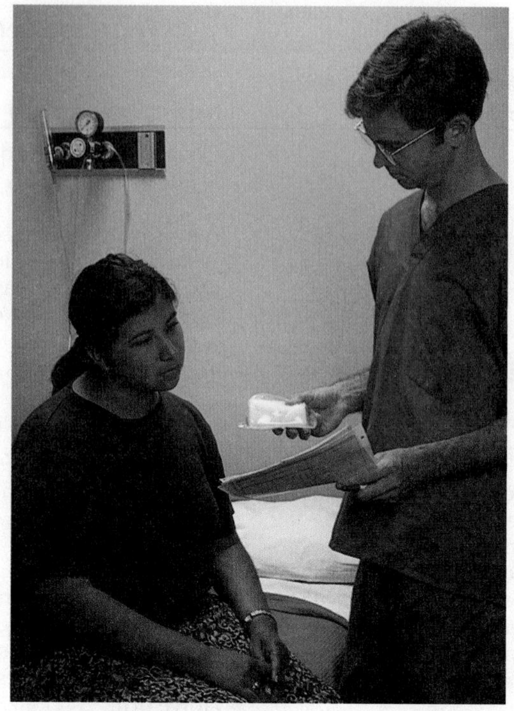

FIGURE 42-18 Reviewing discharge planning instructions.

Get Ready for the NCLEX® Examination!

Key Points

- The time before, during, and after surgery is the perioperative period. It is divided into preoperative, intraoperative, and postoperative phases.
- Perioperative nursing interventions take place before, during, and after surgery.
- The ability to tolerate surgery is influenced by nursing interventions, previous illness, and past surgeries.
- Older adult patients are at surgical risk from their declining physiologic status.
- All medications taken before surgery are automatically discontinued after surgery unless a physician reorders the medications, except for medications for long-term conditions such as phenytoin for seizure control.
- Family members are important in assisting patients with physical limitations and in providing emotional support during the postoperative recovery.
- Preoperative assessment of vital signs and physical findings provides an important baseline for comparing perioperative and postoperative assessment data.
- A patient's feelings about surgery can have a significant effect on relationships with nursing staff and the patient's ability to participate in care.
- Nursing diagnoses of the surgical patient may require interventions during one or all phases of surgery.
- Informed consent should not be obtained if a patient is confused, unconscious, mentally incompetent, or under the influence of sedatives. Know agency policy.
- Structured preoperative teaching positively influences postoperative recovery.
- A routine preoperative checklist is a guide for final preparation of the patient before surgery.
- Nurses in the OR focus on protecting the patient from potential harm.
- Assessment of the postoperative patient centers on the body systems most likely to be affected by anesthesia, immobilization, and surgical trauma.
- Because a surgical patient's condition may change rapidly during immediate postoperative recovery, monitor the patient's status at least every 15 minutes.
- The PACU nurse reports to the nurse on the postoperative unit information pertaining to the patient's current physical status and risk for postoperative complications.
- From the time of admission, plan for the surgical patient's discharge.
- Discharge planning identifies home care measures to promote recovery that involve both patient and family.
- Evaluation of all perioperative care is at times difficult, since the patient may be discharged from the nurse's care before the outcome is certain.

Additional Learning Resources

Go to your Companion CD for an audio glossary, animations, video clips, and more.

evolve Be sure to visit the Evolve site at http://evolve.elsevier.com/Christensen/adult/ for additional online resources.

Review Questions for the NCLEX® Examination

1. The patient has cancer of the larynx and is scheduled for a laryngectomy. This is an example of which type of surgery?
   1. Minor
   2. Elective
   3. Emergency
   4. Major

2. The patient is being discharged, and the nurse is teaching her how to do daily dressing changes at home. The most important point to include in the teaching plan is:
   1. discussion of surgical asepsis.
   2. discussion of hand hygiene.
   3. instruction in sterilization.
   4. demonstration of gloving.

3. To assist the patient in the prevention of postoperative pulmonary complications, preoperatively the nurse should:
   1. ask his physician to prescribe IPPB treatment.
   2. teach him to do leg exercises.
   3. teach him to use an incentive spirometer.
   4. tell him that if he does not cough, he may need to be suctioned.

4. The patient underwent surgery for lysis of adhesions. He is transferred from the PACU to his own room on the surgical floor. During the immediate postoperative period on the surgical floor, measure blood pressure, pulse, and respirations every:
   1. 15 minutes.
   2. 5 minutes.
   3. 20 minutes.
   4. 30 minutes.

5. The nurse is assessing the bowel sounds of her patient who had a suprapubic prostatectomy 2 days ago. To determine that he does not have bowel sounds present, the nurse would need to auscultate each quadrant for:
   1. 1 minute.
   2. 3 minutes.
   3. 10 minutes.
   4. 15 minutes.

6. The patient is recovering from a right lobectomy. The nurse is going to assist in splinting the patient's incision so she can cough and breathe deeply. The most therapeutic administration of an analgesic would be:
   1. after the procedure so she can rest.
   2. 15 minutes before the procedure.
   3. 1 hour before the procedure.
   4. 30 minutes before the procedure.

7. A patient reports being allergic to penicillin. Which question would elicit the most useful information?
   1. When did the reaction occur?
   2. What infection did you have that required penicillin?
   3. What type of allergic reaction did you have?
   4. Did you notify your physician of the allergy?

8. Which patient is at greatest risk for surgical and anesthetic complications?
   1. A 3-year-old patient scheduled for hernia repair
   2. An 80-year-old patient scheduled for exploratory laparotomy
   3. An 18-year-old patient scheduled for emergency appendectomy
   4. A 42-year-old patient scheduled for breast biopsy

9. An alert 75-year-old patient is to undergo elective surgery. The operative permit must be signed in the presence of a witness by:
   1. the patient.
   2. the patient and the patient's spouse.
   3. either the patient or the patient's spouse.
   4. the patient and the surgeon.

10. A nursing intervention to help a patient cope with fear of pain would be to:
    1. describe the degree of pain expected.
    2. explain the availability of pain medication.
    3. inform the patient of the frequency of pain medication.
    4. divert the patient when talking about pain.

11. A patient tells the nurse that "blowing into this tube thing [incentive spirometer] is a waste of time." The nurse explains that the specific purpose of the therapy is to:
    1. directly remove excess secretions from the lungs.
    2. increase pulmonary circulation.
    3. promote lung expansion.
    4. stimulate the cough reflex.

12. When preparing a patient for surgery, the nurse should:
    1. provide sips of water for a dry mouth.
    2. remove the patient's makeup and nail polish.
    3. remove the patient's gown before transport to the OR.
    4. leave all of the patient's jewelry on.

13. A patient who is being prepped for surgery asks the nurse to explain the purpose of the preoperative medications he has been given. The nurse should inform the patient that these particular medications:
    1. reduce preoperative fear.
    2. promote gastric emptying.
    3. reduce body secretions.
    4. facilitate the induction of anesthesia.

14. A patient who receives general or regional anesthesia in an ambulatory surgery center:

1. will remain in the unit longer than a hospitalized patient.
2. is allowed to ambulate as soon as being admitted to the recovery area.
3. must be near the level of preoperative functioning before dismissal.
4. is immediately given liberal amounts of fluid to promote excretion of the anesthesia.

15. After abdominal surgery, a patient is suspected of having internal bleeding. Which finding is most indicative of this complication?

1. Increased blood pressure
2. Incisional pain
3. Abdominal distention
4. Increased urinary output

16. An obese patient is at risk for poor wound healing postoperatively because:

1. ventilatory capacity is reduced.
2. fatty tissue has a poor blood supply.
3. the risk for dehiscence is increased.
4. resuming normal physical activity is delayed.

17. The nurse should ask each patient preoperatively for the name and dosage of all prescription and over-the-counter medications (including herbal remedies) taken before surgery because they:

1. may cause allergies to develop.
2. are automatically ordered postoperatively.
3. may create a greater risk for complications or interact with anesthetic agents.
4. should be taken the morning of surgery with sips of water.

18. A patient who smokes two packs of cigarettes per day is most at risk postoperatively for:

1. infection.
2. pneumonia.
3. hypotension.
4. cardiac dysrhythmias.

19. Family members should be included when the nurse teaches the patient preoperative exercises so that they can:

1. supervise the patient at home.
2. coach the patient postoperatively.
3. practice with the patient while waiting for transport to the OR.
4. relieve the nurse by getting the patient to exercise every 2 hours.

20. When deep breathing and coughing, the patient should be sitting because this position:

1. facilitates expansion of the thorax.
2. is more comfortable.
3. increases the patient's view of the room and is more relaxing.
4. helps the patient to splint with a pillow.

21. The nurse is checking a patient 2 hours after he returns from surgery. Which assessment finding requires immediate attention?

1. The patient's blood pressure has steadily decreased from 144/83 immediately after surgery to 129/71.
2. The patient's skin is warm and dry.
3. The patient vomits, and the emesis is coffee-colored.
4. The patient is drowsy, but responds promptly to voices.

22. A postoperative abdominal surgery patient complains that he "felt something give way" in his incision. On assessing the wound, the nurse notes a large amount of serosanguineous drainage and that wound edges are not approximated. Intestines are protruding from the wound. The nurse immediately:

1. encourages the patient to turn, cough, and deep breathe while splinting the opening.
2. covers the protruding internal organs with sterile gauze moistened with normal saline.
3. paints the open wound with an antimicrobial solution to prevent infection.
4. reinserts the organs and applies a pressure dressing to prevent further organ protrusion.

23. On admission of a patient to the PACU from surgery, the nurse places the highest priority on assessing the:

1. patient's level of consciousness.
2. condition of the surgical site.
3. adequacy of airway and breathing.
4. fluid and electrolyte balance.

24. The patient arrives on the unit after undergoing extensive abdominal surgery. He is awake and alert. He refuses to be repositioned in bed. What should the nurse assess first to determine the reason for the patient's refusal?

1. Consciousness
2. Maturation
3. Knowledge related to complications of immobility
4. Pain

25. The nurse is admitting a patient into the room on the surgical unit after abdominal surgery. There is a 1.5-cm–diameter spot of serosanguineous drainage on the dressing. What should the nurse do at this time?

1. Notify the physician of bleeding from the wound.
2. Note the amount of drainage and continue to monitor.
3. Remove the dressing to check for bleeding from the suture line.
4. Apply gentle pressure to the site for 5 minutes.

chapter 43

Care of the Patient with an Integumentary Disorder

Linda Y. North

http://evolve.elsevier.com/Christensen/foundationsadult

Objectives

Anatomy and Physiology

1. Discuss the primary functions of the integumentary system.
2. Describe the differences between the epidermis and dermis.
3. Discuss the functions of the three major glands located in the skin.

Medical-Surgical

4. Discuss the general assessment of the skin.
5. Discuss the viral disorders of the skin.
6. Discuss the bacterial, fungal, and inflammatory disorders of the skin.
7. Identify the parasitic disorders of the skin.
8. Describe the common tumors of the skin.
9. Identify the disorders associated with the appendages of the skin.
10. State the pathophysiology involved in a burn injury.
11. Identify the methods used to classify the extent of a burn injury.
12. Discuss the stages of burn care with appropriate nursing interventions.
13. Discuss how to use the nursing process in caring for patients with skin disorders.
14. Identify general nursing interventions for the patient with a skin disorder.

Key Terms

alopecia (ăl-ō-PĒ -shē-ă, p. 1330)
autograft (ĂW-tō-grăft, p. 1336)
contracture (kŏn-TRĂK-chŭr, p. 1334)
Curling's ulcer (KŬR-lĭngz ŬL-sĕr, p. 1334)
debridement (dă-BRĒD-mōń, p. 1335)
eschar (ĔS-kăr, p. 1335)
excoriation (ĕks-kŏr-ē-Ā-shŭn, p. 1308)
exudate (ĔKS-ū-dāt, p. 1305)
heterograft (xenograft) (HĔT-ĕr-ō-grăft; ZĒ-nō-grăft, p. 1336)
homograft (allograft) (HŌ-mō-grăft; ĂL-ō-grăft, p. 1336)
keloids (KĒ-loydz, p. 1326)
macules (MĂK-ūlz, p. 1312)
nevi (NĒ-vī, p. 1327)
papules (PĂP-ūlz, p. 1315)
pediculosis (pĕ-dĭk-ū-LŌ-sĭs, p. 1323)
pruritus (proo-RĪ-tŭs, p. 1297)
pustulant vesicles (PŬS-tū-lănt VĔS-ĭ-kŭlz, p. 1312)
rule of nines (p. 1332)
suppuration (sūp-ū-RĀ-shŭn, p. 1313)
urticaria (ŭr-tĭ-KĂ-rē-ă, p. 1317)
verruca (vĕ-RŪ-kă, p. 1327)
vesicle (VĔS-ĭ-kl, p. 1304)
wheals (wēlz, p. 1317)

The skin, or **integument** is a major organ and the outer covering of the body. Together with its appendages—hair, nails, and special glands—it makes up the integumentary system. Skin is essential to life. Society has long held healthy skin in high esteem, probably because it is so visible to others. People spend many hours grooming their hair, cleansing their skin, and manicuring their nails. But beyond its social aspect, the integument is the body's protector, its first line of defense against infection and injury.

ANATOMY AND PHYSIOLOGY OF THE SKIN

FUNCTIONS OF THE SKIN

Although the skin covers the outside of the body, its main function is homeostasis and protection of the internal organs. Each day it is subjected to temperature and humidity changes, trauma, ecchymosis, abrasions, contact with pathogens, and wear and tear. The skin carries out the numerous functions to protect and maintain the body (Box 43-1).

Box 43-1 Functions of the Skin

- Protects from pathogenic organisms and foreign substances; provides a natural barrier against infection
- Regulates temperature
- Prevents excessive water loss (dehydration)
- Aids in excretion of waste products
- Synthesizes vitamin D
- Insulates body and protects from trauma through subcutaneous layer of fat
- Has nerve endings that provide sensory perception to the brain related to pain, heat and cold, touch, pressure, and vibration

Protection

Sensory receptors within the skin receive information about the environment. Messages about heat, cold, pressure, and touch are received and relayed to the central nervous system for interpretation. Healthy skin protects the body from absorbing many chemicals and foreign substances. Additionally, as long as it remains intact, skin provides a barrier to many microorganisms in the environment. Internal organs are cushioned and protected by a subcutaneous layer of adipose (fat) tissue. The skin aids in elimination of waste products, prevents dehydration, and serves as a reservoir for food and water.

Temperature Regulation

Skin assists the body in maintaining a constant temperature under varying internal and external conditions. It allows blood vessels near the surface to constrict when the environment is cold to preserve heat and allows them to dilate when it is hot to release excess body heat. Sweat glands release moisture, which cools the body as it evaporates. A layer of adipose tissue works as an insulator by retaining heat.

Vitamin D Synthesis

Cholesterol compounds in the skin are converted to vitamin D when exposed to the sun's ultraviolet rays. Vitamin D is necessary for healthy bone development. Prolonged exposure to the sun's rays, which is ultraviolet radiation, should be avoided because of the increased risk of developing skin cancer.

STRUCTURE OF THE SKIN

Skin consists of two layers: the outer epidermis and inner dermis, or corium. Beneath these layers of skin lies the subcutaneous layer, or superficial fascia (Figure 43-1).

Epidermis

The **epidermis,** the superficial fascia (avascular layers of the skin), is composed of stratified squamous (from the Latin *squama,* meaning "scale") epithelium. The cells of the epidermis are tightly packed and have no distinct blood supply. The epidermis is divided into layers, or strata: an outer, dead, cornified portion and a deep, living, cellular portion. The inner layer is called the **stratum germinativum;** it is the only layer of the epidermis able to undergo cell division and reproduce itself. It receives its blood supply and nutrition from the underlying dermis through a process called **diffusion.** This provides a constant new supply of cells for the upper layers and enables the skin to repair itself after injury. As these cells push their way to the surface, their internal structures are destroyed and the cells die. When they reach the outermost layer, called the **stratum corneum,** they are flat and the cell structure is filled with a protein called **keratin** (horn). The stratum corneum is sometimes called the horny layer. The keratin makes the cells dry, tough, and somewhat waterproof.

Another layer in the epidermis contains highly specialized cells called **melanocytes.** These cells give rise to the pigment **melanin,** a black or dark brown pig-

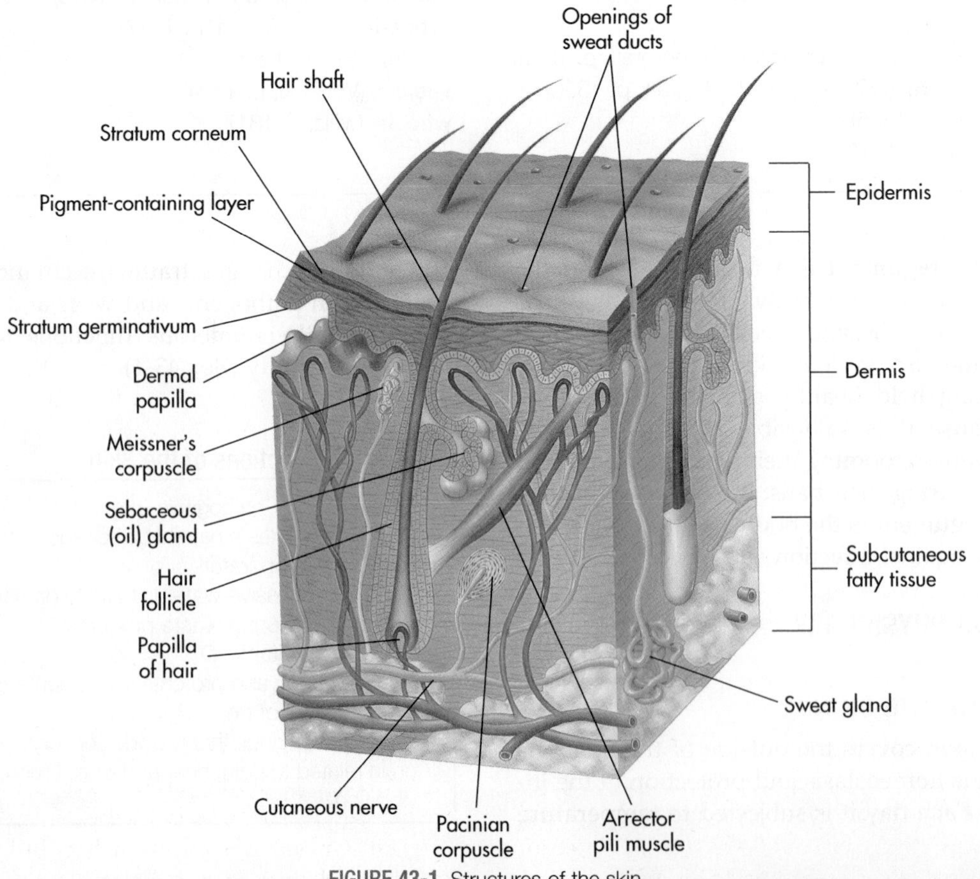

FIGURE 43-1 Structures of the skin.

ment occurring naturally in the hair, the skin, and the iris and choroid of the eye. Melanin is responsible for the skin's color. The greater the concentration of melanin, the darker the skin. Sometimes irregular patches with greater concentrations of melanin occur, producing freckles. The amount of melanin a person has is inherited from the parents. Although skin color is inherited, exposure to the sun and other factors can influence skin color.

Dermis

The **dermis,** or **corium,** is often called the true skin. It is well supplied with blood vessels and nerves and also contains glands and hair follicles. It varies in thickness throughout the body but tends to be thickest in the palms and soles. The dermis is composed of connective tissue with cells scattered among collagen and elastic fibers. The dermis receives strength from the collagen and flexibility from the elastic connective fibers. The cells throughout this layer are bathed in tissue fluid called interstitial fluid. The skin wrinkles with the normal aging process, as the dermis loses some of its elastic connective fibers and the subcutaneous tissue directly beneath it loses some of its adipose tissue. Located in the upper portion of the dermis are small fingerlike projections called **papillae** that project into the lower epidermal layer. Without the dermal papillae, the epidermal layer would be unable to survive.

Subcutaneous Layer

The subcutaneous layer, sometimes called the **superficial fascia,** is the layer of tissue directly beneath the dermis that connects the skin to the muscle surface. This layer is composed of adipose tissue and loose connective tissue. It serves several important functions: (1) stores water and fat, (2) insulates the body, (3) protects the organs lying beneath it, and (4) provides a pathway for nerves and blood vessels. The distribution of subcutaneous tissue throughout the body provides shape and contour. A woman's body usually contains more subcutaneous tissue than a man's; thus her body is softer and more rounded.

APPENDAGES OF THE SKIN

Sudoriferous Glands

The **sudoriferous** (sweat) **glands** are coiled, tubelike structures located in the dermis and subcutaneous layers. The tubes open into pores on the skin surface. Approximately 3 million sweat glands are located throughout the integumentary system. These glands excrete sweat, which cools the body's surface. Sweat is composed of water, salts, urea, uric acid, ammonia, sugar, lactic acid, and ascorbic acid.

Ceruminous Glands

Ceruminous glands are modified sudoriferous glands. They secrete a waxlike substance called **cerumen** and are located in the external ear canal. Cerumen is thought to protect the canal from foreign body invasion.

Sebaceous Glands

The **sebaceous** (oil) **glands** secrete **sebum** (an oily secretion) through the hair follicles distributed on the body. Their function is to lubricate the skin and hair that covers the body. Sebum also inhibits bacterial growth.

Hair and Nails

Hair is composed of modified dead epidermal tissue, mainly keratin. It is distributed all over the body in varying amounts. The root of the hair is enclosed in a follicle deep in the dermis. The shaft of the hair protrudes from the skin. Surrounding the hair follicle is a band of muscle tissue called **arrector pili** (see Figure 43-1). A sensation of cold or fear causes these muscles to contract, making the hair stand upright and dimpling the skin surrounding it. The effect is called piloerection, or "gooseflesh."

Nails are also composed mainly of keratin, but the keratin is more compressed. The base of the nail, the root, is made up of living cells and is mostly covered by the cuticle. Part of the root, the lunula, is exposed and looks like a white crescent. The remainder of the nail is called the **nail body.** It appears pink because of the blood vessels lying immediately beneath it.

ASSESSMENT OF THE SKIN

INSPECTION AND PALPATION

A thorough assessment of the skin helps identify many diseases that result from an outside organism penetrating the skin. However, remember that recognizing skin conditions by inspection takes time and experience.

Begin the assessment by obtaining a careful health history from the patient. Ask the patient about (1) recent skin lesions or rashes, (2) where the lesions first appeared, and (3) how long the lesions have been present. Also ask about a personal or family history of asthma, seasonal rhinitis, or drug allergies. Explore all complaints of pain, **pruritus** (the symptom of itching), tingling, or burning. Ask the patient about personal skin care and about (1) any recent skin color changes: (2) exposure to the sun, with or without sunscreen: and (3) family history of skin cancer.

Assess the skin under natural lighting, and use the senses of sight, touch, and smell while inspecting and palpating the skin. Expose the area to be assessed while maintaining privacy. Remember to wear gloves when inspecting the skin, mucous membranes, and any involved area. In the hospital, the morning bath provides an excellent opportunity to assess the patient's skin without exposure or embarrassment.

Observe the color of the skin. The color depends on many physiologic factors, including the following:

- Amount of hemoglobin in the blood
- Oxygen saturation in the blood
- Amount of substances such as bilirubin, urea, or other chemicals in the blood

- Quality and quantity of blood circulating in the superficial blood vessels
- Amount of melanin in the epidermis

Assessment of specific skin lesions, their appearance, and their location assists the dermatologist in diagnosing skin disorders and the nurse in providing care. Most disorders have only one or two types of lesions. Some of the typical clinical manifestations of skin disorders are shown in Table 43-1.

Assessment also includes the presence of rashes, scars, lesions, or ecchymoses and the distribution of hair. Assess temperature and texture by touch, using

Text continued on p. 1303

Table 43-1 Primary Skin Lesions

DESCRIPTION	EXAMPLES	
MACULE Flat, circumscribed area that is a change in the skin color; <1 cm in diameter	Freckles, flat moles (nevi), petechiae, measles, scarlet fever	Measles[a]
PAPULE Elevated, firm, circumscribed area; <1 cm in diameter	Wart (verruca), elevated moles, lichen planus	Lichen planus[b]
PATCH Flat, nonpalpable, irregularly shaped macule; >1 cm in diameter	Vitiligo, port-wine stains, mongolian spots, café-au-lait spots	Vitiligo[b]
PLAQUE Elevated, firm, and rough lesion with flat top surface; >1 cm in diameter	Psoriasis, seborrheic and actinic keratoses	Plaque[a]

Modified from Thompson, J., & Wilson, S. (1995). *Health assessment for nursing practice.* St. Louis: Mosby.
Sources: [a]Habif, T.P. (1996). *Clinical dermatology* (3rd ed.). St. Louis: Mosby; [b]Weston, W.L., et al. (1996). *Color textbook of pediatric dermatology*. St. Louis: Mosby.

Table 43-1 Primary Skin Lesions—cont'd

DESCRIPTION	EXAMPLES	
WHEAL Elevated irregularly shaped area of cutaneous edema; solid, transient; variable diameter	Insect bites, urticaria, allergic reaction	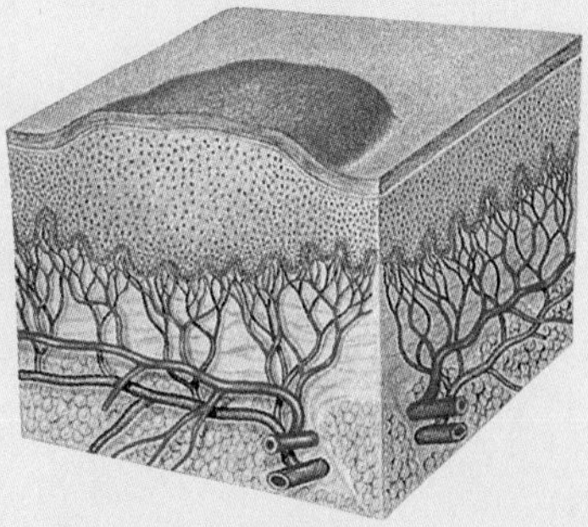 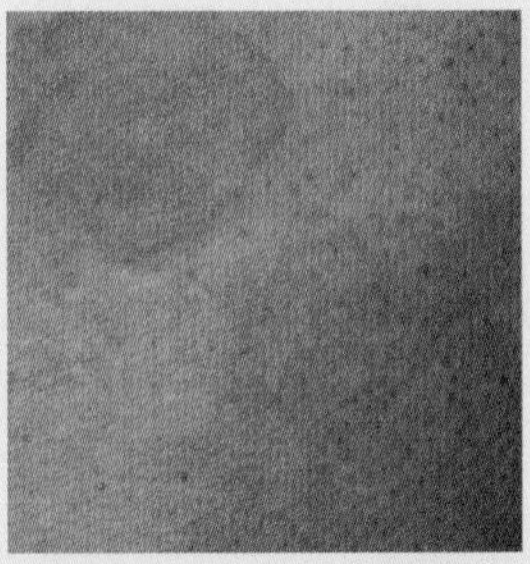 Wheal[c]
NODULE Elevated, firm, circumscribed lesion; deeper in dermis than a papule; 1-2 cm in diameter	Erythema nodosum, lipomas	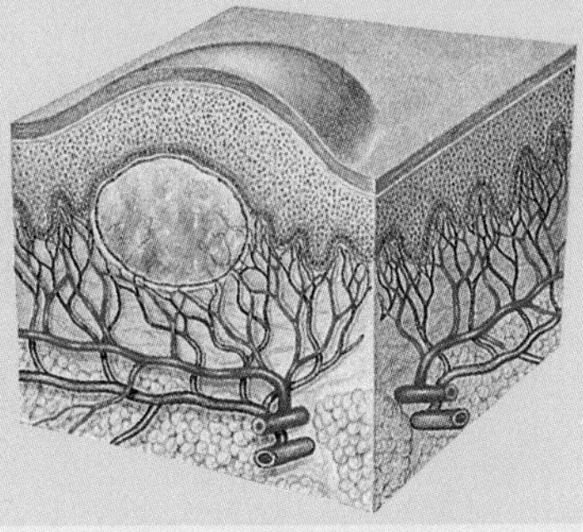 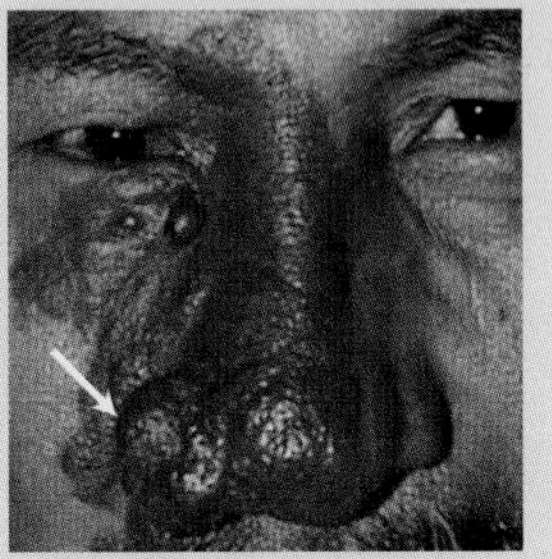 Hypertrophic nodule[d]
TUMOR Elevated and solid lesion; may or may not be clearly demarcated; deeper in dermis; >2 cm in diameter	Neoplasms, benign tumor, lipoma, hemangioma	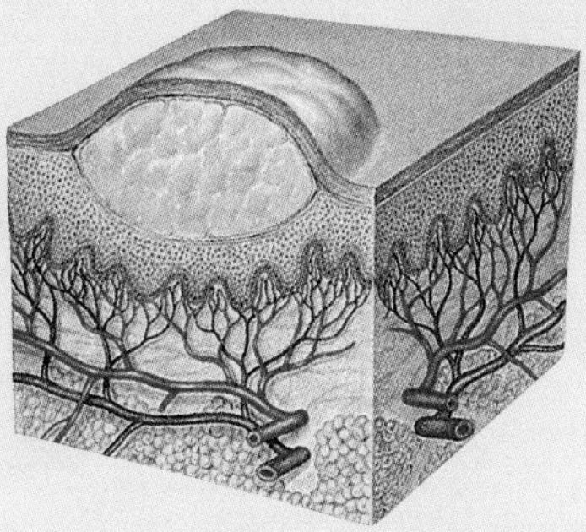 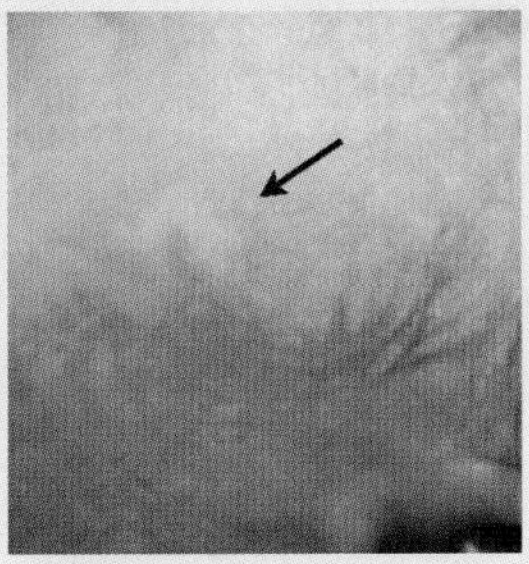 Hemangioma[b]
VESICLE Elevated, circumscribed, superficial, not into dermis; filled with serous fluid; <1 cm in diameter	Varicella (chickenpox), herpes zoster (shingles)	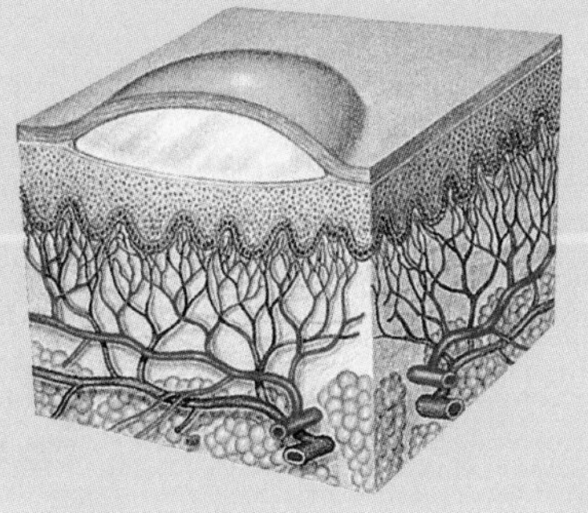 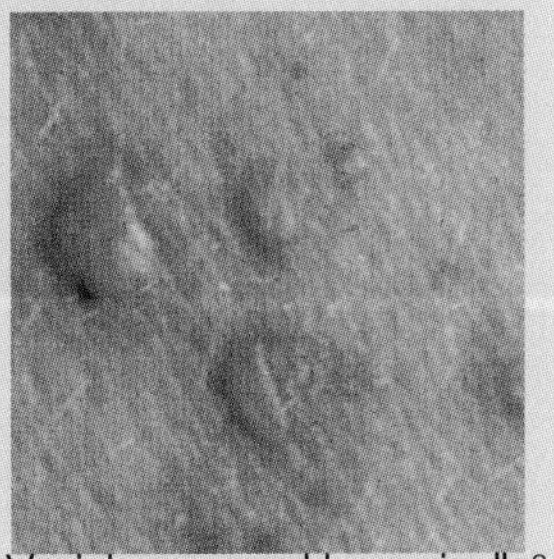 Vesicles caused by varicella[c]

Sources: [b]Weston, W.L., et al. (1996). *Color textbook of pediatric dermatology.* St. Louis: Mosby; [c]Farrar, W.E., et al. (1994) *Infectious diseases* (2nd ed.). London: Gower; [d]Goldman, M.P., & Fitzpatrick, R.E. (1994). *Cutaneous laser surgery: The art and science of selective photo thermolysis.* St. Louis: Mosby.

Continued

Table 43-1 Primary Skin Lesions—cont'd

DESCRIPTION	EXAMPLES	
BULLA Vesicle >1 cm in diameter	Blister, pemphigus vulgaris	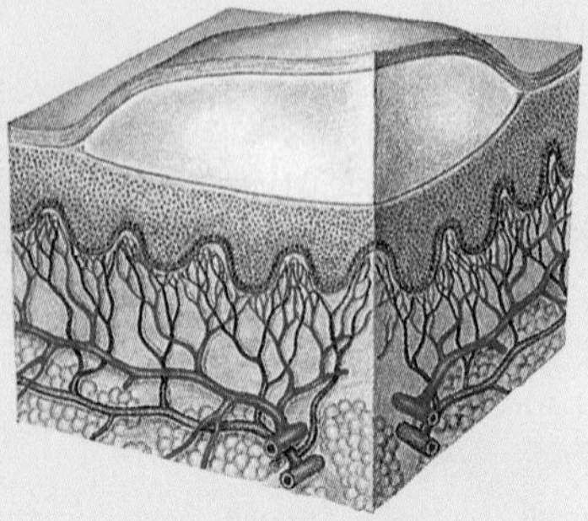 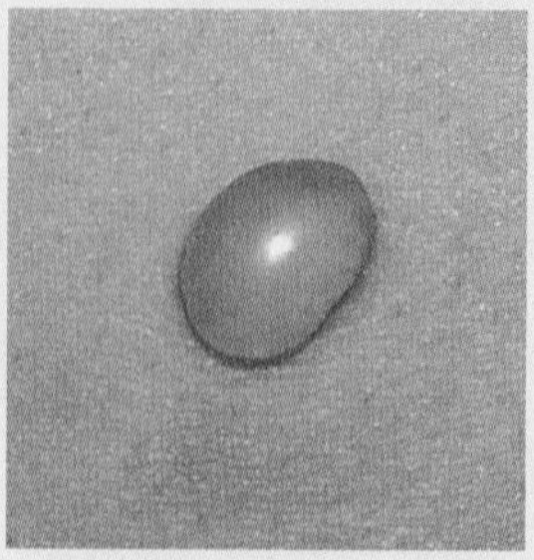 Blister[e]
PUSTULE Elevated, superficial lesion; similar to a vesicle but filled with purulent fluid	Impetigo, acne	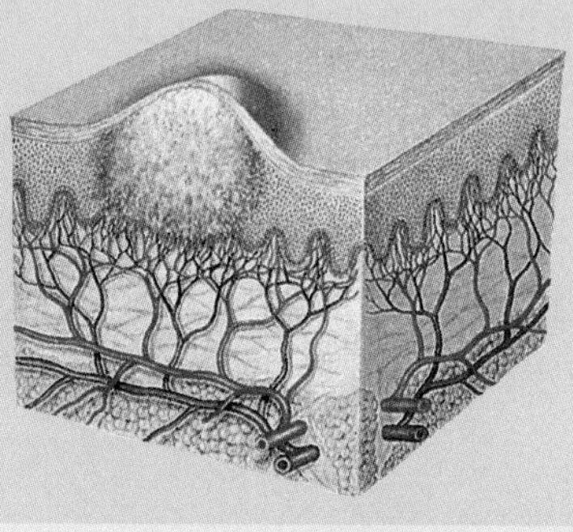 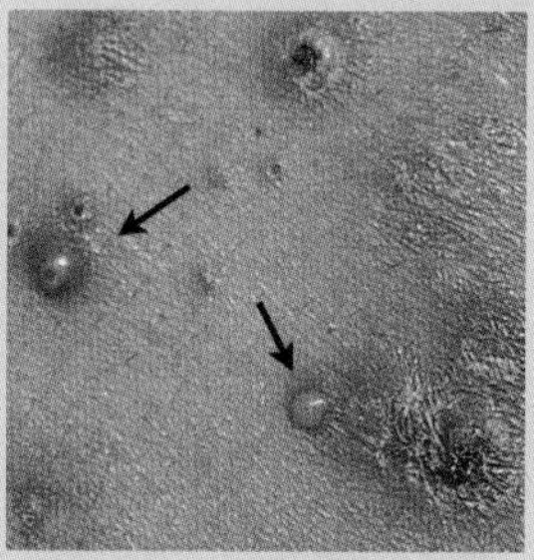 Acne[b]
CYST Elevated, circumscribed, encapsulated lesion; in dermis or subcutaneous layer; filled with liquid or semisolid material	Sebaceous cyst, cystic acne	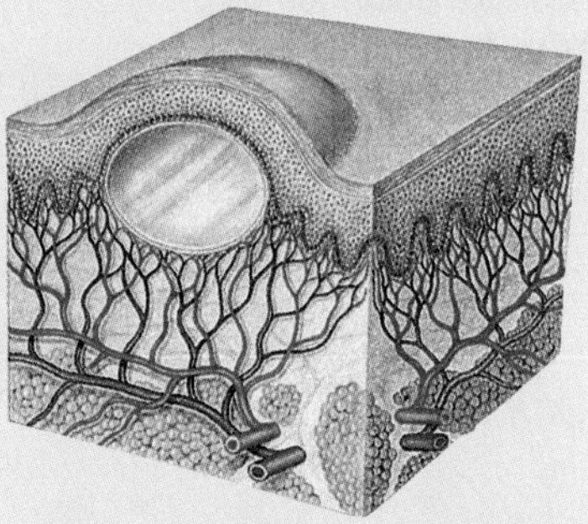 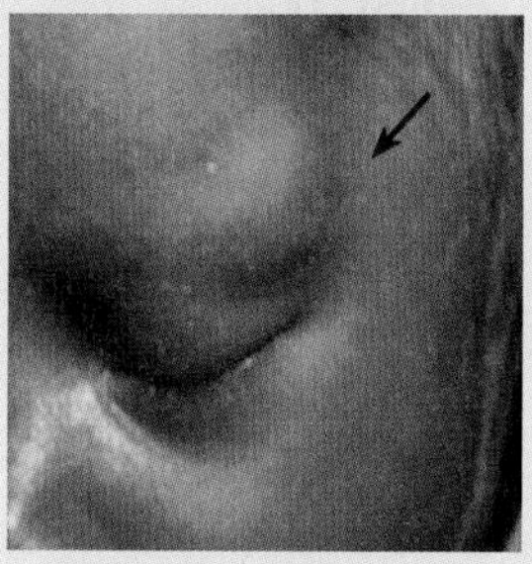 Sebaceous cyst[b]
TELANGIECTASIA Fine, irregular red lines produced by capillary dilation	Telangiectasia in rosacea	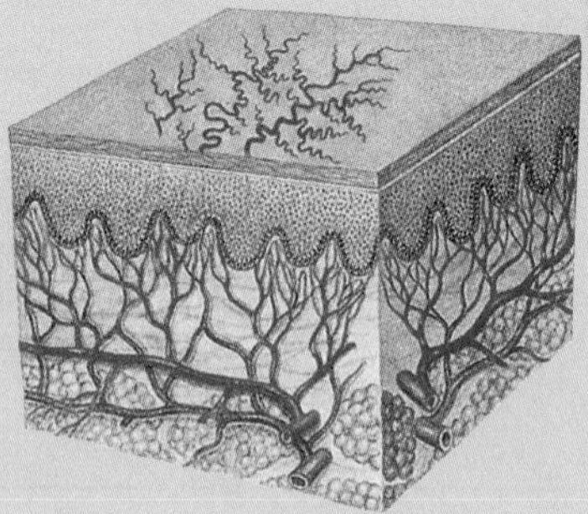 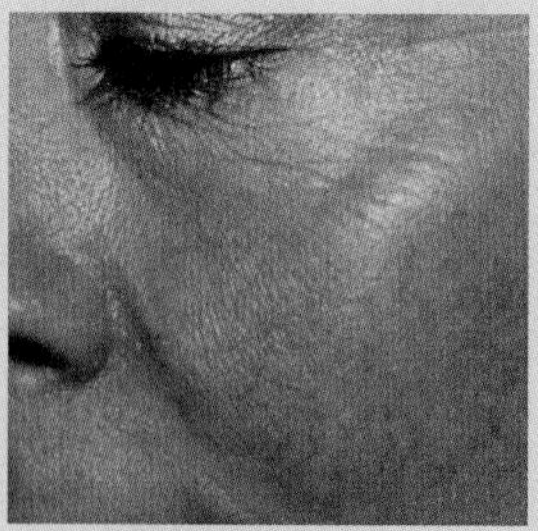 Telangiectasia[d]

Sources: [b]Weston, W.L., et al. (1996). *Color textbook of pediatric dermatology.* St. Louis: Mosby; [d]Goldman, M.P., & Fitzpatrick, R.E. (1994). *Cutaneous laser surgery: The art and science of selective photo thermolysis.* St. Louis: Mosby; [e]White, G.M. (1994). *Color atlas of regional dermatology.* St. Louis: Mosby.

Table 43-1 Primary Skin Lesions—cont'd

DESCRIPTION	EXAMPLES		
SCALE Heaped-up keratinized cells; flaky skin; irregular; thick or thin; dry or oily; variation in size	Flaking of skin with seborrheic dermatitis after scarlet fever, or flaking of skin following a drug reaction; dry skin	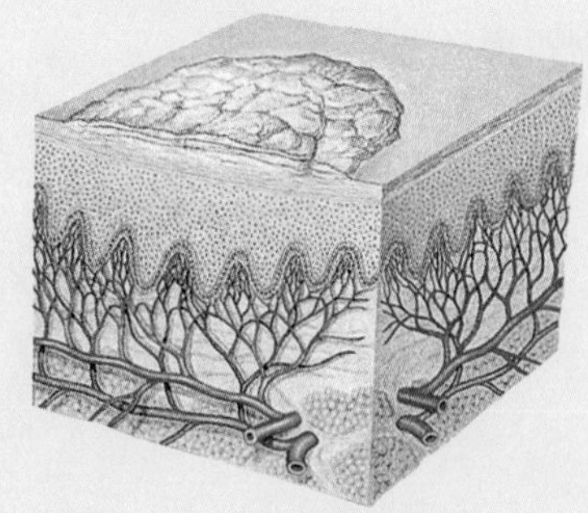	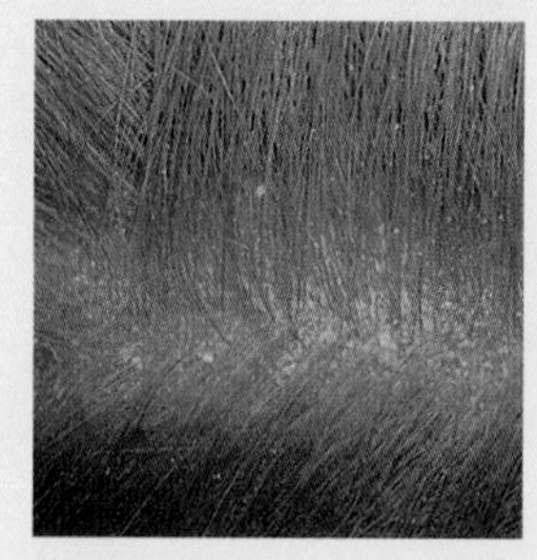 Fine scaling[f]
LICHENIFICATION Rough, thickened epidermis secondary to persistent rubbing, itching, or skin irritation; often involves flexor surface of extremity	Chronic dermatitis	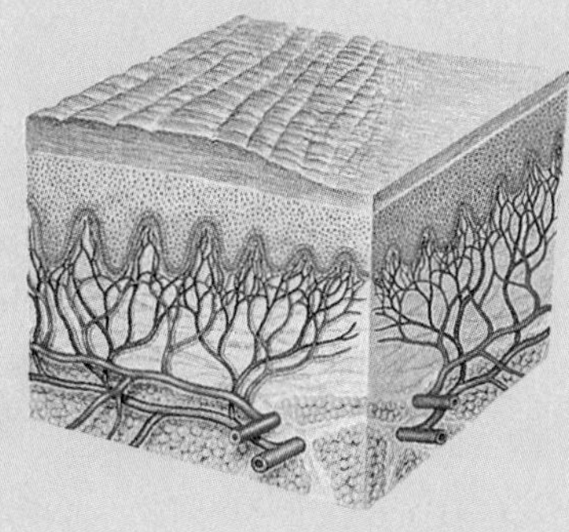	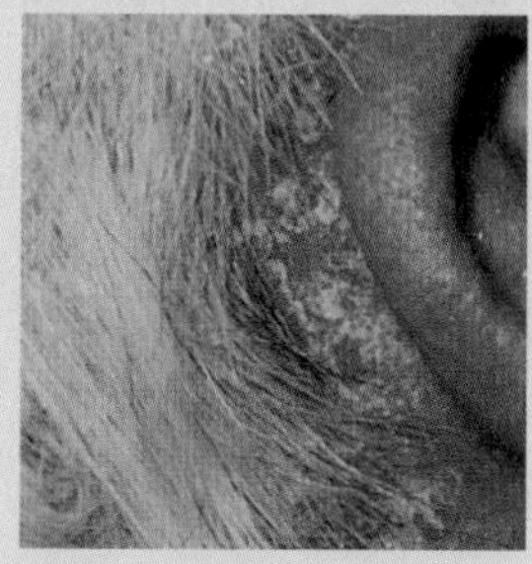 Stasis dermatitis in an early stage[g]
KELOID Irregularly shaped, elevated, progressively enlarging scar; grows beyond the boundaries of the wound; caused by excessive collagen formation during healing	Keloid formation after surgery	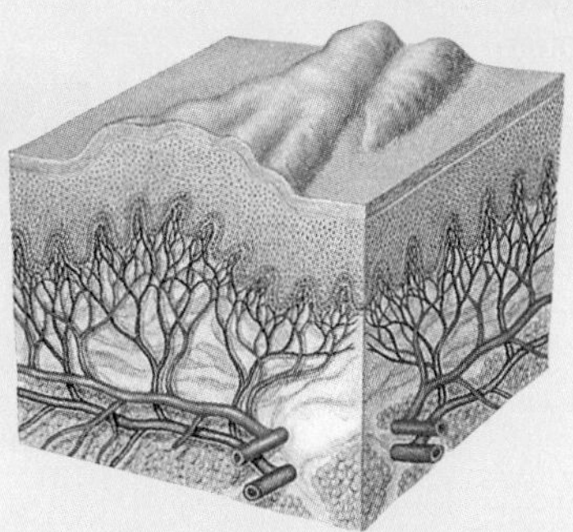	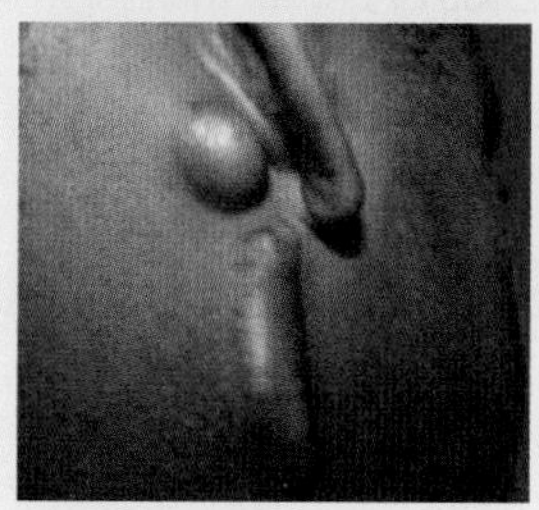 Keloid[b]
SCAR Thin to thick fibrous tissue that replaces normal skin after injury or laceration to the dermis	Healed wound or surgical incision	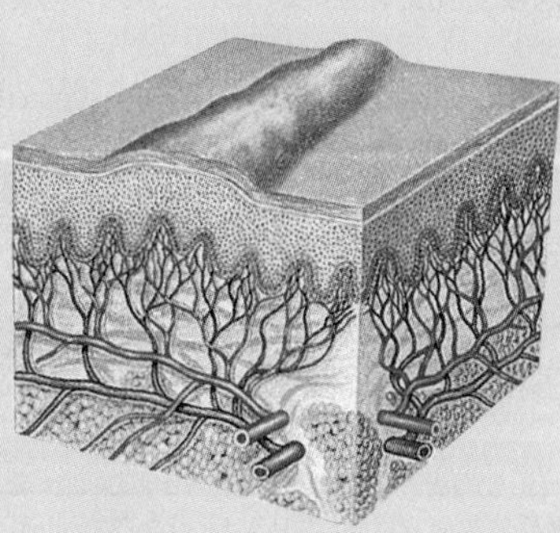	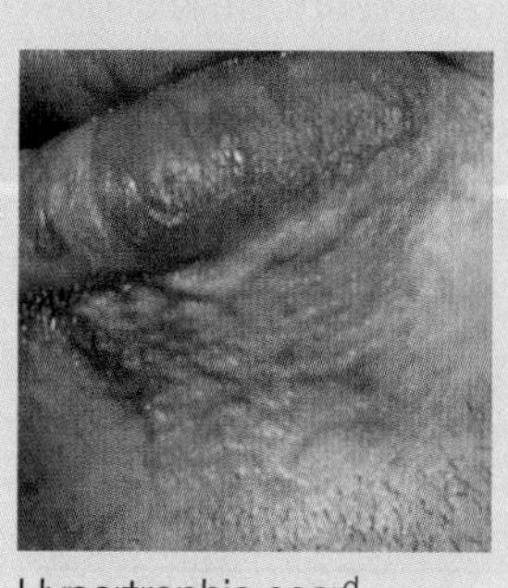 Hypertrophic scar[d]

Sources: [b]Weston, W.L., et al. (1996). *Color textbook of pediatric dermatology.* St. Louis: Mosby; [d]Goldman, M.P., & Fitzpatrick, R.E. (1994). *Cutaneous laser surgery: The art and science of selective photo thermolysis.* St. Louis: Mosby; [f]Baran, R., et al. (1991). *Color atlas of the hair, scalp, and nails.* St. Louis: Mosby; [g]Marks, J.G., Jr., & DeLeo, V.A. (1991). *Contact and occupational dermatitis.* St. Louis: Mosby.

Continued

Table 43-1 Primary Skin Lesions—cont'd

DESCRIPTION	EXAMPLES		
EXCORIATION Loss of the epidermis; linear hollowed-out crusted area	Abrasion or scratch, scabies	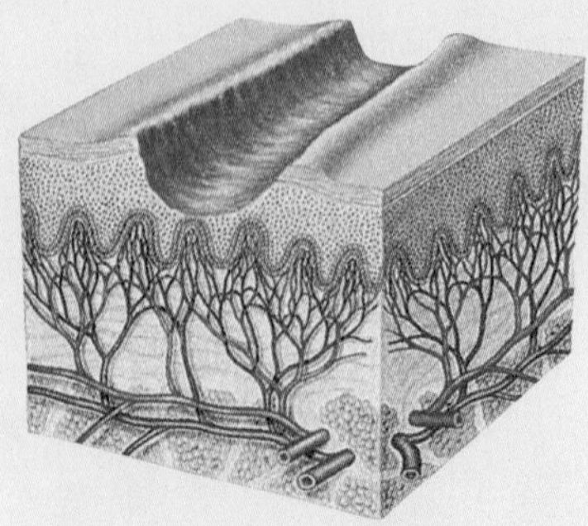	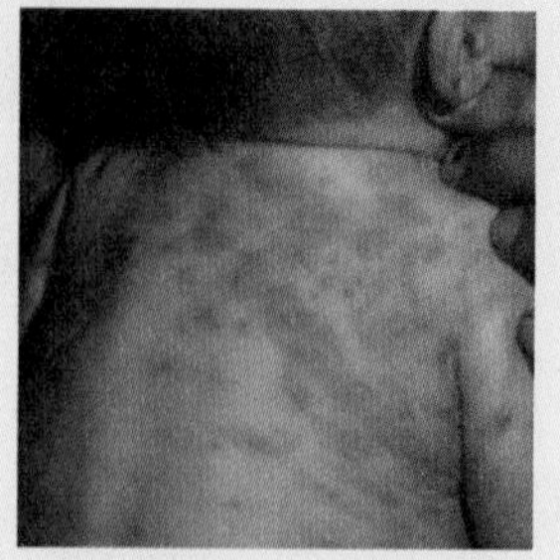 Scabies[b]
FISSURE Linear crack or break from the epidermis to the dermis; may be moist or dry	Athlete's foot, cracks at the corner of the mouth	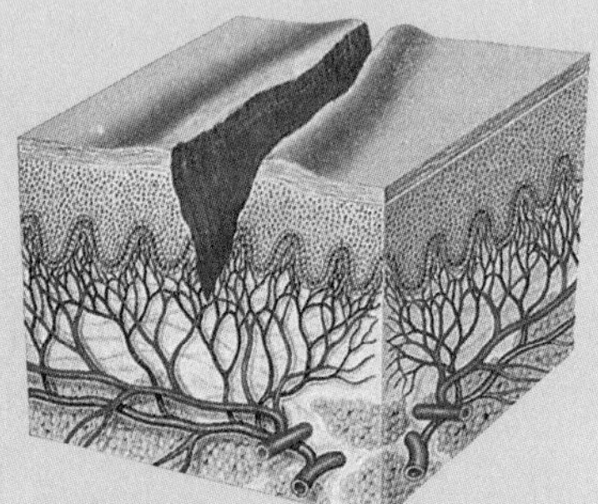	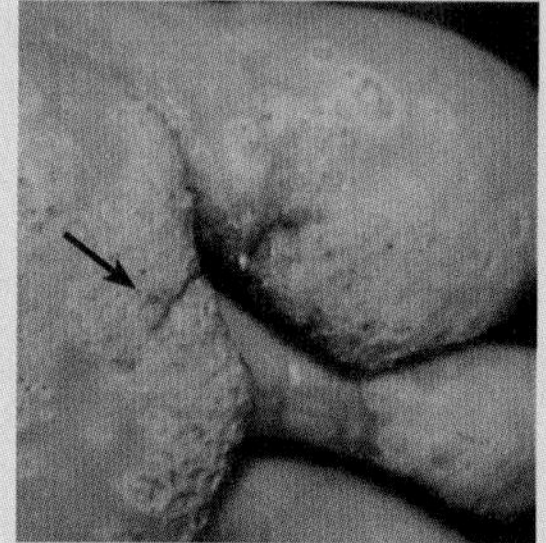 Fissures[d]
EROSION Loss of part of the epidermis; depressed, moist, glistening; follows rupture of a vesicle or bulla	Varicella, variola after rupture	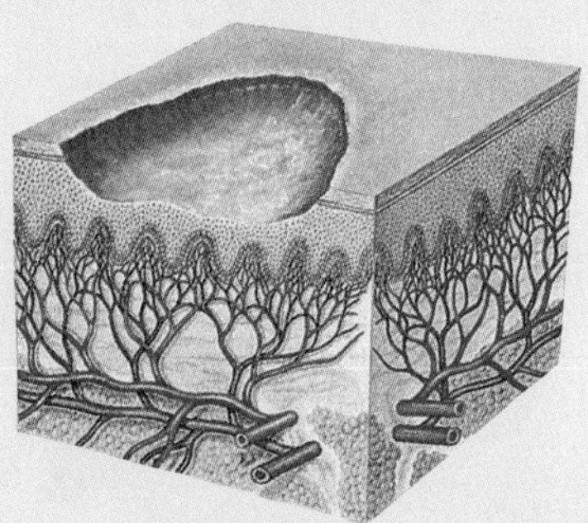	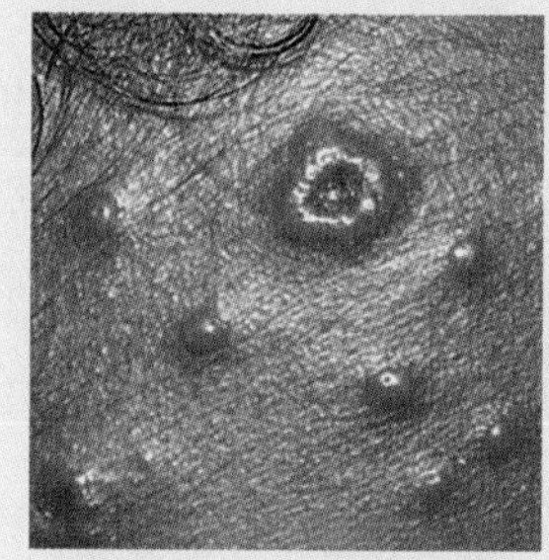 Erosion[h]
ULCER Loss of epidermis and dermis; concave; varies in size	Pressure sores, stasis ulcers	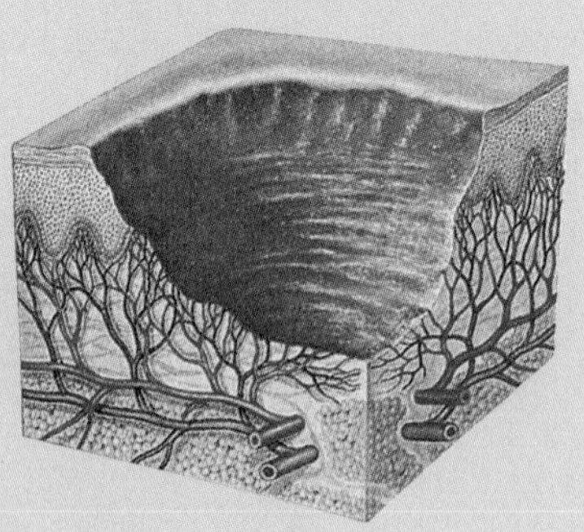	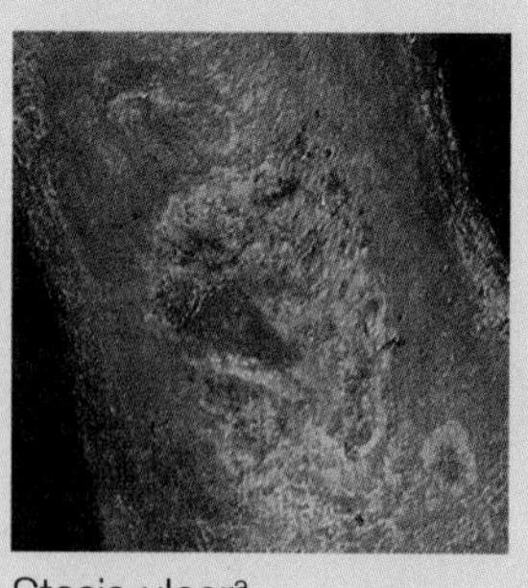 Stasis ulcer[a]

Sources: [a]Habif, T.P. (1996). *Clinical dermatology* (3rd ed.). St. Louis: Mosby; [b]Weston, W.L., et al. (1996). *Color textbook of pediatric dermatology.* St. Louis: Mosby; [d]Goldman, M.P., & Fitzpatrick, R.E. (1994). *Cutaneous laser surgery: The art and science of selective photo thermolysis.* St. Louis: Mosby; [h]Cohen, B.A. (1993). *Pediatric dermatology.* London: Wolfe;

Table 43-1 **Primary Skin Lesions—cont'd**

DESCRIPTION	EXAMPLES
CRUST	
Dried serum, blood, or purulent exudate; slightly elevated; size varies; brown, red, black or tan	Scab on abrasion, eczema Scab[g]
ATROPHY	
Thinning of skin surface and loss of skin markings; skin translucent and paperlike	Striae; aged skin Aged skin[g]

Source: [g]Marks, J.G., Jr., & DeLeo, V.A. (1991). *Contact and occupational dermatitis.* St. Louis: Mosby.

the palms of the hands to compare opposite body areas. For example, feel both legs before concluding that the left leg is cold. Use a cotton-tipped applicator to touch the sole of the foot and assess sensation. Inspect the nails for normal development, color, shape, and thickness. Clubbing (broadening) of the fingertips indicates decreased oxygen (hypoxemia) and should be reported. Inspect the hair for thickness, dryness, or dullness. Assessment also includes inspecting the mucous membranes for pallor or cyanosis. Document profuse sweating or any sign of impaired skin integrity. Examine the ceruminous and sebaceous glands for overactivity or underactivity using appropriate questions, such as, "Tell me how often the physician has had to remove the wax from your ears."

Assessment of Dark Skin

The color of a person's skin, and how dark or light it is, is genetically determined. Dark skin color results from the reflection of light as it strikes the underlying skin pigment. Melanocytes have increased activity and produce large amounts of melanin, which accounts for the darker skin color. This increased melanin forms a natural sun shield, accounting for the lower incidence of skin cancer in people with dark skin.

The structures of dark skin are no different from those of lighter skin, but they are more difficult to assess. Practice and comparison are necessary. Assessment is easier in areas where the epidermis is thin, such as the lips and mucous membranes. Rashes are often difficult to observe and may need to be palpated.

Dark skin is predisposed to certain skin conditions, including pseudofolliculitis, keloids, and mongolian spots. For some persons with dark skin, color cannot be used as an indicator of systemic conditions (e.g., flushed skin with fever) (see Cultural Considerations box).

CHIEF COMPLAINT

When skin lesions are found accompanying a skin disorder, document the exact location, length, width, general appearance, and name. A helpful mnemonic for assessing the chief complaint is to remember the following letters:

- **P:** **P**rovocative and **P**alliative factors (factors that cause the condition)
- **Q:** **Q**uality and **Q**uantity (characteristics and size) of the skin problem
- **R:** **R**egion of the body
- **S:** **S**everity of the signs and symptoms
- **T:** **T**ime (length of time the patient has had the disorder)

An important objective in skin assessment is to identify possible malignancies. The three most common are melanoma, basal cell carcinoma, and squamous cell carcinoma. When assessing growths or

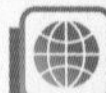

Cultural Considerations

Skin Care

- The darker a person's skin, the more difficult it is to assess for changes in color. Establish a baseline in natural lighting if possible or with at least a 60-watt light bulb.
- Assess baseline skin color in areas with the least pigmentation, such as palms of the hands, soles of the feet, underside of forearms, abdomen, and buttocks.
- All skin colors have an underlying red tone. Pallor in black-skinned individuals is seen as ashen or gray. Pallor in brown-skinned individuals appears as yellowish. Assess pallor in mucous membranes, lips, nailbeds, and conjunctivae of the lower eyelids.
- To assess rashes and skin inflammation in dark-skinned individuals, rely on *palpation* for warmth and *induration* rather than observation.
- Some folk remedies may be misdiagnosed as injuries. Three folk practices of Southeast Asia can leave marks on the body that can be mistaken for signs of abuse or violence. *Cao gio* is the rubbing of the skin with a coin to produce dark blood or ecchymotic strips; it is done to treat a thrombus or the symptoms of the flu. *Bat gio* is skin pinching on the temples to treat headaches or on the neck for a sore throat. The treatment is considered a success if petechiae or ecchymosis appears. *Paua* is the burning of the skin with the tip of a dried weedlike grass. It is believed the burning will cause the noxious element that causes the pain to leave the body.

changes in a mole, ask the following questions, using the mnemonic device **ABCDE:**

A: Is the mole **A**symmetrical?
B: Are the **B**orders irregular?
C: Is the **C**olor uneven or irregular?
D: Has the **D**iameter of the growth changed recently?
E: Has the surface area become **E**levated?

Promptly report a positive finding of any of these characteristics to a physician. After completing the assessment, document the findings. Proper assessment and identification serve as a baseline for evaluating nursing care and determining whether changes are needed.

PSYCHOSOCIAL ASSESSMENT

The person with an integumentary disorder may have a chronic or acute condition. Regardless of the severity, recovery may be lengthy with little visible outward improvement. A person's body image and self-esteem may be affected. Society's reaction to a skin condition has a significant effect on the patient. Personal appearance is a primary concern to many individuals, and others may think the condition is infectious and may socially isolate the patient. An integumentary disorder can have a negative effect on a patient's self-concept because of the value society places on a person's physical characteristics.

Assess the patient's coping abilities by using open-ended questions to encourage him or her to talk and ventilate feelings. Also assess the patient's interaction with family and others. Nonverbal behavior such as covering the involved area and avoiding eye contact may indicate a self-image problem. Validate or correct a patient's knowledge base. Rarely are skin diseases fatal, and few are contagious. Nurses need to work through their own feelings about a patient's skin appearance before they can be a source of encouragement. The nurse's attitude and interventions should be nonjudgmental, warm, and accepting. The nurse must be skilled and knowledgeable about skin care.

A patient with a skin disorder may have a problem with anxiety. Decrease the patient's anxiety by implementing the following interventions:

- Provide patients with consistent information related to their care plan.
- Include the family in the treatment plan. The family may be able to support instructions given, which helps to decrease anxiety.
- Provide positive feedback concerning the patient's efforts and progress, no matter how large or small.
- Refer the patient to a support group as soon as possible (if appropriate).

VIRAL DISORDERS OF THE SKIN

HERPES SIMPLEX

Etiology and Pathophysiology

The herpetovirus *Herpesvirus hominis* is the cause of herpes simplex. Two types of the virus are known:

- Type 1, the most common, causes the common cold sore and is usually associated with febrile conditions. The virus is self-limiting with no cure.
- Type 2 causes lesions in the genital area known as genital herpes. Type 2 is the same virus as type 1 and is discussed with sexually transmitted infections in Chapter 52.

Both types of virus may be transmitted by direct contact with any open lesion. However, in type 2, the primary mode is through sexual contact. The lesions are usually present for 2 to 3 weeks and are most painful during the first week. Complications may be severe if the disease spreads to other body areas.

Clinical Manifestations

Type 1 herpes simplex is characterized by a **vesicle** (circumscribed elevation of skin filled with serous fluid; smaller than 0.5 cm) at the corner of the mouth, on the lips, or on the nose. It is commonly known as a **cold sore** (Figure 43-2). At first the involved area is usually erythematous and edematous. The vesicle then appears, ulcerates, and encrusts. When the vesicle ruptures, it produces a burning pain. The patient experiences general malaise and fatigue. Usual occurrence is during an acute illness or infection.

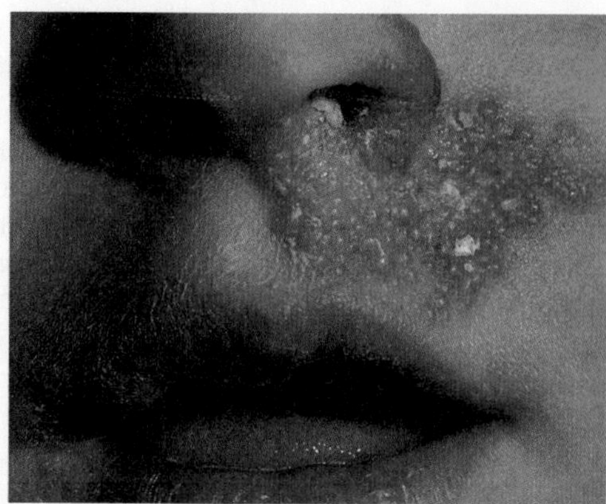

FIGURE 43-2 Herpes simplex.

Type 2, genital herpes, produces various types of vesicles that rupture and encrust, causing ulcerations. The cervix is the most common site in women, and the penis is the most common area in men. Flulike symptoms occur 3 or 4 days after the vesicles erupt. Headache, fatigue, myalgia, fever, and anorexia are common.

Assessment

Assessment primarily involves inspection of the skin. Obtain a complete health history to support assessment data. **Subjective data** include complaints of fatigue along with pruritus and burning pain in the mouth for herpes simplex type 1 and in the genital area for herpes simplex type 2.

Objective data for herpes simplex type 1 include an edematous, erythematous area at the corner of the lip. In herpes simplex type 2, the labia, vulva, or penis will appear edematous and erythematous. The vesicular lesions may rupture and develop a dried **exudate** (fluid, cells, or other substances that have been slowly exuded, or discharged, from cells or blood vessels through small pores or breaks in cell membranes).

Diagnostic Tests

Diagnosis of herpesvirus is made by laboratory assessment of cultures from the lesion. Inspection and health history support the diagnosis. Patients should also be assessed for human immunodeficiency virus (HIV).

Medical Management

Herpesvirus has no cure, but treatment is aimed at relieving symptoms. Acyclovir (Zovirax) is an antiviral agent that can alter the course of the disease. Acyclovir can be administered orally, topically, or intravenously (Table 43-2). These drugs inhibit viral reproduction but are not a cure (Lewis et al., 2007).

Nursing Interventions and Patient Teaching

Nursing interventions primarily focus on treating symptoms and preventing spread of the disease. The patient can use warm compresses to relieve pain and severe pruritus. He or she should keep the lesions dry and avoid direct contact. Analgesics such as acetaminophen (Tylenol) are effective in pain control. The specific nursing diagnoses for herpes are based on assessment data gathered. Type 2 herpesvirus, genital herpes, remains transferable during remission. Teach patients to take precautions such as using condoms during sexual activity (Lewis et al., 2007).

Nursing diagnoses and interventions for the patient with herpes include but are not limited to the following:

Nursing Diagnoses	Nursing Interventions
Pain, related to pruritus	Assess factors that precipitate pruritus. Apply local anesthetic, such as Orabase, for pain. Apply drying agent to lesions. Apply warm compresses. Have patient wear loose-fitting, cotton clothing that does not constrict movement or occlude circulation.
Impaired skin integrity, related to open lesions	Inspect lesions for drainage, color, and location. Wash hands before and after contact. Keep area dry. Administer antiviral agents as ordered. In genital herpes, use of a hair dryer can dry the lesions and promote patient comfort.
Risk for infection, related to skin excoriation	Use body substance precautions. Teach patient proper skin care. Wash hands before and after care. Keep area dry. Administer antiviral drugs as ordered.

Preventing infection remains the top priority when caring for a patient with an open skin lesion. Patient teaching focuses on the principles of medical asepsis and includes specific measures to prevent spread of the disease. Using good hygiene in all areas of care is critical in preventing secondary infections. Include the complications and precipitating factors in patient teaching and discharge planning.

Prognosis

Herpes simplex has no cure. The prognosis for type 1 is healing within 10 to 14 days, and possible recurrence with depression of the immune system. For type 2, lesions are usually present for 7 to 14 days. Unfortunately, 75% of all patients have at least one recurrence, and two thirds have one to five recurrences annually.

Table 43-2 Medications for the Integumentary System

Generic (Trade)	Action	Side Effects	Nursing Implications
Acyclovir (Zovirax)	Antiviral	Topical: Burning, rash, pruritus, stinging Systemic: Headache, seizures, renal toxicity, phlebitis at IV site	Topical: Use glove to apply; cover lesion completely. Systemic: Ensure adequate hydration to prevent crystallization in kidneys; administer IV dose for at least 1 hour
Alpha Keri	Emollient	Local irritation, allergic reactions	For external use only; exercise caution when using in tub to avoid slipping
Aluminum acetate solution (Burow's solution)	Astringent	Local irritation, allergic reactions	For external use only; do not use with occlusive dressings
Antihistamines, including: Diphenhydramine (Benadryl) Hydroxyzine (Vistaril, Atarax)	Blocks histamine at H_1 receptor site, inhibiting many allergic reactions	Drowsiness, dizziness, confusion, dry mouth, urinary retention	If drowsiness occurs, avoid activities that require concentration; avoid using with alcohol or other CNS depressants
Benzoyl peroxide	Antiacne agent	Excessive drying of skin, allergic reactions	Discontinue use if excessive drying or peeling occurs; avoid contact with hair or fabric
Chlorhexidine gluconate (Hibiclens)	Antimicrobial skin cleanser	Irritation, dermatitis, allergic reactions	For external use only; do not use on broken skin unless directed by a physician
Calamine lotion	Astringent	Local irritation	For external use only
Coal tar (Estar-Gel, Psori-Gel, others)	Treatment of pruritic dermatoses, including eczema and psoriasis	Photosensitivity, dermatitis, allergic reactions	Avoid exposure to sunlight for 72 hours after use; may stain clothes and bathtub; for external use only
Corticosteroids (topical), including: Fluocinonide (Lidex) Triamcinolone (Kenalog) Betamethasone (Valisone)	Antiinflammatory agent	Local irritation, maceration, superinfection, atrophy, itching, and drying of skin (more severe local reactions and systemic effects possible with higher doses and potency or when used with occlusive dressings)	Do not use occlusive dressings unless directed by a physician; washing or soaking area before application increases drug penetration
Crotamiton (Eurax)	Scabicidal and antipruritic	Local irritation, allergic reactions	For external use only; do not apply to severely irritated skin
Curel, Eucerin, Lubriderm	Emollient	Local irritation, allergic reactions	For external use only
Fluconazole (Diflucan)	Antifungal	Headache, nausea, vomiting, diarrhea	May elevate liver function test; monitor BUN, creatinine
Griseofulvin (Fulvicin, Grisactin, Grifulvin, others)	Antifungal agent	Hypersensitivity reactions, photosensitivity, nausea, fatigue, mental confusion	Avoid exposure to sunlight; drug absorption increased when given with meals; clinical response may appear only after full course of therapy

BUN, Blood urea nitrogen; *CNS*, central nervous system; *IV*, intravenous; *PT*, prothrombin time; *UVA*, ultraviolet A.

Table 43-2 Medications for the Integumentary System—cont'd

Generic (Trade)	Action	Side Effects	Nursing Implications
Isotretinoin (Accutane)	Antiacne agent	Severe dryness of skin, mouth, eyes, mucous membranes, nose, and nails; skin fragility; epistaxis; joint and muscle pain; nausea; abdominal pain	Absolutely contraindicated in pregnant women or women contemplating pregnancy; women of childbearing age must practice contraception during therapy and 1 month before and after therapy; give drug with meals; do not give vitamin supplements containing vitamin A; avoid exposure to sunlight
Itraconazole (Sporanox)	Antifungal agent	Hypertension, headache, nausea, anorexia	Give with food; check hepatic function; can increase PT level
Lindane (Kwell)	Scabicide, ovicide	Local irritation, dizziness, seizures (rare)	For external use only; avoid applying to open skin lesions
Lubriderm	Emollient	Local irritation, allergic reactions	For external use only; exercise caution when using in tub to avoid slipping
Methoxsalen (Oxsoralen, Oxsoralen-Ultra, 8-MOP)	Skin pigmenting agent	Severe photosensitivity, nausea, nervousness, insomnia, headache, hypopigmentation	Avoid all exposure to sunlight for 8 hours after oral ingestion and for several days after topical application; wear UVA-absorbing sunglasses for 24 hours after oral ingestion; use sunscreens to prevent exposure to sunlight; give agent with food or milk or in divided doses; clinical response may not appear for several months
Povidone-iodine (Betadine)	Topical antimicrobial agent	Local irritation	For external use only; may stain skin and clothing
Pyrethrin (RID, others)	Pediculicide	Local irritation	For external use only; do not use for infestations of eyebrows or eyelashes
Salicylic acid	Keratolytic agent	Local irritation, erythema, scaling	For external use only; may damage clothing, plastic, wood, and other materials on contact
Terbinafine (Lamisil)	Antifungal	Pruritus, local burning, erythema	For external use only; do not use occlusive dressings unless directed by a physician
Tetracycline	Antibacterial agent	Topical: Stinging, burning, slight yellowing of skin may occur Systemic: Nausea, diarrhea, photosensitivity	Topical: Avoid contact with sunlight Systemic: Give on empty stomach; avoid concomitant administration of dairy products, laxatives, antacids, and products containing iron; avoid contact with sunlight; may cause permanent tooth discoloration when used in children
Tolnaftate (Tinactin, Aftate, others)	Antifungal agent	Local irritation	For external use only

BUN, Blood urea nitrogen; *CNS*, central nervous system; *IV*, intravenous; *PT*, prothrombin time; *UVA*, ultraviolet A.

The recurrences, however, are milder and of shorter duration than the primary infection.

HERPES ZOSTER (SHINGLES)

Etiology and Pathophysiology

Herpes zoster, commonly known as **shingles,** is caused by the same virus that causes chickenpox (herpes varicella or herpesvirus type 3). The lesions are located along the nerve fibers of spinal ganglia. The virus causes an inflammation of the spinal ganglia. It is believed that the virus responsible for shingles lies dormant in patients until their resistance to infections has been lowered. The virus then advances to the skin by way of the peripheral nerves. At the skin surface the virus multiplies and forms an erythematous rash of small vesicles along a spinal nerve pathway (Figure 43-3). Sometimes the virus may affect a single nerve such as the trigeminal nerve.

Clinical Manifestations

The eruption of the vesicles is preceded by pain. The rash generally occurs in the thoracic region; the vesicles erupt in a line along the involved nerve. The vesicles rupture and form a crust, and the serous fluid in the vesicle may become purulent. The virus can also affect the lumbar, cervical, or cranial areas. The course of this painful condition runs from 7 to 28 days.

The pain associated with herpes zoster is severe; most patients describe it as burning and knifelike. Extreme tenderness and pruritus occur in the affected area. Patients with herpes zoster request analgesic medications at frequent intervals during the acute episode.

Herpes zoster is usually not permanently disabling to healthy adults. The greatest risk is for patients who have a lowered resistance to infection, such as those receiving chemotherapy or large doses of prednisone. In these patients, with compromised immune systems, the disease could be fatal

Assessment

Assessment of the patient should include both subjective and objective data. A good health history and thorough inspection skills are necessary to gather relevant data.

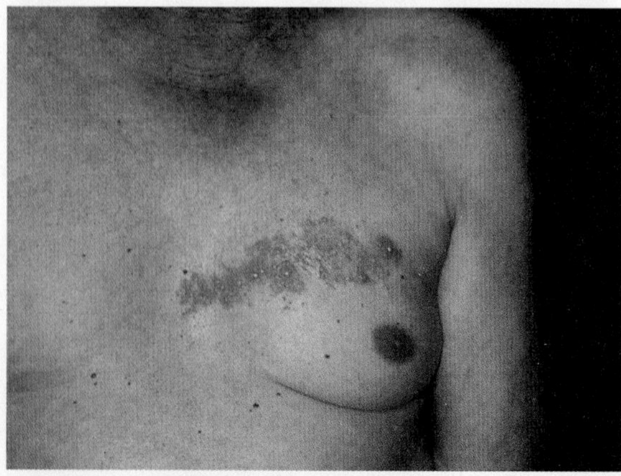

FIGURE 43-3 Herpes zoster.

Subjective data include (1) sharp, burning pain, usually on one side; (2) severe pruritus of the lesions; (3) general malaise; and (4) a history of chickenpox (varicella).

Objective data include (1) evidence of skin **excoriation** (injury to the surface layer of skin caused by scratching or abrasion) related to scratching, (2) patches of vesicles on erythematous skin following a peripheral nerve pathway, and (3) demonstration of tenderness to touch in the involved area. Other objective signs may include frequent requests for analgesics.

Diagnostic Tests

The diagnostic test for herpes zoster is a culture that isolates the virus. Other diagnostic measures are physical examinations and a thorough health history obtained on admission to the health care facility.

Medical Management

Medical interventions are directed at controlling the pain and preventing secondary complications. Analgesics, often opioids, are given for the pain. Steroids may be given to decrease inflammation and edema. Lotions (Kenalog, Lidex) may be used to relieve pruritus, and corticosteroids may be used to relieve pruritus and inflammation. Oral and intravenous acyclovir, when administered early, reduces the pain and duration of the virus. Recovery generally occurs in 2 to 3 weeks. Approximately 20% of patients experience some form of neuralgia following the episode. A vaccine available to prevent herpes zoster called Zostavax is now available. It is recommended for adults over 60 years who have had varicella (chickenpox) (Lewis et al., 2007).

Nursing Interventions and Patient Teaching

Nursing interventions are directed at relieving pain and pruritus and at preventing secondary complications. Tranquilizers such as lorazepam (Ativan) and hydroxyzine HCl (Atarax) are prescribed to decrease the anxiety associated with severe pain. Analgesics are given to control pain. The nurse needs to understand and be able to apply the principles of pain management to provide nursing interventions. Medicated baths and warm compresses may be ordered to soothe the skin. Use aseptic technique when caring for open lesions (Nursing Care Plan 43-1).

Nursing diagnoses and interventions for the patient with herpes zoster include but are not limited to the following:

Nursing Diagnoses	Nursing Interventions
Acute pain, related to inflammation of the involved nerve pathways	Assess pain and pruritus for necessary relief measures. Administer medications for pain and pruritus. Teach stress relaxation techniques, and offer diversional activities.

Continued on p. 1310

Nursing Care Plan 43-1 The Patient with Herpes Zoster

Ms. Lares, a 28-year-old teacher, is admitted with herpes zoster located around her left orbital area. She has several vesicles that have crusted and several vesicles that are still intact. She is complaining of pruritus and pain. She keeps asking the nurse if the lesions will leave a scar.

NURSING DIAGNOSIS ***Impaired tissue integrity related to the open lesions around the left eye***

Patient Goals and Expected Outcomes	Nursing Interventions	Evaluation and Rationale
Patient's tissue integrity will improve as shown by:		
No signs of infection such as erythema, purulent drainage, and elevated white blood cell count during hospitalization	Assess skin, especially eye area, for changes in color, texture, or turgor or increase in lesion size. Assess lesions for signs of infection.Monitor albumin and white blood cell levels as ordered.	The patient showed no signs of erythema or purulent drainage. The patient showed improvement of vesicles.
Remaining skin showing no signs of impairment during hospitalization	Use principles of aseptic technique.	No skin impairment noted in remaining skin
Decrease in the number of lesions within 72 hours	Monitor status of lesions for 12 hours.	The number of lesions increased during the first day of hospitalization but decreased during the next 48 hours.
Patient stating pain level has decreased from a "9" to a "4" within 24 hours	Administer or apply medications as ordered to decrease pain or pruritus. Teach patient importance of using medical asepsis in care of lesions.	Patient stated that pain was a "3" within 24 hours of medication administration.

NURSING DIAGNOSIS ***Disturbed body image, related to location of lesions as manifested by continual remarks to the nurse, "Will these sores leave a scar?"***

Patient Goals and Expected Outcomes	Nursing Interventions	Evaluation and Rationale
The patient will verbalize and demonstrate acceptance of appearance as manifested by: • Verbalizing positive feelings about body image • Participating in normal activities	Assess patient's feelings about personal appearance by encouraging patient to express her feelings. Encourage patient to ask questions about her health problem. Provide reliable information, and reinforce the information already given. Clarify any misconceptions about the care the patient is receiving. Provide privacy, and avoid criticism. Teach patient about the disease and the course of the disease.	The goal was met. The patient stated she believed that lesions would not be permanent. The patient returned to work after dismissal from the hospital before the lesions had completely healed. The goal was met.

Critical Thinking Questions

1. Ms. Lares turns on her call light. She is crying and states she is in severe pain. She describes the pain as a burning, stabbing pain over her left forehead and eye. She rates her pain as a 7 on the pain scale of 0 to 10. She also complains of pruritus. What would be the most appropriate nursing interventions to provide comfort and pain control for Ms. Lares?
2. Ms. Lares tells the nurse that a friend told her she could not visit because she has not had chickenpox. Her friend is afraid she might "catch chickenpox" from Ms. Lares's shingles. Give the accurate patient teaching in response to Ms. Lares' statements.

Nursing Diagnoses	Nursing Interventions
Risk for infection, related to tissue destruction	Assess factors that contribute to infection, such as an immunocompromised patient (one who has decreased white blood cell count). Monitor for signs of infection, such as pyrexia and leukocytosis. Stress aseptic hand hygiene technique. Maintain aseptic technique when providing care. Limit visitors. Don gloves when caring for lesions.

Begin patient teaching by assessing the patient's knowledge and readiness. Areas to cover include (1) methods for controlling pain, (2) application of medication and wet dressings, (3) methods for inhibiting the spread of disease, (4) techniques to prevent secondary infections, and (5) proper diet with vitamin C to promote healing.

Prognosis

The prognosis is generally good; however, older adults are more susceptible to complications such as post-therapy neuralgia, which may persist for several months after the skin lesions have cleared. Evidence indicates that the herpes zoster virus remains latent in the body of a person once infected. A person lacking varicella (chickenpox) immunity can acquire chickenpox from someone who has shingles.

PITYRIASIS ROSEA

Pityriasis rosea is a skin rash that usually affects people between 6 and 30 years of age. The rash begins as a single pink, scaly patch that resembles a large ringworm. It ranges from 1 to 3 inches in diameter.

Etiology and Pathophysiology

Most sources note that pityriasis rosea is caused by a virus. The rash generally disappears without treatment (*Mosby's dictionary of medical, nursing, and health professions*, 8th ed., 2009).

Clinical Manifestations

Pityriasis rosea begins as a single lesion, known as a herald patch, that is scaly, has a raised border, and has a pink center. Seven to 14 days after the initial eruption, smaller matching spots become widespread on both sides of the body. The rash consists of pink oval-shaped spots that are ¼ to ½ inch across. The rash appears mainly on the chest, abdomen, back, groin, and axillae (Figure 43-4).

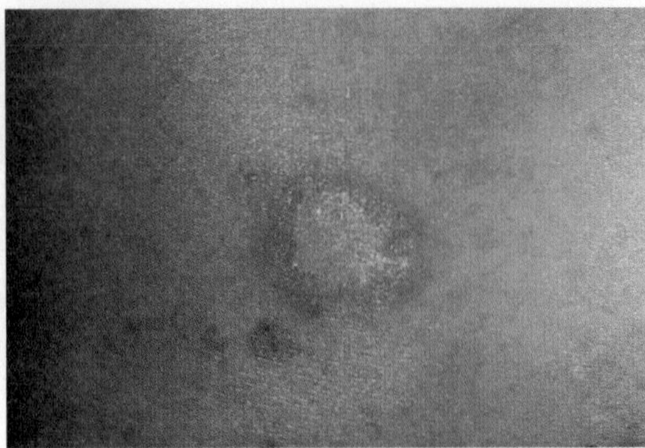

FIGURE 43-4 Pityriasis rosea herald patch.

Assessment

Assessment involves inspecting the skin and gathering a detailed health history. Ask questions related to the objective data.

Diagnostic Tests

Diagnosis of rosea stems from inspection and subjective data from the patient. No specific laboratory tests support a definitive diagnosis.

Medical Management

Generally, rosea requires no treatment, but preventive interventions can control secondary infections related to pruritus. If the skin becomes dry, moisturizing cream may help. For pruritus, the patient should use 1% hydrocortisone cream two or three times a day. Ultraviolet light, such as sunbathing for 30 minutes, shortens the course of pityriasis rosea.

Nursing Interventions

The nursing interventions for pityriasis rosea include symptomatic relief of the symptoms such as pruritus. Analgesics and Aveeno baths may be ordered to help decrease the pain and pruritus. Antihistamines and topical steroids may be used to control the pruritus. Sun exposure aids in the resolution of the lesions.

Prognosis

The disease is thought to be viral. Teach the patient that the disease is self-limiting and resolves in a few weeks.

BACTERIAL DISORDERS OF THE SKIN

CELLULITIS

Etiology and Pathophysiology

Cellulitis, a potentially serious infection, involves the underlying tissues of the skin. Although it is not contagious, the bacteria that cause cellulitis can be spread by direct contact with an open area on a person who has an infection. The most common causes in adults are group A streptococci and *Staphylococcus aureus; Haemophilus influenzae* type B is more common in children. The risk is increased by venous insufficiency or stasis; diabetes mellitus; lymphedema; surgery; malnutrition; substance abuse; presence of another infection; compromised immune function due to HIV; treatment with steroids or cancer chemotherapy; or autoimmune diseases, such as lupus erythematosus.

Cellulitis develops as an edematous, erythematous area of skin that feels hot and tender. It occurs when bacteria enter the body through a break in the skin, such as a cut, scratch, or insect bite that is not cleansed with soap and water. The infection usually affects skin on the lower extremities or face, although cellulitis can occur on any part of the skin. The infection is usually superficial, but cellulitis may spread and become life threatening as the infection invades the deeper tissues, lymph nodes, and bloodstream. Thus it is known by the lay term *blood poisoning*.

Clinical Manifestations

Cellulitis is an infection of the skin and underlying subcutaneous tissues. The affected areas become erythematous, edematous, tender, and warm to the touch. Often a fever accompanies the other symptoms. The first signs and symptoms generally are erythema, pain, and tenderness over an area of skin. These signs and symptoms are caused by bacteria themselves and by the body's attempts to halt the infection. The infected skin may look slightly pitted, like an orange peel. Over time, the area of erythema spreads and small red spots may appear. Vesicles may form and burst, or large bullae may appear on the infected skin. As the infection spreads, nearby lymph nodes may become enlarged and tender (lymphadenitis). Erysipelas is one form of streptococcal cellulitis in which the skin is bright red and noticeably edematous and the edges of the infected area are raised. Edema occurs because the infection occludes the lymphatic vessels in the skin. Most patients with cellulitis feel only mildly ill, but some have fever, chills, tachycardia, headache, hypotension, and confusion.

Assessment

Assessment primarily involves inspection of the skin. Collect a health history to support assessment data. **Subjective data** include complaints of fatigue, tenderness, pain, limited movement of the involved extremity, and general malaise. **Objective data** include edema, erythema, and areas that are warm to touch. Vesicles may be present. An elevated temperature accompanied by tachycardia and leukocytosis often occurs.

Diagnostic Tests

The physician diagnoses cellulitis based on its appearance and signs and symptoms. If a patient is seriously ill, cultures may be needed from blood, purulent exudate, or tissue specimens for laboratory identification of the bacteria. A complete blood count (CBC) reveals leukocytosis. A Gram stain may be done to determine the appropriate antibiotic therapy. Occasionally the physician performs tests to differentiate cellulitis from deep-vein thrombosis of the lower extremity because the signs and symptoms of these disorders are similar. X-ray examination, ultrasound, computed tomography, or magnetic resonance imaging may be used to determine the extent of inflammation and to identify abscess formation.

Medical Management

Prompt treatment with antibiotics can prevent cellulitis from spreading rapidly and reaching the blood and organs. Most cases are treated with antibiotic therapy that is effective against both streptococci and staphylococci. Patients with mild cellulitis may take oral antibiotics. If the patient has rapidly spreading cellulitis, high fever, or other evidence of a serious infection, the physician will order intravenous antibiotics.

Nursing Interventions and Patient Teaching

Nursing interventions involve treating signs and symptoms and preventing spread of the disease. Administer the antibiotic, monitor the patient's progress, assess pain, administer an analgesic, change dressings, and monitor the patient's nutrition and hydration status. The affected body part, when possible, remains immobile and is elevated to help reduce edema. Warm, moist dressings applied to the infected area may relieve discomfort.

Signs and symptoms of cellulitis usually disappear after a few days of antibiotic therapy. However, signs and symptoms often worsen before they improve, probably because the death of the bacteria releases substances that cause tissue damage. When this occurs, the body continues to react even though the bacteria are dead. Antibiotics are continued for a minimum of 10 days. Teach patients that it is important to take the entire prescription of antibiotics and to monitor for signs and symptoms of secondary diseases such as yeast infections. The specific nursing diagnoses for cellulitis depend on the assessment data gathered and the extent of the infection. Analgesics such as acetaminophen or oxycodone-acetaminophen (Percocet) help control the pain and fever associated with cellulitis.

Prognosis

Cure is possible with 7 to 10 days of treatment. Cellulitis may be more severe in people with chronic diseases and those who are susceptible to infection such as those with immunosuppression. Complications from cellulitis include sepsis, meningitis, and lymphangitis.

IMPETIGO CONTAGIOSA

Etiology and Pathophysiology

Impetigo is caused by *S. aureus,* streptococci, or a mixed bacterial invasion of the skin. It is a highly contagious inflammatory disorder, seen at all ages but particularly common in children. The lesions start as **macules** (small, flat blemishes that are flush with the skin surface), develop into **pustulant vesicles** (small, circumscribed elevations of the skin that contain pus), and then rupture and form a dried exudate. The crust is honey colored and easily removed. Under the dried exudate is smooth, red skin (Figure 43-5).

Clinical Manifestations

The exposed areas of the body most often affected are the face, hands, arms, and legs. The pustulant lesions are distributed randomly over the involved area. The honey-colored dried exudate ranges from pinpoint to the size of a nickel or larger. Impetigo is highly contagious to a person who directly contacts the exudate of a lesion. The disease may be spread by touching personal articles, linens, and clothing of the infected person.

Assessment

Subjective data include symptoms of (1) pruritus, (2) pain, (3) malaise, (4) spreading of the disease to different body parts, and (5) other diseases present.

Objective data include all or some of the following: (1) focal erythema; (2) pruritic areas; (3) honey-colored crust over dried lesions; (4) smooth, red skin under the crust; (5) low-grade fever; (6) leukocytosis; (7) positive culture for streptococcus or *S. aureus;* and (8) purulent exudate.

Diagnostic Tests

The diagnosis is made by taking a culture of the exudate and identifying the specific bacterium. Inspection and symptoms are the standard means of identifying the condition.

Medical Management

The physician prescribes systemic antibiotics (such as erythromycin, dicloxacillin, or a cephalosporin) based on the culture and sensitivity test. Topical antibiotics such as mupirocin (Bactroban) have proven effective when started early in the treatment, but most physicians include a systemic antibiotic as well. Retapamulin (Altabax) was approved by the U.S. Food and Drug Administration (FDA) for topical treatment of impetigo (GlaxoSmithKline, 2007). Medical treatment emphasizes the use of antiseptic soaps to remove crusted exudate and cleansing agents to thoroughly clean the involved area before applying an antibiotic cream, ointment, or lotion. A primary goal is preventing glomerulonephritis (inflammation of the glomerulus of the kidney), which may occur after streptococcal infections.

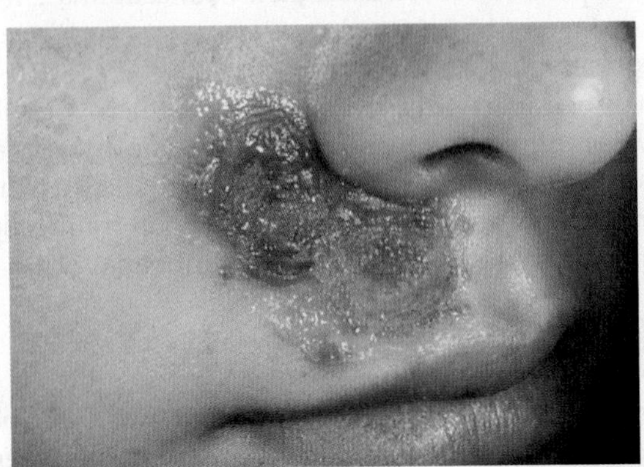

FIGURE 43-5 Impetigo and herpes simplex.

Nursing Interventions and Patient Teaching

Interventions are aimed at disrupting the course of the disease and preventing the spread of infection. Antibiotics are used to arrest the disease process. Systemic parenteral penicillin is one of the most commonly used antibiotics. Ceftriaxone sodium (Rocephin) is widely used as well. Other antibiotics such as cephalosporins may be used. Don gloves and wash the lesions with special cleansing agents, such as povidone-iodine (Betadine) and chlorhexidine gluconate (Hibiclens).

The lesions are usually soaked with an antiseptic solution, and the dried exudate is removed using special instruments. Topical antibiotics are applied several times a day using sterile technique.

Nursing diagnoses and interventions for the patient with impetigo include but are not limited to the following:

Nursing Diagnoses	Nursing Interventions
Impaired skin integrity, related to crusted, open lesions	Inspect lesions every day for drainage, size, and extent of body area covered. Keep area clean and dry. Don gloves when giving direct patient care.
Deficient knowledge, related to the cause and spread of the disease	Assess patient's knowledge level and readiness to learn. Demonstrate appropriate care and application of topical medications. Stress importance of individual personal items, such as linens and towels. Involve family in patient teaching.

Assess the patient's level of knowledge, and instruct the patient and family members in the principles of hygiene. When demonstrating home care techniques, reinforce correct information and stress the importance of preventing the spread of the disease by contact.

Prognosis

With proper treatment the prognosis is good. Emphasize that the patient should take all of the prescribed antibiotic.

FOLLICULITIS, FURUNCLES, CARBUNCLES, AND FELONS

Etiology and Pathophysiology

Folliculitis is an infection of a hair follicle, generally from *S. aureus* bacteria. The infection may involve one or several follicles. It often occurs after men or women shave. A stye is an example of folliculitis.

A **furuncle** (boil) is an inflammation that begins deep in the hair follicles and spreads to the surrounding skin. Irritation is a common predisposing factor to a furuncle. Common locations are the posterior area of the neck, the forearm, buttocks, and the axillae (Figure 43-6).

A **carbuncle** is a cluster of furuncles. It is an infection of several hair follicles that spreads to surrounding tissue. Obesity, poor nutrition, untreated diabetes mellitus, and poor hygiene contribute to the formation of carbuncles.

A **felon** is an infection of the soft tissue under and around an area such as the fingernail. The involved finger becomes erythematous, edematous, and tender to touch.

Clinical Manifestations

The involved area is usually edematous, erythematous, painful, and pruritic. After several days, the infected area becomes localized. The exact area may get shiny, point up; for a furuncle or carbuncle, the center turns yellow. Carbuncles can have four or five cores with spontaneous rupture of the core. The pain stops immediately on rupture. A surgical incision and drainage can be performed if the core does not rupture.

Assessment

Collection of **subjective data** includes asking questions about the patient's general symptoms, such as tenderness and pain with movement. Ask about a family history of diabetes mellitus or the wearing of improperly fitting clothing. Collection of **objective data** includes noting erythema and edema in the involved area. The patient is often overweight and may have poor body hygiene.

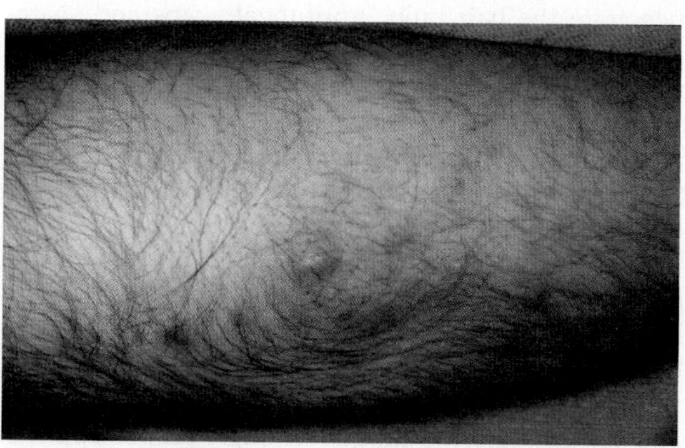

FIGURE 43-6 Furuncle of the forearm.

Diagnostic Tests

Diagnosis is based primarily on a thorough physical examination, health history, and inspection of the area. A culture of the drainage may be done.

Medical Management

Medical treatment is aimed at preventing the spread of infection. Patients in the hospital are isolated, using wound and secretion precautions. Surgical treatment may include draining the lesion and applying topical antibiotics.

Nursing Interventions and Patient Teaching

Warm soaks, two or three times a day, can be used to speed the process of **suppuration** (production of purulent material). When the lesion ruptures, discontinue the soaks to prevent damage of the surrounding skin and spread of the infection. Use good medical asepsis while caring for these patients. In the hospital, follow isolation procedures for drainage and secretion. If the lesion is incised and drained, use sterile technique to apply topical antibiotics. The affected part needs to be immobilized to prevent pain and elevated to decrease the edema.

Nursing diagnoses and interventions for the patient with bacterial disorders include but are not limited to the following:

Nursing Diagnoses	Nursing Interventions
Impaired skin integrity, related to exudates from wound	Assess wound daily for exudates and excoriation. Don gloves when providing care; use correct isolation technique. Apply skin protectant to opening.
Pain, related to edema	Assess area for edema and tenderness. Elevate involved body part above the level of the heart. Apply hot soaks, and immobilize affected part.

Teach patients not to touch the exudate. Meticulous hand hygiene is a must before and after contact with the lesions. Demonstrate good hygiene practices and ask for return demonstrations by the patient and the family. The entire family needs individual toilet items and bath linens and should be encouraged to use bacteriostatic soap and shampoo. Demonstrate proper disposal and cleaning of contaminated articles.

Prognosis

Patients make a full recovery when they follow the treatment plan. A follow-up examination with a physician may be needed to identify any underlying disease process, such as diabetes mellitus.

FUNGAL INFECTIONS OF THE SKIN

Fungal infections, which are known as **dermatophytoses,** are superficial infections of the skin. The most common types are tinea capitis, tinea corporis, tinea cruris, and tinea pedis.

Etiology and Pathophysiology

Tinea capitis is commonly known as ringworm of the scalp. *Microsporum audouinii* is the major fungal pathogen. The fungus is spread by contact with infected articles. Trauma or irritation breaks the skin and facilitates spread of the infection (Figure 43-7).

Tinea corporis is known as ringworm of the body. It occurs on parts of the body with little or no hair.

Tinea cruris is known as jock itch. It is found in the groin area.

Tinea pedis is the most common of all fungal infections. Commonly known as athlete's foot, it occurs between the toes of people whose feet perspire heavily. The fungus can also be spread from contaminated public bathroom facilities and swimming pools.

Clinical Manifestations

Tinea capitis is usually an erythematous, round lesion with pustules around the edges (see Figure 43-7). Temporary alopecia occurs at the site, and infected hairs turn blue-green under a Wood's light (an ultraviolet light).

Tinea corporis produces flat lesions that are clear in the center with erythematous borders. Scaliness also occurs, and pruritus is severe (Figure 43-8).

Tinea cruris has brownish red lesions that migrate out from the groin area. Pruritus and skin excoriation from scratching are found.

Tinea pedis produces more skin maceration than the others. Commonly seen are fissures and vesicles around and below the toes, with occasional discoloration of the infected area.

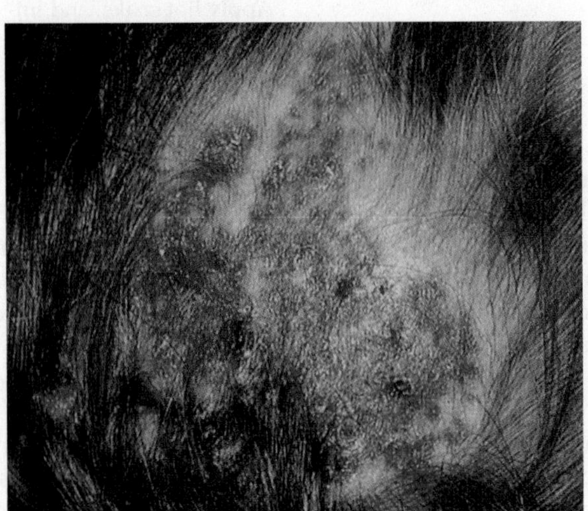

FIGURE 43-7 Tinea capitis.

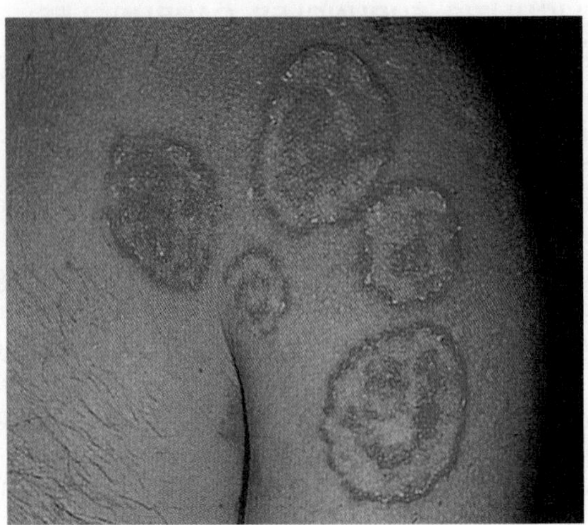

FIGURE 43-8 Tinea corporis.

Assessment

Subjective data include any symptoms of extreme pruritus and tenderness from excoriation of the area. Collection of **objective data** for tinea capitis includes an inspection and location of a round, scaled lesion that has pustules around the edges of the scalp. The involved area is erythematous and has no hair. In tinea corporis, the lesions are flat with clear centers and erythematous borders on nonhairy body parts. In tinea cruris, the groin area reveals brown to red lesions that radiate outward, with skin excoriation from intense scratching. In tinea pedis, fissures between the toes and soft skin are accompanied by vesicular lesions and thick toenails.

Diagnostic Tests

The diagnosis is primarily by visual inspection and, for tinea capitis, use of a Wood's light. The light causes hairs infected by the fungus to become brilliantly fluorescent. No other tests are performed, but a thorough health history supports the diagnosis of all fungal infections of the skin.

Medical Management

Medical treatment involves the use of topical or oral antifungal drugs. Griseofulvin (Fulvicin, Grifulvin) is the most common oral drug given; topical drugs do not penetrate the hair bulb. Antifungal soaps and shampoos are recommended. Antifungal agents such as tolnaftate 1% (Tinactin), miconazole (Lotrimin AF), (Monistat Derm, Desenex), and butenafine (Mentax) can be applied directly. Treatment may last from 2 to 6 weeks. See Table 43-2 for a list of drugs commonly used for fungal and other integumentary infections.

Nursing Interventions and Patient Teaching

Nursing interventions for fungal infections involve two primary principles: (1) protect the involved area from trauma and irritation by keeping it clean and dry, and (2) alleviate the fungus through proper application of medications and warm compresses.

Tinea pedis should be treated with warm soaks using Burow's solution and topical antifungal agents. Excellent foot care is stressed. The feet should be cleaned and dried thoroughly, paying special attention to the toes. Wearing sandals or going barefoot helps decrease foot moisture. Footwear, such as stockings, needs to be of an absorbent material.

A nursing diagnosis and interventions for the patient with fungal infections include but are not limited to the following:

Nursing Diagnosis	Nursing Interventions
Impaired skin integrity, related to: • increased moisture • pruritus	Keep involved area clean and dry. Have patient wear loose-fitting clothing and shoes. Apply medications as directed.

Patient education involves teaching proper skin care and comfort measures to relieve pruritus. Review the medications to be taken and the procedures for the patient to do at home, emphasizing that fungal skin disorders may take months to cure. Stress general information about athlete's foot and clarify the many misconceptions.

Prognosis

Prognosis for recovery is good. Few complications result when treatment is followed.

INFLAMMATORY DISORDERS OF THE SKIN

Superficial infection of the skin is known as **dermatitis.** It can be caused by numerous agents, such as drugs, plants, chemicals, metals, and food. Regardless of the precipitating factor, the lesions associated with dermatitis develop along the same pattern. The nurse first observes erythema and edema, followed by the eruption of vesicles that rupture and encrust. Pruritus is always present, which promotes further skin excoriation.

CONTACT DERMATITIS

Etiology and Pathophysiology

Contact dermatitis is caused by direct contact with agents in the environment to which a person is hypersensitive. The epidermis becomes inflamed and damaged by the repeated contact with the physical and chemical irritants. Common causes of dermatitis are detergents, soaps, industrial chemicals, and plants such as poison ivy.

Clinical Manifestations

Lesions appear first at the point of contact with the irritant. Usually the patient feels burning, pain, pruritus, and edema. The involved area is soon erythematous, with **papules** (small, raised, solid skin lesions less than 1 cm in diameter) and vesicles appearing most often on the dorsal surfaces.

Assessment

Thoroughly research the patient's activities. If necessary, ask the patient to write a log of activities for the 48 hours before development of symptoms.

Collection of **subjective data** usually reveals that the patient has (1) tried a new soap, (2) been traveling and using different personal items, or (3) been working with plants or flowers. The patient may have severe pruritus and difficulty moving the involved area.

Collection of **objective data** should reveal (1) erythema, (2) papules and vesicles that generally ooze and weep a clear fluid, (3) scratch marks resulting from intense pruritus, and (4) edema of the area.

Diagnostic Tests

The primary diagnostic test is an accurate health history to identify the agent. Intradermal skin testing may identify plants and environmental agents, and elimination diets are used to identify food allergies. Elevated serum immunoglobulin E (IgE) levels and eosinophilia support the diagnosis. Both tests are thought to be related to abnormalities of T-cell function.

Medical Management

Medical intervention involves identifying the cause of the hypersensitive reaction. Symptomatic treatment for the inflammation, edema, and pruritus may include application of corticosteroids and the oral administration of antihistamines such as diphenhydramine (Benadryl). If the patient has a history of asthma (reactive airway disease), he or she may have an acute asthmatic episode. Hydroxyzine (Atarax) and inhalation treatments provide prophylactic treatment for asthma.

Nursing Interventions and Patient Teaching

The primary goal is to identify the offensive agent to protect the skin from further damage. Identify the cause by first describing the pattern of the reaction.

Wet dressings, using Burow's solution, help promote the healing process. To prevent infection, use aseptic technique to apply the corticosteroids to the open lesions.

Pruritus is responsible for most of the discomfort. A cool environment with increased humidity decreases the pruritus. Cold compresses may be applied to reduce circulation to the area (vasoconstriction). The patient should take daily baths with an application of oil to cleanse the skin. Fingernails should be cut at the level of the fingertips to decrease excoriation from scratching. Clothing should be lightweight and loose to decrease trauma of the involved area.

Nursing diagnoses and interventions for the patient with inflammation of the skin include but are not limited to the following:

Nursing Diagnoses	Nursing Interventions
Impaired skin integrity, related to scratching	Assess for signs of scratching. Have patient keep fingernails short and wear mittens. Apply medications as directed.
Pain, related to pruritus	Assess degree of pruritus and discomfort every shift. Keep environment cool. Apply cold compresses.

Teach the patient to keep an accurate history of possible predisposing offensive agents. As soon as the primary irritant has been identified, the patient should avoid it, as well as soaps, excessive heat, and rubbing of the area. Any time the skin is exposed to the primary irritant, the affected area should be washed thoroughly. Topical creams may be applied only as directed by a physician.

Prognosis

Removal of the offensive agent results in full recovery. Desensitizing the individual may be necessary if recurrences are frequent.

DERMATITIS VENENATA, EXFOLIATIVE DERMATITIS, AND DERMATITIS MEDICAMENTOSA

Etiology and Pathophysiology

Dermatitis venenata results from contact with certain plants, commonly **poison ivy** and poison oak. The signs and symptoms include mild to severe erythema with pruritus. On first exposure the body undergoes a sensitizing antigen formation. This results in an immunologic change in certain lymphocytes. Subsequent exposure to the antigen causes the lymphocytes to release irritating chemicals, leading to inflammation, edema, and vesiculation. The lesions are mainly found on the body part exposed to the sensitizing agent.

Exfoliative dermatitis can be caused by the infestation of certain heavy metals, such as arsenic or mercury, or by antibiotics, aspirin, codeine, gold, or iodine. The skin sloughs off, and the area becomes edematous and erythematous. Severe pruritus with fever occurs, and most patients require hospitalization. Treatment is individualized. If the cause can be determined, it should be removed or treated appropriately. Careful monitoring is essential to prevent secondary infection, avoid further irritation, and maintain fluid balance.

Dermatitis medicamentosa occurs when people are given a medication to which they are hypersensitive. Any drug can cause a reaction, but the common agents are penicillin, codeine, and iron.

Clinical Manifestations

Clinical manifestations range from mild to severe erythema with vesicular eruptions. In severe reactions, respiratory distress may occur. Any type of lesion may be found.

Assessment

Collection of **subjective data** for dermatitis involves questions about pruritus and a burning pain in the involved area.

Collection of **objective data** reveals lesions that are white in the center and red on the periphery. Vesicles are common in dermatitis venenata. Patients with dermatitis medicamentosa may have severe dyspnea caused by respiratory distress.

Diagnostic Tests

A careful patient history is of prime importance in the diagnosis of dermatitis venenata, exfoliative dermatitis, and dermatitis medicamentosa. A laboratory examination for serum IgE and eosinophilia is ordered.

Medical Management

The medical treatment for dermatitis ranges from therapeutic baths to administration of corticosteroids. The medical treatment is directed at the cause.

Nursing Interventions and Patient Teaching

Pruritus is the primary symptom in all types of dermatitis. Calamine lotion is a common over-the-counter medication used. Therapeutic baths using colloid solution, lotions, and ointments also help relieve the pruritus. Emotional support is necessary. The patient's physical appearance is difficult for the patient and family members to accept.

In dermatitis venenata, instruct the patient to wash the affected part immediately after contact with the offending allergen. After the lesions appear, only cool, open, wet dressings should be used.

In dermatitis medicamentosa, identifying the drug and discontinuing its use are paramount. If the offending allergen cannot be pinpointed, no drugs should be given. Notify the physician. The lesions will disappear after the medication is discontinued. More specific nursing intervention is directed by individual patient symptoms.

Nursing diagnoses and interventions for the patient with dermatitis include but are not limited to the following:

Nursing Diagnoses	Nursing Interventions
Impaired skin integrity, related to crusted, open lesions	Inspect lesions every day for exudate, size, and specific body area involved. Keep area clean and dry. Don gloves when giving direct patient care.

Nursing Diagnoses	Nursing Interventions
Risk for infection, related to break in skin	Assess skin for signs of infection. Identify interventions to prevent or reduce the risk of infection. Monitor vital signs; assess for elevated temperature. Stress medical aseptic hand hygiene technique. Use aseptic technique, and keep involved areas dry when providing care.
Deficient knowledge, related to the cause and spread of the disease	Assess patient's knowledge level and readiness to learn. Demonstrate appropriate care and application of topical medications. Stress importance of individual personal items, such as linens and towels. Involve family in patient teaching.

Advise the patient to wear a medical-alert bracelet or necklace showing the name of the allergen and to notify all health care personnel of the medication allergy.

Prognosis
Full recovery occurs when the offending agent is removed.

URTICARIA

Etiology and Pathophysiology
Urticaria refers to the presence of wheals or hives in an allergic reaction commonly caused by drugs, food, insect bites, inhalants, emotional stress, or exposure to heat or cold. The **wheals** (round elevation of the skin; white in the center with a pale red periphery) (see Table 43-1) of urticaria appear suddenly. Urticaria or hives is caused by the release of histamine in an antigen-antibody reaction.

Clinical Manifestations
The increased histamine causes the capillaries to dilate, resulting in increased permeability. Respiratory involvement may occur.

Assessment
Subjective data include pruritus, edema, a burning pain, and sometimes dyspnea.

Collection of **objective data** identifies transient wheals of varying shapes and sizes with well-defined erythematous margins and pale centers. Intense scratching may be seen, and in some cases respiration may be compromised. Assessment of respiratory status provides a baseline for future assessments.

Diagnostic Tests
A detailed health history is the primary tool to identify the cause of hives. An allergy skin test may be performed using minute quantities of the antigen to identify the allergic substances. A serum examination for IgE elevation may be ordered.

Medical Management
Relief from urticaria can be achieved by administering an antihistamine and sometimes epinephrine. Identification of the cause of the urticaria is important to prevent recurrence.

Nursing Interventions and Patient Teaching
Nursing interventions include helping the patient identify the cause and decreasing the discomfort from the pruritus. Teach the patient about possible causes and prevention methods. Explain medications thoroughly, and demonstrate therapeutic baths. Review the signs and symptoms of an anaphylactic reaction, including shortness of breath, wheezing, and cyanosis.

Prognosis
Patients recover fully when the offending agent is determined and avoided. Compliance with the therapeutic regimen influences the outcome.

ANGIOEDEMA

Etiology and Pathophysiology
Angioedema is a form of urticaria and is caused by the same offenders. It occurs in the subcutaneous tissue, whereas urticaria is a skin and mucous membrane lesion. Angioedema is characterized by local edema of an entire area, such as an eyelid, hands, feet, tongue, larynx, gastrointestinal (GI) tract, genitalia, or lips. Only a single edematous area usually appears at one time.

Assessment
Subjective data include symptoms of burning, pruritus, acute pain if in the GI tract, or respiratory distress if in the larynx.

The collection of **objective data** reveals lesions that have a normal appearance on the outer skin with edema.

Diagnostic Tests
A careful patient history is essential in the diagnosis of angioedema. Patients with a history of allergies are more likely to have angioedema.

Medical Management
Treatment to relieve angioedema may include antihistamine drugs such as diphenhydramine. Epinephrine and corticosteroids such as methylprednisolone (Solu-Medrol) may also be given.

Nursing Interventions

A cold pack or cold compress may be used. Continual respiratory assessment is essential to detect respiratory distress. Tell patients to wear a medical-alert bracelet. Education is the key to preventing recurrent episodes.

Prognosis

With treatment, the prognosis is excellent.

ECZEMA (ATOPIC DERMATITIS)

Etiology and Pathophysiology

Eczema is primarily a disease of infants and is associated with allergies, commonly to chocolate, eggs, wheat, and orange juice. The allergen causes histamine to be released, and an antigen-antibody reaction occurs.

Clinical Manifestations

Papular and vesicular lesions appear and are surrounded by erythema. The vesicles generally rupture, discharging a yellow, tenacious exudate that dries and encrusts. If the lesions become infected, the skin loses its pigment and become shiny with dry scales.

Assessment

Subjective data include pruritus and scratching. Children are generally fussy and irritable, and anorexia is common. The skin is sensitive to touch. A family history of allergies and asthma supports the findings in many cases.

Objective data include vesicles and papules found on the scalp, the forehead, the cheeks, the neck, and the surfaces of the extremities. The involved area is erythematous and dry. Tiny cracks in the epithelium allow fluid to escape and further promote dryness. The primary signs result from the scratching from pruritus. Scales accompanied by dryness in the involved area are a distinguishing characteristic of eczema.

Diagnostic Tests

The diagnosis is generally made during a thorough health history that reveals a family history of eczema, since heredity is a prominent factor. Diet elimination and skin testing may be used to identify the specific substance to which the patient is hypersensitive. IgE serum tests provide data related to allergic response.

Medical Management

Medical treatment involves reducing the amount of allergen exposure. The eruptions and pruritus can be relieved if the aggravating factor is identified and controlled. The primary goal is to break the inflammation cycle.

Hydration of the skin is the key to treatment. The skin is dry because of tiny cracks that allow body fluids to escape. The skin may be hydrated by soaking the affected area in warm water for 15 to 20 minutes and then applying an occlusive ointment to retain the water. Examples of occlusive preparations are petrolatum, corticosteroid ointments, and vegetable shortening. The skin should be patted dry after the bath and the occlusive preparation applied immediately to the damp skin.

Nursing Interventions and Patient Teaching

Nursing interventions are directed toward treatment of symptoms for the eczematous patient. Administer the therapeutic bath and occlusive preparations as directed. Use wet dressings to maximize hydration of the skin. Apply topical steroids to relieve discomfort.

When the lesions begin to heal, a lotion such as Eucerin, Alpha Keri, Lubriderm, or Curel should be applied three or four times a day to add moisture to the skin. Wet wraps and occlusive preparations only hold water already present.

The emotional impact of having eczema ranges from anger to depression. The nurse provides an emotional outlet for these patients. Encourage the patient to share emotions by using effective listening skills and open-ended questions. This provides a means to establishing a therapeutic rapport with the patient.

Before the development of steroids, coal tar products were used to reduce the skin inflammation. Coal tar products do not decrease inflammation as quickly as steroids, but they last longer and have fewer side effects. Therefore coal tar preparations are recommended for chronic eczema. Preparations such as Estar-Gel and Psori-Gel are applied once a day at bedtime with a moisturizer.

Nursing diagnoses and interventions for the patient with eczema include but are not limited to the following:

Nursing Diagnoses	Nursing Interventions
Impaired skin integrity, related to open lesions	Assess skin for signs of secondary infection. Monitor CBC for elevated white blood cell count. Apply ordered medications using medical aseptic technique.
Risk for situational low self-esteem, related to change in body image	Assess patient's mental status. Be an active listener. Encourage verbalization of concerns the patient may be experiencing. Observe interaction with family and staff members and assist in establishing a therapeutic rapport.
Risk for infection, related to open lesion	Report at once the signs of wound infection such as erythema, especially beyond the wound margins. Increasing edema, purulent exudates, change in the description of the pain or increased pain, and increased warmth in the involved area are signs and symptoms of infection.

ACNE VULGARIS

Etiology and Pathophysiology

Acne is an inflammatory papulopustular skin eruption that involves the sebaceous glands; it occurs primarily in adolescents. The exact cause is unknown. However, several factors that may contribute are diet, stress, heredity, and overactive hormones. Hygiene has not been found to be a significant factor in the development of acne.

Acne develops when the oil glands become occluded. At puberty, androgens secreted increase the size of the oil glands, causing the sebum to combine more readily with epithelial cells and bacteria. Sebum may then occlude a hair follicle, forming a comedo (plural, *comedones*). A comedo is a blackhead. It is dark because of the effect of oxygen on sebum, not because of the presence of dirt.

Clinical Manifestations

Acne is found most often on the face, neck, upper chest, shoulder, and back (Figure 43-9). The first symptom is usually tenderness and edema in the area, followed by the comedo. The skin is oily and shiny, and the lesions last up to 10 days. Scarring results from large lesions that are traumatized when the person tries to rupture the comedo.

Assessment

Collection of **subjective data** includes asking the adolescent how acne affects lifestyle: Does it affect your participation in activities or group communication? Most patients acknowledge that acne affects their self-image. Common locations for acne lesions are the face and chin, which are highly visible areas. Lesions increase with emotional upsets and stress.

Collection of **objective data** includes noting the presence of edema in the involved area. Comedones (blackheads) are found on the skin of the face, back, or chest.

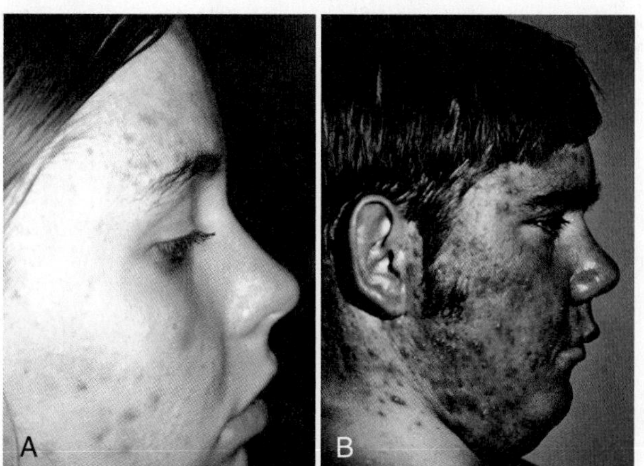

FIGURE 43-9 Acne vulgaris. **A,** Comedones with a few inflammatory pustules. **B,** Papulopustular acne.

Diagnostic Tests

The medical diagnosis is primarily made by inspection of the lesions and a health history that supports the diagnosis. Sometimes blood samples are drawn to measure hormone levels.

Medical Management

The medical management can involve topical, systemic, or intralesional medications. Topical therapy peels away the superficial skin layer to prevent sebum occlusions. A common topical medication is benzoyl peroxide gel (such as Clearasil). Effective topical therapy requires the use of special cleansing agents followed by applications of vitamin A acids, antibiotics, and sulfur-zinc lotions.

Systemic antibiotic therapy, combined with topical therapy, helps decrease the scarring associated with acne. Systemic antibiotics such as tetracycline are used. Isotretinoin (Accutane), a form of vitamin A, is also used frequently. Accutane reduces the sebum production and abnormal keratinization of gland ducts. Accutane must be prescribed with extreme caution in adolescent females because of its destructive effect on fetal development. Depression is a side effect of the drug. Changes in behavior should be noted and the patient referred for assistance. All patients taking the drug must have monthly liver function tests to determine if the drug is hepatotoxic.

Nursing Interventions and Patient Teaching

In planning nursing interventions, be aware that most adolescents do not comply with long-term treatment regimens. Assess and consider what acne means to them. The actual extent of the condition is not as important as the adolescent's feelings. When an adolescent's face constantly has ugly black and white lesions, it is hard to maintain a healthy self-esteem.

In addition to psychological concerns, focus on preventive nursing interventions. The important areas are skin care, compliance, and emotional support. Prevention stresses identification of factors that directly increase acne. Although poor hygiene may not be a cause, cleanliness decreases infection rate and promotes healing. The patient should keep the hands and hair away from the face, wear clothes that do not restrict affected areas, wash the hair daily, and wash the skin two or three times a day with medicated soap. Cosmetics need to be water based, and products that have wax esters should be avoided. Compliance is difficult because improvement is slow. Often 3 weeks of treatment are required before the patient, the family, or friends notice improvement (see Health Promotion box).

Nursing diagnoses and interventions for the patient with acne vulgaris include but are not limited to the following.

Nursing Diagnoses	Nursing Interventions
Impaired skin integrity, related to occluded oil glands	Assess extent of occluded oil glands by inspecting lesions for size, color, and location. Monitor for signs of infection. Wash involved areas two or three times a day. Apply medications to decrease occlusion of oil glands.
Situational low self-esteem, related to physical appearance	Assess primary cause of low self-esteem and depth of feelings. Assess family support. Encourage verbalization of feelings about cosmetic appearance and ways to deal with the situation. Observe nonverbal communication to discover patient's perception of the illness. Stress the importance of not comparing oneself with others. Have patient list current successes and strengths. Give positive reinforcement.
Social isolation, related to decreased self-esteem	Assess extent and feelings of isolation. Assess factors that contribute to sense of helplessness. Listen to and spend time with patient. Involve patient in support group. Focus on patient's strengths.

 Health Promotion

Healthy Skin

- Adequate nutrition (especially fluids; protein; vitamins A, B complex, and C; iron; adequate calories; and unsaturated fatty acids) promotes healthy skin.
- Refrain from smoking to improve skin color and prevent circulation difficulties.
- Drink eight glasses of water per day to help rid the skin of waste products.
- Exercise increases circulation and dilates blood vessels. In addition to the healthy glow produced by exercise, the psychological effects can improve one's appearance and mental outlook. However, caution must be used to protect against overexposure to heat, cold, and sun during outdoor exercise.
- In general, the skin and hair should be washed often enough to remove excess oil and excretions and to prevent odor.
- The use of neutral soaps and avoidance of hot water and vigorous rubbing can noticeably decrease local irritation and inflammation.
- Older adults should avoid using harsh soaps and shampoos because of the increased dryness of their skin.
- Moisturizers should be used after bath or shower, while the skin is still damp, to seal in this moisture.
- Obesity has an adverse effect on the skin. Increased subcutaneous fat can lead to stretching and overheating. Overheating causes an increase in perspiring, which can impair normal or inflamed skin.

Teaching should center on the patient's physical and emotional needs. Address diet, hygiene, stress reduction, makeup, and medications. Coping skills may need to be retaught and counseling referrals made. The extensive treatment time should be covered in minute detail because this disease is chronic and exacerbations will occur. Helping the adolescent communicate about feelings will decrease any long-term effects that acne may have on his or her personality. Patients taking isotretinoin will develop dry skin; teach patients measures to prevent it.

Prognosis

Prognosis for acne is good. However, lasting psychological effects can occur from the scarring that may result. In extreme cases eczema may develop from taking medications for acne, such as isotretinoin.

PSORIASIS

Etiology and Pathophysiology

Psoriasis is a noninfectious skin disorder; it is a hereditary, chronic, proliferative disease involving the epidermis and can occur at any age. No specific predisposing factors are known. The skin cells divide much more rapidly than normal. The normal time for the entire skin to be replaced, through sloughing and generation of new cells, is 28 days; in psoriasis the time may decrease to 7 days. Severe scaling results from the rapid cell division.

Clinical Manifestations

The lesions appear as raised, erythematous, circumscribed, silvery scaling plaques. The primary lesion is papular. The papules become plaques, which are located on the scalp, the elbows, the chin, and the trunk (Figure 43-10). The disease may be classified as mild, moderate, or severe.

Assessment

Collection of **subjective data** initially reveals only mild pruritus. Sometimes patients express feelings of depression, frustration, and loneliness. They report that observers stare and avoid contact with them, increasing their self-consciousness about their appearance.

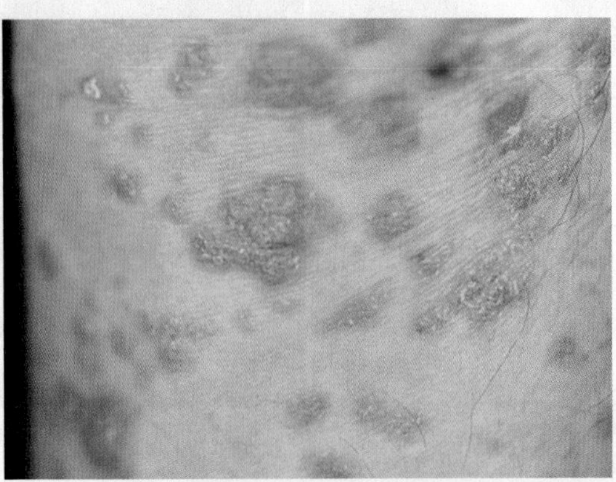

FIGURE 43-10 Psoriasis.

Collection of **objective data** includes observing dull, erythematous, sharply outlined plaques covered with silvery scales on the elbows, the knees, and the scalp. Fingernails can be affected and will show pitting with yellowish discoloration.

Diagnostic Tests

No specific diagnostic tests exist for psoriasis. Primary diagnosis is made by observing the patient and the symptoms displayed.

Medical Management

Medical management is aimed at slowing the proliferation of epithelial layers of the skin. Topical steroids and keratolytic agents are used in occlusive wet dressings to decrease inflammation. Keratolytic agents such as tar preparations and salicylic acid (Calicylic) decrease shedding of the outer layer of the skin. Topical steroids used are hydrocortisone and betamethasone valerate (Valisone).

Another treatment, photochemotherapy, involves the use of a drug enhanced by exposure to light. This therapy combines methoxsalen (Oxsoralen), which is given orally, and the concurrent use of ultraviolet light A (UVA).

Methotrexate and vitamin D reduce epidermal proliferation in some cases. The systemic medications approved by the FDA also include antimetabolite (methotrexate), immunosuppressant (cyclosporine), and retinoid (acitretin). Infliximab (Remicade) is used to control the severe plaque form of the disease (Lewis et al., 2007).

Nursing Interventions and Patient Teaching

Nursing interventions include proper administration of the treatment modality. Additional rest and measures to promote psychological well-being, such as counseling, are necessary. The patient's emotional needs are as important as the physical needs. Because this disease is chronic, encourage the patient to focus on positive attributes.

Nursing diagnoses and interventions for the patient with psoriasis include but are not limited to the following:

Nursing Diagnoses	Nursing Interventions
Impaired skin integrity, related to proliferation of epithelial cells	Assess extent of the scaliness. Administer treatment method correctly. Use medical aseptic technique.
Situational low self-esteem, related to appearance	Assess patient's concept of body. Help patient focus on positive aspects. Discuss with patient ways to conceal obvious lesions.
Social isolation, related to decreased self-esteem	Assess activity pattern and social outlets. Demonstrate ways to conceal lesions with clothes. Involve patient in support group.

The primary points in patient teaching include the nature of the disease, correct application of the treatment modality, and compliance with medical care. Stress that patients should not treat themselves. Inform patients that the disease is not curable.

Prognosis

Psoriasis is a chronic disease. The clinical course is variable, but less than half of the patients have a prolonged remission. Severity ranges from a minimal cosmetic problem to a life-threatening emergency.

SYSTEMIC LUPUS ERYTHEMATOSUS

Lupus is the Latin word for "wolf," used since AD 1230 to describe the cutaneous skin changes that resemble the zygomatic erythema of a red wolf (Figure 43-11). Lupus erythematosus affects the skin and may become systemic. Discoid lupus is an inflammatory condition with skin manifestation that can lead to the autoimmune disease, systemic lupus erythematosus (SLE).

Etiology and Pathophysiology

SLE is an autoimmune disorder characterized by inflammation of almost any body part. It is a chronic, multisystem inflammatory disorder that occurs when the body produces antibodies against its own cells. The resulting antigen and antibody complexes damage connective tissues. SLE is a disease of exacerbations and remissions. It is distinguished by an inflam-

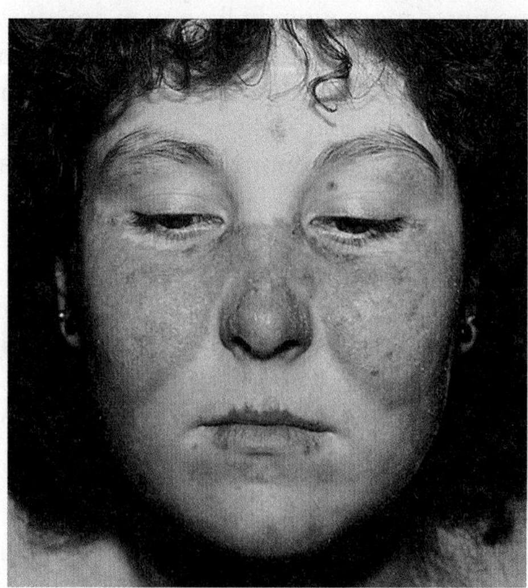

FIGURE 43-11 Systemic lupus erythematosus flare. The classic butterfly rash occurs over the nose and cheek area in 10% to 50% of patients with acute cutaneous lupus erythematosus.

Box 43-2 Pathogenic Conditions and Clinical Manifestations in Body Systems of Persons with Systemic Lupus Erythematosus

MUSCULOSKELETAL
Inflammation of vessels, tendons, and muscle tissue occurs because of deposits of fibrin. Polyarthralgia and polyarteritis occur in approximately 90% to 95% of patients.

GASTROINTESTINAL
Ulceration occurs on mucosal membranes because of degeneration of collagen tissue, with gastrointestinal manifestations of hemorrhage, abdominal pain, pancreatitis, cholecystitis, and bowel infarction.

RENAL
Glomerular sclerosis and glomerulonephritis occur with persistent proteinuria or cellular casts in urine.

HEMATOLOGIC
Cells are destroyed, and interference with coagulation occurs because of circulating antibodies. Anemia, leukopenia, lymphopenia, thrombocytopenia, and elevated erythrocyte sedimentation rate result.

CARDIOVASCULAR
Pericarditis is the most common cardiac manifestation. It often is the first clinical problem the patient manifests. Pericardial rub, commonly associated with pericarditis, can lead to dysrhythmias. Vasculitis in the small vessels may occur.

PULMONARY
Pleurisy and pleural effusions resulting from inflammation of the pleura are relatively common.

INTEGUMENTARY
Classic characteristics include the erythematous butterfly rash over the bridge of the nose and on the cheeks and linear erythema along the eyelids (see Figure 43-11). Other features may include bullae, patchy areas of purpura, urticaria, and subcutaneous nodules.

NEUROLOGIC
Mental and neurologic signs and symptoms occur in 35% to 40% of patients with systemic lupus erythematosus. Signs and symptoms relate to the central nervous system, not to the peripheral nerves. Mental and behavioral changes may occur, as well as seizures, headaches, and strokes.

matory lesion that affects several organ systems: the skin, the joints, the kidneys, and serous membranes.

SLE is a chronic, incurable, and multicausal disease. Although the syndrome's origin is a mystery, increasing evidence suggests that immunologic, hormonal, genetic, and possibly viral factors may contribute to its onset. Genetic predisposition seems to play a role in most cases, coupled with a precipitating agent or factor. The person with SLE has a decreased number of T-suppressor cells; those T-suppressor cells that remain function in a limited manner. Antibodies develop against other antigens.

SLE is most prevalent in women of childbearing age. Nine times more women than men are affected by this disorder, and three times as many blacks as whites are affected. Survival rates have increased to more than 15 years after diagnosis with this disorder. Despite advances in treatment, SLE remains a serious illness.

Clinical Manifestations

Clinical manifestations include oral ulcers, arthralgias or arthritis, vasculitis, rash, nephritis, pericarditis, synovitis, organic brain syndromes, peripheral neuropathies, anemia, leukopenia, thrombocytopenia, coagulopathies, immunosuppression, and dermatitis. Anemia tends to be the most common complication (Box 43-2).

Diagnostic Tests

Diagnosis of SLE may require extensive evaluations over months or years. A detailed history, physical examination, and results of laboratory findings are required to obtain a diagnosis (Lewis et al., 2007). Diagnostic tests for SLE (Box 43-3) often have positive results in the presence of inflammatory disease. No single test is considered conclusive for diagnostic purposes. However, positive results of one or more diagnostic tests along with at least three other criteria lead to the diagnosis of SLE. Criteria for diagnosis include the following:

- Erythematous butterfly rash (see Figure 43-11) over the nose and cheeks and along the eyelids
- Alopecia (hair loss), with frontal alopecia seen more frequently in women

Box 43-3 Diagnostic Tests for Systemic Lupus Erythematosus

- Antinuclear antibody (ANA)
- DNA antibody
- Anti-Sm antibody
- Complement
- Complete blood count (CBC)
- Erythrocyte sedimentation rate (ESR)
- Sedimentation rate (not diagnostic, but used to monitor disease activity and effectiveness of therapy)
- Coagulation profile
- Rheumatoid factor (RF)
- Rapid plasma reagin (RPR)
- Skin and renal biopsy
- C-reactive protein (CRP)
- Coombs' test
- Lupus erythematosus cell preparation (LE cell prep)
- Urinalysis
- Chest radiographic study

- Other skin features, including bullae, patchy areas of purpura, thickening of epidermis
- Photosensitivity
- Oral ulcers
- Polyarthralgias and polyarthritis
- Pleuritic pain, pleural effusion, pericarditis, and vasculitis
- Renal disorders as evidenced by protein or cellular casts in the urine
- Neurologic signs, such as seizures of unknown cause
- Hematologic disorders—such as hemolytic anemia, leukopenia, lymphopenia, or thrombocytopenia—in the absence of other diagnostic reasons
- Immunologic disorder identified with positive lupus erythematosus prep, antinuclear antibody (ANA), or double-stranded DNA
- Positive ANA in the absence of patient use of drugs known to cause drug-induced lupus erythematosus

Medical Management

SLE treatment goals include relief of the symptoms. The outcomes of the medical plan include remission of the disease, early alleviation of exacerbations, and prevention of untoward complications. Additional outcomes include therapeutic management of the signs and symptoms of the syndrome and suppression of inflammation.

Drug therapy includes nonsteroidal antiinflammatory agents, such as acetylsalicylic acid (ASA) and ibuprofen (Motrin); antimalarial drugs (hydroxychloroquine [Plaquenil] or chloroquine); and corticosteroids (such as prednisone) in low doses given several times a day. Methylprednisolone may be used intravenously in cases of exacerbation. Peak amounts of steroids help to achieve remission. The steroid doses are decreased slowly until a maintenance dose is reached. Topical corticosteroid creams are used for the rash of SLE. Antineoplastic drugs such as azathioprine (Imuran), cyclophosphamide (Cytoxan), or chlorambucil (Leukeran) may be used therapeutically to achieve remission or to control signs and symptoms.

Antimalarial drugs (hydroxychloroquine) are used to control discoid and other skin lesions and rheumatic manifestations. Because retinal toxicity may occur at high doses, patients should receive pretreatment and annual ophthalmic examinations.

Antiinfective agents are used both to treat and to prevent infections in the patient with SLE. The specific antibiotic depends on the infection site. Urinary tract infections respond well to ciprofloxacin (Cipro).

Peritoneal dialysis or hemodialysis may be indicated in patients who have moderate to severe renal involvement. Laboratory tests such as assessing blood urea nitrogen (BUN) and serum creatinine provide information regarding kidney function. Analgesics and diuretics may be used to treat symptoms often found in patients with SLE. Supportive therapy—such as a balanced diet, a balance between rest and activity, and reduced exposure to the sun—may also be indicated.

Nursing Interventions and Patient Teaching

Because SLE is a multisymptom disease, a thorough assessment is indicated. Tailor the care plan to include (1) skin care, including teaching avoidance of direct sunlight and use of protective clothing and sunscreen; (2) balance between rest and activity; (3) recognition of signs of exacerbation (i.e., fever, rash, cough, or increasing muscle and joint pain); (4) early recognition of signs and symptoms of infection; (5) stress reduction and management; and (6) balanced nutrition and reduction of sodium intake. Because the disease is one of exacerbation and remissions, each exacerbation will intensify the patient's stress and decrease his or her ability to cope. Provide psychosocial, emotional, and spiritual support for the patient.

Patients with impaired immune system function must endure the consequences of chronic or incurable disease. A caring, gentle, and understanding approach to patient care will help reduce the burden and stress of SLE (Nursing Care Plan 43-2). The nurse's responsibilities in patient education are related to the information needed for the patient to live a normal life. Focus on activity level, prevention of infection, and potential complications.

Prognosis

SLE has no known cure. Management of the disease depends on the nature and severity of the manifestations and the organs affected. Treating SLE earlier in its course has contributed to a better prognosis.

PARASITIC DISEASES OF THE SKIN

PEDICULOSIS

Etiology and Pathophysiology

Pediculosis (lice infestation) is a parasitic disorder of the skin that many associate with poor living conditions and poor personal hygiene. This is not always the case, however; pediculosis can occur anywhere. Lice obtain their nutrition from the blood of their victims. They leave their eggs (nits) on the skin surface attached to the shaft of the hair (Figures 43-12 and 43-13).

Humans have three types of lice: the head louse, the body louse, and the pubic louse. In pediculosis capitis, the head louse attaches itself to the hair shaft and lays 8 to 16 eggs per day. The eggs are visible at the back of the neck as gray, shiny, oval bodies.

In pediculosis corporis, the body louse is found around the neck, waist, and thighs. The louse is generally found in the seams of clothing and causes severe pruritus and pinpoint hemorrhages.

The pubic louse, the parasite involved in pediculosis pubis, does not resemble the head or body louse. It looks like a crab with sharp pincers that attach to the

Nursing Care Plan 43-2 The Patient with Systemic Lupus Erythematosus

Ms. Templeton, age 34, is experiencing an acute exacerbation of systemic lupus erythematosus. She is admitted to the medical unit with severe joint pain, butterfly rash, generalized edema, and Sjögren syndrome.

NURSING DIAGNOSIS *Impaired skin integrity, related to skin rash (butterfly across face), hair loss, skin atrophy, discoid lesions involving other parts of the body*

Patient Goals and Expected Outcomes	Nursing Interventions	Evaluation and Rationale
Patient will verbalize understanding of skin care regimen and positioning schedule	Develop positioning schedule. Use appropriate devices such as air mattress, eggcrate mattress, sheepskin, or foam padding, where indicated.	Patient verbalizes understanding of the purpose of changing positions every 2 hours to prevent skin impairment.
Patient will demonstrate behaviors to promote skin healing	Assess and monitor skin and mucous membranes and describe lesions' size, characteristics, and changes noted. Assess nutritional status and areas at risk for pressure. Measure intake and output. Provide optimum nutrition.	Patient states she understands skin care regimen to promote skin healing.
Patient will experience improved wound and lesion healing	Monitor for signs of infection. Encourage patient to minimize sun exposure by wearing long-sleeved blouses or shirts and wide-brimmed hats and by using sunscreens with a sun protection factor of 15. Teach skin care maintenance.	Patient's skin lesions are beginning to show signs of healing.

NURSING DIAGNOSIS *Disturbed body image, related to baldness and pathologic skin pattern conditions*

Patient Goals and Expected Outcomes	Nursing Interventions	Evaluation and Rationale
Patient will verbalize understanding of altered body image Patient will have a positive, accepting, and realistic body image Patient will perform self-care activities within level of own ability Patient will identify personal community resources that can provide assistance	Assess patient's perception of body image; investigate what aspects are not pleasing and how she perceives changes as deviating from social norms.	Patient states she understands that skin changes and hair loss are part of the disease process of systemic lupus erythematosus.
	Teach patient ways to improve body image (e.g., improving personal hygiene, wearing makeup, changing type of clothes, protecting self from sun). Encourage family members and significant others to maintain open communication with patient. Record emotional changes. Set limits on maladaptive behavior.	Patient talks about importance of open communication with her family and significant other concerning her feelings of body image disturbance.

Critical Thinking Questions

1. Ms. Templeton has painful, edematous joints that greatly decrease her mobility. She has 4+ pitting edema to the lower extremities secondary to the loss of protein through her kidney. What are the most appropriate nursing interventions to decrease Ms. Templeton's pain level and to increase her mobility?
2. On entering the room, the nurse notes Ms. Templeton crying. She says that her lifestyle is severely altered because she is unable to be in the sun to work in her beloved garden. What nursing interventions would be most beneficial?
3. Ms. Templeton confides that she fears that this severe increase in her symptoms will lead to an early death. What initial response to this statement would be of greatest assistance?

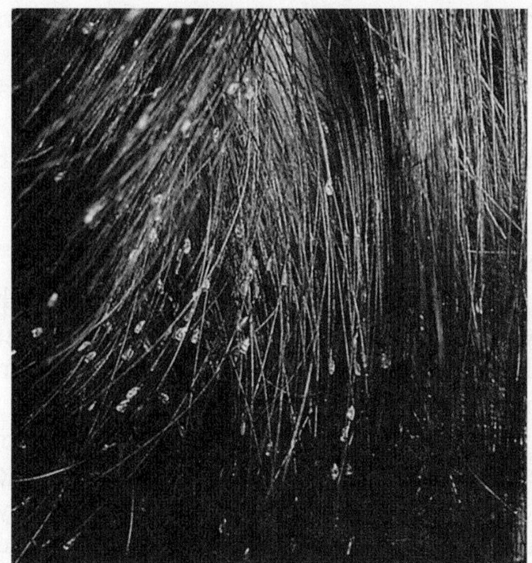

FIGURE 43-12 Eggs of pediculus attached to shafts of hair.

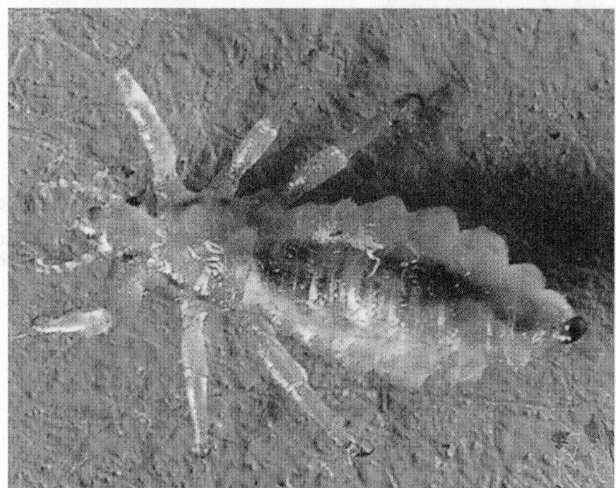

FIGURE 43-13 Lice have six legs and are wingless.

pubic hair. Transmission can be through sexual contact, bed linens, or bath towels.

Clinical Manifestations

Nits or lice can be seen on the body. Pinpoint, raised red macules, pinpoint hemorrhages, and severe pruritus confirm the diagnosis. Excoriation is common because of the intense pruritus.

Assessment

Subjective data include complaints of pruritus in the area involved. Tenderness and difficulty wearing clothes are also noted.

Objective data include erythema, petechiae, and skin excoriation in the area.

Diagnostic Tests

The diagnostic test is a physical examination of the involved area. A health history supports the diagnosis. Removal of the parasite confirms the diagnosis.

Medical Management

A topical pediculicide such as lindane (Kwell) or pyrethrins (RID) is applied in any contaminated area. The specific technique for applying these products varies and should be followed closely to control the lice.

Nursing Interventions and Patient Teaching

The primary nursing intervention involves applying the medication to rid the patient of lice. Identify involved people and appropriate health teaching. Stress the nature and transmission of the disease. Assess each family member for nits, and teach measures to reduce pruritus, such as cool compresses and corticosteroid ointments. Any furniture or nonwashable materials with which the patient has come in contact should be properly cleaned to prevent reinfection. Bed linens should all be washed in hot water and dried in a dryer. Assessment of the patient's emotional needs is also important. Society often associates a lice infestation with poor hygiene practices.

Prognosis

The prognosis is good; proper treatment results in full recovery.

SCABIES

Etiology and Pathophysiology

Scabies is caused by the female itch mite *(Sarcoptes scabiei)*. The mite penetrates the skin and makes a burrow. Once under the skin, the mite lays eggs that mature and rise to the skin surface. Scabies is transmitted by prolonged contact with an infected area. Overcrowded living conditions, poverty, changing sexual behaviors, and world travel have increased the incidence of scabies. Scabies occurs in all age-groups and socioeconomic classes.

Clinical Manifestations

Scabies causes wavy, brown, threadlike lines on the body, especially the hands, arms, body folds, and genitalia (Figure 43-14). Pruritus is severe, and secondary infections are common from the excoriation caused by scratching.

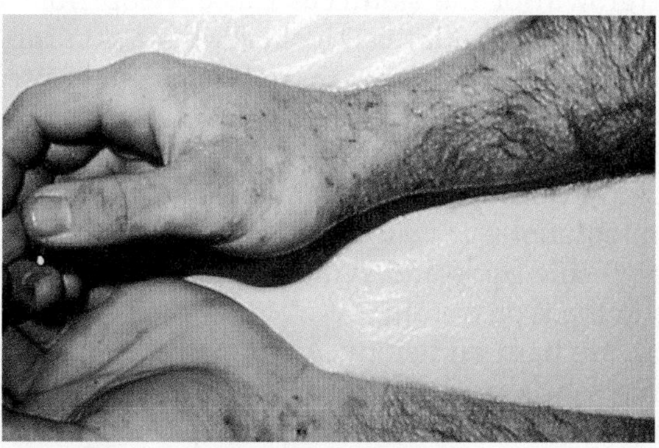

FIGURE 43-14 Scabies.

Assessment

Subjective data include the severe pruritus associated with scabies and the skin excoriation resulting from scratching.

Collection of **objective data** includes finding the wavy brown lines on the body and severe erythema from the scratching.

Diagnostic Tests

The condition can be confirmed by microscopic examination of infected skin. A health history and characteristic signs and symptoms support the diagnosis.

Medical Management

Medical treatment attempts to eliminate the mite and prevent complications. Drug therapy is basically the same as for pediculosis. Two additional drugs used are crotamiton (Eurax) and a 4% to 8% solution of sulfur in petrolatum.

Nursing Interventions and Patient Teaching

Nursing interventions for restoring skin integrity involve using medical aseptic techniques to improve hygiene and to apply medications. Proper application of medication is essential to destroy the parasite. The patient's emotional well-being is another focus of nursing care. Using open-ended questions and listening skills help provide support.

A primary concern is educating family members about the transmission of scabies. Each family member needs to treat the whole body with a scabicide. Clothing, bed linens, and bath articles should be washed in hot water and dried in a dryer. If clothes are line dried, they should be ironed. Stress the importance of compliance with the treatment. Also, teach the family that scabies infestations can happen to anyone. Conveying a nonjudgmental attitude is important.

Prognosis

The prognosis is good; with adequate treatment, full recovery results.

TUMORS OF THE SKIN

Overgrowth of the skin cells can develop from any layer or its appendages. The majority of skin tumors are benign. Many outgrowths or tumors can be predisposing factors for skin cancer.

Etiology, Pathophysiology, and Clinical Manifestations

The specific signs and symptoms of skin tumors relate to the type of tumor. Keloids, which originate in scars, are hard and shiny. Angiomas resemble birthmarks. Warts (verrucae) are located on the arms and hands. Nevi are thought to predispose a person to cancer, and patients become anxious when they notice a color change. Skin cancers may be life threatening and occur wherever exposure to the sun was greatest.

Report any changes in a skin lesion to a physician, including changes in size, color, border, surface, or elevation. Also report the development of pain, bleeding, or pruritus.

Assessment

Collection of **subjective data** includes a good health history. First assess the patient's risk factors, such as lifestyle, occupation, family history, and geographic location.

Collection of **objective data** includes describing the lesion in detail. The size, the location, and any pain are significant factors in determining the type of skin tumor. The lesion's appearance can take several forms.

Diagnostic Tests

The diagnostic test for tumors of the skin is biopsy of the lesion. A health history and visual inspection support the diagnosis.

Medical Management

The primary medical intervention for skin tumors is surgical removal. Other treatment modalities are radiation therapy to decrease the tumor size and application of topical medications such as corticosteroids to decrease the size and inflammation.

Nursing Interventions and Patient Teaching

Patients are understandably concerned about the potential threat of malignancy. Careful explanations of treatments, medications, and tests help decrease anxiety. Nursing interventions center on preparing the patient for the treatment needed. Skin tumors may be a threat to the patient's self-concept. Emotional care is important; encourage the patient to verbalize feelings of fear or anxiety.

Nursing diagnoses and interventions discussed with malignant melanoma are applicable to most skin cancers. Although the tumors previously mentioned are not all malignant, the problems posed are the same until a definitive diagnosis is made.

Discharge instructions include skin care, dressing changes, and follow-up care. Involve the family in teaching so they can support the patient. Discuss the signs and symptoms of infection for patients who have tumors surgically removed.

KELOIDS

Keloids (an overgrowth of collagenous scar tissue at the site of a wound of the skin) are seen more often in blacks than in whites. Collagen tissue becomes raised, hard, and shiny. Keloids usually originate from a scar and can be located anywhere on the body (Figure 43-15). The sternum, the ears, the neck, and the arms are common locations. Keloids are usually surgically ex-

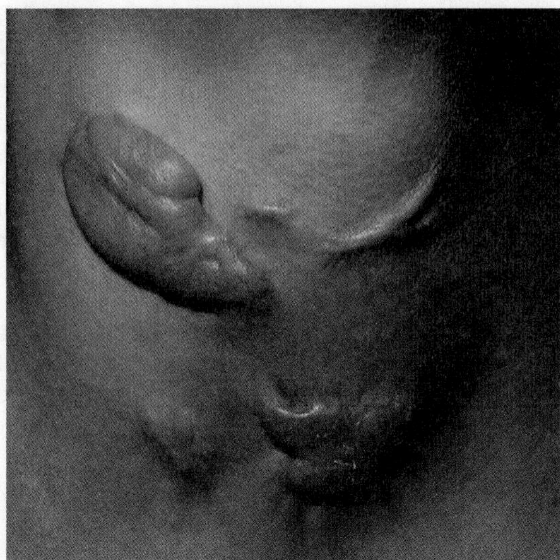
FIGURE 43-15 Keloids.

cised but may recur. Steroids and radiation therapy are two treatment measures.

ANGIOMAS

An angioma develops when a group of blood vessels dilate and form a tumorlike mass. A common angioma is a birthmark, such as the port-wine birthmark. This stain is not elevated and may be found on one side of the face or any part of the body. Treatment involves electrolysis or radiation.

A spider angioma or telangiectasis is associated with liver disease. A group of venous capillaries dilate and branch out like a spider. Spider angiomas usually resolve as the disease improves.

VERRUCA (WART)

A **verruca** is a benign, viral, warty skin lesion with a rough, papillomatous (nipplelike) growth occurring in many forms. Verrucae may occur singly or in groups and are thought to be contagious. Common locations are the hands, arms, and fingers, but warts can occur anywhere on the body. The plantar wart develops on the sole of the foot and is extremely painful. Treatment of warts depends on the type, location, and number. Cauterization, solid carbon dioxide, liquid nitrogen, and preparations of salicylic acid are used to remove warts.

NEVI (MOLES)

Nevi (singular, *nevus;* a pigmented, congenital skin blemish that is usually benign but may become cancerous), or moles, are nonvascular tumors, also called **birthmarks.** There are many types of nevi, and several may become malignant, especially if traumatized. The raised, black nevus is considered one of the most threatening, and removal is recommended to prevent it from becoming malignant. Any change in color, size, or texture or any bleeding or pruritus deserves investigation.

BASAL CELL CARCINOMA

Basal cell carcinoma is one type of skin cancer. Factors related to the development of skin cancer include frequent contact with certain chemicals, overexposure to the sun, and radiation treatment. Fair-skinned people are more likely to develop skin cancer, possibly because they have less melanin on the skin surface.

Basal cell carcinomas arise in the basal cell layer of the epidermis. They are often found on the face and upper trunk and are not noticed by the patient. Metastasis is rare, but underlying tissue destruction can progress to include vital structures. Basal cell carcinoma is usually scaly in appearance. It may be a pearly papule with a central crater and waxy, pearly border.

With early detection and complete removal, the outcome is favorable; however, this type of cancer recurs in 40% to 50% of patients treated (Figure 43-16).

SQUAMOUS CELL CARCINOMA

Squamous cell carcinoma arises in the epidermis. This cancerous neoplasm is a firm, nodular lesion topped with a crust or a central area of ulceration and indurated margins (Figure 43-17). Ten percent of patients have rapid invasion with metastasis by way of the lymphatic system; therefore early detection and treatment are important. Larger tumors are more prone to metastasis.

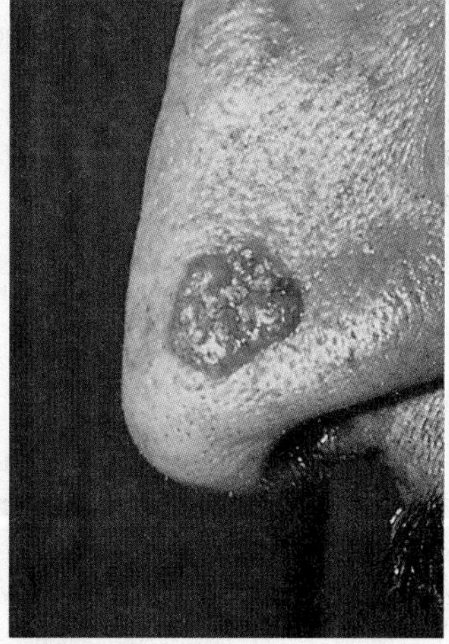
FIGURE 43-16 Basal cell carcinoma.

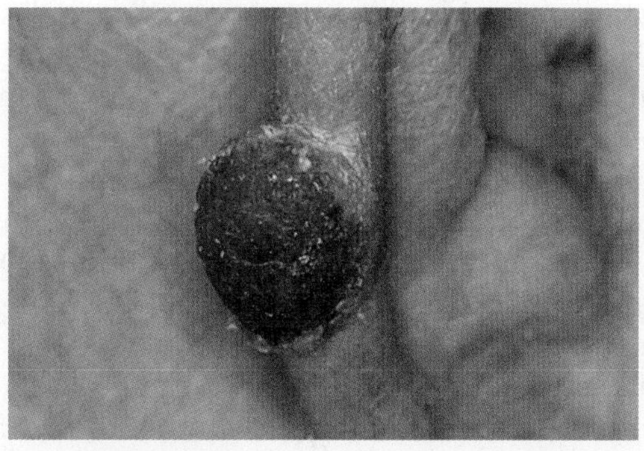
FIGURE 43-17 Squamous cell carcinoma.

Evidence-Based Practice **Skin Cancer Prevention**

Research Summary

What is cancer? More specifically, what is skin cancer? Cancer by definition is an "uncontrolled growth and spread of abnormal cells" (ACS, 2006). Therefore skin cancer is characterized by abnormal skin cells, which can spread and invade other tissues. More importantly, what can we do about skin cancer? As nurses, it becomes our responsibility to assess for and educate our patients about all types of skin cancers, especially for the most serious form called melanoma. There are several risk factors for melanoma. Major factors are positive family history of melanoma, a prior melanoma, and multiple or unusual moles. Other factors include fair complexion/skin that is sensitive to the sun; excessive exposure to the sun (especially before age 18), and the use of tanning beds/booths.

Research has indicated that skin cancer, when detected early and treated properly, is highly curable. Overall survival rates for melanoma at the 5-year mark are 92%, with 98% for localized melanoma; when it is grouped in regional and distant stages, the survival rates dramatically decrease (ACS, 2006). Therefore early intervention is of utmost importance.

Application to Nursing Practice

The results from the research studies have made it a nursing responsibility to screen and intervene for our patients' best interest. It is a necessity that we promote self-screening for all patients and their family members. We must also educate the general public.

- Instruct patients to conduct a complete monthly self-examination of the skin and scalp, noting moles, blemishes, and birthmarks.
- Perform the examination after a bath or shower, including a head-to-toe check.
- Use a well-lit room and mirrors to examine all skin surfaces. If necessary, have the patient ask a family member/significant other to aid in the investigation.
- The ACS (2006) outlines the warning signs of skin cancer using the ABCD mnemonic: *A* is for Asymmetry—look for uneven shape; *B* is for Border irregularity—look for edges that are blurred, notched, or ragged; *C* is for Color—pigmentation is not uniform; blue, black, brown variegated and areas of pink, white, gray, blue, or red are abnormal (Hayes, 2003); and *D* is for Diameter, greater than the size of a typical pencil eraser.
- Teach your patients to contact their health care provider if a skin lesion or mole starts to bleed or ooze or feels different (swollen, hard, lumpy, itchy, or tender to the touch). Especially instruct older adults, who tend to have delayed wound healing.
- Inform your patients of ways to prevent skin cancer by avoiding overexposure to the sun:
  —Wear wide-brimmed hats and long sleeves.
  —Apply broad-spectrum sunscreens with SPF of 15 or greater to protect against ultraviolet B (UVB) and ultraviolet A (UVA) rays approximately 15 minutes before going into the sun and after swimming or perspiring.
  —Avoid tanning under the direct sun at midday (10 AM to 4 PM).
  —Do not use indoor sunlamps, tanning parlors, or tanning pills.
- Inform patients who are on medications that make the skin more sensitive to the sun (e.g., oral contraceptives, antibiotics, antiinflammatories, antihypertensives, immunosuppressives) to take extra precautions when spending time in the sun.
- Inform patients to protect their children from the sun. Severe sunburns in childhood greatly increase melanoma risk later in life (ACS, 2006).
- These interventions will provide the patient with self-screening measures to detect, prevent, and seek early treatment for skin cancer.

From Potter, P.A., & Perry, A.G. (2009). *Fundamentals of nursing: concepts, process, and practice* (7th ed.). St. Louis: Mosby. Data from American Cancer Society (2006). *Cancer facts and figures 2006,* Atlanta: Author; and Hayes, J.L. (2003). Are you assessing for melanoma? *RN,* 66(2), 36.
ACS, American Cancer Society.

Sun-exposed areas, especially the head, neck, and lower lip, are common places of occurrence. The cancer also occurs on sites of chronic irritation or injury (scars, irradiated skin, burns, and leg ulcers).

MALIGNANT MELANOMA

Etiology and Pathophysiology

A malignant melanoma is a cancerous neoplasm in which pigment cells (melanocytes) invade the epidermis, dermis, and sometimes the subcutaneous tissue. Several types of melanoma occur, and they are categorized by location and description. Most melanomas arise from melanocytes in the epidermis, but some may appear in preexisting moles. Melanoma can metastasize to any organ, including the brain and heart.

This is the most deadly skin cancer, and its incidence has doubled in the past two decades, a faster rate of growth than any other cancer (Figure 43-18). The increased occurrence is associated with recreational exposure to the sun (see Evidence-Based Practice box). Heredity is also a factor, and any person who has a large number of moles with a variety of sizes and colors should be monitored. The person who has a history of skin cancer is at greater risk.

Clinical Manifestations

Basically, malignant melanomas are divided into four types: (1) superficial spreading melanomas, (2) malignant lentigo melanomas, (3) nodular melanomas, and (4) acral lentiginous melanomas.

Superficial spreading melanomas are the most common and occur anywhere on the body. These melanomas are slightly elevated, irregularly shaped lesions in a varying hues; common colors are tan, brown, black, blue, gray, and pink. **Lentigo melanomas** are usually found on the heads and necks of older adults. Characteristically these appear as tan, flat lesions that

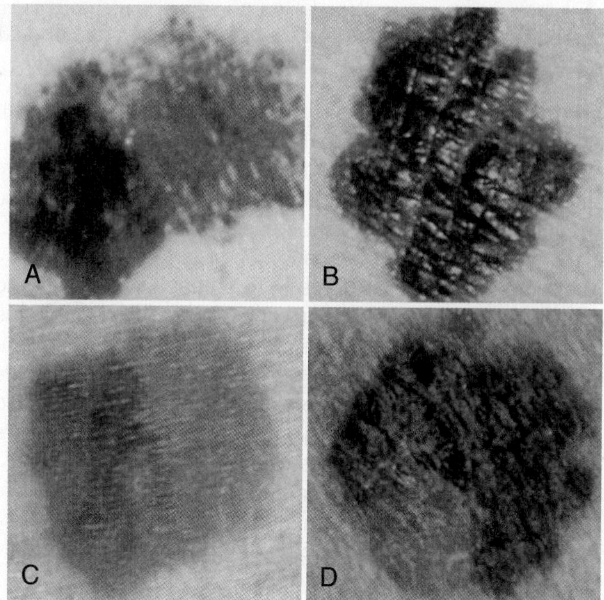

FIGURE 43-18 The ABCDs of melanoma. **A,** Asymmetry (one half unlike the other). **B,** Border (irregularly scalloped or poorly circumscribed border). **C,** Color varied from one area to another; shades of tan and brown, black, and sometimes white, red, or blue; change in shape, size, or color of mole. **D,** Diameter larger than 6 mm as a rule (diameter of a pencil eraser).

change shape and size. **Nodular melanomas** appear as a blueberry-type growth, varying from blue-black to pink. The patient often describes the lesion as a blood blister that fails to resolve. Nodular melanomas grow and metastasize faster than the other types. **Acral lentiginous melanomas** occur in areas not exposed to sunlight and where no hair follicles are present. Common locations are the hands, the soles, and the mucous membranes of dark-skinned people.

Assessment

The collection of **subjective data** should include a thorough health history related to skin cancer. Patients at greatest risk have fair complexions, blue eyes, red or blond hair, and freckles.

Objective data include the location, color, and appearance of the lesions.

Diagnostic Tests

Diagnosis primarily depends on tissue biopsy. The patient is also examined thoroughly for suspicious lesions. Monitor any lesion that is variegated in color, has an irregular border, or has an irregular surface. The tumor thickness at the time of diagnosis is a key factor in the prognosis of malignant melanoma. The two measurements to determine the thickness of the melanoma are Breslow measurement and Clark level. The thicker the tumor, the poorer the prognosis (Lewis et al., 2007).

Medical Management

Medical management depends on the site, level of invasion, thickness of the melanoma, and the patient's age and general health.

A wide, surgical excision of the primary lesion with a margin of normal skin is the treatment of choice. Skin grafts are sometimes needed. Subsequent treatment modalities such as chemotherapy, nonspecific immunotherapy, chemoimmunotherapy, and radiation may be planned, depending on the stage of the disease. Gene therapy is currently being examined as another treatment option (Lewis et al., 2007).

Nursing Interventions and Patient Teaching

The major goals of nursing care include pain relief, reduction of anxiety, and palliative treatment of the disease. Fear of the unknown is a major concern for the patient with a melanoma. Explaining procedures and diagnostic tests in terms that the patient can understand may help decrease anxiety.

Nursing diagnoses and interventions for the patient with melanomas include but are not limited to the following:

Nursing Diagnoses	Nursing Interventions
Pain, related to lesion	Assess pain using the five PQRST variables of the chief complaint. Provide nursing comfort measures, such as back rubs, to decrease pain. Administer pain medication as needed. Teach relaxation techniques.
Anxiety, related to cancer, its treatment, and prognosis	Listen to and accept expression of anger, sadness, and helplessness.

Discharge instructions include wound care, medication, cleansing, and follow-up care. Assess the family's knowledge about the seriousness and treatment of the disease. Explain to the patient the need for regular physical examinations and regular skin self-assessment. Encourage the patient to protect skin from the sun by using sunscreens and protective clothing and by limiting exposure. Stress the use of medical aseptic techniques to prevent a secondary infection.

Prognosis

The key prognostic factor in malignant melanoma is the thickness of the lesion. Individuals with lesions less than 0.76 mm thick have a survival rate of almost 100%, whereas those with lesions 3 mm thick or thicker have survival rates of less than 50%. If the cancer spreads to regional lymph nodes, the patient has a 50% 5-year survival rate. The tumor may metastasize by vascular or lymphatic spread, with rapid movement of melanoma cells to other parts of the body. If metastasis occurs, treatment is largely palliative.

DISORDERS OF THE APPENDAGES

ALOPECIA

Alopecia is the loss of hair. The cause can be aging, drugs such as antineoplastics, anxiety, or disease processes. Unless it is related to aging, alopecia is usually not permanent; the hair usually grows back but can take several months. Any time a patient loses hair, body image and self-esteem are threatened.

HYPERTRICHOSIS (HIRSUTISM)

Hypertrichosis is an excessive growth of hair in a masculine distribution. It can be hereditary or acquired as a result of hormone dysfunction and medications. The treatment is removal by dermabrasion, electrolysis, chemical depilation, shaving, tweezing, or rubbing with pumice. Treatment of the cause usually stops growth of additional hair.

HYPOTRICHOSIS

Hypotrichosis is the absence of hair or a decrease in hair growth. Skin disease, endocrine problems, and malnutrition are associated factors. Treatment involves identifying and treating the cause.

PARONYCHIA

Paronychia is a disorder of the nails. The nails get soft or brittle, and the shape can change as they grow into the soft tissue (ingrown nails). In paronychia, an infection of the nail develops and spreads around the nail, thus giving it the nickname "runaround." The nails are painful as they loosen and separate from the tissue. Wet dressings or topical antibiotics may be used. Sometimes a surgical incision and drainage of the infected area are performed.

BURNS

Etiology and Pathophysiology

Each year more than 1 million people in the United States seek medical attention for burns. About 70,000 of them need to be hospitalized, and one third require extensive care services. An estimated 4500 of these people die annually as a direct result of their burns (CDC, 2009). The incidence of burns has decreased slightly and the number of deaths resulting from burn injury has also decreased (CDC, 2009). This decrease stems from the creation of regional burn centers, a national focus on fire safety, the use of smoke detectors, and occupational safety mandates.

Burns may result from thermal or nonthermal causes. Thermal burns are caused by flames, scalds, and thermal energy (heat). Thermal burns are the most common type of burn injury. Nonthermal burns result from electricity, chemicals, and radiation. Skin destruction depends on the burning agent, the temperature of the burning agent, the condition of the skin before the injury, and the duration of the person's contact with the agent.

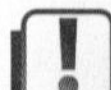 Safety Alert

Prevention of Burns

- The major cause of fires in the home is carelessness with cigarettes. Preventive education is imperative.
- Other causes of burns include hot water from water heaters set higher than 140° F (60° C), cooking accidents, space heaters, combustibles such as gasoline and charcoal lighter fluid, steam from radiators, and chemicals.
- Most burns can be prevented. The nurse as a citizen and health care provider is in a good position to conduct home safety assessments and to educate people about burn injuries before accidents occur. Home safety measures include using smoke alarms and fire extinguishers. Families should have fire drills, and each family member should know where to go and what to do in case of a fire.
- Local fire departments can inform the public of regional fire codes and perform home safety checks.
- Knowledge of potential sources of burn injury allows problem solving for burn prevention.

Teaching people proper use of appliances (e.g., space heaters, electrical cords, wiring, outlets, outdoor grills, and water heaters) can prevent burn injury.

Burns cause dramatic changes in most physiologic functions of the body, beginning in the first few minutes to the first 12 to 24 hours after the burn injury. The burn's effect depends on two factors: the extent of the body surface burned and the depth of the burn injury. The extent of burn is measured in terms of the total body surface area (TBSA) injured. Burns exceeding 20% TBSA result in massive evaporative water losses and fluid loss into the interstitial spaces. Depth depends on the layers of the skin involved.

With any burn injury, a pathophysiologic process ensues. In the damaged area, the capillaries dilate, resulting in capillary hyperpermeability that lasts for about 24 hours. The increased cell permeability causes the fluid to shift from the capillaries into the surrounding tissues (interstitial spaces), resulting in edema and vesiculation (blistering). A larger burned area results in a more rapid shift of fluid from the intravascular area into the interstitial area (sometimes known as *third spacing*). This shift poses the greatest threat to life because the cells become dehydrated. As a result, the body experiences hypovolemic shock and hyperviscosity. Blood pressure and blood flow to the kidneys decrease, symptoms of hypovolemic shock develop, and acute renal failure may result.

The pathophysiology and care of burns may be divided into three stages. The emergent phase, stage 1, is from the onset of the injury until the patient stabilizes. Hypovolemic shock is the major concern for up to 48 hours after a major burn. Stage 2, the intermediate or acute (or diuretic) phase, begins 48 to 72 hours after the burn injury. In this stage the greatest concern is circulatory overload. Circulatory overload may result from the fluid shift back from the interstitial spaces into the capillaries. The acute phase begins when the kidneys excrete large volumes of urine (hence the name *diuretic stage*). Stage 3, the long-term rehabilitation phase, begins at the same time as burn wound treatment. In the third stage, the patient care outcome involves returning the patient to as normal a state as possible. A second outcome is freedom from wound infection.

In a burn injury, usually the greatest fluid loss occurs within the first 12 hours. The proteins, plasma, and electrolytes shift from the vascular compartment to the interstitial compartment. Red blood cells tend to remain in the vascular system, causing increased viscosity of the blood and a falsely elevated hematocrit level. Acute dehydration is present, and renal perfusion is seriously compromised. This fluid shift and the loss of intravascular fluids may lead to the development of burn shock. The rapid loss of fluid places a strain on the heart because the blood volume diminishes and the heart can no longer supply enough blood to perfuse the vital organs. The body responds by increasing the peripheral resistance. Burn shock is characterized by hypotension; decreased urinary output; increased pulse (tachycardia); rapid, shallow respirations (tachypnea); and restlessness. Most deaths from burns result directly from burn shock.

Fluids begin to shift back to the vascular compartment in approximately 48 to 72 hours. Fluid return denotes the end of the hypovolemic stage and the beginning of the diuretic stage. Reabsorption of the interstitial fluid back into the intravascular area causes an increased blood volume. As the blood volume increases, the cardiac output increases, resulting in increased renal perfusion. The result includes diuresis. However, the patient is at risk of fluid overload because of the rapid movement of fluid back into the intravascular space. Carefully monitor the patient's vital signs, urinary output, and consciousness. Patients with preexisting cardiac problems, as well as the very young and very old, run the greatest risk for circulatory overload.

A burn victim may experience smoke inhalation damage from breathing the chemicals produced by the burn. The fumes damage the cilia and the mucosa of the respiratory tract. Alveolar surfactant decreases, and atelectasis can occur. Breathing difficulties may take several hours to appear. While assessing a patient who has sustained any burn to the upper chest, the neck, and the face, consider the patient at high risk for respiratory distress. Signs of respiratory difficulty include a hoarse voice or a productive cough. Other physical findings suggesting an inhalation injury include the following:

- Singed nasal hairs
- Agitation, tachypnea, flaring nostrils, or intercostal retractions
- Brassy cough, grunting, or guttural respiratory sounds
- Erythema or edema of the oropharynx or nasopharynx
- Sooty sputum

Clinical Manifestations

Traditionally, burns were classified as first, second, or third degree (Table 43-3). However, using only the visual characteristics of the burn wound results in an inaccurate description. A more accurate classification is superficial thickness injuries, partial-thickness injuries, and full-thickness injuries; these terms graphically describe the burn and indicate the depth and severity of the tissue injury (Figures 43-19 to 43-21).

Assessment

The nursing assessment includes (1) depth of the burn, (2) causative agent, (3) temperature and duration of contact, and (4) skin thickness. The patient's age and

Table 43-3 Causes and Factors Determining Depth of Burn Injury

DEPTH	CAUSE	APPEARANCE	COLOR	SENSATION
Superficial (first degree)	Flash flame, ultraviolet light (sunburn)	Dry, no vesicles Minimal or no edema Blanches with fingertip pressure, and refills when pressure removed	Increased erythema	Painful
Partial thickness (second degree)	Contact with hot liquids or solids Flash flame to clothing Direct flame Chemicals Ultraviolet light	Large, moist vesicles that increase in size Blanches with fingertip pressure, and refills when pressure removed	Mottled with dull, white, tan, pink, or cherry red areas	Very painful
Full thickness (third degree)	Contact with hot liquids or solids Flame Chemicals Electrical contact	Dry with leathery eschar Charred vessels visible under eschar Vesicles rare, but thin-walled vesicles that do not increase in size may be present No blanching with pressure	White, charred, dark tan Black Red	Little or no pain Hair easily pulls out

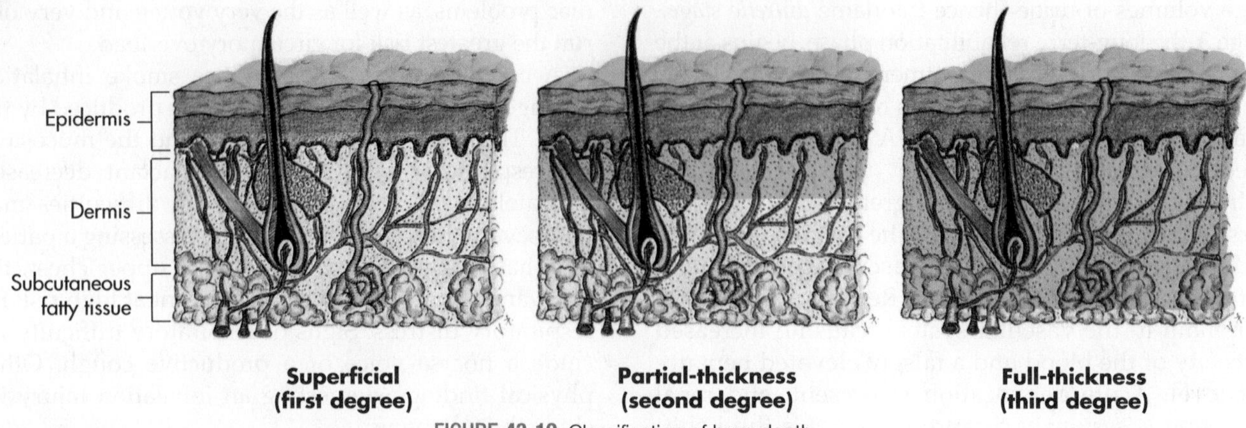

FIGURE 43-19 Classification of burn depth.

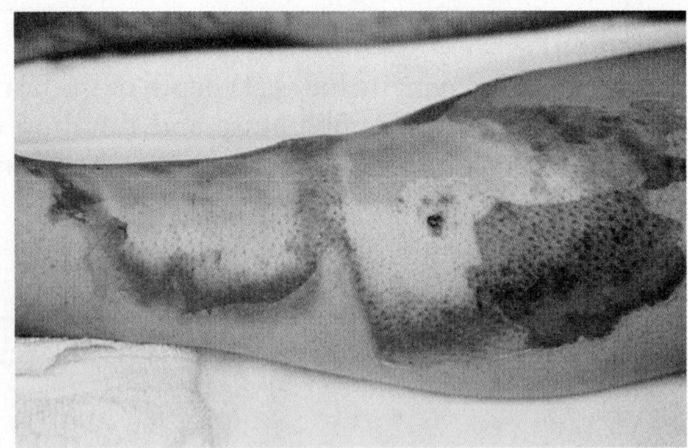

FIGURE 43-20 Superficial partial-thickness injury.

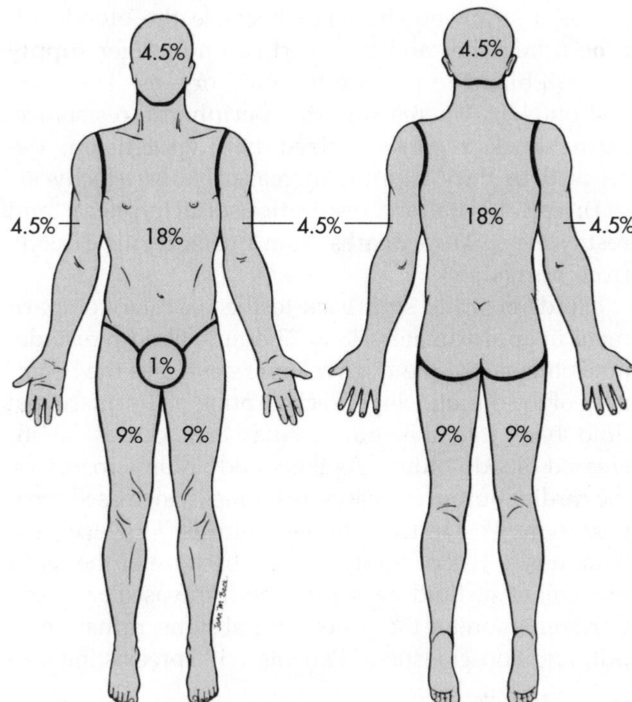

FIGURE 43-22 Rule of nines.

FIGURE 43-21 Full-thickness thermal injury.

other disease processes affect the outcome of the burn. The **rule of nines** determines the TBSA burned (Figure 43-22). The rule of nines divides the body into multiples of nine. The entire head is 9%; the anterior and posterior aspects of the arms are a total of 9% each; the legs are 9% anterior and 9% posterior; the chest and back are 18% each; and the perineum is 1%.

The rule of nines does not take into account the different levels of growth and is not accurate for children.

Collection of **subjective data** reveals the causative agent, other diseases present, the temperature and duration of contact, and the patient's age. If the patient is able to communicate, ask him or her to rate the pain on a scale from 0 to 10.

Objective data include the depth of the burn, the skin thickness involved, the percentage of TBSA burned, the specific location, and any other injuries sustained. Any time a patient has a burn that involves the face, the neck, or the chest, observe for respiratory difficulty. Determine whether the victim has had a tetanus booster in the past 5 years.

The severity of the burn depends on several factors. Major burns require the most skilled nursing interventions. Moderate and minor burns require fewer nursing interventions. Factors determining a major, moderate, or minor burn are the (1) percentage of the TBSA burned, (2) victim's age, (3) specific location of the burn, (4) cause of the burn, (5) other diseases present, (6) depth of the burn, and (7) injuries sustained during the burn (Box 43-4).

Diagnostic Tests

The primary diagnostic test is a physical examination to determine the amount of burned area. Blood assessments—such as those for electrolytes, CBC, serum chemistries, and arterial blood gases—may be done to establish the severity of the dehydration. In inhalation burns, carboxyhemoglobin level is evaluated. Most fatalities occur among survivors with severe asphyxiation or carbon monoxide intoxication. Carbon monoxide (CO) binds to hemoglobin with greater affinity than does oxygen, resulting in tissue hypoxia.

Medical Management

The medical treatment of burns is divided into three phases with differing priorities. Remember that these phases are not always clearly defined and may overlap.

Emergent Phase

The primary concern in the emergent phase is to stop the burning process using the "stop, drop, and roll" technique. Also, removing clothing and shoes from the victim may eliminate the source of the burn to arrest skin damage. Do not apply ice to burns because it can cause rapid vasoconstriction, which may cause more trauma to the tissues by increasing the depth of the burn.

Box 43-4 Classification of Severity of Burns

MAJOR BURN INJURIES

- Greater than 25% total body surface area (TBSA) (greater than 20% in children less than 10 years and adults more than 40 years of age)
- Greater than 10% TBSA, full thickness
- Involvement of face, eyes, ears, hands, feet, perineum
- Electrical burns
- Burns complicated by inhalation injury or major trauma
- Burns in patients with preexisting disease (diabetes, heart failure, or chronic renal failure)

MODERATE BURN INJURIES

- 15% to 25% TBSA in adults, partial thickness (10% to 20% TBSA in children less than 10 years and adults more than 40 years of age)
- Less than 10% TBSA, full thickness
- Burns with no concurrent injury
- Burns in patients with no preexisting disease

MINOR BURN INJURIES

- Less than 15% TBSA in adults (less than 10% in children or older adults)
- Less than 2% TBSA, full thickness
- Burns in patients with no preexisting disease

The second step is to provide an open airway; third is to control bleeding. Fourth, remove all nonadherent clothing and jewelry (rings, watches). Fifth, cover the victim with a clean sheet or cloth. Sixth, transport the victim to the hospital. In the case of a chemical burn, it is important to rinse the skin generously with water to remove all chemicals. Electrical burns have an entry point and an exit point that need to be identified. Most electrical burns result in cardiac arrest, and the patient requires cardiopulmonary resuscitation or astute cardiac monitoring.

During the primary survey assessment, quickly assess the ABCs (airway, breathing, and circulation) and look for life-threatening injuries, such as blunt chest trauma. Assessment of the patient's airway becomes and remains the priority of nursing care. Suspect an inhalation injury, especially if the burn occurred in a closed or confined area. Signs and symptoms of inhalation injury include singed facial hair, black-tinged sputum, soot in the throat, hoarseness, and neck or face burns. Stridor is a life-threatening sign.

CO poisoning is likely if the patient was in an enclosed area. CO displaces oxygen from hemoglobin. Do not rely on pulse oximetry to rule out CO poisoning. Oximeters cannot distinguish between oxyhemoglobin and carboxyhemoglobin. The carboxyhemoglobin level should be measured, when feasible, per blood sample. Early signs of CO poisoning include headache, nausea, vomiting, and unsteady gait. Treatment includes administering 100% oxygen.

Once the patient is in the hospital, the severity of the burn dictates the care given. Perform a thorough assessment every 30 minutes to 1 hour in the emergent phase. Patients with major burns generally are transferred to burn care centers or units for treatment but must be stabilized first. Patients with moderate to severe burns are treated using the following steps:

1. Establish airway. Administer oxygen as ordered. Often the physician inserts an endotracheal tube to ensure a patent airway (Figure 43-23).
2. Initiate fluid therapy. Begin intravenous fluid therapy with Ringer's lactate solution immediately. The amount of fluid given is related to the percentage of TBSA burned. Weigh the patient so the physician can determine the amount of fluids needed.
3. Insert Foley catheter for hourly urinary output. An hourly output of 30 to 50 mL is recommended. Intravenous fluids are given to maintain renal perfusion (Box 43-5).
4. Insert a nasogastric tube to prevent aspiration. Patients with severe burns often develop a paralytic ileus as a result of trauma.
5. Administer analgesics intravenously in small, frequent doses for pain control. Morphine may be used. Any degree of hypovolemia can increase the effects of medications. Carefully assess

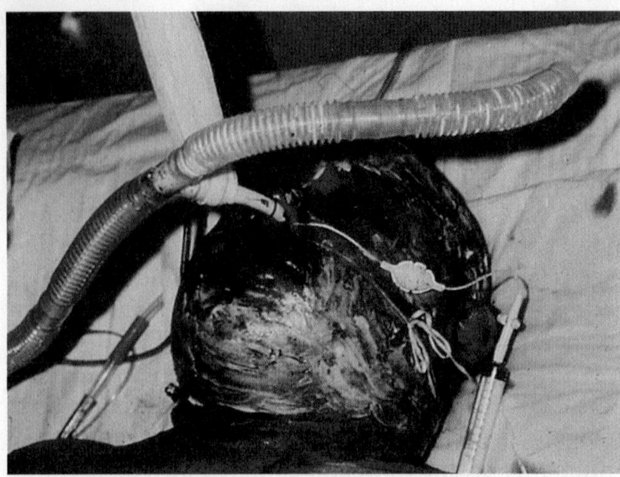

FIGURE 43-23 Endotracheal intubation for patient with severe edema 5 hours after a burn injury.

Box 43-5 Indications for Fluid Resuscitation

- Burns greater than 20% total body surface area (TBSA) in adults
- Burns greater than 10% TBSA in children
- Patient older than 55 or younger than 4 years of age
- Patient with preexisting disease that would reduce normal compensatory responses to minor hypovolemia (cardiac or pulmonary disease, diabetes)
- Electrical burns

the patient's respiratory status when administering morphine.

6. Maintain airway and fluid status, and monitor vital signs.
7. Give tetanus immunization prophylaxis as needed. (Patients who have been immunized against tetanus do not need a tetanus toxoid booster unless the last injection was more than 5 years ago. If the patient has never had a tetanus immunization, administer tetanus serum and active immunization in the emergency department.)

The first 72 hours require diligent medical care. The primary goals in the emergent phase are to maintain respiratory integrity and to prevent hypovolemic shock, which may result in death (Box 43-6).

Box 43-6 Nursing Diagnoses for the Emergent Phase of Burns

- Ineffective airway clearance, related to edema of the respiratory passages
- Deficient fluid volume (dehydration), related to shift of body fluids
- Deficient fluid volume, related to capillary hyperpermeability with fluid moving out of the cells into the interstitial area
- Acute anxiety, related to injury
- Acute pain, related to loss of skin
- Risk for infection, related to impairment of skin integrity
- Impaired skin integrity, related to damage by the burns
- Decreased cardiac output, related to hypovolemia
- Risk for aspiration, related to decreased peristalsis
- Impaired swallowing, related to mucosal edema
- Impaired verbal communication, related to breathing difficulties
- Disturbed sleep pattern, related to hospital environment

Acute Phase

The acute phase begins when fluids shift back to the intravascular compartment, usually 72 hours after the burn. During the acute phase, the patient's metabolism increases. Urinary output also increases as the fluid shifts back into the blood circulation. As the urinary output increases, the edema in the tissues begins to decrease. The acute phase may last from 10 days to months. The two primary treatment goals are treatment of the burn wound and prevention and management of complications. Infection is the most common complication and cause of death after the first 72 hours. Other complications include heart failure, renal failure, **contractures** (shortening or tension of muscles that affects extension), paralytic ileus causing gastric dilation, and **Curling's ulcer** (a duodenal ulcer that develops 8 to 14 days after severe burns on the surface of the body; the first sign is usually vomiting of bright red blood).

Nursing interventions. Prioritizing nursing care using the ABCs remains the most important nursing intervention. After completing the ABCs, gather data in the head-to-toe assessment concerning (1) respiratory pattern, (2) vital signs, (3) circulation, (4) intake and output, (5) ambulation, (6) bowel sounds, (7) inspection of the wound itself, and (8) mental status.

Fluid-reshifting complications may also develop during the acute phase if renal damage has occurred. Monitor the patient for signs of acute renal failure such as elevated serum creatinine and BUN. Heart failure may develop as a result of the rapid increase in blood volume from the return of fluid from the interstitial spaces into the intravascular vessels. The primary goals in the acute phase include proper care of the burn wound to promote healing and prevent infection as well as preventing and treating complications. Assessment for an infection of the burn wound includes observing the wound for increasing erythema, odor, or a green or yellow exudate. Local and systemic infections complicate recovery and increase recovery time (Figure 43-24). Wound cultures and sensitivities help pinpoint the type of organism present and the most effective antibiotic for treatment. Any signs of an infection should be reported.

Once the patient's vital signs and urinary output stabilize and the acute phase begins, complete a nutritional assessment. Provision for adequate nutrition remains a cornerstone of burn care during the acute phase. Increased amounts of protein, calories, and vitamins help repair the damaged tissue; encourage oral

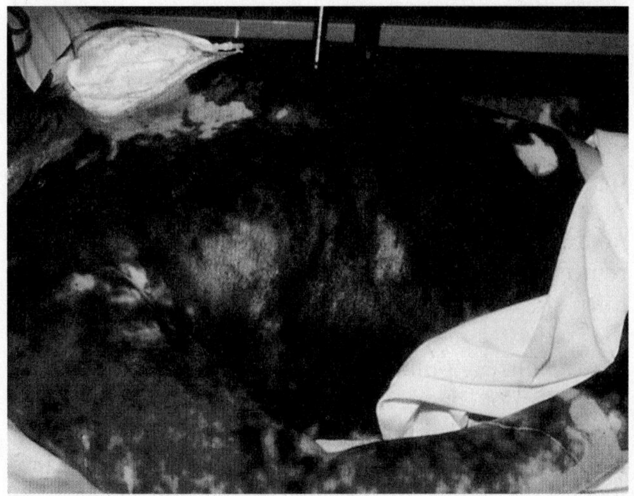

FIGURE 43-24 Postburn *Pseudomonas* infection.

intake of nutrients as soon as possible. The nutritional challenge includes providing enough nutrients to meet the body's increased metabolic requirement. Monitor nutritional status through daily measurement of weight, serum electrolytes, and serum albumin and through urinalysis. Adequate nutrition decreases healing time, whereas weight loss increases healing time. Skin grafts will not be successful unless nutrition is adequate.

Nursing interventions include measures to control pain and to support the patient's psychological well-being. Intravenous opioids in small, frequent doses provide relief from pain, but care must be taken to avoid jeopardizing respiratory integrity. Specific interventions include verbal support, unhurried care, truthful explanations, and effective listening. Excellent communication skills are essential.

Without an intact first line of defense—that is, the skin—the protective mechanisms function abnormally. Thus protective isolation is necessary. Wear gowns, masks, caps, and gloves during each contact with a patient with major burns. Follow strict surgical aseptic technique during dressing changes. Use of proper equipment and cleaning procedures is imperative. Hydrotherapy (e.g., whirlpool) can be a source of infection.

The standard treatment for partial-thickness burns includes debriding the wound, applying topical antibiotics, and changing dressings twice a day. A new treatment for burns includes temporary skin substitutes. Made from a variety of materials, skin substitutes promote faster healing for burn wounds and can eliminate painful dressing changes and minimize scarring. In 1997, TransCyte, a temporary bioengineered skin substitute, became the first such product to be approved by the FDA for burn treatment. TransCyte is designed as an alternative both to silver sulfadiazine (Silvadene) for patients with partial-thickness burns and to cadaver skin for full-thickness burns and deep partial-thickness burns requiring surgical debridement. It is made from neonatal human fibroblast cells. The fibroblasts secrete human derma, collagen, matrix proteins, and growth factors. All of these factors promote wound healing. TransCyte is typically applied only once, thus avoiding the frequent, painful dressing changes. TransCyte provides a temporary covering that helps protect against fluid loss and reduces the risk of infection.

A new and highly successful skin replacement therapy called Integra Dermal Regeneration Template is being used in the treatment of life-threatening, full-thickness or deep partial-thickness burn wounds. Within the first few days of admission, the patient goes to surgery, the wound is debrided, and the Integra artificial skin is applied. The wound is then wrapped with dressings. The artificial skin stimulates regeneration of new dermis by the body. During a second surgical procedure, the artificial skin is removed and replaced by the patient's own autografts (Lewis et al., 2007).

Traditional wound care involves the removal of the eschar that forms. **Eschar** is a black leathery crust (i.e., a slough) that the body forms over burned tissue; eschar can harbor microorganisms and cause infection. It may also compromise circulatory status. An escharotomy is often done to relieve the circulatory constriction (Figure 43-25). Daily **debridement** (removal of damaged tissue and cellular debris from a wound or burn to prevent infection and to promote healing) and special cleansing support regeneration of the tissues. Hydrotherapy softens the eschar to make removal less painful. It also promotes range of motion to decrease contractures.

The specific wound care method depends on the severity of the burn. The open or exposure method may be used for burns of the face, neck, ears, and perineum. The area is cleaned and exposed to air. A hard crust forms, and regeneration of tissue follows.

Proper positioning and range-of-motion exercises (facilitated by the nurse and physical therapist) are vi-

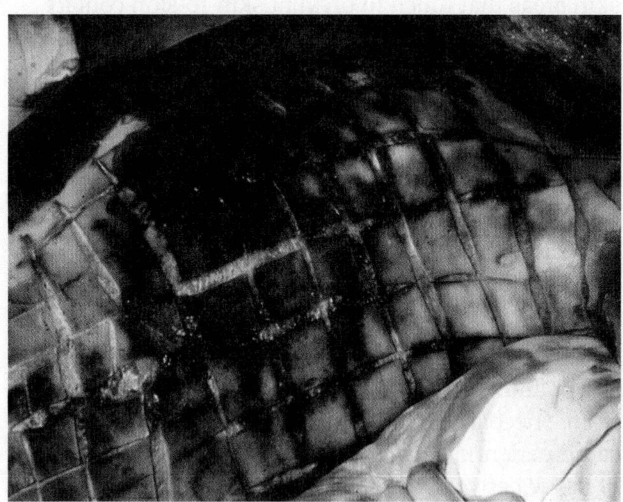

FIGURE 43-25 Grid escharotomy used to alleviate circulatory and pulmonary constriction.

tal for the burn patient's well-being. Special bed equipment is needed to prevent the burn from touching the linens. A bed cradle, a CircOlectric bed, or a Clinitron bed is recommended. Chilling may be controlled by keeping the room temperature at 85° F (29.4° C) and providing lights or heat lamps for additional warmth. Humidity should be between 40% and 50%.

Advantages to the open method are that (1) the wound can be observed more easily, (2) movement in bed is less restricted, (3) circulation of the body part is not restricted, and (4) exercises can be done more easily to prevent contractures. Disadvantages are (1) pain; (2) chilling; (3) contamination of wound by the health care provider; (4) unattractive appearance, which causes emotional distress; and (5) the need for protective isolation precautions for the immunocompromised patient.

Control the pain with intravenously administered opioids in the early days of the acute phase. However, considering the long-term nature of a burn, addiction is a potential problem. Diazepam (Valium) has been found to be effective, but morphine is commonly used.

The closed (or occlusive) method involves cleaning the burn, applying the prescribed medication, and dressing the wound as ordered. Advantages of the closed method are that (1) it protects the burn area from injury, and (2) it prevents contamination of the area by the health care provider. Circulation checks are important with pressure dressings to assess for adequate arterial perfusion to the involved areas.

The topical medications used to hasten healing and prevent infection vary. Topical administration is preferred because the capillaries are coagulated by the burn. Mafenide (Sulfamylon), silver sulfadiazine, and silver nitrate are common drugs used in burn care. Each drug has specific advantages and disadvantages (Table 43-4).

Burn care essentials include a lightweight dressing. A single layer of gauze covered with medication and a single wrap of Kerlix provide adequate coverage. When applying gauze to the burn area, place gauze between skin areas that touch to prevent skin-to-skin contact.

Changing burn dressings is painful; therefore 30 minutes before the procedure, administer an analgesic, either 5 to 10 mg of intravenous morphine sulfate or a sedative. Most dressings are changed after hydrotherapy. Remove all old medication and eschar before applying any new medication. Failure to debride promotes infection, delays healing, and increases scarring.

Skin grafts are used as soon as possible to cover full-thickness burns. Grafting promotes healing and prevents infection. Grafting generally occurs during the first 3 weeks of care. Four types of grafts may be used: (1) an **autograft** (surgical transplantation of any tissue from one part of the body to another location in the same patient), (2) a **homograft (allograft)** (the transfer of tissue between two genetically dissimilar individuals of the same species, such as skin transplant from another person who is not an identical twin [often a cadaver]), (3) a **heterograft (xenograft)** (tissue from another species, such as a pig or a cow, used as a temporary graft), or (4) a synthetic graft substitute. The autograft is permanent, whereas the other types are temporary.

Grafts are applied by either the **pedicle method** (the tissue is left partially attached to the donor site and the other portion of the tissue is attached to the burn site) or the freestanding method (the tissue is completely removed from the donor site and is attached to the burn site).

Graft sites are a nursing challenge. Any movement that results in pulling the graft area can dislodge the graft. Do not change dressings until ordered. The donor site resembles a partial-thickness burn after the graft. Donor site care is as important as care of the burn site. Inspect the donor site for signs of infection, such as erythema and malodor (see Patient Teaching box). Pain is a primary complaint after the graft and should be treated.

The nutritional aspect of burn care is another nursing challenge. Destroyed body proteins and fluid loss present problems as the body increases metabolism to meet the extra demands. Therefore the body requires enough energy to maintain homeostasis while meeting the increased need for repairing the injury.

Burn patients should eat by mouth as soon as their condition permits. Protein requirements are greater than normal. Normal protein intake encompasses 0.8 grams per kilogram of body weight, whereas the burned patient requires 1.5 to 3.2 grams per kilogram of body weight. Thus a normal 150-pound person needs 55 grams of protein per day; if burned, the same person needs 102 to 158 grams of protein, depending on the extent of the burn. Daily caloric requirements range from 2000 calories to more than 6000 calories, depending on the burn. Meeting these enormous requirements requires diligent nursing interventions. Concentrated, high-calorie foods need to be offered frequently. The body also requires additional amounts of vitamins A, B, and C to promote digestion, absorption, and repair of tissue. Increased amounts of calcium, zinc, magnesium, and iron are needed. Vitamin C and zinc aid in wound healing, and added B complex vitamins aid metabolism of the extra protein and

Patient Teaching

Skin Grafts

- Do not remove dressing unless ordered.
- Report changes in the graft (hematoma, fluid collection) to physician.
- Protect grafted skin from direct sunlight with a sunscreen lotion for at least 6 months.
- Keep surface of healed graft moistened daily with skin lotion for 6 to 12 months. (Grafted skin does not perspire; it dries and cracks easily.)
- Wear a strong elastic stocking for 4 to 6 months for grafts on lower extremities.

Table 43-4 Topical Medications for Burn Therapy Skin Grafts

Generic (Trade)	Advantages	Disadvantages
Mafenide (Sulfamylon)	Bacteriostatic against gram-negative and gram-positive organisms Penetrates thick eschar	Metabolic acidosis Pain on application Allergic rash
Silver sulfadiazine (Silvadene)	Broad antimicrobial activity against gram-negative, gram-positive, and *Candida* organisms No electrolyte imbalances Painless and somewhat soothing Not nephrotoxic	With repeated application, skin may develop slimy, grayish appearance, simulating an infection despite negative cultures Prolonged use may cause skin rash and depress granulocyte formation
Silver nitrate	Bacteriostatic effect Lessens pain and eliminates odor Reduces evaporative water loss from burns	Electrolyte imbalances Stains everything it comes into contact with Does not penetrate eschar Pain on application
Nitrofurazone (Furacin)	Inhibits enzymes necessary for bacterial metabolism Broad spectrum of activity Effective against *Staphylococcus aureus* Not absorbed systemically Low incidence of sensitivity	Contact dermatitis in unaffected skin Urine turns a reddish color
Gentamicin sulfate (Garamycin)	Broad antimicrobial activity Painless	Ototoxicity Nephrotoxicity Development of resistant bacterial strains
Neomycin	Broad antimicrobial activity Causes miscoding in the messenger RNA of bacterial cells	Serious toxic effects Ototoxicity Nephrotoxicity
Scarlet red	Nonantiseptic (applied to gauze soaked with oil-based red dye) Drying agent Applied to donor site Promotes epithelialization	No antimicrobial effects Stains and irritates skin Infection may develop beneath scarlet red gauze, which may have systemic effects
Xeroform	Nonantiseptic Debrides and protects donor site Protects graft	Removal may be painful, because it sometimes adheres to wound Neither antiseptic nor antimicrobial
Sodium hypochlorite (Dakin's solution)	Chlorine-based solution that is bactericidal Aids in debriding wounds Aids cleaning of copious drainage	Dissolves blood clots May inhibit clotting May irritate the skin
Sutilains ointment (Travase)	Topical enzymatic agent Dissolves necrotic tissue by proteolytic action Facilitates removal of eschar and purulent drainage	Mild, transient pain on application Paresthesia, bleeding, dermatitis Dressing must be kept moist at all times

RNA, Ribonucleic acid.

carbohydrate intake. Adding oral supplements such as Ensure, Sustacal, and Carnation Instant Breakfast can increase vitamin, mineral, and protein intake. Total parenteral nutrition provides an alternative to oral intake of proteins if the patient is unable to take in adequate nutrients by mouth.

The daily calorie requirement is estimated by the use of the formula (25 kilocalories × body weight in kilograms) + (40 kilocalories × %TBSA burned) = kilocalories per day required. Most burn victims have poor appetites; therefore getting the patient to eat is difficult. Small, frequent feedings of high-calorie, high-protein, low-volume foods are the best way to meet the patient's nutritional needs. Some patients develop Curling's ulcer 8 to 14 days after the burn injury because of increased gastric acidity. The first sign is vomiting of bright red blood. The prophylactic treatment involves intravenous or oral administration of cimetidine (Tagamet), ranitidine (Zantac), omeprazole (Prilosec), or famotidine (Pepcid). See Box 43-7 for nursing diagnoses for the acute phase of burn care.

Rehabilitation Phase

Rehabilitation of the burn patient begins at admission. However, the third phase of burn care begins when 20% or less of the TBSA remains burned. The goal becomes

Box 43-7 Nursing Diagnoses for the Acute Phase of Burns

- Acute anxiety, related to change in body image
- Fear, related to chronic illness
- Chronic pain, related to procedures performed
- Risk for infection, related to open skin wounds
- Imbalanced nutrition: less than body requirements, related to increased metabolic demands
- Social isolation, related to perceived change in body image
- Impaired physical mobility, related to burns
- Self-care deficit in activities of daily living (ADLs), related to area of burn involved
- Deficient knowledge in all areas, related to expected care
- Interrupted family processes, related to long-term hospitalization
- Disturbed body image, related to disfigurement from burns
- Deficient diversional activity, related to confinement during care
- Ineffective coping, related to:
  —Seriousness of injury
  —Perceived role changes
- Powerlessness, related to:
  —Prolonged recovery
  —Loss of income
  —Loss of physical attractiveness

Box 43-8 Nursing Diagnoses for the Rehabilitation Phase of Burns

- Ineffective airway clearance, related to edema of the respiratory passages
- Impaired physical mobility, related to:
  —Splinting
  —Dressings
  —Pain
- Activity intolerance, related to prolonged bed rest
- Anxiety, acute to moderate, related to role change
- Disturbed body image, related to scarring
- Deficient knowledge, related to impaired home maintenance management
- Self-care deficit (in ADLs), related to:
  —Pain
  —Fatigue
- Fear, related to impending surgery
- Risk for disuse syndrome, related to noncompliance
- Post-trauma syndrome, related to the cause of the burn
- Impaired adjustment
- Ineffective coping, related to long-term rehabilitation
- Disturbed personal identity, related to inability to return to previous lifestyle for prolonged period
- Caregiver role strain, related to prolonged recovery period
- Ineffective management of therapeutic regimen, related to complexity and chronicity of rehabilitation
- Anticipatory grieving, related to loss of wellness

to promote independence so the patient may have a productive life. The rehabilitation process addresses both social and physical skills and may take years.

Mobility limitations constitute the major concerns. The patient requires a comprehensive physical therapy program for positioning, skin care, exercise, ambulation, and activities of daily living (ADLs). Contractures remain a concern in the care of a burn patient. Although physical therapists provide most of the rehabilitative care, the nurse assists in providing continuity of care. When planning the care, set realistic, short-term goals to motivate patients to try to achieve more.

Maintaining or restoring the patient's independence remains the primary rehabilitative goal. Given the possibility of a changed body image, encourage the patient to talk about fears and concerns. Working with others such as social workers and counselors, develop a holistic care plan to provide the comprehensive care needed. During visiting hours, assess family interactions. Helping the family cope with the changes in their loved one is a major nursing intervention.

Numerous nursing diagnoses apply to burn victims, encompassing family, patient, and social roles (Box 43-8).

Patient Teaching

Before discharge, the burn patient and family need education. Provide written instructions that are complete, comprehensive, easy to understand, and realistic. Return demonstrations are the best way to determine that learning has taken place. The major topics to cover are (1) wound care, (2) signs and symptoms of complications, (3) dressings, (4) exercises, (5) clothing, (6) ADLs, and (7) social skills (see Home Care Considerations box).

Home Care Considerations

Burns

- Bathe twice a day with mild soap.
- Test the water temperature before getting into the shower because your skin is sensitive to extremes of hot and cold.
- Be certain to clean the tub well before each bath.
- If itching becomes severe, take a lukewarm bath with Alpha Keri lotion added to the bath water.
- Do not use lotions that contain lanolin or alcohol because they will cause blisters.
- Avoid direct sunlight. Wear light clothing to cover areas that have been burned because these areas burn easily.
- Discoloration and scarring are normal during healing. The color of the scar may remain red because of the healing process. Usually within 6 months to a year the scar loses its red color and becomes softer. Normal color to the area may take several months to return.
- Report to the physician:
  —Any signs of infection
  —Fever greater than 101° F (38.3° C)
  —Feeling of inability to cope

Evaluation

Evaluation depends on meeting the stated goals. In evaluating the burn patient, ask the following questions:

- Can the patient take care of self?
- Can the patient ambulate without difficulty?

- Can the patient cope?
- Can the family cope?
- Does the patient have contractures?
- Does the patient understand the treatment process?

Burn care is extensive, and the exact nursing interventions for each patient are individualized. Many times the patient must change vocations, and family relationships change. The degree of scarring—emotionally and physically—cannot be predicted; nor can the patient's acceptance by society.

Prognosis

The outcome for the patient with burns depends on the size of the burn; depth of the burn; the victim's age; the body part involved; the burning agent; and history of cardiac, pulmonary, endocrine, renal, or hepatic disease and other injuries sustained at the time of the burn.

❖ NURSING PROCESS *for the Patient with an Integumentary Disorder*

The role of the licensed practical nurse/licensed vocational nurse (LPN/LVN) in the nursing process as stated is that the LPN/LVN will:

- Participate in planning care for patients based on patient needs
- Review patient care plan and recommend revisions as needed
- Review and follow defined prioritization for patient care
- Use clinical pathways, care maps, or care plans to guide and review patient care

■ Assessment

Assessment of the skin is an important aspect of patient care. Skin changes can reflect specific skin disorders, but they may also alert the nurse to a systemic disorder. Skin assessment allows the identification of obvious and subtle changes in the patient's state of health. Effective skin assessment takes a critical eye and knowledge of the expected normal findings.

Because the skin is usually assessed at the same time as other body systems, nurses tend to underestimate the valuable information that can be obtained. Assessing the skin provides a baseline knowledge of the patient's hygiene measures, nutritional status, circulatory status, and sensory perception. The skin is the first line of defense against infection. Therefore ongoing assessment of the skin is important in the maintenance of health and the prevention of infection.

Assessment of the older adult can be challenging for the health care professional. The normal changes that occur related to aging are important for the nurse to know. The older patient population is growing, as are the opportunities for the student to assess the older patient (see Life Span Considerations box).

Life Span Considerations

Older Adults

Effects of Aging on the Integumentary System

- Physiologic changes make the skin of the older adult more fragile and susceptible to impairment.
- Aging changes include decreases in tissue fluid, subcutaneous fat, and sebaceous secretions. This results in dryness, flaking, pruritus, loss of elasticity, altered turgor, and a wrinkled appearance.
- Hyperkeratotic changes are typically seen in the nails, which make them thick and difficult to care for. Podiatric care is recommended for older adults, particularly those with circulatory impairment.
- Circulatory changes and decreased mobility increase the risk of senile purpura and decubitus ulcers.
- Significant hair and scalp changes can occur with aging:
  —Loss of pigmentation leading to graying
  —Decreased hair thickness or balding
  —Increased incidence of seborrheic dermatitis of the scalp requiring special care
  —Growth of facial hair on women, which can damage self-image
- Localized clusters of melanocytes surrounded by areas of decreased pigmentation result in "age spots."
- The incidence of basal and squamous cell carcinoma increases with age, particularly in individuals who have had excessive sun exposure. Inspect aging skin closely for changes in the appearance of moles or warts.

■ Nursing Diagnosis

Assessment provides data to identify the patient's problems, strengths, potential complications, and learning needs. After defining the diagnoses, start formulating a care plan that meets the patient's needs prioritizing problems from most to least important. Being able to prioritize nursing interventions contributes to a more predictable recovery for the patient. Possible nursing diagnoses that should be considered for the patient with a skin disorder are as follows:

Nursing Diagnoses	Nursing Interventions
Anxiety, related to altered appearance	Assess anxiety level every shift. Observe verbal and nonverbal behavior. Encourage the patient to share feelings. Teach relaxation techniques. Assess patient for pain.
Pain, related to loss of superficial skin layers	Initiate nursing measures to minimize or relieve pain.
Deficient knowledge, related to cause of skin disorder	Assess patient for learning needs daily. Involve patient in setting goals. Use audiovisuals as teaching aids. Evaluate patient's success.

Continued

Nursing Diagnoses	Nursing Interventions
Risk for infection, related to impaired skin integrity	Assess patient daily for risk factors such as abrasions, elevated white blood cell count, and temperature. Implement nursing measures, such as using good hand hygiene and keeping patient's nails trimmed, to decrease risk factors.
Deficient knowledge, related to treatment of pruritus	Assess factors contributing to pruritus. Promote hydration of the skin by having patient avoid hot showers and apply emollients after bathing. Encourage adequate fluid intake. Implement nursing measures to decrease skin irritation, such as avoiding clothes made of rough weave. Encourage patient to stop scratching by rubbing or applying pressure to the area. Administer prescribed medications for pruritus such as corticosteroids and antihistamines.
Risk for trauma, related to excessive scratching	Assess onset and contributing factors of episodes of pruritus. Encourage patient to stop scratching by rubbing or by applying pressure to the involved area.
Social isolation, related to anticipated or actual response of others to disfiguring skin disorders	Encourage patient to discuss feelings of loneliness. Identify available support systems to patient.
Situational low self-esteem, related to disfigured skin	Assess patient's feelings of self-worth by having patient describe feelings about self. Implement nursing measures to assist patient in dealing with body image. Accept feelings of anger or hostility from patient. Suggest clothing to conceal changes in skin integrity.

Expected Outcomes and Planning

When planning patient care, look at the nursing diagnoses and establish the cause of the nursing problem. Determining the cause enables you to develop a care plan that includes nursing interventions to eliminate the cause if possible. Include the patient in this planning. Ascertain the patient's preferences and capabilities. Including the patient is one way to promote compliance. Most skin problems are chronic, and progress is often slow. Also, many patients are older and require more time for healing.

Planning includes the development of realistic goals and outcomes that stem from the identified nursing diagnoses. Establish short- and long-term goals. Examples of measurable goals include the following:

Goal 1: Patient shows no signs of infection in abdominal wound as evidenced by the wound remaining free of erythema, purulent drainage, odor, and localized tenderness.

Goal 2: Patient is able to change dressing correctly as evidenced by the patient following the written guidelines during demonstration.

Goals should have a date when they will be evaluated. Failure to attain a goal means the nurse should reevaluate the chosen interventions and determine why the goals have not been met.

Implementation

When providing nursing interventions related to the skin, (1) include ways to prevent skin problems, (2) provide education in home care management, and (3) provide safety tips for the patient. Patients with skin diseases are usually managed at home and need to be aware of the potential for infection because the skin is not intact (see Box 43-1 and Home Care Considerations box).

Nursing measures for the skin include a variety of simple or complex interventions, including applying medications, dressings, and heat or cold and teaching the patient how to perform these measures at home. The principles of surgical and medical asepsis are important when providing nursing interventions. Also incorporate nutritional guidelines for the patient to follow. Patients need extra nutrients, such as protein, for the building and repair of tissues.

Consider the patient's cultural beliefs, personal values, and economic resources when selecting the appropriate care. More people are using other forms of treat-

Home Care Considerations

Home Care Guidelines for Baths and Soaks

- The water temperature should be comfortable—usually 90° to 100° F (32° to 38° C).
- Dissolve medication completely while tub is filling.
- The soak should last 20 to 30 minutes.
- When oils are added, patients are assisted out of the water to prevent slipping.
- Pat the skin dry, rather than rubbing, to avoid skin irritation.
- Apply creams or ointments immediately after the bath to retain moisture.
- Drain water from the tub before the patient gets out.
- The door should not be locked, and a helper should be within hearing distance.
- Use a bath mat to prevent slipping.
- Hand rails may be needed in the shower or tub.
- A seat may be needed in the shower or tub.
- After a medicated bath, pour 1 cup of bleach into used tub water; let stand 5 minutes; wipe sides and bottom of tub; drain tub, and clean as usual.

ment for integumentary disorders besides traditional medical therapy (see Complementary and Alternative Therapies box). To promote compliance with planned treatment, consider the patient's independence, dignity, privacy, and physical strengths and limitations.

Evaluation

During and after the planned nursing interventions, determine the outcomes. This is an ongoing process of continually trying to establish the most effective care plan.

Economic and home care implications are important. Today patients are being discharged from the health care facility more quickly, and insurance companies are more selective in how they pay for the care and supplies the patient needs. Creativity and critical thinking are important skills to meet the needs of today's patient.

Evaluation involves determining whether the established goals have been met. The nurse and patient evaluate the goals to see whether the criteria for measurement have been met. For example, the goal is that the patient's wound would not become infected, as demonstrated by a lack of erythema, purulent drainage, and odor. If at the end of the designated time frame the wound shows no signs of infection, the goal has been met.

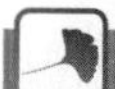

Complementary and Alternative Therapies

Integumentary Disorders

- The management of integumentary disorders is often difficult. Nutritional and herbal approaches to the treatment of skin problems have been shown to be effective for some disorders, often with fewer side effects than with conventional methods.
- Chinese herbs have long been used in Asian countries for the treatment of skin diseases. A landmark study in England showed the effectiveness of Chinese herbs in treating atopic dermatitis. This study was undertaken after dermatologists were impressed by the results in their patients who were also under the care of a Chinese herbalist. Participants in the study who received the active herbal formula reported decreases in the number of lesions and itching, as well as improved sleep.
- A traditional Australian plant remedy, tea tree oil (from *Melaleuca alternifolia*), has been effective in the treatment of acne.
- A topical mixture of the essential plant oils of thyme, rosemary, lavender, and cedarwood, in a carrier of jojoba and grapeseed oils, has been found to have significant effect in the treatment of alopecia areata.
- A published report from Taiwan states that acupuncture has been effective in the treatment of urticaria (hives).

From Sheehan, M.P., Rustin, M.H., Atherton, D.J., et al. (1992): Efficacy of traditional Chinese herbal therapy in adult atopic dermatitis. *Lancet, 340*(8810), 13-17.

Get Ready for the NCLEX® Examination!

Key Points

- The skin, including nails, hair, and glands, makes up the integumentary system.
- The main functions of the integumentary system are protection, temperature regulation, and vitamin D synthesis.
- The two layers of true skin are the epidermis and dermis.
- The layer of tissue directly beneath the skin is the subcutaneous layer; it is composed of adipose tissue and loose connective tissue.
- The sudoriferous (sweat) glands release perspiration through the skin.
- The sebaceous (oil) glands secrete sebum, which lubricates the skin and prevents invasion of bacteria through the skin.
- Any injury to the skin poses a threat to a person's self-concept.
- It is important to establish a therapeutic relationship to meet the patient's psychological needs.
- Most skin disorders are not contagious and are rarely fatal. They are often chronic.
- Sterile technique and isolation techniques are required with any open, draining lesion.
- Wet dressings need to be checked frequently. Constant moisture softens the skin and contributes to skin maceration.
- Medicines must be applied to clean skin.
- The nursing interventions for a skin disorder depend on the cause; however, common problems are decreased skin integrity, risk for infection, lack of knowledge concerning the disease, and ineffective coping.
- A primary nursing intervention is teaching the patient about the mode of transmission of the particular disease.
- The assessment of patients with skin disorders includes collection of both subjective and objective data.
- Wet dressings and baths may be done to soothe, vasoconstrict, debride, or decrease pruritus.
- Before initiating heat and cold therapy, understand normal body responses to local temperature variations, assess the integrity of the body part, determine the patient's ability to sense temperature, and ensure proper operation of equipment.
- Prevent malignant skin diseases by educating the public about causes.
- Burns can be classified by depth and TBSA involved.
- The pathophysiology and care of burns involve three stages: the hypovolemic, or emergent, phase; the acute, or diuretic, phase; and the long-term, or rehabilitation, phase.
- The three phases of burn care overlap, with different goals and nursing interventions in each.
- A primary nursing intervention for the burn patient in the emergent phase is to establish and maintain an open airway.
- The treatment method for a burn patient depends on age, body surface area involved, location, depth, and other diseases present.

- The primary causes of death in burn victims are hypovolemic shock in the first 72 hours and infection during the acute phase.
- Suspect inhalation injury if the burn injury occurred in a closed or confined area.
- A treatment for burns is use of temporary skin substitutes derived from human fibroblast cells.

Additional Learning Resources

Go to your Companion CD for an audio glossary, animations, video clips, and more.

evolve Be sure to visit the Evolve site at http://evolve.elsevier.com/Christensen/adult/ for additional online resources.

Review Questions for the NCLEX® Examination

1. The physician has ordered oral griseofulvin for tinea capitis. The mother asks the nurse why an oral medication is used rather than a cream. The best reply is that:
   1. topical creams do not reach the root of the hair to kill the fungus.
   2. oral medications are more economical.
   3. topical medications cause more pain when applied.
   4. it is more convenient to take the medication once a day rather than applying the cream once a day.
2. The most important nursing intervention for the patient with a skin disorder is:
   1. patient teaching.
   2. prevention of secondary infections.
   3. application of medications.
   4. referral for counseling.
3. The physician instructs a mother to take her child out in the sun for approximately an hour or until the skin turns red (not sunburned). This is a common medical treatment for:
   1. atopic dermatitis.
   2. acne vulgaris.
   3. pityriasis rosea.
   4. psoriasis.
4. Which of the following assessments should the nurse report to the physician immediately for an adult patient with partial-thickness burns over 25% of his body?
   1. Complaints of pain every 4 to 6 hours
   2. Decreasing appetite
   3. Hourly urinary output of 10 to 15 mL
   4. Edema at the IV site
5. The patient has a rash on her back that began about 10 days ago with a raised, scaly border and a pink center. Now she has similar eruptions on both sides of her back. From these signs, the nurse would determine the rash to be:
   1. impetigo contagiosa.
   2. pityriasis rosea.
   3. contact dermatitis.
   4. infantile eczema.
6. A patient complains of a burning pain on his lower thoracic area. On inspection, the area is found to be erythematous and edematous with a cluster of vesicles. The nurse suspects the patient has:
   1. herpes zoster.
   2. herpes simplex.
   3. varicella.
   4. impetigo.
7. A patient complains that he has basal cell carcinoma and is going to die. The nurse knows that:
   1. basal cell carcinoma is rarely terminal.
   2. without proper medication it can result in melanoma.
   3. it is a hereditary disorder caused by decreased melanin.
   4. treatment involves strong chemotherapeutic agents.
8. It is important to teach the patient the warning signs of skin cancer. Which is a warning sign of skin cancer?
   1. Border irregularity
   2. Smooth surface
   3. Decreasing diameter
   4. Mole symmetry
9. A patient has an inhalation burn injury. Which of the following is a medical emergency?
   1. Singed facial hair
   2. Neck or face burns
   3. Pallor
   4. Respiratory stridor
10. Which method of assessing burn size applies only to adults?
    1. Lund-Browder
    2. Rule of nines
    3. Parkland method
    4. Primary survey
11. The nurse just finished an assessment for a patient with SLE. Which of the following clinical manifestations would the nurse expect to find?
    1. Oral ulcers and erythematous rash over the nose and cheeks
    2. Leukocytosis and urticaria
    3. Anemia and jaundice
    4. Diarrhea and hypokalemia
12. The physician has scheduled a debridement for a patient who has partial-thickness burns on his chest and right upper leg. Which nursing intervention is most important?
    1. Ambulate the patient to increase the blood flow to the area.
    2. Administer an opioid analgesic intravenously before the debridement.
    3. Teach the patient to remove the old dressings using clean technique.
    4. Explain to the patient that the procedure will be painful.

13. A patient is admitted with partial- and full-thickness burns on his right lower extremity. Plan for the patient to have a(n):
    1. closed dressing change every 3 hours.
    2. open dressing.
    3. temporary skin cover.
    4. incision and drainage of the wound.

14. A patient is admitted with partial-thickness burns on his upper chest and face. It would be most important for the nurse to initially monitor the patient for:
    1. respiratory problems.
    2. burn shock.
    3. infection of the wound.
    4. cellulitis of the affected area.

15. An electrical burn must be assessed for:
    1. infection.
    2. cardiac irregularities.
    3. burn depth.
    4. hypovolemic shock.

16. A patient is admitted with herpes zoster. The nurse should plan to administer which medication on a frequent basis?
    1. Acyclovir (Zovirax)
    2. Cefaclor (Ceclor)
    3. Acetaminophen (Tylenol)
    4. Cimetadine (Tagamet)

17. The most common symptom of scabies is:
    1. nausea.
    2. nocturnal pruritus.
    3. localized pain.
    4. skin paresthesia.

18. It is most important to assess the adolescent with acne for:
    1. suicidal tendencies.
    2. low self-esteem.
    3. increased intake of fatty foods.
    4. change in weight.

19. A patient with thermal burns over 30% of his body has maintained a urinary output of 250 mL for the past 8 hours. From this information, the nurse might suspect that the:
    1. patient is not improving as expected.
    2. stage of hypovolemic burn shock is resolving.
    3. pain is decreasing.
    4. nutritional status is improving.

20. The patient tells the nurse she has not gone out of the house for weeks because she could not cover the lesions on her face with makeup. The most appropriate nursing diagnosis would be:
    1. Disturbed body image, related to change in personal appearance
    2. Defensive coping, related to lack of social contact
    3. Anxiety, related to the fear of permanent disfigurement
    4. Activity intolerance, related to lack of exercise

21. When inspecting the skin, the nurse remembers that the skin provides a primary:
    1. source for vitamin D storage.
    2. protective device against microorganisms.
    3. means of preventing overhydration.
    4. defense against hyperthermia.

22. When teaching a patient to care for herpes zoster lesions at home, the most important instruction for the nurse to give is:
    1. clean the lesions with sterile saline daily.
    2. wash hands for at least 1 to 2 minutes before applying medication.
    3. report to the physician when the lesions are crusted.
    4. launder all clothes in vinegar.

23. A nurse is reviewing the history for a patient who has been admitted with cellulitis. Which condition would predispose the patient to cellulitis? *(Select all that apply.)*
    1. Malnutrition, substance abuse
    2. Treatment with steroids or chemotherapy
    3. Coronary artery disease
    4. Infectious tonsillitis

24. A parent tells the dermatologist that her daughter seems to be losing interest in school. Which medication could have caused the patient's change in behavior?
    1. Isotretinoin (Accutane)
    2. Minocycline (Minocin)
    3. Tazarotene (Tazorac)
    4. Penicillin

25. A black patient is seen with impending shock after an accident. How would the nurse expect the skin to appear during the assessment of the patient?
    1. Ruddy blue
    2. Generalized pallor
    3. Ashen, gray, or dull
    4. Whitish, blue, or bright

26. The nurse's assessment shows that the patient has a solid, elevated, circumscribed lesion that is less than 1 cm in diameter. In the documentation, the nurse would chart this as a _________.

27. A 28-year-old electrical lineman is brought to the emergency department after coming in contact with a live overhead wire. He has two quarter-size burns on his right hand. He is admitted to the hospital. What is the most important rationale for admission to the hospital?
    1. The skin provides the least resistance to the flow of electricity.
    2. The evident skin injury seldom represents the full extent of the damage.
    3. Ventricular fibrillation may follow within 48 hours after the burns.
    4. Lethal arc burns may develop after a burn.

28. A new student nurse, whose mother recently died from malignant melanoma, asks the faculty member, "What can I do to prevent malignant melanoma from developing?" The best response by the faculty member is:

1. malignant melanoma is a relatively rare type of skin cancer.
2. the patient is at high risk for melanoma because of family history.
3. avoiding excessive sun exposure will decrease risk.
4. individuals with fair skin and blue eyes are at increased risk.

29. The nurse planning the care for a patient who has impetigo expects to administer which topical drug to the patient?

1. Acetaminophen
2. Retapamulin
3. Nystatin
4. Corticosteroids

30. A patient who has developed a severe contact dermatitis of the lower extremities states, "The itching is terrible, I just cannot keep from scratching." Which statement should the nurse include in teaching the patient? *(Select all that apply.)*

1. Take cool or tepid baths several times daily to decrease pruritus.
2. Use cool, wet cloths or dressings to reduce itching.
3. Add oil to the bath water to aid in moisturizing the affected skin.
4. Use an OTC antihistamine with sedative effects to reduce scratching.

31. When teaching home care to a patient with recurrent herpes simplex genitalis infection, it is important to include:

1. the infection is contagious only when lesions are visible.
2. antiviral agents are curative in the majority of cases.
3. the patient will need to take antiviral agents daily for life.
4. the patient will need to use protection even when no lesions are evident.

32. On admission, a patient is noted to have impaired skin integrity related to severe dermatitis. Which nursing intervention to enhance patient comfort should be included when planning the patient's care?. *(Select all that apply.)*

1. Keeping the environment cool
2. Using cool compresses
3. Applying heat for 20 minutes three times per day
4. Using bath oils to decrease dryness

chapter

44

Care of the Patient with a Musculoskeletal Disorder

evolve

Martha E. Spray

http://evolve.elsevier.com/Christensen/foundationsadult

Objectives

Anatomy and Physiology

1. List the five basic functions of the skeletal system.
2. List the two divisions of the skeleton.
3. Describe the location of major bones of the skeleton.
4. Describe the location of the major muscles of the body.
5. List the types of body movements.
6. Describe three vital functions muscles perform when they contract.

Medical-Surgical

7. List diagnostic examinations for musculoskeletal function.
8. Compare medical regimens for patients suffering from gouty arthritis, rheumatoid arthritis, and osteoarthritis.
9. Discuss nursing interventions for rheumatoid arthritis.
10. Describe nursing interventions for degenerative joint disease (osteoarthritis).
11. List at least four healthy lifestyle measures people can practice to reduce the risk of developing osteoporosis.
12. Describe the surgery for arthritis of the hip and knee.
13. Describe nursing interventions for the patient undergoing a total hip or knee replacement.
14. Discuss nursing interventions for a patient with a fractured hip after open reduction with internal fixation and bipolar hip prosthesis (hemiarthroplasty).
15. Discuss the physiology of fracture healing (hematoma, granulation tissue, and callus formation).
16. Describe the signs and symptoms of compartment syndrome.
17. List nursing interventions for a fat embolism.
18. List at least two types of skin and skeletal traction.
19. Compare methods for assessing circulation, nerve damage, and infection in a patient who has a traumatic insult to the musculoskeletal system.
20. List four nursing interventions for bone cancer.
21. Describe the phenomenon of phantom pain.
22. Define lordosis, scoliosis, and kyphosis.

Key Terms

ankylosis (ăng-kĭ-LŌ-sĭs, p. 1360)
arthrocentesis (ăr-thrō-sĕn-TĒ-sĭs, p. 1352)
arthrodesis (ăr-thrō-DĒ-sĭs, p. 1369)
arthroplasty (ĂR-thrō-plăs-tē, p. 1369)
bipolar hip replacement (hemiarthroplasty) (hĕ-mē-ĂR-thrō-plăs-tē, p. 1375)
blanching test (p. 1406)
callus (p. 1380)
Colles' fracture (KŎL-ēz FRĂK-shŭr, p. 1380)
compartment syndrome (p. 1384)
crepitus (KRĔP-ĭ-tŭs, p. 1380)
fibromyalgia (fī-brō-mĭ-ĂL-jă, p. 1367)
kyphosis (kĭ-FŌ-sĭs, p. 1406)
lordosis (lŏr-DŌ-sĭs, p. 1406)
open reduction with internal fixation (ORIF) (p. 1381)
paresthesia (păr-ĕs-THĒ-zē-ă, pp. 1368, 1399)
scoliosis (skō-lē-Ō-sĭs, p. 1406)
sequestrum (sĕ-KWĔS-trŭm, p. 1367)
subluxation (sŭb-lŭk-SĀ-shŭn, p. 1398)
tophi (TŌ-fī, p. 1363)
Volkmann's contracture (VŎLK-mănz kŏn-TRĂK-shŭr, p. 1385)

ANATOMY AND PHYSIOLOGY OF THE MUSCULOSKELETAL SYSTEM

Bones and joints form the framework of the body, and muscles contract and relax to allow movement. All movement of the body is orchestrated by the functioning of the bones, the joints, and the muscles attached to the bones. This chapter discusses the structure and the function of bones and muscles and how they serve the body.

FUNCTIONS OF THE SKELETAL SYSTEM

The human skeletal system is composed of 206 bones. The skeletal system has five basic functions: support, protection, movement, mineral storage, and hematopoiesis.

Support

The skeleton is the the body framework that supports internal tissues and organs.

Protection

The skeleton forms a firm, cagelike structure that protects many internal structures. The cranium (skull) protects the brain, the vertebrae protect the spinal cord, the ribs and the sternum (breastbone) protect the lungs and the heart, and the pelvis protects the digestive and reproductive organs.

Movement

Skeletal muscles are attached to the bones, which enables the bones to provide leverage for movement. As a muscle contracts, it pulls on the bone and movement occurs.

Mineral Storage

The bones serve as a storage area for various minerals, particularly calcium and phosphorus. When the body's intake of these minerals is inadequate, the bones release the minerals.

Hematopoiesis

Hematopoiesis (blood cell formation) takes place in the red bone marrow. The red bone marrow is spongy bone found in the ends of the long bones. A child's bones contain a proportionately larger amount of red bone marrow than an adult's. As a person ages, much of the red bone marrow converts to yellow bone marrow, which is composed of fat cells.

STRUCTURE OF BONES

Bones are classified into four groups, based on their form and shape: long, short, flat, and irregular. Long bones are found in the extremities, short bones are found in the hands and feet, flat bones are found in the skull and sternum, and irregular bones make up the vertebrae (backbone).

ARTICULATIONS (JOINTS)

Bones cannot bend without damage. To allow movement, individual bones articulate (join together) at joint sites (Figure 44-1). Bones are held together by flexible connective tissue. The joint is the point of contact between the individual bones. The structure of the individual bones depends on the function of the area. Every bone in the body (except the hyoid bone, which anchors the tongue) connects, or articulates, with at least one other bone.

Joints perform two important functions: they hold the bones together to form the skeleton, and they allow movement and flexibility of the skeleton.

The most common way to classify joints is according to the degree of movement they permit. There are three types of joints:

1. **Synarthrosis:** no movement
2. **Amphiarthrosis:** slight movement
3. **Diarthrosis:** free movement

A goniometer measures the angle of a joint. It is used to determine the degree of joint mobility (Lewis et al., 2007).

DIVISIONS OF THE SKELETON

The skeleton is divided into the axial and the appendicular skeletons (Box 44-1). The axial skeleton is composed of the skull, hyoid bone in the neck, vertebral column, and thorax (chest). The appendicular skeleton is composed of the upper extremities, lower extremities, shoulder girdle, and pelvic girdle (excluding the sacrum) (Figures 44-2 and 44-3).

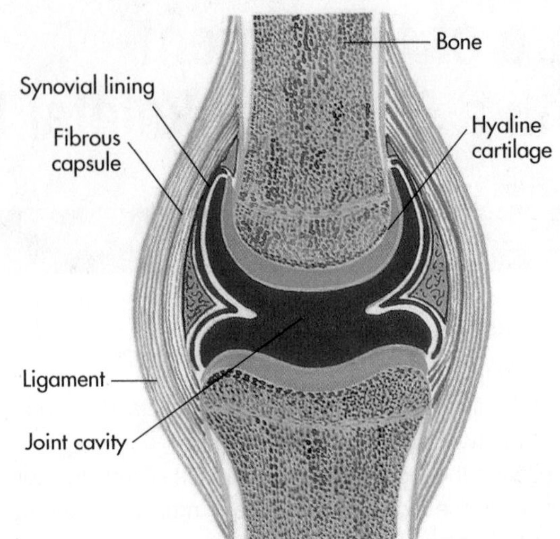

FIGURE 44-1 Structure of a freely movable (diarthrotic) joint. Note these typical features: joint capsule, joint cavity lined with synovial membrane, and articular (hyaline) cartilage covering the end surfaces of the bones within the joint capsule.

Box 44-1 Main Parts of the Skeleton

AXIAL SKELETON	APPENDICULAR SKELETON
Skull	**Upper Extremities**
Cranium	Shoulder (pectoral) girdle
Ear bones	Arms
Face	Wrists
	Hands
SPINE	
Vertebrae	**Lower Extremities**
	Hip (pelvic) girdle
THORAX	Legs
Ribs	Ankles
Sternum	Feet

FUNCTIONS OF THE MUSCULAR SYSTEM

The bones and joints provide the framework of the body, but the muscles are necessary for movement. This motion results from contraction and relaxation of the individual muscles. The body has more than 600 muscles, making up approximately 40% to 50% of the total body weight. They usually act in groups to execute a body movement (Table 44-1).

As muscles contract, they perform three vital functions: motion, maintenance of posture, and production of heat. Contraction also assists in return of venous blood and lymph to the right side of the heart.

All body movements rely on the integrated functioning of the bones, joints, and muscles. Muscle tissue is under voluntary or involuntary control. Voluntary muscle is under conscious control, whereas involuntary muscle tissue responds to internal commands without any conscious control of it. Involuntary motions include activities conducted by the internal organs, such as the heart beating, the gallbladder releasing bile, and the stomach churning food.

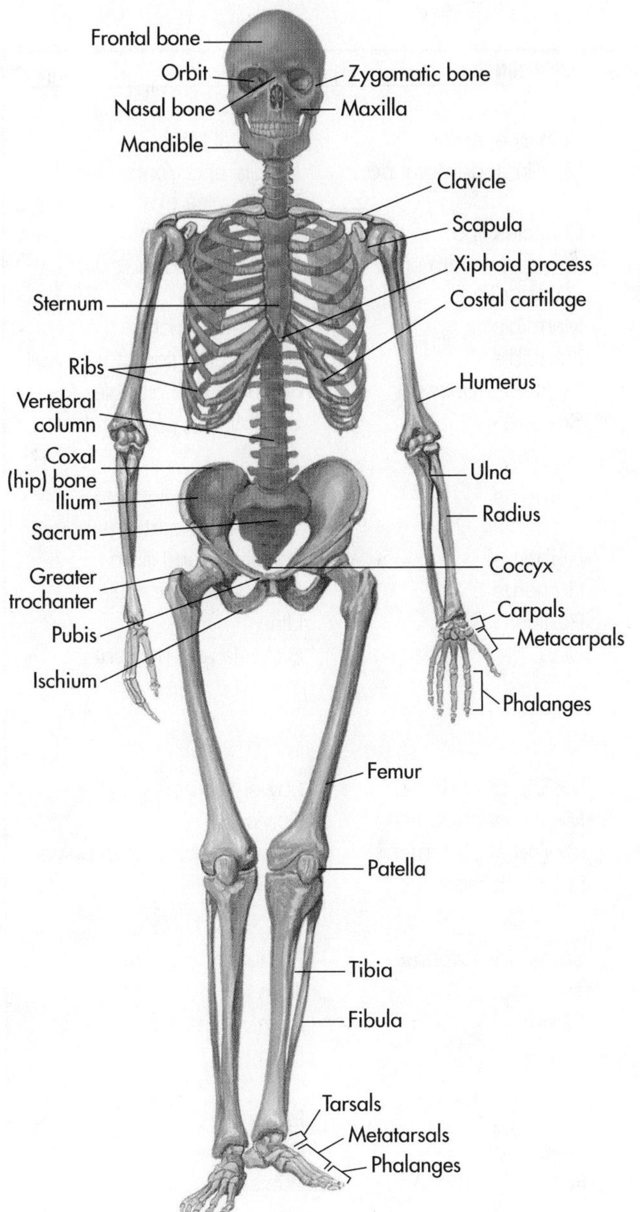

FIGURE 44-2 Skeleton, anterior view. Axial skeleton is shown in blue. Appendicular skeleton is bone colored.

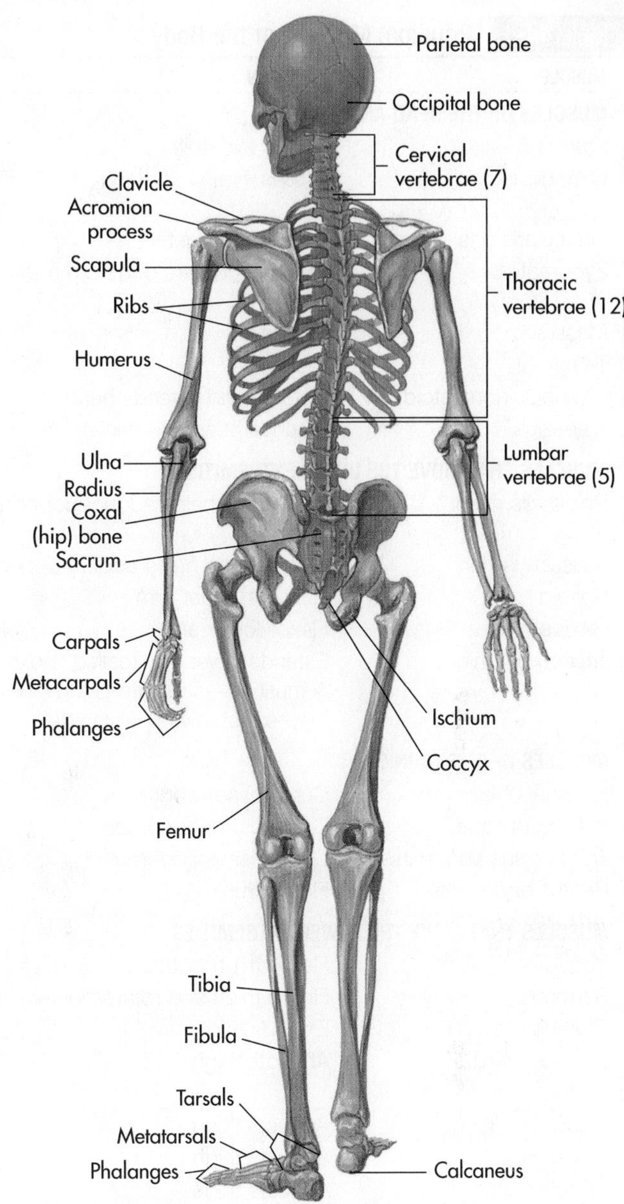

FIGURE 44-3 Skeleton, posterior view. Axial skeleton is shown in blue. Appendicular skeleton is bone colored.

The contraction of certain skeletal muscles gives the body proper posture. These muscles pull on various bones, allowing the body to sit or stand.

As skeletal muscles contract, they produce body heat. Approximately 85% of all body heat is generated by the contraction of the skeletal muscles.

Skeletal Muscle Structure

A skeletal muscle is composed of hundreds of muscle fibers (cells). Each skeletal muscle is surrounded by a covering of connective tissue called the **epimysium.** The epimysium joins with two other inner coverings, the perimysium and the endomysium, and extends beyond the muscle to form a tough cord of connective tissue known as a **tendon.** Tendons anchor muscles to bones. As a muscle contracts, it pulls the corresponding tendon and bone toward it. This is how movement occurs. Tendons in the ankle and wrist are enclosed in **tendon sheaths,** which are sleeves or tubelike structures of connective tissue. Tendon sheaths contain synovial fluid and permit the tendons to slide easily; the sheaths also keep the tendons in place. All the tendons, ligaments, and aponeuroses of the body are composed of connective tissue in various sizes, shapes, and densities. These are collectively known as **fasciae.**

Nerve and Blood Supply

Because of the physical demands placed on the skeletal muscles, they need a constant supply of oxygen and nutrition. They are well supplied with blood vessels that carry oxygen and nutrition to the area and remove the waste products of metabolism.

The skeletal muscles are voluntary, so they need a constant source of information. Nerve cells or fibers continuously send impulses that stimulate the muscle cells. These impulses enter at the neuromuscular junc-

Table 44-1 Principal Muscles of the Body

MUSCLE	FUNCTION	INSERTION	ORIGIN
MUSCLES OF THE HEAD AND NECK			
Frontal	Raises eyebrow	Skin of eyebrow	Occipital bone
Orbicularis oculi	Closes eye	Maxilla and frontal bone	Maxilla and frontal bone (encircles eye)
Orbicularis oris	Draws lips together	Encircles lips	Encircles lips
Zygomaticus	Elevates corners of mouth and lips	Angle of mouth and upper lip	Zygomatic bone
Masseter	Closes jaw	Mandible	Zygomatic arch
Temporal	Closes jaw	Mandible	Temporal region of the skull
Sternocleidomastoid	Rotates and extends head	Mastoid process	Sternum and clavicle
Trapezius	Extends head and neck	Scapula	Skull and upper vertebrae
MUSCLES THAT MOVE THE UPPER EXTREMITIES			
Pectoralis major	Flexes and helps adduct upper arms	Humerus	Sternum, clavicle, and upper rib cartilages
Latissimus dorsi	Extends and helps adduct upper arm	Humerus	Vertebrae and ilium
Deltoid	Abducts upper arm	Humerus	Clavicle and scapula
Biceps brachii	Flexes lower arm	Radius	Ulna
Triceps brachii	Extends lower arm (called "boxer's muscle"—straightens the elbow when a blow is delivered)	Ulna	Scapula and humerus
MUSCLES OF THE TRUNK			
External oblique	Compresses abdomen	Midline of abdomen	Lower thoracic cage
Internal oblique	Compresses abdomen	Midline of abdomen	Pelvis
Transversus abdominis	Compresses abdomen	Midline of abdomen	Ribs, vertebrae, and pelvis
Rectus abdominis	Flexes trunk	Lower ribcage	Pubis
MUSCLES THAT MOVE THE LOWER EXTREMITIES			
Iliopsoas	Flexes thigh or trunk	Ilium and vertebrae	Femur
Sartorius	Flexes thigh and rotates lower leg	Tibia	Ilium
Gluteus maximus	Extends thigh	Femur	Ilium, sacrum, and coccyx
Gluteus medius	Abducts thigh	Femur	Ilium
Adductor group			
Adductor longus	Adducts thigh	Femur	Pubis
Gracilis	Adducts thigh	Tibia	Pubis
Pectineus	Adducts thigh	Femur	Pubis
Hamstring group			
Semimembranosus	Flexes lower leg	Tibia	Ischium
Semitendinosus	Flexes lower leg	Tibia	Ischium
Biceps femoris	Flexes lower leg	Fibula	Ischium and femur
Quadriceps group			
Rectus femoris	Extends lower leg	Tibia	Ischium
Vastus lateralis, intermedius, and medialis	Extends lower leg	Tibia	Femur
Tibialis anterior	Dorsiflexes foot	Metatarsals (foot)	Tibia
Gastrocnemius	Plantar flexes foot	Calcaneus (heel)	Femur
Soleus	Plantar flexes foot	Calcaneus (heel)	Tibia and fibula
Peroneus group			
Peroneus longus and brevis	Plantar flexes foot	Tarsals and metatarsals (ankle and foot)	Tibia and fibula

tion, the point of contact between the nerve ending and the muscle fiber. As a nerve impulse passes through this junction, chemicals are released that cause the muscle to contract.

Usually one artery, two veins, and one nerve penetrate a particular muscle. Each muscle cell comes in contact with several capillaries and a portion of a nerve cell. The muscle cells, in union with the nerve cell that controls them, are called a **motor unit.**

The impulse from the nerve cell must travel across a small gap because the nerve cell and the muscle cell do not directly touch each other. This small gap is called a **synaptic cleft** and is filled with tissue fluid. A special chemical **(neurotransmitter)** travels through the fluid to stimulate the muscle fiber. Acetylcholine is the neurotransmitter for skeletal muscle tissue. An enzyme called **cholinesterase** breaks down the acetylcholine once it has transferred the message. This allows the muscle cell to relax between impulses.

Muscle Contraction

Muscle Stimulus

Muscle cells are governed by the "all or none" law; that is, when a muscle cell is adequately stimulated or shocked, it will contract completely. Because each skeletal muscle is composed of thousands of muscle cells that react to many different nerve cells, the muscle as a whole contracts according to the principle of graded response. The strength of the muscle contraction, therefore, depends on the number of individual muscle cells responding. These muscle responses allow us to tenderly brush a baby's cheek or swat an irritating mosquito.

Muscle Tone

The skeletal muscles are in a constant state of readiness for action. At any given time, several muscle cells within a certain muscle are contracted; the remainder of the muscle cells are relaxed. Muscle tone is necessary for good posture but does not provide movement. To understand the importance of muscle tone, observe an extremity that has become paralyzed; the muscles are flaccid, limp, or atrophied (wasted) and incapable of producing movement because the cells no longer receive stimuli from the nerve fibers.

Types of Body Movements

Some muscles can move some body parts in only two directions, whereas others can move certain body parts in several directions. The body's more common movements include flexion, extension, abduction, adduction, rotation, supination, pronation, dorsiflexion, and plantar flexion (Table 44-2; Box 44-2; Figure 44-4).

Box 44-2 Types of Body Movement

- **Flexion:** A movement allowed by certain joints of the skeleton that decreases the angle between two adjoining bones. For example, bending the arm at the elbow decreases the angle between the humerus and the ulna.
- **Extension** (see Figure 44-4): A movement allowed by certain joints of the skeleton that increases the angle between two adjoining bones. For example, extending the leg increases the angle between the femur and the tibia. If the extension angles more than 180 degrees, the extremity is **hyperextended.**
- **Abduction:** A movement of an extremity away from the midline of the body.
- **Adduction:** A movement of an extremity toward the axis of the body.
- **Rotation:** A movement of a bone around its longitudinal axis (e.g., a pivot motion, such as shaking the head "no").
- **Supination:** A movement of the hand and forearm that causes the palm to face upward or forward.
- **Pronation:** A movement of the hand and forearm that causes the palm to face downward or backward.
- **Dorsiflexion:** A movement that causes the top of the foot to elevate or tilt upward.
- **Plantar flexion:** A movement that causes the bottom of the foot to be directed downward.

Skeletal Muscle Groups

Skeletal muscles are usually classified into two broad categories: axial and appendicular. The axial muscle groups are located on the head, face, neck, and trunk. The appendicular muscle groups are in the extremities. Figures 44-5 and 44-6 show the location of the muscles of the body.

LABORATORY AND DIAGNOSTIC EXAMINATIONS

RADIOGRAPHIC STUDIES

The diagnostic study most often used for determining musculoskeletal system integrity is the radiographic, roentgenographic, or (as it is more commonly known) x-ray examination or diagnostic imaging.

A radiographic examination of a joint reveals fluid, irregularity of the joint with spur formation, or changes

Table 44-2 Muscles Grouped According to Function

PART MOVED	FLEXORS	EXTENSORS	ABDUCTORS	ADDUCTORS
Upper arm	Pectoralis major	Latissimus dorsi	Deltoid and latissimus dorsi contracting together	Pectoralis major
Lower arm	Biceps brachii	Triceps brachii	None	None
Thigh	Iliopsoas and sartorius	Gluteus maximus	Gluteus medius	Adductor group
Lower leg	Hamstrings	Quadriceps group	None	None
Foot	Tibialis anterior	Gastrocnemius and soleus	Peroneus longus	Tibialis anterior

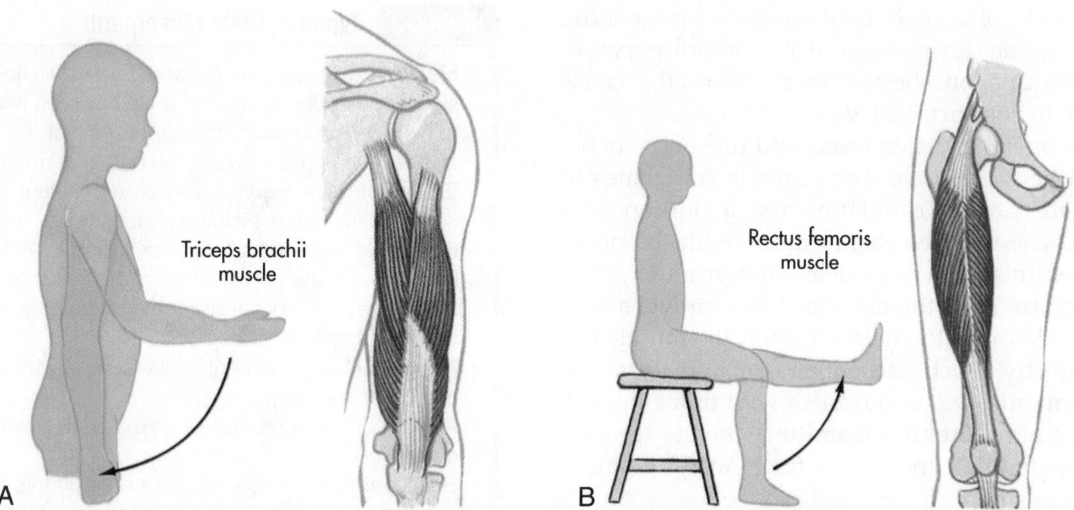

FIGURE 44-4 Extension of the lower arm and lower leg. **A,** When the triceps brachii muscle *(right)* contracts, it extends the lower arm at the elbow joint *(left).* **B,** When the rectus femoris muscle (part of the quadriceps femoris muscle group) *(right)* contracts, it extends the lower leg at the knee joint *(left).*

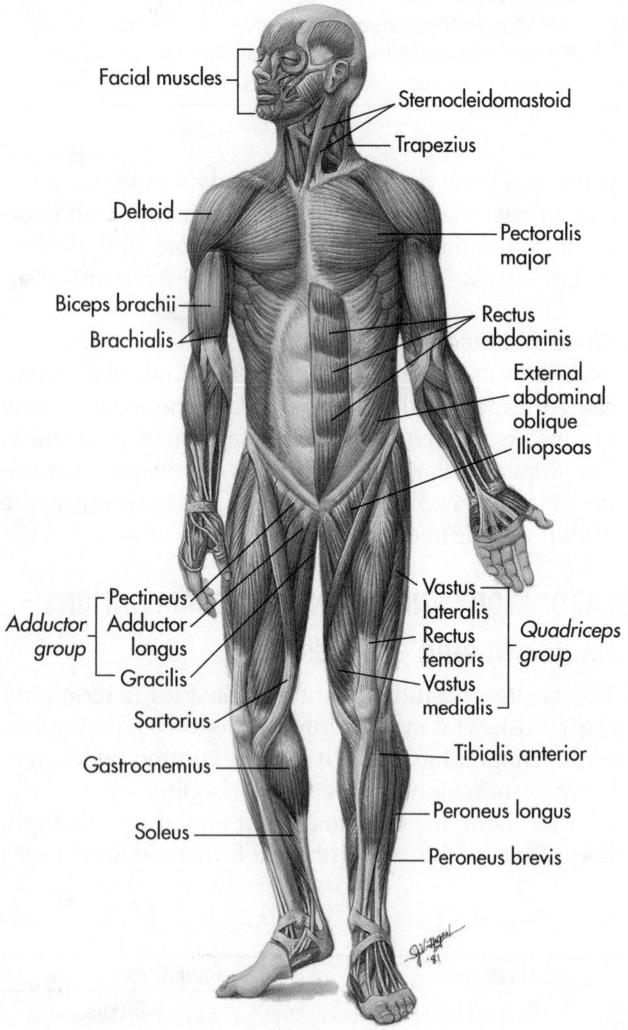

FIGURE 44-5 Anterior view of the body.

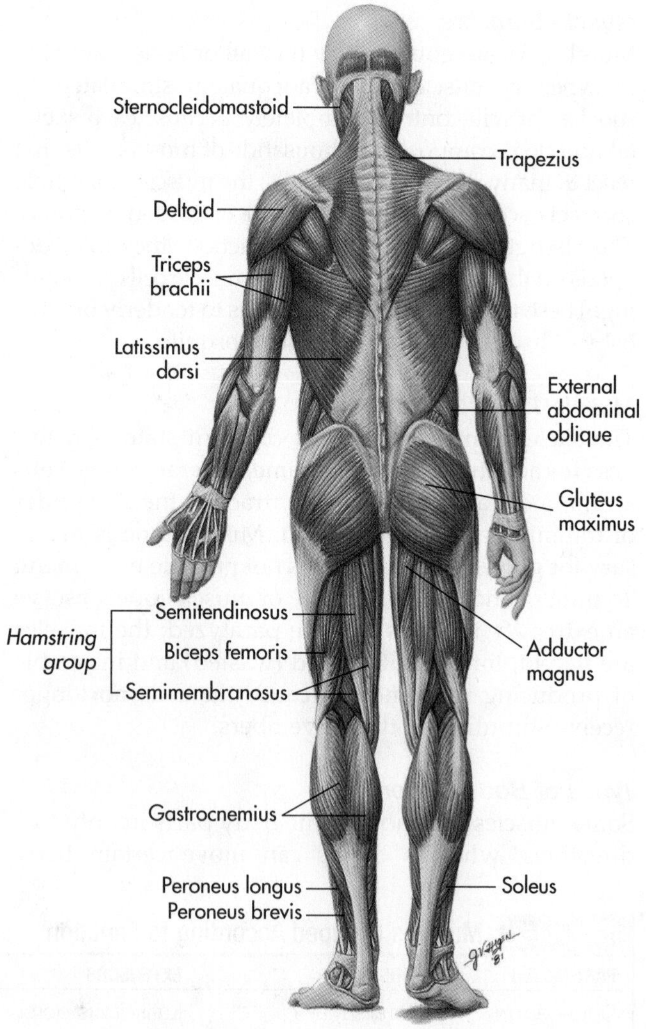

FIGURE 44-6 Posterior view of the body.

in the size of the joint contour. Radiographic examination is used to determine presence of a skeletal fracture. It is important to ask women of childbearing age if there is any possibility that they are pregnant before performing x-ray examinations because pregnant women should not be exposed to radiation except in emergencies because of potential damage to the fetus.

Laminography or **planography** (also called **body section roentgenography**) is useful in locating small cavities, foreign bodies, and lesions that are overshadowed by opaque structures.

Scanography, a method of producing a radiograph of internal body organs using a series of parallel beams that eliminate size distortion, allows accurate measurement of bone length.

Myelogram

Myelographic examination involves injection of a radiopaque dye into the subarachnoid space at the lumbar spine to x-ray the spinal cord and the vertebral column to detect herniated disk syndrome (herniated nucleus pulposus) or spinal tumors. The test involves the same procedure as a lumbar puncture (spinal tap), which is discussed in Chapter 54. Contrast medium causes allergic reactions in patients with allergies to iodine and seafood. Notify the physician about such allergies so that a nonionic contrast agent can be used or medications such as steroids or antihistamines can be given before the examination to minimize any reaction to the radiographic dye.

This examination may involve the entire spine or just the cervical or lumbar area. After the myelogram, oil-based dye is removed through the spinal needle to prevent meningeal irritation. Water-soluble dye is used most often and does not need to be removed; the body absorbs it and excretes it in urine. Inform the patient that the test is performed with the patient on a tilting table that is moved during the test to allow contrast medium to flow up to the cervical area.

The most common discomfort after a myelogram is headache. If water-soluble dye is used, the patient should lie quietly in a semi-Fowler's position for approximately 8 hours. Patient positioning is important to keep the dye in the lower spine. During this time, encouraging fluids helps the body absorb the dye from the spinal column. If oil-based dye is used, the patient rests in a flat position for up to 12 hours. Tell the patient to inform the nurse if he or she has a headache, stiff neck, leg weakness, or difficulty voiding. Rare complications include seizure, infection, drowsiness, severe headache, numbness, and paralysis.

Patients needing a myelogram fear the needle will be inserted into the spinal canal and damage the cord. Inform the patient that the tap is done in the lumbar region of the spine at approximately the fourth or fifth lumbar space (L4-L5). The spinal cord starts at the level of the foramen magnum and ends at the second lumbar space (L2) (lower border of ribcage).

Nuclear Scanning

Nuclear scanning tests are done in the nuclear medicine department, which has scanners or camera detectors that record images on radiographic film. Diagnostic tests use low dosages of radioactive isotopes; precautionary measures that are required for radium therapy are not necessary.

Nursing interventions required when patients are scheduled for nuclear scanning procedures involve (1) obtaining written consent from the patient, (2) informing the patient that the radioactive isotopes will not affect family or visitors, and (3) following the nuclear medicine department's instructions for special preparations for specific scans.

Magnetic Resonance Imaging

Musculoskeletal magnetic resonance imaging (MRI) assists in diagnosing abnormalities of bones and joints and surrounding soft tissue structures, including cartilage, synovium, ligaments, and tendons. The test uses magnetism and radio waves to make images of cross-sections of the body. MRI can give much more detailed pictures of fluid-filled soft tissue and blood vessels than any other test.

In preparation, have the patient remove any metal, such as jewelry, clothing with metal fasteners, glasses, and hair clips. Patients with metal prostheses such as heart valves, orthopedic screws, or cardiac pacemakers cannot undergo MRI.

The standard machine looks like a narrow tunnel which completely encloses the patient. Patients are required to lie still in this machine for 45 to 60 minutes. The patient enters the tunnel head first and may feel some anxiety or claustrophobia. The procedure is painless; however, if the patient is extremely anxious, a sedative is given. Encourage patients to use relaxation techniques, such as imagery, during the test. New MRI machines called open MRI are designed to be less confining and more comfortable than the traditional machine. Because the procedure requires the patient to be motionless, relaxation techniques that require flexing and relaxing the muscles are not appropriate.

After the test, take routine vital sign measurements and allow the patient to resume pretest activities. There are no adverse effects.

Computed Tomography

Body sections can be examined from many different angles using a computed tomography (CT) scanner, which uses a narrow x-ray beam and produces a three-dimensional picture of the structure being studied. The CT scanner is approximately 100 times more sensitive than the radiograph machine and should not be used unnecessarily because of radiation exposure. Iodine contrast dye is sometimes used. CT scan is used for the head and body. It is useful in locating injuries to the ligaments or tendons, tumors of the soft tissue, and fractures in areas difficult to define by other means.

Patient preparation includes (1) having the patient sign a consent form authorizing the examination if not included on the initial hospital consent form, (2) questioning the patient regarding allergies (e.g., iodine and seafood), (3) keeping the patient on NPO (nothing by mouth) status 3 to 4 hours before the test (in case contrast dye is used, since the dye can cause nausea and vomiting), (4) measuring vital signs to be used as a baseline, (5) having the patient void before the test, (6) removing metal articles such as jewelry and hairpins, and (7) telling the patient that he or she must lie still during the test and may feel warm and slightly nauseated for a few minutes when dye is injected.

After the test, observe the patient for delayed allergic reactions (if contrast dye was used). Encourage fluids unless contraindicated. Pretest diet and activity can usually be resumed.

Bone Scan

The bone scan test is especially valuable in detecting metastatic and inflammatory bone disease (osteomyelitis). This test involves the intravenous (IV) administration of nuclides (atomic material) approximately 2 to 3 hours before the test is scheduled. There are no food or fluid restrictions, and patients are encouraged to drink water over the next 1 to 3 hours to aid renal clearance of any radioisotope not picked up by the bone. After the patient has voided, a scanning camera reveals the degree of radionuclide uptake; areas of concentrated nucleotide uptake may represent a tumor or other abnormality. These areas of concentration can be detected days or weeks before an ordinary radiograph reveals a metastatic lesion. The test takes approximately 30 to 60 minutes and requires the patient to lie still.

ASPIRATION

An aspiration procedure is done to obtain a specimen of body fluid. The physician inserts a needle into a cavity with the patient under local anesthesia. This procedure is performed using sterile technique. Commonly the physician takes a biopsy of tissue while doing the aspiration procedure. Nursing interventions are similar for all aspiration tests, with special emphasis on (1) having the consent form signed; (2) reinforcing the physician's explanation of the procedure; (3) encouraging the patient to remain immobile during the procedure; (4) having the patient void before the procedure; (5) maintaining sterile technique; (6) supporting the patient emotionally; (7) applying a sterile pressure dressing to the puncture site and maintaining the dressing until bleeding has stopped; (8) assisting with collecting, labeling, and transporting a specimen to the laboratory immediately; and (9) observing for emotional and physical distress after the procedure.

Synovial Fluid Aspiration

Arthrocentesis is the puncture of a patient's joint with a needle and the withdrawal of synovial fluid for diagnostic purposes. It is helpful in diagnosing trauma, systemic lupus erythematosus, gout, osteoarthritis, and rheumatoid arthritis (RA). It may also be used to instill medications for the patient with septic arthritis or to remove fluid from joints to relieve pain. Normally a patient's synovial fluid is straw colored, clear, or slightly cloudy. If trauma or a disease is present, the synovial fluid appears cloudy, milky, sanguineous, yellow, green, or gray.

After the procedure, provide proper support to the affected extremity. Placing it on a pillow and maintaining joint rest for approximately 12 hours may be indicated. Apply ice to the affected joint for 24 to 48 hours unless otherwise ordered. An antiinfective or corticosteroid may be prescribed. Assess the patient for signs of infection. After the pressure dressing is removed from the site, an adhesive bandage can be used.

ENDOSCOPIC EXAMINATION

For endoscopy, a lighted tube is used to visualize inside a body cavity. Although some procedures require general anesthesia, most require only local anesthesia. Emotional support and complete explanations help relieve the patient's anxiety. Preparation for an endoscopic examination is similar to that for surgical preparation: (1) have the patient sign a consent form; (2) complete a preoperative checklist with special attention to removing jewelry, dentures, and contact lenses; (3) initiate NPO status 6 to 12 hours before the examination; (4) give premedications, such as atropine and a sedative; (5) encourage the patient to void; (6) record vital signs; and (7) maintain bed rest with side rails up after giving the premedication.

Arthroscopy

Arthroscopy is an endoscopic examination that enables direct visualization of a joint. The procedure is used to (1) explore the joint to determine the presence of a disease process, (2) drain fluid from the joint cavity, and (3) remove damaged tissue or foreign bodies.

This examination is most commonly done on the knee joint, with the synovium, articular surfaces, and meniscus (a curved, fibrous cartilage in the knee) visualized through the scope. The procedure involves insertion of a large-bore needle into the suprapatellar pouch and saline instillation into the joint. Arthroscopy can also be done on the hip or shoulder. The patient may be given a general or local anesthetic agent. After the arthroscopic examination, advise the patient to limit activities for several days.

Endoscopic Spinal Microsurgery

Surgeons can perform spinal surgery with less damage to surrounding tissues by passing endoscopic equipment through small incisions. Special scopes enable surgeons to successfully treat spinal column disorders (e.g., herniated disk, spinal stenosis) and spinal deformities (e.g., scoliosis, kyphosis). Spinal microsurgery can be performed with the patient under local anesthesia; discharge occurs after a brief stay. Candidates for microsurgery procedures are evaluated on information obtained from x-ray examinations, MRI scans, CT scans, and bone scans.

ELECTROGRAPHIC PROCEDURE

Electrographic procedures use electrodes to measure electrical activity in specific areas of the body.

Electromyogram

An electromyogram involves insertion of needle electrodes into the skeletal muscles so that electrical activity can be heard, seen on an oscilloscope (an instrument that displays a graphic representation of electron beams), and recorded on paper at the same time. Muscles do not produce an electrical charge at rest, but with neuromuscular disorders unusual patterns can be observed. Nerves can be observed for neuropathy and muscles for myopathy. Electromyography can be used to detect chronic low back pain based on muscle fatigue patterns.

LABORATORY TESTS

Specific laboratory tests are ordered when musculoskeletal disorders are suspected (Table 44-3).

EFFECTS OF BED REST ON MINERAL CONTENT IN BONE

Studies done on people confined to bed rest reveal a loss of body calcium. Immobilization results in bone resorption—the bone tissue becomes less dense. Prolonged bed rest puts the patient at risk for pathologic fractures (Potter & Perry, 2009). This rate of loss over several weeks is a serious concern for an older adult in terms of regaining mobility; it also increases the risk of fracture.

DISORDERS OF THE MUSCULOSKELETAL SYSTEM

INFLAMMATORY DISORDERS

ARTHRITIS

Arthritis is a disease involving an inflammation of the joint. An estimated 50 million Americans are affected by arthritis, and 4 million of these are dependent and unable to work, attend school, or participate in social functions. There are many types of arthritis, but the most common are RA, rheumatoid spondylitis, osteoarthritis (degenerative joint disease [DJD]), and gout

Table 44-3 Laboratory Tests for Musculoskeletal Disorders

NORMAL VALUE	POSSIBLE CAUSE FOR INCREASE OR DECREASE
Calcium: 9.0-10.5 mg/dL	Increased in metastatic tumor to the bone, Addison's disease, Paget's disease of the bone, acromegaly, acute osteoporosis, hyperparathyroidism, vitamin D deficiency, renal failure, malabsorption, and rickets
Phosphorus: 2.5-4.5 mg/dL	Increased in acromegaly, bone metastases, excessive levels of vitamin D, hypocalcemia, renal failure Decreased in acute gout, hypercalcemia, vitamin D deficiency
Vitamin D 25-dihydroxy: 6-52 ng/mL	Increased in vitamin D intoxication Decreased in bowel resection, malabsorption, rickets
Vitamin D_1, 25-dihydroxy: 15-60 pg/mL	Increased in liver disease; bone disease; healing fractures; metastatic tumor in bone; osteogenic sarcoma; osteoporosis; cancer of breast, colon, lung, or pancreas Decreased in severe anemia, folic acid deficiency, pernicious anemia
Alkaline phosphatase: 30-120 units/L	Increased in skeletal muscle injury or myocardial infarction
Myoglobin: 5-70 mcg/dL	Decreased in rheumatoid arthritis
Erythrocyte sedimentation rate (ESR) Males: up to 15 mm/hr Females: up to 20 mm/hr	A nonspecific test used to detect inflammatory, neoplastic, infectious, and necrotic processes Indicates the presence of inflammation as seen in rheumatoid arthritis and rheumatic fever One of the most objective measurements of rheumatoid arthritis severity Increased as the disease worsens Increased in multiple myeloma, acute myocardial infarctions, toxemia, bacterial infections, and gout Decreased in congestive heart failure, sickle cell anemia, polycythemia vera, infectious mononucleosis, degenerative arthritis, and angina pectoris
Lupus erythematosus (LE) preparation: no LE cells seen	Lupus erythematosus, rheumatoid arthritis, scleroderma, and drug sensitivities
Rheumatoid factor (RF): <60 units/mL	An immunoglobulin found in approximately 80% of adults with rheumatoid arthritis; other diseases such as systemic lupus erythematosus may cause a positive RF
Uric acid (blood) Males: 2.1-8.5 mg/dL Females: 2.0-6.6 mg/dL	Increased in patients with gout, kidney failure, alcoholism, leukemia, metastatic cancer, multiple myeloma, or dehydration

(gouty arthritis). See Table 44-4 for a comparison of RA and osteoarthritis.

RHEUMATOID ARTHRITIS

Etiology and Pathophysiology

RA, the most serious form of the arthritis, leads to severe crippling. It is a chronic, systemic disease that affects 3% of the general population. RA can strike anyone; however, some people are more susceptible than others. Of the approximately 6 million Americans who have RA, 75% are women. Although RA can occur at any age, it most often occurs in women of childbearing age. RA is thought to be an autoimmune disorder, although there is evidence of genetic predisposition. Smoking significantly increases the risk of RA in both men and women who are genetically predisposed to the disease.

RA can affect many organ systems (lungs, heart, blood vessels, muscles, eyes, and skin). RA is characterized by a chronic inflammation of the synovial membrane (synovitis) of the diarthrodial joints (also called synovial joints: the freely movable joints in which continuous bony surfaces are covered by cartilage and connected by ligaments lined with synovial membrane).

Clinical Manifestations

RA is believed to involve an immune reaction that will not shut off because of an immune system failure; agents that should protect the body attack joint tissues instead and cause a chronic inflammatory reaction in the synovial membrane. This in turn damages the affected joint and surrounding tissue, possibly leading to gross deformity and loss of function (Figure 44-7).

RA is characterized by periods of remission and exacerbation. Some patients report a precipitating stressful event such as infection, work stress, physical exertion, childbirth, surgery, or emotional upset. During remission the inflammation, pain, stiffness, and edema subside, and progression of tissue damage is halted. (The patient may experience residual joint dysfunction even with remission.)

Table 44-4 Comparison of Rheumatoid Arthritis and Osteoarthritis

	RHEUMATOID ARTHRITIS (RA)	OSTEOARTHRITIS (OA)
Pathophysiology	Inflammation of synovial membrane; destruction of bones, ligaments, tendons, cartilage, and joint capsule.	Degeneration of cartilage from wear and tear; bone spur formation.
Joints most commonly affected	Symmetrical joint involvement noted in wrists, knees, and knuckles.	Often only one side of body affected with changes noted in hands, spine, knees, and hips.
Clinical signs and symptoms	Edema, erythema, heat, pain, tenderness, nodule formation, fatigue, stiffness, muscle aches, and fever. Systemic manifestations occur. Vasculitis (inflammation of blood vessels) may be responsible for a variety of systemic complications, including peripheral neuropathy, myopathy, cardiopulmonary involvement, and ischemic ulcerations of the skin. Potential complications include infection, osteoporosis, and Sjögren syndrome. Dry mouth and decreased tearing occur in Sjögren syndrome.	Localized pain, stiffness, bony knobs of end joints of fingers (Heberden's nodes), edema (not as pronounced as in RA). No systemic involvement is present. Constitutional symptoms such as fatigue or fever are not present. Other organ involvement is absent as well, which is an important differentiation between OA and RA.
Age at onset	Children nearing adolescence. Adults between 20 and 50.	Ages 45-90. Most people have some features with increasing age.
Sex	Females affected more often than males, with a ratio of 3:1.	Males and females affected equally.
Heredity	Familial tendency.	The form with knobby fingers can be hereditary.
Diagnostic tests	Rheumatoid factor (RF) found in serum of about 85% of patients with RA. Erythrocyte sedimentation rate, C-reactive protein, complete blood count, x-rays, examination of joint fluid RF positive in 80% of patients.	X-rays; no specific laboratory abnormalities are useful in diagnosing OA. RF negative.
Treatment	Control inflammation and pain with medications. Balance exercise with rest. Provide joint protection; encourage weight control and stress reduction. Surgically replace joints.	Maintain activity level. Control pain with medication. Encourage exercise, joint protection, weight control, stress reduction. Surgical joint replacement may be necessary.

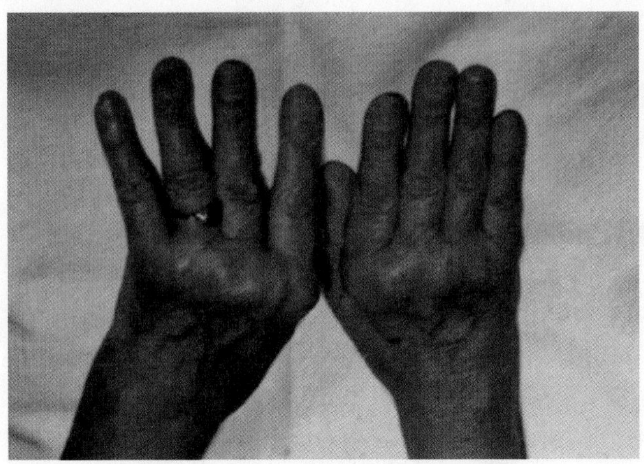

FIGURE 44-7 Rheumatoid arthritis of hands.

Assessment

Collection of **subjective data** includes noting the patient's complaints of malaise, muscle weakness (especially grip strength), loss of appetite, and generalized aching.

Collection of **objective data** includes observing the joints for edema, tenderness, subcutaneous nodules, limitation in range of motion (ROM) (morning stiffness especially), symmetrical joint involvement, and fever.

Diagnostic Tests

No single test is definitive for RA. Diagnosis is based on patient history and physical examination. The four classic symptoms most frequently reported are morning stiffness, joint pain, muscle weakness, and fatigue. Radiographic studies reveal loss of articular cartilage and change in subchondral bone. The following laboratory tests are often used in confirming a diagnosis and in ruling out other diseases:

- Erythrocyte sedimentation rate (ESR): An increase indicates the presence of inflammatory reaction somewhere in body.
- Rheumatoid factor (RF): An elevation indicates abnormal serum protein concentration. Positive RF occurs in approximately 80% of RA patients.
- Antinuclear antibody (ANA) titers and elevated C-reactive protein (CRP): These are seen in some RA patients.
- Latex agglutination test: This test detects presence of the immunoglobulin M version of RF, the anti–immunoglobulin G antibodies.
- Red blood cell count: This detects anemia, which is often present during chronic infection.
- Synovial fluid aspiration: Normal fluid is usually clear and highly viscous; however, when inflammation is present, fluid is cloudy, yellow, and less viscous and contains increased protein.
- Synovial fluid biopsy: The biopsy shows changes in tissue.

Table 44-5 Medications for Rheumatoid Arthritis

Generic (Trade)	Action	Side Effects/Toxic Effects	Nursing Implications
SALICYLATES			
Aspirin, salsalate (Disalicid, Asaphen) Choline salicylate (Arthropan) Choline magnesium trisalicylate (Trillisate)	Antiinflammatory, analgesic, antipyretic; act by inhibiting synthesis of prostaglandins	GI irritation (dyspepsia, nausea, ulcer, hemorrhage) Prolonged bleeding time Exacerbation of asthma (aspirin-sensitive asthma) Tinnitus, dizziness with repeated large doses	Administer drug with food, milk, antacids as prescribed, or full glass of water; may use enteric-coated aspirin. Report signs of bleeding (e.g., tarry stools, bruising, petechiae, nosebleeds).
NONSTEROIDAL ANTIINFLAMMATORY DRUGS (NSAIDs)			
Indomethacin (Indocin)	Analgesic, antiinflammatory	Headache, vertigo, insomnia; confusion, GI irritation, can decrease effect of ACE inhibitors	Give with food, milk, or antacid. Discontinue if CNS symptoms develop and notify physician. Monitor BP. Report signs of bleeding.
Ibuprofen (Motrin, Advil)	Analgesic, antiinflammatory	Same as indomethacin but believed less irritating to GI tract Fluid retention Can cause hypertension	Know that delayed absorption occurs if taken with food. Monitor BP.
Tolmetin sodium (Tolectin)	Analgesic, antiinflammatory	Same as ibuprofen	Give with food or milk.

From Lewis, S.L., et al. (2007). *Medical-surgical nursing: Assessment and management of clinical problems* (7th ed.). St. Louis: Mosby.
ACE, Angiotensin-converting enzyme; *BP*, blood pressure; *CNS*, central nervous system; *GI*, gastrointestinal.

Continued

Table 44-5 Medications for Rheumatoid Arthritis—cont'd

Generic (Trade)	Action	Side Effects/Toxic Effects	Nursing Implications
NONSTEROIDAL ANTIINFLAMMATORY DRUGS (NSAIDs)—cont'd			
Naproxen (Naprosyn)	Analgesic, antiinflammatory	Same as ibuprofen Causes drowsiness	Give with food, milk, or antacid. Tell patient to avoid driving until dosage effect is established.
Meloxicam (Mobic)	Antiinflammatory, analgesic, antipyretic	Dizziness, headache, insomnia, seizures, dysrhythmias, heart failure, hemorrhage, diarrhea, indigestion, nausea, pancreatitis, renal failure, leukopenia, thrombocytopenia, asthma, bronchospasm, angioedema Drug is contraindicated in women who are pregnant or plan to become pregnant.	Monitor BP. Instruct patient to avoid using aspirin or products containing aspirin. Assess patient for history of allergic reactions to aspirin or other NSAIDs before starting drug. Tell patient the drug can be taken without regard to meals. Advise patient to report signs and symptoms of GI ulcers and bleeding. Advise patient to report any skin rash, weight gain, or edema. Alert patient with history of asthma that asthma may recur while taking the drug. Advise patient to avoid alcohol and tobacco products while taking the drug. NSAIDs can cause fluid retention; closely monitor patients with hypertension, edema, or heart failure. Inform patient that consistent pain relief may take several days of drug administration.
Nabumetone (Relafen)	Analgesic, antiinflammatory	Dizziness, anxiety, depression, gastric irritation, edema, prolonged bleeding, rash	Give with meals or antacids. Advise patient to avoid alcohol, aspirin, or aspirin products or acetaminophen without physician's consent. Arthritic relief noted in 1-2 weeks.
Meclofenamate (Meclofen)	Analgesic, antiinflammatory	Gastric irritation, headache, dizziness, edema	Advise patients to avoid aspirin and aspirin products. Give 30 minutes before or 2 hours after eating.
COX-2 INHIBITOR			
Celecoxib (Celebrex)	Analgesic, antiinflammatory	Mild to moderate indigestion, risk of GI bleeding, diarrhea, abdominal pain Has been linked to an increased risk of cardiovascular events, such as MI or stroke (U.S. Food and Drug Administration, 2006)	Give medication orally. It can be taken with or without food. Celebrex is indicated for relief of the signs and symptoms of osteoarthritis and RA. Do not administer to patients who have asthma, urticaria, or allergic reactions to aspirin or other NSAIDs. Do not give to patients who are allergic to sulfonamide. Use cautiously with ACE inhibitors, warfarin, lithium, and furosemide. Monitor patients for signs of GI bleeding.
POTENT ANTIINFLAMMATORY AGENTS			
Adrenocorticosteroids (e.g., prednisone)	Interfere with body's normal inflammatory responses	Fluid retention, sodium retention, potassium depletion, hypertension, decreased healing potential, increased susceptibility to infection, GI irritation, hirsutism, osteoporosis, fat deposits, diabetes mellitus, myopathy Adrenal insufficiency or adrenal crisis if abruptly withdrawn	Give with food, milk, or antacid. Do not increase or decrease dosage without physician supervision. Give in morning if given once a day.

ACE, Angiotensin-converting enzyme; *BP,* blood pressure; *GI,* gastrointestinal; *MI,* myocardial infarction; *NSAIDs,* nonsteroidal antiinflammatory drugs; *RA,* rheumatoid arthritis.

Table 44-5 Medications for Rheumatoid Arthritis—cont'd

Generic (Trade)	Action	Side Effects/Toxic Effects	Nursing Implications
POTENT ANTIINFLAMMATORY AGENTS—cont'd			
Corticosteroids intraarticular injections (methylprednisolone [Depo-Medrol])	Suppression of inflammation and modification of the normal immune response	Decreased wound healing and increased susceptibility to infection	Check injection site for signs of infection. Inform patient joint improvement can last weeks to months. Advise patient to avoid overuse of joint.
SLOW-ACTING ANTIINFLAMMATORY AGENTS			
Antimalarials			
Hydroxychloroquine (Plaquenil)	Antiinflammatory (mechanism unknown); effect not expected to be noted for 6-12 months after beginning therapy	GI disturbances Retinal edema that may result in blindness	Instruct patient to obtain eye examination before beginning therapy and every 6 months thereafter. Monitor CBC.
Gold Salts (IM)			
Gold sodium thiomalate (Myochrysine)	Antiinflammatory; effect not noted for 3-6 months after beginning therapy	Renal and hepatic damage, corneal deposits, dermatitis, ulcerations in mouth, hematologic changes	Monitor urinalysis and CBC before each injection. Report dermatitis, metallic taste in mouth, or lesions in mouth to physician.
Oral gold salts auranofin (Ridaura)	Antirheumatic	Stomatitis (lesions in mouth); thrombocytopenia and leukopenia	Minimize exposure to sunlight and provide meticulous oral hygiene.
Antineoplastic			
Methotrexate (Folex, Rheumatrex, Trexall)	Alters the way the body uses folic acid, which is necessary for cell growth; decreases inflammation	Upset stomach, nausea, vomiting, anorexia, diarrhea, or sore mouth; headache, blurred vision, dizziness	Drug is taken orally or by injection. Monitor vital signs, WBC, platelets, I&O, appetite. Advise patient to avoid pregnancy while on drug and to not get vaccinations without physician's consent. Keep patient well hydrated.
DISEASE-MODIFYING ANTIRHEUMATOID DRUGS (DMARDs)			
Etanercept (Enbrel)	Blocks the normal and inflammatory immune responses seen in RA; binds tumor necrosis factor (TNF), which is involved in immune and inflammatory reactions	Pain at injection site, upper respiratory tract infections and sinusitis; in severe cases, tuberculosis possible	Give twice weekly subcutaneously in the thigh, abdomen, or upper arm. Refrigerate, but never freeze medication. Use with caution in patients with chronic infections. May cause or aggravate systemic lupus erythematosus.
Leflunomide (Arava)	Reduces signs and symptoms of RA and retards structural bone damage	Diarrhea, elevated liver enzymes, alopecia, rash	Medication is taken orally. Monitor urinary output. Do not use with patients with hepatic impairment or positive for hepatitis B or C.
Infliximab (Remicade)	An antibody that binds specifically to proinflammatory enzymes that are produced by the synovial cells	Upper respiratory tract infections, headache, nausea, sinusitis, rash, cough	Administer intravenously at 2 and 6 weeks initially, then every 8 weeks thereafter. Do not give to patients with a clinically active infection.

CBC, Complete blood count; *I&O*, intake and output; *RA*, rheumatoid arthritis; *TNF, tumor necrosis factor; WBC*, white blood cell count.

Continued

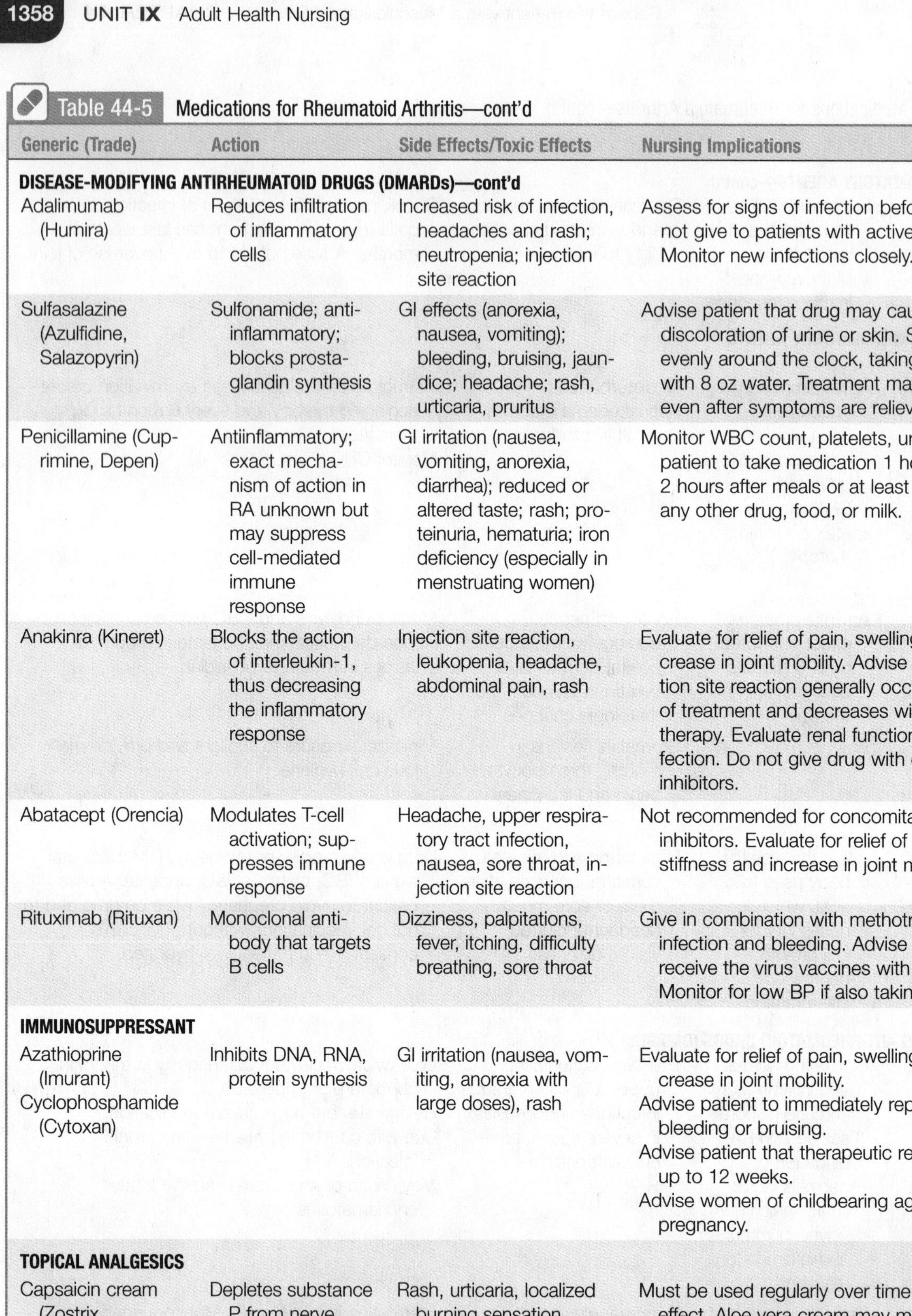

Table 44-5 Medications for Rheumatoid Arthritis—cont'd

Generic (Trade)	Action	Side Effects/Toxic Effects	Nursing Implications
DISEASE-MODIFYING ANTIRHEUMATOID DRUGS (DMARDs)—cont'd			
Adalimumab (Humira)	Reduces infiltration of inflammatory cells	Increased risk of infection, headaches and rash; neutropenia; injection site reaction	Assess for signs of infection before injection. Do not give to patients with active infections. Monitor new infections closely.
Sulfasalazine (Azulfidine, Salazopyrin)	Sulfonamide; anti-inflammatory; blocks prostaglandin synthesis	GI effects (anorexia, nausea, vomiting); bleeding, bruising, jaundice; headache; rash, urticaria, pruritus	Advise patient that drug may cause orange-yellow discoloration of urine or skin. Space doses evenly around the clock, taking drug after food with 8 oz water. Treatment may be continued even after symptoms are relieved. Monitor CBC.
Penicillamine (Cuprimine, Depen)	Antiinflammatory; exact mechanism of action in RA unknown but may suppress cell-mediated immune response	GI irritation (nausea, vomiting, anorexia, diarrhea); reduced or altered taste; rash; proteinuria, hematuria; iron deficiency (especially in menstruating women)	Monitor WBC count, platelets, urinalysis. Advise patient to take medication 1 hour before or 2 hours after meals or at least 1 hour away from any other drug, food, or milk.
Anakinra (Kineret)	Blocks the action of interleukin-1, thus decreasing the inflammatory response	Injection site reaction, leukopenia, headache, abdominal pain, rash	Evaluate for relief of pain, swelling, stiffness; increase in joint mobility. Advise patient that injection site reaction generally occurs in first month of treatment and decreases with continued therapy. Evaluate renal function. Monitor for infection. Do not give drug with other TNF inhibitors.
Abatacept (Orencia)	Modulates T-cell activation; suppresses immune response	Headache, upper respiratory tract infection, nausea, sore throat, injection site reaction	Not recommended for concomitant use with TNF inhibitors. Evaluate for relief of pain, swelling, stiffness and increase in joint mobility.
Rituximab (Rituxan)	Monoclonal antibody that targets B cells	Dizziness, palpitations, fever, itching, difficulty breathing, sore throat	Give in combination with methotrexate. Monitor for infection and bleeding. Advise patient to not receive the virus vaccines with treatment. Monitor for low BP if also taking BP medication.
IMMUNOSUPPRESSANT			
Azathioprine (Imurant) Cyclophosphamide (Cytoxan)	Inhibits DNA, RNA, protein synthesis	GI irritation (nausea, vomiting, anorexia with large doses), rash	Evaluate for relief of pain, swelling, stiffness; increase in joint mobility. Advise patient to immediately report unusual bleeding or bruising. Advise patient that therapeutic response may take up to 12 weeks. Advise women of childbearing age to avoid pregnancy.
TOPICAL ANALGESICS			
Capsaicin cream (Zostrix, Capzasin) 5% lidocaine	Depletes substance P from nerve endings, interrupting pain signals to the brain (Substance P may participate directly or indirectly in the transmission process of certain neurons.)	Rash, urticaria, localized burning sensation, erythema	Must be used regularly over time for maximal effect. Aloe vera cream may moderate burning sensation. Advise patient not to use cream with external heat source (heating pad) because of risk of burns. Available in OTC and prescription strengths. Advise patient to wear gloves when applying cream to other joints and to wash hands; avoid touching damaged or irritated skin, eyes, nose and mouth.

BP, Blood pressure; *CBC,* complete blood count; *DNA,* deoxyribonucleic acid; *GI,* gastrointestinal; *OTC,* over the counter; *RA,* rheumatoid arthritis; *RNA,* ribonucleic acid; *TNF, tumor necrosis factor;* *WBC,* white blood count.

Medical Management

The RA patient benefits from aggressive treatment early in the course of the disease. The medical management of RA is directed toward (1) controlling the disease activity by administering disease-modifying and antiinflammatory drugs (Table 44-5); (2) providing pain relief (see Table 44-5); (3) reducing clinical symptoms in days to weeks with the rapid antiinflammatory effect of methotrexate (Rheumatrex); (4) prolonging joint function (often with physical therapy, traction, and splints); and (5) slowing the progression of joint damage by promoting activities of daily living (ADLs), an exercise program, and weight management.

Advances in cell and molecular biology have influenced the treatment of RA. Current medications actually target the pathophysiology of the disease. Disease-modifying antirheumatoid drugs (DMARDs) offer wider treatment options. These medications target an enzyme known as tumor necrosis factor (TNF). TNF is produced by the synovial cells and other cells of the body and is a proinflammatory substance—that is, it has the ability to produce signs and symptoms of inflammation (see Table 44-5). Complementary therapies to decrease inflammation include capsaicin (Capsin), a nonopioid topical analgesic, fish oil, and antioxidants (vitamins C and E and beta-carotene). Musculoskeletal surgery in the form of joint replacement is another option.

Nursing Interventions and Patient Teaching

Patient education is essential to help the patient and family understand what is happening and what to expect as the disease progresses. Fatigue is a major problem, so sleeping 8 to 10 hours a night and taking a 2-hour nap during the day are recommended. Exercise helps prevent the joints from "freezing" and the muscles from weakening. A typical exercise program calls for two or three 10- to 15-minute daily sessions of "quiet" exercise that gently puts joints through ROM. Heat is often used to relax and soothe muscles. Hot packs, heat lamps, and applications of hot paraffin wax are helpful. Rehabilitation is aimed at helping the patient adapt to physical limitations and promoting normal daily activities.

Nursing diagnoses and interventions for the patient with RA include but are not limited to the following:

Nursing Diagnoses	Nursing Interventions
Pain, related to joint inflammation	Administer prescribed salicylate or nonsteroidal antiinflammatory drugs (NSAIDs). Assist patient with an exercise program prescribed by a physical therapist, including proper body mechanics and use of a walker or cane. During acute stages of disease, encourage patient to rest inflamed joints. Maintain bed rest as ordered; maintain proper body alignment. Assist and teach patient to extend joints as possible and to avoid external rotation of extremities; use sandbags or trochanter rolls. Avoid use of pillow under knees. Immobilize and/or support joints.
Chronic low self-esteem, related to negative self-evaluation about self or capabilities	Encourage patient to express feelings about health problems, progress, and prognosis concerning diagnosis. Encourage patient to explore ways to remain active while experiencing limited mobility (e.g., doing tasks while sitting as opposed to standing or walking).

As with any chronic illness, patient teaching is perhaps the most important aspect of nursing interventions. Patient teaching includes information about joint protection and energy conservation techniques, proper balance of rest and activity, proper use of medications (i.e., names of drugs, dosages, precautions in administration, and side effects or toxic effects), plans for implementation of the exercise program prescribed by the physician or physical therapist, proper application of heat or cold packs, proper use of walking aids, safety measures to prevent injury, basics of good nutrition and importance of avoiding weight gain, and the danger of following programs that promise a "cure."

Prognosis

The course of RA is variable but is most frequently marked by remissions and exacerbations. The prognosis is based on a variety of clinical and laboratory findings. Stage I represents early effects. Stage IV, the terminal category, includes marked joint deformity, extensive muscle atrophy, soft tissue lesions, bone and cartilage destruction, and fibrous or bony ankylosis.

ANKYLOSING SPONDYLITIS

Etiology and Pathophysiology

Ankylosing spondylitis (AKS) is a chronic, progressive disorder of the sacroiliac and hip joints, the synovial joints of the spine, and the adjacent soft tissues. It can affect both sexes but is seen more often in young men. The presence of human leukocyte antigen A and B27 (HLA-B27) in the serum of 90% of whites and 50% of blacks with AKS suggests a hereditary factor. The most common age for onset of AKS is between 15 and 35 years of age. The highest incidence rate is among 25- to 34-year-olds (Lewis et al., 2007). Women develop a milder form of AKS than men, and fusion of the spine is rarely seen. It is sometimes referred to as **rheumatoid spondylitis.**

Clinical Manifestations

AKS involves inflammation of the spine that results in the bones of the spine growing together. This is termed **ankylosis,** the fixation of a joint, often in abnormal position. It usually results from destruction of articular cartilage and subchondral bone.

AKS involves inflammation in which the ligament or tendon attaches to the bone; it does not affect the synovial membrane, as seen in RA. AKS affects joints such as the neck, jaw, shoulders, knees, and hips. The disease process causes the ligaments to become ossified (hardened). The cardiovascular system can be involved, and heart enlargement and pericarditis can occur. If the costovertebral joints are affected, kyphosis can occur and alter respirations. The patient may have difficulty expanding the ribcage while breathing. Many patients with the disease also have inflammatory bowel disease. Vision loss occurs with chronic AKS, and blindness may result from glaucoma and pupil damage.

Assessment

Subjective data include patient complaints of low backache, stiffness, and alternating or bilateral "sciatica pain" that lasts for a few days and then subsides. Pain is more pronounced when the patient is in an erect position. Inactivity exacerbates the pain, and exercise gives relief. Complaints of weight loss, abdominal distention, visual problems, and fatigue are common. AKS is present in 3% to 10% of patients with inflammatory bowel disease.

Collection of **objective data** includes assessment for tenderness over the spine and sacroiliac region. Peripheral joint edema and decreased ROM may be seen. Assessment of vital signs may indicate elevated temperature, tachycardia, and hyperpnea. Respiratory difficulties arise if there is limited expansion of the chest, as is often seen in kyphosis.

Diagnostic Tests

Patients with AKS often have the following laboratory test results: (1) low hemoglobin and hematocrit, indicative of anemia; (2) elevated ESR and CRP, which are common in chronic inflammatory disease; (3) elevated serum alkaline phosphatase levels in patients who are immobilized or have bone resorption; and (4) presence of the HLA-B27 antigen. Radiographic examination often reveals sacroiliac joint and intervertebral disk inflammation with bony erosion and joint space fusion.

Medical Management

The physician usually prescribes oral analgesics and NSAIDs. Etanercept (Enbrel) is a biologic agent that is useful in decreasing symptoms of AKS and improving patient role performance (Lewis et al., 2007). Additional biologic agents, such as infliximab (Remicade) and adalimumab (Humira), may be effective. Exercise programs (swimming and walking) help prevent demineralization of bone.

Surgery may be necessary to replace fused joints (commonly the hip or the knee). Cervical or lumbar osteotomy can be done for severe kyphosis.

Endoscopic microsurgery can be performed on select candidates. In microsurgery, the bone or tissue that is putting pressure on the spinal nerves is removed by using endoscopic equipment placed through small incisions. Most patients leave the hospital within 24 hours and start physical therapy within a few days.

Nursing Interventions and Patient Teaching

Nursing interventions are aimed at maintaining alignment of the spine. Providing a firm mattress, bed board, and back brace helps provide support. Postural and breathing exercises help compensate for the possibility of impaired gas exchange caused by the changes in posture and chest cavity size. Encouraging the patient to lie on the abdomen for at least 15 to 30 minutes four times daily helps extend the spine. Turning and positioning every 2 hours helps prevent pressure sores.

A nursing diagnosis and interventions for the patient with AKS include but are not limited to the following:

Nursing Diagnosis	Nursing Interventions
Chronic low self-esteem, related to body image	Encourage patient to share fears and anxiety about the disease process. Deal with behavior changes: denial, powerlessness, anxiety, and dependence. Be supportive and kind but firm in setting goals. Encourage independence. Be aware of limitations, and encourage discussion of feelings and concerns.

Teach the patient the appropriate use of prescribed medications, postural exercises, and methods of applying heat to back and hips. Promote correct posture and prevent complications by encouraging the patient to use a firm mattress, sleep without a pillow, and do respiratory exercises.

Prognosis

AKS is a chronic disease occurring in persons younger than age 30 that generally burns itself out after a course of 20 years, leaving permanent, irreversible systemic involvement.

OSTEOARTHRITIS (DEGENERATIVE JOINT DISEASE)

Etiology and Pathophysiology

Osteoarthritis is also known as DJD, hypertrophic arthritis, osteoarthrosis, or senescent arthritis. Osteoarthritis is a nonsystemic, noninflammatory disorder that progressively causes bones and joints to degenerate. Almost everyone past 40 years of age has hypertrophic changes in the joints (Box 44-3). The disease is an almost inevitable consequence of aging and is a major cause of severe chronic disability. Osteoarthritis takes two forms: primary (cause is unknown) and secondary (caused by trauma, infections, previous fractures, RA, stress on weight-bearing joints from obesity, or such occupations as coal mining or boxing). A comparison of RA and osteoarthritis is found in Table 44-4.

Clinical Manifestations

This disorder affects the joints of the hand, knee, hip, and cervical and lumbar vertebrae (Figure 44-8). Osteoarthritis appears to be related to aging, but researchers are unclear as to the cause. Nearly all people older than 60 years show osteoarthritic changes, with women being affected more often than men. The disease affects the hands in women more often, whereas in men the hips are affected.

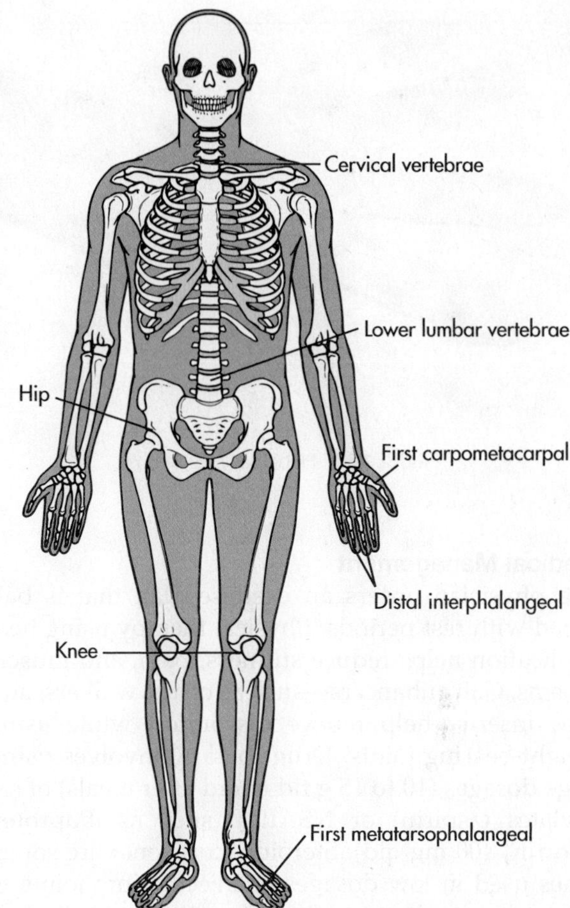

FIGURE 44-8 Joints most frequently involved in osteoarthritis.

Box 44-3 Osteoarthritis

- Osteoarthritis is the most common form of arthritis and the leading cause of disability in people older than age 65. Under age 55, men and women are affected equally. In older individuals, osteoarthritis of the hip is more common in men and osteoarthritis of the interphalangeal joints and the thumb is more common in women. Osteoarthritis occurs more frequently in people who are obese or who experience repetitive stress to the joints.
- More than 70% of total hip and knee replacements are for osteoarthritis.
- Overweight people have a higher risk of knee and hip osteoarthritis.
- Weight-loss programs for overweight older adults lessen symptoms in those with the disease.
- Acetaminophen is recommended by the American College of Rheumatology for osteoarthritis pain because of fewer gastrointestinal and renal side effects compared with other drugs.
- Bicycling and swimming are considered good exercises for people with osteoarthritis of the knee; walking should be done on level ground.
- People with osteoarthritis of the knee or hip should avoid climbing stairs, bending, stooping, or squatting.

Assessment

Collection of **subjective data** includes questioning the patient about pain and stiffness (rest usually relieves pain in the early stages). Past illnesses, surgical procedures, or trauma may be relevant, and information about excessive weight gain and occupation may be significant. Complaints of muscle spasms and reduced grip strength are common.

Collection of **objective data** includes assessment for joint edema, tenderness, instability, and deformity. **Heberden's nodes** appear on the sides of the distal joints of fingers (Figure 44-9), and **Bouchard's nodes** appear on the proximal joints of fingers; these nodes are hard, bony, and cartilaginous enlargements. The patient's gait reveals a limp, especially if the hips or legs are affected.

Diagnostic Tests

There is no specific test to diagnose osteoarthritis. However, radiographic studies, arthroscopy, synovial fluid examination, and bone scans are used to provide information.

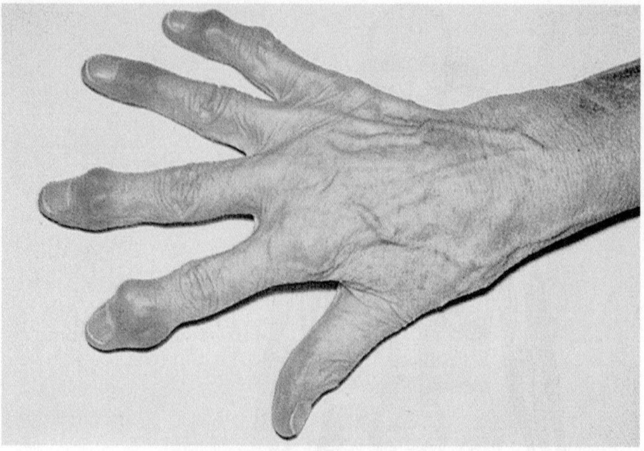

FIGURE 44-9 Heberden's nodes.

Medical Management

The physician orders an exercise plan that is balanced with rest periods. Physical therapy using heat application helps reduce stiffness, pain, and muscle spasms. Gait enhancers—such as canes, walkers, and shoe inserts—help relieve discomfort while using weight-bearing joints. Drug therapy involves using large dosages (10 to 15 g tid to qid after meals) of salicylates (aspirin) or NSAIDs (such as ibuprofen [Motrin] 400 mg qid). Steroids (cortisone) are sometimes used in low dosages or injected into joints to produce immediate pain relief and temporarily halt the destructive process. Patients with hypertension must be screened carefully while taking NSAIDs because certain NSAIDs elevate blood pressure. Patients need to inform their physician so that a safe and effective combination of drugs can be chosen. Indomethacin (Indocin) can decrease the effect of enalapril (Vasotec) (an angiotensin-converting enzyme inhibitor used for hypertension), and the combination of ibuprofen and lisinopril (Prinivil, Zestril) can trigger a hypertensive response. Acetaminophen is commonly used as an analgesic and does not affect the blood pressure. Tramadol hydrochloride (Ultram) is a synthetic analgesic used for moderate to severe pain and can be used for patients taking antihypertensives.

Alternatives to NSAIDs

The discomfort associated with acute or chronic RA, osteoarthritis, gouty arthritis, and AKS may also be decreased through the use of nonpharmacologic measures. Measures such as relaxation techniques, massage therapy, imagery, and therapeutic touch have been proven effective in reducing discomfort and decreasing the need for NSAIDs.

Glucosamine is found in the body as a lubricant and shock absorber necessary for repairing and maintaining healthy joint function. The aging process has been linked to the loss of glucosamine and other substances in the cartilage. Taking supplements to natural glucosamine enables the body to manufacture collagen and proteoglycans and resupply lubricant found in the synovial fluid necessary for restoring healthy cartilage (see Complementary and Alternative Therapies box). Glucosamine supplements have been linked with reductions in articular pain, joint tenderness, and restricted joint movement in people suffering from arthritis. People allergic to shellfish, those with chronic medical problems, or women who are pregnant or lactating should not take supplemental glucosamine without conferring with a health care provider (Lewis et al., 2007).

Surgical intervention, such as osteotomy, may help correct malalignment. Joint replacement may be necessary to replace all or part of the joint's articulating surface. Arthroplasty of the hip and knee is the most common surgical intervention.

Complementary and Alternative Therapies

Musculoskeletal Disorders

- Alternative therapies being considered in the treatment of osteoarthritis include compounds such as glucosamine and chondroitin. These substances appear to provide pain relief, perhaps even slowing the disease process. Glucosamine apparently stimulates cartilage cells to manufacture proteoglycans, whereas chondroitin inhibits enzymes that break down cartilage. Few adverse effects have been seen with glucosamine used up to 3 years.
- Chiropractic adjustment has been effective in patients with some types of back pain. Many insurance companies allow for this form of therapy.
- Other manual healing methods—therapy that includes touch and manipulation of soft tissues or realignment of body parts to correct a dysfunction that affects other body parts—include the following:
  —Massage and other physical healing methods
  —Acupuncture
  —Reflexology (a system of treating certain disorders by massaging the soles of the feet or the palms of the hands)
  —Rolfing (a technique of deep massage intended to realign the body by altering the length and tone of myofascial tissues)

Nursing Interventions and Patient Teaching

Nursing interventions include encouraging the patient to maintain ADLs and adapt to limitations of the disease. Alternating sitting, walking, and standing with periods of rest can help reduce joint discomfort and deterioration. Older patients may be physically capable of turning and moving in bed but may forget to do so because of alteration in their level of orientation. Assist the patient with a weight-reduction plan if obesity is a problem. If splints are used to support a painful joint, assess for neurovascular impairment above and below the site of application. Also check gait enhancers for safety considerations, such as rubber tips on ends, proper size, and patient knowledge about use. If the patient has been taking aspirin over a period of time, gastrointestinal (GI) bleeding may occur. It may be necessary to perform a guaiac test on stool and emesis to determine the presence of occult blood.

As with RA, teaching the person with osteoarthritis about the disease process and the steps to control that process is the most important aspect of nursing interventions. Patient teaching should include the same information as for RA.

Prognosis

Osteoarthritis is a chronic disease that ultimately causes permanent destruction of affected cartilage and underlying bone with variable pain and disability.

GOUT (GOUTY ARTHRITIS)

Etiology and Pathophysiology

Gout is a metabolic disease resulting from an accumulation of uric acid in the blood. It is an acute inflammatory condition associated with ineffective metabolism of purines. Gout can be primary (linked with hereditary factors), secondary (resulting from use of certain medications or complication of another disease), or idiopathic (of unknown origin). It affects men approximately eight times more frequently than women and usually occurs in middle life. It does not occur before puberty in the male or before menopause in the female. For primary disease, it takes approximately 20 years for sufficient urates to accumulate in the body before causing signs and symptoms. Of all people with gout, 85% have a genetic tendency to develop the disease. **Tophi** (calculi containing sodium urate deposits that develop in periarticular fibrous tissue, typically in patients with gout) result in inflammation of the joint; it is unclear why this occurs. Typically the big toes are involved, but other joints can also be affected.

Clinical Manifestations

Onset occurs at night, with excruciating pain, edema, and inflammation in the affected joint. The pain may last a short time but return at intervals, or it may be severe and continuous for 5 to 10 days. The patient may have repeated attacks or only one attack in a lifetime. Tophi are seen around the rim of the ear and can disfigure the ear. Surgical removal may be necessary.

Assessment

Collection of **subjective data** includes noting a complaint of pain occurring at night involving the great toe or other joints. Take a dietary history, with specific questions on consumption of alcohol and foods high in purines, such as organ meats (brain, kidney, liver, and heart), anchovies, yeast, herring, mackerel, and scallops.

Collection of **objective data** includes assessment of joints (especially the great toe) for signs of edema, heat, discoloration (may appear erythematous or purple), and limited movement. Vital sign data may reveal an elevated temperature and hypertension, tachycardia, and tachypnea. Carefully assess urinary output because tophi can form in the kidneys and alter kidney function. Assess the patient for tophi (typically seen on the earlobes, fingers, hands, and toes).

Diagnostic Tests

Laboratory tests used to diagnose gout include serum (see Table 44-3) and urinary uric acid levels (elevation is significant), complete blood count (CBC) (leukocytosis and anemia may be present), and elevated ESR. Radiographic studies reveal cysts and toe bone pockets. Synovial fluid contains urate crystals.

Medical Management

Several drugs are used to treat gout. For acute attacks, colchicine is administered orally or intravenously. The oral dosage is 0.5 mg hourly for 12 doses. The drug is discontinued if GI symptoms develop or pain is not relieved. Indomethacin (Indocin SR) is an affective antiinflammatory drug in treating gout. Corticosteroids can be administered orally, intravenously, or intraarticularly and will relieve signs and symptoms within 12 hours. The physician may order allopurinol (Zyloprim) to decrease the production of uric acid; probenecid (Probalan), inhibits renal tubular resorption of uric acid to increase secretion of uric acid by the kidneys; and sulfinpyrazone (Anturane) to prevent the development of tophi in various parts of the body, including the kidneys. Aspirin inactivates the effect of uricosurics (probenecid), resulting in urate retention, and should be avoided while patients are taking uricosuric drugs.

Nursing Interventions and Patient Teaching

Nursing intervention is aimed at giving medications prescribed by the physician for relief of pain and inflammation. When giving colchicine, it is important to observe for side effects, such as diarrhea, nausea, and vomiting. Increasing the patient's fluid intake to at least 2000 mL daily helps eliminate the excess urinary urates. Approximately 10% to 20% of patients with gouty arthritis have uric acid kidney stones. Carefully document intake and output (I&O). Advise the patient to avoid excessive use of alcohol and consumption of foods high in purine. Maintain bed rest and joint immobilization while the patient is symptomatic. Bed cradles prevent pressure from bed linens on the affected joints.

Nursing diagnoses and interventions for the patient with gout include but are not limited to the following:

Nursing Diagnoses	Nursing Interventions
Pain, related to disease process	Maintain patient in a position of comfort with foot supported and in alignment; place bed cradle over foot; no weight bearing. Apply cold packs as ordered, keeping pressure off joint. Administer analgesics and antigout and antiinflammatory agents as ordered; observe for side effects.
Deficient knowledge, related to lack of information concerning medications and home care management	Provide medication schedule, including name, dosage, purpose, and side effects. Discuss importance of diet, exercise, and rest program. Encourage follow-up visits with physician.

Patient teaching is aimed at giving information about the disease and stressing the importance of keeping the serum uric acid levels within normal range by taking the prescribed medications; following the prescribed diet; and avoiding infections, lack of sleep, and stress. The patient may need to take colchicine, probenecid, and allopurinol as a maintenance dose even when signs and symptoms are not present.

Prognosis
The signs and symptoms are recurrent; episodes become longer each year. The disorder is disabling and, if untreated, can progress to the development of tophi and destructive joint changes.

OTHER MUSCULOSKELETAL DISORDERS

OSTEOPOROSIS

Etiology and Pathophysiology
Osteoporosis is a disorder that results in reduction in the mass of bone per unit of volume. This reduction is sufficient to interfere with the mechanical support function of the bone. The cause of osteoporosis is not completely known. Women between the ages of 55 and 65 years are identified as a high-risk group for postmenopausal osteoporosis, and many researchers believe that this is related to the loss of the female hormone estrogen. An increase of postmenopausal osteoporosis suggests estrogen deficiency is connected with increased bone resorption and sensitivity to parathyroid hormone (substance that weakens bone by increasing calcium movement from bone into extracellular fluid). Senile osteoporosis is seen in people between ages 70 and 85 years and affects twice as many women as men. One in two women compared with one in eight men will have osteoporosis-related fractures in their lifetime (Lewis et al., 2007). Genetic and environmental factors, such as small bone structure and lack of exercise, can contribute to the rate of bone loss. Osteoporosis affects the vertebrae, neck of the femur, pelvis, hands, and wrists. Individuals most at risk for developing osteoporosis are small-framed, white (European descent) or Asian race, nonobese, menopausal women who smoke. Other contributing factors are steroids, anticonvulsants or heparin, diets low in calcium throughout life, excessive caffeine intake, alcoholism, and too much protein in the diet (see Cultural Considerations box).

Clinical Manifestations
The disorder develops slowly, beginning with a complaint of backache. As the disease progresses, the bones become porous and brittle due to a lack of calcium.

Assessment
Collection of **subjective data** includes questioning the patient about lifestyle practices and complaints of pain (low thoracic and lumbar) that worsens with sitting, standing, coughing, sneezing, and straining.

Collection of **objective data** includes assessing the patient for dowager's hump (spinal deformity and height loss that result from repeated spinal vertebral fractures) and increased lordosis, scoliosis, and kyphosis (Figure 44-10). Also assess gait impairment associated with inability to maintain erect posture.

Diagnostic Tests
The physician orders a CBC; serum calcium, phosphorus, and alkaline phosphatase; blood urea nitrogen (BUN); creatinine level; urinalysis; and liver and thy-

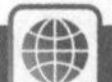

Cultural Considerations

Osteoporosis

- White and Asian women have a higher incidence of osteoporosis than black women.
- Black women have 10% more bone mass than white women.
- Postmenopausal women are at the highest risk regardless of cultural background or ethnic group.
- Black men have dense bones and a low incidence of osteoporosis.
- Hispanic women have a lower incidence of osteoporosis than white women.

From Lewis, S.L., Heitkemper, M.M., Dirksen, S.R., et al. (2007). *Medical-surgical nursing: Assessment and management of clinical problems* (7th ed.). St. Louis: Mosby.

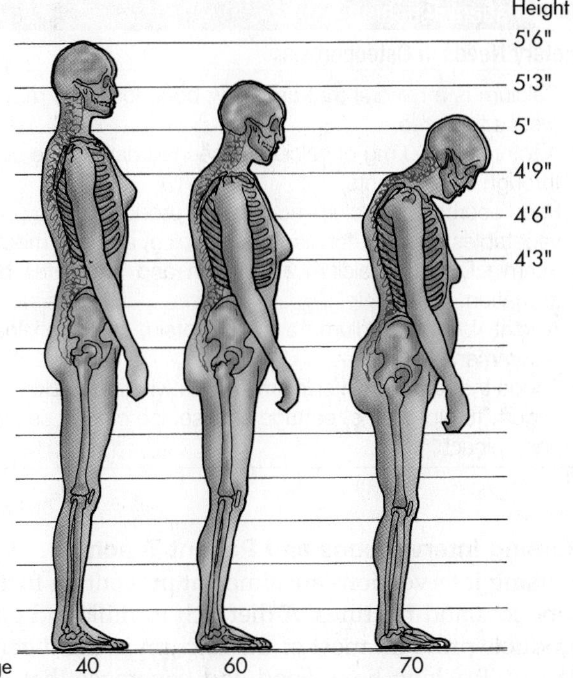

FIGURE 44-10 A normal spine at age 40 years and osteoporotic changes at ages 60 and 70 years. These changes can cause a loss of as much as 6 inches in height and can result in the so-called dowager's hump *(far right)* in the upper thoracic vertebrae.

roid function tests. A bone mineral density (BMD) measurement is recommended for women around the time of menopause. BMD is performed by a dual energy x-ray absorptiometry (DEXA). The BMD test assesses the mass of bone per unit volume, or how tightly the bone is packed. Usually the hip and the spine are measured. The test takes about 10 minutes and has low amounts of radiation. The World Health Organization has defined criteria for adult women as follows:

- Normal bones have a BMD within 1 standard deviation of the young adult average.
- Low bone mass (osteopenia) is 1 standard deviation below the young adult average.
- Osteoporosis is 2.5 standard deviations below the young adult average (www.who.int).

Medical Management

The physician orders a treatment regimen aimed at increasing bone density and retarding bone loss. Calcium supplements that bring the total calcium intake per day to 1,000 mg for men and 1,500 mg for postmenopausal women are recommended (as well as vitamin D, 50,000 international units once or twice per week). Weight-bearing exercise programs to improve muscle tone, such as walking, have been effective in preventing further bone loss and stimulating new bone formation. Treatment may include adequate doses of estrogen. Estrogen will not correct the condition but will help to prevent fractures and may be approved for women at significant risk.

Alendronate (Fosamax), etidronate (Didronel), pamidronate (Aredia), tiludronate (Skelid), and ibandronate (Boniva) are bone resorption inhibitors (Table 44-6). These drugs absorb calcium phosphate crystal in bone and are given orally to treat symptoms of osteoporosis. Administer these drugs first thing in the morning with 6 to 8 ounces of water at least 30 minutes before other medications, beverages, or food. Caution patient to remain upright for 30 minutes after a dose to facilitate passage to stomach and minimize risk of esophageal irritation.

Table 44-6 Medications for Osteoporosis

Generic (Trade)	Action	Side Effects/Toxic Effects	Nursing Implications
Biphosphates: alendronate (Fosamax), risedronate (Actonel), etidronate (Didronel), pamidronate (Aredia), tiludronate (Skelid), ibandronate (Boniva)	Slow bone loss and increase bone density	Difficulty in swallowing, chest pain, severe or recurring heartburn	Administer first thing in the morning with 6-8 oz plain water, 30 minutes before other medications, beverages, or food.
Calcitonin-salmon injection (Miacalcin) or calcitonin-salmon nasal spray (Fortical)	Increases bone mass, particularly in the spine	Injection site reaction, nasal irritation	Monitor for injection site reaction. Advise patient to take medication exactly as directed.
Estrogen receptor modulator: raloxifene (Evista)	Prevents bone loss and spinal fractures	May increase tendency for deep-vein thrombosis, myocardial infarcts, uterine bleeding, and breast abnormalities	Administer without regard to meals.
Parathyroid hormone: teriparatide (Forteo)	Prevents bone loss; promotes bone growth	Increased heart rate or dizziness	Administer subcutaneously into thigh or abdominal wall once daily.

Risedronate (Actonel) is another bone resorption inhibitor. The drug absorbs calcium phosphate crystal in bone and inhibits bone resorption without inhibiting bone formation or mineralization. It is given orally. The patient should sit upright for 30 minutes after a dose to prevent esophageal irritation. Another type of drug used in treating osteoporosis is selective estrogen receptor modulators, such as raloxifene (Evista). These drugs mimic the effect of estrogen on bone by reducing bone resorption.

Teriparatide (Forteo) is a form of parathyroid hormone that is approved for postmenopausal women who are at increased risk for osteoporosis fractures or who cannot use other treatments. The drug prevents sloughing of osteoblasts (bone cells that form new bone) in porous or spongy bones and increases bone mass in the spine and hip. Teriparatide treatment requires a daily subcutaneous injection of the drug and is limited to a 24-month period. The drug must be kept refrigerated. The most common side effects are nausea, dizziness, leg cramps, hypercalcemia, and orthostatic hypotension. The drug is not recommended for patients with an increased risk of osteosarcoma.

Surgical Interventions for Osteoporosis

Women with severe osteoporosis who are unresponsive to an analgesic may be candidates for a surgical procedure to relieve the pain. Vertebroplasty and kyphoplasty are 90% successful in relieving pain from compression fractures of the spine. Vertebroplasty (plastic surgery on a vertebra) involves high-pressure injection of polymethyl methacrylate cement into the spine, which pushes the vertebrae apart. The procedure is done with the patient under a general or local anesthetic. Major complications involve damage to the posterior vertebral walls from the high pressure used to inject the cement and movement of the cement out of vertebral spaces into the spinal canal.

Kyphoplasty (plastic surgery on dowager's hump) involves inserting a balloon into the center of the collapsed vertebrae, which restores the position of the vertebrae and creates a space for injection of polymethyl methacrylate cement. Porous bone is packed around the outside edge. This procedure is less risky than vertebroplasty because the balloon removes the need to use high pressure for the cement placement.

Nursing Considerations

Patients are admitted to the hospital and required to stay up to 23 hours after the procedure. Flat bed rest is ordered for the first 4 hours postoperatively; then patients are allowed to ambulate as able. A small dressing covers the operative site, and antibiotics and steroids are typically ordered for three doses following the procedure.

 **Patient Teaching**

Dietary Needs in Osteoporosis

- Calcium is a mineral that can slow bone loss and may decrease fractures.
- A total of 1,500 mg of calcium is needed daily in the diet or through supplements.
- Food sources of calcium include milk products, many green vegetables, calcium-fortified orange juice, and soy milk.
- Vitamin D helps calcium absorption and stimulates bone formation.
- A diet low in sodium, animal protein, and caffeine is recommended.
- Foods that are high in calcium include whole and skim milk, yogurt, turnip greens, cottage cheese, ice cream, sardines, and spinach.

Nursing Interventions and Patient Teaching

Nursing interventions are aimed at preventing further bone loss and fractures. A diet rich in milk and dairy products provides most of the calcium in the diet (see Patient Teaching box). Food and beverages that contain caffeine also contain phosphorus, which contributes to bone loss. Teach patients relaxation techniques and encourage them to stop smoking. Patients who take estrogen need information about the higher risk for thromboembolism, endometrial cancer, and possibly breast cancer. Hormone replacement must be prescribed at the lowest dose possible and for a short duration. Safety measures, such as side rails, hand rails, bedside commodes with seat elevators, and rubber mats in showers, can help prevent falls in older adults. Efforts are made to keep patients with osteoporosis ambulatory to prevent further loss of bone substance as a result of immobility. Encourage weight-bearing exercise to increase bone density.

A nursing diagnosis and interventions for the patient with osteoporosis include but are not limited to the following:

Nursing Diagnosis	Nursing Interventions
Deficient knowledge, related to issues of home care	Stress importance of activity and rest; provide aerobic management exercise schedule; caution patient to avoid jogging. Advise patient to take recommended medications. Instruct patient in how to maintain a healthy diet.

To prevent osteoporosis, advise women to have an adequate daily intake of calcium and vitamin D; to avoid smoking; to decrease caffeine intake; to decrease excess protein in the diet; and to engage in moderate activity such as walking, bike riding, or swimming at least 3 days a week.

After menopause, the usual recommended daily allowance is 1,000 mg of calcium in postmenopausal women taking estrogen and 1,500 mg in postmenopausal women who are not taking estrogen. Vitamin D, which increases calcium absorption, may be added to the daily regimen of postmenopausal women according to the physician's orders. Encourage the patient to make follow-up visits to the physician for guidance on medication, diet, and exercise regimen.

Prognosis

Osteoporosis is a chronic disorder, but vitamin D and calcium may help stop the rate of bone loss. In postmenopausal women, therapy with estrogen decreases the rate of bone resorption, but does not increase bone formation. Prevention of osteoporosis should begin before bone loss has occurred.

OSTEOMYELITIS

Etiology and Pathophysiology

Osteomyelitis (local or generalized infection of bone and bone marrow) can occur from bacteria introduced through trauma, such as a compound fracture or surgery. Also, bacteria may travel by the bloodstream from another site in the body to a bone, causing an infection. Staphylococci are the most common causative agents. Other invading organisms include *Streptococcus viridians, Escherichia coli, Mycobacterium tuberculosis, Neisseria gonorrhoeae, Pseudomonas* organisms, salmonellae, and fungi (Crowley, 2004).

Bacteria invade the bone, and bone tissue degenerates. If osteomyelitis becomes chronic, the bone tissue often is weak and predisposed to spontaneous fractures. Osteomyelitis can become chronic as a result of inadequate acute treatment. It is either a continuous persistent problem or a process of exacerbations and remissions. Over time, granulation tissue turns to scar tissue. This avascular scar tissue provides an ideal site for continued microorganism growth and is impenetrable to antibiotics.

Clinical Manifestations

The patient with osteomyelitis is subject to contractures in the affected extremity if positioned incorrectly. A new focus of infection can develop months and sometimes years after the initial infection is diagnosed.

Assessment

Collection of **subjective data** includes a complete history of injuries, surgical procedures, and diseases. Assess the patient's complaints of persistent, severe, and increasing bone pain and tenderness, as well as regional muscle spasm. Also inquire about any allergies, especially to medications, because antibiotics are given long term.

Collection of **objective data** includes careful inspection of any wounds. Assess the drainage for color, amount, and odor. Monitor vital signs for signs of infection (temperature elevation, tachycardia, and tachypnea). Note any edema, especially in joints with limited mobility.

Diagnostic Tests

Take a complete history, along with a physical examination. The physician orders radiographic studies and bone scan, CBC (leukocytosis may be present), ESR, and cultures of blood and drainage (if present).

Medical Management

Vigorous and prolonged intravenous antibiotic therapy will be used. Numerous antibiotics may be used depending on the pathogen. These antibiotics may include penicillin, nafcillin (Nafcil), neomycin, cephalexin (Keflex), cefoxitin (Mefoxin), and gentamicin (Garamycin) (Lewis et al., 2007). Parenteral antibiotics are usually necessary for several weeks but may be as long as 3 to 6 months. Bed rest is usually prescribed. For some patients, surgery may be performed to remove a fragment of necrotic bone that is partially or entirely detached from the surrounding or adjacent healthy bone **(sequestrum).**

Nursing Interventions and Patient Teaching

Nursing interventions include gentleness in moving and manipulating the diseased extremity, since pain is severe in the early phase of infection. The affected part may need absolute rest, with careful positioning using pillows and sandbags for good alignment. Often wounds are irrigated with hydrogen peroxide or other antiseptic or antibiotic solution and then covered with a sterile dressing, using strict surgical asepsis. Patients are placed on drainage and secretion precautions. Dietary planning includes a diet high in calories, protein, and vitamins.

Teaching includes information about the signs of infection, such as elevated temperature. Because chronic osteomyelitis may last a lifetime, warn the patient of the recurrence of signs and symptoms. Patients must avoid trauma to the affected bone because pathologic fractures are common.

Prognosis

Acute osteomyelitis may respond to treatment after several weeks. Chronic osteomyelitis may persist for years with exacerbations and remissions.

FIBROMYALGIA SYNDROME

Etiology and Pathophysiology

Fibromyalgia is a chronic syndrome of unknown etiology that causes pain in the muscles, bones, or joints. It is associated with soft tissue tenderness at multiple characteristic sites. It contributes to poor sleep, headaches, altered thought processes, and stiffness or muscle aches. Fibromyalgia affects more women than men, with up to 5% of the population affected. The disorder is more common in people between ages 20 and 50. Fibromyalgia has been referred to as **fibrositis, fibro-**

myositis, myofascial pain syndrome, and **psychogenic rheumatism.** Clinical symptoms of fibromyalgia syndrome (FMS) can overlap those of chronic fatigue syndrome (Hellmann, 2007). It is not considered life threatening and does not cause permanent damage. Stress response appears hyperactive in FMS patients (Lewis et al., 2007).

Clinical Manifestations

Patients with FMS frequently complain of a generalized achiness in axial locations, such as the neck and lower back, accompanied by stiffness that is worse in the morning. Factors that aggravate the condition include cold or humid weather, physical or mental fatigue, excess physical activity, and anxiety or stress.

Patients with FMS also experience irritable bowel syndrome, tension headaches beginning with neck discomfort, **paresthesia** (sensation of numbness or tingling) of the upper extremities with normal nerve conduction studies, and the sensation of edematous hands with no visible signs of edema. Complaints of fatigue are often associated with dysfunctional sleep. Patients complain of nonrestorative or nonrefreshing sleep.

Assessment

Collection of **subjective data** includes questioning the patient about muscle pain, often described as muscle ache; tension or migraine headaches; premenstrual tension; jaw pain; excessive fatigue; anxiety; and depression. Include questions about sensations of numbness, tingling, and perception of insects crawling on or under the skin. Complaints of being forgetful and unable to recall recent information—such as appointments, location of parked car, or how to get to familiar places—are significant.

Collection of **objective data** includes noting periodic limb movement, especially at night, or a persistent need to move the lower extremities day and night. Ask about sleep deprivation and the patient's ability to complete self-care activities.

Diagnostic Tests

No specific laboratory and radiographic tests diagnose FMS. Blood chemistry screening, a CBC, and ESR are normal in patients with FMS. A sleep study may be ordered in patients with a history suggestive of particular types of sleep disturbances; however, sleep study findings are typically normal in FMS patients.

Medical Management

The primary treatment approach includes patient education and reassurance. Inform the FMS patient that this is not a psychiatric disturbance and that symptoms are not uncommon in the general population. Although FMS has no single treatment, combining pharmacologic agents has been helpful. Tricyclic antidepressants are used in the treatment of uncontrollable pain disorders. Benefits of these agents include (1) antidepressant results, (2) antiinflammatory features, (3) central skeletal muscle relaxation, and (4) pain inhibition through suppression of serotonergic and noradrenergic pathways (Table 44-7).

Nursing Interventions and Patient Teaching

Nursing interventions are individualized, holistic, and goal oriented. Management of FMS focuses on functional goals that enable the patient to live as normal a life as possible. Treatment programs include education, exercise, and relaxation techniques. Patients are taught the basic principles of good sleep hygiene (see Patient Teaching box). Exercise programs consist of gentle, progressive stretching, beginning with a muscle warm-up through either gentle exercise or warm baths. Stretching helps release tight muscles. Nonimpact exercise such as swimming, walking, or stationary cycling is helpful.

Table 44-7 Medications for Fibromyalgia Syndrome

Medication	Action
Amitriptyline (Elavil, Endep)	Diminishes local pain and stiffness; improves sleep pattern
Cyclobenzaprine (Flexeril)	Diminishes local pain, improves sleep pattern, and decreases number of tender points
Clonazepam (Klonopin)	Decreases symptoms of constant leg movement, especially at night
Acetaminophen and tramadol	Used together or given alone for management of moderate to severe pain. Binds opioid receptors, inhibits reuptake of norepinephrine and serotonin.
Pregabalin (Lyrica)	An anticonvulsant that decreases pain severity and improves fatigue, sleep, and physical functioning
Tizanidine (Zanaflex)	Eases pain by lowering the substance (P) that participates in the transmission process of certain neurons; improves sleep and physical functioning
Sodium oxybate (Xyrem)	Improves deep sleep and growth hormone levels and helps reduce pain and fatigue
Duloxetine hydrochloride (Cymbalta)	Reduces pain in patients with fibromyalgia with or without having symptoms of major depression

Patient Teaching

Sleep Hygiene

- Maintain regular sleep patterns by going to bed and awaking the same time each day; avoiding long naps, and taking a hot bath within 2 hours of bedtime.
- Control environmental factors by avoiding large meals 2 to 3 hours before bedtime and keeping the sleep environment dark, quiet, and comfortable.
- Exercise regularly each day.
- Recognize how drugs such as nicotine, alcohol, and caffeine affect sleep.

Prognosis

Prognosis is generally excellent.

SURGICAL INTERVENTIONS FOR TOTAL KNEE OR TOTAL HIP REPLACEMENT

Surgical procedures can prevent progressive deformities; relieve pain; improve function; and correct deformities resulting from RA, osteoarthritis, or other disorders. Tendon transplants can replace damaged muscles. Patients with RA may need a synovectomy (excision of synovial membrane) to maintain joint function. An osteotomy (cutting into bone to correct bone or joint deformities) can improve function and relieve pain. **Arthrodesis** (surgical fusion of a joint) can be performed when severe joint destruction has occurred. Total joint replacement **arthroplasty** (repair or refashioning of one or both sides, parts, or specific tissue within a joint) is often required on the elbow, hip, knee, or shoulder joint to restore or increase mobility.

KNEE ARTHROPLASTY (TOTAL KNEE REPLACEMENT)

The knee joint may be replaced to restore motion, relieve pain, or correct deformity. Figures 44-11 and 44-12 show the tibial and femoral components of a knee prosthesis. Nursing interventions for the patient undergoing total knee replacement are shown in Box 44-4 (Figure 44-13).

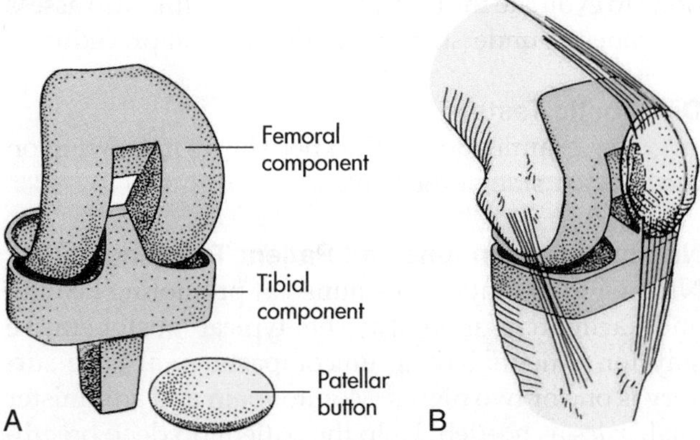

FIGURE 44-11 **A,** Tibial and femoral components of total knee prosthesis. Patellar button, made of polyethylene, protects the posterior surface of the patella from friction against the femoral component when the knee is moved through flexion and extension. **B,** Total knee prosthesis in place.

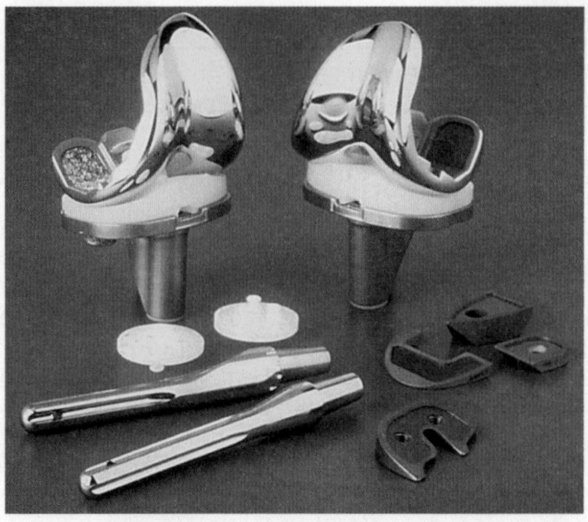

FIGURE 44-12 Total joint replacements: knee.

UNICOMPARTMENTAL KNEE ARTHROPLASTY

Unicompartmental knee replacement is also referred to as partial knee replacement. This modified surgical procedure is performed when only one of the compartments of the knee is affected by arthritic changes. If both sides of the bones in the knee, including the underside of the patella, are damaged, a total knee replacement is necessary (see Figure 44-12).

The knee has three compartments: (1) media, or inside, compartment; (2) lateral, or outside, compartment; and (3) patellofemoral compartment, which is where the kneecap rests. Minimally invasive knee surgery removes only the most damaged areas of cartilage; a small plastic disk replaces the worn cartilage, providing a new cushion between the bones.

The surgery is recommended for select patients ages 50 and older. Patients with RA or lupus erythematosus arthritis are not candidates for the surgery. The long-term benefits of the surgery will last from 5 to 15 years, compared with 20 to 30 years for a total knee procedure. Patients undergoing a unicompartmental knee replacement may eventually need a total knee replacement; at that point, the total knee replacement may be more difficult.

The partial knee surgery involves making a small incision over the knee and exposing the worn-out cartilage. The rough edges of the distal area of the femur and superior area of the tibia are cut flat and cleaned, and the unicompartmental device is put into place. Some of the devices are cemented in place.

Because the kneecap is not disrupted, the patient can resume walking 3 to 4 hours after the operation. There is minimal blood loss and reduced risk of deep-vein thrombosis. The surgery is performed in the hospital with the patient under a spinal block or

Box 44-4 Nursing Interventions for the Patient Undergoing Total Knee Replacement

PREOPERATIVE INTERVENTIONS

Same as for any major surgery (see Chapter 42).

POSTOPERATIVE INTERVENTIONS

1. Positioning
   a. Elevate the operative leg on pillows to enhance venous return for the first 24 hours only. Place pillows with caution to avoid flexing the knee.
   b. The patient may be turned from side to back to side.
2. Wound care
   a. Care of drains (usually Hemovac) as for total hip replacement.
   b. Assess patient for systemic evidence of loss of blood (hypotension, tachycardia) if bulky compression dressing is used because it may hold large quantities of drainage before drainage is visible.
   c. Remove bulky dressings before the patient begins continuous passive motion (CPM) flexion greater than 20 degrees.
3. Activity
   a. Passive flexion in a CPM machine within prescribed flexion-extension limits may be started in the postanesthesia care unit (see Figure 44-13). Patient's leg should remain in machine as much as tolerated (up to 22 hours per day) to facilitate even healing of tissue. The physical therapist increases extension on CPM as patient tolerates. (Once the large bulky dressing is replaced with a smaller dressing, flexion degree is increased.) When CPM is not occurring, patient's leg is extended with no pillow under leg.
   b. Encourage patient to perform active dorsiflexion of the ankles; quadriceps setting; and, after the drain is removed, straight leg–raising exercises.
   c. Patient begins active flexion exercises three or four times a day about the fifth postoperative day.
   d. Light weight bearing with an assistive device may be started as early as the first postoperative day and increased as the patient tolerates.
   e. Sitting in a chair with the leg elevated may be started on the first postoperative day.
   f. Encourage patient to wear a resting knee extension splint (immobilizer) on the operated leg until able to demonstrate quadriceps control (independent straight leg raising).
4. Pain control
   a. For initial control of pain, use opioids (usually with a patient-controlled epidural or patient-controlled analgesia) and positioning; gradually decrease medication to nonopioid analgesics as patient tolerates.
   b. Encourage patient to use cool applications at 40° F continuously on knee.
5. Discharge instructions
   a. Patient must observe partial weight-bearing restriction and use ambulatory aid for approximately 2 months after discharge.
   b. Patient should continue active flexion and straight leg–raising exercises at home.

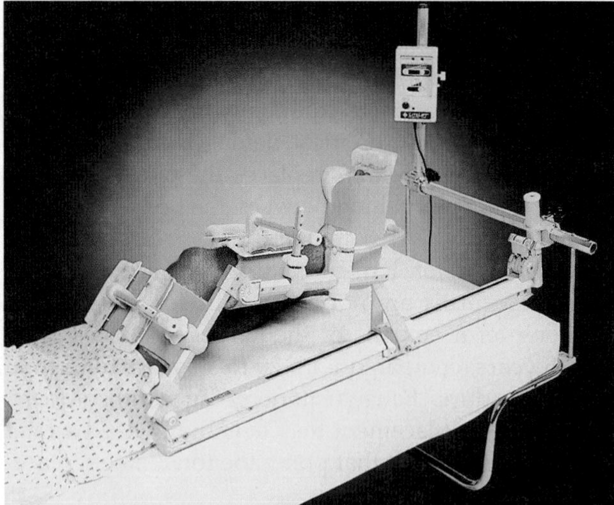

FIGURE 44-13 Continuous passive motion machine.

general anesthetic and takes approximately 60 to 90 minutes.

Assessment

Subjective data include a medical history of home medications, allergies, past surgeries, and significant medical problems such as RA or lupus erythematosus arthritis. Patients with these conditions are not candidates for the surgery. Assess the patient for complaints of pain on one side of the knee with weight bearing. Also gather information on the effectiveness of conservative treatments such as medications, cortisone injections, strengthening exercises, weight loss, and use of gait enhancers.

Objective data include vital signs and weight. Patients who are obese or have significant inflammation are not candidates for the surgery. Blood tests, electrocardiogram (ECG), and chest x-ray examination are done to evaluate the patient's state of health. Also assess the patient's understanding of the surgical procedure.

Diagnostic Tests

An x-ray examination of the knee shows narrowing on the affected side of the joint.

Nursing Interventions and Patient Teaching

Nursing interventions are aimed at promoting healing and facilitating mobility. The typical postoperative stay for patients having unicompartmental knee surgery is one or two nights. Monitor pain and administer analgesics as needed. Help the patient do deep breathing and coughing every 2 hours. Also encourage use of an incentive spirometer. Begin clear liquids and advance to regular diet as tolerated. Monitor IV fluids and antibiotics. Change the dressing as needed.

Patients resume weight bearing 3 to 5 hours postoperatively. Assess their ability to use a gait enhancer such as crutches. The first day after surgery the physical therapist begins teaching basic postoperative exercises. Before discharge, the patient must practice going up and down stairs. Also instruct the patient that prophylactic antibiotics are recommended before routine dental cleaning or any dental procedure up to 2 years following the surgery.

HIP ARTHROPLASTY (TOTAL HIP REPLACEMENT)

Hip arthroplasty, or total hip replacement, is commonly performed when arthritis involves the head of the femur and acetabulum. A Vitallium cup is cemented into the arthritic acetabulum to receive the head of the femur. Total hip replacement was originally developed by John Charnley, a British orthopedic surgeon. Several variations are now practiced, but each uses similar equipment. The Bechtol total hip system involves a white plastic cup cemented in place to replace the damaged acetabulum. A stainless steel or Vitallium ball on a stem replaces the head of the femur, which is surgically removed. The stem is cemented into the femoral canal, and the new head fits precisely into the plastic acetabulum, providing friction-free movement in the joint. The cement used is a soft, surgical bone cement that hardens quickly and stabilizes the prosthesis to prevent erosion of surrounding bone (Figure 44-14).

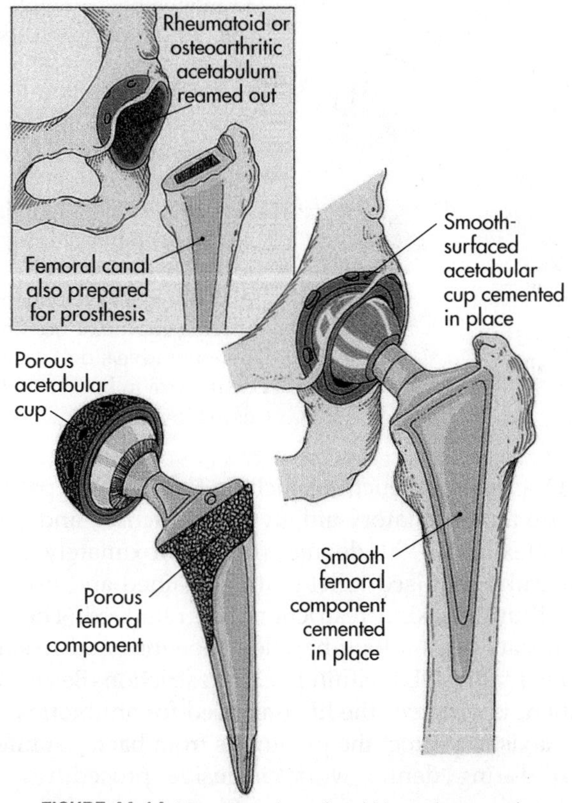

FIGURE 44-14 Hip arthroplasty (total hip replacement).

Assessment

Collection of **subjective data** includes assessing the patient's level of orientation because older adults can become disoriented from a change in the environment (home to hospital setting). Complaints of pain and numbness, tingling, or paresthesia indicate neurovascular impairment.

Collection of **objective data** includes assessment of the patient's compliance with nursing interventions to promote circulation; prevent impairment of skin integrity; and prevent hypostatic pneumonia by such means as coughing, turning (to the unaffected side; additional pillows are used to keep the affected leg abducted), deep breathing every 2 hours, and using an incentive spirometer. Assess vital signs for evidence of excessive bleeding, including hypotension, tachycardia, and tachypnea. Decreased urinary output is indicative of hypovolemia. Carefully assess drainage of the surgical wound at least every 4 hours. Hemovacs or other suction devices are placed in the wound during surgery to provide closed-wound suction. Assess approximation of the incision line and signs of inflammation (erythema, edema, fever, and pain). Also assess traction (if used) for the correct amount of weight, the proper alignment, and maintenance of the affected leg in an abducted position. Look for any reaction to the cement, signs of phlebitis (edema, erythema, and pain), and urinary retention (indwelling catheters may be used for the first 24 to 48 hours).

Nursing Interventions and Patient Teaching

Nursing interventions are aimed at promoting healing and facilitating mobility. Teach the patient to do isometric exercises on the quadriceps and gluteal muscles of the affected extremity by keeping the toes pointed up, flexing the ankles, and flexing and extending the knee of the unaffected extremity. Carefully document the patient's I&O. Apply thigh-high antiembolism stockings before or during surgery. The physician will order a plan of weight bearing and physical therapy; help explain this to the patient.

Additional nursing activities include emptying and recording Hemovac drainage every 4 hours (if ordered) or as needed. Give oxygen at 1 to 2 L per nasal cannula as needed. Instruct the patient in the use of the incentive spirometer every 2 to 4 hours, and help the patient do deep breathing and coughing every 2 hours.

Perform neurovascular checks every hour for 24 hours, then every 2 hours for the next 24 hours, and then every 4 hours. Check vital signs every 4 hours. Also carefully assess the patient for pain control. This includes monitoring patient-controlled epidural (PCE), patient-controlled analgesia (PCA), or oral medications, whichever is prescribed.

Change the dressing using surgical asepsis after 24 to 48 hours as ordered; reinforce the dressing if necessary. Maintain the position of the operative area with a splint, an abduction pillow (Figure 44-15), an immobilizer, or a brace; turn the patient to the unoperated side.

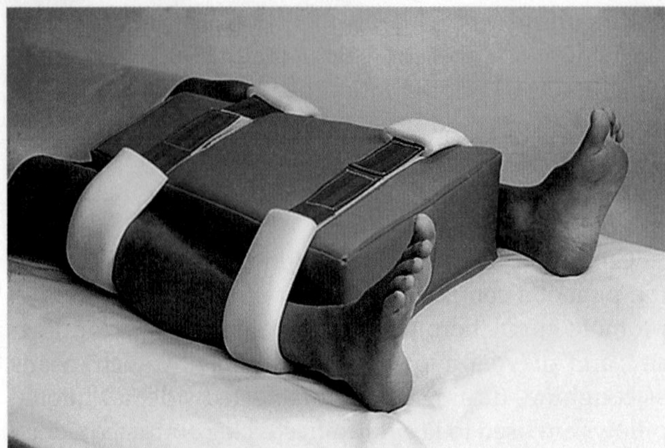

FIGURE 44-15 Maintaining postoperative abduction after total hip replacement.

Begin clear liquids, and advance to regular diet as tolerated. Encourage fluid intake and high-fiber foods (if tolerated) to prevent constipation; administer rectal suppository if needed to empty rectum.

Maintain bed rest for 24 to 48 hours (depending on the security of the replacement prostheses and physician's choice). The patient should be up but not bearing weight on the operative limb after the bed rest order expires. Some physicians may permit touch-down weight bearing. Physical therapy exercises begin on the second postoperative day. The exercises are either active or passive to all joints, excluding the operated joint, and include quadriceps setting, straight leg raising, flexion and extension, or other individually prescribed exercises. The patient should be up with walker or crutches four times daily; increase ambulation as the patient is able with up to 25 pounds of weight bearing on the operative limb, gradually increasing to full weight bearing with crutches or a walker.

Have the patient sit in a chair for only 10 to 15 minutes two or three times daily for the first week, then for 20 to 30 minutes four times daily. The patient should wear antiembolism hose or a pneumatic stocking pump system. Use of a toilet-seat riser prevents hyperflexion of the hip after total replacement.

Nursing diagnoses and interventions for the patient with a total hip replacement include but are not limited to the following:

Nursing Diagnoses	Nursing Interventions
Pain, related to: • preoperative arthritic pain necessitating surgery • postoperative hip incisional pain secondary to bone • soft tissue trauma of surgery	Explain analgesic therapy, including medication, dose, and schedule. If patient is a candidate for PCA or PCE, explain the concept and routine. Respond quickly to pain complaints. Obtain pain rating scale from patient. Instruct patient to request analgesic before pain is severe. Administer analgesics as ordered and per hospital policy or procedure. Encourage use of analgesics 30 to 45 minutes before therapy. Unrelieved pain hinders rehabilitation progress. Provide eggcrate mattress. Change position (within hip precautions) every 2 hours. Document all responses to analgesics.
Impaired physical mobility, related to surgical procedure and discomfort	Allow patient to dangle feet at bedside several minutes before getting out of bed. Reinforce physical therapist's instructions for exercises and ambulation techniques and devices. Maintain weight-bearing status on affected extremity as prescribed. Consistent instructions from interdisciplinary team members promote safe, secure rehabilitation environment. Keep abduction pillow between legs while turning in bed (see Figure 44-15). Do not have the patient lie on the operative side. Maintain the leg in abduction when the patient is lying supine or on the nonoperative side. Use trapeze in bed to assist in mobility.

Discharge instructions include teaching the patient to use an ambulatory aid, avoid adduction, and limit hip flexion to 90 degrees for approximately 2 to 3 months. A raised toilet seat is obtained and used at home until flexion restrictions are removed. The patient may need a long-handled shoehorn and reacher to facilitate ADLs within flexion restriction. Be certain patient is aware of the lifelong need for antibiotic prophylaxis to protect the prosthesis from bacterial infection during dental work, intrusive procedures, or surgery.

FRACTURES

FRACTURE OF THE HIP

Etiology and Pathophysiology

Hip fractures are the most common type of fracture treated in the hospital (see Life Span Considerations box and Health Promotion box). Women may be at a higher risk because of their increased risk for osteoporosis and longer life expectancy compared with men. Fractures of the hip include intracapsular fracture, when the femur is broken inside the joint, and fractures of the femoral head or neck that are contained within the hip capsule (Figure 44-16, *A* to *C*). Intracapsular fractures may disrupt the blood supply to the head of the femur, which subsequently develops avascular necrosis (Figures 44-17 and 44-18). Therefore fractures of the head or proximal femoral neck may be treated with insertion of a femoral prosthesis (Figure 44-19). The more common type of hip fracture is an extracapsular fracture, one that occurs outside the hip joint capsule. These are referred to as intertrochanteric or subtrochanteric fractures (Figure 44-16, *D*). These fractures heal well without vascular necrosis with the use of compression screws or nails because the blood supply to the fracture site comes from the surrounding vessels outside the capsule (see Figures 44-17 and

Life Span Considerations

Older Adults

Musculoskeletal Disorder

- Physiologic changes of aging result in decreased joint flexibility and muscular strength.
- Changes in bone mass, particularly in older women, increase the risk of fractures. Hip fractures and compression fractures of the spine are most common.
- Degenerative joint disease related to "wear and tear" on joints is common. Joint replacement is increasingly common and has done much to improve mobility and the quality of life.
- Changes in the foot can occur from a lifetime of use, poorly fitted shoes, or heredity. Bunions and hammertoe are commonly seen in older adults. These may cause pain and lead to decreased mobility. Encourage older adults to wear properly fitted shoes to reduce discomfort. If discomfort is severe, surgical correction may be necessary.
- Check the homes of older adults for safety hazards such as rugs that could cause falls.
- Older adults should avoid climbing unsteady or uneven surfaces because coordination and balance change with age and falls may result.
- Instruct older adults in the correct use of assistive devices such as canes or walkers. Encourage them to use these regularly to prevent injury.

Health Promotion

Hip Fracture

- Factors that contribute to the incidence of hip fracture in older adults include a propensity to fall, inability to correct a postural imbalance, inadequacy of local tissue shock absorbers (e.g., fat, muscle bulk), and underlying skeletal weakness.
- Factors that increase the risk of older adults falling include gait and balance problems, decreased vision and hearing, diminished reflexes, orthostatic hypotension, and medication use.
- Leading hazards that increase the risk of falls are loose rugs and slippery or uneven surfaces.
- Many falls are associated with getting in or out of a chair or bed.
- Falls to the side, the most common type in the frail elderly, are more likely to result in a hip fracture than forward falls.
- Two important factors influencing the amount of force imposed on the hip are the presence of energy-absorbing soft tissue over the greater trochanter and the state of leg muscle contraction at the time of the fall.
- Many older adults have poor muscle tone, an important factor in the severity of a fall.
- Older women often have osteoporosis and accompanying low bone density, which increases the risk of hip fracture.
- Targeted interventions to reduce hip fractures in older adults include a variety of strategies. Calcium and vitamin D supplementation, estrogen replacement, and drug therapy have been shown to decrease bone loss or increase bone density and decrease the likelihood of fracture. Be vigilant in planning interventions for the older adult that are known to reduce the incidence of hip fracture.

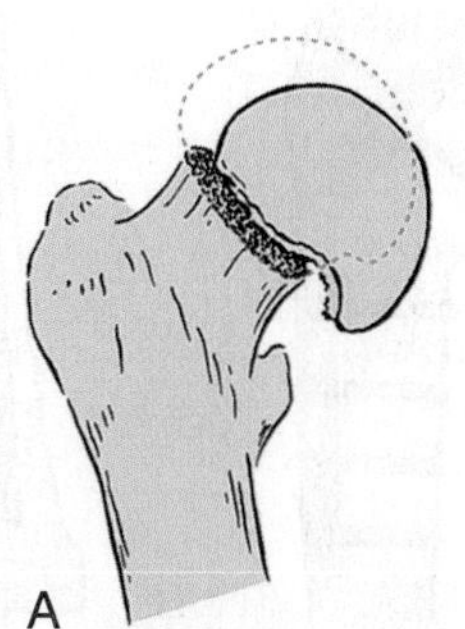

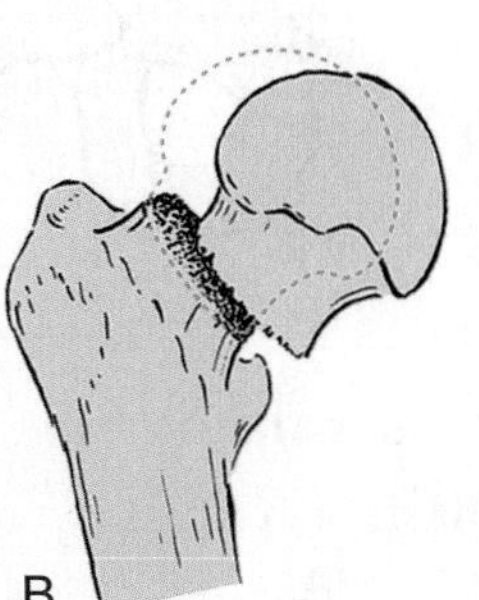

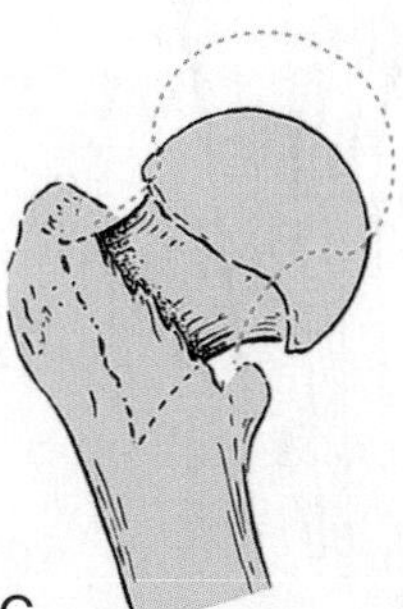

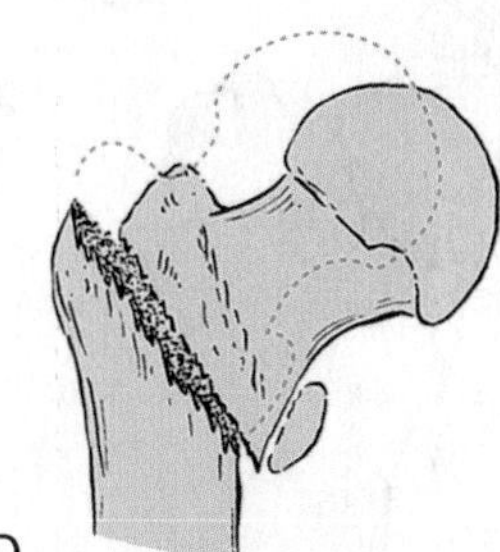

FIGURE 44-16 Fractures of the hip. **A,** Subcapital fracture. **B,** Transcervical fracture. **C,** Impacted fracture of the base of the neck. **D,** Intertrochanteric fracture.

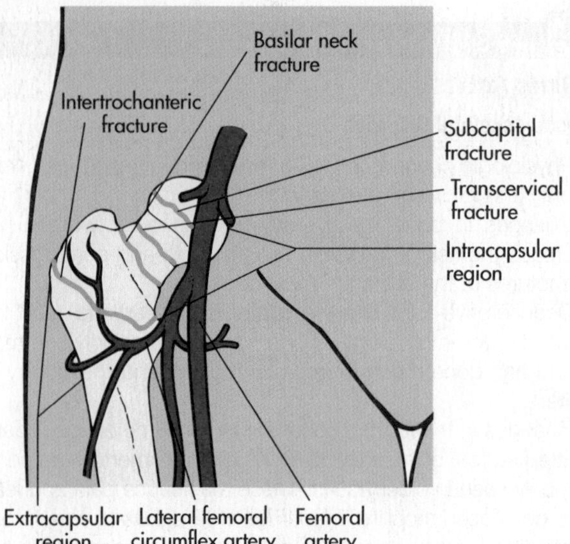

FIGURE 44-17 Femur with location of various types of fractures.

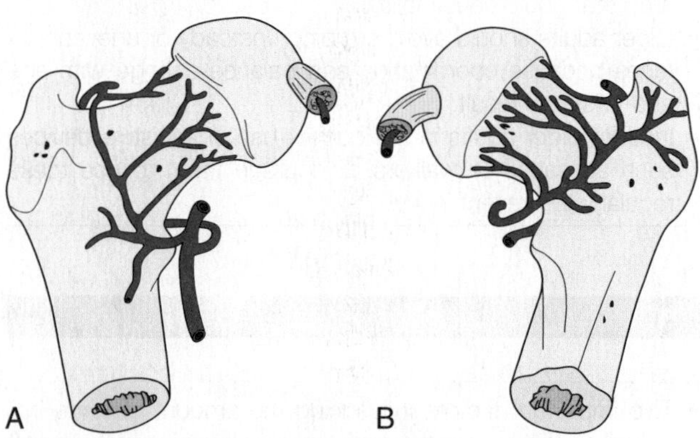

FIGURE 44-18 **A,** Anterior arterial blood supply to hip joint. **B,** Posterior arterial blood supply to hip joint.

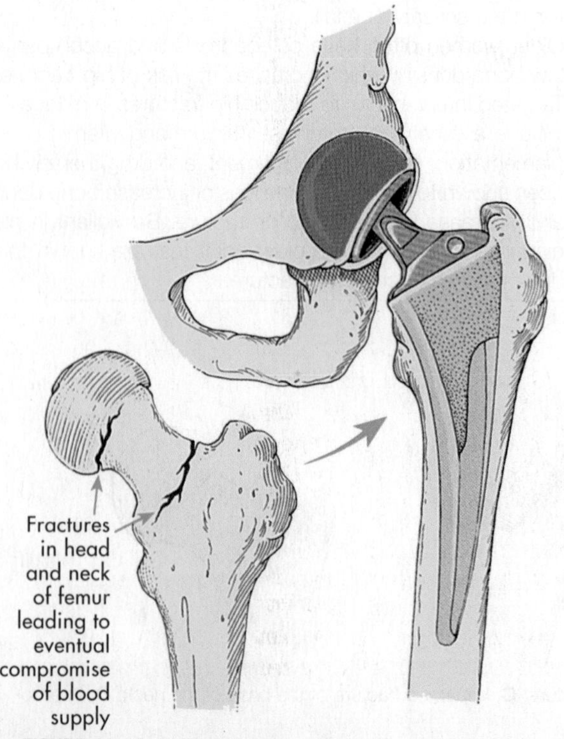

FIGURE 44-19 Bipolar hip replacement (hemiarthroplasty).

44-18). Side plates attached to the nails help maintain a stable reduction while healing progresses (Figure 44-20, *A*). An intertrochanteric fracture occurs below the lesser trochanter and is frequently seen in younger patients suffering from hip trauma (see Figure 44-16, *D*).

Clinical Manifestations

Signs and symptoms of hip fracture are severe pain and tenderness in the region of the fracture site or inability to move the leg voluntarily, and shortening or external rotation of the leg.

Assessment

Subjective data include an accurate history of the events before the injury. Assess the patient's level of orientation. Disorientation can occur, especially in older adults when they are in pain, are anxious, or are in an unfamiliar environment. The patient's medical and surgical history is significant, as is any family history of bone disease. Patients with gastroesophageal reflux disease who are taking antacids or using proton pump inhibitors are at increased risk of hip fractures, since these drugs cause a malabsorption of calcium.

Signs and symptoms of a fracture vary with the type and location of the break. Usually the patient has some degree of discomfort that may be more pronounced with slight movement of the affected part. Most patients complain of pain in the affected leg after sustaining a fractured hip, although patients suffering from an impacted intracapsular fracture have little pain, if any, immediately after the fracture. Assess for edema, tenderness, muscle spasms, deformity, and loss of function. Patients may say they heard a "snap" or "pop" at the time the bone was injured. Impaired sensation may indicate nerve damage from the bone fragments "pinching" or severing the nerve.

Collection of **objective data** includes assessment for soft tissue injury with erythema or ecchymosis noted.

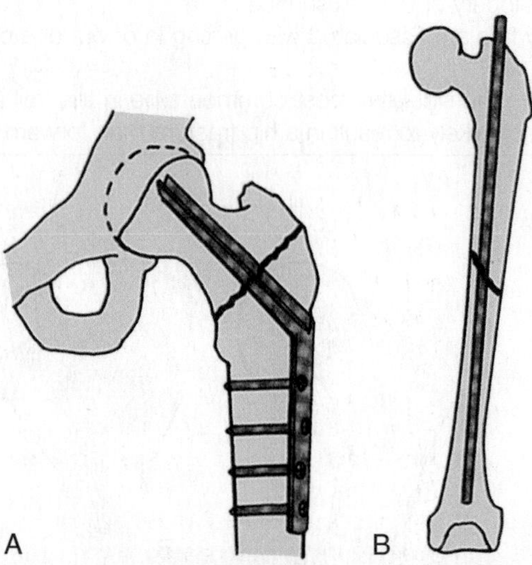

FIGURE 44-20 **A,** Neufeld nail and screws in repair of intertrochanteric fracture. **B,** Küntscher nail (intramedullary rod) used in repair of midshaft femoral fracture.

Look for differences between the injured limb and the uninjured limb. A change in the curvature or length of bone may indicate fracture. The affected leg is shorter, usually externally rotated approximately 90 degrees, and slightly flexed after an extracapsular hip fracture. With an intracapsular fracture, the upper thigh is more edematous than the area below it, and the affected leg is shortened with external rotation. Subtrochanteric fractures cause excessive bleeding into the soft tissue, and the affected leg is shortened and rotated anteriorly. Crepitus may be felt or heard as the broken bone ends rub together. Assess neurovascular status of the extremity (Box 44-5).

Keep the injured part still because movement of a fractured bone can cause additional damage and may turn a closed fracture into an open fracture. Also assess the patient's nutritional status. Both thin and obese patients are at risk for impaired skin integrity if bed rest is ordered. After the fracture is reduced, regularly inspect skin areas in contact with cast edges or traction apparatus for signs of neurovascular compromise. Also note that patients suffering from any trauma are at risk for shock. Treating the shock takes precedence over treating the fracture.

Box 44-5 Circulation Check (Neurovascular Assessment)

- Circulation check is also known as a neurovascular assessment. The mnemonic CMS indicates the need to check circulation, motion, and sensation. The assessment is made on patients following musculoskeletal trauma; postoperatively if damage to nerves and blood vessels is suspected; and after casting, splinting, or bandaging.
- Assess the patient every 15 to 30 minutes for several hours and every 3 to 4 hours thereafter, with proper documentation of the findings.
- **Subjective data** include complaints of numbness or tingling not relieved by flexing the fingers and toes and repositioning the extremity. **Objective data** include cool, pale, or cyanotic skin above or below the altered site; edema; greater than 2 seconds capillary refill time; and absent or diminished pulses.
- Remember the seven Ps when completing the assessment:
  1. Pulselessness
  2. Paresthesia (numbness or tingling sensation)
  3. Paralysis or paresis
  4. Polar temperature
  5. Pallor
  6. Puffiness (edema)
  7. Pain
- Complaints of numbness or tingling may result from general decreased mobility and may be relieved by flexing the fingers and toes and repositioning the extremity. However, if the numbness and tingling are not relieved by these measures and the extremity feels cool to the touch, is slow in capillary refill, has diminished or absent pulses, and appears pale or cyanotic, these are significant symptoms of neurovascular impairment and the findings must be reported immediately.

Diagnostic Tests

Diagnosis is confirmed by radiographic examination of the injured part. Blood tests, such as hemoglobin values, often show decreased laboratory values because of bleeding at the fracture site; the blood glucose level may be elevated because of the stress of the trauma.

Medical Management

Surgical repair is the preferred method of managing intracapsular and extracapsular hip fractures. Surgical treatment enables the patient to get out of bed sooner and decreases the major complications associated with immobility.

The affected extremity may be temporarily immobilized by either Buck's or Russell's traction until the patient's physical condition is stabilized and surgery can be scheduled. The choice of fixation device depends on the fracture location and the potential for avascular necrosis of the femoral head and neck. The use of these devices is called internal fixation. Prosthetic implants, such as the **bipolar hip replacement (hemiarthroplasty)** (see Figure 44-19), are used to replace the femoral head and neck in fractures when the vascular supply to the femoral head may be compromised. A Neufeld nail and screws are used in the repair of intertrochanteric fractures (see Figure 44-20, *A*). A Küntscher nail (intramedullary rod) is used to repair midshaft femoral fractures (see Figure 44-20, *B*). Sliding nails are used in repair of intertrochanteric fractures. Sliding nails usually permit the patient to bear weight to some degree because they "give" slightly without shifting their placement or penetrating the femur. Bone grafts, either autograft (patient's bone) or allograft (cadaver bone), may be used with internal fixation devices when excessive bone is lost at the fracture site. If a stable reduction cannot be achieved, the physician may do an arthroplasty (surgical reconstruction of a joint). Immobilization devices, such as casts or splints, may also be used with open reduction.

Nursing Interventions and Patient Teaching

Nursing interventions for a fractured hip are concerned with preventing shock and further complications. A primary concern is maintaining proper alignment through traction and abduction of the hip when turning a patient with a fractured hip from side to side. Some physicians do not want patients turned onto their sides for several days after surgery; others may order the patient to be turned only on the unoperated side. It is important to know the orders and to educate patients about activity restrictions. Patients who have had internal fixation for a fractured hip should avoid elevating the affected extremity when sitting. Elevate the head of the bed a maximum of 45 degrees to avoid acute flexion of the hip and strain on the fixation device. Instruct the patient *not* to cross the legs because this can adduct the affected extremity and dislocate the hip. Limit weight bearing on the hip by providing walking assists such as a walker or crutches.

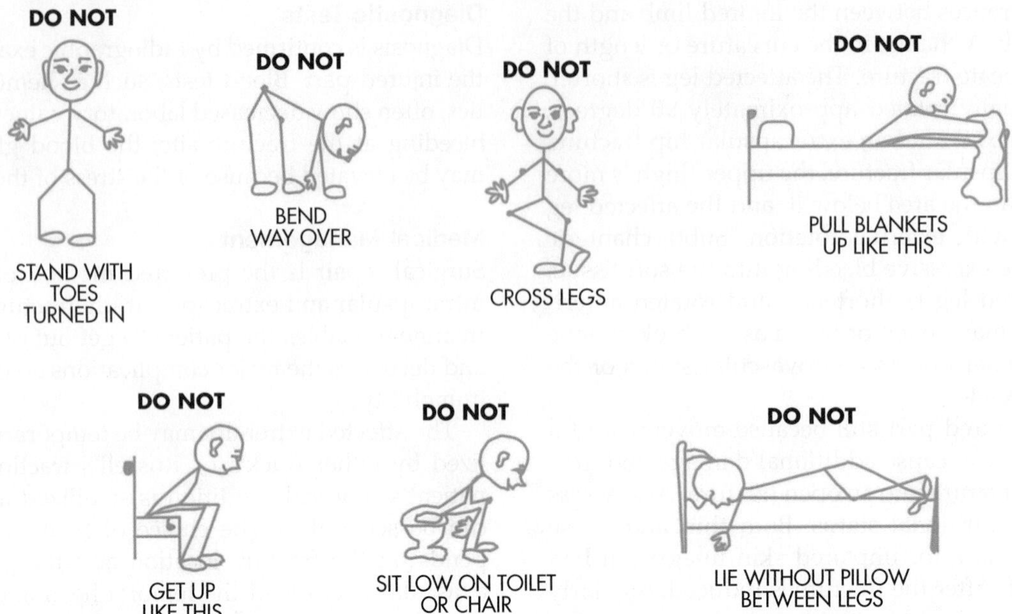

FIGURE 44-21 Instruction sheet for the patient with a bipolar hip replacement (hip prosthetic implant).

Postoperative interventions for a patient with hip fracture repair include wound assessment with special attention to color, amount, and odor of exudate. Assess vital signs, as well as the suture line for approximation of skin edges and intact sutures or staples, at least every 8 hours. Jackson-Pratt drainage tubes or Hemovacs are often used and must be assessed for amount and color of wound drainage at least every 4 hours. Document I&O to help the physician establish the need for IV fluid therapy. Encourage the use of incentive spirometers to aid in adequate respiratory ventilation and prevent pneumonia. Turning and moving the patient on schedule will maintain skin integrity and promote circulation.

Leg manipulation during surgery and immobility afterward place the patient at risk for deep-vein thrombosis and pulmonary embolism. Antiembolism stockings, Ace wraps, or pneumatic compression stockings and foot and leg exercises increase venous flow to the heart. Remove the stockings once each shift to assess for compression points and skin integrity. Anticoagulation therapy with enoxaparin (Lovenox), aspirin, or warfarin (Coumadin) is often prescribed.

Special postoperative instructions regarding proper positioning, sitting, and turning are required for patients who have had a prosthetic implant or bipolar hip replacement (Figure 44-21 and Patient Teaching box on postoperative care of the patient who had a fractured hip). Isometric exercises are done on the quadriceps and gluteal muscles to strengthen the muscles used for walking (see Patient Teaching box on quadriceps setting exercises).

Nursing interventions also involve use of an abduction splint (a wedge-shaped foam bolster or pillow) for 7 to 10 days to ensure postoperative maintenance of leg abduction and to prevent dislocation of the prosthesis. Place the abduction splint between the patient's legs when in a supine position. Turn the patient with the extremities maintained in proper alignment by using the log-rolling procedure with the assistance of at least two nurses. Most physicians order the patient to be turned toward the unoperated side; check each order by the physician. Transfer the patient from bed to chair on the unoperated side by pivoting on the unaffected leg. The injured leg is kept extended forward to avoid extreme hip flexion and possible dislocation of the prosthesis. Provide a chair with a firm, nonreclining seat and arms; elevate the sitting surfaces as necessary with pillows or foam cushions to keep the angle of the hip within the prescribed limits when the patient is sitting. In general, patients who have had *any* kind of internal fixation for a fractured hip should avoid elevation of the operated leg when sitting in a chair, since this puts excessive strain on the fixation device (Nursing Care Plan 44-1).

Patient Teaching

Quadriceps Setting Exercises

Quadriceps and gluteal muscles must be strong for ambulation. The quadriceps muscles stabilize the knee joint. Teach the patient to do the following exercises 10 to 15 times hourly:

- To strengthen quadriceps muscles, push the knee down against the mattress while raising the heel of the foot off the bed; maintain the contraction for a count of five and relax for a count of five.
- For gluteal setting exercises, contract, or "pinch," the buttocks together for a count of five, then relax for a count of five.
- Strengthen the unaffected leg by pushing down against the footboard, holding for a count of five, releasing for a count of five, and repeating.

Nursing Care Plan 44-1 The Patient with a Fractured Hip

Ms. Drake, age 72, fell in her kitchen while removing cookies from the oven. She sustained a subcapital fracture of the right hip. Ms. D. is scheduled in the morning for a bipolar (hemiarthroplasty) prosthesis.

NURSING DIAGNOSIS *Ineffective tissue perfusion, related to vascular injury or interruption of arterial and venous flow secondary to edema*

Patient Goals and Expected Outcomes	Nursing Interventions	Evaluation and Rationale
Patient's circulation will be maintained to fulfill body requirements	Palpate site for warmth. Observe site for color. Apply moderate pressure to nailbed, and subsequently observe speed of capillary refill. Assess pedal pulse bilaterally every 4 hours. Question patient regarding pain and paresthesia in injured part. Apply antiembolism stockings as ordered.	Distal pulses palpable; toes symmetrical, warm, dry, and pink; sensation and mobility intact
	Help and teach patient to cough every 2 hours and deep breathe every hour. Monitor vital signs every 2 to 4 hours.	Able to cough and deep breathe with assistance; oxygen saturation 92%, lungs clear

NURSING DIAGNOSIS *Deficient knowledge, related to home care management*

Patient Goals and Expected Outcomes	Nursing Interventions	Evaluation and Rationale
Patient and/or significant other will demonstrate understanding of home care and follow-up instructions through interactive discussion and return demonstration	Stress importance of prescribed rehabilitation plan of activity, rest, and exercise.	Patient demonstrates ambulation with walker, exercises, transfers, and precautions, verbalizes understanding of discharge instructions and home care.
	Provide diet instructions on type and amount of food to eat, and advise patient to avoid weight gain if applicable.	Discusses correct foods to eat for therapeutic results.
	Discuss medications: name, purpose, schedule, dosage, and side effects.	Verbalizes knowledge of medications for purpose, dosage, side effects and correct schedule to prevent any drug errors.
	Discuss signs and symptoms to report to physician: severe pain; changes in temperature, color, or sensation in extremity; malodorous drainage from wound.	Verbalizes knowledge of need to report abnormalities to the physician including severe pain, abnormal temperature, color or tingling in affected extremity as well as abnormal wound drainage.
	Stress home safety factors such as elimination of throw rugs, use of safety bars on the bathtub, elevated toilet seats.	Discusses home preparations for safety to include: removal of throw rugs, placement of safety bars on bathtub and availability of toilet riser. Safety knowledge will prevent accidents
	Encourage follow-up visits with physician.	Notes the importance of postoperative follow-up visits with physician. Promotes postoperative recovery.

Critical Thinking Questions

1. The first postoperative evening, Ms. Drake is restless and disoriented. What nursing interventions are needed to prevent dislocation of her bipolar hip prosthesis?
2. Ms. Drake is in her third postoperative day, and the nurse notes an erythematous area on her coccyx. What therapeutic measures can prevent skin impairment?
3. On Ms. Drake's third postoperative day, she complains of pain in her right calf when the nurse performs dorsiflexion. What is the most appropriate immediate action by the nurse?

Prognosis

Complications of hip fractures are the most common cause of death after age 75. Hip fractures in older adults are often complicated by other medical conditions such as diabetes mellitus, cardiac problems (e.g., heart failure), and neurologic disorders (e.g., stroke). A large bone such as the hip heals slowly in older patients, and this predisposes them to various complications. They are at high risk for pneumonia, deep-vein thrombosis, fat embolus, pulmonary embolus, impaired skin integrity, urinary retention, constipation, mental disorientation, and depression.

OTHER FRACTURES

Etiology and Pathophysiology

A fracture is a traumatic injury to a bone in which the continuity of the tissue of the bone is broken. Most fractures result from an insult to the bone, such as a forceful blow (twisting or crushing), which places more stress on the bone than it can absorb. Fractures that occur without trauma are referred to as pathologic or spontaneous fractures and can be caused by a weakening of the bone by osteoporosis, metastatic cancer and tumors of the bone, Cushing's syndrome, malnutrition, and complications of long-term steroid therapy.

Fractures may result from (1) direct force, which causes a fracture at the site of the trauma; (2) torsion, as in a twisting injury in which the fracture occurs at a point remote from the trauma (e.g., forceful twisting of the wrist may fracture the arm); or (3) violent contractions involving highly developed muscles (e.g., severe muscle spasms may cause a fracture in a paraplegic patient).

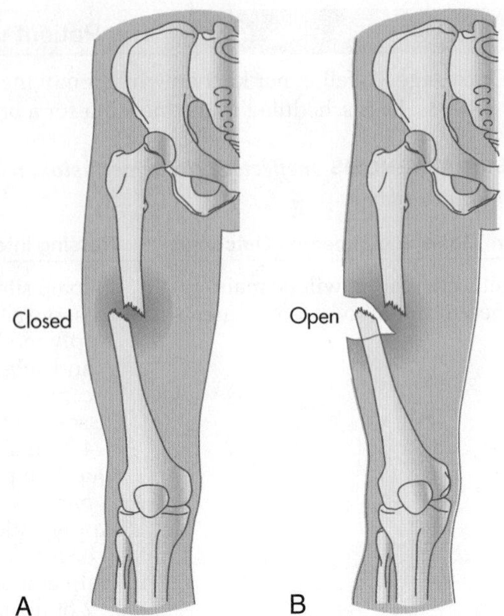

FIGURE 44-22 **A,** Closed fracture. **B,** Open fracture with bone protruding through skin.

The more than 150 types of fractures can be classified in various ways. First, they are described as either closed (simple) or open (compound) (Figure 44-22). In a closed fracture, the bone has not protruded through the skin; in an open fracture, it has. Open fractures are more serious because they involve more soft tissue damage, require surgical treatment to repair, and are prone to infections. A bullet wound (where the injury is directed inward) has fractured a bone is another example of an open fracture. A closed fracture does not involve a break in the

Patient Teaching

Postoperative Care for the Patient Who Had a Fractured Hip

OPEN REDUCTION WITH INTERNAL FIXATION

Teaching for patients who had a fractured hip and received an internal fixation with nails or pins would include the following (see Figure 44-20, *A*):

- Assess patient's ability to understand instructions and limitations.
- Help patient dangle feet at bedside on first postoperative day, then to pivot to chair with no weight on operative leg, or touch-down weight if allowed.
- Stress that the operative foot should be placed on floor but weight should be borne on the unoperative leg (refer to limb as either left or right leg so the patient understands) to maintain safety in care.
- Turn patient every 2 hours; prop with pillows between legs or under the back to maintain position.
- Assist with range-of-motion exercises to maintain muscle strength.
- Help physical therapist walk patient with walker and with limited weight placed on operative limb (if assistance is needed) for comfort and safety.
- Encourage patient and family members to walk together for patient's safety. Instruct family about weight-bearing techniques for clarity and safety.
- If a stable plate and screw fixation is used to repair the fractured hip, the patient should not bear weight for 6 weeks to 3 months to protect the fracture site.
- A telescoping nail fixation allows minimal to partial weight bearing during the first 6 weeks to 3 months.

HIP PROSTHETIC IMPLANT

Teaching for patients who had a fractured hip and received a hip prosthetic implant (hemiarthroplasty) includes the following (see Figure 44-19):

- Avoid hip flexion beyond 60 degrees for approximately 10 days.
- Avoid hip flexion beyond 90 degrees for 2 to 3 months.
- Avoid adduction of the affected leg beyond midline for 2 to 3 months.
- Maintain partial weight-bearing status for approximately 2 to 3 months.
- Avoid positioning on the operative side in bed.
- Maintain abduction of the hip by using a wedge-shaped foam bolster or pillows arranged in a wedge; this will require nursing assistance.

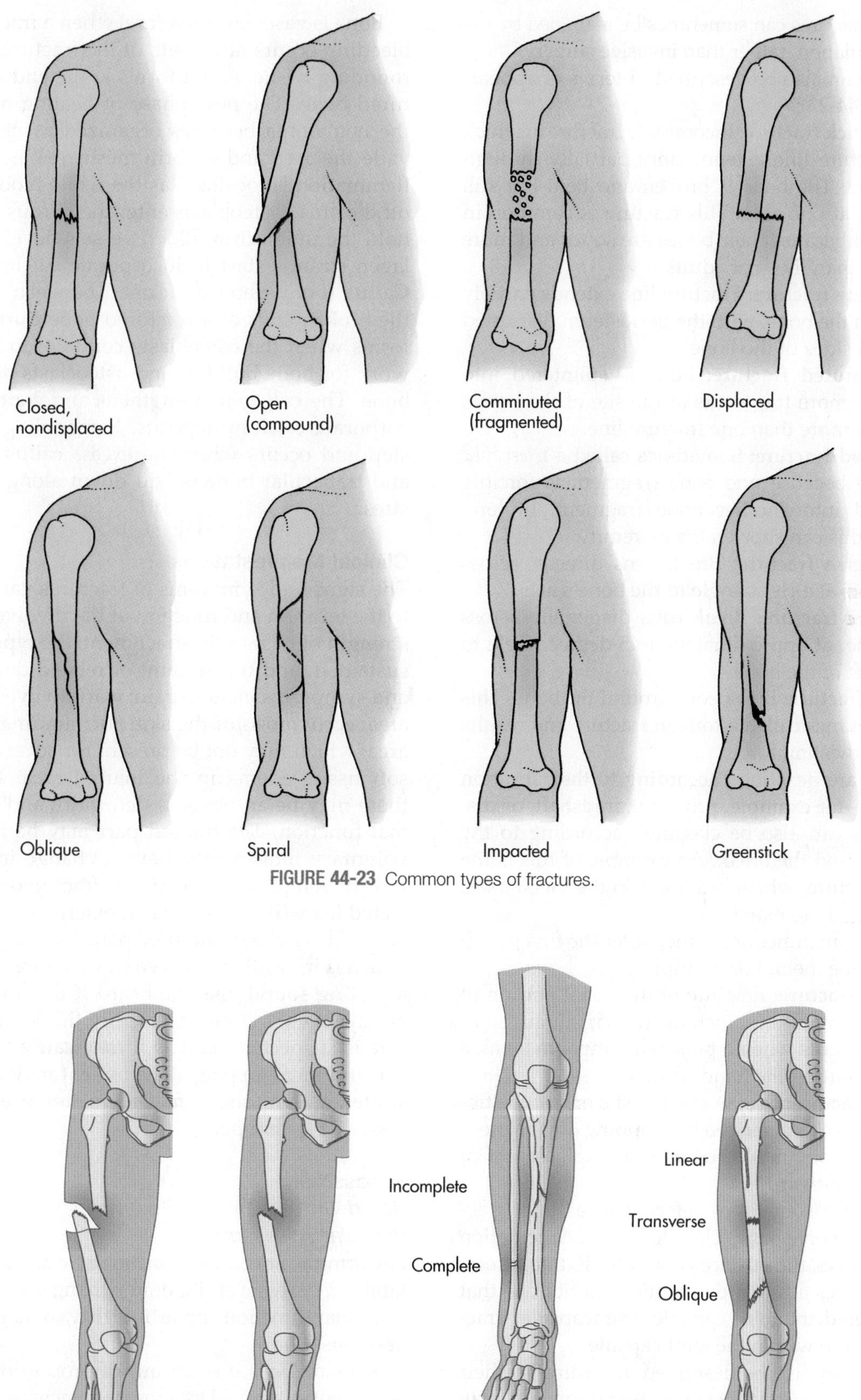

FIGURE 44-23 Common types of fractures.

FIGURE 44-24 Bone fractures. A, Open. B, Closed. C, Incomplete and complete. D, Linear, transverse, and oblique.

skin. These fractures can sometimes be realigned by external manipulation, rather than invasive surgery.

Fractures can also be described in terms of appearance (Figure 44-23):

- **Greenstick fracture:** Incomplete fracture in which the fracture line extends only partially through the bone. The bone is broken and bent but still secured at one side. This fracture is common in children because their bones are softer and more flexible than those of adults.
- **Complete fracture:** Fracture line extends entirely through the bone, with the periosteum disrupted on both sides of the bone.
- **Comminuted fracture:** Bone is splintered into three or more fragments at the site of the break. There is more than one fracture line.
- **Impacted fracture:** Sometimes called a *telescoped* fracture because one bone fragment is forcibly wedged into another bone fragment. In long bones, this can shorten the extremity.
- **Transverse fracture:** Break runs directly across the bone, at a right angle to the bone's axis.
- **Oblique fracture:** Break runs diagonally across the bone, at approximately a 45-degree angle to the shaft of the bone.
- **Spiral fracture:** Break coils around the bone. This is sometimes called a torsion fracture and results from a twisting force.

Fractures are described according to their location on the bone—for example, proximal, midshaft, or distal. Fractures can also be classified according to the force that caused the break. An example of this is the marching fracture, which can occur in the metatarsals as a result of a long march.

Fractures sometimes are named after the first physician to describe them. For example:

- **Colles' fracture:** Fracture of the distal portion of the radius within 1 inch of the wrist joint; commonly occurs when a person attempts to break a fall by putting the hands down.
- **Pott's fracture:** Occurs at the distal end of the fibula and is characterized by chipping off of a piece of the medial malleolus with a displacement of the foot outward.

Fractures are sometimes referred to as joint fractures if they involve or are close to a joint. Articulation fracture involves the surface of a joint. Extracapsular fracture involves a fracture near the joint but one that has not entered the joint capsule. Intracapsular fracture is a fracture within the joint capsule.

Fractures can also be described according to their displacement. Figure 44-24 shows that fragments may be displaced sideways, can override the opposite fractured surface, may angulate or create a bend in the bone, and may rotate away from the fracture site. When a bone is displaced, the bone fragments can cause soft tissue damage. The patient experiences severe pain, edema, and muscle spasms in the early stages of healing.

Bone is vascular; therefore, when a fracture occurs, bleeding occurs at the site of the fracture and in surrounding tissue. A clot forms at the ends of the fractured bone. The next phase of healing occurs when the hematoma becomes organized as fibroblasts invade the area and a fibrin meshwork is formed. Inflammation is localized as the white blood cells wall off the area. Osteoblasts enter the fibrous area to help hold the union firm. Blood vessels develop, and collagen strands start to incorporate calcium deposits. **Callus** (bony deposits formed between and around the broken ends of a fractured bone during healing) forms when the osteoblasts continue to lay the network for bone buildup and osteoclasts destroy dead bone. The collagen strengthens and continues to incorporate calcium deposits. Remodeling is the final step and occurs when the excess callus is resorbed and trabecular bone is laid down along the lines of stress.

Clinical Manifestations

The signs and symptoms of fractures vary according to the location and function of the involved bone, the strength of its muscle attachment, the type of fracture sustained, and the amount of related damage. Signs and symptoms include pain; warmth over the injured area; ecchymosis of the skin surrounding the injured area, which may not be present for several days; and soft tissue edema in the injured area. In addition, there may be an obvious deformity and loss of normal function. The injured part may be incapable of voluntary movements; have a change in the curvature or length of bone (for a fractured hip, the affected leg will be shorter and externally rotated); and have a loss of sensation or paralysis distal to injury, which is indicative of nerve constricture. **Crepitus,** or a grating sound, may be heard if the limb is moved gently (do not attempt to verify this sign when fracture is suspected because it may cause further damage and increase pain). The patient may also demonstrate signs of shock related to tissue injury, blood loss, and severe pain.

Assessment

Rapid Orthopedic and Peripheral Vascular Assessment

Perform the **seven Ps of orthopedic assessment** to establish a baseline and monitor changes in the patient's muscular function, bone integrity, distal circulation, and sensation:

- Pain: Does it seem out of proportion to the patient's injury? Does the pain increase on active or passive motion?
- Pallor
- Paresthesia, or numbness
- Paralysis
- Polar temperature: Is the extremity cold compared with the opposite extremity?
- Puffiness from edema or a hematoma

- Pulselessness: A Doppler ultrasound device may be useful to determine the presence or absence of blood flow if unable to palpate distal pulses

Subjective data include pain at the site of the injury, loss of sensation or movement of the affected part, and cause of injury.

Objective data include warmth, edema, and ecchymosis; obvious deformity; loss of normal function in the injured part; signs of systemic shock; and signs of any circulatory, motor, or sensory impairment.

Diagnostic Tests

An accurate diagnosis of the fracture is made by radiographic examination or fluoroscopy.

Medical Management

Immediate management includes splinting and elevation to prevent edema of the affected part. Preservation of body alignment is also critical. Apply cold packs (during the first 24 hours) to reduce hemorrhage, edema, and pain. Administer analgesics as ordered. Observe the injured part for change in color, sensation, or temperature. Also observe the patient for signs of shock.

Secondary management for a closed fracture begins with optimal reduction: replacing bone fragments in their correct anatomical position. This can be accomplished through (1) closed reduction, which involves manual manipulations—moving bony fragments into position by applying traction and pressure to distal fragments; (2) traction; (3) **open reduction with internal fixation (ORIF),** a surgical procedure allowing fracture alignment under direct visualization while using various internal fixation devices applied to the bone; or (4) immobilization. Immobilization can be achieved through one or a combination of the following: (1) external fixation with a cast or splint; (2) traction; or (3) internal fixation devices such as pins, plates, screws, wires, and prostheses (see Figure 44-20).

For an open fracture, additional measures are taken. The wound undergoes surgical debridement to remove dirt, foreign materials, devitalized tissue, and necrotic bone. Administer tetanus toxoid. Take a culture of the wound and begin treatment with antibiotics. Observe the wound for signs of osteomyelitis, tetanus, or gangrene. Closure of the wound occurs when there is no sign of infection. Reduction and immobilization of the fracture then take place. Finally, observe for and treat any complications.

Nursing Interventions and Patient Teaching

The nursing interventions for patients with fractures are essentially the same as for any surgical patient. The care of the patient in traction and in a cast is discussed later in this chapter. The patient needs a well-balanced diet, but opinions differ on the value of vitamin and mineral supplements in hastening bone repair. Encourage fluids. Exercise of the unaffected joints, muscle-setting exercises, skin care, and elimination are important considerations in patient care. Internal fixation has simplified nursing intervention for many patients with fractures and shortened the period of hospitalization, but many patients require longer periods of hospitalization. If activity is restricted, anticipate and prevent the complications that result from immobility.

Patient teaching includes (1) how to move comfortably in bed; (2) how to transfer safely in and out of bed; (3) weight-bearing restrictions and activity limitations, including how long these need to be observed; (4) proper use of ambulatory assistive devices; (5) how to avoid edema in the affected part by proper elevation; (6) how to control pain or discomfort in the affected part; (7) exercises to perform to maintain strength and enhance circulation; and (8) proper method of cleansing pins, using surgical asepsis per physician's protocol.

Prognosis

Bone production and fracture healing depend on the patient's age and general health. Presence of other systemic diseases complicates the healing process.

FRACTURE OF THE VERTEBRAE

Etiology and Pathophysiology

Injuries such as diving accidents or blows to the head or body can result in fractures of the vertebrae. Patients with osteoporosis and metastatic cancer are at risk for vertebral fractures. Motorcycle and car accidents (especially head-on collisions) occur more frequently with young men (ages 16 to 30 years).

Fractures of the vertebrae may involve the vertebral body, lamina, and articulating processes and may occur with or without displacement. If the fracture has displaced the vertebral structures, pressure may be placed on spinal nerves. The sharp bone fragments may also sever the spinal cord nerves, causing permanent paralysis from the point of injury downward.

Clinical Manifestations

Signs and symptoms of vertebral fracture include pain at the site of the injury; partial or complete loss of mobility or sensation below the level of the injury; and evidence of fracture or fracture dislocation on routine radiographic examination, myelography, or CT scans.

Assessment

Collection of **subjective data** includes assessment for pain (if the fracture has injured the spinal cord, pain may not be present), numbness, tingling, and inability to move extremities from below the level of the trauma site.

Collection of **objective data** includes careful assessment of neurologic function, such as pupillary reaction to light, hand grip, ability to move extremities, level of orientation, vital signs, and reaction to painful stimuli (see Chapter 54). Observe for fecal and urinary retention and for signs of hemorrhage such as hypotension, tachycardia, tachypnea, and decreased renal functioning.

Diagnostic Tests

Radiographic studies are done to determine whether the vertebral bodies are compresssed. A spinal cord injury may result from a fracture or dislocation of a vertebra; if this is suspected, the physician performs a spinal tap to evaluate the spinal fluid. Spinal fluid is normally clear, and the presence of blood indicates trauma (see Chapter 54).

Medical Management

Stable injuries to the vertebrae that are not a threat to spinal cord integrity are treated with pain medication and muscle relaxants. Anticoagulant therapy may be ordered as a prophylaxis for thromboembolic complications. Maintaining erect posture can be enhanced by the use of a back support, corset brace, or a cast. The patient may be allowed to ambulate with assistance (gait enhancers) once discomfort subsides.

Unstable fractures that involve displacement are more serious. Treatment is aimed at fracture reduction through postural positioning and traction. Cranial skeletal traction is used with cervical spine fractures (see Chapter 54). A halo brace (Figure 44-25), an external immobilization device in which a plaster or plastic brace that incorporates metal struts attached to pins is inserted into bone, is used to allow the patient to be mobile. Pelvic traction is used for lumbar spinal fractures. An open reduction may be necessary with internal fixation using a Harrington rod. After this surgical procedure, the patient is placed in a body cast.

Nursing Interventions and Patient Teaching

Nursing interventions are aimed at maintaining the stability of the fracture fixation by (1) log-rolling the patient for position changes; (2) following the correct procedure for turning a patient in a special bed, such as a Stryker frame or Foster bed; (3) elevating the head of the bed no more than 30 degrees; (4) using stabilization devices for the head and back; and assess the continuity of traction (e.g., weights hanging free and ropes not twisted) and skin integrity (e.g., erythema, tenderness, and edema), as well as surrounding traction equipment.

Nursing diagnoses and interventions for the patient with a vertebral fracture include but are not limited to the following:

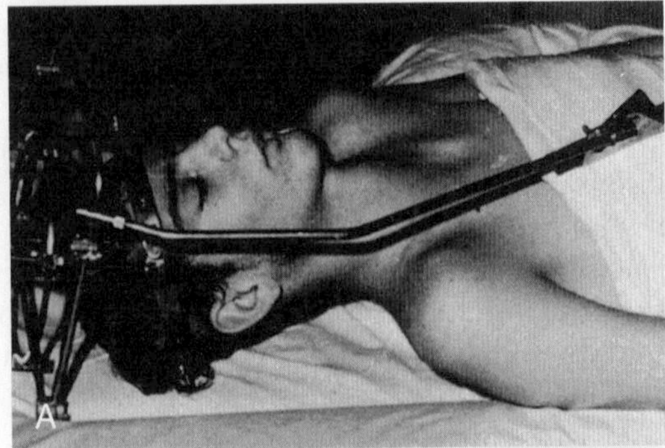

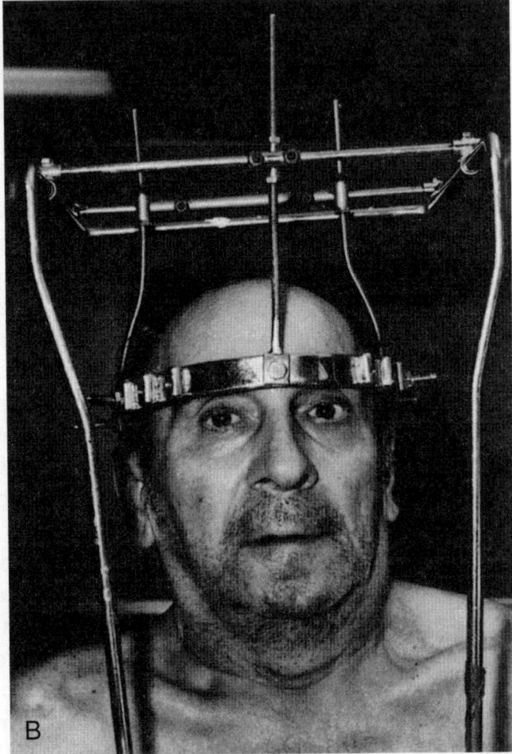

FIGURE 44-25 **A,** Halo attached to body cast. Metal strut will be anchored firmly into body cast with additional plaster. **B,** Metal ring, or halo, that attaches to skull.

Nursing Diagnoses	Nursing Interventions
Powerlessness, related to: • decreased mobility • pain	Use active listening, and permit verbalization of anger and helplessness. Assist patient in identifying coping mechanisms that will reduce feeling of powerlessness; use those that have been successful in the past. Offer positive recognition for increased activity level. Assist patient in identifying areas over which he or she has control. Involve patients in decision-making process for their own care.
Risk for infection, related to immobility and/or surgical intervention	Monitor patient for signs and symptoms of infection (elevated temperature, increased pulse rate, malodorous exudates, erythema, cloudy urine, diminished breath sounds, and crackles and wheezes).

Nursing Diagnoses	Nursing Interventions
Risk for infection, related to immobility and/or surgical intervention—cont'd	Monitor laboratory values (such as CBC) and blood and wound cultures. Protect patient from cross-contamination by practicing good handwashing techniques, maintaining surgical asepsis when changing dressings, and using strict surgical asepsis with catheter care. Encourage coughing, deep breathing, and leg exercises. Encourage use of incentive spirometer. Prevent people with infectious processes from coming in contact with patient.
Impaired physical mobility, related to: • neuromuscular skeletal impairment • pain • discomfort	Maintain bed rest in correct body alignment; avoid lifting or twisting body. Place patient in immobilization device as ordered, such as cervical head halter, skeletal traction, Stryker frame, or Circ-Olectric bed; maintain cervical spine in extension. Assess neurovascular status every 2 hours; monitor pulse, color, temperature, sensation, and mobility of all extremities. Perform passive ROM or assist with and teach active ROM exercises for all extremities every 2 hours. As fracture heals, traction is replaced with cast. Assist patient with ambulation when ordered; monitor for vertigo and weakness; progress slowly.

Patient teaching includes how to support the back by (1) using a firm mattress; (2) sitting in straight, firm chairs (for no longer than 20 to 30 minutes), when allowed; (3) using proper lifting techniques (using the leg muscles, not the back); and (4) doing back exercises to strengthen spinal extensor muscles.

Prognosis

Stable injuries to the vertebrae that are not a threat to spinal cord integrity have an excellent prognosis with full recovery. Unstable fractures are more serious, and prognosis is guarded when spinal cord injury is involved.

FRACTURE OF THE PELVIS

Etiology and Pathophysiology

Most pelvic fractures result from trauma involving great force, such as falls from extreme heights, automobile accidents, or crushing accidents. When trauma is severe enough to fracture the pelvis, vital abdominal organs may also be damaged, such as the bladder, vagina, uterus, liver, spleen, intestines, or kidneys. Because the pelvis has a rich blood supply, a fracture can result in extensive blood loss (as much as 1 to 4 L).

Clinical Manifestations

The patient with a fractured pelvis is unable to bear weight without discomfort. Local tenderness and edema are common at the trauma site. Hematuria (blood in the urine) may result from trauma to the bladder. Hemorrhage is by far the most life-threatening complication to a patient with a pelvic fracture.

Assessment

Subjective data include complaints of pelvic pain or tenderness and backache. Complaints of restlessness, anxiety, and progressive disorientation may be signs of shock.

Collection of **objective data** includes assessment of muscle spasms in the pelvic region; ecchymosis over the pelvis, perineum, groin, or suprapubic area; inability to raise the legs when supine; and external foot rotation on the affected side with noticeable shortening of one leg. Vital sign assessment may indicate shock (hypotension, tachycardia, tachypnea, oliguria, and diaphoresis). Careful observation for fat embolism syndrome is especially pertinent for patients with pelvic fractures. Assess bowel sounds in all four quadrants and document the findings; large bowel and rectal lacerations are possible in patients with pelvic fractures. Assess color and amount of urinary output because of the possibility of laceration of the bladder.

Diagnostic Tests

Abdominal radiographic studies are done with the patient in the supine and lateral positions. CT provides an evaluation of both the bony pelvis and intraabdominal contents. Intravenous pyelogram is performed to determine kidney damage. Interpretation of laboratory values for hemoglobin and hematocrit, urinalysis, and stool for occult blood helps determine whether the patient is bleeding and anemic.

Medical Management

The patient often remains on bed rest for 3 weeks and then walks with crutches for approximately 6 weeks. If the patient has a symphysis pubis fracture and an iliac fracture on the same side, the physician performs surgery. After surgery, skeletal traction is applied for approximately 6 weeks to maintain the leg position. When traction is released, the patient may ambulate without bearing weight for approximately 3 months. For a bilateral fracture of the pelvis, the physician may order a pelvic sling to support the fracture. To treat severe fractures that totally disrupt the pelvic ring and dislocate the sacroiliac joints, the physician may apply an external skeletal fixation device. He or she may also apply a spica or body cast to support the fracture.

Nursing Interventions and Patient Teaching

Nursing interventions involve monitoring the patient for signs of progressive shock (hypotension, tachycardia, tachypnea, and decreased urinary output). Measure the abdominal girth at least every 8 hours for signs of increased abdominal pressure that could result from internal hemorrhaging. Monitor I&O for signs of hypovolemia, laceration of the bladder, and potential kidney trauma. Insert a Foley catheter for monitoring urinary output and color. Implement nursing interventions appropriate for impaired mobility, impaired skin integrity, fluid volume deficit, and pain management.

A nursing diagnosis and interventions for the patient with a pelvic fracture include but are not limited to the following:

Nursing Diagnosis	Nursing Interventions
Risk for ineffective tissue perfusion, related to: • hemorrhage • hypovolemia • shock	Assess for ecchymosis over pelvis and perineum. Monitor vital signs every 15 minutes for evidence of shock until stable. Insert a Foley catheter per physician's order to monitor color and amount of urinary output. Monitor parenteral fluids per physician's order. Provide quiet, therapeutic environment. Administer oxygen per physician's order. Maintain bed rest per physician's order. Monitor bowel sounds and measure abdominal girth to ascertain possible lacerated bowel.

Reinforce the reasons for immobility and not bearing full weight; the patient may be too anxious to hear or understand initial explanations. Also explain measures for dealing with acute pain and changes in medications as pain decreases. In addition, explain turning and moving techniques to prevent skin impairment.

Prognosis

Hemorrhage is by far the most life-threatening complication. The long-term prognosis depends on the severity of the fracture, the patient's age, and the presence of other systemic disorders.

COMPLICATIONS OF FRACTURES

COMPARTMENT SYNDROME

Compartment syndrome is a pathologic condition caused by the progressive development of arterial vessel compression and reduced blood supply to an extremity. Fractures of the forearm or tibia usually precede the onset of muscle edema within the fasciae, which form compartments for the muscles of the forearm and lower leg. With severe trauma, such as fractures or compression of blood vessels as a result of a tight cast or dressing, muscle ischemia (decreased blood supply to the muscles) can occur. Irreversible muscle ischemia can occur within 6 hours as a result of compression of the arteries, nerves, and tendons entering the compartment. Paralysis and sensory loss follow, with contracture and permanent disability of the extremity seen within 24 to 48 hours.

Assessment

Collection of **subjective data** includes pain assessment. Usually the patient complains of sharp pain that increases with passive movement of the hand or foot. The patient experiences deep, unrelenting, progressive, and poorly localized pain unrelieved by analgesics or elevation of the extremity. Numbness or tingling in the affected extremity is common.

Collection of **objective data** includes assessment of the patient's inability to flex the fingers or toes, coolness of the extremity, and absence of pulsation in the affected extremity. Assess skin color for signs of pallor or cyanosis. Gentle palpation of the extremity will reveal slowing of the capillary refill time (blanching). Close monitoring and proper documentation of vital signs are essential (especially temperature to detect signs of tissue necrosis) (see Box 44-5).

Medical Management

Most cases require a fasciotomy (incision into the fascia) to relieve pressure and allow return of normal blood flow to the area. This is done immediately (within 30 minutes). The incision is often left open to heal by granulation (healing by second intention) (Figure 44-26).

Nursing Interventions

Nursing interventions include administration of analgesics with careful documentation of relief ob-

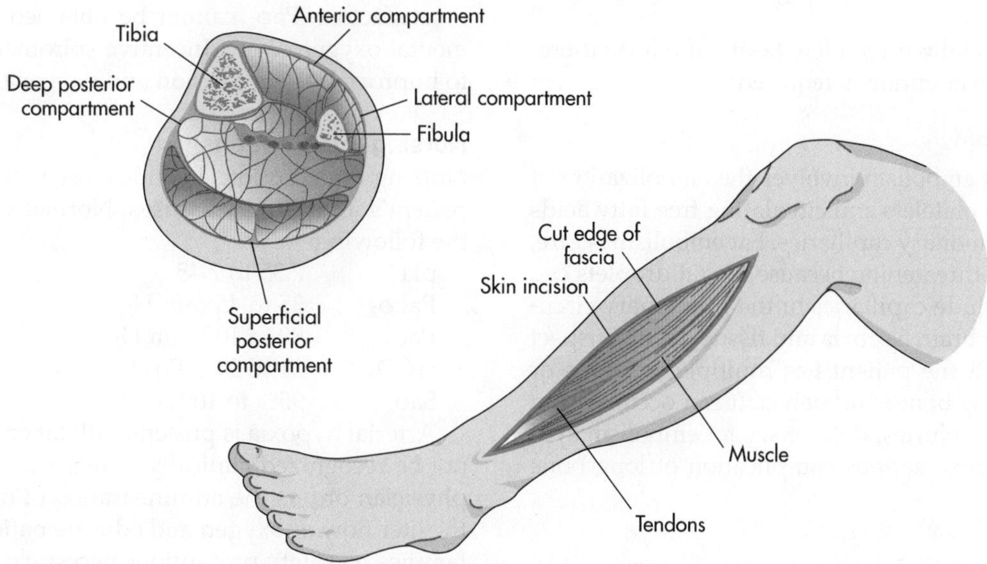

FIGURE 44-26 Compartment syndrome. Often more than one compartment is involved, and anterior compartment is especially vulnerable. Causes include trauma, severe burn, or excessive exercise. A single incision may open more than one compartment.

tained. To slow further circulatory compromise, elevate the affected limb, no higher than heart level, to maintain arterial pressure. Apply cold packs and remove any constricting material, such as an elastic bandage. The most common complication when decompression is delayed is infection as a result of tissue necrosis. Purulent drainage from the dressing is a sign of infection and must be reported immediately. If drainage and secretion isolation are required, provide careful instructions to the patient, who may feel isolated. Encourage patients to express their fears and emotional needs. **Volkmann's contracture** is a permanent contracture (with clawhand, flexion of wrist and fingers, and atrophy of the forearm) that can occur as a result of compartment syndrome. Proper positioning and alignment can reduce the risk of this complication.

Prognosis

Compartment syndrome can result in a permanent contracture deformity of the hand or foot.

SHOCK

Shock can occur as a result of blood loss from a fractured bone (bone is vascular) or from severed blood vessels, seen especially in open fractures. Pain and fear can also cause shock.

Assessment

Collection of **subjective data** includes monitoring the patient's level of consciousness. Restlessness or complaints of anxiety may suggest a decrease in cerebral perfusion, resulting in brain hypoxia. Complaints of weakness and lethargy are common.

Collection of **objective data** includes monitoring vital signs. Typical signs of shock include hypotension, tachycardia, and tachypnea. As shock progresses, hypothermia occurs. The patient may have pale, cool, moist skin. Oliguria (diminished urinary output) is present with shock.

Medical Management

The physician's main concern is restoring blood volume to ensure a rapid return of oxygen to the tissues. Blood volume can be expanded with IV fluids (lactated Ringer's solution or 5% dextrose in normal saline). Whole blood, plasma, or plasma substitutes may also be given. Respiratory assistance may be given by administering oxygen. A central venous catheter may be inserted for accurate monitoring of vital signs to prevent pulmonary edema. Shock trousers may be applied. These are pneumatic trousers designed to counteract hypotension associated with internal or external bleeding and hypovolemia.

Nursing Interventions

Nursing interventions for IV fluid administration include checking (1) the contents and IV flow rate against the physician's orders, and (2) the infusion site for signs of infiltration (erythema, edema, pain, and induration [hardening of tissue]). Monitor the patient's vital signs every 15 minutes until stable. Monitor urinary output every hour. Less than 30 mL of urine per hour indicates decreased renal perfusion. The patient should remain flat in bed. If there are no head injuries, raise the lower extremities slightly to improve venous return. Avoid the Trendelenburg position because it tends to push the abdominal organs against the diaphragm, reducing the effectiveness of heart and lung functions. Keep the patient warm, but avoid external heat. Give nothing by mouth, and avoid sedatives, tranquilizers, and narcotics. Be aware that the patient's family will be anxious and provide them with brief explanations of the patient's condition.

Prognosis

Shock can be fatal within a few hours of injury; therefore immediate attention is required.

FAT EMBOLISM

Pulmonary fat embolism involves the embolization of tissue fat with platelets and circulating free fatty acids within the pulmonary capillaries. Fat embolism is rare, but can be life threatening because the fat droplets can effectively occlude capillaries of the pulmonary circulation, causing brain hypoxia and tissue death. Suspect fat embolism if the patient has multiple fractures or fractures of long bones and pelvis. It can occur within 48 hours of the injuries. Pulmonary fat embolism syndrome is the most serious complication of long bone fractures.

Assessment

Collection of **subjective data** includes assessment of mental disturbances, such as irritability, restlessness, disorientation, stupor, and coma. These symptoms can result from effects of severe hypoxemia. The patient may complain of chest pain, especially on inspiration, and of localized muscle weakness, spasticity, and rigidity.

Collection of **objective data** includes assessing for tachypnea, dyspnea, hypoxemia, and auditory crackles and wheezes in the lung field. As the lung filters and traps embolic material, ventilation is disturbed. Assess the apical pulse to detect dysrhythmias. Patients are placed on cardiac monitoring for observation of dysrhythmias and cardiovascular collapse. Assess the patient for petechiae (especially in the buccal membranes, conjunctival sacs, hard palate, chest, and anterior axillary folds) caused by occlusion of capillaries. The appearance of petechiae on the conjunctiva of the eye, the neck, chest, or axillary region is a typical sign of a fat embolism (Lewis et al., 2007).

Diagnostic Tests

The diagnosis is based on clinical signs and symptoms, which appear within 24 to 48 hours of injury. Blood gases indicate hypoxemia. Hemoglobin and hematocrit laboratory values are decreased. Fat is present in the blood and urine. The sedimentation rate is increased, and the platelet count is decreased.

Medical Management

Treatment for fat embolism is directed at prevention. Careful immobilization of a long bone fracture is probably the most important factor in the prevention of fat embolism. The physician orders the administration of IV fluids to prevent shock and dilute free fatty acids. Use of corticosteroids to prevent or treat fat embolism is controversial. Digoxin is often ordered to increase the patient's cardiac output. Oxygen is administered if the Po_2 is less than 70 mm Hg. Intubation or intermittent positive pressure ventilation may be considered if a satisfactory Pao_2 cannot be obtained with supplemental oxygen alone. Incentive spirometry is ordered to improve lung expansion and oxygenation.

Nursing Interventions

Nursing interventions include close monitoring of the patient's arterial blood gases. Normal values include the following:

pH	7.35 to 7.45
$Paco_2$	35 to 45 mm Hg
Pao_2	80 to 100 mm Hg
HCO_3	21 to 28 mEq/L
Sao_2	95% to 100%

Arterial hypoxia is present with fat emboli and may not be recognized clinically. If hypoxia is present, the physician orders the administration of oxygen. Check the liter flow of oxygen and educate patients and their families on safety precautions necessary when oxygen is administered (e.g., no smoking or use of electrical equipment). Respiratory failure is the most common cause of death. Careful stabilization and immobilization of long bone fractures are important steps in preventing fat embolism syndrome. Careful support when turning and positioning the patient can prevent the manipulation of the fracture and reduce the risk of fat embolism syndrome. Reposition the patient as little as possible before fracture immobilization because of the danger of dislodging more fat droplets into the general circulation. An accurate record of I&O and daily weights is essential to monitor fluid balance.

Prognosis

Fat embolism can be life threatening.

GAS GANGRENE

Gas gangrene is a severe infection of the skeletal muscle caused by gram-positive *Clostridium* bacteria, particularly *Clostridium perfringens,* which may occur in the presence of open fractures and lacerated wounds. These injuries can produce exotoxins that destroy tissue. The onset is usually sudden, generally 1 to 14 days after injury. These organisms are anaerobic (grow and function without oxygen) and spore formers. They are normally found in soil and the intestinal tracts of humans. As the clostridia bacteria invade devitalized tissue (especially where blood supply is diminished), they multiply and produce toxins that cause (1) hemolysis (breakdown of red blood cells and release of hemoglobin); (2) vessel thrombosis; and (3) damage to the myocardium, the liver, the kidneys, and the brain.

Assessment

Collection of **subjective data** includes observation of pain, which is usually sudden and severe at the site of the injury. A characteristic finding is toxic delirium.

Collection of **objective data** includes careful inspection of the skin for gas bubbles at the site of the wound.

The various *Clostridium* species produce a characteristic cellulitis in which gas is present under the skin. This causes crepitation (a crackling sensation when the skin is touched). Observe for signs of infection, including elevated temperature, tachycardia, tachypnea, and edema around the wound. The skin around the wound becomes necrotic and ruptures, revealing necrotic muscle. The wound discharge is thin, watery, and foul smelling. Carefully document the patient's response to antibiotic therapy (e.g., decline in temperature and decrease in amount of wound drainage).

Medical Management

Treatment of gas gangrene involves establishing a larger wound opening to admit air and promote drainage. Antibiotics, such as penicillin G or cephalothin, are ordered intravenously and must be administered as scheduled. Observe the patient for adverse reactions.

Nursing Interventions

Nursing interventions include wound care using strict medical asepsis. Spore-forming bacteria are not destroyed by ordinary disinfecting methods. Therefore all contaminated equipment and linens must be autoclaved. Follow drainage and secretion isolation procedures to prevent the spread of the infection to other patients.

Prognosis

If left untreated, gas gangrene is rapidly fatal. Prompt treatment, including excision of gangrenous tissue and administration of penicillin G intravenously, saves 80% of patients. If massive gangrene develops, amputation is necessary.

THROMBOEMBOLUS

Etiology and Pathophysiology

Thromboembolus is a condition in which a blood vessel is occluded by an embolus carried in the bloodstream from the site of formation of the clot. It is associated with reduced skeletal muscle contractions and bed rest. The person suffering from pelvic and hip fractures is at high risk for this complication.

Clinical Manifestations

The area supplied by an obstructed artery may tingle and become cold, numb, and cyanotic. An embolus in the lungs causes a sudden, sharp thoracic or upper abdominal pain, dyspnea, cough, fever, and hemoptysis.

Assessment

Collection of **subjective data** includes careful investigation of complaints of pain in the lower extremities (especially the calf). A complaint of tenderness over the area is common. The patient may complain of a sharp pain in the thoracic area when an embolus is in the lung.

Collection of **objective data** includes assessing for a positive Homans' sign, which indicates thromboembolus. Homans' sign is pain in the calf of the affected leg on dorsiflexion of the foot. The affected area may be erythematous, warm to touch, and edematous. Assess for differences in leg size (circumference) bilaterally from thigh to ankle. Also observe the patient for dyspnea and blood in the sputum if pulmonary embolus is present. When anticoagulant therapy is ordered, assess for signs of bleeding, such as petechiae, epistaxis, hematuria, hematemesis, and occult or gross blood in the stool.

Diagnostic Tests

A complete history is taken and a physical examination is performed. In addition to checking Homans' sign, obtain a prothrombin time (PT), International Normalized Ratio (INR), D-dimer, and CBC. Diagnostic tests for deep-vein thrombosis may include Doppler ultrasonography or duplex scanning. A spiral CT scan of the lung, a ventilation/perfusion scan, or a pulmonary arteriogram may be ordered to rule out pulmonary embolism.

Medical Management

Treatment includes administration of anticoagulants, such as heparin, enoxaparin or warfarin. A surgical procedure known as thrombectomy (removal of a thrombus from a blood vessel) may be done.

Nursing Interventions

Nursing interventions involve caring for the patient on activity restriction. Many times this involves bed rest with the foot of the bed elevated to aid venous return. Teach the patient to do active exercise, such as dorsiflexion (pointing backward) and plantar flexion (pointing forward) of the toes, several times each hour. This exercise stimulates circulation to the legs. Continuous hot, moist compresses are usually ordered. Antiembolism stockings and intermittent pneumatic compression devices are ordered while the patient is on bed rest and are maintained even after the patient is ambulatory. Assess lung sounds every 4 hours and adhere to the activity ordered. If the patient is receiving anticoagulants, closely monitor PT, INR, and partial thromboplastin times.

Prognosis

Obstruction of the pulmonary artery or one of its branches may be fatal. A thrombus in an extremity usually resolves with treatment, and a favorable prognosis is noted.

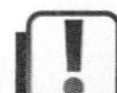
Safety Alert!

Thromboembolus

Never massage a patient's lower extremities. Thromboembolus can be present without clinical signs and symptoms.

DELAYED FRACTURE HEALING

A **delayed union** is a fracture that fails to heal within the usual time. The healing is impaired but has not completely stopped and will eventually repair itself. **Nonunion** is when the ends of the fractured bone fail to unite and produce a stable union after 6 to 9 months. The calcification of cartilage and bone formation do not occur. Bone grafting, prosthetic implant, internal fixation, external fixation, or a combination of these methods can be used to correct the problem of delayed union or nonunion of bone fractures. Physicians are using electrical stimulation as a new method of promoting healing of nonunion fractures. The use of electrical probes on bone stimulates bone production.

Prognosis

Bone production and fracture healing depend on the patient's age and general health. The presence of other systemic diseases complicates the healing process.

SKELETAL FIXATION DEVICES

EXTERNAL FIXATION DEVICES

External fixation devices are used to hold bone fragments in normal position. Casts, skeletal and skin traction, braces, and metal pins are examples of these devices.

Skeletal Pin External Fixation

One external fixation technique immobilizes fractures with pins inserted through the bone and attached to a rigid external metal frame (Figure 44-27). This tech-

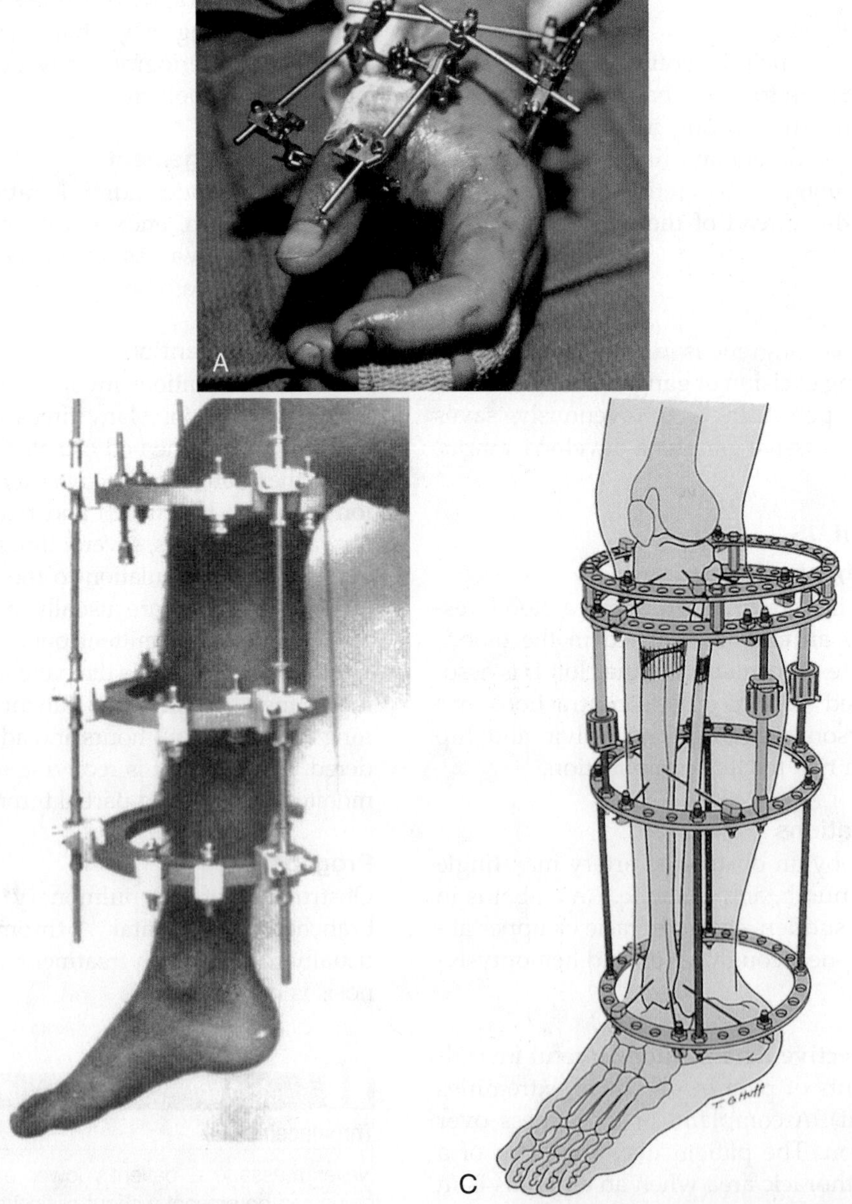

FIGURE 44-27 External fixation apparatuses. **A,** Hoffman. **B,** The Monticello-Spinelli Circular Fixator. **C,** Ilizarov apparatus with corticotomies for lengthening lower leg.

nique is becoming more popular because it provides rigid support of comminuted open fractures, infected nonunions, and infected unstable joints. The patient can use the muscles and joints above and below the fixation. Leaving the fracture open to air has the advantage of visibility of the area and accessibility for wound care.

This procedure is performed with the patient under general anesthesia. Reassure the patient that the pain after the insertion of the pins is minimal. Immediately after the procedure, the extremity is placed in balanced suspension traction to help relieve the edema. Assess the pins that are inserted through the bone at least every 8 hours, with careful observation for signs of infection and loose pins. Remove dried exudate from around the pins once or twice daily with hydrogen peroxide or alcohol, using surgical asepsis. Patients are permitted to ambulate on crutches when soft tissue edema is relieved. They are permitted to shower when the wounds have healed but must avoid salt or chlorinated water to prevent fixator corrosion.

NONSURGICAL INTERVENTIONS FOR MUSCULOSKELETAL DISORDERS

CASTS

Casts are immobilization devices made up of layers of plaster of Paris, fiberglass, or plastic roller bandages. The application is similar to that for an elastic bandage. The type of cast used is indicative of the part of the body immobilized. Examples include (1) short arm cast, which extends from below the elbow to the proximal palmar crease; (2) long leg cast, which extends from the upper thigh to the base of the toes; and (3) spica cast or body cast, which covers the trunk and one or both extremities (Figure 44-28). A cast may be bivalve to relieve pressure. This involves splitting the cast down both sides and securing the pieces so that the extremity is supported (see Skill 44-1, step 8a).

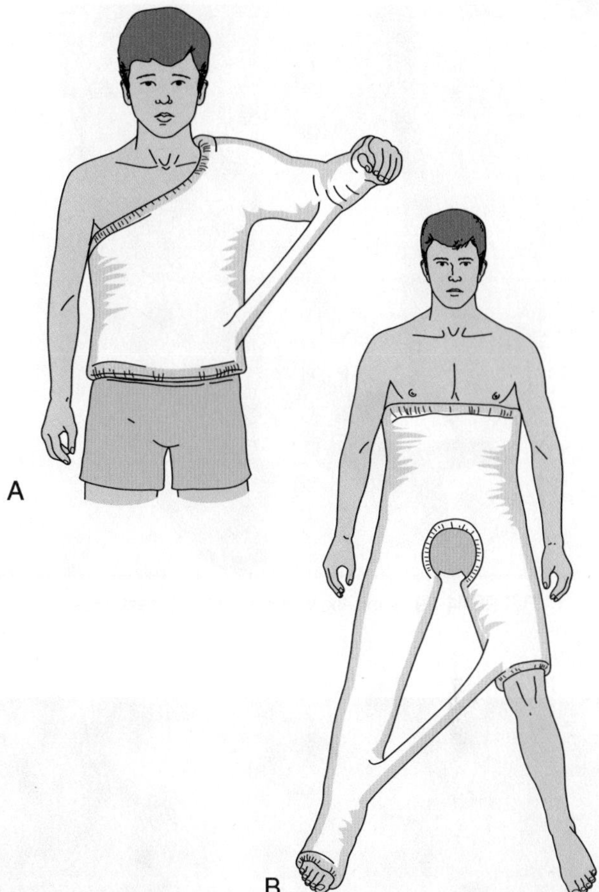

FIGURE 44-28 Spica casts. **A,** Shoulder spica. **B,** One and one-half leg-hip spica.

Casts are applied after the physician has properly aligned the bone through either external or internal fixation. Cast application is relatively painless except for the manipulation of the traumatized extremity. The casting procedure involves the application of a piece of stockinette that covers the length of the extremity and area to be casted, followed by sheet wadding (pressed cotton that comes in rolled bandages), followed by the casting material. Most physicians bring the stockinette up and over the distal and proximal edge of the cast. Inspect these edges for rough pieces of casting that may irritate the skin. Superficial burns can occur as the cast begins to set up, especially if the patient is not appropriately padded or too much fiberglass material is used.

Cast Brace

The cast brace is an alternative appliance to the traditional leg cast. It provides the support and stability of the plaster cast, with additional support and mobility provided by a hinged brace. The appliance is most effective for fractures of the shaft of the femur and permits early ambulation and weight bearing. It is used approximately 2 to 6 weeks after fracture reduction.

Cast bracing is based on the concept that limited weight bearing helps promote the formation of bone. A problem encountered frequently with cast bracing is edema around the knee. Instruct patients to elevate the leg when sitting to promote venous return. A cast shoe or walking heel incorporated into a lower extremity cast permits weight bearing without damaging the cast (Figure 44-29).

Assessment

Nursing assessment is similar regardless of what kind of casting material is used. Perform a neurovascular assessment, including capillary refill, every 15 to 30 minutes for several hours after casting and every 4 hours the first few days (see Box 44-5). Capillary filling time (capillary refill) is a way to assess arterial flow to the extremities; squeeze the patient's nailbeds to produce blanching and observe for the return of color. With normal arterial capillary perfusion, the color returns to normal within 2 seconds (Figure 44-30). Observe the skin at the cast edges for erythema and irrita-

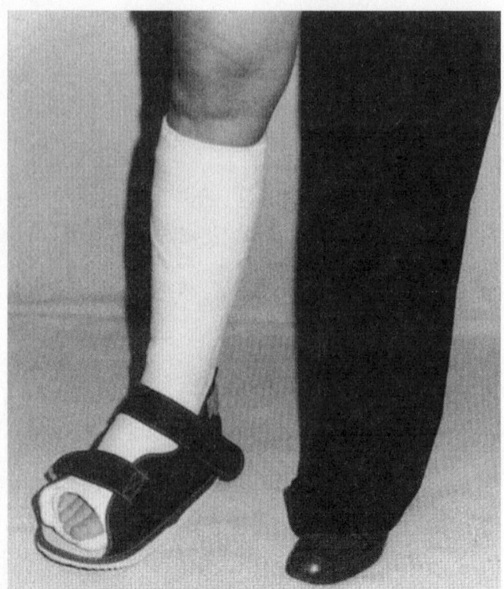

FIGURE 44-29 Short-leg walking cast with cast shoe.

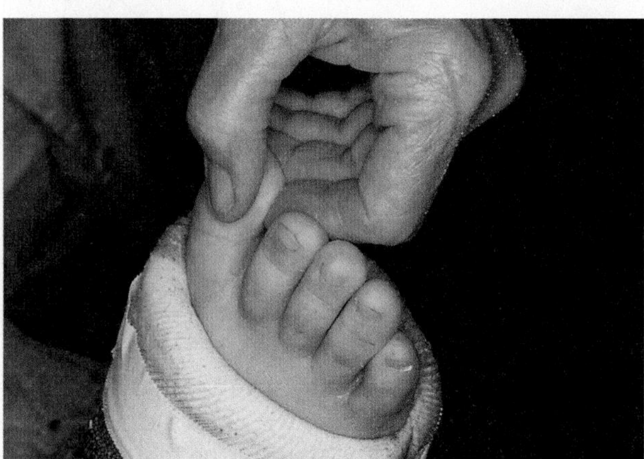

FIGURE 44-30 Capillary refill assessment.

tion. Note any signs of infection, such as odor or drainage coming from under the cast, and document the findings. Assess the patient's ability to use crutches in a three-point gait to establish normal gait and rhythm, and assess crutches for safety by ensuring a proper fit and presence of large, rubber, suction tips on the ends.

Nursing Interventions and Patient Teaching

Nursing interventions for the patient in a cast (Skill 44-1) include patient education on preventing infection, irritation, neurovascular pressure, and misalignment of bone ends. Handle a wet cast gently and support it with the flat of the hand or on pillows to avoid indentations that cause pressure on the skin and lead to skin impairment. Never use the bar in a spica cast as support when turning patient. Turning the patient frequently aids the drying process. If a cast dryer is used, set it on warm, never hot (drying a plaster of Paris cast too quickly from the outside may weaken the cast). Elevating the casted extremity reduces edema (usually elevation is recommended for 24 to 48 hours). Instruct patients using crutches to support their weight on their hands; weight borne on the axillae can damage the brachial plexus nerves (crutch paralysis).

Cast syndrome can occur after the application of a spica (body) cast (see Figure 44-28) and involves acute obstruction of the duodenum. If nausea occurs, place the patient prone to relieve pressure symptoms and alert the charge nurse. Gastric decompression may be necessary, and if conventional measures fail, surgical intervention (duodenojejunostomy—making an opening into the small intestine) may be necessary.

Patient teaching includes information about cleaning around the cast site with a mild soap and rinsing excessive soap so that it does not accumulate around

Skill 44-1 Care of the Patient in a Cast

Nursing Action (Rationale)

1. Patient teaching. *(Ensures patient cooperation; reduces patient anxiety.)*
   a. Explain why the cast is being applied and how it will be applied. *(Sudden movement during procedure could cause injury.)*
   b. Advise the patient that the plaster cast will feel warm as it dries.
   c. Explain the extent of immobilization.
   d. Explain care of the cast and expectations after discharge.
   e. Instruct patient not to insert sharp objects (coat hangers or pencils) under the cast. *(These may abrade the skin and lead to infection.)*
2. Handling the new cast. *(A fiberglass cast dries immediately after application; a plaster extremity cast dries in approximately 24 to 48 hours; a plaster spica or body cast dries in 48 to 72 hours [see Figure 44-29].)*
   a. Support wet cast with the flat of the hands or on pillows. *(Avoids indentations that will cause pressure on underlying skin.)*
   b. Place cotton blankets or other absorbent material under the cast. *(Aids drying of cast.)*
   c. Expose the cast to air as much as possible. *(Aids drying of cast.)*
   d. Turn the patient frequently. *(Aids drying of cast.)*
   e. Use a cast dryer or hair dryer on a warm (not hot) setting. *(Circulates air over the cast.)*
   f. Do not apply paint, varnish, or shellac to the cast. *(Plaster is a porous material that allows air to circulate to the skin.)*

3. Skin care. *(Decreases the chance of skin irritation or tissue injury.)*
   a. Inspect skin at edges of cast and underlying cast for erythema or skin impairment.
   b. Remove plaster crumbs from skin with a washcloth moistened with warm water.
   c. Use creams and lotions sparingly. *(They may soften the skin and cause the cast to stick to the skin.)*
   d. Apply waterproof material around perineal area. *(Prevents soiling of and damage to cast and prevents skin impairment.)*
   e. Attend to patient's complaint of pain under the cast, particularly over bony prominences. *(This may indicate pressure on the skin.)* If discomfort is not relieved by repositioning, report to physician *(Cast pressure may need to be relieved by windowing or bivalving [cutting into halves].)*
4. Turning: Turning to any position is generally permitted as long as the integrity of the cast is not compromised and the patient is comfortable; do not turn by grasping the abductor bar. *(It is not safe transport.)*
5. Toileting for a long leg or hip spica cast.
   a. Use a fracture pan with blanket roll or padding. *(Provides support under the small of the back.)*
   b. Elevate the head of the bed, if permitted, or place the bed in reverse Trendelenburg position. *(Eases procedure.)*
6. Abdominal discomfort: Cast may be "windowed" (an opening cut into it). *(Provides relief of abdominal distention or a port for checking bladder distention.)*
7. Mobilization.
   a. The physician decides whether and how much weight bearing is allowed.
   b. A cast shoe or a walking heel is incorporated into a lower extremity cast (see Figure 44-30). *(Permits weight bearing without damaging the cast.)*
8. Prevention of neurovascular problems: Establish baseline measurements and assess neurovascular status before cast application; palpate distal pulses; assess color, temperature, and capillary refill of the appropriate fingers or toes; assess neurologic function, including sensation and motion in the affected and unaffected extremity. *(Changes in neurovascular status may occur after casting, possibly further compromising already injured tissues. Note the baseline neurovascular status so that those changes, if they occur, can be readily assessed.)*
   a. Perform neurovascular checks every hour for at least 24 hours after cast application to detect difficulty from edema or pressure of cast on nerves or vessels; notify physician of color changes, alterations in sensation, or motion unrelieved by position change; cast may need to be bivalved to relieve pressure (see illustration below).
   b. Elevate affected extremity on pillows. *(Danger of edema is usually 24 to 48 hours.)*
   c. After mobilization of patient with lower extremity or upper extremity cast, avoid keeping extremity in dependent position for prolonged periods. *(Prevents edema.)*
   d. After lower extremity cast is removed, encourage patient to wear elastic stocking and elevate affected leg while at rest until full mobility is regained. *(After immobilization, the involved joints and muscles will be weak and range of motion may be limited. Activity must be resumed slowly. Elastic stockings enhance deep-vein circulation.)*

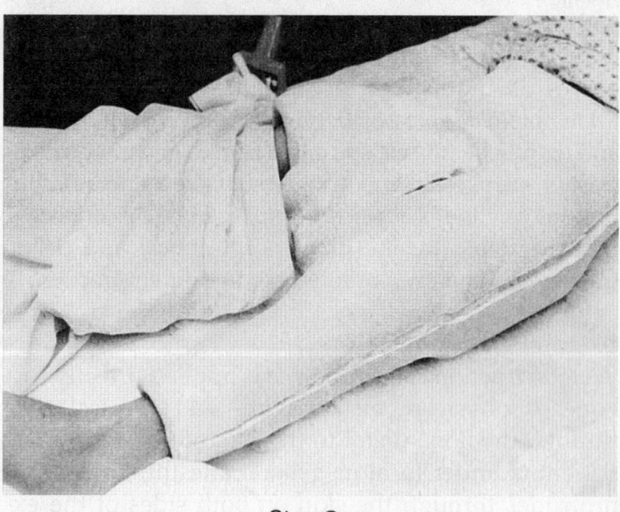

Step 8a

the cast and impair the skin. A synthetic cast can be flushed with water if it becomes soiled. It must be dried afterward to prevent skin impairment and maceration (softening). A synthetic cast can be dried by blotting it with a towel and then using a blow dryer on cool or warm setting in a sweeping motion across the cast. Proper drying may take as long as 1 hour.

Patients often complain of pruritus (itching) of the skin that is covered by a cast (especially after having the cast for a few weeks). Recommend diversional activities when the pruritus begins. Also advise the patient to gently rub the area below and above the cast to decrease the desire to scratch. Warn patients not to stick sharp objects underneath the cast to relieve the pruritus. This may impair the skin and result in serious complications.

CAST REMOVAL

Casts are removed with an electric vibrating saw rather than a cutting saw. Reassure patients that there is little risk of the saw injuring the skin beneath the cast, even though it is noisy and looks like a cutting saw. Cutting the cast can cause a very fine powder or dust to escape into the air. If this powder is inhaled over a period of time, the plaster deposits can build up in the lungs' small air sacs and cause respiratory distress. It is a safe practice for the nurse, the physician, and the patient to wear masks when casts are removed with a cast cutter.

After removal of a cast, eliminate the buildup of secretions and dead skin on the affected extremity by gently washing and applying lotion or cream to the area. This may take several days, but caution the patient against trying to remove the devitalized material rapidly for fear of causing skin impairment. Muscle atrophy is common, especially if the extremity has been casted for several weeks. Reassure the patient that the muscle will regain strength and size with proper exercise through either physical therapy or home exercise programs.

TRACTION

Traction is the process of putting an extremity, bone, or group of muscles under tension by means of weights and pulleys to (1) align and stabilize a fracture site by reducing the fractured part, (2) relieve pressure on nerves as in the case of herniated disk syndrome, (3) maintain correct positioning, (4) prevent deformities, and (5) relieve muscle spasms. The two general types of traction are skeletal and skin. To stabilize a fracture, continuous traction is applied; it must not be disconnected unless ordered by the physician. Cervical and pelvic traction is sometimes ordered as intermittent traction.

Skeletal Traction

Skeletal traction (Figure 44-31) is applied directly to a bone. A physician inserts wires and surgical pins through the bone distal to the fracture site while the patient is under local or general anesthesia. The pin protrudes through the skin on both sides of the extremity, and traction is applied with weights attached to a rope that is tied to a spreader bar. Skeletal traction can be used for fractures of the femur (see Figure 44-31, *A*), tibia (see Figure 44-31, *B*), humerus, and cervical spine (see Chapter 54).

Skin Traction

Skin traction uses weight that pulls on sponge rubber, moleskin, and elastic bandage with adherent or plastic materials attached to the skin below the site of the fracture, with the pull exerted on the limb. Buck's, Russell's, and Bryant's are types of skin traction.

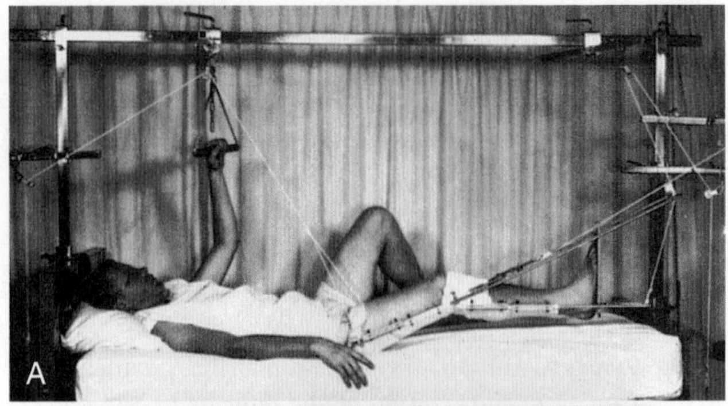

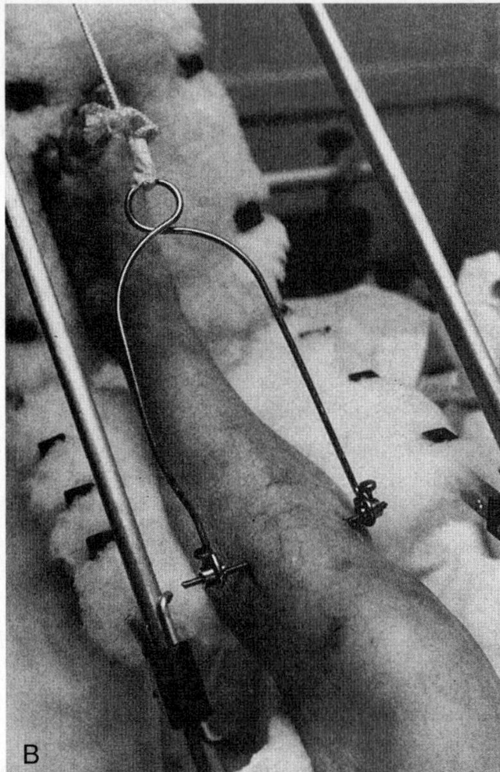

FIGURE 44-31 A, Balanced suspension skeletal traction to the femur. **B,** Tibial pin traction with Steinmann pin used in treatment of distal femoral fracture. The bow attached to the pin provides a place of attachment for the rope that holds the traction weights. The pull exerted by the weight keeps the fracture fragments aligned. Pin sites must be inspected at least daily to detect signs of pin reaction or infection.

Buck's Traction

Buck's traction (Figure 44-32, *C*) is used as a temporary measure to provide support and comfort to a fractured extremity while waiting for more definitive treatment. Traction (pull) is in a horizontal plane with affected extremity. This traction is frequently used to maintain the reduction of a hip fracture before surgery. It can also be used to treat muscle spasms and minor fractures of the lower spine.

Russell's Traction

Russell's traction (Figure 44-32, *B*) is set up similar to Buck's traction. However, a knee sling supports the affected leg. It allows more movement in bed and permits flexion of the knee joint. Russell's traction is commonly used to treat hip and knee fractures.

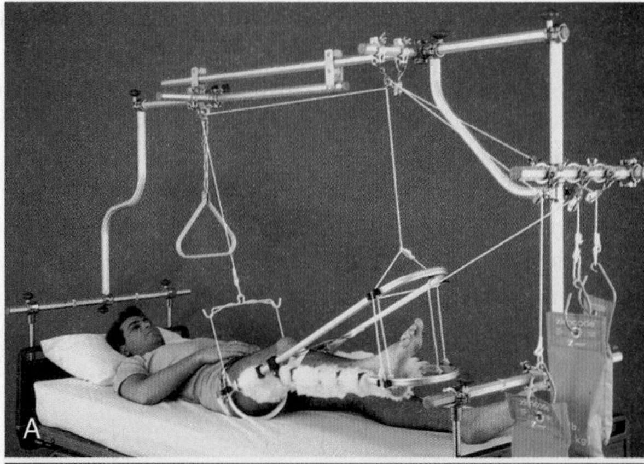

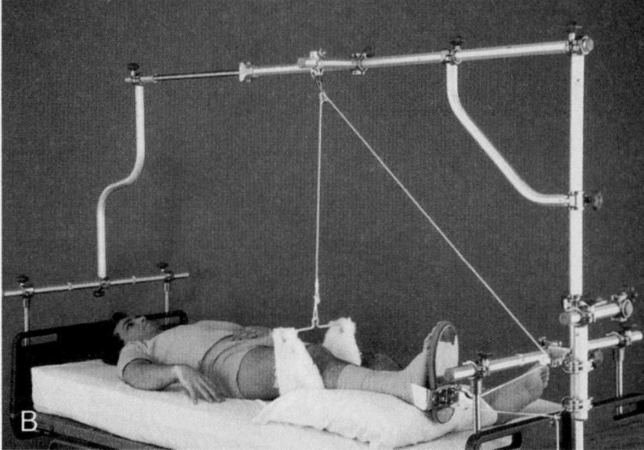

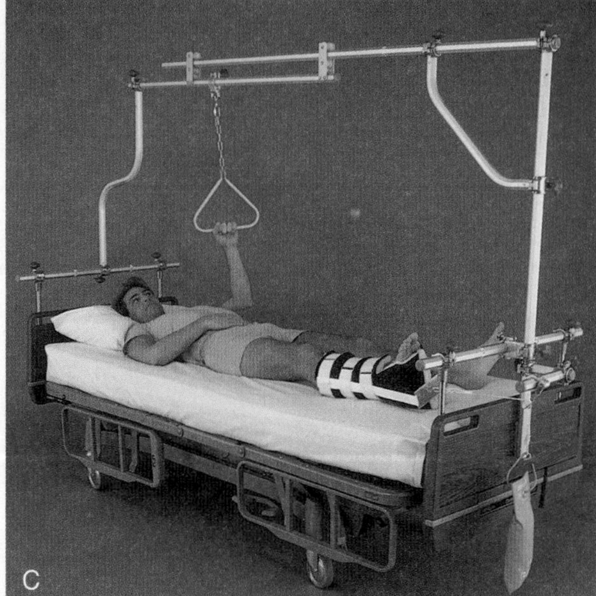

FIGURE 44-32 **A,** Balanced traction with a Thomas ring and a Pearson attachment. **B,** Russell's traction. **C,** Buck's traction.

Nursing Interventions

Nursing interventions of patients in traction include measures to maintain the body in proper alignment and careful assessment of traction equipment. Care of a patient in skeletal traction involves assessment of the pin sites and application of hydrogen peroxide or normal saline per physician's order. Traction care is summarized in Box 44-6.

Box 44-6 Nursing Interventions for the Patient in Traction

- Maintain the patient's body in proper alignment. The force or pull on the extremities should be in alignment with the long axis of the bone.
- Ensure that weights hang freely from the bed and are never removed without a physician's order.
- Question patients as to their understanding of the purpose of the traction, and assess their ability to use a trapeze bar for self-movement. Elevate the foot of the bed to help prevent the patient from sliding down toward the foot of the bed (countertraction).
- Observe the condition of the traction cords, making sure they are not weakened or frayed. All knots used on the rope or cord are to be square knots.
- Center the ropes on the traction pulley.
- Assess, document, and report neurovascular impairment.
- Ensure that weight used is the correct weight as ordered by the physician.
- Carefully observe the skin for signs of impairment. Use sheepskin heel protectors and bed pads to reduce impairment.
- If skeletal traction is used, assess the pin site for signs of infection. Cleanse the pin site every 8 hours with hydrogen peroxide or normal saline, as ordered.
- Assess the distal pulses bilaterally for circulatory integrity of the extremities.
- Inspect for loss of sensation in the dorsal area of the foot with weakness and inversion of the foot (inside surface turned outward).

ORTHOPEDIC DEVICES

Frames can be used for orthopedic patients to assist with turning and positioning while maintaining proper alignment. The **Balkan frame** is a wooden or steel attachment to the hospital bed. It has adjustable pulleys and a trapeze bar attached to an overhead bar.

The **Bradford frame** is made of rectangular steel with two pieces of canvas stretched tightly and laced to the frame. A space is left in the buttocks area for toileting and hygiene.

The **Stryker wedge turning frame** and **Foster bed** are similar and assist in changing the patient's position from supine to prone. Patients may become apprehensive when turned on a frame for fear of falling, so thorough explanations and reassurances are helpful.

The **CircOlectric bed** is a vertical turning bed that can be operated electrically by one person and placed in a variety of positions. Side-to-side movement can be accomplished while maintaining proper positioning if traction is ordered.

The **RotoRest bed** can rock a patient as much as 62 degrees, 17 times per hour. The electric-powered bed can help heal pressure ulcers, prevent venous thrombosis, and reduce kidney stone formation. Orthopedic traction can be attached to the bed, as well as a television set for diversional activity.

Safety Alert!

Crutch Safety

Crutch safety involves:

- Proper measurement (with weight on hands, not axillae, to avoid brachial plexus paralysis); leave a 2-inch width between the axillary fold and the armpiece on the crutches.
- Rubber tips on the ends of the crutches to prevent slippage.
- Adequate muscle strength in the upper extremities to support the patient's weight.

Splints, crutches, and **braces** are used to immobilize and assist with ambulation. There are numerous types of splints and braces, and it is important that the nurse understand the procedure for proper application for each one.

Safety is the first concern when ambulatory devices such as crutches are used. Encourage the patient to do push-ups by pressing the hands against the mattress and lifting the upper body to gain muscle strength. Types of **crutch walking** depend on the number of points making contact with the floor (Figure 44-33).

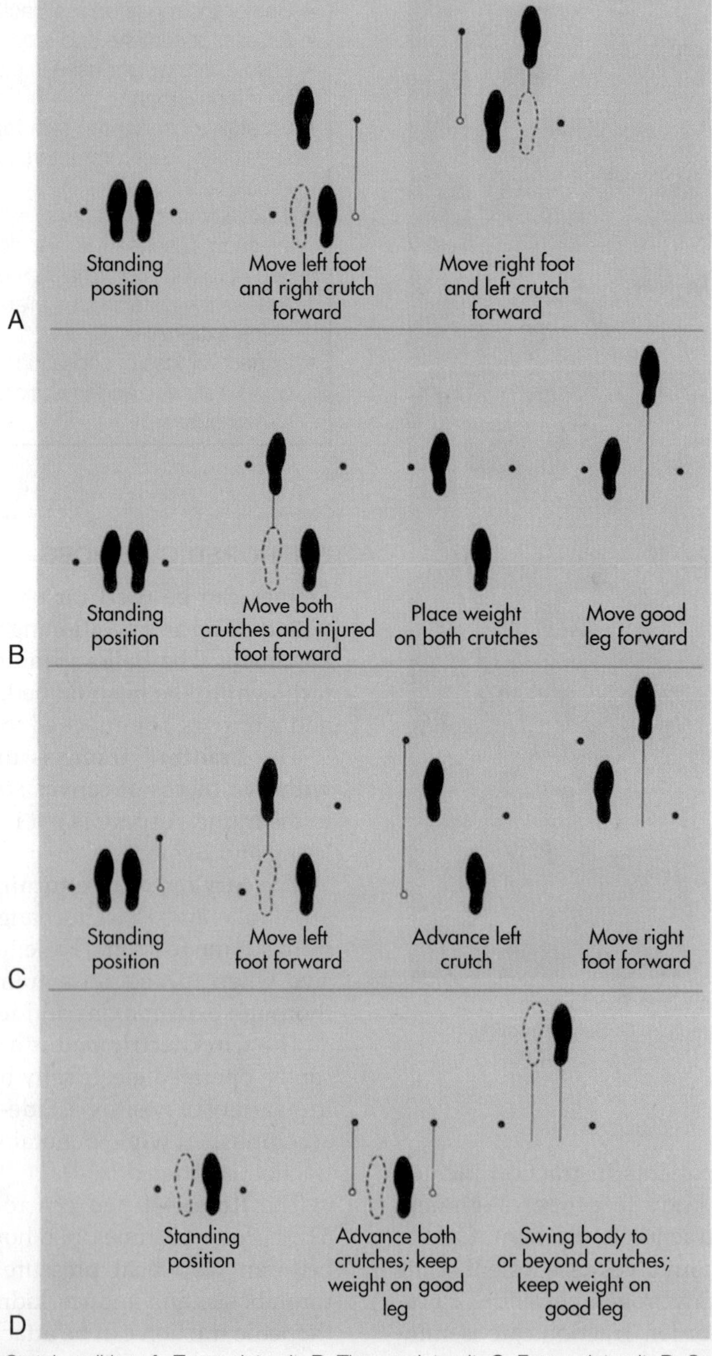

FIGURE 44-33 Crutch walking. **A,** Two-point gait. **B,** Three-point gait. **C,** Four-point gait. **D,** Swing-through gait.

For example, a three-point gait involves two crutch points plus one leg making contact with the floor (patient must have strong arms to support body weight). Instead of a three-point gait, patients may use the four-point gait (slower, but stable) or two-point gait (faster; requires balance). Another type of crutch walking is swing-to or swing-through gait, in which the patient swings the body up to or beyond the two points of the crutch tips. Most crutch walking is taught by a physical therapist (Figure 44-34). However, the nurse monitors the patient's progress.

Older patients are more likely to use **cane walking** for balance and support. Instruct the patient to hold the cane in the opposite hand of the affected extremity and advance the cane at the same time the affected leg moves forward. An effective rubber tip on the point will help prevent slippage (Figure 44-35). Older adults also use walkers to maintain balance. Safety concerns are the same as those for the cane (Figure 44-36).

The Roll-A-Bout walker is a new gait enhancer designed for patients who have an injury below the knee such as a fractured tibia, fibula, ankle, or foot. The Roll-A-Bout allows the patient to distribute weight evenly by placing the knee of the injured leg on the knee pad and propelling the Roll-A-Bout with the unaffected leg (Figure 44-37).

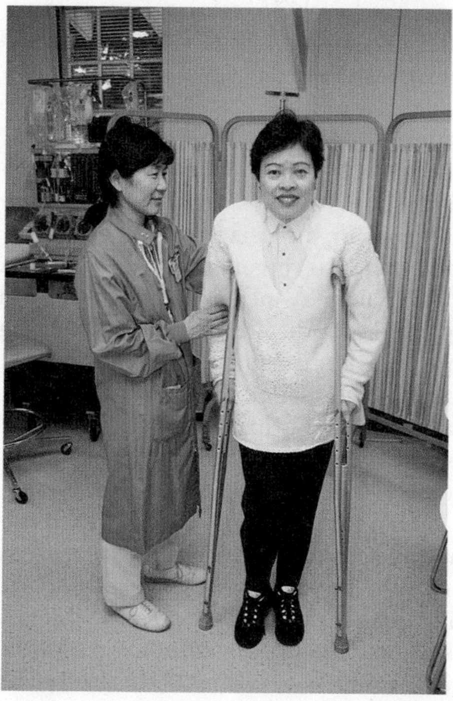

FIGURE 44-34 Assisting the patient with crutch walking. Note how the therapist guards the patient and how the patient's elbows are at no more than 30 degrees of flexion.

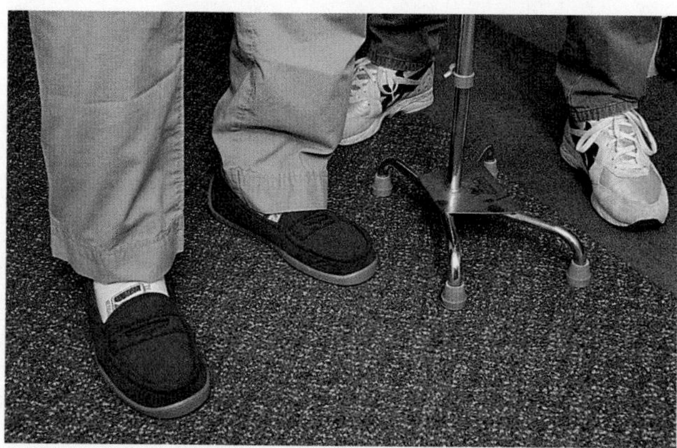

FIGURE 44-35 Quad cane.

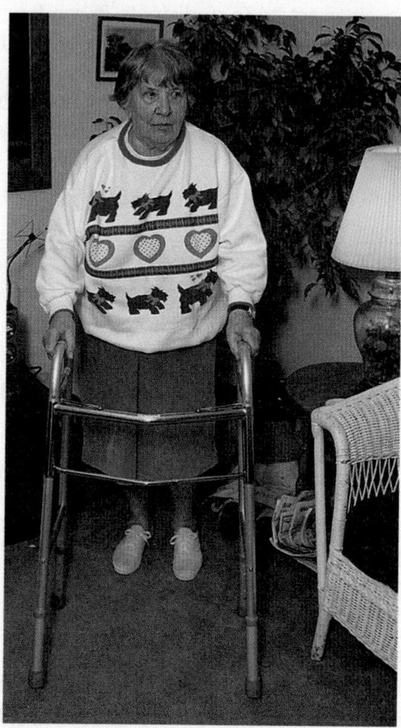

FIGURE 44-36 Patient using a walker.

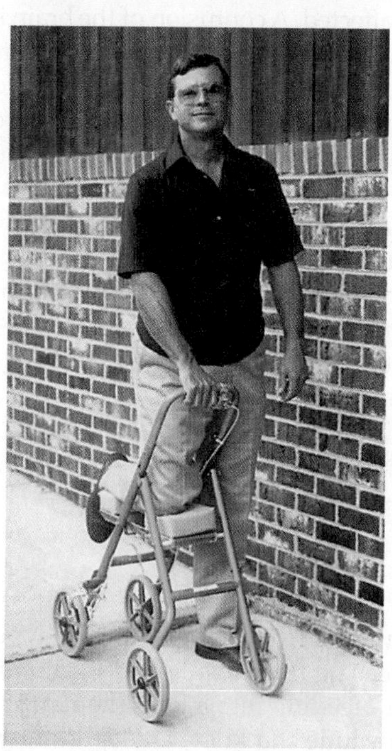

FIGURE 44-37 The Roll-A-Bout walker.

Safety Alert!

Preventing Musculoskeletal Trauma

- Teach patients and community members to take appropriate safety precautions to prevent injuries while at home, at work, when driving, or when participating in sports.
- Be a vocal advocate for personal actions known to reduce injuries such as regularly using seatbelts, driving within posted speed limits, stretching before exercise, using protective athletic equipment (helmets and knee, wrist, and elbow pads), and not combining drinking and driving.
- Encourage older adults to participate in moderate exercise to aid in the maintenance of muscle strength and balance.
- To reduce falls, examine older adults' living environment to rule out the use of scatter rugs, to ensure adequate footwear and lighting, and to clear paths to bathrooms for nighttime use.
- Stress the importance of adequate calcium and vitamin D intake.

TRAUMATIC INJURIES

Traumatic injuries to the musculoskeletal system can occur in all age-groups. However, older adults may have disorders that predispose them to musculoskeletal injuries. The more serious injuries involving fractures are treated in a hospital, whereas the less serious—such as contusions, sprains, or strains—may be treated in an outpatient facility.

CONTUSIONS

Etiology and Pathophysiology

Contusions are the most common soft tissue injury. An injury from a blow or blunt force causes local bleeding under the skin and possibly a hematoma (sac filled with blood). The severity of a contusion depends on the part of the body affected. A contusion of the brain is very serious, whereas a contusion of the arm is less serious. Large areas affected by soft tissue bleeding with slow absorption of the blood have a higher potential of developing into cellulitis (an infection of the subcutaneous tissue).

Medical Management

Most contusions are treated by applying ice bags or cold compresses for 15 to 20 minutes at a time over 12 to 36 hours for the vasoconstricting effects of cold. The involved extremity is elevated to reduce edema and suppress pain.

Prognosis

Prognosis is excellent.

SPRAINS

Etiology and Pathophysiology

Sprains can result from a wrenching or hyperextension of a joint, tearing the capsule and ligaments. A sprain can involve bleeding into a joint (hemarthrosis). Common sites include the knee, ankle, and cervical spine (whiplash). Sprains are often the result of a sudden, twisting injury. Medical management is similar to that for contusions. Treatment usually consists of elevation, compression, ice, and rest of the affected area.

Prognosis

Prognosis is excellent.

WHIPLASH

Etiology, Pathophysiology, and Clinical Manifestations

Injury at the cervical spine, or whiplash, is classified under cervical disk syndrome. Whiplash is caused by an injury that involves hyperextension, which results in compression of the anatomical structures. This type of injury usually occurs as a result of sudden acceleration and deceleration, such as rear-end car collisions that cause violent back-and-forth movements of the head and neck. Symptoms of a whiplash (primarily pain) may not be obvious for a few days or even a week after the injury. Cervical fractures can accompany a whiplash injury.

Assessment

Collection of **subjective data** includes the patient's complaint of pain (the most common symptom), which usually begins in the cervical area but may radiate down the arm to the fingers and increase with cervical motion. The pain may increase sharply with coughing, sneezing, or any radical movement. Other signs and symptoms may be paresthesia (numbness or tingling), headache, blurred vision, decreased skeletal function, and weakened hand grip.

Objective data include edema in the cervical spine region with tightening of the muscles. Vital signs are usually within normal ranges. However, if the assessment findings indicate hypertension with widened pulse pressure and bradycardia, suspect increased intracranial pressure (ICP); report and document the findings immediately. Do a neurologic assessment every 15 to 30 minutes to rule out increased ICP.

Diagnostic Tests

Physical examination and radiographic studies confirm the physician's diagnosis.

Medical Management

Symptoms commonly recur. A medical approach is most often used for treatment of whiplash. Analgesics and muscle relaxants are prescribed, along with intermittent cervical traction. Surgery may be necessary if cervical fracture with displacement occurs. (See Herniation of Intervertebral Disk [Herniated Nucleus Pulposus] later in the chapter.)

Other treatments include special exercises, heat therapy, and administration of mild analgesics as ordered by the physician to control the pain. A soft foam rubber neck brace collar may be used for whiplash injuries to limit head movement.

Nursing Interventions

Nursing interventions include care of the patient with restricted activity to immobilize the cervical vertebrae, decrease irritation, and provide rest for the traumatized area. This is accomplished with cervical traction. If a neck brace is used, carefully inspect the skin around the neck and chin for signs of excoriation.

Prognosis

Prognosis depends on the extent of neurologic involvement. Prognosis is excellent with minor trauma, but because the spinal canal is full of neural tissue in the cervical area, more extensive injury can produce profound disability.

ANKLE SPRAINS

Etiology and Pathophysiology

An ankle sprain is often referred to as a twisted ankle and is caused by a wrenching or twisting of the foot and ankle.

Clinical Manifestations

The ankle area becomes edematous quickly, with spasms of the muscles and pain on passive movement of the joint.

Assessment

Collection of **subjective data** includes assessment of pain and tenderness in the affected ankle that intensifies with movement of the foot or ankle.

Collection of **objective data** includes assessment of the traumatized ankle for signs of edema, limited movement and function of the joint, and ecchymosis of the soft tissue around the ankle.

Diagnostic Tests

A radiographic examination of the injured area is the only accurate way to ensure there is no bone injury.

Medical Management

Surgery may be indicated for severe sprains. The physician sutures torn ligament fibers together. If the ligaments have been torn from the bone, the surgeon reattaches them by drilling small holes in the medial malleolus (rounded bony protrusion on the medial area of the ankle).

Nursing Interventions

The injured area must be elevated and kept at rest. Application of ice for 15 to 20 minutes intermittently for 12 to 36 hours—followed after 24 hours by the application of mild heat for 15 to 30 minutes, four times daily—will promote absorption of blood and fluid from the area. Use compressive dressings and splinting to help support the injured area. A neurovascular assessment is necessary to detect impaired tissue perfusion.

> **! Safety Alert!**
>
> **Strains and Sprains**
>
> A strain and a sprain are not the same. Strains are produced by minute muscle tears and overstretching of tendons, whereas sprains are caused by a twisting of the joint

Prognosis

Prognosis is generally excellent.

STRAINS

Etiology and Pathophysiology

Strains are characterized by microscopic muscle tears as a result of overstretching muscles and tendons. An acute strain results when the muscles and tendons are overstretched in a forceful movement, such as unaccustomed vigorous exercise.

Assessment

Collection of **subjective data** includes noting the patient's complaint of sudden and severe pain away from the joint, which increases with activity. Chronic muscle strain can occur from repeated muscle overuse, and the pain may not appear for several hours. The patient typically complains of soreness, stiffness, and tenderness in the area.

Collection of **objective data** includes observation of stiffness, ecchymosis, and slight edema over the injury site. The most common sites are calf muscles, hamstrings, quadriceps, and the lumbosacral area. Edema can occur rapidly in the muscle and tendon area.

Diagnostic Tests

A radiographic study is necessary to rule out bone trauma.

Medical Management

Surgical repair is necessary if the muscle is completely ruptured. The physician orders analgesics and muscle relaxants. An exercise program is almost always prescribed if the strain is in the lumbosacral region. The exercises are aimed at strengthening the lower abdominal muscles.

Nursing Interventions

Nursing interventions for a strain are similar to those for a sprain. Ice application helps relieve pain, but some physicians prefer heat application rather than ice. Back strains are among the most common strains. If the symptoms worsen, advise the patient to avoid strenuous activities, use a firm chair with rigid back support, avoid wearing high heels, use a firm mattress for sleep, and never sleep on the abdomen. Encourage the patient to do leg exercises to prevent development of thrombosis.

Prognosis

Prognosis is usually favorable.

DISLOCATIONS

Etiology and Pathophysiology

Dislocations usually involve tearing of the joint capsule; **subluxations** (partial or incomplete dislocations) involve stretching of the joint capsule. Both are temporary displacements of bones from their normal position within joints. A dislocation may be (1) congenital (e.g., congenital hip displacement), (2) caused by a disease process, or (3) caused by trauma. A dislocation or subluxation can also be accompanied by stretching and tearing of ligaments and tendons and by fractures. The displaced bone may rupture blood vessels. When subluxation occurs, the joint's articulating (movable) surfaces are partially separated.

Clinical Manifestations

Dislocation may or may not be visible. Sometimes a dislocation changes the length of an affected extremity. Pain and loss of function may be similar to those occurring with a fracture. However, dislocation partially immobilizes a joint, whereas a fracture site typically has abnormal free movement. Common dislocation sites include the shoulder, hip, and knee.

Assessment

Subjective data include the patient's description of the injury and pain. For shoulder dislocation, the patient complains of sensation loss and paresthesia.

Collection of **objective data** includes the assessment of any erythema, discoloration, edema, pain, tenderness, limitation of movement, and deformity or shortening of the extremity. Compare both sides for validation. Neurovascular assessment is important to determine whether vascular or nerve injury is present in the affected area. For shoulder dislocation, assess for an absent radial pulse, hypothermia of the hand, and wrist drop.

Diagnostic Tests

The diagnosis is based on complaints of discomfort, physical examination, and diagnostic radiographic examination of the injured site.

Medical Management

The physician may perform a closed reduction, which corrects the deformity through manipulation of the extremity. Surgical intervention to restore joint articulation is sometimes required.

Nursing Interventions and Patient Teaching

Nursing interventions include (1) reduction of edema and discomfort, (2) immobilization of the injured part to promote healing, and (3) patient education. Ice application is recommended for the first 24 hours after trauma. After 24 hours, heat may be used if there are no indications of bleeding. Elevation of the injured extremity on pillows and the application of elastic bandages help relieve edema. Immobilization of joints may involve application of a splint, sling, or elastic bandage. The air cast or air splint brace is an immobilization device. It is inflatable, is lightweight, and conforms to the extremity's size and shape. When immobilization devices are used, perform a neurovascular assessment frequently (see Box 44-5 and Nursing Diagnoses box below). Administer analgesics as prescribed by the physician. Asking the patient to rate the pain on a scale from 0 to 10 is helpful in determining pain severity. For control of extreme pain, the physician may order an opioid, such as morphine. For moderate to mild pain, ibuprofen or acetaminophen (Tylenol) may be prescribed. Positioning and repositioning the injured part can help reduce discomfort.

Nursing diagnoses and interventions for the patient for neurovascular integrity include but are not limited to the following:

Nursing Diagnoses	Nursing Interventions
Ineffective peripheral tissue perfusion, related to: • injury • treatment	Position extremities in alignment; elevate affected extremity. Carefully monitor distal pulses, capillary refill, and temperature of involved area.
Risk for injury, related to neurovascular impairment	Compare affected extremity with unaffected extremity, using same hand for palpation. Test capillary refill (blanching test). Check each digit for sensation and motion. Document location and characteristics of pain. Palpate pedal, tibial, or radial pulses, and compare with unaffected extremity. Assess for edema with pallor, cyanosis, and coldness. Ask patient to describe sensations. Document all findings.

Promoting an accident-free environment is essential. Areas of preventive medicine to explore with patients include the following:

- Grab bars mounted in the bathroom near the toilet or tub and rubber mats or slip guards in the tub and shower help prevent falls.
- Removing throw rugs and obstacles from the floor can prevent falls.
- A gait enhancer, such as a cane, crutches, or a walker, must be used correctly and with attention to safety precautions, such as using rubber tips

on the points that make contact with the floor to prevent slippage.
- Patients in the hospital are at risk of falling out of bed if their disease, condition, or medication results in disorientation. Carefully assess their level of orientation, keep side rails up, and provide safety reminder devices to prevent self-injury.
- Using a safe ladder when climbing can help prevent a fall.
- Wearing protective clothing while engaging in dangerous work or contact sports is recommended.

Appropriate health teaching should be targeted for people at risk for musculoskeletal diseases, such as osteoporosis, which can predispose them to pathologic or nontraumatic fractures.

Prognosis

Prognosis is generally excellent.

AIRBAG INJURIES

Airbag deployment injuries include chemical burns, ocular trauma, cervical injury, soft tissue injury, and upper extremity and chest trauma. Orthopedic injuries tend to involve the upper extremities, especially the wrist, hand, and elbow. Injuries from airbag deployment can be life threatening in the very young. People at increased risk include older adults and small children. Airbag-induced injuries are associated with a rapid, forceful inflation, lasting less than 1 second from inflation to deflation. Research is continuing to develop safer airbag deployment.

CARPAL TUNNEL SYNDROME

Etiology and Pathophysiology

Carpal tunnel syndrome is a painful disorder of the wrist and hand. It is caused by inflammation and edema of the synovial lining of the tendon sheaths in the carpal tunnel of the wrist. As a result, the tunnel space is narrowed, resulting in compression of the median nerve between the inelastic carpal ligament and other structures in the carpal tunnel (Figure 44-38).

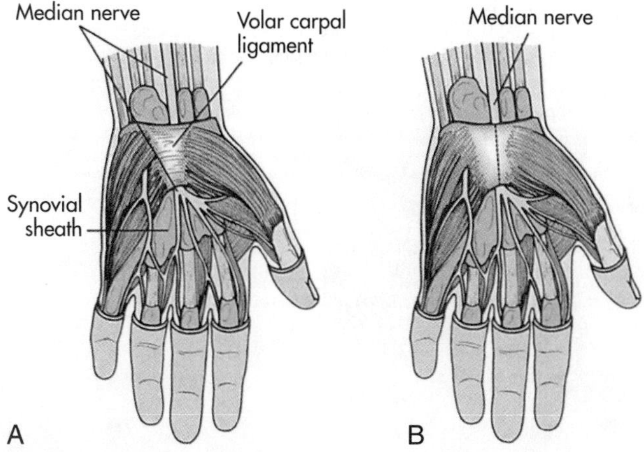

FIGURE 44-38 **A,** Wrist structures involved in carpal tunnel syndrome. **B,** Decompression of median nerve.

The symptoms of **paresthesia** (any subjective sensation such as pricks of pins and needles) and **hypoesthesia** (a decrease in sensation in response to stimulation of the sensory nerves) of the thumb, index, and middle fingers may develop spontaneously or occur as a result of disease or injury.

This condition has a higher incidence in obese, middle-aged women and individuals employed in occupations involving repetitious motions of the fingers and hands (e.g., computing, hairdressing, basket weaving, meat carving, and typing). Carpal tunnel syndrome has become one of the three most common industrial or work-related conditions and is related to increased computer usage. Edema of the tendon sheaths caused by RA can predispose a patient to carpal tunnel syndrome. Curiously, pregnant women may develop the syndrome during their last trimester. The reasons for this are unknown, but it may be related to fluid retention and edema.

Clinical Manifestations

The affected hand has altered ability to grasp or hold small objects. Atrophy of the thenar eminence (the padded area of the palm below the base of the thumb) is noted as the disease progresses. The clinical manifestations also include burning pain, numbness and weakness (especially of the thumb) (Lewis et al., 2007).

Assessment

Subjective data include the patient's description of discomfort, such as burning pain or tingling in the hands relieved by vigorously shaking or exercising the hands. Pain may be intermittent or constant and is often more intense at night. The patient may also complain of numbness (hypoesthesia) of the thumb, index, and ring fingers, especially after prolonged flexion of the wrist; and inability to grasp or hold small objects.

Collection of **objective data** includes assessment of the hand, wrist, or fingers for edema; muscle atrophy; or a depressed appearance of the soft tissue at the base of the thumb on the palmar surface.

Diagnostic Tests

Physical examination reveals deficits in sensory mapping along median nerve innervation pathways; positive Tinel's sign; increased tingling with a gentle tap over the tendon sheath on the ventral surface of the central wrist; edema of the fingers; and thenar surfaces of the palm thinner than normal (wasting). Having the patient hold the wrists against each other in forced palmar flexion for 1 minute can elicit sensory changes of numbness and tingling, which is a positive Phalen's maneuver test (one indication of carpal tunnel syndrome).

An electromyogram shows a weakened muscle response to stimulation. MRI shows compression and flattening of the median nerve, increased signal intensity within the median nerve, and abrupt changes in diameter of the median nerve. A handheld electroneurometer predicts motor latency of the median nerve, which is diagnostic of carpal tunnel syndrome.

Medical Management

If the symptoms are mild and surgery is not a desirable option, an immobilizer such as a splint can be used. Hydrocortisone acetate suspension injected into the carpal tunnel can relieve mild symptoms. Surgery is indicated for severe symptoms with muscle atrophy. The standard surgical treatment is decompression of the median nerve by section of the transverse carpal ligament.

Nursing Interventions and Patient Teaching

Educate the patient about special keyboard pads and mouse devices that may be used to prevent pressure on the medial nerve for computer users. The patient should be encouraged to change body positions and take breaks from activities which promote medial nerve pressure (Lewis et al., 2007).

If surgery is not required, the nurse is involved in the application of an immobilizer to promote comfort. General nursing interventions are use of a wrist cock-up splint to relieve pressure and to lessen wrist flexion, elevation to relieve edema, ROM exercises to lessen sense of clumsiness, and restriction of twisting and turning activities of the wrist.

If surgery is required, postoperative interventions include (1) elevating the hand and arm for 24 hours; (2) implementing and evaluating active thumb and finger motion within limits imposed by the dressing; (3) administering prescribed analgesics as needed; (4) monitoring vital signs (temperature elevation could indicate infection); and (5) checking fingers for circulation, sensation, and movement every 1 to 2 hours for 24 hours.

Encourage patients to use the affected hand in normal activities as soon as 2 to 3 days after surgery.

Prognosis

Mild symptoms of carpal tunnel syndrome are relieved by nonsurgical treatment; severe symptoms require surgical intervention with excellent prognosis. If the patient is pregnant, symptoms are usually relieved after delivery.

HERNIATION OF INTERVERTEBRAL DISK (HERNIATED NUCLEUS PULPOSUS)

Etiology and Pathophysiology

Herniated nucleus pulposus is a rupture of the fibrocartilage surrounding an intervertebral disk, releasing the nucleus pulposus that cushions the vertebrae above and below. This displacement puts pressure on nerve roots. Lumbar and cervical herniations are most common (Figure 44-39). Herniated nucleus pulposus can occur suddenly (from lifting, twisting, or trauma) or gradually (from degenerative changes, as seen with DJD, osteoporosis, aging, and chronic diseases affecting bones). Herniations of the lumbar spine usually affect people 20 to 45 years old; cervical herniations are seen most in people 45 years and older. Men are more prone to this disorder than women.

Clinical Manifestations

Low back pain that occurs with the slightest movement is the most common symptom of lumbar herniation. The pain radiates over the buttock and down the leg, following the sciatic nerve pathway **(radicular pain),** causing numbness and tingling in the affected leg. Neck pain, headache, and neck rigidity are common symptoms of cervical herniations. Complaints of pain in the back radiating down the leg (sciatica) are common. Complaints about activity intolerance and alteration in bowel and bladder elimination (constipation and urinary retention) are significant.

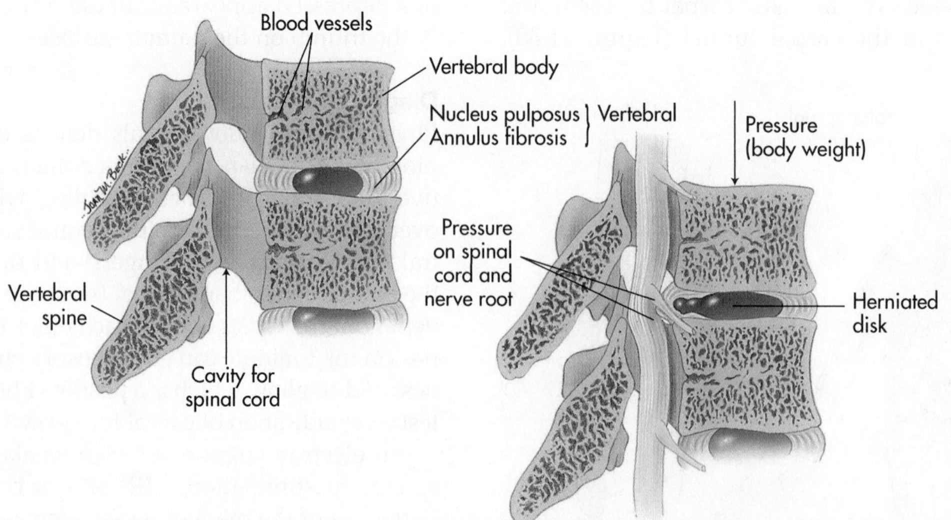

FIGURE 44-39 Sagittal section of vertebrae showing both normal *(left)* and herniated disks.

Assessment

Collection of **subjective data** includes assessing pain and asking patient about measures used for relief and other possible symptoms, such as activity intolerance and altered bowel and bladder function. Pain often gets worse with activity.

Collection of **objective data** includes observing for signs of limited spinal flexibility (limited forward bending) and gait alteration (patient may support weight on one extremity). An ineffective breathing pattern may result from pain and decreased mobility. Assessment includes determination of bowel and bladder elimination and maintenance of traction equipment.

Diagnostic Tests

Obtain a complete history and physical examination. The physician orders radiographic studies, CT, myelography, and electromyelography to determine nerve involvement.

Medical Management

The patient usually follows a 4-week course of conservative therapy such as braces, corset, or belt, local heat or ice, ultrasound and massage, and transcutaneous electrical nerve stimulation (TENS). Drug therapy such as NSAIDs, muscle relaxants, and epidural corticosteroid therapy may be used (Lewis et al., 2007). If the patient demonstrates neurologic deterioration or continued pain, a surgical procedure may be required, such as one of the following:

- **Laminectomy:** Surgical removal of the bony arches or one or more vertebrae performed to relieve compression of the spinal cord caused by bone displacement from an injury or degeneration of a disk or to remove a displaced vertebral disk.
- **Spinal fusion** (arthrodesis; the surgical immobilization of a joint; artificial ankylosis): Removal of the lamina and several herniated nuclei pulposi. A portion of bone taken from the patient's iliac crest or from a bone bank is used as a bone graft in the vertebral spaces.
- **Diskectomy:** Removal of the extruded disk material, often with a microscope. Percutaneous lateral diskectomy—cutting a window around the anulus fibrosus—is performed with the patient under local anesthesia.
- **Artificial disk replacement:** Replacement of a damaged intervertebral disk with an artificial disk called Charité disk. The damaged disk is removed and the Charité disk placed in the spine. The disk allows the natural movement of the spine (U.S. Food & Drug Administration, 2004).
- **Endoscopic spinal microsurgery:** Can be performed with the patient under local anesthesia. Special scopes enable the surgeon to successfully remove herniated disks with minimal damage to surrounding tissues.
- **Chemonucleolysis:** Can be done on patients who have no nerve involvement. The procedure involves administering a local anesthetic agent and then guiding a needle into the nucleus pulposus to inject chymopapain (a drug that dissolves the nucleus pulposus).

Postoperative laminectomy care includes assessing the incision site for signs of infection such as drainage, edema, odor, and temperature elevation. Use of surgical asepsis when changing dressings and handling drainage decreases development of infection. After a chemonucleolysis, carefully assess for signs of allergic reactions to chymopapain, such as urticaria and respiratory difficulties.

Nursing Interventions and Patient Teaching

Nursing interventions are aimed at providing nursing care appropriate for the following nursing diagnoses:

- Anxiety, related to discomfort, fear of unknown, and lifestyle changes
- Pain (back), related to muscle spasms and painful diagnostic tests
- Constipation and impaired urinary elimination, related to pain, analgesics, immobility, and neurologic involvement

Give the patient and family information about procedures and hospital protocol to help reduce their anxiety. Administer the medications prescribed on schedule, and document the effectiveness of the medication. Distraction, heat or ice application (if ordered), and moving (by log-rolling) and positioning the patient every 2 hours (if not contraindicated because of need to maintain traction) can promote patient comfort. Dietary monitoring is important to ensure that the patient maintains a high-protein, iron- and vitamin-enriched diet.

Observe dressing for bleeding or cerebrospinal fluid leakage. Apply antiembolism stockings if ordered. Careful documentation of I&O provides information about bowel and bladder function. Ensure that the patient has voided in the first 8 hours, and use nursing measures to promote voiding before resorting to catheterization. Encourage the patient to sit in a straight, firm chair for no longer than 30 minutes at one time. Monitor the patient for evidence of respiratory distress and paralytic ileus, complications that may occur in laminectomy patients.

Nursing diagnoses and interventions for the patient with herniated disk include but are not limited to the following:

Nursing Diagnoses	Nursing Interventions
Deficient knowledge, related to home care management	Stress importance of rehabilitation plan of activity, rest, and exercise.

Continued

Nursing Diagnoses	Nursing Interventions
Deficient knowledge, related to home care management—cont'd	Provide diet instructions related to type and amount of food and weight maintenance (no gain) if applicable. Discuss medications: name, purpose, schedule, dosage, and side effects. Discuss signs and symptoms to report to physician: severe pain; changes in temperature, color, or sensation in extremity; and malodorous drainage from wound. Encourage follow-up visits with physician.
Powerlessness, related to: • decreased mobility • pain	Use active listening and permit verbalization of anger and helplessness. Assist patient in identifying coping mechanisms that will reduce feeling of powerlessness; use those that have been successful in the past. Offer positive recognition for increased activity level. Assist patient in identifying areas that can be controlled. Involve patient in decision-making process for own care.

The patient may begin activity out of bed as early as 1 day after a simple laminectomy or 2 to 4 days after a laminectomy and fusion. Transfer the patient out of bed with as little time spent in the sitting position as possible. The patient may be permitted to walk as much as tolerated, with assistance if necessary. Braces or corsets, if prescribed, are applied before the patient gets out of bed. Encourage the patient to participate in ADLs within prescribed limits of mobility.

Instruct the patient not to lift or carry anything heavier than 5 pounds (2.25 kg) for at least 8 weeks, not to drive a car until permitted by the surgeon, and to avoid twisting motions of the trunk. Reinforce the importance of follow-up visits to the physician.

Prognosis

With conservative treatment, some patients receive relief of symptoms; if a neurologic pathologic condition develops, surgical intervention is needed. The prognosis is usually favorable.

TUMORS OF THE BONE

Etiology and Pathophysiology

Tumors of the bone may be primary or secondary and may be benign or malignant. As with other types of tumors, the cause of bone tumors is not always known. Carcinoma of the prostate, lung, breast, thyroid, and kidney may metastasize to the bones. **Osteogenic** tumors are primary malignant bone tumors that occur most often in young people.

Osteogenic sarcoma is a fast-growing and aggressive tumor that affects the long bones of the body, particularly the distal femur, the proximal tibia, and the proximal humerus. Osteogenic sarcoma can metastasize to the lungs and to the rest of the body via the bloodstream. It affects males between the ages of 10 and 25 more often than females.

Osteochondroma is the most common benign osteogenic tumor. The incidence is highest in males between 10 and 30 years of age. Osteochondromas can occur as a single tumor or as multiple tumors. They usually affect the humerus, tibia, and femur.

Clinical Manifestations

When healthy bone cells are replaced by cancer cells, the bone's strength is altered and spontaneous fractures can occur. Anemia occurs when cancer invades the long bones and interrupts the manufacture of red blood cells in the bone marrow. Cancerous bone tumors metastasize and invade other bones and lung tissue.

Benign bone tumors can grow large enough to put pressure on blood vessels and nerves. Benign tumors do not spread. However, they may undergo cancerous changes and become malignant.

Assessment

Malignant and benign bone tumors cause pain in the affected bone site. **Subjective data** include complaints of pain, especially with weight bearing. Pain may result from a spontaneous fracture. The patient may also complain of tenderness at the affected site.

Collection of **objective data** includes assessment of the painful part, which may reveal edema and discoloration of the skin.

Diagnostic Tests

Diagnosis is confirmed with radiographic studies, bone scan, bone biopsy, and laboratory studies, such as a CBC (which reveals bone marrow involvement), serum protein levels (elevated in multiple myeloma), and serum alkaline phosphatase level (elevated in osteogenic sarcoma).

Medical Management

The physician evaluates the tumor type, size, and location and plans the treatment accordingly. Larger, symptomatic, benign tumors and malignant tumors require surgical intervention. The surgical procedure depends on the tumor size, location, and extent of tissue involvement. The surgery may involve (1) wide excision or resection, (2) bone curettage, or (3) leg or arm amputation.

Treatment is aimed at destroying or removing the malignant lesion. Amputation of the affected extremity may be necessary. Radiation and chemotherapy may be used before surgery to decrease tumor size or tissue involvement. Limb-salvage surgical procedures in combination with radiation and chemotherapy are being used more frequently for treatment of malignant bone tumors.

Chemotherapy is aimed at destroying cancer cells at both primary and metastatic sites. Patients usually receive chemotherapy in 3- or 4-week cycles. Radiation therapy may be given internally and externally. The nurse must know the safety precautions and side effects of chemotherapy and radiation therapy. (See Chapter 57 for a discussion of care of the patient with cancer.)

Nursing Interventions and Patient Teaching

Preoperatively the patient and family need complete and concise information about procedures and postoperative expectations. Postoperative nursing interventions include (1) performing a neurovascular assessment (see Box 44-5); (2) monitoring vital signs; (3) administering analgesics and evaluating the effectiveness; (4) providing cast care or dressing changes with careful documentation of drainage, odors, and signs of circulation impairment; (5) cooperating with physical and occupational therapists to promote mobility and ADLs; and (6) educating the patient and family about home health care and early detection of tumor recurrence

A nursing diagnosis and interventions for the patient with a bone tumor include but are not limited to the following:

Nursing Diagnosis	Nursing Interventions
Anxiety, related to: • fear of cancer • body image • lifestyle change • possibility of death	Establish therapeutic relationship: acknowledge fear, encourage patient to acknowledge and express feelings. Give accurate information about condition and therapies. Refer patient to other resources when necessary (e.g., social worker, religious counselor).

Prognosis

The prognosis for bone tumors has improved in recent years with the combination of local surgery, chemotherapy, and radiation. Disease-free survival rates for patients whose osteogenic sarcoma is treated with surgery, chemotherapy, and radiation appear to be greater than 50% at 5 years.

AMPUTATION

The amputation of a portion of or an entire extremity may be necessary because of malignant tumors, injuries, impaired circulation (caused by diabetes mellitus or arteriosclerosis), congenital deformities, and infections. Most amputations are elective surgery unless they are related to trauma. Advances in microsurgical techniques enable surgeons to reattach severed extremities. Therefore traumatic amputations can sometimes be reversed by replantation if the severed limb is kept sterile and moist in a plastic bag filled with ice water. (The part should be protected from direct contact with ice; dry ice should not be used.)

Amputation of long bones can result in postoperative anemia. A traumatic or surgical amputation of an extremity can cause serious blood loss. Malignant bone tumors can metastasize via the bloodstream to other body systems.

Preoperative Assessment

Collection of **subjective data** includes questioning the patient about his or her understanding of the injury or disease process. Assess and document complaints of pain and symptoms of neurovascular impairment. Assess the patient's level of orientation, since many amputations occur in the older adult population as a result of impaired circulation.

Collection of **objective data** includes assessment of vital signs (temperature elevation, tachycardia, and tachypnea indicate infection). Assess arterial blood flow by palpation of bilateral pedal pulses and Doppler pressure measurements. Assess wound drainage for color, amount, and presence of odor. Evaluate upper body muscle strength and nutritional status.

Diagnostic Tests

A CBC is done to determine blood dyscrasias, such as anemia and bleeding tendencies, which could increase postoperative complications (such as hemorrhage, delayed wound healing, and disorientation). The physician orders laboratory studies such as BUN, potassium levels, and routine urinalysis. An ECG is performed to detect cardiac dysrhythmias, which are often present in older adult patients.

Medical Management

When the amputation results from traumatic injury to an extremity, the physician's interventions include measures to restore circulating blood volume, control pain, prevent infection in the wound, perform a plastic surgical repair at the amputation site to facilitate the use of a prosthesis, and maintain adequate urinary output.

For elective amputations, the physician assesses the patient's physiologic, psychological, and emotional status. If infection is present in the body (gangrene may occur if circulation is impaired), treatment includes administration of antibiotics, and every attempt is made to control the infection before surgery. The physician discusses the possibility of the patient using a prosthesis. Much of the preoperative preparation focuses on the patient attaining a physical and emotional status conducive to wearing a prosthesis or achieving mobility through the use of a wheelchair or a gait enhancer such as crutches or a walker.

Postoperative Assessment, Nursing Interventions, and Patient Teaching

Collection of **subjective data** includes careful assessment of pain. **Phantom pain** (pain felt in the missing extremity as if it were still present) may occur and be frightening to the patient. Phantom pain occurs because the nerve tracks that register pain in the amputated area continue to send a message to the brain; this is normal.

Collection of **objective data** includes observing for signs of hemorrhage, such as hypotension, tachycardia, tachypnea, pallor, decreased urinary output, restlessness, and progressive loss of consciousness. Monitor and document suction drainage, and assess and protect the remaining extremity. Observe for neurovascular impairment (done hourly in the immediate postoperative period) from tightly applied elastic wraps, dressings, or casts (see Box 44-5).

Nursing intervention is aimed at effective pain management and prevention of deformities (contractures, especially in the joint above the amputation, or abduction deformities are common). Flexion hip contractures can be prevented postoperatively by raising the foot of the bed slightly to elevate the residual extremity (with care taken not to flex the patient's hips by elevating the stump on a pillow), encouraging movement from side to side, and placing the patient in a prone position at least twice a day. This will stretch the flexor muscles. Teach the patient how to strengthen remaining muscles to facilitate mobility and prevent muscle atrophy (push-ups from a prone position and sit-ups from a seated position). Apply elastic wraps to shrink and reshape the residual extremity into a cone and facilitate the proper fit and use of a prosthesis (Figure 44-40). A prosthesis may be fitted as early as 2 or 3 weeks postoperatively. Because many amputations are performed in people between 60 and 70 years of age, observe the patient carefully for pulmonary complications (such as pulmonary embolus) and cardiovascular collapse. Keep suction equipment and oxygen at the bedside.

Patient education concerning phantom-limb sensation, and the fact that it is a normal physiologic response, can help relieve patient fears. The patient may feel pain or other sensations, such as burning, tingling, throbbing, or pruritus in the amputated extremity. These sensations can last for months or decades on a consistent or intermittent basis. Recommend that patients gently rub the residual extremity or take analgesics for relief.

For persistent, severe phantom pain, the following measures may be employed:

- Stump revision with reamputation at a higher level
- Local infiltration of the stump with procaine
- Mechanical percussion by striking the sensitive digital stump against a solid object—believed to shrink neuromas (small tumors that form in the scar tissue of the stump)
- Sympathetic nerve block

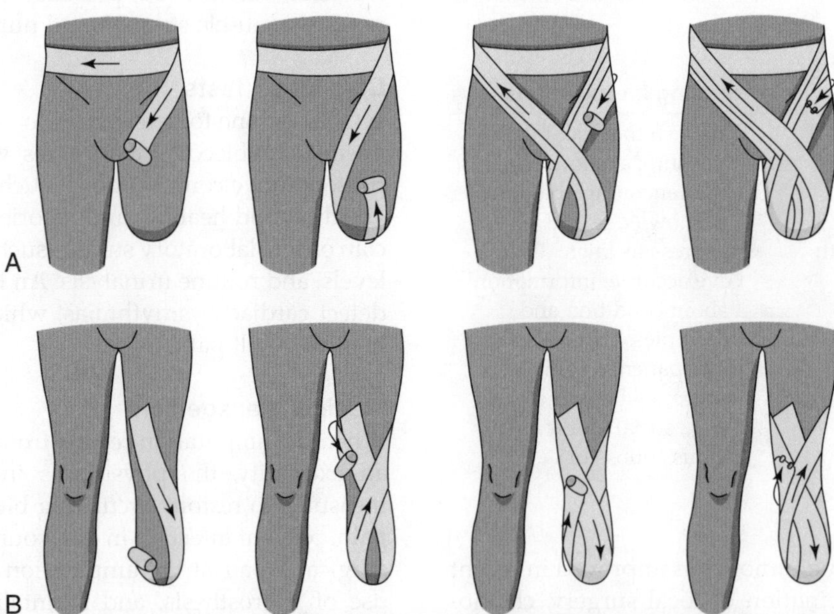

FIGURE 44-40 Correct method of bandaging amputation stump. **A,** Anchor bandage around patient's waist. **B,** Method of bandaging midcalf stump, where bandage need not be anchored around waist.

Encourage the patient to share his or her feelings over the loss of the extremity. Discuss the importance of allowing the grieving process to occur.

Nursing diagnoses and interventions for the patient undergoing an amputation include but are not limited to the following:

Nursing Diagnoses	Nursing Interventions
Disturbed body image, related to loss of limb	Assess effects of amputation on body image. Encourage patient to express feelings of mutilation, grief, anger, and loss to aid adaptation processes. Encourage patient to help with dressing changes and wrapping of stump as able. Teach family member wrapping techniques if necessary to increase competence and independence. Use prescribed pain-management techniques. Encourage family members to walk with patient to maintain strength and social contacts. Encourage grooming and wearing of personal clothing to maintain individuality and personality. Encourage activities for self-care and ambulation to maintain positive outlook and maximum strength. Encourage or arrange for social services consultation for economic and employment aid. Arrange for follow-up care referral to aid rehabilitation.
Impaired physical mobility, related to loss of limb	Assess ability to use remaining limbs. Turn and position on side, back, and abdomen (after 24 hours) to maintain muscle and joint ROM. Teach adduction and extension exercises and help patient perform them every 4 hours to prevent abduction and flexion contractures. Assist with sitting in chair and ambulation with aid as able to maintain muscle strength. Prepare patient for physical therapy, transportation for exercises, and stump wrapping, if appropriate. Encourage family members to walk with patient during initial ambulation periods, accompanied by health professionals, to increase independence. Teach purposes of prone and extension positions to prevent contractures. Assist prosthetist with prosthesis measurements and fitting as needed to aid rehabilitation.

Before discharge, teach the patient and family proper positions, exercises, and ambulation techniques. Also demonstrate stump-wrapping techniques to the patient and family (see Figure 44-40). Explain to them that prolonged phantom pain experiences are unusual and should receive medical attention. Discuss skin care with the patient and family so they can take steps to prevent stump irritation or impairment. Also discuss the signs of a wound infection, and instruct them when it is necessary to call the physician.

Prognosis

The prognosis for successful adaptation to an amputation depends on the patient's age, the condition that resulted in amputation, other systemic disorders, emotional health, and support system.

❖ NURSING PROCESS *for the Patient with a Musculoskeletal Disorder*

The role of the licensed practical nurse/licensed vocational nurse (LPN/LVN) in the nursing process as stated is that the LPN/LVN will:

- Participate in planning care for patients based on patient needs
- Review patient's care plan and recommend revisions as needed
- Review and follow defined prioritization for patient care
- Use clinical pathways, care maps, or care plans to guide and review patient care

■ Assessment

The musculoskeletal system provides protection, support, and movement for the body. Proper function of the musculoskeletal system is closely associated with the proper function of the nervous and circulatory systems. Orthopedics is the branch of medicine that deals with the prevention or correction of disorders involving locomotor structures of the body. Permanent disability and crippling will result if patients with musculoskeletal dysfunction do not receive prompt treatment.

Assess orthopedic function for all patients, especially those who are (1) having difficulty with gait; (2) experiencing muscle weakness; (3) suffering from trauma of soft tissue and bone; (4) unable to move and participate in activities for personal, economic, and social fulfillment; (5) experiencing diseases of the musculoskeletal system; or (6) chronically ill.

Assessment of a patient's mobility includes bone integrity, posture, joint function, muscle strength, gait, pain, and neurovascular disturbances related to pressure. Compare body symmetry. For example, assess both legs for same length and diameter size and for comparable muscle strength. Observe the patient's gait for unsteadiness or irregular movements. Difficult ambulation associated with shortness of breath can indicate cardiovascular or respiratory system difficulties.

Assessment of posture and gait simply involves observing the patient walking. Common posture deformities include lateral (or S) curvature of the spine, known as **scoliosis;** a rounding of the thoracic spine (hump-backed appearance), known as **kyphosis;** and an increase in the curve at the lumbar space region that throws the shoulders back, making the "lordly" or "kingly" appearance known as **lordosis** (Figure 44-41). Rigidity of the spine can result from AKS, in which the vertebrae are fused with loss of mobility, producing a rigid gait or "poker spine" appearance.

Assessment of neurologic and circulatory function is important if the patient has experienced a traumatic injury; damaged blood vessels and nerves can cause permanent disabilities.

Assess the skin for signs of coolness, pallor, sensation, or cyanosis to help determine the patient's circulatory status. A faint or absent pulse in an extremity indicates impaired circulation. Palpating the femoral, popliteal, and dorsalis pedis pulses on both extremities provides pertinent data about the lower extremities. If the pulse is not readily palpated with a light touch of the finger, a Doppler instrument can be used to magnify the sound of the pulsation. The absence of a pulse is serious and must be reported to the charge nurse immediately. Assess the brachial and radial pulses to determine circulation in the upper extremities. Palpating a pulse may be difficult if the patient has a cast or bandage. Reach under the cast or bandage if possible. Assess the pulse in the unaffected extremity for comparison.

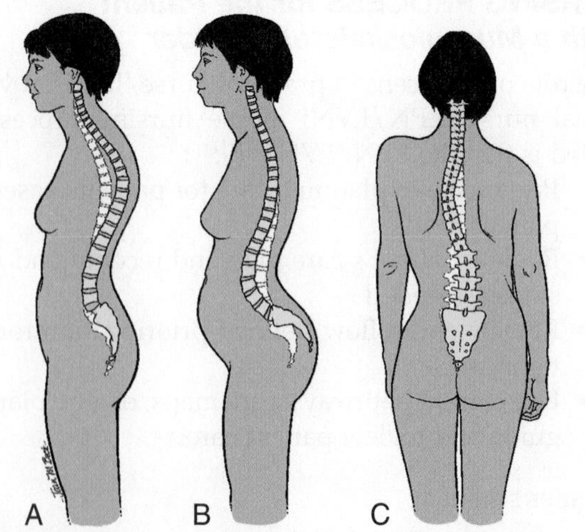

FIGURE 44-41 Abnormal spinal curvatures. **A,** Kyphosis. **B,** Lordosis. **C,** Scoliosis.

The **blanching test** (meaning to whiten or pale) is a test of the rate of capillary refill, which signals circulation status. This is also referred to as a **capillary nail refill test.** Compress each fingernail or toenail of the affected extremity (noting the white color as pressure is applied), release the pressure, and note how quickly the pink color returns to the nailbed. The nailbed color should return to normal within 2 or 3 seconds. If the color is slow to return, circulation is impaired and requires prompt attention (see Box 44-5).

Neurovascular assessments are made on patients with musculoskeletal trauma or damage to nerves and blood vessels resulting from surgery, tight bandages, splints, or casts. Impaired circulation resulting in alteration of nerve function can cause loss of the use of an extremity; this impairment is generally seen in the extremities. See Box 44-5 for information concerning neurovascular (circulation) assessment.

■ Nursing Diagnosis

Nursing assessment establishes the patient's needs regarding mobility. Care of the patient is based on the following nursing diagnoses:

- Impaired physical mobility, related to musculoskeletal impairment
- Impaired bed mobility
- Activity intolerance, related to musculoskeletal impairment
- Ineffective coping
- Anxiety, related to changes in body integrity
- Pain, related to musculoskeletal disorder
- Deficient knowledge regarding therapeutic regimen
- Risk for disuse syndrome

■ Expected Outcomes and Planning

The plan for facilitating mobility must center on improving and restoring performance and preventing deterioration. Nursing interventions help the patient adapt, reduce, or eliminate activities that cause pain.

Consider the amount of assistance needed for ambulation. Assessment of ROM and muscle strength helps decide whether the patient is able to ambulate safely. Ambulation after surgery often requires physical assistance in addition to the use of mobility aids such as walkers, canes, and crutches.

The care plan focuses on accomplishing individual goals and outcomes that relate to the identified nursing diagnoses. Examples of these include the following:

Goal 1: Patient will demonstrate the use of adaptive devices to increase mobility.

Outcome: Patient demonstrates more independence in mobility by meeting self-care needs.

Goal 2: Patient will demonstrate ambulation and state safety precautions before discharge from health care facility.

Outcome: Patient demonstrates ambulation skills and states correct safety precautions before discharge.

Implementation

Improving the patient's mobility requires awareness of physician's orders specific to ambulation. Check mobility aids for the correct size. Educate patients on safety measures, such as rubber tips in good condition on canes. Shoes that are easy to put on, have nonslip soles, and provide foot and ankle support are safer than bedroom slippers or stockings.

Activities need to be alternated with rest periods. Administer analgesics at least 30 minutes before ambulation for patients experiencing pain. Encourage patients to pace themselves. Patient assistance may be necessary to complete ADLs such as ambulating to the bathroom or to a bedside commode.

Specific principles are involved with mobility:

- Bone loss occurs when patients are confined to bed rest.
- The activities of the human body depend on effective interaction between normal joints and the neuromuscular parts that pilot them.
- Muscles, tendons, ligaments, cartilage, and bones all do their share to ensure smooth function.

Nurses working with patient mobility needs must support physical therapy department activities and goals. Assess a patient's perceptions to help determine his or her motivation for mobility independence. For example, when older adults think they are too fragile to walk, they may be afraid of trying. Use a safety belt when a patient's stability is questionable. The belt encircles the patient's waist; grasp the belt in the middle of the back to help the patient stand, gain balance, and ambulate.

Patients may have difficulty coping with mobility aids and perceive them as a visible sign of weakness. Point out that devices to help mobility are not unlike glasses to help eyesight. Mobility aids increase proficiency of activities and promote joint rest and protection.

Evaluation

Evaluate the success of interventions by noting patient's progress during and after ambulation based on stated goals and outcomes. For example, if the patient is not able to walk to the bathroom, a shorter distance may be more practical. The patient may increase mobility by using a bedside commode. When patients are unable to meet expected outcomes, be ready to revise the care plan to promote success. Examples of goals and their corresponding outcomes include the following:

Goal 1: Patient will demonstrate the use of adaptive devices to increase mobility.

Evaluative measure: Patient ambulates within physical environment.

Goal 2: Patient will understand safety precautions concerning use of mobility aids.

Evaluative measures: Patient checks rubber tips on mobility aid and uses equipment correctly.

Get Ready for the NCLEX® Examination!

Key Points

- The skeletal system has five basic functions: support of the body, protection of internal organs, movement of the body, storage of minerals, and blood cell formation.
- The skeleton is divided into the axial and the appendicular skeletons. The axial skeleton is composed of the skull, vertebral column, and thorax. The appendicular skeleton is composed of the upper extremities, lower extremities, shoulder girdle, and pelvic girdle.
- The three types of joints and their movement are (1) synarthrosis: no movement; (2) amphiarthrosis: slight movement; and (3) diarthrosis: free movement.
- Joints hold the bones together and allow movement and flexibility. Differences in the structure determine the amount of flexibility.
- Some of the more common movements that the body produces are flexion, extension, abduction, adduction, rotation, supination, pronation, dorsiflexion, and plantar flexion.
- The bones and joints provide the framework of the body, but the muscles are necessary for movement. Movement results from contraction and relaxation of the individual muscles.
- An ESR is the most objective laboratory test for determining the severity of RA.
- RA affects a young population (ages 30 to 55) with crippling changes in the synovial membrane of the joints.
- Salicylates and NSAIDs are used to treat RA and osteoarthritis.

- Osteoarthritis is a DJD that affects the population older than 40 years of age and causes articular cartilage degeneration.
- Porous and brittle bones caused by a lack of calcium are one of the physiologic changes noted in osteoporosis.
- Osteoporosis-related fractures occur in one in two women, compared with one in eight men, over the course of a lifetime.
- Vertebroplasty and kyphoplasty are surgical procedures used to relieve pain in women with osteoporosis who do not respond to other pain management programs.
- Arthroplasty procedures (such as hip and knee arthroplasty) are commonly performed on patients suffering from severe arthritis.
- Unicompartmental knee arthroplasty, also referred to as partial knee replacement, is performed on patients who have only one of the compartments of the knee affected by arthritis.
- Nursing intervention specific to the care of a patient suffering from a fractured hip involves maintaining abduction of the affected leg.
- Fractured hip fixation devices—such as hip prosthetic implant, plate and screw fixation, and telescoping nail fixation—require some degree of non–weight bearing for 6 weeks to 3 months.
- The use of antacids and proton pump inhibitors increases a patient's risk of hip fractures.
- A significant postoperative nursing intervention for a patient with an amputation is proper care of the stump to facilitate the use of a prosthetic device.
- Herniated nucleus pulposus is seen most often in the cervical and lumbar spinal regions and can be treated surgically (laminectomy and spinal fusion) or medically (medication, traction, and physical therapy).
- Osteogenic sarcoma is a common primary malignant tumor seen in young people; it can metastasize to the lungs.
- Compartment syndrome, shock, fat embolism, gas gangrene, thromboembolus, and osteomyelitis are complications resulting from a fractured bone.
- Petechiae on the conjunctiva of the eye, the neck, the chest, or the axillary region is a typical sign of a fat embolism.
- External fixation devices such as casts, braces, metal pins, and skeletal and skin traction are used to hold bone fragments in normal position.
- Whether the casting material is plaster of Paris or a synthetic material, proper drying, cleansing, handling, and assessing are required to prevent patient complications.
- The nurse caring for a patient in traction is responsible for knowing (1) the purpose of the traction (traction applied for fractures must be continuous), (2) the equipment needed and appropriate safety measures, (3) the amount of weight ordered, and (4) the patient's understanding of the traction.
- Crutches, canes, walkers, and the Roll-A-Bout are used as gait enhancers for patients with altered mobility.
- Crutch walking involving the three-point gait is most commonly used for patients wearing leg casts.

Additional Learning Resources

Go to your Companion CD for an audio glossary, animations, video clips, and more.

evolve Be sure to visit the Evolve site at http://evolve.elsevier.com/Christensen/adult/ for additional online resources.

Review Questions for the NCLEX® Examination

1. The bones serve as storage for which two minerals?
   1. Sodium and potassium
   2. Calcium and phosphorus
   3. Copper and iodine
   4. Magnesium and chloride

2. Hematopoiesis takes place in:
   1. the lymph nodes.
   2. the spleen.
   3. the yellow bone marrow.
   4. the red bone marrow.

3. Movement of an extremity away from the midline of the body is called:
   1. adduction.
   2. pronation.
   3. flexion.
   4. abduction.

4. A 65-year-old patient has been diagnosed with rheumatoid arthritis (RA). A diagnostic test used to confirm RA is:
   1. complete blood count.
   2. erythrocyte sedimentation rate.
   3. prothrombin time.
   4. urinary uric acid level.

5. A clinical sign of gouty arthritis is:
   1. Heberden's nodes.
   2. pathologic fractures.
   3. tophi deposits.
   4. Homans' sign.

6. A 55-year-old patient reveals a postmenopausal history of three previous fractures and daily consumption of caffeine. According to her history, she is at increased risk for:
   1. osteomyelitis.
   2. osteoarthritis.
   3. osteogenic sarcoma.
   4. osteoporosis.

7. An appropriate nursing intervention for a patient suffering from a fractured hip with bipolar hip repair is:
   1. release traction weight every 4 to 6 hours.
   2. maintain abduction of the affected extremity.
   3. maintain adduction of the affected extremity.
   4. encourage active range of motion in the affected extremity.

8. The patient is being discharged after a prosthetic hip implant. She asks when she can begin to bear weight on the affected leg. *(Select the most appropriate response.)*
   1. The patient must not bear weight on the affected leg for 6 to 12 months.
   2. Most patients bear weight in 5 days.
   3. The patient must learn to use a gait enhancer and keep the majority of weight off the unaffected leg.
   4. Most patients require some degree of non–weight bearing for 6 weeks to 3 months.

9. A significant postoperative nursing intervention for a patient with an amputation is:
   1. maintaining abduction of the stump.
   2. elevating the stump with no more than two pillows.
   3. proper stump care to facilitate prosthetic use.
   4. leaving the stump open to air to assess suture site.

10. A 75-year-old retired construction worker has been seeing the physician for complaints of osteoarthritis. Today he is discussing concerns over his condition and asks what has caused his osteoarthritis. An appropriate response would be:
    1. You have osteoarthritis because of the difficult construction work you did for so many years.
    2. Everyone your age has arthritis; you are fortunate you are still able to walk.
    3. The cause of osteoarthritis is unknown. However, almost everyone older than 40 years of age has some changes in their joints.
    4. You probably did not exercise as much as you should have, and you should start vigorous exercising now to prevent further complications.

11. An appropriate nursing intervention for a 32-year-old patient in skeletal traction, would be to:
    1. provide cast care.
    2. cleanse pin sites daily with hydrogen peroxide, and observe for signs of infection.
    3. place patient on drainage and secretion precautions.
    4. encourage patient to sit in a straight, firm chair for no longer than 20 minutes each time.

12. After a fracture of the forearm or tibia, complaints of sharp, deep, unrelenting pain in the hand or foot unrelieved by analgesics or elevation of the extremity indicate which complication?
    1. Fat embolism
    2. Compartment syndrome
    3. Gas gangrene
    4. Cast syndrome

13. A 45-year-old patient suffered a knee injury while playing football. He is scheduled for an arthroscopic examination and asks the nurse to explain the procedure. An appropriate response would be:
    1. Your physician will insert a small scope into your knee joint to visualize the joint for damaged tissue.
    2. The test involves the use of magnetism and radio waves to make images of cross-sections of the body.
    3. The radiographic technician will inject your knee joint with an atomic material and take a radiograph of your affected knee.
    4. The physician will insert needle electrodes into the knee muscle to document electrical activity of the knee.

14. A 51-year-old patient with RA asks if there is a cure. An appropriate response would be:
    1. Yes, new drugs offer a cure.
    2. No, but new drugs can interfere with the body's reaction to inflammation and better control the disease process.
    3. Yes, but the patient must take medication for at least 10 years.
    4. No, most patients with RA also develop osteoarthritis.

15. The patient is scheduled for endoscopic spinal microsurgery to correct a herniated disk. Select the most accurate statement concerning this type of surgery.
    1. Endoscopic spinal microsurgery requires a general anesthetic.
    2. Special scopes are placed through small incisions, causing minimal damage to surrounding tissue.
    3. Patients older than 80 years of age are always candidates for endoscopic spinal microsurgery.
    4. Endoscopic spinal microsurgery is limited to the repair of herniated disks.

16. A 45 year-old patient has a history of lactose intolerance, excessive caffeine intake, and excessive cigarette smoking. The physician orders a bone density index test for her. Select the most appropriate statement concerning information about the test.
    1. The test is also called DEXA and is considered an invasive procedure.
    2. The test involves drawing a small amount of blood to determine your blood calcium level.
    3. The test takes about 10 minutes and involves very low amounts of radiation.
    4. The test is always recommended for women older than 30 years of age.

17. A 62-year-old patient has osteoarthritis of the knee and is seeking information about glucosamine supplements. An appropriate response would be:
    1. Glucosamine is a natural substance in the body, and it is not necessary to take a supplement.
    2. Glucosamine supplements are relatively safe in people younger than 40 years of age.
    3. Studies suggest that glucosamine supplements are helpful in maintaining healthy joint function, with minimal side effects unless you are allergic to shellfish.
    4. A healthy lifestyle with high-impact exercise is more important than taking a supplement.

18. Select the most appropriate nursing assessment for the nursing diagnosis of ineffective tissue perfusion, secondary to fractured hip.
    1. Assess for ecchymosis over pelvis and perineum.
    2. Protect patient from cross-contamination.
    3. Assess for adventitious lung sounds.
    4. Assess distal pulses.

19. A 72-year-old patient has just undergone total hip replacement. She asks why she cannot cross her legs when sitting but must do straight leg–raising exercises. An appropriate response would be:
    1. The exercises help strengthen the leg muscles; crossing your legs puts pressure on the joints and could damage the hip prosthesis.
    2. The exercises keep you from getting too tired while you sit; when you want to cross your legs, it is time to rest.
    3. The exercises strengthen the muscles in your upper legs to help you walk.
    4. The doctor ordered these exercises, but did not order you to cross your legs.

20. Which of the following objective data are found in a patient with compartment syndrome?
    1. Hypotension, tachycardia, and tachypnea
    2. Gas bubbles under the skin
    3. Positive Homans' sign
    4. Absence of pulsation in the affected extremity

21. A 77-year-old patient has persistent complaints of severe back pain related to osteoporosis. She walks with a stooped posture and has a noticeable kyphosis. She has been unresponsive to a traditional pain management program. Based on this information, the patient may be a candidate for:
    1. unicompartmental arthroplasty.
    2. complete bed rest.
    3. kyphoplasty.
    4. injections of Forteo.

22. A 47-year-old patient has signs and symptoms of menopause. She recently fell and fractured her wrist. After doing a bone density test, her physician diagnosed her with osteoporosis. She asks about the benefits of taking estrogen. An appropriate response would be:
    1. Estrogen will not help bone density.
    2. Estrogen can cause cancer of the breast.
    3. Estrogen will not correct the condition but will help to prevent fractures and is approved for women at significant risk.
    4. Forteo is a type of estrogen.

23. A 51-year-old patient exercises routinely. He has been noticing pain on the lateral area of his knee for the past 6 months during and after exercise. The patient is scheduled for unicompartmental knee arthroplasty and asks the nurse to explain the surgery. An appropriate response would be:
    1. The procedure involves replacement of the entire knee joint.
    2. You will need to be in the hospital for approximately 5 days.
    3. You will not need an anesthetic.
    4. Minimally invasive knee surgery removes only the most damaged areas of cartilage, and a small plastic disk replaces the worn cartilage, providing a new cushion between the bones.

24. The patient had a compound fracture of his right femur 2 years before the present admission. His physician suspects osteomyelitis and has informed the patient that tests are needed to confirm the diagnosis. The patient wants to know what tests can be ordered to determine osteomyelitis. An appropriate response would be to describe the specific test(s) for osteomyelitis. *(Select all that apply.)*
    1. Goniometer
    2. BMX
    3. Bone scan
    4. Bone biopsy

25. A construction worker suffered a fracture of the femur 48 hours ago. The nurse notices that he has petechiae on the conjunctiva, chest, neck, and axillae. Petechiae in these locations is a typical sign of:
    1. compartment syndrome.
    2. deep-vein thrombosis.
    3. gas gangrene.
    4. fat embolism.

chapter

45

Care of the Patient with a Gastrointestinal Disorder

evolve

Barbara Lauritsen Christensen

http://evolve.elsevier.com/Christensen/foundationsadult

Objectives

Anatomy and Physiology

1. List in sequence each of the component parts or segments of the alimentary canal and identify the accessory organs of digestion.
2. Discuss the function of each digestive and accessory organ.

Medical-Surgical

3. Discuss the laboratory and diagnostic examinations and give the nursing interventions for patients with disorders of the gastrointestinal tract.
4. Explain the etiology and pathophysiology, clinical manifestations, assessments, diagnostic tests, medical-surgical management, and nursing interventions for the patient with disorders of the mouth, esophagus, stomach, and intestines.
5. Identify nursing interventions for preoperative and postoperative care of the patient who requires gastric surgery.
6. Compare and contrast the inflammatory bowel diseases of ulcerative colitis and Crohn's disease, including etiology and pathophysiology, clinical manifestations, medical management, and nursing interventions.
7. Identify five nursing interventions for the patient with a stoma for fecal diversion.
8. Discuss the etiology and pathophysiology, clinical manifestations, assessment, diagnostic tests, medical management, and nursing interventions for the patient with acute abdominal inflammations (appendicitis, diverticulitis, and peritonitis).
9. Discuss the etiology and pathophysiology, clinical manifestations, assessment, diagnostic tests, medical management, and nursing interventions for the patient with external hernias and hiatal hernia.
10. Differentiate between mechanical and nonmechanical intestinal obstruction, including causes, medical management and nursing interventions.
11. Describe the etiology and pathophysiology, clinical manifestations, assessment, diagnostic tests, medical management, surgical procedures, and nursing interventions for the patient with colorectal cancer.
12. Explain the etiologies, medical management, and nursing interventions for the patient with fecal incontinence.

Key Terms

achalasia (ăk-ăh-LĀ-zē-ă, p. 1425)
achlorhydria (ă-chlŏr-HĪ-drē-ă, p. 1416)
anastomosis (ă-năs-tŏ-MŌ-sĭs, p. 1425)
cachexia (kă-KĔK-sē-ă, p. 1457)
carcinoembryonic antigen (CEA) (kăr-sĭn-ō-ĕm-brē-ĂN-ĭk ĂN-tĭ-jĕn, p. 1457)
dehiscence (dĕ-HĬS-ĕntz, p. 1436)
dumping syndrome (DŬMP-ĭng SĬN-drōm, p. 1432)
dysphagia (dĭs-FĀ-jē-ă, p. 1424)
evisceration (ĕ-vĭs-ĕr-Ā-shŭn, p. 1436)
exacerbations (ĕg-zăs-ĕr-BĀ-shŭnz, p. 1441)
hematemesis (hĕ-mă-TĔM-ĕ-sĭs, p. 1428)
intussusception (ĭn-tŭs-sŭs-SĔP-shŭn, p. 1418)
leukoplakia (lū-kō-PLĀ-kē-ă, p. 1421)
lumen (LŪ-mĕn, p. 1418)
melena (MĔL-ĕh-nă, p. 1428)
occult blood (ŏ-KŬLT, p. 1418)
paralytic (adynamic) ileus (p. 1454)
pathognomonic (păth-ŏg-nō-MŎN-ĭk, p. 1419)
remissions (rĕ-MĬSH-ŭn, p. 1441)
steatorrhea (stĕ-ă-tō-RĒ-ă, p. 1446)
stoma (STŌ-mă, p. 1445)
tenesmus (tĕ-NĔZ-mŭs, p. 1438)
volvulus (VŎL-vū-lŭs, p. 1454)

ANATOMY AND PHYSIOLOGY OF THE GASTROINTESTINAL SYSTEM

DIGESTIVE SYSTEM

Everyone understands that food is necessary for existence, but not (1) what happens to food once it is chewed and swallowed; (2) how food is prepared for its trip to each individual cell; and (3) the many changes that food undergoes, both chemically and physically. This chapter reviews these changes and their effect on the body.

The digestive tract, or alimentary canal, is a musculomembranous tube extending from the mouth to the anus (Figure 45-1). It is approximately 30 feet long. It consists of the mouth, pharynx, esophagus, small intestine, large intestine, and anus. **Peristalsis** is the coordinated, rhythmic, serial contraction of smooth muscle that forces food through the digestive tract, bile through the bile duct, and urine through the ureter. During peristalsis the tract shortens to approximately 15 feet.

Accessory organs aid in the digestive process but are not considered part of the digestive tract. They release

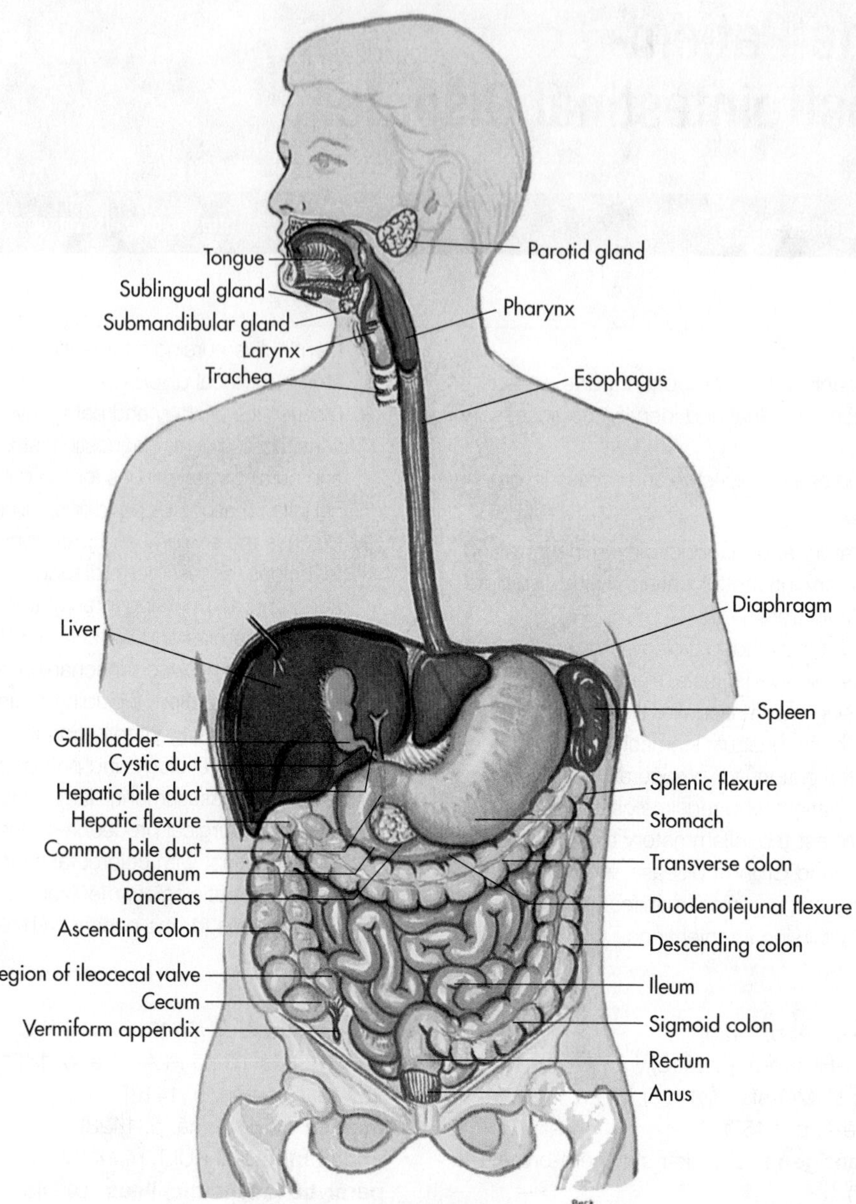

FIGURE 45-1 Location of digestive organs.

chemicals into the system through a series of ducts. The teeth, tongue, salivary glands, liver, gallbladder, and pancreas are considered accessory organs.

Organs of the Digestive System and Their Functions

Box 45-1 lists various organs of the digestive system and the accessory organs involved in digestion.

Mouth

The mouth marks the entrance to the digestive system. The floor of the mouth contains a muscular appendage, the tongue. The tongue is involved in chewing, swallowing, and the formation of speech. Tiny elevations, called **papillae,** contain the taste buds. They differentiate between bitter, sweet, sour, and salty sensations.

Digestion begins in the mouth. Here the teeth mechanically shred and grind the food and the enzymes begin the chemical breakdown of carbohydrates.

Teeth

Each tooth is designed to carry out a specific task. In the center of the mouth are the incisors, which are structured for biting and cutting. Posterior to the incisors are the canines, pointed teeth used for tearing and shredding food. The molars are to the rear of the jaw. These teeth have four cusps (points) and are used for mastication (to crush and grind food).

Salivary Glands

The three pairs of salivary glands are the parotid, submandibular, and sublingual glands (see Figure 45-1). They secrete fluid called **saliva,** which is approxi-

Box 45-1 Organs of the Digestive System

ORGANS OF THE ALIMENTARY CANAL
- Mouth
- Pharynx (throat)
- Esophagus (food pipe)
- Stomach
- Small intestine
  - —Duodenum
  - —Jejunum
  - —Ileum
- Large intestine
- Cecum
- Colon
  - —Ascending colon
  - —Transverse colon
  - —Descending colon
  - —Sigmoid colon
- Rectum
- Anal canal

ACCESSORY ORGANS
- Teeth and gums
- Tongue
- Liver
- Gallbladder
- Pancreas
- Salivary glands
  - —Parotid
  - —Submandibular
  - —Sublingual

mately 99% water with enzymes and mucus. Normally these glands secrete enough saliva to keep the mucous membranes of the mouth moist. Once food enters the mouth, the secretion increases to lubricate and dissolve the food and to begin the chemical process of digestion. The salivary glands secrete about 1000 to 1500 mL of saliva daily. The major enzyme is salivary amylase (ptyalin), which initiates carbohydrate metabolism. Another enzyme, lysozyme, destroys bacteria and thus protects the mucous membrane from infections and the teeth from decay. After food has been ingested, the salivary glands continue to secrete saliva, which cleanses the mouth.

Esophagus

The esophagus is a muscular, collapsible tube that is approximately 10 inches long, extending from the mouth through the thoracic cavity and the esophageal hiatus to the stomach. Digestion does not take place in the esophagus. Peristalsis moves the bolus (food broken down and mixed with saliva, ready to pass to the stomach) through the esophagus to the stomach in 5 or 6 seconds.

Stomach

The stomach is in the left upper quadrant of the abdomen, directly inferior to the diaphragm (Figure 45-2). A filled stomach is the size of a football and holds approximately 1 L. The stomach entrance is the cardiac sphincter (so named because it is close to the heart); the exit is the pyloric sphincter. As food leaves the esophagus, it enters the stomach through the relaxed cardiac sphincter. The sphincter then contracts, preventing reflux (splashing or return flow), which can be irritating.

Once the bolus has entered the stomach, the muscular layers of the stomach churn and contract to mix and compress the contents with the gastric juices and water. The gastric juices are secretions released by the gastric glands. Digestion of protein begins in the stomach. Hydrochloric acid softens the connective tissue of meats,

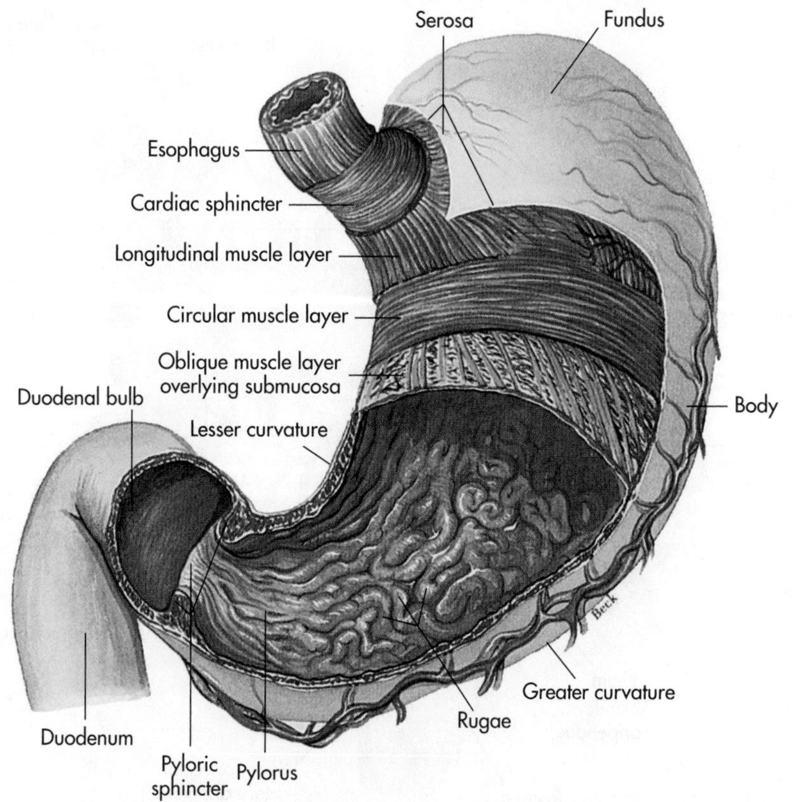

FIGURE 45-2 Stomach. Cut-away sections show muscle layers and interior mucosa thrown into folds called **rugae.**

kills bacteria, and activates pepsin (the chief enzyme of gastric juices that converts proteins into proteoses and peptones). Mucin is released to protect the stomach lining. Intrinsic factor (a substance secreted by the gastric mucosa) is produced to allow absorption of vitamin B_{12}. The stomach breaks the food down into a viscous semiliquid substance called chyme. The chyme passes through the pyloric sphincter into the duodenum for the next phase of digestion.

Small Intestine

The small intestine (see Figure 45-1) is a tube that is 20 feet long and 1 inch in diameter. It begins at the pyloric sphincter and ends at the ileocecal valve. It is divided into three major sections: **duodenum, jejunum,** and **ileum.** Up to 90% of digestion takes place in the small intestine. The intestinal juices finish the metabolism of carbohydrates and proteins. Bile and pancreatic juices enter the duodenum. Bile from the liver breaks molecules into smaller droplets, which enables the digestive juices to complete their process. Pancreatic juices contain water, protein, inorganic salts, and enzymes. Pancreatic juices are essential in breaking down proteins into their amino acid components, in reducing dietary fats to glycerol and fatty acids, and in converting starch to simple sugars.

The inner surface of the small intestine contains millions of tiny fingerlike projections called **villi,** which are clustered over the entire mucous surface. The villi are responsible for absorbing the products of digestion into the bloodstream. They increase the absorption area of the small intestine 600 times. Inside each villus is a rich capillary bed, along with modified lymph capillaries called lacteals. Lacteals are responsible for the absorption of metabolized fats.

Large Intestine

Once the small intestine has finished its specific tasks, the ileocecal valve opens and releases the contents into the large intestine. The large intestine is a tube that is larger in diameter (2 inches) but shorter (5 feet) than the small intestine. It is composed of the cecum; appendix; ascending, hepatic flexure, transverse, splenic flexure, descending, and sigmoid colons; rectum; and anus (Figure 45-3). This is the terminal portion of the digestive tract, which completes the process of digestion. Basically the large intestine has four major functions: (1) completion of absorption of water, (2) manufacture of certain vitamins, (3) formation of feces, and (4) expulsion of feces.

Just inferior to the ileocecal valve is the cecum, a blind pouch approximately 2 to 3 inches long. The vermiform appendix, a small wormlike, tubular structure, dangles from the cecum. To date, no function for the appendix has been discovered. The open end of the cecum connects to the ascending colon, which continues upward on the right side of the abdomen to the inferior area of the liver. The ascending colon then becomes the transverse colon. It crosses to the left side of the abdomen, where it becomes the descending colon. When the descending colon reaches the level of the iliac crest, the

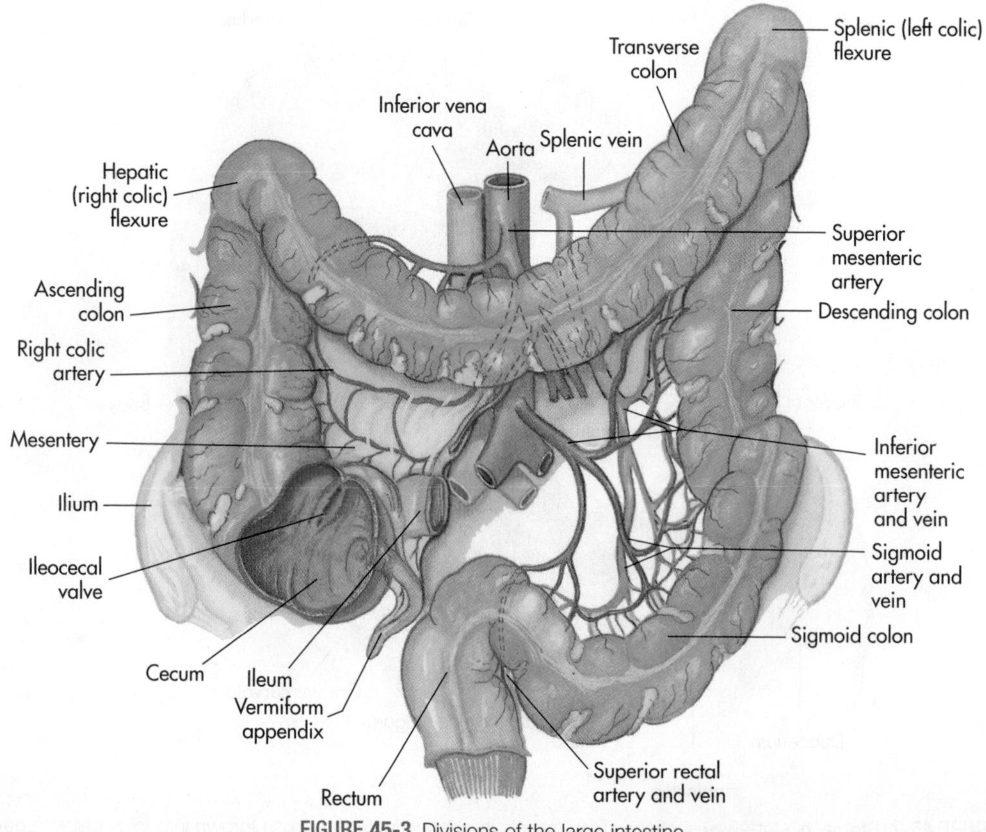

FIGURE 45-3 Divisions of the large intestine.

sigmoid colon begins and continues toward the midline to the level of the third sacral vertebra.

Bacteria in the large intestine change the chyme into fecal material by releasing the remaining nutrients. The bacteria are also responsible for the synthesis of vitamin K, which is needed for normal blood clotting, and the production of some of the B-complex vitamins. As the fecal material continues its journey, the remaining water and vitamins are absorbed into the bloodstream by osmosis.

Rectum

The rectum is the last 8 inches of the intestine, where fecal material is expelled.

ACCESSORY ORGANS OF DIGESTION

Liver

The liver is the largest glandular organ in the body and one of the most complex. In the adult it weighs 3 pounds. It is located just inferior to the diaphragm, covering most of the upper right quadrant and extending into the left epigastrium. It is divided into two lobes. Approximately 1500 mL of blood is delivered to the liver every minute by the portal vein and the hepatic portal artery. The cells of the liver produce a product called **bile,** a yellow-brown or green-brown liquid. Bile is necessary for the emulsification of fats. The liver releases 500 to 1000 mL of bile per day. Bile travels to the gallbladder through hepatic ducts. The gallbladder is a sac about 3 to 4 inches long located on the right inferior surface of the liver. Bile is stored in the gallbladder until needed for fat digestion (Figure 45-4).

In addition to producing bile, the liver's functions include managing blood coagulation; manufacturing cholesterol; manufacturing albumin to maintain normal blood volume; filtering out old red blood cells (RBCs) and bacteria; detoxifying poisons (alcohol, nicotine, drugs); converting ammonia to urea; providing the main source of body heat; storing glycogen for later use; activating vitamin D; and breaking down nitrogenous waste (from protein metabolism) to urea, which the kidneys can excrete as waste from the body.

Pancreas

The pancreas is an elongated gland that lies posterior to the stomach (see Figure 45-4). It is involved in both endocrine and exocrine duties. In this chapter, discussion of the pancreas is limited to its exocrine activities.

Each day the pancreas produces 1000 to 1500 mL of pancreatic juice to aid in digestion. This pancreatic juice contains the digestive enzymes protease (trypsin), lipase (steapsin), and amylase (amylopsin). These enzymes are important because they digest the three major components of chyme: proteins, fats, and carbohydrates. The enzymes are transported through an excretory duct to the duodenum. This pancreatic duct connects to the common bile duct from the liver and gallbladder and empties through a small orifice in the duodenum called the major duodenal papilla, or **papilla of Vater.** In addition, the pancreas contains an alkaline substance, sodium bicarbonate, which neutralizes hydrochloric acid in the gastric juices that enter the small intestine from the stomach.

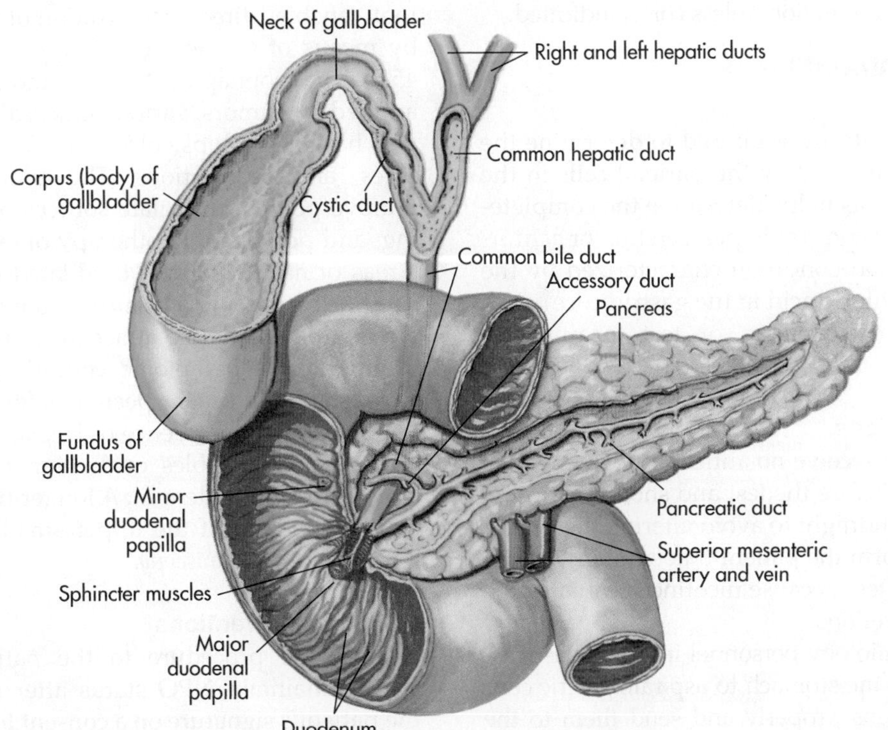

FIGURE 45-4 Gallbladder and bile ducts. Obstruction of the hepatic or common bile duct by stone or spasm occludes the exit of the bile and prevents matter from being ejected into the duodenum.

REGULATION OF FOOD INTAKE

The hypothalamus, a portion of the brain, contains two centers that have an effect on eating. One center stimulates the individual to eat, and the other signals the individual to stop eating. These centers work in conjunction with the rest of the brain to balance eating habits. However, many other factors also affect eating. For example, distention decreases appetite. Other controls in our bodies, lifestyle, culture, eating habits, emotions, and genetic factors all influence intake of food and individual body build.

LABORATORY AND DIAGNOSTIC EXAMINATIONS

UPPER GASTROINTESTINAL STUDY (UPPER GI SERIES, UGI)

Rationale

The upper gastrointestinal study (UGI) consists of a series of radiographs of the lower esophagus, stomach, and duodenum using barium sulfate as the contrast medium. A UGI series detects any abnormal conditions of the upper gastrointestinal (GI) tract, any tumors, or other ulcerative lesions.

Nursing Interventions

The patient should take nothing by mouth (NPO) and avoid smoking after midnight the night before the study. Explain the importance of rectally expelling all the barium after the examination. Stools will be light colored until all the barium is expelled (up to 72 hours after the test). Eventual absorption of fecal water may cause a hardened barium impaction. Increasing fluid intake is usually effective. Give the patient milk of magnesia (60 mL) after the examination unless contraindicated.

TUBE GASTRIC ANALYSIS

Rationale

The stomach contents are aspirated to determine the amount of acid produced by the parietal cells in the stomach. The analysis helps determine the completeness of a vagotomy, confirm hypersecretion or **achlorhydria** (an abnormal condition characterized by the absence of hydrochloric acid in the gastric juice), estimate acid secretory capacity, or test for intrinsic factor.

Nursing Interventions

The patient should receive no anticholinergic medications for 24 hours before the test and should maintain NPO status after midnight to avoid altering the gastric acid secretion. Inform the patient that smoking is prohibited before the test because nicotine stimulates the flow of gastric secretions.

The nurse or radiology personnel inserts a nasogastric (NG) tube into the stomach to aspirate gastric content. Label specimens properly and send them to the laboratory immediately. Remove the NG tube as soon as specimens are collected. The patient may then eat if indicated.

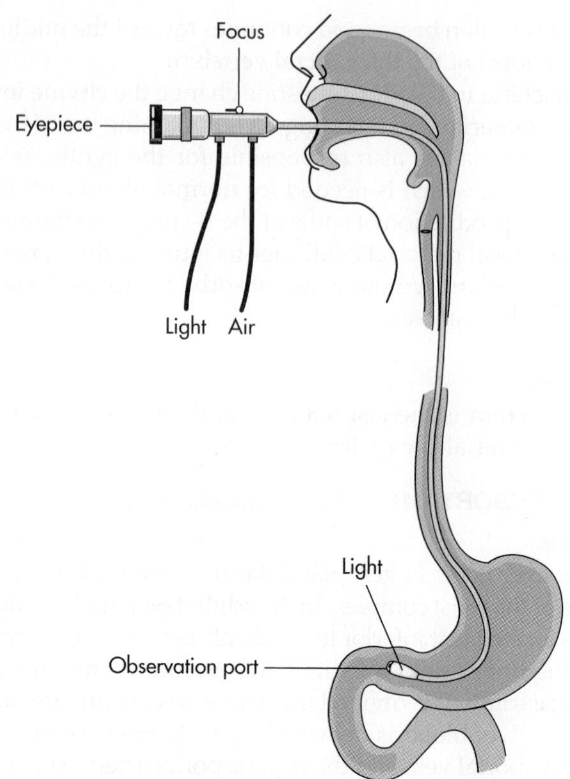

FIGURE 45-5 Fiberoptic endoscopy of the stomach.

ESOPHAGOGASTRODUODENOSCOPY (EGD, UGI ENDOSCOPY, GASTROSCOPY)

Rationale

Endoscopy (from *endo,* within, inward; and *scope,* to look) enables direct visualization of the upper GI tract by means of a long, fiberoptic flexible scope (Figure 45-5). The esophagus, stomach, and duodenum are examined for tumors, varices, mucosal inflammation, hiatal hernias, polyps, ulcers, *Helicobacter pylori,* strictures, and obstructions. The endoscopist can also remove polyps, coagulate sources of active GI bleeding, and perform sclerotherapy of esophageal varices. Areas of narrowing can be dilated by the endoscope itself or by passing a dilator through the scope. Camera equipment can be attached to the viewing lens to photograph a pathologic condition. The endoscope can also obtain tissue specimens for biopsy or culture to determine the presence of *H. pylori.*

Endoscopy enables evaluation of the esophagus, stomach, and duodenum. A longer fiberoptic scope allows evaluation of the upper small intestine. This is referred to as *enteroscopy.*

Nursing Interventions

Explain the procedure to the patient. The patient should maintain NPO status after midnight. Obtain the patient's signature on a consent form and complete a preoperative checklist for the endoscopic examination. The patient is usually given a preprocedure intravenous (IV) sedative such as midazolam (Versed). The patient's pharynx is anesthetized by spraying it with lidocaine hydrochloride (Xylocaine). Therefore do not allow the patient to eat or drink until the gag reflex returns (usually about 2 to 4 hours). Assess for any signs and symptoms of perforation, including abdominal pain and tenderness, guarding, oral bleeding, melena, and hypovolemic shock.

CAPSULE ENDOSCOPY

Rationale

In a capsule endoscopy, the patient swallows a capsule with a camera (approximately the size of a large vitamin) that provides endoscopic evaluation of the GI tract (Figure 45-6). It is commonly used to visualize the small intestine and diagnose diseases (such as Crohn's disease, celiac disease, and malabsorption syndrome). It also helps identify sources of possible GI bleeding in areas not accessible by upper endoscopy or colonoscopy. The camera takes about 57,000 images during an 8-hour examination. The capsule relays images to a data recorder that the patient wears on a belt. After the examination, images are viewed on a monitor.

Nursing Interventions

Dietary preparation is similar to that for colonoscopy. The patient swallows the video capsule and is usually kept NPO until 4 to 6 hours later. The procedure is comfortable for most patients. Eight hours after swallowing the capsule, the patient returns to have the monitoring device removed. Peristalsis causes passage of the disposable capsule with a bowel movement.

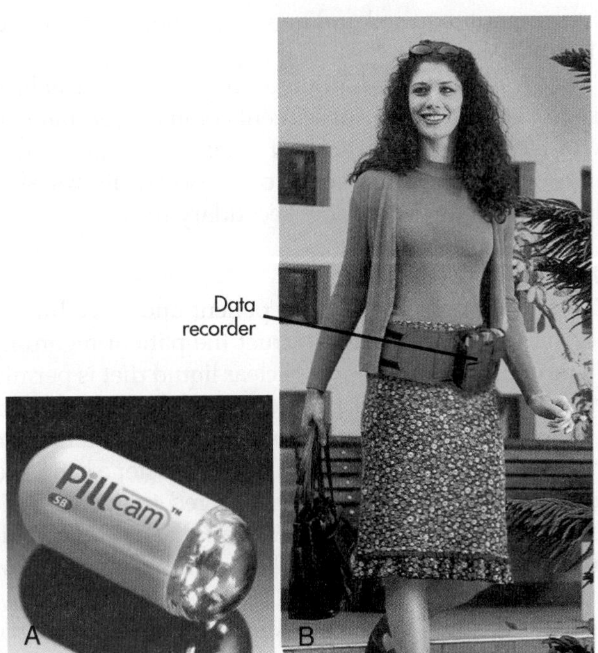

FIGURE 45-6 Capsule endoscopy. **A,** The video capsule has its own camera and light source. After it is swallowed, it travels through the gastrointestinal tract and allows visualization of the small intestine. It sends messages to a data recorder that is worn on a waist belt **B,** During the 8-hour examination, the patient is free to move about. After the test, the images are viewed on a video monitor.

BARIUM SWALLOW AND GASTROGRAFIN STUDIES

Rationale

This barium contrast study is a more thorough study of the esophagus than that provided by most UGI examinations. As in most barium contrast studies, defects in luminal filling and narrowing of the barium column indicate tumor, scarred stricture, or esophageal varices. The barium swallow allows easy recognition of anatomical abnormalities, such as hiatal hernia. Left atrial dilation, aortic aneurysm, and paraesophageal tumors (such as bronchial or mediastinal tumors) may cause extrinsic compression of the barium column within the esophagus.

Diatrizoate meglumine and diatrizoate sodium (Gastrografin) is a product now used in place of barium for patients who are susceptible to bleeding from the GI system and who are being considered for surgery. Gastrografin is water soluble and rapidly absorbed, so it is preferable when a perforation is suspected. Gastrografin facilitates imaging through radiographs, but if the product escapes from the GI tract, it is absorbed by the surrounding tissue. In contrast, if barium leaks from the GI tract, it is not absorbed and can lead to complications.

Nursing Interventions

The patient should maintain NPO status after midnight. Food and fluid in the stomach prevent the barium from accurately outlining the GI tract, and the radiographic results may be misleading. Explain the importance of rectally expelling all barium. Stools will be light colored until this occurs. Eventual absorption of fecal water may cause a hardened barium impaction. Increasing fluid intake is usually effective. Give milk of magnesia (60 mL) after the barium swallow examination unless contraindicated.

ESOPHAGEAL FUNCTION STUDIES (BERNSTEIN TEST)

Rationale

The Bernstein test, an acid-perfusion test, is an attempt to reproduce the symptoms of gastroesophageal reflux. It helps differentiate esophageal pain caused by esophageal reflux from that caused by angina pectoris. If the patient suffers pain with the instillation of hydrochloric acid into the esophagus, the test is positive and indicates reflux esophagitis.

Nursing Interventions

Avoid sedating the patient, since the patient's participation is essential for swallowing the tubes, swallowing during acid clearance, and describing any discomfort during the instillation of hydrochloric acid. The patient is NPO for 8 hours before the examination. Withhold any medications that may interfere with the production of acid, such as antacids and analgesics.

EXAMINATION OF STOOL FOR OCCULT BLOOD

Rationale

Tumors of the large intestine grow into the **lumen** (the cavity or channel within a tube or tubular organ) and are subject to repeated trauma by the fecal stream. Eventually the tumor ulcerates and bleeding occurs. Usually the bleeding is so slight that gross blood is not seen in the stool. If this **occult blood** (blood that is obscure or hidden from view) is detected in the stool, suspect a benign or malignant GI tumor. Tests for occult blood are also called guaiac, Hemoccult, and Hematest.

Occult blood in the stool may occur also in ulceration and inflammation of the upper or lower GI system. Other causes include swallowing blood of oral or nasopharyngeal origin.

Stool may be obtained by digital retrieval by the nurse or physician. However, the patient is usually asked to collect stool in an appropriate container. Obtain a specimen for occult blood before barium studies are done.

Nursing Interventions

Instruct the patient to keep the stool specimen free of urine or toilet paper, since either can alter the test results. The nurse or patient should don gloves and use tongue blades to transfer the stool to the proper receptacle. The patient should keep the diet free of organ meat for 24 to 48 hours before a guaiac test.

SIGMOIDOSCOPY (LOWER GI ENDOSCOPY)

Rationale

Endoscopy of the lower GI tract allows visualization and, if indicated, access to obtain biopsy specimens of tumors, polyps, or ulcerations of the anus, rectum, and sigmoid colon. The lower GI tract is difficult to visualize radiographically, but sigmoidoscopy allows direct visualization. Microscopic review of tissue specimens obtained using this procedure lead to diagnoses of many lower bowel disorders.

Nursing Interventions

Explain the procedure to the patient and have him or her sign a consent form. Administer enemas as ordered on the evening before or the morning of the examination to ensure optimum visualization of the lower GI tract. After the examination, observe the patient for evidence of bowel perforation (abdominal pain, tenderness, distention, and bleeding).

BARIUM ENEMA STUDY (LOWER GI SERIES)

Rationale

The barium enema (BE) study consists of a series of radiographs of the colon used to demonstrate the presence and location of polyps, tumors, and diverticula. It can also detect positional abnormalities (such as malrotation). Barium sulfate assists in visualization of mucosal detail. Therapeutically, the BE study may be used to reduce nonstrangulated ileocolic **intussusception** (infolding of one segment of the intestine into the lumen of another segment) in children.

Nursing Interventions

The evening before the BE, administer cathartics such as magnesium citrate or other cathartics designated by institution policy. Also administer a cleansing enema the evening before or the morning of the BE if directed by physician's order or hospital policy. Milk of magnesia (60 mL) may be ordered after the BE to stimulate evacuation of the barium.

After the BE study, assess the patient for complete evacuation of the barium. Retained barium may cause a hardened impaction. Stool will be light colored until all the barium has been expelled.

COLONOSCOPY

Rationale

The development of the fiberoptic colonoscope has enabled examination of the entire colon—from anus to cecum—in a high percentage of patients. Colonoscopy can detect lesions in the proximal colon, which would not be found by sigmoidoscopy. Benign and malignant neoplasms, mucosal inflammation or ulceration, and sites of active hemorrhage can also be visualized. Biopsy specimens can be obtained and small tumors removed through the scope with the use of cable-activated instruments. Actively bleeding vessels can be coagulated.

A less invasive test than a standard colonoscopy is called virtual colonoscopy. This test uses CT scanning or MRI with computer software to produce images of the colon and rectum. The colon preparation is similar to that for a regular colonoscopic examination. Sedatives are not required and no scope is needed (Lewis et al., 2007).

Patients who have had cancer of the colon are at high risk for developing a subsequent colon cancer; patients who have a family history of colon cancer are also at high risk. For these patients, colonoscopy allows early detection of any primary or secondary tumors.

Nursing Interventions

Explain the procedure to the patient and have him or her sign a consent form. Instruct the patient regarding dietary restrictions: Usually a clear liquid diet is permitted 1 to 3 days before the procedure to decrease the residue in the bowel, and then NPO status is maintained for 8 hours before the procedure. Administer a cathartic, enemas, and premedication as ordered to decrease the residue in the bowel. GoLYTELY, an oral or NG colonic lavage, is an osmotic electrolyte solution that is now commonly used as a cathartic (Box 45-2). It is a polyethylene glycol solution. If it is taken orally, instruct the patient to drink the solution rapidly: 8 ounces (240 mL) every 15 minutes until enough solution has been consumed to make the colonic contents a light yellow liquid. Powdered lemonade may be added to make the oral solution more palatable. If it is given per lavage, it

Box 45-2 GoLYTELY Bowel Preparation

1. Give patient one metoclopramide (Reglan) 10-mg tablet, as prescribed, orally 30 minutes before proceeding with step 2.
2. Administer GoLYTELY solution* (prepared by pharmacy) per physician's orders:
   a. 240 mL orally every 15 minutes *or*
   b. 30 mL/min via nasogastric tube. Use a Travasorb enteral feeding container and a size 10 feeding tube. Administer until stools are clear yellow.
   c. Keep patients warm with heated blankets; they often become chilled after consuming copious amounts of GoLYTELY solution.
   d. Provide a bedside commode for older or weak patients.

*Administer a minimum of 1 gallon of solution over a 2-hour period.

must be given rapidly. Taking the solution slowly will not clean the colon efficiently. Provide warm blankets during the procedure, since many patients experience hypothermia while taking GoLYTELY. Provide a commode at the bedside for older adults and frail patients. Check the patient's stool after the prep to make certain it is light yellow and liquid. A preprocedure IV sedative such as midazolam is often given.

After the colonoscopy, check for evidence of bowel perforation (abdominal pain, guarding, distention, tenderness, excessive rectal bleeding, or blood clots) and examine stools for gross blood. Assess for hypovolemic shock.

STOOL CULTURE

Rationale

The feces (stool) can be examined for the presence of bacteria, ova, and parasites (a plant or animal that lives on or within another living organism and obtains some advantage at its host's expense). The physician may order a stool for culture of bacteria or of ova and parasites (O&P). Many bacteria (such as *Escherichia coli*) are indigenous in the bowel. Bacterial cultures are usually done to detect enteropathogens (such as *Staphylococcus aureus*, *Salmonella* or *Shigella* organisms, *E. coli* O157:H7, or *Clostridium difficile*).

When a patient is suspected of having a parasitic infection, the stool is examined for O&P. Usually at least three stool specimens are collected on subsequent days. Because culture results are not available for several days, they do not influence initial treatment, but they do guide subsequent treatment if bacterial infection is present.

Nursing Interventions

If an enema must be administered to collect specimens, use only normal saline or tap water. Soapsuds or any other substance could affect the viability of the organisms collected.

Stool samples for O&P are obtained before barium examinations. Instruct the patient not to mix urine with feces. Don gloves to collect the specimen, and ensure the specimen is taken to the laboratory within 30 minutes of collection in specified container.

OBSTRUCTION SERIES (FLAT PLATE OF THE ABDOMEN)

Rationale

The obstruction series is a group of radiographic studies performed on the abdomen of patients who have suspected bowel obstruction, paralytic ileus, perforated viscus (any large interior organ in any of the great body cavities), or abdominal abscess. The series usually consists of at least two radiographic studies. The first is an erect abdominal radiographic study that allows visualization of the diaphragm. Radiographs are examined for evidence of free air under the diaphragm, which is **pathognomonic** (signs or symptoms specific to a disease condition) of a perforated viscus. This radiographic study is used also to detect air-fluid levels within the intestine.

Nursing Interventions

For adequate visualization, ensure that this study is scheduled before any barium studies.

DISORDERS OF THE MOUTH

Common disorders of the mouth and esophagus that interfere with adequate nutrition include poor dental hygiene, infections, inflammation, and cancer.

DENTAL PLAQUE AND CARIES

Etiology and Pathophysiology

Dental decay is an erosive process that results from the action of bacteria on carbohydrates in the mouth, which in turn produce acids that dissolve tooth enamel. Most Americans (95%) experience tooth decay at some time in their life. Dental decay can be caused by several factors:

- Dental plaque, a thin film on the teeth made of mucin and colloidal material found in saliva and often secondarily invaded by bacteria
- The strength of acids and the inability of the saliva to neutralize them
- The length of time the acids are in contact with the teeth
- Susceptibility of the teeth to decay

Medical Management

Dental caries is treated by removal of affected areas of the tooth and replacement with some form of dental material. Treatment of periodontal disease centers on removal of plaque from the teeth. If the disease is advanced, surgical interventions on the gingivae and alveolar bone may be necessary.

Nursing Interventions and Patient Teaching

Proper technique for brushing and flossing the teeth at least twice a day is the primary focus for teaching these patients. Plaque forms continuously and must be removed periodically through regular visits to the dentist. Stress the importance of prevention through continual care. Because carbohydrates create an environment in which caries develop and plaque accumulates more easily, include proper nutrition in patient teaching. When the patient is ill, the mouth's normal cleansing action is impaired. Illnesses, drugs, and irradiation all interfere with the normal action of saliva. If the patient is unable to manage oral hygiene, the nurse must assume this responsibility.

Nursing diagnoses and interventions for the patient with dental plaque and caries include but are not limited to the following:

Nursing Diagnoses	Nursing Interventions
Deficient knowledge, related to: • inability to prevent dental caries • periodontal disease	Assess and observe the oral cavity for moisture, color, and cleanliness. Stress importance of meticulous oral hygiene. Explain the need to see a dentist at least yearly for an examination.
Noncompliance, related to hygiene and dietary restrictions	Brush teeth twice daily and as needed with toothpaste or powder, baking soda, or mouthwash. Rinse with water or mouthwash. Cleanse mouth with equal parts of hydrogen peroxide and water as needed for halitosis. Teach the patient about oral hygiene.

Prognosis

The prevention and elimination of dental plaque and caries are directly related to oral hygiene, dental care, nutrition, and heredity. All but heredity are controllable factors. The prognosis is more favorable for people who brush, floss, regularly visit the dentist for removal of affected areas, eat low-carbohydrate foods, and drink fluoridated water.

CANDIDIASIS

Etiology and Pathophysiology

Candidiasis is any infection caused by a species of *Candida,* usually *C. albicans. Candida* is a fungal organism normally present in the mucous membranes of the mouth, intestinal tract, and vagina; it is also found on the skin of healthy people. This infection is also referred to as **thrush** or **moniliasis.**

This disease appears more commonly in the newborn infant, who becomes infected while passing through the birth canal. In the older individual, candidiasis may be found in patients with leukemia, diabetes mellitus, or alcoholism, and in patients who are taking antibiotics (chlortetracycline or tetracycline), are undergoing corticosteroid inhalant treatment, or are immunosuppressed (e.g., patients with acquired immunodeficiency syndrome [AIDS] or those receiving chemotherapy or radiation therapy).

Clinical Manifestations

Candidiasis appears as pearly, bluish white "milk-curd" membranous lesions on the mucous membranes of the mouth, tongue, and larynx. One or more lesions may be on the mucosa, depending on the duration of the infection. If the patch or plaque is removed, painful bleeding can occur.

Medical Management

Nystatin or amphotericin B (an oral suspension) or buccal tablets or fluconazole (Diflucan), half-strength hydrogen peroxide and saline mouth rinses may provide some relief.

Nursing Interventions

Use meticulous hand hygiene to prevent spread of infection. The infection may be spread in the nursery by carelessness of nursing personnel. Hand hygiene, care of feeding equipment, and cleanliness of the mother's nipples are important to prevent spread. Cleanse the infant's mouth of any foreign material, rinsing the mouth and lubricating the lips. Inspect the mouth using a flashlight and tongue blade.

For adults, instruct the patient to use a soft-bristled toothbrush and administer a topical anesthetic (lidocaine or benzocaine) to the mouth 1 hour before meals. Give soft or pureed foods and avoid hot, cold, spicy, fried, or citrus foods.

Prognosis

If the host has a strong defense system and medical treatment is initiated early in the course of the disease, the prognosis is good.

CARCINOMA OF THE ORAL CAVITY

Etiology and Pathophysiology

Oral (or oropharyngeal) cancer may occur on the lips, the oral cavity, the tongue, and the pharynx. The tonsils are occasionally involved. Most of these tumors are squamous cell epitheliomas that grow rapidly and metastasize to adjacent structures more quickly than do most malignant tumors of the skin. In the United States, oral cancer accounts for 4% of the cancers in men and 2% in women. An estimated 35,310 new cases and 7590 deaths from oral cavity and pharynx cancer were expected in 2008. Death rates have been decreasing since the 1970s, with rates declining faster in the 2000s (American Cancer Society (ACS) , Cancer facts and figures, 2008).

Tumors of the salivary glands occur primarily in the parotid gland and are usually benign. Tumors of the submaxillary gland have a high incidence of malignancy. These malignant tumors grow rapidly and may be accompanied by pain and impaired facial function.

Kaposi's sarcoma is a malignant skin tumor that occurs primarily on the legs of men between 50 and 70 years of age. It is seen with increased frequency as a nonsquamous tumor of the oral cavity in patients with AIDS. The lesions are purple and nonulcerated. Irradiation is the treatment of choice.

The tumor seen with cancer of the lip is usually an **epithelioma.** It occurs most frequently as a chronic ulcer of the lower lip in men. The cure rate for cancer of the lip is high because the lesion is apparent to the patient and to others. Metastasis to regional lymph nodes has occurred in only 10% of people when diagnosed. In some instances a lesion may spread rapidly and involve the mandible and the floor of the mouth by direct extension. Occasionally the tumor may be a basal cell lesion that starts in the skin and spreads to the lip.

Cancer of the anterior tongue and floor of the mouth may seem to occur together because their spread to adjacent tissues is so rapid. Because of the tongue's abundant vascular and lymphatic drainage, metastasis to the neck has already occurred in more than 60% of patients when the diagnosis is made. There is a higher incidence of cancers of the mouth and throat among people who are heavy drinkers and have a history of tobacco use (e.g., cigar, cigarette, pipe, chewing tobacco). Also, data show that the mortality rate for males between the ages of 10 and 20 has doubled over the past 30 years as a result of the use of smokeless tobacco (snuff). The combination of high alcohol consumption and smoking or chewing tobacco causes an apparent breakdown in the body's defense mechanism. Predisposing factors include exposure to the sun and wind.

Clinical Manifestations

Leukoplakia (a white, firmly attached patch on the mouth or tongue mucosa) may appear on the lips and buccal mucosa. These nonsloughing lesions cannot be rubbed off by simple mechanical force. They can be benign or malignant. A small percentage develop into squamous cell carcinomas, and biopsy is recommended if the lesions persist for longer than 2 weeks. They occur most frequently between the ages of 50 and 70 years and appear more commonly in men.

Assessment

Collection of **subjective data** includes understanding that malignant lesions of the mouth are usually asymptomatic. The patient may feel only a roughened area with the tongue. As the disease progresses, the first complaints may be (1) difficulty chewing, swallowing, or speaking; (2) edema, numbness, or loss of feeling in any part of the mouth; and (3) earache, facial pain, and toothache, which may become constant. Cancer of the lip is associated with discomfort and irritation caused by a nonhealing lesion, which may be raised or ulcerated. Malignancy at the base of the tongue produces less obvious symptoms: slight dysphagia, sore throat, and salivation.

Collection of **objective data** includes observing for premalignant lesions, including leukoplakia. Unusual bleeding in the mouth, some blood-tinged sputum, lumps or edema in the neck, and hoarseness may be observed.

Diagnostic Tests

Indirect laryngoscopy is an important diagnostic test for examination of the soft tissue. This procedure is especially important for men 40 years of age or older who have dysphagia and a history of smoking and alcohol ingestion. Radiographic evaluation of the mandibular structures is another essential part of the head and neck examination to rule out cancer. Excisional biopsy is the most accurate method for making a definitive diagnosis. Oral exfoliative cytology is used for screening intraoral lesions. A scraping of the lesion provides cells for cytologic examination. The chance for a false-negative finding is about 26%.

Medical Management

Treatment depends on the location and staging of the malignant tumor. Stage I oral cancers are treated by surgery or radiation. Stages II and III cancers require both surgery and radiation. Chemotherapy may also be used when surgery and radiation therapy fail or as the initial therapy for smaller tumors. Treatment for stage IV cancer is usually palliative. The survival rate for patients with oral cancers averages less than 50%.

Small, accessible tumors can be excised surgically. Surgical options include a glossectomy, removal of the tongue; hemiglossectomy, removal of part of the tongue; mandibulectomy, removal of the mandible; and total or supraglottic laryngectomy, removal of the entire larynx or the portion above the true vocal cords.

Large tumors usually require more extensive and traumatic surgery. In a functional neck dissection of neck cancer with no growth in the lymph nodes, the surgeon removes the lymph nodes but preserves the jugular vein, the sternocleidomastoid muscle, and the spinal accessory nerve. In radical neck dissection, all these structures are removed and reconstructive surgery is necessary after tissue resection. Patients may have drains in the incision sites that are connected to suction to aid healing and reduce hematomas. A tracheostomy may also be performed, depending on the degree of tumor invasion.

Because of the location of the surgery, complications can occur. These include airway obstruction, hemorrhage, tracheal aspiration, facial edema, fistula formation, and necrosis of the skin flaps. If the patient has difficulty swallowing, a percutaneous endoscopic gastrostomy (PEG) tube may be inserted to allow for adequate nutritional intake. Neurologic complications can occur because of nerves being severed and manipulated during surgery.

Radiation therapy may involve (1) external radiation by roentgenograms or other radioactive substances or (2) internal radiation by means of needles or seeds. The purpose of radiation therapy is to shrink the tumor. It can be given preoperatively or postoperatively, depending on the physician's preference and the patient's disease process. In more advanced cases, chemotherapy may be combined with radiation postoperatively to make the patient more comfortable. Other treatment options include laser excision.

Nursing Interventions and Patient Teaching

A holistic approach to patient care includes awareness of the patient's level of knowledge regarding the disease, emotional response and coping abilities, and spiritual needs. Nursing interventions must be individualized to the patient—beginning with the preoperative stage, continuing through the postoperative stage, and ending after the patient's rehabilitation in the home environment. Family members, hospice workers, close friends, social workers, and pastoral care staff may provide information and support during this potentially fatal disease.

Nursing diagnoses and interventions for the patient with oral cancer include but are not limited to the following:

Nursing Diagnoses	Nursing Interventions
Imbalanced nutrition, less than body requirements, related to: • oral pain postoperative tissue loss • oral pain (mucous membranes)	Monitor the patient for changes in the character and quantity of mucus after radiation therapy. Provide meticulous oral hygiene. Observe for temporary or permanent loss of taste and the need for alternative routes for nutrition by monitoring daily weights.
Disturbed body image and personal identity, related to: • disfiguring appearance of an oral lesion • reconstructive surgery	Provide alternative methods for communication if radiation therapy results in dysarthria (difficult, poorly articulated speech, resulting from interference in the control over muscles of speech). Provide information to the patient and family to help with difficult decisions related to surgery, radiation, or chemotherapy. Provide support to the patient and family.

Prevention centers on predisposing factors: avoiding excess exposure to sun and wind on the lips, eliminating smoking or chewing tobacco, and eliminating plaque and caries through good oral and dental care. The incidence of cancer of the mouth bears a high correlation to cirrhosis of the liver associated with alcohol intake. Early detection of oral cancer can increase the patient's chance of survival. Any person with a mouth lesion that does not heal within 2 to 3 weeks is urged to seek medical care.

Instruct the patient about preoperative and postoperative care, with full explanations regarding speech loss and alternate methods of nutritional intake. Explanation of tracheostomy care and other tubes the patient may have on discharge relieves anxiety and increases the patient's sense of control over the situation.

Prognosis

Staging and biologic characterization of the neoplasm provide prognostic information. The prognosis of carcinoma in the oral cavity is directly related to the size of the primary tumor, the involvement of regional nodes, and the presence or absence of metastasis. The patient's immunologic response and general condition also influence the prognosis and the choice of therapy.

Carcinomas of the lip can be detected early by the patient, the physician, or the dentist during examination, and the prognosis for cure is good. If the carcinoma is difficult to detect, as on the anterior tongue and the floor of the mouth, it will be in a more advanced stage when detected. The prognosis in such cases is bleak. The 5-year survival rate for cancer of the oral cavity and pharynx is 53% for whites and 34% for blacks (ACS, 2009).

DISORDERS OF THE ESOPHAGUS

GASTROESOPHAGEAL REFLUX DISEASE

Etiology and Pathophysiology

Gastroesophageal reflux disease (GERD) is a backward flow of stomach acid up into the esophagus. Symptoms typically include burning and pressure behind the sternum. Most cases are thought to be caused by the inappropriate relaxation of the lower esophageal sphincter (LES) in response to an unknown stimulus. Symptoms of GERD develop when the LES is weak or experiences prolonged or frequent transient relaxation, conditions that allow gastric acids and enzymes to flow into the esophagus. Reflux is much more common in the postprandial state (after meals); more than 60% of reflux sufferers have delayed gastric emptying. GERD occurs in all age-groups and is estimated to affect up to 45% of the population to some degree, which translates to more than 60 million people. GERD is the most common upper GI problem seen in adults.

Clinical Manifestations

The clinical manifestations of GERD are consistent, but vary substantially in severity. The irritation of chronic reflux produces the primary symptom, which is heartburn **(pyrosis).** The pain is described as a substernal or retrosternal burning sensation that tends to radiate upward and may involve the neck, the jaw, or the back. The pain typically occurs 20 minutes to 2 hours after eating. An atypical pain pattern that closely mimics angina may also occur and must be carefully differentiated from true cardiac disease. The second major symptom of GERD is regurgitation, which is not associated with either eructation or nausea. The individual experiences a feeling of warm fluid moving up the throat. If it reaches the pharynx, a sour or bitter taste is perceived. Water brash, a reflux salivary hypersecretion that does not taste bitter, occurs less commonly.

In severe cases, GERD can produce dysphagia or odynophagia (painful swallowing). Eructation and a feeling of flatulence are other common complaints. Nocturnal cough, wheezing, or hoarseness all may occur with reflux, and it is estimated that more than 80% of adult asthmatics may have reflux. The frequency and severity of reflux episodes usually determine the severity of the symptoms.

Assessment

Subjective data include heartburn, a substernal or retrosternal burning sensation that may radiate to the back or jaw (in some cases the pain may mimic angina); and regurgitation (not associated with nausea or eructation), which causes a sour or bitter taste in the pharynx. Frequent eructation, flatulence, and dysphagia or odynophagia usually occur only in severe cases.

Objective data include nocturnal cough, wheezing, and hoarseness.

Diagnostic Tests

Mild cases of GERD are diagnosed from the classic symptoms, and treatment is initiated based on the presumptive diagnosis. More involved cases may require other screening tools. The gold standard for diagnosis is 24-hour pH monitoring using specially designed probes; such testing accurately records the number, duration, and severity of reflux episodes and is considered to be 85% sensitive. The esophageal motility and Bernstein tests can be performed in conjunction with pH monitoring to evaluate LES competence and the response of the esophagus to acid infusion. The barium swallow with fluoroscopy is widely used to document the presence of hiatal hernia. Endoscopy is routinely performed to evaluate for LES competence, potential scarring and strictures, and the presence and severity of esophagitis, and to rule out malignancy.

Medical Management

In its simplest form, GERD produces mild symptoms that occur infrequently (twice a week or less). In these cases, avoiding problem foods or beverages, stopping smoking, or losing weight may solve the problem. Medication therapy for GERD focuses on improving LES function, increasing esophageal clearance, decreasing volume and acidity of reflux, and protecting the esophageal mucosa. Treatment with antacids or acid-blocking medications called H_2 receptor antagonists—such as cimetidine (Tagamet), ranitidine (Zantac), famotidine (Pepcid), or nizatidine (Axid)—may also be used. More severe and frequent episodes of GERD can trigger asthma attacks, cause severe chest pain, result in bleeding, or promote a narrowing (stricture) or chronic irritation of the esophagus. In these cases, more powerful inhibitors of stomach acid production called proton pump inhibitors, such as omeprazole (Prilosec), esomeprazole (Nexium), pantoprazole (Protonix), rabeprazole (Aciphex), and lansoprazole (Prevacid), may be added to the treatment prescribed. Sucralfate (Carafate) is an antiulcer drug that may be used in GERD patients for its protective properties by forming a complex that adheres to an ulcer. Metoclopramide (Reglan) is used in moderate to severe cases of GERD. It is in a class of drugs called *promotility agents* that increase peristalsis and therefore promote gastric emptying and reduce the risk of gastric acid reflux.

As a last resort, a surgical procedure called **fundoplication** is performed to strengthen the sphincter. The procedure involves wrapping a layer of the upper stomach wall (fundus) around the sphincter and terminal esophagus to lessen the possibility of acid reflux (see Figure 45-16). If GERD is left untreated, serious pathologic (precancerous) changes in the esophageal lining may develop—a condition called **Barrett's esophagus** (esophageal metaplasia**).** In Barrett's esophagus the normal squamous epithelium of the esophagus is replaced by columnar epithelium. Because patients with Barrett's esophagus are at higher risk for esophageal cancer, they may need to be monitored regularly (every 1 to 3 years) by endoscopy and biopsy.

Nursing Interventions and Patient Teaching

Nursing interventions involve educating the patient about diet and lifestyle modifications that may alleviate symptoms of GERD.

Dietary instructions include (1) eat four to six small meals daily; (2) follow a low-fat, adequate-protein diet; (3) reduce intake of chocolate, tea, and other foods and beverages that contain caffeine; (4) limit or eliminate alcohol intake; (5) eat slowly, and chew food thoroughly; (6) avoid evening snacking, and do not eat for 2 to 3 hours before bedtime; (7) remain upright for 1 to 2 hours after meals when possible, and never eat in bed; (8) avoid any food that directly produces heartburn; and (9) reduce overall body weight if needed.

Numerous lifestyle changes are also indicated. Encourage patients who smoke to stop. Cigarette smoking has been associated with decreased acid clearance from the lower esophagus. Advise them to avoid constrictive clothing over the abdomen. They should avoid activities that involve straining, heavy lifting, or working in a bent-over position. Also instruct them to never sleep flat in bed. They should elevate the head of the bed at least 6 to 8 inches for sleep, using wooden blocks or a thick foam wedge.

Prognosis

If GERD is not successfully controlled, it can progress to serious and even life-threatening problems. Esophageal ulceration and hemorrhage may result from severe erosion, and chronic nighttime reflux is accompanied by a significant risk of aspiration. Adenocarcinoma can develop from the premalignant tissue (termed *Barrett's epithelium*). Gradual or repeated scarring can permanently damage esophageal tissue and produce stricture.

CARCINOMA OF THE ESOPHAGUS

Etiology and Pathophysiology

Carcinoma of the esophagus is a malignant epithelial neoplasm that has invaded the esophagus and has been diagnosed as a squamous cell carcinoma or an adenocarcinoma. An estimated 30% to 70% of esophageal cancers are adenocarcinomas; the remainder are squamous cell carcinomas. The incidence of squamous cell esophageal cancer is currently decreasing in the United States, whereas the incidence of adenocarcinoma of the distal esophagus is increasing (Lewis et al., 2007). Risk factors for esophageal cancer include alcohol and tobacco use and possibly longstanding achalasia (an abnormal condition characterized by the inability of a muscle to relax, particularly the cardiac sphincter of the stomach). Environmental carcinogens, nutritional deficiencies, chronic irritation, and mucosal damage have all been considered as causes of esophageal cancer. Another risk factor is Barrett's esophagus. It is estimated that 1 of 200 cases of Barrett's esophagus will progress to esophageal adenocarcinoma (see Health Promotion box).

Unfortunately, because of the location, esophageal cancer is usually at a late stage when discovered; treatment is palliative. Carcinoma of the bronchus, stomach, or breast may metastasize to the esophagus. The prevalent age-group for esophageal cancer is 55 to 70 years. It occurs more commonly in men.

Clinical Manifestations

The most common clinical symptom is progressive **dysphagia** (difficulty in swallowing) over a 6-month period. The patient may have a substernal feeling as though food is not passing through the esophagus.

Assessment

Collection of **subjective data** includes noting that initially the patient may have difficulty swallowing when eating bulky foods such as meat; later the difficulty occurs with soft foods and finally with liquids and even saliva. Another symptom is odynophagia (painful swallowing). Pain is a late symptom and indicates local extension of the malignancy.

Collection of **objective data** includes observing the patient for regurgitation (backward flowing or casting up of undigested food), vomiting, hoarseness, chronic cough, choking, and iron deficiency anemia. Weight loss may be directly related to the tumor or a side effect of treatment or the inability to swallow. When esophageal stenosis (narrowing) is severe, regurgitation of blood-flecked esophageal contents is common. Hemorrhage occurs if the cancer erodes through the esophagus and into the aorta. Esophageal perforation with fistula formation into the lung or trachea sometimes develops. The tumor may enlarge enough to cause esophageal obstruction. The cancer spreads via the lymph system, with the liver and lung being common sites of metastasis (Lewis et al., 2007).

 Health Promotion

Prevention or Early Detection of Esophageal Cancer

- Patients with diagnosed gastroesophageal reflux disease and hiatal hernia need counseling regarding regular follow-up evaluation.
- Health teaching should focus on elimination of smoking and excessive alcohol intake.
- Maintenance of good oral hygiene and dietary habits (intake of fresh fruits and vegetables) may be helpful.
- Patients diagnosed with Barrett's esophagus need to be monitored because this is considered a premalignant condition. Regular endoscopic screening with biopsy is required.
- Encourage patients to seek medical attention for any esophageal problems, especially dysphagia.

Diagnostic Tests

A barium swallow examination with fluoroscopy and endoscopy is used to detect esophageal cancer. An endoscopy with biopsy and cytologic examination provides a highly accurate diagnosis. Endoscopic ultrasonography is an important tool used to stage esophageal cancer. Computed tomography (CT) and magnetic resonance imaging also are used to assess the extent of the disease.

Medical Management

The treatment of esophageal cancer depends on the tumor's location and whether invasion or metastasis has occurred. Tumor staging must be determined to guide patient management. In advanced cases, surgery is palliative to relieve dysphagia and restore continuity of the alimentary tract. An aggressive approach provides excellent palliation (therapy designed to relieve or reduce intensity of uncomfortable symptoms but not to produce a cure), increased longevity, and a chance for a cure. Standard resection seems to give as good a result as a radical procedure.

Radiation therapy may be curative or palliative. Problems associated with radiation therapy include the development of an esophagotracheal fistula (an abnormal passage between two internal organs). Aspiration from the fistula and edema from the radiation are common. Chemotherapeutic agents cisplatin (Platinol), paclitaxel (Taxol), and fluorouracil (5-FU) are currently used in combination with radiation before and/or after surgery. If the tumor is in the upper third of the esophagus, radiation is indicated. A tumor in the lower third is usually resected surgically. Because of the extreme toxicity of these drugs, expect the patient to experience side effects of respiratory and liver dysfunction, nausea and vomiting, leukopenia, and sepsis.

The following four types of surgical procedures can be performed:

1. **Esophagogastrectomy:** Resection of a lower esophageal section with a proximal portion of the stomach, followed by **anastomosis** (surgical joining of two ducts, blood vessels, or bowel segments to allow flow from one to the other) of the remaining portions of the esophagus and stomach
2. **Esophagogastrostomy:** Resection of a portion of the esophagus with anastomosis to the stomach
3. **Esophagoenterostomy:** Resection of the esophagus and anastomosis to a portion of the colon
4. **Gastrostomy:** Insertion of a catheter into the stomach and suture to the abdominal wall; performed when the patient cannot take food orally because inoperable cancer of the esophagus interferes with swallowing

Nursing Interventions and Patient Teaching

Nursing diagnoses and interventions for the patient with esophageal carcinoma include but are not limited to the following:

Nursing Diagnoses	Nursing Interventions
Ineffective breathing pattern, related to: • incisional pain • proximity to the diaphragm	Monitor respirations carefully because of proximity of incision to diaphragm and patient's difficulty in carrying out breathing exercises.
Imbalanced nutrition: less than body requirements, related to: • dysphagia • decreased stomach capacity • anorexia	Monitor intake and output (I&O) and daily weights to determine adequate nutritional intake. Assess which foods patient can and cannot swallow to select and prepare edible foods. Administer tube feedings through gastrostomy, if present.

Discuss with the patient and family all aspects of care, including surgery, radiation, and chemotherapy. Psychological adjustment of the patient who cannot ingest food orally, whether temporary or permanent, is difficult. Step-by-step explanations of all diagnostic tests, medications, procedures, and the treatment plan will help relieve the patient's anxiety. Support the patient with this serious diagnosis by allowing time for questions.

Prognosis

In carcinoma of the esophagus, the disease is usually well advanced by the time symptoms appear. The delay between the onset of early symptoms and when the patient seeks medical advice is often 12 to 18 months. High mortality rates among these patients are affected by the following issues: (1) the patient is generally older; (2) the tumor has usually invaded surrounding structures; (3) the malignancy tends to spread to nearby lymph nodes; and (4) the esophagus is close to the heart and lungs, making these organs accessible to tumor extension.

The esophagus has an extensive lymphatic network, which facilitates the rapid spread of malignant cells to varying local and distant sites. Because esophageal cancer is rarely diagnosed in early stages, the 5-year survival rate is less than 20%. The only prognostic variable is the stage of disease (which underlines the importance of early diagnosis).

ACHALASIA

Etiology and Pathophysiology

Achalasia, also called **cardiospasm,** is an abnormal condition characterized by the inability of a muscle to relax, particularly the cardiac sphincter of the stomach. Although the cause is unknown, nerve degeneration, esophageal dilation, and hypertrophy are thought to contribute to the disruption of the esophagus's normal neuromuscular activity. This results in decreased motility and dilation of the lower portion of the esophagus, along with an absence of peristalsis. Thus little or no food can enter the stomach, and in extreme cases the dilated portion of the esophagus holds as much as a liter or more of fluid. This disease may occur in people of any age, but is more prevalent in those between 20 and 50 years.

Clinical Manifestations

The primary symptom of achalasia is dysphagia. The patient has a sensation of food sticking in the lower portion of the esophagus. As the condition progresses, the patient complains of regurgitation of food, which relieves prolonged distention of the esophagus. The patient may also have substernal chest pain.

Assessment

Observe for loss of weight, poor skin turgor, and weakness.

Diagnostic Tests

Radiologic studies show esophageal dilation above the narrowing at the cardioesophageal junction. The diagnosis is confirmed by manometry, which shows the absence of primary peristalsis. Esophagoscopy is also used to confirm the diagnosis.

Medical Management

Conservative treatment of achalasia includes drug therapy and forceful dilation of the narrowed area of the esophagus. Anticholinergics, nitrates, and calcium channel blockers reduce pressure in the lower esophageal sphincter.

Dilation is done by first emptying the esophagus. Then a dilator with a deflated balloon is passed down to the sphincter. The balloon is inflated and remains so for 1 minute; it may need to be reinflated once or twice.

Box 45-3 Nursing Interventions for the Patient Experiencing Esophageal Surgery

PREOPERATIVE NURSING INTERVENTIONS

1. Encourage improved nutritional status.
   a. Offer a high-protein, high-calorie diet if oral diet is possible.
   b. Total parenteral nutrition may be necessary for severe dysphagia or obstruction.
   c. Gastroscopy tube feedings may be indicated.
2. Give meticulous oral hygiene; breath may be malodorous.
3. Give preoperative preparation appropriate for thoracic surgery.
4. Give prescribed antibiotics before esophageal resection or bypass, as ordered.

POSTOPERATIVE NURSING INTERVENTIONS

1. Promote good pulmonary ventilation.
2. Maintain chest drainage system as prescribed.
3. Maintain gastric drainage system.
   a. Small amounts of blood may drain from nasogastric tube for 6 to 12 hours after surgery.
   b. Do not disturb nasogastric tube (to prevent traction on suture line).
4. Maintain nutrition.
   a. Start clear fluids at frequent intervals when oral intake is permitted.
   b. Introduce soft foods gradually, increasing to several small meals of bland foods.
   c. Have patient maintain semi-Fowler's position for 2 hours after eating and while sleeping if heartburn (pyrosis) occurs.

The preferred surgical approach is a cardiomyotomy. The muscular layer is incised longitudinally down to but not through the mucosa. Two thirds of the incision is in the esophagus, and the remaining one third is in the stomach; this permits the mucosa to expand so that food can pass easily into the stomach.

Nursing Interventions and Patient Teaching

Nursing interventions for esophageal surgery are presented in Box 45-3.

Nursing diagnoses and interventions for the patient with achalasia include but are not limited to the following:

Nursing Diagnoses	Nursing Interventions
Imbalanced nutrition: less than body requirements, related to difficulty swallowing both liquids and solids	Encourage fluids with meals to increase lower esophageal sphincter pressure and push food into stomach. Monitor liquid diet for 24 hours after dilation procedure.
Anxiety, related to continuous dilation process with threat of complications	Monitor for signs of esophageal perforation (chest pain, shock, dyspnea, fever) after dilation. Provide calm, nonstressful environment. Reinforce physician's explanation of disease process. Encourage verbalization of fears; assist patient with identifying stressors and positive coping behaviors.

Discuss home care and follow-up care in preparation for dismissal. Include a family member or support person if possible, and involve the patient as an active participant in the planning. Explain the need for a high-calorie, high-protein diet, and provide printed material describing same. Explain the need to elevate the head while sleeping and to avoid bending and stooping. Discuss medications if prescribed (including name, dosage, time of administration, purpose, and side effects). Discuss methods of avoiding constipation by using high-fiber foods (if tolerated) and natural laxatives. Explain the importance of follow-up care with the physician. Finally, discuss symptoms of recurrence or progression of disease and the need to report these to the physician.

Prognosis

Surgical separation, in addition to bag dilation, permits the return of normal peristalsis in approximately 10% of patients with achalasia.

DISORDERS OF THE STOMACH

GASTRITIS (ACUTE)

Etiology and Pathophysiology

Gastritis is an inflammation of the lining of the stomach. Acute gastritis is a temporary inflammation associated with alcoholism, smoking, and stressful physical problems, such as burns; major surgery; food allergens; viral, bacterial, or chemical toxins; chemotherapy; or radiation therapy. Changes in the mucosal lining interfere with acid and pepsin secretion. Acute gastritis is often a single incident that resolves when the offending agent is removed.

Clinical Manifestations

If the condition is acute, the patient may experience fever, epigastric pain, nausea, vomiting, headache, coating of the tongue, and loss of appetite. If the condition results from ingestion of contaminated food, the intestines are usually affected and diarrhea may occur. Some patients with gastritis have no symptoms.

Assessment

Collection of **subjective data** includes observing for anorexia, nausea, discomfort after eating, and pain.

Collection of **objective data** includes observing for vomiting, hematemesis, and melena caused by gastric bleeding.

Diagnostic Tests

Diagnosis is based on testing the stools for occult blood, noting white blood cell (WBC) differential increases related to certain bacteria, evaluating serum electrolytes, and observing for elevated hematocrit related to dehydration.

Medical Management

If medical treatment is required, an antiemetic—such as prochlorperazine (Compazine), promethazine (Phenergan), or trimethobenzamide (Tigan)—may be prescribed. Antacids and cimetidine (Tagamet) or ranitidine (Zantac) may be given in combination. Antibiotics are given if the cause is a bacterial agent. IV fluids are used to correct fluid and electrolyte imbalances. Patients who experience GI bleeding from hemorrhagic gastritis require fluid and blood replacement and NG lavage.

Nursing Interventions and Patient Teaching

Record the patient's I&O. Withhold foods and fluids orally as prescribed until signs and symptoms subside. Monitor the patient's tolerance to oral feedings and IV feedings as prescribed. Clear liquids are increased to diet as tolerated.

A nursing diagnosis and interventions for the patient with gastritis include but are not limited to the following:

Nursing Diagnosis	Nursing Interventions
Deficient fluid volume, related to vomiting, diarrhea, and blood loss	Keep patient NPO or on restricted food and fluids as ordered, and advance as tolerated. Monitor laboratory data for fluid and electrolyte imbalance (potassium, magnesium, sodium, and chloride). Maintain IV feedings. Record I&O.

Patient education includes explanations of (1) the effects of stress on the mucosal lining of the stomach; (2) how salicylates, nonsteroidal antiinflammatory drugs (NSAIDs), and particular foods may be irritating; and (3) how lifestyles that include alcohol and tobacco may be harmful. Assist the patient in locating self-help groups in the community to deal with these behaviors.

Prognosis

Because of the many classifications and causes of gastritis, prognosis is variable. Generally, prognosis is good in individuals who are willing to change their lifestyles and follow a medical regimen.

PEPTIC ULCERS

Peptic ulcers are ulcerations of the mucous membrane or deeper structures of the GI tract. They most commonly occur in the stomach and duodenum. The term *peptic ulcer* refers to ulcers resulting from acid and pepsin imbalances. Peptic ulcer disease remains a major health problem and affects more men than women. The disease is increasing among older adults, perhaps as a result of the use of NSAIDs. Symptoms are common between the ages of 25 and 50, with peak occurrence at age 40.

The stomach is normally protected from autodigestion by the gastric mucosal barrier. The GI tract has a high cell turnover rate, and the stomach's surface mucosa is renewed about every 3 days. As a result, the mucosa continuously repairs itself except in extreme instances when the cell breakdown surpasses the cell renewal rate. In such cases, peptic ulcers can occur. Peptic ulcers require the presence of gastric acid and result from four major causes: (1) excess of gastric acid (duodenal ulcers); (2) decrease in the natural ability of the GI mucosa to protect itself from acid and pepsin (gastric ulcers); (3) infection with spiral-shaped bacteria *H. pylori;* and (4) gastric injury from NSAIDs, aspirin, or corticosteroids.

Understanding of the factors that contribute to ulcer formation is developing rapidly. The discovery of the bacterium *H. pylori* provided new insight to ulcer formation. *H. pylori* has been identified in more than 70% of gastric ulcer patients and 95% of those with duodenal ulcers. In Western cultures, half of all people over age 50 harbor *H. pylori,* yet most do not develop peptic ulcer disease. Scientists still have to determine what triggers ulcers in those with *H. pylori.*

A common belief is that people exhibiting certain traits such as tenseness or striving for perfection or success are more likely to develop peptic ulcers. Conclusive evidence to support this belief is lacking.

GASTRIC ULCERS

The most common site of a gastric ulcer is in the distal half of the stomach. The cause of gastric ulcer is not clear, but it is related to factors such as diet; genetic predisposition; ingestion of excessive amounts of salicylates or NSAIDs; the use of tobacco; and *H. pylori.* Once the gastric mucosal barrier is damaged, acid secretion is stimulated. Without intervention, the cells die, erosion occurs, and ulcers develop. Gastric mucosal damage can occur in some individuals within 1 hour after the ingestion of acetylsalicylic acid. Reflux of duodenal contents (bile acids) also causes severe gastric mucosal damage. Gastric ulcers may occur on the surface of a gastric tumor because of interference with the blood supply.

PHYSIOLOGIC STRESS ULCERS

Physiologic stress ulcer or stress-related mucosal disease is an acute ulcer that develops after a major physiologic insult such as trauma or surgery. A stress ulcer is a form of erosive gastritis. It is believed that the gastric mucosa of the stomach undergoes a period of transient ischemia in association with hypotension, severe injury, extensive burns, and complicated surgery. The ischemia is due to decreased capillary blood flow or shunting of blood away from the GI tract so that blood flow bypasses the gastric mucosa. This occurs as a compensatory mechanism in hypotension or shock. The decrease in blood flow produces an imbalance between the destructive properties of hydrochloric acid and pepsin and protective factors of the stomach's mucosal barrier, especially in the fundus portion. Multiple superficial erosions result, and these may bleed. Because of the possibility of development of physiologic stress ulcers and high morbidity, patients at risk receive prophylaxis with antisecretory agents, including H_2 receptor blockers and proton pump inhibitors.

DUODENAL ULCERS

Etiology and Pathophysiology

Duodenal ulcers are a group of disorders that may or may not be caused by hypersecretion. Excessive production or excessive release of gastrin or increased sensitivity to gastrin is found in 40% of people with these ulcers. The other 60% have a normal amount of acid production but may lack the buffering ability in the duodenum. Risk factors include *H. pylori* infection, NSAIDs, cigarette smoking, and coffee. Ulceration occurs when the acid secretion exceeds the buffering factors.

Clinical Manifestations

Both gastric and duodenal ulcers may have similar symptoms but differ in timing, degree, or factors that worsen or alleviate the symptoms. Pain is the characteristic symptom and is described as dull, burning, boring, or gnawing; it is located in the midline of the epigastric region.

Assessment

Collection of **subjective data** requires an awareness that in gastric ulcer patients, the pain is closely associated with food intake and usually does not awaken the patient at night, as does the pain experienced by those with duodenal ulcers. Nausea, eructation, and distention are common complaints; these are termed **dyspepsia.** All these subjective symptoms intensify if perforation and obstruction occur.

Collection of **objective data** includes observing for hemorrhage, a common complication with gastric ulcers; more gastric ulcers bleed than do duodenal ulcers. Duodenal ulcers are more likely to have chronic bleeding and are more prone to perforation than gastric ulcers.

When GI bleeding occurs, one sign is vomiting blood **(hematemesis)** that has a coffee-grounds appearance as a result of action of the gastric acid on the hemoglobin molecule. The patient may have **melena** (tarlike, fetid-smelling stool containing undigested blood) that occurs when the blood becomes black and tarry as it passes through the digestive tract. In extreme cases, bright red blood may be passed rectally. Both salicylates and alcohol aggravate bleeding in patients with a history of peptic ulcers.

Bleeding from a gastric ulcer is more difficult to control than bleeding from a duodenal ulcer. Hemorrhage, with accompanying symptoms of shock, occurs when the ulcer erodes into a blood vessel. Surgical intervention is indicated if the patient remains unstable after receiving blood over several hours.

Perforation occurs when the ulcer crater penetrates the entire thickness of the wall of the stomach or duodenum. The release of air, gastric acid, pancreatic enzymes, or bile into the peritoneal cavity causes pain, emesis, fever, hypotension, and hematemesis. Perforation is considered the most lethal complication of peptic ulcer. Bacterial peritonitis may occur within 6 to 12 hours. The severity of the peritonitis is proportional to the amount and duration of the spillage through the perforation.

Gastric outlet obstruction is a complication of peptic ulcer disease that can occur at any time. It occurs more frequently when the ulcer is located close to the pylorus. Symptoms may be relieved by constant NG aspiration of stomach contents. This allows edema and inflammation to subside and permits normal flow of gastric contents through the pylorus.

Diagnostic Tests

Fiberoptic endoscopy can detect both gastric and duodenal ulcers. This is called **esophagogastroduodenoscopy.** Fiberoptic endoscopy is more reliable than barium contrast studies because of the maneuverability of fiberoptic scopes for viewing the entire esophagus and gastric and duodenal mucosa. This procedure also can be used to determine the degree of ulcer healing after treatment. During endoscopy, specimens can be obtained for identification of *H. pylori* or tissue specimens for biopsy. The patient is sedated but remains conscious throughout the endoscopy procedure. Local anesthetics in the throat are used to decrease the gag reflex and minimize pain during the procedure. No liquids or food are allowed for 1 to 2 hours or until the patient can swallow.

In 1996 the U.S. Food and Drug Administration (FDA) approved a breath test to detect *H. pylori.* The test calls for the patient to drink a solution containing carbon 13–enriched urea, a natural, nonradioactive substance. If *H. pylori* infection is present, it breaks down the compound and releases carbon dioxide-13 ($^{13}CO_2$). Thirty minutes after drinking the solution, the patient exhales into a collection bag, which is sent to the manufacturer for analysis. A finding of $^{13}CO_2$ confirms *H. pylori* infection. The test may prove especially useful in determining whether antibiotic therapy eradicated an *H. pylori* infection. Another noninvasive way to confirm *H. pylori* infection is a serum or whole blood antibody test, in particular, immunoglobulin G. This test is approximately 90% to 95% sensitive for *H. pylori* infection but cannot distinguish active from recently treated disease.

Barium contrast studies (UGI) are not as accurate for small lesions but are still commonly used. Testing of feces for occult blood in the intestinal tract is also used for diagnosis.

Medical Management

The physician may order insertion of an NG tube to remove gastric content and blood. Surgery is indicated usually for complications: perforation, penetration, obstruction, or intractability (no longer responding to medical management).

Scar tissue builds up with repeat episodes of ulceration and healing, causing obstruction, particularly at the pylorus. The patient may be seen with gastric dilation, vomiting, and distention. When fluid and electrolyte balance are achieved, surgical intervention is possible.

The primary treatment for peptic ulcers is to reduce signs and symptoms by decreasing or neutralizing normal gastric acidity with drug therapy. The types of drugs most commonly used include the following (Table 45-1).

- **Antacids:** Neutralize or reduce the acidity of stomach contents (e.g., Maalox, Gaviscon, Rolaids, Tums, Mylanta, and Riopan).
- **Histamine (H_2) receptor blockers:** Decrease acid secretions by blocking histamine (H_2) receptors (e.g., cimetidine, ranitidine, famotidine, and nizatidine). Do not give within 2 hours of antacids.
- **Proton pump inhibitors:** Antisecretory agents that inhibit secretion of gastrin by the parietal cells of the stomach (e.g., omeprazole, lansoprazole, pantoprazole, rabeprazole, and esomeprazole).

Table 45-1 Medications for Gastrointestinal Disorders

Generic (Trade)	Action	Side Effects	Nursing Implications
Antacids (aluminum, calcium, and magnesium salts and sodium bicarbonate) (Maalox, Mylanta, Titralac, Alternagel, others)	Neutralizes gastric acid; aluminum and calcium antacids also bind phosphates in renal failure patients	Aluminum: constipation, hypophosphatemia; calcium: constipation, rebound hyperacidity, hypercalcemia; magnesium: diarrhea, hypermagnesemia; sodium bicarbonate: sodium and water retention, alkalosis, rebound hyperacidity	Monitor serum electrolytes with long-term use; do not give antacid simultaneously with other medications because absorption of the other medication may be affected; best to separate administration by 2 hours.
Antispasmodics (including atropine, scopolamine, hyoscyamine, dicyclomine, clidinium) (Donnatal, Bentyl, others)	Anticholinergic agents that decrease GI motility by relaxing GI smooth muscle	Dry mouth and skin, constipation, paralytic ileus, urinary retention, tachycardia, drowsiness, dizziness, confusion, altered vision	Avoid using other CNS depressants or alcohol at the same time; avoid driving or other potentially hazardous tasks until accustomed to sedating effects.
Bismuth subsalicylate (Pepto-Bismol)	Antidiarrheal agent; also used in peptic ulcer disease caused by *Helicobacter pylori*	Fecal impaction, tinnitus	May turn stools dark gray–black; avoid use with aspirin; consult physician if diarrhea is accompanied by high fever or lasts more than 2 days.
Cimetidine (Tagamet)	H_2 receptor antagonist; inhibits gastric acid secretion	Confusion, headache, gynecomastia, bone marrow suppression (rare)	Increases serum levels and clinical effects of oral anticoagulants, theophylline, phenytoin, some benzodiazepines, and propranolol (these medications may require dosage reduction).
Dimenhydrinate (Dramamine, others)	Antiemetic agent; blocks central vomiting center	Drowsiness, dry mouth, constipation	Avoid use with other CNS depressants and alcohol; avoid driving or other hazardous activities until accustomed to sedating effects.

CNS, Central nervous system; *GI*, gastrointestinal;

Continued

Table 45-1 Medications for Gastrointestinal Disorders—cont'd

Generic (Trade)	Action	Side Effects	Nursing Implications
Diphenoxylate with atropine (Lomotil)	Antidiarrheal agent (diphenoxylate: narcotic; atropine: anticholinergic)	Drowsiness, sedation, constipation, dry mouth, urinary retention	Avoid use with other CNS depressants and alcohol; avoid driving or other hazardous activities until accustomed to sedating effects; do not use in infectious diarrhea.
Famotidine (Pepcid)	H_2 receptor antagonist; inhibits gastric acid secretion	Headache, dizziness, constipation, thrombocytopenia (rare)	Unlike cimetidine, does not affect serum levels of hepatically metabolized drugs (warfarin, phenytoin, theophylline).
Kaolin-pectin (Kaopectate)	Antidiarrheal agent	Constipation	Shake well before using.
Ketoconazole (Nizoral)	Antifungal agent	Gynecomastia, impotence, hepatotoxicity, abdominal pain	Requires acid environment for absorption; do not use with antacids, H_2 receptor blockers, or omeprazole; do not use with terfenadine, astemizole, or loratadine (has caused dysrhythmias and death); monitor liver function tests often; monitor serum levels and clinical effects of warfarin, cyclosporine, and theophylline.
Lansoprazole (Prevacid)	Binds to an enzyme in the presence of acid gastric pH, preventing the final transport of hydrogen ions into the gastric lumen	Drowsiness, abdominal pain, diarrhea, nausea	Sucralfate (Carafate) decreases absorption of lansoprazole (take 30 minutes before sucralfate); administer before meals. Assess patient routinely for epigastric or abdominal pain. May cause abnormal liver function tests.
Loperamide (Imodium)	Antidiarrheal agent	Drowsiness, dry mouth, constipation	Monitor for dehydration; do not use in infectious diarrhea.
Mesalamine (Rowasa, Asacol)	GI antiinflammatory agent	Abdominal cramps and gas, rash, headache, dizziness	Swallow tablets whole; give enema at bedtime, retain 10-15 minutes.
Misoprostol (Cytotec)	Prostaglandin analog that acts as gastric mucosal protectant against NSAID-induced ulcers	Diarrhea, nausea, vomiting, flatulence, uterine cramping	Absolutely contraindicated in pregnant women; women of childbearing age must use reliable contraception.
Nizatidine (Axid)	H_2 receptor antagonist, inhibits gastric acid secretion	Drowsiness, headache, dizziness, sweating, thrombocytopenia (rare)	Does not affect serum levels of hepatically metabolized drugs (warfarin, phenytoin, theophylline).
Nystatin (Mycostatin, Nilstat, others)	Antifungal agent, available as oral suspension and topical product	Oral: Nausea, vomiting, diarrhea Topical: Local irritation	Long-term therapy may be needed to clear infection; use for entire course.
Olsalazine (Dipentum)	GI antiinflammatory agent	Diarrhea, abdominal pain and cramps, nausea, allergic reactions, arthralgia, rash, anaphylaxis	Take with food; notify physician if severe diarrhea occurs.
Omeprazole (Prilosec)	Proton pump inhibitor, totally eradicates gastric acid production	Headache, dizziness, abdominal pain, nausea, vomiting, rare bone marrow suppression	Inhibits hepatic metabolism of warfarin, phenytoin, benzodiazepines, and other drugs metabolized by liver; do not crush or chew capsule contents.
Ranitidine (Zantac)	H_2 receptor antagonist; inhibits gastric acid secretion	Headache; abdominal discomfort; granulocytopenia and thrombocytopenia (both rare)	Minimal effect on serum levels of hepatically metabolized drugs (phenytoin, warfarin, theophylline).

CBC, Complete blood count; *NSAID*, nonsteroidal antiinflammatory drug.

Table 45-1 Medications for Gastrointestinal Disorders—cont'd

Generic (Trade)	Action	Side Effects	Nursing Implications
Sucralfate (Carafate)	Gastric mucosal protectant agent; adheres to site of ulcer	Constipation, hypophosphatemia	Do not give with other drugs; coating action may interfere with the absorption of other drugs—separate by 2 hours.
Sulfasalazine (Azulfidine)	GI antiinflammatory agent	Nausea, vomiting, abdominal pain, photosensitivity, rash, Stevens-Johnson syndrome (rare), renal failure, bone marrow suppression (rare), allergic reactions, anaphylaxis	Ensure adequate hydration to prevent crystallization in kidneys; avoid exposure to sunlight; women on oral contraceptives need to use alternative methods because of decreased effectiveness of oral contraceptives; monitor CBC and renal function; take with meals.

- **Mucosal healing agent:** Heals ulcers without antisecretory properties. Sucralfate is a cytoprotective drug. It accelerates ulcer healing, presumably because of the formation of an ulcer-adherent complex that covers the ulcer and protects it from evasion by pepsin, acid, and bile salts.
- **Antisecretory and cytoprotective agent:** Inhibits gastric acid secretion and protects gastric mucosa (misoprostol [Cytotec]). Cytotec is the only drug approved in the United States for the prevention of gastric ulcers induced by NSAIDs and aspirin.

Antibiotic therapy eradicates *H. pylori.* The drugs used include metronidazole (Flagyl), tetracycline, amoxicillin, and clarithromycin (Biaxin). Treatment is typically combined in a therapeutic regimen with other medications, such as bismuth or omeprazole. Another weapon that has entered the battle against *H. pylori* is a combination of bismuth, metronidazole, and tetracycline. Marketed under the brand name Helidac, the medication kit contains a 14-day supply of the three drugs, with each daily dose packaged on a blister card to improve patient compliance.

Among patients whose *H. pylori* is treated with antibiotics, the peptic ulcer recurrence may be as low as 10%. Patients who do not receive antibiotics have a relapse rate of 75% to 90%.

Dietary modification may be necessary to avoid irritating foods and beverages. There is considerable controversy over the therapeutic benefits of a bland diet, since the rationale is not supported by scientific evidence. Therefore it is recommended that the patient eat smaller meals more frequently throughout the day to decrease the degree of gastric motor activity.

Smoking has an irritating effect on the mucosa, increases gastric motility, and delays mucosal healing. Smoking should be eliminated completely or severely reduced. The combination of adequate rest and cessation of smoking accelerates ulcer healing. Because caffeinated and decaffeinated coffee, tobacco, alcohol, and aspirin aggravate the mucosal lining of the stomach and duodenum, educate patients with ulcers about the need for lifestyle change.

Surgical intervention has decreased drastically with more effective diagnosis and medical treatment with antisecretory agents and antibiotics. Approximately 20% of patients with ulcers require surgical intervention. These are patients who are unresponsive to medical management, raising concerns about gastric cancer; patients whose ulcers are drug induced but who cannot be withdrawn from the drugs (e.g., patients with rheumatoid arthritis); or patients who develop complications. Types of surgical procedures include the following:

- **Antrectomy:** Removal of the entire antrum, the gastric-producing portion of the lower stomach, to eliminate the main stimuli to acid production.
- **Gastroduodenostomy (Billroth I)** (Figure 45-7, *A*): Direct anastomosis of the fundus of the stomach to the duodenum; used to remove ulcers or cancer located in the antrum of the stomach.
- **Gastrojejunostomy (Billroth II)** (Figure 45-7, *B*): Closure of the duodenum, and anastomosis of

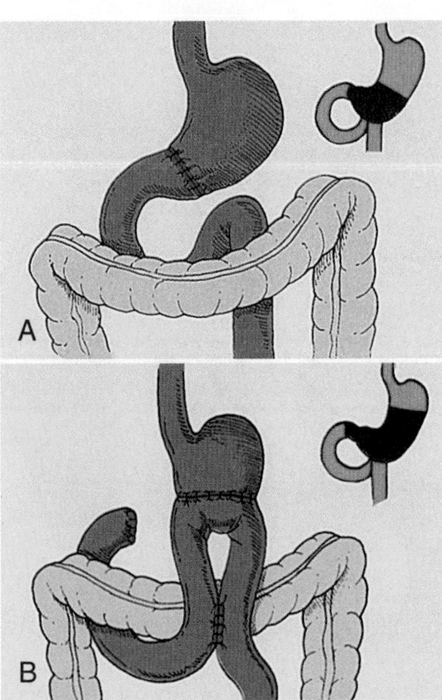

FIGURE 45-7 Types of gastric resections with anastomoses. **A,** Billroth I. **B,** Billroth II.

the fundus of the stomach into the jejunum; used to remove ulcers or cancer located in the body of the fundus.

- **Total gastrectomy:** Removal of the entire stomach; rarely used for patients with gastric cancer.
- **Vagotomy:** Removal of the vagal innervation to the fundus, decreasing acid produced by the parietal cells of the stomach (Figure 45-8); usually done with a Billroth I or II procedure or with a pyloroplasty.
- **Pyloroplasty:** Surgical enlargement of the pyloric sphincter to facilitate passage of contents from the stomach; commonly done after vagotomy or to enlarge an opening that has been constricted from scar tissue. A vagotomy decreases gastric motility and subsequently gastric emptying. A pyloroplasty accompanying vagotomy increases gastric emptying.

The choice of which procedure to use is difficult and depends on physician preference and results of diagnostic testing. Regardless of the procedure selected, postoperative complications are possible. Bleeding may occur up to 7 days after gastric surgery. Abdominal rigidity, abdominal pain, restlessness, elevated temperature, increased pulse, decreased blood pressure, and leukocytosis are all possible indications of postoperative bleeding. Note the amount and type of drainage from the incision. Surgical intervention may be necessary to correct the bleeding.

Dumping syndrome is a rapid gastric emptying causing distention of the duodenum or jejunum produced by a bolus of hypertonic food. Increased intestinal motility and peristalsis and changes in blood glucose levels occur. Patients may report diaphoresis, nausea, vomiting, epigastric pain, explosive diarrhea, borborygmi (noises made from gas passing through the liquid of the small intestine), and dyspepsia. Dumping syndrome is the direct result of surgical removal of a large portion of the stomach and the pyloric sphincter. Approximately one third to one half of patients experience dumping syndrome after peptic ulcer surgery. Treatment includes eating six small meals daily that are high in protein and fat and low in carbohydrates, eating slowly, and avoiding fluids during meals. Treatment also includes (1) anticholinergic agents to decrease stomach motility, and (2) reclining for approximately 1 hour after meals. To increase long-term compliance, reassure patients that following the recommended treatment will decrease symptoms within a few months. The symptoms are self-limiting and often disappear within several months to a year after surgery.

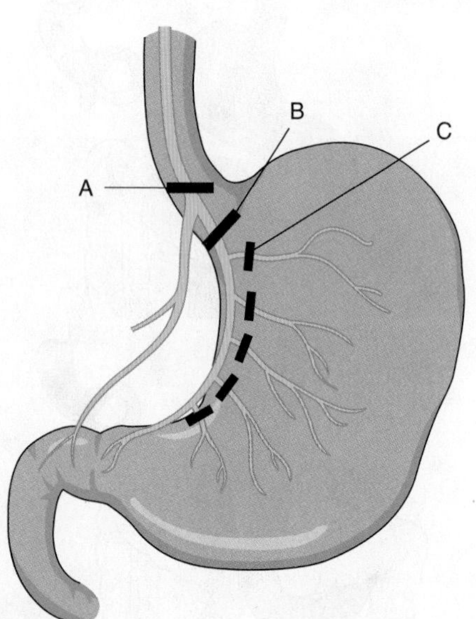

FIGURE 45-8 Types of vagotomies. *A*, Truncal. *B*, Selective. *C*, Proximal or parietal cell.

Several other complications after gastric surgery present serious health threats. Diarrhea is common and usually responds to conservative treatment of controlled diet and antidiarrheal agents. Diphenoxylate with atropine (Lomotil), loperamide (Imodium), paregoric, or codeine is often used. Reflux esophagitis and nutritional deficits—including weight loss, malabsorption, anemia, and vitamin deficiency—can also be life threatening.

Pernicious anemia is a serious potential complication for any patient who has had a total gastrectomy or extensive resections. This is caused by a deficiency of the intrinsic factor, produced exclusively by the stomach, which aids intestinal absorption of vitamin B_{12}. Recommend that all patients with a partial gastrectomy have a blood serum vitamin B_{12} level measured every 1 to 2 years so that replacement therapy of vitamin B_{12} via a monthly injection or via nasal route weekly can be instituted before anemia appears.

Nursing Interventions and Patient Teaching

NG or intestinal tube insertion, irrigation, and intermittent suctioning are often performed while a patient is feeling ill and uncomfortable. In addition to being skilled and knowledgeable in performing these procedures, the nurse is responsible for easing the patient's fears and anxieties. Patient cooperation not only makes the procedures easier but also reduces patient discomfort.

Helping patients through the experience of GI intubation requires understanding of the following points:

- For most patients, NG or intestinal tube placement is a new and frightening experience. Convey the rationale for this therapy to the anxious patient and family. Help them understand that the advantages far outweigh the discomfort.
- Inability to chew, taste, and swallow food and liquids may contribute to patient anxiety during GI intubation.

- A patient with an NG or intestinal tube is usually on NPO status. Occasionally ice chips are allowed.
- An NG or intestinal tube is connected to either continuous or intermittent suctioning, usually at 100 mm Hg for decompression.
- An NG or intestinal tube is a constant irritant to the nasopharynx and nares, requiring frequent care to the mouth and nose.
- A patient with a GI tube may be afraid that moving will dislodge the tube. Implement frequent position changes to enhance tube functioning and prevent complications of immobility.

An NG tube is inserted through the nose, pharynx, and esophagus into the stomach. Various tubes are available, depending on the purpose (Table 45-2).

Nursing interventions depend on the stage of the ulcer disease. The emphasis in patient care should always be on prevention and early detection of pain in the epigastric region, hematemesis, melena, or tenderness and rigidity of the abdomen (see Communication box and Nursing Care Plan 45-1).

Nursing diagnoses and interventions for the specific stages of ulcer care include but are not limited to the following:

Nursing Diagnoses	Nursing Interventions
Deficient knowledge, related to: • medications • diet • signs and symptoms of bleeding, perforation, or gastric outlet obstruction	Provide verbal and written instructions on exact dosage and time intervals for medications and whether medication is taken with or without food. Have dietitian provide instructions on therapeutic diet. Explain that repeat episodes are not uncommon; listen carefully for aggravating factors.
Pain, related to gastric acid on ulceration of gastric or duodenal mucosa	Give prescribed H_2 receptor antagonists (cimetidine, ranitidine, famotidine, or nizatidine) with meals and at bedtime. Give prescribed antacid 1 and 3 hours after meals.

Table 45-2 Purposes of Nasogastric Intubation

PURPOSE	DESCRIPTION	TYPE OF TUBE
Decompression	Removal of secretions and gaseous substances from GI tract; prevention or relief of abdominal distention	Salem sump, Miller-Abbott
Feeding (gavage)	Instillation of liquid nutritional supplements or feedings into stomach for patients unable to swallow fluid	Duo, Dobhoff
Compression	Internal application of pressure by means of inflated balloon to prevent internal GI hemorrhage	Sengstaken-Blakemore
Lavage	Irrigation of stomach in cases of active bleeding, poisoning, gastric dilation, or intestinal obstruction	Ewald, Salem sump

GI, Gastrointestinal.

Communication

Patient with a GI Bleed

Nurse: You look like you are resting better, Mrs. S. How have you been feeling? *(Reaffirming a relationship that was begun yesterday.)*

Patient: Hello, Mrs. F. My stomach pain is much better. The medicine helped.

Nurse: If you are comfortable, perhaps you and your husband have some questions about why you are here. *(Trying to determine whether the patient is receptive to patient teaching. A knowledge deficit was suspected on admission.)*

Patient: I was scared when I started to vomit blood. It has happened before but not this much. Where does the blood come from?

Nurse: You have a diagnosis of GI bleeding with questionable duodenal ulcer. That means you have bleeding in the gastrointestinal system, either in the stomach or in some part of the intestine. Do you understand what I have said so far? *(The nurse begins with the admitting diagnosis and explains one thing at a time, making sure the patient verbalizes understanding before continuing.)*

Patient: Well, I understand where the bleeding is coming from, but why am I bleeding there?

Nurse: We are not sure yet, Mrs. S., but you are scheduled for a procedure that will allow the physician to actually look at the surface of the stomach and a portion of the intestine. It is called an endoscopy, and it will be done tomorrow morning. Did someone explain this to you? *(The nurse answers the patient's question openly and honestly and uses her answer to lead into further patient education.)*

 Nursing Care Plan 45-1 The Patient with Gastrointestinal Bleeding

Mr. Dunne, 33 years of age, is admitted with pain in the epigastric region and copious hematemesis. He appears anxious; his skin is pale, cool, and clammy; and he is breathing rapidly. This patient has a history of recurrent episodes of vomiting blood that has a coffee-grounds appearance. He denies passing blood rectally but admits his stools have changed in consistency.

NURSING DIAGNOSIS *Risk for deficient fluid volume, related to hemorrhage, vomiting, and diarrhea*

Patient Goals and Expected Outcomes	Nursing Interventions	Evaluation
Patient will have normal fluid balance as evidence by balanced intake and output (I&O) within 24 hours, including stable weight. Blood pressure, pulse, and respiratory rate will be within normal limits. Patient will have normal tissue turgor within 24 hours.	Monitor IV and blood transfusion therapy as ordered. Accurately record I&O every hour until stable: emesis, urine, and stool. Document fluid losses for possible imbalance; urinary output less than 30 mL/hr may indicate hypovolemia. Monitor for signs and symptoms of dehydration and fluid and electrolyte imbalance (dry mucous membranes, poor skin turgor, thirst, decreased urinary output, and changes in behavior) every 15 minutes until stable, then every 2 hours. Document characteristics of output. Test all emesis and fecal output for presence of blood as ordered. Prepare to assist with inserting a nasogastric (NG) tube and connecting it to wall suction. Irrigate NG tube with saline as ordered to promote clotting; irrigation removes old blood from the stomach.	Patient has urinary output of 1500 mL for prior 24-hour period. Patient's blood pressure, pulse, and respiratory rate are within patient's pregastrointestinal bleeding baseline levels. Patient's tissue turgor is normal.

NURSING DIAGNOSIS *Anxiety, related to hospitalization and illness*

Patient Goals and Expected Outcomes	Nursing Interventions	Evaluation
Patient will demonstrate decrease in anxiety as evidenced by ability to sleep or rest at frequent intervals, verbalization of feelings, and blood pressure and pulse within normal limits.	Assess physiologic components of anxiety (restlessness, increased pulse and respirations, diaphoresis, and elevated blood pressure) at least every 8 hours. Provide concise explanations for all procedures; prepare patient for surgery if indicated. Develop rapport with patient and family members with each contact.	Patient is sleeping 5 to 6 hours during the night and resting at intervals during the day. Patient verbalizes a feeling of less stress and anxiety. Therapeutic rapport with nurse, patient, and family members is noted.

Critical Thinking Questions

1. Mr. Dunne has an NG tube connected to wall suction that is draining sanguineous fluid. He complains of severe fatigue and epigastric pain. He is pale and drawn, with a hemoglobin level of 5.1 g/dL. Mr. Dunne puts his call light on and requests the nurse to assist him to the bathroom for a bowel movement. What appropriate interventions will ensure Mr. Dunne's safety?
2. During assessment of Mr. Dunne, what signs and symptoms would indicate deficient fluid volume?
3. Mr. Dunne says to the nurse that he fears he may die. He appears anxious and tremulous. What is the most therapeutic approach to help decrease his fears?

Nursing Diagnoses	Nursing Interventions
Pain, related to gastric acid on ulceration of gastric or duodenal mucosa—cont'd	Teach relaxation measures as appropriate. Give prescribed proton pump inhibitors (omeprazole, lansoprazole, pantoprazole, or esomeprazole). Administer antibiotic therapy to eradicate *H. pylori* infections as prescribed. Instruct patient on side effects of antacid drugs (constipation or diarrhea) and importance of contacting physician if this occurs.
Noncompliance, related to: • risk behaviors (use of tobacco or alcohol) • dietary patterns	Assess patient's level of knowledge regarding food and other irritants to mucosal lining. Teach preventive measures, such as quitting smoking. Explain need for small and frequent meals. Caution patient to avoid high-fiber foods, sugar, salt, caffeine, alcohol, and milk. Remind patient to take fluids between meals, not with meals. Explain the need to eat slowly and chew food well. Discuss importance of adequate rest and exercise.
Imbalanced nutrition: less than body requirements, related to preoperative food and fluid restrictions	Maintain NPO status. Connect NG tube to intermittent suction apparatus. Note color and amount of gastric output every 4 hours. Do not reposition tube. Maintain patency of tube by irrigation with measured amounts of saline *only if ordered.* NOTE: After gastrectomy, output is minimal. Monitor parenteral fluids with electrolyte additives as ordered. Measure I&O. When bowel sounds return and flatus is expelled, administer clear liquids as ordered. Progress to small, frequent meals of soft food as ordered. Avoid milk because it may cause dumping syndrome.

It is necessary to form a trusting relationship with the patient with an ulcer because of the severity of the condition and the need for long-term treatment. Include the family in patient education sessions to increase understanding and support, and involve the patient in goal setting to increase compliance (see Home Care Considerations box).

Instruct the patient to seek medical attention immediately if severe and sudden pain occurs. Assist the patient in describing signs and symptoms of weakness, anorexia, nausea, diarrhea, constipation, anxiety, or restlessness. When medications are prescribed, the patient must fully understand (1) the purpose of taking antibiotic therapy to eradicate *H. pylori;* (2) the importance of taking all medications such as H_2 receptor antagonists, antiulcer drugs, prostaglandin E analog, and proton pump inhibitors as prescribed; (3) why the antacids are taken in large doses (30 mL) seven times daily (1 and 3 hours after a meal and at bedtime) or at the specific times ordered; and (4) the known side effects (diarrhea and constipation). Preventive teaching includes identifying high-risk behaviors, such as the use of tobacco, caffeine, and alcohol. Emphasize that the patient should eat six smaller meals daily and avoid any foods that cause noticeable stomach discomfort.

Home Care Considerations

Peptic Ulcer Disease

- The patient who has recurrent ulcer disease after initial healing must learn to live with a chronic disease.
- The patient may be angry and frustrated, especially he or she has faithfully followed the prescribed therapy but failed to prevent the recurrence or extension of the disease process.
- Unfortunately, many patients do not comply with the care plan and experience repeated exacerbations.
- Changes in lifestyle are difficult for most people and may be resisted.
- The patient who is instructed to stop smoking or avoid alcohol may resist.
- The goal should be adhering to the prescribed therapeutic regimen, including nutritional management, cessation of smoking, and decreased use of alcohol and caffeine.
- A patient with chronic ulcers needs to be aware of the complications that may result from the disease, the clinical manifestations indicating their presence, and what to do until the physician can be seen.
- Teach the patient to take all medications as prescribed. This includes both antisecretory and antibiotic drugs. Failure to take prescribed medications can result in relapse.

If surgery is required, explain the procedures thoroughly, including the reasons for them. Explain immediate postoperative care, including deep breathing; coughing; position changes; frequent monitoring of vital signs; IV tubing, NG tubing, catheters, and other drainage tubes; and the use of patient-controlled analgesia (PCA) or other medications for pain relief. The patient's ability to eat normally after healing depends on the type of surgery and when peristalsis returns. Help the patient realize that symptoms often recur and he or she should seek medical care if they do.

Prognosis for Peptic Ulcers

Recurrence of an ulcer may happen within 2 years in about one third of all patients. Among patients whose *H. pylori* is treated with antibiotics, the peptic ulcer recurrence drops to 2%. Patients who do not receive antibiotics have a relapse rate of 75% to 90%. The likelihood of recurrence is lessened by eliminating foods that aggravate the condition. If symptoms recur, the prognosis is better in patients who seek immediate medical treatment and comply with the prescribed regimen.

CANCER OF THE STOMACH

Etiology and Pathophysiology

In the 1940s gastric cancer was the most common malignant disease in the United States, but the incidence has declined significantly. The most common neoplasm or malignant growth in the stomach is adenocarcinoma. The primary location is the pyloric area, but the incidence of proximal tumors appears to be rising. Because of the location, the tumor may metastasize to lymph nodes, liver, spleen, pancreas, or esophagus. Gastric cancer is more common in people 50 to 70 years of age.

Many factors have been implicated in the development of stomach cancer, yet no single causative agent has been identified. Stomach carcinogenesis probably begins with a nonspecific mucosal injury as a result of aging; autoimmune disease; or repeated exposure to irritants such as bile, antiinflammatory agents, or smoking. Other factors include history of polyps, pernicious anemia, hypochlorhydria (deficiency of hydrochloride in the stomach's gastric juice), chronic atrophic gastritis, and gastric ulcer. Because the stomach has prolonged contact with food, cancer in this part of the body is associated with diets that are high in salt, smoked and preserved foods (which contain nitrites and nitrates), and carbohydrates, and low in fresh fruits and vegetables. Whole grains and fresh fruits and vegetables are associated with reduced rates of stomach cancer. Infection with *H. pylori,* especially at an early age, is considered a definite risk factor for gastric cancer.

Clinical Manifestations

The patient may be asymptomatic in early stages of the disease. Stomach cancer often spreads to adjacent organs before any distressing symptoms occur. With more advanced disease, the patient may appear pale and lethargic if anemia is present. With a poor appetite and significant weight loss, the patient may appear cachectic.

Assessment

Subjective data include complaints of vague epigastric discomfort or indigestion, early satiety, and postprandial (after meal) fullness. Ten percent of patients complain of an ulcerlike pain that does not respond to therapy. Anorexia and weakness are also common.

Objective data include weight loss, bleeding in the stools, hematemesis, and vomiting after drinking or eating. Anemia is common. It is caused by chronic blood loss as the lesion erodes through the mucosa or as a direct result of pernicious anemia, which develops when intrinsic factor is lost. The presence of ascites is a poor prognostic sign.

Diagnostic Tests

The tumor is diagnosed by radiographic barium studies (GI series). Endoscopic or gastroscopic examinations with biopsy remain the best diagnostic tool. The stomach can be distended with air during the procedure to stretch mucosal folds. Endoscopic ultrasound and CT scans can be used for staging the disease. Stool examination provides evidence of occult or gross bleeding. Carcinoembryonic antigen (CEA) and carbohydrate antigen 19-9 tumor markers are usually elevated in advanced gastric cancer. Serum tumor markers correlate with the degree of invasion, liver metastasis, and cure rate. Laboratory studies of RBCs, hemoglobin, hematocrit, and serum B_{12} assist in the detection of anemia and determination of severity.

Medical Management

The most therapeutic management of stomach cancer is surgical removal. Unfortunately, the surgery may be done as an exploratory celiotomy to determine involvement or to make the patient more comfortable. The surgical intervention used in treating gastric cancer may be the same procedure used for peptic ulcer disease. A partial or total gastric resection is the choice for an extensive lesion. Surgery for advanced gastric cancer carries high morbidity and mortality rates.

Wound healing may be disrupted by **dehiscence** (a partial or complete separation of the wound edges) or by **evisceration** (protrusion of viscera through the disrupted wound). Dehiscence and evisceration may be caused by problems in suturing the wound or by poor tissue integrity. Excessive coughing, straining, malnutrition, obesity, and infection may also increase the chances of dehiscence. Nursing interventions include instructing the patient to remain quiet and to avoid coughing or straining. Keep the patient in a dorsal recumbent position (on back with knees flexed) to remove stress on the wound. If evisceration occurs, keep the patient on bed rest and loosely cover the protruding viscera with a warm sterile saline dressing. Notify the surgeon immediately because treatment consists of reapproximating the wound edges.

Chemotherapy has greater response and longer survival rates than radiation. Because the radiosensitivity of stomach cancer is low, radiation therapy is of little value. However, it may be used as a palliative measure to decrease tumor mass and temporarily relieve obstruction. The combination of chemotherapy and radiation therapy may be used for patients who are at high risk for disease recurrence after surgery. These treatment modalities are often used with surgery.

Nursing Interventions and Patient Teaching

Provide further clarification about the disease and the surgical intervention to the patient and family. The preoperative preparation includes improving the patient's nutritional status by monitoring total parenteral nutrition and providing supplemental feedings. Postoperative teaching is necessary to relieve anxiety and promote understanding of drainage tubes, feeding tubes, dressing changes, weakness, medications, and other routine care.

Nursing diagnoses and interventions for the patient with cancer of the stomach include but are not limited to the following:

Nursing Diagnoses	Nursing Interventions
Ineffective breathing pattern, related to: • pain • exploration of chest and abdominal cavities • abdominal distention	Place the patient in a semi-Fowler's position to aid ventilation. Encourage and assist with gentle turning and repositioning. Encourage the patient to turn, breathe deeply, and cough at least every 2 hours until ambulating well; splint incision before coughing; use incentive spirometer; and ambulate as soon as possible.
Risk for injury, related to: • aspiration • infection • hemorrhage • anastomotic leak into abdominal cavity • anemia or vitamin deficiency	Monitor closely for elevated temperature, bleeding from incision, pallor, dyspnea, cyanosis, tachycardia, increased respirations, and chest pain. Monitor laboratory results and activity tolerance because of possible anemia. Change dressings using sterile technique.

Because care encompasses so many areas, instruction should be (1) planned according to the patient's needs and level of understanding, (2) given when the patient is free of pain and rested, and (3) communicated both verbally and in print. Explain surgery, chemotherapy, radiation therapy, continued nutritional needs, pain relief, and support groups for psychosocial needs.

Weight loss indicates the need for additional caloric intake and can be measured by monitoring weight and comparing it with the patient's normal weight before illness. Prevent skin excoriation around the feeding tube. Hypermotility or diarrhea that follows radiation therapy can be treated with medication. The debilitated patient and family may require referral for hospice care.

Prognosis

The prognosis for patients with gastric cancer is usually poor. About 60% have clinical findings at the time of diagnosis, resulting in a low cure rate. Only 10% to 20% of patients develop disease confined to the stomach. For patients with lymph node–negative stomach cancer, surgical treatment alone results in a 75% 5-year survival rate. For patients with lymph node–positive cancer, the 5-year survival rate after surgery is 10% to 30%.

DISORDERS OF THE INTESTINES

INFECTIONS

Etiology and Pathophysiology

Intestinal infections are the invasion of the alimentary canal (both the small and large intestine) by pathogenic microorganisms that reproduce and multiply. The infectious agent can enter the body by several routes. The most common way is through the mouth in contaminated food or water. Some intestinal infections occur as a result of person-to-person contact. Fecal-oral transmission occurs through poor hand hygiene after elimination. In active homosexual males, infectious agents can be introduced by single-cell protozoal infections.

Bacterial flora grow naturally in the intestinal tract and help the immune system combat infection. However, long-term antibiotic therapy can destroy the normal flora. The impaired immune response in some individuals delays the body's attempt to destroy invading pathogens.

Infectious diarrhea causes secretion of fluid into the intestinal lumen. *Clostridia*, *Salmonella*, *Shigella*, and *Campylobacter* bacteria are associated with intestinal infections. These bacteria produce toxic substances, and the mucosal cells respond by secreting water and electrolytes, causing an imbalance. The amount of fluid secreted exceeds the ability of the large intestine to reabsorb the fluid into the vascular system.

One strain of *E. coli*—serotype O157:H7—often has a virulent course. Unlike other strains, *E. coli* O157:H7 is not part of the normal flora of the human intestine. Found in the intestines of approximately 1% of food cattle, this strain can, even in small amounts, contaminate a large amount of meat, especially ground beef. It is transmitted in contaminated, undercooked meats such as hamburger, roast beef, ham, and turkey; in produce that has been rinsed with water contaminated by animal or human feces; or by a person who has been handling contaminated food. The bacterium has also been cultured in unpasteurized milk, cheese, and apple juice and can be found in lakes and pools that have been contaminated by fecal matter. Hemorrhagic colitis (which results in bloody diarrhea and severe cramping accompanied by diffuse abdominal tenderness) develops between the second and fourth days. Antidiarrheals should not be given because these medications prevent the intestines from getting rid of the *E. coli* pathogen. Antimotility drugs such as diphenoxylate with atropine or antibiotic therapy is not recommended because they increase the likelihood of developing hemolytic-uremic syndrome, a pathologic condition of the kidney. Poisoning with *E. coli* O157:H7 can be life threatening, particularly in the very young and in older adults. Usually little or no fever is present and the illness resolves in 5 to 10 days. In approximately 2% to 7% of infections, particularly in young children, hemolytic-uremic syndrome occurs and the kidneys fail (Lewis et al., 2007).

Sigmoidoscopic or colonoscopic examination and stool specimens are used to diagnose a type of inflammation or colitis called **antibiotic-associated pseudomembranous colitis** (AAPMC). Immunosuppressed patients and older adults are particularly susceptible. *C. difficile* is a hazardous nosocomial infection because hospitalized patients are often immunosuppressed, antibiotic therapy is common, and the spores can survive for up to 70 days on inanimate objects. *C. difficile* spores have been found on commodes, telephones, thermometers, bedside tables, floors, and other objects in the room, as well as on the hands of health care workers. Health care workers who do not adhere to infection-control precautions can transmit *C. difficile* from patient to patient. Washing hands with soap and water is necessary because antiseptic hand rub does not destroy *C. difficile*. This type of colitis is a complication of treatment with a wide variety of antibiotics, including lincomycin, clindamycin, ampicillin, erythromycin, tetracycline, cephalosporins, and aminoglycosides. A *C. difficile* test is ordered on the stool specimen to aid in the diagnosis of AAPMC in both inpatients and outpatients. Characteristic lesions of AAPMC are identified on tissues obtained through endoscopic examination.

Treatment with antibiotics (especially clindamycin, ampicillin, amoxicillin, and the cephalosporins) inhibits normal bacterial growth in the intestine. This inhibition of normal flora can lead to the overgrowth of other bacteria such as *C. difficile*. Under the right conditions, *C. difficile* produces two toxins, A and B. Both toxins A and B are produced by *C. difficile* at the same time and these toxins cause the tissue damage seen in AAPMC disease. The incidence of *C. difficile* toxin found in the stool ranges from 1% to 2% in a normal population to 10% in hospital inpatients and up to 85% to 90% in patients with proven AAPMC. The *C. difficile* test alone is not conclusive but does aid in the diagnosis of AAPMC.

Because the level of *C. difficile* antigens associated with the disease state may vary, a negative *C. difficile* test result alone may not rule out the possibility of *C. difficile*–associated colitis. Monitor signs and symptoms of the disease such as the duration and severity of diarrhea. These observations, along with the duration of antibiotic treatment and the presence of colitis or pseudomembranes, are all factors the physician must consider when diagnosing AAPMC disease.

The physician treats a mild case of antibiotic-related *C. difficile*–associated diarrhea by simply discontinuing the antibiotic and providing fluid and electrolyte replacement. In more severe cases the physician discontinues the antibiotic and starts antimicrobial therapy; the drug of choice is metronidazole or, if that is ineffective, vancomycin (Vancocin).

Clinical Manifestations

Diarrhea is the most common manifestation of an intestinal infection. The fecal output has increased water content, and if the intestinal mucosa is directly invaded, the feces may contain blood and mucus.

Assessment

Collection of **subjective data** includes noting complaints of diarrhea, rectal urgency, **tenesmus** (ineffective and painful straining with defecation), nausea, and abdominal cramping.

Objective data include a fever greater than 102° F (38.8° C) and vomiting. History taking provides useful information regarding number and consistency of bowel movements, recent use of antibiotics, recent travel, food intake, and exposure to noninfectious causes of diarrhea. Noninfectious diarrhea may be caused by heavy metal poisoning, shellfish allergy, and ingestion of toxins from mushrooms or fish. Diarrhea from noninfectious causes is usually characterized by a short incubation period (minutes to hours after exposure).

Diagnostic Tests

The key laboratory test for patients with intestinal infections is a stool culture. Stools are examined for blood, mucus, and WBCs. A blood chemistry study to monitor changes in the patient's fluid and electrolyte status may be included.

Medical Management

Usually the treatment of intestinal infections is conservative, letting the body limit the infection. Antibiotics are rarely used to treat acute diarrhea, but may be given in cases of prolonged or severe diarrhea with a stool positive for leukocytes. If fluid and electrolyte replacement is necessary to offset the losses from diarrhea, the oral route is usually sufficient. The IV route is indicated if the patient cannot take sufficient fluids orally.

The use of antidiarrheals and antispasmodic agents may actually increase the severity of the infection by prolonging the contact time of the infectious organism with the intestinal wall. Kaolin and pectin (Kaopectate) may be used to increase stool consistency. Bismuth subsalicylate (Pepto-Bismol) can effectively decrease intestinal secretions and decrease the diarrhea volume. These medications require large doses to be effective (30 to 60 mL every 30 minutes to 1 hour), and their use remains controversial.

Nursing Interventions and Patient Teaching

Do a thorough assessment to determine the seriousness of the intestinal infection. Determining the onset of the disease and the number of people exposed is important, since the majority of GI infections are communicable and represent a community health problem. Also assess for fluid imbalance, including measurement of postural changes in blood pressure, skin turgor, mucous membrane hydration, and urinary output.

Nursing diagnoses and interventions for the patient with intestinal infections include but are not limited to the following:

Nursing Diagnoses	Nursing Interventions
Deficient fluid volume, related to excessive losses from diarrhea and vomiting	If oral intake is tolerated, offer apple juice, clear carbonated beverages, clear broth, plain gelatin, and water. If IV feedings are required to maintain intravascular volume, these fluids should have electrolytes added. Maintain accurate I&O.
Imbalanced nutrition: less than body requirements, related to: • decreased intake • decreased absorption	Monitor for decreasing episodes of diarrhea. Monitor blood pressure, tissue turgor, mucous membranes, and urinary output. Monitor weight loss if symptoms are severe.

Instruct the patient to report the number, color, and consistency of bowel movements; abdominal cramping; and pain. Ensure that the patient and family understand the importance of hand hygiene after bowel movements to interrupt the fecal-oral route of transmission. Inform family members responsible for food preparation about the importance of proper methods of food preparation and storage to reduce the growth of infecting organisms.

Prognosis

Intestinal Infections

The body may be able to successfully defend against the infection without intervention. In severe cases, medications and fluid replacement assist the body, and the cure rate is good.

Antibiotic-Associated Pseudomembranous Colitis

The prognosis of AAPMC is better when the disease is diagnosed early and the antibiotics are changed. This allows the normal growth of bacteria in the intestine to resume.

IRRITABLE BOWEL SYNDROME

Etiology and Pathophysiology

Irritable bowel syndrome (IBS) is a disorder with episodes of altered bowel function and intermittent and recurrent abdominal pain. The American Gastroenterological Association (2009) defines IBS as a combination of chronic and recurrent GI symptoms—mainly intestinal pain and disturbed defecation or abdominal distention—that are not explained by structural or biochemical abnormalities; it is a dysfunction of the intestinal muscles (www.gastro.org/wmspage). The syndrome is now thought to result from hypersensitivity of the bowel wall, which leads to disruption of the normal functioning of the intestinal muscles.

IBS is common, occurring in about 10% to 15% of Western populations. A small number of these people (5%) have severe symptoms that are difficult to manage. The cause of IBS may be a low pain threshold to intestinal distention caused by abnormal intestinal sensory neural circuitry.

The patient with IBS may have associated psychological problems. In patients without psychological problems, the symptoms are attributed to spastic and uncoordinated muscle contractions of the colon, usually related to ingestion of excessively coarse or highly seasoned foods. However, there is also (1) a correlation of panic attacks in patients with IBS, and (2) an association of chronic low abdominal (pelvic) pain and a history of childhood sexual abuse.

Clinical Manifestations

Alterations of bowel function include abdominal pain relieved after a bowel movement; more frequent bowel movements with pain onset; a sense of incomplete evacuation; flatulence; and constipation, diarrhea, or both. Stress increases functional diarrhea; usually weight loss does not occur. The physical examination is generally normal, and nocturnal symptoms are rarely present. The symptoms of IBS are deceptive and are frustrating to manage.

Assessment

Subjective data include complaints of abdominal distress, pain at onset of bowel movements, abdominal pain relieved by defecation, and feelings of incomplete emptying after defecation.

Objective data include mucus in stools, visible abdominal distention, and frequent or unformed stools.

Diagnostic Tests

The key to accurate diagnosis of IBS is a thorough history and physical examination. Emphasize symptoms, health history (including psychosocial aspects such as physical or sexual abuse), family history, and drug and dietary history.

Diagnosis of IBS occurs by exclusion. Patients who see the physician with symptoms of intermittent or chronic abdominal pain and altered bowel motility are screened for pathologic conditions such as Crohn's disease, ulcerative colitis, colorectal cancer, diverticulitis, and infections such as salmonella. When no pathologic or structural abnormality is detected, IBS is a probable diagnosis. Symptom-based criteria for IBS have been standardized and are referred to as the **Rome criteria.** Rome II criteria include abdominal discomfort or pain that lasts at least 12 weeks (not necessarily consecutive) within 12 months and that has at least two of the following characteristics: (1) relieved with defecation, (2) onset associated with a change in stool frequency, and (3) onset associated with a change in stool appearance (Lewis et al., 2007).

Medical Management

Diet and Bulking Agents

Increasing dietary fiber increases stool bulk, frequency of passage, and bloating. Adequate fiber is more reliably provided with bulking agents (e.g., Metamucil) than with diet unless the patient is a strict vegetarian. The bulking agents seem to be most effective in treating constipation-predominant IBS, although they may alleviate mild diarrhea. If the patient's symptoms are consistently exacerbated after certain foods, those should be avoided. Advise the patient whose primary symptoms are abdominal distention and increased flatulence to eliminate common gas-producing foods (e.g., broccoli, cabbage) from the diet and to substitute yogurt for milk products to help determine whether he or she is lactose intolerant.

Medication

Anticholinergic drugs relieve abdominal cramps. Milk of magnesia may be prescribed if constipation does not respond to augmented fiber or if the patient cannot tolerate it. Mineral oil, in sufficient doses, is cheaper, "gasless," and generally effective. Opioids can be effective in diarrhea-predominant IBS. Antianxiety drugs may help patients suffering from panic attacks associated with IBS. Antidepressants may be used sparingly for diarrhea-predominant IBS in patients with severe pain who have not responded to other measures. New drug therapies are in development. Drugs that affect serotonin receptors hold promise in the treatment of IBS. Two serotonergic agents have been approved in select patients with IBS: tegaserod (Zelnorm), and alosteron (Lotronex). Because of its serious side effects (e.g., severe constipation, ischemic colitis), alosteron is available only in a restricted access program for women who have not responded to other therapies and in whom other anatomical and chemical abnormalities have been ruled out (Lewis et al., 2007).

Patients with IBS often report higher levels of psychological distress, including anxiety, panic, and depression, which can amplify symptoms and affect treatment response. Psychological nonpharmacologic treatment may include counseling and cognitive-behavioral interventions such as hypnotherapy and progressive muscle relaxation techniques to reduce stress. A significant proportion of patients with IBS had fewer or less severe symptoms after stress-reduction treatment.

Some patients have reported benefits from the use of complementary therapies such as acupuncture, Chinese herbal therapy, chiropractic techniques, and hatha yoga; patients with IBS are significantly more likely (11%) to use alternative remedies such as herbs than are patients with Crohn's disease (4%) (see Complementary & Alternative Therapies box). Although some studies have examined the use of such therapies in the treatment of IBS, clinical trial data are inadequate to determine their efficacy or to recommend any one as the sole therapy in the treatment of the syndrome.

Nursing Interventions and Patient Teaching

Most patients with IBS learn to cope with their symptoms enough to live in reasonable comfort. It is the nurse's role to assist in identifying the 5% of patients with IBS who need management. The nurse's skill in history taking, listening, nutrition planning, and understanding psychological effects on the body can assist the patient in setting goals to manage the disease. Emphasize the importance of keeping a daily log showing diet; number and type of stools; presence, severity, and duration of pain; side effects of medication; and life stressors that aggravate the disorder. This information assists in the diagnosis and treatment of IBS.

Nursing diagnoses and interventions for the patient with an irritable bowel include but are not limited to the following:

Nursing Diagnoses	Nursing Interventions
Pain, related to diet consumed and bowel evacuation	Have patient log the type of food consumed in terms of fiber content, consistency of stool, degree of pain.

Complementary & Alternative Therapies

Irritable Bowel Syndrome

- Traditional Chinese medicine has long been used to treat a variety of gastrointestinal (GI) complaints. Herbal formulas are chosen according to the specifics of the diagnostic patterns of traditional Chinese medicine. Most of the literature about such usage appears in either Chinese or Japanese journals or in textbooks of Chinese medicine, some of which are now available in English translations.*
- Peppermint oil, an herbal extract, has been studied for its use in irritable bowel syndrome. It resulted in significant improvements in symptoms, but the researchers cautioned that study design flaws make a fully positive conclusion difficult.
- Another promising area of research is biofeedback. Also called "psychophysiologic self-regulation," biofeedback is a relaxation training method that gives individuals a greater degree of awareness and control of physiologic function. Computer-based biofeedback equipment gives immediate feedback to the patient on changes in certain parameters, such as muscle electrical activity and skin temperature.
- Similar interventions have used various psychotherapy, stress management, and relaxation exercises, often in combination.
- Herbs that can cause GI upset include milk thistle *(Silybum marianum)*, goldenseal *(Hydrastis canadensis)*, ginger *(Zingiber officinale)*, kelp *(Fucus vesiculosus)*, comfrey *(Symphytum officinale)*, chaparral *(Larrea divaricata)*, cayenne (capsicum), and alfalfa *(Medicago sativa)*.
- Some people find relief from nausea and vomiting through acupuncture or acupressure.
- Some people have found that chiropractic adjustment has improved blood flow to digestive organs and improved digestion.
- Anise has been used to decrease bloating and flatulence and as an antispasmodic. *(Do not confuse with Chinese star anise.)*
- Comfrey is used to treat gastritis.
- Fennel is used to treat mild, spastic disorders of the GI tract, feelings of fullness, and flatulence.
- Queen Anne's lace seeds are used for flatulence, colic, singultus, and dysentery.

Modified from Black, J.M., & Hawks, H.J. (2009). *Medical-surgical nursing: clinical management for positive outcomes.* (8th ed.). Philadelphia: Saunders.
*From Bensoussan, A., Talley N.J., Hing, M. (1998). Treatment of irritable bowel syndrome with Chinese herbal medicine: a randomized controlled trial, *Journal of the American Medical Association, 280*(18):1585.

Nursing Diagnoses	Nursing Interventions
Deficient knowledge, related to the effect of fiber content on spastic bowel	Educate patient regarding the relationship of fiber to both constipation and diarrhea. Teach patient about the use of bulking agents.

IBS involves many personal feelings that the patient must recognize and be comfortable with before a care plan can be established. Therefore it is important to establish a strong relationship with the patient before patient teaching begins. Patient teaching includes diet management and ways to control anxiety in daily living. The goal of patient teaching is to empower the patient to control the disorder. Provide community resources for counseling if psychological problems seem related to increased or decreased elimination accompanied by pain and discomfort.

Prognosis

Approximately 95% of these patients are successfully managed. Compliance with a diet low in residue and a nonstressful daily regimen contributes significantly to a good prognosis.

INFLAMMATORY BOWEL DISEASE

Ulcerative colitis and Crohn's disease are chronic, episodic, inflammatory bowel diseases. These are immunologically related disorders that afflict young adults just beginning their education, careers, and families. These diseases appear more often in women, in the Jewish population, and in the nonwhite population; there seems to be a familial tendency.

The causes of ulcerative colitis and Crohn's disease are unknown. Theories involve both genetic and environmental factors, including bacterial infection, immunologic factors, and psychosomatic disorders. The fact that people with ulcerative colitis commonly have a relative with Crohn's disease and vice versa supports the existence of the common gene. Inflammatory bowel diseases are characterized by **exacerbations** (increases in severity of the disease or any of its symptoms) and **remissions** (decreases in severity of the disease or any of its symptoms).

The two diseases require similar nursing interventions but different surgical interventions and medical treatment. Certain criteria are used to differentiate ulcerative colitis from Crohn's disease (Table 45-3), but the diseases have much in common and cannot be differentiated in about one third of the cases. Patients have been known to have features of both diseases, making a definite diagnosis difficult.

ULCERATIVE COLITIS

Etiology and Pathophysiology

The incidence of ulcerative colitis is twice that of Crohn's disease. Psychosomatic factors may cause, aggravate, or be a result of inflammatory bowel disease. The social isolation and frustration that accompany this chronic illness cause difficulties in effectively coping with daily life.

Ulcerative colitis is confined to the mucosa and submucosa of the colon. The disease can affect segments

Table 45-3 Comparison of Ulcerative Colitis and Crohn's Disease

FACTOR	ULCERATIVE COLITIS	CROHN'S DISEASE
Cause of disorder	Unknown; autoimmune; genetic and environment play a role; various bacteria have been proposed	Unknown; possible cause is an altered immune state; autoimmune; various bacteria have been proposed Genetic and environmental factors play a role
Usual age at onset	Teenage years and early adulthood; second peak in sixth decade	Early adolescence; second peak in sixth decade
Area of involvement	Confined to mucosa or submucosa of the colon	Can occur anywhere along the gastrointestinal tract from the mouth to the anus Most common site is terminal ileum
Area of inflammation	Mucosa and submucosa	Transmural (pertaining to the entire thickness of the wall of an organ)
Characteristics of inflammation	Tends to be continuous, starting at the rectum and extending proximally; limited to the mucosal lining	May be continuous or interspersed between areas of normal tissue; may extend through all layers of the bowel
Character of stools	Blood present No fat 15-20 liquid stools daily	No blood present Steatorrhea (fat in stool) 3-4 semisoft stools daily
Major complication	Toxic megacolon, fistulas, and abscesses (rare)	Malabsorption, bowel obstruction, fistulas, tissue abscesses
Major complaints	Rectal bleeding, abdominal cramping	Right lower abdominal pain with mass present
Reason for surgery	Poor response to medical therapy	Complications
Response to surgery	Removal of the colon cures the intestinal disease, but not extraintestinal symptoms, such as inflammation of joints and liver disease	Indicated to remove diseased areas that do not respond to aggressive medical therapy. Surgery does not cure the disease
Cancer potential	Increased risk after 10 years of disease	Small intestine incidence increased; colon incidence increased, but not as much as in ulcerative colitis
Biopsy findings	Architectural changes consistent with chronic inflammation	Architectural changes consistent with chronic inflammation; may show granulomas
Weight loss	Rare	Cobblestoning of mucosa is common; may be severe
Malabsorption and nutritional deficiencies	Minimal incidence	Common; may be severe; frequent

of the entire colon, depending on the staging (phases or periods in the course of the disease). This disease usually starts in the rectum and moves in a continuous pattern toward the cecum. Although sometimes mild inflammation of the terminal ileum occurs, ulcerative colitis is a disease of the colon and rectum. The inflammation and ulcerations occur in the mucosal layer of the bowel wall. Since it does not extend through all bowel wall layers, fistulas and abscesses are rare. Capillaries become friable and bleed, causing the characteristic diarrhea containing pus and blood. Pseudopolyps are common in chronic ulcerative disease and may become cancerous. With healing and the natural formation of scar tissue, the colon may lose elasticity and absorptive capability.

Clinical Manifestations

Pathologic findings differ, but about 90% of patients with ulcerative colitis have mild to moderately severe disease. Patients with severe ulcerative colitis may have as many as 15 to 20 liquid stools per day, containing blood, mucus, and pus. With severe diarrhea, losses of sodium, potassium, bicarbonate, and calcium ions may occur. Abdominal cramps may occur before the bowel movement. The urge to defecate lessens as scarring within the bowel progresses. This results in involuntary leakage of stool. In mild to moderate ulcerative colitis, diarrhea may consist of two to five stools per day with some blood present.

Complications of ulcerative colitis include toxic megacolon (toxic dilation of the large bowel). This life-threatening complication occurs in less than 5% of patients. The bowel becomes distended and so thin that it could be perforated at any time. Clinical manifestations of toxic megacolon include a temperature of 104° F (40° C) or more and abdominal distention. Among patients who have had chronic ulcerative colitis for 10 to 15 years, 40% to 50% develop carcinoma of the colon with total colonic involvement. Surgical interventions for treatment of this complication are usually necessary.

Assessment

Subjective data include complaints of rectal bleeding and abdominal cramping. Lethargy, a sense of frustration, and loss of control result from painful abdominal cramping and unpredictable bowel movements.

Objective data include weight loss, abdominal distention, fever, tachycardia, leukocytosis, and observation of frequency and characteristics of stools.

Diagnostic Tests

Double-contrast barium enema studies of the intestine, sigmoidoscopy and colonoscopy with biopsy, and stool testing for melena aid the physician in diagnosis. Additional studies include radiologic examination of the abdomen, serum electrolytes and albumin levels, liver function studies, and other hematologic studies.

Medical Management

The medical interventions chosen depend on the phase of the disease and the individual response to therapy. Common treatment modalities include medication, diet intervention, and stress reduction.

Drug Therapy

The four major categories of drugs used are (1) those that affect the inflammatory response, (2) antibacterial drugs, (3) drugs that affect the immune system, and (4) antidiarrheal preparations.

Sulfasalazine (Azulfidine) is the drug of choice for mild chronic ulcerative colitis. Sulfasalazine is broken down by bacteria in the colon into sulfapyridine and 5-aminosalicylic acid (5-ASA). It affects the inflammatory response and provides some antibacterial activity. It is effective in maintaining clinical remission and in treating mild to moderately severe attacks. Newer proportions have been developed to deliver 5-ASA to the terminal ileum and colon (e.g., olsalazine [Dipentum], mesalamine [Pentasa], and balsalazide [Colazal]). These drugs are as effective as sulfasalazine and are better tolerated when administered orally.

Nonsulfa drugs include mesalamine (Rowasa), given by retention enema.

Corticosteroids are antiinflammatory drugs effective in relieving symptoms of moderate and severe colitis; they can be given orally or intravenously if inflammation is severe.

Antidiarrheal agents are recommended over anticholinergic agents because anticholinergic drugs can mask obstruction or contribute to toxic colonic dilation. Loperamide may be used to treat cramping and diarrhea of chronic ulcerative colitis. Azathioprine (Imuran) is also beneficial.

Nutrition Therapy

Diet is an important component in the treatment of inflammatory bowel disease, and a dietitian should be consulted. The goals of diet management are to provide adequate nutrition without making symptoms worse, to correct and prevent malnutrition, to replace fluid and electrolyte losses, and to prevent weight loss. Patients with inflammatory bowel disease must eat a balanced, healthy diet with sufficient calories, protein, and nutrients. Patients can use MyPyramid guidelines to ensure that they get adequate portions from all of the food groups. The diet for each patient is individualized.

Patients with diarrhea often decrease their oral intake to reduce the diarrhea. The anorexia that accompanies inflammation also results in decreases in food intake. Blood loss leads to iron deficiency anemia.

Patients receiving sulfasalazine should receive 1 mg of folate (folic acid) daily, and those receiving corticosteroids need calcium supplements.

Inflammatory bowel disease has no universal food triggers, but patients may find that certain foods initiate diarrhea. A food diary helps them identify problem foods to avoid. Many patients are lactose intolerant and improve when they avoid milk products. High-fat foods also tend to trigger diarrhea. Cold foods and high-fiber foods (cereal with bran, nuts, raw fruit) may increase GI transit. Smoking stimulates the GI tract (increases motility and secretion) and should be avoided. Patients with significant fluid and electrolyte losses or malabsorption may need parenteral nutrition or enteral feedings, such as elemental diets. Elemental diets are high in calories and nutrients, lactose free, and absorbed in the proximal small intestine, which allows the more distal bowel to rest.

Stress Control

Ulcerative colitis is aggravated by stress. Identifying the factors that cause stress is the first step in controlling the disease. Working with the patient to find healthful coping mechanisms is part of the holistic approach in nursing interventions.

Surgical Intervention

If an acute episode does not respond to treatment, if complications occur, or if the risk of cancer becomes greater because of chronic ulcerative colitis, surgical intervention is indicated (Box 45-4). Approximately 25% to 40% of patients with ulcerative colitis need surgery at some time during their illness. Most surgeons prefer a conservative approach, removing only the diseased portion of the colon. The operations of choice may be a single-stage total procto-

Box 45-4 Surgical Interventions for Ulcerative Colitis

- **Colon resection:** Removal of a portion of the large intestine and anastomosis of the remaining segment
- **Ileostomy:** Surgical formation of an opening of the ileum onto the surface of the abdomen, through which fecal matter is emptied
- **Ileoanal anastomosis:** Removal of the colon and rectum but leaving the anus intact, along with the anal sphincter; anastomosis formed between the lower end of the small intestine and the anus
- **Proctocolectomy:** Removal of anus, rectum, and colon; ileostomy established for the removal of digestive tract wastes
- **Kock pouch (Kock continent ileostomy):** Surgical removal of the rectum and colon (proctocolectomy) with formation of a reservoir by suturing loops of adjacent ileum together to form a pouchlike structure, nipple valve, and stoma

colectomy with construction of an internal reservoir and valve (Kock pouch, or Kock continent ileostomy) (Figure 45-9); total proctocolectomy with ileoanal anastomosis with or without construction of an internal reservoir; and temporary ileostomy. In the case of a poor-risk patient, a subtotal colectomy may be performed with ileostomy (Figure 45-10). After the patient's recovery (approximately 2 to 4 months), removal of the rectum or construction of an internal reservoir can be done.

Today some patients view a permanent ileostomy as worse than the disease itself. Surgical procedures do have some risk, and the patient may want to live with the disease and long-term risk of cancer rather than undergo the procedure.

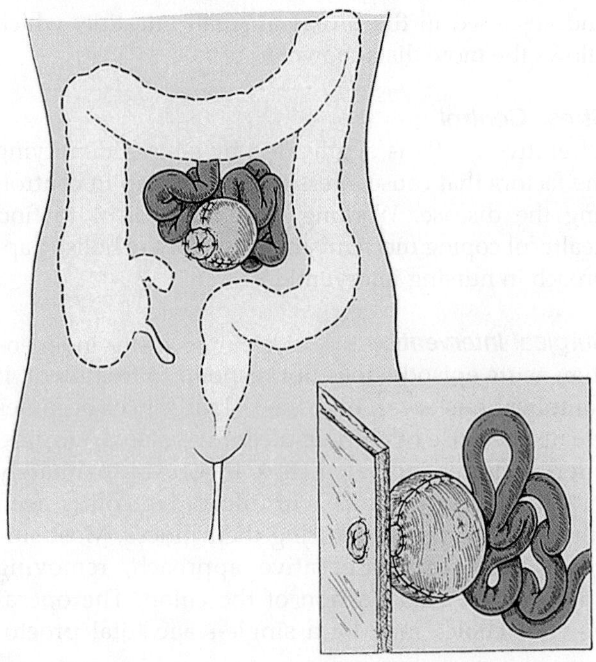

FIGURE 45-9 Kock pouch (Kock continent ileostomy).

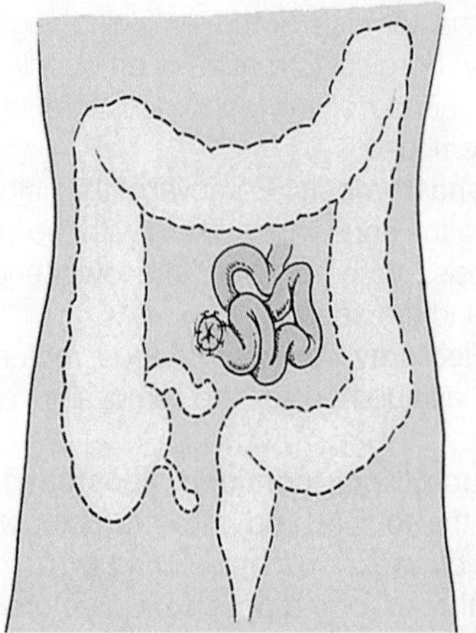

FIGURE 45-10 Ileostomy with absence of resected bowel.

Nursing Interventions

Nursing interventions include a thorough assessment of the patient's bowel elimination, support systems, coping abilities, nutritional status, pain, and understanding of the disease process and treatment required. Patients need a complete understanding of the care plan so they can make informed choices. Prevention of future episodes is a goal for the ulcerative colitis patient.

Preoperative care for these patients includes (1) selecting a stoma site, (2) performing additional diagnostic tests if cancer is suspected, (3) helping the patient accept that previous treatments were unsuccessful in curing the disease, and (4) preparing the bowel for surgery. The bowel is prepared 2 or 3 days preoperatively. A bland to clear liquid diet is ordered, along with a bowel prep of laxatives, GoLYTELY (an oral or NG colonic lavage–electrolyte solution), and enemas (see Box 45-2). Antibiotics, such an erythromycin and neomycin, are given to decrease the number of bacteria in the bowel.

Postoperative nursing interventions depend on the type of procedure performed and the individual's response. Areas of concern are bowel and urinary elimination; fluid and electrolyte balance; tissue perfusion; comfort and pain; nutrition; gas exchange; infection; and, in the case of ostomy construction, assessment of the ileostomy and peristomal skin integrity.

Nursing diagnoses and interventions for the patient with chronic inflammatory bowel disease include but are not limited to the following:

Nursing Diagnoses	Nursing Interventions
Imbalanced nutrition: less than body requirements, related to: • bowel hypermotility • decreased absorption	Provide small frequent meals, which will help patient with poor appetite or intolerance to consume larger amounts. Eliminate foods that aggravate condition.
Powerlessness, related to loss of control of body function	Assist weakened patient with activities of daily living (bathing, oral hygiene, shaving, and other grooming needs). Offer choices to patient, when possible, to provide a sense of control.

Nursing diagnoses for the surgical patient include *risk for ineffective coping, situational low self-esteem*, and *disturbed body image*. Nursing interventions include reinforcing the physician's explanation of the surgical procedure and expected outcomes. Providing reading material and demonstrating the care of an ostomy pouch when the patient seems ready will reduce anxiety. A visitor from the United Ostomy Association can provide hope, as a recovered and productive role model. But do not expect immediate patient accep-

Box 45-5 Postoperative Nursing Interventions for Ulcerative Colitis

1. Monitor nasogastric (NG) suction for patency until bowel function is resumed. Maintain correct wall suctioning. Accurately record color and amount of output. Irrigate NG tube as needed. Apply water-soluble lubricant to nares. Assess bowel sounds, being certain to turn off NG suction during auscultation.
2. Initiate ostomy care and teaching when bowel activity begins. Be sensitive to patient's pain level and readiness for teaching of ostomy care.
3. Observe **stoma** (an artificial opening of an internal organ on the body's surface) for color and size (should be erythematous and slightly edematous). Document assessment (e.g., "stoma pink and viable").
4. Select appropriate pouching system that has skin-protective barrier, accordion flange to ease pressure applied to new incisional site, adhesive backing, and pouch opening no more than 1⁄16 inch larger than the stoma. Stomas change in size over time and should be measured before new supplies are ordered.
5. Empty pouch when it is approximately one third full to prevent breaking the seal, resulting in pouch leakage.
6. Explain that initial dark green liquid will change to yellow-brown as patient is allowed to eat.
7. Teach patient to care for the stoma; this includes having patient look at stoma and gradually assist with emptying, cleaning, and changing pouch. Teach patient that normal grieving occurs after loss of rectal function. Be supportive of patient's concerns.
8. Promote independence and self-care to decrease state of denial.
9. Instruct on follow-up home care, including changing skin barrier (a piece of pectin-based or Karaya wafer with measurable thickness and hydrocolloid adhesive properties) every 5 to 7 days. Using antacids, skin protective paste, and liquid skin barrier may be appropriate if skin excoriation is observed.
10. Patient may shower or bathe with or without pouch on.
11. Patient should avoid lifting objects heavier than 10 pounds until physician says it is allowed.
12. A special diet is not necessary, but patients should drink 8 to 10 glasses of water a day, chew food well, and limit or avoid certain gas-forming foods.
13. Sexual relationships can be resumed when physician feels it is not harmful to the surgical area. Counseling may be appropriate if patient has fear of resuming this activity.

tance of the stoma; acceptance will be gradual. Be supportive and encourage the patient to share fears. Box 45-5 lists postoperative nursing interventions.

Peristomal Area Integrity

Assess the peristomal skin for impaired integrity. Four primary factors contributing to loss of peristomal skin integrity are allergies, mechanical trauma, chemical reactions, and infection.

Allergies to pouches, adhesives, skin barriers, powders and paste, or belts are evident at areas of contact. The skin may appear erythematous, eroded, weeping, and bleeding. Changing the type of pouch, tape, or adhesive may resolve the problem.

Mechanical trauma caused by pressure, friction, or stripping of adhesives and skin barriers can be avoided by changing the pouch less frequently, using adhesive tape sparingly, and wearing a belt only when the patient feels it is necessary. The skin must be protected when the pouch is removed.

The most common chemical irritant is the stool from the stoma. Protect the skin from these digestive enzymes by using skin barriers before applying the pouch. Skin barriers include adhesives (Stomahesive), powders (Stomahesive power), liquid skin barriers (Skin Prep), and caulking paste (Stomahesive paste).

A common cause of infection of the peristomal skin is *Candida albicans*. People who have been taking antibiotics for 5 or more days may be prone to this problem. Treatment is application of nystatin powder or cream, by physician order. Apply a skin barrier over the medicated area to ensure the adhesive sticks.

Patient Teaching

Teach the patient or significant other the appropriate care of the ileostomy or colostomy to foster independence. This includes pouch change, cleansing, irrigation, and skin care. Provide a list of foods that are known to commonly cause constipation, diarrhea, blockage, odors, and flatus. Also, before discharge, give the patient a list of resource people, phone numbers, supplies, and where to obtain them.

Prognosis

The prognosis for patients with chronic ulcerative colitis is directly related to the number of years they have had the disease. The incidence of carcinoma increases when the colon is extensively involved over time. The disease carries a higher mortality rate in patients who have the disease 15 to 20 years.

CROHN'S DISEASE

Etiology and Pathophysiology

Crohn's disease, although not as prevalent as ulcerative colitis, is increasing in incidence. Crohn's disease is characterized by inflammation of segments of the GI tract. It was once thought to be a disease specific to the small intestine and was called regional enteritis. The cause of the disease is not known, but there seems to be a strong association between Crohn's disease and altered immune mechanisms. Both genetic and environmental factors seem to play a role. It commonly occurs during adolescence and early adulthood with a second peak in the sixth decade (Lewis et al., 2007). Crohn's disease can occur anywhere in the GI tract from the mouth to the anus, but occurs most commonly in the terminal ileum and colon. The inflammation involves all layers of the bowel wall. It may involve only one segment of the bowel, or segments of diseased tissue may alternate with healthy tissue. In the early stages of the disease, tiny ulcers form on various parts of the intestinal wall. Over time, horizontal rows of these ulcers fuse with vertical rows, giving the mucosa a cobblestone appearance. Inflammation, fibrosis, and scarring often involving the entire thickness of the intestine are characteristics of Crohn's disease. Patients with Crohn's disease are likely to have a bowel obstruction, fistulas, fissures, and abscesses. In some patients the disease may involve the colon without any changes in the small intestine.

Malabsorption is the major problem when the small intestine is involved, and this contributes to nutritional problems. Megaloblastic (pernicious) anemia results from decreased absorption of vitamin B_{12} in the small intestine. Fluid and electrolyte disturbances with acid-base imbalances can occur, particularly with depletion of sodium or potassium associated with diarrhea or with excessive small intestine drainage through fistulas associated with the pathologic process.

Clinical Manifestations

The manifestations depend largely on the anatomical site of involvement, extent of the disease process, and presence of complications. The onset of Crohn's disease is usually insidious, with nonspecific complaints such as diarrhea, fatigue, abdominal pain, weight loss, and fever. As the disease progresses, the patient experiences weight loss, malnutrition, dehydration, electrolyte imbalance, anemia, and increased peristalsis.

Assessment

Collection of **subjective data** for the patient with Crohn's disease includes noting the patient's list of vague complaints, including weakness, loss of appetite, abdominal pain and cramps, intermittent low-grade fever, sleeplessness caused by diarrhea, and stress. Right-lower-quadrant abdominal pain is characteristic of the disease and may be accompanied by a tender mass of thickened intestines in the same area.

Objective data include complaints of diarrhea—three or four semisolid stools daily, containing mucus and pus but no blood. **Steatorrhea** (excess fat in the feces) may also be present if the ulceration extends high in the small intestine. With small intestine involvement, weight loss occurs from malabsorption. Scar tissue from the inflammation narrows the lumen of the intestine and may cause strictures and obstruction, a frequent complication. Intestinal fistulas are a cardinal feature and may develop between segments of bowel. Cutaneous fistulas, common in the perianal area, and rectovaginal fistulas may occur. Fistulas communicating with the urinary tract may cause urinary tract infections. Poor absorption of bile salts by the ileum may lead to watery stools. Fever and unexplained anemia may also occur.

Diagnostic Tests

A small bowel barium enema is preferred over an upper GI roentgenographic series; small bowel follow-through detects defining mucosal abnormalities such as cobblestoning of the mucosa, fistulas, and strictures of the ileum. The most definitive test to differentiate Crohn's disease from ulcerative colitis is colonoscopy with multiple biopsies of the colon and terminal ileum. The appearance of the mucosa in Crohn's disease can range from normal to severely inflamed, and areas of inflammation may be continuous or interspersed with areas that appear normal. Granulomas in the biopsy specimen confirm the diagnosis of Crohn's disease, but their absence does not rule it out. In contrast, biopsies from a patient with ulcerative colitis show chronic inflammatory changes with no granulomas. Blood tests for anemia may also be ordered. Since an endoscope can enter little of the small intestine, it has not been possible to get a direct view of the ileal inflammation of Crohn's disease. Capsule endoscopy (see Figure 45-6) is used in the diagnosis of small intestine diseases. Thus far, it has been shown to have greater sensitivity than radiography when diagnosing Crohn's disease (Lewis et al., 2007).

Medical Management

Treatment is individualized depending on the patient's age, the location and severity of the disease, and any complications present. Once Crohn's disease has been diagnosed, the patient is started on drug therapy to try to get the disease in remission. Those with mild to moderate disease usually take antiinflammatory agents such as sulfasalazine, mesalamine, olsalazine, or balsalazide. When inflammation is severe, corticosteroids such as prednisone may be prescribed. Patients are weaned off steroids as soon as possible to prevent dependency and long-term complications. Multivitamins and B_{12} injections are often recommended to correct deficiencies.

If first-line therapy fails, treatment with more toxic, second-line drugs becomes necessary. These include immunosuppressive agents such as azathioprine; cyclosporine (Neoral, Sandimmune); methotrexate, or MTX (Folex, Mexate, Rheumatrex); and IV immunoglobin. The FDA approved the use of infliximab (Remicade) for Crohn's disease. It is a monoclonal antibody drug given as a single IV infusion except to those with fistulizing disease, in which case the patient needs two additional infusions. Infliximab works by neutralizing tumor necrosis factor, a protein that causes much of the intestinal inflammation. Infliximab is the only medication specifically indicated for the treatment of Crohn's disease.

Diet intervention, stress reduction, and surgery are also used to manage Crohn's disease.

Diet

Minimize bowel symptoms and diarrhea by excluding from the diet (1) lactose-containing foods in patients suspected of having lactose intolerance; (2) brassica vegetables (cauliflower, broccoli, asparagus, cabbage, and brussels sprouts); (3) caffeine, beer, monosodium glutamate, and sugarless (sorbitol-containing) gum and mints; and (4) highly seasoned foods, concentrated fruit juices, carbonated beverages, and fatty foods.

Diets high in protein (100 g/day) are recommended for patients with hypoproteinemia caused by mucosal loss, malabsorption, maldigestion, or malnutrition. Elemental diets have been shown to induce remission in 90% of patients. Free elemental diets may help patients with diarrhea because they require minimal digestion and reduce stool volume. Such elemental dietary preparations include Criticare, Travasorb HN, and Precision High Nitrogen. Total parenteral nutrition has been shown to be more effective in patients with Crohn's disease than in those with ulcerative colitis.

Medications

Corticosteroids are the preferred medical treatment of active Crohn's disease when the small intestine is involved. Sulfasalazine, olsalazine, mesalamine, and balsalazide are effective in active Crohn's disease, especially when there is colonic involvement. Antibiotics may be used, although no specific infectious agent has been discovered. Metronidazole, ciproflaxin (Cipro), and clarithromycin have been used successfully. Antidiarrheal agents (diphenoxylate with atropine and loperamide) and antispasmodics (Donnatal [atropine, hyoscyamine, phenobarbital, and scopolamine]; and dicyclomine [Bentyl]) have proven effective but are used with caution because of side effects. Biologic drug therapies include monoclonal antibodies to tumor necrosis factor–alpha (infliximab) and to a leukocyte adhesion molecule (natalizumab [Antegren]). Infliximab has been shown to reduce the degree of inflammation; however, not all patients with Crohn's disease respond to infliximab. Natalizumab, on the other hand, works by interrupting the movement of lymphocytes into the endothelial layer of the gut wall and thus decreasing the inflammatory process. Problems with inadequate vitamin B_{12} absorption result when the terminal ileum is resected; lifelong replacement of vitamin B_{12} is then necessary.

Complications of inflammation with fibrous scarring, obstruction, fistula formation in the small intestine, abscesses, and perforation are indications for surgical excision and anastomosis. Resection is the preferred surgery because bypass has a greater failure rate.

Surgical Treatment

About 75% of patients with Crohn's disease eventually require surgery. Although surgery produces remission, recurrence rates are high. Surgical removal of large segments of the small intestine can lead to short-bowel syndrome, a condition in which the absorption surface is inadequate to maintain life and parenteral nutrition is used. Surgery is reserved for emergency situations (excessive bleeding, obstruction, peritonitis) or when medical treatment has failed. The principal surgical technique for Crohn's disease is strictureplasty to widen areas of narrowed bowel. It is sometimes necessary to resect the diseased bowel and anastomose the ends. Unfortunately, the disease commonly recurs at the area of anastomosis. Emergency surgery is necessary when perforation allows bowel contents to drain into the abdominal cavity. In this situation, the purulent exudate is drained, the abdomen is washed out, and the patient has a temporary ostomy. An abscess that is walled off may be surgically drained (Lewis et al., 2007).

Nursing Interventions

In caring for the patient with Crohn's disease, consider nutrition, fluid balance, elimination, medications, psychological aspects, and sexuality. Total parenteral nutrition may be ordered in cases of severe disease and marked weight loss. Tube feedings that allow rapid absorption in the upper GI tract are begun, and then oral intake of a low-residue, high-protein, high-calorie diet is gradually introduced. Vitamin supplements are frequently necessary, and vitamin B_{12} is given when there is a marked loss of ileum. When anemia is present, iron dextran (DexFerrum) is given by Z-track injection because oral intake of iron is ineffective due to intestinal ulceration.

Oral diets of 2500 mL/day to replace fluids and electrolytes lost from diarrhea are not uncommon. Monitor weight for losses or gains. Monitor skin condition and all fluid I&O daily. A urinary output of at least 1500 mL/day is desired.

When a patient is hospitalized, a bedside commode or a bedpan must be accessible at all times because of the urgency and frequency of stools. Emptying the bedpan immediately and deodorizing the room maintain an aesthetic environment. The anal region may become excoriated from frequent stools. Examine the anal area regularly and keep it clean using medicated wipes (Tucks) and sitz baths. These nursing interventions promote comfort and hygiene for the patient.

Most patients with Crohn's disease require emotional support from nurses, physicians, aides, stomal therapists, and others. The onset of the disease (often at 10 to 15 years of age) often occurs before the person has the emotional development and maturity to cope. The support groups sponsored by the Crohn's and Colitis Foundation of America (formerly the National Foundation of Ileitis and Colitis) can play a major role in helping patients. Tranquilizers, antidepressants, and psychology or psychiatry services may be required when managing the disease. Current evidence suggests that Crohn's disease is not caused by psychological stress but that psychiatric disturbances are the result of the disease's symptoms and chronicity.

Nursing diagnoses and interventions for patients with Crohn's disease include but are not limited to the following:

Nursing Diagnoses	Nursing Interventions
Powerlessness, related to exacerbations and remissions	Explore with patient factors that aggravate the disease. Assist patient in listing factors that can be controlled: diet, stressors, medication compliance, self-monitoring of symptoms.
Imbalanced nutrition: less than body requirements, related to: • bowel hypermotility • decreased absorption	Emphasize the importance of weighing daily, following special diets, and assessing energy levels.

Nursing Interventions and Patient Teaching

The patient must understand how diarrhea and rapid emptying of the small intestine affects the body's nutritional needs. This will lead to acceptance of special diets and the ability to retain some personal control of the disease. The patient must also understand the relationship of emotional feelings to Crohn's disease. Identifying resources for emotional support in the family and community and among health professionals will promote coping skills and mental hygiene.

Prognosis

Crohn's disease is a chronic disorder; it has a high rate of recurrence, especially in patients under 25 years of age. The rate of recurrence after surgery is 50% for the first 5 years and 75% in 10 years. Prognosis depends on the extent of involvement, duration of illness, and success of medical interventions. No known therapy will maintain a patient with Crohn's disease in remission.

ACUTE ABDOMINAL INFLAMMATIONS

APPENDICITIS

Etiology and Pathophysiology

Appendicitis is the inflammation of the vermiform appendix, usually acute, which if undiagnosed leads rapidly to perforation and peritonitis. Appendicitis is most likely to occur in teenagers and young adults and is more common in men.

The vermiform appendix is a small tube in the right lower quadrant of the abdomen. The lumen of the proximal end is shared with that of the cecum, whereas the distal end is closed. The appendix fills and empties regularly in the same way as the cecum. However, the lumen is tiny and easily obstructed. The most common causes of appendicitis are obstruction of the lumen by a fecalith (accumulated feces), foreign bodies, and tumor of the cecum or appendix. If it becomes obstructed and inflamed, pathogenic bacteria *(E. coli)* begin to multiply in the appendix and cause an infection with the formation of pus. If distention and infection are severe enough, the appendix may rupture, releasing its contents into the abdomen. The infection may be contained within an appendiceal abscess or may spread to the abdominal cavity, causing generalized peritonitis.

Clinical Manifestations

Light palpation of the abdomen elicits rebound tenderness in the right lower quadrant. The abdomen musculature overlying the right lower quadrant may feel tense as a result of voluntary rigidity. The patient often lies on the back or side with knees flexed in an attempt to decrease muscular strain on the abdominal wall.

Assessment

Subjective data include the most common complaint of constant pain in the right lower quadrant of the abdomen around McBurney's point (halfway between the umbilicus and the crest of the right ileum). The pain may be accompanied by nausea and anorexia.

Objective data include vomiting, a low-grade fever (99° to 102° F [37.2° to 38.8° C]), an elevated WBC count, rebound tenderness, a rigid abdomen, and decreased or absent bowel sounds.

Diagnostic Tests

The physician orders a WBC count with differential. Approximately 90% of patients have a WBC level above 10,000/mm^3 (normal range is 5000 to 10,000/mm^3). Approximately 75% have a neutrophil count greater than 75% (normal range is 60% to 70%). An abdominal CT scan and abdominal ultrasound are excellent diagnostic tools. NeutroSpec imaging is a new technique to diagnose appendicitis. It uses an injection of technetium-labeled anti-CD15 monoclonal antibody that selectively binds to neutrophils at the infection site, labeling these cells with technetium. As a result, physicians can rapidly detect an infection using a gamma camera that records radioactivity. NeutroSpec's advantage over the current standard of care is in vivo labeling of WBCs and a diagnosis in less than 1 hour (Lewis et al., 2007).

Medical Management

Emergency surgical intervention is the treatment of choice for acute appendicitis, or surgery may be performed when a patient is having another abdominal surgical procedure. Because mortality correlates with perforation and peritonitis, and perforation correlates with duration of symptoms, early diagnosis and appendectomy are essential. Antibiotic therapy is given when perforation is likely. Complications include infection, intraabdominal abscess, and mechanical small bowel obstruction (see Safety Alert box).

Nursing Interventions and Patient Teaching

Nursing interventions include following general preoperative procedure. Explain diagnostic tests and possible surgical procedures to relieve anxiety. Maintain

Safety Alert!

Appendicitis

- Encourage the patient with abdominal pain to see a health care provider and to avoid self-treatment, particularly the use of laxatives and enemas.
- The increased peristalsis of laxatives and enemas may cause perforation of the appendix.
- Until the patient is seen by a health care provider, he or she should remain NPO to ensure the stomach is empty in case surgery is needed.
- An ice bag may be applied to the right lower quadrant to decrease the flow of blood to the area and impede the inflammatory process.
- *Heat is never used* because it could cause the appendix to rupture.
- Surgery is usually performed as soon as a diagnosis is made.

bed rest and NPO status, provide comfort measures for pain relief so that symptoms are not masked by medication, and replace fluids and electrolytes. Monitor the temperature, blood pressure, pulse, and respirations and document these every hour because of the threat of perforation with peritonitis.

Administer prescribed opioids after the physician has assessed the patient. Opioids can mask symptoms of acute appendicitis. In some cases an ice bag to relieve pain is given; no heat is applied because this increases circulation to the appendix and could lead to rupture. A cleansing enema is not ordered because of the danger of rupture. General postoperative care is performed.

Nursing diagnoses and interventions for the patient with appendicitis include but are not limited to the following:

Nursing Diagnoses	Nursing Interventions
Deficient fluid volume, related to vomiting	Monitor patient for signs of dehydration and fluid and electrolyte imbalance (poor skin turgor; flushed dry skin; coated tongue; oliguria; confusion; and abnormal sodium, potassium, and chloride levels).
Pain, related to inflammation	Support the patient and the family by listening and by explaining tests and procedures. Administer opioids as soon as indicated after the physician assesses the patient. Monitor for increases in pain, rebound tenderness, and abdominal rigidity. Take vital signs frequently (every 15 minutes).

Patient teaching may include the reason for IV fluids with gradual advancement of the diet from clear liquids to regular diet as peristalsis returns. If antibiotics or oral medications are continued postoperatively, make certain the patient understands the name, purpose, and side effects of each medication. If complications occur, necessitating an NG tube or drainage tubes, tell the patient the reason for these interventions.

Prognosis

The rate of cure through surgical intervention is high in patients with appendicitis. The patient's prognosis is altered if peritonitis complicates this diagnosis.

DIVERTICULOSIS AND DIVERTICULITIS

Etiology and Pathophysiology

Diverticular disease has two clinical forms: **diverticulosis** and **diverticulitis.** Diverticulosis is the presence of pouchlike herniations through the circular smooth muscle of the colon, particularly the sigmoid colon (Figure 45-11). Diverticulitis is the inflammation of one or more of the diverticular sacs.

The incidence of diverticulosis in people older than 50 years of age is increasing, possibly as a result of high luminal pressures from a deficiency of dietary fiber intake and an increase in refined carbohydrates combined with a loss of muscle mass and collagen with the aging process. Penetration of fecal matter through the thin-walled diverticula causes inflammation and abscess formation in the tissues surrounding the colon. With repeated inflammation, the lumen of the colon narrows and may become obstructed. When one or more diverticula become inflamed, diverticulitis results, which is a complication of diverticulosis. This inflammation can lead to perforation, abscess, peritonitis, obstruction, and hemorrhage. Diverticulitis is the most common cause of lower GI hemorrhage.

Clinical Manifestations

When diverticula perforate and diverticulitis develops, the patient complains of mild to severe pain in the left lower quadrant of the abdomen, has a fever, and has an elevated WBC count and sedimentation rate. If the condition goes untreated, septicemia and septic shock can develop. This patient is hypotensive and has

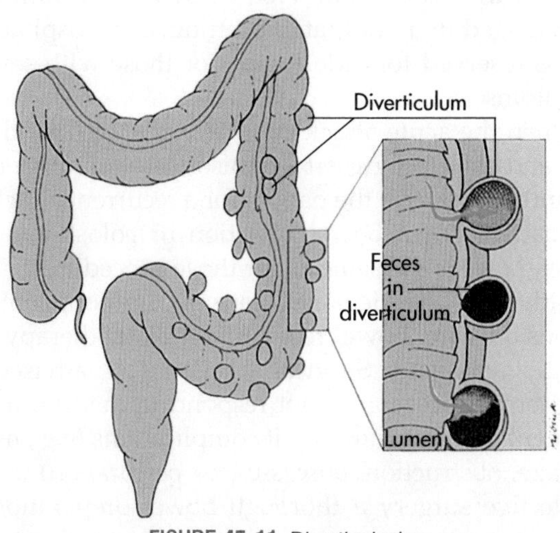

FIGURE 45-11 Diverticulosis.

a rapid pulse. Intestinal obstruction can occur, causing abdominal distention, nausea, and vomiting.

Assessment

Collection of **subjective data** includes an awareness that the patient with diverticulosis may not display any problematic symptoms. Complaints of constipation and diarrhea accompanied by pain in the left lower quadrant are common. Other common symptoms include increased flatus and chronic constipation alternating with diarrhea, anorexia, and nausea.

Objective data include abdominal distention, low-grade fever, leukocytosis, vomiting, blood in the stool, and sometimes a palpable abdominal mass.

Diagnostic Tests

Ultrasound and CT scan with oral contrast are used to confirm the diagnosis and evaluate the severity of the disease. A CBC, urinalysis, and fecal occult blood test should be performed. A barium enema is used to determine narrowing or obstruction of the colonic lumen. Colonoscopy may help rule out polyps or a malignancy. A patient with acute diverticulitis should not have a barium enema or colonoscopy because of the possibility of perforation and peritonitis.

Medical Management

A diet high in fiber, mainly from fresh fruits and vegetables, and decreased intake of fat and red meat are recommended for preventing diverticular disease. High levels of physical activity also seem to decrease the risk.

Weight reduction is important for the obese person. Patients should avoid increased intraabdominal pressure, which may precipitate an attack. Factors that increase intraabdominal pressure are straining at stool; vomiting; bending; lifting; and tight, restrictive clothing.

In acute diverticulitis, the goal of treatment is to allow the colon to rest and the inflammation to subside. Observe the patient for signs of possible peritonitis. Administer broad-spectrum antibiotics as ordered. Monitor the WBC count. Frequently diverticulitis can be managed in an outpatient setting, and hospitalization is reserved for older adults or those with severe symptoms.

When the acute attack subsides, give oral fluids at first and then progress to semisolids. Ambulation is permitted. Observe the patient for a recurrent attack. If the patient has a bowel resection or colostomy, the nursing care is the same as for those procedures.

Although diverticular disease is common, complications are rare. Bowel rest and antibiotic therapy are usually adequate. Surgical treatment is advised if long-term problems do not respond to medical management and is mandatory if complications (e.g., hemorrhage, obstruction, abscesses, or perforation) occur. In elective surgery a thorough bowel preparation is most important. Laxatives, enemas, or intestinal lavage by GoLYTELY (see Box 45-2) are given to cleanse the bowel, depending on the surgeon's preference. Antibiotics are given orally and parenterally.

In cases of perforation, abscess, peritonitis, or fistula, resection of the bowel with a temporary colostomy is needed. Either the one-stage procedure (resection of the affected bowel with anastomosis and no diverting colostomy) or the two-stage procedure (resection of the diseased bowel with diverting colostomy) is performed.

The bowel diversion can be accomplished by Hartmann's procedure (Figure 45-12), in which the descending colon is resected, the proximal end is brought to the abdominal wall surface, and the distal bowel is sealed off for later anastomosis. Other procedures are the double-barrel colostomy, in which the bowel is brought up through the abdominal surface (Figure 45-13), and transverse loop colostomy, in which a loop is formed and the bowel is held in place with a glass rod or a plastic butterfly between the bowel and the abdomen (Figure 45-14). The bowel can be opened at the time of surgery or postoperatively.

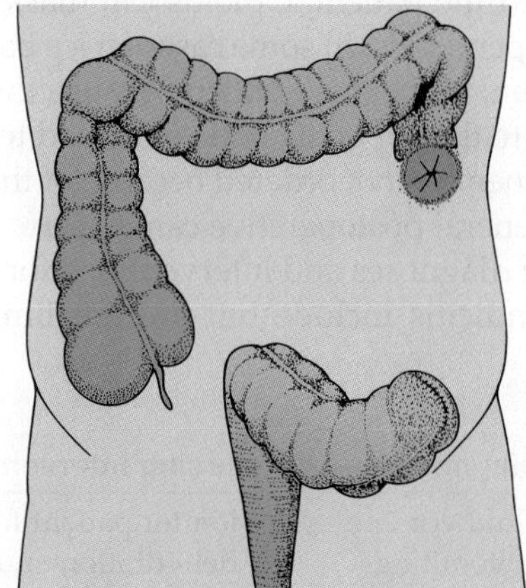

FIGURE 45-12 Hartmann's pouch.

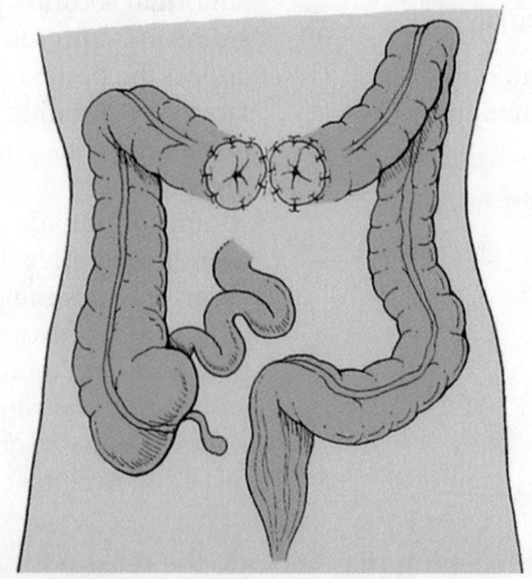

FIGURE 45-13 Double-barrel transverse colostomy.

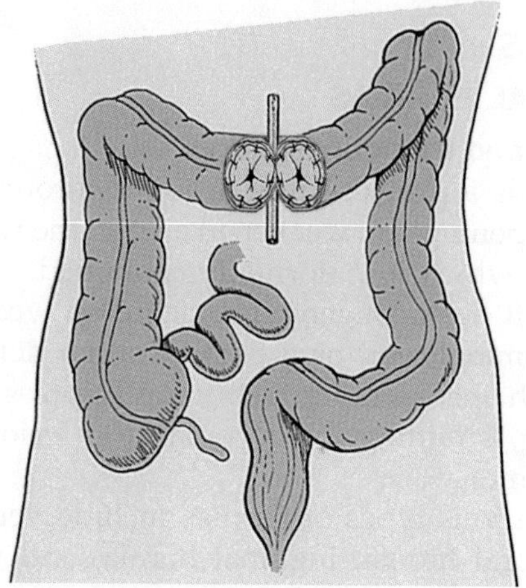

FIGURE 45-14 Transverse loop colostomy with rod or butterfly.

Removal of the affected bowel segment and reanastomosis of the bowel are done during the initial procedure.

Closure of the temporary colostomy is the desired goal in the case of diverticular disease. Usually this takes place 6 weeks to 3 months after the initial surgical procedure. Again, the bowel must be prepared for closure by a liquid diet; laxatives; antibiotics; intestinal lavage as mentioned; and a cleansing colostomy irrigation of the proximal and, in the case of the loop or double-barrel colostomy, distal end of the stoma.

Nursing Interventions and Patient Teaching

Remember that when the distal loop is irrigated, irrigating solution and bowel contents usually return from both the distal opening and rectum, so place the patient on the toilet or bedpan during the procedure.

The return of bowel activity after closure may take several days. The patient will have IV fluids and an NG tube for the first few days postoperatively.

Nursing interventions include patient teaching of the disease process and surgery, if planned. Assess the nutritional status and reinforce the prescribed diet. Determine the nature of the pain the patient is having so that comfort measures or medication can be administered. Include the patient and the family in setting goals for the teaching plan.

Nursing diagnoses and interventions for the patient with diverticular disease include but are not limited to the following:

Nursing Diagnoses	Nursing Interventions
Deficient knowledge, related to disease process and treatment	Instruct patient and family in disease process and signs and symptoms of acute diverticulitis attack.
Imbalanced nutrition: less than body requirements, related to decreased oral intake	Instruct patient about dietary fiber (for prevention) or bland, low-residue diet (for inflammatory phase). Assess daily weights, calorie counts, and I&O. Monitor serum protein and albumin.

When a colostomy is performed, have the patient or family member verbalize and demonstrate understanding of the ostomy care. Do not rush the teaching of colostomy care; wait until the patient is free of pain and receptive to learning. A family member may be taught to help until the patient is able to assume self-care, keeping in mind that the ultimate goal is patient independence. A home care referral may be needed so that the teaching process can continue after discharge.

Prognosis

With diverticulosis, the prognosis is good. Most patients have few symptoms except for occasional bleeding from the rectum. Diverticulitis has a good prognosis, with 30% of patients needing bowel resection of the affected part in acute cases to reduce mortality and morbidity.

PERITONITIS

Etiology and Pathophysiology

Peritonitis is an inflammation of the abdominal peritoneum. This condition occurs after fecal matter seeps from a rupture site, causing bacterial contamination of the peritoneal cavity. Some examples are diverticular abscess and rupture, acute appendicitis with rupture, and strangulated hernia. Peritonitis can also be caused by chemical irritants, such as blood, bile, necrotic tissue, pancreatic enzymes (pancreatitis), and foreign bodies. Ascites that occurs with cirrhosis of the liver provides an excellent liquid environment for bacteria to flourish. Patients who use continuous ambulatory peritoneal dialysis are also at high risk. No matter what the cause, the resulting inflammation response leads to massive fluid shifts (peritoneal edema and adhesions as the body attempts to wall off the infection).

Clinical Manifestations

Generalized peritonitis is an extremely serious condition characterized by severe abdominal pain. The patient usually lies on the back with the knees flexed to relax the abdominal muscles; any movement is painful. Rebound tenderness, muscular rigidity, and spasm are major symptoms of irritation of the peritoneum. The abdomen is usually tympanic and extremely tender to the touch.

Assessment

Collection of **subjective data** includes observing for severe abdominal pain. Nausea and vomiting occur, and as peristalsis ceases, constipation occurs with no passage of flatus. Chills, weakness, and abdominal tenderness (local and diffuse, often rebound) are also manifested.

Collection of **objective data** includes noting a weak and rapid pulse, fever, and lowered blood pressure. Leukocytosis and marked dehydration occur, and the patient can collapse and die.

Diagnostic Tests

A flat plate of the abdomen is ordered to find out whether free air is present under the diaphragm as a result of visceral perforation. A CBC with differential is ordered to determine the degree of leukocytosis. A blood chemistry profile to determine renal perfusion and electrolyte balance is done. Peritoneal aspiration may be performed and the fluid analyzed for blood, bile, pus, bacteria, or fungus. Ultrasound and CT scans may be useful in identifying ascites and abscesses.

Medical Management

Aggressive therapy includes correction of the contamination or removal of the chemical irritant by surgery, and parenteral antibiotics. NG intubation is ordered to prevent GI distention. IV fluids and electrolytes prevent or correct imbalances. Analgesics are provided intravenously via PCA pump. The patient may be placed on total parenteral nutrition because of increased nutritional requirements. Early treatment to prevent severe shock from the loss of fluid into the peritoneal space is essential.

Nursing Interventions and Patient Teaching

Nursing interventions for the patient with peritonitis include the following:

- Place patient on bed rest in semi-Fowler's position to help localize purulent exudate in lower abdomen or pelvis.
- Give oral hygiene to prevent drying of mucous membranes and cracking of lips from dehydration.
- Monitor fluid and electrolyte replacement.
- Encourage deep-breathing exercises; patient tends to have shallow respirations as a result of abdominal pain or distention.
- Use measures to reduce anxiety.
- Use meticulous surgical asepsis for wound care.

Instruct the patient about the importance of ambulation, coughing, deep breathing, use of an incentive spirometer, and leg exercises. If the patient has a draining wound at discharge, teach surgical asepsis for dressing changes. Encourage a nutritious diet. Instruct the patient not to lift more than 10 pounds until the physician approves it. Stress the importance of keeping physician follow-up appointments.

Prognosis

The mortality rate of generalized peritonitis is 40% with the use of antibiotics and intensive support systems. Age, etiology of the peritonitis, and ineffective tissue perfusion negatively affect the prognosis.

HERNIAS

EXTERNAL HERNIAS

Etiology and Pathophysiology

A hernia is a protrusion of a viscus through an abnormal opening or a weakened area in the wall of the cavity in which it is normally contained. Most hernias result from congenital or acquired weakness of the abdominal wall or a postoperative defect, coupled with increased intraabdominal pressure from coughing, straining, or an enlarging lesion within the abdomen.

The various types of hernias include ventral hernia, femoral hernia, inguinal hernia, and umbilical hernia. Ventral, or incisional, hernia is due to weakness of the abdominal wall at the site of a previous incision. It is found most commonly in patients who are obese, who have had multiple surgical procedures in the same area, and who have inadequate wound healing because of poor nutrition or infection. A femoral, or inguinal, hernia is caused by a weakness in the lower abdominal wall opening through which the spermatic cord emerges in men and the round ligament emerges in women.

A hernia may be reducible (able to be returned to its original position by manipulation) or irreducible (or incarcerated; unable to be returned to its body cavity). When the hernia is irreducible, it may obstruct intestinal flow. The hernia is strangulated when it occludes blood supply and intestinal flow. To prevent anaerobic infection in the area, immediate surgical intervention is performed when a hernia strangulates.

Factors such as age, wound infection, malnutrition, obesity, increased intraabdominal pressure, or abdominal distention affect formation of hernias after surgical incisions. Fewer hernias occur with transverse incisions than with longitudinal incisions. Also, upper abdominal incisions are associated with fewer hernias than lower abdominal incisions.

Assessment

Collection of **subjective data** includes palpation of the hernia area, revealing the contents of the sac as soft and nodular (omentum) or smooth and fluctuant (bowel). Never attempt to reduce the sac in the ring because this can lead to complications such as rupture of the strangulated contents.

Both subjective and objective signs and symptoms depend on where the hernia occurs. With an inguinal hernia, the patient may complain of pain, urgency, and a mass in the groin region.

Objective data include a visible protruding mass or bulge around the umbilicus, in the inguinal area, or near an incision; this is the most common objective sign. If complications such as incarceration or strangulation follow, the patient may have bowel obstruction, vomiting, and abdominal distention.

Diagnostic Tests

The diagnosis is aided by palpation of the weakened wall. Radiographs of the suspected area may be ordered.

Medical Management

Hernias that cause no discomfort can be left unrepaired unless strangulation or obstruction follows. Teach the patient to seek medical advice promptly if abdominal pain, distention, changing bowel habits, temperature elevation, nausea, or vomiting occurs. If the hernia can be reduced manually, a truss or firm pad placed over the patient's hernia site and held in place with a belt prevents the hernia from protruding and holds the abdominal contents in place.

Elective surgery for hernia repair may be done because of inconvenience to the patient or constant risk of strangulation. A procedure to close the hernia defect by approximating adjacent muscles or using a synthetic mesh is done on either an inpatient or outpatient basis.

Nursing Interventions and Patient Teaching

Nursing interventions for external hernia require observation of the hernia's location and size and tissue perfusion to the area. The patient may be limited in activity and the type of clothing worn.

Open abdominal surgery may be necessary for the patient with a strangulated hernia. Prepare the patient for a long hospitalization, which may include NG suctioning, IV antibiotics, fluid and electrolyte replacement, and parenteral analgesics until peristalsis returns.

Postoperatively monitor the patient for urinary retention; wound infection at the incision site; and, with inguinal hernia repair, scrotal edema. If scrotal edema is present, elevate the scrotum on a rolled pad, apply an ice pack, and provide a supportive garment (jockstrap or briefs). The patient should deep breathe every 2 hours, but many physicians discourage coughing. Verify the postoperative orders. Teach the patient how to support the incision by splinting the area with pillow or pad. This support, along with analgesics, will help relieve pain.

Nursing diagnoses and interventions for the patient with a hernia include but are not limited to the following:

Nursing Diagnoses	Nursing Interventions
Deficient knowledge, related to disease process	Instruct patient to observe and report hernias that become irreducible or edematous. Instruct patient to report increased pain, abdominal distention, or change in bowel habits. Explain reason to avoid prolonged standing, lifting, or straining. Instruct patient to support weakened area by use of truss or manually as needed (as when coughing).
Ineffective tissue perfusion, related to strangulation or incarceration of hernia	Monitor patient for increased pain, distention, changing bowel habits, abnormal bowel sounds, temperature elevation, nausea, and vomiting. Report changes in appearance and signs and symptoms to physician.

Follow-up care includes teaching the patient to limit activities and avoid lifting heavy objects or straining with bowel movements for 5 to 6 weeks. Also the patient should immediately report to the physician any erythema or edema of the surgical area or increased pain or drainage.

HIATAL HERNIA

A hiatal hernia (esophageal hernia or diaphragmatic hernia) results from a weakness of the diaphragm. Hiatal hernia is a protrusion of the stomach and other abdominal viscera through an opening, or hiatus, in the diaphragm (Figure 45-15). A hiatal hernia is the most common problem of the diaphragm that affects the alimentary tract. It is an anatomical condition, not a disease. This condition occurs in about 40% of the population; most people display few, if any, symp-

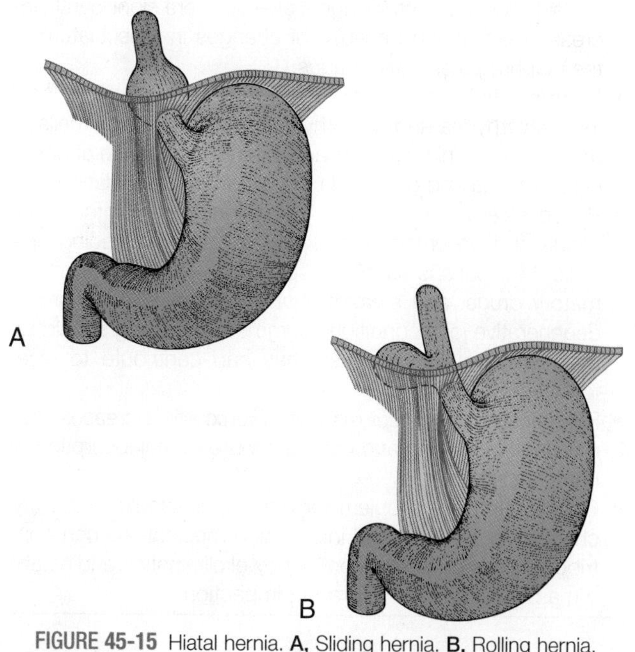

FIGURE 45-15 Hiatal hernia. **A,** Sliding hernia. **B,** Rolling hernia.

toms. The major difficulty in symptomatic patients is gastroesophageal reflux, manifested as pyrosis (heartburn) after overeating. Complications of strangulation, infarction, or ulceration of the herniated stomach are serious and require surgical intervention. Factors contributing to the development of these hernias include obesity, trauma, and a general weakening of the supporting structures as a result of aging (see Life Span Considerations box).

Medical Management

The physician may perform (1) a posterior gastropexy, in which the stomach is returned to the abdomen and sutured in place; or (2) a laparoscopically performed Nissen fundoplication, in which the fundus is wrapped around the lower part of the esophagus and sutured in place (Figure 45-16). The use of laparoscopic techniques has reduced the overall morbidity, complications, and the cost of hospitalization associated with a thoracic or open abdominal approach. However, a thoracic or open abdominal approach may be used in selected cases.

Nursing Interventions

Nursing care of the patient after surgery is similar to that after gastric surgery or thoracic surgery, depending on the procedure performed.

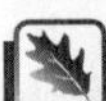 **Life Span Considerations**

Older Adults

Gastrointestinal Disorders

- Loss of teeth and resultant use of dentures can interfere with chewing and lead to digestive complaints.
- Dysphagia is commonly seen in the older adult population and may be caused by changes in the esophageal musculature or by neurologic conditions.
- Hiatal hernias and esophageal diverticuli are significantly increased with aging because of changes in musculature of the diaphragm and esophagus.
- Older adults have decreased secretion of hydrochloric acid (hypochlorhydria and achlorhydria) from the parietal cells of the stomach. This results in an increased incidence of pernicious anemia and gastritis in the older adult population.
- Peptic ulcers are common, but often the symptoms are vague and go unrecognized until there is a bleeding episode. Medications such as aspirin, nonsteroidal antiinflammatory drugs, and steroids that are taken for the chronic degenerative joint conditions common with aging should be used with caution because they can contribute to ulcer formation.
- Frequency of diverticulosis and diverticulitis increases dramatically with aging and can contribute to malabsorption of nutrients.
- Constipation is a problem for many older adults. Inactivity, changes in diet and fluid intake, and medications can contribute to this problem. Monitor bowel elimination and establish a bowel regimen to prevent impaction.

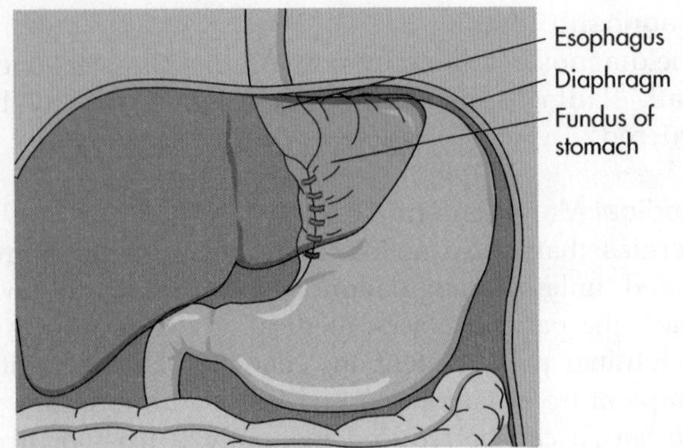

FIGURE 45-16 Nissen fundoplication for hiatal hernia showing fundus of stomach wrapped around distal esophagus and sutured to itself.

Prognosis

The prognosis for hernias is good because surgical intervention is usually successful. The result can be altered if the patient is a poor surgical risk or has other complications.

INTESTINAL OBSTRUCTION

Etiology and Pathophysiology

Intestinal obstruction occurs when intestinal contents cannot pass through the GI tract; it requires prompt treatment. The obstruction may be partial or complete. The causes of intestinal obstruction are classified as mechanical or nonmechanical.

Mechanical Obstruction

Mechanical obstruction may be caused by an occlusion of the lumen of the intestinal tract. Most obstructions occur in the ileum, which is the narrowest segment of the small intestine. Mechanical obstructions account for 90% of all intestinal obstructions. Mechanical obstructions include adhesions (Figure 45-17, *A*) or incarcerated hernias. Adhesions can develop after abdominal surgery. Other causes include impacted feces, diverticular disease, tumor of the bowel, intussusceptions, **volvulus** (Figure 45-17, *B*) (a twisting of bowel onto itself), or the strictures of inflammatory bowel disease. Residues from foods high in fiber, such as raw coconut or fruit pulp, can also obstruct the small bowel.

Nonmechanical Obstruction

Nonmechanical obstruction may result from a neuromuscular or vascular disorder. The cause is something that decreases the muscle action of the bowel and affects the ability of fecal matter and fluid to move through the intestines (Kent, 2007). **Paralytic (adynamic) ileus** (lack of intestinal peristalsis and bowel sounds) is the most common form of nonmechanical obstruction. It occurs to some degree after any abdominal surgery. Other causes include inflammatory responses (e.g., acute pancreatitis, acute appendicitis), electrolyte abnormalities (especially hypokalemia), and thoracic or lumbar spinal

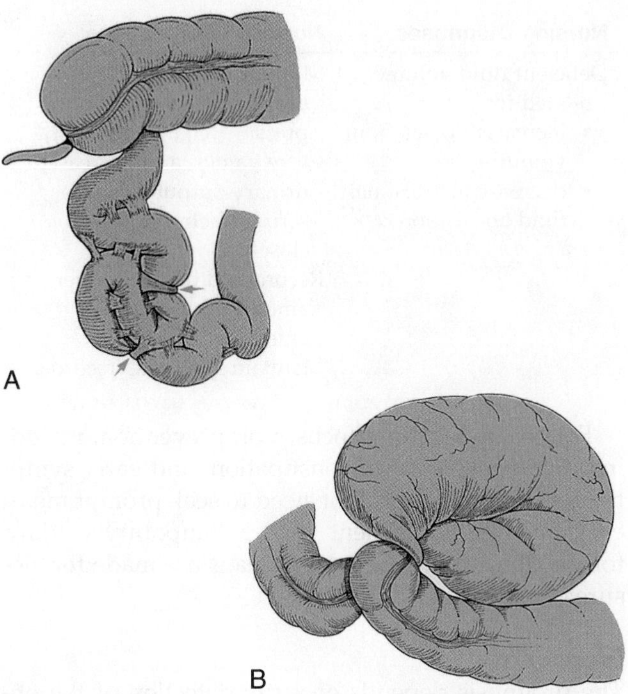

FIGURE 45-17 Intestinal obstructions. **A,** Adhesions. **B,** Volvulus.

trauma from either fractures or surgical intervention. Vascular obstructions are rare and are due to an interference with the blood supply to a portion of the intestines. The most common causes are emboli and atherosclerosis of the mesenteric arteries. The celiac, inferior, and superior mesenteric arteries supply blood to the bowel. Emboli may originate from thrombi in patients with chronic atrial fibrillation, diseased heart valves, and prosthetic valves.

When the small intestine becomes obstructed, it interrupts the normal process of secretion and reabsorption of 6 to 8 L of electrolyte-rich fluid. Large amounts of fluid, bacteria, and swallowed air build up in the bowel proximal to the obstruction. Water and salts shift from the circulatory system to the intestinal lumen, causing distention and further interfering with absorption. As the fluid increases, so does the pressure in the lumen of the bowel. The increased pressure leads to an increase in capillary permeability and extravasation of fluids and electrolytes into the peritoneal cavity. Edema, congestion, and necrosis from impaired blood supply and possible rupture of the bowel may occur. The retention of fluid in the intestine and peritoneal cavity can lead to a severe reduction in circulating blood volume and result in hypotension and hypovolemic shock.

Clinical Manifestations

The signs and symptoms of intestinal obstruction vary with the site and degree of obstruction. During partial or early phases of mechanical obstruction, auscultation of the abdomen reveals loud, frequent, high-pitched sounds. However, when smooth muscle atony (weak, lacking normal tone) occurs, bowel sounds are absent.

Assessment

Subjective data include the pattern of the patient's pain, including onset, frequency, and characteristics. Nausea and the inability to pass flatus are common symptoms. Early complaints of obstruction of the small intestine include spasms of cramping abdominal pain as peristaltic activity increases proximal to the obstruction. As the obstruction progresses, the intestine becomes fatigued, with periods of decreased or absent bowel sounds and increased abdominal pain. Note any history of previous bowel disorders or abdominal surgeries and changes in bowel elimination.

Collection of **objective data** begins with assessing the abdominal surface for evidence of distention, hernias, scars indicating previous surgeries, or visible peristaltic waves. The increased peristaltic activity produces an increase in auscultated bowel sounds. Other objective data include vomiting; signs of dehydration caused by the fluid shift; abdominal distention, tenderness, and muscle guarding; and decreased blood pressure.

Obstruction of the colon causes less severe pain than obstruction of the small intestine, marked abdominal distention, and constipation. The patient may continue to have bowel movements, since the colon distal to the obstruction continues to empty.

Diagnostic Tests

Abdominal x-rays are the most useful diagnostic aids. Flat, upright, and lateral x-rays show gas and fluid in the intestines. Intraperitoneal air (sometimes referred to as free air under the diaphragm) indicates perforation. Radiographic examination reveals the level of obstruction and its cause. Sigmoidoscopy or colonoscopy may provide direct visualization of an obstruction in the colon. CT scans may also be used in diagnosis. Monitor the fluid and electrolyte balance through laboratory test results. Elevated blood urea nitrogen and decreased serum sodium, chloride, potassium, and magnesium are common. The patient's hemoglobin and hematocrit levels may increase because of hemoconcentration associated with the fluid volume deficit.

Medical Management

Treatment is directed toward decompression of the intestine by removal of gas and fluid, correction and maintenance of fluid and electrolyte balance, and relief or removal of the obstruction. Treatment may include the evacuation of intestinal contents by means of an intestinal tube. An NG or nasojejunal tube is inserted and connected to wall suction to decompress the intestine. A long intestinal tube (10 feet [300 cm]) (e.g., Miller-Abbott) may be used instead of an NG tube to decompress the bowel; however, its use is controversial and limited because it is more difficult and time consuming to insert and may not be more effective than an NG tube. Surgical repair is necessary to relieve mechanical obstructions caused by adhesions, volvulus, and strangulated hernias. Restore fluid and electrolyte balance by carefully monitoring IV infusion. Nonopioid analgesics are usually prescribed to avoid the decrease in intestinal motility that often accompanies the administration of opioid analgesics.

Nursing Interventions and Patient Teaching

Unless surgery is indicated, nursing interventions include careful monitoring of fluids and electrolytes, measuring the patient's urinary output, observing the function of tubes used to decompress and relieve distention, and administering analgesics.

For the patient with intestinal obstruction undergoing surgery, preoperative preparation includes explaining the procedure at a level the patient can understand. Provide emotional support for the patient because he or she is experiencing the stressors of pain and vomiting plus the added stressor of emergency surgery.

Postoperative nursing interventions are similar to those for any patient who has had abdominal surgery. Place the patient in a Fowler's position for greater diaphragm expansion. Encourage the patient to breathe through the nose and not swallow air, which would increase distention and discomfort. Encourage deep breathing and coughing. Continue nasointestinal suctioning until bowel activity returns. Assess for bowel sounds and abdominal girth and expulsion of flatus and stool to help determine the return of peristalsis. When the patient is ready to eat, usually within 24 to 48 hours after surgery or at the first sounds of peristalsis, provide a progressive diet as tolerated. Some patients require temporary bowel diversion via a double-barrel or loop colostomy to manage the obstruction.

To manage pain, administer all medications as prescribed. Medications may include opioids or opioid derivatives (note that morphine increases nausea and vomiting and causes constipation [Kent, 2007]).

Nursing diagnoses and interventions for the patient with an intestinal obstruction include but are not limited to the following:

Nursing Diagnoses	Nursing Interventions
Acute pain, related to increased peristalsis	Reposition patient frequently to help intestinal tube advance. Irrigate suction tubing with 30 mL sterile saline to keep tube patent. Explain purpose of all procedures. Provide comfort measures. Administer analgesics as ordered.
Deficient fluid volume, related to: • increased losses from vomiting • decrease in intestinal fluid absorption	Monitor for signs of dehydration, decreased blood pressure, change in laboratory values, and decreased urinary output. Monitor serum electrolyte levels closely. Record and report frequency, amount, and nature of emesis. Maintain strict I&O records.

Follow-up teaching focuses on prevention, including diet, prevention of constipation, and early symptoms of recurrence and the need to seek prompt medical care. For the patient with a temporary ostomy, follow-up care is necessary as plans are made for closure of the stoma.

Prognosis

The prognosis depends on early detection of the obstruction and the type and cause of the obstruction, as well as the success of medical interventions. The prognosis is poorer in patients who develop complications such as hypovolemic shock.

COLORECTAL CANCER

Etiology and Pathophysiology

Malignant neoplasms that invade the epithelium and surrounding tissue of the colon and rectum are the third most prevalent internal cancers in the United States and the second leading cause of cancer deaths.

In the colon, 45% of growths are seen in the sigmoid and rectal areas; 25% in the cecum and ascending colon; and the remaining 30% in the transverse splenic flexure, hepatic flexure, and descending colon. Cancer occurs with the same frequency in men and women, with the highest incidence in people 60 years and older.

The cause of colorectal cancer remains unknown, but certain conditions appear to make patients more susceptible to malignant changes. These conditions are termed *predisposing* or *risk factors.* Fortunately, about 85% of colorectal cancers arise from adenomatous polyps, which can be detected and removed from the rectum and sigmoid colon by sigmoidoscopy or colonoscopy. Some diseases, including ulcerative colitis and diverticulosis, increase the risk of colorectal cancer over time. Recent research has isolated a gene that causes colon cancer in certain families. Hereditary diseases (e.g., familial adenomatous polyposis) account for about 5% to 10% of colorectal cancer cases. Hereditary nonpolyposis colorectal cancer syndrome, also called Lynch syndrome, is the most common inherited form of hereditary colorectal cancer. History taking and regular checkups are important preventive measures.

Other factors implicated in colorectal cancer include lack of bulk in the diet, high fat intake, and high bacterial counts in the colon. It is theorized that carcinogens are formed from degraded bile salts, and the stool that remains in the large bowel for a longer period as a result of too little fiber to stimulate its passage may overexpose the bowel to these carcinogens. Another theory is that the increased transit time for low-fiber foods to pass through the intestine is related to malignancy. These factors have led to diet changes; decreased animal fat, reduced red meat, and increased high dietary fiber found in fruits, vegetables, and bran may have a protective effect and act as a primary preventive measure. Cruciferous vegetables such as cauliflower, broccoli, brussels sprouts, and cabbage may help protect against the malignancy. NSAIDs (e.g., aspirin) also seem to reduce the risk.

Clinical Manifestations

Signs and symptoms of cancer of the colon vary with the location of the growth. During the early stages, most patients are asymptomatic. Clinical manifestations are usually nonspecific or do not appear until the disease is advanced.

Assessment

Subjective data include changes in bowel habits alternating between constipation and diarrhea, excessive flatus, and cramps. Constipation is more likely with descending colon cancer, whereas ascending colon cancer may produce no change in bowel habits. Another complaint may be rectal bleeding (the most common sign of colorectal cancer), with the color varying from dark to bright red, depending on the location of the neoplasm. Later stages of colon cancer may involve subjective symptoms of abdominal pain, nausea, and **cachexia** (weakness and emaciation associated with general ill health and malnutrition).

Collection of **objective data** includes observing for vomiting, weight loss, abdominal distention or ascites, and test results that are compatible with the diagnosis. The most common clinical manifestations are chronic blood loss and anemia.

Diagnostic Tests

Early diagnosis of the tumor, including identification of the type of cells involved, is the most important factor in treating the disease. Digital examination can identify 15% of colorectal cancers. Since half of all cases are found in areas of the colon that are inaccessible by sigmoidoscopy, colonoscopy is considered the gold standard for colorectal cancer screening and the detection and removal of precancerous polyps. Other procedures include endorectal ultrasonography and CT scan of the abdomen and pelvis to localize the lesion or determine its size.

A baseline colonoscopy before age 50 should be performed on those who have a family history of colon cancer. Individuals with known gene mutations need to be monitored with colonoscopy every year.

 Health Promotion

Screening for Colorectal Cancer

Current recommendations from the American Cancer Society for colorectal cancer screening are as follows:

- Annual digital rectal examination should begin at age 50 years.
- Starting at the age of 50 years, fecal testing for occult blood should be done every year.
- Flexible sigmoidoscopy should be performed every 5 years. (Colonoscopy should be done if test results are positive.)
- Colonoscopy should be performed every 10 years.
- Double-contrast barium enema should be performed every 5 years.
- Screening for high-risk patients should begin before age 50, usually with colonoscopy.

American Cancer Society. (2009). *Cancer facts & figures.* Atlanta, GA.

Routine physical examinations should include a digital rectal examination because rectal polyps and cancer can be reached with a finger. The American Cancer Society recommends that a person with no established risk factors receive a fecal occult blood test yearly, a double-contrast enema every 5 years, a sigmoidoscopy every 5 years, or a colonoscopy every 10 years starting at age 50. All positive tests are followed up with colonoscopy (see Health Promotion box). Other laboratory and diagnostic studies include a UGI series, radiologic abdominal series, and barium enema. Hemoglobin, hematocrit, and electrolyte levels are examined, and a blood test is done for **carcinoembryonic antigen (CEA)** (an oncofetal glycoprotein found in colonic adenocarcinoma and other cancers and in nonmalignant conditions) when cancer and metastasis are suspected. Antibodies to this antigen are measured. Because the CEA level can be elevated in benign and malignant diseases, it is not considered a specific test for colorectal cancer. Its use is limited to determining the prognosis and monitoring the patient's response to antineoplastic therapy.

Medical Management

Medical treatment includes radiation, chemotherapy, and surgery. Radiation therapy is often used before surgery to decrease the chance of cancer cell implantation at the time of resection. Radiation can both reduce the size of the tumor and decrease the rate of lymphatic involvement. Radiation before surgery has few side effects but some complications.

Postoperatively those patients at high risk for recurrence or people whose disease has progressed may receive radiation administered over 4 to 6 weeks.

Chemotherapy is given (1) to patients with systemic disease that is incurable by surgery or radiation alone; (2) to patients in whom metastasis is suspected (e.g., when a patient has positive lymph node involvement at the time of surgery); or (3) for palliative therapy to reduce tumor size or relieve symptoms of the disease, such as obstruction or pain. Physician opinion and individual patient response vary regarding use of chemotherapy for colorectal cancer.

Surgical interventions depend on the tumor's location, presence of obstruction or perforation of the bowel, possible metastasis, the patient's health status, and the surgeon's preferences. When obstruction has not occurred, a portion of the bowel on either side of the tumor is removed and an end-to-end anastomosis (EEA) is done between the divided ends. When obstruction of the bowel occurs, the commonly used procedures are as follows:

- One-stage resection with anastomosis.
- Two-stage resection with (1) the ends of the bowel brought to the surface and creation of a temporary colostomy and mucus fistula or Hartmann's pouch (see Figure 45-12); (2) a double-barrel colostomy (see Figure 45-13); or (3) a temporary loop colostomy (see Figure 45-14), for closure later.

Surgical procedures for colorectal cancer include the following:

- **Right hemicolectomy:** Resection of ascending colon and hepatic flexure (Figure 45-18, *A*); ileum anastomosed to transverse colon
- **Left hemicolectomy:** Resection of splenic flexure, descending colon, and sigmoid colon (Figure 45-18, *B*); transverse colon anastomosed to rectum
- **Anterior rectosigmoid resection:** Resection of part of descending colon, the sigmoid colon, and upper rectum (Figure 45-18, *C*); descending colon anastomosed to remaining rectum

In carcinoma of the rectum, the surgeon makes every effort to preserve the sphincter, often with an EEA. The use of EEA staplers allows lower and more secure anastomosis. The stapler is passed through the anus, where the colon is stapled to the rectum. This technique makes it possible to resect lesions as low as 5 cm from the anus. If the surgeon is unable to do an anastomosis, an abdominoperineal resection may be done.

In the abdominoperineal resection, an abdominal incision is made and the proximal sigmoid is brought through the abdominal wall in a permanent colostomy. The distal sigmoid, rectum, and anus are removed through a perineal incision (Figure 45-19). The perineal wound may be closed around a drain or left open with packing to allow healing by granulation. Possible complications are delayed wound healing, hemorrhage, persistent perineal sinus tracts, infections, and urinary tract and sexual dysfunction.

Nutritional status is important because of the threat of infection and a compromised postoperative healing process as a result of constipation, diarrhea, nausea, vomiting, and possible obstruction.

Nursing Interventions and Patient Teaching

Nursing interventions include assessment of bowel and urinary elimination, fluid and electrolyte balance, tissue perfusion, nutrition, pain, gas exchange, infection, and peristomal skin integrity, as discussed previously.

Preoperative Care

The patient has some type of bowel preparation, which usually includes 2 or 3 days of liquid diets; a combination of laxatives, GoLYTELY, or enemas; and oral antibiotics to sterilize the bowel. The antibiotic of choice may be neomycin, kanamycin, or erythromycin; each suppresses anaerobic and aerobic organisms in the colon.

Before surgery, provide instruction in turning, coughing, and deep breathing; use of incentive spi-

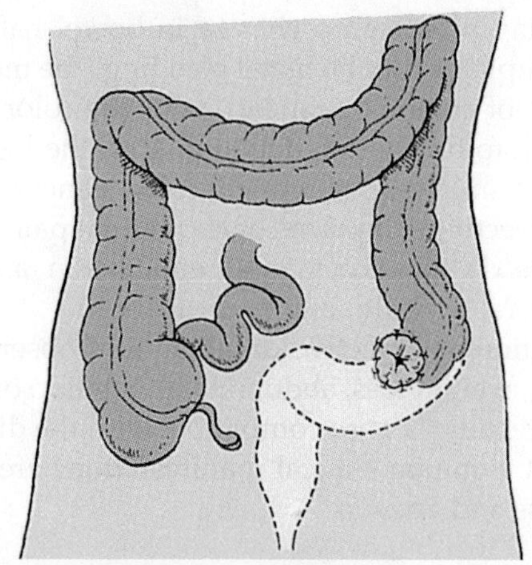

FIGURE 45-19 Descending or sigmoid colostomy.

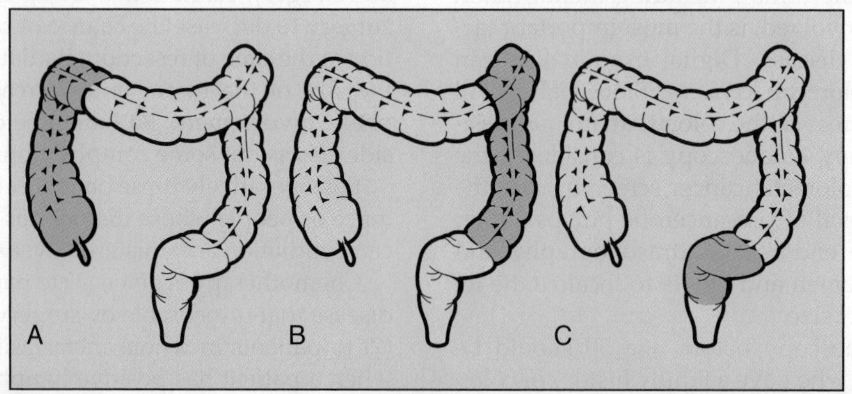

FIGURE 45-18 Bowel resection. **A,** Right hemicolectomy. **B,** Left hemicolectomy. **C,** Anterior rectosigmoid resection.

rometer; wound splinting; and leg exercises. Inform the patient that that he or she will have IV lines, a Foley catheter, possibly an NG tube, a Davol drain, and abdominal dressings after surgery.

If a stoma is planned, the enterostomal therapist should be notified so that the stoma site can be marked before surgery. The stoma should be placed at the best site for the patient.

Postoperative Care

Assess the patient for stable vital signs and return of bowel sounds. Check the dressings for drainage or bleeding and change them as needed per the physician's order. Monitor the NG tube, the Davol drain, and the Foley catheter for flow, amount, and color of output. Keep accurate I&O records to maintain the fluid and electrolyte balance. Other postoperative care includes coughing, deep breathing, early ambulation, adequate nutrition, pain control, and meticulous wound and stoma care.

Paralytic ileus, a common complication of abdominal surgery, produces the classic signs of increased abdominal girth, distention, nausea, and vomiting. Interventions include decompression of the bowel with an NG tube connected to wall suction, NPO status, and increased patient activity.

Long-term complications of abdominal resection with permanent colostomy are urinary retention or incontinence, pelvic abscess, failure of perineal wound healing or wound infection, and sexual dysfunction.

In addition to monitoring the stoma for color, size, location, and the condition of the peristomal skin, watch for possible complications, including necrosis and abscess. Necrosis results from a compromised blood flow to the stoma; the stoma appears pale and dusky to black. Abscess caused by stoma placement too close to the wound, retention sutures, and drains must be assessed promptly. Report all complications promptly to the surgeon and document them in the medical record.

Nursing diagnoses and interventions for the patient with cancer of the colon include but are not limited to the following:

Nursing Diagnoses	Nursing Interventions
Imbalanced nutrition: less than body requirements, related to: • vomiting or anorexia • surgical intervention • depression	Maintain NPO status as ordered. Monitor parenteral fluids. Monitor patency and function of NG tube. Measure I&O. Monitor vital signs and serum electrolytes, hematocrit, and hemoglobin. Provide high-protein, high-carbohydrate, high-calorie, low-residue diet as allowed and tolerated.
Disturbed body image, related to loss of normal body function (colostomy)	Allow time for grieving. Assist patient and family in accepting ostomy. Allow time for and encourage verbalization. Observe for signs of denial, grief, or anger. Answer all questions, and explain treatment and procedure. Provide care in positive manner; always avoid facial expressions connoting distaste. Provide privacy and a safe environment. Encourage self-care and independence when patient demonstrates readiness. Facilitate contact with individuals with similar changes in body image to provide realistic experiences of having ostomy.

The patient with a permanent end colostomy can be taught two forms of colostomy management: (1) emptying and cleansing the pouch as needed and (2) managing colostomy irrigation. In planning patient teaching, consider past bowel habits; location of the colostomy; and the patient's age, general health, and personal preference.

Nerves that control the bladder may be damaged when a large amount of tissue is removed in the abdominoperineal resection. When the Foley catheter is removed after surgery, the patient may be unable to void or empty the bladder completely. If the problem does not resolve, the patient may need a Foley catheter and a urology consultation.

When a large amount of tissue is removed, as in the abdominoperineal resection, the cavity left is a sanctuary for bacteria, increasing the risk of infection. Monitor the drain site for increased pain, erythema, and purulent drainage, and monitor for elevated body temperature. The perineal wound may be closed in one of three ways. The closed wound with a drain to suction has a high risk for abscess formation. The semiclosed wound has either a Davol or Penrose drain left in place, with the drain shortened over time by the physician or nurse. The open wound (in which packing is used and later removed) may need irrigation and sitz baths to facilitate healing. Report to the physician any changes in exudate color and odor and temperature elevation.

Sexual dysfunction of both men and women is related to removal of the rectum. Contributing factors may be partial to complete disruption of the nerve's supply to the genital organs, psychological factors, or decreased activity associated with age. When the nurse and the patient have a comfortable relationship, it is easier to introduce the topic of sex. Exploring the patient's and the partner's fears and providing information on penile prosthesis surgery and simple suggestions to both partners will help decrease anxiety concerning intercourse. Counseling may be necessary if the patient's and the partner's perceptions of body image have been altered. Support groups are available to the cancer patient in most communities. Above all, the nurse's silent communication of touch and eye contact can give the patient a message that he or she is accepted and valued.

Prognosis

The 5-year survival rate is 90% for patients with early localized colorectal cancer and 64% for cancer that has spread to adjacent organs and lymph nodes. Only distant metastases prevent the possibility of a cure.

HEMORRHOIDS

Etiology and Pathophysiology

Hemorrhoids are varicosities (dilated veins) that may occur outside the anal sphincter as external hemorrhoids or inside the sphincter as internal hemorrhoids. This is one of the most common health problems seen in humans, with the greatest incidence from ages 20 to 50 years. Etiologic factors include straining at stool with increased intraabdominal and hemorrhoidal venous pressures. With repeated increased pressure and obstructed blood flow, permanent dilation occurs. Hemorrhoids may be caused by constipation, diarrhea, pregnancy, congestive heart failure, portal hypertension, and prolonged sitting and standing.

Clinical Manifestations

The most common symptoms associated with enlarged, abnormal hemorrhoids are prolapse and bleeding. The bright red bleeding and prolapse usually occur at time of defecation.

Assessment

Subjective data include complaints of constipation, pruritus, severe pain when dilated veins become thrombosed, and bleeding from the rectum that is not mixed with feces.

Collection of **objective data** includes observing external hemorrhoids and palpating internal hemorrhoids. Because bleeding and constipation are signs of cancer of the rectum, all patients with these symptoms should have a thorough examination to rule out cancer.

Diagnostic Tests

Internal hemorrhoids are diagnosed by digital examination, anoscopy, and sigmoidoscopy. External hemorrhoids can be diagnosed by visual inspection and digital examination.

Medical Management

Therapy is directed toward the causes and the patient's symptoms. A high-fiber diet and increased fluid intake prevent constipation and reduce straining, which allows engorgement of the veins to subside. Conservative interventions include the use of bulk stool softeners—such as Metamucil, bran, and natural food fibers—to relieve straining. Topical creams with hydrocortisone relieve pruritus and inflammation, and analgesic ointments, such as dibucaine (Nupercainal), relieve pain. Sitz baths are usually given to relieve pain and edema and promote healing.

Rubber band ligation is a popular and easy method of treatment (Figure 45-20). Tight bands are applied with a special instrument in the physician's office, causing constriction and necrosis. The destroyed tissue sloughs off in about 1 week, and discomfort is minimal. Sclerotherapy (with a sclerosing agent injected at the apex of the hemorrhoid column), cryotherapy (tissue destruction by freezing), infrared photocoagulation (destruction of tissue by creation of a small burn), laser excision, and operative hemorrhoidectomy are additional interventions.

Hemorrhoidectomy, the surgical removal of hemorrhoids, can be performed if other interventions fail to relieve the distressing signs and symptoms. Surgery is indicated for patients with prolapse, excessive pain or bleeding, or large hemorrhoids. In general, hemorrhoidectomy is reserved for patients with severe symptoms related to multiple thrombosed hem-

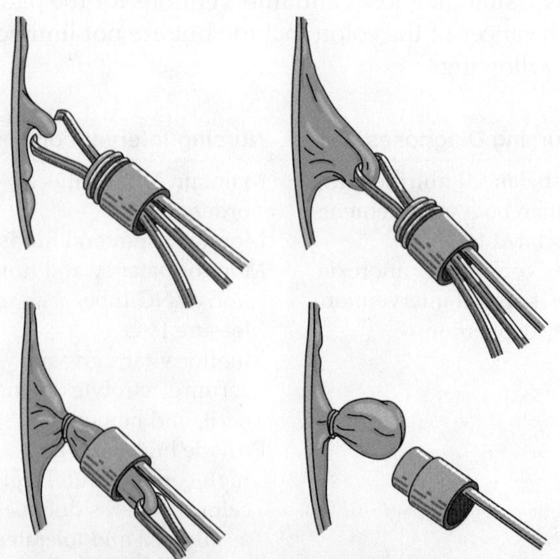

FIGURE 45-20 Rubber band ligation of an internal hemorrhoid.

orrhoids or marked protrusion. Surgical removal may be done by cautery, clamp, or excision. After removal of the hemorrhoid, wounds can be left open or closed, although closed wounds are reported to heal faster. Hemorrhoidectomy is not considered a major procedure, but pain may be acute, requiring opioids and analgesic ointments. Complications include hemorrhage, local infection, pain, urinary retention, and abscess.

Nursing Interventions and Patient Teaching

Rectal conditions can be embarrassing to the patient, and the nurse's direct but concerned attitude can decrease this embarrassment. Assess the knowledge level by asking patients about their condition, what they have been told about treatment, and what treatments have been done before surgery and why.

Observe the patient with a prolapsed hemorrhoid for edema, thrombosis, and ischemia. Ischemic tissue will be dark red to necrotic (black). Explain that a low-bulk diet can produce chronic constipation (see Evidence-Based Practice box).

For the surgical patient, take vital signs frequently for the first 24 hours to rule out internal bleeding. Sitz baths are given several times daily. Early ambulation and a soft diet facilitate bowel elimination. The patient may have a great deal of anxiety concerning the first defecation; open a discussion on this and provide an analgesic before the bowel movement to reduce discomfort. A stool softener such as docusate (Colace) is usually ordered for the first few postoperative days.

Nursing diagnoses and interventions for the patient with hemorrhoids include but are not limited to the following:

Nursing Diagnoses	Nursing Interventions
Pain, related to edema, prolapse, and surgical interventions	Instruct patient to wash anal area after defecation and pat dry. Sitz baths or local heat applied to site may be soothing. Use of local anesthetics (dibucaine ointment or Tucks pads) may give relief. Reinforce need for high-residue diet. Instruct patient on manual reduction of external hemorrhoids. Apply ice packs to hemorrhoids if thrombosed to prevent edema and pain. Use cushion for sitting postoperatively.
Anxiety, related to: • previous experiences • fear of first bowel movement postoperatively • lack of knowledge regarding diet	Establish a supportive relationship with patient. Explain need for high-residue diet. Administer laxatives and oil-retention enema as ordered. Give analgesics before first bowel movement and a sitz bath for pain relief.

Evidence-Based Practice: Treatment of Chronic Constipation in Older Adults

Evidence Summary

The combined effect of decreased activity, change in diet, multiple diseases, and multiple drugs all put older adults at increased risk for constipation. Constipation is diagnosed when a person has two of the following criteria for 12 weeks during the past year: straining, pelletlike stools, sensation of incomplete evacuation, sensation of anal blockage, or using manual maneuvers, all for more than 25% of bowel movements; or having fewer than three bowel movements per week. Data are too limited in the older adult population to recommend one treatment over another. Because constipation in older adults is more likely to be a result of multiple physical and pathologic conditions, there is no consensus that fits all older adults. From a pharmacologic perspective, the ideal drug is selected in terms of effectiveness, tolerance, adverse effects, drug interactions, and cost-effectiveness.

Application to Nursing Practice

- When possible, replace a medication causing constipation with a substitute.
- Encourage older adults to increase physical activity when feasible.
- Give attention to the potential risk of fluid overload in older adult clients with congestive heart failure or renal failure.
- Encourage fiber intake of 20 g/day of wheat bran to start. Observe for bloating and flatulence in older adults.
- Stool softeners are no longer recommended for constipation.
- Fiber and bulk-forming laxatives are the first step in treating constipation in older adults.
- Osmotic laxatives are effective in the treatment of constipation in older adults because they are well tolerated and have no known interactions with other drugs.
- Stimulant laxatives are more effective than placebo, but concern remains regarding their adverse effects on older adults.
- Older adults who have mobility problems often need enemas to avoid an impaction. The tap water enema is the safest for regular use. Glycerol suppositories trigger the defecatory reflex and are sometimes useful in treating older adults.

From Potter, P.A., & Perry, A.G. (2009). *Fundamentals of nursing: concepts, process, and practice.* (7th ed.) St. Louis: Mosby. Adapted from Bosshard, W., Dreher, R., Schnegg, J.F., (2004). The treatment of chronic constipation in elderly people: an update, *Drugs Aging, 21*(14), 911-930.

Advise the patient to include bulk-forming foods in the diet, such as fresh fruits, vegetables, and bran cereals, as well as 8 to 10 glasses of fluid a day unless contraindicated. If the patient is anemic, discuss foods high in iron, such as red meats, liver, and dark green leafy vegetables. Sitz baths are recommended for 1 to 2 weeks postoperatively. Emphasize the need for moderate exercise and a routine time for a daily bowel movement. Also instruct the patient to report any signs of infection or delayed healing.

Prognosis

There are several preferred methods of treatment for hemorrhoids. Both conservative modes of treatment and surgical intervention for hemorrhoids have good prognostic rates.

ANAL FISSURE AND FISTULA

Anal fissure is a linear ulceration or laceration of the skin of the anus. Usually it is the result of trauma caused by hard stool that overstretches the anal lining. The fissure is aggravated by defecation, which initiates spasm of the anal sphincter; pain; and, at times, slight bleeding. If the lesion does not heal spontaneously, the tract is excised surgically.

An anal fistula is an abnormal opening on the cutaneous surface near the anus. Usually this is from a local crypt abscess; it is also common in Crohn's disease. A perianal fistula may or may not communicate with the rectum. It results from rupture or drainage of an anal abscess. This chronic condition is treated by a fistulectomy (removal) or fistulotomy (opening of the fistula tract).

The postoperative care required for repair of an anal fissure or fistula is similar to that for the patient who has had a hemorrhoidectomy.

Prognosis

The prognosis for anal fissures and fistulas is good, whether the patient is treated with conservative measures or with surgical intervention.

FECAL INCONTINENCE

Etiology and Pathophysiology

Fecal incontinence is a complex problem that has a variety of causes. The external anal sphincter may be relaxed, the voluntary control of defecation may be interrupted in the central nervous system, or messages may not be transmitted to the brain because of a lesion within or external pressure on the spinal cord. The disorders that cause breakdown of conscious control of defecation include cortical clouding or lesions, spinal cord lesions or trauma, and trauma to the anal sphincter (e.g., from fistula, abscess, or surgery). Perineal relaxation and actual damage to the anal sphincter are often caused by injury from perineal surgery, childbirth, or anal intercourse. Relaxation of the sphincter usually occurs with the general loss of muscle tone in aging. The normal changes that occur with aging are usually not significant enough to cause incontinence, however, unless concurrent health problems predispose the patient to the disorder.

Normally the contents of the bowel are moved by mass peristaltic movements toward the rectum. The rectum then stores the stool until defecation occurs. Distention of the rectum initiates nerve signals that are transmitted to the spinal cord and then back to the descending colon, initiating peristaltic waves that force more feces into the rectum. The internal anal sphincter relaxes, and if the external sphincter is also relaxed, defecation results. Defecation is a reflex response to the distention of the rectal musculature, but this reflex can be voluntarily inhibited. Voluntary inhibition of defecation is learned in early childhood, and control typically lasts throughout life. The rectum is emptied when the external anal sphincter (under cortical control) relaxes, and the abdominal and pelvic muscles contract.

Reflex defecation continues to occur even in the presence of most upper or lower motor neuron lesions, since the musculature of the bowel contains its own nerve centers that respond to distention through peristalsis. Therefore, even when the patient has motor paralysis, reflex defecation often persists or can be stimulated. Defecation occurs primarily in response to mass peristaltic movements that follow meals or distention of the rectum. Any physical, mental, or social problem that disrupts any aspect of this complex learned behavior can result in incontinence.

Medical Management and Nursing Interventions

Biofeedback training is the cornerstone of therapy for patients who have motility disorders or sphincter damage that causes fecal incontinence. The patient learns to tighten the external sphincter in response to manometric measurement of responses to rectal distention. This technique has been proven effective with alert, motivated patients.

Bowel training is the major approach used with patients who have cognitive and neurologic problems resulting from stroke or other chronic diseases. If a person can sit on a toilet, he or she may be able to defecate automatically given a pattern of consistent timing, familiar surroundings, and controlled diet and fluid intake. This approach allows many patients to defecate predictably and remain continent throughout the day. Surgical correction is possible for a small group of patients whose incontinence is related to structural problems of the rectum and anus.

Patient Teaching

Bowel training requires significant amounts of time and effort on the part of the nursing staff, family, and patient. Incontinence is a major issue in home care and frequently is cited as the most common reason for older adults to be admitted to nursing homes.

To plan the most effective approach, gather specific information concerning the person's general physical and cognitive condition, ability to contract the abdominal and perineal muscles on command, and awareness of the need or urge to defecate. Also collect data about the nature and frequency of the incontinence problem, particularly its relationship to meals or other regular activities.

Teach the family about the training program and how they can assist and support the effort. This includes the importance of providing a high-fiber diet and ensuring that the patient consumes at least 2500 mL of fluid daily. Evaluate the need for a regular stool softener or bulk former. When an optimal time for defecation has been established, usually after breakfast, a glycerin suppository may be inserted to stimulate defecation.

Despite efforts by family members, staff, and patient, fecal incontinence may remain uncontrolled. Efforts then shift to odor control, prevention of skin impairment, and support for the patient's psychological integrity. Commercially available protective briefs are expensive, but they can substantially reduce the burden of care for the family and provide the patient with a sense of security and dignity.

❖NURSING PROCESS *for the Patient with a Gastrointestinal Disorder*

The role of the licensed practical nurse/licensed vocational nurse (LPN/LVN) in the nursing process as stated is that the LPN/LVN will:

- Participate in planning care for patients based on patient needs
- Review patient care plan and recommend revisions as needed
- Review and follow defined prioritization for patient care
- Use clinical pathways, care maps, or care plans to guide and review patient care

Assessment

In caring for the patient admitted with a GI disorder, a thorough, immediate, and accurate nursing assessment is an essential first step. The assessment includes the patient's level of consciousness; vital signs; skin color; edema; appetite; weight loss; nausea; vomiting; and bowel habits, including color and consistency of stools. Assess the abdomen for distention, guarding, and peristalsis. Also obtain a past history of smoking or alcohol use, medications, epigastric or abdominal pain, and acute or chronic stressors and coping–stress tolerance.

Nursing Diagnosis

Assessment provides the data for identifying the patient's problems, strengths, potential complications, and learning needs. Once the diagnoses are defined, assist in formulating a care plan that meets the patient's needs and prioritizing nursing interventions. Possible nursing diagnoses that should be considered for the patient with a GI disorder include but are not limited to the following:

- Activity intolerance
- Anxiety
- Disturbed body image
- Constipation
- Ineffective coping
- Diarrhea
- Fear
- Risk for deficient fluid volume
- Impaired home maintenance
- Ineffective management of therapeutic regimen
- Imbalanced nutrition: less than body requirements
- Pain
- Risk for impaired skin integrity
- Disturbed sleep pattern
- Social isolation
- Ineffective tissue perfusion

Expected Outcomes and Planning

Care planning for the patient with a GI disorder involves looking at the nursing diagnoses and establishing nursing interventions to assist in eliminating the problems. Include the patient in planning to promote compliance with the nursing interventions.

The care plan may be based on one or more of the following goals:

Goal 1: Patient will have no evidence of excoriation around stomal area.

Goal 2: Patient will begin to adjust to disturbed body image.

Implementation

Nursing interventions for the patient with a GI disorder may be simple or complex. Interventions include assessment, monitoring nutritional status, administering medications, promoting health, relieving pain, maintaining skin integrity, managing fluid and electrolyte imbalance, promoting normal bowel elimination patterns, preventing wound infection, health counseling to focus on elimination of smoking and excessive alcohol intake, and patient teaching for enterostomal

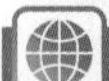
Cultural Considerations

Gastrointestinal Disorders

- Inflammatory bowel disease (Crohn's disease and ulcerative colitis) is more common among whites than blacks and Asian Americans.
- Inflammatory bowel disease is more common among Jewish people and those of Central European origin.
- The incidence of colorectal cancer is higher in the United States and Canada than in Japan, Finland, or Africa.
- The incidence of colorectal cancer is declining in the United States except among black men.

therapy. Cultural considerations are a vital part of nursing interventions for the patient with a GI disorder (see Cultural Considerations box).

Evaluation

Determining the outcomes of the nursing interventions is an ongoing process that helps the nurse establish the most effective care plan. The nurse and the patient evaluate the goals to see whether the criteria for assessment have been met.

Goal 1: Patient will have no evidence of excoriation around stomal area.

Evaluative measure: There is no impairment of skin integrity around stoma.

Goal 2: Patient will begin to adjust to disturbed body image.

Evaluative measures: Patient demonstrates adjustment to disturbed body image by expressing feelings about stoma and is beginning to assume some stoma and pouch care.

Get Ready for the NCLEX® Examination!

Key Points

- The digestive tract begins with the mouth, extends through the thoracic and abdominal cavities, and ends with the anus.
- The major processes of digestion and absorption take place in the small intestine.
- The large intestine is responsible for the preparation and evacuation of the waste products: feces.
- Diet therapy has an important role in the treatment of GI disorders.
- Treatment of esophageal disorders often involves providing the patient with a means of eating, in addition to treating the disorder.
- Common causes of gastric disorders are alcohol, tobacco, aspirin, and antiinflammatory agents.
- Duodenal ulcers are the most common type of peptic ulcer disease.
- A relatively new diagnostic examination is a capsule endoscopy in which the patient swallows a capsule with a camera to visualize the small intestine and diagnose diseases such as Crohn's disease.
- Surgical procedures are available as alternatives to the traditional ileostomy and colostomy.
- A nursing goal for the patient with an ileostomy or a colostomy is fostering patient independence in daily care when the patient demonstrates readiness.
- Keeping the surgical area free of contamination is of primary importance after rectal surgery.
- The approximate location of GI bleeding may be determined by the characteristics of the emesis or the fecal material.
- Explain the purpose of any diagnostic procedure, how the procedure is performed, and the preparation necessary for the procedure, and help the patient understand the results.
- *H. pylori* has been identified in more than 70% of gastric ulcer patients and 95% of those with duodenal ulcers.
- Individuals with inflammatory bowel disease have a greater risk of developing cancer of the bowel.
- Early detection of cancer in the GI system facilitates early treatment and a better prognosis.
- An NG tube is inserted to keep the stomach empty until peristalsis resumes after a general anesthetic or any condition that interferes with peristalsis.
- Effective postoperative care begins with patient teaching during the preoperative period.

Additional Learning Resources

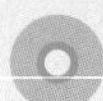

Go to your Companion CD for an audio glossary, animations, video clips, and more.

evolve Be sure to visit the Evolve site at http://evolve.elsevier.com/Christensen/adult/ for additional online resources.

Review Questions for the NCLEX® Examination

1. Because the small intestine needs bile only a few times a day, bile is stored and concentrated in the:
   1. pancreas.
   2. gallbladder.
   3. liver.
   4. small intestine.
2. Although food is digested throughout the alimentary canal, up to 90% of digestion is accomplished in the:
   1. gallbladder.
   2. mouth.
   3. small intestine.
   4. large intestine.
3. The exit from the stomach is called the:
   1. cardiac sphincter.
   2. pyloric sphincter.
   3. lesser curvature.
   4. greater curvature.
4. The intrinsic factor is a gastric secretion necessary for the intestinal absorption of vitamin:
   1. B_1.
   2. B_{12}.
   3. C.
   4. K.
5. Which organ manufactures protease, lipase, and amylase?
   1. Gallbladder
   2. Liver
   3. Pancreas
   4. Salivary gland

6. Paralytic (adynamic) ileus is a functional intestinal obstruction that may result from:
   1. impacted feces, tumor of the colon, or pancreatitis.
   2. electrolyte imbalance, postabdominal surgery, or acute inflammatory reactions.
   3. adhesions or a strangulated hernia.
   4. volvulus, intussusceptions, or electrolyte imbalances.

7. To prepare the patient for endoscopic examination of the upper GI tract, the patient's pharynx is anesthetized with lidocaine (Xylocaine). Nursing interventions for postendoscopic examination include:
   1. allowing fluids up to 4 hours before examination.
   2. withholding anticholinergic medications.
   3. prohibiting smoking before the test.
   4. keeping the patient NPO until the gag reflex returns.

8. A 35-year-old man has been admitted with a diagnosis of peptic ulcers. Which drugs are most commonly used in these patients to decrease acid secretions?
   1. Maalox and Kayexalate
   2. Tagamet and Zantac
   3. Erythromycin and Flagyl
   4. Dyazide and Carafate

9. A patient is scheduled in the morning for a hemicolectomy for removal of a cancerous tumor of the ascending colon. The physician has ordered intestinal antibiotics for her preoperatively to:
   1. decrease the bulk of colon contents.
   2. reduce the bacteria content of the colon.
   3. soften the stool.
   4. prevent pneumonia.

10. A 78-year-old woman was admitted during the evening shift with a tentative diagnosis of cancer of the esophagus. The nurse in her initial assessment finds the patient's major complaint is:
    1. dysphagia.
    2. malnutrition.
    3. pain.
    4. regurgitation of food.

11. Deficient knowledge is a commonly used nursing diagnosis when patients need information regarding their conditions and diagnostic tests. Before a gastroscopy, the nurse should inform the patient that:
    1. fasting for 6 to 8 hours is necessary before the examination.
    2. a general anesthetic will be used.
    3. after gastroscopy, the patient may eat or drink immediately.
    4. admission to the hospital is necessary.

12. In evaluating the care of a young executive admitted with bleeding peptic ulcer, the nurse focuses on nursing interventions. A nursing intervention associated with this type of patient is:
    1. checking the blood pressure and pulse rates each shift.
    2. frequently monitoring arterial blood levels.
    3. observing vomitus for color, consistency, and volume.
    4. checking the patient's low-residue diet.

13. The staff nurse on the surgical floor is aware of pulmonary complications that frequently follow upper abdominal incisions. These are most frequently related to:
    1. aspiration.
    2. pneumothorax if the chest cavity has been entered.
    3. shallow respirations to minimize pain.
    4. not forcing fluids.

14. Which tests can distinguish between peptic ulcer disease and gastric malignancy?
    1. Radiographic GI series
    2. Breath test for *H. pylori*
    3. Serum test for *H. pylori* antibodies
    4. Endoscopy with biopsy

15. A recently approved medication for the treatment of Crohn's disease, infliximab (Remicade), is classified as which type of drug?
    1. Enzyme
    2. Antimetabolite
    3. Alkylating agent
    4. Monoclonal antibody

16. During assessment of the patient with esophageal achalasia, the nurse would expect the patient to report:
    1. a history of alcohol use.
    2. a sore throat and hoarseness.
    3. dysphagia, especially with liquids.
    4. relief of pyrosis with the use of antacids.

17. A nursing intervention that is most appropriate to decrease postoperative edema and pain in the male patient following an inguinal herniorrhaphy is:
    1. applying a truss to the hernial site.
    2. allowing the patient to stand to void.
    3. elevating the scrotum with a support or small pillow.
    4. supporting the incision during routine coughing and deep breathing.

18. The use of nonabsorbable antibiotics as preparation for bowel surgery is done primarily to:
    1. reduce bacterial flora in the colon.
    2. prevent additional formation of ammonia.
    3. prevent postoperative formation of intestinal gas.
    4. stimulate bowel bacteria to increase production of vitamin K.

19. In planning care for the patient with ulcerative colitis, the nurse recognizes that a major difference between ulcerative colitis and Crohn's disease is that ulcerative colitis:
    1. causes more nutritional deficiencies than does Crohn's disease.
    2. causes more abdominal pain and cramping than does Crohn's disease.
    3. is curable with a colectomy, whereas Crohn's disease often recurs after surgery.
    4. is more highly associated with a familial relationship than is Crohn's disease.

20. Which group of medications should be avoided in patients with *E. coli* O157:H7?

1. Antiemetics
2. Antimotility drugs
3. Antilipidemic agents
4. Beta blockers

21. What should a patient be taught after a hemorrhoidectomy?

1. Do not use the Valsalva maneuver.
2. Eat a low-fiber diet to rest the colon.
3. Administer an oil-retention enema to empty the colon.
4. Use a prescribed analgesic before a bowel movement.

22. A medication used to treat *Helicobacter pylori* infection is:

1. erythromycin.
2. neomycin.
3. metronidazole.
4. cefazolin.

23. It is believed that the gastric mucosa of the body of the stomach undergoes a period of transient ischemia in association with hypotension, severe injury, extensive burns, or complicated surgery. This results in the development of what disorder?

1. Crohn's disease
2. Ulcerative colitis
3. Volvulus
4. Stress ulcers

24. In Crohn's disease, major complications that develop due to the granulomatous cobblestone lesions of the small intestine include:

1. malabsorption of nutrients.
2. severe diarrhea of 15 to 20 stools per day.
3. a high probability of developing intestinal cancer.
4. an inability of the body to absorb water.

25. A severe intestinal infection caused by contaminated undercooked beef such as hamburger from a specific pathogenic bacteria present in some cattle is called:

1. *Escherichia coli* O157:H7 intestinal infection.
2. *Clostridium difficile* intestinal infection.
3. Salmonella intestinal infection.
4. *Staphylococcus aureus* infection.

26. After a transverse loop colostomy, the nurse inspects the patient's stoma. The stoma appears mostly pink with some dusky discoloration at the lower border. An appropriate action would be to:

1. clean the area around the stoma and record the observation in the nurses' notes.
2. carefully place a clean pouch over the stoma to prevent any further tissue loss.
3. cover the stoma with a petroleum gauze dressing to prevent any further irritation to the stoma.
4. clean the area around the stoma, apply a clean pouch, and notify the physician about the discoloration.

27. The nurse is teaching a postgastrectomy patient about dumping syndrome. The patient would indicate the need for further instruction if she made which statement?

1. I will lie down after eating a meal.
2. I will eat smaller portions of food, more frequently.
3. I will not drink liquids when I eat.
4. I will avoid fats and increase carbohydrates.

28. The primary medical management for a patient with duodenal ulcers is:

1. gastric resection.
2. antacids, histamine (H_2) receptor blockers, proton pump inhibitors, mucosal healing agents, antibiotic therapy.
3. a diet low in fat and carbohydrates, Rowasa, Imodium.
4. a diet high in protein and milk products, Azulfidine, Dipentum.

29. An 84-year-old patient has a history of a large ventral hernia. He is complaining of nausea, vomiting, abdominal distention, and abdominal pain. A serious complication of a hernia in which the blood supply to the tissue becomes occluded is called a(n):

1. strangulated hernia.
2. hiatal hernia.
3. incarcerated hernia.
4. sliding hernia.

30. Peptic ulcers result from *(Select all that apply.)*:

1. excess of gastric acid or a decrease in the natural ability of the GI mucosa to protect itself from acid and pepsin.
2. invasion of the stomach and/or duodenum by *Helicobacter pylori.*
3. viral infection, allergies to certain foods, immunologic factors, and psychosomatic factors.
4. taking certain drugs, including corticosteroids and antiinflammatory medications.

chapter 46

Care of the Patient with a Gallbladder, Liver, Biliary Tract, or Exocrine Pancreatic Disorder

evolve

Barbara Lauritsen Christensen

http://evolve.elsevier.com/Christensen/foundationsadult

Objectives

1. Discuss nursing interventions for the diagnostic examinations of patients with disorders of the gallbladder, liver, biliary tract, and exocrine pancreas.
2. Explain the etiology, pathophysiology, clinical manifestations, assessment, diagnostic tests, medical management, and nursing interventions for the patient with cirrhosis of the liver, carcinoma of the liver, hepatitis, liver abscesses, cholecystitis, cholelithiasis, pancreatitis, and cancer of the pancreas.
3. Discuss specific complications and teaching content for the patient with cirrhosis of the liver.
4. Define jaundice and describe signs and symptoms that may occur with jaundice.
5. State the six types of viral hepatitis, including their modes of transmission.
6. List the subjective and objective data for the patient with viral hepatitis.
7. Discuss the indicators for liver transplantation and the immunosuppressant drugs to reduce rejection.
8. Discuss the two methods of surgical treatment for cholecystitis and cholelithiasis.

Key Terms

ascites (ă-SĪ-tēz, p. 1472)
asterixis (ăs-tĕr-ĬK-sĭs, p. 1476)
esophageal varices (ĕ-sŏf-ă-JĒ-ăl VĂR-ĭ-sēz, p. 1474)
flatulence (FLĂT-ū-lĕns, p. 1485)
hepatic encephalopathy (hĕ-PĂT-ĭk ĕn-sĕf-ĕ-LŎP-ĕ-thē, p. 1476)
hepatitis (hĕ-pă-TĪ-tĭs, p. 1470)
jaundice (JĂWN-dĭs, p. 1473)
occlusion (ŏ-KLŪ-zhŭn, p. 1489)
paracentesis (păr-ă-sĕn-TĒ-sĭs, p. 1473)
parenchyma (pă-rĕng-KĪ-mă, p. 1472)
spider telangiectases (SPĪ-dĕr tĕl-ăn-jē-ĔK-tĕ-sēz, p. 1472)
steatorrhea (stē-ă-tō-RĒ-ă, p. 1485)

This chapter discusses disorders of the accessory organs of digestion—namely the liver, the gallbladder, and the exocrine pancreas. These organs assist in digestion in various ways. See Chapter 45 for a review of the anatomy and physiology of the liver, the biliary tract, the gallbladder, and the pancreas.

LABORATORY AND DIAGNOSTIC EXAMINATIONS IN THE ASSESSMENT OF THE HEPATOBILIARY AND PANCREATIC SYSTEMS

SERUM BILIRUBIN TEST

Normal values are as follows:

Direct bilirubin: 0.1 to 0.3 mg/dL
Indirect bilirubin: 0.2 to 0.8 mg/dL
Total bilirubin: 0.3 to 1 mg/dL

Rationale

Total serum bilirubin determination measures both direct, or conjugated (water-soluble), and indirect, or unconjugated (water-insoluble), bilirubin. Total serum bilirubin level is the sum of the direct and indirect bilirubin levels. Testing for bilirubin in the blood provides valuable information for diagnosis and evaluation of liver disease, biliary obstruction, and hemolytic anemia. Jaundice, the discoloration of body tissues caused by abnormally high blood levels of bilirubin, is visible when the total serum bilirubin exceeds 2.5 mg/dL.

Nursing Interventions

Keep the patient on nothing by mouth (NPO) status until after the blood specimen is drawn.

LIVER ENZYME TESTS

The normal values are as follows:

- **AST (aspartate aminotransferase; formerly serum glutamic oxaloacetic transaminase [SGOT]):** Adult: 0 to 35 units/L. AST level is elevated in myocardial infarction, hepatitis, cirrhosis, hepatic necrosis, hepatic tumor, acute pancreatitis, and acute hemolytic anemia.
- **ALT (alanine aminotransferase; formerly serum glutamic pyruvic transaminase [SGPT]):** Adult or child: 4 to 36 units/L. ALT level is elevated in hepatitis, cirrhosis, hepatic necrosis, and hepatic tumors and by hepatotoxic drugs.

- **LDH (lactic dehydrogenase):** Adult: 100 to 190 units/L. Values are increased in myocardial infarction, pulmonary infarction, hepatic disease (e.g., hepatitis, active cirrhosis, neoplasm), pancreatitis, and skeletal muscle disease.
- **Alkaline phosphatase:** Adult: 30 to 120 units/L. Alkaline phosphatase level is elevated in obstructive disorders of the biliary tract, hepatic tumors, cirrhosis, hepatitis, primary and metastatic tumors, hyperparathyroidism, metastatic tumor in bones, and healing fractures.
- **Gamma GT (gamma glutamyl transferase):** Male and female older than age 45: 8 to 38 units/L; female younger than age 45: 5 to 27 units/L. Levels are elevated in liver cell dysfunction such as hepatitis and cirrhosis; in hepatic tumors; with the use of hepatotoxic drugs; in jaundice; and in myocardial infarction (4 to 10 days after), heart failure, alcohol ingestion, pancreatitis, and cancer of the pancreas.

Rationale

The liver is a storehouse of many enzymes. Injury or diseases affecting the liver cause release of these intracellular enzymes into the bloodstream, and their levels become elevated. Some of these enzymes are also produced in other organs, and injury or disease affecting these organs will raise the serum level. Therefore, although elevation of these serum enzymes is found in pathologic liver conditions, the test is not specific for liver diseases alone.

Nursing Interventions

Assess the venipuncture site for bleeding.

SERUM PROTEIN TEST

The normal values are as follows:

Total protein: 6.4 to 8.3 g/dL
Albumin: 3.5 to 5 g/dL
Globulin: 2.3 to 3.4 g/dL
Albumin/globulin (A/G ratio): 1.2 to 2.2 g/dL

Rationale

One way to assess the liver's functional status is to measure the products it synthesizes. One of these products is protein, especially albumin. When disease affects the liver cell, the hepatocyte loses its ability to synthesize albumin and the serum albumin level is markedly decreased. Low serum albumin levels may also result from excessive loss of albumin into urine (as in nephrotic syndrome) or into third-space volumes (as in ascites), liver disease, increased capillary permeability, or protein-caloric malnutrition.

Nursing Interventions

Assess the venipuncture site for bleeding.

ORAL CHOLECYSTOGRAPHY

Rationale

The oral cholecystogram (OCG) provides roentgenographic visualization of the gallbladder after the oral ingestion of a radiopaque, iodinated dye. Adequate visualization requires concentration of the dye within the gallbladder. An OCG (also called a gallbladder [or GB] series) is less accurate than a gallbladder ultrasound and is less commonly used for visualizing the biliary tree. OCG will not visualize the biliary tree in the jaundiced patient. Adequate dye concentration depends on the following factors:

- The patient's ingestion of the correct number of dye tablets the evening before the examination
- Adequate absorption of the dye from the gastrointestinal (GI) tract; vomiting or diarrhea preclude absorption of the dye
- Abstinence from food (especially a fatty meal) on the morning of the test
- Uptake from the portal system and excretion of the dye by the liver
- Patency of the cystic duct
- Concentration of the dye within the gallbladder

Nursing Interventions

Before administering the dye, make certain the patient is not allergic to iodine to prevent adverse or allergic reaction. This rarely occurs because the dye is not administered intravenously. If the patient is not allergic to iodine, administer six tablets orally (e.g., iopanoic acid (Telepaque), iodalphionic acid (Priodax), or iprodate (Oragrafin), one every 5 minutes, beginning after the evening meal. The patient is on NPO status from midnight. The patient may be given a high-fat meal or beverage to stimulate emptying of the gallbladder after the test has begun. No other food or fluids are allowed until after the examination.

INTRAVENOUS CHOLANGIOGRAPHY

Rationale

In intravenous cholangiography, intravenously administered radiographic dye is concentrated by the liver and secreted into the bile duct. The intravenous cholangiogram (IVC) allows visualization of the hepatic and common bile ducts and also the gallbladder if the cystic duct is patent. IVC is used to demonstrate stones, strictures, or tumors of the hepatic duct, common bile duct, and gallbladder. IVC is a less commonly used method of visualizing the biliary tree and will not do so in a jaundiced patient.

OPERATIVE CHOLANGIOGRAPHY

In operative cholangiography the common bile duct is directly injected with radiopaque dye. Stones appear as radiolucent shadows, and tumors cause partial or total obstruction of the flow of dye into the duodenum. Visualization of the biliary duct structures provides the surgeon with a "road map" of a difficult anatomical area. This reduces the possibility of inadvertently injuring the common duct.

If common duct stones are suspected, a cholecystectomy as well as a common duct exploration (CDE) must be performed. When intraoperative cholangiography is used routinely, CDE is performed only on those with positive cholangiograms.

T-TUBE CHOLANGIOGRAPHY

Rationale

T-tube cholangiography (postoperative cholangiography) is performed to diagnose retained ductal stones postoperatively in the patient who has had a cholecystectomy and a common bile duct (CBD) exploration to demonstrate good flow of contrast into the duodenum. The test is performed through a T-shaped rubber tube that the surgeon places in the bile duct during the operation. The end of the T-tube exits through the abdominal wall, where dye is injected and radiographic films taken.

Nursing Interventions

Protect the patient from sepsis by connecting the T-tube (if left in place) to a sterile closed-drainage system. If the T-tube is removed, cover the T-tube tract site with a sterile dressing to prevent bacteria from entering the ductal system.

Before administering the dye, ensure that the patient is not allergic to iodine. Preparation of the patient also includes NPO status after midnight and until the examination is completed. Administer a cleansing enema on the morning of the examination, if ordered.

ULTRASONOGRAPHY OF THE LIVER, THE GALLBLADDER, AND THE BILIARY SYSTEM

Rationale

Ultrasonography (ultrasound, echogram) is an imaging technique that visualizes deep structures of the body by recording the reflections (echoes) of ultrasonic waves directed into the tissues. This diagnostic test is not effective in examining all tissue because ultrasound waves do not pass through structures that contain air, such as the lungs, the colon, or the stomach. Although fasting is preferred, it is not necessary for ultrasonography. Because ultrasound requires no contrast material and has no associated radiation, it is especially useful for patients who are allergic to contrast media or are pregnant. Ultrasound is used with increasing frequency to corroborate data already obtained by "questionable positive" cholangiograms, liver scans, and OCGs.

Nursing Interventions

The patient is on NPO status from midnight. If the patient had recent barium contrast studies, request an order for cathartics. Ultrasound cannot penetrate barium, and the study will not be adequate.

GALLBLADDER SCANNING

Rationale

The biliary tract can be evaluated safely, accurately, and noninvasively with the use of intravenous (IV) injection of technetium (^{99}Tc; technetium99m), and positioning the patient under a camera to record distribution of tracer in the liver, the biliary tree, the gallbladder, and the proximal small bowel. The primary use of this study is in the diagnosis of acute cholecystitis. This procedure is superior to oral cholecystography, ultrasonography, and computed tomography (CT) scanning of the abdomen for the detection of acute cholecystitis. Hepatobiliary iminodiacetic acid (HIDA) scanning is also useful for identifying diffuse hepatic disease (such as cirrhosis or neoplasm).

Nursing Interventions

Reassure the patient that exposure to radioactivity is minimal because only a trace dose of the radioisotope is used. The patient is on NPO status from midnight until the examination is complete.

NEEDLE LIVER BIOPSY

Rationale

Needle liver biopsy is a safe, simple, and valuable method of diagnosing pathologic liver conditions. A specially designed needle is inserted through the skin, between the sixth and seventh or eighth and ninth intercostal spaces, and into the liver. The patient lies supine with the right arm over the head. The patient is instructed to exhale fully and not breathe while the needle is inserted. This procedure is often done using ultrasound or CT guidance. A piece of hepatic tissue is removed for microscopic examination. The tissue sample is placed into a labeled specimen bottle containing formalin and sent to the pathology department. Percutaneous liver biopsy is used in the diagnosis of various liver disorders, such as cirrhosis, hepatitis, drug-related reactions, granuloma, and tumor.

Nursing Interventions

Explain the procedure to the patient and obtain the patient's signature on a consent form. Ensure that measurements of platelets, clotting or bleeding time, prothrombin time, and International Normalized Ratio (INR) have been ordered; report any abnormal values to the physician. After the procedure observe the patient for symptoms of bleeding. Monitor vital signs every 15 minutes (two times), then every 30 minutes (four times), and then every hour (four times).

Some pain is common. When leakage involves a large quantity of blood or bile, the peritoneal reaction is great and the resulting pain severe. Assess the patient for pneumothorax (collapsed lung) caused by improper placement of the biopsy needle into the adjacent chest cavity or for bile peritonitis. Immediately report to the physician signs and symptoms of pneumothorax such as shortness of breath, change in respiratory and cardiac rate, or decreased breath sounds on the affected side. Keep the patient lying on the right side for at least 2 hours to splint the puncture site. In this position, the liver capsule is compressed against the chest wall, decreasing the risk of hemorrhage or bile leak.

RADIOISOTOPE LIVER SCANNING

Rationale

This radionuclide procedure is used to outline and detect structural changes of the liver. A radionuclide is given intravenously. Later, a gamma-ray detecting device (Geiger counter) is passed over the patient's abdomen. This records the distribution of the radioactive particles in the liver. The spleen can also be visualized by the detector when technetium 99m sulfur is used.

Nursing Interventions

The patient is on NPO status from midnight. Assure patients that they will not be exposed to a large amount of radioactivity, since only trace doses of isotopes are used.

SERUM AMMONIA TEST

Normal value is 10 to 80 mcg/dL.

Rationale

Ammonia is a by-product of protein metabolism. Most of the ammonia is made by bacteria acting on proteins in the intestine. By way of the portal vein, ammonia goes to the liver, where it is normally converted into urea and then excreted by the kidneys. When the patient has severe liver dysfunction or altered blood flow to the liver, ammonia cannot be catabolized, the serum ammonia level rises, and the blood urea nitrogen level decreases. The serum ammonia level is primarily used as an aid in diagnosing hepatic encephalopathy and hepatic coma. Elevated serum ammonia levels suggest liver dysfunction as the cause of these signs and symptoms.

Nursing Interventions

On the laboratory requisition, list any antibiotics the patient is currently taking. Certain broad-spectrum antibiotics such as neomycin can cause a decreased ammonia level, thus giving inaccurate test results.

HEPATITIS VIRUS STUDIES

A normal laboratory test result will be negative for hepatitis-associated antigen.

Rationale

Hepatitis is an inflammation of the liver caused by viruses, bacteria, and noninfectious causes of liver inflammation. Six viruses, designated A through G, can cause this disease. Hepatitis A and B viruses have been recognized for years, but hepatitis C, D, E, and G viruses were identified more recently (so-called hepatitis F virus was eventually found to be a mutation of hepatitis C virus [HCV]). Hepatitis A, B, and C viruses are the most common viruses that cause hepatitis. Hepatitis D virus is carried by the hepatitis B virus (HBV). Both hepatitis D and E viruses are seen less frequently in the United States than the hepatitis A, B, or C viruses (Pagana & Pagana, 2008). The individual hepatitis viruses can be detected by different antigen and antibody levels, and different incubation periods must be considered.

Nursing Interventions

Use standard precautions and handle the serum specimen as if it were capable of transmitting viral hepatitis. Don gloves when handling any blood or body fluids, and wash hands carefully after handling equipment.

SERUM AMYLASE TEST

Normal value is 60 to 120 Somogyi units/dL, or 30 to 220 units/L (SI units).

Rationale

The serum amylase test is an easily and rapidly performed test for pancreatitis. Damage to pancreatic cells (as in pancreatitis) or obstruction to the pancreatic ductal flow (as in pancreatic carcinoma) causes an outpouring of this enzyme into the intrapancreatic lymph system and the free peritoneum. Blood vessels draining the free peritoneum and absorbing the lymph pick up this excess amylase. An abnormal rise in the serum level of amylase occurs within 2 hours of the onset of pancreatic disease. Because amylase is rapidly cleared by the kidney, serum levels may return to normal within 36 hours. Persistent pancreatitis, duct obstruction, or pancreatic duct leak (e.g., pseudocysts) cause persistent elevated serum levels.

Nursing Interventions

Note on the laboratory requisition whether the patient is receiving intravenous dextrose or any medications, since these can cause a false-negative result.

URINE AMYLASE TEST

The normal value for this study is up to 5000 Somogyi units/24 hr, or 6.5 to 48.1 units/hr.

Rationale

Levels of amylase in the urine remain elevated for 7 to 10 days after the onset of disease. Urine amylase is particularly useful in detecting pancreatitis late in the disease course. This fact is important for diagnosing pancreatitis in patients who have had symptoms for 3 days or longer.

Nursing Interventions

Record the exact time at the beginning and end of the collection period. A 2-hour spot urine or 6-hour, 12-hour, or 24-hour collection can be performed, depending on the physician's order. The collection begins after the patient empties the bladder and discards that specimen. All subsequent urine is collected, including the voiding at the end of the collection period. Keep the specimen on ice or refrigerated until it is sent to the laboratory.

SERUM LIPASE TEST

The normal value is 10 to 140 units/L.

Rationale

Like serum amylase, serum lipase is elevated in acute pancreatitis and is a helpful complementary test because other disorders (e.g., mumps, cerebral trauma, renal transplantation) may also cause an increase in serum amylase. Lipase appears in the bloodstream after damage to the pancreas. The lipase levels rise a little later than amylase levels (4 to 48 hours after the onset of pancreatitis), peak around 24 hours, and remain elevated for at least 14 days. Because lipase peaks later and remains elevated longer than amylase, it is more useful in the diagnosis of acute pancreatitis later in the course of the disease.

Nursing Interventions

Instruct the patient to remain on NPO status from midnight, except for water.

ULTRASONOGRAPHY OF THE PANCREAS

Rationale

With the use of reflected sound waves, ultrasonography of the pancreas provides diagnostic information of this inaccessible abdominal organ. Ultrasound examination of the pancreas is mainly used to diagnose carcinoma, pseudocyst, pancreatitis, and pancreatic abscess. Because abnormalities seen on ultrasound persist from several days to weeks, it can support the diagnosis of pancreatitis even after the serum amylase and lipase levels have returned to normal. Furthermore, follow-up ultrasound study is used to monitor the resolution of pancreatic inflammation and a tumor's response to therapy.

Nursing Interventions

Fluids and food are withheld for 8 hours before the examination, but fasting is not mandatory to obtain accurate results. If the patient's abdomen is distended with gas or if the patient has had a recent barium examination, postpone this study, since gas or barium interferes with sound wave transmission.

COMPUTED TOMOGRAPHY OF THE ABDOMEN

Rationale

CT scan of the abdomen is a noninvasive, accurate radiographic procedure used to diagnose pathologic pancreatic conditions such as inflammation, tumors, pseudocyst formation, ascites, aneurysms, cirrhosis, abscesses, trauma, cysts, and anatomical abnormalities. The recognizable cross-sectional image produced by a CT scan is especially important for studying the pancreas, since this organ is well hidden by the overlying peritoneal organs.

Nursing Interventions

Fluids and food are withheld from midnight until the examination is complete; however, this test can be performed on an emergency basis on patients who have recently eaten. If possible, show the patient a picture of the machine and encourage the patient to verbalize fears because some patients suffer claustrophobia when enclosed in the machine.

ENDOSCOPIC RETROGRADE CHOLANGIOPANCREATOGRAPHY OF THE PANCREATIC DUCT

Rationale

Endoscopic retrograde cholangiopancreatography (ERCP) enables visualization not only of the biliary system but also of the pancreatic duct. The test involves inserting a fiberoptic duodenoscope through the oral pharynx, through the esophagus and the stomach, and into the duodenum (Figure 46-1). Dye is injected for radiographic visualization of the common bile duct and pancreatic duct. ERCP of the pancreas is a sensitive and reliable procedure for detecting clinically significant degrees of pancreatic dysfunction. It can also be used to evaluate obstructive jaundice, remove common bile duct stones, and place biliary and pancreatic duct stents to bypass obstruction. Localized pancreatic duct narrowing indicates tumor. Chronic pancreatitis is demonstrated by multiple areas of ductal narrowing, which can be visualized by ERCP.

Nursing Interventions

Withhold food and fluids for 8 hours before the examination, and obtain the patient's signature on a consent form. Assess prothrombin time and INR before the

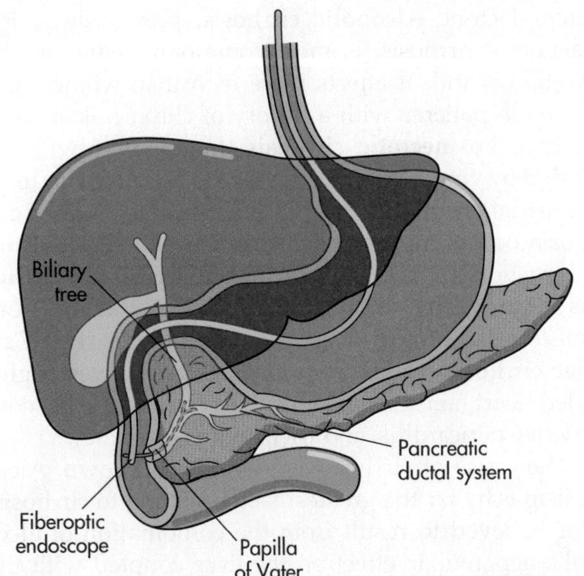

FIGURE 46-1 Endoscopic retrograde cholangiopancreatography (ERCP).

procedure. Tell patients that the test takes approximately 1 to 2 hours, during which time they must lie completely motionless on a hard x-ray table, which may be uncomfortable. After the procedure, keep the patient on NPO status until the gag reflex returns; assess for abdominal pain, tenderness, and guarding. Assess for signs and symptoms of pancreatitis (the most common ERCP complication), including increasingly intense abdominal pain, nausea, fever, chills, vomiting, and diminished or absent bowel sounds. Assess for hypovolemic shock.

DISORDERS OF THE LIVER, BILIARY TRACT, GALLBLADDER, AND EXOCRINE PANCREAS

The liver, the gallbladder, and the exocrine pancreas are all organs that assist with digestion. Review anatomy and physiology of accessory organs of digestion (see Chapter 45) and hepatic portal circulation.

CIRRHOSIS

Etiology and Pathophysiology

Cirrhosis is a chronic, degenerative disease of the liver in which the lobes are covered with fibrous tissue, the **parenchyma** (tissue of an organ, as opposed to supporting or connective tissue) degenerates, and the lobules are infiltrated with fat. The liver tries unsuccessfully to regenerate and, as a result, forms abnormal blood vessels and biliary duct abnormalities (Lewis et al., 2007). The overgrowth of new and fibrous (scar) tissue restricts the flow of blood to the organ, which contributes to its destruction. Hepatomegaly (enlargement of the liver) and, later, liver contraction cause loss of the organ's function.

Cirrhosis is ranked as the ninth leading cause of death in the United States and fourth leading cause of death in people between ages 35 and 54. The highest incidence occurs between ages 40 and 60.

There are several forms of cirrhosis, caused by different factors. **Alcoholic cirrhosis,** previously called Laennec's cirrhosis, is most commonly found in the Western world. It affects more men than women and occurs in patients with a history of chronic alcohol ingestion. **Postnecrotic cirrhosis,** found worldwide, is caused by viral hepatitis, exposure to hepatotoxins (e.g., industrial chemicals), or infection. **Primary biliary cirrhosis** occurs more often in women and results from destruction of the bile ducts. **Secondary biliary cirrhosis** is caused by chronic biliary tree obstruction from gallstones, a tumor, or biliary atresia in children. **Cardiac cirrhosis** results from longstanding, severe right-sided heart failure in patients with cor pulmonale, constrictive pericarditis, and tricuspid insufficiency.

The cause of cirrhosis is not always known. Alcoholism is by far the greatest factor leading to cirrhosis. It is believed to result from the combination of alcohol's hepatotoxic effect on the liver coupled with the common problem of protein malnutrition seen in alcoholics. Cirrhosis of the liver from severe malnutrition without alcoholism has also occurred. Patients with a diagnosis of chronic hepatitis B and C have a 10% to 20% chance of developing cirrhosis of the liver (Lewis et al., 2007).

With repeated insults, the liver progresses through the following stages: destruction, inflammation, fibrotic regeneration, and hepatic insufficiency. Although liver cells have a great potential for regeneration, repeated scarring decreases their ability to be replaced. As the blood supply continues to diminish and scar tissue increases, the organ atrophies.

Functions of the liver are altered in several ways. The liver's ability to synthesize albumin is reduced as a result of liver cell damage. Obstruction of the portal vein as it enters the liver results in portal hypertension—increased venous pressure in the portal circulation caused by compression or by occlusion in the portal or hepatic vascular system. In most instances, portal hypertension that is caused by cirrhosis is irreversible.

This increased pressure causes **ascites** (an accumulation of fluid and albumin in the peritoneal cavity). The damaged liver cannot metabolize protein in the usual manner; therefore protein intake may result in an elevation of blood ammonia levels. Reduced synthesis of protein and the leaking of existing protein result in hypoalbuminemia (reduced protein or albumin level in the blood), which reduces the blood's ability to regain fluids through osmosis. Protein must be present in adequate amounts to create colloidal osmotic pressure and "attract" the fluid to pass back into the blood vessels after it escapes in the capillaries. As fluid leaves the blood and the circulating volume decreases, the receptors in the brain signal the adrenal cortex to increase secretion of aldosterone to stimulate the kidneys to retain sodium and water. The normal liver inactivates the hormone aldosterone, but the damaged liver allows its effect to continue (hyperaldosteronism). Retention of fluid and sodium results in increased pressure in blood vessels and lymphatic channels, resulting in portal hypertension. Ascites is thus a result of portal hypertension, hypoalbuminemia, and hyperaldosteronism.

Hepatic insufficiency gradually causes distention in veins in the upper part of the body, including the esophageal vein. Esophageal varicosities develop and may rupture, causing severe hemorrhage.

Clinical Manifestations

Clinical manifestations of cirrhosis of the liver differ, depending on the stage of the disease. In the early stages the liver is firm and therefore easier to palpate, and abdominal pain may be present because rapid enlargement produces tension on the organ's fibrous covering. Later stages of the disease are characterized by dyspepsia, changes in bowel habits, gradual weight loss, ascites, enlarged spleen, malaise, nausea, jaundice, ecchymosis, and **spider telangiectases** (small, dilated blood vessels with a bright red center point and spiderlike branches). Spider telangiectases occur on the nose, cheeks, upper trunk, neck, and shoulders. These later manifestations are the result of scarring of liver tissue that produces chronic failure of liver function and also fibrotic changes that cause obstruction of the portal circulation.

When enough cells of the liver become involved to interfere with its function and obstruct its circulation, the GI organs and the spleen become congested and cannot function properly. Anemia occurs because of the body's decreased ability to produce red blood cells (RBCs). The cirrhotic liver cannot absorb vitamin K or produce the clotting factors VII, IX, and X. Thus the patient with cirrhosis develops bleeding tendencies.

Assessment

Subjective data in the **early stages** includes the patient's description of flulike symptoms, including loss of appetite, nausea and vomiting, general weakness, fatigue, indigestion, abnormal bowel function (either constipation or diarrhea), flatulence, and abdominal discomfort. The anatomical area most commonly affected is in the epigastric region or the right upper quadrant of the abdomen.

Collection of **subjective data** in the **later stages** includes noting those subjective symptoms listed under early stages, although they are more intense in later stages. The patient may complain of dyspnea, pruritus, and severe fatigue that interfere with the ability to carry out routine activities. Pruritus is a result of an accumulation of bile salts under the skin from the jaundice.

Collection of **objective data** in the **early stages** includes observing low hemoglobin, fever, **jaundice** (yellow discoloration of the skin, mucous membranes, and sclerae of the eyes [scleral icterus], caused by greater than normal amounts of bilirubin in the serum), and weight loss.

Collection of **objective data** in the **later stages** includes noting epistaxis, purpura, hematuria, spider angiomas (telangiectasis), and bleeding gums. Late symptoms are ascites, hematologic disorders, splenic enlargement, and hemorrhage from esophageal varices or other distended GI veins. The patient may also appear mentally disoriented and display abnormal behaviors and speech patterns. Any prolonged interference with gas exchange leads to hypoxia, coma, and ultimately death.

Diagnostic Tests

Many diagnostic tests aid in the diagnosis of cirrhosis. Poor liver functioning may be manifested in abnormal electrolyte values; elevated serum bilirubin, AST, ALT, LDH, and gamma GT; decreased total protein and serum albumin; elevated ammonia; low blood glucose (hypoglycemia) from impaired gluconeogenesis; prolonged prothrombin time; increased INR; and decreased cholesterol levels. Visualization through ERCP (to detect common bile duct obstruction), esophagoscopy with barium esophagography to visualize esophageal varices, scans and biopsy of the liver, and ultrasonography are used to diagnose cirrhosis. **Paracentesis** (a procedure in which fluid is withdrawn from the abdominal cavity) relieves ascites and also provides fluid for laboratory examination.

Medical Management

When possible causes have been identified, the initial treatment is to eliminate these causes, decrease the buildup of fluids in the body, prevent further damage to the liver, and provide individual supportive care. Eliminating alcohol, hepatotoxins (e.g., acetaminophen [Tylenol]), or environmental exposure to harmful chemicals is essential to prevent further damage to the liver. Diet therapy is aimed at correcting malnutrition, promoting the regeneration of functional liver tissue, and compensating for the liver's inability to store vitamins, while avoiding fluid retention and hepatic encephalopathy. A diet that is well balanced, high in calories (2500 to 3000 calories/day), moderately high in protein (75 g of high-quality protein per day), low in fat, low in sodium (1000 to 2000 mg/day), and with additional vitamins and folic acid will usually meet the needs of the patient with cirrhosis and improve deficiencies. A protein-restricted diet may be prescribed for a patient recovering from an acute episode of hepatic encephalopathy.

Antiemetics may be prescribed to control nausea or vomiting. Monitor the patient closely for toxicity, which develops quickly when the poorly functioning liver cannot clear these drugs from the system. Diphenhydramine (Benadryl) or dimenhydrinate (Dramamine) may be given, whereas prochlorperazine maleate (Compazine), hydroxyzine pamoate (Vistaril), or hydroxyzine hydrochloride (Atarax) are contraindicated in severe liver dysfunction.

Later manifestations may be severe and result from liver failure and portal hypertension. Jaundice, peripheral edema, esophageal varices, hepatic encephalopathy, and ascites develop gradually (Figure 46-2).

Complications and Treatment

Ascites is the presence of excessive fluid in the peritoneal cavity. The severity of fluid retention determines the treatment. Initially the patient is placed on bed rest with accurate monitoring of intake and output (I&O). Restrictions are placed on the amount of fluid (500 to 1000 mL) and sodium (1000 to 2000 mg). Diuretic therapy may be added if the diet does not control the ascites and edema. Spironolactone (Aldactone) 300 to 1,000 mg/day may be used to obtain the desired diuresis. Other diuretics may be added, including furosemide (Lasix) or hydrochlorothiazide (HydroDIURIL). Vitamin supplements include vitamin K, vitamin C, and folic acid. Salt-poor albumin

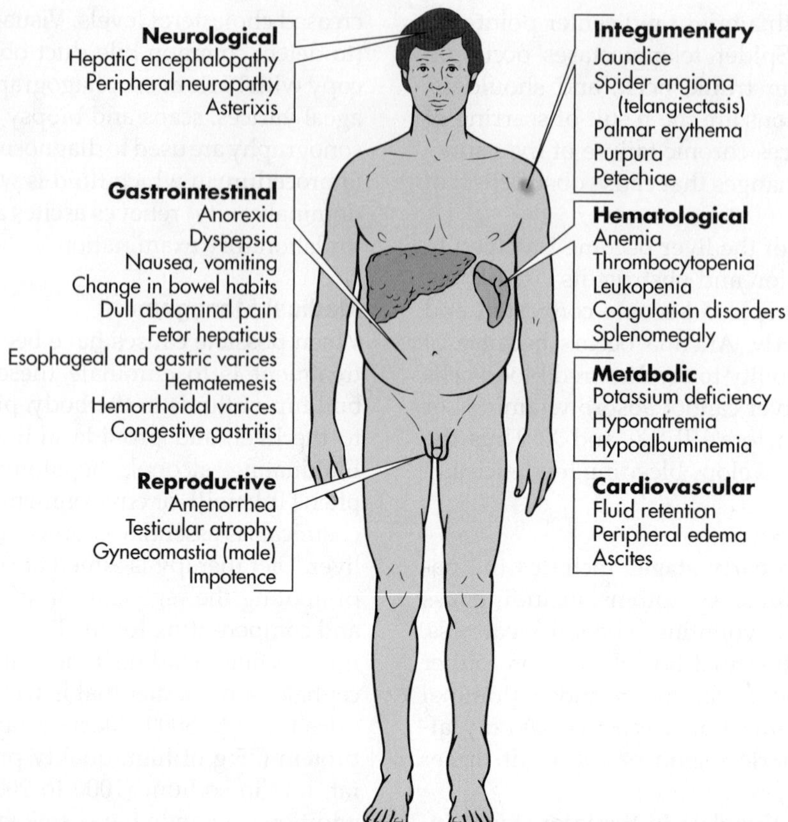

FIGURE 46-2 Systemic clinical manifestations of liver cirrhosis.

may be administered in an attempt to restore plasma volume if the intravascular volume is decreased significantly. Complications of diuretic therapy include plasma volume deficit, decreased renal function, and electrolyte imbalance.

Another method of treatment for ascites and edema is the LeVeen continuous peritoneal jugular shunt (Figure 46-3). This procedure allows the continuous shunting of ascitic fluid from the abdominal cavity through a one-way, pressure-sensitive valve into a silicone tube that empties into the superior vena cava. Monitor the patient carefully for complications, which include congestive heart failure, leakage of ascitic fluid, infection at the insertion sites, peritonitis, septicemia, and shunt thrombosis.

Paracentesis is a temporary method of removing fluid by withdrawing it from the abdominal cavity by either gravity or vacuum. Have the patient void immediately before the procedure to prevent puncture of the bladder. The patient should sit on the side of the bed or be placed in high Fowler's position. An incision is made in the skin, and a hollow trocar, cannula, or catheter is passed through the incision and into the cavity. The fluid is removed over a period of 30 to 90 minutes to prevent sudden changes in blood pressure, which could lead to syncope. Monitor the patient closely for signs of hypovolemia and electrolyte imbalances. Apply a dressing over the insertion site, and observe for bleeding and drainage.

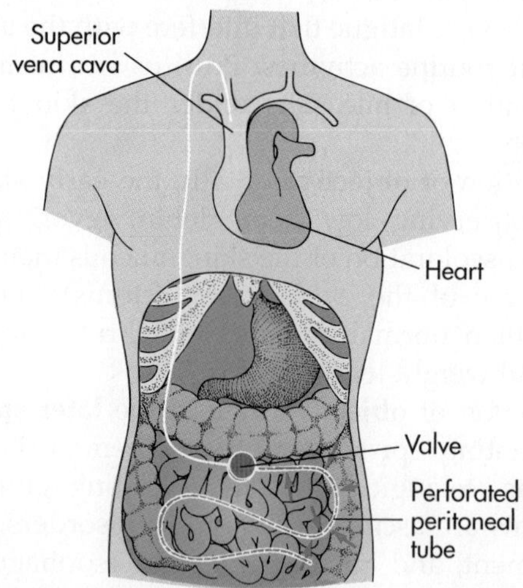

FIGURE 46-3 LeVeen continuous peritoneal jugular shunt.

Esophageal varices (a complex of longitudinal, tortuous veins at the lower end of the esophagus) enlarge and become edematous as the result of portal hypertension. They are susceptible to ulceration and hemorrhage; avoiding this is a main goal of treatment. For patients who have not bled from esophageal varices, prophylactic treatment with nonselective beta blockers (e.g., propranolol [Inderal]) has been shown to reduce the risk of bleeding and bleeding-related deaths. Varices can rupture as a result of anything that increases abdominal venous pressure, such as coughing, sneezing, vomiting, or the Valsalva maneuver. Rupture may occur slowly over several days or suddenly and without pain. An endoscopy may be performed to identify the varices or to rule out bleeding from other sources. Endoscopic therapies include sclerotherapy and ligation of varices.

Therapeutic management of a ruptured esophageal varix is a medical emergency. The patient's airway must be maintained, the bleeding varix controlled, and IV lines established for fluids and blood replacement as needed. The hormone vasopressin (VP), administered intravenously or directly into the superior vena cava, is used to decrease or stop the hemorrhaging. VP produces vasoconstriction of the vessels, decreases portal blood flow, and decreases portal hypertension. Current drug therapy in some institutions is a combination of VP and nitroglycerin (NTG). The NTG reduces the detrimental effects of VP, which are decreased coronary blood flow and increased blood pressure. VP should be avoided or used cautiously in the older adult because of the risk of cardiac ischemia. If the VP drip does not stop or control bleeding, a Sengstaken-Blakemore tube with openings at the tip may be inserted. This triple-lumen tube has a lumen for inflating the esophageal balloon, one for inflating the gastric balloon, and one for gastric lavage (Figure 46-4). The tube is passed through the nose, and the balloon in the stomach, the one in the esophagus, or both are inflated to press against the bleeding vessels and control the hemorrhage. The gastric aspiration is attached to low, intermittent suction. When either balloon is inflated, a Levin tube is passed into the esophagus through the mouth and attached to low suction to drain the saliva that cannot drain into the stomach. The balloon must be deflated periodically to prevent necrosis. Give the patient nothing by mouth and elevate the head of the bed 30 to 45 degrees to help prevent aspiration of stomach contents and help the patient breathe.

Gastric lavage is performed to remove any swallowed blood from the stomach. Some facilities use iced isotonic saline solutions for the lavage to facilitate vasoconstriction. Endoscopic sclerotherapy may also be used to control the bleeding.

Patients suffering from portal hypertension and esophageal varices may benefit from surgical shunting procedures that divert blood from the portal system to the venous system. The portacaval shunt diverts blood from the portal vein to the inferior vena cava. The splenorenal shunt requires the removal of the spleen, and the splenic vein is anastomosed to the left renal vein. The mesocaval shunt involves anastomosis of the

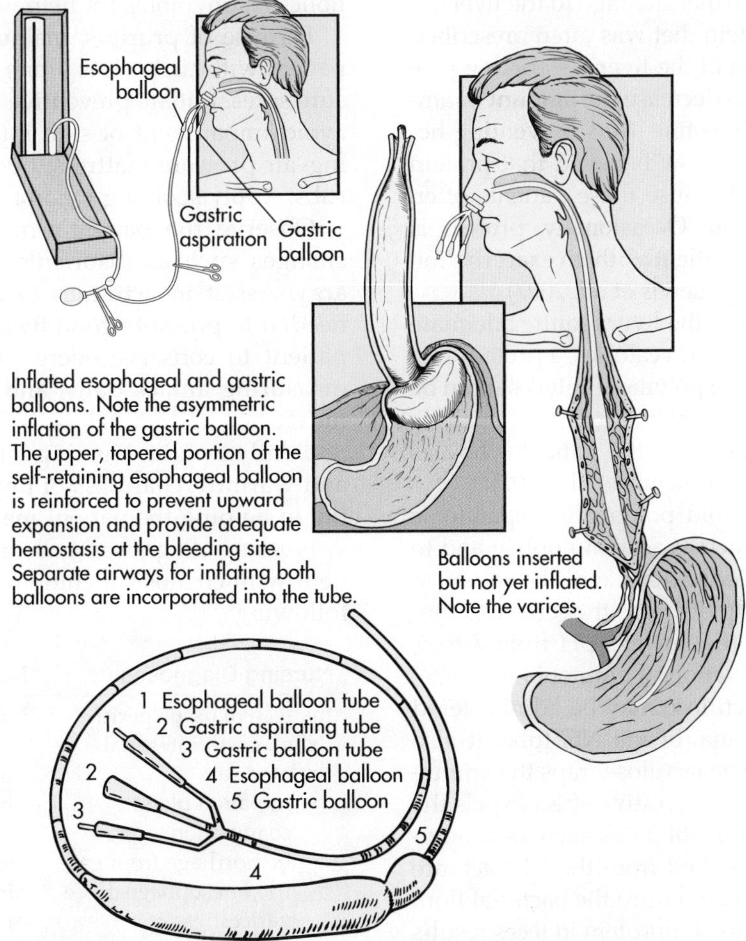

FIGURE 46-4 Esophageal tamponade accomplished with Sengstaken-Blakemore tube.

superior mesenteric vein to the inferior vena cava. These procedures are associated with a high mortality rate. They may be performed in an emergency to control acute esophageal varix bleeding or in a therapeutic situation when a patient has already bled. Complications of surgical shunting procedures are hepatic encephalopathy, GI bleeding, ascites, and liver failure.

Care of the patient who has hemorrhaged from an esophageal varix includes maintenance of oxygen content levels within the blood and administration of fresh frozen plasma and packed RBCs, vitamin K (AquaMEPHYTON), histamine (H_2) receptor blockers such as cimetidine (Tagamet), and electrolyte replacements as needed without fluid overload. Avoid ammonia buildup with the use of cathartics (e.g., lactulose [Chronulac]) and neomycin. Preventing ammonia buildup keeps hepatic encephalopathy from breaking down blood and releasing ammonia in the intestine.

Hepatic encephalopathy is a type of brain damage caused by liver disease and consequent ammonia intoxication. It is thought to result from a damaged liver being unable to metabolize substances that can be toxic to the brain, such as ammonia. The patient's signs and symptoms progress from inappropriate behavior, disorientation, flapping tremors, and twitching of the extremities to stupor and coma. Treatment of the patient with hepatic encephalopathy consists of supportive care to prevent further damage to the liver.

In the past, a low-protein diet was often prescribed for patients with cirrhosis of the liver. Restricting protein intake was thought to decrease the amount of ammonia produced in the intestine, thus preventing hepatic encephalopathy. It is now believed that protein should not be restricted because these patients often have existing malnutrition. Occasionally, protein is decreased in the diet of a patient with an exacerbation of hepatic encephalopathy (Lewis et al., 2007).

Patients with cirrhosis of the liver require adequate carbohydrates. To provide extra calories, a protein-free supplement such as glucose polymer (Polycose) can be used. Other supplemental enteral formulas such as Hepatic-Aid II may be given to the patient who has protein-calorie malnutrition (Lewis et al., 2007).

Teach the patient to avoid potentially hepatotoxic over-the-counter drugs such as acetaminophen and to abstain from alcohol. Medications may be given to cleanse the bowel and help decrease the serum ammonia. Lactulose decreases the bowel's pH from 7 to 5, thus decreasing the production of ammonia by bacteria within the bowel. Lactulose may be administered orally, as a retention enema, or via NG tube. It also functions as a cathartic. The lactulose traps the ammonia in the gut, and the drug's laxative effect expels the ammonia from the colon. Antibiotics such as neomycin, which are poorly absorbed from the GI tract, are given orally or rectally. They reduce the bacterial flora of the colon. Bacterial action on protein in feces results in ammonia production. Because neomycin may cause renal toxicity and hearing impairment, lactulose is frequently preferred.

Asterixis is a hand-flapping tremor in which the patient stretches out an arm and hyperextends the wrist with the fingers separated, relaxed, and extended. A rapid, irregular flexion and extension (flapping) of the wrist occurs in the patient who is acutely ill.

Nursing Interventions and Patient Teaching

Check vital signs every 4 hours, or more often if evidence of hemorrhage is present. Observe the patient for GI hemorrhage as evidenced by hematemesis, melena, anxiety, and restlessness.

Most patients require a well-balanced, moderate, high-protein, high-carbohydrate diet with adequate vitamins. With impending liver failure, protein and fluids are restricted. Sodium restriction is frequently necessary, which can make providing a palatable diet more difficult. Provide frequent oral hygiene and a pleasant environment to help the patient increase food intake.

A major nursing focus for many patients is helping them deal with alcoholism. This requires establishing trust that the health team is interested in the patient's well-being. Patients must admit that they have a drinking problem. Confrontation is sometimes used to help patients accept the problem. Provide information regarding community support programs, such as Alcoholics Anonymous, for help with alcohol abuse.

Because of pruritus, malnutrition, and edema, the patient with cirrhosis is prone to skin lesions and pressure sores. Initiate preventive nursing interventions to avoid impairment of skin integrity, such as alternating–air pressure mattress, frequent turning, and back rubs. Apply soothing lotion to relieve pruritus.

Observe the patient's mental status and report changes such as disorientation, headache, or lethargy. Assist in activities of daily living (ADLs) as needed to promote good hygiene while allowing the patient to conserve energy. Observe for edema by measuring ankles daily, and observe for ascites by measuring abdominal girth. Record an accurate I&O and daily weight. Nursing intervention with concern and warmth regardless of physical changes is essential in helping the patient maintain self-esteem.

Nursing diagnoses and interventions for the patient with cirrhosis include but are not limited to the following:

Nursing Diagnoses	Nursing Interventions
Ineffective tissue perfusion, gastrointestinal, related to: • impaired blood coagulation • hemorrhage from gastric or esophageal varices	Monitor patient for signs of bleeding in the gums and injection sites, decrease in blood pressure, increase in pulse, hematemesis, and melena. Monitor hemoglobin, hematocrit, prothrombin time, and INR.

Nursing Diagnoses	Nursing Interventions
Ineffective tissue perfusion, gastrointestinal, related to: • impaired blood coagulation • hemorrhage from gastric or esophageal varices—cont'd	Monitor parenteral fluids and blood transfusions. Administer vitamin K and neomycin as ordered. Instruct patient to avoid straining with stools and to avoid vigorous tooth brushing. Monitor gastric output (color and consistency).
Acute confusion, related to potential increase of serum ammonia and hepatic coma	Observe frequently for changes in mental status such as lethargy, drowsiness, and confusion. Monitor neurologic status for decreased motor ability. Encourage fluids (if not restricted). Give lactulose as ordered to decrease production of ammonia. Provide a safe environment: side rails up, bed in low position, and safety reminder devices if necessary. Avoid use of sedatives, tranquilizers, and opioids. Occasionally a low-protein diet is ordered until signs and symptoms of hepatic encephalopathy disappear, since ammonia (a breakdown product of protein) is responsible for mental changes (Lewis et al., 2007). Protein is not restricted for prolonged periods because of patient having malnutrition.

The patient with cirrhosis must understand the need for getting adequate rest and avoiding infections. Plan activity around complete bed rest until strength is regained. Turning the patient at least every 2 hours and providing range-of-motion exercises will help avoid infection and prevent thrombophlebitis. Instruct the patient to use a soft-bristled toothbrush, use an electric razor, blow nose cautiously, and avoid straining at stools to prevent bleeding as a result of a lack of vitamin K and certain clotting factors. Avoid soap, perfumed lotion, and rubbing alcohol because they will further dry the skin. For pruritus and dry skin, administer diphenhydramine (Benadryl). Explain the relationship of the therapeutic diet to the diagnosis and the liver's ability to function.

Help the patient and family identify community resources for home health care and alcohol rehabilitation to help them deal with problems that arise after discharge. Because of the seriousness of the disease, the patient and the family need understanding and support throughout the treatment (see Home Care Considerations box).

Prognosis

The prognosis for cirrhosis of the liver is related to the cause of the disease, the patient's general health status, and the extent of the involvement. Fibrosis of the cirrhotic liver cannot be cured, but its progression may be halted or slowed by proper management by the physician, the nurse, the patient, and family members (Nursing Care Plan 46-1). For patients who have recurring problems of hepatic encephalopathy or who are in the late stages of cirrhosis, a liver transplant may be an option (Lewis et al., 2007).

LIVER CANCER

Etiology and Pathophysiology

Primary liver cancer is the seventh most common cancer in men and the ninth most common in women. The type of primary liver cancer seen most frequently is hepatocellular carcinoma; the other primary tumors are cholangiomas or biliary duct carcinomas. Cirrhosis of the liver and infection with hepatitis C or hepatitis B are high-risk factors in primary liver cancer. The increase in cases of primary liver cancer stems from the increased incidence of hepatitis C. In the United States, liver cancer usually occurs in people over 40 years of age.

Metastatic carcinoma of the liver occurs more often than primary liver cancer because of the portal vein circulation with its high rate of blood flow and extensive capillary structure. Malignant cells from other areas of the body migrate to the liver by means of the portal vein (Lewis et al., 2007). Cancer cells often cause hepatomegaly. The tumors can also invade nearby organs and structures such as the gallbladder, the peritoneum, the diaphragm, or the lungs (Lewis et al., 2007).

Home Care Considerations

Cirrhosis of the Liver

- The patient and the family need to understand the importance of continual health care and medical supervision.
- Encourage measures to achieve and maintain remission. These include proper diet, rest, avoidance of potentially hepatotoxic over-the-counter drugs (e.g., acetaminophen [Tylenol]), and abstinence from alcohol.
- Provide information regarding community support programs, such as Alcoholics Anonymous, for help with alcohol abuse.
- Help the patient maintain the highest level of wellness possible and initiate and maintain necessary lifestyle changes.

Nursing Care Plan 46-1 The Patient with Cirrhosis of the Liver

Mr. Kaplan, 49 years of age, is admitted with loss of appetite, generalized edema, pruritus, flappy tremors of the hands, ascites, and lethargy. He appears disoriented. His skin has areas of excoriation caused by scratching and a sallow appearance. His wife states that he has been unable to concentrate, appears confused and listless, and has been eating poorly. Mr. Kaplan has been an alcoholic for the past 18 years. His total bilirubin is 4.5 mg/dL, gamma GT is 65 units/L, total protein is 4.8 g/dL, albumin is 2.8 g/dL, and blood ammonia is 160 mcg/dL. He is demonstrating signs and symptoms of hepatic encephalopathy.

NURSING DIAGNOSIS ***Imbalanced nutrition: less than body requirements, related to anorexia, nausea, and impaired utilization and storage of nutrients, as manifested by lack of interest in food, aversion to eating, inadequate food intake***

Patient Goals and Expected Outcomes	Nursing Interventions	Evaluation/Rationale
Patient will eat 50% of meal Patient will maintain baseline body weight	Monitor weight to determine whether weight loss occurs. Provide oral care before meals to remove foul taste and improve taste of food. Administer antiemetics as ordered to relieve nausea and vomiting. Provide small, frequent meals at times the patient can best tolerate them to prevent feeling of fullness and to maintain nutritional status. Determine food preferences and allow these whenever possible to increase appeal of food for patient.	Patient is eating 50% to 75% of his meals. Patient has no weight loss indicating maintaining satisfactory nutritional balance.

NURSING DIAGNOSIS ***Acute confusion, related to increased formation of ammonia as manifested by inability to concentrate, lethargy, disorientation, and flappy tremors of the hands***

Patient Goals and Expected Outcomes	Nursing Interventions	Evaluation
Patient will be oriented to person, place, time, and purpose	Monitor for hepatic encephalopathy by assessing patient's general behavior, orientation to time and place, speech, and ammonia levels, since liver is unable to convert accumulating ammonia to urea for renal excretion. Encourage fluids (if not restricted), and give laxatives and enemas as ordered to decrease ammonia production. Provide prescribed protein-restricted diet until acute clinical signs and symptoms of hepatic encephalopathy are decreased. Administer lactulose (Chronulac) or neomycin (Mycifradin) as prescribed. Limit physical activity because exercise produces ammonia as a by-product of metabolism. Control factors known to precipitate hepatic coma.	Patient responds appropriately to assessment of person, place, time, and purpose.

Critical Thinking Questions

1. Mr. Kaplan is thrashing about in his bed and has attempted to climb over the side rails. He is disoriented to time and place. What appropriate nursing interventions will ensure Mr. Kaplan's safety?
2. Mrs. Kaplan notes that her husband has a low-protein diet. She confides to the nurse that she thinks he needs more meat, eggs, and cottage cheese to improve his nutrition. What is the most appropriate response?

Clinical Manifestations and Diagnostic Tests

Diagnosing carcinoma of the liver is difficult. In its early stages many of the clinical manifestations (e.g., hepatomegaly, weight loss, peripheral edema, ascites, portal hypertension) are similar to those of cirrhosis of the liver. Other common manifestations include dull abdominal pain in the epigastric or right upper quadrant region, jaundice, anorexia, nausea and vomiting, and extreme weakness. Palpation may reveal an enlarged, nodular liver. Patients frequently have pulmonary emboli. Tests to assist in the diagnosis are a liver scan, ultrasound, CT scan, magnetic resonance imaging, hepatic arteriography, ERCP, and liver biopsy needle. The test for alpha-fetoprotein (AFP) may be positive in hepatocellular carcinoma. AFP helps distinguish primary cancer from metastatic cancer.

Medical Management and Nursing Interventions

Treatment of cancer of the liver is largely palliative. Surgical excision (lobectomy) is sometimes performed if the tumor is localized to one portion of the liver. Only 5% of patients have surgically resectable disease;

usually the cancer is too advanced for surgery when it is detected. Surgical excision or transplant offers the only chance for cure. Medical management is similar to that for cirrhosis of the liver. Chemotherapy may be used, but the response is usually poor. Portal vein or hepatic artery perfusion with 5-fluorouracil (5-FU) may be attempted.

Nursing interventions for the patient with liver carcinoma focus on keeping the patient as comfortable as possible. Because the problems are the same as with advanced liver disease, the nursing interventions discussed for cirrhosis of the liver apply.

Prognosis

The prognosis for cancer of the liver is poor. The cancer grows rapidly, and death may occur within 4 to 7 months as a result of hepatic encephalopathy or massive blood loss from GI bleeding.

HEPATITIS

Etiology and Pathophysiology

Hepatitis is an inflammation of the liver resulting from several types of viral agents or exposure to toxic substances. Rarely, hepatitis is caused by bacteria, such as streptococci, salmonellae, or *Escherichia coli.*

The six types of viral hepatitis are caused by distinct but similar viruses that produce almost identical signs and symptoms but vary in their incubation period, mode of transmission, and prognosis. Hepatitis A (formerly called infectious hepatitis) is the most common form today and is a short-incubation virus (10 to 40 days). Hepatitis B (formerly called serum hepatitis) is a long-incubation virus (28 to 160 days). Hepatitis C has an incubation period of 2 weeks to 6 months (commonly 6 to 9 weeks). Hepatitis D (also called delta virus) causes hepatitis as a coinfection with hepatitis B and may progress to cirrhosis and chronic hepatitis. The incubation period is 2 to 10 weeks. Hepatitis E (also called enteric non-A–non-B hepatitis) is transmitted through fecal contamination of water, primarily in developing countries. It is rare in the United States. The incubation period is 15 to 64 days. Recently hepatitis G virus has been discovered. Hepatitis G virus has been found in blood donors and can be transmitted by transfusion. It frequently coexists with other hepatitis viruses, such as hepatitis C.

Health officials are required by law to report all cases of viral hepatitis to the Centers for Disease Control and Prevention (CDC) in Atlanta. Modes of transmission for the different types of hepatitis are listed in Box 46-1.

! Safety Alert!

Prevention of Acute Viral Hepatitis

HEPATITIS A

- Wash your hands. Hepatitis A virus (HAV) is transmitted when people put something in their mouths that is contaminated with fecal material (called "fecal-oral transmission"). Teach patients the importance of good hand hygiene after using the bathroom or changing a diaper, as well as proper food preparation, to prevent the spread of HAV.
- The best protection against HAV transmission is the two-dose HAV vaccine.

HEPATITIS B

- Wash your hands.
- One of the best preventive measures against hepatitis B virus (HBV) is the HBV vaccine.
- Children younger than 18 years of age are routinely vaccinated today.
- People who are at risk for the virus, such as health care workers, should be vaccinated.
- People who play or work in inner-city parks and playgrounds are at risk for exposure to HBV from litter containers and used needles and syringes. They should be vaccinated, as should men who have sex with men, individuals who use illicit IV drugs, and those who travel to areas with a high infection rate.
- People who are positive for HBV should not donate blood, organs, or tissue.
- Ensure proper disposal of needles.
- Use Standard Precautions when handling blood products.
- Use needleless IV access devices if available.

HEPATITIS C

- Wash your hands.
- Hepatitis C virus is transmitted by needle sharing among illicit IV drug users.
- Other significant risk factors include receipt of clotting factor made before 1987, hemodialysis, receipt of blood or solid organs donated before 1992, maternal-fetal transmission, and multiple or infected sex partners.
- Ensure proper disposal of needles.
- Use standard precautions when handling blood products.
- Use needleless IV access devices if available.

HEPATITIS D

- Modes of hepatitis D virus (HDV) transmission are similar to those of HBV. Sexual transmission of HDV is less efficient than for HBV. Educate patients regarding risky behavior.

HEPATITIS E

- Educate patients to avoid drinking water or beverages with ice in areas with uncertain water quality. They should refrain from eating raw shellfish and avoid raw produce unless it is prepared with purified water.
- Hepatitis E is most often seen in southeastern and central Asia, the Middle East, Africa, and Mexico.

HEPATITIS G

- Hepatitis G has been detected in blood samples in Europe, Asia, and Australia.
- Transmission of hepatitis G virus occurs when tainted injectable drugs are used; tainted blood, organs, or tissues are received through hemodialysis; or unsafe methods are used for tattooing or body piercing.

Box 46-1 Modes of Transmission of the Six Types of Viral Hepatitis

- Hepatitis A spreads by direct contact through the oral-fecal route, usually by food or water contaminated with feces. Up to 50% of all people in the United States have been infected by the time they reach adulthood; most suffer minimal symptoms or none at all. Two or more weeks before symptoms appear, the virus can be found in the bile, blood, and stool. Patients are rarely infectious once they develop jaundice (Durston, 2004).
- Hepatitis B is transmitted by contaminated serum via blood transfusion, contaminated needles and instruments, needlesticks, illicit intravenous (IV) drug use, and dialysis, and by direct contact with body fluids from infected people, such as breast milk and sexual contact. An ever-increasing risk comes from improper disposal of used needles and syringes. Sharing toothbrushes, razor blades, or personal items with an infected person may also lead to exposure.
- Hepatitis C (HCV) is transmitted through needlesticks, blood transfusions, illicit IV drug use, and unidentified means. HCV can also be transmitted by sharing contaminated straws used for snorting cocaine. In the past, hepatitis C could not be detected in banked blood, so it was more easily transmitted through transfusion. The advent of routine blood screening in 1992 greatly reduced the number of cases of transfusion-related hepatitis C.
- Hepatitis D is transmitted the same way as hepatitis B; it appears as a coinfection of hepatitis B.
- Hepatitis E is transmitted by the oral-fecal route; it spreads through the fecal contamination of water.
- Hepatitis G is frequently seen as a coinfection with hepatitis C; it spreads through bloodborne exposure. Hepatitis G has been found in some blood donors and can be transmitted by transfusion. Transmission occurs through contaminated injectable drugs; contaminated blood, organs, or tissues; hemodialysis; or unsafe methods of tattooing or body piercing.

The basic pathologic findings in the six forms of viral hepatitis are identical. A diffuse inflammatory reaction occurs, liver cells begin to degenerate and die, and the liver's normal functions slow down. The outcome may be affected by the virulence of the virus, the liver's preexisting condition, the health care given when the disease is diagnosed, and patient compliance with treatment.

Clinical Manifestations

The clinical manifestations for viral hepatitis vary greatly; some patients are asymptomatic, whereas others develop hepatic failure or hepatic encephalopathy.

Assessment

Subjective data include patients' reports of general malaise, aching muscles, photophobia, lassitude, headaches, and chills. Abdominal pain, dyspepsia, nausea, diarrhea, and constipation are reported also. The patient may complain of pruritus from bile on the skin. The patient complains of tenderness in the liver and remains fatigued for several weeks.

Collection of **objective data** includes observing hepatomegaly, enlarged lymph nodes, weight loss, and rhinitis. Jaundice appears because of the damaged liver's inability to metabolize bilirubin; the resultant signs are yellowish skin, discoloration of the sclera (scleral icterus) and mucous membrane (Figure 46-5), dark tea-colored urine, and clay-colored stools. Relapses are common in the convalescent stage.

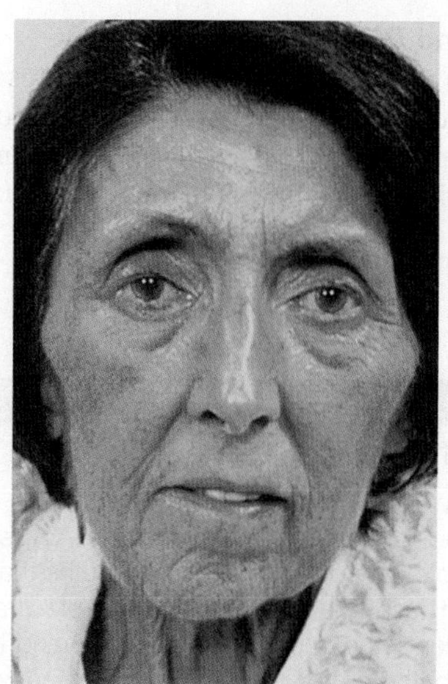

FIGURE 46-5 Severe jaundice.

Diagnostic Tests

Changes in the liver caused by viral hepatitis result in elevated direct bilirubin, gamma GT, AST, ALT, LDH, and alkaline phosphatase levels; a prolonged prothrombin time and increased INR; and, in severe hepatitis, decreased serum albumin. Leukopenia is common in these patients, with a transient neutropenia and lymphopenia, followed by lymphocytosis. Hypoglycemia is present in approximately 50% of patients with hepatitis. Serum is examined for the presence of hepatitis-associated antigen A, B, C, D, or G. A CT of the abdomen reveals hepatomegaly.

Medical Management

Providing supportive therapy for existing signs and symptoms and preventing transmission of the disease are important aspects of treatment of the patient with viral hepatitis. Hospitalization is an option for patients whose bilirubin concentrations in the blood are more than 10 mg/dL and for those with a prolonged prothrombin time and increased INR, but usually patients are cared for at home. Bed rest for several weeks is commonly prescribed.

Drug therapy for chronic hepatitis B focuses on decreasing the viral load, decreasing the rate of disease progression, and monitoring for detection of drug-resistant HBV. At present, several drugs are useful in suppressing viral activity and decreasing viral load in patients with HBV. However, the percentage of patients seroconverting (developing antibodies against the virus) remains relatively low. Lamivudine (Epivir, 3TC), interferon-α, and adefovir dipivoxil (Hepsera) are three drugs being used in the treatment of chronic hepatitis B. Telbivudine (Tyzeka) is a new drug used to treat chronic HBV infection. Telbivudine has been shown to decrease the viral load more effectively than lamivudine and adefovir (Hussar, 2007).

In chronic hepatitis C, drug therapy is also directed at reducing the viral load, decreasing progression of the disease, and promoting seroconversion. Treatment options for HCV are interferon alfa-2b (Intron A), ribavirin (Rebetol), and pegylated interferon alfa-2a (Pegasys). This combination therapy eradicates the virus more effectively than monotherapy. Another treatment option is liver transplantation. In fact half of all liver recipients are HCV positive. Most transplanted livers eventually become infected with HCV, but recipients can increase both quantity and quality of life by avoiding risky behaviors (Durston, 2004).

The patient is not allowed alcohol for at least 1 year and may need supportive care from the community to comply. Most patients tolerate small, frequent meals of a low-fat, high-carbohydrate diet. If the patient is dehydrated, IV fluids are given with addition of vitamin C for healing, vitamin B complex to assist the damaged liver's inability to absorb fat-soluble vitamins, and vitamin K to combat prolonged coagulation time. Avoid all unnecessary medications, particularly sedatives.

Give gamma globulin or immune serum globulin as soon as possible to people who have been in direct contact with a person with hepatitis A during the infectious period (2 weeks before and 1 week after onset of symptoms). The dosage of 0.02 mL/kg of body weight, given intramuscularly, is effective in preventing hepatitis A in 80% to 90% of cases. Currently three vaccines are used to prevent hepatitis A: Havrix, Vaqta, and Avaxim.

Primary immunization consists of a single dose administered intramuscularly in the deltoid muscle. A booster is recommended between 6 and 12 months after the primary dose to ensure adequate antibody titers and long-term protection. However, primary immunization provides immunity within 30 days after a single dose.

Until routine vaccination of children is feasible, people who are at risk for infection should be vaccinated for hepatitis A. This includes people traveling to countries where hepatitis A is endemic; sexually active homosexual and bisexual men; patients with chronic liver disease; injecting drug users; and people at risk for occupational infection, such as those who work with hepatitis A in research laboratory settings.

Individuals who have been exposed to HBV via a needle puncture or sexual contact should be protected with hepatitis B immune globulin. A dose of 0.06 mL/kg of body weight is administered intramuscularly as quickly after exposure as possible. This dose is repeated 1 month later. People identified as being at high risk for developing hepatitis B should be vaccinated if they are not already immune. These people include the following:

- All health care personnel (especially emergency department, operating room, intensive care unit [ICU], and dialysis personnel; phlebotomists; and laboratory technicians)
- People with high-risk lifestyles (drug users, tattoo recipients, homosexual men, and prostitutes)
- Infants born to mothers who are hepatitis B surface antigen positive
- Hemodialysis patients
- Individuals sharing a household with an infected person

The CDC Immunization Practices Advisory Committee (2009) recommends making hepatitis B vaccine a part of routine vaccination schedules for all newborns and adolescents. The protection program consists of three vaccinations: an initial vaccination, a vaccination 1 month later, and a third vaccination 6 months after the first injection. The hepatitis B vaccine has been shown to provide protection for 3 to 5 years in approximately 90% of the people treated. It is hoped that universal vaccination will lead to eventual prevention and control of hepatitis B.

Hepatitis B, C, D, and G are spread through blood transfusions. The blood used should be screened for elevated ALT and anti–hepatitis B core, anti–hepatitis C, anti–hepatitis D, and anti–hepatitis G.

Liver Transplantation

The first human liver transplant was performed in 1963. Liver transplantation has become a practical therapeutic option for many people with end-stage liver disease, generally improving their quality of life. Indications for liver transplantation include congenital biliary abnormalities, inborn errors of metabolism, hepatic malignancy (confined to the liver), sclerosing cholangitis, and chronic end-stage liver disease. Liver disease related to chronic viral hepatitis is the leading indication for liver transplantation. Liver transplants are not recommended for the patient with widespread malignant disease. There are approximately 17,000 people waiting for liver transplants; however, only 6000 transplants are performed annually (Verna & Brown, n.d.; McCaughan et al., 2005).

The major postoperative complications are rejection and infection. Liver transplant candidates must go through a rigorous presurgery screening. However, the liver seems to be less susceptible to rejection than the kidney.

The source of a liver used for transplantation may be a deceased (cadaver) donor or a live donor. The live donor donates only a portion of his or her liver to the recipient. The donor faces potential risks, however, such as biliary problems, hepatic artery thrombosis, wound infection, postoperative paralytic ileus, and pneumothorax (Lewis et al., 2007).

The use of cyclosporine, an effective immunosuppressant drug, has been a major factor in the success rates of liver transplantation. It does not cause bone marrow suppression and does not impede wound healing. Other immunosuppressants used include azathioprine (Imuran), corticosteroids, tacrolimus (Prograf) and mycophenolate mofetil (Cellcept), New agents, including the interleukin-2 receptor antagonists basiliximab (Simulect) and daclizumab (Zenapax), are being used in combination with other immunosuppressive agents to reduce rejection. Other factors in the improved success rate are advances in surgical techniques, better selection of potential recipients, and improved management of the underlying liver disease before surgery.

Patients who have liver disease secondary to viral hepatitis often experience reinfection of the transplanted liver with hepatitis B or C. HCV recurrence as evidenced by histologic damage is almost universal after transplant. Approximately 20% to 30% of patients develop cirrhosis of the transplanted liver by the fifth year posttransplant. Antiviral therapy for HCV initiated posttransplant, even before the development of histologic evidence of recurrence, has failed to alter this recurrence pattern. Approximately 75% of patients survive more than 3 years following transplants (Lewis et al., 2007).

Nursing Interventions and Patient Teaching

The patient who has a liver transplant requires competent and highly skilled nursing interventions, in either an ICU or another specialized unit. Postoperative nursing care includes assessing neurologic status; monitoring for signs of hemorrhage; preventing pulmonary complications; monitoring drainage, electrolyte levels, and urinary output; and monitoring for signs and symptoms of infection and rejection. Common respiratory problems are pneumonia, atelectasis, and pleural effusions. Have the patient use measures such as coughing, deep breathing, incentive spirometry, and repositioning to prevent these complications. Measure and record drainage from the Jackson-Pratt drain, NG tube suctioning, and T-tube, and note the color and consistency of drainage. A critical aspect of nursing interventions after liver transplantation is monitoring for infection. The first 2 months after the surgery are critical. Infection can be viral, fungal, or bacterial. Fever may be the only sign of infection. Emotional support and teaching the patient and family are essential.

The care of the patient with viral hepatitis includes ensuring rest, maintaining adequate nutrition, providing adequate fluids, and caring for the skin. The care of the patient with hepatitis continues over time, and support and patient education are necessary throughout the entire illness.

Preventing transmission of the disease is of primary importance in caring for the patient with viral hepatitis. The patient, family, and health care providers must be knowledgeable about routes of transmission of the virus and take steps to avoid such transmission. Proper personal hygiene and good sanitation, as well as hepatitis A vaccine, will help prevent the spread of hepatitis A. Give patients a thorough explanation of the reasons for the precautions, and instruct them in the proper handling of their own secretions and body wastes and in thorough methods of hand hygiene. Wear gown and gloves when handling excreta, giving enemas, taking rectal temperatures, handling food waste, handling needles, disposing of urine, or carrying out any other procedure or hygiene measure that involves direct contact with the patient's body fluids.

When a patient has hepatitis B, take utmost care in handling syringes, needles, and other instruments that are contaminated with the patient's serum. Use disposable equipment and dishes and take isolation precautions. Maintaining standard precautions while exposed to blood and body fluids such as saliva, semen, and vaginal secretions is essential to prevent the transmission of hepatitis B. Use enteric precautions for 7 days after onset of hepatitis A. Use standard precautions for all patients.

Nursing diagnoses and interventions for the patient with hepatitis include but are not limited to the following:

Nursing Diagnoses	Nursing Interventions
Risk for injury, related to: • poor nutrition • prolonged clotting times	Pad side rails if necessary. Assist weakened patient with activities. Encourage use of electric razor and soft toothbrush.
Imbalanced nutrition: less than body requirements, related to: • anorexia • nausea • vomiting • altered metabolism of nutrients by the liver	Provide diet high in carbohydrates and low in fats, and encourage total fluid intake of 2500 to 3000 mL daily. Monitor I&O. Monitor daily weight. Note color and consistency of stool and color and amount of urine. Administer antiemetics as ordered. Offer support and understanding. Promote adequate rest.

For the patient with viral hepatitis being cared for at home, teach the family necessary precautions. Patients should avoid sexual activity during the acute stage of hepatitis B, C, and D. Patients with hepatitis must wash hands thoroughly after toileting, must disinfect articles soiled with feces (boil 1 minute), and must not prepare foods for others while symptomatic. If possible, the patient should use separate bathroom facilities. Personal care items and drinking glasses should not be shared. The patient's clothes should be laundered separately in hot water. Contaminated items should be disposed of properly.

Inform the patient and family about signs and symptoms associated with hepatitis, including light-colored stools, dark-colored urine, jaundice, fever, GI disturbances, unusual bleeding that might be indicative of a prolonged prothrombin time and increased INR, and tenderness or pain in the abdomen. The danger of alcohol use and its effect on the liver should be clearly understood.

Prognosis

The prognosis of hepatitis differs with the causative agent. Recovery from hepatitis A is high, with a mortality rate of 0.5%. Mortality from hepatitis B has been reported to be as high as 10%. Hepatitis B is a very serious form of hepatitis, often progressing to cirrhosis, chronic hepatitis, liver cancer, and death. Hepatitis C often progresses to chronic hepatitis, cirrhosis, liver cancer, and death. There is a greater risk for hepatitis C infection becoming chronic compared with hepatitis B. Approximately 75% to 80% of patients who acquire HCV go on to develop chronic infection, and 20% develop liver failure. The prognosis of chronic hepatitis C infection has greatly increased the demand for liver transplants. Hepatitis D may progress to cirrhosis and chronic hepatitis. It has a high mortality rate. Hepatitis E has a 10% mortality rate in pregnant women; otherwise it is not believed to be fatal. Hepatitis G infections frequently coexist with other hepatitis infections, such as hepatitis C. However, most hepatitis G infections are not associated with chronic hepatitis; thus hepatitis G virus's association with liver disease is, at this time, uncertain.

Recovery from acute toxic hepatitis is rapid if the hepatotoxin is identified early and removed or if exposure to the agent has been limited. However, the prognosis is poor if the period between exposure and the onset of signs and symptoms is prolonged, since there are no effective antidotes.

LIVER ABSCESSES

If an infection develops anywhere along the GI tract, there is danger of the infecting organisms reaching the liver through the biliary system, portal venous system, or hepatic arterial or lymphatic systems. Most bacteria are promptly destroyed, but occasionally some gain a foothold. If the disease progresses, it can become life threatening. In the past the mortality rate with liver abscesses was 100% because of the vague clinical symptoms, inadequate diagnostic tools, and inadequate surgical drainage. Today medical management is more successful.

Etiology and Pathophysiology

If the body is not successful in destroying bacteria, the bacterial toxins attack neighboring liver cells, and the necrotic tissue produced serves as a protective wall for the organism. Meanwhile, leukocytes migrate into the infected area. The result is an abscess cavity full of a liquid containing living and dead leukocytes and bacteria. Pyogenic (pus-producing) abscesses of this type may be single or multiple.

Clinical Manifestations

Patients with liver abscess are seen with vague signs and symptoms. Fever accompanied by chills, abdominal pain, and tenderness in the right upper quadrant of the abdomen are common complaints.

Assessment

Subjective data include chills, complaints of dull abdominal pain, abdominal tenderness, and discomfort.

Objective data include fever, hepatomegaly, jaundice, and anemia.

Diagnostic Tests

The diagnosis is established by demonstrating a space-occupying lesion in the liver radiographically (radiograph, ultrasound, CT, and liver scan). Amebic (microscopic, single-celled parasite) liver abscess can also be confirmed by amebic serologic examination (laboratory examination of antigen-antibody reaction of amebae in serum).

Medical Management

Usually liver abscesses are managed by medical therapy. Treatment includes IV antibiotic therapy that is specific to the organism identified.

Percutaneous (performed through the skin) drainage of a liver abscess is reserved for patients who do not respond to medical therapy or are at high risk for rupture. Open surgical drainage has been the standard in patients whose liver abscesses have ruptured into the peritoneal space, but some of these patients are now being managed with percutaneous drainage. All patients require a full course of antibiotic therapy.

Nursing Interventions and Patient Teaching

Continuous monitoring and supportive care are indicated because of the seriousness of the patient's condition. Monitoring objective and subjective symptoms is important. Notify the physician if signs and symptoms increase in depth and severity.

The patient's response to drug therapy is determined by a decrease in fever, tenderness and rigidity of the abdomen, chills, and discomfort. If percutaneous or open surgical drainage is instituted, observe the drainage for amount, color, and consistency.

Nursing diagnoses and interventions for the patient with a liver abscess include but are not limited to the following:

Nursing Diagnoses	Nursing Interventions
Risk for imbalanced body temperature, related to infectious state	Check temperature as ordered by physician or as indicated by the patient's worsening condition, and report findings to physician. Encourage fluids to prevent dehydration. Monitor IV fluids. Explain how fever and drainage can deplete fluids in the body. Record I&O. Monitor oral mucous membranes and skin turgor.
Deficient knowledge, related to relationship of infection to nutritional needs	Explain the body's need for added calories and protein to fight infection. Weigh patient daily for weight gain or loss to determine adequate nutritional intake.

In addition to the relationship of infection and nutrition, teach preoperative and postoperative procedures if the patient requires percutaneous or open surgical drainage. A thorough explanation and assessment for the patient's understanding are necessary. The seriously ill patient becomes less anxious as the knowledge base increases and the patient feels more in control of the situation.

Prognosis

The prognosis for patients with liver abscesses was very poor in the past, with a mortality rate of 100%. The prognosis today is much improved because of advanced diagnostic tests, including CT and liver scans, and aggressive medical and nursing interventions.

CHOLECYSTITIS AND CHOLELITHIASIS

Etiology and Pathophysiology

Disorders of the biliary system are common in the United States and are responsible for the hospitalization of more than a half million people a year. The two most common conditions are cholecystitis (inflammation of the gallbladder) and cholelithiasis (presence of gallstones in the gallbladder) (Box 46-2). These two diseases are seen more commonly in women than men; in Native Americans and whites than in Asian Americans and blacks; and in obese people, pregnant women, multiparous women, women who use birth control pills, and people with diabetes.

Box 46-2 Definitions

chole- pertaining to bile
cholang- pertaining to bile ducts
cholangiography radiographic examination of bile ducts
cholangitis inflammation of bile duct
cholecyst- pertaining to gallbladder
cholecystectomy removal of gallbladder
cholecystitis inflammation of gallbladder
cholecystography radiographic examination of gallbladder
cholecystostomy incision into the gallbladder (usually for drainage)
choledocho- pertaining to common bile duct
choledocholithiasis stones in common bile duct
choledochostomy exploration of common bile duct
cholelith- gallstone
cholelithiasis presence of gallstones

Cholecystitis can be caused by an obstruction, a gallstone, or a tumor. More than 90% of cases are caused by gallstones. The exact cause of stone formation in the gallbladder and the common bile duct is not known. However, an alteration in lipid metabolism and the role of female sex hormones are related to the disease. The stones usually occur in multiples but can occur singly (Figure 46-6).

When an obstruction, gallstone, or tumor prevents bile from leaving the gallbladder, the trapped bile acts as an irritant, causing cellular infiltration of the gallbladder wall after 3 to 4 days. A typical inflammatory response occurs, and the gallbladder becomes enlarged and edematous. The vascular occlusion along with bile

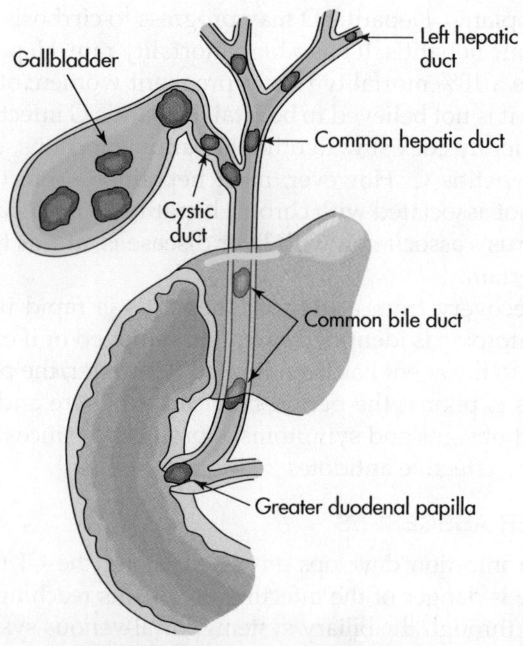

FIGURE 46-6 Common sites of gallstones.

stasis causes the mucosal lining of the gallbladder to become necrotic. Initially the bile in the gallbladder is sterile. The bacterial growth is caused by the ischemia and occurs usually within a few days. The gallbladder is in danger of rupturing and spreading infection to the hepatic duct and liver. When the disease is severe enough to interfere with the blood supply, the gallbladder wall may become gangrenous.

Clinical Manifestations

The condition may be acute, with a sudden onset of indigestion; nausea and vomiting; and severe, colicky pain in the right upper quadrant of the abdomen. The pain may be referred to the right shoulder and scapula. If the condition is chronic, the patient usually has had several milder attacks of pain and a history of fat intolerance. Many patients with gallstones are asymptomatic, and the gallstones are discovered only during an examination for another problem. The patient complains of more severe pain if the gallstones are mobile and moving through the biliary ducts. A gallstone occluding a biliary duct or a stone passing through the ducts may trigger a biliary spasm (Lewis et al., 2007).

Assessment

Subjective data include complaints of indigestion after eating foods high in fat. The pain of acute cholecystitis is abrupt in onset, reaches peak intensity quickly, and remains at that level for 2 to 4 hours. It localizes in the right upper quadrant epigastric region. The pain radiates around the midtorso to the right scapular area. Anorexia, nausea, vomiting, and **flatulence** (excess formation of gases in the stomach or intestine) are also noted. Patients may experience increased heart and respiratory rates and become diaphoretic, leading them to think they are having a heart attack. These symptoms are decreased or absent in patients with chronic cholecystitis.

Objective data include a low-grade fever, increased pulse and respirations, nausea, vomiting, an elevated leukocyte count, mild jaundice, stools that contain fat **(steatorrhea),** and clay-colored stools caused by a lack of bile in the intestinal tract. The urine may be dark amber to tea colored and contain urobilinogen as the kidneys try to remove the excess bilirubin from the bloodstream.

Diagnostic Tests

A number of diagnostic studies are performed to confirm a diagnosis of cholecystitis and cholelithiasis. Fecal studies, serum bilirubin tests, ultrasound of the gallbladder and biliary system, HIDA scan, and OCG may be done. Ultrasound of the gallbladder is 90% to 95% accurate in diagnosing cholelithiasis. HIDA scanning is helpful in assessing the patency of the cystic and common bile ducts. Operative cholangiography—in which the common bile duct is directly injected with radiopaque dye—is frequently done at the time of gallbladder surgery.

Medical Management

If the attack of cholelithiasis is mild, the patient is treated conservatively. Bed rest is prescribed, an NG tube is inserted and connected to low suction, and the patient is placed on NPO status. This allows the GI tract and thus the gallbladder to rest. IV fluids are given to rehydrate the patient and replace drainage from the NG tube.

Antispasmodic and analgesic drugs may be given to decrease pain. Meperidine (Demerol) is commonly used, since it decreases the incidence of spasms of the sphincter of Oddi. Morphine may be used for pain management. Antibiotics may be given (1) prophylactically to prevent infection; (2) to treat an existing infection; and (3) after perforation, should it occur. A diet that is low in fat and cholesterol may be prescribed. Avoidance of spicy foods is also suggested (see Complementary & Alternative Therapies box).

Lithotripsy

Extracorporeal shock wave lithotripsy is used to treat a patient who has mild or moderate symptoms caused by a few stones. The machine discharges a series of shock waves through water or a cushion that breaks the stone into fragments. The natural flow of bile car-

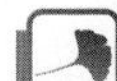

Complementary & Alternative Therapies

Gallbladder, Biliary, and Pancreatic Disorders

- Fresh black root is used as an emetic. The dried root has a gentler action and is used to treat constipation and liver and gallbladder disease and to increase bile flow. Caution patients with gallstones or bile duct obstruction to avoid using it because it may worsen these diseases.
- Blessed thistle is used orally to treat digestive problems such as liver and gallbladder diseases.
- Dandelion is traditionally used as a bile stimulator to treat gallbladder ailments.
- Onion is used as a gallbladder stimulant. It increases the risk of hypoglycemia, so monitor diabetic patients closely.
- Autumn crocus (active ingredient: colchicine) has been used to treat hepatic cirrhosis and primary biliary cirrhosis. Because of the plant's toxicity, internal use is not recommended.
- Papaya (pawpaw) is used to treat pancreatic insufficiency. Patients with a history of Crohn's disease and chronic gastritis should avoid this herb.
- Royal jelly (bee pollen complex) is used in treating liver disease and pancreatitis. Do not confuse royal jelly with bee pollen and honeybee venom. (Royal jelly should be used with extreme caution by patients with asthma because allergic reactions to royal jelly have led to asthma attacks, anaphylaxis, and death.)

ries the stone fragments out of the gallbladder into the intestine for eventual excretion. Nursing intervention after the procedure is similar to that for patients undergoing liver biopsy.

Surgical Intervention

The treatment of choice is cholecystectomy (removal of the gallbladder) with ligation of the cystic duct, vein, and artery. A laparoscopic cholecystectomy and open abdominal cholecystectomy are the two surgical procedures. (See Figure 46-7 for stone retrieval.) A Jackson-Pratt, Penrose, or Davol drain (which promotes drainage and prevents pressure and fluid accumulation under the diaphragm) may be inserted if an open cholecystectomy is performed. If the stones are in the common bile duct and edema is present, a biliary drainage tube, or T-tube, is inserted to keep the duct open and allow drainage of the bile until the edema resolves. The short end of the tube is placed in the common bile duct, and the longer end is brought to the surface through a stab wound (Figure 46-8). The long end is attached to a closed drainage system (bile bag) that is placed below the level of the common bile duct.

The T-tube also provides a route for postoperative cholangiography if desired (T-tube cholangiogram) to assess the patency of the common bile duct. The T-tube is removed 24 hours after the cholangiogram if the edema is resolved and the common bile duct appears normal. The 24-hour period allows the dye to drain out of the common bile duct. If the edema does not resolve in this time, the patient may be discharged with the T-tube in place.

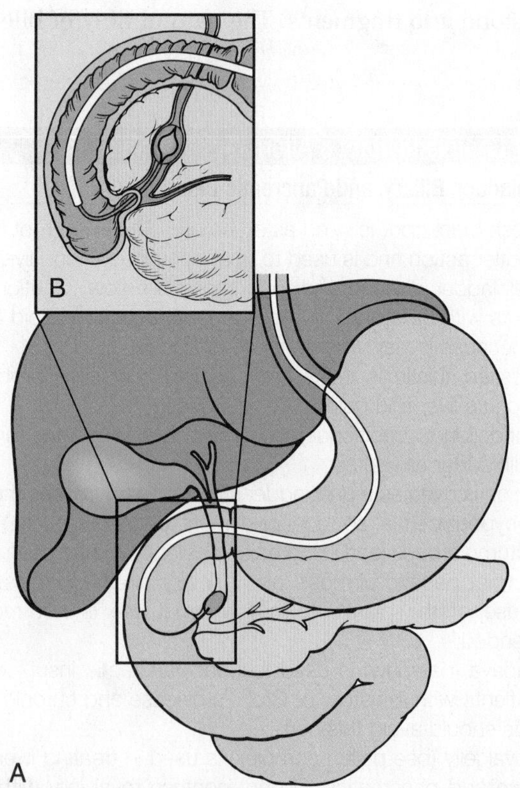

FIGURE 46-7 **A,** During endoscopic sphincterotomy, a flexible endoscope is advanced through the mouth and the stomach until its tip sits in the duodenum opposite the common bile duct. **B,** After widening the duct mouth by incising the sphincter muscle, the physician advances a basket attachment into the duct and retrieves the stone.

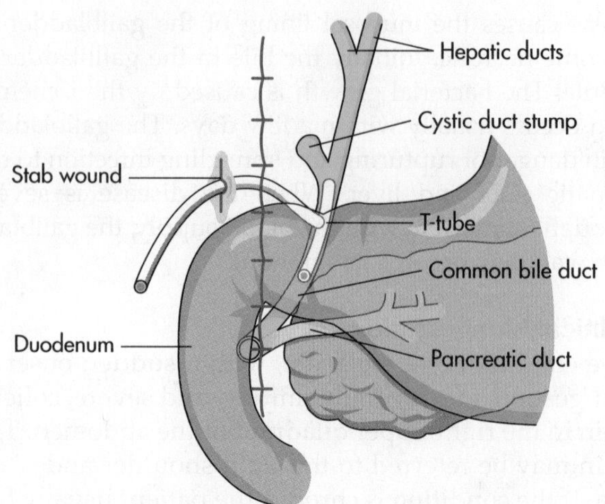

FIGURE 46-8 T-tube in common bile duct.

The most common treatment for cholecystitis and cholelithiasis is done by an endoscopic technique called **laparoscopic cholecystectomy,** which uses a laser or cautery to remove the gallbladder. This procedure replaces the open surgical procedure 80% to 85% of the time. It involves removing the gallbladder through one of four small punctures in the abdomen (a comparatively minor procedure). During surgery, the abdominal cavity is inflated with 3 to 4 L of carbon dioxide to improve visibility. A laparoscope, which has a camera attached, is inserted into the abdomen. The surgeon removes the deflated gallbladder through a laparoscope. If the organ contains so much bile or gallstones that it cannot be collapsed, its contents will be aspirated first. Laparoscopic cholecystectomy offers several advantages over the common open abdominal cholecystectomy, including the following:

- It is less invasive (and thus there is less chance of wound infection or respiratory impairment) and has a shorter healing time and a shorter recuperative time.
- There is no unsightly scar.
- There is less pain and thus more rapid return to normal activities.

When a medical history, physical examination, and blood studies are complete, an ultrasound is done to locate gallstones and detect any dilation of the hepatic bile ducts. If **choledocholithiasis** (stones in common bile duct) is confirmed, a sphincterotomy and stone extraction (see Figure 46-7) are performed before laparoscopic surgery.

It is important to obtain informed consent for endoscopic and open cholecystectomy in case converting from one procedure to the other is necessary. The conversion may be necessary if extensive adhesions, gallstones within the common bile duct, unusual vascular or ductal anatomy, unsuspected pathologic condition of the abdomen, or excessive bleeding complicates the endoscopic procedure.

Postoperative Care for Laparoscopic Cholecystectomy

A small number of patients report minor discomfort at the laparoscopic insertion site or mild shoulder or neck pain resulting from diaphragmatic irritation secondary to abdominal stretching or residual carbon dioxide. Oral analgesics or antiinflammatory agents relieve these symptoms.

Oral liquids and a light meal are given the first night after surgery. The patient has four bandages at the puncture site on the abdomen. Assess vital signs routinely. The patient is ambulatory the first postoperative night.

One out of six patients is discharged the day of surgery. Most patients are discharged the next day. Patients are usually able to resume moderate activity within 48 to 72 hours.

Patient Teaching

Before discharge, patients should be able to eat without difficulty and walk and should have no abdominal distention, evidence of bleeding, or bile leakage. Instruct them to immediately report to the health care provider any severe pain, tenderness in the right upper quadrant, increase in abdominal girth, leakage of bile-colored drainage from the puncture site, increase in pulse, or symptoms of low blood pressure. Patients are usually able to return to work in 3 days and resume full activity after 1 week.

Although there are contraindications for endoscopic cholecystectomies, most patients are treated with this less painful, less expensive procedure.

Nursing Interventions and Patient Teaching

Nursing interventions begin with careful assessment of the characteristics of pain (if it is present) and any signs of jaundice of the skin, sclera, and mucous membrane. Observe the patient's urine and stool for alterations in the presence of bilirubin.

When the patient is treated conservatively, nursing interventions center on keeping the patient comfortable by carefully administering the medications prescribed and monitoring the patient's response to the medication. The patient is on NPO status or on clear liquids. Administer antiemetics if nausea is present. Observe IV infusions for patency, correct rates, and entry sites that are free from erythema and edema. Measure I&O and describe carefully.

Preoperative care includes teaching the patient to turn, cough, and deep breathe and to use an incentive spirometer to facilitate air movement in and out of the lungs to prevent pneumonia and atelectasis. To enable the patient to follow postoperative instructions more easily, teach him or her how to splint the abdomen with the hands, small pillow, or rolled bath blanket before attempting a cough; practice repositioning in the hospital bed; and assume a sitting position from a standing or lying position. If an open cholecystectomy is anticipated, explaining the IV tubing and urinary catheter and their functions will help relieve patient anxiety. The patient should be familiar with any medications that may be used to relieve pain and nausea and should understand that vitamin K and antibiotics may be given preoperatively to prevent hemorrhage and infection.

Postoperative care for open cholecystectomy includes monitoring vital signs and observing dressings frequently and carefully for exudate or hemorrhage. The dressings usually require reinforcement at the drain site. Place the patient in semi-Fowler's position to facilitate drainage. Monitor the Jackson-Pratt, Penrose, or Davol drain for patency. Initially there should be less than 50 mL of serosanguineous exudate during an 8-hour period. Notify the surgeon if the drainage is excessive, contains bile, or is bright red.

The patient needs encouragement to perform deep breathing, cough, and use the incentive spirometer because of the location of the incision. Provide analgesics frequently in the early postoperative period to facilitate movement and deep breathing. Help the patient to dangle the night of surgery and ambulate the first postoperative day. Monitor the patient's neurologic status by checking ability to be aroused easily, orientation to the environment and family, and ability to move extremities equally on command.

Maintain fluid balance with IV therapy; potassium is usually added to compensate for loss from surgery. Check the physician's order before giving ice or clear liquids to the patient, and allow the patient to rinse the mouth frequently.

The nurse is responsible for the care of the T-tube if one is placed. The drainage bag for the T-tube is placed below the level of the common bile duct to prevent the reflux of bile. Position the bag so the tube is not kinked and bile cannot drain from the liver. Frequently check the position of the bag and tube and the color and amount of exudate during the first 24 hours and record the results. Place a gauze roll under the tube, anchoring it to the patient's abdomen and preventing tension and pull on the tube from the weight of the bag. The T-tube drains as much as 500 mL during the first 24 hours. The amount should decrease as the edema resolves and bile begins flowing through the common bile duct. Be careful not to dislodge the T-tube when changing the patient's dressings, as prescribed by the physician.

After oral intake is resumed, the physician may order the T-tube clamped for 1 to 2 hours before meals and unclamped 1 to 2 hours after the patient eats, to aid in the digestion of fat. While the T-tube is clamped, the patient may show signs of distress, including abdominal pain, nausea, vomiting, light brown urine, and clay-colored stools. If distress occurs, unclamp the tube immediately. Increase the time that the T-tube remains clamped as the patient tolerates the procedure. The tube may be left in place for as long as 10 days. The physician removes the tube when the common bile duct is patent for drainage of bile.

Check bowel sounds every 8 hours for the return of peristalsis. Other indicators of the return of peristalsis include expelling flatus, return of appetite, and absence of nausea or vomiting (Madsen et al., 2005). A clear liquid diet is usually ordered immediately or within the first 24 hours postoperatively and increased as tolerated. When solid food is started, it will usually be low in fat. Flatulence or nausea after eating certain foods may persist after surgery; instruct the patient to experiment with different foods.

The patient who undergoes a cholecystectomy must be observed for complications. These include jaundice (from an occluded common duct) and hemorrhage (indicated by decreased blood pressure, increased pulse, and increased exudate at the dressing site). An elevated temperature could indicate peritonitis or wound infection. Pancreatitis may occur after cholecystectomy.

Patients at high risk of not surviving a cholecystectomy may need a cholecystostomy (forming an opening into the gallbladder through the abdominal wall). This can be done using a local anesthetic. The opening provides a means of removing purulent exudate and possibly the stone. It also allows drainage of bile.

Nursing diagnoses and interventions for the patient with open cholecystectomy or cholecystostomy include but are not limited to the following:

Nursing Diagnoses	Nursing Interventions
Ineffective breathing pattern, related to: • pain of high abdominal incision • failure to splint area with coughing and movement	Encourage use of incentive spirometer. Help patient cough and to take 10 deep breaths hourly. Instruct patient on splinting techniques. Turn every 2 hours. Administer analgesics as ordered to facilitate deep breathing and movement. Ambulate as early as possible.
Risk for impaired skin integrity, related to: • wound drainage • accidental obstruction of bile drainage	Maintain patency and prevent tension on T-tube. Promote drainage of T-tube by placing patient in low Fowler's to semi-Fowler's position. Observe, describe, and record amount and character of drainage from T-tube at least every 8 hours. Empty bile bag when half full. Clamp T-tube as ordered by physician 3 to 4 days postoperatively. Reinforce primary dressing and observe exudates; change and apply sterile, dry dressing as ordered; use Montgomery straps to secure if drainage is profuse. Cleanse skin thoroughly at insertion site before applying sterile dressing. Apply skin barriers as needed for added protection.

Dietary teaching is necessary for the patient who is treated conservatively for cholecystitis, as well as the patient who undergoes surgery. The patient who is treated conservatively must continue to avoid fatty foods, including fried foods, cream, whole milk, butter, margarine, peanut butter, nuts, chocolate, pastries, and gravies. For the postsurgical patient, provide instructions to try small amounts of foods that previously caused discomfort and gradually eliminate those that continue to do so. The patient can usually resume a normal diet without difficulty.

The patient should understand that stones may recur elsewhere in the biliary system. Teach the patient to identify the signs of complications that should be reported. These include jaundice caused by occlusion or stricture of a duct, hemorrhage or leakage of bile, elevated temperature, pain, and dietary intolerance associated with another attack. The patient should also be able to demonstrate care of the T-tube, if present on discharge; identify activity restrictions; and identify a date for a return visit to the physician.

Prognosis

To prevent complications from cholecystitis or cholelithiasis, assess the patient for signs and symptoms of gangrenous cholecystitis, subphrenic abscess, pancreatitis, cholangitis, biliary cirrhosis, fistulas, and rupture of the gallbladder with bile peritonitis. A stone occluding the common bile duct (choledocholithiasis) may cause obstructive jaundice (Lewis et al., 2007).

 Life Span Considerations

Older Adults

Gallbladder, Liver, Biliary Tract, or Exocrine Pancreatic Disorder

- The incidence of cholelithiasis increases with aging. Closely observe older adults with histories of this disease for changes in the color of urine and stool or other signs and symptoms of gallbladder problems.
- As the body ages, the number and size of hepatic cells decreases, which results in an overall reduced size and weight of the liver. The liver also has decreased ability to regenerate after injury or from hepatotoxic injury. Also, a transplanted liver takes longer to regenerate in the older patient (Lewis et al., 2007).
- Older adults have a decrease in protein synthesis in the liver and possible changes in the production of enzymes that assist in the metabolism of drugs, particularly anticonvulsants, psychotropics, and oral anticoagulants.
- Be alert to the signs and symptoms of drug toxicity, even when the drugs are administered in normal doses, because the decreased metabolism in the liver can cause an accumulation of the drug.
- The pancreas exhibits ductal hyperplasia and fibrosis with aging, but these changes are not necessarily associated with altered functioning. The output of pancreatic secretions steadily declines after age 40, but related problems with absorption cannot be documented.

With prompt treatment of cholecystitis and cholelithiasis, the prognosis is excellent. Laparoscopic surgery has further decreased the number of complications. The prognosis is not as favorable in patients who develop pancreatitis (see Life Span Considerations box).

PANCREATITIS

Etiology and Pathophysiology

Pancreatitis is an inflammatory condition of the pancreas that may be acute or chronic. The degree of inflammation varies from mild edema to severe hemorrhagic necrosis. Although the exact cause of pancreatitis remains unknown, many predisposing factors have been identified. Acute or chronic pancreatitis is generally the result of damage to the biliary tract (most common in women), alcohol consumption (most common in men), trauma, infectious disease, or certain drugs. Alcoholism and biliary tract disease are the two factors most commonly associated with pancreatitis. Pancreatitis can develop as a postoperative complication in patients who have had surgery of the pancreas, stomach, duodenum, or biliary tract. Pancreatitis can also occur after undergoing ERCP (see Figure 46-1).

In the pathophysiologic process of pancreatitis, the enzymes cannot flow out of the pancreas because of **occlusion** (an obstruction or closing off) of the pancreatic duct (duct of Wirsung) by edema, stones, or scar tissue. The pancreatic enzymes build up and increase pressure within the duct. The duct ruptures, releasing enzymes that begin digesting the pancreas (autodigestion). In chronic pancreatitis, atrophy of the acinar tissue allows replacement of fibrotic tissue, and the pancreas becomes necrotic.

The development of pseudocysts or abscesses in pancreatic tissue is a serious complication. After autodigestion occurs, the pancreas and occasionally surrounding organs form walls around cystic fluid, including pancreatic enzymes, and necrotic debris. These pseudocysts can develop into an abscess.

Clinical Manifestations

Manifestations include severe abdominal pain radiating to the back. The pain is usually located in the left upper quadrant. The pain is sometimes relieved by leaning forward, taking the stomach weight off the pancreas. Jaundice may be noted if the common bile duct is obstructed.

Assessment

Collection of **subjective data** may include noting that patients exhibit extreme symptoms or none at all. It is difficult to distinguish the symptoms of pancreatitis from those of other abdominal disorders. The most specific complaint is abdominal pain (often excruciating) that radiates to the back (Lewis et al., 2007). The pain is caused by the enlargement of the pancreatic capsule, an obstruction, or chemical irritation from enzymes. The pain is usually decreased by flexing the trunk, leaning forward from a sitting position, or by assuming the fetal position. It is increased by eating or lying down. Other complaints include anorexia, nausea, malaise, and restlessness.

Collection of **objective data** includes noting the presence of low-grade fever, leukocytosis, hypotension, vomiting (in 70% to 90% of patients), jaundice if the common bile duct is obstructed, weight loss, steatorrhea, and tachycardia. Bowel sounds may be decreased or absent. Ileus may occur, causing marked abdominal distention. The lungs are frequently involved, with crackles present (Lewis et al., 2007).

Diagnostic Tests

Both acute and chronic pancreatitis are diagnosed by radiologic studies (abdominal CT scan and ultrasound of the pancreas), endoscopy, and laboratory analysis of the pancreatic enzymes in the serum and urine. Laboratory tests reveal an increased level of serum amylase and lipase during the first few days and increased urine amylase thereafter. In acute pancreatitis the level of serum amylase may become elevated early, within 2 to 36 hours. However, the amylase level is not a specific indicator for pancreatitis; abnormal levels also can be seen in cases of perforated peptic ulcer, perforated bowel, and diabetic ketoacidosis. The level of lipase is more specific for diagnosing acute pancreatitis. The lipase level rises in 4 to 8 hours, peaks at 24 hours, and may remain elevated for 14 days. Amylase and lipase levels may be elevated to 5 to 40 times normal (Holcomb, 2007). Leukocytosis, an elevated hematocrit level, hypocalcemia, hypoalbuminemia, and hyperglycemia may also be present. Pancreatic insulin production may be diminished if the islets of Langerhans become infected, and some patients develop diabetes mellitus.

Medical Management

Treatment is medical unless the precipitating cause is biliary tract disease; then surgery may be indicated. Food and fluids are withheld to avoid stimulating pancreatic activity, and IV fluids are administered. The patient is on NPO status, and an NG tube is inserted to decrease pancreatic stimulation, treat or prevent nausea and vomiting, and decrease abdominal distention. A common complaint is constant, severe pain; morphine is used because of its effective control of pain. Meperidine is no longer the drug of choice because of its toxic metabolite, normeperidine, which can cause seizures; all opioids may cause some spasm of the sphincter of Oddi (Holcomb, 2007). Analgesics may be combined with an antispasmodic.

Parenteral anticholinergic medication, such as atropine or propantheline (Pro-Banthine), helps decrease pancreatic activity. This medication is contraindicated in paralytic ileus. Antacids or antihistamine H_2 receptor antagonists, such as cimetidine, may be given to prevent stress ulcers caused by decreased gastric pH. Some physicians prescribe antibiotics to treat secondary infections.

Enteral feeding is begun 24 to 48 hours after the onset of acute pancreatitis and is administered via the jejunum to prevent the release of pancreatic enzymes. Enteral feeding is preferred to the IV route because it is more nutritionally sound, is less costly, and has fewer complications. However, if enteral feeding is not tolerated in 5 to 7 days, the patient may need to be switched to IV feeding.

A clear liquid diet with gradual progression may be started once the patient's pain is under control for at least 24 hours. Notify the health care provider if the patient does not tolerate oral feedings. If pain returns after oral feeding, again place the patient on NPO status for 24 hours or until the pain has ceased (Holcomb, 2007). The diet must be free of alcohol and gastric stimulants, such as coffee. Oral hypoglycemic agents or insulin may be needed if there is destruction of the islets of Langerhans.

Nursing Interventions and Patient Teaching

Determine the presence and location of pain, as well as what aggravates or relieves the pain. Keep the patient as comfortable as possible through proper administration of analgesic medications. The patient is usually on bed rest with bathroom privileges to decrease the flow of pancreatic enzymes. Nutritional needs are met by enteral feeding via the jejunum as long as necessary. If enteral feedings fail, the patient may need parenteral feedings. The patient who is addicted to alcohol may go through withdrawal while in the hospital. Be prepared to protect the patient from injury and provide supportive care to the patient and the family. Carefully monitor all replacement fluids and medications for proper administration.

Nursing diagnoses and interventions for the patient with pancreatitis include but are not limited to the following:

Nursing Diagnoses	Nursing Interventions
Pain, related to stimulation of nerve endings caused by enlargement of pancreatic capsule, obstruction, or chemical irritation from enzymes	Administer medications as prescribed and monitor the response. Restrict diet as necessary to prevent aggravation of pain (eliminate fats, alcohol, caffeine). Use alternative comfort measures: repositioning, positive imagery, and time for listening. Monitor NG tube to wall suction for functioning to prevent abdominal distention.
Imbalanced nutrition: less than body requirements, related to: • anorexia • nausea • vomiting • loss of enzymes necessary for the digestive process	Administer enteral feeding via jejunum as ordered. Weigh patient daily at same time and using same scale. Record I&O, including NG tube suctioning output. Administer antacids and antiemetics as prescribed. Instruct patient to follow a diet that is low in fat and high in protein and carbohydrates when tolerated.
Deficient fluid volume, related to: • decreased oral intake • vomiting • diarrhea • NG suctioning • hemorrhage	Monitor I&O; weigh patient daily. Assess hemodynamic stability: pulse, blood pressure. Assess for signs and symptoms of fluid volume deficit: decreased level of consciousness; poor skin turgor; cool, dry, or clammy skin; and weak peripheral pulses. Assess for signs and symptoms of hemorrhage; assess abdominal girth; monitor NG aspirate for occult or frank bleeding. Monitor for the administration of fluid volume replacement.

The patient remains on a low-fat, high-calorie, high-carbohydrate diet after discharge. Alcohol and beverages or foods containing caffeine are not allowed if full recovery is desired. Ensure that the patient understands the disease process and the severity of the disease and related complications.

Prognosis

The prognosis of pancreatitis depends on the course of the disease and complications, including pseudocysts and abscesses. In most patients, acute pancreatitis is mild, requiring less than 1 week of hospitalization. However, 5% to 25% of patients have a more complicated course. The severity of the disease varies according to the extent of pancreatic destruction. Some patients recover completely; others have recurring attacks. Interestingly, complications can occur with mild, acute, chronic, or severe pancreatitis. Mortality rates for acute necrotizing pancreatitis range from 10% to 50% (Table 46-1).

CANCER OF THE PANCREAS

Although once considered relatively rare, pancreatic cancer is now the fourth leading cause of cancer death in the United States and Canada. According to the American Cancer Society, more than 37,000 Americans

Table 46-1 Medications for Disorders of the Gallbladder, Liver, Biliary Tract, and Exocrine Pancreas

Generic (Trade)	Action	Side Effects	Nursing Implications
Gemcitabine hydrochloride (Gemzar)	Exhibits antitumor activity; indicated as first-line treatment of locally advanced or metastatic adenocarcinoma of the pancreas	Myelosuppression; nausea and vomiting, macular papular pruritic rash	Monitor CBC. Provide antiemetic to control nausea and vomiting. Provide relief measures to control pruritus.
Lactulose (Chronulac, Cephulac)	Acidifies colonic contents, thus decreasing absorption of ammonia from gut; also has cathartic laxative properties; primarily used in hepatic encephalopathy	Nausea, vomiting, diarrhea	Titrate dose to 3-4 loose stools per day; monitor for dehydration; monitor for serum ammonia levels and improved mental status.
Spironolactone (Aldactone)	Competes with aldosterone at receptor sites in distal tubule, resulting in excretion of sodium chloride and water and retention of potassium and phosphate; used in cirrhosis of the liver with ascites	Headache, confusion, diarrhea, bleeding, dysrhythmias, impotence, hypokalemia	Assess electrolytes, sodium, chloride, potassium, BUN, serum creatinine. Weigh daily; monitor I&O. Administer in AM to avoid interference with sleep.
Meperidine (Demerol)	Binds to opiate receptors in CNS; alters perception of and response to painful stimuli, while producing generalized CNS depression; used for biliary pain because morphine may cause spasms of the sphincter of Oddi	Sedation, confusion, respiratory depression, hypotension, bradycardia, nausea, vomiting, urinary retention	Assess type, location, intensity of pain before and 1 hour after administration. If respiratory rate is <10 breaths/min, assess level of sedation.
Propantheline (Pro-Banthine)	Antisecretory and antispasmodic agent; slows GI motility through anticholinergic activity; decreases pancreatic activity	Drowsiness, confusion, dry mouth, constipation, urinary retention, tachycardia, blurred vision	Avoid use with other CNS depressants or alcohol; avoid driving or other activities until accustomed to effects; may cause hypotension when given IV; do not use in patients with Parkinson's disease.
Vasopressin (Pitressin)	Synthetic pituitary agent; antidiuretic effects on kidney; a potent vasoconstrictor; used to treat bleeding esophageal varices	Hypertension; ischemia to heart, mesenteric organs, and kidneys; angina; myocardial infarction; water retention; hyponatremia	Use with caution in older adults and in patients with known coronary artery disease or known CHF; discontinue if chest pain develops; monitor urinary output and serum sodium.
Neomycin (Mycifradin, Myciguent)	Inhibits protein synthesis in bacteria at the level of the 30S ribosome; decreases the number of ammonia-producing bacteria in the gut as part of management of hepatic encephalopathy	Ototoxicity; local stinging, burning; nephrotoxicity	Monitor neurologic status and renal function.

BUN, Blood urea nitrogen; *CBC*, complete blood count; *CHF*, congestive heart failure; *CNS*, central nervous system; *GI*, gastrointestinal; *I&O*, intake and output; *IV*, intravenously.

Continued

Table 46-1 Medications for Disorders of the Gallbladder, Liver, Biliary Tract, and Exocrine Pancreas—cont'd

Generic (Trade)	Action	Side Effects	Nursing Implications
Cholestyramine (Questran)	Binds bile acids in the GI tract, forming an insoluble complex; relief of pruritus associated with elevated levels of bile acids	Nausea, constipation, abdominal discomfort	Assess severity of pruritus and skin integrity.
Pancrelipase (Pancrease, Cotazym)	Increased digestion of fats, carbohydrate, and proteins in the GI tract; treatment of pancreatic insufficiency associated with chronic pancreatitis, pancreatectomy	Diarrhea, nausea, stomach cramps, abdominal pain	Assess patient's nutritional status; monitor stools for high fat content; assess patient for allergy to pork; administer immediately before meals or with meals.

were diagnosed with pancreatic cancer during 2007 and approximately 33,000 Americans died of the disease (American Cancer Society, *Facts and figures,* 2007). A major factor in the high death rate from pancreatic cancer is the difficulty in diagnosing it at an early curable stage. The disease usually occurs after middle age. The risk increases with age, with peak incidence occurring between 65 and 80 years of age.

Etiology and Pathophysiology

The cause of pancreatic cancer is unknown, but it is diagnosed more often in cigarette smokers; people exposed to chemical carcinogens; and people with diabetes mellitus, cirrhosis, and pancreatitis. Diets high in red meat and pork (especially processed meat such as bacon), fat, and coffee are also linked to pancreatic cancer. Obese people are 20% more likely to develop pancreatic cancer (Riehl, 2007).

The cancer may originate in the pancreas or be the result of metastasis from cancer of the lung, the stomach, the duodenum, or the common bile duct. Most often the head of the pancreas is involved and causes jaundice by compressing and obstructing the common bile duct. As the cancer spreads, it may invade the posterior wall of the stomach, the duodenal wall, the colon, and the common bile duct. Biliary obstruction and gallbladder dilation are subsequent complications. It is not uncommon for the tumor to grow rapidly and invade the vascular and lymphatic systems. Many patients live only 4 to 8 months after diagnosis.

Clinical Manifestations

The insidious onset of the disease with initially vague symptoms generally accounts for delays in diagnosis. Abdominal pain occurs in about 85% of the patients. About half the patients develop diabetes mellitus if islet cells are involved.

Assessment

A psychosocial history during patient assessment may reveal at-risk populations such as engineers, coal- and gas-plant employees, chemists, and workers exposed to beta-naphthol and benzidine. **Subjective data** include anorexia; fatigue; nausea; flatulence; a change in stools; and steady, dull, and aching pain in the epigastrium or referred to the back. The pain is usually worse at night.

Objective data include weight loss, often gradual and progressive, which is one of the earliest signs. Jaundice usually is progressive and may occur late. Pruritus accompanies the jaundice. Many patients have recent onset of diabetes mellitus.

Diagnostic Tests

Diagnosis of pancreatic cancer is based on the patient's history, signs and symptoms, and diagnostic studies. Better diagnostic measures are needed for detection of pancreatic cancer because most of the current methods detect only advanced stages. Diagnostic studies include transabdominal ultrasound and CT, duodenal endoscopy to obtain specimens for cytologic examination, ERCP, and pancreatic scans. ERCP is the gold standard for visualization of the pancreatic duct and biliary system. With ERCP, pancreatic secretions and tissues can be collected for analysis of different tumor markers (see Figure 46-1).

The level of the tumor marker cancer-associated antigen CA 19-9 is elevated in patients with pancreatic cancer. It is the most commonly used tumor marker to diagnose pancreatic adenocarcinoma and to monitor the patient's response to treatment. However, CA 19-9 can be elevated in other diseases such as cancer of the gallbladder or in nonmalignant conditions such as acute and chronic pancreatitis, hepatitis, and biliary duct obstruction (Riehl, 2007).

Medical Management

Often, malignant tumors of the pancreas are inoperable by the time they are diagnosed. Treatment of pancreatic cancer is primarily surgical and has been associated with a high mortality rate. Cancer of the head of the pancreas is usually treated by pancreatoduodenectomy; the Whipple procedure involves resection of the antrum of the stomach, the gallbladder, the duodenum, and varying amounts of the pancreas. Anastomoses are constructed between the stomach, the common bile duct and the pancreatic ducts, and the jejunum (Figure 46-9). In most cases, this procedure is performed by surgeons who are specially trained and experienced.

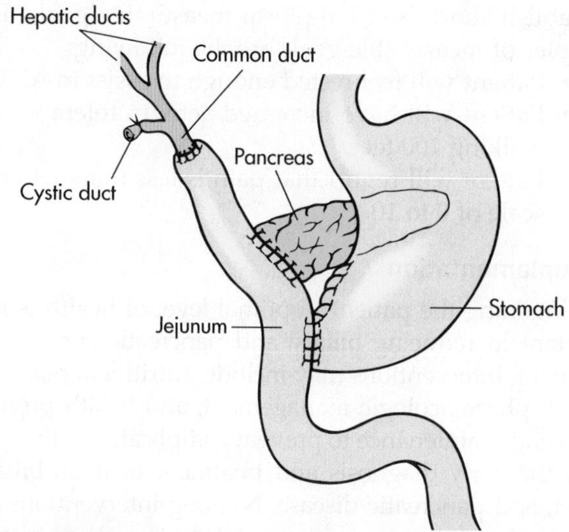

FIGURE 46-9 Whipple procedure, or radical pancreaticoduodenectomy. This surgical procedure involves resection of the proximal pancreas, adjoining duodenum, distal portion of the stomach, and distal portion of the common bile duct. The pancreatic duct, common bile ducts, and stomach are anastomosed to the jejunum.

Another procedure is total pancreatectomy with resection of parts of the GI tract. Subtotal pancreatic resection has complications of postoperative pancreatic fistulas and is not recommended.

Combinations of drugs such as fluorouracil and gemcitabine (Gemzar) may produce a better response than a single chemotherapeutic agent. Gemcitabine is a main treatment for pancreatic cancer that has metastasized. The current role of chemotherapy in pancreatic cancer is limited. Adjuvant therapy—using surgical resection, radiation, and chemotherapy—is believed by some to be the most effective way to manage the almost always fatal cancer of the pancreas.

Nursing Interventions and Patient Teaching

Pancreatic surgery is radical and requires critical care nursing. Postoperative care focuses on maintaining fluid and electrolyte balance, preventing hemorrhage, preventing respiratory complications, and monitoring endocrine and exocrine functions of the pancreas.

Patients with pancreatic cancer may have acute and chronic pain. The patient may receive long-acting opioid analgesics for chronic pain, supplemented by quick-acting opioids for breakthrough pain. A method for providing effective temporary pain relief is to inject corticosteroids and analgesics via a celiac plexus nerve block (Riehl, 2007).

The health care provider caring for the patient with pancreatic cancer must offer compassionate physical and emotional assistance. Refer the patient and the family to social services and support groups. When the patient stops active therapy for the cancer, provide the patient and the family with information about hospice care (Riehl, 2007).

Nursing diagnoses and interventions for patients with cancer of the pancreas include but are not limited to the following:

Nursing Diagnoses	Nursing Interventions
Risk for deficient fluid volume, related to possible hemorrhage and drainage	Maintain patency of GI tubes to relieve distention and compression at the surgical site. Measure I&O and weigh daily. Monitor IV fluid replacement. Assess for signs and symptoms of dehydration (dry mucous membranes, poor skin turgor, oliguria).
Risk for impaired skin integrity, related to drainage from wound	Monitor for excoriation and infection; use skin barriers and disposable postoperative pouches and appliances to prevent enzymatic contact with the skin and to aid in the accurate collection and measurement of pancreatic drainage.

The patient is facing a life-threatening illness, and family members and close friends are important for the patient's well-being. If the patient has an inadequate support system, it is important to use the resources that are available. The hospital chaplain or a personal minister, the social worker, the dietitian, the physician, and the nurse can become a support system. These members of the health care team can provide active listening and a caring attitude for this patient.

Prognosis

The prognosis for patients with cancer of the pancreas is very poor. Median survival after diagnosis is only 5 to 12 months. The 5-year survival rate remains less than 10%. Resection of the tumor improves median survival to 17 to 20 months. Prognosis is related to the tumor's location.

❖NURSING PROCESS *for the Patient with Gallbladder, Liver, Biliary Tract, or Exocrine Pancreatic Disorder*

The role of the licensed practical nurse/licensed vocational nurse (LPN/LVN) in the nursing process as stated is that the LPN/LVN will:

- Participate in planning care for patients based on patient needs
- Review patient's care plan and recommend revisions as needed
- Review and follow defined prioritization for patient care
- Use clinical pathways, care maps, or care plans to guide and review patient care

Assessment

Nursing assessment of the patient with a gallbladder, liver, biliary tract, or exocrine pancreatic disorder must be performed accurately. Perform a head-to-toe assessment. Also assess the patient's knowledge of the disease process, nutritional status, pain, discomfort, current health problems, and signs and symptoms. Note changes in appetite and weight. Measure vital signs, noting any alterations from normal, such as hyperthermia, hypotension, hypertension, tachycardia, or tachypnea. Observe the skin, the sclerae, the mucous membranes, the urine, and the stool for alterations in the presence of bilirubin. Inspect, auscultate, and palpate the abdomen. Document any abdominal tenderness, pain, or abnormal bowel sounds.

Nursing Diagnosis

Assessment provides data for identifying the patient's problems, strengths, potential complications, and learning needs. Nursing diagnoses for patients with disorders of the liver, biliary tract, or exocrine pancreas include but are not limited to the following:

- Activity intolerance
- Ineffective breathing pattern
- Deficient fluid volume
- Impaired home maintenance
- Risk for injury
- Deficient knowledge
- Noncompliance
- Imbalanced nutrition: less than body requirements
- Acute pain
- Chronic pain
- Powerlessness
- Impaired skin integrity
- Acute confusion

Expected Outcomes and Planning

When planning care, look at the nursing diagnosis and establish the cause of the nursing problem. The overall goals for patients with disorders of the gallbladder, liver, biliary tract, and exocrine pancreas include (1) relief of pain and discomfort; (2) stabilization of fluid and electrolyte balance; (3) minimal to no complications; (4) ability to resume normal activities; (5) a return, if possible, to normal pancreatic and liver function without complications; and (6) a return to as normal a lifestyle as possible.

Planning includes the development of realistic goals and outcomes from the identified nursing diagnoses. Establish short- and long-term measurable goals. Examples of measurable goals are the following:

- Patient will feel rested enough to assist in ADLs.
- Patient will have increased activity tolerance by walking 100 feet.
- Patient will report that pain is less than a 4 on a scale of 0 to 10.

Implementation

Maintaining the patient's optimal level of health is important in reducing biliary and pancreatic symptoms. Nursing interventions may include nutritional management, pharmacologic management, and health promotion and maintenance to prevent complications. Encourage the early diagnosis and treatment of liver, biliary tract, and pancreatic disease. Nursing interventions involve supportive care with special attention to nutrition, hydration, skin care, and pain relief.

Evaluation

During and after the planned nursing interventions, determine the outcomes of the interventions. This is an ongoing process of continually trying to establish the most effective care plan.

Evaluation involves determining whether the established goals have been met. Involve the patient in evaluating the goals to see whether the criteria for measurement have been met. Goals and evaluative measures for disorders of the liver, biliary tract, and exocrine pancreas may include the following:

Goal 1: Patient achieves improved activity tolerance.

Evaluative measure: Observe patient exercise.

Goal 2: Patient remains free of bodily injury.

Evaluative measure: Ask patient to list factors that increase the risk of injury.

See Cultural Considerations box.

Cultural Considerations

Gallbladder, Liver, Biliary Tract, or Exocrine Pancreatic Disorder

- Mortality from cirrhosis occurs more frequently among blacks than in other ethnic groups.
- Primary hepatic cancer has a higher incidence among blacks, Asian Americans, and Inuit (Eskimos) than among whites.
- Pancreatic cancer occurs more frequently among blacks and Asian Americans than among whites.
- Whites and Native Americans have a higher incidence of gallbladder disease than blacks and Asian Americans.

Get Ready for the NCLEX® Examination!

Key Points

- Planned nursing interventions must be individualized according to each patient's and family's unique needs.
- The most common cause of cirrhosis of the liver is alcohol ingestion.
- Clinical manifestations of cirrhosis of the liver differ, depending on whether the patient is in the early or later stages of the disease.
- An important aspect of nursing interventions in patients with hepatitis and cirrhosis of the liver is the relief of pruritus.
- Prevention of the spread of viral hepatitis is a primary concern of health care professionals.
- Vaccine is now available to prevent the development of hepatitis A and hepatitis B.
- If an infection develops anywhere along the GI tract, there is danger that the infecting organism may reach the liver through the biliary system, portal venous system, or hepatic arterial or lymphatic system and result in a liver abscess.
- Cholecystectomy (removal of the gallbladder by means of laparoscopic or open abdominal procedure) is one of the most commonly performed surgical procedures.
- Pancreatic disorders may cause diabetes mellitus because of interference with insulin production.
- Clinical manifestations of acute pancreatitis include severe abdominal pain radiating to the back; the pain is sometimes relieved when the patient leans forward, taking the weight of the stomach off the pancreas.
- Tumor markers are used both for establishing the diagnosis of pancreatic adenocarcinoma and monitoring the response to treatment of cancer; CA 19-9 is elevated in pancreatic cancer and is the most commonly used tumor marker.

Additional Learning Resources

Go to your Companion CD for an audio glossary, animations, video clips, and more.

evolve Be sure to visit the Evolve site at http://evolve.elsevier.com/Christensen/adult/ for additional online resources.

Review Questions for the NCLEX® Examination

1. Nurses, as well as other health care providers, are at risk for hepatitis B. For prophylaxis to be most effective in these workers:
   1. prophylaxis must be instituted before exposure.
   2. prophylaxis can be instituted either before or after exposure.
   3. prophylaxis must be instituted after exposure.
   4. prophylaxis instituted before or after exposure is effective forever.

2. Liver needle biopsy is a safe method of diagnosing pathologic liver conditions. However, the nurse must anticipate possible complications, including which nursing diagnosis?
   1. Pain, related to leakage of blood and bile into the peritoneal cavity
   2. Noncompliance of medications, related to testing procedure
   3. Social isolation, related to tissue sample removal for biopsy
   4. Disturbed sleep pattern, related to lack of information on hospital protocol

3. A 78-year-old patient is admitted with common bile duct obstruction related to cancer of the pancreas. Which clinical manifestations would the nurse expect to find? *(Select all that apply.)*
   1. Brown feces
   2. Scleral icterus
   3. Dark, tea-colored urine
   4. Jaundice

4. It is especially important for the patient to cough and breathe deeply postoperatively following an open cholecystectomy because:
   1. the patient is often obese.
   2. the patient usually smokes.
   3. the patient is on bed rest for a prolonged period.
   4. the patient tends to take shallow breaths due to the placement of the incision.

5. In hepatic encephalopathy, when the nurse requests that the patient stretch out the arm and hyperextend the wrist with fingers separated, relaxed, and extended to see whether rapid, irregular flexion and extension (flapping) of the wrist occur, the nurse is assessing for the presence of:
   1. varices.
   2. asterixis.
   3. pruritus.
   4. bacterial toxins.

6. The patient has advanced cirrhosis of the liver with an acute exacerbation of hepatic encephalopathy. What type of food might be limited in his diet?
   1. Fruits
   2. Vegetables
   3. Meats
   4. Carbohydrates

7. Patients with liver abscess are seen with vague signs and symptoms, which are often:
   1. asterixis, ascites, and esophageal varices.
   2. fever accompanied by chills, abdominal pain, and tenderness in the right upper quadrant.
   3. enlarged spleen and spider telangiectases.
   4. constipation; left quadrant abdominal cramping; and loud, high-pitched abdominal sounds on auscultation.

8. A small number of patients who have had a laparoscopic cholecystectomy report mild shoulder pain resulting from:

1. paralytic ileus with mesenteric irritation.
2. incision along the rectus abdominis muscle.
3. diaphragmatic irritation secondary to residual carbon dioxide.
4. spasm of the duct of Wirsung.

9. The patient has been admitted with right upper quadrant pain and has been placed on a low-fat diet. Which of the following trays would be acceptable for her?

1. Whole milk, veal, rice, and pastry
2. Liver, fried potatoes, gelatin, and avocado
3. Skim milk, lean fish, tapioca pudding, and fruit
4. Ham, mashed potatoes, creamed peas, and gelatin

10. Hepatitis types B, C, D, and G are spread mainly through the following: *(Select all that apply.)*

1. Blood transfusions
2. Contaminated needles and instruments
3. Direct contact with body fluids from infected people, such as through breast milk and sexual contact
4. Oral-fecal route

11. In patients with acute pancreatitis, the analgesic meperidine is no longer the opioid of choice because of:

1. paralytic ileus.
2. increased possibility of addiction.
3. urinary retention.
4. its toxic metabolite, normeperidine, which can cause seizures.

12. A patient is scheduled for surgery for a common bile duct exploration. The nurse would expect the patient to return from surgery with:

1. an underwater-seal drainage.
2. a T-tube connected to gravity drainage.
3. a Penrose drain.
4. a nephrostomy tube.

13. Which types of hepatitis now have vaccines for prevention?

1. B only
2. B and D
3. A and B
4. A, B, C, D, E, and G

14. Nursing interventions for the patient with cholecystitis associated with cholelithiasis are based on the knowledge that:

1. the disorder can be successfully treated with oral bile salts that dissolve gallstones.
2. analgesics are usually not necessary to relieve the pain of bile duct spasms during an acute attack.
3. a heavy meal with a high fat content may precipitate the signs and symptoms of the disease.
4. a low-cholesterol diet is indicated to reduce the availability of cholesterol for gallstone formation.

15. Teaching in relation to home management following a laparoscopic cholecystectomy should include:

1. keeping the bandages on the puncture sites for 48 hours.
2. reporting any bile-colored drainage or pus from any incision.
3. using over-the-counter antiemetics if nausea and vomiting occur.
4. emptying and measuring the contents of the bile bag from the T-tube every day.

16. A patient with advanced cirrhosis asks the nurse why his abdomen is so swollen. The nurse's response is based on the knowledge that:

1. a lack of clotting factors promotes the collection of blood in the abdominal cavity.
2. portal hypertension and hypoalbuminemia cause a fluid shift into the peritoneal space.
3. decreased peristalsis in the GI tract contributes to gas formation and bowel distention.
4. bile salts in the blood irritate the peritoneal membranes, causing edema and pocketing of fluid.

17. When caring for a patient with acute exacerbation of hepatic encephalopathy, the nurse may give a lactulose enema, provide a low-protein diet, and limit physical activity. These measures are done to:

1. promote fluid loss.
2. eliminate potassium ions.
3. decrease portal pressure.
4. decrease ammonia production.

18. In planning care for a patient with metastatic cancer of the liver, the nurse includes interventions that:

1. focus primarily on symptomatic and comfort measures.
2. reassure the patient that chemotherapy offers a good prognosis for recovery.
3. promote the patient's confidence that surgical excision of the tumor will be successful.
4. provide information necessary for the patient to make decisions regarding liver transplantation.

19. Patients who receive a liver transplant secondary to viral B or C hepatitis often experience ________________ or ________________ of the transplanted liver.

20. If a patient is scheduled for an ultrasound of the pancreas, which two situations would cause the examination to be postponed?

1. Technetium-99m injected into biliary tract, low serum albumin
2. CT of abdomen, elevated amylase
3. ERCP examination, elevated LDH
4. Abdomen distended with gas, recent barium enema examination

21. The surgical procedure for cancer of the pancreas involves resection of the antrum of the stomach, the gallbladder, the duodenum, and varying amounts of the pancreas. Anastomoses are constructed between the stomach, the common bile and pancreatic ducts, and the jejunum. This procedure is called:

1. Whipple procedure.
2. pancreatectomy.
3. Billroth I.
4. Billroth II.

22. A major factor in the high death rate from pancreatic cancer is: *(Select all that apply.)*

1. difficulty in diagnosing it at an early curable stage.
2. denial on the part of the patient.
3. the majority of cancers have metastasized at the time of diagnosis.
4. tumors starting in the body or tail often remain silent until their growth is advanced.

23. The patient with cirrhosis has bleeding tendencies because the cirrhotic liver cannot:

1. produce RBCs and vitamin K.
2. produce prothrombin; fibrinogen; and clotting factors VII, IX, and X, or absorb vitamin K.
3. produce erythropoietin, reticulocytes, and fibrin.
4. manufacture vitamins E, C, A, and K.

24. Monitoring the color of stools of a patient with hepatitis A is important. The nurse caring for such a patient would expect the stools to be:

1. dark brown.
2. black.
3. clay colored (acholic).
4. green.

25. Laboratory values that are often abnormal in a patient with liver disease include: *(Select all that apply.)*

1. gamma GT.
2. alkaline phosphatase.
3. total bilirubin.
4. CEA, AST.
5. CA 125.

26. A 56-year-old patient has cirrhosis of the liver. He has an accumulation of serous fluid in the abdominal cavity called ascites. The nurse is assisting the physician in the procedure to remove this fluid from his abdominal cavity. This procedure is called an:

1. abdominal paracephalus.
2. abdominal paracentesis.
3. abdominal thoracentesis.
4. abdominal perimetrium.

27. The patient has acute pancreatitis. The diagnostic examination that would probably be ordered would include: *(Select all that apply.)*

1. serum amylase and lipase, ultrasound of pancreas.
2. fecal studies, prothrombin time.
3. CEA, CBC.
4. urine, amylase.

28. The patient was scheduled for a laparoscopic cholecystectomy. Complications developed during surgery, and he underwent an open cholecystectomy with a T-tube inserted into the common bile duct. The purposes of the T-tube are to:

1. decrease abdominal distention and increase peristalsis.
2. improve diaphragmatic expansion and prevent atelectasis.
3. shorten postoperative recovery and hasten healing process.
4. keep the common bile duct open until edema resolves, and allow drainage of bile into drainage bag.

29. The patient has a history of cholelithiasis. He has excruciating pain in the right upper quadrant radiating to the scapula, and severe nausea and vomiting; within a few hours he develops early signs of jaundice. The physician suspects:

1. obstruction choledocholithiasis.
2. cirrhosis of the liver.
3. cancer of the pancreas.
4. asterixis.

chapter

47 Care of the Patient with a Blood or Lymphatic Disorder

evolve

http://evolve.elsevier.com/Christensen/foundationsadult

Barbara Lauritsen Christensen

Objectives

Anatomy and Physiology

1. Describe the components of blood.
2. Differentiate between the functions of erythrocytes, leukocytes, and thrombocytes.
3. Discuss factors necessary for the formation of erythrocytes.
4. Define the white blood cell differential.
5. Describe the blood clotting process.
6. List the basic blood groups.
7. Describe the generalized functions of the lymphatic system and list the primary lymphatic structures.

Medical-Surgical

8. List common diagnostic tests for evaluation of blood and lymph disorders, and discuss the significance of the results.
9. Compare and contrast the different types of anemia in terms of etiology and pathophysiology, clinical manifestations, assessment, diagnostic tests, medical management, nursing interventions, patient teaching, and prognosis.
10. List six signs and symptoms associated with hypovolemic shock.
11. Discuss important issues to cover in patient teaching and home care planning for the patient with pernicious anemia.
12. Discuss the etiology and pathophysiology, clinical manifestations, assessment, diagnostic tests, medical management, nursing interventions, patient teaching, and prognosis for patients with acute and chronic leukemia.
13. Compare and contrast the disorders of coagulation (thrombocytopenia, hemophilia, disseminated intravascular coagulation) in terms of etiology and pathophysiology, clinical manifestations, assessment, diagnostic tests, medical management, nursing interventions, and prognosis.
14. Discuss the etiology and pathophysiology, clinical manifestations, assessment, diagnostic tests, medical management, nursing interventions, patient teaching, and prognosis for the patient with multiple myeloma, malignant lymphoma, and Hodgkin's lymphoma.
15. Discuss the primary goal of nursing interventions for the patient with lymphedema.
16. Apply the nursing process to the care of the patient with disorders of the hematological and lymphatic systems.

KEY TERMS

anemia (ă-NĒ-mē-ă, p. 1505)
aplasia (ă-PLĀ-zhă, p. 1509)
disseminated intravascular coagulation (DIC) (dĭ-SĔM-ĭ-nāt-ĕd, p. 1525)
erythrocytosis (ĕ-rĭth-rō-sī-TŌ-sĭs, p. 1515)
erythropoiesis (ĕ-rĭth-rō-pō-Ē-sĭs, p. 1501)
hemarthrosis (hē-măr-THRŌ-sĭs, p. 1523)
hemophilia A (hē-mō-FĒL-ē-ă, p. 1523)
heterozygous (hĕt-ĕr-ō-ZĪ-gŭs, p. 1513)
homozygous (hō-mō-ZĪ-gŭs, p. 1512)
idiopathic (ĭd-ē-ō-PĂTH-ĭk, p. 1509)
leukemia (lū-KĒ-mē-ă, p. 1518)
leukopenia (lū-kō-PĒ-nē-ă, p. 1517)
lymphangitis (lĭm-făn-GĪ-tĭs, p. 1528)
lymphedema (lĭm-fĕ-DĒ-mă, p. 1529)
multiple myeloma (MŬL-tĭ-pŭl mī-ĕ-LŌ-mă, p. 1527)
myeloproliferative (mī-ĕ-lō-prō-LĬF-ĕr-ă-tĭv, p. 1515)
pancytopenic (păn-sī-tō-PĔN-ĭc, p. 1509)
pernicious (pĕr-NĬSH-ŭs, p. 1508)
Reed-Sternberg cells (rēd-STĔRN-bĕrg, p. 1530)
thrombocytopenia (thrŏm-bō-sīt-ō-PĒ-nē-ă, p. 1522)

ANATOMY AND PHYSIOLOGY OF THE HEMATOLOGIC AND LYMPHATIC SYSTEMS

Transportation and protection are two of the body's most important functions. Without transportation and protection for the cells, the body's homeostasis would be threatened. The systems that provide these vital services for the body are the circulatory and lymphatic systems. This chapter discusses the primary transportation fluid—blood—and presents an overview of the lymphatic system. Blood not only performs vital transportation services, but also provides much of the protection necessary to withstand foreign invaders. The lymphatic system helps maintain fluid balance, and lymphoid tissues help protect the internal environment.

CHARACTERISTICS OF BLOOD

In ancient times, blood was referred to as the "river of life" or "fluid of life." Some people believed it had magical properties. All knew it was necessary to maintain life.

Blood is a viscous (thick), red fluid that contains red blood cells (RBCs), white blood cells (WBCs), and platelets, which are suspended in a light yellow fluid called **plasma.** Plasma constitutes 55% of the blood's volume; the remaining 45% is composed of the blood cells and platelets (Figure 47-1). Blood is slightly alkaline, with a pH range of 7.35 to 7.45. It has a sodium chloride concentration of 0.9%. The average adult blood volume is 5 to 6 L (10½ to 12½ pints).

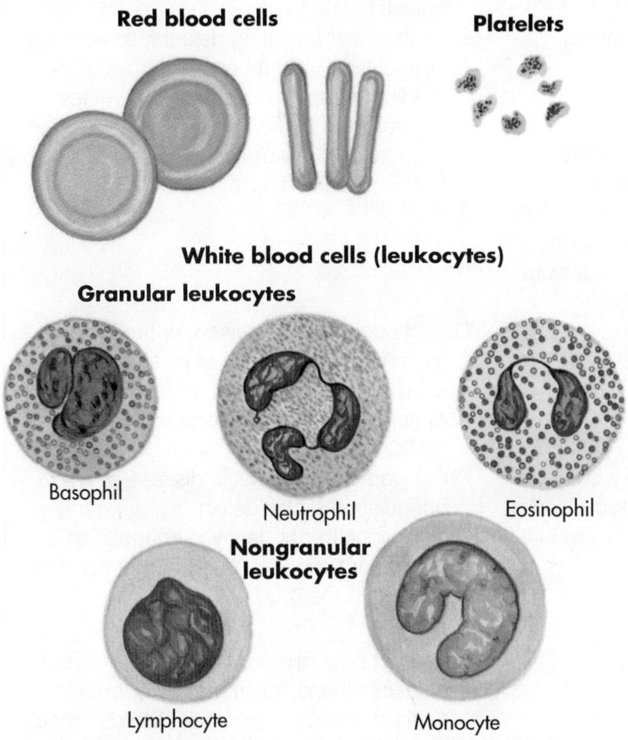

Red blood cells
Platelets
White blood cells (leukocytes)
Granular leukocytes
Basophil
Neutrophil
Eosinophil
Nongranular leukocytes
Lymphocyte
Monocyte

FIGURE 47-1 Human blood cells. There are approximately 30 trillion blood cells in an adult. Each cubic millimeter of blood contains from 4.5 million to 5 million red blood cells, 5000 to 10,000 white blood cells, and 150,000 to 400,000 platelets.

The blood performs three critical functions. First, it transports oxygen and nutrition to the cells and waste products away from the cells, and it transports hormones from endocrine glands to tissues and cells. Second, it regulates the acid-base balance (pH) with buffers, helps regulate body temperature because of its water content, and controls the water content of its cells as a result of dissolved sodium ions. Third, it protects the body against infection with special cells and prevents blood loss with special clotting mechanisms.

The following sections discuss individual components of the blood.

Red Blood Cells

Erythrocytes (RBCs) give blood its rich color. In men, RBCs average approximately 5.5 million/mm^3 of blood; in women, they average approximately 4.8 million/mm^3 (Table 47-1). A mature RBC contains cytoplasm and the red pigment hemoglobin, a compound in the blood that carries oxygen from the lungs to the cells and carbon dioxide away from the cells to the lungs. Erythrocytes are classified according to size, shape, and color. Hemoglobin content is expressed as normochromic or hypochromic anemia, whereas RBC size is usually expressed as macrocytic, microcytic, or normocytic. The normal hemoglobin level is 14 to 18 g/dL for men and 12 to 16 g/dL for women. The average life span of an RBC is 120 days. An erythrocyte is the major cellular element of the circulating blood; its principal function is to transport oxygen and carbon dioxide. Erythrocytes are continuously produced in the red bone marrow,

Table 47-1 Diagnostic Blood Studies

BLOOD TEST	NORMAL VALUES	DESCRIPTION	CLINICAL SIGNIFICANCE
Red blood cells (RBCs)	Males: 4.7-6.1 million/mm^3 Females: 4.2-5.4 million/mm^3	Actual cell count	Increased in dehydration, with polycythemia, at high altitudes, and with hypoxia; decreased in anemia, leukemia, and posthemorrhage
Hemoglobin	Males: 14-18 g/dL Females: 12-16 g/dL	Measure of total amount of hemoglobin (Hgb) in peripheral blood	Increased in polycythemia, dehydration, chronic obstructive lung disease; decreased in anemia and after hemorrhage
Hematocrit	Males: 42%-52% Females: 37%-47%	Measure of the percentage of the total blood volume that is made up by the RBCs	Increased with severe burns, shock, severe dehydration, and polycythemia; decreased with severe blood loss, leukemia, and anemia
Erythrocyte sedimentation rate (ESR)	Male: 0-15 mm/hr Female: 0-20 mm/hr	Rate at which RBCs settle out of a tube of unclotted blood in 1 hour	Increased in tissue destruction; indicates infection when results are compared with elevation in WBC count; a fairly reliable indicator of the course of disease and therefore used to monitor disease therapy, especially for inflammatory autoimmune diseases

Continued

Table 47-1 Diagnostic Blood Studies—cont'd

BLOOD TEST	NORMAL VALUES	DESCRIPTION	CLINICAL SIGNIFICANCE
Reticulocyte count	0.5%-2%	Number of reticulocytes in whole blood	Increased in bone marrow hyperactivity and hemorrhage; decreased in hemolytic disease
Platelet count	150,000-400,000/mm^3	Actual cell count	Increased in granulocytic leukemia; decreased in thrombocytopenia or aplastic anemia
Prothrombin time (PT)	11-12.5 seconds	Rapidity of blood clotting	Detects plasma clotting defects, screens for coagulation, and monitors warfarin (Coumadin) therapy; possible critical values greater than 20 seconds
International Normalized Ratio (INR)	0.7-1.8	World Health Organization has recommended the PT results now include the INR value; many hospitals report PT results in both absolute numbers and INR	Therapeutic INR usually considered to be 2-3.5; possible critical values >3.5
Partial thromboplastin time (PTT)	60-70 seconds	Fibrin clot formation	Detects coagulation defects of the intrinsic system and deficiency of plasma clotting; used for monitoring the appropriate dose of heparin; possible critical values >100 seconds
Bleeding time	1-9 minutes (Ivy method)	Amount of time for a small stab wound to stop bleeding	Prolonged in hemorrhagic disease or with coagulation factor defect
Clotting time	3-9 minutes	Amount of time for blood in a tube to clot	Prolonged with deficiency in coagulation factors or vitamin K; used to monitor anticoagulant therapy
WHITE BLOOD CELLS (WBCs) COUNT WITH DIFFERENTIAL			
WBC	5000-10,000/mm^3	Actual cell count	Increased neutrophils with a number of bacterial infections, inflammatory but noninfectious diseases (collagen disorder, rheumatic fever, and pancreatitis); increased with infectious diseases (usually of bacterial origin) and with trauma or leukemia; decreased by chemotherapy, radiation, aplastic anemia, and agranulocytosis
Neutrophils	60%-70%* 3000-7000/mm^3†		Increased with burns, crushing injuries, diabetic acidosis, and infections; decreased in bone marrow failure following antineoplastic chemotherapy or radiation therapy or in agranulocytosis, dietary deficiencies, and autoimmune diseases
Eosinophils	1%-4%* 50-400/mm^3†		Increased with allergic and parasitic disorders
Basophils	0.5%-1%* 25-100/mm^3†		Increases uncommon; found with some forms of acute leukemia
Lymphocytes	20%-40%* 1000-4000/mm^3†		Increased in infectious mononucleosis, measles, certain viruses, infectious hepatitis, and lymphocytic leukemia; decreased in AIDS, lupus erythematosus, and Hodgkin's disease
Monocytes	2%-6%* 100-600/mm^3†		Increased in the recovery phase of bacterial infections and chronic inflammatory conditions

AIDS, Acquired immunodeficiency syndrome.
*Relative values: expressed as percentage of total WBC.
†Absolute values: expressed in actual numbers × $10^9/mm^3$.

principally in the vertebrae, ribs, sternum, and proximal ends of the humerus and femur.

Erythropoiesis (the process of RBC production) depends on several factors, among them healthy conditions of the bone marrow; dietary substances such as iron and copper, plus essential amino acids; and certain vitamins, especially vitamin B_{12}, folic acid, riboflavin (vitamin B_2), and pyridoxine (vitamin B_6). When the amount of oxygen delivered to the tissues by RBCs is decreased, it triggers the release of an enzyme, the renal erythropoietic factor, in the kidneys. Erythropoietin is carried to the bone marrow, where it initiates the development of mature RBCs. The increased number of RBCs allows more oxygen to be delivered to the tissues, and as a result shuts off the signal to increase RBC production.

A common laboratory test called the **hematocrit** (a measure of the packed cell volume of RBCs, expressed as a percentage of the total blood volume) can tell a great deal about the volume of RBCs in a blood sample. Normally about 42% to 52% of the blood volume in men and 37% to 47% in women consists of RBCs.

If hemoglobin falls below the normal level, as it does in anemia, an unhealthy chain reaction begins: less hemoglobin means less oxygen transported to cells, a slower breakdown and use of nutrients by cells, less energy produced by cells, and decreased cellular function. Understanding the relationship between hemoglobin and energy makes it clear why an anemic person complains of feeling "tired all the time."

White Blood Cells

Unlike erythrocytes, **leukocytes** (WBCs) have nuclei, are colorless, and live from a few days to several years. They are primarily involved in body defenses, such as destruction of bacteria and viruses. They number 5000 to 10,000/mm^3 of blood. Some WBCs can actually leave the bloodstream and move through tissue spaces to fight foreign invaders, such as bacteria. WBCs have two broad categories: granulocytes and nongranulocytes. The three types of granulocytes are neutrophils, eosinophils, and basophils. The nongranulocytes include lymphocytes and monocytes. A **differential white blood cell count** is an examination in which the different kinds of WBCs are counted and reported as percentages of the total examined. They also may be reported as absolute (actual number) (see Figure 47-1).

Because leukocytes respond predictably to symptoms of infection and recovery, they are a reliable gauge of the state of the body's defenses. That is why the differential WBC is such a common blood test. Although the differential WBC cannot, by itself, be used to diagnose a disease or to discriminate between a bacterial and viral infection, it reveals activity that points to occult (hidden) infection or that signals the intensity of chemotherapy.

The granulocytes develop from the red bone marrow and contain granules in their cytoplasm. The granules are demonstrated when the cells are stained with Wright's stain (a chemical solution). **Neutrophils** (granular circulating leukocytes essential for **phagocytosis**—the process by which bacteria, cellular debris, and solid particles are destroyed and removed) ingest bacteria and dispose of dead tissue. Neutrophils are the primary phagocytic cells involved in acute inflammatory response. A mature neutrophil is called a segmental neutrophil, or "seg," because the nucleus is segmented into two to five lobes connected by strands. They also release lysozyme, an enzyme that destroys certain bacteria. The normal value of neutrophils is 60% to 70%.

Mature neutrophils have a short life span (approximately 7 hours), after which they die, along with the bacteria and debris they have engulfed. Bone marrow thus needs to manufacture neutrophils constantly; normally it stores approximately a 6-day supply. Because neutrophils respond in proportion to the severity of the infection, an overwhelming infection may deplete marrow reserves. When this happens, the marrow releases polymorphonuclear leukocytes ("polys") that are in the final stages of development. These immature neutrophils are called bands. When the band count exceeds 8% of the total number of polys, the marrow has used up its reserve. In the differential white count, an increase in the number of band neutrophils is called **bandemia**. Bandemia is seen in patients with serious bacterial infections. The presence of excess bands in the peripheral blood was traditionally called "a shift to the left." This term originated when laboratory reports were handwritten with the immature neutrophils recorded on the left side of paper. This term is still used in some areas (McCarron, 2004).

Eosinophils are WBCs that play a role in allergic reactions and are effective against certain parasitic worms. Normal values of eosinophils are 1% to 4%.

Basophils are WBCs that are essential to the nonspecific immune response to inflammation because they release histamine (vasodilator) during tissue damage or invasion. They have cytoplasmic granules that contain heparin, serotonin, and histamine. If a basophil is stimulated by an antigen or by tissue injury, it releases substances within the granules. This is part of the response seen in allergic and inflammatory reactions. Normal values of basophils are 0.5% to 1%.

Monocytes are WBCs that function like neutrophils; they circulate in the bloodstream and move into tissue, where they engulf foreign antigens and cell debris. Monocytes are the second type of WBC to arrive at the scene of an injury. They are useful in removing dead bacteria and cells in the recovery stage of acute bacterial infections. Normal values of monocytes are 2% to 6%.

Lymphocytes are WBCs that form antibody, a special protein that combats foreign invaders, or antigens. They set up the antigen-antibody process, which protects the body. Lymphocytes have two groups: B cells and T cells. B cells search out, identify, and bind with specific antigens. T cells, when exposed to an antigen, divide rapidly and produce large numbers of new

T cells that are sensitized to that antigen. T cells work together with the B cells to destroy the foreign antigen. Normal values of lymphocytes are 20% to 40%.

Thrombocytes (Platelets)

Thrombocytes, or platelets, are the smallest cells in the blood. They are circular cell fragments that do not contain nuclei. They have a life span of 5 to 9 days and number 150,000 to 400,000/mm^3 of blood (see Figure 47-1). They are produced in the red bone marrow and have a role in the process of hemostasis (the prevention of blood loss). They assist in forming clots, which seal off a break in the continuity of the walls of the blood vessels (Figure 47-2).

Hemostasis

Hemostasis is a body process that arrests the flow of blood and prevents hemorrhage. Three actions take place: (1) vessel spasm, (2) platelet plug formation, and (3) clot formation. When a vessel has a tear or rupture, the smooth muscle in the walls of the vessel causes it to contract. Platelets rush in and attempt to seal the area, which is effective in small vessel tears. The third process, clot formation, is more detailed and occurs in larger injuries. This process can be summarized as follows (see Figure 47-2):

1. Injury
2. Hemorrhage
3. Grouping platelets
4. Thromboplastin released (reacts along with calcium ions)
5. Converts prothrombin to thrombin
6. Links with fibrinogen
7. Formation of fibrin
8. Traps RBCs and platelets
9. Forms clot

Blood Types (Groups)

A person's blood group or type is genetically determined and is inherited from his or her parents. Blood types are determined by the presence or absence of specific antigens on the outer surface of the RBCs. In certain types of blood, the antigens on the RBCs are accompanied by antibodies found in the blood plasma. In the ABO system, every person's blood is one of the following types: type **A,** type **B,** type **AB,** or type **O.**

Forty-one percent of Americans have type A blood. The letter *A* stands for a certain type of antigen in the plasma membrane of the RBCs at birth. A person who is born with type A antigen does not form antibodies to react with it. In other words, this person's blood plasma contains no anti-A antibodies; it does, however, contain anti-B antibodies. For some unknown reason, these antibodies are present naturally in type A blood plasma. The body did not form them in response to the presence of B antigen. In summary, then, in type A blood the RBCs contain type A antigen and the plasma contains anti-B antibodies.

Correspondingly, in type B blood, the RBCs contain type B antigen and the plasma contains anti-A antibodies. In type AB, as its name indicates, the RBCs contain both type A and B antigens, and the plasma contains neither anti-A nor anti-B antibodies. The opposite is true of type O blood: its RBCs contain neither type A nor type B antigens, and the plasma contains both anti-A and anti-B antibodies.

Harmful effects or even death can result from a blood transfusion if antibodies in the recipient's plasma react to the donor's blood and the RBCs become agglutinated. If the donor's blood is type O, and therefore its RBCs do not contain any A or B antigen, the blood cannot be clumped by anti-A or anti-B antibodies. For this reason type O blood is known as **universal**

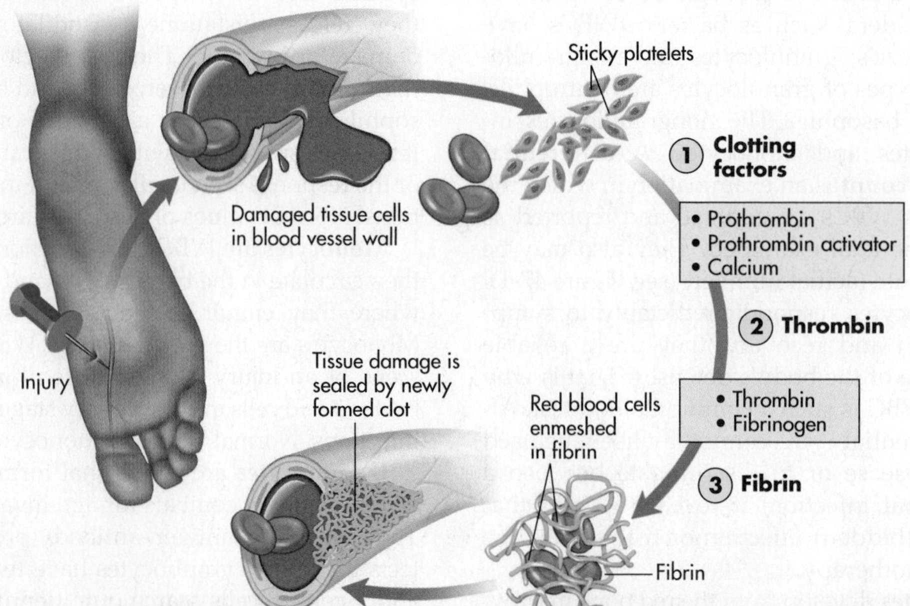

FIGURE 47-2 Blood clotting. The extremely complex clotting mechanism can be distilled into three basic steps: *1,* release of clotting factors from both injured tissue cells and sticky platelets at the injury site; *2,* formation of thrombin; and *3,* formation of fibrin and trapping of red blood cells to form a clot.

donor blood; it can be used in an emergency as donor blood, no matter what the recipient's blood type. Similarly, blood type AB has been called the **universal recipient** blood because it contains neither anti-A nor anti-B antibodies in its plasma. Therefore it does not clump any donor's RBCs containing A or B antigens. In a normal clinical setting, however, all blood intended for transfusion is typed and crossmatched carefully to the blood of the recipient for a variety of factors. Figure 47-3 shows the results of combinations of donor and recipient blood.

Two types of reactions can occur: agglutination and hemolyzation. In agglutination the donor cells clump together because of the antibodies; this occludes arteries and can result in death. In hemolyzation the antibodies cause the RBCs of the recipient to rupture and release their cell contents; this can also lead to death.

Rh Factor

Rh factor is located on the surface of the RBCs. People who have Rh factor are said to be Rh positive; people who do not have Rh factor are said to be Rh negative. Eighty-five percent of humans have Rh factor; 15% do not. Normally, human plasma does not contain Rh antibodies; these develop in response to an individual's receiving the wrong type of blood (i.e., if an Rh-negative person receives Rh-positive blood). Within approximately 2 weeks, Rh antibodies are produced and remain in the blood. If the Rh-negative person then receives more Rh-positive blood, a severe reaction occurs because the Rh-positive antibodies react with the donor blood. The antibodies hemolyze the donor RBCs, causing them to rupture and lose their contents.

Rh incompatibility is seen most commonly in pregnancy. Fortunately, this incompatibility can be prevented. The mother's blood is tested for antibodies, and if they are present, she can receive an intramuscular dose of Rh_o(D) immune globulin (RhoGAM)—a desensitization drug. This enables her to carry the next infant without the potential complications associated with Rh incompatibility.

LYMPHATIC SYSTEM

The lymphatic system is a subdivision of the cardiovascular system. It consists of lymphatic vessels, the lymph fluid, and the lymph tissue. The system has three basic functions: (1) maintenance of fluid balance, (2) production of lymphocytes, and (3) absorption and transportation of lipids from the intestine to the bloodstream.

Lymph and Lymph Vessels

The constancy of the fluid around each body cell can be maintained only if numerous homeostatic mechanisms function together in a controlled and integrated response to changing conditions. The circulatory system plays a key role in bringing many needed substances to cells and then removing the waste products that accumulate as a result of metabolism. This exchange of substances between blood and tissue fluid occurs in capillary beds. Many other substances that cannot enter or return through the capillary walls, including excess fluid and protein molecules, are returned to the blood as lymph.

Lymph is a specialized fluid formed in the tissue spaces and transported by way of lymphatic vessels to eventually reenter the circulatory system. In addition

Recipient's blood		*Reaction with donor's blood*			
RBC antigens	Plasma antibodies	Donor type O	Donor type A	Donor type B	Donor type AB
None (Type O)	Anti-A Anti-B				
A (Type A)	Anti-B				
B (Type B)	Anti-A				
AB (Type AB)	(none)				

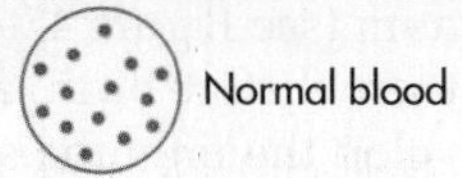

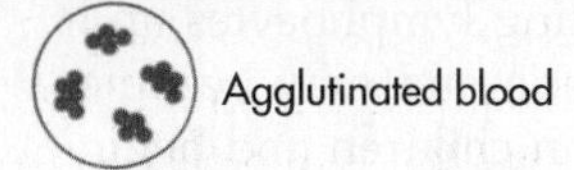

FIGURE 47-3 Results of different combinations of donor and recipient blood. The left columns show the recipient's blood characteristics, and the top row shows the donor's blood type.

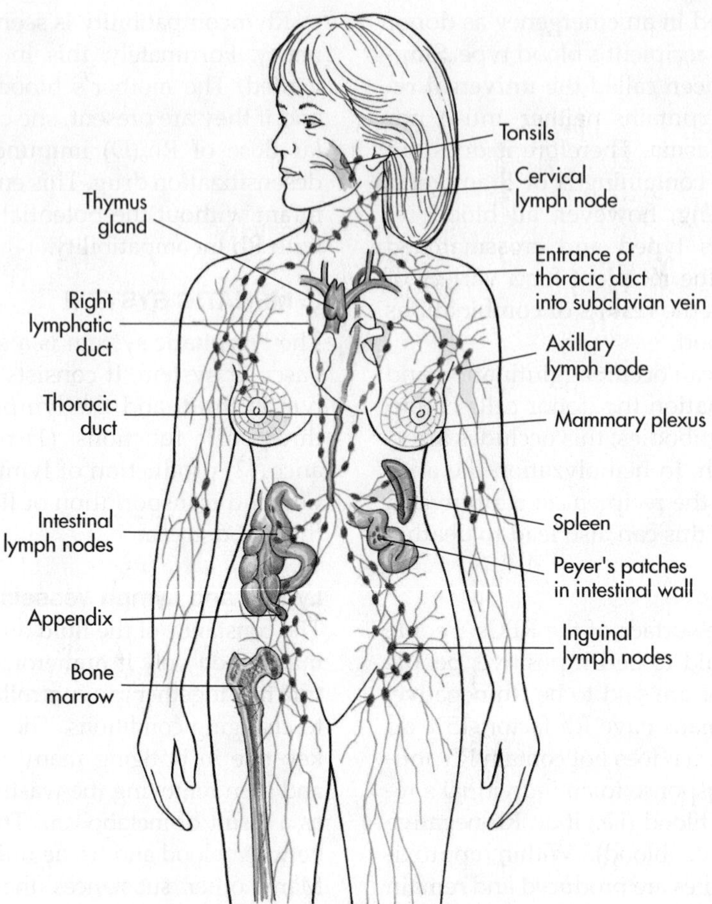

FIGURE 47-4 Principal organs of the lymphatic system.

to lymph and the lymphatic vessels, the lymphatic system includes lymph nodes and lymphatic organs such as the thymus and the spleen (Figure 47-4).

Lymphatic Tissue

Lymph Nodes

Lymph nodes (glands) have two functions: (1) to filter impurities from the lymph (much like an oil filter in a car) and (2) to produce lymphocytes (WBCs). The body contains 500 to 600 lymph nodes. They are small bean-shaped structures, usually appearing in groups. They range from 0.04 to 1 inch (1 to 25 mm) in length. Lymph nodes are most numerous in the axilla, the groin, the abdomen, the thorax, and the cervical regions (see Figure 47-4). The structure of the lymph nodes makes it possible for them to perform two functions: defense and WBC production.

Tonsils

The tonsils are masses of lymphoid tissue embedded in the mucous membrane of the oral cavity and the pharynx. The tonsils protect the body against invasion of foreign substances by producing lymphocytes and antibodies. They also trap bacteria and may become enlarged. The tonsils are larger in children and begin to atrophy (shrink) at about age 7.

Spleen

The spleen is a soft, roughly ovoid, highly vascularized organ located in the left upper quadrant of the abdominal cavity, just below the diaphragm (see Figure 47-4). The spleen is 5 to 6 inches (12.7 to 15.2 cm) long and 2 to 3 inches (5 to 7.6 cm) wide. It contains lymphatic nodules.

The spleen stores 1 pint of blood, which can be released during emergencies, such as hemorrhage, in less than 60 seconds. This large amount of blood gives the spleen its deep purple color. The main functions of the spleen are (1) to serve as a reservoir for blood; (2) to form lymphocytes, monocytes, and plasma cells; (3) to destroy worn-out RBCs; (4) to remove bacteria by phagocytosis (engulfing and digesting); and (5) to produce RBCs before birth (the spleen is believed to produce RBCs after birth only in cases of extreme hemolytic anemia).

Thymus

The thymus is located in the upper thorax posterior to the sternum and between the lungs in the mediastinum (see Figure 47-4). The thymus gland functions in utero (before birth) and a few months after birth to develop the immune system. The thymus is responsible for the development of T lymphocytes in the cell-mediated immune response before they migrate to the lymph nodes and the spleen. At puberty the thymus gland atrophies; it is eventually replaced by fat and connective tissue.

LABORATORY AND DIAGNOSTIC TESTS

Complete Blood Count

The complete blood count (CBC) is an important part of routine screening and hospital admission. It involves several tests, each of which assesses the three major cells formed in the bone marrow. The CBC detects many disorders of the hematological system and provides data for diagnosing and evaluating disorders in other body systems. A CBC includes red and white cell counts, hematocrit and hemoglobin levels, erythrocyte indexes, differential white cell count, and examination of the peripheral blood cells (see Table 47-1). Prepare the patient by explaining that a blood sample will be taken from the hand or arm and evaluated for indicators of infection or anemia in the body.

Erythrocyte Indexes

Erythrocyte indexes are measurements of the size and hemoglobin content of RBCs. This measurement provides information about the average volume or size of a single RBC (mean corpuscular volume [MCV]). Mean corpuscular hemoglobin (MCH) is a measure of the average amount (weight) of hemoglobin within an RBC. Mean corpuscular hemoglobin concentration (MCHC) is a measure of the average concentration or the percentage of hemoglobin within an RBC.

Peripheral Smear

A peripheral smear along with the differential WBC count allows examination of the size, shape, and structure of individual RBCs and platelets. This information is useful in differentiating various forms of anemias and blood dyscrasias. All three hematological cell lines (RBCs, WBCs, platelets) can be examined. When adequately prepared and examined microscopically by an experienced technologist, a smear of peripheral blood is the most informative of all hematological tests.

Schilling Test and Megaloblastic Anemia Profile

The Schilling test is a laboratory blood test for diagnosing pernicious anemia. The test measures the absorption of radioactive vitamin B_{12}, before and after parenteral injection of the intrinsic factor, by examination of the urinary excretion of vitamin B_{12}. Normal findings are excretion of 8% to 40% of radioactive vitamin B_{12} within 24 hours. The Schilling test for pernicious anemia is being replaced by a serum test called **megaloblastic anemia profile,** which measures vitamin B_{12}, methylmalonic acid, and homocysteine levels.

Gastric Analysis

Gastric analysis is an older test for determining pernicious anemia. In pernicious anemia the gastric secretions are minimal and the pH remains elevated, even after injection of histamine.

Radiologic Studies

Radiologic studies for the hematological system involve primarily the use of computed tomography (CT) or magnetic resonance imaging (MRI) for evaluating the spleen, the liver, and the lymph nodes. In the past, lymphangiography with contrast dye was a common procedure for evaluating deep lymph nodes. CT is now the preferred method (Lewis et al., 2007).

Bone Marrow Aspiration or Biopsy

When the diagnosis is not clearly established by peripheral blood smears or further information is needed, bone marrow aspiration or biopsy helps establish the diagnosis and assess treatment response. The most common site for this procedure is the posterior iliac crest. The sternum can also be used, but generally only for aspiration. Normal bone marrow is soft and semifluid and can be removed by aspiration through a needle. Bone marrow aspiration is most commonly performed in people with marked anemia, neutropenia (decreased number of WBCs), acute leukemia, and thrombocytopenia (decreased number of platelets). Cell types, numbers, and maturation are examined. Although complications of bone marrow aspiration are minimal, there is a possibility of penetrating the bone and underlying structures. This hazard is greatest in an aspiration procedure involving the sternum.

DISORDERS OF THE HEMATOLOGIC AND LYMPHATIC SYSTEMS

The hematological and lymphatic systems include the blood and the organs of blood production—the bone marrow and lymphatic tissue. Disorders of blood production, bone marrow, or lymphatic tissues affect virtually all body systems. Disturbances in this delicate balance can produce life-threatening signs and symptoms, severe pain, and incapacitation.

DISORDERS ASSOCIATED WITH ERYTHROCYTES

ANEMIA

Anemia is a disorder characterized by levels of RBCs, hemoglobin, and hematocrit that are below normal range. In hemolytic anemia, increased RBC destruction also occurs. In persons with anemia, insufficient amounts of oxygen are delivered to tissues and cells.

Etiology and Pathophysiology

Anemia can be caused by many factors, including blood loss (hemorrhage), impaired production of RBCs (bone marrow depression), increased destruction of RBCs (hemolysis), or nutritional deficiencies (long-term iron deficiency). Hemorrhage or blood loss accounts for temporary anemia, whereas nutritional deficit can cause long-term iron deficiency anemia. Marrow failure is linked to a disease process, toxic exposure, tumor, or unknown causes. A decrease in RBC production or increased destruction results in a lower number of circulating RBCs. Bone marrow hematopoietic function is unable to produce the needed quantity.

Loss of the oxygen-carrying element in the blood results in a supply/demand imbalance in vital organs. Peripheral circulation compensates by shunting blood to vital organs, thus causing hypoxia in other areas of the body. Rapid hematopoietic effort causes blood cell irregularities (immature RBCs) and inability to produce RBCs, with a resultant decrease in the RBC count.

Clinical Manifestations

Most adults do not experience symptoms until the hemoglobin level is less than 8 g/dL. Older adults, however, may show symptoms with a hemoglobin concentration of less than 10 g/dL. Although each type of anemia has specific signs and symptoms, the decreased oxygen-carrying capacity leads to signs and symptoms that are common in all anemias. These include anorexia, cardiac dilation, disorientation, dizziness, dyspepsia, dyspnea, exertional dyspnea, fatigue, headache, insomnia, pallor (mucous membranes and skin), palpitations, shortness of breath, systolic murmur, tachycardia, and vertigo.

Assessment

Subjective data commonly include expressions of weakness, dyspnea, fatigue, and vertigo. Anorexia and dyspepsia may accompany headache and insomnia, but the patient generally does not link these complaints to the condition unless questioned. In older adult patients with impaired cardiopulmonary reserves, be alert to complaints of chest pain, dyspnea on exertion, palpitations, and dizziness.

Collection of **objective data** includes observing signs of bleeding or shock (hypovolemic anemia). Laboratory values will show a low RBC count and hematocrit and hemoglobin levels. Skin and mucous membranes are pale, and cardiac symptoms are related to anemia. With long-term anemia, the patient may have ulcerations of the extremities.

Diagnostic Tests

Blood studies show RBC count and hemoglobin and hematocrit levels to be below normal. Serum iron, total iron-binding capacity, and serum ferritin levels are below normal. Reticulocyte count is increased because of immaturity of RBCs. A bone marrow study shows a deviation from normal findings. Peripheral blood smears enable identification of abnormalities of shape and color of cells. A megaloblastic anemia profile reveals decreased levels of vitamin B_{12}.

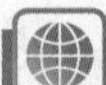
Cultural Considerations

Jehovah's Witness Opposition to Blood Transfusion

The nurse who provides culturally appropriate nursing interventions to a Jehovah's Witness has a number of factors to consider. The paramount concern is that Jehovah's Witnesses are opposed to homologous blood transfusion (blood obtained from a blood bank or through donations). Jehovah's Witnesses believe that receiving blood products from another person carries eternal consequences. However, many (but not all) Jehovah's Witnesses will submit to certain types of autologous blood transfusions (autotransfusion). One type of autologous transfusion that might be acceptable is blood retrieved through induced hemodilution at the start of surgery (blood that is directed to storage bags outside the patient's body).

In addition, some Jehovah's Witnesses permit the use of certain blood volume expanders. Many Jehovah's Witnesses carry a card with the types of blood volume expanders permitted. Ask the patient for this card or, if the patient is unconscious, examine the patient's personal belongings to find this extremely important card.

The consensus of the U.S. Supreme Court has been that a person of adult majority age has the right to refuse treatment but not to withhold a potentially life-saving treatment from a minor child.

Medical Management

Intervention depends on the cause. Correction of the disease process may correct or lessen the anemic condition. Transfusion is appropriate for blood loss; iron and vitamin B_{12} are replaced if these are deficient. Treatment is often specific to the particular anemia (see Cultural Considerations box).

Nursing Interventions and Patient Teaching

Nursing diagnoses and interventions for the patient with anemia include but are not limited to the following:

Nursing Diagnoses	Nursing Interventions
Ineffective tissue perfusion (cardiovascular), related to reduction of cellular components necessary for delivery of oxygen to the cells	Monitor changes in vital signs and in mental alertness. Monitor cardiac rhythms. Monitor hemoglobin, hematocrit, and RBCs. Assess baseline arterial blood gases and electrolytes. Note presence and degree of dyspnea, cyanosis, hemoptysis.
Impaired gas exchange, related to deficient: • RBCs • hemoglobin • hematocrit	Evaluate ability to manage activities of daily living (ADLs), related to oxygen decrease. Assess activity response, dyspnea, and heart rate.

Nursing Diagnoses	Nursing Interventions
Impaired gas exchange, related to deficient: • RBCs • hemoglobin • hematocrit	Observe for cyanosis, hypoxia, and hypercapnia. Maintain bed rest as necessary and provide range-of-motion (ROM) exercise. Monitor oxygen saturations frequently per pulse oximetry. Administer oxygen as ordered. Explain activity-oxygen deficit relationship.
Activity intolerance, related to: • oxygen deficit • secondary to decreased hemoglobin and hematocrit	Plan care to provide optimum rest. Limit environmental stimuli to reduce demands placed on the patient. Assist in identifying factors causing intolerance. Assess ability to perform ADLs, ambulation, and exercise. Assess potential for injury caused by mobility impairment. Teach patient to perform at own rate of ability, to reduce energy expenditure. Monitor hemoglobin and hematocrit levels.

Tailor patient education to the individual conditions and needs.

Hypovolemic Anemia (Blood Loss Anemia)

Etiology and Pathophysiology

Secondary anemia is when deficiencies in RBCs and other components are caused by an abnormally low circulating blood volume from hemorrhage. Blood loss of 1000 mL or more in an adult can be severe. Such a loss is usually related to internal or external hemorrhage caused by a surgical procedure, gastrointestinal (GI) bleeding, menorrhagia, trauma, or severe burns.

Loss of blood decreases the amount of circulating fluid and hemoglobin and thus decreases the amount of oxygen carried to the body tissues. The tissues must have oxygen to survive. The average adult has an approximate total blood volume of 6000 mL (6 L [12 pints]) and can tolerate a loss of up to 500 mL. If the loss approaches 1000 mL, acute complications, such as hypovolemic shock, may occur. The rapidity of blood loss is related to the severity and number of signs and symptoms. The sudden reduction in the total blood volume can lead to hypovolemic shock. RBC count and the hematocrit level drop to half the normal range.

Clinical Manifestations

Signs and symptoms include restlessness; a subtle rise in respiratory rate; weakness; stupor; irritability; and pale, cool, moist skin. Excessive blood loss results in shock. Shock occurs when there is a deprivation of oxygen and nutrients to organs. Hemorrhagic blood loss results in a decrease in blood volume. In shock, vasoconstriction occurs in blood vessels to noncritical organs such as skin, muscles, and intestines. This decreases the blood flow to these organs and shunts blood to the vital organs such as the heart and the brain.

The amount of blood loss affects the heart rate and the blood pressure. In the early stages of shock, when 750 to 1000 mL of blood has been lost, the heart rate is less than 100 bpm with a normal blood pressure. As the blood loss increases to 1000 to 1500 mL, the pulse increases to more than 100 bpm and the patient has orthostatic blood pressure. When the blood loss is 1500 to 2600 mL (about 30% to 40% of the blood volume), the systolic blood pressure decreases to less than 90 mm Hg and the pulse increases to more than 120 bpm. With a blood loss of 1500 to 2000 mL, irreversible end-organ damage can result (Beattie, 2007a).

The patient's clinical signs and symptoms are more important than the laboratory values. Be alert to the patient's expression of pain. Internal hemorrhage may cause pain because of tissue distention, organ displacement, and nerve compression. Pain may be localized or referred. Decreased RBC, hemoglobin, and hematocrit levels may not be evident until several days after severe blood loss has occurred. The severity of the patient's signs and symptoms correlates with the severity of the blood loss.

Assessment

Subjective data commonly include complaints of thirst, weakness, irritability, and restlessness.

Objective data include decreased blood pressure; rapid, weak, thready pulse; and rapid respirations. Cold, clammy skin with pallor is noted. Oliguria is often evident. Mental disorientation and physical collapse with prostration can occur.

Diagnostic Tests

When blood loss is sudden, plasma volume has not yet had a chance to increase, the loss of RBCs is not reflected in laboratory data, and values may seem normal or high for 2 to 3 days. However, once the plasma is replaced, the RBC mass is less concentrated. RBC, hemoglobin, and hematocrit levels are severely decreased, often to half the normal values.

Medical Management

In the case of massive hemorrhage, measures are taken to stop the blood loss and treat for shock and lost volume. Severe hemorrhaging often results in the need for mechanical ventilation. Oxygen therapy restores oxygen that is less available because of decreased hemoglobin in the blood. To replace fluid volume, intravenous (IV) saline is used. In severe fluid volume depletion, a bolus of 2 L of normal saline is given. If hypotension continues or if the hemoglobin is below 6 g/dL, packed RBCs are usually given. It is now recommended to keep the hemoglobin over 7 g/dL. Often platelets, fresh frozen plasma (FFP), or cryoprecipitate is included in the treatment to control hemorrhage (Beattie, 2007a).

Monitor the hemoglobin level to note the effectiveness of the treatment. Be aware that one unit of packed RBCs should increase the hemoglobin by 1 g/dL (Beattie, 2007a). The patient may also need supplemental iron because the availability of iron affects the marrow production of erythrocytes. Oral or parenteral iron preparations are often administered.

Nursing Interventions and Patient Teaching

Monitor blood and fluid restoration and identify blood loss sites to control the bleeding. Keep patients flat and warm. Take vital signs at frequent intervals. Take precautions to prevent injury to a restless or disoriented patient. Measure intake and output (I&O), with careful monitoring of urinary output for oliguria caused by decreased renal perfusion. The decrease in urinary output correlates to the amount of blood lost. If a patient has a blood loss of 1000 to 1500 mL, the urinary output is 20 to 30 mL/hr; with a blood loss of 1500 to 2000 mL, the urinary output is less than 20 mL/hr; and a blood loss of 2000 mL or more would result in anuria (very low urinary output) (Beattie, 2007a).

If hemorrhage is caused by a chronic problem, teach the patient to monitor bleeding amounts and associated factors and to report to the physician immediately for treatment.

Prognosis

Without treatment, death will result. With aggressive treatment, the prognosis is favorable.

Pernicious Anemia

Etiology and Pathophysiology

A **pernicious** disease is one that is capable of causing great injury, destruction, or death. Without treatment, pernicious anemia would be fatal. This type of anemia is the result of a metabolic defect: the absence of a glycoprotein intrinsic factor secreted by the gastric mucosa. Intrinsic secretion fails because of gastric mucosal atrophy. Pernicious anemia is an autoimmune disease in which antibodies in the parietal walls of the stomach prevent the production of the intrinsic factor (Lewis et al., 2007). It is a progressive, megaloblastic, macrocytic anemia primarily affecting older adults. The intrinsic factor is essential for absorption of vitamin B_{12} (cyanocobalamin).

The intrinsic factor is not available to combine with vitamin B_{12}, preventing transport of this necessary vitamin to the ileum (vitamin B_{12} is normally absorbed in the distal ileum). Deficiency of the vitamin affects growth and maturity of all body cells, including RBCs in the marrow. The erythrocyte membrane becomes fragile and ruptures easily. This vitamin is related to nerve myelination; its absence leads to progressive demyelination and degeneration of nerves and white matter.

Clinical Manifestations

Extreme weakness is noted with dyspnea, fever, and hypoxia. As the condition progresses, weight loss is apparent, as is slight icterus (jaundice) with pallor. The skin color may appear a pale lemon-yellow because of the excessive destruction of the RBCs, which causes the bile pigments to increase in the blood serum. The patient experiences edema of the legs, intermittent constipation, and diarrhea.

Assessment

Subjective data include the patient's complaints of palpitations, nausea, flatulence, and indigestion. The tongue is sore and burning. Weakness and difficulty swallowing (dysphagia) may occur. Neurologic symptoms include tingling of the hands and feet and loss of the sense of body position (impaired proprioception).

Collection of **objective data** includes observation of a smooth and erythematous tongue, with infection about the teeth and gums. Cerebral signs include mental disorientation, personality changes, and behavior problems. Severe neurologic impairments can result, including partial or total paralysis from destruction of the nerve fibers of the spinal cord.

Diagnostic Tests

The Schilling test shows malabsorption of vitamin B_{12}. This test is being replaced by the serum megaloblastic anemia profile, which reveals decreased serum levels of vitamin B_{12}, serum methylmalonic acid, and homocysteine. Bone marrow aspiration reveals abnormal RBC development.

The erythrocytes appear large (macrocytic) and have abnormal shapes; serum cyanocobalamin (B_{12}) levels are reduced. A gastric analysis may be done to determine the cause of the vitamin B_{12} deficiency. Pernicious anemia is caused by an absence of intrinsic factor, from either gastric mucosal atrophy or autoimmune destruction of parietal cells of the stomach. This results in a decrease of hydrochloric acid secretion by the stomach. An acidic environment in the stomach is required for the secretion of intrinsic factor.

Medical Management

Oral vitamin B_{12} is ineffective if there is an absence of the intrinsic factor in the stomach or a malabsorption problem in the ileum (Lewis et al., 2007). Cyanocobalamin injections, folic acid supplement, and iron replacement are ordered. If the anemia is severe, the patient may be transfused with packed RBCs. The standard treatment includes initiating vitamin B_{12} replacement therapy; without it, these individuals will die in 1 to 3 years. Treatment is 1,000 units of vitamin B_{12} administered intramuscularly daily for 2 weeks, then weekly until the hematocrit is normal, and finally monthly for life. An intranasal form of cyanocobalamin (Nascobal) is self-administered once weekly. The patient's blood values should return to normal within 2 months of B_{12} therapy. A CBC is necessary every 3 to 6 months to monitor the long-term success of treatment.

Nursing Interventions and Patient Teaching

The nursing interventions depend to some extent on the stage of the disease. A symptomatic approach is appropriate. When the patient is confined to the hospital, check vital signs every 4 hours. Perform special mouth care several times daily. The diet should be high in protein, vitamins, and minerals. Anemic patients are especially sensitive to cold, so additional lightweight, warm blankets may be needed. Interventions should conserve energy and prevent injury.

Nursing diagnoses and interventions for the patient with pernicious anemia include but are not limited to the following:

Nursing Diagnoses	Nursing Interventions
Risk for injury, related to: • sensory and motor losses • alteration in mental status	Use bed rest, with side rails up as needed, to prevent patient fatigue and falls caused by weakness. Assist with ambulation to avoid falls. Use bed cradle or footboard to prevent pressure on lower extremities. Apply heat with extreme caution to avoid burning the skin. If heat therapy is required, evaluate the patient's skin at frequent intervals to detect erythema. Support patient with patience and reassurance to reduce irritability and depression.
Imbalanced nutrition: less than body requirements, related to: • sore mouth and tongue • diarrhea • constipation	Administer vitamin B_{12} and other medications prescribed to promote production of erythrocytes. Encourage diet high in vitamins, iron, and protein to promote production of healthy erythrocytes.
Imbalanced nutrition: less than body requirements, related to: • sore mouth and tongue • diarrhea • constipation	Provide meticulous and frequent oral hygiene to promote improved appetite and prevent infection. Offer small, frequent feedings to prevent digestive overload. Observe for diarrhea or constipation and treat as prescribed to avoid fluid and electrolyte imbalance and discomfort.

To control the disease, the patient must understand the disease process and the importance of lifetime therapy of vitamin B_{12}. Discuss the importance of a diet high in vitamin B_{12}. Adjusting activities when signs and symptoms are present may lessen the patient's stress. The need for assistance with ADLs and for frequent rest periods should be impressed on the patient and significant people involved in the care.

Prognosis

This condition, if untreated, can be considered terminal in 1 to 3 years. With treatment the patient may be asymptomatic. Because the potential for gastric carcinoma is increased in pernicious anemia, the patient should have frequent and careful evaluation for this problem.

Aplastic Anemia

Etiology and Pathophysiology

Aplastic anemia, or **aplasia** (a hematological term for a failure of the normal process of cell generation and development), has two etiologic classifications: **congenital** and **acquired.** Approximately 30% of aplastic anemias that appear in childhood are inherited, caused by chromosomal alterations. Acquired aplastic anemia is directly related to exposure to viral invasion, medications, chemicals (e.g., benzene, insecticides, arsenic, alcohol), radiation, or chemotherapy, in which the hematopoietic tissue is replaced by fatty marrow, causing a defect in RBC production. The causes of 70% of acquired cases of aplastic anemia are **idiopathic** (cause unknown). Aplastic anemia is probably an immune-mediated disease.

Depression of erythrocyte production results in lowered hemoglobin and RBCs. Leukopenia and thrombocytopenia may develop. People with aplastic anemia are usually **pancytopenic**; that is, all three major blood elements (red cells, white cells, and platelets) from the bone marrow are reduced or absent. The incidence of aplastic anemia is low, affecting approximately 4 of every 1 million people.

Clinical Manifestations

The signs and symptoms of aplastic anemia may have an acute onset or develop slowly over several weeks to months. With suppression of all three major blood elements, the patient may have signs and symptoms related to each. For example, suppression of WBCs may result in infection, suppression of RBCs may lead to anemia, or suppression of thrombocytes may cause petechiae (Lewis et al., 2007). Repeated infections with high fevers may occur, along with fatigue, weakness, general malaise, dyspnea, and palpitations. Mortality is high from complications of infection and hemorrhage. Bleeding tendencies are reported: petechiae, ecchymoses, bleeding gums, epistaxis, and GI and genitourinary system bleeding.

Assessment

Subjective data include a history of exposure to chemicals such as insecticides and drugs in addition to a family history of aplastic anemia. Ask the patient about the ability to carry out ADLs without fatigue.

Collection of **objective data** includes monitoring the patient for pallor, signs of infection, and bleeding tendencies. Also, dyspnea and tachycardia may be noted.

Diagnostic Tests

A bone marrow study (aspiration biopsy) shows hypoplastic or aplastic fatty deposits, a decrease in cellular elements with increased yellow marrow (fat content), and depressed hematopoietic activity. The diagnostic findings are especially important because the marrow is hypocellular, with increased yellow marrow, a finding termed *dry tap*. Peripheral blood smears show that blood cells may be normocytic and normochromic.

Medical Management

The cause of aplastic anemia must be identified promptly and removed or discontinued. Bone marrow suppression is expected with certain antineoplastic medications or radiation therapy, and laboratory values should be monitored frequently to maintain control.

Avoid blood transfusions, if possible, to prevent iron overloading and the development of antibodies to tissue antigens. Platelet transfusions that are human lymphocyte antigen (HLA) matched are used to treat serious bleeding in a thrombocytopenic patient. Blood transfusions are used cautiously to minimize the risk of rejection for a bone marrow transplant candidate.

A splenectomy may be required in patients with hypersplenism that is destroying normal platelets. Steroids and androgens are sometimes used to stimulate the bone marrow. Immunosuppressive therapy with antithymocyte globulin and cyclosporine or high-dose cyclophosphamide (Cytoxan) has become important for patients who are not candidates for bone marrow transplantation or hematopoietic stem cell transplant (SCT). Bone marrow transplantation or hematopoietic SCT is the treatment of choice in patients younger than the age of 45 who have a compatible donor. Granulocyte-macrophage colony-stimulating factor (GM-CSF) is used as biologic response modifier treatment for aplastic anemia.

Bone marrow transplant. A bone marrow transplant is indicated in certain cases such as immunodeficient states, cancer, leukemia, and recurrent aplastic anemia. A matched donor and recipient are essential to avoid rejection or complications. Specimens from twins, siblings, or self (autologous) while in remission are preferred.

After emotional and physical preparation of the patient, perform blood studies to set baselines and assess the patient's status. Establish a pathogen-free environment, with the immunocompromised patient placed on reverse isolation (neutropenic precautions). Monitor for fever or infection. The medication therapy used in this preparation may include immunosuppressants, antibiotics, and antianxiety agents.

Bone marrow transplants are used increasingly in hematological malignancies after large doses of chemotherapy or radiation therapy. A limited amount of chemotherapy or radiation can ordinarily be administered because of its toxicity to the bone marrow. When bone marrow is transplanted after these therapeutic modes, much larger therapeutic doses are possible.

Bone marrow is obtained by multiple marrow aspirations under general or spinal anesthesia, usually yielding 500 to 800 mL of marrow. The marrow is cryopreserved (frozen) until it is used. Shortly after chemotherapy (with or without radiation therapy) is completed, the patient receives the donated marrow through an IV catheter. This infusion of marrow is called the **rescue process.** The marrow travels through the bloodstream to the bone marrow, where it begins to manufacture new leukocytes, erythrocytes, and thrombocytes. The infused marrow repopulates the patient's marrow after several weeks. The patient runs a great risk of toxicity, including infections, marrow rejection, and graft-versus-host disease. Medications supporting graft acceptance include cyclosporine (immunosuppressant) and chemotherapy (to prevent graft-versus-host complications).

Splenectomy. Surgical excision of the spleen may be performed to treat blood dyscrasias with splenomegaly, to treat trauma to the spleen, or to remove a diseased spleen. Preoperative assessment includes cardiovascular observation, respiratory function determination, and GI evaluation. Postoperatively, compare these observations with the patient's baseline evaluations, and observe the patient for infection or inflammation. Potential complications include infection, hemorrhage, shock, and paralytic ileus. Maintain parenteral therapy. Use nasogastric (NG) suction if a paralytic ileus develops. Address the patient's postoperative pain. Also maintain movement and use positioning to prevent infection or postoperative pneumonia.

Nursing Interventions and Patient Teaching

Proper observation and care after bone marrow study are essential. Patients with aplastic anemia are highly susceptible to infection; thus nursing interventions should be directed toward prevention. Adhere to strict aseptic techniques for dressing changes and IV site care. To prevent impaired skin and mucous membranes, avoid intramuscular injections and rectal medications or rectal temperatures. Use protective devices, such as an air mattress. In the presence of thrombocytopenia, observe carefully for any signs of bleeding and prevent even the slightest trauma. Monitor the patient's urine and stool for occult or gross blood.

Nursing diagnoses and interventions for the patient with aplastic anemia include but are not limited to the following:

Nursing Diagnoses	Nursing Interventions
Activity intolerance, related to inadequate tissue oxygenation	For hypoxia, place the patient in a sitting position; observe respiration rate, pulse, and dyspnea; observe skin color and temperature; assist with care; plan rest periods; administer oxygen as needed; monitor laboratory values to improve gas exchange. Monitor pulse oximetry levels carefully. Assist with ADLs as needed. Encourage patient to engage in activities on a progressive basis as fatigue decreases in response to therapy. Help patient explore feelings associated with fatigue.
Risk for infection, related to increased susceptibility	Maintain reverse isolation to avoid exposure to pathogen. Observe for increase in temperature, pulse, and respirations as signs of infection. Observe the patient for "sniffles," sore throat, anorexia, and pain on urination. Administer antibiotics as ordered to combat specific pathogens. Encourage mobility, turning, coughing, deep breathing, and increased fluids to reduce susceptibility to infection.

Everyone with aplastic anemia needs to know how to protect themselves from excessive bleeding. Help the patient maintain a balance between rest and activity. Discuss with the patient how to avoid infection, especially of the respiratory or urinary tract (see Safety Alert box).

Safety Alert!

Aplastic Anemia

- Prevent infection.
  - —Use good hand hygiene technique.
  - —Avoid contact with those who have infection.
  - —Avoid sharing eating utensils and bath linens.
  - —Take a bath or shower every day (or every other day if skin is dry); keep perineal area clean.
  - —Use good oral hygiene.
  - —Eliminate intake of raw meats, fruits, or vegetables.
  - —Immediately report signs of infection to physician.
- Prevent hemorrhage.
  - —Observe for signs such as blood in urine or stool and petechiae, and report these to physician.
  - —Use a soft toothbrush or swab for mouth care.
  - —Keep mouth clean and free of debris.
  - —Avoid enemas or other rectal insertions.
  - —Avoid picking or blowing the nose forcefully.
  - —Avoid trauma, falls, bumps, and cuts; avoid contact sports.
  - —Avoid use of aspirin or aspirin preparations (anticoagulant effect).
  - —Use an electric razor.
  - —Use adequate lubrication and gentleness during sexual intercourse.
  - —Avoid intramuscular injections.
- Prevent fatigue.
  - —Take frequent rest periods between ADLs and activity.
  - —Avoid excessive workload or heavy lifting, and ask for assistance with strenuous activity.
  - —Increase time necessary for routine care.
  - —Decrease activity if shortness of breath, dizziness, or sensation of heaviness in extremities occurs.
  - —Report signs of increased fatigue.

Prognosis

The prognosis of untreated aplastic anemia is poor (approximately 75% fatal). However, advances in medical management have improved outcomes significantly in aggressively treated patients. The object of care is to produce remission and prolong survival.

Iron Deficiency Anemia

Etiology and Pathophysiology

Iron deficiency anemia is a condition in which the RBCs contain decreased levels of hemoglobin. The most common cause of iron deficiency anemia is excessive iron loss. In adults the most common source is chronic intestinal or uterine bleeding; however, iron deficiency anemia can also be caused by bleeding from gastric or duodenal ulcers, esophageal varices, hiatal hernias, colonic diverticula, and tumors. The major sources of chronic blood loss are from the GI and genitourinary systems (Box 47-1).

GI bleeding is often not apparent and may exist for a considerable time before being identified. Loss of 50 to 75 mL of blood from the upper GI tract is required for stools to appear as black or melenic. The color results from the iron in the RBCs. Blood losses related to men-

Box 47-1 Causes of Iron Deficiency Anemia

- Iron deficiency may develop from inadequate dietary intake, malabsorption, blood loss, or hemolysis (breakdown of red blood cells).
- Daily iron intake from food and dietary supplements is adequate to meet the needs of men and older women, but it may be inadequate for those with higher iron needs (e.g., menstruating or pregnant women).
- Malabsorption of iron may occur after certain types of gastrointestinal (GI) surgery and in malabsorption syndromes. Iron absorption occurs in the duodenum. Malabsorption of iron may involve disease of the duodenum in which the absorption surface is altered or destroyed.
- Blood loss is a major cause of iron deficiency in adults. The major sources of chronic blood loss are from the GI and genitourinary systems. Common causes of GI blood loss are peptic ulcers, gastritis, esophagitis, diverticulitis, hemorrhoids, and neoplasms. The average monthly menstrual blood loss is about 45 mL and causes the loss of 22 mg of iron.

struation or pregnancy are common causes of iron deficiency anemia in young women. Rarely, excessive losses occur through microhemorrhages into lung tissue or from intestinal parasites. Even without excessive blood loss, iron deficiency anemia can result when the body's demand for iron exceeds its absorption, which commonly occurs in infants, young adolescents, and pregnant women. Less commonly, iron deficiency anemia results from malabsorption of iron caused by diseases such as celiac disease and sprue. Subtotal gastrectomy may lead to iron deficiency caused by **achlorhydria** (loss of hydrochloric acid), occult bleeding, and decreased iron in postgastrectomy diets. Deficiency caused by poor dietary intake is rare in middle-age adults.

Approximately 1 mg of every 10 to 20 mg (5% to 10%) of iron ingested is absorbed in the duodenum. This amount of dietary iron meets the needs of men and older women, but it may be inadequate for people who have higher iron needs (e.g., children, pregnant and lactating women).

Clinical Manifestations

The most common symptoms of iron deficiency anemia are (in order) pallor and glossitis (inflammation of the tongue). Fatigue, weakness, and shortness of breath also often occur. Signs and symptoms typical of angina and heart failure may also occur.

Assessment

Collection of **subjective data** includes noting GI symptoms such as glossitis (manifested by inflammation and soreness of the tongue) and **pagophagia** (the desire to eat ice, clay, or starches). The patient may complain of headache, paresthesia, and a burning sensation of the tongue, all of which are caused by lack of iron in the tissues.

Collection of **objective data** includes noting the signs, including pallor and tachycardia. Fingernails may be fragile and shaped like the head of a spoon with a central depression and raised borders. Mucous membranes of the mouth may be inflamed (stomatitis), and lips may be erythemic with cracking at the angles.

Diagnostic Tests

The peripheral blood counts show that RBC, hemoglobin levels, and hematocrit are decreased; serum iron levels are low.

Medical Management

Administer iron salts such as ferrous sulfate. In 3 weeks the hematocrit level should rise 5% to 15%, and the hemoglobin level should rise to 2 to 5 g/dL. For the body to incorporate 100 mg of iron per day, administer 900 mg/day. Iron is administered orally or by injection. Ascorbic acid has been shown to enhance iron absorption. Food sources of iron include meat, fish, poultry, eggs, green leafy vegetables, whole grains, and dried beans (Box 47-2).

When the patient cannot tolerate oral preparations of iron, parenteral iron therapy is used. The Z-track method of giving iron dextran (DexFerrum) intramuscularly is preferable to prevent skin staining. Iron sucrose (Venofer) is an IV drug frequently used for treatment of iron deficiency anemia.

Nursing Interventions and Patient Teaching

Because treatment is directed toward diagnosis and alleviation of the cause, the patient interview is important. Medication therapy for iron replacement is initiated as ordered. Plan for rest periods when fatigue is present. Education about nutritional needs relative to the condition may prevent this anemia (see Box 47-2).

Explanation of the side effects of iron therapy is essential to alleviate distress and to extend the therapy for the necessary time (see Health Promotion box). The patient must know which signs and symptoms are significant and need to be reported to the physician. Diarrhea or nausea is significant, but black, tarry stools are not (these are to be expected with iron therapy).

Prognosis

The prognosis is usually good with correction of the underlying cause and compliance with the medical treatment.

Sickle Cell Anemia

Etiology and Pathophysiology

Sickle cell anemia is the most common genetic disorder in the United States, predominantly affecting the black population. A sickle cell is an abnormal, crescent-shaped RBC containing hemoglobin S (Hg-S), a defective hemoglobin molecule. This anemia is a severe, chronic, incurable condition that occurs in people **homozygous** (having two identical genes inherited from each parent for a

Box 47-2 Food Sources of Nutrients Needed for Erythropoiesis

IRON
- Organ meats: liver, kidney, heart, and tongue
- Muscle meats, especially dark meat from poultry
- Eggs
- Shellfish
- Whole-grain breads and cereals
- Iron-enriched or iron-fortified breads and cereal
- Dark green vegetables: spinach, Swiss chard, kale, greens (dandelion, beet, and turnip)
- Dried fruits: apricots, dates, figs, prunes, and raisins
- Legumes and nuts

FOLIC ACID
- Green leafy vegetables
- Asparagus, broccoli
- Organ meats: liver
- Meat
- Whole-grain breads and cereals
- Enriched and fortified breads and cereals
- Fish
- Legumes

VITAMIN B_{12}
- Organ meats: liver and kidney
- Muscle meats
- Milk and cheese
- Eggs

AMINO ACIDS
- Eggs
- Meat
- Milk and milk products (cheese, ice cream)
- Poultry
- Fish
- Legumes
- Nuts

VITAMIN C
- Citrus fruits
- Leafy green vegetables
- Strawberries
- Cantaloupe

Health Promotion

Iron Administration

- Iron preparations supplement the body's natural iron stores.
- Dosages are determined by the elemental iron content of the preparation.
- Iron supplements may be contraindicated in peptic ulcer disease.
- Side effects include gastrointestinal (GI) upset (nausea, vomiting), constipation or diarrhea, and green to black stools. Elixir may stain teeth.
- Iron is absorbed best from the duodenum and proximal jejunum. Therefore enteric-coated or sustained-release capsules, which release iron farther down in the GI tract, are counterproductive; they are also more expensive.
- If side effects develop, the dose and type of iron supplement may be adjusted. Some people cannot tolerate ferrous sulfate because of the effects of the sulfate base. Ferrous gluconate may be an acceptable substitute.
- Iron is best absorbed in an acidic environment. To avoid binding the iron with food, iron should be taken about an hour before meals, when the duodenal mucosa is most acidic. Taking iron with vitamin C (ascorbic acid) or orange juice, which contains ascorbic acid, also enhances iron absorption. Gastric side effects, however, may necessitate ingesting iron with meals.
- Do not administer with antacids.
- If a dose is missed, continue with schedule; do not double a dose.
- Iron may interfere with absorption of oral tetracycline antibiotics. Do not take within 2 hours of each other.
- Dilute liquid iron preparations in juice or water, and administer with a straw to avoid staining teeth. Provide oral hygiene after taking.
- Check for constipation or diarrhea. Record color (iron turns stools green to black) and amount of stool.
- Iron is toxic, and caution must be taken to store iron preparations out of a child's reach.

given hereditary characteristic) for Hg-S. Sickle cell crisis is an episode of acute "sickling" of RBCs, which causes occlusion and ischemia in distal blood vessels. Sickling leads to clumping, or aggregation, of these misshapen RBCs, which lodge in small vessels. Sickle cell trait is the **heterozygous** (having two different genes) form of sickle cell anemia whereby the individual has both Hg-S and hemoglobin A (Hg-A) in the RBCs. Patients with sickle cell trait do not have signs or symptoms, but risk passing the disorder on to their children.

Approximately 81% of black Americans have sickle cell trait (about 2 million in the United States), and approximately 1 of every 600 (about 80,000 individuals in the United States) has sickle cell anemia (Lewis et al., 2007). Tissue hypoxia and ischemia occur, causing pain and edema as a result of inflammation. Compared with a normal life span of about 120 days, an RBC affected by sickle cell disease has a life span of only 10 to 20 days (Lewis et al., 2007). Destruction of fragile RBCs thus inhibits the oxygen-carrying function.

Clinical Manifestations

Usually the newborn with sickle cell anemia is asymptomatic for the first 10 to 12 weeks of age, until most of the fetal hemoglobin (Hb-F) has been replaced by Hb-S. However, periods of crisis then occur, accelerating the signs and symptoms. Many people with sickle cell anemia are in reasonably good health the majority of the time. The typical patient is anemic but asymptomatic except during painful episodes. Physical and probably emotional factors (stress) precipitate a painful episode. Physical factors include events that cause dehydration or change the oxygen tension in the body, such as infection, overexertion, weather changes (cold), ingestion of alcohol, and smoking.

Infections are a major complication of sickle cell anemia. Pneumonia, meningitis, influenza, and hepatitis may occur. Loss of appetite and irritability with weakness follow minor infections. Abdominal enlargement with pooling of blood in the liver, spleen, and other organs may accompany jaundice. Joint and back pain is noted, as is edema of the extremities. Complications include multisystem failure, infarctions, hemorrhage, and retinal damage leading to blindness.

Assessment

Collection of **subjective data** begins with assessing the patient's knowledge and feelings about the disease and factors that appear to precipitate crisis or exacerbate signs and symptoms. Fatigue may be reported when anemia is severe. The primary symptom associated with sickling is pain. During the sickle cell crisis, the pain is severe due to tissue ischemia. Aching joints, especially those of the hands and feet, are common complaints. The pain associated with these attacks is often described as deep, gnawing, and throbbing.

Collection of **objective data** includes observing for abdominal enlargement and jaundice, edema of the extremities, and signs of hemorrhage. As a result of the accelerated RBC breakdown, the patient has a characteristic clinical finding of hemolysis (jaundice, elevated serum bilirubin levels).

Diagnostic Tests

Electrophoresis of hemoglobin in a patient with sickle cell anemia is specific for detecting sickle cell crisis or anemia. More than 80% of hemoglobin as shown by electrophoresis is Hg-S, not Hg-A. A stained blood smear detects anemia only. Hematocrit and hemoglobin levels are below normal values. WBCs are increased with infection. Skeletal roentgenograms demonstrate bone and joint deformities and flattening. MRI may be used to diagnose a stroke caused by occluded cerebral vessels from sickled cells.

Medical Management

Sickle cell anemia has no specific treatment. Therapy is usually directed toward alleviating the symptoms that result from complications. For example, chronic leg ulcers may be treated with bed rest, antibiotics, warm saline soaks, mechanical or enzyme debridement, and dressings. Serious infections, such as meningitis, pneumonia, sepsis, and osteomyelitis, must be aggressively treated to prevent death (Lewis at al., 2007). *Haemophilus influenzae,* pneumococcal-conjugated, meningococcal, and hepatitis immunizations should be administered.

Sickle cell crisis may require hospitalization. Oxygen may be administered to alter hypoxia and control sickling. Encourage rest and administer fluids and electrolytes intravenously to reduce blood viscosity and maintain renal function. Use analgesics to treat pain. Sickle cell crisis pain is often undertreated. The nurse needs a clear understanding of the disease process and of current approaches to pain management.

According to pain experts, parenteral morphine and hydromorphone are the preferred opioid analgesics for acute sickle cell crisis pain. Large doses of continuous (rather than prn) opioid analgesics are the mainstay of pain management during the acute phase. Patient-controlled analgesia may be used during an acute crisis. After discharge, patients often continue taking oral opioid analgesics. Health care personnel must overcome their fears of opioid addiction to treat pain optimally and to avoid prolonging its duration. Blood transfusions of packed RBCs should be used cautiously to treat a crisis. Packed RBCs have little role, if any, in treating patients between crises. These patients have an increased need for folic acid, so it is important for them to take daily supplements. Iron therapy generally is not suggested.

Hydroxyurea therapy significantly boosts the production of Hg-F, reduces hemolysis, increases hemoglobin concentration, and decreases sickled cells. An oral antifungal medication is in clinical trials for patients with sickle cell anemia to see if it will decrease sickling and keep the RBCs hydrated by preventing potassium loss (Platt, 2007).

Hematapoietic stem cell transplantation (HSCT) is the only therapy that can cure selected patients with sickle cell anemia. The use of HSCT is limited because of scarcity of appropriate donors, selection of appropriate recipients, and the risks as well as cost effectiveness (Lewis et al., 2007).

Nursing Interventions and Patient Teaching

Supportive treatment depends on signs and symptoms presentation: hydration and analgesia during crises, and dilution of blood with increased fluid intake to reverse sickling. Monitoring the transfusion therapy for evidence of transfusion reaction is vital. Attention to fever and infection is important. Genetic counseling is indicated.

Nursing diagnoses and interventions for the patient with sickle cell anemia include but are not limited to the following:

Nursing Diagnoses	Nursing Interventions
Pain, related to thrombotic crisis	Place patient in proper anatomic alignment, and protect joints. Position patient by slow, gentle handling. Apply warmth with soaks or compresses to relieve discomfort. Give analgesics on a fixed time schedule to maintain a steady serum drug level, which improves pain control, minimizes complications, and decreases anxiety. (A patient-controlled analgesic infusion pump provides a constant, low-dose infusion of an opioid for excellent pain control.)

Nursing Diagnoses	Nursing Interventions
Impaired skin integrity, related to altered circulation to tissues, resulting in hypoxia and inadequate nutrition	Remove constrictive clothing to enhance circulation. Maintain room and body warmth to avoid discomfort or chilling. Initiate ROM exercises; support joints at rest and with movement to stimulate circulation. Palpate for arterial pulses to assess patency of arterial circulation. Monitor blood studies for gas exchange and hematological indicators of adequate tissue perfusion. Place patient on bed rest to decrease resistance to peripheral circulation. Elevate affected parts to enhance venous return. Implement cleaning procedure (use hydrogen peroxide or normal saline solution) to remove drainage and necrotic tissue. Apply sterile dressing or expose affected area to air to promote healing. Apply heat with lamp or cradle as ordered to enhance circulation and healing. Observe response to evaluate effectiveness of therapy. Cut patient's nails and discourage scratching to avoid injury.

Alert the patient to the need for family testing to determine the presence of Hg-S; genetic counseling is available for carriers. Explain how to avoid sickle cell crises: avoid high altitudes, flying in unpressurized planes, dehydration, extreme temperatures, iced liquids, and vigorous exercise; use stress-reduction methods. Patients should not smoke and should protect extremities from injury because of impaired circulation. Patients with sickle cell disease have frequent problems with infections. It is important for the patient to remain current with vaccinations and take prophylactic antibiotics to protect against these infections. Explain that young pregnant women have a high risk for developing pulmonary and/or renal complications. Alert the patient to the signs and symptoms of increased intracranial pressure and to the need to blow the nose gently, avoid coughing, and avoid straining on elimination.

Practice ROM exercises with the patient and encourage regular physical activity to prevent bone demineralization. Explain the need for a balance between rest (physical and mental) and activity, such as ROM and isometric exercises. Also discuss the principles of good nutrition, such as the importance of protein, calcium, vitamins, and adequate fluids. Demonstrate to the patient how to monitor oral intake, urinary output, and urine protein.

Prognosis

Earlier detection, improved treatments, and greater use of immunizations help patients with sickle cell disease live longer, more productive lives (Platt, 2007). Still, the prognosis is guarded. In addition to hemolytic anemia, painful crises with multiple infarctions of most organ systems can occur. With repeated episodes of sickling, there is gradual involvement of all body systems, especially the spleen, the lungs, the kidneys, and the brain. Bone marrow grafts from HLA-identical siblings are providing hope for sickle cell patients.

Polycythemia (Erythrocytosis)

Etiology and Pathophysiology

Two types of polycythemia are **primary polycythemia (polycythemia vera)** and **secondary polycythemia.** Their etiologies and pathophysiology differ, although their complications and clinical manifestations are similar.

Polycythemia vera is a **myeloproliferative** (characterized by excessive bone marrow production) disorder with hyperplasia of bone marrow; it manifests with an increase in circulating erythrocytes **(erythrocytosis)**, granulocytes, and platelets. The condition is a stem cell abnormality of unknown cause. Polycythemia vera develops gradually and is a chronic disease. The average age for the patient is 60 years. It occurs slightly more frequently in men. The patient has blood that is relatively thick and flows more slowly than usual (Lewis et al., 2007). There is also an elevated WBC count with basophilia. Secondary polycythemia is caused by hypoxia rather than by a defect in the development of the RBC. Hypoxia stimulates erythropoietin in the kidneys, which in turn stimulates erythrocyte production. The need for increased oxygen may result from high altitude, pulmonary disease, cardiovascular disease, or tissue hypoxia. Secondary polycythemia is not a pathologic response, but a physiologic response in which the body tries to compensate for a hypoxic problem. In polycythemia vera the pathologic response is a malignancy of the blood cells.

Multiorgan system disease is affected by hyperplastic bone marrow elements. Because of the increased erythrocyte mass, hypervolemia and hyperviscosity (stickiness) of the blood result in congestion of tissues and organs. The sluggish circulatory process results in hypercoagulopathies that predispose patients to infarctions of vital organs.

Clinical Manifestations

Patients with polycythemia vera have increased blood volume and viscosity, which can result in hypertension, angina pectoris, heart failure, and thrombophlebitis

(Platt, 2007). Venous distention and platelet dysfunction cause esophageal varices, epistaxis, GI bleeding, and petechiae. Hepatomegaly and splenomegaly from organ engorgement may contribute to patient complaints of satiety and fullness.

Assessment

Subjective data include patient complaints of sensitivity to hot and cold. Generalized pruritus (often exacerbated by a hot bath) may be a striking symptom and is related to histamine release from an increased number of basophils. Headaches, vertigo, tinnitus, blurred vision, and painful burning of the hands and feet are often present.

Objective data include eczema and dermatologic changes. The skin may develop an erythemic appearance (plethora). Elevated blood pressure accompanies left ventricular hypertrophy and angina.

Diagnostic Tests

Plasma and RBC volume are increased. Elevations are seen in hemoglobin and hematocrit levels, reticulocyte and erythrocyte counts, platelets (thrombocytes), and WBC count with basophilia. Elevated alkaline phosphatase, uric acid, and histamine levels are noted. Bone marrow examination in polycythemia vera shows hypercellularity of RBCs, WBCs, and platelets. The basal metabolic rate (BMR) is increased without thyroid function alteration. Splenomegaly is found in 90% of patients with primary polycythemia but does not accompany secondary polycythemia.

Medical Management

Blood viscosity is decreased by repeated phlebotomy—removal of 500 to 2000 mL of blood until the hematocrit level is maintained at 45% to 48%. The procedure is repeated if hematocrit rises to more than 50%. Once the diagnosis of polycythemia vera is made, treatment is directed toward reducing blood volume and viscosity and bone marrow activity. Myelosuppressive agents such as busulfan (Myleran), hydroxyurea (Hydrea), melphalan (Alkeran), and radioactive phosphorus are often given to inhibit bone marrow activity. Allopurinol may reduce the number of acute gouty attacks.

Nursing Interventions and Patient Teaching

Polycythemia vera is not preventable. However, because secondary polycythemia is generated by any source of hypoxia, problems may be prevented by maintaining adequate oxygenation. Therefore controlling chronic pulmonary disease, stopping smoking, and avoiding high altitudes may be important.

When acute exacerbations of polycythemia vera develop, the nurse has several responsibilities. Judiciously evaluate fluid I&O during hydration therapy to avoid fluid overload (which further complicates the circulatory congestion) and dehydration (which can cause the blood to become even more viscous). If myelosuppressive agents are used, administer the drugs as ordered, observe the patient, and teach the patient about medication side effects.

Assess the patient's nutritional status with the dietitian if necessary to offset the inadequate food intake that can result from GI symptoms of fullness, pain, and dyspepsia. Institute activities, such as active or passive leg exercises and ambulation, to decrease the risk of thrombus formation.

Because of its chronic nature, polycythemia vera requires ongoing evaluation. Phlebotomy may need to be performed every 2 to 3 months, reducing the blood volume by about 500 mL each time. Evaluate the patient for the development of complications.

Nursing diagnoses and interventions for the patient with polycythemia vera include but are not limited to the following:

Nursing Diagnoses	Nursing Interventions
Ineffective tissue perfusion (cardiopulmonary, cerebral, GI, and peripheral), related to: • hyperviscosity of fluid • potential bleeding	Have patient maintain comfortable position. When patient is on bed rest, do not raise knee gatch. Provide active or passive ROM exercises every 2 to 4 hours. Check peripheral pulses and color and temperature of extremities every 4 to 6 hours. Report early signs or symptoms of thrombosis or bleeding to physician. If patient has bleeding tendency, avoid invasive procedures when possible. Avoid trauma; provide soft-bristled toothbrush.
Activity intolerance, related to ischemia	Encourage avoidance of sodium-rich foods to reduce fluid retention. Encourage adequate exercise and mobility to prevent stasis. Explain disease course and signs and symptoms expected.

Educate the patient about this condition if necessary. Emphasize the importance of compliance with the medical and nutritional regimen. Dietary teaching should emphasize avoiding foods that contain iron while increasing the intake of calories and protein (because of BMR increase).

Emphasize that certain signs and symptoms (such as pain, edema, or erythema associated with thrombosis) require medical supervision. Because this is a chronic illness, emotional support is imperative.

Prognosis

Polycythemia vera is a chronic, life-shortening disorder. Although the incidence is small, leukemia and lymphomas develop in some patients with polycythemia vera. This may occur as a result of the chemotherapeutic drugs used to treat the disease or may be secondary to a disorder in the stem cells that progresses to leukemia. The major cause of morbidity and mortality from polycythemia vera is thrombosis. Permanent cure cannot be achieved today, but remission of many years can be produced.

DISORDERS ASSOCIATED WITH LEUKOCYTES

AGRANULOCYTOSIS

Etiology and Pathophysiology

Agranulocytosis is a potentially fatal condition of the blood characterized by a severe reduction in the number of granulocytes (basophils, eosinophils, and neutrophils). The WBC count is extremely low **(leukopenia)**, as is the differential neutrophil count (less than 200/mm^3 [neutropenia]). Normal neutrophil value is 3000 to 7000/mm^3.

Adverse medication reaction or toxicity is the primary cause of agranulocytosis. However, neoplastic disease, chemotherapy, and radiation therapy are often cited as causative. Viral and bacterial infections are possible causes of the condition. Heredity is also considered.

Suppression of the bone marrow by the causative agent reduces the number and production of WBCs. Leukocytes, formed in the bone marrow, provide body protection against microorganisms. This protection is ineffective when bone marrow suppression has occurred.

Clinical Manifestations

Fever, chills, headache, and fatigue are symptoms associated with infection and the inflammatory process. Ulcerations of mucous membranes—mouth, nose, pharynx, vagina, and rectum—are also found. Bronchial pneumonia and urinary tract infections are complications that occur in the later stages.

Assessment

Subjective data include common complaints of fever, extreme fatigue, and prostration. All medications taken, whether prescription or over-the-counter, are considered as possible causes of the condition.

Objective data include fever over 100.6° F (38.1° C). Erythema and pain from ulcerations may occur. Ulcerations are cultured for microorganisms. Lung and bronchial auscultation reveals crackles and rhonchi because of trapped exudates.

Possible causative chemical agents are antibiotics (chloramphenicol, penicillin derivatives, cephalosporins), antiepileptics (phenytoin), antihistamines, antineoplastic drugs (vincristine [Oncovin]), antithyroid drugs (propylthiouracil), diuretics, phenothiazides (chlorpromazine [Thorazine], fluphenazine [Prolixin], promazine [Sparine], prochlorperazine [Compazine]), and sulfonamides and derivatives.

Diagnostic Tests

The levels of leukocytes with neutrophils differential are below normal. A bone marrow study shows depression of activity.

Medical Management

The main objective of treatment is to alleviate the factors responsible for bone marrow depression and prevent or treat infection. Blood cultures may be performed when fever is elevated, and cultures may be ordered if ulceration occurs. Transfusions of packed RBCs are often ordered. Granulocyte colony-stimulating factor (G-CSF) (filgrastim [Neupogen]), pegfilgrastim (Neulasta), and GM-CSF (sargramostin [Leukine, Prokine]) given subcutaneously or intravenously can be used to treat a neutropenic patient. Immunocompromised (neutropenic) precautions may also be instituted.

Nursing Interventions and Patient Teaching

A patient with a compromised WBC system is highly susceptible to life-threatening infections. Nursing interventions are directed toward protecting the patient from potential sources of infection. Monitor the patient conscientiously to detect the earliest signs of infection so that therapy may be initiated promptly. Meticulous hand hygiene by medical and nursing personnel and strict asepsis are mandatory.

A nursing diagnosis and interventions for the patient with agranulocytosis include but are not limited to the following:

Nursing Diagnosis	Nursing Interventions
Risk for infection, related to depressed WBC (leukocyte) production	Maintain scrupulously clean patient environment. Be certain no person with any type of infection is allowed in contact with the patient. Observe for signs and symptoms of infection, such as elevated temperature and chills. Wash hands meticulously and use strict asepsis for procedures. Enforce protective isolation to protect patient from pathogens. Provide high-protein, high-vitamin, high-calorie diet to maintain nutritional status.

Nursing Diagnosis	Nursing Interventions
Risk for infection, related to depressed WBC (leukocyte) production—cont'd	Avoid raw foods, such as sushi, Caesar salad dressing (may have raw eggs), blue cheese, and fruits that cannot be peeled or vegetables that cannot be well cleaned. Encourage patient to take fluids to promote hydration. Monitor heart rate, respirations, blood pressure, and temperature to assess for signs of infection. Observe the patient for extreme fatigue, sore throat or mouth, and fever as signs of infection.
	Monitor WBC count. Use cooling measures (cooling blanket and tepid baths) to reduce fever if present. Administer antibiotics as ordered to combat specific pathogens. Have patient bathe or shower daily. Provide perineal care to maintain hygiene and prevent infection.

In patient teaching, discuss the use of frequent, thorough oral hygiene to treat or prevent mouth and pharyngeal infection. Explain the need to avoid crowds, people with infectious diseases, and cold or hot environments; also teach signs and symptoms of infection and appropriate interventions. Explain the need for a soft, bland diet high in protein, vitamins, and calories. And encourage a balance between rest and activity to prevent fatigue and generalized weakness.

Prognosis

Agranulocytosis is a potentially fatal condition because of the possibility of a life-threatening bacterial infection.

LEUKEMIA

Etiology and Pathophysiology

Leukemia is a malignant disorder of the hematopoietic system in which an excess of leukocytes accumulates in the bone marrow and lymph nodes. The cause, although unknown, is attributed to genetic origin, a virus, people previously treated with radiation, or chemotherapeutic agents that are toxic to bone marrow. A viral cause for human leukemia has been established only for some patients with adult T-cell leukemia (Lewis et al., 2007).

Bone marrow is replaced by rapidly developing white cells with abnormal numbers and forms of immature cells found in the circulation and infiltrated into the lymph nodes, the spleen, and the liver. The increased numbers of WBCs can lead to infiltration and damage to the bone marrow; the lymph nodes; the spleen; and organs, including those of the central nervous system. Leukemic infiltration leads to problems such as hepatomegaly, splenomegaly, lymphadenopathy, bone pain, meningeal irritation, and oral lesions. Hematopoietic function is disturbed by incompetent bone marrow. Increased susceptibility to infection results.

Classification

Leukemias are classified by identifying the type of leukocyte involved, whether it is of myelogenous or lymphocytic origin. Specific leukemia types are further categorized by combining the acute and chronic conditions with the cell type involved. Thus the four major types of leukemia are acute lymphocytic leukemia (ALL), acute myelogenous leukemia (AML), chronic myelogenous (granulocytic) leukemia (CML), and chronic lymphocytic leukemia (CLL). The peak incidence for ALL is between 2 and 9 years of age and in older adults. In AML the peak incidence is around 4 to 5 years of age, in CLL it is between 50 and 70 years of age, and in CML, it is between 25 and 60 years of age (Lewis et al., 2007).

Clinical Manifestations

The clinical manifestations of leukemia vary. Essentially they relate to problems caused by bone marrow failure and the formation of leukemic infiltrates. Bone marrow failure results from (1) bone marrow overcrowding by abnormal cells and (2) inadequate production of normal marrow elements. The patient is predisposed to anemia and thrombocytopenia.

As leukemia progresses, fewer normal blood cells are produced. The abnormal WBCs continue to accumulate. The leukemic cells infiltrate the patient's organs, leading to problems such as splenomegaly, hepatomegaly, lymphadenopathy, bone pain, meningeal irritation, and oral lesions. Enlarged lymph nodes and painless splenomegaly may be the first signs of the disease in some people.

Diagnostic Tests

The WBC count is low, elevated, or excessively elevated. Anemia and thrombocytopenia are noted. Bone marrow biopsy shows immature leukocytes. Chest radiographic examination may show mediastinal node and lung involvement and bone changes. Lymph node biopsy reveals excessive blasts (immature cells). Peripheral blood evaluation and bone marrow examination are the primary methods of diagnosing and classifying the type of leukemia. Further studies such as lumbar puncture and CT scan can be performed to determine the presence of leukemic cells outside of the blood and bone marrow.

Assessment

Subjective data include patient complaints regarding symptoms that may seem unrelated at first. Patients often have pain in bones or joints, fatigue, malaise, decreased activity tolerance, and irritability.

Objective data include those signs listed in clinical manifestations. Infections are common. Occult blood is detected in laboratory specimens of urine and stool. Abnormalities of skin (petechiae, ecchymoses) and mucous membranes (bleeding) may be present.

Medical Management

The goal of treatment is to achieve remission or to control the symptoms. Treatment is aimed at eradicating the leukemia with chemotherapy or bone marrow transplant. Combination chemotherapy is the mainstay for treating leukemia. Multiple drugs are used to (1) decrease drug resistance, (2) minimize the drug toxicity by using multiple drugs with varying toxicities (with lower dosages of each), and (3) interrupt cell growth at multiple points in the cell cycle. Observation for drug toxicity is imperative (Table 47-2).

Table 47-2 Medications for Blood and Lymphatic Disorders

Generic (Trade)	Action	Side Effects	Nursing Implications
Cyanocobalamin (Cobex, vitamin B_{12})	Needed for adequate nerve functioning, protein and carbohydrate metabolism, normal growth, RBC development, and cell reproduction	Flushing, diarrhea, itching, rash, hypokalemia	Assess GI functions and potassium levels at beginning of treatment; stress need for patients with pernicious anemia to return for monthly injections; give intramuscularly only.
Folic acid (B complex vitamin) (Folvite)	Needed for erythropoiesis; increases RBC, WBC, and platelet formation in megaloblastic anemias	Pruritus, rash, general malaise, bronchospasm, slight flushing	Drug may be administered by deep intramuscular, subcutaneous, or intravenous routes; do not mix with other medications in same syringe for intramuscular injections.
Ferrous sulfate (Feosol, Fer-In-Sol)	Replaces iron stores needed for RBC development	Nausea, constipation, epigastric pain, black and red tarry stools, vomiting, diarrhea, discolored urine, staining of teeth	Between-meal dosing is preferable but can be given with some foods, although absorption may be decreased; give tablets with orange juice to promote iron absorption; to avoid staining teeth, give elixir iron preparations through straw; oral iron may turn stools black.
Iron dextran (DexFerrum)	Released into the plasma and carried by transferring to the bone marrow, where it is incorporated into hemoglobin	Stained skin at site of injection, fever, chills, headache, sweating, discolored urine, diarrhea	Administer 0.5-mL test dose by preferred route before therapy; wait at least 1 hour before giving remaining portion.
Desmopressin acetate (DDAVP, Concentraid)	Promotes reabsorption of water by kidneys and increase in plasma factor VIII levels, which increases platelet aggregation, resulting in vasopressor effect	Nasal irritation, congestion, drowsiness, headache, flushing, nausea, abdominal cramps, heartburn, vulval pain, hypertension	Avoid overhydration; assess pulse and blood pressure when giving drug subcutaneously; monitor factor VIII antigen levels and aPTT.
Filgrastim (G-CSF) (Neupogen)	Stimulates proliferation and differentiation of neutrophils	Fever, alopecia, skeletal pain, nausea, vomiting, diarrhea, mucositis, anorexia	Monitor CBC and platelet count before treatment and twice weekly; refrigerate but do not freeze; avoid shaking; store at room temperature for at least 6 hours; discard any vial that has been at room temperature for more than 6 hours.

aPTT, Activated partial thromboplastin time; *CBC,* complete blood count; *G-CSF,* granulocyte colony-stimulating factor; *GI,* gastrointestinal; *RBC,* red blood cell; *WBC,* white blood cell.

Tremendous progress in the treatment of leukemia has been made in recent years with the use of a complex combination of chemotherapeutic drugs and radiation therapy. Bone marrow transplant and HSCT may be the treatment of choice in patients with suitable donors and initial remission of the acute leukemia (see Chapter 57). Before the transplant, the patient's bone marrow cells and leukemic cells must be killed by massive chemotherapy and total body irradiation. The patient may succumb to infection, hemorrhage, or graft-versus-host disease.

In chronic leukemia, which occurs almost exclusively in adults and develops slowly, the desired objectives of treatment depend on the kind of cells involved. Medications commonly used include chlorambucil (Leukeran), hydroxyurea, corticosteroids, and cyclophosphamide. Lymph nodes are often irradiated, and blood transfusion may be given if anemia is severe. Although medications are not curative in chronic leukemia, they help to prolong life (see Table 47-2).

Nursing Interventions and Patient Teaching

Prevent infection by teaching patients about immunocompromised (neutropenic) precautions and the avoidance of infectious agents. Leukopenia (an abnormal decrease in the number of WBCs to less than 5000 cells/mm^3) can be fatal. The usual inflammatory process to control infection is decreased; thus frequent observation for signs and symptoms of infection is necessary. Thrombocytopenia-induced hemorrhage may be life threatening; prevent this condition through safe, gentle care. Control pain through analgesia as ordered and by comfort measures. Coping mechanisms may be strained because of pain, complexities of treatment, side effects and toxicities, change of body image, or fear of death. Support the patient and family by developing a positive nurse-patient-family relationship and referring them to community support groups.

Nurses have contact with a patient 24 hours a day and can reduce feelings of abandonment and loneliness by balancing the demanding technical needs with a humanistic, caring approach. Therefore a nurse faces a special challenge in learning how to meet the intense psychosocial needs of a patient with leukemia while continuing to offer the complex physical care that is usually required. Consult with other health professionals (e.g., psychiatric clinical specialists, oncology clinical specialists, social workers) to help develop the skills required to meet the many needs of a patient with leukemia.

From a physical care perspective, it is challenging to make astute assessments and plan care to help the patient survive the severe side effects of chemotherapy. The life-threatening results of bone marrow suppression (anemia, thrombocytopenia, neutropenia) require aggressive nursing interventions. Additional complications of chemotherapy may affect the patient's GI tract, nutritional status, skin and mucosa, cardiopulmonary status, liver, kidneys, and neurologic system.

Be informed about all drugs being administered, including mechanism of action, purpose, routes of administration, usual doses, potential side effects, safe handling considerations, and toxic effects. In addition, know how to assess laboratory data reflecting the effects of the drugs. Patient survival and comfort during aggressive chemotherapy are significantly affected by the quality of nursing intervention.

Discuss procedures, meaning of treatments, and care plans with the patient and family. Be certain to cover the nature of the disease and previous information given the patient. Community resources for support and information are invaluable for educating the patient and the family. Examine expectations of physical abilities, remission, and future plans. Encourage continuation of the medical regimen and avoidance of situations in which infection can be transmitted. Most patients should receive the pneumococcal vaccine (Pneumovax) at diagnosis and every 5 years and an annual influenza vaccine (Lewis et al., 2007). Medication and diet information is important.

Prognosis

Perhaps more dramatically than in any other malignant disorder, chemotherapy has improved the prognosis of children with ALL. Untreated patients have a median survival time of 4 to 6 months. With current therapy of vincristine and prednisone, plus an anthracycline drug (daunorubicin or doxorubicin [Adriamycin]), the median survival rate is about 5 years, and approximately 50% of children with ALL can now be cured. In AML, remission can be achieved in up to 75% of cases; however, relapse eventually occurs in most cases. Only about 20% to 25% of adults with AML experience a 5-year remission. Overall survival for CLL is variable. When diagnosed in early stages, median survival rate ranges from 10 to 12½ years; when diagnosed in advanced stages, survival is approximately 18 months (Nursing Care Plan 47-1).

DISORDERS OF COAGULATION

Etiology and Pathophysiology

Release of blood from the vascular system results from trauma or vessel damage, vessel inadequacy, disturbance of the function of platelets or clotting factors, or liver disease (impaired clotting mechanisms).

The clotting mechanism is a hemostatic chain reaction. Vasoconstriction inhibits capillary leakage; hematoma compression provides pressure. The body reacts by lowering arterial blood pressure. Any manifestation that alters this process predisposes the body to hemorrhage. The affected mechanism may be vascular, platelet dysfunction, or an alteration in plasma coagulation factor. The disorder may be congenital or acquired, possibly secondary to another disease or to medication toxicity.

Nursing Care Plan 47-1 The Patient with Leukemia

Ms. May is a 26-year-old patient diagnosed with acute lymphocytic leukemia. She is married and the mother of a 3-year-old daughter. Ms. May has been receiving chemotherapy and is immunocompromised, with a differential white blood cell (WBC) count revealing a neutrophil count of 22%. Her hemoglobin is 8.8 g/dL, and her platelets are 55,000/mm^3. Her mouth appears edematous, and she complains of oral tenderness.

NURSING DIAGNOSIS *Risk for infection, related to leukopenia*

Patient Goals and Expected Outcomes	Nursing Intervention	Evaluation/Rationale
Patient or caregiver will identify measures to prevent or control infection	Inspect all body sites for infection at least daily; note and report fever, sore throat, purulent exudate, chills, cough, burning with urination, erythema, edema, tenderness, and pain.	Patient will remain free of infection.
Patient or caregiver will verbalize and report signs and symptoms of infection	Monitor vital signs. Obtain cultures as ordered. Monitor WBC counts and culture reports. Administer antibiotics on time as ordered. Promote and maintain hygiene integrity of skin and mucous membranes. Use aseptic technique in treatments. Teach the patient and family: • Necessity of avoiding crowds or people with infections while WBC count is $<1000/mm^3$ • Personal hygiene measures • Signs and symptoms of infection	Patient demonstrates no signs or symptoms of infection; temperature and WBC count are within normal range.

NURSING DIAGNOSIS *Ineffective coping, related to diagnosis and disease process*

Patient Goals and Expected Outcomes	Nursing Intervention	Evaluation
Patient and family will demonstrate measures to effectively cope by verbalizing role of family, significant others, and support groups in therapeutic coping	Assess coping capabilities of patient and significant others. Discuss disease process and expectations. Alleviate knowledge deficit. Encourage questions and self-expression: listen actively, demonstrate compassion, reassure with touch and personal contact. Assess fear of threat of death: allow time for personal expression and provide one-on-one discussion opportunity.	Patient and family express factors that are causing anxiety and powerlessness.

Critical Thinking Questions

1. What should the nurse do if a visitor with an obvious upper respiratory tract infection is seen approaching Ms. May's room?
2. What nursing interventions would be most appropriate in providing therapeutic oral hygiene for Ms. May?
3. What kind of a bath and activities of daily living would be most beneficial for Ms. May?

Clinical Manifestations

Skin and mucous membrane manifestations include petechiae and ecchymoses. Epistaxis and gingival bleeding are common. Circulatory hypovolemia is noted through hypotension; pallor; cool, clammy skin; and tachycardia. GI tract bleeding is common, with abdominal flank pain caused by internal bleeding. CNS involvement ranges from altered response and malaise to loss of consciousness or affected speech.

Assessment

Subjective data include a history of bleeding after surgical or dental procedures. Exposure to toxic or hazardous agents or to radiation may be revealed. Complaint of headache, extremity pain, and numbness is noted. Medications taken (e.g., aspirin) may lead to suspicion of toxicity.

Collection of **objective data** involves observation of pain on pressure to the abdomen, revealing liver and spleen tenderness and perhaps enlargement. Skin and mucous membranes may have petechiae, ecchymoses, and occasionally hematoma. Emesis and stool may show signs of bleeding. Joint examination reveals motion pain.

Diagnostic Tests

The platelet count is low. The RBC count is low with a decreased hemoglobin level. Coagulation time is altered. Bone marrow studies show abnormal cells.

Medical Management

The underlying cause is assessed and corrected, and replacement transfusions may be ordered. Heparin therapy or medication toxicity is considered as a possible cause. Infections and complications are treated or prevented.

Nursing Interventions

Medical intervention often depends on accurate reporting of signs and symptoms and nursing observations. In coagulation disorders, monitor vital signs to note any signs of hypovolemic shock. Move the patient gently to prevent trauma to the tissues. Monitor IV infusions and transfusions as ordered.

DISORDERS ASSOCIATED WITH PLATELETS

THROMBOCYTOPENIA

Etiology and Pathophysiology

A deficiency of the number of circulating platelets or change in the function of platelets alters the process of coagulation. **Thrombocytopenia** is an abnormal hematological condition in which the number of platelets is reduced to fewer than 150,000/mm^3. Decreased production occurs in aplastic anemia, leukemia, tumors, and chemotherapy. Decreased platelet survival occurs when there is antibody destruction, infection, or viral invasion. Increased platelet destruction is caused by disseminated intravascular coagulation (DIC). Splenomegaly results from entrapment of blood in the spleen.

The most common cause of increased destruction of platelets is **thrombocytopenic purpura,** which may be drug-induced or immune thrombocytopenic purpura. This is the most common acquired thrombocytopenia. It is a syndrome of abnormal destruction of circulating platelets termed *immune thrombocytopenic purpura* (ITP). It was originally termed *idiopathic* (cause unknown) *thrombocytopenic purpura.* However, it is now known that ITP is an autoimmune disease. In ITP, platelets are coated with antibodies. Although these platelets function normally, when they reach the spleen, the antibody-coated platelets are recognized as foreign and are destroyed by macrophages in the spleen. Normal platelets survive 8 to 10 days, but with ITP, platelet survival is an average of 1 to 3 days. If thrombocytopenia is medication induced (Box 47-3), the patient's platelet counts usually return to normal 1 to 2 weeks after the medication is withdrawn. The acute form of ITP is found mostly in children, whereas the chronic form is found among patients of all ages but is more common in 20- to 40-year-old women. It is an autoimmune process caused by the production of an autoantibody (immunoglobulin G) directed against a platelet antigen.

Clinical Manifestations

The major signs of thrombocytopenia that are observable by physical examination are petechiae and ecchymoses on the skin. Petechiae occur only in platelet disorders. The severity of signs and symptoms correlates with the platelet count. As the level drops to less than 100,000/mm^3, the risk for bleeding from mucous membranes and in cutaneous sites and internal organs increases. Significant risk for serious bleeding occurs once the count is less than 20,000/mm^3. When the platelet count is less than 5000/mm^3, spontaneous, potentially fatal CNS or GI hemorrhage can occur.

Box 47-3 Medications with Thrombocytopenic Effects

- Aspirin
- Digitalis derivatives
- Furosemide
- Nonsteroidal antiinflammatory agents (azathioprine, D-penicillamine, phenylbutazone, ibuprofen, indomethacin)
- Oral hypoglycemics
- Penicillins
- Quinidine
- Rifampicin
- Sulfonamides
- Thiazides

Assessment

Collection of **subjective data** includes questioning the patient about recent viral infections (which may produce a transient thrombocytopenia), medications in current use, and the extent of alcohol ingestion.

Collection of **objective data** includes observing the patient's skin for petechiae and ecchymoses. Epistaxis and gingival bleeding may be noted. Signs of increased intracranial pressure caused by cerebral hemorrhage may be detected.

Diagnostic Tests

To ascertain the characteristics of all blood cells, laboratory studies include platelet count, peripheral blood smear, and bleeding time. In addition, a bone marrow analysis is performed to determine the presence of immature platelets. Examination also reveals the presence or absence of primary bone marrow abnormalities, such as neoplastic invasion or aplastic anemia.

Medical Management

Usually, no therapy is needed if the patient has a platelet count of 30,000/mm^3 or greater (Lewis et al., 2007). The primary treatments are corticosteroid therapy to suppress the phagocytic response of splenic macrophages. Corticosteroid therapy also increases the life span of the platelets (Lewis et al., 2007). If the patient does not respond initially to prednisone or requires unacceptably high doses to uphold an adequate platelet count, splenectomy is indicated.

Other treatments may include IV immunoglobulin in the patient who is unresponsive to corticosteroids or splenectomy. Transfusion with platelet concentration may be used in people with thrombocytopenic bleeding. Platelet transfusions are generally not recommended until the count is below 10,000/mm^3 unless the patient is actively bleeding. Each platelet transfusion can be expected to increase a patient's platelets by 10,000/mm^3 (Lewis et al., 2007). Plasmapheresis is used to treat ITP by removing antibodies produced by the autoimmune process.

Immunosuppressive therapy used in refractory cases includes ritaximab (Rituxan), azathioprine (Imuran), cyclosporine, and mycophenolate mofetil (CellCept) (Lewis et al., 2007).

Nursing Interventions and Patient Teaching

Support the medical treatment regimen, using specific interventions for specific disease causes. If medication toxicity is the cause, the medication is discontinued. Prevent infections by meticulous asepsis and gentle handling of the patient. Closely monitor plasma and platelet infusion and whole-blood transfusions for reaction and effects on patients' conditions.

Nursing diagnoses and interventions for the patient with thrombocytopenia include but are not limited to the following:

Nursing Diagnoses	Nursing Interventions
Ineffective tissue perfusion (cerebral, cardiopulmonary, renal, GI, peripheral), related to bleeding	Monitor vital signs and neurologic status. Monitor platelet count. Assess for bleeding and fluid imbalance. Check patient's urine, stool, and emesis for blood. Monitor invasive diagnostic procedure sites for bleeding. Maintain comfort measures and bed rest. Avoid trauma and infection. Monitor patient receiving parenteral fluids and blood components for untoward signs. Monitor potential sites of hemorrhage.
Pain, related to hemorrhage	Assess discomfort and pain level. Assess patient's ability to cope and response to pain. Administer analgesia as ordered and note patient response. Provide education.

The patient must understand the disease process and causative agents to provide self-care and prevent trauma or infection. Provide instructions on signs, symptoms, and preventive measures: avoid trauma, use stool softeners, maintain a high-fiber diet to prevent constipation, check for presence of blood, use a soft toothbrush, and blow nose gently. Stress the importance of notifying the physician of signs and symptoms of bleeding.

Prognosis

The prognosis is variable, depending on the underlying cause. In ITP, treatment may need to be administered for 3 to 4 weeks before a complete response is seen. In chronic ITP, transient remissions occur. Approximately 80% of patients benefit from splenectomy, resulting in a complete or partial remission.

CLOTTING FACTOR DEFECTS

HEMOPHILIA

Etiology and Pathophysiology

Hemophilia, a hereditary coagulation disorder, is characterized by a disturbance of the clotting factors. In **hemophilia A,** the more common type (representing 80% of the total incidence), antihemophilic factor VIII is absent. This factor is essential for conversion of prothrombin to thrombin through thromboplastin component. A decrease in the formation of prothrombin activators occurs as a result of the decrease in clotting factors. Hemophilia B (Christmas disease) exhibits a deficiency of factor IX with an absence of plasma thromboplastin component (a plasma protein), resulting in nonformation of thromboplastin.

Hemophilia is an X-linked hereditary trait that affects mainly males; females are carriers.

In the past the patient with hemophilia was at high risk for being infected with human immunodeficiency virus (HIV) and later developing acquired immunodeficiency syndrome because of the need for cryoprecipitate concentrates, which were potentially contaminated with HIV. Unfortunately, the HIV contamination of blood products caused the majority of hemophilia deaths in the late 1980s (Lewis et al., 2007). Now with viral-detecting processes, donor screening, and heat treatment of factor VIII concentrates (which destroys HIV), the risk of contracting HIV and hepatitis B and C through transfusions is greatly reduced. The use of recombinant replacement factors also is improving long-term survival rates.

Clinical Manifestations

Internal or external hemorrhage occurs with large ecchymoses into tissue—especially muscles, which may show deformity; and joints, which become ankylosed. **Hemarthrosis,** or bleeding into a joint space, is a hallmark of severe disease and usually occurs in the knees, the ankles, the elbows, the shoulders, and the hips. Pain, edema, erythema, and fever accompany hemarthrosis. Small cuts can prove fatal; blood loss from simple dental procedures may be significant.

Assessment

Subjective data include reports by patient and family of incidents of ecchymoses and hemorrhage from even the slightest trauma. Pain is associated with joint motion.

Collection of **objective data** includes noting blood in subcutaneous tissues, urine, or stool and noting edematous or immobile joints.

Diagnostic Tests

Factors VIII and IX are absent or deficient. Coagulation profiles reveal a normal platelet count, bleeding time, prothrombin time, and International Normalized Ratio. The partial thromboplastin time is prolonged. Notify laboratory personnel of the patient's disorder to alleviate further incidents of trauma as a result of diagnostic procedures (e.g., venipuncture).

Medical Management

Care focuses on preventing and treating bleeding and relieving pain. Transfusions and administration of factor VIII or IX concentrate may be prophylactic or used to stop the hemorrhage. Two different clotting factor concentrates made from human plasma can be used. One, cryoprecipitate, is a clotting factor concentrate rich in factor VIII. Its use is waning because of the associated risk, although small, of viral disease transmission. Additionally, home administration of cryoprecipitate is difficult because it must be stored at low temperatures. The second human-derived product, factor VIII concentrate, is most typically used. A wide variety of these products are available; all are freeze-dried concentrates of factor VIII prepared from pooled plasma from thousands of donors. These products are specially treated to inactivate any viral contamination (such as HIV or hepatitis viruses). Factor IX concentrates are prepared in a similar fashion.

Because human plasma products still carry a slight risk of infection transmission and require human donors, scientists have used genetic engineering to manufacture factor VIII. This product, recombinant factor VIII, is advantageous because of viral safety, unlimited supply, and lower cost. Recombinant replacement factor VIII is now commercially available for widespread use.

Nursing Interventions and Patient Teaching

Control hemorrhages in emergency situations by applying pressure and cold to the site. Support and reassurance are imperative. Educate the patient and the entire family because many people may be involved in the patient care. Monitor transfusions of factor VIII concentrate. Supportive care measures include pain management and genetic counseling. Do not give hemophilia patients aspirin because it can further complicate the bleeding tendency.

Nursing diagnoses and interventions for the patient with hemophilia include but are not limited to the following:

Nursing Diagnoses	Nursing Interventions
Ineffective tissue perfusion, related to blood loss from coagulation deficit	Assess for extent of hemorrhage. Prevent further hemorrhage or extension. Monitor vital signs and laboratory reports. Apply cold compresses to bleeding areas. Assess for anxiety, shock, disorientation, and decreased urinary output. Teach safety precautions to prevent trauma. Administer analgesia as ordered. Move patient gently and slowly, supporting joints. Prevent deformity through support, splints, and physical therapy.
Ineffective coping, related to long-term illness	Discuss disease process, altered lifestyle, and acceptance. Suggest genetic counseling. Encourage independence. Encourage compliance with medical regimen. Be an active listener.
Deficient fluid volume, related to bleeding	Monitor vital signs and level of consciousness for evidence of acute hemorrhage. Monitor blood component therapy as ordered to control bleeding. Monitor I&O. Apply ice pack to affected joint or traumatized area to control bleeding. Administer analgesics to relieve joint pain. Assess amount, consistency, and frequency of bleeding: • Nose • Joints • Skin • Stool and urine • Pad counts Monitor laboratory tests to assess degree of blood loss. Avoid trauma, such as falls, bumps, or injections.

Discuss with the patient ways to avoid injury and control bleeding. Also discuss physical activity within limits. Encourage the patient to wear a medical-alert tag. Emergency care teaching includes immobilizing the affected part, applying ice, and notifying the physician. Discuss diet to prevent obesity, which puts excess pressure on joints. Regular dental care and preventive dental and medical measures are important aspects. Overprotection is sometimes a factor to discuss. No aspirin or any other medication should be taken except with the physician's knowledge (Home Care Considerations box).

Prognosis

Before the appearance of the HIV virus, the average life span for a person with hemophilia was near normal. After HIV appeared, the majority of severe hemophiliacs who received clotting factor concentrate before 1984 became seropositive for HIV. Now, with the development of methods to heat-inactivate the virus, the risk of contracting HIV from clotting factor concentrates is almost nil. With the methods to control HIV and hepatitis B and C transmission and the use of recombinant replacement factors, the average life span for a person with hemophilia is once again near normal.

> **Home Care Considerations**
>
> **Hemophilia**
>
> - Home management is a primary consideration for a patient with hemophilia because the disease follows a chronic, progressive course.
> - The quantity and length of life may be significantly affected by the patient's knowledge of the illness and understanding of how to live with it.
> - Refer the patient and family to the local chapter of the National Hemophilia Foundation to encourage association with other individuals who are dealing with the problems associated with hemophilia.
> - Teach the patient with hemophilia to recognize disease-related problems and to learn which problems can be resolved at home and which require hospitalization.
> - Immediate medical attention is required for severe pain or edema of a muscle or joint that restricts movement or inhibits sleep and for a head injury, edema in the neck or mouth, abdominal pain, hematuria, melena, and skin wounds in need of suturing.
> - Daily oral hygiene must be performed without trauma.
> - Aspirin should not be taken because it decreases platelet aggregation.
> - Understanding how to prevent injuries is an important consideration. The patient can learn to participate in noncontact sports (e.g., golf) and wear gloves when doing household chores to prevent cuts or abrasions from knives, hammers, and other tools.
> - The patient should wear a medical-alert tag to ensure that health care providers know about the hemophilia in case of an accident.
> - A person with hemophilia who is mature enough or a family member can be taught to administer some of the factor replacement therapies at home.

VON WILLEBRAND'S DISEASE

Etiology and Pathophysiology

von Willebrand's disease is an inherited bleeding disorder characterized by abnormally slow coagulation of blood and spontaneous episodes of GI bleeding, epistaxis, and gingival bleeding caused by a mild deficiency of factor VIII. It is common during postpartum periods, as menorrhagia, and after surgery or trauma. Although similar to hemophilia, its incidence is not limited to males.

Treatment includes administration of cryoprecipitate containing factor VIII, fibrinogen, or fresh plasma. Desmopressin (DDAVP) is becoming the treatment of choice for patients who have a mild form of hemophilia. This drug is a synthetic of the human antidiuretic hormone, vasopressin. It causes an increase in factor VIII release from storage sites in the body. Desmopressin is often administered prophylactically to patients with mild hemophilia who require surgery or dental extractions. Observation and nursing interventions for hemophilia A and B can easily be adapted to von Willebrand's disease.

Prognosis

The prognosis is usually good.

DISSEMINATED INTRAVASCULAR COAGULATION

Etiology and Pathophysiology

Disseminated intravascular coagulation (DIC) is a grave coagulopathy resulting from the overstimulation of clotting and anticlotting processes in response to disease or injury, including septicemia, obstetric complication, malignancies, tissue trauma, transfusion reaction, burns, shock, and snake bites (Box 47-4). Plasma clotting factors are depleted during widespread clotting within small vessels. This in turn leads to a bleeding disorder and thrombosis. The primary disorder initiates generalized intravascular clotting, which in turn overstimulates fibrinolytic mechanisms. As a result, the initial hypercoagulability is followed by a deficiency in clotting factors with subsequent hypocoagulability and hemorrhaging.

Clinical Manifestations

Bleeding is noted in mucous membranes, venipuncture or surgical sites, GI and urinary tracts, and generally from all orifices. Bleeding ranges from occult to profuse. Dyspnea; hemoptysis (blood-tinged sputum); and diaphoresis with cold, mottled digits are observed.

Assessment

Subjective data include patient complaints of bone and joint pain. Changes in vision occur.

Collection of **objective data** includes observing for occult or obvious bleeding. Purpura on the chest and abdomen, reflecting fibrin deposits in capillaries, is a

Box 47-4 Precipitating Causes of Disseminated Intravascular Coagulation

OBSTETRIC
- Abruptio placentae
- Acute fatty liver of pregnancy
- Amniotic fluid embolism
- Hydatidiform mole (intrauterine mass of grapelike chorionic villi)
- Retained dead fetus
- Retained placenta
- Toxemia

NEOPLASTIC
- Acute leukemias
- Adenocarcinomas
- Carcinomas
- Pheochromocytoma (a vascular tumor of the adrenal medulla)
- Polycythemia vera
- Sarcomas

HEMATOLOGICAL
- Blood transfusion reaction
- Sickle cell crisis
- Thalassemia major (genetic hemolytic anemia; occurs in people of Mediterranean origin)

TRAUMA
- Aspirin poisoning
- Burns
- Fat emboli
- Heatstroke
- Multiple injuries
- Snake bite
- Surgery, particularly if extracorporeal circulation (heart-lung machine) was used
- Transplant rejection

OTHER
- Acute infectious process or sepsis
- Anaphylaxis
- Cirrhosis
- Glomerulonephritis
- Hepatitis
- Necrotizing enterocolitis
- Purpura
- Shock
- Systemic lupus erythematosus

common first sign of DIC. Note the color of skin and mucosa and the presence of petechiae. Abdominal tenderness may be present. GI bleeding, hematuria, pulmonary edema, pulmonary embolism, hypotension, tachycardia, absence of peripheral pulses, decreased blood pressure, restlessness, confusion, seizures, or coma may be present.

Diagnostic Tests

The coagulation profile shows prolonged clotting. The platelet count shows marked thrombocytopenia. Other tests show hypofibrinogenemia and deficits of factors V, VII, VIII, X, and XII.

D-dimer test results are elevated. D-dimer reveals the breakdown of fibrin and is a specific marker for the degree of fibrinolysis in the serum.

Medical Management

In keeping with the medical therapeutic approach, the underlying cause is addressed and corrected and transfusion replacement and cryoprecipitate are ordered. Heparin therapy blocks the subsequent formation of microemboli by inhibiting thrombin activity. It has no effect, however, on existing clots. The goal of administering heparin is to stop the rapid overproduction of microemboli and thus allow for reperfusion of vital organs and replenishment of clotting factor supplies. However, the use of heparin in treating DIC remains controversial. Fibrinolytic inhibitors should be given to adults. This may be dangerous if the thrombotic process has not been previously treated with heparin. Packed RBC transfusion should be initiated to reestablish normal hemostatic potential if the thrombosis is blocked by heparin. FFP is administered to replace other coagulation factors.

Nursing Interventions and Patient Teaching

Protection from bleeding and trauma and pressure to sites of hemorrhage are essential nursing measures. Support and reassurance of the patient may aid in relieving high stress levels. Monitor the patient in a quiet, nonstressful environment. Use padded side rails and foam or cotton swabs for mouth care. Monitor vital signs and administer heparin, blood and FFP transfusions, and cryoprecipitate. Use the blood pressure cuff infrequently to avoid subcutaneous bleeding.

A nursing diagnosis and interventions for the patient with DIC include but are not limited to the following:

Nursing Diagnosis	Nursing Interventions
Risk for injury, bleeding, and fluid deficit, related to: • depleted coagulation factors • adverse effect of heparin (excess heparin, insufficient heparin)	Monitor hematocrit and hemoglobin. Examine skin surface for signs of bleeding; note petechiae; purpura; hematomas; oozing of blood from IV sites, drains, and wounds; and bleeding from mucous membranes.

Nursing Diagnosis	Nursing Interventions
Risk for injury, bleeding, and fluid deficit, related to: • depleted coagulation factors • adverse effect of heparin (excess heparin, insufficient heparin)	Observe for signs of bleeding from GI and genitourinary tracts. Note any hemoptysis or blood obtained during suctioning. Observe for changes in mental status; institute neurologic checklist (mental status changes may occur with the decreased fluid volume or with decreasing hemoglobin). Monitor vital signs. Observe for signs of orthostatic hypotension (drop of greater than 15 mm Hg when changing from supine to sitting position indicates reduced circulating fluids). Avoid intramuscular injections; any needlestick is a potential bleeding site. Apply pressure to oozing site. Prevent trauma to catheter and tubes by proper taping, minimum pulling.

Discuss with the patient and family the signs and symptoms of DIC, and have them repeat this information to the nurse or physician. Teach the patient to self-administer heparin therapy subcutaneously if prescribed. Instruct the patient and family to avoid mechanical trauma, such as from a hard toothbrush, blade razor, rough nose blowing, or contact sports.

Prognosis

Mortality rates from DIC vary, depending on severity. Death is usually a result of either uncontrolled hemorrhage, irreversible end-organ damage, or both.

DISORDER OF PLASMA CELLS

MULTIPLE MYELOMA

Etiology and Pathophysiology

Multiple myeloma, or plasma cell myeloma, is a malignant neoplastic immunodeficiency disease of the bone marrow. Neoplastic plasma cells infiltrate the bone marrow. The tumor destroys osseous tissue, especially in flat bones, causing pain, fractures, and skeletal deformities.

The specific immunoglobulin produced by the myeloma cells is present in the blood and/or urine and is referred to as the monoclonal protein. This protein is a helpful marker to monitor the extent of the disease and the patient's response to treatment. It is measured by serum or urine protein electrophoresis.

Be alert to an older adult patient whose chief complaint is back pain and who has an elevated total serum protein. Evaluate these patients for possible multiple myeloma. It most frequently occurs in patients older than age 40, with a peak incidence around 65 years of age, and affects twice as many men as women. Onset is gradual and insidious; the disease often goes unrecognized for years while the individual experiences frequent, recurrent bacterial infections. This increased susceptibility to infection follows disturbances of antibody formation by abnormal plasma cells. Suppression of normal antibody levels is seen in this plasma cell tumor disease. The incidence of multiple myeloma has increased and now approaches that of Hodgkin's disease.

Clinical Manifestations

The disease process shows a proliferation of malignant plasma cells and development of single or multiple bone marrow tumors. This is followed by bone destruction with dissemination into lymph nodes, liver, spleen, and kidneys.

The skeletal system symptoms typically involve the ribs, the spine, and the pelvis. Osteolytic lesions are seen in the skull, the vertebrae, and the ribs. Vertebral destruction can lead to collapse of vertebrae with ensuing compression of the spinal cord. Patients complain of bone pain that increases with movement. About 30% develop pathologic fractures accompanied by severe pain.

In an individual with multiple myeloma, production of erythrocytes, platelets, and leukocytes is disrupted because the marrow is crowded by the abnormal proliferation of plasma cells. This leads to infection, anemia, and increased potential for bleeding. Calcium and phosphorus drain from bones, leading to hypercalcemia and renal problems. In addition, cell destruction contributes to the development of hyperuricemia, which, along with the high protein levels caused by the myeloma protein, can result in renal failure.

Assessment

Collection of **subjective data** includes assessment of the patient's complaints of pain, especially skeletal pain in the pelvis, the spine, and the ribs.

Collection of **objective data** includes assessing the patient's facial expression for signs of increased pain with movement, the ability to perform ADLs, increased body temperature, increased potential for bleeding, changes in urine characteristics, and effectiveness of medication administration.

Diagnostic Tests

Diagnosis of multiple myeloma is made with radiographic skeletal studies, bone marrow biopsy, and laboratory examination of blood and urine. A monoclonal

(M) antibody protein may be present, as evidenced in serum or urine electrophoresis. Bony degeneration also causes loss of calcium in the bones, eventually causing hypercalcemia. Pancytopenia, hypercalcemia, hyperuricemia, and elevated creatinine may be found. In addition, an abnormal globulin known as Bence Jones protein is found in the urine and can result in renal failure.

Radiographic skeletal examinations reveal widespread demineralization, lytic lesions, and osteoporosis. Lytic lesions may be seen on bone roentgenograms but are not well visualized on bone scans. Bone marrow studies reveal large numbers of immature plasma cells, which normally account for only 5% of marrow population.

Medical Management

Treatment is symptomatic, since multiple myeloma is not curable. Radiation and chemotherapy are initiated to reduce tumor size, impede tumor growth, and produce remission. Radiation is used in small doses. The antineoplastic drugs of choice are the alkylating agents, such as melphalan, cyclophosphamide, chlorambucil, and carmustine (BiCNU). Vincristine, doxorubicin (Adriamycin), and dexamethasone can be added for patients who do not respond to alkylating agents. Bone marrow depression occurs as a side effect; therefore the CBC is monitored during treatment.

Hypercalcemia and pain also should be addressed. Analgesics, orthopedic supports, and localized radiation help reduce the skeletal pain. Hospitalization to administer chemotherapy, corticosteroids, and fluids may be required.

Nursing Interventions and Patient Teaching

Care of the patient with multiple myeloma focuses on relieving pain, preventing infection and bone injury, administrating chemotherapy and radiation, and maintaining hydration. Use ambulation and adequate hydration to treat hypercalcemia, dehydration, and potential renal damage. Fluid intake of 3 to 4 L/day is encouraged to prevent dehydration and maintain a urinary output of 1.5 to 2 L/day. Patients with multiple myeloma with high tumor burdens who receive chemotherapy will have an increased cell lysis and release of uric acid, resulting in hyperuricemia. Adequate hydration and allopurinal (Zyloprim) will help treat hyperuricemia (Lewis et al., 2007). Weight bearing helps the bones reabsorb some calcium, and fluids dilute calcium and prevent protein precipitates from causing renal tubular obstruction.

Because of the potential for pathologic fractures, be careful when moving and ambulating the patient. A slight twist or strain in the wrong area (e.g., a weak area in the patient's bones) may be sufficient to cause a fracture. Attention to the psychosocial, emotional, and spiritual needs is also extremely important.

Nursing diagnoses and interventions for the patient with multiple myeloma include but are not limited to the following:

Nursing Diagnoses	Nursing Interventions
Risk for injury, related to: • osteoporosis • lytic lesions	Protect from bone injury; use log-roll, turning sheet.
Pain, related to disease process	Administer analgesics as ordered (such as nonsteroidal antiinflammatory drugs, acetaminophen, or an acetaminophen-opioid combination). Combination drugs may be more effective than opioids alone in diminishing bone pain.
	Provide comfort measures. Assess contributing factors.
Deficient fluid volume, related to impaired renal function	Increase fluid intake to 3 to 4 L/day. Maintain I&O records.

Teach the patient to avoid traumatic bone injury and infection. Discuss the importance of adequate hydration and review the pain control modalities available. It is also important to identify spiritual resources. Address the patient's understanding of the disease, verbalization of discouragement and hopelessness, and desires for emotional and spiritual support.

Prognosis

This disease is usually progressive and generally fatal. A patient usually lives for approximately 2 years if untreated. With proper therapeutic treatment, the chronic phase of multiple myeloma may last for more than 10 years. Multiple myeloma is seldom cured, but treatment can relieve symptoms, produce remissions, and prolong life.

DISORDERS OF THE LYMPHATIC SYSTEM

LYMPHANGITIS

Etiology and Pathophysiology

Lymphangitis is an inflammation of one or more lymphatic vessels or channels that usually results from an acute streptococcal or staphylococcal infection in an extremity.

Clinical Manifestations

Lymphangitis is characterized by fine red streaks from the affected area in the groin or axilla. The infection is usually not localized, and edema is diffuse. Chills, fever, and local pain accompany headache and myalgia. Septicemia may occur; lymph nodes enlarge.

Medical Management

Administration of penicillin or other antimicrobial drugs controls the infection. Hot, moist heat (soaks or packs) brings comfort.

Nursing Interventions

Aseptic technique promotes healing. Rest and extremity elevation may relieve the pressure.

Prognosis

With treatment, the prognosis is usually good.

LYMPHEDEMA

Etiology and Pathophysiology

Lymphedema is a primary or secondary disorder characterized by the accumulation of lymph in soft tissue and edema. The accumulation of lymph in soft tissue is caused by obstruction, an increase in the amount of lymph, or removal of the lymph channels and nodes. The condition may be hereditary.

If the lymphatic drainage function is disturbed, an inflammatory process may result.

Clinical Manifestations

Massive edema and tightness cause pressure and pain in the affected extremities. It progresses toward the trunk and is aggravated by standing; pressure, as with pregnancy or premenstruation; obesity; and warm, humid environments.

Assessment and Diagnostic Test

Subjective data include complaints of pain and pressure. Medical history of varicosities, pregnancy, or modified radical mastectomy is important.

Collection of **objective data** includes observation of the extremities for edema and palpation of pedal pulses. Lymphangiography is used to differentiate lymphedema from venous disorders.

Medical Management

Diuretics are not prescribed because they remove water from the interstitial spaces and leave the protein. The proteins concentrated in the interstitial spaces then draw the fluid back into the affected area (Holcomb, 2006). Mechanical management includes special massage techniques, compression bandaging, compression pumps, and elastic sleeves or stockings on the affected limb. Diet restrictions include limiting sodium and avoiding spicy foods, which would precipitate thirst. Encourage the patient to consume a healthy diet, maintain a normal body weight, and exercise regularly.

Nursing Interventions and Patient Teaching

The primary goal of care is to increase lymphatic drainage and avoid trauma. Elevation of the extremities while asleep and periodically during the day facilitates drainage. Massage toward the trunk followed by active exercise (e.g., walking) decreases the edema. Advise patients to avoid constrictive clothing, shoes, or stockings (except elastic stockings). Patients with lymphedema are susceptible to infection, so maintain meticulous skin care and make every effort to prevent infections. Discuss precautions they should take to protect the affected area (Holcomb, 2006).

Emotional support for the patient is also important. Address body image disturbance related to the appearance of the lymphedematous extremity. Emphasize that lymphedema need not prevent the individual from engaging in routine activity.

A nursing diagnosis and interventions for the patient with lymphedema include but are not limited to the following:

Nursing Diagnosis	Nursing Interventions
Impaired skin integrity, related to impaired lymphatic drainage	Protect engorged tissues. Consider physical therapy or ROM exercises (aids lymphatic flow). Examine skin for impaired skin integrity. Gently handle affected parts. Apply skin-protecting moisturizers or emollients. Teach application of supportive stockings or elastic sleeves.

Make certain the patient is aware of the condition's progression and cause. If the disorder is long term and ongoing, discuss how to cope with its effects. Explain the rationale behind nursing interventions to enhance the ongoing medical regimen. Encourage the patient to socialize to enhance feelings of well-being.

Prognosis

The prognosis is better when the patient begins treatment early in the course of the disorder (Damsky, 2006). The patient should be referred to a physiatrist (physician specializing in physical medicine and rehabilitation) or another physician experienced in lymphedema diagnosis and treatment and to a physical or occupational therapist or nurse certified by the Lymphology Association of North America (Damsky, 2006).

Lymphedema has no cure, but signs and symptoms can be controlled by compliance with treatment.

HODGKIN'S LYMPHOMA

Etiology and Pathophysiology

Hodgkin's lymphoma, also called Hodgkin's disease, is a malignant disorder characterized by painless, progressive enlargement of lymphoid tissue. It affects males twice as frequently as females, and the age incidence curve is bimodal (two separate populations), with a peak early in life at 15 to 35 years, and a peak later in life at 50 years. The two peaks in incidence may represent separate diseases. The first incident peak suggests a viral cause. Beginning as an inflammatory or infectious process, it develops into a neoplasm. The exact cause is unknown, but Hodgkin's lymphoma is thought to be an immune disorder (T-cell disease).

Hodgkin's lymphoma has no major risk factors, but the disease occurs more frequently in people who have had mononucleosis (an infection caused by the Epstein-Barr virus), have acquired or congenital immunodeficiency syndromes, are taking immunosuppressive drugs after organ transplantation, have been exposed to occupational toxins, or have a genetic predisposition. The presence of HIV increases the incidence of Hodgkin's lymphoma.

Lymphoid tissue enlargement is usually first noticed in the cervical nodes and is characterized by abnormal or atypical cells. **Reed-Sternberg cells** are atypical histiocytes consisting of large, abnormal, multinucleated cells in the lymph nodes found in Hodgkin's lymphoma. These cells increase in number, replacing normal cells. The main diagnostic feature of Hodgkin's lymphoma is the presence of Reed-Sternberg cells in lymph node biopsy specimens.

The disease is believed to arise in a single location (the lymph nodes in 90% of patients) and then spread along adjacent lymphatics. It eventually infiltrates other organs, especially the lungs, the spleen, and the liver. In approximately two thirds of patients, the cervical lymph nodes are affected first. Unless they exert pressure on adjacent nerves, the enlarged nodes are not painful. When the disease begins above the diaphragm, it remains confined to lymph nodes for a variable period. Disease originating below the diaphragm frequently spreads to extralymphoid sites such as the liver.

Clinical Manifestations

Enlargement of the cervical, axillary, or inguinal lymph nodes is most often the initial development. The next most common location is a mediastinal node mass. Anorexia, weight loss, fever, night sweats, malaise, and extreme pruritus are complaints associated with this condition. Night sweats, weight loss, and fever, which are referred to as "B" symptoms, are associated with a worse prognosis (Box 47-5). Low-grade fever may occur. Anemia and leukocytosis follow, with development of respiratory tract infections.

Assessment

Subjective data include the common complaints of malaise and appetite loss. Pruritus is often severe. After the ingestion of even small amounts of alcohol, individuals with Hodgkin's lymphoma may complain of a rapid onset of pain at the site of the disease. The cause for the alcohol-induced pain is unknown. Bone pain occurs later in the disease's course.

Collection of **objective data** includes palpating enlarged cervical and supraclavicular lymph nodes. Splenomegaly, hepatomegaly, and abdominal tenderness are found. Excoriation of skin and evidence of scratching from pruritus are noted. Clinical signs and symptoms vary depending on where the enlarged lymph nodes are located. Involvement in the thoracic area may lead to superior vena cava syndrome with edema of the face, neck, and arms (Lewis et al., 2007).

The patient may develop palpable abdominal masses or interference with renal function as a result of enlarged retroperitoneal nodes. Spinal cord compression causing paraplegia can occur with extradural involvement. If the patient has liver involvement, jaundice may occur (Lewis et al., 2007).

Diagnostic Tests

Peripheral blood studies show anemia (normocytic, normochromic), WBC increase, and an abnormal erythrocyte sedimentation rate. Other blood studies may show hypoferremia caused by excessive iron intake by the liver and the spleen, elevated leukocyte alkaline phosphatase from liver and bone involvement, hypercalcemia from bone involvement, and hypoalbuminemia from liver involvement. Chest radiographic examination may reveal a mediastinal

Box 47-5 Clinical Staging System for Hodgkin's Disease*

STAGE I

- Abnormal single lymph nodes
- Regional or single extranodal site

STAGE II

- Two or more abnormal lymph nodes on the same side of diaphragm
- Localized involvement of extranodal site and one or more lymph node regions on the same side of diaphragm

STAGE III

- Abnormal lymph node regions on both sides of diaphragm
- May be accompanied by spleen involvement
- Now subdivided into lymphatic involvement of the upper abdomen in the spleen (splenic, celiac, and portal nodes) (stage III_1) and the lower abdominal nodes in the periaortic, mesenteric, and iliac regions (stage III_2)

STAGE IV

- Diffuse and disseminated involvement of one or more extralymphatic tissues and/or organs—with or without lymph node involvement; the extranodal site is identified as *H*, hepatic; *L*, lung; *P*, pleural; *M*, marrow; *D*, dermal; *O*, osseous

*Nomenclature used in staging uses a roman numeral (*I* to *IV*) that reflects the location and extent of the disease. *A* and *B* are added after the stage, depending on whether symptoms are present when disease is found. If there are no symptoms at time of diagnosis, add A after staging. If symptoms of night sweats, fever, and weight loss are present, add B after staging (From Lewis, S.L., et al. (2007). *Medical-surgical nursing: assessment and management of clinical problems* (7th ed.). St. Louis: Mosby.

mass. CT or MRI can detect retroperitoneal node involvement. Lymph node biopsy that includes laparoscopy for retroperitoneal nodes is performed. Bone marrow biopsy is an important aspect of staging. A CT scan and an ultrasound examination can indicate an enlarged spleen or liver. The presence of Reed-Sternberg cells remains a hallmark of the presence of Hodgkin's lymphoma.

Positron emission tomography (PET) with or without CT scans is used to assess the response to therapy. PET or CT scans are helpful to note the patient's response to treatment such as observing mediastinal lymphadenopathy; abdominal lymph node enlargement; and liver, spleen, bone, and brain disease (Lewis et al., 2007).

Medical Management

Treatment depends on the staging process (see Box 47-5). The stage of Hodgkin's lymphoma must be established before selecting an appropriate treatment plan. Figure 47-5 illustrates nodal involvement, by stage, in Hodgkin's lymphoma.

Combination chemotherapy is used in some early stages in patients believed to have resistant disease or be at high risk for relapse. Chemotherapy and radiation therapy are used against the generalized forms (stages III and IV). Advances in treatment now enable some stage IIIB and stage IV diseases to be cured with high-dose chemotherapy and bone marrow or peripheral SCT. The site of the disease and the amount of resistant disease after chemotherapy determine the role of radiation in supplementing chemotherapy.

Treatment for Hodgkin's lymphoma involves several drugs. An aggressive treatment approach is required (Lewis et al., 2007). Until recently, a traditional regimen for Hodgkin's disease had been MOPP: mechlorethamine (Mustargen), vincristine, procarbazine (Matulane), and prednisone. Mechlorethamine (also called nitrogen mustard) is one of a group of drugs known as alkylating agents. These can cause serious long-term side effects, such as leukemia, particularly when combined with radiation therapy. Instead of MOPP, oncologists are now choosing a regimen known as ABVD, or they're replacing mechlorethamine with cyclophosphamide to de-

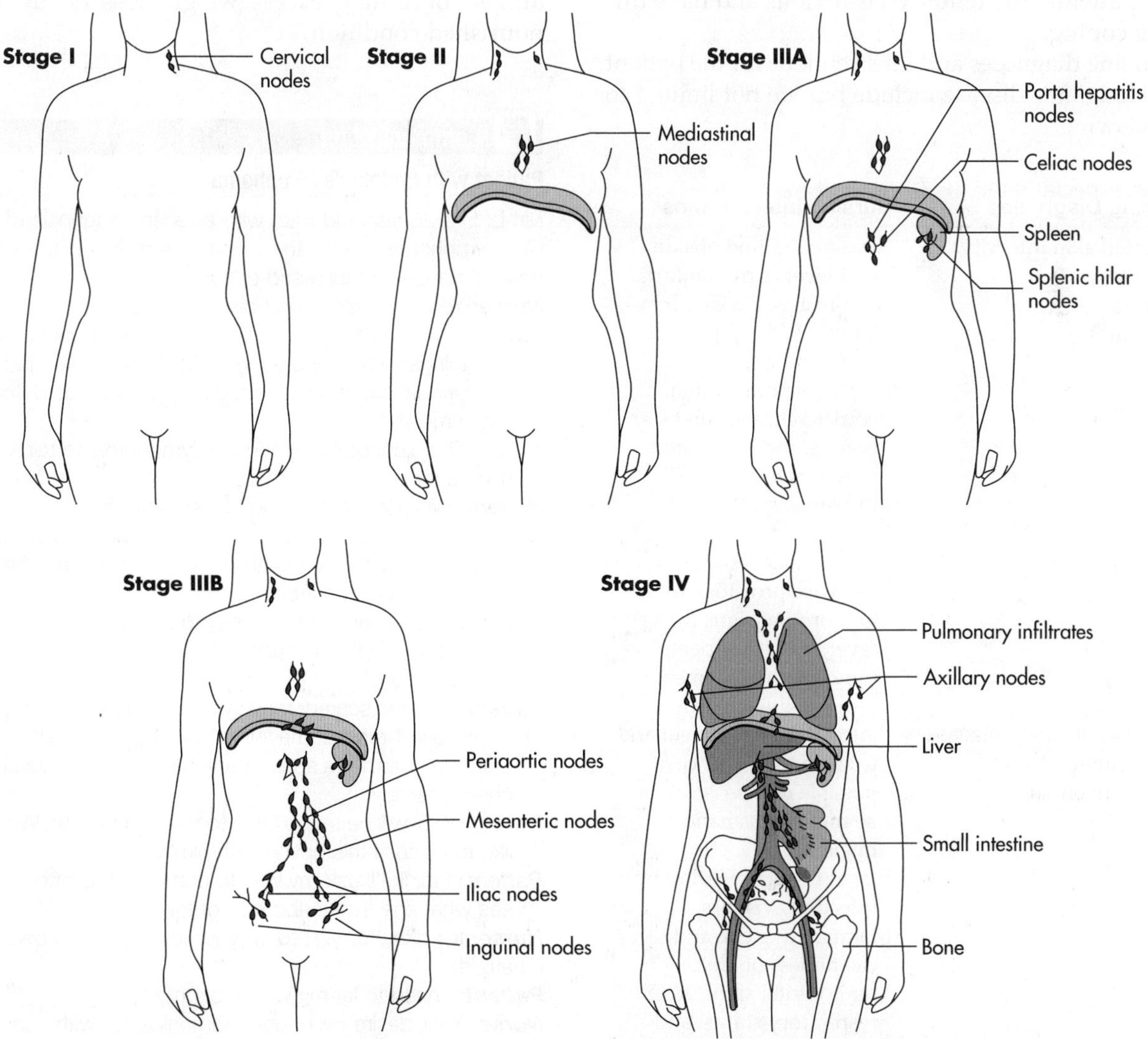

FIGURE 47-5 Nodal involvement by stage in Hodgkin's disease (based on modified Ann Arbor Staging System).

crease the likelihood of long-term complications. ABVD includes doxorubicin, bleomycin (Blenoxane), vinblastine (Velban), and dacarbazine (DTIC-Dome) (Lewis et al., 2007). A biologic response modifier (filgrastim) that stimulates proliferation and differentiation of neutrophils is a treatment option. Filgrastim is used to decrease infection in patients receiving antineoplastics that suppress neutrophil production.

Nursing Interventions and Patient Teaching

Plan care according to the staging level. Awareness of side effects of radiation therapy or chemotherapy is important in preparing the patient to deal effectively with the treatment. Because the survival of patients with Hodgkin's lymphoma depends on their response to treatment, helping the patient deal with the consequences of treatment is extremely important. Comfort measures focus on skin integrity. Soothing baths with an antipruritic medication (as ordered) can be effective. Control fever and perspiration with medication (with attention to increased fluid intake) plus linen changes as necessary to prevent further skin problems. Explain extensive tests to the patient, who tends to be anxious and have difficulty coping.

Nursing diagnoses and interventions for the patient with Hodgkin's disease include but are not limited to the following:

Nursing Diagnoses	Nursing Interventions
Impaired skin integrity, related to: • pruritus • jaundice	Assess condition of skin and level of discomfort. Administer skin care by baths and keep patient clean and dry. Apply calamine lotion, cornstarch, sodium bicarbonate, and medicated powders to relieve pruritus. Maintain adequate humidity and a cool room to decrease pruritus. Monitor vital signs for fever; assess for perspiration and change linen, keeping it wrinkle free.
Risk for infection, related to immune system ineffectiveness	Protect the environment and teach the importance of possible reverse isolation. Use meticulous hand hygiene. Prevent contamination by infectious visitors. Maintain hygiene and cleanliness of area. Monitor vital signs, I&O, respiratory status, and skin integrity.
Anxiety and fear, related to unknown outcome	Instruct patient on symptoms, disease progression, and treatment regimen. Encourage open communication and venting of feelings. Encourage questions and problem solving.

Understanding the disease is important for the patient to perform self-care and retain independence. Fertility issues may be of particular concern because this disease is frequently seen in adolescents and young adults. Help ensure that these issues are addressed soon after diagnosis (Communication box). The effect on the patient's life, as well as on significant others, is a prime consideration in patient attitude and adjustment. Realistic approaches to the illness and therapies are imperative. Referrals for patients seeking counseling for stress management can be helpful. Discuss special nutritional considerations concerning excess weight loss or an undernourished condition.

Communication

Patient with Hodgkin's Lymphoma

Mr. L. is a 25-year-old man with a recent diagnosis of Hodgkin's lymphoma. When the nurse enters Mr. L.'s room, she notes he appears tense and drawn.

Nurse: You seem tense and preoccupied.

Patient: Why did this have to happen to me? I just got married and things were going so well. Dr. S. said I would have to have radiation, then chemotherapy. I've heard that can make me sterile.

Nurse: The diagnosis of Hodgkin's lymphoma certainly is worrisome for you and your wife.

Patient: Why do I feel so sad? I just want to cry.

Nurse: That's a natural response; you're grieving because of the loss of a totally healthy body, and you're concerned over the possibility of being sterile.

Patient: I don't know what to say to my wife.

Nurse: Are you frightened about how she might respond if you become sterile?

Patient: Yes, I'm scared; maybe I won't seem as masculine as I am now. I read somewhere about a man being able to store his sperm in a sperm bank before taking radiation and chemotherapy.

Nurse: Dr. S. will be stopping in to see you tonight. Would you like to discuss this option with him?

Patient: I think I'll ask my wife to come up this afternoon and see what she thinks about all of this.

Nurse: It's okay for you to let your loved ones know you are afraid.

Patient: I need to let my wife know my feelings.

Nurse: Your desire for open communication with your wife is helpful to both of you. I'll stop by and visit with you later.

Prognosis

The prognosis is steadily improving but depends on the stage of the disease. Those diagnosed and treated in stage I or II have a 10-year survival rate near 90%, whereas those in stage III or IV have a 10-year survival rate of more than 50% (Lewis et al., 2007). A serious consequence of the treatment for Hodgkin's lymphoma is the later development of secondary malignancies. The estimated risk of a secondary cancer is approximately 18% at 15 years after treatment for Hodgkin's disease. The most common secondary malignancies are AML, non-Hodgkin's lymphoma (NHL), and solid tumors.

NON-HODGKIN'S LYMPHOMA

Etiology and Pathophysiology

NHLs are a group of malignant neoplasms of primarily B- or T-cell origin affecting all ages. B-cell lymphomas constitute about 90% of NHLs. The condition is starting to be characterized as a neoplasm of the immune system. The cause is unknown, but a herpeslike viral source is suspected. The neoplasms are classified according to different cellular and lymph node characteristics. Patients who receive immunosuppressive agents have a greater chance of developing NHL, probably because the immunosuppressive agents activate tumor viruses. NHL is more common in men older than 60 years of age, whites, and those of Jewish ancestry.

A variety of clinical presentations and courses are recognized, from slowly developing to rapidly progressive disease. Common names for different types of lymphoma include Burkitt's lymphoma, diffuse large B-cell lymphoma, lymphoblastic lymphoma, and follicular lymphoma. Thus NHL comprises a large group of different lymphoid malignancies (Lewis et al., 2007). There is no hallmark pathologic feature in NHL that parallels the Reed-Sternberg cell of Hodgkin's disease. However, all NHLs involve lymphocytes arrested in various stages of development. Tumors usually start in lymph nodes and spread to lymphoid tissue in the spleen, the liver, the GI tract, and the bone marrow. Involvement of lymphoid tissue also results in malabsorption and bone lesions.

NHL is the most commonly occurring hematological cancer and the fifth leading cause of cancer death (Lewis et al., 2007). Each year, approximately 54,000 new cases of NHL are diagnosed and approximately 25,000 deaths occur. As the population ages, the incidence of NHL has increased 2% to 3% per year for at least the past 30 years.

Clinical Manifestations

The method of spread can be unpredictable when NHLs originate outside the lymph nodes. At the time of diagnosis, most patients have widely scattered disease. Painless, enlarged lymph nodes and fever, weight loss, night sweats, anemia, pruritus, and susceptibility to infection may develop. Pressure symptoms in the involved areas are noted. Pleural effusion, bone fractures, and paralysis are complications. Because the disease is usually disseminated when it is diagnosed, other symptoms are present, depending on where the disease has spread (e.g., hepatomegaly with liver involvement).

Assessment

Subjective data include frequent patient complaints of fatigue, malaise, and anorexia.

Collection of **objective data** includes examination of the abdomen for splenomegaly. Enlarged lymph nodes are also evident. Fever, night sweats, and weight loss are usually present.

Diagnostic Tests

A bone scan may reveal fractures, lesions, and tumor infiltration. Blood studies show hypercalcemia and anemia; leukocytosis; and elevated sedimentation rate, platelet count, and alkaline phosphatase level. A Coombs' test yields a positive result for antiglobulin. The patient needs a chest roentgenogram; CT scans of the chest, abdomen, and pelvis; a gallium scan; and possibly a lymphangiogram. Biopsies of lymph nodes, liver, and bone marrow are performed to establish the cell type and pattern. Diagnostic studies used for NHL resemble those used for Hodgkin's disease. Staging, as described for Hodgkin's disease, is used to guide therapy. The International Working Formulation is a useful system for classifying NHL. This system divides each subtype of lymphoma into indolent (low grade), aggressive (intermediate grade), and very aggressive (high grade).

Medical Management

Once the diagnosis is made, the extent of the disease (staging) is determined. Accurate staging is crucial to determine the treatment regimen. The therapeutic regimen for NHLs includes chemotherapy and radiation. Indolent lymphomas have a naturally long course, but are difficult to treat effectively. In contrast, more aggressive lymphomas are more likely to be cured, since they are more responsive to treatment. Some chemotherapy agents used are cyclophosphamide, vincristine, prednisone, doxorubicin, bleomycin, and methotrexate. The monoclonal antibody rituximab (Rituxan) was approved for the treatment of follicular lymphoma. Ibritumomab (Zevalin) is another monoclonal antibody that can be used in patients who are refractory to rituximab or in conjunction with it. Conventional chemotherapy used to treat patients with relapsed, aggressive NHL, who are still responding to salvage chemotherapy, is not as effective as high-dose chemotherapy with autologous (tissue derived from the same individual) hematopoietic stem cells (HSCT).

Patients with lymphoma commonly receive radiation to the chest wall, mediastinum, axillae, and neck—the region known as the "mantle field." Some patients also need radiation to the abdomen; paraaortic area; spleen; and, less commonly, the pelvis.

Chemotherapy is the mainstay of treatment of NHLs that are not localized. High-dose chemotherapy with peripheral blood stem cell or bone marrow transplantation may be indicated. Tumor necrosis factor is being used; it has direct cell toxicity and stimulates the immune system. Interferon is being investigated as a treatment option. Older patients have difficulty tolerating the aggressive chemotherapy treatments. This population is increasing in number, and new approaches are being examined.

Nursing Interventions and Patient Teaching

Supportive care of the patient during radiation and chemotherapy is primary in nursing management. Observation for complications follows. Further intervention is similar to that for Hodgkin's disease.

Explanations of the extensive diagnostic workup and its importance for staging the disease and determining the treatment plan are an important focus of patient teaching during the diagnostic period.

Prognosis

The prognosis is influenced by the staging classification. The prognosis for NHL is generally not as good as that for Hodgkin's disease.

NURSING PROCESS *for the Patient with a Blood or Lymphatic Disorder*

The role of the licensed practical nurse/licensed vocational nurse (LPN/LVN) in the nursing process as stated is that the LPN/LVN will:

- Participate in planning care for patients based on patient needs
- Review patient's care plan and recommend revisions as needed
- Review and follow defined prioritization for patient care
- Use clinical pathways, care maps, or care plans to guide and review patient care

Assessment

Collect data from diverse sources: patient and family observation, physical examination, and diagnostic evaluation results (see Table 47-1).

The **subjective data** collected at the onset of the disease process are generally vague and nonspecific: malaise, fatigue, and weakness. The patient may relate a history of illness, easy bruising, bleeding tendencies with petechiae, and ecchymosis. Integumentary changes (including pruritus, nonhealing cuts and bruises, draining lesions, jaundice, and palpable subcutaneous nodules) may be reported. Edema and tenderness in lymph node regions may be accompanied by pain, sometimes severe. GI complaints are noted, as well as cardiovascular and respiratory changes. Neurologic complaints include headache, numbness, tingling, paresthesias, and behavioral alteration (Life Span Considerations box).

Collection of **objective data** follows a system-by-system approach to confirm patient complaints. Manipulation of joints can reveal stiffness and hematoma and may produce pain. Examination of the oral cavity can reveal lesions, ulcers, signs of bleeding, or gingivitis. Cardiovascular and respiratory assessments include breath and heart sound variations and pain or dyspneic positioning. Note any patient anxiety, and observe for diminished comprehension. Listening and an unhurried interview may reveal many symptoms not previously mentioned.

Nursing Diagnosis

Nursing diagnoses are determined from the assessment, which provides data for identifying the patient's problems, strengths, potential complications, and learning needs. Nursing diagnoses for the patient with a blood or lymphatic disorder include but are not limited to the following:

- Risk for infection
- Injury (trauma), risk for (bleeding, falls)
- Fatigue

Life Span Considerations

Older Adults

Blood or Lymphatic Disorder

- The subjective symptoms of hematological disorders (e.g., fatigue, weakness, dizziness, and dyspnea) may be mistaken for normal changes of aging or attributed to other disease processes commonly seen in older adults.
- The most common blood disorders are forms of anemia.
- Decreased production of the intrinsic factor in an aging gastric mucosa results in increased incidence of pernicious anemia.
- Many older adults suffer from conditions such as colonic diverticula, hiatal hernia, or ulcerations that can cause occult bleeding. Older adults with these conditions should be observed for iron deficiency anemia.
- Age-related problems such as altered dentition, limited financial resources, difficulty in food preparation, and poor appetite resulting from emotional upset or depression can cause an increased incidence of iron deficiency anemia.
- Severe or persistent anemia can place additional stress on the aging or diseased heart.
- Administer blood products with caution because older adults are at increased risk of developing congestive heart failure. Careful assessment of cardiopulmonary function and intake and output is essential.
- Oral administration of iron preparations increases the risk of gastrointestinal (GI) irritation and constipation in older adults.
- Ingestion of large amounts of aspirin and other antiinflammatory medications commonly taken by older adults increases the risk of GI bleeding and can lead to alteration in clotting.
- Chronic lymphocytic leukemia is the most common form seen among older patients. This form of leukemia usually progresses slowly in older adults and is rarely treated.

- Deficient knowledge
- Acute pain
- Chronic pain
- Ineffective tissue perfusion
- Impaired gas exchange
- Activity intolerance
- Ineffective coping
- Impaired skin integrity

Expected Outcomes and Planning

Most patients have more than one nursing diagnosis. Therefore the planning step in the nursing process involves determining the priority for nursing interventions from the list of nursing diagnoses. Use Maslow's hierarchy of needs; that is, assign the highest priority to immediate problems that may be life threatening. For example, impaired gas exchange would have a higher priority than ineffective coping.

Planning includes developing realistic goals and outcomes that stem from the identified nursing diagnosis. Examples of expected patient outcomes for the patient with a blood or lymphatic disorder may include but are not limited to the following:

Goal 1: Patient is free of signs and symptoms of an infection.

Goal 2: Patient has no evidence of bleeding (any bleeding is quickly controlled).

Implementation

The implementation of the nursing process is the actual initiation of the nursing care plan. Patient outcomes and goals are achieved by performance of the nursing interventions. Nursing interventions for the patient with a blood or lymphatic disorder may include the following:

- Place patient in private room; avoid contact with visitors or staff members who have an infection (in the immunocompromised patient).
- Stress careful hand hygiene to patient, significant others, and all caregivers.
- Assist in planning daily activities to include rest periods to decrease fatigue and weakness.
- Provide oxygen for dyspnea or excessive fatigue with exertion.
- Explain the disease process, and stress the importance of continued medical follow-up. Most important is the patient's ability to identify the body's signals that blood abnormalities are present. Petechiae, ecchymoses, and gingival bleeding are the warning signs that one should seek medical attention promptly.

Evaluation

To evaluate the effectiveness of nursing interventions, compare the patient's behaviors with those stated in the expected patient outcomes. Successful achievement of patient outcomes for the patient with a blood or lymphatic disorder is indicated by the following evaluative measures:

- Patient shows no sign of infection; temperature and WBC count are within normal limits.
- Patient has not fallen.
- Patient shows no signs of bleeding (e.g., petechiae, hemorrhage); any bleeding is quickly controlled.
- Patient is able to bathe self in 30 minutes without becoming fatigued.
- Patient is able to correctly explain measures to prevent infection by good hand hygiene techniques and avoidance of people with infectious conditions.
- Patient is able to explain measures to prevent hemorrhage by avoiding traumatic injury and intramuscular injections.
- Patient reports no shortness of breath with activity.

Get Ready for the NCLEX® Examination!

Key Points

- Blood is a thick, red fluid composed of plasma, a light yellow fluid; RBCs; WBCs; and platelets, which are suspended in plasma.
- The blood performs several critical functions: It transports oxygen and nutrients to the cells and waste products away from the cells; it regulates acid-base balance (pH) with buffers; and it protects the body against infection and prevents blood loss with special clotting mechanisms.
- Every person's blood is one of the following blood types in the ABO system of typing: type A, type B, type AB, or type O.
- The lymphatic system is a vast, complex network of capillaries, thin vessels, valves, ducts, nodes, and organs that helps to protect and maintain the internal fluid environment of the entire body by producing, filtering, and conveying lymph and by producing various blood cells.
- The tonsils are composed of lymphoid tissue and are responsible for filtering bacteria.
- The thymus gland is composed of lymphoid tissue in utero (before birth) and the early years of life. It aids in the development of the immune system.
- The spleen is also composed of lymphoid tissue and has many functions, such as filtering out old RBCs, storing a pint of blood, producing antibodies, and phagocytosing bacteria.

- Anemia may be caused by blood loss, impaired RBC production, increased RBC destruction, or nutritional deficiency.
- Shock occurs when organs are deprived of oxygen and nutrients.
- Hypotension, defined as systolic blood pressure of less than 90 mm Hg and tachycardia of more than 120 bpm, occurs with blood loss of 1500 to 2000 mL. By the time blood pressure reaches this point, about 30% to 40% of blood volume may have been lost and end-organ damage may be irreversible.
- Weakness and fatigue are major symptoms of anemia. They result from decreased oxygenation from decreased levels of hemoglobin and increased energy needs required by increased RBC production.
- Ingestion of iron compounds or intramuscular Z-track administration of iron dextran is part of the therapy for iron deficiency anemia.
- Sickle cell anemia is a hemolytic anemia with a genetic basis; a sickle cell crisis occurs when the RBCs become deoxygenated and sickle shaped, thus causing stasis and obstruction of the microvasculature, leading to organ infarction and necrosis.
- Polycythemia vera is characterized by excessive bone marrow production that manifests with an increase in circulating erythrocytes, granulocytes, and platelets. Secondary polycythemia is caused by hypoxia rather than a defect in the development of the RBC.
- Thrombocytopenia is a decrease in the number of circulating platelets and leads to bleeding; people with thrombocytopenia need to learn how to prevent injury and hemorrhage.
- Hemophilia is a hereditary coagulation disorder; hemophilia A is a lack of coagulation factor VIII, and hemophilia B is a lack of factor IX. Maintenance therapy consists of blood factor replacement therapy and prevention of injury.
- DIC is a coagulation disorder characterized initially by clotting and secondarily by hemorrhage. It results from an alteration in the balance between clotting factors and fibrinolytic factors; the person is usually critically ill.
- People with alterations of WBCs are at high risk of infection because leukocytes are a major factor in the body's defense against invading microorganisms.
- The leukemias are malignant disorders characterized by uncontrolled proliferation of WBCs and their precursors; the cause is unknown, but several theories have been proposed.
- Leukemias may be lymphocytic, or myelogenous, and acute or chronic. Acute leukemias have a rapid onset and a short course, if untreated; chronic leukemias have a more insidious onset and longer course. The major therapies for leukemias are chemotherapy and bone marrow transplantation.
- Multiple myeloma is a malignant neoplastic immunodeficiency disease of the bone marrow that affects the plasma cells. The specific immunoglobulin produced by the myeloma cells is present in the blood and urine and is referred to as the monoclonal protein.
- Lymphomas are malignant disorders of the lymphatic system. People with Hodgkin's lymphoma have defective cellular immunity and are therefore at high risk for infection. NHL is a group of lymphoid malignancies. Chemotherapy and radiation are the primary medical treatment for lymphomas.

Additional Learning Resources

Go to your Companion CD for an audio glossary, animations, video clips, and more.

evolve Be sure to visit the Evolve site at http://evolve.elsevier.com/Christensen/adult/ for additional online resources.

Review Questions for the NCLEX® Examination

1. Another name for a red blood cell is:
   1. leukocyte.
   2. monocyte.
   3. erythrocyte.
   4. platelet.

2. The test for a measure of the packed cell volume of red cells expressed as a percentage of the total blood volume is:
   1. hematocrit.
   2. erythrocyte sedimentation rate.
   3. reticulocyte.
   4. differential.

3. The gland that plays a role in the development of the body's immune system is the:
   1. tonsils.
   2. thymus.
   3. spleen.
   4. liver.

4. The compound in the blood that carries oxygen to the cells from the lungs and carbon dioxide away from the cells to the lungs is:
   1. leukocyte.
   2. thrombocyte.
   3. hemoglobin.
   4. erythrocyte.

5. The type of blood that is called the universal donor blood is:
   1. type A.
   2. type B.
   3. type AB.
   4. type O.

6. The spleen is located in which quadrant of the abdominal cavity?
   1. Upper right
   2. Upper left
   3. Lower left
   4. Lower right

7. A patient is immunosuppressed by chemotherapy. She has a WBC count of 1500/mm^3, with neutrophils of 20%. Which statement indicates she understands

home care instructions relating to her immune system?

1. Take antibiotics prophylactically.
2. Take large doses of vitamins.
3. Avoid individuals with infections.
4. Use only sterile bed linens.

8. A patient's platelets have decreased to 18,000/mm^3. The most appropriate nursing intervention is to:

1. provide oral hygiene four times per day.
2. institute bleeding precautions.
3. order a high-protein diet.
4. request an order for oxygen per nasal cannula.

9. A patient's spouse tells the nurse that her husband, who has been admitted to the hospital with advanced leukemia, is talking about dying and expresses fears of death. She asks for suggestions for helping her husband. Which response is best?

1. "Your husband will probably die of another disease before he dies of leukemia."
2. "Your husband is expressing a readiness to be admitted to a hospice."
3. "Talk of death is natural at this time but will diminish as he feels better."
4. "It's normal to want to talk about death; what we can do is be supportive by listening."

10. A 28-year-old man is admitted with fatigue; discomfort; enlarged, painless cervical lymph nodes; and pruritus. A lymph node biopsy leads to the diagnosis of Hodgkin's lymphoma. The abnormal cells noted by the pathologist in Hodgkin's lymphoma are called:

1. Rodem-Lee cells.
2. Bullus-Frendelenburg cells.
3. Reed-Sternberg cells.
4. Stevens-Jorgens cells.

11. A 27-year-old housewife and mother of two children is being seen by the nurse at the health maintenance organization for signs of fatigue. She has a history of iron deficiency anemia. What data from the nursing history indicate that the anemia is not currently managed effectively?

1. Pallor
2. Poor skin turgor
3. Heart rate 68 bpm, weak pulse
4. Respirations 18 breaths/min and regular

12. An important nursing intervention goal to establish for a patient who has iron deficiency anemia is:

1. use birth control to avoid pregnancy.
2. increase fluids to stimulate erythropoiesis.
3. decrease fluids to prevent sickling of RBCs.
4. alternate periods of rest and activity to balance oxygen supply and demand.

13. The nurse instructs a patient about foods rich in iron. Which foods should be included in the diet?

1. Fresh fruit and milk
2. Cheeses and processed lunch meats
3. Dark green leafy vegetables and organ meats
4. Fruit juices and cornmeal bread

14. Which statement by the patient with pernicious anemia would indicate that she understood the teaching?

1. "I'll be glad when I can stop the injections and take only oral medicine."
2. "I'll have to take B_{12} shots for the rest of my life."
3. "After a while I'll no longer need to take shots, just the pills."
4. "I was glad to hear that pills are available to treat me."

15. A patient is admitted with polycythemia vera. He has a hemoglobin value of 20 g/dL. A probable treatment that will be ordered is:

1. whole blood transfusion.
2. platelet transfusion.
3. phlebotomy with removal of 800 mL of blood.
4. vitamin B_{12} injection.

16. Which laboratory finding is a strong indicator of disseminated intravascular coagulation (DIC)?

1. An elevated platelet count
2. An elevated D-dimer test
3. A normal prothrombin time
4. An elevated fibrinogen level

17. In teaching the patient with pernicious anemia about the disease, the nurse explains that it results from a lack of:

1. folic acid.
2. intrinsic factor.
3. extrinsic factor.
4. an RBC enzyme.

18. In addition to the general symptoms of anemia, the patient with pernicious anemia also manifests:

1. neurologic symptoms.
2. coagulation deficiencies.
3. cardiovascular disturbances.
4. a decreased immunologic response.

19. A patient with sickle cell anemia asks the nurse why the sickling crisis does not stop when oxygen therapy is started. The nurse explains that:

1. sickling occurs in response to decreased blood viscosity, which is not affected by oxygen therapy.
2. when red cells sickle, they occlude small vessels, which causes more local hypoxia and more sickling.
3. the primary problem during a sickle cell crisis is destruction of the abnormal cells, resulting in fewer RBCs to carry oxygen.
4. oxygen therapy does not alter the shape of the abnormal erythrocytes but only allows for increased oxygen concentration in hemoglobin.

20. A nursing intervention that is indicated for the patient during a sickle cell crisis is:

1. frequent ambulation.
2. application of antiembolism hose.
3. restriction of sodium and oral fluids.
4. administration of therapeutic doses of continuous opioid analgesics.

21. Hodgkin's lymphoma occurs more frequently in individuals who have:
    1. a history of cancer treated with radiation.
    2. been exposed to nuclear explosions.
    3. had an infection caused by the Epstein-Barr virus.
    4. had an infection of *Helicobacter pylori*.

22. Which statement concerning Hodgkin's lymphoma is correct?
    1. The 10-year survival rate for stage I or II Hodgkin's lymphoma is more than 90%.
    2. The incidence of Hodgkin's lymphoma has increased over the past 20 years.
    3. Hodgkin's lymphoma is considered a difficult form of cancer to treat.
    4. The incidence of Hodgkin's lymphoma in the older adult has increased.

23. A patient with hemophilia is hospitalized with acute knee pain and edema. Nursing interventions include:
    1. wrapping the knee with an elastic bandage.
    2. placing the patient on bed rest and applying ice to the joint.
    3. gently performing ROM exercises to the knee to prevent adhesions.
    4. administering nonsteroidal antiinflammatory drugs as needed for pain.

24. During physical assessment of a patient with thrombocytopenia, the nurse would expect to find:
    1. petechiae and purpura.
    2. jaundiced sclera and skin.
    3. tender, enlarged lymph nodes.
    4. splenomegaly.

25. Which nursing interventions are necessary when caring for a patient who has a WBC of 1800/mm^3? *(Select all that apply.)*
    1. Prevent patient contact with people who have respiratory tract infections or influenza.
    2. Wash hands frequently before and after patient contact.
    3. Report temperature elevation.
    4. Monitor hemoglobin.

26. Which are necessary for the maturation of a red blood cell? *(Select all that apply.)*
    1. Vitamin B_{12}
    2. Folic acid
    3. Renal erythropoietic factor
    4. Capric acid
    5. Iron

27. Choose the correct medical management for the patient with DIC: *(Select all that apply.)*
    1. Addressing and correcting underlying cause
    2. Transfusion replacement
    3. Cryoprecipitate
    4. Administering colony-stimulating factor (filgrastim [Neupogen])
    5. Heparin therapy

28. A young adult with hemophilia A is admitted with uncontrolled bleeding in the left knee joint as a result of a fall from his motorcycle. Which are appropriate nursing interventions and medical management? *(Select all that apply.)*
    1. Applying pressure
    2. Cold applications
    3. Administering cyclophosphamide (Cytoxan)
    4. RBC transfusions
    5. Administering factor VIII concentrate

29. The nurse anticipates that an older adult patient with severe iron deficiency anemia will require which blood product?
    1. Whole blood
    2. Packed red blood cells
    3. Fresh frozen plasma
    4. Frozen red blood cells

30. Acute blood loss can have several serious effects on the body. Serious consequences result when the loss is:
    1. 100 mL.
    2. 300 mL.
    3. 500 mL.
    4. 1000 mL.

31. What is the most important measure in preventing transmission of harmful pathogens to a patient with depressed bone marrow function?
    1. Strict and frequent hand hygiene by all persons having contact with the patient
    2. Placement of the patient in a private room with high-efficiency particulate air filtration
    3. Administration of combinations of prophylactic antibiotics
    4. Creation of a "sterile" environment for the patient with the use of laminar airflow rooms

32. A patient is chronically hypoxic and has an RBC count of 7 million/mm^3, hemoglobin of 20 g/dL, and hematocrit of 50%; his condition would be classified as:
    1. primary polycythemia.
    2. secondary polycythemia.
    3. autoimmune thrombocytopenia.
    4. purpura splenomegaly.

33. The vital signs of a patient who has a blood loss of 1500 to 2000 mL would be: *(Select all that apply.)*
    1. Pulse $>$120 bpm
    2. Pulse $>$100 bpm
    3. Blood pressure normal
    4. Blood pressure $<$90 mm Hg

34. One unit of packed RBCs is expected to raise the hemoglobin level by how many grams per deciliter?
    1. 2 g/dL
    2. 1 g/dL
    3. 0.5 g/dL
    4. 3 g/dL

chapter

48

Care of the Patient with a Cardiovascular or a Peripheral Vascular Disorder

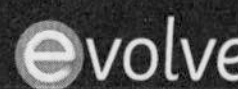

Barbara Lauritsen Christensen

http://evolve.elsevier.com/Christensen/foundationsadult

Objectives

Anatomy and Physiology

1. Discuss the location, size, and position of the heart.
2. Identify the chambers of the heart and their functions.
3. Identify the valves of the heart and their locations.
4. Discuss the electrical conduction system that causes the cardiac muscle fibers to contract.
5. Explain what produces the two main heart sounds.
6. Trace the path of blood through the coronary circulation.

Medical-Surgical

7. List diagnostic tests used to evaluate cardiovascular function.
8. For coronary artery disease, compare nonmodifiable risk factors with factors that are modifiable in lifestyle and health management.
9. Describe five cardiac dysrhythmias.
10. Compare the etiology and pathophysiology, clinical manifestations, assessment, diagnostic tests, medical management, nursing interventions, and prognosis for patients with angina pectoris, myocardial infarction, or heart failure.
11. Specify patient teaching for patients with cardiac dysrhythmias, angina pectoris, myocardial infarction, heart failure, and valvular heart disease.
12. Discuss the purposes of cardiac rehabilitation.
13. Discuss the etiology and pathophysiology, clinical manifestations, assessment, diagnostic tests, medical management, nursing interventions, and prognosis for the patient with pulmonary edema.
14. Compare and contrast the etiology and pathophysiology, clinical manifestations, assessment, diagnostic tests, medical management, nursing interventions, and prognosis for the patient with rheumatic heart disease, pericarditis, and endocarditis.
15. Identify 10 conditions which may result in the development of secondary cardiomyopathy.
16. Discuss the indications and contraindications for cardiac transplant.
17. Describe the effects of aging on the peripheral vascular system.
18. Identify risk factors associated with peripheral vascular disorders.
19. Compare and contrast signs and symptoms associated with arterial and venous disorders.
20. Discuss nursing interventions for arterial and venous disorders.
21. Compare essential (primary) hypertension, secondary hypertension, and malignant hypertension.
22. Discuss the etiology and pathophysiology, clinical manifestations, assessment, diagnostic tests, medical management, and nursing interventions for the patient with hypertension.
23. Discuss the importance of patient education for hypertension.
24. Compare and contrast the etiology and pathophysiology, clinical manifestations, assessment, diagnostic tests, medical management, nursing interventions, and prognosis for patients with arterial aneurysm, Buerger's disease, and Raynaud's disease.
25. Discuss the etiology and pathophysiology, clinical manifestations, assessment, diagnostic tests, medical management, nursing interventions, and prognosis for patients with thrombophlebitis, varicose veins, and stasis ulcer.
26. Discuss appropriate patient education for thrombophlebitis.

Key Terms

aneurysm (ĂN-ŭr-ĭ-zĭm, p. 1595)
angina pectoris (ăn-JĪ-nă PĔK-tŏr-ĭs, p. 1557)
arteriosclerosis (ăr-tē-rē-ō-sklĕ-RŌ-sĭs, p. 1591)
atherosclerosis (ăth-ĕr-ō-sklĕ-RŌ-sĭs, p. 1556)
bradycardia (brăd-ĕ-KĂR-dē-ă, p. 1551)
B-type natriuretic peptide (BNP) (nā'trē-yū-rĕt-ĭk, p. 1547)
cardioversion (kăr-dē-ō-VĔR-zhŭn, p. 1546)
coronary artery disease (CAD) (p. 1556)
defibrillation (dē-fĭb-rĭ-LĀ-shŭn, p. 1553)
dysrhythmia (dĭs-RĬTH-mē-ă, p. 1550)
embolus (ĔM-bō-lŭs, p. 1562)
endarterectomy (ĕnd-ăr-tĕr-ĔK-tō-mē, p. 1594)
heart failure (p. 1568)
hypoxemia (hī-pŏk-SĒ-mē-ă, p. 1546)
intermittent claudication (klăw-dĕ-KĀ-shŭn, p. 1585)
ischemia (ĭs-KĒ-mē-ă, p. 1557)
myocardial infarction (MI) (mī-ō-KĂR-dē-ăl ĭn-FĂRK-shŭn, p. 1562)
occlusion (ō-KLŪ-zhŭn, p. 1562)
orthopnea (ŏr-thŏp-NĒ-ă, p. 1570)
peripheral (pĕ-RĬF-ĕr-ăl, p. 1584)
pleural effusion (PLŪR-ăl ĕ-FŪ-zhŭn, p. 1569)
polycythemia (pŏl-ē-sī-THĒ-mē-ă, p. 1546)
pulmonary edema (PŬL-mō-nă-rē ĕ-DĒ-mă, p. 1576)
tachycardia (tăk-ĕ-KĂR-dē-ă, p. 1550)

ANATOMY AND PHYSIOLOGY OF THE CARDIOVASCULAR SYSTEM

The cardiovascular (circulatory) system is the transportation system of the body. It delivers oxygen and nutrients to the cells to support their individual activities and transports the cells' waste products to the appropriate organs for disposal. This chapter discusses the structure and function of the blood vessels and the heart.

HEART

The heart is a remarkable organ, not much bigger than a fist (Figure 48-1). It is responsible for pumping 1000 gallons of blood every day through the closed circuit of blood vessels. It beats 100,000 times a day and transports the blood 60,000 miles through a network of blood vessels. The heart is a hollow organ composed mainly of muscle tissue with a series of one-way valves.

The heart is located in the chest cavity between the lungs in a region called the **mediastinum** (the mass of organs and tissues separating the lungs; in addition to the heart and its greater vessels, the mediastinum contains the trachea and the esophagus). Two thirds of the heart lies left of the midline. The wider **base** of the heart lies superior and beneath the second rib. The **apex,** or narrow part, of the heart lies inferiorly, slightly to the left between the fifth and sixth ribs near the diaphragm.

Heart Wall

The heart is composed of three layers: **pericardium, myocardium,** and **endocardium.** The pericardium is a two-layered, serous membrane that covers the entire structure. Between the two thin membranes is a serous fluid that allows friction-free movement of the heart as it contracts and relaxes. The pericardium is the outermost layer of the heart. The myocardium forms the bulk of the heart wall and is the thickest and strongest layer of the heart. It is composed of cardiac muscle tissue. Contraction of this tissue is responsible for pumping blood. The endocardium (innermost layer) is composed of a thin layer of connective tissue. This structure lines the interior of the heart, the valves, and the larger vessels of the heart.

Heart Chambers

The heart is divided into a right and left half by a muscular partition called the **septum** (Figure 48-2). The heart has the following four chambers:

1. The **right atrium** is the upper right chamber. It receives deoxygenated blood from the entire body. The superior vena cava returns blood from the head, the neck, and the arms. The inferior vena cava returns blood from the lower body. The coronary vein returns it from the heart muscle to the coronary sinus.
2. The **right ventricle** is the lower right chamber. It receives deoxygenated blood from the right atrium. The right ventricle pumps blood to the lungs via the **pulmonary artery** to release carbon dioxide and receive oxygen.
3. The **left atrium** is the upper left chamber. It receives oxygenated blood from the lungs via the **pulmonary veins.**
4. The **left ventricle** is the lower left chamber. It receives oxygenated blood from the left atrium. It is the thickest, most muscular section of the heart and pumps the oxygenated blood out through the aorta to all parts of the body.

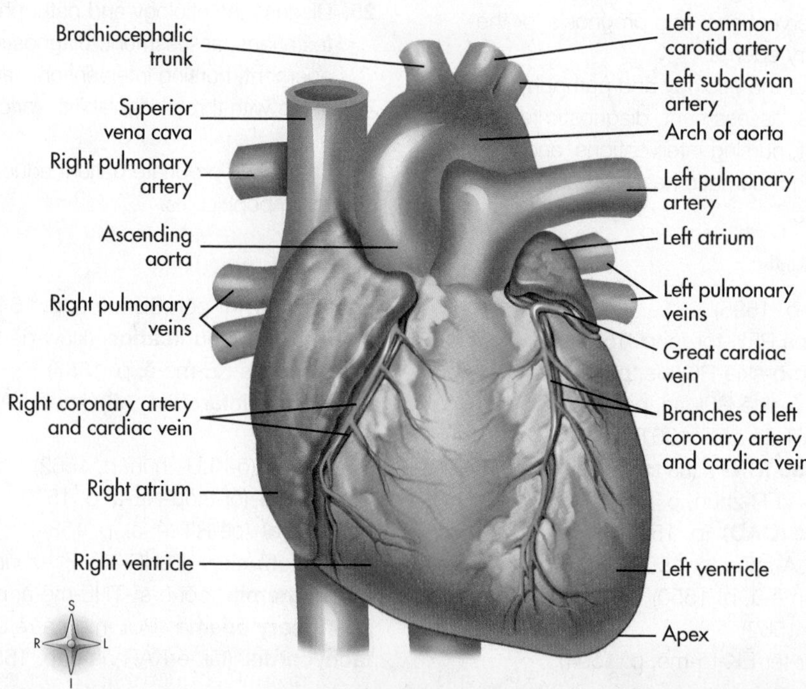

FIGURE 48-1 Heart and major blood vessels viewed from front (anterior).

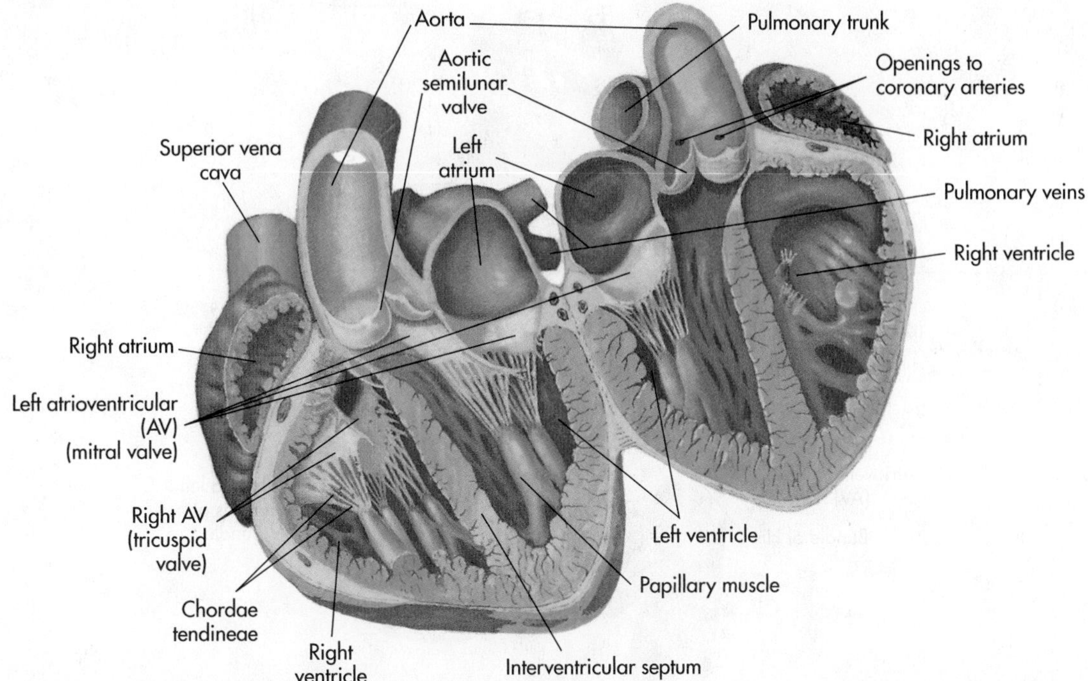

FIGURE 48-2 Interior of the heart. This illustration shows the heart as it would appear if it were cut along a frontal plane and opened like a book. The front portion of the heart lies to the reader's right; the back portion of the heart lies to the reader's left. The four chambers of the heart—two atria and two ventricles—are easily seen.

The heart actually functions as two separate pumps: (1) the right side receives deoxygenated blood and pumps it to the lungs, and (2) the left side receives oxygenated blood from the lungs and pumps it throughout the body.

Heart Valves

Located within the heart are four valves that keep the blood moving forward and prevent backflow. The heart has two **atrioventricular (AV) valves.** They are located between the atrium and the ventricles. The right AV valve, located between the right atrium and the right ventricle, is called the **tricuspid valve** because it contains three flaps, or cusps. The left AV valve is composed of two cusps (bicuspid) and is commonly called the **mitral valve.** It is located between the left atrium and the left ventricle. Both of these valves rapidly close to prevent backflow of blood. Small cordlike structures, **chordae tendineae,** connect the AV valves to the walls of the heart and work with the **papillary muscles** located in the walls of the ventricles to make a tight seal to prevent backflow when the ventricles contract.

The two remaining valves, the **semilunar valves,** are located at the points where the blood exits the ventricles. The **pulmonary semilunar valve** is located between the right ventricle and the pulmonary artery. Blood is pushed out of the right ventricle and travels to the lung via the pulmonary artery. The **aortic semilunar valve** is located between the left ventricle and the aorta. When the left ventricle contracts, the blood is forced into the aorta and the aortic semilunar valve closes. Both of the semilunar valves have three cusps that resemble a half moon, hence the name **semilunar** (see Figure 48-2).

Electrical Conduction System

Heart muscle tissue contains an inherent ability to contract in a rhythmic pattern. This ability is called **automaticity.** If heart muscle cells are removed and placed under a microscope, they continue to beat. In addition, they can respond to a stimulus in the same way that nerve cells do. This unique property is called **irritability.** Automaticity and irritability are two characteristics that affect the functions of the conduction system. Hormones, ion concentration, and changes in body temperature also affect the conduction of messages around the heart, initiation of heartbeat, and coordination of beating patterns between the atria and the ventricles.

The heartbeat is initiated in the **sinoatrial (SA) node,** which is located in the upper part of the right atrium, just beneath the opening of the superior vena cava (Figure 48-3). Because it regulates the heartbeat, the SA node is known as the **pacemaker.** Impulses are passed to the AV node, which is located in the base of the right atrium. The AV node slows the impulses to allow the atrium to complete contraction and to allow the ventricles to fill. The impulses then pass to a group of conduction fibers called the **bundle of His** and divides into right and left branches of AV bundle to travel to smaller branches called the **Purkinje fibers,**

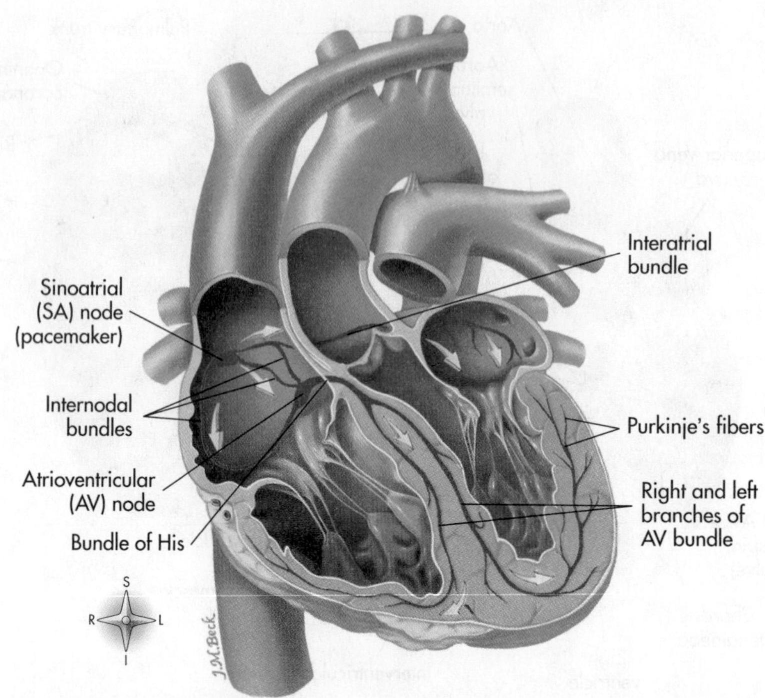

FIGURE 48-3 Conduction system of the heart. Specialized cardiac muscle cells in the wall of the heart rapidly initiate or conduct an electrical impulse throughout the myocardium. The signal is initiated by the SA node (pacemaker) and spreads to the rest of the right atrial myocardium directly, to the left atrial myocardium by way of the bundle of interatrial conducting fibers, and to the AV node by way of the three internodal bundles. The AV node then initiates a signal that is conducted through conduction fibers called the bundle of His and breaks into the right and left branches to travel to smaller branches called the Purkinje fibers, which surround the ventricles.

which surround the ventricles. The message travels rapidly through the ventricles and causes contractions, which empty the ventricles.

IMPULSE PATTERN: SA node → AV node → bundle of His → right and left bundle branches of AV bundle → Purkinje fibers

Cardiac Cycle

The cardiac cycle refers to a complete heartbeat. The two atria contract while the two ventricles relax. When the ventricles contract, the two atria relax. The phase of contraction is called **systole** (Figure 48-4), and the phase of relaxation is called **diastole** (the period between contraction of the atria or the ventricles during which blood enters the relaxed chambers from the systemic circulation and the lungs [Figure 48-5]). Complete diastole and systole of both atria and ventricles constitute a cardiac cycle; this takes an average of 0.8 second.

The heart sounds, **lubb** and **dubb,** are produced by closure of the valves. The first sound, **lubb** (long duration and low pitch), is heard when the AV valves close. The second sound, **dubb** (short duration, sharp sound), is heard when the semilunar valves close. Occasionally a murmur (swishing sound) can be heard. This can be a normal functional phenomenon produced by rapid filling of the ventricles, or it can be an abnormal condition produced by ineffective closure of the valves.

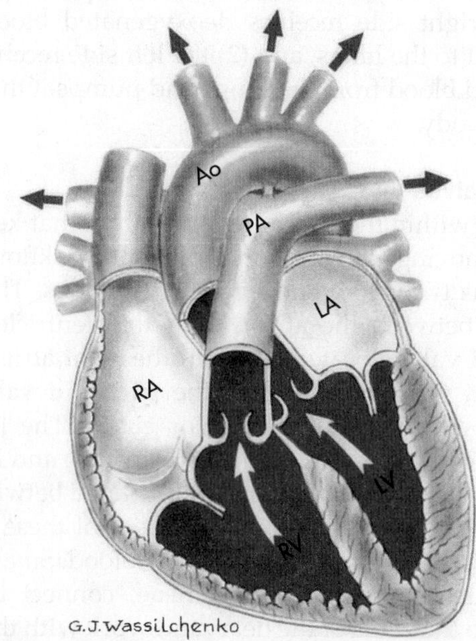

FIGURE 48-4 Blood flow during systole. *Ao,* Aorta; *LA,* left atrium; *LV,* left ventricle; *PA,* pulmonary artery; *RA,* right atrium; *RV,* right ventricle.

BLOOD VESSELS

Three main types of blood vessels are organized to carry blood to and from the heart. **Capillaries** (tiny blood vessels joining arterioles and venules) connect the **arteries** (large vessels carrying blood away from the heart) to the **veins** (vessels that convey blood from the capillaries and return it to the heart). The heart de-

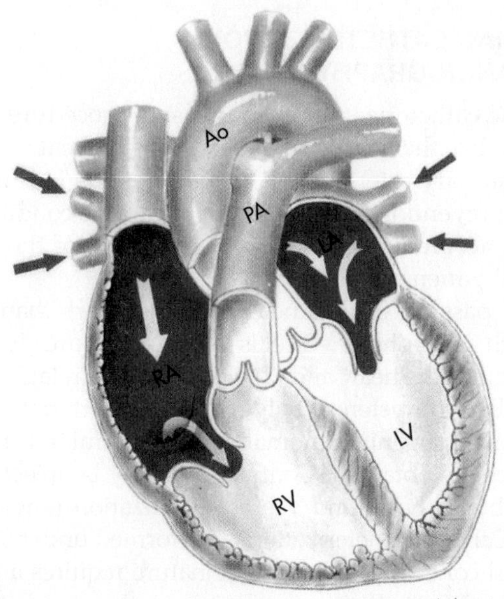

FIGURE 48-5 Blood flow during diastole. *Ao,* Aorta; *LA,* left atrium; *LV,* left ventricle; *PA,* pulmonary artery; *RA,* right atrium; *RV,* right ventricle.

livers the blood to the arteries, which branch into tiny vessels called **arterioles** (blood vessels of the smallest branch of the arterial circulation), which deliver the blood to the tissues. Within the tissues, microscopic vessels (capillaries) form an extensive (50,000 miles) network that allows exchanges of products and byproducts between the tissues and blood. The capillaries then join with tiny veins, or **venules,** that link with the larger veins and return to the heart. The pattern is as follows:

Artery → arteriole → capillary → venule → vein

CIRCULATION

CORONARY BLOOD SUPPLY

To sustain life, the heart must pump blood throughout the body on a continuous basis. As a result, the heart muscle (or myocardium) requires a constant supply of blood containing nutrients and oxygen to function effectively. The delivery of oxygen and nutrient-rich arterial blood to cardiac muscle tissue and the return of oxygen-poor blood from this active tissue to the venous system are called the **coronary circulation** (Figure 48-6).

Blood flows into the heart muscle by way of two small vessels, the right and left coronary arteries, which are the best known of all the blood vessels. The coronary arteries form a crown around the myocardium (see Figures 48-1 and 48-6). The openings into these vessels lie behind the flaps of the aortic semilunar valves (see Figure 48-6). The coronary arteries bring oxygen and nutrition to the myocardium. Once the circulation is completed and the carbon dioxide and waste products have been collected, the blood flows into a large coronary vein and finally into the coronary sinus, which empties into the right atrium. These two main arteries have many tiny branches that serve the heart muscle. If an artery becomes occluded, these branches provide collateral circulation (alternate routes) to nourish the heart muscle. If the occlusion is severe, surgery and other procedures may be needed. These treatments are discussed later in this chapter.

SYSTEMIC CIRCULATION

Systemic circulation occurs when blood is pumped from the left ventricle of the heart through all parts of the body and returns to the right atrium. When the oxygenated blood leaves the left ventricle, it enters the largest artery (1 inch [2.5 cm] in diameter) of the body, the **aorta.** This is the main trunk of the systemic arterial circulation and is composed of four parts: the ascending aorta, the arch, the thoracic portion of the descending aorta, and the abdominal portion of the descending aorta. As the blood flows through the artery branches, the branches become smaller in diameter (arterioles). The blood continues to flow into the capillaries. The capillaries surround the cells and exchange oxygen, nutrients, carbon dioxide, and other waste products. The blood proceeds to the tiny venules, then to the larger veins, and finally returns to the right atrium via the largest vein, the **vena cava** (one of two large veins returning blood from the peripheral circulation to the right atrium of the heart).

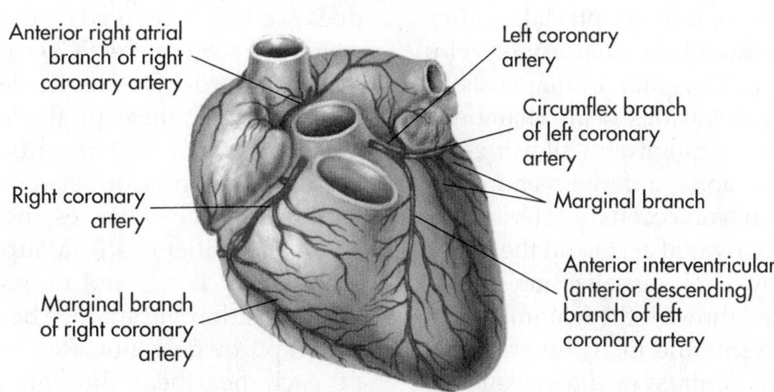

FIGURE 48-6 Arterial coronary circulation (anterior).

The blood is now deoxygenated and needs to be replenished with oxygen. Note that the upper portion of the vena cava (superior vena cava) returns deoxygenated blood from the head, neck, chest, and upper extremities. The inferior vena cava returns deoxygenated blood from parts of the body below the diaphragm.

PULMONARY CIRCULATION

The deoxygenated blood now passes through the pulmonary circulation to pick up the needed oxygen. Blood is pumped from the right atrium to the right ventricle, where it leaves the heart to travel via the pulmonary artery to the lungs. Once the blood reaches the lungs, it travels through arterioles to the capillaries. The microscopic capillaries surround the **alveoli** (air sacs), where oxygen diffuses into the bloodstream. The capillaries then connect with the venules and finally with the four pulmonary veins, which return the oxygenated blood to the left atrium of the heart. It is then pumped to the left ventricle and to the aorta, and systemic circulation is then repeated. The blood circulation pattern is as follows:

Superior or inferior vena cava → right atrium →
tricuspid valve → right ventricle →
pulmonary semilunar valve → pulmonary artery →
capillaries in the lungs → pulmonary veins →
left atrium → bicuspid valve → left ventricle →
aortic semilunar valve → aorta

LABORATORY AND DIAGNOSTIC EXAMINATIONS

A number of diagnostic tests are used to evaluate cardiovascular function. The nursing responsibilities are to physically prepare the patient for diagnostic procedures and to explain the examination to the patient.

DIAGNOSTIC IMAGING

Radiographic examination of the chest provides a film record of heart size, shape, and position and outline of shadows. Lung congestion is also shown, indicating heart failure (HF), perhaps in the earliest stages. Pleural effusion may be noted in left-sided HF.

Fluoroscopy, the action-picture radiograph, allows observation of movement. It is invaluable in pacemaker or intracardial catheter placement.

An **angiogram** is a series of radiographs taken after injection of a contrast medium into an artery or vein. Picturing the circulatory process aids in diagnosis of vessel occlusion, pooling in various heart chambers, and congenital anomalies. Angiography allows x-ray visualization of the heart, aorta, inferior vena cava, pulmonary artery and vein, and coronary arteries.

In an **aortogram,** the abdominal aorta and the major leg arteries are viewed by x-ray visualization after a contrast medium is injected through the femoral artery and into the aorta. Aneurysms and many other abnormalities can be diagnosed. Contrast media to visualize the aortic arch and branches may also be used.

CARDIAC CATHETERIZATION AND ANGIOGRAPHY

Cardiac catheterization is an invasive procedure used to visualize the heart's chambers, valves, great vessels, and coronary arteries. This procedure aids in diagnosis, in prevention of progression of cardiac conditions, and in accurate evaluation and treatment of the critically ill patient.

The passage of a catheter into the heart chambers through a peripheral vessel is used to measure (1) pressure within the heart and (2) blood-volume relationship to cardiac competence. Valvular defects, arterial occlusion, and congenital anomalies are determined. Blood samples are obtained. Contrast dye may be injected to allow better heart and vessel visualization (angiography). Cardiac catheterization is performed under sterile surgical conditions; its invasive nature requires a prior signed consent. Because iodine is in the contrast medium, determine sensitivity to iodine before injection to avoid an allergic reaction. After the procedure, assess circulation to the extremity used for catheter insertion. Check peripheral pulses, color, and sensation of the extremity every 15 minutes for 1 hour and then with decreasing frequency. Observe the puncture site for hematoma and bleeding. Monitor vital signs. Assess for abnormal heart rate, dysrhythmias, and signs of pulmonary emboli (respiratory difficulty). The patient lies supine for a designated period with a compression device over the pressure dressing at the insertion site to prevent hemorrhage.

ELECTROCARDIOGRAPHY

The electrocardiogram (ECG, or EKG) is a graphic study of the electrical activities of the myocardium to determine transmission of cardiac impulses through the muscles and conduction tissue. Each ECG has three distinct waves, or deflections: the **P wave,** the QRS complex, and the **T wave.** When the heart contracts, the electrical activity is called **depolarization. Repolarization** is the relaxation phase. The P wave represents the depolarization of the atria. The QRS complex represents the depolarization of the ventricles. The T wave represents the repolarization of the ventricles. Atrial repolarization is not represented but does occur; it is covered by the large QRS complex and cannot be seen on the ECG tracing.

A standard ECG has 12 electrodes attached to the skin surface to measure the total electrical activity of the heart. Each lead records the electrical potential between the limbs or between the heart and limbs. A conductive gel enhances the contact and transmission. The patient is in a supine position. However, ambulatory ECGs and exercise stress test ECGs require position variation. The machine, an electrocardiograph or galvanometer, records the energy wave of each heartbeat through a vibrating needle on graph paper, which feeds through the machine at a

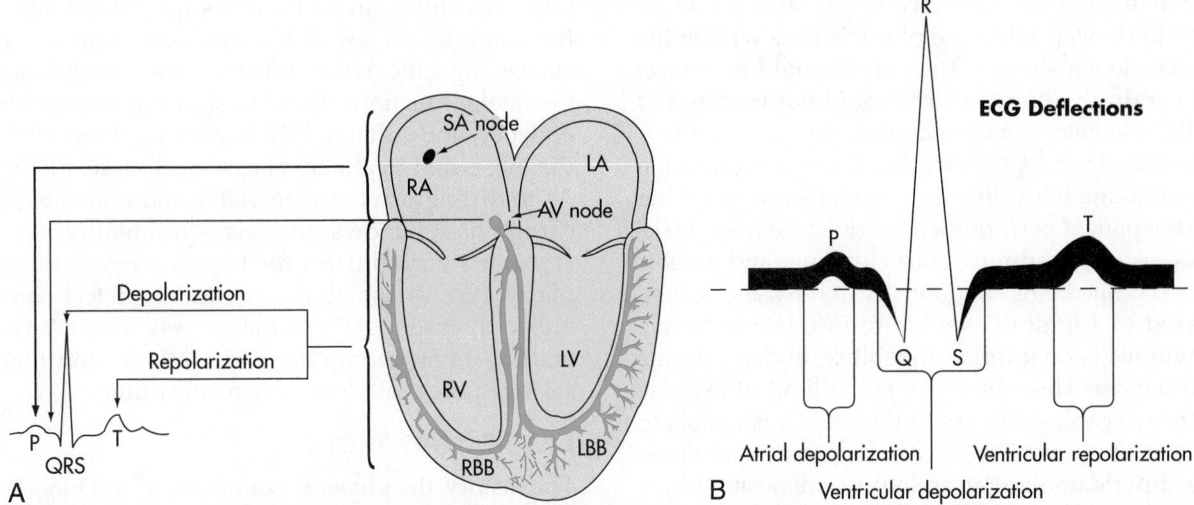

FIGURE 48-7 Normal electrocardiographic (ECG) deflections. **A,** P wave. **B,** Relationship of ECG to cardiac muscle activity. *AV,* Atrioventricular; *LA,* left atrium; *LBB,* left bundle block; *LV,* left ventricle; *RA,* right atrium; *RBB,* right bundle block; *RV,* right ventricle; *SA,* sinoatrial.

standard rate. Each ECG waveform represents a single electrical impulse as it travels through the heart (Figure 48-7).

The ECG tracing is read or interpreted by a cardiac specialist (cardiologist) or by internal medicine specialists, family practitioners, pediatricians, and emergency department practitioners. The reading can also be displayed on the fluorescent screen (oscilloscope) of a cardiac monitor. A graphic tracing may be printed out by the monitor.

Ambulatory ECGs can be used to monitor heart rhythm over prolonged periods—12, 24, or 48 hours—and compared with various activities or symptoms recorded in a diary kept by the patient. A Holter monitor (small portable recorder) is attached to the patient by leads, with a 2-pound tape recorder carried on a belt or shoulder strap. The monitor operates continuously to record the patterns and rhythms of the patient's heartbeat. In conjunction with the diary, the physician can note various events, times, and medication peaks that affect or precipitate dysrhythmias. An ambulatory ECG is particularly useful for patients whose clinical symptoms indicate heart disorders but who may have normal ECG tracings on a resting test.

CARDIAC MONITORS

It is common practice to continuously assess the cardiac electrical activity of patients who are known or suspected to have dysrhythmias or who are prone to develop dysrhythmias or acute cardiovascular symptoms. A cardiac monitor displays information on the electrical activity of the heart transferred via conductive electrodes placed on the chest.

Most monitors provide a visual display of cardiac electrical activity and the correct heart rate. Preset alarms warn of heart rates that exceed or drop below limits considered acceptable for each patient and also warn of dysrhythmias.

Ambulatory patients are increasingly monitored by battery-powered ECG transmitters that do not directly connect the patient to the oscilloscope. This monitoring is called **telemetry,** which is the electronic transmission of data to a distant location. The electrodes placed on the patient's chest are attached to a transmitter the patient carries in a pocket or pouch. The transmitter sends a radio signal to a receiver, usually located at the nurse's station.

Patients need telemetry monitoring for various reasons, including a history of cardiac disease, angina pectoris, suspected dysrhythmias, a change in medications, an electrolyte abnormality, or unexplained syncope. Many of these patients are monitored in a centralized area such as an intermediate care or step-down unit (with monitors at the nurse's station). Remote telemetry means the patient is on a medical-surgical unit and is monitored at a separate location, called the **home unit,** which is usually on a critical care unit. Remote telemetry patients are usually stable. But even a stable patient's condition can change rapidly, and telemetry allows continuous heart monitoring to detect abnormalities.

Attachment to a cardiac monitor does not change a patient's need for nursing interventions. Because the monitoring electrodes are on the anterior thorax (chest) rather than the extremities, the patient is relatively free to carry on usual activities. Pay special attention to the electrode site to ensure a constant tight seal between the electrode and the skin and to note the development of any skin impairment. The conduction gel dries out, even if the pad is sealed; changing electrodes regularly is recommended. Also check the telemetry pack for integrity of the lead wires and test the monitoring device's battery with a battery tester. Inform the monitoring area whenever the patient is moved off the unit for a diagnostic test, since the patient may go outside the monitor's range. Another important safety measure is to ***never*** remove the telemetry device and allow the patient to shower unless the physician has written the order to allow a shower. The patient could be subject to severe dysrhythmia, which would not be detected with the telemetry device removed.

Exercise-stress ECG is another form of monitoring the heart's capability, this time in a laboratory setting while the patient performs a prescribed exercise. Tasks include use of treadmills, stair climbing, and aerobic exercise. While being monitored carefully, the patient is coaxed to a limit of exertion to evaluate ischemia, dysrhythmia, and cardiac capability under extreme circumstances. Thus the test sets the limit of exercise tolerance in cardiac disease. If the patient is unable to tolerate activity, a stress test can be done by administering dipyridamole (Persantine) or adenosine (Adenocard), which mimics the patient's heart under stress or activity.

THALLIUM SCANNING

Thallium 201 is an intracellular ion that is actively transported into normal cells. If the cell is ischemic or infarcted, the thallium will not be picked up. Because the thallium concentrates in tissue with normal blood flow, tissue with inadequate perfusion appears as dark areas on scanning—a "cold spot." The radioisotope is injected intravenously while the patient exercises on a treadmill. Breast tissue in the female can produce artifact, leading to a false-positive result. Using technetium 99m sestamibi instead of thallium can help minimize artifact and thus improve accuracy. In patients who cannot tolerate physical exercise, dipyridamole is given before the thallium to physiologically simulate exercise-induced stress.

ECHOCARDIOGRAPHY

Echocardiography uses high-frequency ultrasound directed at the heart. The echo, or reflected sound, is graphically recorded, outlining size, shape, and position of cardiac structures. This test is used to detect pericardial effusion (collection of blood or other fluid in the pericardial sac), ventricular function, cardiac chamber size and contents, ventricular muscle and septal motion and thickness, cardiac output (ejection fraction), cardiac tumors, valvular function, and congenital heart disorder.

Ejection fraction (EF) of ventricles as demonstrated by an echocardiogram is as follows:

- Normal: greater than 60%
- Moderate HF: 40% to 60%
- Moderate to severe HF: 20% to 40%
- Severe HF (candidate for heart transplant): less than 20%

POSITRON EMISSION TOMOGRAPHY

Positron emission tomography (PET) is a computerized radiographic technique that uses radioactive substances to examine the metabolic activity of various body structures. In PET studies the patient either inhales or is injected with a biochemical radioactive substance. Specific color-coded images reveal organs' metabolic functions. Used to study dementia, stroke, epilepsy, and tumors, PET is proving its merit in the diagnosis and treatment of cardiac disease. PET's ability to distinguish between viable and nonviable myocardial tissue allows physicians to identify the most appropriate candidates for bypass surgery or angioplasty. PET is also able to accurately detect coronary artery disease (CAD), noninvasively, in an asymptomatic patient, prompting early intervention that can salvage potentially ischemic myocardium.

LABORATORY TESTS

The history, the physical examination, and blood studies aid the health care provider in diagnosing and monitoring the cardiovascular disease process. The nurse's responsibility is to prepare the patient by explaining the tests and the preparation required for each test.

Blood cultures to detect growth of bacteria in the blood are crucial to the diagnosis of infective endocarditis.

A **complete blood count** (CBC) is a determination of the number of red and white blood cells per cubic millimeter, as well as the white blood cell differential, platelets, hemoglobin, and hematocrit. Low hemoglobin indicates decreased ability to carry oxygen to the cells and anemia; an elevated white blood cell (leukocyte) count indicates infection or inflammation; and an elevated red blood cell (erythrocyte) count indicates that the body is compensating for chronic **hypoxemia** (an abnormal deficiency of oxygen in the arterial blood) by stimulating red blood cell production by the bone marrow, leading to secondary **polycythemia** (abnormal increase in the number of red blood cells in the blood). Chronic hypoxemia is often noted in HF.

Coagulation studies are useful in monitoring the patient receiving anticoagulant drug therapy, which is prescribed for patients with myocardial infarction (MI). Coagulation studies are also important in patients who have chronic atrial fibrillation or patients with atrial fibrillation who are undergoing **cardioversion** (the restoration of the heart's normal sinus rhythm by delivery of a synchronized electric shock through two metal paddles placed on the patient's chest). Coagulation studies are needed if an MI is diagnosed in case fibrinolytics are needed to dissolve the thrombus. These studies include prothrombin time (PT), International Normalized Ratio (INR), and partial thromboplastin time (PTT).

Erythrocyte sedimentation rate (ESR) is used to monitor or rule out inflammatory infective conditions. The ESR is elevated with MI and infective endocarditis and decreases when healing begins. The ESR also indicates the extent of inflammation and infection in rheumatic fever.

Serum electrolyte tests focus on the body's balance of sodium, potassium, calcium, and magnesium, which are necessary for myocardial muscle function. Sodium (Na^+) helps maintain fluid balance. Potassium (K^+) is required for relaxation of cardiac muscle, and calcium (Ca^{++}) is necessary for contraction of cardiac muscle. Magnesium (Mg^{++}) helps maintain the correct level of electric excitability in the nerves and the muscles, including the myocardium and the cardiac conduction system. The health care provider compares serum electrolyte levels with ECG changes.

Serum lipids are associated with vascular disease, particularly CAD. Cholesterol and triglycerides bound to plasma proteins are found in the blood as lipoproteins. Density levels vary according to the protein-fat ratio. An elevated high-density lipoprotein (HDL) is desired, but low-density lipoprotein (LDL) or very-low-density lipoprotein (VLDL) increases the risk for cardiovascular disease (see Box 48-1, p. 1549).

Arterial blood gases are measured to monitor oxygenation (Pao_2, $Paco_2$) and acid-base balance (pH). This test is useful in patients with unstable cardiac conditions to determine the blood oxygenation process and in evaluation of patients in cardiac failure.

Serum cardiac markers are certain proteins that are released into the blood in large quantities from necrotic heart muscle after an MI. These markers, specifically cardiac serum enzymes and troponin I, are important screening diagnostic criteria for an acute MI. The cardiac enzyme creatine kinase (CK) and its isoenzyme, creatine phosphokinase (CK-MB), have been the gold standard for years. However, CK-MB is also found in skeletal muscle and can be elevated by surgery, muscle trauma, and muscular diseases, so it is not a specific indicator for MI. CK and CK-MB start to rise within 2 to 3 hours after the beginning of an MI, peak in 24 hours, and return to normal within 24 to 40 hours (Nagle, 2002). When cardiac cells die, their cellular enzymes are released into circulation. The increase in serum enzymes that occurs after cell death can demonstrate whether cardiac damage is present and the approximate extent of the damage. Other causes of increased serum enzymes may make the differential diagnosis more difficult.

Troponin I is a myocardial muscle protein released into circulation after a myocardial injury. In the heart there are two subtypes: cardiac-specific troponin T and troponin I. These are sensitive markers that identify very small amounts of myocardial damage. Troponin T appears in the blood 3 to 5 hours after an MI and may remain elevated for up to 21 days. Like CK-MB, troponin T is affected by skeletal muscle injury and renal disease. Troponin I is a sensitive and specific cardiac marker, not influenced by skeletal muscle trauma or renal failure. Troponin I rises 3 hours after MI, peaks at 14 to 18 hours, and returns to normal in 5 to 7 days. Troponin I is useful in diagnosing an MI (Nagle, 2002). The recent ability to measure myocardial contractile proteins (troponins) in serum is a milestone in the diagnosis of acute MI and acute myocardial damage resulting from other causes.

Myoglobin is released into circulation within a few hours after an MI. Although it is one of the first serum cardiac markers that increase after an MI, myoglobin is also present in skeletal muscle, so an increase can be associated with noncardiac causes. In addition, it is rapidly excreted in urine so that blood levels return to normal range within 24 hours after an MI.

B-type natriuretic peptide (BNP) is a neurohormone secreted by the heart in response to ventricular expansion. An elevated BNP of greater than 100 pg/mL indicates HF. BNP is present in the ventricle of the heart and correlates well to left ventricular pressure. The greater the BNP level, the more severe the HF (Pagana & Pagana, 2007).

Homocysteine is an amino acid produced during protein digestion. Normal values range from 4 to 14 μmol/L. Elevated blood levels of homocysteine may act as an independent risk factor for ischemic heart disease, cerebrovascular disease, peripheral arterial disease (PAD), and venous thrombosis. Homocysteine appears to promote the progression of atherosclerosis by causing endothelial damage, promoting LDL deposits, and promoting vascular smooth muscle growth. Homocysteine is an amino acid that plays an important role in blood clotting. An elevated level results in increased platelet aggregation. Screening for elevated homocysteine levels (more than 14 μmol/L) should be considered in patients who have progressive and unexplained atherosclerosis despite normal lipoproteins and who have no other risk factors. It is also recommended in patients with an unusual family history of atherosclerosis, especially at a young age.

Dietary deficiency of vitamins B_6, B_{12}, or folate is the most common cause of elevated homocysteine. Some researchers believe that elevated levels of homocysteine can be treated by administration of vitamins B_6, B_{12}, and folate. Whether this treatment will reduce the incidence of MI remains to be seen (Pagana & Pagana, 2007).

The liver produces **C-reactive protein (CRP)** during periods of acute inflammation. The presence of CRP is a predictor of cardiac events and is emerging as an independent risk factor for CAD. Persons who have diabetes mellitus are already at high risk for developing cardiovascular disease. If a patient has both an elevated CRP and diabetes, his or her risk for a cardiovascular disorder becomes even greater (Pagana & Pagana, 2007).

DISORDERS OF THE CARDIOVASCULAR SYSTEM

Cardiovascular disorders are a major health care problem in the United States. Public awareness, modifications in lifestyles, and improvements in medical treatment have contributed to a decline in overall deaths. The nurse's role in caring for patients with cardiovascular disorders includes being aware of the prevalence of cardiac disease, risk factors, and the disease process; implementing nursing interventions; and patient teaching.

NORMAL AGING PATTERNS

By the time an individual reaches the age of 65 years, physiologic changes have reduced the efficiency of the heart as a pump. Yet the heart still is capable of functioning adequately unless there is underlying cardiac disease (see Life Span Considerations box).

RISK FACTORS

Research has identified risk factors that indicate predispositions to developing cardiovascular disease. The presence of more than one risk factor is associated with an increasing risk of developing cardiovascular disease. Risk factors are classified as those that are nonmodifiable and those that are modifiable.

Nonmodifiable Factors

An important aspect of caring for the patient with a cardiovascular disorder is understanding the risk factors for cardiovascular disease and incorporating them into patient teaching. The nonmodifiable risk factors associated with cardiovascular disorders include the following.

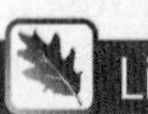

Life Span Considerations

Older Adults

Cardiac Disease

- Changes in the cardiac musculature lead to reduced efficiency and strength, resulting in decreased cardiac output.
- Disorientation, syncope, and decreased tissue perfusion to organs and other body tissues can occur as a result of decreased cardiac output.
- Aging causes sclerotic changes in blood vessels and leads to decreased elasticity and narrowing of the lumen. Arterial disease resulting from the aging process causes hypertension because of the increased cardiac effort needed to pump blood through the circulatory system.
- Progressive coronary artery changes can lead to the development of collateral coronary circulation. This can modify the severity of signs and symptoms seen in MI. Angina symptoms may be less pronounced, and dyspnea may replace angina as a key symptom of acute infarction.
- Heart failure can result from rapid intravenous infusion.
- Edema secondary to heart failure may cause tissue impairment in the immobile older adult. Immobility leads to venous stasis, venous ulcer, and poor wound healing. It also increases the risk of venous thrombosis and embolus formation.
- Older adults with cardiac disease often receive several medications, which are often prescribed at lower doses than for younger adults. Even with lower doses of medications, observe the older adult closely for signs of toxicity, since the rate of drug metabolism and excretion decreases with age.
- Independent older adults with cardiac conditions should receive adequate teaching regarding medication, diet, and warning signs of complications. Encourage them to maintain regular contact with the physician and to seek care at the first sign of problems.

Family History

A family member such as a parent or sibling who has a cardiovascular problem before 50 years of age places the patient at greater risk for developing cardiovascular disease.

Age

Normal physiologic changes that occur with aging and past lifestyle habits increase the patient's risk for developing cardiovascular disease with advancing age. CAD and MI occur most frequently among white, middle-aged men.

Gender

Middle-aged men are at a greater risk of developing cardiovascular disease than women. Although the incidence in men and women equalizes after age 65, cardiovascular disease is a greater cause of death in women than in men. Women develop CAD about 10 years later than men because natural estrogen is believed to have a cardioprotective effect before menopause. The incidence of cardiovascular disease in women 50 years of age and older is increasing. Factors believed to be responsible are increased social and economic pressures on women and changes in lifestyle. Ten times more women die from heart disease than die from breast cancer. The mortality rate for women with CAD has remained relatively constant even though cardiovascular disease remains the leading cause of death. Despite this statistic, only 15% of women consider CAD their greatest health risk. Recent research on CAD has shown that women often do not have the classic signs and symptoms of an acute coronary event (Lewis et al., 2007).

Cultural and Ethnic Considerations

Black men have a higher incidence of hypertension than do white men. Black women have a higher incidence of CAD, with greater severity and higher death rates, than white women (Lewis et al., 2007).

Modifiable Factors

Smoking

Individuals who smoke have a two to three times greater risk of developing cardiovascular disease than nonsmokers. The degree of risk is proportional to the number of cigarettes smoked. Individuals who quit smoking decrease their risk. Tobacco smoke contains nicotine, which causes catecholamine (i.e., epinephrine, norepinephrine) release. Catecholamine release causes tachycardia, hypertension, and vasoconstriction of the peripheral arteries, which in turn increase the work of the heart and result in greater myocardial oxygen consumption (Lewis et al., 2007). Nicotine also increases platelet adhesion, which results in increased risk of embolism (Lewis et al., 2007). The nicotine content of cigarettes causes the production of carbon monoxide, which places a greater demand on the heart and interferes with oxygen supply.

Hyperlipidemia

Hyperlipidemia is elevated concentrations of any or all lipids in the plasma. The ratio of HDL to LDL is the best predictor for the development of cardiovascular disease. Density levels vary according to the protein-fat ratio:

- VLDL contains more fat than protein (primarily triglycerides); triglycerides are the main storage form of lipids and constitute approximately 95% of fatty tissue.
- LDL contains an equal amount of fat and protein (approximately 50%) with moderate amounts of phospholipid cholesterol.

Less than 100 mg/dL	Optimal
100 to 129 mg/dL	Near optimal to above optimal
130 to 159 mg/dL	Borderline high
160 to 189 mg/dL	High
More than 190 mg/dL	Very high

- HDL contains more protein than fat (which serves a protective function, removing cholesterol from tissues). It is suspected that HDL also removes cholesterol from the peripheral tissues and transports it to the liver for excretion. Also, HDL may have a protective effect by preventing cellular uptake of cholesterol and lipids. Low levels (less than 40 mg/dL) are believed to increase a person's risk for CAD, whereas high levels (more than 60 mg/dL) are considered protective (Box 48-1).

A diet high in saturated fat, cholesterol, and calories contributes to hyperlipidemia. Therefore dietary control is an important factor in modifying this risk factor. An overall serum cholesterol level of less than 200 mg/dL is desirable, 200 to 239 mg/dL is borderline high, and more than 239 mg/dL is high.

Change in diet is probably the most important method of lowering cholesterol level. Weight reduction, in overweight patients with abnormal lipid profiles, is an essential element of the dietary intervention. In addition to lowering LDL levels, weight reduction leads to decreases in triglyceride level and blood pressure. A combination of weight reduction and physical exercise improves the lipid profile, with a decrease in

Box 48-1 Cholesterol Numbers: What Do They Mean?

YOUR TOTAL CHOLESTEROL NUMBER A total cholesterol level less than 200 is considered desirable.	**TOTAL CHOLESTEROL** **Desirable:** Less than 200 **Borderline:** 200 to 239 **High:** 240 or greater
HDL CHOLESTEROL NUMBER The higher the HDL cholesterol level, the better, because this means that there are more good lipoproteins to remove adhered cholesterol from the arteries.	**HDL CHOLESTEROL** **Low:** Less than 40 **High:** Greater than 60
LDL CHOLESTEROL NUMBER The higher the number of bad lipoproteins, or LDLs, in the blood, the more likely it is that cholesterol is beginning to adhere to the arteries. Monitor risk factors to assess for probability of development of heart disease.	**LDL CHOLESTEROL** **Optimal:** Less than 100 **Near to above optimal:** 100-129 **Borderline high:** 130-159 **High:** 160-189 **Very high:** Greater than 190

SET LDL CHOLESTEROL GOAL

Once the LDL cholesterol number is known, one can change the diet to help lower the amount of cholesterol in the blood. The table below shows the target LDL cholesterol goal. Reducing the risk factors is important too, so health care providers must make recommendations to assist the patient in maintaining acceptable cholesterol levels.

Risk Factors	***Start Diet Treatment If LDL Cholesterol Is:***	***The LDL Goal Is:***
No heart disease and fewer than two risk factors other than high LDL cholesterol	**160** or more	Less than **160**
No heart disease but two or more risk factors other than high LDL cholesterol	**130** or more	**100** or less
Definite heart disease or arterial disease	**100** or more	Less than **130**

Modified from Third Report of National Cholesterol Education Program (NCEP) Expert Panel on Detection, Evaluation, and Treatment of High Blood Cholesterol in Adults, 2001.
HDL, High-density lipoprotein; *LDL*, low-density lipoprotein.

LDL level, an increase in HDL level, and a decrease in triglyceride levels. Low HDL levels are often familial and only somewhat modifiable.

Cholesterol-lowering drugs are often included in treatment of hyperlipidemia. Cholesterol-lowering drugs are divided into six classes: (1) bile acid sequestrants; (2) nicotinic acid (niacin); (3) statins such as simvastatin (Zocor), pravastatin (Pravachol), and rosuvastatin (Crestor); (4) fibric acid derivatives such as gemfibrozil (Lopid) and probucol (Lorelco); (5) the cholesterol absorption inhibitor ezetimibe [Zetia]; and (6) combination drugs such as ezetimibe and simvastatin (Vytorin) (Cuddy, 2006). Pravastatin reduces the risk of a first MI by about one third in hypercholesterolemic patients with no history of coronary disease. Simvastatin is now allowed by the U.S. Food and Drug Administration (FDA) to add a label statement that the drug can reduce deaths by lowering cholesterol.

Hypertension

Hypertension is blood pressure higher than 140/90 mm Hg, which increases an individual's risk of developing cardiovascular disease. Adhering to medical therapy for control of elevated blood pressure helps to modify the individual's risk.

Diabetes Mellitus

Cardiac disease has been found to be more prevalent in individuals with diabetes mellitus. Diabetes mellitus poses a greater risk than other factors. This is thought to be related to elevated blood glucose levels, which damage the arterial intima and contribute to atherosclerosis. Diabetic patients also have alterations in lipid metabolism and tend to have high cholesterol and triglyceride levels. Medical therapy for regulating blood glucose levels helps to modify the individual's risk.

Obesity

Excess body weight increases the workload of the heart. It also contributes to the severity of other risk factors. A weight-reduction program and maintenance of an ideal body weight help to modify the individual's risk.

Sedentary Lifestyle

Lack of regular exercise has been correlated with increased risk of developing cardiovascular disease. Regular aerobic exercise can improve the heart's efficiency and help lower blood glucose levels, improving the ratio of HDLs to LDLs, reducing weight, lowering the blood pressure, reducing stress, and improving overall feelings of well-being. Some practitioners define regular physical exercise as exercising at least three to five times a week for at least 30 minutes, causing perspiration and an increase in heart rate by 30 to 50 bpm. Walking is one of the best forms of exercise.

Stress

The body's stress response releases catecholamines that increase the heart rate. Catecholamines also affect myocardial cells and may result in cellular damage. The vasoconstriction that occurs may contribute to development of cardiovascular disease. Stress reduction measures may be important in modifying an individual's risk.

Psychosocial Factors

People who develop CAD are more likely to have the coronary-prone, or type A, personality. Type A personality traits include aggressiveness, competitiveness, perfectionism, compulsiveness, and an urgent sense of time. When the type A personality is combined with other risk factors such as age, high lipid levels, and smoking, the risk of heart disease increases.

CARDIAC DYSRHYTHMIAS

A **dysrhythmia** (or arrhythmia) refers to any cardiac rhythm that deviates from normal sinus rhythm. Normal sinus rhythm originates in the SA node and is characterized by the following:

- Rate: 60 to 100 bpm
- P waves: precede each QRS complex (atrial depolarization)
- P-R interval: interval between atrial and ventricular repolarization
- QRS complex: ventricular depolarization
- T wave: ventricular repolarization
- Rhythm: regular

A dysrhythmia is the result of an alteration in the formation of impulses through the SA node to the rest of the myocardium. It also results from irritability of myocardial cells that generate impulses, which is independent of the conduction system. Signs and symptoms of dysrhythmia vary, as does treatment, depending on the type and severity of the dysrhythmia. A short overview of each dysrhythmia follows.

Types of Cardiac Dysrhythmias

Sinus Tachycardia

Sinus **tachycardia** is a rapid, regular rhythm originating in the SA node. It is characterized by a heartbeat of 100 to 150 bpm or more.

Causes of sinus tachycardia include exercise, anxiety, fever, shock, medications, HF, excessive caffeine, recreational drugs, and tobacco use. Tachycardia increases the amount of oxygen delivered to the cells by increasing the amount of blood circulated through the vessels.

Clinical manifestations include occasional palpitations. Many patients are asymptomatic. Other signs and symptoms may include hypotension and angina, if cardiovascular disease is also present.

Medical management is directed at the primary cause. This is a normal rhythm and is not usually caused by a cardiac problem.

Sinus Bradycardia

Sinus **bradycardia** is a slow rhythm originating in the SA node. It is characterized by a pulse rate of less than 60 bpm (or even less than 50 bpm, according to some sources). Causes of sinus bradycardia include sleep, vomiting, intracranial tumors, MI, drugs (especially digitalis toxicity), carotid sinus massage, vagal stimulation, endocrine disturbances, increased intracranial pressure, and hypothermia. When found in association with MI, it is a beneficial rhythm because it reduces myocardial oxygen demand. This may be a normal rate and rhythm for an athlete.

Clinical manifestations include fatigue, lightheadedness, and syncope. Some patients are asymptomatic.

Medical management is directed toward the primary cause of the problem and maintaining cardiac output. Atropine may be prescribed to increase the heart rate. A temporary or permanent implantable pacemaker is sometimes necessary (Figures 48-8 and 48-9).

Supraventricular Tachycardia

Supraventricular tachycardia (SVT) is the sudden onset of a rapid heartbeat. It originates in the atria. It is characterized by a pulse rate of 150 to 250 bpm.

Causes of SVT include drugs, alcohol, mitral valve prolapse, emotional stress, smoking, and hormone imbalance. The cause is typically not associated with heart disease.

Clinical manifestations include palpitations, lightheadedness, dyspnea, and anginal pain.

Medical management first looks at how well the patient tolerates the dysrhythmia and at the overall clinical picture. Then the focus is aimed at decreasing the heart rate and eliminating the underlying cause. Specific treatments may include carotid sinus pressure, adenosine, digoxin (Lanoxin), calcium channel blockers (e.g., diltiazem [Cardizem]), beta-adrenergic blockers, propranolol (Inderal), antidysrhythmics, amiodarone (Cordarone), and cardioversion. Persistent, recurring SVT may ultimately be treated with radiofrequency catheter ablation of the accessory pathway.

Atrial Fibrillation

In atrial fibrillation, electrical activity in the atria is disorganized, causing the atria to fibrillate, or quiver, rather than contract as a unit. Atrial fibrillation is a very rapid production of atrial impulses. The atria beat chaotically and are not contracting properly. It is char-

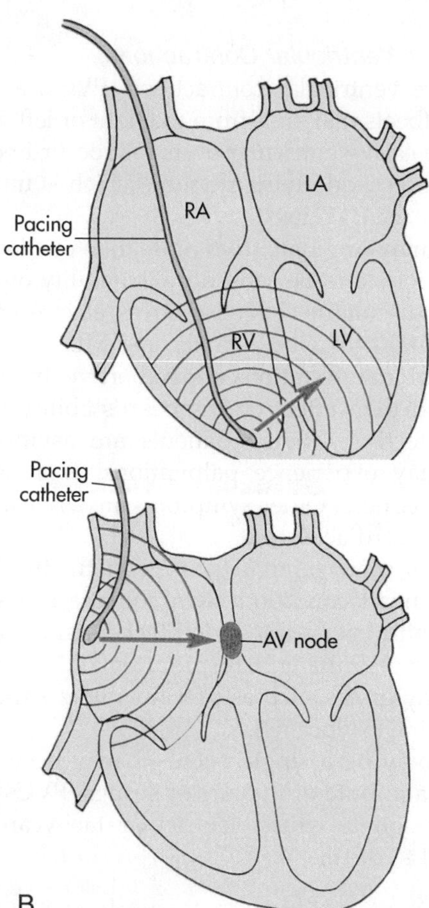

FIGURE 48-8 **A,** Ventricular pacing. Impulses are initiated in ventricle. **B,** Atrial pacing. Impulses are initiated in atrium and travel to ventricles by normal conduction system through the atrioventricular *(AV)* node. *LV,* Left ventricle; *PA,* pulmonary artery; *RA,* right atrium; *RV,* right ventricle.

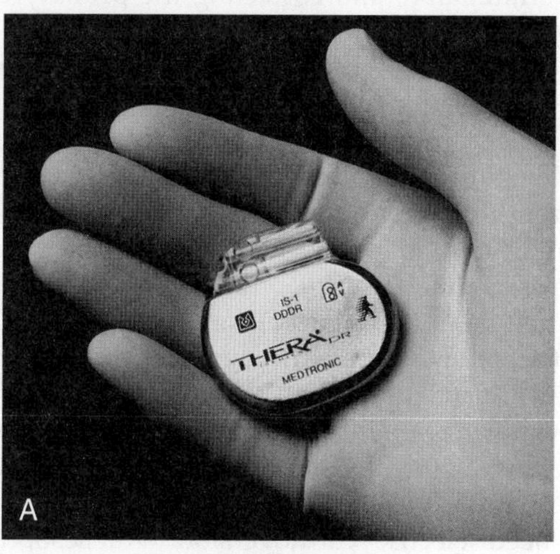

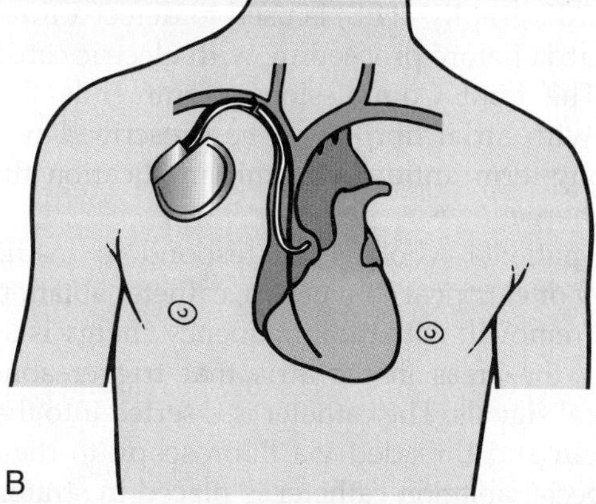

FIGURE 48-9 **A,** A dual-chamber, rate-responsive pacemaker (shown here actual size) from Medtronic, Inc., is designed to detect body movement and automatically increase or decrease paced heart rates based on the level of physical activity. **B,** Cardiac leads, in both the atrium and the ventricle, enable a dual-chamber pacemaker to sense and pace in both heart chambers.

acterized by an atrial rate of 350 to 600 bpm. If untreated, the ventricular response rate may be 100 to 180 bpm.

Causes of atrial fibrillation include cardiac surgery, longstanding hypertension, pulmonary embolism, atherosclerosis, mitral valve disease, HF, cardiomyopathy, congenital abnormalities, chronic obstructive pulmonary disease, and thyrotoxicosis. Clinical manifestations include pulse deficit, palpitations, dyspnea, angina, lightheadedness, syncope, fatigue, change in level of consciousness, and pulmonary edema. Because of ventricular rhythm irregularity and ineffective atrial contractions, decreased cardiac output may be noted, resulting in HF, angina, and shock. Thrombi may form in the atria as a result of ineffective atrial contraction and cause emboli, thus affecting the lungs or periphery (away from the center of the body). An embolized clot may pass to the brain, causing a stroke. Risk of stroke increases fivefold with atrial fibrillation. Risk of stroke is even higher in patients who have structural heart disease, hypertension, and an age over 65 years.

Medical management focuses on treating the irritability of the atria, slowing the ventricular response to atrial stimulation, and correcting the primary cause. The goal of therapy is to prevent atrial thrombi from developing and becoming emboli in the body, such as in the lungs or periphery. Specific treatments for pharmacologic cardioversion may include (1) digitalis; (2) calcium channel blockers such as intravenous (IV) diltiazem (Cardizem) and verapamil (Calan, Isoptin); (3) antidysrhythmics such as procainamide (Procan SR, Pronestyl), amiodarone (Cordarone), dofetilide (Tikosyn), flecainide (Tambocor), or propafenone (Rythmol) (Benz, 2006); and anticoagulants such as heparin or warfarin (Coumadin). Outpatients typically take oral warfarin to maintain anticoagulation. The goal of anticoagulation is to maintain an INR between 2 and 3. If pharmacologic cardioversion fails, the patient may need electric cardioversion. Transesophogeal echocardiography (TEE) is used to detect a thrombus in the atria before proceeding with electric cardioversion. The Joint Commission recommends that patients with atrial fibrillation be prescribed warfarin and long-term antidysrhythmic medication therapy at discharge.

For patients who do not respond to medication therapy or electrical conversion, catheter ablation (cutting or removal) with radiofrequency energy is used to destroy the areas in the atria that trigger abnormal electrical signals. The catheter is inserted into the femoral vein and threaded via fluoroscopy to the heart. The special ablation catheter is placed in strategic areas, and bursts of radiofrequency energy destroy the irritable area (Rocca, 2007; Benz, 2006).

Catheter ablation to treat atrial fibrillation is usually performed on younger patients because of a better response rate and fewer complications than in the older adult. After the catheter ablation procedure, perform neurovascular assessment checks at the peripheral sites distal to the catheter insertion site (Rocca, 2007).

Atrioventricular Block

AV block occurs when a defect in the AV junction slows or impairs conduction of impulses from the SA node to the ventricles. Three types of blocks are seen: first degree, second degree, and third degree. The third-degree block indicates a worsening of the impairment in the AV junction and a complete heart block.

Common causes of AV block include atherosclerotic heart disease (ASHD), MI, and heart failure (HF). Other causes may be digitalis toxicity, congenital abnormality, drugs, and hypokalemia.

Clinical manifestations include no symptoms for first-degree block; vertigo, weakness, and irregular pulse for second-degree block; and hypotension, angina, bradycardia, heart rate often in the 30s, and HF for third-degree block.

Medical management involves evaluating the patient's response and determining the cause of the dysrhythmia. Atropine and isoproterenol may be prescribed. A pacemaker frequently is needed with third-degree block (see Figure 48-8).

Premature Ventricular Contractions

Premature ventricular contractions (PVCs) are abnormal heartbeats that arise from the right or left ventricle. PVCs are early ventricular beats that occur in conjunction with the underlying rhythm, which is unchanged except for the PVC itself.

PVCs may originate from more than one location in the ventricles and be caused by irritability of the ventricular musculature, exercise, stress, electrolyte imbalance, digitalis toxicity, hypoxia, and MI.

Clinical manifestations depend on the frequency of PVCs and their effect on the heart's ability to pump blood effectively. Some patients are asymptomatic; others may experience palpitations, weakness, and lightheadedness. Other symptoms are associated with decreased cardiac output.

Medical management focuses on treating the underlying heart condition. Symptomatic PVCs can be treated with beta-adrenergic blockers such as carvedilol (Coreg), antianginals, propranolol (Inderal), and antidysrhythmics such as procainamide, amiodarone, or lidocaine (Xylocaine).

PVC may be a single event or may occur several times in a minute or in pairs or strings. PVCs that last long enough to cause ventricular tachycardia (VT) may lead to death.

Ventricular Tachycardia

VT occurs when three or more successive PVCs occur. The ventricular rate is greater than 100 bpm (usually 140 to 240 bpm). The rhythm is regular or slightly irregular. Conditions that favor its occurrence include hypoxemia, drug toxicity such as digitalis or quinidine, electrolyte imbalance (e.g., potassium, magnesium), and bradycardia. Repeated and prolonged episodes of VT in the second week after MI may be a warning of ventricular fibrillation and require aggressive evaluation and treatment.

Medical management focuses on intravenously administered procainamide or amiodarone. These drugs depress excitability of cardiac muscle to electrical stimulation and slow conduction in the atria, bundle of His, and ventricles. Lidocaine is used only if acute myocardial ischemia or MI is considered to be the cause of VT. If pharmacologic measures are unsuccessful, the alternative is cardioversion. Catheter ablation can be helpful. Ongoing VT suppression is obtained with oral beta-adrenergic blockers or calcium channel blockers.

Ventricular Fibrillation

Ventricular fibrillation occurs when the ventricular musculature of the heart is quivering. This medical emergency is characterized by rapid and disorganized ventricle pulsation.

The cause is usually myocardial ischemia or infarction. Other causes are untreated VT, electrolyte imbalances, digitalis or quinidine toxicity, and hypothermia. It may also occur with coronary reperfusion after thrombolytic therapy.

Clinical manifestations are the result of no cardiac output and include loss of consciousness, lack of a pulse, decreases in blood pressure and respirations, possible seizures, and sudden death if untreated.

Medical management focuses on providing emergency treatment, including cardiopulmonary resuscitation (CPR), **defibrillation** (the termination of ventricular fibrillation by delivering a direct electrical countershock to the patient's precordium), and medications such as lidocaine or procainamide. Defibrillation is the most effective method of ending ventricular fibrillation and should ideally be performed within 15 to 20 seconds of onset to avoid brain damage from the lack of blood flow.

Assessment

Subjective data for the patient with a cardiac dysrhythmia include the patient's report of symptoms associated with the specific dysrhythmia. Symptoms may include palpitations, skipped beats, nausea, lightheadedness, vertigo, anxiety, dyspnea, fatigue, and chest discomfort.

Collection of **objective data** includes immediate visual observation of the patient when ECG monitoring indicates a dysrhythmia. Signs may include syncope, irregular pulse, tachycardia, and tachypnea. Noting the patient's response to the dysrhythmia is important to plan and implement appropriate nursing interventions. Monitor vital signs and observe for signs of decreased cardiac output.

Diagnostic Tests

ECG monitoring, telemetry, and Holter monitoring are commonly used to confirm the diagnosis of cardiac dysrhythmias.

Medical Management

Treatment varies according to the type of cardiac dysrhythmia (Table 48-1).

Nursing Interventions and Patient Teaching

Nursing interventions focus on symptomatic relief, promotion of comfort, relief of anxiety, emergency action as needed, and patient teaching.

Assess the apical (*not* radial) pulse to obtain an accurate pulse rate when dysrhythmias are present. Because the rhythm is irregular, take the apical pulse for 1 minute. Assess the patient's anxiety and degree of understanding, noting both verbal and nonverbal expressions regarding diagnosis, procedures, and treatments.

Explain the diagnostic and monitoring devices in use. Monitor heart rate and rhythm. Administer antidysrhythmic agents as ordered and monitor response. Maintain a quiet environment; administer sedation or analgesic medication as ordered. Administer oxygen per protocol.

Nursing diagnoses and interventions for the patient with a cardiac dysrhythmia include but are not limited to the following:

Nursing Diagnoses	Nursing Interventions
Pain, related to ischemia	Administer medications as ordered. Teach relaxation techniques. Institute position change and support. Administer prescribed oxygen.
Decreased cardiac output, related to cardiac insufficiency	Monitor heart rate and rhythm. Reduce cardiac workload by encouraging bed rest. Elevate head of bed 30 to 45 degrees for comfort. Restrict activities as ordered; plan care to avoid fatigue. Administer antidysrhythmic agents as ordered. Monitor for signs of drug toxicity.
Ineffective coping, related to fear of and uncertainty about disease process	Assist patient in identifying strengths and coping skills. Supply emotional support. Teach relaxation techniques. Assess coping ability and level of family support. Explain purpose of care as related to specific dysrhythmia.

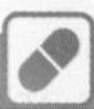

Table 48-1 Medications for Cardiac Dysrhythmias

Generic (Trade)	Action	Nursing Interventions
CARDIOGLYCOSIDE		
Digoxin (Lanoxin)	Used to control rapid ventricular rate in atrial fibrillation and to convert paroxysmal supraventricular tachycardia to normal sinus rhythm Increases cardiac force and efficiency, slows heart rate, increases cardiac output	Monitor apical pulse to ensure rate above 60 bpm (call physician if digoxin held). Monitor for digitalis toxicity (nausea, vomiting, anorexia, dysrhythmias, bradycardia, tachycardia, headache, fatigue, visual disturbance).
ANTIDYSRHYTHMIC		
Procainamide (Pronestyl, Procan SR)	IV solutions given for severe ventricular dysrhythmias Depresses excitability of cardiac muscle to electrical stimulation and slows conduction in atrium, bundle of His, and ventricle, thus increasing refractory period	Observe for new dysrhythmias, dry mouth, blurred vision, bradycardia, hypotension, nausea, anorexia, dizziness, visual disturbances.
Lidocaine (IV)	Suppresses the impulse that triggers dysrhythmias	Monitor heart rate and BP closely.
Disopyramide (Norpace CR)	Provides long-term treatment of premature ventricular contractions, ventricular tachycardia, and atrial fibrillation	Monitor BP and apical pulse.
Adenosine (Adenocard)	Slows conduction through AV node, can interrupt reentry pathways through AV node, and can restore normal sinus rhythm in patients with paroxysmal supraventricular tachycardia (PSVT)	Monitor BP, pulse rate, and respirations. Assess patient for headache, dizziness, gastrointestinal complaints, new dysrhythmias. Do not give caffeine within 4-6 hours of adenosine because caffeine inhibits the effect of the drug.
Amiodarone (Cordarone, Pacerone)	Prolongs duration of action potential and effective refractory period; provides noncompetitive alpha- and beta-adrenergic inhibition; increases P-R and Q-T intervals; decreases sinus rate; decreases peripheral vascular resistance. Used for severe ventricular tachycardia, supraventricular tachycardia, atrial fibrillation, ventricular fibrillation not controlled by first-line agents, cardiac arrest	Observe for headache, dizziness, hypotension, bradycardia, sinus arrest, heart failure, dysrhythmia. Assess BP continuously for hypotension or hypertension. Report dysrhythmia or bradycardia. Monitor for dyspnea, chest pain.
Mexiletine HCl (Mexitil) Propafenone HCl (Rythmol)	Decreases excitability of cardiac muscle	Monitor pulse, BP. Monitor for diarrhea, visual disturbances, respiratory distress.
Tocainide HCl (Tonocard)	Suppresses automaticity of conduction tissue	Notify health care provider if cough, wheezing, or shortness of breath occurs.
BETA-ADRENERGIC BLOCKERS		
Propranolol (Inderal) Sotalol HCl (Betapace) Acebutolol HCl (Sectral) Esmolol HCl (Brevibloc) Metoprolol (Lopressor) Carvedilol (Coreg)	Used to treat supraventricular and ventricular dysrhythmias, persistent sinus tachycardia Decreases myocardial oxygen demand, decreases workload of the heart, decreases heart rate	Monitor heart rate and BP carefully. Use caution with patient with bronchospastic disease. Monitor for bradycardia, hypotension, new dysrhythmias, dizziness, headache, nausea, diarrhea, sleep disturbances.

AV, Atrioventricular; *BP,* blood pressure; *CHF,* congestive heart failure; *HCl,* hydrochloride; *IV,* intravenous.

Table 48-1 Medications for Cardiac Dysrhythmias—cont'd

Generic (Trade)	Action	Nursing Interventions
CALCIUM CHANNEL BLOCKERS		
Verapamil (Calan, Isoptin) Diltiazem HCl (Cardizem)	Treat supraventricular tachycardia and control rapid rates in atrial tachycardia Produce relaxation of coronary vascular smooth muscle, dilate coronary arteries	Use caution in patients with CHF. Monitor apical pulse and BP. Watch for fatigue, headache, dizziness, peripheral edema, nausea, tachycardia. Both verapamil and diltiazem increase the toxicity of digoxin.
INOTROPIC AGENT		
Dobutamine (Dobutrex) (IV) Dopamine (Intropin) (IV)	Used in severe CHF with pulmonary edema Increases myocardial contractility Increases cardiac output, increases BP, and improves renal blood flow	Monitor BP, heart rate, and urinary output continuously during the administration. Palpate peripheral pulses; notify physician if extremities become cold or mottled.
ANTICOAGULANT		
Warfarin (Coumadin)	Used in treatment of atrial fibrillation with embolization to prevent complication of stroke	Assess patient for signs of bleeding and hemorrhage. Monitor prothrombin time and International Normalized Ratio (PT/INR) frequently during therapy. Review foods high in vitamin K. Patient should have consistently limited intake of these foods because these foods will cause levels to fluctuate.

Explain the importance of avoiding or stopping smoking or use of nicotine products. Teach the patient about medication therapy and its purposes, desired effects, and dosage and the side effects to report to the physician. Explain the reason for and method of taking pulse rate and rhythm. Explain the need to avoid exercising beyond the tolerance level, to avoid strenuous or isometric activity, and to check with the physician regarding limitations and allowances. Instruct the patient regarding conserving energy for activities of daily living (ADLs): taking regular rest periods between activities and for 1 hour after meals; when possible, sitting rather than standing while performing a task; and stopping an activity or task if symptoms such as fatigue, dyspnea, or palpitations begin. Stress management is important to promote healing and prevent further cardiac events.

CARDIAC ARREST

The sudden cessation of cardiac output and circulatory process is termed **cardiac arrest.** Conditions leading to cardiac arrest are severe VT, ventricular fibrillation, and ventricular asystole. The absence of an oxygen–carbon dioxide exchange leads to symptoms of anaerobic tissue cell metabolism and respiratory and metabolic acidosis. Thus immediate CPR is necessary to prevent major organ damage. Signs and symptoms of cardiac arrest include abrupt loss of consciousness with no response to stimuli, gasping respirations followed by apnea, absence of pulse (radial, carotid, femoral, and apical), absence of blood pressure, pupil dilation, and pallor and cyanosis.

CPR is initiated by the first person to discover the condition. The aim is to reestablish circulation and ventilation. Prevention of severe damage to the brain, the heart, the liver, and the kidneys as a result of anoxia is of primary concern. Remember the *ABCs* of CPR: **A,** open *Airway*; **B,** restore *Breathing*; and **C,** restore *Circulation*. Resuscitation measures are divided into two components: basic cardiac life support in the form of CPR and advanced cardiac life support (ACLS).

ACLS is a systematic approach to provide early treatment of cardiac emergencies. ACLS includes (1) basic life support, (2) the use of adjunctive equipment and special techniques for establishing and maintaining effective ventilation and circulation, (3) ECG monitoring and dysrhythmia recognition, (4) therapies for emergency treatment of patient with cardiac or respiratory arrest, and (5) treatment of patient with suspected acute MI.

Artificial Cardiac Pacemakers

A pacemaker is made of titanium with computer circuits that control the pacing system; one or more leads are placed into the heart and a lithium battery is used (Sunderlin, 2006). It initiates and controls the heart rate by delivering an electrical impulse via an electrode to the myocardium. These catheter-like electrodes are placed within the area to be paced: right atrium, right ventricle, or both (see Figures 48-8 and 48-9). A permanent pacemaker power source is placed subcutaneously, usually over the pectoral muscle on the patient's nondominant side (Lewis et al., 2007). Most are demand pacemakers, which send electrical stimuli to pace the heart when the heartbeat decreases below a preset rate. Some pacemakers have a single-chamber device with one lead that paces the right atrium or right ventricle; other pacemakers are dual chamber with separate leads that connect to both the right atrium and the right ventricle (Sunderlin, 2006).

Another pacemaker, the biventricular pacemaker, has three leads, one lead for each ventricle and one lead for the right atrium. This device restores normal simultaneous contraction of the ventricles. A biventricular pacemaker significantly improves left ventricular ejection fraction and exercise tolerance. It improves the quality of life for patients with worsening HF (Sunderlin, 2006).

A pacemaker maintains a regular cardiac rhythm by electrically stimulating the heart muscle. It is used when patients experience adverse symptoms because of dysrhythmias that cannot be managed by medications alone. These include second- and third-degree AV block, **bradydysrhythmias** (slow and/or irregular heartbeat), and **tachydysrhythmias** (rapid heartbeat that can be regular or irregular).

An external pacemaker is used in emergency situations on a short-term basis. Temporary pacemakers are used for cardiac support after some MIs or open-heart surgery. A permanent pacemaker is placed when other measures have failed to convert the dysrhythmia or conduction problem. The batteries used in permanent pacemakers today are small, weighing less than 1 ounce, and can last 15 years or more.

Nursing Interventions and Patient Teaching

After placement of a pacemaker, closely monitor heart rate and rhythm by apical pulse and by ECG patterns. Check vital signs and level of consciousness frequently until stable. Observe the insertion site for erythema, edema, and tenderness, which could indicate infection. The patient may be on bed rest with the arm on the pacemaker side immobilized for the first few hours. Discharge teaching includes instructions not to lift the arm on the surgical side over the head for 6 to 8 weeks. The patient needs to refrain from swimming, golfing, and weight lifting until given permission by the health care provider (Sunderlin, 2006).

Inform the patient of the necessity to continue medical management, and advise that he or she wear medical-alert identification and carry pacemaker information. Emphasize the importance of reporting signs and symptoms of pacemaker failure: weakness, vertigo, chest pain, and pulse changes.

Teach the patient to avoid potentially hazardous situations. Each pacemaker manufacturer can provide a list of devices that patients with pacemakers should avoid, such as proximity to high-output electrical generators or large magnets such as an MRI scanner. This may cause interference, placing the pacemaker in a fixed mode and interfering with its functioning. Instruct the patient to move away from any device that may cause untoward symptoms such as vertigo.

The heart rate of the pulse generator for the pacemaker is set according to the patient's clinical condition and the desired therapeutic goal. With rare exceptions, the rate is set between 70 and 80 bpm. If the heart rate falls below the preset level, notify the physician.

Teach the patient how and when to take a radial pulse. The pulse should be taken at the same time each day and when symptoms of vertigo or weakness occur. During patient education, remember to (1) list symptoms to expect and to report to physician, (2) promote understanding of medication administration, (3) explain treatment outcomes, (4) explain importance of maintaining prescribed diet and fluid amounts, and (5) explain importance of not smoking.

Prognosis

The patient can expect to lead a reasonably normal life with full resumption of most activities as prescribed by the physician.

DISORDERS OF THE HEART

CORONARY ATHEROSCLEROTIC HEART DISEASE

The coronary arteries arise from the base of the aorta just below the semilunar valves (see Figure 8-6). These arteries curve and angle to adequately supply the heart muscle with oxygen and nutrients. The shapes, contours, and arrangements of the vessels allow for easy entrapment of substances that interfere with blood flow.

Coronary artery disease (CAD) is the term used to describe a variety of conditions that obstruct blood flow in the coronary arteries. **Atherosclerosis** (a common arterial disorder characterized by yellowish plaques of cholesterol, lipids, and cellular debris in the inner layers of the walls of large and medium-size arteries) is the primary cause of ASHD. The **lumen** (a cavity or channel within any organ of the body) of the vessel narrows as the disease progresses. Blood flow to the heart is obstructed when this process occurs in the coronary arteries.

Atherosclerosis, the basic underlying disease affecting coronary lumen size, is characterized by changes in the intimal lining (the innermost layer) of the arteries. The severity of the disease is measured by the degree of obstruction within each artery and by the number of vessels involved. Obstructions exceeding 75% of the lumen of one or more of the three coronary arteries increase the risk of death.

The basic physiologic changes of the atherosclerotic process result in problems with myocardial oxygen

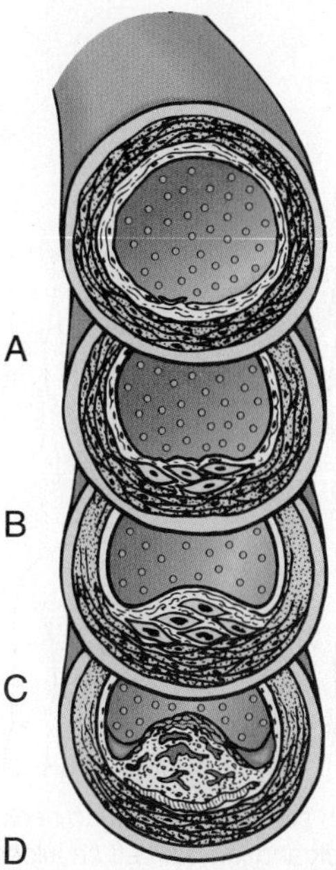

FIGURE 48-10 Progressive development of coronary atherosclerosis. **A,** Injury to intimal wall. **B,** Lipoprotein invasion of smooth muscle cells. **C,** Development of fatty streak and fibrous plaque. **D,** Development of complicated lesion.

supply and demand. When the myocardial oxygen demand exceeds the supply delivered by the coronary arteries, ischemia results (Figure 48-10). The artery walls also become less elastic and less responsive to blood flow (see Cultural Considerations box).

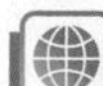 Cultural Considerations

Cardiovascular Disorder

- White, middle-aged men have the highest incidence of coronary artery disease (CAD).
- Blacks, Puerto Ricans, Cubans, and Mexican Americans have a higher incidence of hypertension than white Americans.
- Blacks have an early age of onset of CAD.
- Black women have a higher incidence of CAD than white women.
- Native Americans younger than 35 years of age have a heart disease mortality rate twice as high as that of other Americans.
- Hispanics have a lower death rate from heart disease than non-Hispanics.
- Major modifiable cardiovascular risk factors for Native Americans are obesity and diabetes mellitus.

ANGINA PECTORIS

Etiology and Pathophysiology

Angina means a spasmodic, cramplike, choking feeling. *Pectoris* refers to the breast or chest area. **Angina pectoris** refers to the paroxysmal (severe, usually episodic, increase in symptoms) thoracic pain and choking feeling caused by decreased oxygen or anoxia (lack of oxygen) of the myocardium.

Angina pectoris occurs when the cardiac muscle is deprived of oxygen. Atherosclerosis of the coronary arteries is the most common cause. The narrowed lumina of the coronary arteries are unable to deliver enough oxygen-rich blood to the myocardium. When the myocardial oxygen demand exceeds the supply, **ischemia** (decreased blood supply to a body organ or part, often marked by pain and organ dysfunction) of the heart muscle occurs, resulting in chest pain or angina. Typically angina occurs with an increased cardiac workload brought on by exposure to intense cold, exercise, unusually heavy meals, emotional stress, or any other strenuous activity.

CAD is the nation's number one killer. Many people who die from the disease, however, experience several episodes of unstable angina first. If unstable angina were accurately diagnosed and promptly managed, many deaths and much of the disability associated with CAD could be avoided.

Unstable angina is defined as an unpredictable and transient episode of severe and prolonged discomfort that appears at rest, has never been experienced before, or is considerably worse than previous episodes. It mimics an MI in that the discomfort it causes is often described as tightness or a crushing sensation in the chest, arms, back, neck, or jaw. For some patients, unstable angina is a red flag that an MI will occur.

Clinical Manifestations

Pain is the outstanding characteristic of angina pectoris (Figure 48-11). The patient usually describes the pain as a heaviness or tightness of the chest. At times it is thought to be indigestion. The pain is often substernal (below the sternum) or retrosternal (behind the sternum). Pain may radiate to other sites, or it may occur in only one site. The pain often radiates down the left inner arm to the little finger and also upward to the shoulder and jaw. Patients may also describe it as a pressure or a squeezing sensation, but usually not as a sharp pain. Sometimes a patient experiences posterior thoracic or jaw pain only. The chest pain may be accompanied by other signs and symptoms such as dyspnea, anxiety, apprehension, diaphoresis, and nausea. Symptoms of CAD in women vary and may be more subtle or generalized than in men. Women often report heaviness, squeezing, or pain in the left side of the chest, or pain in the abdomen, arm, mid-back, or scapular region. Women may also complain of palpitations and chest discomfort during rest, during sleep, or with exertion (Cheek, 2008).

The signs and symptoms of angina are often similar to those of MI. Anginal pain is believed to be caused by a temporary lack of oxygen and blood supply to the heart. It is often relieved by rest or medication such as nitroglycerin, which dilates the coronary arteries and increases the flow of oxygenated blood to the myocardium. Nitroglycerin administered sublingually usually relieves angina symptoms but does not relieve the pain from an MI. This is often used as a preliminary diagnostic tool to quickly differentiate angina from an MI.

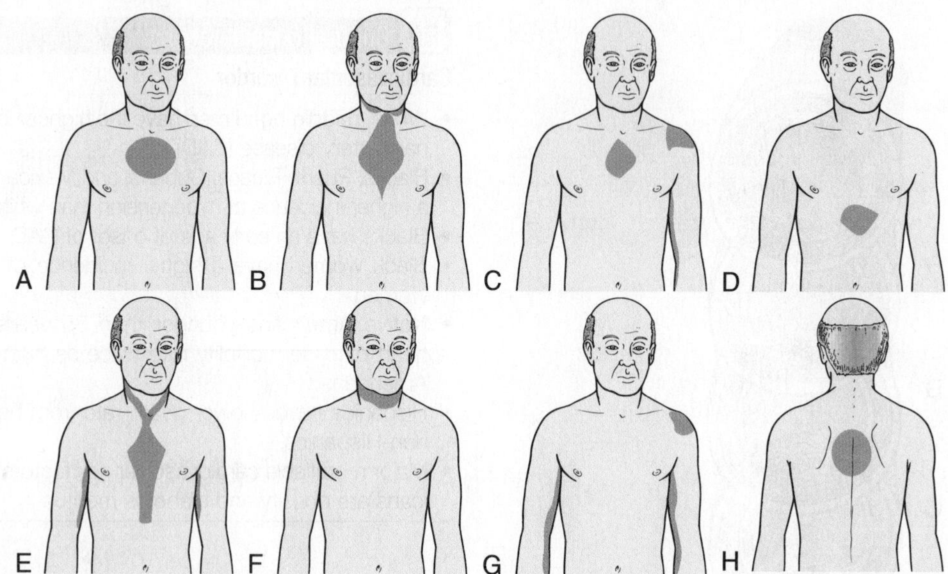

FIGURE 48-11 Sites to which ischemic myocardial pain may be referred. **A,** Upper chest. **B,** Beneath sternum radiating to neck and jaw. **C,** Beneath sternum radiating down left arm. **D,** Epigastric. **E,** Epigastric radiating to neck, jaw, and arms. **F,** Neck and jaw. **G,** Left shoulder and inner aspect of both arms. **H,** Intrascapular.

Assessment

Subjective data include the patient's statements regarding the location, intensity, radiation, and duration of pain. The patient may express a feeling of impending death. Assess precipitating factors that led to the development of symptoms. Determine what relief measures have been used. Identify whether the symptoms have changed in frequency or severity, indicating a worsening of the ischemia.

Collection of **objective data** includes noting the patient's behavior, such as rubbing the left arm or pressing a fist against the sternum. Monitor vital signs and note changes or abnormalities. Increases in pulse rate, blood pressure, and respiratory rate may be noted. Identify the presence of diaphoresis or anxiety.

Diagnostic Tests

The diagnosis of angina pectoris is frequently based on the patient's history. The ECG may reveal ischemia and rhythm changes. Holter monitoring correlates activity with precipitating factors. The exercise stress test determines ischemic changes in a controlled environment. Thallium 201 scanning and PET are used to diagnose ischemic heart disease. Coronary angiography may be done to determine the extent of CAD.

Medical Management

The focus of medical management is to control symptoms by reducing cardiac ischemia. Cardiovascular risk factors are identified and corrected if possible. Precipitating factors—such as exposure to intense cold, strenuous exercise, smoking, heavy meals, and emotional stress—are identified and avoided. Antiplatelet aggregation therapy is a first-line treatment of angina. Aspirin (ASA) is the drug of choice. Low-dose aspirin is indicated for people at risk for CAD who have a calculated 10-year CAD risk of less than 10%. (American Heart Association, 2005). Aspirin, even in low doses (81 mg), is effective in inhibiting platelet aggregation. For patients unable to tolerate aspirin, ticlopidine (Ticlid) or clopidogrel (Plavix) may be given (Lewis et al., 2007). Medication therapy to dilate coronary arteries and decrease the workload of the heart consists of vasodilators (nitrates, especially nitroglycerin); beta-adrenergic blocking agents such as propranolol, metoprolol (Lopressor), nadolol (Corgard), atenolol (Tenormin), and timolol (Blocadren); and calcium channel blockers such as nifedipine (Procardia), verapamil, diltiazem, and nicardipine (Cardene). Give nitroglycerin sublingually for angina. Repeat dose in 5 minutes if pain does not subside. Repeat two or three times at 5-minute intervals. Call physician if pain has not subsided after third nitroglycerin tablet. High-risk, unstable angina patients should be given supplemental oxygen.

Surgical Interventions

Coronary artery bypass graft. Surgical management of the patient with ASHD or CAD may consist of performing a coronary artery bypass graft (CABG) after diagnosis by cardiac catheterization. Any number of grafts can be done, depending on the areas of occlusion in the coronary arteries. Blood flows to the myocardium through the grafts, which bypass the occluded coronary arteries. The grafts are usually taken from sections of the saphenous veins in the legs, or the internal mammary (breast) artery is used.

When the saphenous vein is used for the graft, one end is sutured to the aorta and the other end is sutured to the coronary artery distal to the occlusion. When an internal mammary artery is used, the distal end of this vessel is freed from the anterior chest wall and sutured in place distal to the occlusion in the coronary artery.

Internal mammary arteries are the preferred blood vessels for bypass surgery. A typical procedure involves one or two mammary arteries and saphenous vein grafts. Internal mammary arteries usually last more than 15 years, whereas saphenous vein grafts last an average of 5 to 10 years. Researchers continue to search for alternative blood vessels for CABG surgery (Figures 48-12 and 48-13).

Percutaneous transluminal coronary angioplasty. Another surgical procedure for management of the patient with CAD is percutaneous transluminal coronary angioplasty (PTCA). PTCA is an invasive procedure performed in the cardiac catheterization laboratory. The technique widens the narrowing in a coronary artery without open-heart surgery. *Percutaneous* indicates that the procedure is performed through the skin; *transluminal* means that it is within the lumen of the artery. Patients undergoing PTCA are required to sign a surgical permit for a CABG because of the possibility of complications developing during the procedure that require immediate surgical intervention. Fluoroscopy is used to guide a catheter from the femoral or brachial artery to the coronary arteries to be treated. A balloon is inflated in the catheter once it is positioned (Figure 48-14). The outward push of the balloon against the narrowing wall of the coronary artery reduces the constriction until it no longer interferes with blood flow to the heart muscle. Vessel patency is reestablished by angioplasty (vessel repair). This procedure may take 1 to 2 hours, with the patient usually awake but mildly sedated.

Postprocedure nursing interventions are to continually monitor the patient, as with any surgical recovery. Observe the area of catheter insertion for hemorrhage potential. Monitor the patient in the cardiac care unit, usually for 1 day before dismissal to the medical-surgical unit. The total hospitalization stay is 1 to 3 days compared with the 4- to 6-day stay after open-heart surgery with a CABG; thus PTCA reduces hospital costs. Patients return to work rapidly (approximately 5 to 7 days after PTCA) rather than requiring the 2- to 8-week convalescence common after CABG.

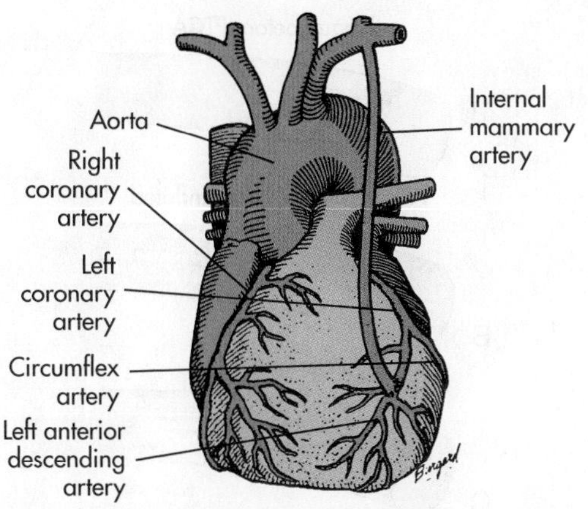

FIGURE 48-13 Coronary artery bypass graft. Internal mammary artery is used; the distal end of this vessel is freed from the anterior chest wall and sutured in place distal to the occlusion in the coronary artery.

Stent placement. Stents are used to treat abrupt or threatened vessel closure after PTCA. Stents are expandable, meshlike structures designed to maintain vessel patency by compressing the arterial walls and resisting vasoconstriction (Figure 48-15). Stents are carefully placed over the angioplasty site to hold the vessel open. Because stents are thrombogenic, the patient must take anticoagulants for at least 3 months. The primary complications from stent placement are hemorrhage and vascular injury. Less common complications are stent thrombosis, acute MI, emergency CABG, and coronary spasms. The possibility of dysrhythmias is always present.

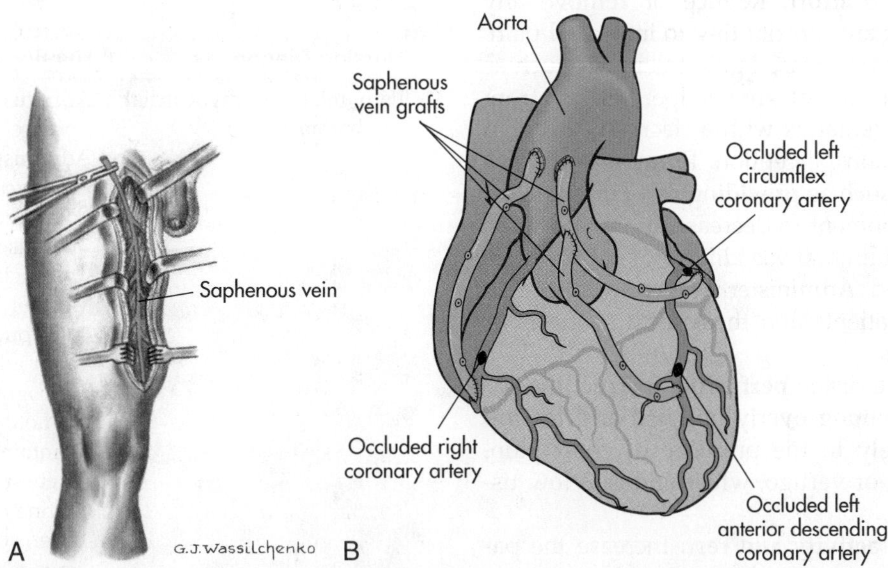

FIGURE 48-12 A, Saphenous vein. **B,** Saphenous aortocoronary artery bypass or revascularization involves taking a piece of saphenous vein from the leg and creating a conduit for blood from the aorta to the area below the blockage in the coronary artery. A triple bypass is illustrated.

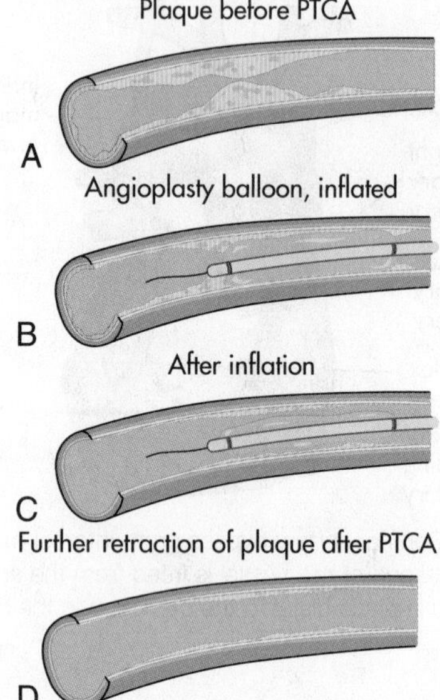

FIGURE 48-14 Percutaneous transluminal coronary angioplasty (PTCA). **A,** Plaque before PTCA. **B,** Inflation of angioplasty balloon. **C,** Plaque after PTCA. **D,** Plaque has retracted even further 6 months after PTCA.

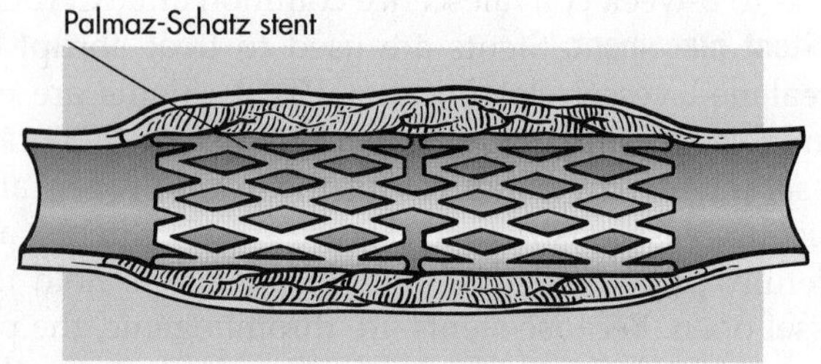

FIGURE 48-15 Palmaz-Schatz stent, an articulated stainless steel mesh deployed by balloon inflation.

Nursing Interventions and Patient Teaching

Nursing interventions are based on the patient's individual needs. They focus on achievement of five major patient outcomes.

First, **promote comfort.** Reduce or remove any known factors that are contributing to increased pain. Assess for causes of decreased pain tolerance, such as anxiety, fatigue, or lack of knowledge. Fatigue from increased oxygen demands with a decreased oxygen supply increases pain perception. Promote measures to reduce fatigue, such as providing rest periods. Provide a calm environment to decrease stress and anxiety. Administer sublingual vasodilators, such as nitroglycerin, as ordered. Administer oxygen for high-risk unstable angina patients and those with cyanosis or respiratory distress.

Second, **promote tissue perfusion.** Instruct the patient to avoid becoming overly fatigued and to stop activity immediately in the presence of chest pain, dyspnea, syncope, or vertigo, which indicate low tissue perfusion.

Third, **promote activity and rest.** Increase the patient's activity tolerance by encouraging slower activity or shorter periods of activity with more rest periods. Most people with angina pectoris are able to tolerate mild exercise such as walking or playing golf, but exertion such as running or climbing stairs rapidly causes pain. Nitroglycerin may be used prophylactically to prevent pain from strenuous activities. Isosorbide mononitrate (Imdur) or isosorbide dinitrate (Isordil) are nitrates that are used for acute treatment of angina attacks (sublingual only) or orally for prophylactic management of angina pectoris. Anginal pain occurs more easily in cold weather. The key is to avoid overexertion.

Fourth, **promote relief of anxiety and a feeling of well-being.** Help the patient reduce the level of anxiety. The patient should minimize emotional outbursts, worry, and tension. People with angina may need continuing help in accepting situations. Supportive family members, a spiritual adviser, business associates, and friends can sometimes be of assistance. Relaxation techniques and music therapy may be beneficial. Peer support groups and behavioral change programs are available. An optimistic outlook helps to relieve the work of the heart. Many people who learn to live within their limitations live out their expected life span despite the disease.

Finally, **teach the patient and the family.** Delay teaching until the patient is ready (see Communication box). The patient needs to be relatively free of pain and anxiety to learn. Promote a positive attitude and active participation of patient and family to encourage compliance. The teaching plan should include information on medications, ways to minimize the events that trigger angina pectoris, effects of exercise on reduction of myocardial oxygen needs, the need to stop smoking because of the vasoconstriction of nicotine, and the need for regular medical follow-up (see Patient Teaching box).

Nursing diagnoses and interventions for the patient with angina pectoris include but are not limited to the following:

Nursing Diagnoses	Nursing Interventions
Pain, related to myocardial ischemia	Administer oxygen as ordered. Administer prescribed nitroglycerin. Repeat every 5 minutes, three times. If pain is unrelieved, notify physician. Monitor blood pressure and pulse before and after administration of nitroglycerin. Promote rest. Maintain diet as ordered; if chest pain occurs while eating or immediately after, advise small feedings rather than two or three large meals.

 Communication

Methods to Decrease Angina Pectoris Attacks

Mrs. M., a patient with angina, has been admitted for further care, diagnosis, and treatment. After the initial nursing assessment, Nurse G. interviews the patient about the course of her anginal episodes. With the data she gathers, Nurse G. will participate in the development of a program to educate Mrs. M. to minimize or control the attacks.

Nurse: I would like to ask you some questions, Mrs. M., about the anginal pain you are experiencing.

Patient: I already told Dr. T. all about those attacks when I visited his office. His nurse, Miss N., has all those records.

Nurse: Yes, I know. Your physician has asked us to help you plan a program for preventing or minimizing these attacks. With the information we gather, we can set goals for your care. We can also identify how angina relates to some of your activities.

Patient: OK, Mrs. G., I would like to understand it better. Perhaps I would be less frightened when it happens. My friend J. told me about her aunt who had angina—she died. That really worries me.

Nurse: We hope to decrease some of your fears, Mrs. M., by helping you understand. First, when do your attacks usually occur?

Patient: Oh, mostly after a real busy day, you know—shopping or gardening or housecleaning. But a few times, I had problems after my sister-in-law visited. She and my husband always seem to get into upsetting discussions. They never got along well. She upsets us both—she criticizes everything!

Nurse: Have you noticed if a big meal is related to the pain?

Patient: No, not really . . . well, only when my sister-in-law is there. We hardly ever eat big meals anymore, except when she comes. She expects to be fed well. My husband and I have cut down a lot. Big meals upset our systems—and then her, that harping on old problems and how she thinks we should run our lives! She upsets me so!

Nurse: Mrs. M., I think we must talk more on how to handle stressful situations like your sister-in-law. But first, could you describe the pain for me? Does it come on suddenly? How long does it last? What does it feel like?

Patient: Oh, no, not all of a sudden. It is just dull at times, like an upset stomach. But then, it travels up in my chest and gets really heavy, like pressure. Sometimes, it makes my face and teeth hurt; and my arm, too—this one [left]—all the way down to my little finger. If it's a really bad attack, I sometimes feel like I am going to vomit.

Nurse: On a scale of 0 to 10, how would you rate most of your angina attacks?

Patient: Probably 5 to 6 would be the average, but sometimes it's a 10.

Nurse: Does your heart beat faster?

Patient: Oh, yes, and I just have to sit down and be quiet or I can't catch my breath. That's when I take the nitroglycerin. I carry it with me all the time now, in this special little container.

Nurse: I see. And how long does it take for the pain to stop after you take the medicine?

Patient: I used to think it took forever, but my husband—he times it for me—says it lasts about 15 to 20 minutes. I relax a little, and it passes.

Nurse: What about the weather, Mrs. M.? Have you noticed that it affects your attacks in any way?

Patient: I don't know if it is all those clothes or the weather, but I get more pains if I get out in the cold.

Nurse: Do you or your husband smoke?

Patient: Not anymore. I gave up cigarettes when this angina started on me. I noticed the difference, too. Now, I can't even stay in a room if people are smoking. I also cut down on coffee when I retired. Dr. T. said that too much caffeine isn't good for the angina. All the good things, they have to go when you get old!

Nurse: Maybe with some understanding of how certain activities and other factors affect your condition, you can find new "good things" that you'll enjoy just as much. We'll talk again soon. There are some effective coping methods to decrease your stress when your sister-in-law visits that we can explore.

Nursing Diagnoses	Nursing Interventions
Pain, related to myocardial ischemia—cont'd	Balance rest with activity. Instruct patient to stop activity at the first sign of chest pain or other symptoms of cardiac ischemia.
Ineffective tissue perfusion, cardiovascular, related to narrowing of coronary arteries	Administer prescribed oxygen. Instruct patient that nitroglycerin may need to be taken before exercise and sexual activity to prevent cardiac ischemia. Encourage less strenuous or shorter periods of activity interspersed with rest. Avoid exercise in cold weather. Take prescribed nitroglycerin before activities that will increase the workload of the heart.

Prognosis

The prognosis for the patient with angina pectoris may be grave. Attacks may be intermittent. With early and aggressive management of angina, mortality rate can be reduced and the disorder can be managed.

Patient Teaching

Angina Pectoris

USING NITRATE MEDICATIONS

- Use nitroglycerin prophylactically to avoid pain known to occur with certain activities.
- Burning sensation on tongue indicates nitroglycerin is activated.
- Throbbing sensation in head and flushing may occur.
- Sit and stand slowly after taking nitroglycerin. Postural hypotension is a side effect of nitroglycerin.
- Place nitroglycerin tablets under the tongue at the onset of anginal pain; second tablet can be taken after 5 minutes and third tablet after another 5 minutes if pain is unrelieved.
- Call physician if pain does not subside after third nitroglycerin tablet; go to nearest emergency department; do not drive yourself.
- Always carry nitroglycerin on your person.
- Store nitroglycerin in a dark bottle and keep in a dry place.
- Replenish nitroglycerin supply every 6 months or before expiration date.
- Remove all old nitrate ointment before application of new cream.
- Place nitroglycerin patches on skin in the morning and remove at bedtime. This prevents development of tolerance and maintains effectiveness.

MINIMIZING PRECIPITATING EVENTS

- Be careful in using medications for erectile dysfunction when using nitrate medications; they could cause severe hypotension.
- Avoid overexertion. Take nitroglycerin before exercise.
- Try to reduce stress and anxiety, which cause blood vessels to constrict.
- Avoid overeating because it places an increased workload on the heart.
- Avoid cold weather (constricts coronary vessels to conserve body heat; hence anginal pain can develop more easily).
- Dress warmly in cold weather.
- Avoid hot, humid conditions (increases workload on the heart).
- Walk downhill and with wind, since walking uphill and against wind increases workload on the heart.
- Stopping smoking is a necessity because of vasoconstriction of arteries from nicotine.

EXERCISING TO REDUCE MYOCARDIAL OXYGEN NEEDS

- Engage in a regular exercise program to improve collateral circulation.
- Exercise conditions heart muscle and can decrease oxygen demand during exertion.
- Space exercise period with rest periods.
- Take nitroglycerin before exertion.

MYOCARDIAL INFARCTION

Etiology and Pathophysiology

Myocardial infarction (MI) is an occlusion of a major coronary artery or one of its branches with subsequent necrosis of myocardium caused by atherosclerosis or an **embolus** (a foreign object, a quantity of air or gas, a bit of tissue, or a piece of a thrombus that circulates in the bloodstream until it becomes lodged in a vessel). An obstruction by atherosclerotic process or an embolus may interrupt the blood supply. Coronary **occlusion** (an obstruction or closing off in a canal, vessel, or passage of the body) is the general term for occlusion of a coronary artery. The occlusion may also be caused by the formation of a thrombus. Eighty percent to 90% of all acute MIs are secondary to thrombus formation. (Lewis et al., 2007). This is generally referred to as a coronary thrombosis. The occlusion leads to tissue ischemia. Ischemia to the myocardium lasting more than 35 to 45 minutes produces cellular damage and necrosis. The ability of the cardiac muscle to contract and pump blood is impaired. The extent of damage to the surrounding tissues depends on the ability to develop collateral circulation. Collateral circulation refers to the development of new vessels in the heart that compensate for the loss of circulation from the occluded artery. The location of the occlusion and the extent of tissue damage affect the patient's response to the injury (Figure 48-16).

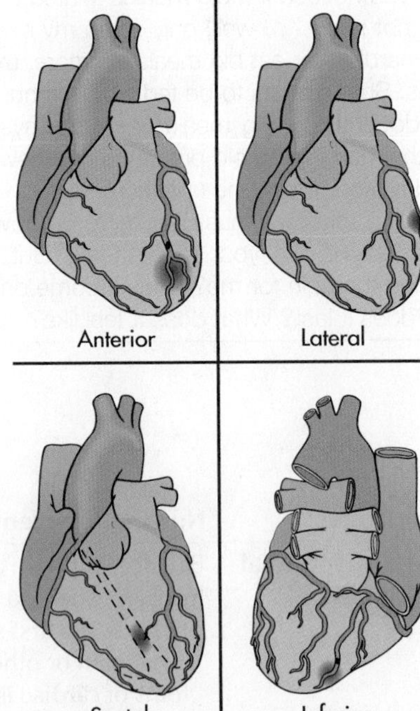

FIGURE 48-16 Four common locations where myocardial infarctions occur.

The body's response to cell death is the inflammatory process. Within 24 hours, leukocytes infiltrate the area. Enzymes are released from the dead cardiac cells and are important diagnostic indicators. (See the discussion on serum cardiac markers, p. 1547.) Phagocytes (neutrophils and monocytes) clear the necrotic debris from the injured area, and by 6 weeks after an MI, scar tissue has replaced necrotic tissue.

Clinical Manifestations

An asymptomatic MI may occur. This is referred to as a *silent MI.* Many of the symptoms of MI are associated with irreversible ischemia, but they are similar to the signs and symptoms of angina pectoris. The symptoms of an MI are more severe and last longer than those of an angina attack. Pain is the foremost symptom of MI (Table 48-2).

The pain location and radiation to other sites are depicted in Figure 48-11. It is often described as crushing or viselike, an oppressive sensation as though a heavy object is sitting on the chest. The pain is retrosternal (behind the sternum) and in the heart region. It often radiates down the left arm and to the neck, jaws, teeth, and epigastric area. It may occur suddenly, or it may build up over a few minutes. It may occur in conjunction with intense emotion, during exertion, or at rest. The pain is prolonged and more intense than anginal pain. It lasts 30 minutes to several hours or longer. It is not relieved by changes in body position, nitroglycerin, or rest. Physicians often tell patients who call complaining of chest pain to take an aspirin (chewable if they have it) and report to the emergency department. Other signs and symptoms that may occur in conjunction with the pain include nausea, dyspnea, dizziness, weakness, diaphoresis, pallor, ashen color, and a sense of impending doom. Early signs and symptoms of an acute MI in women are unusual fatigue, sleep disturbances, shortness of breath, weakness, indigestion, and anxiety. Frequently acute chest pain is not present. With these signs and symptoms, an acute MI can commonly be misdiagnosed as indigestion, gallbladder disease, depression, or anxiety (Sherrod et al., 2007). Table 48-3 provides a comparison of signs and symptoms and the medical management of angina pectoris and MI.

Table 48-2 Signs and Symptoms of Myocardial Infarction

SUBJECTIVE DATA (SYMPTOMS)	OBJECTIVE DATA (SIGNS)
Heavy pressure or squeezing in center of chest behind sternum	Pallor
Pain, retrosternal and in heart region, often radiating down the left arm and to the neck, jaw, and teeth	Erratic behavior
Anxiety	Hypotension, shock
Dyspnea	Cardiac rhythm changes
Weakness, faintness	Vomiting
Nausea	Fever
	Diaphoresis

Assessment

Subjective data include the onset, location, quality, duration, and radiation of pain. The patient may complain of shortness of breath, dizziness, weakness, anxiety, fear, or unusual fatigue. Identify precipitating factors. Inquire about measures the patient has tried to relieve the pain.

Table 48-3 Coronary Artery Disorders

SIGNS AND SYMPTOMS	MEDICAL MANAGEMENT
ANGINA PECTORIS	
Chest pain (substernal, retrosternal), may radiate to neck, jaw, left arm, and shoulder; great anxiety, fear of approaching death; face pale, ashen; pulse variable, usually tense and quick; blood pressure elevated during an attack; usually brought on by exertion, emotional upsets; relieved by rest, nitroglycerin	Avoidance of precipitating factors Reduction of modifiable risk factors Medications: nitrates, beta blockers, calcium channel blockers Oxygen therapy ECG monitoring Aspirin for unstable angina
MYOCARDIAL INFARCTION	
Severe, crushing chest pain; prolonged heavy pressure or squeezing pain in center of chest; may spread to shoulder, neck, arm, fourth and fifth fingers on left hand, teeth, and jaw; may radiate as with angina; not relieved with rest or nitroglycerin; may be associated with dyspnea, diaphoresis, apprehension, nausea, and vomiting; signs and symptoms of cardiogenic shock may develop; the pain is prolonged and more intense than anginal pain In women, these classic symptoms are far less common; most frequent early warning symptoms: unusual fatigue, sleep disturbances, shortness of breath, weakness, indigestion, and anxiety; in one study, only 30% of women reported chest pain, and acute chest pain was absent in 43% (Sherrod et al., 2007).	Relief of pain (oxygen), morphine, and other analgesics ECG monitoring Thrombolytic therapy to dissolve clot Reduction of oxygen demand (rest) Prevention of complications (through use of stool softeners, anticoagulants) Treatment of complications (dysrhythmias, HF) Anticoagulants to prevent further clotting

ECG, Electrocardiogram; *HF*, heart failure.

Collection of **objective data** includes observation of the patient's behavior to detect apprehension and anxiety. Typical vital signs reveal hypotension, pulse abnormalities such as tachycardia or a barely perceptible pulse, and early temperature elevation. Note the presence of diaphoresis; vomiting; ashen color; cool, clammy skin; labored respirations; and cardiac dysrhythmias. If possible, find out about risk factors. A respiratory assessment should also be done.

Diagnostic Tests

Diagnostic tests are used to confirm the diagnosis of MI. Serum tests are initially obtained. Serum cardiac markers (e.g., CK-MB, myoglobin) are released into the vascular system when infarcted myocardial muscle cells die. A sensitive cardiac marker present in serum called **troponin I** has proven useful in detecting ischemic myocardial injury. Troponin I is cardiac specific and therefore a highly specific indicator of an MI. (See the discussion of serum cardiac markers on p. 1547.) An elevated white blood cell count of 12,000 to 15,000/mm^3 is associated with severe infarcts. The increase begins a few hours after the onset of pain and lasts for 3 to 7 days. The ESR rises during the first week and may remain elevated for several weeks.

Twelve-lead ECG findings that indicate MI include ST-segment elevation and the development of Q waves. In time the ST segment returns to normal and the T wave inverts. These ECG changes are important in confirming the diagnosis of MI. Significantly, ECG findings are different for men and women. A woman experiencing an MI is far less likely than a man to have concurrent ST-segment elevation (Cheek, 2008). Thus, she may be misdiagnosed and not receive correct treatment (Cheek, 2008). A chest radiograph is done to note size and configuration of the heart. More complex tests are occasionally done, including cardiac fluoroscopy, myocardial imaging (thallium scan), echocardiogram, PET, and multigated acquisition scanning (MUGA). These tests may be done in conjunction with other tests to diagnose MI and determine the severity of CAD.

Medical Management

Medical management focuses on preventing further tissue injury and limiting the size of the infarction. It is extremely important that a patient with a suspected MI is rapidly diagnosed and treated to preserve cardiac muscle. Intervention is designed to restore cardiac tissue perfusion and reduce the workload of the heart. Promoting tissue oxygenation, relieving pain, preventing complications, improving tissue perfusion, and preventing further tissue damage are all important medical considerations.

Medications such as morphine and diazepam (Valium) are used to alleviate pain and anxiety. A continuous IV infusion of amiodarone may be given to the patient who has frequent PVCs, which may precede ventricular fibrillation. Prophylactic lidocaine is not recommended by the American College of Cardiology practice guidelines for the treatment of acute MI (Singh, 2002). However, lidocaine may be a treatment option for the patient who has sustained VT or ventricular fibrillation. The use of beta-adrenergic blockers such as atenolol, metoprolol, propranolol, nadolol, and carvedilol (Coreg) early in the acute phase of an MI and during a 1-year follow-up regimen can decrease morbidity and mortality. Angiotensin-converting enzyme (ACE) inhibitors may be used after MIs. Their use can help to prevent or slow the progression of HF (Table 48-4). Calcium channel blockers or longer-acting nitrates can be added if the patient is already on adequate doses of beta-adrenergic blockers or cannot tolerate beta-adrenergic blockers. Examples of calcium channel blockers are amlodipine (Norvasc), diltiazem, nifedipine, and verapamil. An example of a long-acting nitrate is isosorbide dinitrate (Antman et al., 2004). Oxygen is prescribed to facilitate cardiac tissue perfusion. Attention is given to respiratory difficulties, fluid overload, and cardiac dysrhythmias.

Medical therapy is also directed toward limiting the size and extent of injury by attempting to reperfuse (reinstitute blood flow to an area that was ischemic) the occluded coronary artery. Fibrinolytic agents such as streptokinase (Streptase), anistreplase, and a tissue plasminogen activator (TPA) such as alteplase are currently used to attempt reperfusion. Thrombolytic therapy is the standard practice in the treatment of acute MI. Thrombolytics salvage heart muscle by minimizing infarct size and maximizing heart function. They lyse (decompose or dissolve) the clot in the occluded coronary artery, reopening the vessel and allowing perfusion of the heart muscle.

Remember the adage, "Time is muscle." Fast action to restore myocardial blood flow limits infarct size, preserves heart tissue, and improves the patient's chance of survival and recovery. To be effective, reperfusion must occur 3 to 5 hours after the onset of symptoms. Myocardial cells do not die instantly. In most patients, it takes approximately 4 to 6 hours for the entire thickness of the muscle to become necrosed. Mortality and infarction size can be significantly reduced if thrombolytic therapy starts within 30 to 60 minutes of symptom onset. Before a thrombolytic is administered, obtain a thorough history. Thrombolytics are not used for patients with active internal bleeding, suspected aortic dissecting aneurysm, recent head trauma, history of hemorrhagic stroke within the past year, or surgery within the past 10 days.

PTCA may be used instead of thrombolytic therapy as a primary treatment in some cases. This involves advancing a balloon-tipped catheter into the lumen of the obstructed coronary artery. The balloon is inflated

Table 48-4 Medications for Myocardial Infarction

Classification	Generic (Trade)	Action
Vasopressors	Dopamine (Intropin)	Raise systemic arterial pressure and cardiac output
Anticoagulants	Heparin Warfarin (Coumadin)	Reduce incidence of clotting
Antiplatelets	Ticlopidine (Ticlid) Aspirin (ASA)	Decrease platelet release of thromboxane, so that vasoconstriction and platelet aggregation are decreased Decrease platelet aggregation
Analgesics	Morphine	Control pain; reduce myocardial oxygen demand
Tranquilizers	Diazepam (Valium)	Decrease anxiety and restlessness
Thrombolytic agents	Streptokinase (Streptase)	Thrombolytic (pertaining to dissolution of blood clots) agents used when acute MI symptoms are less than 6 hours, preferably 30 minutes to 1 hour duration; restore blood flow and therefore limit infarct size in certain patients
Tissue plasminogen activator	Alteplase, recombinant Activase	
Nitrates	Nitroglycerin Isosorbide Atenolol (Tenormin)	Dilate blood vessels by reducing coronary artery spasm, increase coronary artery blood supply, and decrease oxygen demands
Beta-adrenergic blockers	Propranolol (Inderal) Nadolol (Corgard) Metoprolol (Lopressor) Carvedilol (Coreg)	Block beta-adrenergic stimulation and decrease myocardial oxygen demands, thus decreasing myocardial damage; decreases mortality rate
Calcium channel blockers	Nifedipine (Procardia) Diltiazem (Cardizem) Verapamil (Calan, Isoptin) Amlodipine (Norvasc)	Dilate blood vessels, increase coronary artery blood supply, and decrease myocardial oxygen demands
Angiotensin-converting enzyme (ACE) inhibitors	Captopril (Capoten) Enalapril (Vasotec)	Can help prevent ventricular remodeling and prevent or slow the progression of HF Prevent conversion of angiotensin I to angiotensin II Decrease endothelial dysfunction
Salicylates	Aspirin	Decrease platelet adhesion and thus decrease thrombosis formation
Antidysrhythmics	Lidocaine (Xylocaine) IV	Treat ventricular dysrhythmias (rarely used except for ventricular tachycardia)
Stool softeners	Surfak Colace	Reduce straining at stool; prevent constipation produced by decreased mobility and use of constipating narcotics
Diuretics	Furosemide (Lasix)	Control edema
Electrolyte replacement	Slow-K	May be necessary when diuretics are used
Inotropic agents	Digoxin (Lanoxin) Amrinone (Inocor) IV Dobutamine (Dobutrex)	Increase the heart's pumping action (contractility) Indicated when left ventricle failure is present

HF, Heart failure; *MI,* myocardial infarction.

intermittently to dilate the artery and improve blood flow (see Figure 48-14). Along with balloon compression, stents may be used to prevent acute closure and restenosis (see Figure 48-15).

CABG surgery may be considered for patients with multiple vessel disease and when less invasive interventions, such as thrombolysis and PTCA, have failed (see Figures 48-12 and 48-13).

Complications commonly associated with MI include ventricular fibrillation, cardiogenic shock (Table 48-5), HF, and dysrhythmias. Cardiogenic shock, often referred to as pump failure, is characterized by low cardiac output and peripheral vascular system collapse. Left ventricular function is severely decreased, resulting in an inadequate blood supply to the vital organs. Immediate detection and treatment are necessary to prevent irreversible shock and death. Cardiogenic shock proves fatal in 50% to 80% of cases. Other possible complications include ventricular aneurysm, pericarditis, and embolism.

Table 48-5 Cardiogenic Shock

CLINICAL MANIFESTATIONS	SIGNS AND SYMPTOMS	MEDICAL MANAGEMENT	NURSING INTERVENTIONS
Decreased cardiac output Myocardial ischemia Cerebral hypoxia Impaired tissue perfusion Renal circulation decreased Anaerobic metabolism with lactic acidosis Peripheral vascular system collapse Shock	Dysrhythmias, chest pain Anxiety, agitation, restlessness, disorientation Urinary output diminished or absent Lactic acid accumulation in blood Tachycardia, thready pulse, tachypnea Decreased blood pressure Narrowed pulse pressure Cyanosis; cold, moist, pale, clammy skin Decreased peripheral pulses Capillary refill time decreased Hypoactive bowel sounds	Recognition and control of life-threatening signs and symptoms Oxygenation to promote tissue perfusion Parenteral fluid as a volume expander Drug therapy: • Vasopressors: raise arterial blood pressure • Inotropic, cardiac glycoside: (digoxin, Lanoxin) increases cardiac contraction and strengthens and corrects dysrhythmias • Adrenergic drugs: dopamine (Intropin) at therapeutic levels increases cardiac output and blood pressure • Sodium bicarbonate: combats lactic acidosis (given sparingly because it causes fluid retention)	Monitor vital signs every 5 minutes during acute stage and every 1 hour when stabilized. Administer oxygen as ordered. Maintain bed rest to reduce myocardial workload and increase oxygenation. Monitor acid-base balance. Monitor urinary output hourly to determine adequate kidney perfusion. Allow nothing by mouth. Initiate bed rest to minimize energy expenditure. Administer medications as ordered. Provide comfort measures.

Nursing Interventions and Patient Teaching

Administer oxygen per protocol for 24 to 48 hours or longer if pain, hypotension, dyspnea, or dysrhythmias persist. Administer medications as prescribed:

- IV morphine sulfate for relief of pain and anxiety and to produce vasodilation. Morphine also decreases myocardial oxygen demands, reduces contractility, and slows the heart rate. Provisions for comfort and rest are essential to reduce stress and increase myocardial oxygen perfusion.
- Heparin therapy or unfractionated or low-molecular-weight heparin such as enoxaparin (Lovenox) or dalteparin (Fragmin) to inhibit further clotting and prevent reocclusion of the coronary artery after the thrombolytic therapy opens the vessel.
- Antiplatelet agents such as aspirin and ticlopidine to decrease platelet release of thromboxane. These drugs are platelet aggregation inhibitors. Ticlopidine can be ordered for patients allergic to aspirin and should be administered immediately. Clopidogrel inhibits platelet aggregation and is an alternative for patients who cannot use aspirin.
- IV nitroglycerin may help patients with left-ventricular infarctions. It reduces cardiac oxygen demand by relaxing vascular smooth muscle and dilating peripheral vessels; it also dilates coronary vessels, improving blood flow to the heart. Administer beta-adrenergic blockers to inhibit cardiotoxicity of catecholamines.
- Administer lipid-lowering agents such as simvastatin, atorvastatin (Lipitor), or rosuvastatin to prevent elevated cholesterol levels.
- Stool softener as prescribed to prevent rectal straining. The Valsalva maneuver may cause severe changes in blood pressure and heart rate, which may trigger ischemia, dysrhythmias, or cardiac arrest.

To help the post-MI patient minimize straining, offer the use of a bedside commode or nearby bathroom whenever possible. Teach mouth breathing to help decrease the severity of straining to prevent use of the Valsalva maneuver, which is contraindicated in the patient with an MI.

Instruct the patient to avoid excessive fatigue and to stop activity immediately in the presence of chest pain, dyspnea, or faintness. Plan nursing interventions to promote rest and minimize disturbances. Monitor vital signs; document rate and rhythm of pulse.

The patient is usually placed on bed rest with commode privileges for 24 to 48 hours. Assist with ADLs. During this period, sedation with diazepam or an equivalent may be prescribed to relieve anxiety and restlessness and to promote sleep. After the first 24 to 48 hours, encourage the patient to increase activity gradually, depending on the size of the infarction. Continually monitor the patient for signs of dysrhythmias, cardiac pain, and changes in vital signs.

Diet is usually withheld until the patient is stabilized. This is important because of the possible need for cardiac catheterization, PTCA, or a CABG procedure. Liquid diet is progressed as tolerated to regular diet with modifications. A low-fat, low-sodium, easily digested diet is desirable.

Prevention of complications is a primary objective. Antiembolic stockings are used. Continue to assess and report cardiac status, dyspneic condition, and pulse change (rate, rhythm, and volume).

During hospitalization, many patients experience denial, depression, and anxiety. Anxiety varies in intensity, depending on the severity of the perceived threat and the patient's success in coping.

Nursing diagnoses and interventions for the patient with an MI include but are not limited to the following:

Nursing Diagnoses	Nursing Interventions
Acute chest pain, related to myocardial ischemia	Assess original pain and location, duration, radiation, and onset of new symptoms. Administer prescribed analgesics (usually morphine sulfate, which relieves pain, reduces anxiety, causes vasodilation of vascular smooth muscle, and reduces myocardial workload). Maintain bed rest and reduced patient activity. Administer oxygen as prescribed. Record patient's response to pain relief measures. Employ alternative methods of pain relief. Provide calm, restful environment.
Anxiety, related to: • change in health status • fear of death	Assess for signs and verbal expressions of anxiety and coping mechanisms used. Promote restful sleep patterns. Reassure patient by providing education, enlisting family support, and allowing positive and negative expression of feelings. Remain with patient during periods of highest anxiety; offer reassurance; use calm, but concerned voice. Administer antianxiety agents as needed, per physician's order. Initiate relaxation techniques (deep breathing, visual imagery, soft rhythmic music). Encourage participation in cardiac rehabilitation program.
Decreased cardiac output, related to conduction defects (dysrhythmias) and decreased myocardial pumping action	Assess and monitor vital signs every 4 hours. Maintain bed rest with head of bed elevated 30 degrees for first 24 to 48 hours to reduce myocardial oxygen demand. Monitor IV feedings; infuse according to physician's order. Administer prescribed medications such as antidysrhythmics, nitrates, and beta blockers. Auscultate breath sounds and heart rate every 4 hours; increase activity level as prescribed. Palpate for pedal pulses, assess capillary refill, auscultate bowel sounds, assess for pedal or dependent edema every 4 hours, and strictly monitor intake and output (I&O).

Patients and their family members need to be reassured of recovery. More than 85% of patients with an uncomplicated MI return to work. Provide information on the resumption of sexual activities. Once patients with an uncomplicated MI are able to climb two flights of stairs without difficulty, they are usually able to resume sexual activities. Approximately 80% of all postcoronary patients resume sexual activity without serious risks. The other 20% need not abstain totally, but should limit their sexual activity according to their cardiac capacity.

Cardiac Rehabilitation

Before discharge from the hospital, discuss participation in a cardiac rehabilitation program. A monitored exercise program and continuing education are provided with outpatient cardiac rehabilitation. The physician may prescribe cardiac rehabilitation during the inpatient and outpatient phase of recovery after an MI.

Cardiac rehabilitation services are designed to help patients with heart disease recover faster and return to full and productive lives. Cardiac rehabilitation has two major parts:

1. Exercise training to help the patient learn how to exercise safely, strengthen muscles, and improve stamina. The exercise plan is based on the individual's ability, needs, and interests.
2. Education, counseling, and training to help the patient understand his or her heart condition and find ways to reduce the risk of future heart problems. The cardiac rehabilitation team assists the patient in adjusting to a new lifestyle and

dealing with fears about the future. Cardiac rehabilitation may last 6 weeks, 6 months, or longer. Cardiac rehabilitation has lifelong favorable effects (see Health Promotion and Home Care Considerations boxes).

Prognosis

It is imperative that medical care be instituted without delay. Many MI patients not treated before reaching the hospital die. The prognosis also depends on the area and extent of the damage and the presence or absence of complications.

HEART FAILURE

Etiology and Pathophysiology

When the heart is no longer able to pump enough blood to sustain the body's metabolic needs, it is referred to as heart failure or cardiac insufficiency. **Heart failure** (HF) is a syndrome traditionally defined as circulatory congestion as a result of the heart's inability to act as an effective pump. Because many patients suffer pulmonary or systemic congestion with HF, the syndrome was once called **congestive HF** (CHF). However, this term has lost favor because it excludes patients who do not experience congestion. The most recent definition is that HF should be viewed as a neurohormonal problem that progresses as a result of chronic release in the body of

Home Care Considerations

Exercise Program after Myocardial Infarction

- During posthospitalization convalescent period, many patients are encouraged to begin a 2- to 12-week walking program. This is a structured program designed to have the patient walking 2 miles in less than 60 minutes by the end of 12 weeks.
- Encourage patients to work through this program at their own rate until they achieve a pace below a slow jog and their heart rate is below the prescribed rate set by the cardiologist.
- Not all postinfarction patients are physiologically capable of participating in a rigorous exercise program.
- Eventually, most patients are encouraged to participate in a maintenance (lifetime), unsupervised, home-based exercise program designed specifically for them.
- Almost everyone can benefit from some type of cardiac rehabilitation.

Health Promotion

Myocardial Infarction

- Teach the effects of myocardial infarction (MI), the healing process, and the treatment regimen.
- Teach the effect of medications in the treatment of MI.
- Teach the association between risk factors and coronary artery disease (CAD).
- Teach the patient to identify nonmodifiable risk factors.
- Teach the patient to identify modifiable risk factors (especially cigarette smoking and stress). The patient should stop smoking and encourage family and significant others to stop.
- Teach the effect of dietary restrictions on atherosclerotic heart disease or CAD. Recommended daily intake is 2 g sodium, 1500 calories, low cholesterol, and fluid restrictions.
- Limit total fat intake to 25% to 35% of total calories each day. Limit intake of saturated fats to less than 7% of total fat intake. Teach the patient that saturated fats (e.g., shortening, lard, or butter) are solid at room temperature; better sources of fat include vegetable, olive, and fish oils.
- Teach the patient to avoid foods high in sodium, saturated fats, and triglycerides. Review alternative ways of seasoning foods to avoid cooking with salt. Explain the need to limit intake of eggs, cream, butter, and foods high in animal fat. Teach the patient and family how to read labels on foods.
- Teach the patient to eat 20 to 30 g of soluble fiber every day. Foods such as bran, beans, and peas help lower bad cholesterol (low-density lipoprotein).
- Teach the effect of activity on the heart and the need to participate in a progressive activity plan.
- Refer the patient to social support groups as indicated.
- Stress the importance of participating in cardiac rehabilitation services.
- Explain cardiac warning symptoms. Patients and their partners are often unsure which symptoms must be reported. If the patient has a prescription for nitroglycerin, advise him or her to take it when experiencing chest pain and to notify the physician if pain is not relieved within 15 minutes. Other signs to report include shortness of breath, rapid heart rate, dizziness, insomnia, a persistent increase in heart rate or blood pressure, and extreme fatigue after sexual activity.
- Advise the patient on when to resume sexual activity (if appropriate). Explain what is safe and when. The joint guidelines of the American College of Cardiology and the American Heart Association recommend that after an "uncomplicated MI" (meaning that the patient was stable and experienced no complications), sexual intercourse can be resumed in a week to 10 days. However, previous studies have found that patients tend to resume sexual activity more gradually than this. A "complicated MI" means that the patient required cardiopulmonary resuscitation or had hypotension, serious dysrhythmia, or heart failure while hospitalized. Patients with complicated MIs must resume sexual activity more gradually, depending on their tolerance for exercise and activity. Encourage patients to talk to their physicians about resuming sexual activity; the type and extent of damage from the MI might influence recommendations. Most patients have concerns about resuming sexual activity after an MI but may not express them to their nurses. Therefore initiating the conversation is the nurse's responsibility.
- Teach the importance of taking prescribed medications such as beta blockers. The patient who uses beta-adrenergic blockers in the treatment of an acute MI for 1 year after the infarction has a decreased chance of reinfarction and increased survival. Continue with taking lipid-lowering agents such as simvastatin (Zocor), atorvastatin (Lipitor), lovastatin (Mevacor), pravastatin (Pravachol), or rosuvastatin (Crestor).

substances such as catecholamines (epinephrine and norepinephrine). Epinephrine and norepinephrine are hormones of the sympathetic nervous system and produce negative effects on the failing heart and circulatory system.

Circulatory congestion and compensatory mechanisms may occur. HF may develop after an MI, in response to prolonged hypertension or diabetes mellitus, or in relation to valvular or inflammatory heart disease. Other factors associated with HF include infection, stress, hyperthyroidism, anemia, and fluid replacement therapy. HF is the most common diagnosis for the hospitalized patient over 65 years of age. HF affects about 5 million Americans and accounts for 200,000 deaths annually. The increasing prevalence and incidence of HF result from people (1) living longer and (2) being more likely to survive cardiovascular disease.

Because the left ventricle is most often affected by coronary atherosclerosis and hypertension, HF usually begins there. If untreated, the condition progresses to right-sided failure. Right ventricular failure can occur separately from left ventricular failure, but its appearance is more often a consequence of left-sided failure. The signs and symptoms of HF are the result of decreased cardiac output from impaired cardiac pumping power and congestion that involves the pulmonary and/or venous systems (Box 48-2).

Left Ventricular Failure

When the left ventricle is unable to pump enough blood to meet the body's demands, major consequences occur. The first consequences are the signs and symptoms of decreased cardiac output. The second is pulmonary congestion. Increased pressure in the left side of the heart backs up into the pulmonary system, and the lungs become congested with fluid. Fluid leaks through the engorged capillaries and permeates air spaces in the lungs. If during each heartbeat the right ventricle pumps out just one more drop of blood than the left, then within only 3 hours the pulmonary blood volume will have expanded by 500 mL. Pulmonary edema and **pleural effusion** (an abnormal accumulation of fluid in the thoracic cavity between the visceral and parietal pleurae) occur. Signs and symptoms of this condition include dyspnea; orthopnea; pulmonary crackles; wheezing; pink, frothy sputum; and cough.

Right Ventricular Failure

Right ventricular failure occurs when the right ventricle is unable to pump effectively against increased pressure in the pulmonary circulation. Most often the increased pressure is the result of blood backing up from a failing left ventricle, but right ventricular failure can also be a result of chronic pulmonary disease (cor pulmonale) and pulmonary hypertension. The right ventricle's inability to pump blood forward into the lungs results in peripheral congestion and an inability to accommodate all the venous blood that is normally returned to the right side of the heart. Venous blood is reflected backward into the systemic circulation. Increased venous volume and pressure force fluid out of the vasculature into interstitial tissue (peripheral edema). Edema appears in dependent areas of the body such as the sa-

Box 48-2 Classifying and Staging Heart Failure

NEW YORK HEART ASSOCIATION HEART FAILURE CLASSIFICATION

The New York Heart Association classification is a universal gauge of heart failure severity based on physical limitations.

Class I: Minimal
- No limitations.
- Ordinary physical activity does not cause undue fatigue, dyspnea, palpitations, or angina.

Class II: Mild
- Slightly limited physical activity.
- Comfortable at rest.
- Ordinary physical activity results in fatigue, palpitations, dyspnea, or angina.

Class III: Moderate
- Markedly limited physical activity.
- Comfortable at rest.
- Less than ordinary activity causes fatigue, palpitations, dyspnea, or anginal pain.

Class IV: Severe
- Patient unable to perform any physical activity without discomfort.
- Angina or symptoms of cardiac inefficiency may develop at rest. Physical activity increases discomfort.

AMERICAN COLLEGE OF CARDIOLOGY AND AMERICAN HEART ASSOCIATION (ACC/AHA) HEART FAILURE STAGES

Stage A Patient is at high risk for developing heart failure but has no structural disorder of the heart. The patient has a primary condition that is strongly associated with heart failure (such as diabetes mellitus, hypertension, substance abuse, or history of rheumatic fever) but no signs or symptoms of heart failure.

Stage B Patient has a structural disorder of the heart, such as left ventricular remodeling, left ventricular hypertrophy, valvular heart disease, or previous myocardial infarction, but has never developed symptoms of heart failure.

Stage C Patient has past or current symptoms of heart failure associated with underlying structural disease. The patient may display signs of dyspnea or fatigue, but is responding to therapy.

Stage D Patient has end-stage disease and requires specialized treatment strategies that may include mechanical circulatory support, continuous inotropic infusions, heart transplant, or hospice care. These patients are frequently hospitalized and cannot be discharged without symptom recurrence.

The New York Heart Association (NYHA) classification system. Available at www.hearthealthywomen.org. American College of Cardiology and American Heart Association. (ACC/AHA). Heart failure: classification and stages. The AHA/ACC stages of heart failure.

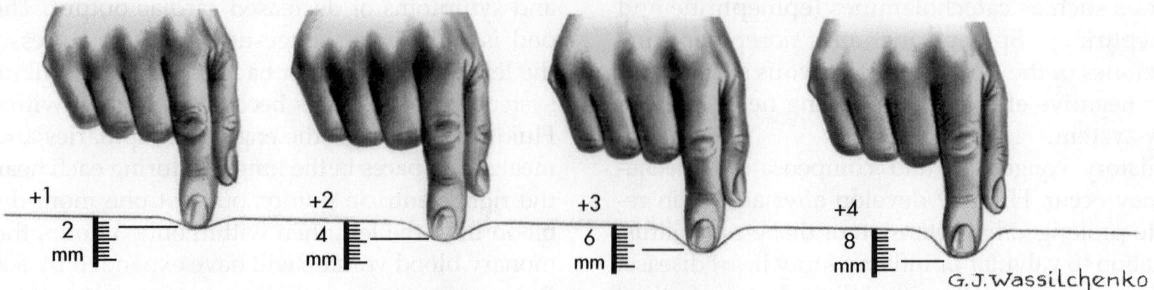

FIGURE 48-17 Scale for pitting edema depth.

Table 48-6 Pitting Edema Scale

SCALE	DEGREE	RESPONSE
1+ Trace	2 mm (0-1/16 inch)	Rapid
2+ Mild	4 mm (0-1/4 inch)	10-15 seconds
3+ Moderate	6 mm (1/4-1/2 inch)	1-2 minutes
4+ Severe	8 mm (1/2-1 inch)	2-5 minutes

crum when supine and the feet and ankles while in an upright position. As right ventricular failure continues, edema may progress to pitting edema and move up the legs into the thighs, external genitalia, and lower trunk. To check for edema, press down on the tissue for several seconds and lift the finger. If the depression does not fill almost immediately, pitting edema is present (Figure 48-17; Table 48-6).

One liter of fluid equals 1 kg (2.2 pounds); a weight gain of 2.2 pounds signifies a gain of 1 L of body fluid. The liver may become congested, and fluid can accumulate in the abdomen (ascites). Distended neck veins may be observed when the patient is sitting.

Clinical Manifestations

Manifestations of HF are those associated with decreased cardiac output, left ventricular failure, and right ventricular failure (Box 48-3).

Assessment

Subjective data include complaints of dyspnea, **orthopnea** (an abnormal condition in which a person must sit or stand to breathe deeply or comfortably) or paroxysmal nocturnal dyspnea (sudden awakening from sleep because of shortness of breath), and cough. The patient may report fatigue, anxiety, weight gain from fluid retention, and edema. Physical symptoms and impaired physical function cause psychosocial stress. Patients with New York Heart Association (NYHA) class III or IV HF are at very high risk for major depression (Artinian, 2003). Document any pain (anginal or abdominal) and the patient's stated ability to perform ADLs.

Collection of **objective data** includes noting presence of respiratory distress, the number of pillows required to breath comfortably while attempting to rest (orthopnea), edema (site, degree of pitting), abdominal distention secondary to ascites, weight gain, adventitious breath sounds, abnormal heart sounds (gallop and murmurs), activity intolerance, and jugular vein distention. Blood flow to the kidneys is diminished, resulting in oliguria. Oxygen deficit in tissues results in cyanosis and general debilitation.

Box 48-3 Signs and Symptoms of Heart Failure

DECREASED CARDIAC OUTPUT
- Fatigue
- Anginal pain
- Anxiety
- Oliguria
- Decreased gastrointestinal motility
- Pale, cool skin
- Weight gain
- Restlessness

LEFT VENTRICULAR FAILURE
- Dyspnea
- Paroxysmal nocturnal dyspnea
- Cough
- Frothy, blood-tinged sputum
- Orthopnea
- Pulmonary crackles (moist popping and cracking sounds heard most often at the end of inspiration)
- Radiographic evidence of pulmonary vascular congestion with pleural effusion

RIGHT VENTRICULAR FAILURE
- Distended jugular veins
- Anorexia, nausea, and abdominal distention
- Liver enlargement with right upper quadrant pain
- Ascites
- Edema in feet, ankles, sacrum; may progress up the legs into thighs, external genitalia, and lower trunk

Diagnostic Tests

Diagnosis is based on presenting signs and symptoms of HF and is confirmed by various diagnostic tests. A chest radiograph reveals pulmonary vascular congestion, pleural effusion, and cardiomegaly (cardiac enlargement). ECG reveals cardiac dysrhythmias. The most noninvasive diagnostic tool for evaluating a patient with HF is an echocardiogram. Echocardiography is done to determine valvular heart disease, presence of pericardial fluid, HF (the percentage of end-diastolic blood volume ejected during systole), and ejection fraction. Pulmonary artery catheterization is done to assess right and left ventricular function.

Exercise stress testing is done to determine activity tolerance and severity of underlying ischemic cardiovascular disease. **Cardiac catheterization** may be performed to detect cardiac abnormalities and underlying cardiovascular disease. **MUGA scanning** is ordered to evaluate cardiac function, ejection fraction, and wall motion abnormalities.

Laboratory tests include electrolytes, sodium, calcium, magnesium, and potassium levels. Blood chemistry will reveal elevated blood urea nitrogen (BUN) and creatinine resulting from decreased glomerular filtration; liver function values (alanine aminotransferase, aspartate transaminase, gamma glutamyltransferase, alkaline phosphatase) will be mildly elevated. **BNP** is a neurohormone secreted by the heart in response to expansion of ventricular volume and pressure overload. With a normal BNP level of less than 100 pg/mL, the patient does not have HF; a level greater than 100 pg/mL is suggestive of HF. Levels greater than 700 pg/mL indicate decompensated HF. A higher level of BNP correlates with an increase in the patient's signs and symptoms of HF. BNP is useful in monitoring chronic HF. Arterial blood gases may reveal hypoxemia and acid-base imbalance.

Medical Management

The objectives of medical management include increasing cardiac efficiency with digoxin and vasodilators (nitroglycerin, isosorbide) for expanded output. Digoxin, a digitalis glycoside that was once the cornerstone of HF treatment, is now used less often and at lower doses. ACE inhibitors such as captopril (Capoten), enalapril (Vasotec), ramipril (Altace), benazepril (Lotensin), lisinopril (Prinivil, Zestril), quinapril (Accupril), and fosinopril (Monopril) decrease peripheral vascular resistance, improve cardiac output, and have proven to extend the lives of patients with HF and lengthen the time between admissions. In January 1999, the Advisory Council to Improve Outcomes Nationwide in Heart Failure (ACTION-HF) recommended that all patients with stable class II or III NYHA HF (see Box 48-2), or stage C or D American College of Cardiology and American Heart Association HF due to left ventricular dysfunction receive a beta blocker to prevent cardiac remodeling. (Remodeling occurs when the left ventricle dilates, hypertrophies, and develops a more spherical shape. The shape change stresses the ventricle walls, increases the magnitude of regurgitation through the mitral valve, and depresses mechanical performance.) Two beta blockers that the FDA has approved to treat HF are carvedilol (an alpha, nonselective beta blocker) and metoprolol. Beta blockers inhibit chronic activation of the sympathetic nervous system. Beta blockers have been so effective at reducing symptoms, improving clinical status, and reducing mortality and hospitalizations that the guidelines identify them as the most significant medications for HF management (Lewis et al., 2007). Angiotensin II receptor blockers such as irbesartan (Avapro), losartan (Cozaar), and valsartan (Diovan) selectively and competitively block the vasoconstrictive and aldosterone-secreting effects of angiotensin, leading to vasodilation. Research for their use in HF is in progress. Angiotensin II receptor blockers are not a substitute for ACE inhibitors unless an ACE inhibitor is clearly not tolerated. In 2001 the FDA approved nesiritide (Natrecor) for the IV treatment of patients with acutely decompensated HF who have shortness of breath (i.e., dyspnea) at rest or with minimal activity. Nesiritide is the first of the drug class called human BNPs. It reduces pulmonary capillary pressure, helps improve breathing, and causes vasodilation with increase in stroke volume and cardiac output (Riggs, 2004).

An additional goal of therapeutic management is to lower oxygen requirements of the body systems; this is accomplished by elevating the head of the bed to 45 degrees or having the patient sit on the edge of the bed with arms resting on the overbed table to reduce myocardial oxygen demand and decrease circulating volume returning to the heart. Oxygen therapy provides oxygen to the tissues if the patient is hypoxic.

Edema and pulmonary congestion are treated with diuretics, a sodium-restricted diet, and restriction of fluid intake. Weigh the patient daily to monitor fluid retention.

Once the workload of the heart is decreased and diuresis of engorged tissues and organs is achieved, the patient's activity level will increase. These objectives are achieved by medication therapy and activity per a physician's orders. Medication therapy with digoxin, ACE inhibitors, thiazide, and loop diuretics is a common initial treatment (Table 48-7).

A biventricular pacemaker can improve symptoms and function, improve quality of life, and decrease hospitalization for patients with HF who also have conduction system disease (Chojnowski, 2007).

The use of an implantable cardioverter-defibrillator can decrease the risk for sudden cardiac death for patients with a family history of sudden cardiac death, life-threatening dysrhythmias, or mild to moderate HF who have an ejection fraction of less than 30% (Chojnowski, 2007).

In acute HF, administration of oxygen and medication should be of first concern. Decreasing oxygen requirements through rest will slow the heart rate and increase cardiac and respiratory reserves. Anxiety produced from the signs and symptoms and the fear of a life-threatening situation can be allayed by reassurance and explanation. Accurate interventions, observation, and reporting reduce the threat of complications such as embolus, thrombophlebitis, MI, and pulmonary edema.

Nursing Interventions

Nursing interventions include measures to prevent disease progression and complications. Monitor vital signs for changes. Note any signs of respiratory distress or pulmonary edema. Carefully monitor signs and symptoms of left-sided versus right-sided HF. Urinary output is typically low, and edema is soft and pitting; legs are elevated to decrease edema.

Also note an increase in abdominal girth and total body weight as indicators of fluid retention, which is common in HF. Auscultate the lung fields to detect presence of crackles and wheezes; also note coughing and complaints of dyspnea. Restful sleep may be possible only in the sitting position or with the aid of extra pillows. Activity intolerance is accompanied by extreme fatigue and anxiety. Assess patients for depression. Explain to patients with HF and depression that the depression is readily treatable and that several approaches to treatment can be used separately or in combination, including pharmacologic therapy, psychosocial and psychotherapeutic interventions, and cardiac rehabilitation.

Table 48-7 Medications for Heart Failure

Generic (Trade)	Action	Nursing Interventions
CARDIAC GLYCOSIDES		
Digitalis preparations, such as digoxin (Lanoxin)	Strengthen cardiac force and efficiency Slow heart rate Increase circulation, effecting diuresis	Monitor apical pulse to ensure rate greater than 60 bpm; monitor for toxicity (nausea, vomiting, anorexia, dysrhythmia, bradycardia, tachycardia, headache, fatigue, and blurred or colored vision).
DIURETICS		
Thiazides, such as chlorothiazide (Diuril), hydrochlorothiazide (Esidrix, Hydrodiuril)	Increase renal secretion of sodium Are safe for long-term use Block sodium and water reabsorption in kidney tubules	Monitor electrolyte depletion; weigh daily to ascertain fluid loss.
Sulfonamides (loop diuretic), such as furosemide (Lasix), bumetanide (Bumex)	Act rapidly for less responsive edema	Administer in AM to prevent nocturia. Monitor for electrolyte depletion. Consider sulfa allergy (furosemide).
Aldosterone antagonist (potassium-sparing), such as spironolactone (Aldactone)	Relieves edema and ascites that do not respond to usual diuretics Blocks sodium-retaining and potassium-excreting properties of aldosterone	Monitor for gastrointestinal irritation and hyperkalemia.
POTASSIUM SUPPLEMENTS		
Potassium (K-Lyte)	Restores electrolyte loss	Monitor blood potassium levels.
SEDATIVES AND ANALGESICS		
Temazepam (Restoril)	Promotes rest and comfort	Monitor rest and sleep benefits.
Morphine	Relieves chest and abdominal pain, reduces anxiety, and decreases myocardial oxygen demands Lessens dyspnea	
NITRATES		
Nitroglycerin (Cardabid)	Dilates arteries, improves blood flow Reduces blood pressure	Monitor blood pressure for hypotension. Monitor for headache and flushing.
ACE INHIBITORS		
Captopril (Capoten) Enalapril (Vasotec) Vamipril (Altace) Benazepril (Lotensin) Lisinopril (Prinivil; Zestril) Quinapril (Accupril) Fosinopril (Monopril) Moexipril (Univasc) Perindopril (Aceon) Trandolapril (Mavik)	Act as antihypertensives and reduce peripheral arterial resistance and improve cardiac output	Observe patient closely for a precipitous drop in blood pressure within 3 hours of initial dose; monitor blood pressure closely. Monitor blood potassium levels.

ACE, Angiotensin-converting enzyme; *CHF*, congestive heart failure; *HF*, heart failure; *I&O*, intake and output.

Table 48-7 Medications for Heart Failure—cont'd

Generic (Trade)	Action	Nursing Interventions
BETA-ADRENERGIC BLOCKERS		
Carvedilol (Coreg)	Directly blocks the sympathetic nervous system's negative effects on the failing heart.	Start at low dose, increasing the dosage slowly every 2 weeks as tolerated by the patient. Monitor blood pressure and notify prescriber of significant change. Monitor pulse: if <50 bpm, hold drug, call prescriber.
Metoprolol (Toprol-XL)	Blocks $beta_2$-adrenergic receptors in bronchial and vascular smooth muscle. Lowers blood pressure by beta blocking effects; reduces elevated rennin plasma levels.	Monitor I&O, weigh daily. Monitor apical or radial pulse before administration. Notify prescriber of any significant changes or pulse <50 bpm.
INOTROPIC AGENTS		
Dobutamine (Dobutrex IV) Dopamine HCl (Intropin IV)	Low-dose dobutamine and low-dose dopamine relatively safe on medical-surgical units; in low doses, dilate renal blood vessels, stimulating renal blood flow and glomerular filtration rate, which in turn promotes sodium excretion, often helping CHF patients improve	Make certain patient is not taking monoamine oxidase (MAO) inhibitors, tricyclic antidepressants, phenytoin (Dilantin), or haloperidol (Haldol). Record accurate I&O; assess for dizziness, nausea, vomiting, headache. Assess vital signs carefully every 15 minutes for first 2 hours, then every 2 hours for following 4 hours, and finally once a shift. Observe carefully for extravasation, tachycardia, bradycardia, angina, palpitations, hypotension, hypertension, azotemia, and anxiety.
HUMAN B-TYPE NATRIURETIC PEPTIDES		
Nesiritide (Natrecor)	New class of synthetic HF drugs; causes arterial and venous dilation, thereby decreasing systemic vascular resistance and pulmonary arterial pressures; decreases blood pressure, promotes better left ventricle ejection, and increases cardiac output; may also promote diuresis; an IV treatment for patients with acutely compensated CHF.	Observe carefully for hypotension. Natrecor should not be used for patients with cardiogenic shock or with a systolic blood pressure <90 mm Hg.

Key Components of Care

The Institute for Healthcare Improvement recommends these components of care for all patients with HF (unless patient cannot tolerate them or unless contraindicated):

- Assess left ventricular systolic function.
- At discharge from hospital (when left ventricular ejection fraction is less than 40%, indicating systolic dysfunction), administer ACE inhibitor or angiotensin.
- At discharge, administer an anticoagulant if the patient has chronic or recurrent atrial fibrillation.
- Encourage smoking cessation.
- Instruct the patient at discharge regarding activity, diet, medication, follow-up appointment, weight monitoring, and what to do if symptoms worsen.
- Provide influenza and pneumococcal immunization.
- At discharge, institute optional beta blocker therapy for stabilized patients with left ventricular systolic dysfunction who have no contraindications.

The new guidelines also advocate a discussion of end-of-life decisions with the patient and the family. Patients should talk with their health care providers about treatment preferences, advance directives, living wills, power of attorney for health care, and life-support issues. Because HF is progressive, patients should make these decisions while they are capable of expressing choices. Hospice services, originally developed to assist cancer patients, are appropriate for the patient with end-stage HF (Nursing Care Plan 48-1; Box 48-4; and Patient Teaching box).

Nursing Care Plan 48-1 The Patient with Heart Failure

Mr. Domrose is a 61-year-old clinical administrator. He was admitted to the hospital with the diagnosis of heart failure. He has a history of hypertension and coronary artery disease. Six months ago he had a myocardial infarction. He has felt tired for the past 3 weeks and has been experiencing increased dyspnea. He has noticed some edema in his ankles and is concerned about gaining 5 pounds in the past week and having an increasing intolerance to exertion. The nursing admission history revealed:

- Mr. Domrose has not been taking his antihypertensive medication regularly. He did not like the side effects and stopped taking the medication, but he was too embarrassed to call his physician.
- Vital signs revealed an elevated blood pressure.
- He has shortness of breath during activities and when lying down.
- Pitting edema is seen on both ankles.
- Crackles are heard bilaterally in the lungs.

NURSING DIAGNOSIS ***Decreased cardiac output, related to cardiac insufficiency***

Patient Goals and Expected Outcomes	Nursing Intervention	Evaluation
Patient will have decreased dyspnea with activities and when lying in bed within 24 hours Patient will have decreased adventitious lung sounds Patient will have oxygen saturations at 91% with prescribed oxygen within 24 hours Patient will have vital signs within acceptable levels within 72 hours Patient will have decreased edema and weight loss of 5 pounds within 72 hours	Maintain initial bed rest with stress-free environment. Maintain semi-Fowler's to high Fowler's position. Explain and encourage gradual increases in activity to prevent a sudden increase in cardiac workload. Monitor respirations, lung sounds, heart sounds, and vital signs every 4 hours. Palpate pedal pulses, and assess capillary refill every 8 hours. Administer digitalis, diuretics, angiotensin-converting enzyme inhibitors, vasodilators, beta blockers, and antihypertensive medication as prescribed. Monitor intake and output and weigh daily. Monitor oxygen saturation with pulse oximetry every 4 hours. Administer prescribed oxygen.	Patient has decreased crackles in lung fields within 24 hours of admission. Patient has an oximetry reading of 91% oxygen saturation with oxygen prescribed within 24 hours of admission. Patient has a heart rate of 80 bpm, respiratory rate of 22 breaths/min, and blood pressure of 148/86 mm Hg within 72 hours of admission. Patient has a weight loss of 5 pounds within 72 hours of admission. Patient has pedal pitting edema decreased to 1+ within 2 days of admission.

NURSING DIAGNOSIS ***Anxiety, related to change in health status, lifestyle changes, fear of death, or threats to self-concept.***

Patient Goals and Expected Outcomes	Nursing Intervention	Evaluation
Patient will verbalize anxieties within 48 hours of admission Patient will demonstrate reduction of anxiety by enjoying periods of rest and sleep undisturbed for 6 hours within 48 hours of admission	Identify coping techniques. Provide information to decrease fears. Identify support systems. Provide calm, relaxing environment. Administer antianxiety medications per physician's orders as needed. Help patient cope with lifestyle changes. He may feel anxious due to changes in body image, family and social roles, and finances. Focus on progress patient is making in managing his condition. Encourage patient to participate in health care decisions, and allow him to release anger and frustration. Allow patient to sleep undisturbed for 6 hours when vital signs are stable.	Patient is verbalizing anger and frustration over current medical conditions within 48 hours of admission. Patient is sleeping 5 to 6 hours per night within 48 hours of admission.

 Nursing Care Plan 48-1 The Patient with Heart Failure—cont'd

Critical Thinking Questions

1. Mr. Domrose is experiencing severe dyspnea, with the presence of crackles bilaterally in all lung fields. His pulse is 108 bpm, and respirations are 33 breaths/min. When performing his morning activities of daily living, what nursing interventions would be most beneficial?
2. On assessing Mr. Domrose's skin, the nurse notes 4+ pitting edema in his lower extremities. A weight gain of 6 pounds in the past 24 hours is also noted. For therapeutic diuresis to occur, what would the medical management include?
3. Mr. Domrose puts his call light on to request assistance to ambulate. The nurse notes subclavicular retractions and cyanosis of his nailbeds. What would be the most appropriate nursing actions?

Box 48-4 Guidelines for Nursing Interventions for the Patient with Heart Failure

- Provide oxygenation.
- Administer oxygen by nasal cannula per protocol as prescribed for dyspnea.
- Patient should be well supported in semi-Fowler's or high Fowler's position.
- Reinforce importance of conservation of energy and planning for activities that avoid fatigue.
- Encourage activity within prescribed restrictions; monitor for intolerance to activity (dyspnea, fatigue, increased pulse rate that does not stabilize).
- Assist with activities of daily living as necessary; encourage independence within patient's limitations.
- Provide diversionary activity that will assist in conservation of energy.
- Monitor for signs of fluid and potassium imbalance; record daily weights, intake and output.
- Provide skin care, particularly over edematous areas; use prophylactic measures to prevent skin impairment.
- Assist in maintaining an adequate nutritional intake while observing prescribed dietary modifications (sodium restrictions).
- Monitor for constipation; give prescribed stool softeners.
- Give prescribed medications:
  —Digitalis (take apical pulse before administration)
  —Diuretics (assess for hypokalemia)
  —Vasodilators, angiotensin-converting enzyme inhibitors, beta blockers
  —Medications to reduce anxiety and promote sleep
- Provide the patient and the family opportunities to discuss their concerns.
- Teach patient about the disorder and self-care.

 Patient Teaching

Heart Failure

- Monitor for signs and symptoms of recurring heart failure and report them to the physician or clinic:
  —Weight gain of 2 to 3 pounds (1 to 1.5 kg) over a short period (about 2 days)
  —Shortness of breath
  —Orthopnea
  —Swelling of ankles, feet, or abdomen
  —Persistent cough
  —Frequent nighttime urination
- Avoid fatigue and plan activity to allow for rest periods.
- Plan and eat meals within prescribed sodium restrictions. Avoid salty foods.
- Avoid drugs with high sodium content (e.g., some laxatives and antacids, Alka-Seltzer); read the labels. Ideally, limit sodium intake to 2 g/day.
- Maintain low-fat diet, with fat intake less than 30% of total calories.
- Eat several small meals rather than three large meals per day.
- Take medications as prescribed.
- If several medications are prescribed, develop a method to facilitate accurate administration.
- When taking digoxin, check own pulse rate daily; report a rate of less than 60 bpm to the physician. Do not take digoxin if pulse is less than 60 bpm.
- Take diuretics as prescribed.
- Weigh self daily at same time.
- Eat foods high in potassium and low in sodium (such as oranges and bananas).
- Take all prescribed medications.
- Report signs of hypotension (lightheadedness, rapid pulse, syncope) to the physician.
- Avoid alcohol when taking vasodilators.
- Reinforce the importance of regular exercise once heart failure is stabilized. Thorough treatment regimen may allow the patient to increase activity level over time. The physician may ultimately recommend 30 to 45 minutes of aerobic exercise three or four times a week to improve patient's well-being.
- Report to the physician for follow-up as directed.

Prognosis
Approximately 10% of patients diagnosed with HF die in the first year, and 50% within 5 years. HF is a chronic condition. With treatment advances, many people now survive for years with damaged hearts. With the advent of ACE inhibitors and new research on the benefits of prescribed exercise, improvement in the quality of life for HF patients is being seen.

PULMONARY EDEMA

Etiology and Pathophysiology
Pulmonary edema (the accumulation of extravascular fluid in lung tissues and alveoli, most often caused by HF) is an acute and extensive, life-threatening complication of HF caused by severe left ventricular dysfunction. Fluid from the left side of the heart backs up into the pulmonary vasculature and results in extravascular fluid accumulation in the interstitial space and alveoli. This causes the patient to "drown" in the secretions.

Clinical Manifestations
The patient exhibits signs of severe respiratory distress when pulmonary edema occurs. Frothy sputum is produced from air mixing with the fluid in the alveoli; the sputum is blood-tinged from blood cells that have exuded into the alveoli.

Assessment
See Box 48-5 for signs and symptoms of pulmonary edema.

Diagnostic Tests
Diagnosis is made by observing signs and symptoms and is supported by chest radiograph and arterial blood gas studies. $Pa{O_2}$ and $Pa{CO_2}$ may reveal respiratory alkalosis or acidosis.

Medical Management
Medical management involves simultaneous interventions to promote oxygenation, improve cardiac output, and reduce pulmonary congestion. Without emergency treatment, respiratory failure may occur (Table 48-8).

Box 48-5 Signs and Symptoms of Pulmonary Edema

- Restlessness
- Vague uneasiness
- Agitation
- Disorientation
- Diaphoresis
- Severe dyspnea
- Tachypnea
- Tachycardia
- Pallor or cyanosis
- Cough production of large quantities of blood-tinged, frothy sputum
- Audible wheezing, crackles
- Cold extremities

Nursing Interventions
Interventions include administering oxygen. Place the patient upright with legs in a dependent position to decrease venous return to the heart, relieving pulmonary congestion and dyspnea. Monitor arterial blood gases and administer drugs as ordered. Auscultate lung sounds often. Provide emotional support; remain with patient. Explain all procedures. Monitor vital signs, fluid I&O, and serum electrolytes.

Nursing diagnoses and interventions for the patient with pulmonary edema include but are not limited to the following:

Nursing Diagnoses	Nursing Interventions
Excess fluid volume, related to fluid accumulation in pulmonary vessels	Administer medications as ordered. Carefully monitor I&O. Weigh patient at same time each day. Assess for edema.
Impaired gas exchange, related to fluid in lungs	Assess for signs of hypoxia, such as restlessness, disorientation, and irritability. Monitor arterial blood gases per physician's order. Administer oxygen per physician's order. Position patient in high Fowler's position with legs in dependent position, or sitting and leaning forward on overbed table to facilitate breathing.
Anxiety, related to fear of suffocation and death	Promote optimal air exchange to decrease anxiety. Assess level of anxiety and coping mechanisms. Deliver nursing interventions in a supportive, kind, and proficient manner. Assess support systems available to patient and mobilize resources.

Prognosis
Pulmonary edema is a grave, life-threatening condition that is usually responsive to aggressive interventions.

VALVULAR HEART DISEASE

Etiology and Pathophysiology
Normal heart valves function to maintain the direction of blood flow through the right atrium, right ventricle, lungs, left atrium, and left ventricle and to the rest of the body. Heart valves operate by passively opening

Table 48-8 Medical Management for Acute Pulmonary Edema

INTERVENTION	RATIONALE
Patient in high Fowler's position or over side of bed with arms supported on bedside table	Promotes expansion of lungs; legs in dependent position causes venous pooling and reduction in venous return (preload)
Morphine sulfate, 10-15 mg IV; titrated	Decreases patient anxiety; relieves pain; slows respirations; reduces venous return; decreases oxygen demand; dilates the pulmonary and systemic blood vessels
Oxygen at 40%-100%; nonrebreather face mask; intubation as needed	Promotes oxygenation; increased tidal volume also promotes removal of secretions from alveoli
Administer sublingual nitroglycerin	Increases myocardial blood flow
Diuretics: furosemide (Lasix), bumetanide (Bumex) (IV)	Reduce pulmonary edema by decreasing the fluid in the lungs and increasing excretion through the kidneys
Insert Foley catheter	Allows patient to rest and conserve energy; monitors urinary output after IV furosemide has been administered.
Inotropic agents: dobutamine (Dobutrex), amrinone (Inocor)	Increase myocardial contractility without increasing oxygen consumption Increase peripheral vasodilation Increase cardiac output
Nitroprusside (Nitropress)	A potent vasodilator; improves myocardial contraction and reduces pulmonary congestion

and closing in response to pressure changes in the heart. The tricuspid valve is located between the right atrium and the right ventricle. The pulmonary semilunar valve allows blood to flow through the pulmonary artery into the lungs. The mitral (bicuspid) valve is located between the left atrium and the left ventricle. The aortic semilunar valve allows blood to flow from the left ventricle into the aorta. Valvular disease occurs when the valves are compromised and do not open and close properly. Two valvular problems are **stenosis,** which is a thickening of the valve tissue, causing the valve to narrow, and **insufficiency,** which occurs when the valve is unable to close completely. Valvular heart disorders include mitral stenosis, mitral insufficiency, aortic insufficiency, aortic stenosis, tricuspid insufficiency, tricuspid stenosis, pulmonary insufficiency, and pulmonary stenosis.

Valvular disorders occur in children, adolescents, and adults, primarily from congenital conditions. Another prominent factor in the development of valvular disease is a history of rheumatic fever. Clinical symptoms of valvular heart disease tend to occur 10 to 40 years after an episode of rheumatic fever. Because the blood volume and workload of the heart are greater on the left than on the right, the mitral and aortic valves are affected more frequently.

Clinical Manifestations

Signs and symptoms seen in valvular disorders are related to decreased cardiac output (Table 48-9).

Assessment

Subjective data include the patient's statement of a history of rheumatic fever and of an inability to perform activities and ADLs without fatigue or weakness. Ask the patient about his or her chest pain, including its quality, duration, onset, precipitating factors, and measures that provide relief. The patient may complain of heart palpitations, lightheadedness, dizziness, or fainting. The history may include a patient statement of weight gain. Dyspnea, exertional dyspnea, nocturnal (nighttime) dyspnea, and orthopnea are often reported, depending on the degree of HF.

Collection of **objective data** includes observing for a heart murmur and noting the character and the presence of any adventitious breath sounds (crackles, wheezes) and edema (pitting or nonpitting).

Diagnostic Tests

The diagnostic tests used to confirm valvular heart disease are chest radiograph, ECG, echocardiogram, and cardiac catheterization.

Medical Management

Medical management includes activity limitations, sodium-restricted diet, diuretics, digoxin, and antidysrhythmics.

When medical therapy no longer alleviates clinical symptoms or when diagnostic evidence exists of progressive myocardial failure, surgery is often performed. The surgery may include the following:

- **Open mitral commissurotomy:** A surgical splitting of the fused mitral valve leaflet for treating stenosis of the mitral valve.
- **Valve replacement:** Replacement of the stenosed or incompetent valve with a bioprosthetic or mechanical valve. Commonly used valves include tilting disks, porcine (pig) heterografts (tissue taken from one species and grafted onto another), homografts (a graft of tissue obtained from a member of the same species as the individual receiving it), and ball-in-cage valves.

Table 48-9 Clinical Manifestations of Valvular Heart Diseases

NURSING DIAGNOSES	CLINICAL MANIFESTATIONS
Mitral valve stenosis	Dyspnea on exertion, hemoptysis; fatigue; palpitations; loud, accentuated S_1; low-pitched, rumbling diastolic murmur; atrial fibrillation on ECG
Mitral valve regurgitation	**Acute**: Generally poorly tolerated, with fulminating pulmonary edema and shock developing rapidly; new systolic murmur **Chronic:** Weakness, fatigue, exertional dyspnea, palpitations; an S_3 gallop
Mitral valve prolapse	Palpitations, dyspnea, chest pain, activity intolerance, syncope; midsystolic click
Aortic valve stenosis	Angina, syncope, dyspnea on exertion, heart failure; normal or soft S_1, diminished or absent S_2
Aortic valve regurgitation	**Acute**: Abrupt onset of profound dyspnea, chest pain, left ventricular failure, and shock **Chronic**: Fatigue, exertional dyspnea, orthopnea, paroxysmal nocturnal dyspnea; water-hammer pulse; heaving precordial impulse; diminished or absent S_1, S_3, or S_4
Tricuspid and pulmonic stenosis	**Tricuspid**: Peripheral edema, ascites, hepatomegaly; diastolic low-pitched murmur **Pulmonic:** Fatigue, loud midsystolic murmur

From Lewis, S.L., et al. (2007). *Medical-surgical nursing: Assessment and management of clinical problems.* (7th ed.). St. Louis: Mosby.
ECG, Electrocardiogram.

Nursing Interventions and Patient Teaching

Nursing interventions focus on assisting with ADLs, relieving specific symptoms associated with decreased cardiac output, and promoting comfort. Administer the prescribed medications (diuretics, digoxin, and antidysrhythmics). Also record I&O, daily weight, respiratory rate and rhythm, auscultation of breath sounds, heart sounds, and blood pressure. Check for capillary perfusion, pedal pulses, and presence of edema. Have the patient consume a sodium-restricted diet for control of edema. Maintain oxygen therapy as prescribed. Discuss with the patient a plan for rest periods, and identify those ADLs that produce fatigue and require assistance.

Nursing diagnoses and interventions for the patient with valvular heart disease include but are not limited to the following:

Nursing Diagnoses	Nursing Interventions
Activity intolerance, related to: • weakness • fatigue • dyspnea	Balance activities with rest periods. Identify fatiguing activities and obtain assistance as needed. Use oxygen as prescribed by physician.
Excess fluid volume, related to decreased cardiac output	Administer prescribed oxygen, digoxin, diuretics, and antidysrhythmics. Monitor I&O. Weigh patient daily. Perform respiratory assessment. Perform cardiovascular assessment. Inspect for presence of edema. Obtain vital signs routinely. Maintain sodium-restricted diet.

Patient teaching focuses on medications, dietary management, activity limitations, diagnostic tests, surgical interventions, and postoperative care as appropriate. Discuss with the patient the disease process and associated symptoms to report to the physician. Explain antibiotic prophylaxis to prevent infective endocarditis. Explain the importance of notifying the dentist, urologist, and gynecologist of valvular heart disease. Patient must remain on higher dosages of warfarin after valve replacement surgery. Carefully monitor PT and INR. Discuss with the patient the need to maintain good oral hygiene and make regular visits to the dentist.

Prognosis

The prognosis for valvular heart disease varies, depending on the specific disease. The prognosis after surgery is fair to good with amelioration (improvement) of signs and symptoms but often without resolution of all abnormalities.

INFLAMMATORY DISORDERS OF THE HEART

All cardiac tissues are susceptible to inflammation, and HF can be a serious and rapid result of the inflammatory process.

RHEUMATIC HEART DISEASE

Etiology and Pathophysiology

Rheumatic heart disease, is the result of rheumatic fever and the clinical manifestation of carditis resulting from an inadequately treated childhood pharyngeal or upper respiratory tract infection (group A β-hemolytic streptococci). By the 1980s rheumatic fever had almost disappeared in developed countries such as the United States. However, it remained common and severe in most developing countries. Antibiotics, especially penicillin, are responsible for the decline in rheumatic fever. A great deal of interest has been generated by a number of "mini-epidemics," with 10 to 75 cases of acute rheumatic fever in a single region. In searching for the cause of the reappearance, researchers have isolated highly virulent strains of the same types of group A streptococci that were prevalent in epidemic rheumatic fever more than 30 years ago (Lewis et al., 2007).

Ineffective treatment of infection results in delayed reaction and inflammation of the cardiac tissues and the central nervous system, joints, skin, and subcutaneous tissues. Ninety percent of patients with rheumatic fever are between 5 and 15 years of age. The onset of rheumatic fever is usually sudden, often occurring in from 1 to 5 symptom-free weeks after recovery from pharyngitis (sore throat) or from scarlet fever. However, rheumatic fever may progress with symptoms and go undiagnosed and untreated. Years later the patient may develop clinical manifestations of valvular heart disease.

Rheumatic heart disease can affect the pericardium, myocardium, or endocardium. The affected tissue develops small areas of necrosis, which heal, leaving scar tissue. The heart valves are typically the most affected by Aschoff's nodules (vegetative growth) and become fibrous and incompetent. With healing, the valves become thickened and deformed. These changes result in valvular stenosis and insufficiency, varying in extent and severity.

Clinical Manifestations

Fever, increased pulse, epistaxis, anemia, joint involvement, and nodules on joints and subcutaneous tissue may be noted. Carditis can develop. When valvular involvement occurs, signs and symptoms are specific to each condition.

Assessment

Collection of **subjective data** may reveal joint pain (polyarthritis) and chest pain. Lethargy and fatigue are also present.

Objective data include skin manifestations of small erythematous circles and wavy lines on the trunk and abdomen that appear and disappear rapidly (erythema marginatum). The nurse may observe involuntary, purposeless movement of the muscles if Sydenham's chorea (St. Vitus' dance), a disorder of the central nervous system, is present. Heart murmur may be auscultated if the patient has carditis with valve involvement. Rheumatic heart disease is characterized by heart murmurs resulting from stenosis or insufficiency of the valves.

Diagnostic Tests

Diagnosis is made through signs and symptoms and supported by laboratory study results. An echocardiogram is done to determine the extent of damage to the valves and myocardium. An ECG shows cardiac dysrhythmia. Cardiac murmurs or friction rub can be heard. No specific diagnostic test exists for rheumatic fever. Sedimentation rate and leukocyte count are elevated. The development of serum antibodies against the streptococci (measured by antistreptolysin-O titer) may occur. CRP, elevated in a specimen of blood, is abnormally high.

Medical Management

Preventive measures are the most effective interventions. Rapid treatment for pharyngeal infection, usually with prolonged antibiotic therapy, is desired. Penicillin is the preferred antibiotic. Prolonged periods of bed rest were recommended, but now the patient without carditis may be ambulatory as soon as acute symptoms have subsided. When carditis is present, ambulation is postponed until HF is controlled. Symptomatic treatment and care are given. Nonsteroidal antiinflammatory drugs (NSAIDs) for joint pain and inflammation are accompanied by application of gentle heat. A well-balanced diet, following the personalized daily food choices and number of servings recommended by the U.S. Department of Agriculture's MyPyramid food planning tool, is supplemented by vitamins B and C and high-volume fluid intake. In some patients, surgical commissurotomy or valve replacement is necessary.

Nursing Interventions and Patient Teaching

Signs and symptoms largely determine the type of nursing interventions. Bed rest during the acute phase is recommended when carditis is present. If the patient has polyarthritis, minimize joint pain by proper positioning. After the acute stage, the child or the adult is treated at home. Review a schedule of daily events with the patient and the parents.

Carry out nursing interventions quickly and skillfully to minimize discomfort and avoid tiring the patient. Throughout the course of the disease, the patient and the family benefit from emotional support and appropriate diversions. Teaching focuses on increasing understanding of the disease process, signs and symptoms, and gradually increasing activity levels. Emphasize the importance of eating a nutritional diet and keeping appointments for medical checkups. Patients with a history of rheumatic fever or evidence of rheumatic heart disease should receive daily prophylactic penicillin by mouth or monthly intramuscular injections of penicillin to prevent streptococcal infection, at least during childhood and adolescence. Patients with evidence of deformed heart valves should be given prophylactic antibiotics before surgery and all dental procedures.

Prognosis

Prognosis depends on involvement of the heart; carditis can result in a serious heart disease, including valvular disease.

PERICARDITIS

Etiology and Pathophysiology

Pericarditis is inflammation of the membranous sac surrounding the heart. It may be an acute or a chronic condition. Bacterial, viral, or fungal infection is associated with acute pericarditis. It may occur as a complication of noninfectious conditions such as azotemia; acute MI; neoplasms such as lung cancer, breast cancer, leukemia, Hodgkin's disease, and lymphoma; scleroderma; trauma after thoracic surgery; systemic lupus erythematosus; radiation; and drug reactions (e.g., from procainamide and hydralazine [Apresoline]). Fibrosis of the pericardial sac develops in the chronic form.

Fibrous constriction and thickening of the pericardium occur gradually, causing compression severe enough to prevent normal filling during diastole. Surgical removal of the pericardium may be necessary to restore normal cardiac output.

Clinical Manifestations

Pericarditis differs clinically from other inflammatory conditions of the heart in that patients often have debilitating pain, much like that of MI. The pain is aggravated by lying supine, deep breathing, coughing, swallowing, and moving the trunk and is alleviated by sitting up and leaning forward. Dyspnea, fever, chills, diaphoresis, and leukocytosis are observed. The hallmark finding in acute pericarditis is pericardial friction rub; grating, scratching, and leathery sounds are detected, although this appears in only about half of cases.

Decreased heart function to the level of cardiac failure can occur when the heart is compressed by excess fluid in the pericardial sac. Normally 15 to 50 mL of fluid are found in the pericardial sac, but with pericarditis 150 to 200 mL or more may develop.

Assessment

Subjective data include the patient's description of muscle aches, fatigue, and dyspnea. Excruciating chest pain is said to originate precordially and radiate to the neck and shoulders with severe and sudden onset.

Collection of **objective data** includes noting expressed substernal chest pain that radiates to the shoulder and neck; such pain is evidenced by orthopneic positioning and facial grimace on inspiration. Elevated temperature accompanies chills and may be followed by diaphoresis. A nonproductive cough is often present. Patients commonly verbalize anxiety, anticipation of danger, or uneasiness. Vital sign changes include a rapid and forcible pulse and rapid, shallow breathing. Pericardial friction rub heart sounds become muffled, and the physician may note a dysrhythmia.

Diagnostic Tests

ECG changes (dysrhythmia) are noted. Echocardiography shows pericardial effusion or cardiac tamponade. Laboratory studies show leukocytosis (10,000 to 20,000/mm^3), and the sedimentation rate is elevated. Blood cultures may be ordered to identify the specific pathogen present. To rule out an MI, cardiac enzyme levels are done. A CRP test used to diagnose bacterial infectious disease and inflammatory disorder may be ordered (Holcomb, 2006). Chest radiographic findings are generally normal or nonspecific in acute pericarditis unless the patient has a large pericardial effusion.

Medical Management

Analgesia for comfort and relief of pain reassures the anxious patient. Oxygen and parenteral fluids are usually given. Antibiotics are used to treat bacterial pericarditis. The physician prescribes salicylates for increased temperature and antiinflammatory agents (e.g., indomethacin) and corticosteroids for a persistent inflammatory process. These medicines require nursing knowledge of troublesome effects and nursing implications for control of this condition. When pericardial effusion restricts heart movement **(cardiac tamponade),** a pericardial tap **(pericardiocentesis)** may be performed to remove excess fluid and restore normal heart function. Surgical intervention—pericardial fenestration (pericardial window) or pericardiocentesis (pericardial tap)—may be performed to provide continuous drainage of pericardial fluid and restore normal heart function. Complications include atelectasis and introduction of infectious agents.

Nursing Interventions

Carefully evaluate vital signs and auscultate lung and heart sounds. Provide supportive measures and observe for complications. Maintain bed rest to promote healing and decrease the cardiac workload. Elevate the head of the bed to 45 degrees to decrease dyspnea. Hypothermia treatment may be necessary to reduce elevated temperature. Remain with the patient if he or she is anxious. Explain all procedures thoroughly.

Nursing diagnoses and interventions for the patient with inflammatory heart conditions include but are not limited to the following:

Nursing Diagnoses	Nursing Interventions
Decreased cardiac output, related to inflammatory process	Maintain bed rest with head of bed elevated to 45 degrees. Assess vital signs every 2 to 4 hours as indicated by patient's condition. Administer medications as ordered. Monitor I&O. Provide planned rest periods.
Pain, related to inflammatory process	Assess and record pain type and quality. Administer analgesics according to need, as ordered. (Pain is what the patient says it is.)

Nursing Diagnoses	Nursing Interventions
	Maintain the patient on bed rest with the head of the bed elevated to 45 degrees and provide a padded overbed table for the patient to rest the arms. Use comfort measures to provide physical and emotional support.
Excess fluid volume, related to ineffective myocardial pumping action	Restrict sodium in diet as prescribed; monitor I&O. Weigh daily; compare values. Administer diuretic therapy as ordered; monitor electrolyte values. Observe respiration and pulse quality. Assess for dyspnea and peripheral edema.

Prognosis

The prognosis is fair in early stages but extremely grave if purulent and fibrinous stages develop.

ENDOCARDITIS

Etiology and Pathophysiology

Endocarditis is an infection or inflammation of the inner membranous lining of the heart, particularly the heart valves. Classified on the basis of cause, it may result from invasion of an organism (**infective endocarditis)** or from injury to the lining. The term **bacterial endocarditis** has been replaced by **infective endocarditis** because causative organisms include fungi, chlamydiae, rickettsiae, viruses, and bacteria. The causative organisms—most commonly *Streptococcus viridans, Streptococcus pyogenes, Staphylococcus aureus, Staphylococcus epidermidis,* and enterococci—are deposited on the heart lining or valves. As the organism embeds into the tissue, a vegetative growth perforates the chambers or valve leaflets. Fibrin and calciferous growths of the vegetation may ulcerate and scar the valves; or the growths may break away, causing emboli, infection, or abscess in organs where they lodge. The loss of portions of vegetative lesions into the circulation results in embolization. Systemic embolization occurs from left-sided heart vegetation, progressing to infarction of an organ (particularly the brain, the kidneys, and the spleen) and limb. Right-sided heart lesions embolize to the lungs. Endocarditis may develop after cardiac surgery, which in itself is traumatic.

People at risk include patients with rheumatic, congestive, or degenerative heart disease. With the increasing use of valve replacement, the incidence of prosthetic valve endocarditis continues to rise. In some cases endocarditis occurs after intrusive procedures such as dental procedures, minor surgery, gynecologic examinations, or insertion of indwelling urinary catheters. People at high risk include those who use illegal IV drugs, which can cause bacteremia from contaminated needles and syringes. Conditions predisposing people to infective endocarditis have changed because of decreasing incidence of rheumatic heart disease, increased recognition and treatment of mitral valve prolapse, the aging population with degenerative heart disease, and IV drug abuse (Lewis et al., 2007).

Clinical Manifestations

Endocarditis occurs in acute or subacute forms. Signs and symptoms progress either rapidly; in dangerous sequence during the acute phase; or gradually in the subacute phase, with damage occurring over a long period.

Assessment

Subjective data include patient complaints of influenza-like symptoms with recurrent fever, undue fatigue, chest pain, headaches, joint pain, and chills.

Collection of **objective data** may reveal the significant signs of petechiae in the conjunctiva, oral mucosa, neck, anterior chest, abdomen, and legs. Splinter hemorrhages (black longitudinal streaks) may occur in the nailbeds. Other signs are nontender macula on the palms and soles, plus tender erythematous, elevated nodules on the pads of the fingers and toes. Microemboli, vasculitis, and embolism are responsible for the development of these signs. They also have the potential to cause serious complications such as stroke and renal or splenic infarction (Holcomb, 2006). Weight loss may occur. Pulse is rapid. Infective endocarditis may cause a murmur, with the aortic and mitral valves most commonly affected.

Diagnostic Tests

ECG changes and chest radiographic examination reveal evidence of HF and cardiomegaly. TEE and digital imaging using two-dimensional transthoracic echograms can detect vegetation or thrombi and abscesses on valves. Laboratory findings indicate leukocytosis, increased ESR, anemia, and hyperglobulinemia. Blood cultures determine the causative organism, and sensitivity tests indicate the antibiotic needed for medical management.

Medical Management

The medical management of the patient with endocarditis includes support of cardiac function, destruction of the pathogen, and prevention of complications.

Embolization, a serious and common complication, can occur. An emboli may go to the brain, the lungs, the coronary arteries, the spleen, the bowel, and the extremities, with catastrophic results. The most frequent embolic events usually occur during the first

2 weeks of acute infective endocarditis. Anticoagulation is not recommended because of the risk of an intracerebral hemorrhage. A patient who was receiving anticoagulation therapy before developing endocarditis may continue therapy as long as neurologic function is carefully monitored (Holcomb, 2006).

Management relies on rest to decrease the heart's workload. Complete bed rest is usually not indicated unless the temperature remains elevated and there are signs of HF. After the blood cultures, massive doses of antibiotics are administered, usually parenterally, to combat the organism. Antibiotic therapy continues often as long as 1 to 2 months. Traditionally this has required a prolonged hospitalization for most patients, but with newer, more versatile antibiotics (and growing economic concerns), outpatient treatment of patients with infective endocarditis is more common.

Prophylactic antibiotic treatment is recommended for individuals who are considered at high risk for developing infective endocarditis. Patients at risk include those with previous valve surgery, preexisting valvular heart disease, or congenital abnormalities. Infective endocarditis precautions involve antibiotic therapy as prescribed by the physician before any invasive procedure such as dental work or minor surgery.

Surgical repair of diseased valves or prosthetic valve replacement may be necessary if the patient's condition is severe. Valve replacement has become an important adjunct procedure in the management of endocarditis. It is used in more than 25% of cases.

Nursing Interventions and Patient Teaching

The nursing interventions are based primarily on the signs and symptoms. Observe for petechiae, location of pain, vomiting, and fever, and report these signs and symptoms if observed.

During the acute phase, maintain the patient on decreased activity and provide a calm, quiet environment. Take vital signs, including apical pulse, every 4 hours. When increased activity or ambulation begins, assess pulse before and after to determine the effects on the heart muscle.

Ensuring adequate nutrition is important. Frequently patients have a decreased appetite because of the disease process. Provide attractive meals with supplemental between-meal nourishment. Promote rest and comfort and prevent further inflammation and infection during hospitalization.

Patient teaching focuses on identifying causes, infective endocarditis precautions, dietary requirements, and gradually increasing activity levels. Also advise the patient on the need for prophylactic antibiotics before any invasive procedure if the patient has preexisting valvular heart disease. Instruct the patient about signs and symptoms that may indicate recurrent infections such as fever, fatigue, malaise, and chills and the need to report any of these signs and symptoms to the physician.

Prognosis

Before the advent of antibiotics, patients with infective endocarditis could be expected to live approximately 1 year; prompt treatment with intensive antibiotic therapy will now cure about 90% of patients with this condition.

MYOCARDITIS

Acute myocarditis is relatively rare. Inflammation of the myocardium may originate from rheumatic heart disease; viral, bacterial, or fungal infection; or endocarditis or pericarditis. In the United States, most significant cases of acute myocarditis are caused by coxsackievirus type B (Holcomb, 2006). However, sometimes the cause may be unknown.

Signs and symptoms vary. The patient may have upper respiratory tract symptoms such as fever, chills, and sore throat; abdominal pain and nausea; vomiting; diarrhea; and myalgia. These generally occur up to 6 weeks before the patient has signs and symptoms of myocarditis, such as chest pain and overt HF with dyspnea (Holcomb, 2006). Cardiac enlargement, murmur, gallop, and tachycardia are typically seen in myocarditis. Cardiomyopathy may develop as a complication. Enlargement of the myocardium may result in dysrhythmias.

Useful tests to help diagnose myocarditis are chest x-ray, ECG, echocardiography, and endomyocardial biopsy (Holcomb, 2006).

Therapy is symptomatic and primarily follows the same approach as that of endocarditis: bed rest, oxygen, antibiotics, antiinflammatory agents, careful assessments, and correction of dysrhythmias.

The goals of treatment are to preserve myocardial function and to prevent HF and other serious complications such as dilated cardiomyopathy. Patients may recover, but may later develop cardiomyopathy. As a result, the disease may have a long, benign course, or it may result in sudden death during exercise.

CARDIOMYOPATHY

Etiology and Pathophysiology

Cardiomyopathy is a term used to describe a group of heart muscle diseases that primarily affect the structural or functional ability of the myocardium. This primary dysfunction is not associated with CAD, hypertension, vascular disease, or pulmonary disease.

When cardiomyopathies are classified by cause, two forms are recognized: primary and secondary. Primary cardiomyopathy consists of heart muscle disease of unknown cause and is classified as dilated, hypertrophic, or restrictive. **Dilated cardiomyopathy,** characterized by ventricular dilation, is the most common type of primary cardiomyopathy. **Hypertrophic cardiomyopathy** results in increased size and mass of the heart because of increased muscle thickness (especially of the septal wall) and decreased ventricular size. In **restrictive cardiomyopathy** the ventricular walls are rigid, thus limiting the ventricles' ability to expand and resulting in impaired diastolic filling (Chojnowski, 2004). Secondary cardiomyopathy has a number of types: (1) infective (viral, bacterial, fungal, or protozoal myocarditis); (2) metabolic; (3) severe nutritional deprivation; (4) alcohol (large quantities consumed over many years leading to dilated cardiomyopathy); (5) peripartum (unexplained cause; may develop in last month of pregnancy or within first few months after delivery); (6) drugs (doxorubicin [Adriamycin] or other medications); (7) radiation therapy; (8) systemic lupus erythematosus; (9) rheumatoid arthritis; and (10) "crack" heart, caused by cocaine abuse.

Cardiomyopathy caused by cocaine abuse is seen more frequently now than ever before. Cocaine causes intense vasoconstriction of the coronary arteries and peripheral vasoconstriction, resulting in hypertension. This can result in increased myocardial oxygen needs and decreased oxygen supply to the myocardium and can lead to acute MI or ischemic cardiomyopathy. Cocaine also causes high circulating levels of catecholamines, which may further damage myocardial cells, leading to ischemic or dilated cardiomyopathy. The cardiomyopathy produced is difficult to treat. Interventions deal mainly with the HF that ensues (Lewis et al., 2007). The prognosis is poor.

Clinical Manifestations

Angina, syncope, fatigue, and dyspnea on exertion are common signs and symptoms. The most common symptom is severe exercise intolerance. The patient may have signs and symptoms of both left-sided and right-sided HF, including dyspnea, peripheral edema, ascites, and hepatic dysfunction.

Diagnostic Tests

Diagnosis of cardiomyopathy is made by the patient's clinical manifestations and noninvasive and invasive cardiac procedures to rule out other causes of dysfunction. Diagnostic studies include ECG, chest radiograph, echocardiogram, CT scan, nuclear imaging studies, MUGA scanning, cardiac catheterization, and endomyocardial biopsy.

Medical Management

Medical management consists of treatment of underlying cause and HF management to slow the progression of the disease and symptoms. Medications may include diuretics, ACE inhibitors, antidysrhythmics, and beta-adrenergic blockers. An automatic internal defibrillator is occasionally implanted. In patients with advanced disease that is not responding to medical treatment, cardiac transplantation should be considered. Educate the patient about avoiding strenuous exercise because of the risk of sudden death.

Cardiac Transplantation

The first heart transplant was performed in 1967. Since that time, heart transplantation has become the treatment of choice for patients with end-stage heart disease who are unlikely to survive the next 6 to 12 months. Patients with cardiomyopathy account for more than 50% of cardiac transplant recipients. Dilated cardiomyopathy is the most common type of cardiomyopathy requiring transplantation. Inoperable CAD is the second most common indication for transplantation, accounting for 40% of candidates (Box 48-6).

Once a patient meets the criteria for cardiac transplantation, the goal of the evaluation process is to identify patients who would most benefit from a new heart. In addition to the physical examination, psychological assessment of candidates is valuable. A complete history of coping abilities, family support system, and motivation to follow through with the transplant and the rigorous transplantation regimen is essential. The complexity of the transplant process may be overwhelming to a patient with inadequate support systems and a poor understanding of the lifestyle changes required after transplant.

Once potential recipients are placed on the transplant list, they may wait at home and receive ongoing medical care if their medical condition is stable. If their condition is not stable, they may require hospitalization for more intensive therapy. Unfortunately, the overall waiting period for a transplant is long, and many patients die while waiting for a transplant.

Donor and recipient matching is based on body and heart size and ABO type. Tissue crossmatching between donor and recipient is generally not done because of difficulty in obtaining good matches and lack of correlation between match and outcome.

Most donor hearts are obtained at locations distant from the institution performing the transplant. The

Box 48-6 Indications and Contraindications for Cardiac Transplantation

INDICATIONS

- Suitable physiologic and chronologic age
- End-stage heart disease that is not responding to medical therapy
- Dilated cardiomyopathy
- Inoperable coronary artery disease
- Vigorous and healthy individual (except for end-stage cardiac disease) who would benefit from procedure
- Compliance with medical regimens
- Demonstrated emotional stability and social support system
- Financial resources available

CONTRAINDICATIONS

- Systemic disease with poor prognosis
- Active infection
- Active or recent malignancy
- Diabetes mellitus type 1, with end-organ damage
- Recent or unresolved pulmonary infarction
- Severe pulmonary hypertension unrelieved with medication
- Severe cerebrovascular or peripheral vascular disease
- Irreversible renal or hepatic dysfunction
- Active peptic ulcer disease
- Severe osteoporosis
- Severe obesity
- History of drug or alcohol abuse or mental illness

maximum acceptable ischemic time for cardiac transplant is 4 to 6 hours.

The recipient is prepared for surgery, and cardiopulmonary bypass is used. The usual surgical procedure involves removing the recipient's heart, except for the posterior right and left atrial walls and their venous connections. The recipient's heart is then replaced with the donor heart, which has been trimmed to match. Care is taken to preserve the integrity of the donor SA node so that a sinus rhythm can be achieved postoperatively.

Immunosuppressive therapy usually begins in the operating room. Regimens vary but usually include azathioprine (Imuran), corticosteroids, and cyclosporine. Cyclosporine was first used in heart transplantation in 1980. Currently it is used with corticosteroids for maintenance immunosuppression. Its use has reduced rejection and also slowed the rejection process so that early treatment can be instituted.

The postoperative care is similar to that of other open-heart surgeries. Endomyocardial biopsies via the right internal jugular vein are performed periodically to detect rejection. In addition, peripheral blood T-lymphocyte monitoring is done to assess the recipient's immune status.

Because the patient is immunosuppressed, nursing interventions involve prevention of infection, which is the leading cause of death in this population. Many deaths from infection occur during augmented immunosuppressive therapy for acute rejection episodes. Provide a great deal of emotional support and teaching for both the patient and the family, since transplantation is a last resort. In addition, the patient is often a long distance from home and significant others.

Advances in surgical technique and postoperative care have improved early survival rates after cardiac transplantation. Attention is directed toward improvements in immunosuppression and management of long-term complications. Nursing management focuses on promoting patient adaptation to the transplant process, monitoring, managing lifestyle changes, and educating the patient and the family. Ongoing data collection and research continue in regard to quality of life, functional level, and rehabilitation of the cardiac transplant recipient (Lewis et al., 2007).

Nursing Interventions and Patient Teaching

Nursing interventions focus on relieving symptoms, observing for and preventing complications, and providing emotional and psychological support. Monitor the response to medications and monitor for dysrhythmias. Teach patients to adjust their lifestyle to avoid strenuous activity and dehydration. Instruct patients to space activities and allow for rest periods.

Prognosis

Most patients have a severe, progressively deteriorating course, and the majority (particularly those older than 55 years of age) die within 2 years of the onset of signs and symptoms. However, improvement or stabilization occurs in a minority of patients. Death is due to either HF or ventricular dysrhythmia. Sudden death resulting from dysrhythmia is a constant threat.

DISORDERS OF THE PERIPHERAL VASCULAR SYSTEM

Peripheral vascular disease is any abnormal condition that affects the blood vessels outside the heart and the lymphatic vessels. The word **peripheral** means pertaining to the outside, surface, or surrounding area. The peripheral vascular system consists of arteries, capillaries, and veins. This system supplies oxygen-rich blood to the upper and lower extremities of the body, and returns blood and carbon dioxide from those areas to the heart and lungs. Disorders of the peripheral vascular system occur when circulation to the upper and lower extremities is compromised.

NORMAL AGING PATTERNS

Degenerative changes occur in the vascular system as part of the normal aging process. These changes affect the walls of the blood vessels and lead to problems in the transport of blood and nutrients to the tissues. The inner walls of the blood vessels (tunica interna) become thick and less compliant. The middle walls of the blood vessels (tunica media) become less elastic. With marked decreases in the elasticity and flexibility of the vessels, peripheral vascular resistance increases, causing a rise in blood pressure and increasing a person's susceptibility to peripheral vascular disease (see Life Span Considerations box).

RISK FACTORS

Risk factors for peripheral vascular disorders are similar to those for cardiovascular disorders. An important aspect of caring for the patient with a peripheral vascular disorder is understanding the risk factors and incorporating them into patient teaching.

Nonmodifiable Factors

Age

As a person ages, arteriosclerotic changes in the peripheral vascular system lead to increased peripheral vascular resistance and decreased blood flow to the tissues.

Gender

Men are more susceptible than women to arteriosclerotic changes. This gender difference decreases after menopause, when the effects of estrogen are no longer present.

Family History

A family history of atherosclerosis increases an individual's risk.

Modifiable Factors

Smoking

Smoking is one of the major contributing factors in the development of peripheral vascular problems. The nicotine in cigarettes causes vasoconstriction and spasms of the arteries, elevates blood pressure, and reduces circulation to the extremities. The carbon monoxide inhaled in cigarette smoke reduces oxygen transport to the tissues.

Hypertension

Increased blood pressure causes wear and damage to the inner arterial walls, resulting in a buildup of fibrous tissue. This in turn leads to further narrowing of the vessel and increased resistance to blood flow.

Hyperlipidemia

An elevation in serum cholesterol and triglycerides contributes to the buildup of plaque inside the blood vessels. The patient should maintain a diet with decreased saturated fat and cholesterol. If serum cholesterol remains elevated, drug therapy must be considered.

Obesity

Excessive body weight and body fat contribute to the severity of other risk factors. Extra weight in relation to bone structure and height places an increased workload on the heart and blood vessels and may contribute to congestion in the venous system.

Lack of Exercise

Decreased activity may compromise the peripheral vascular system because of a lack of muscle tone. The contraction and relaxation of muscles facilitate the return of blood in the veins to the heart and the lungs. A sedentary person does not realize the benefits of regular physical activity, such as weight and stress reduction and improved vascular tone.

Emotional Stress

Stress contributes to increased blood pressure, increased production of cholesterol, and increased vasoconstriction of the blood vessels.

Diabetes Mellitus

Uncontrolled elevated serum glucose levels contribute to the atherosclerotic process, although the exact mechanism by which diabetes mellitus leads to peripheral vascular disorders is unknown. Elevated serum glucose levels result in circulatory disorders.

ASSESSMENT

Arterial Assessment

The first symptom of decreased arterial circulation is pain from arterial insufficiency and ischemia. Arterial insufficiency occurs when not enough blood is available or able to flow through the arteries to body tissues. Ischemia occurs when the tissue does not receive enough oxygen-rich blood to function normally. Ischemic pain in the lower extremities is usually a dull ache in the calf muscles. It is often accompanied by leg fatigue and cramping. The pain is brought on by exercise and relieved by rest. It is referred to as **intermittent claudication** (a weakness of the legs accompanied by cramplike pains in the calves caused by poor circulation of the arterial blood to the leg muscles). Pain may also be felt in the thighs and buttocks. As arterial disease progresses and becomes chronic, pain occurs even at rest. Burning, tingling, and numbness of the legs may occur at night while the patient is lying down.

Other nursing assessments include palpating and comparing pulses in the extremities. Pulses may be weak, thready, or absent in the affected extremity because of decreased blood flow. Several scales are used to measure pulses. To ensure that the patient's pulses are graded the same way each time, all the nurses should use the same scale, such as the following:

0 Absent
+1 Barely palpable, intermittent
+2 Weak, possibly thready, but constantly palpable and with consistent quality
+3 Normal strength and quality
+4 Bounding, easily palpable, may be visible

A Doppler ultrasound device may be needed to check the patient's pulses if pulmonary vascular disease (PVD), low blood pressure, edema, or large amounts of subcutaneous tissue impede the assessment. If a Doppler device is used, record pulsation as **present** or **absent** rather than using the numeric scale. For future reference, use a skin marker to indicate where the pulse is present (Willis, 2001). Check the affected extremity and compare it with the unaffected extremity for color, temperature, skin characteristics, and capillary refill time (Box 48-7).

For a uniform assessment and documentation technique for **veins** and **arteries,** the following mnemonic device, PATCHES, is helpful (Willis, 2001):

P for **pulses:** Assess the patient's affected extremity first. Then assess the apical pulse and bilateral temporal, carotid, brachial, radial, femoral, popliteal, posterior tibial, and dorsalis pedis pulses. Absence of pulses is generally a medical emergency that requires immediate treatment, but in some cases it may be normal. Compare the find-

Box 48-7 Capillary Refill Time

1. Apply pressure to a toenail or fingernail for several seconds until it blanches (the area loses its color).
2. Relieve the pressure.
3. Note the amount of time it takes for the color to return.
   —The color should return almost instantly—in less than 2 seconds.
   —With an arterial disorder, it will take more than 2 seconds for the color to return.

ings with previous ones or correlate them with the patient's signs and symptoms.

A for **appearance:** Note whether the extremity is pale, mottled, cyanotic, or discolored red, black, or brown. Document areas of necrosis or bleeding and the size, depth, and location of ulcers. When assessing ulcers, note whether the edges are jagged or smooth and whether the area is painful to touch.

Shiny skin often marks the presence of edema; a dull appearance may signal inadequate arterial blood supply. Look for superficial veins, erythema, or inflammation anywhere on the affected extremity. Standing allows the saphenous veins to fill, so varicosities in the saphenous system are best evaluated with the patient standing. If a line of color change is present, mark it with a skin marker and monitor for changes in location.

T for **temperature:** If the patient has an arterial problem, the affected extremity will feel cool; if the problem is venous, the extremity will feel normal or abnormally warm. However, problems in arteries and veins are not the only reasons for temperature changes in an extremity; aortoiliac disease, HF, hypovolemia, pulmonary embolism, and other conditions can also affect skin temperature by interfering with peripheral blood flow.

C for **capillary refill:** Capillary refill is normally less than 2 seconds, but it may be extended when the patient has PVD. Press on a nail until the nailbed blanches, then release and count how many seconds it takes for normal color to return. Other sites to check capillary refill are the pads of the toes and fingers, the heel, and the thenar eminence on the palm of the hand proximal to the thumb. Although abnormal capillary refill is not diagnostic in itself, it adds valuable data to the assessment (see Box 48-7).

H for **hardness:** Palpate the extremity to determine whether the tissues are supple or hard and inelastic. Hardness may indicate longstanding PVD, chronic venous insufficiency, lymphedema, or chronic edema. Hardened subcutaneous skin also increases the risk of stasis ulcers.

E for **edema:** Pitting edema frequently indicates an acute process, and nonpitting edema may be seen with chronic conditions, such as venous insufficiency. Assess both extremities for edema and compare and document the findings.

To assess for pitting edema, gently press the skin on the affected extremity for at least 5 seconds. Release and grade pitting as follows: +1, 2-mm indentation; +2, 4-mm indentation; +3, 6-mm indentation; and +4, 8-mm indentation (see Figure 48-17). The most accurate way to determine the degree of nonpitting edema is to measure the circumference of the extremity and compare measurements with the other extremity and subsequent measurements. Measure at the point of edema, and then mark the point with a skin marker so everyone will assess the same area. Accuracy is greatest if the measurements are taken at the same time every day, preferably in the morning before the patient ambulates.

S for **sensation:** Vascular discomfort can originate in arteries, in veins, or in the microcirculation if the patient has diabetes mellitus. In addition to asking the patient about pain, ask if he or she has other abnormal sensations, such as numbness or tingling. Tingling or tenderness can result from peripheral tissue ischemia, and the patient may say the extremity feels abnormally hot or cold (Willis, 2001).

Venous Assessment

Decreased venous circulation leads to edema. When the venous system does not return sufficient blood from the tissues to the heart and the lungs (venous insufficiency), excess fluid is left in the tissues of the affected extremity (edema). Assess for edema in the affected extremity and compare it with the unaffected extremity.

Venous insufficiency may lead to changes in skin pigmentation. Assess the skin for darker pigmentation, dryness, and scaling in the affected extremity. Chronic edema and stasis of blood from venous insufficiency may lead to ulceration of the tissues. These ulcers are referred to as **stasis ulcers.** Peripheral pulses are usually present with venous insufficiency. Pain, aching, and cramping associated with venous disorders are usually relieved by activity and/or elevating the extremity. Refer to Table 48-10 for a comparison of signs and symptoms associated with arterial and venous disorders.

Diagnostic Tests

Diagnostic tests for peripheral vascular disorders include noninvasive procedures and invasive procedures.

Noninvasive procedures include the following:

- **Treadmill test:** This exercise test is used to determine blood flow in the extremities after exercising. It identifies pain associated with exercise such as claudication.
- **Plethysmography:** Plethysmography is used to assess changes in blood volume in the veins of the calf or other body extremities.
- **Digital subtraction angiography**: Initially an IV contrast solution is administered. This allows blood vessels in the extremities to be visualized by radiography using an image intensifier video system and a television monitor.
- **Doppler ultrasound:** A Doppler ultrasound flowmeter measures blood flow in arteries or veins to assess intermittent claudication, obstruction of deep veins, and other disorders of peripheral veins and arteries.

Table 48-10 Comparison of Signs and Symptoms Associated with Arterial and Venous Disorders

SIGNS AND SYMPTOMS	ARTERIAL DISORDER	VENOUS DISORDER
Pain	Aching to sharp cramping; brought on by exercise; relieved by rest	Aching to cramping pain; relieved by activity or elevating extremity
Pulses	Diminished or absent	Usually present
Edema	Usually absent	Usually present; increases at the end of the day and when extremity is in a dependent position
Skin changes	Cool or cold Dry, shiny Hairless Pallor develops with elevation; becomes erythematous with dangling	Warm, thick, and toughened Darkened pigmentation Stasis ulcers

Invasive procedures include the following:

- **Venography:** A contrast medium is administered through a catheter placed in a foot vein. Films are taken to detect filling defects. Venography is the gold standard to assess the condition of the deep leg veins and to diagnose deep-vein thrombosis (DVT). Venography is invasive, is costly, can be unpleasant, and may cause phlebitis. Other diagnostic tests may be used to diagnose DVT.
- **Angiography:** This is done by injection of a contrast medium intravascularly and then visualizing the arteries using radiography.
- **D-dimer:** A serum test. D-dimer is a product of fibrin degradation (change to a less complex form). When a thrombus is present, plasma D-dimer concentrations are usually greater than 1591 ng/mL. The normal range for D-dimer is 68 to 494 ng/mL.
- **Duplex scanning:** This is a combination of ultrasound imaging techniques and Doppler capabilities to determine location and extent of thrombi within veins (most widely used test to diagnose DVT).

HYPERTENSION

Hypertension is considered with peripheral vascular disorders, since it is a risk factor in atherosclerosis, which leads to peripheral vascular disease.

Etiology and Pathophysiology

Normal blood pressure is a reading of less than 120 mm Hg systolic and 80 mm Hg diastolic. Hypertension (or high blood pressure) occurs when a sustained elevated systolic blood pressure is greater than 140 mm Hg and/or a sustained elevated diastolic blood pressure is greater than 90 mm Hg. Stage 1 hypertension is defined as a systolic blood pressure of 140 to 159 mm Hg or a diastolic blood pressure of 90 to 99 mm Hg. Stage 2 and Stage 3 hypertension have been combined into a single category, called stage 2, that is defined as a systolic blood pressure of 160 mm Hg or higher or a diastolic of 100 mm Hg or higher (Wright, 2006). A diagnosis is not based on a one-time elevated blood pressure reading, but on an average of two or more elevated blood pressure readings taken on separate occasions. The guidelines adapted from the Seventh Report of the Joint National Committee on Prevention, Detection, Evaluation, and Treatment of High Blood Pressure, National Institutes of Health, National Heart, Lung, and Blood Institute, May 2003, identify people with a blood pressure of 120 to 139 mm Hg systolic or 80 to 89 mm Hg diastolic as being prehypertensive. People whose blood pressure is in the prehypertensive range are at twice the risk for developing hypertension as people with normal values. The prehypertensive category was created to help patients understand the considerable health risks associated with small increases in blood pressure. Every 20/10 mm Hg increase in blood pressure doubles the risk for cardiovascular events for people ages 40 to 70 (Wright, 2006). Although there is no way of predicting who will develop high blood pressure, hypertension can be detected easily.

Approximately 60 million Americans have hypertension, and an additional 25 million have prehypertension. It has been estimated that up to 30% of the adult population in the United States have undiagnosed hypertension. It is difficult to determine exact numbers because most people are symptom free.

Arterial blood pressure is the pressure exerted by the blood on the walls of blood vessels. Systolic blood pressure is the greatest force caused by the contraction of the left ventricle of the heart. Diastolic blood pressure occurs during the relaxation phase between heartbeats. Blood flow is determined by the amount of blood the heart pumps with each contraction and how fast the heart beats. Peripheral vascular resistance is affected by the diameter of the blood vessel and the viscosity of the blood. Blood flow and peripheral vascular resistance play an important role in regulating blood pressure. Increased peripheral vascular resistance resulting from vasoconstriction, or narrowing of peripheral blood vessels, is a common factor in hypertension.

Vasoconstriction and vasodilation are controlled by the sympathetic nervous system and the renin-angiotensin system of the kidney. Stimulation of the sympathetic nervous system and the release of epinephrine and/or norepinephrine cause blood vessel constriction and increased peripheral vascular resistance. The activation of the renin-angiotensin system occurs with decreased blood flow to the kidney. Renin leads to the formation of angiotensin, which is a potent vasoconstrictor. Angiotensin stimulates the secretion of aldosterone, leading to the retention of sodium and water. The result is an increase in blood pressure.

The two main types of hypertension are **essential (primary)** hypertension and **secondary** hypertension. The incidence of hypertension increases with age and other risk factors.

Essential (Primary) Hypertension

Essential (primary) hypertension makes up 90% to 95% of all diagnosed cases. Although there is no general agreement on the cause of essential hypertension, theories to explain the mechanisms involved include arteriolar changes, sympathetic nervous system activation, hormonal influence (renin-angiotensin-aldosterone system stimulation), genetic factors, greater-than-ideal body weight, sedentary lifestyle, increased sodium intake, and excessive alcohol intake. For a long time many experts believed that an increase in systolic blood pressure was a normal part of aging. In fact, some believed that "100 mm Hg plus the patient's age" was a tolerable systolic blood pressure in the older adult. Treatment for hypertension was based primarily on the diastolic reading, and isolated systolic hypertension (ISH) was often not treated.

Clinical trials have re-emphasized that ISH is believed to raise the risk of cardiovascular disease and stroke (Gennari & Gennari, 2000). ISH is actually a better overall predictor of cardiovascular morbidity and mortality than diastolic pressure. (Diastolic pressure remains the better predictor of CAD in people younger than 45 years.) ISH is defined as an elevated systolic blood pressure of 140 mm Hg or more with a diastolic blood pressure below 90 mm Hg. The value of treating ISH in older patients has only recently been established, but now those findings are widely circulated.

Prognosis

With prolonged untreated essential hypertension, the elastic tissue in the arterioles is replaced by fibrous tissue. This process leads to decreased tissue perfusion and deterioration, especially in the target organs—the heart, the kidney, and the brain. CAD and cerebrovascular accident (stroke), the great causes of death and disability, are much more frequent in those who have elevated blood pressure than in those who are normotensive. With treatment, the prognosis is usually good. Risk factors that contribute to the development of essential hypertension are listed in Box 48-8.

Secondary Hypertension

Secondary hypertension is attributed to an identifiable medical diagnosis. Conditions associated with secondary hypertension are given in Table 48-11.

Box 48-8 Risk Factors for Essential Hypertension

NONMODIFIABLE RISK FACTORS

- **Age:** Risk increased as age advances past 30 years old
- **Gender:** Men more at risk than women
- **Race:** Risk twice as high in blacks as in whites
- **Family history:** Risk increased with a family history of hypertension

MODIFIABLE RISK FACTORS

- **Smoking:** Nicotine constricts blood vessels
- **Obesity:** Associated with increased blood volume
- **High-sodium diet:** Increases water retention, which increases blood volume
- **Elevated serum cholesterol:** Leads to atherosclerosis and narrowing of blood vessels
- **Oral contraceptives or estrogen therapy:** May contribute to elevated blood pressure
- **Alcohol:** Increases plasma catecholamines (biologically active amines, epinephrine, and norepinephrine), which leads to blood vessel constriction
- **Emotional stress:** Stimulates the sympathetic nervous system, which leads to blood vessel constriction
- **Sedentary lifestyle:** Regular exercise helps lower blood pressure over time

Table 48-11 Causes of Secondary Hypertension

CONDITION OR DISORDER	MECHANISM
Renal vascular disease	Kidney disease (glomerulonephritis, renal failure, renal artery stenosis, physiologic changes related to type of disease) affects renin and sodium and results in hypertension
Diseases of the adrenal cortex	Atherosclerotic changes in renal arteries cause increase in peripheral vascular resistance
• Primary aldosteronism	
• Cushing's syndrome	Increase in aldosterone causes sodium and water retention and increases blood volume
• Pheochromocytoma	Increase in blood volume Excess secretion of catecholamines increases peripheral vascular resistance
Coarctation of the aorta	Causes marked elevated blood pressure in upper extremities with decreased perfusion in lower extremities
Head trauma or cranial tumor	Increased intracranial pressure reduces cerebral blood flow and stimulates medulla oblongata to raise blood pressure
Pregnancy-induced hypertension	Cause unknown; generalized vasospasm may be a contributing factor

Prognosis
In most instances, secondary hypertension subsides when the primary disease process is treated or corrected.

Malignant Hypertension
Malignant hypertension is a severe, rapidly progressive elevation in blood pressure (diastolic pressure greater than 120 mm Hg) that causes damage to the small arterioles in major organs (heart, kidneys, brain, eyes). A primary distinguishing finding is inflammation of arterioles (arteriolitis) in the eyes. This type of hypertension is most common in black men under 40 years of age.

Prognosis
Unless medical treatment is successful, the course is rapidly fatal. The most common causes of death are MI, HF, stroke, and renal failure.

Clinical Manifestations
Hypertension is essentially a disease without symptoms until vascular changes occur in the heart, the brain, the eyes, or the kidneys. Longstanding, untreated hypertension can cause target organ damage. Advanced target organ damage may account for left ventricular hypertrophy, angina pectoris, MI, HF, stroke or transient ischemic attack, nephropathy, peripheral arterial disease, or retinopathy. Signs and symptoms usually occur as a result of advanced hypertension. These signs and symptoms may include awakening with a headache, blurred vision, and spontaneous epistaxis (nosebleed).

Assessment
Collection of **subjective data** includes assessing for morning headache in the occipital area and blurred vision. Assess the patient for risk factors (see Box 8-8). Determine the patient's understanding of hypertension, including the definition, meaning of systolic and diastolic readings, complications of hypertension, and possible concerns regarding treatment.

Collection of **objective data** includes measuring the blood pressure in both arms with the patient in supine and sitting positions. Compare the reading with previous blood pressure results. Take two or more blood pressure measurements on two separate occasions. Also measure and record height and weight. Assess and record heart sounds, and palpate and record peripheral pulses.

Diagnostic Tests
Diagnostic tests associated with hypertension evaluate the functions of the brain, the heart, and the kidneys. The results indicate the effects of hypertension on these organs and provide baseline information for future reference. These tests include CBC; serum levels of sodium, potassium, calcium, and magnesium; lipid profile; fasting blood glucose level; creatinine, BUN, urinalysis, and IV pyelography (effect on kidneys); renal arteriography (the gold standard for confirming renal artery stenosis); and chest radiography, ECG, and possible echocardiography (effect on heart).

Medical Management
Medical management is directed at controlling hypertension and preventing complications. The goal in older adults is to keep the blood pressure at less than 140/90 mm Hg. The general goal for younger adults with mild hypertension is to achieve blood pressure of less than 130/80 mm Hg. Treatment is based on the severity of the hypertension, associated risk factors, and damage to major organs. Antihypertensive medications and nonpharmacologic measures are used to lower blood pressure.

Drug Therapy
For stage 1 or 2 hypertension, drug treatments may include the following (Lewis et al., 2007):

- Diuretics (thiazides, loop diuretics, potassium-sparing drugs)
- Beta-adrenergic blockers such as metoprolol, nadolol, propranolol, acebutolol (Sectral), atenolol, bisoprolol (Zebeta), timolol
- ACE inhibitors such as captopril, enalapril, lisinopril
- Angiotensin II receptor blockers such as valsartan, losartan, irbesartan, candesartan (Atacand), telmisartan (Micard)
- Calcium channel blockers such as diltiazem, amlodipine, nifedipine, felodipine (Plendil), verapamil
- Alpha-agonists such as clonidine
- Aliskiren hemifumarate (Tekturna), the first antihypertensive drug that is a direct renin inhibitor; decreases plasma renin activity and inhibits the conversion of angiotensinogen to angiotensin I (Hussar, 2008)

Special considerations include using ACE inhibitors for diabetes mellitus; using ACE inhibitors and diuretics for HF; using beta blockers and ACE inhibitors for MI; using calcium channel blockers and diuretics for blacks; and using diuretics and long-acting calcium channel blockers for older adults with ISH.

Nonpharmacologic Therapy
Nonpharmacologic therapy for hypertension includes the following:

- **Lose excess weight.** Being overweight is associated with increased blood pressure, abnormally high blood lipid levels, diabetes mellitus, and CAD. Limiting calorie intake and increasing physical exercise are the keys to losing weight.
- **Exercise regularly.** Thirty to 45 minutes of aerobic exercise three or four times a week—helps decrease the risk of hypertension and cardiovascular disease.
- **Reduce saturated fat.** A patient with high blood lipid levels may require dietary modification or drug therapy to normalize them. A cardinal

rule is to limit fat intake to less than 30% of total calories. According to the Dietary Approaches to Stop Hypertension (DASH) study, a low-fat diet rich in fruits and vegetables is recommended (www.webmd.com/hypertension-high-blood-pressure/dash-diet).

- **Consume enough potassium, calcium, and magnesium.** Plenty of potassium in the diet helps decrease blood pressure, so eating potassium-rich fruits and vegetables may improve blood pressure control. Administering potassium supplements to a patient who is hypokalemic as a result of diuretic therapy also combats hypertension. A word of caution: Anyone receiving ACE inhibitors or potassium-sparing diuretics should receive potassium supplements only with extreme caution and close monitoring for hyperkalemia. Low dietary calcium and magnesium may contribute to hypertension (www.dashdiet.org); the National Heart, Lung, and Blood Institute suggests consuming adequate amounts of calcium and magnesium but does not recommend supplementation to combat hypertension.
- **Limit alcohol intake.** Excessive alcohol consumption may contribute to hypertension. A man of normal weight should not drink more than 1 ounce of ethanol per day (the equivalent of 24 ounces of beer, 10 ounces of wine, or 2 ounces of 100-proof whiskey). Women and lightweight men should restrict their intake to half this amount.
- **Reduce sodium intake.** High sodium intake can increase blood pressure, especially in blacks, older adult patients with existing hypertension, and patients with diabetes mellitus. It is recommended limiting sodium intake to 2.4 g/day. Encourage your patient to eat unsalted, unprocessed foods and to read labels when shopping.
- **Stop smoking.** Cigarette smoking is one of the leading risk factors for hypertension and heart disease. Smoking also inhibits the effect of antihypertensive medication, so techniques for stopping are an integral part of patient education. Counseling, support groups, and aids to stop smoking are effective. Because many people who stop smoking gain weight, make certain a weight management and exercise program is part of the plan.
- **Use relaxation techniques and stress management.** Stress management and relaxation techniques have also been shown to offset hypertension and its symptoms.

Nursing Interventions and Patient Teaching

The main focus of nursing interventions is to maintain blood pressure management through patient teaching about hypertension, risk factors, and drug therapy. Patient compliance is improved with education about side effects of medications, dietary instruction, exercise, and stress-reduction techniques (Box 48-9).

Box 48-9 Measures to Increase Compliance with Antihypertensive Therapy

- Be certain that patient understands that absence of symptoms does not indicate control of blood pressure; remind patient that symptoms do not occur until advanced stages of the disease.
- Advise patient against abrupt withdrawal of medication; rebound hypertension can occur.
- Encourage patient to discuss unpleasant side effects of medication with a health care professional.
- If remembering to take medications is a problem, discuss alternate ways to remember, such as taking them with certain meals or placing medication in separate containers labeled with times of day.
- Suggest patient participate in an exercise program with a friend or pay for the program (more likely to participate "to get money's worth").
- Include family and significant others in the teaching process to provide support and promote adherence to regimen.
- Explain reason for regular health care follow-up (high blood pressure is a chronic disorder).
- Contact patients who consistently cancel follow-up appointments.

Nursing diagnoses and interventions for the patient with hypertension include but are not limited to the following:

Nursing Diagnoses	Nursing Interventions
Knowledge, deficient, related to: • disease process • therapeutic management	Assess level of understanding. Implement teaching plan for hypertension: • Disease process, risk factors • Prescribed medications and side effects; proper dosage and administration; necessity of taking medication, even when blood pressure readings are normal • Dietary restrictions • Exercise program • Relaxation techniques • Sexual dysfunction as a potential side effect of adrenergic inhibitors • Compliance with therapy and follow-up appointments Encourage the patient to promptly report any problems to health care professionals for counseling.

DISORDERS OF THE ARTERIES

ARTERIOSCLEROSIS AND ATHEROSCLEROSIS

Arteriosclerosis (a common arterial disorder characterized by thickening, loss of elasticity, and calcification of arterial walls, resulting in a decreased blood supply) is the underlying problem associated with peripheral vascular disorders. **Arteriosclerosis** and **atherosclerosis** are frequently used interchangeably.

Atherosclerosis is characterized by yellowish plaques of cholesterol, lipids, and cellular debris in the inner layers of the walls of large and medium-sized arteries. The result is narrowing of the artery and reduced nutrients and oxygen reaching the tissue, resulting in ischemia to the tissue cells. The arterial wall also loses its elasticity and becomes less responsive to change in blood volume and pressure. Once plaque is formed in the arteries, it is thought to be irreversible. Lesions in the arteries formed from plaque may completely occlude an artery. Atherosclerosis can progress to obstruction, thrombosis, aneurysm, and rupture.

When the need for oxygen in the tissues exceeds the supply, ischemia occurs and may result in cell death and tissue necrosis. The degree of reduction in blood flow and oxygen determines the amount of ischemia and necrosis that occurs. Specific peripheral vascular disorders that stem from arteriosclerosis and atherosclerosis are discussed individually in this chapter.

PERIPHERAL ARTERIAL DISEASE OF THE LOWER EXTREMITIES

Etiology and Pathophysiology

PAD of the lower extremities is accompanied by narrowing or occlusion of the intima and the media of the blood vessel walls. Plaque, as a result of the arteriosclerotic process, forms on the internal wall of the blood vessel, causing partial or complete occlusion. The result is little or no blood flow to the affected extremity. The artery is unable to supply blood and oxygen to the tissues whether the patient is exercising or at rest. Thus signs and symptoms associated with tissue ischemia appear.

Patients with PAD have atherosclerosis of the coronary and carotid arteries. The most common arteries affected in PAD of the lower extremities are the iliac, common femoral arteries, and superficial femoral arteries. Patients with diabetes mellitus are especially prone to develop PAD below the knees. Arteries involved are the distal popliteal, anterior tibial, posterior tibial, and peroneal arteries (Figure 48-18) (Lewis et al., 2007).

Clinical Manifestations

The severity of the signs and symptoms of PAD depends on the location and the extent of the atherosclerosis and on the amount of collateral circulation.

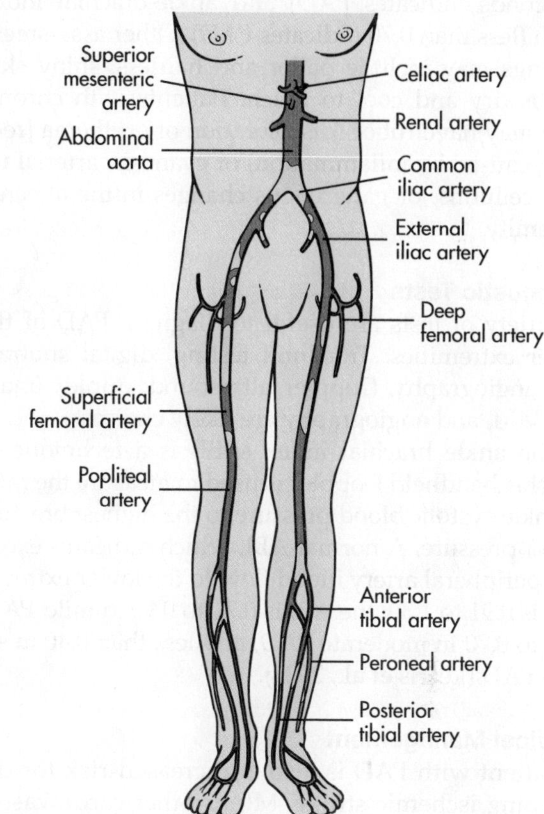

FIGURE 48-18 Common anatomic locations of atherosclerotic lesions *(shown in yellow)* of the abdominal aorta and lower extremities.

Pain is the first symptom that occurs from tissue ischemia. The pain generally occurs in the affected extremity in conjunction with sustained activity (see Table 48-6). This is because the demand of the tissue exceeds the available blood supply. The process of activity → ischemia → pain in an affected extremity is referred to as **claudication.** The pain of claudication subsides with rest; therefore it is frequently referred to as *intermittent claudication* (a weakness of the legs accompanied by cramping pains in the calves caused by poor circulation of the blood to the muscles). A burning pain at rest or at night occurs when the disease process is severe. Symptoms of coldness, numbness, and tingling may be associated with the pain. The signs and symptoms to watch for include the classic five P's of arterial occlusion: **pain, pulselessness, pallor, paresthesia,** and **paralysis.**

Assessment

Collection of **subjective data** focuses on pain associated with intermittent claudication. Does the pain occur with activity, and is it relieved by rest? Does pain occur at rest?

Collection of **objective data** includes assessment of pulses in the affected extremity, which may be weak or absent; comparison with pulses in the unaffected extremity; and assessment of capillary refill (more than

3 seconds indicates PAD) and ankle-brachial index (ABI) (less than 0.70 indicates PAD). Other assessment findings may include pallor and hairless, shiny skin that is dry and cool to touch. Patients with chronic PAD may have rubor (discoloration or erythema [redness] caused by inflammation) or cyanosis, arterial ulcers, cellulitis, or gangrenous changes in the affected extremity.

Diagnostic Tests

A variety of tests are useful to diagnose PAD of the lower extremities. Treadmill testing, digital subtraction angiography, Doppler ultrasound, duplex imaging, MRI, and angiography are likely choices.

The ankle brachial index (ABI) is a technique in which a handheld Doppler is used to measure the ratio of ankle systolic blood pressure to the highest brachial blood pressure. A normal ABI, which indicates excellent peripheral artery blood flow to the lower extremities, is 0.91 to 1.30; the ABI is 0.71 to 0.90 in mild PAD, 0.41 to 0.70 in moderate PAD, and less than 0.40 in severe PAD (Lewis et al., 2007).

Medical Management

A patient with PAD is also at increased risk for developing ischemic stroke, MI, or other cardiovascular problems; therefore the goals of treatment include decreasing the risk of cardiovascular disease and ischemic stroke (Belch, 2003; Treat-Jackson et al., 2003). Smoking cessation is an important aspect of treatment to decrease lower extremity ischemia in PAD and reduce the risk of MI (Belch, 2003; Willigendael et al., 2004).

The most effective oral antiplatelet treatment for patients with PAD is aspirin (160 to 325 mg/day) or clopidogrel (Tran et al., 2004).

ACE inhibitors (e.g., ramipril) are now being prescribed for the patient with PAD regardless of whether they have hypertension or left ventricular dysfunction (Hirsch, 2003). The use of ACE inhibitors decreases cardiovascular risks, improves arterial blood flow to the lower extremities, and improves walking distance (Lewis et al., 2007).

Two drugs approved for use in the United States to specifically treat intermittent claudication are pentoxifylline (Trental) and cilostazol (Pletal). These drugs improve the distance the patient can walk without pain (Lewis et al., 2007).

Fibrinolytics or thrombolytics are useful in dissolving existing thrombi. Urokinase (Abbokinase) is used in most patients with peripheral arterial occlusive disease. Unlike lytic therapy in MI or pulmonary embolism, in peripheral arterial occlusion the drug is administered directly into the thrombus through a central line that contains proximal and distal infusion wires (see Complementary & Alternative Therapies box).

Complementary & Alternative Therapies

Cardiovascular and Peripheral Vascular Disorders

- A number of herbs have been studied for their circulatory effects. Ginkgo biloba has been found to be minimally effective for treating intermittent claudication and decreased cerebral circulation leading to reduced function. Manifestations of decreased cerebral circulation include decreased memory, vertigo, tinnitus, and mood swings with anxiety.
- In the treatment of chronic venous insufficiency, horse chestnut seed extract (HCSE, *Aesculus hippocastanum*) may be equivalent to compression stocking therapy. German health authorities have approved HCSE for the treatment of chronic venous insufficiency, pain and heaviness in the legs, and varicose veins. Gastrointestinal side effects may occur but are uncommon.
- Garlic has been studied for its effects on arteriosclerosis and lipids with varying results. The amount of fresh garlic a person would need to eat for a therapeutic dosage is high and likely to cause gastric upset. Garlic preparations vary widely in terms of their active constituents.
- Patients taking anticoagulants should be cautious regarding the use of herbs, including garlic, ginkgo, angelica, anise, bilberry, devil's claw, goldenseal, licorice root, parsley, and red clover. Although natural, these substances can have potent therapeutic activity. This may in part be due to anticoagulant effects, which may potentiate the action of anticoagulant medications. Be aware if patients are using such substances and monitor any interactions. Not enough controlled research is available to make definite predictions.
- Herbal remedies used to self-treat peripheral vascular disorders include those for hypertension, varicose veins, atherosclerosis, and vascular spasm. Herbs with antihypertensive action include garlic *(Allium sativum)*, hawthorn *(Crataegus oxyacantha)*, kudzu *(Pueraria lobata)*, nettle *(Urtica dioica)*, onion *(Allium cepa)*, purslane *(Portulaca oleracea)*, reishi mushroom *(Ganoderma lucidum)*, and valerian *(Valeriana officinalis)*. Ginkgo biloba has also been used for varicose veins and obliterative arterial disease of the lower extremities. HCSE is used for varicose veins and phlebitis, and valerian is used as an antispasmodic. Antihypertensive spices include basil, black pepper, fennel, and tarragon.

Data from Black, J.M., & Hawks, H.J. (2009). *Medical-surgical nursing.* Philadelphia: Saunders.

Surgical intervention for advanced disease includes embolectomy (removal of embolism) or endarterectomy (surgical removal of the lining of an artery, usually performed on any diseased or occluded major artery, such as the carotid, femoral, or popliteal), arterial bypass (Figure 48-19), PCTA, or amputation. If gangrene is extensive or all major arteries in the extremity are occluded, amputation, although the least desirable end-stage surgical option, may be required.

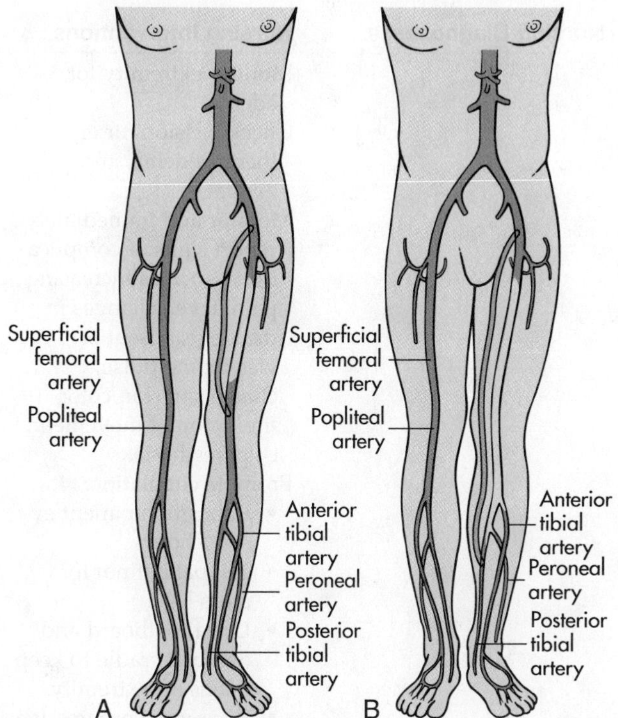

FIGURE 48-19 **A,** Femoral-popliteal bypass graft around an occluded superficial femoral artery. **B,** Femoral posterior tibial bypass graft around occluded superficial femoral, popliteal, and proximal tibial arteries.

Nursing Interventions and Patient Teaching

Nursing interventions are based on assessment findings and nursing diagnoses. Nursing diagnoses and nursing interventions for the patient with PAD of the lower extremities include but are not limited to the following:

Nursing Diagnoses	Nursing Interventions
Activity intolerance, related to: • ischemic pain • immobility	Prevent hazards of immobility by turning, positioning, deep breathing, and performing isometric and range-of-motion exercises. Encourage program of balanced exercise and rest to promote circulation. Instruct the patient to use pain or intermittent claudication as a guide to limiting activity during exercise.
Ineffective tissue perfusion, peripheral, related to decreased arterial blood flow	Place patient's legs in a dependent position relative to the heart to improve peripheral blood flow. Avoid raising feet above heart. Promote vasodilation by providing warmth to extremities and keeping room warm. Teach the patient to avoid vasoconstriction from nicotine, caffeine, stress, or chilling. Teach the patient to avoid constrictive clothing such as garters, tight stockings, or belts. Administer prescribed medications. Teach the patient to avoid crossing the legs.

Prognosis

In advanced disease, ischemia may lead to necrosis, ulceration, and gangrene (particularly of the toes and distal foot) because of the decreased circulation.

ARTERIAL EMBOLISM

Etiology and Pathophysiology

Arterial emboli are blood clots in the arterial bloodstream. They may originate in the heart from an atrial dysrhythmia, MI, valvular heart disease, or HF. Other foreign substances such as a detached arteriosclerotic plaque or tissue may result in arterial emboli. An embolus becomes dangerous when it lodges within and occludes a blood vessel. Blood flow to the area distal to the lodged embolus is impaired, and ischemia occurs. Signs and symptoms depend on the size of the embolus and the amount of circulation that is compromised.

Clinical Manifestations

Sudden loss of blood flow to tissues causes severe pain. Distal pulses are absent, and the affected extremity may become pale, cool, and numb. Necrotic changes may occur. Shock may result if the embolus occludes a large artery.

Assessment

Collection of **subjective data** includes determining the onset of pain and numbness and the location, quality, and duration of these symptoms.

Collection of **objective data** includes assessing pulses in the affected extremity. Compare both extremities to determine skin temperature and color, in addition to pulse volume.

Diagnostic Tests

Doppler ultrasonography and angiography are indicated to obtain a diagnosis.

Medical Management

Medications used to treat obstructed arteries include anticoagulants and fibrinolytics or thrombolytics. Anticoagulants prevent further clot formation and inhibit extension of a clot. Thrombolytics/fibrinolytics dissolve an existing clot. See Table 48-7 for more information on anticoagulants and fibrinolytics.

Endarterectomy (the surgical removal of the intimal lining of an artery) may be the treatment of choice. This involves stripping arteriosclerotic plaque from the intima or inner media of arteries affected by atherosclerosis. Balloon catheters and other instruments are used to accomplish this. Removal of plaque and thrombi increases blood flow and lessens the danger of complications from further emboli or occlusion of an artery.

Embolectomy is another treatment used when larger arteries are obstructed. It is the surgical removal of a blood clot. Surgery must be done within 6 to 10 hours of the event to prevent necrosis and loss of the extremity. Endarterectomy and embolectomy may be done together to deal with the existing emboli and prevent recurrence.

Nursing Interventions and Patient Teaching

Nursing interventions are similar to those for PAD in terms of preventing further arterial problems. During the acute phase monitor the patient for changes in skin color and temperature of the extremity distal to the embolus. Increasing pallor, cyanosis, and coolness of the skin indicate worsening or occlusion of arterial circulation to the extremity. Keep the extremity warm, but do not apply direct heat.

Nursing diagnoses and postoperative nursing interventions for the patient requiring an embolectomy and/or endarterectomy include but are not limited to the following:

Nursing Diagnoses	Nursing Interventions
Ineffective tissue perfusion, peripheral, related to decreased arterial blood flow	Monitor skin color and temperature of affected extremity every hour. Assess sensation and movement in the distal extremity. Assess peripheral pulses and capillary refill in the involved extremity: • Sudden absence of pulse may indicate thrombosis. • Mark location of peripheral pulse with a pen to facilitate frequent assessment. • Use Doppler to monitor whether pulses of involved extremity are nonpalpable and compare with pulses of noninvolved extremity. Monitor extremity for edema. Check incision for erythema, edema, and exudates. Monitor and immediately report signs of complications, such as increasing pain, fever, changes in drainage, absent or weakening pulse, changes in skin color, limitation of movement, or paresthesia. Promote circulation: • Reposition patient every 2 hours. • Tell patient not to cross legs. • Use a footboard and overbed cradle to keep linens off extremity. • Encourage progressive activity when permitted. Avoid sharp flexion in area of graft. Monitor for signs of bleeding secondary to anticoagulation therapy.
Deficient knowledge, related to anticoagulant therapy	Teach patient general action and side effects of prescribed drug; instruct patient to avoid taking anticoagulant medications with aspirin, which also has anticoagulant effect. Instruct patient to take anticoagulant at same time every day and to not stop taking it until advised by physician. Have patient check for signs of bleeding (gums, epistaxis [nosebleed], ecchymosis [bruising], cuts that do not stop bleeding with direct pressure, blood in urine or stool); report promptly to health care professional. Encourage patient to wear a medical-alert bracelet or carry an identification card containing the drug name, drug dosage, and physician's name in case of emergency.

Nursing Diagnoses	Nursing Interventions
	Have patient report for prescribed blood tests (PTT, PT, INR) used to adjust drug dosage.
	Tell patient not to add dark green and yellow vegetables to diet (these contain vitamin K, which counteracts the anticoagulant drug effect). Instruct patient to restrict alcohol intake (increases anticoagulant effect).

Patient teaching is the same as for PAD with an emphasis on anticoagulant therapy.

Prognosis
Prognosis depends on the size of the embolus, the presence of collateral circulation, and the proximity to a major organ.

ARTERIAL ANEURYSM

Etiology and Pathophysiology
An **aneurysm** is an enlarged, dilated portion of an artery that is more than one and a half times the artery's circumference. To be a true aneurysm, the defect must involve all three layers, or tunics (Croce, 2007). Aneurysms may be the result of arteriosclerosis, trauma, or a congenital defect. Aneurysms of the lower extremities commonly affect the popliteal artery. Other areas predominantly affected are the thoracic and abdominal aorta and the coronary and cerebral arteries. The aorta is especially prone to aneurysm and rupture because it is continuously exposed to high pressures. Aortic aneurysms are most common in men in their 60s and 70s, especially if they have ever smoked. Other risk factors are hypertension, atherosclerosis, family history of aortic aneurysm, infarction, and trauma (Croce, 2007). Dissections and ruptures are more likely in the thoracic portion of the aorta than in the abdominal portion. An aneurysm starts with a weakened arterial wall that becomes dilated from blood flow and pressure in the area. The pathologic effect of this condition is differentiated according to shape and site of presentation (Figure 48-20).

Clinical Manifestations
A large pulsating mass may be the only identifiable factor. Clinical signs and symptoms of a thoracic aortic aneurysm depend on its location. If it compresses adjacent structures, it can cause chest pain, shortness of breath, cough, hoarseness, or dysphagia. If it compresses the superior vena cava, the patient may have edema of the face, the neck, and the arms. In the early stages an abdominal aneurysm is unlikely to cause symptoms. As it expands, however, it may cause pain in the chest, the lower back, or the scrotum. A pulsatile, nontender upper abdominal mass may be palpated.

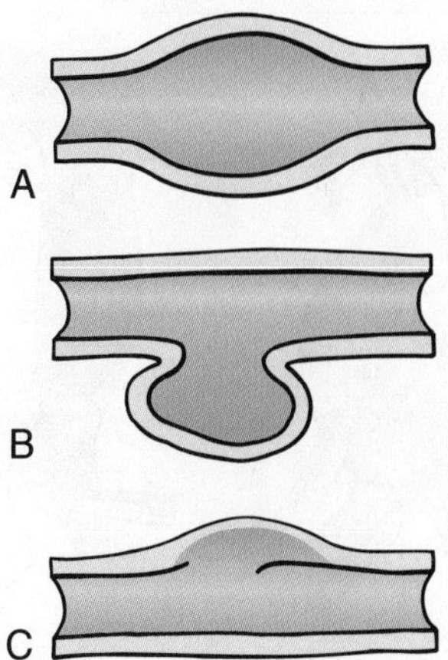

FIGURE 48-20 Types of aneurysms. **A,** Fusiform. **B,** Saccular. **C,** Dissecting.

Assessment
Collection of **subjective data** may reveal no subjective symptoms unless the aneurysm is large and impinges on other structures, causing pain and inequality of pulses. A thoracic aortic aneurysm can result in chest pain, shortness of breath, or dysphagia.

Collection of **objective data** includes palpation of a large, nontender, pulsating mass at the site of the aneurysm.

Diagnostic Tests
Fluoroscopy, chest radiographic studies, CT scan, ultrasound, contrast aortography, arteriography, MRI, and TEE are used to diagnose an aneurysm. It is recommended that all men who have ever smoked have an abdominal aneurysm screening (Croce, 2007).

Medical Management
Aneurysms are monitored for complications such as dissection, rupture, formation of thrombi, and ischemia. Control of hypertension is the first priority of care. An oral beta blocker reduces blood pressure, heart rate, and myocardial contractility. Surgical intervention may be necessary. The blood vessel may be ligated or grafts used to replace the section of the artery that contains the aneurysm or to bypass the aneurysm.

A fusiform or circumferential aneurysm (in which all the walls of the blood vessel dilate more or less equally, creating a tubular swelling) can be removed and repaired with a graft of synthetic fiber, such as Dacron or Teflon, or with a vessel taken from another region of the patient's body. Saccular aneurysms (an aneurysm, usually caused by trauma, that consists of a weak area on only one side of the vessel, causing an outpouching of the vessel wall that is attached to the artery by a narrow neck) can be removed and the vessel then sutured, or a patch graft can be used to replace the deformity (Figures 48-21 and 48-22).

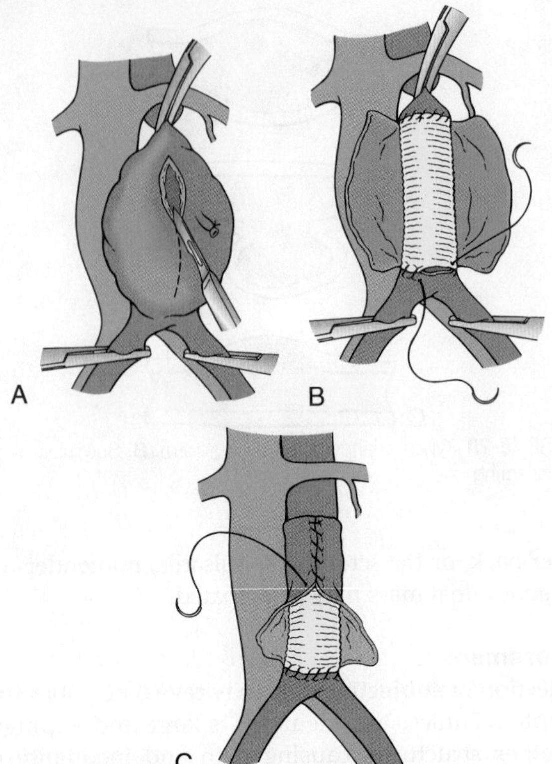

FIGURE 48-21 Surgical repair of an abdominal aortic aneurysm. **A,** Incising the aneurysmal sac. **B,** Insertion of synthetic graft. **C,** Suturing native aortic wall over synthetic graft.

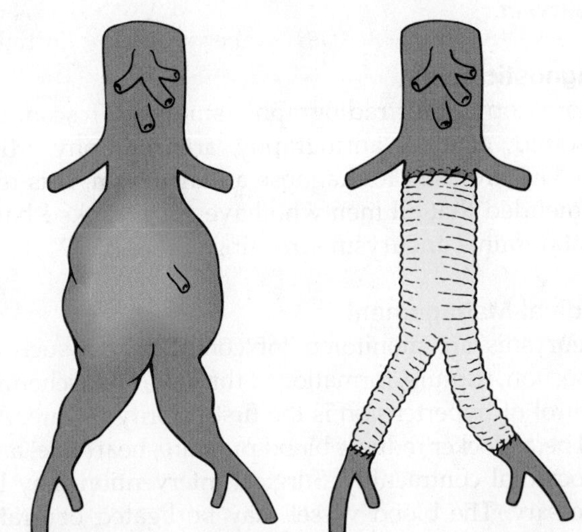

FIGURE 48-22 Replacement of aortoiliac aneurysm with a bifurcated synthetic graft.

In repair of a popliteal aneurysm, popliteal blood flow is enhanced when a homograft (or allograft, tissue transferred between two genetically dissimilar individuals of the same species, such as two humans who are not identical twins) is used.

Nursing Interventions and Patient Teaching

Initial nursing interventions include monitoring the status of an existing aneurysm. Monitor the patient for signs of rupture of the aneurysm, such as paleness, weakness, tachycardia, hypotension, sudden onset of abdominal or chest pain, back pain, or groin pain and a pulsating mass in the abdomen.

Postoperative nursing diagnoses and interventions for the patient with arterial aneurysm include but are not limited to the following:

Nursing Diagnoses	Nursing Interventions
Ineffective tissue perfusion, peripheral, related to decreased arterial blood flow	Assess circulation (especially in extremities) by pedal pulse checks and capillary refill assessments. Be alert for complications.
Anxiety, related to feelings of impending death	Examine coping ability. Provide active listening and genuine interest. Maintain therapeutic environment. Administer antianxiety medications as ordered.

Because aneurysm formation is most commonly associated with atherosclerosis, patient teaching focuses on managing risk factors, including control of hypertension, promotion of tissue perfusion, maintenance of skin integrity, and prevention of infection and injury.

Prognosis

An aneurysm may rupture and cause hemorrhage, resulting in death unless emergency surgical intervention occurs. With surgical intervention, the prognosis is often good.

THROMBOANGIITIS OBLITERANS (BUERGER'S DISEASE)

Etiology and Pathophysiology

Thromboangiitis obliterans (Buerger's disease) is an occlusive vascular condition in which the small and medium-sized arteries become inflamed and thrombotic. The cause is not fully understood, but men between the ages of 25 and 40 years who smoke are most commonly affected by the disorder. Women, however, make up as much as 40% of patients with Buerger's disease. The disorder develops in the small arteries and veins of the feet and hands. Buerger's disease causes inflammation and damage to the arterial walls and is a type of arteritis (Lewis et al., 2007). The wrists and lower legs may also be involved. Occlusion of the arteries leads to ischemia; pain; and, in later stages, infection and ulceration. There is a strong relationship between Buerger's disease and tobacco use. It is thought that the disease occurs only in smokers, and when smoking is stopped, the disease improves.

Clinical Manifestations

The main characteristic is inflammation of vessel walls. The most common symptom is pain with exercise affecting the arch of the foot, also called **instep claudication.** When the hands are involved, the pain is usually bilaterally symmetric (equal). Pain may occur at rest and be frequent and persistent, particularly when the patient also has atherosclerosis. The skin in the affected extremity may be cold and pale, and ulcers and gangrene may be present. Sensitivity to cold is an outstanding clinical manifestation. An early sign of Buerger's disease may be superficial thrombophlebitis.

Assessment

Subjective data include information about pain, claudication, and sensitivity to cold in affected extremities and risk factor assessment.

Objective data include presence of pulses, skin color, and temperature in the affected extremities.

Diagnostic Tests

No diagnostic tests are specific to Buerger's disease. Diagnosis is based on age of onset; history of tobacco use; clinical symptoms; involvement of distal vessels; presence of ischemic ulcerations; and exclusion of diabetes mellitus, autoimmune disease, and proximal source of emboli. Patients with Buerger's disease have a higher level of hematocrit blood viscosity and red blood cell rigidity than patients with PAD (Bozkurt et al., 2004).

Medical Management

Medical management is directed at preventing disease progression. Modifying risk factors and smoking cessation are a major focus. Smoking causes vasoconstriction and decreases blood supply to the extremities. Treatment includes complete cessation of tobacco use in any form (including secondhand smoke and nicotine-replacement products). Tell patients that they have a choice between cigarettes and their affected limbs; they cannot have both. The amputation rate in patients who continue tobacco use is 84%, compared with 30% in patients who discontinue tobacco use (Cooper, 2004). Trauma to the extremities must be avoided. Exercise to develop collateral circulation is encouraged. Surgical intervention, such as amputation of gangrenous fingers and toes, may be indicated. A sympathectomy (a surgical interruption of part of the sympathetic nerve pathways) to alleviate pain and vasospasm may also be performed.

Nursing Interventions and Patient Teaching

Nursing interventions focus on managing risk factors, promoting tissue perfusion, providing comfort measures, and patient teaching. Care of the extremities to prevent necrosis and gangrene includes hydration and cleanliness. Well-fitting shoes and socks alleviate pressure.

The hazards of cigarette smoking and its relationship to Buerger's disease are the primary focus of patient teaching. None of the palliative treatments are effective if the patient does not stop smoking. Nowhere are the cause and effect of smoking so dramatically seen as with Buerger's disease.

Prognosis

Buerger's disease is a chronic condition. Amputation may be necessary if the condition progresses to gangrene with chronic infection and extensive tissue destruction.

RAYNAUD'S DISEASE

Etiology and Pathophysiology

Raynaud's disease is caused by intermittent arterial spasms. Intermittent attacks of ischemia, especially of the fingers, the toes, the ears, and the nose, are caused by exposure to cold or by emotional stimuli. Raynaud's disease is either primary or secondary. The cause of primary Raynaud's is unknown, and the condition is usually mild. When symptoms occur in association with autoimmune diseases, a diagnosis of secondary Raynaud's disease is made. Primary Raynaud's disease usually occurs before 30 years of age, whereas secondary Raynaud's disease usually occurs after age 30. Secondary Raynaud's disease is associated with other conditions such as scleroderma (a relatively rare autoimmune disease affecting blood vessels and connective tissue), rheumatoid arthritis, systemic lupus erythematosus, drug intoxication, and occupational trauma. It usually affects women and is more prevalent during the winter months. The exact cause is unknown, but emotional stress, alterations in the nervous system and immunologic system, and hypersensitivity to cold may play a role in the development of signs and symptoms. Few arterial changes occur initially, but as the disease progresses, the intimal wall thickens and the medial wall hypertrophies.

Clinical Manifestations

The patient typically complains of chronically cold hands and feet. During arterial spasms, pallor, coldness, numbness, cutaneous cyanosis, and burning, throbbing pain occur. Chronic Raynaud's disease may result in ulcerations on the fingers and toes.

Assessment

Collection of **subjective data** includes determining underlying disease processes and evaluating risk factors. The patient may complain of cold hands or feet and a throbbing, aching pain with a tingling sensation (Lewis et al., 2007).

Collection of **objective data** includes assessment of pallor; edema; coldness; blanching; cyanosis; and reactive hyperemia (increased blood in part of the body, caused by increased blood flow), which instigates rubor, following an arterial spasm. Inspect the fingers and toes for ulceration because of circulatory inadequacy and residual waste products.

Diagnostic Tests

A cold stimulation test is used to diagnose Raynaud's disease. Skin temperature changes are recorded by a thermistor attached to each finger. Submerge the patient's hand in an ice water bath for 20 seconds, and record ongoing temperatures. A comparison is made for baseline data.

Medical Management

Medical therapy is aimed at prevention. Drug therapy may be prescribed to reduce pain and promote circulation. Currently the first-line drug therapy involves calcium channel blockers, such as nifedipine and diltiazem, to relax smooth muscles of the arterioles. Nifedipine is preferred over diltiazem because it has a stronger vasodilating effect and less effect on the calcium channels in the conduction system in the heart (Lewis et al., 2007). Biofeedback techniques have been used to increase skin temperature and thereby prevent spasms. Relaxation training and stress management are effective for some patients. Temperature extremes should be avoided. The patient should stop using all tobacco products and avoid caffeine and other drugs with vasoconstrictive effects such as amphetamines and cocaine. Possible surgical interventions include sympathectomy for symptomatic relief. If the disease is advanced, with ulcerations and gangrene, the involved area may have to be amputated.

Nursing Interventions and Patient Teaching

Nursing interventions are similar to those for other arterial disorders: promoting tissue perfusion, maintaining comfort, and preventing injury and infection. Risk factor management includes stress-reduction techniques and smoking cessation.

Nursing diagnoses and interventions stress patient teaching for the patient with Raynaud's disease, including but not limited to the following:

Nursing Diagnosis	Nursing Interventions
Deficient knowledge, related to: • effects of cigarette smoking • stress reduction • avoidance of exposure to cold	Develop teaching plan to include the following: • Effects of smoking on vasoconstriction and arterial blood flow • Techniques for smoking cessation: stop smoking programs, biofeedback, hypnosis • Techniques for stress reduction: massage, imagery, music, exercise, lifestyle changes • Ways of avoiding exposure to cold: layer clothing, wear mittens and warm socks during winter, use caution when cleaning the refrigerator and freezer, wear gloves when handling frozen food, and avoid occupations requiring constant exposure to cold

Prognosis

Raynaud's disease persists but may be controlled by protecting the body and extremities from the cold and using mild sedatives and vasodilators. No serious disability develops, but this condition is sometimes associated with rheumatoid arthritis or scleroderma.

DISORDERS OF THE VEINS

Venous disorders occur when the blood flow is interrupted in returning from the tissues to the heart. Changes in smooth muscle and connective tissue make the veins less distensible. The valves in the veins may malfunction, causing backflow of blood. The major venous disorders are thrombophlebitis and varicose veins (Table 48-12).

THROMBOPHLEBITIS

Etiology and Pathophysiology

Thrombophlebitis is inflammation of a vein in conjunction with the formation of a thrombus. It occurs more frequently in women and affects people of all races. The incidence increases with aging. Other factors associated with thrombophlebitis include venous stasis, hypercoagulability (excessive clotting) of the blood, and trauma to the blood vessel wall. Immobilized patients who have had surgical procedures involving pelvic blood vessel manipulation, such as total hip replacement or pelvic surgery, or patients with MI are prone to thrombophlebitis. Thrombophlebitis develops in deep veins (DVT) or in superficial veins (superficial thrombosis) (Figure 48-23). Thrombophlebitis usually occurs in an extremity, most frequently a leg. Superficial thrombophlebitis is often minor and is treated with elevation, antiinflammatory agents, and warm compresses. DVT is a condition involving a thrombus in a deep vein such as the iliac or femoral veins (Lewis at al., 2007). It is of greater significance and can become dislodged, carried to the lungs in the bloodstream, and cause a pulmonary embolus. Pulmonary embolism is a life-threatening complication.

Clinical Manifestations

Pain and edema occur when the vein is obstructed. The circumference of the calf or thigh may increase. Active dorsiflexion of the foot may result in calf pain. This is referred to as a positive Homans' sign and may indicate thrombophlebitis. Homans' sign is a classic but unreliable sign because it is not specific for DVT and appears in only 10% of DVT patients. Superficial thrombophlebitis may show signs of inflammation such as erythema, warmth, and tenderness along the course of the vein.

Assessment

Subjective data include characteristics of pain in the affected extremity, noting onset and duration and any history of venous disorders.

Table 48-12 Venous Disorders

SIGNS AND SYMPTOMS	MEDICAL MANAGEMENT AND NURSING INTERVENTIONS
THROMBOPHLEBITIS	
Entire extremity may be pale, cold, and edematous. Area along vein may be erythematous and warm to touch. Patient may have Homans' sign: pain in calf on dorsiflexion. Superficial veins feel indurated (hard) and thready or cordlike and are sensitive to pressure. Extremities have difference in circumference.	Maintain bed rest during acute phase. Apply warm, moist heat to reduce discomfort and pain per physician's orders. Elevate extremity, but do not use pillows under the knees, and never bend knees. Assess circulation of the affected extremity, and skin condition and pulses in all extremities. Measure calf circumference daily and record. Use antiembolism stocking on unaffected extremity. Administer heparin or enoxaparin (Lovenox) and warfarin (Coumadin) per physician's orders. Administer fibrinolytics (streptokinase) to resolve the thrombus per physician's orders. Begin exercise program after acute phase per physician's orders.
VARICOSE VEINS	
Veins appear as darkened, tortuous, raised blood vessels; more pronounced on prolonged standing. Legs feel heavy. Patient has fatigue. Patient has pain and muscle cramps. Legs are edematous. Ulcers are seen on skin.	Conservative treatment: • Elevate legs 10-15 minutes at least every 2-3 hours. • Wear elastic stockings. • Unna's paste boot is recommended for older or debilitated person with cutaneous ulcers (see Figure 48-25). • Avoid standing for long periods. • Avoid anything that impedes venous flow, such as garters, tight girdles, crossing the legs, and prolonged sitting. • Reduce weight if obese. • Inject sclerosing solutions for small varicosities. Surgery: • Venous ligation and stripping

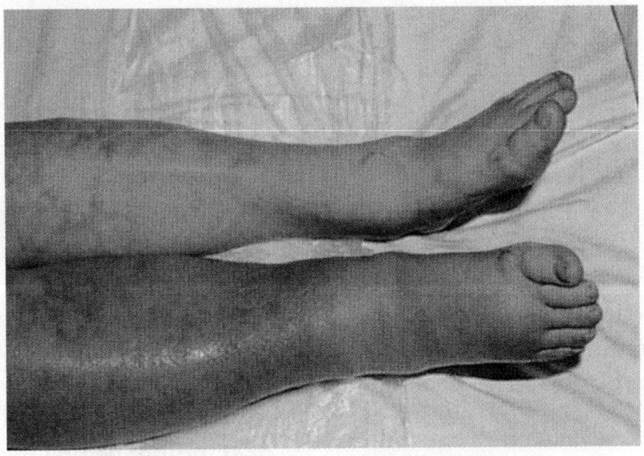

FIGURE 48-23 Deep-vein thrombophlebitis.

Collection of **objective data** includes inspecting the extremity and determining color and temperature (pale and cold if vein is occluded; erythematous and warm if superficial vein is inflamed). Measure both legs for circumference and comparison and to detect edema. If a thrombus involves the inferior vena cava, the lower extremities may become edematous and cyanotic. Involvement of the superior vena cava may result in cyanosis and edema of the arms, the neck, the face, and the back (Lewis et al., 2007).

Diagnostic Tests

Diagnostic tests for DVT include venous Doppler, duplex scanning (the most widely used test), and venogram (phlebogram). A serum D-dimer test will be elevated in DVT. D-dimer is a fibrin degradation fragment that is made from fibrolysis. When a thrombus is undergoing lysis (destruction), it results in increased D-dimer fragments.

Medical Management

Anticoagulant therapy is used for DVT prevention and treatment. For an existing DVT, anticoagulant therapy prevents extension of the clot, development of a new clot, or embolization (embolus traveling through the bloodstream). Anticoagulants do not dissolve a clot. Lysis (destruction) of the clot begins immediately by the body's own fibrinolytic system (Lewis et al., 2007).

Warm compresses may be applied intermittently to the affected extremity. Previously, treatment consisted of bed rest and elevation of the affected area above the level of the heart for 2 to 4 days until the thrombus was stable, therapeutic anticoagulation had occurred, and edema was decreased (Lewis et al., 2007). Current studies report no difference in the incidence of development of a pulmonary embolism in patients with a

Safety Alert!

Patient on Anticoagulant Therapy

1. Teach patient on oral warfarin requirements for frequent follow-up with blood tests (PT, INR) to assess blood clotting and whether change in drug dosage is required.
2. Teach patient side effects and adverse effects of anticoagulant therapy requiring medical attention.
   - Any bleeding that does not stop after a reasonable time (usually 10 to 15 minutes)
   - Blood in urine or stool or black, tarry stools
   - Unusual bleeding from gums, throat, skin, or nose, or heavy menstrual bleeding
   - Severe headaches or stomach pains
   - Weakness, dizziness, mental status changes
   - Vomiting blood
   - Cold, blue, or painful feet
3. Avoid any trauma or injury that might cause bleeding (e.g., vigorous brushing of teeth, contact sports, inline rollerskating).
4. Do not take aspirin-containing drugs or NSAIDs.
5. Limit alcohol intake to small amounts.
6. Wear a medical-alert bracelet or necklace indicating what anticoagulant is being taken.
7. Avoid marked changes in eating habits, such as dramatically increasing foods high in vitamin K (e.g., broccoli, spinach, kale, greens). Do not take supplemental vitamin K.
8. Inform all health care providers, including dentist, of anticoagulant therapy.
9. Correct dosing is essential and supervision may be required (e.g., for patients experiencing confusion).
10. Do not use herbal products that may alter coagulation (see Complementary & Alternative Therapies box).

DVT who were on anticoagulant therapy and who were on bed rest, compared with those allowed to ambulate (Trujillo et al., 2005). Drug therapy may include NSAIDs. DVT usually requires hospital treatment.

Low-molecular-weight heparin (LMWH) is effective for prevention of venous thrombosis and any extension or recurrence. Enoxaparin, and dalteparin are two types of LMWH. LMWH is administered subcutaneously in fixed doses, once or twice daily. LMWH has the practical advantage that it does not require anticoagulant monitoring and dose adjustment. LMWH has a greater bioavailability, more predictable dose response, and longer half-life than heparin with less risk of bleeding complications.

The affected extremity is elevated periodically above heart level to prevent venous stasis and to reduce edema. Specific orders depend on the physician's preference. When the patient ambulates, elastic stockings (antiembolism stockings) are used to compress the superficial veins, increase blood flow through the deep veins, and prevent venous stasis.

Surgery is indicated only when conservative measures have been unsuccessful. A thrombectomy or the **transvenous placement of a grid** or umbrella in the vena cava may be done to prevent the flow of emboli into the lungs. This inferior vena caval interruption device can be inserted percutaneously through superficial femoral or internal jugular veins. When the filter device is opened, the spokes penetrate the vessel walls. The device creates a "sieve-type" obstruction, filtrating clots without interrupting blood flow.

Nursing Interventions and Patient Teaching

Early mobilization is the easiest and most cost-effective method to decrease the risk of DVT. Patients on bed rest need to be instructed to change position, dorsiflex their feet, and rotate ankles every 2 to 4 hours. Ambulatory patients should ambulate at least three times per day. Elastic compression stockings (e.g., thromboembolic disease hose) and/or an intermittent compression device are used for hospitalized patients at risk for DVT. The major emphasis for the patient with thrombophlebitis is preventing complications, promoting comfort, and teaching about the disease and prevention of recurrence.

Nursing diagnoses and interventions for the patient with thrombophlebitis include but are not limited to the following:

Nursing Diagnoses	Nursing Interventions
Ineffective tissue perfusion, peripheral, related to decreased venous blood flow	Confine patient to bed in acute phase. Elevate affected extremity according to physician's orders. Check circulation frequently (monitor pedal pulses, capillary refill). Administer prescribed anticoagulants, and fibrinolytics. Measure calf or thigh circumference daily. Assess site for signs of inflammation and edema. Have patient wear elastic stockings when ambulatory. Implement graded exercise program as ordered.
Deficient knowledge, related to disease process and risk factors	Develop a teaching plan to prevent venous stasis, including the following: • Avoid prolonged sitting or standing; begin weight reduction if obese. • Avoid crossing the legs at the knee and wearing tight stockings or garters. • Elevate legs when sitting. • Do flexion-extension exercises of feet and legs when sitting or lying down to promote circulation and venous return.

Nursing Diagnoses	Nursing Interventions
	• Do not massage extremities because of danger of embolization of clots (thrombus breaking off and becoming an embolus). • Take prescribed medication.

Prognosis

A major risk during the acute phase of DVT is dislodgment of the thrombus, which can migrate to the lungs, causing a pulmonary embolus.

VARICOSE VEINS

Etiology and Pathophysiology

A varicose vein is a tortuous, dilated vein with incompetent valves. The highest incidence of varicose veins occurs in women ages 40 to 60 years. Approximately 15% of the adult population is affected. Causes of varicose veins include congenitally defective valves, an absent valve, or a valve that becomes incompetent. External pressure on the legs from pregnancy or obesity can place a strain on the vessels, and they become elongated and dilated. Poor posture, prolonged standing, and constrictive clothing may also contribute to this problem. The great and small saphenous veins of the legs are most often affected. The vessel wall weakens and dilates, stretching the valves and leaving the vessel unable to support a column of blood. Pooling of blood in the veins or varicosities is the result. Chronic blood pooling in the veins is referred to as **venous stasis.** Hemorrhage can occur if a varicose vein suffers trauma.

Clinical Manifestations

Varicose veins may be primary or secondary. Primary varicosities have a gradual onset and occur in superficial veins. Secondary varicosities affect the deep veins and result from chronic venous insufficiency or venous thrombosis. Often the only symptom is the appearance of darkened veins on the patient's legs. Symptoms include fatigue, dull aches, cramping of muscles, and a feeling of heaviness or pressure arising from decreased blood flow to the tissues. Signs and symptoms such as edema, pain, changes in skin color, and ulceration may occur from venous stasis.

Assessment

Collection of **subjective data** includes gathering information about predisposing factors: a family history of varicose veins, pregnancy, or other conditions that could cause pressure on the veins. Also include symptoms the patient is experiencing such as aches, fatigue, cramping, heaviness, and pain.

Collection of **objective data** includes inspecting the legs for varicosities, edema, color, and temperature of the skin and observing for ulceration.

Diagnostic Tests

Trendelenburg's test is done to diagnose the ability of the venous valves to support a column of blood by measuring venous filling time. The patient lies down with the affected leg raised to allow for venous emptying. A tourniquet is applied above the knee, and the patient stands. The direction and filling time of the veins are recorded both before and after the tourniquet is removed. When the veins fill rapidly from a backward blood flow, the veins are determined to be incompetent.

Medical Management

Mild signs and symptoms may be controlled with elastic stockings, rest periods, and leg elevation. Sclerotherapy consists of injection of a sclerosing solution at the sites of the varicosities. It is done as an outpatient procedure and produces permanent obliteration (complete occlusion of a part) of collapsed veins and good cosmetic results. Elastic bandages are applied for continuous pressure for 1 to 2 weeks. Surgical intervention is indicated for pain, progression of varicosities, edema, stasis ulcers, and cosmetic reasons. Surgery consists of vein ligation and stripping. The great saphenous vein is ligated (tied) close to the femoral junction. The great and small saphenous veins are stripped out through small incisions made in the inguinal area, above and below the knee and the ankle. The incisions are covered with sterile dressings, and an elastic bandage is applied and worn for at least 1 week.

Nursing Interventions and Patient Teaching

Nursing interventions focus on care of the patient after a surgical procedure, including maintaining comfort, maintaining peripheral circulation and venous return, and patient teaching regarding varicosity prevention and maintenance.

Nursing diagnoses and interventions for the patient with varicose veins include but are not limited to the following:

Nursing Diagnoses	Nursing Interventions
Ineffective tissue perfusion, peripheral, related to impaired venous blood return	Monitor for signs and symptoms of bleeding postoperatively. If bleeding occurs, apply pressure to the wound, elevate the leg, and notify the physician. Keep elastic bandage snug and wrinkle free; do not remove bandage for daily dressing change. Encourage deep breathing exercises and early ambulation to facilitate venous return. Encourage dorsiflexion exercises while in bed or sitting to facilitate venous return.

Continued

Nursing Diagnoses	Nursing Interventions
Deficient knowledge, related to disease process and measures to avoid venous stasis and promote venous return	Develop teaching plan to include the following: • Avoid anything that can increase pressure above the knees (crossing the legs, sitting in chairs that are too high, wearing garters and knee-high stockings). • Begin regular exercise to promote venous return by contraction of leg muscles. • Avoid prolonged sitting or standing. • Elevate legs when sitting. • Maintain ideal weight. • Wear elastic stockings for support for activities that require prolonged standing or when pregnant.

Prognosis

Varicosities are chronic conditions; the affected person must know how to prevent venous stasis and encourage venous return.

VENOUS STASIS ULCERS

Etiology and Pathophysiology

Venous stasis ulcers or leg ulcers occur from chronic deep vein insufficiency and stasis of blood in the venous system of the legs. Other causes include severe varicose veins, burns, trauma, sickle cell anemia, diabetes mellitus, neurogenic disorders, and hereditary factors. A leg ulcer is an open, necrotic lesion that results when an inadequate supply of oxygen-rich blood and nutrients reaches the tissue (Figure 48-24). The result is cell death, tissue sloughing, and skin impairment. Decreased circulation to the area contributes to the development of infection and prolonged healing.

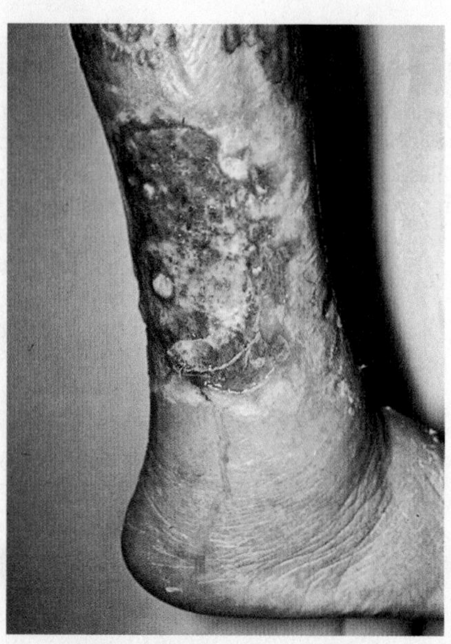

FIGURE 48-24 Venous leg ulcer.

Clinical Manifestations

Patients may report varying degrees of pain, from mild discomfort to a dull, aching pain relieved by elevation of the extremity. The skin is visibly ulcerated and has a leathery appearance and dark pigmentation. Edema may be present. Ulcerations often occur around the medial aspect of the ankle. Pedal pulses are present.

Assessment

Subjective data include onset and duration of pain and successful relief measures. Predisposing factors such as thrombophlebitis, venous insufficiency, and diabetes mellitus are noted.

Collection of **objective data** includes inspection of ulcerated areas: size, location, and condition of skin; color; and temperature. Palpate pedal pulses, and observe for edema.

Diagnostic Tests

Venography and Doppler ultrasonography are used to confirm venous insufficiency and stasis.

Medical Management

Management focuses on promoting wound healing and preventing infection. Diet is important to ensure adequate protein intake, since large amounts of protein in the form of albumin are lost through the ulcers. Also vitamin A and C and the mineral zinc are administered to promote tissue healing. Debridement of necrotic tissue, antibiotic therapy, and protection of the ulcerated area are usual treatments. Debridement can be mechanical, such as applying gauze moistened with saline dressing to the wound. When dry, the dressing is removed, pulling off the debris that has adhered to it. Debridement can also be chemical; enzyme ointments such as fibrinolysin deoxyribonuclease (Elase) are placed over the ulcer to break down necrotic tissue. Surgical debridement using a scalpel is done when other measures are not successful.

Applying compression to the affected area is essential to promote venous ulcer healing and prevent ulcer recurrence. Compression options include elastic wraps, custom-fitted compression stockings, intermittent compression devices, Velcro wraps, and a multilayer bandage system (e.g., Profore) (Wipke-Tevis et al., 2004). An Unna's paste boot can be used to protect the ulcer and provide constant and even support to the area (Figure 48-25). Moist, impregnated gauze is wrapped around the patient's foot and leg. It hardens into a "boot" that may be left on for 1 to 2 weeks, although it may be changed more often if there is copious drainage. It is essential that a patient with a venous leg ulcer has a balanced diet with adequate protein calories and nutrients to promote healing (Lewis et al., 2007).

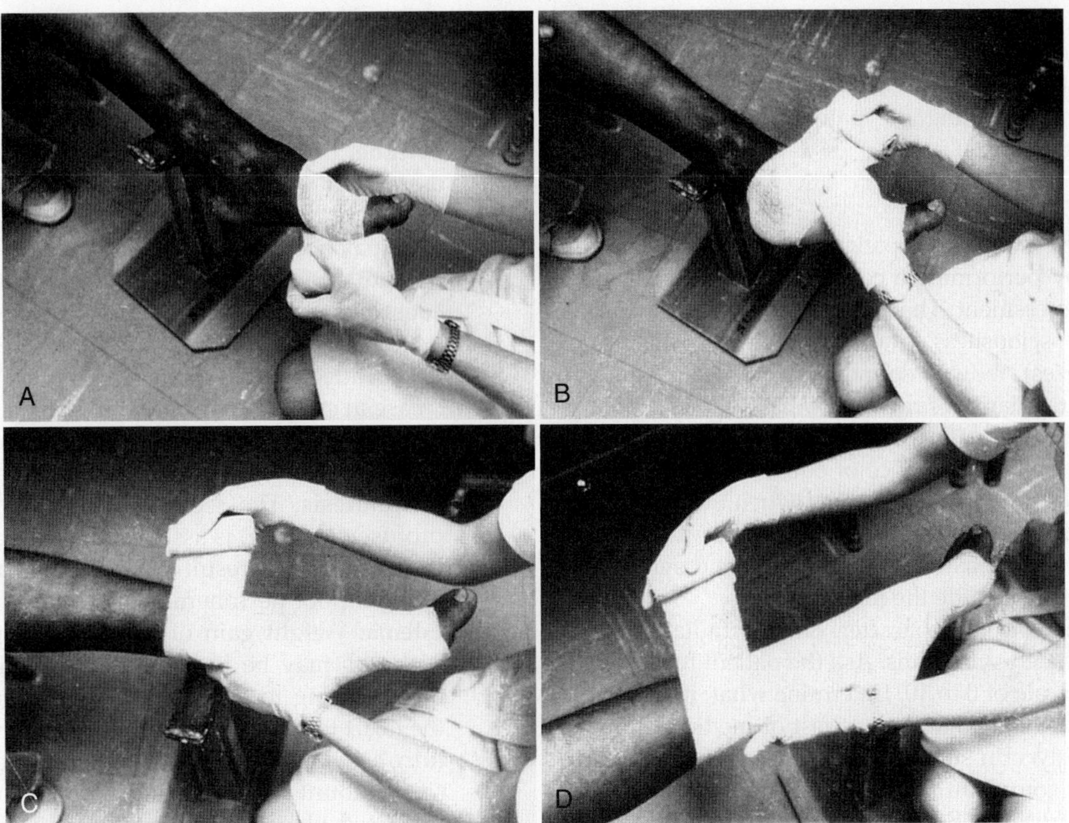

FIGURE 48-25 Nurse applying Unna's paste boot using specially impregnated gauze. Most ulcers are on inferior aspect of patient's foot.

Nursing Interventions and Patient Teaching

Nursing interventions focus on promoting wound healing, promoting comfort, maintaining peripheral tissue perfusion, preventing infection, and patient teaching.

Nursing diagnoses and interventions for the patient with venous stasis ulcers include but are not limited to the following:

Nursing Diagnoses	Nursing Interventions
Impaired skin integrity, related to open ulceration	Perform dressing changes per physician's order, using gauze, moistened with saline, topical drug treatments, and Unna's boot therapy. Assess wound for signs and symptoms of infection. Provide antibiotic therapy as prescribed. Encourage nutritional intake to promote wound healing.
Ineffective tissue perfusion, peripheral, related to insufficient venous circulation	Elevate extremities when sitting or lying to promote venous return and decrease risk of edema and venous stasis. Use overbed cradle to protect extremities from pressure of bed linens. Use cotton between toes to prevent pressure on a toe ulcer. Assess level of discomfort.

Patient teaching focuses on preventing infection, maintaining peripheral tissue circulation, avoiding venous stasis, and providing proper wound care and dressing changes. See previous nursing diagnoses and interventions.

Prognosis

Venous stasis ulcers are a chronic condition caused by chronic venous insufficiency and delayed healing. Most venous ulcers heal with therapy.

❖ NURSING PROCESS *for the Patient with a Cardiovascular Disorder*

The role of the licensed practical nurse/licensed vocational nurse (LPN/LVN) in the nursing process as stated is that the LPN/LVN will:

- Participate in planning care for patients based on patient needs
- Review patient's care plan and recommend revisions as needed
- Review and follow defined prioritization for patient care

- Use clinical pathways, care maps, or care plans to guide and review patient care

Systemic cardiac assessment provides baseline data useful for identifying the patient's physiologic and psychosocial needs.

Assessment

Begin assessment of the patient with a cardiovascular disorder by performing a complete health history and physical assessment. The physical assessment includes level of consciousness, vital signs, lung sounds (crackles, wheezes), bowel sounds, apical heart sounds (strength, regularity of rhythm), pedal pulses, capillary refill, skin color (pallor, cyanosis), turgor, temperature and moisture, and presence of edema. The history includes a description of symptoms, when they occurred, their course and duration, location, precipitating factors, and relief measures. Specific signs and symptoms to be aware of include the following:

- **Pain:** Note the character, quality, radiation, and associated symptoms. Ask the patient to rate pain on a scale of 0 to 10. Determine what, if anything, relieved the pain, such as rest or medication (e.g., nitroglycerin sublingually). Chest pain is the primary complaint when patients have symptoms of heart disease. Some patients with ischemia have pain in the jaw and left shoulder. The patient may describe the pain as dull, sharp, pressure, squeezing, crushing, viselike, grinding, or radiating. Note any factors precipitating the onset. Pain originating from cardiac muscle ischemia (decreased blood supply to a body organ or part) produces anxiety. It may lead to other signs and symptoms such as nausea, vertigo, or diaphoresis. Chest pain is significant in indicating cardiac ischemia or damage.
- **Palpitations:** Characterized by rapid, irregular, or pounding heartbeat, palpitations may be associated with cardiac dysrhythmias (any disturbance or abnormality in a normal rhythmic pattern) or cardiac ischemia. Patients may begin to notice the heartbeat and describe it as "pounding" or "racing." This can be frightening for the patient.
- **Cyanosis:** A bluish discoloration of the skin and mucous membranes caused by an excess of deoxygenated hemoglobin in the blood, cyanosis results from decreased cardiac output and poor peripheral perfusion.
- **Dyspnea:** Dyspnea is characterized by difficulty breathing or shortness of breath. Observe for dyspnea with activity, referred to as **exertional dyspnea,** which is commonly associated with decreased cardiac function.
- **Orthopnea:** Orthopnea is an abnormal condition in which a person must sit or stand to breathe deeply or comfortably.
- **Cough:** The cough may be dry or productive and results from a fluid accumulation in the lungs. The patient may describe it as irritating or spasmodic. Dyspnea may be associated with it. The production of sputum should be observed for frothiness or hemoptysis (see discussion of pulmonary edema).
- **Fatigue:** Exhaustion and activity intolerance are associated with decreased cardiac output. The patient may be unable to perform ADLs. Depression may accompany this or be a result of it.
- **Syncope:** Syncope or fainting is a brief lapse of consciousness caused by transient cerebral hypoxia. It is usually preceded by a sensation of lightheadedness. It can result from a sudden decrease in cardiac output to the brain as a result of dysrhythmia (bradycardia or tachycardia) or decreased pumping action of the heart.
- **Diaphoresis:** The secretion of sweat, especially profuse sweating, is associated with clamminess. Diaphoresis is a result of decreased cardiac output and poor peripheral perfusion.
- **Edema:** Weight gain of more than 3 pounds in 24 hours may be indicative of HF. The mechanism leading to edema in HF is the inability of the heart to pump efficiently or accept venous return, causing retrograde blood flow and an excessive amount of circulating blood volume. This increased blood volume results in increased hydrostatic pressure and an increase of fluid in the interstitial spaces.

Nursing Diagnosis

Assess the patient's cardiovascular system and identify characteristics that reveal a nursing diagnosis. Nursing diagnoses for cardiovascular problems may include the following:

- Activity intolerance
- Anxiety
- Decreased cardiac output
- Ineffective coronary tissue perfusion
- Excess fluid volume
- Impaired gas exchange
- Deficient knowledge (specify)
- Pain

Expected Outcomes and Planning

Plan appropriate interventions to meet the needs of patients with cardiovascular problems. The nurse is in the unique position of ongoing patient monitoring and is able to participate in the development of nursing diagnoses, help select appropriate interventions, and document the care plan. Teaching throughout the hospital stay and when preparing for discharge is important. Reinforcement of good health habits improves the likelihood for compliance with the care plan.

Implementation

Nursing interventions for the patient with a cardiovascular disorder include enhancing cardiac output, promoting tissue perfusion, promoting adequate gas exchange, improving activity tolerance, and promoting comfort. Patient teaching emphasizes adherence to diet and exercise and medication protocols and strategies for balancing activity, getting rest, and reducing stress.

Evaluation

Evaluate the expected outcomes as the final step of the nursing process and determine their effectiveness. Participate in the revision of the plan and nursing interventions when necessary.

Get Ready for the NCLEX® Examination!

Key Points

- The cardiovascular system is composed of the heart, blood vessels, and lymphatic structures.
- The functions of the cardiovascular system are to deliver oxygen and nutrients to the cells and to remove carbon dioxide and waste products from the cells.
- The heart is a large pump (the size of a human fist) that propels blood through the circulatory system.
- The heart is composed of four chambers: two atria and two ventricles.
- There are two coronary arteries; they supply the heart with nutrition and oxygen.
- The electrical pattern of impulse starts with the SA node, which is the pacemaker of the heart; it initiates the heartbeat. This impulse travels to the AV node. From here the impulse travels to a bundle of fibers called the bundle of His and divides into right and left bundle branches and finally to the Purkinje fibers.
- Three kinds of blood vessels are organized for carrying blood to and from the heart: the arteries, the veins, and the capillaries.
- Risk factors for developing CAD are classified as nonmodifiable and modifiable.
- Nonmodifiable risk factors for CAD include advancing age, male gender, black race, and a positive family history of CAD.
- Major modifiable risk factors for CAD include cigarette smoking, hyperlipidemia, stress, obesity, sedentary lifestyle, and hypertension. A diet high in cholesterol and saturated fats contributes to risk.
- An important aspect of caring for the patient with a cardiovascular disorder is understanding the risk factors and incorporating them into patient teaching.
- Major diagnostic tests to evaluate cardiovascular function include chest radiograph, arteriography, cardiac catheterization, ECG, echocardiogram, telemetry, stress test, PET, and thallium scanning.
- Common laboratory examinations to evaluate cardiovascular function are blood cultures, CBC, PT, INR, PTT, ESR, serum electrolytes, lipids (VLDL, LDL, HDL), triglycerides, arterial blood gases, BNP, and serum cardiac markers. Troponin I is a myocardial muscle protein released into circulation after myocardial injury and is useful in diagnosing an MI.
- CAD is the term used to describe a variety of conditions that obstruct blood flow in the coronary arteries.
- When the myocardial oxygen demand exceeds the myocardial oxygen supply, ischemia of the heart muscle occurs, resulting in chest pain or angina.
- Patient teaching to minimize the pain of angina pectoris includes taking nitroglycerin before exertion, eating small amounts rather than two or three larger meals, balancing exercise periods with rest, stopping activity at first sign of chest pain, avoiding exposure to extreme weather conditions, ceasing to smoke, and seeking a calm environment.
- Subjective data of a patient with MI may include heavy pressure or squeezing pressure in the chest, retrosternal pain radiating to left arm and jaw, anxiety, nausea, and dyspnea.
- Objective data for the patient with MI include pallor, hypertension, cardiac rhythm changes, vomiting, fever, and diaphoresis.
- Possible nursing diagnoses for the patient with MI include *pain (acute), tissue perfusion (ineffective), activity intolerance, decreased cardiac output, anxiety,* and *constipation.*
- Cardiac rehabilitation services are designed to help patients with heart disease recover faster and return to full and productive lives. Cardiac rehabilitation improves patient compliance.
- HF leads to the congested state of the heart, lungs, and systemic circulation as a result of the heart's inability to act as an effective pump. The most recent definition is that HF should be viewed as a neurohormonal problem that progresses as a result of chronic release in the body of substances such as catecholamines (epinephrine and norepinephrine). These substances may have toxic effects on the heart.
- It is important to realize that 1 L of fluid equals 1 kg (2.2 pounds); a weight gain of 2.2 pounds signifies a gain of 1 L of body fluid.
- Signs and symptoms of HF with left ventricular failure include dyspnea; cough; frothy, blood-tinged sputum; pulmonary crackles; and evidence of pulmonary vascular congestion with pleural effusion.
- Signs and symptoms of HF with right ventricular failure include edema in feet, ankles, and sacrum, which may progress into the thigh and external genitalia; liver congestion; ascites; and distended jugular veins.
- Medical management of HF includes increasing cardiac efficiency with digitalis, vasodilators, and ACE inhibitors; administering a beta blocker (carvedilol) for mild to moderate HF; lowering oxygen requirements through bed rest; providing oxygen to the tissues through oxygen therapy if the patient is hypoxic; treating edema and pulmonary congestion with a diuretic and a sodium-restricted diet; and weighing daily to monitor fluid retention.
- Nursing interventions for the patient with valvular heart disease include administering the prescribed medications (diuretics, digoxin, and antidysrhythmics); monitoring I&O and daily weight; auscultating breath sounds and heart sounds; taking blood pressure; and assessing capillary perfusion, pedal pulses, and presence of edema.

- Patient teaching for the patient with valvular heart disease includes dietary management, activity limitations, and the importance of antibiotic prophylaxis before invasive procedure.
- Most patients with cardiomyopathy have a severe, progressively deteriorating course, and the majority older than age 55 years die within 2 years of the onset of signs and symptoms.
- PVD is any abnormal condition that affects the blood vessels outside the heart and the lymphatic vessels.
- Arteriosclerosis is the underlying problem associated with PVD.
- Hypertension occurs when there is a sustained elevated systolic blood pressure greater than 140 mm Hg and/or sustained elevated diastolic blood pressure of greater than 90 mm Hg on two or more readings.
- Nursing interventions for hypertension primarily focus on blood pressure management through patient teaching, risk factor recognition, drug therapy, dietary management, exercise, and stress-reduction techniques.
- An aneurysm is an enlarged, dilated portion of an artery and may be the result of arteriosclerosis, trauma, or a congenital defect.
- The hazards of cigarette smoking and its relationship to thromboangiitis obliterans (Buerger's disease) are the primary focuses of patient teaching.
- The two major venous disorders are thrombophlebitis and varicose veins.
- Thrombophlebitis may result in calf pain on dorsiflexion of the foot, which is referred to as a positive Homans' sign. A positive Homans' sign appears in only 10% of DVT patients.
- Patient teaching to avoid thrombophlebitis includes avoid prolonged sitting or standing, avoid dehydration, reduce weight if obese, do dorsiflexion-extension exercises of feet and legs, do not cross legs at the knees, and elevate legs when sitting.

Additional Learning Resources

Go to your Companion CD for an audio glossary, animations, video clips, and more.

evolve Be sure to visit the Evolve site at http://evolve.elsevier.com/Christensen/adult/ for additional online resources.

Review Questions for the NCLEX® Examination

1. The blood that is pumped out of the left ventricle contains:
   1. a full supply of oxygen.
   2. impurities that must be removed by the liver.
   3. a high percentage of carbon dioxide.
   4. all the wastes to be delivered to the organs of excretion.

2. The heart contracts in the following patterns:
   1. right atrium, left atrium, then the ventricles.
   2. both atria, then both ventricles.
   3. right atrium, right ventricle, then the left atrium, left ventricle.
   4. ventricles, then atria.

3. The interior lining of the heart, the valves, and the large vessels of the heart are together called the:
   1. endocardium.
   2. myocardium.
   3. pericardium.
   4. epicardium.

4. Valve flaps prevent the backflow of blood from the pulmonary artery into the:
   1. lung.
   2. right atrium.
   3. right ventricle.
   4. left atrium.

5. The normal period in the heart cycle during which the muscle fibers lengthen, the heart dilates, and the cavities fill with blood, roughly the period of relaxation, is called:
   1. systole.
   2. pulse pressure.
   3. diastose.
   4. diastole.

6. The right atrium receives blood from the:
   1. superior and inferior venae cavae.
   2. pulmonary veins, pulmonary arteries.
   3. superior and inferior venae cavae and coronary sinus.
   4. membranous septum, coronary sinus.

7. When a patient is receiving heparin therapy, the nurse should:
   1. observe him for cyanosis.
   2. remember that a sedimentation rate is ordered for monitoring blood coagulation.
   3. give the injection intramuscularly.
   4. observe emesis, urine, and stools for blood.

8. A 72-year-old patient is admitted to the medical floor with a diagnosis of HF. In HF an increase in abdominal girth, increase in total body weight, and pitting edema are indications of:
   1. fluid retention.
   2. electrolyte imbalance.
   3. disorganized ventricle pulsation.
   4. AV node dysfunction.

9. A 10-year-old patient is diagnosed with rheumatic fever. Of all the manifestations seen in rheumatic fever, the one that can lead to permanent complications is:
   1. Sydenham's chorea.
   2. erythema marginatum.
   3. subcutaneous nodules.
   4. carditis.

10. A 67-year-old patient has a diagnosis of hypertension. She is being dismissed from the hospital. Her teaching should include:
    1. instruction in consuming a bland diet.
    2. instruction of sodium intake up to 4g/day.
    3. encouragement to begin a vigorous exercise program.
    4. education on continuing to take antihypertensive medications as prescribed.

11. An 86-year-old patient is receiving D5½ NS per IV at 83 mL/hr on the electronic infusion pump. It is vitally important that the IV lines of older adult patients be monitored carefully because:
    1. these patients do not get dehydrated very easily.
    2. they may get a fluid overload of the circulatory system.
    3. of the increased risk of infection in the veins.
    4. of the danger of thrombophlebitis developing in the peripheral system.

12. A 34-year-old patient with a history of IV drug use is diagnosed with acute infective endocarditis. Nursing interventions for this patient include:
    1. early ambulation and activity progression.
    2. restricted activity for several weeks.
    3. low-calorie diet.
    4. dilution of blood by increased fluid intake.

13. A 62-year-old patient has a history of angina pectoris. To decrease the pain from angina pectoris, the patient should:
    1. take a cardiac glycoside at first symptom of cardiac pain.
    2. avoid taking more than three or four nitroglycerin pills daily.
    3. take nitroglycerin sublingually qid.
    4. take nitroglycerin sublingually prophylactically before strenuous exercise.

14. A patient has peripheral arterial disorder (PAD) of the lower extremities. Patient teaching for PAD includes:
    1. encouraging the patient to ambulate frequently.
    2. the importance of avoiding exposure to cold and chilling.
    3. teaching self-massage of the legs with lotion.
    4. maintaining a reduced-calorie diet.

15. A 75-year-old patient is diagnosed with heart failure. The nursing diagnosis of *activity intolerance,* related to dyspnea and fatigue, would be appropriate. Choose the appropriate nursing intervention in keeping with this diagnosis.
    1. Plan frequent rest periods.
    2. Allow patient to shower.
    3. Encourage patient to perform all ADLs.
    4. Encourage fluid intake of 3000 L/day.

16. A patient recovering from an MI is being prepared for discharge and should be instructed to:
    1. remain inactive until healing is complete.
    2. remain at home and avoid exposure to cold temperatures.
    3. begin a cardiac rehabilitation program.
    4. perform isometric exercises in a relaxed environment.

17. Dependent edema of the extremities, enlargement of the liver, oliguria, jugular vein distention, and abdominal distention are signs and symptoms of:
    1. right-sided heart failure.
    2. left-sided heart failure.
    3. cardiac dysrhythmias.
    4. valvular heart disease.

18. The primary function of patient teaching after a myocardial infarction is:
    1. explaining the disease process.
    2. assisting the patient in developing a healthy lifestyle.
    3. describing the precipitating causes and onset of pain.
    4. educating the patient on causative factors that initiate cardiac vasoconstriction.

19. An important nursing intervention when caring for a patient with remote telemetry is to:
    1. encourage independence by permitting patient to shower.
    2. never remove telemetry and allow patient to shower unless physician has written an order to allow it.
    3. encourage use of stair climbing, aerobic exercise, and other forms of exertion to promote collateral circulation.
    4. be aware that special microphones, attached to the patient's chest, pick up cardiac sounds produced by pressure changes in the heart.

20. Signs and symptoms of cardiogenic shock include:
    1. warm, dry skin.
    2. decreasing blood pressure and weak, rapid pulse.
    3. flushed face, restlessness.
    4. polyuria and dysuria.

21. Modifiable risk factors for coronary artery disease (CAD) includes?
    1. Diabetes, family history
    2. Family history, smoking
    3. Smoking, heredity
    4. High cholesterol, obesity

22. The name of the neurohormone released from the left ventricle in response to volume expansion and pressure overload that has emerged as the blood marker for the identification of individuals with HF is:
    1. A-type natriuretic peptide (ANP).
    2. troponin I.
    3. B-type natriuretic peptide (BNP).
    4. CPK peptide.

23. The normal range for the above blood marker is:
    1. 0 to 100 pg/mL.
    2. 500 to 900 pg/mL.
    3. 0.003 to 1 pg/mL.
    4. 400 to 500 pg/mL.

24. __________ is a myocardial muscle protein released into circulation after myocardial injury and is useful in diagnosing a myocardial infarction.

25. In the United States, the two beta blocker medications specifically approved for heart failure are carvedilol (Coreg) and:
    1. benazepril (Lotensin).
    2. captopril (Capoten).
    3. long-acting metoprolol (Toprol X-L).
    4. verapamil (Calan).

26. The most useful noninvasive diagnostic tool for evaluating the patient with heart failure is:

1. coronary angiography.
2. echocardiogram.
3. electrocardiogram.
4. thallium scanning.

27. Electrocardiogram findings during an MI:

1. are less likely to show ST-segment elevation in women than in men.
2. always show ST-segment elevation in women, but not in men.
3. always show ST-segment elevation in women and men.
4. are easier to interpret in women than in men.

28. The nursing diagnosis of *decreased cardiac output,* related to loss of myocardial contractility, would be appropriate for the patient who has had an acute myocardial infarction. The correct nursing interventions for this nursing diagnoses would include: *(Select all that apply.)*

1. Assess for and report decreased blood pressure and dysrhythmias.
2. Assess for oliguria.
3. Administer oxygen therapy as ordered.
4. Give opioids sparingly.

29. Heart failure is usually treated with: *(Select all that apply.)*

1. Cardiotonic drugs (digitalis)
2. Diuretic agents
3. Generous fluid intake
4. ACE inhibitors, beta-adrenergic blockers (carvediol), nitrates

30. An invasive procedure in which a catheter from a femoral or brachial artery is placed in the coronary artery and a balloon is inflated against the narrowing wall, thus reducing the arterial constriction, is called:

1. coronary artery bypass graft (CABG) surgery.
2. pacemaker.
3. vectorcardiogram.
4. percutaneous transluminal coronary angioplasty (PTCA).

31. Thrombolytic agents such as streptokinase and tissue plasminogen activators such as alteplase and activase are agents used to dissolve blood clots. These agents are *most* effective in a patient with acute MI signs and symptoms:

1. in the first 24 hours.
2. in the first 30 minutes to 1 hour.
3. in the first 72 hours.
4. in the second 6 hours after an MI.

32. A 74-year-old patient with heart failure is admitted to the hospital because of a weight gain of 12 pounds in the past 2 weeks. After effective results from IV furosemide (Lasix), the patient has lost 8 pounds. This would reflect a loss of how much fluid?

1. 1.6 L
2. 6 L
3. 3.6 or 4 L
4. 2.2 L

33. A patient is admitted with a diagnosis of possible aortic abdominal aneurysm. In assessment for possible complications it is most important to monitor:

1. body temperature.
2. skin turgor.
3. respiratory rate.
4. blood pressure.

34. A 63-year-old patient has Buerger's disease. The most important aspect of patient compliance to decrease signs and symptoms of Buerger's disease is:

1. low-fat diet.
2. weight loss.
3. cessation of tobacco use.
4. keeping extremities warm.

35. An 83-year-old patient is diagnosed with venous stasis ulcers. The medical management includes the use of an Unna's paste boot. An Unna's boot: *(Select all that apply.)*

1. hardens into a "boot" that may be left on for 1 to 2 weeks.
2. is a moist, impregnated gauze wrapped around the patient's foot and leg.
3. applies intermittent external pressure to the lower extremities; it pushes blood from the superficial veins into deep veins.
4. protects the ulcer and provides constant and even support to the area.

36. A 58-year-old patient is admitted with Raynaud's disease. The correct patient teaching information includes: *(Select all that apply.)*

1. avoid cold.
2. warm hands and feet with heating pad.
3. practice stress-reduction techniques.
4. comply with smoking cessation.

37. A patient is admitted with HF and chronic arterial fibrillation. What medication is his physician likely to order to prevent thrombus formation?

1. An ACE inhibitor
2. Nitroglycerin
3. An antihypertensive
4. An anticoagulant

Care of the Patient with a Respiratory Disorder

chapter **49**

evolve

Barbara Lauritsen Christensen

http://evolve.elsevier.com/Christensen/foundationsadult

Objectives

Anatomy and Physiology

1. Differentiate between external and internal respiration.
2. Describe the purpose of the respiratory system.
3. List and define the parts of the upper and lower respiratory tracts.
4. List the ways in which oxygen and carbon dioxide are transported in the blood.
5. Discuss the mechanisms that regulate respirations.

Medical-Surgical

6. Identify those signs and symptoms that indicate a patient is experiencing hypoxia.
7. Differentiate among sonorous wheezes, sibilant wheezes, crackles, and pleural friction rub.
8. Describe the purpose, significance of results, and nursing interventions related to diagnostic examinations of the respiratory system.
9. Describe the significance of arterial blood gas values and differentiate between arterial oxygen tension (PaO_2) and arterial oxygen saturation (SaO_2).
10. Discuss the etiology and pathophysiology, clinical manifestations, assessment, diagnostic tests, medical management, nursing interventions, and prognosis of the patient with disorders of the upper airway.
11. Discuss nursing interventions for the patient with a laryngectomy.
12. Discuss the etiology and pathophysiology, clinical manifestations, assessment, diagnostic tests, medical management, nursing interventions, and prognosis of the patient with disorders of the lower airway.
13. List five nursing interventions to assist patients with retained pulmonary secretions.
14. Differentiate between tuberculosis infection and tuberculosis disease.
15. List four medications commonly prescribed for the patient with tuberculosis.
16. List five nursing assessments or interventions pertaining to the care of the patient with closed-chest drainage.
17. Discuss three risk factors associated with pulmonary emboli.
18. Compare and contrast the etiology and pathophysiology, clinical manifestations, assessment, diagnostic tests, medical management, nursing interventions, and prognosis for the patient with chronic obstructive pulmonary disease, including emphysema, chronic bronchitis, asthma, and bronchiectasis.
19. Differentiate between medical management of the patient with emphysema and the patient with asthma.
20. Discuss why low-flow oxygen is required for patients with emphysema.
21. State three possible nursing diagnoses for the patient with altered respiratory function.

Key Terms

adventitious (ăd-vĕnt-TĪ-shŭs, p. 1615)
atelectasis (ă-tĕ-LĔK-tā-sĭs, p. 1646)
bronchoscopy (brŏng-KŎS-kō-pē, p. 1617)
cor pumonale (kŏr pŭl-mō-NĂ-lē, p. 1657)
coryza (kō-RĪ-ză, p. 1627)
crackles (KRĂK-ŭlz, p. 1615)
cyanosis (sī-ă-NŌ-sĭs, p. 1624)
dyspnea (DĬSP-nē-ă, p. 1614)
embolism (ĔM-bō-lĭz-ŭm, p. 1652)
empyema (ĕm-pī-Ē-mă, p. 1644)
epistaxis (ĕp-ĭ-STĂK-sĭs, p. 1620)
exacerbation (ĕg-zăs-ĕr-BĀ-shŭn, p. 1660)
extrinsic (ĕk-STRĬN-zĭk, p. 1662)
hypercapnia (hī-pĕr-KĂP-nē-ă, p. 1660)
hypoventilation (hī-pō-vĕn-tĭ-LĀ-shŭn, p. 1646)
hypoxia (hī-PŎK-sē-ă, p. 1615)
intrinsic (ĭn-TRĬN-zĭk, p. 1662)
orthopnea (ŏr-thŏp-NĒ-ă, p. 1615)
pleural friction rubs (PLŪ-răl FRĬK-shŭn rŭbz, p. 1615)
pneumothorax (nū-mō-THŌ-răks, p. 1647)
sibilant wheezes (SĬB-ĭ-lănt wēz-ĕz, p. 1615)
sonorous wheezes (sŏ-NŎR-ŭs wēz-ĕz, p. 1615)
stertorous (STĔR-tĕr-ŭs, p. 1621)
tachypnea (tăk-ĭp-NĒ-ă, p. 1646)
thoracentesis (thŏ-ră-sĕn-TĒ-sĭs, p. 1614)
virulent (VĬR-ū-lĕnt, p. 1634)

ANATOMY AND PHYSIOLOGY OF THE RESPIRATORY SYSTEM

For the millions of cells throughout the body to carry out their specialized activities, they must have a continuous supply of oxygen. External respiration, or breathing, is the exchange of oxygen and carbon dioxide between the lung and the environment. As air is inhaled, it is warmed, moistened, and filtered to prepare it for use by the body. The respiratory system works with the cardiovascular system to deliver oxygen to the cells, where it provides energy to carry out metabolism. Internal respiration is the exchange of oxygen and carbon dioxide at the cellular level. Oxygen enters the cells while carbon dioxide leaves them. The gases diffuse across the cell membrane into the bloodstream, which plays the role of transporter. Failure of the respiratory system or cardiovascular system has the same result: rapid cell death from oxygen starvation. Figure 49-1 shows the structure of the respiratory organs.

UPPER RESPIRATORY TRACT

Nose

Air enters the respiratory tract through the nose. The air is filtered, moistened, and warmed as it enters the two nasal openings (nares) and travels to the nasal cavity. The nasal septum separates the nares. This entire area is lined with mucous membrane, which is vascular. The mucous membrane provides warmth and moisture and secretes 1 L of moisture every day.

Lateral to the nasal cavities are three scroll-like bones called **turbinates** or **conchae** (Figure 49-2), which cause the air to move over a larger surface area. This increase in surface area provides more time for warming and moisturizing the air. Lining the nasal cavities are tiny hairs, which trap dust and other foreign particles and prevent them from entering the lower respiratory tract.

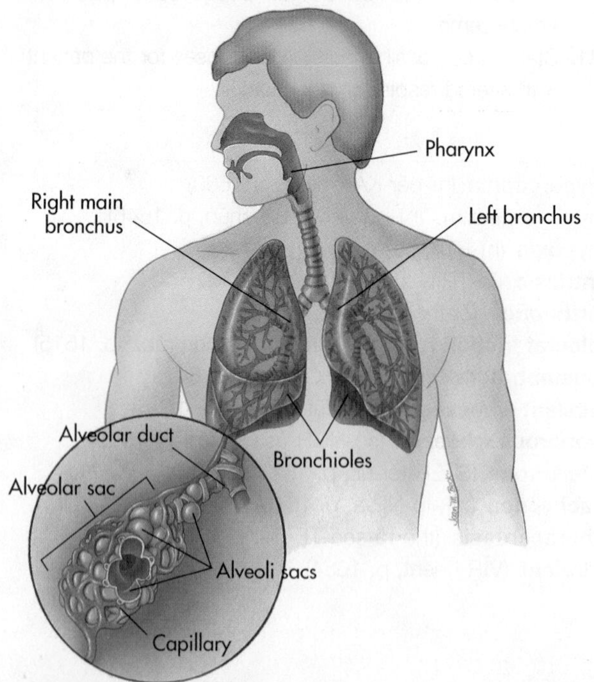

FIGURE 49-1 Structural plan of the respiratory organs showing pharynx, trachea, bronchi, and lungs. Inset shows the grapelike alveolar sacs where the interchange of oxygen and carbon dioxide takes place through the thin walls of the alveoli. Capillaries surround the alveoli.

Communicating with the nasal structures are paranasal sinuses (Figure 49-3). They are called the **frontal, maxillary, sphenoid,** and **ethmoid cavities.** These are hollow areas that make the skull lighter and are believed to give resonance to the voice. They are lined with mucous membranes that are continuous with the nasal cavity. Because of this, nasal infections can cause sinusitis, which is uncomfortable and difficult to treat.

The receptors for the sense of smell are located in the mucosa of the nasal cavities. They are the nerve endings of the olfactory nerve, the first cranial nerve. The nasolacrimal ducts, or tear ducts, communicate with the upper nasal chamber. Hence, when an individual cries, there are copious nasal secretions.

Pharynx

The **pharynx**, or throat (a tubular structure about 5 inches [13 cm] long extending from the base of the skull to the esophagus and situated just in front of the vertebrae), is the passageway for both air and food. At the distal end of the pharynx are three subdivisions: (1) **nasopharynx** (superior portion), (2) **oropharynx** (posterior to mouth), and (3) **laryngopharynx** (directly superior to larynx) (see Figure 49-2).

The eustachian tubes enter either side of the nasopharynx, connecting it to the middle ear. Because the inner linings of the pharynx and the eustachian tube are continuous, an infection of the pharynx can spread easily to the ear. This is common in children. The adenoids (pharyngeal tonsils) are in the nasopharynx, whereas the palatine tonsils are in the oropharynx.

Larynx

The **larynx** (Figure 49-4, *A*), or organ of voice, is supported by nine areas of cartilage and connects the pharynx with the trachea. The largest area of cartilage is composed of two fused plates and is called the **thyroid cartilage,** or **Adam's apple.** It is the same size in girls and boys until puberty, when it enlarges in boys and produces a projection in the neck. The **epiglottis,** a large leaf-shaped area of cartilage, protects the larynx when swallowing. It covers the larynx tightly to prevent food from entering the trachea and directs the food to the esophagus (Figure 49-4, *B*).

The larynx contains the vocal cords. During expiration, air rushes over the vocal cords, causing them to vibrate. This enables speech to occur. The opening between the vocal cords is the glottis.

Trachea

The **trachea** (Figure 49-5), or windpipe, is a tubelike structure that extends approximately 4⅓ inches (11 cm) to the midchest, where it divides into the right and left

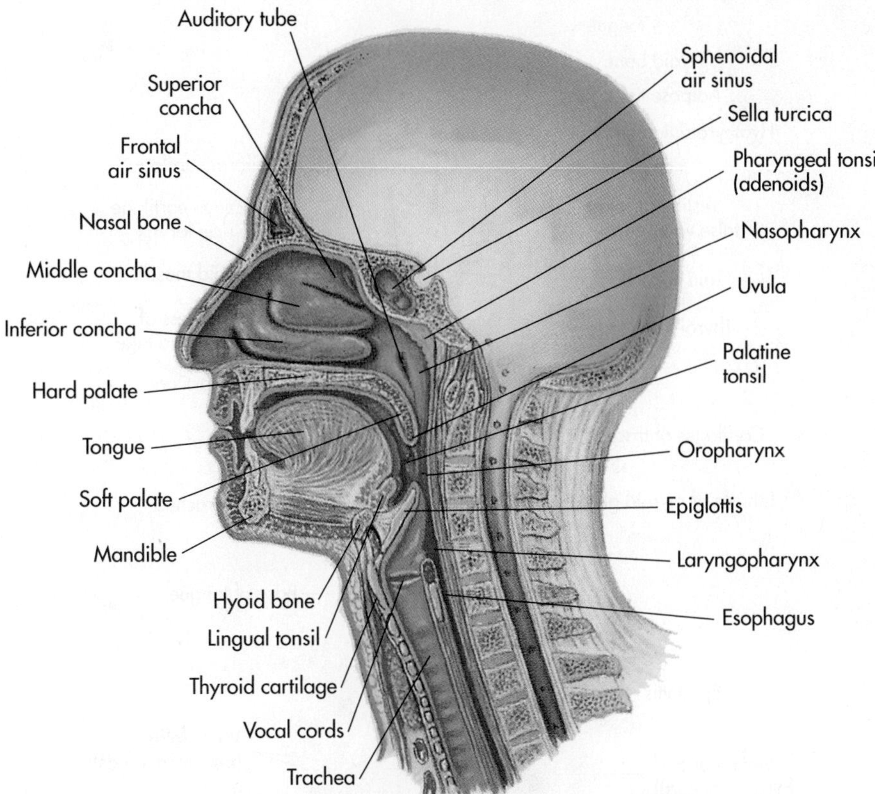

FIGURE 49-2 Sagittal section through the face and the neck.

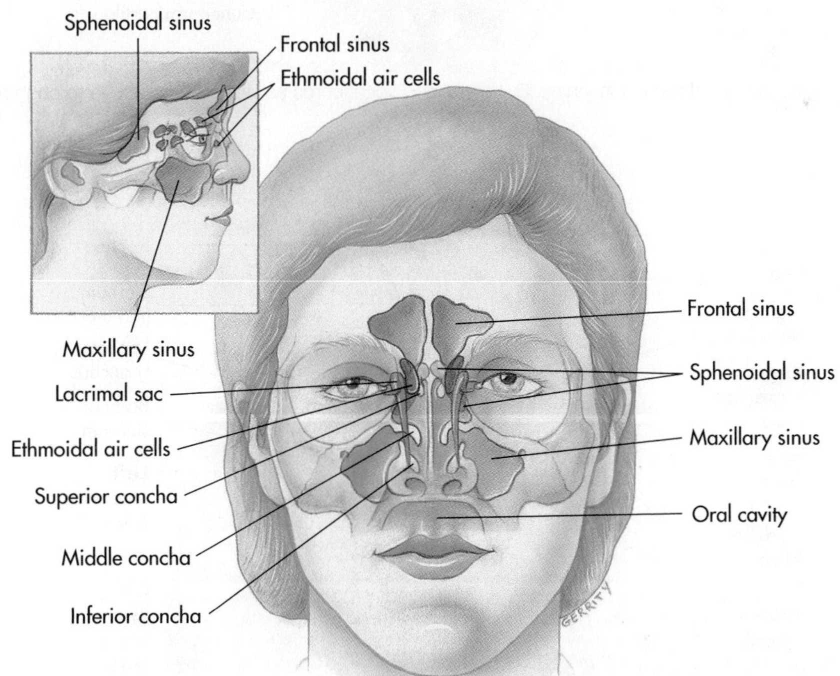

FIGURE 49-3 Projections of paranasal sinuses and oral nasal cavities on the skull and the face. Note the connection between the sinuses and the nasal cavity.

bronchi. It lies anterior to the esophagus and connects the larynx with the bronchi. The ventral (anterior) surface of the tube is covered in the neck by the isthmus (narrow connection) of the thyroid gland. It contains C-shaped cartilaginous rings that keep it from collapsing. The open part of the C-shaped rings lies posterior to the column anterior to the esophagus, which allows the esophagus to expand during swallowing while maintaining patency of the trachea. This is necessary for uninterrupted breathing.

The entire structure is lined with mucous membranes and tiny **cilia** (small, hairlike processes on the

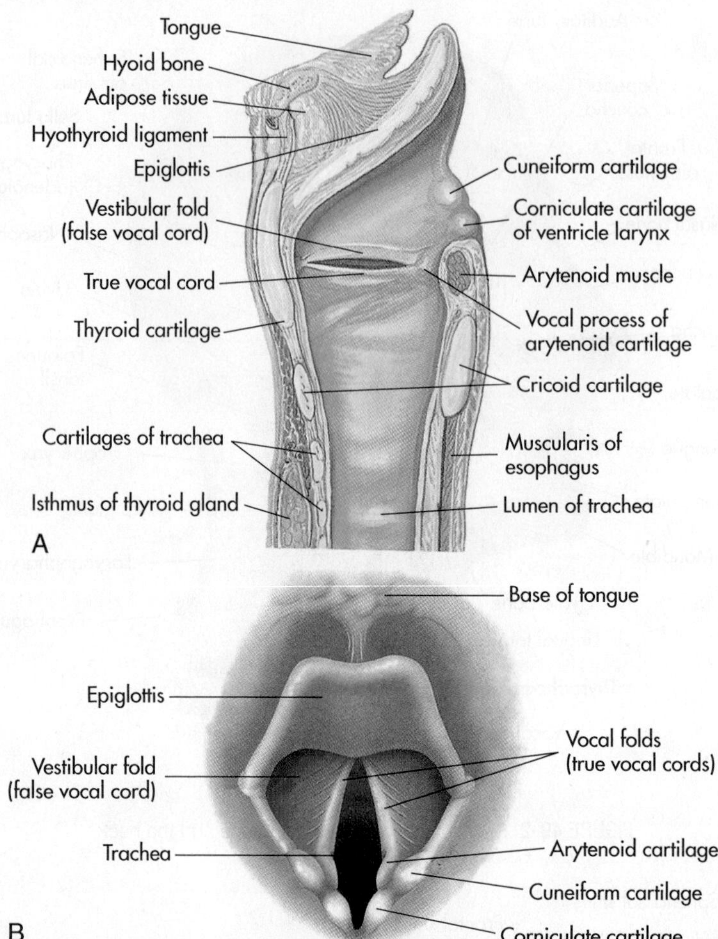

FIGURE 49-4 **A,** Sagittal section through the larynx. **B,** Larynx and vocal cords as viewed from above through a laryngeal mirror.

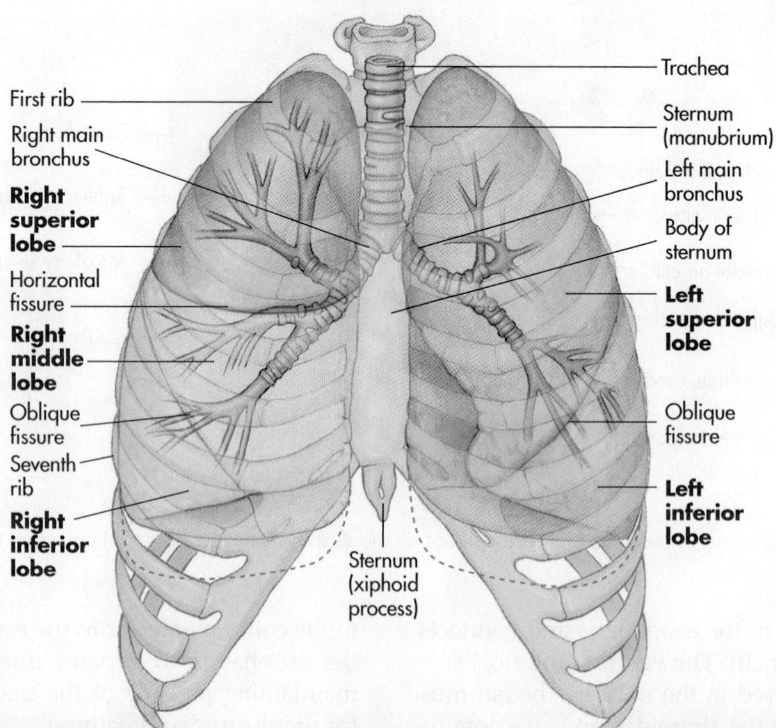

FIGURE 49-5 Projection of the lungs and trachea in relation to ribcage and clavicles. *Dotted line* shows location of dome-shaped diaphragm at the end of expiration and before inspiration. Note that apex of each lung projects above the clavicle. Ribs 11 and 12 are not visible in this view.

outer surfaces of small cells, which produce motion or current in a fluid) that sweep dust or debris upward toward the nasal cavity. Any large particles initiate the cough reflex, which aids in the evacuation of foreign material. Sometimes, because of an airway obstruction, a physician performs a tracheostomy (a surgical opening into the trachea through which an indwelling tube may be inserted). Once this procedure is completed, the individual breathes through the tracheal opening rather than the nose. The opening is below the larynx, so air cannot pass over the vocal cords. The vocal cords cannot vibrate, and speech becomes physiologically impossible.

LOWER RESPIRATORY TRACT

Bronchial Tree

As the trachea enters the lungs, it divides into the right and left bronchi. The right bronchus enters the right lung. It is larger in diameter and more vertical in descent. The left bronchus enters the left lung. It is smaller in diameter and slightly horizontal in position. Because of this design, foreign objects that are aspirated generally enter the right bronchus.

The large bronchi continue to divide into smaller structures called **bronchioles.** These structures divide into smaller, tubelike structures called **terminal bronchioles** or **alveolar ducts.** All these structures are lined with ciliated mucous membrane, as is the trachea. The end structures of the bronchial tree are called **alveoli.** These saclike structures resemble a bunch of grapes. A single grapelike structure is called an alveolus (Figures 49-1 and 49-6). In this terminal structure of the bronchial tree, gas exchange takes place. Each alveolus is surrounded by a blood capillary, where diffusion of carbon dioxide and oxygen occurs. Alveoli are effective in gas exchange, mainly because they are extremely thin walled; each alveolus lies in contact with a blood capillary. In addition, each alveolus is coated with a thin covering of surfactant. Surfactant reduces the surface tension of the alveolus and prevents it from collapsing after each breath (see Figure 49-6).

The lungs contain millions of alveoli; they give shape and form to the lungs. They are filled with air, and lung tissue would float if it was put in water. This tiny, grapelike structure is the most important feature of the respiratory system. It is here that the oxygen diffuses into the cardiovascular system.

MECHANICS OF BREATHING

Thoracic Cavity

The lungs occupy almost all the thoracic cavity except the centermost area, the mediastinum, which contains the heart and the great vessels. This cavity, the interpleural space, is enclosed by the sternum, the ribs, and the thoracic vertebrae.

Lungs

The lungs are large, paired, spongy cone-shaped organs (see Figure 49-5). The right lung weighs approximately 625 g; the left lung weighs approximately 570 g. The right lung contains three lobes; the left lung contains only two lobes. Located approximately 1 inch (2.5 cm) above the first rib is the narrow part (the apex) of each lung. The broad, inferior part (the base) lies in the diaphragm.

The lungs receive their blood supply, which comes directly from the heart, through the pulmonary ar-

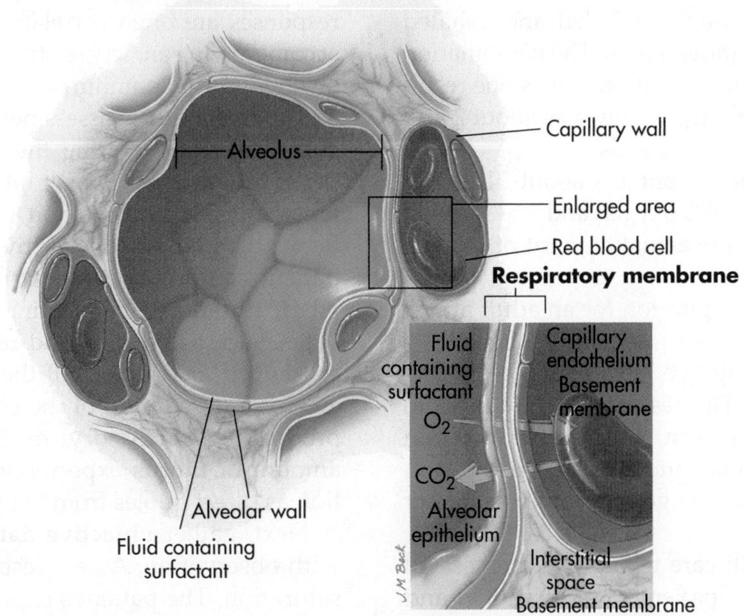

FIGURE 49-6 Each alveolus is continuously ventilated with fresh air. Inset shows a magnified view of the respiratory membrane composed of the alveolar wall (surfactant, epithelial cells, and basement membrane), interstitial fluid, and the wall of a pulmonary capillary (basement membrane and endothelial cells). Carbon dioxide and oxygen diffuse across the respiratory membrane.

teries. By the time the blood reaches the lung capillaries, it is low in oxygen content. Because alveolar air is rich in oxygen, diffusion causes movement of oxygen from the area of high concentration. Carbon dioxide also diffuses between blood and lung capillaries and alveolar air. Blood flowing through the lung capillaries is high in carbon dioxide. After carbon dioxide is diffused into the alveoli and oxygen is diffused into the blood, carbon dioxide leaves the body by expiration of air from the lungs. The blood, now rich in oxygen, returns to the heart for circulation to the body via the pulmonary veins to the left atrium.

The surface of each lung is covered with a thin, moist, serous membrane called the **visceral pleura.** The walls of the thoracic cavity are covered with the same type of membrane called the **parietal pleura.** The pleural cavity around the lungs is an airtight vacuum that contains negative pressure. The air in the lungs is at atmospheric pressure—higher than in the pleural cavity. The negative pressure assists in keeping the lungs inflated. The visceral and parietal pleura produce a serous secretion, which allows the lung to slide over the walls of the thorax while breathing. Usually the body produces the exact amount of serous secretion needed. If too much serous secretion is produced, fluid accumulates in the pleural space; this is called **pleural effusion.** The pleural space becomes distended and puts pressure on the lungs, making it difficult to breathe. The physician may decide to remove the fluid by performing a **thoracentesis**—inserting a needlelike instrument into the pleural space and removing the fluid.

Respiratory Movements and Ranges

The rhythmic movements of the chest walls, ribs, and associated muscles when air is inhaled and exhaled make up the respiratory movements. The combination of one inspiration and one expiration equals one respiration. At rest the normal inspiration lasts about 2 seconds and expiration about 3 seconds.

Room air, when inhaled, contains about 21% oxygen; exhaled air contains 16% oxygen and 3.5% carbon dioxide. This represents the actual amount of oxygen used in a single breath.

The normal range of respiration for an adult at rest is 14 to 20 breaths/min. This rate can be affected by many variables, including age, sex, activity, disease, and body temperature. The respiratory rate is 40 to 60 breaths/min for a newborn, 22 to 24 breaths/min for an early school-age child, and 20 to 22 breaths/min for a teenager. The normal range for women is higher than that for men.

Members of the health care team should assess all factors influencing the patient's respirations and should count the respirations without the patient's awareness to prevent alterations in the breathing pattern.

REGULATION OF RESPIRATION

Nervous Control

The medulla oblongata and pons of the brain are responsible for the basic rhythm and depth of respiration. The body's demands can modify the rhythm. Other parts of the nervous system help coordinate the transfer from inspiration to expiration. Chemoreceptors in the carotid and aortic bodies are specialized receptors. When stimulated by increasing levels of blood carbon dioxide, decreasing levels of blood oxygen, or increasing blood acidity, these receptors send nerve impulses to the respiratory centers, which in turn modify respiratory rates.

Carbon dioxide, which is present in the blood as carbonic acid, is considered the chemical stimulant for regulation of respiration. Therefore the more carbon dioxide in the blood, the more acidic the blood becomes. After exhalation the blood becomes more alkaline. The normal pH of the blood is 7.35 to 7.45—a narrow range. Deviation from this range causes the patient to develop either acidosis or alkalosis.

ASSESSMENT OF THE RESPIRATORY SYSTEM

The function of the respiratory system is gas exchange (oxygen and carbon dioxide) at the alveolar-capillary level. This function depends on the lungs' capability for contraction and expansion, which in turn is influenced by musculoskeletal and neurologic functions.

Physical assessment of the patient's general health always includes the respiratory system. More extensive assessments are required for patients with acute or chronic respiratory or cardiac conditions, those with a history of respiratory impairment related to trauma or allergic reactions, or those who have recently undergone surgery or anesthesia. Because physical and emotional responses are often correlated, also inquire about any accompanying anxiety or stress. This information should be obtained in an unhurried, matter-of-fact manner.

The respiratory assessment includes collection of **subjective data.** During the interview, encourage the patient to describe any symptoms, such as shortness of breath, dyspnea on exertion, or cough. **Dyspnea,** or difficulty breathing, is a subjective experience that only the patient can accurately describe. Data should include onset; duration; precipitating factors; and relief measures, such as position and use of over-the-counter or prescribed medications. If the patient reports a cough, ask for a description of the cough: productive or nonproductive; harsh, dry, or hacking; and color and amount of mucus expectorated. Record this information as direct quotes from the patient when possible.

Next, gather **objective data.** Begin the assessment with observation. Assess respiratory rate and oxygen saturation. The patient's expression, chest movement, and respirations all provide valuable visual clues. At times the patient cannot verbalize distress, but has a wide-eyed, anxious look that reflects the fear of suffocating. Flaring nostrils indicate the patient is struggling to breathe, which is usually a late sign of respiratory distress. Initial observation yields information on the patient's skin color and turgor. Note any obvious respiratory distress, wheezes, or **orthopnea** (an abnormal condition in which a person must sit or stand to breathe deeply or comfortably).

To continue the assessment, auscultate all lung fields, anteriorly and posteriorly, noting the presence of **adventitious** sounds (abnormal sounds superimposed on breath sounds, including sibilant wheezes [formerly called simply **wheezes**], sonorous wheezes [formerly called **rhonchi**], crackles [formerly called **rales**], and pleural friction rubs) (Table 49-1). **Sibilant wheezes** are musical, high-pitched, squeaking or whistling sounds, caused by the rapid movement of air through narrowed bronchioles. **Sonorous wheezes** are low-pitched, loud, coarse, snoring sounds. They are often heard on expiration. **Crackles** are short, discrete, interrupted crackling or bubbling sounds that are most commonly heard during inspiration. Crackles sound like hairs being rolled between the fingers close to the ear. They are thought to occur when air is forced through respiratory passages narrowed by fluid, mucus, or pus. They are associated with inflammation or infection of the small bronchi, bronchioles, and alveoli. **Pleural friction rubs** are low-pitched, grating or creaking lung sounds that occur when inflamed pleural surfaces rub together during respiration.

Also assess chest movement. Note whether the chest expands equally on both sides; chest expansion on one side only may indicate serious pulmonary complications. Look for retraction of the chest wall between the ribs and under the clavicle during inspiration. This can signal late-stage respiratory distress. Be alert for signs and symptoms of **hypoxia** (oxygen deficiency) (Box 49-1).

LABORATORY AND DIAGNOSTIC EXAMINATIONS

A variety of tests are used to evaluate respiratory status and identify respiratory conditions. Other tests include diagnostic imaging, laboratory work, and more invasive measures. Nurses should be familiar with these tests so they can adequately prepare the patient.

CHEST ROENTGENOGRAM

Usually referred to as chest radiographs, chest roentgenograms are an essential diagnostic tool for evaluating disorders of the chest. A chest radiograph provides

Table 49-1 Adventitious Breath Sounds

TYPE	CHARACTERISTICS	COMMENTS
Crackles (rales)	Brief, not continuous; more common in inspiration; interrupted crackling or bubbling sounds, similar to those produced by hairs being rolled between the fingers close to the ear	Caused by fluid, mucus, or pus in the small airways and alveoli.
Fine crackles	As described above; high-pitched, sibilant crackling at end of inspiration	Found in diseases affecting bronchioles and alveoli.
Medium crackles	As described above; medium pitch, more sonorous, moisture sound during midinspiration	Associated with diseases of small bronchi.
Coarse crackles	As described above; loud, bubbly sound in early inspiration	Associated with diseases of small bronchi.
Sonorous wheezes (rhonchi)	Deep, running sound that may be continuous; loud, low, coarse sound (like a snore) heard at any point of inspiration or expiration	Caused by air moving through narrowed tracheobronchial passages (caused by secretions, tumor, spasm); cough may alter sound if caused by mucus in trachea or large bronchi.
Sibilant wheezes (wheezes)	High-pitched, musical, whistlelike sound during inspiration or expiration; sound may be several notes or one, and may vary from one minute to the next	Caused by narrowed bronchioles; bilateral wheeze often result of bronchospasm; unilateral, sharply localized wheeze may result from foreign matter or tumor compression.
Pleural friction rub	Dry, creaking, grating, low-pitched sound with a machinelike quality during both inspiration and expiration; loudest over anterior chest	Sound originates outside respiratory tree, usually caused by inflammation; over the lung fields it suggests pleurisy; over the pericardium it suggests pericarditis with a pericardial friction rub. To distinguish the two, ask the patient to hold the breath briefly. If the rubbing sound persists, it is a pericardial friction rub because the inflamed pericardial layers continue rubbing together with each heartbeat; a pleural rub would stop when breathing stops.

Box 49-1 Signs and Symptoms of Hypoxia

- Apprehension, anxiety, restlessness
- Decreased ability to concentrate
- Disorientation
- Decreased level of consciousness
- Increased fatigue
- Vertigo
- Behavioral changes
- Increased pulse rate; bradycardia as hypoxia advances
- Increased rate and depth of respiration; shallow, slow respirations as hypoxia progresses
- Elevated blood pressure; with continuing oxygen deficiency, decreased blood pressure
- Cardiac dysrhythmias
- Pallor
- Cyanosis (may not be present until hypoxia is severe)
- Clubbing
- Dyspnea

visualization of the lungs, ribs, clavicles, humeri, scapulae, vertebrae, heart, and major thoracic vessels. This test gives information on alterations in size and location of the pulmonary structures and blood flow, and it identifies lesions, infiltrates, foreign bodies, or fluid. A chest radiograph also shows whether a disorder involves the lung parenchyma (the tissue of an organ, as distinguished from supporting or connective tissue) or the interstitial spaces. Chest radiographs can confirm pneumothorax, pneumonia, pleural effusion, and pulmonary edema.

The chest radiographic examination can be performed at different angles for greater clarification. Have the patient wear a hospital gown tied in back. Do not use pins. Any article of clothing containing metal (e.g., a bra with metal hooks) or jewelry must be removed, since the metal produces a shadow on the film.

COMPUTED TOMOGRAPHY

Chest CT Scan

Computed tomography (CT) **scans** of the lungs take pictures of small layers of pulmonary tissue, usually to identify a pulmonary lesion. These views can be diagonal or cross-sectional, with a scanner rotating at various angles. Although this test is painless and noninvasive and results in little radiation exposure, patient teaching is necessary before the procedure to offer explanations and allay anxiety.

Helical or Spiral CT Chest Scan

Helical (also called spiral or volume-averaging) **CT scanning** represents a marked improvement over standard CT scanning. The helical CT scan continuously obtains images. This produces faster and more accurate images. Because the helical CT can scan the abdomen and chest in less than 30 seconds, the entire study can be performed with one breath-hold. Furthermore, when contrast material is used, the entire region can be imaged in just a few seconds after the contrast injection (Pagana & Pagana, 2007).

Pulmonary Angiography (Pulmonary Arteriography)

Pulmonary angiography (pulmonary arteriography) uses a radiographic contrast material injected into the pulmonary arteries to permit visualization of the pulmonary vasculature. Angiography is used to detect pulmonary embolism (PE) and a variety of congenital and acquired lesions of the pulmonary vessels.

When PE is suspected, lung scanning is performed first. If the lung scan is normal, PE is ruled out. If the scan is uncertain however, the diagnosis of PE is questionable because pathologic processes (e.g., emphysema, pneumonia) also may cause abnormalities on the lung scan. Definitive diagnosis for PE may require pulmonary angiography (Pagana & Pagana, 2007).

Ventilation-Perfusion Scan (V/Q Scan)

Ventilation-perfusion (V/Q) scanning is used primarily to check for a PE. An intravenous (IV) radioisotope is given for the perfusion portion of the test, and the pulmonary vasculature is outlined and photographed. For the ventilation portion of the test, the patient inhales a radioactive gas that outlines the alveoli, and another photograph is taken. Normal scans show homogeneous radioactivity. Diminished or absent radioactivity suggests lack of perfusion or airflow (Lewis et al., 2007).

PULMONARY FUNCTION TESTING

Pulmonary function tests (PFTs) are performed to assess the presence and severity of disease in the large and small airways. PFTs include various procedures to obtain information on lung volume, ventilation, pulmonary spirometry, and gas exchange. Lung volume tests refer to the volume of air that can be completely and slowly exhaled after a maximum inhalation **(vital capacity). Inspiratory capacity** is the largest amount of air that can be inhaled in one breath from the resting expiratory level. **Total lung capacity** is calculated to determine the volume of air in the lung after a maximal inhalation. Ventilation tests evaluate the volume of air inhaled or exhaled in each respiratory cycle. Pulmonary spirometry tests evaluate the amount of air that can be forcefully exhaled after maximum inhalation. These tests require the use of a spirometer.

One of the most important tools for diagnosing respiratory diseases is gas exchange, which identifies the capacity for diffusion of carbon dioxide. This component of PFT determines the degree of function in the pulmonary capillary beds in contact with functioning alveoli.

MEDIASTINOSCOPY

Mediastinoscopy is a surgical endoscopic procedure in which an incision is created in the suprasternal notch, allowing the endoscope to be passed into the upper mediastinum. This is performed to gather a sample of lymph nodes for biopsy for tumor diagnosis. Because these lymph nodes receive lymphatic drainage from the lungs, they help diagnose malignant tumors. Tumors in the mediastinum (e.g., thymoma or lymphoma) can also be biopsied through the mediastinoscope (Pagana & Pagana, 2007). This procedure is performed in the operating room, with the patient under general anesthesia.

LARYNGOSCOPY

Laryngoscopy can be performed for either direct or indirect visualization of the larynx. Indirect laryngoscopy is probably the most common procedure for assessing respiratory difficulties; this entails using a laryngeal mirror in the awake patient's mouth for visualization. This procedure can be used for biopsy or polyp excision. Direct laryngoscopy requires local or general anesthesia and exposes the vocal cords with a laryngoscope passed down over the tongue.

BRONCHOSCOPY

Bronchoscopy is performed by passing a bronchoscope into the trachea and bronchi. Using either a rigid bronchoscope or a flexible fiberoptic bronchoscope (the instrument of choice in most cases) allows visualization of the larynx, the trachea, and the bronchi (Figure 49-7). Diagnostic bronchoscopic examination includes observation of the tracheobronchial tree for (1) abnormalities, (2) tissue biopsy, and (3) secretions collected for cytologic (cell) or bacteriologic examination. A local anesthetic agent may be used, but an IV general anesthetic agent is usually given. The patient is treated as a surgical patient.

Nursing interventions for patients after bronchoscopy include (1) keeping the patient on NPO (nothing by mouth) status until gag reflex returns, usually about 2 hours after the procedure; (2) keeping the patient in a semi-Fowler's position and turning on either side to facilitate removal of secretions (unless the physician specifies another position); (3) monitoring the patient for signs of laryngeal edema or laryngospasms, such as stridor or increasing dyspnea; and (4) if lung tissue biopsy is taken, monitoring sputum for signs of hemorrhage (blood-streaked sputum is expected for a few days after biopsy).

SPUTUM SPECIMEN

Sputum samples frequently are obtained for microscopic evaluation, such as Gram stain and culture and sensitivity (Box 49-2). For the range of sputum characteristics, see Box 49-3.

Box 49-2 Guidelines for Sputum Specimen Collection

1. Explain to the patient that the sputum must be brought up from the lungs. Patients who have difficulty producing sputum or who have tenacious sputum may be dehydrated. Encourage fluid intake.
2. Collect the sputum specimen before prescribed antibiotics are started.
3. Collect specimens before meals to avoid possible emesis from coughing.
4. Instruct patient to inhale and exhale deeply three times, then inhale swiftly, cough forcefully, and expectorate into the sterile sputum container. Usually early morning samples are collected on 3 consecutive days.
5. If the patient cannot raise sputum spontaneously, a hypertonic saline aerosol mist may help produce a good specimen. Instruct the patient to take several normal breaths of the mist, inhale deeply, cough, and expectorate.
6. Instruct patient to rinse mouth with water before expectorating into sterile specimen bottle to decrease sputum contamination.
7. Properly label and send to the laboratory without delay.
8. Sputum samples can also be obtained indirectly, such as with nasotracheal suctioning with a catheter or transtracheal aspiration. Take care to ensure that the suction catheters remain sterile. A physician's order must be obtained for endotracheal suctioning.

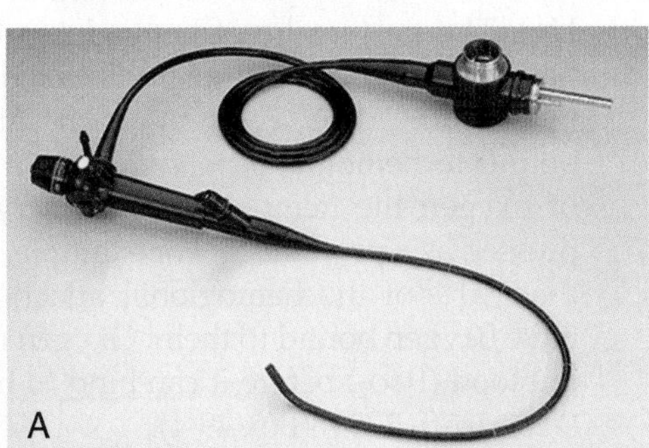

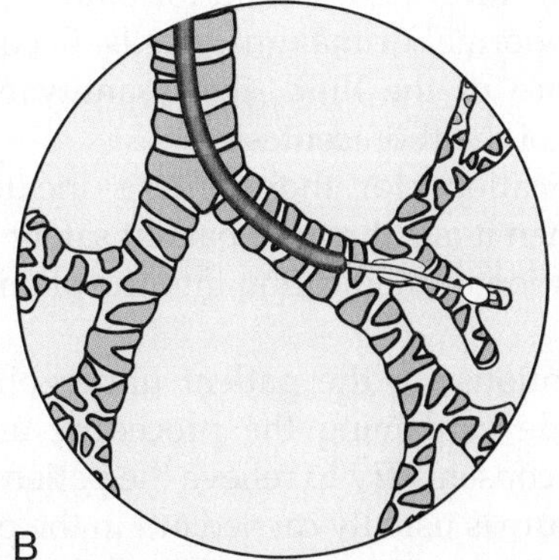

FIGURE 49-7 Fiberoptic bronchoscope. **A,** The transbronchoscopic balloon-tipped catheter and the flexible fiberoptic bronchoscope. **B,** The catheter is introduced into a small airway and the balloon is inflated with 1.5 to 2 mL of air to occlude the airway. Bronchial alveolar lavage is performed by injecting and withdrawing 30-mL aliquots of sterile saline solution, gently aspirating after each instillation. Specimens are sent to the laboratory for analysis.

Box 49-3 Range of Sputum Characteristics

COLOR
- Clear
- White
- Yellow
- Green
- Brown
- Red
- Pink tinged
- Streaked with blood

CONSISTENCY
- Frothy
- Watery
- Tenacious

BLOOD
- All the time
- Occasionally
- Early morning

ODOR
- None
- Malodorous

CYTOLOGIC STUDIES

Cytologic tests can be performed on any body secretion, such as sputum or pleural fluid, to detect abnormal or malignant cells.

LUNG BIOPSY

Lung biopsy may be done transbronchially or as an open-lung biopsy. The purpose is to obtain tissue, cells, or secretions for evaluation. Transbronchial lung biopsy involves passing a forceps or needle through the bronchoscope to obtain a specimen. Specimens can be cultured or examined for malignant cells. Nursing interventions are the same as for fiberoptic bronchoscopy. Open-lung biopsy is used when pulmonary disease cannot be diagnosed by other procedures. The patient is anesthetized, the chest is opened with a thoracotomy incision, and a biopsy specimen is obtained.

THORACENTESIS

Thoracentesis is the surgical perforation of the chest wall and pleural space with a needle for the aspiration of fluid for diagnostic or therapeutic purposes or for the removal of a specimen for biopsy (Figure 49-8). Indications for fluid removal for diagnostic purposes include (1) examining the pleural fluid for specific gravity, white blood cell count, red blood cell count, protein, and glucose; and (2) culturing the fluid for pathogens and checking for abnormal or malignant cells. Record the gross appearance of the fluid, the quantity obtained, and the site of the thoracentesis.

Therapeutic indications for thoracentesis include removal of fluid when it is a threat to patient safety or comfort and instillation of medication into the pleural space.

Nursing interventions for the patient undergoing thoracentesis include explaining the procedure and obtaining a written consent. Try to relieve the patient's anxiety. The procedure is usually carried out in the patient's room. The patient sits on the edge of the bed with the head and arms resting on a pillow placed on an overbed table. If the patient cannot sit up, turn him or her to the unaffected side with the head of the bed elevated 30 degrees.

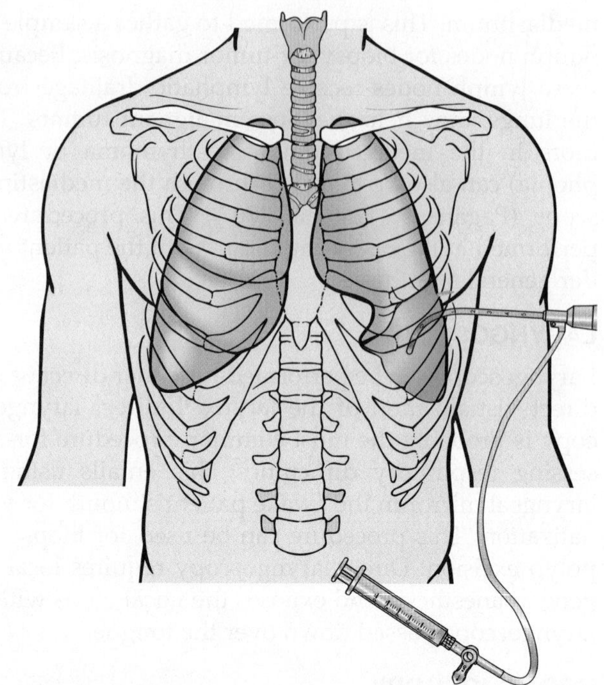

FIGURE 49-8 Thoracentesis. The needle has penetrated the fluid-filled pleural space to remove fluid.

Monitor vital signs, general appearance, and respiratory status throughout the procedure. Usually no more than 1300 mL of pleural fluid should be removed within a 30-minute period because of the risk of intravascular fluid shift with resultant pulmonary edema. After thoracentesis, position the patient on the unaffected side. Label the specimen and send it immediately to the laboratory per physician's orders.

ARTERIAL BLOOD GASES

Blood gas analysis is an essential test in diagnosing and monitoring patients with respiratory disorders. The lungs' ability to oxygenate arterial blood adequately is determined by examination of the arterial oxygen tension (Pao_2) and arterial oxygen saturation (Sao_2). Oxygen is carried in the blood in two forms: dissolved oxygen and oxygen in combination with hemoglobin. The Pao_2 represents the amount of oxygen dissolved in the plasma and is expressed in millimeters of mercury (mm Hg). The percentage of hemoglobin binding sites that have oxygen bound to them is called saturation (Sao_2) (Woodruff, 2006). The Sao_2 is the amount of oxygen bound to hemoglobin in comparison with the amount of oxygen the hemoglobin can carry. The Sao_2 is expressed as a percentage. For example, if the Sao_2 is 90%, then 90% of the hemoglobin attachments for oxygen have oxygen bound to them. Oxygen must first dissolve in blood (Pao_2) before it can bind to hemoglobin (Sao_2) (Woodruff, 2006) (Box 49-4).

The Pco_2 is a measure of the partial pressure of carbon dioxide in the blood. Pco_2 is referred to as the respiratory component in acid-base determination because this value is primarily controlled by the lungs. As the carbon dioxide level increases, the pH de-

Box 49-4 Guidelines for Interpreting Arterial Blood Gas Values

1. Examine each value by itself.
   Normal arterial blood gas values (ABGs)
   - pH: 7.35-7.45
   - $Paco_2$: 35-45 mm Hg
   - Pao_2: 80-100 mm Hg
   - HCO_3^- : 21-28 mEq/L
   - Sao_2: 95%
2. Determine whether the pH reflects acidity or alkalinity.
   - pH ≤7.35 = acidity
   - pH ≥7.45 = alkalinity
3. Which other value corresponds with that condition?
   NOTE: $Paco_2$ reflects respiratory factors; HCO_3^- reflects metabolic factors.
   - Carbon dioxide is a potential acid, so carbon dioxide greater than 45 = more acidity.
   - HCO_3^- is a basic (alkaline) substance, so HCO_3^- greater than 45 = more alkalinity.

   EXAMPLE: A patient with acute exacerbation of chronic obstructive pulmonary disease has the following ABGs:
   - pH: 7.42
   - $Paco_2$: 49 mm Hg
   - Pao_2: 50 mm Hg
   - HCO_3^-: 31 mEq/L
   - Sao_2: 84%

   Because the pH is within a normal range, this is a compensated respiratory problem. The kidneys have increased the amount of bicarbonate they put into the blood to bring the pH to a normal level. The Pao_2 and the Sao_2 are low, indicating hypoxemia.

   EXAMPLE:
   - pH: 7.21
   - $Paco_2$: 58 mm Hg
   - Pao_2: 70 mm Hg
   - HCO_3^-: 24 mEq/L
   - Sao_2: 84%

   The pH is less than 7.35, indicating acidosis. The $Paco_2$ is higher than 45 mm Hg, indicating acidosis. The $Paco_2$ matches the pH, making it a respiratory acidosis. The HCO_3^- is normal, indicating there is no compensation. The $Paco_2$ and the Sao_2 are low, indicating hypoxemia. The full diagnosis for a patient with these ABG results is uncompensated respiratory acidosis with hypoxemia.

Woodruff, D. (2006). Take these 6 easy steps to ABG analysis. *Nursing Made Incredibly Easy!* 4(1):4–7.

creases. Therefore the carbon dioxide level and pH are inversely proportional. The Pco_2 level is elevated in primary respiratory acidosis and decreased in primary respiratory alkalosis. Because the lungs compensate for primary metabolic acid-based derangements, Pco_2 levels are affected by metabolic disturbances as well. In metabolic acidosis the lungs attempt to compensate by "blowing off" carbon dioxide to raise pH. In metabolic alkalosis the lungs attempt to compensate by retaining carbon dioxide to lower pH.

The bicarbonate ion (HCO_3^-) is a measure of the metabolic (renal) component of the acid-base equilibrium. This ion can be measured directly by the bicarbonate value or indirectly by the carbon dioxide content. As the HCO_3^- level increases, the pH also increases; therefore the relationship of bicarbonate to pH is directly proportional. HCO_3^- is elevated in metabolic alkalosis and decreased in metabolic acidosis. The kidneys also compensate for primary respiratory acid-base derangements. For example, in respiratory acidosis, the kidneys attempt to compensate by reabsorbing increased amounts of HCO_3^-. In respiratory alkalosis the kidneys excrete HCO_3^- in increased amounts in an attempt to lower pH through compensation (Table 49-2).

Arterial blood gas (ABG) testing yields definitive information on the patient's respiratory status and metabolic balance. The procedure is performed at the bedside. A heparinized syringe and needle are used to withdraw 3 to 5 mL of arterial blood, usually from the radial artery. Other possible sites include femoral or brachial arteries. After the sample is obtained, place direct pressure on the puncture site for a minimum of 5 minutes to prevent hematoma formation and blood loss. If the patient is taking anticoagulants, maintain pressure for 20 minutes or longer until bleeding stops. Place the capped syringe in a basin of crushed ice and water to preserve the gas and pH levels of the specimen. Send the properly labeled specimen to the laboratory immediately.

Table 49-2 Acid-Base Disturbances and Compensatory Mechanisms

ACID-BASE DISTURBANCE	MODE OF COMPENSATION
Respiratory acidosis	Kidneys retain increased amounts of HCO_3^- to increase pH.
Respiratory alkalosis	Kidneys excrete increased amounts of HCO_3^- to lower pH.
Metabolic acidosis	Lungs "blow off" carbon dioxide to raise pH.
Metabolic alkalosis	Lungs retain carbon dioxide to lower pH.

The blood gas values (see Box 49-4) assess the patient's metabolic (acid-base) status by measuring the pH. Carbon dioxide tension is measured by $Paco_2$ and indicates the patient's ventilation. Oxygen saturation (Pao_2 and Sao_2) is also measured.

PULSE OXIMETRY

Pulse oximetry is a noninvasive method of providing continuous monitoring of Sao_2 (saturation of oxygen) for assessment of gas exchange. The system consists of a probe that looks like a large clothespin and is applied to a finger, a toe, an earlobe, or the bridge of the nose. The noninvasive probe has a light-emitting sensor that shoots narrow beams of red and infrared light through the tissue and a light-receiving sensor that measures the amount of light being absorbed by oxygenated and deoxygenated hemoglobin in pulsating arterial blood. The probe is connected to a computer with a monitor that displays hemoglobin oxygen saturation and pulse rates (Figure 49-9). A pulse oximeter beeps if the patient's Sao_2 registers outside of the limits set according to the physician's order.

For decades, physicians have relied on ABG analysis to evaluate gas exchange and oxygen transport. As valuable as this test is, ABG results reflect a patient's oxygenation status at only one moment in time. Today, pulse oximetry permits continuous, noninvasive monitoring of Sao_2. Oximetry technology allows the nurse to assess minute-to-minute changes in arterial saturations, intervene before hypoxemia produces obvious and serious signs and symptoms, and evaluate the patient's response to treatment. Pulse oximetry alone does not provide data about Pao_2 and acid-base balance. Therefore, ABGs are also needed periodically (Woodruff, 2006).

An Sao_2 of 90% to 100% is needed to adequately replenish oxygen in plasma. The ability of hemoglobin to feed oxygen to the plasma weakens significantly when the Sao_2 drops below 85%. An Sao_2 of less than 70% is considered life threatening.

Arterial oxygen saturation can be quickly and noninvasively determined through pulse oximetry. Severe circulatory problems may diminish the accuracy of the reading. If oximetry results seem questionable, the physician usually orders ABG tests. A pulse oximeter can detect a change within 6 seconds. To get optimal results, remember these points:

- Do not attach the transducer to an extremity that has a blood pressure cuff or arterial catheter in place; these devices reduce blood flow.
- Place the probe over a pulsating vascular bed.
- While the probe is on the patient, protect it from strong light (such as direct sunlight), which can affect the reading.
- Avoid excess patient movement to ensure accuracy.
- Remember that hypothermia, hypotension, and vasoconstriction can affect readings.

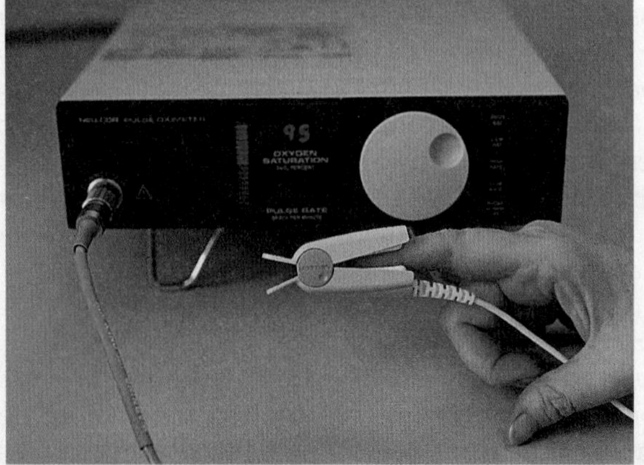

FIGURE 49-9 Portable pulse oximeter with spring-tension digit probe displays oxygen saturation and pulse rate.

DISORDERS OF THE UPPER AIRWAY

EPISTAXIS

Etiology and Pathophysiology

The underlying cause of **epistaxis** (bleeding from the nose) is congestion of the nasal membranes, leading to capillary rupture. This condition is frequently caused by injury and occurs more frequently in men.

Epistaxis can be either a primary disorder or secondary to other conditions. It can be related to menstrual flow in women or hypertension. Other causes include local irritation of nasal mucosa, such as dryness, chronic infection, trauma (e.g., injury, vigorous nose blowing, or nose picking), topical corticosteroid use, nasal spray abuse, or street drug use. If the patient has a disorder that results in a prolonged bleeding time or reduction in platelet counts, this could predispose the patient to epistaxis (Kucik, 2005). Bleeding may also be prolonged if the patient takes aspirin or nonsteroidal antiinflammatory drugs (NSAIDs). A major factor in epistaxis is the many capillaries in the nasal passages.

Clinical Manifestations

The primary observation is bright red blood draining from one or both nostrils. With a severe nasal hemorrhage, adults can lose as much as 1 L of blood per hour, but this loss is not prolonged. Exsanguination (loss of blood to the point at which life can no longer be sustained) from epistaxis is rare.

Assessment

Collection of **subjective data** includes asking the patient to relate the duration and severity of bleeding and identifying precipitating factors, if possible.

Collection of **objective data** involves assessing the presence of bleeding from one or both nostrils. Determine whether the bleeding is occurring in the anterior or posterior portion of the nasal passageway. Assess the patient's blood pressure, temperature, pulse, respirations, and any evidence of hypovolemic shock. Severe bleeding results in a drop in blood pressure, which may cause the bleeding to stop. Hypotension is a late sign of shock.

Diagnostic Tests

A hemoglobin and hematocrit determination will aid in establishing an estimate of the blood loss. Prothrombin time (PT), International Normalized Ratio (INR), and partial thromboplastin time (PTT) assist in identifying contributing factors, such as a bleeding tendency and clotting abnormalities. A rhinoscopy may be performed to locate the bleeding site and possible causes and treatment. This procedure involves inserting a lighted nasal speculum into the nasal cavity.

Medical Management

Epistaxis has many possible treatments, including nasal packing with cotton saturated with 1:1000 epinephrine to promote local vasoconstriction. Cautery can be either electrical (burning [cauterizing] the bleeding vessel) or chemical (applying a silver nitrate stick to the site of the bleeding). Posterior packing of the nasal cavity may be needed. A balloon tamponade may be done by inserting a Foley-like catheter into the nose and inflating the balloon after it is placed posteriorly. Traction is then placed on the catheter to compress the vessel in the area. Also, some physicians prescribe antibiotics (penicillin) after the bleeding is controlled to minimize risk of infection.

Nursing Interventions and Patient Teaching

Nursing interventions include keeping the patient quiet. Place the patient in a sitting position, leaning forward, or in a reclining position with head and shoulders elevated. Apply direct pressure by pinching the entire soft lower portion of the nose for 10 to 15 minutes. Apply ice compresses to the nose and have the patient suck on ice. Partially insert a small gauze pad into the bleeding nostril, and apply digital pressure if bleeding continues. Monitor for signs and symptoms of hypovolemic shock.

Nursing diagnoses and interventions for the patient with epistaxis include but are not limited to the following:

Nursing Diagnoses	Nursing Interventions
Ineffective tissue perfusion, cerebral and/or cardiopulmonary, related to blood loss	Assess vital signs and level of consciousness every 15 minutes and report any changes. Document estimated blood loss.
Risk for aspiration, related to bleeding	Elevate head of bed; place patient in Fowler's position with the head forward; encourage patient to let the blood drain from the nose. Pinch nostrils; have the patient breathe through the mouth; apply ice compresses over the nose (however, the primary benefit of the application of ice is that it requires the patient to remain still); assist patient in clearing secretions. Maintain airway patency. Instruct patient to expectorate any blood or clots rather than swallow them, which could cause nausea and vomiting.

Instruct the patient (and the family, if possible) not to pick, scratch, or otherwise irritate the nares. To prevent recurrent hemorrhage, warn the patient not to blow the nose vigorously and to avoid dryness of the nose. Instruct the patient and the family regarding the risks of foreign objects inserted in the nose (this is especially important in pediatric patients). Encourage the patient to use a vaporizer and saline or nasal lubricants to keep nasal mucous membranes moist. Advise the patient to avoid using aspirin-containing products or NSAIDs, and teach him or her to sneeze with the mouth open.

Prognosis

With treatment, prognosis is good.

DEVIATED SEPTUM AND NASAL POLYPS

Etiology and Pathophysiology

Common conditions that cause nasal obstruction include nasal polyps or a deviated septum caused by congenital abnormality or, more likely, injury. The septum deviates from the midline and can partially obstruct the nasal passageway. Nasal polyps are tissue growths on the nasal tissues that are frequently caused by prolonged sinus inflammation; allergies are often the underlying cause.

Clinical Manifestations

The major manifestations of nasal septal deviations and polyps are **stertorous** (characterized by a harsh snoring sound) respirations, dyspnea, and sometimes postnasal drip.

Assessment

Collection of **subjective data** includes establishing the presence of previous injuries or infections, allergies, and sinus congestion. The patient complains of dyspnea.

Collection of **objective data** involves identifying the condition and its location. Note the rate and character of the patient's respirations.

Diagnostic Tests

Sinus radiographic studies depict the presence of shadowy sinuses when nasal polyps are present. A shift of the nasal septum is evident with a septal defect. A deviated septum may also be seen on visual examination.

Medical Management

These conditions frequently require surgical correction. Nasoseptoplasty is the operation of choice to reconstruct, align, and straighten the deviated nasal septum. A nasal polypectomy is performed to remove the polyps. Actions include nasal packing to control bleeding for 24 hours, and then maintaining nasal mucosa hydration with nasal irrigation of saline or application of a light layer of petroleum jelly to the external nares to prevent drying. Medications include (1) corticosteroids (prednisone), which cause polyps to decrease or disappear; and (2) antihistamines for allergy signs and symptoms, to decrease congestion in both septal deviations and polyps. Antibiotic agents (penicillin) may be used in both conditions to prevent infection. Analgesics (acetaminophen [Tylenol]) may be given to relieve the headache that occurs with septal deviation.

Nursing Interventions and Patient Teaching

Nursing interventions are generally aimed at maintaining airway patency and preventing infection. Postoperative interventions for nasal surgery include monitoring closely for infection or hemorrhage and maintaining patient comfort.

Nursing diagnoses and interventions for the patient with deviated septum or nasal polyps include but are not limited to the following:

Nursing Diagnoses	Nursing Interventions
Ineffective airway clearance, related to nasal exudates	Document patient's ability to clear secretions, and note respiratory status. Elevate head of bed, and apply ice compresses to the nose to decrease edema, discoloration, discomfort, and bleeding. Change nasal drip pad as needed, documenting color, consistency, and amount of exudates.
Risk for injury, related to trauma to bleeding site associated with vigorous nose blowing	Assess and report exudates (as stated above). Instruct patient against blowing nose in immediate postoperative period, since this could increase bleeding, edema, and ecchymosis.

Instruct the patient to contact the physician if bleeding or infection develops. The patient should use nasal sprays and drops judiciously because of the possible rebound effect on nasal mucous membranes. Remind the patient to avoid nose blowing, vigorous coughing, or Valsalva's maneuver (holding the breath and bearing down as if straining during a bowel movement) for 2 days postoperatively. Remind the patient that facial ecchymosis and edema may persist for several days after surgery.

Prognosis

With surgical correction, the prognosis is excellent.

ANTIGEN-ANTIBODY ALLERGIC RHINITIS AND ALLERGIC CONJUNCTIVITIS (HAY FEVER)

Etiology and Pathophysiology

Allergic rhinitis and allergic conjunctivitis (hay fever) are atopic allergic conditions that result from antigen-antibody reactions in the nasal membranes, nasopharynx, and conjunctiva from inhaled or contact allergens. Many infants, children, and adults have these seasonal or perennial conditions, which often result in absences from school and work.

During the antigen-antibody reaction of rhinitis and conjunctivitis, ciliary action slows; mucosal gland secretion increases; leukocyte (eosinophil) infiltration occurs; and, because of increased capillary permeability and vasodilation, local tissue edema results. Common allergens are tree, grass, and weed pollens; mold spores; fungi; house dusts; mites; and animal dander. Some foods, drugs, and insect stings can also cause these reactions.

Clinical Manifestations

Acute ocular manifestations include edema, photophobia, excessive tearing, blurring of vision, and pruritus. Individuals with rhinitis complain of excessive secretions or inability to breathe through the nose because of congestion and/or edema. Otitis media symptoms can occur if the eustachian tubes are occluded. These symptoms occur more in childhood, with the individual complaining of ear fullness, ear popping, or decreased hearing.

Assessment

The initial complaints of seasonal rhinitis and conjunctivitis include severe sneezing, congestion, pruritus, and lacrimation (watery eyes). Cough, epistaxis, and headache may also occur. More chronic signs and symptoms include headache, severe nasal congestion, postnasal drip, and cough. If these are not treated, chronic sufferers eventually develop secondary infections, such as otitis media, bronchitis, sinusitis, and pneumonia.

Diagnostic Tests

In allergic rhinitis, on physical examination the mucosa of the turbines is usually pale because of venous engorgement, which is in contrast to the erythema of viral rhinitis. When symptoms are extremely bothersome, a search for offending allergens may be helpful. This can be done by skin testing or serum radioallergosorbent test.

Medical Management

Treatment goals are to relieve signs and symptoms and prevent infections and other complaints, such as malaise, extreme fatigue, and severe headaches. Avoiding the allergen is effective. Perennial use of antihistamines, intranasal corticosteroids, and leukotriene receptor antagonists such as zafirlukast (Accolate) or montelukast (Singulair) is recommended. Changing from one antihistamine to another seasonally may help impede tolerance to any one medication.

Decongestants may be added and used intermittently for 3 to 5 days if congestion occurs. Common over-the-counter decongestants—such as phenylephrine, pseudoephedrine, chlorpheniramine, and phenylpropanolamine—are contained in familiar products such as Actifed, Triaminic, and Robitussin.

Lodoxamide (Alomide) four times a day is the recommended treatment for mild to moderately severe allergic conjunctivitis.

Long-term, consistent use of topical or nasal corticosteroids is highly recommended. Included are beclomethasone (Vancenase, Beconase), dexamethasone (Decadron, Turbinaire), flunisolide (Nasalide), fluticasone (Flonase), and budesonide (Rhinocort). Corticosteroids require a prescription.

Pressure headaches may require opioid analgesics until signs and symptoms are relieved. Hot packs over facial sinuses offer relief if headache is related to sinus congestion.

Nursing Interventions and Patient Teaching

These illnesses are self-limiting, so focus on health promotion and maintenance teaching to provide for self-care management. Include ways to avoid allergens, self-care management through symptom control, and medication action and usage.

OBSTRUCTIVE SLEEP APNEA

Etiology and Pathophysiology

Obstructive sleep apnea (OSA) is characterized by partial or complete upper airway obstruction during sleep, causing apnea and hypopnea. **Apnea** is the cessation of spontaneous respirations; **hypopnea** is abnormally shallow and slow respirations. Airflow obstruction occurs when the tongue and the soft palate fall backward and partially or completely obstruct the pharynx. The obstruction may last from 15 to 90 seconds. During the apneic period, the patient experiences severe hypoxemia (decreased Pao_2) and hypercapnia (increased $Paco_2$). These changes are ventilatory stimulants and cause the patient to partially awaken. The patient has a generalized startle response, snorts, and gasps, which causes the tongue and soft palate to move forward and the airway to open. Apnea and arousal cycles occur repeatedly, as many as 200 to 400 times during 6 to 8 hours of sleep.

Sleep apnea occurs in 2% to 10% of the population, but is considered underreported. Sleep apnea affects 18 million adults in the United States, but as many as 90% of them are undiagnosed (Dugan, 2007).

Clinical Manifestations and Assessment

Clinical manifestations of sleep apnea include frequent awakening at night, insomnia, excessive daytime sleepiness, and witnessed apneic episodes. The patient's bed partner may complain about loud snoring, sometimes so loud that both people cannot sleep in the same room. Other symptoms include morning headaches (from hypercapnia, which causes vasodilation of cerebral blood vessels), personality changes, and irritability. Systemic hypertension, cardiac dysrhythmias, right-sided heart failure from pulmonary hypertension caused by nocturnal hypoxemia, and stroke are serious complications that may occur.

Symptoms of sleep apnea alter many aspects of a patient's lifestyle. With chronic sleep loss, the patient may have diminished ability to concentrate, impaired memory, failure to accomplish daily tasks, and interpersonal difficulties. Men may experience impotence. Driving accidents are more common in habitually sleepy people. Family life and the patient's ability to maintain employment are also often compromised. As a result, the patient may experience severe depression. Risk factors for OSA include the following (Tate & Tasota, 2002):

- Male gender: About twice as many men as women have OSA.
- Older age: Although younger patients can develop OSA, the incidence increases with age over 65 years, probably because of weight gain and loss of pharyngeal muscle strength.
- Obesity: An obese person's pharynx may be infiltrated with fat, and the tongue and soft palate may be enlarged, crowding the air passages. An obese individual may also have a short, thick neck (more than 17 inches), which increases the susceptibility to obstruction.
- Nasal conditions: Nasal allergies, polyps, or septal deviation decrease the diameter of the pharynx.
- Receding chin: A person with a receding chin may not have enough room in the pharynx for the tongue, thus contributing to obstruction.
- Pharyngeal structural abnormalities: A person with OSA may have enlarged tonsils, an elongated uvula, an especially long tongue, or a soft palate that rests on the base of the tongue. Any of these structural abnormalities can impinge on the airway.

Appropriate referral should be made if problems are identified. Cessation of breathing reported by the bed partner is usually a source of great anxiety because of fear that breathing may not resume.

Diagnostic Tests

Diagnosis of sleep apnea is made during sleep with the use of polysomnography. Electrodes are placed on the patient's scalp, mandibular area, and lateral area of the eyelids. A nasal cannula measures airflow, and pulse oximetry measures Sao_2 (Holcomb, 2006). The patient's chest and abdominal movement, oral airflow, nasal airflow, Spo_2, ocular movement, muscle activity, brain activity, and heart rate and rhythm are monitored, and time in each sleep stage is determined. A diagnosis of sleep apnea requires documentation of multiple episodes of apnea (no airflow with respiratory effort) or hypopnea (airflow diminished 30% to 50% with respiratory effort). Polysomnography may be carried out in a sleep laboratory, or the patient may be taught to attach monitoring leads for a home sleep study.

Medical Management and Nursing Interventions

Mild sleep apnea may respond to simple measures. Instruct the patient to avoid sedatives and alcoholic beverages for 3 to 4 hours before sleep. Referral to a weight loss program may help, since excessive weight exacerbates symptoms. Symptoms resolve in half of the patients with OSA who use an oral appliance during sleep that brings the mandible and tongue forward to enlarge the airway space, thereby preventing airway occlusion. Some individuals find a support group beneficial so they can express concerns and feelings and discuss strategies for resolving problems.

In patients with more severe symptoms, nasal continuous positive airway pressure (nCPAP) may be used. With nCPAP the patient applies a nasal mask that is attached to a high-flow blower (Figure 49-10). The blower is adjusted to maintain sufficient positive pressure (5 to 15 cm H_2O) in the airway during inspiration and expiration to prevent airway collapse. Some patients cannot adjust to exhaling against the high pressure. A technologically more sophisticated therapy, bilevel positive airway pressure (BiPAP), capable of delivering higher pressure during inspiration (when the airway is most likely to be occluded) and lower pressure during expiration, may be helpful and is better tolerated. Although nCPAP is highly effective, compliance is poor even if symptoms of sleep apnea are relieved.

If other measures fail, sleep apnea may be managed surgically. The most common procedures are uvulopalatoplasty, pharyngoplasty (UPP, UPPP, or UP^3) and genioglossal advancement and hyoid myotomy (GAHM). UPPP involves excision of the tonsillar pillars, uvula, and posterior soft palate with the goal of removing the obstructing tissue. GAHM involves advancing the attachment of the muscular part of the tongue on the mandible. When GAHM is performed, UPPP is generally done as well. Symptoms are relieved in up to 60% of patients. Laser-assisted uvulopalatoplasty is a new surgical procedure that has been used to treat OSA (Lewis et al., 2007).

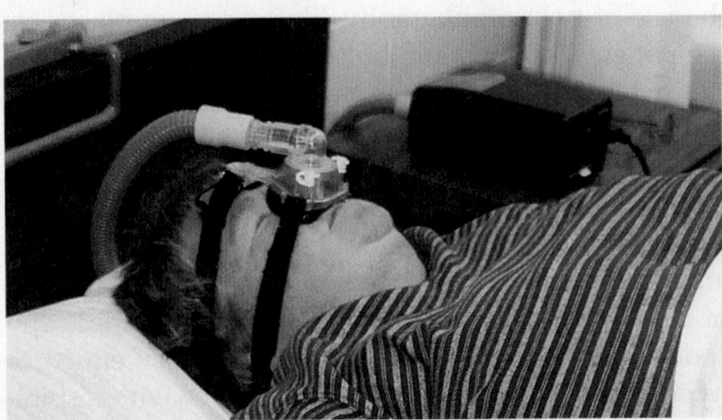

FIGURE 49-10 Nasal continuous positive airway pressure (nCPAP). The patient applies a nasal mask attached to a blower to maintain positive pressure.

UPPER AIRWAY OBSTRUCTION

Etiology and Pathophysiology

Upper airway obstruction is precipitated by a recent respiratory event, such as traumatic injury to the airway or surrounding tissues. Common airway obstructions include choking on food; dentures; aspiration of vomitus or secretions; and, the most common airway obstruction in an unconscious person, the tongue.

Altered physiology includes any condition that could produce airway obstruction, such as laryngeal spasm caused by tetany resulting from hypocalcemia. Another cause may be laryngeal edema caused by injury.

Clinical Manifestations

The main signs are stertorous respirations, altered respiratory rate and character, and apneic periods.

Assessment

Subjective data are limited because a patient is unable to talk when the airway is obstructed. The nurse therefore must make a prompt and accurate assessment of objective data.

Collection of **objective data** includes prompt assessment for the classic sign of choking in which the patient places a hand over throat. Also monitor for signs of hypoxia (an inadequate, reduced tension of cellular oxygen; see Box 49-1), **cyanosis** (slightly bluish, grayish, slatelike, or dark purple discoloration of the skin resulting from excessive amounts of deoxygenated hemoglobin in the blood), stertorous respirations, and wheezing or stridor (harsh, high-pitched sounds during respiration, caused by obstruction). As hypoxia progresses, the respiratory centers in the brain (medulla oblongata and pons) are depressed, resulting in bradycardia and shallow, slow respirations.

Diagnostic Tests

Because this is a medical emergency, no diagnostic tests are needed. This condition is diagnosed by a prompt and accurate assessment.

Medical Management

The patient may require abdominal thrusts (Heimlich maneuver) or an emergency tracheostomy to remove the obstruction. Depending on the cause of the obstruction, an artificial airway may be inserted to maintain patency. Pharyngeal, endotracheal, or tracheal artificial airways may be used.

Nursing Interventions and Patient Teaching

The most immediate nursing intervention is opening the airway and restoring patency. This may be accomplished by properly repositioning the patient's head and neck, or it may require further maneuvers. The head-tilt/chin-lift technique recommended by the American Heart Association minimizes further damage in the presence of a suspected cervical neck fracture. With a foreign body airway obstruction, the Heimlich maneuver is used.

Nursing diagnoses and interventions for the patient with an airway obstruction include but are not limited to the following:

Nursing Diagnoses	Nursing Interventions
Ineffective airway clearance, related to obstruction in airway	Reestablish and maintain secure airway. Administer oxygen as ordered. Suction as needed and assess patient's ability to mobilize secretions. Monitor vital signs and breath sounds closely.
Risk for aspiration, related to partial airway obstruction	Monitor respiratory rate, rhythm, and effort. Assess patient's ability to swallow secretions by elevating the head of the bed. Assess and document breath sounds. Facilitate optimal airway and functional swallowing by elevating head of bed. Note amount, color, and characteristics of secretions Suction as needed.

The goal of education is prevention. Teach the patient and the family how to assess for airway patency. Describe appropriate use of the Heimlich maneuver. Explain the rationale for all treatments and procedures.

Prognosis

With immediate medical and nursing intervention, the prognosis is good; without emergency intervention, the condition is life threatening.

CANCER OF THE LARYNX

Etiology and Pathophysiology

The American Cancer Society (2009) estimated that about 12,290 new cases of laryngeal cancer and about 3,660 deaths due to this disease would occur in 2009.

Squamous cell carcinoma of the larynx is increasing in frequency. Laryngeal cancers occur most often in people older than age 60; 90% of laryngeal cancers occur in men. The incidence appears to be correlated to prolonged tobacco use (cigarettes, pipes, cigars, chewing tobacco, smokeless tobacco) and heavy alcohol use, chronic laryngitis, vocal abuse, and family history. Because of the increase in the number of women who are heavy smokers, their incidence of carcinoma of the larynx is increasing.

Laryngeal cancer limited to the true vocal cords is slow growing because of decreased lymphatic supply; however, elsewhere in the larynx there is an abundance of lymph tissue, and cancer in these tissues spreads rapidly and metastasizes early to the deep lymph nodes of the neck.

Clinical Manifestations

Progressive or persistent hoarseness is an early sign. Any person who is hoarse longer than 2 weeks should seek medical treatment. Signs of metastasis to other areas include pain in the larynx radiating to the ear, difficulty swallowing (dysphagia), a feeling of a lump in the throat, and enlarged cervical lymph nodes.

Assessment

Collection of **subjective data** includes assessing the onset and duration of symptoms. Complaints of referred pain to the ear (otalgia) and difficulty breathing (dyspnea) or swallowing should be noted.

Collection of **objective data** includes examining sputum for blood (**hemoptysis,** or blood expectorated from the respiratory tract).

Diagnostic Tests

Visual examination of the larynx with direct laryngoscopy, with a fiberoptic scope, is done to determine the presence of laryngeal cancer. Other diagnostic tests to detect local and regional spread of laryngeal cancer are CT scan, magnetic resonance imaging (MRI), or positron emission tomography (PET). The patient may also have a chest x-ray study and a CT scan to determine whether there is lung or liver metastasis (Scheich, 2007). A health history helps in making the diagnosis, and a biopsy and microscopic study of the lesion are definitive.

Medical Management

Treatment is determined by the extent of tumor growth. If the tumor is confined to the true cord without limitation of cord movement, then radiation therapy is the best course of treatment. Surgical intervention is considered when extension of the tumor becomes affixed to one of the cords or extends upward or downward from the larynx; surgical options include a total or partial laryngectomy or a radical neck dissection. A partial laryngectomy is done to remove the diseased vocal cord and possibly a portion of thyroid cartilage. This requires placement of a temporary tracheostomy, which is closed when the edema has decreased. A total laryngectomy is performed when the cancer of the larynx is advanced; this requires placement of a permanent tracheostomy. Because the patient can no longer breathe through the nose, the sense of smell is lost. The voice is also absent once the larynx is removed. There is no connection between the patient's mouth and trachea.

A radical neck dissection to remove cervical lymph nodes is often done in conjunction with a total laryngectomy in patients who have a high risk of metastasis to the neck from carcinoma of the larynx. This surgery entails removal of the submandibular salivary gland, the sternocleidomastoid muscle, the spinal accessory nerve, and the internal jugular vein, which results in one-sided shoulder droop.

Chemotherapy using cisplatin and 5-fluorouracil (5-FU) before and after surgery or radiation has achieved a positive response in many cases (Scheich, 2007).

Nursing Interventions and Patient Teaching

Airway maintenance through proper suctioning techniques is important. Assess skin integrity surrounding the tracheal opening; be alert for signs of infection.

Monitor intake and output (I&O) balance and assist with tube feedings as ordered. Explain to the patient that the tube feedings are temporary and that normal eating may begin again when healing occurs in a few weeks. Weigh the patient daily and assess hydration status for the need for additional fluids; note skin turgor and observe for diarrhea.

Because of neck and facial disfigurement and loss of voice, a thorough psychosocial assessment and resultant interventions are beneficial. Encourage communication through writing and facial and hand gestures. Often no one can reassure a patient that speech can be regained as well as a fellow patient who has undergone the same surgical intervention. Many cities have a Lost Chord Club or a New Voice Club, whose members are willing to visit hospitalized patients. A speech therapist should meet with the patient after a total laryngectomy to discuss voice restoration options, including a voice prosthesis, esophageal speech, and an electrolarynx.

Nursing diagnoses and interventions for the patient with a tracheostomy include but are not limited to the following:

Nursing Diagnoses	Nursing Interventions
Ineffective airway clearance, related to secretions or obstruction	Suction secretions as needed. Provide tracheostomy care according to protocol; ensure the availability of emergency equipment (oxygen and tracheostomy tray). Offer small, frequent feedings, and give liquid or pureed food as tolerated to avoid choking. Teach patient stoma protection. Assess respiratory rate and characteristics every 1 to 2 hours. Auscultate lung sounds, monitor Sao_2 every 4 hours. Elevate head of bed 30 degrees or higher. Turn patient and encourage coughing and deep breathing every 2 to 4 hours. Auscultate lung sounds. Provide constant humidity. Suction tracheostomy tube as needed, using aseptic technique; instruct patient to inhale as catheter is advanced. Clean inner cannula of tracheostomy tube every 2 to 4 hours and as needed, using a solution of normal saline and hydrogen peroxide. Suction trachea as needed.
Impaired communication, verbal, related to removal of larynx	Provide patient with implements for communication, including pencil, paper, Magic slate; picture books, or electronic voice device. Keep call signal by patient's hand at all times. If possible, ask patient questions that require only a yes or no response to avoid fatigue and frustration. Refer patient to local support groups and the local chapter of the American Cancer Society. Assist with speech rehabilitation. Review instructions about esophageal and electroesophageal speech. Reinforce need for regular follow-up with speech pathologist and surgeon after discharge.

Explain techniques of airway maintenance, such as oxygen usage, deep breathing, and coughing. Discuss the importance of dietary management in relationship to airway maintenance. Encourage optimal communication through speech rehabilitation and community support groups.

Prognosis

If tumor is limited to the true cord, the cure rate is 80% to 90%. The prognosis in primary supraglottic and subglottic cancer is poorer. The 5-year survival rate is 65%.

RESPIRATORY INFECTIONS

ACUTE RHINITIS

Etiology and Pathophysiology

Acute rhinitis (or acute **coryza**), known as the **common cold,** is an inflammatory condition of the mucous membranes of the nose and accessory sinuses. It is typically characterized by edema of the nasal mucous membrane. The common cold is usually caused by one or more viruses; however, it may become complicated by a bacterial infection. Signs and symptoms usually are evident within 24 to 48 hours after exposure. Sinus congestion causes increased sinus drainage, leading to postnasal drip. The postnasal drip causes throat irritation, headache, and earache. Most people with colds contaminate their hands when coughing or sneezing, thus contaminating everything they touch. Others become infected when touching the telephone, computer, or anything else that has been touched by the person with a cold. Also, many colds are believed to be spread by shaking hands with a person who has a cold.

Clinical Manifestations

An increased amount of thin, serous nasal exudate and a productive cough are two of the most common signs. Sore throat and fever are often present. If the infection remains uncomplicated, it generally subsides in a week.

Assessment

Subjective data include the patient's complaints of sore throat, dyspnea, and congestion of varying duration.

Collection of **objective data** includes noting the color and consistency of the nasal exudate. A visual examination of the throat may reveal erythema, edema, and local irritation. Also document the presence and duration of fever.

Diagnostic Tests

Throat and sputum cultures indicate the presence and nature of microorganisms.

Medical Management

Medical management is aimed at accurate diagnosis and prevention of complications. No specific treatment is available for the common cold. Among the medications used are (1) aspirin or acetaminophen for analgesia and reduction of temperature (aspirin is not used in infants, children, and adolescents because of the danger of developing Reye's syndrome); and either (2) a cough suppressant for a dry, nonproductive cough; or (3) an expectorant for a productive cough. If a secondary bacterial infection is confirmed, an antibiotic agent (e.g., erythromycin) is prescribed (see Complementary & Alternative Therapies box).

Nursing Interventions and Patient Teaching

Nursing interventions are aimed at promoting comfort. Such measures include encouraging fluids and applying warm, moist packs to sinuses.

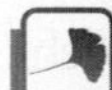
Complementary & Alternative Therapies

Respiratory Disorders

- Herbal medicines for respiratory problems include remedies for nasal discharge and congestion, cough, sore throat, fever and headache, and immunostimulant effects. Ephedra *(Ephedra sinica, Ephedra vulgaris)* is a stimulant and is illegal in some areas. Expectorants include anise *(Pimpinella anisum)*, coltsfoot *(Tussilago farfara)*, and horehound *(Marrubium vulgare)*. Coltsfoot and horehound are also believed to have antitussive action.
- Sore throat remedies include mint (*Mentha piperita* [peppermint], *Mentha spicata*, [spearmint]) and slippery elm *(Ulmus rubra)*. Remedies for the fever and the headache that may accompany colds and influenza include boneset *(Eupatorium perfoliatum)*, feverfew *(Tanacetum parthenium)*, and willow *(Salix purpurea, S. fragilis, S. daphnoides)*.
- Stimulants of the immune system, believed to help ward off colds and flu, include echinacea *(Echinacea angustifolia, E. pallida, E. purpurea)* and goldenseal *(Hydrastis canadensis)*.
- Some interventions that contribute to comfort in patients experiencing dyspnea include the following:
  —Breathing exercises
  —Relaxation therapy
  —Massage
  —Acupuncture
  —Hypnosis
  —Visualization
- Some people believe that reflexology helps relieve congestion.
- Facial massage with diluted aromatic oils is believed by some to open occluded sinuses and relieve congestion. These essential oils include lavender, eucalyptus, peppermint, and tea tree oil.

Nursing diagnoses and interventions for the patient with acute rhinitis include but are not limited to the following:

Nursing Diagnoses	Nursing Interventions
Ineffective airway clearance, related to nasal exudates	Encourage fluids to liquefy secretions and aid in their expectoration. Use vaporizer to moisten mucous membranes and prevent further irritation.
Health-seeking behaviors: illness prevention, related to preventing exacerbation or spread of infection	Remind patient and family of health maintenance behaviors to decrease risk of illness, such as adequate fluid and nutritional management and sufficient rest. Teach importance of hygiene measures to decrease spread of infection.

Teach the patient the correct handwashing technique and proper disposal of tissues used for nasal secretions. Instruct the patient to limit exposure to others during the first 48 hours and to check the temperature every 4 hours.

Prognosis

Signs and symptoms resolve in 2 to 10 days. Even though the common cold does not cause death, its economic importance is vast because it is the greatest cause of absenteeism in industry and schools.

ACUTE FOLLICULAR TONSILLITIS

Etiology and Pathophysiology

Acute follicular tonsillitis can be an acute inflammation of the tonsils. It is the result of an airborne or foodborne bacterial infection, often streptococci. Less frequently, it can also be viral. If it is caused by group A β-hemolytic streptococci, sequelae such as rheumatic fever, carditis, and nephritis must be considered. It appears to be most common in school-age children. Signs and symptoms of tonsillitis include sore throat, fever, chills, and anorexia. The tonsils become enlarged and often contain purulent exudate.

Clinical Manifestations

Acute follicular tonsillitis manifests itself clinically with enlarged, tender cervical lymph nodes. Fever may be present with chills, general muscle aching, and malaise. Laboratory data reveal an elevated white blood cell count.

Assessment

Collection of **subjective data** includes monitoring the severity of throat pain and the possibility of referred pain to the ears. Note headache or joint pain.

Collection of **objective data** includes a visual examination that shows increased throat secretions and enlarged, erythematous tonsils.

Diagnostic Tests

Throat cultures identify the causative microorganism, most commonly β-hemolytic streptococci. A complete blood count (CBC) is done to determine whether the white blood cell count is elevated. Commonly the white blood cell count is 10,000 to 20,000/mm^3.

Medical Management

If antibiotics to which the offending organism is sensitive are administered early, infection subsides. An elective tonsillectomy and adenoidectomy (T&A), where the tonsils and adenoids are surgically excised, is performed in people who have recurrent attacks of tonsillitis. The procedure is usually performed from 4 to 6 weeks after an acute attack has subsided. Either general or local anesthesia is used. Hemostasis is of utmost importance, since the patient can lose a large amount of blood through hemorrhage without demonstrating any signs of bleeding. The physician may be able to control minor postoperative bleeding by applying a sponge soaked in a solution of epinephrine to the site. The patient who is bleeding excessively often is returned to the operating room for surgical treatment to stop the hemorrhage.

Medications used in tonsillitis include analgesics and antipyretics (e.g., acetaminophen) and antibiotic agents (e.g., penicillin). Warm saline gargles are also beneficial.

Nursing Interventions and Patient Teaching

One of the primary nursing goals for acute tonsillitis is to provide meticulous oral care, which promotes comfort and assists in combating infection. Observe and report if the patient swallows frequently, since this is often a subtle but reliable indication of excessive bleeding.

Postoperative care for tonsillectomy includes maintaining IV fluids until the nausea subsides, at which time the patient may begin drinking ice cold clear liquids. The diet is advanced to custard and ice cream and then to a normal diet as soon as possible. Apply an ice collar to the neck for comfort and to reduce bleeding by vasoconstriction. Monitor vital signs to assess for hemorrhage, postoperative fever, or other complications. Comfort measures are important, and emotional support is essential.

Nursing diagnoses and interventions for the patient with acute follicular tonsillitis include but are not limited to the following:

Nursing Diagnoses	Nursing Interventions
Pain, related to inflammation and irritation of the pharynx	Assess degree of pain and need for analgesics. Document effectiveness of medication, and offer analgesic as ordered. Maintain bed rest, and promote rest. Offer warm saline gargles, ice chips, and ice collar as needed.
Risk for deficient fluid volume, related to inability to maintain usual oral intake because of painful swallowing	Assess hydration status by noting mucous membranes, skin turgor, and urinary output. Encourage Popsicles, ice chips, and increased oral intake; cold liquids, sherbet, and ice cream are best tolerated; carbonated drinks may be taken if patient tolerates; avoid offering citrus juices because they may burn the throat.

Nursing Diagnoses	Nursing Interventions
Risk for aspiration, related to postoperative bleeding	Maintain patent airway; keep patient lying on side as much as possible to prevent aspiration.
	Observe for vomiting of dark brown fluid; patient may have "swallowed" blood during surgery.
	Watch for frequent swallowing, which may indicate bleeding; check frequently with flashlight to see if blood is trickling down posterior pharynx.

Instruct the patient (or the family for a child) that the patient should complete the entire course of the prescribed antibiotic. If patient had surgery (T&A), offer dietary instruction regarding appropriate foods and liquids. Tell the patient to avoid attempting to clear the throat immediately after surgery (may initiate bleeding) and to avoid coughing, sneezing, or vigorous nose blowing for 1 to 2 weeks. Most surgeons no longer prescribe aspirin for pain after tonsillectomy, since it increases the tendency to bleed; acetaminophen or another aspirin substitute is usually ordered. Analgesics are usually given orally in liquid form. Remind the patient to avoid overexertion, and make certain that the patient and the family know how to reach the physician in case of increased pain, fever, or bleeding.

Prognosis

Tonsillitis is usually self-limiting, but may have serious complications, such as sinusitis, otitis media, mastoiditis, rheumatic fever, nephritis, or peritonsillar abscess.

LARYNGITIS

Etiology and Pathophysiology

Laryngitis often occurs secondary to other respiratory infections. Laryngeal inflammation is a common disorder that can be either chronic or acute. Acute laryngitis may cause severe respiratory distress in children younger than 5 years of age because the relatively small larynx is subject to spasm when irritated or infected and readily becomes partially or totally obstructed.

Acute laryngitis often accompanies viral or bacterial infections. Other causes include excessive use of the voice or inhalation of irritating fumes. Chronic laryngitis is usually associated with inflammation of laryngeal mucosa or edematous vocal cords.

Clinical Manifestations

Clinical manifestation includes hoarseness of varying degrees or even complete voice loss. The throat feels scratchy and irritated, and the patient may have a persistent cough.

Assessment

Subjective data include the patient reporting progressive hoarseness and a cough that may be productive or may be dry and nonproductive. Attempt to identify any precipitating factors such as excessive voice use or exposure to inhaled irritants.

Collection of **objective data** includes evaluating the patient's voice quality and the characteristics (color, consistency, and amount) of sputum produced.

Diagnostic Tests

Laryngoscopy reveals abnormalities (edema, drainage) of vocal cords and erythematous laryngeal mucosa.

Medical Management

If the laryngitis is due to a virus, there is no specific therapy; if it is bacterial, medications include antibiotics (such as erythromycin or levofloxacin [Levaquin]). Analgesics or antipyretics for comfort, antitussives to relieve cough (such as promethazine [Phenergan] with codeine), and throat lozenges to promote comfort and decrease irritation are useful.

Nursing Interventions and Patient Teaching

General interventions include use of warm or cool mist inhalation via vaporizer. Encourage the patient to rest the voice by limiting verbal communication.

Nursing diagnoses and interventions for the patient with laryngitis include but are not limited to the following:

Nursing Diagnoses	Nursing Interventions
Pain, related to pharyngeal irritation	Assess level of pain, and offer medications to promote comfort.
	Use steam inhalation as ordered.
	Instruct patient on the importance of resting the voice.
Impaired communication, verbal, related to edematous vocal cord	Instruct patient on the importance of resting the voice.
	Provide other means for communication (written word, gestures).
	Anticipate patient's needs whenever possible.

If the patient receives antibiotic agents, instruct him or her to finish the entire prescribed course. Remind the patient of the need to limit use of the voice. Encourage patients who smoke to quit and to limit exposure to irritating fumes.

Prognosis

The prognosis is good in adults. In the infant and young child, respiratory edema can result in respiratory distress.

PHARYNGITIS

Etiology and Pathophysiology

Pharyngitis may be either chronic or acute. It is the most common throat inflammation and frequently accompanies the common cold. Pharyngitis is usually viral but can be caused by β-hemolytic streptococci, staphylococci, or other bacteria. There is increased evidence of gonococcal pharyngitis caused by the gram-negative diplococcus *Neisseria gonorrhoeae.* A severe form of acute pharyngitis often is referred to as **strep throat** because the streptococcus organism is commonly the cause. This disorder is contagious for 2 or 3 days after the onset of signs and symptoms.

Clinical Manifestations

Pharyngitis manifests itself clinically by a dry cough, tender tonsils, and enlarged cervical lymph glands. The throat appears erythematous, and soreness may range from slight scratchiness to severe pain with difficulty swallowing.

Assessment

Subjective data include any reported pharyngeal discomfort, fever, or difficulty swallowing.

Collection of **objective data** includes palpating for enlarged, edematous glands and associated tenderness and noting elevated temperature.

Diagnostic Tests

A rapid step screen is performed to determine the presence of β-hemolytic streptococci. Two throat swabs are obtained so a culture can be performed if the rapid strep screen test is negative (Kamienski, 2007).

Medical Management

Commonly ordered medications include antibiotics, such as penicillin or erythromycin, to (1) treat severe infections; or (2) prevent superimposed infections, particularly in people who have a history of rheumatic fever or bacterial endocarditis. Analgesics and antipyretics, such as acetaminophen, are used to promote comfort.

Nursing Interventions and Patient Teaching

Offer throat rinses or gargles and encourage oral intake. Emphasize the importance of adequate rest and use of a vaporizer to increase humidity.

Nursing diagnoses and interventions for the patient with pharyngitis include but are not limited to the following:

Nursing Diagnoses	Nursing Interventions
Impaired oral mucous membrane, related to edema	Provide warm saline gargles to promote comfort. Assess level of pain and provide medications as ordered. Encourage oral intake of fluids. Offer frequent oral care.
Deficient fluid volume, risk for, related to decreased oral intake as a result of painful swallowing	Observe and record patient's hydration status. Monitor I&O and patient's temperature. Maintain IV therapy if indicated.

Perform and document medication teaching, including the importance of completing the entire prescribed course of antibiotics and any side effects of medications. Instruct the patient to avoid exposure to inhaled irritants and to use preventive measures, such as using a vaporizer and maintaining adequate fluid intake.

Prognosis

Signs and symptoms usually resolve in 4 to 6 days unless secondary complications develop.

SINUSITIS

Etiology and Pathophysiology

Sinusitis can be chronic or acute, involving any sinus area, such as maxillary or frontal. This infection can be either viral or bacterial in origin and often is a complication of pneumonia or nasal polyps. The underlying pathophysiology begins with an upper respiratory tract infection that leads to a sinus infection.

Clinical Manifestations

The patient with sinusitis often complains of a constant, severe headache with pain and tenderness in the particular sinus region, and often has purulent exudate.

Assessment

Subjective data include patient reporting decreased appetite or nausea. The patient may also complain of generalized malaise, headache, diminished sense of smell, and pain in the sinus region when bending forward.

Collection of **objective data** involves assessing vital signs, particularly temperature, and also assessing the character and amount of drainage. Purulent nasal secretions, elevated temperature, facial congestion, and eyelid edema are often noted (Lewis et al., 2007).

Diagnostic Tests

Sinus radiographic studies are frequently done to depict cloudy or fluid-filled sinus cavities. A simple way to diagnose sinusitis is with transillumination. This procedure involves shining a light in the mouth with the lips closed around it; infected sinuses will look dark, whereas normal sinuses will transilluminate. To confirm the diagnosis, a sinus CT scan may be performed.

Medical Management

Nasal windows or other surgical incisions can be created to allow better drainage and removal of diseased mucosal tissue. A common surgical procedure to relieve chronic maxillary sinusitis, the Caldwell-Luc operation, is a radical antrum operation involving the creation of an incision under the lip to remove diseased mucosal and bone tissue.

Medications used to treat sinusitis include antibiotic agents (amoxicillin), analgesics to relieve headache (acetaminophen, possibly with codeine), antihistamines (azatadine [Optimine]) to reduce congestion and secretions, and vasoconstrictors in the form of nasal sprays (oxymetazoline hydrochloride [Afrin]) to reduce local vascular congestion. If symptoms do not resolve in 10 to 14 days, the antibiotic—amoxicillin—should be changed to a broader-spectrum agent such as sulfamethoxazole-trimethoprim (Bactrim) or erythromycin (Lewis et al., 2007).

Nursing Interventions and Patient Teaching

Steam inhalation and warm, moist packs facilitate drainage and promote comfort.

Nursing diagnoses and interventions for the patient with sinusitis include but are not limited to the following:

Nursing Diagnoses	Nursing Interventions
Ineffective breathing pattern, related to nasal congestion	Assess respiratory status frequently, noting any changes; mouth breathing may be necessary because of nasal airway and sinus discomfort.
Pain, related to sinus congestion	Document comfort level. Assess need for analgesics, and document patient response. Elevate head of bed to promote drainage of secretions. Apply warm, moist packs four times a day to promote secretion drainage and provide relief.

The aim of patient education is to prevent recurrence or complications of sinus infection. Instruct the patient to be alert to signs and symptoms of sinusitis so early treatment can be obtained.

Prognosis

Prognosis for uncomplicated sinusitis is good; complications include cavernous sinus thrombosis and spread of infection to bone, brain, or meninges, which can result in meningitis, osteomyelitis, or septicemia.

DISORDERS OF THE LOWER AIRWAY

ACUTE BRONCHITIS

Etiology and Pathophysiology

Usually acute bronchitis is secondary to an upper respiratory tract infection, but it can be related to exposure to inhaled irritants. Inflammation of the trachea and bronchial tree causes congestion of the mucous membranes, which results in retention of tenacious secretions. These secretions can become a culture medium for bacterial growth.

Clinical Manifestations

Acute bronchitis manifests itself with symptoms such as a productive cough, diffuse rhonchi and wheezes, dyspnea, chest pain, and low-grade temperature. Generalized malaise and headache are also common symptoms.

Assessment

Subjective data include the patient's complaints of feeling poorly and experiencing headache and aching tightness in the chest.

Collection of **objective data** includes monitoring vital signs frequently, checking breath sounds, and noting the presence of wheezes or basilar crackles.

Diagnostic Tests

The usual diagnostic aids include a chest radiographic examination to ensure clear lung fields and a sputum specimen to determine the presence of associated bacterial infections.

Medical Management

A quick recovery is promoted by preventing further infectious complications. The physician may order sputum cultures periodically to ascertain that there is no secondary infection.

Medications that are frequently prescribed are cough suppressants (codeine), antitussives (dextromethorphan [Pertussin]), antipyretics (acetaminophen), and bronchodilators (albuterol [Ventolin, Proventil]). Antibiotics such as ampicillin may be ordered to combat or prevent an infectious process.

Nursing Interventions and Patient Teaching

The goal of nursing interventions is to facilitate recovery and prevent secondary infections. Such actions include placing the patient on bed rest to conserve energy, using a vaporizer to add humidity to inhaled air, and increasing fluid intake.

Nursing diagnoses and interventions for the patient with acute bronchitis include but are not limited to the following:

Nursing Diagnoses	Nursing Interventions
Risk for infection, related to retained pulmonary secretions	Assess for signs and symptoms of infection: fever, dyspnea, color and characteristics of sputum production. Administer antipyretics and antibiotics as ordered.

Continued

Nursing Diagnoses	Nursing Interventions
Ineffective airway clearance, related to tenacious pulmonary secretions	Assess patient's ability to move secretions; also note any increase in retained pulmonary secretions. Facilitate airway clearance by elevating head of bed and liquefying secretions by use of humidifier and adequate fluid intake (3000 to 4000 mL/day). Suction as needed. When offering fluids, avoid dairy products, which tend to produce more tenacious secretions.

Instruct the patient on measures that will prevent exacerbation or recurrence of infection. Such measures include increasing oral fluid intake, incorporating rest periods between activities, and recognizing the signs that may indicate worsening infection (purulent sputum and increased dyspnea). Also emphasize the importance of adhering to prescribed medication regimen and using analgesics and antipyretics to reduce fever and malaise. Advise the patient to limit exposure to others, who may spread infection, and to avoid smoking or other irritating fumes.

Prognosis

Prognosis for acute bronchitis is good.

LEGIONNAIRES' DISEASE

Etiology and Pathophysiology

The causative microorganism of legionnaires' disease is *Legionella pneumophila,* first identified in 1976 when it caused a pneumonia outbreak at a convention of the American Legion in Philadelphia. *L. pneumophila* is a gram-negative bacillus not previously recognized as an agent of human disease. This organism thrives in water reservoirs, such as in air conditioners, humidifiers, and whirlpool spas. It is transmitted through airborne routes. The *Legionella* microbe can progress in two different forms: influenza or legionnaires' disease. The latter characteristically results in life-threatening pneumonia that causes lung consolidation and alveolar necrosis. The disease progresses rapidly (less than 1 week) and can result in respiratory failure, renal failure, bacteremic shock, and ultimately death.

Clinical Manifestations

Clinical manifestations include significantly elevated temperature, headache, nonproductive cough, diarrhea, and general malaise.

Assessment

Collection of **subjective data** includes noting the patient's complaints of dyspnea, headache, and chest pain on inspiration.

Objective data include many significant signs associated with this infectious process. A significantly elevated temperature (102° to 105° F [38.8° to 40.5° C]) bears close watching and may require immediate interventions. The patient also has a nonproductive cough with difficult and rapid breathing. Auscultation of lungs reveals crackles or wheezes. Because of the high fever and extreme respiratory effort, tachycardia and signs of shock may be present. Hematuria may develop, indicative of renal impairment.

Diagnostic Tests

Diagnostic tests to confirm *L. pneumophila* infection are cultures of blood, sputum, and pulmonary tissue or fluid. Chest radiographic studies show patchy infiltrates and small pleural effusions.

Medical Management

The physician may need to place the patient on assisted ventilation, which requires intubation through an oral or nasal airway or directly via the trachea. Close observation for disease progression is required. The patient may also require temporary renal dialysis because of acute kidney failure.

To control and compensate for impaired and ineffective respiratory function, the patient requires oxygen therapy, possibly even mechanical ventilation. The patient needs adequate IV fluid therapy to maintain hydration and electrolyte status.

Antibiotic agents (erythromycin) are given intravenously early in the course of the disease and then orally for a prolonged period to treat the infection. Rifampin is also beneficial. Antipyretics are administered to reduce the patient's temperature. The patient may also require vasopressors (dopamine or dobutamine) and analgesics to treat shock signs and promote comfort.

Nursing Interventions and Patient Teaching

Maintain the patient on bed rest, and monitor I&O.

Nursing diagnoses and interventions for the patient with legionnaires' disease include but are not limited to the following:

Nursing Diagnoses	Nursing Interventions
Ineffective tissue perfusion, cardiopulmonary or renal, related to lack of oxygen	Monitor and report signs and symptoms of impending shock (decreased blood pressure and increased pulse). Administer vasopressor drugs as ordered. Maintain hydration status and urinary output. Assess changes in level of consciousness. Assist with acute hemodialysis if indicated.

Nursing Diagnoses	Nursing Interventions
Ineffective breathing pattern, related to respiratory failure	Assess signs and symptoms of respiratory failure. Note respiratory rate, rhythm, and effort. Be alert for cyanosis and dyspnea. Assist with oxygen therapy or mechanical ventilation as ordered. Facilitate optimal ventilation; place patient in semi-Fowler's position if tolerated; suction as needed. Have patient cough and deep breathe every 2 hours if able. Identify associated factors, such as ineffective airway clearance, pain, and altered level of consciousness.

Because of the many alarming actions necessary to treat this disease and its complications, patient and family education is important. Instruct the patient and the family on the purpose of respiratory support (oxygen therapy or ventilator assistance) and how to use these procedures for the greatest benefit. Before their implementation, explain all procedures, including the purpose of hemodialysis and why it is required. Stress the importance of controlling the patient's temperature and fluid and electrolyte status. Offer emotional support to the patient and the family as needed.

Prognosis

Usually the disease is self-limiting, but legionnaires' disease can be severe and fatal. The mortality rate has been 15% to 20% in a few localized epidemics.

SEVERE ACUTE RESPIRATORY SYNDROME

Etiology and Pathophysiology

Severe acute respiratory syndrome (SARS) is an infection caused by a coronavirus. The virus spreads by close contact between people, most likely via droplets in the air. It is possible that SARS may also spread by touching contaminated objects.

Clinical Manifestations

In general, SARS begins with a fever greater than 100.4° F (38° C). Other manifestations may include headache, an overall feeling of discomfort, and muscle aches. Some people also experience mild respiratory symptoms. After 2 to 7 days, SARS patients may develop a dry cough and shortness of breath, difficulty breathing, or hypoxia. About 20% of patients with SARS need intubation and mechanical ventilation (Lewis et al., 2007).

Diagnostic Tests

A chest radiograph is ordered. In the early stages of SARS, the chest radiograph may be normal. In some patients a chest radiograph may later reveal some interstitial infiltrates that progress to a patchy appearance.

A SARS diagnosis can later be made from detection of serum antibodies or positive tissue cultures. Blood specimens for laboratory tests, nasopharyngeal and oropharyngeal swabs, and nasopharyngeal aspirate are obtained. Bronchoalveolar lavage may be used to obtain secretions from the lower respiratory tract. Reverse transcription polymerase chain reaction tests may be done on serum, stool, and nasal secretions.

Initially, the patient's white blood cell count will be normal or low. In about 50% of cases, platelet counts are 50,000 to 150,000/mm^3 (normal range, 150,000 to 400,000/mm^3). Early in the respiratory phase, creatine phosphokinase levels may be as high as 3000 units/L (normal, 5 to 200 units/L) (Parini, 2003).

Additional criteria to establish a diagnosis of SARS include travel within 10 days of symptom onset to an area with current community transmission of SARS—in the recent past, these areas included mainland China (particularly Beijing), Hong Kong, Vietnam, Singapore, Taiwan, and Toronto—or close contact within 10 days of symptom onset with a person suspected of having SARS (Katz & Hirsch, 2003).

Medical Management

Because the disease is severe, treatment is started based on the symptoms before the cause of the illness is confirmed. First, people who are suspected of having SARS are placed in respiratory isolation, including use of an appropriate disposable particulate respirator mask to protect other patients and health care workers. Although no definitive treatment exists, antiviral medications (such as ribavirin) and corticosteroids may be given. Antibiotics will not help with SARS (because it is believed to be caused by a *virus*), but they may be used when the patient also has a bacterial infection.

Nursing Interventions and Patient Teaching

The infection control nurse must notify the local public health department. Respiratory isolation with meticulous hand hygiene is carried out to prevent the spread of SARS. When the patient's respiratory status returns to baseline, he or she is discharged home. The patient can go out in public and return to work 10 days after the fever has resolved and respiratory symptoms are improving or absent (Parini, 2003).

Prognosis

About 80% to 90% of infected people start to recover after 6 to 7 days. However, 10% to 20% go on to develop severe breathing problems and may need mechanical ventilation. The risk of death is higher for this group and appears to be linked to preexisting health conditions. People older than age 40 are more likely to develop severe breathing problems (Lewis et al., 2007).

ANTHRAX

Etiology and Pathophysiology

Anthrax infection is caused by the spore-forming bacterium *Bacillus anthracis.* Found in nature, anthrax most commonly infects wild and domestic hoofed animals. It is spread through direct contact with the bacteria and its spores—dormant, encapsulated bacteria that become active when they enter a living host.

In humans, anthrax gains a foothold when spores enter the body via the skin, intestines, or lungs. It is not contagious by person-to-person contact, so treating family members and others in contact with an infected person is not recommended unless they were exposed to the same source of infection.

Three Types of Anthrax

Anthrax symptoms depend on the initial site of infection. The three types of anthrax are as follows:

1. **Cutaneous anthrax,** the most common type, occurs after bacteria or spores enter the skin through a cut or abrasion. Within several days of exposure, a pruritic reddened macule or papule develops, followed by vesicle formation. The lesion resembles an insect bite at first, until black eschar appears at the center of the lesion and the site becomes edematous. Although a patient may develop bacteremia if the organism enters his or her bloodstream, cutaneous anthrax is rarely fatal if it is treated with antibiotics.
2. **Gastrointestinal anthrax,** the least common type, occurs after ingestion of the organism in contaminated, undercooked food. Spores can germinate in the mouth, the esophagus, the stomach, or the small and large intestines, causing ulcers. Inflammation of the gastrointestinal tract can cause nausea, vomiting, fever, abdominal pain, and diarrhea. Unless treated early, a patient may die from sepsis.
3. **Inhalational anthrax,** seen in global germ warfare, is the most deadly type. It develops when spores are inhaled deeply into the lungs. Immune cells sent to fight the lung infection carry some bacteria back to the lymph system, which spreads the infection to other organs.

Initial symptoms of inhalational anthrax resemble those of the common cold or influenza, except that the patient usually does not develop an increased amount of thin, clear nasal exudate. Subsequent breathing problems may be mistaken for pneumonia, delaying diagnosis. Other severe symptoms, including hemorrhage, tissue necrosis, and lymphedema, are caused by bacterial toxins. Death usually results from blood loss and shock.

Diagnostic Tests

A chest x-ray helps differentiate inhalational anthrax from pneumonia. A widening mediastinum from lymphadenopathy is characteristic of inhalational anthrax infection; infiltrates characterize pneumonia.

No single reliable screening test for anthrax is currently available, although the Mayo Clinic recently announced development of a rapid deoxyribonucleic acid test to identify anthrax in people and the environment. Using standard precautions, obtain specimens for a blood smear and culture and a chest x-ray for anyone with symptoms of inhalational anthrax. A nasal swab is not recommended to diagnose anthrax infection. For a patient suspected of cutaneous anthrax, obtain a culture specimen from the lesion's vesicular fluid. Obtain a stool specimen for culture if intestinal anthrax is suspected.

Medical Management

Antibiotic treatment is indicated for anyone diagnosed with anthrax or exposed to anthrax spores. For both children and adults, ciprofloxacin (Cipro) has been considered the treatment of choice for all three forms of anthrax because of concerns that genetically engineered anthrax strains might resist older antibiotics. Most anthrax strains are susceptible to many other antibiotics, including penicillin and doxycycline (Vibramycin). Concerned about drug resistance, in 2002, health experts in the United States urged health care providers to avoid prescribing antibiotics indiscriminately because of the danger of antimicrobial resistance (www.excellenthealth.com/news011102a.htm).

The Centers for Disease Control and Prevention (CDC) recommend a 60-day course of therapy to ensure eradication of inactive spores and bacteria. An alternative treatment for postexposure prophylaxis is 30 days of antibiotics and three doses of the anthrax vaccine if it is available. (The anthrax vaccine is not currently recommended for the general public in the absence of anthrax exposure.) Consult the U.S. Food and Drug Administration (FDA) and CDC websites for the prescribing information for children and other treatment updates.

TUBERCULOSIS

Etiology and Pathophysiology

In 1882 Robert Koch identified the tubercle bacillus *(Mycobacterium tuberculosis)* as the causative agent for tuberculosis (TB). TB is a chronic pulmonary and extrapulmonary (outside of the lung) infectious disease acquired by inhalation of a dried droplet nucleus containing a tubercle bacillus, coughed or sneezed into the air by a person whose sputum contains **virulent** (capable of producing disease) tubercle bacilli, and inhaled into the alveolar structure of the lung. It is characterized by stages of early infection (frequently asymptomatic), latency, and a potential for recurrent postprimary disease. It most commonly affects the respiratory system, but other parts of the body such as gastrointestinal and genitourinary tracts, bones, joints, nervous system, lymph nodes, and skin may become infected (see Cultural Considerations box).

It is important to differentiate **infection** with TB from **active disease.** Although infection always pre-

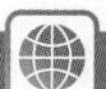 Cultural Considerations

Tuberculosis

- Tuberculosis in the United States tends to be a disease of the older population, urban poor, minority groups, and patients with acquired immunodeficiency syndrome.
- At all ages the incidence of tuberculosis among nonwhites is at least twice that of whites.
- Ethnic groups that have a high incidence of tuberculosis include foreign-born people from Asia, Africa, and Latin America.
- Southeastern Asian, Haitian, and Hispanic immigrants have incidence rates of tuberculosis similar to those of the countries from which they came.

cedes the development of active disease, only about 10% of infections progress to active disease. TB infection is characterized by mycobacteria in the tissue of a host who is free of clinical signs and symptoms and who demonstrates the presence of antibodies against the mycobacteria. TB disease is manifested as pathologic and functional signs and symptoms indicating destructive activity of mycobacteria in host tissue.

A common misconception about TB is that it is easily transmitted. In fact, most people exposed to TB do not become infected. The body's first line of defense, the upper airway, prevents most inhaled TB organisms from ever reaching the lungs. If the inhaled particles are small enough, the organisms can survive in the upper respiratory tract, reach the alveoli, and establish infection. Less commonly, transmission may occur by ingestion or by invasion of the skin or mucous membranes.

TB had been epidemic in the Western world. With the introduction of pharmacologic management in the late 1940s and early 1950s, the prevalence of TB decreased dramatically. TB had been responsible for one third of the deaths of young adults in Europe. After Koch's discovery, improvement in living conditions, sanitation, and the development of effective drug therapy and treatment brought about a steady decline in mortality attributable to TB. Shortly after the centennial of Koch's work, eradication of the disease in the United States by the year 2010 was considered a realistic goal.

Although the overall rate of TB in the United States has declined substantially since 1992, the rates of decrease among foreign-born persons have remained virtually level, with approximately 7000 to 8000 cases per year. In contrast, the number in U.S.-born persons decreased from more than 6000 in 2006. The total number of TB cases reported in the United States in 2006 was 13,779 (CDC, 2007). TB still presents a serious health problem. Most alarming, a growing percentage of new cases of TB are resistant to the drugs that are traditionally used to fight the disease.

TB has been particularly prevalent among people infected with the human immunodeficiency virus (HIV). The status of the host's immune system is the major determinant for the development of active TB. The disease occurs most often in individuals with incompetent immune systems, such as HIV-infected people, older adults, people receiving immunosuppressive therapy, and the malnourished.

Hospitals are a high-risk setting for TB transmission, and health care workers are at high occupational risk for TB infection. Until recently the vulnerability of hospital workers to TB infection had not been emphasized. This complacency is changing with the wide publicity accompanying the increase in TB (Box 49-5).

In the lung, pulmonary macrophages ingest TB bacteria. Macrophages engulf the organisms, but do not kill them. Instead they surround them and wall them off in tiny, hard capsules called **tubercles.** Macrophages activate lymphocytes, and within 2 to 10 weeks, activated lymphocytes usually control the initial infection in the lung and nonpulmonary sites. Nonmultiplying tubercle bacilli can survive more than 50 years in human tissue.

Most people who become infected with the TB organism do not progress to the active disease stage. They remain asymptomatic and noninfectious. They will have a positive tuberculin skin test, and chest radiographs will be negative. These people still retain a lifelong risk of developing reactivation of TB if the immune system is compromised.

Clinical Manifestations

The clinical manifestations are insidious. Generally patients have fever, weight loss, weakness, and a productive cough. Later in the disease, daily recurring fever with chills, night sweats, and hemoptysis is seen.

Assessment

Subjective data include the patient reporting loss of muscle strength and weight loss.

Box 49-5 High-Risk Groups to Screen for Tuberculosis

- People infected with the human immunodeficiency virus
- Close contacts (especially children and adolescents) of people with active infectious tuberculosis (TB)
- People with conditions that increase the risk of active TB after infection, such as silicosis, diabetes, chronic renal failure, history of gastrectomy, weight 10% below ideal body weight, prolonged corticosteroid or other immunosuppressive therapy, some hematologic disorders (e.g., leukemia and lymphomas), and other malignancies
- People born in countries with a high prevalence of TB
- Substance abusers, such as alcoholics, intravenous drug users, and cocaine or crack users
- Residents of long-term care facilities, nursing homes, prisons, mental institutions, homeless shelters, and other congregate housing settings
- Medically underserved low-income populations, including racial and ethnic minorities, homeless people, and migrant workers
- Health care workers and others who provide services to any high-risk group

Collection of **objective data** includes evaluating and recording the amount, color, and characteristics of sputum produced.

Diagnostic Tests

Diagnostic evaluation includes the tuberculin skin test (Mantoux), using purified protein derivative (PPD), to identify people infected with the TB organism. A positive reaction indicates infection 2 to 10 weeks after exposure to the tubercle bacillus. To read the test 48 to 72 hours later, measure and record the subsequent induration (an area of hardened tissue); do not measure the erythema (redness). A negative reaction is less than 5 mm. If the patient is infected with TB (whether active or dormant), lymphocytes recognize the PPD antigen in the skin test and cause a local indurated reaction. Generally, the larger the reaction is, the greater the likelihood that the person is infected with the TB organism. However, a negative reaction does not rule out infection. An infected person whose immune system has been weakened by disease, drugs, or old age may have a limited or negative reaction. If the test is negative and the physician strongly suspects TB, a "second-strength" tuberculin test can be used. If this test is negative, the patient does not have TB.

Other diagnostic tests used to confirm the diagnosis of pulmonary TB are chest radiograph and evaluation of sputum specimens for mycobacterial organisms. Sputum specimens can be rapidly smeared, stained, and screened for the presence of acid-fast organisms. Mycobacteria are one of the few organisms that are characteristically acid fast. Three positive acid-fast smears constitute a presumptive diagnosis of TB and indicate the need for treatment. The diagnosis of TB is confirmed if tubercle bacilli grow in culture, a process that may take 6 to 8 weeks.

QuantiFERON-TB Gold Test

In May 2005 the FDA approved a blood test to aid in the diagnosis of latent TB. This blood test, the QuantiFERON-TB Gold (QFT-G), is more specific for *Mycobacterium* tubercle bacillus than the PPD skin test (Todd, 2006). The advantages of QFT-G are greater specificity and results 24 hours after blood is collected. The PPD skin test requires a 2- to 3-day wait and a return visit to the health care provider (Todd, 2006). Sputum smears and cultures are still done, but the QFT-G offers a quick and reliable diagnosis for the patient and health care provider.

All patients diagnosed with TB must be reported to the public health personnel for appropriate investigation and follow-up care (Todd, 2006).

Medical Management

Drug therapy is the mainstay of TB treatment. Infectiousness declines rapidly once drug therapy is initiated, even before sputum smears become negative. Cough frequently also declines with drug therapy.

TB isolation (acid-fast bacillus [AFB]) is isolation for patients with pulmonary TB who have a positive sputum smear or a chest radiograph that strongly suggests current (active) TB. Laryngeal TB is also included in this isolation category. In general, infants and young children with pulmonary TB do not require isolation precautions because they rarely cough and their bronchial secretions contain few AFB, compared with adults with pulmonary TB. If there is question of infectiousness in the adult TB patient, hospitalized patients usually remain in respiratory isolation during their hospital stay.

Compared with most other infectious diseases, treatment for TB is lengthy, typically 6 to 9 months, and sometimes longer for extrapulmonary disease. If treatment is not continued for a long time, some of the TB organisms survive and the patient is at risk for a relapse.

Treatment therapy now involves multiple drugs to which the organisms are susceptible. If only one drug is given, the patient may become resistant to it. Treatment usually consists of a combination of at least four drugs, each of which helps prevent the emergence of organisms resistant to the others, thus increasing the therapeutic effectiveness. The drugs that are used to treat TB are categorized as first-line drugs and second-line drugs. First-line drugs are isoniazid (INH); rifampin (rifampicin); rifampin and isoniazid (Rifamate), with a fixed combination of 300 mg rifampin and 150 mg isoniazid per capsule; pyrazinamide; ethambutol; and streptomycin. In 1998 the FDA approved rifapentine (Priftin), the first new TB drug to become available in the United States in 10 years. Although it is similar to rifampin, rifapentine has a longer half-life and can be taken less frequently. Second-line drugs are ethionamide, para-aminosalicylate sodium (PAS), cycloserine, capreomycin, kanamycin, amikacin, levofloxacin, ofloxacin, and ciprofloxacin (Table 49-3).

Monitoring patients with TB is critically important; failure to complete prescribed medication treatment is a major factor in the emergence of multi-drug resistance and treatment failures (Todd, 2006). To ensure compliance and to help prevent the development of drug-resistant strains of the tubercle bacillus, in some cases the health care worker may need to watch the patient take the medications; this is referred to as directly observed therapy.

Nursing Interventions and Patient Teaching

If TB is suspected, immediately ask permission to place the patient in AFB isolation precautions. These precautions include the use of isolation rooms with a negative air pressure so that air flows into, rather than out of, the room. Keep doors and windows closed to maintain airflow control. Room air should be exhausted directly to the outside and not recirculated to other rooms. Also included in AFB isolation precautions is the use of high-efficiency particulate respiration masks (because AFB particles pass through standard masks). Although TB is not easily transmitted, it

Table 49-3 Medications for Respiratory Disorders

Generic (Trade)	Action	Side Effects	Nursing Implications
Acetylcysteine (Mucomyst)	Mucolytic agent; also used as antidote in acetaminophen overdose	Nausea, vomiting, rhinorrhea, mucorrhea, bronchospasm	Store product in refrigerator; bad taste may be masked by mixing with soft drink when using as antidote.
Aminophylline	See theophylline	See theophylline	See theophylline
Azatadine (Optimine); also available in numerous combination allergy and cold preparations	Antihistamine; blocks allergic response through histamine receptor blockade	Drowsiness, confusion, dry mouth, constipation, urinary retention, blurred vision, increased viscosity of respiratory secretions	Avoid use with alcohol or other CNS depressants; avoid driving and other hazardous activities.
Short-acting beta$_2$-receptor agonists: albuterol (Proventil, Ventolin), others	Beta$_2$-receptor agonists; cause bronchodilation, cardiac palpitations, angina or chest pain, cardiac dysrhythmias	Anxiety, headache, insomnia, dizziness, restlessness, tachycardia	Use with caution in cardiac disease. Teach patient that paradoxic bronchospasm may occur and to stop drug immediately and call physician. Teach proper use of metered dose inhaler to achieve an excellent therapeutic response.
Long-acting beta$_2$-receptor agonists: salmeterol (Serevent)	Causes bronchodilation; used in prevention of exercise-induced asthma	Tremors, anxiety, insomnia, headache, stimulation, tachycardia, dry mouth, bronchospasm	Avoid use of OTC medications; overstimulation may occur. Use with caution in cardiac disorders, hyperthyroidism, hypertension, and narrow-angle glaucoma.
Corticosteroids: Prednisone (Deltasone), methylprednisolone (Medrol), hydrocortisone (Cortef)	Antiinflammatory agent	Short-term: Sodium and water retention, hypokalemia, hyperglycemia, euphoria	Do not discontinue medication abruptly; dosage must be tapered slowly. Have patient carry identification signaling steroid use. Take with food or milk to minimize upset.
Fluticasone (Flovent) (inhaled corticosteroid)		Long-term: Osteoporosis, increased susceptibility to infection, poor wound healing, bruising, thinning of skin, Cushingoid weight distribution, cataracts, glaucoma, peptic ulcer disease, myopathy, muscle weakness, suppression of endogenous glucocorticoid production	
Epinephrine (Adrenalin, others)	Beta$_1$- and beta$_2$-receptor agonist; causes bronchodilation and cardiac stimulation; alpha$_1$-agonist activity may cause vasoconstriction	Tachycardia, palpitations, angina, chest pain, myocardial infarction, cardiac dysrhythmias, hypertension, restlessness, agitation, anxiety	Use with extreme caution in cardiac disease; do not use OTC cough or cold preparations; do not use discolored preparations.
Ethambutol (Myambutol)	Antitubercular agent	Optic neuritis, blurred vision or decreased visual acuity, hyperuricemia, exacerbation of gout, drowsiness, confusion, GI effects, hepatoxicity, thrombocytopenia	Patient should have baseline visual examination at start of therapy. Emphasize that long-term therapy is required for cure.

GI, Gastrointestinal; *OTC*, over-the-counter.

Continued

Table 49-3 Medications for Respiratory Disorders–cont'd

Generic (Trade)	Action	Side Effects	Nursing Implications
Isoniazid (INH) (Nydrazid, others)	Antitubercular agent	Peripheral neuropathy, hepatotoxicity, SLE-like syndrome, hyperglycemia, bone marrow suppression	Monitor liver function. Emphasize that long-term therapy is required. Instruct patient to report numbness or tingling of extremities.
Leukotriene modifiers; leukotriene receptor antagonists (zafirlukast [Accolate] montelukast [Singulair]); leukotriene synthesis inhibitors (zileuton [Zyflo])	Interferes with the synthesis or blocks the action of leukotrienes, causing both bronchodilator and antiinflammatory effects; for long-term treatment of asthma	Zafirlukast: Hepatic dysfunction, systemic eosinophilia, headache, infection, nausea, asthenia, abdominal pain Montelukast: Tiredness, fever, abdominal pain, dizziness Zileuton: Headache, abdominal pain, asthenia, dyspepsia	Monitor for eosinophilia, worsening pulmonary symptoms, cardiac complications, and neuropathy. Administer after meals for GI symptoms.
Oxymetazoline (Afrin, others)	Vasoconstrictor, used for nasal congestion	Local nasal irritation, dryness, rebound congestion	Do not use for more than 4 consecutive days to minimize rebound congestion.
Para-aminosalicylate sodium (PAS)	Antitubercular agent	Nausea, vomiting, diarrhea, abdominal pain, hypersensitivity reactions, hepatotoxicity, leukopenia, thrombocytopenia	Take with food. Discard if discolored. Use with caution in peptic ulcer disease or congestive heart failure. Emphasize that long-term therapy is required.
Potassium iodide (many; also available in numerous combination preparations)	Expectorant, mucokinetic agent	Hypersensitivity, rash, metallic taste, burning in mouth or throat, GI irritation, headache, parotitis, hyperkalemia	Do not use in pregnant women. Mix with fruit juice to mask taste.
Pyrazinamide (PMS-Pyrazinamide Tebrazid)	Antitubercular agent	Hyperuricemia, exacerbation of gout, hepatotoxicity	Monitor liver function tests and serum uric acid levels; instruct patient not to use alcohol; emphasize that long-term therapy is required.
Rifampin (Rifadin, Rimactane)	Antitubercular agent	Flulike syndrome, hematopoietic reactions, hepatotoxicity, rash, red-orange coloration of body fluids, shortness of breath, heartburn, sore mouth and tongue, dizziness, confusion	Give on empty stomach; emphasize that long-term therapy is required. May accelerate metabolism of other drugs, including theophylline, oral contraceptives, and warfarin. Instruct patient that body fluids may be discolored; may cause permanent staining of soft contact lenses.
Rifapentine (Priftin)	Antitubercular agent	Hepatotoxicity, hyperuricemia, neutropenia, pyuria, proteinuria, rash, anemia, leukopenia, arthralgias, nausea, vomiting, dyspepsia, pseudomembranous colitis	Monitor liver function tests and serum uric acid. Monitor WBC count. Tell the patient that rifapentine may produce red-orange discoloration of body tissues or fluids (e.g., skin, teeth, tongue, urine, feces, saliva, sputum, tears, cerebrospinal fluid). Emphasize importance of not missing any doses.

SLE, Systemic lupus erythematosus; *WBC,* white blood cell.

Table 49-3 Medications for Respiratory Disorders–cont'd

Generic (Trade)	Action	Side Effects	Nursing Implications
Theophylline (Accurbron, Bronkodyl, Theo-Dur) (Aminophylline is a salt of theophylline.)	Bronchodilator	Anxiety, restlessness, insomnia, headache, seizures, tachycardia, cardiac dysrhythmias, nausea, epigastric pain, hematemesis, gastroesophageal reflux, tachypnea	Do not crush sustained-release preparations; contents of pellet-containing capsules may be sprinkled over food. Avoid caffeine; use with caution in peptic ulcer disease or cardiac dysrhythmias. Metabolism is affected by other medications (erythromycin, ciprofloxacin, cimetidine, rifampin); monitor serum concentrations.

is more easily transmitted in closed spaces and in areas with poor ventilation and no environmental controls.

Perhaps the simplest, most effective technique for stopping TB at the source is kindly insisting that patients cover their noses and mouths when coughing or sneezing.

To help the patient comply with the prescribed medication regimen, develop a supportive relationship. Nursing interventions focus on preventing complications and illness transmission.

Nursing diagnoses and interventions for the patient with TB include but are not limited to the following:

Nursing Diagnoses	Nursing Interventions
Ineffective breathing pattern, related to pulmonary infection process	Monitor breathing for evidence of dyspnea or signs and symptoms of pneumothorax. Evaluate degree of respiratory effort and assist as needed. Assess expectorated sputum for hemoptysis. Help immobile patient to turn, cough, and deep breathe every 2 to 4 hours to prevent pooling of secretions.
Risk for infection, (patient contacts), related to viable *M. tuberculosis* in respiratory secretions	Obtain specimen for culture (incorrect collection and handling may destroy or contaminate specimen, thus interfering with diagnostic results). Employ AFB isolation until antimicrobial therapy is successfully initiated for sputum-positive patients to prevent transmission of organisms. Employ drainage and secretion precautions until wounds from patient with extrapulmonary TB stop draining to prevent transmission of organism. Instruct the patient to cough and sneeze into tissue and properly dispose of it to prevent organism transmission.

Teach the patient techniques of proper disposal and handwashing related to coughing and sneezing. These measures will decrease the spread of infection. Explain the vital importance of adhering to the medication regimen as ordered and the need for prolonged treatment. Instruct the patient on medication, dosage, frequency, and possible side effects. Emphasize the need to report hemoptysis, dyspnea, vertigo, or chest pain. Remind the patient to maintain adequate fluid and nutritional intake.

Prognosis

Active TB requires a long course of drug ingestion—6 to 9 months minimum, and often longer—to stop the disease. As many as 50% of patients fail to complete therapy as prescribed. Numerous drug-resistant TB cases have been reported in HIV-infected people. These infections are characterized by rapid disease progression, with 4 to 16 weeks from diagnosis to death and mortality rates of 72% to 89%.

Nonmultiplying tubercle bacilli can survive more than 50 years in human tissue and can be reactivated when the patient has a compromised immune system.

PNEUMONIA

Etiology and Pathophysiology

Pneumonia is an inflammatory process of the respiratory bronchioles and the alveolar spaces that is caused by an infection. It can also be caused by oversedation, inadequate ventilation, or aspiration.

Pneumonia can occur in any season but is most common during winter and early spring. People of all ages are susceptible, but pneumonia is more common among infants and older adults. Pneumonia is often caused by aspiration of infected materials into the distal bronchioles and alveoli. High-risk people include those whose normal respiratory defense mechanisms are damaged or altered (those with chronic obstructive pulmonary disease [COPD], influenza, or tracheostomy and those who have recently had anesthesia); people who have a disease affecting antibody response; people with alcoholism, in whom there is increased danger of aspiration; and people with delayed white blood cell response to infection. Increasingly, nosocomial pneumonia (acquired in the hospital) is a cause of morbidity and mortality (see Health Promotion box).

Pneumonia is a communicable disease; the mode of transmission depends on the infecting organism. Pneumonia is classified according to the offending organism rather than the anatomical location (lobar or bronchial), as was the practice in the past. Pneumonia can be caused by bacteria, viruses, mycoplasma, fungi, and chemicals. Currently, about half of pneumonia cases are caused by bacteria and half by virus. Up to 96% of bacterial pneumonia is caused by four organisms: *Streptococcus pneumoniae* (pneumococcal), hemolytic streptococcus type A, *Staphylococcus aureus,* and *Haemophilus influenzae* type B. Nonbacterial or atypical pneumonia is caused by *Mycoplasma pneumoniae, L. pneumophila* (legionnaires' disease), and *Pneumocystis jiroveci* (formerly *carinii*) pneumonia.

Aspiration pneumonia is frequently called necrotizing pneumonia because of the pathologic changes in the lungs. Aspiration pneumonia occurs most commonly as a result of aspiration of vomitus when the patient is in an altered state of consciousness due to a seizure, drugs, alcohol, anesthesia, acute infection, or shock. Aspiration pneumonia may be acquired through foreign body aspiration or may follow aspiration of toxic materials, such as gasoline or kerosene.

The causative agents of bacterial aspiration pneumonia include *S. aureus, Escherichia coli, Klebsiella pneumoniae, Pseudomonas aeruginosa,* and *Proteus* species.

The pathophysiology of pneumonia depends on the causative agent. Bacterial pneumonia is marked by an alveolar suppurative (process of pus formation) exudate with consolidation of infection. Mycoplasmal and viral pneumonia produce interstitial inflammation with no consolidation or exudate. Fungal and mycobacterial pneumonias are marked by patchy distribution that may undergo necrosis with the development of cavities. Aspiration pneumonia manifests with various physiologic responses depending on the pH of the aspirated substance.

An overview of the pathophysiology is as follows: (1) pulmonary cilia cannot remove accumulating secretions from the respiratory tract; (2) these retained secretions then become infected; (3) inflammation of some part of the respiratory tract develops, leading to a localized edema; and (4) this causes decreased oxygen–carbon dioxide exchange. This process can begin in the bronchi or in the lobe of one lung, and it can become more extensive.

 Health Promotion

Pneumonia

- A number of nursing interventions can help prevent the occurrence of, as well as the morbidity associated with, pneumonia.
- Teach the patient to practice good health habits, such as proper diet and hygiene, adequate rest, and regular exercise, to maintain the natural resistance to infecting organisms.
- Encourage the individual at risk for pneumonia (e.g., the chronically ill, older adult) to obtain both influenza and pneumococcal vaccines.
- In the hospital, identify the patient at risk and take measures to prevent the development of pneumonia.
- Place the patient with altered consciousness in positions that will prevent or minimize the risk of aspiration (e.g., side lying, upright). Turn and reposition the patient at least every 2 hours to facilitate adequate lung expansion and to discourage pooling of secretions.
- The patient who has difficulty swallowing (e.g., stroke patient) needs assistance in eating, drinking, and taking medication to prevent aspiration.
- The patient who has recently had surgery and others who are immobile need assistance with turning and deep breathing measures at frequent intervals and use of incentive spirometer.
- Aspiration pneumonia can occur as a result of nasogastric tube feedings. Always check for correct placement and keep the head of bed elevated to 30 degrees.
- Be careful to avoid overmedication with opioids or sedatives, which can cause a depressed cough reflex and accumulation of fluid in the lungs.
- Before providing food or fluids, ensure the gag reflex has returned to the patient who had local anesthesia to the throat.
- Practice strict medical asepsis and adherence to infection control guidelines to reduce the incidence of nosocomial infections. Health care providers should wash their hands each time before they provide care to a patient. Comply with current Centers for Disease Control and Prevention hand hygiene guidelines.

Clinical Manifestations

Many significant signs and symptoms are seen in pneumonia. A productive cough is common; color and consistency of sputum vary depending on the type of pneumonia present. Severe chills, elevated temperature, and increased heart and respiratory rates may accompany the painful, productive cough (see Life Span Considerations box).

Clinical manifestations depend on the type of pneumonia:

- **Streptococcal, pneumococcal:** Sudden onset; chest pain; chills; fever; headache; cough; rust-colored sputum; crackles and possibly friction rub; hypoxemia as blood is shunted away from area of consolidation; cyanosis; area of consolidation visible on chest radiograph; sputum culture needed to determine causative agent

Life Span Considerations

Older Adults

Respiratory Disorder

- Signs and symptoms of pneumonia are often atypical in older adults. Fever, cough, and purulent sputum may be absent. Generalized signs and symptoms such as lethargy, disorientation, dyspnea, tachypnea, chills, chest pain, and vomiting, as well as an unexpected exacerbation of coexisting conditions, should be viewed with suspicion because they may indicate pneumonia in the older adult.
- Adequate hydration is important for the older person with pneumonia. It helps liquefy secretions and promotes expectoration.
- Many older adults have difficulty expectorating. This slows resolution of congestion and increases the difficulty of obtaining sputum specimens. Because deep breathing and coughing are difficult, the older person may require suctioning to remove respiratory secretions. Perform this with caution, since too-frequent suctioning can stimulate increased production of secretions.
- Older adults, particularly those living in an institution, should have routine skin tests for tuberculosis. Many older adults were exposed to tuberculosis during their childhood and have positive results on skin tests. These individuals should receive routine chest radiographic studies. Older adults who have histories of inactive tuberculosis should be watched for recurrence of active tuberculosis. Signs and symptoms are often vague and include loss of appetite and weight loss.
- Closely watch older immigrants and immunosuppressed older adults for drug-resistant strains of tuberculosis.
- Provided that there is no serious disease of the respiratory tract, the older person is generally able to maintain adequate ventilation and oxygenation. However, changes of aging do have an effect on respiratory function:
  - —Drier mucous membranes and decreased number of cilia affect the older individual's ability to humidify inhaled air and trap debris. This increases the risk for inflammation and irritation of the upper respiratory tract.
  - —Kyphosis and calcification of costal cartilage are common changes. These restrict expansion of the thoracic cavity and lead to a barrel-chested appearance.
  - —Intercostal muscles and the diaphragm lose elasticity, resulting in a decreased ability to breathe deeply and cough.
  - —The elasticity of airways and alveoli decreases, alveoli thicken, and pulmonary blood flow decreases, resulting in an increased risk for impaired gas exchange.
- Years of exposure to air pollution, smoke, and mechanical irritants increase the risk for respiratory disease in older adults, particularly those who have emphysema or chronic bronchitis.
- Inactivity and immobility increase the risk of stasis pooling of respiratory secretions. This increases the risk of pneumonia.
- Neurologic damage as a result of strokes, Parkinson's disease, and other conditions is increasingly common in the older adult. Any neurologic disorder that decreases the gag or swallow reflexes increases the risk of aspiration of fluids and food, with resultant trauma to the respiratory tract.
- Cor pulmonale with right-sided heart failure, as well as left-sided heart failure with pulmonary congestion, are common complications of chronic obstructive pulmonary disease in the older adult.

- **Staphylococcal:** Many of the same signs as streptococcal; sputum copious and salmon colored
- **Klebsiella:** Many of the same signs and symptoms as streptococcal; onset more gradual; more bronchopneumonia (inflammation of the terminal bronchioles and alveoli) visible on chest radiograph; if treatment delayed beyond second day after onset, patient becomes critically ill and mortality rate is high
- **Haemophilus:** Commonly follows upper respiratory tract infection; low-grade fever; croupy cough; malaise; arthralgias; yellow or green sputum
- **Mycoplasmal:** Gradual onset; headache; fever; malaise; chills; cough severe and nonproductive; decreased breath sounds and crackles; chest radiograph clear; white blood cell count normal
- **Viral:** Signs and symptoms generally mild; cold symptoms; headache; anorexia; myalgia (tenderness or pain in muscles); irritating cough that produces mucopurulent or bloody sputum; bronchopneumonic type of infiltration on chest radiograph; white blood cell count usually normal; rise in antibody titers

Assessment

Subjective data include the patient's description of the onset and duration of cough. The patient may complain of fever and night sweats.

Collection of **objective data** includes checking the level of consciousness and vital signs, especially temperature and respirations, every 2 hours or as ordered. Note the color, consistency, and amount of sputum produced. Inspect the thorax to determine the patient's use of accessory muscles (abdominal or intercostal) in respiratory effort, and note any cyanosis or dyspnea. Perform auscultation; the patient will have crackles on inspiration and possibly a pleural effusion.

Diagnostic Tests

Blood and sputum cultures help identify organisms. Collect sputum for culture and sensitivity before starting antibiotic therapy. Chest radiographic studies reveal changes in density, primarily in the lower lobes. White blood cell count is normal or even low in viral or mycoplasmal pneumonia, whereas it is elevated in bacterial pneumonia. Leukocytosis is found in the majority of patients with bacterial pneumonia, usually with a white blood cell count greater than 15,000/mm^3 with a shift to the left. PFTs may be done to determine whether lung volume is decreased, and ABG values are determined to identify altered gas exchange. Pulse oximetry is ordered to monitor oxygen saturation of arterial blood levels. Oximetry is invaluable for rapid and continuous assessment of oxygen needs.

Medical Management

If pus accumulates in the pleural space (empyema), the physician inserts a chest tube for drainage. The physician also prescribes oxygen therapy and physiotherapy (chest percussion and postural drainage). Encourage patients to cough and breathe deeply to maximize ventilatory capabilities.

Commonly prescribed medications include antibiotics (penicillin, erythromycin, cephalosporin, and tetracycline), depending on causative organism and sensitivity. With prompt treatment and appropriate antibiotics, bacterial and mycoplasmal pneumonia patients usually respond to therapy in 48 to 72 hours (Lewis et al., 2007). Currently viral pneumonia has no definitive treatment. Analgesics and antipyretics (acetaminophen or aspirin), expectorants, and bronchodilators are often prescribed. Humidification with a humidifier or a nebulizer if secretions are tenacious and copious is useful. Oxygenation is prescribed if the patient has an oxygen saturation of less than 91%. Venturi mask or nasal cannula is commonly used.

A vaccine is now available for the most common and important bacterial pneumonia, streptococcal (or pneumococcal) pneumonia. Pneumococcal vaccine is indicated primarily for the individual considered at risk who (1) has chronic illnesses such as lung and heart disease and diabetes mellitus, (2) is recovering from a severe illness, (3) is 65 years of age or older, or (4) is in a nursing home or other long-term care facility. This is particularly important because the rate of drug-resistant streptococcal pneumonia is increasing. The vaccine is 50% to 80% effective in preventing pneumococcal disease. The current recommendation is that pneumococcal vaccine is good for the person's lifetime. However, in the immunosuppressed individual or the older adult at risk for development of fatal pneumococcal infection, revaccination should be considered every 5 years. When given in different arms, the influenza vaccine and the pneumococcal vaccine may be administered at the same time.

Nursing Interventions and Patient Teaching

Nursing strategies are aimed at helping the patient conserve energy. Allow rest periods and facilitate optimal air exchange by placing the patient in a high Fowler's position. Place the patient on the side with the "good lung down." This position benefits those with unilateral pulmonary disease, including unilateral pneumonia. In pneumonia and many other pulmonary problems, Pa_{O_2} rises when the healthy lung is dependent (or "good lung down"). When the unimpaired lung is down, this better ventilated lung also is vastly better perfused. Studies have revealed that hypoxia worsened when patients were placed on their back or side with the affected (sick) lung down.

Assess the patient's ability to move secretions. If the patient is unable to expectorate secretions, assist with appropriate measures (such as coughing, positioning, suctioning, and liquefying secretions). Promptly administer bronchodilators, mucolytics, and expectorants as prescribed to dilate bronchioles and remove secretions. Carefully and frequently auscultate the chest for quality of breath sounds and adventitious sounds. Note cough and sputum characteristics and document. Provide hydration to liquefy secretions and replace fluids. Fluid intake of at least 3 L/day is important in the supportive treatment of pneumonia. If oral intake cannot be maintained, IV administration of fluids and electrolytes may be necessary for the acutely ill patient. Fluid intake must be individualized for patients with heart failure.

An intake of at least 1500 calories per day should be maintained to provide energy for the patient's increased metabolic processes. Small, frequent meals are better tolerated by the dyspneic patient.

Nursing diagnoses and interventions for the patient with pneumonia include but are not limited to the following:

Nursing Diagnoses	Nursing Interventions
Ineffective breathing pattern, related to inflammatory process and pleuritic pain	Assess ventilation, including breathing rate, rhythm, and depth; chest expansion; and presence of respiratory distress such as dyspnea, shortness of breath, nasal flaring, pursed-lip breathing, or prolonged expiratory phase and use of accessory muscles. Auscultate lungs for crackles, wheezes, and pleural friction rub. Identify contributing factors such as airway clearance or obstruction problem or weakness. Encourage increased fluid intake to 3 L/day, unless contraindicated, to liquefy secretions for easier expectoration. Maintain patient in position that facilitates ventilation (head of bed in semi-Fowler's position or sitting and leaning forward on overbed table).

Nursing Diagnoses	Nursing Interventions
Impaired gas exchange, related to alveolar-capillary membrane changes secondary to inflammation	Assess patient to identify signs (e.g., restlessness, disorientation, and irritability) that may indicate the body's response to altered blood gas states (hypoxia). If necessary and with physician consultation, administer oxygen by nasal cannula or Venturi mask to maintain oxygen saturations above 90%. Carefully monitor body temperature, which may fluctuate due to alterations in metabolism or infection.

Teach the patient and the family about (1) deep breathing and coughing techniques and the use of an incentive spirometer; (2) the importance of handwashing to prevent the spread of the disease; (3) prescribed medications such as antibiotics, including the purpose, action, dosage, frequency of administration, and side effects; (4) the specific type of pneumonia the patient has, treatment, anticipated response, possible complications, and probable disease duration; (5) the importance of consuming large quantities of fluid; (6) adaptive exercise and rest techniques; and (7) the availability of pneumococcal vaccine. Also inform the patient about changes in health status that must be reported to the health care provider. These include a change in sputum characteristics or color, decreased activity tolerance, fever despite the antibiotics, increasing chest pain, or a feeling that things are not getting better.

Prognosis

Improvement occurs in 48 to 72 hours with appropriate antibiotics in uncomplicated cases (Lewis et al., 2007). The disease usually resolves within 2 to 3 weeks with proper treatment. However, pneumonia is the most common cause of death from infectious disease in North America. It is also the major cause of disease and death in critically ill or older adult patients. Even with treatment with new antimicrobial agents, pneumonia and influenza still remain the seventh leading cause of death in the United States (Lewis et al., 2007).

PLEURISY

Etiology and Pathophysiology

Pleurisy is an inflammation of the visceral and parietal pleura. Pleurisy can be caused by either a bacterial or viral infection. The underlying physiologic change is an inflammation of any portion of the pleura. It may occur spontaneously but more frequently is a complication of pneumonia, pulmonary infarctions, viral infections of the intercostal muscles, pleural trauma, or early stages of TB or lung tumor.

Clinical Manifestations

One of the first symptoms of pleurisy may be a sharp inspiratory pain, often radiating to the shoulder or abdomen of the affected side. The pain is caused by stretching of the inflamed pleura. If pleural effusion develops, pain subsides and fever and dry cough occur. Other signs and symptoms include dyspnea, cough, and elevated temperature.

Assessment

Subjective data include the patient's complaint of chest pain on inspiration. The patient may also report an elevated temperature.

Collection of **objective data** includes assessment of the inspiratory pain, noting its radiation points. Monitor vital signs, especially temperature, every 2 or 4 hours. Monitor and document respiratory rate and rhythm, including dyspnea. On auscultation of the lungs, a pleural friction rub is heard.

Diagnostic Tests

The presence of a pleural friction rub may be considered diagnostic. Chest radiographic examination is of limited value in diagnosing pleurisy unless pleural effusion is present if fluid accumulates.

Medical Management

The physician may inject an anesthetic block around the vertebrae to block the intercostal nerves, thus relieving pain. Prescribed medications may include antibiotics (penicillin) to combat the infection and analgesics (meperidine [Demerol] or morphine) to decrease pain when the patient takes deep breaths and coughs. Antipyretics (acetaminophen) are used for fever. Oxygen may be administered.

Nursing Interventions and Patient Teaching

Position the patient comfortably on the affected side to splint the chest, and apply heat to the area.

Nursing diagnoses and interventions for the patient with pleurisy include but are not limited to the following:

Nursing Diagnoses	Nursing Interventions
Pain, related to stretching of the pulmonary pleura as a result of fluid accumulation	Assess patient's pain level and need for analgesics; administer as needed, documenting effectiveness. Assist with splinting affected side when patient coughs and deep breathes.

Continued

Nursing Diagnoses	Nursing Interventions
Impaired gas exchange, related to pain on inspiration and expiration	Assess patient's level of consciousness, noting any increase in restlessness or disorientation, which may indicate ineffective breathing. Auscultate lungs for wheezes, crackles, and pleural friction rub. Reposition patient every 2 hours to prevent pooling of secretions and to promote optimal lung expansion. Elevate head of bed to facilitate optimal ventilation.

Instruct the patient to be alert to signs and symptoms of exacerbation: purulent sputum production, further increase in temperature, and increased pain. Teach the patient to effectively cough every 2 hours and to splint the affected side.

Prognosis

Prognosis is usually excellent. Complications of atelectasis or secondary infection such as pneumonia may develop.

PLEURAL EFFUSION/EMPYEMA

Etiology and Pathophysiology

Once the pleural lining is inflamed (as in pleurisy), fluid can accumulate in the pleural space. This accumulation of fluid is known as **pleural effusion.** Pleural effusion is rarely a disease by itself but occurs as a secondary problem when the physiologic pressure in the lungs and pleurae is disturbed. If the fluid becomes infected, it is called **empyema,** which is the accumulation of pus in a body cavity, especially the pleural space.

The pathophysiology of pleural effusion lies in the alteration of pressure gradients or surface characteristics of capillaries. Empyema may be acute or chronic. In acute empyema the affected area is inflamed with a thin layer of fluid. If this goes untreated, the fluid thickens and the pleura becomes scarred and fibrosed, losing its elasticity.

Clinical Manifestations

Pleural effusion is generally associated with other disease processes, such as pancreatitis, cirrhosis of the liver, pulmonary edema, congestive heart failure, kidney disease, or carcinoma involving altered capillary permeability. Empyema is usually seen as a result of bacterial infection, as in pneumonia, TB, or blunt chest trauma. The patient may have a persistent fever in spite of receiving antibiotics.

Assessment

Subjective data include patient complaints of dyspnea and air hunger. The patient may also report fear and anxiety related to decreased levels of oxygen.

Collection of **objective data** in both pleural effusion and empyema includes assessment of signs and symptoms of respiratory distress, such as nasal flaring, tachypnea, and decreased breath sounds. Assess breath sounds and vital signs, especially temperature, frequently.

Diagnostic Tests

Effusions or pleural fluid will be evident on chest radiographic examination. Often a thoracentesis (needle inserted into pleural space to aspirate excess fluid) will be done to obtain a specimen for culture to identify the causative agent, and also to relieve dyspnea and discomfort.

Medical Management

Usually this condition requires a thoracentesis to remove fluid from the pleural space. A possible danger from this procedure is removing fluid too rapidly; less than 1300 to 1500 mL at one time is recommended.

A chest tube or tubes may be inserted for continuous drainage of fluid, blood, or air from the pleural cavity and for medication instillation. The tubes are sutured in place and covered with a sterile dressing. To prevent the lung from collapsing, a closed drainage system is used, which maintains the lung cavity's normal negative pressure. Under normal conditions, intrapleural pressure is below atmospheric pressure (approximately 4 to 5 cm H_2O below atmospheric pressure during expiration and approximately 8 to 10 cm H_2O below atmospheric pressure during inspiration). If intrapleural pressure becomes equal to atmospheric pressure, the lungs will collapse. The chest tubes and attached closed drainage system restore normal intrapleural pressure and facilitate expansion of the lung.

With this procedure one or, more commonly, two thoracotomy tubes are inserted into the pleural space and are attached to a closed-system, water-seal drainage. One catheter is inserted through a stab wound in the anterior chest wall; this is referred to as the **anterior tube.** It removes air from the pleural space. The second tube, the **posterior tube,** is inserted through a stab wound in the posterior chest. It is primarily for the drainage of serosanguineous fluid or purulent exudate. The posterior (lower) tube may be larger in diameter than the anterior (upper) tube to prevent it from becoming occluded with exudate or clots (Figure 49-11). The chest tubes are connected to a pleural drainage system with collection, water-seal, and suction control chambers to drain secretions and reestablish negative pressure in the pleural space (Coughlin, 2006) (Figure 49-12).

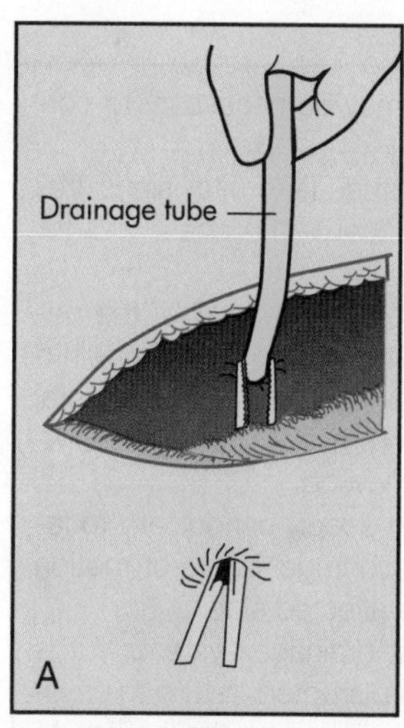

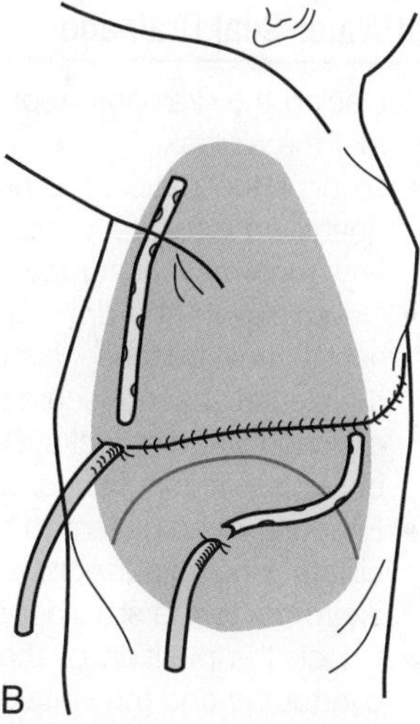

FIGURE 49-11 **A,** Drainage tube inserted into pleural space. **B,** Note that anterior and posterior tubes are placed well into pleural space.

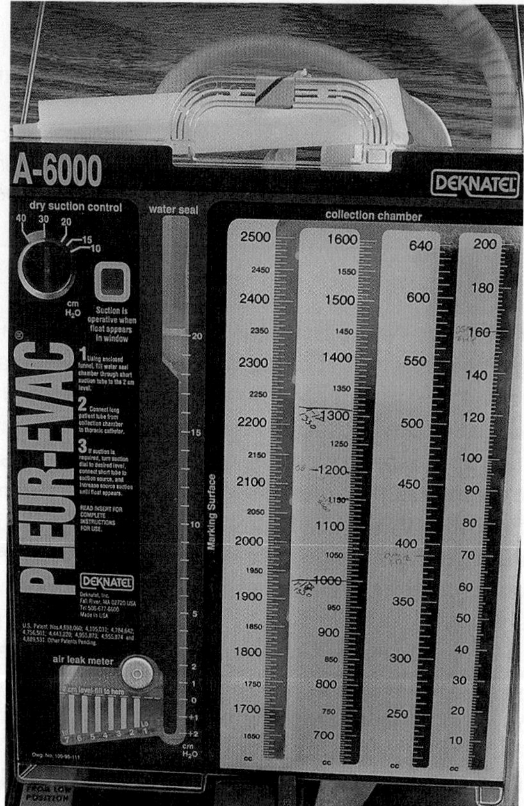

FIGURE 49-12 Pleur-Evac, a disposable, commercial chest drainage system.

Nursing Interventions and Patient Teaching

General nursing measures include placing the patient on bed rest. If the patient is receiving oxygen therapy, provide frequent oral care to keep mucous membranes moist. Also encourage effective coughing and deep-breathing techniques and respiratory treatments. If the patient has had a thoracentesis, apply a large sterile dressing and assess it for drainage, noting the color and amount.

Ensure that patency of the chest tube system is maintained so that it can drain fluid adequately. Areas of concern are the following:

- **Proper system function:** Ensuring that the water in the water-seal chamber fluctuates when suction is applied. There should not be any bubbling in the water seal, since this indicates an air leak.
- **Potential atelectasis resulting from hypoventilation:** Assessing for increased dyspnea; checking chest radiographic studies frequently to compare degree of lung consolidation.
- **Increased air in the pleural space:** Noting any air leaks in the system; ensuring tubing is secure and remains patent.
- **Infection:** Noting an increase in white blood cells, elevated temperature, and presence of purulent drainage.

A patient with a chest tube in place is usually positioned on the unaffected side to keep the tube from becoming kinked; however, the patient may assume any position of comfort in bed. There is no contraindication to ambulation with a chest tube in place, as long as the water-seal bottle remains below the level of the chest. Never elevate the drainage system to the level of the patient's chest, since this would cause fluid to drain back into the pleural cavity. Facilitate coughing and deep-breathing procedures at least every 2 hours and auscultate breath sounds frequently. Document the amount and characteristics of pleural fluid drainage by marking the drainage level on the container at the end of each shift, along with the date and the hour (Box 49-6). Prevent a chest tube from being accidentally removed by paying careful attention to securing connections and positioning drainage tubes. Be careful to keep tubing as straight as possible and coiled loosely. Do not let the patient lie on it. Tubing should never be placed over the side rails.

Administer antibiotic agents as ordered.

Nursing diagnoses and interventions for the patient with pleural effusion or empyema include but are not limited to the following:

Nursing Diagnoses	Nursing Interventions
Impaired gas exchange, related to ineffective breathing pattern	Assess for changes in level of consciousness, such as disorientation, restlessness, or irritability, since these may indicate increasing hypoxia as a result of ineffective breathing. Monitor ABGs and pulse oximetry. Encourage coughing and deep breathing to remove secretions and facilitate lung expansion.

Continued

Box 49-6 Guidelines for Care of Patient with Chest Tubes and Water-Seal Drainage

- Keep all tubing as straight as possible and coiled loosely below chest level. Do not let patient lie on it.
- Keep all connections between chest tubes, drainage tubing, and the drainage collector tight, and tape at connections.
- Keep the water-seal and suction control chamber at the appropriate water levels by adding sterile water as needed because water loss by evaporation may occur.
- Mark the time measurement and the fluid level with a black marker pen on the drainage chamber according to the prescribed orders. Marking intervals may range from every hour to every 8 hours. Any change in the quantity or characteristics of drainage (e.g., clear yellow to serosanguineous) should be reported to the physician and recorded. Record output on chart.
- Observe for air bubbling in the water-seal chamber and fluctuations (tidaling). If no tidaling is observed (rising with inspiration and falling with expiration in the spontaneously breathing patient; the opposite occurs during positive-pressure mechanical ventilation), the drainage system is occluded or the lungs are reexpanded. If bubbling increases, there may be an air leak.
- Bubbling in the water seal may occur intermittently. When bubbling is continuous and constant, the source of the air leak may be determined by momentarily clamping the tubing at successively distal points away from the patient until the bubbling ceases. Retaping tubing connections or replacing the drainage apparatus may be necessary to correct the air leak.
- Monitor the patient's clinical status. Take vital signs frequently, auscultate lungs, and observe the chest wall for any abnormal chest movements.
- Never elevate the drainage system to the level of the patient's chest because this will cause fluid to drain back into the pleural space. Secure the drainage system to the metal drainage stand or racks. Do not empty the drainage chamber unless it is in danger of overflowing.
- Encourage the patient to breathe deeply periodically to facilitate lung expansion, and encourage range-of-motion exercises to the shoulder on the affected side.
- Check the position of the chest drainage system. If it is overturned and the water seal is disrupted, return the system to an upright position and encourage the patient to take a few deep breaths, followed by forced exhalations and cough maneuvers.
- Do not strip or milk chest tubes routinely because this increases pleural pressures.
- If the drainage system breaks, place the distal end of the chest tubing connection in a sterile water container at a 2-cm level as an emergency water seal.
- Chest tubes are not clamped routinely. Clamps with rubber protection are kept at the bedside for special procedures such as changing the chest drainage system and assessment before removal of chest tubes.

Nursing Diagnoses	Nursing Interventions
Impaired gas exchange, related to ineffective breathing pattern—cont'd	Reposition patient every 2 hours to prevent pooling of secretions. Assess for atelectasis.
Self-care deficit, related to mobility restriction	Assess patient's ability to care for self, and assist when needed. Encourage increasing activity level when fever is reduced.

Explain all procedures before their implementation. Prepare the patient emotionally for chest tube insertion. Teach the patient and the family about this condition and the healing process. Instruct the patient on effective coughing and deep-breathing techniques.

Prognosis

The prognosis is variable, depending on the patient's overall health status.

ATELECTASIS

Etiology and Pathophysiology

Atelectasis (the collapse of alveoli, preventing the respiratory exchange of carbon dioxide and oxygen) occurs from occlusion of air (blockage) to a portion of the lung. Atelectasis is a common postoperative complication from a mucous plug resulting from shallow breathing, which interferes with coughing and effective clearance of secretions. All or part of the lung collapses, usually as a result of **hypoventilation** (the condition in which the amount of air that enters the alveoli and takes part in gas exchange is not adequate for the body's metabolic needs), which then leads to bronchial obstruction caused by mucus accumulation. Accumulation of secretions, a foreign body, or a tenacious plug of mucus may completely occlude a bronchus, closing off all air to a portion of the patient's lung. Atelectasis can also result from obstruction of the airway by aspiration of a foreign body or compression of lung tissue caused by emphysema, pneumothorax, or tumor.

The altered physiology depends on the site and the degree of occlusion. If the mainstem bronchus is obstructed, severe ventilatory compromise occurs. When a small bronchiole becomes obstructed, as with secretion accumulation, fewer signs and symptoms are seen because the respiratory system tries to compensate. However, in either case, atelectasis can lead to stasis pneumonia (because the retained secretions are rich in nutrients for the growth of bacteria) and lung damage.

Clinical Manifestations

The patient displays dyspnea, **tachypnea** (an abnormally rapid rate of breathing), pleural friction rub, restlessness, hypertension, and elevated temperature.

Assessment

Subjective data include patient complaints of severe shortness of breath (dyspnea) requiring much effort, which results in fatigue. The patient may also verbalize a feeling of air hunger and resulting anxiety.

Objective data include decreased breath sounds and crackles on auscultation. Assess vital signs frequently because tachycardia and hypertension are present at first, followed by hypotension and bradycardia. Note respiration rate and amount of effort required for breathing. The patient may exhibit altered levels of consciousness caused by hypoxia.

Diagnostic Tests

Serial chest radiographic studies (repeated radiographic examinations of same area done for comparison) demonstrate atelectatic changes. A chest CT scan can detect compression in the airway and may also reveal the underlying pathologic condition contributing to the problem. ABGs reveal a Pao_2 of less than 80 mm Hg initially; this generally improves within the first 24 hours. Pulse oximetry reveals oxygen saturation levels below 90%. $Paco_2$ is normal or low because of hypoventilation. A flexible fiberoptic bronchoscopy may reveal a bronchial obstruction; this procedure can also remove a mucous plug or retained secretions.

Medical Management

Ventilation maintenance with intubation is often required. Incentive spirometry 10 times every hour while awake helps provide visual feedback of respiratory effort. Respiratory therapy with oxygen is ordered. Chest physiotherapy with postural drainage is administered. The patient may require suctioning, coughing, and vigorous respiratory and physical therapy if a mechanical obstruction is present. Prescribed medications may include bronchodilators (albuterol) to facilitate secretion removal, antibiotics to prevent infection, and mucolytic agents (acetylcysteine [Mucomyst]) to reduce viscosity of secretions. A bronchoscope can be used to remove a thick, tenacious secretion or a mucous plug.

Nursing Interventions and Patient Teaching

Postoperatively, remind patients to cough, breathe deeply, use their incentive spirometer, and change positions every 1 to 2 hours. Effective coughing is essential in mobilizing secretions. If secretions are present in the respiratory passages, deep breathing and use of the incentive spirometer often will move them up to stimulate the cough reflex, and then they can be expectorated. Administer analgesics to relieve pain and increase the patient's ability to carry out respiratory exercises and to clear airway passages. Provide emotional support. Encourage early ambulation.

Nursing diagnoses and interventions for the patient with atelectasis include but are not limited to the following:

Nursing Diagnoses	Nursing Interventions
Ineffective airway clearance, related to inability to clear secretions	Assess patient's ability to move secretions, and assist if needed. Encourage use of incentive spirometer 10 times every hour while awake. Encourage coughing and deep breathing every 1 to 2 hours while awake. Encourage adequate hydration to liquefy secretions. Auscultate breath sounds frequently, documenting and reporting any changes. Assess color, consistency, and amount of secretions removed via either coughing or suction.
Ineffective coping, related to invasive medical regimen	Assess the patient's ability to comply with the prescribed regimen and to cooperate with caregivers. Identify patient's emotional support systems.

Instruct the patient on proper techniques for effective coughing and deep breathing and other measures to facilitate optimal air exchange, such as increasing movement and changing position. Medication teaching should address the rationale and side effects of prescribed medications.

Prognosis

Prognosis depends on the patient's age and preexisting illness.

PNEUMOTHORAX

Etiology and Pathophysiology

Pneumothorax is a collection of air or gas in the pleural space, causing the lung to collapse. It can be secondary to a ruptured bleb on the lung surface (as in emphysema) or a severe coughing episode. It can be caused by a penetrating chest injury that punctures the pleural lining, fractured ribs, or injury to the pleura from insertion of a subclavian catheter. A spontaneous pneumothorax can also occur suddenly without an apparent cause (Figure 49-13).

When the pleural space is penetrated, air enters, thus interrupting the normal negative pressure. Consequently the lung cannot remain fully inflated.

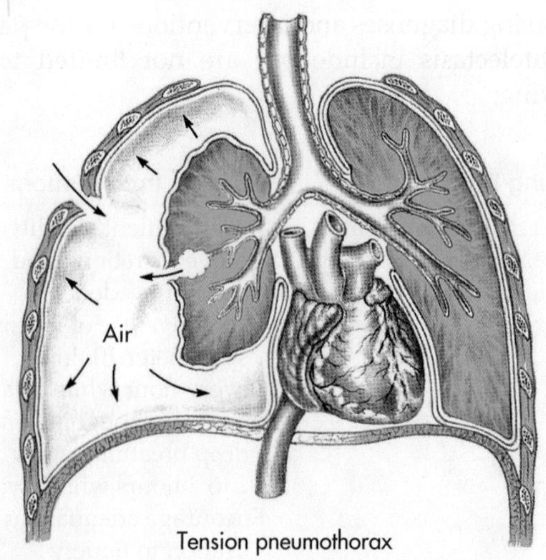

FIGURE 49-13 Pneumothorax (complete collapse of the right lung).

Clinical Manifestations

The patient may be seen with a recent chest injury. He or she will have decreased breath sounds on the affected side and a sudden, sharp, pleuritic chest pain with dyspnea. The patient may be diaphoretic and exhibit an increased heart rate, tachypnea, and dyspnea. Normal chest movements on the affected side cease. With a pneumothorax resulting from penetrating injury, a sucking sound is heard on inspiration.

As intrathoracic pressure increases in the pleural space, the lung collapses. Because lung tissue no longer expands, the mediastinum may shift to the unaffected side (mediastinal shift), which is subsequently compressed. As the intrathoracic pressure increases, cardiac output is altered because of decreased venous return and compression of the great vessels.

Assessment

Collection of **subjective data** includes reporting a precipitating respiratory condition such as COPD, a recent penetrating chest injury, or severe coughing episode. The patient may complain of chest pain, shortness of breath of sudden onset, and feelings of anxiety associated with air hunger.

Collection of **objective data** involves taking frequent vital signs, noting any change in respiratory and cardiac rate and rhythm. A small pneumothorax usually manifests with mild tachycardia and dyspnea. A larger pneumothorax causes reparatory distress, including rapid shallow respirations, air hunger, dyspnea, and oxygen desaturation. Hemoptysis and cough may be present (Lewis et al., 2007). Findings on auscultation are bilaterally unequal breath sounds, with no breath sounds over the affected area. Note color, characteristics, and amount of sputum.

Diagnostic Tests

Chest radiographic examination shows the presence of pneumothorax. ABGs show a decrease in pH and Pao_2, with an increased $Paco_2$.

Medical Management

Surgery may be done to insert a chest tube (thoracotomy). The chest tube is inserted in the fifth and sixth intercostal spaces at the midaxillary line. The chest tube is attached to a water-seal drainage system (see Figures 49-11 and 49-12).

Another approach to correcting a pneumothorax is the use of a Heimlich valve, which is typically used as a stopgap measure until chest tube therapy can be started. The valve attaches to a chest tube and is inserted into the chest. As the patient exhales, air and fluid drain through the valve into a plastic bag. When the patient inhales, however, the flexible tubing in the valve collapses, preventing secretions and air from reentering the pleura.

Nursing Interventions and Patient Teaching

General measures include maintaining airway patency and providing adequate oxygenation. Assess and document patency of the chest tube system, keeping it free from kinks. Note the color and amount of drainage and assess integrity of the drainage system. Monitor blood pressure and place the patient in a high Fowler's position to promote airway clearance and lung expansion. Control pain by administering appropriate analgesics, but avoid the use of respiratory depressants.

Nursing diagnoses and interventions for the patient with pneumothorax include but are not limited to the following:

Nursing Diagnoses	Nursing Interventions
Ineffective breathing pattern, related to nonfunctioning lung	Assess respiratory rate and rhythm, and note any signs of respiratory distress, such as dyspnea, use of accessory muscles, nasal flaring, and anxiety. Provide chest tube care, maintaining secure placement. Facilitate ventilation by elevating head of bed, and administer oxygen as ordered. Suction as needed to remove secretions. Encourage adaptive breathing techniques to decrease respiratory effort. Encourage rest periods interspersed with activities.
Fear, related to feeling of air hunger	Assess patient's feelings of fear related to health concerns and feeling of air hunger. Identify positive coping methods, and support their use. Determine support systems available to patient.

Explain the rationale for treatments (oxygen therapy and chest tube drainage) before their implementation. Reinforce effective breathing techniques and the need for ongoing medical care. Instruct the patient to limit exposure to people who may have infections, such as upper respiratory tract infection or influenza. Advise the patient to not smoke but to drink a lot of fluids, to avoid fatigue and strenuous activity, and to report any signs and symptoms of recurrence (e.g., chest pain, difficulty breathing, or fever) to the physician.

Prognosis

The lung usually reexpands within several days. The physician removes the chest tube when a chest radiograph shows that the lungs are completely expanded.

LUNG CANCER

Etiology and Pathophysiology

The incidence of lung cancer has been steadily increasing during the past 50 years in both men and women. In 1987, cancer of the lung surpassed breast cancer to become the number one cancer killer of women. Thus lung cancer is now the leading cause of death from cancer in both men and women. Lung cancer causes 34% of cancer deaths in men. The American Cancer Society estimated that in 2009 about 219,440 Americans would be diagnosed with lung cancer and 159,390 would die of this devastating disease. Seventy-two percent of people have regional or distant metastases at diagnosis. Tumors may result from metastasis anywhere in the body or may appear as primary tumors. Metastasis from the colon and kidney is common. Metastasis to the lung may be discovered before the primary lesion is known, and sometimes the location of the primary lesion is not determined during the person's life.

Approximately 87% of lung tumors are linked to cigarette smoking. A history of smoking, especially for 20 years or more, is considered to be a prime risk factor. The more cigarettes someone smokes each day, the higher the risk. "Passive smoking" (breathing in sidestream smoke) is qualitatively similar to mainstream smoking; involuntary (secondhand) smoking poses a risk for the development of lung cancer in nonsmokers. Occupational exposures, such as asbestos, radon, and uranium, are also risk factors. It is suspected that air pollutants may increase risk. Most people who develop the disease are older than 50 years of age.

Many studies suggest the importance of certain antioxidant vitamins, especially vitamins A and E, to reduce the risk of developing lung cancer. Studies report that an increased intake of fruits; green and yellow vegetables; and perhaps micronutrients such as total carotenoids, beta-carotene, and vitamins can significantly lower the risk of lung cancer in cigarette smokers as well as nonsmokers (Edmondson, 2007).

The mortality of people with lung cancer depends primarily on the specific type of cancer and the size of the tumor when detected. Lung cancer is classified by microscopic study of the tumor. Treatment is based on the type and extent of the disease, using two major classifications. Small cell lung cancer (SCLC) (oat cell cancer), mixed small cell–large cell carcinoma, and combined small cell carcinoma are the three types of small cell lung cancers (Edmondson, 2007). SCLC is very aggressive and occurs in approximately 20% of patients with lung cancer; non–small cell lung cancer (NSCLC), including adenocarcinoma, accounts for 30% to 32% of lung cancer; squamous cell carcinoma accounts for 30% of lung cancers; and large cell undifferentiated carcinoma occurs in about 9% of cases.

Clinical Manifestations

Lung cancer is insidious because it is usually asymptomatic in the early stages. If the lesion is located peripherally, it produces few symptoms and may not be discovered until visualized on a routine chest radiographic examination. If the peripheral lesion perforates the pleural space, pleural effusion and severe pain will occur. Central lesions originate from a larger branch of the bronchial tree. These lesions cause obstruction and erosion of the bronchus. Signs and symptoms are cough, hemoptysis, dyspnea, fever, and chills. Auscultation may reveal wheezing on the affected side. Phrenic nerve involvement causes paralysis of the diaphragm.

As the disease progresses, metastasis may occur, along with weight loss, fatigue, decreased stamina, and changes in functional status. Pain is unlikely unless the tumor is pressing on a nerve or the cancer has spread to the bones. Primary lung tumors usually metastasize to the liver or to nearby structures, such as the esophagus, the pericardium, skeletal bone, and the brain.

Assessment

Subjective data include the patient's complaints of a chronic cough and of hoarseness. The patient may also report weight loss and extreme fatigue. Interview the patient regarding a family history, especially a history of cigarette smoking and of exposure to occupational irritants.

Collection of **objective data** includes assessing the cough, noting color (especially blood streaked) and consistency of sputum, as well as frequency, duration, and precipitating factors. Also assess the characteristics of the cough (moist, dry, hacking) and effect of body position and identify with the patient what, if anything, helps to relieve the cough. Auscultate the lungs to determine if unilateral wheezing or crackles are present. Invasion of the superior vena cava causes edema of the neck and face and is called **superior vena cava syndrome.**

Diagnostic Tests

Chest radiographic studies and spiral CT scan of the chest are used to identify the location and size of the tumor. MRI may be used along with or instead of spiral CT scans and endobronchial ultrasound. PET may become the standard imaging study to detect lung cancer once enough data are accumulated to confirm its efficacy. When the lesion is on the lung periphery, the physician can obtain specimens via percutaneous fine needle aspiration guided by fluoroscopy or CT. Bronchoscopy with biopsy or brushings for cytologic findings indicates the presence of malignant cells. Sputum cytologic study can identify malignant cells, but results are positive in only 20% to 30% of lung cancer cases. A mediastinoscopy may be done to determine whether the tumor has spread to the lymph nodes. Scalene lymph node biopsy is also done to identify metastasis. This biopsy is performed in the supraclavicular area.

Medical Management

The treatment of lung cancer depends on the type and stage. Unfortunately, most patients are not diagnosed early enough for curative surgical intervention. It is estimated that one third of the patients are inoperable when first seen, and one third are found to be inoperable on exploratory thoracotomy. Of the third who are operable, the surgical mortality is 10% for pneumonectomy and 2% to 3% for lobectomy. A pneumonectomy is the most common surgical treatment. This consists of removing the entire lung. Because there is no lung left to require reexpansion, drainage tubes are usually not necessary. The fluid remaining in that area consolidates eventually, which helps prevent a mediastinal shift. A lobectomy is performed when one lobe is involved rather than the entire lung. If only a portion of a lobe of a lung is involved, a segmental resection is done. Both a lobectomy and a segmental resection require chest tube insertion with water-seal drainage to facilitate lung reexpansion (see Figures 49-11 and 49-12). Video-assisted thoracoscopic surgery allows surgeons to remove tumors through a small keyhole incision in the chest cavity.

Radiation therapy and chemotherapy are often done in conjunction with surgery to enhance recovery for NSCLC. An oral drug called gefitinib (Iressa) has been approved as monotherapy in patients with locally advanced or metastatic NSCLC after failure of first-line treatment with both platinum-based and docetaxel chemotherapies (see Home Care Considerations box). In SCLC, chemotherapy alone or combined with radiation has largely replaced surgery as a treatment of choice because, regardless of staging, SCLC is considered to be metastatic at diagnosis. A large percentage of these patients experience remission; in a few cases the remission has been long lasting. At present about one third of the patients who have surgery experience tumor spread.

Among the promising biologic response modifiers are interferon-α, interleukin-2, interleukin-4, tumor necrosis factor, and monoclonal antibodies. The last are being investigated alone and in combination with radioisotopes, toxins, and standard chemotherapeutic drugs to see if they can identify and destroy cancer cells with specific antigens (Dest, 2000).

Home Care Considerations

Lung Cancer

- If the patient with lung cancer smokes, teach her or him that stopping smoking can improve pulmonary function, minimize postoperative complications, decrease the risk of pneumonia, and improve appetite during treatment.
- The patient who has had a surgical resection of the lung with intent to cure should be followed up carefully after discharge for manifestations of metastasis.
- Instruct the patient and the family to contact the physician if symptoms such as hemoptysis, dysphagia, chest pain, and hoarseness develop.
- For many individuals who have lung cancer, little can be done to significantly prolong their lives.
- Many people with lung cancer require palliative and hospice care. Encourage the patient and his or her family to adjust their expectations and adapt their goals from controlling disease to improving symptom relief.
- Radiation therapy and chemotherapy can provide palliative relief from distressing symptoms.
- Constant pain becomes a major problem, requiring measures to relieve pain.

Nursing Interventions and Patient Teaching

Whether treatment offers comfort or cure, the patient needs comprehensive nursing interventions. From patient education to symptom management to emotional support, nursing care can improve the quality of life and help the patient and the family cope with a frightening diagnosis. Nursing interventions are often directed at postsurgical interventions, including facilitating recovery and preventing complications by promoting effective airway clearance through frequent repositioning, coughing, and deep breathing.

Encourage the use of incentive spirometry. Explain the importance of changing position (to prevent atelectasis) and exercising the legs and feet (to prevent deep-vein thrombosis [DVT]). Administer supplemental oxygen and monitor oxygen saturation levels. If a patient has chest tubes to water-seal drainage, assess for patency, and record the amount, color, and consistency of drainage. Carefully assess lung sounds and record findings. Assess vital signs frequently. After checking routine postoperative vital signs, check the patient every 2 hours until he or she is stable, and then every 4 hours.

Prescribed medications are primarily antineoplastic agents to prevent or reduce tumor growth. Medications are also given for symptomatic relief: opioid analgesics for pain control, antipyretics for fever, and antiemetics for nausea.

Nursing diagnoses and interventions for the patient with lung cancer include but are not limited to the following:

Nursing Diagnoses	Nursing Interventions
Ineffective airway clearance, related to lung surgery	Facilitate optimal breathing by placing patient in a sitting position. Assist with position changes frequently. Promote coughing and deep breathing, providing necessary splinting. Encourage early ambulation to mobilize secretions. Encourage use of an incentive spirometer.
Fear, related to cancer, treatment, and prognosis	Monitor changes in communication patterns with others. Monitor expression of feelings, such as worthlessness, anxiety, powerlessness, abandonment, or exhaustion. Listen and accept expressions of anger without taking it personally. Encourage patient to identify problem, redefine the situation, obtain needed information, generate alternatives, and focus on solutions.

Teach the patient effective coughing techniques. Instruct the patient and the family regarding nutritional needs and importance of maintaining physical mobility. If the patient smokes, encourage him or her to quit; encourage family members to stop also. Encourage the patient to eat a diet high in protein and calories. Instruct the patient and the family regarding signs and symptoms that could indicate recurrence of metastasis, such as fatigue, weight loss, increased coughing or hemoptysis, central nervous system changes, and arm or shoulder pain. Identify resources in the community, such as the American Cancer Society and the American Lung Association, that can assist the patient and the family with information, support groups, and equipment needed.

Prognosis

Only 10% to 15% of lung cancer patients live 5 years or longer after diagnosis. The survival rate is 40% for cases detected in a localized stage; only 20% of lung cancers are discovered that early.

PULMONARY EDEMA

Etiology and Pathophysiology

Pulmonary edema is an accumulation of serous fluid in interstitial lung tissue and alveoli resulting from the following (Lewis et al., 2007):

- Severe left ventricular failure resulting from a weakened myocardium due to a myocardial infarction. The most common cause of pulmonary edema is left-sided heart failure.
- Hypoalbuminemia, hepatic disease, and nutritional disorders.
- Rapid administration of IV fluids (packed red blood cells, plasma, or fluids).
- Altered capillary permeability of lungs: inhaled toxins, inflammation (e.g., pneumonia), severe hypoxia, near drowning.
- Opioid overdose.

Cardiogenic pulmonary edema usually accompanies underlying cardiac disease in which the failure of the left ventricle causes pooling of fluid to back up into the left atrium and into pulmonary veins and capillaries. The most common cause of pulmonary edema is increased capillary pressure from left ventricular failure. As the pulmonary capillary pressure exceeds the intravascular pressure, serous fluid is rapidly forced into the alveoli. Fluid rapidly reaches the bronchioles and bronchi, and patients literally begin to drown in their own secretions. As oxygen decreases, the person shows signs of severe respiratory distress. Pulmonary edema is acute and extensive and may lead to death unless treated immediately.

Clinical Manifestations

The primary signs and symptoms of pulmonary edema are dyspnea and related breathing disturbances. Labored respirations; tachypnea; tachycardia; cyanosis; and, especially, pink (or blood-tinged), frothy sputum are the most obvious signs. The patient may also exhibit restlessness or agitation because of the altered tissue perfusion and resulting hypoxia and respiratory failure.

Assessment

Subjective data include the patient's complaints of severe dyspnea and a feeling of impending death.

Collection of **objective data** involves assessing for signs of respiratory distress, including nasal flaring and sternal retractions with inspiration; rapid, stertorous respirations; hypertension; tachycardia; restlessness; and disorientation. On auscultation the nurse will most likely hear wheezing and crackles. The patient may have a sudden gain weight because of fluid retention; decreased urinary output as a result of retained fluid in the pulmonary vasculature; and a productive cough of frothy, pink sputum.

Diagnostic Tests

Chest radiographic examination reveals fluid infiltrates, indicating alveolar edema, increased pleural space fluid (pleural effusion), and enlarged heart (cardiomegaly). ABGs are altered, with varying Pao_2 and $Paco_2$ levels. The patient may have respiratory alkalosis or acidosis. Sputum cultures are done periodically to rule out a bronchopulmonary infection.

Medical Management

The physician orders oxygen therapy and may intubate the patient for adequate ventilation support. Medications include diuretics to reduce alveolar and systemic edema by increasing urinary output (furosemide [Lasix]). Patients are also given an opioid analgesic, usually morphine sulfate, to decrease respiratory rate; lower the anxiety level; reduce venous return; and dilate both the pulmonary and systemic blood vessels, thus improving the exchange of gases. IV nitroprusside (Nipride) is a potent vasodilator that improves myocardial contraction and reduces pulmonary congestion. Because of its effects on the vascular system, it is the drug of choice for the patient with pulmonary edema. Medications for treatment of heart failure are used to treat underlying cardiac conditions.

Nursing Interventions and Patient Teaching

An important nursing measure is accurate assessment and documentation to identify changes in the patient's condition. This includes assessment of respiratory status and frequent monitoring of cardiac status, I&O, vital signs, ABGs, pulse oximetry, and electrolyte values. Maintain oxygenation therapy as ordered—commonly delivered by Venturi mask at 40% to 70% concentration. Mechanical ventilation may be required; in this case provide the intubated patient with oral and tracheostomy care according to protocol. Facilitate optimal air exchange by placing the patient in a high Fowler's position. Maintain a patent IV line (saline block) for administering prescribed IV medications. IV fluids are usually withheld to prevent adding even more fluid to the overloaded patient.

Nursing diagnoses and interventions for the patient with pulmonary edema include but are not limited to the following:

Nursing Diagnoses	Nursing Interventions
Impaired gas exchange, related to excess fluid in pulmonary vessels interfering with oxygen diffusion	Be alert to any signs indicating altered ventilation, such as restlessness, irritability, disorientation, or apprehension. Monitor ABGs and notify physician of any change. Frequently monitor vital signs, including cardiac rhythm. Administer oxygen therapy as ordered and document patient response. Administer diuretics, bronchodilators, morphine sulfate, cardiotonic glycosides, and other medications as ordered.
Excess fluid volume, related to altered tissue permeability	Assess indicators of patient's fluid volume status, such as breath sounds and skin turgor. Monitor I&O accurately. Monitor electrolyte values closely, and notify physician of alterations. Administer diuretics as ordered, and note patient response. Weigh patient daily on same scale at same time of day with same amount of bed linen and patient clothing. Provide low-sodium diet to prevent excess fluid retention.

Teach the patient effective breathing techniques. Inform the patient and the family about actions, side effects, and dosage of prescribed medications. Instruct the patient and the family about a low-sodium diet and refer them to a dietitian for follow-up. Emphasize the signs and symptoms to observe that would indicate alteration in health, such as productive cough (noting the color and characteristics of sputum), activity intolerance, or dyspnea.

Prognosis

The prognosis for acute pulmonary edema is guarded; it may lead to death unless treated rapidly.

PULMONARY EMBOLISM

Etiology and Pathophysiology

The most common pulmonary perfusion abnormality, pulmonary **embolism** (PE), is caused by the passage of a foreign substance (blood clot, fat, air, tumor tissue, or amniotic fluid) into the pulmonary artery or its branches, with resulting obstruction of the blood supply to lung tissue and subsequent collapse. PE usually occurs in patients identified to be at risk, such as those with prior thrombophlebitis; those who have recently had surgery, been pregnant, or given birth; women who are taking contraceptives on a long-term basis; and those with a history of congestive heart failure, obesity, or immobilization from fracture. Immobilization appears to be a key consideration.

Venous stasis, venous wall injury, and increased coagulability of blood cause the formation of a venous thrombus. The thrombus (usually in the deep veins of the lower extremities) dislodges and travels through the venous circulation; it passes through the right side of the heart and enters the pulmonary artery, where it becomes lodged.

Once an embolus obstructs pulmonary blood flow, a V/Q mismatch develops: an area of lung is ventilated but not perfused. The obstruction hinders oxygenation of the blood. Atelectasis develops, and pulmonary vascular resistance increases. Arterial hypoxia is the result.

Clinical Manifestations

The classic signs and symptoms of dyspnea, hemoptysis, and chest pain occur in less than 20% of patients with a PE, making diagnosis difficult (Lewis et al., 2007). A PE may manifest itself by a sudden, sharp, constant, nonradiating, pleuritic chest pain that worsens with inspiration. Because PE impairs gas exchange, the patient may have acute, unexplained dyspnea. The respiratory rate is rapid. In small areas of infarction, presenting signs and symptoms are a small amount of hemoptysis, pleuritic chest pain, elevated temperature, and increased white blood cell count. In large areas of infarction, symptoms include hypoxia, hemoptysis, hypotension, tachycardia, diaphoresis, and tachypnea. Regional bronchoconstriction, atelectasis, and pulmonary edema develop, along with decreased surfactant production. Lung sounds are diminished, and wheezes may be present.

Assessment

Subjective data include the patient's report of presence and degree of dyspnea and pleuritic chest pain. The patient may complain of a sense of impending doom. Nursing assessment also includes identifying associated risk factors.

Collection of **objective data** involves assessing for pleuritic pain and noting the nature of the patient's cough. Also assess breath sounds and vital signs, and be alert for tachycardia, hypotension, and tachypnea. Auscultation reveals crackles, decreased breath sounds over the affected area, and a pleural friction rub. In assessing the patient's psychological response, document the presence and degree of anxiety, which is often associated with air hunger. Other objective data may include hemoptysis, elevated temperature, increased white blood cell count, and diaphoresis.

Diagnostic Tests

ABGs are significantly altered, indicating hypoxia. The pH remains normal unless respiratory alkalosis develops early from hyperventilation as respiratory drive diminishes. Respiratory acidosis with hypoxemia often follows.

Initially, the chest radiograph is normal. After 24 hours the radiograph may reveal small infiltrates secondary to atelectasis. Chest radiographic examination also shows an enlarged main pulmonary artery. In most cases of PE, the chest radiograph is normal and is useful only to rule out pulmonary edema or pneumothorax.

A helical (or spiral) CT scan of the lung to visualize the pulmonary vasculature is ordered. This new type of noninvasive scan can be performed in a few seconds and is replacing the V/Q scan, although the V/Q scan is still used in smaller facilities where spiral CT is not available. If the V/Q scan result is intermediate or low probability but the physician still suspects a PE based on the patient's signs, symptoms, and risk factors, he or she may order a pulmonary angiogram.

Pulmonary angiogram is the gold standard for detecting PE because it provides a direct anatomical view of the pulmonary vessels to assess perfusion defects. Pulmonary angiography is an invasive procedure that is performed as follows: (1) insert a catheter through the antecubital or femoral vein, (2) advance the catheter to the pulmonary artery, and (3) inject contrast medium. This procedure allows visualization of the pulmonary vascular system and location of the embolus. ABG analysis is important. A D-dimer serum test is drawn. D-dimer is a product of fibrin degradation (a change to a less complex form). When a thrombus or embolus is present, plasma D-dimer concentrations are usually greater than 1591 ng/mL. The normal range for D-dimer is 68 to 494 ng/L. If the D-dimer levels are elevated, a venous ultrasound is indicated to look for a DVT. Positive results from venous ultrasound are helpful in diagnosing DVT.

Medical Management

When multiple PEs are present, an umbrella filter may be placed in the inferior vena cava to retain the emboli, preventing their migration to other parts of the body.

The physician prescribes anticoagulant therapy, for example, oral warfarin (Coumadin) or subcutaneous low-molecular-weight heparin (enoxaparin sodium [Lovenox]) or dalteparin (Fragmin), to prevent clot formation. Initially heparin may be administered intravenously, by way of a continuous infusion on a pump.

Heparin does not dissolve an existing thrombus; its role is to keep it from enlarging and to prevent more thrombi from forming while the body's natural fibrinolytic mechanism lyses (destroys red blood cells) the existing clot. The effectiveness of heparin is determined by monitoring PTT values, which should be maintained at 1½ to 2 times the control (or normal) values. In the event of overheparinization resulting in profound bleeding, the treatment is IV administration of protamine sulfate. Heparin therapy is gradually tapered (it may take several days). Oral anticoagulation (warfarin) is initiated. The patient takes warfarin for up to 1 year. Effectiveness of warfarin therapy is determined by monitoring PT and INR values, with the goal being 1¼ to 1½ times the control (or normal) values. Vitamin

K reverses the effects of warfarin. Fresh frozen plasma may be required in cases of severe bleeding.

A massive PE must be dissolved using thrombolytics such as the tissue plasminogen activator alteplase (Activase).

Nursing Interventions and Patient Teaching

General nursing interventions include applying thromboembolic disease (TED) stockings and elevating the lower extremities. Check peripheral pulses and frequently measure bilateral calf circumference to monitor for occlusion caused by a clot. Slightly elevate the head of the bed, and administer oxygen by mask or nasal cannula to facilitate optimal gas exchange. Promote lung expansion by encouraging the patient to cough and breathe deeply.

Related nursing interventions include assessing for signs of bleeding: epistaxis, hemoptysis, bleeding from gums or rectum, and ecchymosis. Keep the patient adequately hydrated; place the patient on bed rest for the first few days, and gradually increase activity.

Nursing diagnoses and interventions for the patient with PE include but are not limited to the following:

Nursing Diagnoses	Nursing Interventions
Impaired gas exchange, related to alteration in pulmonary vasculature	Assess sensorium and vital signs every 2 hours or as needed, noting any changes indicative of altered oxygenation or ventilation.
	Elevate head of bed 30 degrees to improve ventilation.
	Administer oxygen as ordered.
	Monitor ABGs frequently, reporting any increase or decrease of $Paco_2$ and Pao_2 of more than 10 mm Hg.
Ineffective protection, related to risk of prolonged bleeding or hemorrhage secondary to anticoagulation therapy	Monitor vital signs for indicators of profuse bleeding or hemorrhage resulting from anticoagulant therapy: hypotension, tachycardia, and tachypnea.
	At least once a shift, check stool, urine, sputum, and vomitus for occult blood using agency-approved method for testing.
	At least once a shift, inspect wounds, oral mucous membranes, any entry site of an invasive procedure, and nares for evidence of bleeding.
	To prevent hematoma formation, avoid giving intramuscular injection unless it is unavoidable.
	Teach patient the necessity of using sponge-tipped applicators and mouthwash for oral care to minimize the risk of gum bleeding.
	Instruct patient to shave with an electric rather than a bladed razor.

Medication teaching regarding long-term anticoagulant therapy is a major nursing concern. Patients with recurrent emboli are treated indefinitely; typical anticoagulant therapy continues for at least 3 to 6 months. Oral anticoagulation often becomes a lifelong regimen that bears close monitoring. Assess the patient's present knowledge base and expand on it. Preventive measures are also important, especially in the postoperative period. Teach the patient techniques to reduce venous pooling (which could precipitate thrombophlebitis), such as changing positions and wearing nonrestrictive clothing. Tell the patient to avoid crossing the legs while sitting or lying down and also to avoid standing in one place for a prolonged period, since these activities increase venous pooling. Teach the rationale and application procedure for TED hose. Explain that the patient should put them on in the morning before getting out of bed. Instruct the patient and the family on signs and symptoms of PE to report to the physician, such as chest pain; dyspnea; and blood-tinged sputum or blood in the urine, which could result from anticoagulant therapy.

Prognosis

Early diagnosis and appropriate treatment reduce mortality to 2% to 8%. Untreated PE carries a 30% mortality rate (Thompson et al., 2006). It is one of the most common causes of preventable death in hospitalized patients (Valentine et al., 2006). Although most PEs resolve completely and leave no residual deficits, some patients may be left with chronic pulmonary hypertension.

ACUTE RESPIRATORY DISTRESS SYNDROME

Etiology and Pathophysiology

Acute respiratory distress syndrome (ARDS) is not a disease but a complication that occurs as a result of other disease processes. ARDS has many causes, which result from either a direct or an indirect pulmonary injury. Possible causes include viral or bacterial pneumonia, chest trauma, pulmonary contusion, aspiration, inhalation injury, near drowning, fat emboli, sepsis, or any type of shock. Drug overdoses, renal failure, and pancreatitis are also known causative factors, as are COPD, neuromuscular defects with Guillain-Barré syndrome, and myasthenia gravis. Among these, sepsis is the most common precursor of ARDS.

Regardless of the cause of ARDS, the body's response follows a similar sequence. The surface of the alveolar capillary membrane is altered, causing increased permeability, which then allows fluid to leak into the interstitial spaces and alveoli. This creates pulmonary edema and hypoxia. The alveoli lose their elasticity and collapse, which causes the blood to be shunted through the impaired alveoli, interfering with oxygen transport. The damaged capillaries allow plasma and red blood cells to leak out, resulting in hemorrhage. ARDS is characterized by pulmonary artery hypertension, which results from vasoconstriction.

Clinical Manifestations

ARDS manifests 12 to 24 hours after injury, resulting in lung tissue damage or hypovolemic shock; 5 to 10 days after sepsis development, the patient experiences respiratory distress with altered breath sounds. There may be altered sensorium as a result of an elevated $Paco_2$ and decreased Pao_2. Additional signs are cardiovascular: tachycardia, hypotension, and decreased urinary output.

Assessment

Subjective data include background information and a history of the present illness (obtained from family members, since the patient is usually too ill to give details).

Collection of **objective data** involves being an astute observer of any change in the patient's condition, no matter how small or gradual. Make an accurate and thorough initial assessment so such changes will be quickly recognized. Initial assessment includes identifying and documenting respiratory rate, rhythm, and effort. Note signs of dyspnea, such as nasal flaring, sternal and subclavicular retractions, or cyanosis. Auscultate the lungs and document the presence of crackles or wheezing. Closely observe vital signs. Frequent assessment of the level of consciousness, with particular attention to increased restlessness or lethargy, is necessary.

Diagnostic Tests

PFTs are done to determine the ease or difficulty of oxygen crossing the alveolar capillary membrane. ABGs show definitive changes: Pao_2 is decreased (less than 70 mm Hg), $Paco_2$ is increased (greater than 35 mm Hg), and HCO_3^- is decreased (less than 22 mEq/L). Initially, HCO_3^- increases in an attempt to buffer the elevated $Paco_2$ level, thereby maintaining pH in the normal range. The pH is elevated initially but steadily decreases as the patient's condition deteriorates. A chest radiographic examination depicts thickened bronchial margins and possibly diffuse infiltrates.

Medical Management

The medical plan focuses on supportive treatment by maintaining adequate oxygenation and treating the cause: drug overdose, infections, or inhaled toxins. Medications commonly used to treat associated conditions include corticosteroids, antibiotics, vasodilators like nitroprusside, bronchodilators, mucolytics, and diuretics to treat pulmonary edema, aiding in restoring lung tissues to their normal structure and function. Morphine sulfate is commonly given to sedate restless patients and decrease respiratory rate. When the patient is intubated and ventilator dependent, a neurologic blocking agent, such as pancuronium (Pavulon), may be administered to suppress the patient's own respiratory effort, relying on the controlled ventilator assistance. Positive end-expiratory pressure is the most important ventilator treatment component for the patient with ARDS (Jacobs, 2005). Other medications may include cardiotonic glycosides (digoxin) to enhance cardiac function.

An experimental treatment is being used in which nitric oxide gas is inhaled, causing local vasodilation and maximizing perfusion in ventilated areas of the lungs and often significantly improving oxygenation. Nitric oxide is usually administered via a face mask; if the patient is ventilator dependent, however, the ventilator is the mode of delivery.

Nursing Interventions and Patient Teaching

The goal of nursing interventions is to provide adequate oxygenation and ventilation and to treat the multisystem responses caused by ARDS. Nurses must be knowledgeable about mechanical ventilator settings and effects. Care for intubated patients includes suctioning, providing oral care, and assessing for signs of inadequate ventilation. Closely monitor ABGs and pulse oximetry and report any changes.

To improve gas exchange, frequently reposition the patient from side to side, thus preventing one region of the lung from being in a dependent position for prolonged periods (Jacobs, 2005). Studies suggest some people with ARDS demonstrate a marked improvement in Pao_2 when turned from the supine to prone position. Not all patients respond to prone positioning (Balas, 2000). Also, an accurate, ongoing assessment of cardiac function is important. Be alert for and document any rate or rhythm changes. The registered nurse will notify the physician of any changes.

Assess vital signs and identify elevated temperatures so that cultures can be obtained to treat infections.

Nursing diagnoses and interventions for the patient with ARDS include but are not limited to the following:

Nursing Diagnoses	Nursing Interventions
Impaired gas exchange, related to tachypnea	Monitor ABGs and report any changes. Address any factors that would contribute to restlessness and anxiety, since they increase the body's oxygen demand and exacerbate the patient's already serious condition. Administer oxygen as ordered, assessing and recording patient response. Monitor electrocardiogram (ECG) changes. Report any changes in vital signs and any change in patient's response, no matter how small or gradual.
Ineffective breathing pattern, related to respiratory distress	Assess respiratory rate, rhythm, and effort, being alert to signs of dyspnea. Facilitate optimal ventilation by proper positioning. Maintain airway patency by encouraging frequent coughing and deep breathing, if able, or suctioning as needed.

Teach the patient effective breathing techniques, emphasizing the importance of frequent position changes, coughing, and deep breathing. If the patient is intubated, explain all procedures before their implementation and explain the importance of working with the ventilator and not trying to breathe independently. Reassure the patient that the ventilator will breathe for him or her and that those breaths will be more effective than his or her own. Explain to the patient and the family the importance of using rest and activity appropriately. Also explain the purpose and side effects of all medications.

Prognosis

ARDS affects an estimated 150,000 to 200,000 people each year, with mortality rates of 40% with severe ARDS when trauma is the cause and 55% to 70% when the condition is associated with sepsis.

CHRONIC OBSTRUCTIVE PULMONARY DISEASE

COPD is a progressive and irreversible condition characterized by diminished inspiratory and expiratory capacity of the lungs. It is a chronic respiratory condition that obstructs the flow of air to or from the patient's bronchioles (Figure 49-14). COPD includes emphysema, chronic bronchitis, asthma, and bronchiectasis. All these diseases are characterized by **chronic airflow limitation.** The mantra of the American Lung Association is, "When you can't breathe, nothing else matters." Still, more than 35 million Americans live with chronic lung disease.

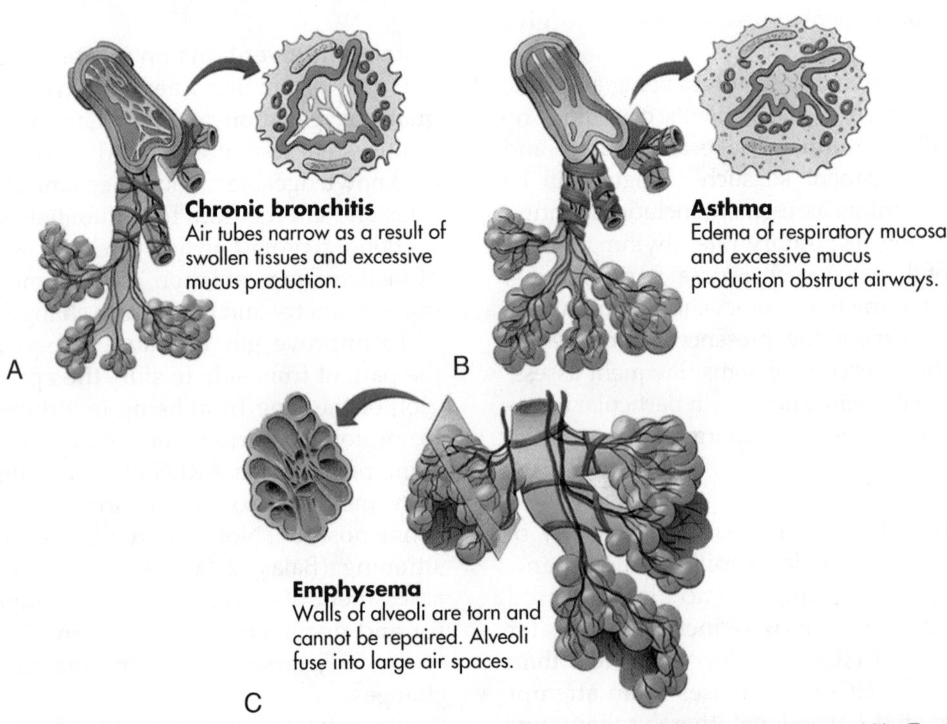

FIGURE 49-14 Disorders of the airways in patients with chronic bronchitis, asthma, and emphysema. **A,** Chronic bronchitis: Excessive amounts of mucus accumulate in the airways, obstructing airflow and impairing ciliary function. **B,** Asthma: Bronchial smooth muscle constricts in response to irritants, resulting in airflow obstruction and wheezing. **C,** Emphysema: Alveoli become overinflated and destructive changes occur in alveolar walls.

EMPHYSEMA

Etiology and Pathophysiology

Emphysema symptoms usually develop when the patient is in his or her 40s, with disability increasing by age 50 to 60. This condition is characterized by changes in the alveolar walls and capillaries: thus emphysema is primarily an **alveolar disease** (see Figure 49-14, C).

Emphysema is an abnormal permanent enlargement of the alveoli distal to the terminal bronchioles, accompanied by destruction of their walls. There is usually an overlap between chronic bronchitis and emphysema. The bronchi, bronchioles, and alveoli become inflamed as a result of chronic irritation. Because of bronchiole lumen narrowing, air becomes trapped in the alveoli during expiration, causing alveolar distention (Figure 49-15). The alveoli then rupture and scar, losing their elasticity. Oxygen in the arterial blood decreases and carbon dioxide increases.

This process is worsened by cigarette smoking and other inhaled irritants. There is a lag of 30 to 35 years, on average, between taking up smoking and onset of signs and symptoms. Cigarette smoking is by far the most common cause of emphysema and chronic bronchitis; 90% of COPD cases are caused by smoking, whereas as few as 25% of smokers develop the disorder. This suggests that genetic susceptibility plays a role in the risk for COPD (Sharma, 2006). Risk factors for emphysema are the same as for chronic bronchitis, with one addition: heredity. An inherited form of emphysema is caused by a deficiency of alpha$_1$-antitrypsin (ATT), a lung protective protein produced by the liver, which acts predominantly by inhibiting neutrophil elastase in the lungs. ATT deficiency accounts for less than 1% of emphysema in the United States.

The patient with emphysema is disabled because all available energy must be used for breathing. COPD can lead to **cor pulmonale,** an abnormal cardiac condition characterized by hypertrophy of the right ventricle of the heart as a result of hypertension of the pulmonary circulation. Cor pulmonale results in edema in the lower extremities and in the sacral and perineal area, distended neck veins, and enlargement of the liver with ascites. Cor pulmonale is a late complication of emphysema.

Normal expiration

Impaired expiration

Reduced airway patency

Easy expiration due to normal elastic recoil of alveolus and open bronchiole

Difficult expiration due to decreased elastic recoil of alveolus and narrowed bronchiole

FIGURE 49-15 Mechanisms of air trapping in emphysema. Damaged or destroyed alveolar walls no longer support and hold airways open. Alveoli lose their property of passive elastic recoil. Both these factors contribute to collapse during expiration.

Clinical Manifestations

The primary symptom of emphysema is dyspnea on exertion, which becomes progressively more severe. Eventually dyspnea occurs at rest. Initially there is little sputum production, but later it becomes copious. The patient eventually appears barrel chested (an increased anteroposterior diameter caused by overinflation) and begins using accessory muscles for breathing (Figure 49-16). Spontaneous pursed-lip breathing and chronic weight loss with emaciation ensue.

Assessment

Subjective data include a history of onset of symptoms. Note the duration and intensity of dyspnea, cough, and sputum production (documenting color and amount). Also determine the patient's reported history of smoking and exposure to inhalants and the family history of respiratory disorders.

Collection of **objective data** includes assessment of presenting signs, such as tachycardia, tachypnea, orthopnea, peripheral cyanosis, and clubbing of fingers. The most outstanding feature of clubbing is a lateral and longitudinal curvature of the nails accompanied by soft tissue enlargement, presenting a bulbous (bulb-

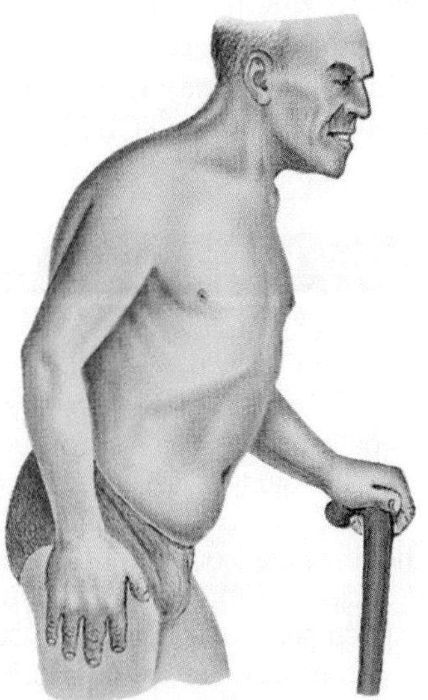

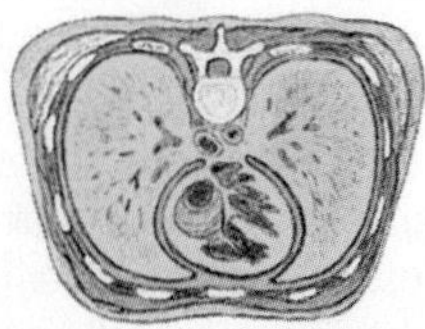

FIGURE 49-16 Barrel chest. Note increase in anteroposterior diameter.

shaped), shiny appearance. This occurs late in the disease. Hypoxemia (especially during exercise) may be present, but hypercapnia does not develop until late in the disease. The person is characteristically underweight, but the exact cause for this is not well understood. One possibility is that the patient is in a hypermetabolic state with increased energy requirements that are partly due to the increased work of breathing. A therapeutic position for the patient with COPD is to lean forward with the head tilted and the arms resting on the patient's legs or a table. Expiration is prolonged as the patient forces his or her breath out through obstructed airways (Crawford, 2008).

Diagnostic Tests

An important goal of the diagnostic workup is to determine the major disease component of COPD, the severity of the disease, and the impact of the disease on the patient's quality of life. A history and physical examination are extremely important.

PFTs are done to measure total lung capacity, which is decreased with COPD. Residual volume is increased, as are compliance and airway resistance. Ventilatory response is decreased. Pulse oximetry is useful in assessing oxygen saturation in arterial blood.

ABGs are usually assessed in the severe stages and are monitored in hospitalized patients with acute exacerbations. ABGs reveal a decreased $Pa{O_2}$ and $Pa{CO_2}$; increased HCO_3^-; and low-normal, elevated, or decreased pH. A chest radiographic examination shows hyperinflation of the lungs, widened intercostal spaces, and flattened diaphragm with increased anteroposterior diameter (barrel chest). Hematological studies are done to determine whether the patient is positive for AAT (an enzyme deficiency causing airway abnormalities resulting in emphysema); this is present in an inherited form of emphysema. CBC reveals elevated erythrocytes and hemoglobin and hematocrit levels (secondary polycythemia, as a compensatory response to chronic hypoxia). This is also a late manifestation of emphysema.

Medical Management

The medical plan includes long-term management with home oxygen therapy and chest physiotherapy as needed. In an acute exacerbation the patient may require mechanical ventilation.

Prescribed medications include bronchodilators such as beta-adrenergic agonists (e.g., short-acting albuterol and long-acting inhaled salmeterol [Serevent]) or theophyllines. Anticholinergics such as ipratropium (Atrovent) are also effective bronchodilators. Bronchodilators enlarge the bronchioles for greater oxygenation and ease of secretion clearance, and corticosteroids decrease pulmonary inflammation and obstruction. Corticosteroids are usually prescribed only during an acute exacerbation because of the many side effects seen in long-term steroid therapy. Antibiotics are frequently ordered to reduce the risk of infection related to retained pulmonary secretions. Diuretics assist with fluid removal. Pulmonary therapy can help mobilize secretions and improve oxygenation.

Many physicians prescribe pulmonary rehabilitation therapy that includes aerobic exercise such as walking. This increases the body's capacity to take up and use oxygen through the sustained rhythmic contraction of large muscle groups. Prescribed exercise training improves aerobic capacity, endurance, and strength; improves and maintains functional performance in day-to-day life; and reduces breathlessness and fatigue during exertion (see Evidence-Based Practice box).

During an acute exacerbation, severe dyspnea can produce considerable anxiety, restlessness, or irritabil-

Evidence-Based Practice The Efficacy of Exercise Training in Patients with COPD

Evidence Summary

Patients with dyspnea often have a difficult time controlling their breathing. Exercise training improves dyspnea and activity tolerance in patients with chronic obstructive pulmonary disease (COPD). This study investigated the impact of exercise training on dyspnea self-management, exercise performance, and health-related quality of life. Researchers randomly placed subjects with COPD into three groups. One group had dyspnea self-management and supervised exercise training. Dyspnea self-management included individualized education about dyspnea management strategies, a home-walking prescription, and daily logs. The other two groups received standard care. Researchers measured outcomes (symptoms) at baseline and every 2 months for a year. Patients measured their symptoms through three questionnaires: Chronic Respiratory Questionnaire (CRQ), Shortness of Breath Questionnaire, and Baseline/Transitional Dyspnea Index. The group with dyspnea self-management and supervised exercise training had improved dyspnea management and activity tolerance.

Application to Nursing Practice

- Using a routine, managed exercise program, such as walking, improves dyspnea.
- Teaching patients how to manage their shortness of breath (dyspnea) during activities helps to improve dyspnea and exercise tolerance.
- Organizing nursing care to use patient's time effectively and avoid interruption helps the patient manage dyspnea and reduces dyspnea-related fatigue.

Reference

Stulbarg, M.S., et al. (2002). Exercise training improves outcomes of a dyspnea self-management program. *J Cardiopulm Rehabil 22*(2), 109.

From Potter, P.A., & Perry, A.G. (2009). *Fundamentals of nursing: concepts, process, and practice.* (7th ed.). St. Louis: Mosby.

ity. Carefully monitor the patient with COPD because of the increased risk for respiratory failure from central nervous system depressants. Careful evaluation for hypoxemia is necessary before a central nervous system depressant is prescribed (see Clinical Pathway 49-1 on Evolve).

Nursing Interventions and Patient Teaching

Nursing interventions are directed toward decreasing the patient's anxiety and promoting optimal air exchange. **Such measures include elevating the head of the bed and administering low-flow (1 to 2 L by nasal cannula) oxygen as ordered.** This is extremely important for COPD patients because a higher flow of oxygen delivery can be dangerous, since it diminishes the brain's respiratory (regulatory) center and can cause respiratory failure. Avoid use of respiratory depressants to ensure adequate alveolar ventilation. Assist with chest physiotherapy, which includes percussion, vibration, and postural drainage. All three techniques help loosen secretions to be expectorated; sometimes it takes several hours after chest physiotherapy before the patient can expectorate loosened secretions. Increasing oral intake of fluids liquefies secretions, thus aiding in their removal. Additionally, the use of a humidifier enhances this process. Allow sufficient rest periods and assist the patient in activities of daily living to prevent a decrease in oxygen saturation levels.

Assist the patient in maintaining nutritional intake by advising rest for 30 minutes before eating. This conserves energy and decreases dyspnea. The patient with emphysema has a markedly increased need for protein and calories to maintain an adequate nutritional status. A high-protein, high-calorie diet should be divided into five or six small meals a day. Oral fluid intake should be 2 to 3 L/day unless contraindicated (e.g., because of congestive heart failure). Instruct the patient to drink fluids between meals, rather than with meals, to reduce gastric distention and pressure on the diaphragm. Perform frequent oral hygiene to freshen the patient's mouth after coughing exercises and before meals.

Cessation of cigarette smoking in the early stages is probably the most significant factor in slowing the progression of the disease and improving pulmonary function. The use of nicotine replacement therapy and the newer, nonnicotine medication bupropion (Zyban) may minimize the effects of nicotine withdrawal. These adjunctive therapies should be combined with other modalities such as support groups, education materials, and behavior modification programs. Regardless of the method used to stop smoking, the most important factor is the patient's commitment.

The patient with COPD should have a vaccination with influenza virus vaccine yearly and a pneumococcal revaccination every 5 years.

Nursing diagnoses and interventions for the patient with emphysema include but are not limited to the following:

Nursing Diagnoses	Nursing Interventions
Ineffective airway clearance, related to narrowed bronchioles	Assess patient's ability to mobilize secretions, intervening as needed. Encourage coughing and deep breathing, frequent position changes, and increased oral intake (up to 2 to 3 L/day). Elevate head of bed; suction as needed. Assist with respiratory treatments. Auscultate lungs, and report any changes in lung sounds.
Activity intolerance, related to imbalance between oxygen supply and demand, secondary to inefficient work of breathing	Organize care so that periods of activity are interspersed with at least 90 minutes of undisturbed rest. Assist patient with active range-of-motion exercises to build stamina and prevent complications of decreased mobility. Monitor patient's respiratory response to activity. Activity intolerance is indicated by excessively increased respiratory rate (e.g., increased more than 10 breaths/min above patient's baseline) and depth, dyspnea, and use of accessory muscles of respiration.

Instruct the patient and the family on (1) the importance of not smoking and of reducing exposure to other inhaled irritants, (2) effective breathing techniques (such as pursed-lip breathing), and (3) relaxation exercises for anxiety control. Teach the patient about the dangers of increased oxygen intake for a patient dependent on hypoxic drive (stimulation of respiration by low PaO_2) for ventilation. Also teach the patient and the family how to prevent infection and symptoms that should be reported to the physician (see Home Care Considerations box, Communication box, and Nursing Care Plan 49-1).

Prognosis

Emphysema is usually irreversible. COPD is the fourth leading cause of death in the United States. COPD affects about 16 million Americans with about 120,000 deaths each year.

 Home Care Considerations

Chronic Oxygen Therapy at Home

- Improved prognosis has been noted in patients with chronic obstructive pulmonary disease who receive nocturnal or continuous oxygen to treat hypoxemia.
- The longer the continuous daily use of oxygen is maintained, the greater the improvement.
- Periodic reevaluations are necessary for the patient who is using chronic supplemental oxygen in the home.
- Home oxygen systems are usually rented from a company that sends a respiratory therapist or pulmonary nurse specialist to the patient's home.
- The therapist teaches the patient how to use the oxygen system, how to care for it, and how to recognize when the supply is running low and needs to be reordered.
- Post "No smoking" warning signs where they can be seen in the home.
- Do not use electric razors, portable radios, open flames, wool blankets, or mineral oils in the area where oxygen is in use.
- Do not allow smoking in the home.

 Communication

Mr. Oden, a 91-year-old, lives at home with his wife of 38 years. He was admitted to the hospital with acute **exacerbation** (an increase in the seriousness of a disease or disorder as marked by greater intensity in the signs or symptoms) of emphysema. Mr. Oden has a 24-year history of emphysema, with progression of signs and symptoms, including exertional dyspnea, expectoration of copious amounts of tenacious mucus, fatigue, and fear of suffocation.

Mr. Oden: Will it always be like this? I'm so short of air.

Ms. Lessing: Are you frightened?

Mr. Oden: I'm not afraid of dying, but I worry about having to fight for my air.

Ms. Lessing: (gently touches Mr. Oden's arm) Try taking slow, deep breaths, and concentrate on remaining calm.

Mr. Oden: Sometimes I can't even get to the bathroom and do my business—much less help my wife with the dishes or even fill the bird feeder.

Ms. Lessing: Do you feel you are becoming a burden?

Mr. Oden: I have to be good to my wife. I want to have something left to give her.

Ms. Lessing: I notice you are breathing more easily. I will be back to check on you, and perhaps we can continue this conversation.

CHRONIC BRONCHITIS

Etiology and Pathophysiology

Chronic bronchitis is characterized by a recurrent or chronic productive cough for a minimum of 3 months a year for at least 2 years. It is caused by physical or chemical irritants and recurrent lung infections. Cigarette smoking is by far the most common cause of chronic bronchitis. Workers exposed to dust, such as coal miners and grain handlers, also are at higher risk. The underlying process is an impairment of cilia, so they can no longer move secretions. Mucous gland hypertrophy causes hypersecretion, altering cilia function (see Figure 49-14, *A*). Excessive mucus is trapped in edematous airways, obstructing airflow. The lining of the bronchial tubes becomes inflamed and eventually scarred. The patient cannot clear tenacious mucus and it becomes a medium for bacteria and infection. This increased airway resistance leads to bronchospasm. The condition results in an altered oxygen–carbon dioxide exchange, hypoxia (an inadequate, reduced tension of cellular oxygen), and **hypercapnia** (greater than normal amounts of carbon dioxide in the blood).

Clinical Manifestations

Primary signs include a productive cough, most pronounced in the mornings (this is often overlooked by cigarette smokers). The patient also has increased dyspnea and use of accessory muscles. A complication of chronic bronchitis is cor pulmonale, which is hypertrophy of the right side of the heart resulting from pulmonary hypertension. Cyanosis develops, often accompanied by right ventricular failure. The patient with chronic bronchitis often has a characteristic reddish blue skin (resulting from chronic hypoxia, which stimulates erythropoiesis, thus resulting in polycythemia, cyanosis, and dependent edema).

Assessment

Subjective data include a detailed history of smoking or exposure to irritants and family history of respiratory disorders. Also determine the patient's current medication and treatment regimen.

Collection of **objective data** includes assessing the patient's productive cough, noting characteristics and amount of sputum. Assess the severity of dyspnea and presence of wheezing, and note the patient's level of restlessness. Also, when checking vital signs, pay special attention to tachycardia, tachypnea, and elevated temperature.

Diagnostic Tests

Chest radiographs taken early in the disease may not show abnormalities; later in the disease they will. An ECG may be normal or show signs indicative of right ventricular failure. An echocardiogram can be used to evaluate right and left ventricular function.

A CBC shows increased erythrocytes, hemoglobin, hematocrit, and white blood cell count. Polycythemia develops as a result of increased production of red blood cells as the body attempts to compensate for chronic hypoxemia. Hemoglobin concentrations may reach 20 g/dL or more. ABG values reveal respiratory acidosis, hypoxia, and hypercapnia. Pulse oximetry is valuable to assess oxygen saturation levels in arterial blood. PFTs will have an alteration that reveals airflow limitation on expiration, increased airway resistance and residual volume, and often electrolyte abnormalities. Monitor oximetry levels on all patients with hypoxia.

Nursing Care Plan 49-1 The Patient with Emphysema

Mr. Oden is a 91-year-old patient admitted with an exacerbation of chronic obstructive pulmonary disease (COPD). His respirations are 32 breaths/min and labored. He has nasal flaring, and his nailbeds are cyanotic. He has a barrel chest and digital clubbing. He states he has a productive cough and "can't get my air." It is noted he expectorates tenacious yellow mucus. He appears anxious during the assessment.

NURSING DIAGNOSIS ***Ineffective airway clearance, related to tenacious secretions and expiratory airflow obstruction***

Patient Goals and Expected Outcomes	Nursing Interventions	Evaluation
Patient will maintain patent airway as evidenced by decreased wheezes, tachypnea, dyspnea, and arterial blood gas (ABG) values within limits (for this patient)	Assess lung sounds every 2 to 4 hours. Encourage turning, coughing, and deep breathing every 2 to 4 hours. Suction as needed. Explain all medications used in inhalation therapy and assist with treatment. Monitor effectiveness. Ensure hydration: oral intake of 2 to 3 L/day to liquefy secretions for easier expectoration.	Patient's respiratory status remains within baseline for this patient. Patient has normal breath sounds on auscultation. Patient is able to expectorate sputum without difficulty.

NURSING DIAGNOSIS ***Ineffective breathing pattern, related to decreased lung expansion secondary to chronic airflow limitations***

Patient Goals and Expected Outcomes	Nursing Interventions	Evaluation
After treatment intervention, patient's breathing pattern will improve as evidenced by patient maintaining respiratory rate within 5 breaths/min of baseline Patient will demonstrate relaxed appearance	Assess for indicators of respiratory distress (agitation, restlessness, decreased level of consciousness, and use of accessory muscles of respiration). Auscultate breath sounds; report a decrease in breath sounds or an increase in adventitious breath sounds. Instruct patient in the use of pursed-lip breathing, which provides internal stability to the airways and may prevent airway collapse during expiration. Administer bronchodilator therapy as prescribed. Monitor patient's response to prescribed oxygen therapy. Be aware that high concentrations of oxygen can depress the respiratory drive in individuals with chronic carbon dioxide retention. Avoid use of respiratory depressants to ensure adequate alveolar ventilation.	Patient's arterial blood gases are within normal values. Patient has absence of adventitious breath sounds. Patient is sleeping for 5 to 6 hours without respiratory distress.

Critical Thinking Questions

1. Mr. Oden turns on his call light and states that he is "unable to get my air." The nurse notes subclavicular retractions and a respiratory rate of 36 breaths/min. His oxygen is flowing at 1 L/min via nasal cannula. What nursing interventions would decrease his dyspnea?
2. While the nurse is performing an assessment on Mr. Oden, he states, "I'm so tired of fighting to breathe that I wish I could just go to sleep and never wake up." What is an appropriate response?
3. During vital signs assessment, the nurse notes that Mr. Oden's temperature is 102° F (38.8° C), the pulse rate is 110 bpm, and the respiratory rate is 44 breaths/min. The nurse knows that Mr. Oden's COPD places him at a high risk for:

Medical Management

The medical plan is aimed at slowing the disease progression and facilitating optimal air exchange by reducing spasms and secretions.

Three main classes of bronchodilators are typically used to treat COPD. To reverse bronchospasm, the health care provider may order beta-adrenergic agonists such as short-acting albuterol and long-acting salmeterol. The theophyllines as well as anticholinergics such as ipratropium are also effective as bronchodilators. Corticosteroids are helpful in reducing airway inflammation. Long-term use of systemic steroids can lead to many adverse reactions, including osteoporosis. Inhaled steroids have fewer systemic effects and are preferred. Mucolytics such as guaifenesin to break up tenacious mucus may be helpful (Wisniewski, 2004). Antibiotic agents (erythromycin) are commonly ordered.

Nursing Interventions and Patient Teaching

Provide adequate hydration to liquefy secretions and aid in their removal. Suction the patient as needed, and provide low-flow oxygen to maintain SaO_2 above 90%. Offer frequent oral hygiene and provide rest periods. The nutritional needs are similar to those of the patient with emphysema.

Nursing diagnoses and interventions for the patient with chronic bronchitis include but are not limited to the following:

Nursing Diagnoses	Nursing Interventions
Ineffective breathing pattern, related to retained pulmonary secretions	Assess degree of dyspnea, noting nasal flaring, sternal retractions, and pursed-lip breathing. Instruct on effective breathing techniques. Suction as needed.
Fatigue, related to increased respiratory effort	Assess degree of fatigue, and use problem-solving techniques with patient to explore ways to decrease fatigue. Provide treatments in calm, unhurried manner. Identify support systems and provide referrals if needed. Encourage adequate periods of rest.

Teach the patient effective breathing techniques, and instruct the patient and the family on avoidance of infection exposure. Instruct the patient to notify the physician at the first sign of a respiratory infection. Usually the best indication of such an infection is a change in the color, consistency, or amount of sputum. Provide medication teaching, including action, rationale, and side effects. Stress the importance of increasing fluid intake, unless contraindicated. Encourage the patient and the family not to smoke. Encourage a patient who smokes to join a smoking cessation program, and teach about prescription and over-the-counter medications to assist with quitting smoking.

Prognosis

Chronic bronchitis is usually irreversible. COPD is the fourth leading cause of death in the United States, after heart disease, cancer, and traumatic injuries.

ASTHMA

Etiology and Pathophysiology

Asthma is a broad clinical syndrome and an airway pathologic condition. It involves episodic increased tracheal and bronchial responsiveness to various stimuli, resulting in widespread narrowing of the airways. Asthma usually improves either spontaneously or with treatment. It is classified as extrinsic or intrinsic. **Extrinsic** means it is caused by external factors, such as environmental allergens (pollen, dust, feathers, animal dander, foods, etc.); **intrinsic** asthma is from internal causes, not fully understood but often triggered by respiratory tract infection. Recurrence of attacks is greatly influenced by secondary factors, by mental or physical fatigue, and by emotional factors.

Asthma can result from an altered immune response or increased airway resistance and altered air exchange. Gastroesophageal reflux disease (GERD) can trigger an asthma attack (Lewis et al., 2007). The actual course of GERD resulting in an asthma attack is unknown, but it is assumed that the gastric acid reflux in the esophagus is aspirated into the lungs, resulting in vagal stimulation and bronchoconstriction (Lewis et al., 2007). An acute asthma attack may be caused by an antigen-antibody reaction in which histamine is released. There are three mechanisms involved (see Figure 49-14, *B*):

- Recurrent, reversible obstruction of airflow in the bronchioles and smaller bronchi secondary to bronchospasm. The muscles around the bronchioles tighten and narrow the air passages.
- Increased capillary permeability resulting in edema of mucous membranes with increased narrowing of airways and increased mucus secretion.
- An acute inflammatory response in the mast cells of the lungs, caused by exposure to an asthma trigger. These cells release histamine and other inflammatory agents. Systemic immune system cells release substances that cause circulating inflammatory cells to migrate to the lungs.

Clinical Manifestations

Mild asthma is manifested by dyspnea on exertion and wheezing. Symptoms are usually controlled by medications. An acute asthma attack usually occurs at night and includes tachypnea, tachycardia, diaphoresis, chest tightness, cough, expiratory wheezing, use of accessory muscles, and nasal flaring. The wheezing sound characteristic of asthma is caused by air forcing its way through the narrowed bronchioles and by vibrating mucus. The patients also has increased anxiety; diaphoresis; and a productive cough of copious, thick mucus. Asthma can be triggered by external factors (e.g., dust, mold, or lint) or precipitated intrinsically by a respiratory tract infection or exercise.

Status asthmaticus is a severe, unrelenting, life-threatening attack that fails to respond to usual treatment and places the patient at risk for respiratory failure. Symptoms of an acute attack are present, and the trapped air leads to exhaustion and respiratory failure. An axiom describes status asthmaticus: "The longer it lasts, the worse it gets, and the worse it gets, the longer it lasts" (Lewis et al., 2007).

Assessment

Subjective data include complaints of anxiety, fear of suffocation, breathlessness, chest tightness, and cough, particularly at night and in the early morning (Lewis et al., 2007).

Collection of **objective data** includes assessing for signs of hypoxia, which may include restlessness, inappropriate behavior, increased pulse and blood pressure, and tachypnea. The patient may assume a "hunched forward" position in an attempt to get more air. Auscultate the lungs for inspiratory and expiratory wheezing. Coughing produces thick, stringy mucus (Lewis et al., 2007).

Diagnostic Tests

To diagnose asthma, the physician orders ABGs and PFTs. The chest radiographic examination reveals lung hyperinflation related to air trapping, and a flat diaphragm related to increased intrathoracic volume. PFTs establish the diagnosis of asthma by determining the reversibility of bronchoconstriction. Normal values for these tests vary, depending on the patient's age, weight, and sex. In an acute asthma episode the patient will not be able to perform a complete pulmonary function study, but the nurse can check the peak expiratory flow rate. ABGs may be ordered during an acute exacerbation of asthma. Pulse oximetry is used to monitor the patient's Sao_2.

Obtain a sputum culture from the patient to rule out any secondary infection. A CBC and differential reveal an increased eosinophil count, which is indicative of an allergic response. If the patient has been taking theophylline, draw a blood sample to determine whether the prescribed dosage is maintained at a therapeutic level; the acceptable therapeutic range is 10 to 20 mcg/mL. This also reduces the risk of complications as a result of toxicity.

Medical Management

Medication management of asthma can be placed in two categories: maintenance therapy and acute (or rescue) therapy. **Maintenance therapy** prevents and minimizes symptoms; the medications are taken on a regular basis. These include the long acting beta$_2$-agonist salmeterol and formoterol (Foradil), which are used prophylactically only; inhaled corticosteroids, such as fluticasone; cromolyn; and theophylline. A combination of fluticasone and salmeterol (Advair Diskus) is also sometimes prescribed.

A recent group of drugs called leukotriene modifiers is now available for the prophylaxis and chronic treatment of asthma. Leukotrienes are chemicals present in the body that are powerful bronchoconstrictors and vasodilators; some also cause airway edema and inflammation, thus contributing to the symptoms of asthma. The two types of leukotriene modifiers are leukotriene receptor antagonists (zafirlukast, montelukast) and leukotriene synthesis inhibitors (zileuton [Zyflo]). These drugs interfere with the synthesis or block the action of leukotrienes. A major advantage is that they have both bronchodilator and antiinflammatory effects. These drugs are not recommended as the only treatment for persistent asthma. A broad range of patients, with mild to severe asthma, can benefit from leukotriene modifiers. Leukotriene modifiers are not indicated for use in the reversal of bronchospasms in acute asthma attacks. They are indicated for the chronic treatment of asthma (see Table 49-1).

Acute (or **rescue**) **therapy** works immediately to relieve symptoms of an asthma attack. The drugs involved include short-acting inhaled beta$_2$-agonist albuterol, metaproterenol (Alupent, Metaprel), and pirbuterol (Maxair) taken by a metered dose inhaler using spacer devices or by a nebulizer; oral or IV corticosteroids; and epinephrine. A study showed that inhaled corticosteroids, given with short-acting beta$_2$-agonists, may be better and faster than IV corticosteroids at treating an acute exacerbation (Miracle & Winston, 2000). Short-acting beta$_2$-agonists quickly relax the muscles around the airway and are the most effective drugs for relieving acute bronchospasms (see Table 49-3). Epinephrine, given subcutaneously or intramuscularly, may be considered in an emergency when symptoms have not been relieved by the use of a beta$_2$-agonist. Epinephrine acts as a bronchodilator. Although the value of administering aminophylline in the treatment of acute asthma has been questioned, IV aminophylline may be considered if the asthma is severe or there is minimal or no response to short-acting inhaled beta$_2$-agonists.

In acute asthma, oxygen therapy should be started immediately and its administration monitored by pulse oximetry and, in severe cases, by measurement of ABGs.

Using a peak flowmeter can help the patient manage asthma. This device measures peak expiratory flow rate—the flow of air in a forced exhalation in liters per minute, which is a good indicator of lung function. Peak flow monitoring measures how well air moves out of the lungs when blown out as hard and fast as possible. Peak flow measurement can help the patient detect early signs of asthma episodes before symptoms occur. Normal peak flow is 80% to 100% of the value predicted for the patient based on height, weight, age, and sex. Severe, persistent asthma is characterized by a peak flow of less than 60% of the value predicted. A severe, life-threatening exacerbation of asthma is characterized by a peak flow of less than 50% of the patient's predicted value.

Once the acute event is over, the medical plan includes identifying precipitating factors and promoting optimal health. Elimination of allergen or countermeasures, such as desensitization or hyposensitization, are desirable.

Nursing Interventions and Patient Teaching

Nursing interventions include administering prescribed medications and ensuring adequate fluid intake and optimal ventilation. To accomplish these goals, incorporate rest periods into activities and interventions; elevate the head of the bed; teach effective breathing techniques, such as pursed-lip breathing and correct use of the peak flowmeter; and provide oxygen therapy as ordered. Monitor vital signs and electrolytes. Kind and empathic emotional support is vital.

Nursing diagnoses and interventions for the patient with asthma include but are not limited to the following:

Nursing Diagnoses	Nursing Interventions
Ineffective breathing pattern, related to narrowed airway	Assess ventilation, and be alert for signs of increasing dyspnea, such as using accessory muscles, nasal flaring, dyspnea, pursed-lip breathing, or prolonged expiration. Maintain position to facilitate ventilation. Administer prescribed medications. Assist with administration of respiratory treatments. Provide care in calm, unhurried manner. Attempt to minimize exposure to dust and other irritants by maintaining clean environment and use of humidifier. Maintain adequate hydration.
Ineffective health maintenance, related to possible allergens in the home	Implement mutual problem solving to explore with patient and family what stimulants may be in home environment, such as allergens. Facilitate allergy testing if needed. Teach the patient and the family importance of avoiding exposure to known irritants.

Educate the patient and the family to identify signs and symptoms and recognize asthma "triggers" and avoid them or lessen their effects to prevent recurrent attacks. Instruct the patient on relaxation techniques to manage anxiety. Stress the importance of health maintenance measures, such as adequate fluid intake and effective breathing techniques. Teach the patient to take prescribed medications correctly and on time, to monitor the peak flowmeter to recognize the early signs of an asthma attack and begin treatment immediately, and to follow the program treatment steps during an attack. The goal is to provide a good control of symptoms with the least possible medication.

Prognosis

Although the incidence of asthma has steadily increased, the mortality and morbidity rates are currently decreasing. There are still more than 4000 deaths per year from asthma (Lewis et al., 2007), which is disheartening, since treatment and education can reduce or eliminate asthma attacks. If status asthmaticus is not reversed, death will ensue.

BRONCHIECTASIS

Etiology and Pathophysiology

Bronchiectasis is a disease characterized by abnormal permanent dilation of one or more large bronchi. This dilation eventually destroys muscular elements and bronchial elastic that support the bronchial wall. Pulmonary muscle tone is gradually lost after one or, more often, repeated pulmonary infections in children and adults. Because of the disease, it is much more difficult to clear mucus from the lungs, and the lungs experience decreased expiratory airflow.

This condition is usually secondary to failure of normal lung tissue defenses (as caused by cystic fibrosis, foreign body, or tumor). It occurs as a complication of recurrent inflammation and infection process that gradually alters the pulmonary structures.

Clinical Manifestations

Signs and symptoms occur after a respiratory tract infection. The late signs and symptoms usually seen are dyspnea, cyanosis, and clubbing of fingers. The patient has paroxysms of coughing on arising in the morning and when lying down. This severe coughing produces copious amounts of foul-smelling sputum. Fatigue, weakness, and a loss of appetite are also noted.

Assessment

Subjective data include the patient's report of difficulty breathing, weight loss, and fever.

Objective data include fine crackles and wheezes in the lower lobes on auscultation. The patient exhibits a prolonged expiratory phase and increased dyspnea. Hemoptysis is seen in 50% of the patients.

Diagnostic Tests

Chest radiographic examination is essentially normal, but inflammation and mediastinal shift may result from overinflation of specific lobes. High-resolution CT scan of the chest is the gold standard for diagnosing bronchiectasis. Sputum cultures can rule out a bacterial infection. PFTs show a decreased forced expiratory volume.

Medical Management

Medical management of bronchiectasis involves treatment of exacerbations with antibiotics. A sputum culture is preferable before treatment with antibiotics, but if a culture is not obtainable, an antibiotic is still prescribed (Lewis et al., 2007).

Oxygen may be ordered at low-flow volume. The patient may require surgery if he or she does not respond to more conservative measures, such as medications, chest physiotherapy, and adequate hydration. If surgery is needed, the affected area is removed (lobectomy).

Medications also include mucolytic agents (acetylcysteine) and bronchodilators.

Nursing Interventions and Patient Teaching

General nursing interventions include using a cool mist vaporizer to provide humidity and increasing oral intake of fluids to aid in secretion removal. Assess vital signs and lung sounds every 2 to 4 hours. Suction the patient as needed and provide assistance in turning, coughing, and deep breathing every 2 hours. Assist with chest physiotherapy.

Nursing diagnoses and interventions for the patient with bronchiectasis include but are not limited to the following:

Nursing Diagnoses	Nursing Interventions
Ineffective airway clearance, related to retained pulmonary secretions	Assess patient's ability to mobilize secretions, assisting as needed. Encourage postural drainage and coughing; suction if needed. Encourage frequent position changes to facilitate secretion mobility and removal. Maintain adequate hydration. Administer mucolytic agents as ordered, and note patient response.
Impaired physical mobility, related to decreased exercise tolerance	Assess patient's activity tolerance, and promote adaptive techniques, such as incorporating rest periods into activities. Promote a gradual increase of activity, noting patient tolerance. Problem solve with patient and family to identify methods of energy conservation and ways to integrate them into lifestyle.

Teach the patient and the family environmental awareness (avoidance of smoke, fumes, and irritating inhalants). Discourage smoking, and advise the patient on appropriate rest and exercise practices. Perform medication teaching, including dosage, rationale, and side effects. Instruct the patient and the family on signs and symptoms of a secondary infection, and ensure the patient knows how to reach the physician after discharge.

Prognosis

Bronchiectasis is a chronic disease. Surgical removal of a portion of the patient's lung is the only cure.

NURSING PROCESS *for the Patient with a Respiratory Disorder*

The role of the licensed practical nurse/licensed vocational nurse (LPN/LVN) in the nursing process as stated is that the LPN/LVN will:

- Participate in planning care for patients based on patient needs
- Review patient's care plan and recommend revisions as needed
- Review and follow defined prioritization for patient care
- Use clinical pathways, care maps, or care plans to guide and review patient care

Assessment

When a patient is admitted with a respiratory disorder, a thorough, immediate, and accurate nursing assessment is an essential first step. The assessment should include the patient's level of consciousness, vital signs, lung sounds (crackles, wheezes, pleural friction rub), and oximetry level. Ask the patient if he or she has shortness of breath, dyspnea on exertion, or cough. If the patient has a cough, ask whether it is productive or nonproductive and the amount and the color of the sputum expectorated. Observe the patient's facial expressions and for signs of respiratory distress such as flaring nostrils, substernal or clavicular retractions, asymmetrical chest wall expansion, and abdominal breathing.

Nursing Diagnosis

Assist in the development of nursing diagnoses. Nursing diagnoses specific to the patient with a respiratory disorder include but are not limited to the following:

- Ineffective airway clearance
- Ineffective breathing pattern
- Impaired gas exchange

- Anxiety
- Activity intolerance
- Imbalanced nutrition: less than body requirements

▪ Expected Outcomes and Planning

The overall goals are that the patient with a respiratory disorder will have (1) effective breathing patterns, (2) adequate airway clearance, (3) adequate oxygenation of tissues, and (4) a realistic attitude toward compliance to treatment. The care plan may include the following goals:

Goal 1: Patient will achieve improved activity tolerance.
Outcome: Patient reports less discomfort with exercise.
Goal 2: Patient will maintain a patent airway.
Outcome: Patient clears airway by coughing.

▪ Implementation

Maintaining the patient's optimal health is important in reducing respiratory symptoms. Nursing interventions may include improving the patient's activity tolerance. This enables the patient to perform activities of daily living while not increasing dyspnea.

▪ Evaluation

Evaluate the expected outcomes and determine their effectiveness. Notify the physician if the patient's respiratory status does not improve immediately.

Goal 1: Patient will achieve improved activity tolerance.
Evaluative measure: Assess patient's exercise tolerance.
Goal 2: Patient will maintain a patent airway.
Evaluative measure: Auscultate lungs after hearing patient cough.

Get Ready for the NCLEX® Examination!

Key Points

- When air is inhaled, it is warmed, moistened, and filtered to prepare it for use by the body.
- The most important structure of the respiratory system is the alveolus, where actual air exchange occurs.
- For breathing to occur, pressure changes must take place within the thoracic cavity.
- The combination of one inspiration plus one expiration equals one respiration, or one respiratory movement.
- The primary function of the respiratory system is to exchange oxygen and carbon dioxide at the alveolar-capillary level.
- The lungs' ability to expand and contract depends on musculoskeletal and neurologic functions, as well as physiologic conditions affecting the respiratory system.
- Activity tolerance is frequently altered as a result of decreased oxygenation-ventilation.
- Anxiety can exacerbate pulmonary disorders, increasing the body's need for oxygen.
- Breathing exercises can improve ventilation.
- Effective breathing techniques include elevating the head and chest to maintain airway patency; deep breathing and coughing exercises to facilitate lung expansion; and pursed-lip breathing to decrease the effort of breathing.
- Adequate fluid intake and humidity help moisten secretions, thus aiding in their clearance.
- A thorough psychosocial assessment and resultant interventions are necessary for the patient with a laryngectomy because of loss of voice and neck and facial disfigurement.
- In May 2005 the FDA approved a new version of a blood test to aid in diagnosing latent TB infection and active TB. It is called QFT-G, and it can be used in place of the traditional PPD skin test. The QFT-G may detect TB with greater specificity than the PPD test.
- SARS is a serious acute respiratory infection caused by a coronavirus.
- People who are suspected of having SARS should be placed in respiratory isolation, including use of an appropriate disposable particulate respirator to protect other patients and health care workers.
- Clinical manifestations of sleep apnea include frequent awakening at night, insomnia, excessive daytime sleepiness, witnessed apneic episodes, morning headaches, personality changes, and irritability.
- Chest drainage serves a twofold purpose: it (1) drains air, blood, or fluid from the pleural space; and (2) restores negative pressure. It requires a water seal to prevent air from reentering the pleural space.
- Techniques used in chest physiotherapy include percussion, vibration, and postural drainage.
- Nursing interventions after thoracic surgery that assist in preventing complications by promoting effective airway clearance are (1) frequent repositioning, (2) coughing, and (3) deep breathing.
- Studies have revealed that hypoxia worsens when patients are placed on their backs or sides with the affected (sick) lung down.
- Low-flow oxygen therapy is required for patients with COPD because higher oxygen concentrations depress the body's own respiratory regulatory centers.
- Hospitals are a high-risk setting for TB transmission, and health care workers are at high occupational risk for TB infection.
- Because PE impairs gas exchange, its hallmark is acute, unexplained dyspnea with abrupt, constant, nonradiating pain that worsens with inspiration.
- Patients with respiratory disorders must reduce exposure to infection, which increases the body's oxygen demands.
- COPD includes emphysema, chronic bronchitis, asthma, and bronchiectasis.

- Transmission of TB is primarily by inhalation of minute droplet nuclei (each containing a single tubercle bacillus) coughed or sneezed by a person whose sputum contains tubercle bacilli.
- Pulse oximetry is a noninvasive method providing continuing monitoring of Sao_2 (saturation of oxygen).

Additional Learning Resources

Go to your Companion CD for an audio glossary, animations, video clips, and more.

evolve Be sure to visit the Evolve site at http://evolve.elsevier.com/Christensen/adult/ for additional online resources.

Review Questions for the NCLEX® Examination

1. Rapid and deeper respirations are stimulated by the respiratory center of the brain when:

1. oxygen saturation levels are greater than 90%.
2. carbon dioxide levels increase.
3. the alveoli contract.
4. the diaphragm contracts and lowers its dome.

2. The tendency of molecules of a substance (gaseous, liquid, or solid) to move from a region of high concentration to one of lower concentration is the passive process at work in the exchange of gases between the blood capillary and alveolar area. This process is called:

1. osmosis.
2. filtration.
3. diffusion.
4. transport.

3. Each alveolus is coated with a thin lipoprotein covering that prevents it from collapsing after each breath; this covering is:

1. LDH.
2. isoenzyme.
3. surfactant.
4. sebum.

4. The walls of the thoracic cavity are lined with a serous membrane composed of tough endothelial cells called:

1. visceral pleura.
2. apneustic serosa.
3. pneumotaxic serosa.
4. parietal pleura.

5. The exchange of oxygen and carbon dioxide in external respiration takes place in the:

1. lungs.
2. bronchioles.
3. capillaries and body cells.
4. alveoli and pulmonary capillaries.

6. A 73-year-old patient is diagnosed with chronic bronchitis. He is very dyspneic and must sit up to breathe. An abnormal condition in which there is discomfort in breathing in any but an erect sitting position is:

1. orthopnea.
2. dyspnea.
3. orthopsia.
4. Cheyne-Stokes.

7. A 45-year-old patient is being evaluated to rule out pulmonary tuberculosis (TB). Which finding is most closely associated with TB?

1. Leg cramps
2. Night sweats
3. Skin discoloration
4. Green-colored sputum

8. The health care workers caring for a patient with active TB, are instructed in methods of protecting themselves from contracting TB. The Centers for Disease Control and Prevention currently recommend that health care workers who care for TB-infected patients:

1. ask the patient to wear a mask while in isolation.
2. wear a surgical mask.
3. wear a small-micron, fitted filtration mask.
4. receive the BCG vaccine.

9. The physician ordered a blood culture and sputum specimen for a patient who has pneumonia. These diagnostic tests should be collected:

1. after initiation of antibiotic therapy.
2. the morning after admission.
3. before initiation of antibiotic therapy.
4. at the first elevated temperature.

10. A 62-year-old patient has just returned to her room after a bronchoscopy. No food or fluids should be given after the examination until:

1. total absence of blood-streaked sputum.
2. the head nurse gives the order.
3. her gag reflex returns.
4. she is up and about and steady on her feet.

11. A patient who was in a motor vehicle accident and has a lacerated pleura secondary to fractured ribs. To promote reexpansion of his lung, what type of thoracic drainage system was used?

1. Open system to promote negative pressure
2. Closed system to maintain the lungs' normal negative pressure
3. Closed system to maintain the lungs' positive pressure
4. Closed system to allow air to enter the pleural cavity for reexpansion

12. A 45-year-old, second-day postoperative patient is recovering from thoracic surgery. A therapeutic nursing intervention would include:

1. helping the patient cough and deep breathe by splinting the anterior and posterior chest.
2. splinting the anterior chest for coughing.
3. placing the patient in a supine position.
4. allowing the patient to sleep uninterrupted for 8 hours.

13. A 71-year-old patient is admitted with an exacerbation of COPD. He has dependent edema, ascites, and dyspnea. A complication that may occur in COPD, in which some of the capillaries surrounding the alveoli are destroyed, resulting in pulmonary hypertension, blood returning to the right side of the heart, and signs and symptoms of right-sided HF, is:

1. pulmonary edema.
2. cor pulmonale.
3. tetralogy of Fallot.
4. acyanotic heart disease.

14. A 52-year-old patient had a laryngectomy due to cancer of the larynx. Discharge instructions are given to the patient and his family. Which response, by written communication from the patient or verbal response by the family, indicates that the instructions need to be clarified?

1. Report swelling, pain, or excessive drainage.
2. The suctioning at home must be a clean procedure, not sterile.
3. Cleanse skin around stoma bid, use hydrogen peroxide and rinse with water, pat dry.
4. It is acceptable to take over-the-counter medications now that condition is stable.

15. Most pulmonary embolisms (PEs) originate from:

1. deep-vein thrombosis (DVT).
2. ventilation/perfusion (V/Q) mismatch.
3. increased pulmonary vascular resistance.
4. right-sided heart failure.

16. Chest pain from pulmonary embolism (PE) typically:

1. radiates to the neck and jaw.
2. is unchanged by deep breathing.
3. is pleuritic and worsens on inspiration.
4. radiates to the abdomen and back.

17. In the treatment of asthma, peak flow monitoring is important to help the patient manage the asthma. Peak flow monitoring measures:

1. the inspiratory capacity of the lungs.
2. the residual volume of the lungs.
3. the vital capacity of the lungs.
4. how well air moves out of the lungs during forceful exhalation.

18. The primary goal for the patient with bronchiectasis is that the patient will:

1. have no recurrence of disease.
2. have normal pulmonary function.
3. maintain removal of bronchial secretions.
4. avoid environmental agents that precipitate inflammation.

19. A patient was seen in clinic for an episode of epistaxis, which was controlled by placement of anterior nasal packing. During discharge teaching, the nurse instructs the patient to:

1. avoid vigorous nose blowing and strenuous activity.
2. use aspirin or aspirin-containing compounds for pain relief.
3. apply ice compresses to the nose every 4 hours for the first 48 hours.
4. leave the packing in place for 7 to 10 days until it is removed by the physician.

20. TB is spread by:

1. contact with clothing, bedding, or food.
2. eating from utensils used by an infected person.
3. inhaling the TB bacteria after a person coughs, speaks, or sneezes.
4. talking with an individual with TB.

21. Which type of medication is used as rescue medication in an acute asthma exacerbation?

1. Methylxanthines
2. Leukotriene modifiers
3. Long-acting beta$_2$-agonists
4. Short-acting beta$_1$-agonists

22. Asthma is best characterized as:

1. an inflammatory disease.
2. a steady progression of bronchoconstriction.
3. an obstructive disease with loss of alveolar walls.
4. a chronic obstructive disorder characterized by mucus production.

23. A patient with COPD asks why the heart is affected by the respiratory disease. The nurse's response to the patient is based on the knowledge that cor pulmonale is characterized by:

1. pulmonary congestion secondary to left ventricular failure.
2. excess serous fluid collection in the alveoli caused by retained respiratory secretions.
3. right ventricular hypertrophy secondary to increased pulmonary vascular resistance.
4. right ventricular failure secondary to compression of the heart by hyperinflated lungs.

24. A patient with TB has a nursing diagnosis of noncompliance. The nurse recognizes that the most common etiologic factor for this diagnosis in patients with TB is:

1. fatigue and lack of energy to manage self-care.
2. lack of knowledge about how the disease is transmitted.
3. little or no motivation to adhere to a long-term drug regimen.
4. feelings of shame and the response to the social stigma associated with TB.

25. Three types of anthrax are:

1. cutaneous, gastrointestinal, inhalational.
2. renal, gastrointestinal, CNS.
3. musculoskeletal, inhalational, adrenal.
4. cutaneous, endocrine, gastrointestinal.

26. To get optimal results from pulse oximetry, which statements are correct? *(Select all that apply.)*

1. Do not attach the transducer to an extremity that has a blood pressure cuff in place.
2. While the probe is in place, protect it from decreased light, which can affect the reading.
3. Place the probe over a pulsating vascular bed.
4. Remember that hypothermia, hypotension, and vasoconstriction can affect readings.

27. *Ineffective airway clearance,* related to tracheobronchial obstruction or secretions, is a nursing diagnosis for a patient with COPD. Which of the following nursing interventions are correct? *(Select all that apply.)*
   1. Offer small, frequent, high-calorie, high-protein feedings.
   2. Encourage generous fluid intake.
   3. Restrict fluid intake to decrease congestion.
   4. Have patient turn and cough every 2 hours; teach effective coughing technique.

28. *Ineffective breathing pattern,* related to decreased lung expansion during an acute attack of asthma, is an appropriate nursing diagnosis. Which nursing interventions are correct? *(Select all that apply.)*
   1. Place patient in a supine position.
   2. Administer oxygen therapy as ordered.
   3. Remain with patient during acute attack to decrease fear and anxiety.
   4. Incorporate rest periods into activities and interventions.
   5. Maintain semi-Fowler's position to facilitate ventilation.

29. The patient with respiratory acidosis demonstrates: *(Select all that apply.)*
   1. disorientation.
   2. pH of less than 7.35.
   3. pH of more than 7.44.
   4. rapid respirations.

30. The appropriate nursing intervention for a 40-year-old patient with active TB, would be to:
   1. place the patient in drainage and secretion precautions.
   2. place the patient in acid-fast bacilli (AFB) isolation precautions.
   3. maintain the patient in enteric isolation.
   4. not use any isolation precautions.

31. Patient teaching after a tonsillectomy and adenoidectomy would include which instruction(s)? *(Select all that apply.)*
   1. Avoid attempting to clear the throat, coughing, and sneezing.
   2. Avoid vigorous nose blowing for 1 to 2 weeks.
   3. Resume foods and fluids as tolerated.
   4. Take aspirin, gr 10, every 4 hours.
   5. Notify the physician in case of increased pain, fever, or bleeding.

32. If the patient has an epistaxis, the correct nursing intervention(s) would be to: *(Select all that apply.)*
   1. place the patient in Fowler's position with the head forward.
   2. place the patient in Fowler's position with the head extended.
   3. compress the nostrils tightly below the bone and hold for 10 minutes or longer.
   4. place ice compresses over the nose.

33. In pulmonary edema, the medical management often include(s): *(Select all that apply.)*
   1. IV fluid infusion at 150 mL/hr.
   2. furosemide (Lasix) IV.
   3. oxygen therapy.
   4. high Fowler's position.
   5. morphine sulfate to decrease respiratory rate.

34. An appropriate nursing diagnosis for a patient with pulmonary edema is *excess fluid volume,* related to altered tissue permeability. Which nursing intervention(s) for this diagnosis are correct? *(Select all that apply.)*
   1. Assess indicators of patient's fluid volume status, such as breath sounds; skin turgor; and pedal, sacral, and periorbital edema.
   2. Monitor intake and output accurately.
   3. Administer diuretics as ordered.
   4. Weigh daily.
   5. Provide regular diet with normal sodium intake.

35. The nurse should educate the patient in the proper techniques to use for the collection of a sputum specimen. Which guideline(s) are correct? *(Select all that apply.)*
   1. Explain to the patient the need to bring the sputum up from the lungs.
   2. Encourage fluid intake.
   3. Collect specimens after meals when patient feels stronger.
   4. Notify staff as soon as specimen is collected so it can be sent to the laboratory without delay.
   5. Place sputum specimen in sterile container.

36. Medical management and nursing interventions of the patient with pulmonary embolism usually include: *(Select all that apply.)*
   1. bed rest.
   2. administration of intravenous heparin per protocol.
   3. elevation of lower extremities.
   4. administration of vitamin K subcutaneously.
   5. oxygen per mask or nasal cannula.

37. A new blood assay test that offers a promising alternative in TB testing is:
   1. QuantiFERON-TB Gold Test.
   2. Relenza Test.
   3. HPV DNA Test.
   4. BNP Test.

chapter

50

Care of the Patient with a Urinary Disorder

evolve

http://evolve.elsevier.com/Christensen/foundationsadult

Alita K. Sellers

Objectives

Anatomy and Physiology

1. Describe the structures of the urinary system, including functions.
2. List the three processes involved in urine formation.
3. Name three hormones and their influence on nephron function.
4. Compare the normal components of urine with the abnormal components.

Medical-Surgical

5. Identify the effects of aging on urinary system function.
6. Appraise the changes in body image created when the patient experiences an alteration in urinary function.
7. Incorporate pharmacotherapeutic and nutritional considerations into the nursing care plan of the patient with a urinary disorder.
8. Prioritize the special needs of the patient with urinary dysfunction.
9. Describe the alterations in kidney function associated with disorders of the urinary tract.
10. Discuss the effect of renal disease on family function.
11. Address patient concerns in teaching about altered sexuality secondary to urinary disorders and treatments.
12. Investigate community resources for support for the patient and significant others as they face lifestyle changes from chronic urinary disorders and treatments.
13. Select nursing diagnoses related to alterations in urinary function.
14. Design culturally sensitive care of the patient with a urinary disorder.

Key Terms

anasarca (ăn-ă-SĂR-kă, p. 1703)
anuria (ă-NŪ-rē-ă, p. 1707)
asthenia (ăs-THĒ-nē-ă, p. 1687)
azotemia (ă-zō-TĒ-mē-ă, p. 1691)
bacteriuria (băk-tēr-ē-Ū-rē-ŭh, p. 1687)
costovertebral angle (CVA) (kŏs-tŏ-VĔR-tĕ-brăl ĂNG-gŭl, p. 1691)
cytologic evaluation (sī-tŏ-LŎJ-ĭk ĕ-văl-ū-Ā-shŭn, p. 1697)
dialysis (dī-ĂL-ĭ-sĭs, p. 1710)
dysuria (dĭs-Ū-rē-ă , p. 1677)
hematuria (hĕm-ă-TŪ-rē-ă, p. 1687)
hydronephrosis (hī-drō-nĕ-FRŌ-sĭs, p. 1693)
ileal conduit (ĭl-ē-ăl KŎN-dū-ĭt, p. 1714)
micturition (mĭk-tū-RĬSH-ŭn, p. 1693)
nephrotoxins (nĕf-rō-TŎK-sĭnz, p. 1716)
nocturia (nŏk-TŪ-rē-ă, p. 1687)
oliguria (ŏl-ĭ-GŪ-rē-ă, p. 1703)
prostatodynia (prŏs-tĕ-tō-DĪN-ē-ă, p. 1690)
pyuria (pĭ-Ū-rē-ă, p. 1687)
residual urine (rĕ-ZĬ-dū-ăl Ū-rĭn, p. 1684)
retention (rē-TĔN-shŭn, p. 1684)
urolithiasis (ū-rō-lĭ-THĪ-ă-sĭs, p. 1693)

ANATOMY AND PHYSIOLOGY OF THE URINARY SYSTEM

Each day, the cells throughout the body metabolize ingested nutrients. This process provides energy for the body and produces waste products. As proteins break down, nitrogenous waste—urea, ammonia, and **creatinine** (a nitrogenous compound produced by metabolic processes in the body)—is produced. The primary function of the kidneys is excretion of these waste products. The kidneys also assist in regulating the body's water, electrolytes, and acid-base balance. The urinary system is probably the most important system in maintaining homeostasis.

The urinary system consists of two kidneys, which produce urine by removing waste, excess water, and electrolytes from the blood; two ureters, which transport urine from the kidneys to the bladder; one bladder, which collects and stores urine; and one urethra, which transports urine from the bladder to the outside of the body for elimination (Figure 50-1). This chapter explores the filtering process, the composition of urine, and the pathway of urine removal from the body.

KIDNEYS

The kidneys lie behind the parietal peritoneum (retroperitoneal), just below the diaphragm on each side of the vertebral column. Kidneys are dark red, bean-shaped organs that are 4 to 5 inches (10 to 12 cm) long, 2 to 3 inches (5 to 7.5 cm) wide, and about 1 inch (2.5 cm) thick. Because of the liver, the right kidney

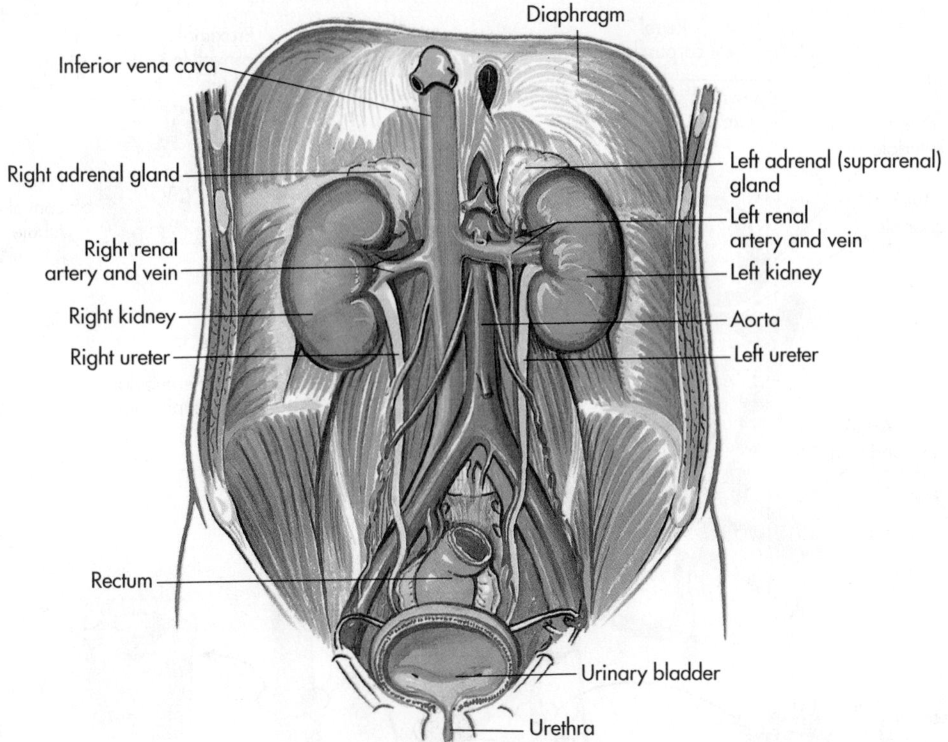

FIGURE 50-1 Locations of urinary system organs.

lies slightly lower than the left. The kidneys are surrounded and anchored in place by a layer of adipose tissue. Near the center of the kidney's medial border is a notch or indentation called the **hilus** where the renal artery enters and the renal vein and the ureter exit the kidney.

The adrenal glands, a part of the endocrine system, sit near the top of each kidney. The adrenal glands secrete hormones that help control blood pressure and heart rate, among other functions. The primary mineralocorticoid secreted by the adrenal cortex is aldosterone. Plasma potassium concentration is the primary regulator of aldosterone. Changes evoked through the adrenal glands create changes in kidney function (see Chapter 51).

Gross Anatomical Structure

The outer covering of the kidney is a strong layer of connective tissue called the **renal capsule.** Directly beneath the renal capsule is the renal **cortex.** It contains 1.25 million renal tubules, which are part of the microscopic filtration system. Immediately beneath the cortex is the **medulla,** which is a darker color. The medulla contains the triangular **pyramids.** Continuing inward, the narrow points of the pyramids **(papillae)** empty urine into the calyces. The **calyces** are cuplike extensions of the renal pelvis that guide urine into the renal pelvis. The **renal pelvis** is an expansion of the upper end of the ureter; the ureter in turn drains the finished product, urine, into the bladder (Figure 50-2).

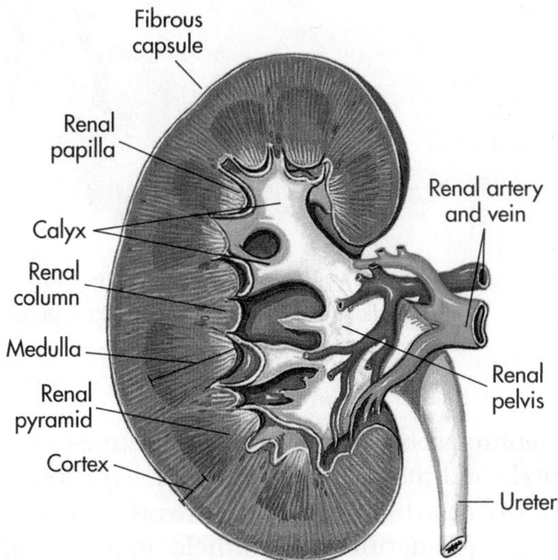

FIGURE 50-2 Coronal section through right kidney.

Microscopic Structure

Nephron

Each kidney contains more than 1 million nephrons. The **nephron** is the functional unit of the kidney, resembling a microscopic funnel with a long stem and two convoluted sections (Figure 50-3). It is responsible for filtering the blood and processing the urine. The nephron has three major functions: (1) controlling body fluid levels by selectively removing or retaining water, (2) assisting with the regulation of the pH of the blood, and (3) removing toxic waste from the blood. Approximately 60 times a day, the body's entire volume of blood is filtered through the kidneys.

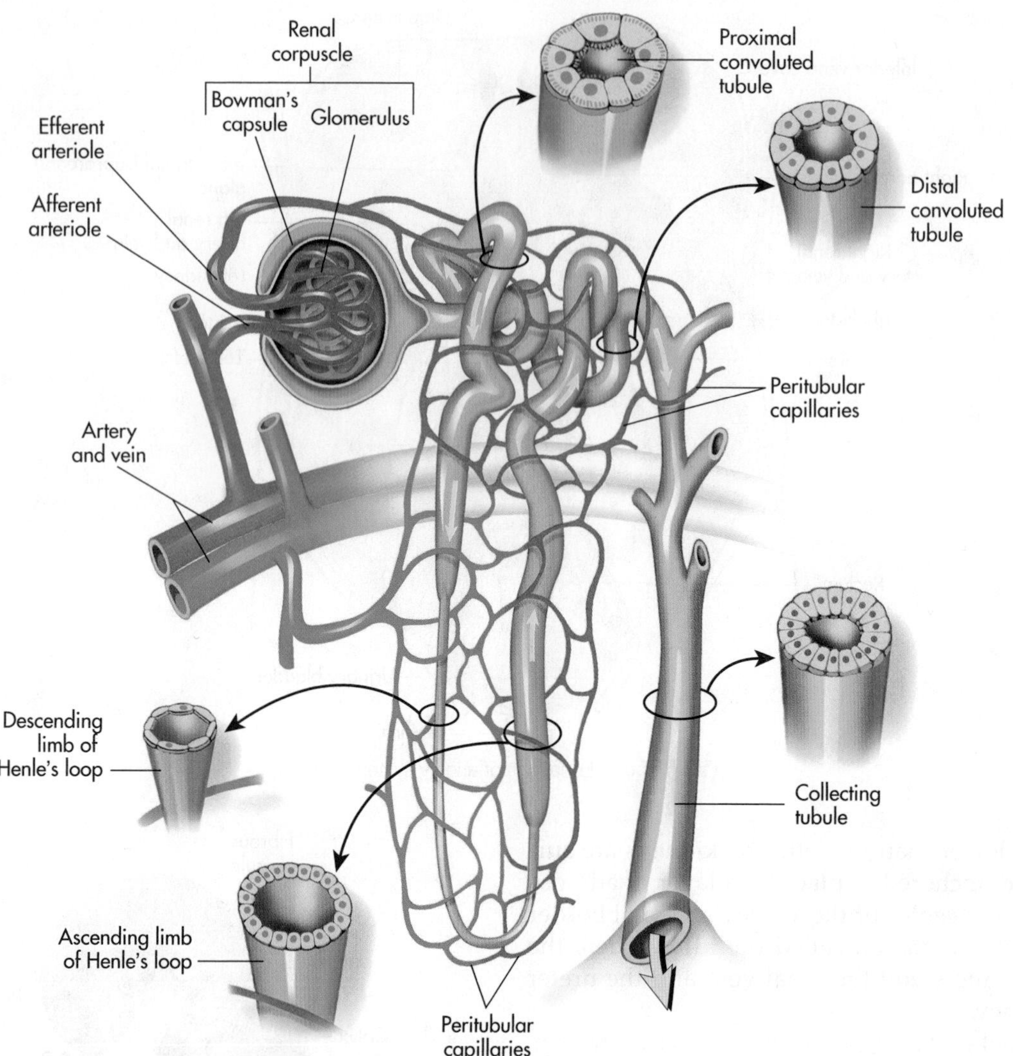

FIGURE 50-3 The nephron unit. Cross-sections from the four segments of the renal tubule are shown. The differences in appearance in tubular cells seen in a cross-section reflect the differing functions of each nephron segment.

A nephron consists of two main structures: the renal corpuscle and the renal tubule. The renal corpuscle is composed of a tightly bound network of capillaries called the **glomeruli** that are held inside a cuplike structure, **Bowman's capsule.** The renal arteries (right and left) branch off the abdominal aorta and enter the kidney at the hilus. The renal arteries continue branching until blood is delivered to the glomerulus by the afferent arteriole. The blood leaves the glomerulus through the efferent arteriole to the peritubular capillary. Blood finally reaches the renal veins and flows into the inferior vena cava.

The renal tubule becomes tightly coiled (at the proximal convoluted tubule), makes a sudden straight drop, and curves back upward like a hairpin (at Henle's loop, or nephron loop) and becomes tightly coiled again (at the distal convoluted tubule). The convoluted tubule terminates at the collecting tubule or duct. Several collecting ducts unite in a pyramid and open at the papilla to empty urine into the associated calyx.

The juxtaglomerular apparatus is the microscopic structure in the kidney, which regulates the function of each nephron. The juxtaglomerular apparatus is named for its proximity to the glomerulus; it is found between the vascular pole of the renal corpuscle and the returning distal convoluted tubule of the same nephron. This location is critical to its function in regulating renal blood flow and glomerular filtration rate. The juxtaglomerular apparatus is where the afferent arterioles come into direct contact with the distal convoluted tubule. The juxtaglomerular apparatus works to regulate systemic blood pressure and filtrate formation.

The specialized cells of the afferent arteriole at this region are called juxtaglomerular cells. These cells contain the enzyme renin and function as mechanoreceptors to sense blood pressure.

The specialized cells of the distal convoluted tubule at the point of contact with the afferent arteriole are the macula densa cells. These cells function as chemoreceptors to sense changes in the solute concentration and flow rate of the filtrate.

When systemic blood pressure decreases, the juxtaglomerular cells have a decreased stretch, which leads to their release of renin (Figure 50-4). Renin release causes the activation of the renin-angiotensin mechanism, which ultimately leads to an increased blood pressure.

Reabsorption begins as soon as the filtrate reaches the tubule system. The filtrate contains important products needed by the body: water, glucose, and ions may be absorbed. In fact, 99% of the filtrate is returned to the body (see Figure 50-4).

In summary, the three phases of urine formation (Table 50-1) and location of the processes are as follows:

1. **Filtration** of water and blood products occurs in the glomerulus of Bowman's capsule.
2. **Reabsorption** of water, glucose, and necessary ions back into the blood occurs primarily in the proximal convoluted tubules, Henle's loop, and the distal convoluted tubules. This process reclaims important substances needed by the body.
3. **Secretion** of certain ions, nitrogenous waste products, and drugs occurs primarily in the distal convoluted tubule. This process is the reverse of reabsorption; the substances move from the blood to the filtrate.

Hormonal Influence on Nephron Function. When the body has suffered increased fluid loss through hemorrhage, diaphoresis, vomiting, diarrhea, or other means, the blood pressure drops. These events decrease the amount of filtrate produced by the kidneys. The posterior pituitary gland releases antidiuretic hormone

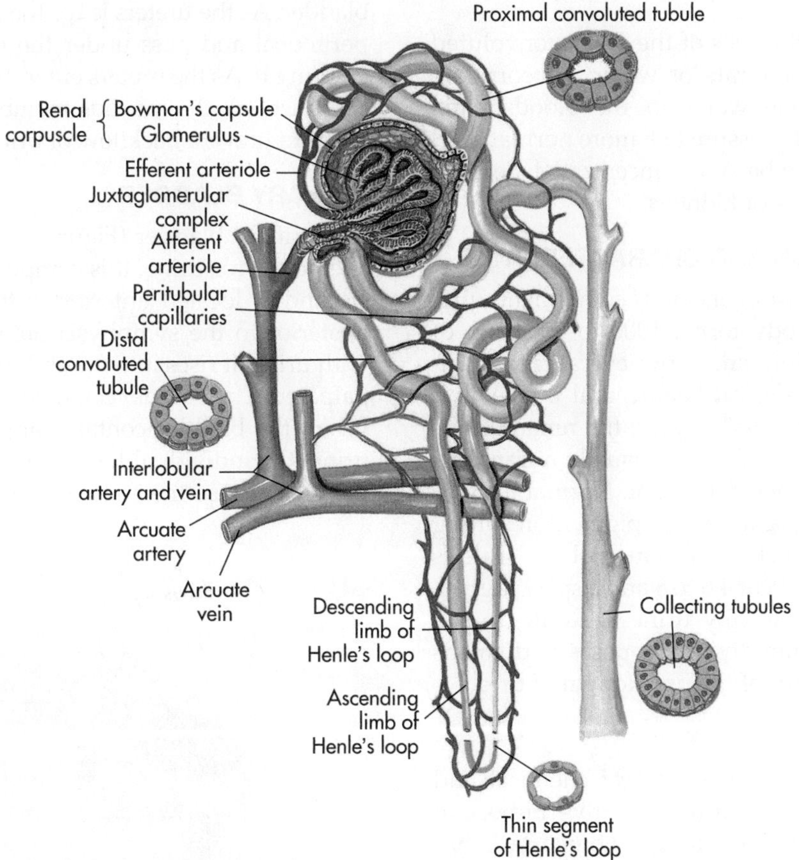

FIGURE 50-4 Cross-section from the four segments of the renal tubule.

Table 50-1 Functions of Parts of the Nephron in Urine Formation

PART OF NEPHRON	PROCESS IN URINE FORMATION	SUBSTANCES MOVED AND DIRECTION OF MOVEMENT
Glomerulus	Filtration	Water and solutes (sodium and other ions, nitrogen wastes, urea, uric acid, creatinine, glucose, and other nutrients) filter through the glomeruli into Bowman's capsule
Proximal convoluted tubule	Reabsorption	Water and solutes
Henle's loop	Reabsorption	Sodium and chloride ions
Distal convoluted and collecting tubules	Reabsorption Secretion	Water, sodium, and other chloride ions Ammonia, potassium ions, urea, uric acid, creatinine, hydrogen ions, and some drugs

Box 50-1 Major Functions of the Kidneys

Urine formation: Glomerular filtration, tubular reabsorption, and secretion; 1000 to 2000 mL of urine formed each day
Fluid and electrolyte control: Maintain correct balance of fluid and electrolytes within a normal range by excretion, secretion, and reabsorption
Acid-base balance: Maintain pH of blood (7.35 to 7.45) at normal range by directly excreting hydrogen ions and forming bicarbonate for buffering
Excretion of waste products: Direct removal of metabolic waste products contained in the glomerular filtrate
Blood pressure regulation: Regulation of blood pressure by controlling the circulating volume and renin secretion
Red blood cell (RBC) production: Secretion of erythropoietin, which stimulates bone marrow to produce RBCs
Regulation of calcium-phosphate metabolism: Regulation of vitamin D activation

(ADH). ADH causes the cells of the distal convoluted tubules to increase their rate of water reabsorption. This action returns the water to the bloodstream, which raises the blood pressure to a more normal level and causes the urine to become concentrated. See Box 50-1 for major functions of kidneys.

URINE COMPOSITION AND CHARACTERISTICS

The word *urine* comes from one of its components, uric acid. Each day, the body forms 1000 to 2000 mL of urine; this amount is influenced by several factors, including mental and physical health, oral intake, and blood pressure. Urine is 95% water; the remainder is nitrogenous wastes and salts. It is usually a transparent yellow with a characteristic odor. Normal urine is yellow because of urochrome, a pigment resulting from the body's destruction of hemoglobin. Urine is slightly acidic, with a pH of 4.6 to 8 and a specific gravity of 1.003 to 1.030. Healthy urine is sterile, but at room temperature it rapidly decomposes and smells like ammonia as a result of the breakdown of urea.

URINE ABNORMALITIES

A urinalysis, which studies the physical, chemical, and microscopic properties of urine, can give important diagnostic information. If the body's homeostasis has been compromised, certain substances may spill into the urine. Some of the more common substances include the following:

- **Albumin** in the urine (albuminuria) indicates possible renal disease, increased blood pressure, or toxicity of the kidney cells from heavy metals.
- **Glucose** (sugar) in the urine (glycosuria) most often indicates a high blood glucose level. The blood glucose level rises above the renal threshold (the point at which the renal tubules can no longer reabsorb), and the glucose spills into the urine.
- **Erythrocytes** in the urine (hematuria) may indicate infection, tumors, or renal disease. Occasionally an individual may have a renal calculus (kidney stone), and irritation produces hematuria.
- **Ketone bodies** in the urine is called ketoaciduria (or ketonuria). It occurs when too many fatty acids are oxidized. This condition is seen with diabetes mellitus, starvation, or any other metabolic condition in which fats are rapidly catabolized.
- **Leukocytes** (white blood cells [WBCs]) are found in urine when there is an infection in the urinary tract.

URETERS

Once the urine has been formed in the nephrons, it passes to the paired ureters. Ureters are actually extensions of the renal pelvis and extend downward 10 to 12 inches (25 to 30 cm) to the lower part of the urinary bladder. As the ureters leave the kidneys, they are retroperitoneal and pass under the urinary bladder before entering it. As the ureters enter the bladder (ureterovesical junction), the mucous membrane folds, acting as a valve to prevent backflow of urine.

URINARY BLADDER

The urinary bladder (Figure 50-5) is a temporary storage pouch for urine. It is composed of collapsible muscle and is located anterior to the small intestine and posterior to the symphysis pubis. As the bladder fills with urine, it rises into the abdominal cavity and can be palpated. The bladder can hold 750 to 1000 mL of urine. When the bladder contains approximately 250 mL of urine, the individual has a conscious desire to urinate. This is because the stretch receptors become activated

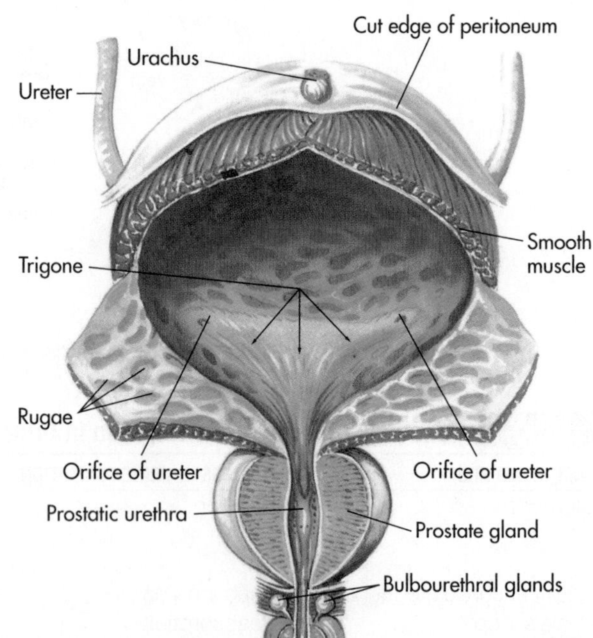

FIGURE 50-5 The male urinary bladder, cut to show the interior. Note how the prostate gland surrounds the urethra as it exits the bladder.

and a message is sent to the spinal cord. A moderately full bladder holds 450 mL (1 pint) of urine.

Two sphincters, the internal and external, control the release of the urine. The internal sphincter located at the bladder neck is composed of involuntary muscle. As the bladder becomes full, the stretch receptors cause contractions, pushing the urine past the internal sphincter. The urine then presses on the external sphincter, which is composed of skeletal or voluntary muscle at the terminus of the urethra.

URETHRA

The **urethra** is the terminal portion of the urinary system. It is a small tube that carries urine by peristalsis from the bladder out of its external opening, the **urinary meatus.** In females it is embedded in the anterior wall of the vagina vestibule and exits between the clitoris and the vaginal opening. The female urethra is approximately ¼ inch in diameter and 1½ inches long. In males the urethra is approximately 8 inches long, passing through the prostate gland and extending the length of the glans penis. In the male the urethra serves two functions: as a passageway for urine and a passageway for semen.

NORMAL AGING OF THE URINARY SYSTEM

With aging the kidneys lose part of their normal functioning capacity; in fact, by 70 years of age, the filtering mechanism is only 50% as efficient as at 40 years. This occurs because of decreased blood supply and loss of nephrons.

In the aging woman the bladder loses tone and the perineal muscles may relax, resulting in stress incontinence. In the aging man the prostate gland may become enlarged, leading to constriction of the urethra. Incomplete emptying of the bladder in both men and women increases the possibility of urinary tract infection (UTI) (see Life Span Considerations box).

Life Span Considerations

Older Adults

Urinary Disorder

- Urinary frequency, urgency, nocturia, retention, and incontinence are common with aging. These occur because of weakened musculature in the bladder and urethra, diminished neurologic sensation combined with decreased bladder capacity, and the effects of medications such as diuretics.
- Urinary incontinence is a leading reason for institutional placement of older adults.
- Urinary incontinence can lead to a loss of self-esteem and result in decreased participation in social activities.
- Older women are at risk for stress incontinence because of hormonal changes and weakened pelvic musculature.
- Older men are at risk for urinary retention because of prostatic hypertrophy.
- Urinary tract infections in older adults are often associated with invasive procedures such as catheterization, diabetes mellitus, and neurologic disorders.
- Inadequate fluid intake, immobility, and conditions that lead to urinary stasis increase the risk of infection in the older adult.
- Frequent toileting and meticulous skin care can reduce the risk of skin impairment secondary to urinary incontinence.

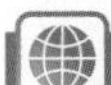

Cultural Considerations

Urinary Disorder

A cultural assessment reflects a dynamic process in which the health care team seeks to understand the patient and gain insights to the meaning of care, health, and well-being. Integral components of a cultural assessment include communication, time orientation, personal space, pain, religious beliefs, taboos, customs, dietary practices, health practices, family roles, and views of death.

Professional discussion of urinary problems requires sensitivity because of the association of the urinary system with the reproductive system and the associated cultural taboos surrounding sexuality. Often the patient's self-image and sexual performance are affected by altered urinary function. Be sensitive to the patient's feelings, guiding the interview to ensure accurate assessment while maintaining the patient's dignity.

LABORATORY AND DIAGNOSTIC EXAMINATIONS

Diagnostic tests for urinary tract conditions include laboratory tests, diagnostic imaging, and endoscopic procedures. Nursing responsibilities vary according to the studies performed. Be aware of specific patient variables that may influence test results: state of hydration, nutritional status, or trauma (see Cultural Considerations box). Prepare patients for diagnostic testing by briefly describing the purpose of the procedure and what the patient can expect to happen.

URINALYSIS

The most common urinary diagnostic study is the urinalysis. Table 50-2 describes normal and abnormal constituents in the urine and possible factors that influence test results. A urinalysis may be done during assessments of other body systems because of the role of the kidneys in maintaining homeostasis. Urine culture and sensitivity may be done to confirm suspected infections, to identify causative organisms, and to determine appropriate antimicrobial therapy. Cultures are also obtained for periodic screening of urine when the threat of a UTI persists. Various reagent strips are available to test urine for abnormal substances. The strips are a quick reference that can be used in a clinical setting or at home. Common substances measured to monitor kidney function include total urine protein, creatinine, urea, uric acid levels, and catecholamines.

Urinalysis is completed on a clean-catch or catheterized specimen. A sterile urine specimen is obtained either by inserting a straight catheter into the urinary bladder and removing urine or by obtaining a specimen from the port of an indwelling catheter via cathe-

Table 50-2 Urinalysis

CONSTITUENT	NORMAL RANGE	INFLUENCING FACTORS
Color	Pale yellow to amber	Diabetes insipidus, biliary obstruction, medications, diet
Turbidity	Clear to slightly cloudy	Phosphates, white blood cells, bacteria
Odor	Mildly aromatic	Medication, bacteria, diet
pH	4.6-8	Stale specimen, food intake, infection, homeostatic imbalance
Specific gravity	1.003-1.030	State of hydration, medications
Glucose	Negative	Diabetes mellitus, medications, diet
Protein	Negative	Renal disease, muscle exertion, dehydration
Bilirubin	Negative	Liver disease with obstruction or damage, medications
Hemoglobin	Negative	Trauma, renal disease
Ketones	Negative	Diabetes mellitus, diet, medications
Red blood cells	Up to 2 LPF	Renal or bladder disease, trauma, medications
White blood cells	0-4 LPF	Renal disease, urinary tract infection
Casts	Rare	Renal disease
Bacteria	Negative	Urinary tract infection

ter port using sterile technique. Because the kidneys excrete substances in varying amounts and rates during a 24-hour period, the nurse may be responsible for collecting a 24-hour urine sample. Discard the first voiding and note the time at the beginning of the 24-hour urine collection. For the next 24 hours collect all urine and place it in a special laboratory container.

SPECIFIC GRAVITY

Specific gravity measures the patient's hydration status and gives information about the kidneys' ability to concentrate urine. Specific gravity is decreased by high fluid intake, reduced renal concentrating ability, diabetes insipidus, and diuretic use. It is increased in dehydration due to fever, diaphoresis, vomiting, diarrhea, and medical conditions such as diabetes mellitus (diabetic ketoacidosis or hyperglycemic hyperosmolar nonketotic coma) and inappropriate secretion of ADH. The value ranges between 1.003 and 1.030, with the lower values suggesting more dilute urine (Pagana & Pagana, 2008).

BLOOD (SERUM) UREA NITROGEN

Blood urea nitrogen (BUN) is a laboratory test used to determine the kidney's ability to rid the blood of non-protein nitrogen (NPN) waste and urea, which result from protein breakdown (catabolism). The acceptable serum range for BUN is 10 to 20 mg/dL. For a more accurate test result, the patient should receive nothing by mouth (NPO) for 8 hours before blood sampling. If the BUN is elevated, institute preventive nursing measures to protect the patient from possible disorientation or seizures.

BLOOD (SERUM) CREATININE

Creatinine is a catabolic product of creatine, which is used in skeletal muscle contraction. The daily production of creatine, and subsequently creatinine, depends on muscle mass, which fluctuates little. Creatinine, as with BUN, is excreted entirely by the kidneys and is therefore directly proportional to renal excretory function. Thus, with normal renal excretory function, the serum creatinine level should remain constant and normal. Only renal disorders (such as glomerulonephritis, pyelonephritis, acute tubular necrosis, and urinary obstruction) cause an abnormal elevation in creatinine.

The serum creatinine test, as with BUN, is used to diagnose impaired kidney function. However, unlike BUN, the creatinine level is affected little by dehydration, malnutrition, or hepatic function. The creatinine level is interpreted in conjunction with the BUN. The acceptable serum creatinine range is 0.5 to 1.1 mg/dL (female) and 0.6 to 1.2 mg/dL (male) (Pagana & Pagana, 2008).

CREATININE CLEARANCE

Creatinine, an NPN substance, is present in blood and urine. Creatinine is generated during muscle contraction and then excreted by glomerular filtration. Levels are directly related to muscle mass and are usually measured for a 24-hour period. During the testing period, the patient avoids excessive physical activity. Draw a fasting blood sample at the onset of testing and another at the conclusion. Discard the initial specimen and start the 24-hour timing at that point. Collect all urine in the 24-hour period because any deviation will alter test results. An elevation in serum levels with a decline in urine levels indicates renal disease. Normal ranges are **serum,** 0.5 to 1.1 mg/dL (female), 0.6 to 1.2 mg/dL (male); **urine,** 87 to 107 mL/min (female), 107 to 139 mL/min (male) (Pagana & Pagana, 2008).

PROSTATE-SPECIFIC ANTIGEN

Prostate-specific antigen (PSA) is an organ-specific glycoprotein produced by normal prostatic tissue. Measurement of PSA has largely replaced that of prostatic acid phosphatase because it is a more accurate test. Test results rise with tissue manipulation; therefore obtain a blood sample before physical examination. Normal range is less than 4 ng/mL. Elevated PSA levels result from prostate cancer, benign prostatic hypertrophy (BPH), and prostatitis.

OSMOLALITY

Assessment of urine **osmolality** (the weight of the solute compared with its own weight) may be preferred over specific gravity. Plasma osmolality may be done in conjunction with the urine sampling when pituitary disorders are suspected. Results provide information on the concentrating ability of the kidney.

KIDNEY-URETER-BLADDER RADIOGRAPHY

A kidney-ureter-bladder (KUB) radiograph assesses the general status of the abdomen and the size, structure, and position of the urinary tract structures. No special preparation is necessary. Explain that the procedure involves changing position on the radiography table, which may be uncomfortably firm. Abnormal findings related to the urinary system may indicate tumors, calculi, glomerulonephritis, cysts, and other conditions.

INTRAVENOUS PYELOGRAM OR INTRAVENOUS UROGRAPHY

Intravenous pyelogram (IVP) or intravenous urography (IVU) evaluates structures of the urinary tract, filling of the renal pelvis with urine, and transport of urine via the ureters to the bladder. It is vital to determine whether the patient has an allergy to iodine (or iodine-containing foods such as iodized salt, saltwater fish, seaweed products, vegetables grown in iodine-rich soils) because it is the base of the radiopaque dye that is injected into a vein for this and other radiologic examinations. If the patient has had an allergic reaction, the physician may order administration of a corticosteroid or an antihistamine before testing or, alternatively, may order ultrasonography.

Because kidneys and ureters are positioned in the retroperitoneal space, gas and stool in the intestines interfere with radiographic visualization. Preparation usually includes eating a light supper, taking a non–gas-forming laxative, and remaining NPO 8 hours before testing. In planning the testing regimen, schedule urography before barium-based studies. When the dye is injected, the patient experiences a warm, flushing sensation and a metallic taste. During the procedure, monitor vital signs frequently. Radiographs are taken at various intervals to monitor movement of the dye. Abnormal findings may indicate structural deviations, hydronephrosis, calculi within the urinary tract, polycystic renal (kidney) disease (PKD), tumors, and other conditions.

RETROGRADE PYELOGRAPHY

Retrograde pyelography involves examination of the lower urinary tract with a cystoscope under aseptic conditions. The urologist injects radiopaque dye directly into the ureters to visualize the upper urinary tract. Urine samples can be obtained directly from the renal pelvis. Additional retrograde studies include the following:

- **Retrograde cystography:** Radiopaque dye is injected through an indwelling catheter into the urinary bladder to evaluate its structure or to determine the cause of recurrent infections.
- **Retrograde urethrography:** A catheter is inserted and dye injected as with the cystography to assess the status of the urethral structure.

VOIDING CYSTOURETHROGRAPHY

Voiding cystourethrography is used in conjunction with other diagnostic studies to detect abnormalities of the urinary bladder and the urethra. Preparation includes an enema before testing. An indwelling catheter is inserted into the urinary bladder, and dye is injected to outline the lower urinary tract. Radiographs are taken, and the catheter is then removed. The patient is asked to void while radiographs are being taken. Some patients experience embarrassment or anxiety related to the procedure and should be given the opportunity to express their feelings. Structural abnormalities, diverticula, and reflux into the ureter may be detected.

ENDOSCOPIC PROCEDURES

Endoscopic procedures are visual examinations of hollow organs using an instrument with a scope and light source. Because of the invasive nature of the procedure, informed consent is necessary, and because the procedure is most often performed in the surgical suite, preoperative preparation is indicated (see Chapter 42). The urologist performs the procedure.

Cystoscopy is a visual examination to inspect, treat, or diagnose disorders of the urinary bladder and proximal structures. Patient preparation includes a description of the procedure. Usually the procedure is carried out using a local anesthetic after the patient has been sedated. Patient safety is paramount when the patient is sedated. The patient is placed in a lithotomy position for the procedure, which may produce embarrassment and anxiety. The thought of a scope being passed while the patient is awake may intensify these feelings. Provide an opportunity for the patient to verbalize feelings.

The scope is passed under aseptic conditions after a local anesthetic is instilled into the urethra. The patient experiences a feeling of pressure as the scope is passed. Continuous fluid irrigation of the bladder is necessary to facilitate visualization. Care after the procedure includes hydration to dilute the urine. Monitor the first voiding after the procedure, assessing time, amount, color, and any **dysuria** (painful or difficult urination). The first voiding is occasionally blood tinged due to the trauma of the procedure.

The urologist can perform a brush biopsy via a ureteral catheter during a cystoscopy. A nylon brush is inserted through the catheter to obtain specimens from the renal pelvis or calyces. Nephroscopy (renal endoscopy) is done using the percutaneous (through the skin) route and provides direct visualization of the upper urinary structures. The urologist can obtain biopsy or urine specimens or remove calculi.

RENAL ANGIOGRAPHY

Renal angiography aids in evaluating blood supply to the kidneys, evaluates masses, and detects possible complications after kidney transplantation. Withhold oral intake the night before the procedure. The procedure requires the passing of a small radiopaque catheter into an artery (usually the femoral artery) to provide a port for the injection of radiopaque dye. Therefore, when the procedure is completed, have the patient lie flat in bed for several hours to minimize the risk of bleeding. Assess the puncture site for bleeding or hematoma, and maintain the pressure dressing at the site. Assess circulatory status of the involved extremity every 15 minutes for 1 hour, then every 2 hours for 24 hours.

RENAL VENOGRAM

A renal venogram provides information about the kidney's venous drainage. Access for the radiopaque catheter is the femoral vein. Monitor the patient afterward for bleeding at the puncture site.

COMPUTED TOMOGRAPHY

A computed tomography (CT) scan differentiates masses of the kidney. Images are obtained by a computer-controlled scanner. A radiopaque dye may be injected to enhance the image. A serum urea and creatinine level are obtained before use of radiopaque dye. The dye is not used if inadequate kidney function is noted. Inform the patient that the table on which he or she is placed and the machine "taking pictures" will move at intervals and that it is important to lie still. The CT body-scanning unit takes multiple cross-sectional pictures at several different sites, creating a three-dimensional map of the renal structure. The adrenals, the bladder, and the prostate may also be visualized.

MAGNETIC RESONANCE IMAGING

Magnetic resonance imaging (MRI) uses nuclear magnetic resonance as its source of energy to obtain a visual assessment of body tissues. The patient requires no special preparation other than removal of all metal objects that might be attracted by the magnet. Patients with metal prostheses (such as heart valves, orthopedic screws, or cardiac pacemakers) cannot undergo MRI.

Emphasize that the examination area will be confining and that a repetitive "pounding" sound will be heard (somewhat like the sound of a muffled jackhammer). MRI can be used for diagnoses of pathologic conditions of the renal system.

RENAL SCAN

A radionuclide tracer substance that will be taken up by renal tubular cells or excreted by the glomerular filtrate is injected intravenously. A series of computer-generated images is then made. The scan provides data related to functional parenchyma (the essential parts of an organ that are concerned with its function). No special preparation is needed. Check facility policy concerning the disposal of the patient's urine for the first 24 hours. Pregnant nurses should refrain from caring for this patient during this time.

ULTRASONOGRAPHY

Ultrasonography is a diagnostic tool that uses the reflection of sound waves to produce images of deep body structures. Inform the patient that a conducting jelly will be applied on the skin over the area to be studied; this improves the transmission of sound waves. The sound waves are high frequency and inaudible to the human ear; the waves are converted into electrical impulses that are photographed for study.

Ultrasonography can visualize size, shape, and position of the kidney and delineate any irregularities in structure. Deviations from normal findings may indicate tumor, congenital anomalies, cysts, or obstructions. No special preparations are necessary.

TRANSRECTAL ULTRASOUND

Transrectal ultrasound instrumentation of the prostate gland provides clear images of prostatic tumors that otherwise might go undiagnosed. Transrectal ultrasound–guided biopsy is performed to obtain samples of prostatic tissue from various areas with minimal discomfort to the patient.

RENAL BIOPSY

The kidney can be biopsied by an open procedure similar to other surgical procedures on the kidney or by the less invasive method of needle biopsy, also called a **percutaneous biopsy.** Tell the patient that he or she may experience pain during the procedure and should follow instructions, such as holding the breath. Bed rest is instituted for 24 hours after the procedure. Mobility is restricted to bathroom privileges for the next 24 hours, and gradual resumption of activities is allowed after 48 to 72 hours.

URODYNAMIC STUDIES

Urodynamic studies are indicated when neurologic disease is suspected of being an underlying cause of incontinence. The studies evaluate detrusor reflex. The patient may experience embarrassment and slight discomfort. During cystometrogram a catheter is inserted into the bladder, then connected to a cystometer, which measures bladder capacity and pressure. The examiner asks the patient about sensations of heat, cold, and urge to void and instructs the patient at times to void and change position.

Cholinergic and anticholinergic medications may be administered during urodynamic studies to determine their effects on bladder function. (A cholinergic drug, such as bethanechol [Urecholine], stimulates the atonic bladder; an anticholinergic drug, such as atropine, brings an overactive bladder to a more normal level or function.)

Associated testing includes rectal electromyography, which involves placement of an electrode; and urethral pressure profile, in which a special catheter connected to a transducer evaluates urethral pressures.

MEDICATION CONSIDERATIONS

The kidneys filter a wide range of water-soluble products from the blood, including medications. The kidneys' effectiveness in removing certain medications from the blood may be affected by various conditions, such as renal disease, changes in the pH of urine, and age. Patients with renal disease are given reduced dosages of medications to minimize further damage or drug toxicity. Alteration in urinary pH affects the absorption rate of certain medications. Older patients may have decreased physiologic functioning, diminishing the kidneys' capacity to excrete drugs. Diminished kidney function interferes with the filtration of water-soluble medications.

The medications included in this discussion are representative of those that directly affect the function of the kidney or are used to treat urinary disorders (Table 50-3).

DIURETICS TO ENHANCE URINARY OUTPUT

Diuretics are administered to enhance urinary output. They achieve this by increasing the kidney's filtration of sodium, chloride, and water at different sites in the kidney. Diuretics are used in the management of a variety of disorders, such as heart failure and hypertension. Diuretics are classified by chemical structure and by the site and type of action on the kidney.

Thiazide Diuretics

Thiazide diuretics act at the distal convoluted tubule to impair sodium and chloride reabsorption, leading to excretion of electrolytes and water. The thiazide diuretic chlorothiazide (Diuril) affects electrolytes to cause hypokalemia (extreme potassium depletion in blood), hyponatremia (decreased sodium concentration in blood), and/or hypercalcemia (excessive amounts of calcium in blood). Hypochloremic alkalosis occurs from a deficiency of chloride. The main uses are management of systemic edema and control of mild to moderate hypertension, although it may take a month to achieve the full antihypertensive effect. Chlorothiazide is contraindicated in anuria.

Loop (or High-Ceiling) Diuretics

Loop, or **high-ceiling, diuretics** act primarily in the ascending Henle's loop to inhibit tubular reabsorption of sodium and chloride. This group is the most potent of all diuretics and may lead to significant electrolyte depletion. These diuretics are effective for use in patients with impaired kidney function.

The loop diuretic furosemide (Lasix) affects electrolytes to cause hypokalemia, hypochloremia, hyponatremia, hypocalcemia (abnormally low blood calcium), and/or hypomagnesemia (decreased magnesium in the blood). The effect on acid-base balance is the development of hypochloremic alkalosis. Furosemide is used in nephrotic syndrome, heart failure, and pul-

Table 50-3 Medications that Affect the Urinary System

Generic (Trade)	Functional Class	Use	Special Considerations
Oxybutynin chloride (Ditropan)	Spasmolytic	Reduces bladder spasms (neurogenic bladder)	Assess voiding pattern.
Bethanechol chloride (Urecholine)	Cholinergic stimulant	Urinary bladder stimulant (urinary retention, neurogenic atony)	Assess for hypotension.
Phenazopyridine (Pyridium, Urogesic)	Nonnarcotic analgesic	Anesthetic on mucosa of urinary tract	Assess decrease in urinary symptoms. Urine may turn red-orange. Report yellowing of sclera.
Flavoxate (Urispas)	Spasmolytic	Relieves nocturia, incontinence, dysuria	Assess decrease of urinary symptoms.
Finasteride (Proscar)	Androgen hormone inhibitor	Prevents benign prostatic hyperplasia	Monitor urinary output. May cause impotence. Pregnant women should avoid handling crushed pills.
Terazosin hydrochloride (Hytrin)	Antihypertensive and benign prostatic hyperplasia agent	In benign prostatic hyperplasia, causes relaxation of smooth muscle and improves urine flow	Assess for hypotension. Assess voiding pattern.

monary edema. Side effects are those associated with rapid fluid loss: vertigo, hypotension, and possible circulatory collapse.

Potassium-Sparing Diuretics

Potassium-sparing diuretics act on the distal convoluted tubule to inhibit sodium reabsorption and potassium secretion. Potassium-sparing diuretics decrease the sodium-potassium exchange. Although the actions of these medications vary, they all conserve potassium that is usually lost with sodium in diuresis. But, because they are weak, they are usually used in combination with other diuretics. Potassium-sparing diuretics are contraindicated in patients who experience hyperkalemia, since further retention of potassium could cause a fatal cardiac dysrhythmia. There are two types of potassium-sparing diuretics: aldosterone antagonists and nonaldosterone antagonists.

The aldosterone antagonist spironolactone (Aldactone) blocks aldosterone in the distal tubule to promote potassium uptake in exchange for sodium secretion. Although it can be used in combination with other diuretics, primarily in the treatment of hypertension and edema, spironolactone is most frequently used for its potassium-sparing quality.

The nonaldosterone antagonist triamterene (Dyrenium) directly reduces ion transportation in the tubule, though it has little diuretic effect. Triamterene is instead used to help limit the potassium-wasting effect of other diuretics.

Osmotic Diuretics

Osmotic diuretics act at the proximal convoluted tubule to increase plasma osmotic pressure, causing redistribution of fluid toward the circulatory vessels. Osmotic diuretics are used to manage edema, promote systemic diuresis in cerebral edema, decrease intraocular pressure, and improve kidney function in acute renal failure (ARF). In ARF, osmotics are used to prevent irreversible failure, but they are contraindicated in advanced states of renal failure.

The osmotic diuretic mannitol (Osmitrol) increases osmolarity of glomerular filtrate; decreases reabsorption of water electrolytes; and increases urinary output, sodium, and chloride, which actually has minimal effect on acid-base balance. Mannitol is used to prevent or treat the oliguric phase of ARF, promote systemic diuresis in cerebral edema, and decrease intraocular pressure. Careful assessment of the cardiovascular system before administering mannitol is essential because of the high risk of inducing heart failure. Avoid extravasation (escape of the medication from the blood vessel into the tissues), which may lead to tissue irritation or necrosis.

Carbonic Anhydrase Inhibitor Diuretics

The **carbonic anhydrase inhibitor diuretic** acetazolamide (Diamox) interferes with the bonding of water and carbon dioxide by the enzyme carbonic anhydrase (present in red blood cells) at the proximal convoluted tubule. Although it has limited usefulness as a diuretic, acetazolamide is used to lower intraocular pressure.

Nursing Interventions

Because patients receiving diuretics often have complicated disease conditions such as heart failure and pulmonary edema, monitor for signs and symptoms of fluid overload: changes in pulse rate, respirations, cardiac sounds, and lung fields. Record daily morning weights for the patient receiving diuretics. Keep accurate intake and output (I&O) records, and document blood pressure, pulse, and respirations four times a day until the medication is regulated and the vital signs stabilize. Assess BUN, serum electrolytes, and urine as ordered. Diet instruction to the patient and the family should include a warning to avoid overuse of salt in cooking or as a table additive. A number of salt substitutes are currently on the market; however, the long-term effects of those potassium preparations are not known and could further complicate the renal patient's condition. The use of most diuretics, with the exception of the potassium-sparing diuretics, requires adding daily potassium sources (e.g., baked potatoes, raw bananas, apricots, or navel oranges). In some cases the physician orders potassium supplements to be taken with the diuretic.

When a diuretic is effective, the serum concentration of other medications may increase as a result. Carefully monitor this potentiating effect to prevent toxicity from other medications. For example, as diuretics effectively decrease the volume of extracellular fluid, the serum level of digoxin may increase proportionately, resulting in digitoxicity. Special care is required in the selection and management of diuretics in the treatment of children, adolescents, and older adults.

MEDICATIONS FOR URINARY TRACT INFECTIONS

Certain antimicrobial agents are administered primarily to treat infections within the urinary tract. The appropriate medication is selected according to Gram-stain sensitivity of the organism. Urinary antiseptics inhibit bacteria growth and are used to prevent and treat urethritis and cystitis. Caution should be used to determine if the patient is pregnant, since all of these agents have not been sufficiently tested for use during pregnancy.

Urinary antiseptics are divided into four groups: quinolones, nitrofurantoins, methenamines, and fluoroquinolones. Examples of each group follow.

Quinolone

Nalidixic acid (NegGram) is used to treat UTIs caused by gram-negative microbes (e.g., *Escherichia coli* and *Proteus mirabilis*). The common side effects are drowsiness, vertigo, weakness, nausea, and vomiting. The use of nalidixic acid is contraindicated in renal impairment.

Nitrofurantoin

Nitrofurantoin compound (Macrodantin) is effective against both gram-positive and gram-negative microbes (e.g., *Streptococcus faecalis, E. coli,* and *P. mirabilis*) in the urinary tract. Common side effects are loss of appetite, nausea, and vomiting.

Methenamine

Methenamine mandelate (Mandelamine) suppresses fungi and gram-negative and gram-positive organisms (e.g., *E. coli,* staphylococci, and enterococci). Acidification of the urine with an acid-ash diet or other acidifiers to a pH of less than 5.5 is necessary for effective action. Methenamine mandelate is used for patients with chronic, recurrent UTIs as a preventive measure after antibiotics have cleared the infection. Although side effects are rare, they include nausea, vomiting, skin rash, and urticaria (hives).

Fluoroquinolone

Norfloxacin (Noroxin) is a broad-spectrum antibiotic effective against gram-positive and gram-negative organisms (e.g., *E. coli, P. mirabilis, Pseudomonas* organisms, *Staphylococcus aureus,* and *Staphylococcus epidermidis*). It is used in the treatment of UTIs, gonorrhea, and gonococcal urethritis. It is administered with a full glass of water 1 hour before or 2 hours after meals or with antacids.

Nursing Interventions

Before administering antibiotics for UTIs, be certain to check all medications the patient is using for potential negative drug interactions. Instruct the patient to take all the medication, even though the symptoms may subside quickly. Hydrate the patient to produce daily urinary output of 2000 mL, unless contraindicated. When indicated, teach the patient to use the acid-ash diet to help maintain a urine pH of 5.5. Soothe skin irritations with cornstarch or a bath of bicarbonate of soda or dilute vinegar. Report continuing signs of infection.

Observe the patient receiving nalidixic acid for visual disturbances and offer appropriate assistance for ambulation or transfer. Monitor the patient receiving nitrofurantoin for signs of allergic response (such as erythema, chills, fever, and dyspnea). If these signs or symptoms develop, discontinue the medication and notify the physician (trial doses of this medication may be used to detect possible allergic reaction before administering full dosage).

NUTRITIONAL CONSIDERATIONS

The nutritional needs of the patient with a urinary tract disorder vary with each disease process. Some general guidelines include provision of food choices and number of servings as recommended by the U.S. Department of Agriculture's MyPyramid nutrition planning tool (www.mypyramid.gov) and daily intake of 2000 mL of water, unless contraindicated. Unique nutritional requirements are discussed with each disorder. Box 50-2 gives an example of dietary modifications for urinary lithiasis. Patients with other systemic diseases, such as diabetes mellitus, require strict adherence to those restrictions as well.

Box 50-2 Acid-Ash and Alkaline-Ash Foods

ACID-ASH FOODS*
Meat, whole grains, eggs, cheese, cranberries, prunes, and plums

ALKALINE-ASH FOODS
Milk, vegetables, fruits (except cranberries, prunes, and plums)

*Acid-ash diets should be supplemented with vitamins C and A and folic acid.

MAINTAINING ADEQUATE URINARY DRAINAGE

Urine clears the body of waste materials and helps balance electrolytes. Conditions that interfere with urinary drainage may create a health crisis. Therefore it is important to reestablish urine flow as soon as possible to prevent the buildup of toxins in the bloodstream. Patients at risk for difficulty with urine elimination include those who have undergone surgical procedures of the bladder, the prostate, or the vagina; patients with primary urologic problems, such as urethral stricture; and those who are critically ill with multisystem problems.

Urinary catheters are used to maintain urine flow, to divert urine flow to facilitate healing postoperatively, to introduce medications by irrigation, and to dilate or prevent narrowing of some portions of the urinary tract. Catheters may be used for intermittent or continuous urinary drainage. Urinary catheters may be introduced into the bladder, the ureter, or the kidney. The type and size of urinary catheter are determined by the location and cause of the urinary tract problem. Catheters are measured by the French (F) system. Urethral catheters range from 14 to 24 F for adult patients. Ureteral catheters are usually 4 to 6 F. The physician always inserts ureteral catheters, whereas the nurse usually inserts indwelling urethral catheters.

TYPES OF CATHETERS

Different types of catheters are used for different purposes (Figure 50-6). The **coudé catheter** has a tapered tip and is selected for ease of insertion when enlargement of the prostate gland is suspected. The coudé catheter is less traumatic during insertion because it is stiffer and more easily controlled than the straight-tip catheter (Potter & Perry, 2009). The **Foley catheter** has

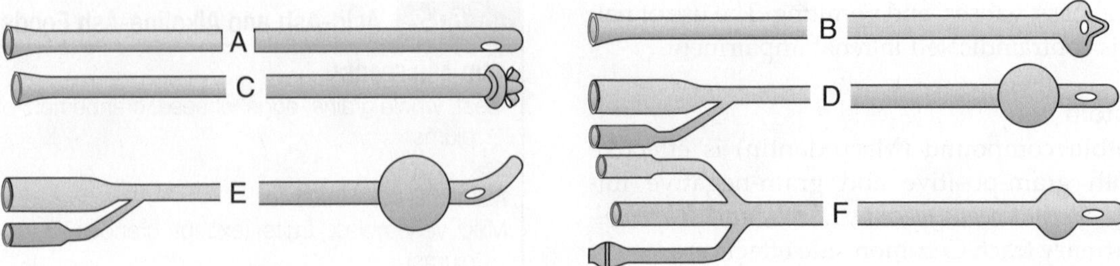

FIGURE 50-6 Commonly used catheters. **A,** Simple urethral catheter. **B,** Mushroom or de Pezzer (can be used for suprapubic catheterization). **C,** Winged-tip or Malecot. **D,** Indwelling with inflated balloon. **E,** Indwelling with coudé tip. **F,** Three-way indwelling (the third lumen is used for irrigation of the bladder).

a balloon near its tip that may be inflated after insertion, holding the catheter in the urinary bladder for continuous drainage. **Malecot** and **de Pezzer,** or **mushroom, catheters** are used to drain urine from the renal pelvis of the kidney. The **Robinson catheter** has multiple openings in its tip to facilitate intermittent drainage. **Ureteral catheters** are long and slender to pass into the ureters. The **whistle-tip catheter** has a slanted, larger orifice at its tip to be used if there is blood in the urine. The **cystostomy, vesicostomy,** or **suprapubic catheter** is introduced by the physician through the abdominal wall above the symphysis pubis. This catheter diverts urine flow from the urethra as needed to treat injury to the bony pelvis, the urinary tract, or surrounding organs; strictures; or obstruction. The catheter is inserted via surgical incision or puncture of the abdominal and bladder walls with a trocar cannula. The catheter is connected to a sterile closed drainage system and secured to avoid accidental removal; the wound is covered with a sterile dressing. When the lower urinary tract has healed, the patient's ability to void is tested by clamping the catheter so the patient can try to void naturally. When the measured residual urine is consistently less than 50 mL, the catheter is usually removed and a sterile dressing is placed over the wound.

An **external (Texas** or **condom)** catheter is not actually a catheter but rather a drainage system connected to the external male genitalia. This noninvasive appliance is used for the incontinent male to minimize skin irritation from urine and to reduce risk of infection from an indwelling catheter. The appliance is removed daily for cleansing and inspecting the skin. Use of the external catheter allows the patient to have a more normal lifestyle.

NURSING INTERVENTIONS AND PATIENT TEACHING

Problems of the urinary tract may be indicative of a primary disorder or may be one of multiple symptoms of complex, chronic disease. Therefore it is important to assess urinary elimination at the time of admission. Because of embarrassment and sociocultural taboos, some patients may be reluctant to share information with the nurse. Often the medical system intensifies this discomfort by repeatedly asking the patient to describe the problem to staff in the laboratory, radiology, and other departments. Discretion during the admission interview and health assessment with strict adherence to Health Insurance Portability and Accountability Act standards enhance patient privacy and comfort.

Nursing interventions for the patient with a urinary drainage system involve a number of principles to prevent and detect infection and trauma:

1. Follow aseptic technique to avoid introducing microorganisms from the environment. Never rest the collecting bag on the floor.
2. Record I&O. For precision monitoring, such as hourly urinary output, add a urometer to the drainage system. If urinary output falls below 50 mL/hr, check the drainage system for proper placement and function before contacting the physician.
3. Adequately hydrate the patient to flush the urinary tract.
4. Do not open the drainage system after it is in place except to irrigate the catheter, and then only with physician orders. It is important to maintain a closed system to prevent UTIs.
5. Perform catheter care twice daily and as needed, using standard precautions. Each institution has a specific protocol for catheter care. Cleanse the perineum with mild soap and warm water, rinse well, and pat dry. At times an antiseptic solution or ointment may be ordered to use at the catheter incision site.
6. Check the drainage system daily for leaks.
7. Avoid placement of the urinary drainage bag above the level of the catheter insertion, which would cause urine to reenter the drainage system and contaminate the urinary tract.
8. Prevent tension on the system or backflow of urine while transferring the patient.
9. Ambulate the patient if possible to facilitate urine flow. If the patient's activity must be restricted, turn and reposition every 1½ hours.
10. Avoid kinks or compression of the drainage tube that may cause pooling of the urine within the urinary tract. Gently coil excess tubing, secure with a clamp or pin to avoid dislodging the catheter, and release the tubing before transferring or repositioning the patient.

11. Gently inspect the catheter entry site for blood or exudate that may indicate trauma or infection. Observe the color and composition of the urine for blood or sediment. During drainage of the collection bag, note the presence of malodor.
12. Collect specimens from the catheter by cleansing the drainage port with alcohol, then withdrawing the urine using a sterile adapter and a sterile 10-mL syringe, using standard precautions. Send the urine specimen immediately to the laboratory.
13. Report and record assessment findings and interventions initiated.

After the urinary catheter is removed, the patient may experience difficulty voiding until bladder tone and sensation return. If the patient complains of urinary retention, stimulate urination by running water, placing the patient's hands in water, or pouring water over the perineum. With the last method, subtract the amount of water used in calculating the correct amount voided. If the patient's condition permits, a woman can sit on a bathroom stool or commode, and a male can stand, to void.

The patient may experience some dribbling of urine after voiding as a result of dilation of the sphincter from the catheter. Record the time, amount, and color of the urinary output.

Nursing diagnoses and interventions for the patient with a urinary catheter include but are not limited to the following:

Nursing Diagnoses	Nursing Interventions
Risk for trauma, related to insertion and maintenance of the catheter	Maintain sterile technique during insertion. Use smallest size catheter possible. Lubricate catheter. Secure catheter to leg, as appropriate. Provide adequate fluids. Administer urinary analgesic as ordered. Allow enough slack in tubing for patient to move about freely while in bed. Inspect insertion site to determine if area is clean and without signs of possible infection or bleeding.
Risk for infection, related to invasive use of catheter	Use aseptic technique and meticulous catheter care. Maintain closed urinary drainage system. Avoid placement of drainage bag above level of catheter insertion (meatus). Avoid reflux of urine. Encourage adequate fluid intake. Administer antimicrobials as ordered. Monitor patient's temperature and the color, odor, and clarity of urine.

Instruct the patient about proper transfer from bed, chair, or stretcher and the principles of catheter care. Encourage fluid intake to flush the urinary system.

Self-Catheterization

Self-catheterization may be the intervention of choice for the patient who experiences spinal cord injury or other neurologic disorders that interfere with urinary elimination. Intermittent self-catheterization promotes independent function. At home there is less risk of cross-contamination than in the hospital, so the catheterization procedure can be safely modified as a clean technique. Still, instruct the patient using strict surgical asepsis in the hospital because of the risk of infection there. Emphasize the need for the patient to be alert for signs and symptoms of infection and to have periodic evaluations by the physician. Follow institutional guidelines for catheter insertion.

Bladder Training

Bladder training involves developing the muscles of the perineum to improve voluntary control over voiding; bladder training may be modified for different problems. In preparation for removal of a urethral catheter, the physician may order a clamp-unclamp routine to improve bladder tone. A patient with stress incontinence can learn to control leakage by performing **Kegel,** or **pubococcygeal, exercises** that tighten the muscles of the perineal floor. The patient can develop awareness of the appropriate muscle group by trying to stop the flow of urine during voiding. Once the patient has identified the correct muscles and the feeling of their contraction, direct her to tighten the muscles of the perineum, hold that tension for 10 seconds, then relax for 10 seconds. The exercises should be done initially in groups of 10, building to groups of 20, four times a day. Because muscle control develops gradually, it may take 4 to 6 weeks to learn to control leakage.

For habit training, establish a voiding schedule. Monitor the patient's voiding for a few days to identify patterns, or schedule voiding times to correlate with the patient's activities. Typical voiding times are on arising, before each meal, and at bedtime. Help the patient void as scheduled. After a few days, evaluate whether the scheduled voiding pattern keeps the patient continent. Modify the schedule until continence is established. Fluid intake and medications may influence voiding patterns (e.g., the patient may need to void 30 minutes after ingesting coffee or furosemide in response to the diuretic effect). Reduction of fluid intake before bedtime may help keep the patient dry during sleep.

PROGNOSIS

The outcome for patients with urinary disorders depends on many variables: age, preexisting health conditions, general health status, complications, compliance, and available family and community support.

DISORDERS OF THE URINARY SYSTEM

ALTERATIONS IN VOIDING PATTERNS

URINARY RETENTION

Etiology and Pathophysiology

Urinary **retention** is the inability to void even with an urge to void. It may be acute or chronic. The patient may not be able to empty the bladder, creating urinary stasis and increasing the possibility of infection.

Urinary retention has a variety of causes: a response to stress; interference with the sphincter muscles during surgery to the perineum; occlusion of the urethra by calculi, infection, or tumor; medication side effects; or perineal trauma secondary to vaginal delivery. With chronic urinary retention the bladder capacity may be exceeded and the urine may overflow the bladder, causing incontinence.

Clinical Manifestations

The signs and symptoms of urinary retention are sometimes vague and easily overlooked. The bladder becomes increasingly distended and may be palpated above the symphysis pubis. Urinary retention may cause the patient considerable discomfort and anxiety.

Assessment

Subjective data include patient complaints of frequency with or without symptoms of burning, urgency, nocturia, and occasionally acute discomfort. Initial symptoms may not seem to be directly associated with urinary retention.

Collection of **objective data** includes assessing urinary bladder distention (palpable ovoid [egg-shaped] bladder arising suprapubically). The patient may void frequently, void small amounts, and have episodes of incontinence. Patients with diminished sensorium, as from spinal cord injury or organic brain disorder, may be restless and irritable without direct complaints about difficulty voiding.

Medical Management

Mechanical methods, such as the use of urinary catheters or the surgical release of obstructions, may be needed to treat urinary retention. Administer urinary analgesics and antispasmodics as prescribed to enhance patient relaxation and comfort.

Nursing Interventions

The primary goal of nursing interventions is the reinstitution of normal voiding patterns. Regardless of the pathologic findings and medical intervention, the nurse can help the patient achieve adequate voiding by providing a private, relaxed environment. Bladder training approaches may assist the patient in emptying the bladder. Warm showers or sitz baths may promote relaxation of the abdominal, gluteal, and sphincter muscles. Provide warm beverages to help the patient relax. If possible, permit the patient whatever position is preferred for voiding: for women, sitting on a commode or bathroom stool is best; for men, standing may be more natural.

When continence is established, the patient may be catheterized intermittently to determine whether the bladder is emptying. Have the patient void and measure the amount. Catheterize the patient immediately after the voiding and measure the amount. The amount retained in the bladder is **residual urine** and should be less than 50 mL. If the underlying pathologic condition remains unchanged, this patient may be at risk for again developing retention. Teach the patient or primary caretaker to observe for signs and symptoms of urinary retention and to notify the physician immediately if they return.

A nursing diagnosis and interventions for the patient with urinary retention include but are not limited to the following:

Nursing Diagnosis	Nursing Interventions
Impaired urinary elimination, related to: • sensory or motor impairment • neuromuscular impairment • mechanical trauma	Establish urinary drainage. Develop a voiding schedule. Teach the patient Kegel exercises. Assist with skin care. Suggest use of protective clothing. Engage patient in social activities. Teach importance of adequate fluid intake. Ensure that patient verbalizes an understanding of factors that alter urinary pattern.

URINARY INCONTINENCE

Urinary incontinence (UI) may be the most common health problem in women. Although stress incontinence is not the only cause of UI, it is the one most frequently mentioned. Stress incontinence is the involuntary loss of urine during physical exertion or when coughing, sneezing, or laughing. Because of embarrassment, stress UI may be underreported, and thus its sociologic and economic influence is impossible to assess. However, UI is a major reason older adults are admitted to long-term care facilities.

Etiology and Pathophysiology

UI is the involuntary loss of urine from the bladder. The patient may be totally incontinent, have dribbling, or experience leakage while lifting or sneezing (stress incontinence). Incontinence may arise as a complication of many disorders, such as UTI, loss of sphincter control, or sudden change of pressure within the abdomen. Incontinence may be permanent, as with spinal cord trauma, or temporary, as with pregnancy. Women with weakened structures of the pelvic floor are prone to stress incontinence. Although incontinence may occur at any age, loss of control of urination is a particular problem for older adults (see Evidence-Based Practice box).

Physical exertion such as heavy lifting, jobs that require long periods of standing, and high-impact sports may increase an individual's risk for UI. UI may also result from physiologic conditions such as obesity, chronic lung disease, smoking, pelvic floor injury, and surgery. Lack of estrogen in postmenopausal women contributes to atrophy of the vaginal and urethral walls with subsequent loss of muscle tone that may result in postvoiding urine retention and possible prolapse of the bladder.

Clinical Manifestations

The cardinal sign of UI is the involuntary loss of urine, which may or may not be the primary reason the patient seeks treatment.

Assessment

Subjective data include information concerning the patient's inability to control the urine. A woman may complain of urine leaking when she coughs, sneezes, lifts heavy objects, or has intercourse.

Collection of **objective data** requires alertness for clues that the patient is experiencing difficulty controlling the flow of urine. Follow the assessment guidelines to clarify the patient's complaints. Although more common in women, UI is a common symptom for men who have BPH and should be included in the assessment.

Medical Management

The management of incontinence depends on the underlying cause. If the problem arises from a disorder within the neck of the bladder, surgical repair may be necessary. Stress incontinence related to sphincter weakness may be treated with collagen implant injections. The patient may require temporary or permanent urinary diversion or management with an indwelling catheter. New appliances and drugs on the market are being used for the control of UI.

The incontinence pessary, which is inserted into the vagina to support the bladder, may help manage episodes of stress incontinence in some women. Close-fitting absorbent pads may be effective in managing mild leakage.

Management of stress incontinence should include behavior modification, pelvic floor muscle therapies, medications, and mechanical devices before resorting to surgical procedures. If these strategies are not effective, surgical interventions offer other treatment options. One procedure is the transvaginal tape sling procedure. The surgeon passes a permanent polypropylene mesh tape, covered by a protective plastic sheath with stainless steel needles attached at each end, through a small incision in the anterior vaginal wall. The U-shaped sling supports the urethra during stress and increased intraabdominal pressure during routine activities. This procedure is not without difficulties. Careful patient teaching is important before any surgical treatment.

Evidence-Based Practice

The majority of older adults have bladder control, but changes due to aging, chronic diseases, and related conditions place them at risk for bladder control problems, especially urinary incontinence and/or frequency. Many persons do not seek treatment because of embarrassment or the mistaken belief that there is no treatment available. In this research study nurses wanted to determine the educational needs of older adults. Focus groups were held in senior centers, churches, and in senior apartment buildings. Questions that guided the discussion included items related to general health and specific questions related to bladder control issues. After the discussion session, the nurses showed the groups a self-help video that included causes of urinary incontinence, treatment, and prevention strategies. The results of the study demonstrated that given the opportunity, older adults will discuss their concerns about bladder control and are willing to learn methods of control.

Although the participants in the focus groups were mainly active older adults in an urban setting, the information gathered was helpful as a starting point for designing educational programs for that population. The participant groups included both men and women and were diverse in ethnicity and race.

Application to Nursing Practice

- Incontinence and/or frequency are experienced by adults of all ages, ethnicities, educational levels, economic status, and health status.
- Many adults wrongly believe that urinary incontinence and/or frequency are an expected part of the aging process and that there are no treatments available.
- Older adults of culturally diverse backgrounds are willing to discuss bladder control issues with nurses.
- Older adults are receptive to different forms of education and are interested in learning.

Reference

Palmer, M.H., & Newman, D.K. (2006). Bladder control: educational needs of older adults, *J Gerontol Nurs, 32*(1), 28.

From Potter, P.A., & Perry, A.G. (2009). *Fundamentals of nursing: concepts, process, and practice.* (7th ed.). St. Louis: Mosby.

Estrogen replacement for the treatment of UI is controversial and its reported effectiveness varies. Topical administration of prednisone and estrogen may help restore turgor and elasticity of the vaginal submucosa. Transdermal oxybutynin (Oxytrol) is effective in reducing the symptoms of an overactive bladder with few side effects. A new self-catheterization system, the Self-Cath Closed System, is available for patients who must maintain intermittent self-catheterization. It is designed for patient convenience and minimization of bacterial contamination. An artificial urinary sphincter is a surgical option to reestablish continence, though there is controversy over its use.

Nursing Interventions

The incontinent patient may reduce fluid intake to decrease voiding, but without adequate fluids, urine may become more concentrated, irritating the bladder mucosa and increasing the urge to urinate. Teach the patient bladder training exercises to improve the tone of the perineal muscles. For the female patient, Kegel exercises are helpful; 10 repetitions, 5 to 10 times a day is suggested to improve muscle tone. Establish a 2-hour schedule for the patient to go to the bathroom. Once continence has been achieved, the goal may be raised to 3 hours.

Incontinence pads of different absorbancy are available in most grocery stores and pharmacies. They can increase the patient's confidence to participate in social activities. Use of protective undergarments may help keep the patient and the patient's clothing dry.

Alcoholic and caffeinated drinks stimulate urgency and urination; advise the patient not to drink too much liquid just before bedtime.

Many patients who are incontinent have low self-esteem. Be supportive by listening, encouraging the patient to express feelings, and providing kind reassurances. Never scold.

NEUROGENIC BLADDER

Etiology and Pathophysiology

Neurogenic bladder means the loss of voluntary voiding control, resulting in urinary retention or incontinence. Neurogenic bladder is caused by a lesion of the nervous system that interferes with normal nerve conduction to the urinary bladder. The lesion may be caused by a congenital anomaly (e.g., spina bifida), a neurologic disease (e.g., multiple sclerosis), or trauma (as in spinal cord injury). The two types of neurogenic bladder are **spastic** and **flaccid.**

Spastic (reflex or automatic) bladder is caused by a lesion above the voiding reflex arc (upper motor neuron) that results in a loss of the urge to void and a loss of motor control. The bladder wall atrophies, decreasing bladder capacity. Urine is released on reflex, with little or no conscious control.

A flaccid (atonic, nonreflex) bladder, caused by a lesion of a lower motor neuron, continues to fill and distend, with pooling of urine and incomplete emptying. Because of the accompanying loss of sensation, the patient may not experience discomfort that would indicate retention.

Clinical Manifestations

Identification of the disease process is the first step in assessing the potential problem of neurogenic bladder. Prevention of complications is a major concern; infection occurs from urinary stasis and repeated catheterization. Retention of urine may lead to backup of urine (reflux) into the upper urinary tract and to the distention of the structures of the urinary tract.

Assessment

Subjective data include patient complaints of diaphoresis, flushing and nausea before reflex incontinence, or infrequent voiding.

Collection of **objective data** involves investigating the urinary status of the patient at risk for neurogenic bladder; this includes patients with a congenital anomaly, a neurologic disease, or a spinal cord injury. The patient with a spastic bladder experiences UI, whereas the patient with a flaccid bladder describes infrequent voiding.

Diagnostic Tests

To assess the type and extent of damage to the urinary tract, chemistry studies monitor change in BUN and creatinine levels. Radiographic studies outline structural changes that occur.

Medical Management

Closely monitor patients identified as at risk for neurogenic bladder. Assess urinary function early in the course of treatment, and give antibiotics to treat signs of infection. The patient is aided by the use of parasympathomimetic medication (e.g., bethanechol) to increase the bladder's contractility. The patient may need to use intermittent self-catheterization or a urinary collection system if continence is not achieved.

Sacral Nerve Modulation (Sacral Neuromodulation) and Stimulation

A number of electronic devices to modulate nerve impulses are being used experimentally and in clinical practice for treating various bladder problems: urinary frequency, urgency, incontinence, chronic pain, and interstitial cystitis (IC).

Sacral nerve stimulation for urinary urge incontinence is the use of a permanently implantable electrical stimulation device to change neuronal activity in the sacral efferent and afferent nerves to reduce urinary urge incontinence. The Interstim device, marketed by Medtronic Inc., delivers continuous low-level electrical impulses to the bladder and urethral sphincters via the sacral nerve. It corrects UI by modulating the neural reflexes, reducing stimulation to an overactive bladder, or boosting stimulation to an underactive one. The action of the impulses is unknown.

Four electrodes are connected to a battery-operated generator. The wire is inserted into the sacral foramen through a 2-cm incision. The end of the wire is tunneled across subcutaneous tissue, exits on the patient's back, and is connected to a temporary generator attached to the outside of the body. The patient tests this temporary implant for 1 to 2 weeks. If the patient achieves 50% continence, a permanent implant is put in place.

Nursing Interventions and Patient Teaching

The management goal for the patient with neurogenic bladder is to establish urinary elimination and prevent complications. Because neurologic function is disturbed, it may not be possible to reinstate normal voiding. The patient with a spastic bladder may be placed on a bladder training program, with self-stimulation used every 2 hours to empty the bladder: The patient tries to initiate voiding using bladder compressions by applying pressure to the abdomen suprapubically or by digital stimulation of the anal sphincter. Residual urine is then measured by catheterization. As the patient becomes more proficient in emptying the bladder, the time between catheterizations is increased until voiding is independent. It is important to educate the patient to be alert for signs of the bladder becoming distended.

Management of the patient with a flaccid bladder is similar. Place the patient on a 2-hour voiding schedule for bladder training. Issues of self-esteem are crucial for this patient to remain in social settings. Provide a supportive, sensitive environment for the patient to discuss ways to adapt to an altered self-image.

INFLAMMATORY AND INFECTIOUS DISORDERS OF THE URINARY SYSTEM

URINARY TRACT INFECTIONS

A UTI is the presence of microorganisms in any urinary system structure. **Bacteriuria** (bacteria in the urine) is the most common of all nosocomial infections; most are associated with the use of urinary catheters. UTIs are common in older patients, related to bladder obstruction, insufficient bladder emptying, decreased bactericidal secretions of the prostate, and increased perineal soiling in women. Immobility, sensory impairment, and multiple organ impairment may increase the chances of infection in older adults. Women are more susceptible to UTIs than men because the urethra is short and proximal to the vagina and rectum.

Etiology and Pathophysiology

UTIs are caused by pathogens that enter the urinary tract, with or without symptoms. Normally the flushing of the urinary tract with urine is sufficient to wash away pathogens. However, some conditions interfere with this process; urinary obstruction, neurogenic bladder, ureterovesical or urethrovesical reflux, sexual intercourse, and catheterization may introduce bacteria into the urinary system. Many chronic health problems predispose the patient to a UTI: diabetes mellitus, multiple sclerosis, spinal cord injuries, hypertension, and renal diseases.

Changes in urinary tract homeostasis allow the concentration of bacteria and increase the risk of infection. The patient with a compromised immune system does not seem to be predisposed to UTI infections, but once the infection is established, that patient has difficulty recovering. Infections of the lower urinary tract increase the risk of infection of the upper urinary tract, especially if untreated.

Gram-negative microorganisms that commonly infect the urinary tract (e.g., *E. coli* and *Klebsiella, Proteus,* or *Pseudomonas* organisms) are usually from the gastrointestinal tract and ascend through the urinary meatus. Normally the body's defenses keep infections in check and clear them from the system before signs and symptoms appear. If there is incomplete emptying of the bladder or reflux of urine, the retained urine supports growth of bacteria.

Clinical Manifestations

The common signs and symptoms associated with UTI are urgency, frequency, burning on urination, and microscopic to gross (visible without aid of microscope) hematuria. UTIs are identified by the location of the infection: urethritis (urethra), cystitis (urinary bladder), pyelonephritis (kidney), and prostatitis (prostate gland). Infections of the bladder are said to be *lower* UTIs, whereas infections of the kidneys are *upper* UTIs.

Assessment

Subjective data include patient complaints of pain or burning on urination, urgency, frequency, and **nocturia** (excessive urination at night). The patient may also have related **asthenia** (a general feeling of tiredness and listlessness). Abdominal discomfort, perineal pain, or back pain may be present, depending on the extent of the disease process and site of infection.

Collection of **objective data** involves palpation of the lower abdomen, which may produce discomfort over the urinary bladder. Urine may be cloudy or blood tinged.

Diagnostic Tests

Urine culture and bacteriologic tests confirm the diagnosis. For patients with recurrent UTIs or systemic disease, more detailed urologic studies, such as an IVP and a voiding cystogram, are completed to assess the extent of involvement and damage to the structures of the urinary tract. Microscopic inspection of the urine often reveals bacteria, **hematuria** (blood in the urine), and **pyuria** (pus in the urine). Prostatitis is confirmed by patient history and culture of prostatic fluid or tissue.

Medical Management

The goal of medical management is to eliminate bacteria from the urinary tract, thereby relieving symptoms, preventing damage to renal structures, and preventing spread of infection to other body systems. The physician prescribes antiinfective medications in either oral or parenteral single or multiple doses, depending on the severity of the infection, microbial sensitivity, cost, and patient tolerance. Urinary antiseptics, such as methenamine mandelate, may be used prophylactically in recurrent infections. Some of these medications are instilled directly into the bladder. If the infection is complicated by obstruction, that obstruction should be removed. For neurogenic bladder or other retention, intermittent catheterization permits urinary drainage (see Complementary & Alternative Therapies box).

Nursing Interventions

Nursing interventions should be supportive, with patient education for adequate hydration and hygiene. Because these infections tend to recur or persist, patient education must include early detection. Comfort measures include a regimen of antiinfective agents, urinary analgesics (e.g., phenazopyridine [Pyridium]), adequate fluid intake, and perineal care. If treatment is effective, the patient should receive relief quickly. Infection may spread from the urinary system to other parts of the body. **Urosepsis** is septic poisoning due to retention and absorption of urinary products in the tissues.

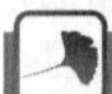 Complementary & Alternative Therapies

Urinary Disorders

- Cranberry (Cranberry Plus, Ultra Cranberry) has been used to prevent urinary tract infections (UTIs), particularly in women prone to recurrent infection. It has also been used to treat acute UTI. Monitor patients for lack of therapeutic effect.
- Echinacea stimulates the immune system and treats UTI. Patients with human immunodeficiency virus infections, including acquired immunodeficiency syndrome, tuberculosis, collagen disease, multiple sclerosis, or other autoimmune disease, should avoid use. Echinacea should not be used in place of antibiotic therapy.
- Sea holly *(Eryngium campestre)* aboveground plant parts have a mild diuretic effect. Roots have an antispasmodic effect. Aboveground parts are used in UTI and prostatitis; roots are used to treat kidney and bladder calculi, renal colic, kidney and urinary tract inflammation, and urinary retention.
- Nettle *(Urtica dioica)* is currently being investigated as an irrigation for the urinary tract and also to treat benign prostatic hypertrophy. Patients with fluid retention caused by reduced cardiac or renal activity should not use this herb.
- Caffeine increases urine production.
- Some believe that acupuncture applied to the abdominal meridian may help relieve cystitis.
- Some advocate massage with diluted rosemary, juniper, or lavender to aid in relieving pain associated with cystitis.

Because of the high incidence of nosocomial UTIs, regular staff in service review of basic procedures for catheter insertion and maintenance is important. Patient education for those who practice self-catheterization should include return demonstration to evaluate the success of maintaining clean technique.

URETHRITIS

Etiology and Pathophysiology

Urethritis, inflammation of the urethra, is classified by the presence or absence of gonorrhea. Nongonorrheal urethritis is called **nonspecific urethritis (NSU).** NSU may be caused by candidal or trichomonal infections in women. Bacteria are present normally in the urethra but do not cause problems unless the integrity of the mucous membrane or tissues is interrupted, as when a catheter is in place or trauma has occurred.

Clinical Manifestations

The clinical manifestations include inflammation of the urethra with pus formation in the mucus-forming glands within the urethral lining. With gonorrheal urethritis, acute infection of the mucous membrane of the urethra causes a purulent exudate from the meatus; the patient feels discomfort, frequency, and burning on urination.

Assessment

Subjective data vary, since the patient may be asymptomatic or may complain of dysuria, urethral pruritus, and urethral discharge. Women may complain of vaginal discharge or vulvar irritation.

Collection of **objective data** includes light palpation of the lower abdomen, which may produce discomfort over the urinary bladder. Inspection of the urethra may reveal purulent exudates or inflammation. Culture and sensitivity may be ordered; follow the institution's procedure.

Diagnostic Tests

Diagnostic tests are usually limited to a Gram stain of the exudate to identify the pathogen.

Medical Management

The first step in medical management is prevention of injury to the urethra during catheterization or sexual intercourse. Treatment is based on identifying and treating the cause and providing symptomatic relief. Drugs that may be prescribed are sulfamethoxazole-trimethoprim (Bactrim, Septra), metronidazole (Flagyl), clotrimazole (Mycelex), and nystatin (Mycostatin). Comfort measures include antibiotics, adequate fluid intake to flush the system, warm sitz baths, and special care of the perineum using clean technique.

Patients with continuous catheter drainage use either a bedside bag or a leg bag for urine collection. Studies are under way to test a drainage system designed with the bag worn around the waist. This experimental drainage system can be maintained closed for 24 hours and offers improvements in ambulation, activities of daily living (ADLs), and social and mental well-being.

Nursing Interventions

Nursing interventions focus on patient education: Avoid sexual activity until the infection clears; take all medications, especially antibiotics, to ensure the infection is resolved; and use condoms for protection from reinfection. Instruct patients with sexually transmitted urethritis to refer their sexual partners for evaluation and testing if they had sexual contact in the 60 days preceding onset of the patient's symptoms or diagnosis.

CYSTITIS

Etiology and Pathophysiology

Cystitis is an inflammation of the wall of the urinary bladder, usually caused by urethrovesical reflux, introduction of a catheter or similar instrument, or contamination from feces. The most common microorganism causing acute cystitis is *E. coli.* Cystitis is most common in women because of the ease of entrance of pathogens through the short urethra, even during voiding. Conflicting data exist about the role of bubble baths, clothing, and hygiene in increasing the risk of cystitis in women. Cystitis in men usually occurs secondary to another infection, such as prostatitis or epididymitis (see Safety Alert box).

Clinical Manifestations

The common signs and symptoms associated with cystitis are dysuria, urinary frequency, and pyuria.

Assessment

Collection of **subjective data** includes assessment of the lower abdomen, which may produce discomfort over the urinary bladder. Patient complaints include burning on urination, dysuria, frequency, urgency, and nocturia.

Collection of **objective data** includes a clean-catch or catheterized urinalysis with culture and sensitivity to aid in confirming the diagnosis and in determining the appropriate treatment.

> **! Safety Alert!**
>
> **Cystitis**
>
> - Teach the woman to cleanse the perineal area anteriorly to posteriorly to prevent contamination of pathogens (especially *E. coli*) from the rectum to the short urethra.
> - Encourage drinking 2000 mL of liquids per day unless contraindicated.
> - Instruct the patient to take all the prescribed medications even though symptoms may subside quickly.
> - Instruct the patient about early detection and testing with Chemstrip LN.

Diagnostic Tests

Microscopic inspection of the urine often reveals bacteria and hematuria. A voiding cystogram may be used to identify reflux of urine into the bladder. Diagnosis is confirmed by a clean-catch, midstream urinalysis that reveals a bacterial count greater than 100,000 organisms/mL.

Medical Management

For cystitis without the complications of obstruction or other underlying pathologic conditions, medical management consists of short-term therapy with an antiinfective agent. If the treatment is effective, the patient should receive relief quickly. A repeat urinalysis 1 to 3 days after initiation of the medication confirms the effectiveness of the intervention.

Nursing Interventions and Patient Teaching

Nursing interventions focus on teaching that these infections tend to recur by either reinfection or persistent infection. Encourage the patient to drink 2000 mL of fluid per day. Record accurate I&O. Include early detection in the teaching. Long-term prophylaxis with low doses of medication may be necessary. A simple urine test, Chemstrip LN, allows the patient to test the urine at the first sign of infection and to call the physician for a prescription.

Prognosis

Successful treatment depends on the patient's ability to adequately flush the urinary tract and completion of the antibiotics prescribed.

INTERSTITIAL CYSTITIS

Etiology and Pathophysiology

IC is a chronic pelvic pain disorder with recurring discomfort or pain in the urinary bladder and surrounding region. It mostly affects middle-age white women. The pathophysiology is unknown, but bacteria do not trigger it. Instead, it seems to be caused by a breech in the bladder's protective mucosal lining that allows urine to seep through to the bladder wall, resulting in pain, inflammation, and small vessel bleeding. The bladder wall is infiltrated by inflammatory cells, resulting in ulceration and scarring of the mucosa, spasm of the detrusor muscle, hematuria, urgency, frequency, and pain on urination.

If a patient has signs and symptoms of a UTI but no bacteriuria, pyuria, or positive urine culture, IC is suspected. Other disorders that produce signs and symptoms similar to those of IC (such as UTI or endometriosis) must be excluded (Lewis et al., 2007). Small bleeding sites may be visualized via endoscopy.

ADLs and personal relationships may be disrupted by voiding patterns; some patients report voiding 60 times a day. IC can affect people of any age or gender, but most patients are women with a median age of 40 years.

Clinical Manifestations

The common signs and symptoms associated with IC are similar to those of cystitis: dysuria, urinary frequency, and microscopic bleeding. IC is characterized by urinary frequency, urgency, suprapubic pain, and dyspareunia (an abnormal pain during sexual intercourse); it is often associated with fibromyalgia and irritable bowel syndrome. Autoimmune, allergic, and infectious etiologies are being studied (Janos & Higgins, 2007).

Assessment

Subjective data include complaints of discomfort over the urinary bladder, dysuria, frequency, urgency, and nocturia.

Collection of **objective data** includes assessment of the lower abdomen, which may produce discomfort over the urinary bladder and the lower quadrants of the abdomen. A clean-catch midstream sample for urinalysis is used to rule out infection. Cystoscopy and tissue biopsy are used to establish a differential diagnosis.

Medical Management

IC is difficult to treat. Medications are prescribed for pain relief and inflammation, including low-dose cyclosporine (Neoral, Sandimmune), doxycycline (Vibramycin), and pentosan polysulfate sodium (Elmiron) (Page et al., 2005).

Amitriptyline (Elavil) and nortriptyline (Aventyl) are two antidepressants that reduce the burning pain and frequency of urination. The only oral medication approved by the FDA to treat the pain or discomfort of IC is pentosan. It improves the bladder's protective mucosal layer and relieves pain from IC by decreasing the irritative effects of urine on the bladder wall. It takes between 4 weeks to 3 months for significant improvement to occur (Page et al., 2005). For immediate relief, a brief course of opioid analgesics may be prescribed (Lewis et al., 2007).

Surgical interventions include studies of the effect of sacral nerve root stimulation via implantation of electrodes; cystectomy, with the creation of a urostomy; and urinary diversion. Some patients continue to experience pain even after surgery.

Nursing Interventions and Patient Teaching

Nursing interventions focus on pain control and comfort measures. Because all medications have side effects, patients must consult their physician before taking any prescription or over-the-counter medication. Pelvic floor exercise may help decrease urgency and nocturia. Patients may be asked to keep a daily bladder diary; this information can be used to make treatment decisions.

Potential dietary irritants include spicy and acidic floods, such as tomatoes, alcohol, citrus fruits, dark chocolate, and coffee. An elimination diet may help identify foods that trigger pain. A complete IC diet, self-management strategies, and other nonmedical management tools are available from the Interstitial Cystitis Association (www.ichelp.com).

IC is often associated with a reduced quality of life. Embarrassment, pain, and inability to manage elimination may lead to withdrawal from business, social, and intimate relationships. The patient and significant others need psychosocial support to face an uncertain outcome.

Prognosis

Only about half of patients with IC recover fully. Until researchers find a cause and an effective treatment, symptoms will continue.

PROSTATITIS

Etiology and Pathophysiology

Prostatitis, defined as inflammation and/or infection of the prostate gland, is actually a group of diseases. Bacterial prostatitis is caused by infectious organisms such as *Pseudomonas* organisms and *S. faecalis* traveling up the urethra. Nonbacterial prostatitis may result from a variety of conditions related to occlusion of the urethra (e.g., enlargement of the prostate gland).

Prostatodynia (pain in the prostate gland) manifests with neither inflammation nor infection but demonstrates the other symptoms typical of prostatitis.

Clinical Manifestations

The signs and symptoms vary in number and intensity. The patient may experience fever; chills; malaise; arthralgia; myalgia; perineal prostatic pain; dysuria; obstructive urinary tract symptoms, including frequency, urgency, dysuria, nocturia, hesitancy, weak stream, and incomplete voiding; low back pain; low abdominal pain; spontaneous urethral discharge; ejaculatory pain; and erectile dysfunction. Chronic bacterial prostatitis may be asymptomatic. Edema of the prostate gland may serve as an obstruction, causing urinary retention as a complication to the prostatitis. Pooling of urine may also foster stone formation. Other complications are epididymitis, pyelonephritis, and bacteremia (the presence of bacteria in the blood). The patient may be asymptomatic, but the symptoms of acute bacterial prostatitis are often the same as those of UTI, with pain in the low back, perineum, or rectum. The condition may become chronic.

Diagnostic Tests

Diagnosis is confirmed by patient history and culture of prostatic fluid or tissue. The expressed prostate secretion (EPS) is considered useful in the diagnosis of prostatitis. EPS is obtained using a premassage and postmassage test. The patient is asked to void into a specimen cup just before and just after a vigorous prostate massage. Prostatic massage (for EPS) should be avoided if acute bacterial prostatitis is suspected, since compression is extremely painful and increases the risk of bacterial spread. Transabdominal ultrasound or MRI may be done to rule out an abscess on the prostate. A urinalysis and urine culture, WBC count, and blood cultures may also be performed.

Assessment

Subjective data include complaints of chills and low back and perineal pain. Chronic bacterial prostatitis causes dysuria; urgency; frequency; nocturia; and pain in the lower abdomen or back, perineum, or genitalia.

Collection of **objective data** involves assessing for elevated temperature and rectal palpation of the prostate gland by the physician, which may reveal it to be firm, edematous, and tender.

Medical Management

If the condition is infectious, management focuses on control of the infection and prevention of the complications of abscess formation or bacteremia. Antibiotics commonly used for acute and chronic bacterial prostatitis include trimethoprim-sulfamethoxazole, ciprofloxin (Cipro), and ofloxacin (Floxin). Doxycycline or tetracycline may be prescribed for patients with multiple sex partners. Antibiotics are usually given orally for up to 4 weeks for acute bacterial prostatitis. However, if the patient has high fever or other signs of impending sepsis, hospitalization and intravenous antibiotics are prescribed. Patients with chronic bacterial prostatitis are given oral antibiotic therapy for 4 to 16 weeks.

Antiinflammatories are the most common agents used for pain control in prostatitis, but these provide only moderate pain relief. Opioid analgesics can be given, but cautiously, since this pain can be chronic. The pain resolves as the infection is treated.

Nursing Interventions and Patient Teaching

Regardless of the pathologic basis, comfort measures used are analgesics, sitz baths, and stool softeners to reduce pain, edema, spasm, and straining pressure in the pelvis.

Teaching includes the medication regimen. Warn the patient with acute prostatitis to avoid sexual arousal and intercourse so the prostate can rest; however, intercourse may be beneficial in the treatment of chronic prostatitis. Follow-up with the physician is crucial because of the likelihood that the disorder will become chronic.

Prognosis

Prostatitis is difficult to cure and requires long periods of antibiotic treatment. Stress the importance of taking all the antibiotics prescribed, even after the initial symptoms have subsided.

PYELONEPHRITIS

Etiology and Pathophysiology

Pyelonephritis is an inflammation of the structures of the kidney—renal pelvis, renal tubules, and interstitial tissue. Pyelonephritis is almost always caused by *E. coli.* The kidney becomes edematous and inflamed, and the blood vessels are congested. The urine may be cloudy and contain pus (pyuria), mucus, and blood. Small abscesses may form in the kidney.

Pyelonephritis is usually seen in association with pregnancy; chronic health problems, such as diabetes mellitus or polycystic or hypertensive renal disease; insult to the urinary tract from catheterization; or infection, obstruction, or trauma. Careful management of these disorders is important to prevent pyelonephritis.

Clinical Manifestations

Acute pyelonephritis may be unilateral or bilateral, causing chills, fever, prostration, and flank pain. Repeated episodes of pyelonephritis lead to a chronic disease pattern, with atrophy of the kidney as the nephrons are destroyed. **Azotemia** (the retention of excessive amounts of nitrogenous compounds in the blood) develops if enough nephrons are nonfunctional.

Assessment

Subjective data in acute pyelonephritis includes a patient who is acutely ill, with malaise and pain in the **costovertebral angle (CVA)** (one of two angles that outline a space over the kidneys). CVA tenderness to percussion is a common finding in pyelonephritis. In the chronic phase the patient may show unremarkable symptoms, such as nausea and general malaise.

Collection of **objective data** includes assessing the patient for signs of infection: elevated temperature, vomiting, and chills. The chronic disease results in systemic signs: elevated blood pressure and gastrointestinal irritation such as vomiting and diarrhea.

Diagnostic Tests

Diagnosis is confirmed by bacteria and pus in the urine, varying degrees of hematuria, WBCs and WBC casts in the urine (indicating involvement of the renal parenchyma), and leukocytosis. A clean-catch or catheterized urinalysis with culture and sensitivity identifies the pathogen and determines appropriate antimicrobial therapy. To prevent spread of infection in the early stages of acute pyelonephritis, imaging examinations such as an IUP or CT scan requiring intrauterine injection of contrast materials are usually not performed. Ultrasound of the urinary system is often done to identify anatomical abnormalities such as renal abscesses, obstructing calculus, or hydronephrosis (Lewis et al., 2007). BUN and creatinine levels of the blood and urine may be assessed to monitor kidney function.

Medical Management

The patient with mild signs and symptoms may be treated on an outpatient basis with antibiotics for 14 to 21 days. Parenteral antibiotics are often given initially in the hospital to establish high serum and urinary medication levels. When initial treatment resolves the acute symptoms and the patient is able to tolerate oral fluids and medications, he or she may be discharged on a regimen of oral antibiotics for an additional 14 to 21 days. Antibiotics are selected according to results of urinalysis culture and sensitivity and may include broad-spectrum medications such as ampicillin or vancomycin combined with an aminoglycoside (e.g., tobramycin [Nebcin], gentamicin [Garamycin]); other treatment options include trimethoprim-sulfamethoxazole and fluoroquinolones such as ciprofloxin and ofloxacin.

Adequate fluids (at least eight 8-ounce glasses per day) are encouraged. Urinary analgesics such as phenazopyridine are helpful. Follow-up urine culture is indicated.

Nursing Interventions and Patient Teaching

Nursing diagnoses and interventions for the patient with pyelonephritis include but are not limited to the following:

Nursing Diagnoses	Nursing Interventions
Risk for infection, related to bacteria in the urinary tract	Monitor urine character and odor. Encourage oral fluids. Instruct patient to void when he or she feels the urge. Encourage perineal hygiene.
Health-seeking behaviors, related to desire for prevention of further renal disease	Assess knowledge level concerning measures to prevent recurrence of symptoms. Discuss personal health habits: diet, exercise. Discuss treatment plan with patient and family.

Teach the patient to identify the signs and symptoms of infection: elevated temperature, flank pain, chills, fever, nausea and vomiting, urgency, fatigue, and general malaise. Also teach the patient indications, dose, length of course, and side effects of the medications. Emphasize the importance of follow-up care with the physician on a routine basis and when signs of infection arise.

Prognosis

Prognosis depends on early detection and successful treatment. Baseline assessment for every patient must include urinary assessment because pyelonephritis can occur as a primary or secondary disorder.

OBSTRUCTIVE DISORDERS OF THE URINARY TRACT

URINARY OBSTRUCTION

Etiology and Pathophysiology

Obstruction at any point within the urinary tract can adversely affect function and alter structure. Causes of obstruction include strictures, kinks, cysts, tumors, calculi, and prostatic hypertrophy. Obstruction may lead to alterations in blood chemistry, infection that thrives as a result of urine stasis, ischemia due to compression, or atrophy of renal tissue.

Clinical Manifestations

The patient may be unaware of any problems at first if the obstruction is partial, allowing urine to drain and kidney function to remain within normal limits. With prostatic hypertrophy the obstructive process may be so gradual that the patient ignores the vague symptom of dull flank pain and seeks medical attention only when urination becomes acutely difficult. Acute pain occurs as the musculature is stretched by increasing pressure from urine accumulation and as muscular contractions increase in an attempt to move urine past the obstruction. This acute pain is called renal colic and is a classic symptom of renal calculi.

Assessment

Subjective data include the patient's cardinal complaint of a sensation of needing to void but only being able to void small amounts. Pain may range from dull flank pain to acute, incapacitating pain. Nausea often accompanies acute pain.

Collection of **objective data** includes noting on physical assessment if the bladder is palpable suprapubically because of urine retention. The affected kidney may also be palpable. Retention with overflow occurs when the patient is unable to completely empty the urinary bladder and it quickly refills, causing the urge to void again. Assess time and amount of voidings.

Diagnostic Tests

As a quick evaluation, the physician may order a KUB radiograph. Renal ultrasonography or IVP provides definitive information about structural changes. Other diagnostic tests may include visual examinations with the aid of endoscopy and a blood chemistry profile.

Medical Management

Initial intervention is aimed at establishing urine drainage and relieving discomfort. Conservative measures include inserting an indwelling catheter and administering an analgesic (usually opioid) and an anticholinergic agent (atropine) to decrease smooth muscle motility. It may be necessary to establish urine drainage surgically by inserting a catheter directly into the bladder through the abdominal wall (suprapubic cystostomy), into a ureter (ureterostomy), or into the kidney (nephrostomy).

Surgical correction of an obstruction in the urinary system may involve a tube, called a stent. Stent insertion is used for patients who are poor operative risks. A meshlike tube or coil-shaped device is inserted through an endoscope into the ureter. The stent holds the tubular structure open to facilitate drainage. Stents may be permanent or temporary. Closely monitor the patient for signs of infection, obstruction, and pain.

Nursing Interventions

After surgery, observe the patient for hemorrhage, provide aseptic care of the surgical site, and provide a safe environment to prevent injury and infection.

Prognosis

The prognosis varies, depending on the cause of the obstruction. If surgical correction is successful, the prognosis is excellent.

HYDRONEPHROSIS

Etiology and Pathophysiology

Hydronephrosis (the dilation of the renal pelvis and calyces) may be congenital or may develop at any time. It can occur unilaterally or bilaterally. Hydronephrosis is caused by obstructions in the lower urinary tract, the ureters, or the kidneys. The location of the obstruction determines whether one or both kidneys are affected.

An obstruction generates pressure from accumulated urine that cannot flow past it. This pressure may cause functional and anatomical damage to the renal system. The renal pelvis and ureters dilate and hypertrophy. This pressure, if prolonged, causes fibrosis and loss of function in affected nephrons. If the condition is left untreated, the kidney may be destroyed.

Clinical Manifestations

Hydronephrosis can occur without any symptoms as long as kidney function is adequate and urine can drain. The amount of pain is proportional to the rate of stretching of urinary tract structures. Slowly developing hydronephrosis may cause only a dull flank pain, whereas a sudden occlusion of the ureter, such as from a calculus, causes a severe stabbing (colicky) pain in the flank. Nausea and vomiting, which often accompany hydronephrosis, are a reflex reaction to the pain and usually subside when the pain is controlled.

Assessment

Subjective data include patient reports of pain, including location, intensity, and character, and nausea. Discuss the patient's voiding pattern: frequency, difficulty starting a stream of urine, dribbling at the end of micturition (voiding), nocturia, and burning on urination. Note any history of obstructive disorders.

Collection of **objective data** includes assessing patients suspected of having hydronephrosis for vomiting, hematuria, urinary output, edema, a palpable mass in the abdomen, bladder distention (detected on palpation), and tenderness over the kidneys or bladder.

Diagnostic Tests

A urinalysis and serum kidney function studies that include measurement of urea and creatinine are obtained. Cystoscopy may be performed with or without retrograde pyelogram. Radiographic examinations may include IVP or IVU, KUB radiograph, CT scan, or ultrasound evaluation. Sometimes a renal biopsy is performed.

Medical Management

Management is usually conservative if the condition is not severe. Surgery relieves the obstruction and preserves kidney function. If the kidney is severely damaged, a nephrectomy may be necessary. If infection is present, antiinfective medications are administered: penicillin in combination with sulfasoxazole (Gantrisin) or sulfamethoxazole-trimethoprim (Bactrim). Opioids, such as morphine and meperidine, in combination with antispasmodic drugs, such as propantheline (Pro-Banthine) and belladonna preparations, are usually necessary to relieve severe, colicky pain.

Nursing Interventions and Patient Teaching

Nursing interventions for the patient with hydronephrosis include administering medications as ordered, monitoring I&O, observing for signs and symptoms of infection, and monitoring vital signs. Encourage the patient to take fluids, and assess the patient for pain. Keep any drainage tubes open and anchored to avoid inadvertent displacement. If a catheter is present, provide catheter care. If surgery has been performed, observe the dressing because drainage of urine may continue for some time. Keep the area clean and dry to avoid excoriation of the skin. Explain all procedures to the patient and the family.

Patient teaching includes explaining the abnormality and the signs and symptoms of infection or obstruction. Describe measures to prevent infection, such as adequate fluid intake, perineal hygiene daily with mild soap and water (drying thoroughly), and regular emptying of the bladder.

Prognosis

Prognosis depends on the degree of urinary system destruction and the need for surgical intervention.

UROLITHIASIS

Urolithiasis (formation of urinary calculi) can develop in any area of the urinary tract. *Urolithiasis* is a general term that encompasses all urinary calculi, but specific names are also used to indicate where they are located or formed: nephrolithiasis (stones in the kidney), ureterolithiasis (stones in the ureter), and cystolithiasis (stones in the bladder). Other descriptive terms are **lithiasis** and **calculi** (the formation of stones).

Etiology and Pathophysiology

Urolithiasis develops from minerals that have precipitated out of solution and adhere, forming stones that vary in size and shape. The event that initiates stone formation remains unknown. However, some individuals are predisposed to urolithiasis: people who are immobile, are hyperparathyroid (calcium leaves the bones and accumulates in the bloodstream), or have recurrent UTIs. Individual history and some foods, nutrients, and medications contribute to development of stones. Thorough assessment and analysis of the composition of the stones guides medical and nursing management.

Clinical Manifestations

Symptoms depend on the stones' size and degree of mobility. The patient with renal colic seeks care immediately, whereas a person with a less mobile stone may not seek assistance until signs of infection or hydronephrosis occur.

Assessment

Subjective data include the patient with mobile calculi complaining of intractable pain (pain that is unrelieved by ordinary medical measures and is usually accompanied by nausea and vomiting). The patient describes the pain as starting in the flank and radiating into the groin, the genitalia, and the inner thigh. The patient with a less mobile stone may develop signs and symptoms associated with UTI secondary to hydronephrosis.

Collection of **objective data** includes assessing for hematuria and vomiting.

Diagnostic Tests

Diagnostic tests include KUB and IVP or IVU radiography, ultrasound, cystoscopy, and urinalysis. Other tests may be ordered to determine stone content, presence of infection, and alterations in blood chemistry that influence stone formation. Twenty-four-hour urine examination may be done to detect abnormal excretion of calcium oxalate, phosphorus, or uric acid.

Medical Management

Antiinfective agents may be administered to treat infection or prophylactically. If stones are not passed, invasive techniques may be indicated (Figure 50-7). Stones in the lower tract can be removed by cystoscopy with stone manipulation or by surgical incision. Terminology describes the location: ureterolithotomy, pyelolithotomy, and nephrolithotomy. Chemolytic agents, either alkylating or acidifying agents, may be instilled to dissolve stones.

Extracorporeal shock wave lithotripsy is an alternative to surgery. The patient is submerged in a special tank of water, and ultrasonic shock waves are used to pulverize the stone. Urine must still be strained, even if a catheter is in place. Renal colic may occur as the patient passes the stone fragments.

Long-term management may include dietary adjustments to alter urine pH or to decrease availability of certain substances that cause stone formation. Moderate reduction of foods containing calcium phosphorus and purine may help when stones are caused by metabolic abnormalities. Foods to avoid include cheese, greens, whole grains, carbonated beverages, nuts, chocolate, shellfish, and organ meat. Daily fluid intake of 2000 mL (unless clinically contraindicated) helps cleanse the urinary tract.

Drug therapy depends on stone composition. In calcium stone formation, sodium cellulose phosphate binds with ingested calcium and prevents its absorption; aluminum hydroxide gel binds with excess phosphorus, allowing intestinal excretion rather than urinary excretion; and allopurinol (Zyloprim) reduces serum urate levels, thereby facilitating reabsorption of urate crystals.

Nursing Interventions and Patient Teaching

Stones are more likely to be passed if the patient remains active and increases fluid intake. If pain is so severe that it requires opioid medication, be cautious when allowing the patient out of bed. If nausea inhibits oral intake, the physician may order supplemental intravenous fluids. All urine is strained. Because stones may be any size, save even the smallest speck for assessment. Encourage fluids and administer analgesics as ordered. Assess urine for possible hematuria. Monitor BUN and creatinine for indications of continuing urinary tract obstruction.

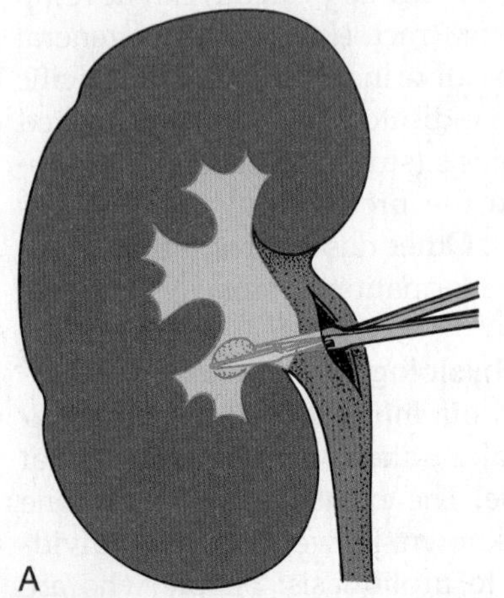

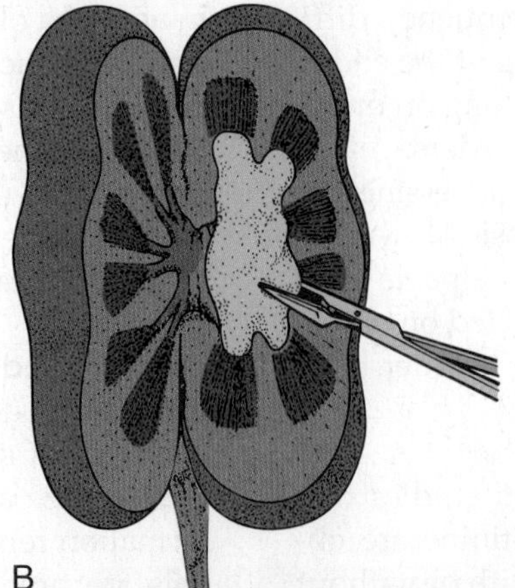

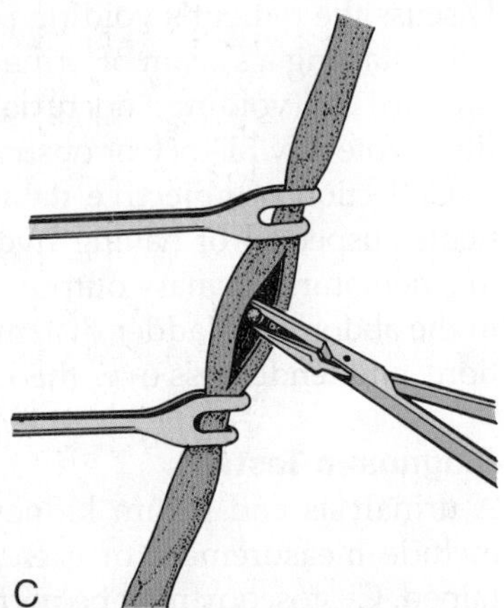

FIGURE 50-7 Location and methods of removing renal calculi from upper urinary tract. **A,** Pyelolithotomy, removal of stone through renal pelvis. **B,** Nephrolithotomy, removal of staghorn calculus from renal parenchyma (kidney split). **C,** Ureterolithotomy, removal of stone from ureter.

Nursing diagnoses and interventions for the patient with urolithiasis include but are not limited to the following:

Nursing Diagnoses	Nursing Interventions
Risk for infection, related to bacteria in the urinary tract	Monitor urine character and odor. Encourage oral fluids. Instruct the patient to void when urge is felt. Encourage perineal hygiene.
Health-seeking behaviors, related to desire for prevention of further renal disease	Assess knowledge level concerning measures to prevent recurrence of symptoms. Discuss personal health habits (diet, exercise). Discuss treatment plan with patient and family.

Discuss the prescribed diet, including fluid intake, and home medications (their purpose, dosage, refills, and side effects). The patient should avoid inactivity by walking frequently. Emphasize the need for follow-up with the physician, including keeping scheduled appointments and reporting difficulty with urination.

Although opinions vary greatly as to benefits of dietary restrictions, the nurse may be responsible for clarifying diet instructions. Encourage a fluid intake of at least 2000 mL in 24 hours, unless contraindicated. People who are calcium stone formers may need to curtail their intake of dietary calcium (dairy products, antacids) to within minimum recommended dietary allowance guidelines. New research on the impact of diet on the development of calcium oxalate kidney stones concludes that restricting consumption of animal protein and salt in combination with normal calcium intake reduces the risk of kidney stones better than the traditional low-calcium diet (Moyad, 2003).

Prognosis

Prognosis is related to the location of the stone and the extent of invasive procedures necessary to remove the stone. A certain population, categorized as "stone formers," is at risk for recurrence.

TUMORS OF THE URINARY SYSTEM

RENAL TUMORS

Etiology and Pathophysiology

The majority of renal tumors are malignant adenocarcinomas, also known as renal cell carcinoma, that develop unilaterally and are often large when first detected. Renal cell carcinoma as a primary malignant tumor appears to arise from cells of the proximal convoluted tubules. This is the tenth most common cancer, accounting for 3% of all cancers in adults, with a median age at diagnosis of 65 years. Twice as many men as women are diagnosed with renal cancer.

No strong risk factors have been identified, although some studies have suggested a relationship to obesity and smoking (American Institute of Cancer Research, 2007). The strongest risk factors appear to be genetic; multifocal renal adenocarcinomas have a hereditary basis, which is being studied intensively. Several multiorgan syndromes are associated with a high risk of renal malignancies; the most prominent is von Hippel–Lindau disease, an autosomally dominant hereditary disease originating from chromosome 3p. von Hippel–Lindau disease is characterized by central nervous system hemangioblastomas, renal adenocarcinomas, and other anomalies.

Because of the isolated anatomical location of the kidney, renal adenocarcinomas can grow large while remaining clinically silent. Most demonstrate a characteristic hypervascularity. Renal adenocarcinomas tend to grow intravascularly within the renal vein and into the inferior vena cava. These tumor thrombi may extend as far as the right atrium, presenting a unique surgical challenge. Although essentially every organ site can be affected, the most common sites of metastases are the lungs, the adrenal glands, the liver, and bones.

Clinical Manifestations

The historic sign and symptom triad of renal adenocarcinoma is hematuria, flank pain, and a flank mass. Most cases with these symptoms are advanced and incurable. Other common signs and symptoms are hypercalcemia, fever, anemia, weakness, and erythrocytosis. Gross hematuria is rarely a sign of renal adenocarcinoma until the malignancy is advanced. Check the patient's home medications for anticoagulant therapy, since this may be the cause of hematuria.

Assessment

Subjective data include a patient history of blood in the urine, which "comes and goes." When the bleeding occurs, there is usually no associated pain. In advanced stages of the illness, the patient experiences weight loss, fatigue, and dull flank pain.

Collection of **objective data** involves a physical assessment that reveals a mass in the patient's flank in the advanced stages of the illness. Hematuria and signs related to systemic metastasis may be obvious.

Diagnostic Tests

Localized adenocarcinoma is being diagnosed in patients who have no signs and symptoms specifically related to the tumor; these tumors are often discovered incidentally during evaluation of other complaints. Patients with gross hematuria should be assessed by a urologist. A cystoscopy followed by an IVP with tomography should be performed.

The vast majority of solid masses are malignant and require definitive evaluation and treatment. Percutaneous biopsy on a solid renal mass is rarely done because it is unlikely to change the future treatment unless there is evidence of advanced disease. A CT (with or without contrast), a chest x-ray, and, in some cases, a bone scan are used to stage renal adenocarcinoma.

Medical Management

Because renal adenocarcinoma is relatively radioresistant, radiation therapy has little or no role in its treatment. Surgery is the sole intervention capable of cure. The standard procedure is radical nephrectomy along with removal of adjacent lymph nodes and tissue. In the patient with renal insufficiency or a solitary kidney, partial nephrectomy (a far more complex procedure) may be indicated.

Nursing Interventions and Patient Teaching

Care of the patient with surgery of the urinary tract is addressed later in this chapter.

Nursing diagnoses and interventions for the patient with renal tumors include but are not limited to the following:

Nursing Diagnoses	Nursing Interventions
Ineffective coping, related to powerlessness	Encourage patient to express feelings. Assist patient in identifying personal strengths and coping skills. Actively listen. Support realistic hope; answer questions honestly.
Decisional conflict, with verbalized uncertainty about choice to have renal surgery	Assess patient's capacity to make decisions. Assess knowledge of procedure. Review outline of surgical procedure and what nursing interventions the patient and significant others can expect postoperatively.
Impaired physical mobility, related to pain and discomfort	Plan activities when pain control is greatest. Encourage active or passive range-of-motion exercises. Assess need for assistive devices.

Instruct the patient about community resources, support groups, and home health care. Emphasize the importance of follow-up care, including following discharge instructions and keeping return appointment.

Prognosis

In most cases of localized renal adenocarcinoma, the 5-year survival rate is more than 60%. The natural history of renal adenocarcinoma is far more unpredictable than that of most solid tumors. Disease may recur more than 15 years after removal of the original primary lesion. Metastatic disease has a poor prognosis and is rarely curable. Metastatic recurrence at a remotely distant time is not uncommon.

RENAL CYSTS

Etiology and Pathophysiology

Acquired renal cysts are simple cysts that must be distinguished from more serious causes of cystic disease. Acquired cysts are usually simple: round and sharply demarcated with smooth walls. They may be single or multiple. Single cysts are isolated and are most often detected incidentally. They are clinically insignificant, but must be distinguished from other more significant cystic renal disorders and renal masses such as renal cell carcinoma. Renal cell carcinoma is typically irregular or multiloculated with irregular walls and areas of unclear demarcation.

Acquired cysts are significant only because patients have a higher incidence of renal carcinoma; whether the cysts become malignant is unknown. For this reason, some physicians periodically screen patients with acquired cysts for renal carcinoma using ultrasonography or CT.

Multiple cysts are most common in patients with chronic renal failure, especially those undergoing hemodialysis. The cause is unknown, but the cysts may be due to compensatory hyperplasia of residually functioning nephrons. A criterion for diagnosis is more than four cysts in each kidney on ultrasonography or CT.

The most significant problems arise with **PKD.** PKD is a genetic disorder characterized by the growth of numerous fluid-filled cysts, which can slowly replace much of the kidney. A patient with longstanding renal insufficiency or a dialysis patient may develop polycystic disease. Kidney function is compromised by the pressure of the cysts on renal structures, secondary infections, and tissue scarring caused by rupture of the cysts. The patient may progress to end-stage renal disease (ESRD).

Clinical Manifestations

Signs and symptoms are influenced by the degree of renal structure involvement. The most common site is the collecting ducts, which fill with urine and/or blood. As the disease progresses, fewer nephrons are available to maintain normal kidney function.

The Bosniak Classification of Renal Cysts classifies lesions according to their character. Class I lesions are simple, benign cysts and do not warrant further workup. Class II lesions are minimally complicated with some features that cause concern. They have smooth, sharp margins; are thicker; and require follow-up scanning. Class III lesions have irregular and thickened walls and multiloculated cysts; they require surgical exploration. Class IV lesions show nonuniform wall thickening and irregular margins; they contain solid components visible on CT. These lesions are clearly malignant, and a total nephrectomy is warranted.

Assessment

Subjective data include the most common symptoms of abdominal and flank pain, followed by headache, gastrointestinal complaints, voiding disturbances, and a history of recurrent UTIs.

Collection of **objective data** involves observation for systemic changes. Closely monitor blood pressure, which is usually elevated, and hematuria. Document patient complaints and response to intervention.

Diagnostic Tests

Diagnosis is established by family history, physical examination, excretory urography, and imaging of cysts on radiographic examination or sonography. Blood chemistry results, such as urea and creatinine levels, are used to monitor the level of kidney function.

Medical Management

PKD has no specific treatment. Medical treatment is aimed at relief of pain and other symptoms. Heat and analgesics may relieve some of the discomfort caused by the enlarging kidneys. If the patient bleeds, discontinue heat and place the patient on bed rest. Hypertension is treated vigorously with antihypertensive agents, diuretics, and fluid and dietary modifications. Because infections are common, antibiotics are often prescribed. As the disease progresses, dialysis or kidney transplantation may be required.

Nursing Interventions

Individual complaints and the severity of the disease process influence nursing interventions. Provide information to patients and family members about the availability of genetic counseling. Emphasize the need to report any changes in health status to the physician.

Prognosis

Prognosis is favorable with a single cyst but guarded with polycystic disease because of its chronic nature.

TUMORS OF THE URINARY BLADDER

Etiology and Pathophysiology

The bladder is the most common site of cancer in the urinary tract. A bladder tumor is an excess growth of cells that line the inside of the bladder, in many cases because the cells were exposed to certain chemicals. Tumors of the urinary bladder range from benign papillomas to invasive carcinomas. Papillomas have the potential to become cancerous and are removed when detected. A noncancerous bladder tumor is usually a small, wartlike growth that does not spread (National Cancer Institute, 2008).

The overall incidence and mortality for bladder cancer have changed little for most racial and ethnic groups over the past 20 years. Recent research has shown black patients were 35% more likely to die of bladder cancer than white patients. Men are more likely to develop bladder cancer than women; cigarette smoking is a major factor (National Cancer Institute, 2008).

Several types of carcinoma arise on the bladder surface. The most common type diagnosed in North America is transitional cell carcinoma (TCC), which can occur anywhere in the urinary tract, but is usually found in the urinary bladder. TCC involves development of a papillary tumor that projects into the bladder lumen and, if untreated, continues into the bladder muscle, where it can metastasize.

Clinical Manifestations

The patient may delay seeking medical attention because the primary sign of bladder cancer is painless, intermittent hematuria.

Assessment

Subjective data include symptoms such as changes in voiding patterns, signs of urinary obstruction, or renal failure, depending on the extent of the disease process.

Collection of **objective data** includes assessing the patient's understanding of current health status, which will aid in planning teaching interventions. Accurately document the time and amount of voiding, including the urine description.

Diagnostic Tests

Diagnostic tests include a urine **cytologic evaluation** (study of cells) and/or one of several available bladder cancer markers. Bladder biopsies are needed to confirm a diagnosis.

Bladder cancer tumors are most commonly staged using the system developed by the American Joint Committee on Cancer. The stage of the tumor is the most important indicator of prognosis and overall survival for invasive tumors. Staging is an assessment of how far the tumor has spread.

Medical Management

Local disease may be treated by removing the tissue by burning with an electric spark (fulguration), laser, instillation of chemotherapy agents, or radiation therapy. Closely monitor these patients with cytologic studies and cystoscopy, since the recurrence rate is as high as 60%. A partial or total cystectomy may be performed to remove invasive lesions. With complete removal of the urinary bladder, urinary diversion is necessary. (See the discussion of the ileal conduit or sigmoid conduit, pp. 1714-1715, and Figure 50-13.)

Nursing Interventions and Patient Teaching

Care of the patient with bladder cancer is influenced by the extent of the disease process, medical treatment, coincidental illness, and the patient's response to treatment. Observe voiding patterns and urine characteristics to monitor response to these therapies. Provide teaching and support so that the patient can return to optimum performance of ADLs. Emphasize the importance of follow-up care for the patient with papillomas.

Prognosis

The prognosis is directly related to the extent of the disease process when diagnosed. Another important aspect in recovery is the patient's adaptability to any changes in urinary elimination as a result of treatment.

CONDITIONS AFFECTING THE PROSTATE GLAND

BENIGN PROSTATIC HYPERTROPHY

Etiology and Pathophysiology

The prostate gland encircles the male urethra at the base of the urinary bladder. It secretes an alkaline fluid that helps neutralize seminal fluid and increases sperm motility. BPH, enlargement of the prostate gland, is common in men older than 50 years of age. The cause is unclear but may be influenced by hormonal changes. The prostate enlarges, exerting pressure on the urethra and vesicle neck of the urinary bladder, which prevents complete emptying.

Clinical Manifestations

The patient has symptoms associated with urinary obstruction. Other clinical manifestations include complications of urinary obstruction, such as UTI, hematuria, oliguria, and signs of renal insufficiency.

Assessment

Subjective data include the patient describing the urine stream as difficult to start, slow, and painful, with complaints of frequency and nocturia. Collectively these symptoms may be referred to as **prostatism** (any condition of the prostate gland that causes retention of urine in the bladder).

Collection of **objective data** involves eliciting information about voiding patterns to aid in determining the severity of the obstruction.

Diagnostic Tests

On rectal examination the physician may palpate the enlarged prostate gland, which has an elastic consistency. The hypertrophied prostate is symmetrically enlarged with a uniform, boggy presentation. Severity of the process can be determined by detecting alterations in blood chemistry, by measuring residual urine, or by cystoscopy or IVP. Cytologic evaluation determines whether the process is benign or malignant.

Medical Management

Treatment is based on the degree of occlusion and on signs and symptoms. Pharmacologic agents such as dutasteride (Avodart) convert testosterone to dihydrotestosterone, a key enzyme in the development and growth rate of prostatic hyperplasia. This medication may take 3 to 6 months to shrink the prostate gland, decreasing its size as much as 25%. Terazosin (Hytrin) is an antihypertensive that dilates arteries and veins and decreases contractions in smooth muscle of the prostatic capsule. This decreases symptoms of prostatic hyperplasia (urinary urgency, hesitancy, nocturia).

Deciding which treatment intervention to choose is difficult. Transurethral resection of the prostate (TURP) is still considered the standard for surgical intervention. The newer, less-invasive treatments are still being evaluated. In general, these treatments are considered to cause less morbidity, but the results are not considered as effective or long lasting as those of TURP.

Transurethral Microwave Thermotherapy

Transurethral microwave thermotherapy (TUMT) is one of various procedures used for the treatment of lower urinary tract symptoms due to BPH. TUMT involves the insertion of a specially designed urinary catheter into the bladder, allowing a microwave antenna to be positioned within the prostate; there, it heats and destroys hyperplastic prostate tissue. The goal of TUMT is to provide a one-time treatment. Candidates for TUMT include persons with moderate-to-severe voiding symptoms due to BPH, those with side effects to medical therapy, those in whom medical therapy has failed, and those who choose to not be treated medically. There are a number of exclusions to the use of TUMT, so all patients require a thorough history and physical examination.

Patients should return to the clinic for follow-up. If a catheter is placed, it can be removed at home or in the clinic. Instruct patients to watch for an inability to void, painful voiding, high fevers, abdominal pain, or other problems. Posttreatment convalescence is relatively rapid, with most patients able to void and recover in less than 5 days at home. Thus some patients return to full activity relatively early (Rubenstein & McVary, 2008).

Transurethral Needle Ablation (TUNA)

Transurethral needle ablation (TUNA) of the prostate is another procedure used to treat BPH. It is performed by placing interstitial radiofrequency needles through the urethra and into the lateral lobes of the prostate, causing heat-induced coagulation necrosis. The tissue is heated to 230° F (110° C) for approximately 3 minutes per lesion. A coagulation defect is created. A comprehensive history and physical examination must be done to determine the benefits of using this procedure. Urethrocystoscopy may be indicated to help select the optimal form of therapy.

Photoselective Vaporization of the Prostate

Photoselective vaporization of the prostate (PVP) using the GreenLight laser is another option for the treatment of BPH. PVP is a safe alternative for patients who are seriously ill, are taking anticoagulants, or have unfavorable anatomy (i.e., a large prostate). The technique employs a laser beam, which emits a visible green light at a wavelength that has shallow tissue penetration and is selectively absorbed by blood. A urologist delivers the laser's energy by way of a thin fiber inserted into the urethra through a 23-F continuous-flow cystoscopy. The GreenLight laser vaporizes the prostate tissue.

Nursing Interventions

Initial management is aimed at relieving the obstruction, usually by insertion of a Foley catheter. Take care to avoid rapid decompression of the bladder to prevent rupture of mucosal blood vessels. Usually no more than 1000 mL of urine should be removed from a distended bladder initially. Follow physician's orders for the individual patient.

Prostatectomy (removal of the prostate gland) is indicated to relieve or prevent further obstruction of the urethra. The physician chooses the surgical approach for the prostatectomy after thorough appraisal of the patient. Preoperatively the physician may order an enema to reduce the possibility of the patient's straining to defecate after surgery, which could cause bleeding. Other preoperative preparations are standard, as noted in Chapter 42. A prostatectomy may be done using any of four surgical techniques (Box 50-3 and Figure 50-8).

With BPH, TURP is the resection most often chosen because it is less invasive and less stressful for the pa-

Box 50-3 Four Prostatectomy Techniques

1. **Transurethral prostatectomy** is done by approaching the gland through the penis and bladder using a resectoscope, a surgical instrument with an electric cutting wire for resection and cautery to resect the lobes away from the capsule (see Figure 50-8, *A*).
2. **Suprapubic prostatectomy** is accomplished by an incision through the abdomen; the bladder is opened, and the gland is removed from above with the finger (see Figure 50-8, *B*).
3. **Radical perineal prostatectomy** requires an incision through the perineum between the scrotum and the rectum (see Figure 50-8, *C*).
4. **Retropubic prostatectomy** requires a low abdominal incision, but the bladder is not opened. The gland is removed by making an incision into the capsule encasing the prostate gland (see Figure 50-8, *D*).

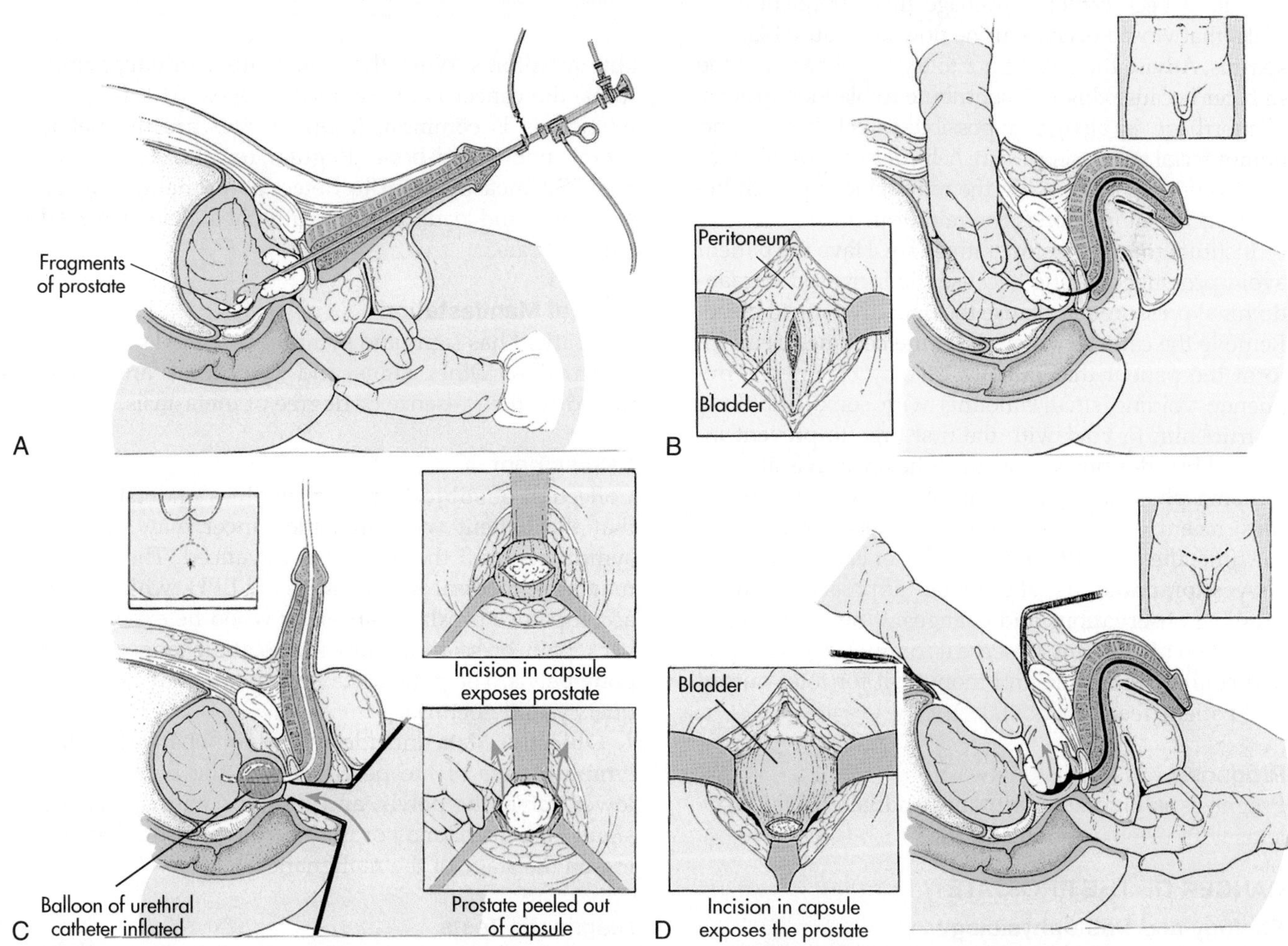

FIGURE 50-8 Four types of prostatectomies. **A,** Transurethral resection of prostate gland by means of resectoscope. Note enlarged prostate gland surrounding urethra and tiny pieces of prostatic tissue that have been cut away. **B,** Suprapubic. **C,** Radical perineal. **D,** Retropubic prostatectomy.

tient, especially the older patient or the patient with coincidental illness. The tissue is removed through the urethra. With this procedure the outer capsule of the prostate gland is left in place, maintaining the continuity between the bladder and the lower urethra (see Figure 50-8, *A*). Care of this patient centers on observing urine characteristics and maintaining patency of the Foley catheter.

The patient who has a TURP may have continuous closed bladder irrigation or intermittent irrigation to prevent occlusion of the catheter with blood clots, which would cause bladder spasms. Inform the patient and the family that hematuria is expected after prostatic surgery. Monitor vital signs and urine color every 2 hours for the first 24 hours to detect early signs of complications. With continuous bladder irrigation the urine will be light red to pink, and with intermittent irrigation the urine will be a clear, cherry red. Continuous irrigation is achieved with a three-way catheter (one lumen for irrigation fluid, one for urine drainage, and one to the retention balloon) or by using two catheters (Foley and suprapubic—one for irrigation fluid and one for urine drainage). The irrigant is an isotonic solution. To determine urinary output, subtract the amount of irrigation fluid used from the Foley catheter output. This is reported as "actual urinary output." Check catheter drainage tubes frequently for kinks that would occlude urine flow and cause bladder spasms. Advise the patient not to try to void around the catheter because this will contribute to bladder spasms. Hemorrhage is always a possibility. Belladonna and opium rectal suppositories are helpful to relieve bladder spasms but are not used in the retropubic approach because rectal stimulation is contraindicated.

Institute routine postoperative care. Have the patient avoid prolonged sitting because the increased intraabdominal pressure may cause the operative site to bleed. Remove the catheter when the urine becomes clear. Inform the patient that initially he may experience frequency, voiding small amounts with some dribbling. Instruct him to void with the first urge to prevent increased bladder pressure against the operative site.

Some physicians may request that samples of the most recent voiding be saved for assessment. Record the time, the amount, and the color of each voiding.

A suprapubic or abdominal approach requires dressing observations and changes. When a suprapubic catheter is present, observe it for unobstructed flow and color of the urine and monitor it for total output (see Patient Teaching box).

Prognosis

Prognosis is favorable without residual effects. Problems with urine dribbling vary.

CANCER OF THE PROSTATE

Etiology and Pathophysiology

Prostatic cancer is common in men older than 50 years of age. This insidious cancer usually starts as a nodule on the posterior portion of the prostate without noticeable symptoms. When the tumor causes urinary symptoms, the cancer is in advanced stages. At this point, metastasis is common; frequent sites are the pelvic lymph nodes and bone. Regular rectal examinations and PSA measurement to detect abnormalities of the prostate gland lead to early treatment and an increased survival rate.

 **Patient Teaching**

Postprostatectomy

Written Instructions with Frequently Asked Questions
- Rest for 48 hours to help prevent postoperative bleeding.
- Do not take aspirin or anticoagulant medications.
- Do not drive for 48 hours.
- Avoid sexual activity for 2 weeks, or as directed by physician.
- If prescribed antibiotics, take medication as prescribed until all are gone.
- Prevent constipation.
- Observe for signs and symptoms of urinary tract infection.
- A list of contact numbers.
- An appointment card for follow-up visit.

Managing Urinary Incontinence
- It usually takes several weeks to achieve urinary continence. Continence may improve for up to 12 months.
- Maintain oral fluids between 2000 and 3000 mL/day (unless contraindicated).

Erectile Dysfunction
- Sexual counseling and treatment options may be necessary if erectile dysfunction becomes a chronic or permanent problem.

Indwelling Catheter
- If the patient goes home with an indwelling catheter, send instructions for the catheter care and local stores where the supplies can be purchased.

Clinical Manifestations

The patient has signs and symptoms related to urinary obstruction. Other signs and symptoms are determined by the presence or degree of metastasis.

Assessment

Collection of **subjective data** involves understanding that the patient with prostatic cancer may have no symptoms until the disease is advanced. The patient may seek medical intervention for BPH, which often accompanies prostate cancer, or when he experiences back pain or sciatica from metastatic changes in the bony pelvis. The patient may complain of dysuria, frequency, and nocturia.

Objective data include metastatic changes in the lymph glands of the pelvis and in the bones of the lower spine, the pelvis, and the hips with associated signs. Hematuria may or may not be present, depending on the stage of the malignancy.

Diagnostic Tests

On rectal examination by the physician, the involved area of the prostate gland feels firm and fixed with hardened nodules typically in the posterior lobe of the gland.

Definitive diagnosis is made by cytologic examination. Prostate cells can be obtained by needle aspiration.

Men should consider a yearly PSA and digital rectal examination starting at age 50 or at age 45 if at high risk (blacks or men with a father or brother diagnosed with prostate cancer at an early age). PSA is greatly increasing the odds of early diagnosis. PSA, normally secreted and disposed of by the prostate, increases in the bloodstream in cancer of the prostate as well as in the harmless condition of BPH. The normal PSA is 0 to 4 ng/mL. It is important to monitor even a slight increase in PSA levels. Elevated PSA levels mean further diagnostic evaluation is needed. When PSA levels are high but a digital examination is normal, transrectal ultrasound is proving increasingly helpful in detecting cancer of the prostate gland too small to be palpated rectally. Other tests, such as a bone scan and serum alkaline phosphatase, are performed to assess the degree of metastasis.

The Gleason Grading System is the most widely used system for grading prostate cancer. Based on microscopic identification of glandular differentiation in tumor cells, tumors are graded from 1 to 5. Grade 1 represents the most well differentiated (most like the original cells), and grade 5 represents the most poorly differentiated (undifferentiated). Gleason grades are given to the two most commonly occurring patterns of cells and added together. The Gleason score, a number from 2 to 10, is used to predict how quickly the cancer will progress. A score of 2 to 4 indicates a slowly growing tumor. Grades 5 to 7 are associated with a more aggressive tumor with a 40% chance of metastasis. Grades 8 to 10 indicate an aggressive tumor with a 75% chance of metastasis (Lewis et al., 2007).

Medical Management

Treatment is based on the stage of the cancer—whether it has spread beyond the wall of the prostate, and to what extent—and the patient's age. In an older man with an estimated remaining life span of 5 to 10 years, controlling the disease with radiation or hormone therapy may be enough. In many cases, particularly in men older than 70 years of age, prostate cancer grows slowly, and hormone therapy can hold the disease at bay for several years.

Localized prostate cancer can be cured by radiation therapy or surgery. A treatment in which radioactive seed implants are placed directly in the prostate gland while sparing the surrounding tissue (rectum and bladder) is called brachytherapy. The seeds are accurately placed with a needle through a grid template guided by a transrectal ultrasound. Brachytherapy is a convenient, one-time outpatient procedure, whereas external radiation can take 5 to 6 weeks (Lewis et al., 2007). The seeds remain in the body, but their radioactivity declines over a period of months. Patients are advised to refrain from having children (or adults) sit in their lap and to avoid intercourse during the first 2 months after therapy. Radiation therapy also is used when the cancer has spread to just outside the gland, in an attempt to destroy cancer cells and shrink the prostate.

The operation to remove the prostate is a radical prostatectomy. Radical prostatectomy by the perineal approach is used in patients with early-stage clinical disease and is considered one of the most effective ways of eradicating the tumor. This procedure involves removing the entire prostate, including the true prostatic capsule, seminal vesicles, and a portion of the bladder neck. The remaining portion of the bladder neck is reanastomosed to the urethra. The retropubic approach is often the first choice because it provides access to the pelvic lymph nodes (pelvic lymphadenectomy) and affords more urinary control and less stricture formation. A third, nerve-sparing prostatectomy procedure uses a retropubic and perineal approach in an attempt to prevent impotence and reduce the likelihood of UI.

The three goals of a radical prostatectomy are removing all the tumor, preserving urine control, and preserving sexual function. Extent of sexual function may not be known for 6 to 12 months postoperatively. The patient needs emotional support related to the cancer and the possibility of impotence after surgery. Preoperative teaching should include an opportunity for the patient and his partner to discuss treatment options and mortality rate.

When the capsule of the prostate gland is removed, as with the perineal approach, the bladder and the lower urethra are no longer connected. The area where these two structures are reconnected is usually supported by placement of a Foley catheter. Extreme care must be taken to avoid placing tension on the catheter, which would disturb the surgical area. The catheter remains indwelling for several postoperative days.

In cases of advanced prostatic cancer, hormonal deprivation therapy may be used in an attempt to alter the tumor growth by blocking androgen (testosterone) production. Hormone deprivation therapy includes estrogens, gonadotropin-releasing hormone analogs, and antiandrogens. Luteinizing hormone–releasing hormone (LHRH) drugs act by causing an initial surge in luteinizing hormone and testosterone, rapidly followed by a decline in testosterone level similar to that achieved by castration. The primary forms of LHRH agonists are leuprolide (Lupron) and goserelin (Zoladex). Alternatives to LHRH agonists include oral nonsteroidal antiandrogens, including bicalutamide (Casodex), flutamide (Eulexin), and nilutamide (Nilandron) (Black & Hawks, 2009). Palliative therapy for patients with metastatic disease also may include orchiectomy (removal of the testes). Bilateral orchiectomy eliminates 95% of testosterone production, a step that is useful in managing metastatic disease. The patient may receive relief from such symptoms as pain or obstruction, but may experience feminization, increased incidence of cardiac disease, thrombophlebitis, pulmonary embolus, and stroke. Additional therapies are instituted to treat these side effects.

Radiation therapy may be used in advanced stages of the illness as primary or palliative treatment. Management of disseminated disease with cytotoxic drugs has been marginally successful.

Because cure for cancer of the prostate is possible only when the tumor is discovered early, it is important to teach all male patients older than the age of 40 to have annual or biannual rectal examinations and yearly PSA serum levels.

Nursing Interventions and Patient Teaching

Postoperative nursing management is similar to that for perineal surgery, with special attention to maintenance of bowel and bladder function while keeping the surgical wound clean and avoiding pressure on the perineum and wound. Adequate fluid intake, modification of dietary selections, and perineal exercises may be used to promote regulation of bowel and bladder function. Take extreme care to prevent trauma to the perineum, which could lead to fistula formation. Rectal temperature-taking, enemas, and use of rectal tubes are therefore forbidden. Also take care not to place tension on the Foley catheter, which would disturb the surgical area. Observe the color of the urine for signs of bleeding. The patient will also have a tissue drain inserted during surgery to promote drainage from the wound in the perineum. Initially there may be a small amount of urine from the drain, but this should cease in 1 or 2 days. Follow surgical asepsis during dressing changes. Irrigation of the perineum may be ordered to cleanse the wound and soothe the patient. Administer comfort measures and analgesics as ordered for pain control in the lower back, pelvis, upper thighs, and operative site.

Nursing diagnoses and interventions for the patient undergoing prostate surgery include but are not limited to the following:

Nursing Diagnoses	Nursing Interventions
Risk for fluid volume, deficient, related to hemorrhage or decreased fluid intake	Monitor signs and symptoms of fluid deficit: decreasing or increasing blood pressure, dyspnea. Observe catheter for urine color and amount. Avoid manipulation of rectum by thermometer or rectal tube.
Ineffective sexuality patterns, related to surgical trauma and altered body function	Encourage verbalization of sexual concerns. Provide privacy with significant other to discuss concerns. Inform physician of patient concerns. Explore professional resources: clergy, sexual counselors.

Because UI may occur postoperatively, teach the patient how to keep himself clean. He may need to discuss feelings of depression about his altered body function. Modifying lifestyle and maintaining confidence are important for his return to preillness function. Discuss alternate expressions of sexuality, the value of sexual counseling, and the possibility of recovering some or all of sexual function after treatment is completed.

Emphasize the need for adequate fluid intake, exercise, and rest. Instruct the patient in pain-relieving measures (e.g., exercise, warmth, and medication). Discuss new pharmacologic agents that act as adjuvants in the treatment of cancer and for pain relief during the postoperative recovery period.

Prognosis

Prognosis is directly correlated to the extent of the disease process when diagnosed. Grading of the tumors (well, moderately, or poorly differentiated) correlates with the prognosis; the more poorly differentiated the tumor, the poorer the prognosis is. Under the Gleason system discussed previously, a low score of 2 through 4 is good; a high score of 7 through 10 is not. The treatment goal for the localized disease process is a cure; palliation is used for the extended disease process.

URETHRAL STRICTURES

Etiology and Pathophysiology

A urethral stricture is a narrowing of the lumen of the urethra that interferes with urine flow. Narrowing may be congenital or acquired. Acquired strictures may be caused by chronic infection, trauma, or tumor or occur as a complication of radiation treatment of the pelvis.

Clinical Manifestations

Signs and symptoms include dysuria, weak stream, splaying (spreading out) of the urine stream, nocturia, and increasing pain with bladder distention. In the presence of infection, fever and malaise may be apparent.

Assessment

Subjective data include patient complaints of difficulty initiating the urine stream and the stream seeming to splay more than usual or even seeming to "fork."

Collection of **objective data** includes assessing for signs that may indicate an infectious process and for information indicating the extent of the stricture and possible presence of an obstruction.

Diagnostic Tests

Diagnosis can be confirmed by a voiding cystourethrogram, which demonstrates stricture. Additional diagnostic studies help evaluate damage caused by the obstruction.

Medical Management

Correction of the stricture may be achieved by dilation with metal sounds or surgical release (internal urethrotomy).

Nursing Interventions

Care includes adequate hydration to decrease discomfort when voiding and monitoring urinary output. Mild analgesics should relieve discomfort. Sitz baths may encourage voiding. Reconstruction of the urethra (urethroplasty) may require temporary urinary diversion. After the procedure a splinting catheter supports the suture line. Take care not to place tension on the catheter.

Prognosis

Prognosis after surgical correction or dilation is favorable.

URINARY TRACT TRAUMA

Etiology and Pathophysiology

Assess any patient with a history of traumatic injury for involvement of the urinary tract. Such injuries may include contusions or rupture of the urinary structures. Also observe a patient who has undergone abdominal surgery for incidental injury sustained during the operation. Traumatic invasion of the urinary tract may be evident in open wounds to the lower abdomen, such as gunshot or stab wounds. Trauma to the bladder can occur from a fractured pelvis. Contusion or laceration of the urethra may lead to urethral stricture and possible impotence in men secondary to soft tissue, blood vessel, and nerve damage.

Clinical Manifestations

Monitor urinary output hourly for amount and color. Report any evidence of hematuria. Assess the patient for abdominal pain and tenderness, which may indicate internal hemorrhage, peritonitis, or seepage of urine into the tissues.

Assessment

Collection of **subjective data** involves understanding that the trauma patient may be unable to relate any symptoms that would aid in the assessment of urinary tract involvement. If the patient is able to respond, asking about signs of hematuria is extremely important.

Collection of **objective data** includes a comprehensive assessment of the trauma patient, reviewing all body systems. Assessment related to the urinary tract includes hourly measurement of I&O; observation of urine character or difficulty voiding; evaluation of complaints of abdominal, flank, or referred shoulder pain; and evaluation of abdominal distention and girth.

Diagnostic Tests

Diagnosis of traumatic involvement of the urinary tract may be aided by KUB radiograph, IVP, urinalysis, excretory urogram, and cystoscopy.

Medical Management

Surgical intervention is necessary for correction of tears or rupture of the urinary tract to reinstate urine flow. If damage is severe, removal of the kidney or the bladder may be necessary with the creation of urinary diversion, as discussed later in this chapter. Management of possible hemorrhage and prevention of infection are necessary both before and after surgery.

Nursing Interventions

Nursing responsibility centers on identifying individuals at risk and detecting variations in assessment findings that indicate trauma to the urinary tract. Document and report all findings.

Prognosis

Prognosis depends on the extent and location of the trauma.

IMMUNOLOGIC DISORDERS OF THE KIDNEY

NEPHROTIC SYNDROME

Etiology and Pathophysiology

Nephrotic syndrome (nephrosis) is characterized by marked proteinuria, hypoalbuminemia, and edema. Several events may precipitate nephrotic syndrome; the primary form of nephrosis occurs in the absence of glomerulonephritis or systemic disease, with the inciting event being an upper respiratory tract infection or allergic reaction.

Nephrotic syndrome is characterized by proteinuria, hypoalbuminemia, hyperlipidemia, and edema. The most common sign is excess fluid in the body. This may take several forms: edema around the eyes, characteristically in the morning; pitting edema over the legs; fluid in the pleural cavity (pleural effusion); or fluid in the peritoneal cavity (ascites).

In nephrotic syndrome, the glomeruli become damaged due to inflammation, so that small proteins, such as albumins, immunoglobulins, and antithrombin, can pass through the kidneys into urine. Physiologic changes in the glomeruli interfere with selective permeability. Blood protein is allowed to pass into the urine (proteinuria), causing a loss of serum protein (hypoalbuminemia). This decreases serum osmotic pressure, thus allowing fluid to seep into interstitial spaces, and edema occurs.

Immune responses, both humoral and cellular, are altered in nephrotic syndrome; as a result, infection is an important cause of morbidity and mortality.

Clinical Manifestations

The patient has severe generalized edema **(anasarca)**, anorexia, fatigue, and altered kidney function.

Assessment

Subjective data include patient complaints of loss of interest in eating, constant fatigue, foamy urine from the presence of protein, and decreased urinary output **(oliguria)**, less than 500 mL in 24 hours.

Collection of **objective data** includes assessing the degree of fluid retention by monitoring daily weight, I&O, respiratory effort, and level of consciousness. The patient may relate problems with "swelling" of the face, hands, and feet. Assess skin integrity to determine special needs.

Diagnostic Tests

Blood chemistry findings include hypoalbuminemia and hyperlipidemia. Renal biopsy provides identification of the type and extent of tissue change. Other diagnostic testing is performed to identify the specific underlying cause.

Medical Management

Medical management depends on the extent of tissue involvement and may include the use of corticosteroids (prednisone); antineoplastic agents for immunosuppressive effect; loop diuretics; and a low-sodium, high-protein diet for therapeutic management of edema. Hypoproteinemia may be treated with normal serum albumin and protein-rich nutrition replacement therapy.

Nursing Interventions and Patient Teaching

Nursing interventions include monitoring fluid balance (weight, measurement of abdominal girth, I&O), maintaining bed rest in the presence of extreme edema (recumbent position may initiate diuresis), and assessing for electrolyte imbalance. Skin care is important, as is a gradual increase in activity as the edema is resolved.

Diet includes protein replacement using foods that provide high biologic value (meat, fish, poultry, cheese, eggs) and restriction of sodium to decrease edema. Blood pressure is often elevated and should be monitored closely for changes.

As the patient begins to convalesce, the teaching plan includes the medication regimen (type, dosage, side effects, and need to finish all prescriptions), nutrition (high protein, low sodium), self-assessment of fluid status (monitor weight, presence of edema), signs and symptoms indicating need for medical attention (increase in edema, fatigue, headache, infection), and the need for follow-up care.

Prognosis

In approximately 25% of children and 50% to 75% of adults who develop nephrosis, the disease progresses to renal failure within 5 years. Other patients (particularly children) may have remissions or chronic nephrotic syndrome. Aside from treating the underlying illness, little can be done to prevent a recurrence of nephrosis.

NEPHRITIS

Nephritis encompasses a number of renal disorders characterized by inflammation of the kidney—involving the glomeruli, tubules, or interstitial tissue—and abnormal function. Included in this group of disorders is acute and chronic glomerulonephritis.

Acute Glomerulonephritis

Etiology and Pathophysiology

The health history commonly reveals that the onset of acute glomerulonephritis was preceded by an infection, such as a sore throat or skin infection (most commonly β-hemolytic streptococci) 2 to 3 weeks earlier, or other preexisting multisystem diseases, such as systemic lupus erythematosus. The infectious disease process triggers an immune response that results in inflammation of glomeruli that allows excretion of red blood cells and protein in the urine. This condition is common in children and young adults.

Clinical Manifestations

Often family members first note that the individual has "swelling" of the face, especially around the eyes. Some patients may be acutely ill with a multitude of symptoms, whereas others may be diagnosed on routine examination with only vague symptoms.

Assessment

Subjective data include symptoms indicative of anorexia, nocturia, malaise, and exertional dyspnea.

Collection of **objective data** includes assessment of skin integrity and general condition of skin; the presence and degree of edema with associated difficulty in breathing on exertion, when recumbent, or as evidenced by changes in lung and heart sounds (unusual heart sounds, crackles over lung fields, distention of neck veins); hematuria with changes in urine color from "cola" to frank sanguineous; or changes in voiding, decrease in amount of urinary output, or dysuria.

Diagnostic Tests

Diagnostic tests reveal elevation of BUN, serum creatinine, potassium, erythrocyte sedimentation rate, and antistreptolysin-O titer. Urinalysis shows red blood cells, casts, and/or protein.

Medical Management

Medical management includes treatment of primary symptoms while preventing complications to cerebral and cardiac function. Serum electrolyte levels (sodium and potassium) may indicate a need to adjust dietary intake of sodium and potassium. Level of consciousness should be monitored when the BUN is elevated. Bed rest and fluid intake adjustments are guided by urinary output until diuresis is adequate.

A prophylactic antimicrobial agent, such as penicillin, may be administered for several months after the acute phase of the illness to protect against recurrence of infection. Diuretics may be prescribed to control fluid retention and antihypertensives to reduce blood pressure.

Nursing Interventions and Patient Teaching

Nursing interventions are guided by individual patient needs, focusing on control of symptoms and prevention of complications. Dietary intake includes pro-

 Health Promotion

The Patient with Nephritis

Activity
- Keep patient on bed rest until edema and blood pressure are reduced.
- Encourage quiet diversional activities.
- Ambulate gradually with assistance.
- Space activity to lessen fatigue.

Fluid Balance Maintenance
- Implement dietary restrictions.
- Monitor intake and output.
- Document reactions to medication.

Diet Therapy
- Restrict protein to decrease nitrogenous wastes.
- Restrict sodium to prevent further fluid retention.
- Increase calories for energy source.

Drug Therapy
- Prophylactic antibiotics
- Antihypertensives
- Diuretics
- Drug interactions, side effects to expect and report

Health Maintenance
- Recovery may be extended.
- Physician will monitor urine for albumin and red blood cells (RBCs).
- Teach early signs of fluid retention.
- Signs and symptoms may resolve and then become worse.
- Normal activities may be resumed after urine is free of albumin and RBCs for 1 month, although the patient is not considered cured until the urine is free of albumin and RBCs for 6 months.
- Report hematuria, headache, edema.

tein restrictions (to decrease blood urea levels), with carbohydrates providing a source of energy.

Monitor I&O and vital signs. Determine the level of activity based on the degree of edema, hypertension, proteinuria, and hematuria, since excessive activity may increase these signs (see Health Promotion box).

Because of the long-term nature of glomerulonephritis, patient teaching is important. Proteinuria and hematuria may exist microscopically even when other symptoms subside. Although fatigue may be present, these patients usually feel well; therefore they often must be convinced of the need to continue prescribed treatment and to return for follow-up care. Explain the nature of the illness and the effect of diet and fluids on fluid balance and sodium retention. Teach about prescribed sodium and fluid restrictions (provide written information regarding sodium content of foods, as necessary). Include information about protein restrictions and carbohydrate sources. Also discuss the medication regimen (dose, frequency, side effects, need to continue per physician instructions). Stress the need to pace activities with rest if fatigue is present; to avoid trauma and infection (which may exacerbate the illness); and to obtain follow-up health care. Teach the patient about the signs and symptoms indicating the need for medical attention (hematuria, headache, edema, hypertension).

Prognosis

The prognosis of acute poststreptococcal glomerulonephritis is generally good; however, some patients develop chronic glomerulonephritis and ESRD, requiring dialysis or kidney transplantation.

Chronic Glomerulonephritis

Etiology and Pathophysiology

With chronic glomerulonephritis there is usually no indication of an inciting event. Occasionally the patient with acute glomerulonephritis progresses to a chronic phase. Because other chronic illnesses (e.g., diabetes mellitus or systemic lupus erythematosus) may mask the symptoms of renal degeneration, many patients do not seek medical attention until kidney function is compromised. Chronic glomerulonephritis is characterized by slow, progressive destruction of glomeruli with related loss of function. The kidneys atrophy (actually decrease in size).

Clinical Manifestations

Signs and symptoms may include malaise, morning headaches, dyspnea with exertion, visual and digestive disturbances, edema, and fatigue. Physical findings include hypertension, anemia, proteinuria, anasarca, and cardiac and cerebral manifestations.

Assessment

Subjective data include patient complaints of fatigue and a decreased ability to perform ADLs as a result of dyspnea and decreasing ability to concentrate. Investigate complaints of morning headaches (their location, pattern, and character), and note the presence of any visual disturbance.

Collection of **objective data** includes clarifying outward manifestations of the headache and respiratory effort that may interfere with daily task performance. Assess mental functioning, irritability, slurred speech, ataxia, or tremors. Carefully assess and document the degree of edema, noting specific location and response to pressure by pressing the fingers into the edematous area and observing for pitting (see Figure 48-17). Note skin color, ecchymoses (irregularly formed hemorrhagic areas of the skin) or rash, dry skin, and scratching. Observe urine color and amount. Monitor vital signs, including a chest assessment for cardiac and pulmonary signs of fluid retention: unusual heart sounds, crackles over lung fields, and distention of neck veins.

Diagnostic Tests

Early disease shows albumin and red blood cells in the urine, although kidney function test results are within normal limits. With advanced destruction of nephrons, the specific gravity becomes fixed and blood levels of

NPN wastes (creatinine and urea) increase. Creatinine clearance may be as low as 5 to 10 mL/min, compared with the normal range of 107 to 139 mL/min in men and 87 to 107 mL/min in women.

Medical Management

Medical management includes control of secondary side effects as discussed with acute glomerulonephritis, with the use of renal dialysis and possible kidney transplantation to provide elimination of wastes from the body.

Nursing Interventions and Patient Teaching

Nursing interventions for the patient with chronic glomerulonephritis represent a special challenge. This patient has already suffered major damage to the kidney filtration system. It is crucial that the patient's condition not be further compromised by infection or other complications. Monitor changes in vital signs and diagnostic tests to aid in choosing proper nursing interventions. Interventions parallel those noted with nephrotic syndrome and acute glomerulonephritis. Chronic glomerulonephritis may progress to ESRD, necessitating related nursing interventions (see Health Promotion box, p. 1708).

Nursing diagnoses and interventions for the patient with chronic glomerulonephritis include but are not limited to the following:

Nursing Diagnoses	Nursing Interventions
Excess fluid volume, related to decreased urinary output	Assess the patient's understanding of therapeutic interventions. Note I&O every hour (or more often). Monitor signs and symptoms of fluid excess: weight gain, hypertension, edema, dyspnea. Provide ice chips for thirst with prescribed diet. Monitor and report abnormal laboratory results.
Activity intolerance, related to kidney dysfunction	Assess level of activity tolerance. Encourage patient to report activities that increase his or her fatigue. Plan activities to minimize fatigue.

Patient teaching focuses on preventive health maintenance, emphasizing a health-promoting lifestyle, with prevention and early treatment of infections.

Prognosis

Some people with minimal impairment in kidney function continue to feel well and show little progression of disease. With other patients the progression of renal deterioration may be slow but steady and end in renal failure. In still others the disease progresses rapidly.

RENAL FAILURE

Renal failure is characterized by the kidneys' inability to remove wastes, concentrate urine, and conserve or eliminate electrolytes. Diabetes mellitus is the most common cause of renal failure, accounting for more than 40% of new cases. Other predisposing concurrent illnesses include burns, trauma, heart failure, volume depletion, and renal disease. Nursing interventions to prevent the development of renal failure include providing adequate hydration, preventing infections, monitoring for signs and symptoms of shock, and teaching drug side effects to report immediately.

ACUTE RENAL FAILURE

Etiology and Pathophysiology

Kidney function may be altered by interference with the kidney's ability to be selective in filtering blood or by an actual decrease in blood flow to the kidneys. ARF can be caused by a number of medical conditions, such as hemorrhage, trauma, infection, and decreased cardiac output.

The course of ARF is divided into phases. In the **oliguric phase,** BUN and serum creatinine levels rise while urinary output decreases to less than 20 mL/hr (less than 400 mL/24 hr). The oliguric phase may last from several days to 4 weeks to several months. Some patients may experience the nonoliguric form, usually caused by nephrotoxic antibiotics, in which urinary output may exceed 2 L/24 hr. In the **diuretic phase,** blood chemistry levels begin to return to normal and urinary output increases to 1 to 2 L/24 hr. The diuretic phase usually lasts 1 to 3 weeks. Return to normal or near-normal function occurs in the **recovery phase.** Recovery begins as the glomerular filtration rate rises. Recovery can take up to 1 year.

Clinical Manifestations

The patient may experience anorexia, nausea, vomiting, edema, and associated signs and symptoms of diminished kidney function.

Assessment

Subjective data include patient reports of lethargy, loss of appetite, nausea, and headache.

Objective data involve physical findings of progression of the disease process. Assess for dry mucous membranes, poor skin turgor, urinary output of less than 400 mL/24 hr, vomiting, diarrhea, and anasarca. Assessment findings may include central nervous system manifestations of drowsiness, muscle twitching, and seizures.

Diagnostic Tests

Physical assessment, history, and elevated blood chemistry tests such as BUN and creatinine (azotemia) confirm the diagnosis. After the patient is stabilized, further studies may be done to assess for residual damage.

Medical Management

Measures include administration of fluids and osmotic preparations to prevent decreased renal perfusion, manage fluid volume, and treat electrolyte imbalances. Renal dialysis may be necessary to manage systemic fluid shifts, especially cardiac and respiratory, and may be effective in removing some nephrotoxins.

Diet should be protein sparing, high in carbohydrates, and low in potassium and sodium. Drug therapy may include diuretics to increase urinary output (e.g., furosemide, hydrochlorothiazide [HydroDIURIL]). Potassium-lowering agents are used to remove potassium through the gastrointestinal tract; sodium polystyrene sulfonate (Kayexalate) is administered orally, per nasogastric tube, or as a retention enema. Antibiotics that are not dependent on kidney excretion are used to eradicate or prevent infection. Whatever combination of drug therapy is used, dosage and administration times require adjustment according to the level of kidney function.

Nursing Interventions and Patient Teaching

Accurately document urinary output to identify the level of kidney function. Azotemia may be revealed by blood chemistry studies. Observe the patient with azotemia for changes in level of consciousness. Closely monitor fluid status, vital signs, and response to therapies. Frequent skin care with tepid water to remove urea crystals will be comforting. Dialysis presents special nursing challenges, discussed later in this chapter.

Teaching includes identifying preventable environmental or health factors contributing to the illness (such as hypertension, nephrotoxic drugs). Teach the patient about activity restrictions, dietary restrictions, and the medication regimen. Provide nutritional support with specialized enteral formulas, which may contain essential amino acids and minerals, in addition to replacement of electrolytes (especially sodium to match insensible loss) and provision of caloric needs. Make a nutritional assessment with appropriate modifications daily.

Stress the need to report signs and symptoms of infection and of returning renal failure to the physician. Emphasize the need for ongoing follow-up care.

Prognosis

Recovery from an episode of ARF depends on the underlying illness, the patient's condition, and careful supportive management given during the period of kidney shutdown. The leading cause of death is infection, such as that of the urinary tract, lungs, and peritoneum. Mortality from fluid overload and acidosis has been reduced as a result of dialysis and other forms of therapy. Patients who survive the acute episode of tubular insufficiency have a chance of recovering kidney function. Although renal tissue may regenerate more completely after toxic injury than ischemia, both forms usually show return to normal or near-normal kidney function.

For those in whom ARF has been caused by glomerular disease or severe infection of renal tissue, the prognosis may not be as favorable. Return of kidney function is determined by the extent of scarring and destruction of functional renal tissue that has occurred during the acute episode of renal failure.

CHRONIC RENAL FAILURE (END-STAGE RENAL DISEASE)

Etiology and Pathophysiology

Chronic renal failure, or ESRD, exists when the kidneys are unable to regain normal function. ESRD develops slowly over an extended period as a result of renal disease or other disease processes that compromise renal blood perfusion. As much as 80% of nephrons may be severely impaired before loss of kidney function is detected. The most common causes of ESRD are pyelonephritis, chronic glomerulonephritis, glomerulosclerosis, chronic urinary obstruction, severe hypertension, diabetes mellitus, gout, and PKD. Whatever the cause, dialysis or kidney transplantation is needed to maintain life.

ESRD represents a significant health problem worldwide, resulting in the death of thousands and financial crisis for patients and their families. The government actively helps defray costs through the Medicare program.

Clinical Manifestations

The onset of signs and symptoms may be so gradual and the signs and symptoms so vague that the patient is unable to identify when the problems started. When questioned, the patient may be able to relate occurrences that seemed insignificant at the time. The clinical picture is usually unique to the individual. Common symptoms are headache; lethargy; asthenia (decreased strength or energy); anorexia; pruritus; elimination changes; **anuria** (urinary output of less than 100 mL/day); muscle cramps or twitching; impotence; characteristic dusky yellow-tan or gray skin color from retained urochrome pigments; and signs and symptoms characteristic of central nervous system involvement, such as disorientation and mental lapses.

Other associated conditions are responsible for many of the symptoms. Azotemia develops as excessive amounts of nitrogenous compounds build in the blood. Anemia occurs when the production of renal erythropoietin is decreased as a result of loss of kidney function. Acidosis, hypertension, and glucose intolerance may be present as a result of the insult to homeostasis.

Assessment

Subjective data include patient complaints of joint pain and edema; severe headaches; nausea; anorexia; intermittent chest pain; weakness; and in particular, fatigue, intractable singultus (hiccups), decreased libido, menstrual irregularities, and impaired concentration. The clinical consequences of renal failure are far reaching, affecting nearly every body system.

Collection of **objective data** involves a nursing assessment that may yield unremarkable results, except for signs and symptoms that support the patient complaints. Uremic encephalopathy affects the central nervous system. Usually the first sign is a reduction in alertness and awareness. The patient exhibits Kussmaul's respirations (abnormally deep, very rapid sighing respirations), and coma develops. The accumulation of urates results in halitosis with a urine odor and "uremic frost" on the skin in the form of a white powder.

Diagnostic Tests

Diagnosis of ESRD is confirmed by elevated BUN of at least 50 mg/dL and serum creatinine levels greater than 5 mg/dL, electrolyte imbalance (including a decreased number of bicarbonate and magnesium and an increased number of potassium, sodium, and phosphatase ions), and other indicators related to the underlying cause. Kidney function studies assess the degree of damage or level of kidney function.

Medical Management

Medical management is instituted to conserve kidney function as long as possible. Renal dialysis is initiated when necessary, and the patient may be prepared for kidney transplantation. Drug therapy may include anticonvulsants to control seizure activity (phenytoin [Dilantin], diazepam [Valium]), antianemics, vitamin supplements to counteract nutritional deficiencies, antiemetics (prochlorperazine [Compazine]), antipruritics (cyproheptadine [Periactin]), and biologic response modifiers to stimulate red cell production (epoetin alfa [Epogen, EPO]) to treat anemia caused by a reduced production of erythropoietin. Iron deficiency anemia must be treated with ferrous sulfate orally or iron dextran (DexFerrum per Z-track intramuscular method) before epoetin alfa will be effective.

Nursing Interventions and Patient Teaching

Nursing interventions focus on restoring homeostasis. Measures to control fluid and electrolyte balance vary greatly, according to individual patient needs. Nutritional therapy is aimed at preserving protein stores and preventing production of additional protein waste products that the kidney would have to clear. High biologic proteins are used to provide the essential amino acids.

The diet is high in calories from carbohydrates and fats from polyunsaturated sources (to maintain weight and spare protein), at least 2500 to 3000 calories daily. Other dietary restrictions are related to the patient's degree of acidosis. Potassium is retained, so foods high in potassium are restricted. Sodium is controlled at a level sufficient to replace sodium loss without causing fluid retention.

Nursing interventions for ARF are also instituted for ESRD. Provide emotional support for the patient who faces role changes and invasive treatments such as dialysis or kidney transplantation. As discussed in the Health Promotion box, fluid balance is of prime importance. The patient may have fluid equal to the amount excreted in the urine plus about 300 to 600 mL to compensate for **insensible** (imperceptible) **fluid loss** (fluid lost through the lungs, perspiration, and feces). Salt substitutes are not advised because most contain potassium. If seizure activity occurs, institute safety measures to protect the patient (Nursing Care Plan 50-1) (see also Chapter 54).

Patient teaching should emphasize food exchanges and fluid intake within restrictions prescribed for that patient. Encourage the patient to increase activity as tolerated; maintain impeccable skin care; prevent infection and injury; and develop coping behaviors to adapt to lifestyle changes for patient, family, and caregiver.

 Health Promotion

The Patient with Renal Failure

Fluid and Electrolyte Balance
- Assess intake and output (hourly may be indicated).
- Weigh daily (same time, same clothing, same scale).
- Assess overt (open to view) signs of hydration status: edema, turgor.
- Assess covert (hidden) signs of hydration status: breath sounds, laboratory studies, and so on.

Nutrition
- Provide prescribed diet.
- Guide patient food selection.
- Plan fluid intake per shift within prescribed limits and according to patient preference.
- Reinforce diet instructions as indicated.

Comfort and Safety
- Provide quiet environment (sound and lighting).
- Space nursing interventions to conserve patient energy.
- Medicate as needed for comfort.
- Provide skin care to alleviate discomfort from pruritus.
- Provide mouth care as needed.
- Maintain asepsis during procedures.
- Prevent exposure to pathogens.

Coping Behaviors
- Listen (to patient and significant others).
- Refer to pastoral care or religious support group.
- Provide private times with significant others.
- Offer interview with social services.

Documentation and Reporting
- Document all relevant findings.
- Maintain open communications with supervisory staff.
- Adjust nursing care plan as indicated to meet changing patient needs.
- Maintain dietary restrictions: food exchange, measuring fluids, food diary.
- Take health promotion–illness prevention measures.

Nursing Care Plan 50-1 The Patient with End-Stage Renal Disease

Mr. Jerrod, a 37-year-old high school basketball coach, visited his family physician with complaints of weight gain, decreasing strength, increasing inability to concentrate, and morning headaches. Physical examination revealed severe hypertension, yellow-gray skin color, and pale mucous membranes. After diagnostic studies reveal chronic glomerulonephritis with end-state renal disease (ESRD), Mr. Jerrod is admitted to the hospital to stabilize his condition.

NURSING DIAGNOSIS *Excess fluid volume, related to compromised renal regulatory mechanism, as evidenced by systemic edema*

Patient Goals and Expected Outcomes	Nursing Interventions	Evaluation
The patient will be able to reduce fluid to precrisis level	Record baseline assessment data. Create chart for patient to monitor: • Daily weight • Intake and output • Edema	Patient is able to complete daily self-monitoring with 1 pound weight loss daily × 3.
The patient will modify diet to exclude foods and fluids that foster sodium, potassium, and water retention	Teach nutritional guidelines for dietary and fluid parameters with scheduling. Evaluate daily or as needed for systemic edema: girth, skin turgor, respiratory rate and quality. Monitor for manifestations of electrolyte imbalance. Teach patient and significant other about the type, cause, and treatment for fluid and electrolyte imbalance, as appropriate.	Patient is able to order daily diet and fluids within prescribed parameters.

NURSING DIAGNOSIS *Powerlessness, related to sudden onset of life-altering illness as evidenced by patient statements: "I've always tried to take care of myself—look where it got me. Nowhere! Now I have to face my own death!"*

Patient Goals and Expected Outcomes	Nursing Interventions	Evaluation
The patient will be empowered to assist in planning own care and in goal achievement	Provide support for the patient. Explain plans and procedures before scheduled times, according to patient's ability to understand. Negotiate with patient when changes are necessary. Accept patient's expression of self and values. Include significant other in planning for the patient's maximum role in self-management. Communicate unique patient planning arrangements for continuity with all treatment team members.	Patient voices a sense that the staff is sensitive to his needs. Patient seems able to plan modifications in work and home schedules to accommodate health needs.

NURSING DIAGNOSIS *Deficient knowledge, related to health education and home maintenance for ESRD*

Patient Goals and Expected Outcomes	Nursing Interventions	Evaluation
The patient will describe the fundamental characteristics of ESRD and treatment options	Assess the amount and depth of the patient's information about ESRD. Collaborate with physician and treatment team in individualizing established institutional protocol for care of the patient with ESRD: 1. What happens when kidneys fail? 2. Treatment options • Hemodialysis • Peritoneal dialysis • Kidney transplantation	Patient is able to correctly answer basic questions about treatment options. Patient is able to correctly answer questions from teaching and is open to pose new questions.

Continued

Nursing Care Plan 50-1 The Patient with End-Stage Renal Disease—cont'd

Patient Goals and Expected Outcomes	Nursing Interventions	Evaluation
The patient will describe the fundamental characteristics of ESRD and treatment options—cont'd	3. Inpatient versus outpatient care 4. Financing treatment 5. Teaching aids 6. Organizations that can help Plan time to listen to the patient's and family's concerns and fears. Allow time for questions and answers and teaching reinforcement each day. Arrange (with patient's permission) opportunity for patient and family to meet with a patient or family who is positively adapting to ESRD. Be consistent in scheduling treatments with primary health care providers. Participate in end-of-life planning, when and if appropriate.	

Critical Thinking Questions

1. Mr. Jerrod complains of loss of appetite and limited food choices. What would be some helpful suggestions to improve his nutritional status?
2. Mr. Jerrod established a therapeutic nurse-patient relationship with the nurse and confided that he is having marital problems partly due to his inability to have a satisfactory sexual relationship with his wife. What would be an appropriate response?
3. The nurse notes Mr. Jerrod's lack of interest in his therapeutic regimen of diet, medications, and fluid restrictions. He states, "What's the use? I will never be well again." What would be some therapeutic interventions?

CARE OF THE PATIENT REQUIRING DIALYSIS

Dialysis is a medical procedure for the removal of certain elements from the blood; the process is based on the difference in their rates of diffusion through an external semipermeable membrane or, in the case of peritoneal dialysis, through the peritoneum. Dialysis mimics kidney function, helping to restore balance when normal kidney function is interrupted temporarily or permanently. Dialysis involves either diffusion of wastes, drugs, and/or excess electrolytes and/or osmosis of water across a semipermeable membrane into a dialysate fluid that is prescribed to meet individual needs. Dialysis is achieved by the process of hemodialysis or peritoneal dialysis.

HEMODIALYSIS

Hemodialysis is used for patients with acute or irreversible renal failure and fluid and electrolyte imbalances. Hemodialysis requires access to the patient's circulatory system to route blood through the artificial kidney (dialyzer) for removal of wastes, fluids, and electrolytes; the blood is then returned to the patient's body. Box 50-4 lists nursing intervention guidelines. Temporary methods include subclavian or femoral catheters or an external shunt placed in the nondominant forearm (Figure 50-9). In ESRD, access can be achieved by constructing a direct or a graft arteriovenous (AV) fistula (Figure 50-10). The AV fistula is preferred for permanent access. Hemodialysis is usually scheduled three times a week for 3 to 6 hours. Patients can be maintained on dialysis therapy indefinitely or while waiting for kidney transplantation.

In a comparative study of the use of daily versus traditional hemodialysis on alternative days, researchers found that more frequent hemodialysis decreased the risk of fatal nonrenal complications of ARF (Schiffl et al., 2002).

Medical Management

Medical management includes continuation of previously instituted therapies. Closely monitor blood levels of drugs excreted by the kidney to maintain therapeutic levels and prevent toxic accumulations. Dose adjustments are affected by glomerular filtration rate, dialysis, vomiting, and doses missed during hospital treatments. Medication may include antihypertensives, cardiac glycosides, antibiotics, and antidysrhythmics. Instruct the patient not to take over-the-counter medications without consulting the physician.

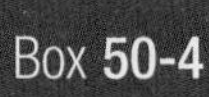

Box 50-4 Nursing Intervention Guidelines for the Patient Undergoing Hemodialysis

PATIENT TEACHING

- Reinforce explanation of dialysis procedure.
- Inform of community resources.
- Explain dietary restrictions.
- Teach about self-care, general information.

MONITORING DURING DIALYSIS

- Maintain asepsis and universal precautions.
- Weigh before and after treatment.
- Obtain vital signs every 30 to 60 minutes (take blood pressure in arm without fistula).
- Maintain orientation (thought processes may be altered).
- Assess for hemorrhage resulting from heparin use during dialysis.
- Monitor equipment (interruption of procedure).

ACTIVITY

- Provide diversions (reading, television, sleep).
- Ensure patient comfort (reclining, sitting, lying).
- Monitor dietary intake (may be hungry or nauseated).

CARE AFTER DIALYSIS OR BETWEEN TREATMENTS

- Schedule fluid intake within restrictions.
- Monitor for signs of fluid and electrolyte imbalance.
- Assess the access site for signs of infection, adequate circulation.
- Post signs regarding location of access site; do not take blood pressure or perform a venipuncture on arm with access site.
- Auscultate arteriovenous fistula for bruit (adventitious sound of venous or arterial origin heard on auscultation); palpate arteriovenous fistula for thrill (abnormal tremor).
- Assess, document, and report changes in general status.
- Provide skin care: bathe with tepid water to remove urea deposit.

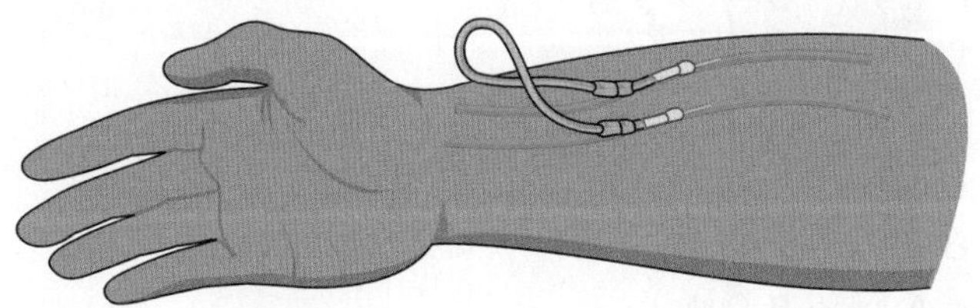

FIGURE 50-9 External arteriovenous shunt.

Nursing Interventions

Nursing interventions are dictated by individual patient conditions, including other acute or chronic problems. Most patients are dialyzed on an outpatient basis. (General nursing intervention guidelines are noted in Box 50-4 and in Nursing Care Plan 50-1.) Psychosocial aspects of care for patients receiving dialysis are illustrated in the Communication box on p. 1712.

Nurses have a key responsibility for maintaining access sites and preventing or managing infection. Use a structured teaching program, with individualized patient teaching strategies to accommodate culture and knowledge level.

PERITONEAL DIALYSIS

Peritoneal dialysis can be performed with a minimum of equipment and by an ambulatory patient. Unlike hemodialysis, peritoneal dialysis is performed four times a day, 7 days a week. One exchange cycle usually requires 30 to 40 minutes. The principle of osmosis and diffusion through a semipermeable membrane is the same as in hemodialysis, but the peritoneum is used as the semipermeable membrane instead of the artificial kidney. Peritoneal dialysis is contraindicated for patients with systemic inflammatory disease, previous abdominal surgery, and chronic back pain, among other conditions.

To facilitate peritoneal dialysis, the physician places a catheter into the peritoneal space under aseptic conditions (Figure 50-11). The dialyzing fluid is instilled for a predetermined period, then drained. The patient with ESRD may be maintained on peritoneal dialysis, continuous ambulatory peritoneal dialysis (CAPD), or continuous cycle peritoneal dialysis (CCPD). Nocturnal intermittent peritoneal dialysis can be done three to five times per week for 10 to 12 hours. The patient is taught how to do the dialysis, which allows for more freedom. Although hemodialysis can also be done at home using strict aseptic technique, it is much more expensive and confining than CAPD.

Nursing Interventions

Common complications associated with peritoneal dialysis guide nursing interventions. Hypotension may occur with excessive sodium and fluid removal. Perito-

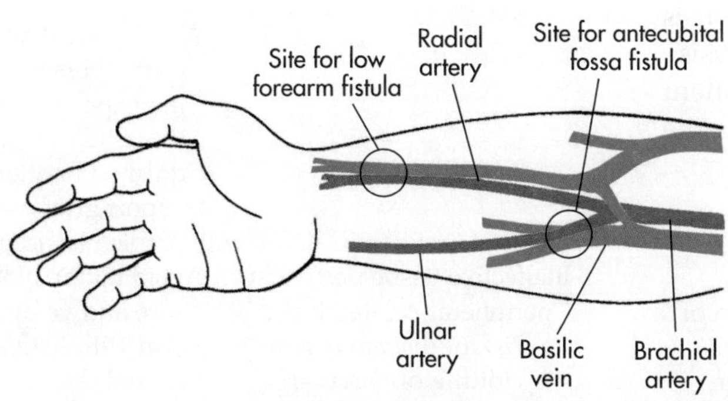

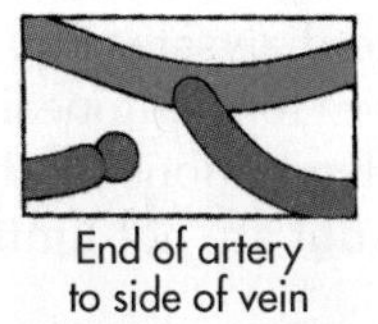

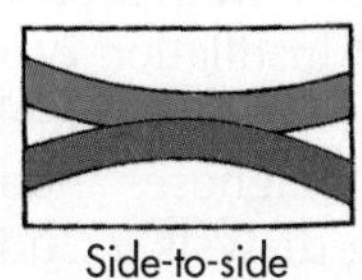

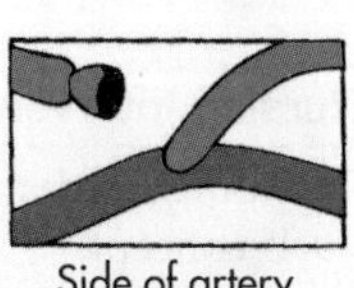

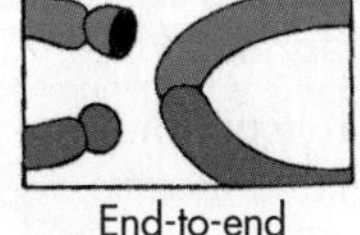

FIGURE 50-10 Internal arteriovenous fistula. Types of fistula construction.

Communication

Psychosocial Aspects of Care for Patients Receiving Dialysis

Mr. Jonas, a student nurse, enters Mr. Klauss's room to complete the initial morning assessment and finds him crying while struggling to get out of bed.

Nurse: Mr. Klauss, what's wrong? (general lead, allows patient to describe)

Patient: Oh, nothing!

Nurse: (therapeutic silence, remains attentive, gives time)

Patient: Nothing is going right. I might as well be dead!

Nurse: What's wrong? (general lead, patient did not answer, encourages description)

Patient: I was trying to get up to take a shower, but I'm so weak I can't get myself out of bed.

Nurse: That must be frustrating. (voicing the implied)

Patient: That's an understatement! Look at me! I'm 37 years old; I should be in my prime but instead I'm gaining weight; can't do my job because I can't concentrate. How am I supposed to feel?

Nurse: It must be frightening to experience all these changes. It would be understandable for you to be scared. (validating feelings)

Patient: I am scared! What if I never get better? I read this article about someone younger than I am who had the same thing and he died when he had to go on dialysis.

Nurse: What do you think will happen to you? (general lead, encourages description without prescribing response)

Patient: Well, I don't know. The doctor keeps avoiding my questions and I see myself being less able to do anything. Maybe I am afraid—afraid of dying.

Nurse: (therapeutic silence, allows time for reflection)

Patient: Well, I never thought I'd say that—being afraid to die. It doesn't seem so frightening to say. I guess I didn't trust myself to be honest with myself or anyone else.

Nurse: Being honest with yourself is an important step to understanding. (pause) It seems, too, that you may not have accurate information about your illness. Let's plan to talk with your doctor about what you can reasonably expect—things you will be able to do, limitations, and things that you can do to enhance your physical and emotional health. (summarizing and goal setting for individualized patient teaching and discharge planning)

Patient: That sounds great, Mr. Jonas. I really do want to do whatever I can to improve my chances of a better life. Would you help me get up to shower?

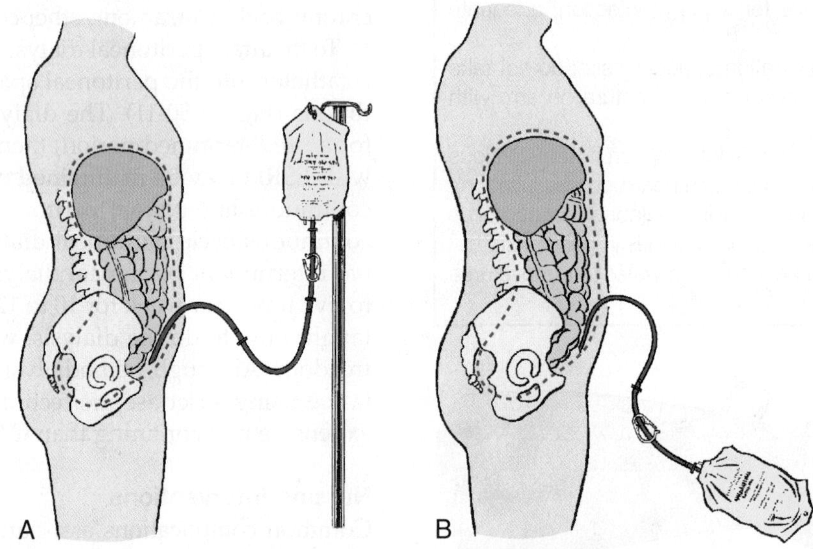

FIGURE 50-11 Peritoneal dialysis. **A,** Inflow. **B,** Outflow.

nitis may arise from sepsis. Pain and hemorrhage may accompany instillation of the dialysate. Box 50-5 lists nursing intervention guidelines for peritoneal dialysis.

Nursing diagnoses and interventions for the patient undergoing dialysis include but are not limited to the following:

Nursing Diagnoses	Nursing Interventions
Ineffective role performance, related to: • chronic illness • treatment side effects	Encourage verbalization of self-concept. Assist in identifying personal strengths. Assist patient and significant others with clarifying expected roles and those that must be relinquished or altered. Support grief work if loss of role has occurred.
Ineffective tissue perfusion, peripheral, related to: • risk of disconnection • clotting of vascular access	Avoid taking blood pressure and venipuncture in arm with fistula or cannula. Auscultate for bruits.

Box 50-5 Nursing Intervention Guidelines for the Patient Undergoing Peritoneal Dialysis

PATIENT TEACHING
- Explanation of procedure
- Signs of complications
- Diet or fluid restrictions
- Medication (schedule in relation to dialysis time)
- Dialysate kept at body temperature to lessen discomfort

MONITORING DURING DIALYSIS
- Weight before and after procedure
- Hemorrhage (smoky, pink, or red-tinged dialysate)
- Type of dialysate (tailored to patient needs)
- Amount and timing of dialysate instillation
- Vital signs

CARE BETWEEN DIALYSES
- Signs of peritonitis (pain, fever, cloudy fluid)
- Strict aseptic care of catheter site
- Weigh daily

Nursing Diagnoses	Nursing Interventions
Ineffective tissue perfusion, peripheral, related to: • risk of disconnection • clotting of vascular access	Observe access site for skin color and condition. After dialysis, inspect needle puncture sites for bleeding.

Prognosis

The patient with effective medical management can be maintained indefinitely on dialysis.

SURGICAL PROCEDURES FOR URINARY DYSFUNCTION

If damage to the urinary system cannot be corrected by medical management, surgical intervention may be necessary for temporary or permanent resection of the affected organ, such as when kidney function is lost. Dialysis is a viable management alternative, but a kidney transplant is preferable. The patient may require a kidney from a live or cadaver donor to replace the damaged kidney. Common surgical interventions and nursing intervention priorities are listed in Table 50-4. Preoperative and intraoperative management measures are the same as for major abdominal surgery with general anesthesia (see Chapter 42). Suggested nursing diagnoses include those for abdominal surgery.

NEPHRECTOMY

Nephrectomy is the surgical removal of the kidney, either a small portion or the entire organ and surrounding tissues. In partial nephrectomy, only the diseased or infected portion of the kidney is removed. Radical nephrectomy involves removing the entire kidney, a section of the ureter, the adrenal gland, and the fatty tissue surrounding the kidney.

Postoperative management for surgical removal of the kidney is based on the prevention and detection of hemorrhage by monitoring vital signs, especially pulse and blood pressure; observation for restlessness and for gastrointestinal complications of nausea, vomiting, and abdominal distention; and establishment of adequate urinary drainage. Record I&O. If the thoracic cavity is opened during surgery, the patient will have chest tubes (see Chapter 49). Pain may compromise respiratory efficiency. Administer analgesics as ordered to facilitate lung expansion and the patient's activity level. Reposition the patient every 2 hours and ambulate as ordered. Change dressings according to the physician's order, and record the amount and color of any drainage. Maintain close surveillance on the function of the remaining kidney.

Patient Teaching

Instruct the patient to avoid heavy lifting, drink 2000 mL of fluid each day (unless contraindicated), monitor output, avoid use of alcohol, and avoid respiratory tract infections and hazardous activities that could damage the remaining kidney.

Prognosis

Complete recovery from nephrectomy is expected in the absence of any complication.

NEPHROSTOMY

A nephrostomy is an incision created between the kidney and the skin to drain urine directly from the renal pelvis. A nephrostomy is performed when an occlu-

Table 50-4 Surgical Procedures for Urinary Dysfunction

SURGICAL INTERVENTION	NURSING INTERVENTION PRIORITIES
Nephrostomy: Surgical procedure in which an incision is made on the patient's flank, so that a catheter can be inserted into the renal pelvis for drainage	Meticulous skin care, assessment for hemorrhage, accurate intake and output (I&O)
Nephrectomy: Surgical removal of the kidney	Assessment for hemorrhage, promotion of respiratory effort, accurate I&O
Cystectomy: Surgical removal of the bladder	Promotion of urinary drainage via ileal conduit, I&O
Ureterosigmoidostomy: Surgical procedure in which a ureter is implanted in the sigmoid colon of the intestinal tract	Meticulous skin care, monitoring of electrolyte imbalance, assessment of signs and symptoms of infection
Cutaneous ureterostomy: Surgical implantation of the terminal ends of the ureter under the skin	Meticulous skin care, assessment of urinary obstruction, accurate I&O

sion keeps urine from passing from the kidney, through the ureter, and into the urinary bladder. Without a way for urine to drain, pressure would rise within the urinary system and damage the kidneys. The most common cause of obstruction is cancer. This procedure can also be used to remove kidney stones.

Catheters are used to drain the wound. Take care to prevent obstruction of the catheters with blood clots postoperatively. Measure and record the amount and nature of drainage from the catheters, and change dressings frequently, keeping the skin clean using surgical sepsis. Turn the patient and position on the affected side as ordered to facilitate drainage and assist in respiratory ventilation. Never clamp a nephrostomy catheter (tube); acute pyelonephritis may result. If ordered by the physician, irrigate a nephrostomy catheter using strict aseptic technique. Gentle instillation of no more than 5 mL of sterile saline solution at one time prevents renal damage.

KIDNEY TRANSPLANTATION

Kidney transplantation is performed as an intervention in irreversible renal failure. The kidney is surgically placed retroperitoneally in the iliac fossa. The renal artery is anastomosed to the recipient's internal or external iliac artery and the renal vein to the recipient's iliac vein. Usually, the kidney begins to function immediately.

Selection of a transplant recipient is based on careful evaluation of the patient's medical, immunologic, and psychosocial status. Usually a recipient is younger than age 70, has an estimated life expectancy of 2 years or more, and is expected to have an improved quality of life after transplantation. Through conservative management and dialysis, the patient's state is as nontoxic as possible. Preoperative nursing intervention is complicated by the patient's fear and anxiety about transplantation and about possible rejection of the implanted organ. The patient is dialyzed until surgery can be satisfactorily completed. In surgery the nonfunctioning kidney remains in place and the donor kidney is positioned in the iliac fossa anterior to the crest of the ileum. The ureter is anastomosed into either the patient's ureter or bladder (Figure 50-12). However, bilateral nephrectomy may be performed before the transplantation procedure for persistent or active bacterial pyleonephritis, uncontrolled renin-mediated hypertension, polycystic kidneys, or rapidly progressive glomerulonephritis.

Postoperatively, assess the patient for signs of rejection and infection: apprehension, generalized edema, fever, increased blood pressure, oliguria, edema, and tenderness over the graft site. An immunosuppressive agent, such as cyclosporine, is used alone or in conjunction with steroids. Cyclosporine is considered an effective drug in suppressing the immune system's efforts to reject tissue while leaving the recipient sufficient immune activity to combat infection. Mycophenolate (CellCept) and tacrolimus (Prograf) are drugs used to prevent rejection of kidney transplants; they are used in combination with corticosteroids. Immunosuppressive therapy increases the risk for infection and possible steroid-induced bleeding.

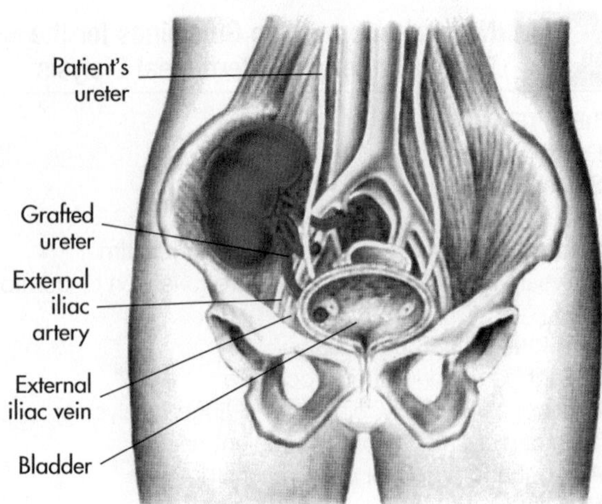

FIGURE 50-12 Kidney transplantation.

Patient Teaching

Postoperative care includes special assessment of kidney function and electrolyte balance. The function of the transplanted kidney is the primary concern after surgery. Home follow-up becomes a life pattern for the transplantation patient. Patient education is extensive: diet, fluids, daily weights, strict I&O measurements, prevention of infection, and avoidance of activities that may compromise the integrity of the urinary tract. Community support groups, sponsored by the American Association of Kidney Patients, help the patient and the family adapt to living with dialysis and transplantation. The National Kidney Foundation has a written protocol for the procurement of organs for donation.

Prognosis

Success of kidney transplantation parallels the individual patient's general health status and compliance with the treatment plan. Transplantation offers the only possibility of return to a normal lifestyle for the ESRD patient. Successful kidney transplantation prolongs and markedly improves quality of life, freeing the patient from the restrictions of dialysis.

URINARY DIVERSION

Several types of procedures are used to divert the flow of urine when required for treatment of bladder cancer, invasive cervical cancer, neurogenic bladder, and congenital anomalies. Often a cystectomy (the surgical removal of the bladder) is performed.

The cystectomy patient presents a unique challenge because of the need to create an artificial port for urine elimination. The most common urinary diversion procedure is the ileal conduit (Bricker's procedure or ileal loop), the ureters are implanted into a loop of the il-

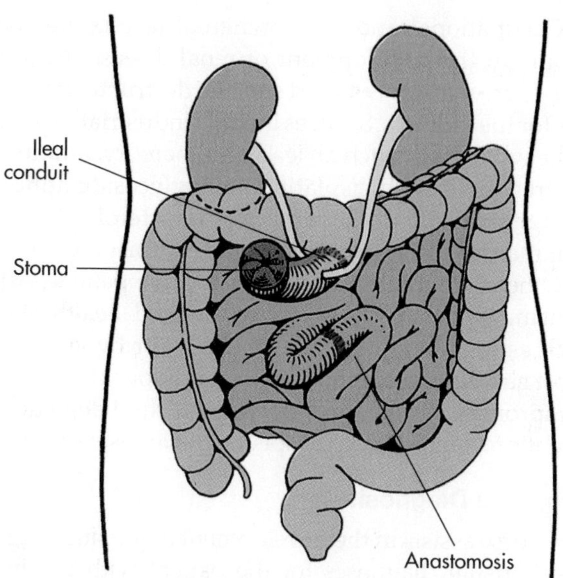

FIGURE 50-13 Ileal conduit or ileal loop.

eum that is isolated and brought to the surface of the abdominal wall (Figure 50-13). Occasionally a segment of the sigmoid colon is isolated and used instead of the ileum to form a sigmoid conduit. Bowel function is maintained with anastomosis of the remaining intestine. A drainage bag (urostomy bag or appliance) is fitted over the stoma to contain the constant drainage of urine. Continuous urine drainage prevents increased pressure within the conduit that would cause backflow to the kidneys, compromise the circulatory integrity of the conduit, or rupture the surgical anastomosis. Decreased urinary output and low abdominal pain may signal the onset of such problems. Complications of this procedure are wound infection, dehiscence, urinary leakage, ureteral obstruction, small bowel obstruction, stomal gangrene or atrophy, pyelonephritis, renal calculi, and compromised respiratory status secondary to incisional pain.

Postoperatively, measure urine flow hourly. Report output less than 30 mL/hr to the physician immediately. A healthy stoma appears moist and pink and may even bleed slightly. Inspect the skin around the stoma daily for signs of bleeding, excoriation, and infection. Mucus is present in the urine from the intestinal secretions. The patient should ingest large quantities of water to flush the ileal conduit. Any odor of urine about the patient may indicate an infection or leak of urine from the drainage bag. Early signs of urinary leakage (indicating a leak in an anastomosis) include increased abdominal girth; fever; and drainage through the incision, tubes, or drains. Ureteral separation from the conduit may cause urine to seep into the peritoneal cavity; observe the patient for signs and symptoms of peritonitis such as fever, abdominal pain and rigidity, and absence of bowel sounds.

Care of the patient with an ileal conduit is a nursing challenge because of the continuous drainage of urine through the stoma.

To change the urostomy bag, remove and drain it. Cleanse the skin with water, and apply the new appliance as outlined in the institution's standards of care. When the peristomal skin is healed, the bag is emptied at 2- to 3-hour intervals. At night a straight drainage tube is connected to a drainage bag. A permanent urostomy bag can be left in place 4 to 7 days if it remains sealed. Recommend that the patient have two bags, so one can be worn while the other is washed. Some patients prefer to use disposable bags. Odor is controlled by using deodorant drops or tablets in the urostomy bag; avoiding odor-producing foods, such as beans, onions, cabbage, asparagus, high-fiber wheat, simple sugars, and milk in the lactose-intolerant patient; and cleansing the urostomy bag with a vinegar and water rinse and thoroughly drying.

The **continent ileal urinary reservoir,** or **Kock pouch,** is created by implantation of the ureters into a segment of the small intestine that has been surgically removed from the rest of the bowel and anastomosed to the abdominal wall. Urine flow is controlled by a nipplelike valve that prevents leakage. To drain urine from the reservoir, the patient inserts a catheter through the valve at regular intervals, thus minimizing the reabsorption of waste materials from the urine and reflux into the ureters (Figure 50-14).

Patient Teaching

Patient teaching centers on the tasks of lifestyle adaptation: care of the stoma, nutrition, fluid intake, maintenance of self-esteem in light of altered body image, modification of sexual activities, and early detection of complications. Patient teaching begins with selecting an appliance, sizing the stoma, and changing the appliances. The home health nurse can assist the patient in modifying care in the home environment and by providing support during this stressful adjustment period (see Home Care Considerations box).

Prognosis

Although the patient may fully recover without recurrence, the day-to-day challenges of managing a urinary diversion are permanent.

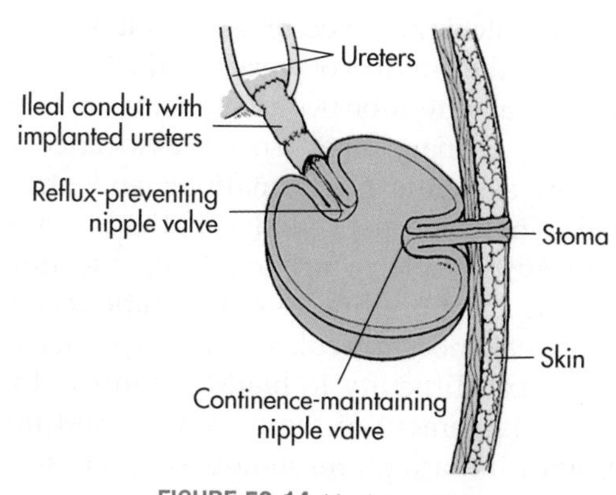

FIGURE 50-14 Kock pouch.

Home Care Considerations

Urinary Diversion Warning Signs

- Provide the patient and significant other with a list of warning signs and symptoms to report to the physician when home. Be certain to compose the list in clear, concise language.
- Keep this list handy and call the physician (phone number _____-__________) if you notice any of the following signs or symptoms:
  —Decrease in urinary output
  —Change in urine color: bloody, cloudy
  —Fever greater than 101° F
  —Change in appearance of stoma: pale color, swelling, "drawing-in" of stoma
  —Skin changes around stoma: redness, burning, breakdown
  —General feeling of weakness
  —Nausea and vomiting
  —Abdominal distention or pain
  —Any other health changes that are new or worse

NURSING PROCESS *for the Patient with a Urinary Disorder*

The role of the licensed practical nurse/licensed vocational nurse (LPN/LVN) in the nursing process as stated is that the LPN/LVN will:

- Participate in planning care for patients based on patient needs
- Review patient's care plan and recommend revisions as needed
- Review and follow defined prioritization for patient care
- Use clinical pathways, care maps, or care plans to guide and review patient care

Assessment

Assessment of the urinary tract is included in baseline data for all patients. The assessment includes **subjective data:** the patient's description of urination patterns and associated sensations, such as complaints of burning or pain on urination or difficulty maintaining the urine stream. Supplement subjective data with **objective data** by assessing for signs of fluid overload or depletion. The skin provides easily assessed clues about the patient's state of hydration. For example, dryness and pruritus (itching) can occur as a result of electrolyte imbalance or the buildup of waste products.

Pay careful attention to assessment of high-risk populations. Urinary disorders are associated with a number of systemic malformations and structural anomalies in newborns. Pediatric patients, especially girls, are susceptible to urinary tract infections because of the short urethra. Geriatric patients may experience weakened musculature and sphincter tone, with resultant difficulty in bladder control. In male patients, enlargement of the prostate gland may interfere with initiating and maintaining an adequate urine stream.

Occupational and environmental factors also contribute to the development of renal disease. Nephrotoxins are substances with specific destructive properties for the kidneys. Sources include industrial exposure to heavy metals, such as lead and mercury, and medical treatment with cisplatin, aminoglycoside antibiotics (gentamicin or kanamycin), nonsteroidal antiinflammatory drugs, or radiopaque contrast media.

Other vulnerable populations include patients experiencing systemic changes from altered health states, such as pregnancy, diabetes mellitus, or hypertension. Most susceptible are those with conditions that directly compromise kidney function: trauma, fluid depletion or retention, and active or suspected renal disease.

Nursing Diagnosis

The nurse assists in the development of nursing diagnoses. Nursing diagnoses for the patient with a urinary disorder include but are not limited to the following:

- Impaired urinary elimination
- Ineffective tissue perfusion: renal
- Acute pain; chronic pain
- Risk for infection
- Risk for deficient fluid volume
- Excess fluid volume
- Ineffective sexuality patterns
- Deficient knowledge

Expected Outcomes and Planning

For the patient with a urinary disorder, the nursing care priority is the short-term goal of reestablishing urinary flow and kidney function. Long-term planning for the patient and the family or significant other focuses on prevention of complications and quick response to recurrent problems. Goals are individualized for each patient and are modified to adapt to the patient's changing health status and urinary elimination management. The care plan may include the following goals:

Goal 1: The patient will achieve control of the elimination of urine.

Outcome: Patient reports effective management of normal patterns of urination.

Goal 2: The patient will practice proper protocol such as drinking adequate fluids and correct methods of perineal cleansing for the female to prevent UTI.

Outcome: Patient reports no signs or symptoms of recurrent urinary difficulty.

Implementation

The nurse will assist patient in bladder training to promote normal patterns of urination. The patient will be educated in importance of drinking 2 to 3 L of water daily (unless contraindicated). Teach the female patient the importance of cleansing from anterior to posterior in the perineal area after a bowel movement to prevent contamination of the urethra with *Escherichia coli.*

■ Evaluation

Evaluation of urinary status is determined by success in attaining expected outcomes. Monitoring of urinary output and character is continual. Because some urinary disorders become chronic, patient involvement in the prevention of complications is vitally important. Avoidance of risk factors and early detection of symptoms are essential to limit damage to the urinary tract.

Goal 1: The patient will experience normal patterns of urinary elimination.

Evaluative measure: Patient reports return to own normal voiding.

Goal 2: The patient will monitor self for early signs and symptoms of recurrent UTI.

Evaluative measure: Patient is able to correctly answer questions about signs and symptoms and appropriate measures to take for treatment.

Get Ready for the NCLEX® Examination!

Key Points

- The kidneys lie retroperitoneally, just below the diaphragm.
- The functioning unit of the kidney is the nephron.
- The kidneys rid the body of wastes and excess electrolytes, maintain water and electrolyte balance, and maintain acid-base balance.
- Kidney function is achieved by the processes of filtration, secretion, and reabsorption.
- Assessment of the urinary tract is included in baseline data for all patients.
- The subject of urinary problems is an embarrassing topic for many patients. Be sensitive to the patient's feelings and be supportive.
- Aging may have a negative influence on urinary function, but many problems can be corrected.
- Hydration status is monitored by daily weights, I&O, laboratory studies, inspection of the skin and mucous membranes, and assessment of the level of consciousness.
- A large percentage of nosocomial infections involve the urinary tract.
- Proper care of urinary catheters decreases the chance of UTIs.
- Surgical intervention may be indicated for urinary dysfunction that cannot be corrected by medical management.
- Dialysis, which mimics kidney function, may be used temporarily or as a long-term therapy.
- Dietary, fluid, and medication modifications may be necessary for the patient with urinary dysfunction.
- Sacral nerve stimulation for urinary urge incontinence is conducted with a permanently implanted electrical stimulation device that changes neuronal activity in the sacral efferent and afferent nerves.

Additional Learning Resources

Go to your Companion CD for an audio glossary, animations, video clips, and more.

evolve Be sure to visit the Evolve site at http://evolve.elsevier.com/Christensen/adult/ for additional online resources.

Review Questions for the NCLEX® Examination

1. When reading the urinalysis report, the nurse recognizes this result as abnormal:

1. turbidity clear.
2. pH 6.0.
3. glucose negative.
4. red blood cells, 15 to 20.

2. After renal angiography, the patient assessment priority is the:

1. blood pressure.
2. respiratory effort.
3. puncture site.
4. urinary output.

3. The nursing care plan includes teaching the patient Kegel exercises. The nurse teaches the patient to alternately tighten and relax which group of muscles?

1. Perineal floor
2. Pubococcygeal
3. Abdominis rectus
4. Detrusor

4. The physician has talked to the patient and his wife about the treatment plan for his bladder cancer. Later, the patient tells the nurse he does not understand what the doctor is going to do. The most appropriate response by the nurse would be:

1. "Okay. I'll explain it to you again."
2. "Make a list of questions for the doctor."
3. "Try not to think about the treatment."
4. "Tell me what you know about the treatment."

5. Which activity would be harmful for the incontinent patient?

1. Restricting fluid intake
2. Drinking only water
3. Fluid intake of 2000 mL/day
4. Restricting acidic fruit juice intake

6. The nurse recognizes that the most common causative organism in pyelonephritis is:

1. *Candida albicans.*
2. *Klebsiella.*
3. *Escherichia coli.*
4. *Pseudomonas.*

7. The most important factor to foster patient compliance with the treatment plan is to provide the patient with:
   1. a set time schedule to follow.
   2. data on success rates.
   3. written information of the plan.
   4. an active role in the planning.

8. When scheduling the administration of furosemide (Lasix), it would be in the patient's best interest to schedule the medication to be given at:
   1. 9 AM.
   2. 12 PM (noon).
   3. 2100.
   4. 12 AM (midnight).

9. In discussion with the patient with ESRD about dietary needs, the nurse recognizes that foods highest in potassium include:
   1. apples, applesauce, grapes, and raisins.
   2. bananas, nuts, and chocolate.
   3. grapefruit, tomatoes, oranges, and bananas.
   4. milk, grapefruit, orange juice, and sugar.

10. Which patient report indicates that phenazopyridine hydrochloride (Pyridium) is being effective?
    1. Decreased bladder spasms
    2. Decrease in burning
    3. Increased urinary output
    4. Increased pain tolerance

11. When calculating actual urinary output during continuous bladder irrigations, the nurse would:
    1. measure and record all fluid output in the drainage bag.
    2. measure the total output and deduct the amount of irrigation solution used.
    3. add the total of all intravenous and irrigation solutions and deduct output.
    4. measure total output and deduct the total intravenous solutions.

12. What statement by the patient indicates the need for further teaching before renal angiography?
    1. "I will miss having breakfast."
    2. "I know the nurse will be checking my pulse after the test."
    3. "I'm glad I don't have to stay in bed after the test."
    4. "I had a test similar to this 3 years ago."

13. The nurse performs a catheterization immediately after the patient voids and obtains 30 mL residual urine. The next step would be to:
    1. document the procedure with outcome data.
    2. continue the catheterization routine after each voiding.
    3. restrict fluid intake after dinner.
    4. immediately notify the physician of the results.

14. Which goal would have priority in planning care of the aging patient with urinary incontinence?
    1. Recognizes the urge to void
    2. Mobility necessary for toileting independently
    3. Episodes of incontinency decrease
    4. Drinks a minimum of 2000 mL of fluid per day

15. The goal for peritoneal dialysis is to:
    1. remove toxins and metabolic waste.
    2. produce rapid fluid shifts.
    3. increase clearance of dialysate flow.
    4. restore normal kidney function.

16. In postoperative care of the patient with an arteriovenous shunt, the nurse should:
    1. secure the shunt with an elastic bandage.
    2. notify the physician if a bruit or thrill is present.
    3. change the shunt if clotting occurs.
    4. use strict surgical asepsis for dressing changes.

17. The teaching priority for the patient with acute renal failure is:
    1. treatment of hyponatremia.
    2. prevention of infection.
    3. maintenance urinary output at 50 mL/hr.
    4. control of caloric intake.

18. The patient with ESRD receiving hemodialysis is at risk for:
    1. sepsis.
    2. renal insufficiency.
    3. anemia.
    4. *Klebsiella* infection.

19. The primary function of the kidney is:
    1. regulation of enzymes.
    2. filtration of water and blood products.
    3. collection of urine from the body.
    4. control of the adrenal glands.

20. The priority short-term goal for disorders of the urinary system is:
    1. patient confidentiality.
    2. privacy.
    3. education for patient and family.
    4. normal patterns of urinary elimination.

21. Assessment of the patient with a urinary disorder may be complicated by:
    1. European practices to withhold personal information.
    2. marital status.
    3. coexisting pathologic condition.
    4. social taboos surrounding sexuality.

22. The nurse making rounds discovers that there is no urine drainage from a postoperative patient's Foley catheter. The first nursing action is to:
    1. ensure patency.
    2. irrigate until clear.
    3. call the physician.
    4. insert larger lumen catheter.

23. Which problem constitutes a medical emergency?
    1. Anuria
    2. Polyuria
    3. Dysuria
    4. Dyspnea

24. The most common cause of renal failure is:

1. trauma.
2. diabetes mellitus.
3. cancer.
4. heart failure.

25. The clinical findings in the oliguric phase of acute renal failure include:

1. BUN and creatinine levels rise.
2. urinary output increases.
3. signs of impending shock.
4. increased blood flow to the kidneys.

26. During postoperative care of the patient with an ileoconduit, which finding represents an emergency?

1. Abdominal pain
2. Presence of mucus in the urine
3. Nausea and vomiting
4. Absence of bowel sounds

27. Choose all of the correct patient teachings for the patient with cystitis.

1. Teach the patient to drink cranberry juice to prevent UTIs.
2. Teach the female patient to cleanse the perineal area from anterior to posterior to prevent rectal *E. coli* contamination of the urethra.
3. Encourage the patient to drink 2000 mL of fluid per day, unless contraindicated.
4. Instruct the patient that it is acceptable to stop taking prescribed medications when symptoms subside.

28. Renal calculi may result from: *(Select all that apply.)*

1. Stasis of urine caused by obstruction or quadriplegia
2. Infections of urinary tract
3. Hyperparathyroidism, which causes increase in calcium metabolism
4. Diabetes mellitus

29. The collection of subjective and objective data for the patient with acute glomerulonephritis could include: *(Select all that apply.)*

1. Periorbital edema
2. Anorexia
3. Hypotension
4. Frankly sanguineous urine

30. Careful preparation of the patient for an IVP is necessary. Nursing interventions would include: *(Select all that apply)*

1. NPO for about 8 hours before examination.
2. Ascertaining whether patient has allergy to magnesium.
3. Giving prescribed non-gas forming laxative.
4. Instructing patient concerning IVP.

31. A patient with diabetes is admitted for evaluation of kidney function because of recent fatigue, weakness, and elevated BUN and serum creatinine levels. While obtaining a nursing history, the nurse identifies an early symptom of renal insufficiency when the patient states:

1. "I get up several times every night to urinate."
2. "I wake up in the night feeling short of breath."
3. "My memory is not as good as it used to be."
4. "My mouth and throat are always dry and sore."

32. A patient diagnosed with ESRD is treated with conservative management, including erythropoietin injections. After teaching the patient about management of ESRD, the nurse determines teaching has been effective when the patient states:

1. "I will measure my urinary output each day to help calculate the amount I can drink."
2. "I need to take the erythropoietin to boost my immune system and help prevent infection."
3. "I need to try to get more protein from dairy products."
4. "I will try to increase my intake of fruits and vegetables."

33. As the nurse reviews a diet plan with a patient with diabetes mellitus and renal insufficiency, the patient states that with diabetes and renal failure there is nothing that is good to eat. The patient says, "I am going to eat what I want; I'm going to die anyway!" The best nursing diagnosis for this patient is:

1. imbalanced nutrition: more than body requirements, related to knowledge deficit about appropriate diet.
2. risk for noncompliance, related to feelings of anger.
3. grieving, related to actual and perceived losses.
4. risk for ineffective health maintenance, related to complexity of therapeutic regimen.

34. The nurse has instructed a patient who is receiving hemodialysis about dietary management. Which diet choices by the patient indicate that the teaching has been successful?

1. Scrambled eggs, English muffin, and apple juice
2. Cheese sandwich, tomato soup, and cranberry juice
3. Split-pea soup, whole-wheat toast, and nonfat milk
4. Oatmeal with cream, half a banana, and herbal tea

35. To determine glomerular filtration rate for a patient with chronic renal disease, the nurse plans to:

1. schedule frequent blood urea nitrogen (BUN) tests.
2. initiate a 24-hour collection of the patient's urine.
3. check the specific gravity on serial urine specimens.
4. use a bladder scanner to check for residual urine.

chapter

51 Care of the Patient with an Endocrine Disorder

evolve

http://evolve.elsevier.com/Christensen/foundationsadult

Barbara Lauritsen Christensen

Objectives

Anatomy and Physiology

1. List and describe the endocrine glands and their hormones.
2. Define the negative feedback system.
3. Explain the action of the hormones on their target organs.
4. Describe how the hypothalamus controls the anterior and posterior pituitary glands.

Medical-Surgical

5. Discuss the etiology and pathophysiology, clinical manifestations, assessment, diagnostic tests, medical management, nursing interventions, patient teaching, and prognosis for patients with acromegaly, gigantism, dwarfism, diabetes insipidus, syndrome of inappropriate antidiuretic hormone, hyperthyroidism, hypothyroidism, goiter, thyroid cancer, hyperparathyroidism, hypoparathyroidism, Cushing's syndrome, and Addison's disease.
6. List four tests used in the diagnosis of hyperthyroidism.
7. Explain how to test for Chvostek's sign, Trousseau's sign, and carpopedal spasms.
8. List two significant complications that may occur after thyroidectomy.
9. Discuss the medications commonly used to treat hyperthyroidism and hypothyroidism.
10. Differentiate between the clinical manifestations of Cushing's syndrome and Addison's disease.
11. Describe the etiology and pathophysiology, clinical manifestations, assessment, diagnostic tests, medical management, nursing interventions, patient teaching, and prognosis for the patient with diabetes mellitus.
12. Differentiate between the signs and symptoms of hyperglycemia and hypoglycemia.
13. Differentiate among the signs and symptoms of diabetic ketoacidosis, hyperglycemic hyperosmolar nonketotic coma, and hypoglycemic reaction.
14. Explain the roles of nutrition, exercise, and medication in the control of diabetes mellitus.
15. Discuss how oral agents work to improve the mechanisms by which insulin and glucose are produced and used by the body.
16. Discuss the two new subcutaneous insulin-enhancing drugs exenatide (Byetta) and pramlintide (Symlin) and their mechanisms of action.
17. Discuss the various insulin types and their characteristics.
18. Describe the correct way to draw up and administer insulin.
19. Discuss the various classes of oral hypoglycemic medications to treat type 2 diabetes mellitus.
20. Discuss the acute and long-term complications of diabetes mellitus.
21. List five nursing interventions that foster self-care in the activities of daily living of the patient with diabetes mellitus.

Key Terms

Chvostek's sign (KHVŎS-tĕks sīn, p. 1734)
dysphagia (dĭs-FĀ-jē-ă, p. 1733)
endocrinologist (ĕn-dō-krĭ-NŎL-ŏ-jĭst, p. 1727)
glycosuria (glī-kōs-Ū-rē-ă, p. 1747)
hirsutism (HĔR-sōōt-ĭszm, p. 1741)
hyperglycemia (hī-pĕr-glī-SĒ-mē-ă, p. 1747)
hypocalcemia (hī-pō-kăl-SĒ-mē-ă, p. 1739)
hypoglycemia (hī-pō-glī-SĒ-mē-ă, p. 1754)
hypokalemia (hī-pō-kă-LĒ-mē-ă, p. 1740)
idiopathic hyperplasia (ĭd-ē-ō-PĂTH-ĭk hī-pĕr-PLĀ-zhă, p. 1725)
ketoacidosis (kē-tō-ă-sĭ-DŌ-sĭs, p. 1747)
ketone bodies (KĒ-tōn bŏd-ēz, p. 1746)
lipodystrophy (lĭp-ō-DĬS-trŏ-fē, p. 1753)
neuropathy (nū-RŎP-ĕ-thē, p. 1758)
polydipsia (pŏl-ē-DĬP-sē-ă, p. 1747)
polyphagia (pŏl-ē-FĀ-jă, p. 1747)
polyuria (pŏl-ē-Ū-rē-ă, p. 1747)
Trousseau's sign (trū-SŌZ sīn, p. 1734)
turgor (TŬR-gŏr, p. 1729)
type 1 diabetes mellitus (tīp 1 dī-ă-BĒ-tēz MĔL-ĭ-tŭs, p. 1745)
type 2 diabetes mellitus (tīp 2 dī-ă-BĒ-tēz MĔL-ĭ-tŭs, p. 1746)

ANATOMY AND PHYSIOLOGY OF THE ENDOCRINE SYSTEM

ENDOCRINE GLANDS AND HORMONES

Glands can be divided into two broad categories: exocrine and endocrine. **Exocrine glands** secrete through a series of ducts (sebaceous and sudoriferous glands of the skin). Their secretions are protective and functional. **Endocrine glands** are ductless; they release their secretions directly into the bloodstream. Their secretions have a regulatory function.

The endocrine system is composed of a series of ductless glands whose work is closely related to the nervous system. Both systems control homeostasis through communication within the systems. The endocrine system communicates more slowly through the use of **hormones,** which are chemical messengers that travel through the bloodstream to their target organ. When the hormone reaches its target, a metabolic change occurs.

The total weight of all the endocrine glands is less than half a pound, yet they have a powerful influence. The slightest change in hormonal levels can upset the metabolic balance of the entire body. Hormones can increase or decrease a normal body process by affecting a target organ. Too much or too little of a given hormone can affect other hormones, and for this reason they are somewhat interrelated. The endocrine glands (Figure 51-1) have a generalized effect on the patient's metabolism, growth, development, reproduction, and many other bodily activities.

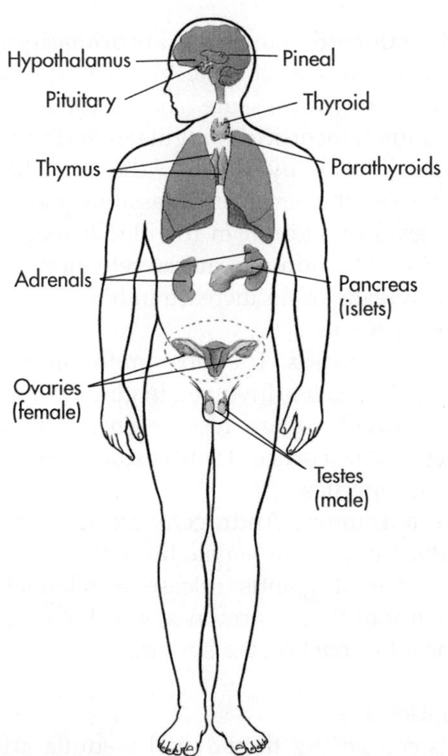

FIGURE 51-1 Location of the endocrine glands in the female and male bodies. Thymus gland is shown at maximal size at puberty.

The amount of hormonal release is controlled by a **negative feedback** (a decrease in function in response to stimuli) system. Information is constantly being exchanged between the target organ and the pituitary gland via the bloodstream regarding the effect of the hormone on the target organ.

Pituitary Gland

The pea-sized **pituitary gland** (hypophysis) is one of the most powerful glands in the body. It has been called the "master gland" because, through the negative feedback system, it controls the other endocrine glands. It works closely with the hypothalamus of the brain and is located in the cranial cavity in a small saddlelike depression in the sphenoid bone. It is divided into two segments, the **anterior pituitary** (adenohypophysis) and the **posterior pituitary** (neurohypophysis). Each segment has specialized hormones. The hypothalamus actually produces the hormones of the posterior pituitary and releases them for storage in the posterior pituitary gland; they are released from here as a result of nerve impulses received from the hypothalamus.

Anterior Pituitary Gland

Six major hormones are secreted by the anterior pituitary gland; the hormones make up about 75% of the gland's total weight. Five hormones are called **tropic** hormones, because they are responsible for the stimulation of other endocrine glands. Prolactin, the remaining hormone, causes the mammary glands to produce milk. These hormones and their functions are shown in Figures 51-2 and 51-3.

Posterior Pituitary Gland

Two hormones are released by the posterior pituitary when the hypothalamus stimulates their release. They are **oxytocin** and **antidiuretic hormone** (ADH) (see Figure 51-2). Oxytocin promotes the release of milk and stimulates uterine contractions during labor. ADH, also called vasopressin, causes the kidneys to conserve water by decreasing the amount of urine produced. ADH/vasopressin also causes constriction of the arterioles in the body and a pressor effect, which results in increased blood pressure.

Thyroid Gland

The **thyroid gland** is butterfly shaped, with one lobe lying on either side of the trachea just below the larynx (Figure 51-4). The lobes are connected by the **isthmus.** The gland is very vascular and receives approximately 80 to 120 mL of blood per minute.

The thyroid gland secretes the hormones **thyroxine** (T_4) and **triiodothyronine** (T_3). Adequate oral intake of iodine is necessary for the formation of thyroid hormones. These hormones regulate three main functions: (1) growth and development, (2) metabolism, and (3) activity of the nervous system. Their function

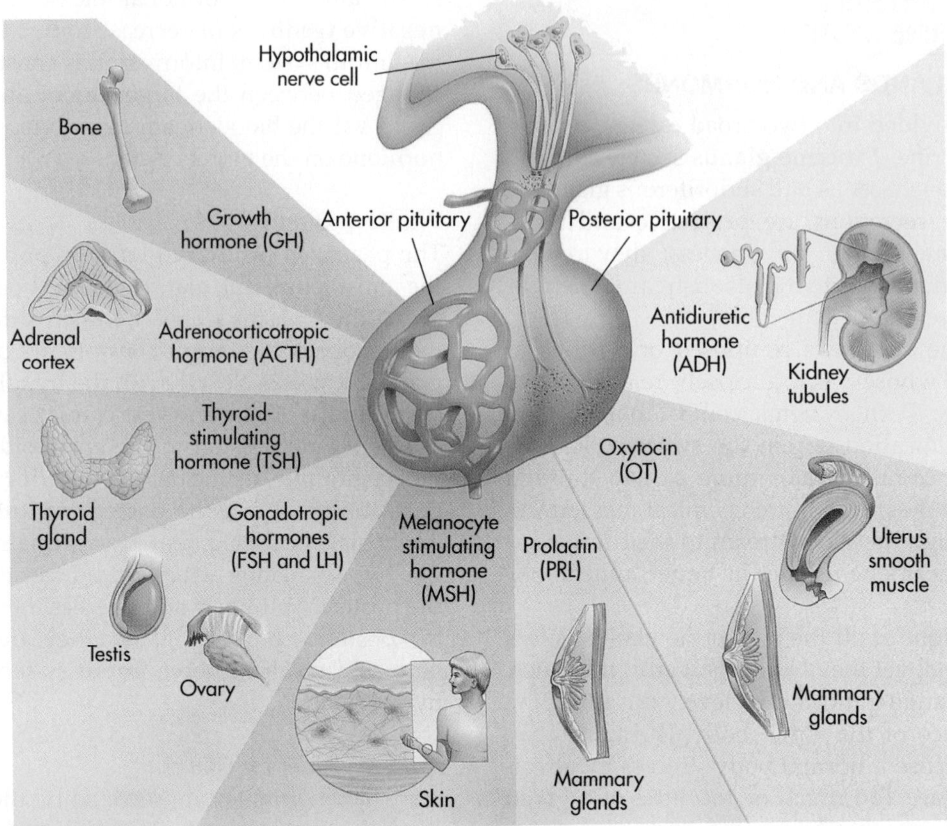

FIGURE 51-2 Pituitary hormones. Principal anterior and posterior pituitary hormones and their target organs.

is controlled by the release of thyroid-stimulating hormone (TSH) from the pituitary gland.

Calcitonin is a hormone also released by the thyroid gland. It decreases blood calcium levels by causing calcium to be stored in the bones.

Parathyroid Glands

The four parathyroid glands are located on the posterior surface of the thyroid gland (see Figure 51-4) and secrete **parathyroid hormone** (PTH, parathormone). As an antagonist to calcitonin from the thyroid, PTH tends to increase the concentration of calcium in the blood. It also regulates the amount of phosphorus in the blood.

The delicate balance of calcium in the blood is extremely important for normal body function. When calcium blood levels are low, the nerve cells become excited and stimulate the muscles with too many impulses, resulting in spasms **(tetany).** When blood calcium levels are abnormally high, heart function becomes impaired; this can result in death. Under the influence of PTH, two changes occur in the kidneys: It increases the reabsorption of calcium and magnesium from the kidney tubules and accelerates the elimination of phosphorus in the urine.

Adrenal Glands

The adrenal glands (suprarenal glands) are small, yellow masses that lie atop the kidneys. Both glands contain an outer section, the adrenal cortex, and a smaller inner section, the adrenal medulla (Figure 51-5).

Adrenal Cortex

The adrenal cortex is divided into three separate layers. Each layer secretes a particular hormone, called a **steroid:**

- **Mineralocorticoids:** These are primarily involved in water and electrolyte balance and indirectly manage blood pressure. Aldosterone, the principal mineralocorticoid, regulates sodium and potassium levels by affecting the renal tubules. It decreases the level of potassium and increases the level of sodium in the bloodstream. The retention of sodium causes retention of water, which leads to an increase in blood volume and blood pressure.
- **Glucocorticoids:** The most important of these is cortisol, which is involved in glucose metabolism and provides extra reserve energy in times of stress. Glucocorticoids also exhibit antiinflammatory properties.
- **Sex hormones:** Androgens are male hormones and estrogens are female hormones. In the adult the adrenal glands release a relatively small amount of these hormones, which have an insignificant impact on the system.

Adrenal Medulla

The cells composing the adrenal medulla arise from the same type of cells as the sympathetic nervous system. Two hormones are released during times of stress: (1) epinephrine (adrenaline), and (2) norepinephrine.

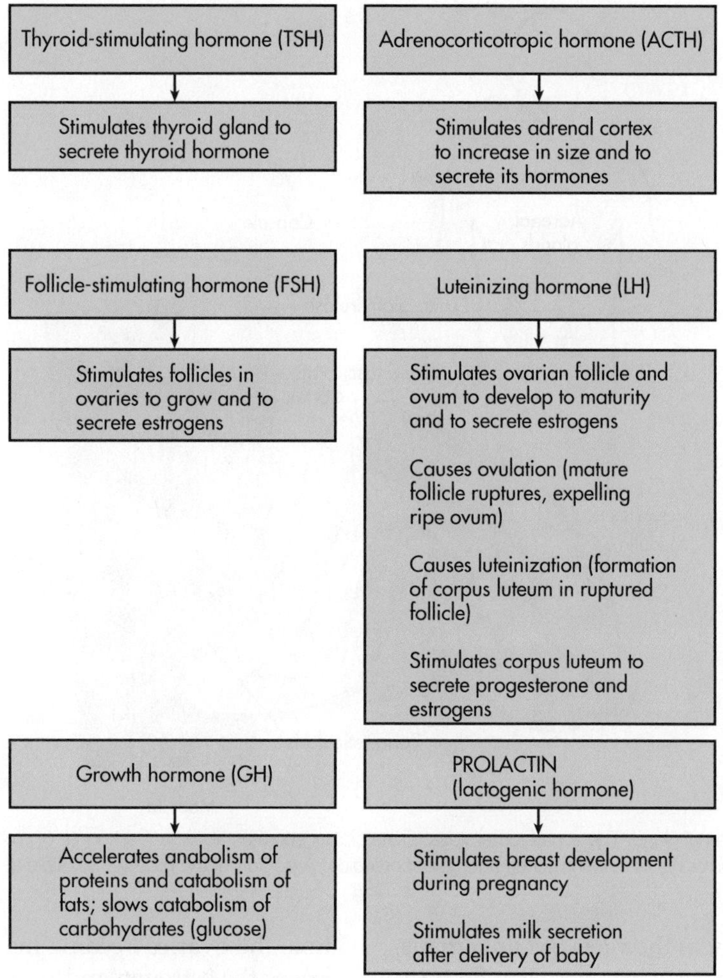

FIGURE 51-3 Names and functions of anterior pituitary hormones.

Posterior of larynx
Epiglottis
Hyoid bone
Larynx
Superior parathyroid glands
Thyroid gland
Inferior parathyroid glands
Trachea

FIGURE 51-4 Thyroid and parathyroid glands. Note their relations to each other and to the larynx and trachea.

They cause the heart rate and blood pressure to increase, the blood vessels to constrict, and the liver to release glucose reserves for immediate energy. This is a systemic preparation of the body for a "fight-or-flight" response needed in times of crisis.

Pancreas

The pancreas is an elongated gland that lies posterior to the stomach. It is an active organ, composed of both exocrine and endocrine tissue. The endocrine tissue of the pancreas contains more than a million tiny clusters

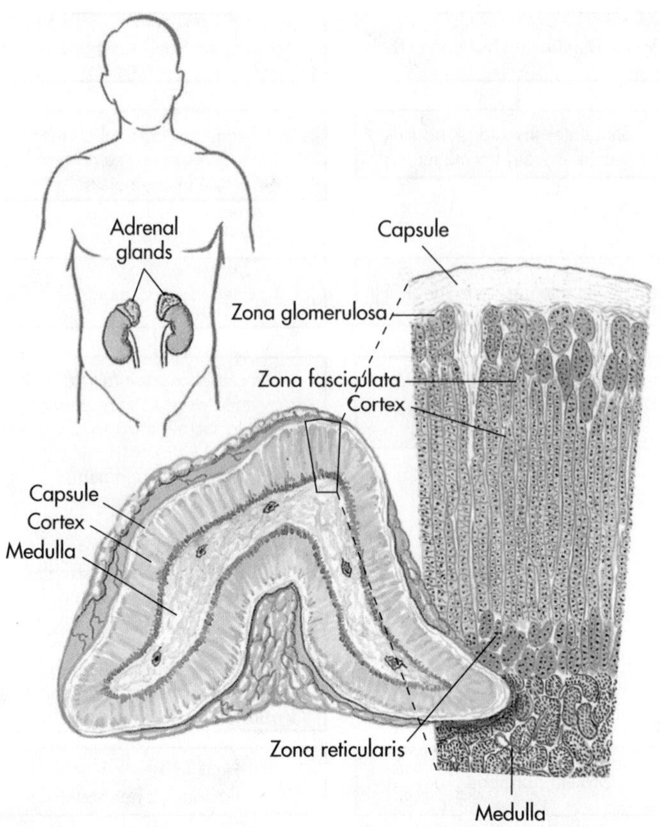

Adrenal glands
Capsule
Zona glomerulosa
Zona fasciculata
Cortex
Capsule
Cortex
Medulla
Zona reticularis
Medulla

FIGURE 51-5 Structure of the adrenal gland. The zona glomerulosa of the cortex secretes abundant amounts of glucocorticoids, chiefly cortisol. The zona reticularis secretes minute amounts of sex hormones and glucocorticoids. A portion of the medulla is visible at the bottom of the illustration.

of cells known collectively as the islets of Langerhans. These cells secrete two major hormones. The first, **insulin,** is secreted by the **beta cells** in response to increased levels of glucose in the blood. Insulin's secretion pattern is a physiologic example of negative feedback between insulin and glucose. Elevated blood glucose levels stimulate the pancreas to secrete insulin. The stimulus for insulin secretion decreases as blood glucose levels decrease. The homeostatic mechanism is considered negative feedback because it reverses the change in blood glucose level. The second pancreatic hormone is **glucagon,** which is secreted by the **alpha cells** in response to decreased levels of glucose in the blood. Insulin and glucagon play a major role in carbohydrate, fat, and protein metabolism.

Female Sex Glands

Deep in the lower abdominal region, lying to the left and the right of the uterus, are two almond-shaped **ovaries,** the major sex glands of the woman. At puberty the ovaries begin producing two hormones: **estrogen** (responsible for the development of secondary sex characteristics, such as axillary hair and pubic hair, and for maturation of the reproductive organs) and **progesterone** (continues the preparation of the reproductive organs that was initiated by the estrogen). (See Chapter 52 for more information.)

The **placenta** is a temporary endocrine gland that forms and functions during pregnancy. During this time the ovaries become inactive and the placenta releases the estrogen and progesterone needed to maintain the pregnancy. (For a more in-depth discussion, refer to Chapter 52.)

Male Sex Glands

Suspended outside the body in the **scrotum,** a saclike structure, are the two oval sex glands called the **testes.** They release the hormone **testosterone,** which is responsible for the development of the male secondary sex characteristics, including axillary, pubic, and facial hair; maturation of the reproductive organs; deepening of the voice; and development of muscle and bone mass. Testosterone is necessary for sperm formation.

Thymus Gland

The thymus gland lies in the upper thorax, posterior to the sternum (see Figure 51-1). It produces the hormone **thymosin,** which plays an active role in the immune system. T lymphocytes (a type of white blood cell) are stimulated to carry out immune reactions to certain types of antigens. The thymus gland programs this information into the T lymphocytes in utero and during the first few months of life.

Pineal Gland

The pineal gland is a small, cone-shaped gland located in the roof of the third ventricle of the brain (see Figure 51-1). It secretes the hormone **melatonin,** which seems to inhibit reproductive activities by inhibiting the gonadotropic hormones. This is particularly important in preventing the sexual maturation of the child's body until adulthood. It is thought to induce sleep, may affect mood, and has an impact on menstrual cycles.

DISORDERS OF THE PITUITARY GLAND (HYPOPHYSIS)

ACROMEGALY

Etiology and Pathophysiology

An overproduction of somatotropin (growth hormone [GH]) in the adult causes acromegaly, a condition that affects an estimated 250 people in the United States each year. The cause may be either (1) idiopathic hyperplasia (an increase in number of cells without a known cause) of the anterior lobe of the pituitary gland or (2) tumor growth. Unfortunately, growth changes that occur in acromegaly are irreversible, even with adequate medical or surgical intervention.

Clinical Manifestations

Manifestations of acromegaly begin gradually, usually in the third or fourth decade of life. Typically an average of 7 to 9 years passes between the initial onset of signs and symptoms and final diagnosis. The subsequent overabundance of GH produces many changes throughout the patient's body, including enlarged cranium and lower jaw, separated and maloccluded teeth, bulging forehead, bulbous nose, thick lips, enlarged tongue, and generalized coarsening of the facial features (Figure 51-6). Enlargement of the tongue results in speech difficulties, and the voice deepens as a result of hypertrophy of the vocal cords. The hands and feet grow larger; the fingertips develop a tufted or clubbed appearance (Lewis et al., 2007). There is enlargement of the heart, the liver, and the spleen. Muscle weakness usually develops. Joints may hypertrophy and become painful and stiff. Male patients may become impotent, and female patients may develop a deepened voice, increased facial hair, and amenorrhea. If a tumor is present, pressure on the optic nerve may cause partial or complete blindness. Severe headaches are common.

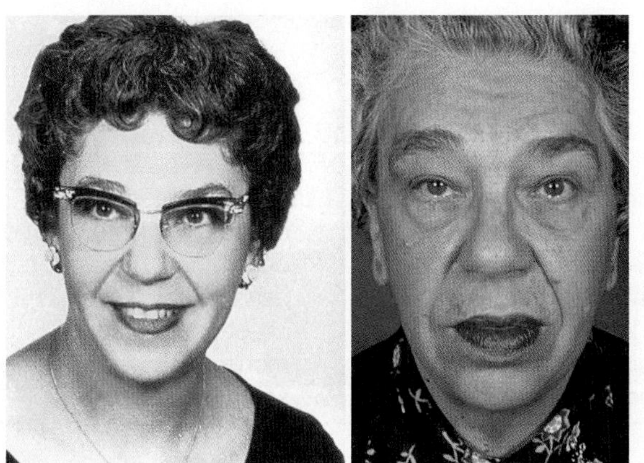

FIGURE 51-6 *Right:* This patient has coarse facial features typical of acromegaly. *Left:* Compare the patient's face many years before she developed the pituitary tumor.

Assessment

Subjective data include headaches or visual disturbances and painful, stiff joints. Evaluate muscle weakness and its effect on the patient's ability to perform activities. Encourage patients to share their emotional responses to sexual problems (such as impotence in men and masculinization in women).

Collection of **objective data** includes ongoing assessment of bone enlargement and joint involvement, evidenced by gait changes and decreasing ability to perform activities. Changes in vital signs that may herald the onset of early heart failure include dyspnea, tachycardia, weak pulse, and hypotension.

Diagnostic Tests

Diagnosis of acromegaly is based on the history and the clinical manifestations, computed tomography (CT) scan, magnetic resonance imaging (MRI), and cranial radiographic evaluation. A complete ophthalmologic examination, including visual fields, is usually performed because a large tumor of the pituitary gland potentially causes pressure on the optic chiasm or optic nerves. Laboratory tests confirm the elevated levels of serum GH and plasma insulin-like growth factor–1. The definitive test for acromegaly is the oral glucose challenge test. Normally GH concentration falls during an oral glucose challenge test, but in acromegaly these levels do not fall (Lewis et al., 2007). Restrict the patient's oral intake for 8 hours before this test.

Medical Management

Medical treatments include dopamine agonists such as cabergoline (Dostinex) and somatostatin analogs (which inhibit GH), such as octreotide (Sandostatin, Sandostatin Depot) (Table 51-1), especially in patients who are not candidates for surgery or radiation therapy. These drugs are used in an attempt to suppress GH secretion. Surgical treatment to remove pituitary tumors associated with acromegaly is accomplished with the transsphenoidal removal of tumor tissue. The goal of transsphenoidal surgery is to remove only the tumor that is causing GH secretion. Irradiation procedures using proton beam therapy have been used to destroy GH-secreting tumors. Proton beam treatment uses very low doses of radiation and therefore is much less destructive to adjacent tissues, such as the hypothalamus and temporal lobes, than conventional radiation therapy.

Nursing Interventions and Patient Teaching

Nursing interventions are mainly supportive. Muscle weakness, joint pain, or stiffness warrant assessment of the ability to perform activities of daily living (ADLs). Headache may impair the patient's ability to socialize and may also impede education. Worsening headaches

Table 51-1 Medications for Endocrine Disorders

Generic/Trade	Action	Side Effects	Nursing Implications
Bromocriptine (Parlodel)	Inhibits prolactin secretion, lowers serum levels of growth hormone, dopamine receptor agonist	Nausea, headache, dizziness, abdominal cramping, orthostatic hypotension	Give with meals to prevent GI effects; change positions carefully to prevent orthostatic hypotension; contraindicated with hypersensitivity to ergot derivatives.
Calcium salts (gluconate, lactate, chloride gluceptate)	Calcium electrolyte replacement	Hypercalcemia, phlebitis, necrosis, and burning at IV site; bradycardia, hypotension, and dysrhythmias with rapid IV administration	Monitor cardiac status and blood pressure and for extravasation when giving intravenously.
Fludrocortisone (Florinef)	Adrenal corticosteroid with mineralocorticoid activity; promotes sodium and water retention	Hypertension, edema, sweating, rash, hypokalemia	Monitor for hypokalemia and fluid retention or depletion; do not discontinue abruptly; patient should carry identification signaling use.
Levothyroxine (Eltroxin, Synthroid, Levothroid) Liothyronine (Cytomel) Liotrix (Thyrolar) Thyroid (Thyrar, Armour Thyroid)	Thyroid hormone replacement	Most side effects due to therapeutic overdose; include anxiety, insomnia, headache, hypertension, tremors, angina, dysrhythmias, tachycardia, menstrual irregularities	Give in morning to minimize insomnia; use caution in older adults or patients with coronary artery disease; monitor for signs of overdose; do not switch brands unless instructed.
Mitotane (Lysodren)	Adrenal cytotoxic agent; reduces production of adrenal steroids	Anorexia, nausea, vomiting, diarrhea, lethargy, somnolence, vertigo, rash	Tell patient to use contraception; instruct patient to use caution when driving or performing tasks requiring alertness; monitor for dehydration.
Potassium iodide (SSKI)	Blocks release of thyroid hormone in thyroid storm and hyperthyroidism; also used as an expectorant	Hypersensitivity reactions, rash, metallic taste, burning in mouth or throat, GI irritation, headache, parotitis, hyperkalemia	Do not use in pregnant women; mix with fruit juice to mask taste.
Somatostatin analogs: octreotide (Sandostatin)	A secretory inhibitory growth hormone suppressant that suppresses secretion of serotonin, gastroenteropancreatic peptides; enhances fluid and electrolyte absorption from the GI tract; used for carcinoid tumors, VIPomas, and high-output fistulas	Nausea, diarrhea, abdominal pain, headache, injection site discomfort, hyperglycemia, hypoglycemia	SubQ route of administration is preferred, but may also be given IV.
Antidiuretic hormone: vasopressin (Pitressin)	Synthetic pituitary hormone with antidiuretic effects on the kidney (used to treat diabetes insipidus); also a potent vasoconstrictor (used to treat bleeding esophageal varices)	Nasal irritation and congestion with nasal preparations; hypertension; ischemia to heart, mesenteric organs, and kidneys; angina; myocardial infarction; water retention; hyponatremia	Use with caution in older adults or patients with coronary artery disease or heart failure; discontinue if chest pain develops; monitor urinary output and serum sodium.

GI, Gastrointestinal; *IV*, intravenous; *subQ*, subcutaneous.

may indicate tumor progression. The diet should be soft and easy to chew, since jaw muscles and the temporomandibular joint may be involved. Encourage the patient to chew thoroughly, and allow adequate time during meals, assisting when necessary. Encourage frequent fluid intake. Nonopioid analgesics may be given for pain relief. Visual impairment may increase the risk of injury for these patients, so take care to prevent them from stumbling into furniture or dropping objects.

As the body changes, the patient may develop problems with self-esteem and may feel physically unattractive. He or she may have difficulty communicating with significant others, which can disrupt individual or family coping methods. Other complications of acromegaly are related to enlargement of the liver, the spleen, and the heart. Cardiac dysrhythmias may develop, and the patient may experience heart failure. Abdominal girth may increase as a result of weight gain and inactivity, and respiratory difficulty may occur.

Nursing diagnoses and interventions for the patient with acromegaly include but are not limited to the following:

Nursing Diagnoses	Nursing Interventions
Disturbed body image, related to enlargement of hands, feet, tongue, jaw, and soft tissue	Convey respect and nonjudgmental acceptance of patient as a person. Help the patient set achievable short-term goals.
Activity intolerance, related to physical weakness	Assess patient's current activity level and priorities for activity performance. Discuss with patient alternate ways of performing activities.

The patient should remain under the supervision of a physician so that any complications can be promptly diagnosed and adequately treated. Teach the patient exercises that can be performed at home, such as active range-of-motion of joints of the extremities and of the neck, to help prevent muscle atrophy and loss of movement.

Prognosis

Even with adequate medical or surgical treatment, the physical changes are irreversible, and the patient is prone to developing complications.

GIGANTISM

Etiology and Pathophysiology

Gigantism usually results from an oversecretion of GH as a result of hyperplasia of the anterior pituitary; this hyperplastic tissue may develop into a tumor. Another possible cause is a defect in the hypothalamus, which directs the anterior pituitary to release excess amounts of GH.

Clinical Manifestations

When overproduction of GH occurs in a child before closure of the epiphyses, there is an overgrowth of the long bones. This results in the attainment of great height, accompanied by increased muscle and visceral development. Weight increases, but body proportions are usually normal. Despite their size, these patients are usually weak. Other kinds of gigantism may be caused by certain genetic disorders or by disturbances in sex hormone production. Once identified, these children should be referred for further medical evaluation and follow-up.

Assessment

Collection of **subjective data** includes assessment of the patient's understanding of the disease process and his or her ability to verbalize emotional responses.

Collection of **objective data** requires frequent measurement of height. Assess the patient's use of adaptive coping measures and family interactions.

Diagnostic Tests

The GH-suppression test (also called the **glucose-loading test**) may be done to evaluate GH levels. In the patient with gigantism, baseline levels of GH are high.

Medical Management

Medical management of children with gigantism may include surgical removal of tumor tissue or irradiation of the anterior pituitary gland, with subsequent replacement of pituitary hormones as indicated. The physician then observes the child for the development of related complications, such as hypertension, heart failure, osteoporosis, thickened bones, and delayed sexual development.

Nursing Interventions and Patient Teaching

Nursing interventions primarily include early identification of children who are experiencing increased growth rates compared with other children their age. The condition causes potential problems with self-image, especially if the child is a preteen who is a great deal taller than peers. Girls usually suffer more emotional trauma in this situation than boys do. Be understanding and compassionate and accentuate the positive aspects of being tall.

Early diagnosis of these patients is essential, since proper medical management can retard the height a child will reach. Stress to the parents the importance of regular visits to the pediatrician or pediatric endocrinologist (a physician who specializes in endocrinology).

Prognosis

With new medical and surgical advances, the expected life span of these patients is longer than it was previously. However, their life expectancy is still shorter than that of the average individual.

DWARFISM

Etiology and Pathophysiology

Hypopituitary dwarfism is a condition caused by deficiency in GH. Most cases are idiopathic, but a small number can be attributed to an autosomal recessive trait. In some cases the patients also lack adrenocorticotropic hormone (ACTH), TSH, and the gonadotropins.

Clinical Manifestations

The most common clinical manifestation of dwarfism is that the child is a great deal shorter than his or her peers. These patients usually appear well proportioned and well nourished but appear younger than their chronologic age. They may have problems with dentition as the permanent teeth erupt, since the jaws are underdeveloped. Sexual development is usually normal but delayed. Many people with hypopituitary dwarfism are able to reproduce normal offspring, unless there is an accompanying deficiency in gonadotropins. Because only a small number of children who experience short stature or delayed growth suffer from dwarfism, a thorough diagnostic workup is crucial.

Assessment

Subjective data include the patient's understanding of the disease process and emotional responses to it. A family history of dwarfism may reveal previously successful coping strategies. Encourage the patient to verbalize feelings. Most of these children display normal intelligence. The child's history usually reveals a normal birth weight. It is important to determine when the child's growth retardation was first noted.

Collection of **objective data** includes regular measurement of height and weight to determine responses to GH and other hormones that may be administered. Compare current height and weight with standard growth charts, and compare the child's growth pattern with that of siblings and other relatives at comparable age periods.

Diagnostic Tests

Diagnostic tests include radiographic evaluation of the wrist for bone age and an MRI or a CT scan to rule out a pituitary tumor. Definitive diagnosis is based on decreased plasma levels of GH. Restrict the patient's oral intake after midnight for this test.

Medical Management

Medical treatment involves replacement of GH by injection and the addition of other hormones as needed to correct deficiencies. If a tumor is the cause of dwarfism, surgery is usually indicated.

Nursing Interventions and Patient Teaching

Exercise particular care to identify children with growth problems. The physician correlates the onset of growth retardation with symptoms of headache, visual disturbances, or behavior changes that might indicate tumor, so be alert for these symptoms. Be careful not to make the parents feel guilty about any delay in seeking medical attention for their child.

Encourage the child to wear age-appropriate clothing and engage in activities with peers, since major problems with self-esteem can occur in dwarfism. Emphasize the child's abilities and strengths instead of his or her physical size.

Prognosis

Most of these patients lead fairly normal lives, and many become parents of normal children. Complications experienced are often of the musculoskeletal and cardiovascular systems.

DIABETES INSIPIDUS

Etiology and Pathophysiology

Diabetes insipidus (*diabetes,* "like a sieve or siphon"; and *insipidus,* "tasteless") is a transient or permanent metabolic disorder of the posterior pituitary in which ADH is deficient. The condition may be either primary or secondary to other conditions, such as head injury, intracranial tumor, intracranial aneurysm, or infarct. Infections such as encephalitis or meningitis have been known to cause diabetes insipidus. Diabetes insipidus occurs when either the secretion or action of ADH goes awry. A decrease in ADH results in electrolyte and fluid imbalances. The imbalances are caused by increased plasma osmolality and increased urinary output.

Clinical Manifestations

Diabetes insipidus is characterized by marked polyuria and intense polydipsia. The urine is very dilute, looking much like water, with a low specific gravity (1.001 to 1.005; the normal range is 1.003 to 1.030). Urinary output may exceed 5 to 20 L/24 hr, whereas the average is 1.5 L/24 hr. Patients typically lose as much as 200 mL of urine an hour for more than 2 consecutive hours. The patient craves cold or iced water and may drink 4 to 20 L of fluid daily, yet may become severely dehydrated and have increased levels of sodium in the blood (hypernatremia). Even when unconscious after surgery or head trauma, these patients continue to produce copious quantities of urine. If untreated, diabetes insipidus can lead to signs and symptoms of hypovolemic shock, including changes in level of consciousness, tachycardia, tachypnea, and hypotension. However, unlike hypovolemic shock, diabetes insipidus causes an increase in urinary output rather than a decrease.

Assessment

Subjective data include the patient's understanding of the relationship of symptoms (such as thirst and polyuria) to the underlying cause. The patient should be able to state the importance of not restricting oral fluids. Assess the severity of thirst. The patient may be embarrassed about the constant need to drink and then empty the bladder and may voluntarily restrict social contacts and work activities. The patient is weak, tired, and lethargic.

Collection of **objective data** includes assessment of skin turgor (the normal resiliency of the skin) and color and specific gravity of the urine. Carefully monitor intake and output (I&O). The skin is dry, turgor is poor, and body weight is lost. Constipation may occur. Weigh the patient daily in the early morning, before breakfast. Determine whether the patient has nocturia.

Diagnostic Tests

Diagnosis is based on clinical manifestations, urine specific gravity, and urine ADH measurement. The urine specific gravity often drops below 1.003, and the serum sodium level increases to more than 145 mEq/L (normal serum sodium level is 135 to 145 mEq/L). The serum osmolality may be greater than 300 mOsm/kg (normal is 280 to 300 mOsm/kg). The fluid deprivation (water deprivation) test may be ordered to determine how well the pituitary is producing ADH and to help rule out other causes. A CT scan and radiographic evaluation of the sella turcica (the "Turkish saddle"–shaped depression in the sphenoid bone that houses the pituitary gland) may be done.

Medical Management

Medical treatment involves intravenous (IV), subcutaneous, intranasal, or oral administration of ADH preparations in the form of desmopressin acetate (DDAVP). Several other drugs are available for ADH replacement, including aqueous vasopressin (Pitressin intramuscular [IM] or intranasal), vasopressin tannate IM, and lypressin (Diapid intranasal). Coffee, tea, and other beverages containing caffeine are usually eliminated from the diet because of their possible diuretic effect. If the patient cannot match the urinary losses through oral intake, he or she is at risk for dehydration and severe hypernatremia. IV fluids of hypotonic saline or dextrose 5% in water are needed.

Nursing Interventions and Patient Teaching

Because of the potential for fluid volume deficiency, carefully monitor the urinary output of pediatric and unconscious patients. Assess skin turgor frequently, along with the condition of oral mucous membranes. Weigh the patient and record I&O daily. Do not limit oral fluids in an effort to reduce urinary output.

Nursing diagnoses and interventions for the patient with diabetes insipidus include but are not limited to the following:

Nursing Diagnoses	Nursing Interventions
Deficient fluid volume, risk for, related to excessive urine production	Assess for signs and symptoms of dehydration (dry oral mucous membranes, poor skin turgor, soft eyeballs, lowered blood pressure, rapid pulse). Monitor electrolyte status carefully. Measure I&O.
Impaired skin integrity, risk for, related to altered state of hydration	Inspect skin for erythema, cyanosis, vesicles, and lesions. Prevent pressure on skin and skeletal prominences by turning and ambulating patient and using sheepskin, eggcrate mattress, or other measures. Increase fluid intake up to 2600 mL/day if possible. Encourage patient to eat food adequate in calories, protein, and vitamin C to promote healthy skin.

Instruct the patient to wear medical-alert jewelry, such as a necklace or bracelet, stating the diagnosis of diabetes insipidus. Stress that the patient must remain under medical supervision for monitoring of the metabolic state, since the condition may worsen with time.

Prognosis

The prognosis depends on the etiology. Patients who survive usually are dependent on medication for the rest of their lives. With proper treatment, most patients can expect to live a relatively normal life.

SYNDROME OF INAPPROPRIATE ANTIDIURETIC HORMONE

Syndrome of inappropriate ADH (SIADH) occurs when the pituitary gland releases too much ADH. In response to ADH, the kidneys reabsorb more water, decreasing urinary output and expanding the body's fluid volume. The patient experiences hyponatremia, hemodilution, and fluid overload without peripheral edema.

Etiology and Pathophysiology

ADH regulates the body's water balance. Synthesized in the hypothalamus, ADH is stored in the posterior pituitary gland. When released into the circulation, it acts on the kidney's distal tubules and collecting ducts, increasing their permeability to water. This decreases urine volume, since more water is reabsorbed and returned to the circulation, which increases blood volume. This syndrome occurs more commonly in older adults.

When the body's system of checks and balances malfunctions—whether from a tumor, medication, unrelated disease process, or some other cause—ADH may be released continuously, causing SIADH.

ADH is released in response to stress. Be alert to patients who have the following risk factors and who are also in pain or undergoing stressful procedures:

- Medications
  - —General anesthetics
  - —Opiates
  - —Barbiturates

—Thiazide diuretics
—Oral hypoglycemics
—Oxytocin

- Malignancies (the most common cause of SIADH; cancerous cells are capable of producing, storing, and releasing ADH):
  —Small cell cancer of the lung
  —Hodgkin's lymphoma, non-Hodgkin's lymphoma, lymphocytic leukemia
  —Prostate cancer
  —Colorectal cancer
  —Duodenal cancer
  —Pancreatic cancer
- Nonmalignant pulmonary diseases
  —Chronic obstructive pulmonary disease
  —Tuberculosis
  —Lung abscess
  —Pneumonia
- Nervous system disorders
  —Head trauma
  —Cerebrovascular thrombosis
  —Cerebral atrophy
  —Acute encephalitis
  —Meningitis
  —Guillain-Barré syndrome
- Miscellaneous
  —Hypothyroidism
  —Lupus erythematosus
  —Adrenal insufficiency

Clinical Manifestations

Clinically, SIADH is characterized by hyponatremia and water retention that progresses to water intoxication. The severity of the patient's condition depends on how hyponatremic he or she becomes and how rapidly fluid accumulates. Most signs and symptoms appear when serum sodium levels fall below 125 mEq/L.

Assessment

Subjective data include vague complaints. Hyponatremia triggers the earliest symptoms, which are nonspecific and could indicate other disorders. These symptoms include weakness, muscle cramps, anorexia, nausea, and headache.

Collection of **objective data** includes assessment for hyponatremia. Hyponatremia may trigger diarrhea. The patient may also be disoriented and irritable and may gain weight. Fluid intake exceeds urinary output. The patient does not develop peripheral edema because excess fluid is accumulating in the vascular system, not in the interstitial spaces.

As water intoxication progresses and serum becomes more hypotonic, brain cells expand (become edematous), so later signs of SIADH are neurologic. The patient becomes progressively lethargic, with marked personality changes. The patient has seizures, and the deep tendon reflexes diminish or disappear altogether.

Diagnostic Tests

The diagnosis of SIADH is made by simultaneous measurements of urine and serum osmolality. Laboratory tests show hyponatremia (sodium less than 134 mEq/L). Serum osmolality is less than 280 mmol/kg (normal is 285 to 295 mmol/kg). The serum is diluted and the urine is concentrated (Lewis et al., 2007). Urine specific gravity is greater than 1.032, and urine sodium is elevated.

Medical Management

The physician orders fluid restriction, initially 800 to 1000 mL/day. However, with severe hyponatremia fluids may be restricted to 500 mL/day. Daily fluid intake should equal fluid output. If fluid restriction is adequate, tests show a gradual increase in serum sodium along with a decrease in body weight.

A hypertonic saline solution (3% to 5%) may be ordered via IV infusion pump at a very slow rate to avoid too rapid a rise in sodium. This is necessary to correct sodium imbalance and to pull water out of edematous brain cells.

The physician may order medications such as demeclocycline (Declomycin), a tetracycline derivative, in a dosage of 300 mg orally four times daily. The physician may also prescribe lithium carbonate. Both drugs interfere with the antidiuretic action of ADH and cause polyuria. Diuretics such as furosemide (Lasix)—40 to 80 mg/day orally in divided dosages or 20 to 40 mg IV daily—may be prescribed, but only if the serum sodium is at least 125 mEq/L, or the drug may promote more loss of sodium. Taking furosemide increases losses of potassium, magnesium, and calcium; supplements may be needed.

Treatment must also be directed at eliminating the underlying problem. Surgical resection, radiation, or chemotherapy may be indicated for malignant neoplasms. If the causative factor is a medication, it is discontinued.

Monitor the loss of potassium and other electrolytes from diuresis, as well as I&O, to prevent hypovolemia.

Nursing Interventions and Patient Teaching

Nursing interventions for SIADH focus on a continual assessment of the patient's condition to determine whether it is improving or deteriorating. Every 3 to 4 hours perform a neurologic examination and assess the patient's hydration status. Auscultate lung sounds every 2 to 4 hours to check for crackles that would indicate overhydration. Document any changes and report them immediately. Carefully observe serum electrolytes, urine sodium, and urine specific gravity because overcorrection can cause hypernatremia. Take a daily weight at the same time and on the same scales. Closely monitor I&O; output is the guide to regulating intake.

The nursing goal is to control the patient's intake and to minimize discomfort. Explain why fluids are being restricted; allow the patient to divide allotted fluids and to choose the fluids, if possible. Supplement the diet with sodium and potassium, especially if diuretics are prescribed. Advise the patient to avoid salty foods (e.g., potato chips or bacon) because they will make the patient more thirsty.

Frequent mouth care is essential to maintain the integrity of oral mucous membranes. Take steps to prevent skin impairment. Inform the patient and family members with simple explanations, such as that pain and anxiety can aggravate SIADH. If nausea is present (because of water intoxication), obtain an order for an antiemetic to be administered 30 minutes before meals.

Nursing diagnoses and interventions for the patient with SIADH include but are not limited to the following:

Nursing Diagnoses	Nursing Interventions
Excess fluid volume, related to decreased urinary output	Obtain daily weight, same scales, same time. Assess and record I&O. Monitor laboratory results. Administer medications as ordered. Maintain dietary and fluid restrictions (fluids should be high in sodium; avoid salty foods). Monitor IV infusions (such as 3% to 5% sodium chloride over several hours).
Risk for impaired oral mucous membrane, related to fluid restrictions of 500 mL/day	Provide frequent oral care; avoid alcohol-based mouthwashes and lemon glycerin swabs. Allow patient to choose fluids and to divide the allotted amount (such as half in morning, one third in evening, and the remainder at night). Offer simple explanation for fluid restrictions. If ordered, administer antiemetics 30 minutes before meals.

Patient teaching should be an ongoing part of nursing care. Be certain the patient understands the treatment plan, the rationale behind it, and the expected outcome. Provide information about signs and symptoms of SIADH, and tell the patient to alert the physician if any changes are noted. SIADH can recur after discharge.

Prognosis

SIADH resulting from an adverse reaction to medication or secondary to a head trauma, is self-limiting. If it occurs as a result of metabolic conditions or tumors, however, it tends to become chronic (Lewis, et al., 2007).

SIADH is potentially dangerous but treatable. If signs and symptoms are recognized early and intervention is appropriate, the prognosis is good; without treatment, coma and death occur.

DISORDERS OF THE THYROID AND PARATHYROID GLANDS

HYPERTHYROIDISM

Etiology and Pathophysiology

Hyperthyroidism—also called **Graves' disease,** exophthalmic goiter, and thyrotoxicosis—is a condition in which there is increased activity of the thyroid gland, with overproduction of the thyroid hormones T_4 and T_3. As a result, all of the patient's metabolic processes are exaggerated. It may occur during pregnancy or in adolescence. Graves' disease occurs most frequently in women in the 20- to 40-year-old age-group. Two percent of the female population is affected by Graves' disease, compared with 0.2% of the male population. Graves' disease is an autoimmune disorder of unknown etiology. It may be caused by genetic factors interacting with precipitating factors such as inadequate iodine, infection, and extreme physical or emotional stress (Lewis et al., 2007).

Clinical Manifestations

Clinical manifestations are numerous and varied, from mild to severe. The patient usually has visible edema of the anterior portion of the neck as a result of enlargement of the thyroid. In severe cases, exophthalmos (bulging of the eyeballs) may occur, usually attributable to periorbital edema (Figure 51-7). Twenty percent to 40% of patients with Graves' disease manifest the classic finding of exophthalmos. The eyeballs are forced outward, resulting in incomplete closure of the eyelids; the exposed corneas become dry with subsequent development of corneal ulcers and loss of vision (Lewis et al., 2007).

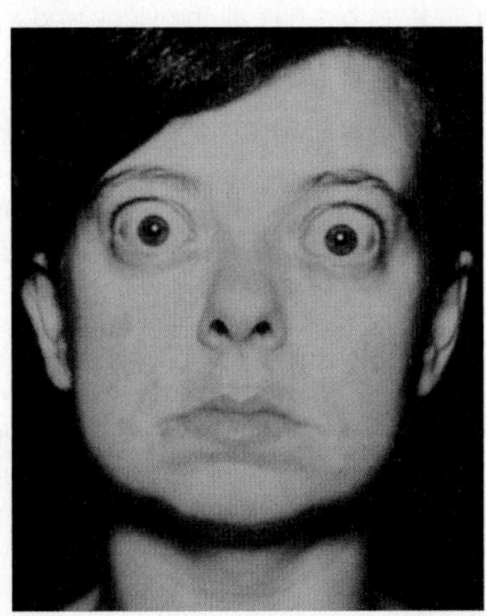

FIGURE 51-7 Exophthalmos of Graves' disease.

Assessment

Subjective data include an inability to concentrate and memory loss. The patient may complain of dysphagia or may be hoarse. There is usually weight loss, even with a voracious appetite. The patient reports feeling nervous, jittery, and excitable and may experience insomnia. These patients are emotionally labile and may overreact to stressful situations.

Objective data include changes in vital signs. The pulse is usually rapid, blood pressure is elevated, and a bruit may be auscultated over the thyroid. The skin is warm and flushed, and the hair is fine and soft. Female patients may cease to menstruate. Elevated body temperature may be accompanied by intolerance to heat, with profuse diaphoresis. Note tremors of the hands. Behavior changes may include hyperactivity and clumsiness. Daily weighing usually shows weight loss.

Diagnostic Tests

Hyperthyroidism is confirmed by a decrease in TSH levels and an elevation of free T_4 (FT_4) levels. Total T_3 and T_4 levels may be evaluated but are not as helpful in the diagnosis. With the radioactive iodine uptake (RAIU) test, the patient demonstrates an uptake of 35% to 95% of the drug (Lewis et al., 2007) (Box 51-1).

Medical Management

Medical management for hyperthyroidism may include administration of drugs that block the production of thyroid hormones, such as propylthiouracil (PTU) or methimazole (Tapazole). PTU must be taken three times per day, but it lowers hormone levels more quickly. Methimazole is usually preferred because only one dose daily is required (Lewis et al., 2007) (Table 51-2). The patient usually begins to notice a decrease in symptoms within 6 to 8 weeks after the dose of the drug. This may be followed after the acute stage by ablation therapy using a therapeutic dose of radioactive iodine (^{131}INaI or ^{125}INaI), based on the patient's age, clinical manifestations, and estimated weight of the thyroid. Ablation therapy using radioactive iodine is the gold standard for treating hyperthyroidism. The goal is to destroy some of the hypertrophied thyroid tissue. Because the therapeutic dose of radioactive iodine is low, no radiation safety precautions are necessary.

An unfortunate outcome of this treatment in most patients is the development of hypothyroidism. Thus the patient must have adequate follow-up medical supervision. If a patient develops hypothyroidism after treatment, levothyroxine therapy will be needed. **^{131}I is not a radiation hazard to the nonpregnant patient but is absolutely contraindicated during pregnancy. Pregnant nurses should not care for this patient for several days after treatment.**

Surgery has fallen out of favor because of possible serious complications, such as hemorrhage, hypoparathyroidism, and vocal cord paralysis. However, surgery may still be indicated for patients who cannot tolerate antithyroid drugs, are not good candidates for radioactive iodine therapy, have a possible malignancy, or have large goiters causing tracheal compression.

Surgical treatment for hyperthyroidism is subtotal thyroidectomy, a procedure in which approximately five sixths of the thyroid is removed. If too much tissue is taken, the gland will not regenerate after surgery and hypothyroidism will result. Surgery is usually delayed, if possible, until the patient is in a normal thyroid (euthyroid) state because of the risk

Box 51-1 Diagnostic Tests for Hyperthyroidism

- **T_3 (serum triiodothyronine):** Measures the T_3 level in the blood. Normal is 65 to 195 ng/dL. As with the thyroxine (T_4 test), the serum T_3 is an accurate measurement of thyroid function. T_3 is less stable than T_4. An elevated T_3 determination is clinically important in the patient who has a normal T_4 level but has all the signs and symptoms of hyperthyroidism. In this patient the test may identify T_3 thyrotoxicosis.
- **T_4 (serum thyroxine):** Measures the T_4 level in the blood. Normal is 5 to 12 mcg/dL. Some medications such as oral contraceptives, steroids, estrogens, and sulfonamides may be withheld for several hours before the T_3 and T_4 tests, but food and fluids are not withheld. Elevated levels of these tests usually indicate hyperthyroidism.
- **Free T_4 (FT_4):** Measures active component of total T_4. Normal values are 1 to 3.5 ng/dL. Because this level remains constant, this is considered a better indication of function than T_4 and is useful in diagnosing hyperthyroidism and hypothyroidism. High FT_4 suggests hyperthyroidism; low FT_4 suggests hypothyroidism.
- **Thyroid-stimulating hormone (TSH):** Measures level of TSH. Normal values are 0.3 to 5.4 mcg/mL. This is considered the most sensitive method for evaluating thyroid disease. It is generally recommended as the first diagnostic test for thyroid dysfunction. TSH is suppressed in hyperthyroidism and elevated in hypothyroidism.
- **Radioactive iodine uptake (RAIU) test:** Radioactive iodine, ^{131}I, is given by mouth to the fasting patient. After 2, 6, and 24 hours, a scintillation camera is held over the thyroid to measure how much of the isotope has been removed from the bloodstream. A hyperactive thyroid may remove 35% to 95% of the drug. This test may be affected by prior ingestion of iodine-containing substances or foods. Obtain a signed consent form for this test. Also note any allergy to iodine on the request form, along with medications currently being taken. No radiation precautions are necessary.
- **Thyroid scan:** ^{131}I is given to the patient either orally or intravenously. If an IV dose is given, the scan may be done in 30 to 60 minutes. A scintillation camera positioned over the patient's thyroid sends images that are received on an oscilloscope and may be printed out on special paper. Obtain a signed consent form for this test. No radiation precautions are necessary.

Table 51-2 Medications Commonly Used to Treat Hyperthyroidism and Hypothyroidism

MEDICATIONS	COMMON SIDE EFFECTS
HYPERTHYROIDISM	
Iodine or iodine products (potassium or sodium iodide with strong iodine solution, potassium iodide, Lugol's solution)	Nausea, vomiting, diarrhea, abdominal pain
Radioactive iodine (^{131}I or ^{125}I)	Sore throat, edema or pain in neck, temporary loss of taste, nausea, vomiting, painful salivary glands
Methimazole (Tapazole), propylthiouracil (PTU)	Rash or pruritus, vertigo, nausea, vomiting, loss of taste, paresthesias, abdominal pain
HYPOTHYROIDISM	
Levothyroxine (Levothroid, Synthroid, Eltroxin, Levo-T, Unithroid) Liothyronine (Cytomel) Liotrix (Thyrolar) Thyroid (Armour Thyroid, Thyrar)	Nervousness, irritability, tremors, insomnia, tachycardia, hypertension, palpitations, cardiac dysrhythmias, vomiting, diarrhea, nausea, appetite changes, weight loss, menstrual irregularities, leg cramps, fever

of excess bleeding during thyroidectomy and postoperative thyroid crisis.

Patients who have only mild hyperthyroidism are rarely admitted to the acute care hospital. They are treated by the physician in an office or clinic setting. However, the hospital nurse may come in contact with the patient because of admission for a different condition and also cares for these patients before and after thyroidectomy.

Nursing Interventions and Patient Teaching

The hyperthyroid patient needs more nutrients because of increased metabolism, so diet therapy usually consists of food high in calories, vitamins (especially the B vitamins), minerals, and carbohydrates. Offer between-meal snacks. Food should be soft and easily swallowed if the patient has **dysphagia** (difficulty swallowing). Coffee, tea, and colas should be avoided because of their stimulant effect.

Preoperative teaching is extremely important for the patient who is scheduled for a thyroidectomy. Keep the environment as stable as possible to prevent emotional strain. Include instructions on how to properly support the head while turning in bed or rising to a sitting or standing position. The nurse (or patient) places both hands behind the head and maintains anatomical position while the rest of the body is being moved. Also teach the patient to deep breathe, but the physician will determine whether coughing is to be done postoperatively, since it strains the suture line. Inform the patient that a period of "voice rest" may be enforced for 48 hours postoperatively and that pencil and paper will be provided for writing notes instead of talking. Do voice checks every 2 to 4 hours, as ordered by the physician. Ask the patient to say "ah" and check for excessive hoarseness or voice change. Slight hoarseness is expected and should not cause alarm. Approximately 12.4% of patients suffer some damage to the laryngeal nerve during surgery, but this is not always permanent.

Postoperative management includes keeping the bed in semi-Fowler's position, with pillows supporting the head and shoulders. Caution the patient to avoid hyperextending the head to prevent excess tension on the incision, which is usually made in a horizontal crease in the anterior neck. Have a suction apparatus and tracheotomy tray available for emergency use. A cool-mist humidifier at the bedside may help soothe the throat and prevent coughing. Check vital signs frequently, with special attention paid to the rate and depth of respirations and observations for any dyspnea (shortness of breath or difficulty breathing) related to edema in the operative site. Before giving any liquid orally, be sure the swallowing and cough reflexes have returned. Be alert for signs of internal or external bleeding; early signs of internal bleeding include restlessness, apprehension, increased pulse rate, decreased blood pressure, and a feeling of fullness in the neck. Later, cyanosis may develop, signaling an obstructed airway; notify the surgeon immediately. Inspect the dressing on the neck frequently for obvious external bleeding. Also check for bleeding at the sides and back of the neck and on top of the patient's shoulders, since oozing blood may pool there as a result of gravity. Most surgeons allow a dressing to be reinforced as needed and loosened slightly if the patient complains that it is too tight.

Postoperatively, the diet initially consists of clear, cool liquids, progressing to soft food as tolerated. This is followed by a regular diet as soon as possible to help the patient regain lost weight and correct any nutritional deficiencies.

Another significant postoperative complication after thyroidectomy is tetany. One possible cause of tetany is the inadvertent removal of one or more of the parathyroid glands during surgery. Another is edema in the operative area, which occludes release of PTH into the bloodstream, resulting in a low serum calcium level (normal serum calcium is 9.0 to 10.5 mg/dL). The symptoms include numbness and tingling in the fingertips and toes and around the mouth. The patient may also have **carpopedal spasms** (muscle spasms in the wrists and feet) and increased pulse, respirations, and blood pressure, accompanied by anxiety and agitation. Laryngeal spasm and stridor may occur. Chvostek's sign is positive (an abnormal spasm of the facial muscles elicited by light taps on the facial nerve in patients who are hypocalcemic), and Trousseau's sign may also be positive (assesses for latent tetany; carpal spasm is induced by inflating a sphygmomanometer cuff on the upper arm to a pressure exceeding systolic blood pressure for 3 minutes; a positive result may be seen in hypocalcemia and hypomagnesemia). If untreated, the condition may progress to convulsions or lethal cardiac dysrhythmias. Emergency treatment of tetany is the IV administration of calcium gluconate, which should always be available postoperatively.

The other serious complication after thyroidectomy is thyroid crisis, or thyroid storm. Fortunately, it occurs rarely and can usually be attributed to manipulation of the thyroid during surgery, which causes the release of large amounts of thyroid hormones into the bloodstream. If thyroid crisis occurs, it usually does so within the first 12 hours postoperatively. In thyroid crisis, all the signs and symptoms of hyperthyroidism are exaggerated. Additionally, the patient may develop nausea, vomiting, severe tachycardia, severe hypertension, and occasionally hyperthermia up to 106° F (41° C). Extreme restlessness, cardiac dysrhythmia, and delirium may also occur. The patient may develop heart failure and die. Diagnostic tests indicate increased FT_4 and decreased TSH.

The three goals of thyroid storm management are (1) to induce a normal thyroid state, (2) prevent cardiovascular collapse, and (3) prevent excessive hyperthermia. Emergency treatment of thyroid crisis includes administration of IV fluids, sodium iodide, corticosteroids, antipyretics, an antithyroid drug (such as PTU or methimazole), and oxygen as needed. Prompt, adequate treatment usually results in dramatic improvement within 12 to 24 hours.

Nursing diagnoses and interventions for the patient having a thyroidectomy include but are not limited to the following:

Nursing Diagnoses	Nursing Interventions
Preoperative	
Risk for hyperthermia, related to increased metabolism	Assess body temperature at regular intervals. Regulate environment (room temperature, linens, clothing) to help keep patient comfortable. Administer acetaminophen as prescribed.
Imbalanced nutrition: less than body requirements, related to increased metabolism	Encourage patient to eat prescribed diet and avoid caffeine. Assess daily weight and food intake.
Postoperative	
Impaired swallowing, related to postoperative edema	Ensure swallowing and cough reflexes are present before oral intake. Encourage patient to drink slowly and chew food thoroughly.
Ineffective breathing pattern, risk for, related to: • postoperative edema • pain	Monitor rate and depth of respirations. Assess breath sounds and skin color. Encourage slow, deep breaths at least once an hour. Position patient to maximize respiratory effort.

Patient education after thyroidectomy includes stressing the importance of follow-up medical supervision. Thyroid function tests are done periodically to check for both hyperthyroidism and hypothyroidism, which occurs in approximately 43% of surgical cases. Before discharge, teach the patient proper care of the incision site and symptoms that might indicate development of an infection, in which case he or she should notify the surgeon immediately. Discuss with the patient the need for a high-calorie, high-protein, high-carbohydrate diet until weight is stable.

Prognosis

With adequate, appropriate medical or surgical treatment, these patients usually have a normal life expectancy. However, exophthalmos, if present, may remain to a lesser degree in some patients.

HYPOTHYROIDISM

Etiology and Pathophysiology

Hypothyroidism is one of the most common medical disorders in the United States, affecting 10% of women and 3% of men older than 65 years of age. It occurs most often in women 30 to 60 years of age and is more common in older adults than previously thought. Hypothyroidism is the clinical state that occurs when the thyroid fails to secrete sufficient hormones, slowing all of the body's metabolic processes. It may be caused by a condition of the thyroid itself or by a failure of the pituitary gland to furnish sufficient TSH for proper stimulation of thyroid secretion. It is sometimes an unfortunate outcome of the medical or surgical treatment of hyperthyroidism. Severe hypothyroidism in adults is called **myxedema** (Figure 51-8). It is characterized by edema of the hands, the face, the feet, and periorbital tissues. Congenital hypothyroidism is called **cretinism** (Figure 51-9) and is estimated to occur in 1 of every 4000 to 5000 newborns. All infants in the United States are screened for decreased thyroid function at birth.

Clinical Manifestations

Clinical manifestations range from mild to severe and depend on the degree of thyroid hormone deficiency present. All the body's metabolic processes slow, resulting in decreased production of body heat, intolerance to cold, and weight gain. Atherosclerotic changes may result in coronary artery disease. Hypothyroidism may have adverse effects on the heart with decreased cardiac output and contractility; the patient experiences decreased exercise tolerance and dyspnea on exertion (Lewis et al., 2007).

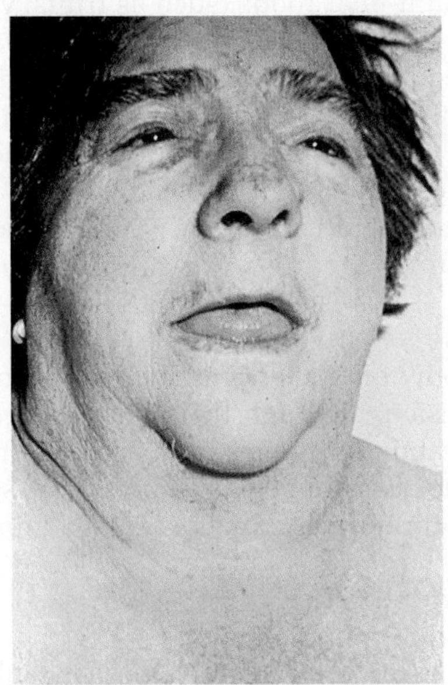

FIGURE 51-8 Person with myxedema.

Assessment

Subjective data include the patient's mental and emotional status, which may include depression, paranoia, impaired memory, and general slowing of thought processes. Speech and hearing may be deficient. The patient is lethargic, forgetful, and irritable. Because of the body's slowed metabolism, cold intolerance, anorexia, and constipation may develop. Both sexes may experience decreased libido and reproductive difficulty. Assess the patient's adaptive coping methods.

Collection of **objective data** includes assessment of the skin and hair. The hair thins and may fall out; the skin becomes thickened and dry. Facial features may enlarge to give the patient an edematous appearance with a masklike facial expression. The voice is characteristically low and hoarse. Decreased metabolism usually causes bradycardia, decreased blood pressure and respirations, and exercise intolerance. The patient has decreased ability to perform activities because of weakness, clumsiness, and ataxia. Assess the respiratory rate after administration of any central nervous system depressant. Evaluate the abdomen for distention, since **myxedema ileus** may occur. Menorrhagia (excessive menstrual flow) is a frequent complaint of women with hypothyroidism. Also inhibition of ovulation with subsequent infertility may occur (Lewis et al., 2007).

Diagnostic Tests

Diagnosis of hypothyroidism is based on the physical examination and history and on appropriate laboratory tests, such as TSH, T_3, T_4, and FT_4 levels. Low levels of T_3, T_4, and FT_4 are the underlying stimuli for TSH.

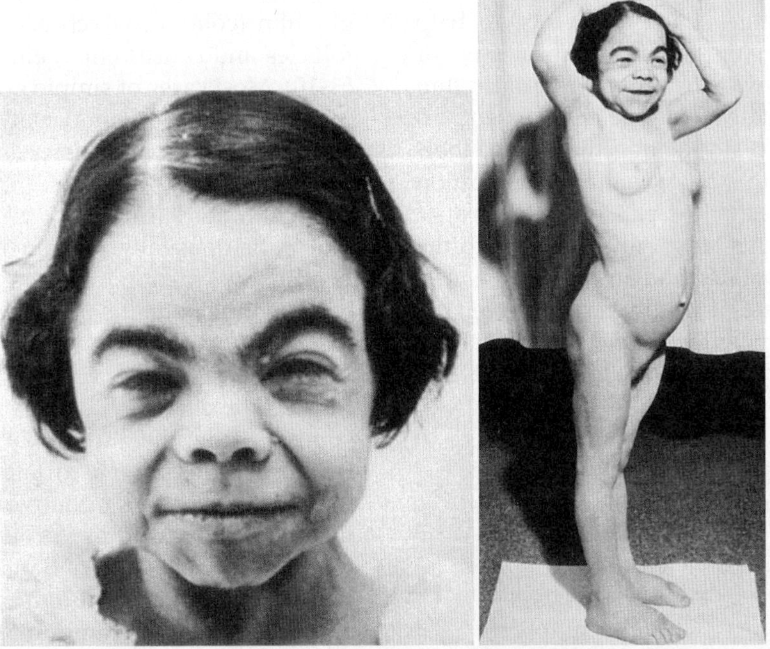

FIGURE 51-9 Adult cretin (33 years old, untreated). Note characteristic cretinoid features: dwarfism (44 inches in height), absent axillary and scant pubic hair, poorly developed breasts, protruding abdomen, and small umbilical hernia.

Therefore a compensatory elevation of TSH occurs in patients with primary hypothyroid states, and low levels of T_3, T_4, and FT_4 are present. Subclinical cases may go undiagnosed for years, so be aware of subtle clues while interviewing and caring for the patient.

Medical Management

The treatment for hypothyroidism is replacement therapy, with desiccated animal thyroid (Armour Thyroid); T_4; or synthetic products, such as levothyroxine (Levothroid, Synthroid, Levo-T, Eltroxin) (see Table 51-2). These drugs are usually given in the morning to enhance utilization of nutrients ingested during the daily meals. The patient initially is given a low dose, with increases as necessary until the desired effect is achieved. A maintenance dose is then established. Early in treatment, monitor hormone levels about every 6 to 8 weeks until the patient's TSH level is normal and at least yearly after that. Watch the patient for adverse effects of drug therapy, which mimic the signs and symptoms of hyperthyroidism. There is usually a dramatic change in the patient within a short time after replacement therapy begins. Lifelong thyroid replacement therapy is usually required.

Nursing Interventions and Patient Teaching

Nursing interventions for the hospitalized severely hypothyroid patient center mainly on symptomatic relief. Keep the room at least 70° to 74° F (21° to 23° C), and be certain the patient is not chilled during the bath or other procedures. Allow extra time for physical care, so the patient does not feel rushed. Keep accurate records of bowel elimination, since constipation may be severe. Stool softeners and bulk laxatives may be ordered. Provide a high-protein, high-fiber, low-calorie diet, and encourage increased fluid intake. The patient should avoid concentrated carbohydrates, such as sweets, to help prevent excess weight gain. Watch for chest pain or dyspnea, accompanied by changes in the rate or rhythm of the heart; this may indicate cardiac involvement. Instruct the patient not to stop taking the thyroid hormone without consulting a physician. This medication must be taken for the rest of the patient's life. Because most hypothyroid patients are more susceptible to the effects of sedatives, hypnotics, and anesthetics, be alert for possible adverse effects if these agents are given.

Nursing diagnoses and interventions for the patient with hypothyroidism include but are not limited to the following:

Nursing Diagnoses	Nursing Interventions
Decreased cardiac output, related to decreased metabolism	Assess pulse, blood pressure, skin color, and temperature. Schedule nursing activities around patient's activity cycle, with rest periods as needed to conserve energy.
Constipation, related to decreased peristaltic action	Assess frequency and character of stools. Encourage increased intake of oral fluids and high-fiber foods.

Regular checkups are essential because drug dosage may have to be adjusted from time to time. The patient and significant other should understand the desired effects and major adverse effects of the medication. Instruct the patient to eat well-balanced meals of high-fiber foods, such as fruits, vegetables, and whole-grain cereals and breads; the patient also needs adequate intake of iodine, in foods such as saltwater fish, milk, and eggs, and increased fluids to prevent constipation. Tell the patient and the family that mental and physical slowness may still be present but should improve with thyroid replacement therapy.

Prognosis

Most hypothyroid patients do well with proper medical supervision, although they will probably have to take medication for the rest of their lives. In children, when T_4 replacement begins before epiphyseal fusion, the chance for normal growth is greatly improved.

SIMPLE (COLLOID) GOITER

Etiology and Pathophysiology

A simple, or colloid, goiter develops when the thyroid gland enlarges in response to low iodine levels in the bloodstream or when it is unable to utilize iodine properly. When the blood level of T_3 is too low to signal the pituitary to decrease TSH secretion, the thyroid gland responds by increasing the formation of thyroglobulin (colloid), which accumulates in the thyroid follicles and causes enlargement of the gland (Figure 51-10). Most cases of simple goiter can be attributed to insufficient dietary intake of iodine, leading to this overgrowth of thyroid tissue.

Clinical Manifestations

The patient usually has no manifestations of overt thyroid dysfunction, and the diagnosis is essentially based on the patient's physical manifestations.

Assessment

Subjective data include the patient's emotional response to the unsightly enlargement of the thyroid. Encourage the patient to talk about his or her feelings. The patient may complain only of symptoms of dysphagia, hoarseness, or dyspnea related to the pressure of the enlarged gland against the esophagus and trachea. Dysphagia may make it difficult to eat and drink adequate amounts. Assess the patient for increasing dyspnea. Determine the patient's understanding of the need for medication, diet therapy, and medical follow-up.

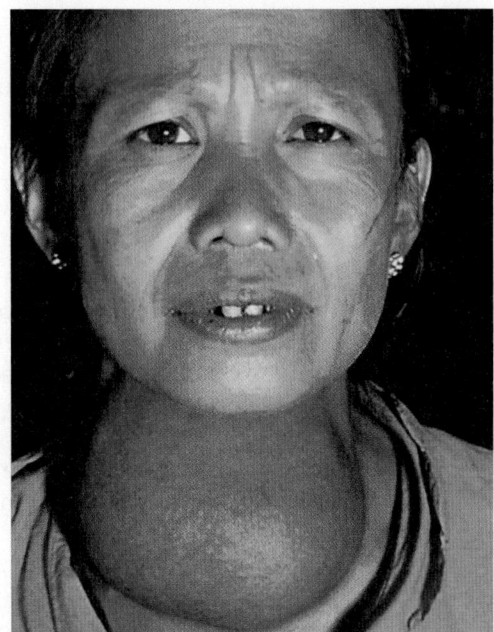

FIGURE 51-10 Simple goiter.

Collection of **objective data** includes assessment of increased goiter size, voice changes, and adequacy of food and fluid intake.

Medical Management

The thyroid may be only slightly enlarged, or it may be so enlarged that surgery must be done to improve respiration or swallowing. Surgery also is sometimes performed for cosmetic effect, since this type of goiter can be unsightly and damage the patient's self-image and self-esteem. If thyroidectomy is done, most of the gland is removed. Medical treatment consists of oral administration of potassium iodide and foods high in iodine.

Nursing Interventions and Patient Teaching

Nursing interventions after thyroidectomy (previously discussed) are aimed at prevention of complications such as bleeding, tetany, and thyroid crisis.

Nursing diagnoses and interventions for the patient with simple (colloid) goiter include but are not limited to the following:

Nursing Diagnoses	Nursing Interventions
Risk for noncompliance, related to therapeutic regimen	Provide opportunities for patient to express feelings about treatment plan. Correct misconceptions and reinforce previous medical instruction. Stress importance of taking prescribed medications, having regular checkups, and avoiding any identified goitrogenic foods.
Risk for disturbed body image, related to altered physical appearance	Develop open and trusting relationship so that the patient will express his or her feelings. Discuss ways to disguise thyroid enlargement (scarves, high collars, makeup).

Stress the importance of adequate dietary intake of iodine by the patient. Medical supervision is recommended at regular intervals.

Prognosis

Most patients can expect to live a normal life after adequate treatment of goiter.

CANCER OF THE THYROID

Etiology and Pathophysiology

Cancer of the thyroid is a relatively rare malignancy, affecting approximately 25 of each 1 million people in the United States each year. However, more cases are expected, since between 1949 and 1960, many infants and children through adolescence were irradiated to shrink enlarged thymus tissue, tonsils, or adenoids and to treat severe cases of acne vulgaris. Cancer of the thyroid occurs more frequently in females and in whites. The incidence rises as age increases. About 75% of malignancies of the thyroid are papillary, well-differentiated adenocarcinomas, a type of cancer that grows slowly, is usually contained, and does not spread beyond the adjacent lymph nodes. Cure rates after thyroidectomy in these cases are excellent. Other cancers, follicular and anaplastic, are more rare and have extremely low cure rates.

Clinical Manifestations

The principal clinical manifestation of thyroid cancer is a firm, fixed, small, rounded, painless mass or **nodule** that is felt during palpation of the gland. Only in rare instances are the symptoms of hyperthyroidism seen.

Assessment

Subjective data include the patient's use of adaptive coping methods to deal with the diagnosis. Also observe the support system provided by the patient's significant others. Assess the patient's understanding of the importance of medical follow-up.

Objective data include progressive enlargement of the tumor area preoperatively, response to ^{131}I therapy, and skin involvement in the neck and torso after radiation therapy.

Diagnostic Tests

Papillary thyroid cancer is suspected when a thyroid scan shows a "cold" nodule, indicating decreased uptake of ^{131}I. Benign adenomas and follicular cancers are usually visualized as "hot" nodules because of their increased uptake of the isotope. Thyroid function tests usually yield normal results. To confirm the diagnosis, a thyroid needle biopsy may be done, but only by a skilled practitioner to avoid seeding of adjacent tissues. Metastasis could result, with the prognosis becoming much more grave.

Medical Management

Treatment of thyroid cancer is a total thyroidectomy, with subsequent lifelong thyroid hormone replacement therapy. If metastasis is present at the time of the initial surgery, a radical neck dissection may be performed. In addition, radiation therapy, chemotherapy, and administration of ^{131}I may be done.

Nursing Interventions and Patient Teaching

Nursing interventions are like those for the patient who has undergone thyroidectomy (see pp. 1733 to 1734). As with a thyroidectomy for noncancerous lesions, the major postoperative complications are respiratory distress, recurrent laryngeal damage, hemorrhage, and hypoparathyroidism.

Nursing diagnoses and interventions for the patient with cancer of the thyroid include but are not limited to the following:

Nursing Diagnoses	Nursing Interventions
Anxiety, related to situational crisis	Encourage patient to discuss feelings about upcoming surgery. Monitor level of anxiety. Maintain a calm environment; try to decrease stressors.
Ineffective coping, related to personal vulnerability in crisis	Help patient identify previously successful coping methods. Teach new coping methods as needed.

Stress the importance of proper medical follow-up to monitor thyroid hormone replacement therapy and to help ensure prompt diagnosis of any metastatic lesions. Before discharge from the hospital, teach the patient proper care of the surgical incision.

Prognosis

The prognosis after treatment for thyroid cancer depends on the type of tumor. For papillary carcinoma the prognosis is excellent; for follicular and anaplastic carcinomas, the prognosis is much less favorable.

HYPERPARATHYROIDISM

Etiology and Pathophysiology

Hyperparathyroidism involves overactivity of the parathyroid glands, with increased production of PTH. The cause of this condition may be a primary hypertrophy of one or more of the tiny parathyroid glands, usually in the form of an adenoma. It may also result from chronic renal failure, pyelonephritis, or glomerulonephritis. Parathyroid carcinoma is a rare condition, with rapid progress and a grave prognosis. Hyperparathyroidism usually occurs in adults between 30 and 70 years of age, and it occurs twice as often in women.

Clinical Manifestations

The primary clinical manifestation is hypercalcemia. This occurs as calcium leaves the bones and accumulates in the bloodstream. As a result, the bones become demineralized, causing skeletal pain, pain on weight bearing, and pathologic fractures (fractures that result from slight or no trauma to diseased bone). The high level of calcium in the blood may lead to the formation of kidney stones.

Assessment

Collection of **subjective data** includes assessment of the severity of skeletal pain, the degree of muscle weakness, and the effectiveness of analgesics. It is important to determine nursing measures that contribute to the patient's comfort and mobility. As neuromuscular function decreases, the patient has generalized fatigue, drowsiness, apathy, nausea, and anorexia; assess the degree of anorexia and nausea. There may be constipation, personality changes, disorientation, and even paranoia. Renal colic and dull back pain may indicate calculus formation.

Collection of **objective data** includes careful observation for any skeletal deformity or abnormal movement of bone that might indicate a pathologic fracture. Observe the urine for quantity and the presence of hematuria and stones. There may be vomiting and weight loss. Hypertension and cardiac dysrhythmias may present significant problems. Changes in the serum calcium level may cause bradycardia and other cardiac irregularities. The level of consciousness may decrease to the level of stupor or coma.

Diagnostic Tests

Radiographic examination may reveal skeletal decalcification. Blood PTH levels are increased, as are alkaline phosphate levels. The patient should receive nothing by mouth for 8 to 12 hours before these tests. The serum calcium level is elevated, whereas the serum phosphorus level is decreased. Bone density measurements may also be used to detect bone loss. Imaging, such as MRI, CT, and ultrasound, may be used to localize the adenoma. A differential diagnosis should be made to rule out multiple myeloma, Cushing's syndrome, vitamin D excess, and other causes of hypercalcemia.

Medical Management

The treatment for hyperparathyroidism is surgical removal of an existing tumor or of one or more parathyroid glands. Normal parathyroid tissue taken from the patient is transplanted in the forearm or near the sternocleidomastoid muscle. This autotransplantation allows the parathyroid tissue to continue to secrete PTH to regulate the concentration of calcium and phosphorus in the blood. If autotransplantation is not possible, or it fails, the patient needs to take calcium replacement for life (Lewis et al., 2007).

Nursing Interventions and Patient Teaching

Preoperative nursing interventions include helping restore fluid and electrolyte balance by encouraging increased oral fluid intake and by carefully monitoring the IV fluid therapy. Monitor the patient's I&O because diuretics may be used. Furosemide is the diuretic of choice. Thiazide diuretics are not used because they decrease renal excretion of calcium and thus increase the hypercalcemic state. Urine may be strained because development of kidney calculi is not uncommon. Daily serum calcium levels may be ordered. The diet should be low in calcium, eliminating milk and other dairy products. Cranberry juice may help promote acidic urine, thereby lessening the possibility of calculus formation. Some antacids are high in calcium and should not be used. Accurately assess the patient's pain and administer prescribed analgesics as needed. Postoperatively, care for the patient in the same manner as after a thyroidectomy, with careful monitoring of I&O. These patients commonly retain fluid in the tissues after surgery and often have decreased urinary output. It is important to avoid overhydration at this point. Assess the patient frequently for signs of **hypocalcemia** (a deficiency of calcium in the blood serum), such as tetany, cardiac dysrhythmias, and carpopedal spasms. If tetany does occur, administer calcium gluconate intravenously.

Nursing diagnoses and interventions for the patient with hyperparathyroidism include but are not limited to the following:

Nursing Diagnoses	Nursing Interventions
Activity intolerance, related to neuromuscular dysfunction	Help patient to identify factors that increase or decrease activity tolerance and to eliminate or reduce painful, fatiguing activities.
	Encourage patient to follow prescribed individualized activity or exercise program.
Acute pain: skeletal, joint; renal colic, related to physiologic variables	Assess factors that cause or worsen pain, and help patient adjust body mechanics or activity.
	Encourage adequate fluid intake while assessing cardiac and urinary output.

Teach the patient the principles of good body mechanics to prevent pathologic fractures during ambulation. Reassure the patient that bone pain should gradually decrease as electrolyte balance is restored and the condition is alleviated. Encourage the patient to participate in mild exercise as prescribed by the physician to regain muscle strength and a feeling of well-being. Teach the patient how to check the urine for stones or blood and how to monitor the pulse for any changes. Evaluate the home environment and develop a plan of changes necessary to prevent accidents.

Prognosis

With proper medical or surgical treatment, the patient can lead a fairly normal life. In patients with parathyroid carcinoma, the prognosis is grave.

HYPOPARATHYROIDISM

Etiology and Pathophysiology

Hypoparathyroidism occurs when there is decreased PTH, resulting in decreased levels of serum calcium. Idiopathic hypoparathyroidism is a rare condition, thought to be either autoimmune or familial in origin. The most common cause is the inadvertent removal or destruction of one or more of the tiny parathyroid glands during thyroidectomy.

Clinical Manifestations

Decreased PTH levels in the bloodstream cause an increased serum phosphorus level and a decreased serum calcium level, resulting in neuromuscular hyperexcitability, involuntary and uncontrollable muscle spasms, and hypocalcemic tetany. Severe hypocalcemia may result in laryngeal spasm, stridor, cyanosis, and an increased possibility of asphyxia. Some patients have calcification of the basal ganglia in the brain, causing a parkinsonian syndrome with bizarre posturing and spastic movements.

Assessment

Collection of **subjective data** includes assessment of neuromuscular activity for symptoms such as dysphagia and numbness or tingling of the lips, fingertips, and occasionally feet and increased muscle tension leading to paresthesias and stiffness. The patient may feel anxious, irritable, or depressed. The patient may experience headaches and nausea. Abdominal or flank pain may occur if a renal calculus attempts to pass down the ureter into the bladder. Assess the effectiveness of narcotics used to relieve renal colic.

Objective data include a positive Chvostek's sign or Trousseau's sign. If laryngeal spasm and stridor occur, cyanosis may appear. Cardiac output may decrease as a result of hypocalcemia, and the patient may develop dysrhythmias. Tetanic spasms of the extremities may be observed.

Diagnostic Tests

Diagnostic laboratory studies confirm the decreased serum calcium and PTH with increased urinary calcium, and increased serum phosphorus with decreased urinary phosphorus. Rule out other possible causes of hypocalcemia, such as vitamin D deficiency, kidney failure, and acute pancreatitis.

Medical Management

The immediate treatment of hypoparathyroid tetany is IV administration of calcium gluconate or calcium chloride (10%). This drug irritates the vessel wall and should always be given slowly, at a rate not to exceed 1 mL/min. The patient may complain of a hot feeling of the skin or tongue. If given too rapidly, IV calcium can precipitate hypotension, serious cardiac dysrhythmias, or cardiac arrest. Thus electrocardiographic monitoring is indicated when administering calcium. Take care that none of the drug escapes the vein and extravasates into the tissues, since sloughing may occur. After the initial IV dose, calcium may be continued in a slow IV infusion until tetany is controlled; then it is given orally. Vitamin D is usually also given orally to increase the absorption and blood level of calcium.

Nursing Interventions and Patient Teaching

Monitor any patient receiving calcium, especially intravenously, for signs of hypercalcemia. The most common clinical manifestations of this are vomiting, disorientation, anorexia, abdominal pain, and weakness. Assess the patient for respiratory distress; renal involvement; and adverse reactions to calcium therapy, such as bradycardia, syncope, and hypotension. Use calcium cautiously in digitalized patients, since it may cause digitalis toxicity. Cimetidine (Tagamet) interferes with normal parathyroid functioning and should be used carefully in these patients. Vitamin D supplements are prescribed to improve the absorption of calcium in the intestinal tract and improve bone resorption in patients with chronic and resistant hypocalcemia. Dihydrotachysterol (Hytakerol) and calcitriol (Rocaltrol) are the preferred medications (Lewis et al., 2007). The diet should contain foods high in calcium, such as dairy products, dark green vegetables, soybeans, tofu, and canned fish with the bones included. Offer high-calcium snacks.

Nursing diagnoses and interventions for the patient with hypoparathyroidism include but are not limited to the following:

Nursing Diagnoses	Nursing Interventions
Risk for injury, related to postoperative hypocalcemia	Assess for signs and symptoms of hypocalcemia (muscle spasms, laryngeal stridor, convulsion). Institute prescribed calcium therapy if needed.
Imbalanced nutrition: less than body requirements, related to calcium intake	Give calcium replacement agents as scheduled. Monitor for Chvostek's and Trousseau's signs. Arrange for dietitian to discuss dietary sources of calcium. Assess patient's intake of high-calcium foods.

Teach the patient the early symptoms of hypocalcemia, with instructions to notify the nurse or physician if they occur. Draw blood levels of calcium and phosphorus periodically while the patient is hospitalized. Teach the patient to monitor the pulse for changes, maintain fluid balance, and use calcium supplements at home. Stress the need for life long treatment and follow-up care, including monitoring calcium levels three or four times a year (Lewis et al., 2007).

Prognosis

For most patients, a fairly normal lifestyle and life expectancy are possible.

DISORDERS OF THE ADRENAL GLANDS

ADRENAL HYPERFUNCTION (CUSHING'S SYNDROME)

Etiology and Pathophysiology

Cushing's syndrome is a spectrum of clinical abnormalities caused by excess corticosteroids, particularly glucocorticoids. This syndrome may be caused by hyperplasia of adrenal tissue resulting from overstimulation by the pituitary hormone ACTH, by a tumor of the adrenal cortex, by ACTH-secreting neoplasms outside the pituitary (such as small cell carcinoma of the lung), and by prolonged administration of high doses of corticosteroids. The body's protective feedback mechanism fails, resulting in excess secretion of the adrenal hormones: glucocorticoids, mineralocorticoids, and sex hormones.

Clinical Manifestations

This overabundance of corticosteroids produces the signs and symptoms commonly associated with Cushing's syndrome, including moon face and buffalo hump. Weight gain, the most common feature, results from accumulation of adipose tissue in the trunk, face, and cervical spine area (Figure 51-11). The arms and legs become thin as a result of muscle wasting. **Hypokalemia** (a condition in which an inadequate amount of potassium, the major intracellular cation, is found in the circulating bloodstream) is usually present. Hyperglycemia occurs because of glucose intolerance (associated with cortisol-induced insulin resistance) and increased glucose release by the liver. The patient usually has protein in the urine and increased urinary calcium

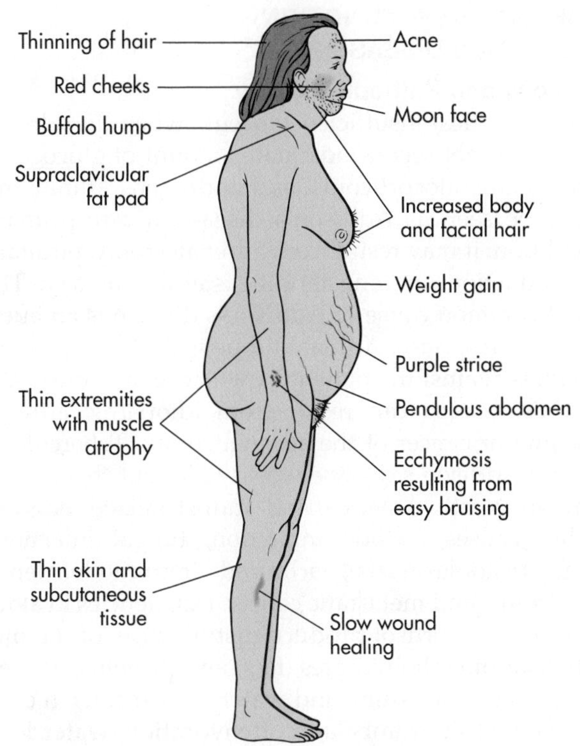

FIGURE 51-11 Common characteristics of Cushing syndrome.

excretion, which may lead to the development of renal calculi. Osteoporosis results from abnormal calcium absorption, and kyphosis may develop. The patient is susceptible to infections, but the symptoms may be masked and the infection not detected until it is life threatening.

Assessment

Collection of **subjective data** includes assessment of the patient's ability to concentrate. Patients may have mood disturbances such as irritability, anxiety, euphoria, insomnia, irrationality, and occasionally psychosis. Depression is common, and the possibility of suicide is an ever-present concern. Be alert to subtle changes in the patient's affect, and keep the environment free from objects with which the patient can inflict self-harm. Patients of both sexes may experience loss of libido and alterations in self-esteem with concerns about sexual dysfunction. Encourage the patient to verbalize concerns about altered body image. Severe backache is often present and may signal a compression fracture of a vertebral body. Assess the severity of back pain and nursing measures that contribute to the patient's comfort. Appetite usually increases. Ensure that the patient understands dietary restrictions and the importance of medical follow-up.

Collection of **objective data** includes observation of the skin for ecchymoses and petechiae. The skin becomes thin and fragile, and wound healing is delayed. The patient may have weight gain and abdominal enlargement, with development of **striae** (a streak or linear scar that often results from stretching of the skin); this increased girth may contribute to difficulty with mobility. Monitor weight, since peripheral edema and associated hypertension are common. Impaired carbohydrate metabolism results in hyperglycemia. Women may experience **hirsutism** (excessive body hair in a masculine distribution), menstrual irregularities, and deepening of the voice. Elevated body temperature may indicate an undetected infection.

Diagnostic Tests

Diagnosis is usually based on the patient's clinical appearance and laboratory test results. Plasma cortisol levels are usually elevated. Plasma ACTH levels may be increased or decreased, depending on the location of a tumor. Skull radiographic evaluation may detect erosion of the sella turcica in the presence of a pituitary tumor. Adrenal angiography aids in diagnosing an adrenal tumor. A 24-hour urine test for 17-ketosteroids and 17-hydroxysteroids shows increased levels. Blood glucose for hyperglycemia and urinalysis for glycosuria are other diagnostic tests associated with but not diagnostic of Cushing's syndrome. Abdominal CT scan and ultrasound may help localize an abdominal tumor.

Medical Management

Treatment is directed toward the causative factor. If an adrenal tumor is present, adrenalectomy is usually indicated for its removal. Pituitary tumors may be irradiated or removed surgically by transsphenoidal microsurgery. If the patient is unable to undergo surgery because of inoperable cancer elsewhere in the body or another preexisting condition, mitotane (Lysodren) therapy may be used. Mitotane alters peripheral metabolism of cortisol, decreases plasma and corticosteroid level, and suppresses cortisol production—essentially providing a "medical adrenalectomy." This cytotoxic agent is toxic to the adrenal glands and is given for at least 3 months, during which time the patient must be monitored for symptoms of hepatotoxicity, such as jaundice, gastrointestinal upset, and pruritus. The diet should be low in sodium to help decrease edema. Reduced calories and carbohydrates help control hyperglycemia, and foods high in potassium help correct hypokalemia. If Cushing's syndrome has developed during the course of prolonged administration of corticosteroids (e.g., prednisone), one or more of the following alternatives may be tried: (1) gradually discontinuing corticosteroid therapy, (2) reducing the corticosteroid dose, and (3) converting to an alternate-day regimen. Gradually tapering the corticosteroids is necessary to avoid potentially life-threatening adrenal insufficiency.

Nursing Interventions and Patient Teaching

Important nursing interventions include gentle handling to prevent skin impairment or excessive ecchymosis and frequent assessment for erythema, edema, or early signs of infection. Encourage the patient to turn frequently and ambulate as tolerated to eliminate undue pressure on bony prominences. Elbow and heel protectors and an eggcrate mattress pad may help prevent decubitus ulcers in the bedridden patient. Encourage the patient to participate as fully as possible in normal ADLs, interspersing personal hygiene tasks with rest periods to prevent overtiring.

Nursing diagnoses and interventions for the patient with Cushing's syndrome include but are not limited to the following:

Nursing Diagnoses	Nursing Interventions
Deficient knowledge, related to therapeutic regimen	Assess patient's understanding of prescribed medication and diet. Encourage patient to wear medical-alert jewelry and carry wallet identification card.
Activity intolerance, related to weakness and immobility	Assess patient's current activity tolerance, and identify priorities for energy expenditures. Plan activity and rest periods with patient.
Risk for infection, related to: • suppression of immune system • lowered resistance to stress	Monitor patient for complaints of pain, purulent exudates, or decrease of function because the usual signs and symptoms of inflammation, such as fever and erythema, may not be present (Lewis et al., 2007). Practice meticulous handwashing before caring for patient.

The patient's mental attitude is extremely important. Encourage verbalization of concerns and watch for the development of depression and suicidal thoughts. Help the patient understand prescribed medications, such as mitotane, as well as possible side effects. It is important for the patient to wear a medical-alert bracelet or necklace and to carry a wallet card stating the diagnosis of Cushing's syndrome. The patient may need to adjust to a major lifestyle change, and the aid of a social worker may be enlisted. Before adrenalectomy, teach the patient the importance of avoiding stress and infections. Postoperative teaching includes proper wound care and the symptoms of Addison's disease, which is sometimes an unavoidable sequela after this type of surgery.

Prognosis

Depending on whether the cause of the disease was benign or malignant and whether the treatment was successful or unsuccessful, the patient with Cushing's syndrome can expect to have major lifestyle changes, possibly with many complications and a shortened life expectancy.

ADRENAL HYPOFUNCTION (ADDISON'S DISEASE)

Etiology and Pathophysiology

Adrenocortical insufficiency occurs when the adrenal glands do not secrete adequate amount of glucocorticoids, mineralocorticoids, and androgens. It may initially be seen as Addison's disease, a rare primary condition; it may result from adrenalectomy, pituitary hypofunction, or longstanding steroid therapy. The most common cause of Addison's disease is an autoimmune response. Adrenal tissue is destroyed by antibodies against the patient's own adrenal cortex. Addison's disease can result from idiopathic adrenal atrophy or cancer of the adrenal cortex. Tuberculosis causes Addison's disease worldwide, but this is now rare in North America and industrialized nations. Other causes include infarction, fungal infections (e.g., histoplasmosis), acquired immunodeficiency syndrome, and metastatic cancer. Deficiencies in aldosterone and cortisol produce disturbances of the metabolism of carbohydrates, fats, and proteins, as well as sodium, potassium, and water. This results in electrolyte and fluid imbalance, dehydration, water loss, and hypovolemia. Adrenal insufficiency most often occurs in adults less than 60 years of age and affects both genders equally.

Clinical Manifestations

Because manifestations are usually not evident until 90% of the adrenal cortex is destroyed, the disease is often advanced before it is diagnosed. Clinical manifestations are directly related to imbalances in adrenal hormones, nutrients, and electrolytes.

Assessment

Subjective data include progressive weakness, fatigue, nausea, anorexia, and craving for salt. Postural hypotension may be associated with vertigo, weakness, and syncope, resulting in reluctance to attempt normal activities. The patient may complain of severe headache, disorientation, abdominal pain, or lower back pain, which could represent early symptoms of adrenal crisis. This patient tolerates stress poorly and feels anxious and apprehensive. It is important to assess emotional status and allow the patient to share feelings about altered self-image. Also assess the patient's overall understanding of the disease process and the importance of medical treatment and follow-up.

Collection of **objective data** includes observation of changes in the color of the mucous membranes and the skin. Skin hyperpigmentation, a common feature, is seen primarily in sun-exposed areas of the body; at pressure points; over joints; and in creases, especially in palmar creases. The patient usually loses weight, often with vomiting and diarrhea. Hypoglycemia may contribute to fatigue; assess the patient's ability to perform ADLs. An abnormally low or abnormally high body temperature, orthostatic hypotension, hyponatremia, and hyperkalemia are signs of impending **adrenal crisis,** a life-threatening emergency caused by insufficient adrenocortical hormones or a sudden sharp decrease in these hormones. Precipitating factors that can trigger an addisonian crisis are stress-producing situations such as infections, surgery, trauma, hemorrhage, psychological stress, sudden withdrawal of corticosteroid hormone replacement therapy, postadrenal surgery, or sudden pituitary gland destruction (Lewis et al., 2007). See Table 51-3 for a comparison of Cushing's syndrome and Addison's disease.

Diagnostic Tests

Laboratory studies show decreased serum sodium, increased serum potassium, and decreased serum glucose. A 24-hour urine specimen shows decreased levels of 17-ketosteroids and 17-hydroxysteroids. Fasting plasma cortisol levels and aldosterone levels are low with an ACTH stimulation test. A glucose tolerance test may yield abnormal results.

Medical Management

Medical treatment involves the prompt restoration of fluid and electrolyte balance and replacement of the deficient adrenal hormones. The most common form of replacement therapy is hydrocortisone, which has both mineralocorticoid and glucocorticoid properties. Glucocorticoid dosage must be increased during times of physiologic stress to prevent addisonian crisis. Fludrocortisone (Florinef) (a mineralocorticoid) is also administered. The diet should be high in sodium and low in potassium.

Treatment for the life-threatening emergency of an addisonian crisis includes shock management, high-dose hydrocortisone replacement therapy, and large volumes of 0.9% saline and 5% dextrose solutions to improve electrolyte imbalances and reverse hypotension (Lewis et al., 2007).

Nursing Interventions and Patient Teaching

Carefully assess the patient's circulatory status, keep accurate I&O records, and record daily weight. Check skin turgor and offer fluids frequently. Monitor vital signs at regular intervals, paying particular attention to temperature and blood pressure. Also monitor the patient for response to prescribed steroid drugs, and promptly report any adverse effects to the physician. Keep the environment as free from stress as possible. Visitors and hospital personnel should be screened for infectious disease and excluded from the patient's room. Continually assess the patient for signs of developing adrenal (addisonian) crisis, manifested by a sudden, severe drop in blood pressure; nausea and vomiting; an extremely high temperature; and cyanosis, progressing to vasomotor collapse and possibly death. The patient should carry an emergency kit at all times with 100 mg of IM hydrocortisone, syringes, and instructions for use. Teach the patient and significant others to give an IM injection in case replacement therapy cannot be taken orally. Also advise the patient that he or she will need extra medications to tolerate periods of physical or emotional stress (Lewis et al., 2007). Patient education is imperative for long-term compliance in the management of Addison's disease.

Nursing diagnoses and interventions for the patient with Addison's disease include but are not limited to the following:

Nursing Diagnoses	Nursing Interventions
Risk for infection, related to altered metabolic processes	Assess environment for stressors. Screen visitors and personnel for contagious disease. Monitor temperature routinely. Stress the importance of taking prescribed medications.

Continued

Table 51-3 Nursing Assessment of Patients with Cushing's Syndrome or Addison's Disease

AREA OF ASSESSMENT	CLINICAL MANIFESTATIONS IN CUSHING'S SYNDROME	CLINICAL MANIFESTATIONS IN ADDISON'S DISEASE
Cardiovascular	Mild to moderate hypertension	Postural hypotension, vertigo, syncope
Neurologic	Impaired memory and concentration, insomnia, irritability	Lethargy, headache
Musculoskeletal	Muscle weakness, muscle wasting in extremities, back and rib pain, kyphosis	Muscle weakness, fatigue, muscle aches, muscle wasting
Integumentary	Thin skin, red cheeks, acne, frequent petechiae and ecchymoses, increased body and facial hair, poor wound healing	Hyperpigmentation, decreased body hair
Self-care and self-concept	Tires easily; insomnia, malaise, negative feelings regarding changes in body	Tires easily; profound weakness, lack of interest in usual activities and relationships
Nutrition and fluid balance	Increased appetite, moderate weight gain, edema, buffalo hump, moon face, obesity of trunk, hyperglycemia; need for decreased salt intake, reduced calories and carbohydrate intake, increased potassium intake	Nausea and vomiting, fluid and electrolyte imbalance, dehydration, weight loss, hypoglycemia; need for increased salt and decreased potassium intake

Nursing Diagnoses	Nursing Interventions
Ineffective tissue perfusion, peripheral, related to electrolyte imbalance	Monitor vital signs and I&O. Have patient make position changes slowly; monitor for vertigo, visual changes.

Before discharge from the hospital, teach the patient the importance of adhering to the prescribed drug therapy; having regular medical checkups; and immediately reporting all illnesses, even a cold, to the physician. Emphasize that stress is one of the major precipitating factors in adrenal crisis, and encourage the patient to minimize stress through cognitive behavior therapy, relaxation therapy, biofeedback, and mental imagery. Other conditions to avoid include overexertion, diarrhea, infection, decreased intake of salt, exposure to cold, and surgery. It is critical that the patient wear a medical-alert bracelet and carry a wallet card stating that the patient has Addison's disease so that appropriate therapy be initiated in case of trauma, accident, or crisis.

Prognosis

With long-term steroid therapy, adequate medical care, and follow-up, this patient has a fair prognosis.

PHEOCHROMOCYTOMA

Etiology and Pathophysiology

A pheochromocytoma is a rare tumor of the adrenal medulla that causes excessive secretion of catecholamines (epinephrine and norepinephrine). These tumors occur most often in adults between 20 and 60 years of age and are almost always benign; only about 10% are malignant. The secretion of excessive catecholamines results in severe hypertension.

Clinical Manifestations

Pheochromocytoma results in severe hypertension because of sympathetic nervous system stimulation. Other classic clinical signs and symptoms include anxiety, severe headache, diaphoresis, tachycardia, and unexplained abdominal or chest pain (Lewis et al., 2007). Hypertensive crisis may occur, during which the blood pressure may fluctuate widely, sometimes as high as 300/175 mm Hg. Signs and symptoms may be triggered by an identifiable factor, such as overexertion or emotional trauma, or they may occur for no apparent reason. Extreme hypertension may result in stroke, kidney damage, and retinopathy. Cardiac damage may occur, resulting in heart failure.

Assessment

Subjective data during a hypertensive crisis include severe headache and palpitations. The patient may feel nervous, dizzy, and dyspneic and may experience paresthesias, nausea, and intolerance to heat. Anxiety is common, and the patient may have trouble sleeping. Question the patient about the occurrence of symptoms in relation to identifiable factors, such as excess stress or overexertion, and identify the coping methods used.

Collection of **objective data** includes frequent measurement of blood pressure and respiratory rate for increases and of pulse for tachycardia. The patient may have tremors, diaphoresis, dilated pupils, glycosuria, and hyperglycemia. Assess responses to prescribed medications.

Diagnostic Tests

The measurement of urinary metanephrines (catecholamine metabolites), usually performed as a 24-hour urine collection, is the simplest and most reliable test. Values are elevated in at least 90% of those with pheochromocytoma. Vanillylmandelic acid (VMA) may also be measured in a 24-hour urine sample. However, this test has more false negatives than that for urine metanephrines. Plasma catecholamines are also elevated. It is preferable to measure serum catecholamines during an "attack." CT scan and MRI of the adrenal glands may help in locating the tumor.

Medical Management

Treatment is usually the surgical removal of the tumor. Surgery is more commonly done via laparoscopic adrenalectomy than via open abdominal incision. Preoperatively, the patient may be given calcium channel blockers such as nicardipine (Cardene) or alpha-adrenergic blocking agents such as phentolamine mesylate (Regitine) or phenoxybenzamine hydrochloride (Dibenzyline) in an effort to control hypertension. Beta blockers (e.g., propranolol [Inderal]) to decrease tachycardia and other dysrhythmias are also used. Metyrosine (Demser) may be given to help inhibit catecholamine production, and the drug must be continued on a long-term basis if the tumor is inoperable.

Nursing Interventions and Patient Teaching

Postoperative care is carried out in the same manner as for any major abdominal surgery, with the following special concerns. If the patient has undergone adrenalectomy, large amounts of hydrocortisone will be given. Watch carefully for fluctuations in blood pressure caused by adrenal manipulation during surgery, with subsequent release of epinephrine and norepinephrine. These fluctuations may be severe and life threatening if cardiovascular collapse occurs. The patient should avoid excess stress and must be allowed adequate time to rest; give sedatives to ensure this. Keep a careful I&O record and administer IV solutions exactly as ordered. Vasopressors and corticosteroids may be given. The diet should be free from stimulants, such as coffee, tea, and soft drinks containing caffeine.

Nursing diagnoses and interventions for the patient with pheochromocytoma include but are not limited to the following:

Nursing Diagnoses	Nursing Interventions
Ineffective tissue perfusion, cardiopulmonary, renal, related to hypertension	Monitor blood pressure and pulse and record I&O. Eliminate smoking and caffeine-containing beverages.
Activity intolerance, related to hypertension	Assist with gradual position changes from lying to sitting or standing. Limit activity, as needed, to prevent increased hypertension.

Follow-up 24-hour urine tests (catecholamine metabolites or VMA) may determine when the levels have returned to normal. The patient is then pronounced cured and may resume normal activities. If the tumor is inoperable, the patient remains under lifelong medical supervision. Stress the importance of compliance with prescribed treatment. The patient should wear medical-alert jewelry and carry a wallet card. Teach the patient self-monitoring of blood pressure and when to call the physician if elevation occurs.

Prognosis

If undiagnosed and untreated, pheochromocytoma may lead to diabetes mellitus, cardiomyopathy, and death. The prognosis after successful removal of the causative tumor is good; for an inoperable tumor, the prognosis depends on adequate medical management of hypertension.

DISORDERS OF THE PANCREAS

DIABETES MELLITUS

Etiology

Diabetes mellitus (DM) (*diabetes,* "like a sieve or siphon"; *mellitus,* "sweet or related to honey") is a systemic metabolic disorder that involves improper metabolism of carbohydrates, fats, and proteins. This is a chronic multisystem disease related to a decrease or absolute lack of insulin production by the beta cells of the islets of Langerhans in the pancreas or by impaired insulin utilization, or both. In nondiabetic people the beta cells are stimulated by increased blood glucose levels; insulin secretion reaches peak levels about 30 minutes after meals and returns to normal in 2 to 3 hours. Between meals or during a period of fasting, insulin levels remain low, and the body uses its supply of stored glucose and amino acids to provide energy for the tissues. The beta cells of the pancreas continuously release insulin into the bloodstream in small amounts. A bolus of insulin is released after the intake of food. The average amount of insulin secreted by the beta cells of the pancreas in an adult is 40 to 50 units every 24 hours. The release of insulin in this systematic manner results in the body maintaining a normal blood sugar between 70 to 120 mg/dL (Lewis et al., 2007). In people with diabetes, the body's insulin supply is either absent or deficient, or target cells resist the action of insulin. There are several types of DM, but in each type, hyperglycemia is the principal clinical manifestation.

Although the exact cause of DM is unknown, a number of factors contribute to its development: genetic predisposition, viruses (such as coxsackievirus B, rubella, and mumps), the aging process, diet and lifestyle, and ethnicity. Obesity is believed to be a major factor. The T lymphocytes may play a role in the autoimmune destruction of the pancreatic insulin-producing cells.

Complications of diabetes are: blindness; nephropathy; amputation of a lower extremity; cardiovascular complications including heart disease, hypertension, and stroke (Lewis et al., 2007).

Types of Diabetes Mellitus

There are two main types of DM: **type 1** and **type 2.** Type 1 was formerly called juvenile diabetes, juvenile-onset diabetes, or insulin-dependent DM. Type 2 was formerly called adult-onset diabetes, maturity-onset diabetes, or non–insulin-dependent DM. Because this disease is becoming more common in children, and because some people with type 2 diabetes use insulin, these terms are no longer appropriate. About 80% to 90% of type 2 diabetes patients are overweight at the time of diagnosis. Other DM patients have conditions such as pancreatitis, genetic syndromes, malnutrition, chemical- or drug-induced disease, and pregnancy. Type 1 and type 2 diabetes have some distinct differences (Table 51-4). In type 1 an autoimmune disease (probably stimulated by a virus) eventually results in destruction of beta cells in the pancreatic islets and results in deficient insulin **production;** the patient retains normal sensitivity to insulin action. Within 5 years of diagnosis, all of the patient's beta cells have been destroyed and no insulin is produced. In type 2 the main problem seems to be an abnormal resistance to insulin **action.**

Regardless of the type of DM, all of these patients have impaired glucose tolerance. Only 5% to 10% of all people with diabetes have type 1. About 90% of people with DM in the United States have type 2, with a high incidence among blacks; Hispanic Americans; and Native Americans, especially members of the Pima tribe. The American Diabetes Association (ADA) estimates that as many as 20.8 million Americans (7% of the population) have DM, and 41 million more people have prediabetes.

Type 1 Diabetes Mellitus

Type 1 diabetes mellitus results from progressive destruction of beta-cell function in the pancreas as a result of an autoimmune process in a susceptible in-

Table 51-4 Comparison of Type 1 and Type 2 Diabetes Mellitus

FACTOR	TYPE 1	TYPE 2
Age at onset	Usually 30 years or younger, but can occur at any age	Usually age 35 years or older, but can occur at any age Incidence is increasing in children
Body weight	Normal or underweight	80% are overweight
Symptoms at onset	Sudden; polyphagia, polydipsia, polyuria, weight loss, weakness, fatigue; glycosuria, hyperglycemia; acidosis, progressing to DKA	Gradual; may be asymptomatic at onset; later, may develop signs and symptoms of type 1; others include slow wound healing, blurred vision, pruritus, boils or other skin infections; vaginal infections in women
Treatment	Diet, exercise, and insulin; may add subcutaneous insulin-enhancing drug (pramlintide [Symlin])	Diet and exercise; or diet, exercise, and oral hypoglycemic agents; or diet, exercise, oral hypoglycemic agents, and insulin during times of illness or stress; may add a subcutaneous insulin-enhancing agent such as exenatide (Byetta) or pramlintide
Incidence of complications	Frequent	Frequent
Psychosocial and sexual concerns	Irritability; disturbed body image; mood swings, depression; menstrual irregularities; decreased libido	Disturbed body image; amenorrhea; decreased libido; poor tolerance to stress

DKA, Diabetic ketoacidosis.

dividual. The pancreatic islets of Langerhans cell antibodies and insulin autoantibodies cause an 80% to 90% reduction in beta cells before hyperglycemia and symptoms occur. Type 1 DM is characterized by autoimmune beta-cell destruction, which is attributed to a genetic predisposition. Genetics plus infection of one or more viral agents and possibly chemical agents are believed to cause type 1 DM. It is not known whether these are the only factors involved. The onset and progression of hyperglycemic signs and symptoms are usually more rapid and acute in type 1 DM than in type 2. Type 1 diabetes may occur at any age, but signs and symptoms usually appear before 30 years of age. The patient is usually thin. The patient often has strongly positive urine ketone tests with hyperglycemia and depends on insulin therapy to prevent ketoacidosis and to sustain life (Lewis et al., 2007). Because they do not produce adequate amounts of endogenous (produced by the body) insulin, patients with type 1 DM must take regular injections of exogenous (from outside the body) insulin or they will die.

Type 2 Diabetes Mellitus

The pathophysiologic factors that have been identified in type 2 diabetes mellitus include (1) decreased tissue (e.g., fat, muscle) responsiveness to insulin as a result of a receptor or postreceptor defects; (2) overproduction of insulin early in the disease, but eventual decreased secretion of insulin from beta-cell exhaustion; and (3) abnormal hepatic glucose regulation. These factors result in what is often referred to as peripheral insulin resistance. This resistance stimulates increased insulin production as a compensatory response, which may also predispose the patient to weight gain. Weight loss for the obese patient with type 2 diabetes tends to reverse this problem. The patient with type 2 diabetes may benefit from oral antidiabetic agents, which increase insulin production, improve cell receptor binding, regulate hepatic glucose production, and delay carbohydrate absorption from the small intestine. Type 2 usually occurs in people who are older than 35 years of age, with about half of the people diagnosed being older than 55 at diagnosis. Eighty percent to 90% of these patients are overweight, with a familial history of diabetes. Patients have few classic symptoms. The patient is usually not prone to ketoacidosis except during periods of stress. Individuals with type 2 diabetes are not dependent on exogenous insulin for survival, but may require it for adequate control of hyperglycemia.

These patients can usually achieve good control of their disease by diet, exercise, and oral hypoglycemics, using insulin only when first diagnosed and during times of illness, surgery, or other periods when the body's insulin level is out of control (Lewis et al., 2007). Most newly diagnosed type 2 diabetic patients have had the disease for as long as 10 years without treatment and have therefore been at risk for serious complications before diagnosis.

Pathophysiology

In normal metabolism the end products of digestion (glucose, fatty acids and glycerol, and amino acids) are absorbed into the venous circulation and carried to the liver, where they may be either used immediately or stored for later use. The liver can change glycerol and fatty acids into glucose, and glucose into triglycerides, as needed. Fatty acids may also be changed into ketone bodies (normal metabolic products, such as β-hydroxybutyric acid and aminoacetic acid, from which acetone may arise spontaneously), which serve as fuel for the muscles and as an energy source for the brain. Glucose is stored in the form of glycogen in the liver. Free glucose in the bloodstream can always be used by the brain and kidney because insulin is not needed for glucose molecules to enter the brain cells or the glomeruli. But insulin must be present for muscle cells and other body cells to utilize glucose. Glycogen can be changed back into glucose as needed by the body for energy. In the patient with diabetes, lack of proper amounts of insulin, or its inadequate utilization, impairs the use of glucose by the body. Thus the excess glucose accumulates in the bloodstream, and **hyperglycemia** (greater than normal amounts of glucose in the blood) exists.

To rid the body of this abnormal amount of glucose, the kidneys excrete it in the urine. This is called **glycosuria** (abnormal presence of a sugar, especially glucose, in the urine), a condition that necessitates an extra amount of water for proper dilution of the urine. The patient thus develops **polyuria** (excretion of an abnormally large quantity of urine) and also **polydipsia** (excessive thirst). Often the patient is unable to drink enough fluid to compensate for polyuria and may become dehydrated. Even though excess glucose is available in the bloodstream, the body tissues cannot utilize it without the help of insulin. Thus the cells are not properly nourished, and **polyphagia** (eating to the point of gluttony) develops. In spite of increased food intake, metabolism remains faulty, and the patient loses weight. Because carbohydrates cannot be utilized properly, proteins and fats are broken down and ketone bodies are used excessively for heat and energy. Because ketone bodies are acid substances, the patient may develop acidosis. Diabetic **ketoacidosis** (DKA) (acidosis accompanied by an accumulation of ketones in the blood), formerly called **diabetic coma,** may develop, and the patient could die. DKA is a severe metabolic disturbance caused by an acute insulin deficiency, decreased peripheral glucose utilization, and increased fat mobilization and ketogenesis.

Clinical Manifestations

The hallmark symptoms of type 1 DM include the three classic "polys": polyuria, polydipsia, and polyphagia. As ketone bodies accumulate in the bloodstream, imbalances of sodium, potassium, and bicarbonate result. People with type 2 DM, most of whom are more than 35 years of age, experience different signs and symptoms. The patient may be asymptomatic in the early stages of the disease, but later may complain of symptoms associated with type 1, plus a number of others. These patients may not seek medical care until a severe complication such as kidney involvement, retinopathy, impotence, neuropathy, or gangrene occurs.

Assessment

Subjective data include hunger, thirst, and nausea. In addition to frequent urination of large amounts, the patient may complain of nocturia, weakness, and fatigue. The patient may have blurred vision, the appearance of halos around lights, and headache. Symptoms such as cold extremities, cramping pain in the calves and feet during exercise or walking, decreased sensation to pain and temperature in the feet, and numbness and tingling of the lower extremities may occur. Symptoms of delayed stomach emptying such as nausea, vomiting, and early satiety (feeling of being full after eating) may develop. Male patients may become impotent. The patient may verbalize negative feelings about his or her body and the ability to cope with the illness. Assess coping methods and knowledge about the disease process. Misunderstandings and lack of interest may result in inadequate skills—such as diet planning, injections, and exercise programs—to manage the necessary diabetic lifestyle. Assess the patient's understanding of the importance of adhering to prescribed medical treatment and obtaining adequate follow-up.

Collection of **objective data** includes assessment of the skin, since slow wound healing, furuncles, carbuncles, and ulcerations are common. Women with DM may experience frequent urinary tract and vaginal infections, and vaginal discharge is often bothersome. In type 1 patients, weight loss and muscle wasting may be seen, but many type 2 patients remain obese. The skin on the lower extremities may appear shiny and thin, with less hair present. The legs and feet may feel cold to the touch, and there may be ulcerated areas. Gangrene of the toes is a dreaded sign. Assess the patient's ability to perform blood glucose testing and proper injection of insulin.

Diagnostic Tests

Diagnosis of DM is made on the basis of clinical manifestations, plus the patient's history and laboratory findings. The patient with random blood glucose greater than 200 mg/dL, a fasting plasma glucose level greater than 126 mg/dL, or a glucose 2-hour postload (75 g anhydrous) level greater than 200 mg/dL should be further evaluated. Blood tests commonly performed include those in Box 51-2.

The ADA recommends self-monitoring of blood glucose (SMBG) instead of urine testing in any patient with DM. This is accomplished in a number of ways. Blood from a fingerstick may be placed on a reagent strip and compared with a color chart, or it may be placed into a reflectance meter. Another type of meter uses a glucose sensor, and test strips are not used; instead, a drop of blood is placed directly into the machine. SMBG is the monitoring tool of choice because it provides an accurate picture of current blood glucose levels (Figure 51-12).

The frequency of monitoring depends on the glycemic goals the patient and health care provider set and the intensity of the treatment regimen. The patient receiving two or more injections of insulin per day may want to test before meals and at bedtime every day. If

Box 51-2 Diagnostic Tests for Diabetes Mellitus

- **Fasting blood glucose (FBG):** After an 8-hour fast, blood is drawn. Normal is 60 to 110 mg/dL of venous blood; 126 mg/dL or greater is considered abnormal.
- **Oral glucose tolerance test (OGTT):** When patient shows overt signs and symptoms of hyperglycemia, polyuria, polydipsia, and polyphagia, together with FBG levels of 126 mg/dL or greater, further OGTTs are usually not warranted. However, whenever OGTTs are used, the accuracy depends on adequate patient preparation and attention to the many factors that may influence the outcome of such tests.
- **Serum insulin:** Absent in type 1 diabetes mellitus (DM); normal to high in type 2 DM.
- **Postprandial (after a meal) blood glucose (PPBG):** Give a fasting patient a measured amount of carbohydrate solution orally, or have the patient eat a measured amount of foods containing carbohydrates, fats, and proteins. Draw a blood sample 2 hours after completion of the meal. Elevated plasma glucose over 160 mg/dL may indicate the presence of DM.
- **Patient self-monitoring of blood glucose (SMBG):** A blood sample is obtained by the fingerstick method, by either the patient or the nurse, and tested using a blood glucose-monitoring device.
- **Glycosylated hemoglobin (HbA_{lc}):** This blood test measures the amount of glucose that has become incorporated into the hemoglobin within an erythrocyte; these levels are reported as a percentage of the total hemoglobin. Because glycosylation occurs constantly during the 120-day life span of the erythrocyte, this test reveals the effectiveness of diabetes therapy for the preceding 8 to 12 weeks. Glycosylated hemoglobin levels remain more stable than plasma glucose levels and are evaluated by a venipuncture every 6 to 8 weeks. Normal HbA_{lc} is approximately 4% to 6% of the total. There is an urgent need to reduce HbA_{lc} values to below 7% to reduce complications. A result greater than 8% represents an average blood glucose level of approximately 200 mg/dL and signals a need for changes in treatment.
- **C-peptide test:** The production of insulin by the beta cells of the pancreas begins with proinsulin with an A chain of amino acids and a B chain of amino acids with a connecting peptide or C-peptide. The C-peptide allows the A and B proinsulin to fold and cleave together, creating the structure of insulin. After the connection has been made, the fusion occurs, creating insulin and a C-peptide by-product. C-peptide then gets secreted into the bloodstream by the pancreas along with insulin. The C-peptide level may be measured in a patient with type 2 DM to see if any insulin is being produced by the body. A newly diagnosed diabetic patient will often use this test to determine whether he or she has type 1 or type 2 DM. Normal values are 0.5 to 2 ng/mL. The patient with type 1 diabetes is unable to produce insulin and therefore has decreased levels of C-peptide; C-peptide levels in type 2 diabetic patients are normal or higher than normal. In type 2 diabetics, the problem seems to be an abnormal resistance to insulin action.

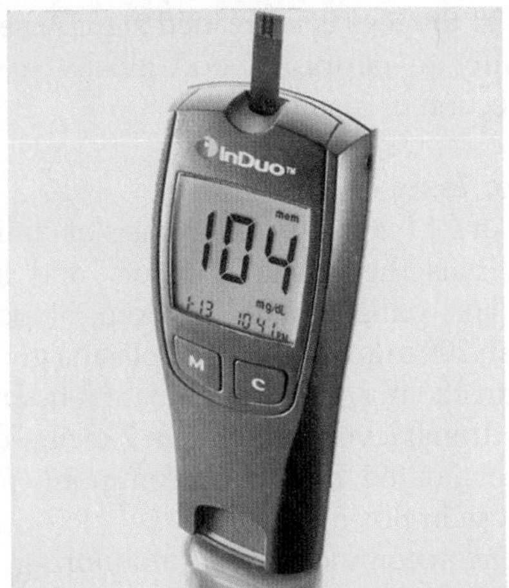

FIGURE 51-12 Glucose sensor for self-monitoring of blood glucose.

glycemic control is relatively stable, the patient may elect to test two or more times a day on certain days of the week. Testing is usually done before meals, but it can be done any time the patient needs to know the way a factor, such as stress, is affecting the blood glucose levels. The frequency of recording SMBG results to guide therapy decision should be jointly determined by the health care provider and the patient.

The technology used for SMBG changes rapidly, with newer and more convenient systems being introduced every year. Blood glucose monitoring technology using a noninvasive spectroscopy—or a laser light on a skin surface such as the forearm or space between finger and thumb—is being researched for possible use in the future. Implantable sensors for continuous glucose monitoring are also being considered in research trials.

Urine testing for ketonuria is a valuable aid in determining the advent of DKA and is recommended for every patient with type 1 diabetes when the patient is experiencing hyperglycemia or acute illness. The amount of acetone is represented by a color change in shades of pink to purple. Acetone testing products include Ketostix and Acetest tablets.

Medical Management

Medical treatment for DM, no matter what type, consists mainly of education, monitoring, meal planning, medication, and exercise. The overall goal is to assist people with diabetes in making changes in nutrition and exercise habits leading to improved metabolic control. Additional goals include the following:

- Maintenance of as near-normal blood glucose levels as possible by balancing food intake with insulin or oral glucose-lowering medications and activity levels.
- Achievement of optimal serum lipid levels.
- Provision of adequate calories for maintaining or attaining reasonable weight for adults and normal growth and development rates for children and adolescents; and for meeting increased metabolic needs during pregnancy, lactation, and recovery from illnesses. Reasonable weight is de-

fined as the weight the patient and health care provider decide is achievable and maintainable in both the short term and the long term. This may not be the same as the usually defined desirable or ideal body weight.
- Prevention and treatment of acute complications such as hypoglycemia and long-term complications such as renal disease, neuropathy, hypertension, and cardiovascular disease.
- Improvement of overall health through optimal nutrition. The U.S. Department of Agriculture's MyPyramid food planning tool (www.mypyramid.gov) summarizes nutritional guidelines and nutrient needs for all healthy Americans and can be used by the patient with diabetes.

It is hoped that the patient will assume a large part of the responsibility for self-care, with emphasis on optimal wellness instead of illness. Since 1921, when Charles Best and Frederick Banting first isolated insulin, medical science has made many dramatic strides in the care of the patient with diabetes, but physicians depend on the help obtained from other members of the health care team, especially nurses. Every newly diagnosed patient must undergo an intensive and extensive education program to learn proper diet, medication routines, SMBG, and the role of exercise. The importance of the nurse as a teacher cannot be overemphasized (see Evidence-Based Practice box).

Diet

Nutritional therapy for the patient with diabetes is aimed at helping to achieve a normal blood glucose level of less than 126 mg/dL and at attaining or maintaining a reasonable body weight, while ensuring proper growth and body maintenance. Nutritional therapy is the cornerstone of care for the person with diabetes. A nutritionally adequate meal plan with a reduction of total fat, especially saturated fat, is important. Monitoring of blood glucose levels, glycosylated hemoglobin, and lipids is essential. Enlist the services of a dietitian for each newly diagnosed diabetic. The menu must be individualized, taking into consideration the patient's age, weight, activity level, lifestyle, ethnic background, and food preferences. Assess the ability to choose and pay for groceries, prepare food, and properly store leftovers to ensure the patient can follow dietary instructions after discharge. If the patient is living with family, educate the person who plans and prepares the meals along with the patient, and teach this person how to accommodate the patient's dietary needs in the family menus. The physician and dietitian decide the proper amounts of each nutrient in the dietary prescription. Dietary treatment, also called **medical nutrition therapy for diabetes,** involves individualized meal plans. Diets are based on ADA recommendations, and patients may obtain additional information and menus from that organization at no cost.

Quantitative diabetic diets, following the food choices and number of servings recommended by the MyPyramid food planning tool, include 45% to 50% of total kilocalories from carbohydrates, 10% to 20% of total kilocalories from proteins, and no more than 30% of total kilocalories from fats. Rigid rules on carbohydrates have softened. Now the emphasis is on the total amount of carbohydrates consumed, rather than on the type. Once it was believed that a simple carbohydrate (sugar) would drive up blood glucose levels, so patients were advised to consume only complex carbohydrates. This has proven inaccurate, however, as: (1) some complex carbohydrates (rice, potatoes, and bread) produce a glycemic response similar to that caused by sucrose (table sugar), and (2) milk and fruit have less effect on blood glucose than most starches. As a result, sugars and complex carbohydrates are counted together as total carbohydrates.

Different carbohydrate foods affect the blood glucose level in different ways; this varying effect is termed the **glycemic index.** So emphasis may be placed not only on the amount of carbohydrate eaten but also on the glycemic index of those foods.

Evidence-Based Practice: Changes in Diabetes Self-Care Behaviors

Evidence Summary

Diabetes self-management is critical, complex, and demanding. In a comparison between diabetes Treatment as Usual (TAU) with the Pathways to Change (PTC) intervention, the PTC group received stage-matched personalized assessment reports, self-help manuals, and newsletters. In addition, individual phone counseling helped determine readiness for self-monitoring of blood glucose (SMBG), healthy eating, and/or smoking cessation. Those in the PTC group were more likely to move into the action stages of those self-care behaviors, such as performing SMBG as instructed, eating more fruits and vegetables, and quitting smoking in order to manage their diabetes.

Application to Nursing Practice

As health care professionals, we need to help patients move through the stages of behavior change. It is important to assess and determine the patient's readiness for change and target messages appropriately. When a patient is not even beginning to think about eating more fruits and vegetables in his or her diet, it is unrealistic to tell the patient to eat at least five fruits and vegetables every day. It would be more appropriate to inform the patient why this is important, have the patient identify a favorite fruit or vegetable, and give one or two simple suggestions as to how to incorporate the fruits or vegetables into his or her diet. By helping patients through the change process, we can reduce long-term complications of diabetes.

Reference

Jones, H., Edwards, L., Vallis, T.M., et al. (2003). Changes in diabetes self-care behaviors make a difference in glycemic control: the Diabetes Stages of Change (DiSC) study, *Diabetes Care*, 26(3):732.

From Potter, P.A., & Perry, A.G. (2009). *Fundamentals of nursing: concepts, process, and practice.* (7th ed.). St. Louis: Mosby.

The **qualitative** diet is unmeasured and more unrestricted, stressing moderation when selecting foods from the MyPyramid food planning tool and reducing the use of simple carbohydrates, saturated fats, and alcohol. This diet may be used for the patient whose blood glucose levels are not extremely high, for the pediatric patient, or for the patient who does not adhere to the ADA diet.

Insulin-dependent patients are usually given midafternoon and bedtime snacks in addition to their regular three meals a day. It is important to evenly distribute food intake throughout the day, taking insulin dosage and exercise into consideration. The patient who plans to engage in strenuous exercise should eat more food, since exercise increases the absorption rate of insulin, thereby enabling muscles to use glucose more effectively.

Exercise

The patient with diabetes should exercise regularly. The physician helps determine the best type of exercise for each patient. Exercise is beneficial not only because it aids in promoting proper utilization of glucose, but also because it is important to the overall functioning of the cardiovascular system and increases the patient's feeling of well-being. Of all the therapies available for treating type 2 diabetes, exercise is probably the least expensive and most cost effective. Exercise can reduce insulin resistance and increase glucose uptake for as long as 72 hours; it also reduces blood pressure and lipid levels. However, it can carry some risks, including hypoglycemia. Patients older than age 40 should have a complete physical examination before beginning a rigorous exercise program. Like medications, exercise can be adjusted to improve blood glucose control. With exercise, motivation is more important than facts and information.

Stress of Acute Illness and Surgery

Both emotional and physical stress can increase the blood glucose level and result in hyperglycemia. However, it is impossible to avoid stress in life situations such as death in the family, job, interviews, and final examinations. These situations may require extra insulin to avoid hyperglycemia.

Common stress-evoking situations include acute illness, pregnancy, and the controlled stress of surgery. The patient with diabetes who has a minor illness such as a cold or the flu should continue drug therapy and food intake. A carbohydrate liquid substitution such as regular soft drinks, gelatin dessert, or beverages such as Gatorade may be necessary. The patient should understand that food intake is important during this time because the body requires extra energy to deal with the stress of the illness.

Blood glucose monitoring should be done every 1 to 2 hours by either the patient or a person who can assume responsibility for care during the illness. Urinary output and the presence and degree of ketonuria should be monitored, particularly when fever is present. Increase fluid intake to prevent dehydration, with a minimum of 4 ounces per hour for an adult.

Instruct the patient to contact the health care provider when the blood glucose level exceeds 250 mg/dL; in such cases, fever, ketonuria, and nausea and vomiting may occur. The health care provider should supervise the necessary adjustments in the treatment regimen during times of stress. Eventually the well-informed patient will be able to make most adjustments independently on the basis of experience.

Surgery is controlled stress, and adjustments in the diabetes regimen can be planned to ensure glycemic control. The patient is given IV fluids and insulin immediately before, during, and after surgery when there is no oral intake. The type 2 diabetic patient receiving oral antidiabetic medications usually has the drugs discontinued 48 hours before surgery and is treated with insulin during the surgical period. Explain to the patient that this is a temporary measure, not a worsening of diabetes.

Medications

Insulin and oral hypoglycemic drugs are the drugs of choice for patients with diabetes. Insulin administration is necessary for all patients with type 1 and patients with type 2 whose condition cannot be controlled by diet, exercise, or hypoglycemic medications alone.

Insulin

Today only biosynthetic insulin is used. In the past, insulin was obtained from the pancreas of cows and pigs. Biosynthetic insulin is produced by genetically altering common bacteria or yeast using deoxyribonucleic acid (DNA) technology. This insulin exhibits chemical and biologic properties identical to those of human insulin produced by human B cells in the pancreas (Figure 51-13). Insulin is a hormone and is most commonly absorbed into the patient's bloodstream. Insulin is given subcutaneously, although IV administration of regular insulin can be done when immediate onset of action is desired. IV regular insulin is mixed in normal saline solution. The amount of solution depends on the institution's protocol.

Insulins differ in regard to onset, peak, action, and duration (Table 51-5). The specific preparation of each

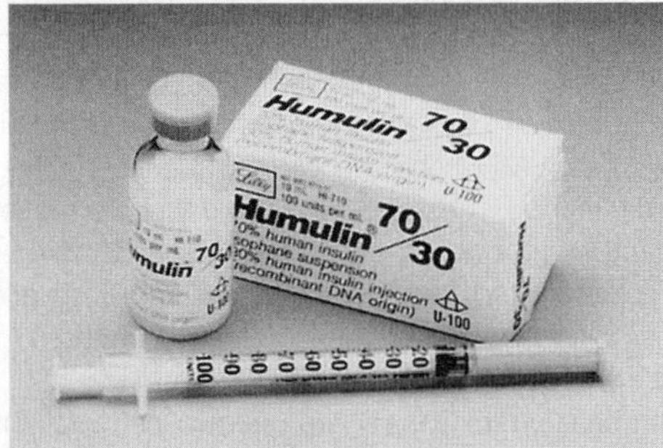

FIGURE 51-13 U/100 insulin and disposable U/100 insulin syringe.

Table 51-5 **Types of Insulin**

TYPE OF INSULIN	SOURCE AND COLOR	INJECTION TIME (BEFORE MEAL)	RISK TIME FOR HYPOGLYCEMIC REACTION	ACTION	START OF ACTION	PEAK ACTION	DURATION
RAPID OR SHORT ACTING							
Lispro (Humalog)	Human Clear	5-15 min	No meal within 30 min	Rapid	15-30 min	1-2 hr	3-4 hr
Aspart (NovoLog)	Human Clear	5-15 min	No meal within 30 min	Rapid	15-30 min	1-3 hr	3-5 hr
Glulisine (Apidra)	Human Clear	5-15 min	No meal within 30 min	Rapid	15-30 min	1-3 hr	3-5 hr
Regular Humulin R Novolin R ReliOn R	Human Clear	30 min	Delayed meal or 3-4 hr after injection	Short	30-60 min	2-4 hr	6-8 hr
MIXED							
Novolog Mix 70/30 (neutral protamine aspart and aspart)	Human Cloudy	15 min	No meal within 30 min	Rapid and intermediate	15-30 min	2-10 hr	12-16 hr
Humalog Mix 75/25 (neutral protamine lispro and lispro)	Human Cloudy	15 min	No meal within 30 min	Rapid and intermediate	15-30 min	2-10 hr	12-16 hr
NPH/regular Mix 70/30 Humulin Mix 70/30	Human Cloudy	30-60 min	Delayed meal or 3-4 hr after injection	Short and intermediate	30-60 min	6-12 hr	18-24 hr
Novolin Mix 70/30	Human Cloudy	30-60 min	Delayed meal or 3-4 hr after injection	Short and intermediate	30-60 min	6-12 hr	18-24 hr
ReliOn N Mix 70/30	Human Cloudy		Delayed meal or 3-4 hr after injection	Short and intermediate	30-60 min	6-12 hr	18-24 hr
NPH/Regular Mix 50/50	Human Cloudy	30-60 min	Delayed meal or 3-4 hr after injection	Short and intermediate	30-60 min	6-12 hr	18-24 hr
Humulin Mix 50/50	Human Cloudy	30-60 min	Delayed meal or 3-4 hr after injection	Short and intermediate	30-60 min	6-12 hr	18-24 hr
INTERMEDIATE ACTING							
NPH (Humulin N, Novolin N, ReliOn N)	Human Milky when mixed	30 min	4-6 hr after injection	Intermediate acting	2-4 hr	6-10 hr	12-16 hr
Lente	Human Milky when mixed	30 min	3-6 hr after injection	Intermediate acting	1-3 hr	6-12 hr	18-26 hr

From Lewis, S.M., et al. (2007). *Medical-surgical nursing: assessment and management of clinical problems.* (7th ed.). St. Louis: Mosby.

Continued

Table 51-5 **Types of Insulin—cont'd**

TYPE OF INSULIN	SOURCE AND COLOR	INJECTION TIME (BEFORE MEAL)	RISK TIME FOR HYPOGLYCEMIC REACTION	ACTION	START OF ACTION	PEAK ACTION	DURATION
LONG ACTING							
Glargine (Lantus) Detemir (Levemir)	Synthetic Clear; do not mix with others	Usually take at 9 PM, once daily*	Starting dose should be 20% less than total daily dose of NPH	Long lasting	1-2 hr	No pronounced peak	24 hr†
Ultralente	Human Milky when mixed	30 min	6 hr after injection	Long lasting	4-6 hr	18 hr	24 hr

Proper timing of insulin and eating if on regular or 70/30 in relationship with blood glucose	Glucose	Primarily Covers
<50 mg/dL = when mealtime is complete	AM: Rapid and short acting	Breakfast to lunch
50-70 mg/dL = at mealtime	AM: NPH or Lente	Lunch to evening meal
70-120 mg/dL = 15 min before mealtime	Noon: Rapid and short	Lunch to midafternoon
120-180 mg/dL = 30 min before meal	PM: Rapid and short acting	Evening meal to bedtime
>180 mg/dL = 45 min before meal	PM: NPH and Lente	Late evening to early morning
	Bedtime: NPH or Lente	Midnight to following morning
	Bedtime: glargine or detemir or Ultralente	Provides continuous coverage

*May take at other times.
†Type 1, once or twice daily; type 2, once daily.

type of insulin is matched with the patient's diet and activity. By adding zinc, acetate buffers, and protamine to insulin in various ways, the onset of activity, peak, and duration times can be manipulated. Different combinations of these insulins can be used to tailor treatment to the patient's specific pattern of blood glucose levels.

Formulas are classified as rapid acting (insulin lispro [Humalog], insulin aspart [NovoLog], insulin glulisine [Apidra]), short acting (regular insulin [Humulin R, Novolin R, ReliOn R]), intermediate acting (NPH insulin [Humulin N, Novolin N, and ReliOn N]), and long acting (glargine [Lantus], detemir [Levemir]). Glargine is used once a day at bedtime and works around the clock for 24 hours. It is a "peakless" insulin that provides a continuous insulin level similar to the slow, steady (basal) secretions of insulin from a normal pancreas. Glargine must not be mixed in the same syringe with other insulins because it will interfere with their action (Figure 51-14).

If hyperglycemia occurs, elevated blood glucose is covered with sliding-scale regular insulin. Premixed combinations are 70/30 (70% NPH and 30% regular) (see Figure 51-13) and 50/50 (50% NPH and 50% regular). Two recent combinations are available: 75/25 (75% lispro protamine [NPH] and 25% lispro [Humalog] [rapid acting], called Humalog mix 75/25) and 70/30 aspart protamine (70% protamine [NPH] and 30% aspart [rapid acting], called Novolog mix 70/30). The premixed insulins are most helpful for those who have stable insulin needs. Timing of insulin action to match food intake can be a challenge, and it tends to be more difficult for people with type 1 diabetes because their only source of insulin is by injection. Regular insulin is prescribed when a rapid onset of glucose-lowering action is needed, such as before meals and during periods of acute illness, surgery, or stress. Only regular insulin can be administered intravenously; thus it is used in emergencies.

A human insulin formula called insulin lispro was approved in June 1996 by the U.S. Food and Drug Administration. Insulin lispro begins to take effect in less than half the time of regular, fast-acting insulin. The products previously on the market must be taken subcutaneously 30 to 60 minutes before a meal; the new formula can be injected 15 minutes before a meal. This timing more closely mimics the body's own hormone activity. Lispro brings the most benefit to people with type 1 diabetes who take short-acting insulin before meals combined with a longer-acting insulin once or twice a day. Two additional rapid-acting insulins, aspart (Novolog) and glulisine (Apidra) with similar onset of action as lispro (Humulog) are also now available. Insulins are commonly used in combination to mimic the normal pancreatic insulin secretion.

When giving insulin, be careful to inject into the **subcutaneous tissue** (space between the fat and muscle layers) only, avoiding depositing the medication directly into the fat or muscle. Insulin administration requires the appropriate syringe. Most commercial insulin is available as U/100, indicating that each milliliter contains 100 units of insulin. U/100 insulin must be used with a U/100-marked syringe. For a user tak-

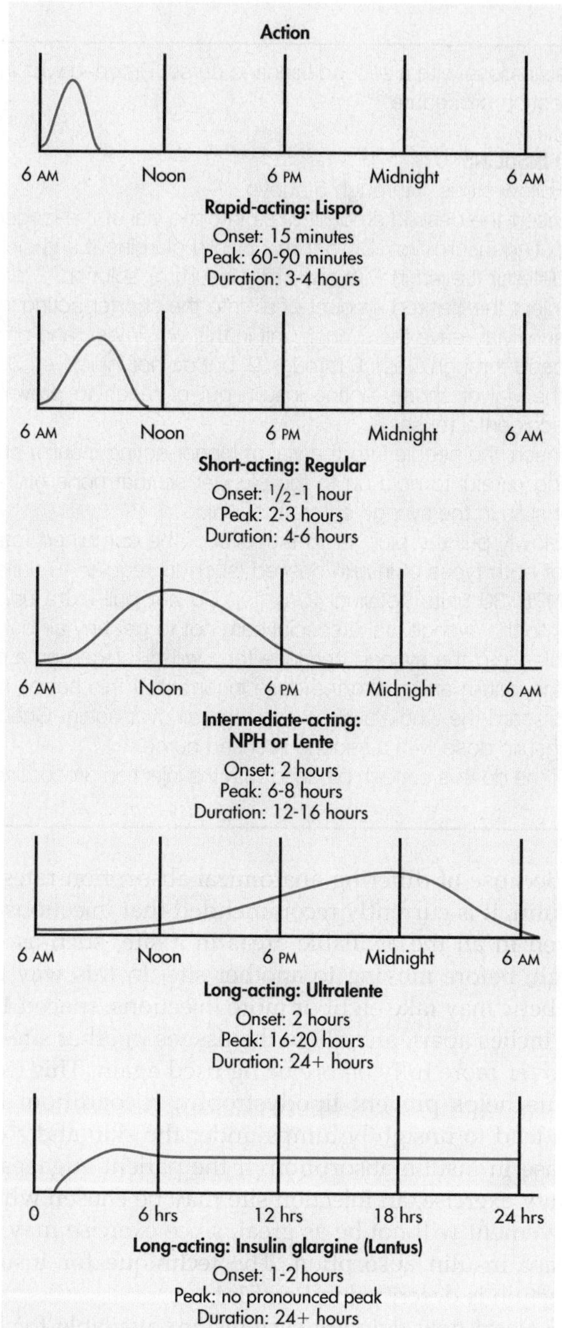

FIGURE 51-14 Commercially available insulin preparations, including onset, peak, and duration of action.

ing smaller doses of insulin, insulin syringes marked for 25, 30, or 50 units are available for use with U/100 syringes. One important distinction is that the 100-unit syringe is marked in 2-unit increments, whereas the 50- and 30-unit syringes are marked in 1-unit increments. Be certain that the patient gets the correct size of syringe and does not switch syringes, thus avoiding serious dosing errors. The Joint Commission now recommends using **units** instead of the abbreviation U on medication orders and medication administration records to decrease errors in dosing.

Insulin pens are another popular method of administering insulin. The pen serves the same function as a needle and syringe but is compact and portable, thus making it more convenient. Insulin pens are handy in that they contain all the necessary parts in one piece, but the user must also attach a needle and discard it after each use (Figure 51-15).

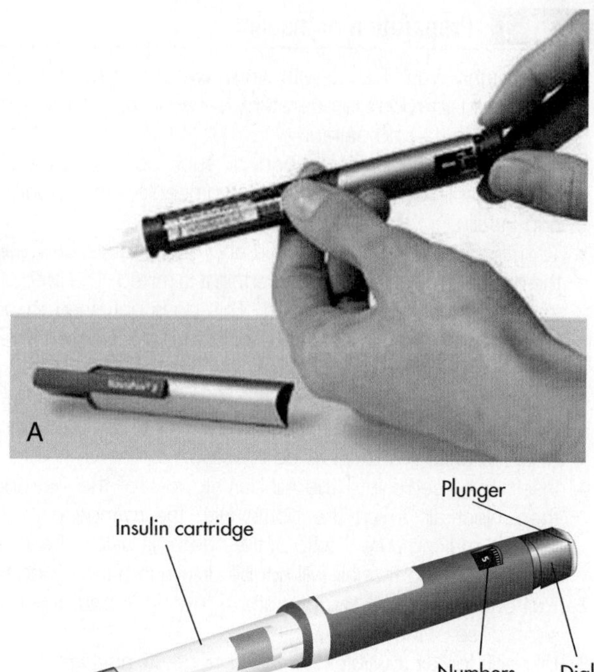

FIGURE 51-15 A NovoPen insulin pen.

Needles are very fine, usually 25 to 32 gauge, to be as atraumatic to the tissue as possible. Disposable needles and syringes are now used in the hospital and the home. An open bottle of insulin currently being used does not have to be refrigerated. In fact, it is now believed that insulin should be administered at room temperature, not straight from the refrigerator, to help prevent insulin **lipodystrophy** (abnormality in the metabolism or deposition of fats; insulin lipodystrophy is the loss of local fat deposits). Extra bottles are stored in the refrigerator. Box 51-3 offers guidelines for preparation of a dose of insulin, one or two types at a time.

Patients who self-inject insulin at home may want to have a family member oversee the procedure. Nurses administering insulin injections must always have another licensed person check and document the dose drawn up in the syringe to prevent medication errors. The patient with diabetes should ideally be taught self-injection technique before discharge from the hospital. However, some patients are unable to perform this because of physical problems, intellectual incapacity, visual disturbances, or age. In these cases, family members or others have to administer the injections. Before discharge, either the patient or the significant other, or both, must display the ability to correctly draw up and inject insulin.

In a newly diagnosed patient, regular or rapid-acting insulin may be injected before each meal. After

Box 51-3 Preparation of Insulin

1. Thoroughly wash hands with warm water and soap. Bring the insulin to room temperature because an injection of cold insulin can be painful.
2. Assemble all equipment needed, such as properly calibrated insulin syringe with a prefitted needle, prep sponge, and insulin.
3. Turn the insulin vial onto its side and gently rotate between the hands several times to be certain it is mixed. The precipitate should be evenly blended. This does not need to be done with regular insulin because it has no precipitate. Never shake insulin vigorously because this creates air bubbles.
4. Clean the rubber stopper on the vial with a prep sponge.
5. Remove the needle cover and draw in the same amount of air as units of insulin to be injected.
6. Insert the needle into the rubber stopper of the vial and then inject air. Invert the bottle with the syringe unit attached, making sure the tip of the needle is below the level of the insulin so that air will not be drawn into the syringe.
7. Pull back slowly on the plunger, a few units past the desired dose of insulin.
8. Inspect for air bubbles in the syringe; if any are seen, gently tap the barrel until they rise to the top, then push back into the vial with plunger to the level of the desired dose of insulin.
9. Holding on to the barrel and plunger, remove the syringe unit and put the needle cover back on. **Always** check insulin dose with a second licensed nurse. Proceed with injection procedure.

TWO INSULINS

1. Follow steps 1 through 5 above.
2. Insert the desired amount of air into the vial of the longer-acting insulin first. Do not mix insulin glargine (Lantus) or detemir (Levemir) with any other insulin or solution.
3. Inject the desired amount of air into the shorter-acting insulin vial; leave the syringe unit in this vial; invert, and proceed through steps 6 through 9, but do not inject yet. Set the vial of shorter-acting insulin out of reach to prevent accidental reuse.
4. Insert the needle into the vial of longer-acting insulin, being careful to hold on to the plunger so that none of the insulin in the syringe enters that vial.
5. Slowly pull the plunger to the level of the combined total of both types of insulin desired (such as regular 10 units, NPH 30 units, totaling 40 units). Do not pull extra units into the syringe. Take special care not to get any air bubbles into the syringe because they will displace some of the insulin and make the dose incorrect. If this happens, discard the whole syringe and start all over again. Check insulin dose with a second licensed nurse.
6. If the dose is correct, proceed with the injection procedure.

reasonable control of hyperglycemia is achieved, the dosage schedule may be changed to once a day, in the morning before breakfast, with the type of insulin being intermediate or long acting (see Figure 51-14 and Table 51-5 for types of insulin). Sometimes patients with DM take two divided doses of insulin, one before breakfast and one before the evening meal. Be alert for signs of hypoglycemia (a less than normal amount of glucose in the blood, usually caused by administration of too much insulin, excessive secretion of insulin by the islet cells of the pancreas, or dietary deficiency) at the peak of action of whatever type of insulin the patient is taking. Instruct the patient to notify a member of the nursing staff if any of the following signs of hypoglycemic (insulin) reaction occur: faintness, sudden weakness, excessive perspiration, irritability, hunger, palpitations, trembling, or drowsiness.

After appropriate blood glucose testing, the patient chooses an injection site. The subcutaneous pocket is the desired layer into which insulin should be injected. Insulin should not be injected into the muscle, because it enters the bloodstream too quickly and could cause hypoglycemia. Site selection is crucial, as is site rotation. The patient may choose sites at the abdomen (except for 2 inches [5 cm] around the navel), the upper arms, the anterior or lateral aspects of the thighs, and the hips or buttocks. The abdomen provides the fastest, least variable absorption, followed by the arms, thighs, and buttocks. Patients may find it easier to keep track of their injection sites by recording each injection on a numbered chart (Figure 51-16).

Because of differing anatomical absorption rates of insulin, it is currently recommended that injections be given in all the available areas in a site, such as the thigh, before moving to another site. In this way the diabetic may take eight or more injections, spaced 1 to 1½ inches apart, and allow the tissues in other sites to recover more fully before being used again. This technique helps prevent lipodystrophy, a condition that can lead to unsightly lumps under the skin and a decrease in insulin absorption. If the patient engages in heavy exercise, an injection site may be chosen where movement will not be as great, since exercise may increase insulin absorption. The technique for insulin injection is described in Box 51-4.

Several new delivery systems are available for patients who find injections emotionally and physically uncomfortable. These include automatic injectors, the jet stream (needleless) injector, the Insuflon indwelling insulin delivery service, and the button infuser.

Another method of insulin administration is continuous subcutaneous insulin infusion using the external infusion pump (Figure 51-17). This small, battery-powered computerized device is worn on the user's body, usually in a pocket or on a belt. It is attached to a thin tube with a needle on the end, which is inserted into the subcutaneous tissue. A continuous, or basal, rate of rapid- or short-acting regular insulin delivery can be programmed, with bolus doses administered as needed. The insulin pump is as close a substitute as available to a healthy, working pancreas. It mimics the pancreas by releasing small amounts of rapid-acting

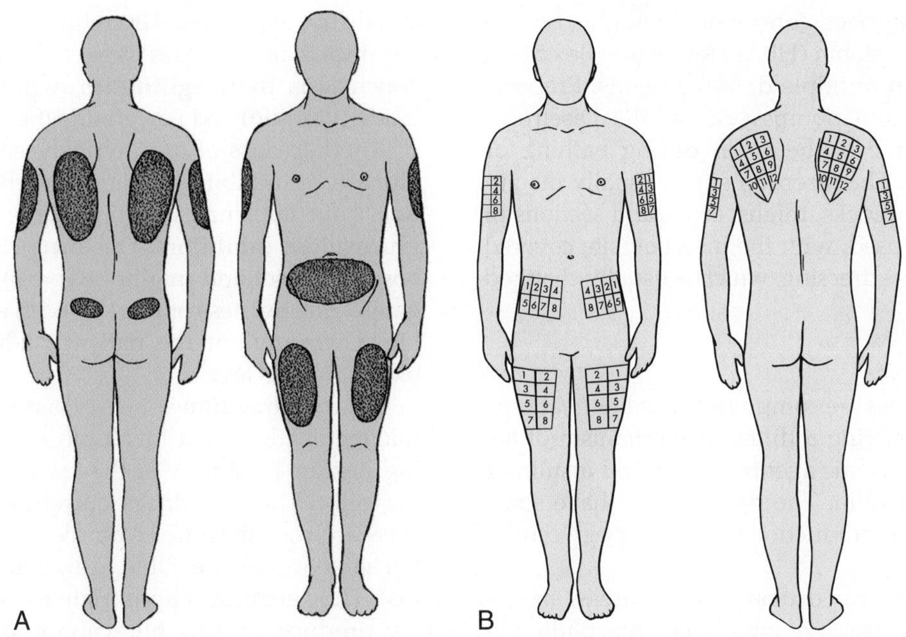

FIGURE 51-16 **A,** Rotation of sites for insulin injections. **B,** Injection diagram to track rotation of injection sites.

Box 51-4 Technique for Insulin Injection

1. Follow the steps in Box 51-3 to prepare the insulin dose.
2. Don disposable gloves.
3. Clean the injection site with a prep swab, using a circular motion. Allow the alcohol to dry. Place the swab between the last two fingers of the hand not used to inject the insulin.
4. Pick up the syringe and remove the needle cover and lay it aside. Hold the syringe like a dart.
5. Using the other hand, gently pinch up at least a 2-inch fold of tissue (not just the skin).
6. Quickly insert the needle into the top (apex) of the fold, entering the subcutaneous tissue. The "soft spot" technique is to insert the needle about 1 inch to the side of the apex of the fold, into softer tissue, entering the pocket. The needle should be inserted at a 90-degree angle unless the patient is very thin and has little subcutaneous tissue. In that case the angle may be reduced by up to 45 degrees to avoid intramuscular injection.
7. Release the skinfold and use that hand to steady the barrel of the syringe.
8. Inject the insulin over a period of 3 to 5 seconds.
9. Place the alcohol swab against the needle hub, at the injection site, and pull the syringe unit straight out in one swift motion. Gently press on the injection site for a few seconds, but do not massage the site.
10. Carefully place the entire unit, uncapped, into the sharps container provided.
11. Record the injection site and insulin dose on a chart, computer, or other documentation sheet. Include the second licensed nurse who witnessed the insulin dose during preparation. Have the nurse witness the dose given. Store insulin and other supplies properly.
12. When instructing patient to self-inject insulin, use the following guidelines (if appropriate):
    —Aspiration does not need to be done before injection.
    —The injection site does not need to be cleansed with alcohol. The use of an alcohol swab by the patient on the site before self-injection is no longer recommended. Routine hygiene such as washing with soap and rinsing with water is adequate (Lewis et al., 2007).

insulin every few minutes. Buffered regular insulin may be substituted in patients unable to use rapid-acting insulin to improve postprandial blood glucose levels and long-term glucose control (Bode et al., 2002). The basal rate is designed to keep the blood glucose level steady between meals and during sleep. When food is eaten, the pump is programmed (at the touch of a button) to deliver a larger quantity of insulin right away to cover the carbohydrate in the meal. This is called a bolus of insulin. The bolus can also be adjusted based on the blood glucose level and planned physical activity. For carefully selected and properly educated patients, the pump offers improved flexibil-

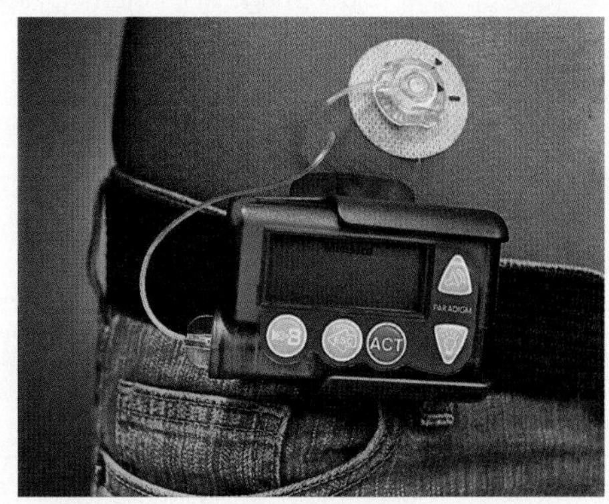

FIGURE 51-17 Medtronic MiniMed insulin pump.

ity in lifestyle, improved control of blood glucose and glycosylated hemoglobin (HbA_{1c}) levels (see Box 51-2), and freedom from multiple daily injections. Properly disassembled insulin pumps such as the Disetronic H-Tron V100 can even be worn during bathing or while swimming. The insertion site is usually the abdomen, but the buttocks, thighs, arms, and sections of the back may be used, with the insertion site covered by a clear occlusive dressing, which is usually changed every other day.

Oral Hypoglycemics

Oral hypoglycemics are compounds used to treat type 2 diabetes, each having a different mechanism of action. Oral hypoglycemic agents are not oral insulin or a substitute for insulin. The patient must have some functioning insulin production for oral hypoglycemics to be effective.

Five classes of oral drugs—sulfonylureas, meglitinides, alpha-glucosidase inhibitors, thiazolidinediones, and biguanide—are available for patients whose insulin production or utilization is inadequate due to type 2 diabetes mellitus (Table 51-6).

Sulfonylureas have blood glucose–lowering effects. They stimulate the pancreas to release insulin. A second generation of sulfonylureas, approved for use in the United States, includes glipizide (Glucotrol XL), glyBURIDE (Micronase, DiaBeta, Glynase), and glimepiride (Amaryl). They are more potent than previous drugs and do not require renal excretion. A class of oral hypoglycemics that stimulates increased insulin release in the pancreas is the **meglitinides,** which includes repaglinide (Prandin) and nateglinide (Starlix).

Another class of oral hypoglycemics lowers blood glucose by inhibiting delay of carbohydrate absorption from the small intestine; these are called **alpha-glucosidase inhibitors.** This drug class includes acarbose (Precose) and miglitol (Glycet). The best way to gauge effectiveness of therapy with acarbose and miglitol is to monitor the patient's 2-hour postprandial blood glucose level.

Thiazolidinediones are a class of oral hypoglycemic medications that lower blood glucose by increasing insulin sensitivity at the insulin receptor sites on the cells. The two drugs currently available in this class are rosiglitazone (Avandia) (which has a potential safety issue; see Table 51-6) and pioglitazone (Actos). They are most appropriate for adults whose bodies produce insulin but cannot use it because of inadequate or ineffective insulin receptor sites.

Metformin (Glucophage) is a **biguanide** glucose-lowering agent. It works primarily by reducing hepatic glucose production and lowers fasting blood glucose levels. It also enhances tissue response to insulin and improves glucose transport into cells. Metformin usually does not promote weight gain and may help improve lipid levels. Metformin is widely used by itself and in combination with a sulfonylurea. Com-

Table 51-6 Five Classes of Oral Hypoglycemics

GENERIC AND BRAND NAME	MECHANICS OF ACTION
SULFONYLUREAS	
Glipizide (Glucotrol, Glucotrol XL) GlyBURIDE (DiaBeta, Micronase, Glynase) Glimepiride (Amaryl)	Insulin secretagogues primarily stimulate the beta cells of the pancreas to release insulin, particularly in the early course of type 2 diabetes mellitus. Sulfonylureas increase the sensitivity to insulin at receptor sites.
MEGLITINIDES	
Repaglinide (Prandin) Nateglinide (Starlix)	Insulin secretagogues, like the sulfonylureas, stimulate the beta cells in the pancreas to increase insulin release. Their effects, which are glucose dependent, decrease when the patient's blood glucose level decreases. Requires functioning pancreatic beta cells.
BIGUANIDE	
Metformin (Glucophage, Glucophage XR, Fotamet, Riomet)	It works primarily by reducing hepatic glucose production and lowers fasting blood glucose levels. It also enhances tissue response to insulin and improves glucose transport into the cells.
ALPHA-GLUCOSIDASE INHIBITORS	
Acarbose (Precose) Miglitol (Glyset)	Metabolized by intestinal bacteria and digestive enzymes; delay carbohydrate absorption from the small intestine.
THIAZOLIDINEDIONES	
Rosiglitazone (Avandia) (use with caution*) Pioglitazone (Actos)	Increases insulin sensitivity at insulin receptor sites on the cell. Thiazolidinediones are most appropriate for adults whose bodies produce insulin but cannot use it because of inadequate or ineffective insulin receptor sites.

Data from Funnel, M., & Barlage, D. (2002). Managing diabetes with "agent oral." *Nursing*, *34*(3):36.

*The U.S. Food and Drug Administration announced a potential safety issue related to the use of rosiglitazone. Patients who are taking rosiglitazone, especially those with underlying cardiac disease or a high risk of myocardial infarction, should consult their diabetic care provider about whether to continue therapy with this medication (Scemons, 2007).

bined glyBURIDE-metformin (Glucovance) is another oral hypoglycemic agent that may be prescribed.

Once an oral drug becomes ineffective, simply substituting rarely works. But combination therapy can be highly effective. For example, oral drugs from two or more classes may be combined, or an oral drug may be combined with a bedtime dose of NPH or glargine insulin or detemir. Metformin and insulin are commonly chosen for combination therapy with sulfonylureas (Funnel & Barlage, 2004).

Other Treatments

Two subcutaneous agents act as adjuncts to insulin therapy, not a replacement for it. Pramlintide (Symlin) is used in type 1 and type 2 DM. It decreases gastric emptying, glucagon secretion, and glucose output from the liver and increases satiety. Exenatide (Byetta) is used only in type 2 DM. It stimulates release of insulin from the pancreatic B cells, decreases glucagon secretion, increases satiety, and decreases gastric emptying (Table 51-7). However, the FDA (2009) warns that it may increase the risk for kidney problems; labeling changes include dosing cautions and contraindications in patients with renal impairment.

Another drug that may be used to treat hypoglycemic reactions in DM is glucagon, a hormone normally secreted by the alpha cells of the pancreas. It stimulates the liver to change stored glycogen into glucose, which is then released into the bloodstream. Glucagon is available in a purified, crystallized form for reconstruction and subcutaneous, IM, or IV administration in the event of loss of consciousness as a result of hypoglycemic reaction. The usual dose is 0.5 to 1 mg for adults, with smaller doses for children. Some form of oral protein and carbohydrate, such as milk and crackers, should be given after the patient regains consciousness. Many people with diabetes carry a commercially prepared kit containing glucagon and concentrated carbohydrate such as candy or glucose gel (see Complementary & Alternative Therapies box).

Selected patients with type 1 DM now have the option of a pancreas transplant. Usually a pancreas transplant is performed on a DM patient who has end-stage renal disease and has already had a kidney transplant or will have one in the near future. A kidney and pancreas transplant are usually done at the same time. Patients who undergo kidney and pancreas transplantation must have lifelong immunosuppression therapy to prevent rejection of the transplants (Lewis et al., 2007).

Table 51-7 Insulin-Enhancing Drugs

CLASSIFICATION	MECHANISM OF ACTION
Pramlintide (Symlin) Subcutaneous	A synthetic form of amylin, a pancreatic hormone that slows gastric emptying and suppresses the release of glucagon and the formation of glycogen in the liver. Used as an adjunct to insulin therapy. Used in type 1 and type 2 diabetics. It carries a black box warning because of potential to cause severe hypoglycemia within 3 hours of administration (Bass, 2007).
Exenatide (Byetta) Subcutaneous	Incretin mimetics. Designed for use in type 2 diabetics. Incretins are gut hormones that promote insulin secretion during a meal, suppress glucagon release, and delay gastric emptying, which effectively reduces postprandial blood sugars. It is not indicated for use with insulin (Bass, 2007).

Complementary & Alternative Therapies

Endocrine Disorders

- Herbal medicines used in the treatment of type 2 diabetes mellitus include aloe vera juice, beans (*Phaseolus* species), bitter gourd, karela *(Momordica charantia)*, black tea *(Camellia sinensis)*, fenugreek *(Trigonella foenum-graecum)*, gurmar *(Gymnema sylvestre)*, macadamia nut, and Madagascar periwinkle *(Catharanthus roseus)*. Effects of these herbs include lowering of blood pressure (fenugreek), boosting of insulin production (gurmar), and increased use of available insulin (black tea).
- Kelp *(Fucus vesiculosus)* may help with weight loss in hypothyroid disorders. Milk thistle *(Silybum marianum)* is used for treatment and prophylaxis of chronic hepatotoxicity, inflammatory liver disorders, and certain types of cirrhosis.
- Yoga may help the patient with diabetes mellitus with diet control and may improve pancreatic function.

Nursing Interventions and Patient Teaching

People with diabetes may be hospitalized as a direct result of their disease process, or they may have a different primary diagnosis. The main focus of nursing interventions must always be on the primary diagnosis, but remember that the patient is also diabetic and is susceptible to a number of complications in addition to all those experienced by nondiabetic patients.

Daily routine for the patient with diabetes includes accurate monitoring of blood glucose levels, either by fingerstick specimens or by laboratory testing. Careful attention to diet is important; note the amount of food eaten at each meal and record it accurately.

If the patient with type 1 DM is ill, is nauseated, or cannot eat for any reason, consult with the physician or primary care provider. Physiologic and psychological stress raises the patient's blood glucose level. Do not withhold insulin in a patient with type 1 DM. Without insulin to promote glucose to enter the cells, the body must seek an alternative source for energy. Fats and protein are used. When these cells break down, ketones are formed. Accumulation of ketones results in ketosis and acidosis. If this situation is not corrected, the patient may develop DKA.

Often the primary care provider recommends providing Popsicles or apple juice, which can compensate for a decrease in calories when a regular diet cannot be consumed. If the patient does not like the types of food on the meal tray, arrange for a dietitian to consult.

Good skin care is essential for the person with diabetes, since poor circulation can lead to the development of skin problems. Compromised skin integrity makes a patient with DM more susceptible to infection. In diabetes, elevated glycosylated hemoglobin in the red blood cells impedes the release of oxygen to the tissues. Elevated blood glucose levels also make some pathogens thrive and proliferate. Vascular changes decrease blood, oxygen, and nutrient supply to the tissues and affect the supply of white blood cells in the area, because if white blood cells do not function properly, phagocytosis is defective (Brozenec, 1998).

Report to the physician any abnormalities such as cuts, scratches, or lesions anywhere on the body, and treat them before infection develops. Special foot care is crucial for this patient, since poor circulation and decreased nerve sensation or **neuropathy** (any abnormal condition characterized by inflammation and degeneration of the peripheral nerves) increase the danger of ulcers or other abnormal lesions developing into gangrene. Many patients seek the services of a podiatrist for their foot care. The patient should thoroughly wash the feet with soap and water every day; dry them thoroughly; and inspect them carefully for cracks, blisters, or foreign objects, paying special attention to the area between the toes. Foot soaks or powders are not recommended. The patient should wear clean socks daily and avoid tight garters. The toenails should be clipped straight across so that the edges do not become ingrown. The nurse should never trim the toenails of a patient with diabetes without a physician's written order. Do not put hot water bottles or heating pads on the feet, since burns may occur and not be felt. The patient should wear sturdy, properly fitting shoes, preferably with wide toe boxes or molded shoes that are less constrictive. Medicare now reimburses patients with DM who have certain conditions for the cost of specially molded shoes. The patient should not go barefoot at any time. Notify the physician immediately of any injury to the toes or feet (see Health Promotion box). Patients with DM are also advised to have an eye examination each year.

Carefully watch the patient who is receiving insulin for development of hypoglycemia, especially when the particular kind of insulin being injected is at its peak of action. Hypoglycemia is seen less frequently in patients receiving oral hypoglycemics, but it can occur.

The emotional aspects of diabetes are numerous, and many patients experience a period of denial after the initial diagnosis. Some patients become depressed. Because this disease affects all age-groups, nursing interventions are tailored to fit the needs of each patient (see Life Span Considerations box). Patients with diabetes must have help in working through their feelings, so be a good listener and supportive at all times. The patient who does not satisfactorily resolve any major problems in accepting the diagnosis of DM may be noncompliant with the treatment plan.

The nurse who supervises the patient in a home setting must encourage the patient to take the prescribed medication faithfully, eat the right kinds of food, test blood or urine correctly, and exercise regularly. If a family member is responsible for the patient's care, ensure that the caregiver is functioning adequately in this role. Some patients live alone and do well caring for themselves, with occasional visits from a home health or public health nurse. Others who have visual disturbances, circulatory problems, or other conditions may need daily visits and more actual nursing intervention, such as help with hygiene, meals, and insulin injections (Nursing Care Plan 51-1).

Health Promotion

Foot Care for the Patient with Diabetes Mellitus

- Wash feet daily with a mild soap and **warm** water. Test water temperature with hands first.
- Pat feet dry gently, especially between toes.
- Examine feet daily for cuts, blisters, edema, erythema, and tender areas. If patient's eyesight is poor, have others inspect feet.
- Use lanolin on feet to prevent skin from drying and cracking. Do not apply between toes.
- Use mild foot powder on feet if perspiring.
- Do not use commercial remedies to remove calluses or corns.
- Cleanse cuts with **warm** water and mild soap, covering with clean dressing. Do not use iodine, rubbing alcohol, or strong adhesives.
- Report skin infections or nonhealing lesions to health care provider immediately.
- Cut toenails even with rounded contour of toes. Do not cut down corners. The best time to trim nails is after a shower or bath.
- Separate overlapping toes with cotton or lamb's wool.
- Avoid open-toe, open-heel, and high-heel shoes. Leather shoes are preferred to plastic ones. Wear slippers with soles. Do not go barefoot. Shake out shoes before putting on.
- Wear clean, absorbent (cotton or wool) socks or stockings that have not been mended. Colored socks must be colorfast.
- Do not wear clothing that leaves impressions or constricts circulation.
- Do not use hot water bottles or heating pads to warm feet. Wear socks for warmth.
- Guard against frostbite.
- Exercise feet daily either by walking or by flexing and extending feet in suspended position. Avoid prolonged sitting, standing, and crossing of legs.

Acute Complications

One of the acute complications of DM is coma, which may be attributed to three different causes. The first type of coma can occur during DKA, which results from inadequate amounts of insulin or from inadequate insulin utilization. The second type, hyperglycemic hyperosmolar nonketotic coma (HHNC), involves no acidosis or ketonemia, but results from excess glucose, diuresis, and dehydration without adequate fluid replacement. The third type may occur during hypoglycemic reaction, which results from an excess amount of insulin with an inadequate amount of glucose present. These three complications are compared and contrasted in Table 51-8. (See also Safety Alert boxes: Emergency Care for Hypoglycemic Reaction and Emergency Care for Hyperglycemic Reaction.)

Another acute complication faced by the patient with diabetes is the development of infections of any kind. Hyperglycemia and ketonemia hinder the phagocytic action of leukocytes. An infection can therefore

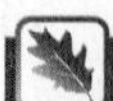

Life Span Considerations

Older Adults

Endocrine Disorder

- Diabetes mellitus is more prevalent in older adults. A major reason for this is that the process of aging involves insulin resistance and glucose intolerance, which are believed to be precursors to type 2 diabetes.
- The classic signs and symptoms of diabetes may not be obvious in older adults.
- Dietary management may be complicated by a variety of functional, social, economic, and financial factors.
- Hormone supplements must be administered with caution.
- Older adult diabetic patients are at increased risk for infection and should be counseled to receive proper immunizations and seek regular medical attention for even minor symptoms. The older adult often has considerable difficulty in managing diabetes.
- Some symptoms of hypothyroidism in the older adult are similar to those in a younger person but are more likely to be overlooked because the symptoms—fatigue, mental impairment, sluggishness, and constipation—are often attributed solely to aging. The older person with hypothyroidism has symptoms unique to the age set, including more disturbances of the central nervous system, such as syncope, convulsions, dementia, and coma. There is often pitting edema and deafness.
- The older patient with hyperthyroidism frequently has manifestations related only to the cardiovascular system, such as palpitations, angina, atrial fibrillation, and breathlessness. Signs and symptoms often attributed to "aging" may actually indicate an endocrine problem.

Nursing Care Plan 51-1 The Patient with Diabetes Mellitus

Ms. Thompson is an obese, 52-year-old married patient with type 2 diabetes mellitus (DM) diagnosed 3 years ago. She was referred to a short-term ambulatory diabetes education program by her physician for instruction on insulin administration because she has not achieved blood glucose control with dietary measures.

Objective data included blood glucose 220 mg/dL, weight 200 pounds, and blood pressure 134/84 mm Hg. Collaborative nursing actions include teaching Ms. Thompson measures that will help her control blood glucose (insulin, diet, and exercise) and how to detect, prevent, and treat hypoglycemic reactions. The nurse reported Ms. Thompson's work schedule to the physician and asked for insulin dosage alterations on weekends. The physician was unaware of her work schedule and stated that blood glucose control could not be optimum with this schedule.

NURSING DIAGNOSIS *Deficient knowledge: self-injections, SMBG, related to lack of exposure*

Patient Goals and Expected Outcomes	Nursing Interventions	Evaluation
Patient will independently self-administer insulin Patient will perform SMBG accurately Patient will use measurements obtained by SMBG to achieve blood glucose less than 126 mg/dL Patient will be able to detect and treat hypoglycemia	Support patient as necessary to self-inject insulin. Observe patient's skill in SMBG; correct as necessary. Review with patient the effect of activity, dietary intake, and insulin on blood glucose. Instruct patient on frequency and timing of SMBG. Review with patient signs and symptoms and treatment measures. Refer to dietitian for modification of diet necessary with insulin and for verification of diet knowledge.	Patient demonstrates safety in drawing up and self-administering insulin. Patient demonstrates accuracy in SMBG. Patient can verbalize the effect of activity, diet, and insulin on blood glucose. Patient can recite signs and symptoms of hypoglycemia and the correct immediate treatment to pursue.

Continued

Nursing Care Plan 51-1 The Patient with Diabetes Mellitus—cont'd

NURSING DIAGNOSIS ***Ineffective health maintenance, related to ineffective coping skills***

Patient Goals and Expected Outcomes	Nursing Interventions	Evaluation
Patient will state at least one change that will improve blood glucose control	Teach patient effects of stress, lack of exercise, and activity pattern on blood glucose. Explore with patient willingness and ability to change behaviors: sleep-activity, coping, and exercise. Engage patient in mutual problem solving; refrain from prescribing. Explore sources for long-term support in learning more effective coping skills; suggest support groups: • For patients with DM • For weight loss and maintaining weight loss • Available at work in health service program Suggest to patient that she seek a trial period on day shift on weekends.	Patient has enrolled in an exercise and weight-reduction program to assist in achieving a reasonable weight and beneficial exercise.

Critical Thinking Questions

1. Ms. Thompson received Humalog 75/25, 25 units subQ at 7:30 AM. She ate her American Diabetes Association diet at breakfast and lunch. At 3:00 PM she complains of being hungry, nervous, and tremulous. What are the immediate nursing interventions?
2. Ms. Thompson states, "I need to lose about 40 pounds, and I'm considering joining a weight-reduction club." What would be some helpful suggestions by the nurse?
3. In discharge planning, the nurse notes that Ms. Thompson has poorly fitting shoes. What would be some important discharge patient teaching for foot care?

Safety Alert!

Emergency Care for Hypoglycemic Reaction

IMMEDIATE TREATMENT: IF CONSCIOUS

- Give patient 10 to 20 g of quick-acting carbohydrate in some form, such as 4 to 6 oz of orange juice or a regular soft drink (not a diet drink); half of a candy bar; commercially prepared concentrated dextrose tablets or glucose paste; one tube Cake Mate icing gel (small); 2 tsp sugar or honey; six jelly beans or gumdrops; five or six LifeSavers or other roll candy; four animal crackers; or one granola bar. Offer another 5 to 20 g of quick-acting carbohydrate in 15 minutes if no relief is obtained.
- Give patient additional food, a longer-acting carbohydrate (e.g., slice of bread, crackers with peanut butter), after symptoms subside.

IMMEDIATE TREATMENT: IF UNCONSCIOUS

- Squeeze one tube of glucagon gel between teeth and gums, in buccal space, or give glucagon 0.5 to 1 mg subQ or IM; get patient to hospital. Hospitalized patients may receive IV bolus of 20 mL of 50% glucose or 50 mL of 20% glucose; glucagon may be given intravenously. Patient may need IV 10% or 20% glucose at 100 mL/hr to follow.

NURSING INTERVENTIONS DURING AND AFTER HYPOGLYCEMIC EPISODE

- Stay with the patient; check vital signs and do fingerstick blood glucose levels.
- Monitor for worsening of condition or relief of symptoms.
- If patient becomes unconscious, administer glucagon buccally, subcutaneously, intramuscularly, or intravenously.
- Be certain patient ingests food such as milk, six crackers with peanut butter, or one slice cheese and six crackers after symptoms end.
- Observe closely for 1 to 2 hours after cessation of symptoms.
- Notify physician about the hypoglycemic reaction.
- Assess reason the reaction may have occurred.

Table 51-8 Comparison of Types of Diabetic Coma

ASSESSMENT	HYPERGLYCEMIC REACTION, DIABETIC KETOACIDOSIS	HYPOGLYCEMIC REACTION	HYPERGLYCEMIC HYPEROSMOLAR NONKETOTIC COMA
Type of diabetes	Type 1	Type 1 or type 2	Type 2
Cause	Inadequate insulin	Too much insulin or oral hypoglycemic agent	Inadequate insulin or oral hypoglycemic agent
Patient history	Omitted or insufficient dose of insulin, physical or emotional stress, gastrointestinal upsets, dietary noncompliance	Reduced food intake, delayed meal, too much exercise	Reduced fluid or food intake with increased urinary output, resulting in severe dehydration
Onset of symptoms	Hours to days	Minutes to hours	Days
Previous diagnosis of having diabetes	Almost always	Yes; on medication	Usually type 2, on hypoglycemic agent
Age of patient	Usually younger patient	Usually younger patient	Usually older adult patient
Appearance of skin	Hot, dry, flushed	Cool, moist	Hot, dry; body temperature elevated
Breath	Fruity (from ketones)	Normal	Normal
Mucous membranes	Dry	Moist	Very dry
Respirations	Deep; may have Kussmaul's respirations (air hunger) as a result of metabolic acidosis	Rapid, shallow	Normal
Neurosensory	Drowsiness to coma	Irritability, tremors, impaired consciousness, personality changes; may lose consciousness	Lethargy, decreased consciousness; may lose consciousness
Blood pressure	Low	Normal	Decreased
Glycosuria and ketonuria	Present	Absent	Glycosuria present; no ketonuria
Polyuria and polydipsia	Present	Absent	Present
Hunger	Absent; may have nausea and vomiting	Present; may be nauseated	Absent
Blood glucose level	Usually 300-800 mg/dL	Usually <50 mg/dL	600-2000 mg/dL; serum osmolality greatly increased
Emergency treatment	Insulin, usually regular	Glucose (oral or IV) or glucagon (subQ, IM, or IV)	Large amounts of intravenous fluids; regular insulin

GI, Gastrointestinal; *IM*, intramuscular; *IV*, intravenous; *subQ*, subcutaneous.

! Safety Alert!

Emergency Care for Hyperglycemic Reaction (Diabetic Ketoacidosis)

USUAL TREATMENT DURING ACUTE STAGE

- Start an IV, using an 18-gauge needle, and begin fluid replacement, usually with 0.9% normal saline 1L/hr, until blood pressure is stabilized and urinary output is 30 to 60 mL/hr. When blood glucose levels approach 250 mg/dL, add 5% dextrose to the fluid regimen to prevent hypoglycemia.
- Give regular insulin (the only kind that can be given intravenously) as a piggyback infusion, using 100 units regular insulin in 500 mL normal saline. Administer the infusion with a pump controller. Adjust the infusion rate to obtain and maintain desired blood glucose levels.
- Determine blood glucose level hourly (SMBG method or venous sample).
- Provide IV replacement of potassium to help move insulin into cells; monitor serum potassium.
- Administer oxygen via nasal cannula or nonrebreather mask.
- Monitor cardiac status, with central venous pressure and Swan-Ganz monitoring if available.
- Insert Foley catheter and monitor I&O hourly.
- Assess vital signs and neurologic status.

NURSING INTERVENTIONS DURING AND AFTER DIABETIC KETOACIDOSIS

- Keep airway patent.
- Maintain patent IV infusion at prescribed rate.
- Keep accurate I&O record.
- Do accurate blood testing for glucose and urine testing for acetone.
- Monitor vital signs frequently, and assess cardiac status on monitor.
- Assess breath sounds for fluid overload.
- Assess level of consciousness frequently, and perform neurologic checks as ordered.
- Assess the cause of DKA.

become more severe and last longer, with poor wound healing taking place. Infection increases the possibility of DKA and makes it harder to control the disease. Patients with diabetes are often hospitalized for treatment of infections that might be handled on an outpatient basis for the nondiabetic patient.

Chronic Complications

Primary chronic complications associated with diabetes are those of end-organ disease, which results from damage to blood vessels (angiopathy) secondary to chronic hyperglycemia (Figure 51-18). Chronic complications of diabetes include blindness, cardiovascular problems, and renal failure.

Diabetes causes more cases of blindness in the United States than any other disease. Diabetic retinopathy involves progressive changes in the microcirculation of the retina, resulting in hemorrhages, scar tissue formation, and various degrees of retinal detachment. Surgical techniques such as laser beam coagulation of retinal vessels may improve vision for selected patients with early diagnosis.

Vascular changes in patients with diabetes, especially capillary changes, contribute to the development of renal sclerosis, often progressing to end-stage renal disease. Many of these patients have to undergo either peritoneal dialysis or hemodialysis as a result. Diabetes contributes to accelerated atherosclerotic changes in the blood vessels, resulting in myocardial infarction, stroke, and gangrene in the lower extremities. Many people with diabetes have to undergo amputation as a result of ischemia to the lower extremities. Additionally, nervous system manifestations (diabetic neuropathy) are commonly seen, which cause pain and decreased sensation in the extremities and contribute to the development of diabetic gangrene.

The patient has pain and paresthesias. The pain—described as burning, cramping, itching, or crushing—is usually worse at night and may occur only at that time. Complete or partial loss of sensitivity to touch and temperature is common. Foot injury and ulcerations may occur without the patient ever having pain. At times the skin becomes so sensitive (hyperesthesia) that even light pressure from bed sheets cannot be tolerated. Many men with diabetes experience problems with impotence or premature ejaculation. Reports of prevalence of impotence among men with diabetes vary from 30% to 60%. Impotence associated with DM is believed to result from damage to the sacral parasympathetic nerves. Patients of either gender may have orthostatic hypotension and bladder or bowel dysfunction.

Neuropathy affecting the autonomic nervous system may also result in gastropathy, a delayed gastric emptying that can produce anorexia, nausea, vomiting, early satiety, and a persistent feeling of fullness. These problems were previously referred to as gastroparesis, a term now reserved for the condition in which the stomach is severely affected and is very slow to empty solid foods. Metoclopramide (Reglan) stimulates gastric emptying and has been used in the treatment of gastroparesis.

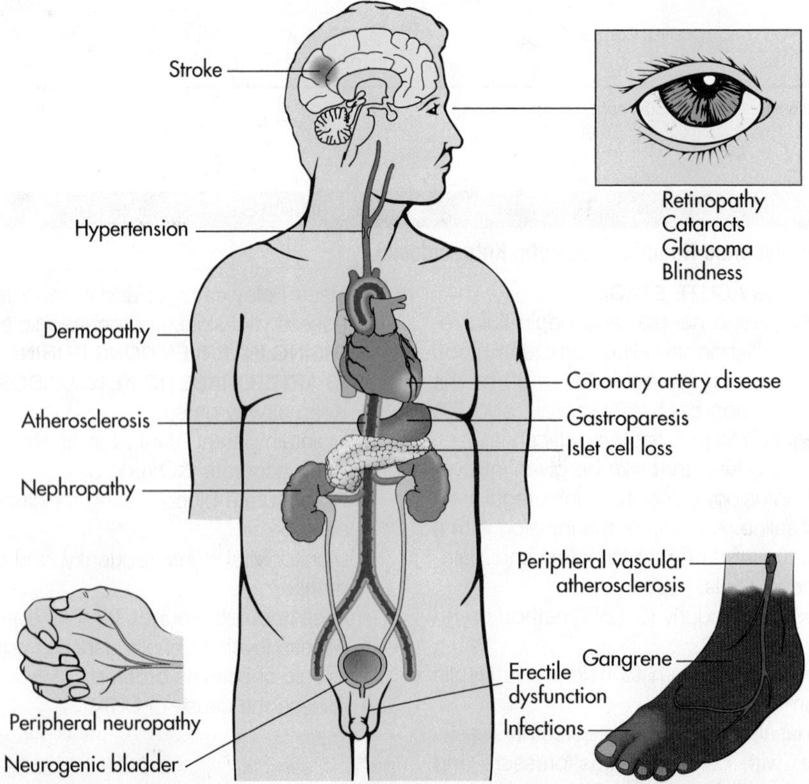

FIGURE 51-18 Long-term complications of diabetes mellitus.

Nursing diagnoses and interventions for the patient with DM include but are not limited to the following:

Nursing Diagnoses	Nursing Interventions
Ineffective therapeutic regimen management, related to health beliefs	Instruct in proper self-injection of insulin; have patient perform return demonstration. Reinforce instructions regarding availability of glucose and glycogen sources. Remove potentially hazardous objects from environment.
Noncompliance (diabetic management, high risk for), related to patient's value system	Establish therapeutic relationship so patient can express negative feelings. Correct misconceptions about trea_tment regimen. Assist patient in setting long-term goals for lifetime optimal disease management. Involve significant others when possible, and encourage communication between them and the patient. Refer patient to appropriate agencies and services (local support groups, ADA).

Education for the person with diabetes has many important aspects, including the proper administration of insulin or oral hypoglycemic medications and their side effects (see Communication box); the signs and symptoms of hyperglycemia and hypoglycemia; methods of testing blood glucose levels and of urine testing for acetone; planning and preparing the prescribed diet; and personal hygiene, emphasizing skin and foot care. Stress the interrelationships of diet, medication, and exercise. Instruct the patient to visit the dentist regularly and an ophthalmologist annually. Because infections and illnesses of any kind could result in loss of diabetic control, instruct the patient to notify the physician at the first sign of any illness. Special plans for travel include taking extra insulin vials and syringes, carrying food and some form of concentrated carbohydrate, and arranging for SMBG or urine testing. Provisions for adequate rest time must be made, since exhaustion can lead to changes in the overall condition.

Before discharge from the hospital, the patient should verbalize an understanding of how to prevent complications and display an interest in maintaining optimal wellness (see Cultural Considerations box). Stress the importance of regular medical checkups. The social aspects of DM cannot be ignored. Patients need to learn about lifestyle adjustment and should wear medical-alert jewelry and carry medical information wallet cards at all times. Decisions such as whether to attempt pregnancy should be thoroughly explored by women with diabetes. Above all, the patient must accept the responsibility for self-care and recognize

Communication

Importance of Proper Foot Care for Patients with Diabetes

Mr. Garcia is a 67-year-old Hispanic American who was diagnosed 18 months ago with type 2 diabetes mellitus. He has done well on a regimen of diet, exercise, and oral hypoglycemic medication (glyBURIDE [DiaBeta], 2.5 mg/day). Three days ago he dropped a brick on his right foot while remodeling his fireplace and was treated in the emergency department. He is being seen today for a follow-up visit with his internist. The office nurse, Mrs. Bloom, will first talk with him and assess his condition.

Nurse: Good morning, Mr. Garcia How are you doing this morning?

Patient: Much better, thank you. My foot still gives me a little trouble when I walk very far, but the swelling is down. I've been watching for red streaks, like they told me to in the emergency department, but so far there is only this scraped place and a bruise on the top of my foot (shows nurse the area).

Nurse: That's good. What kind of treatment are you using for your injured foot?

Patient: I'm washing my foot twice a day with soap and water, putting Neosporin ointment on the scrape, and then putting on a bandage.

Nurse: That sounds as if that should be adequate. Now let me get a close look at both feet (thoroughly examines the injured area, as well as the rest of the right foot, then examines the left foot). The skin on your feet looks a little dry, Mr. Garcia, and your toenails are getting quite thick and long. Do you have any problems cutting them?

Patient: I sure do! It's pretty hard for me to see exactly where I need to clip them sometimes, and I'm afraid I'll cut my toe, so I usually just let them go until my wife can help me. She's scared of cutting me, so she usually doesn't get them short enough.

Nurse: I understand. Proper foot care is important for any patient with diabetes to prevent complications such as infection or tissue injury that could become serious. Dr. Mason usually refers his patients to a podiatrist when they are having problems such as yours. A podiatrist specializes in care of the feet, and can properly trim your toenails as needed, as well as care for any corns or calluses that may develop.

Patient: That sounds like a really good idea. I sure don't want to wind up like my cousin and some other people I've seen, having to have a toe or my whole foot amputated! Can you give me the name of a good podiatrist?

Nurse: Yes, I can (hands pamphlet to Mr. Garcia). This pamphlet stresses the importance of foot care, and on the back page has the names of four podiatrists Dr. Mason recommends. You can choose the one you prefer. Now, I'm going to get Dr. Mason so that he can examine you.

Patient: Thanks, Mrs. Bloom. It's really good not to have to worry about cutting those toenails anymore!

Cultural Considerations

Chronic Conditions

- When dealing with a patient with a chronic condition, identification of the patient's cultural background, values, and beliefs can assist the health care team in identifying appropriate regimens. This is particularly important in a condition such as diabetes mellitus, which may require major lifestyle changes for successful management.
- In assessing patients, it is important to consider the best way to communicate across cultures. For example, Asian and Mexican cultures consider asking a direct question and expecting a direct answer to be ill mannered and rude. Phrasing questions in a more indirect way will foster more effective communication.

that making the right choices can affect life expectancy and quality. A current trend is for hospitals to employ a diabetes nurse specialist to develop and implement patient and staff education (see Home Care Considerations box).

Prognosis

Although the life expectancy for the person with diabetes is usually decreased, current research and recent advances have led to the hope of a much better prognosis. Early diagnosis and prompt, accurate treatment are essential in promoting longevity. Quality of life has been enhanced by better ways to control hyperglycemia and by earlier recognition of developing complications. Life expectancy and quality of life are directly related to glycemic control.

NURSING PROCESS *for the Patient with an Endocrine Disorder*

The role of the licensed practical nurse/licensed vocational nurse (LPN/LVN) in the nursing process as stated is that the LPN/LVN will:

- Participate in planning care for patients based on patient needs
- Review patient's care plans and recommend revisions as needed
- Review and follow defined prioritization for patient care
- Use clinical pathways, care maps, or care plans to guide and review patient care

Assessment

Hormones affect every body tissue and system, causing diverse signs and symptoms of endocrine dysfunction. Endocrine disorders may have nonspecific or specific clinical manifestations. Some specific signs of endocrine dysfunction are the classic "polys" **(polyuria, polydipsia,** and **polyphagia)** in DM and exophthalmos in hyperthyroidism. Specific signs make the assessment easier, whereas nonspecific signs and symptoms, such as tachycardia, fatigue, and depression, are more problematic.

Home Care Considerations

Diabetes Mellitus

- Considering the day of short hospitalization or no hospitalization and the overwhelming amount of information to be learned, home care is a high priority for people with diabetes mellitus.
- Frequently, older adults have difficulty with mobility and changes in vision that may hamper the drawing up of insulin.
- Often there is missing information as to why control cannot be obtained; that missing link may be found during a home visit.
- Diabetes caregivers and home care agencies often team up to provide good care for the older adult.
- Home care personnel network with other community resources to improve the older adult's quality of life or help deal with economic issues.
- Diabetic management should include education in:
  —Motivation
  —Self-monitoring of blood glucose
  —Exercise
  —Nutrition therapy
  —Medications
  —Written treatment plan

Nursing Diagnosis

Nursing diagnoses are determined from careful examination of patient data. Nursing diagnoses for the patient with an endocrine disorder may include but are not limited to the following:

- Deficient knowledge
- Risk for situational low self-esteem
- Disturbed sensory perception
- Risk for deficient fluid volume
- Risk for infection
- Risk for injury
- Sexual dysfunction
- Disturbed body image
- Ineffective coping
- Impaired home maintenance
- Noncompliance
- Imbalanced nutrition: less than body requirements
- Imbalanced nutrition: more than body requirements
- Activity intolerance

Expected Outcomes and Planning

The plan for management of patients with endocrine disorders must center on education to enable patients to understand their disorders, develop a healthy lifestyle, and prevent complications of their disease.

The care plan focuses on accomplishing individual goals and outcomes that relate to the identified nursing diagnoses. Examples of these include the following:

Goal 1: Patient will demonstrate safety in self-injections of insulin.

Evaluation: Patient independently administers insulin injection safely and accurately.

Goal 2: Patient will demonstrate SMBG.

Evaluation: Patient performs SMBG accurately.

Implementation

A major nursing responsibility is to help patients gain self-management skills for their chronic endocrine disorder through teaching and counseling. Self-management skills are probably the major factor in controlling the health problem and maintaining an optimal quality of life. Self-management skills are implemented through education in the disease process, the management of medications, the management of nutrition, and the role of exercise; SMBG; hygiene; the prevention of complications; and assistance with psychological adjustment.

Evaluation

During and after patient educational teaching on self-management skills, assist in evaluating the success of the teaching by noting patient progress based on stated goals and outcomes. For example, when the patient performs SMBG, observe the patient's skill, correct him or her as necessary, and evaluate the patient's technique to ensure accuracy. When patients are unable to meet expected outcomes, be ready to revise the care plan to promote success.

Get Ready for the NCLEX® Examination!

Key Points

- Endocrine glands are ductless glands that release chemicals (hormones) into the bloodstream to regulate body activities.
- The pituitary gland, located in the brain, is the master gland of the endocrine system.
- Hormones have a generalized effect on metabolism, growth and development, and reproduction.
- The endocrine glands regulate themselves by a series of negative feedback messages.
- The hormones secreted by the endocrine glands affect tissues of the entire body, and an imbalance in their levels may contribute to pathologic changes in many different systems.
- Acromegaly and gigantism, disorders of the pituitary gland, result in growth changes that may have a negative effect on the patient's self-image and self-esteem.
- Diabetes insipidus is a disorder of the posterior pituitary and must not be confused with DM, a disorder of the pancreas.
- Clinically, SIADH is characterized by hyponatremia and water retention that progresses to water intoxication. When caring for the patient with hyperthyroidism, provide for adequate rest periods and be sure that fluid and food intake meets the patient's nutritional needs.
- The emotions of the patient with hyperthyroidism are labile, so try to eliminate sources of stress from the environment, to help prevent emotional trauma.
- ^{131}I should not be administered to a pregnant patient because of the risk to the fetus; nurses who are pregnant should not care for these patients.
- The thyroidectomy patient faces three life-threatening postoperative complications: hemorrhage, tetany, and thyroid crisis.
- The patient with hypothyroidism may experience sluggish mental and physical functioning, so be patient and allow adequate time for nursing routines.
- The prognosis for papillary adenocarcinoma of the thyroid is excellent because few of these tumors metastasize.
- When administering IV calcium chloride to any patient, be careful that none of the drug extravasates because tissue sloughing may result.
- The extreme hypertension often seen in patients with pheochromocytoma may result in cerebrovascular accident.
- Depression is common in patients who suffer from Cushing's syndrome; be alert for suicidal thoughts and suicide attempts.
- The four main facets of medical treatment for the patient with DM are diet, SMBG, exercise, and medication.
- Type 1 DM is usually first diagnosed in people younger than 30 years of age; type 2 DM is more commonly found after age 35, and the incidence increases with age.
- As insulin resistance progresses, the pancreas secretes greater amounts of insulin to compensate. This in turn leads to progressive beta-cell failure and a lessening of insulin production. Both beta-cell dysfunction and insulin resistance are required for the development of hyperglycemia, the central metabolic characteristic of type 2 DM.
- The older person with diabetes may have a high blood glucose level before excreting any into the urine because of an increased renal threshold for glucose.
- The diabetic diet must be individualized, taking into consideration many factors, such as age, lifestyle, food preferences, and the ability to cook and store food.
- The person with type 1 DM must have access to a source of quick glucose at all times, in the event of a hypoglycemic reaction.
- Become familiar with the clinical manifestations of DKA, HHNC, and hypoglycemic reaction to properly assess diabetic patients, respond therapeutically, and educate them in self-care.
- Observe patients on insulin therapy and oral hypoglycemic medications during the time of peak action of the medication, and initiate treatment promptly if hypoglycemia develops.
- The nurse must be knowledgeable about the various insulin types and characteristics.
- Two new insulin-enhancing drugs given subcutaneously are pramlintide and exenatide.
- There are five classes of oral hypoglycemic drugs: sulfonylureas, meglitinides, biguanide, alpha-glucosidase inhibitors, and thiazolidinediones.
- DKA can result in seizures, brain damage, or death for the patient with type 1 DM.

Additional Learning Resources

Go to your companion CD for an audio glossary, animations, video clips, and more.

evolve Be sure to visit the Evolve site at http://evolve.elsevier.com/Christensen/adult/ for additional online resources.

Review Questions for the NCLEX® Examination

1. Which of the following hormones is responsible for "fight or flight"?
   1. Estrogen and testosterone
   2. FSH and LH
   3. Epinephrine and norepinephrine
   4. Calcitonin and parathyroid hormone

2. The hormones responsible for blood calcium levels are:
   1. calcitonin and parathyroid hormone.
   2. estrogen and progesterone.
   3. melatonin and follicle-stimulating hormone (FSH).
   4. thyroxine and parathyroid hormone.

3. Which of the following is the master gland of the body?
   1. Thyroid gland
   2. Adrenal gland
   3. Pineal gland
   4. Pituitary gland

4. What hormone is responsible for male secondary sex characteristics?
   1. Estrogen
   2. Progesterone
   3. Testosterone
   4. Adrenaline

5. The patient received ^{131}I yesterday in an attempt to slow the progression of her hyperthyroid condition. For which personnel would participating in her direct bedside care be dangerous?
   1. A 19-year-old first-semester nursing student
   2. A 34-year-old staff nurse who is new to the unit
   3. A 22-year-old aide who is 6 weeks pregnant
   4. A 49-year-old RN just returning from sick leave

6. A 35-year-old patient had a total thyroidectomy. The first night she experienced signs and symptoms of postoperative tetany. The nurse should implement the physician's order and immediately administer:
   1. sodium iodide PO.
   2. potassium chloride IV.
   3. magnesium sulfate IM.
   4. calcium gluconate IV.

7. A 47-year-old mother of three had cranial surgery to remove a pituitary tumor 3 days ago, leaving her with partial left hemiparesis and diabetes insipidus. Which nursing diagnosis is of the greatest priority postoperatively?
   1. Risk for deficient fluid volume, related to excessive loss via the urinary system
   2. Hopelessness, related to development of chronic illness (hemiparesis and diabetes insipidus)
   3. Risk for impaired oral mucous membrane, related to dehydration
   4. Coping, ineffective family: compromised, risk for, related to chronic illness

8. A 34-year-old construction worker was recently diagnosed as having acromegaly. Given the pathophysiology of his condition, the patient's laboratory test results will probably show elevated levels of:
   1. FSH.
   2. LH.
   3. TSH.
   4. GH.

9. While assessing a postoperative thyroidectomy patient, the nurse checks for damage to the laryngeal nerve. Which is most likely to suggest that damage may have occurred?
   1. The patient complains of a slight sore throat.
   2. The patient's voice tone has changed slightly.
   3. The patient is unable to swallow fluids.
   4. The patient is becoming increasingly hoarse.

10. To help a patient newly diagnosed with type 1 diabetes mellitus meet the goal of maintaining blood glucose control, which is the greatest priority in the care plan?
    1. Teach the patient the effect of diet, exercise, and insulin on the blood glucose level.
    2. Refer the patient to the hospital dietitian for intense education about his dietary needs.
    3. Instruct the patient on SMBG, observe return demonstrations, and correct his technique as needed.
    4. Review with the patient the desired effects of his medication, as well as possible side effects.

11. A 22-year-old man has had type 1 diabetes for the past year. Which statement demonstrates his need for more teaching?
    1. "If I want to lose weight, all I have to do is increase my dose of insulin."
    2. "I can have an occasional beer if it's calculated into my diet."
    3. "I will maintain better control of my blood sugar if I eat regular meals."
    4. "It is important that I eat properly, exercise regularly, and take my insulin injections."

12. To meet the goal of preventing injury to a type 1 diabetic patient, which nursing intervention is most important to include in the care plan?
    1. Assess peripheral pulses and capillary refill in the lower extremities.
    2. Instruct the patient in the proper technique for self-injection of insulin.
    3. Stress the importance of keeping the skin on the feet soft and supple.
    4. Remove potentially hazardous objects from the patient's environment.

13. A 45-year-old has been admitted to the hospital unit with the primary medical diagnosis of Addison's disease (adrenal hypofunction). Assessment reveals postural hypotension, fatigue, nausea, vomiting, and

poor skin turgor. Which of these nursing diagnoses is of greatest priority at this time?

1. Risk for infection
2. Risk for imbalanced body temperature
3. Risk for injury
4. Risk for deficient fluid volume

14. A human insulin formula that begins to take effect in less than half the time of regular, fast-acting insulin and more closely mimics the body's own hormone action is:
    1. Humulin R, Novolin R.
    2. lispro (Humalog), aspart (NovoLog).
    3. Humulin N, Novolin N.
    4. Humulin 70/30, Novolin 70/30.

15. The polydipsia and polyuria related to diabetes are caused primarily by:
    1. the release of ketones from cells during fat metabolism.
    2. fluid shifts resulting from the osmotic effect of hyperglycemia.
    3. damage to the kidneys from exposure to high levels of glucose.
    4. changes in RBCs resulting from attachment of excessive glucose to hemoglobin.

16. In planning care for a 78-year-old patient with type 2 diabetes admitted to the hospital with pneumonia, the nurse recognizes that the patient:
    1. must receive insulin therapy to prevent the development of ketoacidosis.
    2. has islet cell antibodies that have destroyed the ability of the pancreas to produce insulin.
    3. has minimal or absent endogenous insulin secretion and requires daily insulin injections.
    4. may have sufficient endogenous insulin to prevent ketosis but is at risk for development of hyperosmolar coma.

17. A diabetic patient takes a combination of regular and NPH insulin twice a day for glucose control. The nurse teaches the patient to be alert for hypoglycemia:
    1. immediately after breakfast and dinner.
    2. immediately after lunch and dinner.
    3. in the late afternoon and at bedtime.
    4. immediately after dinner and at bedtime.

18. The nurse assists the patient with dietary management of diabetes with the knowledge that a diabetic diet is designed:
    1. to be used only for type 1 diabetes.
    2. for use during periods of high stress.
    3. to normalize blood glucose by elimination of sugar.
    4. to help normalize blood glucose through a balanced diet.

19. In teaching a newly diagnosed type 1 diabetic "survival skills," the nurse includes information about:
    1. weight-loss measures.
    2. elimination of sugar from the diet.
    3. need to reduce physical activity.
    4. capillary blood glucose monitoring.

20. An appropriate instruction for the patient with diabetes related to care of the feet is:
    1. use heat to increase blood supply.
    2. avoid softening lotions and creams.
    3. inspect all surfaces of the feet daily.
    4. use iodine to disinfect cuts and abrasions.

21. The oral hypoglycemic that works primarily by reducing hepatic glucose production and lowering fasting blood glucose levels is:
    1. repaglinide (Prandin).
    2. acarbose (Precose).
    3. metformin (Glucophage).
    4. rosiglitazone (Avandia).

22. The types of insulin used in an insulin pump are __________ or __________ insulin.

23. Circle all correct statements.
    1. Regular insulin (Humulin R) has an onset of action of 30 minutes to 1 hour.
    2. Lispro (Humalog) has an onset of action of 15 minutes.
    3. NPH (Humulin N) has an onset of action of 2 hours.
    4. Glargine (Lantus) has an onset of action of 6 to 10 hours.

24. The normal range of serum sodium is:
    1. 10 mEq/L.
    2. 8.9 to 10.1 mEq/L.
    3. 135 to 145 mEq/L.
    4. 8 to 23 mEq/L.

25. In syndrome of inappropriate antidiuretic hormone (SIADH) the body secretes:
    1. too much antidiuretic hormone (ADH).
    2. too little antidiuretic hormone (ADH).

26. Clinically, SIADH is characterized by what? *(Select all that apply.)*
    1. Peripheral edema
    2. Hyponatremia
    3. Water retention
    4. Brain cells becoming edematous

27. In the medical management of SIADH, the physician orders:
    1. increased fluid intake to 3000 mL/day.
    2. fluid restriction to 800 to 1000 mL/day.

28. Choose the correct nursing interventions for SIADH. *(Select all that apply.)*
    1. Daily weight
    2. I&O
    3. Fluid restriction
    4. Foods high in sodium

29. If the diabetic patient engages in increased exercise, his insulin requirement:

1. increases.
2. decreases.
3. remains unchanged.

30. Chvostek's sign, Trousseau's sign, carpopedal spasms, and laryngeal spasms are postoperative complications of total thyroidectomy that indicate:

1. low levels of serum calcium.
2. high levels of serum calcium.
3. low levels of serum sodium.
4. high levels of serum sodium.

31. An appropriate nursing intervention for a patient admitted into the hospital with signs and symptoms of diabetic ketoacidosis is:

1. obtain blood glucose immediately.
2. administer NPH insulin intravenously.
3. give intravenous glucagon.
4. take vital signs every 4 hours.

32. Cushing's syndrome results from what? *(Select all that apply.)*

1. Excessive levels of adrenocortical hormones in plasma
2. Hyperplasia of adrenal tissue from overstimulation of ACTH
3. Overuse of corticosteroid drugs
4. Adrenocortical insufficiency when the adrenal glands do not secrete adequate amounts of glucocorticoids

33. Addison's disease results from:

1. decreased production of parathyroid hormones.
2. excessive secretion of epinephrine and norepinephrine.
3. inadequate secretion of glucocorticoids and mineralocorticoids.
4. overactivity of the parathyroid glands with decreased production of parathyroid hormone.

34. In a patient with pheochromocytoma, the principal clinical manifestation is:

1. darkly pigmented skin and mucous membranes.
2. moonface and buffalo hump.
3. severe hypertension.
4. carpopedal spasms.

35. This blood test measures the amount of glucose that has become incorporated into the hemoglobin within an erythrocyte. This test reveals the effectiveness of diabetes therapy for the preceding 8 to 12 weeks. It is called ____________ or ____________.

36. Good skin care, especially of the feet, is essential for the person with diabetes mellitus because: *(Select all that apply.)*

1. poor circulation can lead to the development of skin problems.
2. elevated glycosylated hemoglobin in RBCs impedes the release of oxygen to the tissues.
3. low blood glucose levels make pathogens thrive and proliferate rapidly.
4. vascular changes decrease blood oxygen and nutrient supply to the tissues and affect the supply of WBCs in the area and thus adversely affect phagocytosis.

37. Urine testing for ____________ is done for a diabetic person with hyperglycemia to determine the potential for DKA.

chapter

52

Care of the Patient with a Reproductive Disorder

Barbara Lauritsen Christensen

evolve

http://evolve.elsevier.com/Christensen/foundationsadult

Objectives

Anatomy and Physiology

1. List and describe the functions of the organs of the male and female reproductive tracts.
2. Discuss menstruation and the hormones necessary for a complete menstrual cycle.

Medical-Surgical

3. Discuss the impact of illness on the patient's sexuality.
4. Discuss nursing interventions for the patient undergoing diagnostic studies related to the reproductive system.
5. Discuss the importance of the Papanicolaou's test in early detection of cervical cancer and mammography as a screening procedure for breast cancer.
6. List nursing interventions for patients with menstrual disturbances.
7. Discuss the etiology and pathophysiology, clinical manifestations, assessment, diagnostic tests, medical management, nursing interventions, patient teaching, and prognosis for infections of the female reproductive tract.
8. Discuss four important points to be addressed in discharge planning for the patient with pelvic inflammatory disease.
9. List four nursing diagnoses pertinent to the patient with endometriosis.
10. Identify the clinical manifestations of a vaginal fistula.
11. Describe the common problems with cystocele and rectocele and the related medical management and nursing interventions.
12. Discuss the etiology and pathophysiology, clinical manifestations, assessment, diagnostic tests, medical management, nursing interventions, patient teaching, and prognosis for cancers of the female reproductive system.
13. Identify four nursing diagnoses pertinent to ovarian cancer.
14. Describe the preoperative and postoperative nursing interventions for the patient requiring major surgery of the female reproductive system.
15. Describe six important points to emphasize in teaching breast self-examination.
16. Compare four surgical approaches for cancer of the breast.
17. Discuss adjuvant therapies for breast cancer.
18. Discuss nursing interventions for the patient who has had a modified radical mastectomy.
19. List several discharge planning instructions for the patient who has undergone a modified radical mastectomy.
20. Discuss the etiology and pathophysiology, clinical manifestations, assessment, diagnostic tests, medical management, nursing interventions, patient teaching, and prognosis for inflammatory disorders of the male reproductive system.
21. Distinguish between hydrocele and varicocele.
22. Discuss the importance of monthly testicular self-examination beginning at 15 years of age.
23. Discuss patient education related to prevention of sexually transmitted infections.

Key Terms

amenorrhea (ă-mĕn-ŏ-RĒ-ă, p. 1782)
candidiasis (kăn-dĭ-DĪ-ă-sĭs, p. 1827)
carcinoma in situ (kăr-sĭ-NŌ-mă ĭn SĪ-tū, p. 1801)
chancre (SHĂNG-kĕr, p. 1825)
Chlamydia trachomatis (klă-MĬD-ē-ă tră-KŌ-mă-tĭs, p. 1827)
circumcision (sĭr-kŭm-SĬZH-ŭn, p. 1820)
climacteric (klī-MĂK-tĕr-ĭk, p. 1787)
colporrhaphy (kŏl-PŎR-ă-fē, p. 1798)
colposcopy (kŏl-PŎS-kŏ-pē, p. 1778)
cryptorchidism (krĭp-TŎR-kĭ-dĭz-ĕm, p. 1821)
culdoscopy (kŭl-DŎS-kŏ-pē, p. 1778)
curettage (KŪ-rĕ-tăhzh, p. 1780)
dysmenorrhea (dĭs-mĕn-ō-RĒ-ă, p. 1782)
endometriosis (ĕn-dō-mē-trē-Ō-sĭs, p. 1796)
epididymitis (ĕp-ĭ-dĭd-ĕ-MĪ-tĭs, p. 1820)
fistula (FĬS-tū-lă, p. 1797)
introitus (ĭn-TRŌ-ĭ-tŭs, p. 1798)
laparoscopy (lă-pă-RŎS-kō-pē, p. 1778)
mammography (măm-MŎG-ră-fē, p. 1780)
menorrhagia (mĕn-ō-RĀ-jă, p. 1782)
metrorrhagia (mĕ-trō-RĀ-jă, p. 1782)
panhysterosalpingo-oophorectomy (păn-HĬS-tĕr-ō-SĂL-pĭng-gō-oof-ō-RĔK-tō-mē, p. 1805)
Papanicolaou (Pap) test (smear) (pă-pĕ-NĬ-kō-lōu tĕst, smēr, p. 1778)
phimosis (fī-MŌ-sĭs, p. 1820)
procidentia (prō-sĭ-DĔN-shă, p. 1798)
sentinel lymph node mapping (SĔN-tĭ-nĕl lĭmf nōd MĂP-ĭng, p. 1810)
trichomoniasis (trĭk-ō-mō-NĪ-ă-sĭs, p. 1826)

Conception and birth are made possible through the dynamics of the normally functioning male and female reproductive systems. Reproduction of like individuals is necessary for the continuation of the species. The male and female sex glands (gonads) produce the gametes (sperm, ova) that unite to form a fertilized egg (zygote), the beginning of a new life.

ANATOMY AND PHYSIOLOGY OF THE REPRODUCTIVE SYSTEM

MALE REPRODUCTIVE SYSTEM

The organs of the male reproductive system include the testes, the ductal system, the accessory glands, and the penis (Figure 52-1). These structures have various functions: (1) producing and storing sperm, (2) depositing sperm for fertilization, and (3) developing the male secondary sex characteristics.

Testes (Testicles)

The two oval **testes** (gonads) are enclosed in the **scrotum,** a saclike structure that lies suspended from the exterior abdominal wall. This position keeps the temperature in the testes below normal body temperature, which is necessary for viable sperm production and storage. Each testis contains one to three coiled seminiferous tubules that produce the sperm cells. After puberty, millions of sperm cells are produced daily. The testes also produce the hormone testosterone. Testosterone is responsible for the development of male secondary sex characteristics.

Ductal System

Epididymis

Sperm (Figure 52-2) produced in the seminiferous tubules immediately travel through a network of ducts called the **rete testis.** These passageways contain cilia that sweep sperm out of the testes into the **epididymis,** a tightly coiled tube structure that lies superior to the testes and extends posteriorly. With sexual stimulation smooth muscle within the walls of the epididymis contract, forcing the sperm along the seminiferous tubules of the testes to the vas deferens.

Ductus Deferens (Vas Deferens)

The **ductus deferens** is approximately 18 inches (46 cm) long and rises along the posterior wall of the testes. As it moves upward, it passes through the inguinal canal into the pelvic cavity and loops over the urinary bladder. The ductus deferens, the nerves, and the blood vessels are enclosed in a connective tissue sheath called the **spermatic cord.** If a man chooses to be sterilized for birth control, it is a simple procedure to make small slits on either side of the scrotum and sever the ductus deferens. This procedure is called a **vasectomy.** It renders the man sterile because sperm can no longer be expelled.

Ejaculatory Duct and Urethra

Behind the urinary bladder, the ejaculatory duct connects with the ductus deferens. The ejaculatory duct is only 1 inch (2.5 cm) long. It unites with the urethra to pass through the prostate gland. Each of the two ejaculatory ducts empties into the prostate urethra. The urethra extends the length of the penis with the urinary meatus. The urethra carries both sperm and urine, but, because of the urethral sphincter, it does not do so at the same time.

Accessory Glands

The ductal system transports and stores sperm. The accessory glands, which produce seminal fluid (semen), include the seminal vesicles, the prostate gland, and Cowper's glands. With each ejaculation (2 to 5 mL

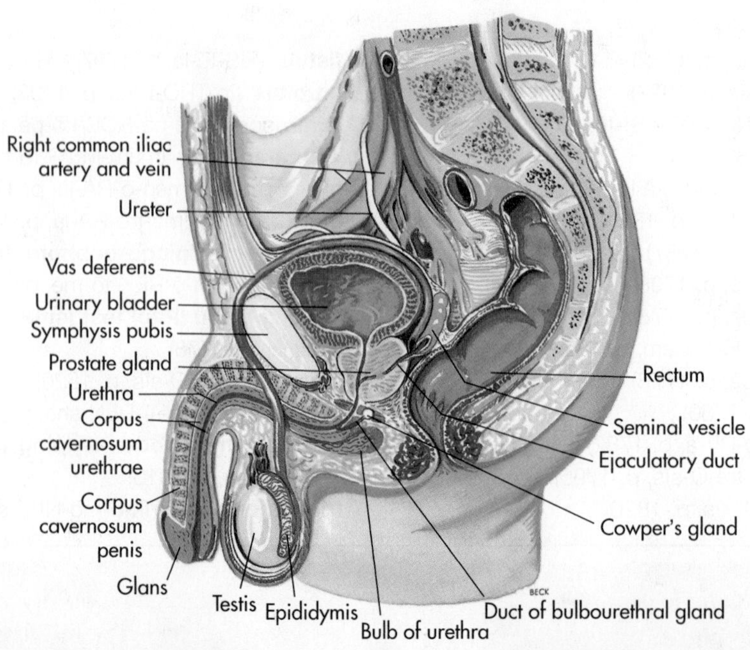

FIGURE 52-1 Longitudinal section of the male pelvis showing the location of the male reproductive organs.

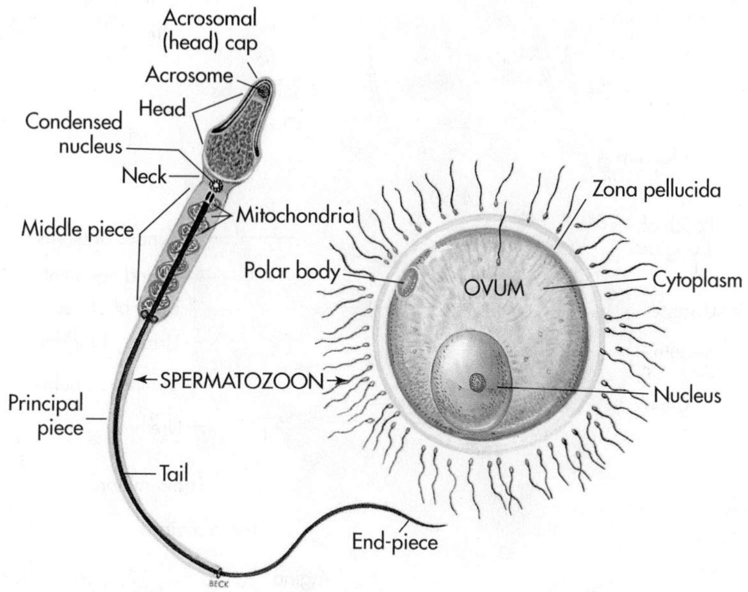

FIGURE 52-2 Male sex cell (spermatozoon) greatly enlarged *(left)*. Female sex cell (ovum) surrounded by sperm at time of fertilization *(right)*.

of fluid), approximately 200 to 500 million sperm are released.

Seminal Vesicles

The **seminal vesicles** are paired structures that lie at the base of the bladder and produce 60% of the volume of semen. The fluid is released into the ejaculatory ducts to meet with the sperm.

Prostate Gland

The single, doughnut-shaped **prostate gland** surrounds the neck of the bladder and urethra. It is a firm structure, about the size of a chestnut, composed of muscular and glandular tissue. The prostate secretes alkaline fluid that contributes to motility of sperm. Smooth muscle of the prostate contracts during ejaculation, expelling semen from the urethra. The ejaculatory duct passes obliquely through the posterior part of the gland. The prostate gland often hypertrophies with age, expanding to surround the urethra and making voiding difficult.

Cowper's Glands

Cowper's glands are two pea-sized glands under the male urethra. They correspond to the Bartholin's glands in women and provide lubrication during sexual intercourse.

Urethra and Penis

The male **urethra** has two purposes: conveying urine from the bladder and carrying sperm to the outside. The cylindrical **penis** is the organ of copulation. The shaft of the penis ends with an enlarged tip called the **glans penis.** The skin covering the penis, called the **prepuce,** or foreskin, lies in folds around the glans. This excess tissue is sometimes removed in a surgical procedure called circumcision to prevent **phimosis** (tightness of the prepuce of the penis that prevents retraction of the foreskin over the glans).

Three masses of erectile tissue, the corpus spongiosum and two copora cavernosa, contain numerous sinuses that fill the shaft of the penis. With sexual stimulation the sinuses fill with blood, causing the penis to become erect. Sexual stimulation concludes with ejaculation, which is brought about by peristalsis of the reproductive ducts and contraction of the prostate gland. After ejaculation, the penis returns to a flaccid state.

Sperm

Spermatogenesis (the process of developing spermatozoa) begins at puberty and continues throughout life. Mature sperm consist of three distinct parts: (1) the head; (2) the midpiece; and (3) the tail, which propels the sperm. Once deposited in the female reproductive system, mature sperm live approximately 48 hours (or in some cases up to 5 days). If they come in contact with a mature egg, the enzyme on the head of each sperm bombards the egg in an attempt to break down its coating (see Figure 52-2). It takes thousands of sperm to break the coating, but only one sperm enters and fertilizes the egg. The remaining sperm disintegrate. Once fertilization takes place, a chemical change occurs making the ova impenetrable for other sperm.

FEMALE REPRODUCTIVE SYSTEM

The organs of the female reproductive system include the ovaries, the uterus, the fallopian tubes, and the vagina (Figure 52-3). These organs, along with a few accessory structures, produce the ovum, house the fertilized egg, maintain the embryo, and nurture the newborn infant. The ability to conceive and nurture this new human being requires the intricate balance of many hormones and the menstrual cycle.

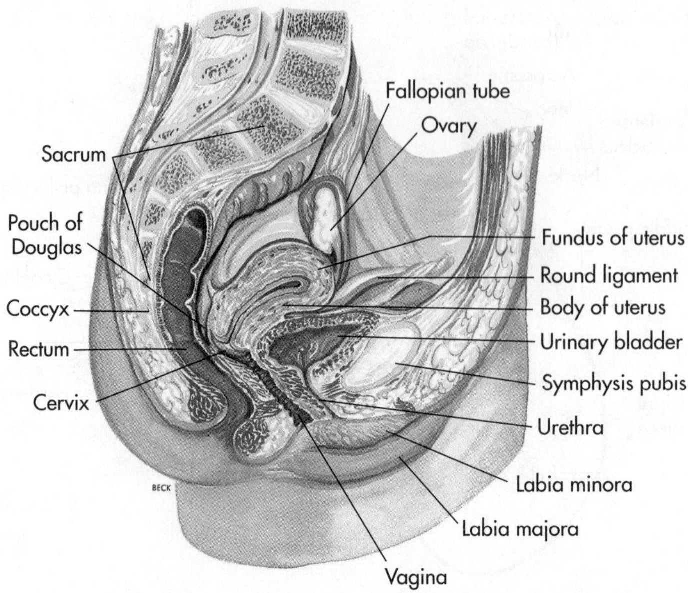

FIGURE 52-3 Longitudinal section of the female pelvis showing the location of the female reproductive organs.

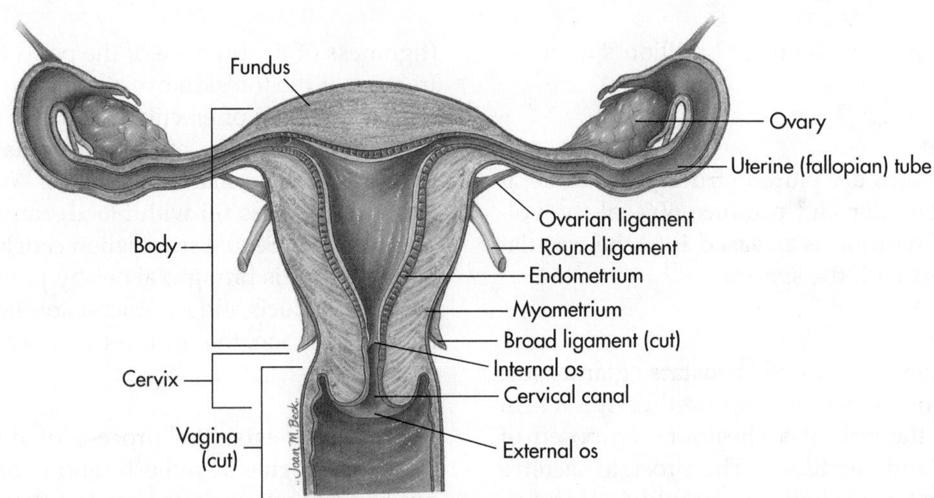

FIGURE 52-4 Sectioned view of the uterus showing relationship to the ovaries and the vagina.

Ovaries

The paired **ovaries** (gonads) are the size and shape of almonds. They are located bilateral to the uterus immediately inferior to the fallopian fimbriae. At puberty they release progesterone and the female sex hormone estrogen, and they release a mature egg during the menstrual cycle. Each ovary contains 30,000 to 40,000 microscopic ovarian follicles.

Fallopian Tubes (Oviducts)

The **fallopian tubes** are a pair of ducts opening at one end into the **fundus** (upper portion of the uterus) and at the other end into the peritoneal cavity, over the ovary. They are approximately 4 inches (10 cm) long with the fimbriae at the distal ends. The entire inner surface of the tubes is lined with cilia. When the graafian follicle of the ovary ruptures and releases the mature ovum, the fimbriae sweep the ovum into the fallopian tube. Fertilization takes place in the outer third of this tube, and the fertilized ovum **(zygote)** is moved through the tube by a combination of muscular peristaltic movements and the sweeping action of the cilia. If the mature ovum is not fertilized, it disintegrates.

Uterus

The **uterus** is shaped like an inverted pear and measures 3 × 2 × 1 inches (7.5 × 5 × 2.5 cm) in the nonpregnant state (Figure 52-4). It is located between the urinary bladder and the rectum and consists of three layers of tissue: (1) endometrium, the inner layer; (2) myometrium, the middle layer; and (3) perimetrium, the outer layer. The uterus is divided into three major portions (see Figure 52-4). The **fundus** (upper, rounded portion) is the insertion site of the fallopian tubes. The larger midsection is the **corpus** (body). The smaller, narrower lower portion of the uterus is the **cervix,** part of which actually descends into the vaginal vault. During pregnancy the uterus is capable of enlarging up to 500 times.

Vagina

The **vagina** is a thin-walled, muscular, tubelike structure of the female genitalia, approximately 3 inches (7.5 cm) long. It is located between the urinary bladder and the rectum. The superior portion articulates with the cervix of the uterus; the inferior portion opens to the outside of the body. The vagina is lined with mucous membrane, responsible for lubrication during sexual activity. The walls of the vagina normally lie in folds called **rugae.** This enables the vagina to stretch to receive the penis during intercourse and to allow passage of the infant during birth.

The external opening of the vagina is covered by a fold of mucous membrane, skin, and fibrous tissue called the **hymen.** For centuries the hymen was a symbol of virginity, but it is now known that rigorous exercise or the insertion of a tampon may tear the hymen. If the hymen does remain intact, it is ruptured by **coitus** (intercourse).

External Genitalia

The reproductive structures located outside the body are the external genitalia, or **vulva.** These structures include the mons pubis, labia majora, labia minora, clitoris, and vestibule (Figure 52-5).

Located superior to the symphysis pubis is a mound of fatty tissue, covered with coarse hair. This structure is the **mons pubis.** Extending from the mons pubis to the perineal floor are two large folds called the **labia majora** (large lips). These protect the inner structures and contain sensory nerve endings and an assortment of sebaceous (oil) and sudoriferous (sweat) glands. Directly under the labia majora lie the **labia minora** (small lips). These are smaller folds of tissue, devoid of hair, that merge anteriorly to form the prepuce of the clitoris. The **clitoris** is comparable to the male penis and is composed of erectile tissue that becomes engorged with blood during sexual stimulation.

The space enclosing the structures located beneath the labia minora is called the **vestibule.** It contains the **clitoris,** the **urinary meatus,** the **hymen,** and the **vaginal opening.**

Accessory Glands

Bilateral to the urinary meatus lie the **paraurethral,** or **Skene's, glands,** the largest glands opening into the urethra. These glands secrete mucus and are similar to the male prostate gland. Bilateral to the vaginal opening are two small, mucus-secreting glands called the greater **Bartholin's glands (vestibular),** which lubricate the vagina for sexual intercourse.

Perineum

The area enclosing the region containing the reproductive structures is referred to as the **perineum.** The perineum is diamond shaped and starts at the symphysis pubis and extends to the anus.

Mammary Glands (Breasts)

The breasts are attached to the pectoral (chest) muscles. Breast tissue is identifiable in both sexes. During puberty, the female breasts change their size, shape, and ability to function. Each breast contains 15 to 20 lobes that are separated by adipose tissue. The amount of adipose tissue is responsible for the size of the breast. Within each lobe are many lobules that contain milk-producing cells; these lobules lead directly to the **lactiferous ducts** that empty into the nipple (Figure 52-6).

The nipple is composed of smooth muscle that allows it to become erect. The dark pink or brown tissue surrounding the nipple is called the **areola.** Milk production does not start until a woman gives birth. At this

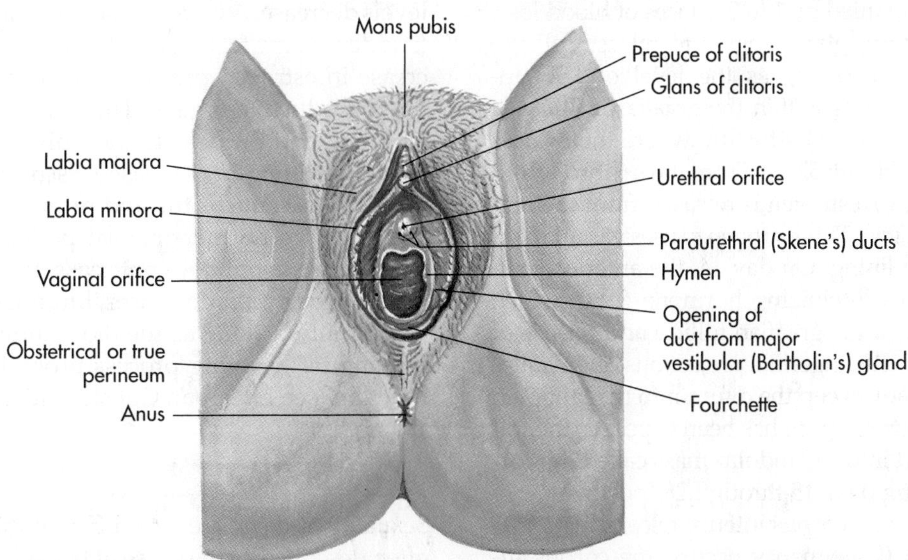

FIGURE 52-5 External female genitalia (vulva).

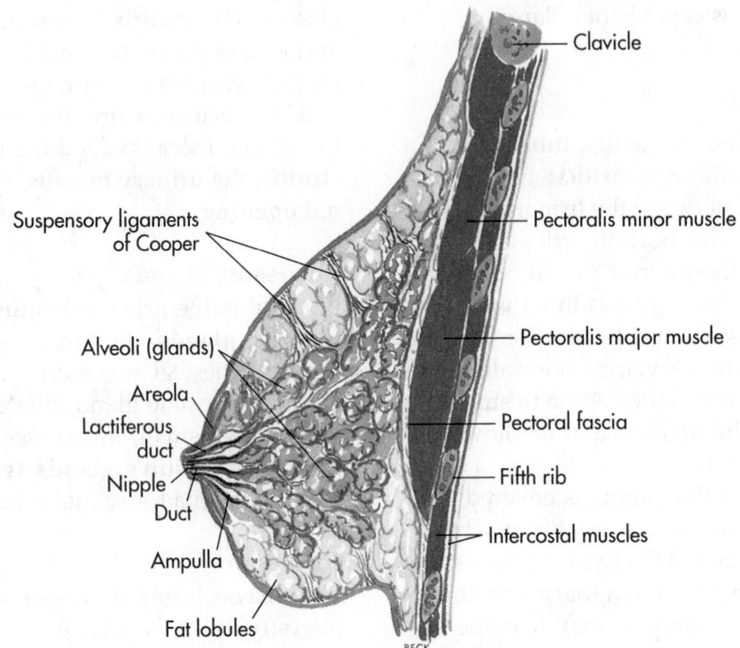

FIGURE 52-6 Lateral view of the breast (sagittal section). The gland is fixed to the overlying skin and the pectoralis muscles by the suspensory ligaments of Cooper. Each lobule of secretory tissue is drained by a lactiferous duct that opens through the nipple.

time, under the influence of prolactin, the milk is formed. The hormone oxytocin allows milk to be released.

Menstrual Cycle

Menarche, the first menstrual cycle, usually begins at approximately 12 years of age. Each month, for the next 30 to 40 years, an ovum matures and is released about 14 days before the next menstrual flow, which occurs on average every 28 days. If fertilization occurs, menstrual cycling subsides and the body adapts to the developing fetus.

Generally, the menstrual cycle is divided into three phases: (1) menstrual, (2) preovulatory, and (3) postovulatory. This discussion uses the example of a 28-day cycle. On days 1 through 5 of the cycle, the endometrium sloughs off, accompanied by 1 to 2 ounces of blood loss. The anterior pituitary gland begins to release follicle-stimulating hormone (FSH); as the level of FSH increases, the egg matures within the **graafian follicle** (a pocket or envelope-shaped structure where the ovaries prepare the ovum [Figure 52-7]). From days 6 through 13 (preovulatory phase), estrogen is released from the maturing graafian follicle. This estrogen causes vascularization of the uterine lining. On day 14, the anterior pituitary gland releases luteinizing hormone (LH), which causes the rupture of the graafian follicle and release of the mature ovum. The fingerlike projections of the fallopian tubes (fimbriae) sweep the ovum into the fallopian tube. Once this mature ovum has been expelled, the follicle is transformed into a glandular mass called the **corpus luteum.** During days 15 through 28 (postovulatory phase), the developing corpus luteum releases estrogen and progesterone. If pregnancy occurs, the corpus luteum continues to release estrogen and progesterone to maintain the uterine lining until the placenta is formed, which then takes over the job of hormonal release. If pregnancy does not occur, the corpus luteum lasts 8 days and then disintegrates. Normally the corpus luteum shrinks and is replaced by scar tissue called **corpus albicans.** At this point the hormone level decreases over several days and menstruation starts again.

EFFECTS OF NORMAL AGING ON THE REPRODUCTIVE SYSTEM

Menopause usually occurs in women between 35 and 60 years of age. The average age is 51. Whether it occurs earlier or later, menopause should not be considered abnormal. Cigarette smoking and living at high altitudes are associated with early menopause. During menopause the menstrual flow ceases and hormone levels decrease. A woman may experience "hot flashes" (sudden warm feelings), which are caused by the decrease in estrogen production. Changes also occur in the reproductive organs. The vagina loses some of its elasticity, and the breasts and vulva lose some adipose tissue, resulting in decreased tissue turgor. The bones may also become brittle and prone to osteoporosis.

Men have no menopausal period. Sperm production decreases but does not cease. In later years, testosterone production decreases, but not dramatically.

Basically, as long as the older individual is healthy, nothing in the aging process prohibits normal sexual function (see Life Span Considerations box).

HUMAN SEXUALITY

Sexuality and sex are two different things. **Sexuality** is often described as the sense of being a woman or a man. It has biologic, psychological, social, and ethical dimensions. Sexuality influences life experiences, and sexual-

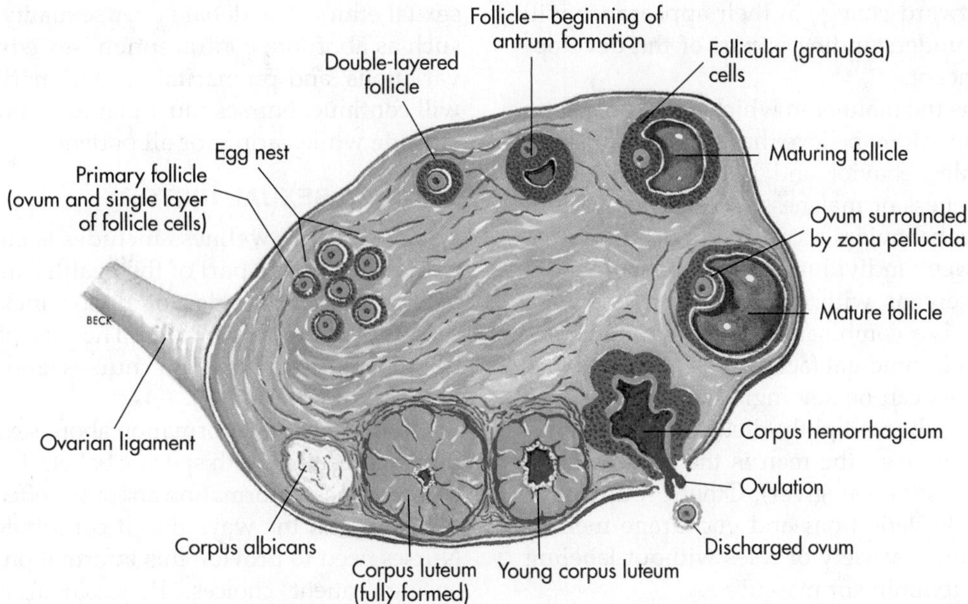

FIGURE 52-7 Mammalian ovary showing successive stages of ovarian (graafian) follicle and ovum development. Begin with the first stage (egg nest) and follow around clockwise to the final stage (corpus albicans).

Life Span Considerations

Older Adults

Reproductive Disorders

WOMEN

- Many older women are reluctant to seek medical care for problems of the reproductive system. This may be related to cultural factors, embarrassment, or lack of knowledge. Routine gynecologic examination should continue as part of the overall physical examination, even after menopause.
- Certain forms of cancer of the reproductive tract are more common with aging. Any vaginal bleeding should be promptly reported to the physician, as should pelvic pain, pruritus, or skin lesions in the genital region.
- Decreased levels of estrogen and systemic diseases, such as diabetes, predispose older women to vaginitis.
- Breast cancer risk increases after 40 years of age. Breast examination should continue throughout the life span. The American Cancer Society (2009a, b) recommends an annual mammogram for women older than 40 years of age. Each woman must make an individualized choice in consultation with her physician.

MEN

- Decreased production of testosterone results in changes in the male reproductive system, but the ability to procreate can continue into the eighth decade. Sexual interest often continues late in life.
- Chronic health problems, such as diabetes mellitus or hypertension, and many kinds of medication result in impotence in older men.
- Prostate enlargement is increasingly common with each decade after 40 years of age. Although this enlargement is usually benign, cancer of the prostate is a serious condition seen in older men. Ultrasonography of the prostate, when combined with rectal examination and prostate-specific antigen testing, is particularly useful in diagnosing prostate cancer.

ity is influenced by life experiences. The term **sex** has a more limited meaning. It usually describes the biologic aspects of sexuality such as genital sexual activity. Sex may be used for pleasure or reproduction. As a result of life's changes or by personal choice, sexual activity may be absent from a person's life for brief or prolonged periods. Some persons may choose to remain celibate.

The process by which people come to know themselves as women or men is not clearly understood. Being born with female or male genitalia and subsequently learning female or male social roles seem to be factors, though these do not explain differences of sexuality and sexual behavior. Such variations are more understandable if the nurse remembers that sexuality is intertwined with all aspects of self.

SEXUAL IDENTITY

Biologic identity, or the differences between men and women, is established at conception and further influenced at puberty by hormones. Gender identity is the sense of being feminine or masculine. As soon as the infant is born (and sometimes before), the outside world labels the child as a girl or boy. Adults adjust their behavior to relate to a female or male infant. These varied patterns of interaction influence the infant's developing sense of gender identity.

Children explore and seek to understand their own bodies. Combining this information with the way in which they are treated, they begin to create an image of themselves as a boy or as a girl. By 3 years of age, children are aware that they will remain boys or girls and that no outward change in their appearance will alter this. This understanding is part of the development of self-concept.

Gender role is the manner in which a person acts as a woman or man. Many believe that society influences female and male behavior and is thus the primary source of femaleness or maleness. Because society encourages certain behaviors according to one's gender, differences between individuals' sexual behaviors develop. Most likely, as with other human behaviors, sexual behavior is a combination of many interacting biologic and environmental factors.

Cultural factors can be key ingredients in defining sex roles. Some cultures tightly dictate roles as feminine or masculine (e.g., the man is the breadwinner, and the woman is the caregiver). Other groups have more flexible role definitions and encourage men or women to explore a variety of roles without labeling the behavior as feminine or masculine.

Sexual orientation is the clear and persistent erotic desire of a person for one sex or the other. There are heterosexual, homosexual, lesbian, and bisexual individuals, but the origins of sexual orientation are still not understood. Biologic theorists describe orientation in genetic terms, meaning it is determined at conception. Psychological theorists attribute orientation to early learning experiences, believing that cognitive processes are the determining factor. Still other theorists state that genetics and environment both play roles in the development of sexual preference.

For some people the inward sense of sexual identity does not match the biologic body. These people are known as transgenders. Researchers do not clearly understand how this mismatch occurs. Transgenders do not see their sexual identity as a choice; it is a clear and persistent orientation dating back to early childhood. In contrast, most homosexual men and women define themselves as satisfied with their gender and social roles; they simply have a persistent desire for their same sex.

A transvestite is most often a heterosexual man who periodically dresses like a woman; however, a transvestite may be a homosexual. Cross-dressing is usually done in private and kept secret even from those who are closest to him.

Because sexuality is linked to every aspect of living, any sexual choice involves personal, family, cultural, religious, and social standards of conduct. Ideas about ethical sexual conduct and emotions related to sexuality form the basis for sexual decision making. The range of attitudes about sexuality extends from a traditional view of sex only within marriage to a point of view that allows individuals to determine what is right. Sexual choices that overstep a person's ethical standard may result in internal conflicts.

Some people may judge sexual decisions as moral or immoral solely on religious standards; others view any private sexual act between consenting adults as moral. People will always have differing beliefs about sexual ethics. The debate over sexuality-related issues such as abortion, contraception, sex education, sexual variations, and premarital or extramarital intercourse will continue. Nurses must maintain a nonjudgmental attitude while caring for all patients.

TAKING A SEXUAL HISTORY

Because overall wellness includes sexual health, sexuality should be a part of the health care program. Yet health care services do not always include sexual assessment and interventions. The area of sexuality can be an emotional one for nurses and patients (see Health Promotion box).

Giving patients information about sexuality does not imply agreement with specific beliefs. Patients need accurate, honest information about the effects of illness on sexuality and the ways that it contributes to wellness. Nurses need to provide this information without influencing patient choices. Professional behavior must guarantee that patients receive the best health care possible without diminishing their self-worth. Promotion of self-education and honest examination of sexual beliefs and values can help in reducing sexual bias.

Although there is no single approach to taking a sexual history, certain principles make it more comfortable for both the patient and the nurse (Box 52-1):

- Obtain the sexual history early in the nurse-patient relationship, which indicates permission for patients to discuss sexual concerns.
- Avoid overreacting or underreacting to a patient's comments; this aids in truthful data collection.
- Use language that the patient understands; both the patient and the nurse may need to define their terms to ensure accurate data gathering.

Health Promotion

Factors that Can Interfere with the Promotion of Sexual Health

- Lack of information
- Conflicting values system (attitudes and beliefs)
- Anxiety (Are specific attitudes, feelings, and actions "normal"?)
- Guilt
- Lack of comfort with sexuality
- Invasion of privacy
- Lack of regard for hospitalized patient's need for time alone with significant other
- Manner in which the patient is touched
- Fear of being judged
- Lack of understanding of the effects of illness and treatment on sexual functioning

Box 52-1 Requirements for Taking a Sexual History

- Provision of privacy—a closed room
- An atmosphere of trust—ensure confidentiality
- Nurses' comfort with their own sexuality
- Nonjudgmental approach

- Move from the less sensitive to the more sensitive areas. This will promote nurse-patient comfort.
- At the end of the sexual history, ask if the patient has additional questions or concerns.

A brief sexual history assessment can be made and included in the nursing history through the use of three questions (Box 52-2). The questions may be adapted to address illness, hospitalization, life events, or any other relevant matter that influences or interferes with sexual health. The questions may also be adjusted to find out what the patient expects to happen as a result of procedures, medications, or surgery. Often the nurse does not need to ask the last two questions because many patients voice their concerns about masculinity, femininity, and sexual functioning without further encouragement.

Nurses may intervene in sexual problems among patient populations through four strategies: (1) educating patient groups likely to have sexual concerns, (2) providing anticipatory guidance throughout the life cycle, (3) promoting a milieu conducive to sexual health, and (4) validating normalcy about sexual concerns.

Several self-help groups and other organizations publish easy-to-read pamphlets on sexuality (see Health Promotion box). These pamphlets can often be purchased for a nominal fee and given to patients. Most pamphlets can be obtained directly from state or local chapters. Contact chapters of other self-help groups about the availability of resources for patients, such as newsletters that address sexuality.

Nurses can also write their own pamphlets for patients. Although this requires some effort, it may provide additional incentive for staff to address sexuality.

ILLNESS AND SEXUALITY

Illness may change a patient's self-concept and result in an inability to function sexually. Medications, stress, fatigue, and depression also affect sexual functioning.

Health Promotion

Self-Help Organizations that Publish Sexuality Pamphlets

- National Multiple Sclerosis Society (www.nationalmssociety.org): *Sexuality and MS*
- Arthritis Foundation (www.arthritis.org): *Living and Loving*
- American Cancer Society (www.cancer.org): *Sexuality for the Man with Cancer; Sexuality for the Woman with Cancer*
- American Diabetes Association (www.diabetes.org): several pamphlets and articles for men and women with diabetes mellitus

Box 52-2 Brief Sexual History

- Has your (illness, pregnancy, hospitalization) interfered with your being a (husband, wife, significant other, father, mother)?
- Has your (abortion, heart attack) changed the way you see yourself as a (woman, man)?
- Has your (colostomy, mastectomy, hysterectomy) changed your ability to function sexually (or altered your sex life)?

Alcohol abuse can lead to a reduced sex drive and inadequate sexual functioning.

Lack of interest or desire for sexual activity often occurs when patients are preoccupied with symptoms of illness. Most often these sexual symptoms disappear as patients recover from the acute phase of illness and resume sexual activity. However, some illnesses—such as diabetes mellitus, end-stage renal disease, prostate cancer, certain types of prostate surgery, spinal cord injuries, and heart disease—may cause patients concern or may result in actual inabilities with sexual function.

Changes in the nervous system, circulatory system, or genital organs may lead to sexual health problems. Spinal cord injuries can interrupt the peripheral nerves and spinal cord reflexes that involve sexual responses. But spinal cord–injured men and women also have reported having satisfying orgasms in spite of complete denervation of all pelvic structures.

Sexual dysfunction of a patient with diabetes mellitus can occur when the disease is not well controlled, but the dysfunction generally disappears when the lack of control is diagnosed and treated. Approximately half of the men who have diabetes mellitus are impotent, generally because of poor control. Sexual counseling is important to (1) provide accurate information about the sexual aspects of the disorder, (2) dispel the patient's incorrect assumptions and expectations, and (3) give advice to improve the patient's sexual self-esteem and dispel the guilt frequently found in both partners.

A mastectomy results in both physical and emotional trauma. In addition to the resultant disfigurement, a patient must also grapple with (1) how to cope with cancer, (2) how the operation will affect her relationship with her spouse or significant other, (3) how to relate to the strangeness of her own body, and (4) how her sex life will be affected. Problems that arise with pelvic irradiation for cancer of the cervix are much harder to treat than those of mastectomy; the entire physiology of the vagina is altered by the radiation, causing a true loss of function. With a mastectomy the only function lost is the ability to nurse an infant. The goal for the patient and her partner is to face the issue in a straightforward manner, acknowledging the diagnosis and discussing their true feelings. If feelings are repressed rather than shared, both the patient and her significant other may suffer. Therapeutic counseling before surgery can aid the patient's and partner's acceptance and recovery after surgery.

LABORATORY AND DIAGNOSTIC EXAMINATIONS

DIAGNOSTIC TESTS FOR WOMEN

A physician performs the pelvic examination, which involves visualization and palpation of the vulva, the perineum, the vagina, the cervix, the ovaries, and the uterine surfaces. During the pelvic examination, specimens are frequently obtained for diagnostic purposes. The bimanual pelvic examination progresses from the visualization and palpation of the external genital organs for edema and irritations to an inspection for abnormalities of the internal organs. To visualize internal organs, the physician inserts a vaginal speculum. The physician may perform a rectovaginal examination to evaluate abnormalities or problems of the rectal area and the posterior internal organs (Box 52-3).

Colposcopy

Colposcopy (*colpo,* vagina or vaginal; and *scopy,* observation) provides direct visualization of the cervix and vagina. Prepare the patient for a pelvic examination and explain the purpose of the procedure. The physician inserts the vaginal speculum, followed by insertion of the colposcope for inspection of the area. The color of the tissue, presence of growths and lesions, and condition of the vascularity are observed and specimens obtained as necessary.

Culdoscopy

Culdoscopy is a diagnostic procedure that provides visualization of the uterus and adnexa (uterine appendages, i.e., the ovaries and fallopian tubes). Explain the purpose and the method of procedure. Prepare the patient for the vaginal operation with preoperative instructions. The patient is given a local, spinal, or general anesthetic. After the anesthetic is administered, the patient is assisted to a knee-chest position. The culdoscope is passed through the vaginal wall in back of the cervix. The area is examined for tumors, cysts, and endometriosis. During the procedure, **conization** (removal of eroded or infected tissue) may be done. This procedure is generally done on an outpatient basis. After the operation, assess for bleeding, assess vital signs, and monitor voiding.

Laparoscopy

Laparoscopy (examination of the abdominal cavity with a laparoscope through a small incision made beneath the umbilicus) provides direct visualization of the uterus and the adnexa. Preparation of the patient includes insertion of a Foley catheter to maintain bladder decompression for an open view. The procedure is done with a general anesthetic. The physician grasps the cervix with forceps and inserts a lighted laparoscope through the incision. Carbon dioxide may be introduced to distend the abdomen for easier visualization. If a biopsy is to be done or organs are to be manipulated, a second incision may be made in the lower abdomen to allow for instrument insertion. The ovaries and fallopian tubes are observed for masses, ectopic pregnancy, adhesions, and pelvic inflammatory disease (PID). Tubal ligations may be done using this procedure. Instruct the patient of the probability of shoulder pain afterward because of carbon dioxide introduced into abdomen.

Box 52-3 Endoscopic Procedures for Visualization of Pelvic Organs

- **Colposcopy:** Visualization of vagina and cervix under low-power magnification
- **Culdoscopy:** Insertion of a culdoscope through posterior vaginal vault into Douglas's cul-de-sac for visualization of fallopian tubes and ovaries
- **Laparoscopy:** Insertion of a laparoscope (with patient under general anesthesia) through small incision in abdominal wall (inferior margin of umbilicus), then insufflation of abdomen with carbon dioxide; permits visualization of all pelvic organs

Papanicolaou (Pap) Test (Smear)

Papanicolaou (Pap) test (smear) (a simple smear method of examining stained exfoliative peeling and sloughed-off tissue or cells) is most widely known for its use in the early detection of cervical cancer. Scrapings of secretions and cells are taken from the cervix and spread on a glass slide. The slide is sprayed with a fixative and sent to the laboratory for analysis. It is important that slides be properly labeled with the date, time of the last menstrual period, and whether the woman is taking estrogens or birth control pills. Instruct patients not to douche, use tampons, use vaginal medications, or have sexual intercourse for at least 24 hours before the examination. Collect careful menstrual and gynecologic history.

The American Cancer Society (ACS) (2009a) highly recommends that every woman begin annual Pap tests within 3 years after becoming sexually active or no later than 21 years of age. Women should be tested every year (regular Pap test) or every 2 years (thin prep Pap test). Women age 30 years or older who have had three normal Pap tests in a row may choose to be screened every 2 to 3 years instead of annually. Women age 70 years or older who have had three or more normal Pap tests in a row and no abnormal test results in the past 10 years may decide to stop having cervical screenings altogether. Also, women who have had a hysterectomy may stop having cervical cancer screenings (unless their surgery was done as a treatment for cervical cancer or precancerous cells).

Thin prep Pap tests may slightly improve the detection of cancers and greatly improve the detection of cervical precancers. Thin prep Pap tests also reduce the number of tests that need to be repeated.

The physician may recommend more frequent testing for women with a history of multiple sexual partners or sexually transmitted infections (STIs), a family history of cervical cancer, or those whose mothers used diethylstilbestrol (DES) during pregnancy.

Table 52-1 provides a comparison of interpretation classifications of the cytologic findings and treatment recommendations. The Bethesda system is preferred because it allows better communication between the

Table 52-1 Pap Test Interpretation Classifications and Action

INTERPRETATION	NUMERICAL SYSTEM	DYSPLASIA CYTOLOGIC CLASSIFICATION	CERVICAL INTRAEPITHELIAL NEOPLASIA (CIN) CLASSIFICATION	BETHESDA SYSTEM*	ACTION
Negative (normal)	Class I	Negative squamous metaplasia	No designation	Negative (normal)	Repeat annually
Probably negative, may indicate infection	Class II	Atypical squamous cells	No designation	Infection Atypical squamous cells Reactive changes	Treat infection, repeat Pap
Suspicious, but not conclusive for malignancy	Class III	Mild dysplasia Moderate dysplasia	CIN I CIN II	Low-grade squamous intraepithelial lesion†	Treat infection, repeat Pap in 8-12 weeks; colposcopy
More suspicious, strongly suggestive of malignancy	Class IV	Severe dysplasia Carcinoma in situ	CIN III	High-grade squamous intraepithelial lesion†	Colposcopy, biopsy, treatment
Conclusive for malignancy	Class V	Invasive carcinoma	Invasive carcinoma	Invasive squamous cell carcinoma	Colposcopy, biopsy, treat with conization, hysterectomy

*The Bethesda system is the preferred system.
†The Bethesda Working Group suggests that "these two new terms encompass the spectrum of terms currently used to delineate the squamous cell precursors to invasive squamous carcinoma, including the grades of CIN, the degree of dysplasia, and carcinoma in situ."

cytologist and the clinician. The Bethesda system evaluates the adequacy of the sample (e.g., satisfactory or not satisfactory for interpretation) and provides a general classification of normal or abnormal and a descriptive diagnosis of the Pap smear. Although the classification system may vary, clinicians agree it is important to monitor Pap smears and ensure proper follow-up, including treatment of vaginal infections and colposcopy if necessary.

Pap tests have long been used to look for cervical cancer and precancerous cells. Cervista 16/18 and Cervista HPV HR are recently introduced tests for detecting the high-risk types of human papillomavirus (HPV) that are most likely to cause cervical cancer by looking for pieces of their deoxyribonucleic acid (DNA) in cervical cells. These DNA-based tests, in conjunction with the Pap test, have been approved by the U.S. Food and Drug Administration (FDA) (2009b) for women ages 30 and over with slightly abnormal Pap test results to find out if more testing or treatment may be needed.

Biopsy

Biopsies are procedures in which samples of tissue are taken for evaluation to confirm or locate a lesion. Tissue is aspirated by special needles or removed by forceps or through an incision.

A **breast biopsy** is performed to differentiate benign or malignant tumors. Breast biopsy is indicated for patients with palpable masses; suspicious areas appearing on mammography; and persistent, encrusted, purulent, inflamed, or sanguineous discharge from the nipples. The biopsy is performed by fine-needle aspiration (FNA); stereotactic or ultrasound core biopsy, under local anesthetic; or surgical biopsy, with general or local anesthetic. In an FNA, fluid is aspirated from the breast and expelled into a specimen bottle. Pressure is placed on the site to stop bleeding, then an adhesive bandage is applied. In an open surgical biopsy, an excisional biopsy is usually performed in a portion of the breast to expose the lesion and then remove the entire mass (Lewis et al., 2007). Another procedure called stereotactic and ultrasound core biopsy is a reliable diagnostic technique to obtain breast biopsy if an abnormal mass is seen on mammogram. A mammogram is used to find the lesion, the skin is anesthetized, and a small superficial incision is made. A biopsy gun device is fired into the lesion and removes a core sample of the mass. Compared with an open surgical biopsy, this procedure produces less scarring, uses only a local anesthesia, has reduced costs, and is done on an outpatient basis (Cleveland Clinic, 2009). Specimens of selected tissue may be frozen and stained for rapid diagnosis. The wound is sutured and a bandage applied. Observe the incision site for bleeding, tenderness, and erythema.

A **cervical biopsy** is done to evaluate cervical lesions and to diagnose cervical cancer. The biopsy is generally done without anesthesia. The colposcope is inserted through the vaginal speculum for direct visualization, the cervical site is selected and cleansed, and tissue is removed. The area is then packed with gauze or a tampon to check the blood flow.

An **endometrial biopsy** is performed to collect tissue for diagnosis of endometrial cancer and analysis for infertility studies. The procedure is generally performed at the time of menstruation when the cervix is dilated and cells are more easily obtained. The cervix is locally anesthetized, a curette is inserted, and tissue is obtained from selected sites of the endometrium.

Other Diagnostic Studies

Conization of the cervix is used to remove eroded or infected tissue or confirm cervical cancer. A cone-shaped section is removed when the mass is confined to the epithelial tissue. After surgery the area is packed with gauze to control bleeding. The patient is observed for bleeding and generally discharged from the hospital the same day.

Dilation and curettage (D&C) (scraping of material from the wall of a cavity or other surface; performed to remove tumors or other abnormal tissue for microscopic study) is a procedure used to obtain tissue for biopsy, to correct cervical stricture, and to treat dysmenorrhea. The patient is placed under general anesthesia, the cervix is dilated, and the inside of the uterus scraped with a curette. Packing may be inserted for hemostasis, and a perineal pad is applied for absorption of drainage. After vaginal packing is removed, instruct the patient to monitor for excessive vaginal bleeding or malodorous drainage.

Cultures and **smears** are collected to examine and identify infectious processes, abnormal cells, and hormonal changes of the reproductive tissue. Specimens collected for smears are prepared by spreading the collected smear on a glass slide and covering it with a second slide or spraying it with a fixative. Handle specimens with aseptic techniques and take care to avoid the transfer and spread of organisms. Cultures are taken from exudates of the breast, the vagina, the rectum, and the urethra. STIs and mastitis are diagnosed by isolation of the causative organisms. Treatment is prescribed according to the results of the culture.

Schiller's iodine test is used for the early detection of cancer cells and to guide the physician in doing a biopsy. An iodine preparation is applied to the cervix, and glycogen, which is present in normal cells, stains brown. Abnormal or immature cells do not absorb the stain. Unstained areas may be biopsied. This method of detection is valuable but not entirely reliable, since normal cells sometimes lack glycogen and malignant tissue sometimes contains glycogen. After the procedure the patient should wear a perineal pad to avoid stains on the clothing.

Radiographic examinations are performed to detect abnormal tissue, locate abnormal structures, and observe patency of ducts.

Hysterograms and **hysterosalpingograms** are studies for visualizing the uterine cavity to confirm (1) tubal abnormalities (adhesions and occlusions), (2) the presence of foreign bodies, (3) congenital malformations and leiomyomas (fibroids), and (4) traumatic injuries. The patient is placed in the lithotomy position. A speculum is inserted into the vagina, a cannula is inserted through the speculum into the cervical cavity, and a contrast medium is injected through the cannula. As the contrast medium progresses through the cavity, the uterus and fallopian tubes are viewed by a fluoroscope and films are taken.

Mammography is radiography of the soft tissue of the breast to allow identification of various benign and neoplastic processes, especially those not palpable on physical examination. **Digital mammography** is a newer technique that allows a clear and more accurate image; it involves digitally coding x-ray images into a computer (Lewis et al., 2007). It is believed that the average breast tumor is present for 9 years before it is palpable. Digital mammography is helpful as a screening procedure. The ACS (2009a, b) recommends baseline mammograms for women between ages 35 and 39, with annual mammograms after age 40.

When the mammography procedure is scheduled, advise the patient to refrain from using body powders, deodorants, and ointments on the breast areas, since this could cause false-positive results. Before the procedure give the patient a gown and ask her to remove jewelry and upper garments. The technician asks the patient to sit or stand in an upright position and rest one breast on the radiographic table. A compressor is placed on the breast, and the patient is asked to hold her breath as an anterior view is taken. The machine is rotated, the breast is again compressed, and a lateral view is taken. This procedure is repeated on the other breast. The patient may be asked to remain until the radiographic films are read.

Because of the greater density of breast tissue, mammography is less sensitive in younger women, which may result in more false-negative results. About 10% to 15% of all breast cancers can only be detected by palpation and cannot be seen on mammography. Even if mammogram findings are unremarkable, all suspicious masses should be biopsied.

Ultrasound is a helpful diagnostic tool to differentiate a benign tumor from a malignant tumor. It is useful in women who have dense breasts with fibrocystic changes. Unlike a mammogram, an ultrasound will not detect microcalcifications (Lewis et al., 2007).

The ACS (2007b) recommends, in addition to annual screening with mammography, the use of magnetic resonance imaging (MRI) for women with a 20% to 25% or greater lifetime risk of developing breast cancer. An MRI is not recommended as a routine screening for all eligible women due to its high cost and greater risk of false positives as compared to mammograms.

In **pelvic ultrasonography,** high-frequency sound waves are passed into the area to be examined, and images are viewed on a screen; this is similar to a radiographic film. Ultrasound is useful in detecting foreign bodies (such as intrauterine contraceptive devices [IUDs]), distinguishing between cystic and solid tumor bodies, evaluating fetal growth and viability, detecting fetal abnormalities, and detecting ectopic pregnancy. Generally it is noninvasive, safe, and painless. Encourage the patient to drink fluids beforehand. Explain that a full bladder is essential to the accuracy of the test.

Tubal insufflation (Rubin's test) involves transuterine insufflation of the fallopian tubes with carbon dioxide. The procedure enables evaluation of the patency of the fallopian tubes and may be part of a fertility study. Tubal insufflation takes approximately 30 minutes and is usually performed on an outpatient basis. If the tubes are open, the gas enters the abdominal cavity. A high-pitched bubbling is heard through the abdominal wall with a stethoscope as the gas escapes from the tubes. The patient may complain of shoulder pain from diaphragmatic irritation. In this case a radiographic film shows free gas under the diaphragm. If the tubes are occluded, gas cannot pass from the tubes, and the patient will not report pain.

All **pregnancy tests,** regardless of method, are based on detection of **human chorionic gonadotropin** (hCG), which is secreted in the urine after the fertilization of the ovum. Regardless of method, it is important to know that the tests do not indicate whether the pregnancy is normal. False-positive results may occur.

Serum CA-125 is a tumor antigen associated with ovarian cancer, since it is positive in 80% of such cases. CA-125 antigen levels in the blood decrease as the cancer cells decrease. CA-125 has been touted as a way to detect primary ovarian cancer, but unfortunately it *does not* do so. CA-125 is useful mainly to signal a recurrence of ovarian cancer and to follow the response to chemotherapy treatment. If chemotherapy causes a progressive decline in CA-125, it is an accurate indicator of a good response and is a good prognostic sign. Other conditions—such as endometriosis, PID, pregnancy, gynecologic cancers, and cancer of the pancreas—may result in an elevation of serum CA-125.

DIAGNOSTIC TESTS FOR MEN

Testicular Biopsy

Testicular biopsy is a means to detect abnormal cells and the presence of sperm. The testing can be done by aspiration or through an incision. The anesthetic used depends on the technique. Postbiopsy care measures consist of scrotal support, ice pack, and analgesic medications. Warm sitz baths for edema may also be helpful. Instruct the patient to call the physician if bleeding or elevated temperature occurs.

Semen Analysis

Semen analysis can be performed to substantiate the effectiveness of a vasectomy, to detect semen on the body or clothing of a suspected rape victim, and to rule out or determine paternity. The procedure is generally one of the first tests performed on men to evaluate fertility. Semen can be collected for testing by manual stimulation, coitus interruptus, or the use of a condom.

Prostatic Smears

Prostatic smears are obtained to detect and identify microorganisms, tumor cells, and even tuberculosis in the prostate. The physician massages the prostate by way of the rectum, and the patient voids into a sterile container prepared with additive preservative. The specimen is collected and a smear is prepared in the laboratory.

Cystoscopy

In **cystoscopy** a man's prostate and bladder can be examined by passing a lighted cystoscope through the urethra to the bladder. Before the procedure, obtain a signed consent form and educate the patient concerning the procedure. The procedure is usually performed without anesthesia, but a local anesthetic may be instilled into the bladder. After the cystoscopy the patient may have pink-tinged urine and frequency and burning on urination. Provide comfort by warm sitz baths, heat, and a mild analgesic (Lewis et al., 2007). Cystoscopy can be done for both men and women to detect bladder infections and tumors.

Other Diagnostic Studies

Other diagnostic studies for men include the rectal digital examination and the **prostate-specific antigen** (PSA), a highly sensitive blood test. PSA, which is normally secreted and disposed of by the prostate, shows up in the bloodstream in cancer of the prostate and in a harmless condition called **benign prostatic hyperplasia** or **prostate enlargement.** The normal PSA is less than 4 ng/mL. Elevated PSA levels in the bloodstream mean something needs to be checked. Even a slight increase in PSA level needs to be closely monitored; referral to a urologist for a biopsy is recommended. Still another study is the alkaline phosphatase (ALP) test. The normal ALP is 35 to 142 units/L for men, and 25 to 125 units/L for women. These specific tests are useful in diagnosing benign prostatic hypertrophy, prostatic cancer, bone metastasis in prostatic cancer, and other disease conditions (Box 52-4).

Box 52-4 Nursing Interventions for the Patient Undergoing Diagnostic Studies

- Explain the examination carefully.
- Provide privacy.
- Obtain a signed consent when necessary.
- Prepare the skin for surgery according to agency protocol.
- Assess the patient for allergies.
- If appropriate, request that the patient partially or completely disrobe and remove all jewelry. Provide gown or drape.
- Give preexamination instructions; instruct the patient to avoid food or drink, if appropriate.
- Encourage verbalization and discussion of fears.
- Administer preexamination medication as ordered by the physician.
- If necessary, advise patients to go without medications for 24 hours. Obtain a medication history.
- If the specimen is to be collected at home, stress the importance of handling all specimens precisely as directed.
- It may be necessary to monitor vital signs.
- Be attentive during examination. Offer support as necessary.
- If appropriate, relay any immediate concerns to the physician.
- Guide patients to follow any postexamination instructions.
- Inform the patient that some discomfort can be expected. Minor discomfort can be relieved by mild analgesics such as aspirin or acetaminophen, but if pain becomes more intense, notify the physician. Most discomfort is temporary.
- When pertinent, tell the patient to rest and to avoid any heavy lifting for 24 hours after the examination as directed by the physician.
- If relevant, advise the patient to avoid douching or intercourse until the site is healed. Consult the physician.
- Caution the patient to report any bleeding from an incisional area.
- Advise the patient to avoid the use of tampons as directed by the physician.
- Tell the patient how to obtain test results.

Health Promotion

Health Teaching for Menstruation

- Knowledge of the physiologic process
- Factors that may alter the menstrual cycle: stress, fatigue, exercise, acute or chronic illness, changes in climate or working hours, and pregnancy
- Personal hygiene
  —Wear pads during early period of heavy flow.
  —Change tampons frequently to decrease risk of toxic shock syndrome.
  —Consult physician if tampons cause discomfort.
  —Take a daily shower for comfort; warm baths may relieve slight pelvic discomfort.
  —Keep perineal area clean and dry; cleanse from anterior to posterior.
  —Wear cotton underwear; remember that nylon pantyhose and tight-fitting slacks retain moisture and should not be worn for extended periods.
  —Feminine hygiene products, such as vaginal sprays and suppositories, may contribute to a feeling of cleanliness.
  —A daily douche is not recommended because it changes the protective bacterial flora of the vagina and predisposes the woman to infection.
- Exercise
  —Exercise is not contraindicated and may help prevent discomfort.
  —Modify exercise if fatigue occurs.
- Diet
  —Restrict salt intake if fluid retention is present.
  —Consult a physician if fluid retention persists after menstruation.
- Discomfort
  —For mild discomfort, take aspirin, acetaminophen (Tylenol), or ibuprofen (Motrin); apply warmth; and rest.
  —For prolonged, severe discomfort, consult a physician.

THE REPRODUCTIVE CYCLE

Menarche

Menarche, the beginning of menses, designates the first menstrual cycle. Menarche occurs in late puberty and indicates that the body is capable of supporting pregnancy. Menarche occurs 2 to 2½ years after breast development (Hockenberry & Wilson, 2007), usually about 9 to 17 years of age, the average age being 12½ years. The menstrual cycle length varies from 24 to 32 days; the average cycle lasts 28 days. The flow lasts from 1 to 8 days; the average is 3 to 5 days. The amount of flow is from 10 to 75 mL; the average is 35 mL per cycle.

Help patients maintain their reproductive and sexual health by instructing or counseling women about personal hygiene. Personal cleanliness is a health habit that should be promoted for all patients and implemented in each care plan. Cleanliness is especially important during menstruation (see Health Promotion box).

DISTURBANCES OF MENSTRUATION

Because of the relationship between the menstrual cycle and the body's mechanisms of hormonal secretion, a decrease or increase in the activity of the hormonal glands can disturb menstruation. The most common disturbances include the following:

- **Amenorrhea:** absence of menstrual flow
- **Dysmenorrhea:** painful menstruation
- Abnormal uterine bleeding
- **Menorrhagia:** excessive bleeding in amount and duration
- **Metrorrhagia:** bleeding between menstrual periods

Another disturbance of the menstrual cycle is premenstrual syndrome (PMS), which is discussed later.

Suggested nursing diagnoses are *anxiety, ineffective coping, fear, pain, deficient knowledge,* and *low self-esteem.* Nursing interventions are based on specific behaviors, symptoms, and treatments.

AMENORRHEA

Amenorrhea (absence of menstrual flow) is normal before puberty, after menopause, during pregnancy, and sometimes during lactation. Menstrual flow may also be absent or suppressed as a result of hormonal abnormalities or surgical interventions such as a hysterectomy (surgical removal of the uterus).

Etiology and Pathophysiology

Amenorrhea is classified as primary when menarche has not occurred by the age of 17 to 18 years. The cause may be a congenital defect. Secondary amenorrhea means menarche has occurred but flow has ceased for at least 3 months or there has been an absence of vaginal fluid for 12 months, coupled with a history of irregular bleeding. Secondary amenorrhea may be due to normal pregnancy; frequent, vigorous exercise, as in female athletes; or an emotional disorder such as depression, anorexia (lack of appetite), or bulimia (an insatiable craving for food, often resulting in episodes of continuous eating followed by purging).

Assessment

Early diagnosis and prompt management are necessary to prevent more serious reproductive and genital problems. Urge the sexually active woman to see a physician as soon as a menstrual period is missed. Maintaining health during pregnancy is vital for both the mother and the fetus. Women who suspect their amenorrhea is caused by menopause can be examined by a physician to confirm this.

Obtaining a family history is important. Assess emotional factors or behaviors that may influence the menstrual cycle. A menstrual history includes (1) the number of periods missed and (2) whether amenorrhea was previously present. Determine recent use of medications and drugs.

Diagnostic Tests

Beyond the preliminary workup and when pregnancy is not a possibility, the diagnostic study for primary and secondary amenorrhea is the same. This study includes a pelvic examination; blood, urine, and hormonal analysis; determination of existing tumors; and a Pap test.

Medical Management

Treatment is based on the underlying cause and must be determined on an individual basis. Hormonal therapy may be needed.

Nursing Interventions and Patient Teaching

A nursing diagnosis and interventions for women with amenorrhea include but are not limited to the following:

Nursing Diagnosis	Nursing Interventions
Ineffective coping, related to lack of menstrual flow	Acknowledge patient's feelings and provide emotional support. Refer to counseling as necessary. Explain diagnostic procedures. Provide information, privacy, and consultation as indicated for sexual concerns.

Encourage patients to comply with treatment, and emphasize the importance of follow-up visits with the physician for treatment, therapy, and evaluation of treatment efficacy.

DYSMENORRHEA

Dysmenorrhea is uterine pain with menstruation, commonly called "menstrual cramps." Primary dysmenorrhea that is not associated with pelvic disorders usually develops when ovulatory function is established (less than 20 years of age) and there is no underlying organic disease. Often it disappears or declines after pregnancy or by a woman's late 20s. Secondary dysmenorrhea is painful menstruation caused by organic disease such as PID or endometriosis and most often occurs in women older than 20 years of age.

Dysmenorrhea is the greatest single cause of absenteeism among women. It is one of the most common health problems for which women seek treatment.

Etiology and Pathophysiology

The causes of dysmenorrhea can be related to endocrine imbalance; an increase in prostaglandin secretions; or chronic illnesses, fatigue, and anemia. A recent theory proposes that dysmenorrhea may be caused by hypercontractility of the uterus resulting from higher-than-normal levels of prostaglandins. Conditions that cause general debilitation, such as inadequate diet and exercise, anemia, and fatigue, are often related to dysmenorrhea.

Assessment

Many women have systemic symptoms of breast tenderness, abdominal distention, nausea and vomiting, headache, vertigo, palpitations, and excessive perspiration. Assess the woman for colicky and cyclic pain and, infrequently, dull pain in the lower pelvis that radiates toward the perineum and back. This pain may be experienced 24 to 48 hours before menses or at the onset of menses. The family history is important, since dysmenorrhea has been reported to be significantly more common among mothers and sisters of women with dysmenorrhea. Secondary dysmenorrhea is suspected if the symptoms begin after 20 years of age. It has been described as a steady or cramping pain and may be specific to the site of pelvic disorder.

Diagnostic Tests

Diagnostic studies to rule out organic causes for dysmenorrhea include pelvic examination, laparoscopy, D&C, and hysterosalpingography.

Medical Management

Treatment of secondary dysmenorrhea is aimed at the cause. Surgical and medication intervention may be appropriate, depending on the severity and underlying causes of dysmenorrhea.

If no organic cause is found, instruct the woman to exercise and eat nutritious foods, especially those high in fiber, to avoid constipation. Local applications of heat and mild analgesics are prescribed. Medications for dysmenorrhea include prostaglandin inhibitors, such as ibuprofen (Motrin, Advil) and naproxen sodium (Anaprox). Oral contraceptives may be used to suppress ovulation by inhibiting prostaglandin levels (Table 52-2).

Nursing Interventions and Patient Teaching

Nursing diagnoses and interventions for women with dysmenorrhea include but are not limited to the following:

Nursing Diagnoses	Nursing Interventions
Deficient knowledge, related to lack of education concerning disease process and treatment	Present information on disease process, procedures to be performed, medications, and treatments. Prepare for informational question-and-answer sessions according to patient needs. Teach procedures patient must know how to perform. Obtain feedback. Be certain learning has taken place; reinforce teaching as needed. Develop a trusting relationship. Involve patient in care.
Pain, related to biologic agent	Assess nature of pain. Observe nonverbal cues. Encourage pain reduction techniques as appropriate. Explore best method for controlling pain (medication, positioning, comfort measures such as back rub or use of heat or cold). Monitor vital signs. Provide quiet environment, calm activities. Promote wellness; discuss with significant other ways in which he or she can assist patient.

Encourage a positive attitude and instruct women to maintain good posture, exercise, and practice good nutrition.

ABNORMAL UTERINE BLEEDING (MENORRHAGIA AND METRORRHAGIA)

Abnormal uterine bleeding may take many forms, including menorrhagia and metrorrhagia.

Menorrhagia is excessive bleeding at the time of the regular menstrual flow. The excessive bleeding can be characterized as an increased duration (more than 7 days), increased amount (more than 80 mL), or both. In younger women it may be attributed to endocrine disturbances, but in older women it usually indicates inflammatory disturbances or uterine tumors. Uterine fibroids (also called leiomyomas) and endometrial polyps are common causes of menorrhagia in women in their 30s and 40s. Emotional or psychological problems may also affect uterine bleeding. The severity of menorrhagia is usually estimated in terms of the number of pads or tampons used in excess of those used for regular menstrual flow.

Metrorrhagia is the appearance of uterine bleeding between regular menstrual periods or after menopause. It merits early diagnosis and treatment because it may indicate cancer or benign tumors of the uterus. Endometrial cancer must be considered for postmenopausal women experiencing spotting.

Diagnosis is made through a routine speculum and pelvic examination. Endometrial biopsy and ultrasonography are also used to diagnose gynecologic causes of menorrhagia and metrorrhagia. Endometrial ablation done by laser or electrosurgical technique has been successful with many patients with menorrhagia.

Nursing interventions include (1) assess for bleeding, pain, vaginal secretions, and psychosocial concerns; (2) encourage the woman to express her feelings; (3) explain the importance of recording dates, type of flow, and number of sanitary pads or tampons used; (4) teach the patient pain-relieving techniques; and (5) explain to the patient the importance of sharing her concerns with her partner.

Table 52-2 Medications for Reproductive Disorders

Generic (Trade)	Action	Side Effects	Nursing Implications
Oral contraceptives: estrogen-progesterone combinations (Ortho Novum, Norlestrin, Ovral, Triphasil)	Inhibits ovulation by suppressing gonadotropins, FSH and LH; alters genital tract to inhibit sperm penetration and inhibit implantation	Nausea, cramps, diarrhea, appetite change, acne, rash, increased BP, thrombophlebitis, edema, dysmenorrhea, bleeding irregularities, depression, fatigue, breast changes, cholestatic jaundice, optic neuritis	Monitor glucose, thyroid function, and liver function tests; check Homans' sign for clot detection; monitor BP; discontinue if patient is pregnant.
Conjugated equine estrogen (Premarin)	Needed for proper functioning of female reproductive systems; affects release of gonadotropins; inhibits ovulation; is involved in adequate calcium use in bone structure	Nausea, peripheral edema, enlargement of breasts, breast tenderness, anorexia, vomiting, diarrhea, headache, thrombophlebitis, dizziness, depression	Notify physician of weight gain of ≥5 lb/wk (patient may need diuretic); monitor BP; check liver function test; check Homans' sign for possible clots; give IV product slowly to prevent flushing.
Butoconazole (Femstat Cream)	Same as clotrimazole	Same as terconazole	Same as clotrimazole.
Clotrimazole (Mycelex-7m, Gyne-Lotrimin, Femcare)	Interferes with fungal DNA replication; binds sterols in fungal cell membrane	Rash, urticaria, stinging, burning, peeling, blistering skin fissures, abdominal cramps, bloating, urinary frequency	Watch for allergic reactions; note therapeutic response (decrease in size and number of lesions); use gloves for application; can be used through menstrual cycle; avoid use of other vaginal creams or suppositories during therapy.
Miconazole nitrate (Monistat-3, Monistat-7)	Same as clotrimazole	Vulvovaginal burning, itching, pelvic cramps, rash, urticaria, stinging, burning, contact dermatitis	Same as clotrimazole.
Tioconazole ointment (Vagistat-1)	Same as miconazole but two to eight times more potent	Vulvovaginal burning, itching, soreness, swelling	Same as clotrimazole.
Metronidazole (Flagyl, Protostat)	Direct-acting amebicide-trichomonacide; binds, degrades DNA in organism	Rash, headache, dizziness, fatigue, convulsions, blurred vision, nausea, vomiting, diarrhea, pseudomembranous colitis, albuminuria, neurotoxicity, metallic taste, disulfiram type of reaction with alcohol	Watch for allergic reactions and superinfection; check stool for parasites; give oral form with food; watch for vision problems; tell patient not to drink alcohol during therapy.
Nystatin (Mycostatin)	Same as clotrimazole	Rash, urticaria, stinging, burning	Same as clotrimazole.
Terconazole (Terazol-7, Terazol-3)	Same as clotrimazole	Vulvovaginal burning, itching, pelvic cramps, rash, urticaria, stinging, burning	Same as clotrimazole.
Topical Nystatin (Nilstat, Mycostatin, Bio-Statin)	Interferes with fungal DNA replication; causes fungal cell membrane permeability	Rash, stinging, burning, urticaria, nausea, vomiting, anorexia, diarrhea	Watch for allergic reaction; use gloves for topical application; for vaginal preparation, tell patient that she may need protective perineal pads.

BP, Blood pressure; *DNA,* deoxyribonucleic acid; *FSH,* follicle-stimulating hormone; *IV,* intravenous; *LH,* luteinizing hormone.

Continued

Table 52-2 Medications for Reproductive Disorders—cont'd

Generic (Trade)	Action	Side Effects	Nursing Implications
Topical amphotericin B (Fungizone cream, lotion, ointment)	Binds to ergosterol, altering cell membrane permeability in susceptible fungi	Urticaria, stinging, burning, dry skin, pruritus, contact dermatitis, staining of nail lesions	Cover lesions completely after cleansing and drying well; use gloves to prevent further infection; watch for allergic reactions; tell patient that it may discolor skin and clothing.
Medroxyprogesterone acetate (Provera, Amen, Cycrin, Depo-Provera)	Inhibits secretion of pituitary gonadotropins, which acts to prevent follicular maturation and ovulation; stimulates growth in mammary tissue	Irregular bleeding, breast tenderness, masculinization of fetus, edema, cholestatic jaundice, thrombophlebitis, anorexia, acne, mental depression, weight gain or loss	Notify physician of weight gain of ≥5 lb/wk; monitor BP at beginning of treatment and periodically thereafter; check liver function test; discontinue if patient is pregnant.
Estradiol transdermal system (Estraderm)	Same as conjugated equine estrogen	Same as conjugated equine estrogen	Same as conjugated equine estrogen.
Testosterone cypionate (Andro-Cyp)	Increases weight by building body tissue; increases potassium, phosphorus, chloride, and nitrogen levels; increases bone development	Acne, flushing, gynecomastia, edema, hypercalcemia, nausea, cholestatic hepatitis, aggressive behavior, headache, anxiety, mental depression, androgenic and anabolic activity	Check weight daily; monitor BP; monitor growth rate in children; check electrolyte (potassium-sodium, chloride, calcium) and cholesterol levels; monitor liver function test.
Danazol (Danocrine)	Synthetic androgen, causes atrophy of endometrial tissue; decreases FSH and LH, which leads to amenorrhea and anovulation	Fluid retention, virilization, androgenic effects, weight gain, amenorrhea, dizziness, headache, rashes, hepatic impairment	Check weight; monitor I&O; check for edema; give with food or milk to decrease gastrointestinal upset.
Acyclovir ointment (Zovirax)	Antiviral agent, interferes with DNA synthesis needed for viral replication	Mild pain with transient burning; stinging, pruritus, rash, vulvitis	Apply ointment q 3 hr or six times daily around the clock; cover all lesions; use gloves for self-protection when applying.

I&O, intake and output.

Women of all ages need to be educated about the importance of follow-up care when abnormal uterine bleeding is initially detected.

PREMENSTRUAL SYNDROME

PMS occurs in 30% to 50% of women between 25 and 45 years of age. It differs from dysmenorrhea because it has no relation to ovulation.

Etiology and Pathophysiology

The etiology and pathophysiology are not well understood. PMS is believed to be related to the neuroendocrine events occurring within the anterior pituitary gland. A loss of intravascular fluid into the body tissues causes water retention, bloating, and weight gain. PMS is thought to have a biologic trigger with compounding psychosocial issues. Some women have a genetic predisposition to PMS. Other proposed causes of PMS include estrogen and progesterone imbalances and nutritional deficiencies of pyridoxine (vitamin B_6) or magnesium. **Premenstrual dysphoric disorder** (PMD-D) is the term applied to a type of PMS that includes a severe mood disorder.

PMS occurs 7 to 10 days before the menstrual period and usually subsides within the first 3 days after the onset of the menstrual flow. Evaluate sodium intake and the use of alcohol, tobacco, and caffeine as possible causes.

Clinical Manifestations

Symptoms are multiple and vary among individuals. Behavioral symptoms include anxiety, mood swings, irritability, lethargy (inactivity), fatigue, sleep disturbances, and depression. Physical symptoms—such as headache, vertigo, backache, breast tenderness, abdominal distention, acne, paresthesia (burning or tingling) of hands and feet, and allergies—appear or may become worse. Many symptoms appear alone or in combination with other symptoms. Some women accept the symptoms as being normal and only seek medical help after the symptoms become severe.

Assessment

Subjective data are specific symptoms experienced by each woman. Ask each patient to maintain a log for three consecutive menstrual cycles and to note symptoms and activities that relate to the menstrual period. The collected information can be analyzed and symptoms treated accordingly.

Objective data pertinent to the syndrome include the inability to perform activities of daily living (ADLs) in the multiple roles of a wife, a mother, and a career person.

Diagnostic Tests

PMS is diagnosed only after eliminating other possible causes for the symptoms. A focused health history and a physical examination are done to identify any underlying conditions, such as thyroid dysfunction, uterine fibroids, or depression, that may account for the symptoms. No definitive diagnostic test is available for PMS. When PMS or PMD-D is a possible diagnosis, a woman keeps a record of her symptoms for two or three menstrual cycles (Lewis et al., 2007). Tests include evaluation of estrogen and progesterone levels to rule out hormonal imbalances and determination of glucose levels; low levels may lead to irritability.

Medical Management

PMS has no single treatment and no specific medication. Some physicians prescribe analgesics, diuretics, and progesterone. Review the patient's diet. The patient should eat a diet high in complex carbohydrates, moderate in protein, and low in refined sugar and sodium, especially during the premenstrual interval. Supplements of vitamin B_6, calcium, and magnesium may be administered as prescribed. She should reduce or eliminate caffeine (in chocolate, tea, coffee, or other beverages), and alcohol and smoking. Encourage regular exercise three or four times a week for 30 minutes, especially during the premenstrual interval. Exercise results in release of endorphins, leading to mood elevation. Techniques for stress reduction include yoga, meditation, imagery, and biofeedback training. Because fatigue may exaggerate PMS symptoms, adequate rest, sleep, and relaxation are helpful. For reducing cramping pain, backache, and headache, prostaglandin inhibitors such as ibuprofen are used. For anxiety, buspirone (BuSpar) taken during the luteal phase of the menstrual cycle has helped some women. Women with PMD-D may benefit from antidepressants, including fluoxetine (Prozac, Sarafem) and tricyclic antidepressants such as amitriptyline (Elavil). Selective serotonin reuptake inhibitors (SSRIs) such as sertraline (Zoloft) have provided significant relief to women with severe PMS (Lewis et al., 2007).

Nursing Interventions and Patient Teaching

A nursing diagnosis and interventions for the woman with PMS include but are not limited to the following:

Nursing Diagnosis	Nursing Interventions
Anxiety, related to PMS	Encourage verbalization of feelings. Acknowledge existence of syndrome and its symptoms. Encourage patient to keep a menstrual symptom diary to document the cycle and nature of the symptoms. Encourage patient to plan activities during the symptom-free part of her cycle. Administer supplements of vitamin B_6, calcium, and magnesium as prescribed. Encourage attending self-help groups and reading self-help literature; group support tends to reduce stress. Provide emotional support in a nonjudgmental and caring manner. Assist in identifying possible sources of anxiety and coping mechanisms.

The patient should take responsibility for following a dietary plan of eating small meals and restricting or eliminating sugar, alcohol, caffeine, and nicotine; this may minimize the symptoms of PMS or PMD-D.

MENOPAUSE

The climacteric is the phase of the aging process of women and men who are making a transition from a reproductive phase to a nonreproductive stage of life. This phase occurs in middle adulthood and marks the onset of physical changes, a decrease in hormone secretion, and the cessation of ovulation and menses. The female climacteric is called **menopause.** Menopause is the normal cessation of menses; menstrual flow appears on an infrequent cycle for a time, usually less than 2 years. However, as long as the menstrual cycle occurs, no matter how infrequently, ovulation continues and the potential for conception exists.

Etiology and Pathophysiology

Menopause is the normal decline of ovarian function resulting from the aging process. Menopause begins in most women between 42 and 58 years of age (the average age being 51) and is characterized by infrequent ovulation, decreased menstrual function, and eventual cessation of the menstrual flow. Factors that have been linked to an earlier age at menopause include higher body mass index; cigarette smoking; and racial, ethnic, and socioeconomic factors (Santoro & Chervenak, 2004). Menopause is a milestone in a woman's life that is embedded in her own personality and her culture (Santoro & Chervenak, 2004).

Menopause may be artificially induced by such procedures as irradiation of the ovaries or surgical removal of both ovaries. Both cause menopause with all its physiologic changes, whereas ovaries left intact after a hysterectomy continue to function provided the woman has not yet reached the age of the climacteric. Menopause also may occur earlier due to illness, side effects of chemotherapy, or drugs.

Decline in ovarian function produces a variety of symptoms, including a decrease in the frequency, amount, and duration of the menstrual flow; spotting; amenorrhea; and **polymenorrhea** (increased number of menstrual periods). Symptoms can last from a few months to several years before menstruation ceases permanently. Menopause is not considered complete until 1 year after the last menstrual period.

Clinical Manifestations

Physical changes that occur in the body do not generally develop until after permanent cessation of menstruation. Changes of the reproductive system include shrinkage of vulval structures, atrophic vulvitis, shortening of the vagina, and dryness of the vaginal wall. A relaxation of supporting pelvic structures results from the decrease in estrogen. Cystitis and urinary frequency and urgency may appear as a result of changes in the urinary system. There is loss of skin turgor and elasticity; increased subcutaneous fat; decreased breast tissue; and thinning of hair of the axilla, the head, and the pubis. About 25% of postmenopausal women develop osteoporosis.

Assessment

Subjective data include a family history. Determine whether family members and significant others are aware of the transition and whether they are supportive. Note emotional illness, if present. Hot flashes caused by glandular imbalances may become prominent. Other symptoms may include fatigue, vertigo, headache, nausea, **dyspareunia** (painful intercourse), palpitations, and chest and neck pain. Some experience a feeling of being unwanted, and some may fear growing old; both feelings could cause depression.

Collection of **objective data** includes an awareness that some patients may display frequent crying spells or outbursts of anger. Explore the use of contraceptives. Assess frequency, amount, and duration of the menstrual flow. Diaphoresis, weight gain, vomiting, and tachycardia may occur.

Diagnostic Tests

Tests include analysis of hormonal levels. Other diagnostic testing may be indicated by specific symptoms. Some examinations are performed to rule out conditions such as cancer.

Medical Management

The status of hormone replacement therapy (HRT) for postmenopausal women has undergone a radical reversal in the past several years. The Women's Health Initiative (WHI), sponsored by the National Institutes of Health, has conducted extensive research on the effects of HRT on women's health. The findings demonstrated that long-term use of an HRT estrogen-progestin combination heightened the risk of ischemic stroke, coronary heart disease, breast cancer that is at a more advanced stage at the time of diagnosis (Chlebowski et al., 2003), ovarian cancer, and thromboembolism. In 2003 further analysis of WHI data found hormone use to increase the risk of cognitive decline in a small percentage of those who receive it (Yeh, 2007).

As a result of these studies, the American Congress of Obstetricians and Gynecologists, the National Institutes of Health (the study's sponsor), and the FDA recommend that women take the lowest effective dose of HRT for the shortest possible time to relieve menopausal symptoms (Akert, 2003).

Nurses are in a good position to apprise their patients of the benefits, risks, and appropriate uses of HRT. HRT is used for short-term treatment of moderate to severe symptoms of menopause, such as hot flashes, night sweats, and vaginal dryness. At present, there are no data that might indicate how long HRT can be taken without the risk of cardiovascular or other adverse effects, and it is not known whether lower dosages lessen the risk of complications. In women with moderate to severe menopausal symptoms, it is assumed that risk can be minimized by providing HRT therapy only until the severe symptoms disappear and using the lowest effective dosage. Low-dose alternatives in HRT include low-dose Prempro, containing either 0.45 mg conjugated estrogens and 1.5 mg medroxyprogesterone, or 0.3 mg conjugated estrogens and 1.5 mg medroxyprogesterone; or low-dose intravaginal estrogen products, such as estrogen topical vaginal cream (Premarin vaginal cream or Estrace) and low-dose vaginal rings. Because of the later diagnosis of breast cancer and colon cancer in women receiving combination HRT, closely scrutinize any abnormal mammogram and screen for colon cancer as part of the follow-up.

Most physicians recommend calcium and vitamin D supplements, which are available in many forms; the generic calcium carbonate products are the most cost effective.

Herbs such as soy or black cohash are used to decrease menopausal symptoms. Patients should consult their health care provider before taking these products (Ulbricht & Basch, 2005).

SSRIs, including the antidepressants paroxetine (Paxil), fluoxetine, and venlafaxine (Effexor), are an effective alternative to HRT in reducing hot flashes, even if the user is not depressed. Also known to relieve hot flashes are clonidine (Catapres), an antihypertensive drug, and gabapentin (Neurontin), an antiseizure drug (Lewis et al., 2007).

Nonhormonal Therapy

To relieve menopausal symptoms without the risks of HRT, several methods to decrease heat produced by the body and promote heat loss have been recommended. Reducing intake of caffeine and alcohol lowers the production of body heat. Suggestions to promote heat loss at night when hot flashes interfere with sleep include increasing air circulation, using light covers and loose-fitting clothing, and placing cool cloths on flushed areas. The daily use of 800 international units of vitamin E has been recommended to reduce hot flashes (Lewis et al., 2007).

Nursing Interventions and Patient Teaching

Education regarding menopause should occur before its onset. Many women appreciate opportunities to discuss menopause. Set up an exercise program that includes both movement and weight bearing to slow bone loss and modify coronary artery disease risk factors (Lewis et al., 2007). Walking is an excellent weight-bearing exercise. Other exercises include bicycling, stationary cycling, and aerobic dancing three or four times per week.

Nursing diagnoses and interventions for the menopausal patient include but are not limited to the following:

Nursing Diagnoses	Nursing Interventions
Situational low self-esteem, related to concerns about femininity, sexuality, and aging	Encourage patient and significant others to verbalize concerns. Confirm accurate information. Correct information related to self-concept issues. Avoid value judgments. Refer patient to couple, family, and sex therapy as appropriate. Provide understanding and support.
Deficient knowledge, regarding patient's physiologic and psychological changes, related to menopause	Explain the process of climacteric and menopause, at a level the patient can understand. Explain importance of keeping fit, eating a well-balanced diet, getting adequate rest and sleep, avoiding stress and fatigue, and continuing contraception until indicated by physician. If estrogen replacement therapy is ordered, inform patient about side effects. Instruct patient to report any vaginal bleeding occurring 6 months or more after last menstrual period. Inform patient of the availability of water-soluble lubricants if needed before coitus.

For patient teaching, emphasize that the climacteric is normal and self-limiting and that menopause is not the end of the patient's sex life. A nutritious diet and weight control will improve physical condition, and an exercise program will promote vitality. Interest and participation in various activities help decrease anxiety and tension. Skin creams and lotions can be used to prevent drying, pruritus, and cracking skin. Encourage the woman to perform breast self-examination (BSE) monthly and monitor calcium intake. Contraceptives should be used for 1 year after the last menstrual period. The patient can obtain a prescription for treatment of pruritus or burning of the vulva. Women can practice Kegel exercises regularly to strengthen pelvic muscles (see Health Promotion box). A water-soluble lubricant, such as KY Jelly, can be used to prevent dyspareunia. Explain the side effects of any medications or hormonal therapy. Emphasize that an annual physical examination is important for maintaining good health.

MALE CLIMACTERIC

Etiology and Pathophysiology

The climacteric is less pronounced in men and often may not even be apparent. The appearance of the climacteric phase is gradual and occurs between 55 and

Health Promotion

Kegel Exercises

Kegel exercises are performed to help strengthen and tighten muscles that support the pelvic organs. These muscles (pelvic floor) are used to stop the flow of urine. To perform Kegel exercises while standing or sitting, tighten the pelvic floor muscles as hard as you can. Hold for 5 seconds, then release. Repeat at least 10 times. This exercise can be done as many as 40 to 50 times each day.

70 years of age. There is a gradual decrease of testosterone levels and seminal fluid production. The impact is largely psychological, possibly because of the recognition of some reduction of sexual activity and interests.

Clinical Manifestations

Manifestations are mostly physiologic changes. Erections require more time and are not as full or firm. The prostate gland enlarges, and secretions diminish; seminal fluid decreases. The physical changes occur as the man grows older, and the most noticeable signs are loss or thinning of hair from the head, chest, axillae, and pubis. There may be some flushing and chilling. Muscle tone is decreased.

Assessment

Collection of **subjective data** reveals that the man is generally at the peak of his career or possibly considering retirement. He interprets his decreased sexual needs as a loss of productivity and sexual power. Therefore the assessment should invite verbalization of emotions with coping mechanisms.

Collection of **objective data** includes assessment of behaviors that may be causing the man stress and concern. Ask him to explore changes he has noted regarding his lifestyle and feelings of loss of self-worth.

Diagnostic Tests

Diagnostic tests include a complete physical examination to rule out abnormalities of structure and function.

Nursing Interventions and Patient Teaching

A nursing diagnosis and interventions for men experiencing male climacteric include but are not limited to the following:

Nursing Diagnosis	Nursing Interventions
Ineffective coping, related to situational crisis (climacteric)	Show understanding and concern. Assist patient in identifying how the problem affects his life and future, his family, and significant others. Encourage patient to talk about factors that could be influencing the way he sees the problem. Assist patient in identifying strengths and coping skills and the nature and strength of situational support. Collect data about current and potential sources of support. Assist patient in planning alternative solutions. Give positive reinforcement.

Inform the patient that the climacteric is normal. Encourage the patient to verbalize his fears and to seek counseling if stress increases.

ERECTILE DYSFUNCTION

Erectile dysfunction (ED) is a man's inability to attain or maintain an erect penis that allows satisfactory sexual performance. Several forms are recognized: (1) functional ED, which has a psychological basis; (2) anatomical ED, which results from a physical defect of genital structures; and (3) atonic ED, which involves disturbed neuromuscular function. Some neurologic abnormalities that affect erectile function are tabes dorsalis, caused by advanced syphilis; congenital spinal cord anomalies, such as spina bifida; spinal cord tumors; amyotrophic lateral sclerosis (Lou Gehrig's disease); multiple sclerosis; or cord compression caused by a herniated disk. Radical prostatectomy often leads to ED. Nerve-sparing surgery can decrease this occurrence.

ED can potentially interfere with a man's self-esteem, relationships, confidence, and sense of well-being. The prevalence alone makes ED a significant condition. About 20 million to 30 million men in the United States experience ED. ED may occur at any age; however, it is estimated that 50% of men between 40 and 70 years old have some degree of ED. ED in younger men is often a result of substance abuse, including alcohol or recreational drugs. Medical conditions that are associated with ED are diabetes mellitus, hypertension, renal disorders, cancer, coronary artery bypass surgery, and organ transplants. Men have a longer life expectancy than in past generations and expect to remain sexually active (Lewis et al., 2007). The nurse can best understand ED by developing a broad understanding of the factors that contribute to the condition.

Medical Management

Medical treatment is based on careful assessment of the causative factors. It is known that medications such as antihypertensives, antidepressants, antihyperlipidemics, diuretics, drugs for Parkinson's disease, marijuana, cocaine, antianxiety agents, and some cardiac agents may cause ED. Illicit or abused substances such as alcohol, cocaine, and nicotine are also known to cause ED. Disease conditions, such as diabetes mellitus or end-stage renal, heart, and chronic obstructive pulmonary disease, may also be causative factors.

A drug named sildenafil citrate (Viagra) is prescribed as an oral therapy for ED. The physiologic mechanism of erection of the penis involves release of nitric oxide in the corpus cavernosum during sexual stimulation. The drug enhances smooth muscle relaxation and the inflow of blood in the corpus cavernosum, thus allowing erection to occur. For most patients, the recommended dosage is 50 mg taken as needed approximately 1 hour before engaging in sexual activity. However, sildenafil may be taken anywhere from a half hour to 4 hours before sexual activity. Sildenafil has been shown to potentiate the hypotensive effects of nitrates; therefore its administration to patients who are using nitrates (either regularly or intermittently) in any form is contraindicated. Tadalafil (Cialis) is another antiimpotence agent for ED contraindicated for concurrent use with nitrates, nitric oxide, or alpha-adrenergic blockers. It should not be used in patients who have unstable angina, recent history of stroke, life-threatening heart failure, uncontrolled hypertension, or myocardial infarction within 90 days. For most patients, the recommended dosage is 10 mg before sexual activity (range 5 to 20 mg; not to exceed one dose in 24 hours). A third antiimpotence agent is vardenafil (Levitra) 10 mg, taken 1 hour before sexual activity (range 5 to 20 mg, no more than once daily). This drug is not to be used with nitrates because of an unsafe decrease in blood pressure, which could result in myocardial infarction or stroke (Skidmore-Roth, 2010).

Mechanical devices are available for the patient with ED. Surgical implantation of a penile prosthesis may be performed as a same-day procedure or may require hospitalization for 5 or more days, depending on the patient and the device used (Figure 52-8).

Nursing Interventions and Patient Teaching

The nurse is responsible for teaching the patient to administer hormonal medication (testosterone) and to watch for side effects. Advise the patient to take oral hormonal replacement drugs with meals to prevent nausea. Inform the patient about signs and symptoms of infection of the implant, including tenderness of the penis, fever, dysuria, and signs of urinary tract infection. Tell the patient to seek medical attention promptly if infection occurs.

INFERTILITY

Etiology and Pathophysiology

Infertility is defined as the inability to conceive after 1 year of sexual intercourse without birth control measures. Primary infertility refers to couples who have never conceived. Secondary infertility refers to couples who have conceived but are now unable to do so.

A woman's age has a significant bearing on her ability to conceive. Women are most fertile between 20 and 29 years of age, whereas men are most fertile in their late teens and early 20s. A man's fertility does not decrease much as he grows older, but a woman's fertility drops dramatically and decreases with menopause.

Infertility may be caused by impaired sperm or ova production or an occlusion in the reproductive system that prevents the sperm and ovum from meeting. Infections of the reproductive tract (such as PID) and STIs (such as syphilis) are frequently associated with infertility. Because the man may be the infertile partner in 40% of the cases of infertility, the quality and quantity of his sperm must be analyzed. The primary causes of infertility in women are tubal insufficiency and ovarian and uterine conditions, such as endometriosis or congenital defects.

Assessment

Collection of **subjective** and **objective data** includes physical examination and health histories for both partners to make the infertility assessment and prepare a treatment plan.

Diagnostic Tests

Specific testing is necessary to rule out systemic diseases such as diabetes mellitus, neoplasms, hepatic and renal diseases, and viral conditions. Genetic defects and disorders of the testes are explored. Diagnostic testing can produce a great deal of anxiety and stress. This testing may continue for fairly long periods with or without favorable results. Male testing is somewhat simpler and usually less expensive than female testing. If there is reason to suspect the man is infertile or sterile, it is appropriate to test him first. Male infertility testing includes semen analysis, which measures the quantity and quality of semen, volume of sperm cells, sperm motility, and sperm density; and endocrine imbalance testing, which explores possible disruption of the pituitary gonadotropins and testosterone production.

Female testing focuses on the ovulation process and function of the reproductive organs. The testing in-

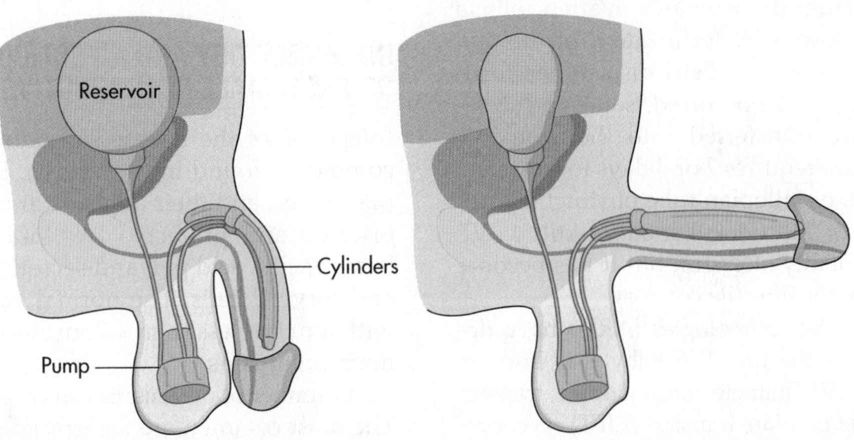

FIGURE 52-8 The Scott inflatable prosthesis has erect and flaccid positions designed to mimic normal erectile function.

cludes (1) basal body temperature to assess ovulation; (2) endometrial biopsy, which confirms ovulation and endometrial cyclic changes; (3) endocrine studies to assess the functioning of the adrenal and thyroid glands with anovulation cycles; (4) Rubin's insufflation test, which determines tubal patency; and (5) hysterosalpingography and hysterography to assess the position and alignment of the reproductive organs.

Male and female interaction studies include (1) Huhner's test, which examines the cervical mucus for motile sperm cells after intercourse, at midmenstrual cycle; (2) immunologic or immunoglobulin (antibody) testing for detection of spermicidal antibodies in the woman's sera; and (3) testing both the man and woman for normalcy of their sex chromosomes.

Medical Management

The management of infertility problems depends on the cause. If infertility is secondary to an alteration in ovarian function, supplemental hormone therapy may be attempted to restore and maintain ovulation. Drugs used to induce ovulation include clomiphene citrate (Clomid), and bromocriptine (Parlodel). These drugs increase the risk for multiple births. When an actual mechanical tubal blockage exists, a reparative microsurgical procedure can be done.

Poor cervical mucus may be a result of chronic cervicitis or inadequate estrogenic stimulation. Careful cauterization of the cervix may eradicate the chronic cervicitis, and the administration of estrogens can improve the quantity and quality of the cervical mucus.

Improving the patient's general health may help, especially when a debilitating or chronic illness is present. Eliminating or reducing psychological stress can improve the emotional climate, making it more conducive to achieving a pregnancy. Education of the couple regarding the probable time of ovulation and appropriate coital technique may also be indicated.

When a couple has not succeeded in conceiving even with infertility management, another option is intrauterine insemination with the partner's or a donor's sperm. If this technique does not succeed, **in vitro fertilization** (IVF) may be used. IVF is the removal of mature oocytes from the woman's ovarian follicle via laparoscopy, followed by fertilization of the ova with the partner's sperm in a Petri dish. When fertilization and cleavage have occurred, some of the resulting embryos are transferred into the woman's uterus. The procedure requires 2 or 3 days to complete and is used in cases of fallopian tube obstruction, decreased sperm count, and unexplained infertility. IVF is costly and emotionally stressful, but it has become an accepted therapy for infertile couples.

Assisted reproductive technologies (ARTs) have developed rapidly since the first IVF baby was born in 1978. ARTs include IVF, gamete intrafallopian transfer (GIFT), zygote intrafallopian transfer (ZIFT), cryopreserved embryo transfer (CPE), and donor oocyte programs. Current research could lead to a rapid expansion of these techniques in the next decade. With the increased knowledge of freezing techniques for embryos (CPE), couples will have increased pregnancy potential. Research is also investigating the replication of normal tubal secretions. This tubal factor is important because the pregnancy rate is higher with GIFT and ZIFT than with IVF. Finally, the development of embryo biopsy and genetic engineering may allow for preconception techniques for those couples with identified genetic abnormalities. It also raises the possibility of gender selection. Thus noncoital reproduction poses many ethical, legal, and social concerns. All decisions related to infertility are influenced by the couple's age, their wishes, and the length of time they have been attempting to conceive.

Nursing Interventions and Patient Teaching

The nurse has a major responsibility for teaching and providing emotional support throughout the infertility testing and treatment period. Feelings of anger, frustration, sadness, and helplessness between partners and between the couple and health care providers may increase as more tests are performed. Infertility can generate great tension in a marriage as the couple exhausts their financial and emotional resources. Few insurance carriers cover the cost of infertility testing or the therapeutic measures associated with infertility. Shame and guilt may arise when other people become involved in such an intimate area of a relationship.

Recognizing and dealing with the psychological and emotional factors that surface can assist the couple in coping with the situation. Encourage couples to participate in a support group for infertile couples and in individual therapy. Continue providing information and emotional support as therapeutic measures are attempted. Give couples ample opportunity to plan what is financially realistic; each GIFT and ZIFT attempt can exceed $10,000 and each IVF treatment costs $4500 to $6000.

Prognosis

Approximately 50% of couples who undergo assessment and treatment for infertility are likely to conceive.

INFLAMMATORY AND INFECTIOUS DISORDERS OF THE FEMALE REPRODUCTIVE TRACT

Infections of the female reproductive tract are most commonly found in the vagina, the cervix, the fallopian tubes, and their adjacent areas. The vagina is lubricated and protected by flora containing Döderlein's bacilli, acid pH, and secretions from the vaginal and cervical cells. The normal vaginal environment, with a pH of less than 4.2, protects against growth of microorganisms.

A number of organisms can cause vaginal infections. The most common are *Escherichia coli, Candida albicans,* and *Trichomonas vaginalis.* Infections are more likely to occur when the flora and the acidity of the vagina are disturbed by medications (birth control pills, antibiotics), stress, malnutrition, douching, aging, and disease. Yeast organisms grow best in an acid pH (−4.7), whereas *Trichomonas* and organisms causing nonspecific vaginitis flourish on a pH that is more alkaline (5+).

Organisms are often introduced from external sources by way of unclean douche nozzles, poor hygiene, inadequate handwashing, neglected nail care, soiled clothing, and intercourse. Vaginal infections can be sexually transmitted and will return unless both partners are treated. Predisposing factors include poor nutrition, inconsistent control of blood glucose levels in those with diabetes mellitus, stress, pregnancy, marked hormonal fluctuations, pH changes, and antibiotics (Lewis et al., 2007).

SIMPLE VAGINITIS

Etiology and Pathophysiology

Vaginitis is a common vaginal infection. It is usually caused by *E. coli,* an organism found in feces and the rectum. It may be caused by staphylococcal and streptococcal organisms, *T. vaginalis* (a flagellated protozoan), *C. albicans* (a yeastlike fungus), and *Gardnerella* bacillus.

Vaginitis is an inflammation of the vagina. If the patient changes perineal pads or tampons infrequently, the vaginal tract and inner groin become irritated. This creates a medium suitable for organism growth. Examination of the vaginal walls will show a profuse foamy (bubbly) exudate if the vaginitis is caused by *T. vaginalis.* If *C. albicans* is the causative agent, a thick, cheeselike discharge results. Bacterial vaginitis produces a malodorous milky discharge.

Clinical Manifestations

The exudate in vaginitis is yellow, white, or grayish white; curdlike; and generally accompanied by pruritus, burning, and edema of the surrounding tissue. Voiding and defecation generally intensify the symptoms.

Assessment

Subjective data include menstrual history, age at menarche, length of cycles, duration and nature of flow, dysfunctions, birth control methods, medications taken, family history of diabetes mellitus, previous vaginal infections, and STIs. Ask about sexual practices and signs of infection in the sex partner. Dysuria may occur as a consequence of local irritation of the urinary meatus.

Collection of **objective data** includes observation for excoriations of the skin caused by scratching, in which case secondary infection may result. Observe the specific type of exudate.

Diagnostic Tests

Diagnostic tests include direct visual examination of the vagina, culture of the organism, and bimanual examination to assess for inflammation of the vagina and its surrounding tissues.

Medical Management

Vaginal infection can be treated by a variety of methods. The major goals of treatment are to (1) cure the infection, (2) prevent reinfection, (3) prevent complications, and (4) prevent infection of the sexual partner(s). Douching is frequently prescribed for treatment, as are local applications of vaginal suppositories, ointments, and creams. Advise the patient to use the medication at bedtime and to remain recumbent for more than 30 minutes after insertion to allow absorption and prevent loss of any medication from the vagina. The patient may require oral medications appropriate to the organism. During treatment the patient should refrain from intercourse or request that her partner use a condom (see Table 52-2).

Nursing Interventions and Patient Teaching

Advise the patient of the importance of handwashing before and after vaginal application of medications. Heat may be applied in the form of douches, perineal irrigations, or sitz baths. Douching too frequently can alter normal vaginal flora. Discourage douching unless specifically prescribed by the health care provider.

Nursing diagnoses and interventions for the patient with vaginitis include but are not limited to the following:

Nursing Diagnoses	Nursing Interventions
Pain, related to vaginal discharge	Flush vagina with acid douche (15 mL white vinegar with 1000 mL water) as ordered. Apply antibiotic creams after douche as ordered. Provide sitz bath for edema.
Risk for infection, related to STIs	Administer medication and treatments as ordered. Teach preventive methods, such as use of condoms. Recommend that partner be checked for infection and treated as necessary to avoid reinfection.

Most patients with vaginal infections are directed to abstain from sexual intercourse during treatment. The male partner's use of a condom until the symptoms of infection disappear may be advised. Also inform the patient that her sexual partner should be treated.

Prognosis

With proper treatment, the prognosis is good.

SENILE VAGINITIS OR ATROPHIC VAGINITIS

This condition occurs in women after menopause and as they age. Low estrogen levels cause the vulva and vagina to atrophy and become susceptible to the invasion of bacteria. The exudate causes pruritus, edema, and skin irritations. Estrogen, vaginal suppositories, and ointments may be prescribed.

CERVICITIS

Cervicitis (infection of the cervix) is one of the most common diseases of the reproductive system. The infection is caused by vaginal infection or STIs, such as *Chlamydia trachomatis* infection, gonorrhea, herpes type 2, or trichomoniasis. The infection often follows childbirth or abortion in which lacerations occur. Therapy is specific to the causative organisms. Symptoms are backaches, whitish exudate, or pink-tinged menstrual discharge and dyspareunia. If cervicitis remains untreated, the tissues are continually irritated and the infection may spread to other pelvic organs. Personal hygiene and frequent warm tub baths can minimize odor and discomfort. Local applications of vaginal suppositories, ointments, and creams are usually prescribed. Drug therapy also includes azithromycin (Zithromax) 1 g orally as single dose or doxycycline (Vibramycin) 100 mg orally twice a day for 7 days; treat the partner with the same drugs (Lewis et al., 2007).

PELVIC INFLAMMATORY DISEASE

PID is any acute, subacute, recurrent, or chronic infection that may involve the cervix (cervicitis), uterus (endometritis), fallopian tubes (salpingitis), or ovaries (oophoritis) and may extend to the connective tissues lying between the broad ligaments.

Etiology and Pathophysiology

The most common causative organisms are *Neisseria gonorrhoeae,* streptococci, staphylococci, chlamydiae, and tubercle bacilli. PID can follow the insertion of a biopsy curette or an irrigation catheter, abortion, pelvic surgery, sexual intercourse, or pregnancy. The condition may occur with or without gonorrheal infection and may be mild or severe.

When conditions or procedures alter or destroy the cervical mucus, bacteria ascend into the uterine cavity. Pelvic examination and movement of the reproductive organs become painful. PID is serious because it may cause adhesions and sterility. Sexually active women with more than one partner are at increased risk for PID.

Clinical Manifestations

Signs and symptoms are temperature elevation, chills, severe abdominal pain, malaise, nausea and vomiting, and malodorous purulent vaginal exudate.

Assessment

Subjective data relate to the severity of the disorder, pain, time of onset, and frequency (primary infection or continuous reinfection). Sexual history, pelvic examinations, and pelvic procedures are important because they may reveal the origin of the pathogen. The patient may complain of lower abdominal and pelvic pain, dysmenorrhea, dysuria, and vulvar pruritus.

Objective data include the patient's knowledge, level of discomfort, and coping mechanisms. Assess the patient for fever and chills and the amount and characteristics of vaginal discharge. The vaginal discharge is purulent to thin and mucoid.

Diagnostic Tests

Diagnostic tests include Gram stains of secretions from the endocervix, urethra, and rectum. Culture and sensitivity testing identifies organisms and is helpful in selecting antibiotics for treatment. Laparoscopic visualization of the pelvic inflammation may be necessary to confirm the extent of infection. Vaginal ultrasonic examinations can aid in diagnosing abscesses and monitoring the treatment and healing process. The leukocyte count and erythrocyte sedimentation rate are elevated.

Medical Management

The goal of treatment is to control and eradicate the infection by preventing it from spreading to other body systems. Treatment includes systemic antibiotics administered intravenously or intramuscularly. The antibiotics of choice are usually cefoxitin (Mefoxin) and doxycycline to provide thorough coverage against the responsible pathogens. The patient must refrain from having intercourse for 3 weeks. The patient's partner(s) must be examined and treated as well. Pain control, rest, and adequate fluid intake are essential to the care. A corticosteroid is often added to the antibiotic treatment to aid in more rapid recovery and improvement in maintaining fertility (Lewis et al., 2007).

Nursing Interventions and Patient Teaching

The patient is usually hospitalized to isolate the organism and plan the treatment. Inform the patient and those assisting with the care of all specific precautions and observe standard precautions. Use goggles if any splashing is likely. Nursing interventions include (1) assessing pain and administering prescribed analgesics as needed; (2) monitoring vital signs and progress of treatment; (3) providing fluids to avoid dehydration; (4) performing palliative measures for comfort such as bathing, changing of perineal pads, personal hygiene, and warm douches; (5) providing patient support with a positive, nonjudgmental attitude; and (6) positioning the patient in Fowler's position to facilitate drainage.

Nursing diagnoses and interventions for the patient with PID include but are not limited to the following:

Nursing Diagnoses	Nursing Interventions
Pain, related to infection process	Manage pain with analgesics as ordered; assess effectiveness of pain-relief measures. Provide comfort measures.

Nursing Diagnoses	Nursing Interventions
Ineffective coping, related to condition	Provide emotional support. Encourage verbalization of feelings. Provide therapeutic environment for patient.
Ineffective health maintenance, related to insufficient knowledge of condition and complications	Teach patient about the significance of PID and the importance of complying with medication therapy.

Discharge planning should include patient teaching and instructions for (1) contacting the physician if a low-grade fever persists or purulent vaginal discharge occurs; (2) understanding the significance of the pelvic inflammatory condition; (3) complying with medication therapy; (4) observing handwashing technique and practices of personal hygiene, such as bathing, avoidance of tampons, frequent changing of perineal pads, and clean clothing; (5) understanding the importance of the sexual partner being examined and treated to avoid recurrence of the PID; and (6) recognizing that intercourse is sometimes painful after PID and that sexual activity should be avoided until advised by a physician.

Prognosis

Women with PID are usually of childbearing age. PID can lead to complications such as adhesions and strictures of the fallopian tubes, infertility, and increased risk of ectopic pregnancy (Lewis et al., 2007). With adequate treatment, the prognosis is good.

TOXIC SHOCK SYNDROME

Etiology and Pathophysiology

Toxic shock syndrome (TSS) is an acute bacterial infection caused by *Staphylococcus aureus.* It usually occurs in women who are menstruating and using tampons (particularly superabsorbent tampons). If the tampon is left in place too long, the bacteria may proliferate and release toxins into the bloodstream, causing TSS. Women at the greatest risk are those who insert tampons with their fingers instead of with inserters, women with chronic vaginal infections, and women with genital herpes. TSS can also occur in nonmenstruating women.

Clinical Manifestations

Often the patient has flulike symptoms for the first 24 hours. Between days 2 and 4 of the menstrual period, the patient may have an elevated temperature (up to 102° F [39° C]), vomiting, dizziness, headache, diarrhea, myalgia, hypotension, and signs suggesting the onset of septic shock. Sore throat, headache, and a red macular palmar or diffuse rash followed by desquamation of the skin, hands, and feet may develop; urinary output is decreased, and the blood urea nitrogen (BUN) level is elevated. Disorientation may occur from dehydration and the release of toxins. Pulmonary edema and inflammation of mucous membranes may occur.

Assessment

Collection of **subjective data** includes determining whether the patient has recently used tampons and how long she used a single tampon before changing it. Obtain information about myalgia, sore throat, headache, and fatigue.

Collection of **objective data** includes assessing for edema. Assess the palms and soles for an erythematous rash. Desquamation and sloughing occur within 1 to 2 weeks after the rash. Note the patient's level of consciousness. Hypotension is a sign of TSS, as are nonpurulent inflammation of the conjunctiva and hyperemia of the oropharynx and vagina.

Diagnostic Tests

There is no definitive test for TSS. However, cervical-vaginal isolates of *S. aureus* are present 90% of the time. Blood tests demonstrate leukocytosis; thrombocytopenia; and elevated levels of bilirubin, BUN, creatinine, serum glutamic-pyruvic transaminase (alanine aminotransferase), serum glutamic-oxaloacetic transaminase (aspartate aminotransferase), and creatine phosphokinase. Blood and urine cultures should be taken along with throat cultures when appropriate.

Medical Management

Treatment of TSS varies because of the range in types and severity of symptoms. Antibiotic therapy is given according to the results of culture and sensitivity tests. Parenteral therapy is given to maintain proper fluid balance. Laboratory data are evaluated for electrolyte imbalance caused by vomiting and diarrhea, elevated BUN suggesting renal involvement, and elevated enzymes suggesting liver dysfunction.

Nursing Interventions and Patient Teaching

When the patient is hospitalized, bed rest is prescribed and antibiotics are administered. Closely monitor vital signs and fluid status. If there is respiratory distress, oxygen therapy is instituted.

Nursing diagnoses and interventions for the patient with TSS include but are not limited to the following:

Nursing Diagnoses	Nursing Interventions
Anxiety, related to TSS	Encourage patient to verbalize fears. Provide quiet, therapeutic environment. Provide support and understanding.

Continued

Nursing Diagnoses	Nursing Interventions
Deficient fluid volume, related to vomiting and diarrhea	Monitor amount, frequency, and characteristics of vomitus and diarrhea. Assess tissue turgor for evidence of dehydration. Assess patient for dry mucous membranes, and monitor parenteral fluids with electrolytes as ordered. Monitor intake and output (I&O).

Because the use of tampons during menstruation has been linked to TSS, advise patients not to use superabsorbent tampons. If tampons are used, they should be alternated with the use of pads. Before it is used, a tampon should be inspected for shedding and other flaws and discarded if any are noted. Tampons should be changed frequently (every 4 hours) and should be inserted carefully to avoid abrasions. Patients who have had TSS should not use tampons. Instruct the patient to wash hands thoroughly before inserting a tampon. Advise women who are menstruating and develop a sudden high fever accompanied by vomiting and diarrhea to seek immediate medical attention. If the woman is wearing a tampon, she should remove it immediately.

Prognosis

TSS is a rare and sometimes fatal disease. The effect of the toxin on the liver, kidneys, and circulatory system makes this a potentially life-threatening condition. Prognosis depends on the severity of the disease and how quickly therapeutic measures to combat shock and renal failure, if present, are instituted.

DISORDERS OF THE FEMALE REPRODUCTIVE SYSTEM

ENDOMETRIOSIS

Etiology and Pathophysiology

Endometriosis is a condition in which endometrial tissue appears outside the endometrial cavity. Endometrial tissue can be found on the ovaries, the fallopian tubes, and the uterus; within the abdominal cavity (the uterovesical peritoneum); and in the vagina (Figure 52-9). Tissue is believed to spread through lymphatic circulation, by menstrual backflow to the fallopian tubes and pelvic cavity, or through congenital displacement of the endometrial cells.

The tissue responds to the normal stimulation of the ovaries; bleeds each month; and forms an endometrial crust, which causes an endometrial cyst. This cyst may rupture and cause further reproduction of tissue.

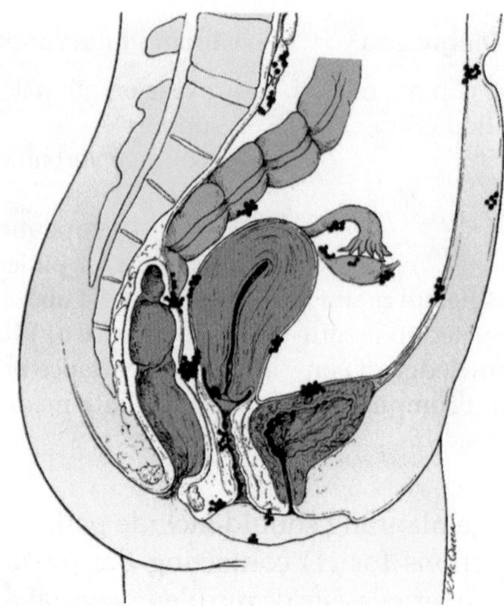

FIGURE 52-9 Common sites of endometriosis.

Clinical Manifestations

Symptoms are lower abdominal and pelvic pain with or without pain in the rectum. It may be unilateral or bilateral and may radiate to the lower back, legs, and groin. Symptoms are more acute during menstruation and subside after menstruation. Some evidence indicates that women have a greater chance (about seven times greater) of developing endometriosis if a sister or mother has it. The highest incidence of endometriosis is among white women 25 to 35 years of age who are in the higher socioeconomic classes and who postpone childbearing until the later reproductive years. Women who have not conceived or lactated are at greater risk.

Assessment

Subjective data include a history of the patient's symptoms, including pelvic pain with menstruation, aching, cramping, a bearing-down sensation in the pelvis, or lower back dyspareunia. The type of pain may indicate cysts that are about to rupture or infected tissue. The patient may reveal a history of menstrual irregularities such as amenorrhea.

Collection of **objective data** involves noting signs such as abnormal uterine bleeding, which appear 5 to 7 days before menses and last 2 or 3 days. Signs may also include infertility.

Diagnostic Tests

Laparoscopy with a biopsy of the lesions may confirm the diagnosis. Regular pelvic examinations are recommended to monitor progression.

Medical Management

Medical treatment consists of high-dose antiovulatory medications to inhibit ovulation and induce a state physiologically similar to pregnancy, thus suppressing menstruation. Synthetic androgens such as danazol (Danocrine) or a gonadotropin-releasing hormone agonist (e.g., leuprolide [Lupron]) may be prescribed to arrest proliferation of the endometrium and prevent ovulation, producing atrophy of the displaced endometrium (Lewis et al., 2007). Occasionally endometriosis spontaneously disappears. It is believed that an interruption of the menstrual cycle will slow the progress of the disorder. Some women who become pregnant are asymptomatic after pregnancy. When involvement is severe, surgery may be necessary. A laparoscopy may be performed to remove endometrial implants and adhesions. Lasers may be used to vaporize the small implants of endometrial tissue. A total hysterectomy, oophorectomy, and salpingectomy may also be done.

Nursing Interventions and Patient Teaching

Reinforce the physician's explanation of the expected results of treatment; instruct the patient regarding the dosage, frequency, and side effects of prescribed medications; and emphasize the importance of regular checkups and of reporting abnormal vaginal bleeding. Also encourage the patient to verbalize her concerns, and assist the patient with comfort measures.

Nursing diagnoses and interventions for the patient with endometriosis include but are not limited to the following:

Nursing Diagnoses	Nursing Interventions
Pain, related to displaced endometrial tissue	Institute comfort measures to cope with pain, such as medications and warm compresses to abdomen.
	Maintain bed rest when pain is most severe.
Sexual dysfunction, related to painful intercourse or infertility	Emphasize importance of communicating fears and concerns that lead to anxiety.

Prognosis

Approximately half of the women with endometriosis are infertile. If a young woman has endometriosis, advise her to have a family early, since the fertility rate is low. Menopause stops the progress of endometriosis.

VAGINAL FISTULA

Etiology and Pathophysiology

A fistula is defined as an abnormal opening between two organs. Vaginal fistulas are caused by an ulcerating process resulting from cancer, radiation, weakening of tissue by pregnancies, and surgical interventions. Vaginal fistulas are named for the organs involved (Figure 52-10). For example, a **urethrovaginal fistula** is an opening between the urethra and the vagina; a **vesicovaginal fistula** is an opening between the bladder and the vagina; and a **rectovaginal fistula** is an opening between the rectum and the vagina.

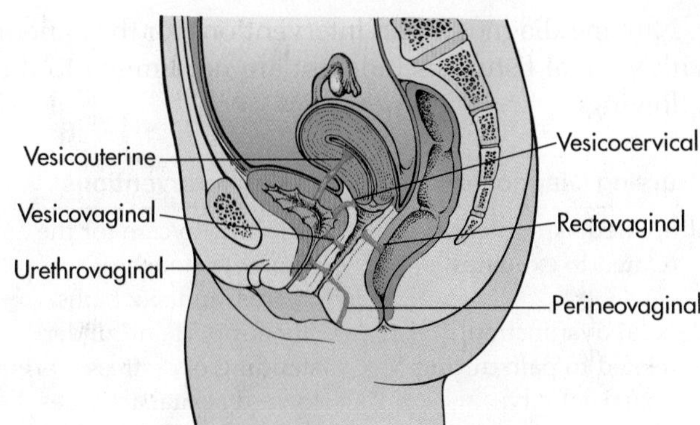

FIGURE 52-10 Types of fistulas that may develop in the vagina and the uterus.

Clinical Manifestations

Fistulas are recognized by their exudate, which has a distinct odor of urine or feces. Generally, a bladder infection is present. The vesicovaginal fistula causes a constant trickling of urine into the vagina; a rectovaginal fistula allows feces and flatus to enter the vagina.

Assessment

Subjective data include the patient's understanding of the exudate that occurs and of any causative factors. The patient reports the presence of urine or feces from the vagina.

Collection of **objective data** includes noting any behaviors that indicate stress, anxiety, and pain. The patient may express feelings of decreased self-esteem because of the condition. Observe for urine or feces on the perineal pad.

Diagnostic Tests

Diagnostic testing includes a methylene blue instillation in the bladder, and an intravenous (IV) pyelogram or cystoscopy to assist in locating the fistula. Pelvic examination is performed.

Medical Management

Healing is promoted by an increase in vitamin C and protein in the diet. The patient is given oral or parenteral antibiotics. If the organ tissue is healthy, a surgical approach is recommended. The surgical approach may be similar to anteroposterior colporrhaphy, which is discussed later in the chapter. Fistulas that are difficult to repair or very large may require urinary or fecal diversion.

Nursing Interventions

Soiling from leakage of urine or stool into the vagina is disturbing for the patient. Sitz baths, deodorizing douches, perineal pads, and protective undergarments are necessary. If the fistula is repaired surgically, insert a Foley catheter postoperatively to prevent strain on the suture line by a full bladder.

Nursing diagnoses and interventions for the patient with vaginal fistula include but are not limited to the following:

Nursing Diagnoses	Nursing Interventions
Impaired skin integrity, related to exudates	Teach how to care for the skin with douches, creams, and sitz baths.
Sexual dysfunction, related to pain during sexual activity	Offer support and understanding of distress toward sexual activities and self-esteem.

Prognosis

Vaginal fistulas may close spontaneously but frequently need to be repaired surgically. If so, 4 to 6 months are required for the inflammation to subside before surgery can be attempted.

RELAXED PELVIC MUSCLES

The most common problems resulting from relaxed pelvic muscles are displaced uterus with prolapse (downward displacement) and procidentia, cystocele, urethrocele, rectocele, enterocele, and malposition of the uterus.

Displaced Uterus

A displaced uterus is usually congenital, but may be caused by childbirth. Normally the uterus lies with the cervix at a right angle to the long axis of the vagina, and the body of the uterus is inclined slightly forward (see Figure 52-3). Backward displacement may be retroversion or retroflexion. Retroversion position places the cervix at the normal axis, but the body of the uterus is directed toward the sacrum. In retroflexion the angle of the body of the uterus is on the cervix. The patient has backache, muscle strain, leukorrheal discharge, and heaviness in the pelvic area. The patient also tires easily. Treatment consists of a pessary (a rubber or plastic doughnut-shaped ring placed in the vagina) and possibly uterine suspension.

Uterine Prolapse

Etiology and Pathophysiology

Prolapse of the uterus through the pelvic floor and vaginal outlet is traditionally rated as first degree (the cervix comes down to the **introitus** [an entrance to a cavity, as in the vaginal introitus]), second degree (the cervix protrudes through the introitus), or third degree (**procidentia** [the entire uterus protrudes through the introitus]) (Figure 52-11). Obstetric trauma, overstretching of the uterine muscle support system, multiple births, coughing, straining, the aging process, and lifting heavy objects contribute to uterine prolapse.

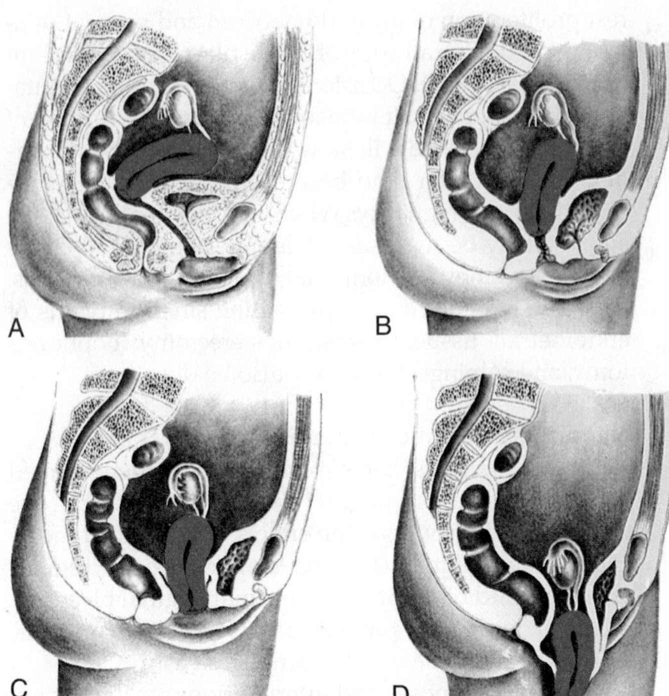

FIGURE 52-11 Uterine prolapse. **A,** Normal uterus. **B,** First-degree prolapse of the uterus. **C,** Second-degree prolapse of the uterus. **D,** Third-degree prolapse of the uterus (procidentia).

Clinical Manifestations

The patient complains of a feeling of "something coming down." She may have dyspareunia, a dragging or heavy feeling in the pelvis, backache, and bowel or bladder problems if cystocele or rectocele is also present. Stress incontinence is a common and troubling problem. When second- or third-degree uterine prolapse occurs, the protruding cervix and vaginal walls are subjected to constant irritation, and tissue changes may occur.

Medical Management

Surgery generally involves a vaginal hysterectomy with anterior and posterior repair of the vagina and underlying fascia. It is also called an **anteroposterior colporrhaphy** (suture of the vagina) (also referred to as anterior posterior colporrhaphy or A&P repair).

When surgery is contraindicated, pessaries are used to provide uterine support. Before insertion of the vaginal pessary, the uterus is manually replaced in its normal position. Once inserted, the pessary holds the cervix in a posterior (anteflexed) position. When the pessary is properly placed, the woman is unaware of its presence and has no difficulty voiding or having intercourse. A variety of pessaries are available for the different degrees of prolapse. Every 3 to 4 months the pessary is cleaned and replaced by the woman, if possible, or by her health care provider. She is also checked for signs of irritation. Pessaries that are unattended for long periods are associated with erosion, fistulas, and an increased incidence of vaginal carcinoma.

Cystocele and Rectocele

Etiology and Pathophysiology

When the tissue, the muscles, and the ligaments that support the uterus and the perineum have been stretched and weakened by childbearing, multiple births, or cervical tears, the organs gradually move into other positions. The relaxation of the tissues, the

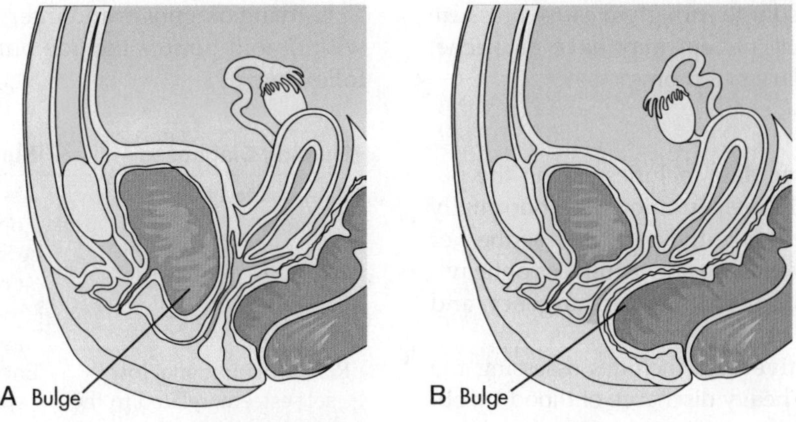

FIGURE 52-12 **A,** Cystocele. **B,** Rectocele.

muscles, and the ligaments of the bladder causes a displacement of the bladder into the vagina. This is referred to as a **cystocele** (Figure 52-12, *A*).

Clinical Manifestations

Clinical symptoms are urinary urgency, frequency, and incontinence; fatigue; and pelvic pressure. A large cystocele prevents complete emptying of the bladder, which leads to bacterial growth and infection.

The relaxation of the supporting tissues to the rectum causes the rectum to move toward the posterior vaginal wall and form a **rectocele** (Figure 52-12, *B*). The rectocele causes constipation, rectal pressure, heaviness, and hemorrhoids.

Medical Management

Cystocele and rectocele are corrected through anteroposterior colporrhaphy, a surgical repair involving shortening of the muscles that support the bladder and repair of the rectocele.

Nursing Interventions and Patient Teaching

An important aspect of preoperative care for colporrhaphy is ensuring as clean an operative area as possible. Patients may be given a cathartic followed by enemas to be sure the bowel is completely empty. A liquid diet for 48 hours before surgery will help keep the bowel empty. A cleansing vaginal douche is given the evening before and the morning of surgery. Postoperative care includes checking vital signs and observing for hemorrhage. A retention catheter is usually inserted into the bladder to keep it empty and prevent pressure on sutures. It is important to keep the fecal residue as soft as possible; some physicians order only liquids for several days, or they may order mineral oil to be given every night. An oil retention enema may be ordered, but cleansing enemas are not given. Carefully clean the patient's perineal area using surgical asepsis.

Encourage early ambulation. Advise the patient against standing for long periods or lifting heavy objects. Coitus must be avoided until healing occurs, usually after about 6 weeks.

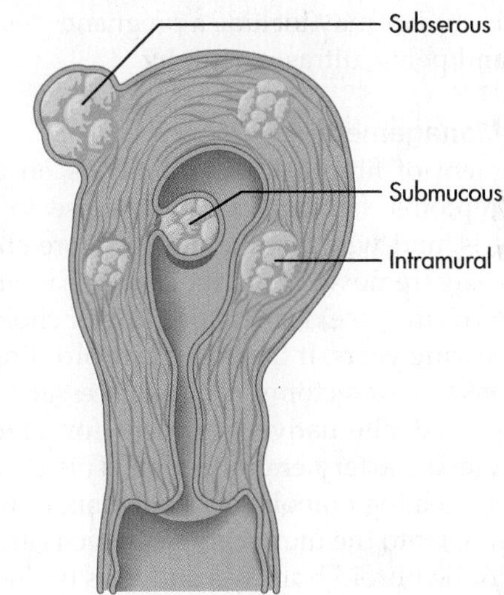

FIGURE 52-13 Leiomyomas. Uterine section showing whorl-like appearance and locations of leiomyomas, which are also called uterine fibroids.

Prognosis

With surgical correction, the prognosis is good.

LEIOMYOMAS OF THE UTERUS

Etiology and Pathophysiology

Leiomyomas (fibroids, myomas) are the most common benign tumors of the female genital tract (Figure 52-13). Fibroids are benign tumors arising from the muscle tissue of the uterus. The causes of leiomyomas is unknown. They seem to depend on ovarian hormones for their growth because of slow growth during reproductive years with atrophy occurring after menopause (Lewis et al., 2007). An estimated 20% to 25% of women over 30 years of age may develop uterine fibroid tumors. The size and number of leiomyomas vary. Most are found in the body of the uterus, but some occur in the cervix or involve the broad ligaments.

Clinical Manifestations

The symptoms are primarily pressure from an enlarging pelvic mass, pain (including dysmenorrhea), abnormal uterine bleeding, and menorrhagia. If the fibroid tumor becomes large enough to cause pressure on other structures, the patient may have backache, constipation, and urinary symptoms.

Assessment

Collection of **subjective data** includes asking the patient about pain with menstruation or abnormally heavy menstrual flow. Have the patient describe her symptoms, which may include pelvic fullness or heaviness, constipation, urinary frequency or urgency, and menorrhagia.

Collection of **objective data** includes assessing the patient for excessively heavy discharge of blood by observing the number and saturation of perineal pads.

Diagnostic Tests

Diagnostic studies may include a pregnancy test, laparoscopy, and pelvic ultrasonography.

Medical Management

The treatment of fibroid tumors depends on the patient's symptoms, her age and how close to menopause she is, and whether she desires more children. **Myomectomy** (removal of uterine myomas while leaving the uterus in place) is the procedure of choice during childbearing years. If there is severe bleeding or an obstruction, a hysterectomy may be necessary. An increasingly used alternative treatment for uterine fibroids is **uterine artery embolization.** This procedure consists of injecting embolic material (small plastic or gelatin beads) into the uterine artery, which carries the material to the fibroid branches and thus occludes the arteries supplying blood to the tumor. Deprived of oxygen and nutrients, the tumor shrinks over time and symptoms diminish (McDaniel, 2007).

Six months after uterine artery embolization, fibroids are typically about 50% smaller in most women, and in 80% to 90% of women, the symptoms are considerably decreased or gone. About 5% of patients experience complications from the procedure, such as infection or permanent cessation of menstrual periods (McDaniel, 2007).

Nursing Interventions and Patient Teaching

Preoperative and postoperative nursing interventions are like those discussed for a patient who undergoes a hysterectomy. Reinforce the physician's explanation of the treatment plan—either a total hysterectomy or pelvic examination at regular intervals to monitor the status of the fibroid tumor. Instruct the patient about the dosage, frequency, and possible side effects of prescribed medications. Tell the patient with menorrhagia to include adequate iron in her diet to prevent iron deficiency anemia from the extra blood loss. Stress the importance of regular checkups to monitor the status of the fibroid tumor, and encourage the patient to express her feelings and assist her with coping mechanisms.

Nursing diagnoses and interventions for the patient with fibroid tumors include but are not limited to the following:

Nursing Diagnoses	Nursing Interventions
Pain, related to fibroid tumors	Assess pain location, onset, and duration. Administer analgesics as ordered. Provide comfort measures as needed.
Risk for situational low self-esteem, related to the presence of fibroid tumors	Encourage verbalization of concerns. Be an active listener.

Prognosis

Fibroid tumors of the uterus tend to disappear spontaneously with menopause. They rarely become malignant. Infertility may result from a myoma that obstructs or distorts the uterus or fallopian tubes. Myomas in the body of the uterus may cause spontaneous abortions; those near the cervical opening may make the delivery of a fetus difficult and may contribute to postpartum hemorrhage.

OVARIAN CYSTS

Etiology and Pathophysiology

Ovarian cysts are benign tumors that arise from dermoid cells of the ovary or from a cystic corpus luteum or graafian follicle.

Clinical Manifestations

Ovarian cysts enlarge and are palpable on examination. They may cause no symptoms, or they may result in a disturbance of menstruation, a feeling of heaviness, and slight vaginal bleeding.

Medical Management

The cysts may be removed by an ovarian cystectomy. Often ovarian cysts are not removed if the patient is not experiencing debilitating symptoms.

Nursing Interventions

If surgery is performed, nursing interventions are similar to those for the patient having an abdominal hysterectomy.

Prognosis

The prognosis is good; ovarian cysts do not become malignant.

CANCER OF THE FEMALE REPRODUCTIVE TRACT

Cancer is the second most common cause of death in women, and malignant tumors of the reproductive tract represent a significant portion of the total number

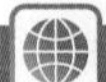 Cultural Considerations

Cancer of Female Reproductive System

- Ovarian cancer is seen more frequently among white women than among black women.
- Japanese women have a low incidence of ovarian cancer. However, second- and third-generation Japanese women in the United States have much higher rates, similar to those of white women born in the United States. Dietary practices may explain this difference.
- Endometrial cancer occurs more frequently among white women than among black women.
- Five-year survival rate for endometrial cancer (all stages combined) is 80% for white women and 55% for black women.
- Cervical cancer has a higher incidence among Hispanic, black, and Native American women than among white women. The mortality rate for cervical cancer is more than twice as high among black women as among white women.
- Jewish-American women have a low incidence of cervical cancer.

of deaths from cancer (see Cultural Considerations box).

Cervical cancer often affects women in their reproductive years. The cancer can be detected in its early stages with a diagnostic Pap test. Endometrial cancer is primarily a disease of women older than 50 years of age, but the incidence among younger women is increasing. Most cases of ovarian cancer occur in women older than 50, but malignant neoplasms of the ovaries may occur at all ages.

CANCER OF THE CERVIX

Cancer of the cervix is a neoplasm that can be detected in the early, curable stage by a Pap test. Cancer of the cervix is usually a squamous cell carcinoma. An estimated 11,270 cases of cervical cancer were diagnosed in 2009. As Pap screening has become more prevalent, preinvasive lesions are detected far more frequently than invasive cancer. An estimated 4070 cervical cancer deaths occurred in 2009. Mortality rates have declined sharply over the past several decades. The five-year relative survival rate for localized stage cervical cancer was 92%, and five-year relative survival rate for all stages of cervical cancer combined was 71% in 2009 (ACS, 2009c).

Etiology and Pathophysiology

Women who become sexually active in their teens are at an increased risk for cancer of the cervix, as are those who have had multiple sexual partners, had partners who had multiple sexual partners, and are of lower socioeconomic status. Cervical cancer risk is closely linked to sexual behavior, to STIs with several strains of HPV, and to smoking. Women who smoke have a 50% higher risk of developing cervical cancer than nonsmokers. Chronic infections and erosions of the cervix are most likely significant in the development of cancer.

Carcinoma in situ is a preinvasive, asymptomatic carcinoma that can only be diagnosed by microscopic examination of cervical cells. Once diagnosed, it can be treated early without radical surgery. Carcinoma in situ of the cervix is essentially 100% curable.

Clinical Manifestations

Most cervical cancer is silent in the early stages and offers few symptoms. The two primary symptoms are leukorrhea and irregular vaginal bleeding or spotting between menses. Bleeding often occurs after coitus or after menopause. Bleeding is slight at first but increases as the disease progresses. The vaginal exudate becomes watery, then increases and becomes dark and bloody with an offensive odor caused by necrosis (death of tissue) and infection of the tumor mass. As the cancer progresses, the bleeding may become constant and may increase in amount. With advanced stages the patient has severe pain in the back, upper thighs, and legs.

Assessment

Subjective data in the early stages of cancer of the cervix are not available, since the woman has no symptoms. If the tumor becomes more invasive, the patient experiences back and leg pain, weight loss, and malaise. Urge women to have regular health appraisals and pelvic examinations so that cancer of the cervix can be detected in its earliest stages.

Collection of **objective data** includes observing the sanitary pads for abnormal vaginal discharge. The vaginal exudate may be watery to dark red and malodorous. Note the number and saturation of the perineal pads. If the tumor becomes more invasive, assess the patient for anemia, fever, and lymphedema.

Diagnostic Tests

Cervical cancer is diagnosed with the following tests: (1) Pap test; (2) physical examination; (3) colposcopy and cervical biopsy; and (4) additional diagnostic studies, such as a computed tomography (CT) scan, chest radiographic evaluation, IV pyelogram, cystoscopy, sigmoidoscopy, or liver function studies to determine the extent of invasion. The ACS (2009a) recommends that cervical cancer screening begin approximately 3 years after a woman begins having vaginal intercourse, but no later than 21 years of age. Traditional Pap tests are less than 100% accurate in screening for cervical cell abnormalities, and false-positive and false-negative results do occur. A newer liquid-based technique, called ThinPrep, can reduce the number of inaccurate Pap tests results.

At or after age 30, women who have had three normal Pap test results in a row may get screened every 2 to 3 years, unless she has certain risk factors, such as human immunodeficiency virus (HIV) infection or a weak immune system. Women age 70 and older who have had three or more normal Pap tests and no abnormal Pap tests in the past 10 years may stop cervical cancer screening. Screening after a total hysterectomy (with removal of the cervix) is not necessary unless the surgery was done to treat cervical cancer or precancer. Women who have had a hysterectomy without removal of the cervix should continue cervical cancer screening at least until age 70 (ACS, 2009).

Medical Management

Gardisil is a vaccine that reduces the incidence of cervical cancer due to infection of HPV types 6, 11, 16, 18. To be effective, the vaccine should be given before a person becomes sexually active. The goal of these vaccines is to reduce the incidence of HPV-related genital disease, including precancerous cervical lesions and cervical cancer. Three injections are given over 6 months. The second dose is given 2 months after the first dose and the third dose 6 months after the first dose (Saslow et al., 2007).

The ACS recommends that the HPV vaccine be routinely given to girls ages 11 to 12 and as early as age 9 at the discretion of physicians. Vaccination is also recommended for females 13 to 18 to catch up on missed vaccine or to complete the vaccination series (Saslow et al., 2007).

Cervarix is a new 3-dose vaccine to prevent cervical cancer, cervical intraepithelial neoplasia (CIN) grades 1, 2, or worse, and adenocarcinoma in situ. It has been approved by the FDA for females 10 to 25 years old, and is undergoing pediatric testing for use in 9-year-old girls. Cervarix is effective against HPV types 16 and 18, but it does not offer coverage against all the other types of HIV infections nor is it effective after exposure to HPV (US FDA, 2009).

Carcinoma in situ is treated by removal of the affected area. A variety of techniques can be used, including electrocautery, cryosurgery (use of subfreezing temperature to destroy tissue), laser, conization, and hysterectomy. **Conization** is the surgical removal of a cone-shaped section of the cervix and is particularly useful in preserving childbearing function.

Early cervical carcinoma can be treated with a hysterectomy or intracavitary radiation (see Chapter 57).

A radical hysterectomy with pelvic lymph node dissection may be required for more extensive lesions. Invasive cervical cancers generally are treated by surgery, radiation, or both, as well as chemotherapy (cisplatin-based) in some cases. Radiation may be external or internal (e.g., cesium, radium). Brachytherapy, or internally implanted radiation into the cervix, is often done. The patient is hospitalized for 48 hours for treatment. The treatment plan is tailored to each patient based on the extent of the disease.

Nursing Interventions and Patient Teaching

Nursing interventions should include verbal reassurance. In advanced cervical cancer, position the patient comfortably; change her position slowly; maintain her body alignment; provide pain-relief measures; change the patient's dressings and sanitary pads often; and assess color, odor, and amount of drainage. Assess the skin for impairment. See nursing interventions for a patient undergoing a hysterectomy.

Nursing diagnoses and interventions for the patient with cancer of the cervix include but are not limited to the following:

Nursing Diagnoses	Nursing Interventions
Impaired urinary elimination related to postsurgical sensorimotor impairment	Connect indwelling catheter to closed gravity drainage. Give meticulous catheter care as indicated. Record color and amount of urinary output. Promote micturition at regular intervals when catheter is removed. Catheterize for residual urine as ordered.
Risk for situational low self-esteem, related to body image change and value of reproductive organs	Encourage discussion with significant others. Relate importance of communicating anything that causes anxiety. Reinforce correct information to correct any misconceptions.
Ineffective tissue perfusion, peripheral, related to: • pelvic surgery • thrombophlebitis	Ensure that bed is not elevated in the knee gatch position. Assess proper placement of antiembolism stockings every 4 hours as ordered. Assist in passive and active leg exercises every shift. Encourage ambulation. Assess legs for erythema, increased tenderness, severe cramping, and positive Homans' sign every shift.

The key to preventing cervical cancer and treating it in the early stages is education. Educate and encourage patients to be responsible for their health by having a yearly Pap test. Education about the HPV vaccine for females is very important. Encourage patients to seek prompt medical assistance for any abnormal vaginal exudate.

Prognosis

The prognosis is good if the cancer is treated in the early stages. It usually takes 2 to 10 years for squamous cell carcinoma to become invasive beyond the basement membrane and metastasize. Therefore early diagnosis and treatment are vital. Survival for those with preinvasive lesions is nearly 100%; 92% of cervical cancer patients survive 1 year after diagnosis, and 71% survive

5 years (ACS, 2009c). When detected at an early stage, invasive cervical cancer has a 5-year survival rate of 92% for localized cancers.

CANCER OF THE ENDOMETRIUM

Etiology and Pathophysiology

Cancer of the endometrium usually affects postmenopausal women. An estimated 42,160 cases of cancer of the uterine corpus (body of the uterus) will be diagnosed in the United States in 2009 (ACS, 2009c). An estimated 7780 deaths were expected for 2009 (ACS, 2009c). Endometrial cancer is usually an adenocarcinoma. The tumor is more likely to be localized, but may spread to the cervix, bladder, rectum, and surrounding lymph nodes. It is the most common malignancy of the female genital tract. Women at increased risk are those with a history of irregular menstruation, difficulties during menopause, obesity, hypertension, or diabetes mellitus; those who have not had children; and those with a family history of uterine cancer. Obesity is a risk factor because adipose cells store estrogen. Women who used estrogen replacement therapy to treat menopausal symptoms are more likely to develop endometrial cancer. Progesterone plus estrogen replacement therapy (HRT) may largely offset the increased risk related to using only estrogen. Also at increased risk for developing endometrial cancer are women at high risk for developing breast cancer as well as those in an advanced stage of breast cancer who are taking tamoxifen (Nolvadex), an antiestrogen drug that blocks estrogen receptors.

The carcinoma in situ is slow growing. Invasion and metastasis occur later, with expansion to the cervix and the myometrium and ultimately to the vagina, the pelvis, and the lungs.

Clinical Manifestations

The first sign of endometrial cancer is abnormal uterine bleeding, usually in postmenopausal women. About 50% of patients with postmenopausal bleeding have cancer of the uterus. In premenstrual or postmenopausal women, any abnormal bleeding or spotting should be reported immediately.

Assessment

Collection of **subjective data** includes assisting the patient in identifying and reporting changes in reproductive or sexual health. The patient may report abdominal pressure, pain, and pelvic fullness. The patient will have a history of postmenopausal bleeding and leukorrhea. Pelvic and back pain and postcoital bleeding are late signs and symptoms.

Collection of **objective data** includes observing the color and amount of vaginal exudate on perineal pads. Assess the patient for enlarged lymph nodes.

Diagnostic Tests

Pelvic and rectal examination and endometrial biopsy are used to diagnose cancer of the endometrium. Any report of abnormal or unexpected bleeding in a postmenopausal woman requires a tissue sample to exclude endometrial cancer. The ACS recommends that an endometrial biopsy be performed at menopause and then periodically in women who are at risk for endometrial cancer (ACS, 2009c). The Pap test is not a reliable diagnostic tool for endometrial cancer, but it can rule out cervical cancer (Lewis et al., 2007).

Medical Management

Treatment of cancer of the endometrium depends on the stage of the tumor and the woman's health. Surgery, radiation, or chemotherapy may be used to remove the tumor and treat metastasis. For early cancer of the endometrium, total abdominal hysterectomy with bilateral salpingo-oophorectomy (TAH-BSO) is done. Intracavitary radiation followed by a TAH-BSO may be done for the early stage of endometrial cancer (stage I). Patients with stage II disease may receive pelvic irradiation to shrink the tumor and help prevent spread. Afterward the patient undergoes a hysterectomy. Patients with stages III and IV disease are uncommon, and treatment is based on the extent of the disease.

Nursing Interventions and Patient Teaching

See the section on interventions for the patient undergoing a hysterectomy; also see Chapter 57 for care of the patient through intracavitary radiation.

Health teaching and follow-up after discharge should emphasize the need for regular physical examination by the physician and the importance of compliance with the prescribed treatment plan.

Prognosis

Cancer of the endometrium is primarily a slow-growing adenocarcinoma. Metastasis occurs late, and the sign of irregular vaginal bleeding often appears early enough to allow for cure of the disease. The 5-year survival rate for all cases of endometrial cancer is about 83% (ACS, 2009c).

CANCER OF THE OVARY

Etiology and Pathophysiology

Ovarian cancer, the fourth most common cause of cancer death in women, is the leading cause of gynecologic death in the United States, following cancer of the uterine corpus. Risk for ovarian cancer increases with age; it occurs most frequently in women between 55 and 65 years of age.

The ACS (2009c) estimated that in 2009, 21,550 women would be diagnosed with ovarian cancer and nearly 14,600 would die of the disease.

In the early stages the tumors are asymptomatic; when detected, they usually have spread to other pelvic organs. Nothing alters the magnitude of risk for ovarian cancer more than genetics. Hereditary ovarian cancer accounts for 5% to 10% of ovarian cancers. In general, the closer the relative with ovarian cancer and the younger the relative at diagnosis, the higher the risk is. Women at increased risk are those who are infertile, anovulatory, nulliparous, and habitual aborters. Because they reduce the number of ovulatory cycles, thus reducing exposure to estrogen, the following practices can reduce the risk of ovarian cancer: oral contraceptive use (greater than 5 years), multiple pregnancies, breastfeeding, and early age of first birth. Other risk factors include a high-fat diet and exposure to industrial chemicals such as asbestos and talc. Ovarian cancer commonly spreads by peritoneal seeding of the cancer cells. Common sites of metastasis are the peritoneum, the omentum, and bowel surfaces.

Clinical Manifestations

In the early stages the symptoms may cause vague abdominal discomfort, flatulence, mild gastric disturbances, pressure, bloating, cramps, sense of pelvic heaviness, feeling of fullness, and change in bowel habits. Pain *is not* an early symptom. As the tumor progresses, abdominal girth enlarges from ascites, and there is flatulence with distention. Other symptoms may include urinary frequency, nausea, vomiting, constipation, menstrual irregularities, and weight loss. The Gynecologic Cancer Foundation, the Society of Gynecologic Oncologists, and the ACS issued the first national consensus statement on ovarian cancer symptoms in June, 2007. This statement mentions that certain symptoms such as bloating, pelvic or abdominal pain, difficulty eating, feeling full quickly, and urinary urgency or frequency are much more likely to occur in women with ovarian cancer than in women without ovarian cancer (ACS, 2007c). Women are strongly advised to see their gynecologist if they experience any of these symptoms almost daily for more than a few weeks.

Assessment

Collection of **subjective data** requires an awareness that cancer of the ovary is difficult to detect. The patient reports symptoms of abdominal discomfort, bloating, fullness, gastric disturbances (nausea, constipation), and urinary frequency.

Collection of **objective data** includes observing any increase in the abdominal girth. The patient may void at frequent intervals because of pressure on the bladder. The patient may be dyspneic due to ascites and pressure on the diaphragm.

Diagnostic Tests

Although detecting ovarian cancer early is difficult, an annual bimanual pelvic examination may help to identify pelvic masses. Because the ovaries are movable and therefore harder to assess, screening for ovarian tumors requires a thorough examination, including bimanual and rectovaginal examination. **Postmenopause palpable ovary syndrome** (a palpable ovary in a woman 3 to 5 years past menopause) may indicate an early tumor. CT scan of the pelvis and abdomen is indicated if an ovarian mass is palpable. Definitive diagnosis of ovarian cancer is usually established by a tumor biopsy at the time of exploratory laparotomy, when staging and tumor debulking take place.

Ovarian cancer is diagnosed by palpation of a pelvic mass and aspiration of ascitic fluid and detection of cancer cells in the fluid. A blood test to determine CA-125 is used to identify women with ovarian cancer. High levels of CA-125 are found in the blood of 80% of women with epithelial ovarian cancer. But although the antigen test can help evaluate a woman's response to cancer treatment, it is controversial as an independent screening tool. Because of the test's lack of specificity and sensitivity, false-positive and false-negative results can occur. Many benign conditions, including endometriosis and fibroid tumors, can raise CA-125 levels above normal.

Vaginal ultrasonography, which also lacks specificity and sensitivity, may be used with pelvic examination and CA-125 antigen testing to follow a woman at increased risk.

Medical Management

Treatment often involves surgery alone or in conjunction with radiation or chemotherapy. Treatment depends on the stage of ovarian cancer (see Chapter 57). Surgery may be a TAH-BSO and omentectomy (excision of portions of the peritoneal folds). In some very early tumors, only the involved ovary is removed, especially in young women who wish to have children. The National Cancer Institute (NCI) issued a clinical announcement suggesting physicians use a combined modality approach after surgical debulking of the tumor: intraperitoneal chemotherapy, administered through a surgically implanted catheter, in addition to the standard IV chemotherapy (NCI, 2006). A gynecologic oncologist or surgical team with expertise in the staging and debulking of ovarian cancer should perform the surgery

Intraperitoneal chemotherapy employs two generic drugs already in widespread use for ovarian cancer: paclitaxel (Taxol) and cisplatin (Platinol). A list of facilities that provide intraperitoneal chemotherapy is available on the NCI website at http://ctep.cancer.gov/highlights/20060105_ovarian.htm.

Nursing Interventions

Nursing interventions for any patient with ovarian cancer include management similar to that for patients undergoing abdominal hysterectomy and receiving chemotherapy and external radiation (see Chapter 57). Because ovarian cancer is generally at an advanced stage when diagnosed, despite the woman's feeling well, support and encouragement to comply with the treatment regimen are important nursing interventions. As the disease progresses, become involved in activities to increase the patient's comfort.

Nursing diagnoses and interventions for the patient with cancer of the ovaries include but are not limited to the following:

Nursing Diagnoses	Nursing Interventions
Fear, related to diagnosis of cancer	Assist patient with recognizing and clarifying fears and with developing coping strategies for those fears. Be an active listener.
Situational low self-esteem, related to body image change and value of reproductive organs	Encourage patient's comments and questions about condition. Encourage discussion with significant others. Provide factual information to correct any misconceptions.

Prognosis

More than 75% of women with ovarian cancer are diagnosed with advanced disease. The 5-year survival rate for all stages is 46%. If diagnosed early and treated while the disease is localized, the 5-year survival rate is 93%. Relative survival rates for more advanced disease are 71% for regional disease and 31% for disease that has spread to distant sites (ACS, 2009c).

HYSTERECTOMY

A hysterectomy involves removal of the uterus, including the cervix. This procedure may be done for many conditions, such as dysfunctional uterine bleeding, endometriosis, malignant and nonmalignant tumors of the uterus and cervix, and disorders of pelvic relaxation and uterine prolapse.

Various terms are used to describe removal of the uterus. A total hysterectomy is removal of the entire uterus. The vagina remains intact, and intercourse is possible even though childbearing is not. Estrogens are still released. Menopause occurs naturally because the ovaries are still present. A total abdominal hysterectomy with bilateral salpingo-oophorectomy (TAH-BSO) is the removal of the uterus, fallopian tubes, and ovaries. It is sometimes called panhysterosalpingo-oophorectomy. A radical hysterectomy also includes removal of the pelvic lymph nodes. If the ovaries are removed in these surgeries, it induces menopause.

VAGINAL HYSTERECTOMY

A vaginal hysterectomy may be done for a prolapsed uterus. It is not used nearly as often as the abdominal approach. The vaginal approach is selected for the patient who cannot tolerate abdominal surgery or prolonged anesthesia. There is no abdominal incision. The patient is placed in a lithotomy position, and the uterus is removed through the vagina. Advantages of the vaginal entrance are that (1) there is no wound dehiscence, (2) there is less pain, (3) complications are less likely, (4) hospitalization is shorter, and (5) there is no abdominal scar. The most important disadvantage is a limited view of the operative field for visualizing intrapelvic and intraabdominal organs. Vaginal hysterectomy is not used in cases of uterine fibroids or enlarged uterine size. Other disadvantages are risk of bleeding and postoperative infection.

ABDOMINAL HYSTERECTOMY

An abdominal hysterectomy is preferred when there is a need to explore the pelvic cavity and when the fallopian tubes and ovaries are to be removed. The three procedures for an abdominal hysterectomy are named according to the extent of the surgery performed. A **subtotal hysterectomy** refers to the removal of the corpus (the midsection or body) of the uterus, leaving the cervical stump in place. Leaving the cervical stump in place may play a role in female sexual pleasure and orgasm. A **total hysterectomy** is the removal of the entire uterus, including the cervix, but leaving the fallopian tubes and ovaries in place. TAH-BSO involves the removal of the entire uterus, the fallopian tubes, and the ovaries.

Nursing Interventions

Preoperative Interventions

When the physician has explained the surgery to the patient, reinforce the explanation and answer any questions. Encourage verbalization of fears. Provide additional preoperative instructions to help the woman prepare for postoperative recovery. Instruct the patient how to turn, cough, and deep breathe.

Before a vaginal or abdominal hysterectomy, the colon is emptied to prevent postoperative distention. The patient may be on a low-residue diet for several days preoperatively. Enemas may be given the evening before surgery. The bladder may be decompressed to prevent trauma during surgery. The indwelling catheter generally remains in place for 1 or 2 days after surgery. An antiseptic vaginal douche may be ordered to decrease microbial invasion of the surgical site.

Surgical preparation of the skin on the abdomen, the pelvis, and the perineum often is performed in surgery. The patient signs a consent form, and oral intake after midnight is restricted. Occasionally, ureteral stents are placed in the ureters for identification and to prevent possible trauma to the ureters during surgery.

Postoperative Interventions

Postoperative nursing interventions focus on monitoring vital signs and preventing urinary retention, intestinal distention, and venous thrombosis. If a retention catheter was inserted, ensure it is kept patent and connected to closed drainage. Perform meticulous catheter care to prevent bladder infection. The indwelling catheter generally remains in place 1 or 2 days postoperatively. If no retention catheter is in place, check the patient frequently for bladder distention; accurately record urinary output. The incidence of urinary retention after a hysterectomy is greater than after any other type of surgery, since some trauma to the bladder is unavoidable. If the patient does not have a catheter and is unable to void, catheterization every 8 hours may be necessary. Occasionally the patient has residual urine, and the physician may order catheterization to check for it; 50 mL or less is within the normal range.

A small up-and-down flush enema may be ordered to help relieve distention. Early ambulation is helpful to return the bowel to normal function. When bowel sounds have returned and flatus is being expelled, the patient is allowed liquids by mouth and a gradual return to solid foods.

Patients undergoing pelvic surgery are susceptible to venous stasis and thrombophlebitis because of trauma to blood vessels. The patient is usually permitted out of bed on the first postoperative day, but encourage the patient to dangle her legs and to sit on the side of the bed before standing and walking to avoid postural hypotension. Encourage the patient to cough, deep breathe, and use an incentive spirometer to prevent postoperative pneumonia and atelectasis. Antiembolism stockings may be used to prevent thrombus or embolus formation, and legs should be exercised frequently when the patient is in bed. Many physicians prescribe intermittent pneumonic compression cuffs for the calves to prevent venous stasis, deep-vein thrombosis, and pulmonary embolism. The patient should avoid bending her knees. This could cause pooling of blood in the pelvic cavity, resulting in stasis in the lower extremities. The patient at risk for thromboembolic disease may receive low-dose heparin or low-molecular-weight enoxaparin (Lovenox) to prevent thrombus formation.

Analgesics such as morphine may be ordered for relief of pain. Slight vaginal drainage may occur for 1 or 2 days, but report any unusual bleeding to the physician. Observe the abdominal dressing on the patient with an abdominal hysterectomy for evidence of hemorrhage. Use surgical asepsis for the dressing change. The patient usually receives IV feedings for the first postoperative day. Carefully monitor the rate of flow and the condition of the IV site.

Nursing diagnoses and interventions for the patient who has had a hysterectomy include but are not limited to the following:

Nursing Diagnoses	Nursing Interventions
Chronic pain, related to metastatic process	Establish trusting relationship with patient. Monitor and document pain characteristics. Administer prescribed analgesics every 3 to 4 hours to control pain. Provide environment conducive to comfort and rest.
Excess fluid volume, related to ascites	Monitor IV fluids. Maintain accurate I&O. Weigh patient daily. Observe for signs of edema. Measure abdominal girth daily.
Compromised family coping, related to poor prognosis	Assess present coping abilities. Encourage and allow time for verbalization of feelings. Support patient's coping strengths, and discuss alternative coping measures. Involve patient and significant others in nursing interventions and procedures.

Patient Teaching

Before discharge, the physician explains to the woman and her partner that they should not have sexual intercourse for 4 to 6 weeks after surgery. With an abdominal incision, there may be further restrictions on heavy lifting (nothing greater than 10 pounds), walking up and down stairs, and prolonged riding in the car. Riding in the car may cause pelvic pooling and development of a thrombus in the legs.

Inform the patient that vaginal drainage is normal for about 2 to 4 weeks after an abdominal hysterectomy. Advise her to avoid wearing any tight clothing such as a girdle or knee-high hose, which might constrict circulation to the surgical site and cause venous stasis.

Several signs and symptoms of infection should be reported to the physician if they occur: (1) erythema, edema, exudate, or increased tenderness along the surgical incision; (2) increased malodorous vaginal exudate; (3) a temperature of 101° F (38.3° C) or more; and (4) any problems with urinating, such as difficulty in starting to void, voiding too often, voiding small amounts, or a burning sensation while urinating (indicative of a bladder infection).

DISORDERS OF THE FEMALE BREAST

FIBROCYSTIC BREAST CONDITION

Etiology and Pathophysiology

Fibrocystic breast condition involves benign tumors of the breasts. It usually occurs in women 30 to 50 years of age and is rare in postmenopausal women. This suggests that the occurrence is related to ovarian activity.

The cysts are characterized by numerous cellular changes, with an abnormal amount of epithelial hyperplasia and cystic formation within the mammary ducts. The cysts rarely become malignant, but the risk of breast cancer does increase for women who have fibrocystic breast condition; therefore observe the cysts carefully.

Clinical Manifestations

Cystic lesions are often bilateral and multiple. The cysts are soft, well differentiated, tender, and freely movable. The lumpiness and tenderness are more apparent before menses.

Diagnostic Tests

The disorder is diagnosed by mammography or ultrasound and confirmed by biopsy. As a therapeutic measure, the cyst is aspirated by needle and syringe to empty the secretions, and the fluid is sent to the laboratory for cytologic examination to rule out a malignancy. Aspiration produces a turbid, nonhemorrhagic, yellow, greenish, or brownish fluid.

Medical Management

When cysts recur in the same area and repeated aspirations are ineffective, surgical excision of the cyst may be done.

Conservative treatment is the usual approach to fibrocystic breast condition. The usefulness of eliminating methylxanthines (in coffee, tea, and cola) from the diet is still controversial, but it is the least expensive therapy. Many women have reported decreased symptoms after altering their diet, even though findings by palpation and mammogram were not significantly changed. Danazol may be prescribed to inhibit FSH and LH production, thereby decreasing ovarian production of estrogen. Danazol may cause weight gain, hot flashes, menstrual irregularities, hirsutism, and deepening of the voice. Vitamin E may also be prescribed, but its efficacy has not been proven.

Nursing Interventions and Patient Teaching

Instruct the patient to perform breast self-examination (BSE) 1 week after menses, to recognize the presence of cysts, and to note any changes.

ACUTE MASTITIS

Acute mastitis is an acute bacterial infection usually caused by *S. aureus* or streptococci. It is most often observed during lactation and late pregnancy. The infection may result from inadequate cleanliness of the breasts, a nipple fissure, or infection in the infant. The breasts are tender, inflamed, and engorged, obstructing the milk flow.

Treatment involves application of warm packs, support of the area with a well-fitting brassiere (which also supplies comfort), and systemic treatment with antibiotics.

CHRONIC MASTITIS

Chronic mastitis tends to develop in women between 30 and 50 years of age and is more common in those who have had children, have had difficulty with inverted and cracked nipples, and have had problems nursing their infants. A traumatic blow to the breasts allows the fat to necrose in the area and form abscesses. Increased fibrosis of the tissue causes cysts to form. The cysts are tender, painful, and palpable on examination. The disorder is generally unilateral and benign and most frequently occurs in obese women. Treatment is the same as for acute mastitis.

BREAST CANCER

Breast cancer is the most common malignancy affecting women in the United States. Approximately 1 of every 8 women will develop breast cancer during her lifetime. The incidence of breast cancer in men is rare (less than 1%). Among men, there are about 1910 new cases of breast cancer and 440 deaths per year. The ACS (2009c) predicted that 194,280 women would be diagnosed with breast cancer in 2009 and that 40,610 would die. Breast cancer ranks second among cancer deaths in women (after lung cancer). Women consider this disease their most serious health problem. Women over 60 years of age have twice the incidence of breast cancer as women ages 45 to 60. In women older than 55, 50% more patients have metastatic disease at presentation than do younger women. Vital to the process of detection are monthly BSEs, breast imaging with digital mammography and MRI or ultrasound to differentiate a cyst from a lesion and to detect small tumors before they can be palpated, and periodic breast examinations by a physician.

Etiology and Pathophysiology

The cause of breast cancer is unknown. The high incidence in women implies a hormonal cause (Box 52-5).

Box 52-5 Predisposing Factors for Women at High Risk for Breast Cancer

- **Gender:** Being a female introduces a high risk.
- **Age:** Higher incidence occurs with women over 40 years of age and in the postmenopausal phase of life. After age 60 the incidence increases dramatically.
- **Race:** White women, in the middle or upper socioeconomic class, are at higher risk
- **Genetics:** The inherited susceptibility genes *BRCA1* and *BRCA2* account for approximately 5% of all cases and confer a lifetime risk in these women, ranging from 35% to 85%.
- **Family history:** This is especially important if diagnosed family member had ovarian cancer, was premenopausal, had bilateral breast cancer, or is a first-degree relative (mother, sister, daughter).
- **Parity** (total number of pregnancies): Risk is decreased for women if birth is before 18 years; it is increased for women who are not sexually active, infertile women, and women who become pregnant for the first time after 30 years of age.
- **Menopause:** Menopause after 55 years of age increases the risk.
- **Obesity:** Weight gain and obesity after menopause increase the risk.
- **Other cancer:** Risk is increased for women who had another cancer such as endometrial, ovarian, or colon; if cancer has appeared in one breast, it is more likely to occur in the other breast.

The primary risk factors are female gender, age older than 50, North American or Northern European descent, a personal history of breast cancer, atypical hyperplasia or carcinoma in situ, two or more first-degree relatives with the disease, and a first-degree relative with bilateral premenopausal breast cancer. Other risk factors include early menarche, a first pregnancy after age 30, natural menopause after age 55, and one or more breast cancer genes. The inherited susceptibility genes, *BRCA1* and *BRCA2*, account for approximately 5% of all cases and confer a lifetime risk in these women ranging from 35% to 85% (Hollingsworth et al., 2004). Recent findings suggest that prophylactic removal of the breasts and/or ovaries in *BRCA1* and *BRCA2* carriers decreases the risk of breast cancer considerably, although not all women who choose this surgery would have developed cancer. Women who consider this option should have an opportunity for counseling before reaching a decision (Hollingsworth et al., 2004). Results of a recent study suggest that women who are overweight are more likely to die from breast cancer. Current data indicate tamoxifen and raloxifene decrease breast cancer risk in women who are at increased risk (Kudachadkar & O'Regan, 2005). With the exception of advancing age and being female, though, most women who develop breast cancer do not have any risk factors for the disease. That is why it is so important to encourage even healthy women to undergo screening examinations.

Breast cancer is usually an adenocarcinoma, arising from the epithelium and developing in the lactiferous ducts; it infiltrates the parenchyma (the tissue of an organ other than the supporting or connective tissue). The cancer occurs most often in women who have not given birth or breastfed a child. It occurs most often in the upper outer quadrant of the breast because this is the location of most of the glandular tissue. A slow-growing breast cancer may take up to 10 or more years to become palpable, or to reach the size of a small pea. Slow-growing lesions are often associated with a lower mortality rate. When referring to estimated growth rate of breast cancer, the term *doubling time* indicates the time it takes malignant cells to double in number. Assuming that the doubling is constant and that the neoplasm originates in one cell, a carcinoma with a doubling time of 100 days may not reach clinically detectable size (1 cm) for 8 years. Rapid-growing cancers have a much shorter preclinical course and a greater tendency to metastasize to regional nodes or more distant sites by the time a breast mass is discovered. In breast cancer, metastasis is by the lymphatic system and bloodstream (Figure 52-14). The most common sites for metastasis are, in order, bones, lungs, pleura, breast site, central nervous system, and liver.

Clinical Manifestations

Breast cancer is detected as a lump or mammographic abnormality in the breast. Breast tumors are usually small, solitary, irregularly shaped, firm, nontender, and nonmobile. There may be a change in skin color, feelings of tenderness, puckering or dimpling (peau d'orange—skin appearance of an orange peel) of tissue, nipple discharge, retraction of the nipple, and axillary tenderness.

More than 90% of breast cancers are detected by the patient. Women should perform BSEs monthly, preferably 1 week after menses. Postmenopausal women should perform a BSE on the same day each month (Figure 52-15). If there are questionable findings, the patient should immediately contact her physician (see Patient Teaching box).

Diagnostic Tests

The essential factors in the early detection of breast cancer are the regular performance of BSE, regular clinical breast examination (CBE), and routine mammography.

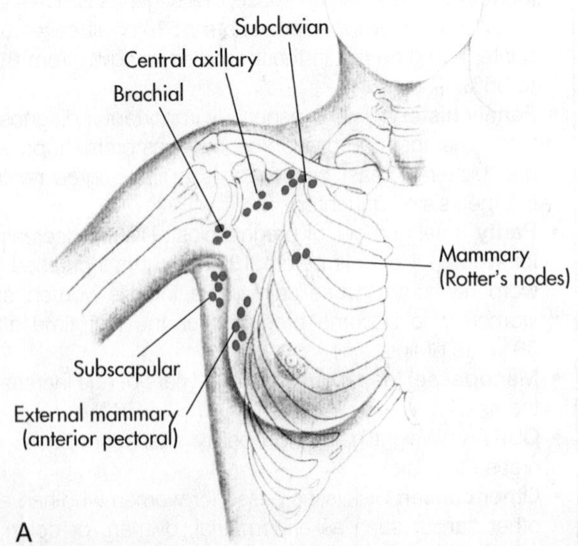

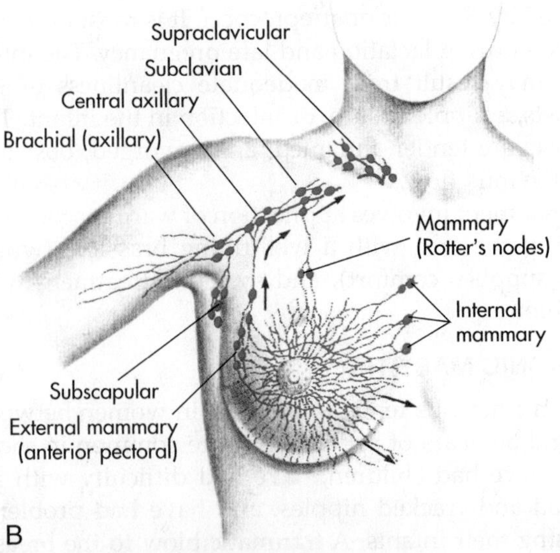

FIGURE 52-14 **A,** Lymph nodes of the axilla. **B,** Lymphatic drainage of the breast.

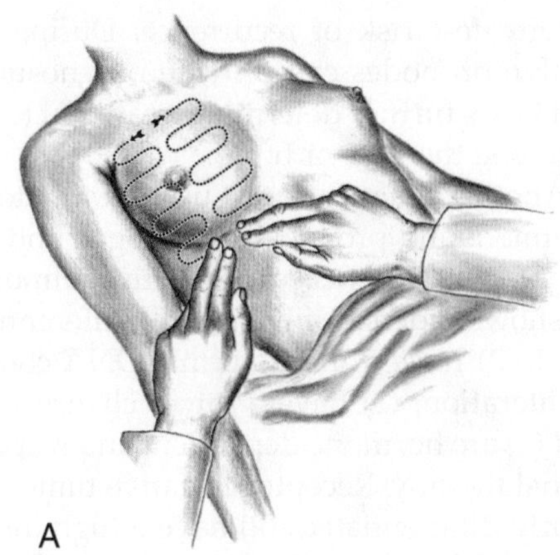

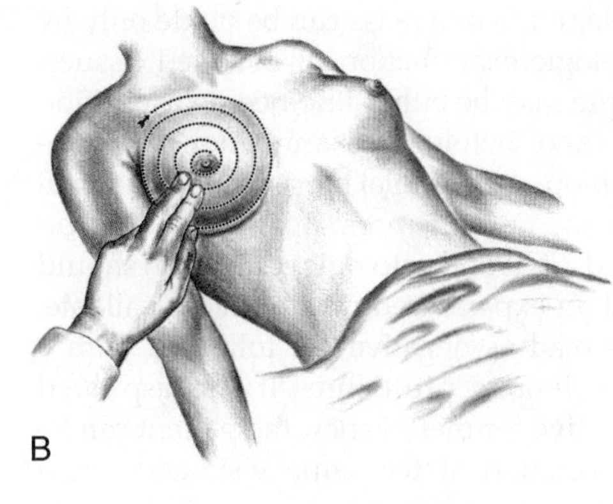

FIGURE 52-15 Methods for palpation. **A,** Back and forth. **B,** Concentric circles.

Patient Teaching

Breast Self-Examination

- The majority of breast lumps are not cancer.
- Cancerous breast lesions are treatable.
- Breasts should be examined by premenopausal women each month, 7 or 8 days after conclusion of the menstrual period when they are least congested, and by postmenopausal women on the same day of each month.
- Visual inspection and palpation should be done.
- Visual inspection should be done when the woman is stripped to the waist and looking in a mirror, using the following arm positions: (1) arms at rest at sides, (2) hands on hips and pressed into hips, (3) contracting chest muscles, (4) hands over the head (torso in upright position), (5) hands over head (torso leaning forward).
- Palpation may be done in the shower when the soap and water help the hands glide over the skin. However, examination of large breasts and axillae is better done in a supine position rather than standing.
- The entire breast should be examined in a systematic way, moving clockwise, with a circular motion, or moving back and forth. Always include the axillae in the examination.
- Do not forget specific examination of the nipple, through compression for discharge, and the areola, through palpation.
- Report any changes to the physician.

The frequency of these examinations is determined by the woman's age, the presence of significant risk factors, and her medical history. Current guidelines accepted by the ACS (ACS, 2009a) regarding breast surveillance practices include the following:

- Monthly BSE starting at 20 years of age.
- Physical examinations of the breast by a trained health professional; CBE every 3 years between 20 and 40 years of age and every year for women 40 and older.
- Screening mammography annually beginning at 40 years of age. If first-degree family member has a history of breast cancer, screening mammogram is recommended at 35 years (ACS, 2007b).
- MRI screening for the following groups of women: women with 20% to 25% or greater lifetime risk of breast cancer, women with a strong family history of breast or ovarian cancer, and women who were treated for Hodgkin's disease and received chest radiation.

New guidelines from the U.S. Preventative Services Task Force (USPSTF) (2009) recommend the following: (1) women age 40 to 49 should not receive routine screening mammography for breast cancer, but these women should decide for themselves when to begin mammography after weighing the risks and benefits; (2) women age 50 to 74 should receive screening mammography every 2 years (instead of annually); (3) routine breast self-examination (BSE) should no longer be taught. The Task Force states that this is not a recommendation against mammography for women in their 40s and BSE, but that there is not enough evidence to prove that women benefit from them. The ACS (2009b) and the American Congress of Obstetricians and Gynecologists (ACOG) (2009) state they will *not* be changing their guidelines.

Several techniques can be used to screen for breast disease or diagnose a suspicious physical finding. Mammography is a radiographic technique used to visualize the internal structure of the breast. Approximately 2 million women have mammograms annually. Mammography can detect tumors that cannot be felt by palpation. The minimum size detectable by physical examination is 1 cm. It takes 10 or more years to grow a tumor this size. Mammography can detect masses of 0.5 cm. Because tumors usually metastasize late in the preclinical course, earlier detection by mammography may prevent metastasis of smaller lesions.

Comparative mammography may show early cancer tissue changes. The diagnostic accuracy of mammography in combination with physical examination has significantly improved early and accurate detection of breast malignancies. In younger women, mammography is less sensitive because of the greater density of breast tissue, resulting in more false-negative results. Mammography will not reveal 10% to 25% of breast cancers. Masses should be biopsied, even if mammogram findings are unremarkable.

Definitive diagnosis of a mass can be made only by means of histologic examination of biopsied tissues. Biopsy technique may be either fine-needle aspiration (FNA) biopsy and cytologic examination or core-cutting needle biopsy, excisional biopsy, and incisional biopsy. Even if the lesion is nonpalpable, an FNA biopsy can be used. FNA and cytologic evaluation should be done only if an experienced cytologist is available, and all lesions read as negative are followed with a more definitive biopsy procedure. If the aspirated specimen is positive for malignancy, the patient can be given this information at the same visit and begin learning about treatment issues.

Improved imaging techniques have reduced the radiation exposure that accompanies mammography to insignificant levels. Therefore the benefits of mammography outweigh the risks from radiation exposure. Ultrasound (echogram, sonogram) can also be used to differentiate a benign cyst (fluid filled) from a malignant mass (solid). An ultrasound will not detect microcalcifications, which are often the only indicators of very small tumors.

Other methods used to help diagnose and stage breast cancer include MRI and positron emission tomography (PET). MRI and PET scans are used to help differentiate between malignant and benign disease in select patients.

A relatively new diagnostic tool used before therapeutic surgery is **sentinel lymph node mapping**, which identifies the first lymph node most likely to drain the cancerous cells. During this procedure a radioactive substance is injected around the breast biopsy site. The patient is then sent to the operating room, where a blue dye is injected as well. The area is then monitored to see which nodes take up the substances. The node that "lights up," containing the most radioactivity and blue dye, is considered the sentinel node and the one most likely to contain cancer cells. The identified node and at least two other nodes are then biopsied to see if they contain tumor cells. If they do not, it is likely that the more distant axillary nodes are cancer free. The nodes can be left intact, reducing the threat of complications such as edema, infection, pain, and loss of function of the arm. Sentinel lymph node dissection has been associated with lower morbidity rates and greater accuracy compared with complete axillary node dissection. National clinical research trials are evaluating whether standard lymph node dissection can be avoided if sentinel lymph node dissection is performed (Lewis et al., 2007). If one or more sentinel lymph nodes are positive for malignant cells, generally an axillary lymph node dissection is recommended (Lewis et al., 2007).

Axillary lymph node involvement is one of the most important prognostic factors in early-stage breast cancer. Metastasis in axillary nodes can be determined by pathologic examination of as few as 6 to 10 nodes. The more nodes involved, the greater the risk of recurrence. Patients with four or more positive nodes have the greatest risk of recurrence. During examination, the lymph nodes can provide prognostic information that helps further determine treatment (chemotherapy, hormone therapy, or both).

Another diagnostic test useful for determining both treatment and prognosis is estrogen and progesterone receptor status. Receptor-positive tumors commonly (1) show evidence of being well differentiated (see Box 57-2), (2) have a more normal DNA content and low proliferation, (3) have a lower chance for recurrence, and (4) are hormone dependent and responsive to hormonal therapy. Receptor-negative tumors (1) are often poorly differentiated, (2) have a high incidence of abnormal DNA content and high proliferation, (3) frequently recur, and (4) are usually unresponsive to hormonal therapy (Lewis et al., 2007).

Medical Management

The intervention for treatment of breast cancer depends on the tumor stage, the patient's age and health, the hormonal status, and the presence of estrogen receptors in the tumor. Radiation, chemotherapy, and surgery alone or in combination are the most common modes of treatment for breast cancer (see Chapter 57).

Staging

After breast surgery and axillary dissection, the staging process is completed. Axillary lymph node dissection or sentinel lymph node mapping is usually performed regardless of the treatment option selected. Examination of nodes provides the most powerful prognostic data currently available. Also, removal of axillary nodes is highly effective in preventing axillary recurrence, aids in decision making regarding adjuvant chemotherapy or hormonal therapy, and eliminates the need for axillary nodal radiation. Radiation of the axilla is equally effective in decreasing the incidence of axillary recurrence (see Figure 52-14).

The most widely accepted staging method for breast cancer is the American Joint Committee on Cancer's TNM system. This system uses tumor size (T), nodal involvement and size (N), and presence of metastasis (M) to determine the stage of disease (Box 52-6). Tumors are classified from stage I to stage IV.

Surgical Intervention

Surgery plays a vital role in the management of breast cancer. Tissue biopsy, inspection and biopsy of lymph nodes in the axillary areas, radiologic examinations, and laboratory reports aid in making the decision to perform surgery.

Because estrogen can affect a tumor's invasive ability, it is suggested to operate on premenopausal women during the menstrual phase, when estrogen levels are lower or opposed by progesterone.

Several surgical options are available for the removal of the breast carcinoma. **Breast conservation surgery**

Box 52-6 TNM System for Staging Breast Cancer

Breast cancer is staged using the TNM (tumor, node, metastasis) system, which categorizes the disease by tumor size and spread, lymph node involvement, and metastasis. The TNM system, which was developed by the American Joint Committee on Cancer and revised in 2003, works this way:

- **Tumor:** A number from **0** to **4** indicates the tumor's size and whether it has spread to nearby tissue. (**Tis** indicates a carcinoma in situ.) Higher numbers indicate a larger tumor or wider spread. For example, a tumor labeled **T1** is 2 cm or smaller; **T4** indicates a tumor of any size that has spread to the chest wall or the skin.
- **Nodes:** A number from **0** to **3** indicates whether the cancer has spread to surrounding lymph nodes and, if so, the number of nodes that are affected. For example, **N1** indicates a spread to one, two, or three lymph nodes under the arm on the same side as the breast cancer.
- **Metastasis: M0** means the cancer has not spread to distant organs; **M1** means the cancer has metastasized to other organs.

All of this information is combined to determine an overall stage of **0** to **IV.**

- **Stage 0:** Refers to carcinoma in situ, in which the tumor is confined to the milk duct or the lobule, no nodes have been affected, and no metastasis has occurred.
- **Stage I:** The tumor is 2 cm or smaller. Lymph nodes are negative. There is no distant cancer spread.
- **Stage IIA:** The tumor is 5 cm or smaller. It may have spread to one, two, or three axillary nodes. There is no distant cancer spread.
- **Stage IIB:** The tumor can be larger than 5 cm. Up to three lymph nodes may be involved, but there is no metastasis to other organs.
- **Stage IIIA:** The tumor may be more than 5 cm and has spread to more than 3 but fewer than 10 lymph nodes. No distant organs are involved.
- **Stage IIIB:** The tumor, regardless of size, has spread to the chest wall or the skin. There is lymph node involvement but no distant metastasis.
- **Stage IIIC:** Refers to any size tumor, including one that has spread to the chest wall or the skin. There is involvement of 10 or more lymph nodes, but no distant metastasis.
- **Stage IV:** The tumor can be any size. There is nodal involvement and metastasis to distant organs.

American Cancer Society (ACS). (2009). *How is breast cancer staged?* Available at www.cancer.org/docroot/CRI/content/CRI_2_4_3x_How_is_breast_cancer_staged_5.asp?mav=cri. Accessed November, 2009; and Lewis, S.L., et al. (2007). *Medical-surgical nursing: assessment and management of clinical problems.* (7th ed.). St. Louis: Mosby.

(termed **lumpectomy**), which conserves the breast, is the removal of a circumscribed area along with the tumor. This surgery is usually done when the tumor is small and located on the peripheral area of the breast. The breast contour and muscle support are preserved if possible. Research has shown that there is no survival advantage in taking the whole breast when the malignancy is confined to just one area and its size is less than 2 cm—as long as adjunctive radiation to the surrounding region, ending with a radiation boost to the tumor bed, is done to destroy any remaining microscopic disease (Mirshahidi, 2004). Axillary nodes are often removed in these breast-sparing procedures as well. Contraindications to lumpectomy or excisional biopsy include two or more separate tumors in separate quadrants of the breast, diffuse microcalcifications, a history of previous radiation to the region, a large tumor-to-breast ratio, a history of collagen vascular disease, large breasts, and a tumor located underneath the nipple.

One of the main advantages of breast conservation surgery and radiation is that it preserves the breast, including the nipple. The goal of the combined surgery and radiation is to maximize the benefits of both cancer treatment and cosmetic outcome while minimizing risks. Disadvantages of this surgery plus radiation include the increased cost over surgery alone and the possible side effects of radiation. Lumpectomy is followed by 6 weeks of radiation.

A **simple mastectomy** is the removal of the entire breast. The skin flap is retained to cover the incised area. Both pectoralis major and pectoralis minor muscles are left intact. The patient has the option of breast reconstruction.

A **modified radical mastectomy** may be performed if the tumor is 4 cm or larger, if it is invasive, or if the patient and physician decide this procedure is in the patient's best interest. In this operation all breast tissue, overlying skin, nipple, and pectoralis minor muscles are removed, as are samples of axillary lymph nodes and fascia under the breast. The pectoralis major muscle remains intact. The patient has the option of breast reconstruction, which can be performed immediately after the mastectomy or can be delayed until postoperative recovery is complete (about 6 months).

Most women diagnosed with early-stage breast cancer (tumors less than 5 cm) are candidates for either lumpectomy and radiation or modified radical mastectomy. Overall 10-year survival with lumpectomy and radiation is about the same as with modified radical mastectomy (Mirshahidi, 2004).

Adjuvant Therapies

Radiation therapy. Depending on the tumor's size, regional spread, and aggressiveness, radiation therapy is often prescribed. Radiation therapy may be used for breast cancer (1) as the primary therapy to destroy the tumor or as a companion to surgery to prevent local recurrence, (2) to shrink a large tumor to operable size, and (3) as the palliative treatment for pain caused by local recurrence and metastasis. Lumpectomy is almost always followed by radiation. Radiation therapy is usually started 2 to 3 weeks after surgery, when the wound is completely healed and the patient can comfortably raise her arm over her head. Contraindications include a diagnosis of breast cancer during the first or second trimester of pregnancy, delayed wound healing, collagen vascular disease, and previous radiation to the same breast.

In **external beam radiation,** the radiation procedure uses an external beam of high-energy protons. The treatments are usually done 5 days a week for 5 to 6 weeks. Adverse effects include fatigue and skin reactions such as burning, erythema, pruritus, dryness, infection, and pain.

Internal radiation, also known as implant radiation or **brachytherapy,** is a new procedure that is an alternative to traditional radiation treatment for early-stage breast cancer. The technique uses a balloon catheter to insert radioactive seeds into the breast after the tumor is removed (at the time of the lumpectomy or shortly thereafter into the tumor resection cavity). The seeds deliver a high dose of concentrated radiation directly to the site where the cancer is most likely to recur. Traditional radiation treatment can take 6 weeks; in contrast, high-dose brachytherapy may require only 5 days (Lewis et al., 2007).

Chemotherapy. Patients who require postsurgical chemotherapy—typically those with lymph node involvement or metastasis to distant organs—receive antineoplastic medications, hormones, a monoclonal antibody, or a combination of these medications. Regimens for node-negative disease (i.e., cancer that has not spread to the lymph nodes) include cyclophosphamide (Cytoxan, Neosar), methotrexate, and 5-fluorouracil (Adrucil, Efudex), referred to as CMF; cyclophosphamide, doxorubicin (Adriamycin), and 5-fluorouracil, or CAF; or doxorubicin and cyclophosphamide, commonly called AC. For those with node-positive disease, the regimens include CAF, AC followed by paclitaxel, doxorubicin followed by CMF, and CMF.

The most common adverse effects of traditional antineoplastic drugs are bone marrow suppression (which causes anemia, thrombocytopenia, and leukopenia), nausea and vomiting, alopecia, weight gain, mucositis, and fatigue. Agents such as filgrastim (Neupogen), which raise leukocyte counts, can combat the threat of infection that accompanies bone marrow suppression. Epoetin alfa (Procrit) is helpful in raising erythrocyte counts to help correct anemia. Other drugs typically ordered for chemotherapy patients are phenothiazines, such as prochlorperazine (Compazine), and serotonin antagonists such as granisetron (Kytril) and ondansetron (Zofran). These drugs prevent or lessen nausea and vomiting (Greifzu, 2004).

Hormonal therapy. Estrogen can promote the growth of breast cancer cells if the cells are estrogen-receptor positive. Hormonal therapy removes or blocks the source of estrogen, thus promoting tumor regression.

Two advances have increased the use of hormonal therapy in breast cancer. First, hormone receptor assays, which are reliable diagnostic tests, have been developed to identify women who are likely to respond to hormonal therapy. The tumor's estrogen and progesterone receptor status can be determined. These assays can predict whether hormonal therapy is a treatment option for women with breast cancer, either at the time of initial therapy or if the cancer recurs. Second, drugs have been developed that can inactivate the hormone-secreting glands as effectively as surgery or radiation. Premenopausal and perimenopausal women are more likely to have tumors that are not hormone dependent, whereas women who are postmenopausal are more likely to have hormone-dependent tumors. Chances of tumor regression are significantly greater in women whose tumors contain estrogen and progesterone receptors.

Estrogen deprivation can occur by destroying the ovaries by surgery or radiation or drug therapy. Hormonal therapy can block or destroy the estrogen receptors. Hormonal therapy is widely used to treat recurrent or metastatic cancer but may also be used as an adjuvant to primary treatment.

Tamoxifen is the hormonal agent of choice in postmenopausal, estrogen receptor–positive women with or without lymph node involvement. Tamoxifen, an antiestrogen drug, blocks the estrogen receptor sites of malignant cells and thus inhibits the growth-stimulating effects of estrogen. It is commonly used in advanced and early-stage breast cancer to prevent or treat recurrent disease. Tamoxifen may also be used to prevent breast cancer in high-risk individuals. Side effects of tamoxifen are minimal but include hot flashes, nausea, vomiting, vaginal discharge, and other effects commonly associated with decreased estrogen. It also increases the risk of blood clots, cataracts, and endometrial cancer in postmenopausal women. Tamoxifen is not used in women desiring continued fertility.

Toremifene (Fareston), an antiestrogen agent similar to tamoxifen, is indicated as first-line treatment for metastatic breast cancer in postmenopausal women with estrogen receptor–positive or estrogen receptor–unknown tumors. Fulvestrant (Faslodex) may be given to women with advanced breast cancer who no longer respond to tamoxifen. This drug slows cancer progression by destroying estrogen receptors in the breast cancer cells. Fulvestrant is given intramuscularly on a monthly basis.

Aromatase inhibitor drugs, which interfere with the enzyme that synthesizes endogenous estrogen, are used to treat advanced breast cancer in postmenopausal women with disease progression. These drugs include anastrozole (Arimidex), letrozole (Femara), vorozole (Rizivor), exemestane (Aromasin), and aminoglutethimide (Cytadren).

Research has shown that letrozole reduced the risk of recurrence of breast cancer among women by 43%. The women in the letrozole study had recently completed (after surgery) the standard 5-year course of tamoxifen, a powerful and widely used drug that eventually loses its effectiveness as, researchers believe, tumors become resistant to it. Until now, breast cancer patients who finished tamoxifen treatment could only wait and hope that their cancer would not recur; however, in up to 20% of such cases, it does recur within 5 years. Letrozole, previously approved by the FDA for advanced breast cancer, offers an exciting new option for extending treatment of early-stage disease (Kudachadkar & O'Regan, 2005). Letrozole, like tamoxifen, works by interfering with the hormone estrogen, which feeds breast cancer cells. Tamoxifen blocks estrogen receptors on the cells, whereas letrozole inhibits the creation of estrogen.

Bisphosphonates, such as pamidronate sodium (Aredia), are being used to delay bone metastases and reduce the occurrence of skeletal problems in patients with advanced breast cancer (Greifzu, 2004). Raloxifene (Evista), used to prevent bone loss, may also reduce the risk of breast cancer without stimulating endometrial growth. Raloxifene acts as an estrogen antagonist at the hormone-sensitive tissues of breast cancer and bone. Additional drugs that may be used to suppress hormone-dependent tumors include megestrol (Megace), DES, and fluoxymesterone (Halotestin) (Lewis et al., 2007).

Monoclonal antibody therapy. A recent drug treatment for breast cancer is the monoclonal antibody trastuzumab (Herceptin). It is used to treat metastatic breast cancer in women who overexpress (i.e., have an excess amount of) a breast cancer cell antigen called HER_2. Up to 30% of patients fall into this category.

Ovarian ablation. Another promising treatment option is **ovarian ablation** by means of a bilateral oophorectomy, which is used in combination with tamoxifen for metastatic disease.

Bone marrow and stem cell transplantation. Autologous (i.e., originating within self) bone marrow or stem cell transplantation combined with high-dose chemotherapy has been used to treat patients with advanced metastatic breast cancer. In this technique, patients donate their own bone marrow or peripheral blood, from which stem cells are harvested. Then they receive high doses of chemotherapy, which causes bone marrow suppression. The patient subsequently undergoes autologous bone marrow or stem cell transplantation to reconstitute or "rescue" their hematopoietic system to start producing hematopoietic blood cells.

Nursing Interventions

The physician discusses with the patient and the family the rationale for the specific surgical approach and the manner of coping with the cosmetic effects of and psychological response to the surgery. Patients will have questions about possible alternatives to standard or modified mastectomy.

The patient may be confused with so many options for therapy and surgical interventions. During this time, play an active role as listener, reinforce information provided by the physician, and encourage the patient to verbalize her concerns and recognize her feelings about the surgery. The emotional preparation of the patient may be more important than the physical preparation. Often she undergoes anticipatory grieving for the loss of a body part.

Preoperative preparation involves patient, support group, and nursing staff so that progressive care can run

Nursing Care Plan 52-1 The Patient Undergoing Modified Radical Mastectomy

Ms. Ceba, age 52, was diagnosed with ductal cell carcinoma of the left breast. She has undergone a left modified radical mastectomy

NURSING DIAGNOSIS *Fear, related to the cancer diagnosis and surgical intervention*

Patient Goals and Expected Outcomes	Nursing Interventions	Evaluation
Patient will be able to state fears Patient will state she has made improvement in coping	Encourage patient to talk about specific fears and feelings about each fear. Provide a calm, supportive environment. Provide information on coping mechanisms. Encourage consultation with resource persons (psychologist, clergy, nurse specialist, Reach to Recovery). Use support of family and significant others. Encourage use of comfort measures, such as music. Encourage patient's comments and questions about surgery and postoperative care.	Patient verbalizes fear, has support of significant others, and expresses confidence in ability to cope.

Continued

Nursing Care Plan 52-1 The Patient Undergoing Modified Radical Mastectomy—cont'd

NURSING DIAGNOSIS *Infection, risk for, related to surgical incision and presence of drain*

Patient Goals and Expected Outcomes	Nursing Interventions	Evaluation
Skin will remain free of signs and symptoms of infection Vital signs and white blood cell (WBC) values will be maintained within normal limits	Assess skin integrity. Instruct patient on signs and symptoms of infection. Assess and report abnormal vital signs and elevated WBC; skin changes; and comfort level. Observe and record amount of exudate. Check drainage tubing for patency. Instruct patient to examine remaining breast once a month. Caution patient to avoid injections, vaccinations, taking of blood pressure, taking of blood samples, or insertion of intravenous line in affected area.	Incision has no erythema or purulent drainage. Temperature remains within normal. WBC remains normal.

NURSING DIAGNOSIS *Body image, disturbed, related to loss of breast through modified radical mastectomy*

Patient Goals and Expected Outcomes	Nursing Interventions	Evaluation
Patient will verbalize acceptance of altered body image as evidenced by absence of weeping, irritability, or verbalization of discomfort with present body; and by the attempting of difficult physical or mental tasks despite limitations Patient will demonstrate interest in her personal appearance Patient will verbalize plans to resume former activities	Encourage patient's comments and questions about surgery, progress, and prognosis. Encourage patient to discuss change in her body with husband or significant other. Reinforce correct information, and provide factual information to correct any misconceptions. Relate importance of communicating anything that causes anxiety. Encourage patient to verbalize and explore feelings regarding impact missing body part might have on patient's functioning as a sexual partner and in activities of daily living. Encourage patient to continue activities associated with femininity, such as fixing hair, using makeup, and wearing own apparel. Encourage patient to look at and touch the changed body part when she is ready. Encourage use of rehabilitation services (Reach to Recovery, Wellness Community).	Patient verbalizes feelings about surgery and change in body image; indicates beginning resolution of negative feelings toward self; and begins to accept altered body image.

Critical Thinking Questions

1. Ms. Ceba confides in her nurse that she feels ugly and unattractive and she refuses to look at her incision. What would be a helpful approach by the nurse?
2. In assessing Ms. Ceba, the nurse notes her holding her left arm guardedly in an adducted position. She does not use it for activities of daily living. What should effective patient teaching include?
3. What should be included in discharge teaching for Ms. Ceba to prevent trauma and infection of her left arm?

continuously from admission through surgery, recovery, and the postoperative period. The initial admission assessment provides data that are helpful for the nurse and patient in planning care. Nursing diagnoses can be developed and a care plan individualized according to the patient's needs (Nursing Care Plan 52-1).

Assess and identify members of the patient's support system to know their strengths and concerns about the pending treatment and interventions. Support does not always need to come from the immediate family and close friends. Outside support and resources can come from co-workers, religious groups, oncology clinicians, psychologists, and Reach to Recovery support groups. It is important to openly discuss the patient's fears; establishing a therapeutic relationship with the patient and family enables this to happen.

Reach to Recovery volunteers are a source of information, encouragement, and support for women with breast cancer. The organization is based on the premise that rehabilitation for the cancer patient should include communication with and support from another who was in a similar situation and learned to cope and resume her normal activities.

Nursing interventions for patients who undergo modified radical mastectomy include monitoring vital signs and observing for symptoms of shock or hemorrhage, since many large blood vessels are involved in the procedure. Drains such as Jackson-Pratt, Davol, or Hemovac may be placed in the axilla to facilitate drainage and prevent formation of a hematoma. Postoperative dressings are usually constrictive and bulky and may tend to impede respiratory effort and cause pain and discomfort. Assess for excessive exudates on the dressing and in the axillary region. Place a smaller, less bulky dressing over the incisional site for the first postoperative day. When the vital signs are stable, place the patient in a 45-degree Fowler's position to promote drainage. Change the position frequently, and encourage deep breathing and coughing.

Some patients may experience incisional pain for several days after surgery and when doing arm exercises. They may complain of numbness and referred pain in the arm of the operative area. The pain radiates to the shoulder and the back because of the severance of the peripheral nerves. Most of the nerves regenerate, but there are cases of residual numbness.

No matter what type of surgery the patient has, pain management and wound care are priorities. Typically a patient will have a patient-controlled analgesia pump with morphine for 12 to 24 hours. She then receives oral analgesics as needed.

Patient Teaching

It is important for the patient to deep breathe and cough to prevent postoperative atelectasis.

Physicians differ in opinion about the best position for the affected arm. Some physicians place the arm in the dressing and place it in a sling for a couple of days postoperatively. Some physicians prefer to avoid slings. If the arm is not restricted by dressings, it may be elevated on a pillow with the hand and wrist higher than the elbow and the elbow higher than the shoulder joint. This will facilitate the flow of fluids through the lymph and venous routes and prevent lymphedema (accumulation of lymph in soft tissues).

Usually the patient is allowed to ambulate on the first postoperative day. She needs assistance in moving out of bed as she learns to maintain balance because of breast removal and bulky dressings.

Instruct the patient not to have any procedures involving the arm on the affected side—blood pressure readings, injections, IV infusion of fluids, or the drawing of blood, which may cause edema or infection. She also needs to guard against infections from burns, needle pricks (sewing), and gardening injuries because defense mechanisms are lessened by the removal of lymph nodes. Removing lymph nodes and channels increases the risk of developing lymphedema, even years after surgery. Referral to physical therapy may be indicated to control lymphedema if it develops. An exercise regimen, built up gradually, can help decrease lymphedema. However, exercise should not be started until the incision has healed completely, which takes up to 2 weeks or at the physician's discretion. Tell the patient to avoid lifting heavy objects with the affected arm for 6 to 8 weeks. Instruct her to avoid sleeping on the involved arm. Clothing on the affected arm should be nonconstricting. Bracelets and watches should be worn on the unaffected arm (Box 52-7).

The longer the edema persists, the more difficult it is to manage. Diuretics and low-sodium diets are often prescribed. If the edema persists, an elastic stockinette is measured for precise fit to avoid venous flow constriction. The sleeve is applied from the wrist to the shoulder and worn when the patient is out of bed. When the patient is sleeping, position the arm to aid venous flow. If the lymphedema is severe, the physician may order Jobst extremity therapy. A pneumomassage sleeve with automatic inflation and deflation can be placed on the arm. The compression pump is strictly contraindicated when there is evidence of acute phlebitis, perivascular lymphangitis, or cellulitis.

Isometric exercises are helpful for increasing the circulation and developing the collateral lymph system. The patient can open and clench fingers and squeeze a rubber ball in the first few postoperative days. This activity provides extension and flexion of the wrist and elbow; it is equivalent to sewing, knitting, typing, and playing piano when at home.

Preventing Muscle Contractures

Specific exercises may be ordered to restore the muscle strength and full range of motion of the affected area. Gentle exercises started early in the postoperative course help to decrease muscle tension and to regain

Box 52-7 Hand and Arm Care after Breast Surgery

PREVENTION OF INFECTION
- Wear gloves when cleaning with harsh detergent.
- Wear gloves when gardening.
- Avoid injections, vaccinations, and venipuncture in involved arm.
- Use cuticle remover rather than cutting cuticles.
- Sew with a thimble.
- Avoid chapped hands; use lanolin cream daily.
- Take care when using equipment that might cut, scrape, or abrade.
- Shave underarms with an electric razor.
- Avoid insect bites; use insect repellent.

PREVENTION OF CONSTRICTING CIRCULATION
- Do not take blood pressure in involved arm.
- Wear loose clothing; avoid tight bra straps or tight sleeves.
- Wear watch or jewelry on uninvolved arm.
- Carry purse on uninvolved arm or shoulder.
- Prevent drag or pull:
  —Carry heavy packages on uninvolved arm.
  —Avoid motions that increase centrifugal force.

PREVENTION OF BURNS
- Wear padded mitts to reach into oven; use potholders.
- Prevent sunburn; use sunscreens with SPF of 15; cover arms during prolonged exposure.
- **Immediately report any signs of erythema, edema, warmth, or pain.**

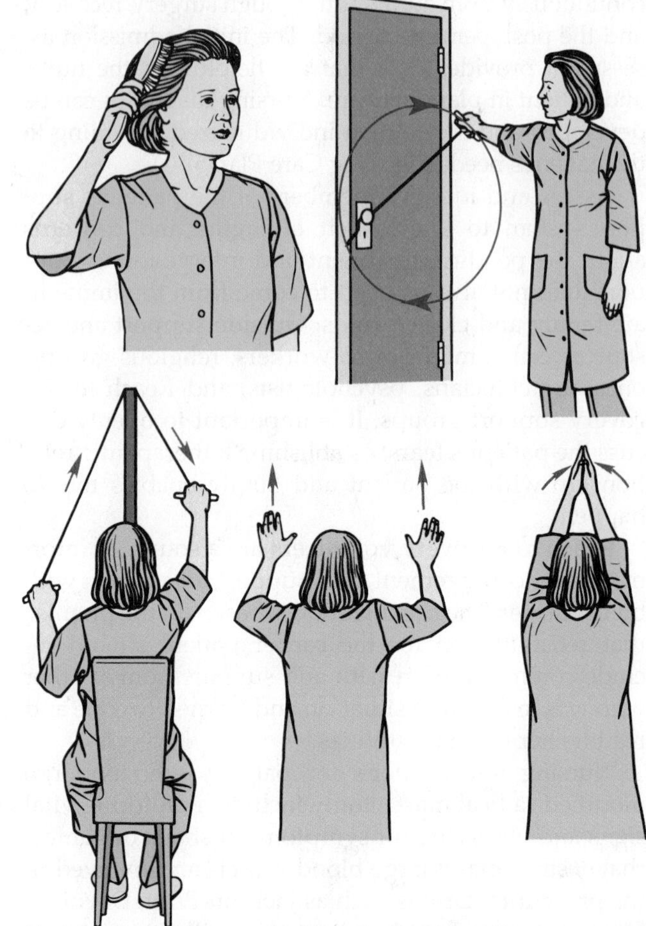

FIGURE 52-16 Exercises after mastectomy.

muscle function more quickly. The nurse or the therapist should instruct the patient and encourage the continuation of the exercises on discharge. Many of the exercises may be incorporated into ADLs as they are resumed (Figure 52-16; Box 52-8). Exercising can be painful, but the patient can meet the challenge with the encouragement of a support group.

Body Image Acceptance

After losing a breast, many patients experience grief over the loss of a body part. This acute grief is like a crisis and may last 4 to 6 weeks or longer. Grief makes the fact of loss real, and the process is essential for personal adaptation to the loss. Assist the patient in finding helpful coping mechanisms.

Initial coping mechanisms often begin to lose effectiveness at about 3 months, and a period of depression ensues. Provide anticipatory guidance for this eventuality. Special nursing interventions, in terms of both psychological support and self-care education, are necessary if the cancer recurs. Participation in a cancer support group is important and has been found to have a clinically significant impact on survival.

When deep breathing exercises are started immediately after surgery and the patient splints the area and exercises her arm, she will recognize the absence of the breast through touch. Dressing changes and incision cleansing with patient involvement make the absence real. Being involved and responsible for the dressing and incision allows a more personal approach to the patient. At this time, the nurse's support is important. Provide a mirror or seat the patient in front of the mirror so she can see the operative site being cleansed and dressed. Be sensitive to the patient and be alert for signs of readiness to become involved in care and accept the loss of the body part. The incisional area may be erythematous and edematous, but the discoloration will gradually lessen and the site will become more comfortable. Encourage her to massage in cocoa butter or a cream to make the incisional line softer. Advise the patient that it takes time to accept the loss and heal both emotionally and physically.

Prosthesis

A breast prosthesis should not be worn unless authorized by the physician. Many breast forms are available. Forms are made of gels, molded silicone, and saline solution. Most forms are covered with soft fabric, are lightweight, and feel like breast tissue. There is a shape for each type of breast, since each body is different and each surgery is different. Forms have been developed that can be fitted for a right or left breast, slanted for the breast that was slanted, or formed with

Box 52-8 Postmastectomy Arm Exercises

CLIMBING THE WALL
1. Stand facing wall with toes 6 to 12 inches from wall.
2. Bend elbows and place palms of hands against wall at shoulder level.
3. Move both hands parallel to each other up the wall as far as possible until incisional pull or pain occurs.
4. Move both hands down to starting position.
5. Goal is complete extension with elbows straight.
6. Activities that use the same action include reaching top shelves, hanging out clothes, washing windows, hanging curtains, and setting hair.

ELBOW PULL-IN
1. Extend arms sideways to shoulder level.
2. Clasp hands behind neck.
3. Pull elbows forward until they touch.
4. Return to position 2.
5. Unclasp hands and extend arms sideways at shoulder level.
6. Lower arms to side.

BACK SCRATCH
1. Place hand of unoperated side on hip for balance.
2. Bend elbow of affected arm, placing back of hand on small of back.
3. Work hand up the back slowly until fingers reach opposite shoulder blade.
4. Lower arm and straighten both arms.

ROPE PULL
1. Attach a rope over a shower rod, a hook, or the top of an open door.
2. Sit on a chair (with door between legs if using a door) and grasp each end of rope.
3. Alternately pull on each end, raising affected arm to a point of incisional pull or pain.
4. The goal is to raise the affected arm almost directly overhead.

an outer curve that simulates the extension of a full breast under the axilla and upward on the chest. It is advisable to have a skilled fitter from a reliable company fit the prosthesis.

A well-fitted brassiere is essential before choosing the shape form. If the woman is active, she may desire a pocket or restraining cup. Some forms can be worn against the skin with no underpadding or bra cups. Most forms can be washed with water and mild detergent to keep them clean and supple. Many prostheses are waterproof and can be worn swimming; when wet, they do not "weigh down" the wearer.

When the patient is being fitted with a prosthesis, the best assurance that the fit is right is when each of the following is observed:

- The brassiere fits snugly around the rib cage.
- The prosthesis fills the bottom of the bra cup.
- The prosthesis projects the same as the remaining breast, with form bulk and nipples in position.
- The breasts are separated when the bra is centered.
- The top of the bra cup is filled and appears like the other breast.

Breast Reconstruction

The patient whose disease is limited to the breast may benefit from reconstructive surgery. The benefits of breast reconstruction include avoidance of an external prosthesis that has potential for slipping, greater choice of clothing (including lower necklines), and loss of self-consciousness about appearance. For many women, breast reconstruction is beneficial in improving self-esteem. Breast reconstruction can provide many women with a renewed sense of wholeness and a return to a normal state. The most important indicators for reconstruction are the patient's motivation and desire for the procedure. The prime determinant for the procedure is the patient's clinical status. Goals for reconstruction are to select the simplest type that meets the patient's needs and expectations and to match the opposite breast in size, shape, and contour.

Breast reconstruction can be performed immediately after surgery or at a later time. An increasing number of women are electing immediate reconstruction; this may prolong the initial hospitalization but eliminates the need for a second hospitalization and contributes to self-esteem. Others wait until they have completed adjuvant chemotherapy or radiation to be certain the area is disease free.

Breast Implant

If the remaining skin is sufficient to cover an implant, surgery may consist of placing a permanent silicone implant under the pectoralis muscle. Possible complications of silicone implants include infection, deflation, a false mammography result, and silicone leaks.

Some researchers have suggested that the silicone filling or the implant covering can lead to autoimmune or connective tissue disease. Although most surgeries have not resulted in complications, differing opinions regarding the safety of breast implants led the FDA (2004) to issue some recommendations in early 1992. Breast implants were permitted after breast cancer surgery because of the offsetting positive contribution to recovery, but a moratorium was imposed on silicone implants solely for cosmetic purposes until data establishing safety could be provided. Many implants are now filled with saline or dextran instead of silicone.

Musculocutaneous Flap Procedure

Breast reconstruction. The musculocutaneous flap has made reconstruction possible for most patients who have undergone mastectomy, even when the pectoralis muscles have been removed or when nerve damage has resulted in muscle atrophy. The flap receives its blood supply from muscle, but it can include an overlying layer of skin. At the same time that this procedure is performed, a silicone or saline breast implant may be inserted; if enough pedicle tissue is available, no implant is needed.

Musculocutaneous flaps are most often taken from the back (latissimus dorsi muscle) or the abdomen (transverse rectus abdominis muscle). When the **latissimus dorsi musculocutaneous flap** is used for reconstruction, a block of skin and muscle from the patient's back is used to replace tissue removed during mastectomy (Figure 52-17, *E*). The **transverse rectus abdominis musculocutaneous (TRAM) flap** is the most frequently used flap operation for breast reconstruction. The rectus abdominis muscles are paired, flat muscles running from the ribcage down to the pubic bone. Arteries inside the muscle branch at many levels, and these branches supply blood to the fat and skin across a large expanse of the abdomen. In the TRAM technique, the surgeon elevates a large block of tissue from the lower abdominal area, but leaves it attached to the rectus muscle (Figure 52-17, *A* to *D*). This tissue is then tunneled under the skin or detached and placed as a "free flap" at the site of the breast reconstruction. The tissue is trimmed and shaped to form a breast mound similar to that of the opposite breast. An implant may be used in addition to the flap to achieve symmetry. The abdominal incision is closed in a fashion similar to that of an abdominal hysterectomy or a "tummy tuck." This surgical procedure can last 2 to 8 hours, with recovery taking 4 to 6 weeks. Complications include bleeding, hernia, and infection (Lewis et al., 2007).

Nipple reconstruction is usually performed as a separate procedure after the breast reconstruction has been completed. Nipple construction is generally from available tissue at the site or harvested tissue from the opposite breast. New techniques allow the nipple to be created from tissue and subcutaneous tissue of the breast mound. Areola reconstruction is provided by obtaining pigmented skin from the upper thigh or by using skin from the lateral chest area.

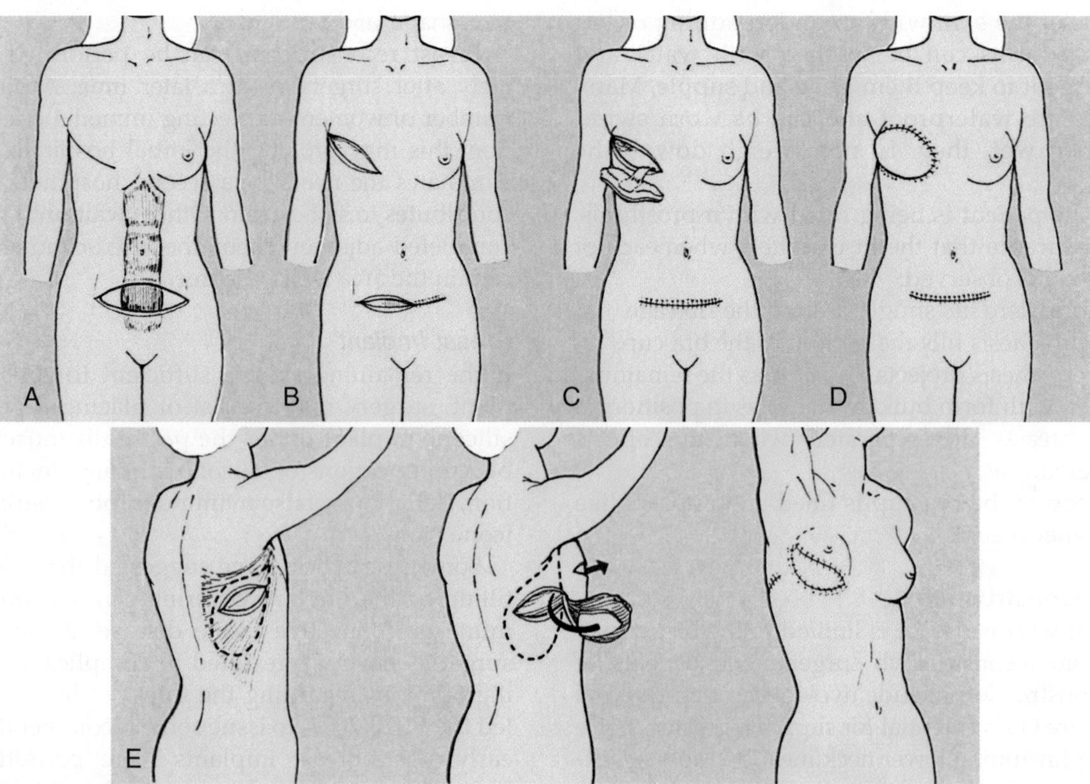

FIGURE 52-17 Transverse rectus abdominis musculocutaneous (TRAM) flap. **A,** TRAM flap is planned. **B,** The abdominal tissue, while attached to the rectus muscle, nerve, and blood supply, is tunneled beneath the abdomen to the chest. **C,** The flap is trimmed to shape the breast. The lower abdominal incision is closed. **D,** Nipple and areola are reconstructed after the breast has healed. **E,** In the latissimus dorsi musculocutaneous flap, a block of skin and muscle from the patient's back is used to replace tissue removed during mastectomy.

Table 52-3 Prognosis and Nodal Involvement in Breast Cancer

LYMPH NODES INVOLVED	METASTATIC RECURRENCE
1-3 nodes	50%-60% metastasis
4-9 nodes	75%-85% metastasis
10 nodes	Even worse prognosis

 Home Care Considerations

Cancer of the Breast

- Explain the follow-up routine to the patient and emphasize the importance of beginning and continuing breast self-examination and annual mammography.
- Symptoms that should be reported to the physician include new back pain, weakness, constipation, shortness of breath, and confusion.
- If adjuvant therapy is to be used, give the woman specific instructions about appointment times and treatment locations.
- If applicable, stress the importance of wearing a well-fitting prosthesis. The return of a normal external appearance is important to most women.
- Often the husband, sexual partner, or family member may need assistance in dealing with their emotional reactions to the diagnosis and surgery for them to effectively support the patient.
- If difficulty in adjustment or other problems develop, counseling may be necessary for women with breast cancer to deal with the emotional component of a modified radical mastectomy and the diagnosis of cancer.

Prognosis

The 5-year relative survival rate for localized breast cancer is 98%, with an 89% 5-year relative survival rate for all stages combined (ACS, 2007a). After the disease spreads beyond the breast, the survival rate drops dramatically. Breast cancer ranks second among cancer deaths in women. The most important prognostic factor is the stage of the disease (see Box 52-6; Table 52-3; Home Care Considerations box).

INFLAMMATORY AND INFECTIOUS DISORDERS OF THE MALE REPRODUCTIVE SYSTEM

PROSTATITIS

Etiology and Pathophysiology

Prostatitis is an acute or chronic infection of the prostate gland. Prostatitis is the most common problem involving the urinary system in men younger than 50 years. Bacterial invasion via the bloodstream and lymphatic channels, ascending from the urethra or descending from the bladder, commonly occurs (Lewis et al., 2007). The causative organisms include *E. coli, Klebsiella, Proteus, Pseudomonas, Streptococcus, N. gonorrhoeae,* and *C. trachomatis.*

Clinical Manifestations

Symptoms include sudden onset of chills and fever. There is urgency and frequency of urination, dysuria (pain when urinating), cloudy urine, perineal fullness, perineal pain, lower back pain, arthralgia (pain in the joints), and myalgia (pain in the muscles). The patient may also have acute urinary retention caused by prostatic edema. On palpation, the gland is tender, edematous, and firm. In chronic prostatitis, many patients may appear asymptomatic, but generally the symptoms are the same as in the acute phase but less intense.

Diagnostic Tests

Diagnosis is based on culture and sensitivity tests of the urethra, prostatic fluid, and urine for organism identification and appropriate antibiotic therapy. Prostatic fluid is collected by prostate massage and expression of fluid. The pH of the fluid is generally elevated. A rectal examination done by the physician reveals gland tenderness and edema.

Medical Management

Medical management includes antibiotic therapy such as ofloxacin (Floxin), ciprofloxacin (Cipro) and sulfamethoxazole-trimethoprim (Bactrim). For patients who have multiple sex partners, doxycycline may be ordered. Oral antibiotics are given for up to 4 weeks for patients with acute prostatitis and 4 to 16 weeks for chronic prostatitis. The most common medications used for pain control are the antiinflammatory agents. Opioids should be used carefully because of the chronic nature of the pain (Lewis et al., 2007). Periodic digital massage of the prostate by the physician to increase the flow of infected prostatic secretions may be performed. Heat may be applied by means of sitz baths.

Nursing Interventions

Nursing interventions primarily focus on symptoms and include (1) a full explanation of antibiotic therapy and the need for compliance with treatment, which may be lengthy in chronic prostatitis; (2) supportive care such as bed rest to relieve strain and pain of the perineum and suprapubic area, sitz baths to promote muscle relaxation, and stool softeners to prevent straining on defecation; (3) monitoring of I&O; (4) bladder drainage with suprapubic catheterization if acute urinary retention develops into acute prostatitis (in acute prostatitis, passage of a catheter through an inflamed urethra is contraindicated); and (5) encouragement of follow-up for evaluation of the inflammation.

Nursing diagnoses and interventions for the patient with prostatitis include but are not limited to the following:

Nursing Diagnoses	Nursing Interventions
Acute pain, related to disease process	Assess type and location of pain; provide analgesics as ordered. Encourage bed rest to promote comfort.

Continued

Nursing Diagnoses	Nursing Interventions
Acute pain, related to disease process—cont'd	Provide nonpharmacologic comfort measures: • Assist patient with assuming comfortable position. • Provide diversional activity. • Provide a restful environment. Instruct patient in necessity of taking prescribed antibiotics and following orders for activity level.
Risk for situational low self-esteem, related to: • fear of impotence • embarrassment	Encourage patient to express feelings. Actively listen. Encourage adaptive coping behaviors.

Prognosis

Recurrent episodes of acute prostatitis may cause fibrotic tissue to form; such fibrosis causes a hardening of the prostate gland that may initially be confused with carcinoma.

EPIDIDYMITIS

Etiology and Pathophysiology

Epididymitis is an infection of the cordlike excretory duct of the testicle, usually secondary to an infectious process (sexually or nonsexually transmitted). It is one of the common infections of the male reproductive tract. The causative organisms are *S. aureus, E. coli*, streptococci, and *N. gonorrhoeae*. The inflammation is associated with urethral strictures, cystitis, and prostatitis.

Symptoms can occur after trauma to the genital area, after instrumentation of the urethra and cystoscopy, and after physical exertion or prolonged sexual activity.

Clinical Manifestations

Severe pain appears suddenly in the scrotum and radiates along the spermatic tube. Edema appears and the patient develops a "duck walk" or "waddling gait" because of the sensitivity and pain that walking stimulates. The scrotal area becomes tender. Pyuria (pus in urine) is present. Chills and fever are noted.

Diagnostic Tests

Diagnostic testing includes examination of the first daily flow of urine and delivery of a midstream specimen to the laboratory to check for pyuria. The epididymis is massaged by the physician, and a fluid expression specimen is sent to the laboratory. Physical examination of the scrotum is performed. Monitor the white blood cell count for leukocytosis.

Medical Management

Medical management includes a regimen of bed rest and support of the scrotum. The use of antibiotics is important for both partners, if the transmission is through sexual contact. Apply cold for relief of edema and discomfort, and administer the appropriate antibiotic. If abscess formation occurs, incision and drainage of the scrotum may be required.

Nursing Interventions

Nursing interventions for patients with epididymitis include (1) bed rest during the acute phase of illness; (2) support of the testicular area, with scrotal support by elevation of the scrotum on a folded towel during bed rest and athletic support when ambulatory; (3) ice compresses to the area in the initial phase to hasten recovery; (4) explanation of the need for compliance with antibiotic therapy until all signs of inflammation have disappeared; and (5) advice to refrain from sexual intercourse during the acute phase.

Prognosis

The infection can be bilateral and may recur. Bilateral epididymitis can cause sterility. Untreated epididymitis leads to necrosis of testicular tissue; in addition, abscesses can form, and septicemia can develop, which can be fatal.

DISORDERS OF MALE GENITAL ORGANS

PHIMOSIS AND PARAPHIMOSIS

Etiology and Pathophysiology

Phimosis is a condition in which the prepuce (foreskin) is too small to allow it to be retracted over the glans. Phimosis is often congenital but may be a result of local inflammation or disease. The condition is rarely severe enough to obstruct the flow of urine but may contribute to local infection because it does not permit adequate cleansing.

Paraphimosis is edema of the retracted uncircumcised foreskin, preventing normal return over the glans (Lewis et al., 2007). If the foreskin is not placed back in the forward position, an ulcer can develop. Paraphimosis can occur when the foreskin remains contracted during perineal cleansing, use of a urinary catheter, or intercourse. Treatment includes warm compresses; occasionally circumcision or dorsal slit of the prepuce is necessary. To prevent this problem, careful cleansing and replacement of the foreskin in the forward position are required (Lewis et al., 2007).

Medical Management

Circumcision may be performed, in which a part of the foreskin is removed, leaving the glans penis uncovered.

Nursing Interventions

After a circumcision a sterile petrolatum gauze dressing is applied and changed after each voiding. Observe the patient for unusual bleeding and obstruction of urine flow.

HYDROCELE

Etiology and Pathophysiology

A hydrocele is an accumulation of fluid between the membranes covering the testicle and the membrane enclosing the testicle. The scrotum slowly enlarges as the fluid accumulates. Diagnosis is fairly simple because the mass can be seen by shining a flashlight through the scrotum (transillumination). Pain occurs if the hydrocele develops suddenly. Most hydroceles occur in men older than 21 years of age, but it can occur in infants and children. The cause is not known, but it may develop as a result of trauma in the area, orchitis (inflammation of the testes), or epididymitis.

Medical Management

No treatment is indicated unless the edema becomes large and uncomfortable, in which case treatment includes aspiration of fluid from the sac or surgical removal of the sac to avoid constriction of the circulation of the testicles. After aspiration the pain is relieved and the scrotum can be examined more easily.

Nursing Interventions

Nursing interventions consist of maintaining bed rest, scrotal support with elevation, ice to edematous areas, and frequent changes of dressings to avoid skin impairment.

Prognosis

With treatment, prognosis is good.

VARICOCELE

Varicocele occurs when the veins within the scrotum become dilated. Obstruction and malfunctioning of the veins cause engorgement and elongation, which do not allow adequate drainage of the blood. The symptoms are a pulling sensation that causes a dull aching and pain accompanied by edema of the scrotal area. The treatment is surgical removal of the obstruction. Persistent varicoceles lead to infertility in 40% to 50% of cases (American Society for Reproductive Medicine Practice Committee, 2006). Nursing interventions include bed rest with scrotal support, ice on the incisional site, and medication for discomfort as ordered.

Ligation of the spermatic vein has been shown to improve semen quality.

CANCER OF THE MALE REPRODUCTIVE TRACT

The more common tumors of the male reproductive tract involve the testis, the prostate gland, and the penis. Most tumors of the male reproductive system are malignant. (See Chapters 50 and 57 for cancer of prostate gland.)

CANCER OF THE TESTIS (TESTICULAR CANCER)

Etiology and Pathophysiology

Testicular cancer is relatively uncommon, accounting for less than 1% of all cancers found in males. However, cancer of the testis is the most common malignancy in men 15 to 35 years of age (NCI, 2009b). The causes are unknown. The incidence of this cancer is higher in men with **cryptorchidism** (failure of testes to descend into the scrotum). Other associated factors are testicular atrophy, orchitis, and scrotal trauma. Most testicular cancers develop from embryonic germ cells. The two types of germ cell cancers are seminomas and nonseminomas. Although seminomas are the most common, they are the least aggressive. Nonseminoma testicular germ cell tumors are rare and very aggressive.

Clinical Manifestations

Testicular cancer may have a slow or rapid onset, depending on the type of tumor. The signs and symptoms of early disease include an enlarged scrotum and a firm, nontender, painless, smooth mass in the testicular area. Some patients complain of a dull ache or heavy sensation in the lower abdomen, perianal area, or scrotum. Acute pain is the presenting symptom in about 10% of patients.

Diagnostic Tests

Palpation of the scrotal contents is the first step in diagnosing testicular cancer. A cancerous mass is firm and does not transilluminate. Ultrasound of the testes is indicated when testicular cancer is suspected (e.g., a palpable mass) or persistent or painful testicular edema is present. If a testicular neoplasm is suspected, obtain blood to determine the serum levels of alpha-fetoprotein, lactate dehydrogenase, and hCG. A chest radiograph and CT scan of the abdomen and pelvis are obtained to detect metastasis.

Medical Management

Radical inguinal orchiectomy is usually the treatment of choice. This is the removal of the testis, epididymis, a portion of the gonadal lymphatics, and their blood supply. The remaining testis provides enough testosterone to maintain the man's sexual characteristics. He may have a lower sperm count and decreased sperm mobility. Surgery is generally followed by radiation or chemotherapy. Often a retroperitoneal lymph node dissection is performed to remove affected nodes and assist in determining the tumor stage. Staging a testicular tumor helps determine treatment.

Nursing Interventions and Patient Teaching

The most important aspect of care of patients who have or are at risk for a tumor of the testis is early detection by testicular self-examination (TSE). Young men should be taught to perform TSE monthly beginning at puberty. Video media and illustrations are available as teaching aids and ideally should be introduced during high school or college physical education classes. Information about TSE is available at the ACS and other websites (Lewis et al., 2007). The examination takes 3 minutes and should be done monthly. The best time to perform a TSE is after a warm shower when the scrotal skin is relaxed. The scrotum is checked for color, contour, and skin breaks. The left side is usually longer because the left testicle is suspended from a longer spermatic cord. Each testicle is gently palpated by grasping the scrotum in the center with the thumb and index finger (see Patient Teaching box; Figure 52-18). Normal testicles are firm but somewhat resilient, smooth, and mobile. If a testicle is indurated (hardened), carcinoma is suspected.

Prognosis

With the advent of tumor markers (which indicate the presence of disease and enable the physician to monitor its response to treatment), early detection, refined surgery, and effective chemotherapy, 99% of the patients obtain complete remission. Survival rates are reduced to 71% when cancer has spread to distant organs of the body, which emphasizes the need for early detection (ACS, 2009a).

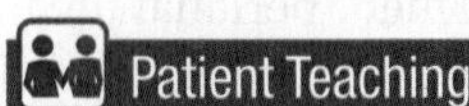

Patient Teaching

Testicular Self-Examination

- Examine the scrotum once a month.
- Perform testicular self-examination after a bath or shower when scrotum is warm and most relaxed.
- Grasp testis with both hands and palpate gently between thumb and index finger. The testis should feel smooth and egg shaped and be firm to touch.
- The epididymis, found behind the testis, should feel like a soft tube (see Figure 52-1 and Figure 52-18).

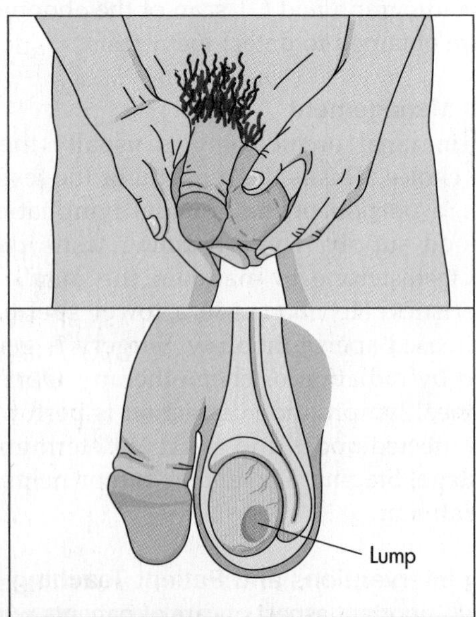

FIGURE 52-18 Testicular self-examination.

CANCER OF THE PENIS

Etiology and Pathophysiology

Cancer of the penis is rare. It generally appears in men older than 50 years of age. Men who have not been circumcised, have not maintained good personal hygiene, or have had STIs are at risk.

Clinical Manifestations

The tumor is painless, and a wartlike growth or ulceration on the glans under the prepuce is present. It is common for metastasis to occur to the inguinal nodes and adjacent organs.

Diagnostic Tests

Biopsy confirms the diagnosis.

Medical Management

Surgical intervention requires removal of as little tissue as possible, but it may be necessary to do a partial or total amputation of the penis and to remove the adjacent tissue and inguinal lymph nodes. When metastasis involves the bladder and rectum, more radical surgery may be needed, and outlets for urinary or fecal elimination are provided by creating an ileal conduit and a colostomy. The surgeon may place a suprapubic catheter into the bladder to drain the urine.

Nursing Interventions

Nursing interventions include providing emotional support. If amputation of the penis is required, the patient faces the psychological trauma associated with the loss of sexuality and the ability to urinate naturally. Monitor urinary output by suprapubic catheter or, if an ileoconduit was performed, monitor urine in the urostomy bag. Elevation of the scrotum controls edema. Provide comfort measures to control pain.

SEXUALLY TRANSMITTED INFECTIONS

Today, despite sweeping advances in the diagnosis and treatment of communicable diseases, the incidence of infections transmitted through intimate or sexual activities continues to increase worldwide. STIs, previously called sexually transmitted diseases or venereal diseases, are infections that are usually transmitted during intimate sexual contact. They may have other routes of transmission (e.g., an infected mother to her newborn), occur with or without symptoms, and have long periods of asymptomatic infectivity.

Any sexually active person may be at risk for an STI. People who have frequent sexual contact with multiple partners are at increased risk. Commonly those most at risk are young, single, urban, poor, male, and homosexual. Because some STIs persist and are infectious for long periods (herpes genitalis, HIV), even people in mutually monogamous sexual relationships are at some risk. The proliferation of HIV since the late 1970s has produced an urgent reason to educate sexually active individuals about the risk of unprotected sexual contact.

Over one million people were living with HIV in the United States at the end of 2006, with an estimated 14,989 HIV-related deaths that year. Of those living with the infection, 278,400 (25%) were adolescent and adult women, and 11,000 were children under the age of 15. The number of new cases in the United States was 56,300, but the epidemic is growing at faster rates among women, people of color, people who live in poverty, and adolescents (CDC, 2006). In addition, treatment has provided major advances in the ability to keep HIV-infected people healthy for longer periods, and the death rate has fallen dramatically (Facts at a Glance, 2004) (see Chapter 56).

These are sobering statistics indeed. The number of people contracting the traditionally defined STIs (e.g., syphilis, gonorrhea) is even greater. Gonorrhea is estimated to infect 250 million people worldwide, and in 2004 more than 330,000 cases were reported in the United States. Annual syphilis incidence is about 50 million cases worldwide; in 2004, the total number of cases was 7980 in the United States. Since 2001, the incidence of syphilis has started to rise among women and men, particularly men who have sex with men (O'Rourke, 2007). No reliable statistics exist for the "new generation" STIs, such as trichomoniasis, herpes simplex virus (HSV), venereal warts, scabies, and others; these are probably even more prevalent now than in the past. In addition, bowel pathogens such as *Salmonella* organisms, amebas, hepatitis B, and hepatitis C may be sexually transmitted.

Despite the physical and emotional discomfort, the possibility of long-term disability (infertility, chronic infectivity), and advances in diagnosis and treatment that sharply decrease the period of infectivity, STIs continue to be among the world's most common communicable diseases. Four main factors are responsible: (1) unprotected sex, (2) antibiotic resistance, (3) treatment delay, and (4) sexual behavior patterns and permissiveness. The following is a discussion of some of the more commonly diagnosed STIs (see Safety Alert box).

GENITAL HERPES

Etiology and Pathophysiology

Genital herpes, or HSV, is an infectious viral disease characterized by recurrent episodes of acute, painful, erythematous, vesicular eruptions (blisters) on or in the genitalia or rectum. The two closely related forms are designated types 1 and 2. Most people are infected in infancy with type 1 during feeding or kissing by adults. There are infrequent recurrences around the lips. HSV 2 is usually acquired sexually after puberty in the genital or anal regions.

! Safety Alert!

Sexually Transmitted Infections

- Teach "safe" sex practices including abstinence, monogamy with an uninfected partner, avoidance of certain high-risk sexual practices, and use of condoms and other barriers to limit contact with potentially infectious body fluids or lesions.
- All sexually active women should be screened for cervical cancer. Women with a history of STIs are at greater risk for cervical cancer than women without this history.
- Inform patients of the new HPV vaccine for girls and women ages 9 to 18 years to prevent HPV infection and the precancerous changes that lead to cervical cancer.
- Instruct patient in hygiene measures, such as washing and urinating after intercourse to destroy many causative organisms.
- Explain the importance of taking all antibiotics as prescribed. Symptoms improve after 1 or 2 days of therapy, but organisms may still be present.
- Teach patient about the need for treatment of sexual partners with antibiotics to prevent transmission of disease.
- Instruct patient to abstain from sexual intercourse during treatment and to use condoms when sexual activity is resumed to prevent spread of infection and reinfection.
- Explain the importance of follow-up examination and reculture at least once after treatment (if appropriate) to confirm complete cure and prevent relapse.
- Allow patient and partner to verbalize concerns to clarify areas that need explanation.
- Instruct patient about symptoms of complications and need to report problems to ensure proper follow-up and early treatment of reinfection.
- Explain precautions to take, such as being monogamous; asking potential partners about sexual history; avoiding sex with partners who use IV drugs or who have visible oral, inguinal, genital, perineal, or anal lesions; using condoms; and voiding and washing genitalia after coitus to reduce the occurrence of reinfection.
- Inform patient regarding state of infectivity to prevent a false sense of security, which might result in careless sexual practices and poor personal hygiene.

Clinical Manifestations

Signs appear as fluid-filled vesicles after the incubation period. In women the vesicles usually occur on the cervix, which is considered the primary site, but may also be seen on the labia, rectum, vulva, vagina, and skin. In men vesicles are found on the glans penis, foreskin, and penile shaft (Figure 52-19). Other lesions may appear on the mouth and anus. Vesicles may rupture and develop into shallow, painful ulcers; they are erythematous with marked edema and tenderness. Lymph nodes may become involved. Initial lesions last from 3 to 10 days, and recurrent lesions have a duration of 7 to 10 days. The primary infection may be accompanied by fever; malaise; myalgia; dysuria; and, in women, leukorrhea. Sites are painful in the presence of fever, stress, or emotional upset or when exposed to

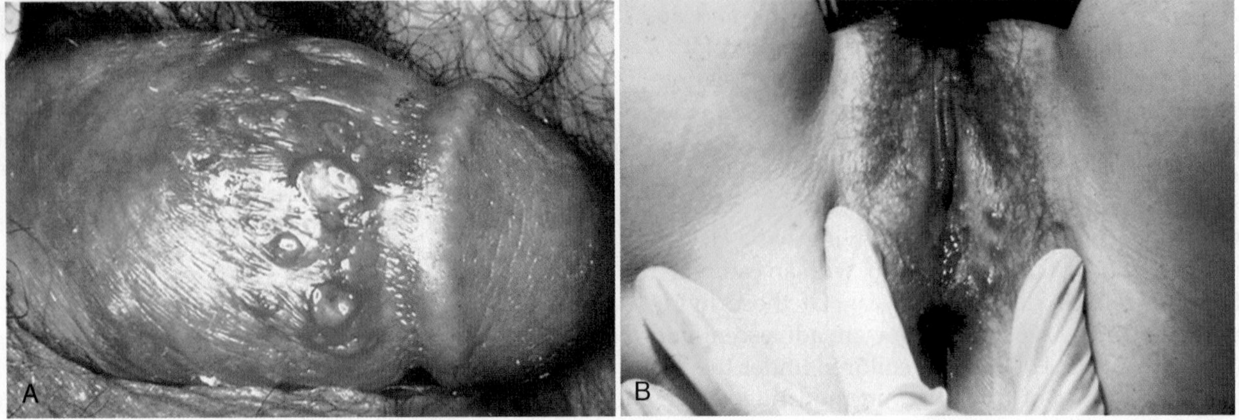

FIGURE 52-19 Herpes simplex virus type 2 in a male and female patient. Vesicular lesions on **A,** penis, and **B,** perineum.

intense heat. Urination may be painful from urine touching active lesions. Complications are rare.

Diagnostic Tests

Diagnosis is based on the physical examination and the patient history. The diagnosis is confirmed by appearance of the virus on tissue cultures. Cultures are more frequently positive when the lesions are from a primary infection versus recurrent infections. The Centers for Disease Control and Prevention (CDC, n.d.) recommend a serum serologic test for HSV 2 in addition to a viral tissue culture. These tests are highly accurate in diagnosing HSV 2 (Lewis et al., 2007).

Medical Management

The skin lesions of genital herpes heal spontaneously unless secondary infection occurs. Encourage symptomatic treatment such as practicing good genital hygiene and wearing loose-fitting cotton undergarments. The lesions should be kept clean and dry. Frequent sitz baths may soothe the area and reduce inflammation. Pain may require a local anesthetic such as lidocaine (Xylocaine) or systemic analgesics such as codeine and aspirin. Advise patients to abstain from sexual contact while lesions are present. However, sexual transmission of HSV has been documented even in the absence of clinical lesions; advise patients to use condoms.

Currently, acyclovir (Zovirax), which inhibits herpetic viral replication, is prescribed for primary infections or for suppression of frequent recurrences (more than six episodes per year). Although not a cure, acyclovir shortens the duration of viral shedding and the healing time of genital lesions and suppresses 75% of recurrences with daily use. Continued use of oral acyclovir for up to 5 years is safe and effective, but it should be interrupted after 1 year to assess the patient's rate of recurrent episodes. Adverse reactions to acyclovir are mild and include headache, occasional nausea and vomiting, and diarrhea. The safety of systemic acyclovir for treatment of pregnant women has not been established. Acyclovir ointment appears to be of no clinical benefit in the treatment of recurrent lesions, either in speed of healing or in resolution of pain. IV Acyclovir is reserved for severe or life-threatening infections in which hospitalization is required for the treatment of CNS infections (meningitis) or pneumonitis. Nephrotoxicity has been observed with high-dose IV use.

Two other antiviral agents are available for the treatment of HSV: valacyclovir (Valtrex) and famciclovir (Famvir). These purine analogs inhibit herpetic viral replication and are prescribed for primary and recurrent infections and to suppress frequent recurrences.

Nursing Interventions and Patient Teaching

Advise the patient to keep genital lesions clean and dry. Hands should be washed thoroughly after touching a lesion. Loose, absorbent underclothing is usually more comfortable than close-fitting clothing. Sitz baths decrease lesional discomfort and enhance urinary and bowel elimination. Teach the patient that sexual intercourse during the active lesion phase increases the risk of transmission and may also be painful. Patients should inform future sexual partners and health care providers of recurring or latent infections. Sexual transmission of HSV has been documented during asymptomatic periods; encourage the use of barrier methods, especially condoms. Inform the patient about the role of stress, poor nutrition, and insufficient rest in recurrences of signs and symptoms. Women patients need a yearly Pap test and should inform their physician in the event of pregnancy so that the disease can be monitored closely; there is a possibility of spontaneous abortion. Provide the patient with nonjudgmental support and with the contact number of the local herpes support group if one exists.

Prognosis

Genital herpes is a recurrent disease with no cure.

SYPHILIS

Etiology and Pathophysiology

The coiled spirochete *Treponema pallidum* causes syphilis. Congenital syphilis occurs in about 1 in 10,000 pregnancies, generally in minority populations. The age-group with the highest incidence is 20 to 40 years. An increase in syphilis rates was noted from 2001 to 2007. In 2007 the total number of cases was 11,466. The increased incidence is mainly among men who have sex with men. The rates increased in whites, blacks, Hispanics, and Asians (CDC, 2007c).

Syphilis is the third most frequently reported communicable disease in the United States, exceeded only by varicella (chickenpox) and gonorrhea. Transmission occurs primarily through sexual contact during the primary, secondary, and latent stages of the disease. In addition to sexual contact, syphilis may be spread through contact with infectious lesions and sharing of needles among drug addicts. Prenatal infection from the mother to the fetus is possible. The organism thrives in the warm parts of the body and can be destroyed by soap and water. The spirochete penetrates intact skin and openings in the mucous membrane of the genital organs, rectum, and mouth.

Clinical Manifestations

Syphilis has four stages—primary, secondary, latent, and tertiary—each with its peculiar signs and symptoms. The signs and symptoms of syphilis include the clean-based chancre (painless erosion or papule that ulcerates superficially with a scooped-out appearance) of primary syphilis to the skin rashes of secondary syphilis. Moist, raised, gray to pink lesions of the genital or perirectal skin; enlarged lymph nodes; fever; fatigue; or infections of the eyes, bones, liver, or meninges may occur. In the late stages of syphilis, dementia, pain or loss of sensation in the legs, and destruction of the aorta occur. Destructive inflammatory masses can appear in any organ. In tertiary or late-stage syphilis the heart and blood vessels (cardiovascular syphilis) and the central nervous system (neurosyphilis) are frequently involved. Tabes dorsalis, paresis, and various psychoses may result.

Diagnostic Tests

Diagnostic tests include the Venereal Disease Research Laboratory (VDRL) slide test and rapid plasma reagin (RPR) test. All patients should be checked for gonorrhea as well.

Medical Management

Therapeutic management of syphilis is aimed at eradication of all syphilitic organisms. However, treatment cannot reverse damage that is already present in the late stage of the disease. Parenteral benzylpenicillin (penicillin G) remains the treatment of choice for all stages of syphilis. The parenteral route provides the highest concentration of antibiotic in the tissues (O'Rourke, 2007). To date, there is no evidence to suggest a decrease in the effectiveness of penicillin against *T. pallidum.* All stages of syphilis should be treated.

Appropriate antibiotic treatment of maternal syphilis before the eighteenth week of pregnancy prevents infection of the fetus. Appropriate treatment after 18 weeks of pregnancy cures both mother and fetus because the antibiotics can cross the placental barrier. Treatment administered in the second half of pregnancy may pose a risk of premature labor. Some authorities recommend hospitalization and fetal monitoring of women at 20 weeks of gestation or later.

Carefully monitor all patients with neurosyphilis, with periodic serologic testing, clinical evaluation at 6-month intervals, and repeated cerebrospinal fluid examinations for at least 3 years. Specific therapeutic management is based on the specific symptoms.

Nursing Interventions

In addition to routine interventions for patients with STIs, monitor for drug reaction to penicillin, stress good handwashing technique, encourage follow-up visits with the physician, and inform the patient that he or she should absolutely not engage in sexual intercourse until cured.

Prognosis

Syphilis can be successfully treated at any stage of the disease, but treatment may be prolonged in latent and tertiary syphilis. Although syphilis can be cured in late stages, damage to the body is more difficult to manage. Untreated syphilis will go from primary to secondary, latent, and eventually tertiary stage.

GONORRHEA

Etiology and Pathophysiology

Gonorrhea is caused by *Neisseria gonorrhoeae,* a gram-negative diplococcoid bacterium, and almost exclusively follows sexual contact. It is the second most commonly reported STI in the United States. (Chlamydial infections are the most common.) Gonorrhea rates remained stable from 1997 to 2000 after a 74% decline from 1975 to 1997. From 2000 through 2004, reported cases of gonorrhea decreased 11.8%, but then the rate increased. More than 358,366 cases of gonorrhea were reported in the United States in 2006 (CDC, 2007b). The highest incidence of gonorrhea occurs in adolescents of all racial and ethnic groups, among blacks, and in persons living in the Southern United States. Most states have laws that permit examination and treatment of minors without the consent of parents (Lewis et al., 2007). Those at risk are sexually active individuals and those who are otherwise susceptible to infections. Gonorrhea is primarily an infection of the genital or rectal mucosa but is not limited to the genital organs; it can infect the mouth and the throat through oral sex with an infected partner. It may also infect the eyes. Three times as many men are infected as women. The incubation period of gonorrhea is 3 to 5 days.

Clinical Manifestations

Some infected men may be asymptomatic after the incubation period but in a short time develop signs and symptoms of urethritis, dysuria, infection with a profuse purulent discharge, and edema of the affected area. Most women remain asymptomatic but may show a greenish yellow discharge from the cervix. Other female signs and symptoms, depending on the infection site, are urinary frequency, purulent discharge from the urethra, pruritus, burning and pain of the vulva, vaginal engorgement and erythema, abdominal pain and distention, muscular rigidity, and tenderness. As the infection spreads, nausea, vomiting, fever, and tachycardia may develop. Other signs and symptoms are pharyngitis, tonsillitis, rectal burning, and purulent rectal discharge. PID, Bartholin's abscess, ectopic pregnancy, and infertility are the main complications of gonorrhea in women (Lewis et al., 2007).

Diagnostic Tests

Diagnosis is determined by cultures from the site of infection to isolate and identify the organism. Cultures of the discharge or secretion can provide a definitive diagnosis after incubation for 24 to 48 hours. An important concern in treatment for gonorrhea is coexisting chlamydial infection (see the discussion of chlamydia for more information). Chlamydia has been documented in up to 45% of gonorrhea cases. It is important to test for syphilis as well.

Medical Management

A history of sexual contact with a partner known to have gonorrhea is considered good evidence for the infection. Because of the short incubation period and high infectivity, treatment is instituted without awaiting culture results, even in the absence of signs or symptoms. Treatment of gonorrhea in the early stage is curative. Traditionally, the drug of choice for gonorrheal therapy was penicillin, but changes have been made because of (1) a rapid increase in the number of cases of gonorrhea caused by resistant strains of *N. gonorrhoeae* and (2) coexisting chlamydial infection.

There is no clinical distinction between infections caused by resistant or sensitive strains of *N. gonorrhoeae*. As a result, ceftriaxone (Rocephin), a penicillinase-resistant cephalosporin, has become part of the treatment plan. The most common treatment for gonorrhea is a single IM dose of ceftriaxone. Cefixime (Suprax) given orally one time is also effective. Other medications that may be used in the treatment of gonorrhea are ciprofloxacin, ofloxacin, and levofloxacin (Levaquin). The high frequency of coexisting chlamydial and gonococcal infections has led to the addition of doxycycline or tetracycline to the treatment plan. The expense of diagnosing chlamydial infection and the sequelae make this strategy cost effective. Patients with coincubating syphilis are likely to be cured by the same drugs.

All sexual contacts of patients with gonorrhea must be treated to prevent reinfection after resumption of sexual relations. The "Ping-Pong" effect of reexposure, treatment, and reinfection will cease only when infected partners are treated simultaneously. Additionally, advise the patient to abstain from sexual intercourse and alcohol for 2 to 4 weeks. Sexual intercourse allows the infection to spread and can retard complete healing as a result of vascular congestion. Alcohol irritates the healing urethral walls. Caution men against squeezing the penis to look for further discharge. Follow-up examination and reculture should be done at least once after treatment, usually in 4 to 7 days. Treat relapse, reinfection, and complications appropriately.

Nurses need to be alert to changes in CDC recommendations. Report the disease to infection control authorities as required by the local health agency.

Nursing Interventions and Patient Teaching

Advise patients that loose, absorbent underclothes, changed frequently after perineal or penile cleansing, enhance comfort. Sitz baths decrease lower abdominal discomfort and dysuria. Obtain laboratory specimens as ordered. Discuss alternative methods of birth control as appropriate. Encourage notification of present and past sexual partners of the diagnosis and stress the need for them to promptly seek medical care. Inform the female that sterility may occur as a result of gonorrhea.

Prognosis

With treatment, gonorrhea is curable. The inflammation may clear up without serious results, or it may become chronic and produce urethral stricture. Complications include prostatitis, epididymitis, orchitis, arthritis, and endocarditis. It can result in sterility in the female. No case of acute gonorrhea in the female should be considered cured until three consecutive negative smears of the cervix and Bartholin's and Skene's glands are obtained. The main cause for infections identified after completed treatment is reinfection, not treatment failure.

TRICHOMONIASIS

Etiology and Pathophysiology

Trichomoniasis is an STI caused by the protozoan *Trichomonas vaginalis,* which affects about 15% of sexually active women and 10% of sexually active men (CDC, 2007d). The incubation period is 4 to 28 days. Trichomoniasis is usually transmitted by sexual intercourse and, at times, by dirty douche nozzles, douche containers, and moist washcloths. Occasionally a newborn develops an infection from an infected mother. *T. vaginalis* thrives when the vaginal mucosa is more alkaline than normal. Frequent douching and use of oral contraceptives and antibiotics raise the normal pH of the vagina, making the woman more vulnerable to trichomoniasis.

Clinical Manifestations

Most men and approximately 70% of women are asymptomatic. The male signs and symptoms are mild to severe transient urethritis, dysuria, frequency of urination, pruritus, and purulent exudate. In women, signs and symptoms include profuse, frothy, gray, green, or yellow malodorous discharge; pruritus; edema; tenderness of vagina; dysuria; frequency of urination; spotting; menorrhagia; and dysmenorrhea. Signs and symptoms may persist for a week to several months and may be more pronounced after menstruation or during pregnancy.

Diagnostic Tests

Diagnosis is based on the microscopic examination of the vaginal discharge that identifies *T. vaginalis.*

Medical Management

Treatment for both men and women is oral metronidazole (Flagyl) in small doses for 7 days or a single large dose. The patient should avoid alcoholic beverages, since alcohol can cause reactions such as disorientation, headache, cramps, vomiting, and possibly convulsions. Metronidazole can cause the urine to turn dark brown (see Table 52-2).

Nursing Interventions and Patient Teaching

Advise the patient to avoid alcohol during treatment; inform patients that their urine may turn dark orange or brown; and counsel patients to avoid douches, sprays, and powders during treatment. Teach the patient how to disinfect douche nozzles, applicators, diaphragms, and the toilet area. Encourage the patient to wear loose-fitting clothing and cotton underwear, to schedule follow-up visits with the physician, and to contact sexual partners so they can get treatment.

Prognosis

With treatment, trichomoniasis is curable. Reinfection is common if sexual partners are not treated simultaneously. Chronic infection may develop in untreated cases.

CANDIDIASIS

Etiology and Pathophysiology

Candidiasis (moniliasis) is a mild fungal infection that appears in men and women. Candidal infections are usually caused by *C. albicans* and *Candida tropicalis.* The fungi are a part of the normal flora of the gastrointestinal tract, mouth, vagina, and skin. The infection often occurs when the glucose level rises from diabetes mellitus or when resistance is lowered from diseases such as carcinoma. Radiation, immunosuppressant drugs, hyperalimentation, antibiotic therapy, and oral contraceptives may predispose individuals to candidiasis. Men and women display signs of scaly skin; erythematous rash; and occasional exudates that appear under the breasts, between the fingers, and in the axillae, groin, and umbilicus.

Clinical Manifestations

If the mother is infected, a newborn can contract thrush during delivery. The infant may display a diaper rash. The infant's nails become edematous and have a darkened, erythematous nail base with purulent exudate. Thrush may appear on the mucous membranes of the infant's mouth as pearly, bluish white "milk-curd" lesions and cause edema and engorgement. The infant may have an edematous tongue that can cause respiratory distress. The adult female patient may have a cheesy, tenacious white vaginal discharge accompanied by pruritus and an inflamed vulva and vagina. The adult male patient has signs of an infected penis with purulent exudate. Systemic infections are indicated by chills, fevers, and general malaise.

Diagnostic Tests

Diagnosis is based on evidence of the *Candida* species on a Gram stain of collected specimens from scraping of the vagina and penis, from pus, and from exudate from the mouth.

Medical Management

Treatment consists of managing any underlying condition, such as controlling diabetes mellitus, discontinuing antibiotics and oral contraceptives. Nystatin (Mycostatin) is effective for superficial candidiasis; topical amphotericin B is effective for skin and nail infections.

Nursing Interventions and Patient Teaching

Emphasize the use of prescribed ointments, sprays, and creams as indicated for each part of the body affected. Teaching includes the method for inserting vaginal suppositories (to be inserted high into the vagina when in a dorsal recumbent position) and remaining on the back for 30 minutes to allow suppository absorption. Patients should encourage sexual partners to have an examination and treatment. Teach good handwashing techniques to avoid reinfection or the transfer of the fungi. Encourage pregnant women to accept treatment to prevent infection of the newborn at the time of delivery.

Prognosis

Candidiasis is curable with the use of the prescribed treatment.

CHLAMYDIA

Etiology and Pathophysiology

Chlamydia trachomatis, a gram-negative, intracellular bacterium, causes several common STIs. Cervicitis and urethritis are most common, but like gonococci, chlamydial organisms also cause epididymitis in men and salpingitis in women. Chlamydial infections are the most commonly occurring STI in the United States. They are responsible for about 20% to 30% of diagnosed PID cases. In 2006 more than 1 million cases of genital chlamydial infections were reported in the United States (CDC, 2007a). It is estimated that about 11,000 women each year become involuntarily sterilized and 36,000 suffer ectopic pregnancies as a result of this organism. Chlamydia incidence is highest in young, promiscuous, indigent, unmarried women who live in the inner city and in those who have a prior history of STIs. Increases in chlamydia rates are more likely a result of better screening and use of more sensitive tests, rather than an increase of the total burden of the disease in the United States (CDC, 2007a). Chlamydia can be transmitted during vaginal, anal, or oral sex.

Although both men and women may have asymptomatic infection, women are more likely to be asymptomatic carriers even with deep pelvic infections, such as infection of the fallopian tubes and PID.

Clinical Manifestations

In men, signs and symptoms may include a scanty white or clear exudate, burning or pruritus around the urethral meatus, urinary frequency, and mild dysuria. Signs and symptoms of cervicitis in women may include one or more of the following: (1) vaginal pruritus or burning, (2) dull pelvic pain, (3) low-grade fever, (4) vaginal discharge, and (5) irregular bleeding. Symptoms of chlamydia may be absent or cause minor discomfort; therefore it has been called a silent disease. Females may develop a PID, which can result in infertility (Lewis et al., 2007). For this reason the CDC (2007a) recommends that all females younger than 25 years of age be routinely screened for chlamydia at their annual gynecologic examination. The CDC further advises annual screening of all women older than 25 years of age with one or more risk factors for the disease (CDC, 2007a).

Diagnostic Tests

The direct fluorescent antibody test provides a ready basis for diagnosis. However, this test is less specific than a culture and may produce false-positive results. Culturing for chlamydial organisms should be done if the laboratory facilities are available. New techniques using nucleic acid amplification promise to surpass culture as the gold standard of chlamydial testing. Treatment can be initiated promptly based on a confirmed diagnosis.

Medical Management

Chlamydial infections respond to treatment with tetracycline, doxycycline, azithromycin, or ofloxacin. For tetracycline, the dosage is 500 mg orally four times a day for at least 7 days. For doxycycline, the dosage is 100 mg two times a day. Doxycycline is more expensive than tetracycline. For ofloxacin, the dosage is 300 mg twice a day. Azithromycin (1 g in a single dose) offers the advantage of ease of administration, but safety for patients younger than 15 years of age has not been established. Alternative regimens include erythromycin, ofloxacin, and levofloxacin. Erythromycin is the drug of choice for use in pregnant patients. If this treatment is not tolerated, amoxicillin is an alternative. Follow-up care includes advising the patient to return if symptoms persist or recur, treating sexual partners, and encouraging the use of condoms during all sexual contact.

Box 52-9 Prevention of Sexually Transmitted Infections

- Reduce the number of sexual partners, preferably to one person.
- Avoid contact with individuals known to be infected or who are at risk of infection.
- Avoid contact with the genital area if signs and symptoms develop.
- Wash the hands and the genital-rectal area before and immediately after having intercourse.
- Pay special attention to washing the foreskin.
- A mouthwash or gargle with hydrogen peroxide (1 part peroxide to 3 parts of water) or Listerine antiseptic may slightly reduce the risk of oropharyngeal sexually transmitted infection (STI).
- Use barrier (condom) contraceptives with new partners.
- Use a water-based lubricant as opposed to an oil-based lubricant.
- Void after intercourse.
- Avoid excess douching.
- If an STI infection is suspected, seek medical help immediately.
- Individuals with multiple sexual partners should have an STI examination twice a year or more if needed.

Because chlamydial infections are closely associated with gonococcal infections, both infections are usually treated concurrently, even without diagnostic evidence.

Nursing Interventions and Patient Teaching

Patients' physical symptoms are often complicated by their emotional responses to STIs. Depression, anger, fear, and guilt need to be addressed if education and treatment are to be effective. Outcome is also influenced by educational and income levels, primary language, health insurance coverage, and support network. Patient education focuses on prevention (Box 52-9).

Prognosis

With treatment, chlamydial infection is curable. Reinfection occurs if sexual partners are not treated simultaneously. Chlamydial infections can be transmitted to infants during delivery, causing conjunctivitis and pneumonia. Poorly treated or untreated chlamydial infection can result in ectopic pregnancy or infertility.

ACQUIRED IMMUNODEFICIENCY SYNDROME

AIDS is the ultimately fatal, advanced stage of a chronic retroviral infection from the HIV virus that gradually destroys the cell-mediated immune system. (For a more detailed discussion on this STI, see Chapter 56.)

FAMILY PLANNING

Advances in drug therapy and family planning technology have made a range of options available for individuals wishing to prevent or plan conception. Birth control planning involves moral, religious, cultural, and personal values, and the nurse should be sensitive to these factors when discussing birth control with patients.

Numerous types of birth control procedures or devices can be employed. The selection of a method should be based on the patient's health, effectiveness of the method, cost, lifestyle, ease of use, and age and parity (total number of pregnancies) of the patient. The patient's willingness to comply with use and the couple's preference are two additional factors taken into consideration when selecting a method of contraception. Reinforce the information given by the physician and encourage patients to seek more information, directing them to the source.

Contraceptive methods and products can be categorized as surgical (Figures 52-20 and 52-21), hormonal, barrier, and behavioral (Table 52-4).

Uterine (fallopian) tubes severed and ligated

FIGURE 52-20 Tubal ligation. Oviduct ligated and severed.

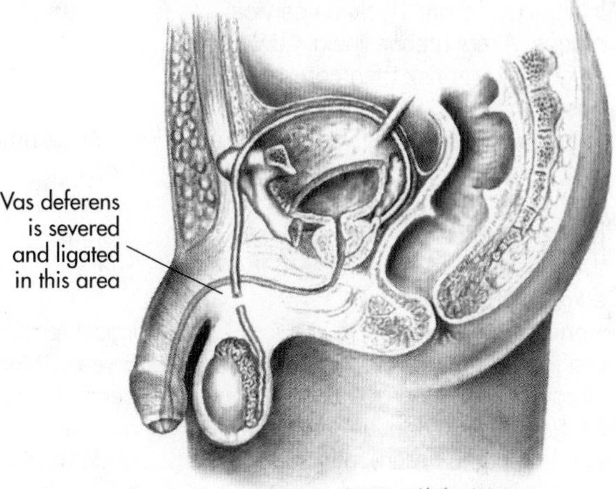

FIGURE 52-21 Vasectomy. Sperm duct severed (and ligated).

Table 52-4 Methods of Birth Control

DESCRIPTION	SIDE EFFECTS AND COMPLICATIONS	PATIENT EDUCATION
TEMPORARY METHODS		
Combined		
Combination pill contains both estrogen and progesterone (standard and low dose). Usually taken on 5th through 25th day of each cycle. Prevents ovulation; causes changes in endometrium; alterations in cervical mucus and tubal transport. Simple and unobtrusive in use. 99% effective. Failure from irregular or incorrect use.	Side effects of weight gain, nausea and vomiting, spotting and breakthrough bleeding, postpill amenorrhea, breast tenderness, headache, chloasma, irritability, nervousness, depression, and decreased libido. Complications of benign liver tumors, gallstones, myocardial infarction, thromboembolism, stroke (smokers >35 years of age at higher risk). Contraindications of history of cardiovascular or liver disease, hypertension, breast or pelvic cancer; use caution with diabetes mellitus, sickle cell anemia. Provides no protection against HIV transmission.	Instruct patient in correct use of pills. Tell patient to take pill same time each day; if forgotten one day, take two next day. Review side effects and contraindications. Explain that the patient should report cramps or edema of legs, chest pain. Discuss need for periodic (every 6-12 months), checkup that involves weight, BP, Pap smear, hematocrit. Review danger signs of drug. Take drug history, asking about use of phenytoin, phenobarbital, antibiotic (ampicillin), which decrease contraceptive action. Inform patient that method is usually not recommended for persons >35 years of age. Discourage smoking.
Morning-after pill (norgestrel and ethinyl estradiol [Ovral]) contains ethinyl estradiol 50 mcg and norgestrel 500 mg. Another use of combined hormonal contraception. 98.4% effective. Creates hostile uterine lining and alters tubal transport.	Nausea for 1-2 days. Does not prevent an ectopic pregnancy. At risk for usual hormonal complications of abdominal pain, chest pain, cough, shortness of breath, headache, dizziness, weakness, leg pain.	Take two Ovral within 72 hours of coitus. Repeat if vomiting occurs. Take second dose 12 hours later. Menses should begin within 2-3 weeks. Start an ongoing method of contraception immediately after menses.

Modified from Lewis S.L., et al. (2007). *Medical-surgical nursing: assessment and management of clinical problems.* (7th ed.). St. Louis: Mosby.
BP, Blood pressure; *HIV,* human immunodeficiency virus.

Continued

Table 52-4 **Methods of Birth Control—cont'd**

DESCRIPTION	SIDE EFFECTS AND COMPLICATIONS	PATIENT EDUCATION
TEMPORARY METHODS—cont'd		
Progestin Only		
Progestin-only pills (POPs or Minipills) are taken daily, with no pill-free days. Preferred for women who are breast-feeding. Does not suppress lactation. Inhibits ovulation. Thickens cervical mucus. Alters uterine lining. Lower cardiovascular risk than combined pills.	Menstrual changes, breakthrough bleeding, prolonged cycles or amenorrhea. Increase in functional cysts of the ovary. Increase in ectopic pregnancy.	Use alternate contraception when starting POPs or if pill is missed. Take pill at same time every day. Keep record of menses and get pregnancy test if 2 weeks late.
Medroxyprogesterone (Depo-Provera, DMPA) is a progestin-only drug given by injection every 3 months. A private, convenient, and highly effective method. Efficacy similar to that of surgical sterilization.	May cause amenorrhea, headaches, bloating, and weight gain. Return of fertility may be delayed for several months.	Return every 3 months for injection. Discontinue method for several months before planning to conceive.
Levonorgestrel (Norplant) is a progestin-only subdermal implant. Six silicone capsules provide protection for 5 years. Continuous, long-term contraception. Failure rate is extremely low. Does not suppress l actation. Pregnancy rate 0.8 per 100 users over 5 years.	Surgical removal of capsules after 5 years. Menstrual irregularities, especially during the first year. Later may cause amenorrhea. May cause abdominal pain, headaches, weight gain.	Is effective after 24 hours. Keep arm dry for 48 hours after insertion. Report arm pain. Implants are soft and flexible and cannot break. Expect some irregular bleeding. Report any other changes. Remove implants in 5 years. Continue to protect against STIs.
Barrier Method		
Diaphragms are dome-shaped latex caps with flexible metal ring (varies in size) covering cervix. Inner surface coated with spermicide before insertion. Provides mechanical barrier to sperm. Available by prescription, fitted by professional. Continuing motivation to use necessary. 87% effective. Failure from improper fitting or placement of device.	Allergy to latex or spermicide.	Demonstrate how to hold, insert, and remove device, using model. Allow for insertion and removal practice sessions. Advise patient that insertion may be just prior to coitus, but removal should be 6-8 hours after coitus. Tell patient to empty bowel and bladder before insertion. Give instructions for cleansing and storing, checking for holes or deterioration. Advise patient that diaphragm must be refitted after pregnancy, weight loss, or weight gain. Advise patient that it is not suitable if severe pelvic relaxation is present.
Cervical caps are rubber thimble-shaped shields covering cervix, held in place by suction. Spermicide in inner surface provides mechanical barrier to sperm. Fitted by professional. Effectiveness similar to that of diaphragm. Failure from dislodgment and improper fit.	Allergy to rubber; or spermicide, possible cervical irritation or erosion from suction.	Provide sufficient time for practice with insertion and removal (more time than for diaphragm). Give instructions for cleaning, storing, and inspecting for damage. Inform patient that it can be used with abnormalities of vaginal canal but not with cervical inconsistencies or PID.
Condoms		
Male: Thin rubber sheath fitting over erect penis, providing mechanical barrier to sperm. Simple method to use. No prescription necessary. 85% effective. Failure from tearing or slipping during coitus. Used with spermicide. Affords some protection against STIs and HIV transmission.	Possible allergy to rubber; possible decrease in sensation and interference with foreplay.	Advise patient to roll sheath along entire penis, leaving slack at end to receive semen. Inform patient that sharp objects (fingernails) may tear condom. Tell patient to hold sheath in place when penis is withdrawn to prevent emptying of sperm in or near vagina.

PID, Pelvic inflammatory disease; *STI,* sexually transmitted infection.

Table 52-4 Methods of Birth Control—cont'd

DESCRIPTION	SIDE EFFECTS AND COMPLICATIONS	PATIENT EDUCATION
TEMPORARY METHODS—cont'd		
Female: Double-ring system fitted into vagina up to 8 hours before intercourse. No prescription necessary. Affords protection against HIV, cytomegalovirus, and hepatitis B.	No significant side effects; generally acceptable to couple.	Discuss insertion, lubrication, and method of removal. More expensive than male condoms.
Other Methods		
Intrauterine devices (IUDs) are inserted into uterus and are flexible objects made of plastic or copper wire (nonmedicated or medicated with substance to alter uterine environment), usually with attached string that protrudes into vagina. Contraception probably provided by inflammatory response in endometrium, preventing implantation. After insertion, no additional equipment necessary. 97% to 99% effective. Failure mainly from undetected expulsion. Most common type used today is Progestasert (contains progestins).	Increased menstrual flow, intramenstrual bleeding and cramping, especially during early months of use; possible complications of ectopic pregnancy, pelvic infection, perforation of uterus, infertility. Undetected expulsion of IUD resulting in pregnancy.	Discuss techniques and experience of insertion and removal. Inform patient that insertion may be more difficult and expulsion and complications greater in nulliparous patients. Instruct patient to check for string in vagina after each period; report to physician if unable to locate. Discuss need for annual pelvic examination and Pap test.
Rhythm method requires periodic abstinence during fertile portion of menstrual cycle. Requires strong motivation, self-control. Complies with all religious doctrines. 60% to 65% effective. Failure from difficulty in determining precise day of ovulation, irregularity of menses.	Inaccurate or incomplete knowledge of menstrual cycle.	Discuss methods to establish baseline menstrual patterns and identify ovulation. Give instructions in use of calendar or basal body temperature method to determine ovulation and fertile period.
PERMANENT		
Tubal sterilization includes a variety of abdominal and vaginal surgical procedures (laparotomy, laparoscopy, culdoscopy) that permanently prevent sperm and ovum from meeting. Crushing, ligating, clipping, or plugging of fallopian tubes (potentially reversible procedure). Nearly 100% (99.96%) effective. Failure due to recanalization of fallopian tubes, erroneous ligation (see Figure 52-20).	Bowel injury, hemorrhage, or infection.	Determine whether temporary contraceptives were used and reason for patient's dissatisfaction. Counsel regarding effects of procedure on physiology and sexual performance. Assist in obtaining written informed consent for procedure. Inform patient that procedure may require short-term hospitalization or can be done on outpatient basis.
Hysterectomy is surgical removal of uterus. 100% effective.	Bladder infection, vascular disorders, infection, hemorrhage, pain, psychological adjustment.	Assess or counsel regarding understanding of extent of surgery, altered physiology, complications, and sexual performance. Hysterectomy only performed for other reasons; sterility is secondary benefit when desired.
Vasectomy is bilateral surgical ligation and resection of ductus deferens.	Hematoma, edema, psychological adjustment (see Figure 52-21).	Inform patient that procedure is usually done as outpatient procedure and takes 15 to 30 minutes. Tell patient that alternative form of contraception is needed until no sperm are seen on examination. Explain that procedure does not affect masculinity.

NURSING PROCESS *for the Patient with a Reproductive Disorder*

The role of the licensed practical nurse/licensed vocational nurse (LPN/LVN) in the nursing process as stated is that the LPN/LVN will:

- Participate in planning care for patients based on patient needs
- Review patient's care plan and recommend revisions as needed
- Review and follow defined prioritization for patient care
- Use clinical pathways, care maps, or care plans to guide and review patient care

Assessment

People with reproductive disorders require skilled assessment by both the nurse and the physician. Assessment occurs through observation of the patient during the patient health history and while doing baseline and continuing assessment of the patient's objective and subjective data.

Health history data should be relevant to the patient's developmental age. Information about reproductive health and sexuality can form a large portion of the collected data. This history is as important as the physical and emotional data in determining appropriate nursing diagnoses and interventions. Data collected about sexual health, sexual relations, birth control methods, STIs, and the use of chemical substances provide an opportunity to clarify any misconceptions or myths revealed during history taking.

Data Collection for Women

Data collection for adolescent and adult women focuses on the reproductive tract and the menstrual, gynecologic, and obstetric history.

The menstrual history encompasses menarche (onset of menstrual flow) through the climacteric (cessation of menstrual cycle), including: (1) age of onset; (2) date of last menstrual flow; (3) usual amount and volume of flow (number of pads used per day); (4) presence of **dysmenorrhea** (painful menstruation), **menorrhagia** (excessive flow), **amenorrhea** (absence of flow), or **metrorrhagia** (excessive spotting between cycles); and (5) other difficulties during menses.

The gynecologic assessment includes data on (1) vaginal discharge (odor, color, frequency, and duration), (2) vaginal pruritus (itching), (3) vaginal irritation with coital activity, (4) date and results of the last Pap test, (5) birth control methods or kinds of contraceptives used, and (6) any family history of cancer of the reproductive system.

If the adolescent or adult woman has conceived, information should be collected as to **gravidity** (number of pregnancies), **parity** (number of births), abortions, miscarriages, and stillbirths. Assessment of the breast includes (1) tenderness of the breast areas; (2) pain; (3) masses in any specific areas; (4) presence of nipple discharge; (5) knowledge and frequency of BSE; and (6) date and results of last mammogram, if applicable.

Data Collection for Men

The data collected from the male adolescent and the adult man include (1) urologic history of voiding difficulties and any discharge from the penis; (2) characteristics of the urine (odor, color, amount, and frequency); (3) information on prostate and testicular problems; (4) frequency of PSA testing, if applicable; (5) masses or lesions on genitalia; (6) frequency of TSE; (7) frequency of professional testicular examination; (8) measures to prevent infections; and (9) birth control method. In addition, note concerns about sexual health voiced by the patient.

Nursing Diagnosis

Possible nursing diagnoses for the patient with a reproductive disorder include but are not limited to the following:

- Anxiety
- Disturbed body image
- Ineffective coping
- Fear
- Deficient fluid volume
- Ineffective health maintenance
- Risk for infection
- Deficient knowledge
- Acute pain
- Chronic pain
- Chronic low self-esteem
- Situational low self-esteem
- Sexual dysfunction
- Impaired skin integrity
- Ineffective tissue perfusion
- Impaired urinary elimination

Expected Outcomes and Planning

Planning is a category of nursing behaviors in which patient-centered goals are established and strategies designed to achieve the goals and outcomes that relate to the identified nursing diagnosis (Table 52-5).

Implementation

The implementation step for the patient with a reproductive disorder is the action-oriented phase of the nursing process in which the nurse initiates and carries out the objectives of the nursing care plan. See Complementary & Alternative Therapies box for additional treatment methods.

Evaluation

Examples of goals and their corresponding evaluative measures include the following:

Goal 1: Patient will be able to cope effectively.

Evaluative measure: Patient verbalizes fears and identifies two strategies for dealing with fear, such as

Table 52-5 Planning and Setting Goals for the Patient with a Reproductive Disorder

NURSING DIAGNOSIS	GOAL	OUTCOME
Coping, ineffective, related to fear of positive diagnosis of breast cancer	Patient will attend cancer support group weekly.	Patient expresses fears of unfavorable outcome.
Knowledge, deficient, regarding postoperative care at home after modified radical mastectomy	Patient will state four postoperative risks before discharge.	Patient verbalizes signs and symptoms of infection. Patient demonstrates exercises for affected arm. Patient verbalizes need to avoid injections and taking of blood or blood pressure in affected arm. Patient verbalizes need to examine remaining breast once a month.

Complementary & Alternative Therapies

Male and Female Reproductive Disorders

MALE REPRODUCTIVE SYSTEM

- Yohimbine *(Pausinystalia yohimbe)* for erectile dysfunction and impotence

FEMALE REPRODUCTIVE SYSTEM

- Biofeedback, therapeutic touch, and acupuncture for primary dysmenorrhea
- Black cohosh *(Cimicifuga racemosa)* for menstrual irregularity, premenstrual syndrome (PMS), and menopausal problems
- Chamomile *(Matricaria recutita, Chamaemelum nobile)* for menstrual cramps
- Chaste tree *(Vitex agnus-castus)* for PMS
- Evening primrose *(Oenothera biennis)* for PMS
- Feverfew *(Tanacetum parthenium)* for menstrual problems
- Sage *(Salvia officinalis)* for menstrual irregularity
- Soybeans and other legumes for their phytoestrogens that may help prevent breast cancer

Modified from Black J.M., & Hawks, H.J. (2009). *Medical-surgical nursing: clinical management for positive outcomes.* (8th ed.). Philadelphia: Saunders.

questioning for clarification and relaxation breathing technique.

Goal 2: Patient will have adequate knowledge regarding postoperative care at home after modified radical mastectomy.

Evaluative measures: Patient states signs and symptoms of wound infection; lists proper arm exercises; verbalizes the need for BSE once per month; and states the need to avoid blood pressure checks, injections, and blood draws in affected arm.

Get Ready for the NCLEX® Examination!

Key Points

- Sperm are produced in the seminiferous tubules and stored in the epididymis.
- Testosterone, the male sex hormone, is responsible for male secondary sex characteristics.
- Seminal fluid is produced in the seminal vesicles, prostate gland, and Cowper's glands.
- The male urethra serves the twofold purpose of conveying urine from the bladder and carrying the reproductive cells and secretions to the outside.
- The uterus consists of three layers of tissue: (1) endometrium, the inner layer; (2) myometrium, the middle layer; and (3) perimetrium, the outer layer.
- In the ovulating female, an egg matures each month in the graafian follicle, which is located in the ovary.
- The menstrual cycle prepares the uterus and causes ovulation to occur each month.
- Because of the relationship between the menstrual cycle and the body's mechanisms of hormonal secretion, a decrease or increase in the activity of the hormonal glands can disturb menstruation.
- Early diagnosis and prompt management are necessary to prevent serious reproductive and genital problems.
- Health teaching for patients with menstrual disturbances includes a knowledge of the physiologic process, factors that alter menstruation, personal hygiene, exercise, diet, and pain management.
- Discharge planning is vital to prevent reinfection after PID.
- Pregnancy is encouraged in the patient with endometriosis, since it will slow the progress of the disorder; infertility is a complication as the condition continues.
- Menarche, the first menstrual cycle, usually begins around the age of 12 years.
- Serum CA-125 is useful mainly to signal a recurrence of ovarian cancer and in following the response to treatment.
- PSA is a highly sensitive blood test that is elevated in cancer of the prostate and in benign prostatic hyperplasia.
- There is no definitive test for TSS. However, cervical-vaginal isolates of *Staphylococcus aureus* are present 90% of the time with TSS.

- Vaginal fistulas are caused by an ulcerating process resulting from cancer, radiation, weakening of tissue from pregnancies, or surgical interventions.
- Correction of cystocele and rectocele is a surgical repair involving shortening of the muscles that support the bladder and repair of the rectocele. This is known as anteroposterior colporrhaphy.
- Screening tests for cervical abnormalities include routine Pap test; ThinPrep, a newer liquid-based technique for Pap tests; and testing for HPV.
- Vaccines are now available that reduce the incidence of cervical cancer due to infection of HPV (types 6, 11, 16, 18).
- A panhysterosalpingo-oophorectomy is the removal of the uterus, the fallopian tubes, and the ovaries.
- In breast cancer patients an axillary lymph node dissection is usually performed regardless of treatment options available. Examination of nodes provides the most powerful prognostic data currently available.
- A relatively new diagnostic tool used before therapeutic surgery for breast cancer is sentinel lymph node mapping, which identifies the first lymph node most likely to drain the cancerous cells.
- Overall 10-year survival with lumpectomy and radiation is about the same as with modified radical mastectomy.
- After losing a breast, many patients experience acute grief that may last 4 to 6 weeks or longer. Grief makes the fact of loss real.
- Caution patients who have undergone a modified radical mastectomy to avoid injections, vaccinations, taking of blood pressure or blood samples, or insertion of IV line in the affected arm.
- Phimosis is a condition in which the prepuce is too small to retract over the glans penis.
- Young men should be taught to perform TSE monthly beginning at 15 years of age for detection of testicular carcinoma.
- Oral acyclovir is prescribed for primary genital herpes to shorten the duration of the healing and suppress 75% of recurrence with daily use.
- Parenteral penicillin remains the treatment of choice for all stages of syphilis. All stages of syphilis should be treated.
- Because of penicillin-resistant strains of *N. gonorrhoeae,* penicillin, the former drug of choice for treatment of gonorrhea, has been changed to ceftriaxone.
- Chlamydial infections respond to treatment with tetracycline, doxycycline, azithromycin, or ofloxacin. Erythromycin is the drug of choice for use in pregnant patients.

Additional Learning Resources

Go to your companion CD for an audio glossary, animations, video clips, more.

evolve Be sure to visit the Evolve site at http://evolve.elsevier.com/Christensen/adult/ for additional online resources.

Review Questions for the NCLEX® Examination

1. A patient visits her physician because of an increase in her abdominal girth and dyspnea during the past month as a result of pressure on her diaphragm. She is diagnosed as having cancer of the ovaries. These two clinical manifestations result from:
   1. development of ascites.
   2. metastasis to the bowel.
   3. dilation of the alveoli.
   4. bladder distention.

2. A 30-year-old premenopausal patient asks the nurse the most appropriate time of the month to do her self-examination of the breasts. The most appropriate reply by the nurse would be:
   1. during her menstruation.
   2. 7 to 8 days after conclusion of the menstrual period.
   3. the same day each month.
   4. the 26th day of the menstrual cycle.

3. A 52-year-old patient has ductal cell carcinoma of the left breast. After a modified radical mastectomy, a Davol drain is in place in the left axillary region. The main purpose of this drain is to:
   1. control numbness of her left incisional site.
   2. improve her ability to perform range-of-motion exercises on her affected side.
   3. facilitate drainage and prevent formation of a hematoma.
   4. prevent postoperative phlebitis in her affected arm.

4. A 35-year-old patient received a vasectomy. Teaching for this patient should include that:
   1. the procedure is reversible if he later changes his mind.
   2. he should abstain from sexual intercourse until the incision is completely healed.
   3. he should apply warm compresses to the scrotum four times a day.
   4. he should return to the physician at regular intervals for sperm counts.

5. A 44-year-old patient is admitted for an abdominal hysterectomy. She is instructed that she will have a Foley catheter in place postoperatively. She asks the nurse how many days she will have the catheter in place. The best response by the nurse would be that:
   1. the indwelling catheter will probably remain in place for 1 week.
   2. the indwelling catheter will be removed after you are fully awake from the anesthesia.
   3. the indwelling catheter will generally remain in place 1 to 2 days after surgery.
   4. the indwelling catheter will remain in place for a few days postdischarge.

6. A 60-year-old patient had a vaginal hysterectomy for a prolapsed uterus. The nurse is aware that patients undergoing pelvic surgery are more susceptible to certain postoperative complications, and thus adjusts postoperative interventions to prevent:
   1. wound dehiscence.
   2. wound infection.
   3. atelectasis and hypostatic pneumonia.
   4. venous stasis and thrombophlebitis.

7. A 49-year-old obese diabetic patient has had a total abdominal hysterectomy. On the second postoperative day, the patient complains of increased pain in the operative site. She states, "It feels like something suddenly popped." With the symptoms presented, it would be likely that when the nurse removes the abdominal dressing she may note that:
   1. the wound has purulent exudate.
   2. dehiscence has occurred.
   3. the wound is indurated and tender.
   4. the wound is well approximated.

8. A 20-year-old patient goes to the physician's office with vaginal pruritus, burning, dull pelvic pain, and purulent vaginal discharge. A diagnostic test reveals she has chlamydia. The nurse goes over the medication schedule carefully with the patient. Another important nursing intervention to achieve satisfactory patient outcome would be to:
   1. encourage her to have her sexual partner(s) seek medical care as soon as possible to avoid reinfection of the patient.
   2. recommend she abstain from sexual contact while lesions are present.
   3. provide social and emotional support because the edematous, draining lymph nodes may be disturbing to the patient's self-image.
   4. educate the patient that the causative organism is a spirochete that gains entrance into the body during intercourse.

9. A 40-year-old patient had a right modified radical mastectomy with wide resection of the axillary lymph nodes. Which interventions are encouraged in the postoperative care for the patient? *(Select all that apply.)*
   1. Encourage turning, coughing, deep breathing, and use of incentive spirometry.
   2. Take blood pressure readings on her right arm.
   3. Assess for excessive exudates on dressings.
   4. Administer an oral analgesic every 4 hours as needed for pain.

10. A 23-year-old man is diagnosed with gonorrhea. Because of statements made in his patient interview, the nurse has established a nursing diagnosis of noncompliance. Which is the most effective way to overcome noncompliance for this patient?
    1. Telephone follow-up
    2. Case finding
    3. Single-dose treatment of ceftriaxone (Rocephin) IM
    4. Extensive patient education program

11. The nurse is teaching a group of teenagers about contraception and sexually transmitted infections (STIs). The nurse asks the students if they know which is the most prevalent STI. They are surprised to learn it is:
    1. syphilis.
    2. chlamydial infection.
    3. gonorrhea.
    4. herpes genitalis.

12. A 73-year-old patient comes to the physician's office with the complaint of constant seepage of feces from her vagina, causing her embarrassment due to soilage and odor. These are signs of:
    1. rectovaginal fistula.
    2. vesicovaginal fistula.
    3. urethrovaginal fistula.
    4. rectocele.

13. The American Cancer Society recommends that women have an annual screening mammography beginning at age:
    1. 21.
    2. 35.
    3. 40.
    4. 52.

14. The first lymph node most likely to drain the cancerous site in a breast cancer patient is known as the:
    1. axillary node.
    2. contaminated node.
    3. primary node.
    4. sentinal node.

15. While discussing risk factors for breast cancer with a group of women, the nurse stresses that the greatest risk factor for breast cancer is:
    1. being a woman over the age of 50.
    2. experiencing menstruation for 40 years or more.
    3. using estrogen replacement therapy during menopause.
    4. having a paternal grandmother with postmenopausal breast cancer.

16. A patient diagnosed with breast cancer has been offered the treatment choice of breast conservation surgery with radiation or a modified radical mastectomy. When questioned by the patient about these options, the nurse informs the patient that the lumpectomy with radiation:
    1. preserves the normal appearance and sensitivity of the breast.
    2. provides a shorter treatment period with fewer long-term complications.
    3. has about the same 10-year survival rate as the modified radical mastectomy.
    4. reduces the fear and anxiety that accompany the diagnosis and treatment of cancer.

17. Postoperatively the nurse teaches the patient with a modified radical mastectomy to prevent lymphedema by:
    1. using a sling to keep the arm flexed at the side.
    2. exposing the arm to sunlight to increase circulation.
    3. wrapping the arm with elastic bandages during the night.
    4. avoiding unnecessary trauma (e.g., venipuncture, blood pressure) to the arm on the operative side.

18. The nurse plans early and frequent ambulation for the patient who has undergone an abdominal hysterectomy to: *(Select all that apply.)*

1. prevent urinary retention.
2. prevent deep-vein thrombosis.
3. relieve abdominal distention.
4. maintain a sense of normalcy.

19. On the second postoperative day, a 63-year-old patient who had an abdominal hysterectomy complains of gas pains and abdominal distention. The patient has not had a bowel movement since surgery. Which nursing intervention will best stimulate peristalsis and relieve distention?

1. Offering carbonated beverages
2. Encouraging ambulation at least qid
3. Administering a 1000 mL soapsuds enema
4. Applying an abdominal binder

20. A 40-year-old patient has a history of multiple births in the past 15 years. She has been hospitalized for surgery to repair a cystocele. The nurse knows a cystocele presents symptoms of:

1. rectal pressure.
2. constipation.
3. hemorrhoids.
4. urinary frequency.

21. The Pap test is done as a diagnostic test for:

1. cervical cancer.
2. cancer of the breast.
3. pelvic inflammatory disease.
4. ovarian cancer.

22. The first significant sign of toxic shock syndrome that a patient will exhibit is:

1. sudden high fever.
2. vaginal hemorrhage.
3. foul vaginal odor.
4. sudden hypertension.

23. Lower abdominal and lower back pain that increases in severity during menstruation is a sign of the following disorder:

1. cervical polyp.
2. ovarian tumor.
3. endometriosis.
4. uterine cancer.

24. Osteoporosis is a disorder commonly seen in postmenopausal women; the dietary supplement recommended to retard this condition is:

1. calcium and vitamin D.
2. phosphorus and vitamin D.
3. vitamins D and C.
4. vitamins A and D.

25. The patient who has had a history of many pelvic inflammatory infections often seeks medical care for:

1. vaginal discharge.
2. infertility.
3. hemorrhage.
4. dyspareunia.

26. The woman at highest risk for toxic shock syndrome is the woman who:

1. experiences multiple sexual contacts.
2. inserts tampons with her fingers.
3. suffers untreated chronic PID.
4. experiences multiple abortions.

27. A 20-year-old patient goes to a neighborhood clinic because she has a purulent vaginal discharge. The physician suspects that the patient has gonorrhea. The nurse instructs the patient to empty her bladder before the pelvic examination. The chief purpose of this instruction is to:

1. prevent possible rupture of a distended bladder.
2. visualize the vaginal canal more easily.
3. aid in assessment of the pelvic organs.
4. enable the pelvic organs to resume their normal position.

28. The patient is to have a Pap smear. The nurse can prepare her for the test by educating her to:

1. use a mild vinegar douche the night before the test.
2. abstain from intercourse 24 hours before the test.
3. take a warm tub bath the night before the test.
4. save a first-voided AM urine specimen.

29. The patient's husband tells the nurse that his wife, who has been diagnosed with inoperable ovarian cancer, is talking about dying and fear of death. He asks the nurse for suggestions to help his wife. Which response by the nurse would be most helpful?

1. "The patient will probably die of another disease before she dies of ovarian cancer."
2. "Talk of death is normal at this time, but will diminish in the future."
3. "The patient is expressing an acceptance of utilizing hospice care."
4. "It is perfectly normal to want to talk about death. It is most helpful to support her by listening."

30. The American Cancer Society recommends that the human papillomavirus (HPV) vaccine against types 6, 11, 16, 18 be routinely given at what age to reduce the incidence of cervical cancer? *(Select all that apply.)*

1. Ages 11 to 12 years
2. Ages 13 to 18 years to catch up on mixed vaccine
3. 24 to 26 years
4. 30 to 35 years

chapter 53

Care of the Patient with a Visual or Auditory Disorder

evolve

Barbara Lauritsen Christensen

http://evolve.elsevier.com/Christensen/foundationsadult

Objectives

Anatomy and Physiology

1. List the major sense organs and discuss their anatomical position.
2. List the parts of the eye and define the function of each part.
3. List the three divisions of the ear and discuss the function of each.
4. Describe the physiologic processes involved in normal vision and hearing.

Medical-Surgical

5. Describe two changes in the sensory system that occur as a result of the normal aging process.
6. Describe age-related changes in the visual and auditory systems and differences in assessment findings.
7. Describe the purpose, significance of results, and nursing responsibilities related to diagnostic studies of the visual and auditory systems.
8. Discuss the refractory errors of astigmatism, strabismus, myopia, and hyperopia, including etiology, pathophysiology, clinical manifestations, assessment, diagnostic tests, medical management, nursing interventions, and patient teaching.
9. Describe inflammatory conditions of the eye, including etiology, pathophysiology, clinical manifestations, assessment, diagnostic tests, medical management, nursing interventions, patient teaching, and prognosis.
10. Discuss Sjögren syndrome, ectropion, and entropion, including etiology, pathophysiology, clinical manifestations, diagnostic tests, medical management, nursing interventions, and prognosis.
11. Compare the nature of cataracts, diabetic retinopathy, macular degeneration, retinal detachment, and glaucoma, including the etiology, pathophysiology, clinical manifestations, assessment, diagnostic tests, medical management, nursing interventions, patient teaching, and prognosis.
12. Discuss corneal injuries, including etiology, pathophysiology, clinical manifestations, assessment, diagnostic tests, medical management, nursing interventions, patient teaching, and prognosis.
13. Describe the various surgeries of the eye, including the nursing interventions and prognosis.
14. Differentiate between conductive and sensorineural hearing loss.
15. Describe the appropriate care of the hearing aid.
16. List tips for communicating with hearing- and sight-impaired people.
17. Identify communication resources for people with visual and/or hearing impairment.
18. Describe major ear inflammatory and infectious disorders, including etiology, pathophysiology, clinical manifestations, assessment, diagnostic tests, medical management, nursing interventions, patient teaching, and prognosis.
19. Discuss noninfectious disorders of the ear, including etiology, pathophysiology, clinical manifestations, assessment, diagnostic tests, medical management, nursing interventions, patient teaching, and prognosis.
20. Describe the various surgeries of the ear, including the nursing interventions, patient teaching, and prognosis.
21. Describe home health considerations for people with eye or ear disorders, surgery, or visual and hearing impairments.
22. Provide patient instructions regarding care of the eye and ear in accordance with written protocol.

Key Terms

astigmatism (ă-STĬG-mă-tĭsm, p. 1847)
audiometry (ăw-dē-ŎM-ĕ-trē, p. 1868)
cataract (KĂT-ă-răkt, p. 1853)
conjunctivitis (kŏn-jŭnk-tĭ-VĪ-tĭs, p. 1850)
cryotherapy (krī-ō-THĔR-ă-pē, p. 1856)
diabetic retinopathy (dī-ă-BĔT-ĭk rĕ-tĭn-NŎP-ă-thē, p. 1854)
enucleation (ē-nū-klē-Ā-shŭn, p. 1865)
exophthalmos (ĕk-sŏf-THĂL-mŏs, p. 1843)
glaucoma (glăw-KŌ-mă, p. 1859)
hyperopia (hī-pĕr-Ō-pē-ă, p. 1847)
keratitis (kĕr-ă-TĪ-tĭs, p. 1851)
keratoplasty (kĕr-ă-tŏ-PLĂS-tē, p. 1865)
labyrinthitis (lăb-ĭ-rĭnth-Ī-tĭs, p. 1875)
mastoiditis (măs-tŏy-DĪ-tĭs, p. 1872)
miotics (mī-ŎT-ĭks, p. 1861)
mydriatic (mĭd-rē-ĂT-ĭk, p. 1844)
myopia (mī-Ō-pē-ă, p. 1847)
myringotomy (mĭr-ĭn-GŎT-ŏ-mē, p. 1881)
radial keratotomy (RĀ-dē-ăl kĕ-ră-TŎT-ŏ-mē, p. 1848)
retinal detachment (RĔ-tĭ-năl dē-TĂCH-mĕnt, p. 1858)
Sjögren syndrome (SHĔR-grĕnz SĬN-drōm, p. 1851)
Snellen's test (SNĔL-ĕnz tĕst, p. 1844)
stapedectomy (stā-pĕ-DĔK-tŏ-mē, p. 1880)
strabismus (stră-BĬZ-mŭs, p. 1847)
tinnitus (TĬ-nī-tĭs, p. 1872)
tympanoplasty (tĭm-pă-nō-PLĂS-tē, p. 1880)
vertigo (VĔR-tĭ-gō, p. 1875)

ANATOMY AND PHYSIOLOGY OF THE SENSORY SYSTEM

The sensory system constantly gathers information through millions of receptors scattered throughout the body and delivers it to the brain for interpretation. This process enables humans to survive safely by enabling them to make appropriate responses to external stimuli. The five major senses are taste, touch, smell, sight, and hearing. The sense of balance (equilibrium) is linked with hearing, since the sensors are located within the ear.

ANATOMY OF THE EYE

The eye, which is only 1 inch (2.5 cm) in diameter, is a marvelous spherical structure that contains 70% of the sensory structures of the body. The optic tracts contain more than 1 million nerve fibers that carry messages from the eye to the brain, where they are interpreted. Only a small portion of the eye is visible externally; the remainder is enclosed in the skeletal bones of the face and cushioned in layers of fat. The bones surrounding the eyeball include the frontal, zygomatic, ethmoid, sphenoid, and lacrimal bones.

ACCESSORY STRUCTURES OF THE EYE

The accessory structures of the eye—eyebrows, eyelashes, eyelids, and lacrimal apparatus—function mainly as protective devices. In addition, six extrinsic eye muscles control gross eye movement and enable the eye to focus on any object in the visual field. The eye muscles are attached to the sclera (or white part of the eye) and move the eye laterally, medially, superiorly, and inferiorly.

The **lacrimal apparatus** (Figure 53-1) manufactures and drains tears to keep the eyeball moist and sweep away debris that might enter the eye. Tears are composed of a watery secretion that contains salt, mucus, and a bactericidal enzyme called **lysozyme.** The lacrimal glands are located superior and lateral to each eye. Blinking causes tears to flow medially to the lacrimal ducts, which empty into the nasolacrimal ducts and drain into the nasal cavity.

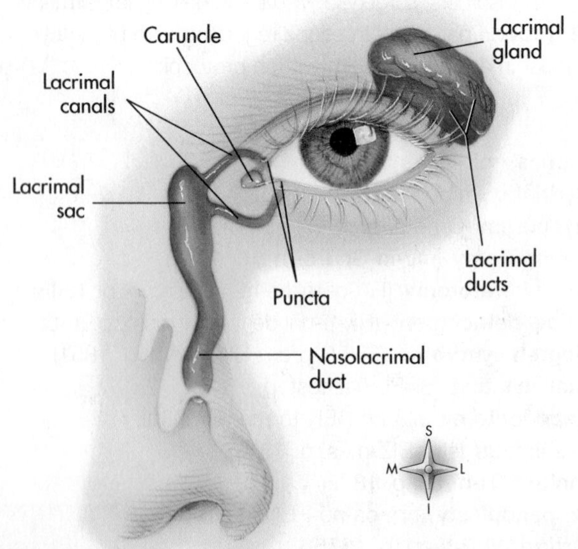

FIGURE 53-1 Lacrimal apparatus.

The **conjunctiva** is a thin mucous membrane that lines the inner aspect of the eyelids and the anterior surface of the eyeball to the edge of the cornea. Sometimes the blood vessels of the conjunctiva become dilated because of irritation or congestion, and the individual is said to have "bloodshot" eyes. The lower conjunctival sac is where eyedrops and eye ointment medication are usually administered.

STRUCTURE OF THE EYEBALL

The eyeball is composed of three layers, or tunics (Figure 53-2). The outermost layer of the eyeball is the fibrous tunic; it is composed of the sclera and the cornea. The **sclera,** or white of the eye, is a thick, white, opaque, connective tissue. The sclera gives shape to the eyeball and, because of its toughness, protects the inner eye structures. Posteriorly it is pierced by the optic nerve.

The **cornea** is the central anterior portion of the sclera. It is transparent and covers the iris, which is the colored portion of the eye. The cornea allows light rays to enter the inner portion of the eye. The cornea is the first part of the eye that refracts (bends) light rays. It is dense, uniform in thickness, and nonvascular, and it projects like a dome beyond the sclera. The cornea is one of the most highly developed, sensitive tissues in the body and is innervated by the trigeminal nerve (cranial nerve V). The avascular cornea obtains oxygen primarily through absorption from the tear film layer that bathes the epithelium. A small amount of oxygen is obtained from the **aqueous humor** (watery fluid in front of the lens in the anterior chamber of the eye) through the endothelial layers. The degree of corneal curvature varies in different individuals and in the same person at different ages. The curvature is more pronounced in youth than in advanced age.

At the junction of the sclera and cornea is a special structure called the canal of Schlemm. This tiny venous sinus at the angle of the anterior chamber of the eye drains the aqueous humor and funnels it into the bloodstream. This aids in controlling intraocular pressure (IOP; the pressure within the eyeball).

The middle layer of the eyeball is the vascular tunic. It contains the choroid, the ciliary body, and the iris. The posterior portion of the vascular tunic is the **choroid,** which is a thin, dark brown membrane that lines most of the internal area of the sclera. It is highly vascular and supplies nutrients to the retina. The anterior portion of the vascular tunic forms the ciliary body, which is an intrinsic muscular ring that holds the lens in place and changes its shape for near or distant vision. The ciliary body also attaches to the iris, a

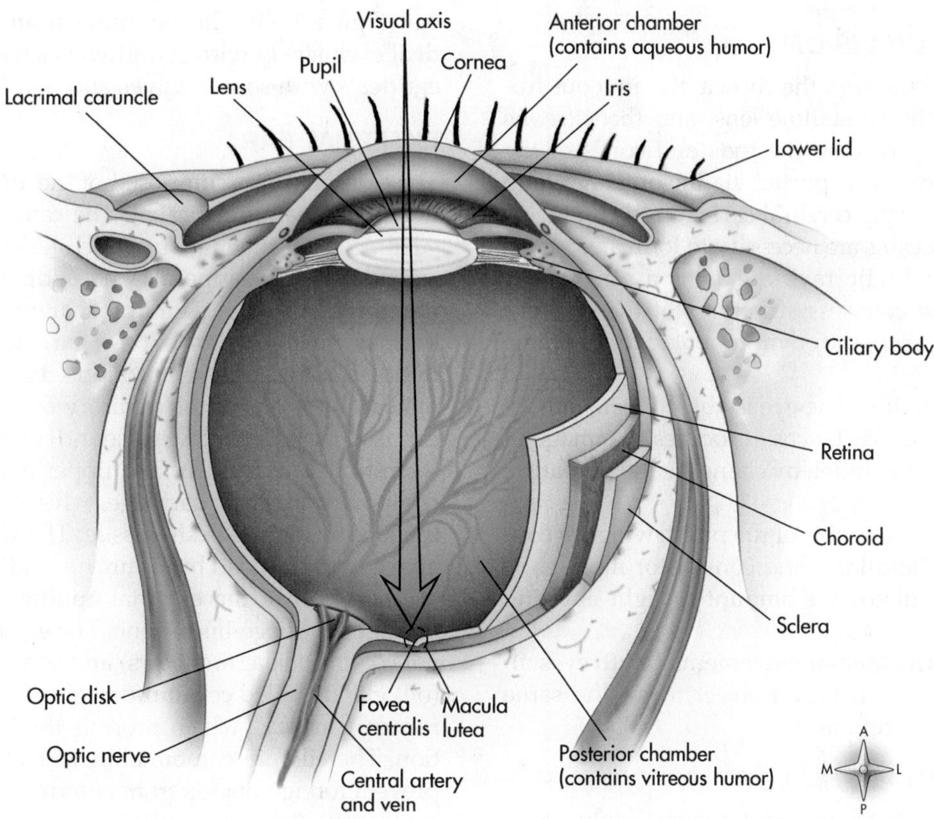

FIGURE 53-2 Horizontal section through the left eyeball. The eye is viewed from above.

pigmented intrinsic muscular ring that resembles a doughnut. Located slightly nasal to the center of the iris is a circular opening called the **pupil.** The iris lies between the cornea and the lens and regulates the amount of light entering the eye through the pupil, much like a camera shutter. Two sets of smooth muscle control the iris, which in turn controls the pupil. In bright light the circular muscle fibers of the iris contract and the pupil contracts; in dim light the radial muscles contract and the pupil dilates. Papillary constriction is a reflex that protects the retina from intense light or that permits more acute near vision.

The innermost tunic of the eye is the **retina,** a 10-layer, delicate, nervous-tissue membrane that receives images of external objects and transmits impulses through the optic nerve to the brain. It lies on the posterior portion of the eyeball. The retina contains specialized sensory cells called **rods** and **cones** (photoreceptors). The rods and cones are scattered throughout the retina except where the optic nerve exits the eye; this area is called the **optic disk** or **blind spot.** Rods are receptors for night vision and are also responsible for peripheral vision. Cones are responsible for day vision. The three kinds of cones are each sensitive to a different color: red, green, or blue. Color pigments that are sensitive to light enable the rods and cones to function. Rods detect only the presence of light, whereas cones detect different wave lengths of color.

The center of the retina is the **fovea centralis,** a pinpoint depression composed only of densely packed cones. The fovea centralis contains the greatest concentration of cones of any area in the retina. This area of the retina provides the sharpest visual acuity and most acute color vision. Surrounding the fovea is the **macula,** an area of less than 1 mm^2 that has a high concentration of cones and is relatively free of blood vessels. Vitamin A is responsible for the production of these color pigments. The absence of these three types of cones causes color blindness, which is an inherited condition found primarily in males.

CHAMBERS OF THE EYE

The eye is divided into the anterior and posterior chambers by the **crystalline lens,** a transparent, colorless structure that is biconvex, enclosed in a capsule, and held in place just behind the pupil by the suspensory ligament. The crystalline lens focuses light rays so that they form a perfect image on the retina. Anterior to the crystalline lens is the anterior chamber, which is filled with **aqueous humor,** a clear, watery fluid similar to blood plasma. The ciliary bodies of the choroid constantly secrete, drain, and replace aqueous humor to maintain normal IOP. Aqueous humor also helps maintain the eyeball's shape, keeps the retina attached to the choroid, and refracts light.

The posterior chamber is filled with **vitreous humor,** a transparent, jellylike substance that gives shape to the eyeball, keeps the retina attached to the choroid, and refracts light. It differs from the aqueous humor in that it is not continuously replaced.

PHYSIOLOGY OF VISION

Light must travel through the cornea, the aqueous humor, the pupil, the crystalline lens, and the vitreous humor and finally reaches the rods and cones of the retina. The image is transported via the optic nerve to the visual center of the cerebral cortex in the brain.

Four basic processes are necessary to form an image:

1. **Refraction:** Light rays are bent as they pass through the colorless structures of the eye, enabling light from the environment to focus on the retina.
2. **Accommodation:** The eye is able to focus on objects at various distances. It focuses the image of an object on the retina by changing the curvature of the lens.
3. **Constriction:** The size of the pupil, which is controlled by the dilator and constrictor muscles of the iris, regulates the amount of light entering the eye.
4. **Convergence:** Medial movement of both eyes allows light rays from an object to hit the same point on both retinas.

ANATOMY AND PHYSIOLOGY OF THE EAR

The external ear (**pinna,** or **auricle**) reveals only a portion of the complex organ of hearing. Within the ear are many structures that enable hearing and interpretation of sound and assist in maintaining equilibrium (balance). Anatomically, from the external structures to the internal structures, the ear has three distinct divisions: the external ear, the middle ear, and the inner ear (Figure 53-3). The external ear and the middle ear deal exclusively with sound waves, whereas the inner ear deals with sound waves and equilibrium.

EXTERNAL EAR

The external ear is composed of the auricle (pinna) and the external auditory canal. The canal is shaped like a small, curved tube (about 1 inch [2.5 cm] in length). It extends into the temporal bone, ending at the **tympanic membrane**—a thin, semitransparent membrane. The tympanic membrane separates the external ear from the middle ear and transmits sound vibrations to the internal ear by means of the auditory ossicles. The external ear is designed to collect sound waves and channel them to the middle ear. The upper part of the pinna is composed of elastic cartilage, whereas the lower part, the lobe, is mainly fleshy tissue. The whole structure is attached to the head by ligaments and muscles.

The walls of the external auditory canal are composed of cartilage-lined bone. The external auditory canal contains cilia (tiny hairs) and specialized sebaceous (oil) glands called **ceruminous glands.** They secrete **cerumen** (earwax), which protects the lining from infection. The cilia, in combination with the cerumen, also prevent foreign objects from entering the ear.

MIDDLE EAR

The middle ear, or tympanic cavity, is a small, air-filled chamber located within the temporal bone. The **eustachian tube,** or auditory canal, is lined with a mucous membrane that joins the nasopharynx and the middle-ear cavity. During swallowing or yawning, the tube

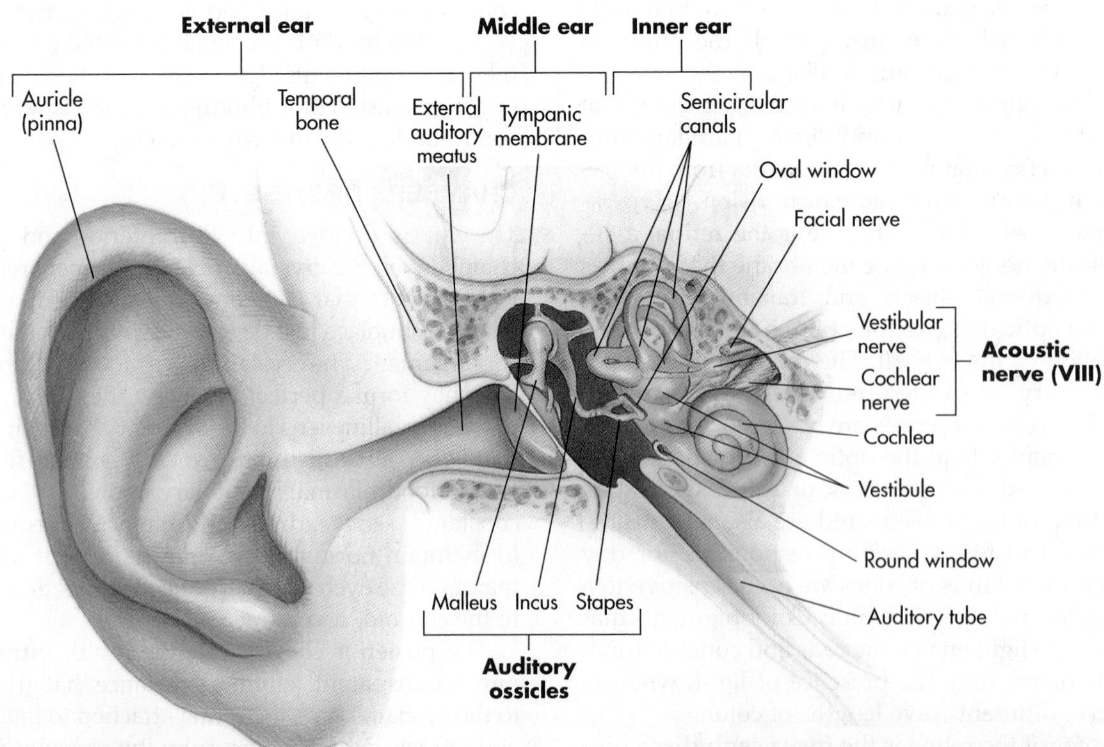

FIGURE 53-3 External, middle, and inner ear. (Not to scale.)

allows air to enter the middle ear, which equalizes the air pressure on either side of the tympanic membrane. Because the pharynx, the eustachian tube, and the middle ear are all covered with a continuous mucous membrane, infection can travel easily from the throat to the middle ear. This is often seen in young children. The posterior wall of the middle ear opens into the mastoid process, an area filled with air spaces, which also aids in equalizing air pressure. Infection of the middle ear, if untreated, can spread to the mastoid process.

Extending along the middle-ear chamber are three small bones (ossicles) that carry sound waves from the external ear to the inner ear. These ossicles are named according to their shape: the **malleus** (hammer), the **incus** (anvil), and the **stapes** (stirrup). The internal surface of the tympanic membrane is connected to the first of these three bones, the malleus. The malleus transfers sound waves to the incus, which in turn transfers them to the stapes. The stapes pushes against the oval window, a small membrane that marks the beginning of the inner ear. When sound waves cause the tympanic membrane to vibrate, that vibration is transmitted and amplified by the ear ossicles as it passes through the middle ear. Movement of the stapes against the oval window causes movement of fluid in the inner ear.

INNER EAR

A very important portion of the ear, the inner ear, or **labyrinth,** is a series of canals (Figure 53-4). Structurally, it contains the bony labyrinth, which is filled with a fluid called **perilymph.** The bony labyrinth has three subdivisions called the **semicircular canal** (associated with the sense of balance), the **vestibule,** and the **cochlea.** The membranous labyrinth is a series of sacs and tubes that contain a thicker fluid called **endolymph.** Endolymph and perilymph conduct sound waves through the inner-ear system.

The **cochlea** resembles a snail's shell and contains the **organ of Corti,** the organ of hearing. It contains many hearing receptors, or hair cells. These cells respond to sound waves by stimulating the cochlear nerve (a branch of the eighth cranial nerve—the vestibulocochlear, or acoustic, nerve), which transmits the message to the brain. These hair cells may become damaged from noise pollution (i.e., high-intensity sounds such as those produced by jet engines, factory equipment, and rock bands). Once these cells are damaged or destroyed, hearing becomes permanently impaired.

Deeper in the inner ear, past the cochlea, is the **vestibule,** or the oval central portion of the bony labyrinth. The vestibule contains receptors that respond to gravity. They provide information on which way is up and which way is down, enabling an individual to remain in an upright position. Extending upward from the vestibule are three semicircular canals responsible for maintaining balance and equilibrium. They contain sensory hair cells and endolymph. The motion of the endolymph stimulates the hair cells, which stimulate the receptors; then the message is sent to the brain for interpretation (see Figure 53-4).

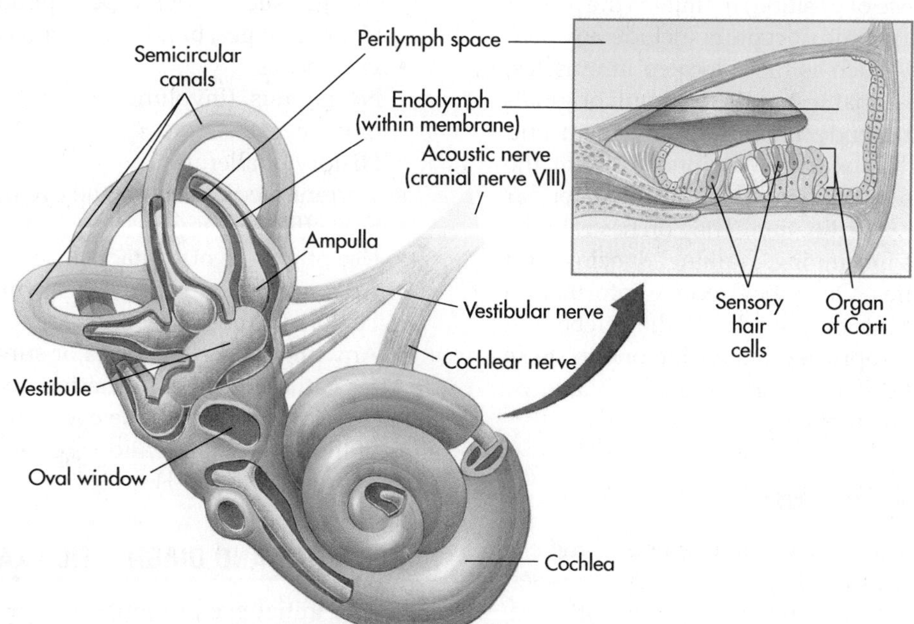

FIGURE 53-4 The inner ear. The bony labyrinth is the hard outer wall of the entire inner ear and includes semicircular canals, the vestibule, and the cochlea. Within the bony labyrinth is the membranous labyrinth *(purple)*, which is surrounded by perilymph and filled with endolymph. Each ampulla in the vestibule contains a crista ampullaris that detects changes in head position and sends sensory impulses through the vestibular nerve to the brain. *Inset* shows a section of the membranous cochlea. Hair cells in the organ of Corti detect sound and send the information through the cochlear nerve. Then vestibular and cochlear nerves join to form the eighth cranial nerve.

OTHER SPECIAL SENSES

TASTE AND SMELL

The tongue of the average adult contains approximately 10,000 taste buds; some are also located on the inner aspect of the cheeks. Certain locations on the taste buds are receptors for four taste sensations, as follow:

1. **Sweet:** Respond to sugar and other sweet substances; located on the tip of the tongue
2. **Sour:** Respond to acid content of foods; located on the sides of the tongue
3. **Salty:** Respond to metal ions within foods; located on the tip of the tongue
4. **Bitter:** Respond to alkaline or basic ions within foods; located on the posterior portion of the tongue

The receptors for the sense of smell (olfactory receptors) are located in the roof, or the upper part of the nasal cavity. On inhalation, an odor comes in contact with the olfactory receptors and the message is sent to the brain. Certain odors are remembered for a long time and stimulate certain memories (e.g., pine scent reminds people of Christmas; talcum powder reminds people of infants). The body is not able to regenerate olfactory cells; once they are damaged, the sense of smell is impaired.

TOUCH

The receptors for touch **(tactile receptors)** are located throughout the integumentary system. They respond to touch, pressure, and vibration.

POSITION AND MOVEMENT

Proprioception (sense of position) maintains the proper position of the body. **Proprioceptors** include any sensory nerve ending—such as those located in muscles, tendons, and joints—that responds to stimuli originating from within the body regarding movement and spatial position. They work in conjunction with the semicircular canals and the vestibule of the inner ear to maintain proper coordination. They orchestrate the body's movements in running, walking, dancing, and many other activities. Once they receive information from the environment, they send it to the cerebellum for interpretation. Proprioceptors enable one to sense the position of the different parts of the body and be aware of the movement of each.

NORMAL AGING OF THE SENSORY SYSTEM

As the individual ages, the crystalline lens of the eye hardens and becomes too large for the eye muscles, thus causing a loss of accommodation. This often results in a need for bifocals or trifocals. The crystalline lens loses some of its transparency and becomes more opaque, and glare begins to become a problem. The lens proteins are vulnerable to biochemical changes and exposure to ultraviolet (UV) light, resulting in cataract development. Hypertension and atherosclerosis lead to retinal vascular changes. Age-related macular degeneration (ARMD) contributes to impaired vision. The pupils become smaller and decrease the amount of light that reaches the retina, resulting in a need for brighter lighting for reading (Lewis et al., 2007).

Impaired hearing can result from age-related changes in the auditory system. A condition called **presbycusis,** a hearing deficit secondary to aging, can occur from numerous sources such as noise, vascular or systemic diseases, poor nutrition, ototoxic drugs, and pollution. These exposures occurring over the life span can damage the delicate hair cells of the organ of Corti, cause calcification of the ossicles of the middle ear, and interfere with sound conduction. Tinnitus (ringing in the ear) may also occur secondary to the aging process.

Visual and hearing losses in the older adult can result in physical and psychosocial problems. Early detection of these helps maintain a more productive lifestyle (Lewis et al., 2007). The remaining senses undergo slight changes that decrease their reaction or threshold time, which results in slower response or diminished sensation (see Life Span Considerations box).

NURSING CONSIDERATIONS FOR CARE OF THE PATIENT WITH AN EYE DISORDER

In caring for the patient with an eye disorder, review the following items:

- Eye pain, pruritus, photophobia, excessive tearing, dryness, floaters, light flashes, scotomas (defect of vision in a defined area of the visual field), halo around lights, diplopia, discharge, visual changes such as depth perception and peripheral vision changes, blind spots, or fading color vision
- Headaches
- Nystagmus (involuntary, rhythmic movements of the eyes)
- History of allergies
- Current medication for the eye disorder
- Side effects of any medications
- Use of glasses or contact lenses
- Adequacy of current eyewear prescription
- Personal habits related to care of eyewear
- Any previous eye injuries or surgeries

After gathering the information and reporting it to the physician, assist with the eye examination. The results of the initial examination are compared with normal findings (Table 53-1).

LABORATORY AND DIAGNOSTIC EXAMINATIONS

After the initial eye examination, the patient may require additional diagnostic testing. The major diagnostic eye tests, including Snellen's test, are explained in Table 53-2. **Amsler's grid test** is used to detect a defect of the macular area of the retina (see Table 53-2). The **tangent screen** evaluates central and peripheral

 Life Span Considerations

Older Adults

Disorders of the Sensory System

- Multiple changes in vision that normally occur with aging include the following:
  —Changes in accommodation, resulting in increased difficulty focusing on close objects (presbyopia), which leads to difficulty reading or doing other close work
  —Decreased color perception and discrimination, particularly with shades of blue, green, and violet
  —Poor adaptation to changes in light, resulting in "night blindness" and increased sensitivity to glare due to increased opacity of the lens and decreased pupil size
  —Alterations in depth perception, leading to increased risk of falls
  —Decreased secretion of tears, resulting in complaints of dryness or pruritus, which leads to a high risk for irritation of the cornea
  —Increased incidence of moving particles or "floaters" that interfere with visually based tasks
- Older adults experience an increased incidence of eye disorders, including cataracts, retinal detachment, macular degeneration, and glaucoma.
- A third of all individuals older than 70 years of age have significant hearing loss.
- Hearing loss in older adults is most often sensorineural (presbycusis) and involves loss of the high frequencies. Hearing loss results in distortion of speech, which can lead to failure to respond to directions or inappropriate behaviors often misinterpreted as disorientation.
- Hearing loss can lead to social isolation when the person cannot understand and participate in normal conversation.
- A decreased number of receptors in the nasal cavities and papillae of the tongue results in changes in smell and taste. Most affected are the sweet and salty tastes.
- Medications often affect the taste of food and can contribute to altered nutrition.

Table 53-1 Normal Findings of the Adult Eye

AREA EXAMINED	FINDINGS
Eyelid	Blink reflex to light or touch intact. Lid margins just above the corneal borders.
Eyeball	Eyeball does not protrude beyond the supraorbital ridge of the frontal bone. The eyeball is usually moist; moisture may be diminished in the older adult.
Conjunctiva	**Palpebral** (eyelid): Pink, uniform blood vessels without discharge. **Bulbar:** Clear, tiny red vessels; in the older adult, the bulbar conjunctiva may lose luster.
Sclera	Generally white; may have yellow-tan dots in a dark-skinned individual.
Cornea	Transparent, smooth, convex. In the older adult, a gray ring around the cornea **(arcus senilis)** may be present as a result of lipid deposits.
Iris	Round, intact, bilateral coloration. In the older adult, color may be paler and shape less regular.
Pupil	Equal, round, reactive to light and accommodation. Response to light is equal bilaterally. In the older adult, constriction response may be slower.
Internal eye (including retina, vessels, and optic disk)	Retina is intact. Vessel structure is intact and bilaterally similar in pattern. Optic disk has well-defined border.
Visual acuity	
Distant vision	20/20 (able to read line 20 of eye chart at a distance of 20 feet)
Near vision	Able to read newspaper print at 14 inches
Peripheral vision	Side vision 90 degrees from central visual axis; upward 50 degrees; downward 70 degrees
Eye movement	Coordinated eye movement bilaterally
Color perception	Able to properly identify colors of major groups: red, blue, and green

fields of vision. The **Goldmann perimetry** test detects and evaluates the progression of glaucoma (an abnormal condition of elevated pressure within the eye because of obstruction of the outflow of aqueous humor), which affects peripheral vision. **Exophthalmometry** measures the degree of forward placement of the eye, known as exophthalmos (an abnormal condition characterized by a marked protrusion of the eyeballs). **Slit-lamp examination** is done to examine the conjunctiva, the lens, the vitreous humor, the iris, and the cornea. **Schirmer's tear** test evaluates the function of the major lacrimal glands (see Table 53-2). **Fluorescein angiography** is used to examine the microvascular structures of the eye, to assess patency of the lacrimal system, and to assess for corneal abrasion.

DISORDERS OF THE EYE

BLINDNESS AND NEAR BLINDNESS

Etiology and Pathophysiology

Blindness is a loss of visual acuity that ranges from partial to total loss of sight. Total blindness is defined as no light perception and no usable vision. Functional blindness is present when the patient has some light perception but no usable vision. It may be congenital or acquired.

Table 53-2 Major Diagnostic Eye Tests

PURPOSE	EQUIPMENT	PROCEDURE	PATIENT TEACHING
Snellen's test*			
Assessment of visual acuity; used as screening test	Snellen's chart; eyepatch or cover	1. Patient stands or sits 20 feet from chart. 2. Patient covers one eye. 3. Ask patient to read above or below the 20/20 line. 4. Repeat step 3 using the other eye. 5. Document findings.	1. Explain test. 2. If findings are abnormal (i.e., other than 20 feet required to read the chart line), encourage patient to seek further eye testing.
Color vision			
Prerequisite for driver's license	Color chart or machine	1. Color dots are reflected on a background of mixed colors. 2. Patient identifies color patterns on the test field. 3. Document findings.	1. Explain procedure. 2. Encourage patient to seek further testing when results indicate inaccurate recognition of color patterns.
Refraction			
Measurement of visual acuity to determine refractory errors such as **myopia** (nearsightedness), **hyperopia** (farsightedness), **presbyopia** (inability to focus on close objects), and **astigmatism** (blurred vision)	Retinoscope or sample lenses	1. Ophthalmologist or optometrist asks patient to indicate clear or blurred vision with each lens change in the retinoscope.	1. Explain procedure. 2. Examiner discusses results with patient and encourages appropriate corrective measures.
Ophthalmoscopy			
Evaluation of underlying structures of the eye; routine screening	Ophthalmoscope; **mydriatic** (causing pupillary dilation) drops to dilate the pupil	1. Apply mydriatic drops (contraindicated in patients with closed-angle glaucoma). 2. As pupil dilation occurs, darken the room. 3. Instruct patient to remain still and focus on a stationary object. 4. Examiner uses ophthalmoscope to view internal eye structure. 5. Document findings.	1. Explain procedure. 2. Instruct patient that effects of the drops will last no longer than 1 hour. 3. Patient requires sunglasses when outside or in brightly lit room until pupils return to normal size. 4. Examiner discusses results with patient and encourages corrective measures.
Tonometry (see Figures 53-11 and 53-12)			
Measurement of intraocular pressure to detect tumors and glaucoma; pressure measured using a Schiøtz or Tono-Pen tonometer, but the most accurate readings are obtained by applanation tonometry	Tonometer (e.g., applanation [see Figure 53-11], Schiøtz [see Figure 53-12]); topical anesthetic may be used	1. Examiner places tonometer on cornea. 2. Obtain pressure readings. 3. Document findings. 4. In applanation tonometry, the surface of the anesthetized cornea is applanated by the tonometer, and the cornea is observed through the biomicroscope (see Figure 53-12). The normal intraocular pressure ranges from 10 to 22 mm Hg.	1. Explain procedure. 2. Encourage patient to relax to avoid false high readings. 3. Eyes are not to be rubbed for approximately 30 minutes to avoid corneal irritation. 4. Contact lenses may be reinserted 2 hours after completion of test.

*Eye chart test for visual acuity: letters, numbers, or symbols are arranged on the chart in decreasing size from top to bottom.

Table 53-2 Major Diagnostic Eye Tests—cont'd

PURPOSE	EQUIPMENT	PROCEDURE	PATIENT TEACHING
Amsler's grid test			
Used to diagnose and monitor macular problems	Handheld card printed with a grid of lines (similar to graph paper)	1. Patient fixates on center dot and records any abnormalities of the grid lines, such as wavy, missing, or distorted areas.	1. Explain test. 2. Regular testing is necessary to identify any changes in macular function.
Schirmer's tear test			
Measures tear volume produced throughout fixed time period; useful in diagnosing keratoconjunctivitis sicca	Strip of lacrimal filter paper	1. Place one end of strip of filter paper in lower cul-de-sac. 2. Measure area of tear saturation after 5 minutes.	1. Explain test. 2. Test may be done with closed or open eyes. 3. Normal results are 10-15 mm of wet paper. Less than 5 mm of wetting within 5 minutes is indicative of keratoconjunctivitis sicca.

The World Health Organization has determined that in the United States approximately 1.3 million people are legally blind (American Foundation for the Blind, 2009). The patient with either total or functional blindness is considered legally blind. Legal blindness refers to individuals with a maximum visual acuity of 20/200 with corrective eyewear and/or visual field sight capacity reduced to 20 degrees. (The normal visual field range is 180 degrees.)

Categories have been established to help determine the exact extent of the vision loss and what assistive measures are appropriate for the individual. These categories range from low vision loss (20/70 to 20/200) to three categories of blindness (20/400, 20/1200, and no light perception).

Congenital blindness results from various birth defects. Acquired blindness in adults occurs as a result of disorders such as diabetic retinopathy, glaucoma, cataracts, and retinal degeneration; acute trauma is also a common cause.

Clinical Manifestations

The degree of vision loss depends on the extent of trauma or disease. Symptoms may include diplopia, pain, presence of floaters and light flashes, and pruritus or burning of the eyes. Additional physical manifestations of the visually impaired patient include loss of peripheral vision; halos (rainbow colors seen around lights); a sense of orbital pressure; bulging of the eye(s); and any difference in the appearance of an eye structure, such as the pupil.

The wide variety of emotions associated with blindness range from fear, anxiety, disorientation, depression, helplessness, and hopelessness to acceptance. The patient may experience poor interpersonal communication skills and coping mechanisms. Because self-care skills may be impaired, a blind individual may prefer isolation, causing additional physical and emotional difficulties.

Assessment

Subjective data include patient complaints of blurred vision as an early symptom of an eye disorder. Determine the onset, the severity, and the duration of symptoms, as well as any factors that relieve them.

Collection of **objective data** may include observations of squinting and rubbing of the eyes. Note the patient's compensation measures, such as use of a magnifying glass. Also determine the use and effectiveness of assistive eyewear.

Medical Management

Corrective eyewear (contact lenses and glasses) is the first method of medical management for a partially sighted individual. If the visual defect results from an inflammatory disorder, medication appropriate to the causative agent is prescribed.

Additional assistive devices for a visually impaired patient include canes, guide dogs, magnifying systems, and telescopic lenses. The patient should be evaluated by an eye specialist to determine which devices are best suited. Some of the more technologically complex devices are expensive and may not be covered by insurance.

Canes are the most frequently used device for the partially or totally blind person. They are lightweight and portable and allow the patient simple maneuvering. The drawback is that canes do not usually help in detecting overhead objects. The newer laser canes provide more information about objects in front and at head and foot levels, but these are not readily available and are expensive. Guide dogs allow the blind person mobility that would otherwise be difficult. Trained dogs steer the patient away from obstacles, both aerial and stationary.

Surgical correction of the visual defect may provide eyesight. New laser surgeries provide excellent results in selected cases. Corneal transplants can restore vision in patients with corneal damage.

Nursing Interventions and Patient Teaching

The nurse might assume that patients who have been blind for years accept their condition, but this is not necessarily the case. Complications of long-term blindness may result in physical and emotional problems. Physically the patient may be malnourished from diminished cooking skills. The patient may also have secondary infections related to poor hygiene. Assistance with activities of daily living (ADLs) is a primary focus of patient care. Allow adequate time for the patient to assist in self-care. Emotional aspects of nursing interventions include appropriate communication (Box 53-1).

Vision loss affects not only the patient but also family, friends, and the community. Patients have different coping mechanisms. Be aware of the services and devices available for the partially sighted or blind person so you can make referrals. With proper rehabilitation, the visually impaired can develop independence and positive self-esteem (Lewis et al., 2007). The main resource for services for the legally blind patient is the state agency for rehabilitation of the blind (Brandt et al., 2008). The American Foundation for the Blind (www.afb.org) lists agencies to assist the partially sighted or blind patient.

For the patient with no functional vision, Braille or audiobooks for reading and a cane or guide dog for ambulation are examples of vision substitution techniques. If a patient has some remaining vision, vision enhancement techniques can help with walking, reading, and carrying out ADLs (Lewis et al., 2007). It is a nursing responsibility to educate, assist, counsel, and prevent complications. A comprehensive approach to care can help the patient successfully adjust to home, work, and society.

Nursing diagnoses and interventions for the patient with blindness or near blindness include but are not limited to the following:

Nursing Diagnoses	Nursing Interventions
Fear, related to blindness	Determine the patient's level of fear.
Risk for injury, related to new environment	Orient the patient to the environment. Use therapeutic touch. Avoid loud sounds that may startle the patient. Use protective devices, such as side rails and canes. Alter surroundings to afford safety (clear passageways, nonslip rugs, etc.).

The patient requires instruction on ambulatory safety. Advise the patient to walk slowly, get verbal clues from the walking companion, and touch objects or borders. The walking companion should precede the patient by about 1 foot, with the patient's hand on the companion's elbow for security (Figure 53-5). For both short- and long-term blindness, describing the surroundings is appropriate.

Box 53-1 Guidelines for Communicating with Blind People

- Announce your presence when entering the room.
- Talk in a normal tone of voice.
- Do not try to avoid common phrases in speech, such as "See what I mean?"
- Introduce yourself with each contact (unless well known to the person).
- Explain any activity occurring in the room.
- Announce when you are leaving the room so the blind person is not put in the position of talking to someone who is no longer there.

Prognosis

Blindness and near-blindness disorders have been reduced as a result of emphasis on early diagnosis and treatment. Laser surgery treatment reduces and limits complications.

REFRACTORY ERRORS

Early childhood vision screening in schools has contributed to early diagnosis and treatment of refractory errors. Permanent visual loss may occur if strabismus and astigmatism are not treated at the preschool level

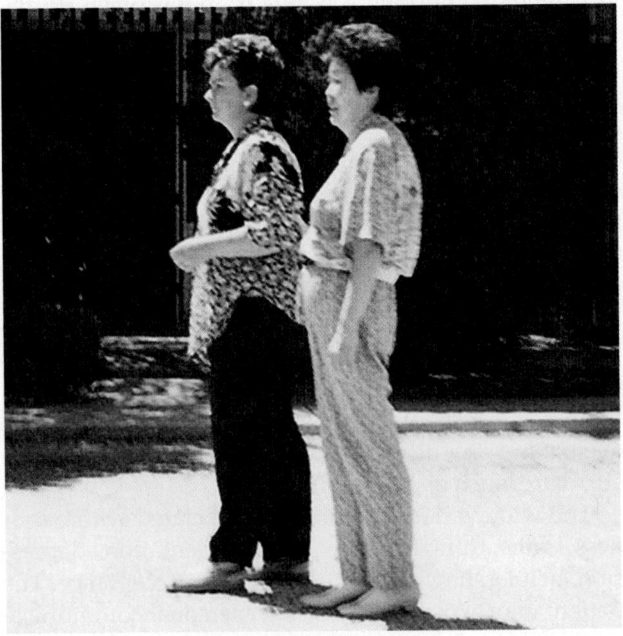

FIGURE 53-5 Sighted-guide technique. The walking companion serves as the sighted guide, walking slightly ahead of the patient with the patient holding the back of the companion's arm.

(Table 53-3). Physician monitoring of intermittent follow-up care is crucial until 10 years of age.

Astigmatism, Strabismus, Myopia, and Hyperopia

Common refractory errors (astigmatism, strabismus, myopia, and hyperopia) are described in Table 53-3.

Diagnostic Tests

Common tests used in the diagnosis of refractory errors include ophthalmoscopy, retinoscopy, visual acuity tests, and refraction tests.

Medical Management

New technology in eyewear significantly reduces refractory error problems in the adult. However, the preferred treatment is surgical correction.

Nursing Interventions and Patient Teaching

The hospitalized patient wearing corrective eyewear requires daily assistance in cleansing and maintenance. Eyeglass lenses are washed daily with a mild or diluted glass cleaner and rinsed before drying with a soft cloth. Check screw fittings to make sure they are secure. Contact lenses are cared for based on the manufacturer's directions. When not in use, place lenses in storage case per protocol. Take safety precautions when corrective eyewear is not worn.

A nursing diagnosis and interventions for the patient with astigmatism, strabismus, myopia, and hyperopia include but are not limited to the following:

Nursing Diagnosis	Nursing Interventions
Risk for injury, related to visual changes	Reinforce physician's instruction. Orient patient to the environment. Remove small, movable objects from the path of the visually impaired patient.

Encourage the patient to see an optometrist or ophthalmologist yearly to keep the eyewear prescription current. Instruct the patient on the use and care of eyewear; complications may result if the patient does not follow use and care instructions.

Myopia

See Table 53-3.

Table 53-3 Common Refractory Errors

DESCRIPTION	ETIOLOGY AND PATHOPHYSIOLOGY	CLINICAL MANIFESTATIONS	ASSESSMENT
Astigmatism			
Defect in the curvature of the eyeball surface	May be hereditary or a muscular deficit Occurs when the light rays cannot be focused clearly on a point on the retina because the spherical curve of the cornea is not equal in all meridians	Blurring of vision	**Subjective data:** Complaints of eye discomfort, difficulty in focusing, blurred vision
Strabismus			
Inability of the eyes to focus in the same direction: commonly called **cross-eyed** **Esotropia:** Eye turns in the direction of the nose **Exotropia:** Eye turns outward	May result from neurologic or muscular dysfunction or may be inherited Only one eye can fix on an object, because axes do not focus simultaneously	Eyeball position is not symmetrical	**Subjective data:** States difficulty in following objects **Objective data:** Only one eye focuses or follows an object
Myopia			
Condition of nearsightedness	Elongation of the eyeball or an error in refraction so that parallel rays are focused in front of the retina	Inability to see objects at a distance	**Subjective data:** Difficulty seeing faraway objects **Objective data:** Snellen's test
Hyperopia			
Condition of farsightedness	May result from error of refraction in which rays of light entering the eye are brought into focus behind the retina	Inability to see objects at close range	**Subjective data:** Difficulty seeing near objects **Objective data:** Snellen's test

Diagnostic Tests

Diagnosis of myopia commonly follows a visit to the physician because of the patient's inability to see distant objects clearly. After routine examinations (see Table 53-3) the patient is assessed for corrective lenses or corrective refractory surgery.

Medical Management

The majority of patients are prescribed corrective eyeglasses or contact lenses. Patients who are unable or unwilling to wear corrective eyewear for occupational or cosmetic reasons may elect surgical correction.

Surgical Management

Refractory surgery is effective in treating the causes of visual problems instead of correcting symptoms. Myopia is the refractive error most commonly corrected by refractive surgery. Patients are selected based on the degree of myopia; the shape of the cornea; and the absence of medical conditions such as severe diabetes, glaucoma, or pregnancy. The usual age for correction is between 20 and 60 years. Radial keratotomy, photorefractive keratotomy, kerotorefractive surgery, and photorefractive keratectomy are procedures for myopia to markedly improve vision and are under continued study for long-term complications.

Keratorefractive surgery (surgery to alter the corneal curvature) is a new method of refractive correction. This surgical category includes a variety of procedures, including making cuts in the cornea or using a laser or a special microsurgical knife to open and replace a flap of corneal tissue.

Radial keratotomy (RK) is a technique in which the surgeon makes partial-thickness radial incisions in the patient's cornea, leaving an uncut optical zone in the center. The patient must evaluate the risk of serious complications, such as operative infection and corneal scarring, when considering this procedure.

Photorefractive keratectomy (PRK) is another procedure that uses an excimer laser to reshape the central corneal surface. It is used primarily to correct myopia but is also used for hyperopia and astigmatism. Evidence suggests that final visual acuity with this procedure is more predictable than with radial keratotomy, at least in the short term. **Laser in-situ keratomileusis (LASIK)** is a procedure in which first a corneal flap is folded back, and then an excimer laser removes some of the internal layers of the cornea. Afterward, the flap is returned to normal position and allowed to heal in place. Evidence supports claims that LASIK creates earlier visual stability in patients with a high degree of myopia than with PRK. Unlike RK, both PRK and LASIK procedures affect the central zone of the cornea (Lewis et al., 2007).

Intacs, which are corneal ring segments, are the newest innovation in refractive procedures. Intacs are two tiny half rings of plastic that are placed between the layers of the cornea around the pupil after the surgeon makes a tunnel-like pathway with a specially designed surgical knife. They can also be removed if necessary, and the effects on refractive error are completely reversed (Lewis et al., 2007).

Nursing Interventions and Patient Teaching

The patient leaves the hospital or clinic shortly after surgery. An eyepatch is placed on the operative site until the next morning. Patients can be up and around at home. Because of visual limitations, patients will need assistance. If the patient experiences pain, the physician prescribes oral analgesics. The patient is photosensitive and may complain of blurred vision initially. The patient is seen the next day for physician follow-up. Postoperative physician checkups are scheduled at 1 week and then monthly for 1 year. A nursing diagnosis and interventions for the patient with myopia are the same as for astigmatism and strabismus errors.

Instruct the patient preoperatively to stop wearing hard contact lenses 1 to 2 days before the surgical evaluation. Encourage rest the first day postoperatively. Inform the patient to notify the patient if pain persists after the first day. Instruct the patient that infection is a rare complication of the procedure. Tell the patient that vision is assessed regularly to evaluate functional vision without corrective eyewear. Advise patients that postoperative visual acuity is not always 20/20 without glasses. The goals of operative interventions are improving the patient's performance of ADLs and allowing him or her to drive a vehicle without glasses during the day. As a result of a slightly dilated pupil, the patient may experience a glare or halos from lights, which may require wearing glasses for night driving.

Hyperopia

Hyperopia is included in Table 53-3.

Diagnostic Tests

Common tests used in the diagnosis of hyperopia include ophthalmoscopy, retinoscopy, visual acuity tests, and refraction tests.

Medical Management

The main treatment for farsightedness is corrective eyewear, either contact lenses or glasses. A variety of lenses are available on the market, including hard, soft, and gas-permeable lenses.

Nursing Interventions and Patient Teaching

Emphasize the importance of proper care of contact lenses (see Health Promotion box). Eyeglasses should properly fit the bridge of the nose to eliminate slippage and an uneven level of each lens.

 Health Promotion

Contact Lens Care

DO

- Wash and rinse hands thoroughly before handling a lens.
- Keep fingernails clean.
- Remove lenses from their storage case one at a time and place on the eye.
- Start with the same lens (left or right) at each insertion.
- Use lens-placement technique learned from eye specialist.
- Use proper lens care products and clean the lenses as directed by the manufacturer.
- Keep the lens storage kit clean.
- Wear lenses daily and follow the prescribed wearing schedule.
- Remove a lens if it becomes uncomfortable.
- Avoid potential corneal abrasions.
- Report any signs of photophobia, dryness, excessive burning, or tearing.
- Keep regular appointments with the eye specialist.
- Remove lenses during sunbathing, showering, or swimming.

DO NOT

- Use soaps that contain cream or perfume for cleansing lenses.
- Let fingernails touch lenses.
- Mix up lenses.
- Exceed prescribed wearing time.
- Use saliva to wet lenses.
- Use homemade saline solution or tap water to wet or clean lenses.
- Borrow or mix lens care solutions.

A nursing diagnosis and interventions for the patient with hyperopia include but are not limited to the following:

Nursing Diagnosis	Nursing Interventions
Deficient knowledge, related to lack of experience with corrective eyewear	Answer all questions the patient may have on eyewear maintenance. Obtain literature on lens care. Encourage physician follow-up as directed.

INFLAMMATORY AND INFECTIOUS DISORDERS OF THE EYE

Hordeolum, Chalazion, and Blepharitis

The most common infections and inflammatory disorders of the lid are listed in Table 53-4.

Diagnostic Tests

The eyelid margin is examined. Culture and sensitivity tests of any drainage may be ordered. Visual disturbances are also noted.

Medical Management

The physician prescribes antiinfective agents and may perform localized incision and drainage of a cyst or stye with the patient under local anesthesia. Warm normal saline compresses are ordered for 10 to 20 min-

Table 53-4 Common Infections and Inflammatory Disorders of the Lid

DESCRIPTION	ETIOLOGY AND PATHOPHYSIOLOGY	CLINICAL MANIFESTATIONS	ASSESSMENT
Hordeolum (stye)			
Acute infection of eyelid margin or sebaceous glands of the eyelashes	Frequently caused by the *Staphylococcus* organism One or more pustules may form	Abscess localized to base of eyelashes, with edema of lid	**Subjective data:** Localized tenderness and pain resulting from edema; pain diminished after pustule ruptures **Objective data:** Raised, erythematous area on eyelid; pustule exudate
Chalazion			
Inflammatory cyst on the meibomian gland at the eyelid margin; may require weeks to develop into a cyst	May be caused by infection; associated with diabetes mellitus, gout, and anemia	Discomfort, mass on eyelid, edema, visual disturbance	**Subjective data:** Pressure felt as eyelid closes over cornea; patient may describe vision changes **Objective data:** Cyst formation; eyelid edema
Blepharitis			
Inflammation of eyelid margins	Ulcerative: Caused by bacterial infection, usually staphylococcal organisms Nonulcerative: Caused by psoriasis, seborrhea, or allergic response	Pruritus, erythema of eyelid, eyelid pain, photophobia Excessive tearing	**Subjective data:** Eye pruritus; lids adhere together during sleep **Objective data:** Eyes erythematous; patient rubs eyes; sensitivity to light; tear spillage

utes two to four times a day. Lid scrubs using no-tear baby shampoo may be ordered.

Nursing Interventions and Patient Teaching

A primary objective of nursing care for the patient with an infectious or inflammatory process of the lids is prevention of the spread of infection. Take care when applying compresses. Hand hygiene is essential before contact with the eye.

Provide instructions on the use of prescribed drops or ointments. Teach the patient about the use of warm compresses and specific hygiene practices, such as keeping hands clean and away from the eyes and replacing mascara after 3 to 6 months because the oils decompose and may harbor bacteria. Caution the patient to avoid irritating fumes or smoke, which may cause rubbing of the eyes, leading to further infection. Discourage the use of eye makeup until all inflammation subsides.

Prognosis

In the majority of patients the inflammatory and infectious phases of these conditions respond favorably to topical antimicrobials. Incision and drainage of cystlike formations result in minimal complications and risk to the patient.

Inflammation of the Conjunctiva

Etiology and Pathophysiology

Conjunctivitis is an inflammation of the conjunctiva caused by bacterial or viral infection, allergy, or environmental factors. It is commonly called **pinkeye.** Although this typically occurs initially in one eye, it spreads rapidly to the unaffected eye.

Acute bacterial conjunctivitis is usually transmitted by the hands after direct contact with a contaminated object. Pneumococcal, staphylococcal, streptococcal, *Haemophilus influenzae,* gonococcal, and chlamydial organisms are the major causative agents. Because of its warmth, moisture, and extensive vascularization, the eye provides the bacteria with an excellent medium for multiplication. Conjunctivitis represents about two thirds of the 1 million cases per year of eye inflammation and infection. The disease is usually self-limiting, leaving no permanent impairment.

Viruses of the respiratory or intestinal tract may result in a secondary infection of the eye. The two most common viral agents are *Chlamydia trachomatis* and type 1 herpes simplex virus (HSV). Trachoma, a highly contagious form of conjunctivitis, is caused by a strain of the *C. trachomatis* virus. Transmission is by direct contact with an ocular discharge. It is rare in the United States but is a major cause of blindness in Asia and in Mediterranean countries.

Clinical Manifestations

Contamination leads to an inflammatory process that produces erythema of the conjunctiva, edema of the lid, and a mucopurulent crusting discharge on the lids and cornea. If untreated, this infection leaves the eyelid scarred with granulations that invade the cornea, resulting in loss of vision.

Assessment

Collection of **subjective data** requires an awareness that, during allergy seasons and exposure to environmental irritants, the patient may report pruritus, burning, and excessive tearing.

Collection of **objective data** includes observing eyes that are erythematous with edema of the lid. Also look for dried exudate.

Diagnostic Tests

The conjunctiva is scraped for bacteria and stained for microscopic examination.

Medical Management

Medical treatment is similar to that for blepharitis.

Nursing Interventions and Patient Teaching

The lid and lashes are cleansed of exudate with normal saline. Warm compresses are applied two to four times a day. When allergies are present, cold saline compresses may be ordered for control of edema and pruritus. Eye irrigations with normal saline or lactated Ringer's solution may be prescribed to remove secretions. Administer topical antibiotics and adrenocortical steroid medications. Eye pads are contraindicated because they enhance bacterial growth.

A nursing diagnosis and interventions for the patient with conjunctivitis include but are not limited to the following:

Nursing Diagnosis	Nursing Interventions
Pain, related to pruritus, secondary to inflammatory process	Apply warm or cold compresses. Administer prescribed eye medications; ensure proper instillation of eyedrops and ointments; administer eye irrigation as prescribed. Administer analgesics as ordered. Assess patient's limitations in visual perception. Implement safety measures as appropriate.

Instruct the patient and the family to avoid contact with the eyes or soiled materials when an infection is present. Individual washcloths and towels are to be used. Tell the patient to wash hands if contact is made with the eyes and before any treatments. Also teach the patient to perform and describe treatments such as irrigations, compresses, and medication administration. The patient should avoid noxious fumes or smoke and should not wear contact lenses during the suppuration period.

Prognosis

Conjunctivitis responds successfully to topical antimicrobials. Patient teaching reduces the risk of continued exposure and reinfection. Although highly contagious, the disease is self-limiting, leaving no chance of permanent visual impairment unless a chronic condition develops.

INFLAMMATION OF THE CORNEA

Etiology and Pathophysiology

Keratitis, an inflammation of the cornea, may result from injury; irritants; allergies; viral infection; or diseases such as congenital syphilis, smallpox, and some nervous disorders. It may be superficial and involve the epithelial layer only or may invade the subepithelial layer and the endothelial membrane. The layers of the eye are innervated, and thus inflammation causes acute pain. Ulcers may form in the eye membrane layers, resulting in scattered scarring of the corneal surface.

Pneumococcal, staphylococcal, streptococcal, and pseudomonal organisms are the most common bacterial causes of keratitis. The viral agent most often responsible for corneal inflammation is HSV. HSV keratitis is a growing problem, especially in immunocompromised patients. Keratitis can be triggered by stress, illness, and exposure to UV light. The condition may be associated with the use of ophthalmologic steroid medications. Overuse or abuse of topical steroids may injure epithelial cells.

Another form of keratitis is acanthamoebic keratitis. The *Acanthamoeba* organism is found in the soil, airborne dust, fresh water, and the noses and throats of healthy humans. This organism is often resistant to antimicrobial agents. Contact lens wearers are more susceptible because traditional cleaning agents for lenses include rinsing with clean or distilled water. People who swim frequently are at greater risk because the organism is not killed by usual methods of disinfection, such as chlorine.

Clinical Manifestations

Severe eye pain is the most common symptom that differentiates this disease from other eye inflammatory diseases. If uncontrolled, keratitis may result in blepharospasms and vision loss. Other symptoms include photophobia, tearing, edema, and visual disturbances.

Assessment

Subjective data include the severity and duration of the pain, the extent of light sensitivity, and any vision loss.

Collection of **objective data** includes assessing the patient for facial grimacing, lacrimation, and photophobia.

Diagnostic Tests

Depending on the causative agent, a variety of diagnostic tests may be ordered, including culture and sensitivity tests, fluorescein staining, and Gram staining. Ophthalmoscopic examination is also performed.

Medical Management

Medical management includes topical antibiotic therapy. Systemic antibiotics may be prescribed for severe cases. Cycloplegic-mydriatic drugs paralyze the ocular muscles of accommodation and dilate the pupil. For viral keratitis, therapy includes corneal debridement followed by topical therapy with vidarabine (Vira-A) or trifluridine (Viroptic) for 2 to 3 weeks. Corticosteroids are contraindicated because they contribute to a longer course, possible deeper ulceration of the cornea, and systemic complications. Drug therapy may also include acyclovir (Zovirax). Analgesics are used to control pain associated with acute inflammation. Pressure dressings may be ordered to relax the eye muscle and decrease discomfort. These dressings are often applied to both eyes because the eyes move together. Warm or cold compresses two to four times daily are prescribed for symptomatic relief. Epithelial debridement of loose tissue may be performed. Surgical management involves a corneal transplant, known as **keratoplasty.**

Nursing Interventions and Patient Teaching

Nursing interventions for keratitis include control of pain, safety, and prevention of complications. Nursing diagnoses and interventions for the patient with keratitis are the same for conjunctivitis. Provide information on self-care of a corneal abrasion. Also teach the patient to wash hands before instilling medication and to prevent infection by not rubbing the eyes. Instruct the patient to note any change in discharge or increase in pain and to notify the physician immediately.

Prognosis

Topical antibiotic, antiviral, or antifungal eyedrops, when begun promptly after diagnosis by culture, result in rapid healing and minimal visual impairment. Chronic keratitis may develop if treatment is delayed. Infection of the cornea can produce corneal ulcer and vision loss as a result of opaque scarring. Keratoplasty may then be indicated.

NONINFECTIOUS DISORDERS OF THE EYE

DRY EYE DISORDERS

Complaints of dry eye, caused by a variety of ocular disorders, are characterized by decreased tear secretion or increased tear film evaporation. Keratoconjunctivitis sicca (dry eyes) is caused by lacrimal gland dysfunction from an autoimmune mechanism. If the patient with keratoconjunctivitis sicca has associated dry mouth, the patient may have primary Sjögren syndrome (an immunologic disorder characterized by deficient fluid production by the lacrimal, salivary, and other glands, resulting in abnormal dryness of the mouth, eyes, and other mucous membranes) (*Mosby's Dictionary of Medicine, Nursing, and Health Professions, 2009*). If the patient has associated rheumatoid arthritis, scleroderma, or systemic lupus erythematosus, the patient has secondary Sjögren syndrome. The patient complains of a sandy or gritty sensation that typically worsens during the day and is better in the morning after eye closure with sleep. Treatment is directed at the underlying cause (Lewis et al., 2007).

Diagnostic Tests

The definitive test for dry eye, a noninfectious disorder of the lacrimal gland, is **Schirmer's test** (see Table 53-2). Normal results are 10 to 15 mm of wet paper.

Medical Management

Medical management for dry eye includes artificial tears replacement. Many nonprescription products are available. They should be used sparingly because preservatives in the drops or overuse can cause further irritation. Punctal plugs (temporary or permanent) may be inserted to close the tear ducts and keep the tears in the eyes longer.

If possible, limit medications that may cause dry eye as a side effect. If an infection accompanies the dry-eye syndrome, antibiotic therapy will be prescribed. Eliminate as many environmental irritants as possible. Filtering machines are available to control pollen and dust levels in the environment. If contact lenses cause local irritation and dry eye, a change in the prescription or type of lens is advised.

Surgical repair of an injured punctal sac by correctly aligning the eyelid margin or by probing an obstructed punctum (opening to the tear duct) to allow for tear reabsorption is the advised method of treatment.

Results of the fluorescein staining test for excessive tear disorder are considered normal if the dye disappears from the lacrimal cul-de-sac within 1 minute.

Nursing Interventions and Patient Teaching

The appropriate nursing diagnosis is *pain*, related to lack of natural eye moisture. Interventions are similar to those for conjunctivitis. Instruct the patient on instilling eye medications, practicing appropriate hygiene, and avoiding irritants.

Prognosis

Eyedrops alleviate the majority of symptoms caused by dry eye. Long-term use of artificial tears results in no adverse reactions. Control of medical conditions minimizes discomfort and complications. Surgical repair of the punctal sac is a safe procedure and has a good prognosis.

ECTROPION AND ENTROPION

Etiology and Pathophysiology

Ectropion and entropion are two noninfectious disorders of the lid causing an abnormal turning of the eyelid margins.

Ectropion is the outward turning of the eyelid margin. In the older patient it is common for the orbicularis oculi muscle to be relaxed. Paralytic ectropion occurs when orbicularis muscle function is disturbed, as with Bell's palsy. Other causes of ectropion are eyelid laceration and burns of the conjunctival tissue.

Entropion is an inward turning of the eyelid. The lower eyelid margin is the most frequently involved. The conjunctival membrane lining the eyelid and part of the eyeball are exposed. Entropion is caused by atrophy of the eyelid tissue, spasms of the orbicularis oculi muscle, or scarring of the tarsal plate (dense connective tissue that stiffens the eyelid) caused by congenital condition or trauma. Varying degrees of atonia commonly exist in the older adult orbicularis.

Clinical Manifestations

Ectropion and entropion are characterized by abnormal direction of the eyelid with tear spillage and corneal dryness.

Assessment

Collection of **subjective data** includes noting the degree of vision loss and determining tear loss and dryness of the cornea.

Collection of **objective data** includes observing the extent to which the patient can perform ADLs and the presence of any eyelid margin inflammation.

Diagnostic Tests

The physician diagnoses these conditions through a visual and ophthalmologic examination.

Medical Management

Medical intervention consists of topical medications to reduce conjunctival and corneal inflammation or drying. Surgery is the preferred treatment. Resection of the tarsal plate, removal of the scarred tissue, or tightening of the orbicularis oculi muscle is the choice for permanent repair.

Nursing Interventions

Interventions for ectropion and entropion involve monitoring the medical treatment and reporting its progress. A nursing diagnosis for the patient with ectropion or entropion is *disturbed sensory perception*, related to edema and exudate. Interventions include assistance in self-care activities, safety measures, observation for infection and inflammation, and medication and dressing treatments as prescribed.

Prognosis

Early diagnosis and treatment of eyelid disorders reduces the risk of conjunctival and corneal inflammation and scarring. Monitoring treatment reduces the need for surgical intervention and minimizes visual disturbances.

DISORDERS OF THE LENS

Cataracts

Etiology and Pathophysiology

A cataract is a crystalline opacity or clouding of the lens. The patient may have a cataract in one or both eyes. If they are present in both eyes, one cataract may affect vision more than the other. The lens is normally clear and transparent. As a person ages, opacification of the lens gradually occurs. About 50% of Americans between 65 and 74 years old have some degree of cataract formation. After 75 years of age, the statistic rises to about 70% of Americans. For Americans older than 65 years, cataract removal is the most common surgical procedure. When a cataract develops, the lens becomes foggy and vision decreases. If a large enough portion of the lens becomes opaque, light cannot reach the retina.

Cataracts may be congenital (e.g., from exposure to maternal rubella) or acquired from systemic disease, trauma, toxins (e.g., radiation or UV light exposure, certain drugs such as systemic corticosteroids or long-term topical corticosteroids), and intraocular inflammation. Most cataracts are age related (senile cataracts). The patient with diabetes mellitus tends to develop cataracts at a younger age than does the patient without diabetes. Smoking has been linked with the development of cataracts. Cataract development is mediated by a number of factors. In senile cataract formation, it appears that altered metabolic processes within the lens cause an accumulation of water and alterations in the fiber structure. These changes affect lens transparency, causing vision changes.

Clinical Manifestations

Cataract symptoms are painless, but include blurred vision, difficulty reading fine print, diplopia, photosensitivity, glare, abnormal color perception, and difficulty driving at night. Glare is due to light scatter caused by the lens opacities, and it may be significantly worse at night when the pupil dilates. The visual decline is gradual, but the rate of cataract development varies from patient to patient. The opacity can be seen in the center of the lens (Figure 53-6).

Assessment

Subjective data include blurred vision, often the first symptom to be expressed by the patient. Note any subjective complaints, such as "hazy" or "fuzzy" vision or abnormal color perception.

Collection of **objective data** involves observing the patient for difficulty in reading, such as noting whether the patient brings a newspaper close to the eyes. Also note sensitivity to light.

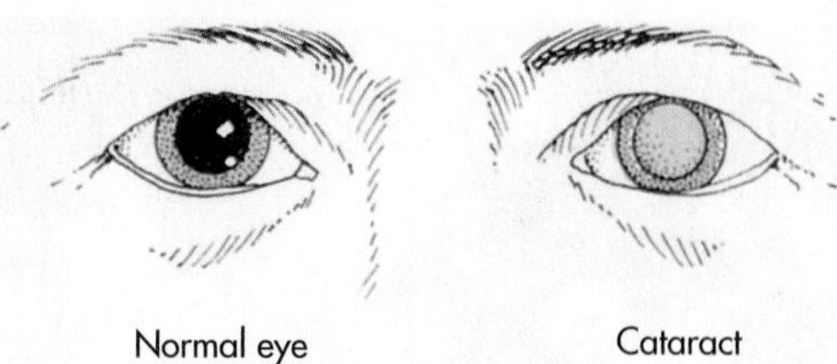

FIGURE 53-6 Cataract, visible in the left eye as white opacity of the lens, is seen through the pupil.

Diagnostic Tests

Diagnosis is based on decreased visual acuity or other complaints of visual dysfunction. The opacity is directly observable by ophthalmoscopic or slit-lamp microscopic examination. A totally opaque lens creates the appearance of a white pupil (see Figure 53-6).

Medical Management

Monitor the patient for changes in vision associated with increasing cataract size. For many patients the diagnosis is made long before they actually decide to have surgery. Often, changing the patient's eyewear prescription can improve the visual acuity, at least temporarily. If glare makes it difficult to drive at night, the patient can drive only during daylight hours and have a family member drive at night. When palliative measures no longer provide an acceptable level of visual function, the patient is an appropriate candidate for surgery. Surgery is the only definitive method of treatment and can be performed at any age. It can be done using a local, topical, or general anesthesia.

There are two methods of surgery: intracapsular and extracapsular extraction. Intracapsular surgery involves removing the lens and its entire capsule. Although some surgeons still perform intracapsular extraction (and it may be necessary in instances of trauma), the intracapsular technique has been largely replaced by extracapsular extraction. In the extracapsular method, the anterior capsule is opened and the lens nucleus and cortex are removed, leaving the remainder capsular bag intact. Healing is rapid with this method.

Phacoemulsification is the most common type of extracapsular cataract extraction (Figure 53-7). This technique uses ultrasound to break up and remove the cataract through a small incision, thereby reducing the healing time and decreasing the chance of complications.

During surgery the physician implants a synthetic (not from a human donor) intraocular lens in the posterior chamber behind the iris. At the end of the procedure, the patient receives injections of subconjunctival corticosteroid and antibiotic medications. Then an antibiotic and corticosteroid ointment is applied

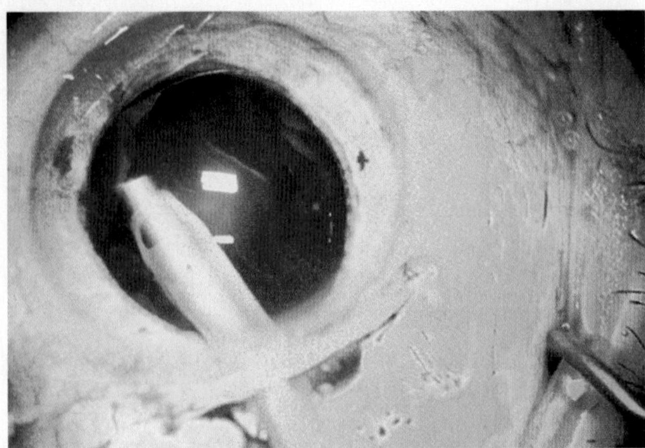

FIGURE 53-7 Phacoemulsification of a cataractous lens through a self-sealing, scleral-tunnel incision. Note the circular opening in the anterior lens capsule.

and the patient's eye is covered with a patch and protective shield. The patch is usually worn overnight and removed during the first postoperative visit. The patient receives a prescription for glasses after the eye is fully recovered (about 6 to 8 weeks postoperatively). Most of the postoperative refractive error is corrected with the intraocular lens, but the patient also needs corrective eyewear for near vision and for residual refractive error (Leyland & Zinicola, 2005). Special contact lenses provide the patient many options for comfort.

Nursing Interventions and Patient Teaching

Preoperative and postoperative nursing care is a primary nursing responsibility (Nursing Care Plan 53-1). Cataract symptoms usually develop slowly and can easily be detected. Encourage patients to have annual examinations, especially if they are age 40 or older. Surgery provides about a 90% success rate of acceptable levels of vision. Unless complications occur, the patient is usually ready to go home within a few hours after the surgery, as soon as the effects of sedative agents have worn off. Postoperative medications usually include antibiotic and corticosteroid drops to prevent infection and decrease the postoperative inflammatory response. Some evidence indicates that postoperative activity restrictions and nighttime eye shielding are unnecessary (American Society of Opthalmic Registered Nurses, 2004). However, many ophthalmologists still instruct the patient to avoid activities that increase IOP, such as bending, stooping, coughing, or lifting. Ophthalmologists may also recommend using an eyeshield over the operative eye at night for protection. Discuss safety measures appropriate to vision alterations, and instruct the patient to notify the physician of any complications such as pain, erythema, drainage, or sudden visual changes. If sudden pain occurs, call the physician (see Communication box and Patient Teaching box).

Prognosis

Gradual loss of lens transparency increases the risk of injury because of vision loss. Carefully monitor patients for degeneration of the lens. The condition may be accompanied by secondary glaucoma, which further reduces visual acuity. Surgical intervention is advised to improve vision. Postoperative complications of cataract surgery are uncommon, but may include infection, hemorrhage, or increased IOP (Lewis et al., 2007). Complications may recur years after cataract surgery and should be reported to the ophthalmologist.

DISORDERS OF THE RETINA

Diabetic Retinopathy

Etiology and Pathophysiology

Diabetic retinopathy is a disorder of retinal blood vessels characterized by capillary microaneurysms, hemorrhage, exudates, and the formation of new vessels and connective tissue. After 15 years with diabetes mellitus, nearly all patients with type 1 and 80% with type 2 have some degree of retinal disease accompanied by nephropathy. The incidence increases in relationship to how long the patient has the disease. The disorder occurs more frequently in patients with longstanding, poorly controlled diabetes mellitus (see Cultural Considerations box).

The initial stage of diabetic retinopathy may last several years. The earliest and most treatable stages often produce no changes in vision. Because of this, the patient with diabetes must have regular dilated eye examinations by an ophthalmologist or specially trained optometrist for early detection and treatment. The blood vessels in the retina begin to widen and become tortuous. Microaneurysms then develop at the periphery, and small hemorrhages develop. These may disappear, but they leave in their place scars that can decrease vision. Increased capillary permeability causes protein exudate.

Cultural Considerations

Hearing and Visual Problems

- Whites have a higher incidence of hearing impairment than blacks or Asian Americans.
- Incidence and severity of glaucoma are greater among blacks than among whites.
- Hispanics have an increased incidence of diabetic retinopathy.
- Native Americans have an increased incidence of otitis media when compared with whites.
- Whites have a higher incidence of macular degeneration than Hispanics, blacks, and Asian Americans.
- Eskimos are susceptible to primary closed-angle glaucoma, resulting from a thicker lens and a shallow chamber angle.
- Native Americans and blacks have a higher incidence of astigmatism than whites.

 Nursing Care Plan **53-1** **The Patient with Cataracts**

Ms. Jakobi is an 82-year-old who lives alone. She has developed bilateral cataracts and is admitted to same-day surgery for right cataract extracapsular procedure with intraocular lens implantation.

NURSING DIAGNOSIS *Risk for injury, related to altered visual acuity*

Patient Goals and Expected Outcomes	Nursing Interventions	Evaluation
Patient will not have any evidence of injury Patient will have a safe environment in which she will avoid injury	**PREOPERATIVE** Instill eyedrops as prescribed wearing clean latex or vinyl gloves. Administer preoperative medications or sedatives as ordered. Explain postoperative procedures to expect, such as patches and eyedrops. **POSTOPERATIVE** Instill mydriatic-cycloplegic and corticosteroid eyedrops as prescribed while wearing clean latex or vinyl gloves. Instruct patient to avoid moving head suddenly, heavy lifting, bending over, coughing, sneezing, vomiting, and straining with elimination, which cause increased intraocular pressure. Maintain prescribed eyepatch or shield in position during specified hours. Instruct patient to avoid lying on the side of the affected eye on the night after surgery. Remove environmental barriers to ensure safety. Keep side rails up at all times. Plan all care with patient: Explain routines of what will happen and when. Visit frequently and announce yourself on entering room. Assist with deep-breathing exercises every 1 to 2 hours while awake. Check with physician for any special positioning or precautions. (If turned, position patient on the unaffected side.) Elevate head of bed 30 degrees as ordered. Assist with and teach active and passive range-of-motion exercises every 4 hours. Provide increased activities and ambulation as ordered; assist as needed. Teach self-care activities, and assist as needed. Instruct family to remove unnecessary furniture and pick up objects that may be blocking pathways. Instruct patient that cataract surgery does not correct nearsightedness or farsightedness. Corrective lenses are still needed for these problems after surgery.	Patient feels secure about upcoming surgery. Patient uses measures to control complications from surgery.

NURSING DIAGNOSIS *Anxiety/fear, related to visual impairment*

Patient Goals and Expected Outcomes	Nursing Intervention	Evaluation
Patient will experience less anxiety and fear	Observe level of patient and family anxiety. Note patient's coping mechanism related to vision loss. Encourage patient and family to vent feelings and concerns. Support patient and family's positive actions toward adapting to visual limitations.	Patient and family display trust and security after venting feelings.

Critical Thinking Questions

1. Ms. Jakobi puts her call light on and tells the nurse that she has severe pain and pressure in her right eye. What should be the initial response by the nurse?
2. What should be included in Ms. Jakobi's discharge planning to minimize the risk of injury to her operative eye?
3. In visiting with Ms. Jakobi, the nurse finds that she enjoys embroidery and knitting. Ms. Jakobi states that she is looking forward to resuming her handiwork. What should be included as appropriate patient teaching?

Communication

Nursing-Patient Dialogue Regarding Postoperative Eye Surgery

Mrs. Betta, age 71, has been experiencing decreasing vision for the past 5 years. She seeks medical attention and is told that surgery is required to correct her condition. While talking to the patient, the nurse senses her reluctance to comply with postoperative treatment.

Patient: I'm too old to go through all the routines that the doctor wants me to. It involves too much.

Nurse: I know that surgery is a concern for you. You must have many emotions right now. It's understandable that you have concerns about your recovery.

Patient: There's so much to think about and remember.

Nurse: The doctor and our staff are here to help make your recovery as easy as possible for you. Tell me what bothers you the most.

Patient: What if I go home and fall? I could reinjure my eye or break something, like my hip.

Nurse: There are several things that you and your family can do to prevent any injury to yourself. The doctor and staff will explain these things very carefully to you.

Patient: I'm afraid I'm too old to learn.

Patient Teaching

After Eye Surgery

- Teach patient and family proper hygiene and eye care techniques to ensure that medications, dressings, and surgical wound are not contaminated during necessary eye care.
- Teach patient and family about signs and symptoms of infection and when and how to report those to allow early recognition and treatment.
- Instruct patient to comply with postoperative restrictions on head positioning, bending, coughing, and Valsalva's maneuver to optimize visual outcomes and prevent increased intraocular pressure.
- Instruct patient to instill eye medications using aseptic techniques and to comply with prescribed eye medication routine to prevent infection.
- Instruct patient to monitor pain and take prescribed medication for pain as directed and to report pain not relieved by prescribed medications.
- Stress the importance of continued follow-up as recommended to maximize potential visual outcomes.

From Lewis, S.L., et al. (2007). *Medical-surgical nursing: Assessment and management of clinical problems.* (7th ed.). St. Louis: Mosby.

As the disease progresses, new blood vessels form on the retina and into the vitreous. These new vessels rupture, causing decreased vision. Some of the blood may be absorbed, which improves vision until another hemorrhage occurs. Significant vision loss eventually occurs as these hemorrhages continue. Vitreous contraction and full detachment can occur as the vessels and surrounding tissue become fibrous.

Clinical Manifestations

Symptoms include microaneurysms, which can only be identified by ophthalmoscopy in the initial stage. In the advanced stages the patient has progressive vision loss and the presence of "floaters," which are minute products of the hemorrhage.

Assessment

Collection of **subjective data** includes assessment of the duration and control of diabetes mellitus. The patient has varying degrees of vision loss, from decreased vision to blindness. Assess the patient's knowledge of therapy.

Collection of **objective data** involves noting that in the early stages there are no symptoms; as the disease progresses, vision is diminished.

Diagnostic Tests

Indirect ophthalmoscopy shows dilated and tortuous vessels and narrowing or obliteration of the arteries. Opacities, hemorrhages, and microaneurysms can be seen. Slit-lamp examination magnifies the lesions.

Medical Management

Surgical intervention includes early photocoagulation, cryotherapy (cryopexy) and/or vitrectomy (see pp. 1866-1867). Photocoagulation uses a laser beam to destroy new blood vessels, seal leaking vessels, and help prevent retinal edema. A vitrectomy or cryotherapy may be performed when photocoagulation is not possible. A topical anesthetic is used in cryotherapy so that a cryoprobe can be placed directly on the surface of the eye. When the probe is properly located, its tip creates a frozen area that extends through the external tissue, then through the eyeball until it reaches a specific point on the retina. Multiple points on the retina can be treated in this way (Lewis et al., 2007).

Nursing Interventions and Patient Teaching

A nursing diagnosis and interventions for the patient with diabetic retinopathy include but are not limited to the following:

Nursing Diagnosis	Nursing Interventions
Fear, related to unfamiliarity with procedure	Determine patient's knowledge of purpose and procedures of photocoagulation, cryotherapy, or vitrectomy.

Home care after surgery for the patient with diabetic retinopathy is the same as for any eye surgery.

Prognosis

The best treatment of diabetic retinopathy is early detection. Frequent eye examinations reduce the complication of vision loss, and modern laser technology is highly effective in reducing further damage to the retina and improving vision.

Age-Related Macular Degeneration

Etiology and Pathophysiology

Age-related macular degeneration (ARMD) of the aging retina is characterized by slow, progressive loss of central and near vision. ARMD is the most common cause of vision loss in people older than 60. A gene responsible for some cases of ARMD has been recently identified. Family history is a major risk factor. Additional risk factors are long-term exposure to UV light, hyperopia, cigarette smoking, and light-colored eyes (Johns Hopkins University, 2004). Nutrition may play a role in the progression of ARMD. The Age-Related Eye Disease Study (AREDS) revealed a dietary supplement of vitamin C, vitamin E, beta-carotene, and zinc slowed the development of advancing ARMD; however, it did not seem to have any effect on people with minimal ARMD or those with no ARMD (National Eye Institute [NEI], National Institutes of Health [NIH], 2008). Studies also indicate that consuming large amounts of dark green, leafy vegetables containing lutein (e.g., spinach, kale) may decrease the risk of developing ARMD (Lewis et al., 2007).

There are two types of macular degeneration. The first, called the **wet type** (also called neovascular macular degeneration), has sudden new vessel growth in the macular region. The macula becomes displaced, and scarring occurs. Because scarred cells no longer register light, vision loss is irreversible. Wet macular degeneration accounts for 10% of cases.

The second, known as the **dry type** (also called nonexudative or nonneovascular macular degeneration), occurs in 90% of cases of macular degeneration. Degenerative changes are the cause. Lipid deposits are followed by slow atrophy of the macular region, including the retina. People with dry ARMD notice that reading and other close-vision tasks become more difficult. In this form the macular cells have wasted or atrophied and simply do not function as well as previously. Patients report that "sometimes I see the image and sometimes it sort of blinks at me, like I have a short circuit."

Clinical Manifestations

The hallmark sign of ARMD is the appearance of drusen in the fundus found on ophthalmoscopic evaluation. Drusen appear as yellowish exudates beneath the retinal pigment of epithelium and represent localized or diffuse deposits of extracellular debris. The main symptom of macular degeneration is gradual and variable bilateral loss of **central vision.** One eye may have a greater loss than the other. Color perception may also be affected.

Assessment

Collection of **subjective data** includes noting that the patient may have difficulty distinguishing colors correctly. Assess for visual disturbances and coping mechanisms for the loss. Macular degeneration develops differently in each person, so the symptoms may vary. However, some of the most common symptoms include (1) a gradual loss of ability to see objects clearly; (2) distorted vision, with objects appearing to be the wrong size or shape or straight lines appearing wavy or crooked; (3) gradual loss of clear color vision; (4) scotomas (blind spots in the visual field); and (5) a dark or empty area appearing in the center of vision.

Collection of **objective data** includes noting the degree to which the patient can centrally view objects.

Diagnostic Tests

Ophthalmoscopy is used to detect opacity, hemorrhage, and new blood vessel formation. The examiner looks for retinal detachment, drusen, and other fundus changes associated with ARMD, and any other abnormalities. Using Amsler's grid test may help define the involved areas (see Table 53-2).

Medical Management

Previously, the treatment for wet ARMD was a laser macular photocoagulation to destroy abnormal blood vessels. Unfortunately, the laser beam also destroyed photoreceptor cells and retinal pigment epithelium, leaving a blind spot from the scarred area in the retina (Lewis et al., 2007). Photodynamic therapy is a new treatment for wet ARMD. This treatment uses intravenous verteporfin (Visudyne) and a "cold" laser. Verteporfin becomes active when exposed to the "cold" laser light wave. This procedure causes deconstruction of abnormal blood vessels but does not cause permanent damage to the retinal pigment epithelium and photoreceptor cells. The specific guidelines when this can be used by patients with wet ARMD are very strict and only about 10% of patients are eligible for treatment (Lewis et al., 2007). Caution patients to avoid direct exposure to sunlight and other intense forms of light for 5 days after treatment (Lewis et al., 2007). There is no treatment for the dry type.

Unfortunately, central vision damaged by macular degeneration cannot be restored. However, since macular degeneration does not damage peripheral vision, low vision aids such as telescopic and microscopic special lenses, magnifying glasses, and electronic magnifiers for close work can be prescribed to help make the most of remaining vision. Often people, with adaptation, can cope well and continue to do most things they were accustomed to doing. **High-dose nutritional supplements** of zinc, beta-carotene, and vitamins C and E have been shown to reduce the risk of progression to advanced ARMD by 25% (NEI, NIH, 2008). A diet rich in fruits and dark green leafy vegetables is also recommended (NEI, NIH, 2008).

Nursing Interventions and Patient Teaching

The patient needs patience and understanding to cope with the continuing loss of sight. Help the patient through the process of accepting loss of sight. Maintaining safety is important because only peripheral vision exists.

A nursing diagnosis and interventions for the patient with macular degeneration include but are not limited to the following:

Nursing Diagnosis	Nursing Interventions
Disturbed sensory perception (visual), related to disease process	Note the extent of visual loss and the level of difficulty with ADLs; assist the patient in developing ways of performing these activities. Determine the patient's support systems and elicit help if available.

Instruct the patient about the disease process, stressing that peripheral vision will be maintained. Provide ways for the patient to maintain as much independence as possible, and help family and friends determine the areas in which to assist.

Prognosis

Early diagnosis of macular degeneration is critical to prevent blindness. Watchful waiting is the only approach to dry macular degeneration. Ophthalmic laser surgery is of limited benefit because of the gradual and progressive course of the disorder. Photocoagulation is preventive, not curative.

Retinal Detachment

Etiology and Pathophysiology

Retinal detachment is a separation of the retina from the choroid in the posterior area of the eye (Figure 53-8). This usually results from a hole in the retina that allows vitreous humor to leak between the choroid and the retina. The immediate cause may be severe trauma to the eye, such as a contusion or a penetrating wound. In most cases, however, retinal detachment is the result of internal changes related to aging and sometimes inflammation of the eye. Retinal detachment may also occur in debilitated patients when there is sudden severe physical exertion. As the detachment progresses, it interrupts the transmission of visual images from the retina to the optic nerve. The result is a progressive loss of vision to complete blindness.

Clinical Manifestations

Symptoms include a sudden or gradual development of flashes of light, followed by floating spots, a "cobweb," a "hairnet," and loss of a specific field of vision.

Assessment

Subjective data include patient complaints of flashing lights unilaterally and floaters. Progressive vision restriction occurs in one area. If the tear is acute and extensive, the patient describes a sensation like a curtain being drawn across the eye. Because the retina does not contain sensory nerves that relay sensations of pain, the condition is painless.

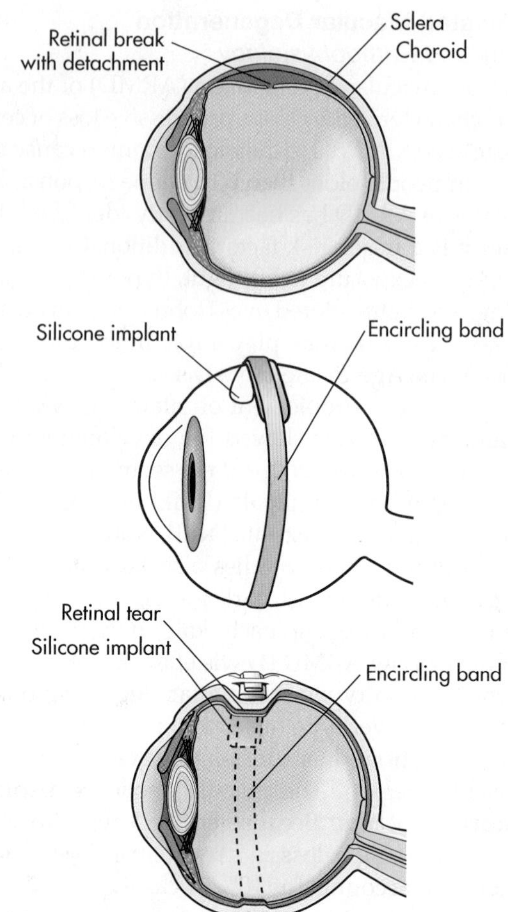

FIGURE 53-8 Retinal break with detachment: surgical repair by scleral buckling technique.

Collection of **objective data** includes observing the patient for the ability to perform ADLs. Also assess the level of anxiety associated with coping.

Diagnostic Tests

Visual acuity measurements should be the first diagnostic procedure with any complaint of vision loss. Indirect and direct ophthalmoscopy is used to detect pallor of the retina and the detachment. Three-mirror gonioscopy provides a magnified view of any retinal lesions. Slit-lamp examination magnifies the lesions. Ultrasound may be useful to identify a retinal detachment if the retina cannot be directly visualized (e.g., when the cornea, lens, or vitreous humor is hazy or opaque).

Medical Management

The treatment of choice is early corrective intervention. One of four procedures may be performed.

Laser photocoagulation burns localized tears or breaks in the posterior portion of the eyeball, eventually sealing the tear or break.

Cryotherapy freezes the borders of a retinal hole with a frozen-tipped probe. The probe is applied to the scleral surface directly over the retinal hole area. The hole seals when the resultant inflammatory process produces scarring.

ElectroDiathermy burns a retinal break using an ultrasonic probe. The probe is applied to the scleral surface directly over the retinal break. Sealing occurs from the resultant inflammatory and scarring process.

Scleral buckling is an extraocular surgical procedure that involves indenting the globe so the pigment epithelium, choroid, and sclera move toward the detached retina. This not only helps seal retinal breaks, but also helps relieve inward traction on the retina. The retinal surgeon sutures a silicone implant against the sclera, causing the sclera to buckle inward. The surgeon may place an encircling band over the implant if there are multiple retinal breaks, if the surgeon cannot locate suspected breaks, or if there is widespread inward traction on the retina (see Figure 53-8). If present, subretinal fluid may be drained by inserting a small-gauge needle to facilitate contact between the retina and the buckled sclera. Scleral buckling is usually accomplished with the patient under local anesthesia. The patient may be discharged on the first postoperative day, or scleral buckling surgery may be performed as an outpatient procedure.

Pneumatic retinopexy. Pneumatic (pertaining to air or gas) **retinopexy** is an intraocular procedure that involves the injection of a gas into the vitreous cavity to form a temporary bubble that closes retinal breaks and places pressure on the separated retinal layers. This bubble is temporary and is combined with treatments of laser photocoagulation or cryotherapy. For several weeks the patient must position the head in a forward position so the bubble is in contact with the retinal break (Lewis et al., 2007).

Nursing Interventions and Patient Teaching

Postprocedure management includes cycloplegic, mydriatic, and antiinfective eyedrops. Eyepatches are applied over only the operative eye or both eyes, providing the required rest of the eye for 1 or 2 days. Safety measures are essential because the eyes are patched.

Depending on the procedures, the position of the head postoperatively may vary. If air is injected into the vitreous, the head is positioned with the unaffected eye upward and the patient lying on the abdomen or sitting forward for 4 to 5 days.

Dark glasses are prescribed after removal of the eye patches to decrease the discomfort of **photophobia** (abnormal sensitivity to light).

A nursing diagnosis and interventions for the patient with retinal detachment include but are not limited to the following:

Nursing Diagnosis	Nursing Interventions
Anxiety, related to visual alterations	Allow the patient the opportunity to discuss feelings and fears about the possible loss of vision. Answer questions honestly and correct any misunderstandings. Explain the reasons for restrictions of activities and for procedures.

Discuss with the patient temporary restrictions of reaching, work, and activity (see Patient Teaching box).

Prognosis

Retinal detachment requires treatment. Reattachment is successful in 90% of cases; the degree of sight restoration depends on the extent and duration of separation. Maximum vision is achieved within 3 months after surgery. Unless replaced, a detached retina slowly dies after several years. Blindness from retinal detachment is irreversible.

GLAUCOMA

Etiology and Pathophysiology

Glaucoma is not one disease, but rather a group of disorders characterized by (1) increased intraocular pressure (IOP) because of obstruction of the outflow of aqueous humor, (2) optic nerve atrophy, and (3) progressive loss of peripheral vision (Figure 53-9). Glaucoma is found in people who are middle-age and older. Approximately 12% to 15% of all blindness in the United States results from glaucoma. One in 50 white people is affected. However, 1 in 10 blacks develops glaucoma. It is seldom seen in people younger than 35 years of age but may occur in infancy.

Open-angle glaucoma, also known as **primary open-angle glaucoma (POAG),** represents 90% of the cases of primary glaucoma. In POAG the outflow of aqueous humor is decreased in the trabecular meshwork. In essence, the drainage channels become occluded, like a clogged kitchen sink. The course of the disease is slowly progressive and results from degenerative changes. It is often bilateral.

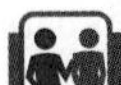 **Patient Teaching**

Retinal Detachment

- Return to sedentary activity in 2 weeks; no heavy lifting or active physical activity for 6 weeks, or as instructed by physician.
- Check with physician about shampooing hair.
- Limit reading for 3 weeks or as instructed by physician.
- Use correct technique for administration of eye medications.
- Report to ophthalmologist any signs of further detachment (flashes of light, increase in floaters, blurred vision).
- Report for medical follow-up visits as instructed.

Slowly rising intraocular pressure

Lens
Cornea
Anterior chamber
Iris
Trabecular meshwork
Canal of Schlemm
Congestion in trabecular meshwork reduces flow
A through canal of Schlemm
Flow of aqueous humor
Posterior chamber
Normal anterior chamber angle

Rapidly rising intraocular pressure

Trabecular meshwork
Canal of Schlemm
Trabecular meshwork and canal of Schlemm blocked, preventing outflow of aqueous humor
B
Closed anterior chamber angle

FIGURE 53-9 **A,** Primary open-angle glaucoma (POAG). Congestion in the trabecular meshwork reduces the outflow of aqueous humor. **B,** Acute angle-closure glaucoma (AACG). Angle between the iris and the anterior chamber narrows, obstructing the outflow of aqueous humor.

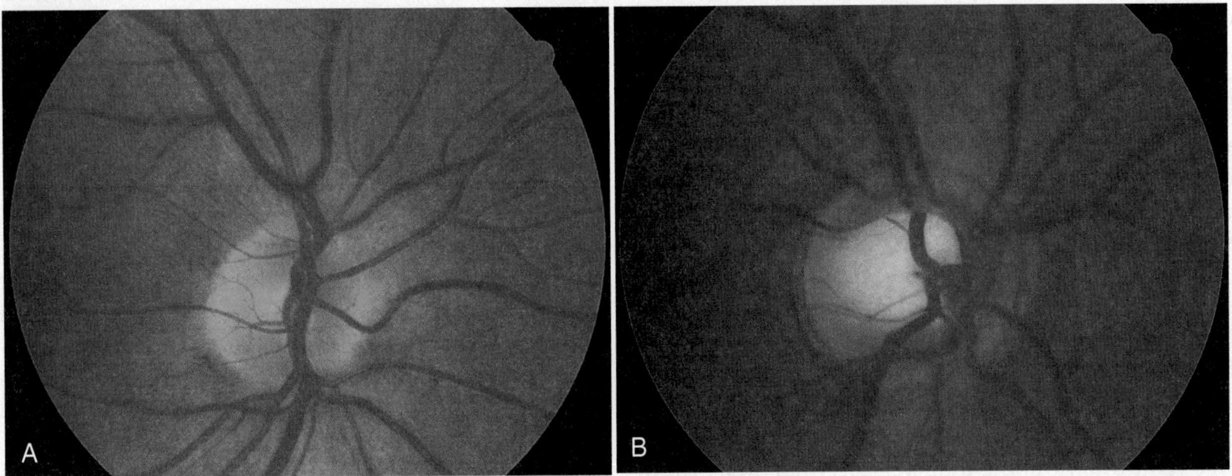

FIGURE 53-10 **A,** In the normal eye, the optic cup is pink with little cupping. **B,** In the glaucomatous eye, the optic disk is bleached and optic cupping is present. (Note the appearance of the retinal vessels, which travel over the edge of the optic cup and appear to dip into it.)

Closed-angle glaucoma, also known as **acute angle-closure glaucoma (AACG),** occurs if there is an abrupt angle change of the iris, causing rapid vision loss and dramatic symptoms. This type of glaucoma represents 10% of the total number of glaucoma cases in the United States.

Clinical Manifestations

In POAG the patient has no signs or symptoms during the early stages of the disease. As the symptoms become apparent, they include loss of peripheral vision (tunnel vision), eye pain, difficulty adjusting to darkness, halos around lights, and inability to detect colors. IOPs are elevated.

AACG produces excruciating pain in or around the eye, decreased vision, and nausea and vomiting. The sclera is erythematous, and the pupil is enlarged and fixed. The patient sees colored halos around lights and has an acute increase in the IOP.

As glaucoma progresses, **optic disk cupping** occurs. This is visible with direct or indirect ophthalmoscopy. The optic disk becomes wider, deeper, and paler (light gray or white). Optic disk cupping may be one of the first signs of chronic open-angle glaucoma. Optic disk photographs are useful for comparison over time to demonstrate an increase in the cup-to-disk ratio and progressive blanching (Figure 53-10).

Assessment

Collection of **subjective data** includes noting the time of day that eye pain occurs. Also assess frequency, intensity, and duration of the pain. Note complaints of peripheral vision loss, maladaptation to darkness, and halos seen around lights. Determine the severity of headaches and presence of nausea and vomiting.

Collection of **objective data** includes noting a need for frequent eyeglass prescription changes. Elevated IOPs are also present.

Diagnostic Tests

Schiøtz tonometry is used to test for IOP (Figure 53-11). A patient with glaucoma would test above the normal range of 10 to 22 mm Hg. IOP is usually between 22 and 32 mm Hg in POAG. IOP may be 50 mm Hg or higher in AACG. Applanation tonometry is also used to measure IOP (Figure 53-12). Visual field studies show a decline in the patient's peripheral vision. Optic disk cupping occurs as glaucoma progresses. Optic disk cupping leads to optic nerve damage.

Medical Management

Keeping the IOP low enough to prevent the patient from developing optic nerve damage is the primary focus of glaucoma therapy.

POAG is medically treated by the use of beta blockers, **miotics** (agents that cause the pupil to constrict), and carbonic anhydrase inhibitors (Table 53-5). A beta blocker, such as betaxolol hydrochloride (Betoptic), reduces IOP. Miotics, such as pilocarpine, constrict the pupil and draw the iris away from the cornea, allowing aqueous humor to drain out of the canal of Schlemm (see Figure 53-9). Carbonic anhydrase inhibi-

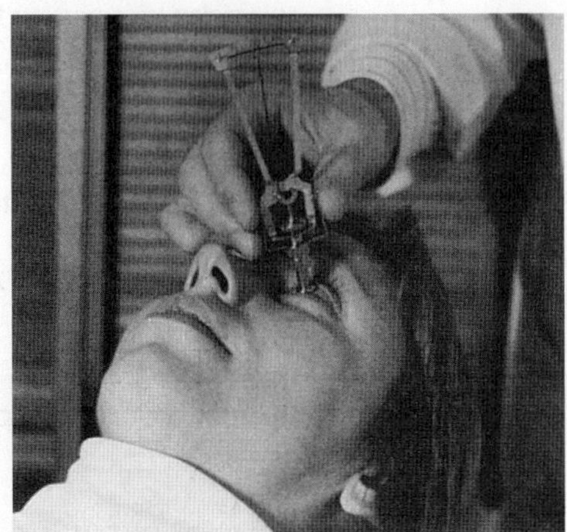

FIGURE 53-11 Measurement of intraocular pressure with the Schiøtz tonometer.

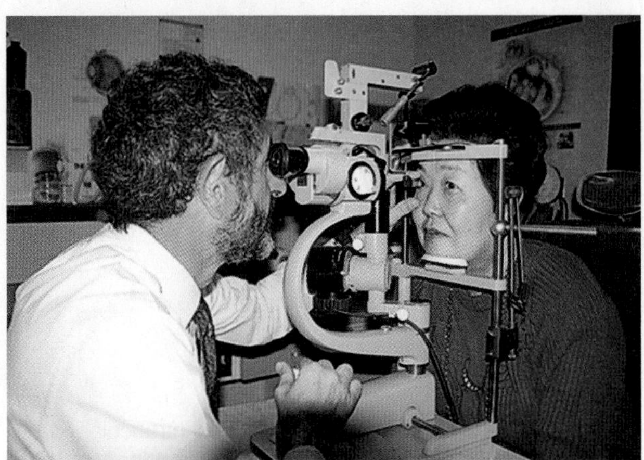

FIGURE 53-12 Applanation tonometry.

Table 53-5 Medications for Eye Disorders

Generic (Trade)	Actions and Uses	Side Effects	Nursing Implications
Sulfacetamide sodium (Sulamyd)	Broad-spectrum bacteriostatic antiinfective agent used in the treatment of ocular infections (conjunctivitis, corneal ulcers, trachoma, and chlamydial infections)	Pruritus, edema, erythema, other eye irritations	It is contraindicated in those with sulfonamide hypersensitivity; purulent exudate may inactivate drug; do not use silver preparations concurrently; comply with full course of treatment; store properly; discard solution if it discolors; warn patient to avoid sharing washcloths and towels with family members.
Betaxolol hydrochloride (Betoptic)	Beta-adrenergic blocking agent that reduces formation of aqueous humor; used for open-angle glaucoma	Insomnia, irritation of eyelids, stinging on instillation, occasional tears, photophobia, systemic effects, possible disorientation, bradycardia, weakness, dyspnea	Know pregnancy cautions; do not touch dropper on eye; keep container tightly closed; determine intraocular pressure 4 weeks after treatment; use cautiously in patients with history of heart failure or with diabetes mellitus.
Timolol maleate (Timoptic)	Beta-adrenergic blocking agent that reduces aqueous humor formation; used for open-angle glaucoma and hypertension; used with caution for patients who have heart conditions	Ocular sensitivity, severe irritation of eye or eyelid, systemic effect of cardiac failure, chest pain, disorientation, diarrhea, dizziness, exacerbation of asthma	It may mask hypoglycemia; measure intraocular pressure after 4 weeks of treatment; avoid abrupt cessation; use cautiously in patients with bronchial asthma and heart conditions; know pregnancy and breastfeeding cautions; keep container tightly closed.

Continued

Table 53-5 Medications for Eye Disorders—cont'd

Generic (Trade)	Actions and Uses	Side Effects	Nursing Implications
Dexamethasone (Decadron)	Decreases inflammation	Local irritation, retardation of corneal healing, blurred vision, eye pain, secondary eye infection	It may mask infection; use only for short term in children; tell patient not to wear contact lens during treatment; shake bottle before using; check with physician before using for future eye conditions; check with physician if condition does not improve in 5-7 days.
Acetazolamide (Diamox)	Lowers intraocular pressure; used for open-angle glaucoma	Diarrhea, weakness, discomfort, urinary frequency, loss of appetite, nausea, vomiting, numbness in hands; contraindicated with severe renal, hepatic, or adrenocortical impairment	Know pregnancy and lactation cautions; give with food; in diabetes, it may increase blood and urine glucose levels; caution patient about drowsiness; monitor intake and output (I&O) and weight daily.
Pilocarpine hydrochloride (Pilocar, Isopto, Carpine)	Reduces intraocular pressure; used for open-angle glaucoma	Muscle tremors, nausea and vomiting, dyspnea, wheezing, bronchial spasms, local irritation	Encourage patient to have periodic intraocular pressure determinations; monitor for blurred vision or changes in vision; use cautiously in bronchial asthma and hypertension; apply light finger pressure on lacrimal sac 1 minute after instillation of drops.
Cyclopentolate hydrochloride (Cyclogyl)	Anticholinergic drug that produces dilation of pupil and temporary paralysis of ciliary muscles; used in glaucoma; a diagnostic agent for angle-closure glaucomas	Ataxia, behavioral disturbances, tachycardia, disorientation, fever	Prevent contamination of dropper; warn patient of increased sensitivity to light and suggest sunglasses; contraindicated in closed-angle glaucoma; use cautiously in older adults.
Mannitol (Osmitrol)	Osmotic diuretic that reduces intraocular pressure; used for glaucoma	Fluid and electrolyte imbalance, chest pain, tachycardia, chills and fever, difficult urination	Administer by intravenous infusion; know pregnancy caution; duration of action is 1-3 hours; monitor vital signs at least hourly and I&O, weight, and potassium levels daily.
Polyvinyl alcohol (Liquifilm Forte)	Tearlike lubricant; used for dry eyes and eye irritations	Headache, burning, blurred vision, eye pain	Teach patient to instill; to avoid contamination of solution, warn patient not to touch tip of container to eye.
Gentamicin sulfate (Garamycin)	Bactericidal antibiotic; used for treatment of blepharitis and conjunctivitis	Pruritus, erythema, edema, ocular discomfort, blurred vision (may occur for few minutes after application)	Comply with full course of therapy; if no improvement occurs after a few days, check with physician.

Patient Teaching

Glaucoma

- Medical supervision is required for the rest of life.
- Eyedrops **must** be continued as long as prescribed even in the absence of symptoms; usually treatment is lifelong.
  —Blurred vision decreases with prolonged use.
  —Avoid driving for 1 to 2 hours after administration of miotics.
- To prevent complications:
  —Press lacrimal duct for 1 minute after eyedrop insertion to prevent rapid systemic absorption.
  —Have reserve bottle of eyedrops at home.
  —Carry eyedrops when away from home.
  —Carry card stating you have glaucoma and the eyedrop solution prescribed.
- Bright lights and darkness are not harmful.
- There is no apparent relationship between vascular hypertension and ocular hypertension.
- Report any reappearance of symptoms immediately to ophthalmologist.
- If admitted to the hospital for a different medical condition, alert the staff of continued need for prescribed eyedrops.
- Avoid the use of mydriatic or cycloplegic drugs (e.g., atropine) that dilate the pupils.

tors, such as acetazolamide (Diamox), decrease the production of aqueous humor. The result is a lowering of IOP. Surgery, which consists of a trabeculectomy or laser trabeculoplasty, is done when medications do not control the pressure. **Trabeculectomy** is the removal of corneoscleral tissue, usually the canal of Schlemm and trabecular meshwork. This produces an increase in the outflow of aqueous humor. Laser trabeculoplasty produces openings in the trabecular meshwork.

AACG is medically treated with osmotic diuretics, such as mannitol; carbonic anhydrase inhibitors; and miotics. Surgical treatment includes a peripheral iridectomy or an iridotomy. A peripheral iridectomy is the removal of part of the iris. The procedure is performed with the patient under local anesthesia. This procedure often restores drainage of the aqueous humor. Postoperatively observe the patient for signs and symptoms of local hemorrhage or excessive pain. An iridotomy is an incision into the iris of the eye to create an opening for aqueous flow. A local or general anesthetic may be used. Postoperatively observe the dressing for signs of drainage.

Nursing Interventions and Patient Teaching

Nursing interventions involve protecting the patient's safety, monitoring compliance to therapy, and reinforcing discharge instructions. Depending on the practice setting, educate individual patients and families, groups of patients, or entire communities about the risk of glaucoma. Let them know that the incidence of glaucoma increases with age and that a comprehensive ophthalmic examination is invaluable in identifying people with glaucoma or those at risk of developing glaucoma. Stress the importance of early detection and treatment in preventing visual impairment. The current recommendation is for an ophthalmologic examination every 2 to 4 years for people between 40 and 64 years of age, and every 1 to 2 years for people 65 years of age or older. Blacks in every age-group should have more frequent examinations because of the increased incidence and more aggressive course of glaucoma in these individuals.

Because of the chronic nature of glaucoma, encourage the patient to follow the therapeutic regimen and follow-up recommendations prescribed by the ophthalmologist (see Patient Teaching box). Provide accurate information about the disease process and treatment options, including the rationale underlying each option. Teach the patient about the purpose, frequency, and technique for administration of prescribed antiglaucoma agents. In addition to verbal instructions, give all patients written instructions that contain the necessary information without being overwhelming. Encourage the patient to comply with the medication regimen by (1) stressing the sight-saving nature of the drops, (2) helping the patient identify the most convenient and appropriate times for medication administration, and (3) advocating a change in therapy if the patient reports unacceptable side effects (Lewis et al., 2007).

Prognosis

Today's method of medical and surgical management provides the patient with an excellent prognosis for a full recovery. Complications are few if care is obtained early in the course of the condition. When the patient ignores glaucoma or is noncompliant with therapy, blindness may occur. Regular eye examinations are required to detect and monitor for increased IOP. Generally, once damage has occurred, the condition is irreversible. Surgery and medication help lessen the complications from glaucoma.

CORNEAL INJURIES

Etiology and Pathophysiology

The cornea is the convex, transparent outermost layer of the eye. It is composed of five layers of tissue and is uniform in nature. The cornea is nonvascular; therefore no bleeding occurs from injury unless subcorneal structures are involved. The cornea is kept moist by tear production and is protected from daily insult by the eyelid. Any wound causes the cornea to become abnormally hydrated and decreases the normal transparency (Lewis et al., 2007).

Foreign bodies are the most common cause of corneal injury. Dust particles, propellants, and eyelashes may lodge in the conjunctiva or cornea. The eyes blink in response to the irritant, and further irritation occurs from the upper lid closing frequently, thus moving the foreign body into deeper layers or a wider area of the cornea.

Burns often occur in the home and workplace. When burns affect the eye, it is a medical emergency. Depending on the chemical causing the burn, the damage may be superficial or deep. Chemical irritants such as acids and alkalis and metal flashes from acetylene blowtorches cause significant pain, depending on the depth of chemical erosion.

Abrasions and lacerations are usually superficial scratches caused by fingernails or clothing. They may be painful, depending on the depth of the abrasion.

Penetrating wounds are the most serious corneal injuries. Eye structures may be injured permanently, resulting in total blindness. Infection may result from the introduction of microorganisms on the penetrating object.

Clinical Manifestations

Foreign bodies produce pain when the eyeball moves or the eyelid moves over the eyeball during blinking. Excessive tearing, erythema of the conjunctiva, and pruritus may occur. Acute pain and burning are the primary symptoms with any topical burn to the eye. Abrasions and lacerations produce mild to severe pain, depending on the depth of corneal involvement. The pain may be transitory and slight, or spasmodic and deep. Penetrating wounds result in varying degrees of pain. If underlying structures are involved, pain may be absent because the nerves have been severed.

Assessment

Foreign Bodies

Subjective data include the time and type of injury. Assess the patient for the degree and severity of eye pain and vision loss. Ask about any first aid treatment provided.

Collection of **objective data** includes observation of the foreign body and extent of damage. When the intracapsular area has been penetrated, fluid leaks from the eye.

Burns

Subjective data include the degree of pain. It is important to assess the substance causing the burn and any first aid treatment that has been provided. Vision loss is determined by the physician.

Collection of **objective data** includes noting the extent of the burn in and around the eye, including eyelashes and eyebrows, and assessing the condition of the eyeball.

Abrasions and Lacerations

Subjective data include the degree of pain after the incident and how the injury occurred. Note treatments used at the time of injury.

Collection of **objective data** includes assessing the degree of damage of the eyeball and surrounding structures and noting any vision loss.

Penetrating Wounds

Subjective data include the time and causative factors related to the injury. Assess presence and severity of pain. Determine whether any first aid treatment was given.

Objective data include the type and size of the penetrating object. Note any fluid leakage from the eye and damage to surrounding structures.

Diagnostic Tests

Tests include visual and ophthalmoscopic examination, fluorescein staining, peripheral vision tests, and slit-lamp examination.

Medical Management

Foreign bodies are medically treated with a flush of normal saline when the object is near the sclera and conjunctiva; it can then be removed by a clean swab or tissue. Cotton is not used, since it may scratch the cornea. If the object is not easily flushed away, the individual must see an ophthalmologist to have the object removed. Antibiotic topical eye ointments are ordered.

Burns are medically treated with a 15- to 20-minute or longer tap water flush immediately after burn exposure. This will help prevent scar formation. Separate the eyelids during the flush procedure. The patient is then treated in a local emergency department or physician's office for follow-up care. Home remedy first aid treatment should not be done. Topical antiinfective agents are ordered for the eye. Abrasions and lacerations of the eye are medically cleaned with a normal saline solution. Antibiotic therapy, usually topical, is prescribed (see Safety Alert box).

Seek medical assistance immediately for eye injuries, chemical eye burns, and foreign bodies that remain in the eye. Immediately after a penetrating wound injury, both eyes should be covered while the patient is transported to the hospital. Both eyes work in synchrony, so covering the unaffected eye prevents it from involuntarily moving with the other eye. A shield reduces further injury but must not touch the foreign object. A Styrofoam cup provides adequate coverage and is readily available. The foreign object should not be removed except by a trained physician.

Nursing Interventions and Patient Teaching

Nursing interventions for foreign bodies include assisting with the required irrigation of the eye. For burns, assist with the flushing process and providing

Safety Alert!

Eye Safety Measures

- Avoid frequent rinsing of eyes with unprescribed solutions.
- Discard any ophthalmic solution that is cloudy or discolored, has been open for longer than 3 months, or contains particles.
- Do not self-treat an eye inflammation with a medication prescribed for a previous eye disorder.
- To avoid eye strain:
  —Use a good light for reading or doing work that requires careful visual focus.
  —When reading or focusing eyes for long periods, look at distant objects for a few minutes at repeated intervals to rest eyes.
- Avoid rubbing eyes.
- Wash hands before and after touching eyes.
- Wear safety glasses when engaging in activities that could injure the eyes. If injury occurs, apply cool compress if no laceration is present; cover if laceration is present.
- Wear dark glasses for prolonged exposure to bright light (such as sunlight, snow, or water).
- Flush eyes immediately for 15 to 20 minutes or longer with cool water when any irritating substances are introduced.
- Do not attempt to remove foreign bodies from the cornea; cover the eye with an eyeshield (e.g., small paper cup) to prevent excessive movement or touching of the eye. Seek medical attention immediately.
- If a speck of dust blows in the eye, pull upper lid over lower lid and let the tears wash the speck to the inner canthus or lower lid, where it may be safely removed. Irrigate the eye with cool tap water, if necessary.

eye medications as ordered. For abrasions and lacerations, assist with cleaning the eye as ordered and providing general first aid.

When a patient has a penetrating wound, note whether the pupil on the affected side becomes irregular in size. This results when the iris of the affected eye moves to occlude the wound area. Infection potential is high; therefore topical and systemic antibiotics are ordered. If the wound is small, self-healing occurs. If the wound is large or deep, enucleation of the eye may be necessary.

Effective and immediate therapy is crucial for any eye injury. If treatment is interrupted, ineffective, or not sustained, permanent eye damage will occur. The most frequent complications include infection, vision disturbances, and blindness. A nursing diagnosis for the patient with an eye injury would be *pain,* acute, related to inflammatory process. (See the discussion on conjunctivitis.)

Ensure that the patient can apply ointments and dressings, if ordered. Instruct the patient in the use of other therapy devices, such as warm or cool compresses. Teach proper handwashing techniques. The patient should wear dark sunglasses if cycloplegic or mydriatic eyedrops are used. Instruct the patient to avoid future episodes with chemical or environmental hazards. Ensure that the patient understands discharge instructions, including the need for follow-up physician visits and symptoms to report. Determine the patient's knowledge about the progress of therapy.

Prognosis

Immediate and appropriate treatment reduces the severity and complications of eye injuries. Monitor the chosen treatment to prevent permanent eye damage and vision problems. Superficial corneal abrasions usually heal without incident. Deeper abrasions or burns may result in permanent visual loss due to scarring.

SURGERIES OF THE EYE

ENUCLEATION

Eye **enucleation** is the surgical removal of the eyeball. It is often necessary after severe eye trauma but may be done for other reasons, such as malignant tumors. Surgical methods vary from removal of the entire eyeball or the eyeball contents to removal of the eyeball and all underlying structures.

Nursing Interventions

The loss of an eye is extremely traumatic for the patient even though the enucleation may be done after severe painful blindness. Be aware of the patient's grieving over the loss of an eye and provide emotional support to the patient and the family (Lewis et al., 2007). Other nursing responsibilities include facilitating a therapeutic dialogue between the physician and patient regarding the exact nature of the surgery.

Postoperatively apply a pressure dressing over the socket of the eye to control hemorrhage. Observe the dressing at least every hour for the first 24 hours. Ask the patient about any pain on the affected side of the head or any headache, which might indicate hemorrhage or infection. Report these findings to the physician immediately. Avoid routine postoperative procedures of coughing and turning on the affected side to prevent sutures from dislodging.

Prognosis

Patients who undergo enucleation surgery are excellent candidates for prosthetic replacements. The wound is adequately healed approximately 6 weeks after the enucleation. An ocularist fits a permanent prosthesis designed to match the remaining eye. The patient must be carefully educated in how to remove, cleanse, and insert the prosthesis (Lewis et al., 2007).

KERATOPLASTY (CORNEAL TRANSPLANT)

Keratoplasty is the removal of the full thickness of the patient's cornea followed by surgical implantation of a cornea from a human donor. It is done to replace a damaged cornea resulting from trauma, ulceration, or congenital deformities. Approximately 40,000 corneal transplants are performed in the United States each year. Improved methods of tissue procurement and preservation, refined surgical techniques, postoperative topical corticosteroids, and careful follow-up have decreased graft rejection. Medications to suppress rejection (e.g., cyclosporine) may be ordered.

Corneal grafts are usually taken within 4 hours after death. An ideal donor is between 25 and 35 years of age and died of injury or acute disease. The corneas of people with chronic or communicable diseases—such as hepatitis, acquired immunodeficiency syndrome, or cancer—are not appropriate for transplantation. The eye banks test donors for human immunodeficiency virus and hepatitis B and C. The donor's eye should have normal light perception and projection. The donor's tissue is best used within 5 days after removal.

The nurse often has the most access to the family when questions of organ donation occur. Responsibilities include notification of appropriate supervisory personnel when an organ donation from a deceased donor is occurring. Keratoplasty is performed with the patient under local or general anesthesia. The transplanted tissue is sutured into place to maintain graft alignment and a watertight wound.

Nursing Interventions

Before surgery encourage the patient to express fears related to surgery. Give instructions in the use of protective eyeglasses if dilation-causing eye medication is used. Prevent injuries by using safety devices and orienting the patient to each new environment. Cleanse and prepare the surgical areas as ordered, usually with an antiseptic solution. Preoperative teaching includes deep breathing and turning to reduce any complications associated with surgery. Coughing is discouraged, since sutures may break. Maintain dietary restrictions, if ordered; a light breakfast may be allowed if the surgery is done with the patient under a local anesthesia. Administer prescribed medications.

After surgery ensure that correct postoperative positioning is maintained; the patient is usually positioned on the back or nonoperated side until the physician allows turning to the operated side. Reinforce activity restrictions as ordered to prevent injury to the eye. Use safety measures until the patient is able to ambulate safely. Anyone coming into the room should announce his or her presence. The patient should avoid bending, lifting, and straining for approximately 1 month to prevent increases in IOP or suture tension.

Progressive activity should be prescribed by the physician. Encourage regular postoperative visits with the eye surgeon. Report any severe or progressive pain to the surgeon immediately, as well as any complaints of erythema, loss of vision, or photophobia that would occur with corneal rejection. Administer systemic and ophthalmic medications. Maintain strict surgical asepsis during dressing changes. Staff, the patient, and the family must wash hands thoroughly before any contact with the eye area. Instruct the patient to avoid the use of such irritants as powder, perfume, and propellants, which might cause sneezing and displacement of sutures. The patient should not rub the eye area to avoid contaminating the site or displacing sutures. Assess the patient's diversional activities; television is usually permitted, but reading is limited because the side-to-side movement of the eyes may loosen the sutures. If an eyepatch or metal eyecup shield is ordered, demonstrate its care. The eyepatch is applied snugly to inhibit the blink reflex and allow the eye to rest. The metal eyeshield is used at night to protect the eye from trauma. Obtain discharge instructions from the physician regarding use of eyewear.

Prognosis

The cornea is avascular; therefore healing is slow. Incidence of infection is increased as a result. The transplanted donor tissue may be rejected. The chances of rejection are reduced if the donor is a family member with similar tissue type.

PHOTOCOAGULATION

Using a laser, the physician directs a small, intense beam of light into a small spot on the retina. The light converts to heat energy, and coagulation of tissue protein occurs; this is called **photocoagulation.** Photocoagulation is a nonsurgical procedure usually performed on an outpatient basis. Without surgical intervention, the structures of the eye remain undisturbed and only the sealing of leaks and destruction of offending tissue occur.

Photocoagulation is useful in diabetic retinopathy to cauterize hemorrhaging vessels. It cannot increase visual acuity but can prevent further loss. Usually no hospitalization or postoperative medical management is required.

Nursing Interventions

Postoperative assessment for patients who have undergone photocoagulation therapy includes assessment of vision. They may have constriction of peripheral fields and a temporary decrease in central vision. A decrease in night vision and a headache from the laser's bright light may also occur.

Prognosis

Photocoagulation is used to prevent eye damage and is not curative. Minimal destruction of tissue occurs with photocoagulation. The procedure is nonsurgical; therefore infection risk is minimal.

VITRECTOMY

A vitrectomy is the removal of excess vitreous fluid caused by hemorrhage and replacement with normal saline. Any scar tissue may also be removed.

Postoperative management includes the prescription of topical eye medication for 4 to 6 weeks. Acetaminophen or acetaminophen with codeine is prescribed for pain management. A pressure patch to the operative eye is placed immediately after surgery. Ice packs to reduce inflammation are ordered.

Nursing Interventions and Patient Teaching

The patient is required to maintain a position on the abdomen or sitting forward resting the nonoperated side of the head on a table to allow air that is in the eye to float against the retina. This position is maintained for 4 to 5 days.

Dark glasses are prescribed postoperatively to decrease the discomfort of photophobia. Postoperative care includes assessing the eyepatch; applying ice packs; monitoring vital signs, especially for fever; and assessing the dressing for bleeding.

Prognosis

The procedure has limited benefits and continues to be investigated as to its benefits versus complications.

NURSING CONSIDERATIONS FOR CARE OF THE PATIENT WITH AN EAR DISORDER

Once the history and general assessment have been completed, focus on assessment of the ear. Additional information would include the following:

- Occurrence of ear drainage, tinnitus, vertigo, wax buildup, pressures, pain, and pruritus
- Other medical diagnoses
- Family history
- Exposure to loud noises
- Behavioral clues indicating hearing loss (Box 53-2)
- History of medications used for ear disorders, specifically those known to be ototoxic
- Current medications for the ear disorder
- Side effects of medications, if any
- Associated speech pattern abnormalities
- Use of assistive hearing devices
- Home remedies that cause ear trauma

Communicate the gathered data to the appropriate personnel and document the findings in the patient record. The next step in the assessment process is to prepare the patient for the initial otoscopic diagnostic evaluation.

LABORATORY AND DIAGNOSTIC EXAMINATIONS

OTOSCOPY

With an otoscope the examiner can visualize the external auditory canal and the eardrum, or tympanic membrane. Normally the tympanic membrane is disk shaped and pearl gray or pale pink. Otoscopy is the initial examination of the ear, performed before other testing. One of the nurse's responsibilities is to explain to the patient the purpose and procedure. Reassure the patient that otoscopy is a painless test requiring only about 1 to 2 minutes, with slight pulling of the ear upward and backward for an adult and down and back for a child.

Box 53-2 Behavioral Clues Indicating Hearing Loss

Any adult who:

- Is irritable, hostile, and hypersensitive in interpersonal relations
- Has difficulty hearing upper-frequency consonants
- Complains about people mumbling
- Turns up volume on television and radio
- Asks for frequent repetition and answers questions inappropriately
- Loses sense of humor, becomes grim
- Leans forward to hear better; face becomes serious and strained
- Shuns large- and small-group audience situations
- May appear aloof and uninterested
- Complains of ringing in the ears
- Has an unusually soft or loud voice
- Repeatedly asks, "What did you say?"

WHISPERED VOICE TEST

General screening regarding the patient's ability to hear can occur with tests using the whispered and spoken voice. To conduct the whispered test, stand 12 to 24 inches (30 to 61 cm) to the side of the patient, exhale, and speak in a low whisper. Then repeat the test using a louder whisper and spoken voice, increasing in loudness. Test each ear, with the patient covering the other ear. Ask the patient to repeat words or numbers or answer questions (Lewis et al., 2007).

TUNING FORK TESTS

The two most common tests using tuning forks are Weber's test and the Rinne test. These tests are used to determine hearing loss and collect data related to the type of loss.

Weber's test is a method of assessing auditory acuity, especially useful in determining whether defective hearing in an ear is a conductive loss caused by a middle ear problem or a sensorineural loss, resulting from a disorder in the inner ear or auditory nerve system. The test is performed by placing the stem of a vibrating tuning fork in the center of the patient's forehead or on the maxillary incisors. The sound is equally loud in both ears if hearing is normal. If the person has a sensorineural loss in one ear, the unaffected ear perceives the sound as louder. When conductive hearing loss is present, the sound is louder in the affected ear, but it does not hear ordinary background noise conducted through the air and receives only vibrations by bone conduction (Figure 53-13).

The **Rinne test** is a method of distinguishing conductive from sensorineural hearing loss. The test is performed with tuning forks placed ½ inch (1.25 cm) from the external auditory meatus and the vibrating stem placed over the mastoid bone. While one ear is tested, the other is masked (Figure 53-14). In sensorineural loss the sound is heard longer by air conduction, whereas in conduction hearing loss the sound is heard longer by bone conduction.

Nursing responsibility in both Weber's test and the Rinne test includes explanation of the purpose and procedure of the tests. Stress that the patient needs to concentrate and use hand signals to indicate the ear in which the sound is heard in Weber's test and when it is no longer heard in the Rinne test. In addition, assure the patient that the test is painless and requires only a few minutes.

Audiometric Testing

Audiometry is a test of hearing acuity. Audiometry is beneficial as a diagnostic test for determining the degree and type of hearing loss and as a screening test for hearing acuity. Various audiometric tests determine the lowest intensity of sound at which an individual can perceive auditory stimulus (hearing threshold), hear different frequencies, and distinguish different speech tones.

Nursing responsibilities include explaining the purpose and procedure of each test and reviewing any required responses by the patient.

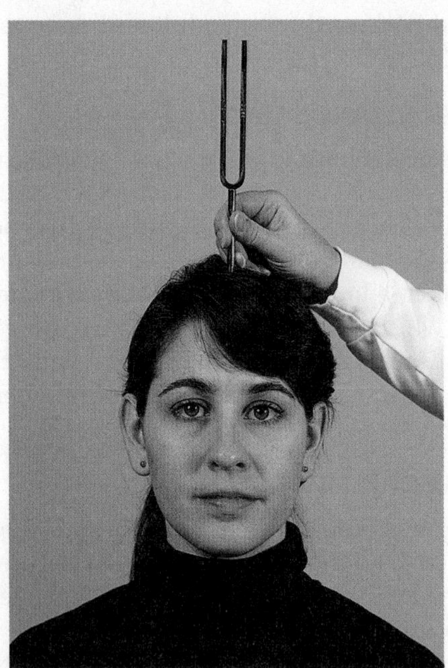

FIGURE 53-13 Weber's tuning fork test.

Vestibular Testing

The auditory and vestibular (balance and equilibrium) systems are closely related. Assess the patient's signs and symptoms carefully to determine whether they originate from balance or hearing loss. The patient needs to describe the symptoms in detail (Lewis et al., 2007).

Problems of the vestibular system may manifest as nystagmus or vertigo. Nystagmus is involuntary, rhythmic movements of the eye. The vibrations may be horizontal, vertical, rotary, or mixed (*Mosby's Dictionary of Medicine, Nursing, and Health Professions*, 2009). Vertigo is a feeling that the person or objects around the person are moving or spinning and is usually accentuated by movement of the head (Lewis et al., 2007). The Romberg and past-point tests are used for patients complaining of dizziness or disequilibrium.

The **Romberg test** measures the patient's ability to perform specific tasks with eyes open and then with eyes closed. The normal response is maintaining balance throughout the entire test. An abnormal response (in which the patient loses balance when standing erect, feet together, eyes closed) indicates loss of the sense of position.

Past-point testing measures the patient's ability to place a finger accurately on a selected point on the body. Inability to correctly perform the test indicates a lack of coordination in voluntary movements.

Explain the purpose and procedure of each test. Institute safety measures to prevent patient injury during the Romberg test if the patient cannot maintain balance.

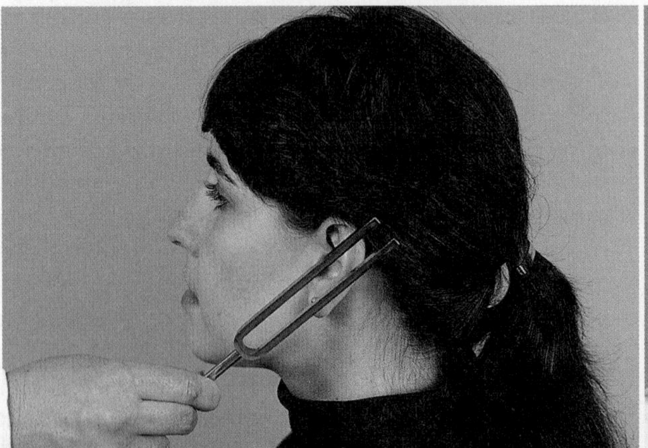

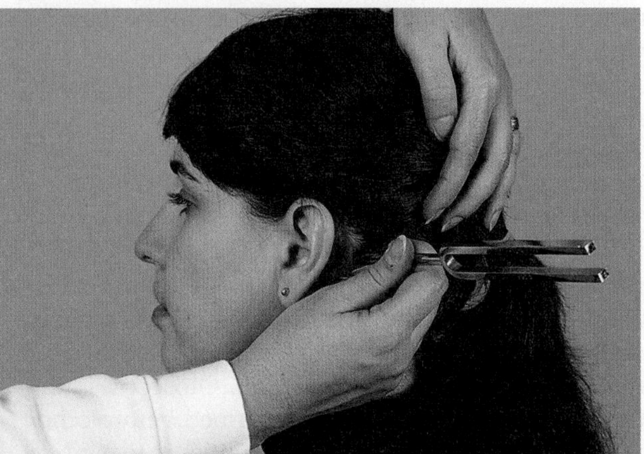

FIGURE 53-14 Rinne tuning fork test.

DISORDERS OF THE EAR

LOSS OF HEARING (DEAFNESS)

Hearing impairment is a state of decreased auditory acuity that ranges from partial to complete hearing loss. It is the most common disability in the United States: 28 million people have a hearing impairment. Among people older than 65 years of age, it is the third most common chronic condition. The quality of life for one third of the adults in the United States between 65 and 75 years of age is decreased because of hearing impairments. Recognition, diagnosis, and early treatment may help prevent further impairment and damage.

The implications of hearing loss are great. Hearing is needed to develop speech and conceptual ability; thus hearing loss may well affect personality development and intelligence-test responses when the hearing impairment is severe and congenital. This may have implications for the person's education and socialization. As hearing loss increases, the person may withdraw socially because of the inability to understand and be understood; this could lead to isolation and depression (see Health Promotion box).

Types of Hearing Loss

There are six types of hearing loss: conductive, sensorineural, mixed, congenital, functional (psychogenic), and central.

In **conductive hearing loss,** sound is inadequately conducted through the external or middle ear to the sensorineural apparatus of the inner ear. Common causes are buildup of cerumen and otitis media with effusion (escape of effusion). Other conditions that may result in conductive hearing loss are foreign bodies, otosclerosis, and stenosis of the external auditory canal. Sensitivity to sound is diminished, but clarity or interpretation of sound is not changed. When increased volume compensates for the loss, then hearing is normal; therefore a hearing aid can be helpful.

In **sensorineural hearing loss,** sound is conducted through the external and middle ear in a normal way, but a defect in the inner ear results in its distortion, making discrimination difficult. This type of hearing loss is usually caused by trauma, infectious processes, presbycusis (hearing loss caused by aging), congenital conditions, or exposure to ototoxic drugs. Destruction of cochlear hair by intense noise may also cause sensorineural loss. Amplifying sound, such as with a hearing aid, will help some people with this type of loss. Many people have an intolerance to loud noise and would not be helped by a hearing aid.

Mixed hearing loss is a combined conductive and sensorineural hearing loss.

Congenital hearing loss is present from birth or early infancy. It can be caused by anoxia or trauma during delivery, Rh incompatibility, or the mother's exposure during pregnancy to syphilis or rubella or use of ototoxic drugs.

Functional hearing loss has no organic cause. It is also known as **psychogenic** or **nonorganic hearing loss.** Functional hearing loss may be caused by an emotional or a psychological factor.

Health Promotion

Facilitating Communication for People with Impaired Hearing

- If the patient wears a hearing aid, make certain it is in place, turned on, and functioning properly.
- Get the person's attention by raising an arm or hand.
- Ask permission to turn off the television or radio or turn down volume.
- Start with the light on your face; this will help the person speech read.
- Face the person when speaking.
- Speech reading is a skill that not all hearing impaired are capable of achieving. Do not assume all hearing impaired can lip read.
- Speak clearly, but do not overaccentuate words.
- Speak in a normal tone; do not shout or raise the pitch of voice. Shouting overuses normal speaking movements and may cause distortion and be too loud for the person with sensorineural damage. If the person has conductive loss only, sometimes making the voice louder without shouting is helpful.
- If the person does not seem to understand what is said, express it differently. Some words are difficult to see in speech reading, such as *white* or *red*.
- Move closer to the person and toward the better ear if the person does not hear you.
- Write out proper names or any statement that you are not sure was understood.
- Do not eat, drink, chew gum, or cover the mouth when talking to a person with limited hearing.
- Observe for inattention that may indicate tiredness or lack of understanding.
- Use phrases rather than one-word answers to convey meaning. State the major topic of the discussion first and then give details.
- Do not show annoyance by careless facial expression; use normal facial expressions. People who are hard of hearing depend more on visual clues for acceptance.
- Encourage the use of a hearing aid if the person has one; allow the person to adjust it before speaking.
- If in a group, repeat important statements and avoid asides to others in the group.
- Avoid the use of the intercommunication system as this may distort sound and cause poor communication.
- Do not avoid conversation with a person who has hearing loss.

Modified from Conover, M., & Cober, J. (1970). Understanding and caring for the hearing impaired. *Nursing Clinics of North America, 5*, 497.

Central hearing loss occurs when the brain's auditory pathways are damaged, as in a stroke or a tumor.

Clinical Manifestations

Clinical manifestations vary, depending on the degree of deafness. Symptoms range from subtle clues, such as requests for repeating information, to more obvious signs of nonresponse.

Assessment

Collection of **subjective data** includes noting the onset and progression of the condition, deficit in one or both ears, family history, history of head trauma, exposure to noise, current medications, visual or speech disorders, and any other ear symptoms.

Collection of **objective data** must include an assessment of behavioral clues that indicate a hearing difficulty (see Box 53-2).

Diagnostic Tests

Conductive hearing loss produces lateralization of sound to the deaf ear in Weber's test. Results of the Rinne test show that sounds transmitted through bone conduction are heard longer than or equal to sounds transmitted through air conduction.

Sensorineural hearing loss produces lateralization of sound to the better ear in Weber's test. Results of the Rinne test show that air-conducted sounds are heard longer than bone-conducted sounds, but not twice as long.

Audiometric testing determines the type of hearing loss and the degree of impairment.

Medical Management

Medical management depends on the type of impairment. Surgical procedures may be required. Hearing aids or cochlear implants may be used when appropriate. Cochlear implantation is performed in individuals with profound bilateral sensorineural hearing loss who receive no measurable assistance from lip reading with a properly fitting hearing aid (see discussion of cochlear implants on p. 1881 and Figure 53-15). The electrical activity of hearing is initiated by hair cells in the organ of Corti and sent to the brain along nerve fibers that make up the auditory nerve. In most deaf individuals, these hair cells are damaged. The goal of cochlear implantation is to bridge the gap created by the hair cell loss and directly stimulate the remaining neurons. Studies have shown that even with complete loss of hair cells, a percentage of cochlear neurons remains (Munson, 2006).

Nursing Interventions

Patients with partial hearing loss may benefit from a hearing aid. Help the patient care for the hearing aid as detailed in Box 53-3.

The hearing aid can only be useful if it is worn. Factors leading to nonuse may include the patient seeing the hearing aid as a sign of disability. Also, the magnification of sound may cause discomfort or irritability.

Box 53-3 Care of the Hearing Aid

DO

- Handle with care.
- Wash earmold or plug daily in mild soap and water, using a pipe cleaner to cleanse the cannula.
- Dry earmold or plug thoroughly before reconnecting it to the receiver.
- Always keep an extra battery and cord available.
- When hearing aid is not in use, turn aid off and open battery compartment.
- If hearing aid whistles, reinsert earmold.
- If hearing aid fails to work:
  —Check the on-off switch.
  —Inspect earmold for cleanliness.
  —Examine battery for tightness of fit.
  —Examine cord plug for tightness of insertion.
  —Examine cord for breaks.
  —Replace battery or cord.
- Check for cracks in tubing or earmold.
- Check to see that earmold and hearing aid are inserted in the correct ear.
- Check that earmold or hearing aid is properly inserted.
- Check that volume control wheel is turned up to appropriate settings.

DON'T

- Put hearing aid on heated surface.
- Wash hearing aid.
- Drop hearing aid.
- Wear hearing aid in bath or shower.
- Wear hearing aid overnight.
- Ignore a hearing aid that is "whistling."
- Use in contact with cream, oil, or hair spray when hearing aid is on.

Therefore it is important to ensure that the hearing aid is used and works properly.

Nursing diagnoses and interventions for the patient with hearing loss include but are not limited to the following:

Nursing Diagnoses	Nursing Interventions
Disturbed sensory perception (auditory), related to disease process	Facilitate communication with the patient by following the interventions provided in the Health Promotion box (p. 1869).
Social isolation, related to loss of hearing	Assess factors that contribute to social isolation. Identify support systems for patient. Identify patient concerns. Establish effective communication.

Patient Teaching

Assist the patient in learning to care for a hearing aid, if prescribed (see Box 53-3). Advise the patient to request that others speak slowly or more clearly and repeat if necessary.

Prognosis

Surgical repair of the injured structures increases the likelihood of restoring partial or complete hearing, especially when implants are used. Complications of surgery are rare. Technical advances have also improved the quality of hearing. Microtechnology has reduced the size of hearing aids until they are almost undetectable.

INFLAMMATORY AND INFECTIOUS DISORDERS OF THE EAR

External Otitis

Etiology and Pathophysiology

External otitis, or otitis externa, is an inflammation or infection of the external canal or the auricle of the external ear. It is sometimes called **swimmer's ear.** External otitis may be acute or chronic.

External otitis can be caused by allergy, bacteria, fungi, viruses, and trauma. Allergic reaction can stem from nickel or chromium in earrings. In addition, chemicals in hair sprays, cosmetics, hearing aids, and medications (especially sulfonamides and neomycin) are common sources of allergy. Common bacterial agents are *Staphylococcus aureus, Pseudomonas aeruginosa,* and *Streptococcus pyogenes.* Frequently the viruses herpes simplex and herpes zoster are implicated. The external ear may also be affected by eczema, psoriasis, and seborrheic dermatitis. Fungi such as *Aspergillus* and *Candida* may also be causes. External otitis is more prevalent during hot, humid weather.

Trauma from cleaning or scratching the ear canal with a foreign object (such as a cotton swab, bobby pin, or finger) may result in irritation and possible introduction of infectious organisms.

Cerumen in the older person becomes dry and hard. Because removal is more difficult, the cerumen may become impacted, causing discomfort and decreased hearing. Certain activities allow moisture to become trapped in the ear, creating a medium for infection; these include using earphones, hearing aids, earplugs, earmuffs, and stethoscopes. Excessive swimming may wash out the protective cerumen, remove skin lipids, and lead to secondary infection.

Malignant external otitis is a rare, lethal form caused by *Pseudomonas* organisms and occurring mostly in patients with diabetes. It is a bone-destroying infection that quickly involves all surrounding ear structures.

Clinical Manifestations

The acute inflammatory or infectious process produces pain with movement of the auricle or chewing, and often the entire side of the head aches. Erythema, scaling, pruritus, edema, watery discharge, and crusting of the external ear may occur. Drainage may be purulent or serosanguineous. If the *Pseudomonas* organism is the cause of the infection, the drainage is green and has a musty smell. Dizziness and decreased hearing may also be present if edema occludes the ear canal. With chronic external otitis there is usually pruritus, but no pain with movement of the auricle. A discharge is also present.

Assessment

Collection of **subjective data** includes determining the onset, duration, and severity of pain, which is crucial to the assessment of inflammatory disease of the ear. An early indication of inflammation or infection of the ear is complaint of ear pain accompanied by patient gently pulling on the pinna. Ask the patient about any home remedies used to treat infections. Also assess knowledge of preventive measures.

Collection of **objective data** includes noting a discharge, which may be watery or yellow and tenacious with a fetid odor. The discharge is black if from a fungal infection. The patient may have a partial loss of hearing or feel like the ear is occluded if the ear canal is edematous or is obstructed by adenoids. Palpation of the external ear may produce pain.

Diagnostic Tests

Obtain a culture of the exudate to identify bacterial, viral, or fungal organisms.

Medical Management

Oral analgesics such as codeine may be used if the pain is severe. Corticosteroids (1% hydrocortisone) may be used to reduce edema to allow antibiotics to penetrate. Insert a wick into the ear canal to prevent loss of medication from the canal and to maintain continuous absorption of the medicine. The physician orders the frequency of the wick change. Antimicrobial agents such as antibiotic or antifungal eardrops may be used. The most commonly used contain 0.5% neomycin or 10,000 units/mL of polymyxin B. Systemic antibiotics are used only if the infection is severe. The specific antibiotic used depends on the results of the culture.

Nursing Interventions and Patient Teaching

Carefully cleanse the ear canal. Heat may be applied to the external ear for pain relief. Implement an adequate method of communication. Instill eardrops.

A nursing diagnosis and interventions for the patient with external otitis include but are not limited to the following:

Nursing Diagnosis	Nursing Interventions
Pain, related to inflammatory process	Apply warm compresses as ordered. Administer prescribed analgesics and instill ordered ear medications.

Ensure that the patient has the information to prevent further infection and can care for the infected ear.

Prognosis

External otitis responds favorably to topical antibiotic and corticosteroid eardrops. Systemic antibiotics are rarely required unless cellulitis is present. Acute external otitis may become a chronic problem. If the infection remains untreated and enters the brain, death can occur. The rare malignant external otitis media has a mortality rate of 50% to 75% unless the condition is treated.

Acute Otitis Media

Etiology and Pathophysiology

Acute otitis media, an inflammation or infection of the middle ear, is the most common disorder of the middle ear. Acute otitis media is most often caused by *Haemophilus influenzae* or *Streptococcus pneumoniae*. Chronic otitis media is usually caused by gram-negative bacteria, such as *Proteus, Klebsiella,* and *Pseudomonas* organisms. In addition, allergy, exposure to cigarette smoke, mycoplasma, and several viruses may be factors.

Otitis media occurs more frequently in children, especially at 6 to 36 months of age, and in the winter and early spring. Children's shorter and straighter eustachian tubes provide easier access of the organisms from the nasopharynx to travel to the middle ear. The patient usually has had a recent upper respiratory tract infection. The infection ascends via the eustachian tube and involves the lining of the entire middle ear. Usually only one ear is affected.

Viral infections frequently cause a serous otitis media. Retraction of the tympanic membrane occurs with a buildup of sterile serous exudate. If there is a secondary bacterial infection, purulent exudate collects behind the tympanic membrane, causing it to bulge. This is called **purulent otitis media.**

Clinical Manifestations

The patient experiences a sense of fullness in the ear and also has severe, deep throbbing pain behind the tympanic membrane. This severe pain may disappear if the tympanic membrane ruptures. Hearing loss, **tinnitus** (a subjective noise sensation heard in one or both ears; ringing or tinkling sounds in the ear), and fever may also be present.

Assessment

For information on collection of **subjective data,** refer to the discussion of external otitis.

Collection of **objective data** is the same as for external otitis, with the exception of noting pain on palpation of the external ear.

Diagnostic Tests

A culture of the purulent drainage is obtained to identify the causative organisms.

Medical Management

Antibiotic therapy is based on results of the culture. Amoxicillin for 10 days is the current therapy of choice in the United States. Analgesics are prescribed for severe pain. Sedatives may be prescribed for children to provide rest and pain relief. Local heat is used, and nasal decongestants are ordered (Table 53-6).

Needle aspiration of secretions collected behind the tympanic membrane may be necessary. Myringotomy—a surgical incision of the tympanic membrane to relieve pressure and release purulent exudate from the middle ear—may be required to prevent spontaneous rupture. A tympanostomy tube may be placed for short- or long-term use. Prompt treatment of an episode of acute otitis media generally prevents spontaneous perforation of the tympanic membrane.

Nursing Interventions and Patient Teaching

Inner-ear pressure may cause discomfort, requiring an analgesic. Sedatives may be ordered for young children.

Hearing loss may also occur. Effective communication is essential. Alert parents of young patients to this fact and enlist their help in monitoring the level of loss.

Chronic otitis media caused by repeated attacks of acute otitis media may result in a permanent perforation of the tympanic membrane. The result is a slight to moderate conductive hearing loss.

A growth called **cholesteatoma** (a mass of epithelial cells and cholesterol in the middle ear) occurs when a tympanic membrane perforation allows keratinizing squamous epithelium of the external auditory canal to enter and grow in the middle ear. Enlargement is slow, but the mass can expand into the mastoid antrum and destroy adjacent structures. Unless removed surgically, a cholesteatoma can cause extensive damage to the structures of the middle ear; erode the bony protection of the facial nerve; create a labyrinthine fistula; or even invade the dura, threatening the brain.

Mastoiditis, an infection of one of the mastoid bones, may develop. It is usually an extension of a middle-ear infection that was untreated or inadequately treated. Immediately report signs of mastoiditis, including earache, fever, headache, malaise, and large amounts of purulent exudate.

A nursing diagnosis and interventions for the patient with otitis media include but are not limited to the following:

Nursing Diagnosis	Nursing Interventions
Impaired skin integrity, related to edema and exudates	Note and report any purulent outer ear exudates. Keep ear clean and dry; use sterile cotton to absorb drainage, if ordered. Monitor temperature and report changes.

Table 53-6 Medications for Ear Disorders

Generic (Trade)	Actions and Uses	Side Effects	Nursing Implications
Carbamide peroxide (Debrox)	Cerumen removal	Contact dermatitis	Do not use if eardrum is perforated or if there is ear discharge; not recommended for children; avoid eyes; reevaluate if edema, erythema, or pain persists; use proper administration technique by allowing drops to enter ear canal; do not touch tip of dropper.
Colistin, neomycin, hydrocortisone, and thonzonium (Coly-Mycin S Otic)	Antibiotic-steroid-detergent used for susceptible disease of external auditory canal, mastoidectomy, and otitis media fenestration	Ototoxicity in prolonged use; contact dermatitis; hypersensitivity, including pruritus, skin rash, erythema, and edema	Do not heat bottle above body temperature; with herpes simplex, do not use if patient is infected; do not use if eardrum is perforated; use for 10 days only; keep dropper from touching skin; check with physician if signs and symptoms worsen or do not improve after 1 week; shake well before using; use cotton plug to keep moist; change plug daily.
Triethanolamine polypeptide oleate (Cerumenex)	Cerumen removal	Contact dermatitis	Fill ear canal; insert cotton plug after 15-30 minutes; irrigate ear canal with warm water.
Amoxicillin trihydrate (Amoxil)	Systemic penicillin antibiotic used in acute otitis media	Anaphylaxis, skin rash, diarrhea	Use caution during pregnancy and lactation; take for full treatment period; consult with physician if no improvement occurs in a few days; take on full or empty stomach; check with physician about treating diarrhea; do not give if patient has penicillin or cephalosporin allergy.
Cefaclor (Ceclor)	Second-generation cephalosporin used to treat amoxicillin-resistant otitis media	Anaphylaxis, skin rash, joint pain; fever, diarrhea, abdominal cramping	Store suspension in refrigerator; give full course of therapy; tell patient not to use alcohol; give on full or empty stomach; do not give if patient has penicillin or cephalosporin allergies.
Meclizine hydrochloride (Antivert)	Anticholinergic antihistamine that acts as antiemetic, antivertigo agent; treatment and prophylaxis; possibly effective for diseases affecting vestibular system	Drowsiness, blurred vision, dry mouth	Use caution during pregnancy and breastfeeding; give with food, water, or milk; tell patient to avoid alcohol and central nervous system (CNS) depressants; not recommended for children under 12.

Continued

Table 53-6 Medications for Ear Disorders—cont'd

Generic (Trade)	Actions and Uses	Side Effects	Nursing Implications
Dimenhydrinate (Dramamine)	Anticholinergic antihistamine used in treatment of vertigo	Blurred vision, drowsiness, shortness of breath, painful urination, disorientation	Antihistamines may inhibit lactation; give no CNS depressants; give with food or milk; use caution during pregnancy in early months.
Antipyrine and benzocaine (Auralgan)	Analgesic; local anesthetic; used for otitis media; adjunct to cerumen removal	Contact dermatitis	Use caution during pregnancy and lactation; date bottle and discard after 6 months from first use; do not use if eardrums are perforated; warm bottle; position patient on side and fill ear canal; use cotton plug; wash dropper before replacing in bottle.
Acetic acid (VoSol hydrochloride otic)	Antibacterial, antifungal, astringent; used for superficial infections of external auditory canal	Contact dermatitis, transient stinging	Clean ear first; use cotton plug for first 24 hours; contact physician if condition worsens or no improvement occurs after 5-7 days; do not wash dropper—doing so may dilute medication.
Trimethoprim-sulfamethoxazole (Bactrim)	Systemic antibacterial; used for acute otitis media; no sulfonamide allergy	Fever, itching, skin rash, photosensitivity, dizziness	Not recommended during lactation or pregnancy; emphasize importance of proper dental care; blood glucose levels may be affected in patients using oral antidiabetic agents; maintain adequate fluid intake; advise patient to avoid sun exposure; complete treatment; with pediatric suspension, shake well.
Polymyxin B, neomycin, bacitracin, and hydrocortisone (Cortisporin)	Antibiotic and steroid used in the same way as Coly-Mycin S; used to treat swimmer's ear	Ototoxicity in prolonged use, contact dermatitis, pruritus, erythema, edema	Use caution during pregnancy and lactation; do not use if eardrum is perforated; keep dropper from touching skin; shake well before using; use cotton plug to keep moist; change plug daily.

Ensure that the patient and parents (if appropriate) are aware of the necessity to complete the entire course of antibiotic therapy. Children are fed upright to prevent nasopharyngeal flora from entering the eustachian tube. Instruct the patient to blow the nose gently, not forcefully. If a myringotomy has been performed, instruct the patient or the parents to change the cotton in the outer ear at least twice a day (see Patient Teaching box).

Prognosis

Middle-ear infections usually resolve completely with antibiotic therapy. Since the advent of treatment with antibiotics, the incidence of severe and prolonged infections of the middle ear has been greatly reduced. Chronic or untreated otitis media may lead to sound transmission hearing loss, which is successfully treated with tympanoplasty.

 Patient Teaching

Ear Infection

PREVENTION OF FURTHER INFECTION

- Protect ear canal during showers (use cotton with petrolatum in external canal or physician-approved earplugs; wear a shower cap over ears).
- Avoid swimming during infection or after a perforated eardrum; avoid swimming in contaminated water when infection is healed.
- Continue antibiotic therapy for prescribed number of days, even when symptoms disappear.
- Get adequate and early treatment of upper respiratory tract infections and allergic conditions.

CARE OF INFECTED EAR

- Use correct eardrop insertion or ear irrigations, as prescribed.
- Wash hands before and after changing cotton plugs to prevent secondary infection.
- Keep external ear clean and dry to protect skin from drainage.

SIGNS REQUIRING MEDICAL ATTENTION

- Fever
- Return of ear pain or discharge

Mastoiditis is difficult to treat and may require antibiotic therapy intravenously for several days. Because children are most often affected, immediate treatment of the infection is crucial. Residual hearing loss may follow the infection. If early decalcification is present, intense antibiotic therapy and myringotomy can usually cure mastoiditis; if it has progressed to further destruction, simple mastoidectomy is necessary.

Labyrinthitis

Etiology and Pathophysiology

Labyrinthitis is an inflammation of the labyrinthine canals of the inner ear. Labyrinthitis is the most common cause of **vertigo** (the sensation that the outer world is revolving about oneself or that one is moving in space). A common cause is a viral upper respiratory tract infection that spreads into the inner ear; other causes include certain drugs and foods. The vestibular portion of the inner ear may be destroyed by streptomycin. Tobacco and alcohol may also be causative factors. A rarer form of labyrinthitis is caused by bacteria. It is usually associated with middle-ear and mastoid infections. Since the advent of antibiotics, bacterial labyrinthitis occurs infrequently.

Clinical Manifestations

Severe and sudden vertigo is the most common symptom of labyrinthitis. Also present are nausea and vomiting, nystagmus, photophobia, headache, and ataxic gait.

Assessment

Subjective data include the frequency and duration of the vertigo and any safety measures taken by the patient during an attack. Assess other symptoms such as hearing ability, ringing in the ears, and nausea. Because fear is associated with the attacks, explore the patient's feelings.

Collection of **objective data** includes noting vomiting and any jerking movement of the eyeballs, unilaterally or bilaterally. Assess the color and moisture of skin to determine the extent of autonomic response.

Diagnostic Tests

Electronystagmography may show a diminished or absent nystagmus with stimulation. Audiometric testing shows a low-tone sensorineural hearing loss.

Medical Management

Labyrinthitis has no specific treatment. Usually antibiotics and dimenhydrinate (Dramamine) or meclizine (Antivert) for vertigo are prescribed. If nausea and vomiting persist, administer parenteral fluids.

Nursing Interventions and Patient Teaching

It is important to note the frequency and degree of vertigo. Administer antibiotics and medications and assess fluid intake to ensure that dehydration does not occur.

Nursing diagnoses and interventions for the patient with labyrinthitis include but are not limited to the following:

Nursing Diagnoses	Nursing Interventions
Risk for injury, related to altered sensory perception (vertigo)	Keep side rails up. Note presence of vertigo before patient ambulates. Supervise ambulation. Caution the patient not to attempt ambulation alone and to call for assistance.
Fear, related to altered sensory perception (vertigo)	Explore patient's feelings about attack. Teach patient concerning actions during an attack (see Patient Teaching box). Reinforce physician's treatment orders.

Instruct the patient about vertigo and how it is treated (see Patient Teaching box).

Prognosis

Labyrinthitis usually resolves itself, with little or no hearing impairment.

Obstructions of the Ear

Etiology and Pathophysiology

Ear canal obstruction is usually caused by impaction or excessive secretion of cerumen or by foreign bodies, including insects. Children often place beans, beads,

Patient Teaching

Vertigo

- Nature of the disorder
  - —Physiologic basis for the vertigo
  - —Avoidance of any known precipitating factors
  - —Rationale for a low-salt diet
- Actions to take during an attack
  - —Lie down immediately, and call for help if necessary at the first signs of an attack.
  - —If driving when an attack occurs, pull over immediately to the curb.
  - —Lie immobile and hold head in one position until vertigo lessens.
- Ask for assistance when ambulating if dizzy.
- Take prescribed medications as instructed even if no recent attacks have occurred; check with physician before discontinuing any medication.
- Seek medical attention for changes in symptoms or in the nature of attacks.

pebbles, and small toys in their ears. Usually those objects are found on routine examination. Obstruction by cerumen can be caused when excessive amounts are produced by overactive glands or from impaction of cerumen in narrow or tortuous ear canals.

Clinical Manifestations

The obstruction may cause the ear to feel occluded. The patient may have tinnitus or buzzing, pain in the ear, and slight hearing loss.

Assessment

Collection of **subjective data** includes interviewing the patient about any possible foreign bodies being introduced into the ear and any home remedies used to remove the object. If the patient is a child, determine risk factors related to ear obstructions, such as beads or nuts.

Collection of **objective data** involves noting any presence of a foreign body in the external ear canal. Observe children for tugging of the pinna.

Diagnostic Tests

Otoscopic examination provides visualization of the cause of the obstruction.

Medical Management

Medical management includes removal of cerumen by irrigation or cerumen spoon. Remove foreign objects with forceps, if possible. Smother insects with drops of an oily substance and remove them with forceps. Medications, such as carbamide peroxide 6.5%, may be used to soften cerumen. Surgical removal of the foreign object may be necessary.

Nursing Interventions and Patient Teaching

Assist with the irrigation of the ear. Instill medications into the ear as ordered.

A nursing diagnosis and interventions for the patient with obstructions of the ear include but are not limited to the following:

Nursing Diagnosis	Nursing Interventions
Disturbed sensory perception (auditory), related to presence of foreign body causing obstruction	Note the presence and amount of hearing impairment and tinnitus. Assure the patient (or parents) that once the obstruction is removed, any hearing loss or tinnitus should disappear.

Inform the patient and parents about the danger of placing objects in the ears. Also reinforce the method for preventing cerumen obstruction by instilling one or two drops of an oily substance at night. This is followed by hydrogen peroxide in the morning and cleaning with a soft cotton wick.

Prognosis

Ear canal obstructions caused by cerumen and foreign bodies resolve completely with treatment. Vertigo may be experienced temporarily until the ear canal dries. The older adult may become disoriented from the cerumen impaction and temporary loss of hearing.

NONINFECTIOUS DISORDERS OF THE EAR

Otosclerosis

Etiology and Pathophysiology

Otosclerosis is a condition characterized by chronic progressive deafness caused by the formation of spongy bone, especially around the oval window, with resulting ankylosis (immobility of a joint) of the stapes. Formation of new bone in adolescence or early adulthood progresses slowly. Gradual replacement of normal bone in the otic capsula by highly vascular otosclerotic bone occurs. This replacement bone is described as spongy. Calcification of the area follows, and the fixation of the footplate of the stapes in the oval window causes tinnitus and then deafness.

Otosclerosis is an autosomal dominant genetic disease. Women are affected twice as often as men. Otosclerosis is bilateral in about 80% of patients. Frequently pregnancy triggers a rapid onset of this condition. Previous ear infections are not believed to be related to otosclerosis.

Clinical Manifestations

The patient with otosclerosis experiences a slowly progressive conductive hearing loss and a low- to medium-pitched tinnitus. The deafness is usually first noted between the ages of 11 and 20.

Assessment

Subjective data include the degree and progression of hearing loss or tinnitus and mild dizziness to vertigo. Assess family history for the disease.

Collection of **objective data** includes assessment of behavioral clues related to hearing loss (see Box 53-2).

Diagnostic Tests

Otoscopy reveals a normal eardrum. A pink blush called **Schwartz's sign** may be seen through the ear; this indicates a high degree of vascularity in active otosclerotic bone. The result of the Rinne test shows sounds transmitted by bone conduction lasting longer than by air conduction in the affected ear. Weber's test results are the reverse from those of normal hearing. Both Weber's test and audiometric testing show a lateralization of sound more to the affected ear. Audiometric testing may show minimal to total hearing loss. Tympanometry may reveal evidence of stiffness in the sound conduction system. Hearing loss ranges from mild in the early stages to total loss in the later stages.

Medical Management

Sodium fluoride with vitamin D and calcium carbonate may be used to stabilize the hearing loss that results from otosclerosis. These agents help retard bone resorption and promote calcification of bony lesions. There is normal inner ear function; therefore amplification of sound by using a hearing aid can be effective (Lewis et al., 2007). Surgical treatment with stapedectomy restores hearing. The ear with poorer hearing is repaired first, and the other ear may be operated on 6 months to a year later. When a stapedectomy is not indicated, an air conduction hearing aid may be prescribed.

Nursing Interventions and Patient Teaching

Nursing diagnoses and interventions of otosclerosis are specific to poststapedectomy care. For patient teaching, see the discussion on ear surgery.

Prognosis

Patients report varying degrees of success with hearing after stapedectomy surgery. For some patients, stapedectomy is successful in permanently restoring hearing. A hearing aid may further enhance sound conduction to more normal levels.

Ménière's Disease

Etiology and Pathophysiology

Ménière's disease is a chronic disease of the inner ear characterized by recurrent episodes of vertigo, progressive unilateral nerve deafness, and tinnitus. Ménière's disease is most common in women between 30 and 60 years of age. The cause is unknown, although occasionally the condition follows middle-ear infection or trauma to the head.

There is an increase in endolymph fluid, either from increased production or decreased absorption. This causes increased pressure in the inner-ear labyrinth. Attacks of severe vertigo, tinnitus, and progressive deafness result from this increased pressure. Usually one ear only is involved.

Clinical Manifestations

The patient experiences recurrent episodes of vertigo with associated nausea, vomiting, diaphoresis, tinnitus, and nystagmus. A sense of fullness in the ear and hearing loss may be present. These attacks last from a few minutes to several hours. Attacks may occur several times a year. Sudden movements often aggravate the symptoms.

Assessment

Collection of **subjective data** includes noting the frequency and severity of the vertigo attack. The patient may complain of tinnitus. Note the patient's history and knowledge of the disorder and circumstances that precipitate an attack. Assess actions taken by the patient during an attack and the degree of relief those actions provide.

Collection of **objective data** includes determining unilateral or bilateral hearing loss. Observe the patient for associated signs during an attack.

Diagnostic Tests

Diagnostic tests are ordered to rule out central nervous system disease. The audiogram demonstrates a mild low-frequency sensorineural hearing loss. Audiologic tuning fork tests show a sensorineural deficit. Vestibular testing shows lack of balance. A glycerol test is performed, in which the patient is given a dose of glycerol orally followed by audiograms over the next 3 hours. A diagnosis of Ménière's disease is made if the patient's speech and hearing improve after taking the glycerol. The improvement is due to the osmotic effect of glycerol that pulls fluid from the inner ear (Lewis et al., 2007).

Medical Management

There is no specific therapy for Ménière's disease. Fluid restriction, diuretics, and a low-salt diet are prescribed in an attempt to decrease fluid pressure. Advise the patient to avoid caffeine and nicotine.

Dimenhydrinate, meclizine, diazepam (Valium), diphenhydramine (Benadryl) and fentanyl with droperidol (Innovar) may be prescribed for use between attacks to reduce the vertigo. In acute attacks the medications may be given intravenously. Atropine is also given for its anticholinergic effect during these acute attacks.

For preservation of hearing, surgical procedures may be performed. Approximately 5% to 10% of the patients with Ménière's disease require surgery. These surgeries and subsequent nursing interventions are discussed in Table 53-7.

Table 53-7 Surgery for Ménière's Disease

TYPE	DESCRIPTION	RESIDUAL	POSTOPERATIVE NURSING INTERVENTIONS
Surgical destruction of labyrinth	Extraction of membranous labyrinth by suction; access to inner ear through external canal (stapes and incus removed)	Destroys remaining hearing	Keep patient on bed rest and NPO until vertigo subsides in 1-3 days. Avoid sudden movement of head for 1-2 weeks. Take action to prevent falls from unsteadiness for 1-3 weeks.
Endolymphatic subarachnoid shunt	Insertion of drain tube from endolymphatic sac into subarachnoid space; access through mastoid	Preserves hearing in 60%-70% of patients	Monitor for vertigo (rare).
Cryosurgery	Application of intense cold to lateral semicircular canals to decrease sensitivity or to create an otic-periotic shunt; access through mastoid	Preserves hearing in 80% of patients	Monitor for dizziness for 2 days. Take action to prevent falls from unsteadiness for 2-3 weeks.
Vestibular nerve section	Dissection of cranial nerve VIII (vestibular portion); access through mastoid or through cranial drilling over roof of internal auditory canal	Preserves hearing in 90% of patients	Same as for surgical destruction of labyrinth.

NPO, Nothing by mouth.

Nursing Interventions and Patient Teaching

Maintain the prescribed low-salt diet and administer diuretics as ordered. Acute vertigo is treated symptomatically with bed rest, sedation, and antiemetics or medications for motion sickness. Nursing interventions are planned to minimize vertigo and provide for patient safety. During an acute attack keep the patient in a quiet, darkened room in a comfortable position. The patient may have some auditory deficit, which requires alternate methods of communication. If the patient's tinnitus becomes distressing, an increase in background noise, such as music, may provide relief. Fluorescent or flickering lights or watching television may exacerbate symptoms and should be avoided. Have an emesis basin available because vomiting is common.

Nursing diagnoses and interventions for the patient with Ménière's disease include but are not limited to the following:

Nursing Diagnoses	Nursing Interventions
Risk for injury, related to sensory-perceptual alterations (vertigo)	Keep side rails up. Assist with ambulation and instruct the patient to call for assistance before attempting to ambulate. Have the patient sit or lie down when vertigo occurs. Have the patient move slowly and avoid turning the head suddenly. Administer medications as prescribed. Position patient on unaffected side. Stand in front of patient and prevent head turning. Avoid bright or glaring lights around patient. Place all needed supplies so that patient does not have to turn head.
Social isolation, related to unpredictable vertigo attacks	Assess factors that contribute to social isolation. Assess feelings of loneliness and abandonment. Identify support systems for patient. Identify patient concerns. Establish effective communication.

Provide information about a low-salt diet and taking diuretics. Warn the patient to avoid reading when vertigo or tinnitus is present. Instruct the patient to avoid smoking to prevent vasoconstriction. The patient should learn to identify precipitating factors and the proper actions to take when an attack occurs: (1) sit or lie down immediately, (2) stop the car and pull over to the side of the road, and (3) keep medication available at all times (Nursing Care Plan 53-2).

 Nursing Care Plan 53-2 **The Patient with Ménière's Disease**

Ms. Luison is a 66-year-old patient admitted with Ménière's disease. She complains of severe dizziness, nausea, vomiting, ringing in the ears, hearing loss, and an unsteady gait. She is accompanied by her husband of 35 years.

NURSING DIAGNOSIS ***Anxiety, related to effect of disorder***

Patient Goals and Expected Outcomes	Nursing Interventions	Evaluation
Patient will experience decreased signs and symptoms of anxiety Patient will control her anxiety	Encourage patient to explore concerns about decreased hearing and effects of vertigo attacks and to take action in relation to the concerns. Explore patient's knowledge of the disorder and correct misunderstandings. Educate patient on strategies that can give her back some control over her life. Suggest keeping an emesis basin, a pillow, a blanket, a car phone, and a large sign with the words "HELP, POLICE" in the car in case of a sudden Ménière's attack. Encourage realistic hope about expected hearing ability as described by physician. Refer patient to necessary support services, such as social worker or audiologist. Refer patient for more information to Vestibular Disorders Association (VEDA; www.vestibular.org).	Patient states that level of anxiety has decreased.

NURSING DIAGNOSIS ***Risk for injury, related to vestibular auditory alterations***

Patient Goals and Expected Outcomes	Nursing Interventions	Evaluation
Patient will describe actions to avoid vertigo Patient will remain free of injury Patient will remain safe from falls	Help patient identify avoidable actions that precipitate vertigo attacks. Encourage patient to move slowly and not turn head suddenly when vertigo is present. If tinnitus is distressing, increase background noises, such as music. If hearing is decreased: • Use measures to facilitate communication with hearing impaired. • Carry wax earplugs; even after losing some hearing, ears are often sensitive to loud noises, which can trigger vertigo. • Refer patient to audiologist, if appropriate. Keep side rails up when patient with vertigo is in bed. Assist with ambulation as needed. Encourage patient to sit or lie down and to remain immobile if signs of dizziness occur. Teach patient to stop car at side of road immediately at first signs of dizziness while driving.	Patient avoids physical environment that could cause injury. Patient does not manifest evidence of injury.

Critical Thinking Questions

1. Ms. Luison states that she would prefer going to the bathroom without the assistance of a nurse. What is an appropriate response by the nurse?
2. Ms. Luison tells the nurse that she is depressed because of her unpleasant symptoms and wonders if she will ever feel well again. What would be a therapeutic reply?
3. The nurse notes an unpleasant odor from Ms. Luison; her hair is unkempt, and she has poor oral hygiene. The nurse is preparing to give her a warm, therapeutic bed bath. Ms. Luison states, "I feel too dizzy to take a bath." What nursing interventions would help promote personal hygiene and patient compliance?

Prognosis

Approximately 75% to 85% of patients experience improvement with medical management and supportive therapy. The remainder of patients may, in time, require surgical intervention. Usually several yearly attacks occur until the disease either resolves itself or progresses to complete deafness in the affected ear.

SURGERIES OF THE EAR

STAPEDECTOMY

Stapedectomy is the removal of the stapes of the middle ear and insertion of a graft and prosthesis, performed to restore hearing in cases of otosclerosis. The stapes that has become fixed is replaced so that vibrations can again transmit sound waves through the oval window to the fluid of the inner ear.

Using a local anesthetic and an operating microscope for visualization, the surgeon removes the stapes and covers the opening into the inner ear with a graft of body tissue. One end of a small plastic tube or piece of stainless steel wire is attached to the graft, while the other end is attached to the two remaining bones of the middle ear, the malleus and the incus.

Nursing Interventions

Postoperative management consists of external ear packing to ensure healing; the packing is left in place for 5 or 6 days. Depending on physician preference, the patient remains in bed for approximately 24 hours and resumes activity gradually. Keep the patient flat with the operative side facing upward to maintain the position of the prosthesis and graft; make certain that the patient is not turned. Headache, nausea, vomiting, and dizziness are expected early in the postoperative period as a result of stimulation of the labyrinth intraoperatively. The patient's hearing does not improve until the edema subsides and the packing is removed by the physician (see Patient Teaching box).

Possible complications of the stapedectomy include infection of the external, middle, or inner ear. Displacement or rejection of the prosthesis or graft may occur, or perilymph fluid may leak around the prosthesis into the middle ear, causing ringing in the ears and vertigo.

Prognosis

During surgery the patient often reports an immediate improvement in hearing in the operative ear. Because of the accumulation of blood and fluid in the middle ear, the hearing level decreases postoperatively but does return to near-normal levels. After stapedectomy, 90% of patients experience an improvement in hearing, in many instances to near-normal levels.

Patient Teaching

After Ear Surgery

- Change cotton in ear daily as prescribed.
- Open mouth when sneezing or coughing and blow nose gently one side at a time for 1 week (to prevent increased ear pressure and infection).
- Keep ear dry for 6 weeks (to prevent infection).
  —Do not wash hair for 1 week.
  —Protect ear when outdoors using two pieces of cotton (use petrolatum jelly on outer ball).
  —Protect ear with shower cap when bathing.
- Wear ear protectors as necessary to prevent exposure to loud noises.
- Follow activity guidelines:
  —No physical activity for 1 week.
  —No exercises or active sports for 3 weeks.
  —Return to work in 1 week (3 weeks for strenuous work).
- Avoid exposure to people with upper respiratory tract infections.
- Avoid airplane flights for at least 1 week (to prevent effects of pressure changes).

TYMPANOPLASTY

Tympanoplasty is any of several operative procedures on the eardrum or ossicles of the middle ear to restore or improve hearing in patients with conductive hearing loss. These operations may be used to repair a perforated eardrum, for otosclerosis, or for dislocation or necrosis of a small bone of the middle ear.

Nursing Interventions

Postoperative management consists of bed rest until the next morning. Elevate the head of the bed 40 degrees, and have the operative side facing upward. Medications include opioid analgesics, otic and oral antibiotics, and meclizine for vertigo.

Postoperatively monitor and report the presence of bleeding; the amount, color, and consistency of drainage; and temperature. Note complaints of vertigo when the patient is getting out of bed; with sudden movements, nausea and vertigo may occur. Possible complications include infection and displacement of the graft.

Nursing diagnoses and interventions for the patient after a tympanoplasty include but are not limited to the following:

Nursing Diagnoses	Nursing Interventions
Impaired physical mobility, related to surgical procedure	Note patient's ability to comply with bed rest order. Keep the patient's operative side up; do not allow the patient to be turned.
Risk for activity intolerance, related to pain and vertigo	Keep side rails up. When movement is allowed, begin gradually. Administer prescribed medications for pain and vertigo as needed. Assist with ambulation to prevent injury.

Prognosis
Hearing will improve if there is no involvement of the ossicles.

MYRINGOTOMY
Myringotomy, also called tympanotomy, is a surgical incision of the eardrum. It is performed to relieve pressure and release purulent exudate from the middle ear. The procedure is done with the patient under either local or general anesthesia. A myringotomy may be performed in one of two ways: (1) using a myringotomy knife, the surgeon makes a curved incision in the drumhead; or (2) a heated wire loop is touched for about 1 second to the drumhead, producing a 2-mm hole.

Nursing Interventions and Patient Teaching
Purulent exudate and fluid may drain immediately, requiring suctioning. Cotton placed in the ear absorbs drainage, which may continue several days. Change the cotton frequently to avoid recontamination of the surgical area. The incision usually heals quickly with little scarring. Hearing is not usually disrupted.

Medications commonly used are tetracycline (Achromycin V) and polymyxin B (Neosporin) eardrops as antiinfective agents. Tylenol with codeine may be used for pain. Monitor for signs of bleeding and reports any occurrence. Note incisional pain or hearing impairment.

Patient teaching involves providing the information in the Patient Teaching box (p. 1880) and ensuring the patient understands.

Prognosis
Once pressure is relieved, hearing is restored to more normal levels unless scarring is present.

COCHLEAR IMPLANT
The cochlear implant is a hearing device for the profoundly deaf. The system consists of a surgically implanted induction coil beneath the skin behind the ear and an electrode wire placed in the cochlea (Figure 53-15). The implanted parts interface with an externally worn speech processor. The system stimulates auditory nerve fibers by an electric current so that signals reach the brainstem's auditory nuclei and ultimately the auditory cortex. The implant is intended for the patient whose sensorineural hearing loss is either congenital or acquired. A small computer changes the spoken words into electrical impulses that are transmitted to the implanted cochlear coil. The ideal candidate is one who became deaf after acquiring speech and language. The adult who was born deaf or became deaf before learning to speak may be considered a candidate for a cochlear implant if she or he has followed an aural-oral educational approach.

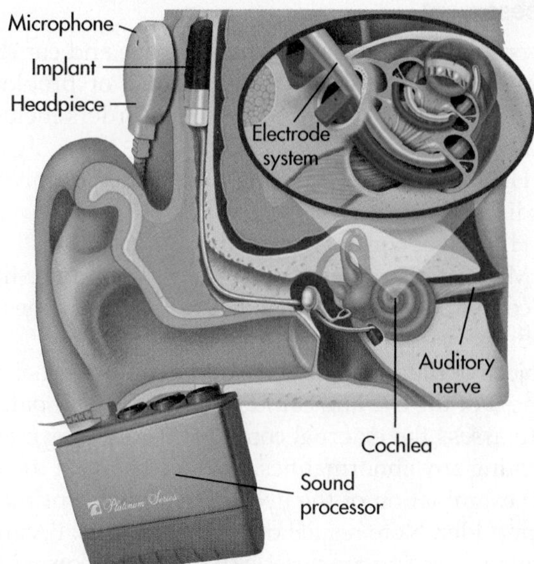

FIGURE 53-15 Cochlear implant.

The implant offers the profoundly deaf the ability to hear environmental sounds, including speech, at comfortable loudness levels. Multichannel cochlear implants also aid in speech production. Extensive training and rehabilitation are essential to receive maximum benefit from these implants. The positive aspects of a cochlear implant include providing sound to the person who heard none, improving the sense of security, and decreasing the feelings of isolation. With continued research, the cochlear implant may offer the possibility of hearing rehabilitation for a wider range of hearing-impaired individuals.

The deaf community is concerned with cultural pride. They believe that life without hearing is healthy and functional and that deafness is not a disease that needs to be cured. The National Association of the Deaf originally opposed use of cochlear implants; it now endorses their use, stating, "cochlear implantation is a technology that represents a tool to be used in some forms of communication, and not a cure for deafness" (Munson, 2006).

❖ NURSING PROCESS *for the Patient with a Visual or Auditory Disorder*
The role of the licensed practical nurse/licensed vocational nurse (LPN/LVN) in the nursing process as stated is that the LPN/LVN will:
- Participate in planning care for patients based on patient needs
- Review patient's care plan and recommend revisions as needed
- Review and follow defined prioritization for patient care
- Use clinical pathways, care maps, or care plans to guide and review patient care

Assessment

The complexity of the assessment for eye and ear disorders depends on the patient's disease or problem. Subjective data for both eye and ear disorders include the following:

- Health history, including any acute or chronic disease
- History of current complaint
- Medications, including prescription, over-the-counter, and home remedies or folk medicines
- Surgery and other treatments

Objective data include the external and internal assessment of the eye and ear. Use inspection and palpation to assess the external components of the eye and ear, noting any abnormalities. Review results of the internal examination of the eye and ear by the primary care provider. Note results of diagnostic tests. Because seeing and hearing are necessary for safety, communication, self-care, and psychosocial interaction, assess these areas as well.

Nursing Diagnosis

Nursing assessment identifies the patient's needs. Care is based on the nursing diagnoses that have been identified. Possible nursing diagnoses include the following:

- Ineffective health maintenance
- Anxiety
- Self-care deficit (specify)
- Fear
- Impaired environmental interpretation syndrome
- Impaired home maintenance
- Impaired social interaction
- Risk for injury
- Risk for loneliness
- Disturbed sensory perception: auditory
- Disturbed sensory perception: visual
- Social isolation

Expected Outcomes and Planning

Impairment of vision or hearing requires a major adjustment in the life of an individual. The patient must adjust to the loss and changes in lifestyle, whether the loss is permanent or temporary. The care plan focuses on achieving specific goals and outcomes that relate to the identified nursing diagnoses. Examples of these include:

Goal 1: Patient will remain free of injury.

Outcome: Patient and family inspect environment for potential hazards related to loss of vision or hearing.

Goal 2: Patient will remain socially active.

Outcome: Patient displays interest in social and recreational activities.

Implementation

Measures used in the care of a patient with vision or hearing loss center around helping the patient remain physically and emotionally safe and secure and ensuring that the patient's needs are communicated and met while adjusting to the loss. Nursing interventions include promoting safety, assisting with ADLs, facilitating communication, and encouraging diversional activity. Also assess readiness to learn and teach health promotion practices (see Patient Teaching boxes throughout this chapter). Consider the patient's culture, beliefs, values, and habits and the special needs of the older adult.

Evaluation

Systematic evaluation requires determining whether expected outcomes have been met. Refer to the goals and outcomes identified when assisting in planning care and evaluating the achievement of the goals. Examples of goals and their evaluative measures include:

Goal 1: Patient will remain free of injury.

Evaluative measure: Ask patient and family to describe what environmental changes need to be made to ensure safety.

Goal 2: Patient will remain socially active.

Evaluative measure: Observe patient participating in social activities.

Get Ready for the NCLEX® Examination!

Key Points

- The five major senses are taste, touch, smell, sight, and hearing and balance.
- The accessory structures of the eye are the eyebrows, the eyelids, the eyelashes, and the lacrimal apparatus.
- The three tunics of the eyeball are the fibrous tunic (sclera), the vascular tunic (choroid), and the retina.
- The two chambers of the eye are the anterior chamber, which contains aqueous humor, and the posterior chamber, which contains vitreous humor.
- Image formation at the retina requires four basic processes: refraction, accommodation, constriction, and convergence.
- The photoreceptors of the retina are the rods and cones. The rods control vision in dim light, and the cones control vision in bright light. The cones are also responsible for color vision.
- Light entering the eye must travel through the cornea, the aqueous humor, the pupil, the crystalline lens, the vitreous humor, and finally the retina.
- The ear is divided into external, middle, and inner ears.
- The external ear flap is called the pinna (auricle); it extends into the external ear canal.
- The middle ear contains the ossicles and the entrance of the eustachian tube and ends with the tympanic membrane.
- The inner ear contains the vestibule, the cochlea, and the semicircular canals.
- The organ of Corti is the organ of hearing; it is located within the cochlea.
- The semicircular canals are responsible for the sense of balance and equilibrium.
- The taste buds differentiate four basic tastes: sweet, sour, salty, and bitter.
- Normal aging causes decreased hearing and sight as a result of normal changes of the structures.
- Individuals who have chronic disease or are older than 40 years of age should be examined yearly to detect eye abnormalities or prescribe changes in therapy.
- Refractory errors include hyperopia (farsightedness), presbyopia (farsightedness related to the aging process), and astigmatism (objects waver).
- Ranges of 20/20 to 20/40 vision are considered normal, whereas 20/200 with correction is defined as legal blindness.
- ARMD is divided into two classic forms: dry (atrophic) and wet (exudative). In dry ARMD, which accounts for 90% of patients with ARMD, the macular cells have wasted or atrophied. Wet ARMD is characterized by the development of abnormal blood vessels in or near the macula.
- Cataracts are an opacity of the lens and may be removed by intracapsular or extracapsular extraction.
- Glaucoma is not one disease, but rather a group of disorders characterized by (1) increased IOP and the consequences of elevated pressure, (2) optic nerve atrophy, and (3) peripheral visual field loss.
- Loss of hearing may result from cerumen buildup, infection, trauma, or use of ototoxic drugs, or it may be a congenital condition.
- Conductive hearing loss is a decrease in amplification, whereas sensorineural hearing loss is interference within the inner ear.
- Prevention of serious complications of ear disorders, such as infections, mastoiditis, and brain abscess, requires early detection and treatment.
- *Injury, risk for,* is the primary nursing diagnosis for the patient experiencing vertigo, which occurs in labyrinthitis and Ménière's disease.
- An essential communication tip for speaking to the hearing impaired is to face the patient and to speak clearly without shouting.
- A cochlear implant is a hearing device for the profoundly deaf. The implanted device is intended for the patient with sensorineural hearing loss.

Additional Learning Resources

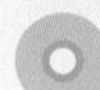

Go to your Companion CD-ROM for an audio glossary, animations, video clips, and more.

evolve Be sure to visit the Evolve site at http://evolve.elsevier.com/Christensen/adult/ for additional online resources.

Review Questions for the NCLEX® Examination

1. The patient is to have a laser treatment to cauterize hemorrhaging vessels caused by diabetic retinopathy. The name of the procedure is:
   1. enucleation.
   2. scleral buckle.
   3. photocoagulation.
   4. trabeculoplasty.
2. The parents of an 11-year-old patient want to know more about their child's conductive hearing loss. The nurse would explain that:
   1. sound is delivered through the external and middle ear, but a defect in the inner ear results in distortion of sound.
   2. sound is inadequately delivered through the external or middle ear to the inner ear.
   3. there is no organic cause, but a functional problem exists.
   4. the brain's auditory pathways are damaged.
3. The patient has impaired hearing. To facilitate communication, the nurse would:
   1. face the patient when speaking.
   2. overaccentuate words to make the communication more effective.
   3. shout to allow the patient to hear.
   4. use one-word answers when speaking.

4. The patient tells the nurse he has dizziness. He states that the doctor used another term. The medical term is:
   1. tinnitus.
   2. labyrinthitis.
   3. sensorineural.
   4. vertigo.
5. The patient is diagnosed with an inner ear problem. The major symptom would be:
   1. echoing.
   2. intense pain.
   3. vertigo.
   4. loss of hearing.
6. Evaluation of the eye as it adjusts to seeing objects at various distances is called:
   1. PERRLA.
   2. refraction.
   3. focusing.
   4. accommodation.
7. The patient has tunnel vision, eye pain, difficulty in adjusting to darkness, halos seen around lights, and failure to detect colors. These indicate:
   1. primary open-angle glaucoma.
   2. cataracts.
   3. entropion.
   4. detached retina.
8. Which of the following would be a safety hazard in the home of a patient who is visually impaired?
   1. Area rug
   2. Room carpeting
   3. Tile floor
   4. Concrete flooring
9. An older adult falls at home, resulting in a blunt injury of an eyeball. The eye is tearing excessively, and the patient complains of a severe stabbing pain as if "something is in my eye!" First aid measures would include:
   1. applying a cool compress three times a day (tid).
   2. lightly covering the eye with a sterile gauze pad.
   3. removing any particles that may be embedded in the eye.
   4. irrigating the eye with tap water.
10. The patient has just had cataract surgery. Important discharge instructions would include: *(Select all that apply.)*
    1. wearing an eyeshield at night on the operative eye.
    2. avoiding bending, stooping, coughing, or lifting.
    3. instilling prescribed eyedrops into the conjunctival sac.
    4. administering an analgesic every 4 hours on a regular basis.
11. Which assessment finding would indicate a need for possible glaucoma testing?
    1. Presence of "floaters"
    2. Colored halos around lights
    3. Intermittent loss of vision
    4. Pruritus and erythema of the conjunctiva
12. While communicating with a patient, you notice a possible hearing deficit in one ear. Which nursing intervention would be appropriate?
    1. Shout in the affected ear.
    2. Speak clearly and in a slightly louder voice toward the patient's face.
    3. Plug the affected ear and shout in the unaffected ear.
    4. Speak more softly than usual in the affected ear.
13. What is the most likely cause of hearing loss in the older adult?
    1. Cerumen buildup
    2. Ossification of the pinna
    3. Low batteries in the hearing aid
    4. Fluid in the ear
14. Patients with permanent visual impairment:
    1. feel most comfortable with other visually impaired people.
    2. may experience the same grieving process that is associated with other losses.
    3. may feel threatened when others make eye contact during a conversation.
    4. usually need others to speak loudly so they can communicate appropriately.
15. A 32-year-old construction worker suffered a penetrating wound to the eye. The best intervention for anyone at the scene to take is to:
    1. gently remove the object.
    2. wipe away the blood and tears.
    3. cover the object with a paper cup and tape.
    4. do nothing; rush to the hospital.
16. A 71-year-old patient complains of being severely dizzy. The nurse should encourage the patient to:
    1. avoid sudden movements.
    2. avoid noises.
    3. increase fluid intake.
    4. lie on affected side.
17. The patient has been blind for the past 10 years. He is hospitalized with heart failure. In the care of a long-term blind individual, it is important to:
    1. keep all items at a distance so he won't bump into them.
    2. schedule a consultation with an occupational therapist to teach activities of daily living.
    3. announce when you enter and leave the room.
    4. initiate a referral to the Department of Health and Human Services.
18. The patient has a family history of cataracts. He asks what symptom would be present if he begins to develop them. The nurse might respond that the first symptoms of a cataract are usually:
    1. pain in the eyes.
    2. blurred vision.
    3. loss of peripheral vision.
    4. dry eyes.

19. The patient has had cataract surgery. Discharge teaching would include:

1. lifting light objects is acceptable.
2. wearing eyepatches for the first 72 hours.
3. bending at the knees and keeping the head straight.
4. bending at the waist is acceptable if done slowly.

20. The patient is scheduled for a stapedectomy. Appropriate postoperative teaching should include:

1. changing cotton from external ear canal hourly.
2. gently blowing both nares simultaneously.
3. teaching patient to open mouth when sneezing or coughing.
4. limiting activities for 3 weeks.

21. A 15-year-old hearing-impaired patient is having problems communicating with the staff. Which behavior would improve communication? *(Select all that apply.)*

1. Overaccentuating words
2. Facing the patient when speaking
3. Speaking in conversational tones
4. Asking permission to turn off television or radio

22. A 76-year-old patient is partially blind. His physician has diagnosed primary open-angle glaucoma. The goal of treatment in glaucoma is to:

1. decrease aqueous humor.
2. increase aqueous humor.
3. decrease discomfort.
4. restore vision.

23. The priority nursing responsibility while caring for a patient with vertigo is:

1. safety.
2. comfort.
3. hygiene.
4. quiet.

24. While cleaning the garage the patient splashed a chemical in his eyes. The initial priority following the chemical burn is to:

1. transport to a physician immediately.
2. cover the eyes with a sterile gauze.
3. irrigate with water for 15 minutes or longer.
4. irrigate with normal saline for 1 to 5 minutes.

25. The patient visits the physician for a routine physical examination that involves testing distance vision. As she faces the Snellen's chart, the nurse instructs the patient to:

1. use both eyes to read the chart.
2. read the chart from right to left.
3. cover one eye while testing the other.
4. use either eye because they will be the same.

26. A 49-year-old patient recently was blinded as a result of an automobile accident. This is her initial ambulation to the bathroom. What precautions should the nurse take when ambulating the patient?

1. Precede the patient with patient's hand on the nurse's elbow.
2. Follow the patient with the patient's hand on the nurse's elbow.
3. Walk in front of the patient, telling of any obstacles.
4. Walk behind the patient with the nurse's hand on the patient's shoulder.

27. The patient comes into the clinic complaining of progressive loss of vision in the center of his visual field. His physician would probably diagnose this condition as:

1. macular degeneration.
2. primary open-angle glaucoma.
3. color blindness.
4. retinal degeneration.

28. After cataract surgery the patient complains of sudden sharp pain in the operative eye. The nurse should immediately:

1. remove the metal eyeshield to relieve pressure.
2. call the physician.
3. administer an analgesic.
4. document complaint of pain on chart.

29. A surgical procedure for the treatment of retinal detachment is:

1. punctal sac repair.
2. radial keratotomy.
3. vitrectomy.
4. scleral buckling.

30. The ______ ______ is a surgically implanted hearing device for the profoundly deaf person whose sensorineural hearing loss is either congenital or acquired.

31. The patient is asked to sign a surgical consent for treatment of otosclerosis. Which statement indicates correct understanding of the procedure?

1. "It involves surgical repair of the external ear."
2. "It means cutting the nerve in my ear."
3. "It cleans the ear canal of wax."
4. "It will help me hear sounds again."

32. The area of most acute vision in which there is the greatest concentration of rods and cones in the retina is the:

1. fovea centralis.
2. optic chiasm.
3. optic disk.
4. ora serrata.

33. Two drugs used in treating open-angle glaucoma are:

1. atropine, Sulamyd.
2. Betoptic, pilocarpine.
3. Decadron, Liquifilm.
4. mannitol, Cyclogyl.

34. The triad of symptoms in Ménière's disease includes:

1. vertigo, sensorineural hearing loss, tinnitus.
2. sensorineural hearing loss, vomiting, nystagmus.
3. tinnitus, headache, vision changes.
4. headache, vertigo, vomiting.

chapter

54

Care of the Patient with a Neurologic Disorder

evolve

http://evolve.elsevier.com/Christensen/foundationsadult

Barbara Lauritsen Christensen

Objectives

Anatomy and Physiology

1. Name the two structural divisions of the nervous system and give the functions of each.
2. List the parts of the neuron, and describe the function of each part.
3. Explain the anatomical location and functions of the cerebrum, the brainstem, the cerebellum, the spinal cord, the peripheral nerves, and cerebrospinal fluid.
4. Discuss the parts of the peripheral nervous system and how the system works with the central nervous system.
5. List the 12 cranial nerves and the areas they serve.

Medical-Surgical

6. List physiologic changes that occur in the nervous system with aging.
7. Explain the importance of prevention in problems of the nervous system, and give several examples of prevention.
8. Identify the significant subjective and objective data related to the nervous system that should be obtained from a patient during assessment.
9. Differentiate between normal and common abnormal findings of a physical assessment of the nervous system.
10. Discuss the Glasgow coma scale
11. List common laboratory and diagnostic examinations for evaluation of neurologic disorders.
12. List five signs and symptoms of increased intracranial pressure, why they occur, and nursing interventions that decrease intracranial pressure.
13. Discuss various neurologic disturbances in motor function and sensory-perceptual function.
14. List four classifications of seizures, their characteristics, clinical signs, aura, and postictal period.
15. Give examples of six degenerative neurologic diseases and explain the etiology, pathophysiology, clinical manifestations, assessment, diagnostic tests, medical management, nursing interventions, and prognosis for each.
16. Discuss the etiology, pathophysiology, clinical manifestations, assessment, diagnostic tests, medical management, nursing interventions, and prognosis for a stroke patient.
17. Differentiate between trigeminal neuralgia and Bell's palsy.
18. Discuss the etiology, pathophysiology, clinical manifestations, assessment, diagnostic tests, medical management, nursing interventions, and prognosis for GBS, meningitis, encephalitis, and AIDS.
19. Explain the mechanism of injury to the brain that occurs with a stroke and traumatic brain injury.
20. Discuss the etiology, pathophysiology, clinical manifestations, assessment, diagnostic tests, medical management, nursing interventions, and prognosis for intracranial tumors, brain trauma, and spinal trauma.
21. Discuss patient teaching and home care planning for the patient with stroke, multiple sclerosis, Parkinson's disease, and myasthenia gravis.

Key Terms

agnosia (ăg-NŌ-zhă, p. 1911)
aneurysm (ĂN-ūr-ĭ-zĭm, p. 1932)
aphasia (ă-FĀ-zē-ă, p. 1895)
apraxia (ă-PRĂK-sē-ă, p. 1925)
ataxia (ă-TĂK-sē-ă, p. 1917)
aura (ĂW-ră, p. 1912)
bradykinesia (brā-dē-kĭ-NĒ-zē-ă, p. 1919)
deep brain stimulation (DBS) (p. 1921)
diplopia (dĭ-PLŌ-pē-ă, p. 1905)
dysarthria (dĭs-ĂHR-thrē-ă, p. 1895)
dysphagia (dĭs-FĀ-jē-ă, p. 1908)
flaccid (FLĂK-sĭd, p. 1896)
Glasgow coma scale (GLĂS-gō KŌ-mă skāl, p. 1894)
global cognitive dysfunction (GLŌ-băl KŎG-nĭ-tĭv dĭs-FŬNK-shŭn, p. 1942)
Guillain-Barré syndrome (GBS) (GĒ-yă bă-RĀ, p. 1939)
hemianopia (hĕm-ē-ă-NŌ-pē-ă, p. 1897)
hemiplegia (hĕm-ē-PLĒ-jă, p. 1909)
hyperreflexia (hī-pĕr-rē-FLĔK-sē-ă, p. 1946)
nystagmus (nĭs-TĂG-mŭs, p. 1917)
paresis (pă-RĒ-sĭs, p. 1896)
postictal period (pōst-ĬK-tăl PĒ-rē-ŏd, p. 1912)
proprioception (prō-prē-ō-SĔP-shŭn, p. 1897)
spastic (SPĂS-tĭk, p. 1896)
stroke (strōk, p. 1930)
unilateral neglect (ū-nĭ-LĂT-ĕr-ăl nĕ-GLĔCT, p. 1897)

ANATOMY AND PHYSIOLOGY OF THE NEUROLOGIC SYSTEM

The nervous system is responsible for communication and control within the body. It interprets or processes the information received and sends it to the appropriate area of the brain or spinal cord, where the response is generated. The nervous system is the body's link with the environment. It works in conjunction with the endocrine system to maintain the body's homeostasis. The nervous system reacts in split seconds, whereas the hormones secreted by the endocrine glands work more slowly in initiating a response. The clinical picture for the patient with neurologic problems is often complex. Understanding these conditions requires knowledge of the anatomy and physiology of the nervous system.

STRUCTURAL DIVISIONS

The nervous system has two main structural divisions. The first division, the central nervous system (CNS), is made up of the brain and the spinal cord. It occupies a medial position in the body and is responsible for interpreting incoming sensory information and issuing instructions based on past experiences. The second component is the peripheral nervous system, which lies outside the CNS.

The peripheral nervous system contains two main divisions: the somatic nervous system and the autonomic nervous system. The somatic nervous system sends messages from the CNS to the skeletal muscles (voluntary muscles). The autonomic system transmits messages from the CNS to the smooth muscle, the cardiac muscle, and certain glands. The autonomic system is sometimes called the **involuntary nervous system** because its action takes place without conscious control.

CELLS OF THE NERVOUS SYSTEM

Two broad categories of cells exist within the nervous system. The first category, the neurons, are the transmitter cells (Figure 54-1). They carry messages to and from the brain and spinal cord. The second category, the neuroglial or glial cells, are the support cells to the neurons. They support and protect the neurons while producing cerebrospinal fluid (CSF), which continuously bathes the structures of the CNS.

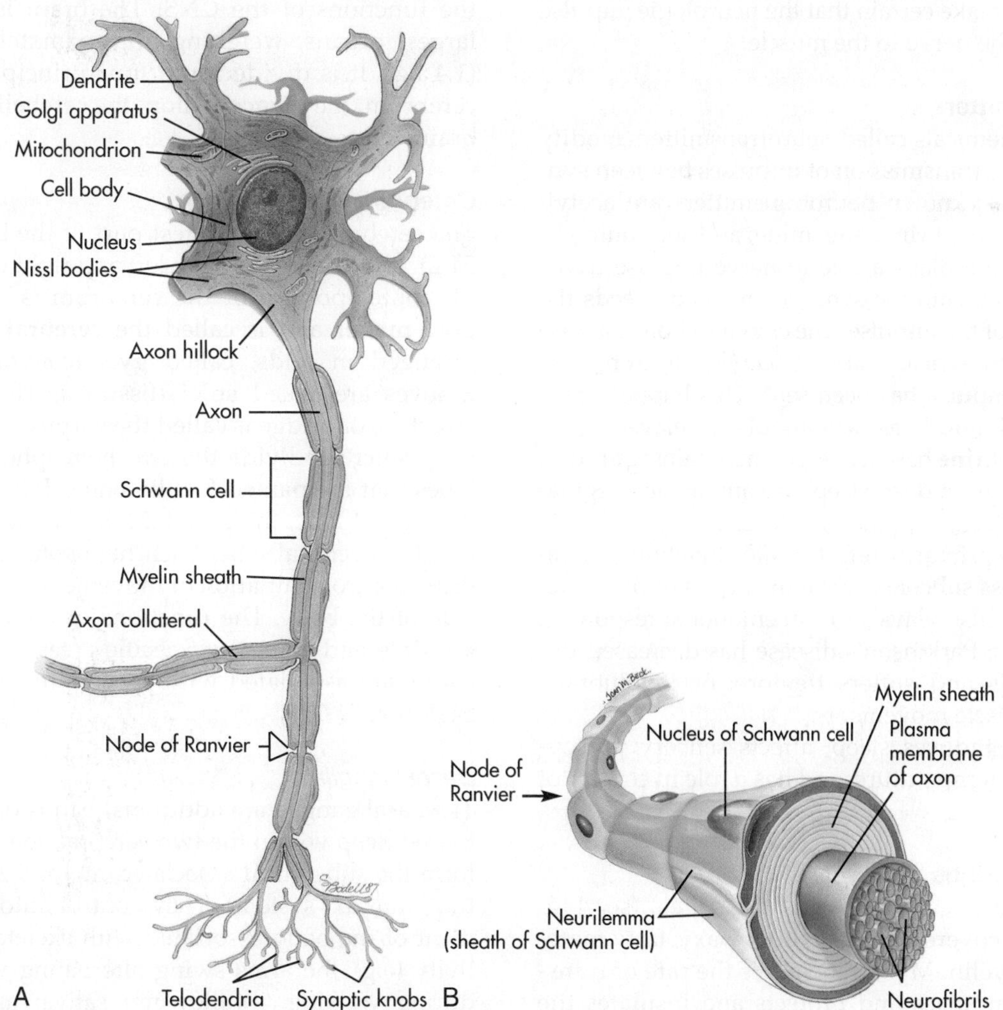

FIGURE 54-1 **A,** Diagram of a typical neuron showing dendrites, cell body, and axon. **B,** Myelinated axon, showing a cross-section of concentric layers of the Schwann cell filled with myelin.

Neuron

A neuron (nerve cell) is the basic cell of the nervous system. It is a separate unit composed of three main structures: the cell body, the axon, and the dendrites. The cell body contains a nucleus surrounded by cytoplasm. The axon is a cylindric extension of a nerve cell that conducts impulses away from the neuron cell body. The dendrites are branching structures that extend from a cell body and receive impulses. Between each neuron is a gap (space) called the synapse, defined as the region surrounding the point of contact between two neurons or between a neuron and an effector organ, across which nerve impulses are transmitted through the action of a neurotransmitter.

All neurons are governed by the "all or none law," which means there is never a partial transmission of a message; the impulse is either strong enough to elicit a response or too weak to generate the message.

Neuromuscular Junction

The area of contact between the ends of a large myelinated nerve fiber and a fiber of skeletal muscle is called the neuromuscular junction. This area of contact is necessary for the body to function. The neurotransmitters act to make certain that the neurologic impulse passes from the nerve to the muscle.

Neurotransmitters

Numerous chemicals called neurotransmitters modify or result in the transmission of impulses between synapses. The best-known neurotransmitters are acetylcholine, norepinephrine, dopamine, and serotonin.

Acetylcholine plays a role in nerve impulse transmission; it spills into the synapse area and speeds the transmission of the impulse. The enzyme cholinesterase is then released to deactivate the acetylcholine once the message or impulse has been sent. This happens rapidly and continuously as each impulse is relayed.

Norepinephrine has an effect on maintaining arousal (awakening from a deep sleep), dreaming, and regulation of mood (e.g., happiness, sadness).

Dopamine primarily affects motor function; it is involved in gross subconscious movements of the skeletal muscles. It also plays a role in emotional responses. A person with Parkinson's disease has decreased dopamine levels and suffers tremors, or involuntary, trembling muscle movements.

Serotonin induces sleep, affects sensory perception, controls temperature, and has a role in control of mood.

Neuron Coverings

Many neuron fibers (axons and dendrites) (see Figure 54-1) are covered with a white, waxy, fatty material called myelin. Myelin increases the rate of transmission of impulses and protects and insulates the fibers. Axons leaving the CNS are wrapped in layers of myelin with indentations called the nodes of Ranvier. These nodes further increase the rate of transmission because the impulse can jump from node to node.

In the peripheral nervous system the myelin is produced by Schwann cells (see Figure 54-1). The outer membrane of the Schwann cells gives rise to another layer called the neurilemma. The neurilemma is important because it helps regenerate injured axons. Thus regeneration of nerve cells occurs only in the peripheral nervous system. Cells damaged in the CNS result in permanent damage (paralysis) because they do not have neurilemma and are not able to regenerate.

CENTRAL NERVOUS SYSTEM

The **CNS**—one of the two main divisions of the nervous system, composed of the brain and the spinal cord—functions somewhat like a computer but is much more complex. The cranium protects the brain, and the vertebral column protects the spinal cord.

Brain

Specialized cells in the brain's mass of convoluted, soft, gray or white tissue coordinate and regulate the functions of the CNS. The brain is one of the largest organs, weighing approximately 3 pounds (1.4 kg). It is divided into four principal parts: the cerebrum, the diencephalon, the cerebellum, and the brainstem.

Cerebrum

The cerebrum is the largest part of the brain (Figure 54-2). It is divided into the left and right hemispheres. The outer portion of the cerebrum is composed of gray matter and is called the **cerebral cortex.** It is arranged in folds, called **gyri** (convolutions); the grooves are called **sulci** (fissures). The connecting structure or bridge is called the corpus callosum. Two deep sulci subdivide the two hemispheres into four lobes that are named for the bones lying over them: the frontal lobe, the parietal lobe, the temporal lobe, and the occipital lobe. Each hemisphere of the cerebrum controls initiation of movement on the opposite side of the body. The functions of the cerebrum are multiple and complex. Specific areas of the cerebral cortex are associated with specific functions (Figure 54-3, Box 54-1).

Basal Ganglia

The basal ganglia are additional bands of gray matter buried deep within the two cerebral hemispheres that form the subcortical associated motor system (the extrapyramidal system). They control automatic movement of the body associated with skeletal muscle activity (e.g., the arms swing alternating with the legs during walking; swallowing; saliva; and blinking) (Lewis et al., 2007).

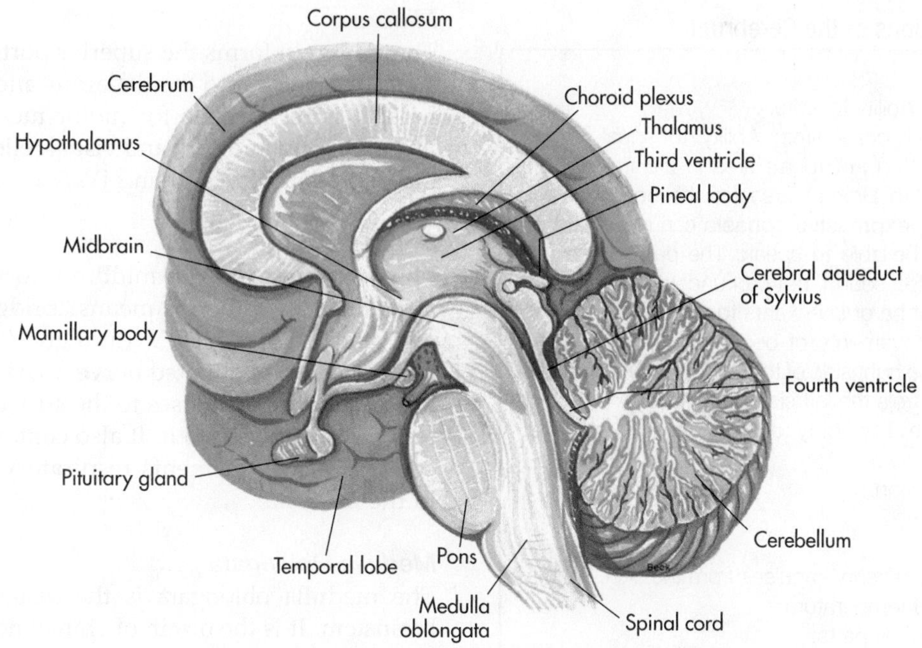

FIGURE 54-2 Sagittal section of the brain (note position of midbrain).

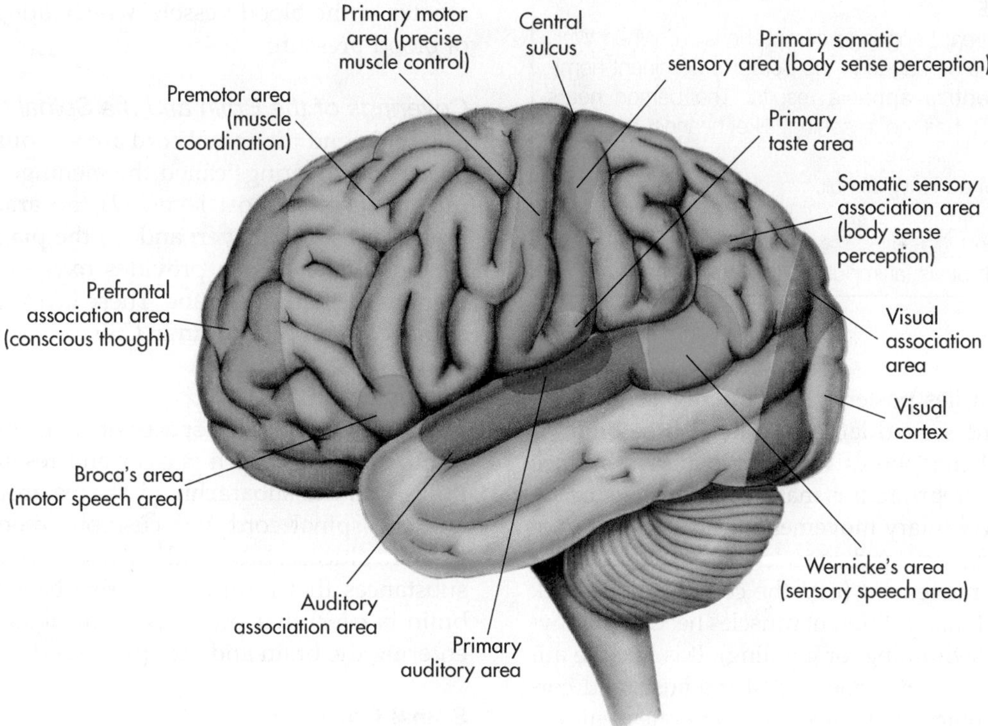

FIGURE 54-3 Cerebral cortex.

Diencephalon

The diencephalon is often called the **interbrain.** It lies beneath the cerebrum and contains the thalamus and the hypothalamus. The thalamus serves as a relay station on the way to the cerebral cortex for some sensory impulses; it interprets other sensory messages, such as pain, light touch, and pressure. The hypothalamus, which lies beneath the thalamus, plays a vital role in the control of body temperature; fluid balance; appetite; sleep; and certain emotions, such as fear, pleasure, and pain. Both the sympathetic and parasympathetic divisions of the autonomic system are under the control of the hypothalamus, as is the pituitary gland. Thus the hypothalamus influences the heartbeat, the contraction and relaxation of the walls of the blood vessels, hormone secretion, and other vital body functions (see Figure 54-2).

Box 54-1 Functions of the Cerebrum

FRONTAL LOBE
- Written speech: Ability to write.
- Motor speech, Broca's area: Ability to speak. Motor speech is mediated in Broca's area in the frontal lobe. When an injury to Broca's area (or the hemisphere in general) occurs, **expressive aphasia** can result and the patient will not be able to speak. The patient can only produce a garbled sound, but can understand language and knows what he or she wants to say.
- Motor ability: Movements of body. The left side of the brain controls the right side of the body, and the right side of the brain controls the left side of the body.
- Intellectualization: The ability to form concepts, personality, emotion, behavior.
- Judgment formation.

PARIETAL LOBE
- Interpretation of sensory impulses from the skin, such as touch, pain, and temperature.
- Recognition of body parts.
- Determination of left from right.
- Determination of shapes, sizes, and distances.

TEMPORAL LOBE
- Wernicke's area: Language comprehension. When Wernicke's area is damaged in the person's dominant hemisphere, **receptive aphasia** results. The person hears sound, but it has no meaning, like hearing a foreign language.
- Integration of auditory stimuli.

OCCIPITAL LOBE
- Interpretation of visual impulses from the retina.

Cerebellum

The cerebellum lies posterior and inferior to the cerebrum and is the second largest portion of the brain. It contains two hemispheres with a convoluted surface much like the cerebrum. It is mainly responsible for coordination of voluntary movement and maintenance of balance, equilibrium, and muscle tone. It coordinates and smoothes movement (e.g., the complex and quick coordination of many different muscles needed in playing the piano, swimming, or juggling). It is like the automatic pilot on an airplane in that it adjusts and corrects the voluntary movement, but operates entirely below the conscious level (Jarvis, 2008). Sensory messages from the semicircular canals in the inner ear send their messages to the cerebellum (see Figure 54-2).

Brainstem

The brainstem is located at the base of the brain and contains the **midbrain,** the **pons,** and the **medulla oblongata** (see Figure 54-2). These structures connect the spinal cord and the cerebrum. The brainstem carries all nerve fibers between the spinal cord and the cerebrum.

Midbrain

The midbrain forms the superior portion of the brainstem. It merges into the thalamus and the hypothalamus. It is responsible for motor movement, relay of impulses, and auditory and visual reflexes. It is the origin of cranial nerves III and IV.

Pons

The pons connects the midbrain to the medulla oblongata; the word pons means "bridge." It is the origin of cranial nerves V through VIII. The pons is composed of myelinated nerve fibers and is responsible for sending impulses to the structures that are inferior and superior to it. It also contains a respiratory center that complements respiratory centers located in the medulla.

Medulla Oblongata

The medulla oblongata is the distal portion of the brainstem. It is the origin of cranial nerves IX and XII. The medulla controls heartbeat, rhythm of breathing, swallowing, coughing, sneezing, vomiting, and hiccups (singultus). A vasomotor center regulates the diameter of the blood vessels, which aids in the control of blood pressure.

Coverings of the Brain and the Spinal Cord

The brain and the spinal cord are surrounded by three protective coverings called the meninges: (1) the dura mater, the outermost layer; (2) the arachnoid membrane, the second layer; and (3) the pia mater, the innermost layer, which provides oxygen and nourishment to the nervous tissue. These layers also bathe the spinal cord and the brain in CSF.

Ventricles

The four ventricles are spaces or cavities located in the brain. The CSF, which is clear and resembles plasma, flows into the subarachnoid spaces around the brain and the spinal cord and cushions them. It contains protein, glucose, urea, and salts; it also contains certain substances that form a protective barrier (the blood-brain barrier) that prevents harmful substances from entering the brain and the spinal cord.

Spinal Cord

The spinal cord is a 17- to 18-inch cord that extends from the brainstem to the second lumbar vertebra. It has two main functions: conducting impulses to and from the brain and serving as a center for reflex actions such as a knee jerk (Figure 54-4). A sensory neuron sends the information to the cord, a central neuron (located within the cord) interprets the impulse, and a motoneuron sends the message back to the muscle or organ involved. Thus a message is sent, interpreted, and acted on without traveling to the brain.

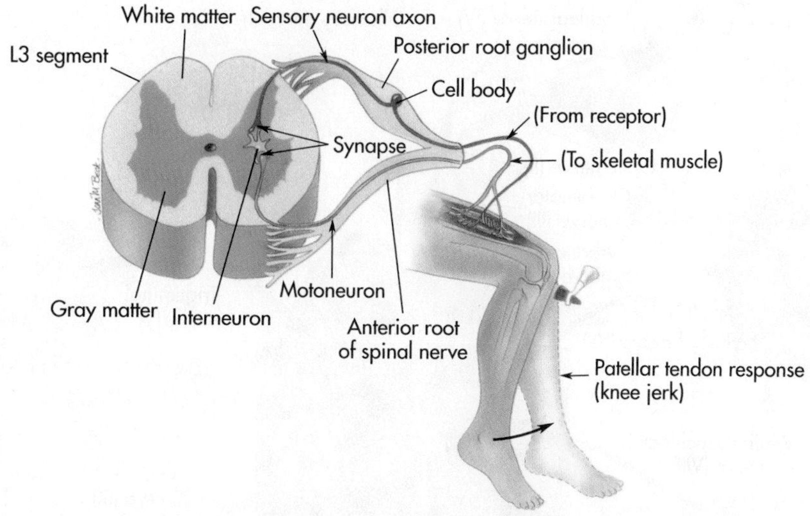

FIGURE 54-4 Neural pathway involved in the patellar reflex.

PERIPHERAL NERVOUS SYSTEM

The **peripheral nervous system** is made up of the motor nerves, the sensory nerves, and ganglia outside the brain and the spinal cord. It is composed of 31 pairs of spinal nerves, 12 pairs of cranial nerves, and the autonomic nervous system.

Spinal Nerves

The 31 pairs of spinal nerves are all mixed nerves. This means that they transmit sensory information to the spinal cord through afferent neurons and motor information from the CNS to the various areas of the body through efferent neurons. The spinal nerves are named according to the corresponding vertebra (e.g., C1, C2).

Cranial Nerves

There are 12 pairs of cranial nerves, which attach to the posterior surface of the brain, mainly the brainstem. Eleven of the pairs conduct impulses between the head, the neck, and the brain; the vagus nerve (X) also serves organs in the thoracic and abdominal cavities (Figure 54-5). Table 54-1 lists the cranial nerves, their impulses, and functions.

Autonomic Nervous System

The autonomic nervous system controls the activities of the smooth muscle, the cardiac muscle, and all glands. The autonomic nervous system is not a separate nervous system but a subdivision of the peripheral nervous system.

It is misleading to think of this system as the automatic system, although most activity is performed on an unconscious level. Its primary function is to maintain internal homeostasis; for example, it strives to maintain a normal heartbeat, a constant body temperature, and a normal respiratory pattern.

To maintain this homeostasis, the autonomic system has two divisions: the **sympathetic nervous system** and the **parasympathetic nervous system.** These two divisions are antagonistic: one slows an action, and the other accelerates the action. These systems function simultaneously, but they are able to dominate each other as the need arises. In times of stress the sympathetic system takes over to prepare the body for "fight or flight." Heartbeat accelerates, blood pressure rises, and adrenal glands increase their secretions. To calm the body after a crisis, the parasympathetic system becomes dominant, slowing the heartbeat and decreasing the blood pressure and adrenal hormone output.

EFFECTS OF NORMAL AGING ON THE NERVOUS SYSTEM

The effects of aging on the nervous system are variable. The changes that occur include a loss of brain weight and a substantial loss of neurons (1% a year after age 50), with the cortex losing cells faster than the brainstem. The remaining cells undergo structural changes. Aging also brings about a general decline in interconnections of dendrites, a reduction in cerebral blood flow, and a decrease in brain metabolism and oxygen utilization. The neurons may contain senile plaques, neurofibrillary tangles, and the age pigment lipofuscin. Older adults often have an altered sleep/wakefulness ratio, a decrease in the ability to regulate body temperature, and a decrease in the velocity of nerve impulses. The blood supply to the spinal cord is decreased, resulting in slower reflexes.

Normal changes in the nervous system associated with aging are *not* the same as senility, organic brain disease, or Alzheimer's disease (AD). Many older people reach old age with no functional deterioration of the nervous system. However, these normal changes may make care or rehabilitation of the older patient a challenge (see Life Span Considerations box).

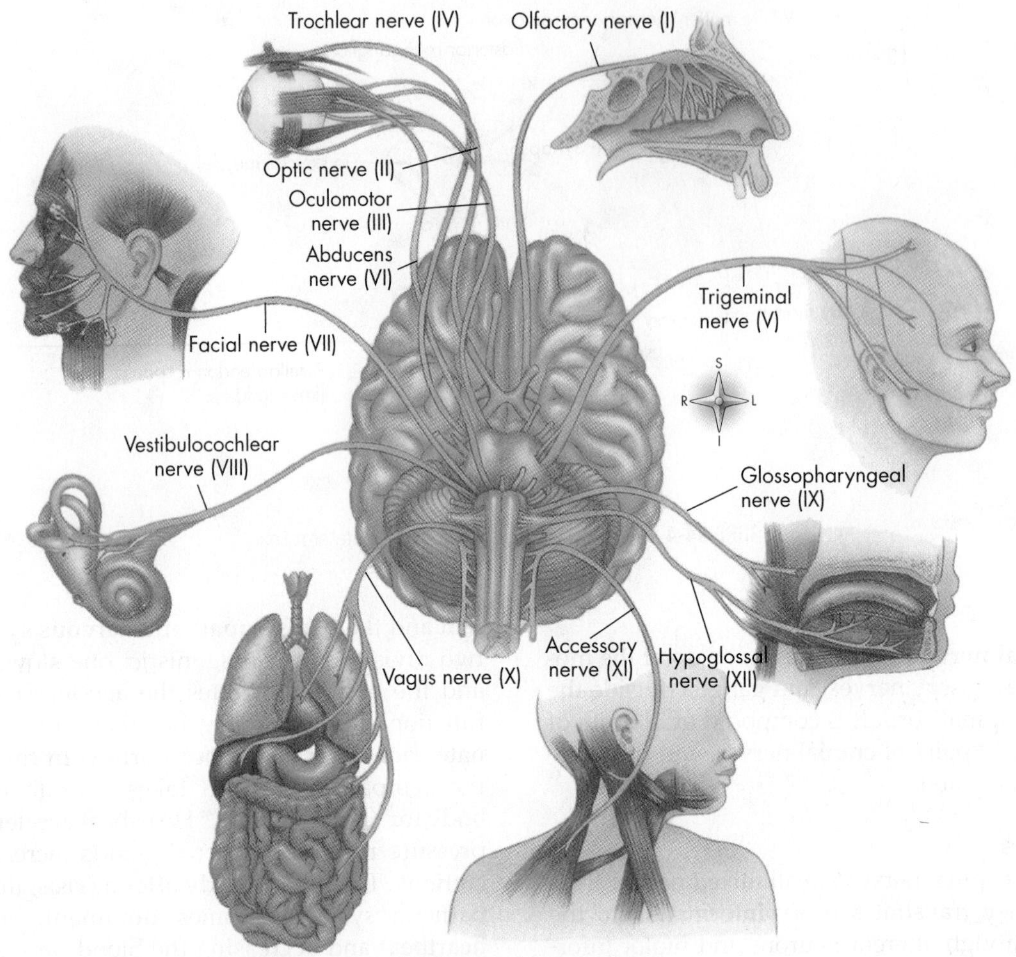

FIGURE 54-5 Cranial nerves.

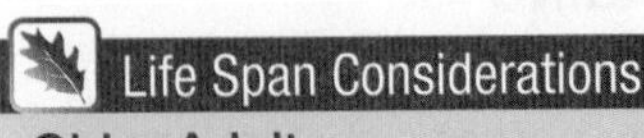

Life Span Considerations

Older Adults

Neurologic Disorder

- As neurons are lost with aging, neurologic function deteriorates, resulting in slowed reflex and reaction time.
- Tremors that increase with fatigue are commonly observed.
- The sense of touch and fine motor coordination diminish with aging.
- Most older people possess the ability to learn, but the speed of learning is slowed. Short-term memory is more affected by aging than long-term memory.
- The incidence of physiologic dementia or organic brain syndrome—including Alzheimer's disease, Pick's disease, and multiinfarct dementia—increases with age.
- The incidence of stroke increases with age. The prognosis is affected by the location and extent of the cerebral damage. Rehabilitation potential after a stroke is often reduced by advanced age and coexisting medical problems.
- Nerve irritation from arthritis, joint injuries, or spinal-cord compression can cause chronic pain or weakness.
- Dementia is not a normal consequence of aging but may be a result of many reversible conditions, including anemia, fluid and electrolyte imbalance, malnutrition, hypothyroidism, metabolic disturbances, drug toxicity, a drug reaction or idiosyncrasy, and hypotension.

PREVENTION OF NEUROLOGIC PROBLEMS

Many conditions of the nervous system have no known cause. Other neurologic problems can be prevented or their effects reduced by modifying lifestyle factors. Neurovascular diseases are in part associated with defined risk factors—the same factors that increase the risk of cardiac disease, including high blood pressure, high blood cholesterol levels, cigarette smoking, obesity, stress, and lack of exercise.

Avoidance of cigarette smoking has been found to decrease the incidence of lung cancer. This is significant for the nervous system, because cancer of the lung often metastasizes to the brain.

Prevention of neurologic problems resulting from trauma is a major challenge. These injuries include spinal cord injury and head injury, which occur frequently in young people. Patient teaching on avoiding such injuries should include avoidance of drug and alcohol use, safe use of motor vehicles (e.g., using automobile seatbelts; wearing helmets with bicycles, motorcycles, and snowmobiles), safe swimming practices (e.g., not diving in shallow water), safe handling and storage of firearms, use of hardhats in dangerous construction areas, and use of protective gear as needed for sports (see Safety Alert box).

Table 54-1 Cranial Nerves

NERVE*		CONDUCTS IMPULSES	FUNCTIONS
I	Olfactory	From nose to brain	Sense of smell
II	Optic	From eye to brain	Vision
III	Oculomotor	From brain to eye muscles	Eye movements, extraocular muscles, pupillary control (pupillary constriction)
IV	Trochlear	From brain to external eye muscles	Down and inward movement of eye
V	Trigeminal Ophthalmic branch Maxillary branch Mandibular branch	From skin and mucous membrane of head to brain; from teeth to brain; from brain to chewing muscles	Sensations of face, scalp, and teeth; chewing movements
VI	Abducens	From brain to external eye muscles	Lateral movement of eye
VII	Facial	From taste buds of tongue to brain; from brain to facial muscles	Sense of taste on anterior two thirds of tongue; contraction of muscles of facial expression
VIII	Acoustic (vestibulocochlear)	From ear to brain	Hearing; sense of balance (equilibrium)
IX	Glossopharyngeal	From throat and taste buds of tongue to brain; from brain to throat muscles and salivary glands	Sensations of throat, taste, swallowing movements, gag reflex, taste posterior one third of tongue, secretion of saliva
X	Vagus	From throat, larynx, and organs in thoracic and abdominal cavities to brain; from brain to muscles of throat and to organs in thoracic and abdominal cavities	Sensations of throat, larynx, and thoracic and abdominal organs; swallowing, voice production, slowing of heartbeat, acceleration of peristalsis
XI	Spinal accessory	From brain to certain shoulder and neck muscles	Shoulder movements (trapezius muscle) and turning movements of head (sternocleidomastoid muscles)
XII	Hypoglossal	From brain to muscles of tongue	Tongue movements

*The first letter of the words in the following sentence are the first letters of the names of cranial nerves: "On Old Olympus's Towering Tops A Finn And German Viewed Some Hops." Many generations of students have used this or a similar mnemonic to help them remember the names of cranial nerves.

Safety Alert!

Preventing Neurologic Injuries

- One of the best ways to prevent head injuries is to prevent car and motorcycle accidents.
- Become active in campaigns that promote safe driving. Speak to driver's education classes regarding the danger of unsafe driving and driving after drinking alcohol or taking drugs.
- The use of seatbelts in cars and the use of helmets for riding on motorcycles are the most effective measures for increasing survival after accidents.
- Individual states have legislation requiring the use of automobile safety devices for both children and adults.
- Recommend the wearing of protective helmets by lumberjacks, construction workers, miners, horseback riders, bicycle riders, snowboarders, and skydivers.
- Encourage swimmers of all ages to refrain from diving into shallow water or areas in which water depth is unknown.

Neurologic diseases, such as meningitis or brain abscess, that occur as a result of infection can sometimes be prevented by prompt treatment of ear and sinus infections. The practice of safe and responsible sex is important, since some neurologically related diseases, such as syphilis and human immunodeficiency virus (HIV) disease, are spread by sexual contact. Safe practices include abstinence, monogamy, and the use of condoms. Treatment for drug abuse, especially intravenous (IV) use, is important, as is the prevention of HIV disease.

ASSESSMENT OF THE NEUROLOGIC SYSTEM

HISTORY

A comprehensive history is essential for diagnosing neurologic disease. This includes specifics about symptoms experienced and the patient's understanding and perception of what is happening. Obtaining information from family members or significant others may also be helpful. Follow the same format routinely to make certain information is complete.

For patients with suspected neurologic conditions, the presence of many symptoms or subjective data may be significant. These include the following.

- Headaches, especially those that first occur after middle age or those that change in character (e.g., headaches that are worse in the morning or awaken a person from sleep)

Table 54-2 Levels of Consciousness

LEVEL	DESCRIPTION
Alert	Responds appropriately to auditory, tactile, and visual stimuli
Disorientation	Disoriented; unable to follow simple commands; thinking slowed; inattentive, flat affect
Stupor	Responds to verbal commands with moaning or groaning, if at all; seems unaware of the surroundings
Semicomatose	Is in impaired state of consciousness, characterized by obtundation and stupor, from which a patient can be aroused only by energetic stimulation
Comatose	Unable to respond to painful stimuli; cornea and pupillary reflexes are absent Cannot swallow or cough Is incontinent of urine and feces Electroencephalogram pattern demonstrates decreased or absent neuronal activity

- Clumsiness or loss of function in an extremity
- Change in visual acuity
- Any new or worsened seizure activity
- Numbness or tingling in one or more extremities
- Pain in an extremity or other part of the body
- Personality changes or mood swings
- Extreme fatigue or tiredness

MENTAL STATUS

Assessment of the neurologic patient's mental status generally includes orientation (person, place, time, and purpose), mood and behavior, general knowledge (such as the names of U.S. presidents), and short- and long-term memory. The patient's attention span and ability to concentrate may also be assessed.

It is important to document mental status in specific terms. For instance, it is better to note "oriented to name, date, hospital, and purpose" than to note simply "oriented." Record actual patient statements. Vary orientation questions because some patients may learn the correct answers through repetition.

Level of Consciousness

Level of consciousness (LOC) is the earliest and most sensitive indicator of the patient's neurologic status. Changes in LOC are a result of impaired cerebral blood flow, which deprives the cells of the cerebral cortex and the reticular activating system (RAS) of oxygen. The RAS is located in the brainstem with neural connections to many parts of the nervous system (Lewis et al., 2007). The RAS is a functional system in the brain essential for wakefulness, attention, concentration, and introspection (*Mosby's Dictionary of Medicine, Nursing, and Health Professions*, 2006). A decreasing LOC is the earliest sign of increased intracranial pressure (ICP). LOC has two components: *arousal* (or wakefulness) and *awareness*. Wakefulness is the most fundamental part of LOC. If the patient can open the eyes spontaneously to voice or to pain, the wakefulness center in the brainstem is still functioning. Awareness, a higher function controlled by the RAS in the brainstem, is the ability to interact with and interpret the environment. Awareness has four components, which are assessed as follows:

1. **Orientation:** Ask questions about orientation to person, place, time, and purpose.
2. **Memory:** Assess short-term memory; do not ask yes or no questions.
3. **Calculation:** Ask a simple math problem (e.g., "If you had $2 and your apple costs $1.25, how many quarters would you get back?").
4. **Fund of knowledge:** Ask the patient to name the president and to tell you what's on the national news.

Restlessness, disorientation, and lethargy may be seen first. Record observations in terms of behavior and signs—not labels such as "disoriented." See Table 54-2 for one method of classifying LOC.

Glasgow Coma Scale

The Glasgow coma scale (Table 54-3) is a quick, practical, and standardized system for assessing the degree of consciousness impairment in the critically ill and for predicting the duration and ultimate outcome of coma, particularly with head injuries. The Glasgow coma scale was developed in 1974 and consists of a three-part neurologic assessment: eye opening, best motor response, and best verbal response.

The stronger the stimulus needed to obtain a response, the lower the patient's score. The number value assigned to each part of the scale is added to yield an objective score. The score for a patient who is not neurologically impaired is 15; the lowest possible score is 3. Generally, any score of 8 or less is commonly accepted as a definition of coma. The scale has a high degree of consistency even when used by staff of varied experience.

FOUR Score Coma Scale

A recently developed scale for assessing coma is the FOUR (Full Outline of UnResponsiveness) Score coma scale (Wijdicks & Bamlet, 2005). It is used to assess patients with neurologic conditions that affect cognitive function such as stroke, craniotomy, and traumatic brain injury. It assesses eye response, motor response,

Table 54-3 Glasgow Coma Scale: Demonstrating Measurement of Level of Consciousness

CATEGORY OF RESPONSE	APPROPRIATE STIMULUS	RESPONSE	SCORE
Eyes Open	• Approach to bedside • Verbal command • Pain	Spontaneous response	4
		Opening of eyes to name or command	3
		Lack of opening of eyes to previous stimuli but opening to pain	2
		Lack of opening of eyes to any stimulus	1
		Untestable	U
Best Verbal Response	• Verbal questioning with maximum arousal	Appropriate orientation, conversant; correct identification of self, place, year, and month	5
		Confusion; conversant, but disorientation in one or more spheres	4
		Inappropriate or disorganized use of words (e.g., cursing), lack of sustained conversation	3
		Incomprehensible words, sounds (e.g., moaning)	2
		Lack of sound, even with painful stimuli	1
		Untestable	U
Best Motor Response	• Verbal command (e.g., "raise your arm, hold up two fingers") • Pain (pressure on proximal nailbed)	Obedience of command	6
		Localization of pain, lack of obedience but presence of attempts to remove offending stimulus	5
		Flexion withdrawal,* flexion of arm in response to pain without abnormal flexion posture	4
		Abnormal flexion, flexing of arm at elbow and pronation, making a fist	3
		Abnormal extension, extension of arm at elbow usually adduction and internal rotation of arm at shoulder	2
		Lack of response	1
		Untestable	U

From Lewis, S.L., et al. (2007). *Medical-surgical nursing: Assessment and management of clinical problems.* (7th ed.). St. Louis: Mosby.
*Added to the original scale by many centers.

brainstem reflexes, and respiration (Table 54-4). Each component is graded on a scale of 0 (worst response) to 4 (best response). The scores are not totaled; therefore there is not a *sum* score in this scale.

The FOUR Score scale may be used as a complementary grading scale, along with the Glasgow coma scale (Wolf & Wijdicks, 2007). The Glasgow coma scale and FOUR Score scale are usually implemented in the intensive care unit.

LANGUAGE AND SPEECH

It is important to assess the language and speech capability of the neurologic patient (see Box 54-1 and Figure 54-3). Speech is a function of the dominant hemisphere, which is on the left side of the brain for all right-handed people and most left-handed people. Aphasia is an abnormal neurologic condition in which the language function is defective or absent because of an injury to certain areas of the cerebral cortex—Broca's area in the frontal lobe and Wernicke's area in the posterior part of the temporal lobe.

Aphasia includes all areas of language, including speech, reading, writing, and understanding. Aphasia has been subdivided as follows:

- **Sensory aphasia, or receptive aphasia:** Inability to comprehend the spoken word or written word. Wernicke's area in the temporal lobe is associated with language comprehension. Pathologic conditions in this area result in receptive aphasia.
- **Motor aphasia:** Inability to use symbols of speech (also called *expressive aphasia*). Broca's area in the frontal lobe mediates motor speech. Pathologic conditions in this area result in expression aphasia.
- **Global aphasia:** Inability to understand the spoken word or to speak. Pathologic conditions in Broca's and Wernicke's areas result in global aphasia.

Anomia is a form of aphasia characterized by the inability to name objects. Dysarthria is difficult, poorly articulated speech that usually results from interference in control over the muscles of speech. The general cause is damage to a central or peripheral nerve.

CRANIAL NERVES

Assessment of cranial nerve function is another important part of the neurologic assessment (see Figure 54-5). The 12 pairs of nerves emerge from the cranial cavity through openings in the skull (see Table 54-1 for specifics of cranial nerve classification and assess-

Table 54-4 FOUR Score Coma Scale

CATEGORY OF RESPONSE	RESPONSE	SCORE
Eye response (E)	Eyelids open or opened, tracking, or blinking to command	4
	Eyelids open but not tracking	3
	Eyelids closed, open to loud noise, not tracking	2
	Eyelids closed, open to pain, not tracking	1
	Eyelids remain closed with pain	0
Brainstem reflexes (B)	Pupil and corneal reflexes present	4
	One pupil wide and fixed	3
	Pupil or corneal reflexes absent	2
	Pupil and corneal reflexes absent	1
	Absent pupil, corneal, and cough reflex	0
Motor response (M)	Thumbs up, fist or peace sign, to command	4
	Localizing to pain	3
	Flexion response to pain	2
	Extensor posturing	1
	No response to pain or generalized myoclonus status epilepticus	0
Respiration (R)	Not intubated, regular breathing pattern	4
	Not intubated, Cheyne-Stokes breathing pattern	3
	Not intubated, irregular breathing pattern	2
	Breathes above ventilator rate	1
	Breathes at ventilator rate or apnea	0

From Wijdicks, E.J., et al. (2005). Validation of a new coma scale, the FOUR score coma scale. *Annals of Neurology, 58*(4), 585.

ment). The cranial nerves are tested in the following ways:

I (olfactory)	Identification of common odors
II (optic)	Testing of visual acuity and visual fields
III (oculomotor)	Testing of ability of eyes to move together in all directions, testing pupillary response
IV (trochlear)	Tested with oculomotor; testing eye movements
V (trigeminal)	Jaw strength and sensation of face, corneal reflex
VI (abducens)	Tested with oculomotor; testing eye movements
VII (facial)	Ability of face to move in symmetry, identification of tastes
VIII (acoustic, or vestibulocochlear)	Testing of hearing through whisper or other means and checking equilibrium and balance
IX (glossopharyngeal)	Identification of tastes
X (vagus)	Gag reflex, movement of uvula and soft palate
XI (spinal accessory)	Shoulder and neck movement
XII (hypoglossal)	Tongue motion

MOTOR FUNCTION

Evaluation of the neurologic patient's motor status detects abnormalities in the normal functioning of nerves and muscles. Motor function disturbances are the most commonly encountered neurologic symptom. In general, the motor status examination includes gait and stance, muscle tone, coordination, involuntary movements, and the muscle stretch reflexes.

Reflexes that are usually tested include biceps, triceps, brachioradialis, quadriceps, gastrocnemius, and soleus muscles. The examiner taps briskly over the muscle with a reflex hammer. The response is noted and graded on a scale, usually from 0 to 4+, with 4+ being hyperreflexic. The most important feature of any reflex pattern is not the absolute value on the scale, but the comparison of one side of the body with the other. Stick figures are commonly used to record the bilateral values.

Damage to the nervous system often causes a serious problem in mobility. A loss of function is called **paralysis;** a lesser degree of movement deficit from partial or incomplete paralysis is called **paresis.**

Injury or disease of motoneurons causes alterations of muscle strength, tone, and reflex activity. The specific signs and symptoms vary according to whether the lesion involves an upper motoneuron or a lower motoneuron. Muscles may be **flaccid** (weak, soft, and flabby and lacking normal muscle tone), with absent deep tendon reflexes, or **spastic** (involuntary, sudden movement or muscular contraction), with increased reflexes. With some muscle problems, the affected muscle shows small, rapid, continuous twitching, called **fasciculations.** Fasciculations are localized, spontaneous, and involuntary without movement of limb. With other problems, clonus (a forced series of alternating contractions and partial relaxation of a muscle) may occur.

SENSORY AND PERCEPTUAL STATUS

The sensory examination is the most difficult part of the neurologic evaluation. Specific alterations in sensation that should be assessed include pain; touch; temperature; and **proprioception,** the sensation pertaining to spatial-position and muscular-activity stimuli originating from within the body or to the sensory receptors that those stimuli activate. This sensation enables one to know the position of the body without looking at it and to recognize objects by the sense of touch.

Unilateral neglect, a condition in which an individual is perceptually unaware of and inattentive to one side of the body, may also occur. Another perceptual problem is **hemianopia,** which is characterized by defective vision or blindness in half of the visual field.

In most clinical settings it is usually not feasible or necessary to complete the total neurologic examination during shift-to-shift assessments of the patient. However, in many settings, such as intensive care units, the neurologic checks may be done as frequently as every 15 minutes. The most important factors include orientation, LOC, bilateral muscle strength, speech, involuntary movements, ability to follow commands, and any abnormal posturing.

LABORATORY AND DIAGNOSTIC EXAMINATIONS

BLOOD AND URINE TESTS

Assessment of the neurologically impaired patient includes a variety of blood and urine tests. A culture of the urine may rule out infection involving the urinary tract. Other urine testing may indicate the presence of diabetes insipidus. Urine drug screens may be done to rule out drug use as a cause of lethargy or to identify specific drugs ingested.

Arterial blood gas (ABG) values may be an important diagnostic tool in monitoring the oxygen content of the blood. The gases may be altered with neurologic diseases such as Guillain-Barré syndrome (GBS), which may affect breathing patterns. Blood tests that are routinely done may help narrow the diagnosis of neurologic disorder.

CEREBROSPINAL FLUID

Examination of the CSF can yield information about many neurologic conditions. Normally CSF contains up to 10 lymphocytes per milliliter. An increase in the number of cells may indicate an infection, such as tuberculosis or a viral infection. Bacterial infections such as tuberculous meningitis often lower the CSF glucose level and chloride levels. A culture or smear examination is done to determine the causative organism in meningitis. Spinal-fluid protein is elevated when a degenerative disease or a brain tumor is present. Blood in the spinal fluid indicates hemorrhage from somewhere in the ventricular system. A protein electrophoresis evaluation may give evidence of neurologic diseases such as multiple sclerosis (MS) (Table 54-5).

Lumbar Puncture

A lumbar puncture is often performed as part of the diagnostic workup of the patient who may have a neurologic problem. It is contraindicated in patients who might have increased ICP, since the withdrawal of fluid may cause the medulla oblongata to herniate downward into the foramen magnum.

A lumbar puncture is done to obtain CSF for examination, to relieve pressure, or to introduce dye or medication. It is a common procedure, done in the patient's room or in the diagnostic imaging department. The procedure takes 10 to 15 minutes. Slight pain and pressure may be felt as the dura is entered. A sharp, shooting pain down one leg may be caused by the needle coming close to a nerve.

The patient is usually positioned on the side with the knee and head flexed at an acute angle. This allows for maximal lumbar flexion and separation of the interspinous spaces. After anesthetizing the area with a local anesthetic, the physician inserts the needle below the level of the spinal cord, at the L4-L5 or L5-S1 interspace (Figure 54-6). The inner needle is removed to allow for drainage and measurement of spinal fluid. The level-of-fluid column in the manometer is used to measure the pressure. The first specimen of spinal fluid may contain blood from slight bleeding at the site of the puncture. This specimen should not be sent for cell count.

Table 54-5 Normal Characteristics of Cerebrospinal Fluid

DETERMINATION	VALUE
Specific gravity	1.007
pH	7.35-7.45
Chloride	120-130 mEq/L
Glucose	50-75 mg/dL
Pressure	80-200 mm H_2O
Total volume	80-200 mL (15 mL in ventricles)
Total protein	15-45 mg/dL (lumbar) 10-25 mg/dL (cisternal) 5-15 mg/dL (ventricular)
Gamma globulin	6%-13% of total protein
Cell count	
Red blood cells	None
White blood cells	0-10 cells (all lymphocytes and monocytes)
Culture and sensitivity	No organisms present
Serology for syphilis	Negative

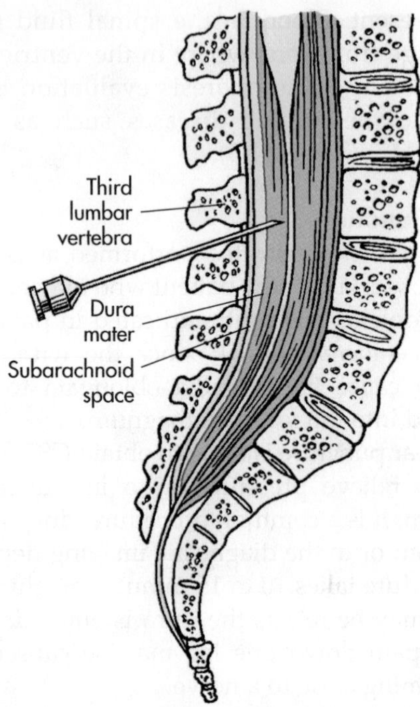

FIGURE 54-6 Position and angle of the needle when lumbar puncture is performed. Note that the needle is in the fourth lumbar interspace below the level of the spinal cord.

After the procedure the patient lies flat in bed for several hours. Assess the site of the puncture for any leakage, as evidenced by moisture on the bandage or around the puncture site. Headache is fairly common and is thought to be caused by the loss of spinal fluid through the dura mater. If a headache develops, bed rest, analgesics, and ice to the head may help. Opioids are usually not helpful.

OTHER TESTS

Routine skull radiographs of the head and vertebral column are useful in ruling out fractures of the skull and cervical vertebrae. Since the development of the computed tomography (CT) scan, skull radiographs are not used as extensively as before.

Computed Tomography Scan

The purpose of the CT scan, also called the **CAT scan,** is to detect pathologic conditions of the cerebrum and spinal cord using a technique of scanning without radioisotopes. No special physical preparation is required for the test. A CT scan takes 20 to 30 minutes if done without contrast medium and about 60 minutes with contrast. The procedure is painless, except for the slight discomfort when an IV line is started for the injection of the contrast dye. The patient may also have some discomfort in lying still and possible feelings of claustrophobia from being positioned in the head holder. If contrast medium is used, document and report to the physician any history of allergy to iodine and seafood, since iodine is present in the contrast medium.

During the procedure the patient lies supine with the head positioned within a rubber head holder to prevent air gaps between the machine and the scalp. The head is scanned in two planes simultaneously and at various angles. Each image that appears is a specific layer of brain tissue. The computer displays a printout that indicates areas of increased density (e.g., tumors or thrombi).

Brain Scan

Like the CT scan, the brain scan's purpose is detecting pathologic conditions of the cerebrum. It uses radioactive isotopes and a scanner. No special physical preparation is required. The procedure takes approximately 45 minutes for the actual scan. The patient is injected with a radioisotope and then lies still while a scanner passes over the brain area. Concentrated areas of uptake are reflected. There are generally no adverse effects from the procedure and only minimal discomfort associated with the IV administration of the radioactive isotopes. If mercury is used as the isotope indicator, a mercurial diuretic (meralluride [Mercuhydrin]) is administered several hours before the procedure to allow a greater concentration of the mercury to circulate to brain tissue, since meralluride minimizes the uptake of mercury by the kidneys. Brain scans are being used less frequently than in the past because of the excellent results obtained from CT scan and magnetic resonance imaging (MRI).

Magnetic Resonance Imaging

MRI uses magnetic forces to image body structures. It is used to detect pathologic conditions of the cerebrum and the spinal cord and in detection of stroke, MS, tumors, trauma, herniation, and seizure. Because MRI yields greater contrast in the images of soft tissue structures than does the CT scan, it is the diagnostic test of choice for many neurologic diseases. Recent advances in MRI techniques include diffusion-weighted imaging and magnetic resonance spectroscopy. Because the scan involves a magnetic force, caution the patient to remove watches, credit cards, and any metal from the clothing before entering the scanning room. Ask the patient about the presence of any metal in the body that would preclude the use of the scan, such as orthopedic appliances, aneurysm clips, and pacemakers.

During the procedure the patient lies supine with the head positioned in a head holder. The test takes 45 to 60 minutes. The procedure is painless, except for the discomfort in lying still and possible feelings of claustrophobia. Warn the patient that the machine makes different and loud noises during the scanning procedure.

Magnetic Resonance Angiography

Magnetic resonance angiography (MRA) uses differential radio waves and magnetic field signals to visualize flowing blood to evaluate extracranial and intra-

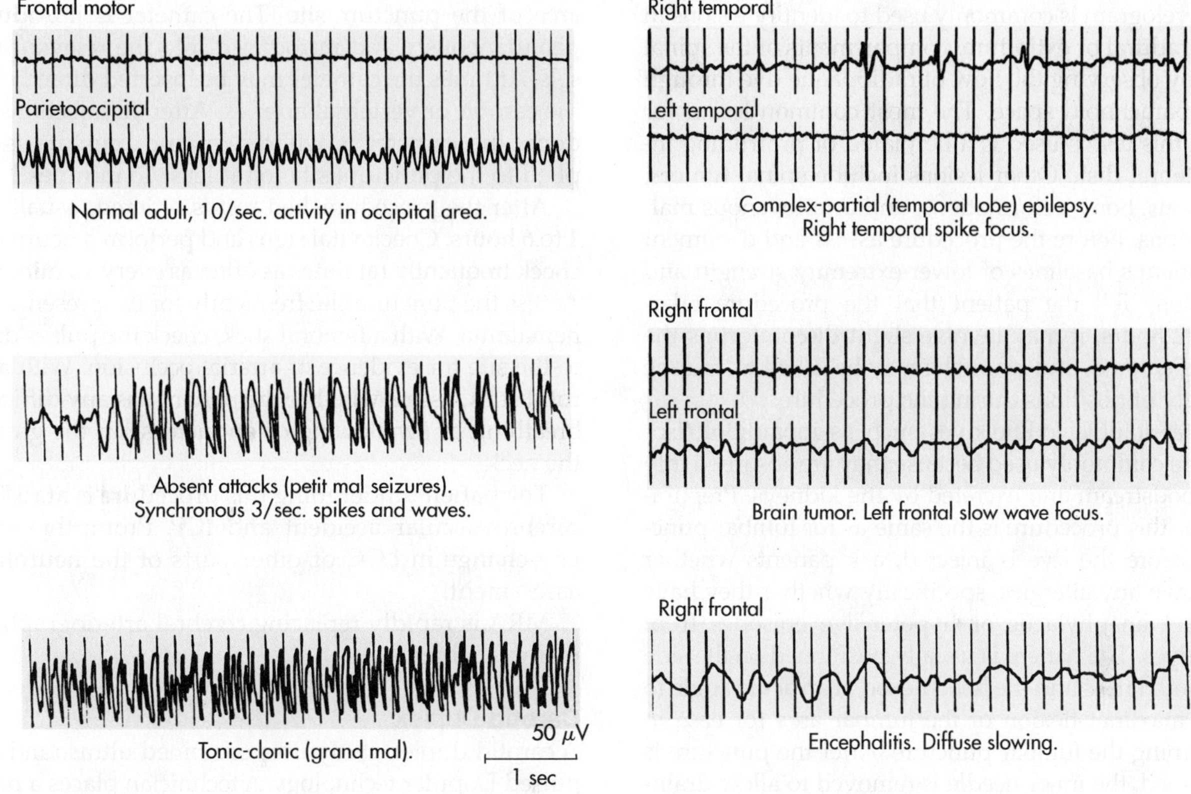

FIGURE 54-7 Tracings of electroencephalogram. The normal tracing is demonstrated, as are several pathologic states.

cranial blood vessels. It is a noninvasive procedure for viewing possible occlusions in arteries. It provides both anatomical and hemodynamic information. It can be used in conjunction with contrast media (contrast-enhanced MRA). MRA is rapidly replacing cerebral angiography in diagnosing cerebrovascular diseases. MRA has been useful in evaluation of the cervical carotid artery and large-caliber intracranial arterial and venous structures.

Positron Emission Tomography Scan

Another evaluative measure that is similar to CT and MRI scans is the positron emission tomography (PET) scan. In this procedure the patient receives an injection of deoxyglucose with radioactive fluorine. The area in question is scanned, and a color composite picture is obtained. Shades of color indicate the level of glucose metabolism, suggestive of a pathologic state. PET scanning provides a noninvasive means of determining biochemical processes that occur in the brain. It is increasingly being used to monitor patients who had a stroke or who have AD, Huntington's disease, tumors, epilepsy, and Parkinson's disease. As with the CT scan, discomfort is minimal. Inform the patient of the need to lie still for the duration of the scan, which is usually about 45 minutes.

Electroencephalogram

The electroencephalogram (EEG) provides evidence of focal or generalized disturbances of brain function by measuring the electrical activity of the brain. Among the cerebral diseases assessed by EEG are epilepsy, mass lesions (e.g., tumors, abscess, hematoma), cerebrovascular lesions, and brain injury. The test requires no special preparation, but encourage the patient to be quiet and rest before the procedure. An exception is a sleep-deprived EEG, where the patient is kept awake the night before the test and the EEG is usually done first thing in the morning. The EEG usually takes about 1 hour to complete. The patient's hair and scalp should be clean. The electrodes are placed on the scalp with collodion in a set pattern to cover all scalp areas. An EEG is painless.

The basic resting rhythm of the EEG is affected by opening the eyes or altering attention. Recordings are sometimes made while the patient is asleep or sleep deprived, when the seizure threshold may be lowered. Comparisons are made of different patterns of the recordings (Figure 54-7). After the test allow the patient to rest. Assist the patient if necessary in washing the hair and removing the collodion from the scalp.

Myelogram

The myelogram is commonly used to identify lesions in the intradural or extradural compartments of the spinal canal by observing the flow of radiopaque dye through the subarachnoid space. The most common lesion for which this test is used is a herniated or protruding intervertebral disk. Other lesions include spinal tumors, adhesions, bony deformations, and arteriovenous malformations. Before the procedure assess and document the patient's baselines of lower-extremity strength and sensation. Tell the patient that the procedure takes about 2 hours, it may involve slight discomfort as the dura is entered, and he or she may be asked to assume a variety of positions during the procedure.

Water-soluble iodine dyes such as iopamidol (Isovue) are commonly used because they are absorbed into the bloodstream and excreted by the kidneys. Preparation for this procedure is the same as for lumbar puncture. Before the dye is injected, ask patients whether they have any allergies, specifically whether they have had any anaphylactic or hypotensive episodes from other dyes. The patient is usually positioned on the side with both knees and the head flexed at an acute angle to allow maximal flexion of the lumbar area for ease in performing the lumbar puncture. After the puncture is performed, the inner needle is removed to allow drainage of CSF, measurement of pressure, and collection of specimens. The dye is instilled and the needle is removed. The patient is then turned to various positions so the spinal cord can be visualized while fluoroscopic and radiopaque films are taken. The patient usually undergoes a CT scan 4 to 6 hours after a myelogram.

After the procedure, observe the puncture site for any leakage of CSF, and assess the strength and sensation of the lower extremities. Headache is fairly common. It may be accompanied by nausea and occasionally by vomiting. The patient should be flat for a few hours.

Angiogram

The angiogram (cerebral arteriography) is a procedure used to visualize the cerebral arterial system by injecting radiopaque material. It allows detection of arterial aneurysms, vessel anomalies, ruptured vessels, and displacement of vessels by tumors or masses.

Before the procedure the patient is usually given clear liquids, although in some institutions all oral intake is restricted. Assess the patient for any allergy to iodine because the dye contains iodine. If the femoral approach is to be used, mark the locations of the bilateral pedal pulses. If the carotid artery is used, measure the neck circumference as part of the baseline data. Immediately before the procedure, measure baseline vital signs and pulses and perform a neurologic check.

The test takes approximately 2 to 3 hours. The patient may experience discomfort in lying still for that time. When the dye is injected, most patients complain of feeling extremely hot and seeing flashes of light. The patient is positioned supine on the radiograph table. A local anesthetic agent is used to anesthetize the area of the puncture site. The catheter is introduced percutaneously and introduced into the relevant vessels. At times the catheter may be inserted directly into the carotid or vertebral arteries. After all injections are done, the catheter is withdrawn and pressure is applied to the puncture site for at least 15 minutes.

After the procedure, bed rest is ordered, usually for 4 to 6 hours. Check vital signs and perform a neurologic check frequently (at times as often as every 15 minutes). Assess the puncture site frequently for the presence of a hematoma. With a femoral stick, check the pulses distal to the site for evidence of arterial occlusion. With a carotid stick, assess whether the patient has any difficulty breathing or swallowing or an increase in the girth of the neck.

The patient undergoing this procedure is at risk for cerebrovascular accident and ICP. Promptly report any change in LOC or other parts of the neurologic assessment.

MRA is rapidly replacing cerebral arteriography in many facilities.

Carotid Duplex

A carotid duplex study uses combined ultrasound and pulsed Doppler technology. A technician places a probe on the skin over the carotid artery and slowly moves the probe along the course of the common carotid to the bifurcation of the external and internal carotid arteries. The ultrasound signal emitted from the probe reflects off the moving blood cells within the vessel. The frequency of the reflected signal corresponds to the blood velocity. This response is amplified and is registered on a graphic record and also as sound. The graphic record registers blood velocity. Increased blood flow velocity can indicate stenosis of a vessel. Carotid duplex scanning is a noninvasive study that evaluates carotid occlusive disease. This study is often ordered when a patient has a transient ischemic attack (TIA).

Electromyogram

An electromyogram (EMG) measures the contraction of a muscle in response to electrical stimulation. It provides evidence of lower motoneuron disease; primary muscle disease; and defects in the transmission of electrical impulses at the neuromuscular junction, such as in myasthenia gravis (MG). There is no special preparation for the test. The test takes approximately 45 minutes for one muscle study. Inform the patient that it is uncomfortable when the electrode is inserted into the muscle and when the electrical current is used. The muscle may ache for a short time after the procedure.

During the test an electrode is inserted into selected skeletal muscles. An electric current is passed through the electrode, and the machine graphs the variations of muscle potentials (voltage). After the procedure assess the patient for signs of bleeding at the site of the electrode insertion. The patient may need an analgesic for discomfort and a rest period.

Echoencephalogram

An echoencephalogram uses ultrasound to depict the intracranial structures of the brain. It is especially helpful in detecting ventricular dilation and a major shift of midline structures in the brain as a result of an expanding lesion. The preparation of the patient, the actual procedure, and aftercare are similar to those of the brain scan.

COMMON DISORDERS OF THE NEUROLOGIC SYSTEM

HEADACHES

Etiology and Pathophysiology

Headache is a common neurologic complaint; its significance and its causes vary. The source of recurring headache should be determined through careful physical examination with appropriate neurologic assessment. Some tumors may produce no symptoms except for headache for a long period.

The exact mechanism of head pain is not known. Although the skull and brain tissues are not able to feel sensory pain, pain arises from the scalp, its blood vessels and muscles, and the dura mater and its venous sinuses. Pain also arises from the blood vessels at the base of the brain and from cervical cranial nerves. Blood vessels may dilate and become congested with blood. Headaches can be classified as vascular, tension, and traction-inflammatory. Vascular headaches include migraine, cluster, and hypertensive headaches. Tension headaches may arise from psychological problems of tension or stress or from medical problems such as cervical arthritis. Traction-inflammatory headaches include those caused by infection, intracranial or extracranial causes, occlusive vascular structures, and temporal arteritis.

Clinical Manifestations

Headache pain may be made worse by stress or tension. Knowledge of the patient's perception of the effect of stress on the pain is important in planning effective interventions.

Migraine headaches are unusual in that prodromal (early signs and symptoms of a developing condition or disease) signs and symptoms occur before the acute attack. These may include visual field defects; unusual smells or sounds; disorientation; paresthesias; and, in rare cases, paralysis of a part of the body. During a migraine headache, signs and symptoms may include nausea, vomiting, sensitivity to light, chilliness, fatigue, irritability, diaphoresis, edema, and other signs of autonomic dysfunction. Abnormal metabolism of serotonin, a vasoactive neurotransmitter found in platelets and cells of the brain, plays a major role. A history of migraine with aura in young women is now known to cause atherosclerosis (deposits, or plaques, containing lipids and lipophages that form within the intima and inner media of large and medium-size arteries). Because each migraine episode decreases cerebral blood flow, damage to the cerebral endothelium from repeated episodes of vasospasm increases the patient's risk for atherosclerosis and stroke (Phillips, 2007).

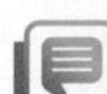 Communication

Nurse-Patient Therapeutic Communication Concerning Patient's Headache

Nurse: Can you describe your problem to me?
Patient: It's a pain in my head.
Nurse: When did this pain start?
Patient: About a month ago.
Nurse: Did anything else happen at that same time?
Patient: My daughter left home for college.
Nurse: How did you feel about that?
Patient: I was really upset. She was my baby. I can't believe that she's gone.
Nurse: Was there anything else that you noticed at the same time? Like an increased temperature or nasal drainage?
Patient: No, I don't think so.
Nurse: What made the headache worse?
Patient: Thinking about my loneliness.
Nurse: What made the headache better?
Patient: Sleeping or taking a Valium.
Nurse: Have you had trouble sleeping or noticed that your appetite was worse?
Patient: I wake up early in the morning. I don't feel much like eating.
Nurse: Have you lost weight?
Patient: About 10 pounds in the last month.
Nurse: Can you tell me what the pain feels like?
Patient: It's a pain that goes through my whole head. It throbs and gets worse in the evening.
Nurse: What do you think is the cause of the headache?
Patient: I guess maybe I'm upset that my daughter left.

Assessment

Subjective data include the patient's understanding of the headache, possible causes, and any precipitating factors. Determine what measures relieve the symptoms and the location, frequency, pattern, and character of the pain. This includes the site of return of the headache, time of day, and intervals between headaches. Also assess the initial onset of the headache, any symptoms that occur before the headache or associated symptoms, the presence of allergies, and any family history of similar headache patterns.

Objective data include any behaviors indicating stress, anxiety, or pain. Changes in the ability to carry out activities of daily living (ADLs), an abnormally raised body temperature, and sinus drainage may be important. Also document abnormalities noted during the physical examination (see Communication box).

Diagnostic Tests

It is important to evaluate headaches that are not transient. Usual testing includes a neurologic examination, a CT scan (MRI or PET scan may also be done), a brain scan, skull radiographs, and a lumbar puncture. A lumbar puncture is not done, however, if there is evidence of increased ICP or if a brain tumor is suspected because quick reduction of pressure produced by removal of the spinal fluid may cause brain herniation. In these situations a CT scan is done first.

Medical Management

Dietary Counseling

Some foods may cause or worsen headaches. These include foods containing tyramine, nitrates, or glutamates (e.g., monosodium glutamate [MSG], often used in the preparation of Chinese foods and on salad bars). Other substances that may provoke headaches include vinegar, chocolate, yogurt, alcohol, fermented or marinated foods, ripened cheese, cured sandwich meat, caffeine, and pork.

Psychotherapy

Patients with headaches may respond to psychotherapy. This does not mean that the headache pain is not physiologic, but counseling can help the patient develop awareness of stress factors and deal with the pain. The patient may need help expressing feelings about intractable headache pain.

Medications

Medications are often used to treat headaches.

Migraine headaches. Acetylsalicylic acid (aspirin) or acetaminophen may help relieve mild or moderate migraine pain. For moderate to severe headaches, the triptans have become the first line of the therapy. Triptans are thought to act on receptors in the extracerebral, intracranial vessels that become dilated during a migraine attack. Stimulating these receptors constricts cranial vessels, inhibits neuropeptide release, and reduces nerve impulse transmission along trigeminal pain pathways.

Eletriptan (Replax) is the seventh triptan to be marketed for treatment of migraine, joining almotriptan (Axert), frovatriptan (Frova), naratriptan (Amerge), rizatriptan (Maxalt), sumatriptan (Imitrex), and zolmitriptan (Zomig). Classified as selective serotonin receptor agonists, these drugs are all indicated to treat acute migraine (with or without aura) in adults. In addition to relieving headache pain, the triptans also relieve the nausea, vomiting, and photophobia associated with acute migraine attack.

Evidence is growing for the role of preventive treatment in the management of migraine headaches (Brandes, 2005; Loder & Biondi, 2005). The decision to initiate prophylactic treatment is individually determined based on frequency and severity of headaches and on any disability due to headaches. Topiramate (Topamax), taken daily, has been shown to be an effective therapy for migraine prevention in adults. Not all patients become pain free on this medication (Lewis et al., 2007). Other preventive drugs for migraine headaches include beta-adrenergic blockers (e.g., propranolol [Inderal], atenolol [Tenormin]), tricyclic antidepressants (e.g., amitriptyline [Elavil]), selective serotonin reuptake inhibitors (e.g., fluoxetine [Prozac]), calcium channel blockers (e.g., verapamil [Isoptin]), divalproex (Depakote), clonidine (Catapres), and thiazides.

Cluster headaches. Because the pain associated with vascular cluster headaches is often severe, narcotic analgesics, sometimes given intramuscularly, are used. Patients with cluster headaches usually feel fine between attacks, so no analgesic is needed during these times.

Tension headaches. Nonnarcotic analgesics are often used to treat tension headaches. These include acetaminophen, propoxyphene, phenacetin, ibuprofen, and aspirin. Narcotics are avoided because these drugs are often subject to abuse; it is much better to counsel patients to develop other ways to relieve headaches.

Nursing Interventions and Patient Teaching

Because stress and emotional upsets may precipitate some headaches and worsen others, the patient requires relaxation and rest. Help the patient with relaxation techniques, planned sleeping hours, and regular rest periods. Alcohol should not be used to relieve tension because it may become addicting and has been found to be a significant cause of cluster headaches. Regular physical exercise may also help prevent headaches, especially ones caused by tension.

If a patient is suffering from a severe headache, plan nursing interventions so that only essential activities take place. Group interventions so that the patient has adequate time to rest.

Comfort Measures

Other treatments that may help a patient with a headache include cold packs applied to the forehead or base of the skull and pressure applied to the temporal arteries. People with migraine headaches are usually most comfortable lying in a dark, quiet room.

Identifying Triggering Factors

Triggering factors associated with severe and recurring headaches may include fatigue, alcohol, stress, seasonal climate changes, hunger, allergies, and menstruation. Help the patient identify these factors, if necessary, through ongoing observation or assessment of the patient's personality, habits, ADLs, career plans, work habits, family relationships, coping mechanisms, and relaxation activities. The patient may keep a diary or journal to help collect this information.

Nursing diagnoses and interventions for the patient with headache include but are not limited to the following:

Nursing Diagnoses	Nursing Interventions
Anxiety, related to pain	Provide quiet environment. Encourage verbalization of concerns. Provide diversional activities.
Acute or chronic pain, related to disease process	Administer prescribed medications. Provide comfort measures. Maintain nonstressful environment. Encourage pain reduction techniques as appropriate: rocking movements, external warmth, breathing patterns.

Teaching is an important part of the nursing intervention of the patient with headaches. Topics include (1) avoidance of factors that trigger headaches; (2) relaxation techniques, including biofeedback; (3) maintenance of regular sleep patterns; (4) medications to be used (including dosage, actions, and side effects); and (5) the importance of follow-up care.

Prognosis

With proper treatment the person with headaches can expect to live a normal life. Changes in lifestyle may need to occur, especially during acute episodes of headache pain. The person may have to adjust to periodic headaches and rest until the headache resolves.

NEUROPATHIC PAIN

Etiology, Pathophysiology, and Clinical Manifestations

Neuropathic pain other than headache is common. Examples include postherpetic neuralgia, phantom limb pain, diabetic neuropathies, and trigeminal neuralgia (Lewis et al., 2007). The transmission of pain is not fully understood, but patients may experience disabling pain either caused by a disorder within the nervous system or caused at a distant part of the body. Neuropathic pain may arise from lesions involving the peripheral cutaneous nerves, the sensory nerve roots, the thalamus, and the central pain tract (lateral spinothalamic) at some level. Each produces characteristic pain. Pain receptors are not adaptable—they are specific for pain only—and pain impulses continue at the same rate as long as the stimulus is present. Pain receptors can be activated by cellular damage, certain chemicals such as histamine, heat, ischemia, muscle spasm, and sensations of cold and pruritus that go beyond a specific level of intensity.

Pain that is described as unbearable and does not respond to treatment is classified as **intractable.** It is chronic and often debilitating and may prevent the patient from functioning in ADLs.

Assessment

The perception of pain is highly subjective. Pain may vary from mild to excruciating. **Subjective data** include the patient's understanding of the pain; any precipitating factors; and measures that relieve stress, including medication. The site, frequency, and nature of the pain are important, as is the patient's usual coping patterns when under stress. Associated symptoms and measures that make the pain worse are important subjective data.

Objective data may be limited when assessing neuropathic pain. Objective factors to assess are behavioral signs indicating pain or stress, a change in the ability to carry out ADLs, muscle weakness or wasting, vasomotor responses (such as flushing), abnormalities of spinal reflexes, and abnormalities noted during the sensory examination.

Diagnostic Tests

Diagnostic tests for the patient in pain may include electrical stimulation, used to define the pain to a greater degree. Psychological testing may be part of the workup. If back or neck pain is present, a myelogram is usually performed.

Medical Management

Nonsurgical Methods of Pain Control

Neuropathic pain sometimes responds to other methods of pain control. These include transcutaneous electrical nerve stimulation and spinal cord stimulation. Both techniques use electrodes applied near the site of pain or on or around the spine (see Chapter 42). The stimulator modifies the sensory input by blocking or changing the painful sensation with a stimulus that is perceived to be less painful or nonpainful. Acupuncture is also used to treat patients with neuropathic pain.

Nerve Block

A nerve block is used to control intractable pain. It involves injecting a local anesthetic, alcohol, or phenol close enough to a nerve to block the conduction of impulses. Sources of pain often treated with a nerve block include trigeminal neuralgia, cancer, and peripheral vascular disease. The effect lasts from several months to several years. Pain and spasticity may also be controlled by means of an epidural catheter. Medication is usually administered continuously.

Medications

Medications are often used to treat patients with neuropathic pain. Anticonvulsant medications such as gabapentin (Neurontin) and carbamazepine (Tegretol) are often useful. Other medications include nonopioid analgesics such as acetaminophen, nonsteroidal antiinflammatory drugs, and acetylsalicylic acid. Opioids do not appear as helpful for neuropathic pain although they are still sometimes used. Antidepressants—such as amitriptyline, doxepin (Sinequan), imipramine (Tofranil-PM), and nortriptyline (Pamelor)—appear to be effective in treating neuropathic pain. The emphasis should be on helping the patient learn various other measures to control the pain.

Surgical Methods of Pain Control

In cases of intractable pain that does not respond to more conservative measures, surgery may be necessary to reduce or eliminate pain. Neurosurgical procedures include neurectomy, rhizotomy, cordotomy, and percutaneous cordotomy. These procedures all have potential complications that need to be considered before the decision is made to perform surgery. For example, a patient who undergoes a cordotomy may have difficulties with postural hypotension, ability to feel hot or cold, and possibly motor and bowel function. Temporary edema of the cord from the procedure may lead to temporary paralysis or leg weakness.

Nursing Interventions and Patient Teaching

Comfort Measures

A patient with neuropathic pain may be uncomfortable and should be assisted to assume a position of comfort. For example, the patient with back pain should avoid movements that cause direct or indirect movement of the spinal cord. The patient may find lying in a supine position uncomfortable. Help the patient find a comfortable position and, if necessary, actively assist the patient in turning or moving. Straining when having a stool can intensify pain, and a stool softener may be needed. Offer prune juice and a high-fiber diet and encourage the patient to drink up to 2000 mL/day or more of fluids.

Promotion of Rest and Relaxation

As with headache, stress and emotional upsets may precipitate or exacerbate neuropathic pain. Facilitate rest and relaxation, with planned sleeping hours and rest periods as needed.

Some patients with pain, especially intractable pain, may respond well to psychotherapy. This does not mean that the pain does not have a physiologic basis, but counseling can help the patient develop awareness of what makes the pain worse and how to cope with the discomfort.

Nursing diagnoses and interventions for the patient with neuropathic pain are the same as those listed previously for headache, with the addition of the following:

Nursing Diagnoses	Nursing Interventions
Risk for disuse syndrome, related to lack of use of a body part as a result of pain	Explain need for regular exercise program to maintain joint mobility; provide range-of-motion (ROM) exercises to all body joints every 2 to 4 hours. Be positive and reassuring in approach.
Feeding, bathing/hygiene self-care deficit, related to pain	Assist with basic ADL needs as necessary, but encourage patient to participate as much as possible. Provide sufficient time for ADLs. Facilitate use of self-help devices as needed. Provide for total hygiene as indicated.

Teaching is an important part of the nursing interventions of the patient with neuropathic pain. Include the factors taught to the patient with headache, and help patient become aware of physical methods such as positioning the body to increase comfort and structuring the home and work setting to minimize stress.

Prognosis

As with headache pain, neuropathic pain can in most cases be treated adequately. Lifestyle changes may be helpful in allowing the person to have a better quality of life.

INCREASED INTRACRANIAL PRESSURE

Etiology, Pathophysiology, and Clinical Manifestations

Increased ICP is a complex grouping of events that occurs because of multiple neurologic conditions. It often occurs suddenly, progresses rapidly, and requires surgical intervention. It is a potential complication in many neurologic conditions and can rapidly lead to death if not treated and reversed.

Increased ICP occurs in patients with acute neurologic conditions such as a brain tumor, hemorrhage, anoxic brain injury, and toxic or viral encephalopathies; it is most commonly associated with head injury. An increase in any one of the contents of the cranium is usually accompanied by a reciprocal change in the volume of one of the others. This is be-

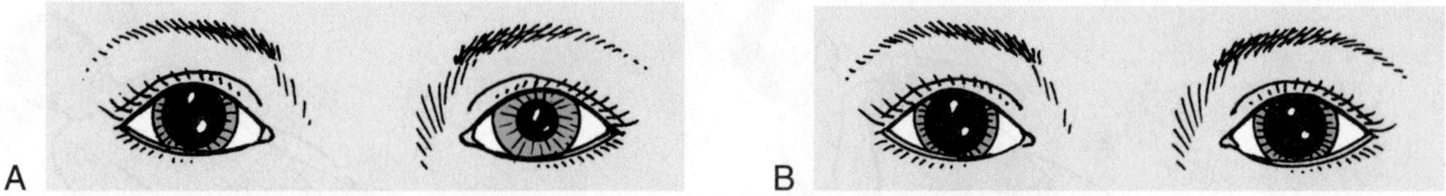

A B

FIGURE 54-8 **A,** Unequal pupils, also called anisocoria. **B,** Dilated and fixed pupils, indicative of severe neurologic deficit.

cause the cranial vault is rigid and nonexpandable. Pressure may build up slowly over weeks or rapidly, depending on the cause. Usually one side of the brain is more involved, but both sides of the brain eventually become involved.

As the pressure increases within the cranial cavity, it is first compensated for by venous compression and CSF displacement. As the pressure continues to rise, the cerebral blood flow decreases and inadequate perfusion of the brain occurs. This inadequate perfusion starts a vicious cycle that causes the Pco_2 to increase and the Po_2 and pH to decrease. These changes cause vasodilation and cerebral edema. The edema further increases the ICP, which causes increased compression of neural tissue and an even greater increase in ICP.

When the pressure buildup is greater than the brain's ability to compensate, pressure is exerted on surrounding structures where the pressure is lower. This movement of pressure is called **supratentorial shift** and can result in herniation. As a result of herniation of the brain, the brainstem is compressed at various levels, which in turn compresses the vasomotor center, the posterior cerebral artery, the oculomotor nerve, the corticospinal nerve pathway, and the fibers of the ascending RAS. The life-sustaining mechanisms of consciousness, blood pressure, pulse, respiration, and temperature regulation are all impaired. A rise in systolic pressure and an unchanged diastolic pressure, resulting in a widening pulse pressure, bradycardia, and abnormal respiration, are late signs of increased ICP and indicate that the brain is about to herniate.

Assessment

Increased ICP must be detected early while it is still reversible. The ability to make accurate observations, interpret observations intelligently, and record observations carefully is most important for the nurse working with patients with increased ICP.

Subjective data for a diagnosis of increased ICP include the patient's understanding of the condition, any visual changes such as diplopia (double vision), a change in the patient's personality, and a change in the ability to think. The diplopia usually results from paralysis or weakness of one of the muscles that controls eye movement. It often occurs fairly early in the process. Nausea or pain, especially headache, is also important. The headache is thought to result from venous congestion and tension in the intracranial blood vessels as the cerebral pressure rises. Headache that occurs with increased ICP usually increases in intensity with coughing, straining at stool, or stooping. It is usually present in the early morning and may awaken the patient from sleep.

Objective data include a change in the LOC, which is the earliest sign of increased ICP. During assessment, it takes more stimulation to get the same response from the patient. Manifestations of a change in the LOC include disorientation, restlessness, and lethargy. Record observations in terms of behaviors and signs and symptoms, not in terms of labels. Pupillary signs may also change with increased ICP. Pupillary responses are controlled by cranial nerve III (oculomotor nerve). The pupils usually change on the same side as the lesion. The first and most subtle clue to trouble is that the pupil reacts, but sluggishly. As the brain herniates, the nerve is compressed—with the top part of the nerve being affected first. The **ipsilateral** pupil (when the lesion is in one hemisphere) remains dilated and is incapable of constricting. The pupil appears larger than that of the affected side and does not react to light. As the ICP increases and both halves of the brain become affected, bilateral pupil dilation and fixation occur. Dilating pupils that respond slowly to light are a sign of impending herniation. A pupil that is fixed and dilated, sometimes called a **blown pupil,** is an ominous sign that *must* be reported to the physician immediately (Figure 54-8).

Changes in the blood pressure and pulse are seen with increasing ICP. Herniation causes ischemia of the vasomotor center, which excites the vasoconstrictor fibers, causing the systolic blood pressure to rise. If the ICP continues to increase, a widening pulse pressure occurs.

Pressure in the vasomotor center also increases the transmission of parasympathetic impulses through the vagus nerve to the heart, causing a slowing of the pulse. A widened pulse pressure, increased systolic blood pressure, and bradycardia are together called **Cushing's response.** It is considered an important diagnostic sign of late-stage brain herniation.

Brain herniation produces respiratory problems that are variable and related to the level of the brainstem compression or failure. The breathing pattern may be deep and stertorous (snorelike) or periodic (Cheyne-Stokes) respirations. **Ataxic** breathing may also occur; this is an irregular and unpredictable breathing pattern with random, shallow, and deep breaths and occasional pauses. It is seen in patients

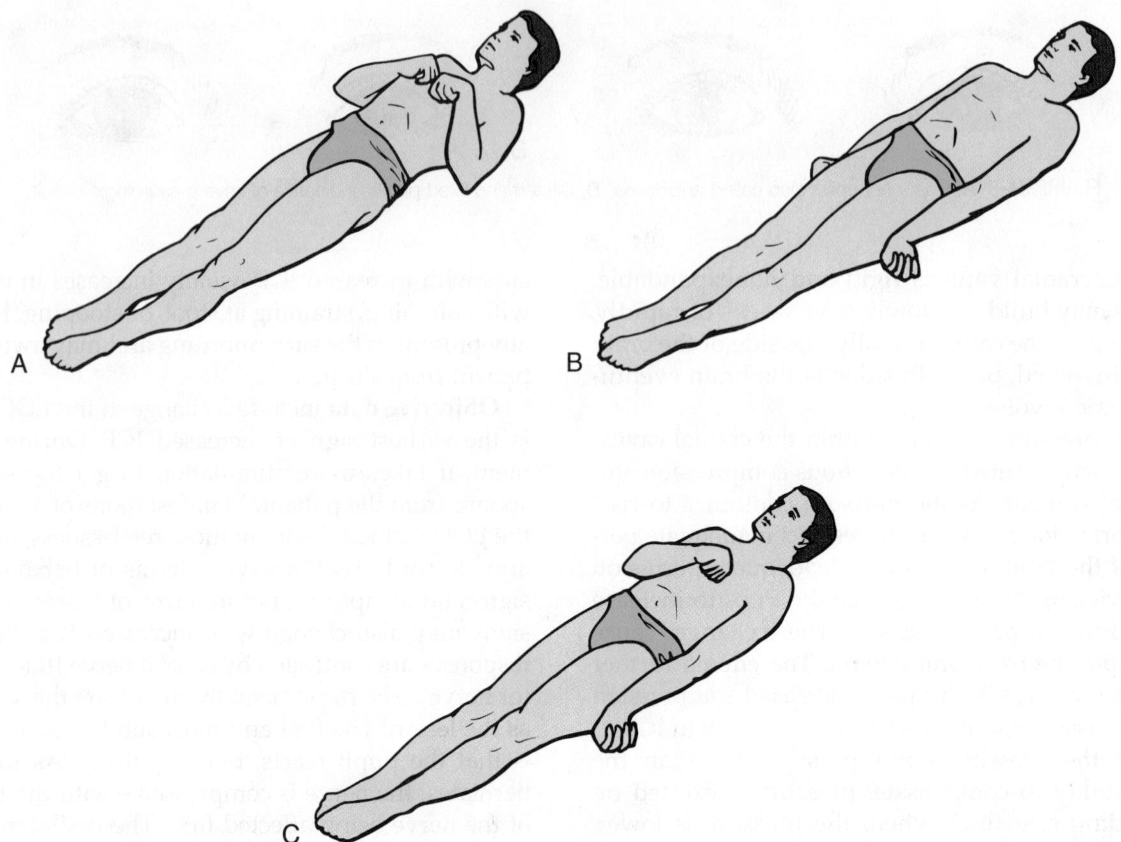

FIGURE 54-9 Decorticate and decerebrate responses. A, Decorticate response. Flexion of arms, wrists, and fingers with adduction in upper extremities. Extension, internal rotation, and plantar flexion in lower extremities. B, Decerebrate response. All four extremities in rigid extension, with hyperpronation of forearms and plantar extension of feet. C, Decorticate response on right side of body and decerebrate response on left side of body.

with medulla oblongata damage. As ICP increases to fatal levels, respiratory paralysis occurs.

Failure of the thermoregulatory center because of compression occurs later with increased ICP. It results in high, uncontrolled temperatures. This hyperthermia increases the metabolism of brain tissue.

Compression of the upper motoneuron pathway (corticospinal tract) interrupts transmission of impulses to the lower motoneuron, and progressive muscle weakness occurs. Babinski's reflex, hyperreflexia, and rigidity are additional signs of decreased motor function. Seizures may occur. Herniation of the upper part of the brainstem may produce characteristic posturing when the patient is stimulated (Figure 54-9). The worsening of motor problems is significant, because it means that the ICP is continuing to increase.

Vomiting and singultus (hiccups) are two objective signs of increased ICP. The vomiting is often projectile and usually not preceded by nausea; this is called unexpected vomiting. Singultus is caused by compression of the vagus nerve (cranial nerve X) as brainstem herniation occurs.

One last objective sign is papilledema, which is detected with the use of an ophthalmoscope (usually by the physician). As ICP increases, the pressure is transmitted to the eyes through the CSF and to the optic disk. As the optic disk becomes edematous, the retina is also compressed. The damaged retina cannot detect light rays. Visual acuity is lessened as the blind spot enlarges. **Papilledema** is also called a **choked disk.**

Diagnostic Tests

Diagnostic studies are aimed at identifying the presence and the underlying cause of increased ICP. The diagnosis of increased ICP is made with CT or MRI, which can show actual structural herniation and shifting of the brain. Because of CT and MRI, the diagnosis of increased ICP has been completely revolutionized and the therapeutic options greatly increased (Lewis et al., 2007).

Most of the time, acute increased ICP is a medical emergency, and diagnostic tests must be done quickly. Other tests include ICP measurement, EEG, cerebral angiography, transcranial Doppler studies, and PET. In general, lumbar puncture is not performed when increased ICP is suspected because of the possibility of cerebral herniation from the sudden release of the pressure in the skull from the area above the lumbar puncture. This can lead to pressure on cardiac and respiratory centers in the brainstem and potentially death (Lewis et al., 2007).

In postoperative or critically ill patients, internal measuring devices are used to diagnose increased ICP. One of the most common measuring devices requires the placement of a hollow screw through the skull into the subarachnoid space. The device is connected to a transducer and oscilloscope for continuous monitoring. Waveforms are produced that indicate the ICP.

Medical Management

The goals of treatment are to identify and treat the underlying cause of increased ICP. Preventing increased ICP may not be possible, but preventing further increases in pressure with resulting damage to the brain is crucial. The medical treatment depends on the cause of the pressure. For example, surgery may be done to remove a tumor. If surgery is not possible, efforts are made to reduce the pressure through drug therapy or other measures.

Ensuring adequate oxygenation to support brain function is the first step in management of increased ICP. Endotracheal intubation may be necessary. Arterial blood gases analysis guides the oxygen therapy. With controlled ventilation, the Pco_2 can be lowered to below normal, which causes a slightly alkalotic pH. The decrease in the Pco_2 and the increase in pH will decrease vasodilation and decrease ICP. The goal is to maintain the Pao_2 at 100 mm Hg.

Mechanical Decompression

Rapidly rising ICP can be relieved by mechanical decompression. This may include a craniotomy, in which a bone flap is removed and then replaced, or a craniectomy, in which a bone flap is removed and not replaced. The craniectomy is often done when pressure is high. Other means of decompression include drainage of the ventricles or any subdural hematoma.

Internal monitoring devices are being used more frequently to diagnose and monitor increased ICP. Three basic monitoring systems are used: the ventricular catheter, the subarachnoid bolt or screw, and the epidural sensor. These monitoring devices produce pressure waves that can be evaluated to indicate the status of ICP.

Medications

Three types of medications are usually administered to patients with increased ICP: osmotic diuretics, corticosteroids, and anticonvulsants. Osmotic diuretics are also called hyperosmolar drugs. They draw water from the edematous brain tissue. An example of this type of medication is mannitol. It begins to reduce increased ICP within 15 minutes, and its effects last for 5 to 6 hours. Loop diuretics such as furosemide (Lasix), bumetanide (Bumex), and ethacrynic acid (Edecrin) may also be used in the management of increased ICP. Continuous midazolam (Versed) and atracurium besylate (Tracrium) infusions are also used.

The corticosteroid that may be given is dexamethasone (Decadron). Corticosteroids are thought to control edema surrounding cerebral tumors and abscesses but appear to have limited value in managing head-injured patients (Lewis et al., 2007). With this drug, monitor blood glucose levels because steroids can affect carbohydrate metabolism and glucose utilization and result in elevated blood glucose levels.

To prevent gastrointestinal ulcers and bleeding, patients receiving corticosteroids should concurrently be given antacids, histamine-receptor blockers (e.g., cimetidine [Tagamet], ranitidine [Zantac]), or proton pump inhibitors (e.g., omeprazole [Prilosex], pantoprazole [Protonix, Protonix I.V.]).

Anticonvulsants are given to prevent seizures. Phenytoin (Dilantin) is the most commonly given drug. It can be given intravenously but usually not intramuscularly because of poor absorption. Fosphenytoin (Cerebyx) is a short-term IV or intramuscular anticonvulsant in current use. Opioids and other drugs that cause respiratory depression are avoided.

Nursing Interventions and Patient Teaching

Therapeutic measures to reduce venous volume include the following:

- Elevate the head of the bed to 30 to 45 degrees to promote venous return.
- Place the neck in a neutral position (not flexed or extended) to promote venous drainage.
- Position the patient to avoid flexion of the hips, the waist, and the neck and rotation of the head, especially to the right. Avoid extreme hip flexion because this position causes an increase in intraabdominal and intrathoracic pressures, which can produce a rise in ICP.
- Instruct the patient to avoid isometric or resistive exercises.
- Restrict fluid intake.
- Implement measures to help the patient avoid the Valsalva maneuver (any forced expiratory effort against a closed airway, such as straining to have a stool). Avoid enemas and laxatives if possible.
- Have a Foley catheter in place if the patient is not alert because of the large amount of urine that is produced.
- Perform suctioning only as necessary and for no longer than 10 seconds with administration of 100% oxygen before and after to prevent decreases in the Pao_2.
- Administer oxygen via mask or cannula to improve cerebral perfusion.
- Use a hypothermia blanket to control body temperature (increased body temperature increases brain damage).

Nursing diagnoses and interventions for the patient with increased ICP may include but are not limited to the following:

Nursing Diagnoses	Nursing Interventions
Ineffective breathing pattern, related to neuromuscular impairment	Maintain patent airway; avoid flexion of neck. Administer oxygen and humidification as ordered. Provide oral nasopharyngeal airway as indicated for managing secretions; suction oropharynx as needed.
Risk for injury, related to physiologic effects of sustained elevation in ICP	Elevate head of bed 30 degrees. Maintain body position; avoid semiprone or prone position. Avoid compression of neck veins. Check blood pressure, pulse, and respiration every 30 minutes. Perform neurologic check every 30 minutes using Glasgow coma scale; report any findings below 8 to physician.

The patient with increased ICP is often unresponsive. Share information about procedures that are being done with the patient and the family. This may help both be as cooperative as possible.

Prognosis

The prognosis for the patient with increased ICP depends on the cause and the speed with which it is treated. The nurse assumes an important role in monitoring the patient for signs and symptoms of increased pressure. After herniation of the brain has begun as a result of pressure, there is little chance for complete reversal without significant brain damage.

DISTURBANCES IN MUSCLE TONE AND MOTOR FUNCTION

Etiology and Pathophysiology

Motor function disturbances are the most commonly encountered neurologic signs and symptoms. Damage to the nervous system often causes serious problems in mobility. An example of this is the patient with cerebral palsy.

Clinical Manifestations

Injury or disease of motoneurons results in alterations of muscle strength, tone, and reflex activity. Muscle tone may be described as **flaccid** (weak, soft, flabby, and lacking normal muscle tone) or **hyperreflexic** (increased reflex actions). The specific clinical manifestations differ according to the location of the neurologic lesion.

Assessment

Subjective data for patients with motor problems include the patient's understanding of the problem and possible causes. Ask about the initial onset of the symptoms; measures that improve symptoms; and the presence of clumsiness, incoordination, or abnormal sensation. If the lesion occurs suddenly, as in traumatic spinal cord injury, subjective symptoms may be minimal. If the motor deficit develops slowly, subjective symptoms may be so subtle that they are at first ignored.

Objective data include coordination, muscle strength, muscle tone, and muscle atrophy. Reflexes are often checked, as well as the presence of clonus or fasciculations and the ability to move muscles. Any abnormal gait is significant, as is a change in the ability to carry out ADLs.

Diagnostic Tests

One of the most common procedures for detecting pathologic conditions of muscle is the EMG. It detects the various types of electrical activity and abnormal patterns that may appear in resting muscle in the presence of disease.

Medical Management

Patients with motor problems may have spasticity. Muscle relaxants may be used to decrease tone and involuntary movements. Some commonly prescribed medications include baclofen (Lioresal), dantrolene (Dantrium), and diazepam (Valium). Baclofen has been used intrathecally to reduce spasticity. Common side effects of these drugs include drowsiness and vertigo. These side effects are increased by the use of alcohol or other depressants.

Some patients may have severe swallowing difficulty **(dysphagia)**. This commonly results from obstructive or motor disorders of the esophagus and is commonly associated with neurologic problems. The patient with dysphagia often requires prefeeding and feeding exercises.

In patients at severe risk for aspiration, a video fluoroscopy with barium may be done when aspiration is suspected. The procedure requires the patient to swallow a small amount of liquid or semisolid barium while a fluoroscopic examination is being done.

For patients with paralysis, the eye on the affected side of the body may need to be protected if the lid remains open and there is no blink reflex. The patient is at high risk for corneal scratches or irritation. Irrigation with a physiologic solution of sodium chloride may be used, followed by eyedrops. An eye pad may be used to keep the eye closed, although an eyeshield is preferable.

Nursing Interventions

Safety Needs

Patients with paralysis have significant safety needs. This includes protection from falling, including the use of side rails when the patient is in bed and a chair restraint when the patient is in a chair, especially if balance cannot be maintained. If the patient also has a sensory problem, which often accompanies paralysis, he or she may not realize when part of the body is in danger. For example, a patient with a stroke may not be aware that a hemiplegic arm is hanging over the side of the wheelchair.

The eye on the affected side of the body should be cleaned and assessed for signs of infection on a regular basis, usually three times a day or more. Also inspect affected body parts for injury.

Regularly inspect the skin over bony prominences for signs of pressure. Paralyzed people are at risk for skin impairment, so teach them to turn themselves in bed and to reposition themselves in the bed or chair independently, if possible. If the patient is unable to turn independently, the nurse carries out this function. Usually the patient is turned from one side to another or from one side to the back to the other side. Repositioning also includes weight shifts, done by the patient or by staff. These weight shifts may include controlled leaning from one side to another or push-ups. If the patient is not able to do the activity, have him or her take responsibility for reminding staff when it is time to do the weight shift.

Inspect paralyzed or weakened areas at least daily for any signs of skin impairment. A mirror is often used to help the patient assess the skin so that he or she is not as dependent on staff or family.

Activity Needs

The extremities of a person who has an acute motor problem may be flaccid at first. Spasticity of muscles develops gradually. The joints then become flexed and fixed in useless, deformed positions unless preventive measures are taken.

Carefully place the extremities in a normal anatomical position to prevent deformity. Counterpositioning may be helpful. In **hemiplegia** (paralysis of one side of the body) the affected upper extremity is pulled inward at the shoulder joint and the wrist drops; in the lower extremity the knee flexes and the foot drops. In counterpositioning, position the patient so that the shoulder and upper arm are in abduction, the elbow is flexed, the wrist is dorsiflexed, the knee is in neutral position, and the foot is dorsiflexed. If the person is supine, place a pillow between the upper arm and the body to hold the arm in abduction. Physical therapists and occupational therapists can provide splints and braces that can aid in positioning (Figure 54-10).

Footboards may be used to prevent footdrop, although some believe that these contribute to increased spasticity and should not be used routinely for patients who have muscle spasms. High-topped tennis shoes or other devices, such as splints or braces, can help prevent footdrop, if therapy is initiated early. In some hospitals, casts are applied to patients' lower extremities to prevent footdrop or to reverse contractures. The presence of the cast impedes spasticity. A sling or hook hemiharness may be useful to support the affected arm to prevent shoulder subluxation.

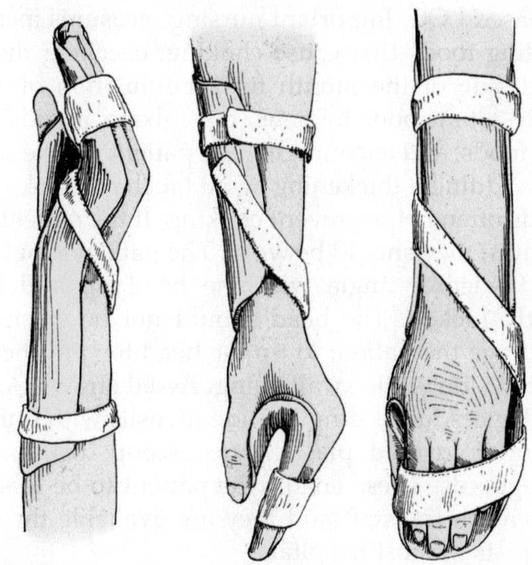

FIGURE 54-10 Volar resting splint provides support to wrist, thumb, and fingers of patient after cerebrovascular accident (stroke), maintaining them in position of extension.

The prone position is excellent for patients who are able to tolerate it. Not only does this position decrease the chance of skin impairment, but it also causes extension of the hip, the knee joints, and the ankles by means of gravity. A pillow placed under the chest may help patients comfortably assume this position.

Positioning of the paralyzed person is extremely important. Complications such as footdrop and flexion contractures of the knee seriously limit mobility. As a result, the level of self-care and independence is diminished. Most joint deformities in a paralyzed person are preventable with early and continuing nursing interventions.

In addition to positioning, interventions for the person with paralysis include ROM exercises to all joints. These may be passive (carried out by the nurse) or active (carried out by the patient). Passive ROM is indicated at least three times daily for all joints that the patient cannot voluntarily move.

Nutritional Needs

Patience and persistence are often necessary in giving food and fluids to the patient with hemiplegia. Aspiration can occur and is related to loss of pharyngeal sensation, loss of oropharyngeal motor control, and decreased LOC. Important nursing measures include avoiding foods that cause choking, checking the affected side of the mouth for accumulation of food and resultant poor hygiene, not mixing liquids and solid foods, and encouraging the patient to take small bites. Adding a thickening agent (such as Thick-It) to liquids often helps prevent choking. If the patient has dentures, they should be worn. The patient should sit at a 90-degree angle with the head up and chin slightly tucked. The head should not be extended; encourage the patient to tip the head toward the unaffected side while swallowing. Avoid straws. Assistive devices for feeding include utensils with universal cuffs, covered plastic cups, scoop dishes, and plate guards. These enable the patient to be less dependent on the staff and they are available through therapists in most hospitals.

Activities of Daily Living

During the acute rehabilitative phases of a motor problem, teach patients with paralysis how to carry out ADLs to the extent that they are able. A variety of devices are available to assist with dressing and grooming (Figures 54-11 and 54-12). The occupational therapist becomes involved in many of these activities, including homemaking. Stress the concept of the rehabilitative team in managing these patients. Teach the patient to compensate for weakness or paralysis. Give the patient the time to do activities on his or her own if able. It is often easier and faster to do things for the patient, but this defeats the purpose of rehabilitation.

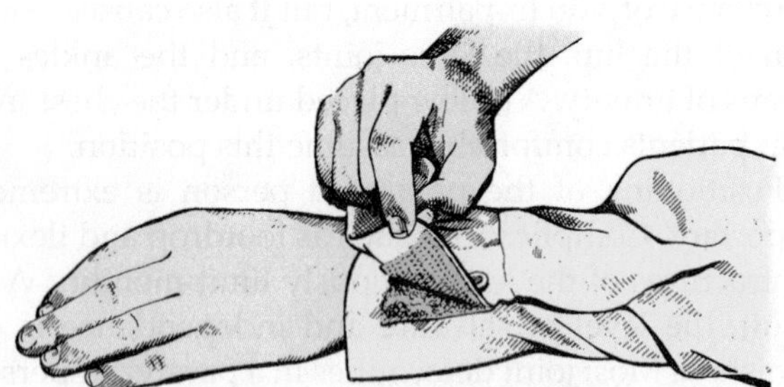

FIGURE 54-11 Velcro shirtsleeve to facilitate closure.

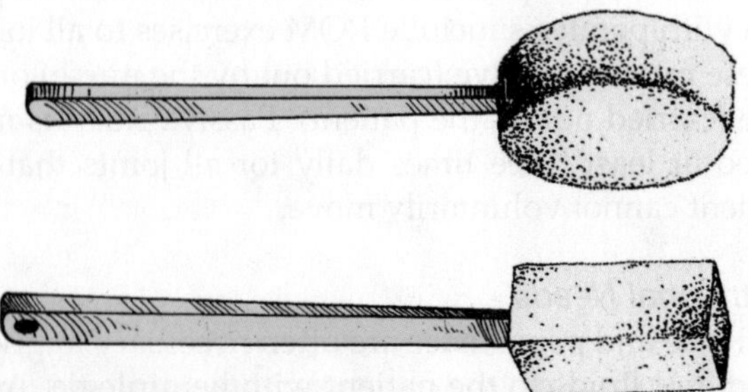

FIGURE 54-12 Long-handled bath sponges.

Psychological Adjustments

The person with paralysis may need assistance in adjusting to body changes. The loss of the ability to function independently is traumatic, and the patient may have fears of rejection, loss of self-esteem, and concerns about the future. A grief reaction similar to that described for a death may occur. At times the patient may relate to the paralyzed part of the body as though it were not a part of him or her and may have nicknames for the body part. To help the patient cope with the loss of function and change in body image, praise the patient for achievements, encourage expression of fears and grief, and help him or her see that there is life after disability. It might be helpful to arrange a visit by someone with the same disability who has been successfully rehabilitated.

Nursing diagnoses and interventions for the patient with alterations in muscle tone and motor function include but are not limited to the following:

Nursing Diagnoses	Nursing Interventions
Impaired physical mobility, related to neuromuscular impairment	Perform active or passive ROM exercise every 4 hours, to all extremities, neck, hands, fingers, wrists, elbows, and knees. Provide physical therapy as ordered (massage and stretching exercises). Maintain planned rest periods. Encourage ambulation to tolerance. Arrange for necessary assistive devices for home care needs.
Risk for disuse syndrome, related to impaired functioning of body part	Perform hand, finger, foot exercises; assist in active and passive ROM exercises every 2 to 4 hours. Assist patient with using supportive devices as indicated (overhead trapeze, braces, walker, cane). Encourage use of involved side when possible. Instruct patient to use unaffected extremity to support weaker side (e.g., lift involved left leg with right leg or lift involved left arm with right arm). Turn every 2 hours.

 Health Promotion

The Patient with a Neurologic Disorder

- **Nutritional-metabolic pattern:** Neurologic problems can result in inadequate nutrition. Problems related to chewing, swallowing, facial nerve paralysis, and muscle coordination could make it difficult for the patient to ingest adequate nutrients.
- **Elimination pattern:** Bowel and bladder problems are often associated with neurologic problems, such as stroke, head injury, spinal cord injury, multiple sclerosis, and dementia. It is important to determine whether the bowel or bladder problem was present before the neurologic event to plan appropriate interventions.
- **Activity-exercise pattern:** Many neurologic disorders can cause problems in the patient's mobility, strength, and coordination. These problems can change the patient's usual activity and exercise patterns.
- **Sleep-rest pattern:** Sleep can be disrupted by many neurologically related factors. Discomfort from pain and inability to move and change to a position of comfort because of muscle weakness and paralysis could interfere with sound sleep.
- **Cognitive-perceptual pattern:** Because the nervous system controls cognition and sensory integration, many neurologic disorders affect these functions. Assess memory, language, calculation ability, problem-solving ability, insight, and judgment.
- **Self-perception–self-concept pattern:** Neurologic disease can drastically alter control over one's life and create dependency on others for daily needs.
- **Role-relationship pattern:** Ask the patient if neurologic problems have led to changes in roles, such as spouse, parent, or breadwinner. These changes can dramatically affect both the patient and significant others.
- **Sexuality-reproductive pattern:** Assess the ability to participate in sexual activity, since many nervous system disorders can affect sexual response.
- **Coping–stress tolerance pattern:** The physical sequelae of a neurologic problem can seriously strain a patient's ability to cope. Often the problem is chronic and may require the patient to learn new coping skills.
- **Value-belief pattern:** Many neurologic problems have serious, long-term, life-changing effects. These effects can strain the patient's belief system and should be assessed

Data from Lewis, S.L., et al. *Medical-surgical nursing: Assessment and management of clinical problems.* (7th ed.). St. Louis: Mosby.

Patient Teaching

Teaching is an extremely important part of caring for the person with motor problems. Appropriate teaching activities include safety needs, skin care, activity (ROM and positioning), medications (dosage, action, times, and side effects), good nutrition, ADLs, bowel and bladder care, and follow-up care. Written instructions reinforce teaching and give the patient something to refer to at home (see Health Promotion box). Prepare family members to assume some of the care for the patient.

DISTURBED SENSORY AND PERCEPTUAL FUNCTION

Etiology and Pathophysiology

The presence of a lesion anywhere within the sensory system pathway, from the receptor to the sensory cortex, alters the transmission or perception of sensory information. The parietal cortex is of major importance in interpretation of sensation. Loss of, decrease in, or increase in sensation of pain, temperature, touch, and proprioception results in difficulty in daily functioning. Any alteration lessens the patient's protection from inadvertent injury.

One specific loss is proprioception, or the ability to know the position of the body and its parts without directly looking at the part. **Agnosia** is a total or partial loss of the ability to recognize familiar objects by sight, touch, or hearing or to recognize familiar people through sensory stimuli as a result of organic brain damage.

Assessment

Subjective data include the patient's understanding of the sensory disturbance, measures that relieve symptoms (including medications), and symptoms that occur with the sensory problem. An example is the person who experiences weakness of a hand and at the same time feels numbness and tingling. Collect information on the onset of the sensory problem and the specific site in the body.

Collection of **objective data** includes noting the patient's ability to perform purposeful movements or to recognize familiar objects.

Medical Management

Refer to medical management for alterations in the patient's muscle tone and motor function.

Nursing Interventions and Patient Teaching

The most important nursing intervention for the patient with sensory dysfunction is teaching the patient protective measures. This includes helping the patient learn to inspect parts of the body that have no feeling or protect sensitive body parts from the discomfort of linen rubbing over them. If a patient has a deficit in one sense, he or she should learn to compensate with another (e.g., the patient who learns to lip read because of a hearing deficit; the patient with hemianopia who is taught to scan the printed page).

A nursing diagnosis and interventions for the patient with a sensory or perceptual problem are the same as those for the patient with a motor problem, with the addition of but not limited to the following:

Nursing Diagnosis	Nursing Interventions
Risk for injury, related to sensory or perceptual disturbances	Maintain safe environment. Teach patient to protect body parts that have decreased sensation. Teach patient to inspect body parts for possible injury. Protect patient from sustaining injury from hot liquid or heating pads.

The teaching for a patient with a sensory deficit is essentially the same as that for the patient with a motor deficit.

OTHER DISORDERS OF THE NEUROLOGIC SYSTEM

Functioning of the neurologic system can be interrupted for a variety of reasons. These include conduction abnormalities, degenerative diseases, vascular problems, infection, tumors, trauma, and cranial and peripheral nerve disorders. Selected disorders in each area are discussed.

CONDUCTION ABNORMALITIES

EPILEPSY OR SEIZURES

Etiology and Pathophysiology

Epilepsy is a group of neurologic disorders characterized by recurrent episodes of convulsive seizure, sensory disturbances, abnormal behavior, LOC, or all of these.

Cases of epilepsy have been recorded throughout history. Seizures occur in all races and affect men and women equally. There is no apparent geographic distribution. In the United States it is estimated that approximately 2.7 million people suffer from active epilepsy, with 200,000 new cases being diagnosed each year (Epilepsy Foundation, 2009). The incidence rates are higher in the first year of life, decline through childhood and adolescence, plateau in middle age, and rise sharply again among older adults. The population within highest prevalence of new-onset epilepsy is those over the age of 60 (Tian et al., 2005).

Clinical Manifestations

Seizures can be classified according to the features of the attack. The types include generalized tonic-clonic (grand mal), absence (petit mal), psychomotor (automatisms), jacksonian (focal), and miscellaneous (myoclonic and akinetic) seizures (Table 54-6).

Epilepsy is associated with paroxysmal, uncontrolled electrical discharges in the neurons of the brain that result in the sudden, violent, involuntary contraction of a group of muscles. The patterns or forms of seizures vary and depend on the area of the brain from which the seizure arises (see Figure 54-7). Seizures occur for a variety of reasons, including cerebral trauma, intracranial infection, brain tumor, vascular disturbances, alcohol intoxication, hypoglycemia, electrolyte imbalance, barbiturate withdrawal, and water intoxication. Although many causes of seizure disorders have been identified, three fourths of all cases are considered idiopathic (without a known cause) (Lewis et al., 2007).

The excessive neuronal discharges may result in a tonic convulsion, with alternate contraction and relaxation of opposing muscle groups. This gives the characteristic tonic-clonic jerking movements of the body. Seizures are followed by a rest period of variable length, called the postictal period (after a seizure). During this period the patient usually feels groggy and acts disoriented. Complaints of headache and muscle aches are common. Usually the patient sleeps after a seizure and may experience amnesia for the event.

When recurrent, generalized seizure activity occurs at such frequency that full consciousness is not regained between seizures, it is called **status epilepticus.** This is a medical emergency and requires medical and nursing interventions. Repeated seizures cause the brain to use more energy than can be supplied; the neurons become exhausted and cease to function, which may result in permanent brain damage or death (Lewis et al., 2007). The nursing interventions always involve ensuring that there is a patent airway and protecting the patient from injury. Medications to stop the seizure activity may be given in high doses that render the patient unconscious. The nurse must then assume total care of the patient's needs. Insert a Foley catheter and an IV line. Intubate the patient if necessary for ventilatory support. Protect the skin from injury. Take care with safety reminder devices if the patient is awake and active so that they do not cause injury if the patient begins to have a seizure.

Assessment

Subjective data include the patient's awareness of the disorder and any precipitating factors. Assess whether an aura preceded the seizure. An aura occurs in about 50% of all patients with generalized tonic-clonic seizures. Aura is a sensation (such as of light or warmth) or emotion (such as fear) that may precede an attack of migraine or an epileptic seizure. An epileptic aura may be psychic, or it may be sensory with olfactory, visual, auditory, or taste hallucinations. The exact character of the aura varies from person to person. Awareness of an aura warns the person of the impending seizure and allows him or her to seek safety and privacy.

Objective data include the number of seizures occurring within a specific time, the character of the seizure, and any behaviors noted and injuries suffered.

Table 54-6 Characteristics of Seizures

INCIDENCE	CHARACTERISTICS	CLINICAL SIGNS	AURA	POSTICTAL PERIOD
GENERALIZED TONIC-CLONIC (FORMERLY KNOWN AS GRAND MAL)				
Most common	Generalized; characterized by loss of consciousness and falling to the floor or ground if patient is upright, followed by stiffening of the body (tonic phase) for 10-20 seconds and subsequent jerking of the extremities (clonic phase) for another 30-40 seconds	Aura Cry Loss of consciousness Fall Tonic-clonic movements Incontinence, cyanosis, excessive salivation, tongue or cheek biting	Yes Flashing lights Smells Spots before eyes (scotomata) Vertigo	Yes Need for 1-2 hours' sleep Headache, muscle soreness commonly felt May not feel normal for several hours or days after a seizure No memory of a seizure
ABSENCE (FORMERLY KNOWN AS PETIT MAL)				
Occurs during childhood and adolescence Frequency decreases as child gets older Rarely continues beyond adolescence	Sudden impairment in or loss of consciousness with little or no tonic-clonic movement Occurs without warning Has tendency to appear a few hours after arising or when person is quiet	Sudden vacant facial expression with eyes focused straight ahead (staring spell) that lasts only a few seconds All motor activity ceases except perhaps for slight symmetric twitching about eyelids Possible loss of muscle tone May have an extremely brief loss of consciousness	No	No
PSYCHOMOTOR (AUTOMATISMS; ALSO CALLED PARTIAL SEIZURES)				
Occur at any age	Sudden change in awareness associated with complex distortion of feeling and thinking and partially coordinated motor activity Longer than absence seizures	Behaves as if partially conscious; may continue an activity that was initiated before the seizure, such as counting out change or picking items from a grocery shelf, but after the seizure does not remember the activity Often appears intoxicated May do antisocial things, such as exposing self or carrying out violent acts Autonomic complaints, such as shivering, lip smacking, repetitive movements that may not be appropriate Urinary incontinence	Yes Complex hallucinations or illusions	Yes Confusion Amnesia Need for sleep
JACKSONIAN-FOCAL (LOCAL OR PARTIAL)				
Occur almost entirely in patients with structural brain disease	Depends on site of focus May or may not be progressive	Commonly begin in hand, foot, or face May end in tonic-clonic seizure	Yes Numbness Tingling Crawling feeling	Yes

Continued

Table 54-6 Characteristics of Seizures—cont'd

INCIDENCE	CHARACTERISTICS	CLINICAL SIGNS	AURA	POSTICTAL PERIOD
MYOCLONIC				
May antedate tonic-clonic by months or years	May be very mild or may have rapid, forceful movements	Sudden, excess jerk of the body or extremities; may be forceful enough to hurl the person to the floor or ground Brief seizures that may occur in clusters No loss of consciousness	No	
AKINETIC				
Not common	Peculiar generalized tonelessness	Falls in flaccid state Unconscious for minute or two	Rarely	No

Describe the seizure as completely as possible, including duration, the patient's movements, whether the patient was incontinent, any cries or sounds that were made, and the level of alertness.

Diagnostic Test

The most common test used to evaluate seizures is the EEG (see Figure 54-7). It allows a specific diagnosis of the seizure.

Medical Management

Medications

In 70% of patients, seizure disorders are controlled by one or more antiseizure drugs (Table 54-7). Therapy is aimed at preventing seizures because cure is not possible. Drugs generally act by stabilizing nerve cell membranes and preventing spread of the epileptic discharge. The choice of medication depends on the type of seizure. Failure to take the prescribed medication or an adequate dose is often the cause of treatment failure. Blood levels may be checked to determine the therapeutic level of the medications taken. The primary goal of antiseizure drug therapy is to obtain maximum seizure control with minimum toxic side effects.

Surgical Therapy

Many patients with epilepsy are unable to control their seizures with medications and are candidates for surgical intervention. All types of epilepsy do not benefit from surgery. Three requirements must be met before surgical intervention can occur: (1) the diagnosis of epilepsy must be confirmed; (2) an adequate trial with drug therapy without therapeutic results must occur; and (3) the type of seizure disorder must be defined. Surgical treatments include removal of small areas of the hippocampus, anterior temporal lobe resection, and disconnective surgery incising through nerve pathways that allow the spread of the seizures. The benefits of surgery are the reduction or cessation of seizures (Lewis et al., 2007).

Activities of Daily Living

Until seizures are controlled, patients should avoid activities such as driving a car, operating machinery, or swimming. Maintaining adequate rest and good nutrition is also important. Alcohol use should be avoided. If the patient is receiving long-term phenytoin therapy, good hygiene practices for the mouth and teeth are important because of the side effect of edematous and enlarged gums (gingival hyperplasia). The patient should wear a medical-alert bracelet or tag (see Patient Teaching box).

 Patient Teaching

The Patient with Seizures

- Explain the need for the patient to continue taking medications even when seizure activity has stopped.
- Teach the patient about medications prescribed, including expected results, time and dosage, and side effects.
- Inform the patient that medical-alert bracelets, necklaces, and identification cards are available. However, the use of these medical identification tags is optional. Some patients have found them beneficial, but others prefer not to be identified as having a seizure disorder.
- Caution the patient to avoid the use of alcohol if taking antiseizure medications.
- Explain the need for good oral hygiene for people taking phenytoin (Dilantin) (a side effect is gingival hyperplasia).
- Stress the importance of adequate rest and a balanced diet.
- Educate about available community resources.
- Explain restrictions concerning driving.
- Explain the importance of follow-up care.
- A tonic-clonic seizure can be treated with first aid; it is not necessary to send the patient to the hospital (or call an ambulance) after a single seizure unless the seizure is prolonged, another seizure immediately follows, or extensive injury has occurred.
- In the event of an acute seizure, protect the patient from injury. This involves supporting and/or protecting the head, turning the patient to one side, loosening any constricting garments, and, if the patient is seated, easing him or her onto the floor.

Table 54-7 Medications for Preventing and Controlling Seizures

Generic (Trade)	Use Related to Seizure Type	Toxic Effects
Phenytoin sodium (Dilantin)	Generalized tonic-clonic, focal, psychomotor	Ataxia, vomiting, nystagmus, drowsiness, rash, fever, gum hypertrophy, lymphadenopathy
Divalproex (Depakote)	Generalized tonic-clonic and myoclonic seizures	Sedation, drowsiness, behavior changes, visual disturbances, hepatic failure
Oxcarbazepine (Trileptal)	Generalized tonic-clonic and partial seizures	Feeling abnormal, headache, dizziness, vertigo, anxiety, burred vision
Phenobarbital (Luminal)	Generalized tonic-clonic, focal, psychomotor	Drowsiness, rash
Primidone (Mysoline)	Generalized tonic-clonic, focal, psychomotor	Drowsiness, ataxia
Ethosuximide (Zarontin)	Absence seizures, psychomotor, myoclonic, akinetic	Drowsiness, nausea, agranulocytosis
Trimethadione (Tridione)	Absence seizures	Rash, photophobia, agranulocytosis, nephrosis
Diazepam (Valium)	Generalized tonic-clonic and status epilepticus, mixed	Drowsiness, ataxia
Carbamazepine (Tegretol)	Generalized tonic-clonic, psychomotor	Rash, drowsiness, ataxia
Valproic acid (Depakene)	Absence seizures	Nausea, vomiting, indigestion, sedation, emotional disturbance, weakness, altered blood coagulation
Clonazepam (Klonopin)	Absence seizures, akinetic, myoclonic, generalized tonic-clonic seizures	Drowsiness, ataxia, hypotension, respiratory depression
Mephenytoin (Mesantoin)	Tonic-clonic, focal, psychomotor	Ataxia, nystagmus, pancytopenia, rash
Gabapentin (Neurontin)	Focal, generalized tonic-clonic in adults	Somnolence, fatigue, ataxia, dizziness, anorexia
Lamotrigine (Lamictal)	Focal, generalized tonic-clonic in adults	Rash, dizziness, tremor, ataxia, diplopia, headache, gastrointestinal upset, Stevens-Johnson syndrome (rare)
Felbamate (Felbatol)	Seizures in children, generalized tonic-clonic seizures in adults; may be used to treat patients whose seizure disorders are refractory to other drugs	Irritability, insomnia, anorexia, nausea, headache; can cause aplastic anemia and hepatic failure
Fosphenytoin sodium (Cerebyx)	Short-term parenteral (IV or IM) in acute generalized tonic-clonic seizures; used for status epilepticus and for preventing and treating seizures during neurosurgery	Dizziness, paresthesia, tinnitus, pruritus, headache, somnolence, ataxia, muscular incoordination, nystagmus, double vision, slurred speech, nausea, vomiting, and hypotension
Topiramate (Topamax), tiagabine (Gabitril), levetiracetam (Keppra), zonisamide (Zonegran)	Indicated for partial seizures and for secondary generalized seizures; currently used as adjunctive therapy	Topiramate: somnolence, dizziness, ataxia, speech disorders and related speech problems, difficulty with memory, paresthesia, diplopia; tiagabine: dizziness, lightheadedness, asthenia (lack of energy), somnolence, nausea, nervousness, irritability, tremor, thinking abnormally, difficulty with concentration or attention

Nursing Interventions and Patient Teaching

Care during a Seizure

The primary goals of the nurse and the family caring for a patient having a seizure are protection from aspiration and injury and observation and recording of the seizure activity. Never leave the patient alone. If the patient is sitting or standing, lower him or her to the floor in an area away from furniture and equipment. Support and protect the head; if possible, turn the head to the side to maintain the airway. If there is time, loosen clothing around the neck. Do not try to restrain the patient during the seizure. Do *not* try to pry open the jaw to place a padded tongue blade. No objects should be placed in the mouth. After the seizure the patient may require suctioning and oxygen. Padded side rails may be used, especially if seizures often occur during sleep.

When a seizure occurs, carefully observe and record details of the event because the diagnosis and subsequent treatment often rest solely on the seizure description. Note all aspects of the seizure: What events preceded the seizure? When did the seizure occur? How long did each phase (aural [if any], ictal, postictal) last? What occurred during each phase?

Nursing diagnoses and interventions for the patient with seizures may include but are not limited to the following:

Nursing Diagnoses	Nursing Interventions
Ineffective airway clearance, related to mucus accumulation in oropharyngeal area during seizure	Place patient in side-lying position to prevent aspiration and ensure airway patency. Suction secretions as needed.
Risk for injury, related to rapid onset of altered state of consciousness and seizure activity	If patient is out of bed during seizure activity, assist to the floor and remove objects that may harm him or her. Provide privacy. Maintain patent airway. After the seizure, inform patient of seizure and reorient if necessary.

Prognosis

Seizure disorders can affect a patient's emotional, economic, and social well-being. Society's attitude has improved, but epilepsy still carries a social stigma. Most states have legal sanctions against driving if one has epilepsy. The inability to maintain a driver's license can negatively affect one's lifestyle (Lewis et al., 2007).

The majority of patients with seizures are able to control them with medications and can lead a fairly normal life. With most seizure disorders, the number and intensity of seizures stay constant. However, in patients who experience a first seizure as a result of a brain tumor or another brain pathologic condition, the prognosis is more uncertain.

DEGENERATIVE DISEASES

The term **degenerative diseases** refers to neurologic disorders in which there is a premature aging of nerve cells, which is caused by suspected metabolic disturbance or for which the cause is unknown. Six diseases are discussed: multiple sclerosis (MS), Parkinson's disease, Alzheimer's disease (AD), myasthenia gravis (MG), amyotrophic lateral sclerosis (ALS), and Huntington's disease.

MULTIPLE SCLEROSIS

Etiology and Pathophysiology

MS is a chronic, progressive, degenerative neurologic disease that affects many people. The cause is unknown, although genetics have been implicated, since there is a higher rate of the disease among relatives. Patients with the first signs and symptoms of MS have a proliferation of a certain type of immune cell called **gamma delta T cells** in their spinal fluid. These cells are not found in patients who have had the disease for a long time. T cells, the "field commanders" of the immune system, usually defend the body from outside attackers. In MS, however, something goes wrong and induces the T cells to attack the body. Myelin damage occurs. The beginning mechanism may be a viral infection early in life that becomes apparent as an immune process later in life. A defective immune response also seems to have an important role in the pathology of MS.

The onset of signs and symptoms is usually between 15 and 50 years of age. Women are affected more often than men. The highest number of people with MS live in the Great Lakes area, the Pacific Northwest, and the North Atlantic states. MS is five times more prevalent in temperate climates between 45 and 66 degrees of latitude.

Multiple foci of **demyelination** are distributed randomly in the white matter of the brainstem, the spinal cord, optic nerves, and the cerebrum. During the demyelination process, the myelin sheath and the sheath cells are destroyed, causing an interruption or distortion of the nerve impulse so that it is slowed or blocked (Figure 54-13). Areas of degeneration show evidence of partial healing, which explains the transitory nature of early signs and symptoms.

Clinical Manifestations

The onset is often insidious and gradual, with vague symptoms that occur intermittently over months or years, thus the disease may not be diagnosed until long after the onset of the first symptom. Because of the wide distribution of areas of degeneration, the variety of signs and symptoms in MS is greater than in other neurologic diseases. These include visual problems, urinary incontinence, fatigue, weakness or incoordination of an extremity, sexual problems such as impotence in men, and swallowing difficulties. The majority of people have early remissions that may last for a year or more. The disease is characterized by chronic, progressive deterioration in some persons and by remissions and exacerbations in others. Exacerbations may be related to fatigue, chilling, or emotional disturbances. With repeated exacerbations, progressive scarring of the myelin sheath occurs, and the overall trend is progressive deterioration in neurologic function.

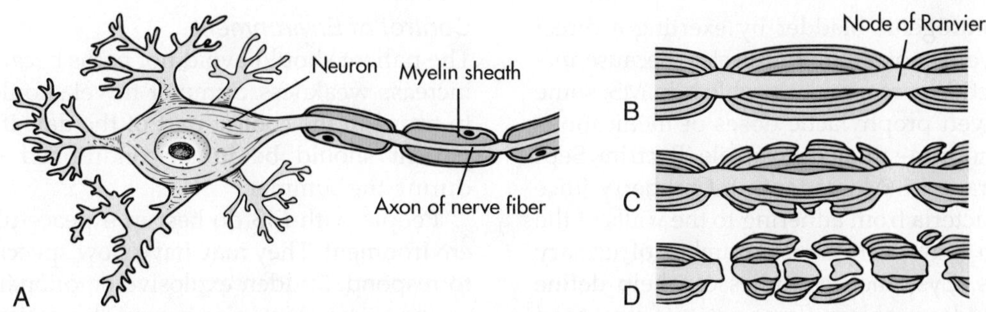

FIGURE 54-13 Pathogenesis of multiple sclerosis. **A,** Normal nerve cell with myelin sheath. **B,** Normal axon. **C,** Myelin breakdown. **D,** Myelin totally disrupted; axon not functioning.

Assessment

Subjective data include the patient's understanding of the disease. Eye problems such as diplopia, scotomata (spots before the eyes), and blindness may be present. The patient may also talk about weakness or numbness of a part of the body, fatigue, emotional instability, bowel and bladder problems, vertigo, or loss of joint sensation. Involvement of the cerebellum can result in ataxia (impaired ability to coordinate movement) and tremor. In men, impotence is significant. Pain is not a common symptom.

Objective data include documented abnormalities in neurologic testing; these may include nystagmus (involuntary, rhythmic movements of the eye; the oscillations may be horizontal, vertical, rotary, or mixed); muscle weakness and spasms; changes in coordination; or a spastic, ataxic gait. Cerebellar signs include ataxia, dysarthria, and dysphagia. There may be evidence of behavior changes such as euphoria, emotional lability, or mild depression. Urinary incontinence and intention tremors of the upper extremities may be present.

Diagnostic Tests

MS has no definitive diagnostic test; diagnosis is based primarily on history and clinical manifestations and the presence of multiple lesions over time as measured by MRI. Examination of the CSF in patients with MS may show elevated gamma globulin, a proliferation of gamma delta T cells in the initial phase, and increased number of lymphocytes and monocytes. A CT scan may show enlargement of the cerebral ventricles. MRI scanning has been helpful in diagnosing MS over time in the presence of multiple lesions; sclerotic plaques as small as 3 to 4 mm in diameter can be detected.

Medical Management

Medications

No specific treatment exists for MS, although many different remedies have been tried. Symptoms are controlled with the use of adrenocorticotropic hormone (ACTH) and corticosteroids such as prednisone (Deltasone) or dexamethasone. These may be given orally, intramuscularly, or intravenously. The effects of ACTH and the steroids on the demyelinating process are unknown, although they probably help by reducing edema and acute inflammation at the site of demyelination. If steroids are used in high doses at the start of an exacerbation, the episode seems to resolve more rapidly. However, these drugs do not affect the ultimate outcome or degree of residual neurologic impairment from the exacerbation. If spasticity is a problem, drugs such as diazepam, dantrolene, and baclofen may help prevent or decrease the spasms. Immunomodulating drugs modify the disease process. Interferon beta-1b (Betaseron), given subcutaneously every other day, is indicated for use in ambulatory patients with relapsing-remitting MS to reduce the frequency of clinical exacerbations. Interferon beta-1a (Avonex) is similar to interferon B-1b in efficacy and is used in similar patient groups with MS. It is given intramuscularly once a week. Interferon beta-1a (Rebif) is administered subcutaneously three times weekly. A new immunomodulator is glatiramer acetate (Copaxone), approved for use in relapsing-remitting MS. Glatiramer is not an interferon, but it is believed to help MS patients by interrupting the inflammatory cycle and preventing the body's immune system from attacking the myelin coating that protects the nerve fiber. It is given subcutaneously daily. Mitoxantrone (Novantrone) is a drug for the treatment of primary-progressive and progressive-relapsing MS. It is an immunosuppressant drug that reduces both B and T lymphocytes. It is given intravenously monthly. Because of cardiac toxicity, it cannot be used for more than 2 to 3 years (Lewis et al., 2007). Many research studies are being conducted in the search for more effective medications to use in the treatment of MS.

Elimination

Urinary frequency and urgency may respond to propantheline (Pro-Banthine). Cholinergic drugs such as bethanechol (Urecholine) can sometimes help the patient with a neurogenic bladder by exerting a direct antispasmodic effect on smooth muscles. Because urinary tract infections are a major problem in MS, some patients are given prophylactic doses of medications such as trimethoprim-sulfamethoxazole (Bactrim, Septra) or nitrofurantoin (Macrodantin). Cranberry juice may prevent bacteria from adhering to the walls of the bladder, which may decrease the number of urinary tract infections. Cystometric studies can help define the specific bladder problem. Some patients may need to be taught self-catheterization.

Encourage the patient to drink adequate fluids (at least 2000 mL/day). If the patient suffers from constipation, a stool softener such as docusate sodium (Colace) may be used, as well as prune juice.

Nursing Interventions

Nutrition

A well-balanced diet with high-fiber foods and adequate fluids is important. Although there is no standard prescribed diet, a high-protein diet with supplemental vitamins is often recommended. Obesity makes it more difficult for the patient to meet daily needs and maintain mobility. The patient who is obese should be referred to the dietitian and be placed on a calorie-restricted diet that will help the patient lose weight slowly, while receiving adequate nutrition.

Skin Care

Teach the patient with MS and/or the caregiver frequent turning to avoid skin impairment. Devices to relieve pressure, such as eggcrate or air mattresses, may be helpful. Because of sensory involvement, the patient may not feel discomfort that signals the need to change position.

Activity

Encourage patients with MS to exercise regularly, but not to the point of fatigue. Physical therapy sometimes improves neurologic dysfunction. Exercise also helps daily functioning for patients with MS not experiencing an exacerbation. Exercise decreases spasticity, increases coordination, and retrains unaffected muscles to substitute for impaired ones (Rietberg et al., 2005). Water exercise is an especially beneficial type of physical therapy. Because of the buoyancy water gives to the body, the patient has more control over the body and is able to perform activities that would be impossible on land (Lewis et al., 2007).

Daily rest periods may be helpful. During an acute exacerbation, patients are often kept as quiet as possible; this includes bed rest.

One side of the body is often more affected than the other. The patient must learn to stabilize the gait by leaning toward the less-involved side. If the foot slaps forward while the patient is walking, teach him or her to put the foot down in a pronounced fashion and roll the weight forward on the side of the foot.

Control of Environment

The patient should avoid hot baths because they often increase weakness. Summer travel should be planned to travel in the coolest part of the day. If possible, the patient should be in air-conditioned surroundings during the summer.

People with MS do best in a peaceful and relaxed environment. They may have slow speech and be slow to respond. Sudden explosive emotional outbursts of crying or laughing also occur. The patient and family need support in dealing with this behavior.

Nursing diagnoses and interventions for the patient with MS may include but are not limited to the following:

Nursing Diagnoses	Nursing Interventions
Risk for powerlessness, related to physical limitations imposed by progressive physical deterioration, loss of body control, and threat to physical integrity	Provide emotional support, thorough explanations, and reassurance. Be alert to emotional changes and mood swings. Encourage the patient's participation and expression of needs and feelings. Maintain planned rest periods. Encourage self-care as indicated. Provide physical care as indicated.
Bathing/hygiene, feeding, toileting self-care deficit, related to limitations in physical mobility imposed by disease process	Administer oral hygiene before meals. Assist with or provide physical hygiene as indicated by physical ability. Maintain appropriate bathing temperatures. Administer oral hygiene every 4 hours and as needed. Catheterize intermittently as indicated; teach self-catheterization when possible. Plan bladder dysfunction program as appropriate for spasticity or flaccidity. Institute bowel control program (establish regular bowel routine, avoid constipation). Assist in dressing and grooming as indicated. Provide nutritious, attractive meals.

Patient Teaching

Teaching is important for both the patient with MS and significant others. In late stages of the disease, the care functions usually are assumed by someone other than the patient. Important points include those for the patient with motor and sensory problems (see pp. 1908-1912). In addition, stress the importance of spacing activities and avoiding temperature extremes and the potential for emotional lability. Make certain that the patient or the family has the address of the nearest MS society or support group.

Prognosis

The prognosis is variable. Some patients have MS for many years with few deficits, whereas other patients quickly become debilitated. The patient's ability to conserve energy and avoid stress may help prevent exacerbations. Exacerbations are treated and may resolve. The average life expectancy after the onset of symptoms is more than 25 years.

PARKINSON'S DISEASE

Etiology and Pathophysiology

Parkinsonism is a syndrome that consists of a slowing down in the initiation and execution of movement **(bradykinesia)**, increased muscle tone (rigidity), tremor, and impaired postural reflexes. Parkinson's disease, a form of parkinsonism, is named after James Parkinson, who, in 1817, wrote a classic essay on "shaking palsy," a disease whose cause is still unknown today. Many other disorders resemble this disease, but their causes are known. These include drug-induced parkinsonism, postencephalitic parkinsonism, and arteriosclerotic parkinsonism. The pathophysiology of these disorders, with the exception of drug-induced parkinsonism, is the same. Damage or loss of the dopamine-producing cells of the substantia nigra in the midbrain leads to depletion, in the basal ganglia, of dopamine that influences the initiation, modulation, and completion of movement and regulates unconscious autonomic movements. In cases of drug-induced parkinsonism, the dopamine receptors in the brain are blocked.

According to the American Parkinson Disease Association, Parkinson's disease affects more than 1 million people in the United States. Symptoms commonly occur after 50 years of age. Peak onset of Parkinson's disease is in the 60s. The average age of the patient with Parkinson's disease is 65 years. There is apparent genetic cause and no known cure. The disease rarely occurs in blacks. Parkinson's disease is more common in men by a ratio of 3:2.

Parkinsonism has many causes. Encephalitis lethargica, or type A encephalitis, has been clearly associated with the onset of parkinsonism. However, the incidence of postencephalitic parkinsonism has dwindled since the 1920s, when there was a large outbreak of this infectious illness. Parkinsonian-like symptoms have occurred after intoxication with a variety of chemicals, including carbon monoxide and manganese (among copper miners) and a product of meperidine-analog synthesis. Drug-induced parkinsonism can follow therapy with reserpine (Hydropres), methyldopa (Aldomet), haloperidol (Haldol), and phenothiazine (Thorazine).

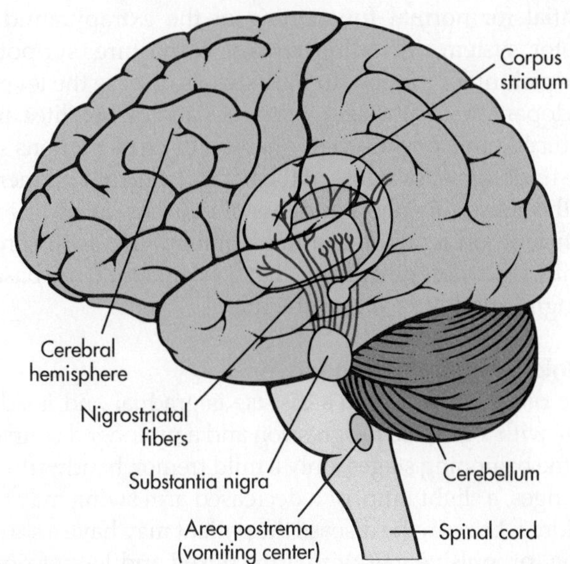

FIGURE 54-14 Nigrostriatal disorders produce parkinsonism. Left-sided view of the human brain showing the substantia nigra and the corpus striatum *(shaded area)* lying deep within the cerebral hemisphere. Nerve fibers extend upward from the substantia nigra, divide into many branches, and carry dopamine to all regions of the corpus striatum.

Although patients with cerebrovascular disease may have parkinsonian-like symptoms, there is little evidence that parkinsonism is caused by arteriosclerosis. Distinguishing arteriosclerosis from true Parkinson's disease is important for prognostic purposes. Patients with arteriosclerosis do not respond as well to treatment and are more likely to experience side effects of drug therapy. Most patients with parkinsonism have the degenerative or idiopathic form, for which the term *Parkinson's disease* is usually reserved.

Other factors linked to Parkinson's disease include reduced estrogen levels and exposure to pesticides, herbicides, industrial chemicals, and metals (mercury, copper, and manganese). Menopausal women who have not received hormone therapy are at risk (McCarron, 2006).

The pathology of Parkinson's disease is associated with the degeneration of the dopamine-producing neurons in the substantia nigra of the midbrain, which in turn disrupts the normal balance between dopamine and acetylcholine in the basal ganglia (Figure 54-14). Major signs and symptoms, such as tremors, muscle rigidity, slowed movements, and impaired balance and coordination, occur when approximately 60% to 80% of dopamine-producing cells have been destroyed. It is believed that there is normally a balance between acetylcholine and dopamine in the basal ganglia. Any shift in the balance of activity (an increase in acetylcholine or a decrease in dopamine) seems to lead to parkinson-like symptoms. Dopamine is a neurotransmitter that is essential for normal functioning of the extrapyramidal motor system, including control of posture, support, and voluntary motion. In Parkinson's disease the levels of dopamine-synthesizing enzymes and metabolites are reduced, and postmortem analysis of cross-sections of the midbrain shows loss of the normal melanin pigment in the substantia nigra and loss of neurons. In addition, deficient amounts of gamma-aminobutyric acid, serotonin, and norepinephrine have been found in basal ganglia and in the substantia nigra.

Clinical Manifestations

The onset of Parkinson's disease is gradual and insidious, with a gradual progression and a prolonged course. In the beginning stages, only a mild tremor, handwriting changes, a slight limp, or a decreased arm swing may be evident. Later in the disease the patient may have a shuffling, propulsive gait with arms flexed and loss of postural reflexes (Figure 54-15). Some patients may have a slight change in speech patterns. None of these alone is sufficient evidence for a diagnosis of the disease.

Because Parkinson's disease has no specific diagnostic test, the diagnosis is based solely on the history, a thorough neurologic examination, and clinical features. A firm diagnosis can be made only when the patient has at least two signs of the classic triad: tremor, rigidity, and bradykinesia (slow or retarded movement). In the early stage of the disease there are subtle changes in cognitive function that can progress to dementia. The ultimate confirmation of Parkinson's disease is a positive response to a low-dose trial of an antiparkinsonian medication, such as carbidopa-levodopa (Sinemet).

Tremor

Tremor, often the first sign, may be minimal initially, so the patient is the only one who notices it. This tremor can affect handwriting, causing it to trail off, particularly toward the ends of words. Parkinsonian tremor is more prominent at rest but disappears when the patient moves; it is aggravated by emotional stress or increased concentration. The hand tremor is described as "pill rolling" because the thumb and forefinger appear to move in a rotary fashion, as if rolling a pill, coin, or other small object. Tremor can involve the hands, diaphragm, tongue, lips, and jaw but rarely causes shaking of the head. Eventually tremors can become so pronounced that the patient cannot hold a newspaper steady enough to read or make a call on a push-button telephone. Unfortunately, in many people a benign essential tremor has mistakenly been diagnosed as Parkinson's disease. Essential tremor occurs during voluntary movement, has a more rapid frequency than parkinsonian tremor, and is often familial.

Rigidity

Rigidity, the second sign of the triad, is the increased resistance to passive motion when the limbs are moved through their range of motion. Parkinsonian rigidity is typified by a jerky quality when the joint is moved, like

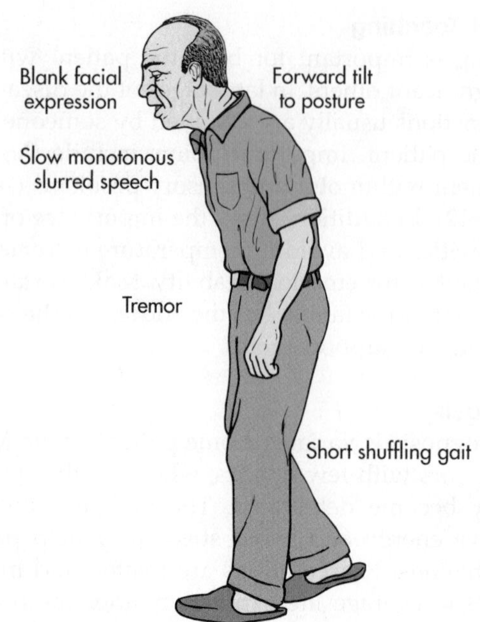

FIGURE 54-15 Characteristic appearance of a patient with Parkinson's disease.

intermittent catches in the movement of a cogwheel. This is termed *cogwheel rigidity.* The rigidity is caused by sustained muscle contraction and consequently elicits a complaint of muscle soreness; fatigue and achiness; or pain in the head, the upper body, the spine, or the legs. Another consequence of rigidity is slowness of movement, since it inhibits the alternating contraction and relaxation of opposing muscle groups (e.g., the biceps and triceps). Simple movements such as tying shoes and rising from a chair become a challenge.

Bradykinesia

Bradykinesia is particularly evident in the loss of automatic movements, which is secondary to physical and chemical alteration of the basal ganglia and related structures in the extrapyramidal portion of the CNS. In the unaffected patient, automatic movements are involuntary and occur subconsciously. They include blinking the eyelids, swinging the arms while walking, swallowing saliva, expressing oneself with facial and hand movements, and making minor postural adjustment. The patient with Parkinson's disease does not execute these movements and lacks spontaneous activity. This accounts for the stooped posture, masked face (deadpan expression), drooling, and shuffling gait (festination) that are characteristic of a person with this disease (see Figure 54-15). The voice softens and loses modulation too, further contributing to communication problems. One may see evidence of bradykinesia in the patient's handwriting. The words become tiny and different from earlier handwriting samples. This is referred to as micrographia (McCarron, 2006). The patient often has a shuffling, propulsive gait that he or she is unable to stop until meeting an obstruction. In addition, there is difficulty initiating movement. Movements such as getting out of a chair cannot be executed unless they are consciously willed.

Assessment

Parkinson's disease starts with subtle symptoms and progresses slowly. **Subjective data** include fatigue, incoordination, judgment defects, emotional instability, anxiety, depression, and heat intolerance. Assess the patient's understanding of the disease.

Objective data include tremor, which is the outstanding sign of the disease. This has been described as a pill-rolling motion of the fingers or a resting tremor. Bradykinesia is present with rigidity and loss of postural reflexes. Muscle rigidity leads to a mask-like appearance of the face; slowed, monotonous speech; and drooling. Dysphagia, or difficulty swallowing, is a common late complication of neurologic degeneration, which poses the risk of choking and aspiration pneumonia. The patient may be constipated. There may be a scaly, erythematous rash, particularly near the ears and eyebrows and in the scalp and nasolabial folds. Moist, oily skin is usually noted. Postural hypotension is prevalent and may be caused by failure of the arterial baroreceptors located in the aortic arch and the internal carotid arteries (McCarron, 2006).

Diagnostic Tests

Parkinson's disease has no firm diagnostic tests. If there is a history of chronic dementia, the CT scan may show cerebral atrophy. The EEG may show minimal slowing, and the upper gastrointestinal evaluation may show decreased motility.

Medical Management

Medications

Treatment for Parkinson's disease is based on easing the signs and symptoms of the disease. Several different drugs have had a dramatic effect on the course of the disease: trihexyphenidyl hydrochloride (Artane), benztropine mesylate (Cogentin), levodopa (Dopar) (the most commonly prescribed medication for Parkinson's disease), amantadine hydrochloride (Symmetrel), carbidopa-levodopa (for 35 years, the gold standard of therapy), selegiline hydrochloride (Eldepryl), ropinirole (Requip), tolcapone (Tasmar), pramipexole (Mirapex), pergolide (Permax), rasagiline (Azilect), and rotigotine (Neupro).

After prolonged treatment with some of the drugs, side effects such as dyskinesia (abnormal involuntary movements) may occur and the medication's effectiveness may decrease. Hospitalization may be helpful, during which time all drugs are withdrawn for a time. This is called a **drug holiday.** The medications are then restarted, and often smaller doses produce favorable results. Complications such as aspiration can occur during this time because withdrawal of the drugs causes immobility and rigidity (Table 54-8). To combat these problems, newer drug classes have been developed.

Surgery

Surgery that involves destroying portions of the brain that control the rigidity or tremor—so-called ablation surgery—has been used for Parkinson's disease for more than 50 years. However, it has been replaced by **deep brain stimulation (DBS).** DBS involves placing an electrode in either the thalamus, globus pallidus, or subthalamic nucleus and connecting it to a generator placed in the upper chest (like a pacemaker). The device is programmed to deliver a specific current to the targeted brain location. DBS can be adjusted to control symptoms and is reversible (the device can be removed). The procedure is nonablative and relatively safe and can improve dyskinesias (an impairment of the ability to execute voluntary movements), gait, rigidity, and tremors. This procedure is often reserved for patients who have developed severe side effects to drug therapy or severe motor complications.

Medications are discontinued several days preoperatively so that signs and symptoms will be at their maximum at the time of surgery.

Another treatment approach for Parkinson's disease involves human fetal dopamine cell transplants into the basal ganglia in an attempt to provide viable dopamine-producing cells to the brain.

Nursing Interventions

Activity Needs

Pay special attention to posture. Lying on a firm bed without a pillow may help prevent the spine from bending forward. Holding the hands folded behind the back when walking may help keep the spine erect and prevent the arms from falling stiffly at the sides. Problems secondary to bradykinesia can be alleviated by relatively simple measures. Advise patients who tend to "freeze" while walking to consciously think about stepping over imaginary or real lines on floor, drop rice kernels and step over them, rock from side to side, lift the toes when stepping, and take one step backward and two steps forward. A patient who has difficulty rising from a sitting position can use a chair that gently propels him or her to an upright position (McCarron, 2006). Do not hurry the patient because it will make the bradykinesia worse.

Nutrition

Diet is of major importance to the patient with Parkinson's disease to avoid malnutrition and constipation. Patients with dysphagia and bradykinesia need appetizing foods that can be easily chewed and swallowed. Food should be cut into bite-sized pieces before it is served. Eating six small meals a day may be less exhausting than eating three large meals. Allow ample time for eating to avoid frustration and encourage independence. When the disease is advanced, aspiration is a real concern. Take care during feeding. Unless the disease is well controlled by medication, drooling can be a problem and increases with general excitement.

Table 54-8 Medications for Disorders of the Neurologic System

Generic (Trade)	Action	Side Effects	Nursing Implications
Amantadine hydrochloride (Symmetrel)	Treats some cases of Parkinson's disease and drug-induced extrapyramidal reactions, although its action in treatment of Parkinson's disease is unknown	Nausea, vomiting, vision changes, dysrhythmias, disorientation, orthostatic hypotension, depression, fatigue	Tell patient to drink no alcohol; administer no CNS depressants; know pregnancy cautions; tell patient not to cease taking medication without conferring with physician and not to deviate from prescribed dosage; for best absorption, instruct patient to take after meals; if orthostatic hypotension occurs, instruct patient not to stand or change positions too quickly.
Baclofen (Lioresal)	Reduces transmission of impulses from spinal cord to skeletal muscles; is antispasticity agent for treatment of spinal spasticity resulting from multiple sclerosis or spinal cord injury	Drowsiness, dizziness, disorientation, lightheadedness, hypotension, urinary frequency, possible increase in blood glucose level	Be aware of pregnancy cautions; give oral form with meals or milk to prevent gastrointestinal distress; watch for increased incidence of seizures in patients with epilepsy; tell patient to avoid activities that require alertness until CNS effects of drugs are known.
Trihexyphenidyl hydrochloride (Artane)	Blocks central cholinergic receptors, helping to balance cholinergic activity of basal ganglia; is antidyskinetic and antiparkinsonian; controls some mild cases as an adjunct to more potent drugs; controls extrapyramidal reactions caused by drugs	Skin rash, eye pain, nervousness, headaches, tachycardia, urinary hesitancy, urine retention, dry mouth, disorientation	Do not give antacids or antidiarrheal agents within 1 hour of giving medication; give with food; caution patient to rise slowly; use cautiously in patients with narrow-angle glaucoma and hypertension; warn patient to avoid activities that require alertness until CNS effects of drugs are known; tell patient to relieve dry mouth with cool drinks, ice chips, and hard candy.
Pyridostigmine bromide (Mestinon)	Inhibits destruction of acetylcholine released from parasympathetic and somatic efferent nerves; causes acetylcholine to accumulate, promoting increased stimulation of receptor; is used in myasthenia gravis and by the oral route for senility associated with Alzheimer's disease	Headache, seizures, bradycardia, hypotension, bronchospasm, increased bronchial secretions	Judging optimum dosage is difficult; monitor and document patient's response after each dose when using for myasthenia gravis; stress importance of taking drug exactly as ordered, on time, and in evenly spaced doses.
Benztropine mesylate (Cogentin)	Blocks central cholinergic receptors, helping to balance cholinergic activity in basal ganglia; is indicated in treatment of mild cases of Parkinson's disease and control of extrapyramidal reactions	Dizziness, drowsiness, depression, orthostatic hypotension, palpitation, tachycardia	Stress importance of following prescribed dosage; discontinue drug slowly; tell patient not to drink alcohol; advise patient of breastfeeding warnings; give with food; tell patient to rise slowly and notify physician of severe allergic reactions; do not give with antacids.
Tacrine hydrochloride (Cognex)	Acts as reversible cholinesterase inhibitor, used for treatment of mild to moderate dementia of Alzheimer's type	Bradycardia, nausea and vomiting, loose stools, ataxia, CNS disturbance, anorexia, agitation, increased serum transaminase levels, jaundice	Know risk of ulcers; monitor liver enzyme weekly for first 18 weeks; increase dosage at 6-week intervals; do not use NSAIDs concomitantly; be aware that it potentiates theophylline.

CNS, Central nervous system; *I&O*, intake and output; *NSAIDs*, nonsteroidal antiinflammatory drugs.

Table 54-8 Medications for Disorders of the Neurologic System—cont'd

Generic (Trade)	Action	Side Effects	Nursing Implications
Levodopa (Dopar, Larodopa)	Antiparkinsonian agent (mechanism of action is unknown); increases balance between cholinergic and dopaminergic activity to allow more normal body movements and alleviate signs and symptoms	Aggressive behavior, involuntary grimacing, head and body movements, depression, suicidal tendencies, orthostatic hypotension, nausea, vomiting, darkened urine, excessive and inappropriate sexual behavior	Do not give to patients with narrow-angle glaucoma; monitor patients receiving antihypertensive and hypoglycemic agents; advise patient to change positions slowly and dangle legs; protect drug from heat, light, moisture.
Carbidopa-levodopa (Sinemet)	Increases levels of dopamine and levodopamine; is antiparkinsonian agent; improves modulation of voluntary nerve impulses transmitted to the motor cortex (lower dosage is needed than with single-dose therapy; efficiency may increase 75% when carbidopa and levodopa are used in combination)	Mental depression, mental changes, nausea and vomiting, orthostatic hypotension, dizziness, uncontrollable body movements	Give with food; give only as directed; effectiveness may take months; warn patient of breastfeeding and pregnancy cautions; caution patient about drowsiness and getting up too fast; lying down may affect control of blood glucose and darken urine.
Selegiline hydrochloride (Eldepryl)	Monoamine oxidase (MAO) inhibitor used as treatment adjunct to levodopa and carbidopa-levodopa; may slow Parkinson's disease and need for increased medication; may prolong life span of people with Parkinson's disease	Severe orthostatic hypotension, increased tremors, chorea, restlessness, grimacing, nausea and vomiting, slow urination, increased sweating, alopecia	Advise patient not to take more than 10 mg/day (there is no evidence that a greater amount improves effectiveness and it may increase adverse reactions); warn patient not to drink alcohol and drink only a little coffee; give with food; tell patient to rise slowly and notify physician of side effects; tell patient not to take over-the-counter cold remedies; monitor blood pressure and respirations.
Donepezil (Aricept)	Improves cholinergic function by inhibiting acetylcholinesterase; anti-Alzheimer's agent; may temporarily lessen some of the dementia associated with Alzheimer's disease, but does not alter the course	Diarrhea, nausea, vomiting, fatigue, headache, ecchymoses, atrial fibrillation, vasodilation	Monitor heart rate (may cause bradycardia); assess cognitive function periodically during therapy; administer in the evening just before bed; may be taken without regard for food.
Memantine (Namenda)	Believed to act as an *N*-methyl-D-aspartate receptor antagonist to decrease glutamate, which is an excitatory neurotransmitter in the CNS; approved for the treatment of moderate to severe Alzheimer's disease; does not prevent or slow neurodegeneration, but found in clinical studies to slow symptom progression	Dizziness, headache, constipation, hypertension, urinary frequency	Monitor I&O; Do not give to patients with severe renal impairment; use cautiously in those with moderate renal impairment; be aware that conditions that increase urine pH, including severe urinary tract infections, lead to decreased excretion and increased serum levels.

When patients are dressed, garments with generous pockets for an ample supply of tissues will help them to be less conspicuous.

Elimination

The patient with Parkinson's disease may feel urgency and hesitancy in voiding. Measures appropriate for the patient with MS also apply to these patients. Chronic constipation may be a real concern. The patient should be on a diet high in fiber and roughage for bulk. Encourage oral fluid intake, and use stool softeners, suppositories, and prune juice if necessary. Mild cathartics such as milk of magnesia are used if required.

Nursing diagnoses and interventions for the patient with Parkinson's disease are the same as those for the patient with MS, with the addition of but not limited to the following:

Nursing Diagnoses	Nursing Interventions
Impaired physical mobility, related to: • rigidity • bradykinesia • akinesia	Assist with ambulation to assess degree of impairment and to prevent injury. Perform active ROM exercises to all extremities to maintain joint ROM, prevent atrophy, and strengthen muscles. Consult physical therapist or occupational therapist for aids to facilitate ADLs and safe ambulation. Teach techniques to assist with mobility by instructing patient to step over imaginary line and rock from side to side to initiate leg movements; these techniques help deal with "freezing" (akinesia) while walking.
Risk for aspiration, related to disease process	Ensure that, when eating, the patient sits at 90-degree angle with head up and chin slightly tucked, avoiding extending the head. Provide soft-solid and thick-liquid diet because these consistencies are more easily swallowed. Consult a speech therapist and a dietitian because they can provide specific plans to improve swallowing. Encourage patient to take small bites. Avoid use of straws.

Patient Teaching

Education for the patient with Parkinson's disease should include the importance of taking medications on the prescribed time schedule. Stress the need for good skin care and keeping active so that the patient remains as mobile as possible. Demonstrate proper ambulation and positioning to the patient and to the family if they will be taking care of the patient. Also teach proper feeding techniques to reduce the risk of aspiration (see Nursing Diagnoses box).

Prognosis

There is no cure for Parkinson's disease. Parkinson's disease is a chronic degenerative disorder with no acute exacerbations. If the patient takes medication as prescribed, signs and symptoms can be controlled for a long period.

Most patients with Parkinson's disease have their needs provided for by family caregivers (e.g., spouse, children). The burden of caregiving increases as the disease progresses. Many caregivers, especially if they are older adults, suffer from deteriorating physical and mental health. Eventually long-term care is often required for the patient with Parkinson's disease (Lewis et al., 2007).

ALZHEIMER'S DISEASE

Etiology and Pathophysiology

AD is a chronic, progressive, degenerative disorder that affects the cells of the brain and causes impaired intellectual functioning. It is a common cause of dementia in the older person and affects men and women in equal numbers. Approximately 4.5 million Americans suffer from AD. It is estimated that 5% of people older than 65 and 50% of those older than age 85 have AD. Alzheimer's may strike people in their 40s and 50s. The cause is unknown, although research has shown a genetic link.

The changes in the brain of patients with AD include plaques in the cortex, neurofibrillary tangles (a tangled mass of nonfunctioning neurons), and loss of connections between cells and cell death (Figure 54-16). This neuronal damage occurs primarily in the cerebral cortex and causes a decrease in brain size. These changes were first discovered in 1907 by the German neurologist Alois Alzheimer.

Homocysteine is a simple amino acid. Research is presenting evidence that, in older adults, elevated plasma levels of homocysteine are associated with a significantly increased risk for AD or another type of dementia. Put in practical terms, the investigators observed that a 5-mmol increment in the plasma homocysteine level increased the risk of AD by 40% (Seshadri et al., 2002). Blood homocysteine levels may be lowered by eating foods rich in folic acid, such as fruits and green leafy vegetables. Clinical trials are under way to determine whether the risk of AD can be reduced by dietary supplements and vitamins that control free radicals (e.g., folic acid, vitamins C and E) and

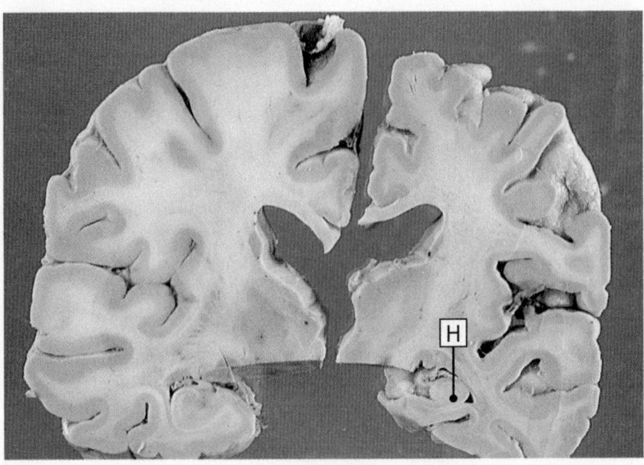

FIGURE 54-16 Effects of Alzheimer's disease on the brain.

those that reduce homocysteine levels (e.g., vitamins B_6 and B_{12}) (National Institute on Aging, 2007).

Studies have shown that individuals who engage in activities that require information processing (e.g., reading, learning a new language, doing crossword puzzles) have a lower risk of developing AD. Dietary patterns, physical activity, leisure activities, and educational achievements may decrease AD risk (National Institute on Aging, 2007).

Clinical Manifestations

The progression of AD is commonly divided into four stages. In the early stage a person with Alzheimer's has relatively mild memory lapses and may have difficulty using the correct word. The attention span is decreased, and there may be disinterest in surroundings. Depression may occur at this time. In the second stage the person has more obvious memory lapses, especially with short-term memory, and usually is disoriented to time. Loss of personal belongings is common, as is confabulating (making up stories) to explain the loss of memory. Patients may lose their ability to recognize familiar faces, places, and objects and may get lost in a familiar environment. Loss of impulse control is common. Behavioral manifestations of AD (e.g., agitation, repetitiveness, wandering, resisting care) result from changes in the brain. A specific type of agitation is termed **sundowning,** in which the patient becomes more confused and agitated in the late afternoon or evening.

The AD patient's behavior is neither intentional nor subject to self-control. Some patients develop psychotic manifestations (i.e., delusions, illusions, hallucinations). By the time a person reaches the third stage, he or she has total disorientation to person, place, and time. Motor problems such as apraxia (an inability to carry out learned sequential movements on command, perform purposeful acts, or use objects properly), **visual agnosia** (inability to recognize objects by sight), and **dysgraphia** (difficulty communicating via writing) interfere with the ability to carry out daily functions. Wandering is common. In the terminal stage, severe mental and physical deterioration is present. Total incontinence is common.

These stages may have some variations. However, all people with AD experience a steady deterioration in their physical and mental status, usually lasting 5 to 20 years until death occurs (Box 54-2).

Assessment

Memory loss is the first symptom usually noticed in AD, combined with the inability to carry out normal activities. Other evidence may be agitation or restlessness. It is important to rule out other conditions such as pernicious anemia, drug reactions, depression, or hormonal imbalances.

Diagnostic Tests

The diagnosis of AD is primarily a diagnosis of exclusion. AD has no specific diagnostic test. A CT scan, EEG, MRI, and PET may be used to rule out other pathologic conditions. A family history of AD is significant. At times the diagnosis can only be confirmed at the time of autopsy.

Medical Management

The care of the patient with AD can be frustrating for the caregiver and the physician because the treatment options are so limited. Often medications make the condition worse. Lorazepam (Ativan) or haloperidol in small doses may be necessary to lessen agitation and unpredictable behavior. Treatment of depression in patients with AD may improve cognitive ability. Depression is treated most often with selective serotonin reuptake inhibitors such as fluoxetine, sertraline (Zoloft), fluvoxamine (Luvox), and citalopram (Celexa). Trazodone (Desyrel), an antidepressant, may help with problems related to sleep but may also cause hypotension. Some antiseizure drugs (neuroleptics), including valproic acid (Depakene) and carbamazepine, tend to act as mood stabilizers and are used to manage behavioral problems (Lewis et al., 2007). Donepezil (Aricept), rivastigmine (Exelon), and galantamine (Razadyne) may have short-term benefit for mild cognitive impairment. Memantine (Namenda) is the first drug approved for the treatment of moderate to severe AD. Memantine does not prevent or slow neurodegeneration, but it was found in clinical studies to slow symptom progression. Many clinical drug trials are trying to find drugs that manage the signs and symptoms of AD while limiting the rate of disease progression. Research shows that the simple addition to a normal diet of large doses of folic acid and vitamin B_{12} will substantially reduce homocysteine levels (Seshadri et al., 2002).

Nursing Interventions and Patient Teaching

Nursing interventions are directed toward maintaining adequate nutrition. This can be a challenge because often the patient will not sit still long enough to eat. Providing finger foods and letting the patient eat while walking may help. Frequent feedings with high

Box 54-2 Early Warning Signs of Alzheimer's Disease

- Memory loss that affects job skills
  - —Frequent forgetfulness or unexplainable confusion at home or in the workplace may signal that something is wrong.
  - —This type of memory loss goes beyond forgetting an assignment, colleague's name, deadline, or phone number.
- Difficulty performing familiar tasks
  - —Most people occasionally become distracted and forget something (e.g., leave something on the stove too long).
  - —People with Alzheimer's disease (AD) may cook a meal but then forget not only to serve it but also that they made it.
- Problems with language
  - —Most people have trouble with finding the "right" word from time to time.
  - —People with AD may forget simple words or substitute inappropriate words, making their speech difficult to understand.
- Disorientation to time and place
  - —Most people occasionally forget the day of the week or what they need from the store.
  - —People with AD can become lost on their own street, not knowing where they are, how they got there, or how to get back home.
- Poor or decreased judgment
  - —Many individuals from time to time may choose not to dress appropriately for the weather (e.g., not bringing a coat or sweater on a cold evening).
  - —People with AD may dress inappropriately in more noticeable ways, such as wearing a bathrobe to the store or a sweater on a hot day.
- Problems with abstract thinking
  - —For the person with AD, this goes beyond challenges such as balancing a checkbook. They may have difficulty recognizing numbers or doing even basic calculations.
- Misplacing things
  - —For many individuals, temporarily misplacing keys, purses, or wallets is a normal albeit frustrating event.
  - —The person with AD may put items in inappropriate places (e.g., eating utensils in clothing drawers) but have no memory of how they got there.
- Changes in mood or behavior
  - —Most individuals experience mood changes.
  - —People with AD tend to exhibit more rapid mood swings for no apparent reason.
- Changes in personality
  - —As most individuals age, they may demonstrate some change in personality (e.g., become less tolerant).
  - —People with AD can change dramatically, either suddenly or over time. For example, someone who is generally easygoing may become angry, suspicious, or fearful.
- Loss of initiative
  - —People with AD may become and remain uninterested and uninvolved in many or all of their usual pursuits.

Adapted from Alzheimer's Association. (2007). Early warning signs. Chicago: Alzheimer's Association. From Lewis, S.M., et al. *Medical-surgical nursing: Assessment and management of clinical problems.* (7th ed.). St. Louis: Mosby.

nutritive value are important. Encourage fluids of at least 2000 mL/day (Nursing Care Plan 54-1).

Safety demands a special mention. Because of memory problems, patients with AD often do dangerous things, such as walking outside while undressed, turning on stoves, wandering away, and setting fires. Measures that the family can take include removing burner controls from the stove at night, double-locking all doors and windows, and keeping the person under constant supervision. Disruptive behavior—including aggressive, agitated behavior—may occur. One frustrating part of the disease is that many patients sleep for only short periods and are awake most of the night.

Most of the time, education is directed at the family, because by the time the condition is diagnosed there is usually serious mental impairment. Help the family set a realistic schedule that also allows them time for rest and relaxation. If necessary, the family may need to consider placing the patient in a long-term care facility. Put the family in touch with the local support group for AD.

Prognosis

Currently no effective treatment is available to stop the progression of AD, which occurs at a variable rate. The course of the disease can span 5 to 20 years. The economic costs of AD in the United States range from approximately $19,000 annually for the care of the person with early disease to $37,000 and more for the person with late disease. Ultimately, most patients die from complications such as pneumonia, malnutrition, and dehydration. Special Alzheimer's units and family and nursing approaches may help the patient stay as productive and safe as possible. The burden on the individual, the family, caregivers, and society as a whole is staggering. Support groups for caregivers and family members have been formed throughout the United States to provide an atmosphere of understanding and to give current information about the disease and related topics such as safety, legal, ethical, and financial issues. Nurses often receive personal and professional satisfaction in participating in such support groups.

MYASTHENIA GRAVIS

Etiology and Pathophysiology

MG is an autoimmune disease of the neuromuscular junction characterized by the fluctuating weakness of certain skeletal muscle groups. MG is an unpredictable neuromuscular disease with lower motoneuron characteristics. MG can occur at any age, but most commonly occurs between the ages of 10 and 65 years. The

 Nursing Care Plan 54-1 **The Patient with Alzheimer's Disease**

Ms. Andrea is a 65-year-old who has been a seamstress. She has a history of progressive memory loss, paranoia, disorientation, and agitation. She was diagnosed as having Alzheimer's disease 2 years ago. Her family kept her at home until 6 months ago, when she was admitted to a long-term care institution. The nursing history indicates that she is incontinent of urine about 50% of the time and expresses a great deal of anxiety, especially around new situations or people. She cries frequently and at times attempts to hit the staff.

NURSING DIAGNOSIS *Anxiety, related to cognitive impairments*

Patient Goals and Expected Outcomes	Nursing Interventions	Evaluation
Patient will demonstrate decreased anxiety as evidenced by decreased outbursts of agitation or crying, the ability to sleep through most of the night, and cooperation with care	Continue to assess presence of anxiety. Comfort patient when she is crying. Provide simple explanation for all procedures. Use calm, undemanding, unhurried approach. Keep nursing interventions consistent and simple. Assist patient in doing relaxation techniques. Maintain consistency of caregiver when able. Minimize patient's choices in care. Encourage patient to exercise. Offer snack at bedtime.	Patient sleeps 5 to 6 hours per night. Patient remains calm with care. Patient experiences decreased episodes of crying or striking out at others.

NURSING DIAGNOSIS *Functional urinary incontinence, related to condition and cognitive impairment*

Patient Goals and Expected Outcomes	Nursing Interventions	Evaluation
Patient will be continent Patient will be free of urinary tract infection	Take patient to bathroom on regular schedule. Encourage adequate fluid intake (at least 2000 mL/day). Determine patient's preference for fluid. Place sign on door indicating "Toilet" or "Bathroom," or with a picture. If patient has urgency, ensure closeness to bathroom. Simplify closures on clothing. Avoid fluids just before bed. Use disposable protective perineal garments (Attends) only as needed.	Patient is free of episodes of incontinence. Patient is free of infection. Patient will void when taken to the bathroom.

Critical Thinking Questions

1. Ms. Andrea continually wanders about the long-term care facility. She is unable to sit at the table for an entire meal. She has lost approximately 20 pounds in the past 3 months. What are some helpful measures to improve her nutritional status?
2. What are some helpful interventions to help Ms. Andrea obtain a better sleep pattern?
3. Ms. Andrea has difficulty in maintaining good personal hygiene. What are some methods for assisting Ms. Andrea in maintaining personal hygiene?

peak age of onset in women is 20 to 30 years. In young people, women are more affected than men, but among older people the distribution between the genders is about equal. Occurrence within families is rare; however, infants of affected mothers may have symptoms at birth. These symptoms usually disappear within several weeks. The incidence is about 14 in every 100,000 population.

With MG, no observable structural change occurs in the muscle or nerve. Nerve impulses fail to pass at the myoneural junction (the space between the nerve ending and muscle fiber), resulting in muscle weakness. MG is caused by an autoimmune process. It is thought to be triggered by antibodies that attack acetylcholine receptor sites at the neuromuscular junction. This attack damages and reduces the number of receptor sites, preventing conduction along the normal pathway at normal conduction speeds. Patients with MG have only about one third as many acetylcholine receptors at the neuromuscular junction as is normal.

About 25% of the patients with MG have been found to have a thymoma, and almost 80% have changes in the cellular structure of the thymus gland.

Clinical Manifestations

MG occurs in both ocular and generalized terms. In ocular MG the signs and symptoms include ptosis (eyelid drooping) and diplopia (double vision). In about 15% of cases, MG remains confined to the eye muscles. The generalized variety may vary from mild to severe signs and symptoms. The patient may complain initially of ptosis and diplopia. Skeletal weakness involving the muscles of the extremities, the neck, the shoulders, the hands, and the diaphragm; dysarthria; and dysphagia may follow. The vocal cords can become weak, and the voice can sound nasal. As the disease progresses, it affects the trunk and lower limbs, leading to difficulty with walking, sustained sitting, and raising the arms over the head. Usually the distal muscles are not as affected as the proximal muscles. Muscle weakness may become so severe that the person cannot breathe without mechanical ventilation. Bowel and bladder sphincter weakness occurs with severe loss of muscle control. Exacerbations of the disease may be initiated by upper respiratory tract infections, emotional tension, and menstruation.

Assessment

Subjective data include the patient's understanding of the disease; complaints of weakness or double vision; difficulty chewing or swallowing; and any bowel or bladder incontinence.

Objective data include any documented muscle weakness on neurologic testing. Nasal-sounding speech may be noted; the voice often fades after a long conversation and breath sounds diminish. Note ptosis of the eyelids and weight loss if there are swallowing problems.

Diagnostic Tests

Because of the slow, insidious onset and occurrence of symptoms with stress, MG sometimes is misdiagnosed as hysteria or neurosis. The diagnosis of MG can be made on the basis of history and physical examination. The simplest diagnostic test for MG is to have the patient look upward for 2 to 3 minutes. If the problem is MG, the eyelids will droop so that the person can barely keep the eyes open. The diagnosis can be made partly on the basis of EMG. The IV anticholinesterase test is a reliable diagnostic test. Edrophonium (Tensilon), a short-acting cholinesterase inhibitor, which decreases the amount of cholinesterase at the neuromuscular junction while making acetylcholine available to muscles, is administered intravenously. The patient response is carefully evaluated. Muscle function improves dramatically after IV injection with Tensilon in a short time with patients who have the illness. Another diagnostic test is serum testing for antibodies to acetylcholine receptors. Acetylcholine receptor antibodies are present in 80% to 90% of patients with generalized myasthenia, so their presence can be used to diagnose the disease.

Medical Management

Medical management includes the use of anticholinesterase drugs such as neostigmine (Prostigmin) and pyridostigmine (Mestinon). These medications promote nerve impulse transmission and effectively alleviate symptoms. Usually the patient is taught how to adjust the dosage depending on symptoms. Corticosteroids may be used as an adjunct therapy. Immunosuppressive medications, including azathioprine (Imuran), cyclosporine (Sandimmune), and cyclophosphamide (Cytoxan), are used because of MG's immune component. Many classes of drugs are contraindicated or must be used with caution in patients with MG; these include anesthetics, antidysrhythmics, antibiotics, quinine, antipsychotics, barbiturates, sedatives, hypnotics, opioids, tranquilizers, and thyroid preparations (Fisher, 2004).

Plasmapheresis as a therapy for MG was first reported in 1976. This procedure involves separation of plasma from blood by a machine called a cell separator, which can be connected to the patient by a vascular cannula. This process removes the antibodies produced by the autoimmune response. Plasmapheresis can yield short-term improvement in symptoms and is indicated for patients in crisis or in preparation for surgery when corticosteroids need to be avoided.

Thymectomy is indicated for almost all patients with a thymoma. For some patients without thymoma, thymectomy may result in improvement in symptoms. Excision of the thymus reduces symptoms of MG in many patients. A thymectomy is a complex surgery, and patients with MG are at high risk for complications from anesthesia.

Another treatment option is the administration of IV immune globulin to reduce the production of acetylcholine antibodies. IV immune globulin is used for a severe relapse of MG.

During exacerbations of the disease, and when the respiratory status is compromised, the patient may require intubation and mechanical ventilation. A tracheostomy may be necessary.

Nursing Interventions and Patient Teaching

Respiratory problems typically occur in patients with MG. Upper respiratory tract infections occur because the patient may not have the energy to cough effectively, and pneumonia or airway obstruction may develop. Aspiration often occurs. During acute episodes of the disease, the patient may require hospitalization. Serial determination of vital capacity, minute volumes, and tidal volumes is made to assess the need for respiratory assistance. The patient may also be taught airway protective techniques during swallowing (e.g.,

 Patient Teaching

Myasthenia Gravis

- Teach the importance of taking medication at the time prescribed and taking it early enough before eating or engaging in activities to obtain maximum relief.
- Explain how to adjust medication dose to maintain muscle strength.
- Caution about medications to avoid.
- Teach importance of seeking medical attention at first sign of an upper respiratory tract infection.
- Explain importance of eating only when sitting up to prevent aspiration.
- Caution patient to avoid crowds in flu and cold season.
- Explain how to adjust to daily activities to allow for leisure activities and rest periods.
- Explain planning to use minimal energy in activities that are essential so that energy may be conserved for activities that the patient enjoys.
- Advise patient to wear a medical-alert bracelet that identifies the patient as having myasthenia gravis.

chin tuck, double swallow). Suctioning is done as needed, and if swallowing becomes impaired, a feeding tube may be necessary.

People with MG may have to change daily patterns of activity. Help the patient and the family plan so that minimal energy is used in activities that are essential to remaining relatively self-sufficient, with energy left for leisure activities. Physical therapy such as ROM exercises may be beneficial for maintaining muscle function.

The patient with MG is usually able to adjust the medication depending on the symptoms. Also, the patient can have much control over preventing respiratory complications. Therefore teaching is important and should include those topics listed in the Patient Teaching box.

Prognosis

MG is a chronic disease. The course is variable with periods of exacerbation and remission. Some cases are mild, but others are severe, with death resulting from respiratory failure. Patients with a thymoma may experience improvement after a thymectomy.

AMYOTROPHIC LATERAL SCLEROSIS

Loss of both upper and lower motoneurons is the major pathologic change in ALS, a rare, progressive neurologic disease that usually leads to death in 2 to 6 years. This disease became known as Lou Gehrig's disease when the famous baseball player was stricken with it in 1939. The onset is between 40 and 70 years of age, and two times as many men as women are affected.

For unknown reasons, motoneurons in the brainstem and spinal cord gradually degenerate in ALS. The dead motoneuron cannot produce or transport vital signals to muscle. Consequently, electrical and chemical messages originating in the brain do not reach the muscles to activate them.

The primary symptoms are weakness of the upper extremities (the hands are often affected first), dysarthria, and dysphagia. However, weakness may begin in the legs. Muscle wasting and fasciculations (muscle twitching) result from the denervation of the muscles and lack of stimulation and use. Death usually results from respiratory tract infection secondary to compromised respiratory function.

Unfortunately there is no cure for ALS. A drug called riluzole (Rilutek) slows the progression of ALS. The drug helps protect motoneurons damaged by the disease and can add 3 months or more to a patient's life.

Multidisciplinary ALS teams at large academic centers such as Johns Hopkins Medical Center and Allegheny University of the Health Sciences are offering renewed hope to these patients. Usually coordinated by a nurse, these programs provide experimental drugs; physical, occupational, and speech therapy; nutritional regimens; and psychological support. Patients in these programs may live 15 years or more after diagnosis—three times the typical life expectancy (Robert Packard Center of ALS Research at Johns Hopkins, 2009).

This illness is devastating because the patient remains cognitively intact while wasting away. The challenge of nursing interventions is to guide the patient in use of moderate intensity, endurance type exercises for the trunk and limbs, since this may help reduce ALS spasticity (Palmieri, 2007c). Support the patient's cognitive and emotional functions by facilitating communication, providing diversional activities such as reading and human companionship, and helping the patient and the family with advanced care planning and anticipatory grieving related to loss of motor function and ultimate death. About 30% of patients with ALS live up to 5 years after diagnosis, and 10% to 20% survive for more than 25 years. However, some patients may die in the first year after diagnosis (Palmieri, 2007c).

HUNTINGTON'S DISEASE

Huntington's disease is a genetically transmitted autosomal dominant disorder that affects both men and women of all races. The offspring of a person with this disease have a 50% risk of inheriting it. The diagnosis often occurs after the affected individual has children. The onset of Huntington's disease is usually between 30 and 50 years of age. In the United States, approximately 25,000 people have Huntington's disease and another 150,000 have a 50/50 chance of developing it.

Diagnosis is based on family history, clinical symptoms, and the detection of the characteristic deoxyribonucleic acid (DNA) pattern from blood samples. People who are asymptomatic but who have a positive family history of Huntington's disease face the dilemma of whether to get tested. If the test is positive, the person will develop Huntington's disease, but at what age and to what extent cannot be determined (Lewis et al., 2007).

Like Parkinson's disease, the pathology of Huntington's disease involves the basal ganglia and the extrapyramidal motor system. However, instead of a deficiency of dopamine, Huntington's disease involves an overactivity of the dopamine pathway. The net effect is an excess of dopamine, which leads to symptoms that are the opposite of those of parkinsonism. The clinical manifestations are characterized by abnormal and excessive involuntary movements (chorea). These are writhing, twisting movements of the face, limbs, and body. The movements get worse as the disease progresses. Facial movements involving speech, chewing, and swallowing are affected and may cause aspiration and malnutrition. The gait deteriorates, and ambulation eventually becomes impossible. Perhaps the most devastating deterioration is in mental functions, which include intellectual decline, emotional lability, and psychotic behavior. Death usually occurs 10 to 20 years after the onset of symptoms.

Because there is no cure, therapeutic management is palliative. Antipsychotic (e.g., haloperidol), antidepressant (fluoxetine, sertraline), and antichorea (clonazepam [Klonopin]) medications are prescribed and have some effect. However, they do not alter the course of the disease.

This disease presents a great challenge to health care professionals. Transplantation of fetal striatal neural tissues into the brain is an experimental treatment that may be effective (Kim, 2004). The goal of nursing management is to provide the most comfortable environment possible for the patient and the family by maintaining physical safety, treating the physical symptoms, and providing emotional and psychological support. Because of the choreic movements, caloric requirements are as high as 4000 to 5000 calories/day to maintain body weight. As the disease progresses, meeting caloric needs becomes a greater challenge when the patient has difficulty swallowing and holding the head still. Depression and mental deterioration can also compromise nutritional intake. Genetic counseling is important. DNA testing can be done on fetal cells obtained by amniocentesis or chorionic biopsy. Genetic testing can determine whether a person is a carrier. No test is available to predict when symptoms will develop.

VASCULAR PROBLEMS

Interference with function because of vascular conditions is a common neurologic impairment.

STROKE

Etiology and Pathophysiology

Stroke (or "brain attack") is an abnormal condition of the blood vessels of the brain, characterized by hemorrhage into the brain or the formation of an embolus or thrombus that occludes an artery, resulting in ischemia of the brain tissue normally perfused by the damaged vessels. The term *brain attack* is increasingly used to describe stroke. This term communicates the urgency of recognizing the clinical manifestations of a stroke and treating a medical emergency, just as one would with a heart attack.

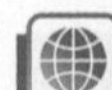

Cultural Considerations

Stroke

A high mortality rate from strokes exists among black men, possibly as a result of the high frequency of hypertension, obesity, and diabetes mellitus in this group. Thrombotic strokes are twice as common among blacks as among whites. Hemorrhagic strokes are three times more common among blacks than among whites. Hispanics, Native Americans, and Asian Americans have a higher stroke incidence than whites.

After the onset of a stroke, immediate medical attention is crucial to reduce disability and death (Lewis et al., 2007). Stroke is the most common disease of the nervous system. It is estimated that 700,000 people in the United States suffer a stroke annually. It is ranked as the third leading cause of death in the United States, with about 160,000 deaths annually. Strokes affect people in all age-groups, but most are between 75 and 85 years of age. Strokes leave many people with serious, long-term disability. Of those who survive, 50% to 70% are functionally independent, and 15% to 30% live with permanent disability. Common long-term disabilities include hemiparesis, inability to walk, complete or partial dependence in ADLs, aphasia, and depression (see Cultural Considerations box).

Strokes are classified as ischemic or hemorrhagic, based on the underlying pathophysiologic findings. Ischemic strokes are thrombotic and embolic. These account for 85% of strokes. The remaining 15% are hemorrhagic strokes, which result from bleeding into the brain tissue itself (Figure 54-17). Many underlying factors also contribute: atherosclerosis, heart disease, hypertension, kidney disease, peripheral vascular disease, and diabetes mellitus. Other risk factors include family history of stroke, obesity, high serum cholesterol, cigarette smoking, stress, cocaine use, and a sedentary lifestyle. Newer low-dose oral contraceptives have lower risks for stroke than early forms of birth control pills, except in those individuals who are hypersensitive and smoke. Hypertension is the single most important modifiable risk factor. Stroke risk can be reduced by up to 42% with appropriate treatment of hypertension. Atrial fibrillation is the most important treatable cardiac-related risk factor (Phillips, 2007). Atrial fibrillation is responsible for about 15% to 20% of all strokes. The risk for stroke in people with diabetes mellitus is four to five times higher than the general population. Carotid artery stenosis, also called carotid artery disease, is defined as the narrowing of the carotid arteries that supply blood to the brain, usually from plaque buildup (atherosclerosis) in the inner lining of the artery. It is responsible for 80% of the 500,000

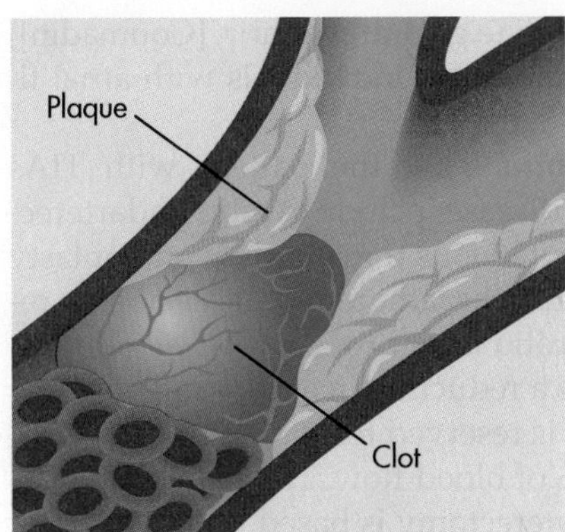

A **Thrombotic stroke.** Cerebral thrombosis is a narrowing of the artery by fatty deposits called *plaque*. Plaque can cause a clot to form, which blocks the passage of blood through the artery.

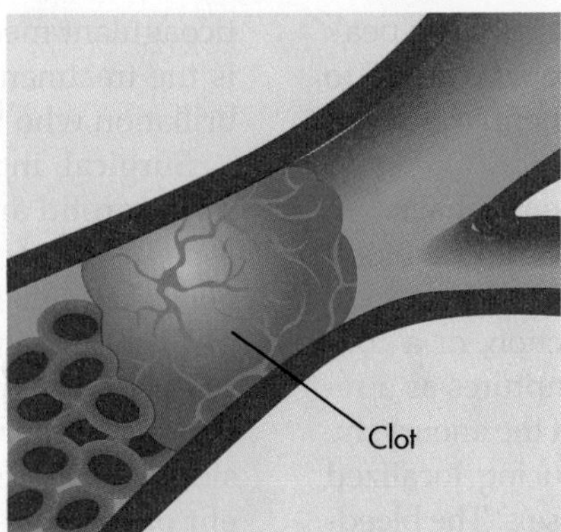

B **Embolic stroke.** An embolus is a blood clot or other debris circulating in the blood. When it reaches an artery in the brain that is too narrow to pass through, it lodges there and blocks the flow of blood.

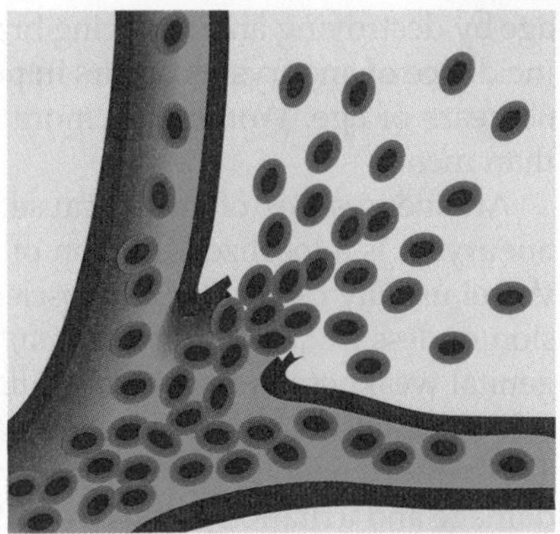

C **Hemorrhagic stroke.** A burst blood vessel may allow blood to seep into and damage brain tissues until clotting shuts off the leak.

FIGURE 54-17 Three types of stroke.

TIAs that affect patients annually (Phillips, 2007). In 2002 data from the Women's Health Initiative (longitudinal intervention trial in middle-age women) showed an increased risk of stroke in women taking estrogen plus progestin compared with those not receiving hormone replacement therapy. These data suggest that postmenopausal hormone replacement therapy does not protect against stroke (Women's Health Initiative, 2002).

Clinical Manifestations

A stroke can have an effect on many body functions, including motor activity, elimination, intellectual function, spatial perception, personality, affect, sensation, and communication. The functions affected are directly related to the artery involved and the area of brain it supplies. Permanent damage can result from a stroke because of anoxia of the brain. The vessel most commonly affected is the middle cerebral artery. The patient may be unconscious and may experience seizures as a result of generalized ischemia and the brain's response to abrupt hypoxia.

Ischemic Stroke

Deficient blood flow to the brain from a partial or complete occlusion of an artery results in an ischemic stroke. Ischemic strokes are divided into **thrombotic** and **embolic** and account for about 80% of all strokes (National Institute of Neurological Disorders and Stroke, n.d.).

Thrombotic Stroke

Thrombosis is the most common cause of stroke, and the most common cause of cerebral thrombosis is atherosclerosis. Additional disease processes that cause thrombosis are hypertension or diabetes mellitus, both of which accelerate the arteriosclerotic process. Additional risk factors associated with thrombotic strokes include coagulation disorders, polycythemia vera, arteritis, chronic hypoxia, and dehydration. In 30% to 50% of individuals, thrombotic strokes have been preceded by a TIA. Stroke resulting from thrombosis is seen most often in the 60- to 90-year-old age-group. Thrombosis occurs in relation to injury of a blood vessel wall and formation of a blood clot. The lumen of the blood vessel becomes narrowed, and if it becomes occluded, infarction occurs. Thrombosis develops readily where atherosclerotic plaques have already narrowed blood vessels. Thrombi usually occur in larger vessels, especially the internal carotid arteries.

Symptoms of this type of stroke tend to occur during sleep or soon after arising. This is thought to result partly because recumbency lowers blood pressure, which can lead to brain ischemia. Postural hypotension may also be a factor. Neurologic signs and symptoms frequently worsen for the first few hours after a stroke and peak in severity within 72 hours as edema increases in the infarcted areas of the brain.

Embolic Stroke

Embolism is the second most common cause of stroke. People who have a stroke resulting from embolism are usually younger. The emboli most commonly originate from a thrombus in the endocardial (inside) layer of the heart, often caused by rheumatic heart disease, mitral stenosis and atrial fibrillation, myocardial infarction, infective endocarditis, valvular prostheses, and atrial septal defects. Less common causes of emboli include air, fat from long bone (femur) fractures, amniotic fluid after childbirth, and tumors. The embolus travels upward to the cerebral circulation and lodges where a vessel narrows or bifurcates. They most frequently occur in the midcerebral artery.

Hemorrhagic Stroke

Hemorrhagic stroke accounts for approximately 15% of all strokes and result from bleeding into the brain tissue or subarachnoid space. The bleed causes damage by destroying and replacing brain tissue. The peak incidence of aneurysms occurs in people who are 35 to 60 years of age. Women are more frequently affected than men.

An aneurysm is often the cause of hemorrhage. An **aneurysm** is a localized dilation of the wall of a blood vessel usually caused by atherosclerosis and hypertension or, less frequently, by trauma, infection, or a congenital weakness in the vessel wall. It ruptures as a result of a small hole that occurs in a part of the aneurysm. The hemorrhage spreads rapidly, producing localized damage and irritation to the cerebral vessels. The bleeding usually stops when a plug of fibrin platelets is formed. The hemorrhage begins to absorb within 3 weeks. Recurrent rupture is a risk 7 to 10 days after the initial hemorrhage. The patient with intracerebral hemorrhage has no forewarning; has rapid, severe symptoms; and has a poor prognosis for recovery. Fifty percent of patients die soon after the stroke. Only about 20% are functionally independent after 6 months.

Transient Ischemic Attack

TIA refers to an episode of cerebrovascular insufficiency with temporary episodes of neurologic dysfunction lasting less than 24 hours and often less than 15 minutes. Most TIAs resolve within 3 hours. TIAs may be caused by microemboli that temporarily occlude the blood flow. TIAs often occur in patients with carotid artery stenosis. The most common deficits are contralateral weakness of the lower face, hands, arms, and legs; transient dysphasia; numbness or loss of sensation; temporary loss of vision of one eye; or a sudden inability to speak. Other symptoms may include tinnitus, vertigo, blurred vision, diplopia, eyelid ptosis, and ataxia. Between attacks the neurologic status is normal.

A TIA should be considered a forerunner of a stroke. After a TIA the health care provider orders a complete workup to rule out carotid artery stenosis. Duplex ultrasonography is the primary noninvasive test for carotid artery stenosis. If a patient is symptomatic and duplex ultrasound findings are abnormal, MRA or contrast-enhanced CT angiography (CTA) may be ordered to confirm the diagnosis and classify the severity of the carotid artery stenosis (Phillips, 2007). Evaluation must be done to confirm that the signs and symptoms of a TIA are not related to other brain lesions, such as a developing subdural hematoma or an increasing tumor mass. CT of the brain without contrast media is the most important initial diagnostic study.

The major importance of TIAs is that they warn the patient of an underlying pathologic condition. At least one third of patients who experience TIAs will have a stroke in 2 to 5 years. The patient is given medications that prevent platelet aggregation, such as aspirin, ticlopidine (Ticlid), dipyridamole (Persantine), and clopidogrel (Plavix). Aspirin is the most frequently used antiplatelet agent, commonly at a dose of 81 to 325 mg/day. An anticoagulant medication (e.g., oral warfarin [Coumadin]) is the treatment of choice for individuals with atrial fibrillation who have had a TIA.

Surgical interventions for the patient with TIAs from carotid artery disease include carotid endarterectomy (CEA) or percutaneous transluminal angioplasty and stenting. In CEA the atheromatous lesion is removed from the carotid artery to improve blood flow. CEA surgery causes a reduction in stroke and vascular death. This surgery is reserved for patients with occlusions of 70% to 99% of blood flow. The long-term benefit of carotid endarterectomy is based on the severity of the preoperative stenosis. In patients with stenosis of 30% or less, surgery actually increases the risk for an ipsilateral stroke in the first 5 years postoperatively. There has been no proven effect within 5 years when the stenosis is 31% to 40% and only a marginal improvement in patients with 50% to 69% stenosis. However, the greatest benefit occurs when the stenosis is 70% or more (Phillips, 2007).

Percutaneous transluminal angioplasty is the insertion of a balloon to open a stenosed artery to permit increased blood flow. This procedure is used to treat patients with clinical manifestations related to stenosis in the vertebrobasilar or carotid arteries and their branches. The risk of the angioplasty procedure is the possibility of dislodging emboli, which can travel to the brain or retina.

Assessment

Subjective data include the description of the onset of symptoms; the presence of headache; any sensory deficit, such as numbness or tingling; the inability to think clearly; and visual problems. In the case of a hemorrhage, the headache may be described as sudden and explosive. Assess the patient's ability to understand the condition.

Objective data include hemiparesis or hemiplegia, any change in the LOC, signs of increased ICP, respiratory status, and aphasia. The exact clinical picture varies, depending on the area of the brain affected (Figure 54-18). A lesion on one side of the brain affects motor function on the opposite (contralateral) side of the brain. When the middle cerebral artery is affected, as is most common, the signs and symptoms seen include contralateral paralysis or paresis, contralateral sensory loss, dysphasia or aphasia if the dominant hemisphere is involved, spatial-perceptual problems, changes in judgment and behavior if the nondominant hemisphere is involved, and **contralateral (homonymous) hemianopia** (Figure 54-19).

In right-handed people and in most left-handed people, the left hemisphere is dominant for language skills. Language disorders affect expression and comprehension of written and spoken words. When a stroke damages the dominant hemisphere of the brain, the patient may experience **aphasia** (total loss of comprehension and use of language). Strokes affecting

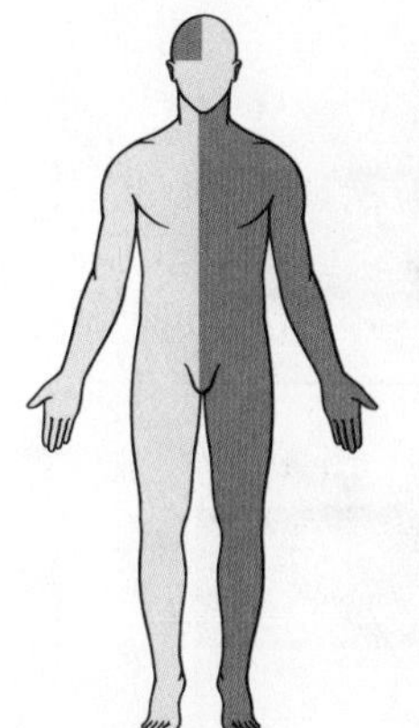

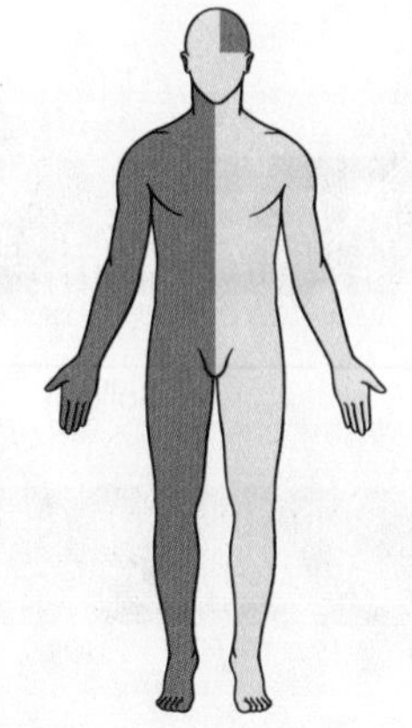

Right brain damage
(Stroke on right side of the brain)
- Paralyzed left side: hemiplegia
- Left-sided neglect
- Spatial-perceptual deficits
- Tends to deny or minimize problems
- Rapid performance, short attention span
- Impulsive, safety problems
- Impaired judgment
- Impaired time concepts

Left brain damage
(Stroke on left side of the brain)
- Paralyzed right side: hemiplegia
- Impaired speech/language aphasias
- Impaired right/left discrimination
- Slow performance, cautious
- Aware of deficits: depression, anxiety
- Impaired comprehension related to language, math

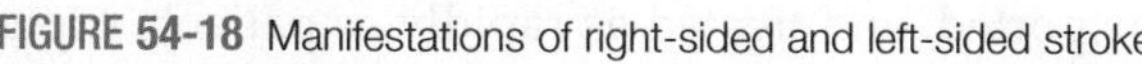

FIGURE 54-18 Manifestations of right-sided and left-sided stroke.

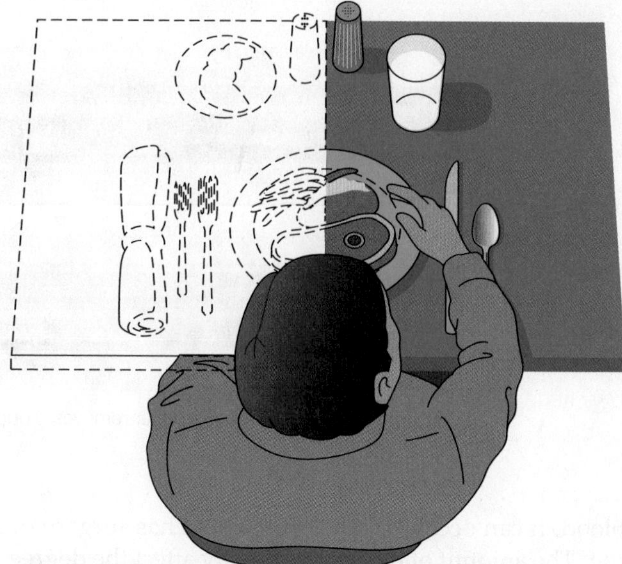

FIGURE 54-19 Spatial and perceptual deficits in stroke. Perception of a patient with homonymous hemianopsia shows that food on the left side is not seen and thus is ignored.

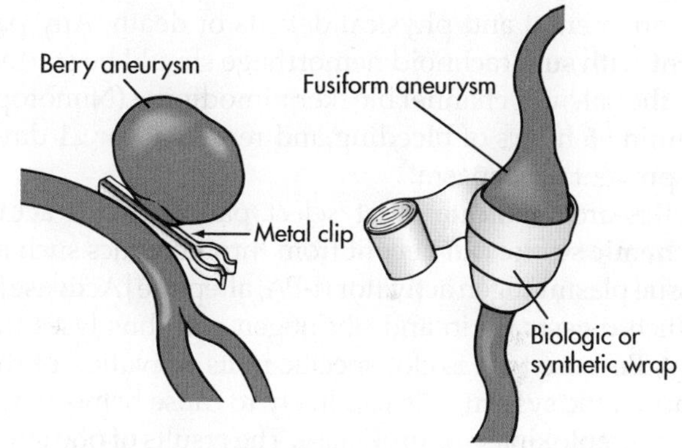

FIGURE 54-20 Clipping and wrapping of aneurysms.

Broca's areas of the brain cause difficulty in speaking and writing, or **expressive aphasia** (Lewis et al., 2007) (see Figure 54-3 and Box 54-1). If a patient has a stroke that affects Wernicke's center in the brain, he or she will have **receptive aphasia,** that is, difficulty comprehending the spoken and written language (Lewis et al., 2007).

A stroke patient may experience **dysarthria,** which is difficult or poorly articulated speech. Dysarthria is a result of deficits in the muscular control of speech and not in a pathologic condition of the Broca's area that is involved in speech production (Lewis et al., 2007). Some stroke patients experience a combination of aphasia and dysarthria.

Diagnostic Tests

Noncontrast CT is the primary test used to diagnose a stroke. CT can indicate the size and location of the lesion and differentiate between ischemic and hemorrhagic stroke. For optimal results, the CT scan should be obtained within 25 minutes and read within 45 minutes of arrival at the emergency department. If the stroke is ischemic and is less than 3 hours old, the CT will appear normal because the brain structure with or without blood flow appears the same in a noncontrast CT scan. If the CT scan appears normal with no sign of hemorrhage, the patient qualifies for fibrinolytic therapy (Lewis et al., 2007). CTA provides visualization of vasculature. MRI is used to determine the extent of brain injury. MRI has greater specificity than CT. PET is also useful in assessing the extent of tissue damage by showing the brain's metabolic activity. After TIAs, a cerebral angiogram may be done. Doppler, CTA, or MRA studies of the carotid arteries should be performed. The results of these noninvasive carotid artery studies determine whether the more invasive cerebral angiogram is performed.

Medical Management

If the patient has had a hemorrhagic stroke as a result of an aneurysm, surgery may be necessary to prevent a rebleed. The surgery consists of performing a craniotomy; tying off or clipping the aneurysm; and removing the clot to prevent rebleeding into the brain (Figure 54-20). An aneurysm often causes vasospasm in the brain as blood in the subarachnoid space becomes an irritant. Vasospasm narrows blood vessels in the brain, decreasing perfusion to the areas they supply with

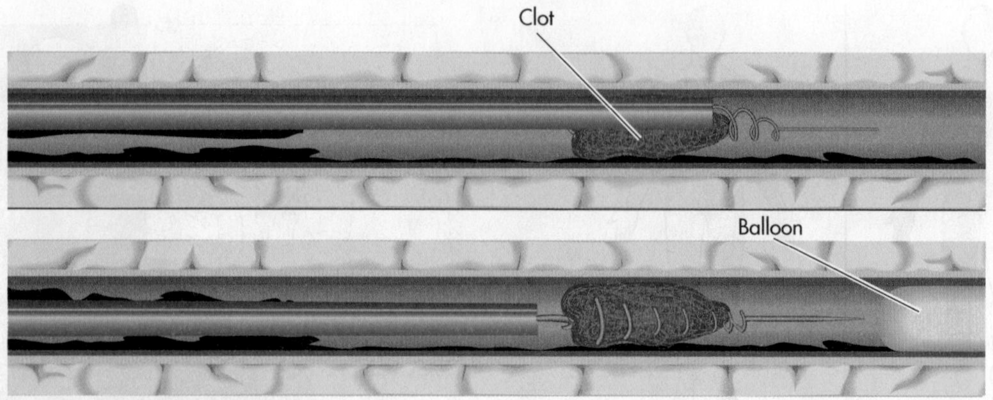

FIGURE 54-21 The MERCI Retriever removes blood clots in patients who are experiencing ischemic stroke.

blood. It can occur whether the patient has surgery or not. The amount of blood can directly affect the degree of vasospasm.

Vasospasm typically occurs in 30% to 60% of cases between postoperative days 4 and 12. The mortality rate is as high as 50%. If it is not treated rapidly, it can cause cerebral ischemia or cerebral anoxia, leading to severe mental and physical deficits or death. Any patient with subarachnoid hemorrhage should be started on the calcium channel blocker nimodipine (Nimotop) within 96 hours of bleeding and receive it for 21 days to prevent vasospasm.

Research indicates that select patients with **acute ischemic stroke** can benefit from thrombolytics such as tissue plasminogen activator (t-PA, alteplase [Activase]), which digests fibrin and fibrinogen and thus lyses the clot. Because t-PA is clot specific in its activation of the fibrinolytic system, it is less likely to cause hemorrhage than streptokinase or urokinase. The results of one landmark study have revealed that selected patients who are treated within 3 hours of the onset of symptoms are at least 30% more likely than patients who do not receive timely treatment to recover with little or no disability after 3 months. **Time lost is brain lost.** Although thrombolysis improves the chance of recovery by up to 30%, only 2% to 3% of ischemic stroke patients receive it. That is largely because of the limited therapeutic window (Barker, 2006).

In the summer of 2004, the U.S. Food and Drug Administration approved the first mechanical device for endovascular embolectomy: Mechanical Embolus Removal in Cerebral Ischemia (MERCI) Retriever. This device is used to remove blood clots inside the brain and can be used up to 8 hours after acute stroke onset (Barker, 2006). The MERCI Retriever is a tiny corkscrew device that uses a microcatheter inserted through a femoral artery balloon catheter (Figure 54-21). Under x-ray guidance, the balloon catheter is maneuvered until it reaches the clot in the artery in the brain. Once the clot is entrapped, the balloon catheter is inflated to temporarily prevent forward flow while the blood clot is withdrawn. The clot is enclosed in the balloon catheter and removed from the body. The balloon is deflated and blood flow is restored to the brain (Lewis et al., 2007).

It is important to educate patients about the risk factors associated with stroke and to instruct them to dial 911 immediately if they or someone else shows signs of stroke. Immediate treatment in the nearest hospital gives patients the best chance for improved outcomes—whether treatment is within 3 hours for t-PA or within 8 hours for the MERCI Retriever (Barker, 2006).

Patients with stroke symptoms need to be triaged, transported, and treated as rapidly as patients experiencing an acute myocardial infarction. In administration of thrombolytic drugs, the single most important factor is timing. Patients are screened carefully before treatment is initiated. This includes blood tests for coagulation disorders, recent history of gastrointestinal bleeding, and a CT or MRI scan to rule out hemorrhagic stroke. In patients with acute ischemic stroke, thrombolytic therapy increases short-term mortality, increases (but not a statistically significant amount) symptomatic or fatal intracranial hemorrhage, decreases long-term death rate, and decreases dependence in terms of ADLs. The decision to use thrombolytic therapy should be based on a discussion of the risks and benefits with the patient and the family. Some patients would accept a high risk of death from hemorrhage in an attempt to improve their chances of escaping permanent aphasia or dependency. Others prefer to avoid interventions that carry significant risk (Lewis et al., 2007). Patients with stroke caused by thrombi and emboli (ischemic strokes) may also be treated with platelet inhibitors and anticoagulants (after the first 24 hours if treated with t-PA) to prevent the formation of more clots. Common anticoagulants include heparin, enoxaparin (Lovenox), and warfarin. Platelet inhibitors include aspirin, ticlopidine, clopidogrel, and dipyridamole.

Drugs to reduce ICP, such as dexamethasone, may be given. Suppositories such as bisacodyl (Dulcolax) are generally prescribed to be given daily or every other day. However, some physicians order stool softeners, laxatives, or enemas.

Fluids may be restricted for the first few days after a stroke in an effort to prevent edema of the brain. The patient is fed IV fluids, or a nasogastric or gastrostomy tube may be inserted and tube feedings begun.

The length of time the patient remains in bed depends on the type of stroke suffered, deficits noted, and the physician's judgment in regard to early mobilization. Some physicians prescribe fairly long periods of rest after strokes, whereas others believe in early mobilization—1 or 2 days after the accident occurred.

Nursing Interventions

Carefully monitor the patient's neurologic status. The neurologic assessment includes the Glasgow coma scale (see Table 54-3), LOC, pupillary responses, extremity movement and strength, facial symmetry, speech, and vital signs. A decrease in the LOC may indicate increasing ICP (Lewis et al., 2007). Interventions in the initial phase are directed toward preventing neurologic deficits (see Clinical Pathway 54-1 on Evolve).

Because nutrition is a concern and the patient may have difficulty swallowing at first, tube feedings and IV fluids may be necessary. See the section on motor and sensory problems for a discussion of techniques to assist in feeding the patient with dysphagia.

If the patient is responsive after the onset of the stroke, help the patient assume as much self-care as possible. This includes teaching the patient one-handed dressing techniques and one-handed feeding techniques if motor deficits have occurred. It is important to reinforce teaching by other members of the patient's health team.

The patient with a stroke may be incontinent at first. Remove the urinary catheter (if there is one) as soon as possible to prevent urinary tract infection and delayed bladder retraining. Because of the lower incidence of urinary tract infections, an intermittent catheterization program may be used for patients with urinary retention. Place the patient on a bladder training program to assist in regaining continence. This usually includes taking the patient to the bathroom every few hours and encouraging fluids (at least 2000 mL/day), with the majority given between 8 AM and 7 PM. Assess the patient's normal bowel pattern before the stroke and include this in the nursing care plan if possible. If the patient has difficulty with communication, a picture of a bathroom or toilet can be useful.

Return of motor impulses and movement in involved extremities occurs in stages, lasting from hours to months. Recovery may also halt at a specific stage and progress no further. Return of function is significant for functional use of extremities but also increases the possibility of contractures. Appropriate nursing interventions to prevent contractures include passive exercise, active exercise, strength building of the unaffected side, and early ambulation to promote the return of muscle function.

One way to position the patient with a stroke is the **Bobath approach,** designed to normalize muscle tone by providing as many sensations of normal muscle tone, posture, and movement as possible. The goal of the treatment is to redirect short-term memory toward an appreciation of normal movement of the paralyzed side by incorporating techniques of weight bearing, counterrotation, and protraction of the shoulder girdle and pelvis. The reader is referred to a rehabilitation nursing text for further description of this technique. Nurses in rehabilitation settings are often taught this approach.

Patients may experience a loss of proprioception with a stroke. Neurologic deficits of apraxia and agnosia (a total or partial loss of the ability to recognize familiar objects or people) may also occur. Assist the patient with activities by repeating directions and demonstrating care. If the patient has hemianopia, which is common, approach the patient from the nonparalyzed side for care. Teach the patient to scan past midline to the side with the deficit. These patients may also fail to recognize that they have a paralyzed side. This is called **unilateral neglect** (described earlier). Teach the patient to inspect this side of the body for injury and to protect it from harm. These patients often show poor judgment and may move impulsively or unsafely. Observe for this and take safety precautions if needed until the patient can learn to compensate for this lack of judgment. Patients who have had a stroke may have difficulty controlling their emotions. Emotional responses may be exaggerated or unpredictable. Depression and feelings associated with changes in body image and loss of function can make this worse. Patients may also be frustrated by mobility and communication problems.

To foster the patient's self-esteem, always treat the patient as an adult, not as a child. Praise and reinforce the patient's successful efforts and gains in self-care.

Communication Problems

Many stroke patients have speech problems, including dysarthria and aphasia. A speech pathologist evaluates and treats the patient with language disorders. The patient may be frustrated and should be approached in an unhurried manner. Often the patient does much better with communication when not feeling pressured to speak. Giving the patient a communication board may be helpful. Wait for the patient to communicate, rather than prompting or finishing the sentence before the patient has a chance to find the appropriate word. Inability to articulate does not mean that the patient has decreased cognitive abilities.

Nursing diagnoses and interventions for the patient who has had a stroke include but are not limited to the following:

Nursing Diagnoses	Nursing Interventions
Impaired verbal communication, related to ischemic injury	Speak slowly and distinctly. Ask questions that can be answered by yes or no (or by signals). Try to anticipate patient needs. Provide a call signal within reach of the unaffected hand. Begin speech therapy as soon as possible.
Imbalanced nutrition: less than body requirements, related to impaired ability to swallow	Provide IV fluids and tube feedings as prescribed during the initial period. Refer to speech therapist for assessment of swallowing problems. Assess ability to swallow before initiating feedings. Position patient with head elevated and turned to unaffected side during feedings. Provide foods initially that are easier to swallow (soft foods, except for mashed potatoes). Thin liquids are often difficult to swallow and may promote coughing. Thicken liquids with a commercially available thickening agent (Thick-It). Do not use milk products because they tend to increase the viscosity of mucus and increase salivation. Use a training cup for fluids as necessary. Do not use a straw. Inspect mouth for food trapped in cheek pockets. Be patient when feeding patient and provide directions for swallowing as needed. Ensure that meals are unrushed and nonstressful. Encourage patient to feed self as soon as possible; provide self-help devices as necessary. Provide scrupulous oral hygiene after meal because food may collect on the affected side of the mouth.

Patient Teaching

Teaching for a patient with a stroke should include techniques to compensate for the deficits suffered as a result of the stroke. In this the nurse functions as part of the rehabilitation team. Begin rehabilitation at the time of admission to the acute care facility. The patient will probably attend occupational and physical therapy and perhaps speech therapy. Depending on the patient's status, the patient's rehabilitation potential, and available resources, the patient may be transferred to a rehabilitation facility or unit.

If the patient is receiving medications (e.g., for hypertension or anticoagulation), teach the patient and the family about side effects and the dosing schedule. Discuss plans for follow-up. Also teach the patient's family techniques to enhance safety and communication. If the patient has a problem with dysphagia, teach the family appropriate communication techniques. Because of the chronicity of caring for the stroke patient, caregivers are at high risk for stress. Referral to an appropriate stroke support group is needed. Write instructions for the patient or the family to refer to after discharge. Most rehabilitation centers also include therapeutic leaves as a way to test the family's skills and knowledge. Each pass or leave has specific goals; obtain feedback from the family about additional teaching that may be needed. Also educate the family and the patient about perceptual problems associated with stroke and techniques to compensate for these deficits (e.g., writing down instructions for the patient who has trouble carrying out an activity alone).

Prognosis

The prognosis for patients with a stroke depends on the size of the lesion in the brain and the patient's premorbid status. More than 160,000 deaths occur in the United States each year as a result of strokes. Of those who survive, 50% to 70% are functionally independent; however, 15% to 30% have a permanent disability. The most frequent long-term disabilities include hemiparesis, inability to ambulate, aphasia, depression, and complete or partial dependence in ADLs. In 2005 the cost of stroke was estimated to be $56.8 billion per year in the United States (Lewis et al., 2007). With therapy, significant functional gains can be made, even when paralysis or weakness continues. Many patients are able to return home and remain independent after a stroke. With new medical treatment for selected patients, using t-PA for thrombolysis or mechanical clot removal, the prognosis is greatly improved.

CRANIAL AND PERIPHERAL NERVE DISORDERS

TRIGEMINAL NEURALGIA

Etiology and Pathophysiology

Trigeminal neuralgia is one specific kind of peripheral nerve problem. It is caused by degeneration of or pressure on the trigeminal nerve (cranial nerve V), and its etiology is unknown. It is also called **tic douloureux.** It

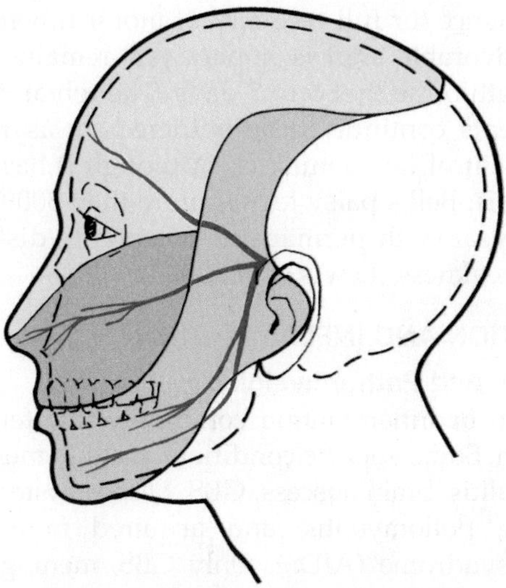

FIGURE 54-22 Pathway of trigeminal nerve and facial areas innervated by each of the three main divisions of this nerve.

usually affects people in middle or late adulthood and is slightly more common in women. The pathophysiology is not fully understood.

Clinical Manifestations

Trigeminal neuralgia is characterized by excruciating, knifelike, or lightninglike shock in the lips, upper or lower gums, cheek, forehead, or side of the nose. The pain radiates along one or more of the three divisions of the fifth cranial nerve (Figure 54-22). The fifth cranial nerve has both motor and sensory branches. In trigeminal neuralgia the sensory (or afferent) branches, primarily the maxillary and mandibular branches, are involved. The pain typically extends only to the midline of the face and head because this is the extent of the tissue supplied by the offending nerve. The attacks are usually brief, lasting only seconds to 2 to 3 minutes, and are generally unilateral. Recurrences are unpredictable; they may occur several times a day or weeks or months apart. Areas along the course of the nerve are known as **trigger points,** and the slightest stimulation of these areas may initiate pain. People with trigeminal neuralgia try desperately to avoid triggering them. Precipitating stimuli include chewing, toothbrushing, a hot or cold blast of air on the face, washing the face, yawning, or even talking.

Medical Management

Antiseizure medications such as carbamazepine, phenytoin, valproate, gabapentin, oxcarbazepine (Trileptal), lamotrigine (Lamictal), and topiramate are the drugs of choice for the treatment of trigeminal neuralgia pain. Absolute alcohol injected into the peripheral branches of the trigeminal nerve provides relief for weeks to months. Biofeedback, acupuncture, and megavitamins are other therapies used.

Permanent relief of pain is obtained only by surgery that involves inserting a fine needle through the cheek and injecting an alcohol solution or surgically resecting the sensory root of the trigeminal nerve. This is not always successful. Within 24 hours after a fifth nerve resection, many patients develop herpes simplex of the lips (cold sores). Usually these lesions heal in approximately 1 week.

Box 54-3 Comfort Measures for Patients with Trigeminal Neuralgia

- Keep room free of drafts, moderate temperature.
- Avoid walking briskly to bedside of patient.
- Place bed out of traffic area to prevent jarring of bed.
- Avoid touching the patient's face.
- Do not urge patients to wash or shave the affected area or to comb the hair during acute attack.
- Stress the importance of hygiene, nutrition, and oral care and convey understanding if previous oral neglect is apparent.
- Provide lukewarm water and soft cloths and cotton saturated with solutions that do not require water for cleaning the face.
- A warm mouthwash or small, soft-bristled toothbrush assists in promoting oral care.
- When analgesia is at its peak, conditions are optimum for instructing in matters of hygiene. Many patients, however, prefer to execute their own care as they fear inadvertent injury at the hands of someone else.
- Avoid hot or cold liquids, which trigger pain.
- Puree food and ensure that it is lukewarm. If necessary, suggest that food be taken through a straw.

Nursing Interventions

It is common for patients with trigeminal neuralgia not to have eaten properly for some time because eating causes pain. They may be undernourished and dehydrated. They may not have washed, shaved, or combed the hair for some time. Oral hygiene often has been neglected. Measures to increase comfort for patients before surgery or for patients being treated nonsurgically are listed in Box 54-3.

Prognosis

The acute pain seldom lasts more than a few seconds or 2 or 3 minutes, but it is excruciating. The onset of pain can occur at any time during the day or night and may recur several times daily for weeks at a time. Some patients have more or less continuous discomfort and sensitivity of the face. Although this condition is considered benign, the severity of the pain and the disruption of lifestyle can result in almost total physical and psychological dysfunction or even suicide. Permanent relief of pain is obtained only by surgery.

BELL'S PALSY (PERIPHERAL FACIAL PARALYSIS)

Etiology and Pathophysiology

Bell's palsy is thought to be caused by an inflammatory process involving the facial nerve (cranial nerve VII) anywhere from the nucleus in the brain to the periphery. Although the exact etiology is not known, there is evidence that reactivated herpes simplex virus (HSV) may be involved in the majority of cases. The reactivation of the HSV causes inflammation, edema, ischemia, and eventual demyelination of the facial nerve, creating pain and disturbances in motor and sensory function. Any of the three branches of the facial nerve may be affected. The disorder can be unilateral or bilateral. It can affect any age-group, but is more common in the 20- to 60-year-old age range.

Clinical Manifestations

With Bell's palsy there is usually an abrupt onset of numbness, stiffness, or drawing sensation of the face. Unilateral weakness of the facial muscles usually occurs, resulting in a flaccidity of the affected side of the face with inability to wrinkle the forehead, close the eyelid, pucker the lips, smile, frown, whistle, or retract the mouth on that side. The face appears asymmetric, with drooping mouth and cheek. Other symptoms include loss of taste, altered chewing ability, reduction of saliva on the affected side, pain behind the ear on the affected side, and ringing in the ear or other hearing loss.

Medical Management

Bell's palsy has no specific therapy. Electrical stimulation or warm moist heat along the course of the nerve may help. Stimulation may maintain muscle tone and prevent atrophy. Corticosteroids, especially prednisone, are started immediately, preferably before paralysis is complete. When the patient improves to the point that the corticosteroids are no longer necessary, they should be tapered off over a 2-week period. Because HSV is implicated in approximately 70% of cases of Bell's palsy, treatment with acyclovir (Zovirax), alone or in conjunction with prednisone, is used. Additional antiviral agents to treat HSV, including valacyclovir (Valtrex) and famciclovir (Famvir), have also been used in the management of Bell's palsy.

Nursing Interventions

Protection of the eye when the eyelid does not close is important. To prevent drying of the cornea, instill artificial tears frequently while the patient is awake. Apply an ointment with use of an impermeable eyeshield at night to facilitate retention of moisture (Lewis et al., 2007). Massage of the affected areas is sometimes recommended. Active facial exercises may be prescribed for 5 minutes three times a day. These include wrinkling the brow and forehead, closing the eyes, and puffing out the cheeks.

Prognosis

Some 85% of patients recover fully in weeks or months, although recovery may take as long as a year. Recovery of taste is the first sign of improvement; if it occurs within the first week, it signals a good chance for full recovery of motor function. Another favorable sign is if paralysis remains incomplete within the first 5 to 7 days. The remaining 15% of patients continue to be bothered by asymmetric movement of facial muscles. Although it has a good prognosis, Bell's palsy leaves more than 8000 Americans a year with permanent, potentially disfiguring facial weakness (Lewis et al., 2007).

INFECTION AND INFLAMMATION

Etiology and Pathophysiology

Infection or inflammation commonly interferes with function. Some specific conditions include meningitis, encephalitis, brain abscess, GBS, herpes zoster, neurosyphilis, poliomyelitis, and acquired immunodeficiency syndrome (AIDS). Only GBS, meningitis, encephalitis, brain abscess, and AIDS are discussed in this chapter.

The nervous system may be affected by a variety of organisms and may suffer from toxins of bacteria and viruses. These toxins reach the nervous system from a variety of sources, including adjacent bones, blood, or lymph. Meningitis can occur as a result of an invasive procedure such as surgery.

Assessment

Subjective data include a history of infection, such as an upper respiratory tract infection, and discomfort such as headache or stiff neck. The initial onset of symptoms, difficulty in thinking, and weakness may be important. Assess the patient's understanding of the condition.

Objective data include behavioral signs indicating discomfort or disorientation and an inability to carry out ADLs. Physical assessment may reveal abnormalities; fever, vomiting, abnormal CT results, seizures, altered respiratory patterns, tachycardia, or meningeal irritation. Also assess the patient's LOC and orientation.

Diagnostic Tests

Many of the infections of the nervous system can be diagnosed by examining the CSF. A CT scan or an EEG may also be done.

Nursing Interventions and Patient Teaching

Nursing diagnoses and interventions for the patient with an infection or inflammation are the same as those for the patient who has had a stroke, with the addition of but not limited to the following:

Nursing Diagnoses	Nursing Interventions
Hyperthermia, related to inflammatory response to CNS infection	Assess temperature every 2 hours and as needed. Provide cooling measures as needed; avoid cooling to point of shivering.

Nursing Diagnoses	Nursing Interventions
	Administer antipyretics and antibiotics as ordered. Monitor parenteral fluids as ordered. Control exposure to extremes in temperature. Assess temperature, pulse, and respiration every 2 hours as indicated.
Acute confusion, related to neurophysiologic response to infection	Introduce self to patient and establish rapport to prevent agitation. Relate date, time of day, and recent activities. Speak in kind tone, using short, simple sentences. Maintain a therapeutic environment.

Education for the patient with an infection includes teaching about the disease process, the treatments involved, and the expected outcomes. If the patient is seriously ill, the initial teaching involves the family. Other aspects of teaching for motor and sensory problems may also be relevant for the patient with an infection or inflammation, depending on the signs and symptoms demonstrated.

GUILLAIN-BARRÉ SYNDROME (POLYNEURITIS)

Etiology and Pathophysiology

Guillain-Barré syndrome (GBS) is also called **acute inflammatory polyradiculopathy** or **postinfectious polyneuritis.** It is an acute, rapidly progressing, and potentially fatal form of polyneuritis. It results in widespread inflammation and demyelination of the peripheral nervous system. The disease affects people of all ages and is seen equally in men and women. It affects 1.5 people in 100,000 each year. The etiology is unknown, but it is thought to be an autoimmune reaction involving the peripheral nerves. GBS often follows a viral infection, trauma, surgery, viral immunizations, or HIV infection. Other pathogens include *Campylobacter jejuni* (precedes the syndrome in about 30% of cases), mycoplasma, pneumoniae, cytomegalovirus, Epstein-Barr virus, and varicella-zoster virus (Lewis et al., 2007).

The peripheral nervous system is composed of 31 pairs of spinal nerves, 12 pairs of cranial nerves, and various plexuses and ganglia. Each nerve cell, or neuron, is composed of several parts, including the axon. Responsible for transmitting nerve impulses, axons are wrapped in segments of insulation called the myelin sheath, which is composed of Schwann cells.

In GBS the antibodies attack the Schwann cells, causing the sheath to break down (a process called demyelination) and the uninsulated portion of the nerve to become inflamed. Nerve conduction is interrupted, causing the classic signs of muscle weakness, tingling, and numbness. These signs begin in the legs or feet and work their way upward, perhaps because the signals to and from the legs are most vulnerable because they have to travel the longest distance. The demyelination is self-limiting. Once it stops, the Schwann cells rebuild the lost insulation. Remyelination, and therefore recovery, occurs in reverse; it starts at the top of the body and proceeds downward.

Clinical Manifestations

There is variation in the pattern of the onset of weakness and in the rate of progression of signs and symptoms. The progression may stop at any point. The patient may have difficulty swallowing, breathing, and speaking if cranial nerves VII, IX, and X are involved. Symmetric muscle weakness and lower motoneuron paralysis are present. The paralysis usually starts in the lower extremities and moves upward to include the thorax, the upper extremities, and the face. Respiratory failure may occur if the intercostal muscles are affected. Fluctuating blood pressure may occur as a result of effects on the autonomic nervous system.

Diagnostic Tests

GBS is diagnosed by elimination of other reasons for the signs and symptoms and by the characteristic muscle weakness. A CT scan may be ordered to rule out tumors or stroke. Changes in the respiratory status may aid in the diagnosis. A lumbar puncture is done. CSF in patients with GBS commonly has elevated protein levels. The physician may order a nerve conduction velocity study to test for slow impulse transmission. Electromyography and nerve conduction studies are markedly abnormal. A history of a recent infection is considered important.

Medical Management

Once GBS is suspected, hospitalization is essential. The patient's condition can rapidly deteriorate into paralysis that affects the respiratory muscles.

Adrenocortical steroids are used to treat the signs and symptoms of GBS. It has also been found that therapeutic plasmapheresis (the removal of unwanted or pathologic components from the patient's blood serum by means of a continuous-flow separator) in the first 2 weeks of GBS leads to decreased severity and length of symptoms. An alternative to plasmapheresis is IV immunoglobulin (Sandoglobulin). Patients receiving high-dose immunoglobulin need to be well hydrated and have adequate renal function.

Patients who develop respiratory failure require mechanical ventilation and may require a tracheostomy. ABG monitoring and pulmonary function tests are used to assess the respiratory status. If the patient has severe paralysis and is expected to have a long recovery period, a gastrostomy tube may be placed to provide adequate nourishment.

Nursing Interventions

Closely monitor respiratory function. If the patient requires mechanical ventilation, be aware that cognition (the mental faculty or process by which knowledge is acquired) is not impaired and that the patient requires reassurance. The patient may also need to be fed intravenously or through a nasogastric tube. Attention to the prevention of complications, such as contractures, pressure ulcers, and loss of ROM, is important to allow complete recovery. Initiate physical therapy early in the course of the disease to prevent contractures. Administer medication to help reduce neuropathic pain, such as gabapentin or a tricyclic antidepressant such as amitriptyline. Assess the patient's vital signs and motor strength frequently. Monitor the patient for signs of hypoxia.

Prognosis

Of the people suffering from GBS, 85% regain complete function. Only 20% of patients have weakness at 1 year and only 5% have severe permanent disability. The recovery period may vary from weeks to years. Those not recovering completely have some degree of permanent neurologic deficit. Generally, recovery from the disease occurs in the reverse order of how the paralysis or weakness occurred.

MENINGITIS

Etiology and Pathophysiology

Meningitis is an acute infection of the meninges. It is usually caused by one of several organisms, including pneumococci, meningococci, *Neisseria meningitidis,* staphylococci, streptococci, *Haemophilus influenzae,* and viral aseptic agents. The bacteria in the subarachnoid space cause an inflammatory reaction in the pia mater, arachnoid and pus accumulation in the CSF and possible injury to nervous tissue.

Meningitis can be classified as bacterial (septic), or viral (aseptic). The incidence of bacterial meningitis is higher in fall and winter when upper respiratory tract infections are common. Pathologic changes that can occur include hyperemia of the meningeal vessels, edema of brain tissue, increased ICP, a generalized inflammatory reaction with exudation of white blood cells into the subarachnoid spaces, and associated hydrocephalus (in infants) caused by exudate occluding the ventricles.

Clinical Manifestations

Two abnormal signs that occur with meningitis are **Kernig's sign** (the inability to extend the legs completely without extreme pain) and **Brudzinski's sign** (flexion of the hip and knee when the neck is flexed). The onset of meningitis is usually sudden and is characterized by severe headache, stiffness of the neck, irritability, malaise, and restlessness. The patient develops nausea and vomiting; delirium; and increased temperature, pulse rate, and respirations.

Diagnostic Tests

A CT of the head is ordered to rule out increased ICP. A lumbar puncture to obtain CSF is performed, unless ICP is increased. The CSF is sent to the laboratory to identify the pathogen responsible for causing the meningitis.

Medical Management

Rapid diagnosis and treatment are crucial in caring for the patient with bacterial meningitis. When meningitis is suspected, cultures are collected and diagnosis is confirmed. Treatment of meningitis includes multiple antibiotics given intravenously over a 2-week period. Medication options include ampicillin, penicillin, piperacillin, and third-generation cephalosporin (usually ceftriaxone [Rocephin] or cefotaxime for treating bacterial meningitis). Corticosteroids (dexamethasone) are given intravenously to decrease ICP. Anticonvulsants are given to prevent seizures. Aseptic (viral) meningitis is treated with supportive therapy, such as maintaining bed rest, ensuring fluid and electrolyte balance, and providing rest and comfort measures (Lower, 2007).

Nursing Interventions

Respiratory isolation is required until the pathogen can no longer be cultured from the nasopharynx. This is usually accomplished after 24 hours of effective antibiotic therapy. Other nursing interventions include the general care given a critically ill patient who may be irritable, disoriented, and unable to take fluids. Dehydration is common, and the patient almost always has an IV line. Keep the room darkened and noise to a minimum because any increase in sensory stimulation may cause a seizure. If the patient is disoriented, take safety precautions. Vigorously manage fever because it increases cerebral edema and the frequency of seizures. In addition, neurologic damage may result from an extremely high temperature over a prolonged time. Acetaminophen may be used to reduce fever. However, if the fever is resistant to acetaminophen, more vigorous means are necessary, such as an automatic cooling blanket (Lewis et al., 2007).

Prophylactic antibiotic therapy for family and friends in close contact with a patient with bacterial meningitis may be recommended to destroy the causative bacteria that may have colonized in the nasopharynx.

Some forms of bacterial meningitis can be prevented by vaccination. The pneumococcal vaccine may be given to adults age 65 and older and other high-risk adults. The meningococcal vaccine is effective against *N. meningitidis* and is recommended for patients ages 11 to 12 and college freshmen living in dormitories. The *H. influenzae* vaccine has significantly decreased meningitis caused by this organism in children (Lewis et al., 2007).

Prognosis

With most cases of meningitis, the prognosis for complete recovery is good. The prognosis depends on the speed with which antibiotics are administered. With severe cases of meningitis, residual neurologic damage or death may occur.

ENCEPHALITIS

Encephalitis is an acute inflammation of the brain and is usually caused by a virus. Many different viruses have been implicated in encephalitis; some are associated with certain seasons of the year and endemic to certain geographic areas. Epidemic encephalitis is transmitted by ticks and mosquitoes. Nonepidemic encephalitis may occur as a complication of measles, chickenpox, or mumps.

Encephalitis is a serious, sometimes fatal disease. Overall mortality rate ranges from 5% to 20%, with the highest mortality rate in encephalitis caused by HSV and the eastern and Venezuelan equine viruses. Unfortunately, HSV encephalitis is the most common form of viral encephalitis. Cytomegalovirus encephalitis is a common complication in patients with AIDS.

Manifestations resemble those of meningitis, but they have a more gradual onset. They include headache, high fever, seizures, and a change in LOC. Early diagnosis and treatment of viral encephalitis are essential for favorable outcomes. Brain imaging techniques such as MRI and PET, along with viral studies of CSF, allow for earlier detection of viral encephalitis.

Medical management and nursing interventions are symptomatic and supportive. Cerebral edema is a major problem, and diuretics (mannitol) and corticosteroids (dexamethasone) are used to control it. The disease is characterized by diffuse damage to the nerve cells of the brain, perivascular cellular infiltration of glial cells, and increasing cerebral edema. The sequelae of encephalitis include mental deterioration, amnesia, personality changes, and hemiparesis.

Acyclovir or vidarabine (Vira-A) are used to treat encephalitis caused by HSV infection. Acyclovir has fewer side effects than vidarabine and is often the preferred treatment. Use of these antiviral agents has been shown to reduce mortality rates from 70% to 30%, although neurologic complications may not be reduced. Long-term symptoms include memory impairment, epilepsy, anosmia, personality changes, behavioral abnormalities, and dysphasia. For maximal benefit, antiviral agents should be started before the onset of coma.

WEST NILE VIRUS

West Nile virus (WNV) has been commonly found in humans and birds and other vertebrates in Africa, Eastern Europe, western Asia, and the Middle East, but it was not documented in the United States until 1999. The virus can infect humans, birds, mosquitoes, horses, and some other animals.

The principal route of human infection with WNV is through the bite of an infected female mosquito. Mosquitoes become infected when they feed on infected birds. When the virus is injected into humans by a mosquito, it can multiply and possibly cause illness. The incubation period ranges from 3 to 14 days. Most people who become infected with the virus do not have any type of illness. Those who develop West Nile fever have flulike manifestations of fever, headache, back pain, myalgia, and anorexia, lasting only a few days and without any long-term health effects. It is estimated that 1 in 150 people infected with WNV develops encephalitis or meningitis, a more severe form of the disease. **WNV meningitis** is usually associated with a sudden onset of febrile illness, headache, chills, neck pain, and sometimes confusion. Patients with **WNV encephalitis** often have fever; headache; altered LOC; disorientation; behavioral and speech disturbances; and other neurologic signs such as hemiparesis, seizures, and coma. Advanced age is the most significant risk factor contributing to death from infection; conditions such as immunosuppression are also contributing factors (Bender, 2003). Even in areas where the virus is circulating, however, few mosquitoes are infected with the virus. The chances of becoming severely ill from any one mosquito bite are extremely small.

The current standard for diagnosing WNV is by testing blood or CSF with the immunoglobulin M (IgM) antibody capture enzyme-linked immunosorbent assay (ELISA) and immunoglobulin G indirect ELISA. The IgM test may not be positive when symptoms first occur; however, it becomes positive in most infected people within days of symptom onset. Someone recently vaccinated against yellow fever or Japanese encephalitis also will have a positive IgM antibody test result.

WNV cannot be transmitted through casual contact such as touching or kissing a person who has the disease. However, in a small number of cases, the virus has been transmitted through blood transfusion, organ transplantation, breastfeeding, and pregnancy (from mother to fetus).

One can reduce the risk of becoming infected with WNV by applying insect repellent to exposed skin. Choose an insect repellent that contains *N,N*-diethyl-3-methylbenzamide (DEET) and one that provides protection for the amount of time to be spent outdoors. Also spray clothing because mosquitoes can bite through thin clothing. Wearing long-sleeved shirts, long pants, and socks while outdoors can reduce the risk. Take special precautions from April to October, the months when mosquitoes are most active.

DEET is the gold standard in currently available over-the-counter insect repellents. DEET was developed in 1946 by the U.S. Army for use by military personnel in insect-infested areas. It has been used worldwide for more than 40 years and has a remarkable safety profile. Toxic reactions can occur, and they are usually linked to misuse of the product, such as massive exposure due to chronic use. Reports of greatest concern involve encephalopathy caused by DEET exposure. Most adverse reactions, though, are less serious, involving eye irritation and inhalation irritation (related to spraying repellent in the eyes or inhaling it).

DEET has been classified as a group D carcinogen (not classifiable as a human carcinogen). For casual use, a 10% to 35% concentration provides adequate protection. The American Academy of Pediatrics recommends limiting DEET repellents to a 30% maximum concentration when used on infants and children. DEET is not recommended for use in children younger than 2 months (Centers for Disease Control and Prevention, 2008).

Other means of decreasing the mosquito population and thus decreasing the possibility of transmission of the WNV include the following (Overstreet, 2004):

- Limit outdoor activities between dusk and dawn.
- Place mosquito netting over infant carriers or strollers when outdoors.
- Keep swimming pools, outdoor saunas, and hot tubs clean and properly chlorinated. Remove standing water from pool covers.
- Store any containers that may become filled with standing water, such as cans, flowerpots, or trash cans, indoors.
- Install or repair window and door screens so that mosquitoes cannot get indoors.

If WNV infection is confirmed, treatment is supportive, intended to manage symptoms, such as headache, fever, and nausea. In more severe cases, patients may need intensive therapy, often involving hospitalization for IV fluids, airway management, respiratory support, and prevention of secondary infections such as pneumonia. To manage WNV encephalitis, the patient may receive interferon alfa-2_b, steroids, antiseizure medications, or osmotic diuretics.

Approximately 80% of WNV infections are asymptomatic. Infected people have a transient viremia, making transmission of the virus via donated blood, organs, or tissue possible. As with many viruses, contact with the blood of an infected person could lead to transmission of the virus; therefore use the same standard precautions as with all patients.

Since July 2003, more than 2.5 million blood donations have been screened for WNV. As of September 16, 2003, the Centers for Disease Control and Prevention's surveillance system reported that 601 viremic donations had been identified. Two cases of blood transfusion–associated WNV infection were detected in the United States in 2003—one in Texas and one in Nebraska. Both people were receiving care, including blood transfusions, for other serious health conditions. They developed encephalitis from the WNV infection; both recovered (Goldrick, 2003).

BRAIN ABSCESS

Brain abscess is an accumulation of pus within the brain tissue that can result from a local or a systemic infection. Direct extension from ear, tooth, mastoid, or sinus infection is the primary cause. Other causes for brain abscess formation include septic venous thrombosis from a pulmonary infection, infective endocarditis, skull fracture, and a nonsterile neurologic procedure. Streptococci and staphylococci are the primary infective organisms.

Clinical manifestations are similar to those of meningitis and encephalitis and include headache and fever. Signs of increased ICP may include drowsiness, confusion, and seizures. Focal symptoms may be present and reflect the local area of the abscess. For example, visual field deficits or psychomotor seizures are common with a temporal lobe abscess, whereas an occipital abscess may be accompanied by visual impairment and hallucinations.

Antimicrobial therapy is the primary treatment for brain abscess. Other manifestations are treated symptomatically. If drug therapy is not effective, the abscess may need to be removed if it is encapsulated. In untreated cases the mortality rate approaches 100%. Seizures occur in approximately 30% of the cases. Nursing interventions are similar to those for management of meningitis or increased ICP. If the abscess is removed surgically, nursing interventions are similar to those described under intracranial tumors.

Other infections of the brain include subdural empyema, osteomyelitis of the cranial bones, epidural abscess, and venous sinus thrombosis after periorbital cellulitis.

ACQUIRED IMMUNODEFICIENCY SYNDROME

Etiology and Pathophysiology

AIDS is a disease that has serious implications for the nervous system, with more than 80% of advanced HIV disease patients having neurologic signs and symptoms. Patients develop neurologic signs and symptoms either from infection with HIV itself or as a result of associated infections. See Chapter 56 for a discussion of advanced HIV disease (AIDS).

Clinical Manifestations

Patients with AIDS may have AIDS dementia complex (ADC), which is known as subacute encephalitis. They may exhibit difficulty concentrating or a recent memory loss, which may progress to a **global cognitive dysfunction** (generalized impairment of intellect, awareness, and judgment). Patients may also experience opportunistic infections such as meningitis, HSV, cytomegalovirus, toxoplasmosis, and cryptococcal meningitis. Primary malignant lymphomas of the CNS may also develop.

Diagnostic Tests

The diagnostic tests used to determine whether a neurologic problem is related to AIDS include serologic studies, analysis of CSF through a lumbar puncture, CT scan, and MRI. At times, a cerebral biopsy may be necessary to make the differential diagnosis.

Medical Management

Treatment of the patient with neurologic problems related to AIDS depends on the infection. Methods of treatment include administration of antiviral, antifungal, and antibacterial agents. Radiation has been used on the affected part of the brain. Experimental therapies, including iron dextran (DexFerrum), have been tried. Dehydration or shock is treated with fluid volume expanders. Seizures are controlled with diazepam, phenytoin, or fosphenytoin. Mortality remains high despite aggressive therapy.

Nursing Interventions

The patient is likely to be disoriented and may need to be reoriented frequently. Safety measures such as padded side rails may be necessary to prevent injury to the patient, who may have seizures. The patient may experience pain and have difficulty sleeping. Administer medications as needed and structure activities to avoid waking the patient. Visual problems may also be associated with the disease; be careful to orient the patient to nursing interventions.

Most patients with AIDS experience depression and a sense of powerlessness about the disease. They may isolate themselves from others. Encourage patients to talk about their fears and concerns, help them find emotional support, and refer them to a support group. Above all, maintain a nonjudgmental attitude, regardless of how the patient contracted the disease.

The patient may be incontinent of bowel and bladder. Encourage an active bowel and bladder program. If the patient has diarrhea, keep the rectal area as clean and dry as possible and administer antidiarrheals if ordered. The patient may also have nausea. Offer foods that the patient likes in small, frequent meals. Tube feedings or total parenteral nutrition may be needed if the patient agrees.

Prognosis

The prognosis for the patient with AIDS is terminal, often within a short time. Currently, little can be done to substantially lengthen life. After a patient experiences neurologic complications, AIDS is usually fairly well advanced.

BRAIN TUMORS

Etiology and Pathophysiology

Brain tumors include both benign and metastatic lesions. All areas and structures of the brain can be affected. Primary brain tumors, or **neoplasms,** form when changes occur in the genetic structure of normal brain cells (neurons and glial cells). Changes may be caused by a genetic predisposition, an environmental trigger, or both; the causes of most primary brain tumors are unknown. Most benign tumors affect the meninges, whereas most malignant tumors affect the glial cells (Palmieri, 2007b). These tumors include gliomas, meningiomas, pituitary tumors, and neuromas. Metastatic tumors also occur frequently in the brain. Brain tumors are named for the tissues from which they arise.

Assessment

Subjective data include the patient's understanding of the diagnosis, changes in personality or judgment, and abnormal sensations or visual problems. The patient may complain of unusual odors with tumors of the temporal lobe. Also assess headache, nausea or hearing loss, or the inability to carry out daily activities. Patients with brain tumors usually experience headaches as a prominent early symptom. The headache is usually intermittent, moderate to severe, associated with nausea or vomiting, and typically worse in the morning. The patient may also have paresis, diplopia, or weakness (Palmieri, 2007c).

Objective data include motor strength, gait, the level of alertness and consciousness, and orientation. Assess the pupils for response and equality. In some patients, the initial sign of a brain tumor is new-onset seizures; about half of patients have seizure activity at some time during their illness. Other troubling signs of a brain tumor are cognitive changes in memory, speech, concentration, and communication. The patient's family may notice changes in intellectual function, personality, and behavior (Palmieri, 2007b). Speech impairments, cranial nerve abnormalities, and signs and symptoms of increased ICP are also significant.

Diagnostic Tests

No one procedure is entirely diagnostic of brain tumors, but a CT scan is often the basis for the diagnosis. Other tests that may be performed include the brain scan, MRI, PET scans, and the EEG. Arteriography may also be done.

Medical Management

The general method of treatment for brain tumors includes surgical removal when feasible, radiation, and chemotherapy. The choice of therapy is determined by the tumor type and site. A combination of methods is often used. The blood-brain barrier may limit the effectiveness of chemotherapy when used as adjuvant therapy or to treat tumor recurrence (Palmieri, 2007c).

Surgery

A surgical opening through the skull is called a **craniotomy.** After removing the bone, the surgeon makes an incision into the meninges and removes the tumor. The removed bone is carefully preserved and may be replaced at the end of surgery if there is no indication of infection or increased ICP. The removal of part of the skull without replacement is called **craniectomy.** Recent advances have been made in the use of intracranial endoscopy.

Nursing Interventions

Preoperative preparation of both the patient and the family is important. Specific fears may be related to a permanent change in appearance, dependency, and possible death. A baseline neurologic assessment is important. Explain treatments and procedures, including shaving the hair. Usually hair is shaved in the operating room. It is then given to the patient, who may choose to have it made into a wig. Prepare the family for the patient's appearance after surgery.

Postoperative care is determined by the patient's condition. Most patients spend one or two nights in an intensive care unit under close nursing observation with frequent neurologic checks. Assess the patient carefully for indications of increased ICP. The patient may have residual motor or sensory problems as a result of the tumor or surgery.

Nursing diagnoses and interventions for the patient with a brain tumor are the same as those for the patient who has had a stroke, with the addition of but not limited to the following:

Nursing Diagnoses	Nursing Interventions
Disturbed sensory perception: visual, auditory, kinesthetic, tactile, related to compression or displacement of brain tissue	Maintain method of communication. Provide for social environment. Provide orientation and appropriate level of stimuli.
Acute confusion, related to: • altered circulation • destruction of brain tissue	Protect patient from self-injury. Provide soft safety reminder devices as indicated. Assist patient in self-care activities. Speak in kind tone using short, simple sentences. Give one direction at a time. Relate date, time of day, and recent activities. Maintain a therapeutic environment. Keep equipment and personal possessions in same place. Encourage socialization.

Prognosis

The outlook for the patient with a brain tumor depends on whether the tumor is benign or malignant and on its size and location. Tumors that infiltrate the brain usually result in a decreased life span. With radiation and chemotherapy, patients with malignant tumors may live longer.

TRAUMA

Interference with neurologic function can occur as a result of trauma. Parts of the nervous system commonly subjected to trauma include the brain, the spinal cord, and peripheral nerves. Only the first two are discussed in this chapter.

HEAD INJURY

Etiology and Pathophysiology

The term *head trauma* is used primarily to signify craniocerebral trauma, or head injury, which includes an alteration in consciousness, no matter how brief. Head injury is the second most common cause of neurologic injuries and the major cause of death between ages 1 and 35. Previously, the most common causes of head injury in the United States were motor vehicle collisions and falls. Deaths from motor vehicle collisions and falls have decreased; however, firearm-related head injury death rates have increased. Head injury can result from recreational injuries, sports-related trauma, and assaults. The incidence of traumatic brain injury is twice as high in males as in females (Lewis et al., 2007).

Craniocerebral trauma may result in injury to the scalp, skull, and brain tissues. Injuries vary from minor scalp wounds to concussions and open fractures of the skull with severe damage to the brain. The amount of obvious damage is not indicative of the seriousness of the trouble. Effects of severe head injury include cerebral edema, sensory and motor deficits, and increased ICP.

Injuries to the brain can result from direct or indirect trauma to the head. Indirect trauma is caused by tension strains and shearing forces transmitted to the head by stretching the neck. Direct trauma occurs when the head is directly injured. Indirect trauma results in an **acceleration-deceleration** injury, with rotation of the skull and its contents. Bruising or contusion of the occipital and frontal lobes, the brainstem, and the cerebellum may occur.

Clinical Manifestations

Head injuries may be open or closed. Open head injuries result from skull fractures or penetrating wounds. The amount of injury with this type of wound is determined by the velocity, mass, shape, and direction of the impact. A skull fracture (linear, comminuted, depressed, or compound) may also occur. Fractures of the base of the skull are more serious because they are near the medulla.

Closed head injuries include concussions (a violent jarring of the brain against the skull), contusions, and lacerations. Lacerations of the scalp bleed profusely because of the vascularity in the region. Hemorrhage resulting from craniocerebral trauma may occur in the scalp or the epidural, subdural, intracerebral, and intraventricular areas. Epidural and subdural hematomas require careful and continuous observation. Epidural hematomas resulting from arterial bleeding form as blood collects rapidly between the dura and skull. If lethargy or unconsciousness develops after the patient regains consciousness, an epidural hematoma may be suspected and needs immediate treatment.

A subdural hematoma forms as venous blood collects below the dura. Because the bleeding is under venous pressure, the hematoma formation is relatively slow. The clot causes pressure on the brain surface and displaces brain tissue. If a patient who has been conscious for several days after head injury loses consciousness or develops neurologic signs and symptoms, suspect a subdural hematoma. Subdural hematomas may be classified as acute, subacute, or chronic.

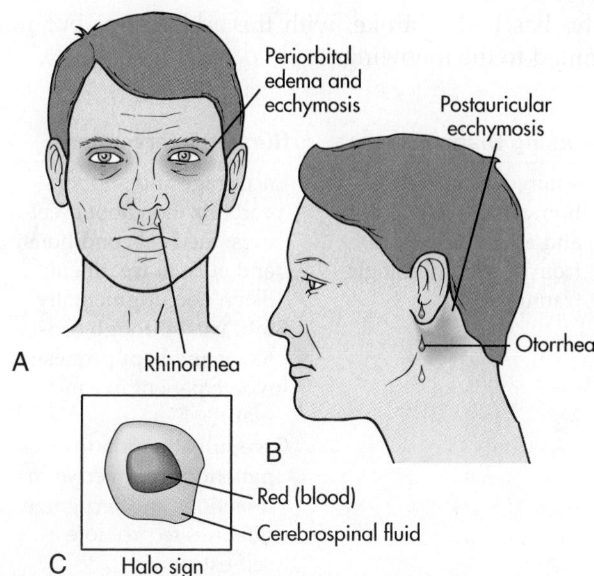

FIGURE 54-23 **A,** Raccoon eyes and rhinorrhea. **B,** Battle's sign (postauricular ecchymosis) with otorrhea. **C,** Halo or ring sign.

Assessment

Subjective data include the patient's understanding of the injury and the resulting pathologic processes. Determine how the injury happened and whether the patient has headache, nausea, or vomiting. Note abnormal sensations and a history of LOC and of bleeding from any orifice.

Objective data include the status of the respiratory system, level of alertness and consciousness, and size and reactivity of the pupils; check these frequently. Also assess the patient's orientation, motor status, vital signs, bleeding or vomiting, and abnormal speech patterns. The presence of **Battle's sign** (a small hemorrhagic spot behind the ear) usually indicates a fracture of a bone of the lower skull (Figure 54-23).

Diagnostic Tests

CT, MRI, and PET scans are the primary diagnostic imaging examinations in assessing soft tissue injuries.

Medical Management

Immediate care of the patient with a head injury is directed toward lifesaving measures and the maintenance of normal body function until recovery is ensured. It is extremely important to maintain a patent airway and ensure adequate oxygenation. Suctioning may be necessary (but never through the nose because of the possibility of a skull fracture), along with the administration of oxygen. Check ABG levels. Stabilize the cervical spine; assume neck injury with head injury until diagnostic examination proves otherwise.

Medications are used to reduce cerebral edema and increased ICP, which are common problems in patients with head injuries. Medications include mannitol and dexamethasone. Pegorgotein, a scavenger of oxygen-derived free radicals, has been used experimentally. Codeine or other analgesics that do not depress the respiratory system are used for pain control. Anticonvulsants may be given to prevent seizures. Take measures to control elevated temperatures, since hyperthermia increases brain metabolism, resulting in brain damage.

Nursing Interventions

Check the patient's ears and nose carefully for signs of blood and serous drainage, which indicate that the meninges are torn and spinal fluid is escaping. *Do not* attempt to clean out the orifice. If there is evidence of drainage from the nose, the patient should not cough, sneeze, or blow the nose. If there is a question about whether drainage is CSF, Tes-Tape will show a positive reaction for glucose. Meningitis is a possible complication when communication with the meninges and the nose or ears occurs.

The patient with a head injury often shows a loss of memory and loss of initiative. Behavioral problems associated with a lack of judgment and restlessness may also occur. Restlessness may be caused by the need for a change of position, pain, or the need to empty the bladder. These patients require firm but gentle care, with specific guidelines for what behavior is allowed. Medications to decrease agitation may be needed. It is not helpful to argue with patients, but redirecting their attention may help. Memory aids such as a log book or written schedule can assist with orientation.

The length of convalescence depends on the amount of brain damage and how rapid the recovery is. Many patients with head injury recover physically but have behavioral and psychological problems that make it difficult for them to function independently.

A nursing diagnosis and interventions for the patient with a head injury are the same as for the patient who has had a stroke, with the addition of but not limited to the following:

Nursing Diagnosis	Nursing Interventions
Impaired social interaction, related to cognitive and affective deficits from neurophysiologic trauma	Encourage and support verbalization about feelings, medical conditions, and current treatment; listen nonjudgmentally. Build trust through consistency and kept promises. Involve patient in care plan. Give full attention to patient during verbal interactions and recognize qualities to promote self-esteem.

Patient Teaching

A patient with a mild head injury may be seen in the emergency department but not be admitted to the hospital. Teach the patient about observations for complications such as increased drowsiness, nausea, vomiting, worsening headache or stiff neck, seizures, blurred vision, behavioral changes, motor problems, sensory disturbances, or decreased heart rate. Teaching for patients with a head injury who have residual deficits severe enough to require rehabilitation is similar to that needed for patients with motor or sensory problems.

Prognosis

The outcome for a patient with a head injury is often unpredictable. The extent of damage or recovery is not positively correlated with the amount of damage seen in surgery or on CT scan. Even minor head injuries can have residual effects. The person with a head injury is more prone to injuries and problems related to the brain damage.

SPINAL CORD TRAUMA

Etiology and Pathophysiology

Spinal cord injury from accidents is a common and increasing cause of serious disability and death. Approximately 10% of traumatic injuries to the nervous system involve the spinal cord. Most people involved with spinal cord injuries are men between 18 and 25 years of age. Automobile, motorcycle, diving, surfing, and other athletic accidents and gunshot wounds are major causes of spinal cord injury.

The soft tissue of the spinal cord is protected by the vertebral column. Injuries to this column include a simple fracture, compressed or wedge fracture, comminuted or burst fracture, or dislocation of the vertebrae (Figure 54-24). As a result, the cord is often damaged. Severe traumatic lesions of the spinal cord may result in total transection of the spinal cord or tearing

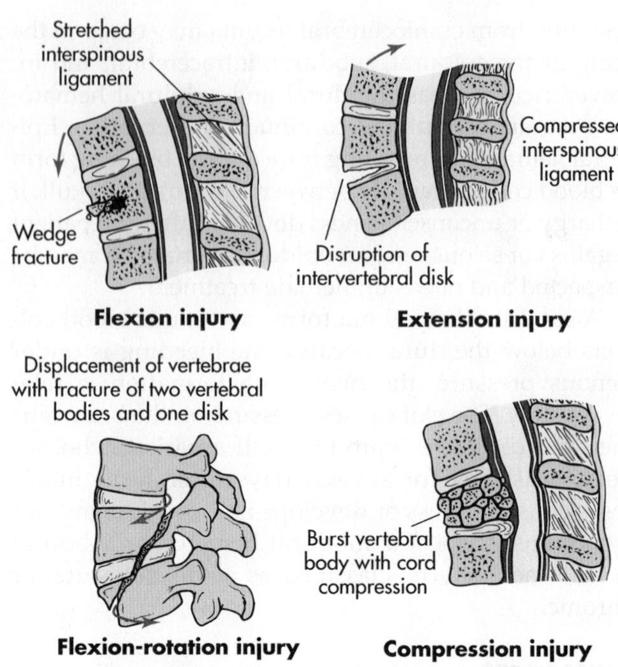

FIGURE 54-24 Mechanisms of spinal injury.

of the cord from side to side at a particular level, with a complete loss of spinal cord function. This total transection is also called a **complete cord injury.** With this type of injury, all voluntary movement below the level of the trauma is lost. A partial transection, or **incomplete injury,** of the cord may also occur. Tetraplegic patients (formerly referred to as quadriplegic) are those who sustain injuries to one of the cervical segments of the spinal cord. Paraplegic patients are those whose lesions are confined to the thoracic, lumbar, or sacral segments of the spinal cord. The signs and symptoms of an incomplete injury vary (Table 54-9).

Clinical Manifestations

Initially, in most spinal cord injuries, there is a period of flaccid paralysis and a complete loss of reflexes below the level of trauma. Sensory and autonomic functions are also lost. The loss of systemic sympathetic vasomotor tone may result in vasodilation, increased venous capacity, and hypotension. This is called areflexia, or spinal shock, and is temporary. During this time the patient may need temporary respiratory support.

One important complication of spinal cord injury is autonomic dysreflexia or **hyperreflexia,** a neurologic condition characterized by increased reflex actions. It occurs in patients with cord injuries at the sixth thoracic vertebra or higher and most commonly in patients with cervical injuries. Autonomic dysreflexia is an abnormal cardiovascular response to stimulation of the sympathetic division of the autonomic nervous system; the condition occurs as a result of stimulation of the bladder, large intestine, or other visceral organs (Figure 54-25). The clinical signs include severe bradycardia, hypertension (systolic blood pressure up to 300 mm Hg),

Table 54-9 Functional Level of Spinal Cord Injury and Rehabilitation Potential

LEVEL OF INJURY	MOVEMENT REMAINING	REHABILITATION POTENTIAL
TETRAPLEGIA		
C1-C3		
Often fatal injury, vagus nerve domination of heart, respiration, blood vessels, and all organs below injury	Movement in neck and above, loss of innervation to diaphragm, absence of independent respiratory function	Ability to drive electric wheelchair equipped with portable ventilator by using chin control or mouth stick, headrest to stabilize head; computer use with mouth stick, head wand, or noise control; 24-hour attendant care, able to instruct others
C4		
Vagus nerve domination of heart, respirations, and all vessels and organs below injury	Sensation and movement in neck and above; may be able to breathe without a ventilator	Same as C1-C3
C5		
Vagus nerve domination of heart, respirations, and all vessels and organs below injury	Full neck, partial shoulder, back, biceps; gross elbow, inability to roll over or use hands; decreased respiratory reserve	Ability to drive electric wheelchair with mobile hand supports; indoor mobility in manual wheelchair; able to feed self with setup and adaptive equipment; attendant care 10 hr/day
C6		
Vagus nerve domination of heart, respirations, and all vessels and organs below injury	Shoulder and upper back abduction and rotation at shoulder, full biceps to elbow flexion, wrist extension, weak grasp of thumb, decreased respiratory reserve	Ability to assist with transfer and perform some self-care; feed self with hand devices; push wheelchair on smooth, flat surface; drive adapted van from wheelchair; independent computer use with adaptive equipment; attendant care 6 hr/day
C7-C8		
Vagus nerve domination of heart, respirations, and all vessels and organs below injury	All triceps to elbow extension, finger extensors and flexors, good grasp with some decreased strength, decreased respiratory reserve	Ability to transfer self to wheelchair; roll over and sit up in bed; push self on most surfaces; perform most self-care; independent use of wheelchair; ability to drive car with powered hand controls (in some patients); attendant care 0-6 hr/day
PARAPLEGIA		
T1-T6		
Sympathetic innervation to heart, vagus nerve domination of all vessels and organs below injury	Full innervation of upper extremities, back, essential intrinsic muscles of hand; full strength and dexterity of grasp; decreased trunk stability, decreased respiratory reserve	Full independence in self-care and in wheelchair; ability to drive car with hand controls (in most patients); independent standing in standing frame
T6-T12		
Vagus nerve domination only of leg vessels, GI and genitourinary organs	Full, stable thoracic muscles and upper back; functional intercostals, resulting in increased respiratory reserve	Full independent use of wheelchair; ability to stand erect with full leg brace, ambulate on crutches with swing (although gait difficult); inability to climb stairs
L1-L2		
Vagus nerve domination of leg vessels	Varying control of legs and pelvis, instability of lower back	Good sitting balance; full use of wheelchair; ambulation with long leg braces
L3-L4		
Partial vagus nerve domination of leg vessels, GI and genitourinary organs	Quadriceps and hip flexors, absence of hamstring function, flail ankles	Completely independent ambulation with short leg braces and canes; inability to stand for long periods

From Lewis, S.L., et al. (2007). *Medical-surgical nursing: assessment and management of clinical problems.* (7th ed.). St. Louis: Mosby.
GI, Gastrointestinal.

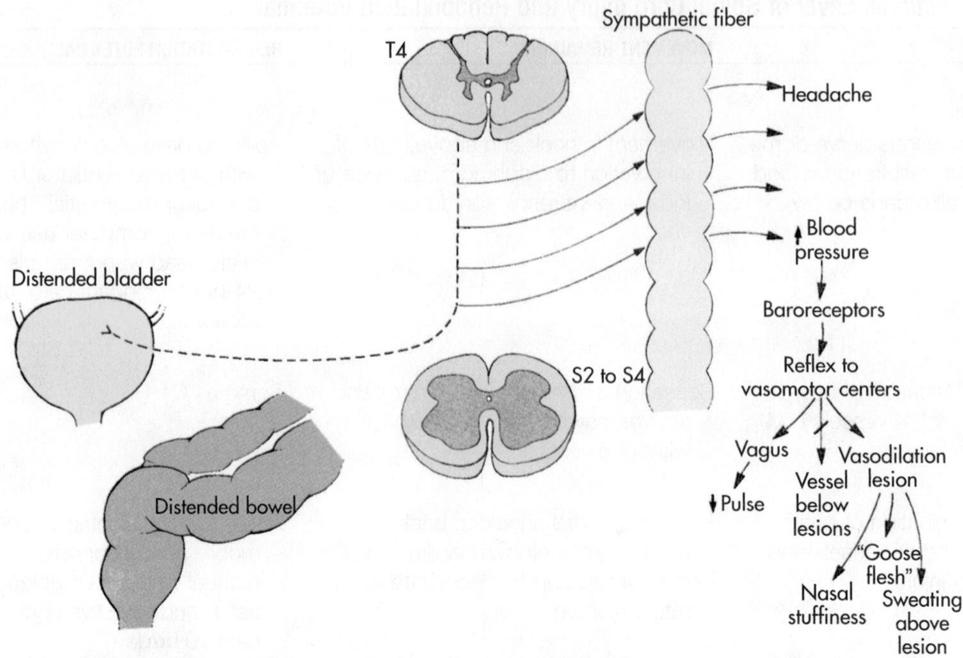

FIGURE 54-25 Pictorial diagram of cause of autonomic hyperreflexia (dysreflexia) and results.

diaphoresis, "goose flesh," flushing (above the level of the lesion), dilated pupils, blurred vision, restlessness, nausea, severe headache, and nasal stuffiness. Patients tend to develop individual signs and symptoms of this condition and are soon able to recognize them. The most common causes of this condition include a distended bladder or a fecal impaction. It is a medical emergency that requires immediate treatment to prevent a stroke, blindness, or death (Box 54-4).

In most cases of spinal cord injury, men experience impotence, decreased sensation, and difficulties with ejaculation. Impaired fertility is common. The experience of orgasm is described as different than before the injury. Women with spinal cord injury are able to continue to perform sexually, although perception of sexual pleasure is usually altered.

Box 54-4 Emergency Care for Autonomic Dysreflexia or Hyperreflexia

- Unless contraindicated, place patient in sitting position to decrease blood pressure.
- Check patency of catheter for kinking. If catheter is occluded, insert new catheter immediately.
- Check rectum for impaction.
- If it is necessary to remove impaction, use an anesthetic ointment.
- Administer ganglionic blocking agent such as hexamethonium or a vasodilator such as nitroprusside (Nipride) as ordered if conservative measures are not effective.
- Continue monitoring blood pressure.
- Send urine for culture if no other cause is found; urinary tract infection can lead to symptoms of autonomic dysreflexia.

Assessment

Subjective data include information about the nature of the injury, any dyspnea, and unusual sensations. The presence of pain, any loss of consciousness, and the absence of sensation on sensory examination are important to assess.

Objective data include the level of alertness and consciousness; orientation; pupil size and reactivity; motor strength; skin integrity; and bowel and bladder status, including distention. Assess for other injuries, such as fractured bones or head injury.

Diagnostic Tests

Radiographs are often taken first to detect any cervical vertebra fracture or displacement. A spinal tap or myelogram may also be done to detect occlusion. A CT scan and MRI may help rule out spinal cord injury.

Medical Management

Immediate care after spinal cord injury is directed toward realignment of the bony column in the presence of fractures or dislocations. This may involve simple immobilization, skeletal traction, or surgery for spinal decompression. Skeletal traction may include Crutchfield tongs (Figure 54-26), halo traction (see Chapter 44), or a Stryker or Foster frame. Bracing may be used for thoracic or lumbar injuries. Often surgical decompression is not performed until after a period of skeletal traction if the injury involves the cervical region. In patients seen within 8 hours of injury, high-dose methylprednisolone is given.

Nursing Interventions and Patient Teaching

Throughout all stages of hospitalization of the patient with a spinal cord injury, nursing and medical interventions are directed toward restoring structural or body

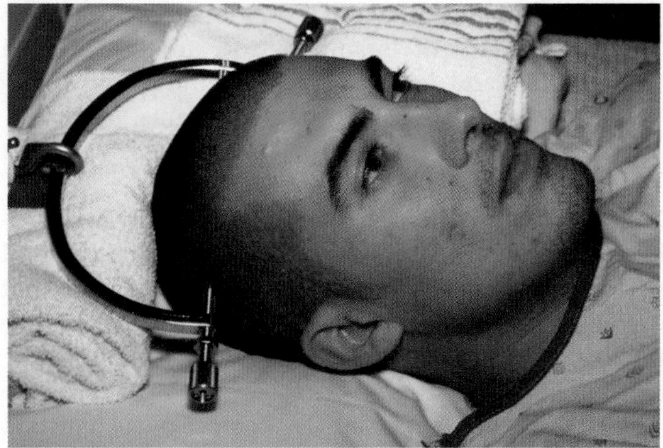

FIGURE 54-26 Patient with Crutchfield tongs inserted into skull to hyperextend.

integrity. All efforts are taken to ensure that the skin is intact, that contractures do not develop, and that ROM is maintained. Early mobilization is important. When patients, especially those with tetraplegia, begin to sit up, it may be necessary to wrap the legs with thromboembolism stockings to encourage venous return. Slowly increasing the angle of sitting up is essential to prevent hypotension. A recliner wheelchair is usually necessary.

Usually a Foley catheter is inserted initially; later bladder training is started (see Chapter 50). Chronic indwelling catheterization increases the risk of infection. Intermittent catheterization should begin as early as possible. This helps maintain bladder tone and decreases the risk of infection. Encourage fluid intake of more than 2000 mL/day. Encourage cranberry juice to decrease renal calculi formation.

Patients are usually started on a bowel program early in their hospital stay. At first, bisacodyl suppositories are given at regular intervals (usually every other night). This is followed by digital stimulation to promote peristalsis. The goal is to eliminate the need for suppositories. Other aids to bowel programs are the use of adequate fluids (usually at least 3000 to 4000 mL/day, unless contraindicated), stool softeners, and prune juice.

Nursing diagnoses and interventions for the patient with a spinal cord injury are the same as those for the patient with a motor or sensory problem, with the addition of but not limited to the following:

Nursing Diagnoses	Nursing Interventions
Autonomic dysreflexia, related to neurophysiologic trauma to spinal cord above sixth thoracic vertebra	See Box 54-4 for emergency interventions.
Impaired urinary elimination, related to sensory-motor impairment	Check carefully for voiding and for distention of bladder. Teach patient intermittent self-catheterization if indicated. Teach patient Crede's maneuver as indicated. Use Foley catheter if indicated; administer meticulous aseptic technique in changing catheters. Teach patients signs of infection. Encourage patient to have a genitourinary checkup at least yearly. Maintain fluid intake of 3000 to 4000 mL/day unless contraindicated. Use adult perineal protector for incontinency, if necessary.

Teaching of the patient with a spinal cord injury includes education about autonomic dysreflexia and about sexual functioning after spinal cord injury. Other teaching points are found in the sections of this chapter dealing with the patient with motor or sensory problems.

Prognosis

In cases of a complete spinal cord injury, there is almost no chance of return of any function. However, the paraplegic or tetraplegic patient can live a satisfying life with adaptations and assistance. Today, with improved treatment strategies (specifically, intermittent catheterization), even the very young patient with a spinal cord injury can anticipate a long life. The prognosis for life is generally only about 5 years less than for people of the same age without spinal cord injury. Take care to prevent infections, such as urinary tract or respiratory tract infections. With patients with incomplete cord lesions, the amount of function regained is variable and often unpredictable.

NURSING *PROCESS for the Patient with a Neurologic Disorder*

The role of the licensed practical nurse/licensed vocational nurse (LPN/LVN) in the nursing process as stated is that the LPN/LVN will:

- Participate in planning care for patients based on patient needs
- Review patient's plan of care and recommend revisions as needed
- Review and follow defined prioritization for patient care
- Use clinical pathways, care maps, or care plans to guide and review patient care

Assessment

People with neurologic deficits require skilled assessment by both a nurse and a physician. Assessment includes observing the patient during the patient history. Nursing assessment is an ongoing process and should be tailored to meet the patient's needs. For example, hourly neurologic checks will not be as detailed as the initial assessment.

While interviewing the patient, obtain data about subjective complaints, such as pain, dizziness, or vision difficulties. Also assess the ability to speak and reason. Observations may also include vital signs, data about gait, symmetry of body parts, evidence of pain, or seizure activity. During ongoing assessments, data are usually obtained about pupil size, level of alertness, ability to perform motor tasks, changes in LOC, and ability to speak. Because subtle changes in neurologic status can often be the first sign of a complication, be alert for small changes in the neurologic assessment and report these to the proper person.

Nursing Diagnosis

Nursing assessment helps identify the patient's needs for care and observation. The actual care of the patient is then based on the nursing diagnoses that have been identified. Possible nursing diagnoses for a patient with a neurologic disorder include but are not limited to the following:

- Autonomic dysreflexia
- Impaired verbal communication
- Compromised family coping
- Risk for disuse syndrome
- Risk for falls
- Grieving
- Risk for infection
- Deficient knowledge
- Impaired memory
- Impaired physical mobility
- Imbalanced nutrition: less than body requirement
- Acute pain
- Chronic pain
- Bathing/hygiene self-care deficit
- Feeding self-care deficit
- Toileting self-care deficit
- Impaired swallowing
- Acute confusion
- Ineffective tissue perfusion (cerebral)

Expected Outcomes and Planning

The plan for providing neurologic assessment and care should focus on the type of deficit the patient is experiencing and possible complications. Consider a patient's preferences and mental status. The type of care required determines the supplies and equipment needed. Schedule necessary care around tests and procedures and the patient's need for rest.

The care plan focuses on achieving specific goals and outcomes that relate to the identified nursing diagnosis. Examples of these include the following:

Goal 1: Patient's cerebral perfusion will be maintained.

Outcome: Patient remains awake, alert, and oriented; coma scale score remains the same or improves.

Goal 2: Patient will maintain optimal nutrition.

Outcome: Patient maintains or attains optimal weight, and laboratory values indicating nutritional health are within normal limits.

Implementation

Nursing interventions for the patient with a neurologic disorder include those that maintain cerebral perfusion and other functioning, as well as those that prevent complications such as decubitus, falls, or contractures. Certain principles guide nurses in providing neurologic care:

- The neurologic system is a complex system that produces a wide variety of neurologic signs and symptoms.
- Identical disorders may result in different sets of signs and symptoms in different patients.
- The maintenance of cerebral perfusion is of utmost importance.
- The patient with a neurologic illness is prone to complications.
- Disorders of the nervous system produce physical problems and a wide variety of cognitive difficulties.

While providing care to meet the patient's specific challenges, also assess the patient's readiness to learn. At times the family must receive the primary teaching because the patient is unable to understand. Consider the patient's preferences and background in delivering care. Encourage the patient to be as independent as possible and give appropriate feedback. Preserve the patient's dignity and privacy whenever possible. Also consider the special needs of older patients (see Life Span Considerations box, p. 1892).

Evaluation

Evaluate the success of planned interventions during and after care is given. The process is ongoing and dynamic because the patient's condition often changes. Always be ready to revise the care plan as needed. For example, if a patient has new episodes of confusion after surgery, notify the physician, increase safety measures, and assess more frequently.

Ongoing systematic evaluation requires determining whether specific outcomes have been met. The evaluation is specific to measure the goals identified. Examples of goals and their corresponding evaluative measures include the following:

Goal 1: Patient will be free of infection.

Evaluative measure: Assess patient for any signs of infection such as increased temperature, frequency of urination, erythematous incision, elevated white blood cell count, or confusion.

Goal 2: Patient will remain clear and oriented in thought processes.

Evaluative measure: Ask patient to respond to orientation questions. Observe ability to engage in conversation and to carry out care activities.

Get Ready for the NCLEX® Examination!

Key Points

- The nervous system is the body's link with the environment. It allows the interpretation of information and appropriate action.
- The two main structural divisions of the nervous system are the CNS and the peripheral nervous system.
- The CNS is composed of the brain and the spinal cord.
- The peripheral nervous system is composed of the nerve cells lying outside of the CNS. It is divided into the somatic nervous system and the autonomic nervous system.
- A nerve cell is composed of three parts: the dendrite, the cell body, and the axon.
- The brain and the spinal cord are protected by the bony coverings (skull and vertebral column), the CSF, and the three meninges (pia mater, arachnoid, and dura mater).
- The cerebrum is the largest part of the brain and contains five major areas: motor, sensory, visual, speech, and auditory. The cerebrum governs the ability to reason and make judgments.
- The diencephalon lies beneath the cerebrum and contains the thalamus and hypothalamus. The thalamus serves as a relay station. The hypothalamus has several roles, such as temperature control, water balance, and appetite.
- The cerebellum is the second largest portion of the brain and is responsible for coordination of skeletal muscles and maintenance of balance and equilibrium.
- The peripheral nervous system is composed of the cranial nerves, the spinal nerves, the somatic nervous system and the autonomic nervous system.
- The autonomic nervous system contains two subdivisions: the sympathetic nervous system and the parasympathetic nervous system. The sympathetic nervous system speeds things up, and the parasympathetic nervous system slows things down.
- Normal changes of aging are not the same as senility, AD, or organic brain damage.
- The source of any headache should be determined through neurologic testing because it may be a symptom of a serious pathologic condition.
- A lumbar puncture should not be done if there is evidence of increased ICP because of the danger of brain herniation.
- Any increase in the volume of one of the contents of the cranium (brain, blood vessels, and CSF) results in increased ICP because the cranial vault is rigid and does not expand.
- Classic signs of increased ICP include restlessness, disorientation, headache, contralateral hemiparesis, an ipsilaterally dilated pupil, and visual changes that include blurring and diplopia.
- Nursing intervention measures can significantly influence ICP.
- Epilepsy is a transitory disturbance in consciousness or in motor, sensory, or autonomic functions with or without loss of consciousness, caused by sudden, excessive, and disorderly electrical discharges of the brain.
- Early signs and symptoms of MS are usually transitory.
- Stroke, or "brain attack," is the most common disease of the nervous system and can be caused by thrombus, embolus, or hemorrhage. The term *brain attack* is used to describe stroke and communicates the urgency of recognizing stroke signs and symptoms and treating their onset as a medical emergency, just as one would with a myocardial infarction.
- The MERCI device can be used for up to 8 hours after acute stroke onset to remove blood clots from arteries deep inside the brain.
- Helpful nursing interventions for the patient with AD include using nonverbal cues or demonstrations as adjuncts to verbal cues, providing few choices, and not hurrying the patient.
- Trigeminal neuralgia (tic douloureux) is characterized by excruciating, burning pain that radiates along one or more of the three divisions of the fifth cranial nerve.
- With Bell's palsy, there is usually an abrupt onset of numbness, a feeling of stiffness, or a drawing sensation of the face.
- Of the people suffering from GBS, 85% regain complete function.
- Approximately 80% of patients with advanced HIV disease (AIDS) have neurologic symptoms that result from infection from HIV itself or from associated complications of the disease.
- Many patients with head injury may recover physically, but they will have behavioral and psychological problems that make it difficult for them to function independently.
- The signs and symptoms of intracranial tumors result from both local and general effects of the tumor.
- Autonomic dysreflexia in the patient with spinal cord injury is a medical emergency that demands quick nursing interventions.
- The first sign of increased ICP may be a declining state of consciousness.
- It is important to document patients' behaviors in terms of what is seen, not what is inferred.
- It is estimated that 1 in 150 people infected with WNV will develop encephalitis or meningitis, a more severe form of the disease.

Additional Learning Resources

Go to your Companion CD for an audio glossary, animations, video clips, and more.

evolve Be sure to visit the Evolve site at http://evolve.elsevier.com/Christensen/adult/ for additional online resources.

Review Questions for the NCLEX® Examination

1. A patient is admitted to the hospital with the diagnosis of transient ischemic attack. What normal change of aging would the nurse expect to see in this 90-year-old man?
   1. Increased sense of touch
   2. Diminished long-term memory
   3. Increased reflex time
   4. Decreased fine motor coordination

2. A 35-year-old patient is being seen for complaints of headache, which she has experienced for the past month. Her physician wants to rule out a brain tumor. In this case, what diagnostic test is contraindicated?
   1. Brain scan
   2. PET scan
   3. Lumbar puncture
   4. Electroencephalography

3. A nurse in the emergency department of her community hospital is teaching a group of sixth graders how to prevent head and spine injuries. Teaching would include all but:
   1. use of helmets for bicycles, motorcycles, and skateboarding.
   2. use of a lumbar support for sports activities.
   3. safe handling and storage of guns.
   4. use of seatbelts and shoulder harnesses in a car.

4. A 70-year-old with back pain is scheduled to have a myelogram in the morning to rule out a pathologic condition of the spine. In preparing him for the procedure, what information is important to share?
   1. His mental status will be assessed frequently.
   2. He may be asked to change positions during the procedure.
   3. He will be able to ambulate immediately after the test.
   4. Strength of the lower extremities will be assessed frequently.

5. The nursing assessment of an 80-year-old who has had a stroke found that she had difficulty swallowing. A videofluoroscopy with barium was performed to rule out aspiration. The rehabilitation team in the skilled nursing facility determined that she can eat a soft diet with one-to-one supervision. Which is important to prevent aspiration?
   1. Tipping the head toward the unaffected side while swallowing
   2. Extending the head during swallowing
   3. Mixing solids and liquids to facilitate swallowing
   4. Encouraging the patient to take large bites to make swallowing easier

6. A 12-year-old student has a history of generalized tonic-clonic seizures. The school nurse educates his classmates about his seizure activity by telling them:
   1. he will be normal immediately after the seizure.
   2. it is important to place a tongue blade in his mouth during the seizure.
   3. his desk should be placed in a corner of the room by himself.
   4. he may cry out at the beginning of a seizure.

7. The patient was involved in a snowmobile accident. On admission to the emergency department, he is receiving oxygen and is intubated. His Glasgow coma scale score is 6. About 10 minutes after arrival, he is noted to have a widened pulse pressure, increased systolic blood pressure, and bradycardia. These signs are considered an important diagnostic sign of late stage increased ICP. Together they are known as:
   1. anisocoria.
   2. supratentorial shift.
   3. Cushing's response.
   4. medullary reflex.

8. A 76-year-old who has had Parkinson's disease for the past 6 years has now been admitted to a nursing home. The nurse doing the admission interview and assessment notices which characteristic sign of the disease?
   1. Bradykinesia
   2. Increased postural reflexes
   3. Sensory loss
   4. Intention tremor

9. A 13-year-old student is admitted to the pediatric unit with possible meningitis. The nurse finds that the patient cannot extend her legs completely without experiencing extreme pain. The nurse knows that this is an indication of meningitis and is called:
   1. Brudzinski's sign.
   2. Battle's sign.
   3. Kernig's sign.
   4. Cosgrow's sign.

10. A patient is diagnosed with Bell's palsy as indicated by a feeling of stiffness and a drawing sensation of the face. What is important to teach her about the disease?
    1. There is a heightened awareness of taste, so foods must be bland.
    2. There may be an increased sensitivity to sound.
    3. The eye is susceptible to injury if the eyelid does not close.
    4. Drooling from increased saliva on the affected side may occur.

11. What is the first nursing intervention for a patient with autonomic dysreflexia?
    1. Sit the patient upright, if permitted.
    2. Check for bowel impaction.
    3. Give medication as ordered.
    4. Place the patient in supine position.

12. When teaching the patient with Parkinson's disease, which response would indicate the need for further education?
    1. "If I miss an occasional dose of the medication, it doesn't matter much."
    2. "I need to exercise at least some every day."

3. "I need to be sitting straight up with my chin slightly tucked so I won't choke when I eat or drink."
4. "I should eat a diet high in fiber and roughage to decrease my constipation."

13. Important nursing interventions for a patient with sensory dysfunction are: *(Select all that apply.)*
    1. teaching the patient protective measures in relation to the sensory deficit.
    2. inspecting parts of the body that have no feeling to ascertain any impairment of skin integrity.
    3. having the patient practice scanning the printed page.
    4. keeping the patient warm with the use of heating pads.

14. When injury to the spinal cord is in the cervical region, the resultant complication would be:
    1. tetraplegia.
    2. hemiplegia.
    3. paraplegia.
    4. paresthesia.

15. The nurse determines that a patient is unconscious when the patient:
    1. has cerebral ischemia.
    2. responds only to painful stimuli.
    3. is unaware of self or environment.
    4. does not respond to verbal stimuli.

16. The nurse plans care for the patient with increased intracranial pressure with the knowledge that the best way to position the patient is to:
    1. keep the head of the bed flat.
    2. maintain the head of the bed at 30 degrees.
    3. increase the head of the bed's angle to 30 degrees with patient on left side.
    4. use a continuous-rotation bed to continuously change patient position.

17. During admission of a patient with a severe head injury to the emergency department, the nurse places the highest priority on assessment for:
    1. patency of airway.
    2. presence of a neck injury.
    3. neurologic status with the Glasgow coma scale.
    4. cerebrospinal fluid leakage from the ears or nose.

18. The primary goal of nursing interventions after a craniotomy is:
    1. preventing infection.
    2. ensuring patient comfort.
    3. avoiding need for secondary surgery.
    4. preventing increased intracranial pressure.

19. A right-handed patient with right-sided hemiplegia and aphasia resulting from a stroke most likely has a lesion in the:
    1. left frontal lobe.
    2. right brainstem.
    3. motor areas of the right cerebrum.
    4. medial superior area of the temporal lobe.

20. A patient experiencing TIAs is scheduled for a carotid endarterectomy. The nurse explains that this procedure is done to:
    1. promote cerebral flow to decrease cerebral edema.
    2. reduce the brain damage that occurs during a stroke-in-evolution.
    3. prevent a stroke by removing atherosclerotic plaques obstructing cerebral blood flow.
    4. provide a circulatory bypass around thrombotic plaques obstructing cranial circulation.

21. A 69-year-old patient has been admitted to the medical floor with a diagnosis of Parkinson's disease. His nursing interventions will include: *(Select all that apply.)*
    1. encouraging activities to increase his speed for doing ADLs.
    2. care during feeding to prevent aspiration.
    3. providing means for disposal of facial tissues.
    4. diet high in fiber and generous fluid intake.

Matching

Column A	Column B
22. _____ MRI	A. Optic disk is edematous "choked disk"
23. _____ Myelography	B. Involuntary rhythmic movement of the eyes; oscillations that are horizontal, vertical, or mixed
24. _____ Babinski's sign	C. Use of magnetic forces to image body structures
25. _____ Nystagmus	D. Backward flexion of the great toe due to an abnormal CNS condition
26. _____ Papilledema	E. Diagnostic procedure done to identify tumors of the spinal cord or herniated nucleus pulposus by observing flow of Amipaque dye

27. Which sign or symptom of late-stage increased intracranial pressure should the LPN/LVN be aware of? *(Select all that apply.)*
    1. Increase in systolic blood pressure
    2. Widening of pulse pressure
    3. Bradycardia
    4. Unequal pupils that react slowly to light
    5. Tachycardia

28. The nursing interventions that would be appropriate and beneficial to a patient who has had a stroke with right-sided hemiplegia and expressive aphasia include: *(Select all that apply.)*
    1. stating questions so that the patient can verbalize freely to articulate his needs.
    2. encouraging self-help, such as bathing.
    3. remaining calm and conversing in an intelligent manner.
    4. performing ROM to all extremities every shift.

29. The nurse is teaching patients with potential aspiration problems airway protective techniques during swallowing. Which procedures should be taught? *(Select all that apply.)*
   1. Chin tuck
   2. Double swallow
   3. Full Fowler's position
   4. Use of a straw
   5. Soft or pureed foods

30. The pathophysiology of myasthenia gravis is caused by:
   1. myelin sheath breakdown.
   2. degeneration of the dopamine-producing neurons in the midbrain.
   3. antibodies attacking the acetylcholine receptors, damaging them, and reducing their number.
   4. inflammation of cranial nerve VII.

31. A graphic recording of the electrical conduction activities of the brain that is a helpful diagnostic tool for a patient with seizures is called:
   1. ECG.
   2. MRI.
   3. PET.
   4. EEG.

32. The condition that involves cranial nerve VII that results in tenderness to the posterior ear, followed by paralysis of the facial muscles unilaterally with ptosis of the eyelid and mouth pulled to the opposite side of the face, is:
   1. trigeminal neuralgia.
   2. Bell's palsy.
   3. Romberg.
   4. proprioception.

33. Two of the more effective therapies that lead to faster recuperation for the patient with Guillain-Barré syndrome are:
   1. Avonex and Betaseron.
   2. thymectomy and Zarontin.
   3. Depakote and Zarontin.
   4. plasmapheresis and intravenous immune globulin.

34. Select patients with acute ischemic stroke can benefit from:
   1. IV Tensilon in the first 3 hours.
   2. anticholinesterase in the first 3 hours.
   3. thrombolytics such as t-PA in the first 3 hours.
   4. intravenous immune globulin in the first 3 hours.

35. The primary goals of the nurse and the family caring for a patient having a seizure include: *(Select all that apply.)*
   1. protection from aspiration.
   2. protection from injury.
   3. recording of seizure activity.
   4. gently restraining to prevent injury.

36. Parkinson's disease is caused by:
   1. myelin sheath pathologic condition.
   2. damage or loss of the dopamine-producing cells of the midbrain, leading to dopamine depletion in the basal ganglia.
   3. depletion of the neurotransmitter acetylcholine resulting in muscular weakness.
   4. presence of atheroma in arterial walls.

37. A nonablative surgical treatment in selected patients with Parkinson's disease in which stimulation wires are placed in the thalamus, globus pallidus, or subthalamic nucleus to improve dyskinesias, rigidity, bradykinesia, tremor, and overall motor function is:
   1. deep brain stimulation.
   2. MERCI retriever.
   3. vagal nerve stimulation.
   4. disconnection surgery.

chapter 55

Care of the Patient with an Immune Disorder

Barbara Lauritsen Christensen

evolve

http://evolve.elsevier.com/Christensen/foundationsadult

Objectives

1. Differentiate between natural and acquired immunity.
2. Compare and contrast humoral and cell-mediated immunity.
3. Explain the concepts of immunocompetence, immunodeficiency, and autoimmunity.
4. Review the mechanisms of immune response.
5. Discuss five factors that influence the development of hypersensitivity.
6. Identify the clinical manifestations of anaphylaxis.
7. Outline the immediate aggressive treatment of systemic anaphylactic reaction.
8. Discuss the two types of latex allergies and recommendations for preventing allergic reactions to latex in the workplace.
9. Discuss selection of blood donors, typing and crossmatching, storage, and administration in preventing transfusion reaction.
10. Explain an immunodeficiency disease.
11. Discuss the cause of autoimmune disorders.
12. Explain plasmapheresis in the treatment of autoimmune diseases.

Key Terms

adaptive immunity (ă-DĂP-tĭv ĭ-MŪ-nĭ-tē, p. 1956)
allergen (ĂL-ĕr-jĕn, p. 1958)
anaphylactic shock (ăn-ĕ-flăk-tĭc, p. 1962)
antigen (ĂN-to-jĕn, p. 1957)
attenuated (ă-TĔN-ū-āt-ĕd, p. 1959)
autoimmune (ăw-tō-ĭ-MŪN, p. 1966)
autologous (ăw-TŎL-ŏ-gĕs, p. 1965)
cellular immunity (SĔL-ū-lĕr ĭ-MŪ-nĭ-tē, p. 1958)
humoral immunity (HŪ-mŏr-ĕl ĭ-MŪ-nĭ-tē, p. 1957)
hypersensitivity (hī-pĕr-sĕn-sĭ-TĬV-ĭ-tē, p. 1960)
immunity (ĭ-MŪ-nĭ-tē, p. 1956)
immunization (ĭm-ū-nĭ-ZĀ-shŭn, p. 1957)
immunocompetence (ĭm-ū-nō-KŎM-pĕ-tĕns, p. 1955)
immunodeficiency (ĭm-ū-nō-dĕ-FĬSH-ĕn-sē, p. 1966)
immunogen (ĭm-Ū-nō-jĕn, p. 1958)
immunology (ĭm-ū-NŎL-ŏ-jē, p. 1956)
immunosuppressive (ĭm-ū-nō-sū-PRĔ-sĭv, p. 1965)
immunotherapy (ĭm-ū-nō-THĔR-ă-pē, p. 1959)
innate immunity (ĭ-NĀT ĭ-MŪ-nĭ-tē, p. 1956)
lymphokine (LĬM-fō-kīn, p. 1957)
plasmapheresis (plăz-mă-fĕ-RĒ-sĭs, p. 1967)
proliferation (prō-lĭf-ĕ-RĀ-shŭn, p. 1957)

NATURE OF IMMUNITY

The human body exists in an environment of antagonistic forces that are constantly attacking and threatening its integrity. In response to these onslaughts, the body exhibits a wide array of adaptations to protect against external and internal harmful agents. This chapter deals with those mechanisms.

The word ***immune*** is derived from the Latin word *immunis,* meaning "free from burden." Immunology is an evolving science that essentially deals with the body's ability to distinguish self from nonself. The body makes this distinction through a complex network of highly specialized cells and tissues that are collectively called the **immune system.** The immune system (also called the **host defense system**) is critical to our survival.

The immune system has three main functions: (1) to protect the body's internal environment against invading microorganisms by destroying foreign antigens and pathogens thus preventing the development of infections (Lewis et al., 2007); (2) to maintain homeostasis by removing damaged cells from the circulation, thereby maintaining the body's various cell types in an unchanged and uniform form (Lewis et al., 2007); and (3) to serve as a surveillance network for recognizing and guarding against the development and growth of abnormal cells. Abnormal cells (mutations) are constantly being formed in the body but are recognized as abnormal cells and are destroyed (Lewis et al., 2007). When the immune system responds appropriately to a foreign stimulus, the body's integrity is maintained; this is called **immunocompetence.**

Immunocompetence is the immune system's ability to mobilize and use its antibodies and other responses to stimulation by an antigen. If the immune response is too weak or too vigorous, homeostasis is disrupted, causing a malfunction in the system. This is called **immunoincompetence.** With disruption of the homeostatic balance of the immune system, a number of diseases develop. Inappropriate immune responses are classified into four categories: (1) hyperactive responses against environmental antigens (e.g., allergy); (2) inability to protect the body, as in immunodeficiency disorders (e.g., acquired immunodeficiency syndrome [AIDS]); (3) failure to recognize the body as self, as in autoimmune disorders (e.g., systemic lupus erythematosus); and (4) attacks on beneficial foreign tissue (e.g., organ transplant rejection or transfusion reaction).

Immunity is the quality of being insusceptible to or unaffected by a particular disease or condition. Immunity has two major subclassifications: innate (natural) and adaptive (acquired) (Figure 55-1). Innate immunity is nonspecific, whereas adaptive immunity is specific. The study of the immune system is **immunology.**

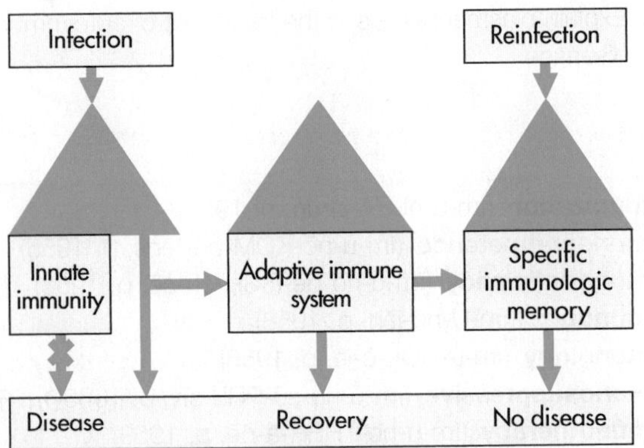

FIGURE 55-1 When an infectious agent enters the body, it first encounters elements of the innate immune system. These may be sufficient to prevent disease; if not, a disease will result and the adaptive immune system is activated. The adaptive immune system helps the patient recover from the disease and establishes a specific immunologic memory. After reinfection with the same agent, no disease results. The individual has acquired immunity to the infectious agent.

INNATE, OR NATURAL, IMMUNITY

The body's first line of defense, **innate immunity,** provides physical and chemical barriers to invading pathogens and protects against the external environment. The innate system is composed of the skin and mucous membranes, cilia, stomach acid, tears, saliva, sebaceous glands, and secretions and flora of the intestine and vagina. These organs, tissues, and secretions provide biochemical and physical barriers to disease. The first line of defense provides nonspecific immunity to the individual (Table 55-1).

ADAPTIVE, OR ACQUIRED, IMMUNITY

If the components of innate or natural immunity fail to prevent invasion or to destroy a foreign pathogen, the adaptive, or acquired, immune response assists in the battle. This is the body's second line of defense against disease. **Adaptive immunity** provides a specific reaction to each invading antigen and has the unique ability to remember the antigen that caused the attack. The adaptive immune system is composed of highly specialized cells and tissues, including the thymus, the spleen, bone marrow, blood, and lymph (Figure 55-2). Adaptive immunity includes both humoral and cell-mediated immunity. The adaptive immune system's specificity (i.e., being specific) results from the production of antibodies in the cells. Antibodies develop naturally after infection or artificially after vaccinations.

The cells of the immune system are the macrophages (any phagocytic cell involved in defense against infection) and the lymphocytes. When organisms pass the epithelial barriers, phagocytes become activated. Phagocytes also migrate through the bloodstream to the tissues for the body's second line of defense against disease. Phagocytes engulf and destroy microorganisms that pass the skin and mucous membrane barri-

Table 55-1 Innate (Natural) and Adaptive (Acquired) Immunity

CHARACTERISTICS	INNATE (NATURAL)	ADAPTIVE (ACQUIRED)
Physical barriers	Physical defense: skin and mucous membranes Mucous membranes line body cavities such as the mouth and stomach. These cavities secrete chemicals (saliva and hydrochloric acid) that destroy bacteria. Cilia, tears, and flora of the intestine and vagina also provide natural protection.	None
Response mechanisms	Nonspecific: Mononuclear phagocytic system; inflammatory response	Specific immune response: Humoral immunity, cellular immunity
Soluble factors	Chemical defense: Lysozyme, complement, acute phase proteins, interferon	Antibodies, lymphokines
Cells	Phagocytes, natural killer (NK) cells	T cells, B cells
Specificity	None	Present
Memory	None	Present

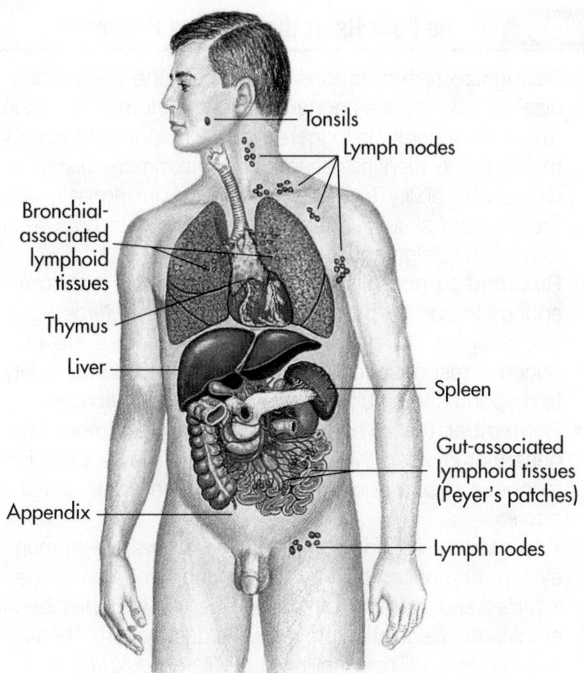

FIGURE 55-2 Organization of the immune system.

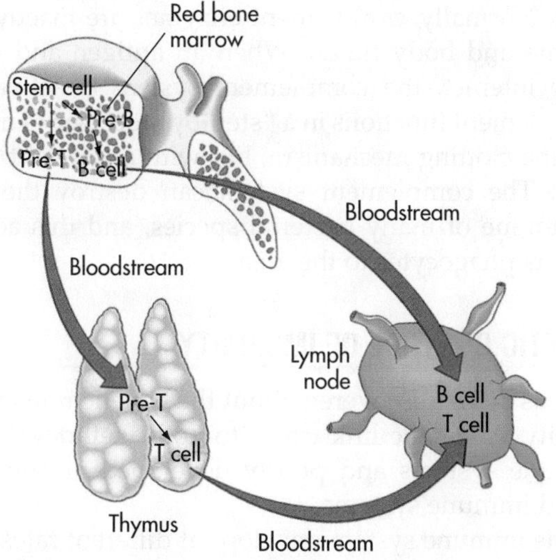

FIGURE 55-3 Origin and processing of B and T cells. B and T cells originate in red bone marrow. B cells are processed in the red marrow, whereas T cells are processed in the thymus. Both cell types circulate to other lymph tissues. B cells produce antibodies to destroy specific foreign antigens (humoral immunity). T cells attack and destroy antigens (cell-mediated immunity).

ers. These cells also assist in the immune response by carrying antigens to the lymphocytes.

Lymphocytes include the T and B cells (Figure 55-3) and the large, granular lymphocytes also known as **natural killer,** or NK, cells. Approximately 70% to 80% of the lymphocytes are T-cell lymphocytes. When activated, T cells release a substance called lymphokine. **Lymphokine** attracts macrophages to the site of infection or inflammation and prepares them for attack. T cells cooperate with the B cells to produce antibodies but do not produce antibodies themselves. T cells are responsible for cell-mediated immunity and protect the body against viruses, fungi, and parasites. T cells also provide protection in allografts (transfer of tissue between two genetically dissimilar individuals of the same species) and against malignant cells.

B cells make up approximately 20% to 30% of the lymphocyte population. B cells trigger the production of antibodies and proliferate (increase in number) in response to a particular **antigen** (a substance recognized by the body as foreign that can trigger an immune response). An antigen is usually a protein that causes the formation of an antibody and reacts specifically with that antibody. B cells migrate to the peripheral circulation and tissues and eventually are filtered from the lymph and stored in the lymphoid tissue of the body.

The initial formation of B cells does not require antigen stimulation or any other environmental stimulus. However, B-cell **proliferation** (reproduction or multiplication of similar forms) depends on antigen stimulation. B cells are responsible for humoral immunity. B cells produce antibodies and protect against bacteria, viruses, and soluble antigens.

HUMORAL IMMUNITY

Humoral immunity (one of the two forms of immunity that respond to antigens, such as bacteria and foreign tissue) is mediated by the B cells. B cells produce antibodies in response to antigen challenge. On first exposure to a given antigen, a primary humoral response is initiated. This response is generally slow compared with subsequent antigen exposures. When a second exposure occurs, memory B cells cause a quick response, regardless of whether the first exposure was to an antigen or to immunization. **Immunization** is a process by which resistance to an infectious disease is induced or increased.

Antigen is presented to the T-helper cell population by the macrophages. T lymphocytes can be categorized into T-helper (CD_4) and T-suppressor (CD_8) cells. An antigen is taken to the B cells and, assisted by T-helper cells, the B cells initiate production of antibodies. T-suppressor cells maintain the humoral response at a level appropriate for the stimulus.

Antibodies produced by one's own body are said to provide active immunity. An example of active immunity is a person who has been vaccinated against rubeola (red measles). In contrast, temporary, or passive, immunity is provided by antibodies that are formed by one person in response to a specific antigen and administered to another person. An example of passive immunity is hepatitis B immune globulin administered after exposure to hepatitis B virus in a nonimmune person.

Even though humoral immunity is mediated by the B-cell population, T-helper cells and T-suppressor cells are vital to the immunocompetent person. **Immunocompetence** is the ability of an immune system to mobilize and deploy its antibodies and other responses to stimulation by an antigen. Both the number and functions of the helper and T-suppressor cells help determine the strength and persistence of an immune response. The normal ratio of T-helper cells to T-suppressor cells in the body is 2:1. When this ratio is disrupted, autoimmune and immunodeficient diseases occur. Factors that may weaken immunocompetence include the aging process, viruses, radiation, and chemotherapeutic drugs (*Mosby's Dictionary of medicine, nursing, and health professions*, 2009).

Exposure to antigen and response with antibody may activate either (1) the humoral complement (one of the 25 complex enzyme serum proteins) system, which results in breakdown of the bacteria and release of lysosomes to destroy bacteria; or (2) the antigen-antibody reaction, which results in mast cells releasing histamine, which produces the symptoms of allergy. When symptoms of allergy occur, antigen is referred to as **allergen** (a substance that can produce a hypersensitive reaction in the body but may not be inherently harmful). When immunity results, antigen is referred to as **immunogen** (any agent or substance capable of provoking an immune response or producing immunity).

CELLULAR IMMUNITY

Cellular immunity, also called **cell-mediated immunity** (the mechanism of acquired immunity characterized by the dominant role of small T cells), results when T cells are activated by an antigen. Whole cells become sensitized in a process similar to that which stimulates the B cells to form antibodies. Once these T cells have been sensitized, they are released into the blood and body tissues, where they remain indefinitely. On contact with the antigen to which they are sensitized, they attach to the organism and destroy it. Cellular immunity is involved in resistance to infectious diseases caused by viruses and some bacteria.

Cellular immunity is of primary importance in (1) immunity against pathogens that survive inside cells, including viruses and some bacteria (e.g., *Mycobacterium* organisms); (2) fungal infections; (3) rejection of transplanted tissues; (4) contact hypersensitivity reactions; (5) tumor immunity; and (6) certain autoimmune diseases (Box 55-1).

Hypersensitivity reactions are cell-mediated responses of the body (Box 55-2).

Box 55-1 The Four Rs of the Immune Response

- **Recognize** self from nonself: Normally the body recognizes its own cells as nonantigenic; therefore an immune response generally is triggered only in response to agents that the body identifies as foreign. Autoimmune disorders disrupt the ability to differentiate self from nonself, and the immune system attacks the body's own cells as if they were foreign antigens.
- **Respond** to nonself invaders: The immune system responds in part by producing antibodies that target specific antigens for destruction. New antibodies are produced in response to new antigens. Deficits in the ability to respond can result in immunodeficiency disorders.
- **Remember** the invader: The ability to remember antigens that invaded the body in the past allows a quicker response if subsequent invasion by the same antigen occurs.
- **Regulate** its action: Self-regulation allows the immune system to monitor itself by "turning on" when an antigen invades and "turning off" when the invasion has been eradicated. Regulation prevents the destruction of healthy or host tissue. The inability to regulate could result in a chronic inflammation and damage to the host tissue.

COMPLEMENT SYSTEM

The word ***complement*** became part of the terminology of immunology at the turn of the nineteenth century, when researchers recognized that blood plasma contained a substance necessary to complete the destruction of bacteria. The complement system includes approximately 25 serum enzymatic proteins that interact with one another and with other components of the innate (natural) and adaptive (acquired) immune systems. Normally, complement enzymes are inactive in plasma and body fluids. When an antigen and antibody interact, the complement system is activated. Complement functions in a "step-by-step" series much like the clotting mechanism, but with a different purpose. The complement system can destroy the cell membrane of many bacterial species, and this action attracts phagocytes to the area.

GENETIC CONTROL OF IMMUNITY

More is being discovered about the genetic role in immunity. A genetic link exists to both well-developed immune systems and poorly developed or compromised immune systems.

The immune system develops at different rates and at different times in fetal and early life. Bone marrow serves as an important mechanism of producing stem cells and all the other cells involved in the immune response.

EFFECTS OF NORMAL AGING ON THE IMMUNE SYSTEM

With advancing age, there is a decline in the immune system. The primary clinical evidence for this immunosenescence is the high incidence of tumors in older adults. Older adults are also more susceptible to infections (such as influenza and pneumonia) from pathogens that they were relatively immunocompetent against earlier in life.

Aging does not affect all aspects of the immune system. The bone marrow is relatively unaffected by increasing age. However, aging has a pronounced ef-

Box 55-2 Review of the Mechanisms of Immune Response

- The skin and mucous membranes are natural barriers to infectious agents. When these barriers are crossed, the immune response begins in the immunocompetent host.
- The first time an antigen enters the body, the antigen is processed by macrophages and presented to lymphocytes. Responses of B cells to the antigen in humoral immunity require interaction with T-helper cells, which assist B cells in responding to the antigen by proliferating, synthesizing, and secreting the appropriate antibody. Antigens are then neutralized by antibodies or can form immune complexes or be phagocytosed by macrophages or neutrophils.
- Humoral immunity responds to antigens such as bacteria and foreign tissue. Humoral immunity is the result of the development and continuing presence of circulating antibodies in the plasma. Humoral immunity consists of antibody-mediated immunity. *Humoral* means body fluid, and antibodies are proteins found in plasma. Therefore the term *humoral immunity* is used.
- Cellular immunity is the primary defense against intracellular organisms, including viruses and some bacteria (e.g., mycobacteria).
- In cellular immunity the antigen is processed by macrophages and recognized by T cells. T cells produce lymphokines, which further attract macrophages and neutrophils to the site for phagocytosis, or cytotoxic killer T cells can respond directly.
- Immunodeficiency is an abnormal condition of the immune system in which cellular or humoral immunity is inadequate and resistance to infection is decreased. The immunodeficiency diseases are sometimes classified as B-cell (antibody) deficiencies, T-cell (cellular) deficiencies, and combined T- and B-cell deficiencies.
- Hypersensitivity reaction is an inappropriate and excessive response of the immune system to a sensitizing antigen. The antigen stimulant is an allergen. Humoral reactions, mediated by the circulating B lymphocytes, are immediate such as anaphylactic hypersensitivity. Cellular reactions, mediated by the T lymphocytes, are delayed cell-mediated hypersensitivity reactions.

fect on the thymus, which decreases in size and activity. These changes in the thymus are probably a primary cause of immunosenescence. Both T and B cells show deficiencies in activation, transit time through the cell cycle, and subsequent differentiation. However, the most significant alterations seem to involve T cells. As thymic output of T cells diminishes, the differentiation of T cells in peripheral lymphoid structures increases. Consequently, there is an accumulation of memory cells rather than new precursor cells responsive to previously unencountered antigens.

Delayed hypersensitivity response, as determined by skin testing with injected antigens, is frequently decreased or absent in older adults. The clinical consequences of a decline in cell-mediated immunity are evident. Older adults have an increased risk of death from cancer (see Life Span Considerations box).

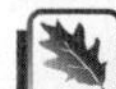

Life Span Considerations

Older Adults

Immune Disorder

- Older adults are at increased risk for inflammation and infections resulting from changes in natural defense mechanisms.
- Pathogens are able to enter through breaks in fragile, dry skin, increasing the risk of skin infections.
- Decreased movement of respiratory secretions increases the risk of respiratory tract infections.
- Decreased production of saliva and gastric secretions increases the risk of gastrointestinal infections.
- Decreased tear production increases the risk of eye inflammation and infections.
- Structural changes in the urinary system that lead to urinary retention or stasis increase the risk of urinary tract infection.
- Signs and symptoms of infection tend to be more subtle than in younger individuals. Because older adults have decreased body temperature, fever may be more difficult to detect. Changes in behavior such as lethargy, fatigue, disorientation, irritability, and loss of appetite may be early signs of infection.
- Immune system functioning declines with advanced age. Research is continuing.
- The older adult's immune system continues to produce antibodies; therefore immunization for diseases such as pneumonia and influenza is recommended.
- Older adults who have chronic illnesses are generally at increased risk for infection.

IMMUNE RESPONSE

There are two ways of helping the body to develop immunity: **immunization** and **immunotherapy.** The theory behind immunization is that controlled exposure to a disease-producing pathogen develops antibodies while preventing disease. The first immunization is credited to Edward Jenner (1796), who observed that individuals who had had cowpox became immune to the disease. The idea of administering "attenuated [weakened] microbes" developed, and the scientific approach was applied by Louis Pasteur. Vaccines and toxoids are altered, or **attenuated** (the process of weakening the virulence of a disease organism), to reduce their power without affecting their ability to stimulate the production of antibodies. After immunization the immune system mounts a greater response to a second encounter with an antigen. The vaccine, or toxoid, stimulates humoral immunity, which provides protection from disease for months to years.

Immunotherapy (a special treatment of allergic responses that administers increasingly large doses of the offending allergens to gradually develop immunity) consists of injecting a person with a very diluted antigen (allergen) to which the patient has a type I hypersensitivity. The strength of the dilution is increased as weekly injections are given over a 1- to 3-year period. The theory is that immunotherapy assists the individual in building tolerance to the allergen without developing fever or increased signs and symptoms. ***Desensitization*** is another term used for immunotherapy. It is indicated for patients with clinically significant disease for whom avoidance of the allergen or treatment with medication is inadequate. It is considered safe in properly selected patients but is a lengthy, expensive process with a potential for severe anaphylaxis.

Immunotherapy may be co-seasonal, preseasonal, or perennial. Perennial therapy is most widely accepted because it allows for a higher cumulative dose, which produces a better effect. Perennial therapy usually begins with 0.05 mL of a 1:10,000 dilution and increases to 0.5 mL in a 6-week period. In the next series the amount given again decreases to 0.05 mL while the dilution lessens to 1:1000. The amount increases each week until a 0.5-mL dose is given. The next cycle begins with a 0.05-mL dose of 1:100 dilution, increasing to 0.5 mL over another 6-week period. Perennial therapy is administered subcutaneously. Observe the patient for at least 20 minutes after administration because a hypersensitivity reaction or anaphylaxis may occur.

The treatment protocol for anaphylaxis with immunotherapy is generally accepted to be 0.2 to 0.5 mL of 1:1000 epinephrine hydrochloride (Adrenalin Chloride) subcutaneously every 20 minutes for three doses.

Most patients begin immunotherapy at the physician's office, and subsequent weekly injections are given until the maintenance level is reached. Home administration by the patient or a family member is acceptable once maintenance level is reached. Interrupted regimens because of illness may place the patient at risk for reaction. Consult the physician before administering a dose of diluted allergen if the patient's maintenance immunotherapy was interrupted by illness or other factors.

DISORDERS OF THE IMMUNE SYSTEM

Immune system failure occurs in several ways and expresses itself in mild to severe form. The system can malfunction at many points while attempting to provide the body with protective defense. It is thought that failures occur because of genetic factors, developmental defects, infection, malignancy, injury, drugs, or altered metabolic states.

The severity of altered immune response disorders ranges from mild to chronic to life threatening. The disorders are categorized as follows:

1. **Hypersensitivity** disorder involves allergic response and tissue rejection.
2. **Immunodeficiency** disease involves altered and failed immune response.
3. **Autoimmune** disease involves extensive tissue damage resulting from an immune system that seemingly reverses its function to one of self-destruction.

See Box 55-1 for the four Rs of the immune response.

HYPERSENSITIVITY DISORDERS

Etiology and Pathophysiology

Hypersensitivity is an abnormal condition characterized by an excessive reaction to a particular stimulus. **Hypersensitivity reaction** is an inappropriate and excessive response of the immune system to a sensitizing antigen. **Hypersensitivity disorders** arise when harmless substances (such as pollens, danders, foods, and chemicals) are recognized as foreign. The body mounts an immune response in much the same way it does to any foreign protein. The result, however, differs. The host becomes sensitive after first exposure and on subsequent exposure exhibits a hypersensitivity reaction. Chronic exposure leads to chronic allergy response, which ranges from mild to incapacitating signs and symptoms.

Hypersensitivity disorders are believed to be caused by a genetic defect that allows increased production of immunoglobulin E (IgE; a humoral antibody) with release of histamine and other mediators from mast cells and basophils. Humoral reactions, mediated by the circulating B lymphocytes, are immediate. Cellular reactions, mediated by the T lymphocytes, are delayed hypersensitivity reactions. Exposure to antigen may occur by inhalation, ingestion, injection, or touch (contact). Signs and symptoms caused by histamine release include vasodilation, edema, bronchoconstriction, mucus secretion, and pruritus. Reaction may be local (gastrointestinal, skin, respiratory, conjunctival) or systemic (anaphylaxis). The exact mechanism and pathway of these inflammatory responses are not clearly understood.

A combination of interrelated factors occurs that increases the severity of symptoms (Box 55-3). The disorders that result from hypersensitivity, which are discussed in other chapters, are urticaria, angioedema, allergic rhinitis, allergic conjunctivitis (hay fever), atopic dermatitis, and asthma. Approximately 40% of all cases of asthma are related to an allergic response (Global Institute of Asthma, 2004).

Assessment

Assessment should involve predominantly the integumentary, gastrointestinal, respiratory, and cardiovascular systems. Be aware of the seasonal nature of the complaints.

Subjective data include pruritus, nausea, and uneasiness.

Box 55-3 Factors Influencing Hypersensitivity

- **Host response to allergen:** The more sensitive the individual, the greater the allergic response is.
- **Exposure amount:** Generally, the more allergen the individual is exposed to, the greater the chance of severe reaction is.
- **Nature of the allergen:** Most allergic reactions are precipitated by complex, high-molecular–weight protein substances.
- **Route of allergen entry:** Most allergens enter the body via gastrointestinal and respiratory routes. Injections of venoms and medications hold a more severe threat of allergic response.
- **Repeated exposure:** Generally, the more the individual is exposed, the greater the response is.

Objective data include sneezing, excessive nasal secretions, lacrimation, inflamed nasal membranes, skin rash or areas of raised inflammation, diarrhea, cough, wheezes, impaired breathing, and hypotension.

Hypersensitivity illnesses are diagnosed largely through patient history and physical examination. The most important diagnostic tool is a detailed history, listing (1) onset, nature, and progression of signs and symptoms; (2) aggravating and alleviating factors; and (3) frequency and duration of signs and symptoms. Assess environmental, household, and occupational factors. Common offenders include pollens, spores, dusts, food, drugs, and insect venoms. Many but not all offenders are seasonal. Signs and symptoms generally vary from mild upper respiratory tract manifestations, such as sneezing and excessive nasal secretions, to watery, itching eyes. Skin signs and symptoms are often eczema-like or urticarial (hives). Diarrhea may be a gastrointestinal complaint in some individuals. More severe signs and symptoms include those of the lower respiratory tract, such as coughing, wheezing, chest discomfort, breathing difficulties, and shock, which could be followed by cardiovascular collapse and respiratory arrest. The complete history assists in an accurate diagnosis (see Health Promotion box).

The physical examination should include a thorough assessment of the skin, the middle ear, the conjunctiva, the nasooropharynx, and the lungs.

Diagnostic Tests

Laboratory studies are usually not necessary unless allergic signs and symptoms are severe and protracted. A complete blood count (with differential to identify the type of white blood cells that are elevated), skin testing, total serum IgE levels, and a specific IgE level for a particular allergen may be ordered. The latter test is called radioallergosorbent test (RAST).

 **Health Promotion**

Assessing the Patient with Allergies

- Obtain a comprehensive history that covers family allergies, past and present allergies, and social and environmental factors, especially the physical environment.
- Identify the allergens that may have triggered a reaction.
- Determine the time of year that an allergic reaction occurs as a clue to a seasonal allergen.
- Obtain information about any over-the-counter or prescription medications used to treat allergies.
- In addition to identification of the allergen, find out about the clinical manifestations and course of allergic reaction.
- Ask about pets, trees, and plants on the property; air pollutants; and floor coverings, houseplants, and cooling and heating systems in the home and workplace.
- Have the patient keep a daily or weekly food diary with a description of any untoward reactions.
- Screen for any reaction to medication.
- Review questions about the patient's lifestyle and stress level in connection with allergic symptoms.

Medical Management

Treatment of hypersensitivity disorders includes (1) symptom management with medications, (2) environmental control, and (3) immunotherapy.

The most effective treatment is environmental control, which includes avoidance of the offending allergen. Pollens are seasonal and can be avoided at season peaks with air conditioning and limited time spent outdoors. Mold spores can be reduced by maintaining dry conditions and using air filters. House dust can be controlled by damp dusting, use of air filters, and decreased use of carpet and overstuffed furniture. Most other offending allergens (food, drugs, chemicals, and stinging insects) can simply be avoided.

Medications are used to treat and alleviate signs and symptoms. Antihistamines compete with histamine by attaching to the cell surface receptors and blocking histamine release. Antihistamines therefore must be initiated soon after exposure or taken on a regular basis. Drowsiness, mucous membrane dryness, and occasionally central nervous system excitation are side effects of the earlier antihistamines. Examples of these include pseudoephedrine (Actifed), diphenhydramine (Benadryl) chlorpheniramine (Chlor-Trimeton), and brompheniramine (Brovex). Nonsedating antihistamines include cetirizine (Zyrtec), loratadine (Claritin), and fexofenadine (Allegra). The nonsedating antihistamines are more desirable for those who experience drowsiness with antihistamine use (Table 55-2).

Leukotriene inhibitors are agents that significantly reduce symptoms of an allergic reaction caused by the release of leukotrienes from mast cells and basophils. Three are currently available in the United States: montelukast (Singulair) and zafirlukast (Accolate) act

Table 55-2 Medications for Immune Disorders

Generic (Trade)	Action	Side Effects	Nursing Implications
Diphenhydramine (Benadryl)	Antihistamine	Drowsiness, confusion, nasal stuffiness, dry mouth, photosensitivity, urine retention	Use cautiously with central nervous system depressants, including alcohol; give with food; it is a safe hypnotic for older adults; tell patient to avoid driving or hazardous activity due to drowsiness.
Loratadine (Claritin)	Nonsedating antihistamine	Slight sedation (more common with increased doses)	Store in tight container at room temperature. Teach patient and family to avoid driving or other hazardous activities if drowsiness occurs.
Fexofenadine (Allegra)	Nonsedating antihistamine	Headache, drowsiness, blurred vision, hypotension, bradycardia, tachycardia, dysrhythmias (rare), urinary retention, pancytopenia	
Dexamethasone (Decadron)	Corticosteroid		Do not use for extended period; use cautiously with patients with diabetes or peptic ulcers.
Flunisolide (AeroBid)	Corticosteroid (inhaled)	Headache, transient nasal burning, epistaxis, nausea, vomiting	Not effective for acute episodes; use regularly; teach care and cleaning of inhaler; if symptoms do not improve in 3 weeks, consult physician.
Epinephrine (Adrenalin Chloride, Sus-Phrine, EpiPen)	Bronchodilator	Nervousness, tremor, headache, hypertension, tachycardia, ventricular fibrillation, stroke	Do not use with monoamine oxidase inhibitor; use cautiously in patients with hyperthyroidism, hypertension, diabetes, and heart disease.

as leukotriene-receptor blockers, and zileuton (Zyflo) inhibits the production of leukotrienes.

Nursing Diagnoses

Nursing diagnoses for patients with hypersensitivity include (1) *risk for injury,* related to exposure to allergen; (2) *activity intolerance,* related to malaise; and (3) *risk for infection,* related to inflammation of protective mucous membranes.

Patient Teaching

Patient teaching should revolve around the specific diagnosis. Advise the patient with seasonal allergies to avoid offending allergens, and ensure he or she understands the therapeutic medication plan. Focus on health promotion and health teaching for self-care management (see Safety Alert box).

Safety Alert!

Treating the Patient with a Hypersensitivity Reaction

- List all of a patient's allergies on the chart, the nursing care plan, and the medication record.
- After an allergic disorder is diagnosed, therapeutic treatment is aimed at reducing exposure to the offending allergen; treating the symptoms; and, if necessary, desensitizing the person through immunotherapy.
- All health care workers must be prepared for the rare but life-threatening anaphylactic reaction, which requires immediate medical and nursing interventions.
- Instruct the patient to wear a medical-alert bracelet listing the particular drug allergy.
- For a patient allergic to insect stings, commercial bee sting kits contain epinephrine and a tourniquet. Teach the patient to apply the tourniquet and self-inject the subcutaneous epinephrine. The patient should wear a medical-alert bracelet and carry a bee sting kit whenever going outdoors.

ANAPHYLAXIS

Etiology and Pathophysiology

The most severe IgE-mediated allergic reaction is anaphylaxis, or systemic reaction to allergens. **Anaphylaxis,** or anaphylactic shock, is an acute and potentially fatal hypersensitivity (allergic) reaction to an allergen (Lewis et al., 2007). The allergens causing anaphylaxis include (1) venoms; (2) drugs, such as penicillin and aspirin; (3) contrast media dyes; (4) insect stings (such as bees and wasps); (5) foods such as eggs, shellfish, and peanuts; (6) latex; and (7) vaccines.

The hypersensitivity reaction results in a sudden severe vasodilation as a consequence of the release of certain chemical mediators from mast cells. The vasodilation causes an increase in capillary permeability, which causes fluid to seep from the vascular space into the interstitial space (Lewis et al., 2007).

Clinical Manifestations

In anaphylaxis the reaction occurs rapidly after exposure, from seconds to a few minutes. A massive release of mediators initiates events in target organs throughout the body. Skin and gastrointestinal signs and symptoms may occur, although respiratory and cardiovascular signs and symptoms predominate. Fatal reactions are associated with a fall in blood pressure, laryngeal edema, and bronchospasm, leading to cardiovascular collapse, myocardial infarction, and respiratory failure. Anaphylactic reactions are classified as mild, moderate, and severe.

Assessment

Early recognition of signs and symptoms and early treatment may prevent severe reactions and even death. Generally, the more rapid the onset, the more severe the outcome is. The patient may have a feeling of uneasiness that increases to a sense of foreboding and then a fear of impending death. The skin may or may not be involved. Urticaria, pruritus, and angioedema may be present in mild and moderate anaphylaxis, whereas cyanosis and pallor may be seen in severe reactions. Upper respiratory signs and symptoms range from congestion and sneezing to edema of the lips, the tongue, and the larynx with stridor and occlusion of the upper airways. Lower respiratory signs and symptoms occur soon thereafter and include bronchospasm, wheezing, and severe dyspnea. Gastrointestinal signs and symptoms increase from nausea, vomiting, and diarrhea to dysphagia and involuntary stools. The patient may have cardiovascular signs and symptoms, such as tachycardia and hypotension. Signs and symptoms may worsen, and the patient may display coronary insufficiency, vascular collapse, dysrhythmias, shock, cardiac arrest, respiratory failure, and death.

Medical Management

Immediate aggressive treatment is the goal in anaphylaxis. At the first sign, 0.2 to 0.5 mL of epinephrine 1:1000 is given subcutaneously for mild symptoms. It may be repeated at 20-minute intervals as prescribed by the physician. Epinephrine produces bronchodilation and vasoconstriction and inhibits the further release of chemical mediators of hypersensitivity reactions from mast cells. The effects of epinephrine take only a few minutes (Lewis et al., 2007). Epinephrine 1:10,000, 0.5 mL IV at 5- to 10-minute intervals, may be administered for severe reaction as prescribed by the physician. Diphenhydramine 50 to 100 mg may be given intramuscularly or intravenously as indicated for allergic signs and symptoms. If moderate to severe signs and symptoms occur, IV therapy with volume expanders and vasopressor agents such as dopamine (Intropin) may be initiated to prevent vascular collapse, and the patient may be intubated to prevent airway obstruction. Oxygen may be administered by nonrebreather mask. Intubation or a tracheostomy may be required for oxygen delivery if progressive hypoxia exists. Place the patient in a recumbent position and elevate the legs. Keep the patient warm.

Nursing Interventions and Patient Teaching

Nursing interventions begin with assessing respiratory status, including dyspnea, wheezing, and decreased breath sounds. Also assess circulatory status, including dysrhythmias, tachycardia, and hypotension. Monitor vital signs continually. Other assessments include (1) intake and output (I&O); (2) mental status, including anxiety, malaise, confusion, and coma; (3) skin status, including erythema, urticaria, cyanosis, and pallor; and (4) gastrointestinal status, including nausea, vomiting, diarrhea, and incontinence.

The diagnosis is most often made by a history of signs and symptoms. Looking at and listening to the anxious patient should be leading clues in suspecting anaphylaxis. Question the patient about recent exposure to known antigens that cause anaphylaxis (Box 55-4). Most laboratory studies are not beneficial.

Box 55-4 Common Allergens Causing Anaphylaxis

DRUGS	VENOMS	FOODS
Vaccines	Honeybees	Milk
Allergen extracts	Wasps	Peanuts
Enzymes	Hornets	Brazil nuts
Penicillins		Cashew nuts
Sulfonamides		Shellfish
Cephalosporins		Egg albumin
Dextrans		Strawberries
Hormones		Chocolate
Contrast media		
Anesthetic agents		

Nursing diagnoses and interventions for the patient with anaphylaxis include but are not limited to the following:

Nursing Diagnoses	Nursing Interventions
Ineffective breathing pattern, related to: • edema • bronchospasm • increased secretions	Maintain airway. Administer high-flow oxygen via nonrebreather mask. Endotracheal intubation or a tracheostomy will be established for oxygen delivery if progressive hypoxia exists. Administer prescribed medications. Keep the patient warm. Monitor vital signs. Suction if necessary. Anticipate intubation with severe respiratory distress.
Decreased cardiac output, related to: • increased capillary permeability • vascular dilation	Monitor IV fluid infusions as ordered. Monitor vital signs. Monitor I&O. Obtain complete allergy history. Document signs and symptoms, interventions, and response.

Reassure the patient during procedures. After the event, teach the patient about avoidance of the allergen, advise him or her to wear or carry medical-alert identification, and teach the patient to prepare and administer epinephrine subcutaneously.

Prognosis
If the signs and symptoms are left untreated, anaphylaxis can lead to death in a relatively short time.

LATEX ALLERGIES
Allergies to latex products have become an increasing problem, affecting patients and health care professionals. The increase in allergic reactions has coincided with the sharp increase in glove use after the introduction of universal precautions against infectious diseases in 1987. It is estimated that 8% to 17% of health care workers regularly exposed to latex are sensitized. The more frequent and prolonged the exposure, the greater likelihood of developing a latex allergy. In addition to gloves, latex-containing products used in health care include blood pressure cuffs, stethoscopes, tourniquets, IV tubing, syringes, electrode pads, oxygen masks, tracheal tubes, colostomy and ileostomy pouches, urinary catheters, anesthetic masks, and adhesive tape.

Latex proteins can become aerosolized through powder on gloves and can result in serious reactions when inhaled by sensitized individuals; therefore all health care agencies are advised to use powder-free gloves. Certain food proteins are similar to some proteins in rubber; therefore an allergic reaction to latex may also result in an allergic reaction to some foods. Bananas, avocados, kiwi, tomatoes, water chestnuts, peaches, grapes, and apricots are the most common foods to result in an allergy if one is allergic to latex (Lewis et al., 2007).

Types of Latex Allergies
Two types of latex allergies that can occur are **type IV allergic contact dermatitis** and **type I allergic reactions.** Type IV contact dermatitis is caused by the *chemicals used in the manufacturing process of latex gloves.* It is a delayed reaction that occurs within 6 to 48 hours. Typically the person first has dryness, pruritus, fissuring, and cracking of the skin, followed by erythema, edema, and crusting at 24 to 48 hours. Chronic exposure can lead to thickening and hardening of the skin, scaling, and hyperpigmentation. The dermatitis may extend beyond the area of physical contact with the allergen.

A type I allergic reaction is a response to the *natural rubber latex proteins* and occurs within minutes of contact with the proteins. These types of allergic reactions can range from skin erythema, urticaria, rhinitis, conjuctivitis, or asthma to full-blown anaphylactic shock. Systemic reactions to latex may result from exposure to protein via various routes, including the skin, mucous membranes, inhalation, or blood.

Nursing Interventions
The identification of patients and health care workers sensitive to latex is crucial in preventing adverse reactions. Collect a thorough health history and history of any allergies, especially for patients with any complaints of latex contact symptoms. However, not all latex-sensitive individuals can be identified, even with a thorough history. Risk factors include long-term exposure to latex products (e.g., health care personnel, individuals who have had multiple surgeries, rubber industry workers) and a history of hay fever, asthma, and allergies to certain foods (e.g., avocados, guava, kiwi, bananas, water chestnuts, hazelnuts, tomatoes, potatoes, peaches, grapes, apricots, peanuts).

The National Institute for Occupational Safety and Health (NIOSH) has published recommendations for preventing allergic reactions to latex in the workplace.* In summary, they include the following:

- Use nonlatex gloves for activities that are not likely to involve contact with infectious materials (e.g., food preparation, housekeeping).
- Use powder-free gloves with reduced protein content.

*U.S. Department of Health and Human Services, National Institute for Occupational Safety and Health. (1997). *Preventing allergic reactions to natural rubber latex in the workplace.* US DHHS/NIOSH Pub. No. 97-135.

- Do not use oil-based hand creams or lotions when wearing gloves.
- After removing gloves, wash hands with mild soap and dry thoroughly.
- Frequently clean work areas that are contaminated with latex-containing dust.
- Know the signs and symptoms of latex allergy, including skin rash; hives; flushing; itching; nasal, eye, or sinus symptoms; asthma; and shock.
- If symptoms of latex allergy develop, avoid direct contact with latex gloves and products.
- People who have a latex allergy should wear a medical-alert bracelet and carry an epinephrine pen.

Use latex precaution protocols for patients identified as having a positive latex allergy test or a history of signs and symptoms related to latex exposure. Many health care facilities have created latex-free product carts that can be used for patients with latex allergies (Lewis et al., 2007).

TRANSFUSION REACTIONS

Transfusion reactions are a hypersensitivity disorder, best illustrated by reactions that occur with mismatched blood. Preventing transfusion reaction requires careful selection of blood donors, followed by careful typing and crossmatching of blood from donor to recipient. Storage of blood and administration protocol are critical. Refrigerate blood and blood components at specific temperatures until a half hour before administration. Administer blood within 4 hours of removal from refrigeration, and blood components within 6 hours. Donor and recipient numbers are specific and must be thoroughly checked and the patient identified with an armband. Administer all blood and blood products through microaggregate filters. Monitor for adverse effects.

Transfusion reactions are labeled mild, moderate, and severe. The most severe reactions occur within the first 15 minutes, moderate reactions occur within 30 to 90 minutes, and mild reactions may be delayed to late in the transfusion or hours to several days after transfusion.

Mild transfusion reaction signs and symptoms include dermatitis, diarrhea, fever, chills, urticaria, cough, and orthopnea. Treatment includes (1) stopping the transfusion; and (2) administering saline, steroids, and diuretics as ordered. Transfusion may continue at a slower rate. In moderate reactions—in which fever, chills, urticaria, and wheezing occur after the first 30 minutes of administration—stop the transfusion and continue with saline. Antihistamines and epinephrine may be given. The physician decides whether to continue the transfusion. With severe reaction stop the transfusion and give saline to provide venous access. Return the blood or blood product and tubing to the laboratory for immediate testing if any type of reaction occurs. Further nursing responsibilities after a blood transfusion reaction include (1) following hospital protocol for collecting required blood and urine specimens to assess for hemolysis, (2) filling out a transfusion reaction record, and (3) documenting the transfusion reaction on the appropriate form on the patient's chart (Lewis et al., 2007).

The best method for preventing transfusion reaction is **autologous** (pertaining to a tissue occurring naturally and derived from the same individual) transfusion, or use of one's own blood, for replacement therapy. The blood can be frozen and stored for as long as 3 years. Usually the blood is stored without being frozen and is given to the person within a few weeks of donation.

DELAYED HYPERSENSITIVITY

Delayed hypersensitivity reactions occurring 24 to 72 hours after exposure are mediated by T cells accompanied by release of lymphokines. Delayed reaction contact dermatitis, such as after contact with poison ivy, is one example. Tissue transplant rejection, another example, is discussed here.

Transplant Rejection

Transfer of healthy tissue or organs from a donor to a recipient has been done for many years. The immune process that protects the body from foreign protein is the same process at work in tissue transplant rejection. Knowledge of the function of the immune system enabled medical experts to find a way to control the rejection process. Now the body is prepared before tissue transplant to decrease the chances of rejection.

Autograft, or transplantation of tissue from one site to another on an individual, is successful. It is used after trauma, especially on full-thickness burns, and in reconstructive surgery. **Isograft** is transfer of tissue between genetically identical individuals (e.g., identical twins). **Allograft** is transplantation of tissue between members of the same species. Because few humans are born with an identical sibling, allograft is the most common form of tissue transplant.

Antigenic determinants on the cells lead to graft rejection via the immune process. Therefore antigenic determinants in recipient tissue and donor tissue are matched as closely as possible before transplantation. Tissue matching leads to a better chance of success.

Tissue rejection does not occur immediately after transplantation. It takes several days for vascularization to occur. Seven to 10 days after blood supply is adequately established, sensitized lymphocytes appear in sufficient numbers for sloughing to occur at the site.

Graft rejection is slowed through use of chemical agents that interfere with the immune response. Included are corticosteroids, cyclosporine (Neoral, Sandimmune), and azathioprine (Imuran). This is referred to as **immunosuppressive** therapy (the administration of agents that significantly interfere with the immune system's ability to respond to antigenic stimulation by inhibiting cellular and humoral immunity).

Infection is a threat to the immunosuppressed patient. Meticulous aseptic technique is required when caring for these individuals. Prophylactic antibiotic therapy may be advisable, and good skin care is necessary. Limit the frequency of bedside visits for both staff and family. Do not allow people with infection near the patient.

IMMUNODEFICIENCY DISORDERS

The first evidence of immunodeficiency (an abnormal condition of the immune system in which cellular or humoral immunity is inadequate and resistance to infection is decreased) disease is an increased susceptibility to infection. The problem can manifest as recurrent or chronic infection. Unusually severe infection with complications or incomplete clearing of an infection may also indicate an underlying immunodeficiency.

Defects in genes leading to immunodeficiency provide a hereditary link to the diseases. Many diseases are believed to be associated with immunodeficiency. These diseases include AIDS, agammaglobulinemia, and multiple myeloma, which are discussed elsewhere in the text.

When the immune system does not adequately protect the body, an immunodeficient state exists. The immunodeficiency disorders involve an impairment of one or more immune mechanisms: (1) phagocytosis, (2) humoral response, (3) cell-mediated response, (4) complement, and (5) a combined humoral and cell-mediated deficiency. Immunodeficiency disorders are primary if the immune cells are improperly developed or absent, and secondary if the deficiency is caused by illnesses or treatment. Primary immunodeficiency disorders are rare and often serious, whereas secondary disorders are more common and may be less severe.

PRIMARY IMMUNODEFICIENCY DISORDERS

The basic categories of primary immunodeficiency disorders include (1) phagocytic defects, (2) B-cell deficiency, (3) T-cell deficiency, and (4) a combined B-cell and T-cell deficiency.

SECONDARY IMMUNODEFICIENCY DISORDERS

Drug-induced immunosuppression is the most common type of secondary immunodeficiency disorder. Immunosuppressive therapy is prescribed for patients to treat a wide variety of chronic diseases, including inflammatory, allergic, hematologic, neoplastic, and autoimmune disorders. Immunosuppressive therapy is also used to prevent rejection of a transplanted organ. Some of these immunosuppressive drugs are cyclosporine, mycophenolate mofetil (CellCept), and azathioprine. Immunosuppression is also a serious side effect of cytotoxic drugs used in cancer chemotherapy. Generalized leukopenia often results, leading to a decreased humoral and cell-mediated response. Therefore secondary infections are common in immunosuppressed patients.

Stress may alter the immune response. This effect involves interrelationships between the nervous, endocrine, and immune systems.

A hypofunctional immune system exists in young children and older adults. Immunoglobulin levels decrease with age and therefore lead to a suppressed humoral immune response in older adults. Thymic involution occurs with aging, along with decreased numbers of T cells. The incidence of malignancies and autoimmune diseases increases with aging and may be related to immunologic deterioration.

Malnutrition also alters cell-mediated immune responses. When protein is deficient over a prolonged period, the thymus gland atrophies and lymphoid tissue decreases. In addition, susceptibility to infections increases.

Radiation destroys lymphocytes either directly or through depletion of stem cells. As the radiation dose is increased, more bone marrow atrophies, leading to severe pancytopenia and severe suppression of immune function.

Surgical removal of lymph nodes, thymus, or spleen can suppress the immune response. Splenectomy in children is especially dangerous and may lead to septicemia from simple respiratory tract infections.

Hodgkin's lymphoma greatly impairs the cell-mediated immune response, and patients may die from severe viral or fungal infections. Viruses, especially rubella, may cause immunodeficiency by direct cytotoxic damage to lymphoid cells. Systemic infections can place such a demand on the immune system that resistance to a secondary or subsequent infection is impaired.

AUTOIMMUNE DISORDERS

Autoimmune disorders entail the development of an immune response (autoantibodies or cellular immune response) to one's own tissues; thus these disorders are failures of the tolerance to "self." Autoimmune disorders may be described as an immune attack on the self and result from the failure to distinguish "self" protein from "foreign" protein.

For some unknown reason, immune cells that are normally unresponsive (tolerant to self-antigens) are activated. Both T cells and B cells can have tolerance to self-antigens. Therefore an alteration in T cells alone or in both B cells and T cells can produce autoantibodies and autosensitized T cells to cause pathophysiologic tissue damage. The particular autoimmune disease depends on which self-antigen is involved.

Autoimmune diseases tend to cluster so that a given person may have more than one (e.g., rheumatoid arthritis and Addison's disease), or the same or related autoimmune diseases may be found in other members of the family. This observation has led to the concept of genetic predisposition to autoimmune disease.

As a person ages, the probability of failure in any system occurs. The pathophysiology of autoimmune responses is not clearly understood. Nevertheless, many illnesses are now believed to be in this classification. Included are pernicious anemia, Guillain-Barré syndrome, scleroderma, Sjögren's syndrome, rheumatic fever, rheumatoid arthritis, ulcerative colitis, male infertility, myasthenia gravis, multiple sclerosis, Addison's disease, autoimmune hemolytic anemia, immune thrombocytopenic purpura, type 1 diabetes mellitus, glomerulonephritis, and systemic lupus erythematosus. These conditions are discussed elsewhere in the text.

PLASMAPHERESIS

Plasmapheresis is the removal of plasma that contains components causing, or thought to cause, disease. When plasma is removed, it is replaced by substitution fluids such as saline or albumin. Therefore the term ***plasma exchange*** more accurately describes this procedure.

Plasmapheresis has been used to treat autoimmune diseases such as systemic lupus erythematosus, glomerulonephritis, myasthenia gravis, thrombocytopenic purpura, rheumatoid arthritis, and Guillain-Barré syndrome. The rationale is to remove pathologic substances present in plasma. Many disorders for which plasmapheresis is being used are characterized by circulating autoantibodies (usually of the immunoglobulin G [IgG] class) and antigen-antibody complexes. Immunosuppressive therapy prevents recovery of IgG production, and plasmapheresis prevents antibody rebound.

In addition to removing antinuclear antibodies (an autoantibody that reacts to nuclear material) and antigen-antibody complexes, plasmapheresis may also remove inflammatory mediators (e.g., complement) that are responsible for tissue damage. In the treatment of systemic lupus erythematosus, plasmapheresis is usually reserved for the patient in an acute attack who is unresponsive to conventional therapy.

Plasmapheresis involves the removal of whole blood through a needle inserted in one arm and circulation of the blood through a cell separator. The separator divides the blood into plasma and its cellular components by centrifugation or membrane filtration. Plasma, platelets, white blood cells, or red blood cells can be separated selectively. The undesirable component is removed, and the remainder is returned to the patient through a needle in the opposite arm. The plasma is generally replaced with normal saline, lactated Ringer's solution, fresh frozen plasma, plasma protein fractions, or albumin. When blood is manually removed, only 500 mL may be taken at one time. However, with the use of apheresis procedures, more than 4 L of plasma can be pheresed in 2 to 3 hours.

As with administration of other blood products, be aware of side effects associated with plasmapheresis. The most common complications are hypotension and citrate toxicity. Hypotension is usually the result of vasovagal reaction or transient volume changes. Citrate is used as an anticoagulant and may cause hypocalcemia, which may manifest as headache, paresthesias, and dizziness. See text for complete coverage of various autoimmune disorders.

Get Ready for the NCLEX® Examination!

Key Points

- The two major forms of immunity are innate (natural) and acquired (adaptive).
- T lymphocytes, B lymphocytes, and macrophages are the three major cells active in acquired immunity.
- B lymphocytes produce antibodies. T lymphocytes do not produce antibodies, but assist the B cell. T lymphocytes release lymphokines.
- Macrophages trap, process, and present antigen to T lymphocytes.
- Autoimmune disorders are failures of the tolerance to "self."
- Plasmapheresis is used to treat autoimmune diseases such as systemic lupus erythematosus, glomerulonephritis, myasthenia gravis, thrombocytopenic purpura, rheumatoid arthritis, and Guillain-Barré syndrome.
- Infection is a primary threat to the immunosuppressed patient. Aseptic technique is required when caring for these patients. Good skin care is necessary.
- Careful selection of blood donors and careful typing and crossmatching of blood are important to prevent transfusion reaction.
- Early recognition of signs followed by early treatment may decrease the severity of allergic reaction.
- The five factors influencing hypersensitivity response are host response to allergen, exposure amount, nature of the allergen, route of allergen entry, and repeated exposure.
- Two types of latex allergies are type IV allergic contact dermatitis and type I allergic reactions. Type IV is caused by the chemicals used in the manufacturing process of latex gloves, whereas type I allergic reaction is a response to the natural rubber latex proteins.

Additional Learning Resources

Go to your Companion CD for an audio glossary, animation, video clips, and more.

evolve Be sure to visit the Evolve site at http://evolve.elsevier.com/Christensen/adult/ for additional online resources.

Review Questions for the NCLEX® Examination

1. Immune disorders that result from failure of the tolerance to "self" responding immunologically to one's own antigens are known as:
   1. immunodeficiency disorders.
   2. hypersensitivity disorders.
   3. desensitization disorders.
   4. autoimmune disorders.

2. A nurse is caring for a patient who had a kidney transplant. What should be included in the care of a patient with a suppressed immune system?
   1. Prophylactic antibiotic therapy
   2. Meticulous aseptic technique
   3. Restriction of all visitors
   4. Antineoplastic medication administration

3. Which statement describes innate, or natural, immunity?
   1. The body's first line of defense against disease, which protects locally against the external environment
   2. The body's second line of defense against disease, which protects the internal environment
   3. Mediated by B cells to produce antibodies in response to antigenic challenge
   4. An immunity that is specific

4. The nurse is caring for a patient with a history of numerous allergies. What is the most important teaching concept?
   1. Immunotherapy regimen
   2. Avoidance of the allergen
   3. Antihistamine administration
   4. Adrenaline administration

5. Humoral immunity is mediated by:
   1. T cells.
   2. B cells.
   3. macrophages.
   4. myeloblasts.

6. Cellular immunity develops when which cells are activated by an antigen?
   1. T cells
   2. B cells
   3. Neutrophils
   4. Monoblasts

7. Desensitization is another term for:
   1. autoimmune disorders.
   2. adaptive immunity.
   3. immunotherapy.
   4. immunodeficiency disease.

8. After a bee sting, the patient's face becomes edematous and she begins to wheeze. Based on this assessment, the nurse would be prepared to administer:
   1. aminophylline.
   2. Benadryl.
   3. epinephrine.
   4. Valium.

9. The nurse gave an intramuscular penicillin injection to a patient. What would be a sign of a systemic anaphylactic response?
   1. Increased blood pressure
   2. Bradycardia
   3. Urticaria
   4. Wheezing

10. A 38-year-old patient is receiving 2 units of packed red blood cells at 125 mL/hr. Fifteen minutes after the start of the blood transfusion, the nurse notes the following vital signs: pulse 110 bpm, respirations 28 breaths/min, blood pressure 98/58 mm Hg, and temperature 101° F. The patient is shivering. The nurse's next action would be to:
    1. slow the infusion rate.
    2. stop the infusion.
    3. administer aspirin as ordered for elevated temperature.
    4. report the findings to the nurse manager.

11. A 72-year-old patient is admitted to the hospital with a diagnosis of immunodeficiency disease. The primary nursing goals would be to:
    1. reduce the risk of the patient developing an infection.
    2. encourage the patient to provide self-care.
    3. plan nutritious meals to provide adequate intake.
    4. encourage the patient to interact with other patients.

12. The patient tells the nurse he is overwhelmed. There is so much he must do to keep his new kidney functioning, and then rejection may still occur. Which nursing diagnosis is appropriate?
    1. Ineffective coping
    2. Disturbed body image
    3. Impaired adjustment
    4. Situational low self-esteem

13. What is the correct nursing intervention for anaphylaxis? *(Select all that apply.)*
    1. Assess vital signs every 4 hours.
    2. Assess respiratory status frequently.
    3. Maintain patent airway.
    4. Administer epinephrine 1:1000, 0.2 to 0.5 mL subQ, as ordered.

14. The patient comes to the clinic for his weekly allergy injection. He missed his appointment the week before because of a family emergency. Which action is appropriate in administering the patient's injection?
    1. Administer the usual dosage of the allergen.
    2. Double the dosage to account for the missed injection the previous week.
    3. Consult with the physician about decreasing the dosage for this injection.
    4. Reevaluate the patient's sensitivity to the allergen with a skin test.

15. The nurse advises a friend who asks him to administer his allergy injections that:

1. it is illegal for nurses to administer injections outside of a medical setting.
2. he is qualified to do it if the friend has epinephrine in an injectable syringe provided with his extract.
3. avoiding the allergens is a more effective way of controlling allergies and allergy shots are not usually effective.
4. immunotherapy should only be administered in a setting where emergency equipment and drugs are available.

16. A patient is undergoing plasmapheresis for treatment of systemic lupus erythematosus. The nurse explains that plasmapheresis is used to:

1. remove T lymphocytes in her blood that are producing antinuclear antibodies.
2. remove normal particles in her blood that are being damaged by autoantibodies.
3. exchange her plasma that contains antinuclear antibodies with a substitute fluid.
4. replace viral-damaged cellular components of her blood with replacement whole blood.

17. Type I allergic reaction to latex is a response to the _________ _________ _________ _________.

18. The most common allergens that cause an anaphylactic reaction include: *(Select all that apply.)*

1. leafy green vegetables.
2. bees, wasps.
3. shellfish.
4. peanuts.

19. Which illness is believed to be an autoimmune disorder? *(Select all that apply.)*

1. Rheumatoid arthritis
2. Lung cancer
3. Systemic lupus erythematosus
4. Guillain-Barré syndrome

chapter

56 Care of the Patient with HIV/AIDS

evolve

http://evolve.elsevier.com/Christensen/foundationsadult

Craig E. Nielsen

Objectives

1. Describe the agent that causes HIV disease.
2. Provide the definition of AIDS given in January 1993 by the Centers for Disease Control and Prevention.
3. Explain the differences between HIV infection, HIV disease, and AIDS.
4. Describe the progression of HIV infection.
5. Discuss how HIV is and is not transmitted.
6. Describe patients who are at risk for HIV infection.
7. Discuss the pathophysiology of HIV disease.
8. List signs and symptoms that may be indicative of HIV disease.
9. Discuss the laboratory and diagnostic tests related to HIV disease.
10. Discuss the issues related to HIV antibody testing.
11. Describe the multidisciplinary approach in caring for a patient with HIV disease.
12. List opportunistic infections associated with advanced HIV disease (AIDS).
13. Discuss the nurse's role in assisting the HIV-infected patient with coping, grieving, reducing anxiety, and minimizing social isolation.
14. Implement a care plan for the patient with AIDS.
15. Discuss the importance of adherence to HIV treatment.
16. Discuss the use of effective prevention messages in counseling patients.
17. Define the nurse's role in the prevention of HIV infection.

Key Terms

acquired immunodeficiency syndrome (AIDS) (ĭm-ū-nō-dĕ-FĬSH-ĕn-sē, p. 1980)
adherence (ăd-HĔR-ĕns, p. 1996)
CD_4^+ lymphocyte (LĬM-fō-sīt, p. 1978)
Centers for Disease Control and Prevention (CDC) (p. 1970)
enzyme-linked immunosorbent assay (ELISA) (ĭm-ū-nō-ZŎR-bĕnt, p. 1983)
HIV disease (p. 1980)
HIV infection (p. 1980)
human immunodeficiency virus (HIV) (p. 1970)
Kaposi's sarcoma (kă-PŌS-sĕz săr-KŌ-mă, p. 1970)
opportunistic (ŏp-pŏr-tū-NĬS-tĭk, p. 1972)
phagocyte (făg-ō-SĬT-ĭk, p. 1980)
***Pneumocystis jiroveci* (formerly *carinii*) pneumonia (PCP)** (nū-mō-SĬS-tĭs kă-RĬN-ē, p. 1970)
retrovirus (rĕ-trō-VĪ-rŭs, p. 1978)
seroconversion (sĕr-ō-kŏn-VĔR-zhŭn, p. 1976)
seronegative (sĕr-ō-NĔG-ă-tĭv, p. 1983)
vertical transmission (p. 1975)
viral load (p. 1975)
virulent (VĬR-ū-lĕnt, p. 1971)
Western blot (p. 1983)

NURSING AND THE HISTORY OF HIV DISEASE

As early as 1979, physicians in New York and California were noting cases of *Pneumocystis jiroveci* (formerly *carinii*) pneumonia (PCP), an unusual pulmonary disease caused by a fungus and primarily associated with people who have suppressed immune systems. These physicians also noted an increase in the number of people with Kaposi's sarcoma, a rare cancer of the skin and mucous membranes characterized by blue, red, or purple raised lesions seen mainly in Mediterranean men. The interesting thing was that these two diseases were occurring at alarming rates in clusters of young homosexual men whose immune systems were failing. Researchers at the Centers for Disease Control and Prevention (CDC), a division of the U.S. Public Health Service in Atlanta that investigates and controls various diseases, soon learned that this immune disorder was also affecting injecting drug users and hemophiliacs. They later learned that it also affected heterosexual men and women.

The origins of human immunodeficiency virus (HIV) remain somewhat obscure, and why HIV gave rise to the acquired immunodeficiency syndrome (AIDS) pandemic only in the twentieth century has not yet been determined. The earliest case of HIV infection has been dated to 1959. It was identified in the Democratic Republic of Congo by using different methods of molecular clock analysis. It has also been estimated that HIV began to radiate from its source around the 1930s (Buonaguro et al., 2007). The escalating pandemic likely resulted from the combination of significant cultural and sociobehavioral changes, the use of nonsterile needles for parenteral injections and vaccinations, and the unintended contamination of products used for medical treatments.

HIV/AIDS has been recognized as a clinical syndrome since the early 1980s. But several researchers have identified patients who might have fit the CDC's Case Surveillance definition before this time. For example, the unusual and rapid death of a 15 year-old black boy from aggressive disseminated Kaposi's sarcoma suggests he might be the first confirmed case of HIV infection in the United States (Garry et al., 1988). This patient from St. Louis had no international travel experience, which suggests that other individuals were HIV infected as well. This also suggests that HIV has existed in some form in the United States since at least the 1960s.

HIV is known as **zoonotic,** an organism that has been able to cross from an animal species to humans. A similar virus was noted in primates (called simian immunodeficiency virus) and likely crossed into humans with the hunting and consumption of these animals in Africa. Other examples of zoonotic transmission include severe acute respiratory distress syndrome, anthrax, and Hantavirus and West Nile virus (World Health Organization [WHO], 2009). HIV began to spread in the middle to late 1970s, but because of the long incubation period, in most countries the viral epidemic progressed undetected. When the virus began causing widespread disease in the 1980s, it provoked fear among laypeople and health care providers alike. It was also an exciting time for health care workers because they knew they were seeing a new pathogen with a route of transmission not completely understood. In spite of the stigmas and fears that emerged (which still exist to some extent today), nurses were at the forefront providing care. Nurses met the challenges of providing and coordinating services, organizing community-based organizations, teaching about prevention, and helping patients deal with a terminal disease.

In June 1981, the CDC published a notation about some patients with signs and symptoms that later would be attributed to AIDS (CDC, 1981). The signs and symptoms listed were related to the development of opportunistic infections (OIs). Since that time, AIDS has become known as one of the most challenging infectious diseases of the twentieth and twenty-first centuries. In 1982, the CDC stated that blood and other body fluids may transmit the disease, and they issued a statement about using precautions with other people's body fluids.

In 1983 French researchers isolated the virus believed to be responsible for AIDS, and they called it lymphadenopathy-associated virus (Barré-Sinoussi et al., 1983). One year later an American scientist claimed the discovery of the etiologic agent and named it the human T-cell lymphotropic virus type III (Gallo et al., 1984). Other researchers discovered viruses that appeared to be the same or close members of the same family. In 1986 the International Committee on Taxonomy of Viruses renamed the virus, calling it the human immunodeficiency virus (HIV). In that same year a second and distinctly different strain of the virus was discovered in West Africa. Researchers believed that this strain may have been present in West Africa for many years. The scientific names assigned to distinguish the two viruses are HIV-1 and HIV-2.

The discovery of a second HIV strain was both major and alarming, since it was the first clue that HIV could change its appearance and mutate rapidly. This capability for rapid mutation, often referred to as genetic promiscuity, has become the trademark of this virus. It represents an immense challenge for scientists as they search for treatment and vaccine strategies. HIV-1 is found worldwide and is the prevalent strain in most places, including the United States, Europe, and Central Africa. HIV-1 and HIV-2 are both spread in the same ways and have similar signs and symptoms. Both of these viral strains also result in OIs. Whereas most HIV-1 infected people develop profound immunodeficiency and high viral loads, resulting in death, most HIV-2 infected people act as long-term nonprogressors (Rowland-Jones & Whittle, 2007). Patients diagnosed with HIV-2 tend to be less infectious during the initial stage of the infection than those diagnosed with HIV-1. As the HIV-2 infection progresses, the patient's ability to infect other people increases. The prevalence rate of HIV-2 is higher in parts of Africa and in the countries surrounding Africa. This is thought to be related to commercial trading relationships and immigration. There are increased reports of cases in the United States of HIV-2, mainly in refugees and immigrants from countries with HIV-2.

HIV-1 is much more virulent (toxic) than HIV-2. People diagnosed with HIV-2 tend to have a normal life span when compared with their uninfected population cohort. Also, in contrast to HIV-1, HIV-2 does not result in higher mortality risks in patients between the ages of 55 and 80 years old (Rowland-Jones & Whittle, 2007). Patients infected with HIV-2 develop problems with immunodeficiency more slowly. However, HIV-2 patients who are malnourished, without adequate access to health care, and without clean water have an increased mortality risk when compared with a healthier HIV-2 infected patient.

Since the first cases of AIDS were reported in 1981, the CDC has revised the case definition three times in response to improved laboratory and diagnostic methods (CD_4^+ and viral test results), additional clinical conditions, increased knowledge of the natural history of HIV disease, and improved clinical management (CDC, 2006). The current definition (Table 56-1), used by all states and U.S. territories, allows the disease to be consistently monitored for public health purposes. Because HIV selectively infects and destroys cells that display

Table 56-1 Diagnostic Criteria for AIDS

1993 CLASSIFICATION SYSTEM FOR HIV INFECTION IN ADOLESCENTS AND ADULTS			
	CLINICAL CATEGORIES		
CD_4^+ CELL CATEGORIES*	A: ASYMPTOMATIC, PGL, ACUTE HIV INFECTION	B: SYMPTOMATIC, NOT (A) OR (C) CONDITIONS	C: AIDS-INDICATOR CONDITIONS
1. ≥500/mm³	A1	B1	C1
2. 200-499/mm³	A2	B2	C2
3. <200/mm³	A3	B3	C3

CLINICAL CATEGORY A CONDITIONS	CLINICAL CATEGORY B CONDITIONS	CLINICAL CATEGORY C CONDITIONS
• Asymptomatic HIV infection • Persistent generalized lymphadenopathy (PGL) • Acute primary HIV illness (acute retroviral or seroconversion illness)	• Bacillary angiomatosis • Candidiasis, oropharyngeal (thrush) • Candidiasis, vulvovaginal; persistent, frequent, or poorly responsive to therapy • Cervical dysplasia (moderate or severe) or cervical carcinoma in situ • Constitutional symptoms, e.g., severe fever (101.3° F [38.5° C]) or diarrhea lasting more than 1 month • Herpes zoster (shingles) involving at least two distinct episodes or more than one dermatome • Idiopathic thrombocytopenic purpura • Listeriosis • Oral hairy leukoplakia • Pelvic inflammatory disease, particularly if complicated by tubo-ovarian abscess • Peripheral neuropathy	• Candidiasis of bronchi, trachea, or lungs • Candidiasis, esophageal • Cervical cancer, invasive • Coccidioidomycosis, disseminated or extrapulmonary • Cryptococcus, extrapulmonary • Cryptosporidiosis, chronic intestinal (>1 month's duration) • Cytomegalovirus (CMV) disease (other than liver, spleen, or nodes) • CMV retinitis • Encephalopathy, HIV related • Herpes simplex; chronic ulcer(s) (>1 month's duration); or bronchitis, pneumonitis, or esophagitis • Histoplasmosis, disseminated or extrapulmonary • Isosporiasis, chronic intestinal (>1 month's duration) • Kaposi's sarcoma • Lymphoma, Burkitt's (or equivalent term) • Lymphoma, primary of brain • *Mycobacterium avium* complex or *Mycobacterium kansasii,* disseminated or extrapulmonary • *Mycobacterium tuberculosis,* any site • *Mycobacterium,* other identified or unidentified species, disseminated or extrapulmonary • *Pneumocystis jiroveci* (formerly *carinii*) pneumonia • Pneumonia, recurrent • Progressive multifocal leukoencephalopathy • Salmonella septicemia, recurrent • Toxoplasmosis of brain • Wasting due to HIV

People with AIDS-indicator conditions (A3, B3, C1, C2, and C3) are currently reportable to local health departments in every state and U.S. territory. The red categories incorporate the AIDS surveillance case definition; these categories are AIDS indicators.
*According to the lowest, most accurate count, not the most recent count.

CD_4^+ molecules on their surface (primarily lymphocytes), the new definition includes all HIV-infected people who have CD_4^+ counts of 200 cells/mm³ or fewer (as opposed to the normal 600 to 1200 cells/mm³). These revisions to the AIDS surveillance case definition took into account the advances in diagnostic methods and treatment to provide more accurate information on the numbers of life-threatening **opportunistic** (caused by normally nonpathogenic organisms in a host whose resistance has been decreased by such disorders as HIV disease) illnesses and deaths among HIV-infected individuals.

It was not until 1987, after the CDC reported three cases of occupationally acquired HIV infection in health care providers, that guidelines called universal blood and body fluid precautions, or standard precautions, were developed for the prevention of occupational exposure. This forever changed the way health care personnel protect themselves and others from the spread of bloodborne pathogens. That same year, the Association of Nurses in AIDS Care was established to address the needs of individuals with HIV disease and to provide a professional forum for nurses, who often faced discrimination for providing care to HIV-infected patients.

By now, a broad spectrum of individuals, including children and adults and people from all socioeconomic groups, is affected by this disorder (see Life Span Considerations box). Nurses have been instrumental in establishing education and treatment standards, in collaboration with community-based organizations. Today, nurses comprise the largest group of health care providers who care for individuals with HIV disease, stressing the importance of prevention and influencing policymakers. HIV nursing has imparted lessons that can be useful in other patient populations as well: the importance of patient education, adherence to medical regimens, prevention, and health-promoting behaviors.

SIGNIFICANCE OF THE PROBLEM

Disease Burden

Throughout the world, HIV is one of the leading causes of death and results in more deaths than any other disease caused by infection. As of 2007, approximately 33.2 million people were infected with HIV. Approximately 2.5 million living with this infection were children, and 2.5 million new diagnoses were made that year—7400 new cases each day. More than 2 million people die every year due to AIDS. Almost all of those people living with HIV reside in countries with low or middle incomes.

Sub-Saharan Africa has been hit especially hard (WHO, 2008). This region contains more than 65% of the world's HIV population and accounts for 76% of the total mortality rate attributed to AIDS (Henry J. Kaiser Family Foundation, 2007). It is estimated that by the year 2010, 18 million children in that region will lose both of their parents to AIDS. Death related to AIDS is largely associated with poor health care access for prevention and treatment services (Henry J. Kaiser Family Foundation, 2007). During the past 2 years the number of people infected with HIV has declined. This decreasing infection rate is thought to be related to increased access to antiretroviral treatments. Managing and treating this disease will remain a challenge for years to come, especially in the sub-Saharan region of Africa.

In the United States approximately 56,000 new cases of HIV are diagnosed each year (Hall et al., 2008). More than 1 million people in the United States are currently living with HIV/AIDS (Henry J. Kaiser Family Foundation, 2007). Between 2003 and 2006, the number of new HIV/AIDS cases in the United States stabilized, while the number of people who were living with the disease increased. At the end of 2006, almost 500,000 people were infected and living with HIV/AIDS (CDC, 2008). California, Florida, and New York accounted for most of the patients with AIDS diagnoses (CDC, 2008).

Life Span Considerations

Older Adults

HIV Disease

- Approximately 7.5% of the total AIDS cases reported through the end of 2006 were people age 55 or older at the time of diagnosis (CDC, 2006). This figure does not include individuals who are HIV positive. Although still a relatively small percentage, the number of individuals in the older adult population with HIV/AIDS is increasing steadily.
- Improved treatments and prophylactic medications are contributing to individuals with HIV disease living longer, making the disease one of a chronic nature.
- A decrease in the immune system's ability to fight infection as efficiently in older adults leads to faster progression of HIV disease and increased complications.

TRENDS AND MOST AFFECTED POPULATIONS

Beginning in 1996 the use of *highly active antiretroviral therapy* (HAART) greatly increased among persons with HIV infection in the United States. Since that time, fewer people have developed AIDS (CDC, 2009a). New HIV and AIDS cases affect varied racial groups, ethnic groups, geographic areas, and demographic populations. This epidemic has affected non-white people, women, heterosexuals, and intravenous drug users. However, people with HIV are living longer (CDC, 2008).

Men who have sex with other men (MSM) comprise the biggest proportion of HIV/AIDS patients, accounting for 71% of the total number of HIV infections in adult and adolescent males (CDC, 2007). The HIV infection rates of MSM decreased from 71% in 1983 to 44% in 1996. A prediction was made that this rate would continue to decrease to approximately 25% (Holmberg, 1996). Instead of decreasing, however, new HIV infections for MSM have stayed about the same. Despite media campaigns to educate MSM about high-risk behaviors, many believe that HIV is now a chronic and treatable disease, and this has led to an increase in high-risk sexual behaviors (Holmberg, 1996).

During the first 25 years of this epidemic, the distribution of new cases based on ethnicity and race changed (see Cultural Considerations box). Hispanics and blacks have been disproportionately infected with HIV. In 2006, although blacks made up only 13% of the population in the United States, they accounted for almost half of the total number of HIV/AIDS cases that were diagnosed. Black adults and adolescents are 10 times more likely to be diagnosed with AIDS than

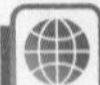

Cultural Considerations

HIV Disease

- Since 1990 the number of Hispanics living in the United States has increased by 58%. This population increase is not the result of immigration, but of increases in fertility because the population is young. Future population growth is taking place in areas with the highest rates of HIV seroprevalence. Hispanics experience a higher seroprevalence rate than whites, and as a result, HIV prevention education is important. Although Hispanics comprise only 13% of the total U.S. population, they represented 19% of the AIDS cases diagnosed in 2006—almost three times that of whites.
- Barriers to prevention include difficulty providing care in a nonthreatening environment where health care providers are viewed as authorities.
- Undocumented residents, including Hispanics, are reluctant to seek HIV care because this condition disqualifies them for U.S. legal residency and they fear deportation. Additionally, nearly 80% of Hispanics are members of the Catholic church, which has historically been opposed to sex outside marriage, men having sex with men, and artificial birth control. These beliefs complicate prevention efforts that stress the use of condoms.
- Because of the deportation threat, recognize that Hispanic-American patients may not share important health information.
- Assessment and interventions should be sensitive to language and cultural differences.
- Provide a safe, supportive environment for assessment and treatment, and advocate for patients who need treatment, regardless of ability to pay for services or residency status.

white adults and adolescents. The primary risk factor for black men who developed HIV is sexual contact. In 2005, black MSM were much more likely to be infected with HIV. Another risk factor is when black men engage in high-risk heterosexual behavior (CDC, 2009a).

Some black men who engage in sex with other men identify themselves as heterosexuals because of the stigma and homophobia issues. Many black MSM are secretive about their homosexuality or choose not to identify their sexual orientation. This phenomenon is known as keeping it on the "down low." Prevention programs are challenged when people do not identify themselves as engaging in risky behaviors or having increased risk factors.

The number of women who have been infected is growing. In 2005 females accounted for 26% of new HIV/AIDS diagnoses, and most of the females were black (CDC, 2007c). HIV was the leading cause of mortality in black women between 25 and 34 years of age. Black women are 23 times more likely to be diagnosed with AIDS than white women. Young people between 15 and 24 years old make up 40% of the new diagnoses (CDC, 2007d). Most people are diagnosed between 25 and 44 years of age. In 2007, an estimated one half of all people infected with HIV/AIDS did not receive appropriate health care, and 25% were not yet diagnosed (Henry J. Kaiser Family Foundation, 2007).

During 2006, Hispanics accounted for almost 20% of the total number of HIV/AIDS cases in the United States (CDC, 2007b). Many socioeconomic and cultural factors have contributed to this epidemic and associated prevention challenges in the U.S. Hispanic and Latino communities. The primary risk factor for developing HIV in Hispanic men and women is sex with men. Hispanics also have higher rates than non-Hispanic whites of other sexually transmitted infections (STIs), including chlamydia, gonorrhea, and syphilis (CDC, 2007b). Transient Hispanic populations often have difficulty receiving access to health care because of social structure, language barriers, and migration patterns (CDC, 2008). The predicaments caused by poverty lead to limited access to appropriate health care, housing, and HIV prevention. All of these factors may directly or indirectly increase risk factors for HIV infection in the Hispanic population.

In 1996 researchers falsely predicted that HIV cases would increase for injecting drug users (Holmberg, 1996). The biggest increase in new HIV cases has occurred in heterosexual populations. In 1983 heterosexuals made up 5% of new HIV cases. In 2006 that number grew to 36% (CDC, 2008). Drugs that are not injected also affect the spread of HIV because drug users often engage in high-risk behaviors when they are under the influence (CDC, 2008).

As treatment for HIV has advanced, the progression from HIV to AIDS has slowed, resulting in a decreased mortality rate for those infected with HIV. Data from 2006 indicates that, although AIDS cases have remained stable, the death rate has decreased (CDC, 2008). Advanced treatment options mean that people are living longer after their AIDS diagnoses. Unfortunately, in countries where HIV-infected people are without adequate access to health care, HIV infection is still one of the leading causes of death.

TRANSMISSION OF HIV

Despite significant research into the modes of transmission of HIV, considerable fear and misinformation about HIV transmission, perhaps more than for any other disease, still exists. It is imperative that health care providers and patients be knowledgeable about modes of transmission and behaviors that put them at risk for HIV infection. Modes of transmission have remained constant throughout the course of the HIV pandemic. Health care providers also need to remember that transmission of HIV occurs through sexual **practices,** not sexual **preferences.**

The patterns in the spread of HIV changed considerably during the first two decades of the epidemic in the United States. Worldwide, sexual intercourse is by far the most common mode of HIV transmission, but in the United States, as many as one half of all new HIV infections are now associated either directly or indirectly with injection drug use—that is, using

HIV-contaminated needles to inject drugs or having sexual contact with an HIV-infected drug user. Overall, compared to the 1980s, HIV infection is spreading fastest in the United States among young people, injecting drug users, women, blacks, and Hispanics. The number of estimated pediatric AIDS cases diagnosed each year has declined since 1992. This decline is associated with the increased compliance with universal counseling and testing of pregnant women and the use of zidovudine (Retrovir, ZDV, AZT) by HIV-infected pregnant women and their newborn infants.

HIV is an **obligate virus,** meaning it must have a host organism to survive. The virus cannot live long outside the human body. HIV transmission depends on the presence of the virus, the infectiousness of the virus, the susceptibility of the uninfected host, and any conditions that may help put the person at risk. HIV is transmitted from human to human through infected blood, semen, cervicovaginal secretions, and breast milk. If these infected fluids are introduced into an uninfected person, the potential for HIV transmission exists. In addition to the aforementioned body fluids, HIV is also found in pericardial, synovial, cerebrospinal, peritoneal, and amniotic fluids. Vertical transmission of HIV, or transmission from a mother to a fetus, can occur during pregnancy, during delivery, or through postpartum breastfeeding (transmitted in the breast milk). Conditions that affect the likelihood of infection include the duration and frequency of exposure, the amount of virus inoculated, the virulence of the organism, and the host's defense capability (immune system). Although HIV has been found in other body fluids such as saliva, urine, tears, and feces, there has been no evidence that these substances are capable of transmission, unless the fluids contain visible blood.

HIV is generally transmitted by **behaviors** and not by casual contacts, such as hugging, dry kissing, shaking hands, or sharing food and utensils. HIV is not transmitted by animals or insects; coughing or sneezing; or sharing objects such as pencils, computer keyboards, or telephones. The three most common modes of HIV transmission are anal or vaginal intercourse, contaminated injecting drug equipment and paraphernalia, and transmission from mother to child.

Once infected, an individual is capable of transmitting HIV to others at any time throughout the disease spectrum, even when the host appears healthy and has no obvious signs of immune destruction. In HIV infection the viral load (amount of measurable HIV virions in the blood) is highest immediately after infection and during the later stages of the disease (Figure 56-1). During these periods, unprotected exposure (through sexual behaviors or blood) to an infected individual increases the likelihood that transmission will occur. However, it is important to remember that HIV can be transmitted during the entire disease spectrum.

SEXUAL TRANSMISSION

Sexual transmission of HIV remains the most common mode of transmission in the world today and is responsible for the majority of the world's total AIDS cases. Sexual activity provides the potential for the exchange of semen, cervicovaginal secretions, and blood. The sexual orientation or sexual practices of an individual are irrelevant in HIV transmission. Factors that are important are the presence of HIV in one or both partners and the occurrence of behaviors that puts one or both partners at risk for transmission. Some individuals become infected with HIV after a single unprotected sexual encounter, whereas others remain free from infection after hundreds of such encounters.

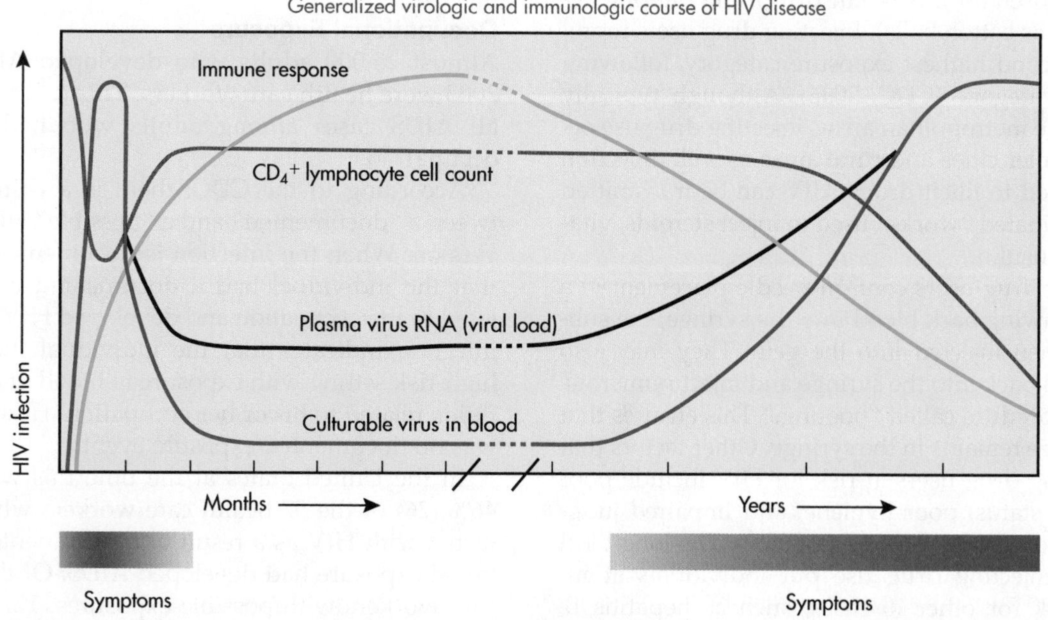

FIGURE 56-1 Viral load in the blood and the relationship to CD_4^+ lymphocyte cell count over the spectrum of HIV disease. *RNA*, Ribonucleic acid.

Although the majority of HIV transmissions in the United States occur in the MSM category via receptive anal intercourse, heterosexual transmission via anal intercourse is becoming increasingly prevalent. Heterosexual couples may prefer this method of sexual expression or use it because it eliminates the risk of pregnancy. Unfortunately, the most risky sexual activity is unprotected receptive anal intercourse. Because the rectum is generally tighter and less well lubricated than the vagina, the rectal mucosa may be torn, providing an excellent portal for the virus to enter the bloodstream.

During any form of sexual intercourse (anal, vaginal, oral), the risk of infection is considerably higher for the receptive partner, although infection can be transmitted to an insertive partner as well. The receptive partner generally has prolonged exposure to semen (National Institute of Allergy and Infectious Diseases, 2006). Other factors that may increase the risk of sexual transmission include ulcerating genital diseases, such as herpes simplex virus (HSV) and syphilis; chancres secondary to STIs; intact (uncircumcised) foreskin; sex that is "rough"; and immunosuppression due to drug use, including the use of nicotine and alcohol. Infection risk for HIV can also be increased during intercourse when the infected partner has a high viral load. An increased viral load is often found in the primary and late stages of infection (Klimas et al., 2008). Oral-genital transmissions have been reported but are considered rare, and experts disagree on whether this constitutes an actual mode of transmission.

PARENTERAL EXPOSURE

Injecting Drug Use

HIV may be transmitted by exposure to contaminated blood through the accidental or intentional sharing of injecting equipment and paraphernalia. Such equipment includes syringes, needles, cookers (spoons or bottle caps used for mixing the drug), and filtering devices (such as cotton balls). Injecting drug users represent the second highest exposure category, following the MSM category (CDC, 2006). Although typically seen in large metropolitan areas, injecting drug use occurs in smaller cities and rural areas as well. Injection is not limited to illicit drugs; HIV can be transmitted via contaminated "works" used to inject steroids, vitamins, and insulin.

Injecting drug users confirm needle placement in a vein by drawing back blood into the syringe; the substance is then injected into the vein. They may also draw blood back into the syringe and inject numerous times, a procedure called "booting." This ensures that no substance remains in the syringe. Other factors that put injecting drug users at risk for HIV include poor nutritional status, poor hygiene, and impaired judgment due to mood-altering substances. The long-term effects of injecting drug use put individuals at increased risk for other diseases, such as hepatitis B, hepatitis C, and other bloodborne illnesses.

Blood and Blood Products

Since 1985, blood banks in the United States have screened all donated blood for HIV-1 antibodies, and since 1992 they have also screened for HIV-2. Blood banks have also implemented procedures to find blood donors who might be at high risk for being infected with HIV. Blood from donors who are deemed high risk or that tests positive for HIV is discarded. In addition to HIV, blood is currently screened for HTLV-1, HTLV-2, hepatitis B virus, syphilis, and hepatitis C virus.

Every year, a small number of blood donations come from donors who are infected with HIV but in whom the HIV antibody was undetected. When a blood donor has not yet undergone **seroconversion** (a change in serologic test results from negative to positive as antibodies develop in reaction to an infection), the current HIV antibody test is unable to detect the infection. In the past there was a 22-day window where the donor could donate HIV-infected blood that would not be detected by the HIV-1 and HIV-2 antibody test. Since 1995, however, blood has also been screened for HIV-1 p24 antigen. With this addition, this window has been reduced to 16 days. In 1999, another test called the nucleic acid amplification test was introduced. This test detects HIV-1 ribonucleic acid (RNA) and has reduced the window again to only 11 days. By 2003, after 25 million donations, only three people were infected with HIV after receiving a blood product transfusion. The blood came from two separate donors, and the blood tested negative for HIV with all currently available HIV tests (Donnegan, 2003).

Before 1985, people who received replacement clotting factors for blood coagulation difficulties had an increased risk of contracting HIV. Since 1985, a recombinant technique is used to manufacture the clotting factors or the clotting factors are treated with chemicals or heated to kill the HIV.

Occupational Exposure

Almost 25,000 adults who developed AIDS before 2003 were health care workers. This represents 5% of all AIDS cases among adults who had a known occupation.

According to the CDC, there is a distinction between a "documented" and a "possible" HIV seroconversion. When the infection is documented, it means that the individual had a documented exposure related to the occupation and developed HIV. A possible infection indicates that the individual worked in a high-risk setting with exposure to blood or other body fluids related to his or her occupation. However, there was no documented exposure event.

In the United States at the time this was written, 46% (26) of the 57 health care workers who were infected with HIV as a result of a documented occupational exposure had developed AIDS. Of those health care workers with possible exposures, 121 of 138 developed AIDS (Sepkowitz & Eisenberg, 2005). Of all health care workers with HIV, most did not have a documented exposure, and the source of their infection is thought to be from high-risk sexual behavior.

Most of the health care workers who have been infected with HIV are nurses. The second largest group is laboratory clinicians, and the third largest group is physicians (nonsurgical). Other health care workers with possible exposures included emergency medical technicians, health care aides, housekeepers, and maintenance workers. Most of the infections occurred after a needlestick injury with resulting puncture wound. There is thought to be some underreporting of exposures because it is voluntary. If a health care worker does have a needlestick resulting in exposure to a known HIV-infected person, the risk for contracting HIV is low, at just about 0.3%.

As of this writing, the last new HIV case involving a possible exposure to an HIV/AIDS patient was in 2000 (CDC, 2007f). Some cases are still being investigated.

Needlesticks that occur when a health care worker is exposed to known HIV-infected persons are known as percutaneous exposure. If the exposure involves a hollow-bore needle filled with blood that is placed in the patient's vein or artery, then the transmission risk of HIV is increased. Also, the transmission risk is increased if the health care worker suffers a deep injury at the time of the exposure. Scalpels, suture needles, and smaller gauge injection needles also pose a risk for transmission, but it is much smaller. If only the mucous membranes are exposed during the incident, then the risk for seroconversion is only 0.09%. There is a small risk for seroconverting if the health care worker's skin is not intact and is exposed to blood or body fluids.

Unfortunately, postexposure antiviral therapy given to health care workers after a documented exposure may result in severe hepatitis that may require a liver transplant. Some health care workers have died after documented or possible exposure to HIV, but that number has not been reported at this time.

PERINATAL (VERTICAL) TRANSMISSION

HIV infection can be transmitted from a mother to her infant during pregnancy, at the time of delivery, or after birth through breastfeeding. In the United States, it is estimated that approximately 30% of infected mothers will transmit HIV to their infants, with approximately 50% to 70% of the transmissions occurring late in utero or intrapartum. For unknown reasons, the rate of vertical transmission varies around the world; the rate in France is around 11%, but it is nearly 50% in parts of Africa. Factors such as the stage of maternal HIV disease (it is more likely to be transmitted during the initial and later stages of infection, when more of the virus is circulating in the mother's blood and body fluids), a decreased CD_4^+ count or high viral load, the presence or absence of STIs, and the mother's nutritional status all play a role in vertical transmission. Factors that increase the risk of transmission during delivery include extreme prematurity; complicated pregnancies leading to extended labor; the mixing of maternal and fetal blood; newborn ingestion of maternal blood, amniotic fluid, or vaginal secretions; skin excoriation in the newborn; and being the first child born in a multiple gestation.

In 1994 the AIDS Clinical Trials Group (ACTG) 076 study demonstrated that a plan of zidovudine therapy started after the 14th week of gestation, given intravenously to the mother during delivery and including zidovudine syrup given to the infant after birth, reduces the risk of HIV transmission by 67% (Perinatal HIV Guidelines Working Group, 2001). The long-term effects of zidovudine or combination therapy are not known, but anecdotal evidence suggests that polydactyly (the congenital presence of more than the normal number of fingers and toes) and ventricular septal defect may be caused by zidovudine. It is difficult to determine whether these defects are caused by in utero exposure to the drug or whether the incidence is the same as in the general population. Children who received zidovudine in the womb and for the first 6 weeks of life are closely monitored by authorities to document any long-term side effects.

In addition to drug therapy, substantial advances have been made in understanding the pathophysiology, treatment, and monitoring of HIV infection. These advances have resulted in changes in the standard of care for individuals, including pregnant women, with HIV infection. More aggressive combination drug regimens that provide maximal viral suppression are now recommended. Although pregnancy alone is not a reason to defer treatment, the use of anti-HIV drugs during pregnancy requires special consideration. Unfortunately, no long-term data regarding the long-term effects on the fetus exist. Because of this, offering antiretroviral therapy (ART) to HIV-infected women—whether to primarily treat HIV infection or to reduce the likelihood of perinatal transmission—should be accompanied by a discussion of the known and unknown short- and long-term benefits and potential risks. Because of the findings of ACTG 076, zidovudine should be a part of this treatment regimen.

An HIV-positive pregnant woman should be given this information to make an informed decision about treatment options. Current recommendations call for routine HIV counseling and voluntary HIV testing of pregnant women and those women considering pregnancy. However, there are no legal requirements that a woman take zidovudine during pregnancy or that she be tested for HIV antibodies.

The HIV transmission rates from mother to child have been reduced due to several recommended interventions. This includes ART, formula feeding, and cesarean section. In developed countries, this number has decreased from 25% (without interventions) to less than 2%. In countries where ART is not available and mothers continue to breastfeed, by age 2 the infection rate for babies born to HIV-infected mothers can be as high as 25%. Infants born to HIV-infected mothers have positive HIV antibody results as long as 15 to 18 months after birth. This is caused by maternal antibodies that cross the placenta during gestation and remain in the infant's circulatory system. An earlier diagnosis of HIV infection can be made by doing an HIV viral culture or by measuring the amount of HIV RNA or viral load through a technique called polymerase chain reaction (PCR) or branched chain DNA testing (bDNA).

PATHOPHYSIOLOGY

HIV is classified as "slow" retrovirus or a lentevirus. After infection with these types of viruses, a long time passes before specific signs and symptoms appear. HIV requires cells for replication. The virus takes over the host cell and reproduces viral copies of itself. Retroviruses are made of RNA. Most organisms' genetic material is made up of deoxyribonucleic acid (DNA). The retrovirus uses an enzyme called reverse transcriptase to make its RNA change to DNA. This process allows the virus to be incorporated into the host's genetic material (Smith & Daniel, 2006).

HIV can cross over into the host at the dendritic immune cells that are located in the mucosal layer of the vulva, the vagina, the rectum, and the penis. The exterior layer of the dendritic cell passes the virus into the interior portion of the cell. The HIV virus is released into the lymphatic system via tissue or lymph nodes. Then the virus binds to a CD_4^+ lymphocyte (a type of white blood cell; a protein on the surface of cells that normally helps the body's immune system combat disease), where it can travel farther into the lymphatic system and begin the initial infectious cycle (Lekkerkerker et al., 2006).

When the viral particle attaches to the host cell's CD_4^+ receptor and coreceptor (CCR5 or CXCR4), this is the first step in replication of the virus (see Figure 56-1). The HIV virion enters the host cell when the virus binds with the cell. After binding to the cell, coreceptors are needed to continue the fusion process and to allow the viral particle to eject two copies of the virus's RNA. Inside the cell, HIV reverse transcriptase changes the viral RNA into DNA. A full copy of this DNA is created and broken down into smaller more functional pieces that are moved to the nucleus of the cell (Smith & Daniel, 2006). The HIV DNA moves into the nucleus of the cell, where viral integrase helps insert it into the DNA of the host. The inserted virus is called a **provirus.** After activation, the cell makes a new copy of HIV by using viral proteins. Afterward, there is an abnormal amount of immune activation, and this perpetuates the progress of the HIV infection because it creates more CD_4^+ cells that will be under attack by HIV and will eventually exhaust the immune system (Potter et al., 2007). The number of CD_8^+ T cells that are activated at this time is directly related to an increased risk of developing advanced HIV infection, or AIDS. However, the HIV can remain dormant for years if the CD_4^+ cell remains inactivated (Potter et al., 2007). It has been difficult to completely control HIV because of its ability to remain undetected. Patients with HIV are advised to continue taking their antiretroviral medications.

New viral proteins are created when the infected CD_4^+ cell converts DNA into RNA. This process is called **transcription.** The process relies on the host cell and the viral genetic material. The new RNA is called messenger RNA (mRNA), and it is returned from the nucleus back into the cytoplasm. In the cytoplasm, mRNA is used as a template to begin making HIV protein. This process is called **translation.** The protein sequence of the mRNA is changed back into RNA, and this makes up the outer envelope and inner core of HIV. After translation the genetic materials become smaller and smaller pieces of viral material. The viral protease chunks the genetic products into smaller pieces so that they can infect more CD_4^+ host cells. This HIV protease is specific to this virus and is targeted by a class of medications called protease inhibitors that is used to manage HIV. The envelope's viral proteins are joined together inside the host cell's membrane, with the core proteins, RNA, and enzymes just inside the membrane.

HIV then "buds" by pinching off this cell (Smith & Daniel, 2006). One infected CD_4^+ cell has the ability to quickly make thousands of cell copies. The CD_4^+ cell dies due to this replication process. As time goes on, so many CD_4^+ cells are destroyed that the immune system becomes dysfunctional and OIs develop within the host.

INFLUENCES ON VIRAL LOAD AND DISEASE PROGRESSION

HIV replicates quickly after entering the host body. It can rapidly produce billions of copies, which infect CD_4^+ cells and the lymphatic system. The viral load of the host during the early stage of the infection can be extremely high and increases transmission risk to others who are exposed. The severity and progression of the infection are related to the host's infection with other STIs, age, and immune response (Fletcher & Klimas, 2007). Basic host immune defenses (cellular and humoral) help limit replication and slow progression of HIV. Unfortunately, these immune responses cannot completely eliminate HIV from the host. The host can remain healthy appearing even when infected with the virus (Table 56-2). Some patients live with the virus for at least 10 years without any treatment and appear healthy. They are referred to as long-term nonprogressors. When HIV patients who were also coinfected with another type of virus took ART, their CD_4^+ count was low (Cheng et al., 2007). When older people do not use ART, their rate of disease progression is much faster than in younger people. It is thought to be related to more pathogen exposure over their life, an increased number of memory CD_4^+ cells (which are tar-

Table 56-2 Types of White Blood Cells and their Involvement in HIV Disease

WHITE BLOOD CELL (WBC) TYPE	DESCRIPTION OF FUNCTION	ROLE IN HIV DISEASE
Neutrophils	Neutrophils normally constitute 50%-75% of all circulating leukocytes and are capable of phagocytosis. Important in the inflammatory response and the first line of defense against infection. Short life span.	Neutropenia (decreased WBC) commonly occurs in advanced HIV disease. Drug-induced neutropenia is common, especially with drugs used to treat PCP, toxoplasmosis, CMV retinitis or colitis, and with NRTI usage.
Monocytes, macrophages	Constitute about 3%-7% of all WBCs. Macrophages are distributed throughout tissue and are capable of phagocytosis. Involved in the inflammatory response. Capable of processing antigens for presentation to T cells. They have CD_4^+ receptors.	Monocytes and macrophages serve as a reservoir for HIV. When activated by stimulation with interferon (inflammatory response), they produce neopterin. Neopterin levels are increased in HIV disease.
Basophils, mast cells	Basophils and mast cells are involved in acute inflammation; breakdown of mast cells releases histamine and other factors.	In HIV infection, may inhibit leukocyte migration.
T-helper cells (CD_4^+ or T_4 cells)	T-helper cells contain CD_4^+ receptors. They are considered the "conductor" of the immune system because of their secretion of cytokines, which control most aspects of the immune response.	Major target of HIV. Progressive infection gradually destroys the available pool of T-helper cells so that the overall CD_4^+ cell count drops. Lower CD_4^+ cell counts correspond with more immunodeficiency and the onset of opportunistic infections. Infection with HIV can impair T-helper cell function without killing the cell.
Cytotoxic T cells or cytotoxic T lymphocytes (CTL, CD_8^+ cell)	Cytotoxic T cells contain CD_8^+ receptors and produce cytokines in a more limited fashion than CD_4^+ cells. They regulate viral and bacterial infections and are involved in direct killing of target cells by binding to them and releasing a substance that can perforate the cell membrane.	Increase in HIV infection. Represent the cellular response to infection. The strength of this initial cellular response has been shown to predict progression to AIDS (i.e., better cell response equals slower disease progression). Cytotoxic T cells kill T-helper cells infected with HIV.
Natural killer (NK) cells	Large granular lymphocytes involved in cell-mediated immune response. Target cells are coated with antibody that binds to receptors on the surface of NK cells, allowing the NK cell to attach to the target cell and kill them. NK cells kill target cells by releasing a substance that triggers lysis (breakdown of cell wall) of cell.	Retain normal counts and normal structure in patients with HIV infection, but they are functionally defective.
B cells	B cells produce antibodies specific to an antigen. They are capable of being stimulated by T-helper cells.	B cells are involved in the humoral response to HIV infection and produce a variety of antibodies against HIV. Present throughout the course of HIV disease.

CMV, Cytomegalovirus; *NRTI,* nucleoside reverse transcriptase inhibitor; *PCP, Pneumocystis jiroveci* (formerly *carinii*) pneumonia.

geted by HIV), and fewer numbers of naïve CD_4^+ cells. Older people tend to have a harder time keeping up with the demand to produce more CD_4^+ cells.

Many factors can increase HIV disease progression. People who use drugs and engage in high-risk sexual behavior are less likely to employ prevention methods. Depression may impair their use of resources to help manage their infection (Kalichman, 2008). Poor coping mechanisms and high levels of emotional stress have a negative impact on HIV disease progression (Ironson & Hayward, 2008; Leserman, 2008; Temoshok et al., 2008).

The virus can make amazing numbers of copies of itself daily (Ho et al., 1995; Wei et al., 1995). HIV contained in the plasma of blood has a half-life of less than 2 days. While the virus continues to replicate, many millions of CD_4^+ cells are produced and destroyed each day. The viral load in the patient's blood determines how quickly the CD_4^+ cells are destroyed.

The HIV viral load in the blood can remain low or difficult to detect for weeks or even months after the initial exposure and infection (Figure 56-2). When the immune system responds, the viral load decreases

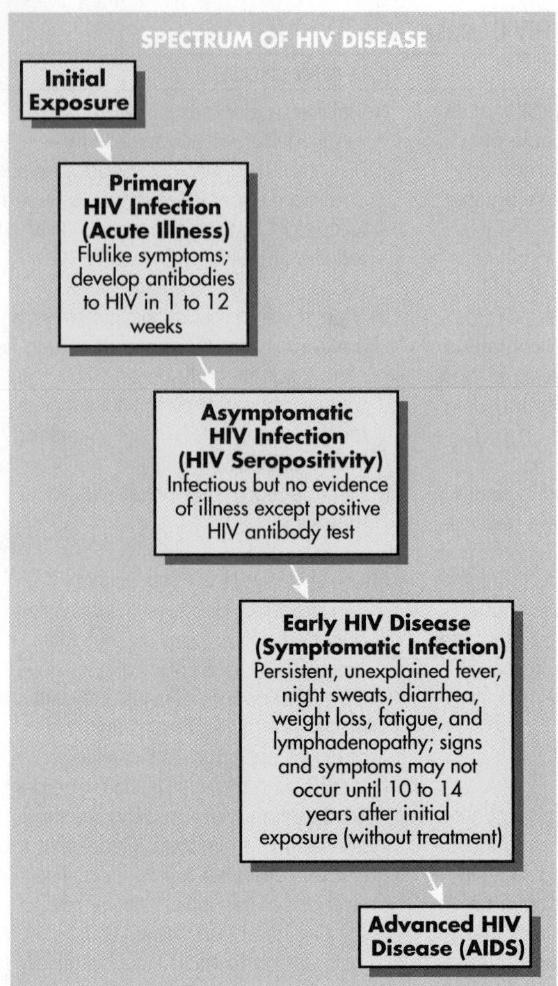

FIGURE 56-2 Spectrum of HIV disease and associated signs and symptoms at various stages of the disease process.

quickly as the body effectively contains the infection. Normally, antigens that are deemed as foreign intermingle with B cells. At this stage, antibodies are produced. T cells start a cellular-based immune response. In the early stages of the infection, the antibodies are able to reduce the viral load. T cells are beckoned to the lymph nodes where the virus is trapped (see Table 56-2). The virus replicates in the lymph system (nodes, tissue, spleen, and tonsils).

The lymphatic system carries the infection from one site to another. During this time, the HIV-infected person does not have any signs or symptoms. Over time, the lymphatic system is damaged by the HIV. The virus enters the blood, which increases the rate of disease progression. The body is not able to mount an adequate response to new infections. The immune system damage can be seen when examining B-cell dysfunction, but more important CD_4^+ cells are destroyed and their levels depleted (see Figure 56-1).

As the CD_4^+ cells are destroyed, the immune system fails. Immune dysfunction can occur when the CD_4^+ lymphocytes fall below 500 cells/mm^3 of blood. When the level falls below 200 cells/mm^3, severe immune system dysfunction is apparent. This results in the development of possibly fatal OIs in the host.

Monocytes can be infected by HIV because some of them also have CD_4^+ receptors. When the monocyte is infected, it can change into a phagocyte. When a **phagocyte** (cell that ingests and digests bacteria) is infected with HIV, it merely works as a factory to create more HIV. This infected phagocyte can rupture due to a normal local inflammatory response. When this happens, the HIV is spread even deeper into the body. In this way, the skin, the lungs, bone marrow, the central nervous system, and lymph nodes become directly infected.

SPECTRUM OF HIV INFECTION

The term **HIV disease** (the state in which HIV enters the body under favorable conditions and multiplies, producing injurious effects), encompasses the immune system progressive dysfunction that **HIV infection** produces within the host. HIV disease replaces the previous term *AIDS-related complex* (ARC). **Acquired immunodeficiency syndrome (AIDS)** (the end stage of HIV infection, in which the infected person has a CD_4^+ count of 200 cells/mm^3 or fewer) occurs as the disease progresses and the body is severely damaged by OIs (Table 56-3). At this stage, the host can no longer protect itself and the body is injured (see Figure 56-2). The CD_4^+ count is less than or equal to 200 cells/mm^3. People can live for years with the infection before they develop any signs or symptoms of HIV. The signs and symptoms include night sweats, weight loss, diarrhea, unexplainable fevers, and fatigue. The viral course of HIV depends on host factors. The host has an increased risk of morbidity and mortality when he or she has inadequate health care access, is of lower socioeconomic status, or is under the care of a health care provider with minimal experience dealing with HIV.

Progression from the early stages of HIV to end-stage HIV varies greatly. Three patterns have been found: typical progressors, long-term nonprogressors, and rapid progressors. In the typical progression pattern, people develop signs and symptoms several years after seroconverting. Many do not know they have been infected with HIV and can infect others. Long-term nonprogressors develop signs and symptoms at least 10 years after seroconverting. Long-term nonprogressors are rare. Their illness progression is thought to take longer because their immune response is very intense, so their viral load is lower. Also, there are genetic differences in their receptors (CCR5) on CD_4^+ lymphocytes that make it difficult for the HIV to attach. This allows their CD_4^+ and CD_8^+ cells to be maintained at near normal levels.

Approximately 5% to 10% of people who are infected with HIV are rapid progressors. These people move from being infected with HIV to an AIDS diagnosis within 3 years. Several common factors are found in rapid progressors: their cytotoxic T cells (CD_8^+) are dysfunctional and unable to contain HIV, the level of virus remains very high throughout the infection, and HIV antibodies are minimal.

Table 56-3 **Proper Terms Related to HIV and AIDS**

MISLEADING PHRASES	MORE ACCURATE PHRASES
High-risk groups	High-risk behaviors
Infected with AIDS	HIV infection
AIDS test	HIV antibody test
AIDS positive	HIV positive
AIDS victim or patient	Person living with HIV or AIDS
AIDS carrier	HIV-infected person

The term *AIDS* has been defined for surveillance and reporting purposes; it is not used alone to diagnose serious disease caused by HIV infection (see Table 56-3).

ACUTE RETROVIRAL SYNDROME

Viral replication occurs during the acute infection period. The viral load peaks in millions of copies of virus per milliliter of plasma. The decline of virus occurs right before the appearance of detectable antibodies that can be measured in the blood. The viral set point, or stabilizing of the viral load, is then reached 4 to 6 months after exposure. This viral set point is important, and some researchers believe it to be a prognostic indicator of long-term survival; that is, the lower the viral set point, the longer the individual will survive with HIV disease. Postexposure prophylaxis (PEP), begun as soon as possible after exposure, may help lower this viral set point. This theory is demonstrated in health care personnel who initiate PEP medications after an exposure and do not seroconvert.

Seroconversion is the development of antibodies from HIV, which takes place approximately 5 days to 3 months after exposure (generally within 1 to 3 weeks). This process is accompanied by a flulike or mononucleosis-like syndrome consisting of fever, night sweats, pharyngitis, headache, malaise, arthralgias, myalgias, diarrhea, nausea, and a diffuse rash prominent on the trunk. These symptoms last approximately 1 to 2 weeks, although some symptoms may last for several months. Seroconversion illness occurs in approximately 89% of HIV-infected people. HIV antibodies appear in 95% of people within 3 months, and 99% seroconvert within 6 months. The viral load during the period of seroconversion is extremely high, with a short-term drop in CD_4^+ cells. The CD_4^+ level quickly returns to normal as the immune system mounts an attack against the viral infection, resulting in viral loads existing at nearly undetectable levels in the blood. In most people the acute retroviral illness is mild and may be mistaken for a cold or other minor viral infection (Table 56-4).

EARLY INFECTION

The median time between HIV infection and the development of end-stage HIV disease, or AIDS, in an untreated individual is anywhere from 10 to 14 years (Figure 56-3). This phase of HIV disease is sometimes called the asymptomatic phase, because the HIV-infected individual looks and feels healthy. Some individuals have vague symptoms indicative of a viral infection, including fatigue, headaches, low-grade fever, and night sweats. Because many of the symptoms of early infection are nondescript, a diagnosis of HIV infection might not be made. Consequently, individuals may continue to engage in risky sexual and drug-using behaviors. Although seemingly healthy, the HIV-infected individual is capable of transmitting HIV to others. Lack of knowledge of one's HIV antibody status puts one at risk for earlier development of more advanced disease, since changes in behaviors, such as those that promote health, are not instituted. Furthermore, if an individual is aware of the virus, early intervention with antiretroviral medications may prolong the asymptomatic phase and prevent progression to AIDS.

Table 56-4 **Primary HIV Infection: Signs and Symptoms**

SIGNS AND SYMPTOMS	% OF PATIENTS EXPERIENCING
Fever	96
Adenopathy	74
Pharyngitis	70
Rash*	70
Myalgias	54
Diarrhea	32
Headache	32
Nausea and vomiting	27
Hepatosplenomegaly	14
Weight loss	13
Thrush	12
Neurologic symptoms†	12

*Erythematous maculopapular rash on face and trunk, sometimes extremities, including palms and soles. Some have mucocutaneous ulceration involving mouth, esophagus, or genitalia.
†Aseptic meningitis, meningoencephalitis, peripheral neuropathy, facial palsy, Guillain-Barré syndrome, brachial neuritis, cognitive impairment, or psychosis.

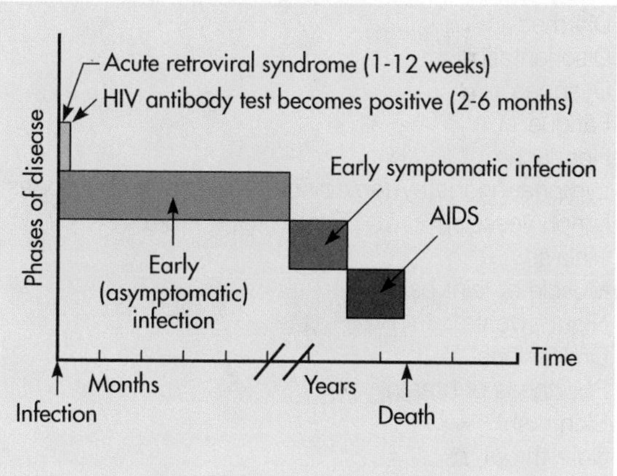

FIGURE 56-3 Timeline for the spectrum of HIV infection. This timeline represents the course of the illness from the time of infection to the clinical manifestations of it in an untreated individual.

EARLY SYMPTOMATIC DISEASE

The early symptomatic phase of HIV infection occurs when the CD_4^+ cell count drops below 500 cells/mm^3. Early symptoms include constitutional problems such as persistent, unexplained fevers; recurrent drenching night sweats; chronic diarrhea; headaches; and fatigue. These signs and symptoms become severe enough to affect activities of daily living (ADLs). A physical examination may reveal persistent generalized lymphadenopathy (PGL); recurrent or localized infections; and neurologic manifestations, such as numbness and tingling or weakness in the extremities (Box 56-1).

One of the most common infections seen in individuals with early symptomatic disease is oral candidiasis (thrush), a fungal infection rarely seen in healthy adults (Figure 56-4). Other infections that signal immune dysfunction include varicella-zoster virus, or shingles; persistent vaginal candidiasis (yeast infections); and increased frequency of oral or genital HSV outbreaks. Oral hairy leukoplakia (OHL), a condition related to the Epstein-Barr virus, and oral thrush are early indicators of HIV disease and prognostic markers for disease progression. Because of this, dental health professionals are key individuals in case finding for early HIV disease.

PGL is defined as two or more enlarged lymph nodes (1 cm or greater), located in places other than the inguinal region, that persist for at least 3 months. PGL may be present for many years before an individual progresses to an AIDS diagnosis.

Neurologic manifestations of HIV disease occur in more than 90% of individuals who are infected. Neurologic symptoms include peripheral neuropathies, headaches, aseptic meningitis, cranial nerve palsies, and myopathies. These conditions may be caused by the HIV infection itself or may be side effects related to antiretroviral medications.

Several cofactors may influence a more rapid progression of HIV disease. Very young children and very old adults progress more quickly. Concurrent infections such as HSV, cytomegalovirus (CMV), or Epstein-Barr virus affect progression. Drug and alcohol use, including smoking, may suppress the immune system. Malnutrition is also known to affect immune function, but further study relative to HIV is needed.

Box 56-1 Signs and Symptoms of HIV Infection

- Abdominal pain
- Chills and fever
- Cough (dry or productive)
- Diarrhea
- Disorientation
- Dyspnea
- Fatigue
- Headache
- Lymphadenopathy (any disorder of the lymph nodes or lymph vessels)
- Malaise
- Muscle or joint pain
- Night sweats
- Oral lesions
- Shortness of breath
- Skin rash
- Sore throat
- Weight loss

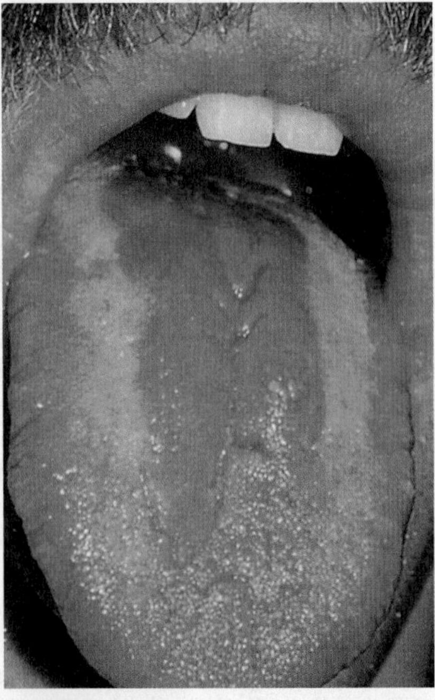

FIGURE 56-4 Oral candidiasis, or thrush, manifests with a whitish, curdlike substance on the tongue or inside the mouth.

AIDS

AIDS is the term used to describe the end stage, or terminal phase, of the spectrum of HIV infection. The CDC has developed specific diagnostic criteria that must be applied to make this diagnosis (see Table 56-1). These conditions are more likely to occur with severe immunosuppression. As HIV disease progresses, the CD_4^+ lymphocyte cell count decreases, and the ratio of CD_4^+ to CD_8^+ cells (T-helper cells to T-suppressor cells), which is normally 2 to 1, gradually shifts, resulting in more CD_8^+ than CD_4^+. The amount of virus detectable in the blood increases rapidly and remains high despite pharmacologic interventions. The number of white blood cells (WBCs) may also decline, and the person's reactivity to skin tests, such as purified protein derivative tuberculin, is decreased or absent. An individual is said to be anergic if no skin response is noted.

Without treatment, the median time from an AIDS diagnosis to death averages 1⅓ years, although this varies greatly. With the advent of more effective antiretroviral and opportunistic disease prophylaxis, the life span of an HIV-infected individual is unpredictable. Morbidity in people with advanced HIV disease also varies widely. Some people are severely ill and become terminal rather quickly, whereas others only have to make minor adjustments in their lifestyle to cope with medical regimens or physical symptoms, such as fatigue or pain. Significant advances in the management of HIV disease have made it resemble a chronic illness. The effects of therapy on mortality have been significant, with a leveling off of new AIDS cases reported to the CDC every year. This can be attributed to effective prophylaxis for OIs and to the development of HAART.

LABORATORY AND DIAGNOSTIC EXAMINATIONS

Strong evidence shows that early intervention postpones the onset of severe immunosuppression. Encourage individuals at risk for HIV infection to seek HIV antibody testing, and educate them in how to decrease the risk of HIV transmission.

HIV ANTIBODY TESTING

Patients need to understand the implications of an HIV antibody test (Box 56-2):

- The individual's blood is tested with enzyme-linked immunosorbent assay (ELISA) or enzyme immunoassay (EIA), antibody tests that detect the presence of HIV antibodies. If the EIA is positive for HIV, then the same blood is tested a second time. If the second EIA is positive, a more specific confirming test such as the Western blot is done. Blood that is reactive or positive in all three steps is reported to be HIV positive.
- Tests with indeterminate results are repeated at a later date, generally in 4 to 6 weeks. Consistently indeterminate results require the use of a viral culture or the measurement of viral load using a bDNA, a reverse transcriptase–polymerase chain reaction (RT-PCR), or nucleic acid sequence–based amplification (NASBA) laboratory measures.
- The series of laboratory tests confirms the presence of antibodies to HIV but does not mean the person has AIDS. The tests are not diagnostic of AIDS. AIDS is diagnosed according to the 1993 CDC definition.
- A seronegative (the state of lacking HIV antibodies as confirmed by blood test) test is not an assurance that the individual is free of HIV infection, since seroconversion may not yet have occurred.
- A seronegative test does not mean that an individual is free from risk of infection. If an individual continues to engage in risky behaviors, such as unprotected sexual intercourse or use of contaminated needles or drug paraphernalia, transmission may occur (Box 56-3).

Box 56-2 Tests Used to Detect HIV Infection

ANTIBODY DETECTION TESTS

Screening Tests
- Enzyme-linked immunosorbent assay (ELISA)
- Agglutination assays
- Oral fluid test
- Urine screening test

Confirmatory Test
- Western blot (interpreted by a pathologist)
- Indirect immunofluorescent antibody assay
- Radioimmunoprecipitation assay (RIPA)

ANTIGEN DETECTION TESTS (P24 ANTIGEN)

HIV Viral Load Tests/ Nucleic Acid Determination Assays
- Reverse transcriptase–polymerase chain reaction (RT-PCR)
- Branched chain DNA (bDNA)
- Nucleic acid sequence–based amplification (NASBA)

Viral Culture Method
- HIV culture

ACTIVATED IMMUNE MARKERS
- Neopterin
- β_2-microglobulin
- Absolute CD_4^+ cell count
- CD_4^+ percentage
- CD_8^+ percentage
- CD_4^+/CD_8^+ ratio

CD_4^+ CELL MONITORING

Monitoring CD_4^+ cells is one of the laboratory parameters used to track the progression of HIV disease. As the disease progresses, the number of CD_4^+ cells decreases. The more significant the loss, the more severe immunosuppression becomes. The CD_4^+ count is the best marker for the immunodeficiency associated with HIV infection. As such, the CD_4^+ count is used in making decisions about antiretroviral and prophylactic drug therapy and in evaluating specific complaints relative to the risk for contracting particular OIs. For example, *Mycobacterium avium* complex and CMV infections are rare in patients with CD_4^+ counts greater than 50 cells/mm^3. PCP and cryptococcosis are unusual in patients with CD_4^+ counts greater than 200 cells/mm^3. The CD_4^+ count is not a perfect surrogate marker of immunodeficiency, and factors such as the patient's clinical status must always be taken into account.

The CD_4^+ cell count reflects the number of CD_4^+ cells per cubic millimeter (or per microliter) of blood. It does not indicate the total number of CD_4^+ cells in the body. Millions of new CD_4^+ cells are produced daily and cleared by normal body processes (unrelated to the virus). The absolute CD_4^+ count can vary greatly in the same individual depending on the time of day the blood is drawn; which laboratory is used; and the presence of acute illness or other factors, such as alcohol. Therefore continue to use the same laboratory, draw blood at the same time of day, and avoid testing on days when the patient is acutely ill or under abnormal stress. When using the CD_4^+ count to make important treatment decisions, such as initiating prophylaxis for OIs, draw two separate samples a few weeks apart.

VIRAL LOAD MONITORING

The ability to detect HIV viral load measurements in plasma is a significant advancement in the monitoring of HIV disease. Viral load or burden refers to a quantitative measure of HIV viral RNA in the peripheral circulation, or the level of virus in the blood.

At present, three quantitative assay tests are available to measure viral load levels: NASBA, RT-PCR, and bDNA. Even very small numbers of infected cells can be detected by identifying virions. These tests can only be used to identify HIV. These tests are helpful

Box 56-3 Pretest and Posttest Counseling Associated with HIV-Antibody Testing

GENERAL GUIDELINES

- People who are being tested for HIV are commonly fearful of the test results; therefore carry out the following steps:
  —Establish rapport with the patient.
  —Assess patient's ability to understand counseling.
  —Determine the patient's access to support systems.
- Explain the following benefits of testing:
  —Testing provides an opportunity for education that can decrease the risk of new infections.
  —Infected patient can be referred for early intervention and support programs.
- Discuss the following negative aspects of testing:
  —Breaches of confidentiality have led to discrimination.
  —A positive test affects all aspects of the patient's life (personal, social, economic) and can raise difficult emotions (anger, anxiety, guilt, thoughts of suicide).

PRETEST COUNSELING

- Determine the patient's risk factors and when the last exposure risk occurred. Individualize counseling according to these parameters.
- Provide education to decrease future risk of exposure.
- Provide education that will help the patient protect sexual and drug-sharing partners.
- Discuss problems related to the delay between infection and an accurate test:
  —Testing needs to be repeated at intervals for 6 months after each possible exposure.
  —The patient needs to abstain from further risky behaviors during that interval.
  —The patient needs to protect partners during that interval.
- Discuss the possibility of false-negative tests, which are most likely to occur during the window period.
- Explain that a positive test shows HIV infection, not AIDS.
- Explain that the test does not establish immunity, regardless of the results.
- Assess support systems; provide telephone numbers and resources as needed.
- Discuss patient's personally anticipated responses to test results (positive and negative).
- Outline assistance that will be offered if the test is positive.

POSTTEST COUNSELING

- If the test is negative, reinforce pretest counseling and prevention education. Remind patient that test needs to be repeated at intervals for 6 months after the most recent exposure risk.
- If the test is positive, understand that the patient may be in shock and not hear what is said.
  —Provide resources for medical and emotional support, and help the patient get immediate assistance.
  —Evaluate suicide risk and follow up as needed.
  —Determine need to test others who have had risky contact with the patient.
  —Discuss retesting to verify results. This tactic provides hope for the patient, but more important it keeps the patient in the system. While waiting for the second test result, the patient has time to think about and adjust to the possibility of being HIV infected.
  —Encourage optimism:
    - Remind patient that treatments are available.
    - Review health habits that can improve the immune system.
    - Arrange for patients to speak to HIV-infected people who are willing to share and assist the newly diagnosed patients during the transition period.
    - Reinforce that an HIV-positive test means the patient is infected, but a positive test does not necessarily mean that the patient has AIDS.

Modified from Bradley-Springer, L.A., & Fendrick, R. (1994). *HIV instant instructor cards.* El Paso, Tex: Skidmore-Roth.

when trying to identify HIV in people who have a negative ELISA (antibody) test.

Important characteristics include the following:

- In all clinical stages of illness, HIV viral detection techniques identify measurable viral RNA copies in the plasma of most HIV-infected individuals.
- Viral load can provide significant information used to predict the course of disease progression, initiate ART, measure the degree of antiretroviral effect achieved, and note the failure of a drug regimen.
- Plasma HIV RNA levels fall dramatically after effective ART.
- Detection of HIV RNA levels in plasma does not indicate whether any virus is present in lymphoid or other tissues.

Viral load and CD_4^+ cell counts are distinct markers that provide different information. Viral load can predict disease progression and long-term clinical outcome; CD_4^+ cell measurements can indicate the damage sustained by the immune system (the loss of CD_4^+, or T cells) and the short-term risk for developing OIs. Each is an independent predictor of clinical outcome, and when used in combination they can give a more complete indication of clinical status, treatment response, and prognosis. A metaphor used by John Coffin describes the asymptomatic, infected patient as a train rushing along a track, heading for a bridge that has been destroyed. The time the crash will occur is determined by two variables: (1) where the train is at this instant (CD_4^+), and (2) how fast it is going (viral load) (Coffin, 1996).

A baseline determination of viral burden is recommended, with subsequent measurements every 3 to 4 months, in conjunction with CD_4^+ cell monitoring and clinical evaluations such as a history and physical examination. Guidelines will continue to be revised as the implications of viral measurement evolve and its interpretation and use become better understood. In the future, OI prophylaxis may be based on viral load as well as CD_4^+ cell counts.

RESISTANCE TESTING

Drug resistance to HAART can make effective treatment of HIV challenging. In North America and Europe, approximately, 6% to 16% of HIV has at least one resistant mutation (Yerly et al., 2007). HIV mutates easily, and this makes it hard to treat and contain. After multiple genetic mutations, the replication of HIV is "sloppy," which makes it more resistant to medication treatment and has prevented the development of an effective vaccine. ART resistance is based in the patients' inability to adhere to ART protocols. Assay tests are available that can detect HIV genetic mutations that result in ART resistance. Results of these tests are available in less than a month. A list of ART-resistant mutations has been developed by the International AIDS Society–USA. Phenotyping is available to help estimate how well the specific virus will respond to treatment in people who have been on ART for a long time. To perform phenotyping, the patient must have a high viral load (Panel on Antiretroviral Guidelines for Adults and Adolescents, 2008).

During the acute stage of HIV, resistance testing can be important so that appropriate ART can be used to prevent extensive replication of HIV. Some health care providers identify baseline genetic mutations before starting ART. A patient-specific ART regimen can be created to avoid medications that would not work. When patients are resistant to some medications used in ART, they may have cross-resistance issues with other ART medications. Resistant HIV strains are found in people who have undergone ART as well as in other people who are newly infected and often treatment naïve. Resistance to some ART drugs and the ability to transmit resistance to newly infected people are important issues for public health officials who are battling to control and prevent HIV.

OTHER LABORATORY PARAMETERS

Hematological abnormalities are common in HIV infections and may be caused by the HIV itself, by OIs, or by drug or radiation therapy. A decreased WBC count is often seen, usually in conjunction with lymphopenia (decreased lymphocytes). Thrombocytopenia (decreased platelet count) may be caused by antiplatelet antibodies. Anemia is related to the chronic disease process and to HIV invasion of the bone marrow; it is a common adverse effect of antiretroviral agents.

Alterations in liver function tests are not uncommon. Abnormalities may be caused by viral hepatitis, alcohol abuse, OIs, neoplasms, or medications. Early identification of hepatitis B and hepatitis C viral infections is important because these infections may follow a more serious course in the patient with HIV disease. Patients who are HIV positive are often also positive for hepatitis B, since both infections are bloodborne and sexually transmitted. In addition, about one fourth of HIV-infected people in the United States are coinfected with hepatitis C, one of the most important causes of chronic liver disease.

Syphilis testing is important because syphilis is more complicated and aggressive in the HIV-infected individual. It is also more difficult to treat with standard therapies and more likely to advance quickly to neurosyphilis. If a person is positive for syphilis, begin assessment and treatment immediately.

THERAPEUTIC MANAGEMENT

Therapeutic management of the HIV-infected patient focuses on monitoring HIV disease progression and immune function, preventing the development of opportunistic diseases, initiating and monitoring ART, detecting and treating opportunistic diseases, managing symptoms, and preventing complications of treatment.

HIV-positive individuals need to be linked to various points of intervention, depending on their individual needs. Individuals often deny the infection, neglect their mental and physical health, and continue behaviors that put themselves and others at risk. Interventions need to be sustained and reinforced; the emotional impact of such devastating news ("you are HIV positive") can overshadow any initial information or education provided. Stress safer behaviors and the need for medical and emotional support, such as assistance in family planning, treatment for substance abuse, treatment for STIs, treatment for tuberculosis, and immunizations.

A transdisciplinary care approach is most appropriate for patients with HIV disease because of their complex medical and psychosocial needs. The HIV-infected individual should be the primary member of this team, working along with a physician who specializes in HIV/AIDS, a social worker, a case manager, a dietitian, and a nurse. Other team members may include a dentist, a primary care provider (medical doctor, doctor of osteopathy, nurse practitioner, or physician assistant), a mental health worker, a substance abuse counselor, a nontraditional therapist (such as a massage therapist or acupuncturist), and the individual's family and significant other.

PHARMACOLOGIC MANAGEMENT

Opportunistic Diseases Associated with HIV

Probably the most difficult aspect of the medical management of HIV is dealing with the many opportunistic diseases that develop as the immune system degenerates. Although it is usually impossible to totally eradicate opportunistic diseases, the use of antiretrovirals and prophylactic interventions can control their emergence or progression. However, these regimens must continue throughout the patient's life, or the disease will return. Advances in the diagnosis and treatment of opportunistic diseases have contributed significantly to increased life expectancy and decreased morbidity. Table 56-5 lists common opportunistic diseases associated with HIV disease. Table 56-6 lists common prophylactic regimens in the HIV-infected individual.

Antiretroviral Therapy

Combination active retroviral therapy (ART) is an important component in the management of HIV infection (Table 56-7). In 1987 zidovudine was the only medication available to treat patients with HIV disease, but now the U.S. Food and Drug Administration (FDA) has approved 20 antiretroviral medications (Table 56-8). Six different classes of ART are used to prevent the viral replication process. There are integrase inhibitors, fusion inhibitors, CCR5 antagonists, NRTIs and NtRTIs (nucleoside and nucleotide reverse transcriptase inhibi-

Table 56-5 Common Opportunistic Diseases Associated with HIV/AIDS

ORGANISM OR DISEASE	CLINICAL MANIFESTATIONS	DIAGNOSTIC TESTS	TREATMENT
RESPIRATORY SYSTEM			
Pneumocystis jiroveci (formerly *carinii*) pneumonia (PCP)	Fever, night sweats, nonproductive cough, progressive SOB	Chest radiograph, induced sputum for culture, bronchoalveolar lavage	Trimethoprim-sulfamethoxazole, dapsone + pyrimethamine + leucovorin, clindamycin, atovaquone, pentamidine, steroids, trimetrexate, folinic acid
Cryptococcus species	Pneumonia, fever, cough, malaise	Sputum culture, serum antigen assay	Fluconazole, itraconazole, amphotericin B
Histoplasmosis	Pneumonia, fever, cough	Sputum culture, serum antigen assay	Amphotericin B, itraconazole, fluconazole
Mycobacterium tuberculosis	Productive cough, fever, night sweats, fatigue, weight loss	Chest radiograph, sputum for AFB stain and culture, skin test	Isoniazid, ethambutol, rifabutin, pyrazinamide, streptomycin, azithromycin, clarithromycin
Coccidioidomycosis	Fever, weight loss, cough	Sputum culture, serology	Amphotericin B, fluconazole, itraconazole
Herpes simplex virus (HSV) I	Vesicular eruptions on tracheobronchial mucosa	Viral culture or PCR	Acyclovir, famciclovir, valacyclovir
Toxoplasma gondii	Fever, SOB, nonproductive cough	Antibody test	See Neurological System section
Rhodococcus equi	Chest pain, productive cough, SOB, fever, hemoptysis	Culture from sputum or bronchoalveolar lavage	Vancomycin + imipenem + ciprofloxacin with or without rifampin, erythromycin
Aspergillosis	Fever, cough, SOB, chest pain, hemoptysis, occasional CNS symptoms	Stain of respiratory secretions of biopsy	Amphotericin B, itraconazole
INTEGUMENTARY SYSTEM			
HSV-I	Vesicular eruptions on mouth	Viral culture or PCR	Acyclovir, foscarnet, famciclovir, valacyclovir
HSV-II	Vesicular eruptions around perianal area	Viral culture or PCR	Acyclovir, foscarnet, valacyclovir, famciclovir
Varicella-zoster virus (VZV)	Shingles: erythematous macules, rash, pain, pruritus	Viral culture	Acyclovir, foscarnet, valacyclovir
Kaposi's sarcoma	Firm, flat, raised, or nodular, hyperpigmented, multicentric lesions	Biopsy of lesions	HAART, radiation, chemotherapy, alpha-interferon, palliative care, bleomycin, daunorubicin
Bacillary angiomatosis	Erythematous papules and nodules	Biopsy of lesions	Erythromicin, doxycycline, clarithromycin, azithromycin
EYE			
Cytomegalovirus (CMV) retinitis	Lesions on the retina, blurred vision, loss of vision	Ophthalmoscopic examination	Valganciclovir, foscarnet, cidofovir

Table 56-5 Common Opportunistic Diseases Associated with HIV/AIDS—cont'd

ORGANISM OR DISEASE	CLINICAL MANIFESTATIONS	DIAGNOSTIC TESTS	TREATMENT
EYE—cont'd			
HSV-I	Blurred vision, corneal lesions, acute retinal necrosis	Ophthalmoscopic examination, culture	Acyclovir, foscarnet, famciclovir, valacyclovir
VZV	Ocular lesions, acute retinal necrosis	Ophthalmoscopic examination, culture	Acyclovir, foscarnet, valacyclovir, famciclovir
Toxoplasma gondii	Visual field defects	Antibody test	See Neurological System section
GASTROINTESTINAL SYSTEM			
Cryptosporidium muris	Watery diarrhea, abdominal pain, weight loss, nausea, fever	Stool examination	Antidiarrheals, paromomycin, azithromycin
CMV	Stomatitis, esophagitis, gastritis, colitis, bloody diarrhea, pain, weight loss	Endoscopic visualization, culture, biopsy; rule out other causes	Valganciclovir, foscarnet, cidofovir
HSV-I	Vesicular eruptions on tongue, buccal, pharyngeal, or perioral esophageal mucosa	Viral culture or PCR	Acyclovir, foscarnet, famciclovir, valacyclovir
Candida albicans	Whitish yellow patches in mouth, esophagus, GI tract	Microscopic examination of scraping from lesion	Nystatin, clotrimazole, ketoconazole, fluconazole, itraconazole, amphotericin B
Mycobacterium avium complex (MAC)	Watery diarrhea, weight loss, fever, fatigue, night sweats, anemia, ↑LDH, ↓alkaline phosphatase	Small bowel biopsy with AFB stain and culture Blood cultures	Azithromycin or clarithromycin + rifabutin, ofloxacin, rifampin, clofamizine, rifabutin amikacin, ciprofloxacin, ethambutol
Isospora belli	Diarrhea, weight loss, nausea, abdominal pain	Stool examination	Trimethoprim-sulfamethoxazole, pyrimethamine + folic acid
Salmonella species	Gastroenteritis, fever, diarrhea	Blood and stool culture	Ampicillin, amoxicillin, ciprofloxacin, trimethoprim-sulfamethoxazole
Kaposi's sarcoma	Diarrhea, hyperpigmented lesions of mouth and GI tract, GI bleeding	GI series, biopsy	Radiation, chemotherapy, HAART
Non-Hodgkin's lymphoma	Abdominal pain, fever, night sweats, weight loss	Lymph node biopsy	Chemotherapy, HAART
NEUROLOGIC SYSTEM			
Toxoplasma gondii	Cognitive dysfunction, motor impairment, fever, headache, seizures, ↓LOC, hemiparesis	MRI, CT scan, toxoplasma serology	Pyrimethamine + leucovorin + sulfadiazine, clindamycin, azithromcycin, clarithromycin
Jamestown Canyon virus	Progressive multifocal leukoencephalopathy, mental and motor declines	MRI, CT scan, brain biopsy, autopsy	No proven therapy, but HAART may help, IV alpha-interferon or cytosine arabinoside
Cryptococcal meningitis	Cognitive impairment, motor dysfunction, fever, seizures, stiff neck, nausea and vomiting	CT scan, serum antigen test, CSF analysis	Amphotericin B + 5-flucytosine, fluconazole, itraconazole
CNS lymphomas	Cognitive dysfunction, motor impairment, aphasia, seizures, personality changes, headache	MRI, CT scan	Radiation, chemotherapy

Table 56-6 Opportunistic Illness Prophylaxis Guidelines

PROBLEM	INDICATION	PREVENTIVE REGIMENS FIRST CHOICE	ALTERNATIVE CHOICES	COMMENTS
STRONGLY RECOMMENDED AS STANDARD OF CARE				
Pneumocystis jiroveci (formerly *carinii*) pneumonia (PCP)	CD_4^+ cell count <200/mm^3 or CD_4^+ % <14%, presence of oral thrush or other AIDS-defining illness	Trimethoprim-sulfamethoxazole (TMP-SMX), 1 DS tablet/day; consider desensitization protocol for patients with non–life-threatening allergy	Dapsone, aerosolized pentamidine, atovaquone	May stop if CD_4^+ cell count >200/mm^3 for 3 months; check patients receiving dapsone for G6PD deficiency
Mycobacterium tuberculosis	Skin test (PPD) ≥5 mm or prior positive skin test	Isoniazid + pyridoxine for 9 months	Rifampin 600 mg qid for 6 months	Rule out active or extrapulmonary disease, which requires multidrug therapy; remember that a negative PPD in the presence of HIV does not exclude a diagnosis of tuberculosis
Toxoplasma gondii	CD_4^+ cell count <100/mm^3, and positive IgG antibody; check for antibodies soon after diagnosis	TMP-SMX, 1 DS tablet qid	Dapsone + pyrimethamine	If using dapsone, check for G6PD deficiency; may stop if CD_4^+ cell count >200/mm^3 for at least 3 months
Mycobacterium avium complex	CD_4^+ cell count <50/mm^3	Azithromycin 1,200 mg once each week; or clarithromycin 500 mg po bid	Rifabutin 300 mg po every day or; azithromycin 1,200 mg once weekly	
Varicella zoster virus (VZV)	Significant exposure to chickenpox or shingles for patients who have no history of either illness	Varicella zoster immune globulin IM ≤96 hours after exposure	VZV vaccine not well studied, though undergoing trials	
GENERALLY RECOMMENDED				
Streptococcus pneumoniae	CD_4^+ cell count ≥200/mm^3	Pneumovax every 5-6 years		
Hepatitis B virus	All susceptible patients	Hepatitis B vaccine series	Combination hepatitis A and B vaccine (Twinrix)	Provide as soon as possible during course of infection; antibody response is optimal with CD_4^+ cell count >200/mm^3
Influenza	All patients before influenza season	Inactivated trivalent influenza vaccine, dosed each year	Oseltamivir 75 mg po qid; rimantidine 100 mg po bid, or amantadine 100 mg po bid (active against influenza A only)	
Hepatitis A virus (HAV)	All susceptible patients at risk for HAV infection: illicit drug users, men who have sex with men, hemophiliacs, chronic liver disease	Hepatitis A vaccine (2 doses)		Combination vaccine available for hepatitis A and hepatitis B (Twinrix)

G6PD, Glucose-6-phosphate dehydrogenase; *IgG,* immunoglobulin G; *PPD,* purified protein derivative.

tors), NNRTIs (nonnucleoside reverse transcriptase inhibitors), and protease inhibitors. Each class of medication interrupts HIV at different stages of the infectious process. When health care providers prescribe three drugs from at least two different classes, this is called HAART (highly active antiretroviral therapy).

Scientists have found that the most effective medication regimen is the use of **cocktails** (at least two, but generally three or more compounds given together). Using medication combinations makes it much more difficult for the virus to develop resistance to the drugs. Such intervention may also slow the progression from asymptomatic or mildly symptomatic HIV infection to a more advanced disease. Recent developments include therapies that can dramatically reduce the quantity of circulating virus in the blood; in many cases, blood cir-

Table 56-7 Pros and Cons of Highly Active Antiretroviral Therapy (HAART)

PROS	CONS
• Minimize chance of emergence of resistant virus • May play a role in the reduction of HIV transmission • Slows disease progression • Improves quality of life	• Drugs can be toxic • Frequent side effects • Complexity of drug and dosing regimens • Impact of nonadherence on treatment failure • Expensive

Table 56-8 Medications for HIV Disease (Antiretrovirals)

Generic (Brand)	Side Effects	Comments
NUCLEOSIDE REVERSE TRANSCRIPTASE INHIBITORS (NRTIs, NUCLEOSIDE ANALOGS, "NUKES")		
Zidovudine (ZDV, Retrovir) 300 mg po q12h	Anemia, fever, malaise, headache, rash, nausea, insomnia, myalgia, confusion, agitation, seizures, bone marrow suppression, anemia, granulocytopenia, thrombocytopenia, hepatomegaly	Side effects, such as headache and nausea, typically resolve within 1 month. Bone marrow suppression side effects occur after long-term use (6 months to 2 years). Treat anemia with blood transfusions or erythropoietin (Procrit); consider treating granulocytopenia or neutropenia with colony-stimulating factor, such as filgrastim (Neupogen).
Didanosine (ddI, Videx) >60 kg: 400 mg/day <60 kg: 250 mg/day po, or if used with tenofovir (Viread)	Pancreatitis, painful peripheral neuropathy (dose related and reversible), nausea, abdominal pain, diarrhea, rash, hyperglycemia, hyperuricemia, hepatic failure, headache, insomnia, seizures, thrombocytopenia	Take on an empty stomach 2 hours apart from other drugs, such as dapsone, itraconazole, or ketoconazole. Need alkaline environment for absorption. Avoid use with H_2 blockers, alcohol, and proton pump inhibitors (PPIs). Do not cut, crush, or chew.
Stavudine (Zerit, d4T) >60 kg: 40 mg po q12h <60 kg: 30 mg po q12h	Painful peripheral neuropathy, elevations in AST/ALT anemia, headache, rash, abdominal pain, diarrhea, nausea, vomiting, myalgia	Crosses the blood-brain barrier. Use in combination therapy Decrease dosage in patients with impaired renal function. Monitor for lactic acidosis.
Lamivudine (3TC, Epivir) 300 mg/day or 150 mg po q12h	Neutropenia, rash, insomnia, fever, headache, fatigue, diarrhea, vasculitis, photophobia, paresthesias	Generally well tolerated, with most patients reporting no side effects. Pancreatitis has been reported in 15% of children taking lamivudine. Never use alone, since HIV develops resistance rapidly. Typically used with zidovudine, stavudine, abacavir, or didanosine.
Abacavir (Ziagen, ABC) 300 mg po q12h or 600 mg/day po	Nausea, vomiting, headache, fatigue, rash	About 3% of people develop a hypersensitivity, which results in flulike symptoms. Life-threatening development of Stevens-Johnson syndrome may occur; stop drug immediately and do not rechallenge, since death may occur. Avoid alcohol (increases abacavir levels in blood). No dietary restrictions. Check for HLA-B5701 type before initiating therapy.

Continued

Table 56-8 Medications for HIV Disease (Antiretrovirals)—cont'd

Generic (Brand)	Side Effects	Comments
NUCLEOSIDE REVERSE TRANSCRIPTASE INHIBITORS (NRTIs, NUCLEOSIDE ANALOGS, "NUKES")—cont'd		
Emtricitabine (FTC, Emtriva) 200 mg/day po	Headache, diarrhea, nausea, rash, lactic acidosis, "fatty liver"	No food restrictions; also active against hepatitis B virus infection. Do not combine with lamivudine.
Tenofovir (TDF, Viread) 300 mg/day po	Mild side effects, some nausea, vomiting, loss of appetite, potential for renal failure, bone mineral density loss	Do not combine with lamivudine and abacavir. Take tenofovir 2 hours before or 1 hour after didanosine. No food restrictions.
COMBINATION MEDICATIONS		
Zidovudine plus lamivudine plus abacavir (Trizivir, T2V) 1 tablet po q12h	See zidovudine, lamivudine, and abacavir	Combination of 300 mg zidovudine, 150 mg lamivudine, and 300 mg abacavir. No food restrictions. Monitor for rash.
Tenofovir plus emtricitabine (Truvada, TRV) 1 tablet/day	See emtricitabine and tenofovir	No food restrictions.
Abacavir plus lamivudine (Epzicom, EP2) 1 tablet/day	See abacavir and lamivudine	No food restrictions. Blood levels may be increased by trimethoprim-sulfamethoxazole (Bactrim, Septra); do not take with zalcitabine or stavudine.
Zidovudine plus lamivudine (Combivir, CBV) 1 tablet q12h	See zidovudine and lamivudine	Do not take with zalcitabine or stavudine. Combination of 300 mg zidovudine and 150 mg lamivudine; significantly reduces the number of pills a patient has to take.
Tenofovir plus emtricitabine plus efavirenz (Atripla) 1 tablet po q24h	See tenofovir, emtricitabine, and efavirenz	Take on an empty stomach, preferably at bedtime.
NUCLEOTIDE REVERSE TRANSCRIPTASE INHIBITORS (NtRTIs)		
Tenofovir (Viread, TDF) 300 mg/day po	Renal insufficiency and failure; lactic acidosis	
NONNUCLEOSIDE REVERSE TRANSCRIPTASE INHIBITORS (NNRTIs)		
Nevirapine (Viramune, MP) 200 mg/day po for 14 days, then 200 mg po q12h	Rash, thrombocytopenia, fever, headaches, nausea	Use in combination therapy. Report any new rash immediately; rash may progress to Stevens-Johnson syndrome, which may result in death.
Delavirdine (Rescriptor, DLV) 400 mg po q8h	Rash, elevated liver function tests	Use in combination therapy.
Efavirenz (Sustiva, EFV) 600 mg once daily (initially at bedtime)	Initial dizziness, insomnia, transient rash, vivid dreams, nightmares, difficulty concentrating	This drug may cause hyperlipidemia; monitor cholesterol and triglycerides regularly. Take on an empty stomach. Contradicted in pregnancy.
Etravirine (Intelence, ETV) 200 mg po q12h	Skin rash, lipid abnormalities, elevated liver enzymes	Give after meals; multiple drug-drug interactions.
PROTEASE INHIBITORS		
Ritonavir (Norvir, RTV) 600 mg po q12h or used as boosting agent with other protease inhibitors	Nausea, vomiting, diarrhea, circumoral paresthesias (numbness and tingling), peripheral paresthesias, taste perversions, asthenia (weakness), increased liver enzymes, elevated cholesterol and triglyceride levels	Because of side effects, institute dose escalation. Start with 300 mg po q12h and increase by 100 mg every 3-4 days until at full dose of 600 mg po q12h. Take with food to decrease gastrointestinal side effects. Ritonavir has many drug interactions: benzodiazepines, opiates, long-acting nonsedating antihistamines (terfenadine [Seldane], astemizole [Hismanal], loratadine [Claritin]), antidysrhythmics, calcium channel blockers, rifabutin, clarithromycin levels increased by 80%. Medication must be refrigerated.

Table 56-8 Medications for HIV Disease (Antiretrovirals)—cont'd

Generic (Brand)	Side Effects	Comments
PROTEASE INHIBITORS—cont'd		
Indinavir (Crixivan, DV) 800 mg po q8h, or 1,200 mg po q12h	Headache, nausea (for the first few weeks), kidney stones, (signs include kidney pain, fever, abdominal tenderness, and painful urination), asymptomatic elevation of bilirubin and liver enzymes	Take on an empty stomach (1 hour before or 2 hours after meal); recommend six to eight glasses of water per day; take 1 hour before or after didanosine; ketoconazole increases indinavir levels by 60%; should not be used with rifampin. Taken in combination with nucleoside analogs or NNRTIs.
Nelfinavir (Viracept, NFV) 1,250 mg po q12h	Diarrhea most common side effect	Can be taken without regard to food. Use in combination with nucleoside analogs or NNRTIs. Manage diarrhea with antidiarrheals (atropine-diphenoxylate [Lomotil] or loperamide [Imodium]) and increased fiber in diet.
Lopinavir plus ritonavir (Kaletra, LPVr) 2 pills q12h	Diarrhea, nausea, headaches, lipid abnormalities	Combination drug of 400 mg lopinavir and 100 mg ritonavir. Can be taken without regard to food. Dose of lopinavir should be increased to three tablets twice a day if taken with efavirenz or nevirapine.
Atazanavir (Reyataz, ATZ) 300 to 400 mg/day (2 capsules) po	High levels of bilirubin, nausea, headache, rash, stomach pain, vomiting, diarrhea, tingling in hands or feet, depression, changes in heart rhythm	Take with food. If taken with didanosine, take 2 hours before or after atazanavir. Efavirenz and tenofovir lower levels of atazanavir (take with ritonavir to compensate). Do NOT take PPIs (e.g., omeprazole [Prilosec], esomeprazole [Nexium]). Take H_2 blockers such as famotidine (Pepcid) and ranitidine (Zantac) 12 hours apart from atazanavir.
Saquinavir (Invirase, SQV) hard gel capsule 1,000 mg (5 capsules) plus 100 mg ritonavir q12h	Minimal nausea, diarrhea, vomiting, headache, fatigue	Take up to 2 hours after a full meal. Take with high-fat food. Refrigerate in hot climates. Give with 100 mg ritonavir.
Fosamprenavir (Lexiva, FPV) 1,400 mg (two 700-mg tablets) bid; may be combined with ritonavir: 1,400 mg fosamprenavir plus 200 mg ritonavir once daily, or 700 mg fosamprenavir plus 100 mg ritonavir bid	Nausea, diarrhea, vomiting, rash, numbness around mouth, abdominal pain	No food restrictions. Less than 1% of people get serious skin reactions, including Stevens-Johnson syndrome. No other side effects seem to be serious. The diarrhea in most cases can be controlled with over-the-counter medications. Fosamprenavir can increase triglycerides (a blood fat). However, it might cause less of an increase in cholesterol than other protease inhibitors. Fosamprenavir is a sulfa drug; do not administer to patients who are allergic to sulfa drugs.
Darunavir (Prezista, DRV) 600 mg po with 100 mg ritonavir q12h	Diarrhea, lipid abnormalities, nausea, vomiting	Give with food. Use with caution in patients with sulfa allergy. Monitor lipid profile regularly.
Tipranavir (Aptivus, TPV) 500 mg po with 200 mg ritonavir q12h	Intracranial hemorrhage (rare), lipid abnormalities, diarrhea	Use with caution in patients with hepatitis; monitor lipid profile.

Continued

Table 56-8 Medications for HIV Disease (Antiretrovirals)—cont'd

Generic (Brand)	Side Effects	Comments
FUSION INHIBITORS		
Enfuvirtide (T-20, Fuzeon) 90 mg (1 mL) injected subQ bid in the upper arm, thigh, or abdomen (for patients weighing >94 pounds [42.6 kg])	Skin reactions where drug is injected, ranging from redness and itching to hard lumps; headache, pain and numbness in feet or legs, dizziness, loss of sleep	Almost everybody who uses enfuvirtide gets a skin reaction, ranging from mild (slight redness) to itching, swelling, pain, hardened skin, or hard lumps. Each reaction might last up to a week. With two injections each day, reactions might occur at several spots at the same time. Long-term adherence is poor because of side effects (skin).
INTEGRASE INHIBITOR		
Raltegravir (Isentress, RAL) 400 mg po q12h	Uncommon, but renal dysfunction, anemia, hepatitis described	Very well tolerated. Some drug-drug interactions.

culating levels become undetectable. Protease inhibitors directly reduce the ability of HIV to replicate, or make copies of itself inside cells. As increasing numbers of therapeutic agents and clinical trial results become available, decisions about ART have become increasingly complex. For now, these combination therapies offer optimism for successful disease management and improvements in the quality and duration of life.

It is important to administer anti-HIV medications around the clock. For example, a medication ordered three times per day should be given as close to every 8 hours as possible, not three times while the patient is awake. When medications are not given regularly, the drug levels in the blood fall low enough to allow HIV to develop resistance. This is a critical teaching point to communicate to patients.

Considerations for antiretroviral therapy include the following:

- Previous antiretroviral experience may affect the efficacy of a proposed therapy, since the HIV may have become resistant to those medications taken by the patient in the past (e.g., zidovudine, lamivudine).
- Certain combinations of antiretrovirals may reverse the resistance to a single drug. Recycling drugs previously taken can sometimes lead to improved viral suppression. Incorrect dosing (timing) or usage (missed doses) can cause drug resistance.
- Drug incompatibilities, similar side effect profiles, and toxicities must be considered when choosing a regimen.
- Consider the individual's commitment and ability to adhere to complex drug regimens. Inadequate adherence can lead to drug resistance and, ultimately, to drug failure. Stress this point to the patient. Adherence is paramount to survival and success of treatment.

Opinions differ as to when to initiate ART. The increasing number of antiretroviral agents and rapid evolution of new information have introduced extraordinary complexity into the treatment of HIV-infected people. A provider with expertise in HIV should supervise the care. Treatment should be offered to all patients with acute HIV syndrome (seroconversion illness), those within 6 months of HIV seroconversion, and all patients with symptoms credited to HIV infection. In general, treatment should be offered to individuals with fewer than 350 CD_4^+ cells/mm^3 or plasma HIV viral loads exceeding 30,000 copies/mL (bDNA method) or 55,000 copies/mL (PCR method).

Health care providers are beginning to start ART on patients with higher CD_4^+ counts than before. This strategy results in fewer prescribed medications, that are taken less often, and fewer side effects. The U.S. Public Health Service has provided guidelines for health care providers to help with decision making regarding ART. Also, the National Institutes of Health's treatment strategies have helped decrease morbidity and mortality rates for HIV-infected patients (Panel on Antiretroviral Guidelines for Adults and Adolescents, 2008).

Current HIV treatment is aimed at preventing the immune system damage that results from HIV replication. If HIV replication can be halted, then viral mutation can be prevented, and drug resistance issues can be decreased. ART is aimed at limiting viral loads to undetectable levels. With early ART, the patient's CD_4^+ counts will remain normal for a longer time. It is better to start ART when CD_4^+ counts are higher because they will drop less and recover more quickly (Paredes et al., 2000). The recommendation to treat an asymptomatic patient should be based on the patient's willingness and readiness to begin therapy; the degree of existing immunodeficiency as determined by the CD_4^+ cell count; the risk of progression as determined by the CD_4^+ cell count and viral load; the potential benefits and risks of initiating therapy; and the likelihood, after counseling and education, of adherence to the prescribed treatment regimen. Once the decision has been made to begin ART, the goal should be maximal and durable suppression of viral load, restoration or preservation of immunologic function, improvement in quality of life, and reduction of HIV-related morbidity and mortality.

Clinical trials being conducted by the ACTG and the National Institutes of Health in conjunction with universities, pharmaceutical companies, and other agencies may be important considerations for people with HIV disease. Patients may be able to participate in clinical trials or may benefit from the results of such research studies. Benefits include access to new and potentially effective treatments for HIV disease before they are released to the public, and the chance to have physician visits and laboratory work paid for by the research study.

Alternative and Complementary Therapies

People with HIV disease often use nontraditional or complementary therapies, such as massage, acupuncture or acupressure, and biofeedback. Some patients use nutritional supplements or herbal remedies with the hope of alleviating the side effects of the disease and the medications. Many patients prefer these therapies because of the limitations or side effects of approved drugs, mistrust of the health care system, easier access, lack of adequate insurance coverage, or the high cost of anti-HIV medications. These alternatives are best used in conjunction with approved therapeutic intervention.

Encourage patients to use complementary therapies as long as they do not cause undue harm and are not part of quackery medicine, which tends to drain financial resources. Warn patients about unproven drugs and the potential for fraud and quackery in a manner that does not discount their efforts at self-care. Patients may need guidance to avoid expensive and particularly dangerous forms of alternative treatments. However, remember that alternative forms of therapy may be beneficial and should always be thoroughly explored. An open relationship and good communication with the patient build trust, creating a positive atmosphere for addressing difficult issues. They also reinforce the philosophy that the patient is an important member of the health care team.

Vaccine Development

Unfortunately, a vaccine for HIV is not yet available. This is because the virus easily mutates, many different viral strains exist, and poor adherence to ART has led to drug resistance issues. However, with greater understanding of the immune response to HIV and more effective ways to administer antigens, an aggressive push to create a vaccine is currently under way. Since the mid-1980s, many trials of possible vaccines have been performed with thousands of healthy people (WHO, 2006). Almost $700 million each year has been spent on this type of research (International AIDS Vaccine Initiative, 2005). Researchers have taken many approaches: live attenuated vaccinations, live recombinant vaccines, and subunit vaccines. The results have left the researchers surprised and disappointed. One initially promising study involving a vaccine that was supposed to increase cellular immune function (with an adenovirus used in place of HIV) showed that the vaccine offered no protection against HIV and in fact increased viral infection rates (Sekaly, 2008) (see Heath Promotion Box).

NURSING INTERVENTIONS

Establish a comfort level in interacting with people with HIV disease. Treat patients in a nonjudgmental, empathic, and caring manner regardless of their sexual practices or history of drug use. Your attitudes, values,

Health Promotion

Healthy People 2010

OBJECTIVE 13-05: THE NUMBER OF HIV/AIDS CASES THAT ARE NEWLY DIAGNOSED IN ADULTS AND ADOLESCENTS WILL DECREASE.

When obtaining health histories from any client, ask questions regarding safety of sex practices and sexual activities.

- All patients should be assessed for bloodborne pathogen and sexually transmitted disease exposures.
- All patients should be encouraged to know their HIV status.
- All patients should know their partner's HIV status.
- Patients should be educated about sex practices that are "safer."
- Injection drug users should be referred to support groups and rehabilitation programs.
- Patients should be provided with culturally appropriate and age-specific educational resources that promote HIV prevention.
- Seek assistance from community-based groups when disseminating educational resources.
- HIV-infected people should be educated about ways to prevent transmitting the infection by:
  —Avoiding sharing any item that could be contaminated with the patient's blood (razors, toothbrushes, etc.)
  —Not donating any body fluid or tissues
  —Notifying all health care providers about HIV status
  —Cleaning any body fluid that has spilled on an inanimate object with freshly mixed bleach and water solution (10 parts water to 1 part bleach)

OBJECTIVE 21.11: THE PERIOD OF TIME BETWEEN HIV INFECTION AND DEVELOPING AIDS, AND BETWEEN THE DIAGNOSIS OF AIDS AND DEATH, WILL INCREASE.

- Asymptomatic HIV-infected people should continue to receive regular evaluation by health care providers.
- Education must focus on the importance of adhering to antiretroviral therapy.
- HIV-infected people should work to improve the function of their immune system by eating nutrient-dense foods with the appropriate amount of calories and vitamins. Diet should be high in protein and low in fat content. They should reduce stress levels in all areas of life and get adequate amounts of exercise and rest.
- HIV-infected people should practice safer sexual practices to protect themselves and their partners.
- HIV-infected women should not get pregnant.

and beliefs should not interfere with the care of a patient with HIV disease. Patients are aware when their caregiver is not comfortable dealing with HIV disease. Knowledge of HIV transmission and competence in standard precautions and body substance isolation will minimize the fear of caring for HIV-infected patients. Box 56-4, Table 56-9, and Box 56-5 list appropriate nursing assessments, activities, and interventions for HIV infection and disease.

Nursing diagnoses and interventions for the patient with HIV disease include but are not limited to the following:

Nursing Diagnoses	Nursing Interventions
Risk for caregiver role strain, related to advancing disease in care receiver and inadequate caregiver coping patterns	Assess needs and capabilities of patient and caregiver. Assess factors that contribute to caregiver strain. Develop supportive and trusting relationship with caregiver. Enlist the help of family members, significant others, and friends to assist caregiver. Encourage interaction in support groups for caregivers. Teach stress reduction techniques to caregiver. Encourage caregiver to attend to own personal and health care needs.
Diarrhea, related to: • gastrointestinal infections • malabsorption • medication side effects	Document quantity, quality, and frequency of stools. Monitor intake and output, vital signs, and daily weight. Assess for skin impairment. Administer antidiarrheals on a routine schedule. Encourage increased electrolyte-rich fluid intake (fruit juices, Gatorade, Pedialyte). Encourage high-protein, high-calorie, and low-residue diet.

Box 56-4 Nursing Assessment of the Patient with HIV Infection

SUBJECTIVE DATA

Important Health Information

Past health history: Route of infection, risk factors, history of hepatitis or other sexually transmitted infections, frequent viral infections, parasitic infections, tuberculosis, alcohol and drug use, foreign travel

Medications: Use of immunosuppressive drugs

Functional Health Patterns

Health perception–health management: Chronic fatigue, malaise, weakness

Nutritional-metabolic: Unexplained weight loss; low-grade fevers, night sweats; anorexia, nausea, vomiting; oral lesions, bleeding, ulcerations; abdominal cramping; lesions of lips, mouth, tongue, throat; sensitivity to acidic, salty, or spicy foods; problems with teeth or bleeding gums, difficulty swallowing; skin rashes or color changes, lesions (painful or nonpainful), blisters; nonhealing wounds, pruritus

Elimination: Persistent diarrhea, constipation, painful urination

Activity-exercise: Muscle weakness, difficulty with ambulation; cough, shortness of breath

Cognitive-perceptual: Headaches, stiff neck, chest pain, rectal pain, retrosternal pain; blurred vision, photophobia, loss of vision, diplopia; confusion, forgetfulness, attention deficit, changes in mental status, memory loss; hearing impairment, personality changes, paresthesias; hypersensitivity in feet

Sexuality-reproductive: Lesions on genitalia (internal or external), pruritus, or burning in vagina or on penis; painful sexual intercourse; changes in menstruation; vaginal or penile discharge

OBJECTIVE DATA

General: Vital signs, weight, general status, diaphoresis

Eyes: Exudate, retinal lesions or hemorrhage, papilledema, pupillary response, extraocular muscle movements

Oral: A variety of mouth lesions, including blisters (herpes simplex virus–1 lesions), white-gray patches (*Candida* organisms), painless white lesions on lateral aspects of tongue (oral hairy leukoplakia), discolorations (Kaposi's sarcoma), gingivitis, tooth decay or loosening

Neck: Enlarged lymph nodes, nuchal rigidity, enlarged thyroid

Throat: Redness or white patchy lesions

Integumentary: Impaired skin integrity and skin turgor; general appearance; lesions, eruptions, discolorations; enlarged lymph nodes, bruises, cyanosis, dryness, delayed wound healing, alopecia

Respiratory: Crackles or rhonchi, dyspnea, cough (productive or nonproductive, color and amount of sputum), wheezing, tachypnea, intercostal retractions, use of accessory muscles

Lymphatic: Generalized lymphadenopathy

Abdominal: Tenderness, masses, enlarged liver or spleen, hyperactive bowel sounds

Genitourinary-rectal: Lesions or discharge, abdominal pain denoting pelvic inflammatory disease, difficult or painful urination

Neuromuscular: Aphasia, ataxia, lack of coordination, sensory loss, tremors, slurred speech, memory loss, apathy, agitation, social withdrawal or isolation, pain, inappropriate behavior, changes in level of consciousness, depression, seizures, paralysis, coma

Table 56-9 Nursing Activities in HIV Disease

LEVELS OF CARE AND GOALS	ASSESSMENT	INTERVENTIONS
HEALTH PROMOTION AND MAINTENANCE		
Prevention of HIV infection Early detection of HIV infection	Risk factors: What behavioral, social, physical, emotional, pathologic, and immune factors place patient at risk? Does patient need to be tested?	Educate patient, including knowledge, attitudes, and behaviors, with an emphasis on risk reduction to: • General population (cover general information) • Individual patient (specific to assessed need) Empower patient to take control of prevention measures. Provide HIV-antibody testing with pretest and posttest counseling.
ACUTE INTERVENTION		
Promotion of health and limitation of disability Successful management of problems caused by HIV infection	Physical health: Is patient experiencing problems? Mental health status: How is the patient coping? Resources: Does the patient have family and social support? Is patient accessing community services? Is money and insurance a problem? Does patient have access to spiritual support?	Provide case management. Educate regarding HIV, the spectrum of infection, options for care, signs and symptoms to watch for. Educate regarding immune enhancement and harm reduction. Establish long-term, trusting relationship with patient, family, and significant others. Refer to needed resources. Provide emotional and spiritual support. Provide care during acute exacerbations: recognition of life-threatening developments, life support, rapid intervention with treatments and medications, patient and family emotional support during crisis, comfort and hygiene needs. Develop resources for legal needs: discrimination prevention, wills and powers of attorney, child care wishes. Empower patient to identify needs, direct care, seek services.
CHRONIC AND HOME MANAGEMENT		
Maximizing quality of life Resolution of life and death issues	Physical health: Are new symptoms developing? Is patient experiencing drug side effects or interactions? Mental health status: How is patient coping? What adjustments have been made? Finances: Can patient maintain health care and basic standards of living? Family, social, and community supports: Are these supports available? Is patient using supports in an effective manner? Spirituality issues: Does patient desire support from an established religious organization? Are spirituality issues private and personal? What assistance does patient need?	Continue case management. Educate regarding treatment options. Empower patient to continue to direct care and to make desires known to family members and significant others. Continue physical care for chronic disease process: treatments, medications, comfort and hygiene needs. Refer to resources that will assist in meeting identified needs. Promote health maintenance measures. Assist with end-of-life issues: resuscitation orders, funeral plans, estate planning, child care continuation.

Box 56-5 Nursing Interventions for the Patient with HIV Infection or HIV Disease

PREVENT INFECTION
- Wash hands frequently and use skin lubricants for patient and caregiver to prevent skin breakdown.
- Use a gentle liquid soap (such as Castile); avoid bar soaps, which may irritate skin.
- Provide for daily showering or basin bath; avoid tub bath if rashes are present; avoid extremely hot temperatures.
- Use a separate washcloth for lesions.
- Use soft toothbrushes; nonabrasive toothpaste; and mouth rinses with sodium bicarbonate, saline, or lemon and hydrogen peroxide before meals and at bedtime.
- Use measures to prevent skin impairment, such as turning sheets, air mattresses.
- Elevate and support areas of edema.
- Observe biopsy sites and intravenous insertion sites daily for signs of infection.
- Change dressings at least every other day; avoid plastic occlusive dressings.
- Avoid sources of microbes, such as plants or ingestion of uncooked fresh fruits and vegetables.
- Carry out measures to prevent spread of infection: use gloves for contact with bodily secretions, double plastic bags to dispose of bodily secretions, use bleach and water (1:10) for cleaning contaminated areas.

MODIFY ALTERATIONS IN BODY TEMPERATURE
- Administer prescribed antibiotics, intravenous fluids, or antipyretics.
- Encourage fluid intake of more than 2500 mL/day.
- Maintain daily intake and output records.
- Weigh daily.
- Provide tepid sponge baths and linen changes as necessary.
- Instruct patient in deep-breathing and coughing exercises to prevent atelectasis and additional fever.

PROMOTE GOOD NUTRITION
- Provide instruction for high-calorie, high-protein, high-potassium, low-residue diet.
- Encourage high-calorie, high-potassium snacks.
- Suggest foods that are easy to swallow (gelatin, yogurt, puddings) when dysphagia is present.
- Advise patient to avoid foods that are spicy or acidic, rare meats, and raw fruits and vegetables.
- Provide oral care before patient eats.
- Encourage patient to get out of bed and sit up for meals if possible.
- Avoid odors by aerating room.
- Make appropriate dietary consultations.

PROMOTE SELF-CARE
- Assess realistic functional ability.
- Plan, supervise, and assist with activities of daily living as necessary.
- Encourage patient to be as active and independent as possible.
- Assist patient with range-of-motion exercise to prevent contractures.
- Provide equipment such as assistive eating devices, walkers, and commodes to promote patient independence.
- Pace activities and schedule rest periods to prevent fatigue.

PROVIDE COUNSELING
- Assess and support patient coping mechanisms.
- Explore with patient and significant others normalcy of grief.
- Assist patient and significant others in acknowledging and planning for anticipated losses.
- Provide information as desired and necessary, depending on patient's ability to understand.
- Suggest appropriate religious support.
- Facilitate participation in support groups or individual counseling as appropriate.

Health care needs can be unpredictable and assessment difficult because of the clinical diversity of HIV infection. HIV disease may require alternating periods of long-term and acute care. The patient may fear isolation from the community or family and friends because of the social stigma associated with HIV disease.

The disease primarily affects young people who are at the most productive time in their lives, a time when they are expected to take control. For this reason, they often want an active role in the decision-making and planning stages of their care. Patients may experience bouts of serious, debilitating illness, then recover enough to function effectively for an unpredictable amount of time. People with HIV disease often prefer to stay at home as long as possible, and some prefer to die at home. But long-term care in an inpatient setting (e.g., long-term care facility) is not compatible with the social needs of the young patient. Prolonged care is expensive, and many patients with HIV disease do not have health insurance; alternative care is an important consideration. Church and community-based organization volunteers, such as AIDS project workers, provide support and care services for patients and families. Friends, family, and significant others are also important resources to be considered when planning care for the patient with HIV disease.

ADHERENCE

As Dr. Margaret Chesney has noted, with regard to HIV disease, "There is no point in medical history where we have ever expected any patient to adhere to a regimen this complex, as an ambulatory patient, for an indefinite period of time." **Adherence** (following a prescribed regimen of therapy or treatment for disease) to a prescribed regimen is paramount to survival and the success of treatment. The nurse is in a unique position to help patients adapt and maintain vigilance in their treatment. Help patients understand that ART is a lifelong, complex undertaking. The ability to incorporate anti-HIV treatment into a lifestyle is affected by multiple factors, including treatment knowledge or misinformation, underlying psychiatric or psychological pathologic conditions, physical status, family and caregiver support, health care views, socioeconomic status, culture, fear of side effects, denial, and skills (memory, impaired function) necessary to carry out a medical regimen.

Patients with higher level of motivation to take their medications as ordered can have much better outcomes compared with patients who are less compliant. Drug resistance to ART can occur over a weekend of missing doses. Typical adherence to ART is poor even when patients only have to take one or two pills each day. One study performed by the Veterans Administration indicated that only 76% of that population was up to date with their drug refills (Braithwaite et al., 2007).

Strategies to increase adherence include assessing your level of comfort with HIV, learning to listen, having knowledge and skills, giving permission to grieve and feel sad, acknowledging frustration and helplessness, providing a safe environment, and seeking expert assistance as needed. All of these can help patients incorporate this difficult treatment into their lifestyles (Table 56-10).

PALLIATIVE CARE

The WHO defines palliative care as helping patients and families deal with possibly fatal illnesses and quality-of-life issues. Palliative care's focus is on preventing and relieving suffering by quickly identifying and treating pain. Palliative care also focuses on all physical, spiritual, psychological, and social issues that affect the patient or the family (WHO, 2008a).

Palliative care is not seen as hastening the dying process or postponing death. Nurses realize that death is a natural process of life, but others may believe that a patient's death signifies the failure of medicine. The goal of palliative care is to address physical, psychological, social, spiritual, and existential needs of patients with progressive, life-threatening illnesses, with the overall goal of improving the quality of life. Most hospice programs use a palliative care approach, understanding that impending death means a shift from curing to caring. Remember that the goal is to relieve suffering through pain and symptom management at *any* point in the patient's disease process. Not surprisingly, care for dying people in the United States often does not meet the needs or expectations of the patient or family.

Palliative care for the patient with HIV disease is different from the care provided to a patient with a cancer diagnosis. Patients are treated for the chronic debilitating conditions associated with HIV disease, but also for superimposed acute exacerbations of OIs and related symptoms. Intravenous therapy, blood transfusions, and antibiotic usage may be considered palliative in the end stage of HIV disease because these interventions keep the patient comfortable and help maintain quality of life. In AIDS care, short-term aggressive, curative therapy is often important in treating acute infections such as pneumonia, while the overall goal remains palliation.

The complex needs of patients with HIV disease require a multidisciplinary team of physicians, nurses, social workers, dietitians, physical therapists, and clergy. The nurse is the "voice and advocate" for the patient who may or may not be able to communicate his or her treatment desires. Because of this unique role, it is important to be comfortable discussing treatment issues and options with patients, as well as respecting their decisions. Families and significant others of patients with end-stage HIV disease can experience what is called **disenfranchised grief,** which occurs when a loss is not openly acknowledged, publicly mourned, or socially supported (Sherman, 2001). Symptoms such as pain, fatigue, anorexia, fever, shortness of breath, diarrhea, and insomnia are common. Become familiar with the causes and interventions necessary to alleviate these symptoms. Remember that symptoms such as pain are a subjective experience and must be treated appropriately until the patient indicates the treatment has worked. Although this phase of life is difficult for both patient and nurse, many nurses express significant satisfaction with these interactions, relationships, and their outcomes.

As the HIV pandemic has changed over time with health care providers using ART and aggressive approaches to treatment, fewer HIV-infected people are requiring hospice or palliative care. However, some

Table 56-10 Factors Related to Nonadherent Behavior

FACTOR	EXAMPLES
Psychosocial factors	Locus of control Ineffective communication Mental health problems Trust Internal conflict, social stress, stigma Paternalistic behavior of the health care provider
Medications and treatments	Complex regimens Inconvenient dosing schedules Skepticism about treatment effectiveness
Cultural issues	Lack of understanding of cultural influences Differing worldview
Substance use	Continuing substance use Lack of social support Tenuous living arrangements Negative view of addiction

Modified from Crespo-Fierro, M. (1997). Compliance/adherence and care management in HIV disease. *Journal of the Association of Nurses in AIDS Care, 8*(4), 43-54.

patients are not diagnosed with HIV until they are in later stages of the disease process. These patients may choose palliative or hospice care instead of treatment.

PSYCHOSOCIAL ISSUES

People who have been diagnosed with HIV deal with a more complex set of psychosocial issues than people diagnosed with another long-term or fatal disease. Often, they are uncertain, fearful, depressed, and isolated. HIV can be treated, but it is incurable and contagious. Many people feel isolated and abandoned by friends and family because of the stigma associated with HIV. Most patients are diagnosed at an early age and do not have adequate resources to pay for the treatment. When ART is initiated when CD_4^+ counts are over 350 cells/mm^3, the cost of care over an HIV-infected person's life is approximately $620,000. When ART is initiated when CD_4^+ are under 200 cells/mm^3, the cost of care over the patient's lifetime is $567,000 (Schackman et al., 2006). The patient may be struggling with homosexuality and issues related to family acceptance. The patient may be trying to raise a family with limited resources and inadequate emotional support. Some patients are dealing with drug abuse.

Nurses and health care providers must be empathic during contact with these patients. Listening is an important skill to help convey compassion. Use therapeutic communication skills to further develop rapport with this patient. Help the patient plan and decide about health care options. The patient has the right to be supported even when the decision seems imprudent.

Assisting with Coping

Individuals who have been exposed to HIV infection, but who are without any symptoms or complications, live with uncertainty, anxiety, denial, and hopefulness (Box 56-6). The nurse's role in this stage of the disease process is to provide continued education about HIV disease and prevention and to assist in realistic goal setting. Make every effort to include the patient and the support system in planning care. Early in the care process, assess past coping styles and support systems, and continually reevaluate these issues. Encourage healthy patterns of coping, such as talk therapy, relaxation, and meditation. Relationships with family, friends, and significant others should be maintained, and in fact may become stronger during the HIV crisis. However, prior family conflicts amongst family members may get worse due to the stress of the illness. Families with poor communication skills are at particular risk for this outcome.

Box 56-6 Psychological Crisis Intervals in the Course of HIV Disease

- Diagnosis of HIV infection
- Viral load testing
- Increases in viral load
- Initiation of antiretroviral therapy
- Signs of treatment failure
- Adding prophylaxis therapies (e.g., *Pneumocystis jiroveci* [formerly *carinii*] pneumonia)
- Occurrence of opportunistic illnesses
- Change in antiretroviral treatment regimen
- Illness or death in support networks
- New treatment advances

As HIV disease progresses through the clinical complications of infections and cancers, patients experience multiple losses, including the loss of energy; a self-care deficit requiring assistance with ADLs; and the loss of independence, employment, finances, and hope. The reality of death emerges. Nursing interventions should focus on a philosophy of facing life a day at a time and living each day to its fullest. This may be a time for strengthening personal and spiritual relationships and resolving any conflicts.

Anxiety and depression can become chronic, ultimately interfering with daily functioning, relationships, communication, and even the ability to make even simple decisions. Although anxiety and depression are normal with a significant health care threat, refer patients to mental health professionals for possible pharmacologic or verbal counseling when these feelings affect daily functioning for more than 3 months. Assess patients with HIV disease and depression regularly for suicidal ideation, since this phenomenon occasionally occurs in terminally ill patients. Early recognition of depression and anxiety is critical because most cases respond to medications, psychotherapy, or a combination.

Severe anxiety can cause individuals to believe they have no control over the events in their lives. Helping the patient develop a schedule of activities may decrease anxiety and feelings of powerlessness. Explore opportunities for spiritual support and comfort. Community support groups for patients and significant others may contribute to healthy coping. Arrange to spend time with the patient and the support system, in hopes this will decrease anxiety and promote better coping.

Empathic listening and helping patients find meaning in life are critical nursing interventions. Assisting families and significant others in providing support to the terminally ill patient despite their own anger and grief is a unique nursing challenge. Such care, although emotionally draining, can provide great satisfaction.

Minimizing Social Isolation

The psychosocial aspects of HIV infection are devastating. Although it is treatable, no cure exists which promotes denial, fear, depression, and anger (much as a cancer diagnosis does). The social stigma of homosexuality or injection drug use, and the fact HIV is primarily an STI, cannot be underestimated. The first stressful issue a newly diagnosed person must face is disclosure of HIV status. A tremendous fear of family, significant others, and friends reacting with anger, rejection, or abandonment is a real concern. On occasion, families and friends of the newly diagnosed individual have misinformation and unfounded fears. This can result in abandonment, though this is uncommon. Should this occur, assist the patient in identifying other sources of support or refer him or her to a mental health provider familiar with HIV infection. In larger cities, support groups for both patients and significant others can help. HIV-infected individuals who have been exposed through contaminated blood or women with HIV contracted from homosexual or heterosexual spouses may feel anger and hostility. These patients are usually supported by their families and friends, but can be isolated by other people who do not understand that HIV is not unique to MSM.

Assisting with Grieving

Many patients diagnosed with HIV infection benefit simply from listening and exploring in detail the feelings, unfounded fears, and treatment options. On the other hand, many of them need the more structured support found in therapeutic relationships or formal support groups. Significant others and family members also may need assistance to provide support to their loved one. Formal counseling can help a patient address issues such as continued employment, health insurance concerns, preparations for disability, and feelings related to death. Referral to medical or clinical social workers and appropriate community agencies is part of the nurse's responsibility in addressing psychosocial needs. For some patients, referral to clergy is another option for counseling.

CONFIDENTIALITY

Respect for the patient's right to confidentiality is particularly important for the patient with HIV disease. The diagnosis needs to be carefully protected and shared only with caregivers who need to know for the purpose of assessment and treatment.

Do health care providers have a right to know a patient's HIV status? The answer to that depends on the circumstances. If the question is whether a phlebotomist needs to know so he or she can wear two pairs of latex gloves, then the answer is no. But if it concerns whether an oncoming shift nurse needs to know so he or she can develop an appropriate care plan, then the answer is yes. Ancillary personnel such as laboratory or radiograph technicians, dietary personnel, and housekeeping staff generally do not need to know a patient's diagnosis. The use of standard precautions by all staff members for all patients all the time simplifies this issue. Knowing a patient's HIV status merely provides a false sense of security; for every patient who is known to be HIV positive, there are an additional four to seven whose seroconversion status is unknown (perhaps even to the patient).

The patient should be in control of who is told of the diagnosis. Have the utmost respect for the patient's right to confidentiality, meaning ***never*** discuss the patient or the diagnosis at mealtime, during breaks, in the elevator with co-workers, or with friends or family.

DUTY TO TREAT

A nurse's professional obligation to treat patients in need transcends concerns about the patients' diseases or conditions. As infectious disease health care providers note, it is not the known HIV-infected patient who is of concern; the patient whose HIV or infectious status is not known presents the greatest risk. If a nurse's primary concern is personal safety, the nurse needs to reexamine his or her commitment to the profession. The patient with HIV disease can provide valuable lessons in issues related to infectious disease control, the stereotyping of patients, and an understanding of the dedication of health care providers.

ETHICAL AND LEGAL PRINCIPLES

- The Rehabilitation Act of 1973 and the Americans with Disabilities Act (ADA) prohibit discrimination against the handicapped and the disabled. People with HIV infection or AIDS are included under these acts.
- Refusal to treat or care for people who are HIV infected or have AIDS, when that refusal is not based on a medical judgment, is as unethical as discrimination based on race, gender, or other characteristics.
- Health care professionals may not pick and choose their patients, if they are true to their oaths to provide care to all those in need.

ACUTE INTERVENTION

Early intervention after detection of an HIV infection can promote health and limit or delay disability. Because the course of HIV is extremely variable, assessment is of primary importance. Nursing interventions are tailored to any patient needs noted during assessment. The nursing assessment of HIV disease should focus on the early detection of constitutional symptoms, opportunistic diseases, and psychosocial problems (Box 56-7).

HIV disease progression may be delayed by promoting a healthy immune system. Useful interventions for the HIV-infected patient include (1) nutritional changes that maintain lean body mass, increase weight, and ensure appropriate levels of vitamins and micronutrients; (2) elimination of smoking and drug use; (3) elimination or moderation of alcohol intake; (4) regular exercise; (5) stress reduction; (6) avoidance of exposure to new infectious agents; (7) mental health counseling; (8) involvement in support groups; and (9) safer sexual practices.

Teach the patient to recognize clinical manifestations that may indicate progression of the disease; this

Box 56-7 Conducting a Risk Assessment

Risk assessment specific to HIV and sexually transmitted infections (STIs), as well as bloodborne diseases, is crucial in health care delivery today. Perform regular risk assessments on all patients and when evaluating any new patient. Determine sexual and drug use risks along with other risks during routine history taking.

KEY QUESTIONS TO ASK

- Any "yes" responses require further assessment and evaluation
  - —"Have you ever had a blood transfusion? Have you ever received any other kind of blood product? Before 1985?"
  - —"Do you now or have you ever shared injection equipment?"
  - —"Are you now or have you ever been sexually active?"

KEY POINTS TO CONSIDER

- Begin by assuring confidentiality and telling the patient why asking these questions is important:
  - —"I am going to ask some personal questions. I ask all of my patients these questions so I can provide better care. All of your responses will be kept confidential. Is it OK to proceed?"
- Ask direct questions about specific behaviors:
  - —"When was the last time you . . .?"
  - —"How often do you . . .?"
  - —"Have you ever exchanged sex for money or drugs?"
- Exploratory questions may help (especially with adolescents and young adults):
  - —"Do your friends use condoms?"
  - —"What happens at parties?"
  - —"How easy is it to get drugs?"
- Honest responses may be more forthcoming if the behaviors are normalized:
  - —"Some of my patients who use drugs inject them. Do you inject drugs or other substances?"
  - —"Sometimes people have anal intercourse. Have you ever had anal intercourse?"

DRUG USE ASSESSMENT

- It is important to be nonjudgmental and nonmoralistic:
  - —Injection drug use is illegal in the United States and many patients are afraid to be honest unless trust is established.
- Start with less threatening questions:
  - —"What over-the-counter or prescription medications are you taking?"
  - —"How often do you use alcohol? Tobacco?"
  - —"Have you ever used drugs from a nonmedical source?"
  - —"Have you ever injected any kind of drug?"
- Do not assume anything.
  - —Drug use occurs in all socioeconomic strata. Do not forget that people inject substances such as insulin, steroids, and vitamins. Any sharing, even one time, can result in HIV exposure.
- Look for other clues in the history and physical examination, including antisocial behavior, recurrent criminal arrests, and needle tracks.
- If there is a positive history of drug injection use, get more information:
  - —"Do [did] you share needles or other equipment?"
  - —"Is [was] the equipment you use(d) clean? How did you know it was clean?"
  - —"What drugs did you inject?"

SEXUAL RISK ASSESSMENT

- Direct and nonjudgmental questions work best:
  - —"Do you have sex with men, women, or both?"
  - —"Do you have oral sex? Vaginal sex? Anal sex?"
  - —"What do you know about the sexual activities of your partners?"
  - —"What do you do to protect yourself during sex?"
  - —"Do you use condoms? How often?"
  - —"Have you ever had sex with someone you didn't know or just met?"
- Ask for an explanation of sexual practices:
  - —"When you say you had sex, what exactly do you mean?"
  - —"I don't know what you mean; could you explain . . .?"
- Do not assume anything.
  - —Marriage does not always mean an individual is monogamous or heterosexual.
  - —People who identify as homosexual may also have heterosexual sex.
- Use specific terms:
  - —Use "men who have sex with men" or "women who have sex with women" instead of gay.
  - —Some men do not consider themselves "gay" if they practice anal insertive intercourse, but their receptive partners are considered to be gay (can be culturally related).

CLINICAL RISK ASSESSMENT

- Assess the patient for constitutional signs, history of chronic infection and HIV, and associated problems:
  - —Headaches
  - —Diarrhea
  - —Fatigue
  - —Shingles
  - —History of STI, hepatitis, or tuberculosis
  - —Fever, chills, night sweats
  - —Skin lesions
  - —Weight loss
  - —Oral thrush
  - —Generalized lymphadenopathy

Modified from Mountain Plains AIDS Education and Training Center. (2009). *HIV risk assessment, a quick reference guide.* Denver: Author.

will ensure that prompt medical care is initiated. Early manifestations that need to be reported include unexplained weight loss, night sweats, diarrhea, persistent fever, swollen lymph nodes, OHL, oral candidiasis (thrush), and persistent vaginal yeast infections. Additionally, the patient should report unusual headaches, changes in vision, nausea and vomiting, and numbness or tingling in the extremities. Give the patient as much information as needed to make health care decisions. These decisions will dictate the appropriate medical and nursing interventions.

Nursing interventions become more complicated as the patient's immune system deteriorates and new problems arise to compound existing difficulties. The nursing focus should be on quality-of-life issues and symptom management, rather than on issues regarding a cure.

When opportunistic diseases develop, provide symptomatic nursing interventions, education, and emotional support. For example, an acute case of PCP requires intensive nursing interventions, including monitoring the respiratory status, administering medications and oxygen, positioning the patient to facilitate breathing, managing anxiety, promoting nutritional support, and helping the patient conserve energy to decrease oxygen demand. Because advanced HIV disease can lead to death, emotional support for the patient, caregiver, or significant other is particularly important (see Nursing Care Plan 56-1, p. 2004).

Diarrhea is often a long-term problem for HIV-infected people. Damage to the intestinal villi, malabsorption, infections of the gastrointestinal tract, and the side effects of medications all contribute to a large number of patients developing diarrhea. Nursing interventions include recommending dietary interventions (Table 56-11), encouraging adequate fluid intake to prevent dehydration, instructing the patient about skin care, and managing excoriation around the perianal area. In some cases, administer antidiarrheals to help control diarrhea and prevent further complications. Recommend the use of incontinence products to prevent soiling of the clothes and bed linens. In addition, assess for factors that may trigger the diarrhea, such as anxiety, medications, or lactose intolerance.

Wasting and Lipodystrophy Syndromes

AIDS wasting has been a common clinical manifestation of HIV disease since early in the epidemic. Wasting is due to disturbances in metabolism, which interfere with the effective use of nutrients, resulting in the loss of lean (muscle) body mass, often without reduction of body fat. This loss of lean body mass is a primary cause of functional decline in wasting, resulting in increased risk of OIs, reduced quality of life, and reduced survival.

The causes of wasting are most likely multifactorial. Food intake may be inadequate because of mechanical difficulties (e.g., thrush or esophageal ulcers), loss of appetite (e.g., side effect of medications or neurologic disease), or psychological factors such as depression and anxiety. The patient may also have decreased absorption in the intestine due to infections and a damaged mucosal barrier, which may lead to diarrhea. Some patients stop eating to decrease the number of bowel movements per day.

Wasting disturbs self-concept and self-image and can be one of the most difficult consequences of HIV infection to accept. Useful interventions for these disturbances include creating an atmosphere of acceptance and reassurance, encouraging a focus on past accomplishments and personal strengths, and facilitating the use of positive affirmations.

Decreased levels of testosterone have been reported in HIV-infected men. Testosterone has two distinct biologic properties: virilizing activity (androgenic effect) and protein building (anabolic effect). Because testosterone is an anabolic hormone, a deficiency may cause a loss of body cell mass, contributing to HIV wasting. The role of gonadotropic hormones in women with wasting has not been studied sufficiently. Women who are wasted tend to lose a lot of body fat, but body cell mass is not significantly decreased. Conversely, men tend to lose a significant amount of lean body mass (e.g., skinny arms and legs), with preservation of fat, particularly in the truncal area.

With the advances in HIV treatment and OI prophylaxis, serious malnutrition is less evident. However, nutrition does not return to normal after anti-HIV treatment begins. A syndrome of increased truncal obesity (visceral, abdominal), subcutaneous fat loss on the extremities and face (also called lipoatrophy), and metabolic abnormalities such as hyperlipidemia and insulin resistance has been reported in both men and women.

The management of wasting and lipodystrophy is difficult and generally requires multiple nursing interventions. Assess for and document the presence of diminished appetite and weight. Encourage nutritional supplementation (see Table 56-9) and increased protein intake, provide enteral supplements (through nasogastric or gastric tubes if necessary), and assist with total parenteral nutrition when needed. Administering medications to stimulate appetite, such as dronabinol (Marinol), can help. Unfortunately, these medications tend to increase body fat and not lean muscle mass. Testosterone (anabolic steroid) can be administered by mouth, intramuscularly, or transdermally to increase lean body mass and weight. The effect of testosterone can be enhanced by a low-weight resistance-training program (e.g., weightlifting), which maintains muscle tone and improves appetite.

Nutrition counseling is vital to ensure that individuals with HIV disease maintain a well-balanced diet, including supplements if necessary. The dietitian can assist in counseling, provide the patient with high-protein and high-calorie diets, and suggest meal plans

Table 56-11 Nutritional Management: HIV Infection

CONDITION	DIETARY RECOMMENDATION	INTERVENTION
Diarrhea	Lactose-free, low-fat, low-fiber, and high-potassium foods	Avoid dairy products, red meat, margarine, butter, eggs, dried beans, peas, raw fruits and vegetables. Cooked or canned fruits and vegetables provide needed vitamins. Eat potassium-rich foods such as bananas and apricot nectar. Discontinue foods, nutritional supplements, and medications that may make diarrhea worse (Ensure, antacids, stool softeners). Avoid gas-producing foods. Serve warm, not hot, foods. Plan small, frequent meals. Drink plenty of fluids between meals.
Constipation	High-fiber foods	Eat fruits and vegetables (beans, peas), cereal, and whole wheat breads. Gradually increase fiber. Drink plenty of fluids. Exercise.
Nausea and vomiting	Low-fat foods	Avoid dairy products and red meat. Plan small, frequent meals. Prepare nonodorous foods. Eat dry, salty foods. Serve food cold or at room temperature. Drink liquids between meals. Avoid gas-producing, greasy, spicy foods. Eat slowly in a relaxed atmosphere. Rest after meals with head elevated. Take antiemetics 30 minutes before meals.
Candidiasis	Soft or pureed foods	Serve moist foods. Drink plenty of fluids. Avoid acidic and spicy foods. Use straw and tilt head back and forth when drinking. To decrease discomfort, eat soft foods, such as puddings and yogurt.
Fever	High-calorie, high-protein foods	Use nutritional supplements. Increase fluid intake.
Altered taste	Diet as tolerated	Try herbs and spices. Marinate meat, poultry, and fish. Serve food cold or at room temperature. Drink plenty of fluids. Add salt or sugar. Introduce alternative protein sources.
Anemia	High-iron foods	Eat organ meats and raisins. Drink orange juice when taking iron supplements to facilitate absorption.
Fatigue	High-calorie foods	Cook in large quantities and freeze in meal-size packets. Use microwave and convenience foods. Use easy-to-fix snack foods. Use social support system to assist with meal planning and preparation. Access in-home homemaker services and Meals-on-Wheels programs.

that fit the patient's lifestyle. Smaller, more frequent meals can be less overwhelming than larger meals. Of course, teaching about food safety is of paramount concern because enteric infections (e.g., cryptosporidiosis, microsporidiosis, and amebas) in HIV disease are often not treatable or are relapsing. In some cases, enteral or parenteral feeding becomes necessary.

Management of elevated triglycerides and lipids (cholesterol) is becoming common in HIV disease. As in other patient populations, these elevations can lead to cardiovascular disease and, in some cases, diabetes. Lipid-lowering agents such as the statins may be effective in treating this complication. However, because the liver metabolizes many of the antilipid agents, it is important to choose a statin that is safer than those that must pass through the liver to be activated; safer anticholesterol drugs include pravastatin (Pravachol), fluvastatin (Lescol), and possibly atorvastatin (Lipitor). A program of diet, exercise, and medications can safely lower lipids and reduce the chances of a cardiovascular event.

Insulin resistance or diabetes sometimes respond to oral hypoglycemic agents (e.g., metformin or rosiglitazone [Avandia]). In some cases, the anti-HIV therapy needs to be changed to a protease-sparing combination. Managing diet, stopping smoking, losing weight, and exercising can help control the elevated blood glucose that can occur with the use of anti-HIV medications. Studies are being conducted to determine the appropriate interventions for HIV-infected individuals who are experiencing fat redistribution body changes.

Unfortunately, as with any overwhelming viral infection, HIV infection increases the patient's metabolic needs. This hypermetabolism and consequent higher energy expenditure frequently exceed the number of calories taken in by the patient. Malnutrition, weight loss, and generalized wasting are common problems in patients with HIV disease (Nursing Care Plan 56-1). As many as 70% to 90% of patients with HIV disease experience wasting. When a patient's weight is reduced to 60% of his or her ideal body weight, death can occur, regardless of the underlying condition. Malnutrition may influence morbidity and mortality in several ways. Malnutrition contributes to wasting, and wasting hastens the negative immune consequences of HIV infection. HIV wasting contributes to slower recovery from infection, impaired wound healing, increased risk of secondary infection, and decreased cardiac and respiratory function. Thus wasting can lead to an earlier death. The weight loss associated with HIV disease is often severe and debilitating, producing a vicious cycle of anorexia, malnutrition, loss of tissue mass, muscle wasting, profound fatigue, and increased susceptibility to infections and drug interactions. Although typically seen in later stages of HIV disease, malnutrition and wasting can occur in the early stages of HIV infection.

Neurologic Complications

HIV-Associated Cognitive Motor Complex

HIV-associated cognitive motor complex (previously known as AIDS dementia) is the term preferred by the WHO and the American Academy of Neurology to describe a common central nervous system complication of HIV disease. It occurs in 20% to 33% of all adults and as many as 50% of children with end-stage disease (AIDS). This condition is a complex combination of signs and symptoms, including dementia; impaired motor function; and, at times, characteristic behavioral changes that resemble those accompanying a stroke or head trauma. The disease generally does not cause alterations in the level of consciousness or psychiatric disturbances. It is usually described as a triad of cognitive, motor, and behavioral dysfunction that slowly progresses over a period of weeks to months. The cognitive changes primarily involve a mental slowing and inattention. Patients typically lose their train of thought and complain of slowed thinking. They may miss appointments and find themselves making lists of tasks and chores that need completing. The symptoms of motor dysfunction ordinarily develop after those of cognitive impairment. They include poor balance and coordination (e.g., falling and tripping, dropping things); slower hand activities (e.g., writing, eating); and, ultimately, leg weakness that can limit ambulation. The diagnosis of this type of dementia can be made by conducting a simple physical examination, neurologic testing, magnetic resonance imaging and computed tomography examinations, and cerebrospinal fluid analysis.

Nursing interventions for neurocognitive dysfunction include the administration of anti-HIV and psychotropic medications (cautiously). Supervision of the patient, which includes a home safety assessment, is imperative. Ensure that orientation cues such as clocks and calendars are present, hallways and living areas are brightly lit, walkways are clear of electrical cords or throw rugs, and potentially dangerous objects (e.g., knives, poisons) are safely stored.

Caring for patients with dementia is a collaborative effort between the health care provider and family. It is advisable to seek advice from a social worker, the home health care department, and a psychologist in developing a plan to care for an impaired individual.

AIDS-dementia complex (ADC), caused by HIV infection in the brain, is a common neurologic disorder associated with HIV. Dementia symptoms are sometimes reversible if a treatable cause can be diagnosed. Treatable causes include dehydration, depression, and medication toxicity or side effects. Clinical manifestations of ADC include cognitive, behavioral, and motor abnormalities. Symptoms of ADC include decreased ability to concentrate, apathy, depression, social withdrawal, personality changes, confusion, hallucinations, altered levels of consciousness, and slowed response rates. ADC can lead to coma. Nursing interventions are focused on patient safety and caregiver support.

Peripheral Neuropathy

Neuropathies are diseases that affect the peripheral nervous system. They can affect sensory, motor, or autonomic nerves. The causes of neuropathies can be related to HIV disease itself or, more frequently, the side effects of many anti-HIV medications (e.g., stavudine [d4T, Zerit], zalcitabine [ddC, Hivid], and didanosine [ddI, Videx]). Symptoms include numbness, localized tingling, hypesthesia (diminished sensitivity to stimulation) or anesthesia, loss of vibration and position sense (proprioception), and decreased or increased sensitivity to pain. In most cases, patients complain of numbness in the fingers, the hands, and the feet and pain on walking. Patients may also experience autonomic neuropathy. Symptoms such as mild positional hypotension, cardiovascular collapse, and chronic diarrhea suggest autonomic neuropathy.

As new HIV medications with less neurotoxic side effects become available, fewer people are experiencing peripheral neuropathy. Older ART medications caused painful peripheral neuropathy, and people who have taken these medications in the past may develop this problem later.

 Nursing Care Plan 56-1 **The Patient Who Is HIV Positive**

Ms. James is a 20-year-old who comes to the emergency department, accompanied by her mother, with complaints of severe vomiting and recent weight loss of 10 pounds. Ms. James went to the 24-hour clinic and learned that she is approximately 8 weeks pregnant and, because of risk factors for HIV exposure, gave informed consent for HIV antibody testing. The clinic determined that she is HIV positive by ELISA and Western blot testing. Ms. James is tearful and reluctant to answer questions about her recent HIV diagnosis and positive pregnancy test. She states she could not be HIV positive because she has had sexual intercourse only with her boyfriend of 5 years. Additionally, Ms. James is concerned about telling her mother about her HIV status and the pregnancy because she lives with her mother, who is also taking care of her sick elderly grandmother. Ms. James does not have a job and depends on family members to help her meet financial obligations and needs. Ms. James feels the added burden to her mother would "be too much" and is considering leaving home to live in a shelter.

NURSING DIAGNOSIS ***Risk for caregiver role strain, related to advancing disease in care receiver, inadequate caregiver coping pattern***

Patient Goals and Expected Outcomes	Nursing Interventions	Evaluation
Caregiver will use available community and personal resources Caregiver will be able to complete necessary caregiving tasks Caregiver will receive effective support	Assess needs and capabilities of patient and caregiver. Assess factors that contribute to caregiver strain (unrealistic expectations, poor insight, inability to use resources, unsatisfactory relationship with care receiver, insufficient financial and psychosocial resources). Develop supportive and trusting relationship with caregiver. Enlist help of other family members or friends to assist. Teach caregiver to perform care activities in a safe, efficient, and energy-conserving manner. Teach stress-reduction techniques. Encourage caregiver to attend to own personal and health needs.	The caregiver provides safe, supportive care to the HIV-infected patient. The caregiver acknowledges the need for personal support and accesses resources in family and community. The caregiver shares frustrations about difficulty of caring for a significant other. The caregiver receives assistance from family members and/or professional caregivers.

NURSING DIAGNOSIS ***Imbalanced nutrition: less than body requirements, related to chronic infections and/or malabsorption, nausea, vomiting, diarrhea, fatigue, or side effects of medications as evidenced by 10% or greater loss of ideal body mass***

Patient Goals and Expected Outcomes	Nursing Interventions	Evaluation
Patient's weight will remain stable Patient's nutritional intake will exceed metabolic needs Patient will regain lost weight	Assist with diagnosis of underlying opportunistic infections. Assess patient's knowledge of optimal nutritional intake. Increase protein, calorie, and fat intake. Offer nutritional supplements (Carnation Instant Breakfast, Boost, Sustacal, etc.). Schedule procedures that are painful, stressful, or nauseating so they do not interfere with mealtimes. Provide the patient with several small meals throughout the day as opposed to three large meals. Provide referrals to dietitians, social workers, and case managers. Weigh patient daily.	Patient's weight remains stable or increases. Patient reports increased energy level. Patient is able to complete activities of daily living. Patient experiences increase in lean muscle mass.

Critical Thinking Questions

1. Ms. James is tearful and asks the nurse if there is any treatment to prevent her baby from becoming HIV positive. What should be included in the nurse's information to Ms. James?
2. Ms. James asks the nurse if she can legally require her boyfriend to be tested for HIV. What is the most appropriate response?
3. Ms. James asks the nurse when she will develop AIDS now that she is HIV positive. What is the correct answer?

Management of Opportunistic Infections

With the advent of effective ART and better understanding of OI prophylaxis, the frequency of OIs has decreased dramatically. OIs still occur in severely immunocompromised patients, so become familiar with the recognition, treatment, and prophylaxis of these diseases. OIs are typically seen in individuals who are nonadherent to their antiretroviral regimen, nonadherent to OI prophylactic regimens, or at the end stage of HIV disease, and in individuals who do not consistently access the health care system. (See Tables 56-5 and 56-6 for common OIs, treatment, and prevention.)

Health Promotion

Because patients with HIV disease are living longer, more productive lives, attention to the promotion of health and healthy behaviors is important (see Health Promotion box). Encourage patients to eat well-balanced meals, stop or at least reduce the number of cigarettes smoked, get adequate sleep and rest periods if possible, use stress-reduction modalities (e.g., biofeedback, referral for counseling), obtain dental care regularly, and keep scheduled appointments with all health care providers. Attention to comorbid conditions, such as hypertension and diabetes, helps minimize additional health problems. Encourage patients to get all immunizations and keep them up to date; female patients should regularly receive gynecologic care. If hospitalizations are necessary, encourage the patient and the significant other(s) to participate in treatment decision making, and arrange for home care follow-up if indicated.

Although some pets can pose risks for transmission of OIs, they are, overall, therapeutic for the patient and healing. Only minor modifications need to be made for pet-owning HIV-infected people (e.g., birdcage and cat litter box cleaning). If possible, arrange pet visits to the hospital or care facility if a long separation is anticipated; do not dismiss the idea of benefit because this practice is not acceptable at your health care facility. Speak with managers and supervisors to obtain permission, or help develop policies and procedures that allow the visitation of pets.

> **Health Promotion**
>
> **The Patient Infected with HIV**
>
> - Remind patients that a positive diagnosis is not an immediate "death sentence." Patients are living increasingly longer after diagnosis because of medications, more specialized care, and decreased morbidity and mortality related to opportunistic diseases.
> - Stress the importance of health-promoting behaviors to reduce the risk of comorbidity.
> - Encourage patients to maintain good nutritional status by eating regular, well-balanced meals that are high in protein and calories. Increased protein is necessary for cell and tissue repair, especially in patients who may be hypermetabolic.
> - Encourage patients to limit their intake of alcoholic beverages and avoid the use of illicit or recreational drugs.
> - Encourage patients to maintain an adequate sleep schedule.
> - Encourage patients to use stress-reduction practices, such as biofeedback, massage, or progressive relaxation. They should also engage in relaxing or pleasurable activities.
> - Advise patients to use safer sexual practices to avoid reinfection and exposure to other sexually transmitted infections.
> - Encourage patients to establish an exercise regimen that includes aerobic activity as well as low-resistance weightlifting if possible.
> - Most important, support patients in setting short- and long-term goals and assist them in achieving those goals.

PREVENTION OF HIV INFECTION

HIV disease is **preventable.** However, prevention takes the cooperation and efforts of public health care providers, medical providers, nurses in all specialties, families, communities, churches, and schools (Box 56-8). Education on prevention is the only truly effective "vaccine" available to curb the HIV pandemic. Many patients admitted to acute care facilities have unrecognized HIV disease or are at risk for HIV infection. Assess each patient's risk and counsel those at risk about HIV testing, the behaviors that put them at risk, and how to reduce or eliminate those risks. Today, every nurse is an HIV nurse, meaning that all nurses are responsible for teaching patients methods to reduce the risk of transmission. Nurses must be able to discuss behaviors related to sexual activity and substance use in a nonjudgmental way (e.g., condom application, using clean "works"). Establish rapport with patients before asking sensitive, explicit questions related to behaviors typically not discussed.

Harm-reduction education is a fundamental element of HIV prevention methods. Harm reduction does not completely eliminate the risk of HIV transmission, but it minimizes the social harms and costs associated with certain behaviors. For example, asking patients to quit smoking two packs of cigarettes per day all at once almost always results in failure. With a harm-reduction approach, suggest that the patient reduce the number of cigarettes smoked from 40 to 30 a day. Although the ultimate goal is for the patient to stop smoking altogether, the patient has at least reduced the risk of long-term effects by limiting the number of cigarettes smoked. The same is true for HIV prevention. Encouraging patients to use protective barriers 50% of the time (although not ideal) still results in a reduced risk of HIV transmission.

HIV TESTING AND COUNSELING

An important part of preventing HIV transmission is HIV screening tests and follow-up education and counseling (see Box 56-3). However, do not coerce patients into having an HIV screening test. The process of helping patients make the decision about whether to undergo testing and how to be tested is called **test**

Box 56-8 Prevention Options

SEXUAL

No Risk

- Abstinence from sexual contact in which there is exchange of semen, vaginal secretions, or blood.
- Partners who are in a mutually monogamous (the state of having one mate) relationship in which neither partner is at risk of infection through injecting drug use, and in which neither partner was previously exposed to HIV.

Reduced Risk

- Limiting the number of partners, even though a potential risk exists if there was sexual contact with only one infected partner.
- Protective measures through consistent and correct use of latex condoms with a spermicide in every act of sexual intercourse in which there would be exchange of semen, vaginal secretions, or blood. The correct use of condoms is as follows:
  —Put on the condom as soon as erection occurs and before any sexual contact (anal, vaginal, oral).
  —Leave space at the tip of the condom.
  —Use only water-based lubricants.
  —Hold the condom firmly to keep it from slipping off; withdraw from partner immediately after ejaculation.

INJECTING DRUG USE

No Risk

- Stop the use of injectable drugs. Provide drug treatment opportunities.
- If drugs are going to be injected, use sterile needles and equipment.

Reduced Risk

- If needles and equipment are going to be shared, follow instructions on cleaning.
- Fill the syringe with sodium hypochlorite 5.25% (Clorox) bleach two times; empty two times. Fill the syringe with clean water two times; empty two times.

PERINATAL

No Risk

- Avoidance of pregnancy is the only certain way to prevent transmission of HIV to a fetus or infant.
- Counsel a woman of childbearing age of unknown HIV status about behaviors that would put her and her partner or spouse at risk for HIV infection. If risk factors are determined in either case, counsel both individuals about testing for HIV.

Reduced Risk

- Adherence to barrier birth control measures, including use of condoms, to avoid pregnancy.
- Use of antiretroviral therapy given during pregnancy and to infant for first 6 weeks of life.

decision counseling. Nurses and health care providers should counsel their patients before and after HIV testing. HIV tests require informed consent per state law before drawing blood. The informed consent is always accompanied by an explanation about the testing and implications of results. Also explain the limitations of the test.

HIV testing that is performed early in the disease is important for increasing survival rates of HIV-infected patients and preventing the transmission to others through high-risk behaviors. The U.S. Public Health Service published guidelines in 1987 regarding testing for people who were at high risk for becoming infected with HIV. Guidelines from the CDC in 2006 mandated that all patients in health care agencies be informed about HIV screening and then screened for HIV. However, these patients are allowed to refuse the test. Offer HIV antibody testing to all patients, regardless of patient-specific risk factors. Also, test results should be made available rapidly to the patient so education could be given to the patient, if needed. The CDC's recommendations state that informed consent is not needed. However, patients may opt out of testing if they wish. In rare emergency situations where health care providers need to know a patient's HIV status to make a decision regarding health care and the patient is unable to speak, the patient may be tested without his or her consent.

More people with HIV can be identified with the current push for routine HIV screening. The FDA approved the use of ELISA for routine use during blood bank screenings. ELISA can identify antibodies for HIV-1 and HIV-2. Researchers who recently performed a study in Cameroon found that ELISA was highly sensitive even with wide variations in the genetic makeup of the HIV (Lee et al., 2007). The FDA has approved four rapid tests for HIV. Multispot and Oraquick can detect HIV-1 and HIV-2. Uni-Gold Recombigen and Reveal can only identify HIV-1 (Greenwald et al., 2006). These four tests are not yet available without a physician's order.

HIV antibody testing may take place in a physician's office or at designated HIV counseling and testing sites. Many patients feel more comfortable being tested by someone who knows their medical and social history, but others prefer to be tested in a location where they are unknown. Be aware of the various options for HIV antibody testing in your state or community in order to advise patients appropriately.

HIV antibody testing can be done one of two ways: confidentially or anonymously. In **confidential testing,** patients provide identifying information, including a name; an address; and often demographic information such as age, sex, race, and occupation. Using this information, care providers can locate and provide information to an individual who does not return for the test results or counseling. All records are strictly confidential, and testing in physicians' offices, clinics, and hospitals is conducted in a confidential manner. Health care providers who share or use this information inappropriately can be sued for negligence and invasion of privacy, and they may be disciplined by licensing boards for unauthorized disclosure or breach of confidentiality. Inform patients that the results of their HIV antibody test will be linked to the patient's medical record.

In **anonymous testing,** individuals are not asked to provide identifying information. Records are kept through assigned numbers, and the patient must retain this number to receive test results. It is not possible to locate and provide information to an individual who does not return for test results and counseling. In either form of testing, the nurse can perform pretest and posttest counseling.

RISK ASSESSMENT AND RISK REDUCTION

Testing for HIV is an important part of the public health response to HIV disease. Risk assessment should be patient centered, a joint process between the nurse and patient. The patient should take "ownership" of the risk for HIV infection. Assess patients for indications of risky behaviors, such as STIs. However, a patient will not get tested unless he or she perceives a need for testing and feels safe doing so. Help the patient assess the risks by asking some basic questions:

- Have you ever had a transfusion or used clotting factors? Was it before 1985?
- Have you ever shared needles, syringes, or other injecting equipment with anyone?
- Have you ever had a sexual experience in which your penis, vagina, rectum, or mouth came into contact with another person's penis, vagina, rectum, or mouth?

A positive response to any of the above questions requires further exploration with the patient. Be prepared to refer the patient to centers that provide testing and counseling services. All testing should include pretest and posttest counseling (see Boxes 56-3 and 56-7).

HIV infection in women has been frequently overlooked for several reasons. In the United States, the disease initially occurred mostly in men, and treatment models were developed accordingly. Providers did not assess the risks for women, and women did not seek testing and counseling because of denial or ignorance; thus interventions have not been implemented effectively. Heterosexual transmission of HIV in women surpassed injecting drug use as a vector for HIV transmission in the second decade of this pandemic and globally continues to be the highest risk factor in women (Dole, 2001). The 1993 CDC case definition includes at least one female-specific disease: cervical carcinoma. Women now need to be assessed for different manifestations, such as vaginal candidiasis, a common presenting condition for HIV-positive women.

BARRIERS TO PREVENTION

HIV prevention has numerous barriers, not the least of which is a denial of risk, an attitude that "it won't happen to me." Because the virus initially infected the MSM population in the United States, many other subpopulations have ignored their risks. Fear, misunderstanding, and the potential for social isolation and social stigma are significant barriers. Some individuals are so fearful that they no longer give blood or eat at a restaurant if they think a homosexual food handler works there. Such reactions reinforce the need for consistent, accurate information about the virus, the risks of transmission, and HIV disease itself.

Cultural and community attitudes, values, and norms can affect the success of prevention efforts. A community may be opposed to HIV/AIDS education in the local school district because of the fear that values will be compromised. Those values may include views on sexuality, abstinence, the use of condoms, the use of drugs, and the provision of instructions on cleaning needles and syringes. Community organizations, churches, educators, and leaders can determine the community's expectations or norms. Cooperative efforts are essential for successful prevention of HIV transmission. The issues related to the HIV epidemic—sex, drug use, death, and homosexuality—are not easy issues for most cultures or communities.

Fear of alienation and discrimination are significant additional barriers to prevention. In some cases, individuals are reluctant to even pick up a pamphlet about HIV because they fear someone will believe they are gay or using illicit drugs. Some people will not go to a physician or to a testing and counseling site for HIV testing for fear of being seen. This fear is very real, particularly in rural parts of the country. Fear of discrimination includes fear of losing family, friends, prestige, job, housing, and insurance. Fortunately, many states have statutes to protect individuals with HIV disease from discrimination. Protection is also afforded by the ADA.

REDUCING RISKS RELATED TO SEXUAL TRANSMISSION

When patients have acute HIV and high viral loads, they are 10 times more likely to transmit HIV during sexual intercourse than during the chronic stage of HIV. Infection risk is also increased when sex is forceful or mucosal membranes are disrupted (often associated with STIs). Most HIV infections are transmitted during the primary stage of the infection. This is when most people are unaware of their infection because they are asymptomatic. Men are less likely to be infected with HIV during heterosexual intercourse than women. Women have more mucosal surface that can be exposed to infected body fluids when compared to men (National Institute of Allergy and Infectious Diseases, 2006). Male circumcision can also minimize a male's risk of becoming infected with HIV via heterosexual intercourse, according to the WHO (2009a).

Safer sexual activities reduce the risk of exposure to HIV through semen and cervicovaginal secretions. Abstaining from all sexual activity is the most effective way to accomplish this goal. Limiting sexual behavior to activities in which the mouth, penis, vagina, or rectum do not come into contact with the partner's mouth, penis, vagina, or rectum is also safe, since there is no contact with blood, semen, or cervicovaginal secretions. These activities may include massage, masturbation, mutual masturbation, telephone or cyber sex, and many other activities. Insertive sex is considered safe only in a mutually monogamous relationship with a partner who is not infected with, or at risk of becoming infected with, HIV. The problem with mutual monogamy is that both partners need to follow all of the rules all of the time. Unfortunately, cases of HIV infection occur in individuals who are not aware that their partner has not remained monogamous. Serial monogamy (maintaining a monogamous relationship, often including unprotected intercourse, with one partner for a short time, followed by another relationship, and then another) still presents an increased risk of HIV exposure (Box 56-9).

ART can be provided to people who have been exposed to HIV through unwanted sexual intercourse (rape) or via injecting drugs. The U.S. Department of Health and Human Services has developed some recommendations regarding these types of nonoccupational exposures. When a person has been exposed to body fluids from an HIV-infected person during high-risk activity less than 72 hours before seeking treatment, the exposed person should receive a 28-day supply of HAART. This is recommended even if the HIV-infected source of the exposure has a viral load that is undetected. However, if the activity is deemed to be low-risk exposure to body fluids, or if the exposed person seeks health care after the 72-hour window, ART is not recommended. Examine cases on an individual basis to determine the need for PEP, counseling, treatment, and education about preventing future exposures (CDC, 2005a).

The use of barriers reduces the risk of contact with HIV during sexual activity. Barriers should be used when engaging in sexual activity with a partner whose HIV status is not definitely known or with a partner who is known to be infected with HIV. The most commonly used barrier is the male condom. Although not 100% effective, when used correctly and consistently, male condoms are very effective in the prevention of HIV transmission. Other barriers include female condoms and latex dental dams. Female condoms consist of a vinyl sheath with two spring-form rings. The smaller ring is inserted into the vagina and holds the condom in place internally. The larger ring surrounds the opening to the condom. It keeps the condom in place externally while also protecting the external genitalia. The use of the female condom is complicated and cumbersome, and practice may be necessary to use this method effectively. Female condoms can also be used for anal sex, in both men and women. Dental dams or microwave-safe plastic wrap can be used to cover the external genitalia or anus during oral sexual activity ("rimming"). Although the risk of HIV transmission is significantly reduced with the use of latex

Box 56-9 Risk of HIV Transmission Associated with Sexual Practices

HIGH RISK (IN DESCENDING ORDER OF RISK)
- Receptive anal intercourse with ejaculation (no condom)
- Receptive vaginal intercourse with ejaculation (no condom)
- Insertive anal intercourse (no condom)
- Insertive vaginal intercourse (no condom)
- Receptive anal intercourse with withdrawal before ejaculation
- Insertive anal intercourse with withdrawal before ejaculation
- Receptive vaginal intercourse (with spermicidal foam, no condom)
- Insertive vaginal intercourse (with spermicidal foam, no condom)
- Receptive anal or vaginal intercourse (with a condom)*
- Insertive anal or vaginal intercourse (with a condom)*

SOME RISK (IN DESCENDING ORDER OF RISK)
- Oral sex with men with ejaculation
- Oral sex with women
- Oral sex with men with preejaculate fluid (precum)
- Oral sex with men, no ejaculation or precum
- Oral sex with men (with a condom)

NO RISK
- Masturbating with another person without touching one another
- Hugging, massage, dry kissing, frottage (rubbing against each other)
- Masturbating alone
- Abstinence

UNRESOLVED ISSUES
- The role of preejaculate in transmission
- The protection offered by covering female genitalia with a dental dam during oral sex
- The risk of transmission with wet kissing (French kissing) (though unlikely)

Modified from Schram, N.R. (1990). Redefining safer sex, *Focus 5*(7):3. In D.E. Grimes & R.M. Grimes (1994). *AIDS and HIV infection.* St. Louis: Mosby.
*Risk lower if no ejaculation and/or spermicidal foam used.

barriers, other STIs, such as human papillomavirus, warts, and HSV, can still be transmitted.

REDUCING RISKS RELATED TO DRUG ABUSE

The use of illicit or recreational drugs can cause immunosuppression, malnutrition, and emotional difficulties. Although using illicit drugs can increase one's risk for acquiring an HIV infection, drug use itself is not to blame. The major risks of HIV transmission are related to sharing injecting equipment and having unsafe sexual experiences while under the influence of mood-altering chemicals. Essentially, one can reduce the risk of HIV infection by not using drugs. If drugs are injected, equipment should not be shared with others. Sexual activity should not be engaged in while under the influence of any drug, including alcohol, that impairs decision making.

Abstaining from drugs is not always a viable option for a user who has no access to drug treatment services or chooses not to quit. The risk of HIV for these individuals can be eliminated if they can find alternatives to injecting, such as smoking, snorting, or ingesting drugs. Risk can also be eliminated if the user does not share injecting equipment, including needles, syringes, cookers, cotton, and rinse water. The safest tactic is for the user to have ready access to sterile equipment. Many states have laws that prohibit over-the-counter sale of needles and syringes, such as diabetic supplies. Some communities have needle exchange programs that supply sterile equipment to users to help reduce the risk of HIV transmission. The fear that needle exchange programs will result in increased illicit substance use has led to a lack of community support. However, studies have shown that in communities where exchange programs have been established, drug use does not increase and rates of HIV infection are controlled (Wodak & Cooney, 2006).

Cleaning the equipment before use decreases the risk for those who must share equipment, particularly in "shooting galleries." To clean the equipment, rinse used needles and syringes twice with tap water (using fresh tap water each time). Then fill syringes with full-strength household bleach, shake for 30 seconds, and squirt clean; repeat the bleaching process. Then rinse the equipment twice with tap water. This process takes time and may be difficult for a person experiencing drug withdrawal and in need of drugs.

REDUCING RISKS RELATED TO OCCUPATIONAL EXPOSURE

As previously discussed, the risk of acquiring HIV through occupational exposure is low. The CDC and Occupational Safety and Health Administration have instituted policies to protect employees from exposure to blood and other potentially infectious fluids (CDC, 2005b). The use of standard precautions and body substance isolation has been shown to reduce the risk of bloodborne pathogens, the risk of transmission of other diseases between the patient and the health care worker, and the risk of transmission between patients. Hand hygiene in the form of handwashing still remains the single most effective means of preventing the spread of infection.

Epidemiologic and laboratory studies suggest that several factors might affect the risk of HIV transmission after an occupational exposure. In a retrospective study conducted by the CDC of health care workers who had percutaneous exposure to HIV, the risk of HIV infection was found to be increased with exposure to a larger quantity of blood from the source patient as indicated by (1) a device visibly contaminated with the patient's blood, (2) a procedure that involved a needle being placed directly in a vein or artery, or (3) a deep injury. The risk is also increased for exposure to blood from a patient with terminal illness, possibly reflecting the higher viral load of the patient late in the course of HIV disease (CDC, 2001). Information about primary HIV infection (seroconversion) indicates that a systemic infection does not occur immediately. This leaves a brief window of opportunity during which initiation of antiretroviral PEP might prevent or inhibit systemic infection by limiting the proliferation of the virus in the initial target cells or lymph nodes.

For best prophylactic effect, PEP must be initiated within 36 hours—but preferably **within 1 to 4 hours**—of the exposure. Depending on the type of exposure and many other variables, either a two- or three-drug regimen is chosen (CDC, 2005a, b). In addition to possible exposure to an antiretroviral-resistant strain of HIV, other factors that might contribute to failures include a high titer or large volume of inoculum exposure, delayed initiation or short duration of PEP, and factors related to the exposed health care personnel (e.g., immune status).

Completion of a 4-week course of therapy after an occupational exposure is fundamental. The medications used have many side effects, and health care workers may stop PEP prematurely because of these. It is important to consult with experts in occupational exposure if side effects (headache, nausea, vomiting, diarrhea) become unbearable. The use of PEP regimens has been associated with new-onset diabetes mellitus, hyperglycemia, hypertriglyceridemia, pancreatitis, elevated lipids (cholesterol, low-density lipoproteins), and kidney stones. Despite these serious side effects, the exposed health care worker must continue therapy for 4 weeks, or until it is determined that the source patient is not HIV infected.

Hospitals or agencies should have policies that specifically address occupational HIV exposure, since chemoprophylaxis needs to occur immediately—even before testing the source patient's and health care worker's blood for HIV or other bloodborne pathogens. Serial testing of the health care worker for HIV occurs at baseline, 6 weeks, 3 months, and 6 months after the exposure.

Maintaining confidentiality for both the exposed health care worker and the source patient is of utmost importance. Many states and health care organizations have separate, distinct consent forms that are required before HIV antibody testing can be performed. Only in rare circumstances, such as the inability to give consent, can HIV antibody testing be completed without the patient's informed consent. Many ethical and legal issues surround HIV antibody testing, so be informed of the applicable laws in the state in which you practice. In many states, charges of assault and battery can be brought against health care workers who perform HIV testing against a patient's will. Appropriate counseling and referrals should be made for the health care worker and patient when HIV testing is indicated.

OTHER METHODS TO REDUCE RISK

Instruct HIV-infected people not to give blood, donate organs, or donate semen for artificial insemination. They should not share razors, toothbrushes, or other household items that may contain blood or other body fluids. They should also avoid infecting sexual and needle-sharing partners, consider using birth control measures, and eliminate breastfeeding to avoid spreading the virus to infants.

OUTLOOK FOR THE FUTURE

As we enter the third decade of the HIV pandemic, much has been learned about transmission of the virus and ways to prevent infection. With no cure in sight, prevention of infection through education, prevention of mother-to-child transmission, and in some cases PEP or preexposure prophylaxis can limit the effect this disease has on the human population.

The dynamics of the pandemic have changed dramatically as well. In the United States, HIV has the characteristics of any other chronic illness, in that it (1) has no cure, (2) continues throughout the patient's life, (3) causes increasing physical disability and dysfunction if not treated, and (4) ultimately results in significant morbidity and mortality. Chronic diseases are characterized by acute exacerbations of cyclic problems that compound each other. Despite a significant decrease in the number of OIs, new complications have emerged. Health care providers today must address body composition changes, cardiac disease, neuropathies, and the long-term effects of the very medications that have kept HIV at bay.

Since the discovery of HIV, significant advances have occurred in knowledge about the viral cycle, resulting immune response, and disease progression of HIV. New medication treatments are very effective and can help the host manage the disease by limiting replication of the virus. This can allow the immune system to continue to function. Survival rates of patients who have been diagnosed with late-stage HIV (and have access to HAART and are being cared for by health care providers with expertise in dealing with HIV) has increased dramatically. Patients who previously would have become disabled, quit jobs, and tended to end-of-life decisions are now reevaluating goals, returning to work, and rediscovering relative health. Now, couples who are serodiscordant have the option of having children with the use of sperm "washing" and in vitro fertilization.

In no other disease has there been such a rapid understanding and attempts at developing therapies as with HIV infection The HIV research arena has provided insight into other diseases and scientific fields, including virology, immunology, and oncology. At this point, though, scientists' ability to develop new therapies depends on the individual being nearly 100% adherent to regimens that are sometimes quite toxic. Adherence is poor even when therapy consists of only one pill per day. Even though treatment options for HIV have advanced, there is still a wide variation in disease progression. As research continues, it will be interesting to determine how psychological and social stressors alter immune system responses.

HIV has become a disease whose face is represented by women and people of color. Underdeveloped countries in Africa and Southeast Asia have been hardest hit; in fact, many villages have been destroyed because of HIV. The global threat of HIV is enormous, with nurses playing a key role in the care and treatment of HIV-infected individuals. For the best possible outcomes, always seek guidance from HIV specialists when treating an individual with HIV disease because the care is very complex, and multiple needs arise.

The field of HIV and AIDS nursing changes frequently, and nurses must constantly refresh their base of knowledge. Resources include local AIDS service organizations and state and regional AIDS education and training centers. As new therapies emerge, the nurse is in a unique position to educate patients and the public regarding what is undoubtedly the most challenging infectious disease discovered in the twentieth century.

Get Ready for the NCLEX® Examination!

Key Points

- HIV, a retrovirus, is the agent that causes HIV disease and AIDS.
- Education on prevention is the only "vaccine" for preventing HIV disease and AIDS.
- Women and people of color constitute the fastest-growing segment of the population with HIV disease.
- AIDS is the end stage of HIV infection.
- When HIV enters the body, its primary target is the immune system.
- HIV is transmitted by three major routes: (1) anal and vaginal intercourse, (2) injecting drugs with contaminated needles or works, and (3) from infected mother to child.
- Blood, semen, vaginal secretions, and breast milk are the body fluids that most readily transmit HIV.
- Assess each patient's risks for HIV infection and counsel those at risk about testing, behaviors that put them at risk, and how to eliminate or reduce those risks.
- A positive HIV antibody test does not mean the patient has AIDS.
- A multidisciplinary care approach in which the patient is a primary member of the team is the most appropriate method of caring for patients with HIV disease because of their complex needs.
- As HIV infection progresses, the immune system loses its ability to fight infectious agents and cancer cells.
- Encourage patients at risk for HIV infection to know their HIV status.
- Whether or not signs and symptoms are present, a person infected with HIV virus can transmit the virus.
- Barriers to HIV prevention include denial, fear, misinformation, and cultural and community norms.
- CD_4^+ counts are important markers of disease progression and the status of the immune system.
- The stigma of HIV disease, because of its association with drug use, homosexuality, and sexual transmission, is a major concern.
- The 1993 expanded case definition of AIDS includes all HIV-infected people who have CD_4^+ T-lymphocyte counts of less than 200 cells/mm^3; includes all people who have one or more of three clinical conditions (pulmonary tuberculosis, recurrent pneumonia, or invasive cervical cancer); and retains the 23 clinical conditions listed in the 1987 AIDS case definition.
- Measuring viral load in the blood assesses effectiveness of therapy and possibly adherence.
- Adherence to medications is essential.

Additional Learning Resources

Go to your free Companion CD for an audio glossary, animations, video clips, and more

evolve Be sure to visit the companion Evolve site at http://evolve.elsevier.com/Christensen/adult/ for additional online resources.

Review Questions for the NCLEX® Examination

1. The virus responsible for causing the majority of HIV disease and AIDS is:

1. human immunodeficiency virus type 1.
2. human immunodeficiency virus type 2.
3. African immunodeficiency virus type 1.
4. *Pneumocystis jiroveci* (formerly *carinii*) deficiency virus.

2. Vertical transmission of HIV occurs from:

1. male to female.
2. female to male.
3. father to child.
4. mother to child.

3. The nurse is assessing a patient who has requested HIV testing. What would be considered to be the most risky behavior?

1. Dry kissing a casual date
2. Sharing a soda with an infected person
3. Swimming with an infected person
4. Having more than three sex partners in a year

4. What would be the most likely route of transmission of HIV?

1. From infected female to noninfected male
2. From infected male to noninfected female
3. From infected father to child
4. From infected mother to child

5. An 8-year-old is diagnosed with hemophilia. His mother is upset about the risk of her son acquiring HIV from blood products. What would be the nurse's best response?

1. "All blood and blood products are screened for bloodborne diseases, so it is impossible for J. to be infected."
2. "Many blood products are treated with heat or chemicals to inactivate the HIV virus."
3. "We can talk about this if the patient requires transfusions or blood products."
4. "All blood donors are asked about HIV status and risk factors before giving blood."

6. The storage area in which HIV reproduces in the human body is:

1. lymph glands.
2. muscle tissues.
3. bone marrow.
4. B cells.

7. A 34-year-old patient comes to the clinic requesting HIV testing. He is a gay man with two significant others in his lifetime. His lover was recently diagnosed with HIV. The patient asks the nurse how long it will take before the infection will show up in him. The best response would be:
   1. "Antibodies usually are detected in the blood within 4 to 12 weeks of exposure."
   2. "It takes at least a year to know if you will be infected with HIV."
   3. "You'll have to ask your doctor the next time you go in for an appointment."
   4. "We don't know how long it will take to seroconvert to being HIV positive."

8. The patient is concerned that he may be infected with HIV. Which symptom would alert the nurse to further assess the patient?
   1. Night sweats
   2. Rash on the legs only
   3. Constipation
   4. Pruritus

9. The HIV factory of the human body is:
   1. infected CD_4^+ cells.
   2. infected macrophages.
   3. infected sweat glands.
   4. infected parotid glands.

10. The patient is diagnosed with symptomatic HIV disease. The nurse would assess her regarding which of the following?
    1. T-cell count greater than 800/mm^3
    2. WBC greater than 20,000/mL
    3. Thrush
    4. Weight gain

11. Which diagnostic procedure is used to confirm a diagnosis of AIDS?
    1. ELISA test
    2. CD_4^+ counts
    3. B-cell count
    4. Western blot test

12. The patient is diagnosed with HIV disease. She visits the physician today for her prescriptions. The nurse would expect the physician to order:
    1. tenofovir and emtricitabine (Truvada).
    2. efavirenz (Sustiva).
    3. lopinavir and ritonavir (Kaletra).
    4. combination of these drugs.

13. The nurse should instruct the patient with HIV to follow which diet?
    1. High calorie, high fiber, low protein
    2. Low calorie, low fiber, high protein
    3. High calorie, high protein, low residue
    4. Low calorie, high fiber, high protein

14. The progression of HIV disease is predictable in all patients. True or False?

15. HIV disease is diagnosed when the CD_4^+ cell count is 200 cells/mm^3 or fewer. True or False?

16. HIV disease in men who have sex with men is decreasing. True or False?

17. Ninety-nine percent seroconversion of exposed individuals occurs within 6 months of the exposure. True or False?

18. An HIV-infected person may appear to be healthy. True or False?

19. It is not possible to become infected with HIV after one unprotected sexual encounter. True or False?

20. Most of the children infected with the HIV virus were infected during pregnancy. True or False?

21. The most common opportunistic infection and malignant neoplasm in the patient with advanced HIV disease (AIDS) are:
    1. streptococcal pneumonitis, myeloma.
    2. *Pneumocystis jiroveci* (formerly *carinii*) pneumonia, Kaposi's sarcoma.
    3. *Streptococcus pneumoniae,* malignant melanoma.
    4. *Mycoplasma,* pneumonitis, Kaposi's sarcoma.

22. For most people who are HIV positive, marker antibodies are usually present 10 to 12 weeks after exposure. The development of these antibodies is called:
    1. immunocompetence.
    2. seroconversion.
    3. immunodeficient.
    4. viral load.

23. The expanded definition for AIDS is that the person will:
    1. have the HIV virus present.
    2. have a dysfunction of the immune system and be HIV positive.
    3. be HIV positive and have an opportunistic disease.
    4. be HIV positive with CD_4^+ lymphocyte count less than 200/mm^3.

24. "Why should I use condoms? They don't work," retorts a young gay patient being treated for his third sexually transmitted infection. The nurse's most appropriate response would be:
    1. "Condoms may not provide 100% protection, but when used correctly and consistently with every act of sexual intercourse, they reduce your risk of getting infected with HIV or other sexually transmitted infections."
    2. "You are correct: condoms don't always work. So your best protection is to limit your number of partners."
    3. "Condoms do not provide 100% protection, so you should always discuss with your sexual partners their HIV status or ask if they have any STIs."
    4. "Condoms do not provide 100% protection, but when used with a spermicide, you can be assured of complete protection against HIV and other STIs."

25. The patient has been advised to be tested for HIV because of multiple sexual partners and intravenous illicit drug use. The nurse should make certain that the patient understands the test by informing him that:

1. the blood is tested with the highly sensitive test called the Western blot, then with ELISA.
2. the blood is tested with ELISA; if positive, it is tested again with ELISA and then the Western blot.
3. a series of HIV tests are performed to determine whether the patient has AIDS.
4. if the HIV tests are seronegative, the patient can be assured that he is not infected.

26. When the human immunodeficiency retrovirus enters the body, it attacks primarily which cells, resulting in an immunocompromised status?

1. T-cell lymphocytes
2. B-cell lymphocytes
3. Neutrophils
4. Monocytes

27. A 21-year-old patient has been treated for chlamydia and has a history of recurrent vaginal herpes. What would be the most appropriate action by the nurse?

1. Counsel the patient about her sexual and drug use history, risk reduction measures, and HIV testing.
2. Refer the patient to a family planning clinic.
3. Counsel the patient about testing for HIV and what the test results mean.
4. Counsel the patient about abstinence and a monogamous relationship.

28. If a person is infected with HIV and has not seroconverted to the HIV-specific antibody and will not test HIV antibody positive, this is referred to as:

1. a "window-period."
2. negative CD_4^+ count.
3. positive CD_4^+ count.
4. viral load.

29. In people who are HIV positive, the highest viral load is seen:

1. at seroconversion time with CD_4^+ count less than 500/mm^3.
2. in symptomatic phase of HIV spectrum.
3. at seroconversion time and in advanced HIV disease (AIDS).
4. None of the above

30. The purpose of doing a viral load study once every 3 to 4 months in the HIV-positive person is to determine:

1. the CD_4^+ count.
2. the progression of the disease.
3. effectiveness of the medication regimen.
4. the results of the Western blot test.

31. The physician asks the nurse to talk with a patient about how HIV is transmitted. Which route of transmission should be discussed with the patient?

1. Receiving blood, donating blood
2. Food, water, air
3. Sexual intercourse, sharing needles, mother-to-child transmission
4. Dirty toilets, swimming pools, mosquitoes

32. The patient asks the nurse, "How does HIV cause AIDS?" The nurse's response should be:

1. "HIV attacks the immune system, a system that protects the body from foreign invaders, making it unable to protect the body from organisms that cause diseases."
2. "HIV breaks down the circulatory system, making the body unable to assimilate oxygen and nutrients."
3. "HIV attacks the respiratory system, making the lungs more susceptible to organisms causing pneumonia."
4. "HIV attacks the digestive system, decreasing the absorption of essential nutrients and resulting in weight loss and fatigue."

33. The pathophysiology of advanced HIV disease results from: *(Select all that apply.)*

1. T-helper lymphocytes decreasing.
2. T-suppressor lymphocytes dominating.
3. profound immunosuppression.
4. B lymphocytes unable to help with infection and antibody formation.
5. T-helper lymphocytes increasing.

34. People at high risk for contracting HIV virus include: *(Select all that apply.)*

1. a monogamous partner.
2. homosexuals.
3. drug users.
4. heterosexual partners of homosexuals or bisexuals.
5. prostitutes.

chapter

57 Care of the Patient with Cancer

evolve

http://evolve.elsevier.com/Christensen/foundationsadult

Barbara Lauritsen Christensen

Objectives

1. Discuss the incidence of cancer as one of the leading causes of death in the United States.
2. Compare the three most common sites for cancer in men and women.
3. Discuss development, prevention, and detection of cancer.
4. List seven risk factors for the development of cancer.
5. Discuss the American Cancer Society's recommendations for preventive behaviors and screening tests for men and women.
6. State seven warning signs of cancer.
7. Explain common reasons for delay in seeking medical care when a diagnosis of cancer is suspected.
8. Define the terminology used to describe cellular changes, characteristics of malignant cells, and types of malignancies.
9. Describe the pathophysiology of cancer, including the characteristics of malignant cells and the nature of metastasis.
10. Describe the process of metastasis.
11. Define the systems of tumor classification: grading and staging.
12. List common diagnostic tests used to identify cancer.
13. Explain why biopsy is essential in confirming a diagnosis of cancer.
14. Describe nursing interventions for the individual undergoing surgery, radiation therapy, chemotherapy, bone marrow transplantation, or peripheral stem cell transplantation.
15. Describe the major categories of chemotherapeutic agents.
16. Explain the etiology, pathophysiology, clinical manifestations, diagnostic tests, medical management, nursing interventions, and prognosis for tumor lysis syndrome.
17. Discuss six general pain relief guidelines for the patient with advanced cancer.

Key Terms

alopecia (ăl-ō-PĒ-shē-ă, p. 2032)
autologous (aw-TŎL-ō-gŭs, p. 2036)
benign (bē-NĪN, p. 2021)
biopsy (BĪ-ŏp-sē, p. 2022)
cachexia (kă-KĔK-sē-ă, p. 2037)
carcinogen (kăr-SĬN-ō-jĕn, p. 2015)
carcinogenesis (kăr-sĭn-ō-JĔN-ĕ-sĭs, p. 2015)
carcinoma (kăr-sĭ-NŌ-mă, p. 2021)
differentiated (dĭf-ĕr-ĔN-shē-ā-tĕd, p. 2021)
immunosurveillance (ĭm-ū-nō-sĕr-VĀ-lĕns, p. 2021)
leukopenia (lū-kō-PĒ-nē-ă, p. 2028)
malignant (mă-LĬG-nănt, p. 2021)
metastasis (mĕ-TĂS-tă-sĭs, p. 2021)
neoplasm (NĒ-ō-plăzm, p. 2021)
oncology (ŏn-KŎL-ŏ-jē, p. 2014)
palliative (PĂL-ē-ā-tĭv, p. 2025)
Papanicolaou's test (smear) (pă-pĕ-NĬ-kō-lūz tĕst, smēr, p. 2022)
sarcoma (săr-KŌ-mă, p. 2021)
stomatitis (stō-mă-TĪ-tĭs, p. 2032)
thrombocytopenia (thrŏm-bō-sīt-ō-PĒ-nē-ă, p. 2032)
tumor lysis syndrome (TŪ-mŏr LĪ-sĭs SĬN-drōm, p. 2035)

ONCOLOGY

Oncology is the sum of knowledge about tumors; it is the branch of medicine concerning the study of tumors. Oncology nursing is the care of people with cancer.

Until the appearance of acquired immunodeficiency syndrome (AIDS), probably no other medical diagnosis produced as much fear as a diagnosis of cancer. Cancer is feared far more than heart disease. The word *cancer* is viewed as synonymous with death, pain, and disfigurement. However, attitudes toward cancer have not kept pace with advances in the treatment and control of cancer. Education of health care professionals and the public is essential to promote more positive and realistic attitudes about cancer and cancer treatment (Lewis et al., 2007). The American Cancer Society (ACS) indicates that in the United States men have a 1 in 2 lifetime risk of developing cancer; for women, the risk is 1 in 3. The leading cancer sites for the male are prostate, lung, colon, and rectum. The leading cancer sites for the female are breast, lung, colon, and rectum (ACS, 2008a). Of every five deaths in the United States, one is from cancer, making it the second leading cause of death (heart disease is the most common).

Cancer is not one disease, but a group of more than 200 diseases characterized by the uncontrolled and unregulated growth and spread of abnormal cells.

 Life Span Considerations

Older Adults

Cancer

- More cases of cancer occur among older adults than people of any other age-group.
- The incidence of cancer increases with aging, possibly as a result of decreased effectiveness of the immune system and changes in deoxyribonucleic acid.
- The types of cancers seen in older adults are prostate, lung, breast, and colorectal cancer. Cancers of the skin, urinary bladder, vagina, and vulva are seen primarily in older adults. Chronic lymphocytic leukemia and multiple myeloma are seen more frequently in older adults than in younger people.
- Many early signs and symptoms of cancer may be misdiagnosed as normal changes of aging. Stress the importance of routine medical screening and self-examination.
- Because of fear or experience, older adults may adopt a fatalistic frame of mind after hearing the diagnosis of cancer. Use of the terms *tumor* or *growth* may be more acceptable.
- The type of treatment for cancer should be based on the older person's wishes and overall state of health. Older individuals, their family members, and significant others should be presented with all options so that they can make informed decisions regarding treatment.

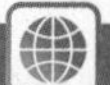 Cultural Considerations

Cancer

- Blacks have a higher incidence of cancer than whites.
- The death rate from the four most common cancers (lung, colorectal, breast, prostate) is higher among minorities (except Asian Americans) than among whites.
- Asian Americans have the lowest death rate from cancer of any ethnic group.
- Black men have almost twice the rate of prostate cancer as white men and are more than twice as likely to die from the disease.
- Hispanic women have the highest rate of invasive cervical cancer of any group other than Vietnamese, and twice the incidence rate of non-Hispanic white women.
- Although black women are less likely than white women to develop breast cancer, they are more likely to die from the disease if they develop it.
- Native Americans have a lower incidence of cancer than any other group in the United States but have the poorest survival rate when they do get cancer.

Source: American Cancer Society. (2008). *Cancer facts and figures.* Atlanta: American Cancer Society.

Early detection and prompt treatment can cure some cancers and slow the progression of others. If not detected and controlled, cancer can result in death. Overall, it affects people of all ages, but most cases (76%) are diagnosed in those over the age of 55 (see Life Span Considerations box). Cancer incidence is higher in blacks than in whites and other minority groups (see Cultural Considerations box). An estimated 30% of Americans now living will experience cancer at some point in their lives. In 2006, 564,830 Americans died from cancer, which is more than 1500 persons per day (ACS, *Cancer facts and figures,* 2009).

The death rate from all cancers combined has decreased by 2.6% per year among men and by 1.8% per year among women since 2002. Cancer death rates have been decreasing since 1991 in men and since 1992 in women. Compared to the peak rates in 1990 for men and 1991 for women, the cancer death rate for all sites combined in 2004 was 18.4% lower in men and 10.5% lower in women (ACS, 2009). The 5-year survival rate is now 65%.

Lung cancer is the leading cause of cancer-related death in both men and women. Other cancers, such as breast and prostate, occur more often than lung cancer, but they have better cure and survival rates because of early detection and treatment (Figures 57-1 and 57-2).

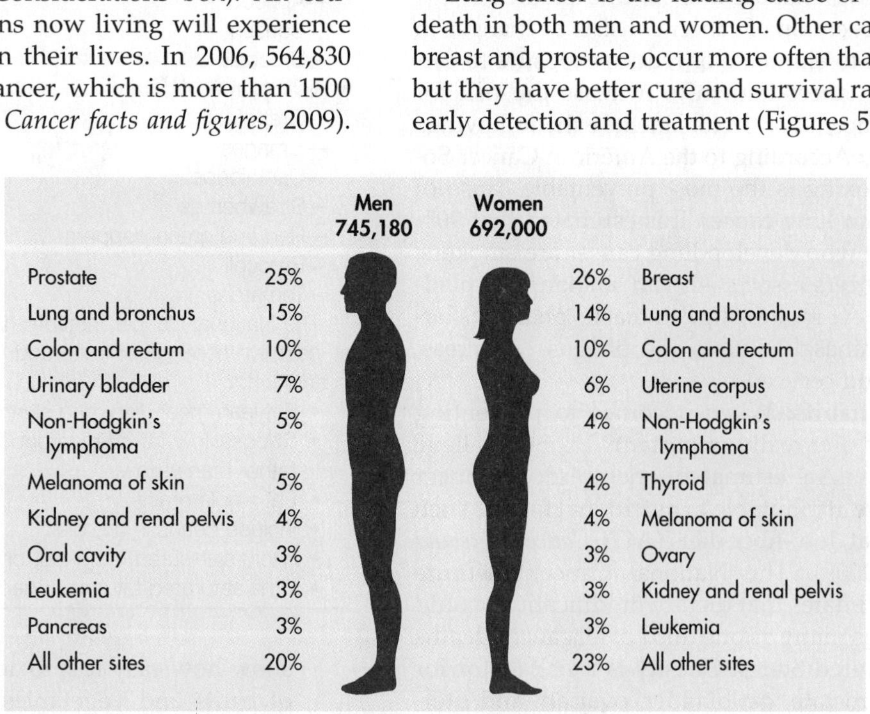

FIGURE 57-1 Estimated cancer cases in the United States (2008 estimates). Excludes basal and squamous cell skin cancers and in situ carcinomas except urinary bladder.

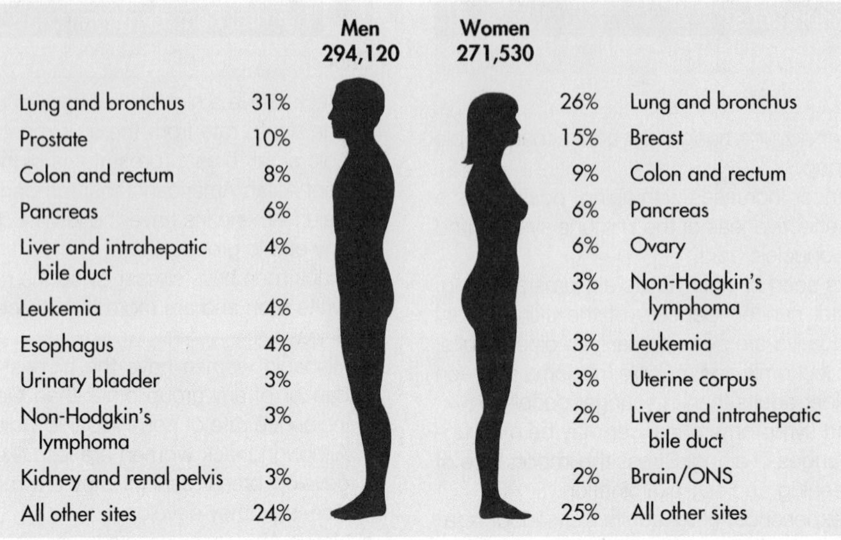

FIGURE 57-2 Estimated cancer deaths in the United States (2008 estimates). Excludes basal and squamous cell skin cancers in situ carcinomas except urinary bladder.

DEVELOPMENT, PREVENTION, AND DETECTION OF CANCER

Carcinogenesis is the process by which normal cells are transformed into cancer cells. Although numerous theories have been proposed to explain it, no single cause has been accepted. The exact cause of most human cancers is still unknown, but most types are likely to have multiple causes. It is not known how many tumors have a chemical, environmental, genetic, immunologic, or viral origin. Cancers may arise spontaneously from causes that are thus far unexplained.

Primary prevention of cancer consists of changes in lifestyle habits to eliminate or reduce exposure to **carcinogens,** substances known to increase the risk for developing cancer. Risk factors include the following:

- **Smoking:** According to the American Cancer Society, smoking is the most preventable cause of death from lung cancer. It is estimated that 90% of people who develop lung cancer are smokers. Other cancers associated with smoking are bladder, kidney, mouth, lip, stomach, pharynx, larynx, paranasal sinuses, esophagus, pancreas, uterus, and cervix.
- **Dietary habits:** When it comes to preventing cancer, is diet really important? Experts believe that it is. An estimated one third of cancer deaths are attributable to nutritional factors such as high-fat, low-fiber diets (ACS, *Cancer facts and figures,* 2009). The National Cancer Institute (NCI) estimates that dietary modifications could prevent as many as one third of all cancer deaths in the United States. Obesity is a risk factor for breast, prostate, gallbladder, ovarian, and uterine cancer (National Cancer Institute, 2004). Diet also plays a role in the development of colon, rectal, and breast cancer. The NCI has launched a program called "5 a Day for Better Health" to show how easy it is to add at least five servings of fruits and vegetables to the daily diet as a way of reducing the risks of cancer (see Health Promotion box). Fruit and vegetable consumption may protect against cancers of the mouth and pharynx, esophagus, lung, stomach, and

Health Promotion

Foods to Reduce Cancer Risk

- Vegetables from the cabbage family, such as:
  —Broccoli
  —Cauliflower
  —Brussels sprouts
  —All types of cabbage and kale
- Vegetables and fruits high in beta-carotene, such as:
  —Carrots
  —Peaches
  —Apricots
  —Squash
  —Broccoli
- Rich sources of vitamin C, such as:
  —Grapefruit
  —Oranges
  —Cantaloupe
  —Strawberries
  —Red and green peppers
  —Broccoli
  —Tomatoes

The National Cancer Institute has recommended including at least five servings of fruits and vegetables in the daily diet. In addition:

- Eat lean meat, fish, and skinned poultry.
- Choose low-fat dairy products, including white cheese rather than yellow.
- Eat whole grains.
- Include beans in the diet.
- Avoid salt-cured, smoked, or nitrite-cured foods.
- Limit saturated fat and added sugars.

colon and rectum. However, consumption has seen little improvement since the mid-1990s. Less than one in four adults was eating the recommended servings in 2005 (ACS, 2009). At present only 20% of the U.S. population consumes five daily servings of fruits and vegetables.
- **Ultraviolet (UV) radiation:** Excessive exposure to the sun's UV rays is a factor in the development of basal and squamous cell skin cancers and melanoma. Sunlamps and tanning booth beds also emit UV rays and have the same risks as sunlight. (In addition, the effects of radiation commonly used for medical diagnosis and treatment are known to be carcinogenic. Exposure should be limited and monitored.)
- **Environmental and chemical carcinogens:** Some of these include fumes from rubber and chlorine and dust from cotton, coal, nickel, chromate, asbestos, and vinyl chloride. There is a greater incidence of bladder cancer among people who live in urban areas and among those who work with dyes, rubber, or leather.
- **Smokeless tobacco:** Use of smokeless tobacco increases the risk of cancer of the mouth, larynx, pharynx, and esophagus. Long-term snuff users have as much as a 50-fold greater risk of cheek and gum cancers.
- **Frequent heavy consumption of alcohol:** Alcohol may result in oral cancer and cancer of the larynx, throat, esophagus, and liver.

HEREDITARY CANCERS

About 90% of cancers are not inherited. Hereditary cancers arise from germline mutations. They are diagnosed usually 15 to 20 years earlier than cancers that are not inherited. Often, several relatives have the same or related cancers. They are more likely to be bilateral, and the same person may have multiple cancers. These multiple cancers are often seen in unusual organ combinations, such as breast and sarcoma, breast and thyroid, leukemia and brain tumors. Hereditary cancers are characterized by precursor lesions, such as polyps in colorectal cancer and dysplastic nevi in melanoma (Lewis et al., 2007).

GENETIC SUSCEPTIBILITY

For many years scientists have searched for genetic patterns in the most common cancer sites. Only 10% of cancers have an etiology of a strong genetic link (Tannock et al., 2005). The following patterns have emerged:
- The incidence of postmenopausal breast cancer is three times higher and the incidence of premenopausal breast cancer is five times higher in women with a family history of this disease. If a female has genes *BRCA1* or *BRCA2*, she has a 40% to 80% risk of having breast cancer during her lifetime. Of all women who develop breast cancer, 95% do not carry these genes (Tannock et al., 2005). Breast cancer is rare in Asian women and common in white women.
- The incidence of lung cancer is greater in smokers with a family history of this disease than in smokers without a family history of the disease.
- The incidence of leukemia is greater in an identical twin of a person with the disease.
- Neuroblastoma occurs with increased frequency among siblings.
- Colon cancer is more likely to occur in women who have a history of breast cancer.

CANCER RISK ASSESSMENT AND GENETIC COUNSELING

When an individual or family is suspected of having a mutation in a cancer-causing gene, a cancer risk assessment is performed. This is the first step toward identifying hereditary cancer predisposition. The assessment begins with a comprehensive family history, included information on first-, second-, and third-degree relatives. Next obtain medical records to confirm the cancer diagnoses identified in the family history. The records usually requested include pathology reports, autopsy reports, death certificates, and discharge summaries from hospitalizations. Confirmation of cancer diagnoses through medical record analysis provides the patient with the most accurate risk analysis possible.

Genetic counseling is an essential component of the genetic evaluation. It is comprehensive and includes obtaining informed consent and proving education, health promotion, and support to individuals and families facing the uncertainty of hereditary cancer and cancer syndromes.

CANCER PREVENTION AND EARLY DETECTION

Prevention and early detection of cancer includes recognition of cancer's warning signals (Box 57-1). The American Cancer Society advises specific preventive behaviors and screening tests for men and women (Table 57-1). The nurse plays a prominent role in prevention and detection of cancer. Early detection and prompt treatment are directly responsible for increased survival rates in patients with cancer (see Health Promotion box). It is reported that 65% of patients who are diagnosed with cancer today will be alive 5 years after diagnosis.

Box 57-1 Cancer's Seven Warning Signals

If you have a warning signal, see your physician.
1. **C**hanges in bowel or bladder habits
2. **A** sore that does not heal
3. **U**nusual bleeding or discharge
4. **T**hickening or lump in breast or elsewhere
5. **I**ndigestion or difficulty swallowing
6. **O**bvious change in warts or moles
7. **N**agging cough or hoarseness

Table 57-1 Cancer Prevention and Early Detection in Women and Men

The American Cancer Society recommends that all people get a cancer-related checkup every 3 years between the ages of 20 and 40, and every year thereafter. This checkup, depending on a person's age, might include examinations for cancer of the skin, thyroid, mouth, and lymph nodes. Screening for colorectal cancer begins at age 50. For women, examination for cancer of the ovaries begins at age 20, and screening for breast cancer begins at age 40. For males, examination for testicular cancer begins at puberty, and screening for prostate cancer begins at age 50.

PREVENTIVE BEHAVIORS	SCREENING TESTS
MEN AND WOMEN **Colorectal Cancer** • Follow screening guidelines to remove adenomatous polyps before they become cancer. • Get at least 30 minutes of physical activity on most days. • Achieve and maintain a healthy weight. • Eat plenty of fruits, vegetables, and whole-grain foods, and limit intake of high-fat foods. • Quit smoking.	Beginning at age 50, a person should follow one of the four screening options below: • Yearly fecal occult blood test (FOBT) • Stool DNA tests (SDNA) • Flexible sigmoidoscopy every 5 years • Yearly FOBT plus flexible sigmoidoscopy every 5 years Of the options above, the American Cancer Society prefers yearly FOBT combined with flexible sigmoidoscopy every 5 years, or one of the following examination schedules: • Double-contrast barium enema every 5 years • Colonoscopy every 10 years • CT colonography (also known as virtual colonoscopy) every 5 years Talk to physician about beginning screening earlier and/or more often if a patient has any of the following risk factors: • Strong family history of colorectal cancer or polyps (cancer of polyps in a first-degree relative younger than 60 or in two first-degree relatives of any age). NOTE: A first-degree relative is a parent, sibling, or child. • Known family history of colorectal cancer syndromes. • Personal history of colorectal cancer or adenomatous polyps. • Personal history of chronic inflammatory bowel disease.
Skin Cancer • Stay out of the sun, especially between 10 AM and 4 PM. • Wear a broad-brimmed hat, a shirt, and sunglasses when out in the sun. • Use sunscreen with an SPF of 15 or higher; reapply it often. • In addition to seeking shade, the American Cancer Society recommends the "Slip! Stop! Slap! Wrap!" method of prevention: *Slip* on a shirt, *Slop* on 15 SPF (or higher) sunscreen, *Slap* on a hat, and *Wrap* on sunglasses before any exposure to the sun. • Do not use tanning beds or sunlamps. • Protect young children from excessive sun exposure. • Check your skin regularly for abnormal or changing areas, especially moles, and have them examined by a physician.	• Skin examination —Older than age 20: Every 3 years —Older than age 40: Every year • Self-examination (monthly) —Become familiar with any moles, freckles, or other abnormalities on the skin; use a mirror or have a family member or close friend look at areas one cannot see (ears, scalp, lower back). —Check for changes once a month; show any suspicious or changing areas to the physician.
Lung Cancer • Quit smoking. • Encourage those you live with or work with to quit. • If you smoke, let your physician know if you develop any of the following symptoms (some may have causes other than cancer): —A cough that does not go away —Chest pain, often aggravated by deep breathing —Hoarseness —Weight loss and loss of appetite —Bloody or rust-colored sputum —Shortness of breath —Fever without a known reason —Recurring infections such as bronchitis and pneumonia —New onset of wheezing	No screening tests have been found to be effective; cancer is usually found on x-ray examination, but there are often no symptoms. • Talk to the physician about possible screening if one has any of the risk factors listed below: —Smoke tobacco —Work around asbestos —Exposed to radon —Exposed to uranium —Exposed to arsenic —Exposed to vinyl chloride —Smoke marijuana —Regularly exposed to secondhand smoke

Table 57-1 Cancer Prevention and Early Detection in Women and Men—cont'd

PREVENTIVE BEHAVIORS	SCREENING TESTS
WOMEN	
Cervical Cancer • Abstain from sex or practice safer sex using barrier protection each time you have intercourse. • Quit smoking. • Eat a diet rich in fruits and vegetables. • Watch for and report signs and symptoms (although all of these can have other causes): —Abnormal uterine bleeding or spotting —Abnormal vaginal discharge —Pain during intercourse	• Have a yearly pelvic examination with Papanicolaou's (Pap) test beginning at age 18 or when sexually active, whichever is earlier. • A vaccine is approved for females aged 9 to 19 years to reduce cervical-related neoplasia and cervical cancer resulting from HPV types 16 to 18. Three vaccines are given over 6 months. • Beginning at age 30, after three or more consecutive satisfactory normal yearly examinations, the conventional or liquid-based Pap test may be screened every 2 or 3 years at the physician's discretion. • Alternatively, every 3 years the following should be performed: conventional or liquid-based cytology and cervical cancer screening with human papillomavirus DNA testing (American Cancer Society, 2007).
Breast Cancer • Follow recommended guidelines for early detection of breast cancer. • Talk with your physician about the risks and benefits of hormone replacement therapy for your risk of cancer and other diseases (like heart disease and osteoporosis). • Get at least 30 minutes of physical activity on most days. • Achieve and maintain a healthy weight. • Eat plenty of fruits, vegetables, and whole-grain foods, and limit intake of high-fat foods. • Decrease your alcohol intake.	**Ages 20 to 39** • Breast self-examination each month • Clinical breast examination by health care professional every 3 years **Ages 50 and over** • Mammogram every 2 years (U.S. Preventive Services Task Force, 2009) • Clinical breast examination by a health care professional, near the time of the mammogram • Breast self-examination every month • If woman is at increased risk (e.g., genetic tendency or family history), consult health care provider about benefits and limitations of baseline mammogram before age 50 and additional examinations such as breast ultrasound and MRI (ACS, 2007).
Endometrial Cancer • Watch for and report any abnormal uterine spotting or bleeding. • Use oral contraceptives for many years. • Talk with your physician about the risks and benefits of hormone replacement therapy for your risk of cancer and other diseases (like heart disease and osteoporosis). • If taking hormone replacement therapy with your uterus still intact, take estrogen with progesterone.	**Average risk:** • Talk with the physician especially at the time of menopause, about the risks and symptoms of endometrial cancer. • Report any vaginal bleeding or spotting to your physician.
Ovarian Cancer • Use oral contraceptives for several years. • Watch for and report signs and symptoms (although all of these can have other causes): —Abdominal swelling —Vaginal bleeding —Back or leg pain —Chronic stomach pain • Talk with your physician about the risks and benefits of hormone replacement therapy and your risks of cancer and other diseases, like heart disease and osteoporosis.	There are no effective and proven tests for early detection of ovarian cancer. • As part of one's health maintenance, undergo a periodic and thorough pelvic examination as directed by the physician.

Continued

Table 57-1 Cancer Prevention and Early Detection in Women and Men—cont'd

PREVENTIVE BEHAVIORS	SCREENING TESTS
WOMEN—cont'd **Ovarian Cancer—cont'd** • Talk with your physician about having your ovaries removed, if you are at high risk. (This surgery causes sudden menopause.)	
MEN **Prostate Cancer** • Eat a diet low in fat and high in vegetables, fruits, and grains. • Get at least 30 minutes of physical activity on most days. • Achieve and maintain a healthy weight.	Men should consider a yearly prostate-specific antigen (PSA) blood test and digital rectal examination starting at age 50 or at age 45 if at high risk (black men, or those with a father or brother diagnosed with prostate cancer at a young age).
Testicular Cancer • Eat a balanced diet which includes fresh fruits and vegetables. • Participate in a regular exercise program. • Learn and practice testicular self-examination.	Teach the male at puberty to perform a monthly testicular self-examination. Monthly self-examination should continue throughout the life span. Males at high risk are those with a history of an undescended testis or a previous testicular tumor.

Health Promotion

Prevention and Detection of Cancer

- Reduce or avoid exposure to known or suspected carcinogens and cancer-promoting agents, including cigarette smoke and sun exposure.
- Eat a balanced diet that includes vegetables (green, deep yellow, and orange), cruciferous vegetables (cabbage, broccoli, cauliflower and Brussels sprouts), fresh fruits, allium vegetables (onion and garlic), nuts, legumes, soy products, whole grains, and adequate amounts of fiber. Reduce the amount of fat and preservatives, including smoked and salt-cured meats. Limit the consumption of processed and red meats.
- Exercise regularly. The American Cancer Society recommends that adults engage in at least 30 minutes of moderate to vigorous physical activity, above usual activities, on five or more days per week.
- Obtain adequate, consistent periods of rest (at least 6 to 8 hours per night).
- Have a health examination on a regular basis that includes a health history, a physical examination, and specific diagnostic tests for common cancers in accordance with the guidelines published by the American Cancer Society (www.cancer.org) (see Table 57-1).
- Eliminate, reduce, or change the perceptions of stressors and enhance the ability to effectively cope with stressors.
- Enjoy consistent periods of relaxation and leisure.
- Know the seven warning signs of cancer (see Box 57-1). (These actually indicate fairly advanced disease.)
- Learn and practice self-examination (e.g., skin examination, breast self-examination, testicular self-examination).
- Seek immediate medical care if you notice a change in what is normal for you and if cancer is suspected. Early detection of cancer has a positive effect on prognosis.

Beginning in high school, all women should be taught to perform breast self-examination (BSE) each month, 2 or 3 days after the menstrual period ends. After menopause, a woman should choose a specific day to help her remember, such as the first day of each month. A woman needs to become familiar with the appearance and feel of her breasts. This will help her identify any change from one month to the next. Any abnormality—such as discharge from the nipples; puckering, dimpling, peau d'orange (skin appearance of an orange peel, or scaling of the skin; and the palpation of a lump or thickness)—is significant. (See Chapter 52 for instructions on BSE.) Teach BSE to all patients (men and women), emphasizing that any identifiable problem should be brought to the attention of a physician. Any delay is a waste of valuable time if cancer is present.

Teach males, beginning at puberty, to check the scrotum for enlargement, thickening, or the presence of a lump in the testicles. This should be done monthly, after a warm bath or shower. Emphasize that a physician must be contacted to determine the significance of any changes from the normal, smooth consistency of the testes (see Chapter 52). Some symptoms of testicular cancer include a lump in or enlargement of either testicle, a heavy feeling in the scrotum, dull aching in either the groin or the lower abdomen, fluid collection in the scrotum, and tenderness or enlargement of the breasts (this results from hormones produced by cancer cells) (National Cancer Institute, 2007).

Advise men over age 50 to have a prostate-specific antigen (PSA) test and rectal examination once a year. Symptoms of blood in the urine, difficulty starting to urinate, a weak flow of urine, or other urination problems should be reported to the physician.

A common reason for delay in diagnosing cancer is that early malignant changes do not produce pain. Cancer may be insidious at the onset, and it may be far advanced before the individual has any symptoms.

PATHOPHYSIOLOGY OF CANCER

CELL MECHANISMS AND GROWTH

The basic unit of structure and function in all living things is the **cell.** The adult human body contains approximately 60,000 billion cells. Although there are many different types of cells, all of them have certain common characteristics. For example, all cells need nourishment to maintain life, and all cells use almost identical nutrients. All cells use oxygen, which combines with fat, protein, or carbohydrates to release the energy needed for cells to function. The mechanisms for changing nutrients into energy are generally the same in all cells, and all cells deliver their end product of chemical reactions into the nearby fluids.

Most cells are able to reproduce. When cells are destroyed, the remaining cells of the same type reproduce until the correct number has been replenished. This orderly replacement of cells is governed by a control mechanism that stops when the loss or damage has been corrected. Dynamic, active, and orderly, the healthy cell is a small powerhouse, laboratory, factory, and duplicating machine, perfectly copying itself over and over. Our immune system helps us from developing cancer by destroying the abnormal cells. Occasionally our immune system fails to recognize these abnormal cells and cancer develops.

Cancer cells are not subject to the usual restrictions placed on cell proliferation by the host. When malignant cells change, they become unlike parent cells; they are not differentiated, or recognizable as being the same in size or shape as normal cells. Cancer cells can divide and multiply, but not in a normal manner. Instead of limiting their growth to meet specific needs of the body, they continue to reproduce in a disorderly and unrestricted manner. The cellular features of cancer cells are a local increase in the number of cells, loss of normal cellular arrangement, variation in cell shape and size, increased nuclear size, increased miotic activity, and abnormal mitosis and chromosomes.

Proliferation is not always indicative of cancer, however. Abnormal cellular growth is classified as nonneoplastic growth and neoplastic growth. The four common nonneoplastic growth patterns are hypertrophy, hyperplasia, metaplasia, and dysplasia. Though not neoplastic conditions, these may precede the development of cancer. **Anaplasia** means "without form" and is an irreversible change in which the structures of adult cells regress to more primitive levels.

Neoplasm is the term for uncontrolled or abnormal growth of cells. Neoplasms may be **benign** (not recurrent or progressive; nonmalignant) or **malignant** (growing worse and resisting treatment, as in cancerous growths [Table 57-2]). The growths are also called **tumors,** which means swelling or enlargement. They may be localized or invasive. Benign tumors may become serious because their increased size damages surrounding tissues, as in a benign brain tumor. Malignant neoplasms may progress and destroy surrounding tissues. They may also metastasize from the primary site of origin to distant sites.

Table 57-2 General Characteristics of Neoplasms

BENIGN TUMORS	MALIGNANT TUMORS
Slow, steady growth	Rate of growth varies—usually rapid
Remains localized	Metastasizes
Usually contained within a capsule	Rarely contained within a capsule
Smooth, well defined; movable when palpated	Irregular; more immobile when palpated
Resembles parent tissue	Little resemblance to parent tissue
Crowds normal tissue	Invades normal tissue
Rarely recurs after removal	May recur after removal
Rarely fatal	Fatal without treatment

Metastasis is the process by which tumor cells spread from the primary site to a secondary site. Once cancer cells have moved to another area of the body, secondary tumors may grow in that area. Metastasis can occur by (1) direct spread of tumor cells by diffusion to other body cavities or (2) circulation by way of blood and lymphatic channels.

In addition to the identified carcinogenic factors that may cause malignant cellular changes, certain viruses have been suspected. There is also evidence to suggest that certain genetic factors result in a predisposition to the development of cancer.

The body's immune system is responsible for recognizing and destroying malignant cells. The immune system may be weakened by cancer-producing substances, tumor cells, and the aging process. Some T cells are responsible for **immunosurveillance** (the immune system's recognition and destruction of newly developed abnormal cells). When a cell becomes malignant, it carries a tumor-specific antigen on its membranes that is recognized by the body as nonself and destroyed. If T-cell function is suppressed by age, drugs (e.g., corticosteroids), poor nutrition, alcohol, serious infections, or certain disease processes (e.g., neoplastic invasion of bone and lymph tissue), the risk of cancer increases. To suppress T-cell rejection of a transplanted organ, steroids and other drugs are given. The resultant loss of immunosurveillance increases the risk of certain cancers.

DESCRIPTION, GRADING, AND STAGING OF TUMORS

Cancers are described according to the original site of the primary tumor. **Carcinoma** is the term used for malignant tumors composed of epithelial cells, which

Box 57-2 TNM Cancer Staging Classification System

T SUBCLASSES: PRIMARY TUMOR

T_x	Tumor cannot be adequately assessed
T_0	No evidence of primary tumor
T_{is}	Carcinoma in situ
T_1-T_4	Progressive increase in tumor size and involvement

N SUBCLASSES: REGIONAL LYMPH NODES

N_x	Regional lymph nodes cannot be assessed
N_0	No regional lymph node metastasis
N_1-N_4	Increasing involvement of regional lymph nodes

M SUBCLASSES: DISTANT METASTASIS

M_x	Not assessed
M_0	No (known) distant metastasis
M_1-M_4	Distant metastasis present, specify site(s)

HISTOPATHOLOGY

G_1	Well-differentiated grade; cells differ slightly from normal cells (mild dysplasia)
G_2	Moderately well-differentiated grade; cells are more abnormal (moderate dysplasia)
G_3	Poorly differentiated grade; cells are very abnormal (severe dysplasia)
G_4	Undifferentiated; cells are immature and primitive (anaplasia); cells difficult to determine

From American Joint Committee for Cancer. (1992). *AJCC manual for staging of cancer.* (4th ed.). Philadelphia: Lippincott.

tend to metastasize. Carcinomas originate from embryonal ectoderm (skin and glands) and endoderm (mucous membrane linings of the respiratory tract, gastrointestinal [GI] tract, and genitourinary tract). Sarcoma refers to malignant tumors of connective tissues; they originate from embryonal mesoderm, such as muscle, bone, or fat, usually manifesting as a painless swelling. Sarcoma may affect bone, bladder, kidneys, liver, lungs, parotids, and spleen. **Lymphomas** and **leukemias** originate from the hematopoietic system.

A tumor may be named for its location, its cellular makeup, or the person by whom it was identified.

Grading of Tumors

Tumors are classified grade 1 to grade 4 by the degree of malignancy. Grade 1 is the most differentiated (most like the parent tissue) tumor and the least malignant. Grade 4 is the least differentiated (unlike parent tissue) tumor and the most malignant (Box 57-2).

Extent of Disease Classification

Classifying the extent and spread of disease is termed **staging.** This classification system is based on a description of the extent of the disease rather than on cell appearance. Although staging for different types of cancer has similarities, there are many differences, based on a thorough knowledge of the natural history of each specific type of cancer.

Clinical Staging

The clinical staging classification system determines the extent of the disease process of cancer by stages:

- **Stage 0:** Cancer in situ
- **Stage I:** Tumor limited to the tissue of origin; localized tumor growth
- **Stage II:** Limited local spread
- **Stage III:** Extensive local and regional spread
- **Stage IV:** Metastasis

TNM Classification System

The **TNM classification system** represents the standardization of the clinical staging of cancer. This classification system is used to determine the extent of the disease process of cancer according to three parameters: tumor size (T), degree of regional spread to the lymph nodes (N), and metastasis (M) (see Box 57-2). This system is used to direct treatment, predict prognosis, and contribute to cancer research by ensuring reliable comparison of different patients.

Bethesda System

Exfoliative (pertaining to the shedding of something) cytology (e.g., Papanicolaou's test [smear] [Pap]) is a means of studying cells that the body has shed during the normal sequence of growth and replacement of body tissues. If cancer is present, cancer cells are also shed. The method is most commonly used to detect cancers of the cervix, but it may be used for tissue specimens from any organ.

The results of the Pap test, as given by the **Bethesda system** (the preferred system), are as follows:

- **Negative:** Normal (formerly class I)
- **Probably negative:** May indicate infection, atypical squamous cells, or reactive changes (formerly class II)
- **Suspicious, but not conclusive for malignancy:** Low-grade squamous intraepithelial lesion (formerly class III)
- **More suspicious, strongly suggestive of malignancy:** High-grade squamous intraepithelial lesion (formerly class IV)
- **Conclusive for malignancy:** Invasive squamous cell carcinoma (formerly class V)

DIAGNOSIS OF CANCER

BIOPSY

People who show signs of cancer should undergo diagnostic testing to confirm or rule out the diagnosis. The only definitive way to determine the presence of malignant cells is to perform a tissue biopsy (the removal of a small piece of living tissue from an organ or other part of the body for microscopic examination; used to confirm or establish a diagnosis, establish prognosis, or follow the course of a disease).

In general, the purpose of a biopsy is to obtain a sample of tissue for pathologic examination. The three

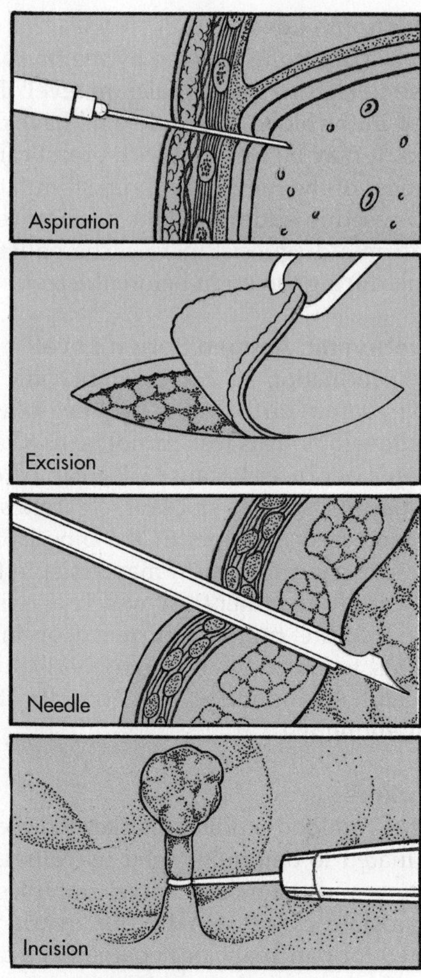

FIGURE 57-3 Types of biopsy.

types of biopsy are incisional, excisional, and needle aspiration (Figure 57-3). **Incisional** biopsy is the removal of a portion of tissue for examination, such as the bite biopsy performed during endoscopy. **Excisional** biopsy is the removal of the complete lesion, with little or no margin of surrounding normal tissue removed, as in polypectomy. Another example of excisional biopsy is the dissection of peripheral lymph nodes, such as those of the axilla for staging of breast cancer or those of the peritoneal region for staging of various abdominal cancers. **Needle aspiration** biopsy is the aspiration of fluid or tissue by means of a needle (breast biopsy is performed with an aspiration needle). Transcutaneous aspiration biopsy has eliminated most of the exploratory laparotomies for diagnosing metastatic cancer of the liver or for primary inoperable pancreatic cancer. Organs accessible to thin-needle biopsy under guidance of palpation include breasts, skin, thyroid gland, prostate, palpable lymph nodes, and salivary glands.

ENDOSCOPY

Cells or tissue can also be obtained using an **endoscope** to directly visualize an internal structure through a body cavity or a small incision. Endoscopes are rigid or flexible tubes containing a magnifying lens and a light. Endoscopes vary in diameter and length according to the structure being examined. The bronchoscope is used to visualize the tracheobronchial tree; upper GI endoscopy allows direct visualization of the upper GI tract (esophagus, stomach, duodenum); the colonoscope is used to visualize the entire colon; and the sigmoidoscope is used to examine the sigmoid colon, the rectum, and the anus.

DIAGNOSTIC IMAGING

Other diagnostic studies determine the depth of the specific lesion and identify other structures that may have been invaded. These include radiographs and scanning procedures. Commonly ordered radiographic studies are the chest radiograph, mammography, bone scan, GI series, barium enema, and intravenous pyelogram.

Bone scanning involves several steps. Before the scan, a radioactive material is injected into a vein in the arm. The patient is encouraged to drink water over the next 1 to 3 hours to aid renal clearance of any radioisotope not picked up by the bone. Areas of concentrated uptake may represent a tumor or an abnormality. These areas of concentration can be detected days or weeks before an ordinary radiograph could reveal a lesion. Bone scanning is indicated to detect metastatic tumors. All malignancies capable of metastasis may reach the bone, especially malignancies of breasts, kidneys, lungs, prostate, thyroid gland, and urinary bladder.

Tomography is the special technique of making multiple radiographic films at different depths of a specific area, organ, or structure. The details of each thin section can be clearly visualized.

Computed Tomography

Computed tomography (CT) scan uses radiographs and a computed scanning system to record images of specific structures at different angles. The entire body can be scanned to detect any abnormal lesion. CT scan is especially helpful in detecting small lesions that were missed by radiographs or tomography.

Radioisotope Studies

Radioisotope studies require the injection or ingestion of a radioactive substance. A scanning device is used to identify the distribution of the substance in different areas of the body. Concentration of the radioisotope in a specific organ, such as the thyroid gland or the brain, identifies a tumor in that location (may be primary or metastatic).

Ultrasound Testing

Ultrasound is a noninvasive procedure using high-frequency sound waves to examine internal structures. As a transducer is moved over the area being studied, an ultrasound beam is directed through the tissues and reflects back to the transducer. The sound waves are converted into electrical impulses, which produce an image on a display screen. Ultrasound can show the size, consistency, and shape of the structure being studied. It is most helpful in distinguishing between cystic and solid tumors. Ultrasound is not used to examine bones or air-filled organs. The procedure is painless. People having ultrasonography feel the transducer moving over their skin and may need to hold their breath for brief periods and remain still during the procedure.

Magnetic Resonance Imaging

Magnetic resonance imaging (MRI) is a painless diagnostic procedure that does not involve any exposure to radiation. The person reclines on a narrow surface that moves into a cylindrical tunnel containing magnetic coils; radiofrequency energy waves produce signals that are processed by a computer and displayed as images on a video monitor. The images can be recorded on film or magnetic tape for permanent storage. This test is currently used in the diagnosis of intracranial and spinal lesions and of cardiovascular and soft tissue abnormalities. The procedure also provides information about changes within the cells of soft tissues, arteries, veins, the brain, and the spinal column.

During the test the person having MRI must not have any metallic materials on the body, including jewelry. MRI cannot be done on patients with metallic implants, such as a pacemaker, orthopedic nail, or aneurysm clip.

During the test the patient can talk to those performing the test by means of a microphone placed inside the scanner tunnel. The patient will hear the sound waves thumping on the magnetic field and must lie still while the test is being done; it may take more than an hour to obtain the images needed.

Position Emission Tomography

Positron emission tomography (PET) is useful in many aspects of oncology. A radioactive chemical is given to the patient just before PET scanning. A PET scan can demonstrate glucose metabolism, oxygenation, blood flow, and tissue perfusion for any designated area. Alterations in the normal metabolic process in pathologic conditions are diagnosed during a PET scan (Pagana & Pagana, 2007).

PET is useful to visualize fast-growing tumors and to specify their anatomical location. PET also helps note tumor response to therapeutic intervention, identify a recurrence of a tumor after surgical intervention, and assist in differentiating a tumor from other abnormal conditions such as an infection (Pagana & Pagana, 2008). PET is extremely useful in visualizing regional and metastatic extension of a specific tumor. Oncologic staging is more accurate with PET than CT scan. PET is also used to determine the specific site to perform a biopsy of a suspected tumor (Pagana & Pagana, 2008).

LABORATORY AND DIAGNOSTIC EXAMINATIONS

Measurement of Alkaline Phosphatase Blood Levels

Alkaline phosphatase is elevated if there is metastasis to the bone or liver.

Serum Calcitonin Level

Calcitonin is a hormone secreted by the thyroid gland in response to a rising serum calcium level. The level is increased in the blood of people who have cancer of the thyroid. It may be elevated with breast cancer and oat cell cancer of the lung. Calcitonin stimulation testing may be used in addition to the baseline level testing to confirm a diagnosis. Instruct the patient to not eat or drink during the night before the test.

Carcinoembryonic Antigen Serum Level

Normally, production of carcinoembryonic antigen (CEA) stops before birth, but it may begin again if a neoplasm develops. This test cannot be used as a general indicator of cancer because CEA can be elevated for other reasons, such as smoking cigarettes. CEA is found in increased amounts in the blood of people with colorectal cancer. The test may assist in the evaluation of cancer treatment, in which a rising CEA level may indicate tumor recurrence or metastatic disease. This test is used less frequently today because research has found it less accurate than was previously thought.

Blood Markers

Many different blood studies (markers) are currently being evaluated to determine their usefulness in cancer screening and diagnosis. Three examples are the PSA for prostate cancer, CA-125 for ovarian cancer, and CA-19-9 for pancreatic or hepatobiliary cancer.

PSA is a biologic marker, specific for cellular activity in the prostate gland. PSA, the gold standard tumor marker for prostate cancer, is increasingly important in the diagnostic assessment and follow-up of patients with the disease. PSA also plays an important role in staging prostate cancer and in monitoring for recurrence. The American Cancer Society began recommending its use for screening asymptomatic men in November 1992.

Although PSA levels are usually elevated when cancer is present, PSA alone does not diagnose prostate cancer. Other common conditions, such as benign enlargement of the prostate, can also elevate PSA. The finding of elevated PSA requires further evaluation to assess the cause of the high levels. This may involve transrectal ultrasonography (TRUS) of the prostate gland.

The PSA assay requires a physician's interpretation. No specific level of PSA signals the presence or absence of prostate cancer. The PSA test is produced by different manufacturers, and the different products yield different results. Men with benign prostatic enlargement have different normal levels than men with normal prostate glands.

In 1987, to determine what role PSA might play in screening asymptomatic men, the American Cancer Society undertook its National Prostate Cancer Detection Project, a long-term study of 2425 men at 10 clinical centers across the United States. This study looked at the impact of PSA and two other screening methods—digital rectal examination (DRE) and TRUS—alone and in combination in the early detection of prostate cancer.

The American Cancer Society currently recommends that asymptomatic men older than the age of 40 be screened for prostate cancer via DRE; men older than age 50 should undergo annual PSA and DRE. Men who are at high risk for prostate cancer (black men or men with a first-degree relative, such as a father or brother, diagnosed with prostate cancer at a young age) should begin annual PSA testing at age 45 (ACS, 2009). If the result of either is suspicious, further evaluation is necessary.

A PSA is done by collecting a sample of the patient's blood before prostate palpation. The normal range for a man over the age of 40 is 0 to 4 ng/L. Even a small increase in a PSA test level needs to be carefully evaluated. Although the PSA is used to screen for prostate cancer, it is used most widely to determine the effectiveness of cancer treatment and to assess the recurrence of prostate cancer. A rising PSA after surgery for cancer of the prostate suggests recurrence.

CA-125 is a cancer antigen detected in the blood and peritoneal ascites. The normal range is 35 units/mL. CA-125 may be elevated in gynecologic cancers (including ovarian cancer) and cancer of the pancreas. A monoclonal antibody has been developed that reacts with this antigen, giving physicians a method to measure the amount of CA-125 in blood samples. This test is used mainly to signal a recurrence of ovarian cancer. It is not a way to detect primary ovarian cancer, since other conditions—such as endometriosis, hepatitis, pelvic inflammatory diseases, or pregnancy—may increase CA-125 levels in the blood.

A tumor marker, **CA-19-9** antigen, is used in the diagnosis, monitoring of a patient's response to therapeutic intervention, and surveillance of the patient with pancreatic or hepatobiliary cancer. CA-19-9 is elevated in 70% of patients with pancreatic cancer and 65% of patients with hepatobiliary cancer. CA-19-9 is not an effective screening tool for pancreatic or biliary tumors in the general population because of its lack of sensitivity and specificity (Pagana & Pagana, 2008).

Stool Examination for Occult Blood

The cause of blood in the stool must be identified to rule out the possibility of cancer. The **guaiac test** is commonly used to detect occult (hidden) blood in the stools. Other commonly used tests for occult blood in the stool are **Hematest, Occultest,** and **Hemoccult test.** Early detection self-tests are available for home use. If blood is found, the person should seek immediate medical attention. For accurate test results, it is essential that the person not ingest red meat, turnips, melons, aspirin, or vitamin C for 4 days before the test.. The test must be performed on three consecutive bowel movements. Urge people to follow through with diagnostic tests recommended by their physician as a result of preliminary examinations and laboratory tests.

CANCER THERAPIES

SURGERY

By the time it is decided that surgery is needed to remove a cancerous lesion, cancer cells may already have spread to other areas. The goal of surgery is to remove all malignant cells; this may include removal of the tumor, surrounding tissue, and regional lymph nodes. Surgery in conjunction with chemotherapy and/or radiation therapy may increase the destruction of cancer cells. The effects of cancer drugs and radiation treatments administered before, during, and after surgery are being investigated. A surgical cure may result from a well-isolated lesion removed in the very early stages, as in cancer of the skin, testicle, breast, or cervix. Surgery may be performed for many reasons: preventive, diagnostic, curative, and **palliative** (therapy designed to relieve uncomfortable symptoms, but that does not produce a cure).

Polyps in the colon may be removed during a colonoscopy before malignant changes occur. Occasionally, prophylactic mastectomy is done to prevent breast cancer in those identified to be at increased risk because of their family history or other factors. If the cancerous lesion has already metastasized, surgery may provide palliation by relieving some of the associated problems, such as obstruction, ulceration, hemorrhage, and pain. The pituitary, adrenal glands, ovaries, or testes may be surgically removed to help control the growth and spread of malignancies caused by hormonal stimulation.

A radical surgical approach to operable tumors is no longer routinely used because of more sensitive and accurate diagnosing methods, a greater variety of surgical procedures, more sophisticated staging techniques, and more available advanced treatment options. The more conservative surgical management of breast cancer (i.e., lumpectomy instead of total mastectomy) is an excellent example of this trend.

Reconstructive surgery may be needed to improve body functions and appearance after some types of surgery, such as modified radical mastectomy. Breast reconstruction is an option for women whose disease and treatment enable the surgeon to implant a prosthesis or to transplant tissue from other areas of the body to recreate a more natural-looking breast. When this is anticipated, preoperative counseling by the surgeon and the nurse helps the patient consider the long-range outcome instead of the immediate surgical procedure.

The use of laser beams as an alternative for some oncology surgical procedures is increasing. The laser beam vaporizes tissue with little bleeding and low risk of infection. Currently the major uses of laser surgery are in ophthalmology, gynecology, urology, neurosurgery, and otolaryngology. The chief discomfort while undergoing laser surgery is that the person must lie very still while the laser is in use.

Communication

Nurse-Patient Therapeutic Dialogue Prior to Modified Radical Mastectomy

Nurse: Good afternoon, Mrs. Snyder My name is Jill, and I will be your nurse this evening. How are you feeling? (introduction and general lead)

Patient: I'm feeling all right now. It's tomorrow I'm dreading.

Nurse: You're dreading tomorrow? (restatement)

Patient: Yes. My doctor told me he has to remove my entire breast. I dread the thought that I'll look so different.

Nurse: You're anxious about the fact that you may look different. (reflection)

Patient: I'll be embarrassed to undress in front of my husband. He may think I'm no longer attractive.

Nurse: Have you had a chance to discuss your feelings with your husband? (clarification)

Patient: No, he's out of town but will be back tonight. I guess I could talk to him then. Maybe he will accept it better than I think.

Nurse: We'll talk more after you've had a chance to talk to him about your feelings. Is there anything else on your mind that you'd like to talk about now? (showing acceptance and general lead)

Nursing Interventions

If you are not present when the physician explains recommendations for care, ask the physician what he or she has told the patient and the family. This is essential to be able to reinforce the information given. Patients and families are usually frightened and may not remember all that the physician has explained to them.

Patients should have confidence and trust in those responsible for their care. Positive feelings and attitudes promote relaxation and help reduce anxiety and fear (see Communication box). Encourage the patient to ask the physician any questions concerning potential risks of a given treatment. A patient needs to feel comfortable with the decision to follow through with the physician's recommendations.

The following are nursing guidelines to ensure that patients get the information they need:

- Be present when patient and physician are discussing treatment decisions.
- If necessary, clarify explanations of treatments, including benefits and side effects, and help the patient formulate questions and voice concerns. Address patient or family concerns and questions concerning alternative treatments.
- Afterward, talk to the patient and the family about the information the physician presented; assess their understanding of the treatment, as well as their goals and needs.
- Report any apparent misunderstandings, unrealistic expectations, or other problems to the physician.
- Communicate with the patient to verify that his or her questions were answered.
- Accept and support the patient's choice, regardless of personal opinion.

Preparing the patient for a surgical procedure must include an explanation of what to expect postoperatively. Preoperative teaching is discussed in Chapter 42.

Whatever the surgical procedure, the patient's nutritional status, both before and after surgery, has been found to be a significant factor in the amount of surgery that can be tolerated, the rate of recovery, the patient's role performance, and the adequacy of wound healing.

When surgery may result in a changed body image, as in mastectomy, laryngectomy, or the formation of an ostomy, the patient may benefit from talking with another person who has undergone the same type of surgery. The American Cancer Society sponsors support groups and prepares volunteers to visit patients who need these types of surgical procedures. Reach to Recovery; the Lost Chord Club; I Can Cope; Look Good, Feel Good; and a local chapter of the United Ostomy Associations of America are some of the special groups available in some local communities.

RADIATION THERAPY

Radiation therapy can be used to cure or control cancer that has spread to local lymph nodes or to treat tumors that cannot be removed. Radiation may be used preoperatively to reduce the size of a tumor. Postoperative radiation may be indicated to destroy malignant cells not removed by surgery. Radiation may also be used to slow the growth of malignant tumors.

Radiation may be delivered externally or internally. External therapy may be directed toward superficial lesions or toward deeper structures within the body. Because malignant cells lack the capacity for repair, more cancer cells than normal cells are damaged by radiation, and normal cells are able to recover better. However, normal cells do have a maximum dose of radiation that they can tolerate before irreversible damage occurs. Treatment plans are designed to minimize the radiation dose to normal structures. Meticulous planning and recording of the dose are essential.

External Radiation Therapy

When external radiation is planned, the specific area on the body is marked to indicate the port at which external radiation will be directed. These markings must not be washed off. If the area becomes wet while bathing, the skin should be patted with an absorbent towel. Help the patient understand the need to protect this area. Also instruct the patient to avoid using any ointments, lotions, or powder on this area. The physician may approve specific lotions or creams for drying skin. Tell the patient to protect the radiated area from direct sunlight and to avoid applications of heat or cold because these would increase erythema, drying, and pruritus of the skin, which is common over an irradiated area.

Encourage a diet high in protein and calories and a fluid intake of 2 or 3 L/day. Reassure the person undergoing radiation therapy that lethargy and fatigue are common during treatment, and that frequent rest periods are helpful.

Some 60% of all people with cancer are treated with radiation therapy at some point. For many of these, radiation therapy is the only therapy needed to destroy the cancer.

Internal Radiation Therapy

Radioactive implant (brachytherapy) is the insertion of **sealed radioactive materials** temporarily or permanently into hollow cavities, within body tissues, or on the body's surface. The radioactive source delivers a specific radiation dose continuously over hours or days. A highly concentrated radiation dose is delivered in or near a tumor. This technique is generally combined with a course of external radiation therapy to increase the dosage to a specific site. Certain organs, such as the uterus and vagina, are natural receptacles for the placement of an applicator that can be loaded with radioactive material. Radioactive needles, wires, seeds, beads, or catheters may be inserted directly into tumor tissue.

Unsealed internal radiation is administered intravenously or orally, so that it is distributed throughout the patient's body. Take special precautions to prevent exposure to radiation from direct contact with the patient or any body tissue or fluid (Box 57-3). In general, assemble materials and plan ahead to provide several nursing interventions at the same time on entering the patient's room. Stand as far away as possible from the site where an internal radiation device is in the patient's body. Limit the time needed for close contact near the irradiated site. If direct, prolonged care is needed, wear a lead apron.

Children younger than 18 years of age and pregnant women should not be allowed to visit implant patients. Advise approved visitors to limit visits to 10 minutes and to stand as far away from the patient as possible.

When cancer of the cervix is treated with the use of an applicator containing a radioactive material, the applicator is placed in the vagina. The following special nursing measures are indicated:

1. Place "Radiation in Use" sign on the patient's door.
2. Prevent dislodgment. Keep the patient on strict bed rest. Instruct the patient not to turn from side to side or onto the abdomen. Do not raise the head of the bed more than 45 degrees.
3. Do not give a complete bed bath while the applicator is in place, and do not bathe the patient below the waist. Do not change bed linen unless necessary.
4. Encourage the patient to do active range-of-motion (ROM) exercises with both arms and mild foot and leg exercises to minimize the hazards of immobility. Patient wears antiembolism stockings (thromboembolic disease hose) or pneumatic compression boots.
5. Monitor vital signs every 4 hours, observing for elevations in temperature, pulse, and respirations. Report to the physician a temperature higher than 100° F (37.7° C).
6. Observe for and report any rash or skin eruption, excessive vaginal bleeding, or vaginal discharge.
7. Keep accurate intake and output record. Encourage a fluid intake of at least 3 L/day. An indwelling catheter is in place to reduce the size of the bladder and decrease the effects of radiation on the bladder. Check to be sure it is draining well.
8. Serve diet as ordered—usually a low-residue diet to minimize peristalsis and bowel movement, which might lead to dislodgment of the applicator.
9. Check position of applicator every 4 hours.
10. Keep long-handled forceps and a special lead container in the patient's room for use by the radiologist, should the implant become dislodged. Never touch a dislodged applicator or any other materials that have fallen out of the patient. These may contain the radioactive sources. Any bed linens, dressings, or pads that have been changed for the patient must be checked with a radiation survey meter before they are removed from the patient's room.
11. After the applicator is removed, the indwelling catheter is usually removed, and a douche and enema are generally prescribed.
12. Precautions are no longer needed after removal of the applicator. Encourage ambulation and gradual resumption of activities.
13. Sexual intercourse is usually delayed for 7 to 10 days.
14. Instruct the patient to notify the physician of nausea, vomiting, diarrhea, frequent or painful urination, or a temperature more than 100° F (37.7° C).

CHEMOTHERAPY

Chemotherapy drugs are used to reduce the size or slow the growth of metastatic cancer. Most chemotherapeutic agents work by interfering with the cells' **replication** process (ability to multiply or reproduce). These drugs damage the cell and cause cellular death. Both malignant and normal cells are affected by chemotherapy. Cells that multiply rapidly, such as cells of the **hematopoietic system,** the **hair follicles,** and the **GI system,** are affected the most. The majority of the side effects from chemotherapeutic agents result from the destruction of normal cells in these systems (Table 57-3).

Hematopoietic System

Leukopenia

Leukopenia (reduction in the number of circulating white blood cells [WBCs] due to depression of the bone marrow) is a common problem for patients receiving chemotherapy. It can lead to life-threatening

Box 57-3 Instructions for Nursing Interventions for Patients Treated with (Unsealed Internal Radiation) ^{131}I for Thyroid Cancer

Spend as little time as possible for ordinary nursing care. The patient must be as self-sufficient as possible. The patient is radioactive and exposes the nurse to radiation while caring for the patient. The radioactive ^{131}I leaves the patient through urine and perspiration. Therefore the patient contaminates everything he or she touches and can spread contamination to the nurse in this way.

PRECAUTIONS TO REDUCE EXPOSURE TO THE NURSE

a. Limit the time spent in the room. Work quickly and enter only as necessary.
b. When in the room, maintain as much distance from the patient as possible. A few feet of distance makes a lot of difference in the amount of exposure to the nurse.
c. Wear shoe covers and disposable, fluid-proof gloves, and avoid contact with all surfaces in the room.
d. When leaving the room:
   1. Wash hands with gloves on.
   2. Remove one shoe cover at the door, step that foot out, and drop that shoe cover into the trash.
   3. Remove the other shoe cover and step that foot out and drop that shoe cover into the trash.
   4. Remove gloves and drop them into the trash.
   5. Do not remove shoe covers or gloves from the room. All trash must stay in the room.
e. Always wear the dosimeter while in the room and log the exposure you receive at each visit. The dosimeter, log, and instructions are kept outside the door.
   1. No visitors are allowed.
   2. The patient is confined to the room.
   3. Nothing is to leave the room unless checked for contamination and released by the radiation safety officer (RSO)/designee. All trash and laundry are to remain in the special containers.
   4. Pregnant, nursing, or nuclear medicine personnel will not enter the area.
   5. Shoe covers and fluid-proof disposable gloves (nonsterile type) are to be worn when entering the room. Gowns will be available.
   6. The dosimeter is to be worn in the room, and exposure is to be logged when leaving the room.
   7. All clothes and bed linens used by the patient should be placed in the laundry bag provided and should be left in the patient's room to be checked by the RSO/designee.
   8. No housekeeping is allowed until the room is officially released.
   9. Food is delivered only by nursing. It is delivered to the door and picked up by the patient. Mail, flowers, and other items are delivered in the same way.
   10. Whenever possible, only disposable items may be used in the care of these patients. These items should be placed in the designated waste container. Contact the RSO/designee for proper disposal of the contents of the designated waste container.
   11. Except in emergencies, urine collection or blood draws are not allowed after the patient has been dosed with ^{131}I. The urine and blood are radioactive.
   12. The patient is to flush the toilet three times after each use, and males should sit down to void.
   13. If the nurse helps to collect the excreta, disposable gloves should be worn. Afterward, hands should be washed with the gloves on and again after the gloves are removed. The gloves should be placed in the designated waste container for disposal by the RSO/designee.
   14. Utmost precautions must be taken to see that no urine or vomitus is spilled on the floor or the bed. If any part of the patient's room is suspected to be contaminated, notify the RSO/designee in the Nuclear Medicine Department.
   15. If a nurse, attendant, or anyone else knows or suspects that his or her skin or clothing, including shoes, is contaminated, notify the RSO/designee immediately. The potentially contaminated person should remain in an area adjacent to the patient's room and should not walk about the hospital. If the hands become contaminated, wash them immediately with soap and water.
   16. If a therapy patient should need emergency surgery or should die, notify the RSO or the Nuclear Medicine Department immediately.
   17. Vomiting within 24 hours after oral administration, urinary incontinence, or excessive sweating within the first 48 hours may result in contamination of linen and floor. In any such situation, or if radioactive urine or feces is spilled during collection, call the RSO/designee. Meanwhile, handle all contaminated material with disposable gloves and avoid spreading contamination.
   18. All vomitus must be kept in the patient's room for disposal by the RSO/designee only if the patient has vomited over the bed or the surrounding area. Otherwise, it will be flushed down the toilet with at least three volumes of water or more after it. Feces need not be routinely saved unless ordered on the chart. The same toilet should be used by the patient at all times, and it should be well flushed (at least three times).
   19. The patient may not be discharged without prior approval of the RSO/designee. The room may not be remade, used, or entered by unauthorized people until released by the RSO. Nothing may leave the room unless it is checked for contamination and released by the RSO.

Courtesy Great Plains Regional Medical Center Nuclear Medicine Department, North Platte, Nebraska.

 Table 57-3 Medications for Chemotherapy

Drug and Class	Mode of Action	Disease for Which Commonly Used	Common Side Effects
ALKYLATING AGENTS			
Cyclophosphamide (Cytoxan)	Interferes with DNA replication, cell-cycle nonspecific	Leukemia, breast, lymphoma, lung, ovarian, myeloma	Myelosuppression, alopecia, hemorrhagic cystitis, nausea, vomiting, cardiotoxicity
Cisplatin (Platinol)	Interferes with DNA replication, cell-cycle nonspecific	Testicular, ovarian, lung, cervical, head and neck	Nephrotoxicity, neurotoxicity, nausea, vomiting, ototoxicity
Carboplatin (Paraplatin)	Interferes with DNA replication, cell-cycle nonspecific	Ovarian, leukemia, lung	Myelosuppression, nausea, vomiting, nephrotoxicity, neurotoxicity
Chlorambucil (Leukeran)	Interferes with DNA replication, cell-cycle nonspecific	Lymphoma, chronic lymphocytic leukemia	Myelosuppression, sterility, stomatitis, pulmonary infiltrates
ANTITUMOR ANTIBIOTICS			
Bleomycin (Blenoxane)	Inhibits DNA and RNA synthesis, cell-cycle nonspecific	Testicular, cervical, Hodgkin's lymphoma	Anaphylaxis, nausea, vomiting, rash, pulmonary fibrosis, alopecia, stomatitis
Doxorubicin (Adriamycin)	Inhibits DNA and RNA synthesis, cell-cycle nonspecific	Breast, endometrial, leukemia, Hodgkin's melanoma, lymphoma	Myelosuppression, cardiotoxicity, extravasation, nausea, vomiting, alopecia, stomatitis, red urine (24-48 hours)
Mitoxantrone (Novantrone)	Inhibits DNA and RNA synthesis, cell-cycle nonspecific	Hodgkin's lymphoma, leukemia, breast cancer	Myelosuppression, cardiotoxicity, nausea, vomiting, blue urine (immediate to 24 hours)
ANTIMETABOLITES			
Cytarabine (Ara-C, Cytosar)	Damages cell in S phase, cell-cycle specific	Leukemia, lymphoma	Myelosuppression, neurotoxicity, rash, nausea, vomiting, stomatitis, alopecia, anaphylaxis
Fludarabine (Fludara)	Damages cell in S phase, cell-cycle specific	Leukemia (chronic lymphocytic leukemia, hairy cell), low-grade lymphoma	Myelosuppression, CNS toxicity, visual disturbance, nausea and vomiting, renal damage (tumor lysis syndrome)
Fluorouracil (5-FU)	Damages cell in S phase, cell-cycle specific	Breast, colorectal, liver, endometrial, esophageal, pancreatic, bladder	Myelosuppression, nausea, vomiting, stomatitis, alopecia, diarrhea
Gemcitabine (Gemzar)	Damages cell in S phase, cell-cycle specific	Pancreatic, lung	Myelosuppression, fatigue
Methotrexate (MXT, amethopterin)	Damages cell in S phase, cell-cycle specific	Breast, lymphoma, leukemia, bladder, head and neck, esophageal	Myelosuppression, diarrhea, oral and GI ulcerations, pulmonary infiltrates, nausea and vomiting
HORMONAL AGENTS			
Corticosteroids (dexamethasone [Decadron], hydrocortisone [Solu-Cortef], methylprednisolone [Solu-Medrol, Medrol], prednisone)	Alter hormonal environment that promotes cancer growth	Used in many chemotherapy disease protocols	Fluid and electrolyte disturbances, neuromuscular imbalances, changes in appetite and energy, requires glucose and insulin adjustment
Megestrol (Megace)	Alters hormonal environment that promotes cancer growth	Breast, prostate	Menstrual changes, hot flashes, nausea, vomiting, headache, weight gain, edema

CNS, Central nervous system; *DNA*, deoxyribonucleic acid; *GI*, gastrointestinal; *RNA*, ribonucleic acid.

Continued

Table 57-3 Medications for Chemotherapy—cont'd

Drug and Class	Mode of Action	Disease for Which Commonly Used	Common Side Effects
HORMONAL AGENTS—cont'd			
Leuprolide (Lupron)	Alters hormonal environment that promotes cancer growth	Prostate	Impotence, testicular atrophy, hot flashes, gynecomastia, peripheral edema
Tamoxifen (Nolvadex)	Competes with estrogen for binding sites in breast and other tissues	Breast	Vaginal bleeding, hot flashes, rash, hypercalcemia, peripheral edema
VINCA ALKALOIDS			
Etoposide (VP-16)	Inhibits cell division, cell-cycle specific	Lung, testicular, leukemia, lymphoma, small cell carcinoma of the lung	Myelosuppression, nausea, vomiting, diarrhea, fever, hypotension, phlebitis, alopecia
Vinblastine (Velban)	Inhibits cell division, cell-cycle specific	Testicular, Hodgkin's, lung, lymphoma, bladder, renal	Myelosuppression, extravasation, nausea, vomiting, alopecia, loss of deep tendon reflex
Vincristine (Oncovin)	Inhibits cell division, cell-cycle specific	Leukemia (acute lymphocytic leukemia, chronic myelogenous leukemia)	Extravasation, alopecia, stomatitis, constipation, peripheral neuropathy, optic atrophy
Vinorelbine (Navelbine)	Inhibits cell division, cell-cycle specific	Breast, lung, Hodgkin's, head and neck	Myelosuppression, alopecia, injection site reaction (phlebitis), nausea, anorexia, constipation, peripheral neuropathy
MISCELLANEOUS ANTINEOPLASTIC AGENTS			
Asparaginase (Elspar)	Cell-cycle specific (G phase)	Acute lymphocytic leukemia	Nausea, vomiting, chills, headache, CNS depression, abdominal pain, anaphylaxis
Paclitaxel (Taxol)	Mitotic inhibitor	Breast, lung, ovarian	Myelosuppression, dyspnea, hypotension, alopecia, cardiotoxicity, peripheral neuropathy, anaphylaxis
Docetaxel (Taxotere)	Miotic inhibitor	Breast, lung, ovarian	Myelosuppression, fluid retention, mucositis, phlebitis, vomiting, diarrhea, anaphylaxis
Topotecan (Hycamtin)	Interrupts DNA synthesis	Lung, breast, esophagus, tumor, lymphoma	Myelosuppression, nausea, vomiting, diarrhea, fever, fatigue, alopecia, elevated liver enzymes
Irinotecan (CPT-11, Camptosar)	Interrupts DNA synthesis	Colorectal, pancreatic	Severe diarrhea, myelosuppression, nausea and vomiting

infections. Normal value for WBCs is 5000 to 10,000/mm^3. A total WBC less than 4000/mm^3 is leukopenia. Lack of neutrophils, the type of WBC most often suppressed in the differential WBC count, is called **neutropenia.** Normal value for neutrophils is 60% to 70%, or 3000 to 7000/mm^3. The neutrophil count is less than 1000/mm^3 in neutropenia and less than 500/mm^3 in severe neutropenia. A patient with severe neutropenia should be placed on neutropenic precautions. Without enough neutrophils, the body's first line of defense collapses, opening the way for pneumonia, septicemia, or other potentially overwhelming infections.

Protect the patient against pathogens, monitor the patient for signs of infection, and respond aggressively if an infection occurs. Monitor the patient's vital signs every 4 hours and notify the physician if temperature starts to rise. A temperature of 100.4° F (38° C) or more is considered a sign of impending infection (see Safety Alert box).

Safety Alert!

Neutropenic Precautions

- Monitor for fever and neutrophil count to identify signs of and potential for infection.
- Evaluate for presence of chills. Take vital signs every 4 hours because fever may be the only indication of infection and septic shock.
- Report temperature elevations of more than 100.4° F (38° C) to the health care provider immediately so that antibiotic therapy can be initiated promptly to avoid the rapidly lethal effects of infection.
- Institute good hand hygiene technique with antiseptic solution for all people in contact with patient; place patient in private room; limit or screen visitors and hospital staff members with colds or potentially communicable illness to prevent transmission of harmful pathogens to patient.
- Teach patient necessary personal hygiene techniques (e.g., hand hygiene, oral care, skin hygiene, pulmonary hygiene, and potential infection risks).
- Avoid invasive procedures (e.g., venipuncture, urinary catheter) as much as possible.
- Administer hematopoietic growth factors (e.g., granulocyte colony-stimulating factors [G-CSFs] such as filgrastim [Neupogen] or pegfilgrastim [Neulasta]) to increase patient's WBC count and reduce infection risk during periods of neutropenia. Maintain neutropenic diet (avoid fresh fruits and vegetables because of presence of microscopic pathogens in uncooked produce). Discourage fresh flowers or live plants in the room. Mites, gnats, and other microscopic organisms could be a potential source of infection for the patient.

Take the following systematic approach to assessing the patient for infection.

Assessing the mouth. Stomatitis (inflammation of the oral mucosa) is one of the most common complications of chemotherapy and can lead to severe swallowing problems and systemic infections. Use a penlight and tongue blade to look for lesions, ulcers, or white plaque.

Teach the patient the importance of performing regular, but gentle, mouth care. Have the patient use a soft toothbrush and rinse the mouth with normal saline or sodium bicarbonate solution every 2 to 4 hours. A sponge-tipped applicator (Toothette) may help prevent bleeding gums, a common adverse effect of chemotherapy and radiation.

To reduce the risk of an oral *Candida* infection, the physician may order prophylactic antifungal medications such as an oral nystatin (Mycostatin) suspension, clotrimazole (Lotrimin) lozenges, or fluconazole (Diflucan). A soft or liquid diet may also be ordered

Assessing the skin. A rash or eruption may indicate that the patient has an infection or is predisposed to one. Bacteria may flourish in skinfolds, such as in the groin and axillae, so clean these areas twice a day with soap and water. Water-soluble moisturizers may be used to keep the patient's skin from drying. To prevent cuts, advise the patient to shave with an electric razor.

Vascular access sites are common gateways to infection. Monitor central and peripheral intravenous (IV) catheters carefully. Check for edema, drainage, erythema, or pain around catheter entry sites. Organisms can also grow along catheter tracts and infect the blood, resulting in septicemia. Signs and symptoms of a catheter tract infection include tenderness around the catheter site and referred pain in the shoulder.

Administer oral drugs whenever possible. Try to avoid subcutaneous or intramuscular injections because they can cause abscesses in patients with neutropenia. Excessive bleeding is also a risk for these patients because of the potential for associated decreases in platelets and other formed elements in the blood.

Puncturing the skin is sometimes unavoidable, as when the patient needs a bone marrow biopsy. After a biopsy, carefully assess the site, swab it with an antibacterial solution (such as povidone-iodine [Betadine]), and apply an occlusive dressing until the skin heals.

Assessing for pulmonary function. Many neutropenic patients with lung infections do not have common signs and symptoms, such as sputum production or infiltrates demonstrable on chest radiographs. Therefore be alert for other indications of an impending infection, including changes in lung sounds, respiratory rate and rhythm, and breathing effort. The patient may also complain of pain during inspiration or expiration.

To help prevent a lung infection, encourage the patient to perform deep-breathing and coughing exercises and to be as active as possible. Use of an incentive spirometer can help by maximizing ventilatory capacity.

Assessing urinary and bowel function. Changes in urinary function can also warn of infection in a neutropenic patient. Assess for decreased urinary output, changes in the urine's odor or color, hematuria, or glycosuria. The patient may also complain of urinary frequency, urgency, or pain.

To reduce the risk of urinary tract infection, avoid bladder catheterization. If catheterization is absolutely indicated, follow strict aseptic technique when inserting the catheter and perform catheter care according to the agency's guidelines.

Also routinely assess the patient's bowel function. Assess stool samples for color, consistency, and the presence of blood, and ask the patient to report any changes in bowel habits.

Does the patient need to strain when defecating? If so, the physician may prescribe a stool softener such as docusate (Colace). Straining can cause ulcerations or fissures in the rectum, creating ports of entry for bacteria. Avoid enemas, rectal medications, and rectal thermometers, which can break the mucosal lining. Be aware that neutropenia predisposes a patient to rectal abscesses. If the patient complains of perirectal pain, notify the physician immediately.

Medical management. A breakthrough in treating patients with neutropenia is commercially made colony-stimulating factors (CSFs), the only therapy that can actually prevent or manage neutropenia. The two types of CSFs are G-CSF (filgrastim, pegfilgrastim) and granulocyte-macrophage colony-stimulating factors (GM-CSF) (sargramostim [Leukine, Prokine]). These CSFs are given subcutaneously or intravenously. Although CSFs are extremely expensive, they are used prophylactically for patients at increased risk for neutropenia, such as those with a history of developing severe or prolonged neutropenia after chemotherapy.

Anemia

Anemia is a reduction in the number of circulating red blood cells (RBCs), hemoglobin, or volume of packed RBCs (hematocrit) due to depression of the bone marrow. Normal values are as follows:

	Male	Female
Erythrocytes (RBCs)	4.7 to 6.1 million/mm^3	4.2 to 5.4 million/mm^3
Hemoglobin	14 to 18 g/dL	12 to 16 g/dL
Hematocrit	42% to 52%	37% to 47%

Hemoglobin levels of 10 to 14 g/dL indicate mild anemia, 6 to 10 g/dL indicate moderate anemia, and less than 6 g/dL indicate severe anemia. Fatigue is a major problem for persons with anemia because of the decreased oxygenation to tissues from the decreased hemoglobin. For the hospitalized patient, plan to balance activities and rest to prevent increased oxygen expenditure and hypoxemia. Persons at home need to plan activities of daily living to allow rest periods.

Recombinant human erythropoietin, or epoetin alfa (EPO; Epogen, Procrit), was initially approved by the U.S. Food and Drug Administration (FDA) in 1987 for management of chronic anemia associated with end-stage renal disease. In 1993 the FDA approval was expanded to include management of chemotherapy-related anemia. EPO is given subcutaneously or intravenously.

Transfusion of packed RBCs is indicated if there is evidence of cardiac decompensation or if low hemoglobin levels are combined with low platelet counts. The transfusion improves oxygen-carrying capacity, which provides for more efficient use of blood components and less risk of volume overload.

Thrombocytopenia

Thrombocytopenia is a reduction in the number of circulating platelets due to the depression of the bone marrow. Normal platelet values are 150,000 to 400,000/mm^3. When the platelet count is less than 20,000/mm^3, spontaneous bleeding can occur. Platelet transfusions may be necessary.

Patient teaching measures to prevent injury and hemorrhage due to decreased platelets include (1) use soft toothbrush or swab for mouth care; (2) keep mouth clean and free of debris; (3) avoid intrusions into rectum (such as rectal medications or enemas); (4) use electric shaver; (5) apply direct pressure for 5 to 10 minutes if any bleeding occurs; (6) avoid contact sports, elective surgery, and tooth extraction; (7) avoid picking or blowing nose forcefully; (8) avoid trauma, falls, bumps, and cuts; (9) avoid use of aspirin or aspirin preparations; and (10) use adequate lubrication and gentleness during sexual intercourse.

Integumentary System

Alopecia

Alopecia is loss of hair due to the destruction of hair follicles. It may occur by two mechanisms. If the hair roots are atrophied, alopecia occurs readily. The hair falls out either spontaneously or during hair combing, often in large clumps. If the hair shaft is constricted because of atrophy or necrosis, the hair will break off very near the scalp. The root remains in the scalp, and a patchy, thinning pattern of hair loss occurs. Hair loss may also occur on other parts of the body. Loss of leg, arm, pubic, axillary, and facial hair is less common than loss of eyebrows and eyelashes.

The pattern and extent of hair loss cannot be accurately predicted for a given patient. When treatment is given with a drug known to cause alopecia, tell the patient that severe hair loss can begin within a few days or weeks of treatment and that partial or complete baldness can quickly ensue. Drug-induced alopecia is never permanent. The patient may experience a change in hair color or texture when the hair grows back. Occasionally, hair growth may return while chemotherapy treatment continues. Because hair loss is temporary, and the drugs are necessary to control or cure the cancer, most patients tolerate the hair loss with minimal distress. However, many patients have difficulty adjusting to the change in body image due to hair loss.

To meet the patient's needs, provide an education program, written materials, and educational sessions with a hair stylist. Inform the patient about health care measures for scalp protection, such as using gentle shampoos; avoiding hair dryers, curling irons, permanents, and hair coloring; protecting the scalp in winter and summer (cold or heat loss); and wearing protective covering when outdoors. The patient with long or thick hair may wish to trim or cut hair short to delay hair loss as long as possible. Provide sincere concern and emotional support for the patient.

Gastrointestinal System

Stomatitis

Stomatitis is a mouth inflammation due to destruction of normal cells of the oral cavity. It may range from erythema of the oral mucosa to mild or severe ulceration. Methotrexate, 5-fluorouracil (5-FU), doxorubicin, dactinomycin, and bleomycin are the chemotherapeutic drugs that most frequently cause stomatitis. Patients may also develop a superimposed fungal infection of the mouth and esophagus, and oral nystatin or fluconazole is usually prescribed. Good mouth care is important.

Viscous lidocaine (Xylocaine) is used when stomatitis becomes intolerable. Light topical application can decrease pain so the patient may eat and drink. Usually a soft or liquid diet is encouraged to help maintain nutritional status.

Nausea, Vomiting, and Diarrhea

Nausea, vomiting, and diarrhea are disorders of the GI tract caused by the excessive breakdown of normal GI cells. Nausea and vomiting are among the most uncomfortable and distressing side effects of chemotherapy. The onset and duration vary greatly among patients and with the drug given. For the ambulatory patient, nausea may interfere with the ability to continue daily work. Persistent vomiting may result in fluid and electrolyte imbalance, general weakness, and weight loss. Decline of nutritional status renders the patient more susceptible to infection and perhaps less able to tolerate therapy. Such physiologic symptoms can accompany or precipitate psychological responses such as depression and withdrawal. Every effort must be made to minimize chemotherapy-induced nausea and vomiting.

Antiemetics vary in success. Tetrahydrocannabinol (THC) (a chemical found in marijuana) taken in pill form produces an antiemetic effect in some patients who have not benefited from the commonly prescribed prochlorperazine (Compazine). Metoclopramide (Reglan), ondansetron (Zofran), and granisetron (Kytril) are often helpful for people receiving chemotherapy, and lorazepam (Ativan) may produce a relaxed state during which an individual is less sensitive to nausea-inducing stimuli (Table 57-4). The patient may receive antiemetics orally,

Table 57-4 Medications for Symptom Control of Cancer Treatment

Generic (Brand)	Action	Side Effects	Nursing Implications
Ondansetron (Zofran)	Antiemetic	Headache, diarrhea, constipation, abdominal pain, transient increase in aspartate aminotransferase (AST) or alanine aminotransferase (ALT)	Dilute intravenous dose with D_5W or NaCl and give total dose (approximately 32 mg) 30 minutes before chemotherapy. Give 8 mg po before chemotherapy and three times a day for 2 days.
Granisetron (Kytril)	Antiemetic	Headache, constipation, somnolence, diarrhea, mild changes in blood pressure	Administer dose over 5-minute period, beginning 30 minutes before chemotherapy. Give once a day in a 5-minute infusion, or give 2 mg po 1 hour before chemotherapy and 1 mg bid for 2 days.
Metoclopramide (Reglan)	Antiemetic	Drowsiness, extrapyramidal reactions, restlessness, dysrhythmias, anxiety	Administer IV dose 30 minutes before administration of chemotherapeutic agent. Administer oral doses 30 minutes before meals and at bedtime.
Prochlorperazine (Compazine)	Antiemetic	Extrapyramidal symptoms, orthostatic hypotension, ocular changes (blurred vision), dry mouth, constipation, urine retention, photosensitivity	Use cautiously with other CNS depressants (e.g., alcohol) and medications that decrease blood pressure, as well as patients with liver disease. Decrease dose in older adults. Do not exceed recommended dose. Protect from light.
Diphenoxylate with atropine (Lomotil)	Antidiarrheal	Sedation, dizziness, dry mouth, urinary retention, rash	Watch for physical dependence. It should work within 48 hours. Give naloxone as antidote for respiratory depression.
Morphine (Roxanol, MS Contin)	Opioid analgesic	Decreased respiratory rate, euphoria, seizures, physical dependence, hypotension, bradycardia, miosis, drowsiness, dizziness, urinary retention, constipation, rash	Use cautiously with other CNS depressants (e.g., alcohol). Monitor respirations, heart rate, and mental status closely. Have naloxone available as antidote. Do not give sustained-release tablets for acute pain.
Hydromorphone (Dilaudid)	Opioid analgesic	Decreased respiratory rate, euphoria, seizures, physical dependence, hypotension, bradycardia, miosis, drowsiness, dizziness, urinary retention, constipation, rash	Use cautiously with other CNS depressants (e.g., alcohol). Monitor respirations, heart rate, and mental status closely. Have naloxone available as antidote. Do not give sustained-release tablets for acute pain. Have Dilaudid-HP (10 mg/mL) available for chronic pain.

GI, Gastrointestinal; *NaCl*, sodium chloride.

Continued

Table 57-4 Medications for Symptom Control of Cancer Treatment—cont'd

Generic (Brand)	Action	Side Effects	Nursing Implications
Naproxen (Naprosyn, Anaprox)	Nonsteroidal antiinflammatory agent	Agranulocytosis, headache, dizziness, drowsiness, peripheral edema, visual disturbances, GI upset (occult blood loss and peptic ulcers), prolonged bleeding time, tinnitus	Concurrent use of alcohol, acetylsalicylic acid, and steroids increases chance of GI bleeding. It may interact with warfarin sodium (Coumadin). Avoid use in patient allergic to acetylsalicylic acid. Give with food. Advise patient that it may take 4 weeks to show benefit.
Diphenhydramine (Benadryl)	Antihistamine; may also be used for antiemetic and sedation purposes	Drowsiness, dry mouth	Anticholinergic effect; used as an antiemetic.
Metoclopramide (Reglan)	Antiemetic	Restlessness, dry mouth, delayed gastric emptying, gastroesophageal reflux	Assess patient for nausea, vomiting, abdominal distention, and bowel sounds before and after administration
Amitriptyline (Elavil)	Tricyclic antidepressant	Tremors, orthostatic hypotension, urinary retention	Use in combination with narcotics in neuropathies and postherpetic neuralgia (especially with burning pain). Therapeutic effect takes 2 to 3 weeks.
Dexamethasone (Decadron)	Antiinflammatory and immune modifier	Hyperglycemia, mood swings, depression	Effective as antiemetic in chemotherapy: immunosuppression, palliation of selected neoplasms.
Lorazepam (Ativan)	Antianxiety agent, antiemetic	Drowsiness, headache, diarrhea, respiratory depression	Smoking decreases effectiveness. Decreases nausea, especially when given before and during chemotherapy.

intramuscularly, rectally, or intravenously, as well as via pumps in patient-controlled analgesia.

The development and use of the 5-HT_3 antagonists (ondansetron, granisetron) has resulted in effective antiemetic therapy. Prevention of nausea and vomiting increases patient comfort while decreasing or eliminating anxiety and fear. These antiemetics are given before chemotherapy and afterward, as directed by the physician. The drugs have mild side effects and can be used safely in the outpatient setting. Metoclopramide, a dopamine antagonist, has proven effective in controlling mild to moderate nausea and vomiting. Metoclopramide blocks dopamine receptors in the chemoreceptor trigger zone of the central nervous system, stimulates motility of the upper GI tract, and accelerates gastric emptying (see Table 57-4).

Changes in bowel habits commonly occur but usually do not require intervention. If diarrhea becomes marked or persistent, an antidiarrheal medication such as diphenoxylate with atropine (Lomotil) may be prescribed.

Nursing Interventions

Combinations of chemotherapy agents, as well as chemotherapy combined with other treatments, have increased the number of cures, remissions, and palliative outcomes. Many of the problems experienced by people undergoing chemotherapy are the same as those that may result from radiation therapy (depending on the target site and amount of radiation). Help the patient realize that some of the problems are the result of therapy and not a sign that the cancer is getting worse.

Nursing diagnoses and interventions for the patient undergoing chemotherapy include but are not limited to the following:

Nursing Diagnoses	Nursing Interventions
Impaired tissue integrity: oral mucous membrane, related to: • stomatitis (inflammation of the mouth) • xerostomia (decreased salivation)	Assist with frequent, careful oral hygiene and hydration; use very soft toothbrush. Provide meticulous mouth care. Administer prescribed antifungal medication such as fluconazole. Give soothing oral lozenges, ice chips, and frequent sips of ice water; avoid hot beverages; use lip balm for dryness.

Nursing Diagnoses	Nursing Interventions
Imbalanced nutrition: less than body requirements, related to: • anorexia (from changes in taste and smell) • nausea and vomiting • dysphagia (difficulty swallowing) • aspiration • diarrhea • malabsorption • cachexia (general ill health and malnutrition, marked by weakness and emaciation, usually associated with a serious disease such as cancer)	Provide adequate, easily digestible, soft, bland diet; avoid spicy foods. Keep room free of odors and clutter. Administer prescribed antiemetic medications. Give small, frequent, highly nutritional meals to meet the extra demands created by energy used by malignant cells; allow extra time to eat.
Risk for infection, related to: • weakened immune system • leukopenia	Protect against infections, especially from other people. Advise patient to avoid crowds. Observe and promptly report to physician any signs of inflammation at injection sites or insertion sites of any peripheral or central IV lines; report any temperature greater than 100° F (37.7° C). Use sterile technique whenever possible. Initiate reverse isolation as indicated. Monitor temperature, leukocyte count. Discourage fresh-cut flowers. Avoid indwelling catheters and performing rectal procedures or examinations. Administer antibiotics as prescribed.

Tumor Lysis Syndrome

Tumor lysis syndrome (TLS) is an oncologic emergency with rapid lysis of malignant cells.

Etiology and Pathophysiology

TLS may occur spontaneously in patients with inordinately high tumor burdens. However, it is usually a result of chemotherapy or, less commonly, radiation therapy. It may occur anywhere from 24 hours to 7 days after antineoplastic therapy is initiated. Patients most at risk are those who have large tumor cell burdens (e.g., high-grade lymphomas) or markedly elevated WBC level (acute leukemias). TLS is also seen in chronic lymphocytic leukemia and metastatic breast cancer.

The syndrome develops when chemotherapy or irradiation causes the destruction (or lysis) of a large number of rapidly dividing malignant cells. As malignant cells are lysed, intracellular contents are rapidly released into the bloodstream. This results in high levels of potassium (hyperkalemia), phosphate (hyperphosphatemia), and uric acid (hyperuricemia). These conditions, plus secondary hypocalcemia, all put the patient at risk for renal failure and alterations in cardiac function.

Clinical Manifestations

Early signs include nausea, vomiting, anorexia, and diarrhea; these may be accompanied by muscle weakness and cramping. Later signs may progress to tetany, paresthesias, seizures, anuria, and cardiac arrest.

Diagnostic Tests

TLS is diagnosed by observation of the signs and symptoms and by confirmation of abnormal laboratory values. Early symptoms of TLS may not be readily apparent, and clinical manifestations appear rapidly; the syndrome is most frequently detected by abnormalities in blood chemistry. Serum potassium, phosphate, calcium, and uric acid are diagnostic. Other important values include serum creatinine, blood urea nitrogen, and urine pH.

Medical Management

The best way to treat TLS is to prevent it by recognizing the patient population who is at risk and initiating prophylactic measures before beginning antineoplastic therapy. This includes pretreatment **hydration** to maintain a urinary output of 150 mL/hr. Hydration should begin 24 to 48 hours before treatment and continue for at least 72 hours after treatment. **Diuretics** may be used to promote the excretion of phosphate and uric acid, to prevent volume overload, and to promote the excretion of potassium in the urine. **Allopurinol** prevents uric acid formation. It is begun a few days before treatment and should be continued for 3 to 5 days after treatment is completed. **Sodium bicarbonate** is used to maintain an alkaline urine (pH over 7) to prevent uric acid crystallization. Cation-exchange resins, such as kayexalate, are used to bind with potassium so it can be excreted through the bowel. **Calcium gluconate** is given intravenously to correct hypocalcemia. Cardiac monitoring is required. Phosphate-binding gels, such as aluminum hydroxide, are given to form an insoluble complex that is excreted by the bowel. When these measures are not successful, renal dialysis may be necessary.

Nursing Interventions

Nursing interventions include identifying patients at risk for TLS and initiating hydration 24 to 48 hours before chemotherapy. Administer allopurinol before and during chemotherapy to maintain alkaline urine. Assess medications for those that contain phosphate or spare potassium and discuss discontinuation with physician. Monitor potassium, phosphorus, calcium, and uric acid levels. Also assess patient for signs and symptoms of TLS, including the following:

- **Hyperkalemia:** electrocardiographic changes, muscle weakness, twitching, paresthesia, paralysis, muscle cramps, nausea, vomiting, lethargy, and syncope
- **Hyperphosphatemia:** azotemia, oliguria, hypertension, and renal failure
- **Hypocalcemia:** electrocardiographic changes (heart block, dysrhythmias, and cardiac arrest), tetany, confusion, and hallucinations
- **Hyperuricemia:** renal failure, nausea, vomiting, flank pain, gout, and pruritus

If hyperuricemia is detected, administer diuretics, sodium bicarbonate, cation-exchange resins, and phosphate-binding gels as appropriate. Monitor intake and output and notify physician if urinary output is less than 100 mL/hr. Monitor urine pH and maintain at greater than 7 with sodium bicarbonate. Prepare the patient and family for dialysis if other measures are not effective.

Prognosis

Successful treatment of TLS depends on preventing renal failure. TLS typically resolves within 7 days, once appropriate treatment is initiated.

Chemotherapy has proven effective in treatment of many cancer patients. Many cancer patients can be cured with chemotherapy, whereas others experience cancer-free intervals or control of cancer pain. Learn about each drug being administered to anticipate the expected side effects and plan the nursing interventions needed.

Follow safety guidelines in preparing and administering chemotherapeutic agents because they may be absorbed into the skin or inhaled. The major types of chemotherapeutic agents used to treat cancer are given in Table 57-3.

BIOTHERAPY

The observation of interactions between the immune system and malignant cells led to the development of therapies that could manipulate this natural process. Traditionally, this field has been known as immunotherapy. It has led to the modern era of biotherapy. Since the 1980s, biotherapy, or biologic therapy, has emerged as an important fourth modality for treating cancer. **Biotherapy** may be defined as treatment with agents derived from biologic sources or affecting biologic responses.

Biologic response modifiers (BRMs) work through three major mechanisms. The first mechanism increases, restores, or modifies the host defenses against the tumor (CSFs, filgrastim, erythropoietin, GM-CSFs). The second mechanism uses agents that are directly toxic to tumors (interleukins, bacille Calmette-Guérin vaccine [BCG]). The third mechanism modifies the tumor biology (interferons alpha, beta, and gamma).

Most of these therapies are intramuscular or subcutaneous injections and need to be given over an extended time. Compliance and motivation are important considerations when monitoring these patients. Side effects common to BMRs include fatigue, flulike symptoms, leukopenia, nausea, and vomiting.

Health care professionals must understand these therapies to help give the cancer patient the best chance available. These therapies and research are leading to the development of gene therapy today; this will lead to improved cancer therapy in the future.

BONE MARROW TRANSPLANTATION

Bone marrow transplantation is the process of replacing diseased or damaged bone marrow with normally functioning bone marrow. Bone marrow transplants (BMTs) are used in the treatment of a variety of diseases and offer a chance for long-term survival.

Stem cell transplants are being used in some solid tumor cancers, such as high-risk breast cancer. Bone marrow harvests are becoming less frequent because many centers have turned to peripheral stem cell transplants for hematopoietic support after high-dose chemotherapy (Lewis et al., 2007).

Most transplantation bone marrow is obtained by multiple needle aspirations from the posterior iliac crest while the patient is under general or spinal anesthesia. The anterior iliac crest and sternum may also be used. The amount of marrow extracted ranges from 600 to 2500 mL for the average adult. After processing, the marrow is given to the patient intravenously through a transfusion bag, or it can be frozen (cryopreservation). Marrow may be kept for 3 or more years. When the bone marrow is infused, it is via a central line without a filter over 1 to 4 hours.

Bone marrow may be removed from an individual for personal use (**autologous,** indicating something that has its origin within an individual, especially a factor present in tissues or fluids) at a later time. Alternatively, an individual may be given **allogenic** bone marrow (meaning the transplant came from someone else). Three types of allogenic BMTs are (1) **syngeneic** (donation from the patient's identical twin), (2) **related** (donation from a relative, usually a sibling), and (3) **unrelated** (donation from a nonrelative). The patient is at increased risk for developing infection during the process of transplant because the immune defenses are weakened. These patients are cared for in special bone marrow units so they can be monitored closely.

Interventions to prevent infections include protective isolation or laminar airflow rooms; prophylactic systemic antibiotics and antiviral agents (primarily acyclovir); and routine cultures of blood, urine, throat, and stool. Despite these and other interventions, the patient can become septic in hours, with multisystem failure.

Survival after bone marrow transplantation depends on the patient's age, remission, and clinical status at the time of transplantation.

PERIPHERAL STEM CELL TRANSPLANTATION

An emerging and promising alternative to BMT is peripheral stem cell transplant (PSCT). This procedure is based on the fact that peripheral or circulating stem cells are capable of repopulating the bone marrow. PSCT is a type of transplant that differs from BMT primarily in the method of collection of stem cells. Because there are fewer stem cells in the blood than in the bone marrow, mobilization of stem cells from the bone marrow into the peripheral blood can be done using chemotherapy or hematopoietic growth factors, such as GM-CSF and G-CSF.

The donor's blood is collected via pheresis, in which the person is attached to a cell separator machine that removes peripheral stem cells and then returns the blood to the person. This procedure, called **leukapheresis,** usually takes 2 to 4 hours. In autologous transplants the stem cells are purged to kill any cancer cells and then frozen and stored until used for transplantation. Although many of the same steps (harvesting, intensive chemotherapy, reinfusion) of BMT are used in PSCT, the hematologic recovery period in PSCT is shorter, and fewer, less severe complications are seen (Lewis et al., 2007).

NURSING INTERVENTIONS

Communicate genuine concern for cancer patients by reinforcing information explained to patients by their physicians regarding the expectations of their specific treatments. Patients may become discouraged by toxic side effects and other problems they experience while undergoing conventional cancer therapies. Allow extra time to listen to patients with cancer express their feelings, and encourage them to follow the guidelines of conventional medical practice that offer the most hope.

ADVANCED CANCER

PAIN MANAGEMENT

Patients with cancer may have pain at any point during the course of the disease and its treatment. In fact, of the 4 million people throughout the world who die from cancer each year, 70% experience pain as a primary symptom. Unfortunately, many people believe that pain is an early symptom of cancer and do not seek diagnosis until pain occurs. In fact, pain is almost always a late symptom and indicates tumor obstruction, pressure on the nerves, invasion of bone, phantom sensation, peripheral neuropathy, and neuralgia.

It is estimated that 85% of patients with cancer pain can be managed effectively with appropriate therapy. The American Cancer Society, the American Pain Society, the World Health Organization, the Oncology Nursing Society, and many other organizations consider pain control a major issue in the management of a person with cancer.

One of the many challenges in caring for the patient with pain is the assessment. Accept the definition of pain as whatever the person experiencing the pain says it is, existing whenever the patient says it does. It is extremely important not to be judgmental concerning the patient's complaints of pain.

Cultural and religious practices in one's family play an important role in the perception of pain or suffering as a weakness. Some families tend to minimize pain. Other cultures expect the expression of pain; therefore they may have a greater overt expression of pain.

Opioids used in the management of cancer pain include morphine (the prototype), hydromorphone (Dilaudid), fentanyl, and methadone. Sustained-release morphine in an oral form, such as MS Contin, Oramorph SR, Avinza, Kadian, or Roxanol SR, is particularly effective in the management of the terminally ill person with pain. Administering opioids via transdermal method, inhalation, IV drips, intrathecally, and epidurally enhances the analgesic effect. Avoiding the peaks and valleys of pain relief with bolus injections provides more constant pain relief. The need for around-the-clock dosage is clear. Fixed dosage schedules with adequate doses for pain relief provide more constant blood levels and predictable pain relief. Some patients have breakthrough pain that requires additional doses, but the fixed dosage schedule should be maintained. Monitor and treat any opioid side effects such as constipation, vomiting, and respiratory and central nervous system depression.

In addition to opioids, valuable nonopioid analgesics used in the treatment of certain levels of cancer pain are acetaminophen; aspirin; and nonsteroidal antiinflammatory drugs, such as ibuprofen, indomethacin, and naproxen.

Patient self-control methods include distraction, massage, relaxation, biofeedback, hypnosis, and imagery. Many patients find that self-care measures enhance the effectiveness of other prescribed pain interventions. Adequate rest, sleep, diversion, and other meaningful activities also help manage the patient's pain. The patient with advanced cancer often experiences cachexia, a profound state of ill health, and malnutrition, marked by weakness and emaciation. Positioning, giving meticulous skin care, offering nutritious fluids and foods, and using other comfort measures to promote relaxation and rest will help to reduce pain and severe fatigue.

The nurse's unique role in pain management involves acting as link between the patient and the health care team, spending time with the patient, assessing the patient's response to the pain and its management, and educating the patient and the family. In addition, be able to articulate a concise pain assessment as well as anticipate and address patient, family, and health care provider misconceptions about pain management. For example, many patients and their families have opioid phobia, the irrational and undocumented fear that even the appropriate use of opioids causes addiction. This fear of addiction among both health care providers and the public seems to be a major reason for the undertreatment of pain. Understand and be able to state why opioids are needed for terminally ill patients. Appropriate use of pain management strategies enables patients and families to accept the therapeutic value of drugs such as opioids. Ensure that patients are not subjected to severe suffering from potentially controllable pain.

General guidelines for the use of pain relief measures are (1) use a variety of pain relief measures; (2) use pain relief measures before the pain becomes severe; (3) include pain relief measures that the patient believes will be helpful; (4) determine the patient's ability or willingness to participate actively in the use of pain relief measures; (5) rely on patient behavior to indicate pain severity rather than relying on known physical stimuli; (6) encourage the patient to try a pain relief measure at least two times before abandoning it as ineffective; (7) have an open mind as to what may relieve the patient's pain, including nonpharmacologic measures; and (8) keep trying to relieve the pain; do not become discouraged and do not stop working with the patient.

Fear and anxiety increase as a result of pain. Many cancer patients believe increased pain is a sign their condition is worsening and death is imminent. Pain increases their fear, and the cycle of pain continues. The most effective pain relief is probably a combination of (1) appropriate pain relief methods, (2) the opportunity to make personal and spiritual peace if there are unresolved conflicts in relationships with others, and (3) someone to listen and offer comfort.

NUTRITIONAL THERAPY

Nutritional problems that most frequently occur in the patient with cancer are malnutrition, anorexia, altered taste sensation, nausea, vomiting, diarrhea, stomatitis, and mucositis. These problems can be caused by a combination of factors, including drug toxicity, effects of radiation therapy, tumor involvement, recent surgery, emotional distress, or difficulty with ingestion or digestion of food. If the patient is inadequately nourished, the normal cells will not be able to recover from the effects of therapy, and the immune system will be depressed because of depletion of protein stores.

Malnutrition

The patient with cancer usually experiences protein and calorie malnutrition characterized by fat and muscle depletion. Encourage the patient to eat foods that increase protein intake and facilitate repair and regeneration of cells, as well as high-calorie foods that provide energy and minimize weight loss.

Suggest to the physician the need for a nutritional supplement as soon as a 5% weight loss is noted or the patient has the potential for protein and caloric malnutrition. Monitor albumin and prealbumin levels. Once a 10-pound (4.5-kg) weight loss occurs, it is difficult to maintain the nutritional status. Instruct the patient to use nutritional supplements in place of milk when cooking or baking. Nutritional supplements can be easily be added to scrambled eggs, pudding, custard, mashed potatoes, cereal, and cream sauces. Packages of instant breakfast can be used as indicated or sprinkled on cereals, desserts, and casseroles. If the malnutrition cannot be treated with dietary intake, it may be necessary to use enteral or parenteral nutrition as an adjunct nutritional measure.

Anorexia

The anorexia experienced by a patient with cancer is a challenging problem. An intervention may be effective one day and ineffective the next. Continual assessment and intervention are necessary to successfully manage this problem. Adopt the philosophy that something can be done to prevent or minimize anorexia, evaluate each intervention, and continue to use those interventions that have been successful in the past. Megestrol (Megace) is used in cachexia anorexia to stimulate the appetite.

Altered Taste Sensation

Cancer cells are believed to release substances that resemble amino acids and stimulate the bitter taste buds. The patient may also experience an alteration in the sweet, sour, and salty taste sensations. Meat may taste bitter. At this time the physiologic basis of these varied taste alterations is unknown. Instruct the patient with an altered taste problem to avoid foods he or she dislikes. Frequently the patient may feel compelled to eat certain foods because they are "healthy." Advise the patient to experiment with spices and other seasoning agents to mask the taste alterations. Lemon juice, onion, mint, basil, and fruit juice marinades may improve the taste of certain meats and fish. Bacon bits, onion, and pieces of ham may enhance the taste of vegetables. Just adding more spice or seasoning agent is usually not an effective way to enhance the taste.

COMMUNICATION AND PSYCHOLOGICAL SUPPORT

The patient and the family may become irritable and angry with caregivers when the patient is suffering and has progressive problems. Understand that these feelings are not directed toward the caregivers personally but have emerged from the circumstances associated with the patient's disease. A display of anger toward the staff may be caused by deep-seated frustration or anxiety. Understanding and continued warm, responsive caring are the best approaches. The patient may not hear the explanations that are given when feelings are at a high level. Listening and administering kind, gentle nursing care may communicate more effectively than words. Touch may also be appropriate, letting the patient know that someone else is aware of the emotional distress being experienced.

Nurses are able to make cancer's effects less traumatic through sensitivity and creativity. Understand how much each patient needs a sense of control; some need it more than others. The health care system encourages dependency by stripping away most traces of a patient's identity. An adult is told when to get out of bed, have a drink, wash up, and even urinate. Be aware of what is happening to the patient and provide as many avenues of patient control as possible. Learn the art of talking to patients, not *at* patients.

Psychological support of the patient is an important aspect of cancer care. Because of the effectiveness of cancer treatment, many patients with cancer are cured or their disease is controlled for long periods. Thus emphasis must be placed on maintaining an optimal quality of life after the diagnosis of cancer. A positive attitude of patient, family, and caregivers toward cancer and cancer treatment has a significant positive effect on the quality of life that the patient experiences. A positive attitude may also influence the patient's prognosis.

Most people view the diagnosis of cancer as a crisis. Cancer affects the quality of life of all cancer patients in some way. Four quality-of-life factors affecting cancer patients and their families are social, psychological, physical, and spiritual (American Cancer Society, 2008a). The most common concerns voiced by the patient are (1) fear of recurrence, (2) chronic or acute pain, (3) sexual problems, (4) fatigue, (5) guilt for delaying screening or treatment, (6) behavior that may have increased the risk for cancer, (7) changes in physical appearance, (8) depression, (9) sleep problems, (10) change in role performance, and (11) being a financial burden on their loved ones (American Cancer Society, 2008a).

Coping with these fears exposes the patient to a range of emotions and behaviors: shock, anger, denial, bargaining, depression, helplessness, hopelessness, rationalization, acceptance, and intellectualization. These behavioral patterns may occur at any time during the process of cancer. However, some patterns appear to occur more frequently or at a greater intensity at certain specific stages of the disease process. The following factors may determine how the patient will cope with the diagnosis of cancer:

- **Ability to cope with stressful events in the past** (e.g., loss of job, major disappointment): Ask how the patient has coped with stressful events to gain an understanding of the patient's coping patterns, their effectiveness, and the usual coping time frame.
- **Availability of significant others:** The patient who has effective support systems tends to cope more effectively than the patient who does not.
- **Ability to express feelings and concerns:** The patient who is able to express feelings and needs and who seeks and asks for help appears to cope more effectively than the patient who internalizes feelings and needs.
- **Age at the time of diagnosis:** Age determines the coping strategies to a great degree. For example, a young mother with cancer has different concerns than a 70-year-old woman with cancer.
- **Extent of disease:** Cure or control of the disease process is usually easier to cope with than the reality of terminal illness.
- **Disruption of body image:** Disruption of the body image (e.g., radical neck dissection, alopecia, mastectomy) may intensify the psychological effect of cancer.
- **Presence of symptoms:** Symptoms such as fatigue, nausea, diarrhea, and pain may intensify the psychological effect of cancer.
- **Experience with cancer:** If experiences with cancer have been negative, the patient will probably view the present status as negative.
- **Attitude associated with cancer:** A patient who feels in control and has a positive attitude about cancer and cancer treatment is better able to cope with the diagnosis and treatment than one who feels hopeless, helpless, and out of control.

To facilitate the development of a hopeful attitude about cancer and to support the patient and the family during the various stages of the process of cancer, continue to be available, especially during difficult times. Exhibit a caring attitude, and listen actively to fears and concerns. Maintain a relationship based on trust and confidence; be open, honest, and caring in the approach. Use touch to exhibit caring; a squeeze of the hand may at times be more effective than words.

Provide essential information regarding cancer and cancer care. Provide relief from distressing symptoms. Assist the patient in setting realistic, reachable short- and long-term goals. Assist the patient in maintaining usual lifestyle patterns. Above all, maintain hope, which is the key to effective cancer care. Hope varies, depending on the patient's status—hope that the symptoms are not serious, hope that the treatment is curative, hope for independence, hope for relief of pain, hope for a longer life, or hope for a peaceful death. Hope provides control over what is occurring and is the basis of a positive attitude toward cancer and cancer care (Lewis et al., 2007) (see Evidence-Based Practice box).

TERMINAL PROGNOSIS

Coping with the multiple problems associated with advanced cancer can lead to a sense of helplessness and hopelessness in spite of all efforts. The patient and the family may look forward to death as a relief from unrelenting suffering.

Most patients with advanced cancer know that they are dying. They recognize attempts to avoid the truth and may distrust and feel hostile toward the person who makes such attempts. Honesty and openness are

Evidence-Based Practice: The Burden of Illness for Cancer Survivors

Evidence Summary

A group of researchers wanted to learn about the burden of illness among cancer survivors. They studied more than 1800 cancer survivors, as well as individuals without cancer (control group) who were matched with cancer survivors by age, sex, and educational attainment. The study examined several measures of burden or stress, including a person's sense of utility or feeling useful, a perception of overall health, and days lost from work. The results of the study showed that cancer survivors had poorer outcomes across all measures: lower utility, higher levels of lost productivity, and more likely to report their health as fair or poor when matched with control subjects.

Application to Nursing Practice

As a nurse, learn to assess the many ways in which cancer affects the lives of patients who are survivors. Because cancer causes long-term effects, spend time assessing patients' symptoms, the effects of symptoms on lifestyle and self-care ability, the effects on patient relationships, the patients' ability to remain productive and successful in their jobs, their economic security, and their physical well-being. Patients' self-perceptions are also important to understand when you attempt any intervention that requires the patient to be motivated and involved.

Reference

Yabroff, K.R., et al. (2004). Burden of illness in cancer survivors: findings from a population-based national sample, *J Natl Cancer Inst 96*(17):1322.

From Potter, P.A., & Perry, A.G. (2009). *Fundamentals of nursing: concepts, process, and practice.* (7th ed.). St. Louis: Mosby.

the best approaches. Most patients surprise caregivers by expressing relief at a willingness to discuss what is foremost in their minds: their imminent death.

Spiritual activities may provide mental and emotional strength in spite of physical deterioration. The patient may ask the nurse to read the Bible or to pray with him or her, or the patient may request that a minister, priest, or rabbi visit. Spiritual strength may help the patient and the family cope with the continuing problems encountered in the cancer experience.

The hospital social worker assists the patient and family in planning for home care. Arrangements for any special supplies and equipment are made before discharge. The nurse plays a major role in teaching the patient and at least one family member or significant other how to continue any special care needed at home, such as dressing changes, irrigations, the management of a feeding tube, or the care of a central venous line for administration of parenteral nutrition or medications.

Throughout the hospital stay, take advantage of time available to promote self-care to the greatest extent possible. Assess the patient's readiness to learn and ability to actively participate in self-care. If necessary, consult advanced clinical nursing specialists to provide individualized guidelines for teaching patients. Include plans for patient education in the nursing care plan. Document evidence of the patient's comprehension of and ability to handle self-care, and plan for any assistance needed from others. Continuity of care is the goal in discharge planning. Hospice services can be arranged in most communities for those who have advanced cancer. There are freestanding hospices, hospices within a hospital or skilled nursing facility, or at-home arrangements. The primary focus of a hospice is enhancing the patient's quality of life, not prolonging it. Efforts are directed toward relief from pain and other problems. Skilled professional care and voluntary support services are provided to assist the patient and the family in living life to the fullest each day.

Get Ready for the NCLEX® Examination!

Key Points

- It is currently estimated that one of every five people in the United States will get cancer. The 5-year survival rate is 65%.
- There is strong evidence that what people eat or drink or their lifestyle habits may predispose them to the development of cancer.
- The American Cancer Society recommends specific preventive behaviors and screening tests for cancer prevention and early detection for men and women.
- It is imperative for the person to perform self-examination to detect any changes and report them to the physician immediately.
- It is important to have periodic physical examinations and to seek medical attention promptly if one of the warning signs of cancer develops.
- A common reason for a delay in diagnosing cancer is that early malignant changes are not accompanied by pain.
- Seeking medical attention when warning signs occur is also frequently delayed because people fear the possible diagnosis of cancer and hope the signs and symptoms will just go away.
- The diagnosis of cancer has a profound effect on family members, as well as on the patient. They experience shock, disbelief, denial, anger, fear, anxiety, and a sense of helplessness.
- Most of the side effects from chemotherapeutic agents result from the destruction of normal cells from the hematopoietic system, hair follicles, and the GI system.
- TLS is an oncologic emergency that occurs in cancer patients with heavy tumor burdens after they receive chemotherapy or irradiation, which causes rapid lysis of malignant cells.

- The American Cancer Society sponsors organized support groups for individuals with the same types of cancer; some of these are Reach to Recovery; the Lost Chord Club; I Can Cope; Look Good, Feel Good; and the Ostomy Club. Prepared volunteer visitors are available in most communities to visit a newly diagnosed patient.
- Spiritual strength assists the patient and the family in coping with the problems experienced as a result of cancer. Based on the patient's preference, religious counsel may be helpful.
- The American Cancer Society, the American Pain Society, the World Health Organization, and the Oncology Nursing Society consider pain control a major issue in the management of a person with cancer.
- The concept of rehabilitation should be applied in planning care for the patient with cancer to promote the highest level of functioning possible.

Additional Learning Resources

Go to your Companion CD for an audio glossary, animations, video clips, and more.

evolve Be sure to visit the Evolve site at http://evolve.elsevier.com/Christensen/adult/ for additional online resources.

Review Questions for the NCLEX® Examination

1. The patient has mouth pain 10 days after receiving chemotherapy. On inspection, the nurse finds the inside of the mouth is erythematous, edematous, and dry. The most likely problem is:
   1. candidiasis.
   2. hypercalcemia.
   3. stomatitis.
   4. esophagitis.
2. The patient has metastatic breast cancer with involvement in her L5 vertebral body. She is paralyzed from the waist down with incontinence of stool and urine. She is undergoing radiation therapy for spinal cord compression. What is an appropriate nursing diagnosis?
   1. Risk for disturbed body image, related to alopecia
   2. Risk for deficient fluid volume, related to stool incontinence
   3. Risk for impaired skin integrity, related to prolonged immobility and incontinence
   4. All of the above
3. A 58-year-old patient with colon cancer is receiving combined radiation and chemotherapy. He has diarrhea; this is related to the:
   1. diagnosis.
   2. patient's inability to eat and drink during treatment.
   3. treatment's irritating effect on the mucosa of the GI tract.
   4. fluid and electrolyte imbalance.
4. The current recommendation for first-time baseline mammogram in asymptomatic women is:
   1. at the onset of menopause.
   2. that it is not necessary if the patient has had a previous biopsy.
   3. at ages 35 to 39.
   4. at age 50.
5. What are considered cancer-screening activities? *(Select all that apply.)*
   1. Performing a risk factor assessment and physical examination
   2. Giving a patient instructions for performing the test for fecal occult blood
   3. Instructing a patient in self-examination of the skin or oral cavity
   4. Laboratory examinations for CA-125 and CA-19-9
6. The patient has terminal lung cancer. To maintain optimal pain control, oral analgesics generally should be given:
   1. at scheduled intervals.
   2. every 2 hours.
   3. as required.
   4. in relation to the patient's activity level.
7. Cancer prevention and health promotion behaviors for patients with cancer:
   1. will not decrease the risk of developing a second malignancy.
   2. will not be affected by personal choices related to diet and smoking.
   3. are increasingly important with the growing population of cancer survivors.
   4. would include only routine physical examinations.
8. The patient has been diagnosed with stage I breast cancer. She is receiving adjuvant chemotherapy and radiation therapy following a lumpectomy. Which point about alopecia should not be made? *(Select all that apply.)*
   1. Chemotherapy-related hair loss is reversible and temporary.
   2. All chemotherapeutic agents result in alopecia.
   3. Hair that grows back may have a different texture and color.
   4. Gentle shampooing is recommended.
9. A 61-year-old patient is receiving chemotherapy. The patient becomes anemic and has petechiae and ecchymoses scattered over her upper trunk, especially her arms. What side effect is the patient experiencing?
   1. Bone marrow suppression
   2. Cardiac suppression
   3. Liver toxicity
   4. Pulmonary toxicity

10. Before the insertion of a cervical implant, the nurse tells the patient what to expect while it is in place. Which statement is accurate?
    1. "Nurses will always be available, but they will spend only a short time at your bedside."
    2. "Personal cleanliness is essential, so you will be given a complete bed bath each day."
    3. "Pain or discomfort is a common side effect of this type of radiation."
    4. "Your bed linens will be completely changed each day to minimize radioactive contamination."

11. A 24-year-old patient has been receiving chemotherapy for acute lymphoblastic leukemia. Which statement indicates that he understands discharge teaching concerning leukopenia?
    1. "I am cured and have no limitations."
    2. "My family can catch leukopenia, so I need to be careful to not get too close to any of them."
    3. "I should avoid close contact with people who might give me an infection."
    4. "I need to be careful not to cut myself when shaving because I may not be able to stop the bleeding."

12. A 42-year-old patient has palpated a small lump on her left breast during her monthly BSE. She has scheduled an appointment with her physician. Which test will be used to make a definite diagnosis of a benign or malignant tumor of her breast?
    1. Biopsy
    2. Mammography
    3. Tomography
    4. Ultrasound

13. The nurse educator is discussing the importance of the reduction of carcinogens in primary prevention of cancer. Which risk factor is considered significant in numerous types of cancer?
    1. Diet low in fat
    2. Occasional moderate use of alcohol
    3. High pollen count in the environment
    4. Smoking

14. A therapeutic approach by the nurse to assist a terminally ill cancer patient in the management of his pain is that:
    1. antiinflammatory agents are effective analgesics for severe pain.
    2. opioids should be withheld because they are addictive.
    3. pain is what the patient says it is.
    4. one can increase one's tolerance for pain.

15. Which statement by a chemotherapy patient who has a low WBC count, a low platelet count, and a hemoglobin measurement of 5.6 g/dL, would indicate the need for further teaching?
    1. "I check my mouth and teeth after each meal."
    2. "I've been very constipated and need an enema."
    3. "My husband and I have been using a vaginal lubrication before intercourse."
    4. "My lips are dry and cracking. I need some lubricant."

16. Which is a biologic modifier that is a breakthrough in treating patients with neutropenia and is used prophylactically for patients at risk for neutropenia?
    1. Lymphopenic stimulating factor (LSF)
    2. Erythropoietic stimulating factor (ESF)
    3. Neutropenic stimulating factor (NSF)
    4. Colony-stimulating factor (CSF)

17. According to the American Cancer Society, what would have the greatest influence in reducing the risk of lung cancer?
    1. Five fruits and vegetables a day
    2. Yearly chest radiograph for those 50 years and older
    3. Cessation of smoking
    4. Reduction of environmental and chemical carcinogens

18. Aggressive chemotherapy to decrease the growth of rapidly progressive malignant tumors causes destruction of a large number of rapidly dividing malignant cells and increases the risk of which complication? (The drug allopurinol and hydration help control the metabolic complication that may occur.) ______

19. The nursing diagnosis of *imbalanced nutrition: less than body requirements* is often seen in chemotherapy patients as a result of:
    1. impaired tissue integrity, related to damage to integumentary tissue.
    2. alopecia and leukopenia.
    3. stomatitis, anorexia, vomiting, and diarrhea.
    4. myelosuppression.

20. What points are important in educating the patient and the family in prevention of constipation? *(Select all that apply.)*
    1. Opioids may cause constipation, so laxatives must be given with opioids.
    2. Patients who are not eating continue to produce waste in the bowel and get impacted with feces.
    3. High fluid intake should be maintained.
    4. The patient should have a bowel movement at least every day.
    5. If possible, eating foods high in fiber is helpful.

21. A patient has a vaginal radiation implant in place. The nurse would:
    1. instruct her to turn from side to side for comfort.
    2. restrict fluid intake to prevent bladder distention.
    3. promote intake of a high-residue diet to prevent constipation.
    4. monitor vital signs every 4 hours and report temperature greater than 100° F.

22. In the nursing interventions of a patient receiving external radiation therapy for a malignancy, the nurse must remember to:
    1. vigorously scrub the areas of entry of "ports" marked by the radiologist.
    2. apply some form of ointment with a metallic base to the area of entry each time the patient goes for radiation treatments.

3. instruct the patient to avoid irritating the "ports" by not lying on that part of the body and not wearing constricting clothing.
4. isolate the patient so he or she will not expose others to radiation.

23. The patient has a history of oat cell carcinoma of the lung and is being treated with chemotherapy. His WBC count is 2.5/mm^3. The nurse's primary concern would be:
    1. prevention of hemorrhage.
    2. prevention of infection.
    3. prevention of dehydration.
    4. prevention of electrolyte imbalance.

24. A 63-year-old patient has a diagnosis of cancer of the prostate gland with metastasis and is experiencing cachexia. This state is best described by which characteristic?
    1. Poor health, malnutrition, weakness, and emaciation
    2. Increased appetite and nervousness
    3. Irritability and anger
    4. Depression, fear, and anxiety

Matching

25. ______	Carcinogen	A. Reduction of WBCs
26. ______	Mammography	B. Radiographic examination of the breast
27. ______	Pathogenesis	C. The development of morbid conditions or of disease
28. ______	Thrombocytopenia	D. Decrease in platelets
29. ______	Leukopenia	E. Any agent or substance that causes cancer

30. Metoclopramide (Reglan) is an antiemetic that is helpful in preventing chemotherapy-induced emesis. Choose all the correct answers that describe its action.
    1. Blocks dopamine receptors in chemoreceptor trigger zone of CNS
    2. Accelerates gastric emptying
    3. Blocks the effects of serotonin at 5-HT$_3$ receptor sites
    4. Stimulates motility of the upper GI tract

31. The destruction of cancer cells results in the release of what factors into systemic circulation? *(Select all that apply.)*
    1. Linoleic acid
    2. Potassium
    3. Uric acid
    4. Phosphorus

32. The TNM staging classification stages cancer according to:
    1. absence of atypical or abnormal cells.
    2. cytology suggestive of but not conclusive for malignancy.
    3. tumor size, lymph node involvement, any metastasis.
    4. cytology conclusive for malignancy.

33. The medication of choice for pain control in the hospice setting is usually:
    1. ibuprofen.
    2. morphine.
    3. meperidine.
    4. codeine.

34. Using the TNM staging classification system, a tumor staged as T4N3M1 would mean:
    1. no evidence of primary tumor, lymph node involvement, or distant metastasis.
    2. carcinoma in situ, regional lymph node involvement, and metastasis to one site.
    3. large tumor, lymph node involvement, and distant metastasis.
    4. medium-sized tumor, no lymph node involvement, and distant metastasis.

chapter 58

Professional Roles and Leadership

evolve

Elaine Oden Kockrow and Barbara Lauritsen Christensen

http://evolve.elsevier.com/Christensen/foundationsadult

Objectives

1. Discuss the three methods of applying for a job.
2. Describe what it is possible to expect from an interview for a new job.
3. Describe the "night shift survival guide."
4. Discuss confidentiality.
5. List the advantages of membership in professional organizations.
6. Discuss career opportunities for the licensed practical nurse or licensed vocational nurse (LPN/LVN).
7. Discuss mentoring.
8. Explain the organizational position and the role of the charge nurse.
9. Discuss the guidelines for being an effective leader.
10. Discuss styles of leadership that are options for nurses to use.
11. Discuss the duties of a nurse team leader.
12. Identify strategies for burnout prevention.
13. Discuss nurse practice acts.
14. Identify three important functions of a state board of nursing.
15. List four possible reasons for a state board of nursing to revoke a nursing license.
16. Discuss the Computerized Adaptive Testing (CAT) for the National Council Licensure Examination (NCLEX) for the LPN/LVN candidate (NCLEX-PN® examination).
17. Identify two reasons why an evaluation is important.
18. Discuss the place and the nature of telephone manners in professionalism.
19. Discuss delegating nursing tasks.
20. Discuss the use of computers in nursing.
21. List the three types of physicians' orders, and discuss the legal aspects of each.
22. List three ways to ensure accuracy when transcribing physicians' orders.
23. List the pertinent data necessary to compile an effective change-of-shift report.
24. Discuss the importance of malpractice insurance.
25. Discuss the chemically impaired nurse.

Key Terms

advancement (p. 2051)
articulate (p. 2049)
burnout (p. 2066)
career (p. 2045)
contract (p. 2048)
endorsement (p. 2056)
interview (p. 2048)
negligence (p. 2058)
nurse practice act (p. 2057)
reciprocity (rĕs-ĭ-PRŎS-ĭ-tē, p. 2057)
resignation (p. 2051)
résumé (p. 2046)
role (p. 2045)
transcribe (p. 2069)

FUNCTIONING AS A GRADUATE

Today's health care system is volatile, and the job market has never been so competitive. For that reason, you need to take charge of your future. The significant investment you make in yourself to become a licensed practical nurse or licensed vocational nurse (LPN/LVN), the valuable work you do for the public, and the uncertainty of the times make it necessary for each of you to think through your future carefully and "map" a course for your career (a profession for which one trains and that is undertaken as a permanent calling) (Box 58-1). As an LPN/LVN, you are too valuable a resource to wander aimlessly through a career in nursing.

The role (a socially expected behavior pattern associated with an individual's function in social groups) of a graduate nurse will be exciting and challenging. The LPN/LVN is a valuable member of the health care team and functions in many settings. This chapter provides some guidelines for being a conscientious nurse while assuming this new role. Many opportunities are available to choose from. Methods to obtain a job include letter of application, résumé, and interview.

Box 58-1 Eight-Step Career Planning Tool

1. **Take Stock**—the most important step of the career-planning process
   a. Read, listen, watch, learn—find out as much as possible about the trends in health care.
   b. Assess your professional strengths and weaknesses honestly and objectively.
   c. Ask yourself if you hold certain beliefs that have any potential to undermine your attitude; such beliefs—myths, even—sometimes interfere with job performance and satisfaction.
2. **Explore the Options**
   a. Consider what kind of nursing positions are likely to enhance your strengths.
   b. Discuss your options with a mentor.
3. **Gather More Information**
   a. Attend health care job fairs.
   b. Research different nursing positions.
   c. Visit with colleagues who are doing the kinds of work you are interested in doing.
   d. Call nurse recruiters.
   e. Read professional journals and newspapers.
4. **Narrow Your Focus**
   a. Take into account the education and skills required for each position.
   b. Evaluate the responsibilities involved in each position.
   c. Consider salary range, days and hours, travel time, and availability of that job in your area.
5. **Make a Decision**—list the pros and cons of each position, and narrow the field to two or three possibilities.
6. **Get Specific**—learn as much as you can about other finalists.
   a. Obtain additional training if needed.
   b. Investigate the possibility of tuition reimbursement.
   c. Find out if on-the-job training is available.
7. **Map Your Strategy**
   a. Record each step of your strategy.
   b. Develop a résumé.
   c. Develop interviewing skills.
   d. Practice interviewing by role-playing with a mentor or friend.
8. **Manage Your Career**—periodically review where you are in your career and your life; choose a special date each year (e.g., your birthday) to make your reassessment.

Remember: Successful careers do not happen accidentally. You make choices and changes along the way.

FINDING AND OBTAINING A JOB

Letter of Application

It is always best to customize the letter of application. Type it neatly, and make sure the spelling is correct. Keep it brief simple, and direct. Its objective is to introduce yourself, announce your interest in employment, briefly state your qualifications, and express your availability. You will find a sample letter of application in Figure 58-1.

Your cover letter necessarily requires a thorough discussion of your qualifications. Although some applicants will choose the third person (he or she) as a creative approach to presenting their qualifications, potential employers sometimes find this voice disconcerting. In general, using the first person (I) voice is preferable (Box 58-2).

Résumé

The **résumé** (a summary of educational and professional experiences, including activities and honors) is a one- or two-page written document that contains certain information about you, your education, and your experience. It is a brief outline of your personal and professional life.

Box 58-2 Guidelines for Writing Letters of Application

1. Include your full address above the date of your letter.
2. Address the letter appropriately. If you are responding to a classified advertisement that provides a return box only, use the address given and the salutation Sir/Madam. If you have learned about a position through your school office or through a friend, you will probably be able to learn the name of the person in charge of employment. In this case, include the name in the inside address as follows:

   Mr. Thomas L. Leeper
   Personnel Manager
   The Azzaro Corporation
   3689 Wilson Street
   Atlanta, GA 30315

   The proper salutation is this (note the colon at the end):

   Dear Mr. Leeper:
3. In the first paragraph, state your interest. Address and satisfy the basic job requirement printed in the advertisement:

   The nursing position that you advertised in the *Atlanta Times* on Monday, June 2, is of interest to me.

   or

   Miss Cathie Royer, the placement counselor at Greenville College, has suggested that I apply for the nursing position that is available in your facility.
4. In the second paragraph refer to your résumé, which you will enclose. Use this paragraph to highlight the main points of your education and experience.
5. In the final paragraph of your application, indicate your interest in a personal interview and the times you are available.
6. The complimentary close is fine to leave at a simple *Sincerely.* Include your signature above your typewritten name, and indicate the enclosure.

(return address) 1402 Iowa Avenue
Chariton, IA 69101
(date) April 12, 2009

Mr. Todd Fye (inside address)
Personnel Manager
Broadlawns General Hospital
1915 Hickman Road
Des Moines, IA 50318

Dear Mr. Fye: (salutation)

I am interested in the position of LPN on a surgical unit for which you advertised an opening in the *Des Moines Tribune* on Sunday, March 10.

I will graduate on May 16 from North Central Iowa College and will take the LPN licensure examination in May. Throughout my education, I have maintained a keen interest in medical-surgical nursing. In addition, I worked part-time as a nurse assistant on a surgical floor at St. Francis Hospital in Ames for a year while I was in nursing school. My resume is enclosed for further information about my background and experience.

I am a highly motivated individual and perform well in stressful situations. I am energetic, systematic, organized, and efficient and provide quality nursing care to patients. I am enthusiastic about my career in nursing and look forward to reviewing my qualifications with you.

I will be in Des Moines on Friday, April 17, and if it is convenient for you, I would like to talk with you then about this position. You can reach me by phone at (506) 827-1032. I look forward to hearing from you.

(complimentary close) Sincerely,

Angela Fisher
Angela Fisher

Enclosure

FIGURE 58-1 Sample letter of application.

It communicates your concrete skills and interests. You become a bundle of marketable skills, not a job title. A concise, comprehensive, well-prepared résumé will impress future employers; therefore it should be well organized, neat, and accurate. Guard against being too wordy—use only short bulleted sentences no more than four words long, if possible. Prepare a résumé that is basic, is properly arranged, and contains the most recent information. Be certain to use a variety of action words and self-descriptive words. There are several types of résumés—keep yours brief and informative (Box 58-3). The employer is seeking the employee with the most potential for the job. The résumé is likely to be the first, or one of the first, means by which the employer gains an impression of you: Make it a good one. A sample résumé is presented in Figure 58-2.

Box 58-3 Guidelines for Writing a Winning Résumé

1. Include your name, telephone number, and complete address.
2. Use high-quality paper: acid-free 100% cotton 24-lb paper in a neutral shade such as white, light gray, or buff.
3. Use a matching 9 × 12 envelope (not a No. 10 letter-size envelope) so you are able to send your letter of application flat, without folding it, with your résumé.
4. Aim for a clean, uncluttered look.
5. Put the most important information near the top, where it will be easy to find.
6. Choose a font that is easy to read.
7. Limit yourself to one page if possible.
8. Do not use a photocopy of your résumé.
9. Label each section clearly.
10. Put work experience in one category and education in another.
11. Cover work experience first.
12. List jobs you have held in reverse chronologic order, beginning with the most recent. Do the same for schools and degrees in your education section.
13. Be positive.
14. Be honest and accurate.
15. List references if the job posting requires it. Be sure to contact references before submitting the résumé to ensure that person will provide a positive reference.

LINDA PATTERSON 2777 EAST EIGHTH TRENTON, MO 64683	PHONE: (816) 359-8888
JOB OBJECTIVES:	Staff LPN interested in operating room, post-anesthesia care unit, or home health care.
EDUCATION:	North Central Missouri College, Trenton, MO 64683 Licensed Practical Nurse: Graduation: May 2008; License, 2008
	Kirksville Health Center, Kirksville, MO 63501 Advanced Cardiac Life Support, 2009 Advanced Fluid and Electrolyte Course, 2010
EXPERIENCE:	St. Francis Hospital, Marceline, MO 64668, August 2004 to July 2005, Nurse Assistant
	Brookfield Nursing Center, Brookfield, MO 64628, January 2000 to July 2004, Nurse Assistant
	Grim-Smith Hospital, Kirksville, MO 63501, June 1998 to December 2000, Nursing Assistant
HONORS AND ACTIVITIES:	North Central Missouri College: Dean's Honor Roll, Class Secretary; Intramural sports.
	High School: Member, National Honor Society; Class President; Who's Who Among American High School Students; Girls' State delegate; Member, concert and marching band; Softball; Basketball
	Community: Girl Scout; Community Betterment; Youth Leadership Award from the governor — 2008; Extension Club President
REFERENCES:	Available upon request

FIGURE 58-2 Sample résumé.

Personal Interview

The **interview** (a meeting of people face to face, as for evaluating or questioning a job applicant) is important; make every effort to ensure its success (Box 58-4). First impressions are sometimes incorrect, and whether they are positive or negative, they have a lasting effect. Prepare carefully for the interview, and make a good impression (Box 58-5).

For a good working relationship, it is best if your skills and nursing care values are in harmony with the objectives of the job description (Box 58-6, Table 58-1).

CONTRACTS AND STARTING OUT

A **contract** is a promise or a set of promises between two or more people that creates a legal relationship between them and a legal obligation that one or more of

Box 58-4 Preparing for a Successful Interview

1. Build contacts—Employers fill 90% of all jobs through personal contacts.
2. Know the institution—Learn everything possible about the institution to which you are applying.
3. Take your personal inventory—Record your strengths.
4. Write or review your résumé—Prepare or update your work history and professional accomplishments.
5. Rehearse questions and answers—Four standard interview questions are:
   a. Would you tell me about yourself?
   b. What are your major strengths and weaknesses?
   c. What are your plans?
   d. What does your specialty or position involve?
6. Make a good impression—You only have a very short time to make a good impression.
7. Understand the goal—Interviewers will need to determine four things about a job applicant: qualifications, attitude, adaptability, and affordability.
8. Market yourself—Think of a job interview as a sales pitch; you are assertively promoting yourself and your skills.
9. Answer effectively—How you answer a question is often more important than what you say.
10. Practice role-playing—Have different friends practice interviewing with you; tape these role-plays, and use a video camera or cassette player and review the tape.

Box 58-5 Steps to a Successful Interview

1. Be well groomed. Dress conservatively and appropriately. "Businesslike" dress for men requires a suit or sports coat and tie; women's proper attire is a suit or dress.
2. Arrive at the interview 10 minutes earlier than the appointment; if there is a receptionist or secretary, identify yourself, and give the name of the person you are to see.
3. Be cheerful and polite.
4. Be knowledgeable about the position for which you are applying.
5. Be patient while waiting for an interview.
6. Smile and give your name distinctly when greeting the interviewer.
7. Use a firm handshake.
8. Address interviewer by name, using Mr., Mrs., or Ms.
9. Have extra copies (three) of your résumé and a neatly typed list of references.
10. Do not slouch or fidget—sit upright and be attentive. Do not chew gum or smoke.
11. Maintain eye contact with the interviewer.
12. Allow the interviewer to take the initiative; be an attentive listener.
13. Put purses or portfolios on the floor beside you, not in your lap. Do not move the interview chair. Avoid looking at your watch. Scan the interviewer's office as you first enter for something to comment about.
14. Answer questions concisely. Try to make the interview interesting and informative. Use the time effectively.
15. Be prepared to be interviewed by a group or committee or to have the interview recorded. Look at each member of the interview team. Shake hands with each one, using their name.
16. **Articulate** (speak clearly, distinctly, and to the point; present yourself with clarity and effectiveness).
17. Be factual.
18. Avoid being critical.
19. Convey genuine interest and enthusiasm.
20. Avoid discussing personal problems unless they are applicable to the job.
21. Be prepared to relate qualifications and experiences.
22. Inquire as to job description, work schedule, and fringe benefits.
23. If requested, state salary desired; if salary offered is unacceptable, do not mislead the interviewer.
24. Inquire about starting salary, pay increases, and maximum salary allowed.
25. If asked, indicate your preference of positions (if more than one position is open, or if the interviewer invites you to "dream a little").
26. Look for clues when the interview is over. Usually an employer will ask, "Do you have any more questions?" This is probably a good time to say, "No thank you, but I enjoyed our interview and hope that you will consider me for the position with your company." Hold any questions not covered until this time.
27. Express appreciation for the interview.
28. Suggest when and where you might be contacted, if necessary.
29. Send additional information promptly on request.
30. Be aware that most beginning nursing positions require rotating shifts, even night shifts and working every other weekend. Many facilities require that you have medical-surgical experience before they will assign you to a specialty area such as obstetrics or pediatrics.
31. Follow up the interview with a thank-you letter within 48 hours.

Box 58-6 Common Interview Questions

1. Are you a competitive person?
2. You've changed jobs frequently. Why?
3. Have you ever been fired?
4. Do you prefer working with others or independently?
5. What are your travel or relocation limitations?
6. How do you prefer people to criticize you, and how do you criticize others?
7. How many hours per week do you think someone should spend on the job?
8. What do you know about the company?
9. Why do you want to work for us?
10. You may be overqualified or too experienced for the position we have to offer.
11. What important trends do you see in our industry?
12. Tell me about yourself.
13. What are your three most important accomplishments thus far in your career?
14. Give an example of your creativity.
15. How do you define success?
16. What did you like best about your last job?
17. Is your present (or past) income commensurate (in proportionate to or adequate) with your abilities?

Table 58-1 What an Interviewer Can and Cannot Ask

CAN ASK	CANNOT ASK
Job-related criminal convictions	Criminal arrest or non–job-related criminal convictions
Hobbies	Financial or credit status
Community or social activities	Sexual preferences
Future professional goals	Marital status
Education	Age
Work experience	Color
Strengths and weaknesses	Religious beliefs
Reason(s) for leaving your previous job	Race
Reason(s) you think you are qualified	Creed
Reason(s) for applying for this job	Nationality

them has to fulfill. The usual contract the LPN/LVN will encounter is the employment contract. Although it is desirable to have a written employment contract, an oral employment contract will in some cases be binding on the nurse and the employer. Under the employment contract, it is the nurse's obligation to perform nursing functions with the skill and knowledge of an LPN/LVN in accordance with the standards of the profession and any additional qualifications the nurse claimed to possess. The employer is responsible for providing a safe working environment, sufficient and competent fellow workers, and safe equipment. Failure on the part of the nurse or the employer to perform these duties is a breach of contract. It is possible for breach of contract to result in a lawsuit seeking a court to order the breaching party to perform the obligations of the contract or to pay money to the party who suffered damage because of the breach. However, because the contract is one for personal services, a nurse will usually not be forced to work for the employer. Rather, the nurse will possibly be liable for money damages to an employer for breach of contract.

The employment contract properly specifies the length of the contract period; hours the nurse is to work; salary; vacation; sick leave pay; medical, maternal, disability, and liability insurance coverage; educational benefits; and any other benefits or working conditions that the nurse and employer agree on. The employment contract is possible to terminate legally, without a breach, by completion of all obligations under the terms of the contract or by consent of all parties to the termination.

New employees usually find that facilities provide orientation programs. Many facilities also require newly graduated nurses to take exams or tests to determine medication and math skills.

Recent graduates are also often required to serve a period of internship or residency before acquiring the status of a benefit-earning member of the staff.

An internship helps with the transition to graduate nurse. Some facilities provide a mentor to assist the new graduate during this internship period.

Ask about these probationary policies when discussing salary and benefits.

KEEPING YOUR JOB

Getting a job is important, but doing a good job and keeping your job are equally important. This is what you need to do to keep your job. Here are some specific tips:

- Keep current and competent.
- Look and act professional.
- Be on time and ready to start at the beginning of the shift.
- Be organized.
- Do not spend time with personal phone calls.
- Take only the allotted time for lunch and breaks.
- Work hard and give the best care possible.
- Be a good leader and a good follower.
- Help others when you can.
- Stretch yourself—do not be satisfied with doing the minimum.
- Display a positive attitude and flexibility. Avoid being influenced by negative people.
- Respect your patients, their family members, your co-workers, and your supervisors.

Encountering Problems

If you encounter a problem, follow the chain of command. Be aware of the organizational chart. Be aware of the grievance procedure if you think you are being treated unfairly. Remember that any problem is best resolved by communication at the most basic level. Do not let the situation get out of hand. Be calm and objective in your approach. Above all, **listen carefully** to what the parties involved are saying. If you are ultimately obliged to file a grievance, follow the procedure carefully. Know your agency policy.

Work Schedule

Today's nursing profession offers any nurse who wishes to work the opportunity to do so.

Schedules are flexible. There are part-time and full-time options, straight evenings or straight nights, weekends only, shared jobs, flex time, 12-hour shifts, and 10-hour shifts.

Employers have offered many incentives to encourage nurses to work. Nurses who work just weekends work 2 to 3 days every weekend. You will be paid a large bonus for choosing to do so, usually time and a half; for example, 36 hours' pay for 24 hours worked. If you work in a shared job situation, you will share a single full-time position with another nurse, thus allowing for more free time. Nurses working flex time are sometimes allowed to set their own hours, which permits them to fit their work schedule around family responsibilities. Some nurses working only part-time receive a full-time wage, especially if working weekends.

Nurses working the 12-hour shift usually work three 12-hour shifts per week, with most employers considering this a full-time position. Twelve-hour shifts are from 7 AM to 7 PM. These nurses are usually required to work every other weekend.

You are likely to find the much less common 10-hour shift in home care, clinics, and industries.

There remains, of course, the 8-hour shift. Nursing goes on around the clock to ensure continuity of care for all patients.

There is a growing concern over mandatory overtime. If there are no nurses available for the oncoming shift, those who worked the preceding shift are obliged to remain on duty. Some hospitals have been forced to turn away patients because they did not have adequate staffing. As nurses express their concerns and negotiate to improve patient care and working conditions, salaries will continue to improve and nursing shortages to ease.

As a new graduate, you will perhaps be required to work either the evening or night shift until an opening on the day shift becomes available.

If required to work the night shift, follow the "night shift survival guide" (Box 58-7).

ADVANCEMENT

Advancement (a rise in rank or importance, a promotion, progress, improvement) is a possible result of additional preparation or additional experience. Sometimes you will gain it by learning the position more thoroughly and by assuming new and greater responsibilities. Advancements, together with the difficulties and obstacles that they bring, stimulate interest and enthusiasm. They are usually based on a person's qualifications, behavior, performance, and preparation.

LPN/LVN to RN Programs

Many community colleges and private schools have programs that offer LPNs/LVNs a specialized program that leads to obtaining a registered nurse (RN) license. These programs usually last about 1 year and build on the education the student obtained in the LPN/LVN program.

In other cases the LPN/LVN will have the chance to enroll in a generic RN program but will, in certain instances, "test out" of certain course requirements. There are programs such as the associate's degree and bachelor's degree RN programs. Colleges vary in their admission requirements and offer differing credits for previous education. Chapter 1 discusses other ways to progress from the LPN/LVN qualification to the RN.

Refresher courses are a good idea when nurses have not been actively employed in nursing for several years. The nurse whose license has lapsed or has been revoked, or who is on inactive licensure status for some time, will sometimes be required to take a refresher course to obtain relicensure. In addition, graduates who do not pass the licensure exam in the first two or three attempts will sometimes be required to take a refresher course before taking the exam again. A refresher course often includes several hours of clinical experience as well as theory classes.

Box 58-7 Night Shift Survival Guide

STAYING ALERT AT WORK

- Sleep and eat well before your shift.
- Eat balanced meals, combining complex carbohydrates with some protein and moderate amounts of fat.
- Wear a digital watch on 24-hour international time to prevent disorientation.
- Eat or drink something warm if hormonal changes make you feel especially chilled.

GETTING TO SLEEP

- Make your sleeping area cool, comfortable, quiet, and dark, with blackout shades or blinds, a sleep mask, earplugs, or a white noise machine. Unplug the phone and turn down the doorbell.
- Stop drinking coffee at least 4 hours before you plan to go to sleep, and avoid eating large, greasy meals after work.
- Don't use alcohol or a sedative to get to sleep. Try herbal teas and warm milk instead.
- Allow at least an hour to unwind after work. Eat breakfast, watch a morning show, read, go for a walk, or take a warm bath. Try to follow the same routine every day.

BALANCING YOUR LIFE

- Eat right, exercise regularly, and get outside for some fresh air.
- Take short naps as needed, especially before driving home from work.
- Maintain strong family and social relationships.

Sources: American College of Emergency Physicians. (2003). *Circadian rhythms and shift work*. Available at www.acep.org/practres.aspx?id=30560; Grossman, V.G. (1997). Defying circadian rhythm: The emergency nurse and the night shift. *Journal of Emergency Nursing*, *23*(6), 602; and Perkins, L.A. (2000). Is the night shift worth the risk? *RN*, *64*(8), 65.

TERMINATING EMPLOYMENT

Resigning from a position properly is another skill that you will need to have as an LPN/LVN. Employers will sometimes question a résumé that reflects frequent job changes; therefore it is in your best interest to remain at the first place of employment at least 1 year. If this is impossible, follow the proper **resignation** (the act of resigning to give up a position of employment) procedure. A verbal statement and a written resignation, providing at least a two-week notice, will often be beneficial in obtaining your next position. If the facility has a formal resignation form, complete it neatly and legibly. If the expectation is that you supply a letter of resignation, keep it brief and courteous. In concise terms, state your reason for leaving. Address the letter to your immediate supervisor or employer, and deliver it in a sealed envelope (Figure 58-3).

TRANSITION FROM STUDENT TO GRADUATE

KNOW YOUR ROLE

Sometimes it is difficult to clearly understand the exact responsibilities of each health team member. No one has yet written job descriptions to fit some of the new roles in the field. The LPN/LVN is responsible to an RN or to the physician. The role of the LPN/LVN, like the roles of others associated with health care, is constantly changing. As the services of health care facilities reach out to meet the increasing demand of the population, the role of the LPN/LVN does not remain static. Many technical and scientific changes in the health care system have resulted in a

406 Martin Lane
Edinburg, MO 64683
December 7, 2009

Mr. David Torres, RN
Director of Nurses
Memorial Hospital
Edinburg, MO 64683

Dear Mr. Torres:

Because of unforeseen circumstances, I must resign my position as staff LPN on 1-E. My husband has been transferred to another city, and I must seek employment there.

I would like my resignation to be effective as of December 30, 2009.

I would appreciate it if I could have my accrued benefits added to my terminal salary check.

I thank you for all the courtesies extended to me during my employment. The staff has been helpful, and I have enjoyed my 4 years of employment at Memorial Hospital. I hope that in the future I can seek employment again at this facility.

Sincerely,

(provide signature)
Mrs. Karma Baumberger, LPN

FIGURE 58-3 Sample letter of resignation.

multiplicity and complexity of functions placed on nurses' job descriptions. In light of these developments, it is incumbent on those who work with patients to keep an unwavering eye on their principal concern, the human being. Patients quickly recognize nurses who have a genuine concern for their individual needs. Your enthusiasm and zest for nursing are clearly evident in the personalized quality of care you give. Stay focused on the patient and the patient's needs.

CONFIDENTIALITY

Consider as confidential all information the patient gives. The information is acceptable to exchange with other members of the health care team only in the performance of your duties. Release of information to anyone other than the health care team without the consent of the patient is a violation of the right to privacy. Box 58-8 lists important reminders concerning confidentiality (see also Chapter 2).

Box 58-8 Confidentiality Reminders

1. Discuss patient information only in conferences or reports. Be mindful of conversations in the cafeteria and at the nurses' station.
2. Keep confidential all information gathered from medical records, reports, or conferences.
3. Be nonjudgmental in observations of patients, hospital staff, family members, or other personnel.
4. Do not store patient statistics on any retrievable or permanent computer system unless authorized.
5. Do not keep or copy any patient information except when necessary for required report. All notes are necessary to destroy after submitting required report.
6. Never copy any original medical records for any reason unless a physician orders it done.
7. Do not leave a patient chart where unauthorized people are able to access it.
8. It is generally not the nurse's responsibility to release patient information to the police, media, relatives, or visitors.
9. Familiarize yourself with how patient information is to be handled within the facility.
10. You are ethically obligated to treat information about your patient as confidential.
11. Be aware of the actions of unlicensed personnel with whom you work. If necessary, teach others the importance of safeguarding a patient's privacy.

Remember:
WHAT YOU SEE HERE,
WHAT YOU HEAR HERE,
WHILE YOU ARE HERE,
LET IT STAY HERE,
WHEN YOU LEAVE HERE.

ROLE OF THE LICENSED PRACTICAL NURSE OR LICENSED VOCATIONAL NURSE IN THE COMMUNITY

The LPN/LVN participates in activities that promote the community's positive attitude toward health care. You will use community resources to promote a better understanding of the health services available to the general public and promote and participate in community health projects and other health-oriented activities such as maternal and child health clinics, disabled children clinics, mental health clinics, blood pressure clinics, and community health fairs.

PROFESSIONAL ORGANIZATIONS

If you want a voice in your vocation, you will do well to join the professional organizations of its members. No organization has the power to be any more active or effective than its members. Some professional organizations provide opportunities for continuing education to their members and associated allied health staff.

Two national organizations exist to support and meet the needs of the LPN/LVN: the National Association for Practical Nurse Education and Service (NAPNES) and the National Federation of Licensed Practical Nurses (NFLPN).

The purpose of NAPNES, founded in 1941, is to promote an understanding of practical nursing schools and continuing education for the LPN/LVN. The organization also developed a position on the education of the practical nurse and defines ethical conduct and publishes standards of practical and vocational nursing practice. The *Journal of Practical Nursing* is the official publication, and *NAPNES Forum* is the newsletter that informs members of activities. Membership is open to students, graduates, faculty, and others who are interested in the practical or vocational nurse. NFLPN, founded in 1949, serves the interests of the LPN/LVN. It restricts membership to only LPN/LVN students and graduates. It informs members of the most current issues of interest and makes available to its members malpractice, personal liability, health, and accident insurance. The NFLPN also lobbies on both the state and national levels for issues that are of interest and concern to its members. The *Licensed Practical Nurse* is the official publication. For further information about NAPNES, visit www.napnes.org or write to NAPNES, 1940 Duke Street, Suite 200, Alexandria, VA 22314. For further information about NFLPN, visit www.nflpn.org or write to NFLPN, 605 Poole Drive, Garner, NC 27529.

Members who constitute these two organizations all share the common goals of the LPN/LVN.

CONTINUING EDUCATION

The health care system is changing daily as a result of rapidly developing technology, and it is critical to keep current on nursing trends and issues. More excellent opportunities to learn new nursing skills are available to the nurse than ever. Facilities are offering employees continuing education (Box 58-9) through seminars or workshops using tools like current videos, journals,

Box 58-9 Continuing Education

- **Orientation to the facility:** Provides an opportunity to learn about variations in routine plus a review of selected previously learned information and skills if you have been out of nursing for a while.
- **Inservice education:** Information chosen to meet specific needs within a facility. Attendance at some inservice programs, such as a yearly update on bloodborne pathogens, is required. You are permitted to offer employers suggestions for content. Usually a specified amount of time is required for inservice programs, such as 1 hour a month or three times a year, according to the agency policy. Depending on the credentials of the instructor, continuing education credits are sometimes available.
- **Workshops:** Forum in which to present information and practice what is taught. Workshops provide excellent opportunities to learn new skills. The length varies according to the content. Some agencies pay the workshop fee or expenses if the topic is specific to and enhances your nursing skills. Workshops are also a major source of continuing education credits required by many states as a part of relicensure.
- **Continuing education classes:** Sometimes called field services in the vocational system. There are often classes on complex nursing skills such as intravenous therapy, physical assessment, licensed practical nurse or licensed vocational nurse (LPN/LVN) charge nurse, mental health concepts, nursing process for LPNs/LVNs and so on. Many vocational schools and community colleges will provide any course you are interested in if you request it and there are enough potential students to make up the required minimum enrollment. Many of these classes provide continuing education credits as opposed to course credit. You receive a certificate if you have completed coursework satisfactorily.
- **Sharing information:** One of the most valuable benefits of continuing education classes is the opportunity to get together with other working LPNs/LVNs. You discover similarities in challenges and satisfactions. You share ideas on how to deal with difficult situations in the work setting. It is a good idea to keep a running record of all inservice programs, seminars, and workshops offered, including dates, credits, and topics, for future reference. Ask your employer to include these records in your file at your place of employment, as well as keeping copies for yourself.

textbooks, and computers. Nurses are utilizing the Internet to obtain the most recent nursing information.

To renew nursing licenses, some states require a given number of hours per year in continuing education units (CEUs). This is to improve the quality of patient care by educating nurses on the most recent trends in nursing interventions. Not all continuing education opportunities are accepted by all state boards of nursing for renewal of licensure. You are responsible for acquiring the required number of CEUs and for ensuring that you attained them from approved providers.

CERTIFICATION OPPORTUNITIES

It is a good idea for LPNs/LVNs to take advantage of the knowledge available from certification (a process in which an individual or an institution, agency, or education program is evaluated and recognized as meeting certain predetermined standards) seminars or self-guided study courses. Knowledge is the basis for improved nursing skills and safety in patient care. In many states or agencies, certification is also the basis for salary increases and advancement.

Certification in Managed Care

An intensive 2-day seminar prepares the LPN/LVN to take the examination. On successful completion of the examination, you are certified and entitled to the extended title of certified managed care nurse (CMCN). Plans for establishing a recertification mechanism are under way.

Certification in Pharmacology

NAPNES pharmacology certification requirements vary according to the individual nurse or sponsoring agency. If desired, the LPN/LVN has the option of taking the challenge examination without benefit of a course. Courses are available, however, and some sponsoring agencies mandate the course as an initial step. Recertification is required every 5 years, and continuing education requirements vary from 48 to 120 CEUs.

Certification in Long-Term Care

NAPNES and the National Council of State Boards of Nursing (NCSBN) developed this home study certification program. It covers pharmacology, aging, pediatrics, and key topics that enhance nursing competence. Once you successfully complete the certification examination, you receive a certificate and pin and are entitled to the extended title of certified in long-term care (CLTC). Eligibility requirements for certification are an LPN/LVN license in the United States or its territories and 2000 hours of long-term care practice within the past 3 years.

Certification in Addiction

The National Nursing Society on Addiction is developing a certification program for LPNs/LVNs. Plans are to confer the extended title of certified in addiction licensed practical nurse (CALPN) on those who successfully complete the program.

Further Education

LPNs/LVNs who wish to pursue further education will possibly receive credit for education. There are now progressive LPN/LVN-to-RN programs throughout the United States, making it possible for an LPN/LVN to become an RN in a shorter period of study (see Chapter 1). There are various names for these programs, such as **career ladder, upper mobility, level I** and **level II, III,** and **accelerated/associate degree nursing program.** Coordinators of these programs plan them carefully to avoid duplication of content. Programs vary, so thorough investigation is warranted. The state board of nursing is an excellent source of information about programs in each area.

MEN IN NURSING

Many men have commented on the various reasons for becoming nurses, including the desire to help and care for people, make a significant contribution to society, and educate patients on health care issues. An additional reason many men cite for choosing this path is their lack of desire for the traditional role of physician. Unfortunately, stereotyping has not disappeared, and some individuals still believe that it is somehow not right for men to be nurses. On the other hand, we know that most patients are receptive to male nurses providing care, although female patients tend to prefer that female nurses complete personal aspects of their care.

Data from a study conducted in 2004 by the U.S. Department of Health and Human Services (US DHHS) show that only 5.8% of the 2.9 million RNs in the United States were men. However, this number is 14.5% higher than the 2000 number. This survey also showed that that one third of nurses in the military were men. Also, 83% of male nurses reported being content in their role as a nurse and would encourage other males to become nurses, citing the personal and professional rewards they had gained in the nursing role (Hart, 2004).

Experts have formulated a useful recommendation for male nurses: Don't feel you have to prove yourself and try to fit into some stereotypical ideal. Rather, emphasize the positive personal characteristics that make you a good nurse (Weber & Roman, 2008).

LICENSURE EXAMINATION

TEST PREPARATION

Some nursing programs administer an exit exam before graduation that will provide the graduate with an estimated likelihood of passing the National Council Licensure Examination for Practical Nurses (NCLEX-PN®) Examination. Do not consider the exit exam as pass or fail, but as a good indicator of how much preparation for the NCLEX-PN you will need for success.

Review courses are available to assist the graduate nurse in preparing for the NCLEX-PN. Before you sign up, evaluate which course will be most beneficial to you. In considering a review course, remember the objective is not primary learning, but review.

- Plan ahead, and make an intelligent decision regarding a review course.
- Carefully evaluate your need for a review course.
- Look for a course that uses faculty from outside your school.
- Know the course modality. Some are taught via video.
- Consider the cost; most review courses cost about $200 to $250.
- Know the following: how long the course will last, where the course is held, the size of the class, and when the course is offered.

Review books are available to aid the new graduate in preparing for the NCLEX-PN Examination. It is important to select a review book that meets your study needs. Nursing faculty, friends with review books, the school library, and the bookstore are all sources of information regarding review books. Plan on purchasing a review book while you are still in school. Review books undergo revision about every 3 years. A comprehensive review is available online at www.learningext.com. For more information, go to the National Council of the State Boards of Nursing (NCSBN) website at www.ncsbn.org.

Sometimes graduates do not understand that completing the required hours of theory and clinical practice does not automatically make them eligible to take the examination. Most state boards require a criminal background check prior to granting permission for an applicant to take the NCLEX-PN Examination. If there is a question as to the moral character of the applicant, an individual state board hearing will sometimes take place. A person who is knowledgeable about the applicant will sometimes write a recommendation as to the applicant's moral character. Often there will be a request to a nurse educator to submit such a letter to the state board of nursing. The state board has the authority to accept or reject an applicant to sit for the national licensure. It is necessary that the director of the school of nursing recommend the graduate to sit for the national licensure.

Each state enforces its own nurse practice act that addresses various issues, including licensure. The board of nursing in the jurisdiction where the candidate will take the NCLEX-PN Examination approves the candidate's application. The state board of nursing has the authority to refuse any graduate the right to take the examination.

There are at least 200 testing stations in 150 geographic markets nationwide. The candidate receives a ticket of admission from the Educational Testing Service (ETS) Data Center. The candidate also receives information that describes the test, the protocol for making an appointment for the examination, and a list of available centers and their toll-free numbers. Testing is offered 15 hours a day, 6 days a week. The center schedules an appointment for a 5-hour time slot within 30 days of the call.

TAKING THE TEST

The NCSBN adopted computerized adaptive testing (CAT) for the NCLEX Examination in 1994. The maximum time length for administration of the NCLEX-PN Examination is 5 hours. Some candidates are able to complete the exam in less time.

CAT test centers are quiet and comfortable, with specially designed workstations to enhance security while providing a personal testing environment. The examinee sits at an individual computer or terminal and answers questions that appear on the screen. Test staff maintain security by directly observing the testing session, in addition to continuous monitoring by video camera and audiotaping. The proctor is able to observe all candidates simultaneously and continuously during testing without entering the room, which eliminates the noise and movement of people moving about the room.

In April 2005, test administrators revised the test format by introducing **alternate items** (previously known as innovative items and "next-generation" NCLEX-PN Examination items). An alternate-item format is an examination item that takes advantage of new technology and uses a format to assess candidate ability other than the standard one of four multiple-choice options with one correct response. Possible alternate-item formats include questions with multiple correct responses, fill-in-the-blank questions (including calculation and ordered-response item types), and items asking a candidate to identify an area, picture, or graphic. It is important to note that all NCLEX-PN Examination item formats, including current standard multiple-choice items, will sometimes include charts, tables, or graphic images; the intent of these new alternate-item formats is to assess each candidate's ability to function in a mature, more efficient world and with more fidelity than is possible with standard multiple-choice items.

Each test unfolds in an interactive way as the individual proceeds through the material, but each one covers the same subject content (each test is based on the test plan). The goal of CAT is to determine competence based on the difficulty of questions, not on how many questions are answered correctly. The interactive computerized format makes it possible to match the test questions posed to each examinee to the individual's demonstrated competence level. This makes for greater efficiency in the testing process: The computer poses only those questions that will offer the best measurement of the candidate's competence, rather than a one-size-fits-all set that includes questions not relevant to a given individual's situation.

How does it work? First of all, testing experts have ascertained the difficulty level of each of the thousands of questions in the computer's item bank by trying them out on thousands of candidates and then statistically analyzing the results. In the actual testing situation, the computer uses a candidate's answers to calculate a competence estimate based on the known level of difficulty. It then scans through the test item bank, classified by test plan area and level of difficulty, and determines the question that will most precisely and appropriately measure the candidate in the next test plan area. It presents this selection on the computer screen as the successive test question to the candidate. This process continues, creating as it goes an examination tailored to the individual's knowledge and skills and at the same time fulfilling all NCLEX-PN Examination test plan requirements.

Picture the full range of questions all lined up, from easiest to hardest. If asked the easiest questions, most candidates will get most of them right. If asked only the hardest, they will probably get most wrong. Going from easy to hard as the examination progresses, there will come a point at which each candidate is answering 50% of the questions correctly. Questions further along the difficulty continuum are likely to receive wrong answers (that is, although some will be right, more will be wrong), and easier questions are likely to receive correct answers. The goal of CAT is to find that point, which is different for everyone. That point is the competence level.

The minimum number of questions for the NCLEX-PN Examination is 85 (60 "real" questions and 25 "try-out" questions). The try-out questions are not counted toward the competence level of the candidate. If a candidate is able to answer the difficult questions correctly, there is no point wasting time giving a lot of easy questions. Likewise, if the candidate is not able to answer the easy ones correctly, there is no point continuing with the difficult ones since the candidate is unlikely to be able to answer them. In fact, the computer often has enough data to make a decision after less than the minimum of 60 questions, but a minimum of 60 scored questions is necessary to ensure coverage of the test plan. It is important that the candidates get the opportunity to answer several questions in each of the test plan content areas.

So after the candidate has answered 85 questions, the computer compares the competence level with the passing standard and determines (1) whether the candidate is clearly above the passing standard (the candidate passes), (2) whether the candidate is clearly below the passing standard (the candidate fails), or (3) whether the competence level is not clear. If it is not clear whether the candidate has passed, the computer continues to ask questions. The computer stops asking questions when the competence level is clearly above or clearly below the passing standard, when the maximum number of questions has been answered (265 for RN and 205 for practical nurse [PN]), or when the candidate runs out of time.

Of the candidates whose examinations end early, many more pass than fail. More than half of the people taking the maximum number of questions pass. Almost half of the people who run out of time pass.

There is no random selection of candidates to get a long examination. The length of the NCLEX-PN Examination is based on the performance of the candidate on the examination.

People who are accustomed to knowing most of the answers on tests sometimes find a CAT test difficult, because they will only know the answers to about half the questions. However, it is in fact possible that these candidates are doing quite well: Since they are answering the most difficult questions in the item bank, even 50% correct scores a high competence level.

The most current and complete information about the NCSBN and the NCLEX-PN Examination is available from its website at www.ncsbn.org.

AFTER THE TEST

The test scores are pass or fail. Test administrators print score reports and send them to the board of nursing in each jurisdiction within 24 hours. Each board of nursing schedules its own notification timetable; thus a candidate no longer needs to wait 6 to 8 weeks for examination results. Most test results are received in about 1 week.

Forty-six states allow students who have failed their licensure exam to retest after waiting 45 days. Additional guidelines from the state board of nursing include the number of times a candidate is allowed to retest before being required to seek re-education, and the amount of time allowed from graduation from nursing school to taking the licensure exam.

On successful completion of the examination, you have the right to practice as an LPN/LVN. After receiving the LPN/LVN license, you are responsible for renewing it and keeping the state board informed of any changes of address, name, and employment (i.e., active or inactive) status. Without a license, it is not legal for you to practice nursing. Licensure permits people to offer special skills to the public, but it also provides legal guidelines for protection of the public.

ENDORSEMENT AND RECIPROCITY

The NCLEX-PN Examination makes it possible for you to practice nursing in states other than the one in which you first qualify (see Chapter 2). If you move after you have successfully passed the examination and fulfilled the educational requirements, it is necessary to apply for a license or temporary practice permit before practicing nursing. Licensure that transfers this way from one state to another is called **endorsement** (a statement of recognition of the license of a health practitioner in one state by another state; the applicant needs to meet the current state's licensing requirements). Some states called this licensure reciprocity. This is a mutual agreement to exchange privileges, dependence, or relationships, such as, for example, an agreement between two governing bodies to accept the credentials of caregivers licensed in the other's state. True reciprocity means that an individual licensed in one state can automatically receive licensure in the other, even if the licensing requirements of the states differ.

Nurse Licensing Compact and Mutual Recognition

To date, 19 states have adopted mutual recognition licensure, or an interstate compact. Those states (known as **compact states**) are as follows:

- Arizona
- Arkansas
- Colorado
- Delaware
- Idaho
- Iowa
- Kentucky
- Maine
- Maryland
- Mississippi
- Nebraska
- New Hampshire
- New Mexico
- North Carolina
- North Dakota
- Rhode Island
- South Dakota
- Tennessee
- Texas
- Utah
- Virginia
- Wisconsin

Because mutual recognition licensure is based on the primary state of residence, every nurse is required to declare his or her primary state of residence. The primary state of residence is defined as a declared, fixed, permanent, and principal home for legal purposes (domicile). Indicators of a domicile include, but are not limited to, where real property is located and where the person pays state taxes, votes, and is licensed to operate a motor vehicle.

For example, if your primary state of residence is Nebraska and your nursing practice is totally confined to the state of Nebraska—that is, you do not physically leave the state to care for patients and you do not use technology (telephone, computer interface, interactive closed circuit television) to assess or provide advice to patients living outside of Nebraska—this does not affect how you are licensed.

If you travel with a patient from one state to the other or to Canada, the license you have in your possession is valid for the length of the stay in the other state or Canada.

If your primary state of residence is Nebraska and the state (or states) in which you practice is on the list of compact states, you are entitled to practice in that state based on your license after Nebraska's effective date and the other compact state's effective date have passed. Make sure to maintain your Nebraska license on active status. After Nebraska and the other compact state's effective dates have passed, you will no longer need to maintain a license in the other compact state.

If your primary state of residence is Nebraska but the state in which you practice is not on the list of compact states, you will need to maintain a license in the other state. If your primary state of residence is Nebraska but you practice in one or more states that are on the compact state list and one or more states that are not on the compact state list, you are permitted to practice in the compact states based on your Nebraska license, but you must maintain a license in any states that are not on the list. Also consider maintaining your Nebraska license in anticipation of other states' adopting mutual recognition licensure.

If you are on active duty in the armed forces or employed by the U.S. Public Health Service, the U.S. Department of Veterans Affairs, or any other federal institution, it is necessary to meet the licensure requirements of those federal institutions. The nurse licensure compact does not supersede the federal requirements and thus will not necessarily affect your licensure status. However, you are still required to declare your primary state of residence. If you are a federal employee and you hold a second, civilian, job in nursing, the compact does not apply to the civilian position and you will need to obtain licensing by the usual route of applying to the state board of nursing. Some states that do not accept mutual recognition still require endorsement or reciprocity.

State boards of nursing differ, so contact the board of nursing in the state where you are seeking licensing for the specific requirements of that state.

NURSE PRACTICE ACTS

The nurse practice act is a statute enacted by the legislature of any of the states or by appropriate officers of the districts or possessions.

A nurse practice act is the licensing law. It defines the title and the regulations governing the practice of nursing. The act delineates the legal scope of the practice of nursing within the geographic boundaries. Its provisions assist the nurse in staying within the legal scope of nursing practice in each state. Some states have separate governing boards for professional and practical or vocational nursing. The nurse practice act defines the regulations for practical nursing and includes requirements for an approved school of nursing. It also states the requirements for licensure and conditions for which a license may be revoked or suspended (see Chapter 2).

STATE BOARD OF NURSING

The state board of nursing consists of members who represent the different levels of nursing and who are appointed by the governor. The purpose of the board is to protect the public by administering the nurse practice act. The board is responsible for approving schools of nursing and renewing and issuing licenses.

The board has the authority to suspend or revoke a license. Some of the conditions under which a nurse's license is sometimes suspended or revoked because of inability to perform competently are drug addiction, alcohol abuse, and lack of mental or physical well-being. A nursing license is also revoked at times for **negligence** (the commission of an act that a prudent person would not have done or the omission of a duty that a prudent person would have fulfilled, resulting in injury or harm to another person; proof is necessary that other prudent members of the same profession would ordinarily have acted differently under the same circumstances) in patient care, endangering a patient's life, or failing to comply with the standard and requirements of the nurse practice act of the state in which the nurse is practicing (see Chapter 2).

MENTORING AND NETWORKING

A mentor is a nurse with more experience and knowledge who is willing to assist a novice to learn the skills of the profession through counseling, role modeling, and teaching. Nurses need to demonstrate caring behaviors for themselves, each other, and patients. Mentoring is a high-order form of professional caring.

Most nurses are fortunate if they have one or two mentors throughout their careers. This does not commonly happen. The reality is that there are few committed mentors in nursing.

Identification of a mentor is your first challenge. Locate someone who demonstrates both interest in your area and the behaviors you want to achieve. Evaluate how receptive to questions the person seems and whether he or she seems likely to take time to explain and clarify information as you are learning and developing.

A good mentor meets the following criteria:

- Has an interest in the same clinical practice you are interested in learning
- Demonstrates a high level of skill in your area of interest
- Is receptive to questions from you and others
- Integrates teaching into questions or explanations

Most professionals are aware of the need to mentor the less experienced people on a health care team. Because of nursing's history, however, nurses do not always know how to go about mentoring because they have not seen many role models for this behavior.

Sometimes mentors are not available. In this situation, try being your own mentor.

The following are five self-mentoring strategies that are possible for all professionals to use in making a transition:

- Interact with people. Ask questions, listen, and clarify what you know with others to enhance your understanding.
- Discover and use references. Read books and journal articles.
- Observe others who are knowledgeable and insightful.
- Enroll in educational programs, especially those that include skill practices.
- Determine solutions for yourself, reflect on them, and work through them on your own.

There are other strategies such as networking, which is an effective method for informing people about your goals, concerns, or desires in an informal manner. Start networking with members of your facility, who will sometimes be able to advise you because they hear of jobs before they are posted.

It is impossible to know ahead of time which networking contact will be your best reward. That is why you should form several alliances to promote your work as a nurse.

Your career in nursing has the potential to be rich in experience with others, information, and opportunity if you consciously decide to develop a network system (Box 58-10). It is most important for you to have a desire to move ahead. Everyone has to be willing to both give and take for the system to be successful. It is necessary for individuals in the network system to have a positive self-concept and believe that they can contribute to others' needs (*Mosby's Dictionary of Medicine, Nursing, and Health Professions,* 2009).

CAREER OPPORTUNITIES

Never before has nursing been so exciting; today the new graduate has an unprecedented variety of job opportunities available. The options will require considerable thought for you to make the correct decision. The job opportunities for the LPN/LVN have expanded and now extend beyond those in the long-term care facility and the hospital.

Many believe that it is better for the LPN/LVN to seek employment first in a hospital or long-term care facility with a subacute unit. This provides the opportunity to sharpen your skills and solidify your knowledge base. Later, if you want to explore job opportunities in other settings, you have a broader base on which to build. However, this depends on your goals and your personal situation. If you know that you can only work days and that you need weekends off, a physician's office or clinic will perhaps be preferable for your first job.

HOSPITALS

Employment of LPNs/LVNs in hospital settings today is at record high levels. Because of health care economics, hospitals are responsible for providing quality care as economically as possible. Under the supervision of an RN, the LPN/LVN is legally able to provide most bedside care to patients in the hospital setting. Since the LPN/LVN salary is less than that of the RN, it

Box 58-10 Tips from New Nurses

When you are making the transition from student to graduate nurse then the following tips may help prepare you for the challenges ahead:

- Unexpected things will happen and you won't be prepared. Know where the crash cart is located and where the items are on it. Learn the emergency procedure for your facility.
- Nursing is a stressful profession, so make sure you have someone to vent to without compromising patient confidentiality.
- Make sure you receive a comprehensive report on your patient before you see him or her. Keep this report with you or within easy access and protect patient confidentiality.
- Have all your facts together and try to troubleshoot the situation before you call the patient's health care provider. If you are unsure what information the health care provider might want, ask another nurse; don't be afraid to ask for assistance.
- If possible, spend your first 6 months to 1 year on a hospital medical-surgical unit. Even though you don't plan to work on such a unit long term, the experience you gain will be invaluable.
- Be flexible and learn to prioritize your patients. If you get bogged down, ask another nurse to help you for a few minutes.
- Watch for the nurses who have the shameful habit of "eating their young." These nurses seem to enjoy making new nurses feel uncomfortable and doubt themselves. Don't take it personally; seek out those who are interested in assisting you.
- Read the policy and procedure manual thoroughly and pay close attention to things that are specific to your job description. It's your responsibility to decide if you are legally allowed to perform a task, so visit your state board of nursing's website and stay within your scope of practice.
- Don't gossip or spread rumors about co-workers. Talk with the co-worker if you have a problem and if that doesn't resolve the problem, talk to your supervisor.
- Know everything about the medication you are giving your patient. Make use of a current drug guide, either there on the unit or your personal digital assistant (PDA).
- Document, document, document. "If it isn't documented, then it wasn't done." Your documentation should also support your patient's diagnosis.
- You'll get a great deal of on-the-job training; don't refuse to do anything that you don't know how to do, are uncomfortable doing, or haven't been taught to do. No one can observe and perform every nursing skill. Ask if you can participate in or watch different activities, such as starting an IV or inserting a urinary catheter.
- Most nurses and physicians are excellent teachers and are happy to share their knowledge. Take notes as you ask questions so you aren't asking the same questions over again.
- Don't be forced to do something that isn't in the patient's best interest. You are the patient's advocate, and it's your duty to speak for him or her. It's not so much about "how you feel," but about standards of care and what's best for the patient.

Wright, J. (2008). Tips for new nurses. *LPN 2008,* 4(2):20, 21.

makes economic sense to employ a number of LPNs/LVNs. It also makes sense because the LPN/LVN is prepared to give excellent bedside care. This is his or her specialty (Figure 58-4).

The LPN/LVN has gained access to areas of the hospital that only RNs staffed previously. These areas include coronary care, intensive care, emergency department, surgery scrub, outpatient surgery, and pediatrics. Policies vary by facility and by localities. In the hospital setting, the LPN/LVN has responsibility for supervising nursing assistants. The overall management of a unit is the responsibility of an RN.

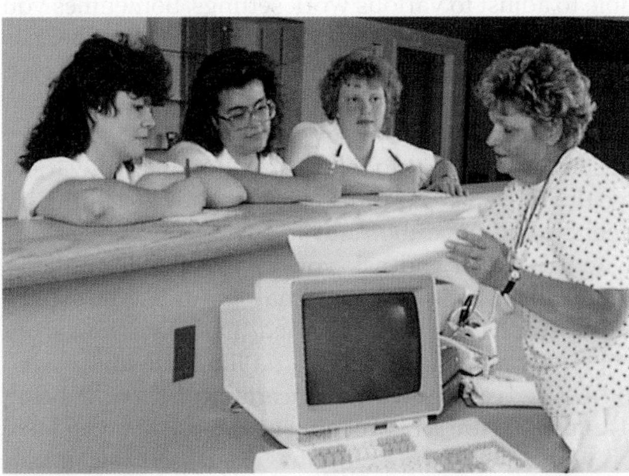

FIGURE 58-4 Various positions on the health care team are available in the hospital setting.

Salaries in a hospital setting typically include shift differential and extra pay for holidays and perhaps weekends. Benefits tend to be good in hospitals. Some provide for 12-hour shifts and special schedule plans such as a 3-day weekend work schedule. In some, you will have the opportunity to function on hospital committees. There are sometimes some unique positions such as working in infection control or employee health, but these will not give the LPN/LVN the chance of advancing to charge positions in the hospital setting.

There are a number of different types of hospitals to consider. Some have a wide range of services, and some are more specialized. Some focus only on pediatric patients, and others have only mental health patients. Hospitals also exist that have only rehabilitation patients. Some have a lot of outpatient services, and others include a long-term care unit. Some operate a home health service. Others will perhaps have a hotel facility for individuals from out of town who require extensive testing. Some hospitals operate in conjunction with a university and are the site of a great deal of teaching and research. Some hospitals are trauma centers. Some have specialties such as orthopedics, specialized surgeries, or testing that are not available at other local hospitals that draw patients from surrounding areas. Some even have a helicopter service for emergency patients.

LONG-TERM CARE FACILITIES

The LPN/LVN is the backbone of long-term care facilities. You have the opportunity to advance to charge nurse and supervisory capacity with RN supervision. You will perhaps also serve in staff development, recruitment, and all types of committee work. Your management and leadership skills have ample opportunity for development in the long-term care setting.

Salaries are typically higher in long-term care facilities than in hospitals, but not in all situations. Typically, shift differential pay and scheduling alternatives are possible. Benefit packages also tend to be good in the long-term care setting.

Many positive changes have occurred in the facilities that were previously called nursing homes. The long-term care facility is just that—a facility for those who require long-term care. Hospitals no longer are an option for patients past the most acute period. Alternatives include rehabilitation hospitals if patients meet the qualifications, home health, or a long-term care facility. Residents will be of any age, although the majority continue to be in the older age-group. Units vary in the level of care they provide. Some provide care that in years past was only possible in the hospital setting. Some have special units earmarked for acquired immunodeficiency syndrome (AIDS) or patients with Alzheimer's disease. Some have rehabilitation units for stroke and orthopedic patients. Physical, speech, occupational, and other therapies are available. Many patients receive therapy and are able to return home.

HOME HEALTH

The degree to which home health opportunities are available to LPNs/LVNs varies in different parts of the United States. The LPN/LVN is capable of providing much of the care required, but RN supervision has to be available. The advantages of home health care are a more relaxed atmosphere, decreased patient load, and a primarily daytime schedule. Home health is the wave of the future. Health care in the home setting is much less costly for insurance companies.

Pay is often on a per case basis, and there is reimbursement for travel expenses. The salary is often good for individuals who put in a lot of hours. Continuity of care and a degree of independence are advantages of this type of position. There is also scheduling flexibility, which is hard to find in other positions.

PHYSICIAN'S OFFICE OR CLINIC

Many physicians choose to employ an LPN/LVN for their office because they prefer to have the assistance of someone with that educational background. Some of the skills required will not be included in the LPN/LVN educational program. These include laboratory testing, electrocardiograms, and other testing. In some cases the physician will teach these skills; there are also specific classes to take to learn them. In a small office, computer skills and perhaps insurance coding and billing skills are necessary. The LPN/LVN has the potential to become the vital right arm of the physician in the office setting. Supervision of other office personnel will sometimes be required.

Salary in offices tends to be lower than that in hospitals and long-term care facilities. Often the benefits package will not be as complete as in the other settings. However, the schedule of primarily days with minimal weekends is a definite advantage. There is an opportunity to focus on prevention in these settings, and opportunities for patient teaching are also available. Less manual dexterity is required, which might be advantageous for some individuals.

INSURANCE COMPANIES

Many insurance companies employ LPNs/LVNs in their preadmission and claims departments. These positions are office positions with few manual dexterity requirements. Companies usually require prior experience in medical-surgical nursing. Salary tends to be lower than in hospitals and long-term care facilities. However, the schedule is usually days, with no holidays or weekend work required.

TEMPORARY AGENCIES

There are opportunities to work for staffing agencies. These agencies provide nurses to meet the staffing needs in a variety of health care facilities. The salary is usually very good, but sometimes the benefits package is limited. You need to be a highly flexible person to be able to adjust to various work settings. Sometimes you will end up working primarily in one facility that has frequent staffing needs. However, you will still be on different units within the facility.

Advantages of employment with a temporary agency are the right to refuse and the wealth of variety available. When you are employed by a temporary agency, you have the right to say no on a given day when they call and ask you to work. This provides more flexibility in your personal schedule. The experiences you have are more varied than when you work every day at the same facility on the same unit.

A disadvantage is the uncertainty of work being available. There will probably be times when you have no work. Perhaps a facility has decreased census and therefore decreased staffing needs. It tends to be hard to budget with no guarantee of a specific number of hours per week. Another disadvantage is that you are not a constant part of a particular work group. You are always an outsider.

TRAVEL OPPORTUNITIES

After you have had some experience, consider exploring opportunities to travel and work for specified periods in areas in need of nurses through a type of temporary agency with an expanded area of service. These agencies match employers' needs with nurses' experience and interest in living in that area for a time. Lodging is provided in addition to salary. This affords nurses who have the flexibility to travel the chance to visit an area and work there for a while.

PHARMACEUTICAL SALES

After you have some experience, pharmaceutical sales is a field of possible interest. These companies usually require experience in specific areas and an expertise in science and pharmacology. Salary is usually based on sales. There is no direct patient care. You will make contacts with physicians, pharmacists, and nurses in various clinical settings to present the advantages of products and to teach about side effects and precautions.

OTHER MEDICAL SALES

Opportunities are also available for nurses with companies selling medical supplies. Responsibilities and compensation are similar to those in pharmaceutical sales. Sometimes nurses in this line of work do in-service programs at facilities to demonstrate product use. Products vary widely, from such items as incontinence products to surgical equipment.

OUTPATIENT HOTELS

In some areas, opportunities sometimes become available in hotel settings owned by a hospital. The patient-guests stay in the hotel while they undergo testing before surgery. The nurse is available for patient teaching and to assist the guests in any preparation required for the tests. The nurse is also available in case of an emergency. Salary and benefits are the same as those of the hospital.

THE MILITARY

Opportunities are available for the LPN/LVN in military service. Use of the LPN/LVN is increasing in the military just as it is in civilian life. Active duty and the reserves are options. If you are interested, your local recruiter will be able to provide all of the necessary information. Benefits in the military are generous. One major benefit is in the area of educational opportunities. You have the possibility of getting assistance to help you repay loans or for tuition for additional education.

ADULT DAYCARE

Some communities may provide adult daycare facilities that require nursing supervision. These facilities are designed for individuals who require medical supervision while their family members work or take a break from the responsibility of care. The pace is relaxed, and the schedule is excellent. Many nurses find it to be a rewarding experience to work in a facility providing this kind of service to the adults and their family members who need it.

SCHOOLS

Opportunities come up in some communities to work as a school nurse. Health screening, emergency care, and health teaching are the major responsibilities. The nurse perhaps functions in one school or travels to different schools. Working only during the school year is an advantage for the nurse who would like to be off summers and is in a financial position to permit this.

PUBLIC HEALTH

There will sometimes be opportunities for LPNs/LVNs with the public health department in your community. Responsibilities usually include working in clinics and home visits. The nurse will sometimes also participate in health inspections. Teaching is a major area of responsibility. The focus is on prevention. Day schedules are usually available. Salaries tend to be lower than in hospitals and long-term care facilities.

OUTPATIENT SURGERY

Work in a large number of outpatient facilities is available, especially for outpatient surgery. The LPN/LVN is sometimes employed to prepare patients for surgery, as a scrub nurse, or to work in the recovery room under the supervision of an RN. This is typically a Monday-through-Friday position. Some facilities are freestanding and others part of a hospital complex.

PRIVATE DUTY

The private duty nurse gives total care to one patient. The setting for the private duty nurse changes from patient to patient, but basically the job description is the same. This type of nursing is totally independent nursing care service. Private duty nursing takes place in the hospital, the home, or other facility and while traveling abroad or in the United States. When doing private duty nursing, you accept not only the patient but the family as well. You are paid directly by the patient or responsible person. When the setting for private duty nursing is in a health care facility, you are expected to follow the policies and procedures of that facility.

When doing private duty nursing, you are legally responsible for your own actions. If you ever have any doubt about an order or procedure, obtain clarification from the physician before carrying out the order or procedure. It is important to keep charts carefully. In the home, set up a type of record in which you are able to list necessary items, such as medications given, vital signs, and the conditions of the patient. This home record will sometimes be requested by and released to the physician. You will return any narcotics not used to the physician before you leave the case.

The major problems of private duty nursing are the irregular assignments and the economic aspects. In private duty nursing, there is no certainty of work or payment. However, because today there are so many unfilled demands for private duty nurses, the availability of cases presents fewer problems for the LPN/LVN.

If you choose this field of nursing, it is advisable to remember that you will be responsible for the payment of your Social Security, as well as your federal, state, and city taxes. This means that you have to keep continuous, accurate records of your days worked and payments received.

An advantage of private duty nursing is that you have the option of working as many days as you like, and the opportunity to accept a case for as long a period as you desire. You have more freedom and fewer restrictions in your workday.

GOVERNMENT (CIVIL SERVICE)

Some LPNs/LVNs work in a Veterans Administration hospital or other government hospitals. Advantages are good salary, fringe benefits, and good insurance and retirement plans. The disadvantage is that the ratio of nurses to patients is sometimes steep.

INDUSTRY

The focus in industrial nursing is on promoting wellness and preventing accidents. There is an emphasis on safety, and usually the nurse is first aid oriented. As an industrial nurse, you will perhaps do physical assessment, health surveys, insurance form preparation, and health education, as well as nursing intervention for patients injured in industrial accidents. The LPN/LVN will work under the supervision of an RN or a physician. Depending on the size of the industrial site, this type of nursing sometimes offers shifts and benefits different from those of other career opportunities.

In this field of nursing you have to have patience, understanding, observational skills, and current first aid techniques and principles. You need organizational skills and the ability to keep neat records. It is important to be able to adjust to all types of situations and people.

REHABILITATION

This field requires responsibility for guiding the patient toward health and independence. Advantages are steady employment, a less formal environment, and an opportunity to provide good care.

PSYCHIATRY

Psychiatric nursing requires a psychologically mature person (not necessarily mature in years) to handle the responsibilities of the job. The setting for this type of nursing varies from an open unit in a general hospital to outpatient clinics, mental health agencies, psychiatric hospitals, or other institutions. Advantages are a good salary and advancement in leadership areas.

HOSPICE

Hospice nursing offers the opportunity to care for terminally ill patients in either an institution or a home setting, usually under the auspices of home health nursing. The qualifications for hospice nurses are to have a clear understanding of their own feelings concerning death and to understand the philosophy of the hospice setting. The nurse closely supports the patient and family without interfering with family interpersonal relationships. Advantages of hospice nursing are steady employment, an environment that is less formal, and opportunities to provide good bedside care that is concerned with pain relief and comfort measures. Disadvantages are always caring for dying patients and the possibility of having to travel to more than one home each shift (see Chapter 40).

POTENTIAL OPPORTUNITIES

Potential opportunities include Head Start programs—these are designed for very young children. There are also weight-loss clinics, where the nurse functions as a support person or counselor. Camp programs are available in some areas. The head nurse will perhaps be an RN, but LPNs/LVNs are often employed to assist. The cases range from poison ivy or poison oak, insect or snake bites, fractures, lacerations, and various infections. Camp nursing is often a summertime position, which leaves you to either seek different employment the rest of the year or further your education.

LEADERSHIP AND MANAGEMENT

Leadership is the art of getting others to want to do something you are convinced has to be done. One root of the word *lead* means "to go." Leaders typically have a vision of where to go—a direction in which they influence others to follow. Leaders are the ones who show the way and have a grasp of the big picture.

Management is closely related. The word *management* comes from a word meaning "hand." Managers handle the day-to-day operations to achieve a desired outcome. Successful organizations require both leadership and management (see Coordinated Care box for responsibilities of the nurse manager).

Leadership is an important factor in determining the effectiveness of any undertaking. Styles refer to the approach or manner a leader uses to influence the behavior of others in various situations. Leadership

 Coordinated Care

Supervision

RESPONSIBILITIES OF THE NURSE MANAGER

- Assist staff in establishing annual goals for the unit and the systems needed to accomplish goals.
- Monitor professional nursing standards of practice on the unit.
- Develop an ongoing staff development plan, including one for new employees.
- Recruit new employees (interview and hire).
- Conduct routine staff evaluations.
- Establish yourself as a role model for positive customer service (customers include patients, families, and other health care team members).
- Submit staffing schedules for the unit.
- Conduct regular patient rounds and help solve patient or family complaints.
- Establish and implement a quality improvement plan for the unit.
- Review and recommend new equipment needs for the unit.
- Conduct regular staff meetings.
- Conduct rounds with physicians.
- Establish and support necessary staff and interdisciplinary committees.

styles relate to the amount of control or freedom the manager allows the group. Styles range from total control by the manager to extreme permissiveness. The most common styles are autocratic, democratic, and laissez-faire.

AUTOCRATIC STYLE

The autocratic leader retains all authority and responsibility and is concerned primarily with tasks and goal accomplishment. This type of leader assigns clearly defined tasks and establishes one-way communication with the group. The autocratic leader is firm, insistent, and dominating. Such a leader stresses prompt, orderly performance and uses power to intimidate or pressure those who fail to adhere to expectations. This leader displays little trust or confidence in employees and therefore makes all the decisions. Because employees generally fear this type of manager, there tends to be some stifling of individual initiative and creativity.

The autocratic style of leadership is sometimes appropriate to a situation. In situations in which immediate action is required and there is no time for group decisions, the autocratic leader is able to take quick action. Autocratic leaders excel in times of crisis (e.g., cardiac arrest) and in situations of disorder (e.g., natural disaster); they often have the reputation for being able to get difficult assignments completed.

DEMOCRATIC STYLE

The democratic style is a people-centered approach that allows employees more control and individual participation in the decision-making process. The emphasis is on team building and a spirit of collaboration through the joint effort of all team members. Democratic leaders function to facilitate goal accomplishment while stressing the self-worth of each individual. These leaders treat each staff member as an adult and expect the same in return. Criticism focuses on behaviors, not on personality, and its purpose is to promote growth and development of the staff.

The democratic style works best with mature employees who work well together as groups. This style sometimes does not work as well with ancillary staff, who in many cases will need more direction. The group decision-making process sometimes seems slow and frustrating to those who expect prompt action on an issue. Disagreements are more likely, and sometimes require more time to resolve. This style tends to demand more of the leader, but many value it for the sake of the growth and development of the staff it facilitates. The results of the democratic leadership style in health care settings are evident in shared governance (an organized, systematic approach to decision making that enables nurses at all levels to participate), self-directed work teams, and quality improvement staff committees.

LAISSEZ-FAIRE STYLE

This leadership style is often referred to as the "free-run style," or permissive leadership. This type of leader relinquishes control completely and chooses to avoid responsibility by delegating all decision making to the group. Laissez-faire leaders want everyone to feel free to "do their own thing," and as a result there is no sense of direction unless provided by the group or an informal leader. This style sometimes works well with highly motivated professional groups (e.g., a research staff); however, it seldom works well in health care settings because of the complexity of the work environment.

SITUATIONAL LEADERSHIP

Situational leadership as a comprehensive approach to the issue of management takes into account the style of the leader, the maturity of the group, and the situation at hand. Supporters of situational leadership contend that no single leadership style is best but rather that the best style for the manager to use is contingent on the maturity level of the employees or group and the situation at hand.

The more managers adapt their leadership styles to work situations and the needs and abilities of staff, the more effective the managers will be. Situational leadership theorists identify four typical styles for leaders. The leader will at times use all four styles all at once, depending on the size of the work group, the maturity of the staff, and the situations the work group encounters. The four styles are directing, coaching, supporting, and delegating:

- **Directing:** The leader provides specific instructions and supervises the accomplishment of tasks. There is high directive and low supportive behavior. Leaders give detailed instructions; state specific expectations; enforce rules and policies; and tell employees what to do, how to do it, and when to do it. This style applies with new employees, employees with repeated performance problems, and crisis work situations.

- **Coaching:** The leader monitors the accomplishment of tasks while also explaining decisions, asking for feedback or suggestions, and recognizing good performance. There is high directive and high supportive behavior. Typically, leader and staff have jointly developed a work plan.
- **Supporting:** The leader supports the efforts of others, facilitates their goal accomplishment, and shares responsibility for decision making. There is high supportive and low directive behavior. The leader is willing to try new ideas of staff and uses consensus decision making (a group process involving all participants, with the outcome being a decision that all members are able to agree with and support) to choose a course of action. The leader values growth and not perfection, collaboration and not competition.
- **Delegating:** The leader gives the responsibility for decision making and problem solving to mature staff who have demonstrated their competence. There is low supportive and low directive behavior. The leader recognizes that there is more than one right way to do things and gives authority to staff that matches their level of responsibility.

The approach of gradually giving up control and giving increasing decision-making authority to staff is in keeping with modern management theory regarding staff empowerment. This management technique fosters the growth of others and facilitates their development so that they become progressively less dependent on the leader. Staff become able to know when they will be able to make decisions confidently on their own, such as intervening and resolving patient and family complaints, dealing with unclear medical orders from a physician, or resolving conflicts between fellow staff nurses.

The cornerstone of situational leadership theory is the flexibility of the manager in adapting to the needs of the individual or the work group. In a typical work setting, the manager will perhaps be directive in dealing with staff who are in orientation, while acting as a coach for those on another shift who are more experienced but still need some guidance. The supporting style will likely be apparent as the manager works with a staff practice committee and assists members in solving a problem with another department. A manager who relies on seasoned staff nurses to monitor quality-of-care issues and to regularly report results of studies is using the delegating style to promote staff development. It is important to carefully assess developmental level or job maturity of staff and match it with the appropriate leadership style. The situational leadership style is growth producing for both manager and staff.

TEAM LEADING

Sometimes an LPN/LVN receives the assignment of assuming the role of team leader. This role entails assisting and guiding the nursing team in providing care for a select group of patients. The team leader assigns patients to each team member and takes responsibility for the delivery of care to patients, as well as for supervision of all members of the team, including nursing assistants. Duties of a team leader include the following:

- Receiving reports on assigned patients
- Making assignments for team members
- Making rounds and assessing all assigned patients
- Giving team members a report on assigned patients
- Assisting in administering medications and treatments
- Providing time in the early part of the shift to have a conference with team members on priority patients (those with the most urgent needs) to keep everyone informed of progress in patient care, provide continuity of care, and allow the team member to answer questions and resolve problems

An advantage of team nursing is the collaborative style that encourages each member of the team to help others (see Coordinated Care box on effective leadership).

TIME MANAGEMENT

Using time to good advantage will be of great value. Learn effective time management skills, and practice them frequently until they become fully developed. These skills will help you manage not only at work but also in daily living (see Coordinated Care box on prioritization and time management). Manage your time so that you are able to accomplish both what you are *required* to do and what you *want* to do.

ANGER MANAGEMENT

Besides providing income, work provides you with the opportunity to be recognized for what you do, to belong to a group, and to display your competence (Figure 58-5). When any of these needs are threatened in the course of the workday or you feel like a victim in the workplace with lack of control, you have the potential to get angry. Anger is not automatically bad. Anger gives you a cue that something is wrong. If your anger is justified, it has some power to help you get your needs met by stimulating you to action. Harassment and discrimination are examples of situations in which anger is justified. If your anger is unjustified, or

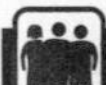

Coordinated Care

Leadership

GUIDELINES FOR EFFECTIVE LEADERSHIP

1. Keep notepad and pencil with you (document on notepad pertinent information that will possibly be relevant later). Also have available a pocket calculation guide on drug doses and intravenous (IV) drip rate.
2. Develop your own system of abbreviations for your information, but use only standard abbreviations on legal documents.
3. Make patient rounds as soon as report is over. If you are to be responsible for the direct care of a certain number of patients, make certain you are able to document accurate information concerning their conditions. Note on your "pocket notes" date and time, and briefly state what you observe or hear. This is helpful if the patient's condition changes.
4. Check all equipment and supplies that you will be responsible for during your shift. It is acceptable to assign these duties to another responsible person if available. These checks are good to make part of the routine and will assist in the proficiency of the staff.
5. Everyone performs best when the team works together and each member receives recognition for individual performance.
6. Keep informed of the events within the facility.
   a. Attend necessary meetings.
   b. Become familiar with rules and regulations of the facility in which you work.
   c. Learn what surveys or inspections will be conducted.
   d. Learn where the policy and procedure documents are kept; also ensure that they receive proper updates and are in a central area.

Coordinated Care

Prioritization

PRINCIPLES OF TIME MANAGEMENT

Goal Setting

Review the patient's goals of care for the day and the goals you have for activities such as completing documentation, attending a patient care conference, giving the staff report on time, or preparing medications for administration.

Time Analysis

Reflect on how you use your time. While working in a clinical area, keep track of how you use your time in different activities. This will often provide valuable information and reveal how well organized you really are.

Priority Setting

Schedule the priorities that you have established for patients within set time frames. Determine the best time for activities such as conducting teaching sessions, planning ambulation, and providing times for rest.

Interruption Control

Everyone needs time to socialize or to discuss issues with colleagues. However, do not let this interrupt important patient care activities. Use time during reports, meal breaks, or team meetings to the best advantage. Also, plan time to assist colleagues so that it complements your patient care schedule.

Evaluation

At the end of each day, take time to think about how effectively you used your time. If you are having difficulties, discuss them with a more experienced colleague.

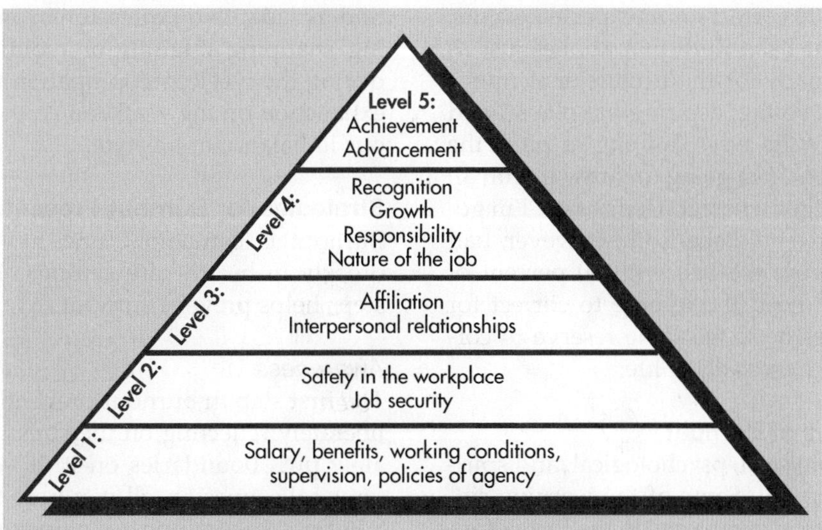

FIGURE 58-5 Howlett's hierarchy of work motivators.

Box 58-11 Personal Anger Management Techniques

1. Learn your personal signs that let you or others know that you are becoming angry. Pay attention to what you are thinking and feeling.
2. How you appraise events causes the anger response. Change irrational thoughts to rational thoughts.
3. If your heart is pounding, take deep breaths.
4. If you feel tension in a body area, rub the area for a few seconds.
5. When angry, speak slowly and in a lower tone of voice, acknowledge how you feel, and take a time-out.
6. View a stimulus to anger as a problem. Use the problem-solving process to arrive at a solution. The key to successful problem solving is to identify the real issue and solve it. What is the problem? Avoid spending precious time on finding solutions for what is not really the problem. The nursing process is an excellent problem-solving method. You have been using it throughout your LPN/LVN program. The nursing process lends itself to solving resident or patient problems and staff problems. The nursing process also works at home, as well as in the clinical area.

Box 58-12 Symptoms of Burnout

PHYSICAL
- Fatigue
- Changes in sleeping, eating
- Lack of energy
- Loss of interest in sex

PSYCHOLOGICAL
- Irritability
- Hypersensitivity
- Frustration
- Negative outlook
- Forgetting

SPIRITUAL
- Loss of commitment
- Loss of meaning
- Loss of integrity

displayed inappropriately, it has the potential to get you and others in trouble (Box 58-11).

BURNOUT

Physical, emotional, and spiritual exhaustion among caregivers is sometimes called **burnout.** Nurses are at high risk for burnout because they care. The road to burnout often begins insidiously (subtly). It occurs more often in people who have excessive expectations of themselves and who feel they need to do everything right, and nurses are especially prone to this characteristic. So strong is the need to be the exemplary nurse, the model parent, and the expert clinician that the compulsion to do the highest quality job takes over at the expense of health and well-being.

The need to be perfect does not allow for error or the necessary reserve to correct for unexpected events. There is a story about Babe Ruth that applies just as well to a good approach for the professional nurse. Babe was coaching a young, aspiring ballplayer, and he asked the boy how he was planning to pitch the ball. The boy answered, "I'm going to throw it with all my might and get it right where it needs to go. I'm going to give it 110 percent." Babe Ruth, however, had different advice: "Throw the ball with 80 percent of your might. You will need the reserve to correct for any mistakes." Nurses need the same reserve to correct for the inevitable curveballs of life.

Signs and Symptoms of Burnout

Box 58-12 identifies physical, psychological, and spiritual symptoms of burnout. Some of the warning signals of stress are physical symptoms in the form of increased smoking, drinking, or eating; skipping meals; eating compulsively on the run; and sleep disturbances. The potential burnout victim begins to feel emotionally drained, constantly tired, "like a robot," or in a constant state of hyperarousal, in which much of life seems irritating.

Conscientiousness becomes confused with the fear of losing control. It becomes increasingly difficult to delegate responsibility because of the fear that others will perhaps not do a task as well. Time begins to slip away, and the nurse finds little time for replenishing the self. Nor is there time for others (e.g., family or friends). Every demand on one's time seems like an intrusion. The person is always tired and preoccupied with work. Emotional pleasures become a thing of the past.

Self-needs become buried by rationalizations, such as "As soon as I get the unit staffed . . ." or "As soon as I get my degree. . . ." Despite working harder and enjoying it less, the nurse feels alone and isolated, misunderstood, and unappreciated. Repressed self-needs find maladaptive expression in overeating, overspending, snapping at family, or avoiding friends. Insomnia during the week, preoccupation with tasks, and utter exhaustion on the weekend or days off suggest a serious imbalance in lifestyle.

Strategies for Burnout Prevention

Burnout is contagious and has potential to spread quickly in health care settings. Taking the following steps helps prevent burnout.

Awareness

The first step in burnout prevention is awareness. Deliberately reflecting on the stress in your life immediately puts boundaries on it. If you are in doubt, ask your colleagues to tell you how they experience you. Solutions become possible once you define the problem appropriately.

Balance

The second and perhaps most important step is restoring balance to your life. A **healthy balance** among work, family, leisure, and lifelong learning enhances personal judgments, satisfaction, and productivity. Actively scheduling time for each of these activities is the only way to achieve balance. Anything else falls short of the mark. Good intentions will never cure burnout. Only deliberate actions will provide relief.

Choice

People experiencing the burnout syndrome usually do not think they have any choice other than to keep doing what they have been doing, but life is a series of choices and negotiations. All human beings have choices, and the choices we make create the fabric of our lives. Refusing to delegate work because someone else is not able to do it as well and not going to dinner with friends because you have too much work to do are choices on your part.

Detachment

Detachment differs from disengagement. With disengagement, there is a withdrawal of emotional energy. Detachment allows full emotional involvement in a task or relationship, but not to the degree that it compromises your quality of life, values, or needs. It means focusing on a job or project to the best of your ability and then, at the end of the day or the time designated to the project, dropping it completely. Saying to yourself that something is "sufficient for the day" is a stress management strategy that puts boundaries on life tasks.

Altruistic Egoism

Potential burnout victims generally put everyone and everything ahead of themselves. They ignore their own needs or take them for granted. **Altruistic egoism** simply means paying as much attention to your own personal needs as you do to the needs of others. Although this seems obvious, many nurses consider attention to their own needs as being selfish. Nothing is further from the truth. In the long run, a balance between self-needs and the needs of others enhances the quality of care you are able to give to others.

Focus

People who are focused achieve their goals. Those who are not will sometimes reach a goal, but usually it takes longer and is not as certain. Focusing full energy on one thing at a time and finishing one project before starting another has several benefits: It is more likely that you will enjoy each activity more, and your full attention will make for a better product. A powerful contributor to the development of burnout is having several unfinished projects all demanding similar space in your mind.

Goals

This step is closely aligned with focus, with an emphasis on outcome. An excellent burnout prevention strategy is identifying goals that are realistic, achievable, and in line with your personal values. If you want to go to New York, you do not buy a ticket to California. The same is true of life. Knowing where you want to go and what it takes to get there enhances your chances of success. It is important to know where you do want to go with your life and to have a realistic sense of what you will find when you get there.

Hope

People who feel burned out experience helplessness and hopelessness about changing their situation. The despair that accompanies emptiness and futility is possible to reverse by simply seeking out connections with empathic others. Their advice and caring support, even in one encounter, has considerable power as an antidote to inner emptiness. It is important, however, to seek support from people who will work with you on developing solutions and not in commiserating (sympathizing) with how horrible the situation is. A solution-focused, rather than problem-oriented, approach is essential to the development of hope.

Integrity

The final step in reversing burnout is to restore your personal integrity (wholeness). Burnout always leads to some loss of personal integrity in the sense that you ignore or devalue important values. When you begin to forget who you are and instead become what everyone else expects of you, you are in trouble. Reclaim yourself! Burnout is possible to reverse by taking responsibility for yourself and doing what you believe is important. Take the risk to be all that you are as well as all you can be.

DELEGATION

Delegation of tasks is an important aspect of patient care. Delegation of care refers to the act of making another individual responsible for a specific task. One of the benefits of delegation is that licensed personnel are allowed more time to focus on higher-level tasks (see Coordinated Care box on effective delegation).

It is imperative to understand that delegation involves clearly communicating all aspects of the delegated care to the person completing the task. Equally important is that the nurse takes into account the job description, the legal responsibility, the educational level, the ability, and the licensure of the person he or she is delegating to complete care. The staff member performing the care has to be able to perform tasks independently, and have the ability and knowledge to complete the task (see Coordinated Care box on the five rights of delegation). It is important not to assign care to an unqualified staff member. For example, a

 Coordinated Care

Delegation

EFFECTIVE DELEGATION

- **Identify the task:** Know whether the task is legal to delegate. You retain responsibility for assessment of the patient's nursing care needs.
- **Analyze the skill and knowledge needed to accomplish the task:** Consider whether the task is within the scope of the assignee's education and ability, whether the circumstances are appropriate to delegate the specific task, whether directions and other communications have been sufficient, and how much direct supervision is needed. Know whether the person is able to properly and safely perform the task without jeopardizing the patient's welfare and whether the task requires professional nursing judgment. Instruct the unlicensed person in the delegated task, or verify the person's competency to perform the nursing task through knowledge of individual characteristics, education, or training. Validate the person's understanding.
- **Assign the task:** Provide clear and concise details about the task, including the time frame and the expected outcome, the purpose of the task, and any limitations in responsibility or authority for accomplishing the task.
- **Periodically evaluate the delegation of tasks:** Let the assignee complete the task with occasional follow-up and feedback. Adequately supervise the performance of the delegated nursing task. Do NOT delegate a task if you feel uncomfortable about someone else having control over how it will be completed.

From Harkreader, H., et al. (2007). *Fundamentals of nursing: caring and clinical judgment.* (3rd ed.). Philadelphia: Saunders.

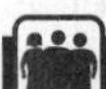 Coordinated Care

Delegation

THE FIVE RIGHTS OF DELEGATION

Right Task

The right task is one you delegate for a specific patient, such as tasks that are repetitive, require little supervision, are relatively noninvasive, have results that are predictable, and pose only minimal risk.

Right Circumstances

Consider the appropriate patient setting, available resources, and other relevant factors. In an acute care setting, patients' conditions often change quickly. Good clinical decision making is necessary to determine what to delegate.

Right Person

The right person is delegating the right tasks to the right person for performance on the right patient.

Right Direction (Communication)

Give a clear, concise description of the task, including its objective, limits, and expectations. It is essential for communication to be ongoing between the registered nurse (RN) and assistive personnel during a shift of care.

Right Supervision

Provide appropriate monitoring, evaluation, intervention as needed, and feedback. It is essential that assistive personnel feel comfortable asking questions and seeking assistance.

Modified from National Council of State Boards of Nursing. (1995). *Delegation: Concepts and decision-making process.* Chicago: Author; National Council of State Boards of Nursing. (1997). *The five rights of delegation.* Chicago: Author; and American Nurses Association (ANA) and National Council of State Boards of Nursing (NCSBN). (2006). *Joint statement on delegation.* Available at www.ncsbn.org/pdfs/joint_statement.pdf.

properly trained nursing assistant will have the capability to perform vital signs on patients and report the findings to the nurse; however, the nursing assistant is not responsible for determining the need for prn medication based on the vital signs.

It is essential for nurses to be aware that accountability remains with the delegating nurse in many situations. A major advantage of delegation is that tasks are completed in a more timely manner when all staff are working together to reach the common goal for the patient (Harkreader et al., 2007).

COMPUTERS IN HEALTH CARE

The computer is the most common and visible example of technology in health care. Continued advances in computer technology have drastically changed how nurses do their work, and will continue to do so. Computers have provided the technology for voice-activated charting, customized nursing care plans, assessment of acuity levels, and reminders to staff of treatments and medication schedules. Computer technology has aided in ordering supplies, equipment, diagnostic tests, and medications. Computers have assisted in developing clinical pathways and care maps. Computer programs have provided quick access to looking up drug incompatibilities and food interactions, treatment modalities, and suggested interventions related to specific nursing diagnoses.

The widespread use of computer technology in health care poses many concerns. Questions about how to maintain confidentiality of the patient's medical record and how to protect the integrity of the system are already big concerns. It remains to be seen what effect an even temporary failure of the system on which the nursing staff is totally dependent will have on their ability to carry out scheduled medications and treatment plans.

Being proficient in using current computer technology in health care settings today does not guarantee success in the future. New programs, new systems, and new applications will require continued education and training.

TRANSCRIBING PHYSICIANS' ORDERS

Physicians' orders are written, telephoned, or verbal. The physician records written orders on the chart. Some facilities employ ward clerks, ward secretaries, or unit secretaries to transcribe the physician's orders.

But in long-term care facilities, there usually are no unit secretaries. In facilities that do employ unit secretaries, the secretaries usually do not work at night. Therefore in many facilities, one expectation of you will be to transcribe the order from the patients' record. There will be times when the order will be difficult to read. **NEVER GUESS.** If in doubt, get a second opinion. Also, if the written order does not read like a "routine order" or if it is a little different from usual, check with the physician or another responsible person. It is imperative to check on the written order before carrying out the order. If in doubt about the physician's order, always recheck for clarity (Figure 58-6).

The physician is in charge of directing the patient care, and nurses carry out the physician's orders for care, unless the nurse believes that the orders are in error or will be harmful to the patient. In this case, it is necessary to contact the physician to confirm or clarify the orders. If the nurse still believes the orders to be inappropriate, the appropriate procedure is to immediately contact the nursing supervisor and put in writing why the orders are not being carried out. A nurse who carries out an erroneous or inappropriate order is at risk to be held liable for harm experienced by the patient. Nurses are responsible for their actions regardless of who told them to perform those actions.

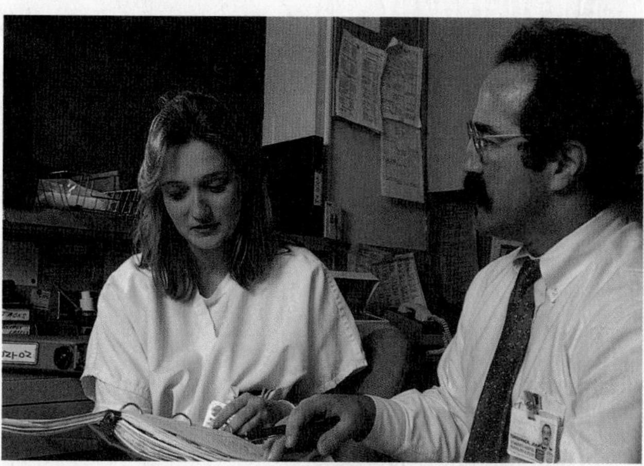

FIGURE 58-6 Clarifying the physician's order.

The policies for verbal or telephone orders vary in different facilities. Be certain to check the policy of the facility for the LPN/LVN regarding accepting verbal or telephone orders. Orders given by telephone or verbal communication are more subject to error. If you are responsible for accepting this type of order, be certain of its accuracy. Clarify the order by repeating it back to the person giving it, and document that you did so. This gives both people a chance to hear the order. Always write a telephone or verbal order immediately. If it is given too rapidly, ask the giver to repeat it, more slowly. When the correct spelling of a medication is questionable, refer to a list of commonly ordered medications or to the *Physicians' Desk Reference* (PDR). Be cautious about medications that look alike when written, have similar spelling, or sound alike. Several medications sound alike but have very different actions (e.g., Xanax and Zantac; Xanax is an antianxiety agent, and Zantac is a histamine antagonist for the treatment of ulcers).

When you **transcribe** (to write or type a copy of) from physicians' orders, there are a number of precautions to use to prevent errors.

Medication Safety Alert!

Precautions for Transcribing Orders

The following information applies to all physicians' orders:

1. Check that written orders correspond correctly to the intended chart.
2. If there is more than one order, read through all orders before beginning.
3. Process stat orders first. (A stat order instructs you to give a single dose of medication immediately and only once.)
4. If there is some confusion during a telephone order, have another nurse listen for clarification.
5. When taking telephone or verbal orders, write the order on the order sheet, read the order back to the person giving it, and document that you read the order back.

The following items are basic guidelines and sometimes vary from one facility to another. Know agency policy.

6. Order the medication needed from the pharmacy; include date, patient's name, room number, time, medication, route of administration, dosage, and frequency.
7. Record the orders in the required areas, such as Kardex, Medex, or medication card. Be certain to include the date.
8. It is sometimes necessary to write a stat medication on a card of a different color. Write STAT on the card, and also write the room number, the patient's name, the drug dose, the route, and the time. Pay special attention to stat orders—and make sure to destroy the card after the order is given and recorded. Stat orders are essential to carry out immediately, not at the next routine time for medication administration or procedure performance.
9. Make very certain that all orders have been carried out and recorded in the proper record. (Have a second nurse verify for accuracy until you gain experience.)
10. Check off each order on the physicians' order sheet and sign it with your name or initials.
11. Make sure to notify those nurses responsible for administering medications of any new order.
12. Most facilities use a sign that indicates a new order. Sometimes you will place a red flag on each chart, or perhaps the physician places the chart in a specific place, such as on the unit secretary's desk.
13. Preferably the charge nurse has the assignment of examining all patients' charts for new orders. This is required during each shift.
14. When your facility uses computers, follow agency policy. Most agencies will have their own computer-based program or procedure.

When there is an order to discontinue or change a medication, take the steps in the Medication Safety Alert below (this procedure will vary in different facilities).

Orders requiring transcription are diet, preoperative and postoperative instructions, all medical treatments, activity, procedures, medications, diagnostic imaging and other diagnostic studies, and laboratory tests. When a patient undergoes surgery, all preoperative orders are automatically canceled. The physician has to rewrite the orders postoperatively if continuation of the orders is desired. Many physicians have routine postoperative orders, which have been prepared beforehand. This sheet is placed in the patient's chart, and the orders are transcribed as discussed. There will be a procedure for each order according to the facility's policy. When transcribing any order, follow completely through all steps one order at a time, and then check it off on the order sheet.

Many facilities now use computers. Transcribe orders onto the computer per agency policy. The nurse transcribing the orders remains responsible for indicating on the sheet of physicians' orders that the transcription has taken place. Some agencies use a stamp followed by the nurse's legal signature. Often, many institutions now have orders faxed to various departments (such as diagnostic imaging, dietary, or pharmacy) to be filled.

When you transcribe orders, record the time and sign your full name on each order. When appropriate, complete the proper requisition slip. As a charge nurse, report any new orders or changes to other staff members to facilitate optimum care for the patient.

After the physician writes new medication orders, it is necessary to obtain the drugs from the pharmacy. Usually you will send the carbon copy of the physician's order sheet to the pharmacy, by computer or fax. The pharmacist is responsible for providing the correct medications and delivering them to the nursing unit.

In acute care settings, each patient on the nursing unit has a medication bin or drawer that contains all the medications for a 24-hour period. Many times this is in a medication cart that it is possible to push from room to room to facilitate administration of medications at routine times. The cart is kept locked when not attended (Figure 58-7). In some settings the medications are kept in a locked cabinet in the patient's room. Narcotic (opioid) analgesics are sometimes distributed from a computerized system (Figure 58-8).

Some drugs may be distributed as floor stock. Floor stock are medications that are distributed to the nursing unit in bulk (either individually wrapped or in bottles). Generally, medications that are appropriate for floor stock are those that physicians tend to prescribe routinely on an as-required (prn) basis. Examples of these medications are stool softeners, antacids, and antipyretics. Newer medication dispensing systems, such as computer-assisted or electronic devices, are variations of unit-dose and floor stock systems. For example, the MedStation (Cardinal Health Pyxis Products, San Diego, Calif.) has the capacity to carry a variety of medications, housed in individual compartments that the nurse can access after requesting the medication from a computerized screen. The MedStation often houses medications that are frequently used, such as floor stock and narcotics. All medications

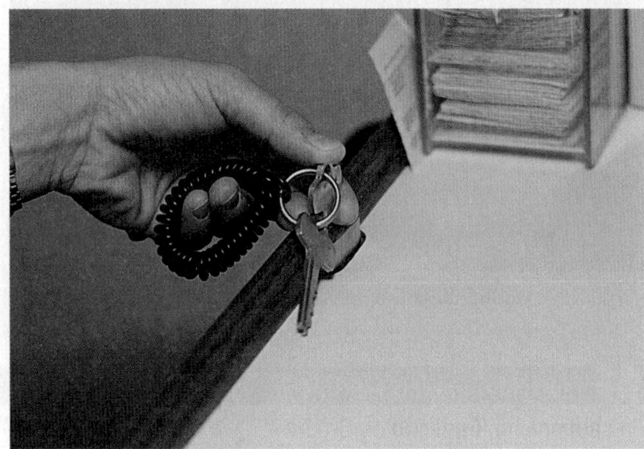

FIGURE 58-7 The medication cart is kept locked when a nurse is not in attendance.

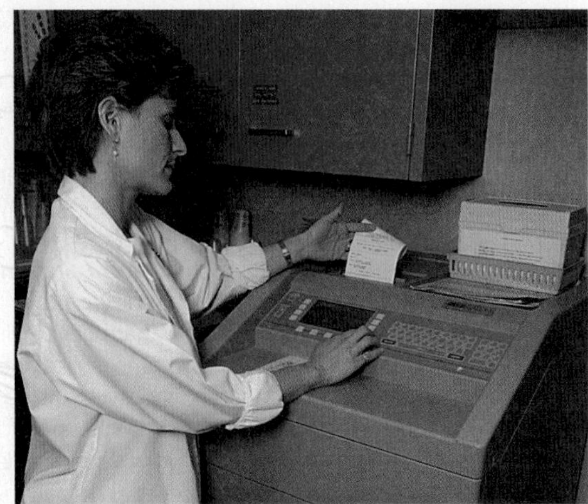

FIGURE 58-8 Computerized system for narcotics distribution.

Medication Safety Alert!

Procedure for Discontinuing or Changing a Medication

1. Mark the old medication order off the Kardex or Medex by crossing through with a highlighter marking pen. If it is an order change, write a new order.
2. Notify the nurse responsible for carrying out new orders about discontinued and newly ordered medications.
3. See that the old medication card is destroyed, if a medication card is issued.
4. Check off the order on the physicians' order sheet.

nurses retrieve from the MedStation are necessary to record in the system's computer. The Sure-Med Unit Dose Center (Baxter Healthcare Corp., Deerfield, Ill.) provides single doses of floor stock medications. (See Chapter 23 for more detailed discussion of medication administration.)

CHANGE-OF-SHIFT REPORT

As an LPN/LVN, you will often be responsible for giving a change-of-shift report. The purpose of the change-of-shift report is to provide the next shift with pertinent information about the patient. The quality of nursing care the patient receives is contingent on how well each shift communicates with the others.

You will sometimes give the change-of-shift report in person and sometimes by audiotape recording or by making rounds from patient to patient (Figure 58-9). You will give oral reports in a conference room with nurses from both shifts participating. When using an audiotape, record the report before the end of the shift. This allows the nurses who are preparing to leave to finish last-minute tasks while the oncoming staff listens to the report. It is beneficial to allow time for clarification or updates before the nurses rotating off leave the unit. Giving reports in person or on rounds allows immediate feedback. Make sure to maintain confidentiality.

The following material will assist you in organization of data for a more efficient and accurate report.

Before beginning the report, plan your communication. Be cognizant of what you want to express. Consider your choice of words. Be precise. Use accepted medical and nursing terminology. Practice pronouncing difficult vocabulary.

Before beginning the report, write down all necessary information, such as vital signs, type of intravenous (IV) fluids, rate of infusion, and credit left in IV bottles and continuous bladder irrigations. Report the condition of the IV site. Record the patient's appetite, intake, and output for feces, urine, and gastric secretions. Report output from drainage tubes, such as Davols, Hemovacs, T-tubes, Malecot drains, and closed-chest tubes. Report color of all body excretions. Have information regarding analgesics you gave, the time of administration, and the effect. Record the amount of patient-controlled analgesia (PCA) used. Write down narcotic credits from the PCA. Write down the assessment results of your patient's lung sounds, bowel sounds, abdomen (soft or distended), and condition of the skin—report abnormal color and turgor for dehydration or edema. Note circulatory checks if pertinent, as well as presence or absence of pedal pulses. If the patient has a bruit, report it. Note dressing changes, amount and color of exudate, and the condition of the incision. Note any abnormal signs and symptoms, such as dyspnea, tachycardia, or abnormal mental status or level of consciousness. Note neurologic deficits, such as flaccid extremity, drooping side of face, hemianopia, or difficulty swallowing (dysphagia).

Once all of these data are compiled, use the Kardex, the worksheet, or the nursing care plan and begin the report (Boxes 58-13 and 58-14). Be systematic.

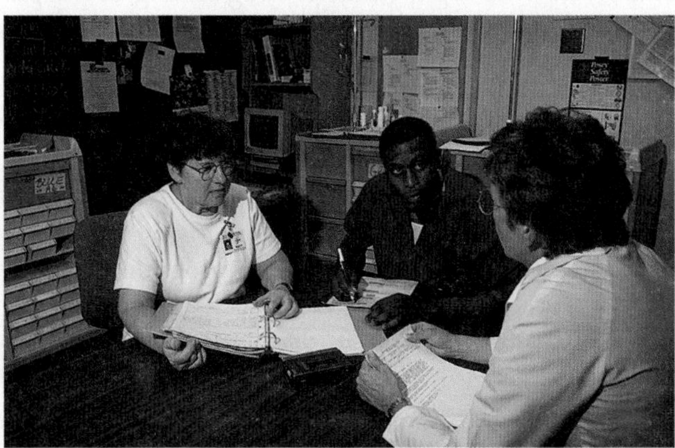

FIGURE 58-9 Giving a change-of-shift report.

Box 58-13 Information for Change-of-Shift Report

1. State patient's room and bed number, name, age, physician, all diagnoses, and date of surgery if patient is postoperative.
2. Summarize patient's day (or evening or night).
3. Report all pertinent nursing care.
4. Describe change in patient's condition. Usually, most facilities report only abnormal vital signs except for first postoperative day, when the last set of vital signs is given.
5. Report special medications, intravenous (IV) solutions, infusion rate, and IV credits. State time, method, and dosage of analgesics given and the effect.
6. Report all intakes and outputs.
7. Report status of lungs and bowel sounds.
8. Report mental status and level of consciousness.
9. Report circulatory checks, pedal pulses, and skin abnormalities in turgor or color.
10. State diagnostic procedure, such as computed tomography scans, x-ray studies, magnetic resonance imaging, endoscopy, proctoscopy, thoracentesis, and surgery. Report diet changes, special permits, preoperative procedures, daily weights, activity status, Accuchecks, Hematest for stools, clean-catch urine for analysis or culture and sensitivity (C&S), sputum specimen for C&S, respiratory therapy, and physical therapy orders. Report all nursing interventions, such as dressings, packs, ostomy care, and oxygen.
11. Discuss patient and family education.
12. Note other services, such as social services, pastoral care, and discharge planning.
13. State any pertinent information helpful in patient care.
14. Report "no code" status.
15. Present the report in an unbiased, nonjudgmental manner.

Box 58-14 Sample of a Change-of-Shift Report

348[A] Mabel Lauritsen, age 87, patient of Dr. Bernard, in with heart failure and stasis ulcer of the right leg. She is alert and cheerful, has had a comfortable day. She has a slight decrease of the edema in her lower extremities. Received an additional 40 mg of Lasix orally at 10 AM; weight is 165 lb, down 10 lb since admission 2 days ago. Vital signs unremarkable except BP 168/100 mm Hg. Has an IV of D_5W with 20 mEq of KCl infusing at 60 mL per hr with a credit of 600 mL. IV site in right forearm is without edema or erythema. Has been up about 1 hour today. Appetite has been good. Received Bancap tablets two at 1400 (2 PM) for pain in right leg. Intake 480 mL IV, 350 mL oral; voided 650 mL of clear, amber urine. Lung sounds clear except for fine crackles in base of right lung. She is expectorating a small amount of clear mucus. No dyspnea noted. Bowel sounds present; abdomen soft. Had moderate amount soft brown stool. Pedal pulses 21/min bilaterally. Has a 2 to 3-cm stasis ulcer of right leg treated with whirlpool and Betadine dressing. The dressings are to be changed four times per day; TED hose are on. There is an order for Hematest of stools ×3, clean-catch urine for C&S, and a chest x-ray. She is to be NPO after midnight for surgery at 9 AM for debridement of the ulcer of her right leg. A preoperative consent form is needed. Social services will be seeing the patient and her daughter Ann Zahrt for discharge planning a few days after surgery.

BP, Blood pressure; *C&S,* culture and sensitivity (testing); *D_5W,* dextrose 5% in water solution; *IV,* intravenous; *KCl,* potassium chloride; *NPO,* nothing-by-mouth status; *TED,* thromboembolic disease.

MALPRACTICE INSURANCE

Malpractice insurance for nurses is becoming increasingly important in a society that has become lawsuit conscious. Paying for the defense of a lawsuit and any possible judgment is beyond the ability of most people. To protect their employees and themselves against any legal and financial consequences that have potential to arise from provision of services, institutional employers carry malpractice liability insurance. However, because individuals are responsible for their own actions, it is still possible for an employee (for example, you as a nurse) to be sued personally. This is true even in states in which charitable immunity, the protection of nonprofit hospitals from legal liability, applies.

A separate, personal malpractice insurance policy over and above your employer's policy is a wise investment that some consider essential. There are at least three reasons why it is a good idea for nurses to carry their own liability insurance. First, if you or your employer are co-defendants and the court finds you liable and the cost of the settlement exceeds your employer's policy limits, it is possible that you will be required to pay the excess out of your own pocket.

Second, it is possible for your employer's insurance company to sue you if they believe they incurred a loss because of your actions.

Third, many employee policies are claim based rather than occurrence based. A claims-based policy covers claims made while the policy is in effect. If your employer discontinues this policy and a claim is made later (which often happens), you will not have coverage. An occurrence-based policy provides coverage if the incident occurs within the policy period, no matter when the claim arises. If the policy is allowed to lapse and a suit is filed for an incident that occurred during the policy period, coverage is in place.

For personal protection against crimes against you, make certain your employer carries a policy of liability insurance that covers you. Find out the exact nature and the limits of the coverage it gives you. Then, with a knowledgeable expert, determine what additional amounts (dollar value) and type (occurrence or claims based) of personal coverage it is best for you to carry, and purchase a policy accordingly. (See Chapter 2 for further discussion of liability and professional liability insurance.)

CHEMICALLY IMPAIRED NURSES

The number of nurses who are illegally using drugs and abusing alcohol will continue to increase. Some of the excuses so many nurses give for resorting to using drugs, alcohol, or both include job-related stress, inability to cope with changes in the workplace, overwhelming personal responsibilities, a feeling of frustration and helplessness in their personal and professional lives, and easy access to drugs.

The American Nurses Association (ANA) has developed and recommended to state boards of nursing a Model Disciplinary Diversion Act that includes a voluntary treatment and rehabilitation program for addicted nurses. It is expected that more state boards of nursing will include these recommendations in their nurse practice acts in the future, just as more and more employers will begin random drug testing of people who provide health care services.

It is your responsibility to yourself, your family, and your patients to avoid the abuse of nonprescription medications. If you or someone you know does become addicted to drugs or alcohol, the only option is to seek immediate assistance. Referring yourself or someone else to your state board of nursing for voluntary treatment and a rehabilitation program may not only save a career, it may save a life. See Chapter 36 for further discussion of chemically dependent nurses.

Get Ready for the NCLEX® Examination!

Key Points

- Today's health care system is volatile, and the job market has never been so competitive. As an LPN/LVN, you need to take charge of your own future.
- A well-prepared résumé broadens interview opportunities.
- An interview is important; make every effort to guarantee a successful one.
- Learning does not cease after graduation.
- The new graduate has a variety of available job opportunities. Each option requires considerable thought.
- A mentor is a nurse with more experience and knowledge who is able and willing to assist a novice nurse to learn the skills of the profession.
- Nursing goes on around the clock to ensure continuity of care for all patients.
- LPNs/LVNs are legally liable for their actions; therefore they need to understand the legal framework within which they are practicing.
- Endorsement or reciprocity enables you to practice in another state without retaking the NCLEX-PN.
- The National Council of State Boards of Nursing has adopted the CAT for the NCLEX-PN.
- The nurse practice act is the licensing law.
- It is a good idea for the LPN/LVN to take advantage of the knowledge available from certification seminars or self-guided study courses.
- The main function of a state board of nursing is to ensure safety for the consumer of nursing services.
- Licensure permits people to offer special skills to the public, but it also provides legal guidelines for protection of the public.
- Leadership skills are more important in nursing today than ever before.
- Although no one leadership style is best, the overall approach of a leader has to foster the growth of others and facilitate their development so that they become less dependent on the leader.
- The more nurse managers adapt their leadership styles to work situations and the needs and abilities of staff, the more effective they will be as managers.
- The key to successful problem solving is to identify the real issue and solve it.
- Continued advances in computer technology will drastically change how nurses do much of their work.
- Follow the correct procedure for transcribing physicians' orders.
- The physician is in charge of directing the patient's care, and nurses carry out the physician's orders, unless they believe that the orders are in error or will be harmful to the patient.
- The purpose of the change-of-shift report is to accurately communicate pertinent patient information from one shift to another.
- Burnout occurs more often in people who have excessive expectations of themselves and who feel that they need to do everything right. Nurses are especially prone to this characteristic.
- Malpractice insurance for nurses is becoming increasingly important in a society that has become lawsuit conscious.

Additional Learning Resources

Go to your Companion CD for an audio glossary, animations, video clips, and more.

evolve Be sure to visit the Evolve site at http://evolve.elsevier.com/Christensen/foundations/ for additional online resources.

Review Questions for the NCLEX® Examination

1. LPNs/LVNs know that the function of the state board of nursing is to:
   1. establish certain nursing procedures in the hospital.
   2. renew and issue licenses and suspend or revoke a license.
   3. separate schools of nursing in the state.
   4. establish inservice programs in the hospital.

2. The following organizations are totally committed to practical and vocational nursing and its continuing education:
   1. NAPNES and NFLPN
   2. NPANES and NLN
   3. NLN and ANA
   4. ANA and NFLPN

3. The LPN/LVN license permits:
   1. giving first aid.
   2. recommending a particular physician.
   3. supervising care in a long-term care facility.
   4. rendering safe nursing service to the public.

4. The primary purpose of states' requiring nurses to be licensed to practice nursing is to:
   1. protect the LPN/LVN employer and the nurse.
   2. provide legal guidelines to protect the public.
   3. protect the patient and employer.
   4. protect the LPN/LVN from malpractice.

5. A new nurse wants to join a professional organization. The national organization for LPNs/LVNs is:
   1. ANA.
   2. NLN.
   3. NAPNES.
   4. NRN.

6. The type of leadership skill that sometimes stifles individual initiative and creativity is:
   1. democratic style.
   2. autocratic style.
   3. situational style.
   4. laissez-faire style.

7. The style of leadership that works well with highly motivated professional groups but seldom works well in health care settings is:
   1. autocratic style.
   2. situational style.
   3. laissez-faire style.
   4. democratic style.

8. The style of leadership that takes into account the style of the leader, the maturity of the groups, and the circumstances at hand is called:
   1. autocratic style.
   2. situational style.
   3. democratic style.
   4. laissez-faire style.

9. The LPN/LVN knows that the following physician orders take priority:
   1. prn orders.
   2. one-time-only orders.
   3. routine orders.
   4. stat orders.

10. The physician's order that is the least subject to error is:
    1. written.
    2. telephone.
    3. verbal.
    4. transcribed.

11. An LPN/LVN is contemplating which field of nursing he will enter. Several options are available to him. He is aware that in private duty nursing:
    1. he always has to work fixed hours and days.
    2. he will care for three or four patients.
    3. the pay is the same as for an RN.
    4. he is directly responsible to the individual employer for salary and schedule.

12. A statute enacted by the legislature of any of the states to delineate the legal scope of the practice of nursing within the geographic boundaries of the jurisdiction is called the:
    1. NLN Act.
    2. nurse practice act.
    3. NCLEX Act.
    4. JCOAH Act.

13. It is 1430, time for the change-of-shift report. During a change-of-shift report, the nurse:
    1. repeats gossip about specific patients.
    2. drinks coffee and visits with colleagues.
    3. identifies nursing diagnoses.
    4. gives her impression of the patient.

14. Every nurse giving a change-of-shift report has to realize it is important to:
    1. evaluate results of nursing interventions.
    2. discuss various opinions about the patient.
    3. criticize the patient's behavior.
    4. discuss the patient's finances.

15. Which statement best reflects the autocratic style of leadership?
    1. "Everyone knows their work assignment, so let's not meet together unless we have an unexpected crisis."
    2. "Let's discuss this case study thoroughly and decide on a plan of action as a group."
    3. "I'll consider each of your requests, and then give you the guidelines for establishing new acuity ratings for our patients."
    4. "I'll try to pair you in comparable work teams, and we'll evaluate the success of this approach in 2 weeks."

16. Time management skills for the nurse include:
    1. meeting all of the patient's major needs in the early morning hours.
    2. anticipating possible interruptions by therapists.
    3. doing each of the patient's assessments and treatments individually at separate times.
    4. leaving each day unplanned to allow for adaptations in treatments.

17. Select the strategy that will allow the nurse to practice situational leadership.
    1. Tell subordinates what to do.
    2. Put subordinates first before the policies of the long-term care facility.
    3. Seek input from employees for emergency situations during the actual situation.
    4. Evaluate the circumstances in the work environment and vary leadership style to meet the occasion.

18. To settle a conflict, it is suggested that the nurse focus on:
    1. developing a compromise solution to solve the conflict.
    2. investigating what the conflict parties want to achieve as an outcome.
    3. identifying the real issues and solving them.
    4. limiting the number of possible solutions to the conflict.

19. What is the primary area for LPN/LVN jobs in the United States and Canada?
    1. Doctors' offices and clinics
    2. Temporary help agencies
    3. Long-term care facilities
    4. Hospital-based medical units

20. Why become certified in other areas after becoming an LPN/LVN?
    1. The certifications are designed to increase nursing knowledge and skill.
    2. The nurse will be able gradually to assume the work of an RN without becoming an RN.
    3. Use of the extended title(s) will improve the nurse's status among other employees and peers.
    4. Unless the state board of nursing acknowledges the certification, it serves no purpose.

21. Which is a function of the LPN/LVN?

1. Teaching professional and practical nursing students
2. Providing direct patient care
3. Being in charge in various health care settings
4. Directing nurses and other personnel who are employed in the hospital setting

22. The NCLEX-PN® Examination measures:

1. the LPN/LVN student's ability to compete in the job market.
2. the LPN/LVN student's entry-level competencies.
3. the LPN/LVN student's proficiency-level competencies.
4. success of the nursing program.

23. What will a new graduate include on a résumé?

1. Person to notify in an emergency
2. Grade transcripts from nursing schools
3. Only current work experience
4. Education history

24. What is a quality of an effective mentor?

1. One who is inconsistent
2. One who is unaccountable
3. One who is inaccessible
4. One who is informative

25. What will the nurse wish to consider when obtaining malpractice insurance?

1. Malpractice insurance is becoming less important for the nurse in today's health care environment.
2. If the employer has a claims-based policy in force, a personal policy is not necessary.
3. Most employers carry insurance for the employee, which will more than cover any expenses that will be incurred.
4. A separate personal malpractice insurance policy over and above the employer's policy is a wise investment.

26. How does the impaired nurse use alcohol and/or other drugs?

1. To separate from work responsibilities
2. To treat an inherited condition
3. To self-medicate for fear and anger
4. To understand what patient's experience is like

appendix

A Common Abbreviations

evolve

http://evolve.elsevier.com/Christensen/foundationsadult

° C	degrees Centigrade
° F	degrees Fahrenheit
ʒ	dram
@*	at
♀	female
♂	male
>*	greater than
<*	less than
↑	increase
↓	decrease
1°	primary
2°	secondary
Δ	change
$\overline{aa}$	indicating equal amounts of each
ABGs	arterial blood gases
ac	before meals
ad lib	freely as desired
ADL	activities of daily living
ama, AMA	against medical advice
AND	allow natural death
BE	barium enema
bid	two times a day
BP	blood pressure
BRP	bathroom privileges
BUN	blood urea nitrogen
$\bar{c}$	with
cap	capsule
CBC	complete blood count
cc*	cubic centimeter
CDC	Centers for Disease Control and Prevention
cm	centimeter
c/o	complains of
CO	carbon monoxide
CO_2	carbon dioxide
CPR	cardiopulmonary resuscitation
CT	computed tomography
D_5W	5% dextrose in water
dL	deciliter
DNR	do not resuscitate
Dx, dx	diagnosis
ECG, EKG	electrocardiogram
EEG	electroencephalogram
elix	elixir
ER	emergency room
ESR	erythrocyte sedimentation rate
ETOH	ethyl alcohol
F$\bar{ʒ}$	fluid ounce
FUO	fever of unknown origin
Fx, fx	fracture; fractional urine test
g, gm, Gm	gram
GI	gastrointestinal
gr	grain
gt; gtt	drop; drops
GTT	glucose tolerance test
h, hr	hour
H&P	history and physical examination
HCT, Hct	hematocrit
Hgb	hemoglobin
HIV	human immunodeficiency virus (AIDS)
hs	at bedtime
I&O	intake and output
IDDM	insulin-dependent diabetes mellitus
IM	intramuscular
IV	intravenous
IVP	intravenous push; intravenous pyelogram
IVU	intravenous urogram
K	potassium
kg	kilogram
KUB	kidney, ureters, and bladder (radiograph)
KVO	keep vein open
L	liter
LOC	laxative of choice; level of consciousness
m	meter
mcg, μg*	microgram
mg	milligram
mL	milliliter

*On The Joint Commission's Lists of Dangerous Abbreviations, Acronyms, and Symbols (see Appendix B).

mm	millimeter
mm Hg	millimeters of mercury
MRI	magnetic resonance imaging
Ndx	nursing diagnoses
NPO	nothing per os, nothing by mouth
O_2	oxygen
OD	optical density; overdose
O.D.	right eye
O.S.	left eye
O.U.	both eyes
oz, ℥	ounce
pc	after meals
PERRLA	pupils equal, round, and reactive to light and accommodation
pH	hydrogen ion concentration (acidity and alkalinity)
PO, po	orally, per os
prn	as often as necessary, when required
q	every
qd*	every day
qh	every hour
qid	four times a day
qod*	every other day
ROM	range of motion
Rx	take; treatment
s̄	without
SC, SQ, Sub-Q, subQ	subcutaneous
ss	half
SSE	soapsuds enema
stat	immediately
tid	three times a day
TKO	to keep open
TLC	tender loving care
TPN	total parenteral nutrition
TPR	temperature, pulse, and respirations
U*	unit
IU*	international unit
WBC	white blood cell, white blood count

appendix

B The Joint Commission's Lists of Dangerous Abbreviations, Acronyms, and Symbols

evolve

http://evolve.elsevier.com/Christensen/foundationsadult

A "minimum list" of dangerous abbreviations, acronyms, and symbols has been approved by The Joint Commission (TJC). Beginning March 5, 2009 the items in Table 1 must be included on each accredited organization's Do Not Use list:

Table 1 Minimum Do-Not-Use List of Abbreviations

ABBREVIATION	POTENTIAL PROBLEM	PREFERRED TERM
U (for unit)	Mistaken as *zero (0)*, *four (4)*, or cc	Write *unit*
IU (for international unit)	Mistaken for IV (intravenous) or 10 (ten)	Write *international unit*
Q.D., Q.O.D., Q.I.D. (Latin abbreviations for once daily, every other day, and 4 times daily)	Mistaken for each other The period after the "Q" can be mistaken for an "I," and the "O" can be mistaken for "I"	Write *daily, every other day,* and *4 times daily*
Trailing zero (X.0 mg) (NOTE: prohibited only for medication-related notations) Lack of leading zero (.X mg)	Decimal point is missed	Never write a zero by itself after a decimal point (X mg), and always use a zero before a decimal point (0.X mg)
MS MSO_4 $MgSO_4$	Confused for one another Can mean morphine sulfate or magnesium sulfate	Write *morphine sulfate* or *magnesium sulfate*

Additional abbreviations, acronyms, and symbols for *possible* future inclusion in the official "Do Not Use" list are provided in Table 2.

Table 2 Additional Abbreviations to Avoid

ABBREVIATION	POTENTIAL PROBLEM	PREFERRED TERM
Greater than (>) Less than (<)	Mistaken for the letter "L" or the number "7" (seven)	Write "greater than" or "less than"
Abbreviations for drug names	Mistaken for abbreviations for similar drugs	Write out full drug names
Apothecary units	Confused with metric units Uncommon term	Use metric units
@	Mistaken for the number "2" (two)	Write "at"
cc	Mistaken for U (units)	Write "ml" or "milliliters" or "mL" (preferred)
µg	Mistaken for mg (milligrams)	Write "micrograms" or "mcg"

Recommended precautions: Two nurses must double-check the following before administration: heparin, insulin, parental chemotherapeutic agents, patient-controlled analgesia, and epidural pumps.

Health Insurance Portability and Accountability Act (HIPAA) privacy requirements: Patient information concerning name, age, diagnosis, and so forth should not be posted. Charts and medication records must be kept in confidential area.

Also, the Institute for Safe Medication Practices (ISMP) has published a list of dangerous abbreviations relating to medication use that it recommends should be explicitly prohibited. This list is available on its website, www.ismp.org (revised 2007).

appendix C

Laboratory Reference Values*

evolve

http://evolve.elsevier.com/Christensen/foundationsadult

Reference Intervals for Hematology

TEST	CONVENTIONAL UNITS	SI UNITS
Acid hemolysis (Ham test)	No hemolysis	No hemolysis
Alkaline phosphatase, leukocyte	Total score, 14-100	Total score, 14-100
Cell counts		
Erythrocytes		
Males	4.6-6.2 million/mm^3	4.6-6.2 × 10^{12}/L
Females	4.2-5.4 million/mm^3	4.2-5.4 × 10^{12}/L
Children (varies with age)	4.5-5.1 million/mm^3	4.5-5.1 × 10^{12}/L
Leukocytes, total	4500-11,000/mm^3	4.5-11.0 × 10^9/L
Leukocytes, differential counts*		
Myelocytes	0%	0/L
Band neutrophils	3%-5%	150-400 × 10^6/L
Segmented neutrophils	54%-62%	3000-5800 × 10^6/L
Lymphocytes	25%-33%	1500-3000 × 10^6/L
Monocytes	3%-7%	300-500 × 10^6/L
Eosinophils	1%-3%	50-250 × 10^6/L
Basophils	0%-1%	15-50 × 10^6/L
Platelets	150,000-400,000/mm^3	150-400 × 10^9/L
Reticulocytes	25,000-75,000/mm^3	25-75 × 10^9/L
Coagulation tests	(0.5%-1.5% of erythrocytes)	
Bleeding time (template)	2.75-8.0 min	2.75-8.0 min
Coagulation time (glass tube)	5-15 min	5-15 min
D-Dimer	<0.5 mcg/mL	<0.5 mg/L
Factor VIII and other coagulation factors	50%-150% of normal	0.5-1.5 of normal
Fibrin split products (Thrombo-Welco test)	<10 mcg/mL	<10 mg/L
Fibrinogen	200-400 mg/dL	2.0-4.0 g/L
Partial thromboplastin time, activated (aPTT)	20-25 sec	20-35 sec
Prothrombin time (PT, Pro-time, International normalized ratio [INR])	12.0-14.0 sec	12.0-14.0 sec
Coombs' test		
Direct	Negative	Negative
Indirect	Negative	Negative
Corpuscular values of erythrocytes		
Mean corpuscular hemoglobin (MCH)	26-34 pg/cell	26-34 pg/cell
Mean corpuscular volume (MCV)	80-96 μm^3	80-96 fL
Mean corpuscular hemoglobin concentration (MCHC)	32-36 g/dL	320-360 g/L
Haptoglobin	20-165 mg/dL	0.20-1.65 g/L
Hematocrit		
Males	40-54 mL/dL	0.40-0.54
Females	37-47 mL/dL	0.37-0.47
Newborns	49-54 mL/dL	0.49-0.54
Children (varies with age)	35-49 mL/dL	0.35-0.49

*Conventional units are percentages; SI units are absolute cell counts.
SI, International System of Units.

Continued

*From Rakel, R.E., & Bope, E.T. (2009). *Conn's current therapy* 2009. Philadelphia: Saunders.

Reference Intervals for Hematology—cont'd

TEST	CONVENTIONAL UNITS	SI UNITS
Hemoglobin		
Males	13.0-18.0 g/dL	8.1-11.2 mmol/L
Females	12.0-16.0 g/dL	7.4-9.9 mmol/L
Newborns	16.5-19.5 g/dL	10.2-12.1 mmol/L
Children (varies with age)	11.2-16.5 g/dL	7.0-10.2 mmol/L
Hemoglobin, fetal	<1.0% of total	<0.01 of total
Hemoglobin A_{1C}	3%-5% of total	0.03-0.05 of total
Hemoglobin A_2	1.5%-3.0% of total	0.015-0.03 of total
Hemoglobin, plasma	0.0-5.0 mg/dL	0.0-3.2 μmol/L
Methemoglobin	30-130 mg/dL	19-80 μmol/L
Erythrocyte sedimentation rate (ESR)		
Wintrobe		
Males	0-5 mm/hr	0-5 mm/hr
Females	0-15 mm/hr	0-15 mm/hr
Westergren		
Males	0-15 mm/hr	0-15 mm/hr
Females	0-20 mm/hr	0-20 mm/hr

Reference Intervals* for Clinical Chemistry (Blood, Serum, and Plasma)

ANALYTE	CONVENTIONAL UNITS	SI UNITS
Acetoacetate plus acetone		
Qualitative	Negative	Negative
Quantitative	0.3-2.0 mg/dL	30-200 μmol/L
Acid phosphatase, serum (thymolphthalein monophosphate substrate)	0.1-0.6 units/L	0.1-0.6 units/L
ACTH (see Corticotropin)		
Alanine aminotransferase (ALT, serum (SGPT)	1-45 units/L	1-45 units/L
Albumin, serum	3.3-5.2 g/dL	33-52 g/L
Aldolase, serum	0.0-7.0 units/L	0.0-7.0 units/L
Aldosterone, plasma		
Standing	5-30 ng/dL	140-830 pmol/L
Recumbent	3-10 ng/dL	80-275 pmol/L
Alkaline, phosphatase (ALP), serum		
Adult	35-150 units/L	35-150 units/L
Adolescent	100-500 units/L	100-500 units/L
Child	100-350 units/L	100-350 units/L
Ammonia nitrogen, plasma	10-50 μmol/L	10-50 μmol/L
Amylase, serum	25-125 units/L	25-125 units/L
Anion gap, serum calculated	8-16 mEq/L	8-16 mmol/L
Ascorbic acid, blood	0.4-1.5 mg/dL	23-85 μmol/L
Aspartate aminotransferase (AST), serum (SGOT)	1-36 units/L	1-36 units/L
Base excess, arterial blood, calculated	0 ± 2 mEq/L	0 ±2 mmol/L
Bicarbonate		
Venous plasma	23-29 mEq/L	23-29 mmol/L
Arterial blood	21-27 mEq/L	21-27 mmol/L
Bile acids, serum	0.3-3.0 mg/dL	0.8-7.6 μmol/L
Bilirubin, serum		
Conjugated	0.1-0.4 mg/dL	1.7-6.8 μmol/L
Total	0.3-1.1 mg/dL	5.1-19.0 μmol/L
Calcium, serum	8.4-10.6 mg/dL	2.10-2.65 mmol/L
Calcium, ionized, serum	4.25-5.25 mg/dL	1.05-1.30 mmol/L
Carbon dioxide, total, serum or plasma	24-31 mEq/L	24-31 mmol/L
Carbon dioxide tension (P_{CO_2}), blood	35-45 mm Hg	35-45 mm Hg
β-Carotene, serum	60-260 mcg/dL	1.1-8.6 μmol/L
Ceruloplasmin, serum	23-44 mg/dL	230-440 mg/L

*Reference values may vary depending on the method and sample source used.

Reference Intervals for Clinical Chemistry (Blood, Serum, and Plasma)—cont'd

ANALYTE	CONVENTIONAL UNITS	SI UNITS
Chloride, serum or plasma	96-106 mEq/L	96-106 mmol/L
Cholesterol, serum or EDTA plasma		
Desirable range	<200 mg/dL	<5.20 mmol/L
Low-density lipoprotein (LDL) cholesterol	60-180 mg/dL	1.55-4.65 mmol/L
High-density lipoprotein (HDL) cholesterol	30-80 mg/dL	0.80-2.05 mmol/L
Copper	70-140 mcg/dL	11-22 μmol/L
Corticotropin (ACTH), plasma, 8 AM	10-80 pg/mL	2-18 pmol/L
Cortisol, plasma		
8:00 AM	6-23 mcg/dL	170-630 nmol/L
4:00 PM	3-15 mcg/dL	80-410 nmol/L
10:00 PM	<50% of 8:00 AM value	<50% of 8:00 AM value
Creatine, serum		
Males	0.2-0.5 mg/dL	15-40 μmol/L
Females	0.3-0.9 mg/dL	25-70 μmol/L
Creatine kinase (CK), serum		
Males	55-170 units/L	55-170 units/L
Females	30-135 units/L	30-135 units/L
Creatinine kinase MB isoenzyme, serum	<5% of total CK activity <5% of ng/mL by immunoassay	<5% of total CK activity <5% of ng/mL by immunoassay
Creatinine, serum	0.6-1.2 mg/dL	50-110 μmol/L
Erythrocytes	145-540 ng/mL	330-120 nmol/L
Estradiol-17β, adult		
Males	10-65 pg/mL	35-240 pmol/L
Females		
Follicular	30-100 pg/mL	110-370 pmol/L
Ovulatory	200-400 pg/mL	730-1470 pmol/L
Luteal	50-140 pg/mL	180-510 pmol/L
Ferritin, serum	20-200 ng/mL	20-200 mcg/L
Fibrinogen, plasma	200-400 mg/dL	2.0-4.0 g/L
Folate, serum	3-18 ng/mL	6.8-4.1 nmol/L
Follicle-stimulating hormone (FSH), plasma		
Males	4-25 mU/mL	4-25 units/L
Females, premenopausal	4-30 mU/mL	4-30 units/L
Females, postmenopausal	40-250 mU/mL	40-250 units/L
Gastrin, fasting, serum	0-100 pg/mL	0-100 mg/L
Glucose, fasting, plasma or serum	70-115 mg/dL	3.9-6.4 nmol/L
γ-Glutamyltransferase (GGT), serum	5-40 units/L	5-40 units/L
Growth hormone (hGH), plasma, adult, fasting	0-6 ng/mL	0-6 mcg/L
Haptoglobin, serum	20-165 mg/dL	0.20-1.65 g/L
Immunoglobulins, serum (see table of Reference Intervals for Tests of Immunologic Function)		
Iron, serum	75-175 mcg/dL	13-31 μmol/L
Iron-binding capacity, serum		
Total	250-410 mcg/dL	45-73 μmol/L
Saturation	20%-55%	0.20-0.55
Lactate		
Venous whole blood	5.0-20.0 mg/dL	0.6-2.2 mmol/L
Arterial whole blood	5.0-15.0 mg/dL	0.6-1.7 mmol/L
Lactate dehydrogenase (LD), serum	110-220 units/L	110-220 units/L
Lipase, serum	10-140 units/L	10-140 units/L
Lutropin (LH), serum		
Males	1-9 units/L	1-9 units/L
Females		
Follicular phase	2-10 units/L	2-10 units/L
Midcycle peak	15-65 units/L	15-65 units/L
Luteal phase	1-12 units/L	1-12 units/L
Postmenopausal	12-65 units/L	12-65 units/L
Magnesium, serum	1.3-2.1 mg/dL	0.65-1.05 mmol/L
Osmolality	275-295 mOsm/kg water	275-295 mOsm/kg water

EDTA, ethylenediaminetetraacetic acid.

Continued

Reference Intervals for Clinical Chemistry (Blood, Serum, and Plasma)—cont'd

ANALYTE	CONVENTIONAL UNITS	SI UNITS
Oxygen, blood, arterial, room air		
Partial pressure (Pao_2)	80-100 mm Hg	80-100 mm Hg
Saturation (Sao_2)	95%-98%	95%-98%
pH, arterial blood	7.35-7.45	7.35-7.45
Phosphate, inorganic, serum		
Adult	3.0-4.5 mg/dL	1.0-1.5 mmol/L
Child	4.0-7.0 mg/dL	1.3-2.3 mmol/L
Potassium		
Serum	3.5-5.0 mEq/L	3.5-5.0 mmol/L
Plasma	3.5-4.5 mEq/L	3.5-4.5 mmol/L
Progesterone, serum, adult		
Males	0.0-0.4 ng/mL	0.0-1.3 mmol/L
Females		
Follicular phase	0.1-1.5 ng/mL	0.3-4.8 mmol/L
Luteal phase	2.5-28.0 ng/mL	8.0-89.0 mmol/L
Prolactin, serum		
Males	1.0-15.0 ng/mL	1.0-15.0 mcg/L
Females	1.0-20.0 ng/mL	1.0-20.0 mcg/L
Protein, serum, electrophoresis		
Total	6.0-8.0 g/dL	60-80 g/L
Albumin	3.5-5.5 g/dL	35-55 g/L
Globulins		
α_1	0.2-0.4 g/dL	2.0-4.0 g/L
α_2	0.5-0.9 g/dL	5.0-9.0 g/L
β	0.6-1.1 g/dL	6.0-11.0 g/L
γ	0.7-1.7 g/dL	7.0-17.0 g/L
Pyruvate, blood	0.3-0.9 mg/dL	0.03-0.10 mmol/L
Rheumatoid factor	0.0-30.0 IU/mL	0.0-30.0 kIU/L
Sodium, serum or plasma	135-145 mEq/L	135-145 mmol/L
Testosterone, plasma		
Males, adult	300-1200 ng/dL	10.4-41.6 nmol/L
Females, adult	20-75 ng/dL	0.7-2.6 nmol/L
Pregnant females	40-200 ng/dL	1.4-6.9 nmol/L
Thyroglobulin	3-42 ng/mL	3-42 mcg/L
Thyrotropin (hTSH), serum	0.4-4.8 μIU/mL	0.4-4.8 mIU/L
Thyrotropin-releasing hormone (TRH)	5-60 pg/mL	5-60 ng/L
Thyroxine (FT_4), free, serum	0.9-2.1 ng/dL	12-27 pmol/L
Thyroxine (T_4), serum	4.5-12.0 mcg/mL	58-154 nmol/L
Thyroxine-binding globulin (TBG)	15.0-34.0 mcg/mL	15.0-34.0 mg/L
Transferrin	250-430 mg/dL	2.5-4.3 g/L
Triglycerides, serum, after 12-hr fast	40-150 mg/dL	0.4-1.5 g/L
Triiodothyronine (T_3), serum	70-190 ng/dL	1.1-2.9 nmol/L
Triiodothyronine uptake, resin (T_3RU)	25%-38%	0.25-0.38
Troponin I	0.05-0.50 ng/mL	0.05-0.5 ng/mL
Urate		
Males	2.5-8.0 mg/dL	150-480 μmol/L
Females	2.2-7.0 mg/dL	130-420 μmol/L
Urea, serum or plasma	24-49 mg/dL	4.0-8.2 nmol/L
Urea, nitrogen, serum or plasma	11-23 mg/dL	8.0-16.4 nmol/L
Viscosity, serum	1.1-1.8 × water	1.1-1.8 × water
Vitamin A, serum	20-80 mcg/dL	0.70-2.80 mcmol/L
Vitamin B_{12}, serum	180-900 pg/mL	133-664 pmol/L

SI, International System of Units.

Reference Intervals for Therapeutic Drug Monitoring (Serum or Plasma)*

ANALYTE	THERAPEUTIC RANGE	TOXIC CONCENTRATIONS	PROPRIETARY NAME(S)
ANALGESICS			
Acetaminophen	10-40 mcg/mL	>150 mcg/mL	Tylenol Datril
Salicylate	100-250 mcg/mL	>300 mcg/mL	Aspirin Bufferin
ANTIBIOTICS			
Amikacin	20-30 mcg/mL	Peak >35 mcg/mL Trough >10 mcg/mL	Amkin
Gentamicin	5-10 mcg/mL	Peak >10 mcg/mL Trough >2 mcg/mL	Garamycin
Tobramycin	5-10 mcg/mL	Peak >10 mcg/mL Trough >2 mcg/mL	Nebcin
Vancomycin	5-35 mcg/mL	Peak >40 mcg/mL Trough >10 mcg/mL	Vancocin
ANTICONVULSANTS			
Carbamazepine	5-12 mcg/mL	>15 mcg/mL	Tegretol
Ethosuximide	40-100 mcg/mL	>250 mcg/mL	Zarontin
Phenobarbital	15-40 mcg/mL	40-100 ng/mL (varies widely)	Luminal
Phenytoin	10-20 mcg/mL	>20 mcg/mL	Dilantin
Primidone	5-12 mcg/mL	>15 mcg/mL	Mysoline
Valproic acid	50-100 mcg/mL	>100 mcg/mL	Depakene
ANTINEOPLASTICS AND IMMUNOSUPPRESSIVES			
Cyclosporine A	150-350 ng/mL	>400 ng/mL	Sandimmune
Methotrexate, high-dose, 48 hr	Variable	>1 μmol/L, 48 hr after dose	
Sirolimus (within 1 hr of 2-mg dose)	4.5-14 ng/mL	Variable	Rapamune
Sirolimus (within 1 hr of 5-mg dose)	10-28 ng/mL	Variable	Rapamune
Tacrolimus (FK-506), whole blood	3-20 mcg/L	>15 mcg/L	Prograf
BRONCHODILATORS AND RESPIRATORY STIMULANTS			
Caffeine	3-15 ng/mL	>30 mcg/mL	Elixophyllin
Theophylline (aminophylline)	10-20 mcg/mL	>30 mcg/mL	Quibron
CARDIOVASCULAR DRUGS			
Amiodarone (obtain specimen more than 8 hr after last dose)	1.0-2.0 mcg/mL	>2.0 mcg/mL	Cordarone
Digoxin (obtain specimen more than 6 hr after last dose)	0.8-2.0 mcg/mL	>2.4 ng/mL	Lanoxin
Disopyramide	2-5 mcg/mL	>7 mcg/mL	Norpace
Flecainide	0.2-1.0 mcg/mL	>1 mcg/mL	Tambocor
Lidocaine	1.5-5.0 mcg/mL	>6 mcg/mL	Xylocaine
Mexiletine	0.7-2.0 mcg/mL	>2 mcg/mL	Mexitil
Procainamide	4-10 mcg/mL	>12 mcg/mL	Pronestyl
Procainamide plus NAPA (*N*-acetyl procainamide)	8-30 mcg/mL	>30 mcg/mL	
Propranolol	50-100 ng/mL	Variable	Inderal
Quinidine	2-5 mcg/mL	>6 mcg/mL	Cardioquin Quinaglute
Tocainide	4-10 ng/mL	>10 ng/mL	Tonocard
PSYCHOPHARMACOLOGICAL DRUGS			
Amitriptyline	120-150 ng/mL	>500 ng/mL	Elavil Triavil
Bupropion	25-100 ng/mL	Not applicable	Wellbutrin
Desipramine	150-300 ng/mL	>500 ng/mL	Norpramin
Imipramine	125-250 ng/mL	>400 ng/mL	Tofranil
Lithium (obtain specimen 12 hr after last dose)	0.6-1.5 mEq/L	>1.5 mEq/L	Lithobid
Nortriptyline	50-150 ng/mL	>500 ng/mL	Aventyl Pamelor

*Values may vary depending on the method and sample collection device used. Always consult the reference values provided by the laboratory performing the analysis.

Reference Intervals* for Clinical Chemistry (Urine)

ANALYTE	CONVENTIONAL UNITS	SI UNITS
Acetone and acetoacetate, qualitative	Negative	Negative
Albumin		
Qualitative	Negative	Negative
Quantitative	10-100 mg/24 hr	0.15-1.5 μmol/day
Aldosterone	3-20 mcg/24 hr	8.3-55 nmol/day
δ-Aminolevulinic acid (δ-ALA)	1.3-7.0 mg/24 hr	10-53 μmol/day
Amylase	<17 units/hr	<17 units/hr
Amylase-to-creatinine clearance ratio	0.01-0.04	0.01-0.04
Bilirubin, qualitative	Negative	Negative
Calcium (regular diet)	<250 mg/24 hr	<6.3 nmol/day
Catecholamines		
Epinephine	<10 mcg/24 hr	<55 nmol/day
Norepinephine	<100 mcg/24 hr	<590 nmol/day
Total free catecholamines	4-126 mcg/24 hr	24-745 nmol/day
Total metanephrines	0.1-1.6 mg/24 hr	0.5-8.1 μmol/day
Chloride (varies with intake)	110-250 mEq/24 hr	110-250 mmol/day
Copper	0-50 mcg/24 hr	0.0-0.80 μmol/day
Cortisol, free	10-100 mcg/24 hr	27.6-276 nmol/day
Creatine		
Males	0-40 mg/24 hr	0.0-0.30 mmol/day
Females	0-80 mg/24 hr	0.0-0.60 mmol/day
Creatinine	15-25 mg/kg/24 hr	0.13-0.22 mmol/kg/day
Creatinine clearance (endogenous)		
Males	110-150 mL/min/1.73 m^2	110-150 mL/min/1.73 m2
Females	105-132 mL/min/1.73 m^2	105-132 mL/min/1.73 m2
Cystine or cysteine	Negative	Negative
Dehydroepiandrosterone		
Males	0.2-2.0 mg/24hr	0.7-6.9 μmol/day
Females	0.2-1.8 mg/24hr	0.7-6.2 μmol/day
Estrogens, total		
Males	4-25 mcg/24 hr	14-90 nmol/day
Females	5-100 mcg/24 hr	18-360 nmol/day
Glucose (as reducing substance)	<250 mg/24 hr	<250 mg/day
Hemoglobin and myoglobin, qualitative	Negative	Negative
Hemogentisic acid, qualitative	Negative	Negative
17-Hydroxycorticosteroids		
Males	3-9 mg/24 hr	8.3-25 μmol/day
Females	2-8 mg/24 hr	5.5-22 μmol/day
5-Hydroxyindoleacetic acid		
Qualitative	Negative	Negative
Quantitative	2-6 mg/24 hr	10-31 μmol/day
17-Ketogenic steroids		
Males	5-23 mg/24 hr	17-80 μmol/day
Females	3-15 mg/24 hr	10-52 μmol/day
17-Ketosteroids		
Males	8-22 mg/24 hr	28-76 μmol/day
Females	6-15 mg/24 hr	21-52 μmol/day
Magnesium	6-10 mEq/24 hr	3-5 mmol/day
Metanephrines	0.05-1.2 ng/mg creatinine	0.03-0.70 mmol/mmol creatinine
Osmolality	38-1400 mOsm/kg water	38-1400 mOsm/kg water
pH	4.6-8.0	4.6-8.0
Phenylpyruvic acid, qualitative	Negative	Negative
Phosphate	0.4-1.3 g/24 hr	13-42 mmol/day
Porphobilinogen		
Qualitative	Negative	Negative
Quantitative	<2 mg/24 hr	<9 μmol/day
Porphyrins		
Coproporphyrin	50-250 mcg/24 hr	77-380 nmol/day

*Values may vary depending on the method used.
SI, International System of Units.

Reference Intervals for Clinical Chemistry (Urine)—cont'd

ANALYTE	CONVENTIONAL UNITS	SI UNITS
Uroporphyrin	10-30 mcg/24 hr	12-36 nmol/day
Potassium	25-125 mEq/24 hr	25-125 mmol/day
Pregnanediol		
Males	0.0-1.9 mg/24 hr	0.0-6.0 μmol/day
Females		
Proliferative phase	0.0-2.6 mg/24 hr	0.0-8.0 μmol/day
Luteal phase	2.6-10.6 mg/24 hr	8-33 μmol/day
Postmenopausal	0.2-1.0 mg/24 hr	0.6-3.1 μmol/day
Pregnanetriol	0.0-2.5 mg/24 hr	0.0-7.4 μmol/day
Protein, total		
Qualitative	Negative	Negative
Quantitative	10-150 mg/24 hr	10-150 mg/day
Protein-to-creatinine ratio	<0.2	<0.2
Sodium (regular diet)	60-260 mEq/24 hr	60-260 mmol/day
Specific gravity		
Random specimen	1.003-1.030	1.003-1.030
24-hr collection	1.015-1.025	1.015-1.025
Urate (regular diet)	250-750 mg/24 hr	1.5-4.4 mmol/day
Urobilinogen	0.5-4.0 mg/24 hr	0.6-6.8 μmol/day
Vanillylmandelic acid (VMA)	1.0-8.0 mg/24 hr	5-40 μmol/day

Reference Intervals for Toxic Substances

ANALYTE	CONVENTIONAL UNITS	SI UNITS
Arsenic, urine	<130 mcg/24 hr	<1.7 μmol/day
Bromides, serum, inorganic	<100 mg/dL	<10 mmol/L
Toxic symptoms	140-1000 mg/dL	14-100 mmol/L
Carboxyhemoglobin, blood	Saturation, percent	
Urban environment	<5%	<0.05
Smokers	<12%	<0.12
Symptoms		
Headache	>15%	>0.15
Nausea and vomiting	>25%	>0.25
Potentially lethal	>50%	>0.50
Ethanol, blood	<0.05 mg/dL, <0.005%	<1.0 mmol/L
Intoxication	>100 mg/dL, >0.1%	>22 mmol/L
Marked intoxication	300-400 mg/dL, 0.3%-0.4%	65-87 mmol/L
Alcoholic stupor	400-500 mg/dL, 0.4%-0.5%	87-109 mmol/L
Coma	>500 mg/dL, >0.5%	>109 mmol/L
Lead, blood		
Adults	<20 mcg/dL	<1.0 μmol/L
Children	<10 mcg/dL	<0.5 μmol/L
Lead, urine	<80 mcg/24 hr	<0.4 μmol/day
Mercury, urine	<10 mcg/24 hr	<150 nmol/day

SI, International System of Units.

Reference Intervals for Tests Performed on Cerebrospinal Fluid

TEST	CONVENTIONAL UNITS	SI UNITS
Cells	<5 mm^3; all mononuclear	<5 × 106/L; all mononuclear
Protein electrophoresis	Albumin predominant	Albumin predominant
Glucose	50-75 mg/dL (20 mg/dL less than in serum)	2.8-4.2 mmol/L (1.1 mmol/L less than in serum)
IgG		
Children <14 yr	<8% of total protein	<0.08 of total protein
Adults	<14% of total protein	<0.14 of total protein
IgG index	0.3-0.6	0.3-0.6
Oligoclonal banding on electrophoresis	Absent	Absent
Pressure, opening	70-180 mm H_2O	70-180 mm H_2O
Protein, total	<15-45 mg/dL	150-450 mg/L

SI, International System of Units.

Reference Intervals for Tests of Gastrointestinal Function

TEST	CONVENTIONAL UNITS
Bentiromide	6-hr urinary arylamine excretion >57% excludes pancreatic insufficiency
β-Carotene, serum	60-250 ng/dL
Fecal fat estimation	
Qualitative	No fat globules seen by high-power microscope
Quantitative	<6 g/24 hr (>95% coefficient of fat absorption)
Gastric acid output	
Basal	
Males	0.0-10.5 mmol/hr
Females	0.0-5.6 mmol/hr
Maximum (after histamine or pentagastrin)	
Males	9.0-48.0 mmol/hr
Females	6.0-31.0 mmol/hr
Ratio: basal/maximum	
Males	0.0-0.31
Females	0.0-0.29
Secretion test, pancreatic fluid	
Volume	>1.8 mL/kg/hr
Bicarbonate	>80 mEq/L
D-Xylose absorption test, urine	>20% of ingested dose excreted in 5 hr

Reference Intervals for Tests of Immunologic Function

TEST	CONVENTIONAL UNITS	SI UNITS
AUTOANTIBODIES, SERUM, ADULT		
Anti-CCP antibody	0-19 units	
Anti-dsDNA antibody	0-40 international units	0-40 international units
Antinuclear antibody	<1:40	
Rheumatoid factor (total IgG, IgA, IgM)	0-30 mg/dL	
COMPLEMENT, SERUM		
C3	85-175 mg/dL	0.85-1.75 g/L
C4	15-45 mg/dL	150-450 mg/L
Total hemolytic (CH_{50})	150-250 units/mL	150-250 units/mL
IMMUNOGLOBULINS, SERUM, ADULT		
IgA	70-310 mg/dL	0.70-3.1 g/L
IgD	0.0-6.0 mg/dL	0.0-60 g/L
IgE	0.0-430 mg/dL	0.0-430 mg/L
IgG	640-1350 ng/dL	6.4-13.5 mcg/L
IgM	90-350 mg/dL	0.90-3.5 g/L

Anti-CCP, Anticyclic citrullinated peptide; *dsDNA*, double-stranded DNA; *Ig*, immunoglobulin; *SI*, International System of Units.

Reference Intervals for Lymphocytes Subsets, Whole Blood, Heparinized

ANTIGEN(S) EXPRESSED	CELL TYPE	PERCENTAGE (%)	ABSOLUTE CELL COUNT
CD2	E rosette T cells	73-87	860-1880
CD3	Total T cells	56-77	140-370
CD3 and CD4	Helper-inducer cells	32-54	550-1190
CD3 and CD8	Suppressor-cytotoxic cells	24-37	430-1060
CD3 and DR	Activated T cells	5-14	70-310
CD16 and CD56	Natural killer (NK) cells	8-22	130-500
CD 19	Total B cells	7-17	140-370

Helper-to-suppressor ratio: 0.8-1.8.

Reference Values for Semen Analysis

TEST	CONVENTIONAL UNITS	SI UNITS
Volume	2-5 mL	2-5 mL
Liquefaction	Complete in 15 min	Complete in 15 min
pH	7.2-8.0	7.2-8.0
Leukocytes	Occasional or absent	Occasional or absent
Spermatozoa		
Count	60-150 × 10^6 mL	60-150 × 10^6 mL
Motility	>80% motile	>0.80 motile
Morphology	80%-90% normal forms	>0.80-0.90 normal
Fructose	>150 mg/dL	>8.33 mmol/L

SI, International System of Units.

appendix D

Answers to Review Questions for the NCLEX® Examination

evolve

http://evolve.elsevier.com/Christensen/foundationsadult

Chapter 1
1. 3
2. 4
3. 3
4. 4
5. 1
6. 3
7. 2
8. 3
9. 1
10. 2
11. 4
12. 3
13. 1
14. 2
15. 1
16. 2
17. 4

Chapter 2
1. 3
2. 2
3. 1
4. 4
5. 3
6. 4
7. 2
8. 1
9. 2
10. 3
11. 2
12. 1
13. 4
14. 1
15. 4
16. 2

Chapter 3
1. 3
2. 4
3. 2
4. 2
5. 3
6. 2
7. 4
8. 4
9. 1
10. 2
11. 2
12. 1
13. 2
14. 2
15. 1
16. 2
17. 1
18. 4
19. 3
20. 3

Chapter 4
1. 2
2. 2
3. 3
4. 2
5. 2
6. 4
7. 2
8. 4
9. 4
10. 4
11. 2
12. 3
13. 4
14. 1
15. 2
16. 4
17. 4
18. 1
19. 4
20. 4
21. 2
22. 2
23. 1
24. 2
25. 1
26. 2
27. 3
28. 1
29. 2
30. 1

Chapter 5
1. 3
2. 1
3. 3
4. 3
5. 2
6. 1
7. 2
8. 1
9. 2
10. 2
11. 1
12. 3
13. 3
14. 1
15. 2
16. 1, 2, 4
17. 3
18. 2

Chapter 6
1. 2
2. 3
3. 2
4. 3
5. 3
6. 1
7. 1
8. 4
9. 3
10. 4
11. 2
12. 1
13. 2
14. 2
15. 1
16. 3
17. 3
18. 4
19. 2
20. 2
21. 3
22. 3
23. 3
24. 2

Chapter 7
1. 1
2. 4
3. 3
4. 2
5. 1
6. 3
7. 1
8. 4
9. 3
10. 4
11. 4
12. 1
13. 4
14. 1
15. 2
16. 1
17. 2
18. 4
19. 2
20. 2
21. 1
22. 4

Chapter 8
1. 2
2. 3
3. 2
4. 2
5. 3
6. 3
7. 2
8. 4
9. 3
10. 2
11. 2
12. 3
13. 3
14. 1
15. 4
16. 2

Chapter 9
1. 4
2. 2
3. 4
4. 4
5. 2
6. 3
7. 2
8. 4
9. 4
10. 3
11. 2
12. 3
13. 2
14. 2
15. 3
16. 3
17. 3
18. 2
19. 1, 2, 4
20. 4
21. 3
22. 2
23. 2
24. 2
25. 4
26. 3
27. 4
28. 3
29. 3
30. 2
31. 3
32. 1
33. 1

Chapter 10
1. 4
2. 3
3. 4
4. 2
5. 2
6. 4
7. 1
8. 1
9. 1
10. 2
11. 4
12. 2
13. 1
14. 3
15. 2
16. 3
17. 1
18. 3
19. 2
20. 3
21. 3
22. 3
23. 2
24. 3
25. 3
26. 4
27. 1

Chapter 11
1. 4
2. 1
3. 4
4. 4
5. 1
6. 4
7. 2
8. 4
9. 1
10. 3
11. 1
12. 4
13. 3
14. 2

Chapter 12
1. 1
2. 3
3. 1
4. 3
5. 4
6. 4
7. 2
8. 3
9. 4
10. 1
11. 1
12. 1
13. 1
14. 3
15. 2
16. 2
17. 3
18. 4
19. 3
20. 2
21. 3
22. 2

23. 1
24. 2

Chapter 13
1. 4
2. 4
3. 1
4. 3
5. 4
6. 3
7. 4
8. 1
9. 4
10. 3
11. 3
12. 1
13. 4
14. 3
15. 3
16. 2
17. 3
18. 2
19. 1
20. 1

Chapter 14
1. 3
2. 1
3. 2
4. 1
5. 4
6. 4
7. 4
8. 3
9. 4
10. 1
11. 4
12. 2
13. 3
14. 1
15. 3

Chapter 15
1. 3
2. 1
3. 2
4. 1
5. 3
6. 2
7. 1
8. 4
9. 4
10. 1
11. 2
12. 2
13. 2
14. 4
15. 1
16. 3
17. 2
18. 1
19. 1
20. 4

Chapter 16
1. 3
2. 1
3. 3
4. 1
5. 3
6. 4
7. 2
8. 4
9. 1
10. 2
11. 2
12. 3
13. 3
14. 4
15. 1
16. 3
17. 3
18. 1, 4

Chapter 17
1. 1
2. 3
3. 1
4. 3
5. 1
6. 3
7. 2
8. 4
9. 3
10. 1
11. 4
12. 4
13. 1
14. 1
15. 4
16. 3
17. 2
18. 4

Chapter 18
1. 3
2. 4
3. 2
4. 4
5. 1
6. 2
7. 4
8. 1
9. 1
10. 4
11. 3
12. 3
13. 4
14. 1
15. 4
16. 3
17. 3
18. 3
19. 2
20. 4
21. 2
22. 2
23. 1
24. 1
25. 2
26. 1
27. 3
28. 2
29. 2

Chapter 19
1. 1
2. 2
3. 4
4. 1
5. 2
6. 4
7. 3
8. 2
9. 1
10. 1
11. 1
12. 2
13. 2
14. 1
15. 3
16. 4
17. 2
18. 1
19. 4
20. 3
21. 2
22. 1
23. 1

Chapter 20
1. 2
2. 4
3. 2
4. 3
5. 3
6. 2
7. 2
8. 1
9. 1
10. 2
11. 3
12. 4
13. 2
14. 3
15. 2
16. 2
17. 4
18. 3
19. 3
20. 3
21. 2
22. 3
23. 4
24. 2
25. 4
26. 3
27. 1
28. 4
29. 2
30. 1
31. 2
32. 2
33. 3
34. 1

Chapter 21
1. 3
2. 3
3. 3
4. 2
5. 1
6. 3
7. 2
8. 4
9. 1
10. 3
11. 2
12. 1
13. 2
14. 3
15. 3
16. 2
17. 1
18. 3
19. 1
20. 4
21. 2
22. 4
23. 1
24. 3

Chapter 22
1. 1
2. 1
3. 1
4. 1
5. 3
6. 4
7. 1
8. 2
9. 3
10. 3
11. 1
12. 3
13. 2
14. 3
15. 1 liter
16. 3
17. 1, 2, 3
18. 2
19. 4
20. 1
21. 7.35 to 7.45
22. 2

Chapter 23
1. 1
2. 2
3. 1
4. 3
5. 2
6. 2
7. 1
8. 4
9. 3
10. 4
11. 1
12. 3
13. 4
14. 2
15. 1
16. 2
17. 3
18. 1
19. 4
20. 1
21. 4
22. 3
23. 3
24. 4
25. 4
26. 4
27. 4
28. 3
29. 4
30. 4
31. 3
32. 1

Chapter 24
1. 2
2. 4
3. 2
4. 3
5. 4
6. 1
7. 4
8. 3
9. 3
10. 1
11. 4
12. 1
13. 30, 2
14. 100
15. 3
16. 3

Chapter 25
1. 2
2. 3
3. 3
4. 3
5. 1
6. 2
7. 4
8. 1
9. 1
10. 3
11. 4
12. 3
13. 2
14. 2
15. 2
16. gravida
17. primagravida
18. multigravida
19. viability
20. 3
21. 1
22. 4
23. 2
24. 2

Chapter 26
1. 3
2. 4
3. 1
4. 2
5. 3
6. 2
7. 3
8. 4
9. 2
10. 4
11. 1
12. 1
13. 1
14. 4
15. 1
16. FL
17. FL

18. TL
19. TL
20. FL

Chapter 27
1. 2
2. 4
3. 1
4. 3
5. 3
6. 2
7. 3
8. 1
9. 4
10. 2
11. 4
12. 2
13. 1
14. 2
15. 1
16. 1
17. 2
18. Bonding
19. Enface
20. Engrossment
21. Taking-In

Chapter 28
1. 3
2. 1
3. 4
4. 2
5. 3
6. 1
7. 2
8. 4
9. 2
10. 3
11. 4
12. 3
13. 2
14. 4
15. 4
16. 3
17. Preventing hemorrhage
18. Multifetal pregnancy
19. Cesarean birth
20. Postpartum depression

Chapter 29
1. 1, 2, 3
2. 3
3. 2
4. 2
5. syrup of ipecac
6. rear
7. 40
8. 2
9. 3
10. 1, 2, 4
11. 1, 3
12. 4

Chapter 30
1. 2
2. 3
3. 3
4. 3
5. 4
6. 2
7. 2
8. 3
9. 3
10. 3
11. 3
12. 3
13. 4
14. 5th
15. 3
16. 1
17. 2
18. 1
19. 2, 3, 4
20. scoliosis
21. 4

Chapter 31
1. 3
2. 1
3. 2
4. 1
5. 1
6. 1
7. 2
8. 1
9. 4
10. 1
11. 1
12. 4
13. 2
14. 2, 3, 4
15. 4
16. 2
17. 3
18. 2
19. 3
20. 2
21. 2
22. 1
23. 2
24. 1

Chapter 32
1. 3
2. 2
3. 4
4. 3
5. 1, 2, 4
6. suicidal tendencies
7. 2
8. 4
9. 4
10. 1
11. 1
12. 3
13. 2
14. 3
15. 1, 2, 3
16. 2
17. 2

Chapter 33
1. 1
2. 4
3. 2
4. 4
5. 1
6. 2
7. 4
8. 1
9. 3
10. 3
11. 1
12. 2
13. 3
14. 4
15. 3
16. 2
17. 4

Chapter 34
1. 2
2. 3
3. 3
4. 2
5. 4
6. 1
7. 3
8. 2
9. 1
10. 4
11. 2
12. 3
13. 1
14. 4
15. 4
16. 3
17. 2
18. 3
19. 2
20. 3
21. 3
22. 1

Chapter 35
1. 2
2. 2
3. 2
4. 1
5. 4
6. 1
7. 2
8. 3
9. 1
10. 4
11. 2
12. 1
13. 4
14. 3
15. 2
16. 3
17. 1
18. 4
19. 2
20. 4
21. 4
22. 1
23. 3
24. 3
25. 1
26. 2
27. 4
28. 1
29. 2

Chapter 36
1. 2
2. 4
3. 1
4. 2
5. 3
6. 2
7. 1
8. 3
9. 2
10. 2
11. 1
12. 3
13. 4
14. 2
15. 2
16. 3
17. 3
18. 2
19. 3
20. 3

Chapter 37
1. 2
2. 3
3. 2
4. 3
5. 3
6. 2
7. 2
8. 1, 2, 3
9. 1
10. 3
11. 2
12. 1
13. 2
14. 4
15. telemonitoring
16. 2, 3

Chapter 38
1. 2
2. 2
3. 4
4. 4
5. 1
6. 1
7. 1
8. 1
9. 4
10. 3
11. 2

Chapter 39
1. 1, 2, 3, 4, 5
2. 3
3. 1
4. 3
5. 1
6. 1
7. 3
8. 3
9. 3
10. 1
11. 3
12. 2
13. 4
14. 4

Chapter 40
1. 1
2. 2
3. 1
4. 3
5. 3
6. 3
7. 2
8. 3
9. 3
10. 2
11. Medical Director
12. Pain
13. 3
14. 3
15. 1
16. 1, 3
17. 3
18. 1, 2, 3

Chapter 41
1. 2
2. 3
3. 1
4. 4
5. 2
6. 4
7. 1
8. 3
9. 2
10. 2
11. 3
12. 4
13. 3
14. 2
15. e
16. d
17. a
18. c
19. b
20. f
21. k
22. a
23. i
24. b
25. g
26. c
27. j
28. d
29. e
30. h

Chapter 42
1. 4
2. 2
3. 3
4. 1
5. 1
6. 4
7. 3

8. 2
9. 1
10. 2
11. 3
12. 2
13. 4
14. 3
15. 3
16. 2
17. 3
18. 2
19. 2
20. 1
21. 3
22. 2
23. 3
24. 4
25. 2

Chapter 43

1. 1
2. 2
3. 3
4. 3
5. 2
6. 1
7. 1
8. 1
9. 4
10. 2
11. 1
12. 2
13. 3
14. 1
15. 2
16. 1
17. 2
18. 2
19. 2
20. 1
21. 2
22. 2
23. 1, 2
24. 1
25. 3
26. papule
27. 2
28. 3
29. 2
30. 1, 2, 4
31. 4
32. 1, 2, 4

Chapter 44

1. 2
2. 4
3. 4
4. 2
5. 3
6. 4
7. 2
8. 4
9. 3
10. 3
11. 2
12. 2
13. 1
14. 2
15. 2
16. 3
17. 3
18. 4
19. 1
20. 4
21. 3
22. 3
23. 4
24. 3, 4
25. 4

Chapter 45

1. 2
2. 3
3. 2
4. 2
5. 3
6. 2
7. 4
8. 2
9. 2
10. 1
11. 1
12. 3
13. 3
14. 4
15. 4
16. 3
17. 3
18. 1
19. 3
20. 2
21. 4
22. 3
23. 4
24. 1
25. 1
26. 4
27. 4
28. 2
29. 1
30. 1, 2, 4

Chapter 46

1. 1
2. 1
3. 2, 3, 4
4. 4
5. 2
6. 3
7. 2
8. 3
9. 3
10. 1, 2, 3
11. 4
12. 2
13. 3
14. 3
15. 2
16. 2
17. 4
18. 1
19. Reinfection, cirrhosis
20. 4
21. 1
22. 1, 3
23. 2
24. 3
25. 1, 2, 3
26. 2
27. 1, 4
28. 4
29. 1

Chapter 47

1. 3
2. 1
3. 2
4. 3
5. 4
6. 2
7. 3
8. 2
9. 4
10. 3
11. 1
12. 4
13. 3
14. 2
15. 3
16. 2
17. 2
18. 1
19. 2
20. 4
21. 3
22. 1
23. 2
24. 1
25. 1, 2, 3
26. 1, 2, 3, 5
27. 1, 2, 3, 5
28. 1, 2, 4, 5
29. 2
30. 4
31. 1
32. 2
33. 1, 4
34. 2

Chapter 48

1. 1
2. 2
3. 1
4. 3
5. 4
6. 3
7. 4
8. 1
9. 4
10. 4
11. 2
12. 2
13. 4
14. 2
15. 1
16. 3
17. 1
18. 2
19. 2
20. 2
21. 4
22. 3
23. 1
24. Troponin I
25. 3
26. 2
27. 1
28. 1, 2, 3
29. 1, 2, 4
30. 4
31. 2
32. 3
33. 4
34. 3
35. 1, 2, 4
36. 1, 3, 4
37. 4

Chapter 49

1. 2
2. 3
3. 3
4. 4
5. 4
6. 1
7. 2
8. 3
9. 3
10. 3
11. 2
12. 1
13. 2
14. 4
15. 1
16. 3
17. 4
18. 3
19. 1
20. 3
21. 4
22. 1
23. 3
24. 3
25. 1
26. 1, 3, 4
27. 1, 2, 4
28. 2, 3, 4, 5
29. 1, 2, 4
30. 2
31. 1, 2, 3, 5
32. 1, 3, 4
33. 2, 3, 4, 5
34. 1, 2, 3, 4
35. 1, 2, 4, 5
36. 1, 2, 3, 5
37. 1

Chapter 50

1. 4
2. 3
3. 1
4. 4
5. 1
6. 3
7. 4
8. 1
9. 3
10. 2
11. 2
12. 3
13. 1
14. 1
15. 1
16. 4
17. 2
18. 3
19. 2
20. 4
21. 4
22. 1
23. 1
24. 2
25. 1
26. 4
27. 1, 2, 3
28. 2, 3
29. 1, 2, 4
30. 1, 3, 4
31. 1
32. 1
33. 3
34. 1
35. 2

Chapter 51

1. 3
2. 1
3. 4
4. 3
5. 3
6. 4
7. 1
8. 4
9. 4
10. 1
11. 1
12. 4
13. 4
14. 2
15. 2
16. 4
17. 3
18. 4
19. 4
20. 3
21. 3
22. Regular or rapid acting
23. 1, 2, 3
24. 3
25. 1
26. 2, 3, 4
27. 2
28. 1, 2, 3
29. 2
30. 1
31. 1
32. 1, 2, 3
33. 3
34. 3
35. Glycosylated hemoglobin (HgA_{1c})
36. 1, 2, 4
37. ketonuria

Chapter 52

1. 1
2. 2

3. 3
4. 4
5. 3
6. 4
7. 2
8. 1
9. 1, 3, 4
10. 3
11. 2
12. 1
13. 3
14. 4
15. 1
16. 3
17. 4
18. 2, 3
19. 2
20. 4
21. 1
22. 1
23. 3
24. 1
25. 2
26. 2
27. 3
28. 2
29. 4
30. 1, 2

Chapter 53

1. 3
2. 2
3. 1
4. 4
5. 3
6. 4
7. 1
8. 1
9. 2
10. 1, 2, 3
11. 2
12. 2
13. 1
14. 2
15. 3
16. 1
17. 3
18. 2
19. 3
20. 3
21. 2, 3, 4
22. 1
23. 1
24. 3
25. 3
26. 1
27. 1
28. 2
29. 4
30. Cochlear implant
31. 4
32. 1
33. 2
34. 1

Chapter 54

1. 4
2. 3
3. 2
4. 2
5. 1
6. 4
7. 3
8. 1
9. 3
10. 3
11. 1
12. 1
13. 1, 2, 3
14. 1
15. 2
16. 2
17. 1
18. 4
19. 1
20. 3
21. 2, 3, 4
22. C
23. E
24. D
25. B
26. A
27. 1, 2, 3, 4
28. 2, 3, 4
29. 1, 2, 3, 5
30. 3
31. 4
32. 2
33. 4
34. 3
35. 1, 2, 3
36. 2
37. 1

Chapter 55

1. 4
2. 2
3. 1
4. 2
5. 2
6. 1
7. 3
8. 3
9. 4
10. 2
11. 1
12. 1
13. 2, 3, 4
14. 3
15. 4
16. 3
17. Natural rubber latex proteins
18. 2, 3, 4
19. 1, 3, 4

Chapter 56

1. 1
2. 4
3. 4
4. 2
5. 2
6. 1
7. 1
8. 1
9. 1
10. 3
11. 4
12. 4
13. 3
14. False
15. True
16. True
17. True
18. True
19. False
20. False
21. 2
22. 2
23. 4
24. 1
25. 2
26. 1
27. 1
28. 1
29. 3
30. 2
31. 3
32. 1
33. 1, 2, 3, 4
34. 2, 3, 4, 5

Chapter 57

1. 3
2. 3
3. 3
4. 3
5. 1, 2, 3
6. 1
7. 3
8. 1, 3, 4
9. 1
10. 1
11. 3
12. 1
13. 4
14. 3
15. 2
16. 4
17. 3
18. Tumor lysis syndrome
19. 3
20. 1, 2, 3, 5
21. 4
22. 3
23. 2
24. 1
25. E
26. B
27. C
28. D
29. A
30. 1, 2, 4
31. 2, 3, 4
32. 3
33. 2
34. 3

Chapter 58

1. 2
2. 1
3. 4
4. 2
5. 3
6. 2
7. 3
8. 2
9. 4
10. 1
11. 4
12. 2
13. 3
14. 1
15. 3
16. 2
17. 4
18. 3
19. 3
20. 1
21. 2
22. 2
23. 4
24. 4
25. 4
26. 3

References and Suggested Readings

Chapter 1 The Evolution of Nursing

American Nurses Association (ANA). (2002a). *Nursing's agenda for the future: a call to the nation,* Washington, DC, Author.

American Nurses Association (ANA). (2002b). *The center for ethics and human rights*. Available at http://nursingworld.org/ethics. Accessed October, 2009.

American Nurses Association (ANA). (2004). *Nursing: scope and standards of practice,* Washington, DC: Author.

Dochterman, J.M., & Grace, H.K. (2009). *Current issues in nursing*. (6th ed.). St. Louis: Mosby.

Donahue, M.P. (1996). *Nursing: the finest art*. (2nd ed.). St. Louis: Mosby.

Elkin, M.K., Perry, A.G., & Potter, P.A. (2007). *Nursing interventions and clinical skills*. (4th ed.). St. Louis: Mosby.

Frantz, A. (1998). Nursing pride: Clara Barton in the Spanish-American War. *American Journal of Nursing*, 98(10):39-41.

Hill, S.S., & Howlett, H.A. (2005). *Success in practical nursing: personal and vocational issues*. (4th ed.). Philadelphia: Saunders.

Keenan, E. (2001). Oh, how things have changed . . . , *Nursing*, 31(11):32hn6.

Metules, T. (1998). Pins and pinning—the traditions continue, *RN*, 61(12):49-50.

Mosby's dictionary of medicine, nursing, and health professions. (2009). (8th ed.). St. Louis: Mosby.

Nightingale, F. (1860). *Notes on nursing: what it is and what it is not*. London: Harrison & Sons.

Potter, P.A., & Perry, A.G. (2007). *Basic nursing: essentials for practice*. (6th ed.). St. Louis: Mosby.

Potter, P.A., & Perry, A.G. (2009). *Fundamentals of nursing: concepts, process, and practice*. (7th ed.). St. Louis: Mosby.

Server, S. (1998). The story of the lamp. *American Journal of Practical Nursing*, 5(1).

Shiller, J. (2007). Reflection on caring: the pin. *RN*, 70(9):72, 2007.

Chapter 2 Legal and Ethical Aspects of Nursing

Aiken, T.D. (2004). *Legal, ethical, and political issues in nursing* (2nd ed.). Philadelphia: F.A. Davis.

Aiken, T.D. (2008). *Legal and ethical issues in health occupations*. (2nd ed.). Philadelphia: Saunders.

Anderson, P.S., & Commons, D. (2007). Medical futility: a nurse's viewpoint. *American Nurse Today*, 2(2).

Battaglia, S.K. (2003). HIPAA compliance requires facilities to have privacy policy. *Nursing Homes Long Term Care Management*, 51(1):30.

Black, H.C. (2008). *Black's law dictionary*. (9th ed.). St. Paul, Minn.: West.

Brooke, P.S. (2006). So you've been named in a lawsuit. What happens next? *Nursing*, 36(7):44-48.

Brown, L.A. (2002). Your state board of nursing: friend or foe? *Nursing 2002*, 32(12):48.

Canadian Nurses Association. (2002). *Code of ethics for nursing*. Ottawa, Ont.: Author.

Croke, E. (2003). Nurses, negligence and malpractice. *American Journal of Nursing*, 103(9):54.

Dochterman, J.M., & Grace, H.K. (2005). *Current issues in nursing*. (7th ed.). St. Louis: Mosby.

Edelman, C.L., & Mandle, C.L. (2006). *Health promotion throughout the lifespan*. (6th ed.). St. Louis: Mosby.

Giger, J.M., & Davidhizar, R.E. (2007). *Transcultural nursing: assessment and intervention*. (5th ed.). St. Louis: Mosby.

Hughes, R.G. (2004). Avoiding the near misses. *American Journal of Nursing*, 104(5):81.

Husted, G.L., & Husted, J.H. (2005). *Ethical decision making in nursing*. (4th ed.). St. Louis: Mosby.

Leonard, C. (2004). A person's right to active or passive euthanasia. *Journal of Practical Nursing*, (Spring):12.

Levine, C. (2006). HIPAA and talking with family caregivers. What does the law really say? *American Journal of Nursing*, 106(8):51.

Mason, D.J. (2004). When silence kills. *American Journal of Nursing*, 104(12):11.

Olson, D. (2007). Unwanted treatment. What are the ethical implications? *American Journal of Nursing*, 107(9):51.

Reising, D.L., & Allen, P.N. (2007). Protecting yourself from malpractice claims. *American Nurse Today*, 2(2):39.

Roman, L. (2007). 4 nurse attorneys tell you how to stay out of legal hot water. *RN*, 70(1):26-31.

Additional Resources

American Association of Legal Nurse Consultants (AALNC), 401 N. Michigan Ave. Chicago, IL 60611, 877-402-2562.

American Association of Nurse Attorneys (TAANA), 877-53TAANA. taana@taana.org. Available at www.taana.org. Accessed November, 2009.

LPN Boards of Nursing and nursing associations (LPN link). Available at www.NurseLaw.com/education.php. Accessed November, 2009.

Chapter 3 Communication

Ackley, B.J., & Ladwig, G.B. (2008). *Nursing diagnosis handbook: an evidence-based guide to planning care*. (8th ed.). St. Louis: Mosby.

Carpenito-Moyet, L.J. (2008). *Handbook of nursing diagnosis*. (12th ed.). Philadelphia: Lippincott Williams & Wilkins.

Harkreader, H., Hogan, M.A., & Thobaben, M. (2007). *Fundamentals of nursing: caring and clinical judgment*. (3rd ed.). Philadelphia: Saunders.

Perry, A.G., & Potter, P.A. (2009). *Clinical nursing skills and techniques*. (7th ed.). St. Louis: Mosby.

Potter, P.A., & Perry, A.G. (2009). *Fundamentals of nursing: concepts, process, and practice*. (7th ed.). St. Louis: Mosby.

Pullen, R. (2007). Tips for communicating with a patient from another culture. *Nursing 2007*, 37(10):48-49.

Riley, J.B. (2008). *Communication in nursing*. (6th ed.). St. Louis: Mosby.

Roman, L. (2007). Finding the words. How to handle difficult conversations. *RN 2007*, 70(3):34-38.

Smith, L.S.S. (2007). Speaking up for medical language interpreters. *Nursing 2007*, 37(2):48-49.

Sullivan, R., & Ferriter, A. (2008). Preventing life-threatening communication breakdowns. *Nursing 2008*, 38(2):17.

Chapter 4 Vital Signs

Ackley, B.J., & Ladwig, G.B. (2009). *Nursing diagnosis handbook*. (7th ed.). St. Louis: Mosby.

Barkauskas, V.H., et al. (2006). *Mosby's medical, nursing, and allied health dictionary*. (7th ed.). St. Louis: Mosby.

Beard, R.M., & Day, M.W. (2008). Fever and hyperthermia, learn to beat the heat. *Nursing 2008*, 38(6): 28.

Beare, P., & Myers, J. (2006). *Principles and practice of adult health nursing*. (5th ed.). St. Louis: Mosby.

Bulechek, G.M., Butcher, H.K., & Dochterman, J.M. (2008). *Nursing interventions classification (NIC)*. (5th ed.). St. Louis: Mosby.

Editorial. (2007). Now hear this: how to identify heart sounds. *LPN 2007*, 3(1):4.

Editorial. (2007). Take care with tympanic temperature readings. *Nursing 2007*, 37(4):52.

Elkin, M.K., Perry, A.G., & Potter, P.A. (2007). *Nursing interventions and clinical skills*. (4th ed.). St. Louis: Mosby.

Giger, J.M., & Davidhizar, R.E. (2007). *Transcultural nursing: assessment and intervention*. (5th ed.). St. Louis: Mosby.

Maddox, T., & Parker, D.M. (2006). Don't let hypertension sneak by you. *Nursing Made Incredibly Easy!* 4(1):9.

Moorhead, S., Johnson, M., Maas, M., et al. (2008). *Nursing outcomes classification (NOC)*. (4th ed.). St. Louis: Mosby.

Mosby's dictionary of medicine, nursing, and health professions. (2009). (8th ed.). St. Louis: Mosby.

North American Nursing Diagnosis Association International (NANDA-I). (2009). *NANDA-I nursing diagnoses: definitions and classification 2009-2011*. Oxford, United Kingdom: Author.

National High Blood Pressure Education Program (NHBPEP). National Heart, Lung, and Blood Institute; Natural Institutes of Health, the Seventh Report of The Joint Commission on Detection, Evaluation and Treatment of High Blood Pressure. *JAMA*, 298(19): 2560, 2003.

Perry, A.G., & Potter, P.A. (2009). *Clinical nursing skills and techniques*. (7th ed.). St. Louis: Mosby.

Potter, P.A., & Perry, A.G. (2007). *Basic nursing: essentials for practice*. (6th ed.). St. Louis: Mosby.

Potter, P.A., & Perry, A.G. (2009). *Fundamentals of nursing: concepts, process, and practice*. (7th ed.). St. Louis: Mosby.

Seidel, H.M., Ball, J.W., Dains, J.E., et al. (2007). *Mosby's guide to physical examination*. (6th ed.). St. Louis: Mosby.

Thomas, J., & Feliciana, C. Measuring BP with a Doppler device. *Nursing*, 33(7):52-53. 2003.

Tucker, S.M., et al. (2008). *Patient care standards: collaborative planning and nursing interventions*. (9th ed.). St. Louis: Mosby.

United States Environmental Protection Agency (EPA). (2005). What should I do if I have a mercury spill? Available at www.epa.gov/epawaste/hazard/tsd/mercury/index.htm. Accessed December, 2009.

Chapter 5 Physical Assessment

American Heart Association (2007). *Heart disease and stroke statistics*. Available at www.americanheart.org/downloadable/heart. Accessed February, 2007.

Barkauskas, V., Baumann, L.C., & Darling-Fisher, C. (2006). *Health and physical assessment*. (4th ed.). St. Louis: Mosby.

Bermis, P.A. (2005). *Abdominal pain and abdominal emergency*. Available at www.nursingceu.com/courses/index_ncea.html.

Elkin, M.K., Perry, A.G., & Potter, P.A. (2007). *Nursing interventions and clinical skills*. (4th ed.). St. Louis: Mosby.

Estes, M. (2002). *Health assessment and physical examination*. (2nd ed.). New York: Delmar.

Fitzpatrick, J.B., & Shinners, M.C. (1996). How to make assessing as easy as ABC. *Nursing*, 26(8):51.

Geissler, E. (2006). *Cultural assessment*. (4th ed.). St. Louis: Mosby.

Harkreader, H., Hogan, M.A., & Thobaben, M. (2007). *Fundamentals of nursing: care and clinical judgment*. (3rd ed.). St. Louis: Mosby.

Jarvis, C. (2008). *Physical examination and health assessment*. (5th ed.). Philadelphia: Saunders.

Khan, N.A., Rahim, S.A., Anand, S.S., et al. (2006). Does the clinical examination predict lower extremity peripheral arterial disease? *Journal of the American Medical Association*, (295):536.

Lewis, S.L., Heitkemper, M.M., Dirksen, S.R., et al. (2007). *Medical-surgical nursing: assessment and management of clinical problems*. (7th ed.). St. Louis: Mosby.

Lower, J. (2002). Facing neuro assessment fearlessly. *Nursing 2002*, (2):58.

Madsen, D., Sebolt, T., Cullen, L., et al. (2005). Listening to bowel sounds: an evidence-based practice project. *American Journal of Nursing*, 105(12):40.

McCormick, M. (2007). Every breath you take: making sense of breath sounds. *Nursing Made Incredibly Easy!* 5(1):7-11.

McCraig, L., & Burt, C. (2005). *Advance data from vital and health statistics* (No. 358, 2005). Atlanta: Centers for Disease Control and Prevention.

Mody, L., Sun, R., & Bradley, S.F. (2006). Assessment of pneumonia in older adults: effect of functional status. *Journal of the American Geriatric Society*, (54):1062.

Mosby's dictionary of medicine, nursing, and health professions. (2009). (8th ed.). St. Louis: Mosby.

Movius, M. (2006). What's causing that gut pain? *RN*, 69(7):25.

Perry, A.G., & Potter, P.A. (2009). *Clinical nursing skills and techniques*. (7th ed.). St. Louis: Mosby.

Potter, P.A., & Perry, A.G. (2009). *Fundamentals of nursing: concepts, process, and practice*. (7th ed.). St. Louis: Mosby.

Schutte, D. (2006). Alzheimer disease and genetics. *American Journal of Nursing*, 106(12):40.

Seidel, H.M., Ball, J.W., Dains, J.E., et al. (2007). *Mosby's guide to physical examination*. (6th ed.). St. Louis: Mosby.

Thomas, C.L. (2005). *Taber's cyclopedic medical dictionary*. (20th ed.). Philadelphia: F.A. Davis.

Thompson, J.M., McFarland, G., Hirsch, J., et al. (2009). *Mosby's clinical nursing*. (7th ed.). St. Louis: Mosby.

Timby, B. (2008). *Fundamental skills and concepts in patient care*. (9th ed.). Philadelphia: Lippincott-Raven.

Tucker, S.M., Cannobio, M.M., Paquette, E.V., et al. (2007). *Patient care standards: collaborative planning and nursing interventions*. (7th ed.). St. Louis: Mosby.

U.S. Department of Health and Human Services. (2000). *Healthy People 2010*. (Conference Edition). Washington, DC: U.S. Government Printing Office.

Walker, B. (2004). Assessing gastrointestinal. *Nursing 2004*, (34):48.

Weber, J. (2005). *Nurse's handbook of health assessments*. (5th ed.). Philadelphia: Lippincott.

Weber, J., & Kelly, J. (2006). *Health assessment in nursing*. (3rd ed.). Philadelphia: Lippincott.

Wilson, S., & Giddens, J. (2008). *Health assessment for nursing practice*. (4th ed.). St. Louis: Mosby.

Chapter 6 Nursing Process and Critical Thinking

Ackley, B.J., & Ladwig, G.B. (2007). *Nursing diagnosis handbook*. (8th ed.). St. Louis: Mosby.

Alfaro-LeFevre, R. (2009a). *Critical thinking and clinical judgment: a practical approach*. (4th ed.). St. Louis: Mosby.

Alfaro-LeFevre, R. (2009b). *Applying nursing process: a tool for critical thinking*. (7th ed.). Philadelphia: Wolters Kluwer/Lippincott Williams & Wilkins.

American Nurses Association (ANA). (1998). *Standards of clinical practice*. Washington, DC: Author.

American Nurses Association (ANA). (2003). *Nursing's social policy statement*. Washington, DC: Author.

American Nurses Association (ANA). (2004). *Nursing: scope and standards of practice*. Washington, DC: Author.

Berman, A., Snyder, S., Kozier, B., et al. (2008). *Kozier and Erb's fundamentals of nursing: concept, process, and practice*. (8th ed.). Upper Saddle River, NJ: Pearson/Prentice Hall.

Bulechek, G.M., Butcher, H.K., & Dochterman, J.M. (2008). *Nursing interventions classification (NIC)*. (5th ed.). St. Louis: Mosby.

Carpenito-Moyet, L.J. (2008a). *Handbook of nursing diagnosis*. (12th ed.). Philadelphia: Lippincott Williams & Wilkins.

Carpenito-Moyet, L.J. (2008b). *Nursing diagnosis: application to clinical practice*. (12th ed.). Philadelphia: Lippincott Williams & Wilkins.

Craven, R.F., & Hirnle, C.J. (2007). *Fundamentals of nursing: human health and function*. (5th ed.). Philadelphia: Lippincott Williams & Wilkins.

Daniels, R., Nosek, L.J., & Nicoll, L.H. (2007). *Contemporary medical-surgical nursing*. Clifton Park, NY: Thompson Delmar Learning.

Doenges, M.E., & Moorhouse, M.F. (2008a). *Application of nursing process and nursing diagnosis: an interactive text for diagnostic reasoning*. (5th ed.). Philadelphia: F.A. Davis.

Doenges, M.E., Moorhouse, M.F., & Murr, A.C. (2008b). *Nurse's pocket guide: diagnoses, prioritized interventions, and rationales.* (10th ed.). 2008, Philadelphia: F.A. Davis.

Doenges, M.E., Moorhouse, M.F., & Murr, A.C. (2008c). *Nursing diagnosis manual: planning, individualizing, and documenting client care.* (2nd ed.). Philadelphia: F.A. Davis.

Gordon, M. (1994). *Nursing diagnosis: process and application*. (3rd ed.). St. Louis: Mosby.

Gordon, M. (2002). *Manual of nursing diagnosis.* (10th ed.). St. Louis: Mosby.

Jarvis, C. (2008). *Physical examination and health assessment*. (5th ed.). Philadelphia: Saunders.

Johnson, M., Dochterman, J.M., & Moorhead, S. (2006). *NANDA, NOC, & NIC linkage: nursing diagnosis, outcomes & intervention.* (2nd ed.). St. Louis: Mosby.

Kostovich, C.T., Poradzisz, M., Wood, K., et al. (2007). Learning style preference and student aptitude for concept maps. *Journal of Nursing Education*, 46(5):225-231.

Moorhead, S., Johnson, M., Maas, M., et al. (2008). *Nursing outcomes classification (NOC)*. (4th ed.). St. Louis: Mosby.

National League for Nursing. (2000). *Think tank on critical thinking.* New York: Author.

North American Nursing Diagnosis Association (NANDA). (2005). *Nursing diagnoses: definitions and classification 2005-2006*. Philadelphia: NANDA.

North American Nursing Diagnosis Association International (NANDA-I). (2009). *NANDA-I nursing diagnoses: definitions and classification 2009-2011*. Oxford, United Kingdom: Author.

Potter, P.A., & Perry, A.G. (2009). *Fundamentals of nursing: concepts, process, and practice.* (7th ed.). St. Louis: Mosby.

Sparks, S.M., & Taylor, C.M. (2008). *Nursing diagnosis reference manual*. (7th ed.). Springhouse, PA: Springhouse.

Taylor, J., & Wros, P. (2007). Concept mapping: a nursing model for care planning. *Journal of Nursing Education*, 46(5):211-216.

Volk, S. (2007). The use of NANDA, NIC, and NOC in an electronic documentation system. *DNA Report*, 32(2), 7-7. Retrieved May 19, 2008 from CINAHL database.

Wilkinson, J.M., & Ahern, N.R. (2009). *Prentice Hall nursing diagnosis handbook with NIC interventions and NOC outcomes*. (9th ed.). Upper Saddle River, NJ: Pearson/Prentice Hall.

Wilkinson, J.M., & Van Leuven, K. (2007). *Fundamentals of nursing: theory, concepts, & applications*, Philadelphia: F.A. Davis.

Chapter 7 Documentation

American Nurses Association (ANA). (1997). *NIDSEC standards and scoring guidelines*. Washington, DC: Author.

Austin, S. (2006). Ladies and gentlemen of the jury. *Nursing 2006*, 36(1):56.

Bulechek, G.M., Butcher, H.K., & Dochterman, J.M. (2008). *Nursing interventions classification (NIC)*. (5th ed.). St. Louis: Mosby.

Dortch, T. (2007). Document it! The importance of accurate charting. *LPN 2007*, 3(4):25.

Editorial. (2002). Comparing charting systems. *Nursing*, 32(8):81.

Editorial. (2007a). Charting check up: documenting health situations. *LPN 2007*, 3(6):9.

Editorial. (2007b). Charting check up: do you know what's on the "do not use" list? *LPN 2007*, 3(1):25.

Editorial. (2007c). Charting check up: your patient wants to see his medical records. *LPN 2007*, 3(5):4.

Elkin, M.K., Perry, A.G., & Potter, P.A. (2007). *Nursing interventions and clinical skills*. (4th ed.). St. Louis: Mosby.

Gordon, M. (2006). *Manual of nursing diagnosis*. (11th ed.). St. Louis: Mosby.

Harkreader, H., Hogan, M.A., & Thobaben, M. (2007). *Fundamentals of nursing: care and clinical judgment*. (3rd ed.). St. Louis: Mosby.

Heleda, T., Czar, P., & Mascara, C. (2005). Information security and confidentiality. In T. Heleda, P. Czar, & C. Mascara (Eds.), *Handbook of informatics for nurses and health care professionals* (3rd ed.). Upper Saddle River, N.J.: Pearson Prentice Hall.

Iyer, P.W., & Camp, N.H. (2004). *Nursing documentation: a nursing process approach*. St. Louis: Mosby.

The Joint Commission on Accreditation of Healthcare Organizations (JCAHO). (1999a). *Standards for the accreditation of home care*. Chicago: Author.

The Joint Commission on Accreditation of Healthcare Organizations (JCAHO). (2003). *Standards for the accreditation of home care*. Chicago: Author.

The Joint Commission on Accreditation of Healthcare Organizations (JCAHO). (2005). *Standards for the accreditation of hospitals*. Chicago: Author.

Marrelli, T.M. (2008). *Nursing documentation handbook*. (4th ed.). St. Louis: Mosby.

Mosby's dictionary of medicine, nursing, and health professions. (2009). (8th ed.). St. Louis: Mosby.

Perry, A.G., & Potter, P.A. (2009). *Clinical nursing skills and techniques*. (7th ed.). St. Louis: Mosby.

Potter, P.A., & Perry, A.G. (2007). *Basic nursing: essentials for practice*. (6th ed.). St. Louis: Mosby.

Potter, P.A., & Perry, A.G. (2009). *Fundamentals of nursing: concepts, process, and practice*. (7th ed.). St. Louis: Mosby.

Smith, L. (2007a). Chart smart documenting culturally competent psychosocial nursing diagnosis. *Nursing 2007*, 37(1):70.

Smith, L. (2007b). Chart smart documenting with photographs. *Nursing 2007*, 37(8):20.

Smith, S.S. (2007). Chart smart documenting use of an interpreter. *Nursing 2007*, 37(7): 25.

Springhouse. (2006). *Chart smart: the A-Z guide to better nursing documentation*, Springhouse, PA: Author.

Springhouse. (2007). *Charting: an incredibly easy pocket guide*. Philadelphia: Lippincott Williams & Wilkins.

Chapter 8 Cultural and Ethnic Considerations

Carson, V.B. (1989). *Spiritual dimensions of nursing practice*, Philadelphia: Saunders.

Dapice, A.N. (2006). The medicine wheel. *Journal of Transcultural Nursing*, 17:251-260.

D'Avanzo, C., & Geissler, E. (2007). *Pocket guide to cultural health assessment*. (4th ed.). St. Louis: Elsevier.

Eason, J.A. (2006). Cultural exchange. *RN 2006*, 69(5):62.

Giger, J.M., & Davidhizar, R.E. (2007). *Transcultural nursing: assessment and intervention*. (5th ed.). St. Louis: Mosby.

Harkreader, H., Hogan, M.A., & Thobaben, M. (2007). *Fundamentals of nursing: care and clinical judgment*. (3rd ed.). St. Louis: Mosby.

Meiner, S.E., & Lueckenotte, A.G. (2006). *Gerontologic nursing*. (3rd ed.). St. Louis: Mosby.

Mosby's dictionary of medicine, nursing, and health professions. (8th ed.). (2009). St. Louis: Mosby.

Nelma, L.W., & Gorski, J. (2006). The role of the African traditional healer in women's health. *Journal of Transcultural Nursing*, 17(4):184.

North American Nursing Diagnosis Association International (NANDA-I). (2009). *NANDA-I nursing diagnoses: definitions and classification 2009-2011*. Oxford, United Kingdom: Author.

Obermyer, M.V. (2006). Are you a culturally competent preceptor? *Nursing 2006*, 36(6):54-55.

Potter, P.A., & Perry, A.G. (2007). *Basic nursing: essentials for practice*. (6th ed.). St. Louis: Mosby.

Potter, P.A., & Perry, A.G. (2009). *Fundamentals of nursing: concepts, process, and practice*. (7th ed.). St. Louis: Mosby.

U.S. Census Bureau. (2007). *State and county quick facts*. Available at http://quickfacts.census.gov/gfd/states/00000.html. Accessed October, 2009.

U.S. Department of Commerce, Bureau of the Census. (2007a). *Population profiles of the United States. Internet update*. Washington, DC: U.S. Government Printing Office.

U.S. Department of Commerce, Bureau of the Census. (2007b). *Transcultural and multicultural health links.* Washington, DC: U.S. Government Printing Office.

Wells, J.N., & Cagle, C.S. (2006). Building on Mexican-American cultural values. *Nursing 2006*, 36(7):20-21.

Chapter 9 Life Span Development

Ahmann, E. (2006). Supporting fathers' involvement in children's health care. *Pediatric Nursing*, 32(1):88-90.

Anbarghalami, R., Yang, L.T., Van Sell, S.L., et al. (2007). When to suspect child abuse. *RN*, 70(4):35-38.

Bartlett, R., Holditch-Davis, D., & Belyea, M. (2007). Problem behaviors in adolescents. *Pediatric Nursing*, 33(1):13-18.

Butler, F., & Zakari, N. (2005). Grandparents parenting grandchildren: assessing health status, parental stress, and social supports. *Journal of Gerontological Nursing*, 31(3):43-54.

Di-Maria-Ghalili, R., & Amella, E. (2005). Nutrition in older adults. *American Journal of Nursing*, 105(3):40-50.

Faircloth, C. (2005). Aging bodies: images and everday experience. *Contemporary Gerontology*, 11(4):176-181.

Hascup, V. (2005). Nearing death awareness. *Advance for Nurses*, 5(24):25-26.

Henry, L. (2005). Childhood obesity: what can be done to help today's youth? *Pediatric Nursing*, 31(1):13-16.

Herzberger, S. (2005). Depressed teens: a thorny problem. *Advance for Nurses*, 5(23):29-30.

Horodynski, M., & Stommel, M. (2005). Nutrition education aimed at toddlers: an interventional study. *Pediatric Nursing*, 31(5):364-372.

Howard, P. (2005). Parents belief about children and gun safety. *Pediatric Nursing*, 31(5):400-403.

Jachna, C., & Forbes-Thompson, S. (2005). Osteoporosis: health beliefs and barriers to treatment in an assisted living facility. *Journal of Gerontological Nursing*, 31(1):25-30.

Malloy, P., Wang, J., Peng, L., et al. (2006). Palliative care education for pediatric nurses. *Pediatric Nursing*, 32(6):555-561.

Pringle-Specht, J. (2005). 9 Myths of incontinence in older adults. *American Journal of Nursing*, 105(6):58-68.

Skybo, T. (2005). Witnessing violence: biopsychosocial impact on children. *Pediatric Nursing*, 31(4):263-269.

Thompson, D. (2005). Safe sleep practices for hospitalized infants. *Pediatric Nursing*, 31(5):400-403.

U.S. Department of Health and Human Services. (2002). *Healthy People 2010.* Washington, DC: Author.

Chapter 10 Loss, Grief, Dying, and Death

Archer, M. (2008). A quilt creating an end-of-life program that works. *RN*, April, pages 38-44.

Babus, A. (1975). The dying patient's bill of rights. *American Journal of Nursing*, 75:99.

Bielochek, G.M., Butcher, H.K., Dochterman, J.M. (2008). *Nursing interventions classification (NIC).* (5th ed.). St. Louis: Mosby.

Bowlby, J. (1980). *Attachment and loss, Vol. 3. Loss, sadness and depression.* New York: Basic Books.

Darrach, B. (1992). The war on aging. *Life Magazine*, 15(10):32-43.

Davidovic, M. (2003). The privilege to be old. Gerontology 49(5):335.

Ebersole, P., Touhy, T., Hess, P., et al. (2008). *Toward healthy aging: human needs and nursing response.* (7th ed.). St. Louis: Mosby.

Editorial. (2007). Patient education advanced directives. *LPN 2007*, 3(4):42.

Elkin, M.K., Perry, A.G., & Potter, P.A. (2007). *Nursing interventions and clinical skills.* (4th ed.). St. Louis: Mosby.

Ferszt, G.G., & Leveilee, M. (2006). How to distinguish between grief and depression. *Nursing*, 36(9):59.

Furman, J. (2004). Healing the mind and spirit as the body fails. *Nursing*, 43(4):50.

Giger, J.M., & Davidhizar, R.E. (2007). *Transcultural nursing: assessment and intervention.* (5th ed.). St. Louis: Mosby.

Harkreader, H., Hogan, M.A., & Thobaben, M. (2007). *Fundamentals of nursing: care and clinical judgment.* (3rd ed.). St. Louis: Mosby.

Hockenberry, M.J., & Wilson, D. (2007). *Wong's nursing care of infants and children.* (8th ed.). St. Louis, Mosby.

Kapel, S. (1974). Dying boy's letter pleads for empathy. *Kansas City Times*, March 8.

Kouch, M. (2006). Managing symptoms for a "good death." *Nursing 2006*, 36(11):58.

Kouch, M. (2007). End of life care: helping patients rest easy. *LPN 2007*, 3(4):37.

Kübler-Ross, E. (1969). *On death and dying.* New York: Macmillan.

Kübler-Ross, E. (1995). *Death is of vital importance, on life, death, and life after death.* New York: Station.

Kübler-Ross, E. & Kessler, D. (2006). *On grief and grieving: finding the meaning of grief through the fine stages of loss.* New York: Scribner.

Meiner, S.E., & Lueckenotte, A.G. (2006). *Gerontologic nursing.* (3rd ed.). St. Louis: Mosby.

Moorhead, S., Johnson, M., & Maas, M. (2008). *Nursing outcome classification (NOC).* (4th ed.). St. Louis: Mosby.

Mosby's dictionary of medicine, nursing, and health professions. (2009). (8th ed.). St. Louis: Mosby.

NANDA Conference 2007-2008. Organized by Doenges and Moorehouse's Diagnostic Divisions, as seen on pages 2656-2657 of *Taber's Cyclopedia Medical Dictionary.* (20th ed.). 2007.

Patient Education Series. (2006). Advanced directives. *Nursing 2006*, 36(9):43.

Perry, A.G., & Potter, P.A. (2009). *Clinical nursing skills and techniques.* (7th ed.). St. Louis: Mosby.

Potter, P.A., & Perry, A.G. (2007). *Basic nursing: essentials for practice.* (6th ed.). St. Louis: Mosby.

Potter, P.A., & Perry, A.G. (2009). *Fundamentals of nursing: concepts, process, and practice.* (7th ed.). St. Louis: Mosby.

Recer, P. (2000). Showing your age? Quality-control genes at fault, study finds, *San Francisco Examiner*, March 31.

Ryan, P.W. (2004). The gift of life. *American Journal of Nursing*, 99(4):80.

Schlessinger, D. (2000). Alleles and aging: the effects of different forms of genes on aging and longevity. *Generations*, 24(1): 36.

Ufema, J. (2006). Insights on death and dying. Death bed experiences. Angels among us. *Nursing 2006*, 36(6):30.

Ufema, J. (2006). Insights on death and dying. Katrina aftermath, unique grieving needs. *Nursing 2006*, 36(8):22.

Ufema, J. (2006). Insights on death and dying. Surviving spouses deciding when to die. *Nursing 2006*, 36(8):22.

Ufema, J. (2006). Insights on death and dying. Views on dying. At war with death. *Nursing 2006*, 36(6):30.

Ufema, J. (2008). Insights on death and dying. Death anniversary private remembrance. *Nursing 2008*, 38(2):18.

Ufema, J. (2008). Insights on death and dying. Dying mom's request. Raising Amy's boys. *Nursing 2008*, 38(2):18.

Ufema, J. (2008). Insights on death and dying. Terminal weaning protocol for peaceful death. *Nursing 2008*, 38(2):18.

Varcarolis, E.M., & Halter, M.J. (2009). *Foundations of psychiatric mental health nursing: a clinical approach.* (6th ed.). Philadelphia: Saunders.

Werden, J.W. (1982). *Grief counseling and grief therapy.* New York: Springer.

Chapter 11 Admission, Transfer, and Discharge

Ackley, B.J., & Ladwig, G.B. (2009). *Nursing diagnosis handbook.* (7th ed.). St. Louis: Mosby.

Austin, S. Walk a fine line if your patient wants to leave AMA, *Nursing 2006*, 36(12):48, 206.

Chart Smart. (2006). (ed.2)., Philadelphia: Lippincott Williams & Wilkins.

Charting check up, before you say good-bye: discharge summaries. *LPN 2008*, 4(1):4.

Complete guide to documentation (2nd ed.). (2008). Amsterdam: Wolters Kluwer.

Elkin, M.K., Perry, A.G., & Potter, P.A. (2007). *Nursing interventions and clinical skills.* (4th ed.). St. Louis: Mosby.

Giger, J.M., & Davidhizar, R.E. (2007). *Transcultural nursing: assessment and intervention.* (4th ed.). St. Louis: Mosby.

Harkreader, H., Hogan, M.A., & Thobaben, M. (2007). *Fundamentals of nursing: care and clinical judgment*. (3rd ed.). St. Louis: Mosby.

Joint Commission on Accreditation of Healthcare Organizations (JCAHO). (2003). *Comprehensive accreditation manual for hospitals, the official handbook*. Oakbrook Terrace, Ill.: Author.

The Joint Commission (TJC). (2008). *Comprehensive accreditation manual for hospitals: the official handbook (CAMH)*. Chicago: Author.

Katz, M.J. (2006). Save time? Do a 5-minute initial assessment. *RN*, 69(3):43.

Maslow, A.H. (1954). *Motivation and personality*. New York: Harper & Row.

Mosby's dictionary of medicine, nursing, and health professions. (2009). (8th ed.). St. Louis: Mosby.

North American Nursing Diagnosis Association International (NANDA-I). (2009). *NANDA-I nursing diagnoses: definitions and classification 2009-2011*. Oxford, United Kingdom: Author.

Perry, A.G., & Potter, P.A. (2009). *Clinical nursing skills and techniques*. (7th ed.). St. Louis: Mosby.

Potter, P.A., & Perry, A.G. (2007). *Basic nursing: essentials for practice*. (6th ed.). St. Louis: Mosby.

Potter, P.A., & Perry, A.G. (2009). *Fundamentals of nursing: concepts, process, and practice*. (7th ed.). St. Louis: Mosby.

Smith, S.L. (2006). Chart Smart. Documenting discharge planning. *Nursing 2006*, 36(6):18.

Chapter 12 Medical-Surgical Asepsis and Infection Prevention and Control

Association of Perioperative Registered Nurses (APRN). (2005). *Standards, recommended practices, and guidelines*. Denver: Author.

Boyce, J.M., Pittet, D., HICPAC/SHEA/APIC/IDSA Hand Hygiene Task Force, & the CDC Healthcare Control Practices Advisory Committee. (2002). Guideline for hand hygiene in health-care settings. *Infection Control and Hospital Epidemiology*, 23(12 Suppl):S3-S40.

Centers for Disease Control and Prevention (CDC). (n.d.). *Personal protective equipment (PPE) in health care settings*. Available at www.cdc.gov/ncidod/dhqp/ppe.html. Accessed December, 2009.

Centers for Disease Control and Prevention (CDC), & Hospital Infection Control Practices Advisory Committee. (2002b). *Guidelines for hand hygiene in health care settings*. Available at www.cdc.gov/handhygiene. Accessed December, 2009.

Centers for Disease Control and Prevention (CDC). (2005). *Updated U.S. Public Health Service guidelines for the management of occupational exposure to HIV and recommendations for postexposure prophylaxis*. Washington, D.C.: Author.

Centers for Disease Control and Prevention (CDC). (2006). *Management of multi-drug-resistant organisms in health care settings*. Available at www.cdc.gov/ncidod/dhqp/pdf/ar/mdroGuideline2006.pdf. Accessed December, 2009.

Centers for Disease Control and Prevention (CDC). (2007). *Guideline for isolation precautions: preventing transmission of infectious agents in health care settings*. Available at http://www.cdc.gov/ncidod/dhqp/gl_isolation.html. Accessed December, 2009.

Cooper, E. (2008).Vancomycin-resistant Enterecocci (VRE). How you can stop the spread of this drug–resistant organism. *RN 2008*, 71(2):27-31.

Delahanty, K.M., & Myers, F.E., III. (2007). Infection control survey report. *Nursing 2007*, 37(16):36-38.

Dent, M. (2004). Hospital-acquired pneumonia: the gift that keeps on taking. *Nursing*, 34(2):48.

Editorial. (2002). Infection control—hospital nursing. Infection collection. *Nursing*, 32(5):32hn8.

Elkin, M.K., Perry, A.G., & Potter, P.A. (2007). *Nursing interventions and clinical skills*. (4th ed.). St. Louis: Mosby.

Grant, P. (2004). Making the most of your infection control professional. *Nursing*, 32(5):32hn5.

Harkreader, H., Hogan, M.A., & Thobaben, M. (2007). *Fundamentals of nursing: care and clinical judgment*. (3rd ed.). St. Louis: Mosby.

Institute for Bio Security. Available at http://bioterrorism.slu.edu. Accessed December, 2009.

Jensen, P.A., Lambert, L.A., Iademarco, M.F., et al. (2005). Guidelines for preventing the transmission of *Mycobacterium tuberculosis* in health-care settings. *MMWR Morbidity and Mortality Weekly Report*, 54:RR-17.

Klein, E., et al. (2008). Staph aureus. Infections up in the United States. *Nursing 2008*, 38(2):35.

Kuehnert, M.J., Hill, H.A., Kupronis, B.A., et al. (2005). *Methicillin-resistant*–Staphylococcus aureus *hospitalizations, United States*. Available at www.cdc.gov/ncidod/EID/vol11no06/04-0831.htm. Accessed July, 2009.

Lewis, S.L., Heitkemper, M.M., Dirksen, S.R., et al. (2007). *Medical-surgical nursing: assessment and management of clinical problems*. (7th ed.). St. Louis: Mosby.

Monahan, F.D., Sands, J.K., Neighbors, M., et al. (2007). *Phipps' medical-surgical nursing: health and illness perspectives*. (8th ed.). St. Louis: Mosby.

Mosby's dictionary of medicine, nursing, and health professions. (2009). (8th ed.). St. Louis: Mosby.

North American Nursing Diagnosis Association International (NANDA-I). (2009). *NANDA-I nursing diagnoses: definitions and classification 2009-2011*. Oxford, United Kingdom: Author.

Oriola, S. (2006). *C. difficile*: a menace in hospitals and homes alike. *Nursing 2006*, 36(8):14-15.

Overstreat, M. (2007). Infection prevention, detecting and preventing West Nile Virus. *LPN 2007*, 37(6):11-13.

Pagana, K.D., & Pagana, T.J. (2007). *Diagnostic and laboratory test reference*. (7th ed.). St. Louis: Mosby.

Potter, P.A., & Perry, A.G. (2007). *Basic nursing: essentials for practice*. (6th ed.). St. Louis: Mosby.

Potter, P.A., & Perry, A.G. (2009). *Fundamentals of nursing: concepts, process, and practice*. (7th ed.). St. Louis: Mosby.

Rebmann, T. (2006). Infection prevention: the basics of hand hygiene. *LPN 2006*, 2(6):21-23.

Rebmann, T. (2007). Protect yourself, protect your patients: the essentials of personal protective equipment (PPE). *Nursing Made Incredibly Easy!* 30-39.

Rebmann, T. (2008). Infection protection. Dress up for safety with personal protective equipment (PPE). *LPN 2008*, 4(2):6-13.

Rhinehart, E. (2004). Revised CDC isolation guideline takes home care into account. *Caring*, 23(9):22-27.

Rushing, J. (2006). Wearing personal protective gear. *Nursing 2006*, 36(10):56-57.

Sack, K. (2007). *Deadly bacteria found to be more common*. Available at www.nytimes.com/2007/10/17/healthy17infect.html?_R+1&oref+slogin.

Siegel, J., et al. *Guidelines for isolation: preventing transmission of infectious agents in healthcare settings*. Centers for Disease Control and Prevention. Available at www.cdc.gov/nicd/hip/isguide.htm. Accessed August 4, 2004.

Siegel, J.D., Rhinehart, E., Jackson, M., et al., & Healthcare Infection Control Practices Advisory Committee. (2007). *Guideline for isolation precautions: preventing transmission of infectious agents in healthcare settings*. Available at www.cdc.gov/ncidod/dhqp/pdf/isolation2007.pdf. Accessed July, 2009.

Snow, M. (2006). Combating infection. Preventing salmonella infection. *Nursing 2006*, 36(9):17.

The Joint Commission (TJC). (2009). *National patient safety goals*. Available at www.jointcommission.org/patientsafety/nationalpatientsafetygoals. Accessed December, 2009.

Wood, S., et al. (2007). What you need to know about asepsis. *Nursing 2007*, 37(3):46-51.

United States Department of Labor, Occupational Safety and Health Administration (OSHA). *Respiratory precautions*. Available at www.osha.gov/pls/oshaweb/owadisp.show_document?p_table=STANDARDS&p_id=12716. Accessed July, 2009.

Chapter 13 Surgical Wound Care

Ackley, B.J., & Ladwig, G.B. (2009). *Nursing diagnosis handbook*. (7th ed.). St. Louis: Mosby.

Baranoski, S. (2008). Choosing a wound dressing, Part I. *Nursing 2008*, 28(1):60, 61.

Baranoski, S. (2008). Choosing a wound dressing, Part II. *Nursing 2008*, 38(2):14, 15.

Beare, P., & Myers, J. (2006). *Principles and practice of adult health nursing*. (6th ed.). St. Louis: Mosby.

Beattie, S. (2007). Bedside emergency: wound dehiscence. *RN 2007*, 70(6):34.

Bulechek, G.M., Butcher, H.K., & Dochterman, J.M. (2008). *Nursing interventions classification (NIC)*. (5th ed.). St. Louis: Mosby.

Centers for Disease Control. (1985). Guidelines for prevention of surgical wound infection. *Atlanta Center for Disease Control*, 1955:1-10.

Editorial. (2007). A fount of wound irrigation tips. *Nursing Made Incredibly Easy!* 5(1):14-15.

Editorial. (2007). Wound watch; tips for proper wound irrigation. *LPN 2007*, 3(4):27-28.

Editorial. (2008). Assessing the nutritional status of wound care patients. *LPN 2008*, 4(3):23-36.

Elkin, M.K., Perry, A.G., & Potter, P.A. (2007). *Nursing interventions and clinical skills*. (4th ed.). St. Louis: Mosby.

Frantz, R.A. (2006). Uncover the clues to wound infection. *Nursing Made Incredibly Easy!* 4(5):10.

Giger, J.M., & Davidhizar, R.E. (2007). *Transcultural nursing: assessment and intervention*. (5th ed.). St. Louis: Mosby.

Glenn, Y. (2006). Tape sensitivity: avoiding a sticky situation. *LPN 2006*, 2(6):10, 11.

Glenn, Y. (2006). When your patient is sensitive to tape. *Nursing 2006*, 36(1):17.

Gray, M., & Weir, D. (2007). Prevention and treatment of moisture associated skin damage (maceration) in periwound skin. *Journal of Wound, Ostomy, and Continence Nursing*, 34(2):153.

Harkreader, H., Hogan, M.A., & Thobaben, M. (2007). *Fundamentals of nursing: care and clinical judgment*. (3rd ed.). St. Louis: Mosby.

Hess, C.T. (2004). *Clinical guide to wound care*. (65th ed.). Philadelphia: Lippincott, Williams & Wilkins.

Hunter, S., Thompson, P., Langemo, D., et al. Understanding wound dehiscence. *Nursing 2007*, 37(9):29.

KCI USA. The VAC—vacuum-assisted closure—guidelines for use. *Physician and caregiver reference manual*. Product information, San Antonio, Tex: KCI USA.

Langemo, D., Anderson, J., Hanson, D., et al. (2007). Understanding palliative wound care. *Nursing 2007*, 37(1):18, 21.

Langemo, D., & Hanson, D. (2007). Sizing up your patient's wounds. *LPN 2007*, 3(1):29-30.

Mendez-Eastman, S. (2007). Giving stubborn wounds a helping hand. *Nursing Made Incredibly Easy!* 5(5):18.

Moorhead, S., Johnson, M., Maas, M., et al. (2008). *Nursing outcomes classification (NOC)*. (4th ed.). St. Louis: Mosby.

North American Nursing Diagnosis Association International (NANDA-I). (2009). *NANDA-I nursing diagnoses: definitions and classification 2009-2011*. Oxford, United Kingdom: Author.

Odom-Forren, J. (2006). Preventing surgical site infections. *Nursing 2006*, 36(6):59-63.

Perry, A.G., & Potter, P.A. (2009). *Clinical nursing skills and techniques*. (7th ed.). St. Louis: Mosby.

Potter, P.A., & Perry, A.G. (2007). *Basic nursing: essentials for practice*. (6th ed.). St. Louis: Mosby.

Potter, P.A., & Perry, A.G. (2009). *Fundamentals of nursing: concepts, process, and practice*. (7th ed.). St. Louis: Mosby.

Sardina, D. (2007). Managing and preventing skin tears. *LPN 2007*, 3(5):27.

Sarvis, C. (2006a). Marjolin's ulcer: when healing goes awry. *Nursing 2006*, 36(4):27.

Sarvis, C. (2006b). Post-operative wound care. *Nursing 2006*, 36(12):56.

Sarvis, C. (2007). Using antiseptics to manage infected wounds. *Nursing 2007*, 37(12):20.

Schweon, S. (2006). There's a move about to reduce the number of surgical site infections: are you doing all you should? *RN 2006*, 69(8):37-41.

Springhouse. (2007a). *LPN expert guides: wound care*. Philadelphia: Lippincott Williams & Wilkins.

Springhouse. (2007b). *Wound care facts made incredibly quick!* Philadelphia: Lippincott Williams & Wilkins.

Springhouse. (2007c). *Wound care made incredibly easy!* (2nd ed.). Philadelphia: Lippincott Williams & Wilkins.

Wound Care Strategies, Inc. Available at www.woundcarestrategies.com. Accessed December, 2009.

Chapter 14 Safety

American Society for Microbiology. (n.d.). *Biological weapons control and bioterrorism preparations: information and resources*. Available at www.asmusa.org/pcsrc/bioprep.htm.

Bailes, B.K., & Fasano, N. (1986). The left-handed patient: is there a difference? *Journal of Practical Nursing*, 36(3):28.

Beare, P., & Myers, J. (2006). *Principles and practice of adult health nursing*. (6th ed.). St. Louis: Mosby.

Blocks, M. (2007). Practical solutions for safe patient handling. *LPN 2007*, 3(4):20.

Bulechek, G.M., Butcher, H.K., & Dochterman, J.M. *Nursing interventions classification (NIC)*. (5th ed.). St. Louis: Mosby.

Centers for Disease Control and Prevention (CDC). (1999). *NIOSH alert: preventing needlestick injuries in health care settings*. Cincinnati, OH: Department of Health and Human Services, DHHS Publication No. (NIOSH) 200-208.

Centers for Disease Control and Prevention (CDC). (2001). U.S. Public Health Service guidelines for the management of occupational exposure to HBV, HCV, HIV. Recommendations for past exposure prophylaxis. *MMWR Morbidity and Mortality Weekly Report*, 50(RRII):1-42.

Centers for Disease Control and Prevention (CDC). (n.d.a). *Emergency preparedness and response*. Available at www.bt.cdc.gov. Accessed December, 2009.

Centers for Disease Control and Prevention (CDC). (n.d.b). *The National Institute for Occupational Safety and Health (NIOSH)*. Available at www.cdc.gov/niosh. Accessed December, 2009.

Centers for Disease Control and Prevention (CDC). Home and Recreational Safety. (2007). *Falls among older adults: an overview*. Available at www.cdc.gov/HomeandRecreationalSafety/Falls/adultfalls.html. Accessed December, 2009.

Elkin, M.K., Perry, A.G., & Potter, P.A. (2007). *Nursing interventions and clinical skills*. (4th ed.). St. Louis: Mosby.

Environmental Protective Agency. *Radioactive waste disposal: an environmental perspective*. Available at www.epa.gov/radiation/docs/radwaste. Accessed December, 2009.

Fischer, R.A. (2007). Prevent fires when using oxygen cylinder regulators. *Nursing 2007*, 37(1):20.

Gulanick, M., et al. (2006). *Nursing care plans: nursing diagnoses and interventions*. (6th ed.). St. Louis: Mosby.

Gustafson, S.E. (2007). Assess for fall risk, intervene and bump up patient safety. *Nursing 2007*, 37(12):24.

Harkreader, H., Hogan, M.A., & Thobaben, M. (2007). *Fundamentals of nursing: care and clinical judgment*. (3rd ed.). St. Louis: Mosby.

Hendrick, A. (2007). Predicting patient falls. *American Journal of Nursing*, 107(11):50.

Hockenberry, M.J., & Wilson, D. (2007). *Wong's nursing care of infants and children*. (8th ed.). St. Louis: Mosby.

Jasniewski, J. (2006). Drug file, help your patient avoid medication-related falls. *LPN 2006*, 2(6):4.

Jasniewski, J. (2006). Putting a lid on medication related falls. *Nursing 2006*, 36(6):22.

Joint Commission on Accreditation of Healthcare Organizations (JCAHO). National Patient Safety Goals. (2007). *2007 Hospital/critical access hospital national patient safety goals*. Available at www.jointcommission.org/PatientSafety/NationalPatientSafetyGoals/07_hap_cah_npsgs.htm. Accessed December, 2009.

Lowdermilk, D.L., & Perry, S.E. (2007). *Maternity and women's health care.* (9th ed.). St. Louis: Mosby.

Madden, A.M. (2008).Question of the month; should nurses be finger printed and subject to background checks. *RN 2008,* 70:12.

Metules, T., & Bauer, J. (2007). JCAHO's patient safety goals: a practical guide. Part 1. *RN 2007,* 69(12):21-26.

Mosby's dictionary of medicine, nursing, and health professions. (8th ed.). (2009). St. Louis: Mosby.

North American Nursing Diagnosis Association International (NANDA-I). (2009). *NANDA-I nursing diagnoses: definitions and classification 2009-2011.* Oxford, United Kingdom: Author.

Patient Safety. (2007). Whither do they wander and how can you intervene? *Nursing 2007,* 34(4):14.

Persell, D., et al. (2002). Preparing for bioterrorism. *Nursing 2002,* 32(2):36.

Potter, P.A., & Perry, A.G. (2007). *Basic nursing: essentials for practice.* (6th ed.). St. Louis: Mosby.

Potter, P.A., & Perry, A.G. (2009). *Fundamentals of nursing: concepts, process, and practice.* (7th ed.). St. Louis: Mosby.

Rafter, R.H., & Keown, S. (2006). Aim high: achieving JCAHO's National Patient Safety Goals. *LPN 2006,* 2(6):18.

Ridge, R. (2006). Focusing on JCAHO National Patient Safety Goals. *Nursing 2006,* 36(11):14.

Roman, L. (2006). Professional update. Safe patient lifting is now the law in WA. *RN 2006,* 69(6):17.

Roman, L. (2007). Professional update. CMS tightens rule on restraints and seclusion. *RN 2007,* 70(5):16.

Rushing, J. (2007). Helping a patient who is visually impaired. *Nursing 2007,* 37(8):29.

Taschner, M.A. (2008). Responding to a fire emergency. *Nursing 2008,* 38(5):44-47.

Week, S.K., et al. (2004). A search for ways to prevent a patient from falling. *American Journal of Nursing,* 104(4):72A.

What you must know about new patient safety standards. (2001). *RN 2001,* 64(6):24hf1.

Wong, D.L., Perry, S.E., Hockenberry, M.J., et al. (2006). *Maternal child nursing care.* (3rd ed.). St. Louis: Mosby.

Chapter 15 Body Mechanics and Patient Mobility

Ackley, B.J., & Ladwig, G.B. (2005). *Nursing diagnosis handbook.* (6th ed.). St. Louis: Mosby.

Alitzer, L. (2004). Compartment syndrome. *Orthopedic Nursing,* 23(6):391.

Anderson, D.M., et al. (2006). *Nursing, and allied health dictionary.* (7th ed.). St. Louis: Mosby.

Beare, P., & Myers, J. (2006). *Principles and practice of adult health nursing.* (5th ed.). St. Louis: Mosby.

Converso, A., & Murphy, C. (2004). Winning the battle against back injuries. *RN 2004,* 67(2):53.

deWit, S.C. (2009). *Fundamental concepts and skills for nursing.* (3rd ed.). Philadelphia: Saunders.

Elkin, M.K., Perry, A.G., & Potter, P.A. (2007). *Nursing interventions and clinical skills.* (4th ed.). St. Louis: Mosby.

Giger, J.M., & Davidhizar, R.E. (2007). *Transcultural nursing: assessment and intervention.* (5th ed.). St. Louis: Mosby.

Harkreader, H., Hogan, M.A., & Thobaben, M. (2007). *Fundamentals of nursing: care and clinical judgment.* (3rd ed.). St. Louis: Mosby.

Johnson, M., Dochterman, J.M., & Moorhead, S. (2006). *NANDA, NOC, & NIC linkage: nursing diagnosis, outcomes, & intervention.* (2nd ed.). St. Louis: Mosby.

Kozier, B., et al. (2004). *Fundamentals of nursing concepts, process and practice.* (7th ed.). Upper Saddle River, NJ: Prentice Hall.

Meiner, S.E., & Lueckenotte, A.G. (2006). *Gerontologic nursing,* (3rd ed.). St. Louis: Mosby.

Millsaps, C. (2006). Pay attention to patient positioning. *RN 2006,* 69(1):59.

Monahan, F.D., Sands, J.K., Neighbors, M., et al. (2007). *Phipps' medical-surgical nursing: health and illness perspectives.* (8th ed.). St. Louis: Mosby.

Occupational Safety and Health Administration (OSHA). (2001). Individual factors and epidemiology of work-related musculoskeletal disorders. *OSHA proposed ergonomic standard appendix 1.*

Performing passive range of motion exercises. (2006). *Nursing 2006,* 36(3):50.

Perry, A.G., & Potter, P.A. (2009). *Clinical nursing skills and techniques.* (7th ed.). St. Louis: Mosby.

Potter, P.A., & Perry, A.G. (2007). *Basic nursing: essentials for practice.* (6th ed.). St. Louis: Mosby.

Potter, P.A., & Perry, A.G. (2009). *Fundamentals of nursing: concepts, process, and practice.* (7th ed.). St. Louis: Mosby.

Pullen, R.L., Jr. (2008). Smooth patient transfers: part I transferring a patient from a bed to a stretcher. *Nursing 2008,* 28(1):43.

Pullen, R.L., Jr. (2008). Smooth patient transfers: part II transferring a patient from a bed to a wheelchair. *Nursing 2008,* 38(2):46.

Pullen, R.L., Jr. (2008). Smooth patient transfers: part III using a hydraulic lift. *Nursing 2008,* 38(3):54.

U.S. Department of Veterans Affairs (VA). (2005). *Safe patient handling and movement.* Available at www.visn8.med.va.gov/patientsafety center/safePtHandling/default.asp. Accessed December, 2009.

Chapter 16 Pain Management, Comfort, Rest, and Sleep

Acello, B. (2000). Meeting JCAHO standards for pain control. *Nursing,* 30(3):52.

American Pain Society (APS). (1995). *Principles of analgesic use in the treatment of acute and chronic pain: a concise guide to medical practice.* (2nd ed.). Glenview, IL: Author.

Barkauskas, V., Baumann, L.C., & Darling-Fisher, C. (2006). *Health and physical assessment.* (4th ed.). St. Louis: Mosby.

Beare, P., & D'Arcy, Y. (2007). Managing pain in a patient who's drug-dependent. *Nursing 2007,* 37(3):36.

Berry, P.H., & Dahl, J.L. (2000). The new JCAHO pain standards: implications for pain management nurses. *Pain Management Nursing,* 1(1):3-12.

D'Arcy, Y. (2007a). Managing pain with nonpharmologic therapies. *LPN 2007,* 3(5):10.

D'Arcy, Y. (2007b). Safe pain relief at the push of a button. *Nursing Made Incredibly Easy!* 5(5):9-12.

D'Arcy, Y. (2006). Which analgesic is right for my patient? *Nursing 2006,* 36(7):50.

Dart, R.C., Erdman, A.R., Olson, K.R., et al. (2006). Acetaminophen poisoning: an evidence-based consensus guideline for out-of-hospital management. *Clinical Toxicology,* 44(1):1-18.

Elkin, M.K., Perry, A.G., & Potter, P.A. (2007). *Nursing interventions and clinical skills.* (4th ed.). St. Louis: Mosby.

Geissler, E. (2007). *Cultural assessment.* (4th ed.). St. Louis: Mosby.

Good, M., et al. (2002). Relaxation and music reduce pain after gynecologic surgery. *Pain Management Nursing,* 3(2):61-70.

Hockenberry, M.J., & Wilson, D. (2007). *Wong's nursing care of infants and children.* (8th ed.). St. Louis, Mosby.

Ignatavicius, D.D., & Workman, M.L. (2006). *Medical-surgical nursing: patient-centered collaborative care.* (6th ed.). Philadelphia: Saunders.

Keller, D. (2006). Pain relievers. *RN,* 69(4):22.

Lewis, S.L., Heitkemper, M.M., Dirksen, S.R., et al. (2007). *Medical-surgical nursing: assessment and management of clinical problems.* (7th ed.). St. Louis: Mosby.

Manno, M. (2006). Preventing adverse drug events. *Nursing,* 36(3):56.

Mayer, D.M., et al. (2001). Speaking the language of pain. *American Journal of Nursing,* 101(2):44.

McCaffery, M. (2002a). Teaching your patient to use the pain rating scale. *Nursing,* 32(8):17.

McCaffery, M. (2002b). Your patient is in pain. Here's how you respond. *Nursing,* 32(10):35.

McCaffery, M., & Pasero, C. (2003). *Pain: clinical management.* (3rd ed.). St. Louis: Mosby.

Meinhart, N.T. ,& McCaffery, M. (1983). *Pain: a nursing approach to assessment and analysis.* New York: Appleton-Century-Crofts.

Melzack, R. (1983). *Pain measurement and assessment*. New York: Raven.

Merritt, S. (2000). Putting sleep disorders to rest. *RN*, 63(7):26.

Mosby's dictionary of medicine, nursing, and health professions. (2009). (8th ed.). St. Louis: Mosby.

Pasero, C. (2003). Epidural analgesia for postoperative pain. *American Journal of Nursing*, 103(10):62.

Pasero, C., & McCaffery, M. (2001). Hydromorphone. *American Journal of Nursing*, 101(2):22.

Perry, A.G., & Potter, P.A. (2009). *Clinical nursing skills and techniques*. (7th ed.). St. Louis: Mosby.

Potter, P.A., & Perry, A.G. (2007). *Basic nursing: essentials for practice*. (6th ed.). St. Louis: Mosby.

Potter, P.A., & Perry, A.G. (2009). *Fundamentals of nursing: concepts, process, and practice*. (7th ed.). St. Louis: Mosby.

Shepler, S., et al. (2007). Helping older patients avoid medication mishaps. *LPN*, 3(4):7.

Siedlecki, S. (2004). Assessing chronic pain. *Nursing*, 34(5):18.

Smith, D. (2007). Managing acute acetaminophen toxicity. *Nursing*, 37(1):58.

Tucker, S.M., Cannobio, M.M., Paquette, E.V., et al. (2007). *Patient care standards: collaborative planning and nursing interventions*. (7th ed.). St. Louis: Mosby.

Selected Websites

American Nurses Association. (n.d.). *Position statement on pain management and control of distressing symptoms in dying patients*. Available at www.nursingworld.org/readroom/position/ethics/etpain/htm. Accessed May 7, 2006.

American Pain Foundation. (n.d.). *Pain facts: an overview of American pain surveys*. Available at www.painfoundation.org. Accessed May, 2006.

American Pain Society. (2003). *Principles of analgesic use in the treatment of acute and cancer pain*. (5th ed.). Glenview, IL: American Pain Society. Available at www.ampainsoc.org/pub.principles.htm. Accessed May 20, 2006.

American Pain Society (APS). Available at www.ampainsoc.org. Accessed September, 2005.

American Society of Pain Management Nurses. Available at www.aspmn.org. Accessed September, 2005.

American Society of Pain Management Nursing and American Pain Society. (2004). *Consensus statement: the use of "as needed" range orders for opioid analgesics in the management of acute pain*. Available at www.ampainsoc.org/advocacy/range.htm. Accessed May 20, 2006.

Joint Commission on Accreditation of Health Care Organizations. (2001). *Pain—current understanding of assessment, management, and treatments*. Available at www.ampainsoc.org/ce/downloads/npc/npc.pdf. Accessed October, 2009.

The Joint Commission (TJC). Available at www.jointcommission.org. Accessed December, 2009.

Chapter 17 Complementary and Alternative Therapies

American Holistic Nurses Association (AHNA). (2007). *Holistic nursing: scope and standards of practice*. Silver Spring, Md.: American Nurses Association.

Basch, E.M., & Ulbright, C.E. (2005). *National standard herb and supplement handbook*. St. Louis: Mosby.

Black, J.M., & Hawks, H.J. (2009). *Medical-surgical nursing: clinical management for positive outcomes*. (8th ed.). Philadelphia: Saunders.

Editorial. (2002). Understanding St John's wort. *Nursing*, 32(3):81.

Editorial. (2004). More Americans than ever use CAM, says CDC. *Nursing*, 34(9):73.

Editorial. (2005). Understanding chiropractic practice. *Nursing*, 35(1):73.

Editorial. (2006). Research supports the use of ginseng in fighting colds. *RN*, 69(1).

Editorial. (2007). Get familiar with glucosamine. *Nursing 2007*, 37(10):29.

Editorial. (2007). Herbs at a glance: grape seed extract. *Nursing 2007*, 37(10):20.

Editorial. (2007). How herbal products increase surgical risks. *Nursing 2007*, 37(9):24-25.

Jackson, R., Lacroix, A.Z., et al. (2006). Calcium plus vitamin D supplementation and the risk of fractures. *New England Journal of Medicine*, 35(4):669.

Lai, J.S., et al. (1993). Cardiorespiratory responses of tai chi chuan practitioners and sedentary subjects during cycle ergometry. *Journal of the Formosa Medical Association*, 92(10):894.

Li, F., et al. (2001). An evaluation of the effects of tai chi exercise on physical function among older persons: a randomized controlled trial. *Annals of Behavioral Medicine*, 23(2):139.

Li, F., et al. (2004). Tai chi and self-rated quality of sleep and daytime sleepiness in older adults: a randomized controlled trial. *Journal of the American Geriatric Society*, 52(6):892.

Lorenzo, P. (2003). Complementary therapies—they're not without risk. *RN*, 66(1):65.

Miller, S. (2006). Vitamins and minerals. *RN 2006*, 69(10):37-43.

Mills, S., & Bone, K. (2005). *The essential guide to herbal safety*. St. Louis: Mosby.

Mitzel-Wilkinson, A. (2000). Massage therapy as a nursing practice. *Holistic Nursing Practice*, 14(2):48.

Moraffaghi, Z., et al. (2006). Effects of therapeutic touch on blood hemoglobin and hematocrit levels. *Journal of Holistic Nursing*, 24(1):41.

National Center for Complementary and Alternative Medicine. *Herbs at a glance*. http://nccam.nih.gov/health/herbsataglance.htm.

National Center for Complementary and Alternative Medicine (NCCAM). Available at http://nccam.nih.gov.

Novey, D. (2000). *Clinician's complete reference to complementary and alternative medicine*. St. Louis: Mosby.

Potter, P.A., & Perry, A.G. (2009). *Fundamentals of nursing: concepts, process, and practice*. (7th ed.). St. Louis: Mosby.

Rakel, D.P. & Faass, N. (2006). *Complementary medicine in clinical practice*. Sudbury, Mass.: Jones & Bartlett.

Skidmore-Roth, L. (2006). *Mosby's handbook of herbs and natural supplements*. (3rd ed.). St. Louis: Mosby.

Song, R., et al. (2003). Effects of tai chi exercise on pain, balance, muscle strength, and perceived difficulties in physical functioning in older women with osteoarthritis: a randomized clinical trial. *The Journal of Rheumatology*, 30(9):2039.

Taylor, E.J., & Oultau, F.H. (2002). Use of prayer among persons with cancer. *Holistic Nursing Practice*, 16(3):46.

Yang, Y., Zhiqiang, F., & Schlageal, R. (2008). *Taijiquan: the art of nurturing—the science of power*. (2nd ed.). Champaign, Ill: Zhenwu.

Chapter 18 Hygiene and Care of the Patient's Environment

Ackley, B.J., & Ladwig, G.B. (2009). *Nursing diagnosis handbook*. (7th ed.). St. Louis: Mosby.

Anderson, D.M., et al. (2006). *Mosby's medical, nursing, and allied health dictionary*. (7th ed.). St. Louis: Mosby.

Anderson, J. (2007). What you can learn from a comprehensive skin assessment. *Nursing*, 37(4):65-66.

Ayello, E.A., & Lyder, C.H. (2007). Protecting patients from harm: preventing pressure ulcers in hospital patients, 2007. *Nursing*, 13(10):36.

Baldwin, K.M. (2006). Damage control: preventing and treating pressure ulcers. *Nursing Made Incredibly Easy!* 4(1):13-26.

Baraaoski, S. (2006). Pressure ulcers: a renewed awareness. *Nursing 2006*, 36(8):36-41.

Barrick, A.L., et al. (2002). *Bathing without a bathtub—personal care of individuals with dementia*. New York: Springer.

Black, J. (2006). Saving the skin during kinetic bed therapy, 2006. *Nursing*, 36(10):17.

Bulechek, G.M., Butcher, H.K., & Dochterman, J.M. (2008). *Nursing interventions classification (NIC)*. (5th ed.). St. Louis: Mosby.

Duhon, J. (2007). Taking the pressure out of pressure ulcer therapy. *RN 2007*, 70(2):25-31.

Duimel-Peeters I. (2005). Preventing pressure ulcers with massage? *American Journal of Nursing*, 105(8):31, 33.

Elkin, M.K., Perry, A.G., & Potter, P.A. (2007). *Nursing interventions and clinical skills*. (4th ed.). St. Louis: Mosby.

Giger, J.M., & Davidhizar, R.E. (2007). *Transcultural nursing: assessment and intervention*. (5th ed.). St. Louis: Mosby.

Glenn, Y. (2006). When your patient is sensitive to tape. *Nursing 2006*, 36(1):17.

Hanson, D., & Thompson, P. (2007). Measuring wounds. *Nursing 2007*, 37(2):18-21.

Harkreader, H., Hogan, M.A., & Thobaben, M. (2007). *Fundamentals of nursing: care and clinical judgment*. (3rd ed.). St. Louis: Mosby.

Hopkins, A., et al. (2006). Patient stories of living with a pressure ulcer. *Journal of Advanced Nursing*, 56(4):245-353.

Jarvis, C. (2008). *Physical examination and health assessment*. (5th ed.). Philadelphia: Saunders.

The Joint Commission. Available at www.thejointcommission.org.

Kozier, B., et al. (2004). *Fundamentals of nursing concepts, process and practice*. (6th ed.). Upper Saddle River, NJ: Prentice Hall.

Mascolo, L. (2006). Skin care team improves assessment and documentation. *Nursing 2006*, 36(10):66-67.

Moorhead, S., Johnson M., Maas, M., et al. (2008). *Nursing outcomes classification (NOC)*. (4th ed.). St. Louis: Mosby.

National Pressure Ulcer Advisory Panel. *Updated staging system*. Available at www.npuap.org/pr2.htm. Accessed August 26, 2009.

North American Nursing Diagnosis Association International (NANDA-I). (2009). *NANDA-I nursing diagnoses: definitions and classification 2009-2011*. Oxford, United Kingdom: Author.

Potter, P.A., & Perry, A.G. (2007). *Basic nursing: essentials for practice*. (6th ed.). St. Louis: Mosby.

Potter, P.A., & Perry, A.G. (2009). *Fundamentals of nursing: concepts, process, and practice*. (7th ed.). St. Louis: Mosby.

Rasin, J., & Barrick, A.L. (2004). Bathing patients with dementia—concentrating on the patient's needs rather than the task. *American Journal of Nursing*, 104(3):30-34

Reddy, M., et al. (2006). Preventing pressure ulcers: a systematic review. *Journal of the American Medical Association*, 296(8): 974-984.

Slotts, N.A. (2007). Predicting pressure ulcer risk. *American Journal of Nursing*, 107(11):40-48.

Spilsbury, K., et al. (2007). Pressure ulcers and their treatment and effects on quality of life; hospital inpatient perspectives. *Journal of Advanced Nursing*, 57(5):494-504.

Zulkowski, K., & Ratliff, C. (2006). Perineal dermatitis or pressure ulcer: how can you tell? *Nursing 2006*, 36(12):22-23.

Chapter 19 Specimen Collection and Diagnostic Examination

Ackley, B.J., & Ladwig, G.B. (2009). *Nursing diagnosis handbook*. (7th ed.). St. Louis: Mosby.

Anderson, D.M., et al. (2006). *Mosby's medical, nursing, and allied health dictionary*. (7th ed.). St. Louis: Mosby.

Brege, D.J. (2007). Take a look inside the blood vessels with angiography. *Nursing Made Incredibly Easy 2007*, 5(6):14-18.

Brege, D.J. (2008). Action stat: contrast reaction. *Nursing 2008*, 38(3):72.

Centers for Disease Control and Prevention (CDC). (2005). Updated U.S. public health service guidelines for the management of occupational exposures to HIV and recommendations for past exposure prophylaxis. Washington, DC: Author.

Craven, R.F., & Hirnle, C.J. (Eds.). (2007). *Fundamentals of nursing skills*. Philadelphia: Lippincott Williams & Wilkins.

Dale, L. (2006). Making a point about alternate site blood glucose sampling. *Nursing 2006*, 36(2):52.

Davis, K. (2004). Need urine from a catheter system? Forget the needle. *Nursing 2004*, 34(12):64.

Editorial. (2007). Disciplining diagnostics: take a look inside the lungs with bronchoscopy. *Nursing Made Incredibly Easy!* 5(2):11-12.

Elkin, M.K., Perry, A.G., & Potter, P.A. (2007). *Nursing interventions and clinical skills*. (4th ed.). St. Louis: Mosby.

Ellis, J.R., & Bentz, P.M. (Eds.). (2007). *Modules for basic nursing skills*. Philadelphia: Lippincott Williams & Wilkins.

Goldich, G. (2006). Understanding the 12-lead ECG Part I. *Nursing 2006*, 36(11):36-41.

Goldich, G. (2006). Understanding the 12-lead ECG Part II. *Nursing 2006*, 36(11):36-41.

Gonzales, F. (2004). How will your patient respond to contrast media? *Nursing 2004*, 34(1):32hn1.

Infusion Nurses Society (INS). (2006). Infusion nursing standards of practice. *Journal of Infusion Nurses Society*, 29(1 Suppl):S1-S92.

Kruger, A. (2007). Photo-guide. Need help finding a vein. *Nursing 2007*, 37(6):39-41.

LPN expert guide: wound care. (2007). Philadelphia: Lippincott, Williams & Wilkins.

North American Nursing Diagnosis Association International (NANDA-I). (2009). *NANDA-I nursing diagnoses: definitions and classification 2009-2011*. Oxford, United Kingdom: Author.

Occupational Safety and Health Administration. (1991). Occupational exposure to bloodborne pathogens. Final Rule 29CR7 1919:10:30. *Federal Register*, 56, 64, 175.

Occupational Safety and Health Administration. (2001a). Enforcement procedures for the occupational exposure to bloodborne injury, final rule. *Federal Register*, 66:5318.

Occupational Safety and Health Administration (2001b). Needlestick safety and prevention act. *Public Law 106-430*.

Ott, L.K. (2008). Eye on diagnostics: assessing blood flow with CT angiography. *Nursing 2008*, 28(1):26.

Pagana, K.D., & Pagana, T.J. (2007). *Mosby's diagnostic and laboratory test reference*. (8th ed.). St. Louis: Mosby.

Perry, A.G., & Potter, P.A. (2009). *Clinical nursing skills and techniques*. (7th ed.). St. Louis: Mosby.

Potter, P.A., & Perry, A.G. (2007). *Basic nursing: essentials for practice*. (6th ed.). St. Louis: Mosby.

Rushing, J. (2006). Clinical do's and don'ts: assisting with bone marrow aspiration and biopsy. *Nursing 2006*, 36(3):68.

Rushing, J. (2006). Clinical do's and don'ts: assisting with thoracentesis. *Nursing 2006*, 36(12):8.

Rushing, J. (2007). Clinical do's and don'ts: assisting with lumbar puncture. *Nursing 2007*, 37(1):23.

Rushing, J. (2007). Clinical do's and don'ts: obtaining a throat culture. *Nursing 2007*, 37(3):20.

Rushing, J. (2007). Clinical do's and don'ts: obtaining a wound culture specimen. *Nursing 2007*, 37(11):20.

Schock, L., & Whitman, K. (2007). Maintaining liver function. *Nursing 2007*, November, 22-23.

Wound care made incredibly easy. (2nd ed.). (2006). Philadelphia: Lippincott, Williams & Wilkins.

Wound watch, three techniques for collecting wound specimens. (2008). *LPN 2008*, 4(1), 24-25.

Chapter 20 Selected Nursing Skills

Ackley, B.J., & Ladwig, G.B. (2009). *Nursing diagnosis handbook*. (7th ed.). St. Louis: Mosby.

American Association of Blood Banks. (2007). *Standards for blood banks and transfusion services*. (23rd ed.). Bethesda, Md.: American Association of Blood Banks.

Arbique, J., & Arbique, D. (2007). Reducing the risk of nerve injuries. *Nursing 2007*, 37(11):20-21.

Beattie, S. (2006). Back to basics with O_2 therapy. *RN*, 69(9):37-40.

Boyce, J.M., & Pittet, D.; Healthcare Infection Control Practices Advisory Committee, & HICPAC/SHEA/APIC/IDSA Hand Hygiene Task Force. (2002). Guideline for hand hygiene in health-care settings. Recommendatons of the Healthcare Infection Control Practices Advisory Committee and the HICPAC/SHEA/APIC/IDSA

Hand Hygiene Task Force. *Infection Control and Hospital Epidemiology,* 23(12 Suppl):S3-S40.

Crumm, E. Can a bloodless surgery program work in a trauma setting? *Nursing 2007,* 37(3):54-56.

Davis, M.M., & Johnston, J. (2008). Maintaining supplemental O_2 during transport. *American Journal of Nursing,* 108(8):35.

Editorial. (2007). Skill building: now to apply an ostomy pouch. *LPN 2007,* 3(3):20-22.

Editorial. (2008). Calculating IV infusion rates. *Nursing 2008,* 4(3): 21-22.

Elkin, M.K., Perry, A.G., & Potter, P.A. (2007). *Nursing interventions and clinical skills.* (4th ed.). St. Louis: Mosby.

Frey, A.M., & Schears, G.J. (2006). What's the best way to secure a catheter? *Nursing 2006,* 36(9):30-31.

Giger, J.M., & Davidhizar, R.E. (2007). *Transcultural nursing: assessment and intervention.* (5th ed.). St. Louis: Mosby.

Guthrie, D., Dreher, D., & Munson, M. (2007). What you need to know about PICC, Part 1. *Nursing 2007,* 37(8):18.

Guthrie, D., Dreher, D., & Munson, M. (2007). What you need to know about PICC, Part 2. *Nursing 2007,* 37(8):14-15.

Hadaway, L.C. (2006). Tips using implanted ports safely. *Nursing 2006,* 36(8):66-67.

Harkreader, H., Hogan, M.A., & Thobaben, M. (2007). *Fundamentals of nursing: care and clinical judgment.* (3rd ed.). St. Louis: Mosby.

Hyland, J.M. (2004). Basics of ostomies. *Gastroenterology Nursing,* 25(6):241.

Infusion Nurses Society (INS). (2000). Local complication of nursing interventions on peripheral veins. *Journal of Infusion Nursing,* 23(3):167.

Infusion Nurses Society (INS). 220 Norwood Park South. Norwood, MA 02052.

Infusion Nurses Society. (2006). Infusion nursing standards of practice. *Journal of Intravenous Nursing, 29*(1S):S59.

Jacobs, B. (2006). IV rounds using an infusion pump safely. *Nursing 2006,* 36(10):24.

Krueger, A. (2007). Need help finding a vein? *Nursing 2007,* 37(6): 39-41.

Lewis, S.L., Heitkemper, M.M., Dirksen, S.R., et al. (2007). *Medical-surgical nursing: assessment and management of clinical problems.* (7th ed.). St. Louis: Mosby.

Marders, J. (2005). Sounding the alarm for IV infiltration. *Nursing 2005,* 3(1):22.

Metules, T.J. (2007). Hands on help. Hot and cold packs. *RN 2007,* 70(1):45-48.

Mosby's dictionary of medicine, nursing, and health professions. (8th ed.). (2009). St. Louis: Mosby.

Movreau, N.L. (2004). Tips for inserting an IV in an older patient. *Nursing 2004,* 34(7):18.

North American Nursing Diagnosis Association International (NANDA-I). (2009). *NANDA-I nursing diagnoses: definitions and classification 2009-2011.* Oxford, United Kingdom: Author.

O'Grady, N.P., Alexander, M., Dellinger, E.P., et al.; Centers for Disease Control and Prevention (CDC). (2002). Guidelines for the prevention of intravascular catheter-related infection. *MMWR Morbidity and Mortality Weekly Report,* 51(RR-10):1-29.

Overstreet, M. (2004). How does a peg tube stay in? *Nursing,* 34(6):21.

Potter, P.A., & Perry, A.G. (2007). *Basic nursing: essentials for practice.* (6th ed.). St. Louis: Mosby.

Potter, P.A., & Perry, A.G. (2009). *Fundamentals of nursing: concepts, process, and practice.* (7th ed.). St. Louis: Mosby.

Pullen, R.L., Jr. (2004). Inserting an indwelling urinary catheter in a male patient, *Nursing 2004,* 34(7):24.

Pullen, R.L., Jr. (2004). Measuring gastric residual volume. *Nursing 2004,* 34(4):18.

Pullen, R.L., Jr. (2005). Tips for using dry heat therapy. *Nursing 2005,* 35(12):18.

Pullen, R.L., Jr. (2006). Teaching your patient to irrigate a colostomy. *Nursing 2006,* 36(4):22.

Pullen, R.L., Jr. (2007). Replacing a urostomy drainage pouch. *Nursing 2007,* 37(6):14.

Regan, E.N., & Dallachiesa, L. (2009). How to take care of a patient with a tracheostomy. *Nursing 2009,* 39(8):34-39.

Rosenthal, K. (2004). It's not magic! The tricks to cannulating difficult veins. *Nursing Made Incredibly Easy!* 2(2):4-7.

Rosenthal, K. (2004). Phlebitis: an irritating complication. *Nursing Made Incredibly Easy!* 2(1):62-63.

Rosenthal, K. (2004). Selecting the best IV site for an obese patient. *Nursing,* 34(11):14.

Rosenthal, K. (2005). Avoiding bad blood–key steps to safe transfusion. *Nursing Made Incredibly Easy!* 3(5):20.

Rosenthal, K. (2006). IV essentials: the why's and wherefores of IV fluids. *Nursing Made Incredibly Easy!* 4(3):8-11.

Rosenthal, K. (2006). IV rounds: what you need to know about ports. *Nursing 2006,* 36(1):20-21.

Rosenthal, K. (2007). Intravenous fluids: the why's and wherefores. *Nursing 2006,* 36(7):26.

Rosenthal, K. (2007). IV rounds: are you up to date with the infusion nursing standards? *Nursing 2007,* 37(7)15.

Rosenthal, K. (2007).What's new in the infusion nursing standards? *Nursing Made Incredibly Easy!* 5(1):12-13.

Rushing, J. (2004). Inserting an indwelling urinary catheter in a female patient. *Nursing 2004,* 34(8):22.

Rushing, J. (2006). Clinical do's and don't's: caring for your patient with a suprapubic catheter. *Nursing 2006,* 36(7):32.

Schmelzer, M., et al. (1993). Say nope to soap. *American Journal of Nursing,* 93(3):21.

Smeltzer, S.C., Bare, B.G., Hinkle, J.L., et al. (2007). *Brunner and Suddarth's textbook of medical-surgical nursing.* (11th ed.). Philadelphia: Lippincott Williams and Wilkins.

Smith, S.F., Duell, D.J., & Martin, B.C. (2004). *Clinical nursing skills—basic to advanced skills.* (6th ed.). Upper Saddle River, NJ: Prentice Hall.

U.S. Food and Drug Administration. (2003). *Reports of blue discoloration and death in patients receiving the dye FDA blue #1.* Available at www.cfsan.fda.gov/dms/col-ltr2.html.

Weaner, R., & McDonald, M. (2006). What you need to know about infusing platelets. *Nursing 2006,* 36(6): 26-27.

Weitzel, T., et al. (2008). Up front. Doing it better: to cath or not to cath? *Nursing 2008,* 38(2):20-21.

Chapter 21 Basic Nutrition and Nutrition Therapy

American Academy of Pediatrics. (2001). American Academy of Pediatrics Committee on Nutrition policy statement: the use and misuse of fruit juice in pediatrics. *Pediatrics,* 107(5):1210.

American Congress of Obstetricians and Gynecologists. (2004). Practice bulletin no. 52: nausea and vomiting of pregnancy. *Obstetrics and Gynecology,* 103:803.

American Congress of Obstetricians and Gynecologists. (2005). ACOG Committee Opinion #315: Obesity in pregnancy. *Obstetrics and Gynecology,* 106:671.

American Diabetes Association. (2008). Position statement: nutrition recommendations and interventions for diabetes. *Diabetes Care,* 31 (suppl. 1):S61.

American Diabetes Association. (n.d.). *Diabetes basics.* Available at http://www.diabetes.org/diabetes-basics/. Accessed December, 2009.

American Dietetic Association. (2006). Nutrition intervention in the treatment of anorexia nervosa, bulimia, nervosa, and other eating disorders. *The Journal of the American Dietetic Association,* 106(12):2073.

American Dietetic Association. (2008). Dietary guidance for healthy children aged 2 to 11 years. *The Journal of the American Dietetic Association,* 108(6):1038.

American Dietetic Association. (2008). Nutrition and lifestyle for a healthy pregnancy outcome. *The Journal of the American Dietetic Association,* 108:553.

American Heart Association Nutrition Committee; Lichtenstein, A.H., Appel, L.J., Brands, M., et al. (2006). Diet and lifestyle recommendations revision 2006: a scientific statement from the American Heart Association Nutrition Committee. *Circulation*, 114:82-96.

American Heart Association. (n.d.). *Diet and lifestyle recommendations*. Available at www.americanheart.org/presenter.jhtml?identifier=851. Accessed August, 2009.

Bessesen, D.H. (2008). Update on obesity. *Journal of Clinical Endocrinology and Metabolism*, 93:2027.

Buchwald, H., Avidor, Y., Brauwald, E., et al. (2004). Bariatric surgery: a systematic review and meta-analysis. *Journal of the American Medical Association*, 292(14):1724.

Butte, N., Cobb, K., Dwyer, J., et al. (2004). The Start Healthy Feeding Guidelines for infants and toddlers. *Journal of the American Dietetics Association*, 104(3):442.

Center for Science in the Public Interest. (2007). *Caffeine content of food & drug*. Available at www.cspinet.org/new/cafchart.htm. Accessed July, 2008.

Centers for Disease Control and Prevention (CDC). (2008). *Overweight and obesity*. Available at www.cdc.gov/nccdphp/dnpa/obesity. Accessed July, 2008.

Daniels, J. (2006). Obesity: America's epidemic. *American Journal of Nursing*, 106(1):40.

Elkin, M.K., Perry, A.G., & Potter, P.A. (2007). *Nursing interventions and clinical skills*. (4th ed.). St. Louis: Mosby.

Grundy, S.M., Cleeman, J.I., Daniels, S.R., et al. (2005). Diagnosis and management of the metabolic syndrome. *Circulation*, 112(17):2735-2752.

Institute of Medicine. (1990). *Nutrition during pregnancy. Part I weight gain and Part II nutrient supplements*. Washington, DC: National Academies Press.

Institute of Medicine, Food and Nutrition Board. (1997). *Dietary reference intakes for calcium, phosphorus, magnesium, vitamin D, and fluoride*. Washington, DC: National Academies Press.

Institute of Medicine, Food and Nutrition Board. (1998). *Dietary reference intakes for thiamin, riboflavin, niacin, vitamin B_6, folate, vitamin B_{12}, pantothenic acid, biotin, and choline*. Washington, DC: National Academies Press.

Institute of Medicine, Food and Nutrition Board. (2000a). *Dietary reference intakes: applications in dietary assessment*. Washington, DC: National Academies Press.

Institute of Medicine, Food and Nutrition Board. (2000b). *Dietary reference intakes for vitamin C, vitamin E, selenium, and carotenoids*. Washington, DC: National Academies Press.

Institute of Medicine, Food and Nutrition Board. (2001). *Dietary reference intakes for vitamin A, vitamin K, arsenic, boron, chromium, copper, iodine, iron, molybdenum, nickel, silicon, vanadium, and zinc*. Washington, DC: National Academies Press.

Institute of Medicine, Food and Nutrition Board. (2003). *Dietary reference intakes: guiding principles for nutrition labeling and fortification*. Washington, DC: National Academies Press.

Institute of Medicine, Food and Nutrition Board. (2004). *Dietary reference intakes for water, potassium, sodium, chloride, and sulfate*. Washington, DC: National Academies Press.

Institute of Medicine, Food and Nutrition Board. (2005). *Dietary reference intakes for energy, carbohydrate, fiber, fat, fatty acids, cholesterol, protein, and amino acids (macronutrients)*. Washington, DC: National Academies Press.

Klein, S., Allison, D.B., Heymsfield, S.B., et al. (2007). Waist circumference and cardiometabolic risk: a consensus statemement from Shaping America's Health: Association for Weight Management and Obesity Prevention; NAASO, The Obesity Society; the American Society for Nutrition; and the American Diabetes Association. *The American Journal of Clinical Nutrition*, 85:1197-1202.

Mozaffarian, D., Katan, M.B., Ascherio, A., et al. (2006). *Trans* fatty acids and cardiovascular disease. *The New England Journal of Medicine*, 354(15): 1601-1613.

National Eating Disorders Association. (n.d.). *Health consequences of eating disorders*. Available at www.nationaleatingdisorders.org/p.asp?WebPage_ID=286&Profile_ID=41143. Accessed December, 2009.

National Institutes of Health, National Heart, Lung, and Blood Institute. (2001). *The DASH diet*. NIH publication no. 01-4082. Washington, DC: U.S. Government Printing Office.

National Institutes of Health, National Heart, Lung, and Blood Institute. (2001). *Third report of the National Cholesterol Education Program (NCEPP) expert panel on detection, evaluation and treatment of high blood cholesterol in adults (ATP III) executive summary*. NIH publication no. 01-3670. Washington, DC: U.S. Government Printing Office.

Oranzo, J., & Scott, J.G. (2004). Diagnosis and treatment of obesity in adults: an applied evidence-based review. *The Journal of the American Board of Family Practice*, 17:359.

Parkes, E. (2006). Nutritional management of patients after bariatric surgery. *The American Journal of the Medical Sciences*, 331(4):207.

Peters, R.M., & Flack, J.M. (2004). Hypertensive disorders of pregnancy. *Journal of Obstetric, Gynecologic, and Neonatal Nursing*, 33:209.

Pitkin, R.M. (2007). Folate and neural tube defects. *American journal of clinical nutrition*, 85(1):2855S.

Schaible, U.E., & Kaufmann, S.H. (2007). Malnutrition and infection: complex mechanisms and global impacts. *PLoS Medicine*, 4(5):e115.

Theuwissen, E., & Mensink, R.P. (2008). Water-soluble dietary fibers and cardiovascular disease. *Physiology & Behavior*, 94(2):285.

Toth, P.P. (2005). The "good cholesterol:" high-density lipoprotein. *Circulation*, 111:e89.

U.S. Department of Agriculture. (n.d.). USDA national nutrient database for standard reference, release 22. Available at U.S. Department of Health and Human Services and U.S. Department of Agriculture. (2005). *Dietary guidelines for Americans*. (6th ed.). Washington, DC: U.S. Government Printing Office.

U.S. Department of Health and Human Services, U.S. Department of Agriculture. (2005). *Nutrition and your health: dietary guidelines for Americans*. Available at www.health.gov/dietaryguidelines. Accessed July, 2008.

Vainer, V. (2008). Treatment modalities of obesity: what fits whom? *Diabetes Care*, 31(suppl. 2):S269.

Weickert, M.O., et al. (2008). Metabolic effect of dietary fiber consumption and prevention of diabetes. *Journal of Nutrition*, 138(3): 439.

Wheeler, M. (2003). Nutrient database for the 2003 exchange lists for meal planning. *Journal of the American Dietetic Association*, 103(7): 894.

World Health Organization. (2001). *Global burden of protein-energy malnutrition in the year 2000*. Available at www.who.int/healthinfo/statistics/bod_malnutrition.pdf. Accessed September, 2009.

Chapter 22 **Fluids and Electrolytes**

Ackley, B.J., & Ladwig, G.B. (2005). *Nursing diagnosis handbook*. (6th ed.). St. Louis: Mosby.

Barkauskas, V., Baumann, L.C., & Darling-Fisher, C. (2006). *Health and physical assessment*. (4th ed.). St. Louis: Mosby.

Bixby, M. (2006). Third-spacing: where has all the fluid gone? *Nursing Made Incredibly Easy!* 4(5):42-53.

Burger, C. (2004. Hypokalemia—averting crisis with early recognition and intervention. *American Journal of Nursing*, 104(11):61.

Diehl-Oplinger, L. (2004). Choosing the right fluid to counter hypovolemic shock. *Nursing*, 34(3):42.

Editorial. (2002). Incredibly easy, understanding hypokalemia. *Nursing 2002*, 32(3):54.

Elkin, M.K., Perry, A.G., & Potter, P.A. (2007). *Nursing interventions and clinical skills*. (4th ed.). St. Louis: Mosby.

Gahart, B.L., & Nazareno, A.R. (2010). *2010 Intravenous medications: a handbook for nurses and health professionals*. St. Louis: Mosby.

Goertz, S. (2006). Gauging fluid balance with osmolality. *Nursing 2006*, 36(10):70.

Hayes, D. (2004). What happens when sodium and water are off kilter? *Nursing Made Incredibly Easy!* 2(1):42.

Lewis, S.L., Heitkemper, M.M., Dirksen, S.R., et al. (2007). *Medical-surgical nursing: assessment and management of clinical problems*. (7th ed.). St. Louis: Mosby.

Monahan, F.D., Sands, J.K., Neighbors, M., et al. (2007). *Phipps' medical-surgical nursing: health and illness perspectives.* (8th ed.). St. Louis: Mosby.

Mosby's dictionary of medicine, nursing, and health professions. (2006). (7th ed.). St. Louis: Mosby.

Pagana, K.D., & Pagana, T.J. (2006). *Diagnostic testing and nursing implications.* (6th ed.). St. Louis: Mosby.

Potter, P.A., & Perry, A.G. (2009). *Fundamentals of nursing: concepts, process, and practice.* (7th ed.). St. Louis: Mosby.

Springhouse. (1997). *Fluids and electrolytes made incredibly easy.* Springhouse, PA: Springhouse.

Thibodeau, G., & Patton, K. (2008). *Structure and function of the human body.* (13th ed.). St. Louis: Mosby.

Thompson, J.M., et al. (2005). *Mosby's clinical nursing.* (6th ed.). St. Louis: Mosby.

Weldy, N.J. (2008). *Body fluids and electrolytes: a programmed presentation.* (10th ed.). St. Louis: Mosby.

Chapter 23 Mathematics Review and Medication Administration

Ackley, B.J., & Ladwig, G.B. (2009). *Nursing diagnosis handbook.* (7th ed.). St. Louis: Mosby.

American Diabetes Association. (2004). Insulin administration. *Diabetes Care,* 27(Suppl 1):S106-109.

Brown, M., & Mulholland, J. (2008). *Drug calculations: process and problems for clinical practice.* (8th ed.). St. Louis: Mosby.

Caesar, B., et al. (2006). Reducing medication errors by using applied technology. *Nursing 2006,* 36(3):24.

Capriotti, T. (2005). Changes in inhaler devices for asthma and COPD. *MedSurg,* 14(3):185.

Clark, J.B., et al. (2008). *Pharmacologic basis of nursing practice.* (8th ed.). St. Louis: Mosby.

Clayton, D., & Stock Y.N. (2008). *Basic pharmacology for nurses.* (14th ed.). St. Louis: Mosby.

Cohen, H., et al. (2003). Getting to the root of medication errors: survey results. *Nursing,* 33(9):36.

Colihan, K. (2008). *Hands-only CPR gets thumbs up.* Available at www.webmd.com/heart-disease/news/20080331/hands-only-cpr-gets-thumbs-up. Accessed December, 2009.

Dison, N. (2009). *Simplified drugs and solutions for nurses.* (14th ed.). St. Louis: Mosby.

Ebersole, P., Touhy, T., Hess, P., et al. (2008). *Toward healthy aging: human needs and nursing response.* (7th ed.). St. Louis: Mosby.

Editorial. (2007). Skill building-easy does it. Administering rectal suppositories and ointments. *LPN 2007,* 4(3):4.

Editorial. (2004a). JCAHO says watch your p's and q's. *Nursing 2004,* 34(3):55.

Editorial. (2004b). The dosage calculation two-step. *Nursing Made Incredibly Easy!* 2(2).

Editorial. (2003a). Incredibly easy: ins and outs of giving drugs transmucosally. *Nursing 2003,* 33(8):84.

Editorial. (2003b). The ins and outs of giving drugs transmucosally. *Nursing 2003,* 33(8):84.

Editorial. (2002). Giving Z-track injections. *Nursing 2002,* 32(9):81.

Elkin, M.K., Perry, A.G., & Potter, P.A. (2007). *Nursing interventions and clinical skills.* (4th ed.). St. Louis: Mosby.

Gahart, B.L., & Nazareno, A.R. (2010). *2010 Intravenous medications: a handbook for nurses and health professionals.* St. Louis: Mosby.

Giger, J.M., & Davidhizar, R.E. (2007). *Transcultural nursing: assessment and intervention.* (5th ed.). St. Louis: Mosby.

Grissinger, M., & Globus, N. (2004). How technology affects your risk of medication errors. *Nursing,* 34(1):35.

Hockenberry, M.J., & Wilson, D. (2007). *Wong's nursing care of infants and children.* (8th ed.). St. Louis, Mosby.

Ignatavicius, D.D. (2000). Asking the right questions about medication safety. *Nursing,* 30(9):51.

Ignatavicius, D.D., & Workman, M.L. (2006). *Medical-surgical nursing: patient-centered collaborative care.* (6th ed.). Philadelphia: Saunders.

Institute for Safe Medication Practices (ISMP). (2006). *Suppository stories, medication safety alert 2006.* Available at www.ismp.org/consumers/suppository.asp.

Jarvis, C. (2008). *Physical examination and health assessment.* (5th ed.). Philadelphia: Saunders.

The Joint Commission. (2005). National safety goals and requirements: hospital. Available at www.jointcommission.org/GeneralPublic/NPSG/05_gp_npsg.htm. Accessed September 15, 2009.

Kee, J., & Hayes, E. (2007). *Pharmacology: a nursing process approach.* (5th ed.). St. Louis: Saunders.

Kling, L. (2003). Subcutaneous insulin technique. *Nursing Standard,* 17(34):45.

Lewis, S.L., Heitkemper, M.M., Dirksen, S.R., et al. (2007). *Medical-surgical nursing: assessment and management of clinical problems.* (7th ed.). St. Louis: Mosby.

Lilley, L., & Harrington, S. (2007). *Pharmacology and the nursing process.* (4th ed.). St. Louis: Mosby.

McConnell, E.A. (2000). Administering subcutaneous heparin. *Nursing,* 30(6):17.

McKenry, L.M., & Salerno, E. (2008). *Mosby's pharmacology in nursing.* (23rd ed.). St. Louis: Mosby.

Metules, T., et al. (2007). JCAHO's patient safety goals: preventing med errors. *RN,* 70(1):39-43.

Meyer, T. (2004). Calculating drug dosages accurately. *American Journal of Nursing,* 104(11):13.

Miller, D. (2000). To crush or not to crush. *Nursing,* 30(2):51.

Myers, J. (2006). *Quick medication administration references.* (5th ed.). St. Louis: Mosby.

Nicoll, L.H., et al. (2002). Intramuscular injection: an integrative research review and guideline for evidence-based practice. *Applied Nursing Research,* 16(2):149.

Occupational Health and Safety Administration. (2009). Bloodborne pathogens and needlestick prevention. Hazard recognition. Available at www.osha.gov/SLTC/bloodbornepathogens/recognition.html. Accessed December, 2009.

Otto, S. (2008). *Mosby's pocket guide to intravenous therapy.* (6th ed.). St. Louis: Mosby.

Perry, A.G., & Potter, P.A. (2009). *Clinical nursing skills and techniques.* (7th ed.). St. Louis: Mosby.

Pope, B. (2002). How to administer subcutaneous and intramuscular injections. *Nursing,* 32(1):50.

Potter, P.A., & Perry, A.G. (2007). *Basic nursing: essentials for practice.* (6th ed.). St. Louis: Mosby.

Potter, P.A., & Perry, A.G. (2009). *Fundamentals of nursing: concepts, process, and practice.* (7th ed.). St. Louis: Mosby.

Pullen, R. (2003). Managing IV patient-controlled analgesia. *Nursing,* 33(7):24.

Rodger, M.A., et al. (2000). Drawing up and administering intramuscular injections: a review of the literature. *Journal of Advanced Nursing,* 31(3):574.

Rubin, D.K., et al. (2005). How do clients determine that their metered dose inhaler is empty? *Chest,* 126(4):1134.

Rushing, J. (2007). Administering eye drops. *Nursing,* 37(5):18.

Schulmeister, L. (2007). Stuck on you: transdermal drug patches. *Nursing Made Incredibly Easy!* 5(2):17-19.

Skidmore-Roth, L. (2009). *Mosby's 2009 nursing drug reference.* St. Louis: Mosby.

Chapter 24 Emergency First Aid Nursing

American Academy of Pediatrics, Committee on Injury, Violence and Poison Preventions. (2003). Poison treatment in the home. *Pediatrics,* 112(5):1182-1185.

American Heart Association (AHA). (2006). *BLS for healthcare providers.* Available at www.americanheart.org/cpr. Accessed December, 2009.

American Society for Microbiology. (n.d.). *Biological weapons control and bioterrorism preparations: information and resources.* Available at www.asmusa.org/pcsrc/bioprep.htm.

Beattie, S. (2006). In from the cold-hypothermia. *RN 2006,* 69(11):22.

Bessen, H.A. (2008). Hypothermia. In J.E. Tintinalli, G.D. Kelen, & S.J. Stapczynski (Eds.). *Emergency medicine: a comprehensive study guide.* (7th ed.). New York: McGraw-Hill.

Brettler, S.J. (2004). Traumatic brain injury. *RN 2004, 67*(4):32.

Bryant, R.A. (2008). *Acute and chronic wounds: nursing management.* (4th ed.). St. Louis: Mosby.

Causey, A.L., Nichter, M.A. (2008). Near-drowning. In J.E. Tintinalli, G.D. Kelen, & S.J. Stapczynski (Eds.). *Emergency medicine: a comprehensive study guide.* (7th ed.). New York: McGraw-Hill.

Clark, R., et al. (2008). Arthropod bites and stings. In J.E. Tintinalli, G.D. Kelen, & S.J. Stapczynski (Eds.). *Emergency medicine: a comprehensive study guide.* (7th ed.). New York, McGraw-Hill.

Craig, K. (2006). Understanding the new AHA guidelines, Part I. *Nursing*, 36(4):53.

Craig, K. (2006). Understanding the new AHA guidelines, Part II. *Nursing*, 36(5):52.

DeBoer, S. (2004). Prehospital and emergency department burn care. *Critical Care Nurses Clinic of North America*, 16(1):61.

Editorial. (2007). Emergencies in the field: focusing on eye emergencies. *Nursing*, 37(2):46.

Emergency Nurses Association. (2005). *Position statement family presence at the bedside during invasive procedures and resuscitation.* Available at www.ena.org/SiteCollectionDocuments/Position%20Statements/Family_Presence_-_ENA_PS.pdf. Accessed December, 2009.

Emergency Nurses Association (ENA) & American College of Emergency Physicians (ACEP). (2004). *Standardized ED triage scale and acuity categorization.* Available at www.ena.org/SiteCollectionDocuments/Position%20Statements/Standardized_ED_Triage_Scale_and_Acuity_Categorization_-_ENAACEP.pdf. Accessed December, 2009.

Ganahl, B.H. (2009). Triage. In J. Fultz & P.A. Sturt (Eds.). *Mosby's emergency nursing reference.* (4th ed.). St. Louis: Elsevier.

Hockenberry, M.J., & Wilson, D. (2007). *Wong's nursing care of infants and children.* (8th ed.). St. Louis, Mosby.

Hurley, M. (2007). Antidote on board to fight bioterrorism. *RN*, 70(4):61.

Kilpatrick, J. (2002). Nuclear attacks. *RN*, 65(5):46.

Kress, T. (2004). Identifying carbon monoxide poisoning. *Nursing*, 34(1):68.

Laskowski-Jones, L. (2006a). First aid for amputation. *Nursing*, 36(4):50.

Laskowski-Jones, L. (2006b). First aid for bleeding wounds. *Nursing*, 36(9):50.

Laskowski-Jones, L. (2006c). First aid for burns. *Nursing*, 36(1):41.

Laskowski-Jones, L. (2006d). First aid for sprains. *Nursing*, 36(8):48.

Laskowski-Jones, L. (2006e). Responding to trauma, your priorities in the first hour. *Nursing*, 36(9):52.

Laskowski-Jones, L. (2006f). Responding to trauma. *Nursing*, 36(9): 52.

Lewis, S.L., Heitkemper, M.M., Dirksen, S.R., et al. (2007). *Medical-surgical nursing: assessment and management of clinical problems.* (7th ed.). St. Louis: Mosby.

Mills, A.C., & McSweeney, M. (2005). Primary reasons for ED visits and procedures performed for patients who saw nurse practitioners. *Journal of Emergency Nursing*, 31:145.

Newberry, L. (Ed.). (2007). *Sheehy's emergency nursing: principles and practice.* (6th ed.). St. Louis: Mosby.

Occupational Health and Safety Administration. (2005). *Best practices for hospital-based first receivers of victims from mass casualty incidents involving the release of hazardous substances.* Available at www.osha.gov/dts/osta/bestpractices/html/hospital_firstreceivers.html. Accessed December, 2009.

Potter, P.A., & Perry, A.G. (2007). *Basic nursing: essentials for practice.* (6th ed.). St. Louis: Mosby.

Proehl, J.A. (2004). Emergency accidental amputation: a frightening injury requiring quick action. *American Journal of Nursing*, 104(2):50.

Pruitt, W.C. (2004). Manual ventilation by one or two rescuers. *Nursing*, 34(11):43.

Rebmann, T., et al. (2002). Are you prepared for a bioterrorist attack? *Nursing*, 32(9):32hnl.

Ressel, G.W. (2004). AAP releases policy statement on poison treatment in the home. *American Family Physician*, 69(3):741.

Rice, K., et al. (2006). Learning from Katrina. *Nursing*, 36(4):44.

Rutenberg, C. (2008). How to recognize life threatening emergencies over the phone. *Nursing*, 21:56hnl.

Rzucidlo, S.E., & Shirk, B.J. (2004). Pediatric patients: children are not just little adults. *RN*, 67(6):36.

Scholle, C. (2006). How a rapid response team saves lives. *Nursing*, 36(1):35.

Snyder, M.L. (2005). Learn the chilling facts about hypothermia. *Nursing*, 35:32hnl.

Sturt, P.A. (2009). Toxicologic conditions. In J. Fultz, & P.A. Sturt (Eds.). *Mosby's emergency nursing reference.* (5th ed.). St. Louis: Elsevier.

Thompson, J. (2007). Katrina's aftermath: how our disaster plan was tested. *RN*, 70(8):36.

U.S. Environmental Protection Agency (EPA). (n.d.). *Understanding radiation. Health effects.* Available at www.epa.gov/radiation/understand/health_effects.html. Accessed December, 2009.

Chapter 25 Health Promotion and Pregnancy

Ackley, B.J., & Ladwig, G.B. (2009). *Nursing diagnosis handbook.* (7th ed.). St. Louis: Mosby.

Blackburn, S. (2003). *Maternal, fetal, and neonatal physiology: a clinical perspective.* (2nd ed.). St. Louis: Saunders.

Bulechek, G.M., Butcher, H.K. & Dochterman, J.M. (2008). *Nursing intervention classification (NIC).* (5th ed.). St. Louis: Mosby.

Giger, J.N., & Davidhizar, R.E. (2008). *Transcultural nursing: assessment and intervention.* (5th ed.). St. Louis: Mosby.

Lamondy, A.M. (2007). Managing hyperemesis gravidarum. *Nursing 2007*, 37(2):66-68.

Lowdermilk, D.L., & Perry, S.E. (2007). *Maternity and women's health care.* (9th ed.). St. Louis: Mosby.

May, K. (1980). A typology of detachment and involvement styles adopted during pregnancy by first time expectant fathers. *Western Journal of Nursing Research*, 2(2):444-461.

May, K. (1982). Three phases of father involvement in pregnancy, *Nursing research*, 31(6):337-342.

Mercer, R. (1995). *Becoming a mother*. New York: Springer.

Moorhead, S., Johnson, M., Maas, M., et al. (2008). *Nursing outcomes classification (NOC).* (4th ed.). St. Louis: Mosby.

Mosby's dictionary of medicine, nursing, and health professions. (8th ed.). (2009). St. Louis: Mosby.

Murray, S.S., et al. (2001). *Foundations of maternal-newborn nursing.* (3rd ed.). Philadelphia: Saunders.

North American Nursing Diagnosis Association International (NANDA-I). (2009). *NANDA-I nursing diagnoses: definitions and classification 2009-2011.* Oxford, United Kingdom: Author.

Olds, S., et al. (2007). *Maternal-newborn nursing and women's health care.* (8th ed.). Upper Saddle River, NJ: Prentice Hall.

Pagana, K.D., & Pagana, T.J. (2007). *Mosby's diagnostic and laboratory test reference.* (8th ed.). St. Louis: Mosby.

Pillitteri, A. (2003). *Maternal & child health nursing: care of the childbearing and childrearing family.* (4th ed.). Philadelphia: Lippincott Williams & Wilkins.

Rubin, R. (1975). Maternal tasks in pregnancy. *Maternal Child Nursing Journal*, 4(3): 145-153.

Schlef, C. (2000). *Mosby's maternal-newborn patient teaching guides.* St. Louis: Mosby.

Seidel, H.M., Ball, J.W., Dains, J.E., et al. (2007). *Mosby's guide to physical examination.* (6th ed.). St. Louis: Mosby.

Thompson, J., et al. (1998). Embryonic stem cell lines derived from human blastocyst, *Science*, 282:1145.

Tucker, S.M., et al. (2004). *Patient care standards: collaborative planning and nursing interventions.* (8th ed.). St. Louis: Mosby.

Wong, D.L., et al. (2006). *Maternal-child nursing care.* (3rd ed.). St. Louis: Mosby.

Chapter 26 Labor and Delivery

Ackley, B.J., & Ladwig, G.B. (2005). *Nursing diagnosis handbook.* (6th ed.). St. Louis: Mosby.

American College of Nurse-Mid-Wives. (n.d.). *Midwifery strategies for liability risk reduction pre-term labor and delivery.* Available at www.midwife.org/liability_risk_reduction_preterm.cfm. Accessed February 13, 2008.

Bulechek, G.M., Butcher, H.K., & Dochterman, J.M. (2008). *Nursing intervention classification (NIC).* (5th ed.). St. Louis: Mosby.

D'Avanzo, C., & Geissler, E. (2003). *Pocket guide to cultural health assessment.* (3rd ed.). St. Louis: Mosby.

Documentation in maternal-neonatal nursing. (2008). *LPN 2008,* 4(3): 4-12.

Giger, J.M., & Davidhizar, R.E. (2008). *Transcultural nursing: assessment and intervention.* (5th ed.). St. Louis: Mosby.

Gilbert, E.S., & Harmon, J.S. (2006). *Manual of high-risk pregnancy and delivery.* (4th ed.). St. Louis: Mosby.

Lowdermilk, D.L., & Perry, S.E. (2007). *Maternity and women's health care.* (9th ed.). St. Louis: Mosby.

Marshall, K.M., & Baker, J. (2006). Are patients in labor satisfied with PCEA? *Nursing 2006,* 36(6):18.

Martin J., Hamilton, B., et al. (2005). Births: final data for 2003. *National vital statistics report,* 54(2):1-116.

Maternal and neonatal nursing. (2007). *Nursing made incredibly easy.* (2nd ed.). Philadelphia: Lippincott Williams & Wilkins.

McKinney, E.S., James, S.R., Murray, S.S., et al. (2008). *Maternal-child nursing.* (3rd ed.). St. Louis: Saunders.

Mennick, F. (2006). Cesarean section on demand. *American Journal of Nursing,* 106(6):19-20.

Moorhead, S., Johnson, M., Maas, M., et al. (2008). *Nursing outcomes classification (NOC).* (4th ed.). St. Louis: Mosby.

Mosby's dictionary of medicine, nursing, and health professions. (8th ed.). (2009). St. Louis: Mosby.

Newton, P. (2004). The doula's role during L & D. *RN 2004,* 67(3):34-37.

North American Nursing Diagnosis Association International (NANDA-I). (2009). *NANDA-I nursing diagnoses: definitions and classification 2009-2011.* Oxford, United Kingdom: Author.

Pagana, K.D., & Pagana, T.J. (2007). *Mosby's diagnostic and laboratory test reference.* (8th ed.). St. Louis: Mosby.

Pillitteri, A. (2007). *Maternal & child health nursing: care of the childbearing and childrearing family.* (5th ed.). Philadelphia: Lippincott Williams & Wilkins.

Ricci, S.S. (2007). *Essentials of maternity newborn and women's health nursing.* Philadelphia: Lippincott Williams & Wilkins.

Skidmore-Roth, L. (2008). *Mosby's nursing drug reference.* (21st ed.). St. Louis: Mosby.

Tucker, S.M., Cannobio, M.M., Paquette, E.V., et al. (2007). *Patient care standards: collaborative planning and nursing interventions.* (7th ed.). St. Louis: Mosby.

Wong, D.L., et al. (2006). *Maternal-child nursing care.* (3rd ed.). St. Louis: Mosby.

Chapter 27 Care of the Mother and Newborn

Ackley, B.J., & Ladwig, G.B. (2005). *Nursing diagnosis handbook.* (6th ed.). St. Louis: Mosby.

American Academy of Pediatrics Task Force on Circumcision. (1999). Circumcision policy statement. *Pediatrics,* 103(3):686-693.

Biancuzzo, M. (2003). *Breastfeeding the newborn: clinical strategies for nurses.* (2nd ed.). St. Louis: Mosby.

Boxoky, I., & Corwin, E. (2002). Fatigue as a predictor of post-partum depression. *Journal of Obstetrics, Gynecologic, and Neonatal Nursing,* 31(4):436.

Britt, R. (2002). Epidural analgesia during labor: lower the risk. *Nursing 2002,* 32(6):78.

Cerrate, P.L. (2001). Complementary therapies update. *RN,* 64(9):19.

D'Avanzo, D., & Geissler, E. (2003). *Pocket guide to cultural assessment.* (3rd ed.). St. Louis: Mosby.

Dickason, E.J., et al. (2002). *Maternal-infant nursing care.* (4th ed.). St. Louis: Mosby.

Giger, J.M., & Davidhizar, R.E. (2003). *Transcultural nursing: assessment and intervention.* (4th ed.). St. Louis: Mosby.

Hockenberry, M.J., & Wilson, D. (2007). *Wong's nursing care of infants and children.* (8th ed.). St. Louis, Mosby.

Juretschke, L. (2000). Apgar scoring: its use and meaning for today's newborn. *Neonatal Network,* 19(1):17.

Lowdermilk, D.L., & Perry, S.E.. (2004). *Maternity nursing.* (8th ed.). St. Louis: Mosby.

Mache, J. (2001). Analgesia for circumcision: effects on newborn behavior and maternal-infant interactions. *Journal of Obstetric, Gynecologic and Neonatal Nursing,* 30(5):507.

McKinney, E.S., James, S.R., Murray, S.S., et al. (2008). *Maternal-child nursing.* (3rd ed.). St. Louis: Saunders.

Mosby's dictionary of medicine, nursing, and health professions. (8th ed.). (2009). St. Louis: Mosby.

Murray, S.S., et al. (2001). *Foundations of maternal-newborn nursing.* (3rd ed.). Philadelphia: Saunders.

North American Nursing Diagnosis Association International (NANDA-I). (2009). *NANDA-I nursing diagnoses: definitions and classification 2009-2011.* Oxford, United Kingdom: Author.

Pagana, K.D., & Pagana, T.J. (2006). *Mosby's manual of diagnostic and laboratory tests.* (3rd ed.). St. Louis: Mosby.

Pagana, K.D., & Pagana, T.J. (2008). *Mosby's diagnostic and laboratory test reference.* (9th ed.). St. Louis: Mosby.

Ruchala, P. (2000). Teaching new mothers: priorities of nurses and postpartum women. *Journal of Obstetric, Gynecologic, and Neonatal Nursing,* 29(3):265.

Stachowicz, T.L. (2001). Breast-feeding basics: how to help your patient and your baby get off to a good start. *Nursing,* 31(7):32hn8.

Tucker, S.M., et al. (2004). *Patient care standards: collaborative planning and nursing interventions.* (8th ed.). St. Louis: Mosby.

Wong, D.L., et al. (2002). *Maternal-child nursing care.* (2nd ed.). St. Louis: Mosby.

Chapter 28 Care of the High-Risk Mother, Newborn, and Family with Special Needs

Ackley, B.J., & Ladwig, G.B. (2009). *Nursing diagnosis handbook.* (7th ed.). St. Louis: Mosby.

Arias, E., MacDorman, M.F., Strobino, D.M., et al. (2003). Annual summary of vital statistics—2002. *Pediatrics,* 112(6):1215-1230.

Ballard, J., et al. (1979). A simplified score for assessment of fetal maturations of newly born infants. *Journal of Pediatrics,* 95(5p+1):769-774.

Brown-Gutlouz, H. (2006). About ectopic pregnancy. *Nursing 2006,* 36(8):70.

Fink, J.L. (2006). Diabetes in pregnancy and beyond. *RN 2006,* 69(5):26-30.

Giger, J.M., & Davidhizar, R.E. (2008). *Transcultural nursing: assessment and intervention.* (5th ed.). St. Louis: Mosby.

Gilbert, E.S., & Harmon, J.S. (2006). *Manual of high-risk pregnancy and delivery.* (4th ed.). St. Louis: Mosby.

Halditch-Davis, D. (2005). If only they could talk. *American Journal of Nursing,* 105(12):75.

Juretschke, L. (2005). Kernecterus: still a common concern. *Neonatal Network,* 24(2):7-19.

Korby, J. (2004). Abruptio placentae. *Nursing,* 34(2):96.

Lowdermilk, D.L., & Perry, S.E. (2007). *Maternity and women's health care.* (9th ed.). St. Louis: Mosby.

McKinney, E.S., James, S.R., Murray, S.S., et al. (2008). *Maternal-child nursing.* (3rd ed.). St. Louis: Saunders.

Montgomery, K.S. (2003). Health promotion for pregnant adolescents. *MCN: The American Journal of Maternal/Child Nursing,* 7(5):432.

North American Nursing Diagnosis Association International (NANDA-I). (2009). *NANDA-I nursing diagnoses: definitions and classification 2009-2011.* Oxford, United Kingdom: Author.

Pagana, K.D., & Pagana, T.J. (2008). *Mosby's diagnostic and laboratory test reference.* (9th ed.). St. Louis: Mosby.

Seidel, H.M., Ball, J.W., Dains, J.E., et al. (2007). *Mosby's guide to physical examination.* (6th ed.). St. Louis: Mosby.

Skidmore-Roth, L. (2010). *Mosby's 2010 nursing drug reference.* (23rd ed.). St. Louis: Mosby.

Snow, M. (2008). On alert for post-partum *C. sardelli* infection. *Nursing 2008*, 38(1):10.

Tough, S.C., Newburn-Cook, C., Johnston, D.W., et al. (2002). Delayed childbearing and its impact on population rate changes in lower birth weight, multiple birth, and preterm delivery. *Pediatrics*, 109(3):399-403.

White, H., & Bourrier, D. (2005). Caring for a patient having a miscarriage. *Nursing 2005*, 35(7):18-19.

Wolfberg, A., et al. (2005). Postevacuation hcg levels and risk of gestational traphoblastic neoplasia in women with complete molar pregnancy. *Obstetrics and Gynecology*, 106(3):548-552.

Wong, D.L., et al. (2006). *Maternal-child nursing care.* (3rd ed.). St. Louis: Mosby.

Zinkus, J., et al. (2007). Gestational diabetes: a danger to mother and baby. *LPN 2007*, 3(3):36-43.

Chapter 29 Health Promotion for the Infant, Child, and Adolescent

American Academy of Pediatrics (AAP). (2000). Guiding principles for managed care arrangements for the health care of newborns, infants, children, adolescents, and young adults. *Pediatrics*, 105(1):132.

American Academy of Pediatrics (AAP). (2004). *Committee on nutrition: pediatric nutrition handbook.* (5th ed.). Elk Grove Village, IL: Author.

American Academy of Pediatrics (AAP). (2005). Committee on environmental health: lead exposure in children: prevention, detection and management. *Pediatrics*, 116(4):1036-1046.

American Academy of Pediatrics (AAP). (2008). *Car safety seats: a guide for families*. Available at www.aap.org/family/carseatguide.htm.

American Academy of Pediatrics (AAP), & Committee on Infectious Diseases. (2004). Recommended childhood immunization schedule—United States, January–December. *Pediatrics*, 105(1):148.

American Academy of Pediatrics, Committee on Public Education. (2001). Media violence, *Pediatrics*, 108(5):1222-1226.

American Dietetic Association (ADA). (2004). Position of the American Dietetic Association: dietary guidance for healthy children. *Journal of the American Dietetic Association*, 194(4):660.

Briggs, M., et al. (2003). Nutrition services: an essential component of comprehensive school health programs. *Journal of the American Dietetic Association*, 103(4):505.

Cantor, J. (2000). Media violence. *Journal of Adolescent Health*, 27S:30-34.

Carroll, S.T., et al. (2002). Tattoos and body piercing as indicators of adolescent risk-taking behaviors. *Pediatrics*, 109(6):1021.

Centers for Disease Control and Prevention (CDC). (2005). *Healthy youth! Coordinated school health programs*. Available at www.cdc.gov/healthyyouth/cshp/index.htm. Accessed May, 2005.

Chalupka, S. (2005). Tainted water on tap. *American Journal of Nursing*, 105(11):40.

Crowley, A., et al. (2005). A model pre-school vision and hearing screening program. *American Jounal of Nursing*, 105(6):52.

Drago, D.A. (2005). Kitchen scalds and thermal burns in children 5 years and younger. *Pediatrics*, 115(1):10-16.

Erickson, L., et al. (2005). A review of a preventable poison: pediatric lead poisoning. *Journal of the Society of Pediatric Nurses*, 104(4):171.

Granbaum, J., et al. (2004). Youth risk behaviors surveillance, *MMWR Morbidity and Mortality Weekly Report*, 53(55-2):1.

Grossman, D. (2000). Teaching kids to kill. *National Forum*, 80(4): 10-14.

Hamilton, J.T. (2000). *The economic market for violent television*. Princeton, NJ: Princeton UP.

Herman, J.W. (2001). Pediatric nursing and *Healthy People 2010:* a call to action. *Pediatric Nursing*, 27(1):82.

Hockenberry, M.J., & Wilson, D. (2007). *Wong's nursing care of infants and children*. (8th ed.). St. Louis: Mosby.

Hoff, J.T., et al. (2003) *National Survey of adolescent and young adult sexual health knowledge, attitudes and experiences*. Menlo Park, Calif.: Henry Kaiser Family Foundation.

Hornor, G. (2005). Physical abuse: recognition and reporting. *Journal of Pediatric Health Care*, 19(1):4.

Johnson, C.F. (2008). Abuse and neglect of children. In R. Behrman, (Ed.). *Nelson's textbook of pediatrics.* (18th ed.). Philadelphia: Saunders.

Laraque, D. (2004). Committee on injury, violence and poison prevention: injury risk of nonpowder guns. *Pediatrics*, 114(5):1357-1361.

LaSala, K.B., & Todd, S.J. (2000). Preventing youth use of tobacco products: the role of nursing. *Pediatric Nursing*, 26(2):143.

Logan, D., Carlini-Marlatt, B. (2004). *Smoking and adolescence: some issues on prevention and cessation*. Available at www.mentorfoundation.org/pdfs/prevention_perspectives/5.pdf. Accessed December, 2009.

MaCue, M. (2001). Child safety seats work. *Journal of the Society of Pediatric Nurses*, 6(2):87.

Maes, L., et al. (2003). Can the school make a difference? a multianalysis of adolescent risk and health behavior. *Social Science and Medicine*, 56(3):517.

McColgan, M., et al. (2005). Internet poses multiple risks to children and adolescents. *Pediatrics Annals*, 34(4):405.

National Association of School Nurses. (2007). *Expert committee recommendations on the assessment, prevention and treatment of child and adolescent overweight and obesity*. Available at www.ama-assn.org/ama1/pub/upload/mm/433/ped_obesity_recs.pdf. Accessed December, 2009.

National Institute of Allergy and Infectious Diseases (NIAID). (2009). *Human papilloma virus (HPV) and genital warts*. Available at http://www3.niaid.nih.gov/topics/genitalWarts. Accessed December, 2009.

Paoletti, J. (2007). Tipping the scales, what nurses need to know about the children's obesity epidemic. *RN 2007*, 70(11):35-40.

Perry, L., et al. (2002). Adolescent vegetarians: how well do their dietary patterns meet the *Healthy People 2010* objectives? *Archives of Pediatric and Adolescent Health*, 156(5):426.

Putnam, F.W. (2003). Ten-year update review: child sexual abuse. *Journal of the American Academy of Child and Adolescent Psychiatry*, 42(3):269.

Saewyc, E., et al. (2004). Suicidal ideation and attempts in North America school based surveys: are bisexual youth at increasing risk? *Journal of Adolescent Health*, 34(2):138.

Schmitt, B.D. (2004). Toilet training: getting it right the first time. *Contemporary Pediatrics*, 21(3):105-108.

Treacy, V., et al. (2004). Breaking sexuality taboos. *Pediatric Nursing*, 16(2):19.

U.S. Department of Health and Human Services. (2000). *Healthy People 2010: Understanding and improving health, objectives for improving health, tracking Healthy People 2010.* Washington, DC: U.S. Government Printing Office.

U.S. Department of Health and Human Services. (2008). *The national survey on drug use and health report*. Available at www.oas.samhsa.gov/nsduhLatest.htm. Accessed October 20, 2009.

U.S. Department of Health and Human Services, U.S. Department of Agriculture. (2005). *Nutrition and your health: dietary guidelines for Americans*. Available at www.health.gov/dietaryguidelines. Accessed July, 2008.

U.S. Food and Drug Administration (FDA). (2009). *Cervarix. Product information: package insert*. Available at www.fda.gov/downloads/BiologicsBloodVaccines/Vaccines/ApprovedProducts/UCM186981.pdf. Accessed November, 2009.

Chapter 30 Basic Pediatric Nursing Care

American Academy of Pediatrics (AAP). (2003). Consent for emergency medical services for children and adolescents. *Pediatrics*, 111(3):703-705.

American Academy of Pediatrics (AAP). (2002). Guidelines for monitoring and management of pediatric procedures. *Pediatrics*, 110(4): 836.

American Academy of Pediatrics (AAP) & Task Force on Sudden Infant Death Syndrome. (2005). Controversies regarding the sleeping environment, and new variables to consider in reducing risk, *Pediatrics* 116(5):1245-1255.

American Nurses Association (ANA). (2003). *Nursing's social policy statement*. Silver Springs, MD: Nursesbooks.org.

Anderson, S.L., et al. (2005). Adolescent patients and their confidentiality: staying within legal bounds. *Contemporary Pediatrics*, 22(7):54.

Bald, M. (2002). Ambulatory blood pressure monitoring in children and adolescent. *Minerva Pediatrics*, 54(1):13.

Banitalebi, H., et al. (2002). Measurement of fever in children—is infrared tympanic thermometry reliable? *Tidsskrift for den Norske Laegeforening*, 122(28):2700.

Board, R., et al. (2003). Stressors and symptoms of mothers and children in the PICU. *Journal of Pediatric Nursing*, 18(3):195.

Bowinkel, J., et al. (2005). Sedating patients for radiologic studies. *Pediatric Annals*, 34(8):650-656.

Bryant, R., et al. (2008). Acute and chronic wounds. *Nursing management*, (4th ed.). St. Louis: Mosby.

Centers for Disease Control and Prevention (CDC). (2009). *Preventing teen pregnancy: an update in 2009*. Available at www.cdc.gov/reproductivehealth/adolescentreprohealth/aboutTP.htm. Accessed October 21, 2009.

Chambers, C., et al. (2005). Faces scales for the measurement of postoperative pain intensity in children following minor surgery. *Clinical Journal of Pain*, 21(3):277-285.

Clark, J.A., et al. (2002). Discrepancies between direct and indirect blood pressure measurements using various recommendations for arm cuff selection. *Pediatrics*, 110(5):920.

Clinical and Laboratory Standards Institute. (n.d.). *Blood collection via capillary puncture in infants*. Available at www.phlebotomypages.com/phleb_infants.htm. Accessed March, 2006.

Cook, I., et al. (2006). Ventrogluteal area—a suitable site for intramuscular vaccination of infants and toddlers. *Vaccine*, 24(13):2403-2408.

Cook, I.F., & Murtagh, J. (2006). Ventrogluteal area—a suitable site for intramuscular vaccination of infants and toddlers. *Vaccine*, 24(13):2403-2408.

Diggle, L., & Deeks, J. (2000). Effect of needle length on incidence of local reaction to routine immunization in infants aged 4 months: randomized control trial. *British Medical Journal*, 321(7266):931.

Ellis, J.A., et al. (2002). Pain in hospitalized pediatric patients: how are we doing? *Clinical Journal of Pain*, 18(4):262.

El Radhi, A.S., et al. (2003). Do antipyretics prevent febrile convulsions? *Archives of Disease in Childhood*, 88(7):641.

Gad, L., et al. (2005). Optimized use of EMLA cream in children–secondary publication: a randomized, prospective, controlled comparison of two application regimens, *Ugeskv Laeger*, 167(4):404-407.

Gerard, L.L., Cooper, C.S., Duethman, K.S., et al. (2003). Effectiveness of lidocaine lubricant for discomfort during pediatric urethral catheterization. *Journal of Urology*, 170:564-567.

Gilbert, H.C., & Green, C.R. (n.d.). *JCAHO's Pain Initiative–New Opportunities/New Risks*. Available at www.asahq.org/Newsletters/2000/11_00/gilbert.htm. Accessed October, 2009.

Goldman, L.R., et al. (2001). Technical report: mercury in the environment: implications for pediatrics. *Pediatrics*, 108(1):197.

Hockenberry, M.J., & Wilson, D. (2007). *Wong's nursing care of infants and children*. (8th ed.). St. Louis: Mosby.

Houlder, L.C. (2000). The accuracy and reliability of tympanic thermometry compared to rectal and axillary sites in young children. *Pediatric Nursing*, 26(3):311.

IPPM, Gold, R., et al. (1989). Adverse reactions to diphtheria, tetanus, pertussis-polio vaccination at 18-months of age. Effect of injection site and needle length. *Pediatrics*, 83(5):679-682.

Luffy, R., et al. (2003). Examining the validity, reliability, and preference of three pediatric pain measurement tools in African-American children. *Pediatric Nursing*, 29(1):54.

Quality, equipment holds key to infection control. (2006). *Education Management*, 18(2):19-21.

Robertson, J., & Robertson, J. (1990). *Separation and the very young*. Free Association Books: London.

Rogers, T.A. (2004). The use of EMLA cream to decrease venipuncture pain in children. *Journal of Pediatric Nursing*, 19(1):33.

Sparks, L. (2001). Taking the ouch out of injections for children. *MCN: The American Journal of Maternal/Child Nursing*, 26(2):72.

Spitz, R.A. (1945). Hospitalism: an inquiry into the genesis of psychiatric conditions in early childhood. *Psychoanalytic Study of the Child*, 1:53-74.

Thompson, E. (2007). *Introduction to maternity and pediatric nursing*. (5th ed.). Philadelphia: Saunders.

Tillett, J. (2005). Adolescents and informed consent in ethical and legal issues. *Journal of Perinatal and Neonatal Nursing*, 19(2):1120-1121.

Wong, D. (2003). Topical anesthetics: two products for pain relief during minor procedures. *American Journal of Nursing*, 103(6):45.

Chapter 31 Care of the Child with a Physical Disorder

Albright, A.I., et al. (2003). Long-term intrathecal baclofen therapy for severe spasticity of cerebral origin. *Journal of Neurosurgery*, 98(2):291.

American Academy of Otolaryngology—Head and Neck Surgery. (2000). 2000 clinical indicators compendium. *Bulletin*, 19:6.

American Academy of Pediatrics (AAP), Committee on Genetics. (1999). Folic acid for prevention of neural tube defects. *Pediatrics*, 104(2 pt 1):325-327.

American Academy of Pediatrics (AAP), Task Force on Infant Sleep Position and Sudden Infant Death Syndrome. (2000). Changing concepts of SIDS: implications for infant sleeping environment and sleep positions. *Pediatrics*, 105(3):650-656.

American Academy of Pediatrics (AAP), Committee on Fetus and Newborn. (2003). Apnea, sudden infant death syndrome, and home monitoring. *Pediatrics*, 111(4):914.

American Academy of Pediatrics (AAP), Committee on Infectious Diseases. In L. Pickering (Ed.). (2003). *2003 redbook: report of the committee on infectious diseases*. (26th ed.). Elk Grove Village, Ill: Author.

American Academy of Pediatrics (AAP), Committee on Nutrition. (2004). *Pediatric nutrition handbook*. (5th ed.). Elk Grove Village, Ill: Author.

American Academy of Pediatrics (AAP). (2005). Chronic abdominal pain in children. *Pediatrics*, 115(3):812-815.

American Academy of Pediatrics (AAP). (2005). Policy statement: breastfeeding and the use of human milk, *Pediatrics*, 115(2):496-506.

American Academy of Pediatrics (AAP), Committee on Infectious Disease. (2005). Recommended childhood and adolescent immunization schedule: United States, 2005. *Pediatrics*, 115(1):182-186.

American Academy of Pediatrics (AAP), The Task Force on Sudden Infant Death Syndrome. (2005). The changing concept of sudden infant death syndrome: diagnostic coding shifts, controversies regarding sleeping environment, and new variables to consider in reducing risk. *Pediatrics*, 116(5):1245-1255.

American Diabetes Association (ADA). (2001). Report of the expert committee on the diagnosis and classification of diabetes mellitus. *Diabetes Care*, 24(suppl):S5-S20.

American Diabetic Association (ADA). (2005). Care of children and adolescents with Type I diabetes. *Diabetic Care*, 28:186-212.

Anabwani, M., et al. (2005). Treatment of human immunodeficiency virus (HIV) in children using antiretroviral drugs. *Seminars in Pediatric Infectious Disease*, 16:116-124.

Anderson, M., et al. (2005). Sudden infant death syndrome and prenatal maternal smoking: rising attributed risk in the back to sleep era. *BMC Medicine*, 3(1):4.

Ashwal, S., et al. (2004). Practice parameter: diagnostic assessment of the child with cerebral palsy: report of the quality standards subcommittee of the American Academy of Neurology. *Neurology*, 62(6): 851-863.

Baucom, B. (2006). Help stamp out this lingering menace. *RN*, 69(4):43.

Block, R., et al. (2005). Committee on child abuse and neglect and committee on nutrition (AAP): Failure to thrive as a manifestation of child neglect. *Pediatrics*, 116(5):1234-1237.

Boguniewicz, M. (2005). Atopic dermatitis: beyond the itch that rashes. *Immunology and Allergy Clinics of North America*, 25(2):333-351.

Bolton-Maggs, P., et al. (2004). The child with immune thrombocytopenic purpura: is pharmacotherapy or watchful waiting the best initial management? *Pediatric Hematology and Oncology*, 26(2):146-151.

Brodsky, R., et al. (2005). Aplastic anemia. *Lancet*, 365:1647-1656.

Brosnan, C. (2001). Type 2 diabetes in children and adolescents: an emerging disease. *Journal of Pediatric Health Care*, 15(4):187-193.

Browne, T.R., & Holmes, G.L. (2004). *Handbook of epilepsy*. (3rd ed.). Philadelphia: Lippincott, Williams & Wilkins.

Brown-Guttouz, H. (2007). Intussusception. *Nursing*, 37(2):80.

Buchanan, G.R., DeBaun, M.R., Quinn, C.T., et al. (2004). Sickle cell disease, *Hematology*, 2004:35-47.

Centers for Disease Control and Prevention (CDC). (1994). Revised classificiation system for HIV infection in children. *MMWR Recomm Rep* 43(RR-12):1-10.

Centers for Disease Control and Prevention (CDC). (1999). Prevention of varicella: recommendations fo the advisory committee on immunization practices (ACIP). *MMWR Recomm Rep* 48(RR-6): 1-5.

Chavez-Bueno, S., et al. (2005). Respiratory syncytial virus: old challenges and new approaches. *Pediatric Annals*, 34(1):62-68.

Cystic Fibrosis Foundation. (2006). *Patient registry 2006 annual report*. Bethesda, Md: Author.

Dover, G.J., Platt, O.S. (2009). Sickle cell disease. In S.H. Orkin, D.E. Fisher, & A.T. Look (Eds.). *Nathan and Oski's hematology of infancy and childhood*. (7th ed.). Philadelphia: Saunders.

Fickert, N. (2006). Taking a closer look at acute otitis media in kids. *Nursing*, 36(4):20.

Frank, G., Mahoney, H.M., & Eppes, S.C. (2005). Musculoskeletal infections in children. *Pediatrics Clinics of North America*, 52(4):1083-1106.

Gilmore, A., Gilmore, A., Thompson, G.H. (2003). Common childhood foot deformities. *Consult Pediatr*, 2(2):63-71.

Goldrick, B. (2005). Emerging infections-pertussis on the rise. *American Journal of Nursing*, 105(1):69.

Golub, T., et al. (2006). Acute myelogenous leukemia. In P. Pizza, & D. Poplack (Eds.). *Principles and practices of pediatric oncology*. (5th ed.). Philadelphia: Lippincott.

Green, L., et al. (2003). Primary care of children with cerebral palsy. *Clinical Family Practice*, 5(2):1.

Gribbons, D., Zahr, L.K., & Opas, S.R. (1995). Nursing management of children with sickle cell disease. *Journal of Pediatric Nursing*, 10(4): 232-242.

Hahn, R.G., Knox, L.M., & Forman, T.A. (2005). Evaluation of poststreptococcal illness. *American Family Physician*, 71(10):1949-1954.

Hockenberry, M.J., & Wilson, D. (2007). *Wong's nursing care of infants and children*. (8th ed.). St. Louis: Mosby.

Huh, P., et al. (2006). Diagnostic method for differentiating external hydrocephalus from simple subdural hygroma. *Journal of Neurosurgery*, 105(1):65-70.

Jick, H., et al. (2004). Antidepressants and the risk of suicidal behaviors. *Journal of the American Medical Association*, 292(3):338-343.

Kahn, J.L., Binns, H.J., Chen, T., et al. (2002). Persistence and emergence of anemia in children during participation in the special supplemental nutrition program for women, infants, and children. *Archives of Pediatric and Adolescent Medicine*, 156:1028-1032.

Kemp, J.S., et al. (2000). Unsafe sleep practices and an analysis of bed sharing among infants dying suddenly and unexpectedly: results of a 4-year study of SIDS and related deaths. *Pediatrics*, 106(3):e41.

Kemper, K.J., & Gardiner, P. (2008). Herbal medicine. In R. Behrman (Ed.). *Nelson's textbook of pediatrics*. (18th ed.). Philadelphia: Saunders.

Kennedy, M. (2006). SIDS: More guidelines, more controversy. *American Journal of Nursing*, 106(1).

Kiess, W., et al. (2003). Type 2 diabetes mellitus in children and adolescents: a review from a European perspective. *Hormone Research*, 59(Suppl 1):77.

Kliegman, R.M., Behrman, R.E., Jenson, H.B., et al. (2007). *Nelson's textbook of pediatrics*. (18th ed.). Philadelphia: Saunders.

Kumar, K., et al. (2005). Treatment, outcomes and cost of care in children with idiopathic thrombocytopenic purpura. *American Journal of Hematology*, 78:181-187.

Kwiatkowski, J.L., West, T.B., Heidary, N., et al. (1999). Severe iron deficiency anemia in young children, *Journal of Pediatrics*, 135(4): 514-516.

Lambros, K., et al. (2005). Management of the child with a learning disorder. *Pediatric Annals*, 34(4):275-287.

Lewis, K. (2005). New pertusis vaccine for adolescent. *Prevention Bulletin*, 19(3):1.

Liu, A., et al. (2008). Childhood asthma. In R.M. Kliegman, R.E. Behrman, & H.B. Jenson, H.B., et al. (Eds). *Nelson's textbook of pediatrics*. (18th ed.). Philadelphia: Saunders.

Malloy, M.N. (2002). Trends in postneonatal aspiration deaths and reclassification of SIDS: impact of the "back to sleep" program. *Pediatrics*, 109(4):661-665.

Manco-Johnson, M. (2005). Hemophilia management: optimizing treatment based on patient needs. *Current Opinions in Pediatrics*, 17(3):6.

Margolin, E., et al. (2006). Acute lymphoblastic leukemia. In P.A. Pizzo, & D. Poplack. (Eds). *Principles and practices of pediatric oncology*. (5th ed.). Philadelphia: Lippincott.

McKinney, E.S., James, S.R., Murray, S.S., et al. (2008). *Maternal-child nursing*. (3rd ed.). St. Louis: Saunders.

McWhorter, J.W., et al. (2003). The obese child: motivation as a tool for exercise. *Journal of Pediatric Health Care*, 17(1):11.

Merchant, R.G. (2005). Prevention of mother-to-child transmission of HIV—an overview. *Indian Journal of Medical Research*, 121:489-501.

Mesich, H.M. (2005). Understanding the debate and maximizing infant safety. *MCN—Maternal Child Nursing*, 30(1):30-37.

Milla, P. (2004). Motor disorders including pyloric stenosis. In W.A. Walker, et al. (Eds.). *Pediatric gastrointestinal disease: pathophysiology, diagnosis, management*. (4th ed.). Hamilton, Ont.: B.C. Decker.

Mohan, K., Saroha, V., Sharma, A. (2004). Investigated occlusion therapy in children for strabismus. *Journal of Pediatric Ophthalmology Strabismus*, 41(2):89-95.

Montgomery, R.R. (2009). Hemophilia and von Willebrand disease. In S.H. Orkin, D.E. Fisher, & A.T. Look (Eds.). *Nathan and Oski's hematology of infancy and childhood*. (7th ed.). Philadelphia: Saunders.

Mueller, N.E. (1999). The epidemiology of Hodgkin's disease. In P.N. Mauch, J.O. Armitage, & V. Diehl (Eds.). *Hodgkin's disease*. Philadelphia: Lippincott, Williams & Wilkins.

National Heart, Lung, and Blood Institute (NHLBI), National Institute of Health (NIH). (2007). *Guidelines for the diagnosis and management of asthma (EPR-3)*. Available at www.nhlbi.nih.gov/guidelines/asthma. Accessed December, 2009.

Olohan, K., & Zappitelli, D. (2003). The insulin pump. *American Journal of Nursing*, 103(4):48-56.

Paradise, J.L. (2002). Tonsillectomy and adenotonsillectomy for recurrent throat infections in moderately affected children. *Pediatrics*, 110:15.

Peterson, P. (2007). Recognizing and treating seizure disorder in children. *LPN*, 3(6).

Petty, R., et al. (2006). International league of association of rheumatology classification of juvenile idiopathic arthritis: second revision. *Journal of Rheumatology*, 31(2):390-392.

Pichichero, M. (2005). Meningococcal immunization update: a new conjugated vaccine, consult. *Pediatrics*, 116:263-267.

Pizzo, P., & Poplack, D. (2006). *Principles and theories of pediatric oncology*, Philadelphia: Lippincott, Williams & Wilkins.

Plotnik, L.P. (2003). The next step in blood glucose monitoring? *Pediatrics*, 111(4):885.

Ramchandani, N. (2004). Type 2 diabetes in children. *American Journal of Nursing*, 104(3):65.

Selekman, J. (2006). Changes in the screening for tuberculosis in children. *Pediatric Nursing*, 32(1):73-75.

Stephenson, M. (2003). Type 2 diabetes: a growing epidemic in children. *Infectious Disease in Childhood*, 16(4):34.

Thompsen, V. (2008). *Strabismus: all about vision*. Available at www.allaboutvision.com. Accessed April, 2008.

Urrutia-Rojos, X. et al. (2006). Prevalence of risk for Type 2 diabetes in school children. *Journal of School Health*, 76(5):189-194.

Weinstein, J.L. (2003). Advances in the diagnosis and treatment of neuroblastoma. *Oncologist*, 8(3):278-292.

White, K.C. (2005). Anemia is a poor indicator of iron deficienty among toddlers in the United States: for heme the bell tolls, *Pediatrics*, 115(2):315-320.

Williams, H. (2005). Atropic dermatitis. *New England Journal of Medicine*, 35(22):2314-2324.

Wisniewski, A. (2007). Hydrocephalus. *LPN*, 3(1).

Wood, R. (2005). Allergic rhinitis. In R.A. Hoekelman, R. Hoekelman, H. Adam, et al. (Eds.). *Primary pediatric care*. (5th ed.). St. Louis: Mosby.

Wyllie, R., & Hyams, J.S. (2006). *Pediatric gastrointestinal and liver disease: pathophysiology, diagnosis, management*. (3rd ed.). Philadelphia: Saunders.

Chapter 32 Care of the Child with a Mental or Cognitive Disorder

Afzal, N., Murch, S., Thirrupathy, K., et al. (2003). Constipation with acquired megarectum in children with autism. *Pediatrics*, 112(41): 939-942.

Allegretti, C.M. (2002). The effects of a cochlear implant on the family of a hearing impaired child. *Pediatric Nursing*, 28(6):614.

American Academy of Pediatrics (AAP). (2000). Clinical practice guidelines: diagnosis and evaluation of the child with attention-deficit/hyperactivity disorder. *Pediatrics*, 105(5):1158-1170.

American Academy of Pediatrics (AAP). (2001). Clinical practice guideline: treatment of the school-aged child with attention-deficit/hyperactivity disorder. *Pediatrics*, 108(4):1033-1044.

Anbarghalami, R., Yang, L.T., Van Sell, S.L., et al. (2007). When to suspect child abuse. *RN*, 70(6):10.

Autism Research Institute. (2005).*Treatment option for mercurylmetal toxicity in autism and related developmental disabilities: consensus position paper.* San Diego: Author.

Borowsky, I.W., Ireland, M., & Resnick, M.D. (2001). Adolescent suicide attempts: risks and protectors. *Pediatrics*, 107(3):485-493.

Centers for Disease Control and Prevention. (2004). Youth risk behavior surveillance—United States, 2003. *MMWR Morbidity and Mortality Weekly Report*, 53(SS02):1-96.

Centers for Disease Control and Prevention (CDC). (2006). *How common are autism spectrum disorders?* Available at www.cdc.gov/ncddd/autism/asd-common.html. www.cdc.gov/ncbddd/autism/addm.html. Accessed November, 2009.

Filipek, P.A., Accardo, P.J., Ashwal, S., et al. (2000). Practice parameters: screening and diagnosis of autism. Report of the Quality Standards Subcommittee of the American Academy of Neurology and the Child Neurology Society. *Neurology*, 55(2):468-479.

Giardino, A., & Finkel, M.A. (2005). Evaluating child sexual abuse. *Pediatric Annals*, 34(5):382-394.

Hockenberry, M.J., & Wilson, D. (2007). *Wong's nursing care of infants and children*. (8th ed.). St. Louis: Mosby.

Holte, L. (2003). Early childhood hearing loss: a frequently overlooked cause of speech and language delay. *Pediatric Annals*, 32(7):461-465.

Johnson, C.P., Kastner, T.A., American Academy of Pediatrics, Committee/Section on Children with Disabilities. (2005). Helping families raise children with special health care needs at home. *Pediatrics*, 115(2):507-511.

Kliegman, R.M., Behrman, R.E., Jenson, H.B., et al. (2007). *Nelson textbook of pediatrics*. (18th ed.). Philadelphia: Saunders.

Kubra, M., & Gulati, S. (2003). Mental retardation, *Indian Journal of Pediatrics*, 70(2):153-158.

Lambros, K.M., & Leslie, L.K. (2005). Management of the child with a learning disorder. *Pediatric Annals*, 34(4):275-287.

Miller, L. (2006). *Sensational kids: hope and help for children with sensory processing disorder*. New York: G.P. Putnam's Sons.

Muhle, R., Trentacoste, S.V., & Rapin, I. (2004). The genetics of autism. *Pediatrics*, 113(5):e475-e486.

Murphy, K. (2007). The skinny on eating disorders. *Nursing Made Incredibly Easy!* 5(3):40-48, 49, 62.

National Centers for Injury Prevention and Control. (n.d.). *Child maltreatment: facts at a glance*. Available at www.cdc.gov/violenceprevention/pdf/CM-DataSheet-a.pdf. Accessed November, 2009.

National Down Syndrome Society. (2003). *Down syndrome: myths and truths*. Available at www.ndss.org/index.php?option=com_content&view=article&id=59&Itemid=76. Accessed November, 2009.

National Institutes of Health (NIH). (2007). Largest-ever search for autism genes reveals new clues, *NIH News*. Available at www.nih.gov/news/pr/feb2007/nimh-18.htm. Accessed November, 2009.

Pace, B. (2001). Down syndrome. *Journal of the American Medical Association*, 285(8):1112.

Parker, S.K., Schwartz, B., Todd, J., et al. (2004). Thimerosal-containing vaccines and autistic spectrum disorder: a critical review of published original data. *Pediatrics*, 114(3):793-804.

Pfeuffer, M. (2008). Understanding the world of children with autism. *RN*, 71(2):40.

Pinto-Martin, J., Souders, M.C., Giarelli, E., et al. (2005). The role of nurses in screening for autistic spectrum disorder in pediatric primary care. *Journal of Pediatric Nursing*, 29(3):163-169.

Riley, J. (2007). Do you know how to recognize child abuse? *Nursing Made Incredibly Easy!* 5(2):54-61.

Sivberg, B. (2003). Parents' detection of early signs of their children having an autism spectrum disorder. *Journal of Pediatric Nursing*, 18(6):433.

Thompson, S. (2005). Accidental or inflicted? *Pediatric Annals*, 34(5): 312.

Thorne, A. (2007). Are you ready to give care to a child with autism? *Nursing*, 37(5):59-61.

U.S. Department of Health and Human Services (US DHHS), Administration for Children and Families, Administration on Children, Youth and Families, Children's Bureau, Office on Child Abuse and Neglect. (2006). *Child neglect: a guide for prevention, assessment, and intervention*. Available at www.childwelfare.gov/pubs/usermanuals/neglect/neglect.pdf. Accessed November, 2009.

VanRipen, M. (2003). A change of plans: the birth of a child with Down syndrome doesn't have to be a negative experience. *American Journal of Nursing*, 103(6):71.

Walzman, S.B., et al. (2002). Delayed implantation in congenitally deaf children and adults. *Otology and Neurology*, 23(3):333.

WebMD.com. (2007). *Understanding autism—the basics*. Available at www.webmd.com/brain/autism/understanding-autism-basics.

Ylisaukko-Oja, T., Rehnström, K., Vanhala, R., et al. (2005). MECP2 mutation analysis in patients with mental retardation. *American Journal of Medical Genetics*, 132A(2):121-124.

Chapter 33 Health Promotion and Care of the Older Adult

Administration on Aging (AoA). (2001). Older Americans Act. American Indian Elders. Available at www.aoa.gov. Accessed November 2, 2009.

Agency for Healthcare Research and Quality (AHRQ). (2007). *Choosing pain medicine for osteoarthritis*. AHRQ Publication Number 06(07)-Eltc009-3. Available at http://effectivehealthcare.ahrq.gov/index.cfm/search-for-guides-reviews-and-reports/?pageaction=displayproduct&productID=4&returnpage=. Accessed November, 2009.

Alzheimer's Association. (2006). *Ethical issues in Alzheimer's disease: assisted oral feeding and tube feeding*. Chicago, Ill: Author.

American Elder Care Research Organization. (n.d.). *Disturbing statistics about long term care in the U.S.* Available at www.payingforseniorcare.com/longtermcare/statistics.html. Accessed November, 2009.

Baier, B. (2006). The medicine prescription drug benefit. *American Journal of Nursing*, 106(6):66.

Brager, R. (2004). Is polypharmacy hazardous to your older patient's health? *Nursing 2004*, 34(4)32hn1.

Capezuti, E. (2004). Building the science of falls—prevention research. *Journal of the American Geriatric Society*, 52(3):461-462.

Danter, J.H. (2003). Put a realistic spin on geriatric assessment. *Nursing 2003*, 33(12):52.

Dimaria-Ghalili, R., Guenter, P.A. (2008). The mini nutritional assessment. *American Journal of Nursing*, 108(2):50-59.

Ebersole, P., & Hess, P. (2005). *Gerontological nursing and healthy aging*. (2nd ed.). St. Louis: Mosby.

Ebersole, P., Touhy, T., Hess, P., et al. (2008). *Toward healthy aging: human needs and nursing response*. (7th ed.). St. Louis: Mosby.

Elkin, M.K., Perry, A.G., & Potter, P.A. (2007). *Nursing interventions and clinical skills*. (4th ed.). St. Louis: Mosby.

Engberg, S.J., Bender, M.A., & Stilley, C.S. (2003). Kegels and communication. *American Journal of Nursing*, 103(7):93-94.

Fick, D.M., Hodo, D.M., Lawrence, F., et al. (2007). Recognizing delirium superimposed on dementia: assessing nurses' knowledge using case vignettes. *Journal of Gerontological Nursing*, 33(2):40-47.

Fick, D., & Mion, L.C. (2008). How to try this: delirium superimposed on dementia. *American Journal of Nursing*, 108(1):52-60.

Fielo, S.B. (2001). The mystery of sleep: how nurses can help the elderly. *Nurse Spectrum*.

Flaherty, J.H. (2008). Insomnia among hospitalized older persons. *Clinics in Geriatric Medicine*, 24(1):51-67.

Fulmer, T. (2007). Fulmer spices: a framework of six "marker conditions" can help focus assessment of hospitalized patients. *American Journal of Nursing*, 107(10):40.

Galvin, J.E., Roe, C.M., Powlishta, K.K., et al. (2005). The AD8: a brief informant interview to detect dementia. *Neurology*, 65(4): 559-564.

Gerber, L. (2008). Help your older patient blossom socially. *Nursing*, 38(2):24-25.

Graf, C. (2006). Functional decline in hospitalized older adults. *AJN*, 106(1):58.

Greenberg, S. (2007). The geriatric depression scale: short-form. *AJN*, 107(10):60.

Grogan, T. (2006). Keep your older patients out of medication trouble. *Nursing*, 36(9):44.

Hamdy, R.C., et al. (2006). *Alzheimer's disease: a handbook for caregivers*. (5th ed.). St. Louis: Mosby.

Hazzard, W.R., Blass, J., Halter, J., et al. (2003). *Principles of geriatric medicine and gerontology*. (5th ed.). New York: McGraw Hill.

Johnson, C. (2008). Hospital screening for dementia. *American Journal of Nursing*, 108(1):72A.

Kaasalainen, S. (2007). Pain assessment in older adults with dementia: using behavioral observation methods in clinical practice. *Journal of Gerontological Nursing*, 33(6):6-10.

Kennedy, M.S. (2003). Why so many feeding tubes in nursing homes? *American Journal of Nursing*, 103(10):17.

Lewis, S.L., Heitkemper, M.M., Dirksen, S.R., et al. (2007). *Medical-surgical nursing: assessment and management of clinical problems*. (7th ed.). St. Louis: Mosby.

Linton, A., & Lach, H. (2007). *Matteson & McConnell's gerontological nursing concepts and practice*. (3rd ed.). St. Louis: Saunders.

Maas, M.L., Buckwalter, K., Hardy, M., et al. (2001). *Nursing care of older adults: diagnoses, outcomes, and interventions*. St. Louis: Mosby.

Mau, K. (2006). Reaching and teaching older adults. *Nursing*, 38(2): 24-25.

Maze, L. (2008). Stroke: an all-out assault on the brain. *LPN*, 4(3):37.

McCance, K.L., & Huether, S.E. (2009). *Pathophysiology: the biological basis for disease in a adults and children*. (6th ed.). St. Louis: Mosby.

McGee, M., & Jensen, G.L. (2000). Nutrition in the elderly. *Journal of Clinical Gastroenterology*, 30(4):372.

Meiner, S.E., & Leuckenotte, A.G. (2006). *Gerontologic nursing*. (3rd ed.). St. Louis: Mosby.

Miller, J.Q. (2006). Parkinson's disease. In R.J. Ham, P. Sloane, G. Warshaw, et al. (Eds.). *Primary care geriatrics: a case-based approach*. (5th ed.). St. Louis: Mosby.

Murphy, K. (2007). Is your older patient depressed? *Nursing*, 37(6):22.

National Center for Health Statistics. (2007). Hyattsville, MD: U.S. Department of Health and Human Services.

National Institute of Neurological Disorders and Stroke (NINDS). (2007). *NINDS swallowing disorders information page*. Available at www.ninds.nih.gov/disorders/swallowing_disorders. Accessed November, 2009.

Neyhart, B., & Gibbs, L.M. (2006). Osteoporosis. In R.J. Ham, P. Sloane, G. Warshaw, et al. (Eds.). *Primary care geriatrics: a case-based approach*. (5th ed.). St. Louis: Mosby.

Nnodim, J., & Alexander, N. (2005). Assessing falls in older adults. *Geriatrics*, 69(10):24-29.

Ozminkowski, R.J., Wang, S., & Walsh, J.K. (2007). The direct and indirect costs of untreated insomnia in adults in the United States. *Sleep*, 39(3):263-273.

Palmer, J., & Metheny, N.A. (2008). Preventing aspiration in older adults with dysphagia. *American Journal of Nursing*, 108(2):40-48.

Peterson, J.A. (2001). Osteoporosis overview. *Geriatric Nursing*, 22(1):17.

Porter-O'Grady, T. (2001). Into the new age: the call for a new construct for nursing. *Geriatric Nursing*, 22(1):12.

Potter, P.A., & Perry, A.G. (2009). *Fundamentals of nursing: concepts, process, and practice*. (7th ed.). St. Louis: Mosby.

Puentes, W.J. (2000). Using social reminiscence to teach therapeutic communication skills. *Geriatric Nursing*, 21(6):315.

Ramsey, D., Smithard, D., & Kalra, L. (2005). Silent aspiration: what do we know? *Dysphagia*, 29(3):218-225.

Randall, R.L. (2006). Can polypharmacy reduction efforts in an ambulatory setting be successful? *Clinical Geriatrics*, 14(7):33-35.

Sauer, J. (2002). Highlights from 27th international stroke conference, San Antonio, Feb 7-9, 2002. *Medscape Neurology and Neurosurgery*, 4(1).

Seidel, H.M., Ball, J.W., Dains, J.E., et al. (2007). *Mosby's guide to physical examination*. (6th ed.). St. Louis: Mosby.

Stanton, M.W., & Rutherford, M.K. (2006). The high concentration of U.S. health care expenditures. Rockville (MD): Agency for Healthcare Research and Quality; 2005. *Research in Action* Issue 19. AHRQ Pub. No. 06-0060.

Sullivan, M. (1987). Atrophy and exercise. *Journal of Gerontological Nursing*, 13(7):26.

Thorsdottir, I., Jonsson, P.V., Asgeirsdottir, A.E., et al. (2005). Fast and simple screening for nutritional status in hospitalized, elderly people. *Journal of Human Nutrition and Dietetics*, 18(1):53-60.

United Nations Population Division. (n.d.). *World population prospects, the 2002 revision*. Available at www.un.org/esa/population/publications/wpp2002/WPP2002-HIGHLIGHTSrev1.PDF. Accessed November, 2009.

U.S. Census Bureau. (n.d.). *The 2007 statistical abstract: the national data book*. Available at www.census.gov/compendia/statab/2007/2007edition.html. Accessed November 2, 2009.

U.S. Department of Health and Human Services. (2008). *Healthy People 2010: national health promotion and disease prevention objectives*. Washington, DC: U.S. Government Printing Office.

van Haastregt, J., van Rossum, E., Dederiks, J.P., et al. (2000). Preventing falls and mobility problems in community-dwelling elders: the process of creating a new intervention. *Geriatric Nursing*, 21(6): 309-314.

Williams, C.M. (2002). Using medications appropriately in older adults. *American Family Physician*, 66(10):1917-1924.

Chapter 34 Basic Concepts of Mental Health

Archer, D. (2004). Exploring nonverbal communication. Available at http://nonverbal.ucsc.edu/index.html. Accessed November, 2009.

Bulechek, G.M., Butcher, H.K., & Dochterman, J.M. (2008). *Nursing international classification (NIC)*. (5th ed.). St. Louis: Mosby.

Fortinash, K.M., & Holoday-Worret, P.A. (2004). *Psychiatric mental health nursing*. (3rd ed.). St. Louis: Mosby.

Giger, S.N., & Davidhizar, R.E. (2008). *Transcultural nursing: assessment and intervention*. (5th ed.). St. Louis: Mosby.

Marmer, S.S. (2003). Theories of the mind and psycho-pathology. In R.E. Hales, & S.L. Yudofsky (Eds). *Textbook of clinical psychiatry*. (4th ed.). Washington, DC: American Psychiatric Publishing.

Moorhead, S., Johnson, M., Maas, M., et al. (2008). *Nursing outcomes classification (NOC)*. (4th ed.). St. Louis: Mosby.

North American Nursing Diagnosis Association International (NANDA-I). (2009). *NANDA-I nursing diagnoses: definitions and classification 2009-2011*. Oxford, United Kingdom: Author.

Townsend, M.C. (2008). *Essentials of psychiatric mental health nursing*. (4th ed.). Philadelphia: F.A. Davis.

Varcarolis, E.M., & Halter, M.J. (2009). *Foundations of psychiatric mental health nursing: a clinical approach*. (6th ed.). Philadelphia: Saunders.

Weber, D. (2006). Is it more than just stress? *RN*, 69(3):53.

Chapter 35 Care of the Patient with a Psychiatric Disorder

American Psychiatric Association (APA). (2000). *Diagnostic and statistical manual of mental disorders (DSM-IV-TR)*. (4th ed.). Washington, DC: Author.

Captain, C. (2006). Is your partner a suicide risk? *Nursing 2006*, 36(8):43-47.

Fortinash, K.M., & Holoday-Worret, P.A. (2008). *Psychiatric mental health nursing*. (4th ed.). St. Louis: Mosby.

Hodgson, B.B., & Kizior, R.J. (2010). *Saunder's nursing drug handbook 2010*. Philadelphia: Saunders.

Keltner, N.L., & Folks, D.G. (2005). *Psychotropic drugs*. (4th ed.). St. Louis: Mosby.

McGlotten, S. (2003). Attempted suicide. *Nursing*, 33(4):96.

Morrison-Valfre, M. (2008). *Foundations of mental health care*. (4th ed.). St. Louis: Mosby.

Mosby's dictionary of medicine, nursing, and health professions. (8th ed.). (2009). St. Louis: Mosby.

Murphy, K. (2005). The separate reality of bipolar disorder and schizophrenia. *Nursing Made Incredibly Easy!* 3(3):6-18.

Murphy, K. (2006). Managing the ups and downs of polar disorder. *Nursing 2006*, 36(10):58-63.

Murphy, K. (2006). Square pegs: managing personality disorders. *Nursing Made Incredibly Easy!* 4(4):34-35.

Natural Medicines Comprehensive Database. (n.d.). Available at www.naturaldatabase.com. Accessed November, 2009.

Neason, K. (2006). PTSD: Help patients break free. *RN*, 69(10):30-35.

Skidmore-Roth, L. (2009). *Mosby's handbook of herbs and natural elements*. (4th ed.). St. Louis: Mosby.

Stoner, SC., & Dubisar, B. (2006). Psychotropics. *RN 2006*, 69(7): 31-37.

Townsend, M.C. (2003). *Nursing diagnoses in psychiatric nursing: a pocket guide for care plan construction*. (5th ed.). Philadelphia: F.A. Davis.

Townsend, M.C., & Pederson, D.D. (2007). *Essentials of psychiatric mental health nursing*. (4th ed.). Philadelphia: F.A. Davis.

Uko-Ekpenyong, G. (2006). Improving medication adherence with orally disintegrating tablets. *Nursing 2006*, 36(9):20-21.

Varcarolis, E.M., & Halter, M.J. (2009). *Foundations of psychiatric mental health nursing: a clinical approach*. (6th ed.). Philadelphia: Saunders.

Wichowski, H. (2004). Your patient has schizophrenia—handle with care. *Nursing 2004*, 34(11):32ln1.

Woods, A. (2003). Depression. *Nursing 2003*, 33(3):54.

Chapter 36 Care of the Patient with an Addictive Personality

Alcoholics Anonymous. (1976). New York: Alcoholics World Service, Inc.

American Society of Addiction Medicine. (n.d.). Available at www.asam.org. Accessed October, 2009.

Bulechek, G.M., Butcher, H.K., & Dochterman, J.M. (2008). *Nursing interventions classification (NIC)*. (5th ed.). St. Louis: Mosby.

Davidson, D., Palfai, T., Bird, C., et al. (1999). Effects of naltrexone on alcohol self-administration in heavy drinkers. *Alcoholism, Clinical and Experimental Research*, 23(2):195.

Doe, J. (2003). My journey through addiction. *Nursing 2003*, 33(1): 32hn6.

Federation of State Medical Boards of the United States. (1998). *Model guidelines for the use of controlled substances for the treatment of pain*. Available at www.painpolicy.wisc.edu/domestic/model.htm. Accessed December, 2009.

Fortinash, K.M., & Holoday-Worret, P.A. (2008). *Psychiatric mental health nursing*. (4th ed.). St. Louis: Mosby.

Giger, J.N., & Davidhizer, R.E. (2008). *Transcultural nursing: assessment and intervention*. (5th ed.). St. Louis: Mosby.

Jennings-Ingle, S. (2007). Sobering up to alcohol withdrawal syndrome. *LPN 2007*, 3(5):40-48.

Jennings-Ingle, S. (2007). The sobering facts of alcohol withdrawal. *Nursing Made Incredibly Easy!* 5(1):50-60.

Kelly, A.E., & Saucier, J. (2004). Is your patient suffering from alcohol withdrawal? *RN 2004*, 62(2):27.

Keltner, N.L., Folks, D.G., Palmer, C.A., et al. (1998). *Psychobiological foundations of psychiatric care*. St. Louis: Mosby.

Moorhead, S., Johnson, M., Maas, M., et al. (2008). *Nursing outcomes classification (NOC)*. (4th ed.). St. Louis: Mosby.

National Council of State Boards of Nursing. (2000) *HIPDB and NPDB questions and answers*. Available at www.ncsbn.org. Accessed September, 2005.

National Institute on Drug Abuse. (n.d.). Available at www.nida.nih.gov. Accessed October, 2009.

National Institute on Drug Abuse. (n.d.). *Club drugs*. Available at www.clubdrugs.org. Accessed December, 2009.

North American Nursing Diagnosis Association International (NANDA-I). (2009). *NANDA-I nursing diagnoses: definitions and classification 2009-2011*. Oxford, United Kingdom: Author.

Ries, R.K., Miller, S.C., Fiellin, D.A., et al. (2009). *Principles of addiction medicine*. (4th ed.). Philadelphia: Lippincott, Williams, & Wilkins.

Science News Daily. Available at www.sciencedaily.com.

Touhy, T.A., & Jett, K. (2009). *Ebersole and Hess' gerontological nursing and healthy aging*. (3rd ed.). St. Louis: Mosby.

Townsend, M.V. (2008). *Essentials of psychiatric mental health nursing*. (4th ed.). Philadelphia: F.A. Davis.

U.S. Department of Health and Human Services (US DHHS). (2000). *Healthy People 2010: national health promotion and disease prevention objectives*. Washington, DC: U.S. Government Printing Office.

Varcarolis, E.M., & Halter, M.J. (2009). *Foundations of psychiatric mental health nursing: a clinical approach*. (6th ed.). Philadelphia: Saunders.

Chapter 37 Home Health Nursing

Baiada, M., & Freedman, A. (2003). Searching for the heart of home care. The Bayada Way Project. *Caring*, 22(5):10.

Bolch, E. (2004). America's health care system in crisis: the case for telemedicine. *Caring*, 23(7):6.

Case Management Society of America (CMSA). (n.d.). *What is a case manager?* Available at www.cmsa.org/Home/CMSA/WhatisaCaseManager/tabid/224/Default.aspx. Accessed December, 2009.

Centers for Disease Control and Prevention (CDC). (n.d.). The burden of chronic diseases and their risk factors. Available at www.cdc.gov/nccdphp/burdenbook2004. Accessed December, 2009.

Centers for Disease Control and Prevention (CDC). (2007). *HIV/AIDS surveillance report, 2005*. Vol. 17. Rev. ed. Atlanta: U.S. Department of Health and Human Services, Centers for Disease Control and Prevention. Also available at www.cdc.gov/hiv/topics/surveillance/resources/reports.

Centers for Medicare & Medicaid Services. (n.d.). Available at www.cms.hhs.gov/homehealthpps. Accessed October, 2009.

Clemen-Stone, S., McGuire, S.L., & Gerber Eigsti, D. (2002). *Comprehensive community health nursing*. (6th ed.). St. Louis: Mosby.

Federal Interagency Forum on Aging-Related Statistics. (2004). *Older Americans 2004: key indicators of well-being*. Washington, DC: U.S. Government Printing Office.

Frantz, A. (2001). Evaluating technology for success in home care. *Caring*, 20(7):10-12.

Gabriel, B. (2004). Telemedicine then and now. *Caring*, 23(7):20.

Gent, R., Strauss, S.G., Webb, T., et al. (2001). Feeling the effects of PPS: one year later. *Caring*, 20(11):18-19.

Giger, J.M., & Davidhizar, R.E. (2007). *Transcultural nursing: assessment and intervention*. (5th ed.). St. Louis: Mosby.

Horstman, P., & Ferretti, A. (2001). Habitat for Humanity. *American Journal of Nursing*, 101(8):63-65.

Jaffe, M., & Skidmore-Roth, L. (2005). *Home health nursing assessment and care planning*. (5th ed.). St. Louis: Mosby.

Keintz, C. (2004). A model of preparedness: state associations partner for disaster response. *Caring*, 23(9):10.

Kinsella, A. (2003). Home telehealth program planning. *Caring*, 22(8):16.

Lewis, S.L., Heitkemper, M.M., Dirksen, S.R., et al. (2007). *Medical-surgical nursing: assessment and management of clinical problems*. (7th ed.). St. Louis: Mosby.

Marrelli, T., & Hilliard, L. (2002). *Home health and clinical paths: effective care planning throughout the continuum*. (2nd ed.). St. Louis: Mosby.

Monks, K. (2008). *Pocket guide to home health care*. (3rd ed.). Philadelphia: Saunders.

National Association for Home Care and Hospice (NAHC). (n.d.). Available at www.nahc.org. Accessed December, 2009.

National Health Ministries. (2004). *Parish nursing*. Available at www.pcusa.org/health/usa/parishnursing. Accessed June 15, 2005.

O'Sullivan, A., & Siebert, C. (2004). Occupational therapy and home health—a perfect fit. *Caring*, 23(5):10.

Rice, R. (2006). *Home care nursing practice concepts and application*. (4th ed.). St. Louis: Mosby.

Rice, R. (2008). *Handbook of home health nursing procedures*. (4th ed.). St. Louis: Mosby.

Siegel, S., & Strausbaugh, M. (n.d.). *Guidelines for isolation: preventing transmission of infectious agents in healthcare settings*. Available at www.cdc.gov/ncidod/dhqp/pdf/guidelines/Isolation2007.pdf. Accessed December, 2009.

St. Pierre, M., & Dombi, W.A. (2000). Home health PPS: new payment system, new hope. *Caring*, 19(11):6.

Stanhope, M., & Knollmueller, R. (2008). *Handbook of community and home health nursing: tools for assessment, intervention, and education*. (5th ed.). St. Louis: Mosby.

Stanhope, M., & Lancaster, J. (2007). *Community and public health nursing*. (6th ed.). St. Louis: Mosby.

Wehrman, P., & Bennet, D. (2002). Hi-tech and hi-touch: combining state-of-the-art technology with state-of-the-art home health care. *The Remington Report*, 19(2):28.

Wright, K. (2003). Planning for positive clinical and financial returns for telemonitoring. *Caring*, 22(10):45.

Resources

Home Healthcare Nurses Association, 202-546-4754. Available at www.hhna.org. Accessed December, 2009.

National Association for Home Care, 202-547-7424. Available at www.nahc.org. Accessed December, 2009.

Chapter 38 Long-Term Care

Administration on Aging (AoA). (2004). *A profile of older Americans*. Available at www.aoa.gov/AoARoot/Aging_Statistics/Profile/index.aspx. Accessed December, 2009.

Alzheimer's Association. (n.d.). Available at www.alz.org. Accessed December, 2009.

Bulechek, G.M., Butcher, H.K., & Dochterman, J.M. (2008). *Nursing intervention classification (NIC)*. (5th ed.). St. Louis: Mosby.

Caregivers USA. (2004). *Residential care facilities*. Available at www.caregivers-usa.org/facility/. Accessed September, 2008.

Centers for Disease Control and Prevention (CDC). (2004). *Home health patients according to age, sex and diagnosis: United States*. Available at www.cdc.gov/nchs/data/nhhcsd/curhomecare00.pdf. Accessed December, 2009.

Centers for Disease Control and Prevention (CDC), National Center for Health Statistics. (2004). *Living arrangements by age, sex, and race/hispanic origin: United States*. Available at http://209.217.72.34/aging/TableViewer/tableView.aspx. Accessed September, 2005.

Centers for Healthy Aging. c/o National Council on Aging. (n.d.). www.ncoa.org/contact. Accessed September, 2008.

Geiger, J.N., & Davidhizar, R.E. (2008). *Transcultural nursing assessment and intervention*. (5th ed.). St. Louis: Mosby.

Long-Term Care Education.com. (2004). *Definition of the types of residential care*. Available at www.longtermcareeducation.com. Accessed September, 2008.

Lucas, J.A., et al. (2002). *Adult day health services: a review of the literature*. Available at www.cshp.rutgers.edu. Accessed September, 2008.

Medicare.gov. (2007). *Alternatives to nursing home care*. Available at www.medicare.gov/Nursing/Alternatives.asp. Accessed December, 2009.

Moorhead, S., Johnson, M., Maas, M., et al. (2008). *Nursing outcomes classification (NOC)*. (4th ed.). St. Louis: Mosby.

National Adult Day Services Association, Inc. (2008). *Adult day services: overview and facts*. Available at www.nadsa.org/adsfacts/default.asp. Accessed December, 2009.

National Center for Assisted Living (2006). *Assisted living resident profile*. Available at www.ahcancal.org/ncal/resources/Pages/ResidentProfile.aspx. Accessed December, 2009.

National Center for Assisted Living (2009). *Assisted living state regulatory review*. Available at www.ahcancal.org/ncal/resources/Pages/StateRegulatoryReview.aspx. Accessed December, 2009.

National Hospice and Palliative Care Organization. (2004). *What is hospice and palliative care?* Available at http://www.nhpco.org/i4a/pages/index.cfm?pageid=4648. Accessed December, 2009.

North American Nursing Diagnosis Association International (NANDA-I). (2009). *NANDA-I nursing diagnoses: definitions and classification 2009-2011*. Oxford, United Kingdom: Author.

O'Neill, P.A. (2002). *Caring for the older adult: a health promotion perspective*. Philadelphia: Saunders.

Potter, P.A., & Perry, A.G. (2007). *Basic nursing: essentials for practice*. (6th ed.). St. Louis: Mosby.

Potter, P.A., & Perry, A.G. (2009). *Fundamentals of nursing: concepts, process, and practice*. (7th ed.). St. Louis: Mosby.

Rantz, M., Popejoy, L., & Zwygart-Stauffacher, M. (2001). *The new nursing homes: a 20-minute way to find great long-term care*. Minneapolis: Fairview Press.

Sahyoun, N.R., Pratt, L.A., Lentzner, H., et al. (2001). The changing profile of nursing home residents: 1985-1997. *Aging Trends, No. 4*. Hyattsville, NC: National Center for Health Statistics.

U.S. Department of Health and Human Services (US DHHS). (2000). *Healthy People 2010: national health promotion and disease prevention objectives*. Washington, DC: U.S. Government Printing Office.

U.S. Department of Health and Human Services (US DHHS). (2004). *Health care in America: trends in utilization*. Hyattsville, NC: National Center for Health Statistics.

U.S. Department of Health and Human Services (US DHHS). (n.d.) *Healthy People: what are its goals?* Available at www.healthypeople.gov/About/goals.htm. Accessed December, 2009.

U.S. Department of Health and Human Services (US DHHS). Administration on Aging (AoA). (2003). *A statistical profile on hispanic older Americans aged 65*. Available at www.aoa.gov/AoARoot/Aging_Statistics/Minority_Aging/Facts-on-Hispanic-Elderly-2008.aspx. Accessed December, 2009.

Chapter 39 Rehabilitation Nursing

American Psychiatric Association (APA). (1980). *Diagnostic and statistical manual of mental disorders*. (3rd ed.). Washington, DC: American Psychiatric Press.

American Psychiatric Association (APA). (2000). *Diagnostic and statistical manual of mental disorders*. (4th ed., Text rev.). Washington, DC: American Psychiatric Press.

Arlinger, S. (2003). Negative consequences of uncorrected hearing loss—a review. *International Journal of Audiology*, 42(Suppl 2): 2S17-S20.

Association of Rehabilitation Nurses. (n.d.). Available at www.rehabnurse.org. Accessed October, 2009.

Bisson, J., & Andrew, M. (2005). Psychological treatment of post-traumatic stress disorder (PTSD). *Cochrane Database Systems Review*, 18(2):CD003388.

Bostrom, C.E., & Schwecke, L.H. (2007). Anxiety-related disorders, somatoform, and dissociative disorders. In N.L. Keltner, C.E. Bostrom, & L.H. Schwecke (Eds.). *Psychiatric nursing*. (5th ed.). St. Louis: Mosby.

Bradley, R., Greene, J., Russ, E., et al. (2005). A multidimensional meta-analysis of psychotherapy for PTSD. *American Journal of Psychiatry*, 162(2):214-227.

Broome, M., & Rollins, J. (1999). *Core curriculum for the nursing care of children and their families*. Pitman, NJ: Jannetti.

Burks, K.J. (1999). A nursing practice model for chronic illness. *Rehabilitation Nursing*, 24(5):197.

Clark, C.C. (1997). Posttraumatic stress disorder: how to support healing. *American Journal of Nursing*, 97(8):27-33.

Commission on Chronic Illness. (1957). Chronic illness in the United States. In L. Braslow, (Ed.). *Chronic illness in the United States*, vol. 1. Cambridge, Mass: Harvard University Press.

Cook, P. (1999). *Supporting sick children and their families*. London: Harcourt.

Cross T., Bazron, B., Dennis, K., et al. (1989). *Towards a culturally competent system of care, volume I*. Washington, D.C.: Georgetown University Child Development Center, CASSP Technical Assistance Center.

Danielson, C., & Hamel-Bissell, B. (1993). *Families, health, and illness: perspectives on coping and intervention*. St. Louis: Mosby.

Easton, K. (1999). *Gerontological rehabilitation nursing*. Philadelphia: Saunders.

Edwards, P.A. (2000). *The specialty practice of rehabilitation nursing: a core curriculum*. (4th ed.). Skokie, IL: Association of Rehabilitation Nurses.

Edwards, P.A., Hertzberg, D.L., Hays, S.R., et al. (1999). *Pediatric rehabilitation nursing*. Philadelphia: Saunders.

Elsayed, N.M. (1997). Toxicology of blast overpressure. *Toxicology*, 121:1-15.

Elsayed, N.M., & Gorbunov, N.V. (2006). Pulmonary biochemical and histological alterations after repeated low level blast overpressure exposures. *Toxicological Sciences*, 95(1):289-296.

Emerson, R.W. (2003). *Selected writings of Ralph Waldo Emerson*. New York: Signet Classics.

Ferguson, A.D., Richie, B.S., & Gomez, M.J. (2004). Psychological factors after traumatic amputation in landmine survivors: The bridge between physical healing and full recover. *Disability and Rehabilitation*, 26(14-15):931-938.

Glass, A.J. (1969). Introduction. In P.G. Bourne (Ed.). *The psychology and physiology of stress*, pp. xiv-xxx. New York: Academic Press.

Gordon, W.A., Brown, M., Sliwinski, M., et al. (1998). The enigma of "hidden" traumatic brain injury. *Journal of Head Trauma Rehabilitation*, 13:39-56.

Haworth, S.K., & Dluhy, N.M. (2001). Holistic symptom management: modeling the interaction phase. *Journal of Advanced Nursing*, 36(2):302.

Hoeman, S. (2000). *Rehabilitation nursing: process and application*. (3rd ed.). St. Louis: Mosby.

Leavitt, R.L. (2001). *Cross-cultural rehabilitation: an international perspective*. Philadelphia: Saunders.

Lubkin, I.M., & Larsen, P.D. (Eds.). (2006). *Chronic illness: impact and interventions*. (6th ed.). Sudbury, Mass: Jones & Bartlett.

Merck Institute on Aging and Health. (2002). *The state of aging and health in America*. Available at www.agingsociety.org/agingsociety/publications/state/index.html. Accessed December, 2009.

Mosby's dictionary of medicine, nursing, and health professions. (8th ed.). (2009). St. Louis: Mosby.

Nathenson, P. (1999). *Integrating rehabilitation and restorative nursing concepts into the MDS*. Glenview, Ill: Association of Rehabilitation Nurses.

Neal, J.N., & Guilett, S.E. (2004). *Care of the adult with a chronic illness or disability: a team approach*. St. Louis: Mosby.

Nelson, A.L. (2008). Polytrauma: a new frontier in rehabilitation nursing. *Rehabilitation Nursing*, 33(5):191-192.

Nolan, M., & Nolan, J. (1999). Rehabilitation, chronic illness and disability: the missing elements in nurse education. *Journal of Advanced Nursing*, 29(4):958.

Orem, D.E. (2001). *Nursing concepts of practice*. (6th ed.). St. Louis: Mosby.

Pivar, I. (2006). Helping the soldier to recognize, understand and manage grief reactions. National Center for PTSD. VAKN Continuing Education Program. Palo Alto, Ca: VA, Palo Alto.

Potter, P.A., & Perry, A.G. (2007). *Basic nursing: essentials for practice*. (6th ed.). St. Louis: Mosby.

Redman, B.K. (2001). *The practice of patient education*. St. Louis: Mosby.

Rehabilitation Nursing Foundation of the Association of Rehabilitation Nurses. (1995). *Rehabilitation nursing: directions for practice*. (3rd ed.). Skokie, Ill: Association of Rehabilitation Nurses.

Rolland, J. (1994). *Families, illness, and disability*. New York: Basic Books.

Rumpler, C.H. (2008). How do you intervene in posttraumatic stress disorder symptoms associated with traumatic injury? *Rehabilitation Nursing*, 33(5):187-188.

Schwecke, L.H. (2007). Models of working with psychiatric patients. In N.L. Keltner, C.E. Bostrom, & L.H. Schwecke (Eds.). *Psychiatric nursing*. (5th ed.). St. Louis: Mosby.

Scott, S.G., Vanderploeg, R.D., Belanger, H.G., et al. (2005). Blast injuries: evaluating and treating the postacute sequelae. *Federal Practitioner*, 22(1):66-75.

Sheldon, L., Barrett, R., & Ellington, L. (2006). Difficult communication in nursing. *Journal of Nursing Scholarship*, 38(2):141-142.

Stein, D.J., Davidson, J.R.T., Seedat, S., et al. (2003). Paroxetine in the treatment of post-traumatic stress disorder: pooled analysis of placebo-controlled studies. *Expert Opinion on Pharmacotherapy*, 4(10):1829-1838.

Stryker, R.P. (1977). *Rehabilitative aspects of acute and chronic nursing care*. (2nd ed.). Philadelphia: Saunders.

U.S. Department of Health and Human Services (US DHHS). (2000). *Healthy People 2010*. (Conference Edition). Washington, DC: U.S. Government Printing Office.

Warden, D. (2006). Military TBI during the Iraq and Afghanistan wars. *Journal of Head Trauma Rehabilitation*, 21(5):398-402.

World Health Organization (WHO). (1980). *International classification of impairment, disabilities, and handicaps: a manual classification relating the consequences of disease*. Geneva, Switzerland: Author.

Wrightman, J.M., & Gladish, S.L. (2001). Explosions and blast injuries. *Annals of Emergency Medicine*, 37:664-687.

Chapter 40 Hospice Care

Clark, D. (2002). *Cicely Saunders, founder of the modern day hospice movement*. New York: Oxford University Press.

Claxton-Oldfield, S., Claxton-Oldfield, J., & Rishchynski, G. (2004). Understanding of the term "palliative care": a Canadian survey. *American Journal of Hospice & Palliative Care*, 21(2):105.

Dahlin, C. (2004). Oral complication at the end of life. *American Journal of Nursing*, 104(7):40.

Editors. (2004). The state of hospice in America—looking back, looking forward. *Caring*, 23(2):44.

Esper, P. (2000). Pain management in patients with advanced malignancies. *Home Health Care Consultant*, 7(10):11.

Ferrell, B.R., & Coyle, N. (2005). *Textbook of palliative nursing*. New York: Oxford University Press.

Giger, J.M., & Davidhizar, R.E. (2007). *Transcultural nursing: assessment and intervention*. (5th ed.). St. Louis: Mosby.

Gordon, A. (2001). End of life issues. *Caring*, 20(21):6.

Harper, B. (2000). Hospice and palliative care: a vision for the new millennium. *Journal of Hospice and Palliative Nursing Care*, 2(1):21.

Haughney, A. (2004). Nausea and vomiting in end-stage cancer. *American Journal of Nursing*, 104(11):40.

Heffler, S., Smith, S., Keehan, S., et al. (2003). Health spending projections for 2002-2012. *Health Affairs*. Available at http://content.healthaffairs.org/cgi/content/abstract/hlthaff.w3.54v1. Accessed December, 2009.

Hospice Foundation of America. (n.d.). *Be a hospice volunteer.* Available at www.hospicefoundation.org/pages/page.asp?page_id=53134. Accessed October, 2009.

Kacela, X. (2004). Religious maturity in the midst of death and dying. *American Journal of Hospice & Palliative Care*, 21(3):203.

Knowlton, C. (2004). Collaborative pharmacy practice enters hospice care. *Caring*, 23(6):26.

Lewis, S.L., Heitkemper, M.M., Dirksen, S.R., et al. (2007). *Medical-surgical nursing: assessment and management of clinical problems.* (7th ed.). St. Louis: Mosby.

Lorenz, K., & Asch, S. (2004). Hospice admission practices: where does hospice fit in the continuum of care? *Journal of the American Geriatric Society*, 52:725.

May, V., Onarcan, M., Olechowski, C., et al. (2004). International perspectives on the role of home care and hospice in aging and long-term care. *Caring*, 23(1):14.

McCaffery, M., & Pasero, C. (2007). *Pain: clinical management.* (4th ed.). St. Louis: Mosby.

Morita, T., Tsunoda J., Inoue, S., et al. (2000). Terminal sedation for existential distress. *American Journal of Hospice and Palliative Care*, 17(3):189.

Morrison, R., & Meier, D. (2004). Palliative care. *New England Journal of Medicine*. 350:2582.

Naik, A., & Dehaven, M. (2004). Short stays in hospice. *Caring*, 20(2):10.

National Consensus Project. (2004). *Clinical practice guidelines for palliative care.* Available at www.nationalconsensusproject.org/Guidelines_Download.asp. Accessed December, 2009.

Rich, S. (2005). Providing quality end-of-life care. *Journal of Cardiovascular Nursing*, 20:141.

Schmidt, L. (2003). Pediatric end of life care: coming of age? *Caring*, 22(5):20.

Trueman, C. (2003). Raising the bar of excellence in home care and hospice. *Caring*, 22(3):24.

World Health Organization (WHO). (n.d.). *Palliative care.* Available at www.who.int/cancer/palliative/en. Accessed October, 2009.

Wrede-Seaman, L. (2001). Treatment options to manage pain at the end of life. *Journal of Hospice and Palliative Care*, 18(2):89.

Resources

Hospice and Palliative Nurses Association, 412-787-9301. Available at www.hpna.org. Accessed December, 2009.

Hospice Education Institute, 207-255-8800. Available at www.hospiceworld.org. Accessed December, 2009.

Hospice Foundation of America, 800-854-3402. Available at www.hospicefoundation.org. Accessed December, 2009.

National Association for Home Care and Hospice, 202-547-7424. Available at www.nahc.org. Accessed December, 2009.

National Consensus Project for Quality Palliative Care. Palliative Care Clinical Practice Guidelines. Available at www.nationalconsensusproject.org. Accessed December, 2009.

National Hospice and Palliative Care Organization, 703-837-1500. Available at www.nhpco.org. Accessed December, 2009.

Palliative Care Educational Resources Team (PERT). Educational resources for delivering end-of-life care in nursing homes. Available at www.swedishmedical.org/PERT/links.htm. Accessed December, 2009.

Chapter 41 Introduction to Anatomy and Physiology

Herlihy, B., & Maebius, N.K. (2008). *The human body in health and illness.* Philadelphia: Saunders.

Jarvis, C. (2008). *Physical examination and health assessment.* (5th ed.). Philadelphia: Saunders.

Langford, R.W., & Thompson, J.M. (2008). *Mosby's handbook of diseases.* (4th ed.). St. Louis: Mosby.

Lewis, S.L., Heitkemper, M.M., Dirksen, S.R., et al. (2007). *Medical-surgical nursing: assessment and management of clinical problems.* (7th ed.). St. Louis: Mosby.

Memmler, R.L., et al. (2008). *Structure and function of the human body.* (9th ed.). Philadelphia: Lippincott.

Monahan, F.D., Sands, J.K., Neighbors, M., et al. (2007). *Phipps' medical-surgical nursing: health and illness perspectives.* (8th ed.). St. Louis: Mosby.

Mosby's dictionary of medicine, nursing, and health professions. (2009). (8th ed.). St. Louis: Mosby.

Patton, K.T., & Thibodeau, G.A. (2008). *Mosby's handbook of anatomy and physiology.* St. Louis: Mosby.

Petti, K. (2007). *Anatomy and physiology.* (6th ed.). St. Louis: Mosby.

Swisher, L. (2008). *Structure and function of the body.* (13th ed.). St. Louis: Mosby.

Thibodeau, G.A., & Patton, K.T. (2007). *Anatomy and physiology.* (6th ed.). St. Louis: Mosby.

Thibodeau, G.A., & Patton, K.T. (2008). *Structure and function of the body.* (13th ed.). St. Louis: Mosby.

Thibodeau, G.A., & Patton, K.T. (2009). *The human body in health and disease.* (5th ed.). St. Louis: Mosby.

Thompson, J.M., McFarland, G.K., Hirsch, J.E., et al. (2001). *Mosby's clinical nursing.* (5th ed.). St. Louis: Mosby.

Chapter 42 Care of the Surgical Patient

Ackley, B.J., & Ladwig, G.B. (2009). *Nursing diagnosis handbook.* (7th ed.). St. Louis: Mosby.

Beattie, S. (2007). Wound dehiscence. *RN*, 70(6):34-38.

Bulechek, G.M., Butcher, H.K. & Dochterman, J.M. (2008). *Nursing interventions classifications (NIC).* (5th ed.). St. Louis: Mosby.

Blaney-Koen, L. (2007). Safe surgery a patient's guide. *Journal of Patient Surgery*, 3(1):56.

Centers for Disease Control and Prevention (CDC). (2002). *Guideline for hand hygiene in healthcare settings.* Available at www.cdc.gov/handhygiene. Accessed November, 2009.

Cofer, M. (2005). Unwelcome companion to older patients: postoperative delirium. *Nursing*, 35(1):32.

Crum, E., & Valinti, J. (2007). Can a bloodless surgery program work in a trauma setting? *Nursing*, 37(3):54-56.

D'Arcy, Y. (2006). How to care for a surgical patient with chronic pain. *Nursing*, 36(3):17.

Daniels, S.M. (2007). Improving hospital care for surgical patients. *Nursing*, 37(8):36-42.

Dunn, D. (2006). Age smart care. Preventing perioperative complications in older adults. *Nursing Made Incredibly Easy!* 4(3):30-41.

Elkin, M.K., Perry, A.G., & Potter, P.A. (2007). *Nursing interventions and clinical skills.* (4th ed.). St. Louis: Mosby.

Giger, J.M., & Davidhizar, R.E. (2007). *Transcultural nursing: assessment and intervention.* (5th ed.). St. Louis: Mosby.

Harkreader, H., Hogan, M.A., & Thobaben, M. (2007). *Fundamentals of nursing: care and clinical judgment.* (3rd ed.). St. Louis: Mosby.

Hunter, S., Thompson, P., Langemo, D., et al. (2007). Understanding wound dehiscence. *Nursing*, 37(9):28, 30.

The Joint Commission (2009a). *Universal protocol.* Available at www.jointcommission.org/PatientSafety/UniversalProtocol/up_facts.htm. Accessed November, 2009.

The Joint Commission. (2009b). *Universal protocol for preventing wrong site, wrong procedure and wrong person surgery.* Available at www.jointcommission.org/PatientSafety/NationalPatientSafetyGoals. Accessed November, 2009.

Lewis, S.L., Heitkemper, M.M., Dirksen, S.R., et al. (2007). *Medical-surgical nursing: assessment and management of clinical problems.* (7th ed.). St. Louis: Mosby.

McCaffery, M., Grimm, M.A., Pasero, C., et al. (2005). On the meaning of "drug seeking." *Pain Management Nursing*, 6(4): 122-136.

McCaffery, M., & Pasero, C. (1999). *Pain: clinical manual.* (2nd ed.). St. Louis: Mosby.

Monahan, F.D., Sands, J.K., Neighbors, M., et al. (2007). *Phipps' medical-surgical nursing: health and illness perspectives.* (8th ed.). St. Louis: Mosby.

Moorhead, S., Johnson, M., Maas, M., et al. (2008). *Nursing outcomes classification (NOC).* (4th ed.). St. Louis: Mosby.

Mosby's dictionary of medicine, nursing, and health professions. (2009). (8th ed.). St. Louis: Mosby.

Nichols, R.L. (2001). Preventing surgical site infections: a surgeon's perspective. *Emerging Infectious Diseases*, 7(2):220-224.

North American Nursing Diagnosis Association International (NANDA-I). (2009). *NANDA-I nursing diagnoses: definitions and classification 2009-2011*. Oxford, United Kingdom: Author.

Occupational Safety and Health Administration (OSHA). (n.d.). *Healthcare wide hazards: infection*. Available at www.cdc.gov/handhygiene. Accessed November, 2009.

Odom-Forren, J. (2006). Preventing surgical site infections. *Nursing 2006*, 36(16):59-64.

Pagana, K.D., & Pagana, T.J. (2008). *Mosby's diagnostic and laboratory test reference*. (9th ed.). St. Louis: Mosby.

Patient education series. (2007). *Nursing*, 37(8):43.

Pearce, J.M. (2006). Documenting preoperative education. *Nursing*, 36(8):71.

Potter, P.A., & Perry, A.G. (2007). *Basic nursing: essentials for practice*. (6th ed.). St. Louis: Mosby.

Potter, P.A., & Perry, A.G. (2009). *Fundamentals of nursing: concepts, process, and practice*. (7th ed.). St. Louis: Mosby.

Ridge, R.A. (2008). Doing it right to prevent wrong-site surgery. *Nursing*, 38(3):24,25.

Rothrock, J.C. (2007). *Alexander's care of the patient in surgery*. (13th ed.). St. Louis: Mosby.

Sarvis, C. (2006). Postoperative wound care. *Nursing*, 36(12):56-57.

Schwartz, A., Jr. (2006). Learning the essentials of epidural anesthesia. *Nursing*, 36(1):44-50.

Skidmore-Roth, L. (2010). *Mosby's 2010 nursing drug reference*. (23rd ed.). St. Louis: Mosby.

Tabor, W. (2007). Cutting edge of robtic surgery. *Nursing*, 37(2):48-50.

Chapter 43 Care of the Patient with an Integumentary Disorder

Anderson, L.M. (2005). Atopic dermatitis: More than a simple skin disorder. *Journal of the American Academy of Nurse Practitioners*, 17(7):249, 251.

Aschenbrenner, D.S. (2007). A new topical ointment for impetigo. *American Journal of Nursing*, 107(9):31.

Black, J.M., & Hawks, H.J. (2009). *Medical-surgical nursing: clinical management for positive outcomes*. (8th ed.). Philadelphia: Saunders.

Bresett, J. (2006). Would you suspect this skin eating infection? *RN*, 69(3):31-35.

Burn Care Central. (2007). *Nursing Made Incredibly Easy!* 5(4):17-20.

Centers for Disease Control and Prevention (CDC). (2009). Fire deaths and injuries: fact sheet. Available at www.cdc.gov/HomeandRecreationalSafety/Fire-Prevention/fires-factsheet.html. Accessed November, 2009.

DeBoer, S., Felty, C., Seaver, M. (2004). Burn care in EMS. *Emergency Medical Services*, 33(2):69, 72, 87.

Dulak, S.B. (2006). Stop: the assault on the skin in HIV. *RN*, 69(6):25-30.

GlaxoSmithKline (GSK). (2007). *SGK announces FDA approval of Altabax (retapamulin ointment), 1%*. Available at www.gsk.com/media/pressreleases/2007/2007_04_12GSK1014.htm. Accessed November, 2009.

Hess, C.T. (2003). Treating a fungal rash. *Nursing*, 33(9):9.

Hockenberry, M.J., & Wilson, D. (2007). *Wong's nursing care of infants and children*. (8th ed.). St. Louis, Mosby.

Holcomb, S.S. (2006). Nonmelanoma skin cancer. *RN*, 36(6):56-58.

Kent, H. (2000). PDT effective for inflammatory, viral skin lesions. *Dermatology Times*, 22(8):19.

Kleinpell, R. (2003). The role of the critical care nurse in the assessment and management of the patient with severe sepsis. *Critical Care Nursing Clinics of North America*, 15(1):27.

Lee, M., & Kalb, R.E. (2008). Systemic therapy for psoriasis. *Dermatology Nursing*, 20(8):105-108.

Lewis, S.L., Heitkemper, M.M., Dirksen, S.R., et al. (2007). *Medical-surgical nursing: assessment and management of clinical problems*. (7th ed.). St. Louis: Mosby.

Linton, A.D. (2007). *Introduction to medical surgical nursing*. (4th ed.). Philadelphia: Saunders.

McCance, K.L., & Huether, S.E. (2010). *Pathophysiology: the biologic basis for disease in adults and children*. (6th ed.). St. Louis: Mosby.

Melnyk, B.M., & Ebling, A.M. (2001). Effectiveness of oral antibiotics and topical retinal therapy in the treatment of acne in adolescents. *Pediatric Nursing*, 27(4):41.

Monahan, F.D., Sands, J.K., Neighbors, M., et al. (2007). *Phipps' medical-surgical nursing: health and illness perspectives*. (8th ed.). St. Louis: Mosby.

Mosby's dictionary of medicine, nursing, and health professions. (2009). (8th ed.). St. Louis: Mosby.

Mower-Wade, D., & Kang, T.M. (2004). Sepsis: when defense turns deadly. *Nursing 2004*, 34(7):30.

Novatnack, E. (2007). Shingles: what you should know. *RN*, 70(6):27-32.

Nowlin, A. (2006). The delicate business of burn care. *RN*, 69(1):51-58.

Quillen, T.F. (2004). Easing the heartbreak of psoriasis. *Nursing*, 34(11):18.

Quillen, T.F. (2007). Myths and facts ... about shingles. *Nursing*, 7:29-32.

Roy, D.E., & Stotts, N.A. (2002). Targeting cellulitis. *Nursing*, 32(12):32.

Sheridan R., & Tompkins, R. (2004). What's new in burns and metabolism. *Journal of the American College of Surgeons*, 198:243.

Stalbow, J. (2004). Preventing cellulitis in older people with persistent lower limb edema. *British Journal of Nursing*, 13(12):725.

Chapter 44 Care of the Patient with a Musculoskeletal Disorder

American Academy of Orthopaedic Surgeons (AAOS). (2006). *Total hip replacement*. Available at http://orthoinfo.aaos.org/fact/thr_report.cfm?thread_ID=504&topcategory=Joint% 20Replacement. Accessed October, 2009.

American Association of Hip and Knee Surgeons (AAHKS). *Minimally invasive and small incision joint replacement surgery: What surgeons should consider.* Available at www.aahks.org/member/resources/MIS_Surgeons.pdf. Accessed October, 2009.

American Society for Surgery of the Hand (ASSH). *Wrist arthroscopy*. Available at www.assh.org/Public/HandConditions/Pages/Wristarthroscopy.aspx. Accessed October, 2009.

Bergstrom, I., Freyschuss, B., & Landgren, B.M. (2005). Physical training and hormone replacement therapy reduce the decrease in bone mineral density in peri-menopausal women: a pilot study. *Osteoporosis International*, 16(7):823-828.

Bezaitis, A. (2008). Successful strategies for fall prevention. *AgingWell*. 1(1):28-31.

Bonner, S. (2007a). Fixate on pin site care. *Nursing Made Incredibly Easy!* 5(4):22-25.

Bonner, S. (2007b). TKO knee pain with total knee replacement. *Nursing Made Incredibly Easy!* 5(2):30-39.

Brookhart, M.A., Avorn, J., Katz, J.N., et al. (2007). Gaps in treatment among users of osteoporosis medications: the dynamics of noncompliance. *American Journal of Medicine*, 120(3):251-256.

Capo, J.T., Swan, K.G., Jr., & Tan, V. (2006). External fixation techniques for distal radius fractures. *Clinical Orthopaedics and Related Research*, 445(3):30-41.

Centers for Disease Control and Prevention. National Center for Injury Prevention and Control. Division of Unintentional Injury Prevention. (2007). *Falls among older adults: an overview*. Available at www.cdc.gov/HomeandRecreationalSafety/Falls/adultfalls.html. Accessed October, 2009.

Chou, R., Qaseem, A., Snow, V., et al. (2007). Diagnosis and treatment of low back pain pain: a joint clinical practice guideline from the American College of Physicians and the American Pain Society. *Annals of Internal Medicine*, 147(7):478-491.

Cleveland Clinic. (2007). *Osteomyelitis*. Available at http://my.clevelandclinic.org/disorders/osteomyelitis/hic_osteomyelitis.aspx. Accessed October, 2009.

Crowley, L.V. (2004). *An introduction to human disease: pathology and pathophysiology considerations*. Sunbury, Mass: Jones & Bartlett.

D'Arcy, Y. (2006a). Phantom limb pain: what it is, how to treat it. *LPN*, 2(6):15-17.

D'Arcy, Y. (2006b). Treating pain after a total joint replacement. *Nursing*, 36(5):26-28.

D'Arcy, Y. (2007). Latest pain relief a combination of new and old. *The Nurse Practitioner*, 32(1):11-12.

D'Arcy, Y. (2008). Getting a grip on neuropathic pain. *LPN*, 4(2):14-19.

Dell, D.D. (2007). Getting the point about fibromyalgia. *Nursing*, 36(2):61-64.

Dubuisson, W.C. (2009). Orthopedic measures. In A.G. Perry & P.A. Potter, *Clinical nursing skills and techniques*. (7th ed.). St. Louis: Mosby.

Editorial. (2007). The path to managing neuropathic pain. *Nursing Made Incredibly Easy!* 5(1):26-29.

Geerts, W.H., Pineo, G.F., Heit, J.A., et al. (2004). Prevention of venous thromboembolism: the Seventh ACCP Conference on Antithrombotic and Thrombolytic Therapy. *Chest*, 126(3 Suppl):338S-400S.

Goldenberg, D.I., Burckhardt, C., & Crofford, L. (2006). Management of fibromyalgia syndrome. *Journal of the American Medical Association*, 292(19):2388-2395.

Gowall, B. (2007). Joint surgery paving the way to a smooth recovery. *RN*, 70(1):37.

Habel, M. (2006). Fibromyalgia: looking good and feeling awful. *Nursing Spectrum*, 15(12):17-18.

Hairon, N. (2007). Improving falls prevention and standards of fracture care. *Nursing Times*, 103(47):23-24.

Helmann D., & Stone, J.H. (2007). Arthritis and musculoskeletal disorders. In L. Tierney, S.J. McPhee, & M.A. Papadakis (Eds.): *Current medical diagnosis and treatment*. (44th ed.). New York: McGraw-Hill.

Hendrich, A. (2007). Predicting patient falls. *American Journal of Nursing*, 107(11):50-58.

Holcomb, S. (2006). Osteoporosis. *Nursing*, 36(4):48-49.

Kelly, A.M. (2006). Managing osteoarthritis pain. *Nursing*, 36(11): 20-21.

Keskin, D., Borman, P., Ersöz, M., et al. (2008). The risk factors related to falling in elderly females. *Geriatric Nursing*, 29(1):58-63.

Kneale, J., & Davis, P. (2005). *Orthopaedic and trauma nursing*. (2nd ed.). Edinburgh, London: Churchhill Livingstone.

Leavitt, F., & Katz, R.S. (2006). Distraction as a key determinant of impaired memory in patients with fibromyalgia. *Journal of Rheumatology*, 33(1):127-132.

Lewis, S.L., Heitkemper, M.M., Dirksen, S.R., et al. (2007). *Medical-surgical nursing: assessment and management of clinical problems*. (7th ed.). St. Louis: Mosby.

Majithia, V., & Geraci, S. (2007). Rheumatoid arthritis: diagnosis and management. *American Journal of Medicine*, 129(2):936-939.

Mauck, K.F., & Clarke, B.L. (2006). Diagnosis, screening, prevention and treatment of osteoporosis. *Mayo Clinic Proceedings*, 81(15): 662-672.

Mayo Clinic staff (n.d.). *Phantom pain*. Available at www.mayoclinic.com/health/phantom-pain/DS00444. Accessed October, 2009.

McCarberg, B., & D'Arcy, Y. (2007). Target pain with topical peripheral analgesics. *The Nurse Practitioner*, 32(7):44-49.

National Institute of Arthritis and Musculoskeletal and Skin Disease (n.d.). *Arthritis*. Available at www.niams.nih.gov/Health_Info/Arthritis/default.asp. Accessed October, 2009.

National Institute on Aging. (2008). *Osteoporosis: the bone thief*. Available at www.nia.nih.gov/HealthInformation/Publications/osteoporosis.htm. Accessed October, 2009.

Olson, A. (2007). Osteoporosis detection. *The Nurse Practitioner*, 32(6):20-27.

Patkar, A., Masand, P.S., Krulewicz, S., et al. (2007). A randomized, controlled, trial of controlled release paroxetine in fibromyalgia. *The American Journal of Medicine*, 120(5):448-454.

Potter, P.A., & Perry, A.G. (2009). *Fundamentals of nursing: concepts, process, and practice*. (7th ed.). St. Louis: Mosby.

Ricks, E. (2007). Wrist arthroscopy. *AORN Journal*, 86(2):181-188.

Seabolt, J. (2007). Bone up on osteoporosis. *LPN*, 3(6):30-37.

Seabolt, J. (2008). An overview of osteomyelitis. *LPN*, 4(2):45-48.

Smeltzer, S.C., Bare, B.G., Hinkle, J.L., et al. (2007). *Brunner & Suddarth's textbook of medical-surgical nursing*, (11th ed.). Philadelphia: Lippincott, Williams and Wilkins.

Springhouse. (2007). *Surgical care made incredibly visual!* Philadelphia: Lippincott Williams & Wilkins.

Sweeney, J., & Ardisson, M. (2006). What's fat embolism? *Nursing*, 36(11):22.

Sze, P.-C., Cheung, W.H., Qin, L., et al. (2008). Biomechanical study of an anthropometrically designed hip protector for older Chinese women. *Geriatric Nursing*, 29(1):64-69.

Taylor, J. (2007). What's happened to pain management. *Nursing Times*, 103(48):18-19.

U.S. Food and Drug Administration (FDA). (2006). *FDA Talk Paper: FDA approved artificial disc: another alternative to treat low back pain*. Available at www.fda.gov/MedicalDevices/ProductsandMedicalProcedures/DeviceApprovalsandClearances/PMAApprovals/ucm110875.htm. Accessed November, 2009.

Webb, R. (2007). Bone up proton pump inhibitors and fracture risk. *Nursing*, 37(10):60-61.

Yeom, H., Fleury, J., & Keller, C. (2008). Risk factors for mobility limitation in community-dwelling older adults: a social ecological perspective. *Geriatric Nursing*, 29(2):133-140.

Chapter 45 Care of the Patient with a Gastrointestinal Disorder

Abdel-Rahman, W.M., Mecklin, J.P., Peltomäki, P. (2006). The genetics of HNPCC: application to diagnosis and screening. *Critical Reviews in Oncology/Hematology*, 58(3):208-220.

Ackley, B.J., & Ladwig, G.B. (2009). *Nursing diagnosis handbook*. (7th ed.). St. Louis: Mosby.

Agrawal, J., & Syngal, S. (2005). Colon cancer screening strategies. *Current Opinions in Gastroenterology*, 21(1):59.

Alspach, J. (2006). *Core curriculum for critical care nursing*. (6th ed.). Philadelphia: Saunders.

American Cancer Society (ACS). (2007). *Cancer facts and figures 2007*. Atlanta: Author.

American Cancer Society (ACS). (2008). *Cancer facts and figures 2008*. Atlanta: Author.

American Cancer Society (ACS). (2009). *Cancer facts and figures 2009*. Available at www.cancer.org/docroot/STT/STT_0.asp. Accessed November, 2009.

American Gastroenterological Association (AGA). Available at www.gastro.org. Accessed October, 2009.

Amerine, E. (2007). Preventing and managing acute diverticulitis. *Nursing*, 37(9):56.

Austin, N. (2007). Spores, babies and alcohol. A nurses battle with *C. diff. RN*, 70(3):39-43.

Baker, D.E. (2005). Rationale for using serotonergic agents to treat irritable bowel syndrome. *American Journal of Health-System Pharmacology*, 62(7):700-711.

Barkauskas, V., Baumann, L.C., & Darling-Fisher, C. (2006). *Health and physical assessment*. (4th ed.). St. Louis: Mosby.

Black, J.M., & Hawks, H.J. (2009). *Medical-surgical nursing: clinical management for positive outcomes*. (8th ed.). Philadelphia: Saunders.

Brush, K. (2007). Abdominal compartment syndrome. *Nursing*, 37(7):37.

Carlo, J.T., DeMarco, D., Smith, B.A., et al. (2005). The utility of capsule endoscopy and its role for diagnosing pathology in the gastrointestinal tract. *American Journal of Surgery*, 190(6):886.

Chan, H.L., Wu, J.C., Chan, F.K., et al. (2001). Is non-*Helicobacter pylori*, non-NSAID peptic ulcer a common cause of upper GI bleeding? *Gastrointestinal Endoscopy*, 53:438.

Deglin, J., & Vallerand, A. (2005). *Davis' drug guide for nurses*. (13th ed.). Philadelphia: Davis.

Dicken, B.J., Bigam, D.L., Cass, C., et al. (2005). Gastric adenocarcinoma review and considerations for future directions. *Annals of Surgery*, 241(1):27.

Ebersole, P.E., Touhy, T.A., Hess, P., et al. (2008). *Toward healthy aging: human needs and nursing response.* (7th ed.). St. Louis: Mosby.

Elkin, M.K., Perry, A.G., & Potter, P.A. (2007). *Nursing interventions and clinical skills.* (4th ed.). St. Louis: Mosby.

Freeman, L. (2007). Responding to small-bowel obstruction. *Nursing*, 37(5):56.

Fry, D. (2007). Exposing the source of peptic ulcer disease. *LPN*, 3(3):6.

Gabriel, S. (2006). Bariatric surgery basics, getting to the heart of a weighty matter. *Nursing Made Incredibly Easy!* 4(1):43.

Gallagher, S. (2004). Taking the weight off with bariatric surgery. *Nursing*, 34(3):59.

Greenwald, B. (2005). Comparison of three stool tests for colorectal cancer screening. *Medsurg Nursing*, 14:292.

Hahn, J. (2007). The bottom line on hemorrhoids. *Nursing Made Incredibly Easy!* 5(5):13.

Hara, A.K., Leighton, J.A., Heigh, R.I., et al.: (2006). Crohn disease of the small bowel: preliminary comparison among CT enterography, capsule endoscopy, small bowel follow-through, and ileoscopy. *Radiology*, 238(1):128-134.

Harris, H. (2006). *C. difficile*, attack to killer diarrhea. *Nursing Made Incredibly Easy!* 4(3):13.

Heitkemper, M., & Jarrett, M. (2005). Overlapping conditions in women with irritable bowel syndrome. *Urologic Nursing*, 25:25-30.

Hill, R. (2007). Conquering constipation. *LPN*, 3(4):48.

Hirano, I., Richter, J.E.; Practice Parameters Committee of the American College of Gastroenterology. (2007). ACG practice guidelines: esophageal reflux testing. *American Journal of Gastroenterology*, 102(3):668.

Jarvis, C. (2008). *Physical examination and health assessment.* (5th ed.). Philadelphia: Saunders.

Johanson, J.F. (2004). Options for patients with irritable bowel syndrome: contrasting traditional and novel serotonergic therapies. *Neurogastroenterology and Motility*, 16(6):701-711.

Kang, J.Y., Meville, D., Maxwell, J.D. (2004). Epidemiology and management of diverticular disease of the colon. *Drugs & Aging*, 21(4):211, 2004.

Karlowicz, D. (2004). An endoscopic approach to GERD. *RN*, 66(12):56.

Kent, V. (2007). Caring for a patient with a bowel obstruction. *LPN*, 3(5):31.

Lawrence, B. (2007). Esophogeal pH monitoring goes wireless. *Nursing*, 37(10):26.

Legnani, P., & Kornblut, A. (2005). Video capsule endoscopy in inflammatory bowel disease 2005. *Current Opinions in Gastroenterology*, 21:438.

Lewis, S.L., Heitkemper, M.M., Dirksen, S.R., et al. (2007). *Medical-surgical nursing: assessment and management of clinical problems.* (7th ed.). St. Louis: Mosby.

Livingston, C.D., Jones, H.L., Jr., Askew, R.E., Jr., et al. (2001). Laparoscopic hiatal hernia repair in patients with poor esophageal motility or paraesophageal herniation, *The American Surgeon*, 67:987, 2001.

Matthew, C.G., & Lewis, C.M. (2004). Genetics of inflammatory bowel disease: progress and prospects *Human Molecular Genetics*, 13:R161, 2004.

Memmler, R.L., et al. (2008). *Structure and function of the human body.* (9th ed.). Philadelphia: Lippincott.

Monahan, F.D., Sands, J.K., Neighbors, M., et al. (2007). *Phipps' medical-surgical nursing: health and illness perspectives.* (8th ed.). St. Louis: Mosby.

Mosby's dictionary of medicine, nursing, and health professions. (2009). (8th ed.). St. Louis: Mosby.

Pagana, K.D., & Pagana, T.J. (2008). *Mosby's diagnostic and laboratory test reference.* (9th ed.). St. Louis: Mosby.

Perry, A.G., & Potter, P.A. (2009). *Clinical nursing skills and techniques.* (7th ed.). St. Louis: Mosby.

Potter, P.A., & Perry, A.G. (2007). *Basic nursing: essentials for practice.* (6th ed.). St. Louis: Mosby.

Sansbury, L.B., Millikan, R.C., Scroeder, J.C., et al. (2005). Use of nonsteroidal anti-inflammatory drugs and risk of colon cancer in a population-based, case-control study of African-Americans and whites. *American Journal of Epidemiology*, 162(6):548-558.

Seidel, H.M., Ball, J.W., Dains, J.E., et al. (2007). *Mosby's guide to physical examination.* (6th ed.). St. Louis: Mosby.

Smeltzer, S.C., Bare, B.G., Hinkle, J.L., et al. (2007). *Brunner & Suddarth's textbook of medical-surgical nursing*, (11th ed.). Philadelphia: Lippincott, Williams and Wilkins.

Thibodeau, G.A., & Patton, K.T. (2007). *Anatomy and physiology.* (6th ed.). St. Louis: Mosby.

Thibodeau, G.A., & Patton, K.T. (2008). *Structure and function of the body.* (13th ed.). St. Louis: Mosby.

Thibodeau, G.A., & Patton, K.T. (2009). *The human body in health and disease.* (5th ed.). St. Louis: Mosby.

Thompson, J.M., McFarland, G.K., Hirsch, J.E., et al. (2001). *Mosby's clinical nursing.* (5th ed.). St. Louis: Mosby.

Tucker, S.M., Cannobio, M.M., Paquette, E.V., et al. (2007). *Patient care standards: collaborative planning and nursing interventions.* (7th ed.). St. Louis: Mosby.

Vglente, S. (2007). Keep *C. difficile* infection at bay. *Nursing*, 37(10):56.

Walker, B. (2004). Assessing gastrointestinal infections. *Nursing*, 34(5):48.

Young-Fadok, T., et al. *Treatment of acute diverticulitis and clinical manifestations of colonic diverticular disease.* Available at www.uptodate.com. Accessed July 8, 2007.

Additional Resources

Crohn's and Colitis Foundation of America, 386 Park Ave. South, 17th Floor, New York, NY 10016-8804. 800-932-2423 or 212-685-3440. Information hotline: 800-343-3637. Available at www.ccfa.org. Accessed November, 2009.

United Ostomy Association, 19772 MacArthur Blvd., Suite 200, Irvine, CA 92612-2405. 800-826-0826. Available at www.uoaa.org. Accessed November, 2009.

Chapter 46 Care of the Patient with a Gallbladder, Liver, Biliary Tract, or Exocrine Pancreatic Disorder

Ackley, B.J., & Ladwig, G.B. (2009). *Nursing diagnosis handbook.* (7th ed.). St. Louis: Mosby.

American Cancer Society (ACS). (2007). *Cancer facts and figures 2007.* Atlanta: Author.

American Cancer Society (ACS). (2007). Detailed guide: pancreatic cancer. Available at www.cancer.org/docroot/CRI/CRI_2_3x.asp?dt=34. Accessed October, 2009.

Black, J.M., & Hawks, H.J. (2009). *Medical-surgical nursing: clinical management for positive outcomes.* (8th ed.). Philadelphia: Saunders.

Boyer, M.J. (2008). *Study guide to Brunner and Suddarth's textbook of medical-surgical nursing.* (11th ed.). Philadelphia: Lippincott.

Centers for Disease Control and Prevention (CDC). (2009). *Recommended immunization schedule for persons aged 1 through 6 years.* Available at www.cdc.gov/vaccines/recs/schedules/downloads/child/2009/09_0-6yrs_schedule_pr.pdf. Accessed November, 2009.

Centers for Disease Control and Prevention (CDC), & National Center for Infectious Diseases. (2008). *Viral hepatitis.* Available at www.cdc.gov/hepatitis/index.htm. Accessed October, 2009.

Durston, S. (2004). The ABCs and more of hepatitis. *Nursing Made Incredibly Easy!* 2(4):22-32.

Editorial. (2007). Function junction: testing your patient in liver function. *Nursing Made Incredibly Easy!* 5(1):17-19.

Giger, J.M., & Davidhizar, R.E. (2007). *Transcultural nursing: assessment and intervention.* (5th ed.). St. Louis: Mosby.

Holcomb, S. (2007). Stopping the destruction of acute pancreatitis. *Nursing*, 37(6):43.

Hussar, D. (2007). New drugs07, part 2. *Nursing*, 37(8):46.

Jacobson, I. (2006). Therapeutic options for chronic hepatitis B: considerations and controversies. *American Journal of Gastroenterology,* 101:51.

Jones, S. (2003). When the liver fails: new help and hope. *RN,* 66(11):33.

Lewis, S.L., Heitkemper, M.M., Dirksen, S.R., et al. (2007). *Medical-surgical nursing: assessment and management of clinical problems.* (7th ed.). St. Louis: Mosby.

Madsen, D., Sebolt, T., Cullen, L., et al. (2005). Listening to bowel sounds: an evidence-based practice project. *American Journal of Nursing,* 105(12):40.

McCarron, K. (2007). Jaundice: more than meets the eye. *Nursing Made Incredibly Easy!* 5(3):25.

McCaughan, G.W., Koorey, D.J., & Strasser, S.I. (2005). Liver transplantation for viral hepatitis, *Hospital Medicine,* 66(1):8-12.

Monahan, F.D., Sands, J.K., Neighbors, M., et al. (2007). *Phipps' medical-surgical nursing: health and illness perspectives.* (8th ed.). St. Louis: Mosby.

Mosby's dictionary of medicine, nursing, and health professions. (2009). (8th ed.). St. Louis: Mosby.

Pagana, K.D., & Pagana, T.J. (2008). *Mosby's diagnostic and laboratory test reference.* (9th ed.). St. Louis: Mosby.

Pellegrino, A. (2006). Looking at liver cancer. *Nursing,* 36(10), 52.

Perry, A.G., & Potter, P.A. (2009). *Clinical nursing skills and techniques.* (7th ed.). St. Louis: Mosby.

Phillips, R.A. (2006). Acute pancreatitis: inflammation gone wild. *Nursing Made Incredibly Easy!* 4(5):18-28.

Potter, P.A., & Perry, A.G. (2007). *Basic nursing: essentials for practice.* (6th ed.). St. Louis: Mosby.

Potter, P.A., & Perry, A.G. (2009). *Fundamentals of nursing: concepts, process, and practice.* (7th ed.). St. Louis: Mosby.

Riehl, M. (2007). Help your patient cope with pancreatic cancer. *Nursing,* 37(4):54.

Seidel, H.M., Ball, J.W., Dains, J.E., et al. (2007). *Mosby's guide to physical examination.* (6th ed.). St. Louis: Mosby.

Shaheen, N., Hansen, R.A., Morgan, D.R., et al. (2006). The burden of gastrointestinal and liver diseases. *American Journal of Gastroenterology,* 101(9):2128-2138.

Thibodeau, G.A. & Patton, K.T. (2007). *Anatomy and physiology.* (6th ed.). St. Louis: Mosby.

Thibodeau, G.A. & Patton, K.T. (2008). *Structure and function of the body.* (13th ed.). St. Louis: Mosby.

Thibodeau, G.A., & Patton, K.T. (2009). *The human body in health and disease.* (5th ed.). St. Louis: Mosby.

Thompson, J.M., McFarland, G.K., Hirsch, J.E., et al. (2001). *Mosby's clinical nursing.* (5th ed.). St. Louis: Mosby.

Tucker, S.M., Cannobio, M.M., Paquette, E.V., et al. (2007). *Patient care standards: collaborative planning and nursing interventions.* (7th ed.). St. Louis: Mosby.

Venes, D. (2009.) *Taber's cyclopedic medical dictionary.* (21st ed.). Philadelphia: Davis.

Verna, E.C., & Brown, R.S., Jr., (n.d.). *Liver transplantation for hepatitis C virus infection.* Available at www.uptodate.com/patients/content/topic.do?topicKey=~aJJa1SKQK2jouT&selectedTitle=3~150&source=search_result. Accessed November, 2009.

Chapter 47 Care of the Patient with a Blood or Lymphatic Disorder

Ackley, B.J., & Ladwig, G.B. (2009). *Nursing diagnosis handbook.* (7th ed.). St. Louis: Mosby.

Aster, J. (2005). Diseases of white blood cells, lymph nodes, spleen and thymus. In V. Kumar, A. Abbas, N. Fausto, et al., (Eds.): *Robbins and Cotran pathologic basis of disease,* Philadelphia: Elsevier.

Baehner, R. (n.d.) *Overview of neutropenia.* Available at www.uptodate.com. Version 13.2. Accessed June 20, 2006.

Barkauskas, V., Baumann, L.C., & Darling-Fisher, C. (2006). *Health and physical assessment.* (4th ed.). St. Louis: Mosby.

Beattie, S. (2007a). Bedside emergency-hemorrhage. *RN,* 70(8):32-36.

Beattie, S. (2007b). Hands-on-help, bone marrow aspiration and biopsy. *RN,* 70(2):41.

Black, J.M., & Hawks, H.J. (2009). *Medical-surgical nursing: clinical management for positive outcomes.* (8th ed.). Philadelphia: Saunders.

Borton, D. (1996). WBC count and differential. *Nursing,* 26:11.

Burruss, N., & Holz, S. (2005). Managing the risks of thrombocytopenia. *Nursing,* 35:32hn5.

Canellos, G. (2004). Lymphoma: present and future challenges. *Seminars in Hematology,* 41(suppl 17):26.

Damsky, D. (2006). Caring for a patient with lymphedema. *Nursing 2006,* 36(6):49.

Deglin, J., & Vallerand, A. (2009). *Davis's drug guide for nurses.* (17th ed.). Philadelphia: Davis.

Deitch, E. (2006). Intensive care management of the trauma patient. *Critical Care Medicine,* 34(9):2294.

Geiter, H. (2003). Disseminated intravascular coagulopathy. *Dimensions of Critical Care Nursing,* 22(3):108.

Giger, J.M., & Davidhizar, R.E. (2008). *Transcultural nursing: assessment and intervention.* (5th ed.). St. Louis: Mosby.

Hebbel, R. (2005). Pathobiology of sickle cell disease. In R. Hoffman, B. Furie, E. Benz, et al. (Eds.), *Hematology: basic principles and practice.* (4th ed.). Philadelphia: Saunders.

Holcomb, S.S. (2006). Putting the squeeze on lymphedema. *Nursing Made Incredibly Easy!* 4(2):26-34.

Kim, M.J., McFarland, G.K., & McLane, A.M. (1989). *Pocket guide to nursing diagnoses.* (3rd ed.). St. Louis: Mosby.

Lewis, S.L., Heitkemper, M.M., Dirksen, S.R., et al. (2007). *Medical-surgical nursing: assessment and management of clinical problems.* (7th ed.). St. Louis: Mosby.

Lipschitz, D. (2003). Medical and functional consequences of anemia in the elderly. *Journal of the American Geriatrics Society,* 51(suppl 3):510.

March, J.C. (2005). Management of acquired aplastic anemia. *Blood Reviews,* 19:143.

Mauch, P. (2006). *Staging and selection of treatment modality in patients with Hodgkin's disease.* Available at www.uptodate.com. Accessed June 20, 2006.

McCarron, K. (2004). Deciphering diagnostics. Clues in the blood: know your CBCs. *Nursing Made Incredibly Easy!* 5(3):13-17.

MedlinePlus. (2009). *Sickle cell anemia.* Available at www.nlm.nih.gov/medlineplus/sicklecellanemia.html. Accessed October, 2009.

Monahan, F.D., Sands, J.K., Neighbors, M., et al. (2007). *Phipps' medical-surgical nursing: health and illness perspectives.* (8th ed.). St. Louis: Mosby.

Montoya, V.L, Wink, D., Sole, M.L. (2004). Anemia, what lies beneath. *Nursing Made Incredibly Easy!* 2(1):37-45.

Mosby's dictionary of medicine, nursing, and health professions. (2009). (8th ed.). St. Louis: Mosby.

Munson, B. (2005). Myths and facts . . . about polycythemia vera. *Nursing,* 35(5):28.

North American Nursing Diagnosis Association International (NANDA-I). (2009). *NANDA-I nursing diagnoses: definitions and classification 2009-2011.* Oxford, United Kingdom: Author.

Pagana, K.D., & Pagana, T.J. (2008a). *Diagnostic testing and nursing implications: a case study approach.* (6th ed.). St. Louis: Mosby.

Pagana, K.D., & Pagana, T.J. (2008b). *Mosby's diagnostic and laboratory test reference.* (9th ed.). St. Louis: Mosby.

Perry, A.G., & Potter, P.A. (2009). *Clinical nursing skills and techniques.* (7th ed.). St. Louis: Mosby.

Platt, A. (2007). How much do you know about sickle-cell disease? *LPN,* 3(4):32.

Portielje, J.E., Westendorp, R.G., Kluin-Nelemans, H.C., et al. (2001). Morbidity and mortality in adults with immune thrombocytopenic purpura. *Blood,* 97:2549.

Potter, P.A., & Perry, A.G. (2007). *Basic nursing: essentials for practice.* (6th ed.). St. Louis: Mosby.

Redaelli, A. (2005). A systematic literature review of the clinical and epidemiological burden of acute lymphoblastic leukemia (ALL). *European Journal of Cancer Care,* 14:53.

Robinson, P. (2005). Is surgery safe for a patient with hemophilia? *Nursing,* 35:32.

Seidel, H.M., Ball, J.W., Dains, J.E., et al. (2007). *Mosby's guide to physical examination.* (6th ed.). St. Louis: Mosby.

Seiter, K. (2002). Treatment of acute myelogenous leukemia in the elderly patients. *Clinical Geriatrics,* 10:41.

Skidmore-Roth, L. (2010). *Mosby's 2010 nursing drug reference.* (23rd ed.). St. Louis: Mosby.

Stone, R., O'Donnell, M.R., & Sekeres, M.A. (2004). Acute myeloid leukemia. *American Society of Hematology,* 1:98.

Thibodeau, G.A., & Patton, K.T. (2007). *Anatomy and physiology.* (6th ed.). St. Louis: Mosby.

Thibodeau, G.A., & Patton, K.T. (2008). *Structure and function of the body.* (13th ed.). St. Louis: Mosby.

Thompson, J.M., McFarland, G.K., Hirsch, J.E., et al. (2001). *Mosby's clinical nursing.* (5th ed.). St. Louis: Mosby.

Weiss, G., & Goodnough, L.T. (2005). Anemia of chronic disease. *New England Journal of Medicine,* 352(10):1011-1023.

Chapter 48 Care of the Patient with a Cardiovascular or a Peripheral Vascular Disorder

Agruss, J.C., & Garrett, K. (2006). The stealth factor in cardiovascular disease risk. *Nursing Made Incredibly Easy!* 4(2):51-55.

American College of Obstetrics and Gynecologists (ACOG) Women's Health Care Physicians. (2004). Coronary artery disease. *Obstetrics and Gynecology,* 104(4 Suppl):415.

American Heart Association. (2005). *2005 heart and stroke facts statistics.* Dallas: Author.

Antman, E.M., Anbe, D.T., Armstrong, P.W., et al. (2004). ACC/AHA guidelines for the management of patients with ST-elevation myocardial infarction: a report of the American College of Cardiology/American Heart Association Task Force on Practice Guidelines (Committee to Revise the 1999 Guidelines for the Management of Patients with Acute Myocardial Infarction). *Circulation,* 110(9):e82-292.

Bartley, M. (2006). Keeping thromboembolism at bay. *Nursing,* 36(10), 36.

Belch, J.J., Topol, E.J., Agnelli, G., et al. (2003). Critical issues in peripheral arterial disease detection and management: a call to action. *Archives of International Medicine,* 163(8):884-892.

Bentz, B. (2006). Gaining control over A-fib. *RN,* (12):35.

Black, J.M., & Hawks, H.J. (2009). *Medical-surgical nursing: clinical management for positive outcomes.* (8th ed.). Philadelphia: Saunders.

Bozkurt, A.K., Koksal, C., & Ercan, M. (2004). The altered hemorheologic parameter in thromboangitis obliterans: a new insight, *Clinical and Applied Thrombosis/Hemostasis,* 10:45.

Calianno, C., & Holton, S.J. (2007). Fighting the triple threat of lower extremity ulcers. *Nursing,* 37(3):57-63.

Cheek, D. (2006). New respect for the humble endothelium. *Nursing,* 36(3):44.

Cheek, D. (2008). Women's heart disease: what's new? *Nursing,* 38(1):36.

Chojnowski, D. (2004). Putting together the pieces of cardiomyopathy. *Nursing Made Incredibly Easy!* 2(3):18-28.

Chojnowski, D. (2006). Managing systolic heart failure. *Nursing,* 36(7):36.

Chojnowski, D. (2007). Protecting patients from harm: taking aim at heart failure. *Nursing,* 37(11):50-55.

Cooper, L.T. (2004). Long-term survival and amputation risk in thromboangitis obliterans (Buerger's disease). *Journal of the American College of Cardiologists,* 44:2410.

Cotter, J., Bixby, M., & Morse, B. (2006). Helping patients who need a permanent pacemaker. *Nursing,* 36(8):50-54.

Craig, K. (2006). Heart attack. *Nursing,* 36(5):43.

Croce, H. (2007). Aortic problems. *RN,* 70(3):26.

Cuddy, P. (2006). Lipid lowerers. *RN,* 69(8):27.

Fink, A. (2006). Endocarditis after valve replacement surgery. *American Journal of Nursing,* 106(2):40.

Gahan, L. (2005). Using compression therapy for venous insufficiency. *Nursing,* 35(12):24.

Giger, J.M., & Davidhizar, R.E. (2008). *Transcultural nursing: assessment and intervention.* (5th ed.). St. Louis: Mosby.

Hayes, D. (2007). New guidelines for preventing infective endocarditis. *Nursing,* 37(8):22.

Hirsch, A.T., & Duprez, D. (2003). The potential role of angiotension-converting enzyme inhibition in peripheral arterial disease. *Vascular Medicine,* 8:273-278.

Hobbs, R.E. (2003). Using BNP to diagnose, manage, and treat heart failure. *Cleveland Clinics Journal of Medicine,* 70(4):333.

Holcomb, S. (2006). Carditis hearts afire. *Nursing Made Incredibly Easy!* 4(4):14-24.

Hussar, D. (2008). New drugs. *Nursing,* 38(2):49.

Irwin, G. (2007). How to protect a patient with aortic aneurysm. *Nursing,* 37(2):36.

Iyer, P.W., & Camp, N.H. (2007). *Nursing documentation: a nursing process approach.* (5th ed.). St. Louis: Mosby.

Kasper, D.L., Braunwald, E., Hauser, S., et al. (2004). *Harrison's principles of internal medicine.* (16th ed.). New York: McGraw-Hill.

Lackey, S. (2006). Suppressing the scourge of AMI. *Nursing,* 36(5):36.

Langford, R., & Thompson, J. (2008). *Mosby's handbook of diseases.* (4rd ed.). St. Louis: Mosby.

Lewis, S.L., Heitkemper, M.M., Dirksen, S.R., et al. (2007). *Medical-surgical nursing: assessment and management of clinical problems.* (7th ed.). St. Louis: Mosby.

McCarron, K. (2006). Puzzled about atherosclerosis? *Nursing Made Incredibly Easy!* 4(6):11-14.

McFarland, G., & McFarland, E. (2005). *Nursing diagnosis and intervention: planning for patient care.* (5th ed.). St. Louis: Mosby.

Miller, J. (2007). Keeping your patient hemodynamically stable. *Nursing,* 37(5):36.

Moriarty, M. (2004). Heart disease. *RN,* 67(1):33.

Mosby's dictionary of medicine, nursing, and health professions. (2009). (8th ed.). St. Louis: Mosby.

Moz, T. (2007). Cardiovascular disease: the heart of the matter. *LPN,* 3(2):35.

National Heart, Lung and Blood Institute. Available at www.nhlbi.nih.gov. Accessed November, 2009.

Nienaber, C., & Eagle, K. (2003). Aortic dissection: new frontiers in diagnosis and management. Part II: therapeutic management and follow-up. *Circulation,* 108(5):772.

Pagana, K.D., & Pagana, T.J. (2008). *Mosby's diagnostic and laboratory test reference.* (9th ed.). St. Louis: Mosby.

Palatnik, A. (2005). And the beat goes on. *Nursing Made Incredibly Easy!* 3(1):30-41.

Pence, C., et al. (2005). Anticoagulation self-monitoring. *American Journal of Nursing,* 105(10):62.

Pope, B. (2004). What's at the heart of your patient's chest pain? *Nursing Made Incredibly Easy!* 8:18.

Riggs, J. (2004). New therapies for heart failure. *RN,* 67(3):29.

Riggs, J. (2006). Too pooped to pump: managing chronic heart failure. *Nursing Made Incredibly Easy!* 4(1):28-39, 41, 42.

Roca, J. (2007). Responding to atrial fibrillation. *Nursing,* 37(4):37.

Roman, L., & Metules, T.J. (2007). Door-to-balloon time: the race is on. *RN,* 70(2):35-38.

Shatzer, M., & Saul, L. (2004). What does BNP tell you? *Nursing Made Incredibly Easy!* 2(3):7.

Sherrod, M.M., Albarez, Y., Brookshire, A., et al. (2007). A woman's worst enemy. *American Nurse Today,* 2(2):26.

Sunderlin, M. (2006). Keeping pace with cardiac devices. *RN,* 69(7):40.

Thibodeau, G.A. & Patton, K.T. (2008). *Structure and function of the human body.* (13th ed.). St. Louis: Mosby.

Thibodeau, G.A., & Patton, K.T. (2009). *The human body in health and disease.* (5th ed.). St. Louis: Mosby.

Thomas, C.L. (2009). *Taber's cyclopedic medical dictionary.* (21st ed.). Philadelphia: Davis.

Thompson, J.M., McFarland, G.K., Hirsch, J.E., et al. (2001). *Mosby's clinical nursing.* (5th ed.). St. Louis: Mosby.

Tran, H., & Anand, S.S. (2004). Oral antiplatelet therapy in cerebrovascular disease, coronary artery disease, and peripheral artery disease. *Journal of the American Medical Association*, 292:1867-1874.

Treat-Jackson, D., & Walsh, M.E. (2003). Treating patients with peripheral arterial disease and claudication. *Journal of Vascular Nursing*, 21:5-14, 2003.

Trujillo-Santos, J., Perea-Milla, E., Jimenez-Puente, A., et al. (2005). Bedrest or ambulation in the initial treatment of patients with acute deep vein thrombosis or pulmonary embolism: findings from RIETE registry. *Chest*, 127:1631-1636.

Tucker, S.M., Cannobio, M.M., Paquette, E.V., et al. (2007). *Patient care standards: collaborative planning and nursing interventions*. (7th ed.). St. Louis: Mosby.

Turka, J. (2006). Is this on the level? *Nursing Made Incredibly Easy!* 4(4):7, 9.

Turner, L. (2006). Keeping warfarin therapy in balance. *Nursing*, 36(11):43.

U.S. Department of Health and Human Services, National Institutes of Health, & National Heart, Lung and Blood Institute. (2003). *The seventh report of the Joint National Committee on Prevention, Detection, Evaluation, and Treatment of High Blood Pressure*, Bethesda, Md.: Author.

Willigendael, E.M., Teijink, J.A., Bartelink, M.L., et al. (2004). Influence of smoking on increase and prevalence of peripheral arterial disease. *Journal of Vascular Surgey*, 40:1158.

Willis, K. (2001). Gaining perspective on peripheral vascular disease. *Nursing*, 31:2.

Wipke-Tevis, D.D., & Sae-Sia, W. (2004). Caring for vascular leg ulcers: a best approach practice update. *Home Healthcare Nurse*, 22(4):237.

Wright, J. (2006). Cardiovascular meds. *RN*, 69(5):33.

Xu, Y., & Whitmer, K. (2006). C-reactive protein and cardiovascular disease in people with diabetes. *American Journal of Nursing*, 106(8):66.

Chapter 49 Care of the Patient with a Respiratory Disorder

American Cancer Society (ACS). (2009). *Cancer facts and figures*. Available at www.cancer.org/downloads/STT/500809web.pdf. Accessed November, 2009.

American Lung Association. (2007). *Chronic obstructive pulmonary disease*. Available at www.lungusa.org/lung-disease/copd. Accessed November, 2009.

Astle, S. (2007). Taking your patient off of a ventilator. *RN*, 70(5):34.

Balas, M. (2009). Prone positioning of patients with acute respiratory distress syndrome: applying research to practice. *Critical Care Nurse*, 20(1), 24-36.

Barkauskas, V., Baumann, L.C., & Darling-Fisher, C. (2006). *Health and physical assessment*. (4th ed.). St. Louis: Mosby.

Bauldoff, G.S., & Diaz, P.T. (2006). Improving outcomes for COPD patients. *Nurse Practitioner*, 31(8):26-28.

Beattie, S. (2007). Bedside emergency. *RN*, 70(7):34.

Black, J.M., & Hawks, H.J. (2009). *Medical-surgical nursing: clinical management for positive outcomes*. (8th ed.). Philadelphia: Saunders.

Carr, E. (2005). Nursing care of the patient with head and neck cancer. In J. Itano, & K. Taoka, (Eds.):, *Core curriculum for oncology nursing*. (4th ed.). St. Louis: Elsevier.

Centers for Disease Control and Prevention (CDC). (2006). *Reported TB in U.S.* U.S. Department of Health and Human Services, Atlanta: Author.

Coughlin, A. (2007a). Coping with COPD. *Nursing Made Incredibly Easy!* 5(6):40.

Coughlin, A. (2007b). Helping patients cope with COPD. *LPN*, 3(3):46.

Coughlin, A., & Parchinsky, C. (2006). Go with the flow of chest tube therapy. *Nursing*, 36(3):36.

Crawford, A., & Harris, H. (2008). *COPD: help your patients breathe easier*. Available at http://rn.modernmedicine.com/rnweb/article/articleDetail.jsp?id=482654. Accessed November, 2009.

Deglin, J., & Vallerand, A. (2009). *Davis's drug guide for nurses*. (17th ed.). Philadelphia: Davis.

Dest, V. (2000). Oncology today: lung cancer. *RN*, 63(5):32.

Dest, V. (2006). Lung cancer, the battle continues. *RN*, 69(11):30.

Dugan, M. (2007). A tale of sleep apnea. *Nursing Made Incredibly Easy!* 5(3):28-37.

Edmondson, D. (2008). Smoke out lung cancer. *LPN*, 4(1):39, 2008.

ExcellentHealth.com. (n.d.). *Anthrax drugs*. Available at www.excellenthealth.com/news011102a.htm. Accessed November, 2009.

Giger, J.M., & Davidhizar, R.E. (2008). *Transcultural nursing: assessment and intervention*. (5th ed.). St. Louis: Mosby.

Global initiative for chronic obstructive lung disease. (n.d.). Available at http://goldcopd.com. Accessed November, 2009.

Goldrick, B. (2004). 21st-century emerging and reemerging infections. *American Journal of Nursing*, 104(1):67.

Goldrick, B. (2005). Emerging infections—update TB in the United States. *American Journal of Nursing*, 105(7):85.

Holcomb, S.S. (2006). The stuffy head blues. *Nursing Made Incredibly Easy!* 4(2):64.

Ignatavicius, D.D., & Workman, M.L. (2006). *Medical-surgical nursing: patient-centered collaborative care*. (6th ed.). Philadelphia: Saunders.

Jacobs, M. (2005). Ease the stress of managing ARDS. *Made Incredibly Easy!* 3(1):6.

Jacobs, M., & Meyer, T. (2006). The push is on in pulmonary hypertension. *Made Incredibly Easy!* 4(3):42-52.

Jeffries, M. (2007). Helping your patient combat lung cancer. *Nursing*, 37(12):36.

Kamangar, N., Nikhanj, N.S., & Sharma, S. (2006). *Chronic obstructive pulmonary disease*. Available at www.emedicine.com/med/topic373/htm. Accessed November, 2009.

Kamienski, M. (2007). When sore throat gets serious. *American Journal of Nursing*, 107(10):35.

Kattan, M., et al. (2005). Asthma outcomes: you get what you pay for. *Journal of Allergy and Clinical Immunology*, 116(5):1058-1063.

Katz, J., & Hirsch, A. (2003). When global health is local health (SARS). *American Journal of Nursing*, 103(12):75.

Koschel, M. (2004). Pulmonary embolism. *American Journal of Nursing*, 104(6):46.

Kucik, C.J., et al. (2005). Management of epistaxis. *American Family Physician*, 71:305.

Langford, R., & Thompson, J. (2008). *Mosby's handbook of diseases*. (4th ed.). St. Louis: Mosby.

Lewis, S.L., Heitkemper, M.M., Dirksen, S.R., et al. (2007). *Medical-surgical nursing: assessment and management of clinical problems*. (7th ed.). St. Louis: Mosby.

Manno, M. (2005). Managing mechanical ventilation. *Nursing*, 35(12):36, 2005.

McCarron, K. (2006). Puzzled about the state of airlessness? (Atelectasis). *Nursing Made Incredibly Easy!* 4(10):60.

McFarland, G., & McFarland, E. (2007). *Nursing diagnosis and intervention: planning for patient care*. (5th ed.). St. Louis: Mosby.

Miracle, V., & Winston, M. (2000). Take the wind out of asthma. *Nursing*, 30(8):34.

Monahan, F.D., Sands, J.K., Neighbors, M., et al. (2007). *Phipps' medical-surgical nursing: health and illness perspectives*. (8th ed.). St. Louis: Mosby.

Mosby's dictionary of medicine, nursing, and health professions. (2009). (8th ed.). St. Louis: Mosby.

Otto, S. (2005). *Oncology nursing*. (5th ed.). St. Louis: Mosby.

Pagana, K.D., & Pagana, T.J. (2008). *Mosby's diagnostic and laboratory test reference*. (9th ed.). St. Louis: Mosby.

Parini, S. (2003). Severe acute respiratory syndrome. *Nursing*, 33(9):96.

Potter, P.A., & Perry, A.G. (2007). *Basic nursing: essentials for practice*. (6th ed.). St. Louis: Mosby.

Potter, P.A., & Perry, A.G. (2009). *Fundamentals of nursing: concepts, process, and practice*. (7th ed.). St. Louis: Mosby.

Price, S., & Wilson, L. (2007). *Pathophysiology: clinical concepts of disease processes.* (7th ed.). St. Louis: Mosby.

Pruitt, B. (2006). Weaning patients from mechanical ventilation. *Nursing*, 36(9):36.

Pruitt, B. (2007a). Clearing the air with chest tubes. *LPN*, 3(5):50.

Pruitt, B. (2007b). Fending off influenza. *Nursing*, 37(10):44.

Pruitt, B., et al. (2006). Ventilation associated pneumonia. *Nursing*, 36(2):36.

Ruppel, G. (2007). *Manual of pulmonary function testing.* (9th ed.). St. Louis: Mosby.

Rushing, J. (2007). Clinical do's and don'ts—managing a water-seal chest drainage unit. *Nursing*, 37(12):12.

Scheff, B. (2006). Avian influenza. *Nursing*, 37(5):51.

Schiech, L. (2007). Looking at laryngeal cancer. *Nursing*, 37(5):50.

Schleder, B. (2004). Keeping hospital bugs at bay: how you can protect your patients from noscomial pneumonia. *Nursing Made Incredibly Easy!* 2(2):36-42.

Seidel, H.M., Ball, J.W., Dains, J.E., et al. (2007). *Mosby's guide to physical examination.* (6th ed.). St. Louis: Mosby.

Skidmore-Roth, L. (2010). *Mosby's 2010 nursing drug reference.* (23rd ed.). St. Louis: Mosby.

Swearingen, P.L. (2007). *Manual of medical-surgical nursing.* (6th ed.). St. Louis: Mosby.

Tate, T.J., & Tasota, F. (2002). More than a snore: recognizing the danger of sleep apnea. *Nursing*, 32(8):46.

Thibodeau, G.A., & Patton, K.T. (2008). *Structure and function of the body.* (13th ed.). St. Louis: Mosby.

Thibodeau, G.A., & Patton, K.T. (2009). *The human body in health and disease.* (5th ed.). St. Louis: Mosby.

Thompson, B.T., et al. (2006). *Clinical manifestations of and diagnostic strategies for acute pulmonary embolism.* Available at www.uptodate.com.

Thompson, J.M., McFarland, G.K., Hirsch, J.E., et al. (2001). *Mosby's clinical nursing.* (5th ed.). St. Louis: Mosby.

Todd, B. (2006). The Quantiferon-TB Gold Test. *American Journal of Nursing*, 106(6):33.

Valentine, K.A., et al. (2006). *Treatment of acute pulmonary embolism.* Available at www.uptodate.com.

Wisniewski, A. (2004). When air is rare—helping patients with chronic bronchitis or emphysema breathe easier. *Nursing Made Incredibly Easy!* 2(1):20-27, 35.

Woodruff, D. (2006). Take these 6 easy steps to ABG analysis. *Nursing Made Incredibly Easy!* 4(1):4-7.

Chapter 50 Care of the Patient with a Urinary Disorder

Abrams, A.C. (2006). *Clinical drug therapy.* (8th ed.). Philadelphia: Lippincott.

Ackley, B.J., & Ladwig, G.B. (2009). *Nursing diagnosis handbook.* (7th ed.). St. Louis: Mosby.

Adam, L., Kassouf, W., & Dinney, C. (2005). Clinical applications for targeted therapy in bladder cancer. *Urologic Clinics of North America*, 32(2):239-246.

American Institute of Cancer Research (AICR). (2007). *Concerns over the increasing incidence of kidney cancer.* Available at www.elements-4health.com/concerns-over-the-increasing-incidence-of-kidney-cancer.html. Accessed November, 2009.

Aparicio, A., et al. (2005). The current and future application of adjuvant systemic chemotherapy in patients with bladder cancer following cystectomy. *Urologic Clinics of North America*, 32(2):217-230.

Barton-Burke, M., & Gustason, C. (2007). Sexuality in women with cancer. *Nursing Clinics of North America*, 42(4):531-554.

Berry, A. (2006). Helping children with nocturnal enuresis. *American Journal of Nursing*, 106(8):56-64.

Beuscart-Azephir, A., Pelayo, S., Anceaux, F., et al. (2005). Impact of CPOE on doctor-nurse cooperation for the medication ordering and administration process. *International Journal of Medical Informatics*, 74(7-8):629-641.

Black, J.M., & Hawks, H.J. (2009). *Medical-surgical nursing: clinical management for positive outcomes.* (8th ed.). Philadelphia: Saunders.

Breiterman-White, R. (2005). Functional ability of patients on dialysis: the crital role of anemia. *Nephrology Nursing Journal*, 32(1):79-82.

Bruner, D., & Calvano, T. (2007). The sexual impact of cancer and cancer treatments in men. *Nursing Clinics of North America*, 42(4):555-580.

Burrows-Hudson, S. (2005). Chronic kidney disease: an overview. *American Journal of Nursing*, 105(2):40-50.

Campbell, B. (2006). Bladder cancer. *Nursing*, 36(4):54-64.

Campoy, S., & Elwell, R. (2005). Pharmacology & CKD. *American Journal of Nursing*, 105(9):60-72.

Chang, S., & Cookson, M. (2005). Radical systectomy for bladder cancer: the case for early intervention. *Urologic Clinics of North America*, 32(2):147-155.

Coca, S., Krumholz, H., Garg, A., et al. (2006). Underrepresentation of renal disease in randomized controlled trials of cardiovascular disease. *Journal of the American Medical Association*, 296(11): 1377-1384.

Collins, K. (2009). *Concerns over kidney cancer grow.* Available at www.aicr.org/site/News2?page=NewsArticle&id=14447&news_iv_ctrl=0&abbr=pr_hf_. Accessed November, 2009.

Costantini, L., Beanlands, H., McCay, E., et al. (2008). The self-management experience of people with mild to moderate chronic kidney disease. *Nephrology Nursing Journal*, 35(2):147-156.

Curtin, R., Johnson, H., & Shatell, D. (2004). The peritoneal dialysis experience: insights from long-term patients. *Nephrology Nursing Journal*, 31(6):615-625.

De Geest, S., Schäfer-Keller, P., Denhaerynck, K., et al. (2006). Supporting medication adherence in renal transplantation (SMART): a pilot RCT to improve adherence to immunosuppressive regimens. *Clinical Transplantation*, 20:359-368.

Editorial. (2007). Fast facts about loop diuretics. *Nursing*, 37(10): 56hn7-56hn8.

Eeles, R., Kote-Jarai, Z., Giles, G.G., et al. (2008). Multiple newly identified loci associated with prostate cancer susceptibility. *Nature Genetics*, 40:316-321.

Ficorelli, C., & Weeks, B. (2006). Facing up to prostate cancer. *Nursing*, 36(5):66-67.

Frey, K., Ed. (2008). *Surgical technology for the surgical technologist.* (3rd ed.). Clifton Park, NY: Delmar Cengage.

Gesek, F., & Desmond, J. (2008). Improved patient outcomes in chronic kidney disease: optimizing vitamin D therapy. *Nephrology Nursing Journal*, 35(2S):5A-23S.

Gilchrist, K. (2007). BPH. *LPN*, 3(1):32-39.

Goldstein, S.L, Graham, N., Warady, B.A., et al. (2008). Measuring health-related quality of life in children with ESRD: performance of the generic and ESRD-specific instrument of the pediatric quality of life inventory. *American Journal of Kidney Diseases*, 51(2):285-297.

Greenlings-Coppin, C., Porzolt, F., Autenrieth, M., et al. (2006). Targeted therapy for advanced renal cell carcinoma (Protocol). *Cochrane Data Base of Systematic Reviews*, Issue 2, Art. No. CD006017. DOI:101002/14651858.CD006017.

Hautmann, R., & Stein, J. (2005). Neobladder with prostatic capsule and seminal-sparing cystectomy for bladder cancer: a step in the wrong direction. *Urologic Clinics of North America*, 32(2):177-185.

Hedayati, T., & Keegan, M. (2009). *Prostatitis.* Available at http://emedicine.medscape.com/article/785418-overview. Accessed November, 2009.

Herr, H. (2005). Surgical factors in the treatment of superficial and invasive bladder cancer. *Urologic Clinics of North America*, 32(2): 157-164.

Hinds, A. (2004). Obstructive uropathy: considerations for the nephrology nurse. *Nephrology Nursing Journal*, 31(2):166.

Hlebovy, D. (2006). Hemodailysis special interest group networking session: fluid management: moving and removing fluid during hemodialysis. *Nephrology Nursing Journal*, 33(4):441-446.

Israel, G., & Bosniak, M. (2003). Renal imaging for diagnosis and staging of renal cell carcinoma. *Urologic Clinics of North America*, 30(3):499-514.

Jamison, R., Hartigan, P., Kaufman, J.S., et al. (2008). Effect of homocysteine lowering on mortality and vascular disease in advanced chronic kidney disease and end-stage renal disease. *Journal of the American Medical Association*, 298(10):1163-1170.

Janos, V., & Higgins, L. (2007). Interstitial cystitis. *ADVANCE for Nurse Practitioners*, 15(3):55-57.

Jemal, A., Siegal, R., Ward, E., et al. (2006). *Cancer statistics*. Available at http://caonline.amcancersoc.org/cgi/content/abstract/56/2/106. Accessed November, 2009.

Johns Hopkins Children's Center. (2006). *Kidney stones occurring more often in children*. Available at www.hopkinschildrens.org/Kidney-Stones-Occuring-More-Often-in-Children.aspx. Accessed November, 2009.

Karch, A. (2008). *2009 Lippincott's nursing drug guide*. Philadelphia: Lippincott.

Kessler, T., Burkhard, F., & Studer, U. (2005). Clinical indications and outcomes with nurse-sparing cycstectomy in patients with bladder cancer. *Urologic Clinics of North America*, 32(2):165-175.

Khera, M., & Lipshultz, L. (2007). The role of testosterone replacement therapy following radical prostatectomy. *Urologic Clinics of North America*, 34(4):549-553.

Kidney Disease Outcomes Quality Initiative (KDOQI). (2007). Clinical practice guidelines and clinical practice recommendations for diabetes and chronic kidney disease. *American Journal of Kidney Diseases*, 49(suppl2):2.

Koivula, B., & Minielly, B. (2006). The Canadian introduction to the Greenlight laser. *Canadian Operating Room Nursing Journal*, 24(1):30-34.

Kontak, J., & Campbell, S. (2003). Prognostic factors in renal cell carcinoma. *Urologic Clinics of North America*, 30(3):467-480.

Krebs, L. (2007). Sexual assessment: research and clinical. *Nursing Clinics of North America*, 42(4):515-529.

Legg, V. (2005). Complications of chronic kidney disease. *American Journal of Nursing*, 105(6):40-50.

Leibovich, B., Pantuck, A., Bui, M., et al. (2003). Current staging of renal cell carcinoma. *Urologic Clinics of North America*, 30(3):481-498.

Lewis, S.L., Heitkemper, M.M., Dirksen, S.R., et al. (2007). *Medical-surgical nursing: assessment and management of clinical problems*. (7th ed.). St. Louis: Mosby.

Lilley, L., Harrington, S., & Snyder, J. (2007). *Pharmacology and the nursing process*. (5th ed.). St. Louis: Mosby, Inc.

Lu, D.F., McCarthy, A.M., Lanning, L.D., et al. (2007). A descriptive study of individuals with membranoproliferative glomerulonephritis. *Nephrology Nursing Journal*, 34(3):295-303.

Mahoney, C. (2007). Should patients eat during dialysis? *Nursing*, 37(10):57-58.

Matsuoka, S., Tominaga, Y., Uno, N., et al. (2006). Surgical significance of undescended parathyroid gland in renal hyperparathyroidism. *Surgery*, 139(6):815-820.

MayoClinic.com.(2009). *Urinary incontinence*. Available at http://mayoclinic.com/health/urinary-incontinence/DS00404. Accessed November, 2009.

McCarley, P., & Salai, P. (2005). Cardiovascular disease in chronic kidney disease. *American Journal of Nursing*, 105(4):40-53.

Medtronic, Inc. (n.d.). *About overactive bladder*. Available at www.medtronic.com/your-health/overactive-bladder/index.htm. Accessed November, 2009.

Middelton, L., & Essick, M. (2003). Inherited urologic malignant disorders: nursing implications. *Urologic Nursing*, 23(1):15-29.

Miller, D., Macdonald, D., Kolnacki, K., et al. (2004). Challenges for nephrology nurses in the management of children with chronic kidney disease. *Nephrology Nursing Journal*, 31(3):287.

Monoharan, M., & Soloway, M. (2005). Optimal management of the T1G3 bladder cancer. *Urologic Clinics of North America*, 32(2):133-145.

Moore, P., Farney, A., Sundberg, A., et al. (2006). Experience with dual kidney transplants from donors at the extremes of age. *Surgery*, 140(4):597-606.

Morgentaler, A. (2007). Testosterone replacement therapy and prostate cancer. *Urologic Clinics of North America*, 34(4):555-563.

Moyad, M. (2003). Calcium oxalate kidney stones: another reason to encourage moderate calcium intakes and other dietary changes. *Urologic Nursing*, 23(4):310.

Mulders, P., Bleumer, I., & Oosterwijk, E. (2003). Tumor antigens and markers in renal call carcinoma. *Urologic Clinics of North America*, 39(3):455-465.

Muruve, N., Steinbecker, K., & Willard, T.B. (2008). *Transurethral needle ablation of the prostate*. Available at www.emedicine.com/MED/topic3069.htm. Accessed November, 2009.

National Cancer Institute (NCI). (2008). *Bladder cancer*. Available at www.cancer.gov/cancertopics/pdq/treatment/bladder/Patient. Accessed November, 2009.

National Kidney Foundation (NKF). (2004). *Sexuality and chronic kidney disease*. Available at www.kidney.org/atoz/content/sexuality.cfm. Accessed November, 2009.

Nicholson, L., & Smith, D. (2007). Dysfunctional elimination syndrome. *ADVANCE for Nurse Practitioners*, 15(3):27-32.

Nieder, A., & Taneja, S. (2003). The role of partial nephrectomy for renal cell carcinoma. *Urologic Clinics of North America*, 30(3):529-542.

O'Donnell, M. (2005). Practical applications of intravesical chemotherapy and immunotherapy in high-risk patients with superficial bladder cancer. *Urologic Clinics of North America*, 32(2):121-131.

Pagana, K.D., & Pagana, T.J. (2008). *Mosby's diagnostic and laboratory test reference*. (9th ed.). St. Louis: Mosby.

Page, S., Rosenberg, M., & Hazzard, M. (2005). Interstitial cystitis: current diagnosis and management strategies, *ADVANCE for Nurse Practitioners*, 13(12):18.

Palmer, M.H., & Newman, D.K. (2006). Bladder control: educational needs of older adults, *Journal of Gerontologic Nursing*, 32(1):28.

Pasche, B. (2006). A new strategy in the war on renal cell cancer. *Journal of the American Medical Association*, 295(21):2537-2538.

Pavkov, M., Bennett, P.H., Knowler, W.C., et al. (2006). Effect of youth-onset type 2 diabetes mellitus on incidence of end-stage renal disease and mortality in young and middle-aged Pima Indians. *Journal of the American Medical Association*, 296(4):421-426.

Pelusi, J. (2006). Sexuality and body image. *American Journal of Nursing*, 106(3suppl):32-38.

Phillips, M. (2007). *Berry & Kohn's operating room technique*. (11th ed.). St. Louis, Mosby.

Pilkey, R., Morton, A., Boffa, M., et al. (2007). Subclinical vitamin K deficiency in hemodialysis patients. *American Journal of Kidney Disease*, 49(3):432-439.

Polt, C. (2006). Taking the pressure off for women with stress incontinence. *Nursing 2006*, 36(2):49-51.

Potter, P.A., & Perry, A.G. (2009). *Fundamentals of nursing: concepts, process, and practice*. (7th ed.). St. Louis: Mosby.

Purcell, W., Manias, E., Williams, A., et al. (2004). Accurate dry weight assessment: reducing the incidence of hypertension and cardiac disease in patients on hemodialysis. *Nephrology Nursing Journal*, 31(6):631-638.

Rossi, S., Ed. (2004). *Australian medicine handbook*. Adelaide: Australian Medicines Handbook.

Rubenstein, J., & McVary, K.T. (2008). *Transurethral microwave thermotherapy of the prostate (TUMT)*. Available at http://emedicine.medscape.com/article/449623-followup. Accessed November, 2009.

Saccomano, S., & DeLuca, D. (2008). Managing acute renal failure. *Men in Nursing*, 3(2):32-42.

Schiffl, H., Lang, S.M., & Fischer, R. (2002). Daily hemodialysis and the outcome of acute renal failure. *New England Journal of Medicine*, 346(5):305.

Shiller, J., & Gonzalez, R. (2007). Green light laser: BPH treatment shows promise. *RN*, 70(11):28-32.

Smith, J. (2008). *Robotic versus open radical prostatectomy: "What is the real story?"* Available at http://www1.gotomeeting.com/en_US/island/webinare/registration0Post.temp1Z_sid=12178969%3A. Accessed May 3, 2008.

Stafford, H.S., Saltzstein, S.L., Shimasaki, S., et al. (2008). Oncology: adrenal/renal/upper tract/bladder. *Journal of Urology*, 179(5):1704-1708.

Stewart, M. (2006). Narrative literature review: sexual dysfunction in the patient on hemodialysis. *Nephrology Nursing Journal*, 33(6):631-641.

Stratta, R., Sundberg, A., Rohr, M., et al. (2006). Optimal use of older donors and recipients in kidney transplantation. *Surgery*, 139(3): 324-333.

Thomas-Hawkins, C., & Zazworsky, D. (2005). Self-management of chronic kidney disease. *American Journal of Nursing*, 105(10): 40-49.

U.S. Department of Agriculture (USDA). (2009). *MyPyramid*. Available at www.mypyramid.gov. Accessed November, 2009.

Uzzo, R., Cairns, P., Al-Saleem,T., et al. (2003). The basic biology and immunobiology of renal cell carcinoma: considerations for the clinician. *Urologic Clinics of North America*, 39(3):423-436.

Vasavada, S., & Rackley, R. (2006). How effective is pharmacotherapy for overactive bladder? *Patient Care*, January 1, 2006. Available at www.modernmedicine.com/modernmedicine/Urology/How-effective-is-pharmacotherapy-for-overactive-bl/ArticleStandard/Article/detail/283042. Article now available only to registered Modern Medicine members.

Vaughn, D., & Malkowicz, S. (2005). Neoadjuvant chemotherapy in patients with invasive bladder cancer. *Urologic Clinics of North America*, 32(2):231-237.

Vogel, S., & Rossert, J. (2005). A clinical review of antibody-mediated pure red cell aplasia. *Nephrology Nursing Journal*, 32(1):17-27.

Wijeysundera, D., Karkouti, K., Dupuis, J.Y., et al. (2007). Derivation and validation of simplified predictive index for renal replacement therapy after cardiac surgery. *Journal of the American Medical Association*, 297(16):1801-1809.

Wilmoth, M. (2007). Sexuality: a critical component of quality of life in chronic disease. *Nursing Clinics of North America*, 42(4):507-514.

Wilson, R.T., Silverman, D.T., Fraumeni, J.F., Jr., et al. (2008). *New malignancies following cancer of the urinary tract*. Available at http://seer.cancer.gov/publications/mpmono/Ch11_Bladder.pdf. Accessed November, 2009.

Wood, L., & Manchen, B. (2007). Sorafenib: a promising new targeted therapy for renal cell carcinoma. *Clinical Journal of Oncology Nursing*, 11(5):649-656.

Chapter 51 Care of the Patient with an Endocrine Disorder

American Diabetes Association. (2006). Standards of medical care for patients with diabetes mellitus. *Diabetes Care*, 29(suppl 1):54-542.

American Diabetes Association. (2007a). *Insulin pumps*. Available at www.diabetes.org/living-with-diabetes/treatment-and-care/medication/insulin/insulin-pumps.html. Accessed November, 2009.

American Diabetes Association. (2007b). Standards of medical care in diabetes. *Diabetes Care*, 30(suppl 1):540-541.

Anthony, M. (2006). When the blood glucose level takes a dive. *Nursing Made Incredibly Easy!* 4(6):15-17.

Appel, S. (2005). Sizing up metabolic syndrome. *Nursing*, 35(12):20.

Aschenbrenner, D. (2005). New drug for diabetes approved. *American Journal of Nursing*, 105(7):25.

Barkauskas, V., Baumann, L.C., & Darling-Fisher, C. (2006). *Health and physical assessment*. (4th ed.). St. Louis: Mosby.

Bass, A., Will, T., Todd, M., et al. (2007). The latest tools for patients with diabetes. *RN*, 70(6):39-43.

Bauer, J. (2006). Drug update: manufacturer breathes new life into delivery of insulin. *RN*, 69(31):64.

Black, J.M., & Hawks, H.J. (2009). *Medical surgical nursing: clinical management for positive outcomes*. (8th ed.). Philadelphia: Saunders.

Bode, B., Weinstein, R., Bell, D., et al. (2002). Comparison of insulin aspart with buffered regular insulin and insulin lispro in continuous subcutaneous infusion: a randomized study in type 1 diabetes. *Diabetes Care*, 25(3):439-444.

Brozenec, S. (1998). *Coping with multisystem complications*. St. Louis: Mosby.

D'Arcy, Y. (2007). Getting a grip on neuropathic pain. *LPN*, 4(2):14.

Davidson, M., Mehta, A.E., Siraj, E.S. (2006). Inhaled human insulin: an inspiration for patients with diabetes mellitus? *Cleveland Clinic Journal of Medicine*, 73(6):569-578.

Funnel, M., & Barlage, D. (2002). Managing diabetes with "agent oral." *Nursing*, 34(3):36.

Gattullo, B. (2007). Diabetic retinopathy. *Nursing*, 37(7):51.

Griffing, G.T., Odeke, S., Nagelberg, S.B. (2009). *Addison's disease*. Available at http://emedicine.medscape.com/article/116467-diagnosis. Accessed November, 2009.

Hieronymus, L., & O'Connell, B. (2004). Diabetes basics: managing hyperglycemia. *Diabetes Self-Management*, 21(6):44, 46-48.

Holcomb, S.S. (2005). Detecting thyroid disease. *Nursing*, 35(10): 4-8.

Holcomb, S.S. (2007). A delicate balance: keeping thyroid hormones in check. *LPN*, 3(2):46.

Hussar, D. (2007). New drugs-insulin glulisine and insulin determir. *Nursing*, 37(2):52.

Hypoglycemia Support Foundation. Available at www.hypoglycemia.org. Accessed November, 2009.

Jacques, S. (2004). Diabetes under control: diabetes and depression. *American Journal of Nursing*, 104(9):56.

Jones, H., Edwards, L., Vallis, T.M., et al. (2003). Changes in diabetes self-care behaviors make a difference in glycemic control: the Diabetes Stages of Change (DiSC) study, *Diabetes Care* 26(3):732-737.

Levine, A., & Brennan, A.P. (2007). Rethinking sliding-scale insulin: one hospital's efforts in the ICU and elsewhere. *American Journal of Nursing*, 107(10):74-79.

Lewis, S.L., Heitkemper, M.M., Dirksen, S.R., et al. (2007). *Medical-surgical nursing: assessment and management of clinical problems*. (7th ed.). St. Louis: Mosby.

LoBiondo-Wood, G., & Haber, J. (2009). *Nursing research: methods and critical appraisal for evidence-based practice*. (7th ed.). St. Louis: Mosby.

Maddox, T., & Parker, D.M. (2006). Going up? Rapid ACTH screening. *Nursing Made Incredibly Easy!* 4(3):62-53.

McCance, K.L., & Huether, S.E. (2010). *Pathophysiology: the biologic basis for disease in children and adults*. (6th ed.). St Louis: Mosby.

Medical Letter, Inc. (2006). Drugs for hypothyroidism and hyperthyroidism. *Treatment Guidelines from Medical Letter*, 44(4):17, 2006.

Monahan, F.D., Sands, J.K., Neighbors, M., et al. (2007). *Phipps' medical-surgical nursing: health and illness perspectives*. (8th ed.). St. Louis: Mosby.

Mosby's dictionary of medicine, nursing, and health professions. (2009). (8th ed.). St. Louis: Mosby.

National Diabetes Education Program. Available at www.ndep.nih.gov. Accessed November, 2009.

Pagana, K.D., & Pagana, T.J. (2008). *Mosby's diagnostic and laboratory test reference*. (9th ed.). St. Louis: Mosby.

Perry, A.G., & Potter, P.A. (2009). *Clinical nursing skills and techniques*. (7th ed.). St. Louis: Mosby.

Potter, P.A., & Perry, A.G. (2007). *Basic nursing: essentials for practice*. (6th ed.). St. Louis: Mosby.

Ridge, R. (2007). Boosting insulin safety. *Nursing*, 37(2):14.

Scemons, D. (2007). Are you up-to-date on diabetes medications? *Nursing*, 37(7):45.

Skidmore-Roth, L. (2010). *Mosby's 2010 nursing drug reference*. St. Louis: Mosby.

Thibodeau, G.A., & Patton, K.T. (2008). *Structure and function of the body*. (13th ed.). St. Louis: Mosby.

Thibodeau, G.A., & Patton, K.T. (2009). *The human body in health and disease*. (5th ed.). St. Louis: Mosby.

Thompson, J.M., McFarland, G.K., Hirsch, J.E., et al. (2001). *Mosby's clinical nursing*. (5th ed.) .St. Louis: Mosby.

Tierney L., McPhee, S.J., Papadakis, M.A. (2007). *Current medical diagnosis and treatment*. (44th ed.). New York: McGraw-Hill.

U.S. Food and Drug Administration (US FDA). (2009). *Byetta (exenatide)—renal failure*. Available at www.fda.gov/Safety/MedWatch/SafetyInformation/SafetyAlertsforHumanMedicalProducts/ucm188703.htm. Accessed November, 2009.

Watts, S.A., Anselmo, J. (2006). Nutrition for diabetes—all of day's work. *Nursing*, 36(6):45-48.

White, R. (2007). Insulin pump therapy (continuous subcutaneous insulin infusion). *Primary Care*, 34(4):845.

Whiteman, K. (2006). ACTH stimulation: testing the adrenals. *Nursing*, 36(7):24.

Wilson, S.F., & Gidden, J.F. (2009). *Health assessment for nursing practice*. (4th ed.). St Louis: Mosby.

Wright, M., & Appel, S.J. (2007). Inhaled insulin: breathing new life into diabetes therapy. *Nursing*, 37(1):46.

Chapter 52 Care of the Patient with a Reproductive Disorder

Ackley, B.J., & Ladwig, G.B. (2009). *Nursing diagnosis handbook*. (7th ed.). St. Louis: Mosby.

Akert, J. (2003). Hormone replacement therapy, *RN*, 66(12):40.

American Cancer Society (ACS). (2007a). *Cancer facts and figures, 2007*. Available at www.cancer.org/downloads/STT/CAFF-2007PWsecured.pdf. Accessed November, 2009.

American Cancer Society (ACS). (2007b). Guidelines for breast screening with MRI as an adjunct to mammography. *CA: A Cancer Journal for Clinicians*, 57:75-89.

American Cancer Society (ACS). (2007c). *Ovarian cancer has early symptoms*. Available at www.cancer.org/docroot/NWS/content/NWS_1_1x_Ovarian_Cancer_Symptoms_The_Silence_Is_Broken.asp. Accessed November, 2009.

American Cancer Society (ACS). (2008a). *Cancer facts and figures*, 2008. Available at www.cancer.org/docroot/stt/content/stt_1x_cancer_facts_and_figures_2008.asp. Accessed November, 2009.

American Cancer Society (ACS). (2008b). *Cancer statistics*. Atlanta: Author.

American Cancer Society (ACS). (2009a). *American Cancer Society guidelines for the early detection of cancer*. Available at www.cancer.org/docroot/PED/content/PED_2_3X_ACS_Cancer_Detection_Guidelines_36.asp?sitearea=PED. Accessed November, 2009.

American Cancer Society (ACS). (2009b). *American Cancer Society responds to changes to USPSTF mammography guidelines*. Available at www.cancer.org/docroot/MED/content/MED_2_1x_American_Cancer_Society_Responds_to_Changes_to_USPSTF_Mammography_Guidelines.asp?sitearea=MED. Accessed November, 2009.

American Cancer Society (ACS). (2009c). *Cancer facts and figures*. Available at www.cancer.org/downloads/STT/500809web.pdf. Accessed November, 2009.

American Cancer Society (ACS). (2009d). *How is breast cancer staged?* Available at www.cancer.org/docroot/CRI/content/CRI_2_4_3X_How_is_breast_cancer_staged_5.asp?rnav=cri. Accessed November, 2009.

American Congress of Obstetricians and Gynecologists (ACOG). (2004). *Menopausal bleeding*. Available at www.acog.org/publications/patient_education/bp162.cfm. Accessed November, 2009.

American Congress of Obstetricians and Gynecologists (ACOG). (2009). *Response of the American Congress of Obstetricians and Gynecologists to new breast cancer screening recommendations from the U.S. Preventive Services Task Force*. Available at www.acog.org/from_home/Misc/uspstfResponse.cfm. Accessed November, 2009.

American Society for Reproductive Medicine Practice Committee (ASRM). (2006). *Report on varicocele and infertility*. Available at www.asrm.org/Media/Practice/Report_on_varicocele.pdf. Accessed November, 2009.

Aschenbrenner, D. (2004). Hormone replacement therapy (HRT): what should you tell patients about it now? *American Journal of Nursing*, 104(6):51.

Balzer-Riley, J. (2008). *Communication in nursing*. (6th ed.). St. Louis: Mosby.

Barkauskas, V., Baumann, L.C., & Darling-Fisher, C. (2006). *Health and physical assessment*. (4th ed.). St. Louis: Mosby.

Barton, D., & Loprinzi, C.L. (2004). Making sense of the evidence regarding nonhormonal treatments for hot flashes. *Clinical Journal of Oncology Nursing*, 8:39.

Black, J.M., & Hawks, H.J. (2009). *Medical-surgical nursing: clinical management for positive outcomes*. (8th ed.). Philadelphia: Saunders.

Carroll, C. (2006). Sorting out breast biopsy options. *Nursing*, 36(3):70.

Centers for Disease Control and Prevention (CDC). (2006). *New estimates of U.S. HIV prevalence, 2006*. Available at www.cdc.gov/hiv/topics/surveillance/resources/factsheets/prevalence.htm. Accessed November, 2009.

Centers for Disease Control and Prevention (CDC), Division of STD Prevention. (2007a). *Sexually transmitted diseases surveillance, 2007: chlamydia*. Available at www.cdc.gov/std/stats07/chlamydia.htm. Accessed November, 2009.

Centers for Disease Control and Prevention (CDC), Division of STD Prevention. (2007b). *Sexually transmitted diseases surveillance, 2007: gonorrhea*. Available at www.cdc.gov/std/stats07/gonorrhea.htm. Accessed November, 2009.

Centers for Disease Control and Prevention (CDC), Division of STD Prevention. (2007c). *Sexually transmitted diseases surveillance, 2007: syphilis*. Available at www.cdc.gov/std/stats07/syphilis.htm. Accessed November, 2009.

Centers for Disease Control and Prevention (CDC), Division of STD Prevention. (2007d). *Sexually transmitted diseases surveillance, 2007: trichomoniasis*. Available at www.cdc.gov/STD/Trichomonas/STDFact-Trichomoniasis.htm. Accessed November, 2009.

Centers for Disease Control and Prevention. (CDC). (2008). HIV prevalence estimates—United States, 2006. *MMWR Mortality and Morbidity Weekly Report*, 57(39):1073-1076.

Centers for Disease Control and Prevention (CDC). (n.d.). *Sexually transmitted diseases: genital herpes—CDC fact sheet*. Available at www.cdc.gov/std/herpes/STDFact-herpes.htm. Accessed November, 2009.

Chlebowski, R., Hendrix, S.L., Langer, R.D., et al. (2003). Influence of estrogen plus progestin on breast cancer and mammography in healthy postmenopausal women: the Women's Health Initiative Randomized Trial. *Journal of the American Medical Association*, 289:3243-3253.

Cleveland Clinic. (2009). *Image guided biopsy*. Available at http://my.clevelandclinic.org/services/biopsy/hic_Minimally_Invasive_Breast_Biopsy.aspx. Accessed November, 2009.

Cullen, P., & Cameron, C. (2006). Progress towards an effective syphilis vaccine: the past, present, and future. *Expert Review of Vaccines*, 5(1):65.

Deglin, J., & Vallerand, A. (2008). *Davis's drug guide for nurses*. (16th ed.). Philadelphia: Davis.

Elkin, M.K., Perry, A.G., & Potter, P.A. (2007). *Nursing interventions and clinical skills*. (4th ed.). St. Louis: Mosby.

Editorial. (2005). Who should use hormone therapy? *Nursing Made Incredibly Easy!* 3(1):64.

Facts at a glance. (n.d.). *Regional/global HIV/AIDS statistics*. Available at www.statehealthfacts.org. Accessed November, 2009.

Ficorelli, C. (2007). Untangling the complexities of male infertility. *Nursing*, 37(1):24.

Gardner, J. (2006). What you need to know about genital herpes. *Nursing*, 36(10):26.

Giger, J.M., & Davidhizar, R.E. (2007). *Transcultural nursing: assessment and intervention*. (5th ed.). St. Louis: Mosby.

Greifzu, S. (2004). Breast cancer. *RN*, 67(2):35.

Hockenberry, M.J., & Wilson, D. (2007). *Wong's nursing care of infants and children*. (8th ed.). St. Louis, Mosby.

Holcomb, S. (2008). Assessing the cause of postmenopausal bleeding. *LPN*, 4(2):50.

Hollingsworth, A.B., Singletary, S.E., Morrow, M. et al. (2004). Current comprehensive assessment and management of women at increased risk for breast cancer. *American Journal of Surgery*, 187(3):349-362.

Katz, A. (2005). Sexuality and hysterectomy: finding the right words: responding to patients'concerns about the potential effects of surgery. *American Journal of Nursing*, 105(12):65-68.

Kudachadkar, R., O'Regan, R.M. (2005). Aromatase inhibitors as adjuvant therapy for post menopausal patients with early stage breast cancer. *CA: A Cancer Journal for Clinicians*, 55(3):145-163.

Lehman, M. (2007). It whispers, so listen—ovarian cancer. *RN*, (10):28.

Lewis, J.H., Rosen, R., & Goldstein, I. (2005). Erectile dysfunction. *Nursing*, 35:64.

Lewis, S.L., Heitkemper, M.M., Dirksen, S.R., et al. (2007). *Medical-surgical nursing: assessment and management of clinical problems*. (7th ed.). St. Louis: Mosby.

Mahoney, S.F., & Armstrong, A. (2005). Accurate diagnosis of postmenopausal bleeding. *Nursing*, 30(8):61-63.

Martin, V. (2006). Shining a light on ovarian cancer, the hidden tumor. *Nursing Made Incredibly Easy!* 4(6):28-37.

McCaffery, M., & Pasero, C. (1999). *Pain: clinical manual*. (2nd ed.). St. Louis: Mosby.

McDaniel, C. (2007). Uterine fibroid embolization: the less invasive alternative. *Nursing*, 37(7):26-27.

Memmler, R.L., et al. (2008). *Structure and function of the human body*. (9th ed.). Philadelphia: Lippincott.

Mirshahidi, H. (2004). Managing early breast cancer. *Postgraduate Medicine*, 116:23.

National Cancer Institute (NCI). (2006a). *Clinical announcement: intraperitoneal chemotherapy for ovarian cancer*. Available at http://ctep.cancer.gov/highlights/docs/clin_annc_010506.pdf. Accessed November, 2009.

National Cancer Institute (NCI). (2006b). *NCI issues clinical announcement for preferred method of treatment for advanced ovarian cancer*. Available at www.cancer.gov/newscenter/IPchemotherapyQandA. Accessed November, 2009.

National Cancer Institute (NCI). (2009a). *A closer look: does mammography sometimes detect too much breast cancer*? Available at www.cancer.gov/ncicancerbulletin/102009/page6. Accessed November, 2009.

National Cancer Institute (NCI). (2009b). *Factsheet: testicular cancer: questions and answers*. Available at www.cancer.gov/cancertopics/factsheet/Sites-Types/testicular. Accessed November, 2009.

National Institutes of Health (NIH). (n.d.). *Women's Health Initiative hormone therapy study: menopausal hormone therapy information*. Available at www.nih.gov/PHTindex.htm. Accessed November, 2009.

O'Rourke, E. (2007). Syphilis, still a public health danger. *RN*, 70(7):26.

Pagana, K.D., & Pagana, T.J. (2008). *Mosby's diagnostic and laboratory test reference*. (9th ed.). St. Louis: Mosby.

Park, A. (2007). Breast-cancer basics: diagnosis and treatment keep changing: here's what you need to know now. *Time*, 170(16):46.

Potter, P.A., & Perry, A.G. (2009). *Fundamentals of nursing: concepts, process, and practice*. (7th ed.). St. Louis: Mosby.

Santoro, N., & Chervenak, J.L. (2004). The menopause transition. *Endocrinology and Metabolism Clinics of North America*, 33:627.

Saslow, D., Castle, P.E., Cox, J.T., et al. (2007). American Cancer Society guideline for human papillomavirus (HPV) vaccine use to prevent cervical cancer and its precursors. *CA: A Cancer Journal for Clinicians*, 57(1):7-28.

Seidel, H.M., Ball, J.W., Dains, J.E., et al. (2007). *Mosby's guide to physical examination*. (6th ed.). St. Louis: Mosby.

Skidmore-Roth, L. (2010). *Mosby's 2010 nursing drug reference*. (23rd ed.). St. Louis: Mosby.

Snow, M. (2007). HPV vaccine: new treatment for an old disease. *Nursing*, 37(3):67.

Thibodeau, G.A. & Patton, K.T. (2007). *Anatomy and physiology*. (6th ed.). St. Louis: Mosby.

Thibodeau, G.A. & Patton, K.T. (2008). *Structure and function of the body*. (13th ed.). St. Louis: Mosby.

Thompson, J.M., McFarland, G.K., Hirsch, J.E., et al. (2001). *Mosby's clinical nursing*. (5th ed.).St. Louis: Mosby.

Timby, B.K., & Lewis, L.W. (2008). *Fundamental skills and concepts in patient care*. (9th ed.). Philadelphia: Lippincott.

Ulbricht, C.E., & Basch, E.M. (2005). Natural standard herb and supplement reference: evidence based clinical reviews. St. Louis: Mosby.

U.S. Food and Drug Administration (FDA). (2009a). *Cervarix. Product information: package insert*. Available at www.fda.gov/downloads/BiologicsBloodVaccines/Vaccines/ApprovedProducts/UCM186981.pdf. Accessed November, 2009.

U.S. Food and Drug Administration (FDA). (2009b). *FDA approved first DNA test for two types of human papillomavirus: agency also approved second DNA test for wider range of HPV types*. Available at www.fda.gov/NewsEvents/Newsroom/PressAnnouncements/ucm149544.htm. Accessed November, 2009.

U.S. Food and Drug Administration (FDA). (2004). *Timeline of breast implant activities*. Available at www.fda.gov/MedicalDevices/ProductsandMedicalProcedures/ImplantsandProsthetics/BreastImplants/ucm064242.htm. Accessed November, 2009.

U.S. Preventive Services Task Force (USPSTF). (2009). *Screening for breast cancer*. Available at www.ahrq.gov/clinic/USpstf/uspsbrca.htm. Accessed November, 2009.

Villa, I.I., Costa, R.L., Petta, C.A., et al. (2005). Prophylactic quadrivalent human papillomavirus (types 6, 11, 16, and 18) L1 virus-like particle vaccine in young women: a randomized double-blind placebo-controlled multicentre phase II efficacy trial. *Lancet Oncology*, 6(5):271-278.

Weaver, C. (2007). Compassionate care for the mastectomy patient. *Nursing Made Incredibly Easy!* 5(6):36.

Yeh, I.T. (2007). Post menopausal hormone replacement therapy: endometrial and breast effects. *Advances in Anatomic Pathology*, 14(1):17.

Additional Resource

American Cancer Society. Available at www.cancer.org. Accessed November, 2009.

Chapter 53 Care of the Patient with a Visual or Auditory Disorder

Albert, D., Miller, J.W., Azar, D.T, et al. (2008). *Albert and Jakobiec's principles and practice of ophthalmology*. (3rd ed.). Philadelphia: Saunders.

American Foundation for the Blind. (2009). *Facts and figures on Americans with vision loss*. Numbers of legally blind Americans. Available at www.afb.org/Section.asp?SectionID=15&DocumentID=4398#legal. Accessed December, 2009.

American Society of Ophthalmic Registered Nurses (ASORN). (2004). *Core curriculum for ophthalmic nursing*. (3rd ed.). Dubuque, Iowa: Kendall/Hunt.

Ball, K. (2007). *The perioperative challenge*. (5th ed.). St. Louis: Mosby.

Black, J.M., & Hawks, H.J. (2009). *Medical-surgical nursing: clinical management for positive outcomes*. (8th ed.). Philadelphia: Saunders.

Brandt, J.T., et al. (2008). Community resources for the ophthalmic practice. In D. Albert, J.W. Miller, D.T. Azar, et al. (Eds.), *Albert and Jakobiec's principles and practice of ophthalmology*. (3rd ed., vol. 5). Philadelphia: Saunders.

Burke, M., & Walsh, M. (2009). *Gerontologic nursing*. (5th ed.). St. Louis: Mosby.

Corell, C. (2007). New outlook for age-related macular degeneration. *Nursing*, 37(3):27.

Gallagher, R.P., & Lee, T.K. (2006). Adverse effects of ultraviolet radiation: a brief review. *Progress in Biophysics and Molecular Biology*, 92(1):119-31.

Giger, J.M., & Davidhizar, R.E. (2007). *Transcultural nursing: assessment and intervention*. (5th ed.). St. Louis: Mosby.

Hard of Hearing Advocates. Available at www.hohadvocates.org. Accessed November, 2009.

Jaffe, M., & Skidmore-Roth, L. (2005). *Home health nursing*. (5th ed.). St. Louis: Mosby.

Johns Hopkins University. (2004). New strategies for preventing vision loss. *John Hopkins Medical Letter*, 15:4.

Lewis, S.L., Heitkemper, M.M., Dirksen, S.R., et al. (2007). *Medical-surgical nursing: assessment and management of clinical problems*. (7th ed.). St. Louis: Mosby.

Leyland M., & Zinicola, E. (2003). Multifocal versus monofocal intraocular lenses after cataract extraction. *Cochrane Data Base of Systematic Reviews*, Issue 3., Art No. CD003169.

Mayo Clinic staff. *Cataracts*. Available at www.mayoclinic.com/health/cataracts/DS00050. Accessed November, 2009.

McGwin, G., Jr., Gewant, H.D., Modjarrad, K., et al. (2006). Effect of cataract surgery on falls and mobility in independently living older adults. *Journal of the American Geriatric Society*, 54(7):1089-1094.

Monahan, F.D., Sands, J.K., Neighbors, M., et al. (2007). *Phipps' medical-surgical nursing: health and illness perspectives.* (8th ed.). St. Louis: Mosby.

Monk, H. (2005). Bring common eye emergencies into focus. *Nursing*, 35(12):46.

Monk, H. (2006). Presbyopia and cataract. *LPN*, 2(6):27.

Monk, H. (2007). Glaucoma and macular degeneration. *LPN*, 3(10):47.

Mosby's dictionary of medicine, nursing, and health professions. (2009). (8th ed.). St. Louis: Mosby.

Munson, B. (2006). Now, listen up! Understanding hearing loss and deafness. *Nursing Made Incredibly Easy!* 4(2):38.

National Eye Institute (NEI). National Institutes of Health (NIH). (2008). *Age-Related Eye Disease Study: results.* Available at www.nei.nih.gov/amd. Accessed November, 2009.

National Institute on Deafness and other Communication Disorders. (n.d.). *Cochlear implants.* Available at www.nidcd.nih.gov/health/hearing/coch.asp. Accessed November, 2009.

National Institutes of Health (NIH), & National Eye Institute. (2006). *Cataract: what you should know.* NIH Publication No. 03-201. Bethesda, MD: Author.

Novak, J.C., & Broom, B.L. (2008). *Ingalls and Salerno's maternal and child health nursing.* (11th ed.). St Louis: Mosby.

Potter, P.A., & Perry, A.G. (2009). *Fundamentals of nursing: concepts, process, and practice.* (7th ed.). St. Louis: Mosby.

Pullen, R. (2006). Spin control, caring for a patient with inner ear disease. *Nursing*, 36(5):48.

Rosenthal, B. (2009). *Age-related macular degeneration (AMD): an overview.* Available at www.healthandage.com/?q=archive/2233. Accessed November, 2009.

Rothrock, J. (2007). *Alexander's care of the patient in surgery.* (13th ed.). St. Louis: Mosby.

Seidel, H.M., Ball, J.W., Dains, J.E., et al. (2007). *Mosby's guide to physical examination.* (6th ed.). St. Louis: Mosby.

Skidmore-Roth, L. (2010). *Mosby's 2010 nursing drug reference.* (23rd ed.). St. Louis: Mosby.

Thibodeau, G.A., & Patton, K.T. (2007). *Anatomy and physiology.* (6th ed.). St. Louis: Mosby.

Thibodeau, G.A., & Patton, K.T. (2008). *Structure and function of the body.* (13th ed.). St. Louis: Mosby.

Thompson, J.M., McFarland, G.K., Hirsch, J.E., et al. (2001). *Mosby's clinical nursing.* (5th ed.). St. Louis: Mosby.

Zhou, B. Wang, B. (2006). Pegaptanib for the treatment of age-related macular degeneration. *Experimental Eye Research*, 83(3):615-619.

Additional Resources

"The Aging Eye," a special report, is available from Harvard Health Publications, P.O. Box 421073, Palm Coast, FL 32142-1073. E-mail: harvardpro@palmcoastd.com.

American Academy of Ophthalmology, P.O. Box 7424, San Francisco, CA 94120-7424. Available at www.aao.org. Accessed November, 2009.

American Academy of Otolaryngology, Head and Neck Surgery, *Meniere's disease.* Available at www.entnet.org/HealthInformation/menieresDisease.cfm. Accessed November, 2009.

American Foundation for the Blind, 15 West 16th St., New York, NY 10011. A list of free brochures.

American Optometric Association Communications Division, 243 North Lindbergh Blvd., St. Louis, MO 63141. Free brochures on eye care for the elderly.

Captioned Films for the Deaf, 800-237-6213.

The EAR Foundation. Available at www.earfoundation.org. Accessed November, 2009.

Glaucoma Research Foundation. Available at www.glaucoma.org. Accessed November, 2009.

Macular Degeneration Partnership. Available at www.amd.org. Accessed November, 2009.

MD support. Available at www.mdsupport.org/support.html. Accessed November, 2009.

National Eye Institute, 2020 Vision Place, Bethesda, MD 20892. 301-496-5248. Available at www.nei.nih.gov. Accessed November, 2009.

National Eye Institute, Office of Scientific Reporting, Bldg. 31, Rm. 6A32, Bethesda, MD 20205. A list of free brochures on eye disorders.

National Institute on Deafness and Other Communication Disorders Balance Disorders. Available at www.nidcd.nih.gov/health/balance/balance_disorders.htm. Accessed November, 2009.

National Institute to Prevent Blindness, 79 Madison Ave., New York, NY 10016. Free pamphlets on specific diseases affecting the eye.

Vision Foundation, 2 Mt. Auburn St., Watertown, MA 02172. Free vision inventory list.

Vestibular Disorders Association (VEDA). Available at www.vestibular.org. Accessed November, 2009.

Chapter 54 Care of the Patient with a Neurologic Disorder

Alexander, D. (2007). Controlling pain, facing the pain of trigeminal neuralgia. *Nursing*, 37(11):18.

Alverzo, J. (2007). Improving stroke outcomes. *American Journal of Nursing*, 107(110):72B.

Alzheimer's Disease Education and Referral Center, 800-438-4380. Available at www.alzheimers.org. Accessed November, 2009.

American Parkinson Disease Association. Available at www.apdaparkinson.org. Accessed November, 2009.

American Stroke Association. Available at www.strokeassociation.org/presenter.jhtml?identifier=1200037. Accessed November, 2009.

Avalos-Bock, S. (2005). West Nile virus and the U.S. blood supply. *American Journal of Nursing*, 105(2):34.

Awakenings. Available at www.parkinsonsdisease.com.

Baldwin, K. (2006). It's a knock-out punch. *Nursing Made Incredibly Easy!* 42(2):11.

Barker, E. (2006). A new weapon to combat stroke. *RN*, 69(3):26.

Beattie, S. (2007). Bedside emergency, unconscious patients. *RN*, 70(9):32.

Bender, K. (2003). West Nile virus: a growing challenge. *American Journal of Nursing*, 103(6):32.

Black, J.M., & Hawks, H.J. (2009). *Medical-surgical nursing: clinical management for positive outcomes.* (8th ed.). Philadelphia: Saunders.

Brandes, J.L. (2005). Practical use of topiramax for migraine prevention. *Headache*, 45 (suppl 1):566.

Centers for Disease Control and Prevention (CDC). (2008). *Division of vector-borne infectious diseases: West Nile virus.* Available at www.cdc.gov/ncidod/dvbid/westnile/index.htm. Accessed November, 2009.

Czaplinski, A., Yen, A.A., & Appel, S.H. (2006). Amyotrophic lateral sclerosis: early predictors of prolonged survival. *Journal of Neurology*, 253(11):1428-1436.

Deuschl, G., Schade-Brittinger, C., Krack, P., et al. (2006). A randomized trial of deep-brain stimulation for Parkinson's disease. *The New England Journal of Medicine*, 355:896-908.

Editorial. (2004). Drug for migraine: eletriptan hydrobromide (Replax). *Nursing*, 34(2):58.

Epilepsy Foundation. (n.d.). *Epilepsy and seizure statistics.* Available at www.epilepsyfoundation.org/about/statistics.cfm. Accessed November, 2009.

Fagley, M. (2007). Taking charge of seizure activity. *Nursing*, 37(9):42.

Fisher, D. (2004). Help your patient manage myasthenia gravis. *Nursing Made Incredibly Easy!* 2(1):28-35.

Giger, J.M., & Davidhizar, R.E. (2007). *Transcultural nursing: assessment and intervention.* (5th ed.). St. Louis: Mosby.

Goetz, C. (2007). *Textbook of clinical neurology.* (3rd ed.). Philadelphia: Saunders.

Goldrick, B. (2003). Keeping West Nile virus at bay. *Nursing*, 33(8):44.

Goldstein, L.B., Adams, R., Alberts, M.J., et al. (2006). Primary prevention of ischemic stroke: a guideline from the American Heart Association/American Stroke Association Stroke Council, *Stroke*, 37(6):1583-1633.

Gusa, D., Miers, A., & Wijdicks, E. (2007). More than meets the eye. *RN*, 70(12):43-47.

Hayes, D. (2006). Viral meningitis in adults. *Nursing*, 36(2):64.

Hess, D., & Highes, M. (2005). Multiple sclerosis: when to suspect—keys to diagnosis. *Consultant*, 45(8):844-852.

Jarvis, C. (2008). *Physical examination and health assessment*. (5th ed.). Philadelphia: Saunders.

Kim, S.U. (2004). Human neural stem cells genetically modified for brain repair in neurological disorders. *Neuropathology*, 24:159.

King, K., & Olson, D.M. (2007). What you should know about neurogenic shock. *American Nurse Today*, 2(2):36, 2007.

Lawes, R. (2007). Uncovering the layers of meningitis and encephalitis. *Nursing Made Incredibly Easy!* 5(4):26-35.

Lewis, S.L., Heitkemper, M.M., Dirksen, S.R., et al. (2007). *Medical-surgical nursing: assessment and management of clinical problems*. (7th ed.). St. Louis: Mosby.

Loder, E., & Biondi, D. (2005). General principles of migraine management: the changing role of prevention. *Headache*, 45(suppl 1):533.

Lower, J. (2007). Fearlessly facing neurologic evaluation. *LPN*, 3(2):11.

Mathews, C. (2007). Getting ahead of acute meningitis and encephalitis. *Nursing*, 37(11):36-39.

Mauk, K. (2006). Heeding TIAs: stroke's early warning system. *Nursing*, 36(5):20.

McCarron, K. (2006). The shakedown on Parkinson's disease. *Nursing Made Incredibly Easy!* 4(6), 2006.

Michael J. Fox Foundation for Parkinson's Research. Available at www.michaeljfox.org. Accessed November, 2009.

Mosby's dictionary of medicine, nursing, and health professions. (2009). (8th ed.). St. Louis: Mosby.

Nadalo, L.A., & Walters, M.C. (2009). *Carotid artery, stenosis*. Available at http://emedicine.medscape.com/article/417524-media. Accessed November, 2009.

National Guideline Clearinghouse. (n.d.). *Practice guidelines for the management of bacterial meningitis*. Available at www.guidelines.gov/summary/summary.aspx?doc_id=5946. Accessed November, 2009.

National Institute of Neurological Disorders and Stroke. (n.d.a). *Know stroke. Know the signs. Act in time*. Available at www.ninds.nih.gov/disorders/stroke/knowstroke.htm. Accessed November, 2009.

National Institute of Neurological Disorders and Stroke. (n.d.b). *Parkinson's disease: hope through research*. Available at www.ninds.nih.gov/disorders/parkinsons_disease/detail_parkinsons_disease.htm.

National Institute of Neurological Disorders and Stroke. (n.d.c) Available at www.ninds.nih.gov. Accessed November, 2009. Accessed November, 2009.

National Institute on Aging. (2007). *Progress report on Alzheimer's disease*. Available at www.nia.nih.gov/Alzheimers/Publications/ADProgress2007. Accessed November, 2009.

Nowlin, A. (2006). The dysphagia dilemma: how you can help. *RN*, 69(6):44-48.

Overstreet, M. (2004). When mosquitoes attack—an update on West Nile virus. *Nursing Made Incredibly Easy!* 2(3):42-45.

Pagana, K.D., & Pagana, T.J. (2008). *Mosby's diagnostic and laboratory test reference*. (9th ed.). St. Louis: Mosby.

Palmieri, R. (2006). Cerebral artery stenosis paves the way for a stroke. *Nursing*, 36(6):36-41.

Palmieri, R. (2007a). Piecing together the puzzle of Guillain-Barré syndrome. *Nursing Made Incredibly Easy!* 5(6):52-55.

Palmieri, R. (2007b). Responding to primary brain tumor. *Nursing*, 37(1):36.

Palmieri, R. (2007c). Unraveling the mystery of amyotrophic lateral sclerosis. *LPN*, 3(3):29.

Patient education series. (2007). Alzheimer's disease. *Nursing*, 37(6):50.

Phillips, R. (2007). Treating carotid artery stenosis to prevent stroke. *Nursing Made Incredibly Easy!* 5(1):41.

Rice, R. (2008). *Home health nursing practice*. (5th ed.). St. Louis: Mosby.

Rietberg, M.B., Brooks, D., Uitdehaaga, B.M., et al. (2005). Exercise therapy for multiple sclerosis. *Cochrane Data Base of Systematic Reviews*, Issue 1, Art. No. CD003980.

Schutte, D.L. (2006). Alzheimer disease and genetics. *American Journal of Nursing*, 106(12):40-48.

Serdans, B. (2005). A nurse with dystonia chooses DBS. *American Journal of Nursing*, 105(9):54.

Seshadri, S., Beiser, A., Selhub, J., et al. (2002). Plasma homocysteine as a risk factor for dementia and Alzheimer's disease. *New England Journal of Medicine*, 346:476.

Smith, M., & Buckwalter, K. (2005). Behaviors associated with dementia. *American Journal of Nursing*, 105(7):40-53.

Spinal Cord Information Network. (2009). *Spinal cord injury: facts and figures at a glance*. University of Alabama at Birmingham. Available at www.spinalcord.uab.edu/show.asp?durki=119513. Accessed November, 2009.

Parkinson's Disease Foundation. Available at www.pdf.org. Accessed November, 2009.

Thomure, A. (2006). Helping your patient manage Parkinson's disease. *Nursing*, 36(8):20.

Tian, G.F., Amzi, H., Takano, T., et al. (2005). An astrocytic basis of epilepsy. *Nature Medicine*, 11:973.

U.S. Food and Drug Administration (FDA). (2003). *Memantine approved for Alzheimer's disease*. FDA Patient Safety News: Show #22. Available at www.accessdata.fda.gov/psn/printer.cfm?id=182. Accessed November, 2009.

Weir, C.J., Muir, S.W., Walters, M.R., et al. (2003). Serum urate as an independent predictor of poor outcome and future vascular events after acute stroke. *Stroke*, 34(8):1951.

Wijdicks, E.F. (2006). Clinical scales for comatose patients: The Glasgow Coma Scale in historical context and the new FOUR score. *Reviews in Neurological Diseases*, 3(3), 109.

Wijdicks, E.F., & Bamlet, W.R., et al. (2005). Validation of a new coma scale: the FOUR Score. *Annals of Neurology*, 58(4), 585.

Wolf, C.A., Wijdicks, E.F., Bamlet, W.R., et al. (2007). Further validation of the FOUR score coma scale by intensive care nurses. *Mayo Clinic Proceedings*, 82(4):435-438.

Chapter 55 Care of the Patient with an Immune Disorder

American Autoimmune Related Diseases Association. Available at www.aarda.org. Accessed November, 2009.

Barkauskas, V., Baumann, L.C., & Darling-Fisher, C. (2006). *Health and physical assessment*. (4th ed.). St. Louis: Mosby.

Black, J.M., & Hawks, H.J. (2009). *Medical-surgical nursing: clinical management for positive outcomes*. (8th ed.). Philadelphia: Saunders.

Colletti, M., et al. (2002). Immunologic system. In J.M. Thompson, G.K. McFarland, J.E. Hirsch, et al., (Eds.): *Mosby's clinical nursing*. (5th ed.). St. Louis: Mosby.

Durston, S. (2006). Caring for the immune compromised patient. *LPN*, 2(4):31.

Durston, S. (2007). Uncompromising immunocompromised patient care. *Nursing Made Incredibly Easy!* 5(4):52-61.

Global Initiative for Asthma (GINA). *Guidelines. 2004 Update: workshop report, global strategy for asthma management and prevention*. Available at www.ginasthma.org/GuidelineItem.asp:intId-987. Accessed November, 2009.

Gulanick, M., & Myers, J.L. (2006). *Nursing care plans: nursing diagnoses and interventions*. (6th ed.). St. Louis: Mosby.

Hayden, M. (2004). In defense of the body: how the immune system protects us from harm. *Nursing Made Incredibly Easy!* 2(3):30-41.

Hoffman, R., Benz, E.J., Jr., Shattil, S., et al. (2004). *Hematology: basic principles and practice*. (4th ed.). Philadelphia: Churchill Livingstone.

Immune Deficiency Foundation (IDF). (2007). *IDF guide for nurses: on immune globulin therapy for primary immunodeficiency diseases.* Available at www.primaryimmune-org/pubs/book_nurse/nurses_guide_pdf. Accessed November, 2009.

Lewis, S.L., Heitkemper, M.M., Dirksen, S.R., et al. (2007). *Medical-surgical nursing: assessment and management of clinical problems.* (7th ed.). St. Louis: Mosby.

Lupus Foundation of America. Available at www.lupus.org. Accessed November, 2009.

Male, D., Brostoff, J., Roth, D., et al. (2006). *Immunology.* (7th ed.). St. Louis: Mosby.

Monahan, F.D., Sands, J.K., Neighbors, M., et al. (2007). *Phipps' medical-surgical nursing: health and illness perspectives.* (8th ed.). St. Louis: Mosby.

Mosby's dictionary of medicine, nursing, and health professions. (2009). (8th ed.). St. Louis: Mosby.

National Institute of Allergy and Infectious Diseases. (2009). *The immune system.* Available at http://www3.niaid.nih.gov/topics/immuneSystem. Accessed November, 2009.

Pagana, K.D., & Pagana, T.J. (2008). *Mosby's diagnostic and laboratory test reference.* (9th ed.). St. Louis: Mosby.

Potter, P.A., & Perry, A.G. (2007). *Basic nursing: essentials for practice.* (6th ed.). St. Louis: Mosby.

Pullen, R. (2007a). Managing cutaneous vaxculitis in a patient with lupus erythematosus. *Dermatology Nursing,* 19(2):21.

Pullen, R. (2007b). Understanding systemic lupus erythematosus. *LPN,* 3(6):41.

Rooney, J. (2005). Systemic lupus erythematosus. Unmasking a great imitator. *Nursing,* 35(11):54.

Rote, N.S. (2010). Alternations in immunity and inflammation. In K.L. McCance, & S.E. Huether, *Pathophysiology: the biologic basis for disease in adults and children.* (6th ed.). St. Louis: Mosby.

Scherf, R., & White-Reid, K. (2008). Giving intravenous immunoglobulin. *RN,* 71(1):29-34.

Seidel, H.M., Ball, J.W., Dains, J.E., et al. (2007). *Mosby's guide to physical examination.* (6th ed.). St. Louis: Mosby.

Shearer, W., & Fleisher, T. (2007). The immune system. In N.F. Adkinson, W. Busse, B. Bochner, et al. (Eds.), *Middleton's allergy: principles and practice.* (7th ed.). Philadelphia: Mosby.

Thompson, J.M., McFarland, G.K., Hirsch, J.E., et al. (2002). *Mosby's clinical nursing.* (5th ed.). St. Louis: Mosby.

Venes, D. (2009.) *Taber's cyclopedic medical dictionary.* (21st ed.). Philadelphia: Davis.

Wysocki, L. (2007). Anaphylaxis doesn't have to be a shock. *Nursing Made Incredibly Easy!* 5(6):9-13.

Chapter 56 Care of the Patient with HIV/AIDS

AIDS Education Global Information System, (2002). *CDC fact sheet: human Immunodeficiency virus type 2.* Available at: www.aegis.com/default.asp?req=http://www.aegis.com/pubs/cdc_fact_sheets/2002/HIV-2.html. Accessed November, 2009.

Andrews G, Skinner D, & Zuma K. (2006) Epidemiology of health and vulnerability among children orphaned and made vulnerable by HIV/AIDS in sub-Saharan Africa. *AIDS Care* 2006;18:269-276.

Barré-Sinoussi, F., Chermann, J.C., Rey, F., et al. (1983). Isolation of a T-lymphotropic retrovirus from a patient at risk for acquired immune deficiency syndrome (AIDS), *Science,* 220(4599): 868-871.

Black, J.M., & Hawks, H.J. (2009). *Medical-surgical nursing: clinical management for positive outcomes.* (8th ed.). Philadelphia: Saunders.

Braithwaite, R.S., Kozal, M.J., Chang, C.C., et al. (2007). Adherence, virological and immunological outcomes for HIV-infected veterans starting combination antiretroviral therapies. *AIDS,* 21:1579-1589.

Buonaguro, L., Tornesello, M.L., & Buonaguro, F.M., (2007). Human immunodeficiency virus type 1 subtype distribution in the worldwide epidemic: pathogenetic and therapeutic implications, *Journal of Virology,* 81(19):10209-10219.

Centers for Disease Control (CDC). (1981). MMWR: recommendations and reports. *MMWR: Morbidity and Mortality Weekly Report,* 30 (RR-21):1-3.

Centers for Disease Control and Prevention (CDC). (1998). *Human immunodeficiency virus type 2.* Available at www.cdc.gov/hiv/resources/factsheets/hiv2.htm. Accessed November, 2009.

Centers for Disease Control and Prevention (CDC). (2001). Updated U.S. Public Health Service guidelines for the management of occupational exposures to HBV, HCV, and HIV and recommendations forpostexposure prophylaxis. *MMWR: Morbidity and Mortality Weekly Report,* 50(RR-11):1.

Centers for Disease Control and Prevention (CDC). (2005a). Antiretroviral postexposure prophylaxis after sexual, injection-drug use, or other nonoccupational exposure to HIV in the United States. *MMWR: Morbidity and Mortality Weekly Report,* 54(RR-02):1-20.

Centers for Disease Control and Prevention (CDC). (2005b). Updated U.S. Public Health Service guidelines for the management of occupational exposures to HIV and recommendations for postexposure prophylaxis. *MMWR: Morbidity and Mortality Weekly Report,* 54(RR-09):1-17.

Centers for Disease Control and Prevention (CDC). (2006). Revised recommendations for HIV testing of adults, adolescents, and pregnant women in health-care settings. *MMWR: Morbidity and Mortality Weekly Report,* 22:55(RR-14):1-17.

Centers for Disease Control and Prevention (CDC). (2007a). *HIV/AIDS Surveillance Report, 2005.* Atlanta: US Department of Health and Human Services.

Centers for Disease Control and Prevention (CDC). (2007b). *HIV/AIDS among women.* Available at www.cdc.gov/hiv/topics/women/resources/factsheets/women.htm. Accessed November, 2009.

Centers for Disease Control and Prevention (CDC). (2007c). *HIV/AIDS among youth.* Available at www.cdc.gov/hiv/resources/factsheets/youth.htm. Accessed November, 2009.

Centers for Disease Control and Prevention (CDC). (2007d). *Sexually transmitted siseases surveillance, 2006.* Atlanta: U.S. Department of Health and Human Services.

Centers for Disease Control and Prevention (CDC). (2007e). *Surveillance of occupationally acquired HIV/AIDS in healthcare personnel, as of December, 2006.* Available at www.cdc.gov/ncidod/dhqp/bp_hcp_w_hiv.html. Accessed November, 2009.

Centers for Disease Control and Prevention (CDC). (2008). *HIV/AIDS surveillance report, 2006.* Available at www.cdc.gov/hiv/topics/surveillance/resources/reports/. Accessed November, 2009.

Centers for Disease Control and Prevention (CDC). (2009a). *HIV/AIDS among gay and bisexual men.* 2007. Available at www.cdc.gov/nchhstp/newsroom/docs/FastFacts-MSM-FINAL-508COMP.pdf. Accessed November, 2009.

Centers for Disease Control and Prevention (CDC). (2009b). *HIV/AIDS surveillance report,* Available at www.cdc.gov/hiv/topics/surveillance/resources/reports/index.htm#surveillance. Accessed November, 2009.

Cheng, D.M., Nunes, D., Libman, H., et al. (2007). Impact of hepatitis C on HIV progression in adults with alcohol problems. *Alcoholism, Clinical and Experimental Research,* 31(5):829-836.

Donnegan, E. (2003). *Transmission of HIV by blood, blood products, tissue transplantation and artificial insemination.* Available at http://hivinsite.ucsf.edu/InSite?page=kb-00&doc=kb-07-02-09. Accessed November, 2009.

Fletcher, M.A., & Klimas, N.G. (2007). Cytotoxic lymphocytes. In G. Fink, (Ed.), *Encyclopedia of stress.* (2nd ed.) Oxford: Academic Press.

Gallo, R.C., Salahuddin, S.Z,. Popovic, M., et al. (1984). Frequent detection and isolation of cytopathic retroviruses (HTLV-III) from patients with AIDS and at risk for AIDS. *Science,* 224 (4648):500-503.

Garry, R.F., Witte, M.H., Gottlieb, A.A., et al. (1988). Documentation of an AIDS virus infection in the United States in 1968, *Journal of the American Medical Association,* 260(14): 2085-2087.

Greenwald, J.L., Burstein, G.R., Pincus, J., et al. (2006). A rapid review of rapid HIV antibody tests. *Current Infectious Disease Report,* 8(2):125-131.

Hall, H.R., Song, R., Rhodes, P., et al. (2008). Estimation of HIV incidence in the United States, *Journal of the American Medical Association*, 300(5):520-529.

Henry J. Kaiser Family Foundation (2007). *The global HIV/AIDS epidemic. HIV/AIDS policy fact sheet, November 2007*. Available at www.kff.org/hivaids/upload/3030-103.pdf. Accessed November, 2009.

International AIDS Vaccine Initiative. (2005). *Tracking funding for preventive HIV vaccine research & development: estimates of annual investments and expenditures, 2000-2005*. International AIDS Vaccine Initiative. Available at www.iavi.org/lists/iavipublications/attachments/bf4f74f0-95b1-446c-9da9-78ca1bb40ecf/hvmrtwg_tracking_funding_for_preventive_hiv_vaccine_research_and_development_2006_eng.pdf. Accessed November, 2009].

Ironson, G., & Hayward, H. (2008) Do positive psychosocial factors predict disease progression in HIV? A review of the evidence. *Psychosomatic Medicine*, 70(5):546-554.

Joint United Nations Programme on HIV/AIDS (UNAIDS) & World Health Organization (WHO). (n. d.). *AIDS epidemic update report update*. Available at www.unaids.org/en/KnowledgeCentre/HIVData/EpiUpdate/EpiUpdArchive. Accessed November, 2009.

Kalichman, S.C. (2008). Co-occurrence of treatment nonadherence and continued HIV transmission risk behaviors: implications for positive prevention interventions. *Psychosomatic Medicine*, 70(5): 593-597.

Klimas, N., Koneru, A.O., & Fletcher, M.A. (2008). Overview of HIV. *Psychosomatic Medicine*, 70(5):523-530.

Lee, S., Wood, O., Tang, S., et al. (2007). Detection of emerging HIV variants in blood donors from urban areas of Cameroon. *AIDS Research and Human Retroviruses*, 23(10):1262-1267.

Lekkerkerker A.N., van Kooyk Y., & Geijtenbeek T.B. (2006). Viral piracy: HIV-1 targets dendritic cells for transmission. *Current HIV Research*, 4(2):169-176.

Leserman, J. (2008). Role of depression, stress, and trauma in HIV disease progression. *Psychosomatic Medicine*, 70(5):539-545.

National Institute of Allergy and Infectious Diseases. National Institutes of Health (NIH). (2009). *HIV infection in women*. Available at http://www3.niaid.nih.gov/topics/HIVAIDS/Understanding/Population+Specific+Information/womenHiv.htm. Accessed November, 2009.

Panel on Antiretroviral Guidelines for Adult and Adolescents (2008). *Guidelines for the use of antiretroviral agents in HIV-1-infected adults and adolescents*. Available at www.aidsinfo.nih.gov/ContentFiles/AdultandAdolescentGL.pdf. Accessed November, 2009.

Paredes, R., Mocroft, A., Kirk, O., et al. (2000). Predictors of virological success and ensuing failure in HIV-positive patients starting highly active antiretroviral therapy in Europe: results from the EuroSIDA study. *Archives of Internal Medicine*, 24(160):1123-1132.

Perinatal HIV Guidelines Working Group (2008). *Public Health Service Task Force recommendations for use of antiretroviral drugs in pregnant HIV-infected women for maternal health and interventions to reduce perinatal HIV transmission in the United States*. Available at aidsinfo.nih.gov/ContentFiles/PerinatalGL.pdf. Accessed November, 2009.

Potter, S.J., Lacabaratz, C., Lambotte, O., et al. (2007) Preserved central memory and activated effector memory CD4+ T-cell subsets in human immunodeficiency virus controllers: an ANRS EP36 study. *Journal of Virology*, 81(24):13904-13915.

Rowland-Jones, S., & Whittle, H.C. (2007). Out of Africa: what can we learn from HIV-2 about protective immunity to HIV-1? *Nature Immunology*, 8(4):329-331.

Schackman, B.R., Gebo, K.A., Walensky, R.P., et al. (2006). The lifetime cost of current human immunodeficiency virus care in the United States. *Medical Care*, 44(11):990-997.

Sekaly, R.P. (2008). The failed HIV Merck vaccine study: a step back or a launching point for future vaccine development? *Journal of Experimental Medicine*, 205(1):7-12.

Sepkowitz, K.A., & Eisenberg, L. (2005). *Occupational deaths among healthcare workers*. Available at www.cdc.gov/ncidod/EID/vol11no07/04-1038.htm. Accessed November, 2009.

Sherman, D. (2001). Palliative care. In C.A. Kirton, D. Talotta, & K. Zwolski (Eds.), *Handbook of HIV/AIDS nursing*. St. Louis: Mosby.

Smith, J., & Daniel, R. (2006). Following the path of the virus: the exploitation of host DNA repair mechanisms by retroviruses. *ACS Chemical Biology*, 1(4):217-226.

Temoshok, L.R., Wald, R.L., Synowski, S., et al. (2008). Coping as a multisystem construct associated with pathways mediating HIV-relevant immune function and disease progression. *Psychosomatic Medicine*, 70(5):555-561.

Wodak, A., & Cooney, A., (2006). Do needle syringe programs reduce HIV infection among injecting drug users: a comprehensive review of the international evidence. *Substance Use and Misuse*, 41(6-7):777-813.

World Health Organization (WHO). (2006). *State of the art of new vaccines: research and development*. 2006. Available at www.who.int/vaccines-documents/DocsPDF06/814.pdf. Accessed November, 2009.

World Health Organization (WHO). (2007). *Male circumcision for HIV prevention*. Available at www.who.int/hiv/topics/malecircumcision/en/index.html. Accessed November, 2009.

World Health Organization (WHO). (2008). *WHO definition of palliative care*. Available at www.who.int/cancer/palliative/definition/en. Accessed November, 2009.

World Health Organization (WHO). (2009). *Initiative for Vaccine Research (IVR): zoonotic infections*. Available at www.who.int/vaccine_research/diseases/zoonotic/en/index.html. Accessed: June 15, 2009.

Yerly, S., von Wyl, V., Ledergerber, B., et al. (2007). Transmission of HIV-1 drug resistance in Switzerland: a 10-year molecular epidemiology survey. *AIDS*, 21(18):2223-2229.

Chapter 57 **Care of the Patient with Cancer**

Ackley, B.J., & Ladwig, G.B. (2009). *Nursing diagnosis handbook*. (7th ed.). St. Louis: Mosby.

Alfaro-Lefevre, R. (2007). *Critical thinking in nursing: a practical approach*. (4th ed.). St. Louis: Mosby.

American Cancer Society (ACS). (2003). *Tamoxifen and raloxifene to reduce breast cancer risk: questions and answers*. Available at www.cancer.org/docroot/CRI/content/CRI_2_6Xtamoxifen_ and_Raloxifene_Question_and_Answers_5.asp. Accessed May, 2008.

American Cancer Society (ACS). (2008a). *Cancer statistics*. Atlanta: Author.

American Cancer Society (ACS). (2008b). *Understanding chemotherapy*. www.cancer.gov/cancertopics/chemo-side-effects/understandingchemo. Accessed November, 2009.

American Cancer Society (ACS). (2009). *Cancer facts and figures*. Available at www.cancer.org/downloads/STT/500809web.pdf. Accessed November, 2009.

American Cancer Society (ACS). (n.d.). *Kidney cancer*. Available at www.cancer.gov/cancertopics/types/kidney. Accessed November, 2009.

American Cancer Society. (n.d.). *Testicular cancer*. Available at www.cancer.gov/cancertopics/types/testicular. Accessed November, 2009.

Balzer-Riley, J. (2008). *Communication in nursing*. (6th ed.). St. Louis: Mosby.

Barkauskas, V., Baumann, L.C., & Darling-Fisher, C. (2006). *Health and physical assessment*. (4th ed.). St. Louis: Mosby.

Black, J.M., & Hawks, H.J. (2009). *Medical-surgical nursing: clinical management for positive outcomes*. (8th ed.). Philadelphia: Saunders.

Calle, E.E., Rodriguez, C., Walker-Thurmond, K., et al. (2003). Overweight, obesity, and mortality from cancer in a prospectively studied cohort of US adults. *New England Journal of Medicine*, 348(17):1625-1638.

Cantril, C. (2004). Emergency tumor lysis syndrome. *American Journal of Nursing*, 104(4):49.

Carroll, C. (2006). Sorting out breast biopsy options. *Nursing*, 36(3):70.

Correa, P. (2003). *Helicobacter pylori* infection and gastric cancer. *Cancer Epidemiology, Biomarkers, and Prevention*, 12(3):238S.

Coyne, B. (2004). Chemo's toll on memory. *RN*, 67(4):40.

Curtis, C. (2006). Improving the care of cancer survivors. *American Journal of Nursing,* 106(3):48.

D'Arcy, Y. (2005). Conquering pain: have you tried these new techniques? *Nursing,* 35(3):36-41.

Dell, D.D. (2005). Battling breast cancer. *Nursing Made Incredibly Easy!* 3(5):4-20.

Dest, V. (2006a). Cancer therapies. *RN,* 69(6):31.

Dest, V. (2006b). Lung cancer, the battle continues. *RN,* 69(11):30.

Edmondson, D. (2008). Smoke out lung cancer. *LPN,* 4(1):39.

Freedman, G.M., & Anderson, P.R. (2003). Routine mammography is associated with earlier stage disease and greater eligiblity for breast conservation in breast carcinoma patients age 40 years and older. *Cancer,* 98(5):918.

Giger, J.M., & Davidhizar, R.E. (2007). *Transcultural nursing: assessment and intervention.* (5th ed.). St. Louis: Mosby.

Gordon, M. (2009). *Manual of nursing diagnosis.* (11th ed.). St. Louis: Mosby.

Held-Warmkessel, J. (2005). Managing three critical cancer complications. *Nursing,* 35(1):58.

Higdon, M.L., & Higdon, J.A. (2006). *Treatment of oncologic emergencies.* Available at www.aafp.org/afp/20061201/1873.html. Accessed November, 2009.

Jeffries, M. (2007). Helping your patient combat lung cancer, *Nursing,* 37(2):36-41.

Kehoe, C. (2007). Getting to know oncologic emergencies. *Nursing Made Incredibly Easy!* 5(5):49-56.

Lehman, M. (2007). *It whispers, ovarian cancer.* Available at www.rnweb.com, 28, 2007.

Lewis, S.L., Heitkemper, M.M., Dirksen, S.R., et al. (2007). *Medical-surgical nursing: assessment and management of clinical problems.* (7th ed.). St. Louis: Mosby.

Lilley, L., Harrington, S., & Snyder, J. (2007). *Pharmacology and the nursing process.* (5th ed.). St. Louis: Mosby, Inc.

Mayo Clinic staff. (2009). *Chemotherapy.* Available at www.mayoclinic.com/health/chemotherapy/MY00536. Accessed November, 2009.

McCaffery, M., & Pasero, C. (2007). *Pain: clinical manual.* (4th ed.). St. Louis: Mosby.

Mee, C.L. (2007). Hospice care. *Nursing,* 37(11):43.

Monahan, F.D., Sands, J.K., Neighbors, M., et al. (2007). *Phipps' medical-surgical nursing: health and illness perspectives.* (8th ed.). St. Louis: Mosby.

Mosby's dictionary of medicine, nursing, and health professions. (2009). (8th ed.). St. Louis: Mosby.

National Cancer Institute (NCI). (n.d.a). *Cancer health disparities.* Available at www.cancer.gov/cancertopics/types/disparities. Accessed November, 2009.

National Cancer Institute (NCI). (n.d.b). *Renal cell cancer treatment (PDQ): health professional version.* Available at www.cancer.gov/cancertopics/pdq/treatment/renalcell/healthprofessional. Accessed November, 2009.

National Cancer Institute (NCI). (n.d.c). *Targeted cancer therapies.* Available at www.cancer.gov/cancertopics/factsheet/Therapy/targeted. Accessed November, 2009.

National Comprehensive Cancer Network. (2006). *Breast cancer treatment guidelines for patients: Version VIII.* Available at www.nccn.org/patients/patient_gls_english/_breast/contents/asp. April 2008.

National Guidelines Clearinghouse. (n.d.). *Management of breast cancer in women: a national clinical guideline.* www.guideline.gov/summary/summary.aspx?doc_id=8510. Accessed November, 2009.

Netherbee, S. (2006). New weapons to snuff out kidney cancer. *Nursing,* 36(12):59.

Ngo-Metzger, Q., McCarthy, E.P., Burns, R.B., et al. (2003). Older Asian American and Pacific Islanders dying of cancer use hospice less frequently than older white patients. *American Journal of Medicine,* 115(1):47.

Otto, S. (2005). *Oncology nursing.* (5th ed.). St. Louis: Mosby.

Pagana, K.D., & Pagana, T.J. (2008). *Mosby's diagnostic and laboratory test reference.* (9th ed.). St. Louis: Mosby.

Shinn, S. (2004). Cervical cancer. *Nursing,* 34(5):36.

Skidmore-Roth, L. (2010). *Mosby's 2010 nursing drug reference.* (23rd ed.). St. Louis: Mosby.

Smeltzer, S.C., Bare, B.G., Hinkle, J.L., et al. (2007). *Brunner & Suddarth's textbook of medical-surgical nursing,* (11th ed.). Philadelphia: Lippincott Williams and Wilkins.

Tannock, I.F., Hill, R., Bristow, R., et al. (2005). *The basic science of oncology.* (4th ed.). New York: McGraw-Hill.

Taylor, D.S., & Penny, A.S. *Oncologic emergencies.* Available at www.emedicine.com/ped/topic2590.htm. Accessed November, 2009.

Thompson, J.M., McFarland, G.K., Hirsch, J.E., et al. (2001). *Mosby's clinical nursing.* (5th ed.). St. Louis: Mosby.

Tucker, S.M., Cannobio, M.M., Paquette, E.V., et al. (2007). *Patient care standards: collaborative planning and nursing interventions.* (7th ed.). St. Louis: Mosby.

U.S. Department of Health and Human Services. (n.d.). *Tracking Healthy People 2010.* Washington, DC: U.S. Government Printing Office.

U.S. Food and Drug Administration (US FDA). (2006). *FDA approves new treatment for gastrointestinal and kidney cancer.* Available at www.fda.gov/NewsEvents/Newsroom/PressAnnouncements/2006/ucm108583.htm. Accessed November, 2009.

Weaver, C. (2007). Compassionate care for the patient with a mastectomy. *Nursing Made Incredibly Easy!* 5(6):26.

Workman, L. (2002). Breast cancer—new strategies to beat an old enemy. *Nursing,* 32(10):58.

Chapter 58 Professional Roles and Leadership

American Nurses Association (ANA). (2008). *Nursing: scope and standards of practice.* Washington, DC: American Nurses Association.

Ayers, D.M., & Montgomery, M. (2008). Delegating the right way. *Nursing 2008,* 38(4):56hnl.

Bidigare, C. (2006). Camp nursing. *RN 2006,* 69(1):41-43.

Eason, J.A. (2007). Sweet fun in the summer time. *RN 2007,* 70(4):52-54.

Eason, J.A. (2008). Traveling south—or west—for the winter. *RN 2008,* 71(2):22.

Editorial. (2006a). Career choices made incredibly easy. *Nursing Made Incredibly Easy!* 4(2):59.

Editorial. (2006b). Nurses in white. *Nursing 2006,* 26(6):44.

Editorial. (2006c). White uniforms. *Nursing 2006,* 36(2):43.

Editorial. (2007). What are you worth: LPN salary survey. *LPN 2007,* 3(4):20-21.

Elkin, M.K., Perry, A.G., & Potter, P.A. (2007). *Nursing interventions and clinical skills.* (4th ed.). St. Louis: Mosby.

Ericksen, A.B. (2007). Earning survey. How does it add up? *RN 2007,* 70(10):42-48.

Hansen, R., & Jackson, M. (2008). *Clinical delegation skills: a handbook for professional practice.* (4th ed.). St. Louis: Mosby.

Harkreader, H., Hogan, M.A., & Thobaben, M. (2007). *Fundamentals of nursing: care and clinical judgment.* (3rd ed.). St. Louis: Mosby.

Hart, K. (2004). Breathrough to nursing national survey results. *Imprint,* 52(2):30-34.

Jackson, C.M. (2008). Fighting words. *RN 2008,* 71(2):56.

McVay, S. (2007). Conflict resolution: turning a negative into a positive. *LPN 2007,* 3(2):9-10.

Mee, C. (2006). Nursing 2006 salary survey. *Nursing 2006,* 36(10):46-51.

Metules, T. (2007). Tips to avoid burnout. *RN 2007,* 70(4):9.

Mosby's dictionary of medicine, nursing and health professions. (8th ed.). (2009). St. Louis: Mosby.

National Council of State Boards of Nursing (NCSBN). (n.d.). Available at www.ncsbn.org. Accessed December, 2009.

National Council of State Boards of Nursing: (n.d.). *The five rights of delegation.* Available at www.ncsbn.org.

National League for Nursing (NLN). (n.d.). Available at www.nln.org.

Nebraska Department of Health and Human Services, Regulation and Licensure, Credentialing Division. Lincoln, Neb.

Nolan, S., & Roman, L.M. (2008). Nursing M & M reviews. Learning from our outcomes. *RN 2008,* 71(1):37-40.

Pettengill, E. (2007). Career options—the other side of nursing. *RN 2007*, 70(11):17.

Potter, P.A., & Perry, A.G. (2007). *Basic nursing: essentials for practice.* (6th ed.). St. Louis: Mosby.

Potter, P.A., & Perry, A.G. (2009). *Fundamentals of nursing: concepts, process, and practice.* (7th ed.). St. Louis: Mosby.

Riley, J.B. (2008). *Communication in nursing.* (6th ed.). St. Louis: Mosby.

Roman, L. (2007). There's no business like your own business. *RN 2007*, 70(9):38-43.

Roman, L. (2008). Nursing shortage. *RN 2008*, 71(3):34-41.

Samuels, J. (2008). Expanding your options. *RN 2007*, 70(7):22-23.

Schroeder, S.J. (2006). Picking up the pace: a new template for shift report. *Nursing 2006*, 36(10):22-23.

Seago, J.A., et al. How can LPN's ease the nursing shortage? *LPN 2007*, 3(1):16-17.

Seave, R.J. (2006). Don't call me doctor. *RN 2006*, 69(8):35.

Sirata, T. (2007). Improving the nurse/physician relationship. *LPN 2007*, 3(5):14-18.

Sirata, T. (2007). Nurse/physician relationships. Improving or not? *Nursing 2007*, 37(1):52-55.

Steppie, S. (2008). Mentoring matters. *LPN 2008*, 4(3):19-20.

Stermer, D. (2008). Fitness makeover 2008: the real world. *RN 2008*, 71(2):47-50.

VanSell, S. (2008). Changing your practice. *RN 2008*, 71(3):9.

Vonfrolio, L.G. (2006). Don't blame the shortage. *RN 2006*, 69(6):68.

Weber, D. (2006). Where spirituality and health care meet. *RN 2006*, 69(9):53-54.

Weber, D., & Roman, L. (2008). Finding their niche. *RN 2008*, 71(2): 34-39.

Weiss, B. (2004). Taking on the night shift. *RN 2004*, 67(8):59.

Weiss, Barbara. No need to stress. *RN 2006*, 69(5):53-54.

Wright, J. (2008). Tips for new nurses. *LPN 2008*, 4(2):20, 21.

Illustration Credits

Chapter 1

1-1, from the Dolan Collection, *Nursing Times* photograph. **1-2, 1-8,** courtesy of the National Library of Medicine, National Institutes of Health, Bethesda, Maryland. **1-3,** from Jamieson, E.M., et al. (1966). *Trends in nursing history.* Philadelphia: Saunders. **1-6, 1-7,** from Lindeman, C.A., & McAthie, M. (1999). *Fundamentals of contemporary nursing practice.* Philadelphia: Saunders.

Chapter 2

2-1, courtesy of Great Plains Regional Medical Center, North Platte, Nebraska. **2-2,** from Potter, P.A., & Perry, A.G. (2005). *Fundamentals of nursing: concepts, process, and practice.* (6th ed.). St. Louis: Mosby.

Chapter 3

3-2, 3-4, from Potter, P.A., & Perry, A.G. (2009). *Fundamentals of nursing: concepts, process, and practice.* (7th ed.). St. Louis: Mosby. **3-3,** from Leahy, J.M., & Kizilay, P.E. (1998). *Foundations of nursing practice: a nursing process approach.* Philadelphia: Saunders.

Chapter 4

4-1, 4-2, courtesy of Great Plains Regional Medical Center, North Platte, Nebraska. **4-3, 4-4, 4-5, 4-12, 4-13,** from Potter, P.A., & Perry, A.G. (2009). *Fundamentals of nursing: concepts, process, and practice.* (7th ed.). St. Louis: Mosby. **4-6, 4-9, *A, B,* 4-14, 4-15, *A, B,*** from Elkin, M.K., et al. (2008). *Nursing interventions and clinical skills.* (4th ed.). St. Louis: Mosby. **4-8, 4-11, 4-18, *A, B, C,*** from Sorrentino, S.A. (2008). *Mosby's textbook for nursing assistants.* (7th ed.). St. Louis: Mosby. **4-16,** courtesy of Critikon, Inc., Tampa, Florida. **Skill 4-1, step 7d,** from Potter, P.A., & Perry, A.G. (2009). *Fundamentals of nursing: concepts, process, and practice.* (7th ed.). St. Louis: Mosby.

Chapter 5

5-1, from Elkin, M.K., et al. (2008). *Nursing interventions and clinical skills.* (4th ed.). St. Louis: Mosby. **5-3,** from Jarvis, C. (2008). *Physical examination and health assessment.* (5th ed.). Philadelphia: Saunders. **5-4, 5-5, 5-6, 5-8, 5-9, 5-10, 5-12,** from Seidel, H.M., et al. (2006). *Mosby's guide to physical examination.* (6th ed.). St. Louis: Mosby. **5-7,** modified from Stresmeyer, J.K. Pulmonary assessment: a four-step approach. *American Journal of Nursing,* 93(8):22, 1993. **5-11,** from Thompson, J.M., & Wilson, S.F. (1996). *Health assessment for nursing practice.* St. Louis: Mosby.

Chapter 6

6-1, modified from Potter, P.A., & Perry, A.G. (2005). *Fundamentals of nursing.* (6th ed.). St. Louis: Mosby. **6-2,** redrawn from Maslow, A.H. (1970). *Motivation and personality.* Upper Saddle River, NJ: Prentice-Hall.

Chapter 7

7-1, 7-3, 7-9, courtesy of Great Plains Regional Medical Center, North Platte, Nebraska. **7-10,** from Potter, P.A., & Perry, A.G. (2009). *Fundamentals of nursing: concepts, process, and practice.* (7th ed.). St. Louis: Mosby.

Chapter 8

8-1, 8-2, from Leahy, J.M., & Kizilay, P.E. (1998). *Foundations of nursing practice: a nursing process approach.* Philadelphia: Saunders. **8-3,** from Harkreader, H., & Hogan, M.A. (2007). *Fundamentals of nursing: caring and clinical judgment.* (3rd ed.). Philadelphia: Saunders. **8-4,** U.S. Census Bureau.

Chapter 9

9-2, from Wong, D.L.(1995). *Whaley & Wong's nursing care of infants and children.* (5th ed.). St. Louis: Mosby. **9-3, 9-4, 9-6, 9-8, 9-11, 9-14,** from Hockenberry, M.J., et al. (2007). *Wong's nursing care of infants and children.* (8th ed.). St. Louis: Mosby. **9-13,** from Jarvis, C. (2008). *Physical examination and health assessment.* (5th ed.). Philadelphia: Saunders. **9-15, 9-16, 9-18, 9-19,** from Leahy, J.M., & Kizilay, P.E. (1998). *Foundations of nursing practice: a nursing process approach.* Philadelphia: Saunders. **9-17,** courtesy of the American Society on Aging.

Chapter 10

10-1, 10-2, from Potter, P.A., & Perry, A.G. (2009). *Fundamentals of nursing: concepts, process, and practice.* (7th ed.). St. Louis: Mosby. **Unn fig 10-1, *A-E,*** from Sorrentino, S.A. (2008). *Mosby's textbook for nursing assistants.* (7th ed.). St. Louis: Mosby.

Chapter 11

11-1, 11-2, 11-3, 11-4, 11-5, 11-6, courtesy of Great Plains Regional Medical Center, North Platte, Nebraska.

Chapter 12

12-4, from Beeching, N.J., Cheesbrough, J. (1993). *Illustrated case histories in infectious disease.* London: Mosby-Wolfe. **12-5, 12-10, 12-12,** from Potter, P.A., & Perry, G.A. (2009). *Fundamentals of nursing.* (7th ed.). St. Louis: Mosby. **12-6, 12-7, 12-8,** copyright © 1997–2007 Brevis Corporation. Courtesy Brevis Corporation, Salt Lake City, Utah. **12-9, 12-11,** from Elkin, M.K., et al. (2008). *Nursing interventions and clinical skills.* (4th ed.). St. Louis: Mosby. **Skill 12-1, step 8, step 10; Skill 12-2 step 6, step 7; Skill 12-3, step 5, step 6; Skill 12-6, step 3d, step 3e(1), step 3e(2), step 3f, step 3g(1), step 3g(2); Skill 12-8, step 3a4; Skill 12-9, step 3, step 4, step 6, step 7, step 8, step 9,** from Elkin, M.K., et al. (2008). *Nursing interventions and clinical skills.* (4th ed.). St. Louis: Mosby. **Skill 12-1, step 16; Skill 12-4, step 2, step 5; Skill 12-9, step 10,** from Potter, P.A., & Perry, A.G. (2009). *Fundamentals of nursing: concepts, process, and practice.* (7th ed.). St. Louis: Mosby. **Skill 12-3, step 4,** from Cole, G. (1996). *Fundamental nursing: concepts and skills.* (2nd ed.). St. Louis: Mosby. **Skill 12-8, step 3a3,** from Harkreader H., et al. (2007). *Fundamentals of nursing: caring and judgment,* (3rd ed.). Philadelphia: Saunders. **Skill 12-9, step 11, step 12, step 13,** from Sorrentino, S.A. (2009). *Mosby's textbook for nursing assistants.* (7th ed.). St. Louis: Mosby.

Chapter 13

13-1, from Lewis, S.L., et al. (2007). *Medical-surgical nursing: assessment and management of clinical problems.* (7th ed.). St. Louis: Mosby. **13-2, 13-3, 13-4, 13-5, 13-7,** from Elkin, M.K., et al. (2008). *Nursing interventions and clinical skills.* (4th ed.). St. Louis: Mosby. **13-6,** from Potter, P.A., & Perry, A.G. (2006). *Basic nursing: essentials for practice.* (6th ed.). St. Louis: Mosby. **13-8,** from Potter, P.A., & Perry, A.G. (2009). *Fundamentals of nursing: concepts, process, and practice.* (7th ed.). St. Louis: Mosby. **13-9,** from Beare, P.G., & Myers, J.L. (1998). *Adult health nursing.* (3rd ed.). St. Louis: Mosby. **13-10,** Courtesy of Kinetic Concepts, Inc. (KCI), San Antonio, Texas. **Skill 13-1, step 9, step 11, step 14a, step 14b; Skill 13-2, step 13; Skill 13-5, step 17; Skill 13-6, step 6; Skill 13-9, step 5a(2), step 5b, step 5c,** from Potter, P.A., & Perry, A.G. (2009). *Fundamentals of nursing: concepts, process, and practice.* (7th ed.). St. Louis: Mosby. **Skill 13-3, step 6, step 11a, step 11b, step 11c; Skill 13-4, step 13; Skill 13-9, step 5d,** from Elkin, M.K., et al. (2008). *Nursing interventions and clinical skills.* (4th ed.). St. Louis: Mosby. **Skill 13-5, step 9,** from Perry, A.G., & Potter, P.A. (2010). *Clinical nursing skills and interventions.* (7th ed.). St. Louis: Mosby. **Skill 13-7, step 2, step 12, step 14, step 18,** Courtesy of Kinetic Concepts, Inc. (KCI), San Antonio, Texas.

Chapter 14

14-1, 14-2, courtesy of Great Plains Regional Medical Center, North Platte, Nebraska. **14-4,** courtesy of Alert-Care, Mill Valley, California. ***14-6, A, B, C,*** modified from Sorrentino, S.A. (2004). *Assisting with patient care.* (2nd ed.). St. Louis: Mosby. **Skill 14-1, step 6a(4), step 6b(1), step 6c(4), step 6d(1),** from Potter, P.A., & Perry, A.G. (2009). *Fundamentals of nursing: concepts, process, and practice.* (7th ed.). St. Louis: Mosby. **Skill 14-1, step 15a, step 15b, step 15c, step 15d,** from Elkin, M.K., et al. (2008). *Nursing interventions and clinical skills.* (4th ed.). St. Louis: Mosby.

Chapter 15

15-1, from Potter, P.A., & Perry, A.G. (2009). *Fundamentals of nursing: concepts, process, and practice.* (7th ed.). St. Louis: Mosby. **15-2, 15-6,** Box 15-2 unnumbered figures, from Sorrentino, S.A. (2004). *Assisting with patient care.* (2nd ed.). St. Louis: Mosby. **15-3, 15-4, 15-5,** from Potter, P.A., & Perry, A.G. (2006). *Basic nursing: essentials for practice.* (6th ed.). St. Louis: Mosby. Table 15-4 **figures,** from Potter, P.A., & Perry, A.G. (2006). *Fundamentals of nursing: concepts, process, and practice.* (6th ed.). St. Louis: Mosby. **Skill 15-1, step 9a, step 9g, step 9h; Skill 15-3, step 13c, step 13f, step 13h,** from Potter, P.A., & Perry, A.G. (2006). *Basic nursing: essentials for practice.* (6th ed.). St. Louis: Mosby. **Skill 15-1, step 9f; Skill 15-2, step 8; Skill 15-3, step 9f(2), step 14f,** from Elkin, M.K., et al. (2008). *Nursing interventions and clinical skills,* (4th ed.). St. Louis: Mosby. **Skill 15-1, step 9i,** from Seidel, H.M., et al. (2006). *Mosby's guide to physical examination.* (6th ed.). St. Louis: Mosby. **Skill 15-3, step 9f(4), step 12e, step 13j(7), step 13j(8),** from Sorrentino, S.A. (2004). *Assisting with patient care.* (2nd ed.). St. Louis: Mosby. **Skill 15-3, step 11e,** from Perry, A.G., & Potter, P.A. (2010). *Clinical nursing skills and techniques.* (7th ed.). St. Louis: Mosby.

Chapter 16

16-1, from Leahy, J.M., & Kizilay, P.E. (1998). *Foundations of nursing practice: a nursing process approach.* Philadelphia: Saunders. **16-3,** courtesy of Great Plains Regional Medical Center, North Platte, Nebraska. **16-4, 16-5, 16-6,** from Potter, P.A., & Perry, A.G. (2005). *Fundamentals of nursing: concepts, process, and practice.* (6th ed.). St. Louis: Mosby.

Chapter 17

17-1, 17-3, from Potter, P.A., & Perry, A.G. (2009). *Fundamentals of nursing: concepts, process, and practice.* (7th ed.). St. Louis: Mosby. **17-2,** from Leahy, J.M., & Kizilay, P.E. (1998). *Foundations of nursing practice: a nursing process approach.* Philadelphia: Saunders.

Chapter 18

18-1, 18-2, 18-3, 18-5, 18-7, 18-10, from Potter, P.A., & Perry, A.G. (2009). *Fundamentals of nursing: concepts, process, and practice.* (7th ed.). St. Louis: Mosby. **18-4,** Courtesy Laurel Wiersma, RN, MSN, Clinical Nurse Specialist, Barnes-Jewish Hospital, St. Louis, Missouri. In Potter, P.A., & Perry, A.G. (2009). *Fundamentals of nursing.* (7th ed.). St. Louis: Mosby. **18-8, 18-9,** from Elkin, M.K., et al. (2008). *Nursing interventions and clinical skills.* (4th ed.). St. Louis: Mosby. **Skill 18-1, step 8e, step 8h, step 8i, step 8r, step 8u, step 14f; Skill 18-2, step 9c, step 10c; Skill 18-3, step 9a; Skill 18-4, step 9e, step 9g, step 10c, step 10d,** from Potter, P.A., & Perry, A.G. (2009). *Fundamentals of nursing: concepts, process, and practice.* (7th ed.). St. Louis: Mosby. **Skill 18-1, step 10e; Skill 18-2, step 9a, step 9d; Skill 18-3, step 10e; Skill 18-4, step 9b; Skill 18-5, step 8i, step 8j, step 8m, step 8o, step 8q, step 8r, step 9g; Skill 18-6, step 11(b), step 11(c),** from Elkin, M.K., et al. (2008). *Nursing interventions and clinical skills.* (4th ed.). St. Louis: Mosby.

Chapter 19

19-1; 19-3; 19-4; 19-5; 19-6, *B*; 19-8; 19-10, *D, E*, from Elkin, M.K., et al. (2008). *Nursing interventions and clinical skills.* (4th ed.). St. Louis: Mosby. **19-2, 19-10, *C*,** from Potter, P.A., & Perry, A.G. (2009). *Fundamentals of nursing: concepts, process, and practice.* (7th ed.). St. Louis: Mosby. **19-6, *A*; 19-7; 19-10, *A, B*,** from Zakus, S.M. (1995). *Clinical procedures for medical assistants.* (3rd ed.). St. Louis: Mosby. **19-10, *C*,** from Potter, P.A., & Perry, A.G. (1997). *Fundamentals of nursing: concepts, process, and practice.* (4th ed.). St. Louis: Mosby. Table 19-1 figures, **bone marrow, fiberoptic endoscope,** from Phipps, W.J., et al. (2007). *Medical-surgical nursing: concepts and clinical practice.* (8th ed.). St. Louis: Mosby. Table 19-1, figure, **flexible fiberoptic bronchoscope,** courtesy of American Cystoscope Makers, Inc., Pelham, New York. Table 19-1, figures, **CT scan, endoscopy, lumbar puncture, MRI,** from Elkin, M.K., et al. (2008). *Nursing interventions and clinical skills.* (4th ed.). St. Louis: Mosby; Table 19-1, figure, **proctoscopy,** from Potter, P.A., & Perry, A.G. (2009). *Fundamentals of nursing: concepts, process, and practice.* (7th ed.). St. Louis: Mosby. Table 19-1, figures, **liver biopsy, paracentesis,** from Pagana, K.D., & Pagana, T.J. (2009). *Mosby's diagnostic and laboratory test reference.* (9th ed.). St. Louis: Mosby. Table 19-1, figure, thoracentesis, from Beare, P.G., & Myers, J.L. (1998). *Adult health nursing.* (3rd ed.). St. Louis: Mosby. **Skill 19-1, step 11; Skill 19-2, step 2; Skill 19-3, step 7a; Skill 19-5, step 2, step 14, step 16, step 17a, step 17b; Skill 19-7, step 8a; Skill 19-8, step 9f; Skill 19-9, step 14, step 18; Skill 19-13, step 17a(10), step 17a(11), step 17b(1), step 17b(6); Skill 19-14, step 10b(1),** from Elkin, M.K., et al. (2008). *Nursing interventions and clinical skills.* (4th ed.). St. Louis: Mosby. **Skill 19-6, step 8, step 9,** from Sorrentino, S.A. (2008). *Mosby's textbook for nursing assistants* (7th ed.). St. Louis: Mosby. **Skill 19-10, step 8,** from Grimes, D. (1991). *Mosby's clinical nursing series: infectious diseases.* St. Louis: Mosby. **Skill 19-14, step 10b,** from Sorrentino, S.A. (2004). *Assisting with patient care.* (2nd ed.). St. Louis: Mosby.

Chapter 20

20-1, 20-2, 20-3, 20-5, 20-6, 20-15, 20-19, 20-20, 20-22, 20-23, 20-24, 20-25, 20-26, from Elkin, M.K., et al. (2008). *Nursing interventions and clinical skills.* (4th ed.). St. Louis: Mosby. **20-4,** from Potter, P.A., & Perry, A.G. (2009). *Fundamentals of nursing: concepts, process, and practice.* (7th ed.). St. Louis: Mosby. **20-7, 20-8, 20-9, 20-10,** from Perry, A.G., Potter, P.A (2010). *Clinical nursing skills and interventions.* (7th ed.). St. Louis, Mosby. **20-18,** from Lewis, S.L., et al. (2007). *Medical-surgical nursing: assessment and management of clinical problems.* (7th ed.). St. Louis: Mosby. **20-21,** from Potter, P.A., & Perry, A.G. (2006). *Basic nursing: essentials for practice.* (6th ed.). St. Louis: Mosby. **Unn figure 20-1,** from Potter, P.A., & Perry, A.G. (2006). *Basic nursing: essentials for practice.* (6th ed.). St. Louis: Mosby. **Skill 20-1, step 10; Skill 20-3, step 5; Skill 20-7, step 4, step 7, step 8a(3), step 8, step 11, step 12, step 7; Skill 20-9, step 9, step 11, step 13d, step 15; Skill 20-11, step 7; Skill 20-12, step 5b, step 12, step 16a, step 16b(3), step 18, step 20a(5); Skill 20-15, step 2; Skill 20-17, step 8, step 27, step 28; Skill 20-22, step 2,** from Elkin, M.K., et al. (2008). *Nursing interventions and clinical skills.* (4th ed.). St. Louis: Mosby. **Skill 20-5, step 4,** from Ignatavicius, D.D., & Workman, M.L. (2009). *Medical-surgical nursing across the health care continuum.* (6th ed.). Philadelphia: Saunders. **Skill 20-6, step 8b(1), *A*, step 8b(1), *B*, step 8b(2), *A*, step 8b(2), *B*, step 8b(3), *A*, step 8b(3), *B*; Skill 20-8, step 8a, step 8a(4), step 8a(5), step 8b, step 8b5, *A*; Skill 20-12, step 13; Skill 20-17, step 12; Skill 20-25, step 7,** from Potter, P.A., & Perry, A.G. (2009). *Fundamentals of nursing: concepts, process, and practice.* (7th ed.). St. Louis: Mosby.

Chapter 21

21-1, from U.S. Department of Agriculture, Center for Nutrition Policy and Promotion, April 2005, CNPP-15. **21-2,** from Mahan, L.K., & Escott-Stump, S. (2008). *Krause's food, nutrition, and diet therapy.* (12th ed.). Philadelphia: Saunders. **21-5,** from Potter, P.A., & Perry, A.G. (2009). *Fundamentals of nursing: concepts, process, and practice.* (7th ed.). St. Louis: Mosby. **21-6,** courtesy of Rolin Graphics. In Potter, P.A., & Perry, A.G. (2009). *Fundamentals of nursing,* (7th ed.). St. Louis: Mosby. **Skill 21-1, step 10a, *A*, step 12a, step 13a(3), step 13b(1), step 13c(1),** from Elkin, M.K., et al. (2008). *Nursing interventions and clinical skills.* (4th ed.). St. Louis: Mosby. **Skill 21-1, step 10a, *B*, step 10b,** from Potter, P.A., & Perry, A.G. (2009). *Fundamentals of nursing: concepts, process, and practice.* (7th ed.). St. Louis: Mosby.

Chapter 22

22-1, from Phipps, W.J., et al. (2007). *Medical-surgical nursing: health and illness perspectives.* (8th ed.). St. Louis: Mosby. **22-2, 22-3,** redrawn from Long, B.C., et al. (1993). *Medical-surgical nursing: a nursing process ap-*

proach (3rd ed.). St. Louis: Mosby. **22-4,** from Lewis, S.L., et al. (2007). *Medical-surgical nursing: assessment and management of clinical problems.* (7th ed.). St. Louis: Mosby. **22-5,** from Thibodeau, G.A., & Patton, K.T. (2005). *The human body in health and disease.* (4th ed.). St. Louis: Mosby. **22-6,** from Potter, P.A., & Perry, A.G. (2009). *Fundamentals of nursing: concepts, process, and practice.* (7th ed.). St. Louis: Mosby. **Table 22-4 figures,** from Thibodeau, G.A., & Patton, K.T. (2004). *Structure and function of the body.* (12th ed.). St. Louis: Mosby.

Chapter 23

23-1, from Berhman, R.E., & Kliegman, R.M. (2007). *Nelson's textbook of pediatrics.* (18th ed.). Philadelphia: Saunders. **23-2; 23-19; 23-20; 23-22, *A, B*; 23-23,** from Potter, P.A., & Perry, A.G. (2009). *Fundamentals of nursing: concepts, process, and practice.* (7th ed.). St. Louis: Mosby. **23-3, *A*,** courtesy of Great Plains Regional Medical Center, North Platte, Nebraska. **23-3, *B*,** courtesy of Barnes-Jewish Hospital, St. Louis, Missouri. In Elkin M.K., et al. (2008). *Nursing interventions & clinical skills.* (4th ed.). St. Louis: Mosby. **23-4; 23-5; 23-15, *C*; 23-16, *C*; 23-18, *C*; 23-21; 23-22, *C, D*,** from Elkin, M.K., et al. (2008). *Nursing interventions and clinical skills.* (4th ed.). St. Louis: Mosby. **23-6; 23-7; 23-12; 23-13; 23-15, *A, B*; 23-16, *A, B*; 23-17; 23-18, *A, B*,** from Clayton, B.D., & Stock, Y.N. (2007). *Basic pharmacology for nurses.* (14th ed.). St. Louis: Mosby. **23-11,** from Potter, P.A., & Perry, A.G. (2006). *Basic nursing: essentials for practice.* (6th ed.). St. Louis: Mosby. **Skill 23-1, step 5; Skill 23-2, step 13; Skill 23-6, step 13; Skill 23-7, step 14a; Skill 23-13, step 10b(1), step 10b(2); Skill 23-17, step 10,** from Potter, P.A., & Perry, A.G. (2009). *Fundamentals of nursing: concepts, process, and practice.* (7th ed.). St. Louis: Mosby. **Skill 23-7, step 14b; Skill 23-8, step 14,** from Clayton, B.D., & Stock, Y.N. (2007). *Basic pharmacology for nurses.* (14th ed.). St. Louis: Mosby. **Skill 23-10, step 14a, step 14b; Skill 23-13, step 10c(6); Skill 23-16, step 11,** from Elkin, M.K., et al. (2008). *Nursing interventions and clinical skills.* (4th ed.). St. Louis: Mosby.

Chapter 24

24-1, 24-13, from Lewis, S.L., et al. (2007). *Medical-surgical nursing: assessment and management of clinical problems.* (7th ed.). St. Louis: Mosby. **24-3, 24-4, 24-5, 24-6, 24-7, 24-8, 24-9, 24-11,** from Sorrentino, S.A. (2008). *Mosby's textbook of nursing assistants.* (7th ed.). St. Louis: Mosby. **24-12,** from Kidd, P.S., & Stuart, P.A. (1996). *Mosby's emergency nursing reference.* St. Louis: Mosby. **24-14, 24-15,** from Henry, M.C., & Stapleton, E.R. (1997). *EMT prehospital care.* (2nd ed.). Philadelphia: Saunders. **24-16,** from Sheehy, S.B., & Lombardi, J. (1995). *Manual of emergency care.* (4th ed.). St. Louis: Mosby. **Skill 24-1, step 7; Skill 24-2, step 4; Skill 24-3, step 1, *A, B*,** from Henry, M.C., & Stapleton, E.P. (1997). *EMT prehospital care.* (2nd ed.). Philadelphia: Saunders.

Chapter 25

25-1, 25-2, 25-5, from Wong, D.L., et al. (2006). *Maternal-child nursing care.* (3rd ed.). St. Louis: Mosby. **25-3,** courtesy of Marjorie Pyle, RNC, LifeCircle, Costa Mesa, California. **25-4,** courtesy of Marjorie Pyle, RNC, LifeCircle, Costa Mesa, California. In Lowdermilk, D.L., & Perry, S.E. (2007). *Maternity and women's health care.* (9th ed.). St. Louis: Mosby. **25-6, 25-8,** from Lowdermilk, D.L., & Perry, S.E. (2007). *Maternity and women's health care.* (9th ed.). St. Louis: Mosby. **25-7,** from McKinney, E.S., et al. (2009). *Maternal-child nursing.* (3rd ed.). Philadelphia: Saunders. Table 25-1 figures, from Lowdermilk, D.L., & Perry, S.E. (2007). *Maternity and women's health care.* (9th ed.). St. Louis: Mosby.

Chapter 26

26-1; 26-2, *A, B, C*, from Lowdermilk, D.L., & Perry, S.E. (2007). *Maternity and women's health care.* (9th ed.). St. Louis: Mosby. **26-3; 26-4; 26-6; 26-7; 26-9; 26-12; 26-13; 26-15; 26-16, *A*; 26-17; 26-20; 26-22; 26-23,** from Lowdermilk, D.L., & Perry, S.E. (2007). *Maternity and women's health care.* (9th ed.). St. Louis: Mosby. **26-5,** from Novak, J.C., & Broom, B.L. (1995). *Ingalls & Salerno's maternal and child health nursing.* (8th ed.). St. Louis: Mosby. **26-16, *B*, 26-18,** from Tucker, S.M. (2009). *Pocket guide to fetal monitoring and assessment.* (6th ed.). St. Louis: Mosby. **26-8, 26-10, 26-11, 26-14, 26-19, 26-21,** from Wong, D.L., et al. (2006). *Maternal-child nursing care.* (3rd ed.). St. Louis: Mosby. **Unn figure 26-1,** from Lowdermilk, D.L., & Perry, S.E. (2007). *Maternity and women's health care.* (9th ed.). St. Louis: Mosby.

Chapter 27

27-1, 27-6, from Lowdermilk, D.L., & Perry, S.E. (2007). *Maternity and women's health care.* (9th ed.). St. Louis: Mosby. **27-3,** from Elkin, M.K., et al. (2008). *Nursing interventions and clinical skills.* (4th ed.). St. Louis: Mosby. **27-4, 27-7, 27-8,** from Lowdermilk, D.L., & Perry, S.E. (2007). *Maternity and women's health care.* (9th ed.). St. Louis: Mosby. **27-5, *B, C, D*; 27-9; 27-11, *B, C, D*,** courtesy of Marjorie Pyle, RNC, LifeCircle, Costa Mesa, California. **27-10,** from McKinney, E.S., et al. (2009). *Maternal-child nursing.* (3rd ed.). Philadelphia: Saunders. **27-11, *A*,** courtesy of Kim Malloy, Knoxville, Iowa. **27-13, 27-14,** from Murray, S.S., & McKinney, E.S. (2006). *Foundations of maternal-newborn nursing.* (4th ed.). Philadelphia: Saunders. Table 27-4 figure, **moro reflex,** from Wong, D.L., et al. (2006). *Maternal-child nursing care.* (3rd ed.). St. Louis: Mosby. Table 27-4 figures, **tonic neck reflex, step reflex, Babinski reflex, palmer grasp reflex, plantar grasp reflex,** from Murray, S.S., & McKinney, E.S. (2006). *Foundations of maternal-newborn nursing.* (4th ed.). Philadelphia: Saunders. Table 27-4 figure, **pull to sit,** from Jarvis, C. (2008). *Physical examination and health assessment.* (5th ed.). Philadelphia: Saunders; Table 27-4 figure, **gallant reflex,** from Lowdermilk, D.L., & Perry, S.E. (2007). *Maternity and women's health care.* (9th ed.). St. Louis: Mosby.

Chapter 28

28-1, from Hamilton, P.M. (1989). *Basic maternity nursing.* (6th ed.). St. Louis: Mosby. **28-2, 28-3, 28-4, 28-5, 28-6, 28-8,** from Wong, D.L., et al. (2006). *Maternal-child nursing care.* (3rd ed.). St. Louis: Mosby. **28-7,** from Seidel, H.M., et al. (2003). *Mosby's guide to physical examination.* (5th ed.). St. Louis: Mosby. **28-9, *A*,** from *Perinatal assessment of maturation.* National Audiovisual Center, Washington DC. **28-9, *B*,** modified from Battaglia, F.C., & Lubchenco, L.O. A practical classification of newborn infants by weight and gestational age. *Journal of Pediatrics,* 71(2):59-63, 1967. **28-10,** from Ballard, J.L., et al. New Ballard Score, expanded to include extremely premature infants. *Journal of Pediatrics,* 119(3):417-423, 1991. **28-11,** from Novak, J.C., & Broom, B.L. (1995). *Ingalls & Salerno's maternal and child health nursing.* (8th ed.). St. Louis: Mosby.

Chapter 29

29-4, 29-5, 29-6, department of Health and Human Services, Centers for Disease Control and Prevention, Atlanta, Georgia. **29-7,** from Swartz, M.H. (2005). *Textbook of physical diagnosis: history and examination.* (4th ed.). Philadelphia: Saunders.

Chapter 30

30-1, 30-2, 30-3, 30-4, 30-5, 30-7, 30-8, 30-9, from Hockenberry, M.J. (2009). *Wong's essentials of pediatric nursing.* (8th ed.). St. Louis: Mosby. **30-6,** from Hockenberry, M.J., & Wilson, D. (2007). *Wong's nursing care of infants and children.* (8th ed.). St. Louis: Mosby. **30-10,** from Lowdermilk, D.L., & Perry, S.E. (2007). *Maternity and women's health care.* (9th ed.). St. Louis: Mosby. **30-12, 30-13, 30-14, 30-15, 30-16,** from Wong, D.L., et al. (2006). *Maternal-child nursing care.* (3rd ed.). St. Louis: Mosby. **30-17, *B*,** courtesy of Marjorie Pyle, RNC, LifeCircle, Costa Mesa, California. In Lowdermilk, D.L., & Perry, S.E. (2007). *Maternity and women's health care.* (9th ed.). St. Louis: Mosby.

Chapter 31

31-1, from Lowdermilk, D.L., & Perry, S.E. (2007). *Maternity and women's health care.* (9th ed.). St. Louis: Mosby. **31-2, 31-4, 31-5, 31-6, 31-7, 31-8, 31-9, 31-13, 31-14, 31-17, 31-18, 31-19, 31-21, 31-22,** from Hockenberry, M.J. (2009). *Wong's essentials of pediatric nursing.* (8th ed.). St. Louis: Mosby. **31-10,** from McCance, K.L., & Huether, S.E. (2006). *Pathophysiology: the biologic basis for disease in adults and children.* (5th ed.). St. Louis: Mosby. **31-11,** from Center for Attitudinal Healing, Tiburon, California. **31-12, 31-16, 31-23,** from Ashwill, J.W., & Droske, S.C. (2007). *Nursing care of children: principles and practice.* (3rd ed.). Philadelphia: Saunders. **31-15,** courtesy of Paul Vincent Kuntz, Texas Children's Hospital, Houston, Texas. In Hockenbery, M.J., et al. (2005). *Wong's essentials of pediatric nursing.* (7th ed.). St. Louis: Mosby. **31-20,** courtesy of Harry C. Shirkey, Fort Thomas, Kentucky. **31-24,** from Thompson, J.M., et al. (1997). *Mosby's clinical nursing.* (4th ed.). St. Louis: Mosby. **31-25, 31-27, 31-28, 31-30,** from Wong D.L., et al. (2006). *Maternal-child nursing care.* (3rd ed.). St. Louis: Mosby. **31-26,** from Zitelli, B.J., & Davis, H.W. (2007). *Atlas of pediatric physical diagnosis.* (5th ed.). St. Louis: Mosby. **31-29,** from Bowden, V.P., et al. (1998). *Children and their families: the continuum of care.* Philadelphia: Saunders.

Chapter 32

32-1, from Hockenberry, M.J. (2009). *Wong's essentials of pediatric nursing.* (8th ed.). St. Louis: Mosby.

Chapter 33

33-1, from Sorrentino, S.A. (2008). *Mosby's textbook for nursing assistants.* (7th ed.). St. Louis: Mosby. **33-2, 33-12,** from Lewis, S.L., et al. (2007). *Medical-surgical nursing: assessment and management of clinical problems.* (7th ed.). St. Louis: Mosby. **33-3, 33-4, 33-6, 33-10, 3-11, 33-13,** from Elkin, M.K., et al. (2008). *Nursing interventions and clinical skills.* (4th ed.). St. Louis: Mosby. **33-7; 33-8, *A*,** from Monahan, F.D., et al. (2007). *Phipps' medical-surgical nursing: health and illness perspectives.* (8th ed.). St. Louis: Mosby. **33-9,** from Barkauskas, V.H., et al. (2002). *Health and physical assessment.* (3rd ed.). St. Louis: Mosby.

Chapter 34

34-1, from Lewis, S.L., et al. (2007). *Medical-surgical nursing: assessment and management of clinical problems.* (7th ed.). St. Louis: Mosby. **34-2,** from "The Rake in Bedlam," c.1735. From the series titled *The Rake's Progress,* copyright © The British Museum, London, England. **34-4,** from Varcarolis, E.M. (2006). *Foundations of psychiatric mental health nursing.* (5th ed.). Philadelphia: Saunders.

Chapter 36

36-1, illustration by Lee Hoffman. **36-2,** from National Institute on Drug Abuse, Bethesda, Maryland, 1999, National Institutes of Health.

Chapter 37

37-1, from Potter, P.A., & Perry, P.G. (2009). *Fundamentals of nursing: concepts, process, and practice.* (7th ed.). St. Louis: Mosby. **37-2,** photo by Marilu Halamandaris, *Caring* magazine, National Association for Home Care. **37-3,** from Lewis, S.L., et al. (2007). *Medical-surgical nursing: assessment and management of clinical problems.* (7th ed.). St. Louis: Mosby.

Chapter 38

38-3, from Leahy, J.M., & Kizilay, P.E. (1998). *Foundations of nursing practice: a nursing process approach.* Philadelphia: Saunders.

Chapter 39

39-1, from Leahy, J.M., & Kizilay, P.E. (1998). *Foundations of nursing practice: a nursing process approach.* Philadelphia: Saunders.

Chapter 40

40-1, from Harkreader, H., & Hogan, M.A. (2007). *Fundamentals of nursing: caring and clinical judgment.* (3rd ed.). Philadelphia: Saunders.

Chapter 41

41-1, 41-2, 41-3, 41-4, 41-5, 41-6, 41-9, 41-13, from Thibodeau, G.A., & Patton, K.T. (2008). *Structure and function of the body.* (13th ed.). St. Louis: Mosby. **41-7,** from Herlihy, B., & Maebius, N.K. (2007). *The human body in health and illness.* (3rd ed.). Philadelphia: Saunders. **41-8, 41-10, 41-11,** from Thibodeau, G.A., & Patton, K.T. (2007). *Anatomy and physiology.* (6th ed.). St. Louis: Mosby.

Chapter 42

42-1, 42-6, 42-9, 42-12, 42-17, 42-18, from Harkreader, H., & Hogan, M.A. (2007). *Fundamentals of nursing: caring and clinical judgment.* (3rd ed.). Philadelphia: Saunders. **42-2,** from Cole, G. (1996). *Fundamental nursing: concepts and skills.* (2nd ed.). St. Louis: Mosby. **42-3, 42-4, 42-7, 42-16,** from Elkin, M.K., et al. (2007). *Nursing interventions and clinical skills.* (4th ed.). St. Louis: Mosby. **42-5,** from Potter, P.A., & Perry, A.G. (2006). *Basic nursing: essentials for practice.* (6th ed.). St. Louis: Mosby. **42-8,** from Meeker, M.H., & Rothrock, J.C. (1999). *Alexander's care of the patient in surgery.* (11th ed.). St. Louis: Mosby. **42-10, 42-14,** courtesy of Great Plains Regional Medical Center, North Platte, Nebraska. **42-11,** from Lewis, S.L., et al. (2007). *Medical-surgical nursing: assessment and management of clinical problems.* (7th ed.). St. Louis: Mosby. **42-13,** from Potter, P.A., & Perry, A.G. (2009). *Fundamentals of nursing.* (7th ed.). St. Louis: Mosby. **Skill 42-1, step 14,** from Sorrentino, S.A. (2008). *Mosby's textbook for nursing assistants.* (7th ed.). St. Louis: Mosby. **Skill 42-2, step 9a, step 10c; Skill 42-3, step 10; Skill 42-4, step 17, step 20,** from Potter, P.A., & Perry, A.G. (2009). *Fundamentals of nursing.* (7th ed.). St. Louis. Mosby. **Skill 42-3, step 8,** from Elkin, M.K., et al. (2007). *Nursing interventions and clinical skills.* (4th ed.). St. Louis: Mosby.

Chapter 43

43-1, from Thibodeau, G.A., & Patton, K.T. (2005). *The human body in health and disease.* (4th ed.). St. Louis: Mosby. **43-2, 43-7, 43-8, 43-13, 43-18,** from Habif, T.P. (2004). *Clinical dermatology.* (4th ed.). St. Louis: Mosby. **43-3, 43-4, 43-5, 43-6, 43-10, 43-17,** courtesy of the Department of Dermatology, School of Medicine, University of Utah. **43-9** from Weston, W.L., et al. (2007). *Color textbook of pediatric dermatology.* (4th ed.). St. Louis: Mosby. **43-11,** from Habif, T.P., et al. (2005). *Skin disease: diagnosis and treatment.* (2nd ed.). St. Louis: Mosby. **43-12,** from Baran R., et al. (1991). *Color atlas of the hair, scalp, and nails.* St. Louis: Mosby. **43-14,** courtesy of Department of Dermatology, University of North Carolina at Chapel Hill. **43-15,** from Zitelli, B.J. & Davis, H.W. (2007). *Atlas of pediatric physical diagnosis.* (5th ed.). St. Louis: Mosby. **43-16,** from Belcher, A.E. (1992). *Cancer nursing.* St. Louis: Mosby. **43-19,** from Hockenberry, M. J., & Wilson, D. (2007). *Wong's nursing care of infants and children.* (8th ed.). St. Louis: Mosby. **43-20, 43-21,** courtesy of Intermountain Burn Center, University of Utah. **43-22,** from Thibodeau, G.A., & Patton, K.T. (2007). *Anatomy and physiology.* (6th ed.). St. Louis: Mosby. **43-23, 43-24, 43-25,** courtesy of Burn Center, Cleveland Metropolitan General Hospital, Cleveland, Ohio.

Chapter 44

44-1, 44-4, from Thibodeau, G.A., & Patton, K.T. (2008). *Structure and function of the body.* (13th ed.). St. Louis: Mosby. **44-2, 44-3, 44-5, 44-6, 44-22, 44-24, 44-39, 44-41,** from Thibodeau, G.A., & Patton, K.T. (2005). *The human body in health and disease.* (4th ed.). St. Louis: Mosby. **44-7, 44-8,** from Kamal, A., & Brocklehurst, J.C. (1991). *Color atlas of geriatric medicine.* (2nd ed.). St. Louis: Mosby. **44-9, 44-17, 44-25,** from Lewis, S.L., et al. (2007). *Medical-surgical nursing: assessment and management of clinical problems.* (7th ed.). St. Louis: Mosby. **44-10, 44-23, 44-34,** from Ignatavicius, D.D., & Workman, M.L. (2009). *Medical-surgical nursing across the healthcare continuum.* (6th ed.). Philadelphia: Saunders. **44-11, 44-16, 44-20, 44-31, *B*; Skill 44-1, step 8a,** from Monahan, F.D., et al. (2007). *Phipps' medical-surgical nursing: health and illness perspectives.* (8th ed.). St. Louis: Mosby. **44-12, 44-15, 44-32,** courtesy of Zimmer, Inc., Warsaw, Indiana. **44-13,** courtesy of Orthologic Corporation, Phoenix, Arizona. **44-18, 44-31, *A*,** modified from Mourad, L. (1991). *Orthopedic disorders.* St. Louis: Mosby. **44-26, 44-29,** courtesy of Dr. Henry Bohlman, Cleveland, Ohio. **44-27, 44-40,** from Beare, P.G., & Myers, J.L. (1998). *Adult health nursing.* (3rd ed.). St. Louis: Mosby. **44-28, *A*,** from Stryker Howmedica Osteonics, Inc. Mahway, New Jersey. **44-28, 44-38,** from Thompson, J.M., et al. (2002). *Mosby's clinical nursing.* (5th ed.). St. Louis: Mosby. **44-30,** from Elkin, M.K., et al. (2008). *Nursing interventions and clinical skills.* (4th ed.). St. Louis: Mosby. **44-33,** from Harkness, G.A., & Dincher, J.R. (1999). *Medical-surgical nursing: total patient care.* (10th ed.). St. Louis: Mosby. **44-34, 44-36,** from Potter, P.A., & Perry, A.G. (2006). *Basic nursing: essentials for practice.* (6th ed.). St. Louis: Mosby. **44-35,** from Elkin, M.K., et al. (2004). *Nursing interventions and clinical skills.* (3rd ed.). St. Louis: Mosby. **44-37,** courtesy of Roll-a-Bout Corporation, Frederica, Delaware.

Chapter 45

45-1, 45-2, 45-4, from Thibodeau, G.A., & Patton, K.T. (2007). *Anatomy and physiology.* (6th ed.). St. Louis: Mosby. **45-3,** from Thibodeau, G.A., & Patton, K.T. (2008). *Struc-*

ture and function of the body. (13th ed.). St. Louis: Mosby. **45-5, 45-20,** from Monahan, F.D., et al. (2007). *Phipps' medical-surgical nursing: health and illness perspectives.* (8th ed.). St. Louis: Mosby. **45-6,** from Lewis, S.L., et al. (2007). *Medical-surgical nursing: assessment and management of clinical problems.* (7th ed.). St. Louis: Mosby. **45-8, 45-12, 45-13, 45-14, 45-16,** from Beare, P.G., & Myers, J.L. (1998). *Adult health nursing.* (3rd ed.). St. Louis: Mosby.

Chapter 46

46-1, courtesy of Olympus America, Inc., Melville, New York. **46-2, 46-4, 46-7, 46-9,** from Lewis, S.L., et al. (2007). *Medical-surgical nursing: assessment and management of clinical problems.* (7th ed.). St. Louis: Mosby. **46-3, 46-8,** from Beare, P.G., & Myers, J.L. (1998). *Adult health nursing.* (3rd ed.). St. Louis: Mosby. **46-5,** from Kamal, A., & Brockelhurst, J.C. (1991). *Color atlas of geriatric medicine.* (3rd ed.). St. Louis: Mosby. **46-6,** from Monahan, F.D., et al. (2007). *Phipps' medical-surgical nursing: health and illness perspectives.* (8th ed.). St. Louis: Mosby.

Chapter 47

47-1, 47-4, from Thibodeau, G.A., & Patton, K.T. (2007). *Anatomy and physiology.* (6th ed.). St. Louis: Mosby. **47-2, 47-3,** from Thibodeau, G.A., & Patton, K.T. (2007). *The human body in health and disease.* (3rd ed.). St. Louis: Mosby. **47-5,** from Belcher, A.E. (1992). *Mosby's clinical nursing series: blood disorders.* St. Louis: Mosby.

Chapter 48

48-1 from Thibodeau, G.A., & Patton, K.T. (2004). *Structure and function of the human body.* (12th ed.). St. Louis: Mosby. **48-2, 48-3,** from Thibodeau, G.A., & Patton, K.T. (2007). *Anatomy and physiology.* (6th ed.). St. Louis: Mosby. **48-4, 48-5, 48-6, 48-17,** from Canobbio, M. (1990). *Mosby's clinical nursing series: cardiovascular disorders.* St. Louis: Mosby. **48-9, *A*,** courtesy of Medtronic, Inc., Minneapolis, Minnesota. **48-9, *B*, 48-10, 48-11, 48-12, *B*, 48-16, 48-19, 48-20, *A*, *B*, 48-21, 48-23,** from Lewis, S.L., et al. (2007). *Medical-surgical nursing: assessment and management of clinical problems.* (7th ed.). St. Louis: Mosby. **48-12, *A*,** from Urden, L.D., et al. (2006). *Thelan's critical care nursing: diagnosis and management.* (5th ed.). St. Louis: Mosby. **48-13, 48-25,** from Monahan, F.D., et al. (2007). *Phipps' medical-surgical nursing: health and illness perspectives.* (8th ed.). St. Louis: Mosby. **48-14,** from Beare, P.G., & Myers, J.L. (1998). *Adult health nursing.* (3rd ed.). St. Louis: Mosby. **48-15,** from *Heart disease and stroke,* 2:99, 1993. Copyright American Heart Association. **48-23, 48-24,** from Kamal, A., & Brockelhurst, J.C.: *Color atlas of geriatric medicine.* (3rd ed.). St. Louis: Mosby–Year Book, Europe.

Chapter 49

49-1, 49-2, 49-3, 49-4, 49-6, from Thibodeau, G.A., & Patton, K.T. (2008). *Structure and function of the body.* (13th ed.). St. Louis: Mosby. **49-5,** from Thibodeau, G.A., & Patton, K.T. (2005). *The human body in health and disease.* (4th ed.). St. Louis: Mosby. **49-7, *A*,** courtesy of Olympus America, Melville, New York. **49-7, *B*,** from Meduri, G.U., et al. Protected bronchoalveolar lavage. *American Review of Respiratory Disease,* 143:855, 1991, official journal of the American Thoracic Society, copyright American Lung Association. **49-8,** from Lewis, S.L., et al. (2007). *Medical-surgical nursing: assessment and management of clinical problems.* (7th ed.). St. Louis: Mosby. **49-9, 49-12,** from Potter, P.A., & Perry, A.G. (2009). *Fundamentals of nursing.* (7th ed.). St. Louis: Mosby. **49-13,** from Wilson, S., & Thompson, J. (1991). *Mosby's clinical nursing series: respiratory disorders.* St. Louis: Mosby. **49-14,** from Lewis, S.L., et al. (1996). *Medical-surgical nursing: assessment and management of clinical problems.* (4th ed.). St. Louis: Mosby. **49-15,** from McCance, K.L., & Huether, S.E. (2006). *Pathophysiology: the biologic basis for disease in adults and children.* (5th ed.). St. Louis: Mosby.

Chapter 50

50-1, 50-2, 50-3, 50-5, from Thibodeau, G.A., & Patton, K.T. (2007). *Anatomy and physiology.* (6th ed.). St. Louis: Mosby. **50-6,** from Lewis, S.L., et al. (2007). *Medical-surgical nursing: assessment and management of clinical problems.* (7th ed.). St. Louis: Mosby. **50-7, 50-9,** from Beare, P.G., & Myers, J.L. (1998). *Adult health nursing.* (3rd ed.). St. Louis: Mosby. **50-10, 50-11,** from Tucker, S., et al. (1996). *Patient care standards: collaborative practice planning guides.* (6th ed.). St. Louis: Mosby. **50-12,** from Belcher, A.E. (1992). *Cancer nursing.* St. Louis: Mosby. **50-14,** from Thibodeau, G.A., & Patton, K.T. (2008). *Structure and function of the body.* (13th ed.). St. Louis: Mosby.

Chapter 51

51-1, 51-2, 51-4, from Thibodeau, G.A., & Patton, K.T. (2008). *Structure and function of the body.* (13th ed.). St. Louis: Mosby. **51-5,** from Thibodeau, G.A., & Patton, K.T. (2007). *Anatomy and physiology.* (6th ed.). St. Louis: Mosby. **51-6,** courtesy of the Group for Research in Pathology Education. **51-7, 51-8,** from Seidel, H.M., et al. (2003). *Mosby's guide to physical examination.* (5th ed.). St. Louis: Mosby. **51-9,** from Schneeburg, N.G. (1979). *Essentials of clinical endocrinology.* St. Louis: Mosby. **51-10,** courtesy of L.V. Bergman & Associates, Inc., Cold Springs, New York. **51-14, 51-15, *A*, *B*, 51-17, 51-18,** from Lewis, S.L., et al. (2007). *Medical-surgical nursing: assessment and management of clinical problems.* (7th ed.). St. Louis: Mosby. **51-16,** from Potter, P.A., & Perry, A.G. (2003). *Basic nursing: essentials for practice.* (5th ed.). St. Louis: Mosby.

Chapter 52

52-1, 52-2, 52-3, 52-5, 52-6, 52-7, from Thibodeau, G.A., & Patton, K.T. (2007). *Anatomy and physiology.* (6th ed.). St. Louis: Mosby. **52-4,** from Thibodeau, G.A., & Patton, K.T. (2008). *Structure and function of the body.* (13th ed.). St. Louis: Mosby. **52-8, 52-18, 52-19,** from Beare, P.G., & Myers, J.L. (1998). *Adult health nursing.* (3rd ed.). St. Louis: Mosby. **52-10,** from Herbst, A.L., et al. (1998). *Comprehensive gynecology.* (3rd ed.). St. Louis: Mosby. **52-12, 52-16,** from Lewis, S.L., et al. (2007). *Medical-surgical nursing: assessment and management of clinical problems.* (7th ed.). St. Louis: Mosby. **52-13,** redrawn from Novak, E.R., & Woodruff, J.D. (eds.). (1967). *Novak's gynecologic and obstetric pathology.* (6th ed.). Philadelphia: Saunders. (In K.L. McCance, & S.E. Huether [Eds.]. [1998]. *Pathophysiology: the biologic basis for disease in adults and children.* [3rd ed.]. St. Louis: Mosby.) **52-11, 52-14, 52-15,** from Seidel, H.M., et al. (2003). *Mosby's guide to physical examination.* (5th ed.). St. Louis: Mosby. **52-17,** from Belcher, A.E. (1992). *Cancer nursing.* St. Louis: Mosby. **52-20, 52-21** from Lowdermilk, D.L., et al. (2007). *Maternity and women's health care.* (9th ed.). St. Louis: Mosby.

Chapter 53

53-1, from Thibodeau, G.A., & Patton, K.T. (2007). *Anatomy and physiology.* (6th ed.). St. Louis: Mosby. **53-2, 53-3,** from Thibodeau, G.A., & Patton, K.T. (2008). *Structure and function of the body.* (13th ed.). St. Louis: Mosby. **53-4,** from Thibodeau, G.A., & Patton, K.T. (2005). *The human body in health and disease.* (4th ed.). St. Louis: Mosby. **53-5, 53-7, 53-8, 53-10, 53-12,** from Lewis, S.L., et al. (2007). *Medical-surgical nursing: assessment and management of clinical problems.* (7th ed.). St. Louis: Mosby. **53-6,** from Lowdermilk, D.L., et al. (2007). *Maternity and women's health care.* (9th ed.). St. Louis: Mosby. **53-9** from Havener, W.H. (1997). *Synopsis of ophthalmology.* St. Louis: Mosby. **53-11,** from Monahan, F.D., et al. (2007). *Phipps' medical-surgical nursing: health and illness perspectives.* (8th ed.). St. Louis: Mosby. **53-13, 53-14,** from Seidel, H.M., et al. (2003). *Mosby's guide to physical examination.* (5th ed.). St. Louis: Mosby. **53-15,** from Lemmi, F.O., & Lemmi, C.A.E. (2000). *Physical assessment findings CD-ROM.* Philadelphia: Saunders.

Chapter 54

54-1, ***A, B,*** **54-2,** from Thibodeau, G.A., & Patton, K.T. (2007). *Anatomy and physiology.* (6th ed.). St. Louis: Mosby. **54-3, 54-5,** from Thibodeau, G.A., & Patton, K.T. (2005). *The human body in health and disease.* (4th ed.). St. Louis: Mosby. **54-4,** from Thibodeau, G.A., & Patton, K.T. *Anthony's textbook of anatomy and physiology.* (18th ed.). St. Louis: Mosby. **54-6,** from Elkin, M.K., et al. (2004). *Nursing interventions and clinical skills.* (4th ed.). St. Louis: Mosby. **54-7,** from Long, B., et al. (1993). *Medical-surgical nursing: a nursing process approach.* (3rd ed.). St. Louis: Mosby. **54-8, 54-22, 54-25,** from Monahan, F.D., et al. (2007). *Phipps' medical-surgical nursing: health and illness perspectives.* (8th ed.). St. Louis: Mosby. **54-9** from Rudy, E.B. (1984). *Advanced neurological and neurosurgical nursing.* St. Louis: Mosby. **54-10,** from Hoemann, S.P. (1996). *Rehabilitation nursing: process and application.* (2nd ed.). St. Louis: Mosby. **54-11, 54-12,** from Dittmar, S.S. (1989). *Rehabilitation nursing: process and application.* St. Louis: Mosby. **54-13, 54-14, 54-15, 54-16, 54-17, 54-18, 54-19, 54-20, 54-21, 54-23, 54-24,** from Lewis, S.L., et al. (2007). *Medical-surgical nursing: assessment and management of clinical problems.* (7th ed.). St. Louis: Mosby. **54-26,** courtesy of Michael S. Clement, MD, Mesa, Arizona.

Chapter 55

55-2, from Grimes, D. (1991). *Infectious diseases.* St. Louis: Mosby. **55-3,** from Thibodeau, G.A., & Patton, K.T. (2007). *Anatomy and physiology.* (6th ed.). St. Louis: Mosby.

Chapter 56

56-4, redrawn from Gottfried, S.S. (1993). *Human biology.* Sudbury, Mass: Jones & Bartlett. **56-4,** from Friedman-Kien, A.E., & Cockerell, C.J. (1996). *Color atlas of AIDS.* (2nd ed.). Philadelphia: Saunders.

Chapter 57

57-1, 57-2 from *2008 estimated U.S. cancer cases.* © 2004, American Cancer Society, Inc., Surveillance Research. **57-3,** from Belcher, A.E. (1992). *Cancer nursing.* St. Louis: Mosby.

Chapter 58

58-4, from Polaski, A.L., & Warner, J.P. (1994). *Saunders' fundamentals for nursing assistants.* Philadelphia: Saunders. **58-5,** from Hill, S.S. & Howlett, H.S. (2009). *Success in practical/vocational nursing: from student to leader.* (6th ed.). Philadelphia: Saunders. **58-6,** from Leahy, J.M., & Kizilay, P.E. (1998). *Foundations of nursing practice: a nursing process approach.* Philadelphia: Saunders. **58-7, 58-8, 58-9,** from Elkin, M.K., et al. (2008). *Nursing interventions and clinical skills.* (4th ed.). St. Louis: Mosby.

Glossary

Pronunciation of Terms*

The markings ¯ and ˘ above the vowels (a, e, i, o, and u) indicate the proper sounds of the vowels.

When ¯ is above a vowel, its sound is long, that is, exactly like its name. For example:

ā as in āpe
ē as in ēven
ī as in īce
ō as in ōpen
ū as in ūnit

The ˘ marking indicates a short vowel sound, as in the following examples:

ă as in ăpple
ĕ as in ĕvery
ĭ as in ĭnterest
ŏ as in pŏt
ŭ as in ŭnder

*From Chabner, D. (2004). *The language of medicine.* (7th ed.). Philadelphia: Saunders.

A

ABCs Mnemonic for assessing status of emergency patients: *A*irway, *B*reathing, *C*irculation; used in one- or two-rescuer CPR.

abduction Movement of an extremity away from the midline of the body.

ablation Amputation or excision of any part of the body; removal of a growth or harmful substance.

abuse Misuse, as of an addictive substance such as alcohol, tobacco, nicotine, and so forth.

accountability Being answerable for one's own actions.

accreditation Process whereby a professional association or nongovernmental agency grants recognition to an institution or agency for demonstrated ability in a special area of practice.

achalasia Abnormal condition characterized by the inability of a muscle, particularly the cardiac sphincter of the stomach, to relax.

achlorhydria Abnormal condition characterized by the absence of hydrochloric acid in the gastric secretions.

acid-base balance Homeostasis of the hydrogen ion (H^+) concentration in the body fluids.

acquired heart disorder Abnormality occurring after birth that compromises heart function.

acquired immunodeficiency syndrome (AIDS) Acquired condition that impairs the body's ability to fight infection; the end stage of the continuum of HIV infection, in which the infected person has a CD_4^+ (lymphocyte) count of 200 cells/mm^3 or fewer.

acrocyanosis Peripheral cyanosis; the blue discoloration of the hands and feet in most infants at birth that may persist for 7 to 10 days.

active listening Giving full attention and a concerted effort to understand the message being sent.

active transport The movement of materials across the membrane of a cell by means of chemical activity, which allows the cell to admit larger molecules than would otherwise be able to enter.

activities of daily living (ADLs) Those activities of daily life, such as toileting, bathing, dressing, and grooming, that promote maintenance of functional abilities and independence in the environment.

actual nursing diagnosis Statement of a health problem that a nurse is licensed and competent to treat.

acupressure Complementary and alternative medicine therapy that uses gentle pressure at points on the body; used primarily for prevention and relief of symptoms of muscle tension.

acupuncture Complementary and alternative medicine therapy that stimulates certain points on the body by insertion of special needles to modify the perception of pain, normalize physiologic functions, and to treat or prevent disease.

acute Having a short and relatively severe course; a disease process characterized by a relatively short duration of signs and symptoms that are usually severe and begin abruptly.

acute coryza Acute rhinitis, also known as the common cold; an inflammatory condition of the mucous membranes of the nose and accessory sinuses.

acute pain Intense, unpleasant sensation of short duration, lasting less than 6 months.

adaptation Adjustment to changing life situations by using various strategies.

adaptive immunity Protection that provides a specific reaction to each invading antigen and has the unique ability to remember the antigen that caused the attack.

addiction Excessive use or abuse of a substance or practice, displayed by psychological disturbance, decline of social and economic function, and uncontrollable consumption, indicating dependence.

addictive personality One who exhibits a pattern of compulsive and habitual use of a substance or practice to cope with psychological pain from conflict and anxiety.

adduction Movement of an extremity toward the axis of the body.

adenosine triphosphate A substance produced in the mitochondria from nutrients and is capable of releasing energy that in turn enables the cell to work.

adherence Following a prescribed regimen of therapy or treatment for disease.

adjuvant Additional, as in additional drug or treatment.

admission Entry of a patient into a health care facility.
adoptive family Family unit with adoptive children who are chosen and taken into the family by legal process and raised as the family's own.
adult daycare A community-based program designed to meet the needs of functionally or cognitively impaired adults through an individualized plan of care.
advance directives Signed and witnessed documents providing specific instructions for health care treatment in the event that the person is unable to make those decisions personally at the time they are needed.
advancement Rise in rank or importance; a promotion, progress, improvement.
adventitious Abnormal sounds superimposed on breath sounds.
adverse drug reaction A harmful, unintended reaction to a drug administered at a normal dosage.
advocate A person who acts on behalf of another person.
affect External manifestation of inner feeling or emotions, often reflected by facial expression.
against medical advice (AMA) Charting notation when a patient leaves a health care facility without a physician's order for discharge.
ageism Process of systematic stereotyping of and discrimination against people because of their advanced age.
aggressive communication Interacting with another in an overpowering and forceful manner to meet one's own needs at the expense of others.
agnosia Total or partial loss of the ability to recognize familiar objects or people through sensory stimuli; results from organic brain damage.
agonist Drug that produces a predictable response at the intended site of action.
agoraphobia An anxiety disorder characterized by a fear of being in an open, crowded, or public place, such as a field, tunnel, bridge, congested streets, or busy stores, where escape may be difficult or help unavailable if anxiety incapacitates the sufferer. If untreated the sufferer often refuses to leave the home.
air embolism An abnormal circulatory condition in which air travels through the bloodstream and becomes lodged in a blood vessel.
akinesia Abnormal state of motor and psychic hypoactivity.
Alcoholics Anonymous (AA) Nonprofit organization founded in 1935 consisting of abstinent alcoholics helping other alcoholics to become and stay sober through group support.
alcoholism Addiction to alcohol.
alignment Relationship of various body parts to one another.
allergen A substance that can produce a hypersensitive reaction in the body but that is not necessarily inherently harmful.
allopathic medicine Traditional or conventional Western medicine.
alopecia Loss of hair resulting from destruction of hair follicles.
alpha-fetoprotein (AFP) Antigen present in the human fetus; can be used to evaluate fetal development.
altered cognition A decrease or lack of cognitive ability to receive, process, and send information.
alternative therapies Nontraditional therapies that may include the same interventions as complementary therapies but that often become the primary treatment modalities that replace allopathic (nontraditional) medicine. Examples are exercise, massage, acupuncture, and herbalism.
Alzheimer's disease A presenile dementia that is characterized by confusion, memory failure, disorientation, restlessness, agnosia, speech disturbances, inability to carry out purposeful movements, and hallucinosis. Also called *senile dementia—Alzheimer's type (SDAT).*
amblyopia Lazy eye; reduction or dimness of vision, especially when there is no apparent pathologic condition of the eye.
amenorrhea Absence of menstrual flow.
amino acids Building blocks out of which proteins are constructed; the end products of protein digestion.
amniocentesis Obstetric procedure in which a small amount of amniotic fluid is removed for laboratory analysis; usually performed between the 16th and 20th weeks of gestation to aid in the diagnosis of fetal abnormalities.
amniotomy Artificial rupture of the fetal membranes (AROM).
amotivational cannabis syndrome Following the use of cannabis and characterized by decreased goal-directed activities, abrupt mood swings, abnormal irritability, etc.
anabolism The building aspect on which the energy released from catabolism allows the cells to build more complex, usable forms of nutrients; the building and repairing phase of metabolism; opposite of catabolism.
anaphylactic shock Severe, life-threatening hypersensitivity reaction to a previously encountered antigen.
anasarca Severe, generalized edema.
anastomosis Surgical joining of two ducts or blood vessels to allow flow from one to the other.
anatomy The study, classification, and description of structures and organs of the body.
anemia Blood disorder characterized by red blood cell, hemoglobin, and hematocrit levels below normal range.
anesthesia Absence of sensation (*an-*meaning "without," and *-esthesia* meaning "awareness or feeling").
aneurysm A localized dilation of the wall of a blood vessel, usually caused by atherosclerosis, hypertension, and less commonly by a congenital weakness in a vessel wall.
angina pectoris Paroxysmal thoracic pain and choking feeling caused by decreased oxygen (anoxia) of the myocardium.
anion Negatively charged ion that, when in solution, is attracted to the positive electrode.
ankylosis Fixation of a joint, often in an abnormal position, usually resulting from destruction of articular cartilage and subchondral bone.
anorexia nervosa A psychoneurotic disorder characterized by a prolonged refusal to eat; self-imposed starvation.
antagonist Drug that will block the action of another drug.
antepartal First stage of the maternity cycle; also known as the prenatal or antenatal period.
anterior fontanelle A diamond-shaped space covered by tough membranes between the bones of an infant's cranium. The posterior fontanelle is triangular.
anticipatory grief Expectation of or preparation for the loss of one of more valued or significant objects; accomplishment of part of the grief work before the actual loss.
anticipatory guidance Psychological preparation of a patient for an event expected to be stressful, as in the preparation of a child for surgery by explaining what will happen and what it will feel like. It is also used to prepare parents for normal growth and development of their children.
antigen A substance recognized by the body as foreign that can trigger an immune response.
antioxidant Chemical or other agent that delays or prevents the breakdown of a substance by oxygen.

antiseptic A substance that tends to inhibit the growth and reproduction of microorganisms; may be used on humans.
anuria Urinary output of less than 100 to 250 mL in 24 hours.
anxiety Condition in which an individual experiences a vague feeling of apprehension resulting from a real or perceived threat to the self.
aphasia Abnormal neurologic condition in which language function is defective or absent because of an injury to certain areas of the cerebral cortex.
apical pulse Heartbeat as measured with the bell or disk of the stethoscope placed over the apex of the heart; represents the actual beating of the heart. Most authentic of all pulses.
aplasia In hematology, a failure of the normal process of cell generation and development.
approved program Program that meets minimum standards established by the state agency responsible for overseeing education programs.
apraxia Impairment of the ability to perform purposeful acts; inability to use objects properly.
aromatherapy An alternative therapy that uses essential oils produced from plants to provide health benefits.
arteriosclerosis Common arterial disorder characterized by thickening, loss of elasticity, and calcification of arterial walls, resulting in a decreased blood supply.
arthrocentesis Puncture of a joint with a needle to withdraw fluid; performed to obtain synovial fluid for diagnostic purposes.
arthrodesis Surgical fusion of a joint.
arthroplasty Surgical repair or refashioning of one of both sides, parts, or specific tissues within a joint.
articulate Speak clearly, distinctly, and to the point; present yourself with clarity and effectiveness.
ascites An accumulation of fluid and albumin in the peritoneal cavity.
asepsis Free of pathogenic microorganisms.
assertive communication Interaction that takes into account the feelings and needs of the receiver.
assessment Evaluation or appraisal of a condition; includes observing, gathering, verifying, and communicating pertinent data, usually information pertaining to the patient.
assisted living Residential care whereby the adult patient rents a small one-bedroom or studio apartment and can receive personal care services, for example, for bathing, dressing, eating, etc.
asterixis Hand-flapping tremor usually induced by extending the arm and dorsiflexing the wrist; frequently seen in hepatic coma.
asthenia General feeling of tiredness and listlessness.
astigmatism Defect in the curvature of the eyeball surface.
ataxia Abnormal condition characterized by impaired ability to coordinate movement.
atelectasis Collapse of lung tissues, preventing the respiratory exchange of carbon dioxide and oxygen.
atherosclerosis A common arterial disorder characterized by yellowish plaques of cholesterol, lipids, and cellular debris in the inner layer of the walls of large and medium-sized arteries.
atony Lack of normal tone or strength.
attention-deficit/hyperactivity disorder (ADHD) A group of behaviors—hyperactivity, inattentiveness, and impulsivity—that appear early in a child's life, persist throughout childhood and adolescence, and may extend into adulthood.
attenuation The process of weakening the degree of virulence of a disease organism.
attitude In obstetrics, the relationship of fetal body parts to one another.
audiometry Testing of hearing acuity.
auditors People appointed to examine patient charts and health records to assess the quality of care.
aura Sensation, as of light or warmth, that may precede the onset of a migraine or an epileptic seizure. An epileptic aura may be psychic, or it may be sensory with olfactory, visual, auditory, or taste hallucinations.
auscultate/auscultation To listen for sounds within the body to evaluate the condition of the heart, lungs, pleura, intestines, or other organs or to detect fetal heart sounds.
autism A complex developmental disorder of brain function accompanied by a broad range and severity of intellectual and behavioral deficits that impairs the child's ability for appropriate social interaction, communication skills, and behavior.
autocratic family pattern Family unit with unequal relationships; parents attempt to control with strict, rigid rules and expectations.
autograft Surgical transplantation of any tissue from one part of the body to another location in the same individual.
autoimmune/autoimmunity Immune response (autoantibodies or cellular immune response) to one's own tissues.
autologous Something that has its origin within an individual, especially a factor present in tissues or fluids.
autolysis Self-dissolution or self-digestion in tissues or cells by enzymes in the cells.
autopsy Examination performed after a person's death to confirm or determine the cause of death.
axilla Underarm area or armpit.
azotemia Retention of excessive amounts of nitrogenous compounds in the blood.

B

bacteriuria Presence of bacteria in the urine.
ballottement Technique of palpating an organ or floating structure by bouncing it gently and feeling it rebound. Ballottement of a fetus within the uterus is a probable objective sign of pregnancy.
bandage A strip or roll of cloth or other material that may be wound around part of the body in a variety of ways for multiple purposes.
basal metabolic rate (BMR) Amount of energy used by the body at rest to maintain vital functions such as respiration, circulation, temperature, peristalsis, and muscle tone.
base of support Area on which an object rests; a stance with feet slightly apart.
basic life support (BLS) The role of cardiopulmonary resuscitation (CPR) and emergency cardiac care (ECC) that prevents circulatory or respiratory function or both in the emergency treatment of a victim of cardiac or respiratory arrest.
bedpan Device for receiving feces or urine from patients confined to bed; may be used for specimen collection.
behavior Manner in which a person acts or performs; any or all of the activities of a person, including physical actions, that are observed directly, and mental activity, which is inferred and interpreted. Kinds of behavior include abnormal, automatic, invariable, and variable.
benign Not recurrent or progressive; opposite of malignant.

bereavement Common depressed reaction to the death of a loved one.

bereavement overload The individual's experience of an initial loss compounded with an additional loss, before resolution of the initial loss.

bicarbonate A main anion of the extracellular fluid.

binder Bandage made of large pieces of material to fit a specific body part (e.g., abdominal or breast binder).

biographic data Relating to the facts and events of a person's life.

biologic death Results from permanent cellular damage caused by a lack of oxygen.

biomedical health belief system A belief that health and illness are controlled by a series of physical and biochemical processes that can be analyzed and manipulated by humans. Primary health belief in the United States.

biopsy The removal of a small piece of living tissue from an organ or another part of the body for microscopic examination to confirm or establish a diagnosis, estimate a prognosis, or follow the course of a disease.

bioterrorism Use of biologic agents to create fear and threat in a terrorist act.

bipolar hip replacement (hemiarthroplasty) Prosthetic implant used to replace the femoral head and neck in hip fractures when the vascular supply to the femoral head is or may become compromised.

birth defect (congenital anomaly) Any abnormality present at birth, particularly a structural one that may be inherited genetically, acquired during gestation, or inflicted during parturition (process of giving birth).

bladder training Development of the use of the muscles of the perineum to improve voluntary control over voiding.

blanching test A test of the rate of capillary refill; blanching means to cause to become pale by applying digital pressure.

blastocyst Embryonic form that is a spheric mass of cells having a central fluid-filled cavity (blastocele) surrounded by two layers of cells; the outer layer forms the placenta, and the inner layer later forms the embryo.

blended (reconstituted) family Family unit formed by parents who bring unrelated children from prior marriages into a new, joint living situation. Also known as a stepfamily.

blood pressure Pressure exerted by the circulating volume of blood on the arterial walls, veins, and chambers of the heart.

body mass index (BMI) An estimate used to determine if a person may be at health risk because of excessive weight.

body mechanics Physiologic study of the muscular actions and the functions of muscles in maintaining the posture of the body.

body surface area (BSA) Total area exposed to the outside environment.

bonding See *parent-child attachment.* Emotional attachment between parent and child.

borborygmi Loud, gurgling sounds that accompany increased motility of the bowel.

botulism An often fatal food poisoning that results from ingestion of the toxin produced by the bacillus *Clostridium botulinum.*

bradycardia Slow rhythm characterized by a pulse rate of fewer than 60 beats per minute.

bradykinesia An abnormal condition characterized by slowness of voluntary movements and speech.

bradypnea A slow respiratory rate of fewer than 12 breaths per minute.

brain death Irreversible form of unconsciousness characterized by a complete loss of brain function while the heart continues to beat. The legal definition of this condition varies from state to state.

Braxton Hicks contractions Irregular tightening of the pregnant uterus that begins in the first trimester and increases in frequency, duration, and intensity as pregnancy progresses. Near term, strong Braxton Hicks contractions are often difficult to distinguish from real labor.

bronchoscopy Visual examination of the larynx, trachea, and bronchi using a standard rigid, tubular metal bronchoscope or a narrower, flexible fiberoptic bronchoscope.

brown fat Source of heat unique to the neonate that is capable of greater thermogenic (heat-producing) activity than ordinary fat. Deposits are formed around the adrenal glands, kidneys, and neck; between scapulas; and behind the sternum, and they remain for several weeks after birth.

bruit Abnormal swishing sound heard over organs, glands, and arteries.

bruxism Teeth-grinding.

B-type natriuretic peptide (BNP) A neurohormone secreted by the heart in response to ventricular expansion.

buccal In or directed toward the cheek.

buffer Chemical system that circulates through the body in pairs, neutralizing excess acids or bases by contributing of accepting hydrogen ions; can be considered chemical sponges.

bulimia nervosa An eating disorder involving an insatiable craving for food, often resulting in continual eating followed by periods of depression, self-deprivation, and/or purging; also called *bulimia.*

burnout Physical, emotional, and spiritual exhaustion among caregivers.

burping Belching, or eructation.

C

cachexia General ill health and malnutrition marked by weakness and emaciation; usually associated with a serious disease such as cancer.

calcium Silvery yellow metal; the most abundant mineral in the body; a positively charged ion, known as a cation.

callus Bony deposits formed between and around the broken ends of a fractured bone during healing.

candidiasis Mild fungal infection that appears in men and women; usually caused by *Candida albicans* and *C. tropicalis.*

cannabis Marijuana.

canthus Angle at the medial and lateral margins of the eyelid (inner or outer corners of the eye).

carcinoembryonic antigen (CEA) Oncofetal glycoprotein antigen found in colonic adenocarcinoma and other cancers; also found in nonmalignant conditions.

carcinogen Substance known to increase the risk for the development of cancer.

carcinogenesis Various factors that are possible origins of cancer.

carcinoma The term used for a malignant tumor composed of epithelial cells; it displays a tendency to metastasize.

carcinoma in situ Preinvasive, asymptomatic carcinoma that can be diagnosed only by microscopic examination of cervical cells.

cardiac arrest Sudden cessation of functional circulation.

cardiopulmonary resuscitation (CPR) Basic emergency procedure for life support, consisting of artificial respiration and manual external cardiac massage.

cardioversion Restoration of the heart's normal sinus rhythm by delivery of a synchronized electric shock through two metal paddles placed on the patient's chest.

career A profession for which one trains and is undertaken as a permanent calling.

carrier Person or animal who harbors and spreads an organism, causing disease in others but does not itself become ill.

case management The assignment of a health care provider to oversee the case of an individual patient.

catabolism Breakdown or destructive phase of metabolism. Catabolism occurs when complex body substances are broken down to simpler ones; opposite of anabolism.

cataract Opacity or clouding of the lens.

catheterization Introduction of a rubber or plastic tube through the urethra and into the bladder.

cation Positively charged ion that, when in solution, is attracted to the negatively charged electrode.

CD_4^+ lymphocyte A type of white blood cell; a protein on the surface of cells that normally helps the body's immune system combat disease.

cell The fundamental unit of all living tissue.

cellular immunity Acquired immunity characterized by the dominant role of small T lymphocytes; also called *cell-mediated immunity.*

Centers for Disease Control and Prevention (CDC) Federal agency that provides facilities and services for investigation, identification, prevention, and control of disease; headquartered in Atlanta, Georgia.

cephalocaudal Growth and development that proceeds from the head toward the feet. The infant's head is large compared with the rest of the body.

cephalopelvic disproportion The head of the fetus is larger than the pelvic outlet. Also referred to as pelvic disproportion.

cerclage Technique that uses suture material to constrict the internal os of the cervix. Aids in preserving the pregnancy.

certification Process in which an individual or institution, agency, or educational program is evaluated and recognized as meeting certain predetermined standards.

cerumen Yellowish or brownish waxy secretion produced by vestigial apocrine sweat glands in the external ear canal; earwax.

chancre Painless erosion of a papule that ulcerates superficially with a scooped-out appearance.

chart (health care record) Legal record that is used to meet many demands of the health accreditation, medical insurance, and legal systems.

charting Process of recording information on a patient's chart.

charting by exception Recording only new data or changes in patient status or care; charting the exceptions to the previously recorded data.

charting, documenting, or recording Process of noting data in a patient record, usually at prescribed intervals.

chelation therapy In toxicology, use of a compound to group a toxic substance and make it inactive and thus nontoxic. Chelating agents are used in the treatment of metal poisoning.

chevron A method of applying tape to secure an intravenous line; a narrow piece (½-inch wide) of sterile tape is placed under hub of catheter with adhesive side up and then criss-crossed over the hub to form an inverted V. This method is no longer frequently used.

Cheyne-Stokes respiration An abnormal pattern of respiration characterized by alternating periods of apnea and deep, rapid breathing.

child maltreatment Physical and emotional neglect, and physical, emotional, and sexual abuse of children.

children with special needs Infants and children with congenital abnormalities, malignancies, gastrointestinal diseases, and central nervous system anomalies.

chiropractic therapy Nontraditional therapy that includes manipulation of the musculoskeletal system.

Chlamydia trachomatis A gram-negative intracellular bacterium that causes several common sexually transmitted diseases.

chloride Negatively charged extracellular anion; a salt of hydrochloric acid.

cholesterol Fat-soluble sterol found in animal fats and oils, organ meats, and egg yolk.

chorionic villi Tiny vascular protrusions of the chorionic surface that project into the maternal blood sinuses of the uterus and help form the placenta. This occurs when conception has occurred.

chromosomes Threadlike structures in the nucleus of a cell that function in the transmission of genetic information.

chronic Developing slowly and persisting for a long period, often for the remainder of an individual's life.

chronic illness An irreversible presence, accumulation, or latency of disease states or impairments that involve the total human environment for supportive care, function, and prevention of further disability.

chronic pain Pain lasting longer than 6 months; can be as intense as acute pain; can be continuous or intermittent.

chronologic age Age of an individual expressed as time elapsed since birth.

Chux Waterproof, disposable underpad.

Chvostek's sign Abnormal spasm of the facial muscles elicited by light taps on the facial nerve in patients who are hypocalcemic; seen in tetany.

circumcision Surgical procedure in which a part of the foreskin is removed, leaving the glans penis uncovered.

circumorbital Around an orbit; often referring to the eye.

clarifying Restating the patient's message in a manner that asks the patient to verify that the message received is accurate.

claudication Weakness of the legs accompanied by cramp-like pain in the calves caused by poor circulation of the blood to the leg muscles.

climacteric Phase of the aging process marking the transition from the reproductive phase to a nonreproductive stage of life.

clinical death Occurs when heartbeat and respiration have ceased.

clinical pathway Multidisciplinary plan that schedules clinical interventions over an anticipated time frame for high-risk, high-volume, high-cost types of cases.

closed posture A formal, distant stance, generally with the arms and possibly the legs tightly crossed.

closed question Focused question that seeks a particular answer (e.g., yes or no).

club drugs Drugs taken for euphoric effect at parties, concerts, dance clubs, raves.

code System of notification that allows information to be transmitted rapidly.

cognitive impairment Significantly subaverage general intellectual functioning; existing concurrently with deficits in adaptive behavior and manifested during developmental period (formerly referred to as mental retardation).

collaborative problem Actual or potential health problem (complication) that focuses on the pathophysiologic response of the body of which nurses are responsible and accountable for identification and treatment in collaboration with the physician.

collagen Fibrous insoluble protein found in connective tissue, including skin, bone, and ligaments.

Colles' fracture A fracture of the distal portion of the radius within 1 inch of the joint of the wrist.

colostrum Breast fluid that may be excreted from the second trimester of pregnancy onward but is most evident in the first 2 or 3 days after birth and before the onset of true lactation. This thin yellowish fluid is rich in proteins and calories, in addition to antibodies and lymphocytes.

colporrhaphy Surgical correction of cystocele and rectocele by shortening the muscles that support the bladder and repair the rectocele.

colposcopy Examination of the cervix and vagina using a colposcope.

Commission on Accreditation of Rehabilitation Facilities (CARF) A not-for-profit, private, international standards–setting and accreditation body. Its mission is to promote and advocate delivery of quality rehabilitation. It is governed by a board of trustees who are responsible for accreditation decisions. Surveyors are peers involved in administrative or professional positions within an organization that is eligible for CARF accreditation.

communication Use of words and behaviors to construct, send, and interpret messages.

compartment syndrome Pathologic condition caused by progressive development of arterial compression and reduced blood supply to an extremity. Increased pressure from external devices (casts, bulky dressings) causes decreased blood flow, resulting in ischemic tissue necrosis; most often occurs in the extremities.

compatibility Quality or state of existing together in harmony.

complementary therapies/complementary and alternative therapies Therapies that are used in addition or as a complement to nontraditional therapies. Examples are exercise, massage, reflexology, acupuncture, and herbalism.

comprehensive rehabilitation plan An overall individualized plan of care that is initiated within 24 hours of admission and ready for review and revision by the team within 3 days of admission for each individual; a planned, orderly sequence of services for a disabled individual designed to help the patient realize maximum potential.

compress A soft pad, usually made of cloth, used to apply heat, cold, or medication to the surface of a body area, or over a wound to help control bleeding.

compulsion Irresistible, repetitive, irrational impulse to perform an act that is usually contrary to one's ordinary judgments or standards yet results in overt anxiety if not completed.

conception (fertilization) Beginning of pregnancy.

concrete operational phase Phase of Piaget's theory in which thoughts become increasingly logical and coherent so that the child is able to classify, sort, and organize facts while still being incapable of generalizing or dealing with abstractions; occurs between 7 and 10 years of age.

conflict Mental struggle, either conscious or subconscious, resulting from the simultaneous presence of opposing or incompatible thoughts, ideas, goals, or emotional forces, such as impulses, desires, or drives.

congenital heart disease (CHD) An abnormality or anomaly of the heart, present at birth.

conjunctivitis Inflammation of the conjunctiva.

connotative meaning Reflects the individual's perception or interpretation of a given word.

conscious sedation Administration of central nervous system depressant drugs and/or analgesia to relieve anxiety and/or provide amnesia during surgical, diagnostic, or interventional procedures.

contamination Condition of being soiled, stained, touched, or otherwise exposed to harmful agents by the entry of infectious or toxic material into a previously clean or sterile environment; making an object potentially unsafe for use as intended.

continuing care retirement community Offers complete range of housing and health care accommodations from independent to 24-hour skilled nursing care.

continuity of care Continuing of established patient care from one setting to another.

contract Promise or a set of promises between two or more people that creates a legal relationship between them and a legal obligation that one or more of them must fulfill.

contracture Abnormal, usually permanent condition of a joint characterized by flexion and fixation and caused by atrophy and shortening of muscle fibers.

contusion An injury that does not break the skin, is caused by a blow, and is characterized by edema, discoloration, and pain.

coping responses Voluntary patterns of behavior used to relieve stress or anxiety.

cor pulmonale Abnormal cardiac condition characterized by hypertrophy of the right ventricle of the heart as a result of hypertension of the pulmonary circulation.

coronary artery disease (CAD) Variety of conditions that obstruct blood flow in the coronary arteries.

coryza Acute inflammation of the mucous membranes of the nose and accessory sinuses, usually accompanied by edema of the mucosa and nasal discharge.

costovertebral angle Pertaining to a rib and a vertebra; one of two angles that outline a space over the kidneys.

cotyledon One of the 15 to 28 visible segments of the placenta on the maternal surface, each made up of fetal vessels, chorionic villi, and intervillous space.

crackle(s) Short, discrete, interrupted crackling or bubbling adventitious breath sounds heard on auscultation of the chest, most commonly upon inspiration. They are produced by passage of air through the bronchi that contain secretions of exudate or are constricted by spasms or thickening; usually heard during inspiration; formerly called rales.

crepitus Sound that resembles the crackling noise heard when rubbing hair between the fingers or throwing salt on an open fire. It is associated with gas gangrene, the rubbing of bone fragments, or the crackles of a consolidated area of the lung in pneumonia.

crime Breaking of any law; an offense to society that is punishable.

crisis Time of change or turning point in life when patterns of living must be modified to prevent disorganization of the person or family.

cryosurgery Procedure to "freeze" the border of a retinal hole with a frozen-tipped probe.

cryotherapy A procedure in which a topical anesthetic is used so that a cryoprobe can be placed directly on the surface of the eye.

cryptorchidism Failure of testes to descend into the scrotum.

cue Word, phrase, or symptom that indicates the nature of something perceived. Cues are grouped to assist the nurse in interpretation of data, as in formulating the patient's plan of care.

culdoscopy Diagnostic procedure that provides visualization of the uterus and adnexa (uterine appendages that include the ovaries and fallopian tubes).

cultural competence Awareness by the nurse of his or her own cultural belief practices and an understanding of the limitations that these beliefs put on the nurse when dealing with those from other cultures. This understanding should give the nurse the ability to react to others with openness to and understanding and acceptance of cultural differences between them.

cultural healing beliefs Beliefs that reflect a specific culture's orientation to health and illness.

culture (1) A set of learned values, beliefs, customs, and practices that are shared by a group and passed from one generation to another. (2) A laboratory test involving cultivation of microorganisms or cells in a special growth medium.

cumulative A drug that builds up in the body; can lead to a toxic or even lethal (deadly) effect.

curative treatment Aggressive care with the goal and intent of curing the disease and prolonging life at all costs.

curettage Scraping of material from the wall of a cavity or other surface; performed to remove tumors or other abnormal tissue for microscopic study.

Curling's ulcer Duodenal ulcer that develops 8 to 14 days after severe burns on the surface of the body; the first sign is usually vomiting of bright red blood.

currant jelly stools Feces mixed with blood and mucus from the intestinal mucosa.

customs Habitual practices; the usual way of acting under given circumstances.

cyanosis Slightly bluish, gray, slatelike, or dark purple discoloration of the skin resulting from the presence of abnormally reduced amounts of oxygenated hemoglobin in the blood.

cyclothymic disorder A pattern that involves repeated mood swings of hypomania and depression but are less intense than with bipolar disorder. There are no periods of "normal function" with this condition. It is thought to be a muted version of bipolar disorder.

cytology/cytologic evaluation Study of cells and their formation, origin, structure, biochemical activities, and pathology.

cytoplasm "Living matter"; a substance that exists only in cells, composed largely of a gel-like substance that contains water, minerals, enzymes, and other specialized materials.

D

database Large store or bank of information, as in forming the patient's nursing diagnosis.

death Cessation of life.

debridement Removal of damaged cellular tissue from a wound or burn to prevent infection and promote healing.

deciduous teeth Set of 20 teeth that normally appear during infancy.

deep brain stimulation (DBS) Involves placing an electrode in either the thalamus, globus pallidus, or subthalamic nucleus and connecting it to a generator placed in the upper chest (like a pacemaker).

defecation Elimination of bowel waste.

defense mechanisms Unconscious, intrapsychic reactions that offer protection to the self from stressful situations.

defibrillation The termination of ventricular fibrillation by delivering a direct electrical countershock to the precordium.

defining characteristics Clinical signs and symptoms that a problem exists.

dehiscence Partial or complete separation of a surgical incision or rupture of a wound closure.

deinstitutionalization Release of institutional psychiatric patients to be treated in the community setting.

delirium An acute, organic mental disorder characterized by confusion, disorientation, clouding of consciousness, incoherence, fear, anxiety, excitement, and often illusions and hallucinations. Symptoms are of short duration and reversible with treatment of the underlying cause. An example may be fever or electrolyte imbalance.

delirium tremens (DTs) An acute psychotic reaction that is a complication of alcohol withdrawal.

delusion A persistent, aberrant belief or perception held inviolable by a person despite evidence to the contrary.

dementia A slow, progressive, organic mental disorder characterized by chronic personality disintegration, deterioration of intellectual capacity and function, and memory loss that leads to confusion, disorientation, and stupor. An example is Alzheimer's disease.

democratic family pattern Family style in which the adult members are considered equal and children are treated with respect and recognized as individuals.

dendrite Branching process that extends from the cell body of a neuron and receives impulses.

denominator Bottom number of a fraction.

denotative meaning The commonly accepted definition of a particular word.

dentures Artificial teeth not permanently fixed or implanted.

deposition Out-of-court, under-oath statement of a witness.

depressant A drug that depresses the central nervous system, such as alcohol, sedative-hypnotic medications, and opioid analgesics.

depression An emotional disorder brought on by an imbalance of the neurotransmitter serotonin in the brain, which brings about exaggerated feelings of sadness, melancholy, emptiness, worthlessness, and frustration. Fatigue, inability to concentrate, short-term memory loss, and sleep pattern disturbance, as well as slowed body functions, can be seen with this disorder.

descent In obstetrics, the downward progress of the presenting part belonging to the fetus. The amount of progress measured by comparing the lowest point of the presenting part with the ischial spines of the mother.

detoxification Removal of poisonous effects of a substance from a patient.

development Gradual process or change and differentiation from a simple to a more advanced level of complexity.

diabetes mellitus (See type 1 diabetes mellitus; type 2 diabetes mellitus.)

diabetic retinopathy Disorder of retinal blood vessels characterized by capillary microaneurysms, hemorrhage, exudates, and formation of new vessels and connective tissue.

diagnose To identify a disease or condition by a scientific evaluation of physical signs, symptoms, history, laboratory tests, and procedures.

diagnosis-related group (DRG) System that classifies patients by age, diagnoses, and surgical categories; used to predict the use of hospital resources, including the length of stay.

dialysis Medical procedure for the removal of certain elements from the blood or lymph by virtue of the difference in their rates of diffusion through an external semipermeable membrane or, in the case of peritoneal dialysis, through the peritoneum.

diaphoresis The secretion of sweat, especially the profuse secretion of sweat.

diastole The period of time between contractions of the atria or the ventricles, during which blood enters the relaxed chambers from the systemic circulation and the lungs.

diastolic pressure The second number recorded in the blood pressure reading; represents the minimum level of blood pressure measured between the contractions of the heart.

dietary fiber Generic term for nondigestible chemical substances in plants.

differentiated Describes a tumor that is most like the parent tissue.

differentiation Process of cellular development in which unspecialized cells or tissues are systematically modified to achieve specific and characteristic physical forms, physiologic functions, and chemical properties.

diffusion A process in which solid particles in a fluid move from an area of higher concentration to an area of lower concentration.

dilemma Situation requiring a choice between two equally desirable or undesirable alternatives.

diplopia Double vision.

direct Coombs' test Laboratory blood test to detect autoantibodies against red blood cells, which can cause cellular damage. These antibodies result in hemolytic anemia. Normal findings: negative, no agglutination.

disability Any restriction or lack (resulting from an impairment) of an ability to perform an activity in the manner or within the range considered normal for a human being.

disaster manual Written agency instructions specifying departmental responsibilities, chain of command, callback procedures for the receipt and management of casualties, and policies related to the overall management of supplies and equipment.

disaster situation Uncontrollable, unexpected, psychologically shocking event.

discharge Release of a patient from a health care facility.

discharge planning Schedule of events often planned by a multidisciplinary team leading to the return of a patient from hospital confinement to life at home or another health care setting.

disease Any disturbance of a structure or function of the body; a pathologic condition of the body.

disengagement stage Period of family life when the grown children depart from the home. In some family units this stage is brief because the adult children return to live in the family home.

disinfectant A chemical that can be applied to objects to destroy microorganisms.

disinfection Process by which pathogens, but not necessarily their spores, are destroyed.

disorientation Mental confusion characterized by inadequate or incorrect perceptions of place, time, and identity.

disoriented Having lost awareness or perception of space, time, or personal identity and relationships.

disseminated intravascular coagulation (DIC) Acquired hemorrhage syndrome of clotting, cascade overstimulation, and anticlotting processes.

diuresis Secretion and passage of large amounts of urine.

dizygotic Of or pertaining to twins from two fertilized ova.

Do not resuscitate (DNR) A note written in a patient's record and signed by a qualified attending physician instructing the staff of the institution not to attempt to resuscitate the patient in the event of cardiac or respiratory failure. Also called *no code.*

documenting Process of adding information to the chart, usually at prescribed intervals.

dominant group Group of people exercising authority or influence; ruling or prevailing group.

Dorothea Dix A retired teacher who was appalled by the care of the mentally ill. In 1841, she began her crusade for placing individuals with mental illnesses in specially built hospitals. Her efforts brought millions of dollars toward developing mental hospitals in the United States.

dorsal Toward the back.

dorsal (supine) Lying horizontally on the back.

dorsal recumbent Supine position with patient lying on the back, with head, shoulders, and extremities moderately flexed and legs extended.

dorsiflexion Bending or flexing backward, as in upward bending of the fingers, wrist, foot, or toes.

double bagging Infection control practice of placing a bag of contaminated items into another bag that is clean and held outside the isolation room by a second staff member.

Down syndrome A congenital condition characterized by varying degrees of cognitive disability and multiple physical defects.

drainage Free flow or withdrawal of fluids from a wound or cavity by some sort of system (such as a urinary catheter or T-tube).

DRG See *diagnosis-related group.*

drip factor A method that is used to deliver measured amounts of intravenous solutions at specific flow rates based on the size of drops of the solution.

drug interaction Modification of the effect of a drug when administered with another drug.

dullness Low-pitched thudlike sound upon percussion of the body.

dumping syndrome Combination of profuse perspiration, nausea, vertigo, and weakness experienced by patients who have had a subtotal gastrectomy; symptoms are felt soon after eating, when the contents of the stomach empty too rapidly into the duodenum.

durable power of attorney A written determination that appoints another person to make decisions in the event of the patient's incompetence. Usually completed by a patient while still able to function.

dysarthria Difficult, poorly articulated speech resulting from interference in the control over the muscles of speech.

dysfunctional grieving Unresolved grief or complicated mourning.

dysmenorrhea Painful menstruation.

dysphagia Difficulty swallowing.

dyspnea Shortness of breath or difficulty in breathing; may be caused by disturbances in the lungs, certain heart conditions, and hemoglobin deficiency.

dysrhythmia Any disturbance or abnormality in a normal rhythmic pattern, specifically irregularity in the normal rhythm of the heart; also called *arrhythmia.*

dysuria Painful or difficult urination.

E

ecchymosis Discoloration of an area of the skin or mucous membrane caused by the extravasation of blood into the subcutaneous tissues. Also called a *bruise.*

eclampsia Most severe form of pregnancy-induced hypertension (also referred to as gestational hypertension [GH]), characterized by toxic and grand mal convulsions, coma, hypertension, albuminuria, and edema.

ectoderm Outer layer of embryonic tissue that gives rise to skin, nails, and hair.

ectopic pregnancy Implantation of the fertilized ovum outside the uterine cavity in, for example, the abdomen, fallopian tubes, or ovaries.

edema Abnormal accumulation of fluids in interstitial spaces of tissue; a combining form meaning swelling.

effacement Thinning and shortening of the cervix as it is stretched and dilated by the fetus. This occurs during late pregnancy, labor, or both.

electrocardiogram (ECG) Graphic representation of electrical impulses generated by the heart during a cardiac cycle.

electrolyte Substance that is sometimes called a mineral or salt; develops tiny electrical charges when dissolved in water and breaks up into particles known as ions.

embolism An abnormal circulatory condition in which an embolus (e.g., a foreign substance, blood clot, fat, air, or amniotic fluid) travels through the bloodstream and becomes lodged in a blood vessel.

embolus A foreign object, quantity of air or gas, bit of tissue or tumor, or a piece of thrombus that circulates in the bloodstream until it becomes lodged in a vessel.

emergency medical services (EMS) National network of services coordinated to provide aid and medical assistance from primary response to definitive care, involving personnel trained in the rescue, stabilization, transportation, and advanced treatment of traumatic or medical emergencies.

empathy Ability to recognize and, to some extent, share the emotions and states of mind of another and to understand the meaning and significance of that person's behavior.

empyema Accumulation of pus in a body cavity, especially the pleural space, as a result of infection.

en face position Position in which the adult's face and the infant's face are approximately 8 inches apart, as when the mother holds the infant up in front of her face or when she nurses the infant.

endarterectomy Surgical removal of the intimal lining of an artery.

endocrinologist Physician who specializes in endocrinology.

endoderm Innermost cell layer; from the endoderm arises the lining of cavities and passages of the body and covering for most internal organs.

endogenous Growing within the body; originating from within the body, or produced from internal causes, such as a disease caused by the structural or functional failure of an organ or system.

endometriosis Condition in which endometrial tissue appears outside the uterus.

endorphin Any one of the neuropeptides composed of many amino acids, elaborated by the pituitary gland and acting on the central and peripheral nervous systems to reduce pain.

endorsement Statement of recognition of the license of a health practitioner in one state by another.

enema The instillation of a solution into the rectum of the sigmoid colon for the purpose of evacuating the bowel or introducing a medication.

engagement Fixation of the presenting part of the fetus in the maternal pelvis. The lowest part of the presenting part is at or below the level of the ischial spines.

engagement/commitment stage Period when the couple prepares for marriage and becomes free of parental domination.

engorgement Process of swelling of the breast tissue brought about by an increase in blood and lymph supply to the breast; occurs around 48 hours postpartum and usually reaches a peak between the third and fifth days.

enteral Within, or by way of, the intestine.

enteral nutrition Administration of nutrients into the gastrointestinal tract; usually referred to as tube feeding.

enteric-coated Encasement of a tablet in a candylike-coated shell to prevent medications from being absorbed in the stomach; absorption takes place in the intestine.

enucleation Surgical removal of the eyeball.

enzyme-linked immunosorbent assay (ELISA) Antibody test that uses a rapid enzyme immunochemical assay method to detect HIV antibodies.

epididymitis Infection of the cordlike excretory duct of the testicles.

episiotomy Surgical incision of the perineum at the end of the second stage of labor to facilitate delivery and avoid laceration of the perineum.

epistaxis Hemorrhage from the nose; nosebleed.

epistaxis digitorum Self-inflicted local digital trauma (i.e., from nose-picking).

erythema Redness or inflammation of the skin or mucous membranes resulting from dilation and congestion of superficial capillaries. Examples are mild sunburn, nervous blushes, injury resulting from trauma or infection.

erythematous Pertaining to erythema (redness).

erythroblastosis fetalis Hemolytic anemia in newborns resulting from maternal-fetal blood group incompatibility, especially involving the Rh factor and ABO blood groups.

erythrocytosis Abnormal increase in the number of circulating red blood cells.

erythropoiesis The process of red blood cell production.

eschar Black, leathery crust; a slough that the body forms over burned tissue.

esophageal varices A complex of longitudinal, tortuous veins at the lower end of the esophagus.

essential nutrient Carbohydrates, proteins, fats, minerals, vitamins, and water necessary for growth, normal function, and body maintenance. These substances must be supplied by food; they are not synthesized by the body in the quantities required for normal health.

establishment stage Period in a couple's life between their wedding and the birth of their first child.

ethical dilemma Situation that does not have a clear correct or incorrect answer.

ethics The way one should behave; how a person ought to act.

ethnic stereotype A fixed concept of how all members of an ethnic group act or think.

ethnicity A group of people who share a common social and cultural heritage based on traditions, national origin, and physical and biologic characteristics. They often share social practices such as language, religion, dress, music, and food.

ethnocentrism A perception that the practices and beliefs of one's own culture are superior to those of other cultures.

etiology The study of all factors that may be involved in the development of a disease; the cause of disease.

euthanasia Deliberately bringing about the death of a person who is suffering from an incurable disease or condition; can be done actively or passively.

evaluation The determination made about the extent to which the established outcomes have been achieved in the nursing care plan.

evisceration Protrusion of an internal organ through a disrupted wound or surgical incision.

exacerbation An increase in the seriousness of a disease or disorder; marked by greater intensity in the signs or symptoms of the patient being treated.

excoriation Injury to the surface layer of skin caused by scratching or abrasion.

exogenous Outside the body; originating outside the body or produced from external causes, such as a disease caused by a bacterial or viral agent foreign to the body.

exophthalmos An abnormal condition characterized by a marked protrusion of the eyeballs.

expectant stage The period of family life that begins when conception occurs and continues through the pregnancy.

expectorate To eject mucus, sputum, or fluids from the trachea and lungs by coughing or spitting.

expressive aphasia A physiologic condition in which an individual is unable to communicate a desired message.

expulsion Having the tendency to drive out or expel.

extended family A family group consisting of the biologic parents, their children, the grandparents, and other family members.

extension Movement allowed by certain joints of the skeleton that increases the angle between two adjoining bones.

external rotation Occurs as the head and body move through the birth canal, using the same maneuvers as the head. The shoulders are delivered similarly to the fetal head, with the anterior shoulder pressing under the symphysis pubis, which again acts as a leverage point and assists in delivery of the posterior shoulder.

extracellular Fluid outside the cells of the body.

extravasation The escape of fluids into surrounding tissue.

extremes Outer terms of the proportion. Very severe or drastic.

extrinsic Caused by external factors.

exudate Fluid, cells, or other substances that have been slowly exuded or discharged from body cells or blood vessels through small pores or breaks in cell membrane.

F

failure to thrive The abnormal retardation of growth and development of the infant resulting from conditions that interfere with normal metabolism, appetite, and activity.

family-centered care Philosophy of care that recognizes the family as the constant in the child's life and holds that systems and personnel must support, respect, encourage, and enhance the strengths and competence of the family.

febrile Body temperature above normal.

feces Waste from the intestine; bowel movement (BM).

fetal lie Relationship existing between the long axis of the fetus and the long axis of the mother.

fetal position The relationship of the occiput, sacrum, chin, or scapula on the presenting part of the fetus to its location in the front, back, or sides of the maternal pelvis.

fetal presentation The part of the fetus that enters the pelvis first and lies over the inlet; head, face, feet, or shoulders.

fetopelvic disproportion Also referred to as cephalopelvic disproportion—the head of the fetus is larger than the pelvic outlet.

fibromyalgia A musculoskeletal chronic pain syndrome of unknown etiology that causes pain in muscles, bones, or joints.

filtration The transfer of water and dissolved substances from an area of higher pressure to an area of lower pressure.

fistula Abnormal opening between two organs.

fixative Any substance used to preserve gross or histologic specimens of tissue for examination.

flaccid Weak, soft, and flabby; lacking normal muscle tone.

flagellation Whiplike movement.

flail chest Two or more ribs fractured in two or more places resulting in instability in part of the chest wall with associated hemothorax, pneumothorax, and pulmonary contusion.

flatness Soft, high-pitched, flat sound produced by performing percussion over tissue such as muscle tissue.

flatulence Excess formation of gases in the stomach or intestine.

flatus Air or gas in the intestine that is passed through the rectum.

flexion Movement of certain joints that decreases the angle between two adjoining bones.

focus charting Expansion of the data and need columns in nurses' notes to include topics concerning the whole patient, such as behavior or treatment and response. The charting format is data, action, response (DAR).

focused assessment Concentration of attention on the part of the body where signs and symptoms are localized or most active in order to determine their significance.

focusing A communication technique used when more specific information is needed to accurately understand the patient's message.

folk health belief system Belief that health and illness are controlled by supernatural forces. May use native healers, plants, religious rituals, and prayers.

fomite Nonliving material, such as bed linens, stethoscope, needles, and many other objects that may host and transfer pathogenic microorganisms.

fontanelle Broad area or soft spot consisting of a strong bond of connective tissue between an infant's cranial bones.

formal operational thought phase Piaget's phase that begins during adolescence, permitting abstract reasoning and systematic scientific problem solving.

foster family Family unit that cares for, supervises, and nurtures children whose parents are unable to care for them.

functional assessment The assessment of the functional status of the patient, which is the ability of an individual to perform normal, expected, or required activities of daily living.

functional disease May be manifested as an organic disease, but careful examination fails to reveal evidence of structural or physiologic abnormalities.
functional limitation Any loss or ability to perform tasks and obligations of usual roles and normal daily life.

G

gate control theory Suggests that pain impulses can be regulated or even blocked by gating mechanisms located along the central nervous system.
gateway drug A drug, for example, alcohol, that is the first drug of abuse, later followed by other drugs.
gauge A standard or scale of measurement.
genupectoral Patient kneels so weight of body is supported by knees and chest.
gerontologic rehabilitation nursing Specialty practice that focuses on the unique requirements of elderly rehabilitation patients.
gestational diabetes mellitus (GDM) Disorder characterized by an impaired ability to metabolize carbohydrates, usually caused by a deficiency of insulin; occurs in pregnancy and disappears after delivery but in some cases returns years later.
gestures Movements used to emphasize the idea being communicated.
Glasgow coma scale A quick, practical, standardized system for assessing the degree of conscious impairment in the critically ill; also used for predicting the duration and ultimate outcome of coma, primarily in patients with head injuries.
glaucoma An abnormal condition of elevated pressure within an eye because of obstruction of the outflow of aqueous humor.
global cognitive dysfunction Generalized impairment of intellect, awareness, and judgment.
glomerulonephritis Inflammation of the glomeruli of the kidney.
glycogen Polysaccharide that is the major carbohydrate stored in animal cells.
glycosuria Abnormal presence of sugar, especially glucose in the urine.
glycosylated hemoglobin This test produces an accurate long-term index of the patient's average blood glucose level by measuring the patient's glycohemoglobin (GHB). Glycohemoglobin is a minor hemoglobin that makes up 4% to 8% of the total hemoglobin. It is a combination of hemoglobin and blood glucose. This test can have a blood sample drawn at any time because it is not affected by short-term variations. This test reflects the average blood sugar level for the 100- to 120-day period before the test.
goal The purpose to which an effort is directed.
Good Samaritan law Legal stipulation for protection of those who give first aid in an emergency situation.
Goodell's sign Softening of the uterine cervix; a probable sign of pregnancy.
Gowers' sign Classic sign of Duchenne's muscular dystrophy; the child positions on all fours and uses the hands to walk up the thighs.
graduated Container that has interval markings of measurement.
granulation Soft, pink, fleshy projection consisting of capillaries surrounded by fibrous collagen that slowly fills the incision during process of healing.
gravida A pregnant woman.
grief A pattern of physical and emotional responses to bereavement, separation, or loss; a natural response to loss.
grief therapy Mental treatment aimed at helping an individual deal with the pain of loss; a program in assisting the bereaved to cope with their loss.
grief work Adaptation process of mourning a loss.
group therapy Provides a caring, emotionally supportive atmosphere for a patient in a recovery program.
growth Increase in the size of an organism or any of its parts.
gynecomastia Development of abnormally large mammary glands in a male that sometimes may secrete milk. When observed in the newborn, it is in response to maternal hormones; may be noted in either sex of the newborn.

H

hallucination A sensory experience without a stimulus trigger that occurs in the waking state. It can occur in any of the senses.
hallucinogen A drug that alters perception and thinking.
handicap A disadvantage for a given individual resulting from an impairment or disability that limits or prevents the fulfillment of a role that is normal for the particular individual.
harlequin sign Rare color change of no pathologic significance occurring between the longitudinal halves of the newborn's body; when the infant is placed on one side, the dependent half is noticeably pinker than the superior half.
Hazard Communication Act Requires hospitals to inform employees about the presence of or potential for harmful exposures and how to reduce the risk of exposures.
health A condition of physical, mental, and social well-being and the absence of disease or other abnormal conditions.
health care facility Agency or institution that provides health care.
health care system The complete network of agencies, facilities, and all providers of health care in a specific geographic area.
Healthcare Integrity and Protection Data Bank (HIPDB) National data bank created in 1999 to which federal and state agencies report all final adverse actions taken against a health care provider.
heart failure (HF) Syndrome characterized by circulatory congestion due to the heart's inability to act as an effective pump; it should be viewed as a neurohormonal problem in which pathology progresses as a result of chronic release in the body of substances such as catecholamines (epinephrine and norepinephrine).
Hegar's sign Softening of the isthmus of the uterine cervix early in gestation; a probable sign of pregnancy.
Heimlich maneuver An emergency procedure for dislodging a bolus of food or other obstruction from the trachea to prevent asphyxiation.
hemarthrosis Bleeding into a joint space, a hallmark of severe disease usually occurring in the knees, ankles, and elbow.
hematemesis Vomiting blood.
hematuria Blood in the urine.
hemianopia Defective vision or blindness in half of the visual field.
hemiplegia Paralysis of one side of the body.
Hemoccult test Detects occult (hidden) blood feces.
hemophilia A Hereditary coagulation disorder; caused by a lack of antihemophilic factor VIII, which is needed to convert prothrombin to thrombin through thromboplastin component.

hemoptysis Expectorating blood from the respiratory tract.

hemothorax Collection of blood into the pleural space.

hepatic encephalopathy A type of brain damage caused by a liver disease and consequent ammonia intoxication.

hepatitis Inflammation of the liver resulting from several causes, including several types of viral agents or exposure to toxic substances.

herbal therapy An alternative therapy that uses herbs to provide health benefits.

heterograft (xenograft) Tissue from another species, used as a temporary graft.

heterozygous Having two different genes.

high-risk pregnancy Condition in which the life or health of the mother or infant is jeopardized by a disorder coincidental with or unique to pregnancy.

HIPAA The most recent federal law governing patient privacy is the Health Insurance Portability and Accountability Act (HIPAA) of 1996, which went into effect on April 14, 2003. It mandates national standards for protecting all verbal or documented health information from improper alteration, access, or loss. The goal is to ensure the security and privacy of this data.

hirsutism Excessive body hair in a masculine distribution.

HIV disease Symptomatic human immunodeficiency virus (HIV) infection that is not severe enough for a diagnosis of acquired immunodeficiency syndrome (AIDS); symptoms of HIV disease are persistent unexplained fever, night sweats, diarrhea, weight loss, and fatigue.

HIV infection State in which HIV enters the body and, under favorable conditions, multiplies, producing injurious effects to the body.

holistic Pertaining to the total patient care that considers the physical, emotional, social, economic, and spiritual needs of the person.

holistic health belief system Belief that forces of nature must be kept in natural balance or harmony.

holistic health care A system of comprehensive or total patient care that considers the physical, emotional, social, economic, and spiritual needs of the person; the response to the illness and the effect of the illness on the person's ability to meet self-care needs.

Homans' sign Early sign of thrombophlebitis of the deep veins of the calf in which there are complaints of pain when the leg is in extension and the foot is dorsiflexed.

home health agency An organization that provides health care in the home.

home health care Services that enable individuals of all ages to remain in the comfort and security of their homes while receiving health care.

homeostasis A relative constancy in the internal environment of the body, naturally maintained by adaptive responses that promote healthy survival.

homograft (allograft) The transfer of tissue between two genetically dissimilar individuals of the same species, such as a skin transplant between two humans who are not identical twins.

homosexual family Family group made up of same-sex adults who share bonds of emotional commitment and roles of childrearing.

homozygous Having two identical genes, inherited from each parent, for a given hereditary characteristic.

hospice From the Latin word *hospitum,* meaning hospitality; a resting place for travelers on a difficult journey; philosophy of care that provides support to terminally ill people and their families.

host A person or group who, because of risk factors, may be susceptible to disease or illness; an organism in which another, usually parasitic, organism is nourished and harbored.

huffing Typically in a group setting, breathing in solvents from a cloth, paper, or plastic bag.

human immunodeficiency virus (HIV) An obligate virus; a retrovirus that causes AIDS.

humoral immunity One of the two forms of immunity that respond to antigens such as bacteria and foreign tissue. It is mediated by B cells.

humoral theory A theory dating back to Hippocrates. He viewed mental illness as an imbalance of humors (the fundamental elements of the world: air, fire, water, and earth). Each basic element was represented in the body by certain fluids: blood, yellow bile, black bile, and phlegm.

hydramnios Abnormal condition of pregnancy characterized by an excess of amniotic fluid.

hydrogenation Process in which hydrogen is added to vegetable oil to make it more solid and stable to rancidity.

hydronephrosis The dilation of the renal pelvis and calyces.

hygiene The science of health and its maintenance; system of principles for preserving health and preventing disease.

hyperbilirubinemia An excess of bilirubin in the blood of the newborn.

hypercapnia Greater than normal amounts of carbon dioxide in the blood.

hyperextension Position of maximum extension; extreme or abnormal stretching.

hyperglycemia A greater than normal amount of glucose in the blood.

hyperopia Farsightedness; inability to see objects at close range.

hyperreflexia Neurologic condition characterized by increased reflex reactions.

hypersensitivity An abnormal condition characterized by an excessive reaction to a particular stimulus.

hypertension Occurs when the elevated blood pressure is above normal.

hyperthermia Condition of abnormally high body temperature.

hypertonic A solution of higher osmotic pressure.

hypocalcemia A deficiency of calcium in serum.

hypoglycemia A lower than normal amount of glucose in the blood; usually caused by administration of too much insulin, excessive secretion of insulin by the islet cells of the pancreas, or dietary deficiency.

hypokalemia A condition in which an inadequate amount of potassium, the major intracellular cation, is found in the circulatory bloodstream.

hypomanic episode The early phase of a manic episode when symptoms are not severe.

hypotension Occurs when the blood pressure is below normal.

hypothermia Condition of abnormally low body temperature.

hypotonic A solution of lower osmotic pressure.

hypoventilation An abnormal condition of the respiratory system that occurs when the volume of air is not adequate for the metabolic needs of the body.

hypoxemia An abnormal deficiency of oxygen in the arterial blood.

hypoxia An inadequate, reduced tension of cellular oxygen.

I

idiopathic Cause unknown.
idiopathic hyperplasia Increase, without any known cause, in the number of cells.
idiosyncratic An individual's unique hypersensitivity to a particular drug.
ileal conduit Ureters are implanted into a loop of the ileum that is isolated and brought to the surface of the abdominal wall.
illness An abnormal process in which aspects of the social, emotional, or intellectual condition and function of a person are diminished or impaired.
illusion A false interpretation of an external sensory stimulus, usually visual or auditory, such as a mirage in the desert or voices on the wind.
imagery Visualization techniques to create mental images to evoke physical changes in the body, improve perceived well-being, and enhance self-awareness.
immobility Inability to move around freely, caused by any condition in which movement is impaired or therapeutically restricted.
immunity The quality of being unsusceptible to or unaffected by a particular disease condition.
immunization A process by which resistance to an infectious disease is induced or increased.
immunocompetence/immunocompetent The ability of an immune system to mobilize and deploy its antibodies and other responses to stimulation by an antigen.
immunodeficiency An abnormal condition of the immune system in which cellular or humoral immunity is inadequate and resistance to infection is increased.
immunogen Any agent or substance capable of provoking an immune response or producing immunity.
immunology Study of the immune system; the reaction of tissues of the immune system of the body of antigenic stimulation.
immunosuppression/immunosuppressive Administration of agents that significantly interfere with the ability of the immune system to respond to antigenic stimulation by inhibiting cellular and humoral immunity.
immunosurveillance The immune system's recognition and destruction of newly developed abnormal cells.
immunotherapy A special treatment of allergic responses; involves the administration of increasingly larger doses of the offending allergens to gradually develop immunity.
impaction Condition of being tightly wedged into a part, such as eruption of a tooth blocked by other teeth; the presence of a large or hard fecal mass in the rectum or colon which the patient is unable to pass.
impairment Any loss or abnormality of psychological, physical, or anatomic structure or function.
implantation Embedding of the fertilized ovum in the uterine mucosa.
implementation The phase of the nursing process that includes ongoing activities of data collection, prioritization, and performance of nursing intervention and documentation.
incentive spirometry A procedure in which a device (spirometer) is used at the bedside at regular intervals to encourage a patient to breathe deeply.
incision Surgical cut produced by a sharp instrument to create an opening into an organ or space in the body.
incompetent cervix Passive and painless dilation of the cervix during the second trimester of pregnancy; it is variable and exists as a continuum that is determined in part by cervical length.
incontinence The inability to control urination or defecation.
indirect Coombs' test Laboratory blood test that detects circulating antibodies against red blood cells (RBC). The test can detect Rh antibodies in maternal blood and is used to anticipate hemolytic disease of the newborn.
induration Hardening of a tissue, particularly the skin, because of edema, inflammation, or infiltration by neoplasm. May be seen with an IV infiltrate.
infarct Localized area of necrosis in tissue, a vessel, or an organ resulting from tissue anoxia; caused by an interruption in the blood supply to an area.
infection Caused by an invasion of microorganisms such as bacteria, viruses, fungi, or parasites that produce tissue damage.
infection control The policies and procedures of a hospital or other health care facility to minimize the risk of nosocomial or community-acquired infection spreading to patients or other members of the staff.
infectious process Condition caused by the invasion of the body by pathogenic microorganisms.
infiltration The process whereby a fluid passes into the tissues.
inflammation Protective response of body tissues to irritation, injury, or invasion by disease-producing organisms. The cardinal signs include erythema, edema, heat, and loss of function.
inflammatory response A tissue reaction to injury.
informed consent Permission obtained from the patient to perform a specific test or procedure.
informed consent doctrine A legal doctrine that requires the patient to fully understand any proposed treatment and consent to it; this document gives the competent adult the choice to accept or reject any treatment modalities.
inhalant A volatile chemical that can alter thinking and feeling when inhaled.
innate immunity The body's first line of defense; provides physical and chemical barriers to invading pathogens and protects the body against the external environment.
inquest A legal inquiry into the cause or manner of a death.
inspection Visual examination of the external surface of the body and of its movements and posture, including observation of moods and all responses and nonverbal behaviors.
instrumental activities of daily living (IADLs) Daily tasks that are more complex than ADLs, such as shopping or using the telephone.
intelligence quotient (IQ) Index of relative intelligence determined through the subject's answers to arbitrarily chosen questions.
interdisciplinary When health care professionals work together as a team to meet the needs of a patient.
interdisciplinary hospice team Multiple-professional health team, such as physicians, nurses, social workers, and pastors, working together in caring for the terminally ill patient.
interdisciplinary rehabilitation team Team that collaborates to identify an individual's goals and is characterized by a combination of expanded problem solving beyond discipline boundaries and discipline-specific work toward goal attainment.
interdisciplinary team A diverse team of professionals from several disciplines who collaborate to optimize care and decrease fragmentation services.

intermittent claudication A weakness of the legs accompanied by cramplike pains in the calves; caused by poor arterial circulation of the blood to the leg muscles.

intermittent venous access device (also called *heparin* or *saline lock*) An intravenous infusion device with a male adapter covered by a rubber diaphragm for intermittent intravenous therapy.

internal rotation In obstetrics, when the largest diameter of the fetal head aligns with the largest diameter of the pelvis. This allows the fetal head to progress through the maternal pelvis.

interstitial Fluid between the cells or in the tissues of the body.

interview Meeting people face to face, as for evaluating or questioning a job applicant.

intracellular Fluid inside the cells of the body.

intraoperative Pertaining to a period of time during a surgical procedure.

intrapartal Period that begins with the onset of labor and ends with the delivery of the placenta; also called *perinatal.*

intravascular Fluid or plasma within the vessels of the body.

intravenous (IV) Pertaining to the inside of a vein, as of a thrombus, or an injection, infusion, or catheter.

intrinsic Caused by internal factors.

introitus An entrance to a cavity (e.g., the vaginal introitus).

intussusception Infolding of one segment of the intestine into the lumen of another segment; occurs in children.

involution Reduction in size of the uterus after delivery and return to its normal size.

ion Electronically charged particle resulting from the breakdown of an electrolyte; negatively or positively charged.

irrigation A gentle washing of an area with a stream of solution delivered through an irrigating syringe.

ischemia Decreased blood supply to a body organ or part; often marked by pain and organ dysfunction.

isolation precautions Practices of infection control to reduce or eliminate the transmission of pathogens; precautions include wearing protective apparel such as gowns, gloves, and masks and following the procedure for double bagging.

isotonic Having equal tension designating or of a salt solution. Having the same osmotic pressure as blood.

J

jargon Commonplace language or terminology unique to people in a particular work setting.

jaundice Yellowish discoloration of the skin, mucous membranes, and sclera of the eyes caused by greater than normal amounts of bilirubin in the blood.

joint Any one of the connections between bones.

K

Kaposi's sarcoma (KS) Rare cancer of the skin or mucous membranes; characterized by blue, red, or purple raised lesions and seen mainly in middle-aged Mediterranean men and those with HIV disease.

Kardex/Rand A card system used to consolidate patient orders and care needs in a centralized, concise way.

keloids Overgrowths of collagenous scar tissue at the site of a skin wound.

keratitis An inflammation of the cornea.

keratoplasty Excision of the corneal tissue, followed by surgical implantation of a cornea from another human donor.

kernicterus Abnormal toxic accumulation of bilirubin in central nervous system tissue caused by hyperbilirubinemia (an excess of bilirubin in the blood of the newborn).

ketoacidosis Acidosis accompanied by an accumulation of ketone in the blood resulting from faulty carbohydrate metabolism.

ketone bodies Normal metabolic products, β-hydroxybutyric and aminoacetic acid, from which acetone may spontaneously arise.

kick count Daily counting of fetal movements felt in 1 hour while the mother is resting.

kilocalorie Unit that denotes the heat expenditure of an organism and the fuel or energy value of food; often abbreviated kcalorie or kcal.

Korotkoff sounds Sounds heard while measuring blood pressure when using a sphygmomanometer and stethoscope.

kyphosis An abnormal condition of the vertebral column; characterized by increased convexity in the curvature of the thoracic spine.

L

labia majora Two large folds of tissue extending from the mons pubis to the perineal floor; lip.

labia minora Smaller fold of tissue covered by the labia majora; lip.

labile Liable to change; unstable. As in unstable blood pressure.

labyrinthitis Inflammation of the labyrinthine canals of the inner ear.

lactation Function of secreting milk from the breasts for the nourishment of an infant or breastfeeding child.

lanugo Downy, fine hair characteristic of the fetus between 20 weeks of gestation and birth; most noticeable over the shoulders, forehead, and cheeks, but found on nearly all parts of the body except for the palms of the hands and the soles of the feet.

laparoscopy The examination of the abdominal cavity with a laparoscope through a small incision beneath the umbilicus.

law The reference of a rule, principle, or regulation established and made known by a government to protect or restrict the people affected.

Legg-Calvé-Perthes disease A disorder caused by decreased blood supply to the femoral head that results in epiphyseal necrosis or degeneration of the femoral head followed by regeneration or calcification.

leukemia Malignant disorder of the hematopoietic system in which an excess of leukocytes accumulates in the bone marrow and lymph nodes.

leukopenia An abnormal decrease in the number of white blood cells to fewer than 5000 cells/mm^3 due to depression of the bone marrow.

leukoplakia A white patch in the mouth or on the tongue.

liability A legal concept that holds a person legally responsible for harm caused to another person or property.

licensure The granting of permission by a competent authority (usually a government agency) to an organization or individual to engage in a practice or activity that would otherwise be illegal.

lichenification Hypertrophy of the epidermis, resulting in rough, thickened, leatherlike skin.

life expectancy Average number of years an individual will probably live.

lightening Sensation of decreased abdominal distention produced by uterine descent into the pelvic cavity as the fetal presenting part settles into the pelvis. It usually occurs 2 weeks before the onset of labor in nulliparas.

Linda Richards Practiced in the 1880s and has been credited as the first psychiatric nurse.

lipids Group name for organic substances of a fatty nature, including fats, oils, sterols (such as cholesterol), phospholipids, waxes, and related compounds.

lipodystrophy Abnormality in the metabolism or deposition of fats. Insulin lipodystrophy is the loss of local fat deposits in diabetic patients as a complication of repeated insulin injections.

lipoprotein A protein-and-lipid molecule that facilitates transport of lipids in the bloodstream.

lithotomy Incision of a duct or organ, especially the bladder, for removal of a stone.

lithotomy position Position assumed by the patient lying supine with the hips and knees flexed and the thighs abducted and rotated externally.

living will A legal document drawn up by a person who is not yet near death detailing how much medical care he or she wants to receive if terminally ill.

LOC Level of consciousness.

lochia Vaginal discharge during the puerperium consisting of blood, tissue, and mucus; following childbirth.

long-term care The range of services—physical, psychosocial, spiritual, social, and economic—needed to help people attain, maintain, and regain their optimum level of functioning.

lordosis An increase in the curve at the lumbar space region that throws the shoulder back, making the appearance "lordly or kingly."

loss When any aspect of self is no longer available to a person, that person suffers loss.

lumen Space within an artery, vein, intestine, or tube such as a needle or catheter.

lymphangitis Inflammation of one or more lymphatic vessels or channels; usually results from an acute streptococcal or staphylococcal infection in an extremity.

lymphedema Primary or secondary disorder characterized by the accumulation of lymph in soft tissue and edema.

lymphocytes White blood cells that occur in two forms—B cells and T cells.

lymphokine One of the chemical factors produced and released by T lymphocytes that attract macrophages to the site of infection or inflammation and prepare them for attack.

M

macules Small, flat, discolored blemishes; flush with the skin surface.

magnesium The second most abundant cation in the intracellular fluid of the body.

malignant Growing worse, resisting treatment; said of cancerous growths. Also tending or threatening to produce death; harmful.

malpractice (in law) Professional misconduct; behavior that fails to meet the standard of care.

mammogram X-ray examination of the breast; use of radiography of the breast to diagnose breast cancer.

mammography Radiography of the soft tissue of the breast to allow identification of various benign and neoplastic processes.

managed care A health care system that involves administrative control over primary health care services in a medical group practice. Redundant facilities and services are eliminated, and costs are reduced. Health education and preventive medicine are emphasized.

mania A state characterized by an expansive emotional state, extreme excitement, excessive elation, hyperactivity, flight of ideas, increased psychomotor activity, and sometimes violent, destructive, and self-destructive behavior.

Martha Mitchell Nurse educator and clinical specialist in psychiatric mental health nursing, appointed to the President's Commission on Mental Health, established in 1978.

mastoiditis Infection of one of the mastoid bones.

matriarchal family patterns A style in which the female assumes primary dominance in areas of child care and homemaking; also called *matrilocal*.

maturational loss A loss from normal life transitions.

means Inner terms of the proportion; halfway between extremes.

meconium First stools of the infant; viscid, dark greenish brown, almost black; sterile; odorless.

Medicaid A federally funded, state-operated program of medical assistance to people with low income; authorized by Title XIX of the Social Security Act.

medical asepsis A group of techniques that inhibit the growth and spread of pathogenic microorganisms. Sometimes referred to as clean technique.

medical diagnosis The identification of a disease or condition by scientific evaluation of physical signs, symptoms, history, laboratory tests, and procedures.

medical nutrition therapy The use of specific nutrition services to treat an illness, injury, or condition.

Medicare A federally funded national health insurance for certain people older than 65 years of age.

medicine The art and science of the diagnosis, treatment, and prevention of disease and the maintenance of good health.

melena Abnormal, black, tarry stool containing digested blood.

membrane Thin sheet of tissue that serves many functions in the body; it covers surfaces, lines and lubricates hollow organs, and protects and anchors organs and bones.

meniscus Curved upper surface of a column of liquid as in a mercury column.

menorrhagia Excessive menstrual flow.

mental health One's ability to cope with and adjust to the recurrent stresses of everyday living.

mental illness May be evidenced by behavior that is conspicuous, threatening, and disruptive of relationships or that deviates significantly from behavior that is considered socially acceptable. It is a manifestation of dysfunction (behavioral, psychological, and biologic).

meridians Channels of energy.

mesoderm Embryonic middle layer of germ cells giving rise to all types of muscles, connective tissue, bone marrow, blood lymphoid tissue, and all epithelial tissue.

metabolite Substance produced by metabolic action.

metastasis The process by which tumor cells spread to distant parts of the body.

metrorrhagia Excessive spotting between cycles.

microorganism Any tiny (usually microscopic) entity capable of carrying on living processes; kinds of microorganisms include bacteria, fungi, protozoa, and viruses; seen only by a microscope.

micturition Urination.

midstream urine specimen Urine collected after voiding is initiated and terminated before voiding is complete—midstream.
milliequivalent (mEq) Number of grams of soluble substance dissolved in 1 mL of normal solution.
mind-body link Connection between the physiologic and the mental as applied to healing.
minimal encouragement A subtle communication technique that communicates to the patient that the nurse is interested and wants to hear more.
minimum data set (MDS) A part of the patient assessment instrument (PAI) that incorporates many of the same assessment factors as a functional assessment tool and requires input from nursing and social services within a specific time frame.
minority group A racial, religious, ethnic, or political group smaller than and differing from the larger, controlling group in a community or nation.
miotic Causing constriction of the pupil of the eye.
mitosis Type of cell division of somatic (i.e., nonreproductive) cells in which each daughter cell contains the same number of chromosomes as the parent cell.
mobility A person's ability to move around freely in his or her environment.
monozygote Originating or coming from a single fertilized ovum, such as identical twins.
morbidity An illness or an abnormal condition or quality; the rate at which an illness occurs in a particular area of population.
mores Accepted traditional customs, moral attitudes, or manners of a particular social group.
mortality The condition of being subject to death; number of deaths in a specific population, usually expressed as deaths per 1000, 10,000, or 100,000.
mortician Person trained in the care of the dead.
morula Development stage of the fertilized ovum in which there is a solid mass of cells resembling a mulberry.
mourning Reaction activated by a person to assist in overcoming a great personal loss.
multiaxial system A system that classifies mental disorder; used by most hospitals and health care professionals in the United States. Various disorders and descriptive references are outlined.
multidisciplinary rehabilitation team Team characterized by discipline-specific goals, clear boundaries between disciplines, and outcomes that are the sum of each discipline's efforts.
multidisciplinary setting A group of health care workers who are members of different disciplines, each one providing specific services to the patient.
multiple myeloma A malignant neoplastic immunodeficiency disease of the bone marrow; the tumor is composed of plasma cells.
mummification Mortification producing a dry, hard mass.
mydriatic Causing pupillary dilation.
myeloproliferative The excessive production of bone marrow elements.
myocardial infarction An occlusion of a major coronary artery or one of its branches; it is caused by atherosclerosis or an embolus resulting in necrosis of a portion of cardiac muscle.
myopia Condition of nearsightedness; inability to see objects at a distance.
myringotomy A surgical incision of the tympanic membrane to relieve pressure and release purulent exudate from the middle ear.

N

NANDA-I North American Nursing Diagnosis Association–International.
narrative charting Traditional system of charting in which the nurse documents in story form all pertinent patient observations, care, and responses in the nurse's notes section of the patient's records.
nasal cannula A device for delivery of oxygen by way of two small tubes that are inserted into the nares.
nasogastric tube A pliable tube that is inserted through the patient's nasopharynx and into the stomach.
negligence Failure to act as a responsible prudent person would act in the given situation; applies to professional and laypeople.
neoplasm Uncontrolled or abnormal growth of cells.
neoplastic Any abnormal growth of new tissue, benign or malignant.
nephrotoxin Substances with specific destructive properties for the kidneys, such as certain antibiotics, heavy metals, solvents, and chemicals.
neural tube Tube formed from the fusion of the neural folds from which the brain and spinal cord arise.
neuropathy Any abnormal condition characterized by inflammation and degeneration of the peripheral nerves.
neurosis A term describing difficulty with stress that causes mild interpersonal disorganization. There is no loss of reality perception; the individual has insight that he or she has a problem.
neurotoxic Toxic or damaging to the brain.
nevi Pigmented, congenital skin blemishes that are usually benign but may become cancerous.
Nissen fundoplication A surgical procedure to wrap the fundus of the stomach around the distal esophagus to prevent reflux of the stomach contents to the esophagus.
nitrogen balance Difference between intake and output of nitrogen in the body. If intake is greater, a positive nitrogen balance exists and anabolism occurs. If output is greater, a negative nitrogen balance exists and catabolism occurs. When nitrogen intake equals output, the body is in zero nitrogen balance.
nocturia Excessive urination at night.
nonmaleficence Ethical principle meaning "to do no harm."
Non–rapid eye movement (NREM) One of two highly individualized sleeping states divided into four stages through which a sleeper progresses during a typical sleeping cycle; represents three fourths of a period of typical sleep.
nontherapeutic communication Communication techniques, both verbal and nonverbal, that hinder the nurse-patient relationship.
nonverbal communication The transmission of messages without the use of words.
nosocomial infection An infection acquired in a hospital or any other health care facility; an infection acquired at least 72 hours after admission.
noxious A stimulation of the sensory nerve endings that is harmful, injurious, or detrimental to physical health.
nuchal rigidity Pain and stiffness of the neck when flexed.

nuclear family A family unit consisting of the biologic parents and their offspring.
nucleus Largest organelle within the cell; it is responsible for cell reproduction and control of the other organelles.
numerator Top number of a fraction.
nurse practice act A statute enacted by the legislature of any of the states or by the appropriate officers of the district's possessions. The act delineates the legal scope of the practice of nursing within the geographic boundaries of jurisdiction.
nursing bottle caries Tooth decay caused by bottle feeding during sleep.
nursing care plan Plan of care based on a nursing assessment and a nursing diagnosis; lists nursing actions necessary to meet a patient's needs.
nursing diagnosis A clinical judgment about individual, family, or community responses to actual or high-risk (potential) health problems or life processes.
nursing health history Data collected about the patient's level of wellness, changes in life patterns, sociocultural role, and mental and emotional reactions to illness.
nursing intervention Activity performed by nurses that should promote the achievement of the desired patient outcome.
nursing notes The form on the patient's chart on which nurses record their observations, care given, and the patient's responses.
nursing physical assessment Identification by a nurse of the needs, preferences, and abilities of a patient. Assessment provides the scientific basis for a complete nursing care plan.
nursing process Systematic method by which nurses plan and provide care for patients.
nursing-sensitive outcomes The results or outcomes of nursing interventions. These outcomes or indicators are influenced by nursing and can be used to judge effectiveness of care and determine best practices.
nutrient density Nutrients relative to calories.
nutrient-dense foods Foods providing a high quantity of one or more nutrients in a small number of calories is nutrient dense.
nystagmus Involuntary, rhythmic movement of the eyes. Oscillations may be horizontal, vertical, rotary, or mixed.

O

obesity Abnormal increase in the proportion of fat cells, mainly in the viscera and subcutaneous tissues of the body; grossly overweight.
objective data Of or pertaining to a clinical finding that is observed, palpated, or auscultated. Laboratory findings, as well as radiologic and other studies, are included; observable and measurable signs.
obsession Refers to the persistent thought or idea with which the mind is continually and involuntarily preoccupied and that suggests an irrational act.
obsessions Thoughts that are recurrent, intrusive, and senseless. These thoughts are anxiety producing and distressing in that they are uncontrollable.
occlusion An obstruction or closing off in a canal, vessel, or passage of the body.
occult Hidden.
occult blood Blood that is hidden or obscured from view.
Occupational Safety and Health Administration (OSHA) Federal agency responsible for monitoring safety and health standards in the workplace.
oligohydramnios Abnormally small amount or absence of amniotic fluid; often indicative of fetal urinary tract defect.
oliguria A diminished capacity to form and pass urine (less than 500 mL in 24 hours); result is that the end products of metabolism cannot be excreted efficiently.
Omnibus Budget Reconciliation Act (OBRA) Federal legislation that mandates specific standards governing the care of older adults in U.S. nursing facilities and prohibits routine use of safety reminder devices (SRDs; restraints) in nursing homes.
oncology The sum of knowledge regarding tumors; the branch of medicine that deals with the study of tumors.
one-way communication A structured form of communication in which the sender is in control.
open-ended question A question that does not require a specific response and allows the individual to elaborate freely on a subject.
open posture A relaxed stance with uncrossed arms and legs while facing another individual.
open reduction with internal fixation (ORIF) A surgical procedure allowing fracture alignment under direct visualization while using various internal fixation devices applied to the bone.
opportunistic Disease characteristic caused by a normally nonpathogenic organism in a host whose resistance has been decreased by a disorder such as AIDS.
oral hygiene Care of the oral cavity (mouth).
organ A group of several different kinds of tissue arranged so that they can work together to perform a special function.
organic disease Results in a structural change in an organ that interferes with its functioning.
orthopnea An abnormal condition in which a person must sit or stand to breathe deeply or comfortably.
orthopneic Pertaining to the posture assumed by the patient sitting up in bed at a 90-degree angle; patient may also lean forward supported by a pillow or over a bed table.
orthostatic hypotension A drop of 25 mm Hg in systolic pressure and a drop of 10 mm Hg in diastolic pressure when moving from a lying to sitting position.
osmosis Passage of water across a selectively permeable membrane; the water moves from a less concentrated solution to a more concentrated solution.
outcome Description of the specific measurable behavior (outcome criteria) that the patient will be able to exhibit after the nursing interventions.
oxytocin Hormone produced in the hypothalamus and stored in the posterior pituitary gland; when needed, promotes the release of breast milk and stimulates uterine contractions during labor.

P

pain assessment An evaluation of the factors that alleviate or exacerbate a patient's pain.
palliative Designed to relieve pain and distress and to control the signs and symptoms of disease; not designed to produce a cure.
palliative care Preventing, relieving, reducing, or soothing symptoms of disease or disorders without effecting a cure. Extends the principles of hospice care to a broader population that could benefit from comfort care earlier in their illness or disease process.

palpation A technique used in physical examination in which the examiner feels the texture, size, consistency, and location of certain parts of the body with the hands.
pancytopenia Deficient condition of all three major blood elements (red cells, white cells, and platelets); results from the bone marrow being reduced or absent.
panhysterosalpingo-oophorectomy Removal of the uterus, fallopian tubes, and ovaries; also called total abdominal hysterectomy with bilateral salpingo-oophorectomy.
panic disorder An anxiety disorder that exhibits a sudden onset of acute, extreme anxiety. Feelings of terror and intense apprehension are accompanied with physical manifestations such as dyspnea, palpitations, sweating, trembling, and dizziness. An attack may last for several minutes and may be triggered again in certain situations.
Papanicolaou test (Pap smear) A simple smear method of examining stained exfoliative cells; used most commonly to detect cancers of the cervix.
papules Palpable, circumscribed, red solid elevations in the skin; smaller than 0.5 cm.
para- A combining form meaning "similar, beside." Also a combining form meaning a woman who has given birth to children in a number of pregnancies (e.g., nonpara, unipara, bipara).
paracentesis A procedure in which fluid is withdrawn from the abdominal cavity.
paralytic (adynamic) ileus Most common type of intestinal obstruction; a decrease in or absence of intestinal peristalsis and bowel sounds that may occur after abdominal surgery.
paraphilia Sexual perversion or deviation. One of three main clusters of sexual and gender identity disorders.
paraphrasing A communication technique that involves restating the patient's message in the nurse's own words to verify that the nurse's interpretation of the message is correct.
parenchyma Tissue of an organ as distinguished from supporting or connective tissue.
parent-child attachment (bonding) Initial phase in a relationship characterized by strong attraction and a desire to interact.
parenteral Pertaining to treatment other than through the digestive system.
parenteral nutrition Administering nutrients by a route other than the alimentary canal, such as intravenously.
parenthood stage Begins at the birth or adoption of the first child.
paresis A lesser degree of movement deficit from partial or incomplete paralysis.
paresthesia Any subjective sensation, such as a prickling "pins and needles" feeling or numbness.
passive listening Receiving a message without any response or indication of understanding.
passive transport The movement of small molecules across the membrane of a cell by diffusion; no cellular energy is required.
patency A condition of being opened and unblocked.
pathogenic Capable of causing disease.
pathognomonic Sign or symptom specific to a disease condition.
patient A recipient of a health care service, usually thought of as a recipient who is ill or hospitalized.
patient assessment instrument (PAI) A method of patient assessment and care plan development prescribed by OBRA in 1987.
patient-controlled analgesia (PCA) A drug delivery system that dispenses a preset intravenous dose of an opioid analgesic into a patient's vein when the patient pushes a switch on an electric cord.
patriarchal family pattern A family style in which the male assumes the dominant role.
pediatric rehabilitation nursing Specialty practice that focuses on the care of children with disabilities or other chronic conditions and their families.
pediculosis Lice infestation.
peer assistance program Administers contract agreements requiring a nurse to undergo treatment and monitoring to keep his or her license in good standing.
peer review An appraisal by professional co-workers (of equal status) or the way an individual nurse conducts practice, education, or research.
percent Hundredths; symbolized as %.
percussion Using fingertips to tap the body's surface to produce vibration and sound.
percutaneous Through the skin or mucous membrane.
perinatal Period during pregnancy that begins with the onset of labor and ends with delivery of the placenta; sometimes called intrapartal.
perineal care Care given to the genitalia.
perioperative Entire surgical inpatient period occurring immediately before, during, and immediately after surgery.
peripheral Pertaining to the outside, surface, or surrounding area of an organ, other structure or fluid of vision.
pernicious Capable of causing great injury or destruction; deadly, fatal.
pernicious anemia A progressive megaloblastic, macrocytic anemia, affecting mainly older people, that results from a lack of intrinsic factor essential for the absorption of vitamin B_{12}.
personal hygiene Self-care measures that people use to maintain their health.
personality Refers to the relatively consistent set of attitudes and behaviors particular to an individual; it consists of a pattern of mental, emotional, and behavioral tracts of a person.
phagocytes White blood cells that are able to surround, engulf, and digest microorganisms and cellular debris.
phagocytic Refers to the ingestion and digestion of bacteria.
phagocytosis The process that permits a cell to surround or engulf any foreign material and digest it.
pharmaceuticals Drugs, or drug-based products or preparations.
pharmacology Study of drugs and their actions on the living body.
phimosis A condition in which the prepuce is too small to allow retraction of the foreskin over the glans penis.
phobia An anxiety disorder characterized by obsessive, irrational, and intense fear of a specific object or activity.
phosphorus Chiefly, an intracellular anion in fluid of the body.
phototherapy Treatment for hyperbilirubinemia and jaundice in the newborn that involves the exposure of light; accelerates the excretion of bilirubin in the skin, decomposing it by photooxidation.
physiologic jaundice Jaundice usually occurring 48 hours or later after birth, gradually disappearing by the 7th to 10th day; caused by the normal reduction in the number of red blood cells. The infant is otherwise well.
physiology Explanation of the processes and functions of the various structures of the body and how they interrelate.
pica Craving to eat nonfood substances.

pinocytosis The process by which extracellular fluid is ingested by the cells.
placebo effect Positive response to treatment.
placental barrier Obstruction, boundary, or separation provided by the placental tissue between the fetal and maternal circulation; substances of small size, excluding blood cells, may cross this barrier.
planning In the five-step nursing process, a category of nursing behavior in which a strategy is designed for the achievement of the goals of care for an individual patient, as established in assessing and analyzing. Planning includes developing and modifying a care plan for the patient, cooperating with other personnel, and recording relevant information.
plasmapheresis Removal of plasma that contains components causing or thought to cause disease. Also called *plasma exchange* because when the plasma is removed, it is replaced by substitution fluids such as saline or albumin.
pleural effusion An abnormal accumulation of fluid in the thoracic cavity between the visceral and parietal pleurae.
pleural friction rub Low-pitched, grating, or creaking lung sounds that occur when inflamed pleural surfaces rub together during respiration.
pleural space The potential space between the visceral and parietal layers of the pleurae.
***Pneumocystis jiroveci* (formerly *carinii*) pneumonia (PCP)** An unusual pulmonary disease caused by a parasite that is primarily associated with people who have suppressed immune systems, especially in people with AIDS.
pneumothorax A collection of air or gas in the pleural space, causing the lung to collapse.
poisoning The condition or physical state produced by the ingestion, injection, inhalation, or exposure of a poisonous (toxic) substance.
polycythemia Abnormal increase in the number of red blood cells in the blood.
polydactyly Excessive number of digits (finger or toes).
polydipsia Excessive thirst.
polyphagia Eating to the point of gluttony.
polyuria Excretion of an abnormally large quantity of urine.
POMR See *problem-oriented medical record.*
postictal period A rest period of variable length after a tonic-clonic seizure.
postmortem care Care of the body after death.
postoperative Pertaining to a period of time after surgery.
postpartal The final stage of the maternity cycle; from Latin *post,* "after."
potassium The dominant intracellular cation.
potentiation When one drug increases the action or effect of another drug.
preeclampsia An abnormal condition of pregnancy characterized by the onset of acute hypertension after the 24th week of gestation.
pregnancy-induced hypertension (PIH) A disease encountered during pregnancy or early in the puerperium, characterized by increasing hypertension, albuminuria, and generalize edema (also called *gestational hypertension [GH]*).
prenatal Before birth; occurring or existing before birth; referring to both the care of the woman during pregnancy and the growth and development of the fetus.
preoperational thought stage Piaget's phase of child development during the period of 2 to 7 years of age, when the child focuses on the use of language as a tool. The child has the emerging ability to reason.
preoperative Pertaining to a period of time before surgery.
presbycusis A normal loss of hearing acuity, speech intelligibility, auditory threshold, and pitch associated with aging.
presbyopia Defect in vision in advancing age involving loss of accommodation or recession of near vision; due to loss of elasticity of crystalline lens.
priapism Persistent penile erection.
primary caregiver One who assumes ongoing responsibility for health maintenance and therapy for the ill.
primary (deciduous) teeth Baby teeth that normally appear during infancy.
primary intention A wound that has been made surgically and has little tissue loss; skin edges are close together and minimal scarring results.
problem Any health care condition that requires diagnostic, therapeutic, or educational action.
problem list Prioritized master list of the patient's active, inactive, temporary, and at-risk medical or other problems; serves as an index to the rest of the record.
problem-oriented medical record (POMR) Method of recording data about the health status of a patient in a problem-solving system. Parts included are the database, problem list, initial plan, and progress notes.
procidentia Protrusion of the entire uterus through the introitus.
prodromal Early sign of a developing condition or disease.
prolactin A hormone secreted from the anterior pituitary gland that is responsible for stimulating milk production in the mammary alveolar cells.
proliferation Reproduction or multiplication of similar forms.
pronation Palm of the hand turned down.
prone Lying face down on the abdomen.
proportion Shows that the relationship between two ratios has equal value.
proprioception Sensation pertaining to stimuli originating from within the body regarding spatial position and muscular activity stimuli or to the sensory receptors that those stimuli activate. This sensation gives one the ability to know the position of the body without looking at it and the ability to "know objectively the sense of touch."
prostatodynia Pain in the prostate gland.
prosthesis Artificial replacement for a missing body part.
proximodistal Growth and development that moves from the center toward the outside. The infant gains control of the shoulders before developing control of the hands and fingers.
pruritus The symptoms of itching; an uncomfortable sensation leading to the urge to scratch; scratching often leads to secondary infection. Some causes of pruritus are allergy, infection, elevated serum urea, jaundice, and skin irritation.
pseudomenstruation Discharge of blood-tinged mucus from the vagina of the newborn, which occurs in response to maternal hormones.
psychoactive drugs Drugs that make the user feel good but have the potential to be abused or addicting.
psychogenic Relating to causes that are emotional, psychological, or nonorganic in origin.
psychosis Any major disorder characterized by gross impairment in reality testing; the affected person exhibits moderate to severe personality disintegration.
psychosocial A combination of psychological and social factors.

puerperium Period of time after the third stage of labor and lasting until involution of the uterus takes place, usually about 3 to 6 weeks.

pulmonary edema Accumulation of extravascular fluid in lung tissues and alveoli; caused most commonly by left-sided heart failure.

pulse A rhythmic beating or vibrating movement; regular recurrent expansion and contraction of an artery produced by waves of pressure caused by the ejection of blood from the left ventricle of the heart as it contracts.

pulse deficit A condition that exists when the radial pulse rate is less than the ventricular rate as auscultated at the apex of the heart.

pulse pressure Difference between the systolic and diastolic blood pressures, usually 30 to 40 mm Hg.

pulverized Crushed to a powder.

purulent Producing or containing pus.

pustulant vesicles Small, circumscribed pus-containing elevations of the skin.

pyuria Pus in the urine.

Q

Qi Life force.

quality assurance/assessment/improvement In health care, any evaluation of services provided and the results achieved as compared with accepted standards.

quality of life A measure of the optimum energy that endows a person with the power to cope successfully with the full range of challenges encountered in the real world.

R

RACE A formula to enable nurses to be prepared when safety is threatened by fire; *R*escue the patient, sound the *A*larm, *C*onfine the fire, *E*xtinguish or *E*vacuate.

race A group of people who share biologic and physical characteristics.

racism Any ethnocentric activity—cultural, individual, or institutional, deliberate or not—that is based on a belief in the superiority of one racial group over other racial groups; the oppression of, thus maintaining control over, these groups.

radial keratotomy Microscopic incisions on the surface of the cornea outside the optical area. These eight spokelike incisions flatten the cornea to a more normal curvature, thus reducing or eliminating myopia.

range of motion (ROM) Normal movement that any given joint is capable of making. Any body action involving the muscles, joints, and natural directional movements.

rapid eye movement (REM) One of the two highly individualized sleeping states that follows NREM state. May last from a few minutes to a half an hour and alternate with NREM periods; dreaming occurs during this time.

ratio Relationship of one number or quantity to another number or quantity.

raves All-night parties or "trances"; often the scene of club drug use.

receiver The individual or individuals to whom a message is conveyed.

receptive aphasia A physiological condition in which an individual cannot recognize or interpret the message being received.

receptors Molecules that recognize or respond to specific invaders.

reciprocity Mutual agreement to exchange privilege, dependence, or relationships as an agreement between two governing bodies to accept the credit of caregivers licensed in each state. True reciprocity means that individuals licensed in one state can automatically receive licensure in the next, even if the licensure requirements of the states differ.

recording Process of adding written information to the chart, usually at prescribed intervals.

Reed-Sternberg cells Atypical histiocytes; large, abnormal, multinucleated cells in the lymphatic system, found in Hodgkin's lymphoma.

referred pain Pain that is felt at a site other than in the injured or diseased organ or part of the body.

reflecting A communication technique that assists the patient to "reflect" on inner feelings and thoughts rather than seeking answers or advice from someone else.

reflexology A form of complementary and alternative medicine based on the premise that zones and reflexes in different parts of the body correspond to all parts, glands, and organs of the entire body. In reflexology it is thought that the entire body can be reached by applying pressure to specific areas on the feet.

relaxation The state of generalized decreased cognitive, physiologic, or behavioral arousal.

remission A decrease in the severity of a disease or any of its symptoms.

reservoir Any natural habitat of a microorganism that promotes growth and reproduction.

resident assessment instrument (RAI) A comprehensive tool that includes the minimum data set, resident assessment protocols, and guidelines for functional assessment of the resident.

residential care A care setting for older adults, providing a wide range of services, such as assisted living and continuing care.

residual urine Urine remaining in the urinary tract after voiding.

residue Bulk in the colon that includes undigested food, fiber, bacteria, body secretions, and cells.

resignation Act of resigning; giving up a position of employment.

respirations The taking in of oxygen, its use in the tissues, and the giving off of carbon dioxide; the act of breathing (i.e., inhaling and exhaling).

respite Period of relief from responsibilities for the care of a patient.

restating A communication technique that involves the nurse repeating to the patient what the nurse believes to be the main point that the patient is trying to convey.

restitution In obstetrics, the turning of the fetal head to the left or right after it has completely emerged from the introitus of the vagina as it assumes a normal alignment with the infant's shoulders.

restorative nursing care Basic concepts of physical therapy for maintenance of functional mobility and physical activity.

résumé A summary of educational and professional experiences, including activities and honors, to be used in seeking employment for biologic citations on professional meeting programs or related purposes; curriculum vitae.

retention The inability to void even in the presence of an urge to void.

retinal detachment Separation of the retina from the choroid in the posterior of the eye.

retrovirus Lentivirus that contains reverse transcriptase, which is essential for reverse transcription (the production of a deoxyribonucleic acid [DNA] molecule from a ribonucleic acid [RNA] model).

risk nursing diagnosis A clinical judgment that an individual, family, or community is more vulnerable to develop the problem than others in same or similar situation.

role A socially expected behavior pattern associated with an individual's function in various social groups.

rule of nines Division of the body into multiples of nine; used to determine the total body surface area (BSA) involved in burn trauma.

S

safety reminder device (SRD) Any one of numerous devices used to immobilize a patient; formerly referred as a restraint.

sanguineous Pertaining to blood.

sarcoma Malignant tumor of connective tissues such as muscle or bone; usually presents as a painless swelling.

satiety Feeling of fullness and satisfaction from food.

savants Children with autism who excel in particular areas such as art, music, memory, mathematics, or perceptual skills such as puzzle building.

schema Innate knowledge structure that allows a child to organize his or her mind.

schizophrenia Any one of a large group of psychotic disorders characterized by gross distortion of reality, disturbances of language and communication, and disorganized and fragmented thought, perception, and emotional reaction.

school avoidance Repeated absence from school of a child who is physically healthy.

school violence Anything that physically or psychologically injures schoolchildren or damages school property.

scoliosis Curvature of the spine usually consisting of two curves: the original abnormal curve and a compensatory curve in the opposite direction.

secondary intention Healing that occurs when skin edges of the wound are not close together or when pus is formed.

self-concept How an individual views the self; pertains to personal identity, body image, role, and self-esteem.

semi-Fowler's position The position a patient assumes while lying in bed; the head of the bed is raised to about 30 degrees, and the foot of the bed is raised slightly.

sender The person conveying a message.

senescence stage The last stage of the life cycle that requires the older adult to cope with a long range of changes.

senile The state of physical and mental deterioration associated with aging.

senility Pertaining to or characteristic of old age or the process of aging.

sensitivity A laboratory method of determining the effectiveness of antibiotics. A report of resistance means that the antibiotic is not effective in inhibiting the growth of a pathogen, whereas use of an effective antibiotic results in a sensitive report.

sensorimotor stage The developmental phase of childhood encompassing the period from birth to 2 years of age, according to Piaget's psychology. In this stage, an infant's knowledge of the work comes about primarily through sensory impressions and motor activities.

sensory deprivation An involuntary loss of physical awareness caused by detachment from external sensory stimuli.

sentinel lymph node mapping Diagnostic tool used before therapeutic surgery, which identifies the first lymph node most likely to drain cancerous cells; used in axillary lymph node biopsy, specifically in breast cancer staging.

separation anxiety Fear and apprehension caused by separation from familiar surroundings and significant people.

sequestrum A fragment of necrotic bone that is partially or entirely detached from the surrounding or adjacent healthy bone.

seroconversion The development of detectable levels of antibodies; a change in serologic tests (e.g., ELISA and Western blot) from negative to positive as antibodies develop in reaction to an infection.

seronegative Negative result on serologic examination. The state of lacking HIV antibodies; confirmed by blood tests.

serosanguineous Thin, red exudate composed of serum and blood.

serotonin syndrome A potentially life-threatening condition that can occur as a result of an interaction between an selective serotonin reuptake inhibitor (SSRI) and another serotonergic agent.

serous Thin, watery exudate composing the serum portion of blood.

shearing forces Applied forces or pressure exerted against the surface and layers of the skin as tissue slides in opposite but parallel planes.

shock Abnormal condition of inadequate blood flow to peripheral tissues, with life-threatening cellular dysfunction, hypotension, and oliguria.

sibilant wheeze Musical, high-pitched, squeaking, or whistlelike sound caused by the rapid movement of air through narrowed bronchioles.

sickled cell Erythrocyte whose characteristic round shape has altered to an elongated crescent shape.

sign An objective finding as perceived by the examiner; a sign can be seen, heard, measured, or felt by the examiner.

Sims' position Lying on the left side with the right knee and thigh drawn upward toward the chest; the chest and abdomen are allowed to fall forward.

single-parent family Family group that occurs when one parent leaves the nuclear family because of divorce, separation, desertion, or death. May also be the result of unwed parents living alone or the decision of a single person to adopt a child.

singultus Hiccup.

situational loss Loss occurring suddenly in response to a specific external effect.

Sjögren syndrome Dry eye syndrome; an immunologic disorder characterized by low fluid production by lacrimal (tear), salivary, and other glands, resulting in abnormal dryness of mouth, eyes, and other mucous membranes.

skilled nursing facility Houses a subacute unit with a stronger rehabilitative focus and shorter length of stay than a long-term facility.

Snellen's test Eye chart test for visual acuity; letters, numbers, or symbols are arranged on the chart in decreasing size from top to bottom.

SOAPE Charting format used in POMR. Components include subjective data *(S)* reported by the patient; objective data *(O)* acquired by inspection, percussion, auscultation, and palpation and by tests, usually measurable findings; assessment *(A)* of the problem; plan *(P)* of care; and evaluation *(E)* of the patient's response to the treatment plan.

SOAPIER Same as SOAPE charting except that intervention *(I)* and revision *(R)* are added. Interventions are specific actions carried out, and revisions are the changes to be made to the original plan.

social contract family/cohabitation Unmarried couple living together and sharing roles and responsibilities similar to those of the nuclear family structure.

society A nation, community, or broad group of people who establish particular aims, beliefs, or standards of living and conduct.

sodium The most abundant electrolyte in the body; the major extracellular electrolyte; it is a cation.

somatization A disorder characterized by recurrent, multiple, physical complaints and symptoms for which there is no organic cause.

sonorous wheeze Low-pitched, loud, coarse, snoring sound.

souffle cup Ungraduated, disposable paper cup.

spastic Involuntary, sudden movements or muscular contractions with increased reflexes.

specimen A small sample of something, intended to show the nature of the whole, such as a urine specimen.

sphygmomanometer Device for measuring arterial blood pressure.

spider telangiectases Dilated superficial arterioles.

spinal cord injury (SCI) An injury in which the spinal cord is compressed by fractures or displaced vertebrae, bleeding, or edema.

spore The reproductive cell of some microorganisms such as fungi or protozoa. These cells are highly resistant to heat and chemicals. Under proper environmental conditions they may revert to an actively multiplying form of bacterium (e.g., gas gangrene or tetanus).

stages of dependence The three characteristic stages of dependence, which are chronic, incurable, and progressive.

standard precautions A set of guidelines set forth by the CDC to reduce the risk of transmission of bloodborne pathogens and pathogens for moist body substances. These precautions promote handwashing and use of gloves, masks, eye protection, and gowns when appropriate for patient contact. These precautions are designed to reduce the risk of transmission of microorganisms from both recognized and unrecognized sources of infection.

standardized languages A structured vocabulary that provides nurses with a common means of communication.

standards of care Those acts that are permitted to be performed or prohibited from being performed by a prudent person working within the limits of the training, licensing, experience, and conditions existing at the time of the duty to give care.

stapedectomy The removal of the stapes of the middle ear and insertion of a graft and prosthesis.

steatorrhea Excessive fat in the feces.

stereotype A generalization about a form of behavior, an individual, or a group.

sterilization A process by which all microorganisms, including their spores, are destroyed.

stertorous Pertaining to a respiratory effort that is strenuous and struggling, which provokes a snoring sound.

stethoscope Instrument placed against patient's body to hear heart, lung, or bowel sounds.

stimulants Drugs that affect the central nervous system.

stoma Combining form meaning a mouth or opening.

stomatitis Inflammation of the mouth due to destruction of normal cells of the oral cavity that may result from infection by bacteria, viruses, or fungi from exposure to certain chemicals or drugs, vitamin deficiency, or systemic inflammatory disease.

strabismus Condition in which the eyes are unable to focus in the same direction; commonly called *cross-eyed.*

street drugs Substances (drugs) sold to users illegally by drug dealers and that are manufactured without strict controls, illegally obtained prescription drugs, or drugs not approved for use in the United States.

stress The nonspecific response of the body to any demand made on it.

stressor A situation, activity, or event that produces stress.

stridor Harsh sound made during respirations; high pitched and resembling the blowing of wind; due to obstruction of air passages.

stroke An abnormal condition of the blood vessels of the brain characterized by hemorrhage into the brain; formation of an embolus or thrombus resulting in ischemia of the brain tissues normally perfused by the damaged vessels. The sequelae depend on the location and extent of ischemia.

subacute unit Institutional setting that provides a less expensive alternative to acute care; a bridge between acute care and long-term care.

subculture A group that shares many characteristics with the primary culture but has characteristic patterns of behavior and ideals that distinguish it from the rest of a cultural group.

subjective data Symptoms; verbal statements provided by the patient. That which arises from within or is perceived by the individual and related to the examiner.

sublingual Under the tongue.

subluxation Partial dislocation.

sundowning syndrome Sometimes referred to as nocturnal delirium. Manifested by increased disorientation and agitation only during the evening and nighttime. Seen more often in older adults.

supination Kind of rotation that allows the palm of the hand to turn up.

supine Being in the horizontal position, lying face upward.

suppuration To produce purulent material.

surfactant Lipoprotein necessary for normal respiratory function that prevents alveolar collapse (atelectasis); may be necessary for preterm infants.

surgery Branch of medicine concerned with diseases and trauma requiring operative procedures.

surgical asepsis A group of techniques that destroy all microorganisms and their spores (sterile technique).

surveillance Exercise of continuous scrutiny of and watchfulness over the distribution and spread of infections and factors related thereto, of sufficient accuracy and completeness to be effective control.

symptom Subjective indication of a disease or a change in condition as perceived by the patient.

syncope A transient loss of consciousness due to inadequate blood flow to the brain (fainting).

syndactyly Malformation of digits, commonly seen as a fusion of two or more toes to form one structure.

syndrome nursing diagnosis Used when a cluster of actual or risk nursing diagnoses are predicted to be present in certain circumstances.

synergistic Action of two or more substances or organs to achieve an effect of which each is capable.

system An organization of varying numbers and kinds of organs arranged so that they can work together to perform complex functions for the body.

systolic The number or reading that represents ventricles contracting, forcing blood into the aorta and pulmonary arteries. In blood pressure readings, it is the higher of the two readings.

T

tachycardia An abnormal condition in which the myocardium contracts regularly but at a rate greater than 100 beats per minute.

tachypnea An abnormally rapid rate of breathing.

Tai chi/Taiji Martial arts practice that emphasizes relaxing the body and focusing the mind; Tai chi movement is performed slowly, accentuating the intention, mechanics, accuracy, and precision of motion.

temperature Relative measure of sensible heat or cold.

tenesmus Persistent, ineffectual spasms of the rectum or bladder, accompanied by the desire to empty the bowel or bladder.

teratogen Any substance, agent, or process that interferes with normal prenatal development, causing the formation of one or more developmental abnormalities in the fetus.

teratogenic agent See *teratogen.*

terminal illness An advanced stage of disease with no known cure and poor prognosis.

terrorism Use or threats of violence by individuals or organized groups using biological, chemical, or nuclear weapons against society or government for political gain.

tertiary intention Healing that occurs by primary intention with delayed suturing of a wound in which two layers of granulation tissue are sutured together.

tetanus toxoid Active agent prepared from detoxified tetanus toxin that produces an antigenic response in the body, conferring permanent immunity to tetanus infection.

thanatologist One who studies dying and death.

thanatology The study of dying and death.

therapeutic Beneficial.

therapeutic communication A form of communication that facilitates the formation of a positive nurse-patient relationship.

therapeutic diet A diet used as a medical treatment.

therapeutic massage The manipulation of the soft tissues of the body to assist with healing.

third-party payers Entities (persons or elements) other than the giver or receiver of service responsible for payment (e.g., Medicare or an insurance company).

thoracentesis The surgical perforation of the chest wall and pleural space with a needle for the aspiration of fluid for diagnostic or therapeutic purposes.

thrill Fine vibration sensation along the artery, which is palpated by the examiner.

thrombocytopenia An abnormal hematologic condition in which the number of platelets is reduced to fewer than $100{,}000/mm^3$.

thrombus Of or pertaining to a clot.

tinnitus A subjective noise sensation in one or both ears; ringing or tinkling sound in the ear.

tissue An organization of many similar cells that act together to perform a common function.

titrate Slowly increasing the amount of drug to find the therapeutic dose.

tolerance A state that develops as the amount and frequency of use of an addicting substance increases to achieve the same effect.

tophi Calculi containing sodium urate deposits that develop in periarticular fibrous tissue; typically found in patients with gout.

topical application Applied to the skin.

TORCH (*T*oxoplasmosis, *O*ther, *R*ubella virus, *C*ytomegalovirus, and *H*erpes simplex viruses) Group of agents that can infect the fetus or the newborn infant, causing a constellation of morbid effects called TORCH syndrome.

total parenteral nutrition (TPN) The administration of a hypertonic solution into a large central vein, usually the superior vena cava, via a catheter threaded through either the subclavian or internal jugular vein.

tourniquet Constricting device applied to control bleeding.

toxicologic analysis Scientific study of poisons, their detection, and their effects.

tracheostomy A surgical opening into the trachea through which an indwelling tube may be inserted; created by a tracheotomy.

traditional (block) chart Conventional patient chart broken down into sections or blocks; included are admission data, physicians' orders, history and physical examination, nursing care plan, nurses' notes and graphics, progress notes, and test data.

transcribe To write or type a copy.

transcultural nursing An integration of the nurse's understanding of culture into all aspects of nursing care.

transcutaneous electrical nerve stimulation (TENS) A type of pain control that is managed with a pocket-sized, battery-operated device that provides a continuous, mild electrical current to the skin via electrodes.

transdisciplinary rehabilitation team Team characterized by the blurring of boundaries between discipline and by cross training and flexibility to minimize duplication of effort toward individual goal attainment.

transfer Moving a patient from one unit to another (intra-agency transfer) or moving a patient from one health care facility to another (interagency transfer).

traumatic brain injury Head injury classified as either penetrating or closed; may also be classified as mild, moderate, severe, or catastrophic.

Trendelenburg A position in which the patient is lying supine with the head lower than the body with body and legs elevated and on an incline.

triage Process of classifying a group of patients as to the severity of injury and need of care.

trichomoniasis A sexually transmitted disease caused by the protozoan *Trichomonas vaginalis.*

trimester One of the three periods of approximately 3 months into which pregnancy is divided.

Trousseau's sign A test for latent tetany in which carpal spasms are induced by inflating a sphygmomanometer cuff on the upper arm to a pressure exceeding systolic blood pressure for 3 minutes; used in hypocalcemia and hypomagnesemia.

tube feeding Administration of nutritionally balanced liquefied food or formula through a tube inserted into the stomach, duodenum, or jejunum by way of nasoenteric or a feeding ostomy.

tumor lysis syndrome Oncologic emergency that occurs with rapid lysis of malignant cells; most frequently associated with chemotherapy treatment. It is most commonly a result of treatment-related malignant cell death in patients with large tumor cell burdens.

turgor The normal resiliency of the skin caused by the outward pressure of the cells and interstitial fluid; may be assessed as increased or decreased skin turgor.

two-way communication A form of communication that requires that both the sender and the receiver participate equally in the interaction.

tympanic Membranous eardrum.

tympanoplasty One of several operative procedures on the eardrum or ossicles of the middle ear designed to restore or improve hearing in patients with conductive hearing loss.

tympany A high-pitched drumlike sound produced by performing percussion over a hollow organ such as the stomach.

type 1 diabetes mellitus Condition in which impaired glucose tolerance results because of destruction of beta cells in the pancreatic islets; results in deficient insulin production, but the patient retains normal sensitivity to insulin action; also called insulin-dependent diabetes mellitus.

type 2 diabetes mellitus Condition in which impaired glucose tolerance results from an abnormal resistance to insulin action; also called non–insulin-dependent diabetes mellitus.

U

ultrasonography The process of imaging deep structures of the body by measuring and recording the reflection of pulsed or continuous high-frequency sound waves. Also called *sonography.*

umbilicus Point on the abdomen at which the umbilical cord joined the fetus. In most adults it is marked by a depression.

unassertive communication A style of communication in which the sender sacrifices legitimate personal rights to meet the needs of the receiver, often resulting in feelings of resentment.

unilateral neglect Condition in which an individual is perceptually unaware of and inattentive to one side of the body.

urinal A device for receiving urine; may be used with male or female; may be used for specimen collection.

urinary catheter A hollow, flexible tube that can be inserted into the bladder through the meatus and urethra to withdraw urine or instill medication or an irrigant.

urolithiasis Formation of urinary calculi.

urticaria Itching skin eruption characterized by welts of varying sizes with well-defined inflamed margins and pale centers (also called *hives*).

uterine inertia Absence or weakness of uterine contractions during labor.

V

Vacutainer Container used in blood collection.

value clarification A process of self-inspection to identify one's own beliefs, morals, and values.

values Individual's intrinsic (or personal) beliefs about the importance of a particular idea, object, or custom that will influence behavior.

variance The unexpected event that occurs during the use of a clinical pathway; can be positive or negative.

vasoconstriction When the lumen of the blood vessel narrows, thus hindering blood flow and resulting in less edema.

vasodilation When the lumen of the blood vessel widens, thus increasing the blood flow.

vastus lateralis muscle Located in the anterior (front) of thigh, this site is preferred for injections in children.

vector A living carrier for transmission of microorganisms.

vegan Vegetarian whose diet excludes all foods of animal origin.

vehicle The means by which organisms are carried about.

venipuncture Most common method of drawing a blood sample, involving inserting a hollow-bore needle into the lumen of a large vein.

ventral Facing forward; the front of the body.

verbal communication A form of communication that involves the use of spoken or written words or symbols.

verdict Decision rendered based on the facts of a case, evidence and testimony presented, credibility of witnesses, and laws pertaining to the case.

vernix caseosa Protective, gray-white fatty substance of cheesy consistency covering the fetal skin at birth.

verruca Benign, viral, warty skin lesion with a rough, papillomatous (nipplelike) growth.

vertical transmission Transmission of HIV from a mother to a fetus; can occur during pregnancy, during delivery, or through postpartum breastfeeding.

vertigo The sensation that the outer world is revolving about oneself or that one is moving in space.

vesicle Circumscribed elevation of skin filled with serous fluid.

villi Short vascular processes or protrusions clustered over the entire mucous surface of the small intestine.

viral load Amount of measurable HIV virions.

virulent Having the power to produce disease; of or pertaining to a very pathogenic or rapidly progressive condition.

visual analog scale An objective means of assessing pain severity; it consists of a straight line, representing a continuum of intensity, and has visual descriptors at each end.

vital signs Measurement of temperature, pulse, respiration, and blood pressure.

Volkmann's contracture A permanent contracture with clawhand, flexion of wrist and finger, and atrophy of the forearm; can occur as a result of compartment syndrome.

volvulus Twisting of the bowel on itself, causing intestinal obstruction.

W

weaning Gradually eliminating breast- or bottle feedings, replaced by cup and table feeding.

wellness A dynamic state of health in which an individual progresses toward a higher level of functioning, achieving an optimum balance between internal and external environments.

wellness nursing diagnosis A clinical judgment about an individual, group, or community in transition from a specific level of wellness to a higher level of wellness.

Western blot A laboratory blood test to detect the presence of antibodies to a specific antigen; used in diagnosing HIV.

Wharton's jelly Gelatinous tissue that remains when the embryonic body stalk blends with the yolk sac within the umbilical cord.

wheals Irregularly shaped, elevated areas, white in the center with a pale red periphery, with superficial localized edema; vary in size (hives, mosquito bite).

wheeze Adventitious breath sounds that have a whistling or sighing sound resulting from narrowing of the lumen of a respiratory passageway. May be heard both on inspiration and expiration. Wheezes characteristically clear on coughing.

Y

yoga Holistic system of mind-body connection that includes control of the body through correct posture and breathing, control of the emotions and mind, and meditation and contemplation.

Z

zygote Cell formed by the union of two reproductive cells; the fertilized ovum resulting from the union of a sperm and ovum from the time it is fertilized until, as a blastocyst, it is implanted in the uterus.

Index

Page numbers followed by b indicate boxes; f, figures; t, tables.

E

F

G

Q

R

S

U

V

W

W

NANDA International–Approved Nursing Diagnoses 2009–2011

Activity intolerance
Activity intolerance, Risk for
Activity planning, Ineffective
Airway clearance, Ineffective
Allergy response, Latex
Allergy response, Risk for latex
Anxiety
Anxiety, Death
Aspiration, Risk for
Attachment, Risk for impaired parent/infant/child
Autonomic dysreflexia
Autonomic dysreflexia, Risk for
Behavior, Risk-prone health
Bleeding, Risk for
Body image, Disturbed
Body temperature, Risk for imbalanced
Bowel incontinence
Breastfeeding, Effective
Breastfeeding, Ineffective
Breastfeeding, Interrupted
Breathing pattern, Ineffective
Cardiac output, Decreased
Cardiac perfusion, Risk for decreased
Cardiac tissue perfustion, Risk for ineffective
Caregiver role strain
Caregiver role strain, Risk for
Cerebral tissue perfusion, Risk for ineffective
Childbearing process, Readiness for enhanced
Comfort, Readiness for enhanced
Comfort, Impaired
Communication, Impaired verbal
Communication, Readiness for enhanced
Conflict, Decisional
Conflict, Parental role
Confusion, Acute
Confusion, Chronic
Confusion, Risk for acute
Constipation
Constipation, Perceived
Constipation, Risk for
Contamination
Contamination, Risk for
Coping, Compromised family
Coping, Defensive
Coping, Disabled family
Coping, Ineffective
Coping, Ineffective community
Coping, Readiness for enhanced
Coping, Readiness for enhanced community
Coping, Readiness for enhanced family
Death syndrome, Risk for sudden infant
Decision making, Readiness for enhanced
Denial, Ineffective
Dentition, Impaired
Development, Risk for delayed
Diarrhea
Dignity, Risk for compromised human
Distress, Moral
Disuse syndrome, Risk for
Diversional activity, Deficient
Electrolyte imbalance, Risk for
Energy field, Disturbed
Environmental interpretation syndrome, Impaired
Failure to thrive, Adult
Falls, Risk for
Family processes: alcoholism, Dysfunctional
Family processes, Interrupted
Family processes, Readiness for enhanced
Fatigue
Fear
Fluid balance, Readiness for enhanced
Fluid volume, Deficient
Fluid volume, Excess
Fluid volume, Risk for deficient
Fluid volume, Risk for imbalanced
Gas exchange, Impaired
Gastrointestinal motility, Dysfunctional
Gastrointestinal motility, Risk for dysfunctional
Gastrointestinal tissue perfusion, Risk for ineffective
Glucose level, Risk for unstable
Grieving
Grieving, Complicated
Grieving, Risk for complicated
Growth and development, Delayed
Health maintenance, Ineffective
Health management, Ineffective self
Health management, Readiness for enhanced self
Health-seeking behaviors
Home maintenance, Impaired
Hope, Readiness for enhanced
Hopelessness
Hyperthermia
Hypothermia
Identity, Disturbed personal
Immunization status, Readiness for enhanced
Incontinence, Functional urinary
Incontinence, Overflow urinary
Incontinence, Reflex urinary
Incontinence, Stress urinary
Incontinence, Urge urinary
Incontinence, Risk for urge urinary
Infant behavior, Disorganized
Infant behavior, Risk for disorganized
Infant behavior, Readiness for enhanced organized
Infant feeding pattern, Ineffective
Infection, Risk for
Injury, Risk for
Injury, Risk for perioperative-positioning
Insomnia
Intracranial adaptive capacity, Decreased
Jaundice, Neonatal
Knowledge, Deficient
Knowledge, Readiness for enhanced
Lifestyle, Sedentary
Liver function, Risk for impaired
Loneliness, Risk for
Maternal/Fetal dyad, Risk for disturbed
Memory, Impaired
Mobility, Impaired bed
Mobility, Impaired physical
Mobility, Impaired wheelchair
Nausea
Neglect, Self
Neglect, Unilateral
Noncompliance
Nutrition: less than body requirements, Imbalanced
Nutrition: more than body requirements, Imbalanced
Nutrition, Readiness for enhanced
Nutrition: more than body requirements, Risk for imbalanced
Oral mucous membrane, Impaired
Pain, Acute
Pain, Chronic
Parenting, Readiness for enhanced
Parenting, Impaired
Parenting, Risk for impaired
Peripheral neurovascular dysfunction, Risk for
Peripheral tissue perfusion, Ineffective
Poisoning, Risk for
Post-trauma syndrome
Post-trauma syndrome, Risk for
Power, Readiness for enhanced
Powerlessness
Powerlessness, Risk for
Protection, Ineffective
Rape-trauma syndrome
Relationship, Readiness for enhanced
Religiosity, Impaired
Religiosity, Readiness for enhanced
Religiosity, Risk for impaired
Relocation stress syndrome
Relocation stress syndrome, Risk for
Renal perfusion, Risk for ineffective
Resilience, Impaired individual
Resilience, Readiness for enhanced
Resilience, Risk for compromised
Role performance, Ineffective
Self-care, Readiness for enhanced
Self-care deficit, Bathing/hygiene
Self-care deficit, Dressing/grooming
Self-care deficit, Feeding
Self-care deficit, Toileting
Self-concept, Readiness for enhanced
Self-esteem, Chronic low
Self-esteem, Situational low
Self-esteem, Risk for situational low
Self-mutilation
Self-mutilation, Risk for
Sensory perception, Disturbed
Sexual dysfunction
Sexuality pattern, Ineffective
Shock, Risk for
Skin integrity, Impaired
Skin integrity, Risk for impaired
Sleep deprivation
Sleep, Readiness for enhanced
Sleep pattern, Disturbed
Social isolation
Social interaction, Impaired
Sorrow, Chronic
Spiritual distress
Spiritual distress, Risk for
Spiritual well-being, Readiness for enhanced
Stress overload
Suffocation, Risk for
Suicide, Risk for
Surgical recovery, Delayed
Swallowing, Impaired
Therapeutic regimen management, Ineffective family
Thermoregulation, Ineffective
Tissue integrity, Impaired
Tissue perfusion, Ineffective
Transfer ability, Impaired
Trauma, Risk for
Urinary elimination, Impaired
Urinary elimination, Readiness for enhanced
Urinary retention
Vascular trauma, Risk for
Ventilation, Impaired spontaneous
Ventilatory weaning response, Dysfunctional
Violence, Risk for other-directed
Violence, Risk for self-directed
Walking, Impaired
Wandering